TRAUMA
Critical Care

VOLUME 2

TRAUMA

Critical Care

VOLUME 2

edited by

William C. Wilson, MD, MA

Clinical Professor
Director of Anesthesiology Critical Care Program
Department of Anesthesiology and Critical Care
University of California, San Diego School of Medicine
La Jolla, California
Director of Trauma Anesthesia
Associate Director Surgical Intensive Care Unit
UC San Diego Medical Center
San Diego, California, U.S.A.

Christopher M. Grande, MD, MPH

Executive Director
International TraumaCare (ITACCS)
Baltimore, Maryland, U.S.A.

David B. Hoyt, MD, FACS

John E. Connolly Professor and Chairman
Department of Surgery
University of California, School of Medicine
Irvine, California
UC Irvine Medical Center
Orange, California, U.S.A.

informa

healthcare

New York   London

Informa Healthcare USA, Inc.
52 Vanderbilt Avenue
New York, NY 10017

© 2007 by Informa Healthcare USA, Inc.
Informa Healthcare is an Informa business

No claim to original U.S. Government works
Printed in the United States of America on acid-free paper
10 9 8 7 6 5 4 3

International Standard Book Number-10: 0-8247-2920-X (Hardcover)
International Standard Book Number-13: 978-0-8247-2920-2 (Hardcover)

Library of Congress Cataloging-in-Publication Data

Trauma / edited by William C. Wilson, Christopher M. Grande, David B. Hoyt.
    p. ; cm.
   Includes bibliographical references and index.
    ISBN-13: 978-0-8247-2919-6 (hardcover : v. 1 : alk. paper), ISBN-10: 0-8247-2919-6 (hardcover : v. 1 : alk. paper)
    ISBN-13: 978-0-8247-2920-2 (hardcover : v. 2 : alk. paper), ISBN-10: 0-8247-2920-X (hardcover: v. 2 : alk paper) 1. Wounds and injuries
   --Treatment. 2. Surgical emergencies. 3. Critical care medicine . I. Wilson, William C. II. Grande, Christopher M. III. Hoyt, David B.
   [DNLM: 1. Wounds and Injuries. 2. Critical Care. 3. Emergencies. WO 700 T7735 2007]

RD93.T67136 2007
617.1--dc22   2007005815

Visit the Informa Web site at
www.informa.com

and the Informa Healthcare Web site at
www.informahealthcare.com

Editors

William C. Wilson, MD, MA
Clinical Professor
Director of Anesthesiology Critical Care Program
Department of Anesthesiology and Critical Care
University of California, San Diego School of Medicine
La Jolla, California
Director of Trauma Anesthesia
Associate Director Surgical Intensive Care Unit
UC San Diego Medical Center
San Diego, California, U.S.A.

Christopher M. Grande, MD, MPH
Executive Director
International TraumaCare (ITACCS)
Baltimore, Maryland, U.S.A.

David B. Hoyt, MD, FACS
John E. Connolly Professor and Chairman
Department of Surgery
University of California, School of Medicine
Irvine, California
UC Irvine Medical Center
Orange, California, U.S.A.

Volume 2 Associate Editors

Bruce Potenza, MD, FACS

Associate Professor of Surgery
Director of Burns, Division of Trauma, Burns and Critical Care
Department of Surgery, University of California San Diego
La Jolla California
Director Burn Unit
UC San Diego Medical Center
San Diego, California, U.S.A.

Joseph F. Rappold, MD, FACS

Associate Professor of Surgery
Director, Division of Trauma and Critical Care
Department of Surgery
Naval Medical Center San Diego
San Diego, California, U.S.A.
Past Naval Medical Commander
Fallujah and Ramadi, Iraq

Anne J. Sutcliffe, BSc, MB ChB

Consultant in Anaesthesia and Critical Care
Department of Anaesthesia
Alexandra Hospital
Redditch, UK

Theodore E. Warkentin, MD, FACP, FRCPC

Professor of Medicine
Departments of Medicine, and Pathology and Molecular Medicine
McMaster University
Associate Head, Transfusion Medicine
Hamilton Regional Laboratory Medicine Program
Hematologist, Hamilton Health Sciences
Hamilton, Ontario, Canada

Volume 2 Section Editors

Section A: Basic Science Review

Rahul Jandial, MD

Resident, Division of Neurosurgery
UC San Diego Medical Center
San Diego, California
Research Associate
Burnham Institute for Medical Research
La Jolla, California, U.S.A.

Section B: Analgesia, Sedation, and Neuromuscular Blockade

Todd Dorman, MD, FACS

Associate Professor
Departments of Anesthesiology and Critical Care Medicine
Internal Medicine, Surgery and Nursing
Johns Hopkins School of Medicine
Director of the Division of Adult Critical Care Medicine
Co-Director of the Surgical Intensive Care Units
Medical Director of the Adult Postanesthesiology Care Units
Medical Director of Respiratory Care Services
Johns Hopkins Medical Center
Baltimore, Maryland, U.S.A.

Section C: Monitoring Considerations for Trauma and Critical Care

Jose´ A. Acosta, MD, FACS

Associate Professor
Division of Trauma and Critical Care
Department of Surgery
Naval Medical Center San Diego
San Diego, California, U.S.A.

Section D: Neurological Injuries and Considerations

Lawrence F. Marshall, MD

Professor of Surgery and Chief
Division of Neurological Surgery
Director, Neurological Surgery Residency Program
Department of Surgery
UCSD Medical Center
San Diego, California, U.S.A.

Section E: Cardiovascular Considerations in Critical Care

William J. Mazzei, MD

Clinical Professor and Vice Chair for Clinical Affairs
Department of Anesthesiology
University of California, San Diego School of Medicine
La Jolla, California
Medical Director of Perioperative Services
Chief Anesthesiology for Liver Transplantation
UC San Diego Medical Center
San Diego, California, U.S.A.

Charles E. Smith, MD, FRCPC

Professor of Anesthesiology
Case Western Reserve University
Director, Cardiothoracic Anesthesia
MetroHealth Medical Center
Cleveland, Ohio, U.S.A.

Section F: Pulmonary Considerations in Critical Care

Jonathan L. Benumof, MD

Professor of Anesthesiology
Director of Airway Management Training
Department of Anesthesiology
University of California San Diego
La Jolla California
Chief Division of Airway Management
UC San Diego Medical Center
San Diego, California, U.S.A.

Section G: Gastrointestinal Considerations in Critical Care

David B. Hoyt, MD, FACS

John E. Connolly Professor and Chairman
Department of Surgery
University of California, School of Medicine
Irvine, California
UC Irvine Medical Center
Orange, California, U.S.A.

Section H: Renal, Fluid, Electrolyte, and Acid–Base Considerations

David M. Ward, MD, FRCP

Professor of Medicine
Division of Nephrology and Hypertension
Department of Medicine
UC San Diego School of Medicine
La Jolla, California
Director of Clinical Nephrology, Dialysis & Apheresis Programs,
UC San Diego Medical Center
San Diego, California, U.S.A.

Section I: Infectious Disease and Antibiotic Considerations

Dennis G. Maki, MD

Ovid O. Meyer Professor of Medicine
Head, Section of Infectious Diseases, Department of Medicine
University of Wisconsin Medical School
Attending Physician, Center for Trauma and Life Support
Hospital Epidemiologist
University of Wisconsin Hospital and Clinics
Madison, Wisconsin, U.S.A.

Charles L. James, PharmD, FCSHP, BCPS
Associate Clinical Professor of Medicine and Pharmacy
Division of Infectious Diseases, Departments of Pharmacy and Medicine
UC San Diego School of Medicine
Course Chief, Medical Microbiology and Infectious Disease Therapeutics
UCSD, Skaggs School of Pharmacy and Pharmaceutical Sciences
La Jolla, California
Infectious Disease Pharmacy Specialist
Directory Emergency Preparedness Pharmacy Practice
Co-director Antibiotic Utilization Team
UC San Diego Medical Center
San Diego, California, U.S.A.

Section J: Hematological Disorders in Trauma and Critical Care

Theodore E. Warkentin, MD, FACP, FRCPC
Professor of Medicine
Departments of Medicine, and Pathology and Molecular Medicine
McMaster University
Associate Head, Transfusion Medicine
Hamilton Regional Laboratory Medicine Program
Hematologist, Hamilton Health Sciences
Hamilton, Ontario, Canada

Section K: Endocrine and Autocrine Disorders in Critical Illness

Greet Van den Berghe, MD, PhD
Professor and Chair
Department of Intensive Care Medicine
University Hospital Gasthuisberg
Catholic University of Leuven
Leuven, Belgium

Section L: Psychological Support and Physical Rehabilitation

Catherine McCoy-Hill, RN, MSN, CCRN, CNS, ANP
Assistant Professor
Director Critical Care Nursing Education
School of Nursing
Azusa Pacific University
Azusa, California, U.S.A.

Section M: Ethical Considerations and End of Life Care

Anne J. Sutcliffe, BSc, MB ChB
Consultant in Anaesthesia and Critical Care
Department of Anaesthesia
Alexandra Hospital
Redditch, UK

Section N: Miscellaneous Trauma and Critical Care Considerations

Joseph F. Rappold, MD, FACS
Associate Professor of Surgery
Director, Division of Trauma and Critical Care
Department of Surgery
Naval Medical Center San Diego
San Diego, California, U.S.A.
Past Naval Medical Commander
Fallujah and Ramadi, Iraq

This book is dedicated to the trauma victims, as well as the doctors, nurses, prehospital personnel, and other members of the trauma team who tirelessly strive to provide optimum care for their recovery.

Foreword

From my recent perspective as the 17th surgeon general of the United States, along with my prior experiences as a trauma surgeon, combat experienced U.S. Army Special Forces medical specialist, paramedic, police officer, and registered nurse, I have witnessed numerous developments over the last three decades in the fields of trauma and critical care. Despite these significant advances, trauma remains the chief cause of death and disability of individuals between 1 and 44 years of age; hence, much work remains to be done.

Trauma is a worldwide phenomenon with profound public health implications and numerous existent challenges, including the need for an increased emphasis on accident prevention; overcoming barriers to care for the indigent, the elderly, and rural populations; and streamlining and improving disaster response effectiveness.

This two-volume book provides comprehensive coverage of all realms of modern trauma management, including the important aforementioned areas of care, which continue to impact the outcomes for these vulnerable populations.

Volume 1 focuses on initial management and is divided into sections that mirror the continuum of care, including prehospital, resuscitation suite, and perioperative management. The prehospital section includes chapters on trauma mechanisms, epidemiology, scoring and triage, and transport. The authors acknowledge that optimal management algorithms for this early phase of care can differ based on the setting (urban/rural) and the prevailing geographical, political, and financial conditions. Hospital-based components of management (e.g., primary survey, secondary survey, etc.) are meticulously reviewed, including specific chapters on the critical elements of care (e.g., airway management, fluid therapy, etc.). The perioperative section details the anesthetic and surgical priorities, but surgical technical details are minimized in favor of global management guidelines, which are important to all members of the care team. Important trauma-related conditions are also fully reviewed.

Volume 2 encompasses the critical care management of trauma and other surgical conditions. These topics are arranged in sections according to organ systems, with each chapter dedicated to a specific lesion or critical illness condition. Recent evidence-based principles are fully characterized, including the management of abdominal compartment syndrome, tight glucose control, adrenal suppression, and thromboembolism, etc. In addition, chapters covering post-traumatic stress disorder, family centered care, rehabilitation, and palliation at the end of life provide a breadth of coverage not present in other trauma books.

Chapters in both volumes are co-authored by experts from complimentary specialties, with surgeons, anesthesiologists, emergency medicine physicians, and pulmonologists involved throughout. Specialty sections are written by medical or surgical sub-specialists with extensive trauma and critical care experience. Interdisciplinary collaboration is further evident with chapters co-authored or edited by experienced nurses, pharmacists, and social workers, as well as occupational, physical, and respiratory therapists, among others.

The editors are eminently qualified and have succeeded in producing an authoritative and comprehensive book on trauma. Drs. Wilson, Grande, and Hoyt have each conducted important research and have published and lectured extensively on numerous trauma-related topics over the last two decades. They have assembled a superb table of contents and an expert array of contributors and associate editors. The editors have also insured that recommendations are evidence based where possible. Accordingly, the novice will learn in depth about the scientific basis of the guidelines provided here, and the expert will be updated on the latest thinking in trauma management.

In summary, this two-volume book is an extremely valuable contribution because of the importance of the subject, the fact that the topic has not been so comprehensively covered in one book until now, and because of the wisdom and insight of the editors.

Vice Admiral Richard Henry Carmona, MD, MPH, FACS
17th Surgeon General of the United States of America

Foreword

The modern-day management of trauma is multidisciplinary and requires teamwork. The specialists involved include emergency physicians, anesthesiologists, radiologists, surgeons, toxicologists, and critical care specialists along with paramedics, nurses, and technical staff.

Those involved in the management of trauma have a need for a comprehensive book that spans the entire spectrum of trauma management by all specialists, including prehospital, perioperative, and critical care. This two-volume book, edited by Wilson, Grande, and Hoyt, does precisely that. Along with a superbly designed table of contents, the editors have recruited a world-class group of contributors from all specialties to write the chapters. The editors are abundantly qualified to oversee a work of this magnitude in terms of academic and intellectual strength, as well as in terms of clinical expertise.

Volume 1 covers the areas of prehospital, emergency department, and perioperative management. Other important trauma-related conditions (e.g., alcohol and drug intoxication, burns, near drowning, environmental conditions) and management of unique populations of trauma patients (e.g., pediatric, geriatric, and obstetric) are also reviewed by experts in this volume. In addition to reviewing the key conditions, this volume contains clear guidelines for medical and surgical decision making in the various stages of care.

In Volume 2, the critical care management of trauma is reviewed. This volume proceeds in a logical systems-based presentation of the conditions and complications commonly encountered in a modern trauma or surgical intensive care unit. All of the evidence-based measures recommended to improve outcomes in critically ill patients are included. In addition, emerging topics such as the remote evaluation and management of trauma and critical illness are introduced.

As the only book to cover the full spectrum of trauma management, this two-volume set is strongly recommended for all students and clinically active physicians engaged in the management of trauma and surgical critical care.

Peter J. F. Baskett, BA, MB, BCh, BAO,
FRCA, FRCP, FCEM
Consultant Anaesthetist Emeritus, Frenchay Hospital
and the Royal Infirmary, Bristol, U.K.
Editor-in-Chief, Resuscitation
Past President, International Trauma Anaesthesia
and Critical Care Society

Three decades ago, as an impressionable resident physician-in-training at the University of Washington in Seattle, I was asked to respond with the city's emergency medical services personnel on 9-1-1 emergency calls. Working out of the Harborview Emergency-Trauma Center, I soon began to recognize how the outcomes of those with severe injury are often determined, for better or for worse, in the first few minutes after injury. After accompanying hundreds of patients from the incident scene, in the back of ambulances, in the emergency centers, and in operating rooms and intensive care units, I soon learned that a continuity of optimized care must be stewarded by an integrated team of experts from many disciplines. In turn, I have always stressed that an interdependent "chain of survival/recovery" had to be created with each link being strong and solidly connected to each other. I have been fortunate to train, perform research, and provide care in all of those arenas, and thus appreciate the tremendous expertise and demands required of each team member at each and every link.

This two-volume book (edited by Wilson, Grande, and Hoyt) is, in many ways, the first book to examine that entire spectrum of trauma care. Accordingly, as an emergency medicine physician originally trained in surgical critical care and trauma fellowships to challenge sacred cows with clinical trials, and as a prehospital care trauma specialist who has since spent many a night responding to out-of-hospital 9-1-1 incidents, I am now honored to write a foreword for this book. For those of us who have come to understand the chain of care and the impact of early decision making on long-term outcomes, this book is a tremendous gift.

Volume 1 discusses many of the areas with which I am quite familiar, namely the initial treatment priorities in prehospital care, the resuscitation suite, and the perioperative period. These chapters are very current, including recent citations emphasizing the need for only a few assisted rescue breaths in conditions of severe circulatory impairment, while also minimizing initial intravascular fluid infusion in the face of internal injuries resulting from penetrating trauma. Associated conditions known to confound initial trauma care are also expertly reviewed.

Volume 2 covers the critical care management of trauma and the other emergency surgical conditions commonly encountered in modern surgical intensive care units. Recent evidence-based principles of care are provided for virtually every condition for which such data exist. In addition, there are chapters focusing on the patient's transition to recovery following the critical care period, including physical, occupational, and psychological rehabilitation. For example, it addresses screening and treatment of posttraumatic stress disorder.

Complementing the breadth of material, the chapters are co-written by experts from all of the relevant pivotal specialties, ranging from resuscitologists, emergency medicine doctors, anesthesiologists, and orthopedists to the spectrum of surgeons, intensivists, psychiatrists, and rehabilitation experts. In addition, the co-authors hail from around the globe, emphasizing the international appeal, perspective, and orientation of this extremely inclusive, contemporary book.

Finally, I should also say that the editors are exceptionally well qualified for a book of this magnitude. They are all experienced investigators, authors, and international lecturers on the many topics covered. In summary, this two-volume book should be considered as mandatory reading for every clinician actively involved in the care and management of trauma patients.

Paul E. Pepe, MD, MPH, FACEP, FCCM
Professor of Surgery, Medicine, Public Health
and Riggs Family Chair in Emergency Medicine,
University of Texas Southwestern Medical Center
and the Parkland Emergency Trauma Center
Director, City of Dallas Medical Emergency Services
for Public Safety, Public Health, and Homeland Security
Dallas, Texas, U.S.A.

Foreword

Physicians involved in the care of injured patients come from many different disciplines and are sometimes called "traumatologists." Emergency medical services personnel, emergency physicians, anesthesiologists, surgeons, intensivists, and hospital administrators are all concerned with a broad spectrum of trauma management. This two-volume book, edited by Wilson, Grande, and Hoyt, joins relatively few such comprehensive books on this subject and describes management of the trauma patient from a multidisciplinary standpoint, and emphasizes the anesthesiologist's physiologic perspective.

Internationally, the anesthesiologist is often the resuscitation or reanimation physician, with major responsibilities in the ambulance and in the evaluation area of hospitals, often without a specific trauma service. The table of contents reflects an international group of contributors assembled by the editors to author the chapters. The editors have ensured academic and intellectual strength and clinical expertise. They are to be commended for achieving such attention to detail in the first edition.

Dr. William C. Wilson, a trauma anesthesiologist and intensivist, is internationally recognized in the areas of trauma airway management, respiratory gas exchange, thoracic anesthesia, and monitoring. As editor-in-chief, Dr. Wilson's editorial leadership is evident in the clear organization of the book, fluency of the writing, and balance of coverage.

Dr. Christopher Grande, a clinically active trauma anesthesiologist and intensivist, is the executive director of International Trauma Care (ITACCS). He has published extensively in the area of trauma anesthesia and critical care for decades. Doctor Grande's editorial influence is evidenced by the expert international coverage of many topics.

Dr. Hoyt is a world-renowned trauma surgeon and surgical intensivist. He has been an active leader of numerous prestigious surgical trauma organizations, including past president of the American Association for the Surgery of Trauma and the Shock Society, as well as chairman of the American College of Surgeons Committee on Trauma.

He is the current president of the Pan American Trauma Society. Dr. Hoyt's experience and wisdom are reflected in his careful editorial oversight of this comprehensive two-volume treatise on trauma care.

Volume 1 covers the areas of prehospital care, resuscitation, perioperative management, and associated trauma conditions. It is logically organized, covering the key conditions, and provides clear guidelines for medical and surgical decision making, including global operative considerations. However, by design, esoteric technical details of surgical procedures are omitted in favor of general management concepts and principles supported by recent literature. Other important trauma-related conditions (e.g., alcohol and drug intoxication, burns, near drowning, etc.) and management of unique populations (e.g., pediatric, geriatric, and obstetric) are also reviewed in Volume 1.

Volume 2 covers the critical care management of trauma and is a logical, systems-based presentation of the problems commonly encountered in a modern intensive care unit. This volume reviews medical conditions, the role of psychological factors, the family, rehabilitation, and ethics. In addition, emerging topics such as remote evaluation and management are introduced.

Because of the fundamental importance of the subject matter along with the editorial review, this two-volume set represents a compelling resource in the management of trauma and is highly recommended for all clinicians with primary responsibility for resuscitation and management of trauma patients.

Kenneth L. Mattox, MD, FACS
Professor and Vice Chair
Michael E. DeBakey Department of Surgery
Baylor College of Medicine
Chief of Surgery
Ben Taub General Hospital
Houston, Texas, U.S.A.

Preface

OVERVIEW OF BOTH VOLUMES

Trauma is the leading cause of death in the young (ages 1-44) in the United States and the chief reason for lost years of productive life among citizens living in industrialized countries. Despite the enormous importance of the subject matter, no single text has yet been published that fully covers all phases of trauma management.

The purpose of this book is to bring together in one source a description of modern clinical management principles for the care of the trauma patient. This two-volume set, *Trauma, Volume 1: Emergency Resuscitation, Perioperative Anesthesia, Surgical Management and Trauma, Volume 2: Critical Care,* thoroughly encompasses the entire spectrum of trauma management from the prehospital phase through critical care and rehabilitation.

A comprehensive table of contents, at the front of each volume, encapsulates the organization of the entire book (providing a macroscopic view), and also details the sections and sub-headings within each chapter (providing a microscopic view). The extensive index at the back of the book is organized to provide expeditious referral to specific pages that cover the subject matter of interest. The reader is encouraged to utilize both the very detailed table of contents and the index as needed to quickly locate topics.

Each chapter in this work incorporates important features that greatly enhance information communication and learning. The chapters are generously illustrated with figures and tables to facilitate synthesis of important concepts. In addition, key points are highlighted within the text and are summarized at the end of each chapter for quick review. Care has been taken to minimize redundancy by maximizing appropriate cross-referencing throughout. Another useful aspect of each chapter is the Eye to the Future section, which reviews emerging concepts and new research findings likely to impact clinical management.

The contributors to these volumes are both authoritative (having performed original research and authored numerous publications on their subject matter) and have extensive clinical experience. The authorship considered as a whole is truly international, with contributors from all continents. Furthermore, both civilian and military considerations are reviewed whenever relevant. The majority of chapters have multi-specialty co-authorship by experts in trauma surgery, trauma anesthesiology, emergency medicine, and numerous other medical and surgical specialties. In addition, chapters have multidisciplinary involvement by experts in physical medicine, rehabilitation, nursing, and pharmacy, among other disciplines. The scientific soundness is further insured by the multiple layers of editorial oversight; every chapter has been reviewed by at least three experts in the field (principal, associate and section editors). The high level of scientific accuracy and the reader-friendly nature of these two volumes are expected to facilitate learning in order to improve the care provided to trauma patients around the globe.

OVERVIEW OF VOLUME 2

Volume 2 is comprised of 74 chapters that are organized into sections beginning with a basic science review emphasizing the concepts most relevant to the practice of critical care. A section on analgesia, sedation, and neuromuscular blockade begins the clinical management portion of the volume. A review of the important monitoring principles of relevance to trauma critical care is provided next. The core of this volume is comprised of sections covering management considerations for surgical and trauma critical care conditions. These sections and chapters are grouped according to the systems affected, including neurological, cardiovascular, pulmonary, gastrointestinal, renal, infectious diseases, hematological, as well as endocrinological disorders and the systemic inflammatory response syndrome (SIRS). Sections are also provided covering physical and psychological rehabilitation, ethical concerns, and other topics, including techniques for conducting rounds, remote management, the economics of trauma, and severity of illness scoring.

Woven throughout this text are current diagnostic, monitoring, and organ support strategies recognized to improve outcomes in critically ill trauma patients. These concepts include: early enteral nutrition; aggressive monitoring and treatment of pain, agitation, and delirium; and prophylaxis against such complications as thromboembolism, stress ulcers, pressure sores, and ventilator-associated pneumonia. Newly emphasized guidelines such as tight glucose control with intensive insulin therapy, lung protective strategies of mechanical ventilation, early goal-directed therapy for sepsis, and other evidence-based recommendations are also provided where such data exist. The recognition that rehabilitation begins upon admission and that the consequences of early management decisions can impact long-term outcomes are also emphasized.

William C. Wilson, MD, MA
Christopher M. Grande, MD, MPH
David B. Hoyt, MD, FACS

Acknowledgments

The editors would like to express gratitude to our families and loved ones for their unwavering support during the many years of planning and production of this book. Without their sacrifices, encouragement, and love, this two-volume book could not have been completed.

The associate editors and numerous section editors have likewise sacrificed time from their families and other professional responsibilities during their dedicated work on this important project. We cannot over express our gratitude for their contributions, or for our delight in the superb job accomplished by these gifted experts. Due to their diligence, this book has achieved a level of editorial oversight seldom found in multi-authored books.

Essential to the production of this work was the superb administrative assistance provided by Paul Hobson and Bertha Englund. Paul, in particular, must be acknowledged for his dedicated support, working weekends and late into many evenings throughout the process of chapter formatting and editing. In addition, the contributions made by Linda Kesselring, Jan Bailey, and Sereyrathana Keng during the early stages of this project were critical to the ultimate success of the book. The excellent administrative support of Linda Collins throughout the project was likewise essential.

Also vital to the development of this book has been the assistance of ITACCS (International TraumaCare), whose membership has contributed numerous chapters, and whose leadership has supported this project throughout its development.

Finally, we would like to acknowledge the expert assistance provided by our publishers at Informa Healthcare. The professionalism of this organization has been superb, starting at the top with Sandra Beberman, and throughout the publication process with the able assistance of Vanessa Sanchez and Joe Stubenrauch. The professionals at the Egerton Group (Joanne Jay and Paula Garber) were likewise essential to the production of this book. In particular, Mrs. Garber, editorial supervisor, must be commended for providing excellent attention to detail, a strong work ethic, and calm, kind leadership throughout the typesetting and final editing. Geoffrey Greenwood must also be acknowledged for helping us initiate this project many years ago. Each of these individuals has served to kindly and expertly assist our navigation through the ardors of the publication process, and we are grateful to them all.

William C. Wilson, MD, MA
Christopher M. Grande, MD, MPH
David B. Hoyt, MD, FACS

Contents

SECTION B: ANALGESIA, SEDATION, AND NEUROMUSCULAR BLOCKADE
Section Editor: Todd Dorman

**SECTION C: MONITORING CONSIDERATIONS FOR TRAUMA AND
CRITICAL CARE**
Section Editor: José A. Acosta

SECTION E: CARDIOVASCULAR CONSIDERATIONS IN CRITICAL CARE
Section Editors: William J. Mazzei and Charles E. Smith

SECTION F: PULMONARY CONSIDERATIONS IN CRITICAL CARE
Section Editor: Jonathan L. Benumof

SECTION I: INFECTIOUS DISEASE AND ANTIBIOTIC CONSIDERATIONS
Section Editors: Dennis G. Maki and Charles L. James

SECTION K: ENDOCRINE AND AUTOCRINE DISORDERS IN CRITICAL ILLNESS
Section Editor: Greet Van den Berghe

SECTION L: PSYCHOLOGICAL SUPPORT AND PHYSICAL REHABILITATION
Section Editor: Catherine McCoy-Hill

64. Providing Family-Centered Care 1143
Catherine McCoy-Hill and William C. Wilson

65. Post-traumatic Stress Disorder in Trauma and Critical Care 1155
Robert Stone, Catherine McCoy-Hill, Troy L. Holbrook, William C. Wilson, and David B. Hoyt

Omaran Abdeen   Division of Nephrology and Hypertension, Department of Medicine, UC San Diego Medical Center, and VA Medical Center, San Diego, California, U.S.A.

José A. Acosta   Division of Trauma and Critical Care, Department of Surgery, Naval Medical Center San Diego, San Diego, California, U.S.A.

Shamsuddin Akhtar   Department of Anesthesiology, Yale University School of Medicine, New Haven, Connecticut, U.S.A.

Eric R. Amador   Department of Anesthesia, Stanford University Medical Center, Stanford, California, U.S.A.

Niren Angle   Department of Surgery, UC San Diego Medical Center, San Diego, California, U.S.A.

Devashish J. Anjaria   Division of Trauma, Burns, and Critical Care, Department of Surgery, UC San Diego Medical Center, San Diego, California, U.S.A.

Donald M. Arnold   Section of Transfusion Medicine, Department of Medicine, McMaster University, Hamilton, Ontario, Canada

Henry E. Aryan   Division of Neurosurgery, Department of Surgery, UC San Diego Medical Center, San Diego, California, U.S.A.

Ahmed Fikry Attaallah   Department of Anesthesiology, West Virginia University, Morgantown, West Virginia, U.S.A.

Benjamin I. Atwater   Department of Anesthesiology, UC San Diego School of Medicine, San Diego, California, U.S.A.

Vishal Bansal   Division of Trauma, Burns, and Critical Care, Department of Surgery, UC San Diego Medical Center, San Diego, California, U.S.A.

Michael Berrigan   Department of Anesthesiology and Critical Care Medicine, George Washington University Hospital, Washington, D.C., U.S.A.

Tareg Bey   Department of Emergency Medicine, UC Irvine Medical Center, Irvine, California, U.S.A.

Sangeeta N. Bhatia   Department of Electrical Engineering and Computer Science, Massachusetts Institute of Technology, Cambridge, Massachusetts, U.S.A.

Janice Bitetti   Department of Anesthesiology and Critical Care Medicine, George Washington University Hospital, Washington, D.C., U.S.A.

Grant V. Bochicchio   Department of Surgery, University of Maryland School of Medicine, Baltimore, Maryland, U.S.A.

Marie L. Borum   Division of Gastroenterology and Liver Diseases, Department of Medicine, George Washington University, Washington, D.C., U.S.A.

Michael Bouvet   Department of Surgery, UC San Diego Medical Center, San Diego, California, U.S.A.

James Gordon Cain   Department of Anesthesiology and Critical Care Medicine, University of Pittsburgh, Pittsburgh, Pennsylvania, U.S.A.

Paul A. Campbell   Department of Medicine and Anesthesiology, UC San Francisco Medical Center, San Francisco, California, U.S.A.

Enrico M. Camporesi   Department of Anesthesiology and Critical Care, University of South Florida College of Medicine, Tampa, Florida, U.S.A.

Kenneth D. Candido   Department of Anesthesiology, Northwestern University Medical School, and Department of Respiratory Care, Northwestern Memorial Hospital, Chicago, Illinois, U.S.A.

A. Sue Carlisle   Department Anesthesiology and Critical Care Medicine, UC San Francisco Medical Center, San Francisco, California, U.S.A.

Shobana Chandrasekar   Department of Anesthesiology, Baylor College of Medicine, Houston, Texas, U.S.A.

Lakhmir Chawla   Department of Anesthesiology and Critical Care Medicine, George Washington University Medical Center, Washington, D.C., U.S.A.

William C. Chiu   Department of Surgery, R Adams Cowley Shock-Trauma Center, Baltimore, Maryland, U.S.A.

Jua Choi   Department of Nutrition, UC San Diego Medical Center, San Diego, California, U.S.A.

Jonathan B. Cohen   Department of Anesthesiology and Critical Care, University of South Florida College of Medicine, Tampa, Florida, U.S.A.

Raul Coimbra   Division of Trauma, Burns, and Critical Care, Department of Surgery, UC San Diego Medical Center, San Diego, California, U.S.A.

John B. Cone   Department of Surgery, University of Arkansas, Little Rock, Arkansas, U.S.A.

Donnelle L. Crouse   Division of Trauma, Burns, and Critical Care, Department of Surgery, UC San Diego Medical Center, San Diego, California, U.S.A.

Terence M. Davidson   Department of Otolaryngology–Head and Neck Surgery, UC San Diego Medical Center, and San Diego VA Healthcare System, San Diego, California, U.S.A.

Peter J. Davis   Departments of Anesthesiology, Critical Care Medicine, and Pediatrics, Children's Hospital of Pittsburgh, Pittsburgh, Pennsylvania, U.S.A.

Tercio de Campos   Division of Trauma, Burns, and Critical Care, Department of Surgery, UC San Diego Medical Center, San Diego, California, U.S.A.

Charles D. Deakin   Department of Anesthesia, Southampton University Hospitals NHS Trust, Southampton, U.K.

Todd Dorman   Departments of Anesthesiology, Adult Critical Care Medicine, and Surgery, School of Medicine, Johns Hopkins University, Baltimore, Maryland, U.S.A.

Ulrike B. Eisenmann Department of Anesthesiology and Critical Care, UC San Diego Medical Center, San Diego, California, U.S.A.

Ahmed Elrefai Department of Anesthesiology, INOVA Fairfax Hospital, Falls Church, Virginia, U.S.A.

Christopher R. Entwisle Division of Gastroenterology and Liver Diseases, Department of Medicine, George Washington University, Washington, D.C., U.S.A.

Henri R. Ford Department of Surgery, University of Southern California School of Medicine, Children's Hospital Los Angeles, Los Angeles, California, U.S.A.

Richard Ford Department of Respiratory Care, UC San Diego Medical Center, San Diego, California, U.S.A.

Samme Fuchs Department of Nutrition, UC San Diego Medical Center, San Diego, California, U.S.A.

Thomas Genuit Department of Surgery, R Adams Cowley Shock-Trauma Center, Baltimore, Maryland, U.S.A.

Eugene Golts Department of Surgery, UC San Diego Medical Center, San Diego, California, U.S.A.

Michael A. Gropper Department of Anesthesia and Critical Care Medicine, UC San Francisco Medical Center and the UCSF Cardiovascular Research Institute, San Francisco, California, U.S.A.

Cristina Guerra Department of Trauma and Critical Care Surgery, Alamogordo, New Mexico, U.S.A.

Rukaiya K. Hamid Department of Anesthesiology, UC Irvine Medical Center, Irvine, California, U.S.A.

Leland H. Hanowell Department of Anesthesia, Stanford University Medical Center, Stanford, California, U.S.A.

Tarek Hassanein Division of Hepatology and Liver Transplantation, Department of Medicine, UC San Diego Medical Center, San Diego, California, U.S.A.

J. C. Heygood Division of Occupational Therapy, Department of Rehabilitation Services, UC San Diego Medical Center, San Diego, California, U.S.A.

Troy L. Holbrook Department of Family and Preventative Medicine, UC San Diego Medical Center, San Diego, California, U.S.A.

David B. Hoyt Department of Surgery, UC Irvine Medical Center, Irvine, California, U.S.A.

Samuel A. Hughes Department of Neurosurgical Surgery, Oregon Health and Science University, Portland, Oregon, U.S.A.

Doug Humber Department of Pharmacy, UC San Diego Medical Center, San Diego, California, U.S.A.

Judith C. F. Hwang Department of Anesthesiology, UC Davis Medical Center, Sacramento, California, U.S.A.

Irving "Jake" Jacoby Hyperbaric Medicine Center, Department of Emergency Medicine, UC San Diego Medical Center, San Diego, California, U.S.A.

Farivar Jahansouz Department of Pharmacy, UC San Diego Medical Center, San Diego, California, U.S.A.

Charles L. James Division of Infectious Diseases, Departments of Medicine and Pharmacy, UC San Diego Medical Center, San Diego, California, U.S.A.

Rahul Jandial Division of Neurosurgery, UC San Diego Medical Center, San Diego, and the Burnham Institute for Medical Research, La Jolla, California, U.S.A.

Christopher Junker Department of Anesthesiology and Critical Care Medicine, George Washington University Hospital, Washington, D.C., U.S.A.

Abdallah Kabbara Department of Anesthesia, MetroHealth Medical Center, Cleveland, Ohio, U.S.A.

Lewis J. Kaplan Section of Trauma, Critical Care, and Surgical Emergencies, Yale University School of Medicine, New Haven, Connecticut, U.S.A.

Matthew H. Katz Department of Surgery, UC San Diego Medical Center, San Diego, California, U.S.A.

John A. Kellum Departments of Critical Care Medicine and Medicine, University of Pittsburgh, Pittsburgh, Pennsylvania, U.S.A.

Robert R. Kirby University of Florida College of Medicine, and the Malcom B. Randall VA Medical Center, Gainesville, Florida, U.S.A

Theo N. Kirkland Division of Infectious Diseases, Departments of Pathology and Medicine, UC San Diego School of Medicine, San Diego, California, U.S.A.

Erik B. Kistler Department of Anesthesiology and Critical Care, UC San Diego Medical Center, San Diego, California, U.S.A.

W. Andrew Kofke Department of Anesthesia, University of Pennsylvania Hospital, Philadelphia, Pennsylvania, U.S.A.

Jeanne Lee Division of Trauma, Burns, and Critical Care, Department of Surgery, UC San Diego Medical Center, San Diego, California, U.S.A.

Sung Lee Division of Cardiology, Department of Medicine, George Washington University Hospital, Washington, D.C., U.S.A.

Michael L. Levy Division of Neurosurgery, Department of Surgery, UC San Diego Medical Center, San Diego, California, U.S.A.

Ludwig H. Lin Department of Anesthesiology and Critical Care Medicine, UC San Francisco Medical Center, San Francisco, California, U.S.A.

Emilio B. Lobato Department of Anesthesiology and Critical Care Medicine, University of Florida College of Medicine, Malcolm B. Randall VA Medical Center, Gainesville, Florida, U.S.A.

John M. Luce Department of Medicine and Anesthesia, UC San Francisco School of Medicine, San Francisco General Hospital, San Francisco, California, U.S.A.

Eugenio Lujan Department of Anesthesiology and Critical Care Medicine, Naval Medical Center San Diego, San Diego, California, U.S.A.

Colin F. Mackenzie Department of Anesthesiology, University of Maryland School of Medicine, Baltimore, Maryland, U.S.A.

Peter Mair Department of Anesthesia and Intensive Care Medicine, Division of Cardiovascular Anesthesia, University of Innsbruck School of Medicine, Innsbruck, Austria

Debra L. Malone Department of Surgery, University of Maryland School of Medicine, R Adams Cowley Shock-Trauma Center, Baltimore, Maryland, U.S.A.

Gerard R. Manecke, Jr. Section of Cardiothoracic Anesthesia, Department of Anesthesiology, UC San Diego Medical Center, San Diego, California, U.S.A.

Jason Marengo   Department of Surgery, UC San Diego Medical Center, San Diego, California, U.S.A.

Rhonda K. Martin   Division of Hepatology and Liver Transplantation, Department of Medicine, UC San Diego Medical Center, San Diego, California, U.S.A.

Michael A. Matthay   Departments of Medicine, Anesthesia, and Critical Care Medicine, UC San Francisco Medical Center, and the UCSF Cardiovascular Research Institute, San Francisco, California, U.S.A.

Catherine McCoy-Hill   School of Nursing, Azusa Pacific University, Azusa, California, U.S.A.

Amy A. McDonald   Department of Surgery, MetroHealth Medical Center, Case Western Reserve University, Cleveland, Ohio, U.S.A.

Brian McGrath   Department of Anesthesiology and Critical Care Medicine, George Washington University School of Medicine, Washington, D.C., U.S.A.

Ravindra Mehta   Division of Nephrology and Hemodialysis Services, Department of Medicine, UC San Diego Medical Center, San Diego, California, U.S.A.

Douglas N. Mellinger   Division of Cardiothoracic Surgery, Department of Surgery, UC San Diego Medical Center, San Diego, California, U.S.A.

Pedro Alejandro Mendez-Tellez   Departments of Anesthesiology, Adult Critical Care Medicine, and Surgery, School of Medicine, Johns Hopkins University, Baltimore, Maryland, U.S.A.

Dieter Mesotten   Department of Intensive Care Medicine, University Hospital Gasthuisberg, Catholic University of Leuven, Leuven, Belgium

Sara Minasyan   Department of Surgery, UC San Diego Medical Center, San Diego, California, U.S.A.

Anushirvan Minokadeh   Department of Anesthesiology and Critical Care, UC San Diego Medical Center, San Diego, California, U.S.A.

Benoit Misset   Department of Medicine and Anesthesiology, UC San Francisco Medical Center, San Francisco, California, U.S.A.

Tobias Moeller-Bertram   Section of Pain Management, Department of Anesthesiology, UC San Diego Medical Center, and VA Medical Center, San Diego, California, U.S.A.

A. R. Moossa   Department of Surgery, UC San Diego Medical Center, San Diego, California, U.S.A.

Lena M. Napolitano   Department of Surgery, University of Michigan School of Medicine, Ann Arbor, Michigan, U.S.A.

Srdjan Nedeljkovic   Department of Anesthesiology and Critical Care Medicine, Brigham and Women's Hospital, Harvard University School of Medicine, Boston, Massachusetts, U.S.A.

Shelley Nehman   Department of Surgery, University of Maryland School of Medicine, Baltimore, Maryland, U.S.A.

Philippa Newfield   Department of Anesthesiology, UC San Francisco, Children's Hospital of San Francisco, San Francisco, California, U.S.A.

Quyen T. Nguyen   Department of Otolaryngology–Head and Neck Surgery, UC San Diego Medical Center, and San Diego VA Healthcare System, San Diego, California, U.S.A.

Eric S. Nylen   Department of Endocrinology, George Washington University, VA Medical Center, Washington D.C., U.S.A.

Kerrie Olexa   Division of Physical Therapy, Department of Rehabilitation Services, UC San Diego Medical Center, San Diego, California, U.S.A.

Joanne Ondrush   Department of Anesthesiology and Critical Care Medicine, George Washington University Hospital, Washington, D.C., U.S.A.

Steven L. Orebaugh   Department of Anesthesiology, University of Pittsburgh Medical Center, Pittsburgh, Pennsylvania, U.S.A.

Eamon O'Reilly   Department of Surgery, Naval Medical Center San Diego, San Diego, California, U.S.A.

Lucia Palladino   Department of Anesthesiology and Critical Care Medicine, George Washington University Hospital, Washington, D.C., U.S.A.

Joel R. Peerless   Department of Surgical Critical Care, MetroHealth Medical Center, Case Western Reserve University, Cleveland, Ohio, U.S.A.

Linda Pelinka   Department of Anesthesia and Critical Care, Lorenz Boehler Trauma Center, Vienna, Austria

Eleni Pentheroudakis   Department of Emergency Medicine, Drexel University College of Medicine, Philadelphia, Pennsylvania, U.S.A.

William T. Peruzzi   Department of Anesthesiology, Northwestern University Medical School, and Department of Respiratory Care, Northwestern Memorial Hospital, Chicago, Illinois, U.S.A.

Paul Picton   Department of Anesthesiology, University of Michigan School of Medicine, Ann Arbor, Michigan, U.S.A.

Bruce Potenza   Division of Trauma, Burns, and Critical Care, Department of Surgery, UC San Diego Medical Center, San Diego, California, U.S.A.

Faisal Qureshi   Department of Surgery, University of Southern California School of Medicine, Children's Hospital Los Angeles, Los Angeles, California, U.S.A.

Joseph F. Rappold   Division of Trauma and Critical Care, Department of Surgery, Naval Medical Center San Diego, San Diego, California, U.S.A.

Agnes Ricard-Hibon   Department of Anesthesiology and Critical Care Medicine, Beaujon University Hospital, Clichy, France

Leland S. Rickman   Division of Infectious Diseases, Departments of Medicine and Pharmacy, UC San Diego Medical Center, San Diego, California, U.S.A.

José Manuel Rodríguez-Paz   Departments of Anesthesiology, Adult Critical Care Medicine, and Surgery, School of Medicine, Johns Hopkins University, Baltimore, Maryland, U.S.A.

David M. Roth   Section of Cardiothoracic Anesthesia, Department of Anesthesiology, UC San Diego Medical Center, San Diego, California, U.S.A.

Sacha Salzberg   Department of Cardiothoracic Surgery, Mount Sinai School of Medicine, New York, New York, U.S.A.

Ramon Sanchez   Sections of Cardiothoracic Anesthesia and Liver Transplantation, Department of Anesthesiology, UC San Diego Medical Center, San Diego, California, U.S.A.

Daniel Scheidegger   Department of Anesthesiology, University of Basel School of Medicine, Basel, Switzerland

Hans W. Schweiger   Department of Anesthesiology and Critical Care, University of South Florida College of Medicine, Tampa, Florida, U.S.A.

Michael G. Seneff   Department of Anesthesiology and Critical Care Medicine, George Washington University Medical Center, Washington, D.C., U.S.A.

Ahmet Can Senel   Department of Anesthesiology and Critical Care Medicine, George Washington University Medical Center, Washington, D.C., U.S.A.

Nitin Shah   Department of Anesthesiology and Critical Care, Long Beach VA Hospital, Long Beach, California, U.S.A.

Shamik Shah   Division of Nephrology and Hypertension, Department of Medicine, UC San Diego Medical Center, San Diego, California, U.S.A.

Niten Singh   Division of Vascular Surgery, Department of Surgery, USUHS Medical Center, Bethesda, Maryland, and the Madigan Army Medical Center, Tacoma, Washington, U.S.A.

Elizabeth H. Sinz   Departments of Anesthesiology and Neurosurgery, Penn State College of Medicine, Penn State University Hospital, Hershey, Pennsylvania, U.S.A.

Charles E. Smith   Department of Anesthesiology, MetroHealth Medical Center, Case Western Reserve University, Cleveland, Ohio, U.S.A.

Jan Stange   Division of Gastroenterology, Department of Internal Medicine, University of Rostock School of Medicine, Rostock, Germany

John K. Stene   Department of Anesthesiology, Penn State College of Medicine, Penn State University Hospital, Hershey, Pennsylvania, U.S.A.

Marc E. Stone   Department of Anesthesiology, Mount Sinai School of Medicine, New York, New York, U.S.A.

Robert Stone   Department of Psychiatry, Post Traumatic Stress Disorder Unit, Oregon State Hospital, Salem, Oregon, U.S.A.

Martin Straznicky   Section of Cardiothoracic Anesthesia, Department of Anesthesiology, UC San Diego Medical Center, San Diego, California, U.S.A.

Anne J. Sutcliffe   Department of Anesthesia and Critical Care, Alexandra Hospital, Redditch, U.K.

Mark A. Swancutt   Departments of Microbiology and Medicine, Southwestern Medical Center, Dallas, Texas, U.S.A.

Hoi Sang U   Division of Neurosurgery, Department of Surgery, UC San Diego Medical Center, San Diego, California, U.S.A.

Jeffrey S. Upperman   Division of Pediatric Surgery, Department of Surgery, University of Southern California School of Medicine, Children's Hospital Los Angeles, Los Angeles, California, U.S.A.

Greet Van den Berghe   Department of Intensive Care Medicine, University Hospital Gasthuisberg, Catholic University of Leuven, Leuven, Belgium

Ilse Vanhorebeek   Department of Intensive Care Medicine, University Hospital Gasthuisberg, Catholic University of Leuven, Leuven, Belgium

Daniel P. Vezina   Division of Cardiovascular Anesthesiology, Department of Anesthesiology, and the Division of Cardiology, Department of Medicine, University of Utah School of Medicine, and the VA Medical Center, Salt Lake City, Utah, U.S.A.

Theodore E. Warkentin   Departments of Pathology and Molecular Medicine, McMaster University School of Medicine, and the Transfusion Medicine Service, Hamilton Health Sciences, Hamilton, Ontario, Canada

Jon C. White   Department of Surgery, VA Medical Center, George Washington University, Washington, D.C., U.S.A.

Jeanine P. Wiener-Kronish   Departments of Medicine, Anesthesia, and Critical Care Medicine, UC San Francisco Medical Center, and the UCSF Cardiovascular Research Institute, San Francisco, California, U.S.A.

William C. Wilson   Department of Anesthesiology and Critical Care, UC San Diego Medical Center, San Diego, California, U.S.A.

Todd N. Witte   Division of Gastroenterology and Liver Diseases, Department of Medicine, George Washington University, Washington, D.C., U.S.A.

Michael J. Yanakakis   Department of Anesthesia and Perioperative Care, UC San Francisco Medical Center, San Francisco, California, U.S.A.

Charles J. Yowler   Department of Surgery, MetroHealth Medical Center, Case Western Reserve University, Cleveland, Ohio, U.S.A.

1

Neurophysiology Review

Paul Picton
Department of Anesthesiology, University of Michigan School of Medicine, Ann Arbor, Michigan, U.S.A.

Charles D. Deakin
Department of Anesthesia, Southampton University Hospitals NHS Trust, Southampton, U.K.

INTRODUCTION

Pathophysiological principles underpin the modern management of trauma and head injury. It is vital that healthcare professionals have a good understanding of neurophysiology and pathophysiology and are able to interpret the many monitoring parameters now available in order to offer best management.

In this chapter, the most important physiological principles relevant to the management of trauma patients, in general, and to head injury, in particular, will be discussed. Some important anatomy will be included. The pathophysiological response to injury of the central nervous system (CNS) will be outlined, which continues to be an area of intense research. Some pharmacological and therapeutic interventions will be discussed where relevant, and some monitoring techniques will be briefly considered.

APPLIED ANATOMY

The nervous system may be divided anatomically into the CNS, the peripheral nervous system (PNS), and the autonomic nervous system (ANS). The CNS is further divided into brain, brainstem, and spinal cord. The cerebrospinal fluid (CSF) system provides a buffer against movement for the CNS, and the blood–brain barrier provides for some separation of the CNS from the systemic environment.

Brain

The brain has a mass of approximately 1500 g and is contained within a noncompliant bony vault: the skull. It is formed of the four major lobes (frontal, parietal, temporal, and occipital), the thalamus, the hypothalamus, the basal ganglia, brainstem, and the cerebellum (Fig. 1). A relatively thin stratum of neurons on the surface of the cerebrum and cerebellum comprise the portions known as the cerebral and cerebellar cortex. Each geographical region of the brain, and its associated structures, serve specific neurological functions. Accordingly, destructive lesions to discrete regions will result in characteristic clinical findings (Table 1).

Four Major Lobes (Frontal, Parietal, Temporal, and Occipital)

The frontal lobes are responsible for motor and various elements of intellectual and emotive function. The precentral gyrus, the primary motor cortex, is located immediately anterior to the central sulcus. The motor complex is somatotopically organized (Fig. 2) so that stimulation of the medial portion causes muscle contraction in the lower limb and trunk, stimulation of the middle portion causes muscle contraction in the upper limb, and stimulation of the most lateral portion causes muscle contraction in the head and neck. Immediately anterior to the primary motor cortex is the premotor cortex that is also somatotopically organized, but here stimulation at various points results in patterns of movement rather than individual muscle or muscle group contraction (1,2). Destructive lesions of the frontal lobe cause intellectual impairment, personality change, and contralateral motor dysfunction (3). An important speech region known as Broca's area is found within the frontal lobe (see subsequently).

The parietal lobes are located above the temporal lobes between the frontal and occipital lobes. The primary sensory cortex is located in the postcentral gyrus and like the primary motor cortex is somatotopically represented (Fig. 3) (4). Destructive lesions of the parietal lobes result in contralateral sensory dysfunction, apraxia, a failure to recognize faces or surroundings, and homonymous visual field defects (3).

The temporal lobes are situated inferior to the parietal lobes. Destructive lesions result in acalculia, confusional states, and homonymous visual field defects (3). Alexia and agraphia may result from either temporal or parietal lobe injuries. Also, auditory associations may be impaired when Wernicke's area is injured (see subsequently).

The occipital lobes contain the primary visual cortex. Destructive lesions result in visual field and visuo-spatial defects and disturbances in visual recognition (3).

Cerebral Cortex

The cerebral cortex forms a 2- to 5-mm surface layer of the brain, which is organized into six horizontal layers. The neurons of layers I, II, and III form connections with other parts of the ipsilateral or contralateral cerebral cortex. The neurons in layer IV receive sensory input from the thalamus. Projections to the brainstem and spinal cord take origin from cell bodies located in layer V, and corticothalamic fibers arise from layer VI (5,6).

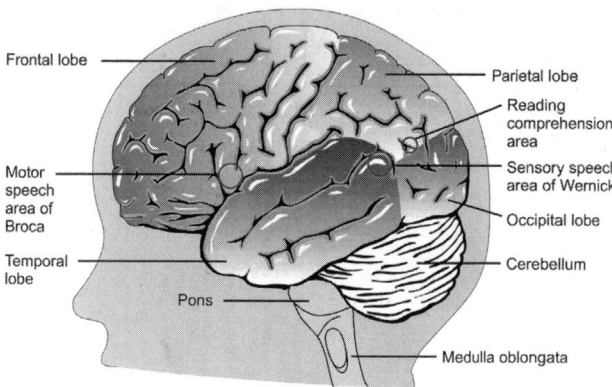

Figure 1   Major anatomical brain regions illustrated in the lateral view of the left hemisphere.

Thalamus, Hypothalamus, and the Basal Ganglia

The thalamus forms a relay station between the periphery and cerebral cortex. The hypothalamus provides a link between the nervous and endocrine systems. Together with a portion of the basal ganglia, these pathways form the limbic system, which controls emotion and physiologic drives (7,8).

Table 1   Regions of the Brain, Their Primary Functions, and the Result of Destructive Lesions

Brain region	Primary function	Result of destructive lesion
Frontal lobe	Motor	Contralateral hemiparesis
	Intellect	Intellectual impairment
	Personality	Personality change
	Motor aspects of speech (Broca's area)	Expressive dysphasia
Parietal lobe	Primary sensory	Contralateral sensory dysfunction
		Apraxia
		Homonymous visual field defects
Temporal lobe	Hearing	Acalculia
	Language	Alexia
	Perception	Agraphia
		Homonymous visual field defects
Temporal-parietal	Speech comprehension (Wernike's area)	Receptive dysphasia
Occipital lobe	Primary visual	Visual field defects
		Disturbances of visual recognition
Thalamus	Relay station	Signal disruption
	Memory	Disruption of long-term memory
Limbic system	Emotion and drives	Emotional instability/ dysfunction
Cerebellum	Motor coordination	Ipsilateral loss of motor coordination

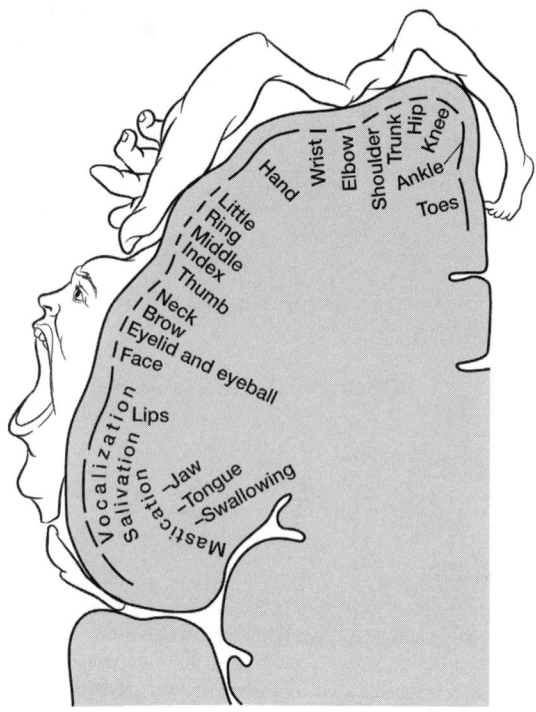

Figure 2   The motor homunculus showing somatotopical representation of the primary motor cortex.

Cerebellum and Cerebellar Cortex

The cerebellum consists of a three-layered cortex and four paired nuclei. The vermis divides the cerebellum in the sagittal plane and is organized in a somatotopical fashion. The cerebellum and a portion of the basal ganglia are vital for the control and co-ordination of movement (9,10).

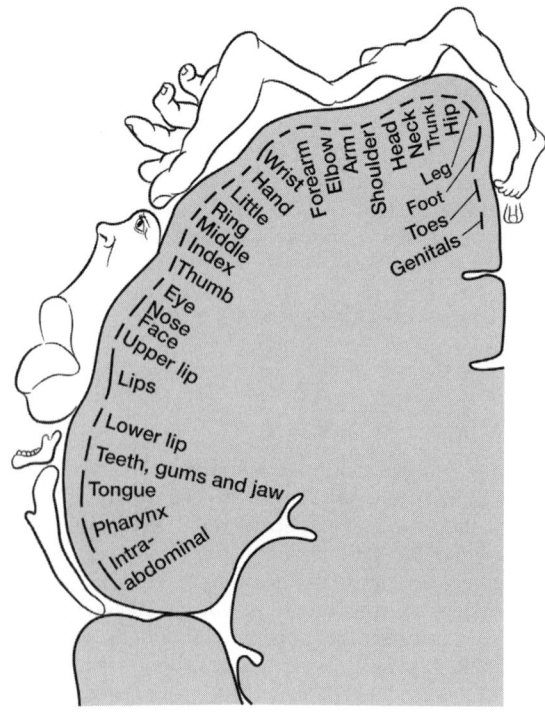

Figure 3   The sensory homunculus showing somatotopical representation of the primary sensory cortex.

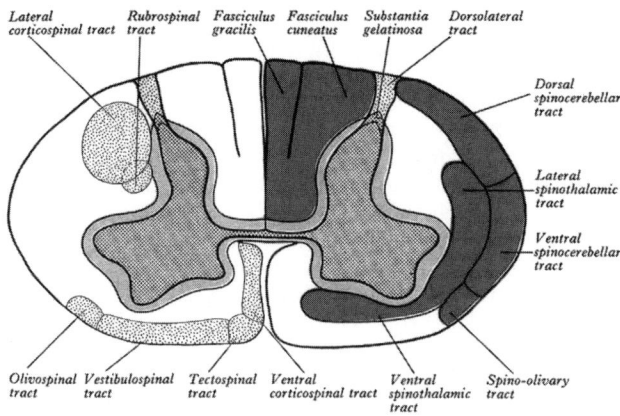

Figure 4 Cross-section of the spinal cord showing the main ascending (*dark gray*) and descending (*stippled*) pathways. The ventral portion of the cord is shown on the bottom of the figure, and the dorsal portion is shown on the top of the figure.

Brainstem

The brainstem consists of the midbrain, pons, and medulla oblongata. It contains vital centers for respiratory and cardiovascular control, the reticular activating system, and the cranial nerve nuclei. It maintains consciousness, the sleep–wake cycle, and spontaneous ventilation. Descending and ascending pathways pass through the brainstem.

Spinal Cord

The spinal cord is approximately 45 cm long in the adult, terminating inferiorly in the conus medularis at approximately L1/L2; although there is considerable variation. The lumbar and sacral roots have a progressively longer course from the spinal cord to reach their corresponding intervertebral foramina and collectively form the cauda equine (11).

In transverse section, the cord consists of a central canal, a pericentral zone of gray matter, and an outer zone

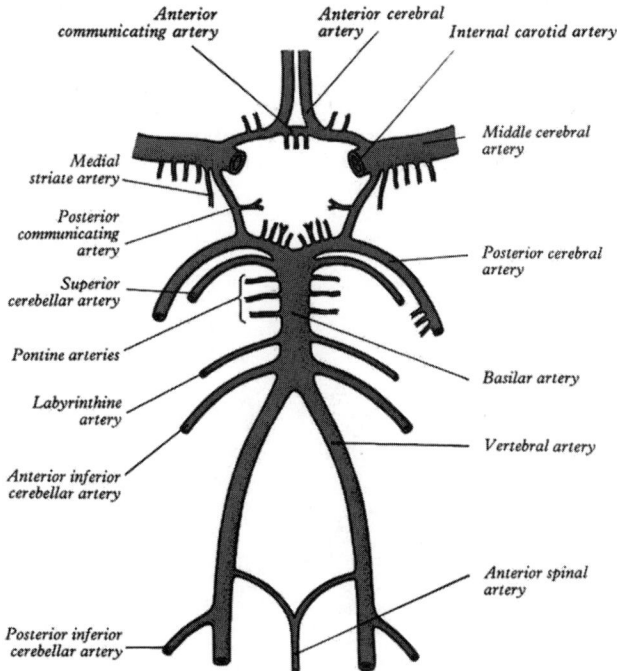

Figure 5 Circle of Willis—the major blood supply to the brain.

of white matter. In the white matter, definite ascending and descending tracts are formed (Fig. 4). The function of the individual tracts is outlined in Table 2.

Arterial Supply and Venous Drainage of the Central Nervous System

Brain and Brainstem

☞ **The blood supply of the brain derives from the Circle of Willis.** ☞ The paired internal carotid arteries (ICAs) divide into anterior cerebral arteries (ACAs) and middle cerebral arteries (MCAs) and provide 70% of cerebral blood supply. The basilar artery is formed by the union of the paired vertebral arteries, dividing into the two posterior cerebral arteries (PCAs) to provide the remaining 30% of cerebral blood flow (CBF). The anterior communicating artery joins the two ACAs, and the posterior communicating artery joins the ICA with the PCA. This anastomosis forms the Circle of Willis (Fig. 5) (12). The ACA supplies the medial portions of the cerebral hemispheres, the MCA supplies the lateral portions, and the PCA supplies the occipital and inferior portions of the temporal lobe (13). The brainstem derives its blood supply from the vertebrobasilar system.

Venous blood drains from the brain cortex and subcortical medullary substance into superficial cerebral veins, and subsequently into the dural venous sinus network. The veins of the brain, as well as the dural sinus system, are entirely devoid of valves. The venous dural sinuses collect blood from the superficial and deep cerebral veins, as well as the skull, and represent the major drainage pathway of the cranial cavity. The venous dural sinuses drain into the jugular bulb and internal jugular vein, which empties into the superior vena cava on the right side, and the innominate vein on the left (13). In most individuals, one of the two internal jugular veins is dominant (receiving most of the dural sinus flow), usually the right one, hence the best site for jugular venous saturation monitoring.

Spinal Cord

The spinal cord blood supply emanates from the larger and more important anterior spinal artery (formed by the union

Table 2 Name and Function of Major Spinal Cord Tracts

Tracts	Name	Function
Ascending (sensory)	Fasciculus gracilis	Contralateral touch, vibration, and proprioception of lower limb
	Fasciculus cuneatus	Contralateral touch, vibration, and proprioception of upper limb
	Spinothalamic	Contralateral pain and temperature
	Spinocerebellar	Transmit ipsilateral proprioceptive information to the cerebellum
Descending (motor)	Lateral corticospinal	Primary motor (75–90%)—crossed
	Ventral corticospinal	Primary motor (10–25%)—uncrossed
	Vestibulospinal	Transmit vestibular information to the motor system

of a branch from each vertebral artery) and the posterior spinal arteries (bilateral vessels which take origin from the inferior cerebellar arteries). The anterior blood supply is supplemented by a series of radicular branches most of which are small but some offer significant flow, particularly the radicularis magna, also known as the "artery of Adamkiewicz" (Fig. 6) (14).

Venous drainage of the spinal cord and vertebral column is complex, with numerous free anastamoses between two primary networks of veins (internal and external). The internal veins drain the spinal cord, and correspond to the arteries in their distribution, forming a

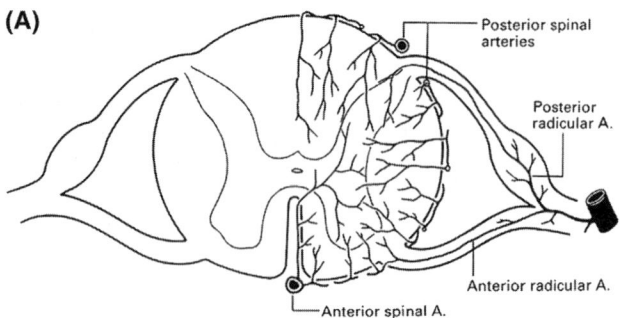

(A)

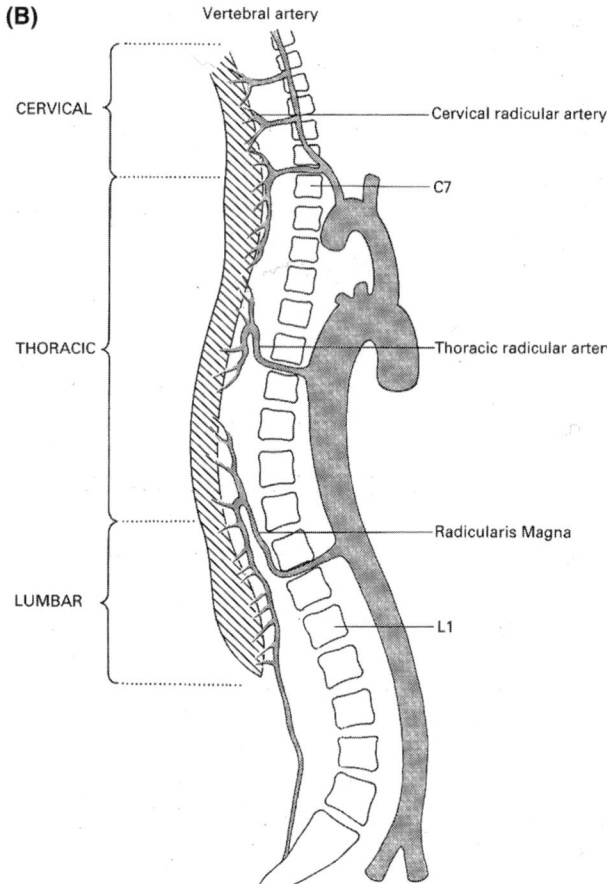

(B)

Figure 6   Blood supply to the spinal cord. (**A**) Transverse section demonstrating contributions from the anterior, posterior, and radicular spinal arteries. (**B**) Lateral schematic view illustrating the contribution of the radicular branches. The thoracic radicular artery, and especially the radicularis magna ("artery of Adamkiewicz") are particularly important.

tortuous pattern in the pia matter surrounding the spinal cord. The venules empty into the anterior and posterior spinal veins, which drain above and below as well as segmentally into anterior and posterior radicular veins (adjacent to each nerve route as it exits the foramen). The external venous plexus drains the vertebral bodies (anterior) and laminae (posterior) and empties segmentally into the intervertebral veins. Here, there is anastomosis with the segmental drainage from the spinal cord. Therefore, changes in intrathoracic pressure or cerebral spinal fluid pressure may produce variations in cord blood volume and flow characteristics. Under various conditions, including surgery, placement of epidural fluids, pregnancy, and spinal trauma, the venous flow may become congested or alter its characteristics, making the cord more vulnerable to ischemia.

Cerebrospinal Fluid System

The CSF system is comprised of the interconnecting ventricles, cisterns, and the subarachnoid space (Fig. 7). The two lateral ventricles communicate with the third ventricle via the interventricular foramina of Monro, and the third ventricle communicates with the fourth via the cerebral aqueduct of Sylvius. The fourth ventricle communicates with the basal cisterns via the bilateral formina of Luschka and via the foramen of Magendie to the subarachnoid space. The intracranial ventricular system contains approximately 150 mL of CSF that, having the same specific gravity as CNS tissue, provides a buffer against movement and trauma (i.e., the brain essentially floats). Also, by changing the volume of CSF, it provides a pressure buffer against any expanding lesion within the cranium (14,15).

The bulk of CSF production occurs in the choroid plexuses of the four ventricles at a constant rate of approximately 500 mL/day, which allows for approximately four turnovers in 24 hours. The CSF circulates through the system to be eventually absorbed into the sagittal venous sinus via multiple arachnoid villi. The absorption rate determines both CSF volume and pressure (16). The normal intracranial pressure (ICP) ranges from 1 to 15 mmHg (i.e., 1–20 cm H_2O).

When compared to plasma, the CSF contains lower glucose, potassium, and protein and greater sodium, chloride, and hydrogen ion concentrations (Table 3). There are no red blood cells and few white blood cells. The CSF

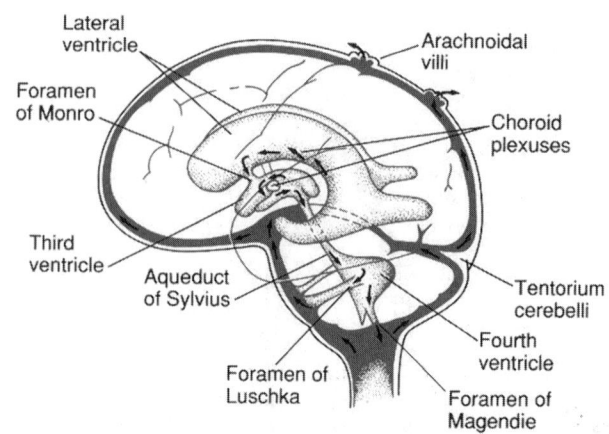

Figure 7   The cerebral ventricular system.

Table 3 Comparison of Plasma and Cerebrospinal Fluid Constituents

	Plasma	CSF
Na$^+$ (mmol/L)	134–146	146–148
K$^+$ (mmol/L)	3.4–5.0	2.8–3.1
HCO$_3^-$ (mmol/L)	22–32	23–24
Cl$^-$ (mmol/L)	98–104	120–28
pH (pH units)	7.35–7.45	7.30–7.35
Glucose (mmol/L)	3.9–6.2	2.7–4.2
WBC (mm^3)	5–10^3/mm^3	<5/mm^3
Protein (g/L)	63–78	0.15–0.45
IgG (g/L)	5.4–16.1	<0.05

Abbreviations: CSF, cerebrospinal fluid; WBC, white blood cell count; Ig, immunoglobulin.

is in direct communication with the CNS extracellular fluid, and hence their compositions are the same (3).

Blood–Brain Barrier

The blood–brain barrier is formed by tight junctions between endothelial cells of CNS capillaries and, to a lesser extent, by astrocyte function. The movement of substances into the brain is restricted, and hence the composition of CSF and CNS extracellular fluid (CNS ECF) is not the same as ECF, elsewhere in the body. It is virtually impermeable to plasma proteins and large nonlipid-soluble molecules. It is slightly permeable to electrolytes and highly permeable to lipid-soluble substances, water, oxygen, and carbon dioxide (16,17).

Cellular Elements

The key cellular elements of the CNS are neurons and their supporting glial cells. The adult human CNS is estimated to contain more than 100 billion neurons.

Despite considerable variability in neuronal morphology they all consist of three basic elements: the cell body, dendrites, and a single axon. Generally speaking, they are organized into two systems: afferent and efferent. The afferent neurons bring impulses inward for processing. For example, the sensory system is responsible for information reception regarding touch, temperature, pain, position, taste, smell, hearing, and sight. The efferent system includes all of the out going impulses (e.g., the motor system, which controls and co-ordinates movement). Neuronal function is dependent on rapid communication between neurons. This occurs via synapses. The synapses are junctions that may be chemical or electrical, the former comprising the vast majority. Presynaptic neuronal depolarization causes calcium-dependent synaptic vesicle/synaptic terminal membrane interaction and the subsequent release of neurotransmitter into the synaptic cleft (a 10–30 μ space between the synaptic terminal and postsynaptic neuron). Electrical synapses consist of low resistance gap junctions between neurons. Electrical communication occurs, allowing rapid signal transfer (18).

Glial cells outnumber neurons approximately ten to one. They have a supporting role and consist of several different types. The star-shaped astrocytes function to maintain the local environment within the CNS and secrete various regulatory factors. Oligodendrocytes ensheath neuronal processes, and are hence responsible for CNS myelination. Microglia have a predominantly phagocytic role. Ependymal cells separate neurons from the ventricular system (17,19).

Autonomic Nervous System

The ANS has efferents to visceral organs, blood vessels, and secretory glands. ☞ **Although influenced by higher brain centers, such as the limbic cortex, the ANS operates to control the homeostatic environment in a purely reflex fashion.** ☞ Cardiac output (Q̇), arterial blood pressure, bronchiolar tone, gastrointestinal motility, urinary bladder function, sexual function, sweating and body temperature, and many other systems are influenced. It is conventionally divided into two systems: the sympathetic and the parasympathetic (Fig. 8), which differ anatomically, physiologically, and pharmacologically. Each has pre- and postganglionic neurons. Preganglionic neurons have cell bodies located in either the brainstem or spinal cord and synapse with postganglionic neurons located in ganglia via thinly myelinated axons. Postganglionic neurons send unmyelinated fibers to visceral effector cells (20–22).

Sympathetic (Thoraco-Lumbar)

The sympathetic chain is a ganglionated nerve trunk, extending from the base of the skull to the coccyx in close approximation to the spinal cord. Postganglionic branches from the sympathetic chain are unmyelinated, tend to run a long course, and may be divided into somatic and visceral groups. Somatic fibers, distributed by spinal nerves, supply the skin and sweat glands. Visceral fibers to the head and neck ascend with the internal carotid and vertebral arteries. Thoracic organs are supplied from local plexuses, and abdominal organs are supplied from the celiac, hypogastric and pelvic plexuses.

The cell bodies of preganglionic neurons are located in the intermediolateral horn of the spinal cord from segments T1-L2. The small segmental myelinated axons leave the spinal cord in the anterior primary rami and pass into the sympathetic chain at the same level via the white rami communicans. The axons then take one of three paths: (*i*) terminate in the sympathetic chain, at its level of origin; (*ii*) ascend or descend in the sympathetic chain, before synapsing at a different level; or (*iii*) exit the sympathetic chain without synapsing and terminate in paravertebral ganglion via splanchnic nerves. Sympathetic preganglionic neurons are generally short (23). Sympathetic innervation follows a segmental pattern. The spinal segments responsible are approximately as follows: head and neck, T1-2; upper limb, T2-7; thorax, T1-4; abdomen, T4-L2; lower limb, T11-L2 (24).

The adrenal medulla forms an important part of the sympathetic nervous system. It is supplied with a rich plexus of preganglionic fibers that pass directly through the celiac plexus. These fibers terminate in contact with medullary cells and stimulate the release of epinephrine and norepinepherine into the bloodstream from where they act at effector sites in a hormonal fashion (21,22). Sympathetic stimulation generally increases cardiovascular activity and arousal while reducing other visceral activity. This forms the "fight or flight" response.

Parasympathetic (Cranio-Sacral)

The parasympathetic system is less widely distributed. The bulk of innervation is to the body cavity viscera. There is no supply to skeletal muscle or skin. Preganglionic fibers are long and myelinated, whereas postganglionic fibers are short and are unmyelinated. Preganglionic fibers arise from a cranial and a sacral component.

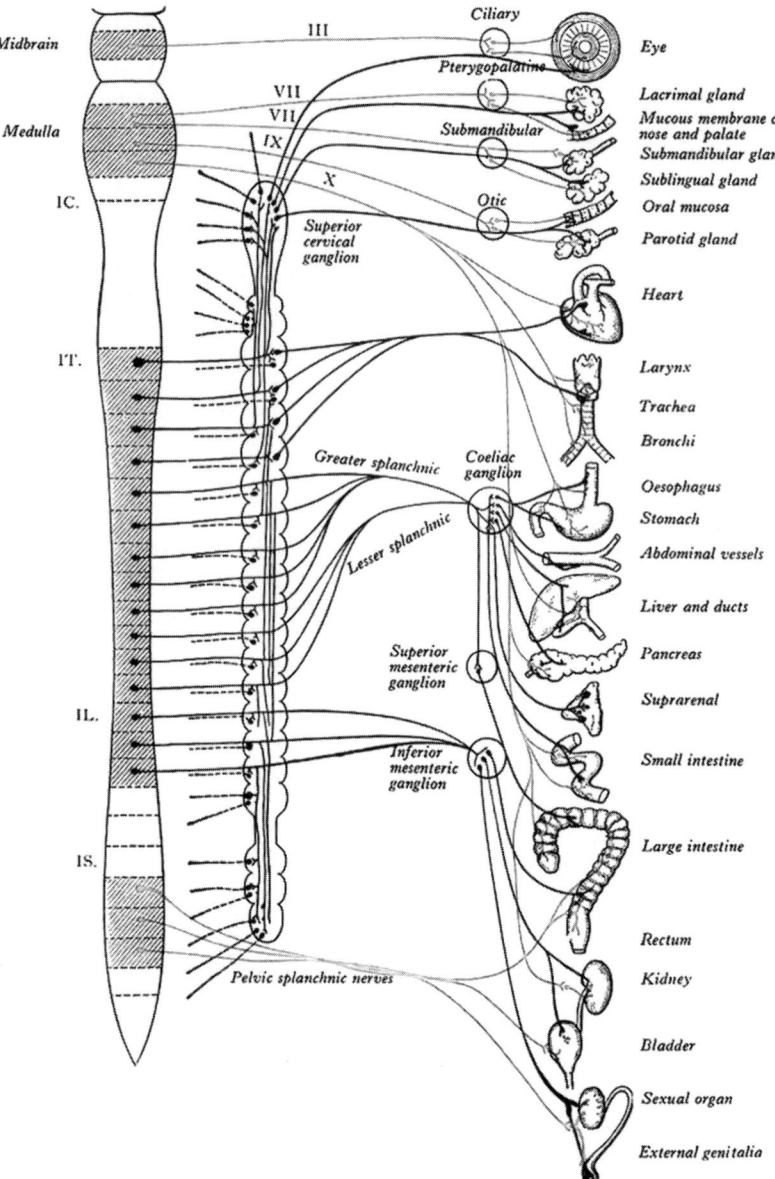

Figure 8 The efferent pathways of the autonomic nervous system. The sympathetic pathways are shown in bold lines, and the parasympathetic pathways are shown in thin lines.

Cell bodies of the cranial outflow are located in brainstem nuclei of the cranial nerves III, VII, IX, and X. Fibers are then distributed with these nerves. Fibers from III, VII, and IX are relayed via four ganglia close to the effector sites: III, the ciliary ganglion; VII, the pterygopalatine and submandibular ganglia; IX, the otic ganglion. The vagal outflow (X) has the most widespread and most important distribution. Fibers terminate in tiny ganglia that lie in visceral walls.

Cell bodies of the sacral outflow are located at sacral segments S2-4 from where their fibers leave in the anterior primary rami. Fibers from the anterior primary rami join to form the pelvic splanchnic nerves that pass through the pelvic plexus to synapse on tiny ganglia in the walls of the pelvic viscera (24). Postganglionic fibers synapse with effector organ cells. Parasympathetic stimulation is generally inhibitory to the heart and lungs and stimulatory to the gastrointestinal system. It also provides a "mechanism for emptying" (21,22).

Neurotransmission (Cholinergic vs. Adrenergic) and Receptor Subtypes

All preganglionic neurons and postganglionic parasympathetic neurons secrete acetylcholine as a neurotransmitter. Cholinergic receptors are subdivided into muscarinic and nicotinic. At both sympathetic and parasympathetic ganglia, postsynaptic membranes have nicotinic acetylcholine receptors. In addition, the neuromuscular junction (NMJ) of skeletal muscle is nicotinic (see Volume 2, Chapter 6). Nicotinic receptors are so named because nicotine is agonist and curare antagonist. Muscarinic receptors are located on all effector cells stimulated by postganglionic parasympathetic neurons. Muscarine has agonist and atropine antagonist actions at these receptors.

Sympathetic postganglionic neurons secrete norepinepherine as a neurotransmitter and are referred to as adrenergic, in all cases except for three (piloerector muscles, sweat glands, and some blood vessels) which secrete acetylcholine and are muscarinic.

Adrenergic receptors are subdivided into α- and β-receptors. Norepinepherine has greater action at alpha receptors. Epinephrine has approximately equal action at both types. Effector tissue response to catecholamines is determined by the type and density of the receptors expressed by that tissue.

Receptors are further subdivided into pre- (α_2) and post- (α_1) junctional receptors. The α_1 stimulation causes vasoconstriction, contraction of gut and bladder sphincters, and dilation of the iris. The α_2 stimulation results in vasodilation, and centrally located receptors are important in the perception of pain.

β-receptors are also subdivided into two types: β_1 and β_2. The β_1-receptors are located on the heart and have positive inotropic and chronotropic effects. The β_2-receptors mediate bronchodilation, skeletal muscle vasodilation, uterine relaxation, and glycogenolysis (24).

Autonomic Tone

It is appropriate to view the often-opposing actions of the sympathetic and parasympathetic nervous systems as a means of co-ordinating visceral activity. The basal rate of activity of the ANS allows a single division to exert a change in the function of an effector organ. For example, baseline sympathetic tone constricts systemic arterioles to approximately half of their maximum diameter. A decrease in sympathetic tone will result in vasodilation, and an increase in sympathetic tone in vasoconstriction (22).

Location of Higher Intellectual Brain Functions
Speech and Language

☞ **Almost all right-handed people and 70% of left-handed individuals have speech and language centers located in the left cerebral hemisphere.** ☞ The location of the speech and language centers designate hemisphere dominance. Two centers for speech are classically described: Broca's area located in the dominant frontal lobe and Wernicke's area located in the dominant temporoparietal zone. A lesion in Broca's area causes expressive dysphasia or aphasia; comprehension is preserved, but fluency is compromised. A lesion in Wernicke's area causes receptive dysphasia or aphasia; comprehension is compromised, but fluency of speech is preserved. However, the spoken words are often incorrect, and the affected patient speaks in muddled jargon (2,25).

Memory

Memory formation is incompletely understood. It may result from changes in synapse structure or in altered pathways. Lesions in the hippocampus cause anterograde amnesia and disrupt short-term memory, whereas those in the thalamus and cortex disrupt long-term memory (2).

PHYSIOLOGY
Impulse Generation
Membrane Structure

Membranes form a permeability barrier to most water-soluble molecules, separate cells from one another, and divide compartments within cells. All cell membranes are composed of a lipid bilayer, approximately 10 nm in depth, with phospholipids and proteins being their major constituents. Phospholipid molecules have polar, usually choline- containing, hydrophilic heads and hydrophobic fatty acid chains as tails. Membrane proteins are either intrinsic, which traverse the lipid bilayer, or extrinsic, which are located on the membrane surface. Membrane proteins form ion channels and receptors and also function as enzymes. A small amount of glycolipid exists on the outer surface of cell membranes that has important receptor function and constitutes antigens (26).

Transport Across Membranes

The transfer of molecules across membranes is either passive (energy independent) or active (energy dependent). Active transport requires more oxygen (O_2) and glucose utilization.

Passive Transfer (Diffusion and Osmosis)

Passive transfer of solutes occurs across cell membranes principally by diffusion (simple or facilitated), as molecules travel from an area of high concentration to an area of lower concentration. Diffusion results from the continuous random movement of molecules in the fluid state, resulting from the normal kinetic motion of matter.

Simple diffusion occurs without binding to specific proteins. Water-soluble molecules cross via membrane channels or junctions within the lipid bilayer. Lipid-soluble substances are able to pass directly through. In general terms, the rate of diffusion of a substance across a plasma membrane is directly proportional to its lipid solubility (27). The rate of diffusion may be described in the terms of Graham's law (i.e., "The rate of diffusion of a substance is inversely proportional to the square root of its molecular weight") (28), and by Fick's law (Equation 1), which states that the rate of diffusion is proportional to the surface area of the membrane and the concentration difference across a membrane and inversely proportional to the thickness of the membrane (26,28).

$$\text{Diffusion} = DA_{surface}\Delta C\ T_{membrane} - 1 \qquad (1)$$

where D is the diffusion coefficient of a substance through a particular membrane; $A_{surface}$, the surface area; ΔC, the concentration difference; and $T_{membrane}$, the membrane thickness.

Facilitated diffusion requires binding to a specific carrier protein within the membrane. Conformational change occurs within the carrier protein, and both substance and protein move through the membrane in a nonenergy-dependent process. The substance is released on the other side of the membrane. The rate of diffusion is limited by the rate of conformational change of the carrier protein. Movement is only possible down a concentration gradient. An important example is the transport of glucose into cells (26,27,29).

Osmosis is the movement of water across a semipermeable membrane from a higher to a lower concentration (of water). The osmotic pressure of a solution is the pressure that must be applied in order to prevent the movement of water into that solution. Osmotic pressure is described in terms of the number of particles per unit volume of fluid. Changes in the osmotic pressure gradient across cell membranes cause them to swell or shrink (26,27).

Active Transfer (Energy Dependent)

Active transport is an energy-dependent process that moves a substance against its electrochemical gradient. It relies on the presence of a transmembrane carrier protein and can be primary or secondary.

Primary active transport is linked directly to the cellular breakdown of a high-energy phosphate compound, usually adenosine triphosphate (ATP). An important example is the sodium–potassium pump. Three sodium ions are moved out of the cell for every two potassium ions moved in. Binding of the ions to the carrier protein activates ATPase that cleaves a molecule of ATP to release the required energy. The pump is vital to maintain the normal resting negative electrical potential inside cells and for regulating cell volume (30). A further example is calcium ATPase found on cell plasma membranes and on those of intracellular vesicles in which calcium is concentrated. Calcium is a key second messenger, and the maintenance of a low baseline intracellular calcium concentration and the facility for its rapid control are vital to normal cellular function (26,27).

Secondary active transport utilizes the energy derived from the electrochemical gradient of a substance transported by primary active transport. It may be cotransport, the secondary substance moving in the same direction as the primary substance, or countertransport, the secondary substance moving in the opposite direction to the primary substance. Glucose and amino acids may be cotransported with sodium, whereas calcium and hydrogen ions may be countertransported with sodium (26,27,31).

Resting Membrane Potential

The cytoplasm of all cells is electronegative, relative to extracellular fluid, and hence a potential difference exists across plasma membranes. This is termed the resting potential. Neurons and myocytes have the capability of electrical impulse generation. They are termed excitable tissues.

The resting potential is dependent upon ionic equilibria and the selective permeability of the plasma membrane. Ionic equilibrium exists when the two "forces" acting on charged particles (i.e., the concentration gradient and the electrical potential difference) balance. This is described mathematically for a single univalent ion X^+ (such as potassium) by the Nernst equation (Equation 2).

$$\text{EMF(millivolts)}_{X+} = -61 \log[X_i^+]/[X_o^+] \quad (2)$$

where EMF_{X+} is the electromotive force acting on X^+; $[X_i^+]$, the concentration of X^+ inside the cell; and $[X_o^+]$, the concentration of X^+ outside the cell.

Plasma membranes are essentially impermeable to anionic protein molecules and selectively permeable to ions. At rest, the membrane is approximately one hundred times more permeable to potassium than to sodium. Therefore, at rest, potassium makes the most significant contribution to the resting potential. The Nernst equation represents the potential due to a single ion (the Nernst potential for potassium is -90 mV), but in reality, other ions contribute to the resting potential, which approximates to -70 mV. The overall membrane potential (which reflects the inside compared to outside concentrations for all of the clinically significant ions) is represented mathematically by the Goldman equation (which provides a value close to -70 mV when normal intracellular and extracellular ion concentrations are present) (32,33).

Action Potential

The action potential can be considered in three stages: depolarization, repolarization, and propagation. In nervous

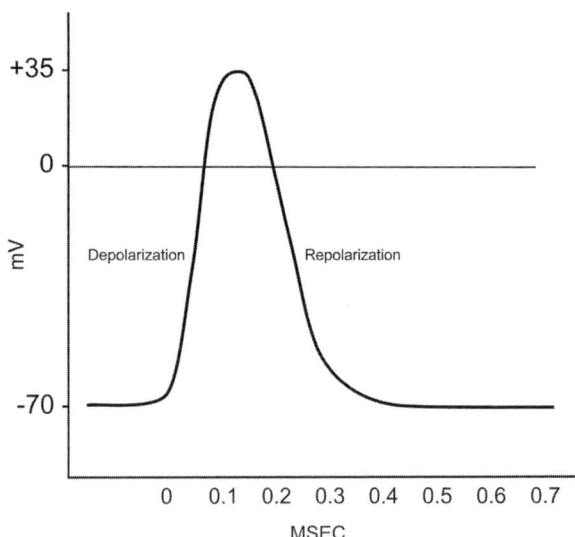

Figure 9 The action potential, showing the resting potential (-70 mV), depolarization and repolarization.

tissue, it occurs extremely rapidly (<1 msec) in an "all or nothing" fashion (Fig. 9).

Depolarization

An initial stimulus, for example, the action of a neurotransmitter on a postsynaptic membrane, causes the membrane potential to increase towards zero. If sufficiently large, the threshold potential is reached (approximately -55 mV), and voltage-gated sodium channels open. Sodium conductance increases by a factor of about 5000, sodium moves inward down both electrical and concentration gradients, and the membrane potential reaches $+35$ mV (34).

Repolarization

Voltage-gated sodium channels are inactivated (a process initiated simultaneously with channel opening, but at a slower rate), which halts the influx of sodium. Voltage-gated potassium channels open fractionally after sodium channel opening, allowing the efflux of intracellular potassium, and the membrane potential returns toward its normal resting potential. The sodium–potassium pump then restores intracellular resting sodium and potassium concentrations in an energy-dependent process (35).

Propagation

Depolarization at a single point of a neuronal membrane causes a change in potential in adjacent membrane of sufficient magnitude to open voltage-gated sodium channels, therefore creating a "wave" of depolarization. The electrical impulse travels unidirectionally because the previously depolarized section remains refractory to further stimulation until its resting state has been at least partially restored (32,35).

Metabolism

✍ **The brain is one of the most metabolically active organs in the body and requires a constant supply of O₂ and glucose.** ✍ It has a mass of 1500 g (2% body weight), and receives 15% $\dot{Q}$, yet accounts for more than 20% of the total body O₂ consumption ($\dot{V}O_2$), and 25% of the total body glucose utilization. The extraction ratio for oxygen is approximately 50% and that of glucose approximately 10%. Although glial cells comprise approximately 50% of the brain, they consume less than 10% of cerebral energy (36).

Aerobic and Anaerobic Metabolism

Glycolysis and subsequent oxidative phosphorylation of glucose (60 mg/100 g/min) to water and carbon dioxide is by far the most important energy pathway in the brain (37). Thirty-eight molecules of ATP are formed per molecule of glucose. The ATP is vital for normal neuronal function, and having no significant energy store, the brain is extremely sensitive to any derangement in the supply of oxygen or metabolic substrate (38).

In the absence of O_2, the metabolism of glucose via the glycolytic pathway is very inefficient: only two molecules of ATP are formed per molecule of glucose (39).

SjO_2, $AVDO_2$, and $CMRO_2$

The SjO_2 is the percentage oxygen saturation of jugular venous blood. It normally varies between 55% to 65% (40,41). The $AVDO_2$ is the arterio-venous oxygen difference. It is calculated as the measured difference between the O_2 content of arterial and jugular bulb venous blood. It represents a ratio of metabolism to blood and $\dot{D}O_2$. The normal value is 6.3 vol% (42). The $CMRO_2$ is the cerebral metabolic rate for oxygen. It is normally 3.5 mL/100 g/min (43). It decreases by 6% per degree Celsius fall in brain temperature.

There is coupling between CBF and $\dot{V}O_2$. This represents metabolic autoregulation. Normal aerobic metabolism, glucose consumption, and $\dot{V}O_2$ lead to normal CO_2 production ($\dot{V}CO_2$) that mediates normal cerebral microcirculatory diameter, and hence blood flow. If $CMRO_2$ decreases, $\dot{V}CO_2$ decreases, and hence CBF and oxygen delivery ($\dot{D}O_2$) decrease. The converse is true. If CBF falls and the $CMRO_2$ remains unchanged, then the oxygen extraction and $AVDO_2$ will increase, and be reflected in a decreased SjO_2 (44). The $AVDO_2$ can increase to a maximum of double the normal value (39).

Brain Parenchymal Gas Tensions

The determination of brain tissue O_2 (Brain-$P_{ti}O_2$) and CO_2 partial pressures is problematic. Human studies in normal brain do not exist. Normal values inferred from animal studies have estimated brain tissue oxygen at 25–30 mmHg with a PaO_2 of 102–104 mmHg (39), and that for carbon dioxide at 55 mmHg (45). A change in CO_2 tension results in a change in extracellular pH that profoundly affects neuronal function, and is tightly controlled.

Brain capillary O_2 tension decreases from arterial to venous ends, as a result of oxygen extraction. Most models assume that each capillary supplies a cylindrical volume of tissue and that O_2 freely diffuses into the tissues along the radial axis. The available O_2 is less than the arterial supply and depends on the diffusion pressure of O_2, being the difference in oxygen tension between capillary and mitrochondria. Similarly, the Brain-$P_{ti}O_2$ levels are lowest at the venous ends, hence forming more vulnerable regions. During normal resting conditions, some tissue O_2 diffuses back into the capillary. This O_2 surplus helps initially to meet any increase in tissue demand without the need for increasing CBF (46,47).

In models of global cerebral ischemia, Brain-$P_{ti}O_2$ changes with cerebral perfusion pressure (CPP) and is almost linearly coupled to local CBF. During systemic hypoxia, Brain-$P_{ti}O_2$ falls with SaO_2 accompanied by a compensatory increase in CBF. $CMRO_2$ falls steadily with Brain-$P_{ti}O_2$ until the ischemic threshold is reached, at which point $CMRO_2$ falls steeply, indicating exhausted compensatory increases in oxygen extraction during ischemia or CBF during systemic hypoxia (48).

Patients undergoing craniotomy for mass lesions and aneurysm surgery (ventilated with $FIO_2 = 0.4$) had a Brain-$P_{ti}O_2$ value of 48 ± 13 mmHg measured (49). The Brain-$P_{ti}O_2$ falls in parallel with other parameters of brain oxygenation (50), and may increase to > 130 mmHg in patients ventilated with 100% oxygen (45). Although Brain-$P_{ti}O_2$ <25 to 30 mmHg probably indicates impaired brain oxygenation, the anaerobic threshold for Brain-$P_{ti}O_2$ is in the order of 20 mmHg (39) (providing an intracellular pO_2 somewhat greater than 1 mmHg) (47).

Following traumatic brain injury (TBI), both depth and duration of tissue hypoxia are independent predictors of poor prognosis (51,52). Following severe stroke in humans, therapeutic measures which decrease ICP and increase CPP have been associated with an increase in Brain-$P_{ti}O_2$ (53). Also, pattern changes in Brain-$P_{ti}O_2$ graphical plots may predict imminent herniation syndrome in this patient population (53). Before Brain-$P_{ti}O_2$ can be used clinically as targeted treatment, significant additional research needs to be conducted in normal and abnormal neurological states.

Intracranial Pressure
The Monro-Kellie Doctrine

The volume of the adult cranial cavity remains constant: the skull is a noncompliant bony vault of fixed dimensions. ☛ **For ICP to remain constant (normal = 1–15 mmHg), the sum of the volumes of the intracerebral components must remain constant (54).** ☛ The main intracerebral components are brain parenchyma (intracellular volume and interstitial volume), CSF, and cerebral blood volume (CBV). Therefore, if the volume of one component increases, the volume of another must decrease, otherwise ICP will increase (39). This forms the central idea of the Monro-Kellie doctrine (55,56).

The first line of compensation for increasing ICP is usually a decrease in CSF volume. As discussed earlier, the rate of CSF formation remains constant, and in order to decrease CSF volume, the rate of absorption must increase.

Approximately 5% of intracerebral volume is occupied by blood (roughly 60 mL), most of which is contained within the venules whose diameter remains fairly constant despite changes in other physiological variables. Arterial diameter does vary (80–160% baseline), which results in a corresponding change in CBV, ICP, and CPP (57). If CBF autoregulation is intact (see subsequently) an increase in CPP will result in cerebral vasoconstriction to keep CBF constant and a decrease in CBV and ICP.

Measurement of Intracranial Pressure

The measurement of ICP is an important and now routine part of the management of severe head injury. The "gold standard" measuring device is the fluid-filled intraventricular catheter called a ventriculostomy (see Volume 2, Chapter 7). It is reliable, cost-effective, allows for periodic rezeroing and the withdrawal of CSF (for ICP control and CSF analysis). The catheter can sometimes block or leak. Alternatives include solid-state (pressure-sensitive resistors) and fiberoptic transducers that are usually placed within the parenchyma. Values correlate well with fluid-filled systems.

The major drawback is drift in ICP reading over time. Overall, indwelling ICP monitoring devices have an infection rate in the order of 7% and a hemorrhage rate of approximately 3% (58).

Cerebral Perfusion Pressure and Intracranial Pressure

A true measure of CPP would naturally be mean arterial pressure (MAP)—cerebral venous pressure. However, cerebral venous pressure is not easily measured. ICP is the closest measurable variable to cerebral venous pressure, and thus the surrogate, used clinically. The CPP is therefore best represented by MAP − ICP (13). ICP is profoundly linked to CBF: as ICP increases, CPP must fall for any given MAP (39).

Cerebral Blood Flow

It is vital to understand the physiological control of CBF, since its therapeutic manipulation is a key feature in neurotrauma management. Normal CBF is 50 mL/100 g/min (4,20,1). Reversible loss of electrical activity occurs with flows less than 23 mL/100 g/min (ischemic threshold), and sodium–potassium ATPase pump failure occurs at flows less than 18 mL/100 g/min. Prolonged hypoperfusion results in infarction (39).

Autoregulation

Autoregulation is the intrinsic ability of an organ to maintain a constant blood flow in the face of changing perfusion pressure, and is particularly well developed in the brain. As outlined earlier, CPP = MAP − ICP. ☞ **A normal value for CPP is approximately 70 mmHg.** ☞ Autoregulation

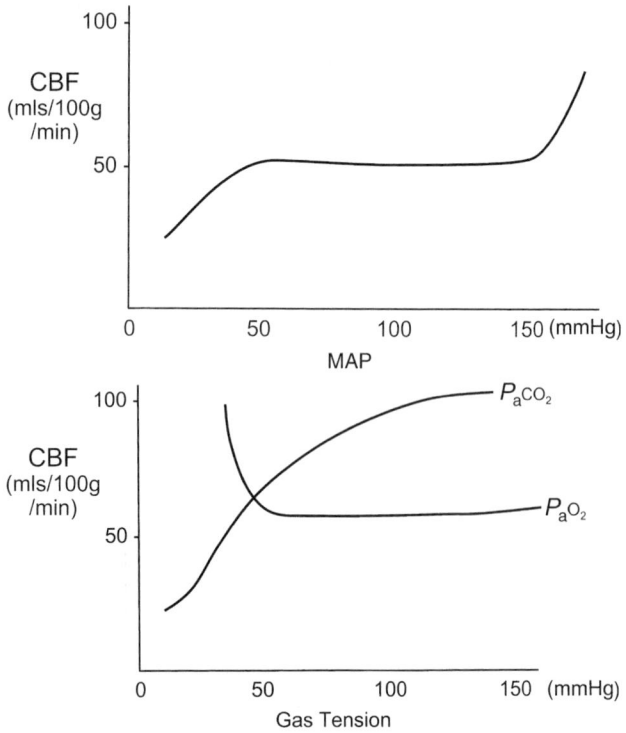

Figure 10   Regulation of cerebral blood flow with mean arterial blood pressure (MAP) (*upper graph*) and gas tensions for carbon dioxide (PaCO₂) and oxygen (PaO₂) (*lower graph*).

operates between MAPs 50 and 150 mmHg (Fig. 10) (13,37,39,59). As MAP increases, cerebral arteriolar diameter decreases, cerebrovascular resistance (CVR) increases, and CBF is maintained. The brain is protected against ischemia during hypotension and from cerebral edema during hypertension. Outside the normal operating range, CBF varies more directly with CPP (13,37). Below the lower limit of autoregulation, oxygen extraction is initially increased but once maximal, further decreases in CPP result in cerebral hypoxia. The CVR reaches a minimum below the lower limit of autoregulation. If CPP reduces still further, there is a sharp rise in CVR subsequent upon cerebral vessel collapse and consequent severe ischemia. At CPP above the upper limit of autoregulation, forceful vasodilation may occur, resulting in a marked fall in CVR, blood–brain barrier damage, and cerebral edema (21).

The mechanism for autoregulation is likely to be a combination of myogenic, metabolic, and neurogenic factors. The myogenic process involves an inverse variation in arteriolar diameter in response to a changing transmural pressure gradient (13). The response occurs within seconds and is most effective at high CPP (39). Metabolic mechanisms involve increasing concentrations of by-products (CO₂, H⁺, and K⁺), as CBF fails to meet metabolic demands and is most effective at low CPP (13,59). The limits of autoregulation are under the dynamic control of the ANS (sympathetic discharge shifts the autoregulation curve to the right) and are affected by the renin–angiotensin system and some disease states. Chronic hypertension shifts the autoregulation curve to the right. Accordingly, hypotension and the associated fall in CPP is less well tolerated in the hypertensive population (21).

Effect of Carbon Dioxide Tension

PaCO₂ is one of the most powerful factors affecting CBF (Fig. 10) (59,60). ☞ **Within the range PaCO₂ 25–60 mmHg, vasodilation and hence CBF increases linearly with PaCO₂ (13,28).** ☞ Outside the quoted range, maximal vasoconstriction/vasodilation occurs and no further decrease/increase in CBF is possible.

The vasodilation caused by hypercapnia blunts the response of vasoconstriction seen as CPP increases. The autoregulatory plateau is narrowed, shifted upwards, and rendered more pressure passive (59).

Effect of Oxygen Tension

Arterial oxygen tension has little effect on CBF within the normal PaO₂ range (37). Very high PaO₂ (>300 mmHg) can cause cerebral vasoconstriction. Breathing 100% oxygen causes a 10% reduction in CBF (13). At approximately PaO₂ of 60 mmHg, cerebral vasodilation begins to occur, and CBF increases rapidly as PaO₂ falls below this value (Fig. 10) (13,37).

Neurogenic Control

Cerebral blood vessels are richly innervated, and it seems likely that neurogenic mechanisms provide a means of rapid CBF control (13,59). Sympathetic vasoconstrictor fibres arise from the superior cervical and stellate ganglia. Nerve endings secrete norepinepherine, serotonin, and neuropeptide Y and provide a means of protecting the brain from high CPP during systemic hypertension caused by sympathetic stimulation. Cholinergic parasympathetic fibers take origin from the sphenopalatine, internal carotid, and otic ganglia (13). Sensory innervation via the first division of the trigeminal nerve and innervation from an intrinsic nerve supply also have a role (59). Cerebral blood vessels also express opiate receptors that may be important in the control of CBF during stress (13).

Measurement of Cerebral Blood Flow

The Kety-Schmit method, based on the Fick principle, uses nitrous oxide or radio isotope as a tracer and is a cumbersome procedure. It does, however, directly measure flow. Single-photon emission computed tomography (SPECT), positron emission tomography (PET), angiography with magnetic resonance imaging, and stable xenon-enhanced computed tomography (sXe-CT) are other measures of CBF, which are research tools and not suitable for bedside use (60). Transcranial Doppler, jugular bulb oximetry (SjO$_2$), and near-infrared cerebral spectroscopy (NIRS) measure variables related to CBF, but not flow itself (61–63). Jugular continuous thermodilution provides a direct measure of CBF and has been used successfully at the bedside (60).

States of Brain Activity
Consciousness and Unconsciousness

Consciousness depends upon interaction between the cerebral hemispheres and the brainstem reticular activating system. It is defined as awareness of self and environment. Unconsciousness is therefore unawareness of self and environment and may be seen as a continuum from confusion (reduced awareness and disorientation) to coma (unrousable unresponsiveness). Although the Glasgow Coma Scale (GCS) was designed to grade the severity and prognosis of traumatic head injury, it is now used almost universally to grade the depth of unconsciousness from all causes (64).

Sleep

Sleep is defined as a recurrent state of unconsciousness from which one can be readily aroused by sensory stimuli. There are two components: slow wave sleep and rapid eye movement (REM) sleep.

Slow wave sleep is usually deep, with progressive slowing and an increase in amplitude on electroencephalogram (EEG). There is slowing of heart and respiratory rates, decreased peripheral vascular resistance, decreased muscle tone, and decreased metabolic rate.

REM sleep is characterized by a rapid, low-voltage EEG, with bursts of large phasic potentials associated with increases in heart rate, respiratory rate, and body temperature. Cerebral metabolic rate may increase by 20% and CBF also increases. There is marked muscular relaxation. Dreams occur during REM sleep and are often remembered. REM sleep occurs in a cyclical fashion every one to two hours and lasts up to one hour. There is considerable variation between individuals (65).

Seizures

A seizure is uncontrolled, excessive neuronal discharge, the motor consequences of which are termed convulsions. Epilepsy is a continuing tendency to have seizures and is classified according to the pattern of seizure activity. ☞ **The cerebral metabolic rate is markedly increased during seizure activity (13).** ☞ Increased metabolic activity in injured brain can cause cell injury and death. Accordingly, seizures should be promptly treated (benzodiazepines are often used first line). Seizure prophylaxis is widely

employed in the first couple of weeks following severe TBI (phentoin is the most common first line chain) (66). However, the duration of prophylaxis, the relative need in the setting of concomitant sedation, and the most efficacious agents are all subjects of controversy (67).

Anesthesia

Anesthesia may be defined as a drug-induced, reversible loss of awareness and pain sensation. With increasing depth of anesthesia, there is slowing of EEG activity and a progressive increase in amplitude. Periods of isoelectricity interspersed with bursts of activity occur (burst suppression), and finally isoelectricity remains constant (68).

Brainstem Death

Brainstem death is a state of irreversible apneic coma. The diagnosis must be made with certainty. Rigid criteria must be fulfilled, which in most countries are based on U.K. or U.S. guidelines (69). Brainstem death is always followed by asystole within days, which almost always is preceded by an isoelectric EEG (70).

PATHOPHYSIOLOGY
Gross Pathology

The major mechanisms of TBI are positive pressure, negative pressure, brain laceration, and shear caused by direct impact or acceleration/deceleration (71).

TBI may be classified as primary or secondary and focal or diffuse. Primary injury is that which occurs at the time of impact and includes fracture, contusion, and hemorrhage. It is influenced only by prevention. Secondary brain injury is that which develops after the time of impact and includes ischemia, hypoxia, and the consequences of raised ICP. Its severity can be limited by prompt and appropriate medical and/or surgical intervention.

Focal brain injury is limited to a specific location and includes contusion and hematoma, whereas diffuse injury is more uniform throughout the brain, for example, diffuse axonal injury (DAI) and diffuse subarachnoid hemorrhage.

Contusion

A contusion is essentially a traumatic intracerebral hemorrhage resulting from mechanical injury to small-caliber vessels, that may, if severe, progress to necrosis. It typically occurs at the site of impact (coup) or at a point opposite the site of impact (contra coup) caused by brain movement within the skull.

Hemorrhage

☞ **Hemorrhage usually presents as a space-occupying lesion, with increased ICP, and when severe, as brain or brainstem herniation.** ☞ Extradural hematomas are caused by tearing of meningeal arterial vessels and separate the dura from the skull. The classic "lucid interval" may be seen. Subdural hematomas are usually caused by rupture of the veins that bridge the subdural space. Subarachnoid hemorrhage is the most common form of vascular injury seen following TBI and although usually minor, it may be life threatening.

Intracerebral hemorrhage is caused by rupture of vessels within brain parenchyma (72). When numerous small hemorrhages are scattered throughout the brain, the term "diffuse vascular injury" is applied. It is uncommon, seen in only the most severe TBI (73).

Diffuse Axonal Injury

DAI is a direct consequence of physical injury to the brain axons, caused by rotational acceleration/deceleration of the brain (71,74). It is characterized by axonal damage scattered throughout the brain that produces a clinical spectrum from mild-to-severe neurological impairment. The distribution of damaged axons is not uniform, but occurs predominantly throughout the corpus callosum, fornix, internal capsule, midline grey, cerebellar follicles and brainstem (75). Using conventional microscopy, axonal swellings are demonstrable at approximately 15 hours post injury (72). Evidence of axonal injury may be demonstrated much earlier, however, by more sophisticated techniques (76). DAI is really a pathological diagnosis. However, certain magnetic resonance imaging (MRI) findings (e.g., petechia along axon tracts) correlate with the pathologic findings.

Only with severe injury are axons sheared at the moment of impact. This is termed "primary axonotomy." More commonly, axons undergo a series of changes, resulting in axonal disruption after the moment of injury, a process termed "secondary axonotomy." Secondary axonotomy follows a sequence of events. At impact, there is transient depolarization, abnormal ionic flux, and abnormal axonal permeability. There is subsequent interruption of axoplasmic transport with the accumulation of cytoskeletal components and organelles (three to six hours). Axons and mitochondria then swell, secondary to calcium accumulation. Finally, the proximal axonal segment separates and the distal segment undergoes Wallerian degeneration (usually by 24 hours) (72,73,75).

Cell Death

Cell death is conventionally divided into two main types: necrosis and apoptosis, which differ both morphologically and biochemically. Hybrid forms of cell death with features of both are also seen (77).

Necrosis

Necrosis is triggered by abnormal physiology or extrinsic insults, for example, hypoxia, ischemia, trauma, and toxins. In normothermic patients, three to five minutes of arrest can cause necrosis of certain brain cells. The hippocampal region of the brain is one of the least tolerant to ischemia. Necrosis results from defective ion transport, ATP depletion, swelling and degeneration of organelles, loss of membrane integrity, cellular dissolution, and an accompanying acute inflammatory response. The process is usually complete within 24 hours and is more rapid with more severe insults (77). The mechanisms of necrotic death will be considered subsequently.

Apoptosis

Apoptosis is a process of programmed cell death that has a vital role in normal development, and is just now becoming understood. Approximately 50% developing sensory and spinal motor neurons die by apoptosis. The earliest changes occur in the nucleus. The chromatin condenses followed by nucleolar disintegration. The cytoplasm then condenses, the cell shrinks and the plasma membrane remains intact. The cell then fragments into membrane bound "apoptic bodies," which are phagocytosed by neighboring cells.

An inflammatory response does not occur (77,78). The time course is similar to that seen in necrosis.

The mechanisms of apoptosis may be divided into intrinsic (arising from mitochondria) and extrinsic (initiated by the binding of "death factors"), both converging on the caspase pathway. The caspases are a family of proteases that are fundamental to the process of apoptosis. Activation of the caspase pathway causes amplification of the apoptic signal, amplification of the caspase cascade, altered cellular morphology, disables repair processes, inactivates survival signals, and produces a signal for phagocytosis. However, caspase-independent apoptosis is recognized, and caspase activation is not an absolute requirement (78). The bcl-2 proto-oncogene family have a regulatory role (77). Excitatory amino acids, changes in intracellular calcium, and free radicals can induce apoptosis. In fact, all of the mechanisms traditionally considered to be triggers of necrosis can trigger apoptosis if the correct conditions apply.

Hybrid Necrosis–Apoptosis/Necrosis–Apoptosis Spectrum

☞ **Neuronal apoptosis and necrosis may be occurring simultaneously in the injured brain.** ☞ For example, although the features of ischemia and trauma are typically necrotic, apoptosis does occur in some neuronal groups and glial cells following ischemic injury, especially in the developing nervous system (77). Apoptosis also occurs alongside necrosis, following TBI, and can form a significant portion of neuronal loss (79). Apoptotic neurons have been identified at the site of injury, remote from the site of injury, and in contusions. Morphological features of both necrosis and apoptosis can occur in the same neuron. It is likely that the nature and intensity of an insult defines whether injured neurons undergo necrosis or apoptosis (80). Intracellular ATP concentrations may be a determinant of cell death route. If sufficient ATP is present, an injured neuron will have the metabolic capability to initiate the apoptotic cascade, whereas if deplete, necrosis will occur (81). Calcium influx during excitotoxicity may influence apoptosis and necrosis in opposing ways. The development of apoptosis may be inversely related to the intracellular calcium concentration at a critical point in the injury process. This forms the "calcium set point" hypothesis (79,82,83). Apoptosis may provide a protective mechanism, following TBI; since an inflammatory response is not initiated, surrounding cells are not damaged and therefore neuronal loss may be limited (79).

Mechanisms of Cell Death

The mechanisms of cell death are complex, diverse, and interdependent, but will be considered under specific headings.

Excitotoxicity

☞ **Excitotoxicity is the uncontrolled release of excitatory amino acids, causing massive sodium and calcium influx, further amino acid release, and ATP depletion culminating in cell death.** ☞ Glutamate is by far the most important and most studied excitatory amino acid. Normally, extracellular concentrations of glutamate are extremely low, subsequent upon reuptake by neurons and glia and intact cellular metabolic function that maintains a concentration gradient of glutamate between the intracellular (millimolar) and extracellular (micromolar) compartments (84).

The broad triggers of excitotoxicity include hypoxia, hypoperfusion, and TBI. Following TBI, the initial release of glutamate may occur secondary to neuronal depolarization on impact, direct membrane disruption, reverse function of glutamate pumps in neurons and glia, and the reversal of ionic gradients (85). Both CSF and extracellular levels of glutamate quickly reach toxic levels (85–87). Glutamate acts at three main sites: G-protein coupled receptors, α-amino-3-hydroxy-5-methy-4-isoxazole proprionic acid (AMPA) receptors, and N-methyl-D-aspartate (NMDA) receptors. The G-protein, coupled receptor activation causes intracellular calcium release. The AMPA receptor activation mediates fast excitation mainly via sodium entry. The NMDA receptor activation causes calcium influx. Membrane depolarization results, allowing further calcium entry, via voltage-gated calcium channels, sodium entry and excessive activation of Na^+, K^+ ATPase causing cellular ATP depletion. Elevated intracellular calcium levels result in further glutamate release, activates calcium-dependent enzyme systems, and increase oxidative stress. A vicious spiral results in cellular swelling, cytotoxic edema, and cell death (88). Calcium accumulation lasts approximately four days postinjury, the duration showing some proportionality to injury severity (89). There is also evidence that nitric oxide mediates at least some of the neurotoxicity of glutamate (90,91).

NMDA receptor activation not only affects calcium flux, but also that of potassium. Changes in potassium flux influence metabolic pathways in favor of hyperglycolysis, resulting in lactate accumulation. This may represent an attempt to re-establish normal homeostasis and ionic gradients. Glycolysis continues for approximately one hour postinjury, after which injured brain enters a state of metabolic depression with an accompanying decrease in CBF. Excitotoxicity may therefore be seen in terms of a neurochemical and metabolic cascade (89).

Oxidative Stress

During TBI, hypoxia, hypoperfusion and reperfusion, free radicals, and other strong oxidants are formed to which the brain is particularly vulnerable. Free radicals include superoxide, the hydroxyl radical, and the nitric oxide radical. Other strong oxidants include singlet oxygen and hydrogen peroxide. They affect the brain by causing NADH depletion, lipid peroxidation, interfering with mitochondrial ATP production, and activating neutrophil-mediated inflammation (88). The free-radical scavenging effects of mannitol may benefit patients with traumatic brain injuries; these and other effects of this antioxidant osmotic diuretic are further delineated later.

Calcium-Sensitive Enzyme Activation

Intracellular calcium accumulation, following TBI, results in the activation of several calcium-sensitive enzyme systems: lipases, kinases, phosphatases, and proteases. Calpain (a family of calcium-activated intracellular proteases) activation appears to be a particularly important step in the pathogenesis of cellular injury. Calpains have some selectivity for the lysis of cytoskeletal proteins, calmodulin-binding protein, signal transduction enzymes, membrane proteins, and transcription factors. Unchecked pathological activation has profound effects on both neuronal structure and function (92,93).

The Role of Mitochondria

Mitochondria are pivotal in calcium homeostasis and may be a source of reactive oxygen species. The exact mechanisms by which mitochondria participate in apoptosis and necrosis remains to be fully elucidated. Mitochondria actively accumulate calcium in response to excitotoxicity; subsequent mitochondrial swelling and lysis may be the primary cause of cell death. Inflammation and mechanical stress may also result in mitochondrial damage. Cell death proteins are released from mitochondria following TBI and induce apoptosis (94).

Inflammation

There is increasing evidence that inflammation contributes to the pathogenesis of TBI. Following TBI, both tumor necrosis factor alpha (TNFα) and interleukin 1β (IL-1β) are expressed in the brain. Both are important in the initiation and propagation of the acute inflammatory response. The principal adhesion molecules necessary for leukocyte recruitment (ICAM 1 and VCAM) are rapidly upregulated following TBI. Neutrophils appear first, followed by macrophages. The resulting inflammatory response causes bystander cell damage and death and promotes edema formation (95).

Gene Expression

Apolipoprotein E (APOE) is a lipoprotein produced by glial cells that may have a role in transporting lipids to injured neurons. There are three human isoforms: ε2, ε3, and ε4. TBI may trigger β amyloid precursor protein (βAPP) deposition that forms part of the acute phase response. It appears that βAPP deposition is more marked in those who express APOE ε4, leading to a worse outcome and an increased risk of developing Alzheimer's disease following TBI (96).

Chaperones (a group of proteins involved in the folding and intracellular transport of damaged proteins), immediate early genes (e.g., *c*-fos, *c*-jun and jun-*B*), and growth factors (e.g., nerve growth factor and insulin-like growth factor) are expressed following TBI and probably influence repair (93).

Raised Intracranial Pressure

☞ **A sustained rise in ICP above 20 mmHg, following severe head injury, is a highly significant predictor of poor outcome (97).** ☞ Although CPP is generally held as the critical parameter, the direct effects of raised ICP remain detrimental even when CPP is maintained at normal levels. The causes of raised ICP include intracranial mass (tumor or hematoma), hydrocephalus, increased intravascular volume (arterial or venous), and cerebral edema (cytogenic or vasogenic).

Initially, as intracerebral volume rises, CSF and blood are displaced to maintain ICP at normal levels in a "compensated state." As intracranial volume rises further, an "uncompensated state" is reached where a small rise in volume causes a disproportionate rise in pressure (Fig. 11) (39). The CNS ischemic reflex and/or herniation syndromes may then occur.

The CNS ischemic reflex is an intense sympathetic discharge activated by low CPP probably secondary to increasing CO_2 tension at the vasomotor center. The Cushing reflex is a special form of the former, triggered by raised ICP.

Herniation syndromes are shifts in brain tissue through rigid skull openings caused by raised ICP.

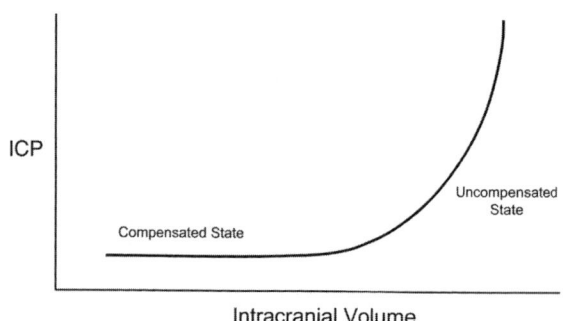

Figure 11 Relation between intracranial pressure (ICP) and volume (elastance curve).

Other CNS components are compressed. The most common herniation syndromes are central, uncal, cingulate, upward cerebellar, and tonsillar.

Uncal: The medial uncus and hippocampal gyrus are forced over the edge of the tentorium, compressing the ipsilateral occulomotor nerve (unilateral dilating pupil) and brainstem (causing unconsciousness and contralateral hemiparesis). *Tonsillar*: The cerebellar tonsils descend through the foramen magnum, compressing the brainstem and causing respiratory arrest (98).

Changes in Cerebral Circulation Following Traumatic Brain Injury

Changes in CBF, autoregulation, and vasoreactivity are critical factors in the development of secondary injury following brain trauma. Alterations occur at both macro- and microvascular level.

Cerebral Blood Flow

σ⁺ **Most severely head-injured patients show a trimodal pattern of change in CBF: an initial decline, a period of relative hyperemia (high CBF relative to cerebral metabolism), flow again decreases (37).** σ⁺ CBF decreases early after TBI, often to extremely low levels; the degree of impairment in CBF increases with injury severity (41,99). In fact, there is postmortem evidence of cerebral ischemia in most patients who die from TBI (41). Vasospasm occurs in up to 40% of severe head injuries, causes a marked decrease in CBF, and is a predictor of poor outcome (37,100). In the region of contusions or hematomas, CBF is decreased even further than globally (101). Hyperemia can result in vasogenic cerebral edema with raised ICP; both extremely high as well as extremely low CBF results in poor prognosis (102).

Autoregulation and Vasoreactivity

Autoregulation is often disrupted or abolished following severe TBI not only in injured areas, but also in areas remote from the injury; changes in CPP are paralleled by changes in CBF (103,59). Therefore, at low CPP, compensatory vasodilation does not occur and ischemia may result. At high CPP, compensatory vasoconstriction does not occur and vasogenic cerebral edema and vascular injury may result. Furthermore, CBF may become uncoupled from cerebral metabolism (41). Impaired autoregulation is not only limited to severe head injury; it has been described in patients at six days, following mild head injury (104).

The cerebrovascular response to carbon dioxide is usually but not always preserved (105,106). A state of "dissociated vasoparalysis" therefore, frequently occurs.

Mechanisms

Changes in the equilibrium of endothelin-1 (vasoconstriction) and nitric oxide (vasodilation) both acting at a microvascular level are thought to account, at least in part, for the alterations seen in CBF and autoregulation. It is probable that other vasoactive substances (acetylcholine, serotonin, vasopressin, angiotensin, and cytokines) also have a significant role (107). Vasospasm, which occurs at a macrovascular level, is probably related to the release of hemoglobin breakdown products into the CSF (41).

Physiological Basis of Treatment Models

Increased morbidity and mortality, following TBI, are strongly related to hypotension (systolic BP <80 mmHg) and low CPP postinjury (107,108). The minimum CPP and the benefits of increasing it above this threshold remain controversial. Head injury management can be considered under three headings: traditional management, CPP management, and Lund therapy.

The traditional and well-established management of severe head injury involves avoiding hypoxia and hypotension with early ICU and neurosurgical intervention. ICP is monitored and controlled in a stepwise fashion, and secondary brain injury is limited (41).

Autoregulation may be altered but not lost, and this is the basic pathophysiological requirement in CPP management (109). The CPP management strategy, now incorporated into head injury guidelines, is based on the central theme of a "vasodilatory cascade" (110,111). A decrease in MAP or increase in ICP causes a fall in CPP, followed by cerebral vasodilation. Cerebral vasodilation causes an increase in CBV that, in the poorly compliant brain, further increases ICP and decreases CBF in a vicious circle. The aim of management is to increase MAP and break the cycle (108).

Lund therapy is a more controversial approach (108,112,113). The aim is to reduce microvascular pressure gradients and hence minimize edema formation. Colloid osmotic pressure is maintained and systemic blood pressure reduced.

Metabolic and Neuroendocrine Complications of Traumatic Brain Injury
Cerebral Metabolism

Immediately following TBI, there is a short-lived but intense period of hyperglycolysis, as neurons attempt to normalize membrane gradients. This is followed by a profound state of metabolic depression (sometimes to half normal) that may be longstanding. This phase may be secondary to hypoxia, hypoperfusion, and mitochondrial dysfunction (114).

Basal Metabolic Rate

σ⁺ **Following TBI, a hypermetabolic and hypercatabolic state ensues.** σ⁺ This persists for at least two weeks. There is a marked increase in calorific requirement (to approximately 140% baseline) and nitrogen wasting (triple normal fasting levels) (115,116). Glucose stores are rapidly depleted, and amino acids become the major substrate for gluconeogenesis. A patient can lose approximately 1 kg/day muscle mass if the situation goes unchecked, resulting in severe protein/energy malnutrition. The process is driven by massive stress hormone and cytokine release (117). Calorific requirement may be decreased to 100% expected if the patient is paralyzed and sedated. Current guidelines recommend the provision of 140% resting metabolic expenditure in nonparalyzed and 100% resting metabolic expenditure in paralyzed patients (118). The mode of nutritional support has no effect on neurological outcome.

Syndrome of Inappropriate ADH Secretion

TBI stimulates excessive anti diuretic hormone (ADH) release, which when prolonged, produces the syndrome of inappropriate ADH (SIADH) secretion. This is characterized by hyponatremia and decreased plasma osmolality with urine osmolality greater than serum osmolality. The free water retained promotes cerebral edema formation.

Diabetes Insipidus

Diabetes insipidus (DI) is caused by inflammation, edema, ischemia, and infarction or direct traumatic destruction of the posterior pituitary. It is characterized by polyuria with low urinary sodium, hypernatremia, and high serum osmolality. Hypertonic coma can ensue. Although usually transient in patients who recover from their brain injury, DI may become permanent (119). Vasopressin (1–5 units/hr) or ddAVP (1–4 μg/12 hr) is usually administered to treat DI.

Disturbed Glucose Metabolism

Diabetes mellitus may occur secondary to the increased secretion of insulin antagonists following trauma. Following TBI, glucose response to insulin is subnormal (113). Nonketotic hyperglycemia may be seen. ✍ **Serum glucose must be closely controlled towards normal following TBI, because hyperglycemia is strongly associated with worse outcome (120).** ✍

Hypothalamic and Pituitary Injury

Loss of normal thermoregulation is a sensitive marker of hypothalamic dysfunction. Severe damage to the lower pituitary stalk or anterior pituitary causes low levels of all anterior pituitary hormones. No response to their respective releasing factors is seen.

Hypothalamic injury causes dissociated adrenocorticotrophic hormone (ACTH)-cortisol levels, hypothyroidism [with preserved thyroid stimulating hormone (TSH) response to TSH-releasing harmone (RH)], low gonadotropins (with preserved response to gonadotropin-RH), variable growth hormone levels, and hyperprolactinemia. Damage to both structures causes a mixed pattern (119,121).

Spinal Cord Pathophysiology

The mechanism of spinal cord injury (SCI) is usually direct compression from fracture/dislocation of the vertebral column or disc rupture. The spinal cord is extremely vulnerable to injury without the capacity to regenerate. SCI leads to well-recognized clinical patterns, defined by the loss or impairment of motor/sensory modalities below the level of the injury. Total lesions above C3 result in the total loss of ventilatory function. Lesions above T1 cause sympathetic paralysis, resulting in distributive shock; bradycardia may also result secondary to unopposed vagal tone (see Volume 1, Chapter 26 and Volume 2, Chapter 13 for additional information).

Excitotoxicity, inflammation, necrosis, and apoptosis all occur after SCI and result in axonal loss, to which the term "diffuse axonal injury" may be applied (122–125).

Corticosteroids have proved effective in improving functional outcome in patients following SCI (126–128).

Drugs, Anesthesia, Intensive Care, and Neuroprotection
Anesthesia and Intensive Care
Basic Interventions

Laryngoscopy, intubation, extubation, pain and awareness all increase ICP and MAP. Positive pressure ventilation, positive end expiratory pressure (PEEP), coughing and straining, head down posture, and tight endotracheal tube ties increase central venous pressure, intracerebral venous pressure, and hence ICP.

Drugs

When using any drugs in the context of TBI, it is important to consider the effect that agent has on the cerebral circulation, ICP, and cerebral metabolic rate. A summary of the most commonly used agents is presented in Table 4. Etomidate (decreases $CMRO_2$ and maintains CPP) is the induction drug of choice in patients with TBI and other possible injuries. Barbiturates, mannitol, and hypertonic saline are often employed as ongoing therapy in the ICU, and will be considered in more detail.

Barbiturates. Barbiturates (thiopentone, phenobarbital) are general anaesthetic induction agents and anticonvulsants. They produce marked CNS depression, acting predominantly at inhibitory gamma amino butyric acid (GABA) receptors, and a marked reduction in cerebral metabolic rate that remains coupled to CBF. Cerebral vascular resistance is increased, CBV decreased, and therefore, ICP is also decreased. In the context of TBI, cerebral extracellular concentrations of lactate, glutamate, and aspartate are reduced, which provide neuroprotective benefit (129,130).

The use of high-dose barbiturates is recommended to treat refractory elevated ICP. It is effective at lowering ICP and decreasing mortality in this setting. The use of prophylactic barbiturates is not indicated (124).

Mannitol. Mannitol is an osmotic diuretic widely used for ICP control following TBI (131). Mannitol has two distinct effects on the brain (rheological and osmotic) and theoretically an antioxidant effect. Concerning rheology, there is plasma expansion, reduced blood viscosity, increased CBF, and increased cerebral $\dot{D}O_2$. The osmotic effects are delayed for 15 to 30 minutes and persist for over six hours. Once osmotic gradients are established between plasma and intracellular fluid, intracellular volume reduces and ICP is also therefore reduced. Mannitol may also provide beneficial antioxidant effects due to its free-radical scavenger properties. Mannitol may theoretically accumulate in areas of the brain where the blood–brain barrier is disrupted, causing a reverse shift of fluid and elevation in ICP. It may also cause renal failure when serum osmolality is allowed to exceed 330 mosm/L. Mannitol is recommended in most neurosurgical guidelines for the control of ICP following TBI (132). Uncertainty exists over the optimal treatment regimen, and its usefulness if given at other stages of TBI management (e.g., prehospital) (133).

Hypertonic Saline. If hypertonic saline is used for volume replacement following TBI, smaller volumes are required to maintain cardiovascular stability when compared to standard crystalloid solutions. There is decreased ICP and improved CBF and $\dot{D}O_2$. Cortical water in uninjured brain is decreased, improving intracranial compliance (134). Hypertonic saline also has vasoregulatory, neurochemical (extracellular glutamate concentration may be reduced)

Table 4 Cerebral Circulatory Effects of Sedatives, Analgesics, and Other Agents

	CBF	ICP	CMRO$_2$	CSF production	Autoregulation	CO$_2$ reactivity
Intravenous anesthetics						
Thiopental	D	D	D	N	N	N
Etomidate	D	D	D	D	N	N
Propofol	D	D	D	N	I	N
Ketamine	I[a]	I[a]	I[a]	N	N	N
Midazolam	D	D	D	N	N	N
Inhaled agents						
Nitrous oxide	I	I	I	N	N	N
Halothane	I	I	D	N	Impaired	N
Enflurane	I	I	D	I	Impaired	N
Isoflurane	I	I	D	N	Impaired	I
Sevoflurane	I	I	D	N	Impaired	N
Desflurane	I	I	N	N	Impaired	N
Xenon	I	I	?	?	?	?
Opioid analgesics (ventilation controlled)						
Morphine	N	N	N	N	N	N
Fentanyl	N	N	N	N	N	N
Alfentanil	D	D (bolus I)	?D	N	N	N
Remifentanil	D	D	?D	N	N	N
Opioid analgesics (spontaneous ventilation)						
All opioids	I	I	?N	N	N	N
Muscle relaxants						
Succinylcholine	I	I	?I	N	N	N
Non-depolarizing	N	N	N	N	N	N
Diuretics						
Mannitol	N[c]	D	N	D	N	N
Furosamide	N	D	N	D	N	N
Others						
Hydralazine	I	I	N	N	Impaired	N
Glyceryl trinitrate	I	I	N	N	Impaired	N
Sodium nitroprusside	I	I	N	N	Impaired	N
Nimodipine	I	I	N	N	N	N
Lidocaine	D	D	N[b]	N	N	N
α_2-Agonists	D	D	?	?	?	?
Anticholinergics	N	N	N	N	N	N
Anticholinesterases	N	N	N	N	N	N

Note: CO$_2$ reactivity is the slope of the graph relating CBF to changes in arterial carbon dioxide tension.
[a]Effects modified by pretreatment with sedatives.
[b]Decreases with large doses.
[c]Increases initially.
Abbreviations: CBF, cerebral blood flow; CSF, cerebrospinal fluid; D, decreased; I, increased; ICP, intracranial pressure; N, no effect; ?, unknown.

and immunomodulatory properties. It is better excluded via the blood–brain barrier than mannitol and does not possess osmotic diuretic properties. Accordingly, volume depletion and hypotension, rebound effects seen with mannitol, are avoided. The main concerns are osmotic demyelination syndrome (especially in previously hyponatremic patients), renal insufficiency, hemorrhage, coagulopathy, and red cell lysis (135). Meta-analysis of TBI patients treated with hypertonic saline-dextran has shown a marked survival benefit (136). Randomized controlled trials investigating the role of hypertonic saline in fluid resuscitation, following TBI, are currently underway (137).

Hyperventilation

The potential benefits of hyperventilation are cerebral vasoconstriction for ICP control. However, CSF pH changes are short-lived, as bicarbonate is removed from

the CSF to re-establish equilibrium (138). A further disadvantage is vasoconstriction that may reduce CBF to ischemic thresholds (139). The use of prophylatic hyperventilation (PaCO$_2 \leq 35$ mmHg) should be avoided during the first 24 hours, following severe TBI (140). Hyperventilation is used only for the treatment of elevated ICP as an acute temporising measure (141). Randomized controlled trials to assess target PaCO$_2$, timing and duration of hyperventilation are warranted (142).

Neuroprotection

Neuroprotection encompasses pharmacological and other interventional strategies that limit/prevent neuronal damage, reduce secondary injury processes, or promote regeneration, following TBI. The interval between the time of injury and the development of the complete pathological process represents a window of opportunity for such strategies to be employed. Understanding the pathological mechanisms of cell death and damage allows for the application of neuroprotective therapies, which target specific points in the injury cascade.

Targeting Excitotoxicity

Many strategies have focused on limiting glutamate excitotoxicity. This may be achieved by decreasing glutamate release, preventing neurotransmission, or promoting the effects of inhibitory neurotransmitters (143).

Agents that block sodium or calcium channels reduce glutamate release. Riluzole, lubelazole, phenytoin, and fosphenytoin are among those agents studied (143,144).

The NMDA receptor antagonists (e.g., ketamine, phencyclidine, dizolcipine, and dextromethorphan) have shown promise in laboratory work (145). Magnesium causes voltage-dependent NMDA receptor blockade and may prove beneficial (143).

GABA is the main inhibitory neurotransmitter in the CNS that offers balance against the excitatory glutamate system. GABA agonists (vigabatrin, diazepam) are beneficial during experimental ischemia (146).

Targeting Calcium and Mitochondria

Calcium plays a key role in the evolution of TBI. Calcium channel blockers have been used in an attempt to prevent cerebral vasospasm after injury, and hence maintain CBF. The evidence for their use is unconvincing and side effects may outweigh benefits. A subgroup of patients with traumatic subarachnoid hemorrhage may benefit (147). Mitochondria have significant calcium-buffering capacity in the noninjured system. This capacity is lost early in the injury cascade. Cyclosporin A may delay or prevent mitochondrial dysfunction and attenuate the intracellular calcium rise (148). Calcium-sensitive proteases are another potential target. Blockade of the caspase pathway may, in particular, be useful in limiting apoptic cell death (143).

Targeting Inflammation

Inflammation is a complex process involving the interaction of multiple molecular systems and causes widespread damage within the CNS following injury. Corticosteroids, aminosteroids, and free-radical scavengers have been investigated for their potential neuroprotective effects.

Corticosteroids act as both immunosuppressant and free-radical scavenger (143). Despite a quarter of a century of intense investigation, a beneficial role for corticosteroids in improving outcome following TBI has not been established. Their use is not currently recommended for this purpose (149,150).

Aminosteroids (e.g., tirilazad mesylate) have been shown to limit lipid peroxidation in laboratory animals. Currently there is no evidence to support their routine use following TBI (151).

Other potential therapies aimed at reducing free-radical formation and lipid peroxidation include superoxide dismutase, catalase, and vitamin E (143).

Sex Hormones

There is some evidence that sex hormones in males (progesterone and estrogen) reduce excitotoxicity, are antioxidant, reduce inflammation, provide neurotrophic support, and enhance neuronal regeneration, following TBI (152). Estradiol exerts a profound protective effect against ischemia if treatment precedes insult; it may act in part via genomic mechanisms (13).

Other Potential Agents

Preliminary findings indicate that activation of adenosine A1 receptors ameliorates trauma-induced central neuronal death. Adenosine may play a role in several steps of the injury cascade (154). Nitric oxide affects both excitotoxicity and microvascular tone, following TBI. Nitric oxide synthase inhibitors represent a potential strategy (143).

Hypothermia

With decreasing temperature, cerebral metabolic rate, CBF, and ICP decrease. In the context of TBI, there is decreased glutamate release, decreased free-radical production, and there maybe improved neuronal tolerance to insults (155). Despite encouraging results from small trials, there is no evidence that hypothermia is beneficial and the risk of pneumonia is increased. The use of this treatment modality is not recommended outside of controlled trials (156).

Shortfalls in Neuroprotection

Despite enormous experimental promise, the results of clinical studies have been disappointing. TBI is a complex disorder within a heterogeneous group of patients. Problems may arise with the timing of therapy, and animal models may not represent a true reflection of the pathophysiological processes involved in human TBI. The idea that a single agent will offer significant improvement may be over simplistic. For such a complex process, multimodal treatment may be required.

EYE TO THE FUTURE

Although the basic principles of neurophysiology and neuropathophysiology have been unraveled, our understanding of cerebral function and the response to injury remain limited. The effects of hypoxia and hypotension on morbidity and mortality are clear, and the importance of early optimization of DO_2 and CPP in head injury is well established. Some areas of controversy still exist (157). Mannitol is recommended for the control of ICP, but uncertainty exists regarding the optimal treatment regime and its usefulness at other stages of TBI management. Hyperventilation is used as a short-term treatment for acutely raised ICP. Randomized controlled trials to assess target $PaCO_2$, timing and duration of hyperventilation are warranted. Hypertonic treatment improves CBF and reduces infarct size, following rat cortical vein occlusion (158). The use of hypertonic saline for fluid resuscitation in TBI patients has shown significant promise; controlled trials are currently underway.

Secondary brain injury occurs almost without exception in patients with severe head injury. The goal of ameliorating secondary injury must begin with a deeper understanding of the molecular pathways of the pathophysiological process. The future of neurophysiology lies at a molecular level. As this chapter has made clear, there are large numbers of molecules involved in normal and pathological responses whose exact role remains to be elucidated. The response to injury is a complex integrated cascade, the modification of which is likely to involve an understanding of all processes rather than the action of individual molecules.

Many agents which target excitotoxicity, including riluzole, lubelazole, phenytoin, ketamine, phencyclidine, magnesium, and GABA agonists, have shown promise in laboratory and/or animal work. Cyclosporin A may delay or prevent mitochondrial dysfunction. New pharmacological agents with neuroprotective effects continue to be discovered (159,160); further research is required. Despite intense research over nearly 25 years, corticosteroids have not found a role in TBI management. However, aminosteroids, superoxide dismutase, catalase, and vitamin E may prove to be useful in the limitation of free-radical formation and lipid peroxidation. Indeed, the immune system plays a vital role in both injury and recovery, and posttraumatic vaccination to boost repair mechanisms may be an option for the future (161).

With the sequencing of the human genome, it is also likely that genetic influences will be shown to have a strong bearing on the outcome from head injury, and with this may come the ability to alter the genetic response to neuropathophysiology (162).

The development of cell replacement therapies (cell lines transplanted into injured CNS in order to provide repair) may represent a further opportunity for late intervention, following TBI (163).

However, prevention is better than cure, and changes in society infrastructure to reduce death and injury from head trauma will remain the biggest single factor in reducing the burden of head injury on society.

SUMMARY

The nervous system may be divided anatomically into the CNS, the PNS, and the ANS. The CNS is further divided into brain, brainstem, and spinal cord. The CSF system provides a buffer against movement for the CNS, and the blood–brain barrier provides for some separation of the CNS from the systemic environment. The brain is contained within a noncompliant bony vault: the skull.

Normal physiology is a complex, tightly regulated process, based on the generation of action potentials. The action potential involves depolarization, repolarization, and propagation to create a wave of depolarization. Pathological processes that alter the resting potential of the cell membrane can have profound effects on the generation of action potentials. Alterations in cellular metabolism also affect neurophysiological processes. The brain is one of the most metabolically active organs in the body. It has a mass of 1500 g (2% body weight), receives 15% $\dot{Q}$ and uses 20% and 25% total body oxygen and glucose consumption, respectively. The extraction ratio for oxygen is approximately 50% and that of glucose approximately 10%. Delivery of oxygen and metabolites to the brain tissue is dependent upon adequate CBF, which in turn is related to CPP. Autoregulation through myogenic responses, oxygen tension, carbon dioxide tension, and neurogenic control regulates CBF. Pathological processes resulting in increased intracranial volume increase ICP, reducing CPP and $\dot{D}O_2$. Hypotension also reduces CPP and below a MAP of 50 mmHg, autoregulation fails.

Both primary (initial insult) or secondary (due to ischemia), and focal or diffuse damage occurs, following TBI. Injury is often a combination of primary damage to neurons and supporting glia, with hemorrhagic injury. Cell death is conventionally divided into two main types: necrosis and apoptosis, which differ both morphologically and biochemically. Hybrid forms of cell death with features of both are also seen. Mechanisms of cell death are complex and diverse. However, nearly all modes of cell death result in the final common pathway of calcium influx across a damaged cell membrane, resulting in the disruption of mitochondrial and cellular homeostasis. Release of excitatory amino acids, oxidative stress, and calcium-sensitive enzyme activation are all mechanisms resulting in cell death. TBI causes variations in gene expression that have a bearing on pathogenesis, repair, and ultimately recovery. Apolipoprotein, chaperone, and growth factor expression have been identified as important genes in inflammation and repair from neurotrauma.

Changes in blood flow are an important mechanism in the pathophysiology of TBI. Most severely head-injured patients show a trimodal pattern of change in CBF: an initial decline, a period of relative hyperemia, and finally a decrease in flow. This latter decrease is often to extremely low levels, the degree of impairment in CBF increasing with injury severity. In the region of contusions or hematomas, CBF is decreased even further than globally. Current recommendations for the management of cerebral hemodynamics are based on maintaining adequate CPP, which results in maintenance of CBF irrespective of ICP.

TBI also disrupts metabolic and neuroendocrine pathways. Immediately following TBI, there is a short-lived, but intense, period of hyperglycolysis, as neurons attempt to normalize membrane gradients. This is followed by a profound state of metabolic depression that may be longstanding. Eventually, a hypermetabolic and hypercatabolic state ensues. Glucose stores are rapidly depleted, and amino acids become the major substrate for gluconeogenesis. A patient can lose approximately 1 kg/day muscle mass if the situation goes unchecked, resulting in severe protein/energy malnutrition. Current guidelines recommend the provision of 140% resting metabolic expenditure in nonparalyzed and 100% resting metabolic expenditure in paralyzed patients. A SIADH secretion is common, due to excessive ADH release. The free water retained promotes cerebral edema formation. Glucose metabolism may also be disturbed, with diabetes mellitus occurring secondary to the increased secretion of insulin antagonists, following trauma. Hyperglycemia is associated with a worse outcome following head injury.

The mechanism of SCI is usually direct compression from fracture/dislocation of the vertebral column or disc rupture. The spinal cord is extremely vulnerable to injury without the capacity to regenerate. SCI leads to well-recognized clinical patterns, defined by the loss or impairment of motor/sensory modalities below the level of the injury. Corticosteroids have proved effective in improving functional outcome in patients, following SCI.

KEY POINTS

- The blood supply of the brain derives from the Circle of Willis.
- Although influenced by higher brain centers, such as the limbic cortex, the autonomic nervous system operates to control the homeostatic environment in a purely reflex fashion.
- Almost all right-handed people and 70% of left-handed individuals have speech and language centers located in the left cerebral hemisphere.
- The brain is one of the most metabolically active organs in the body and requires a constant supply of O_2 and glucose.

☞ For ICP to remain constant (normal = 1–15 mmHg), the sum of the volumes of the intracerebral components must remain constant.

☞ A normal value for CPP is approximately 70 mmHg.

☞ Within the range $PaCO_2$ 25–60 mmHg, vasodilation and hence cerebral blood flow increases linearly with $PaCO_2$ (13).

☞ The cerebral metabolic rate is markedly increased during seizure activity.

☞ Hemorrhage usually presents as a space-occupying lesion, with increased ICP, and when severe, as brain or brainstem herniation.

☞ Neuronal apoptosis and necrosis may be occurring simultaneously in the injured brain.

☞ Excitotoxicity is the uncontrolled release of excitatory amino acids, causing massive sodium and calcium influx, further amino acid release, and ATP depletion culminating in cell death.

☞ A sustained rise in ICP above 20 mmHg, following severe head injury, is a highly significant predictor of poor outcome.

☞ Most severely head-injured patients show a trimodal pattern of change in CBF: an initial decline, a period of relative hyperemia (high CBF relative to cerebral metabolism), flow again decreases.

☞ Following TBI, a hypermetabolic and hypercatabolic state ensues.

☞ Serum glucose must be closely controlled following TBI, because hyperglycemia is strongly associated with worse outcome.

☞ Secondary brain injury occurs almost without exception in patients with severe head injury.

REFERENCES

1. Gray H, Williams PL, Bannister LH. Nervous system. In: Williams PL, ed. Gray's Anatomy. The Anatomical Basis of Medicine and Surgery. 38th ed. New York, NY: Churchill Livingstone, 1995:901–1398.
2. Cortical and brainstem control of motor function. In: Guyton AC & Hall JE, eds. Textbook of Medical Physiology. 10th ed. Philadelphia, PA: W.B. Saunders Company, 2000:634–646.
3. Clarke CRE. Neurological disease. In: Kumar PJ, Clark ML, eds. Clinical Medicine. 4th ed. Philadelphia, PA: W.B. Saunders, 1998:1007–1104.
4. Willis, WD Jr. General sensory system. In: Berne RM, Levy MN, eds. Principles of Physiology. 3rd ed. St. Louis, MO: Mosby, 1999:78–94.
5. Levitt P, Barbe MF & Eagleson KL. Patterning and specification of the cerebral cortex. Annu Rev Neurosci 1997; 20:1–24.
6. The cerebral cortex; intellectual functions of the brain; and learning and memory. In: Guyton AC & Hall JE, eds. Textbook of Medical Physiology. 10th ed. Philadelphia, PA: W.B. Saunders Company, 2000:663–677.
7. Mega MS, Cummings JL, Salloway S, Malloy P. The limbic system: an anatomic, phylogenetic and clinical perspective. J Neuropsychiatry Clin Neurosci 1997; 9:315–330.
8. Behavioral and motivational mechanisms of the brain-the limbic system and hypothalamus. In: Guyton AC, Hall JE, eds. Textbook of Medical Physiology. 10th ed. Philadelphia, PA: W.B. Saunders Company, 2000:678–688.
9. Garwicz M, Ekerot CF, Jorntell H. Organizational principles of cerebellar neuronal circuitry. News Physiol Sci 1998; 13:26.
10. The cerebellum, the basal ganglia, and overall motor control. In: Guyton AC, Hall JE, eds. Textbook of Medical Physiology.10th ed. Philadelphia, PA: W.B. Saunders Company, 2000:647–662.
11. Ellis H, Feldman S, Harrop-Griffiths AW. The vertebral canal and its contents. In: Ellis H, Feldman S, eds. Anatomy for Anaesthetists. 7th ed. Oxford, UK: Blackwell Science, 1997:101–142.
12. Giray H, Williams PL, Bannister LH. Cardiovascular system. In: Williams PL, ed. Gray's Anatomy: The Anatomical Basis of Medicine and Surgery. 38th ed. New York, NY: Churchill Livingstone, 1995:1451–1626.
13. Moss E. The cerebral circulation. Br J Anaesth, CEPD Rev 2001; 1(3):67–71.
14. Cerebral blood flow; the cerebrospinal fluid; and brain metabolism. In: Guyton AC & Hall JE, eds. Textbook of Medical Physiology. 10th ed. Philadelphia, PA: W.B. Saunders Company, 2000:709–717.
15. Greitz D, Greitz T, Hindmarsh T. A new view on the CSF-circulation with the potential for pharmacological treatment of childhood hydrocephalus. Acta Paediatr 1997; 86:125.
16. Willis, WD Jr. Cellular organization. In: Berne RM, Levy MN, eds. Principles of Physiology. 3rd ed. St. Louis, MO: Mosby, 1999:68–77.
17. Ermisch A, Brust P, Kretzschmar R, Ruhle HJ. Peptides and blood-brain barrier transport. Physiol Rev 1993; 73:489–527.
18. Guyton AC, Hall JE. Organization of the nervous system; basic functions of synapses and transmitter substances. In: Guyton AC, Hall JE, eds. Textbook of Medical Physilogy. 10th ed. Philadelphia, PA: W.B. Saunders Company, 2000:512–527.
19. Gehrmann J, Matsumoto Y, Kreutzberg GW. Microglia: intrinsic immunoeffector cell of the brain. Brain Res Rev 1995; 20:269–287.
20. Willis, WD Jr. Autonomic nervous system and its control. In: Berne RM, Levy MN, eds. Principles of Physiology. 3rd ed. St. Louis, MO: Mosby, 1999:134–141.
21. Ellis H, Feldman S, Harrop-Griffith AW. The autonomic nervous system; and the adrenal medulla. In: Guyton AC, Hall JE, eds. Textbook of Medical Physiology. 10th ed. Philadelphia, PA: W.B. Saunders Company, 2000:697–708.
22. Dampney RA. Functional organization of central pathways regulating the cardiovascular system. Physiol Rev 1994; 74:323–364.
23. Ellis H, Feldman S, eds. The autonomic nervous system. Anatomy for Anaesthetists. 7th ed. Oxford, UK: Blackwell Science, 1997:237–254.
24. Calvey TN, Williams NE, eds. Drugs and the autonomic nervous system. Principles and Practice of Pharmacology for Anaesthetists. 3rd ed. Oxford, UK: Blackwell Science, 1997:414–447.
25. Willis, WD Jr. Higher functions of the nervous system. In: Berne RM, Levy MN, eds. Principles of Physiology. 3rd ed. St. Louis, MO: Mosby, 1999:142–146.
26. Kutchai HC. Cellular membranes and transmembrane transport of solutes and water. In: Berne RM, Levy MN, eds. Principles of Physiology. 3rd ed. St. Louis, MO: Mosby, 1999:4–18.
27. Guyton AC, Hall JE, eds. Transport of substances through the cell membrane. Textbook of Medical Physilogy. 10th ed. Philadelphia, PA: W.B. Saunders Company, 2000:40–51.
28. Davies PD, Parbrook GD, Kenny GNC, eds. Diffusion and osmosis. Basic Physics and Measurement in Anaesthesia. 4th ed. Oxford, UK: Butterworth Heinemann, 1995: 89–102.
29. Carruthers A. Facilitated diffusion of glucose. Physiol Rev 1990; 70:1135.
30. Mercer RW. Structure of the Na,K-ATPase. Int Rev Cytol 1993; 137C:139.
31. Christensen HN. Role of amino acid transport and countertransport in nutrition and metabolism. Physiol Rev 1990; 70:43.
32. Guyton AC, Hall JE, eds. Membrane potentials and action potentials. Textbook of Medical Physilogy. 10th ed. Philadelphia, PA: W.B. Saunders Company, 2000:52–66.
33. Kutchai HC. Ionic equilibria and resting membrane potentials. In: Berne RM, Levy MN, eds. Principles of Physiology. 3rd ed. St. Louis, MO: Mosby, 1999:19–28.
34. Armstrong C, Hille B. Voltage-gated ion channels and electrical excitability. Neuron 1998; 20:371.

35. Kutchai HC. Generation and conduction of action potentials. In: Berne RM, Levy MN, eds. Principles of Physiology. 3rd ed. St. Louis, MO: Mosby, 1999:29–38.

36. Siesjo BK. Cerebral circulation and metabolism. J Neurosurg 1984; 60:883–908.

37. Matta BF, Menon DK. Management of acute head injury. Part I: pathophysiology and initial resuscitation. In: Kaufman L, Ginsburg R, eds. Anaesthesia Review 13. New York, NY: Churchill Livingstone, 1997:163–178.

38. Zauner A, Doppenberg E, Woodward JJ, et al. Multiparametric continuous monitoring of brain metabolism and substrate delivery in neurosurgical patients. Neurol Res 1997; 19: 265–273.

39. Zwienenburg M, Muizelaar JP. Cerebral perfusion and blood flow in neurotrauma. Neurological Research 2001; 23:167–174.

40. Ferring M, Berre J, Vincent JL. Induced hypertension after head injury. Intensive Care Med 1999; 25:1006–1009.

41. Finfer SR, Cohen J. Severe traumatic brain injury. Resuscitation 2001; 48:77–90.

42. Obrist WD, Langfitt TW, Jaggi JL, Cruz J, Gennarelli TA. Cerebral blood flow and metabolism in comatose patients with acute head injury. J Neurosurg 1984; 61:241–253.

43. Martin NA, Patwardhan RV, Alexander MJ, et al. Characterization of cerebral hemodynamic phases following severe heat trauma: hypoperfusion, hyperemia and vasospasm. J Neurosurg. 1997; 87(1):9–19.

44. Cruz J. The first decade of continuous monitoring of jugular bulb oxyhaemoglobin saturation: Management strategies and clinical outcome. Crit Care Med 1998; 26:344–351.

45. Mass AI, Fleckenstein W, de Jong D, Wolf M. Effect of increased ICP and decreased cerebral perfusion pressure on brain tissue and cerebrospinal fluid oxygen tensions. In: Avezaat CJ, Van Eijdhoven JH, Maas AI, Trans JT, eds. Intracranial Pressure. 8th ed. NewJersey, USA: Springer-Verlag, 1993:233–237.

46. Sakoh M, Gjedde A. Neuroprotection in hypothermia linked to redistribution of oxygen in brain. Am J Physiol Heart Circ Physiol. 2003; 285:H17–H25.

47. Mintun MA, LundstromBN, SnyderAZ, et al. Blood flow and oxygen delivery to human brain during functional activity: theoretical modeling and experimental data. Proc Natl Acad Sci 2001; 98:6859–6864.

48. Scheufler K-M, Rohrborn H-J, Zentner J. Does tissue oxygen-tension reliably reflect cerebral oxygen delivery and consumption? Anesth. Analg. 2002; 95(4):1042–1048.

49. Meixensberger J, Dings J, Kuhnigk H, Roosen K. Studies of tissue PO2 in normal and pathological human brain cortex. Acta Neurochir 1993; 59(suppl):58–63.

50. Sarrafzadeh AS, Kiening KL, Bardt TF, Schneider GH, Unterberg AW, Lanksch WR. Cerebral oxygenation in contusioned vs. nonlesioned brain tissue: Monitoring of PtiO2 with Licox and Paratrend. Acta Neurochir 1998; 71(suppl):186–189.

51. Van den Brink WA, van Santbrink H, Steyerberg EW, et al. Brain oxygen tension in severe head injury. Neurosurgery 2000; 4:868–876.

52. van Santbrink H, Maas AI, Avezaat CJ. Continuous monitoring of partial pressure of brain tissue oxygen in patients with severe head injury. Neurosurgery 1996; 38:21–31.

53. Steiner T, Pilz J, Schellinger P, et al. Multimodal online monitoring in middle cerebral artery territory stroke. Stroke 2001; 32:2500–2506.

54. Ekstedt J. CSF hydrodynamic studies in man. 2. Normal hydrodynamic variables related to CSF pressure and flow. J Neurol Neurosurg Psychiatry 1978; 41:345–353.

55. Monro A. Observations on the structure and function of the nervous system. Edinburgh; 1783.

56. Kellie G. On death from cold, and on congestions of the brain. An account of the appearances observed in the dissection of two of the three individuals presumed to have perished in the storm of 3rd November 1821; with some reflections on the pathology of the brain. Trans Med Chir Soc Edinburgh 1824; 84–169.

57. Kontos HA, Wei EP, Navari RM, Levasseur JE, Rosenblum WI, Patterson JL Jr. Responses of cerebral arteries and arterioles to acute hypotension and hypertension. Am J Physiol 1978; 243:H371–H383.

58. Vinas FC. Bedside invasive monitoring techniques in severe brain-injured patients. Neurological Res 2001; 23:157–166.

59. Paulson OB, Strandgaard S, Edvinsson L. Cerebral autoregulation. Cerebrovasc Brain Metab Rev 1990; 2:161–192.

60. Melot C, Berre J, Moraine JJ, Kahn RJ. Estimation of cerebral blood flow at bedside by continuous jugular thermodilution. J Cereb Blood Flow Metab 1996; 16:1263–1270.

61. Aaslid R, Markwalder TM, Nornes H. Noninvasive transcranial doppler ultrasound recording of flow velocity in basal cerebral arteries. J Neurosurg 1982; 57:769–774.

62. Prough DS. Brain monitoring. In: Taylor RW, Shoemaker WC, eds. Critical Care. State of the Art. Anaheim, CA: The Society of Critical Care Medicine, 1991:157–196.

63. Simonson SG, Piantadosi, CA. Near infrared spectroscopy for monitoring tissue oxygenation in the critical care setting. Curr Opin Crit Care 1995; 1:217–223.

64. Myburgh JA, Oh TE. Disorders of consciousness. In: Oh TE, ed. Intensive Care Manual. 4th ed. Oxford, UK: Butterworth Heinmann, 1997:375–380.

65. Atkinson RS, Rushman GB, Davies NJH. Physiology. In: Atkinson RS, Rushman GB, Davies NJH, eds. Lee's Synopsis of Anaesthesia. 11th ed. Oxford, UK: Butterworth-Heinemann, 1993: 3–49.

66. Chang BS, Lowenstein DH. Practice parameter: antiepileptic drug prophylaxis in severe traumatic brain injury. Report of the quality standards subcommittee of the American academy of neurology. Neurology 2003; 60:10–16.

67. Latronico N, Cagnazzi E, Chang BS, Lowenstein DH. Antiepileptic drug prophylaxis in severe traumatic brain injury. Neurology 2003; 61:1161–1162.

68. Willatts S, Logan SD. Physiology of the nervous system. In: Aitkenheah AR, Smith G, eds. Textbook of Anaesthesia. 3rd ed. Oxford, UK: Churchill Livingstone, 1996:47–76.

69. Oh TE. Brain death. In: Oh TE, ed. Intensive Care Manual. 4th ed. Oxford, UK: Butterworth Heinmann, 1997:412–415.

70. Pallis C. Prognostic significance of a dead brainstem. Br Med J 1983; 286:123–124.

71. King IA. Fundamentals of impact biomechanics: part I-biomechanics of the head, neck, and thorax. Ann Rev Biomed Eng 2000; 2:55–81.

72. Finnie JW. Animal models of traumatic brain injury: a review. Aust Vet J 2001; 79(9):628–633.

73. Povlishock JT. Pathophysiology of neural injury: therapeutic opportunities and challenges. Clin Neurosurg 2000; 46:113–126.

74. Strich SJ. Diffuse degeneration of the cerebral white matter in severe dementia following head injury. J Neurosurg Psychiat 1956; 19:163–185.

75. Maxwell WL, Povlishock JT, Graham DL. A mechanistic analysis of nondisruptive axonal injury: a review. J Neurotrauma 1997; 14(7):419–440.

76. Blumbergs PC, Scott G, Manavis J, Wainwright H, Simpson DA, McLean J. Topography of axonal injury as defined by amyloid precursor protein and the sector scoring method in mild and severe closed head injury. J Neurotrauma 1995; 12(4):565–572.

77. Martin LJ, Al-Abdulla NA, Brambrink AM, Kirsch JR, Sieber FE, Portera-Cailliau C. Neurodegeneration in excitotoxicity, global cerebral ischaemia, and target deprivation: a perspective on the contributions of apoptosis and necrosis. Brain Res Bull 1998; 46(4): 281–309.

78. Bredesen DE. Apoptosis: overview and signal transduction pathways. J Neurotrauma 2000; 17(10):801–810.

79. Zipfel GJ, Babcock DJ, Lee J-M, Choi DW. Neuronal apoptosis after CNS injury: the roles of glutamate and calcium. J Neurotrauma 2000; 17(10):857–869.

80. Raghupathi R, Graham DI, McIntosh TK. Apoptosis after traumatic brain injury. J Neurotrauma 2000; 17(10):927–938.

81. Tsujimoto Y. Apoptosis and necrosis: intracellular ATP levels as a determinant of cell death modes. Cell Death Differ 1997; 4:429–434.

82. Koike T, Martin DP, Johnson EM. Role of Ca2+ channels in the ability of membrane depolarization to prevent neuronal death induced by trophic-factor deprivation: evidence that levels of internal Ca2+ determine nerve growth factor dependence of sympathetic ganglion cells. Proc Natl Acad Sci 1989; 86:6421–6425.

83. Lee JM, Zipfel GJ & Choi DW. The changing landscape of ischaemic brain injury mechanisms. Nature 1999; 6738(suppl):A7–A14.

84. Danbolt NC. The high affinity uptake system for excitatory amino acids in the brain. Prog Neurobiol 1994; 44:377–396.

85. Brown JIM, Baker AJ, Konasiewicz SJ, Moulton RJ. Clinical significance of CSF glutamate concentrations following severe traumatic brain injury in humans. J Neurotrauma 1998; 15(4):253–263.

86. Stover JF, Morganti-Kossmann MC, Lenzlinger PM, Stocker R, Kempski OS, Kossman T. Glutamate and taurine are increased in ventricular cerebrospinal fluid of severely brain-injured patients. J Neurotrauma 1999; 16(2):135–142.

87. Bullock R, Zauner A, Woodward JJ, Myseros J, Choi SC, Ward JD et al. Factors affecting excitatory amino acid release following severe human head injury. J Neurosurg 1998; 89:507–518.

88. Juurlink BH, Paterson PG. Review of oxidative stress in brain and spinal cord injury: suggestions for pharmacological and nutritional management strategies. J Spinal Cord Med 1998; 21(4):309–334.

89. Hovda DA, Lee SM, Smith ML, et al. The neurochemical and metabolic cascade following brain injury: moving from animal models to man. J Neurotrauma 1995; 12(5):903–906.

90. Dawson VL, Dawson TM, London ED, Bredt DS, Snyder SH. Nitric oxide mediates glutamate neurotoxicity in primary cortical cultures. Proc Natl Acad Sci USA 1991; 88:6368–6371.

91. Chabrier PE, Demerle-Pallardy C, Auguet M. Nitric oxide synthases: targets for therapeutic strategies in neurological diseases. CMLS Cell Mol Life Sci 1999; 55:1029–1035.

92. Kampfl A, Postmantur RM, Zhao X, Schmutzhard E, Clifton GL, Hayes RL. Mechanisms of calpain proteolysis following traumatic brain injury: implications for pathology and therapy: a review and update. J Neurotrauma 1997; 14(3):121–134.

93. Dutcher SA, Michael DB. Gene expression in neurotrauma. Neurolog Res 2001; 23:203–206.

94. Fiskum G. Mitochondrial participation in ischaemic and traumatic neural cell death. J Neurotrauma 2000; 17(10):843–855.

95. Anthony DC, Blond D, Dempster R, Perry H. Chemokine targets in acute brain injury and disease. Prog in Brain Res 2001; 132:507–524.

96. Samatovicz RA. Genetics and brain injury: apolipoprotein E. J Head Trauma Rehabil 2000; 15(3):869–874.

97. Marmrou A, Anderson RL, Ward JD, Choi SC, Young HF. Impact of ICP instability and hypotension on outcome in patients with severe head trauma. J Neurosurg 1991; 75:S59–S66.

98. Greenberg MS, Coma Lakeland, FL. In: Greenberg MS, ed. Handbook of Neurosurgery. 5th ed. Lakeland, FL: Greenberg Graphics, Inc, 2001:118–127.

99. Chan K-H, Miller JD, Dearden NM. Intracranial blood flow velocity after head injury: relationship to severity of injury, time, neurological status and outcome. J Neurol Neurosurg Psychiatry 1992; 55:787–791.

100. Lee JH, Martin NA, Alsina G, et al. Hemodynamically significant cerebral vasospasm and outcome after head injury: a prospective study. J Neurosurg 1997; 87:221–233.

101. Salvant JB, Muizelaar JP. Changes in cerebral blood flow and metabolism related to the presence of subdural hematoma. Neurosurg 1993; 33:387–393.

102. Bouma GJ, Muizelaar JP. Cerebral blood flow, cerebral blood volume, and cerebrovascular reactivity after severe head injury. J Neurotrauma 1992; 9:S333–S348.

103. Bouma GJ, Muizelaar JP. Relationship between cardiac output and cerebral blood flow in patients with intact and with impaired autoregulation. J Neurosurg 1990; 73:368–374.

104. Strebel S, Lam AM, Matta BF, Newell DW. Impaired cerebral autoregulation after mild brain injury. Surg Neurol 1997; 47:128–131.

105. Paulson OB, Olesen J, Christensen MS. Restoration of autoregulation of cerebral blood flow by hypocapnia. Neurology 1972; 22:286–293.

106. Cold GE. Cerebral blood flow in acute head injury. The regulation of cerebral blood flow and metabolism during the acute phase of head injury, and its significance for therapy. Acta Neurochir Suppl (Wien) 1990; 49:1–64.

107. Petrov T, Rafols JA. Acute alterations of endothelin-1 and iNOS expression and control of brain microcirculation after head trauma. Neurol Res 2001; 23:139–143.

108. Robertson CS. Management of cerebral perfusion pressure after traumatic brain injury. Anesthesiology 2001; 95:1513–1517.

109. Rosner MJ, Daughton S. Cerebral perfusion pressure management in head injury. J Trauma 1990; 30:933–941.

110. Rosner NJ, Rosner SD, Johnson AH. Cerebral perfusion pressure: management protocol and clinical results. J Neurosurg 1995; 83:949–962.

111. The Brain Trauma Foundation. The American Association of Neurological Surgeons. The Joint Section on Neurotrauma and Critical Care. Guidelines for cerebral perfusion pressure. J Neurotrauma 2000; 17(6/7):507–511.

112. Grande PO, Asgeirsson B, Nordstrom CH. Physiologic principles for volume regulation of a tissue in a rigid shell with application to the injured brain. J Trauma 1997; 42:S23–S31.

113. Eker C, Asgeirsson B, Grande PO, Schalen W, Nordstrom CH. Improved outcome after severe head injury with a new therapy based on the principles for brain volume regulation and preserved microcirculation. Crit Care Med 1998; 26:1881–1886.

114. Xiong Y, Peterson PL, Lee CP. Alterations in cerebral energy metabolism induced by traumatic brain injury. Neurol Res 2001; 23:129–138.

115. Young B, Ott L, Norton J, Tibbs P, Rapp R, McClain C, et al. Metabolic and nutritional sequelae in the non steroid treated head injury patient. J Neurosurg 1985; 17:784–791.

116. Duke JH Jr, Jorgensen SD, Broell JR. Contribution of protein to caloric expenditure following injury. Surgery 1970; 68:168–174.

117. Pepe JL, Barba CA. The metabolic response to acute traumatic brain injury and implications for nutritional support. J Head Trauma Rehabil 1999; 14(5):462–474.

118. The Brain Trauma Foundation. The American Association of Neurological Surgeons. The Joint Section on Neurotrauma and Critical Care. Nutrition. J Neurotrauma 2000; 17(6/7):539–547.

119. Yuan X-Q, Wade CE. Neuroendocrine abnormalities in patients with traumatic brain injury. Frontiers in Neuroendocrinology 1991; 12(3):209–230.

120. Lam AM, Winn RH, Cullen BF, Sundling N. Hyperglycemia and neurological outcome in patients with head injury. J Neurosurg 1991; 75:545–551.

121. Segal-Lieberman G, Karasik A, Shimon I. Hypopituitarism following closed head injury. Pituitary 2000; 3:181–184.

122. Panter SS, Yum SW, Faden AI. Alteration in extracellular amino acids after traumatic spinal cord injury. Ann Neurol 1990; 27:96–99.

123. Popovich PG. Immunological regulation of neuronal degeneration and regeneration in the injured spinal cord. Prog Brain Res 2000; 128:43–58.

124. Kakulas BA. A review of the neuropathology of human spinal cord injury with emphasis on special features. J Spinal Cord Med 1999; 22:119–124.

125. Beattie MS, Farooqui AA, Bresnahan JC. Review of current evidence for apoptosis after spinal cord injury. J Neurotrauma 2000; 17(10):915–925.

126. Bracken MB, Shepard MJ, Collins WF, et al. A randomized controlled trial of methylprednisolone or naloxone in the treatment of acute spinal-cord injury. N Engl J Med 1990; 322:1405–1461.

127. Bracken MB, Shepard MJ, Holford TR, et al. Administration of methylprednisolone for 24 or 48 hours or tirilazad mesylate for 48 hours in the treatment of acute spinal cord injury. Results of

the third national acute spinal cord injury randomized controlled trial. JAMA 1997; 277:1597–1604.

128. Bracken MB, Shepard MJ, Holford TR, et al. Methylprednisolone or tirilazad mesylate administration after acute spinal cord injury: 1-year follow up. Results of the third national acute spinal cord injury randomized controlled trial. J Neurosurg 1998; 89:699–706.

129. Rhoney DH, Parker D Jr. Use of sedative and analgesic agents in neurotrauma patients: effects on cerebral physiology. Neurol Res 2001; 23:237–259.

130. The Brain Trauma Foundation. The American Association of Neurological Surgeons. The Joint Section on Neurotrauma and Critical Care. Use of barbiturates in the control of intracranial hypertension. J Neurotrauma 2000; 17(6/7):527–530.

131. Jeevaratnam DR, Menon DK. Survey of intensive care of severely head injured patients in the United Kingdom. BMJ 1996; 312:994–997.

132. The Brain Trauma Foundation. The American Association of Neurological Surgeons. The Joint Section on Neurotrauma and Critical Care. Use of mannitol. J Neurotrauma 2000; 17(6/7): 521–525.

133. Schierhout G, Roberts I. Mannitol for acute traumatic brain injury (Cochrane Review). In: The Cochrane Library, Issue 1, 2002. Oxford: Cochrane Database Syst Rev 2000;(2): CD 001049.

134. Shackford SR, Zhuang J, Schmoker J. Intravenous fluid tonicity: effect on intracranial pressure, cerebral blood flow, and cerebral oxygen delivery in focal brain injury. J Neurosurg 1992; 76: 91–98.

135. Doyle JA, Davis DP, Hoyt DB. The use of hypertonic saline in the treatment of traumatic brain injury. J Trauma 2001; 50:367–383.

136. Wade CE, Grady JJ, Kramer GC, Younes RN, Gehlsen K, Holcroft JW. Individual patient cohort analysis of the efficacy of hypertonic saline/dextran in patients with traumatic brain injury and hypotension. J Trauma 1997; 42(5): S61–S65.

137. The Brain Trauma Foundation. The American Association of Neurological Surgeons. The Joint Section on Neurotrauma and Critical care. Resuscitation of blood pressure and oxygenation. J Neurotrauma 2000; 17(6/7):471–478.

138. Muizelaar JP, Marmarou A, Ward JD, et al. Adverse effects of prolonged hyperventilation in patients with severe head injury: a randomized clinical trial. J Neurosurg 1991; 75:7 31–739.

139. Menon DK, Minhas PS, Matthews JC, Downey SP, Parry DA, Kendall IV, et al. Blood flow decreases associated with hyperventilation in head injury result in ischaemia. J Cereb Blood Flow Metab 1999; 19:S372.

140. The Brain Trauma Foundation. The American Association of Neurological Surgeons. The joint section on Neurotrauma and Critical Care. Hyperventilation. J Neurotrauma 2000; 17(6/7):513–520.

141. Provencio JJ, Bleck TP, Connors AF Jr. Critical care neurology. Am J Respir Crit Care Med 2001; 164(3):341–345.

142. Schierhout G, Roberts I. Hyperventilation therapy for acute traumatic brain injury (Cochrane Review). In: The Cochrane Library, Issue 1, 2002. Oxford: Cochrane Database Syst Rev 2000;(2): CD 000566.

143. Verma A. Opportunities for neuroprotection in traumatic brain injury. J Head Trauma Rehabil 2000; 15(5):1149–1161.

144. Fisher M. Potentially effective therapies for acute ischemic stroke. Eur Neurol 1995; 35:3–7.

145. Haghighi SS, Johnson GC, de Vergel CF, Vergel-Rivas BJ. Pretreatment with NMDA receptor antagonist MK801 improves neurophysiological outcome after an acute spinal cord injury. Neurol Res 1996; 18:509–515.

146. Abel MS, McCandless DW. Elevated gamma-aminobutyric acid levels attenuate the metabolic response to bilateral ischemia. J Neurochem 1992; 58:740–744.

147. Langham J, Goldfrad C, Teasdale G, Shaw D, Rowan K. Calcium channel blockers for acute traumatic brain injury (Cochrane Review). In: The Cochrane Library, Issue 1, 2002. Oxford: Update Software. Cochrane Database Syst Rev 2003; (4) CD000565.

148. Okonkwo DO, Buki A, Siman R, Povlishock JT. Cyclosporin A limits calcium-induced axonal damage following traumatic brain injury. Neuroreport 1999; 10:353–358.

149. The Brain Trauma Foundation. The American Association of Neurological Surgeons. The Joint Section on Neurotrauma and Critical Care. Role of steroids. J Neurotrauma 2000; 17(6/7):531–535.

150. Alderson P, Roberts I. Corticosteroids for acute traumatic brain injury (Cochrane Review). In: The Cochrane Library, Issue 1, 2002. Oxford: Cochrane Database Syst Rev 2000;(2): CD 000196.

151. Roberts I. Aminosteroids for acute traumatic brain injury (Cochrane Review). In: The Cochrane Library, Issue 1, 2002. Oxford: Cochrane Database Syst Rev 2000;(4): CD 001527.

152. Stein DG. Brain damage, sex hormones and recovery: a new role for progesterone and estrogen? Trends in Neurosci 2001; 24(7):386–391.

153. Wise PM, Dubal DB, Wilson ME, Rau SW. Estradiol is a neuroprotective factor in in vivo and in vitro models of brain injury. J Neurocytol 2000; 29:401–410.

154. Phillis JW, Goshgarian HG. Adenosine and neurotrauma: therapeutic perspectives. Neurol Res 2001; 23:183–189.

155. Marion DW, Penrod LE, Kelsey SF, et al. Treatment of traumatic brain injury with moderate hypothermia. N Eng J Med 1997; 336 (8):540–546.

156. Gadkary CS, Alderson P, Signorini DF. Therapeutic hypothermia for head injury (Cochrane Review). In: The Cochrane Library, Issue 1, 2002. Oxford: Cochrane Database Syst Rev 2002;(1): CD 001048.

157. Naredi S, Koskinen LO, Grande PO, et al. Treatment of traumatic head injury-U.S./European guidelines or the Lund concept. Crit Care Med 2003; 31(11):2713–2714.

158. Heimann A, Takeshima T, Alessandri B, Noppens R, Kempski O. Effects of hypertonic/hyperoncotic treatment after rat cortical vein occlusion. Crit Care Med 2003; 31(10):2559–2560.

159. Darlington CL. Dexanabinol: a novel cannabinoid with neuroprotective properties. I Drugs 2003; 6(10):976–979.

160. Zhou F, Hongmin B, Xiang Z, Enyu L. Changes of mGluR4 and the effects of its specific agonist L-AP4 in a rodent model of diffuse brain injury. J Clin Neurosci 2003; 10(6):684–688.

161. Kipnis J, Nevo U, Panikashvili D, et al. Therapeutic vaccination for closed head injury. J Neurotrauma 2003; 20(6):559–569.

162. Hiraiwa M, Liu J, Lu AG, et al. Regulation of gene expression in response to brain injury: enhanced expression and alternative splicing of rat prosaposin (SGP-1) mRNA in injured brain. J Neurotrauma 2003; 20(8):755–765.

163. Royo NC, Schouten JW, Flup CT, Shimizu S, Marklund N, Graham DI et al. From cell death to neuronal regeneration: building a new brain after traumatic brain injury. J Neuropathol Exp Neurol 2003; 62(8):801–811.

2

Pulmonary Physiology Review

Shamsuddin Akhtar

Department of Anesthesiology, Yale University School of Medicine, New Haven, Connecticut, U.S.A.

INTRODUCTION

Atmospheric air is a mixture of oxygen (O_2, 20.95%), nitrogen (N_2 78.09%), argon (0.93%), carbon dioxide (CO_2, 0.03%), and water vapor (0–2%). For practical purposes we usually assume O_2, 21% and N_2, 79% and ignore the contributions from CO_2 and argon. The degree of humidification determines the water vapor pressure and proportional dilution of other gases.

In order for the cells to utilize the O_2 in the atmosphere, it has to be transported efficiently to the tissues and cells (Fig. 1) (1). The first step is inspiration and ventilation, the transfer of atmospheric air (or gases) to the alveoli, where it is brought in close proximity to the blood to allow efficient gas exchange, with the subsequent movement of alveolar air back to the outside. Ventilation is closely coupled with adequate perfusion of the alveoli. The interaction of ventilation and perfusion [ventilation-perfusion ($\dot{V}/\dot{Q}$) relationship] ultimately determines the gas exchange in the lungs. The transport of O_2 requires reversible binding of O_2 to hemoglobin (Hb), which is then unloaded at the tissues. The O_2 flows through its concentration gradient to the extracellular space and cells. Intracellular concentrations of O_2 also varies within the cell, and the mitochondrial pO_2 is 1–0.6 mmHg. The process of ventilation is tightly regulated by neural and nonneural mechanisms. Furthermore, interaction of the circulatory system with the respiratory system adds another level of fine-tuning and complexity to the process of perfusion, ventilation, and ventilation-perfusion interaction. Pulmonary function does not remain static throughout life. Significant differences in respiratory physiology are evident in neonates and the elderly. There are alterations in pulmonary physiology during pregnancy as well. Lungs also have very important nonpulmonary metabolic and humoral functions.

MECHANICS OF RESPIRATION
Lung Volumes and Capacities

The diaphragm is the most important muscle used for breathing. Contraction of the diaphragm forces the abdominal contents downward and forward, which increases the vertical diameter of the chest cavity. In addition the intercostal muscles lift the rib margins outward and upward, increasing the transverse diameter of the thorax. During normal tidal breathing, the diaphragm moves about 1 cm, while under forced inhalation and exhalation it can move up to 10 cm (2). The contraction of the internal intercostal muscles also increases the lateral and anteroposterior diameters of the thorax because of the "buckle-handle" movement of the ribs. Exhalation is passive during quiet breathing. However,

during active expiration (e.g., exercise, voluntary hyperventilation), abdominal muscles play the most active role. The internal intercostal muscles also assist by pulling the ribs down and inward ("reverse buckle-handle").

Normal breathing volume (tidal volume, V_T) is about 7 mL/kg. Vital capacity (VC) is the maximum volume of gas exhaled after maximal inspiration. In health, the VC is about 70 mL/kg. Residual volume (RV) is the gas that remains in the lung even after maximal exhalation. However, the amount of gas that remains in the lung at end exhalation during normal tidal breathing (or apnea) is referred to as the functional residual capacity (FRC) and is the combination of RV and expiratory reserve volume (ERV) (Fig. 2). ☞ **The FRC has important clinical significance as it is the major reservoir of oxygen in the body and is directly related to the time till desaturation following apnea. In addition, the FRC is inversely proportional to the degree of shunt (see below).** ☞ The FRC changes significantly with posture (1). In the standing healthy individual the FRC is about half the VC (or about 35 cc/kg). FRC and RV cannot be measured by simple spirometry. They can be measured using any of the three techniques: (*i*) N_2 washout technique; (*ii*) gas dilution technique using helium or; (*iii*) body plethysmography (1).

Minute Ventilation (Alveolar Ventilation and Dead Space)

The exhaled total ventilation or minute volume (V_E) is equal to volume of gas exhaled per minute. Thus total ventilation is equal to V_T × number of breaths (f) in a minute.

$$\dot{V}_E = V_T \times f \tag{1}$$

Not all the gas that is inhaled (or exhaled) participates in alveolar gas exchange. However, they do participate in warming and humidification of air, or exchange of highly soluble gases (e.g., ethyl alcohol). There is a fraction of the gas that traverses the nose, pharynx, larynx, trachea, bronchi, and bronchioles and does not participate in gas exchange of O_2 and CO_2; this is termed the anatomic dead space. Furthermore, a certain proportion of alveoli are not adequately perfused, although they may be adequately ventilated; this is termed the alveolar dead space. ☞ **Alveolar ventilation ($\dot{V}_A$) is referred to as the gas that participates in gas exchange; the amount of ventilation that is wasted is referred to as physiologic dead space ventilation ($\dot{V}_D$).** ☞

$$\dot{V}_E = \dot{V}_A + \dot{V}_{D_{physiol}} \tag{2}$$

The volume per minute of alveolar ventilation is critical, because it determines the amount of air presented to

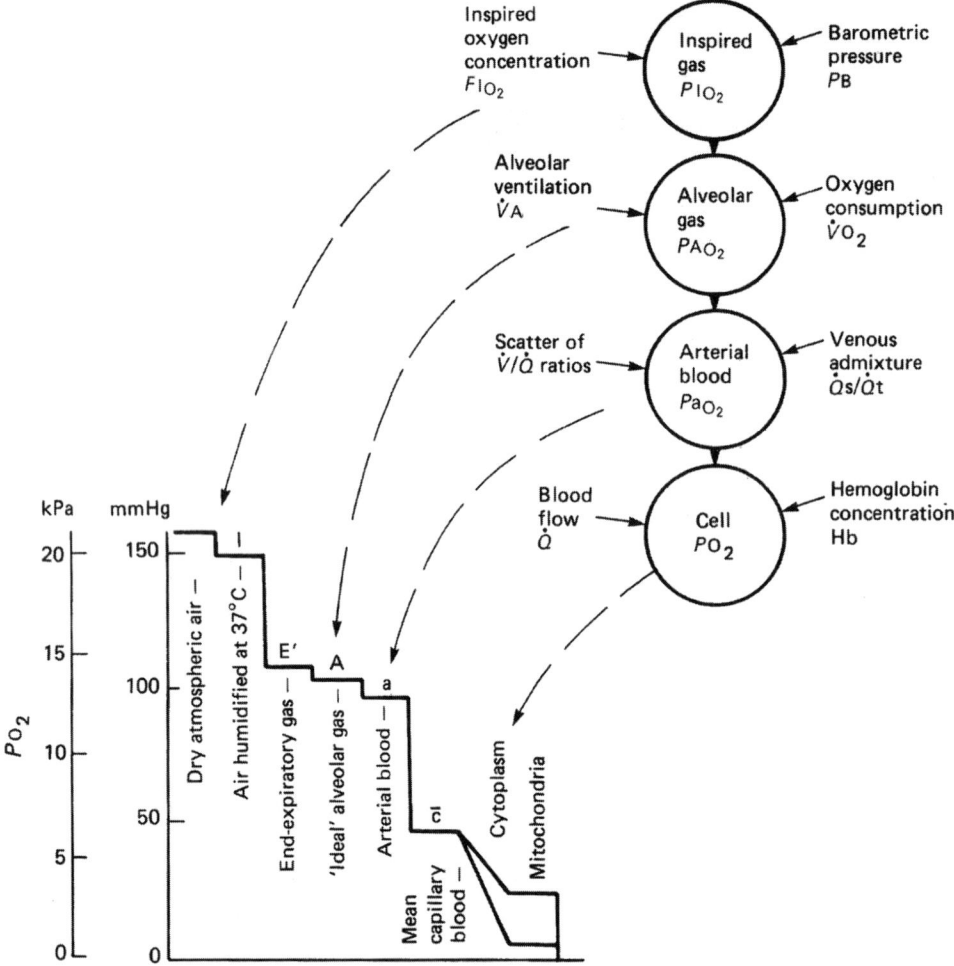

Figure 1   *Left*: The oxygen cascade with PO_2 falling from the level in the ambient air down to the level in mitochondria. *Right*: A summary of the factors influencing oxygenation at different levels in the cascade. *Source*: From Ref. 1.

alveoli into which CO_2 can be added and from which O_2 can be removed.

Dead space can be measured by nitrogen washout technique (Fowler's method) (3). Since this method measures the volume of conducting airways down to the midpoint of the transition from dead space to alveolar gas it is called anatomic dead space ($\dot{V}_{D_{anat}}$). It is dependent on

the geometry of the rapidly expanding airways and reflects morphology of the lung. The other method of calculating dead space is by using Bohr's equation, which is based on the assumption that all CO_2 comes from the alveolar gas, and none from the dead space.

$$\dot{V}_D/\dot{V}_E = P_ACO_2 - P_ECO_2/P_ACO_2 \qquad (3)$$

Bohr's method measures the volume of the lung that does not eliminate CO_2 and is more of a functional measurement. It is referred to as physiologic dead space ($\dot{V}_{D_{physiol}}$). Physiologic dead space ventilation consists of wasted ventilation in conducting airways (anatomic dead space ventilation, $\dot{V}_{D_{anat}}$) and wasted ventilation of nonperfused alveoli (alveolar dead space ventilation, $\dot{V}_{D_{alv}}$) as shown in Equation 4.

$$\dot{V}_{D_{physiol}} = \dot{V}_{D_{anat}} + \dot{V}_{D_{alv}} \qquad (4)$$

$$\dot{V}_A = \dot{V}_E - (\dot{V}_{D_{physiol}}) \qquad (5)$$

$$\dot{V}_A = \dot{V}_E - (\dot{V}_{D_{anat}} + \dot{V}_{D_{alv}}) \qquad (6)$$

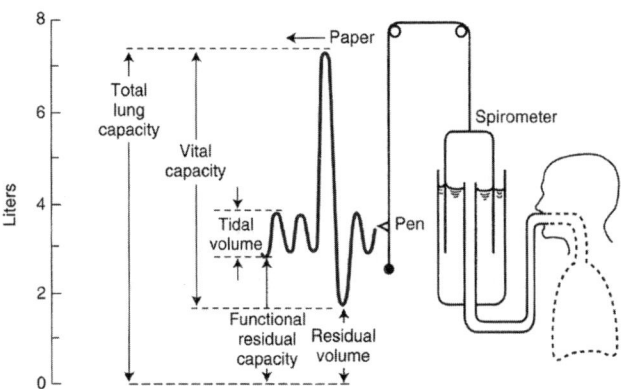

Figure 2   Lung volumes. Note that residual volume (and thus total lung capacity and functional residual capacity) cannot be measured with the spirometer. *Source*: From Ref. 2.

In normal subjects, the alveolar dead space ventilation is small and volume of anatomic dead space and physiologic dead space are nearly the same. The $\dot{V}_{D_{physiol}}$ is frequently expressed as a fraction of the tidal volume (e.g., V_D/V_T). The normal V_D/V_T (dead space to tidal volume ratio) is 0.2 to 0.35 (2). In patients with lung disease, physiologic dead space may be considerably larger due to increased alveolar dead space ventilation. In normal patients, V_{Dalv} can be increased during mechanical ventilation when excessive tidal volumes or positive end-expiratory pressure (PEEP) is applied, as well as by conditions that decrease the cardiac output ($\dot{Q}$) during normal tidal breathing.

Lung Compliance

The lung can be regarded as an elastic chamber, which is connected to the atmosphere by a tube. Thus, the amount of ventilation depends on the compliance of the chamber and resistance of the tube. The elasticity of the lung originates from the basic component of the lung "skeleton," which is a continuous network of elastin fibers. The collagen fiber network also contributes to this elasticity. Change in the ratio of collagen with elastin contributes to decreased compliance with aging (4).

Lung compliance, which is a measure of its distensability, is defined as the change in lung volume per unit change in transmural pressure gradient (i.e., between the alveolus and pleural space), $\Delta V / \Delta P$ = compliance. Normal compliance is $100 \, mL/cm/H_2O$. Stiff lungs have low compliance. Under experimental conditions one can evaluate lung compliance without the effect of the chest wall by developing pressure-volume (P-V) curve at inflation and deflation (Fig. 3). As is evident from the Figure 3, the inflation and deflation curves are not identical and the difference is described as hysteresis. Furthermore, even at zero pressure around the lung, a certain volume of air is held in the alveoli due to closure of small airways. The volume of gas required to be in the lung to keep the small conducting airways open is referred to as the "closing volume." It is difficult to measure compliance in spontaneously breathing patients. However, in mechanically ventilated patients, lung compliance can be readily measured. Furthermore, compliance can be used clinically to monitor respiratory function and severity of disease.

There are many factors that affect lung compliance. Foremost, lung compliance is related to lung volume. At high or low lung volumes the lung compliance is low (Fig. 3). Compliance is greatest at mid lung volume (i.e., FRC). If the alveoli collapse in the lower zones, the compliance at low lung volumes is particularly poor. This partly explains the utility of PEEP. It improves ventilation by pushing the system to a favorable part of the P-V curve, thus decreasing $\dot{V}/\dot{Q}$ mismatch during pathological states. Posture changes lung volume, and hence, alters lung compliance. Pulmonary blood vessels also contribute to the stiffness of the lung. Increased pulmonary venous congestion, as in congestive heart failure, decreases lung compliance. Hypoventilation without periodic deep breaths leads to atelectasis, and may also lead to decreased compliance. Emphysema increases pulmonary compliance. However, in most other pulmonary pathologies (pulmonary fibrosis, acute lung injury, consolidation, collapse, vascular engorgement, fibrous pleurisy) pulmonary compliance is decreased.

The total compliance of the lung and the chest wall is determined by the P-V curve in vivo (Fig. 4). The chest wall has a tendency to expand, while the lungs, due to their elastic recoil, tend to collapse. This creates a negative intrapleural pressure. The balance where tendency to collapse matches the tendency to expand is the FRC of the

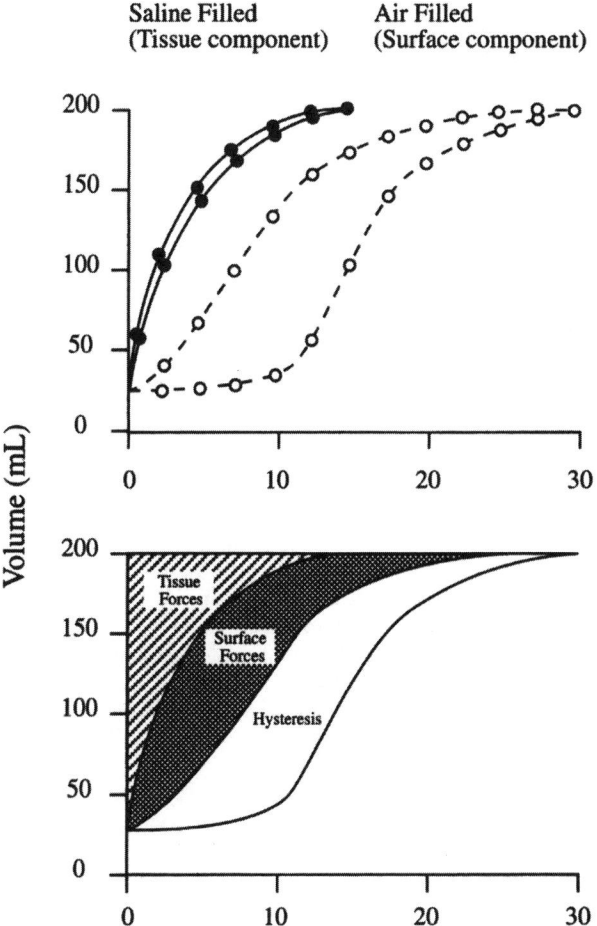

Figure 3 Compliance (volume/pressure) curves of lungs filled with saline and with air (*upper panel*). The vertical axis units are mL of volume; the horizontal axis units are cm H_2O pressure. The amount of force required to expand the tissue, surface forces, and hysteresis are shown in the *bottom panel*. *Source*: Modified from Ref. 2.

lung. Mathematically, the total compliance is not strictly additive. Rather, they are related by the following formula:

$$1/C_T = 1/C_L + 1/C_{CW} \qquad (7)$$

where C_T is the total compliance of the lung and chest wall; C_L is the compliance of the lung; C_{CW} is compliance of the chest wall. ☞ **The formula for compliance is analogous to the mathematical formula used to calculate capacitance in electronics.** ☞

Resistance from the surface forces at the alveolar gas/liquid interface also impact on the elastic property of the lung. Other factors that can impede ventilation are collectively described as nonelastic resistance. They are: (*i*) frictional resistance to gas flow through the airways; (*ii*) frictional resistance from deformation of thoracic tissues (visco-elastic tissue resistance); and (*iii*) inertia associated with movement of gas and tissues. Work done in overcoming nonelastic resistance is usually wasted as heat, while the work done in overcoming the elastic resistance is stored as potential energy and utilized in recoil of the chamber.

Another important component affecting elasticity of the lungs is surfactant. The phospholipids component

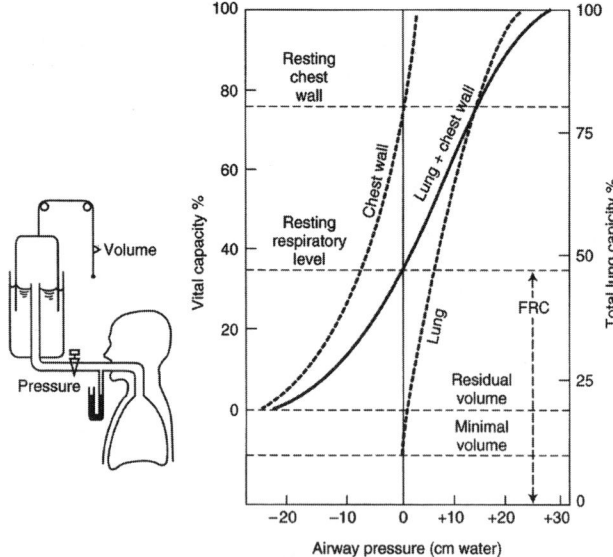

Figure 4 Relaxation pressure-volume curve of the lung and chest wall. The subject inspires (or expires) to a certain volume for the spirometer, the tap is closed, and the subject then relaxes his respiratory muscles. The curve for lung + chest wall can be explained by the addition of the individual lung and chest wall curves. *Source*: From Ref. 2.

(90%) of the surfactant favorably alters the surface tension at the alveolar gas interface, while the protein component (10%) provides stability to the molecule and is responsible for its immunological properties (5,6). If not for the surfactant, surface tension would make the small alveoli empty into a large alveolus. In the presence of surfactant, surface tension in the smaller alveoli decreases, as the molecules of surfactant are pushed closer, which helps to maintain their patency. Lack of surfactant is the major cause of respiratory distress syndrome in premature infants.

Airway Resistance

The second factor that significantly affects the ventilation (flow of gases) is the size of the airways. Airway resistance is the pressure difference between the alveoli and mouth, divided by a flow rate. Flow of gases in the airways is a mixture of turbulent and laminar flow. Flow is mostly turbulent in large airways and becomes near laminar in smaller airways (7). Flow of gas in the lungs can be demonstrated by developing flow-volume loops. Over most of the lung volume, flow rate is independent of effort and is due to dynamic compression of the airways by intrathoracic pressure. Maximal flow decreases with lung volume (Fig. 5), as the difference between alveolar and intrapleural pressure (driving pressure) decreases, the airways become narrower. Driving pressure is also reduced if compliance is increased. One common pulmonary function test is the measurement of forced expiratory volume in one second (FEV_1). The other is forced expiratory flow between 25% and 75% of the volume ($FEF_{25-75\%}$). The FEV_1 is normally 80% of forced vital capacity (FVC). The ratio of FEV_1/FVC is decreased with increase in airway resistance or a reduction in elastic recoil of the lung as seen in emphysema. In restrictive lung disease, the FEV_1/FVC ratio is not altered, however, the flow-volume curve is significantly changed (Fig. 6) (8).

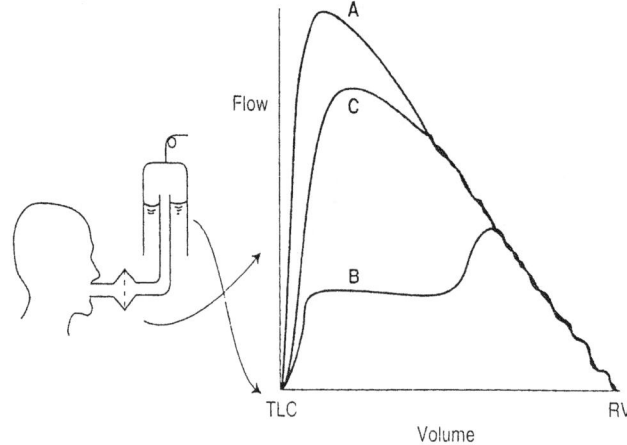

Figure 5 Flow-volume curves. (**A**) Maximal inspiration was followed by a forced expiration. (**B**) Expiration was initially slow and then forced. (**C**) Expiratory effort was submaximal. In all three, the descending portions of the curves are almost superimposed. *Source*: From Ref. 2.

Based on Poiseuilli's equation (resistance $\alpha \ 1/radius^4$), decreasing the radius by half would increase the resistance by 16-fold. This would lead one to believe that the major part of the airway resistance lies in the very narrow airways. However, this has been disproven by direct measurements (9). Major resistance lies in the medium-sized, seventh generation airways, while only 20% is attributable to airways less than 2 mm in diameter (about eight generation) (2).

☞ **Factors that affect airway resistance include lung volume, bronchial smooth muscle tone, carbon dioxide, and the density/viscosity of the inhaled gas.** ☞ Airways are imbedded in the lung tissue and are held open by traction. Thus, low lung volume decreases the diameter of the

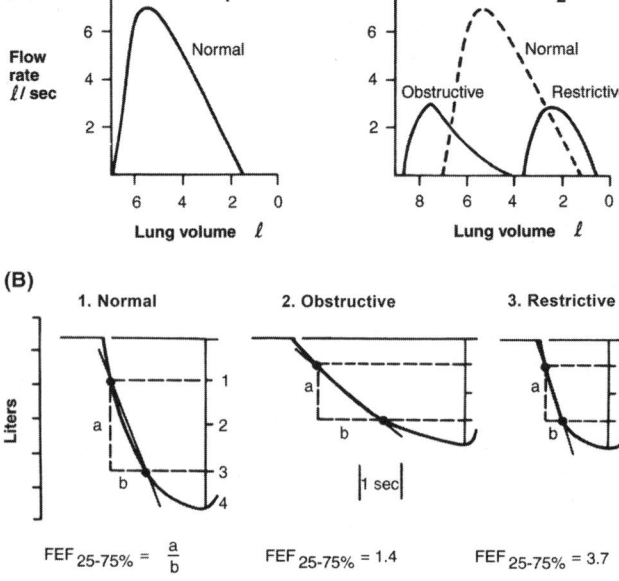

Figure 6 (**A**) Calculation of forced expiratory flow ($FEF_{25-75\%}$) from a forced expiration. (**B**) Expiratory flow-volume curves: (1) normal, (2) obstructive, and (3) restrictive patterns. *Source*: From Ref. 8.

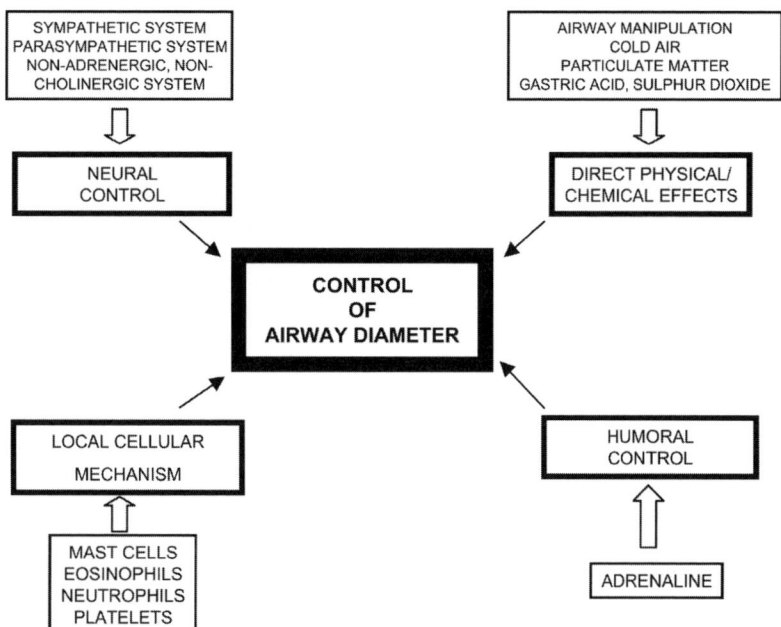

Figure 7 Factors that control bronchial smooth muscle contraction and airway diameter.

airways and increases airway resistance. Bronchial smooth muscle contraction controls the diameter of the airway and itself is controlled by many factors (Fig. 7). Sympathetic stimulation via $\beta2$-adrenergic receptor activation relaxes airway smooth muscle, while parasympathetic stimulation and acetylcholine increase bronchoconstriction. There are also many other mediators that impact on airway smooth muscle contraction. A fall in the CO_2 of alveolar gas also causes contraction of airway smooth muscle. The exact mechanism is not known. The density and viscosity of inspired gases offers resistance to flow. This is the rationale for using HELIOX (mixture of helium and O_2) in deep dives and acute bronchoconstriction, as it offers less resistance than O_2 or air, due to decreased density.

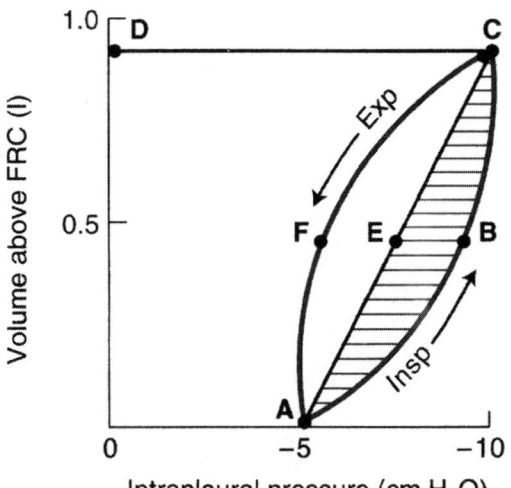

Figure 8 Pressure-volume curve of the lung showing the inspiratory work done overcoming elastic forces (area 0ACD0) and viscous forces (hatched area ABCEA). *Source*: From Ref. 2.

Work of Breathing

Work done in moving the lung and chest wall can be represented as pressure (P) × volume (V). This is represented on P-V curve (Fig. 8). The total area represents the total work done in each respiratory cycle. It includes work done to overcome airway, tissue, surface, and elastic resistances. In physical terms the efficiency of the system is believed to be 5% to 10% and significant amount of work is dissipated as heat (2).

The higher the rate of breathing, airway resistance or the inspiratory flow rate, the greater the viscous work of breathing, while with larger tidal volume and slower respiratory rate there is increased elastic work of breathing. Abnormal breathing patterns also increase the percentage of $\dot{V}O_2$ that is spent on the work of breathing. For example, the $\dot{V}O_2$ for quiet breathing is about 5% of the total resting O_2 utilization, which can increase to 30% with hyperventilation.

PULMONARY CIRCULATION

✄ **Blood flow has to be closely coupled to adequate ventilation to allow for optimal exchange of O_2 and CO_2.** ✄ The amount of blood flow through the pulmonary circulation is the same as through the systemic circulation. However, pulmonary pressures and pulmonary vascular resistance (PVR) are significantly lower. Mean pressure in the pulmonary artery is 15 mmHg, which is six times less than in the aorta (100 mmHg). Pulmonary vascular resistance is about eight times less (100 dynes/sec/cm⁵) than the systemic circulation.

Factors Affecting Regional Pulmonary Blood Flow

Normal pulmonary circulation is also able to accommodate significant changes in cardiac output (Q̇) (e.g., from 6 to 25 L with exercise) without significant changes in PVR. The exact pressure in pulmonary capillaries is uncertain, and is thought to be somewhere between pulmonary artery and venous pressure. It also varies throughout the lung due to hydrostatic effects of gravity. Furthermore, as

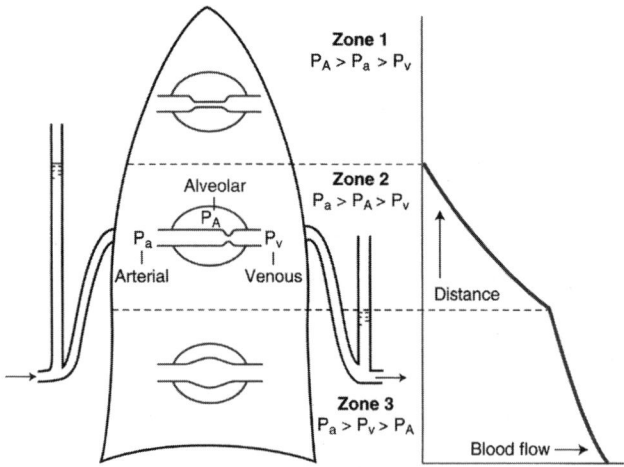

Figure 9 Zones of West, an explanation of the uneven distribution of ventilation and blood flow in the lung, based on the pressures within the alveolus (P_A), the pulmonary artery (Pa), and the pulmonary veins (Pv). *Source*: From Ref. 2.

pulmonary capillaries are embedded in the lung parenchyma and have minimal independent structural support. Their caliber is significantly affected by arterial, alveolar, and venous pressure. Collectively, these four variables (arterial, alveolar, venous pressure, and gravity) determine the blood flow in any particular region of the lung.

Zones of West

Classically, lung can be divided into three zones based on the abovementioned pressures and the effect of gravity (Fig. 9) (10).

Zone 1: It is the upper third of the lung, where alveolar pressure (P_A) exceeds arterial pressure (P_a), and pulmonary venous pressure (P_v). Both ventilation (Fig. 10A) and blood flow (Fig. 10B) are decreased. However, ventilation is slightly greater than flow, thus Zone 1 has relatively high $\dot{V}/\dot{Q}$.

Zone 2: It is the middle third of the lung, where P_a exceeds P_A. However, P_v is still lower than P_A, resulting in some impediment to blood flow.

Zone 3: It is the lower third of the lung, where P_a and P_v exceed P_A, allowing capillaries to be patent and permitting best perfusion of the three zones. In normal circumstances, as discussed earlier, the lower portion is also the best ventilated. This allows for appropriate perfusion and ventilation matching and efficient gas exchange (Fig. 10).

However, there is slightly less ventilation than perfusion (i.e., a zone of low $\dot{V}/\dot{Q}$). The absolute position of the zones changes with posture; for example, Zone 3 becomes the most dependent zone in the supine patient.

Factors Affecting Pulmonary Vascular Resistance

Based on simplification of pulmonary blood flow, pulmonary vascular resistance (PVR) can be calculated using Ohm's law (E = IR). Thus, PVR equals driving pressure divided by $\dot{Q}$. Many factors affect PVR. These include $\dot{Q}$, perfusion pressure and lung volume. There are also other factors that control PVR by active constriction and relaxation of the smooth muscle. There is some evidence to suggest that pulmonary vasculature is modulated by pulmonary endothelium and is normally kept in state of vasodilation by nitric oxide (11). PVR is also modulated by hypoxia, metabolic and neuro-humoral factors (1).

Cardiac Output/Perfusion Pressure

Since capillaries have minimal structural independence, they can collapse easily. However, with increased $\dot{Q}$ or perfusion pressure, they expand. Two processes occur simultaneously. There is either recruitment of collapsed capillaries or distension of existing open capillaries. The later process seems to be more important in vivo (1,12,13). Paradoxically, this can lead to decrease in pulmonary vascular resistance with increase in pulmonary arterial or venous pressures.

Lung Volume

PVR is significantly influenced by lung volume. PVR is lowest at FRC (Fig. 11) and increases with higher or lower volume than FRC. At higher lung volume, increase in PVR is thought to be due to compression of intraparenchymal blood vessels, while at lower lung volume it is thought to be due to the compression of extraparenchymal vessels at the hila (2).

Hypoxia

☞ **Unlike systemic vessels, pulmonary vessels constrict in response to hypoxia, hypercarbia, and acidosis.** ☞ This phenomenon of hypoxic pulmonary vasoconstriction (HPV) is mediated predominantly by alveolar hypoxia, with some influence of mixed venous PO_2. When pulmonary blood flow is plotted against alveolar PO_2, the shape of the curve is very similar to the O_2-dissociation curve. P_{50} of the curve is around 30 mmHg with marked vasoconstriction happening at 70 mmHg. Short-term regional HPV can be a

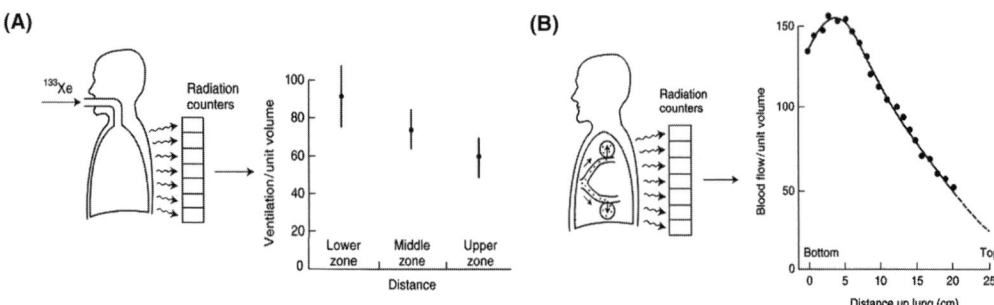

Figure 10 Distribution of ventilation and perfusion and gas exchange down the upright lung. (**A**) Measurement of regional differences in ventilation with radioactive xenon. (Note that the ventilation decreases from the lower to upper regions of the upright lung.) (**B**) Measurement of the distribution of blood flow in the upright human using radioactive xenon. (Note the small flow at the apex.)

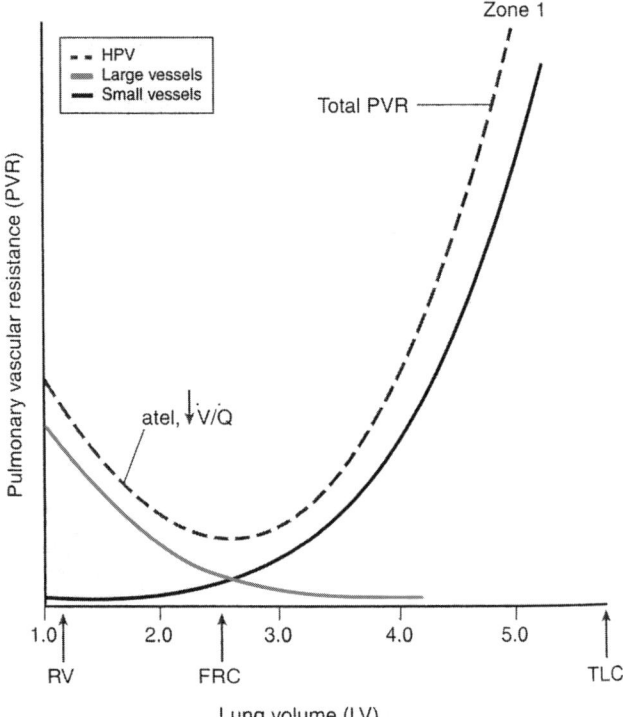

Figure 11 Total pulmonary vascular resistance relates to lung volume as an asymmetric U-shaped curve. The trough of the curve occurs when lung volume equals functional residual capacity. Total pulmonary resistance is the sum of the resistance in small vessels (increased by increasing lung volume) and the resistance in large vessels (increased by decreasing lung volume). The end point for increasing lung volume (toward total lung capacity) is the creation of zone 1 conditions, and the end point for decreasing lung volume (toward residual volume) is the creation of low ventilation-perfusion ($\dot{V}_A/\dot{Q}$) and atelectatic (atel) areas that demonstrate hypoxic pulmonary vasoconstriction.

beneficial means of diverting blood away from the poorly ventilated areas of the lung and would optimize $\dot{V}/\dot{Q}$ relationships. However, chronic or intermittent hypoxia leads to pulmonary hypertension (e.g., altitude), with its deleterious clinical effects. The mechanism of HPV is unclear. Mechanisms involving nitric oxide inhibition, prostacyclin (PGI_2) and endothelin have been proposed (14). Other proposed mechanisms suggest involvement of O_2-sensitive K^+ channels or adenosine triphosphate (ATP)-sensitive ion channels (15). Current consensus suggests that it is probably multifactorial in origin.

Metabolic and Humoral Control

Both respiratory and metabolic acidosis augment HPV, while respiratory or metabolic alkalosis cause pulmonary vasodilation and reduce or abolish HPV. Many humoral factors are involved in control of pulmonary vascular tone. Some of these are locally mediated (autocrine/paracrine) humoral factors (Table 1). Others circulate through the cardiovascular system and interact with the pulmonary vasculature. Circulating epinephrine tends to increase PVR, as does 5-hydroxytryptamine (5HT), which is released from activated platelets. This may be one of the reasons pulmonary hypertension can occur following pulmonary embolism.

Neural Control

Pulmonary vasculature is supplied by sympathetic, para-sympathetic and nonadrenergic, noncholinergic nerves (NANC). The sympathetic system plays little role at rest. However, it is activated via peripheral chemoreceptor in response to hypoxia. α1-adrenergic stimulation causes vasoconstriction, while β2-adrenergic stimulation and α2-adrenergic stimulation are involved in vasodilatation. As for cholinergic nerves, their activation via acetylcholine causes pulmonary vasodilatation via activation of endothelium and NO-dependent mechanisms. In the lung most NANC nerves are vasodilatory (and exert their effect) via NO or peptide pathways (14).

GAS EXCHANGE IN THE LUNG
Ventilation-Perfusion Relationship in the Lung

As mentioned before, for optimal exchange of gases to occur, ventilation and perfusion should be matched. For example, no gas exchange would occur if one lung was ventilated and the other lung is only perfused. One can consider the relationship between ventilation and perfusion in terms of

Table 1 Local Tissue (Autocrine/Paracrine) Molecules Involved in Active Control of Pulmonary Vascular Tone

Molecule	Subtype (abbreviation)	Site of origin	Site of action	Response
Nitric oxide	NO	Endothelium	Sm. muscle	Vasodilation
Endothelin	ET-1	Endothelium	Sm. muscle (ET-A receptor)	Vasoconstriction
	ET-1	Endothelium	Endothelium (ET-B receptor)	Vasodilation
Prostaglandin	PGI_2	Endothelium	Endothelium	Vasodilation
Prostaglandin	$PGF_2\alpha$	Endothelium	Sm. muscle	Vasoconstriction
Thromboxane	TXA_2	Endothelium	Sm. muscle	Vasoconstriction
Leukotriene	LTB_4–LTE_4	Endothelium	Sm. muscle	Vasoconstriction

Abbreviations: sm. muscle, pulmonary arteriole smooth muscle cell; ET-A receptor, endothelin–1 receptor located on the smooth muscle cell membrane; ET-B receptor, endothelin–1 receptor located on the endothelial cell membrane.
Source: From Ref. 90.

ventilation-perfusion ratio (V̇/Q̇). As each quantity is measured in liters/min, considering ventilation to be 4 L/min and perfusion 5 L/min, we get a ratio of 0.8. Thus, if ventilation/perfusion was uniform in all alveoli, each alveolus V̇/Q̇ ratio would be 0.8. However, V̇/Q̇ ratios are not uniformly distributed. Though ventilation and perfusion increase with decreasing height, in upright position, each does not change to the same extent. Blood flow per unit lung volume increases by 11% per centimeter descent through the lung, while ventilation decreases less dramatically (Fig. 10) (2). There are also more alveoli in the lower part of the lung. Thus, V̇/Q̇ ratios decrease down the lung.

As shown in (Fig. 12), in a young adult, ventilation and perfusion are mainly confined to alveoli with V̇/Q̇ ratio in the range of 0.5–2.0. However, in older individuals the V̇/Q̇ ratio widens significantly (ratio 0.3–5.0). Also, blood flows through the areas which are poorly ventilated (due to dependency and airway closure), V̇/Q̇ ratio can be in the range 0.01–0.03. Furthermore in disease states, the V̇/Q̇ ratios can alter significantly and give rise to hypoxemia (vide infra).

Shunt, Dead Space, and Effect of V̇/Q̇ Inequality on Overall Gas Exchange

Shunt and dead space are essentially two extremes of V̇/Q̇ mismatch. When there is no ventilation in the presence of perfusion (V̇/Q̇ ratio = 0), it is called shunt. Conversely, when there is no blood flow in fully ventilated alveoli (V̇/Q̇ = infinity), it is functionally $V_{Dalveolar}$. In the shunt region, alveolar pO_2 and PCO_2 would be the same as mixed venous blood (e.g., PO_2 = 42 mmHg), while in the dead space areas the alveolar gas partial pressure would be unchanged from the inspired gas. As described above in vivo, V̇/Q̇ ratios are unevenly distributed throughout the lung and so is the concentration of alveolar gas in different regions of the lung. The concentration of gases impacts the saturation of arterial blood. Thus, the final PO_2 is dependent on the combined value of concentration of O_2 from all the regions of the lung. To simplify, one can consider a

three-compartment model of gas exchange (Riley), where the final gaseous concentration is reflective of blood coming from the areas of shunt, dead space, and ideal alveolar gas exchange (Fig. 13) (16). Increasing shunt causes hypoxemia, as the proportion off blood not oxygenated is increased, while increasing dead space should cause an increase in CO_2. However, due to tightly controlled negative feedback and near linear CO_2/ventilatory curve, hyperventilation effectively blows off the excess CO_2. It is difficult to compensate for hypoxemia with hyperventilation, as increasing O_2 concentration in the alveoli, which are on the flat part of the O_2-dissociation curve, does little to increase the overall O_2 saturation and content. Areas of low V̇/Q̇ ratios contribute to hypoxemia by behaving functionally as areas of shunt. However, with supplemental O_2 it is possible to mitigate their effects, unlike in true significant shunt situation (>30%), it is difficult to improve hypoxemia with 100% FiO_2. Normal shunt is less than 5%, however, it can increase significantly in acute lung injury (ALI), adult respiratory distress syndrome (ARDS), atelectasis, lobar pneumonia, and lung collapse.

Diffusion of Gases: The Blood–Gas Barrier

All gases move across the alveolar wall by passive diffusion. Diffusion through the tissues follows Fick's law, which states that rate of transfer is (*i*) proportional to tissue area, (*ii*) the difference in partial pressure between two sides, (*iii*) the diffusion constant (which is dependent on the solubility and inversely proportional to the square root of the molecular weight of the gas) and (*iv*) inversely proportional to the thickness of the tissue. Lung with its large surface area (50–100 m^2) and minimal thickness 0.3 μm in many areas is ideally suited for diffusion (1,2).

☞ **Under typical resting conditions, the RBC PO_2 virtually reaches that of alveolar gas when it is about one-third of the way along the capillary.** ☞ Thus, under resting conditions the O_2 transfer is perfusion limited. However, when diffusion properties of the lung is impaired, the

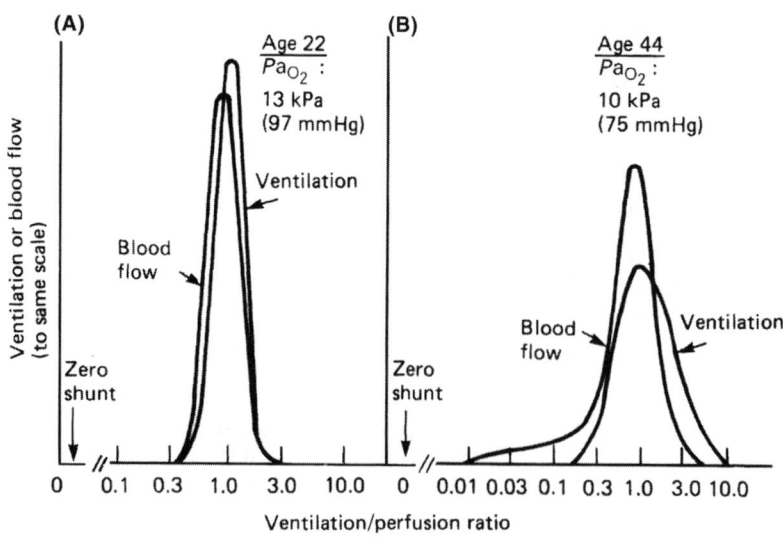

Figure 12   The distribution of ventilation and blood flow in relation to ventilation/perfusion ratios in two normal subjects. (**A**) A male aged 22 years with typical narrow spread and no measurable intrapulmonary shunt or alveolar dead space. This accords with high arterial PO_2 while breathing air. (**B**) The wider spread in a male aged 44 years. Note in particular the "shelf" of blood flow distributed to alveoli with V̇/Q̇ ratios in the range 0.01–0.3. There is still no measurable intrapulmonary shunt or alveolar dead space. However, the appreciable distribution of blood flow to underperfused alveoli is sufficient to reduce the arterial P_aO_2 to 10 kPa (75 mmHg) while breathing air. *Source*: From Ref. 1.

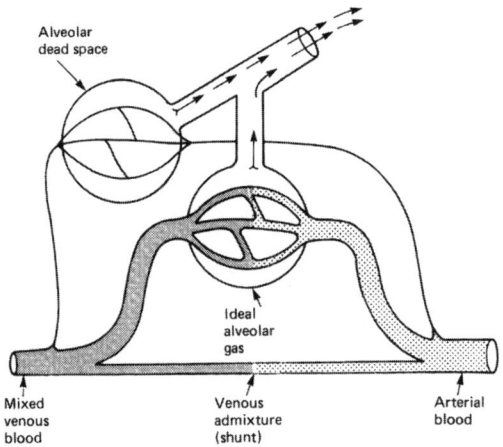

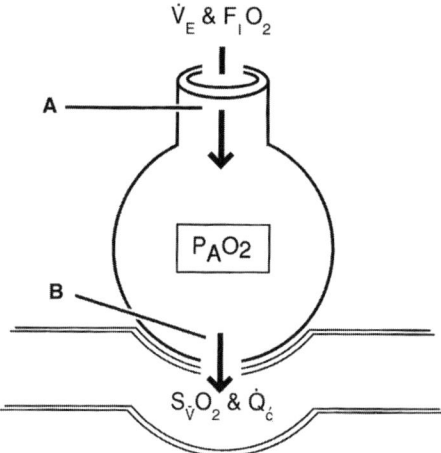

Figure 13 Three-compartment (Riley) model of gas exchange. The lung is imagined to consist of three functional units comprising alveolar dead space, "ideal" alveoli, and venous admixture (shunt). Gas exchange occurs only in the "ideal" alveoli. The measured alveolar dead space consists of true alveolar dead space together with a component caused by $\dot{V}/\dot{Q}$ scatter. The measured venous admixture consists of true venous admixture (shunt) together with a component caused by $\dot{V}/\dot{Q}$ scatter. Note that "ideal" alveolar gas is exhaled contaminated with alveolar dead space gas, so it is not possible to sample "ideal" alveolar gas. *Source*: From Ref. 1.

Figure 14 Alveolar oxygen tension (P_AO_2) is determined from the dynamic equilibrium established between the alveolar oxygen deliver (*arrow A*) and the alveolar oxygen extraction (*arrow B*). Alveolar oxygen delivery is a function of the minute ventilation ($\dot{V}_E$) and the inspired oxygen fraction (F_IO_2). Alveolar oxygen extraction is a function of the pulmonary arterial oxygenation status ($S\bar{V}O_2$) and the capillary blood from ($\dot{Q}c$). *Source*: From Ref. 19.

blood PO_2 does not reach the alveolar value by the end of the capillary, which suggests diffusion limitation.

It would be incorrect to assume that all resistance to movement of O_2 resides in the barrier between the blood and gas. Another factor that has to be taken into account is the combination of O_2 with Hb. Though the reaction is very fast (0.2 seconds), it is still an important rate-limiting step as oxygenation of pulmonary blood is extremely fast (17). Thus, actual diffusing capacity of the lung is made up of two components, that due to the diffusion process itself, and the other attributed to the time taken for O_2 to react with Hb. Though the capacity for gas exchange is referred to as diffusion capacity of the lung, some prefer to denote it as "transfer capacity," to emphasize that factors other than diffusion also play a part in effective transfer of gases. Since transfer of carbon monoxide is diffusion dependent, clinically, it has been used to measure diffusing capacity of the lung (DL_{CO}) (18). There are many factors that affect diffusing capacity. Some effect by changes in the area of the membrane, alteration in diffusion barrier itself, or factors related to uptake by hemoglobin. Other factors like gender, exercise, racial origin, and smoking also influence diffusion capacity (1).

Alveolar Gas Composition
Saturation of Hb with O_2 is dependent on PaO_2 as determined by O_2 dissociation curve. PaO_2 is dependent on alveolar partial pressure of O_2 (P_AO_2). The level of alveolar O_2 tension reflects a balance of two processes: (*i*) O_2 entry within the alveoli and (*ii*) O_2 removal from the alveoli by the capillary blood (Fig. 14) (19). O_2 entry within the alveoli is determined by the alveolar ventilation ($\dot{V}_A$) and the fraction of inspired O_2 (F_IO_2). But O_2 is also carried away in exhaled air. The air leaving alveoli has the alveolar O_2 concentration (F_AO_2). Thus, net O_2 entering the alveolus

is given by $V_A \times (F_IO_2 - F_AO_2)$. O_2 removal is governed by $\dot{V}O_2$. In steady-state situations, O_2 entering the alveolus and $\dot{V}O_2$ are equal. Writing the relationship as a conservation-of-mass equation, taking into account the barometric pressure and water vapor pressure and converting to partial pressure, one obtains the equation:

$$P_IO_2 - P_AO_2 = \dot{V}O_2/\dot{V}_A(PB - 47) \qquad (8)$$

However, CO_2 occupies space within the alveoli and is also a byproduct of $\dot{V}O_2$. The quantities of $\dot{V}O_2$ and $\dot{V}CO_2$ are linked. If the respiratory quotient (RQ) is equal, then the decrease in PO_2 from inspired to alveolar air is exactly the same as the increase in PCO_2 from zero to the alveolar level. Thus:

$$P_IO_2 - P_AO_2 = P_ACO_2 \qquad (9)$$

Rearranging

$$P_IO_2 - P_ACO_2 = P_AO_2 \qquad (10)$$

Since, P_ACO_2 is very similar to P_aCO_2, one can write:

$$P_IO_2 - P_aCO_2 = P_AO_2 \qquad (11)$$

However, in vivo, RQ < 1, $\dot{V}CO_2$ is less than $\dot{V}O_2$. A more complete form of alveolar gas equation that accounts for the change in gas volume is:

$$P_AO_2 = P_IO_2 - PaCO_2[F_IO_2 + (1 - F_IO_2/R)] \qquad (12)$$

For typical normal values (R = 0.8; $F_IO_2 = 0.21$; $P_IO_2 = 150$ mmHg; $PaCO_2 = 40$ mmHg), P_AO_2 turns out to be about 102 mmHg. In clinical situations, when interpreting blood gases it is useful to estimate P_AO_2 as alveolar-arterial PO_2 differences increase significantly in situations of increased shunt and $\dot{V}/\dot{Q}$ mismatch. Another way to denote abnormalities in gas exchange is to calculate ratio between arterial PO_2 and inspired O_2 (P_aO_2/F_IO_2).

GAS TRANSPORT BETWEEN LUNGS AND TISSUES
Oxygen Delivery Concepts

$\dot{D}O_2$, also known as O_2 transport, is the product of $\dot{Q}$ and O_2 Content. The respiratory and cardiovascular systems are series linked to carry out their important functions of $\dot{D}O_2$ to and CO_2 removal from the tissues. $\dot{D}O_2$ increases and decreases as the metabolic needs dictate over a wide range. Indeed there is a capacity for increasing the $\dot{D}O_2$ 30-fold from rest to heavy exercise. The functional links in the $\dot{D}O_2$ chain are as follows: (i) ventilation and ventilation with respect to perfusion; (ii) diffusion of O_2 across the alveolar epithelium, through the interstitial space, and across the capillary endothelium into the blood; (iii) chemical reaction of O_2 with Hb; (iv) $\dot{Q}$ of arterial blood; and (v) transport of blood to tissues and release of O_2 (Table 2). In healthy patients the system has abundant reserve and is seldom stressed, except with exercise. Accordingly, the first signs and symptoms of cardiopulmonary disease often present during exercise. The content of O_2 in the arterial blood is directly related to the concentration and saturation of hemoglobin, and a very small amount that is dissolved in plasma (as per Equation 13).

$$O_2 \text{ Content} = Hb \times 1.34 \times sat + 0.003 \times PO_2 \quad (13)$$

Determinants of O_2 Delivery

$\dot{D}O_2$ is dependent on two factors, namely, O_2 content and $\dot{Q}$. O_2 content is dependent on Hb concentration and its percentage saturation (SaO_2) with minimal addition from the dissolved amount of O_2 in the plasma, which is dependent on the PaO_2. Decreased O_2 delivery to the tissues will result if there is decrease in $\dot{Q}$ (stagnant hypoxia), decreased hemoglobin (anemic hypoxia), or decreased saturation of hemoglobin (anoxic hypoxia) or combination thereof. Finally, the tissues may not be able to utilize the O_2 delivered to it because malfunction of oxidative enzymes (cytotoxic hypoxia e.g., due to cyanide). Under physiological conditions the body compensates for the fall of one parameter with changes in the other. For example, a fall in hemoglobin is compensated by increase in $\dot{Q}$, or chronic hypoxia is compensated by increase in hemoglobin concentration (altitude). Decrease in PaO_2 ultimately

decreases SaO_2 which would decrease O_2 content and $\dot{D}O_2$ even if Hb concentration and $\dot{Q}$ are kept constant.

Structural Biology of Hemoglobin

Hemoglobin is the major protein of the RBC. It allows transport of O_2 from the lungs to the tissues and return CO_2 from the tissue to the lungs [20]. Hemoglobin is a protein tetramer consisting of 574 AA. Hb consists of a protein part, the globin, and a component that binds to oxygen, the heme group. Both components interact with each other in that the protein controls the O_2 binding properties of heme, which in turn reports the absence or presence of oxygen to its protein environment [21,22].

O_2 is a nonpolar molecule and therefore its solubility in the polar water phase of the extra- and intracellular space of the human body is very poor. The fact that the heme part is literally embedded in the globin part of Hb is biologically very important. Normally, ferrous iron, even if bound within the heme group, reacts with O_2 irreversibly to yield ferric heme. When embedded in the folds of the globin chain, ferrous heme is protected in such a way that its reaction with O_2 is reversible. This type of situation is unique and occurs because of the amino acid histidine, which donates a negative charge to the iron and helps create a loose bond with O_2 [22].

Hemoglobin consists of four polypeptide chains, two identical alpha subunits with 141 AAs and two identical beta subunits with 146 AAs. The surface of the Hb tetramer is studded with many polar residues that are all hydrated, which contributes to the high solubility of Hb. Erythrocytes are densely packed with Hb (5 mmol/L), each of which contains 300 million molecules of tetrametric Hb, and four times as many O_2 binding sites [21]. This increased solubility of Hb and potential to bind O_2 increases the capacity of blood to transport O_2 70 times more than if it was being transported only in the dissolved form.

O_2–Hemoglobin Disassociation Curve

The main function of Hb is the reciprocal transport of O_2 and CO_2 between tissue and lungs. The relationship between the fractional saturation of Hb with O_2 (SaO_2) and PaO_2 under equilibrium conditions is the familiar O_2 hemoglobin dissociation curve (oxy-heme curve) of Hb (Fig. 15). Its position is often represented by the value of P_{50}, the PO_2 at half saturation. ☞ **Increased O_2 affinity shifts the oxy-heme curve to the left (i.e., reduces P_{50}), while decreased O_2 affinity**

Table 2 Functional Capacities and Potential Maximum Oxygen (O_2) Transport of Each Link in the O_2 Transport Chain in Normal Humans[a] at Sea Level

Link in chain	Functional capacity in normal humans	Theoretic maximal O_2 transport capacity
Ventilation	200 L/min (MVV)	$0.030 \times MVV = 6.0$ L O_2/min
Diffusion and chemical reaction	$87 \dfrac{mLO_2/\ min}{mmHg\ O_2\ gradient}$	$DL_{O_2} = 6.1$ L O_2/min
$\dot{Q}$	20 L/min	
O_2 extraction (a-v O_2 difference)	75% (16 mL O_2/100 mL or 0.16)	$0.16 \times \dot{Q} = 3.2$ L O_2/min

[a]Hemoglobin = 15 g/dL; physiologic dead space in percentage of tidal volume = 0.25; partial alveolar pressure of oxygen >110 mmHg.
Abbreviations: $\dot{Q}$, cardiac output; MVV, maximum voluntary ventilation.
Source: From Ref. 91.

$$CO_2 + H_2O \overset{CA}{\rightleftharpoons} H_2CO_3 \rightleftharpoons H^+ + HCO_3^-$$

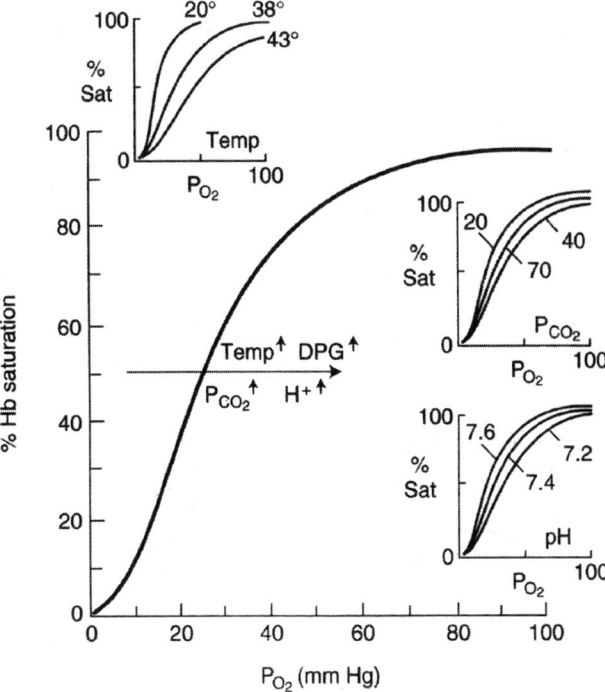

Figure 15 Rightward shift of the oxyhemoglobin dissociation curve is caused by increase of H^+ PCO_2, temperature, and 2,3 diphosphoglycerate. In addition to the normal oxyhemoglobin dissociation curve, the family of curves that result from changes in temperature (Temp), PCO_2, and pH are shown. *Source*: From Ref. 2.

shifts the oxy-heme curve to the right (i.e., increases P_{50}). ☞ Many different models have been proposed to explain the binding of O_2 to Hb. It has been difficult experimentally to prove one model or the other in its entirety (23,24). However, the two-state model proposed by Monod (24), which is based on the two confirmations for hemoglobin corresponding to deoxygenation and oxyhemoglobin, has been most successful. According to the two-state model the hemoglobin can exist in either R (relaxed, oxygenated) or T (tense, deoxygenated) conformation, each with its unique O_2 affinity. Deoxygenated (T state) has low O_2 affinity while the R state (oxygenated state) has O_2 affinity, which is about 100 to 150 times higher than that of T state (23). Of fundamental importance in this model is that the T state is physically constrained by salt and hydrogen bonds to a much greater degree than is the R state. With successive oxygenation of the heme groups, some of these bonds break, the stability of T structure decreases, accompanied by release of the constraints and increase in O_2 affinity. This transition accounts for the cooperativity with oxygenation and sigmoid shape of the oxy-heme curve. The equilibrium between the T state and R state is influenced by a number of other "effector molecules." These small molecules react with Hb at non-heme sites in such a way as to stabilize the T conformation. The overall reactivity of a mixture of R and T conformation depends on the R-T equilibrium.

Factors Affecting Oxy-Heme Curve

The three major effector molecules that alter the binding of O_2 to hemoglobin include: 2,3 diphyosphoglycerate (2-3 DPG), the hydrogen ions and CO_2. The oxy-heme curve is also very sensitive to temperature shifting rightward with increasing temperature (25). Other molecules that decrease O_2 affinity include Cl^- and ATP, but their physiological roles are minor. 2-3 DPG: 2-3 DPG is present in normal human RBCs and is a metabolic intermediate in the glycolytic pathway. Its concentration within the RBC is approximately 5 mmol/L, which is 1:1 ratio with Hb (26). It binds to deoxyhemoglobin much more tightly than to oxyhemoglobin. In the normal arterial O_2 oxygenation condition, the presence of 2-3 DPG helps in the transfer of O_2 to the tissue. However, in conditions of diminished O_2 availability (anemia, hypoxia), 2-3 DPG levels increase and oxy-heme curve is shifted to the right (Fig. 15). Bohr observed that when pH was lowered (or PCO_2 was raised) the O_2 affinity of the blood decreased. Though qualitatively the effects of pH and increased PCO_2 are similar, they are separate, and the effect of pH (now called the "Bohr effect") is much stronger than the CO_2 in lowering the O_2 affinity. H^+ shifts the R-T equilibrium towards T, stabilizing T conformation, thus decreasing O_2 affinity (27).

CO_2-Binding

CO_2 can bind to the alpha-amino groups of amino acids. This decreases their O_2 affinity. CO_2 binding is diminished in the presence of 2,3-DPG, as both 2-3 DPG and CO_2 compete for the B-chain amino-terminal amino groups (27).

Other RBC properties that affect DO_2 include: (*i*) the rates of binding of physiologic ligands (O_2, CO_2, H^+, 2,3 DPG); (*ii*) buffering capacity; (*iii*) the barrier of diffusion presented by the RBC membrane; (*iv*) the layer of unstirred plasma immediately surrounding it; and (*v*) hematocrit-dependent blood viscosity.

O_2, CO_2, and Hb interact in a very complex way in blood to regulate the position and shape of the oxy-heme curve. The flux of O_2 into the pulmonary capillary blood is proportional to the diffusing capacity of the lung, which is dependent on the membrane component of diffusing capacity and the reaction rate with Hb, and is also proportional to the difference in alveolar and capillary O_2 concentrations. The CO_2 affects the O_2 affinity in two ways: (*i*) as an allosteric effector of the Hb-O_2 reaction, and; (*ii*) by its effect on the intracellular pH. Thus there are a multitude of effects that determine the actual in vivo shape and position of the RBC oxy-heme curve. H^+, perhaps the strongest physical effector, is regulated by PCO_2 and by the buffering capacity of the Hb. Buffering by Hb is in turn determined by Hb concentration and by the degree of O_2 saturation. O_2 saturation is determined by the PO_2 and O_2 affinity of Hb. Thus, exact quantification of multiple effects in the determination of gas exchange by blood is extremely difficult (23).

Carbon Monoxide Effect on O_2 Transport

As early as the 17th century, carbon monoxide (CO) was recognized as a potentially life-threatening gas. The toxicity is due to the very high affinity of CO for oxygen carrier proteins Hb and myoblobin (28). CO is not only present in O_2-poor environments (caves, ruins), smoke, and automobile engine exhaust, but is also produced in minute amounts physiologically. It is produced through the catabolism of hemoglobin when protoporphyrin is degraded to biliverdin by the heme-oxygenases in the spleen, liver, and the brain.

Physiologically, CO is an activator of guanylcyclase and could be a transmitter like NO (29). In the heart and skeletal muscle it can be oxidized to CO_2. Normally, the blood CO concentration does not exceed 1% to 2% of the blood CO-carrying capacity and consequently it does not interfere with blood CO_2 transport. Its levels are increased in smokers (5%/pack), and symptoms of toxicity become evident at 15% to 20% (30).

Carbon monoxide disturbs $\dot{D}O_2$ in essentially three ways decreasing the functional amount of hemoglobin, altering the oxy-heme curve, and binding to myoglobin and the electron transport chain.

CO binds chemically like O_2 to the divalent iron atom of the heme in the Hb. However, the affinity of CO is 200 to 250 times greater than that for O_2. CO has an intrinsic affinity for "isolated heme rings," which is about 1500 times more than that of O_2 (31). However, the globin molecule imposes thermodynamic constraints on the bonding, which reduces the intrinsic affinity of the CO for the heme. Binding CO to the heme decreases the number of heme groups available to bind to the O_2, functionally decreasing the O_2 content for the same amount of Hb (CO anemia).

In addition to decreasing the amount of functional Hb available for O_2, CO increases the O_2 affinity for Hb (32,33). Increasing concentration of CO shifts the ODC curve to the left as the P_{50} for O_2 is decreased. Dissociation of O_2 from heme is decreased at the tissue level, which translates to decreased O_2 supply to the tissue. Furthermore, with increasing levels of CO, the O_2 content is also decreased. It has been shown that tissue oxygenation is hindered more by a decrease in functional Hb through CO anemia, than by a reduction of equal percentage of the Hb concentration (i.e., simple anemia). Furthermore, CO binds 20 times more avidly to myoglobins than O_2, while the affinity for cytochrome c is the same as for O_2 (28). The difference in affinity to different heme proteins is thought to be related either to the differences in the chemical structure of the protein part of the molecule or due to the effects of other molecules (H^+, CO_2, 2-3 DPG) that alter the O_2 affinity more than CO

affinity. Changes in oxidative phosphorylation have been shown, though quantitative measurements of the impact of CO binding to myoglobin and cytochrome c has been difficult.

Carbon Dioxide Transport

Although CO_2 has an aqueous solubility approximately 20 times that of O_2, it is still considered relatively insoluble in aqueous solution. ☞ **CO_2 is transported in the blood primarily in three different forms, namely: (*i*) physically dissolved in blood; (*ii*) bound to amino groups of proteins (e.g., hemoglobin), as carbamate compounds; and (*iii*) as bicarbonate ions.** ☞ The relative contribution of each of these forms to overall transport is dependent on PCO_2, hydrogen ion concentration, 2,3-DPG concentration and degree of saturation of Hb (34). The relative contributions of each form of CO_2 to resting gas exchange are listed in Table 3 (35).

Pathways of CO_2 Transport

CO_2 in solution: CO_2 dissolved in physical solution accounts for only 5% of the CO_2 content of arterial or venous blood, which is not sufficient to transport CO_2 generated by tissue metabolism. However, it plays an important role in CO_2 transport and exchange, as access to bicarbonate and carbamate pools is achieved only through dissolved CO_2. Molecular CO_2 is lipid soluble and can cross cell membranes instantaneously. CO_2 diffuses across the normal pulmonary membrane with the same speed as inert gases. However, the time required for completion of CO_2 exchange in the lung capillary is dependent on rate of conversion of HCO_3 and carbamate to CO_2.

Bicarbonate Pathway: Hydration of CO_2 produces carbonic acid (H_2CO_3), which is almost completely ionized to H^+ and HCO_3 ions. Bicarbonate ions can further dissociate into H^+ and carbonate ions, but in vivo little carbonate is formed because the pH of this reaction is >10.0. The hydration of CO_2 to H_2CO_3 occurs naturally and is a very slow process. Similarly, the reverse reaction, dissociation of H_2CO_3 to CO_2 and water, is also a slow process. Both reactions require a catalytic enzyme, carbonic anhydrase, which is present in the cells and virtually absent from the plasma. RBCs contain the highest concentration of carbon anhydrase while lower levels of the isoenzyme have been noted in capillary endothelium of the lung (36).

Carbamate Compounds: CO_2 and hydrogen ions reversibly bind to unchanged amino groups of proteins and form carbamic acid. The formation of carbamate compounds is markedly pH-dependent and increases with decreasing acidity. The concentration of carbamates in plasma is approximately 0.6 mM, and plasma carbamates have no appreciable role in the CO_2 exchange. However, carbamates formation by beta-amino groups of Hb is an important factor in CO_2 exchange. Release of O_2 by Hb in the tissues is accompanied by increased binding of CO_2 to beta-amino groups. Conversely, oxygenation of Hb in the lung promotes release of CO_2 bound as carbamate. Earlier studies suggested that this behavior accounted for 27% of all CO_2 excreted in the lungs. However, recent studies taking into account the role of 2,3–DPG suggest that oxylabile carbamate account for only 10% of the total CO_2 exchange (37).

CO_2 Dissociation Curve

CO_2 dissociation curve is linear when plotted on a logarithmic axis. The slope of this relationship is essentially constant and is profoundly affected by concentration of Hb in the blood.

Table 3 Contributions to CO_2 Transport and Exchange from Different Pathways

	Arterial content		Arteriovenous difference	
	(mL/dL blood)	(% of Total)	(mL/dL blood)	(% of Total)
Plasma				
Dissolved CO_2	1.51	3.1	0.20	4.7
Bicarbonate	30.01	62.1	2.07	48.7
Carbamate	0.67	1.4	0.00	0.00
CO_2 content	32.19	66.6	2.27	53.4
Erythrocyte				
Dissolved CO_2	0.93	1.9	0.16	3.8
Bicarbonate	12.58	26.0	1.29	30.3
Carbamate	2.67	5.5	0.53	12.5
CO_2 content	16.18	33.4	1.98	46.6

Note: Concentrations are expressed in mL/dL of blood. Arterial pH and PCO_2 are 7.40 and 40.0 mmHg, respectively. Corresponding venous values are 7.37 and 46.0 mmHg.
Source: From Ref. 35.

Hemoglobin is the major nonbicarbonate buffer in the blood and is essential to buffer the protons released during ionization of carbonic acid. Although the total quantity of CO_2 contained in all forms in the plasma is twice as great as in the RBCs (table 3), plasma proteins have only one-eighth the buffering power of intracellular hemoglobin (35). Furthermore, Hb serves as a source of protons for the reversal of reactions which converts bicarbonate and carbamate into CO_2, when it reaches the lung. RBCs play a key role in enhancing blood's ability to carry CO_2. It is because of three characteristics of RBCs: (*i*) large internal buffering capacity of RBC; (*ii*) presence of intracellular carbonic anhydrase; and (*iii*) ability to exchange bicarbonate across the RBC membrane (38).

One other factor that significantly affects the CO_2 dissociation curve is oxygenation. The Haldane Effect describes the influence of oxygenation on the CO_2 dissociation curve. It accounts for one-half of CO_2 excretion at rest (39).

REGULATION OF BREATHING

Breathing is a complex process. It is governed by a multitude of control systems hierarchically arranged to regulate ventilation and the pattern of breathing so as to meet optimally the prevailing metabolic needs. Furthermore, the control system also allows the pattern of breathing to automatically adapt to other activities like changes in posture, speech, voluntary movement, and exercise. This section begins by describing the origin of respiratory rhythm and basic organization of the efferent pathways that bring about respiration (neural control of breathing). This basic respiratory rhythm is then modulated by inputs from the cortex, pons, hypothalamus and peripheral inputs from airways and lungs (nonchemical influences on respiration). The metabolic needs of the body are gauged by changes in the pCO_2, pH, and pO_2 and described as the chemical control of breathing (Fig. 16).

Neural Control of Breathing

The medulla is the major respiratory center where the respiratory pattern is initiated and various voluntary and involuntary demands on respiratory activity are coordinated. **Autonomous respiratory pattern is generated in the medulla by synchronized activity of six distinct neuronal groups (central pattern generator, CPG).** CPG is governed by a combination of excitatory and inhibitory neurotransmitters. These neurotransmitters subsequently modulate potassium and calcium channels, which lead to depolarization and/or hyperpolarization of neurons. The excitatory neurotransmitters include amino acids like glutamate, which can activate fast-activating ion channels like N-methyl D-aspartate (NMDA) receptors or nonNMDA receptors, which are slow reacting receptors and mediate their effects via G-proteins. Inhibitory neurotransmitters include γ-amino butayric acid (GABA) and glycine, which act through $GABA_A$ receptors and specific glycine receptors, respectively (40). Furthermore, the CPG is affected by neuro-modulators which modify the CPG output, but are not primarily involved in rhythm generation. These include agents like opioids, acetylcholine, and substance P, to name a few (Fig. 17). Furthermore, there are other neurons in the medulla involved in respiratory control. These are divided into two groups, namely, (*i*) dorsal respiratory neurons and (*ii*) the ventral respiratory neurons. They have numerous interconnections. The dorsal respiratory group neurons are primarily concerned with the timing of the respiratory cycle. While the ventral respiratory group of neurons is composed of four nuclei, each is involved with a specific aspect of ventilatory control, for example, function of pharyngeal muscles, larynx and tongue, force of contraction of inspiratory muscles, expiratory muscles (41).

The output from the CPG converges on the motor anterior horn cells, which control the inspiratory and

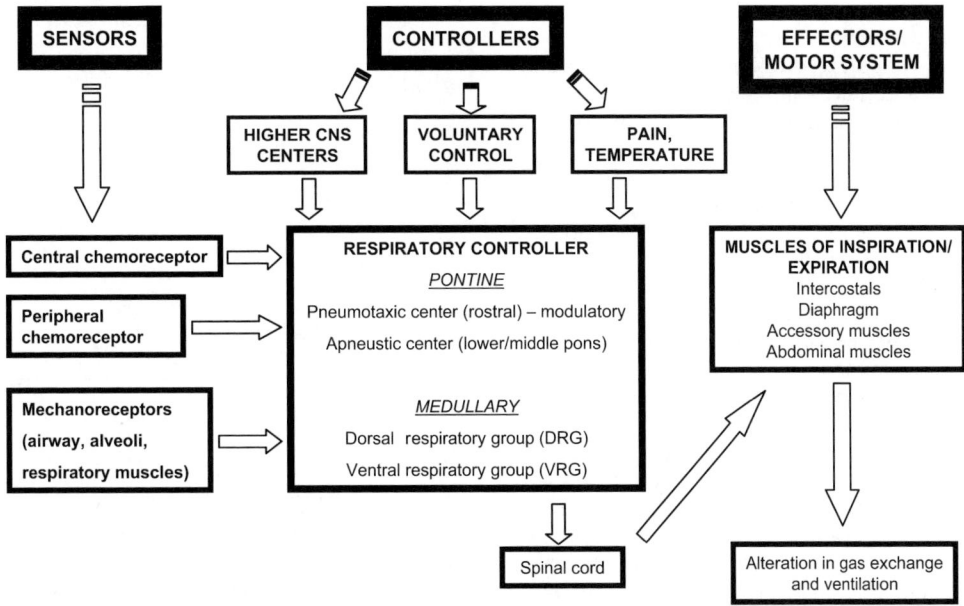

Figure 16 Regulation of breathing is accomplished by a complex interactive system of sensors, controllers, and effector systems. Although there is voluntary override of the breathing system at rest, involuntary systems regulate most breathing and become more dominant when extreme conditions of exercise or disease are present.

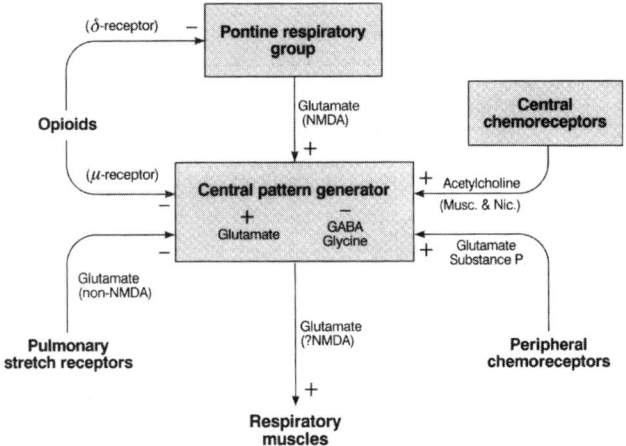

Figure 17 Neurotransmitters and neuromodulators in the respiratory center. Boxes indicate functional neuronal groups and bold type represents other influences on the respiratory center. Substances involved in neurotransmission are shown with the most likely receptor subtype, in parentheses, if known. +indicates excitatory effect increasing respiratory activity; −indicates inhibitory activity decreasing respiration. *Source*: From Ref. 1.

expiratory muscles. The synchronized firing of CPG neurons leads to activation of specific respiratory muscle groups. Alterations in the rate at which spontaneous neuronal activity increases or decreases and the point at which the next group of neurons are activated, allows for infinite variations in respiratory patterns and adjustment to constantly changing needs (1,41).

Two other sources also converge on respiratory motor neurons. These include direct input from the cortex and non-respiratory reflexes (swallowing, cough, hiccups etc.). These integrated inputs are responsible for voluntary control of breathing and execution of a multitude of involuntary reflexes (Fig. 16) (42).

Chemical Control of Breathing
The effect of O_2 and CO_2 on respiration was first described by Pfluger in 1868 and later classified by Haldane and Priestly in 1905 (43). Changes in pCO_2 and pO_2 are sensed by central and peripheral chemoreceptors, respectively, which subsequently trigger an appropriate ventilatory response. Influence of CO_2 and O_2 on respiratory control is described followed by discussion of a combined responses of these gases to control of breathing.

Effect of CO$_2$ on Ventilatory Response (1)
Alveolar ventilation is extremely sensitive to changes in pCO_2. Changes in pCO_2 are sensed by "central chemoreceptors," which are located in the medulla. They are separate from the respiratory neurons but are very close to the respiratory center. MRI and positron emission tomography (PET) scanning techniques during CO_2-stimulated breathing have confirmed that the surface of the anterior medulla is the primary site of chemosensitive neuronal activity (44). Though other areas of the brain (other regions in the medulla, midline pons, small areas in cerebellum, and limbic system) are also stimulated, their contribution in control of respiration is unclear (45,46). About 85% of the total respiratory response to inhaled CO_2 originates in the medullary chemoreceptors.

A rise in arterial pCO_2 causes an approximate equal rise in cerebrospinal fluid (CSF) pCO_2, which is about 10 mmHg more than the arterial pCO_2. Blood-brain-barrier (BBB) is permeable to CO_2. In the short term, increased CO_2 permeates through the BBB; it gets hydrolysed to carbonic acid, which dissociates to yield hydrogen ions. This leads to a fall in the CSF pH, which stimulates to respiratory neurons indirectly through the stimulation of receptors in the chemosensitive area. The precise mechanism by which a change in pH causes stimulation of neurons in the chemosensitive area is not established. However, there is some evidence to suggest that M_2 muscarinic receptors may be involved (47). Also, the response to respiratory acidosis is more than for metabolic acidosis, for the same change in pH. If the pCO_2 in CSF is increased, the pH returns to normal over the course of many hours, as a result of changes in the CSF bicarbonate levels. Compensatory changes in CSF bicarbonate and restoration of its pH are evident not only in chronic respiratory acidosis, but also occur in respiratory alkalosis, chronic metabolic acidosis and alkalosis (48). Direct changes in the bicarbonate concentration of CSF also lead to changes in ventilation. For example, after intracranial hemorrhage CSF pH and bicarbonate levels fall, which causes hyperventilation (49).

Respiratory depth and rate increase with rise in pCO_2 until a steady state of hyperventilation is achieved after a few minutes. Within acceptable experimental conditions the ventilatory response to CO_2 is linear. Under normal conditions ($pO_2 = 90$ mmHg) the slope of the curve is 2 L/min/mmHg while the intercept (apneic threshold) is at 36 mmHg. As depicted in Figure 18, the slope of the curve changes with changes in arterial pO_2. Furthermore, the apneic threshold will be altered in the presence of acid-base changes. It should be kept in mind that the pCO_2/ventilation response curve is the response of the entire respiratory system to the challenge of altered

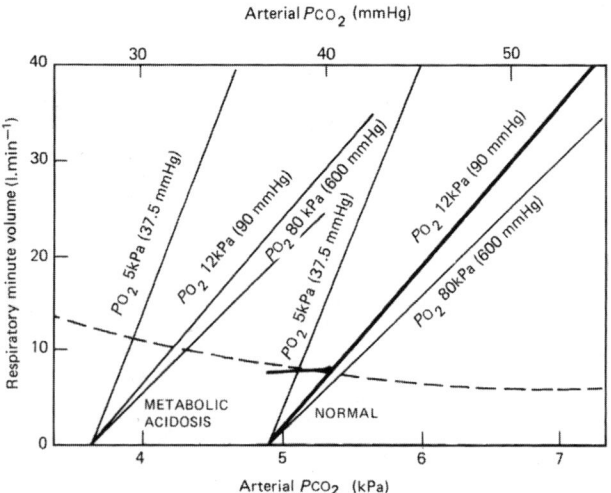

Figure 18 Two fan-shaped families of curves of PCO_2/ventilation response curves at different values of PO_2. The right-hand fan is at normal metabolic acid-base state (zero base excess). The left-hand fan represents metabolic acidosis. The broken line represents the PCO_2 produced by the indicated ventilation for zero inspired PCO_2, at basal metabolic rate. The intersection of the broken curve and any response curve indicates the resting PCO_2 and ventilation for the relevant metabolic acid-base state PO_2. The heavy curve is the normal response. *Source*: From Ref. 1.

pCO_2. The CO_2 response curve will be altered by changes in the sensitivity of the central chemoreceptors, partial neuromuscular blockade, anesthetic drugs, opioids, obstructive, and restrictive lung disease. Inhalational anesthetics decrease the sensitivity to CO_2 responsiveness by altering the slope of the pCO_2/ventilatory response curve and displace the curve to the right (50). The initial respiratory response to elevated pCO_2 is extremely rapid and takes place in just a few minutes. With sustained hypercapnia the minute ventilation continues to increase for an hour before reaching a plateau and can be sustained for eight hours (51). As pCO_2 is raised to pCO_2 (100–200 mmHg), a point of maximal ventilatory response is reached beyond which respiratory fatigue and CO_2 narcosis intervenes.

Influence of O_2 on Respiratory Control
☞ The central chemoreceptors play an important role in monitoring pCO_2, while the peripheral chemoreceptors which reside in the carotid body respond predominantly to changes in pO_2. ☞ The peripheral chemoreceptor also responds to a rise in pCO_2, H^+ ion concentration, temperature, fall in perfusion pressure, and chemicals (52). The response to changes is rapid (within one to three seconds), is processed by glomus cells and relayed by afferent fibers in the glossopharyngeal nerves. Type I glomus cells are predominantly involved in sensing of hypoxemia. Hypoxemia of glomus cells leads to decrease in ATP and release of calcium from the mitochondria. Furthermore, oxygen-sensitive K^+ channels and heme-based intracellular proteins also respond to changes in local pO_2 (53). Neurotransmitters that have been described in the carotid bodies include dopamine, noradrenaline, acetylcholine, substance P, and enkephalins. Dopamine (acting via D_2 receptors) and clonidine (α_2 receptor antagonist) reduce ventilatory response to acute hypoxia. However, no single receptor blocker prevents the hypoxic ventilatory response completely.

Peripheral chemoreceptors respond to decrease in pO_2 and not to decrease in O_2 content (1). There is minimal stimulation in anemia, carboxyhemoglobinemia, and methhemoglobinemia. Acidemia, either secondary to metabolic or respiratory acidosis causes stimulation, which can lead to hyperventilation. Quantitatively, the response of peripheral chemoreceptors to increase in pCO_2 is one-sixth that of central chemoreceptors. However, the response is very rapid. Oscillations in pCO_2 within the respiratory cycle are detected by peripheral chemoreceptors and discharge rates are altered accordingly. Hypoperfusion of carotid bodies (systolic BP <60 mmHg) and increase in temperature causes stimulation and leads to hyperventilation. Nicotine, acetylcholine, doxapram, and almitrine stimulate ventilation directly, while cyanide and carbon monoxide increase ventilation by inhibiting the cytochrome system, which prevents oxidative metabolism. Hypoxia also has a direct effect on the respiratory center. Central respiratory neurons are depressed by hypoxia, and apnea follows severe medullary hypoxia whether due to ischemia or to hypoxemia. Phrenic motor nerve activity becomes silent when medullary pO_2 falls to about 13 mmHg. More intense hypoxia can cause resumption of the abnormal pattern of breathing possibly by activation of the gasping center.

Integrated Effects of pCO_2, pH, and pO_2 on Respiratory Control
Though the effects of pCO_2, pH, and pO_2 on the respiratory control have been described independently, they are integrated in vivo. The acute hypoxic response is enhanced at elevated pCO_2, while the responses to both acute and prolonged hypoxia are depressed by hypocapnia. When pCO_2 is not controlled during hypoxic ventilation, hypoxia-induced hyperventilation immediately gives rise to hypocapnia and attenuates the ventilatory response to hypoxia. Similarly, changes in PO_2 alter the slope of the ventilatory response curve, while metabolic acidosis pushes the curve to the left and makes ventilatory response more sensitive to changes in pCO_2 (Fig. 18) (1,54).

Nonchemical Pulmonary Reflexes
In addition to neural and chemical control of breathing, ventilation is significantly modulated and affected by pulmonary reflexes. These reflexes can result in a myriad of responses, from apnea, to alterations in airway caliber, to hemodynamic effects.

HEART–LUNG INTERACTIONS

Because the heart and great vessels lie within the thorax, the respiratory system is the milieu within which the heart must function. Q is determined by the heart rate (HR) and stroke volume. Stroke volume is in turn dependent on preload, afterload, and contractility. Conceivably, effect on any one or more of these components would change Q. The major mechanical interactions of respiration and circulation are produced by changes in pleural and alveolar pressure (55). Changes in these pressures affect the circulation by producing changes in preload and afterload of the right and left ventricle (55). The magnitude of both preload and afterload is determined by a complex interaction of the heart and blood vessels. Discussion of all these changes is beyond the scope of this chapter, and the reader is referred to other references for full discussion (55). It is important to understand that it is the static recoil pressure of the systemic or pulmonary circulation relative to the right or left atrial pressure that provides the driving pressure that returns the blood to the heart (the resistance to venous return) and not the conventional vascular resistance (56). The magnitude of this static recoil is determined by blood volume and the elastic properties of the blood vessels. Increase in blood volume increases static recoil and thus increases preload.

Effect of Pleural Pressure on Preload and Afterload
Because the right heart is surrounded by pleural pressure and the systemic vessels are not, a decrease in pleural pressure (e.g., during inspiration) reduces the right atrial pressure relative to the static recoil pressure of the systemic circulation, thus increasing venous return. The overall effect on preload is modified by systemic vascular compliance, accompanying changes in abdominal pressure, and the collapse of the extrathoracic venae cava.

Increase in pleural pressure (e.g., positive pressure ventilation) results in increased intrathoracic pressure and pressure around a portion of the heart and circulation. It is thought that this decreases the overall transmural pressure (intraluminal—intrathoracic pressure) across the wall of the ventricle. The transmural LV pressure is the measure of afterload. Intraluminal pressure approximates aortic pressure (as long as there is no obstruction to aortic outflow and no significant variation in intrathoracic pressure) and provides a good estimate of the afterload. However, if intrathoracic pressure fluctuates considerably

(+20 to −60 mmHg), transmural LV pressure and afterload can alter significantly. Hemodynamic benefits of positive pressure ventilation in patients with severe heart failure are attributable to decrease in preload and afterload with mechanical ventilation.

Effect of Alveolar Pressure on Preload and Afterload

When lung volume is constant, any change in pleural pressure is accompanied by an approximately equal change in alveolar pressure. However, with any change in lung volume there is a change in alveolar pressure, relative to pleural pressure as determined by the static recoil of the lung. The effect of changes in alveolar pressure to preload and afterload becomes more complicated with varying effects on right and left cardiac chambers. The effect of an increase in alveolar pressure relative to pleural pressure is also different in zone II versus zone III states. With increasing alveolar pressure in zone II, there is a steady-state increase in right ventricular afterload (due to increase in back pressure from ejection) and transient decrease in LV preload. This can be seen in an asthmatic attack where large increase in lung volume gives rise to marked increase in right ventricular afterload (57). In zone III, there is a transient increase in RV afterload, but also in LV preload, which causes no significant steady-state changes.

Effect of Positive End Expiratory Pressure on Cardiac Function

Positive end expiratory pressure causes significant effect on the cardiac function (58). These include: (*i*) reduced venous return, secondary to increased pleural presure; (*ii*) increased right ventricular load, secondary to increased lung vascular resistance; (*iii*) decreased LV load secondary to rise in pleural pressure; and (*iv*) reflex changes in heart rate, systemic vascular resistance and perhaps cardiac contractility, caused by inflation reflexes and secondarily by changes in vascular pressures.

Reflex Effects of Lung Inflation on Hemodynamics

Cardiovascular effects of changes in pleural and alveolar pressure have been described earlier. However, there are also direct reflex cardiovascular effects secondary to lung inflation. The lungs are significantly innervated by the vagus nerve (59). Cardiovascular response to low level of lung inflation (<10 mmH$_2$O) and higher level of lung inflation is different. Low level of inflation decreases systemic vascular resistance (SVR) and has variable effect on HR (60). Static inflation of the lungs to distending pressures of 15 mmH$_2$O depresses cardiovascular function. The reflex effect includes decrease in HR, arterial pressure, Q̇, cardiac contractility, systemic vascular resistance. The afferent limb of the reflex arc is the ipsilateral vagus nerve (61). These reflexes play a role in normal physiology (sinus arrhythmia) and possibly during pathological conditions and mechanical ventilation of the lungs.

RESPIRATORY PHYSIOLOGY AT EXTREMES OF AGE AND PREGNANCY

With the first few breaths changes occur in the cardiopulmonary system, which allow the fetus adapt to the extrauterine environment. Significant anatomical and functional differences in the respiratory system are notable in the neonates compared to adults. Furthermore, respiratory function continues to change with advancing age and alterations in the respiratory system are also evident during pregnancy. Salient changes in the respiratory system in neonates, the elderly, and during pregnancy are discussed.

Respiratory Changes in the Elderly
Structural Alterations in the Upper and Lower Airways

With advancing age, structural changes occur both in upper and lower airways. There is loss of pharyngeal support. In addition, the protective airway reflexes of coughing and swallowing are depressed. Mean pulmonary artery pressure increases by 30%, and the pulmonary vascular resistance increases by 80% between age 20 and 70 years (62). Part of the pulmonary vascular changes results from a decline in the volume of the pulmonary capillary bed. Additionally, there is a progressive age-related decrease in surface area of at least 30% occurring from age 20 to the age of 70 years (63). Dilatation of the respiratory bronchioles and alveolar ducts (ductectasia) leads to increase in anatomical dead space. Molecular changes in protein structure leads to increased proteolysis of elastin, which leads to decreased elastic recoil. Though the absolute elastin content is not altered, the ratio of collagen to elastin is. There is increased interstitial collagen, which probably contributes to increased O$_2$ diffusing capacity (4).

Changes in Respiratory Mechanics and Lung Volume

The elastic properties of the lung and thoracic wall gradually change by aging. The chest wall becomes stiffer due to calcification of ribs and vertebral joints, while the lung parenchyma loses elastic recoil. The volume-pressure curve of the aged total system (lung + thorax) is flatter and shows less compliance. Loss of elastic recoil leads to increased overall tension, which can contribute to an increased pulmonary vascular resistance.

With aging, tidal volume decreases and respiratory frequency increases slightly; abdominal contribution to tidal breathing increases. The total lung capacity (TLC) does not change considerably, when corrected for age-related decreases in height. However, changes in chest wall and lung lead to barrel-like appearance of chest and flattened diaphragm.

FEV$_1$ (forced expiratory volume in one second) decreases annually by 30 mL. Closing capacity (CC), the volume at which the elastic recoil of the lungs becomes insufficient to support small bronchioles (<1 mm), reaches FRC in the erect 60 year old. In supine position, FRC equals CC at age of 44 years (Fig. 19) (64). Vital capacity is significantly decreased, however, FRC does not change.

The diaphragmatic efficiency in the elderly is also impaired by a significant loss of muscle mass. Though the reduction in diaphragmatic strength is small (10–20%), maximum pressures generated by full inhalation and expiration are significantly decreased. FEV$_1$/FVC ratio may be as low as 65% to 55% in apparently healthy individuals. The work of breathing may be elevated by 30% during exercise.

Impaired Efficiency of Gas Exchange

Arterial oxygenation is progressively impeded with increasing age (65); whereas V̇CO$_2$ is less affected by aging in the absence of disease. Oxygen tension decreases progressively with aging (approximately 5 mmHg per decade from the age of 20 years), with significant drop between ages 40 and 75 years. Thereafter, arterial O$_2$ tension remains stable at about 83 mmHg. The drop in O$_2$ tension is primarily

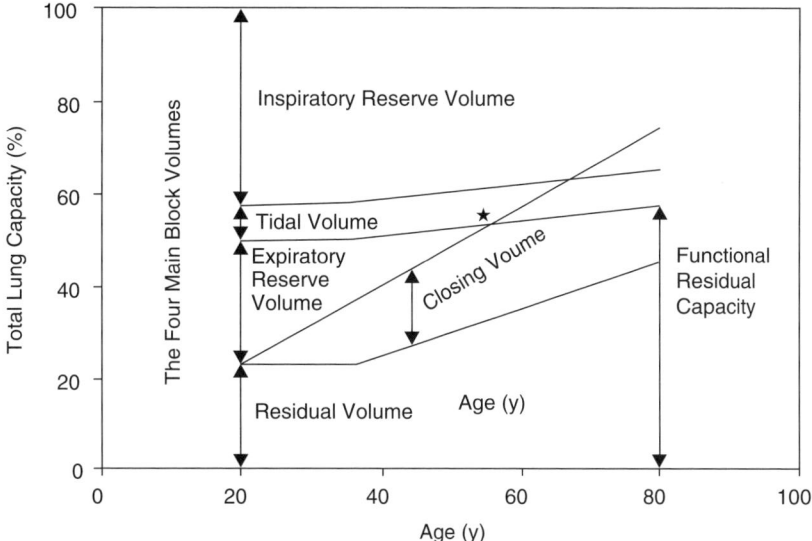

Figure 19 Changes in lung volumes with aging (*erect position*). Residual volume (RV) (5–10% per decade) and functional residual capacity (FRC = ERV + RV) (1–3% per decade) gradually increase by aging, while expiratory and inspiratory reserve volumes (ERV, IRV) and thus vital capacity (VC = ERV + IRV) decrease. Specific (height-adapted) total lung capacity does not change with aging. *Source*: From Ref. 4.

due to alterations in $\dot{V}/\dot{Q}$ mismatch (Fig. 12) (66). Loss of hypoxic pulmonary vasoconstriction and hypocapnic bronchoconstriction prevents fine-tuning of ventilation/perfusion balance. Cumulatively, $\dot{V}/\dot{Q}$ mismatch and loss of functional alveolar surface significantly decreases the diffusing capacity (0.24 mLO$_2$/mmHg/yr in men and 0.16 mLO$_2$/mmHg/yr in women) (67).

Alterations in Ventilatory Drive
Respiratory response to hypoxemia and hypercapnia is roughly decreased by 50% in the 70-year old healthy individual (68). This is due to reduced central nervous system (CNS) activity, and reduced neuronal output to respiratory muscles. In the elderly, the response to hypoxemia during rapid eye movement (REM) sleep is profoundly impaired.

Clinical Implications
☞ **Age-related loss of pharyngeal muscle support leads to an increased propensity for upper airway obstruction. Furthermore, loss of dentition make establishment of patent airway by bag and mask more difficult.** ☞ Loss of protective reflexes makes the elderly more prone to aspiration. Four vital capacity breaths prior to induction of anesthesia may not be sufficient to provide adequate preoxygenation as vital capacity is significantly decreased in the elderly (69). Impaired gas exchange makes them more prone to hypoxemia. Furthermore, in the elderly, response to chemical (hypoxia, hypercapnia) and mechanical stress (increased airway resistance) is significantly reduced in the presence of small amounts of opioids, benzodiazepines, and inhalational anesthetic agents.

Respiratory Changes in the Neonate
Structural Alterations in the Upper and Lower Airways
Neonates are obligate nasal breathers and have a small pharynx and a large tongue (70). The larynx is located anteriorly and slightly higher in the neck. The epiglottis is

mobile. The cricoid cartilage is the narrowest portion of the trachea. At full term all major elements of the lungs are fully formed, but, the number of alveoli present is only about 15% of the lung (71). Division of saccules into alveoli continues following birth and is believed to be complete by two years of age (1,71).

Changes in Respiratory Mechanics and Lung Volume
The chest wall of the neonate is highly compliant compared to the adult (where compliance of chest wall and the lung is nearly equal) (1,71,72). Most of the impedance to expansion is due to the lung and is dependent on the presence of surfactant in the alveoli. Though a small amount of surfactant is present at 24 weeks, significant synthesis of surfactant does not begin until 34 to 36 weeks. Compliance is about one-twentieth that of an adult and resistance is about 15 times greater (1). As in the elderly, the diaphragm is not as dome shaped as in adults. The lower portion of the rib cage has large anteroposterior and lateral diameters. As a result, the diaphragmatic insertions are spread out, limiting range of lengths of the diaphragmatic fibers.

Minute ventilation of a neonate is about twice that of an adult. This is due to significant respiratory rate 25–40/min, while the tidal volume, corrected for weight is not significantly different. Vital capacity is half of an adult when corrected for weight, while the functional residual capacity is not significantly different. Dead space is close to half that of tidal volume and shunt is about 10% immediately after birth.

Impaired Efficiency of Gas Exchange
The single most important difference in respiratory parameters that distinguishes pediatric patients from the adult is $\dot{V}O_2$. In the neonate, the $\dot{V}O_2$ is >6 mL/kg/min, which is about twice that of the adult. Increased demand is maintained by increased alveolar ventilation (vide supra). Because of increased shunt, the alveolar/arterial difference

is about 25 mmHg, which is about twice that in adults. PCO_2 is slightly decreased to 30–36 mmHg.

Alterations in Ventilatory Drive
Adult hypoxic ventilatory responses are not fully developed in the neonates (73). In normal babies under two months of age, there may be an excess of 200 apneic episodes and 50 minutes of periodic breathing per day, with short-lived desaturations (74). Though the ventilatory response to CO_2 seems to be similar to adults, the response is depressed in REM sleep (75).

Clinical Implications
Presence of large head, large tongue, floppy epiglottis, and anterior larynx requires slightly different maneuvering to achieve tracheal intubation (70). The size of the endotracheal tube (ET) tube also needs to be gauged to the cricoid cartilage rather than to laryngeal opening to avoid trauma to the trachea. High $\dot{V}O_2$, along with a relatively low total volume of FRC, predisposes neonates to develop hypoxia quickly, after apnea. Though cardiovascular responses to hypoxia (bradycardia, vasoconstriction) are well developed in the neonates, compensatory responses to hypoxia/hypercarbia are not fully developed (73). Thus neonatal hypoventilation is very likely after administration of respiratory depressant drugs and anesthesia.

Respiratory Changes During Pregnancy
Structural Alterations in the Upper and Lower Airways
Several physiological changes occur during pregnancy that affect respiratory function (76,77). Fluid retention causes edema throughout airway mucosa. This causes difficult nasal breathing. Furthermore, edema of the upper airway increases the propensity of bleeding even with minimal trauma and makes airway management more difficult.

Changes in Respiratory Mechanics and Lung Volume
Lung volume does not change until about the fifth month of gestation. The diaphragm becomes displaced cephalad by the expansion of the uterus in the abdomen (78). This leads to decrease in residual volume and expiratory reserve volume by 20%. FRC also decreases significantly. However, vital capacity, FEV_1, and maximal breathing capacity are normally unchanged.

Increase in $\dot{V}_E$ is one of the earliest and most dramatic changes in pulmonary function. The $\dot{V}_E$ is increased about 50% above nonpregnant levels during the first trimester and is maintained for the remainder of the pregnancy. It is thought to be centrally mediated due to increased levels of progesterone which can rise sixfold during pregnancy. Increase in $\dot{V}_E$ is due to increase in tidal volume with slight increase in respiratory rate. Airway resistance decreases by 35%.

Impaired Efficiency of Gas Exchange
Increase in blood volume contributes significantly to increase in O_2 delivery. Though total O_2 consumption is increased by 15% to 30% it is attributed to increased demands of the fetus, uterus, and placenta and not significantly different when expressed per kilogram of body weight. **Due to the increase in alveolar ventilation, which is more than the increase in $\dot{V}O_2$, the P_AO_2 is higher than normal, and the**

$PaCO_2$ decreases to 30 mmHg during the first trimester of pregnancy whereas pH remains normal.

Alterations in Ventilatory Drive
The hyperventilation observed during the pregnancy is attributable to progesterone level. The mechanism is assumed to be a sensitization of the central chemoreceptors. Pregnancy gives rise to three-fold increase in slope of PCO_2/ventilation response curve (79). The hypoxic ventilatory response is also increased two-fold (80).

Clinical Implications
Airway edema, swelling and easy propensity to bleed contribute significantly to difficulty in airway management in a parturient. Furthermore, the significant decrease in FRC and increased $\dot{V}O_2$ contribute to quicker development of desaturation and hypoxemia (77). Adequate denitrogenation requires longer period of breathing 100% O_2. For preoxygenation to be beneficial to the fetus, it should be performed for about six minutes to allow for adequate maternal-fetal equilibrium (77).

NONPULMONARY FUNCTIONS OF THE LUNG

The lungs primary function is gas exchange. However, due to its significant surface area and capillary network, it is an ideal organ to perform other functions. Some nonpulmonary functions are as follows: (i) *Filtration*: Thrombi are cleared most rapidly from the lungs than other organs. The lung possesses a well-developed proteolytic enzyme system, which dissolves small clumps of fibrin and platelets (81). Plasmin activator from pulmonary endothelium converts plasminogen to plasmin, which converts fibrin to fibrin degradation products. (ii) *Processing of compounds*: Table 4 shows the effects on various hormones while passing through the pulmonary circulation (81,82). Some pass through the circulation unchanged, others are activated (angiotensin I to angiotensin II, arachidonic acid), while many are inactivated. Lungs not only process endogenously produced substances, but metabolize a number of chemicals utilizing the mixed function oxidases and cytochrome P-450 systems as seen in the liver. Furthermore, the process involving the conjugation with glucuronide and glutathione also takes place in the lung. (iii) *Release of inflammatory mediators*: histamine, endothelium, and arachidonic acid derivatives are released from the lung following immunological activated by inhaled allergens. Some animal studies have demonstrated the presence of clusters of peptide and amine-secreting cells in the lung tissue (83). The cells degranulate in the presence of hypoxia, however, their function a significance is still not known. (iv) *Host defenses*: The lungs are exposed to the environment and are constantly being bombarded with pathogens. Lungs have developed an elaborate network of minimizing and handling of pathogens. Larger particles >5 μm are filtered in the nose and upper pharynx. The mucociliary layer helps to trap particles between 1 and 5 μm, while particles <1 μm reach the alveoli. Local host defenses are provided by macrophages, neutrophils, and lymphocytes. They protect the tissues in the short term, but chronic long-term inflammation can cause significant destruction or remodeling of tissues. This can lead to alterations in ventilation/perfusion and ultimate gas exchange.

Table 4 Effect on Hormones by Passage Through the Pulmonary Circulation

Molecule	Effect of compound passing through pulmonary circulation		
	Activated	Unchanged	Inactivated
Amines		Dopamine Epinephrine Histamine	5-Hydroxytryptamine Norepinephrine
Peptides	Angiotensin I	Angiotensin II Oxytocin Vasopressin	Bradykinin Atrial naturetic peptide Endothelins
Ecosanoids	Arachidonic acid	PGI_2 PGA_2	PGD_2 PGE_1, PGE_2 $PGF_{2\alpha}$ Leukotrienes
Purine derivatives			Adenosine ATP, ADP, AMP

Abbreviations: ATP, adenosine tri-phosphate; ADP, adenosine diphosphate; AMP, adenosine monophosphate; PGI_2, prostacyclin; PGA_2, prostaglandin A_2; PGD, prostaglandin D; PGE_1, prostaglandin E_1; PGE_2, prostaglandin E_2; $PGF_{2\alpha}$, prostaglandin.
Source: Modified from Ref. 92.

RESPIRATORY ADJUSTMENT IN HEALTH AND DISEASE

For significant range of O_2 extraction, $\dot{V}O_2$ is independent of supply (Fig. 20) (84). However, below a critical $\dot{D}O_2$ level, $\dot{V}O_2$ begins to diminish and is directly dependent upon the supply of O_2. In critical illness, "supply dependency" is observed at a much higher $\dot{D}O_2$ level (Fig. 20) than occurs at baseline conditions. This observation leads some to believe and suggest that increasing $\dot{D}O_2$ to supramaximal levels could improve outcomes in critically ill patients. However, this has not been proven conclusively (85).

Respiratory failure is defined as a failure of maintenance of normal arterial blood gas tension. Hypoxia due to cardiac and other extrapulmonary forms of shunting are excluded. As mentioned before, saturation of Hb with O_2 is dependent on PaO_2, which is dependent on alveolar P_AO_2. Alveolar P_AO_2 under normal conditions is dependent on the balance of two factors: (*i*) amount of O_2 entering the lung, which is determined by alveolar ventilation and concentration of O_2 (F_IO_2), and, (*ii*) O_2 leaving the alveoli, which is determined by Q and O_2 saturation of mixed venous (PvO_2) (Fig. 13). This presumes that there is no impediment to diffusion of O_2 across the alveoli to the blood. If Q and PvO_2 are kept constant and $\dot{V}/\dot{Q}$ is matched the two factors that would significantly affect PAO_2 are alveolar ventilation and fractional inspired concentration. Breathing a hypoxic mixture of gas (accidental, smoke inhalation), and low F_IO_2 (as at high altitude) would lead to hypoxia even if ventilation is maintained. More often it is the decreased ventilation, in combination with $\dot{V}/\dot{Q}$ mismatching and shunting, that causes decreased PaO_2. Decreased PaO_2 with or without increases in $PaCO_2$ is described as acute hypoxic respiratory failure. The pathophysiologic reasons for acute hypoxic respiratory failure are reviewed in Volume 2, Chapter 23.

Management of acute hypoxemic respiratory failure (AHRF) requires mechanical ventilation. The parameters of mechanical ventilation are determined predominantly by the pathophysiologic process. For example, in situations of ventilatory failure secondary to neuromuscular dysfunction (myopathy, neuropathy, neuromuscular blockade) adequate $\dot{V}_E$ with low F_IO_2 would suffice. However, in situations of acute lung injury, where $\dot{V}/\dot{Q}$ mismatch and shunts predominate as the major pathophysiologic process, ventilatory parameters that keep the alveoli open (PEEP), improve $\dot{V}/\dot{Q}$ ratio, and increase F_IO_2 will be required (see Volume 2, Chapter 27). Increased F_IO_2 is able to improve PaO_2 (and SaO_2) in states where $\dot{V}/\dot{Q}$ mismatch is the primary pathophysiology, while it has limited effect in situations where there is a large shunt. If the shunt is more than 30% of the Q, O_2 supplementation has less effect in improving the PaO_2. However, decreasing the F_IO_2 will drastically lower the PaO_2 due to the effect on alveoli that are participating in gas exchange.

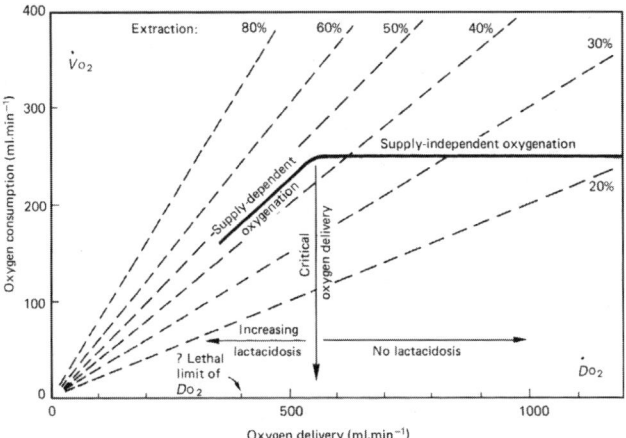

Figure 20 For an otherwise healthy subject, the thick horizontal line shows the extent to which oxygen delivery can be reduced without reducing oxygen consumption and causing signs of cellular hypoxia (supply independent oxygenation). Below the postulated critical delivery, oxygen consumption becomes supply-dependent and there are signs of hypoxia. *Source*: From Ref. 1.

EYE TO THE FUTURE

Technological advancements are significantly contributing to our understanding of biological processes. Completion of the human genome project has been a major development and is fueling research at a level which was incomprehensible a decade ago. Evaluation of gene activation and responses to specific stimuli, which was studied one gene at a time, is now being studied at the whole genome level using microarray and other technologies. Currently data is being generated at unprecedented levels adding to the understanding and complexities of biological processes. It is also being recognized that the evaluation of proteins (proteomics) and interaction of proteins and genes (interactomes) are equally important. Variations in biological responses are being linked to differences in specific genes. Alterations in nucleotide composition of genes, single nucleotide polymorphisms (SNPs), are being linked to variations in biological activity and pathological predispositions.

One area of pulmonary physiology that has seen great advancement in our understanding in the last decade is pulmonary vascular physiology. This is also an area where these new gene-based technologies are likely to be employed. The pulmonary vasculature is affected by many pathological processes (chronic obstructive pulmonary disease, acute respiratory distress syndrome, collagen vascular disease, pulmonary embolism, etc.), which lead to secondary pulmonary hypertension, culminating in acute and chronic right heart failure. Pulmonary hypertension and right heart failure are difficult to treat. Better understanding of mechanisms that lead to pulmonary hypertension are the focus of significant research. The exact mechanism of hypoxic pulmonary vasoconstriction, which is central to the development of acute and chronic pulmonary hypertension, continues to remain elusive (86,87). The recently described role of carbon monoxide in oxygen sensing/transduction mechanism in carotid glomus cells adds a new dimension to possible mechanisms of oxygen-sensing and hypoxic ventilatory control (88). Similar pathways may be involved in hypoxic pulmonary vasoconstriction; however, that remains to be determined.

Elucidation of the mechanisms by which the pulmonary vascular system is formed, maintained, or disrupted during development and disease represents a major challenge in contemporary lung biology. Though it is appreciated that processes involving cellular proliferation, differentiation, and apoptosis need to be carefully coordinated, knowledge of the underlying cellular and molecular mechanisms involved is limited. Discovery of homeobox genes represents a definitive advance in this area (89). However, the specific role of these genes in lung organogenesis and tissue remodeling is in its infancy. Many research initiatives are currently active to develop a systematic approach to biological processes integrating molecular, cellular, and interactive processes.

As molecular biology techniques have progressed, so have advances in the complexity and accessibility of imaging techniques. It is now possible to study physiological and pathological phenomenon noninvasively in vivo in animals and humans. High-resolution computed tomography (CT) scans and PET scanning are helping us test long-held hypotheses and theories. Functional MRI techniques are allowing us to better delineate areas of the brain responsible for specific physiological functions. Such studies will help us understand respiratory control mechanisms and sleep-related disorders.

SUMMARY

The primary purpose of the respiratory system is to facilitate the uptake of O_2 in the alveoli, where it combines with hemoglobin and is transported throughout the body by the circulatory system, while at the same time removing CO_2 which has been transported from the tissues to be exhaled via the alveoli. These functions are achieved by intricate coordination of the upper and lower airways, alveoli, pulmonary blood flow, respiratory muscles, metabolic sensors, and medulla-based neural control centers.

Cardiac and respiratory functions are also closely integrated with numerous feedback mechanisms designed to match ventilation with perfusion. The lungs and the heart are the only organs that receive full $\dot{Q}$. Accordingly, the lungs are anatomically well situated to perform many of the secondary (nonpulmonary) functions. The list of nonpulmonary functions continues to grow. Pulmonary and nonpulmonary functions adapt to constantly changing needs of the body. They also vary significantly with age and pregnancy. Understanding the basic physiological mechanisms involved in pulmonary and nonpulmonary functions of the lungs is the key to appreciating pathophysiology of respiratory disorders and rational management of respiratory function following trauma, resuscitation, perioperative management, and critical care.

KEY POINTS

- The FRC has important clinical significance as it is the major reservoir of oxygen in the body and is directly related to the time to desaturation following apnea. In addition, the FRC is inversely proportional to the degree of shunt.
- Alveolar ventilation ($\dot{V}_A$) is referred to as the gas that participates in gas exchange; the amount of ventilation that is wasted is referred to as physiologic dead space ventilation ($\dot{V}_D$).
- The formula for compliance is analogous to the mathematical formula used to calculate capacitance in electronics.
- Factors that affect airway resistance include lung volume, bronchial smooth muscle tone, carbon dioxide, and the density/viscosity of the inhaled gas.
- Blood flow has to be closely coupled to adequate ventilation to allow for optimal exchange of O_2 and CO_2.
- Unlike systemic vessels, pulmonary vessels constrict in response to hypoxia, hypercarbia, and acidosis.
- Under typical resting conditions, the RBC PO_2 virtually reaches that of alveolar gas when it is about one-third of the way along the capillary.
- Increased O_2 affinity shifts the oxy-heme curve to the left (i.e., reduces P_{50}), while decreased O_2 affinity shifts the oxy-heme curve to the right (i.e., increases P_{50}).
- CO_2 is transported in the blood primarily in three different forms, namely: (*i*) physically dissolved in blood; (*ii*) bound to amino groups of proteins (e.g., hemoglobin), as carbamate compounds; and (*iii*) as bicarbonate ions.
- Autonomous respiratory pattern is generated in the medulla by synchronized activity of six distinct neuronal groups (central pattern generator, CPG).
- The central chemoreceptors play an important role in monitoring pCO_2, while the peripheral chemoreceptors which reside in the carotid body respond predominantly to changes in pO_2.
- Age-related loss of pharyngeal muscle support leads to an increased propensity for upper airway obstruction. Furthermore, loss of dentition makes establishment of patent airway by bag and mask more difficult.

☞ Due to the increase in alveolar ventilation, which is more than the increase in $\dot{V}O_2$, the P_AO_2 is higher than normal, and the $PaCO_2$ decreases to 30 mmHg during the first trimester of pregnancy whereas the pH remains normal.

REFERENCES

1. Lumb AB. Nunn's Applied Respiratory Physiology. 5th ed. Oxford: Butterworth-Heinemann, 2000.
2. West JB. Respiratory Physiology; The Essentials. 6th ed. Philadelphia: Lippincott Williams and Wilkins; 1999.
3. Fowler W. Lung function studies II. The respiratory dead space. Am J Physiol 1948; 154:405–416.
4. Zaugg M, Lucchinetti E. Respiratory function in the elderly. In: Silverstein J, ed. Geriatric Anesthesia. Philadelphia: W.B. Saunders, 2000:47–58.
5. van Gold L, Batenburg J, Robertson B. The pulmonary surfactant system: biochemical aspects and functional significance. Physiol Rev 1988; 68:374–455.
6. Hamm H, Kroegel C, Hohlfeld J. Surfactant: a review of its functions and relevance in adult respiratory disorders. Respir Med 1996; 90:251–270.
7. Burwell D, Jones J. The airways and anesthesia- 1: Anatomy, physiology and fluid mechanics. Anaesthesia 1996; 51:849–857.
8. West JB. Pulmonary Pathophysiology; the essentials. 5th ed. Baltimore: Williams and Wilkins; 1997.
9. Pedley TJ, Schroter RC, Sudlow MF. Energy losses and pressure drop in models of human airways. Respir Physiol 1970; 9(3):371–386.
10. West JB, Wagner P. Ventilation-perfusion relationships. 2nd ed. New York: Raven Press; 1997.
11. Cooper CJ, Landzberg MJ, Anderson TJ, Charbonneau F, Creager MA, Ganz P, et al. Role of nitric oxide in the local regulation of pulmonary vascular resistance in humans. Circulation 1996; 93(2):266–271.
12. Marshall B, Marshall C. Pulmonary Cirulation During Anaesthesia. Amsterdam: Kluwer, 1992.
13. Johnson RL, Jr., Hsia CC. Functional recruitment of pulmonary capillaries. J Appl Physiol 1994; 76(4):1405–1407.
14. Barnes PJ, Liu SF. Regulation of pulmonary vascular tone. Pharmacol Rev 1995; 47(1):87–131.
15. Archer S, Michelakis E. The mechanism(s) of hypoxic pulmonary vasoconstriction: potassium channels, redox O(2) sensors, and controversies. News Physiol Sci 2002; 17(4):131–137.
16. Riley R, Cournard A. "Ideal" alveolar air and the analysis of ventilation perfusion relationships in lung. J Appl Physiol 1949; 1:825–849.
17. Staub N. Alveolar-arterial oxygen tension gradient due to diffusion. J Appl Physiol 1963; 18:673–680.
18. American Thoracic Society. Single-breath carbon monoxide diffusing capacity (transfer factor). Recommendations for a standard technique—1995 update. Am J Respir Crit Care Med 1995; 152(6 Pt 1):2185–2198.
19. Shapiro B, Peruzzi W, Kozelowski-Templin R. Clinical Application of Blood Gases. St. Louis: Mosby, 1994.
20. Bauer C. Structural Biology of Hemoglobin. 2nd ed. Philadelphia: Lippincott-Raven, 1997.
21. Perutz MF. Regulation of oxygen affinity of hemoglobin: influence of structure of the globin on the heme iron. Annu Rev Biochem 1979; 48:327–386.
22. Jaenicke R. Folding and association of proteins. Prog Biophys Mol Biol 1987; 49(2-3):117–237.
23. Winslow R, Vandegriff K. Oxygen-Hemoglobin dissociation curve. 2nd ed. Philadelphia: Lippincott-Raven, 1997.
24. Monod J, Wyman J, Changeux J.-P. On the nature of allosteric transitions; a plausible model. J Mol Biol 1965; 12:88–118.
25. Benesch RE, Benesch R, Yu CI. The oxygenation of hemoglobin in the presence of 2,3-diphosphoglycerate. Effect of tempera-

ture, pH, ionic strength, and hemoglobin concentration. Biochemistry 1969; 8(6):2567–2571.
26. Benesch R, Benesch RE. Intracellular organic phosphates as regulators of oxygen release by haemoglobin. Nature 1969; 221(181):618–622.
27. Perrella M, Kilmartin JV, Fogg J, Rossi-Bernardi L. Identification of the high and low affinity CO2-binding sites of human haemoglobin. Nature 1975; 256(5520):759–761.
28. Haab P, Durand-Arczynska W. Carbon Monoxide Effect on Oxygen Transport. 2nd ed. Philadelphia: Lippincott-Raven, 1997.
29. Verma A, Hirsch DJ, Glatt CE, Ronnett GV, Snyder SH. Carbon monoxide: a putative neural messenger. Science 1993; 259(5093):381–384.
30. Piantadosi CA. Carbon monoxide poisoning. N Engl J Med 2002; 347(14):1054–1055.
31. Collman JP, Brauman JI, Halbert TR, Suslick KS. Nature of O2 and CO binding to metalloporphyrins and heme proteins. Proc Natl Acad Sci USA 1976; 73(10):3333–3337.
32. Zwart A, Kwant G, Oeseburg B, Zijlstra WG. Human whole-blood oxygen affinity: effect of carbon monoxide. J Appl Physiol 1984; 57(1):14–20.
33. Hlastala MP, McKenna HP, Franada RL, Detter JC. Influence of carbon monoxide on hemoglobin-oxygen binding. J Appl Physiol 1976; 41(6):893–89.
34. Klocke R. Carbon Dioxide Transport. 2nd ed. Philadelphia: Lippincot-Raven, 1997.
35. Klocke R. Carbon dioxide transport. In: Farhi L, Tenney S, eds. Handbook of Physiology. Bethseda: American Physiological Society, 1987:173–179.
36. Zhu XL, Sly WS. Carbonic anhydrase IV from human lung. Purification, characterization, and comparison with membrane carbonic anhydrase from human kidney. J Biol Chem 1990; 265(15):8795–8801.
37. Bauer C, Schroder E. Carbamino compounds of haemoglobin in human adult and foetal blood. J Physiol 1972; 227(2):457–471.
38. Klocke RA. Rate of bicarbonate-chloride exchange in human red cells at 37 degrees C. J Appl Physiol 1976; 40(5):707–714.
39. Grant BJ. Influence of Bohr-Haldane effect on steady-state gas exchange. J Appl Physiol 1982; 52(5):1330–1337.
40. Bianchi AL, Denavit-Saubie M, Champagnat J. Central control of breathing in mammals: neuronal circuitry, membrane properties, and neurotransmitters. Physiol Rev 1995; 75(1):1–45.
41. von Euler C. Neural organization and rhythm generation. In: Crystal RG, West JB, Weibel ER, Barnes PJ, eds. The Lung: Scientific Foundations. 2nd ed. Philadelphia: Lippincott-Raven, 1997:1711–1724.
42. Farber N, Pagel P, Waltier D. Pulmonary pharmacology. In: Miller R, ed. Anesthesia. 5th ed. Philadelphia: Churchill Livingstone, 2000:125–146.
43. Haldane J, Priestley J. The regulation of lung ventilation. J Physiol (Lond) 1905; 32:225–266.
44. Gozal D, Hathout GM, Kirlew KA, et al. Localization of putative neural respiratory regions in the human by functional magnetic resonance imaging. J Appl Physiol 1994; 76(5):2076–2083.
45. Corfield DR, Fink GR, Ramsay SC, et al. Evidence for limbic system activation during CO2-stimulated breathing in man. J Physiol 1995; 488(Pt 1):77–84.
46. Corfield DR, Fink GR, Ramsay SC, et al. Activation of limbic structures during CO2-stimulated breathing in awake man. Adv Exp Med Biol 1995; 393:331–334.
47. Dev NB, Loeschcke HH. A cholinergic mechanism involved in the respiratory chemosensitivity of the medulla oblongata in the cat. Pflugers Arch 1979; 379(1):29–36.
48. Mitchell R, Carman C, Severinghaus J, Richardson B, Singer M, Snider S. Stability of cerebrospinal fluid pH in chronic acid-base disturbances in blood. J Appl Physiol 1965; 20:443–452.

49. Froman C, Smith AC. Hyperventilation associated with low pH of cerebrospinal fluid after intracranial haemorrhage. Lancet 1966; 1(7441):780–782.

50. Eger E. Desflurane (Suprane): A Compendium and Reference. Nutley, NJ: Anaquest, 1993.

51. Tansley JG, Pedersen ME, Clar C, Robbins PA. Human ventilatory response to 8 h of euoxic hypercapnia. J Appl Physiol 1998; 84(2):431–434.

52. Lahiri S. Physiological responses: Peripheral chemoreceptors and chemoreflexes. In: Crystal RG, West JB, Weibel ER, Barnes PJ, eds. The Lung: Scientific Foundations. 2nd ed. Philadelphia: Lippincott-Raven, 1997:1747.

53. Peers C. Potassium channels in carotid body Type I cells and their sensitivity to hypoxia. In: Lopez-Barneo J, Weir E, eds. Oxygen Regulation of Ion Channels and Gene Expression. Armonk: Futura Publishing Company, 1998:145.

54. Weil JV, Byrne-Quinn E, Sodal IE, et al. Hypoxic ventilatory drive in normal man. J Clin Invest 1970; 49(6):1061–1072.

55. Scharf SM, Sharon SC, eds. Heart-Lung Interaction in Health and Disease. New York: Marcel Dekker Inc., 1989.

56. Permutt S, Caldini P. Regulation of cardiac output by the circuit: venous return. In: Baan J, Noodergraff A, Raines J, eds. Cardiovascular System Dynamics. Cambridge: MIT Press, 1978:465–479.

57. Permutt S. Relation between pulmonary arterial pressure and pleural pressure during the acute asthmatic attack. Chest 1973; 63(suppl):25–28.

58. Lloyd T. Mechanical heart-lung interaction. In: Scharf SM, Cassidy S, eds. Heart-Lung Interaction in Health and Disease. New York: Marcel Dekker Inc., 1989:309–336.

59. Kaufman M, Cassidy S. Reflex effects of lung inflation and other stimuli on the heart and circulation. In: Scharf SM, Cassidy S, eds. Heartlung interaction in health and disease. New York: Marcel Dekker Inc., 1989:339–363.

60. De Burgh Daly M, Hazzledine JL, Ungar A. The reflex effects of alterations in lung volume on systemic vascular resistance in the dog. J Physiol 1967; 188(3):331–351.

61. Cassidy SS. Stimulus-response curves of the lung inflation cardio-depressor reflex. Respir Physiol 1984; 57(2):259–268.

62. Davidson WR, Jr., Fee EC. Influence of aging on pulmonary hemodynamics in a population free of coronary artery disease. Am J Cardiol 1990; 65(22):1454–1458.

63. Kenney R. The respiratory and cardiovascular systems. In: Physiology of Aging. Chicago: Mosby, 1989.

64. Jones RL, Overton TR, Hammerlindl DM, Srpoule BJ. Effects of age on regional residual volume. J Appl Physiol 1978; 44(2):195–199.

65. Cerveri I, Zoia MC, Fanfulla F, et al. Reference values of arterial oxygen tension in the middle-aged and elderly. Am J Respir Crit Care Med 1995; 152(3):934–941.

66. Kronenberg RS, Drage CW, Ponto RA, Williams LE. The effect of age on the distribution of ventilation and perfusion in the lung. Am Rev Respir Dis 1973; 108(3):576–586.

67. Neas LM, Schwartz J. The determinants of pulmonary diffusing capacity in a national sample of U.S. adults. Am J Respir Crit Care Med 1996; 153(2):656–664.

68. Kronenberg RS, Drage CW. Attenuation of the ventilatory and heart rate responses to hypoxia and hypercapnia with aging in normal men. J Clin Invest 1973; 52(8):1812–1819.

69. Valentine SJ, Marjot R, Monk CR. Preoxygenation in the elderly: a comparison of the four-maximal-breath and three-minute techniques. Anesth Analg 1990; 71(5):516–519.

70. Stoelting R, Dierdorf S. Diseases common to the pediatric patient. In: Stoelting R, Dierdorf S, eds. Anesthesia and Co-existing Disease. New York: Churchill Livingstone, 1993:579–630.

71. Merkus PJ, ten Have-Opbroek AA, Quanjer PH. Human lung growth: a review. Pediatr Pulmonol 1996; 21(6):383–397.

72. Cotes J. Lung Function: Assessment and Application in Medicine. Oxford: Blackwell Scientific Publications, 1993.

73. Marcus CL, Glomb WB, Basinski DJ, Davidson SL, Keens TG. Developmental pattern of hypercapnic and hypoxic ventilatory responses from childhood to adulthood. J Appl Physiol 1994; 76(1):314–320.

74. Richards JM, Alexander JR, Shinebourne EA, et al. Sequential 22-hour profiles of breathing patterns and heart rate in 110 full-term infants during their first 6 months of life. Pediatrics 1984; 74(5):763–777.

75. Cohen G, Xu C, Henderson-Smart D. Ventilatory response of the sleeping newborn to CO2 during normoxic rebreathing. J Appl Physiol 1991; 71(1):168–174.

76. Elkus R, Popovich J, Jr. Respiratory physiology in pregnancy. Clin Chest Med 1992; 13(4):555–565.

77. Stoelting R, Dierdorf S. Physiologic changes and diseases unique to the parturient. In: Anesthesia and Coexisting Diseases. New York: Churchill Livingstone; 1993:539–578.

78. Norregaard O, Schultz P, Ostergaard A, Dahl R. Lung function and postural changes during pregnancy. Respir Med 1989; 83(6):467–470.

79. Garcia-Rio F, Pino JM, Gomez L, Alvarez-Sala R, Villasante C, Villamor J. Regulation of breathing and perception of dyspnea in healthy pregnant women. Chest 1996;110(2): 446–453.

80. Moore LG, McCullough RE, Weil JV. Increased HVR in pregnancy: relationship to hormonal and metabolic changes. J Appl Physiol 1987; 62(1):158–163.

81. Lumb AB. Non-respiratory functions of the lung. In: Nunn's Applied Respiratory Physiology. 5th ed. oxford: Butterworth Heinemann, 2000:306–315.

82. de Wet C, Moss J. Metabolic functions of the lung. In: Breen P, ed. Respiration in Anesthesia: Pathophysiology and Update. Philadelphia: W.B. Saunders, 1998:181–199.

83. Gosney JR. The endocrine lung and its response to hypoxia. Thorax 1994; 49(suppl):S25–S26.

84. Wood LDH. The respiratory system. In: Hall JB, Schimdt GA, Wood LDH, eds. Principles of Critical Care. 1st ed. New York: McGraw-Hill Inc., 1992:3–25.

85. Gattinoni L, Brazzi L, Pelosi P, et al. A trial of goal-oriented hemodynamic therapy in critically ill patients. SvO2 collaborative group. N Engl J Med 1995; 333(16):1025–1032.

86. Moudgil R, Michelakis ED, Archer SL. Hypoxic pulmonary vasoconstriction. J Appl Physiol 2005; 98:390–403.

87. Waypa GB, Schumacker PT. Hypoxic pulmonary vasoconstriction: redox events in oxygen sensing. J. Appl Physiol 2005; 98:404–414.

88. Williams SE, Wootton P, Masson HS, et al. Hemoxygenase-2 is an oxygen sensor for a calcium-sensitive potassium channel. Science 2004; 306:2093–2097.

89. Jones PL. Homeobox genes in pulmonary vascular development and disease. Trends Cardiovascul Med 2003; 13:336–345.

90. Wilson WC. Benumof JL: Respiratory physiology and respiratory function during anesthesia. In: Miller RD, ed. Miller's Anesthesia. 6th ed. Philadelphia, PA: Elsevier Churchill Livingstone, 2005:685.

91. Cassidy SS. Heart-lung interactions in health and disease. Am J Med Sci 1987; 30:451–461.

92. Lumb AB. Non-respiratory functions of the lung. In: Lumb AB, ed. Nunn's Applied Respiratory Physiology, 5th ed. London: Butterworths, 2000:309.

3

Cardiovascular Physiology Review

Gerard R. Manecke, Jr. and David M. Roth

Section of Cardiothoracic Anesthesia, Department of Anesthesiology,
UC San Diego Medical Center, San Diego, California, U.S.A.

INTRODUCTION

A firm knowledge of cardiovascular physiology is necessary for the effective management of the critically ill. A complex interplay between compromised hemodynamic status, metabolic derangement, and preexisting cardiovascular disease is often present (Fig. 1). Thus, an appropriate diagnosis and treatment require an understanding of the cardiovascular signs and symptoms of acute catastrophic illness, as well as those associated with preexisting cardiovascular disease. Patients requiring intensive care and/or resuscitation frequently are unable to provide a complete history or cooperate for a comprehensive physical examination. Thus, the skillful use of the physiologic data, both invasive and noninvasive, is essential.

This chapter reviews the fundamentals of cardiovascular physiology directly applicable to the anesthetic and intensive care management of critically ill trauma victims. The relationships between physiologic processes and hemodynamic data are emphasized, since these are important components of critical care to some extent. First, the heart's pumping mechanism is presented. Mechanical functions of the myocardium and vasculature are reviewed, as are the effects of vascular tone on cardiac filling and performance. Second, cardiac myocyte metabolism, with particular emphasis on myocardial oxygen balance, is discussed, followed by reviews of cellular electrophysiology, cardiac electrical conduction, and a discussion of common mechanisms for dysrhythmia development. Finally, the physiologic aberrations associated with representative traumatic conditions are briefly presented. These include massive blood loss (hypovolemia), cardiac tamponade, pneumothorax, cardiac contusion, and head trauma. Although these clinical examples are presented in detail elsewhere in this book, they are presented in this instance to illustrate the application of physiologic principles to the clinical arena. It is hoped that these brief discussions will encourage the reader to approach the cardiovascular problems in patients who are critically ill from a "physiologic perspective."

THE PUMPING MECHANISM OF THE HEART AND MECHANICS OF THE VASCULAR SYSTEM
The Flow of Blood in the Cardiovascular System

In 1628, the great English physician William Harvey provided the first modern description of the human circulatory system (1,2). As he described, it consists of two pumps and a system of vessels and capillaries arranged in series (Fig. 2). The left side pump (left ventricle) ejects blood to the systemic circulation, whereas the right side pump (right ventricle) ejects blood under relatively low pressure (approximately 1/6 systemic) to the pulmonary vasculature. Amazingly, the two pumps are housed in the same unit, functioning in a completely synchronous manner. The atria and the ventricles are adjacent to one another, sharing the septae that separate them. Thus, changes in geometry and function on one side have profound effects on the other. ☞ **Cardiac contraction is a complex three-dimensional event.** ☞ Each ventricle ejects its volume in a remarkably complex way, with concentric contraction (short axis), a rotating "wringing" motion, long axis contraction with downward movement of the mitral and tricuspid annuli, and contraction of the papillary muscles (3–5). With papillary muscle contraction, the atrio ventricular valvular leaflets become properly aligned in order to prevent regurgitation.

The performance of the heart is under local, humoral, and neural control. Intrinsic response to chamber filling, hormonal influence, and autonomic innervation combine to provide the mechanisms for the heart's response to changes in demand.

Local Control of Cardiac Function

The most significant local factor is chamber filling, which is related to the diastolic ventricular compliance and "venous return." The mechanism by which the myocardium increases its performance (stroke work) in response to increased diastolic volume is known as the Frank-Starling mechanism. ☞ **The Frank-Starling mechanism causes enhanced myocardial performance when cardiac filling is increased.** ☞ Stretch of myocardial fibers caused by increased chamber volume causes increased contractile force. This increased force results from improved alignment of actin and myosin filaments in the sarcomeres (Fig. 3), which results in the ejection of the extra volume, enhanced myocardial contractility, and increased myocardial oxygen consumption. This mechanism has a limit, however. The slope of the ventricular function curve depends on baseline myocardial performance. When volume is added, the curve eventually reaches a plateau, above which increases in performance do not occur (Fig. 4).

Increase in afterload (impedance to ejection) usually represents a rise in systemic vascular resistance (SVR). ☞ **The healthy heart responds favorably to meet the demand of increased SVR, without exhibiting a decrease in output until the mean arterial pressure (MAP) is greater than 160 mmHg (6).** ☞ When under physiologic stress and varying loading conditions, however, the heart can become quite sensitive to changes in afterload. Indeed, in the clinical setting, pharmacologic manipulation of afterload can be an effective

PREEXISTING DISEASE   TRAUMA

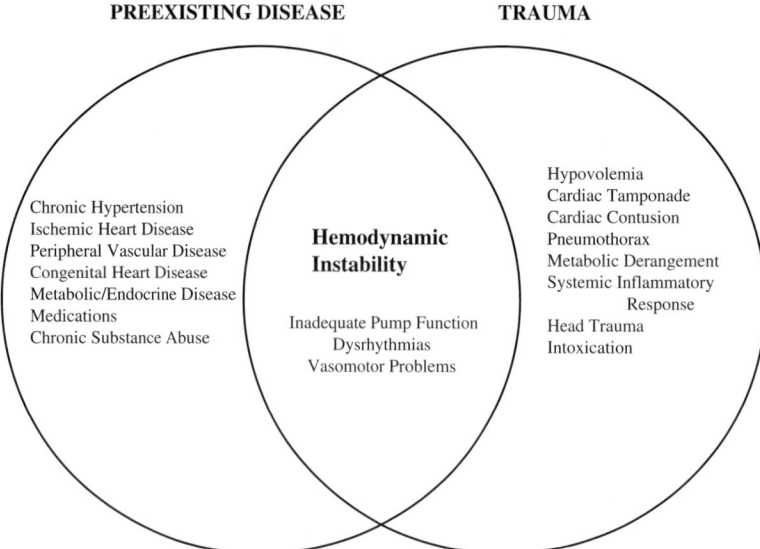

Chronic Hypertension
Ischemic Heart Disease
Peripheral Vascular Disease
Congenital Heart Disease
Metabolic/Endocrine Disease
Medications
Chronic Substance Abuse

**Hemodynamic
Instability**

Inadequate Pump Function
Dysrhythmias
Vasomotor Problems

Hypovolemia
Cardiac Tamponade
Cardiac Contusion
Pneumothorax
Metabolic Derangement
Systemic Inflammatory
       Response
Head Trauma
Intoxication

Figure 1   The interrelationship between preexisting cardiovascular disease and cardiovascular compromise resulting from trauma.

means of influencing cardiac function. For example, in the setting of high afterload, vasodilation can significantly augment cardiac output without increasing myocardial oxygen consumption (7–9). ☞ **Although vasodilation will augment cardiac output in the setting of high SVR, it may also decrease perfusion pressure to the needy tissue beds, including the coronary arteries.** ☞

In the interpretation of hemodynamic monitoring data, it must be remembered, "pressure is not analogous to volume." For example, when interpreting the central venous pressure (CVP), we tend to equate a high CVP to a "full" right atrium and ventricle, and a low pressure as an "empty" heart. In reality, a high CVP can be obtained in several clinical situations where the heart is actually empty (e.g., tamponade, noncompliant right ventricle, etc.).

The relationship between venous return and right atrial pressure is shown in Figure 5. When the heart fails and $\dot{Q}$ falls below venous return, right atrial pressure rises. In Figure 5, the venous return curve is flat for right atrial pressures less than zero. As the right atrial pressure increases (at a fixed capillary tone, intravascular volume, $\dot{Q}$, and contractility), the venous return decreases.

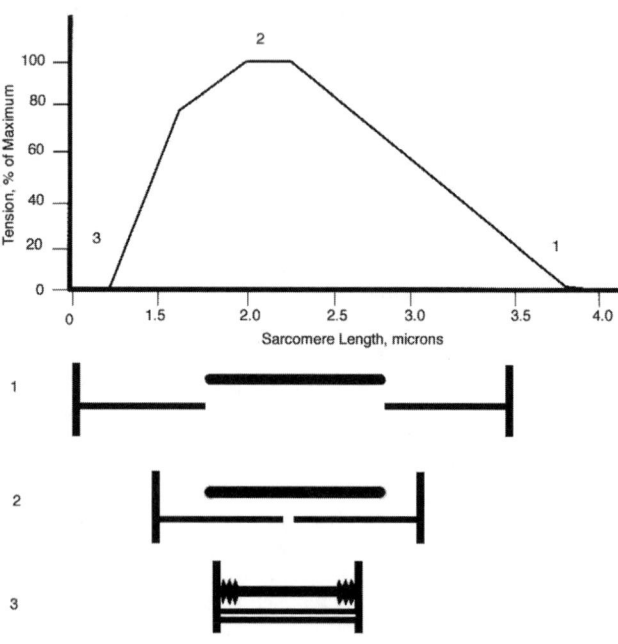

Figure 3   The Frank-Starling mechanism: force of contraction depends upon sarcomere length. Improvement in performance associated with volume administration results from a transition from area "3" to area "2." Area "1" occurs when excessive stretching of fibers causes inadequate overlap of actin and myosin filaments. This overstretch condition (Area 1) seldom occurs in vivo in mammalian species. However, it can be seen in the laboratory (e.g., frog muscle prep). *Source*: From Ref. 44.

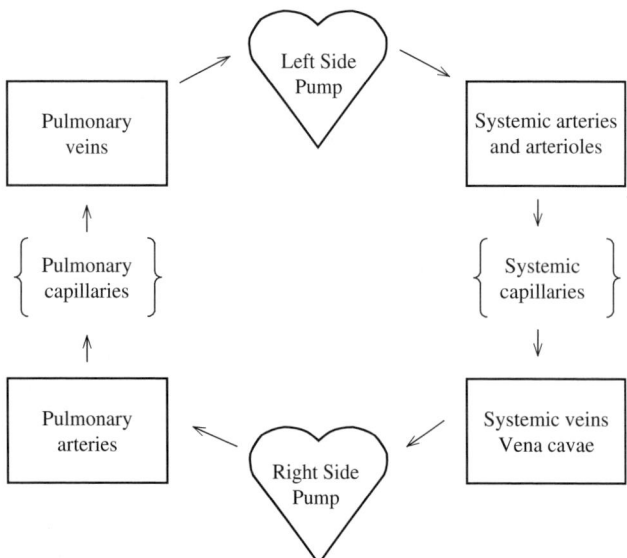

Figure 2   A schematic of the cardiovascular system, illustrating that the right and left sides of the circulation are arranged in series.

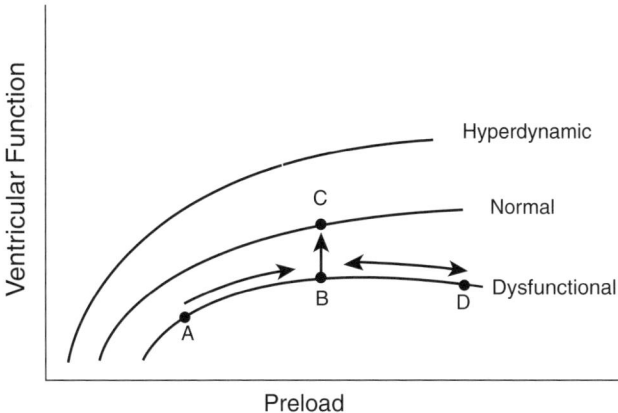

Figure 4 The Frank-Starling mechanism at work in the intact circulatory system. Movement from A to B results from volume loading in hypovolemia, B to D from volume overload in the dysfunctional heart, and B to C from inotropic support. *Source*: From Ref. 45.

However, under the same steady-state conditions of contractility, the addition of one liter of blood to the system would result in an increased $\dot{Q}$ and venous return (Fig. 5). Pressure may often be useful as surrogate measurement for volume or filling, but there are numerous clinical situations in which this relationship breaks down. Examples, such as cardiac tamponade and tension pneumothorax, are discussed later.

The Cardiac Work Loop: "Pressure Work" and "Volume Work"

Ohm's law (Equation 1) for electricity can be applied to the global mechanics of the cardiovascular system:

$$E = I * R \qquad (1)$$

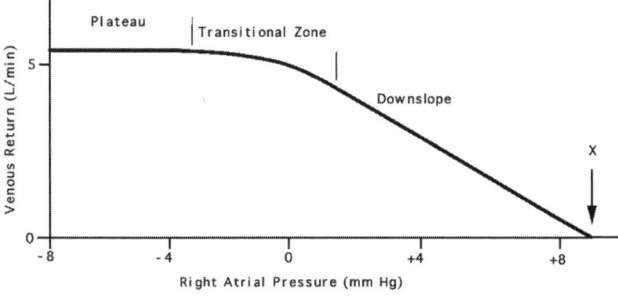

Figure 5 The interplay between right atrial pressure and venous return. Venous return is a function of venous capacitance, intravascular blood volume, cardiac output, and right atrial pressure. When venous capacitance, intravascular blood volume, and cardiac output are all stable and normal, venous return decreases linearly as the right atrial pressure increases above zero. When the pressure in the atrium becomes equal with the mean systemic venous pressure (point x), venous return ceases. If the cardiovascular system was augmented with a transfusion of one liter of blood (e.g., in a 70-kg patient, goes from 5 to 6 L), the cardiac output would increase as would the venous return. The new point x (at which venous return would diminish to zero) might be as high as 16 mmHg. *Source*: From Ref. 10.

where E is the voltage, I the current, and R the resistance. If one considers pressure in the vascular system to be analogous to voltage, and flow analogous to current, then Equation 2 results for the vascular system:

$$\Delta P = \dot{Q} * R \qquad (2)$$

where ΔP is the pressure drop across the system, $\dot{Q}$ the flow through the system, and R the resistance to blood flow through the system. The formulae for calculating the pulmonary vascular resistance (PVR) and SVR are simply algebraic modifications of the aforementioned formula:

$$R = \frac{\Delta P}{\dot{Q}} \qquad (3)$$

In Equation 3, Ohm's law is restated in an algebraic equation that is the solution to obtain the resistance. In clinical practice the resistance calculated this way is either PVR or SVR.

$$PVR = \frac{MPAP - P_{pao}}{\dot{Q}} \qquad (4)$$

Equation 4 is the formula used to provide the solution for PVR. In this situation the ΔP is mean pulmonary artery pressure (MPAP) deducted from pulmonary artery occlusion pressure (P_{pao}). When calculated this way, results are expressed as Wood's units.

$$PVR = \frac{MPAP - P_{pao}}{\dot{Q}} * 80 \qquad (5)$$

(units in dynes cm^{-5}sec^{-1})

Equation 5 converts the units into dynes cm^{-5} sec^{-1} by multiplying Equation 4 by 80.

$$SVR = \frac{MAP - CVP}{\dot{Q}} * 80 \qquad (6)$$

Equation 6 solves for SVR. MAP, CVP, and 80 is the multiplied conversion factor required to yield the standard units (dynes cm^{-5} sec^{-1}).

☞ **The pulmonary vascular system is a low-pressure, high-compliant network in health, with pressures approximately 1/10 systemic.** ☞ A normal cardiac work loop is shown in Figure 6. The amount of work the heart does in one cycle is the "stroke work," and can be calculated by determining the area of the work loop. This could be estimated by drawing a similar rectangle and multiplying the change in x axis (volume) by the change in y axis (pressure).

$$\text{Work} = \text{energy} = \text{pressure} * \text{volume} \qquad (7)$$

Thus, one component of the cardiac work provides pressure generation, and the other volume ejection (Equation 7). In hemodynamic management, it is often necessary to balance these two factors. For instance, if most of the heart's energy is invested in pressure generation, then there may not be sufficient flow to support the oxygen requirements of the body. Likewise, if the heart generates high volume but very low pressure (as occurs in low SVR states), the pressure generated may not be sufficient for adequate peripheral perfusion to organs such as the brain, liver, kidneys, or the myocardium itself.

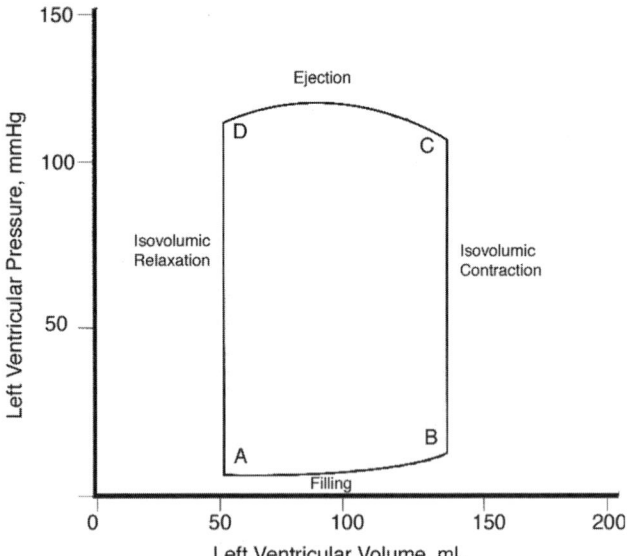

Figure 6 The left ventricular cardiac work loop. The area inside the shape A-B-C-D equals the work performed by the left ventricle during one cycle. At "A," the mitral valve opens. At "B" the mitral valve closes and the ventricle begins to contract. At "C" the aortic valve opens, and at "D" the aortic valve closes.

The Effect of Respiration on Circulatory Mechanics

It has long been known that systemic blood pressure varies during each respiratory cycle. During spontaneous inspiration, blood pressure (BP) normally decreases. This is because the highly compliant pulmonary venous bed expands during enlargement of the chest cavity, and pulmonary venous pressure drops causing decreased venous return to the left side of the heart. Simultaneously, the venous return to the right side of the heart increases because of the negative intrathoracic pressure. When pathologic processes occur which impede cardiac filling, such as cardiac tamponade and constrictive pericarditis, this normal drop in BP with inspiration is exaggerated. The resultant drop of more than 10 mmHg is called "pulsus paradoxus" (11,12).

As Figure 7 indicates, this decrease is accompanied by the concomitant decrease in CVP and pulmonary artery pressure (PAP). When patients receive positive pressure ventilation, a reciprocal phenomenon occurs. Positive intrathoracic pressure "squeezes" pulmonary venous blood into the left side of the heart, initially raising systemic BP and left

ventricular output. This notion is supported by the echocardiographic demonstration that both transmitral early flow and pulmonary venous flow increase during mechanical inspiration (13). The rise in intrathoracic pressure is also thought to decrease left ventricular afterload, thereby facilitating the flow of blood to the periphery (14). Simultaneously, venous return to the right side is decreased.

If the increased intrathoracic pressure is sustained for a couple of additional beats, the BP drops, reflecting the decrease in right sided venous return and increased right ventricular afterload. The magnitude of cyclical variation in BP variation reflects the filling of the heart, and can be used in the assessment of volume status (15). Figure 8 depicts the respiratory variation in arterial blood pressure with positive pressure ventilation. "Δ Up" refers to the rise in systolic pressure above baseline during positive pressure inspiration, and "Δ down" refers to the drop in pressure below baseline that occurs with the next couple of heart beats.

☞ The "Δ down" component of the systolic blood pressure variation with ventilation is quite sensitive in detecting hypovolemia. ☞ In many patients it is possible to use the "Δ down" as a surrogate for PCWP (16). Caution should be exercised, however, since such variations may also depend on other factors such as ventilatory pressure, ventilatory volume, and vasodilator therapy (17,18). The ventilation-induced changes in BP, pulmonary artery pressure, and CVP have led clinicians to make these pressure measurements at the "end-exhalation" point of the ventilatory cycle (19). This minimizes the effect of ventilation, as well as allows for consistency between measurements.

Neural Control of Cardiovascular Function

The heart (and entire cardiovascular system) responds to autonomic influences from both the sympathetic and parasympathetic nervous systems.

The parasympathetic innervation of the heart is via the vagus nerve, which profoundly affects automaticity in the sinoatrial (SA) node, as well as conduction and automaticity in the atrioventricular (AV) node. The vagus nerve (cranial nerve X) originates at the floor of the fourth ventricle as the dorsal vagal nucleus, sending afferent and efferent fibers through the medulla. It receives efferent fibers from the vasomotor center in the brainstem, and its end-organ ganglionic synapses are muscarinic.

The primary cardiovascular influences of the vagus nerve are to decrease heart rate and decrease conduction through the AV node. Also, particularly strong vagal

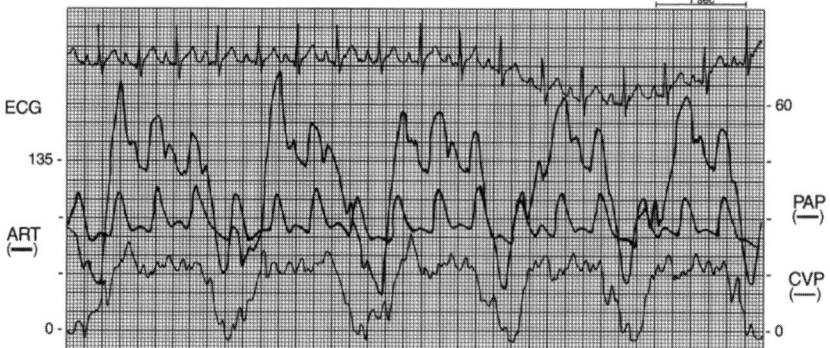

Figure 7 Spontaneous forceful inspiration causes simultaneous decreases in arterial pressure, pulmonary artery pressure, and central venous pressure. *Abbreviations*: ART, arterial pressure; CVP, central venous pressure; ECG, electrocardiogram; PAP, pulmonary artery pressure. *Source*: From Ref. 19.

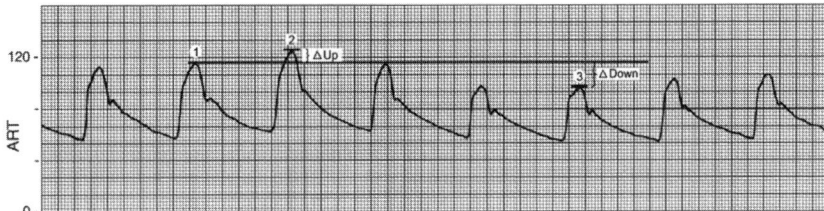

Figure 8 Variation in arterial blood pressure with positive pressure ventilation. "1" is at baseline, "Δ Up" is the rise in systolic pressure during a positive pressure breath, and "Δ Down" is the decrease in systolic pressure occurring after a positive pressure breath. *Abbreviation*: ART, arterial pressure. *Source*: From Ref. 19.

stimulation can have a negative inotropic effect on both the atria and the ventricles. The parasympathetic system exerts relatively minor influences on vascular tone.

Sympathetic innervation of the heart is via the "cardiac accelerator fibers," which exit from the thoracolumbar sympathetic chain at spinal vertebral levels T1–T4. These postganglionic neurons release norepinephrine, primarily causing stimulation of the cardiac β_1 receptors. The β_1 receptors have dramatic positive chronotropic and inotropic effects on the heart, via a cyclic adenosine monophosphate (AMP) mediated mechanism. ☞ **The heart and vasculature are under the constant influence of the autonomic nervous system. The resulting cardiac output and systemic blood pressure continuously reflect the intravascular blood volume and the relative parasympathetic and sympathetic "tone."** ☞

Cardiovascular stress, central nervous system activity, anesthesia, and other exogenous substances can profoundly alter the respective "tones" of both the sympathetic and parasympathetic systems.

Humoral Control of Cardiovascular Function

Under stressful circumstances, catecholamines (epinephrine and norepinephrine) are released into the circulation by the adrenal medulla. Epinephrine has primarily β agonist activities, although in high concentrations it exhibits α activity as well. The β_1 receptors are found in the heart and mediate positive inotropic, chronotropic, and dromotropic (conduction) activities. The β_2 receptors are found throughout the peripheral vasculature, mediating vasodilatation. Norepinephrine is a potent α and β agonist. Stimulation of peripheral α receptors (α_1) causes vasoconstriction whereas central α receptor agonism yields a decrease in the sympathetic output from the central nervous system. The preponderance of effect of norepinephrine is on the peripheral α receptors. The α_1 and α_2 receptors have been discovered in the coronary vasculature, located primarily in the epicardial conduit vessels (20,21). Under normal circumstances, these receptors appear to have little effect on coronary vascular tone. However, they may be important in mediating coronary vasoconstriction in patients with ischemic heart disease or vasospastic angina (21). Although minor increases in coronary vascular tone may occur after administration of alpha adrenergic agonists (22), a current Medline search reveals no reports of vasospastic ischemia precipitated by the clinical use of α_1 or α_2 agonists.

CARDIAC CELLULAR PHYSIOLOGY
Cellular Homeostasis and Excitation–Contraction Coupling

Cardiac muscle exhibits characteristics of both smooth and striated muscle. Morphologically it is more similar to striated muscle, but differs from it in that it exhibits intrinsic automaticity and a longer action potential. The mechanism of cardiac muscle contraction is similar to that of skeletal muscle, and has been reviewed in detail in numerous physiology texts (23).

Contraction depends on a mechanism consisting of actin and myosin filaments as well as an interlacing sarcoplasmic reticulum (Figs. 9 and 10). Depolarization of the sarcoplasmic reticulum causes intracellular calcium release, which results in interaction of the myosin and actin filaments. This interaction, regulated by troponin I, T, and C, as well as tropomyosin, involves the swiveling of the myosin heads, and results in the sliding of actin and myosin filaments past one another. This process is known as "excitation–contraction coupling." The subsequent breakage of the actin–myosin linkage requires energy [adenosine triphosphate (ATP)], as does the calcium pump maintaining the intracellular sarcoplasmic calcium gradient. ☞ **When a myocardial energy deficit occurs, actin and myosin bridges fail to break, resulting in inability of the muscle to relax.** ☞ This is one of the mechanisms for diastolic dysfunction (stiffness) and, ultimately, the mechanism for the rigor mortis to set in. The entire process of excitation–contraction coupling is modulated by a complex G-protein system, which involves cyclic guanosine monophosphate (GMP), cyclic AMP, protein kinase A, and troponin.

When energy or oxygen deficits occur, homeostatic and excitation–contraction coupling mechanisms break down. This results in cellular acidosis and cardiac failure (systolic and diastolic). It is also important to remember that the heart lives in the same metabolic milieu as the rest of the body. ☞ **Metabolic derangements resulting from abnormalities such as sepsis, systemic inflammatory response, hypovolemia, and diabetes can have devastating effects on the myocardium as well as other organs and tissues.** ☞ Obviously, cardiac dysfunction resulting from these aberrations responds best to their correction, when possible.

Myocardial Oxygen Balance

The myocardium is designed for endurance, beating approximately 42 million times per year. Although it is magnificently efficient, it functions with a very high oxygen requirement. The heart extracts a maximal amount of oxygen from the coronary arterial blood, resulting in coronary sinus oxygen content of only 10 mg/dL. For this reason, it is extremely sensitive to perturbations in its oxygen supply/demand relationship. The left ventricular myocardium receives blood supply during diastole only, so its perfusion is dependent upon diastolic time. Coronary

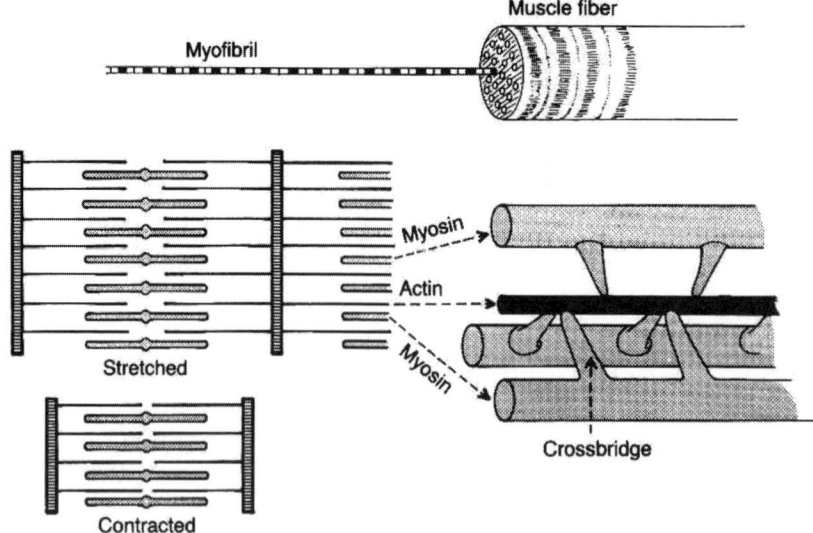

Figure 9   Muscle contraction results from actin and myosin filaments sliding past one another. This "sliding filament" mechanism is dependent upon formation of actin–myosin crossbridges, swiveling of the myosin filaments, and subsequent breakage of the crossbridges. *Source*: From Ref. 45.

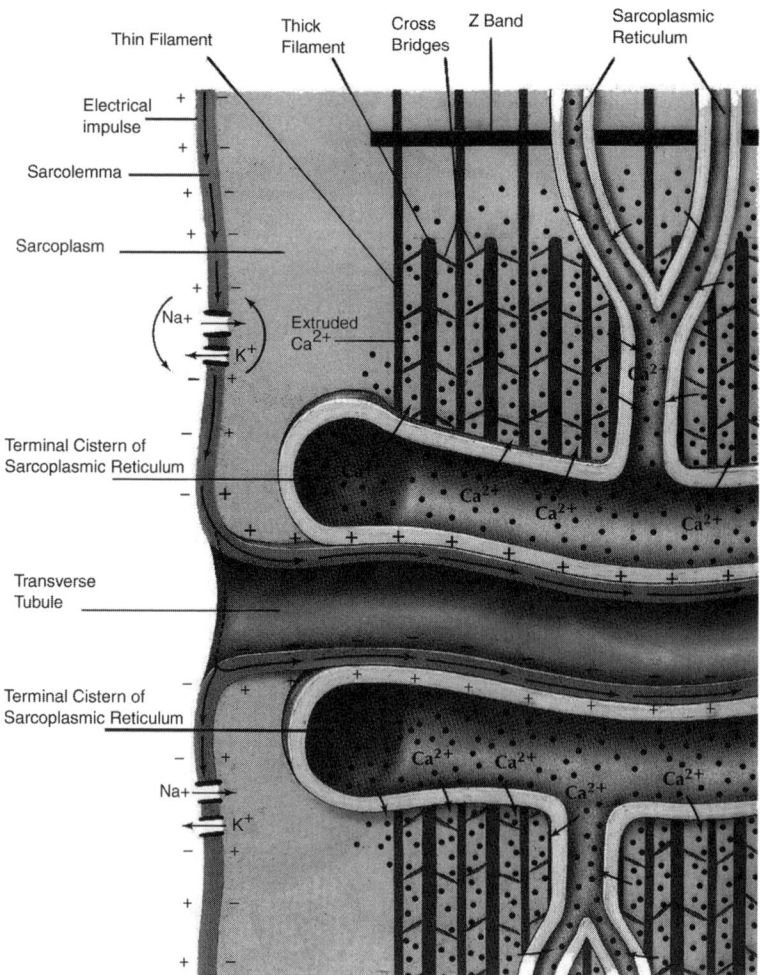

Figure 10   The anatomic physiologic relationships between the sarcolemma, sarcoplasmic reticulum, and contractile mechanism. *Source*: From Ref. 47.

perfusion pressure (CPP) for the left ventricular myocardium can be estimated using the formula:

$$CPP = DBP - LVEDP \qquad (8)$$

where DBP is the diastolic blood pressure and LVEDP the left ventricular end diastolic pressure. Autoregulatory mechanisms maintain constant coronary blood flow when the perfusion pressure is between 50 and 150 mmHg. When coronary stenoses occur, however, autoregulatory mechanisms may break down, leaving coronary perfusion completely dependent on driving pressure (Fig. 11).

Tachycardia and bradycardia have opposite effects on coronary artery perfusion. Left ventricular perfusion occurs almost exclusively during diastole. An increase in heart rate will decrease the diastolic (coronary artery perfusion) time while increasing the amount of ATP used per minute (increased beats/min), because energy is required for each heart beat. ✒ **Accordingly, the heart rate is by far the most significant factor in myocardial oxygen balance.** ✒ The determinants of myocardial oxygen supply and demand are summarized in Table 1.

The aspect to be kept in mind is that, some of the very factors that are associated with enhanced myocardial performance, such as increased preload, increased contractility, and increased heart rate, cause an increase in oxygen demand. Even decreased afterload, which is a favored means of enhancing myocardial performance without increasing myocardial work, can cause oxygen balance problems by decreasing CPP. Thus, therapeutic maneuvers designed to enhance cardiac performance must always be undertaken with the concomitant effects on oxygen balance in mind. Likewise, efforts to decrease myocardial work such as beta blockade administration, and to increase CPP (peripheral vasoconstriction with vasopressin or α_1 agonists) may precipitate a significant decrease in systemic perfusion. ✒ **In trauma and critical care management, a constant effort is made to balance the metabolic needs of the systemic tissues with the metabolic needs of the myocardium.** ✒

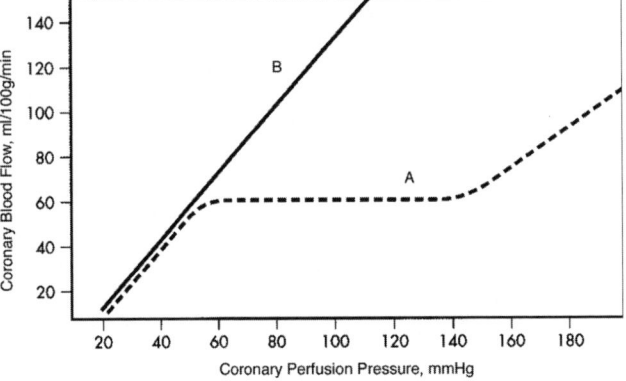

Figure 11 Autoregulation normally maintains constant coronary blood flow between perfusion pressures of 50 and 150 mmHg (**A**). When coronary stenoses occur, coronary blood flow becomes completely pressure dependent (**B**). *Source*: From Ref. 44.

Table 1 The Determinants of Myocardial Oxygen Supply and Demand

Oxygen supply	Oxygen demand
1/Heart rate (duration of diastole)	Heart rate
$CPP = P_{CA} - P_{Lvi}$	Preload
Coronary patency	Afterload
Oxygen delivery	Contractility
Oxygen availability	Basal metabolic rate
Myocardial blood flow distribution	Activation energy

Note: "Activation energy" refers to the energy required for myocardial relaxation. During systole the P_{Lvi} exceeds the P_{CA} and blood actually flows retrograde out of the heart muscle through the coronary arteries and into the aorta, whereas during diastole the pressure in the aorta (and coronary arteries) is far greater than the P_{Lvi} promoting perfusion of the left ventricular myocardial tissues.

Abbreviations: CPP, coronary artery perfusion pressure; P_{CA}, coronary artery pressure (the aortic blood pressure can be used as a surrogate for this value when the coronary arteries are without placque/stenosis >70%); P_{Lvi}, left ventricular intracavetary pressure.

CARDIAC ELECTROPHYSIOLOGY

The heart contains cells that have intrinsic electrical automaticity resulting from spontaneous depolarization. These cells, which include the nodal cells (SA and AV), conduction fibers, and Purkinje fibers, make up the cardiac electrical system. The automaticity, together with the conduction characteristics and anatomical configuration of the "wiring," combine to produce atrioventricular contraction which is automatic, sequential, and coordinated.

Cellular Electrophysiology and the Cardiac Action Potential

Nodal cells have a resting membrane potential of -55 mV, which is maintained primarily by a potassium concentration gradient across the cell membrane. The effect of this concentration gradient on the transmembrane potential is quantified by the Nernst equation (Equation 9):

$$EMF = -61 * \log \frac{[K_i]}{[K_o]} \qquad (9)$$

where EMF is the electromotive force in millivolts. As with other cells, the inside of the cell membrane is negative relative to the outside. The potassium gradient is maintained by a Na^+-K^+-ATPase membrane pump. Nodal cells are unique in that they depolarize because of a slow inward calcium flux, rather than a rapid conductance of sodium (Fig. 12). This is because voltage-dependent sodium gates are inoperative at this relatively high (less negative) resting membrane potential. Automaticity of the cells results from the spontaneous "phase 4 depolarization," which is caused primarily by steady background calcium conductance (T-Ca^{2+} channels) (24,25) as well as sodium leakage. This raises the membrane potential to -40 mV, at which time L-Ca^{2+} channels open fully.

Repolarization results from outward potassium flux ("delayed rectifier"). Ionic concentrations are restored by membrane ion pumps. The action potentials of SA nodal cells are similar to those of AV nodal cells, except the phase 4 depolarization of SA nodal cells is more rapid.

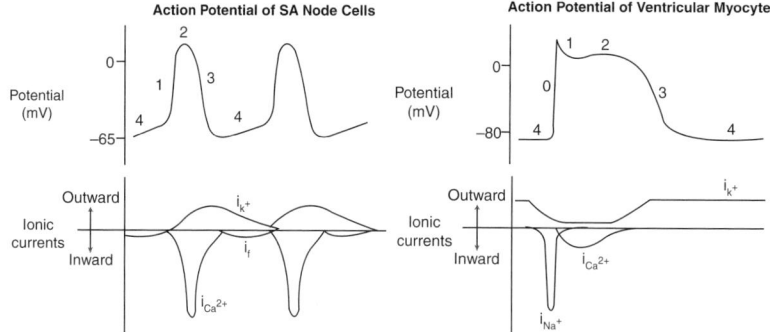

Figure 12   The action potential morphologies of nodal cells and ventricular myocytes. Nodal cells exhibit phase 4 depolarization, which likely results from gradual sodium leak and calcium influx. Phase 1 is caused by calcium influx. Ventricular myocytes exhibit a "phase 0," resulting from rapid sodium influx. Phase 2 represents a balance between calcium influx and potassium efflux, and phase 3 repolarization is caused by unopposed potassium efflux. *Abbreviation*: SA, sinoatrial. *Source*: From Ref. 47.

Thus, under normal circumstances, the SA node is the instigator of cardiac electrical activity. The conducting fibers, Purkinje fibers, and ventricular muscle cells all exhibit a fast Na+ influx (phase 0 depolarization) followed by a plateau. The rapid depolarization results in rapid action potential propagation. These cells normally exhibit very slow phase 4 depolarization. To illustrate the rate of beats per minute, SA nodal spontaneous rate is typically 60 to 100 beats per minute (BPM), AV nodal rate 40 to 60 BPM, and ventricular escape rate 30 to 40 BPM.

The Normal Cardiac Conduction System

The cardiac conduction system consists of the SA nodal cells, internodal pathways, left and right bundle branches, and the Purkinje fibers. This arrangement is depicted in Figure 13. The action potential initiated at the SA node is propagated via the internodal fibers to the AV node. Branches of the internodal fibers depolarize the atrium, resulting in atrial contraction and the "P" wave on the electrocardiogram (ECG) trace. From the AV node, the action potential travels

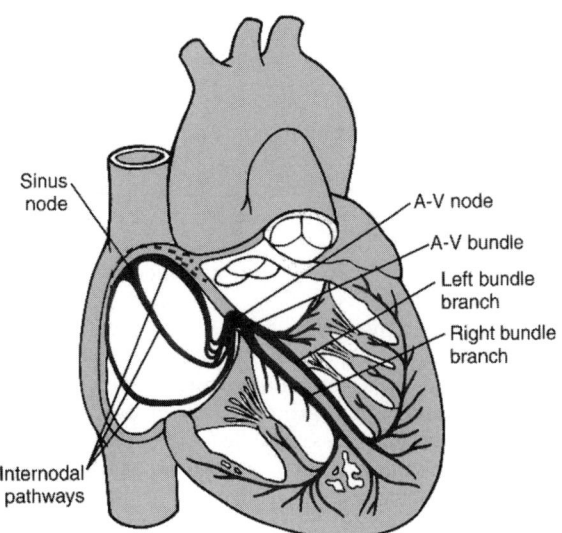

Figure 13   The cardiac conduction system. Action potentials are generated at the sinus node, travel via internodal pathways to the A-V node, and then are distributed to the ventricles via the left and right bundle branches. *Source*: From Ref. 46.

along the common His bundle, the right and left bundle branches, and Purkinje fibers to the ventricular muscle. The depolarization pattern of the ventricles results in the "QRS" complex seen on the ECG trace.

Repolarization of the ventricles, resulting from outward potassium flux, results in the "T" wave. The direction of current at various points in the cycle causes the characteristic morphologies in each lead. The 12-lead ECG trace demonstrates these morphologies and allows anatomic placement of electrical abnormalities.

The Pathophysiology of Common Dysrhythmias

Two common mechanisms of cardiac dysrhythmias are reentry and ectopic foci. Reentry results from slowing of conduction along one of the two divergent electrical paths (changes depicted in Fig. 14). If a conducting pathway branches, and the diverging branches reconnect, then under conditions of conduction slowing (or blockade) in one limb of a bifurcating pathway, the conduction can proceed to retrograde through the previously blocked pathway and reenter the initial pathway. This process sets up a "circus" movement through the loop of cardiac tissue. A further prerequisite for this condition is a pathway circuit long enough to allow the completion of the refractory period (in the initially blocked limb of the circuit) prior to the return of the impulse. This "circus" movement or "reentry" phenomenon is thought to be the mechanism for a wide variety of tachydysrhythmias, including atrial fibrillation, atrial flutter, and ventricular fibrillation (26,27).

Ectopic foci usually occur at irritable areas of myocardium or conduction. These areas can result from myocardial ischemia, infarction, cardiac contusion, and mechanical irritation. Ectopic foci may result in premature atrial contractions, premature ventricular contractions, and reentrant dysrhythmias (28). ☛ **Various electrolyte abnormalities, such as hypokalemia (29,30) and hypomagnesemia (31), particularly when they occur together (32), as well as hypocalcemia (33) increase the likelihood of cardiac dysrhythmias.** ☛ Enhanced atrial and ventricular excitability and prolonged Q-T interval are often part of the pathogenesis. For example, hypocalcemia causes prolongation of the Q-T interval, and hypokalemia potentiates dysrhythmias caused by Q-T prolongation (34). Q-T prolongation predisposes to the "R on T" phenomenon, which leads to reentry dysrhythmias.

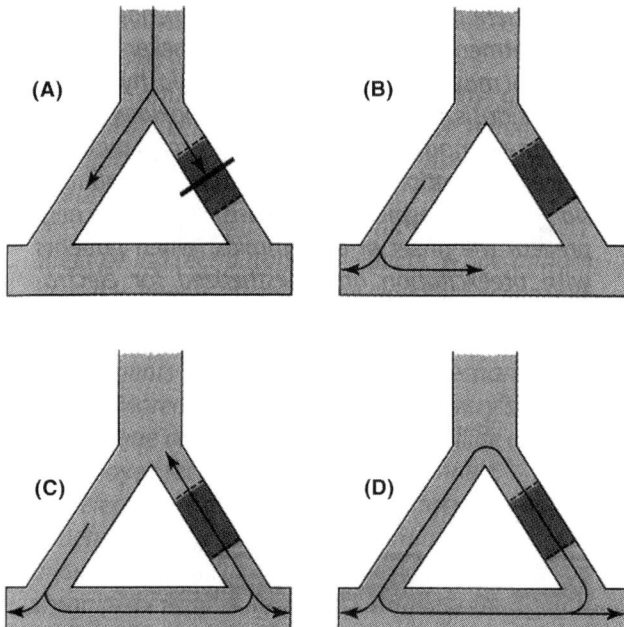

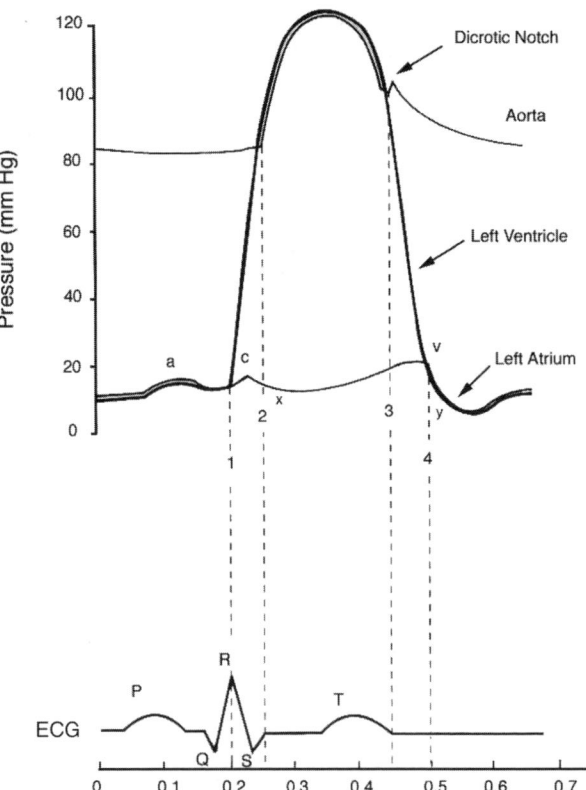

Figure 14 The mechanism of reentry. The figure demonstrates four conditions (**A–D**) required for reentry. (**A**) Two pathways with differing conductivity (or refractory periods) that can form a closed electrical loop. (**B**) Unidirectional block in one pathway (*dark stippled area*). (**C**) Sufficient length in the circuit, or slow enough conduction, to allow recovery of previously blocked pathway. (**D**) Passage through blocked pathway and "reentry" into the initially open pathway sets in motion the "circus" rhythm. *Source*: From Ref. 48.

Figure 15 The cardiac cycle. Electrocardiographic (ECG) changes are shown below, and the pressure tracings for the left atrium, left ventricle, and aorta are shown above. 1 refers to the beginning of isovolumic ventricular contraction, 2 the opening of the aortic valve, 3 the closure of the aortic valve, and 4 the diastole. a, c, v, x, and y signify the components of the venous waveform (see text), and P, Q, R, S, and T refer to the components of the ECG waveform. *Source*: From Ref. 19.

When dysrhythmias occur in trauma victims, every effort should be made to correct electrolyte and acid base abnormalities, aggressive antidysrhythmic treatment should be undertaken, and clinical suspicion for myocardial contusion should increase. Combinations of abnormalities, for example hypokalemia with hypomagnesemia, can be particularly troublesome.

THE CARDIAC CYCLE AND THE CENTRAL VENOUS WAVEFORMS

Understanding the information obtained from invasive intravascular monitors such as transesophageal echocardiography, CVP, and pulmonary capillary wedge pressure (PCWP) requires familiarity with the timing of events in the cardiac cycle (Fig. 15). Left and right ventricular ejections result in the systemic arterial and pulmonary arterial waveforms respectively. The dicrotic notch results from closure of the semilunar valve (aortic, pulmonic).

Pressure changes in the heart and vasculature are preceded by their associated ECG tracing (Fig. 16). The venous pressure wave in the right atrium and superior vena cava result from mechanical events on the right side of the heart (right ventricle, tricuspid valve), and the venous waveforms of the left atrium and PCWP result from the left side (left ventricle, mitral valve).

Atrial depolarization results in atrial contraction, which in turn causes the "a" wave of the central venous waveforms. Right atrial contraction, which produces the "a" wave on the

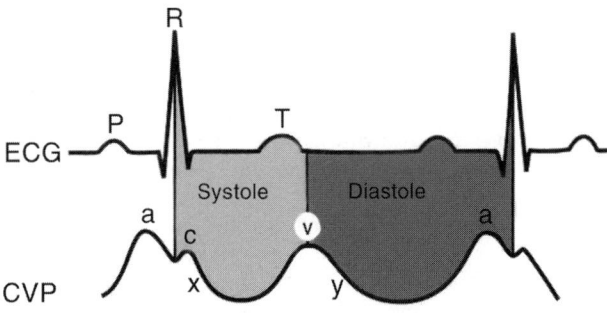

Figure 16 The cardiac cycle and genesis of "a," "c," and "v" waves. The "a" wave is caused by atrial contraction. The "c" wave is caused by the bulging of the atrioventricular (AV) valve into the atrium during isovolemic ventricular contraction. The "v" wave is caused by passive venous filling of the right atrium prior to the opening of the AV valve. The "x" descent is due to ventricular decompression following the opening of the ventricular outlet (which allows the AV valve to retract back toward the ventricle). The "y" descent is due to the opening of the AV valve. Mechanical pressure events in the right atrium are slightly delayed relative to the electrical events in the electrocardiogram. *Abbreviations*: CVP, central venous pressure; ECG, electrocardiogram; P, atrial depolarization; R, ventricular depolarization; T, ventricular repolarization. *Source*: From Ref. 19.

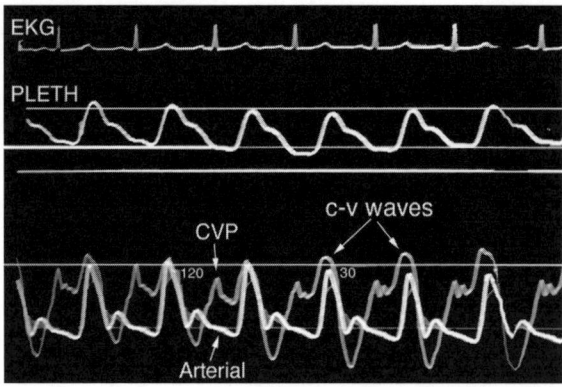

Figure 17 The electrocardiograph tracing, plethysmograph, arterial, and central venous waveforms obtained from a patient with severe tricuspid regurgitation as noted on transesophageal echocardiography. Notice the "c-v" waves of regurgitation precede the systemic arterial upstroke. This illustrates that regurgitant waves are a systolic event. The arterial upstroke in this patient is delayed because of poor cardiac performance. The CVP tracing is in gray tone, the arterial in white. The traces overlap because the CVP scale is 30 mmHg, and the arterial is 120 mmHg. *Abbreviations*: CVP, central venous pressure; EKG, electrocardiograph tracing; PLETH, plethysmograph.

CVP waveform, precedes left atrial contraction. This is because the sinus node is in the wall of the right atrium adjacent to the superior vena cava, and atrial depolarization spreads from that point across the right atrium to the left atrium. Isovolemic ventricular contraction causes a retrograde bulging of the AV valve, resulting in the "c" wave. Ventricular ejection results in release of this "bulging" pressure (x descent). The "v" wave occurs at the juncture between systole and diastole. To understand this wave, one must consider three things.

First, atrial filling occurs primarily during ventricular systole. By the time ventricular diastole occurs, the atrium is essentially full. Second, in early ventricular diastole, the AV valve is still closed. Third, ventricular contraction is three dimensional, with shortening along the long axis (base to apex) being an important component. During systole, the AV valve annulus moves downward, and it rapidly moves upward during early ventricular diastole. It is likely that this upward annular movement against a full atrium causes the "v" wave. The "y" descent occurs when the AV valve opens and allows the blood previously held entirely in the atrium to enter the ventricle and hence transiently decrease the atrial pressure.

One should note that the "v" wave should not be confused with the pathologic "c-v" waves associated with AV valvular regurgitation. Regurgitant "c-v" waves occur earlier in the cycle, and are a continuation of the "c" wave. Figure 17 shows the regurgitant "c-v" wave with the concomitant arterial pressure trace to emphasize the timing and pathophysiology.

THE PATHOPHYSIOLOGY OF CONDITIONS COMMONLY ASSOCIATED WITH TRAUMA
Hypovolemia
Massive blood loss and multiple trauma tend to go "hand in hand." Compensatory physiologic mechanisms, however, may either obscure the diagnosis or cause the clinician to

underestimate the severity of the situation. These mechanisms are mediated primarily by the sympathetic nervous system.

Baroreceptors, located in most of the major arteries, are found in particular abundance at the bifurcation of the carotid arteries (carotid sinus). The baroreceptor reflex is a negative feedback loop. An increase in arterial pressure causes an increase in the firing of the baroreceptor afferent fibers. These afferents travel via the vagus nerve to the glossopharyngeal nerve. These fibers ultimately signal the tractus solitarius in the medullary portion of the brainstem. This causes a decrease in sympathetic vasoconstrictor response, as well as an increase in vagally mediated parasympathetic output.

When BP drops, baroreceptor afferents are inhibited, resulting in activation of the medullary vasoconstrictor center. Sympathetic output from the central nervous system then causes increase in heart rate (β stimulation) and α_1-mediated vasoconstriction. This vasoconstriction serves to maintain BP and distribute blood flow to the vital organs (brain, heart, splanchnic circulation). In otherwise healthy individuals, this mechanism maintains homeostasis until a large portion (30–40%) of the blood volume has been lost.

Medications causing vasodilatation or sympatholysis, for example, anesthetics, narcotics, beta blockers, can thwart this mechanism, resulting in catastrophic hemodynamic compromise. **Elderly patients and/or patients chronically receiving beta blockade may not mount a dramatic tachycardic response to hypovolemia or stress.** This is because of the effects of age and beta blockade on the baroreceptor reflexes and sympathetic nervous system responsiveness (35–37). Also, elderly patients, particularly those with chronic hypertension, may have a decreased central compartment volume of distribution, leading to a decreased capacitance vessel response to hypovolemia (38).

Cardiac Tamponade
Cardiac tamponade can result from blunt trauma or stab wound to the chest. Typically, there is leakage of blood from the aortic root or one of the cardiac chambers into the pericardial sac. This leakage, if under pressure, can cause rapid accumulation of blood around the heart. As the pressure in the pericardium rises, cardiac diastolic expansion is impeded. The diagnosis should be considered in the presence of Beck's triad (jugular venous distension, muffled heart sounds, and hypotension). Figure 18 depicts the complex interrelationship between impaired diastolic function, decreased BP Q̇, and impaired myocardial perfusion that results from the accumulation of pericardial fluid.

Cardiac tamponade triggers the same sympathetic response as hypovolemia (tachycardia and vasoconstriction), but can usually be differentiated from hypovolemia by the presence of high filling pressures (or distended neck veins, in the absence of central monitoring). Diagnosis can be rapidly confirmed by transesophageal echocardiography (TEE) as described in Volume 2, Chapter 21. Drainage of the pericardial fluid usually results in rapid improvement. In contrast to chronic pericardial effusions, which can be managed by subxiphoid window and pericardiocentesis, traumatic effusions are best treated by thoracotomy or median sternotomy, since the site of injury needs to be evaluated and repaired.

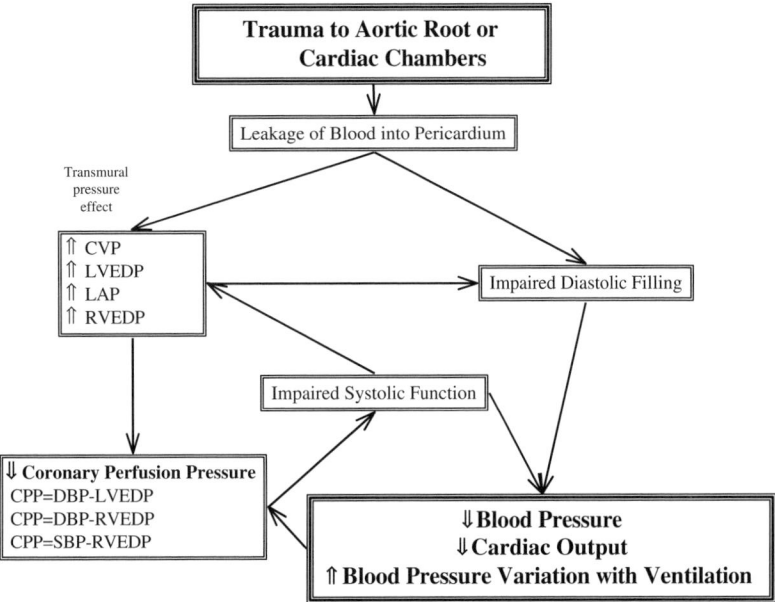

Figure 18 The physiologic events of cardiac tamponade, leading to shock. *Abbreviations*: CVP, central venous pressure; CPP, coronary perfusion pressure; DBP, diastolic blood pressure; LAP, left atrial pressure; LVEDP, left ventricular end-diastolic pressure; RVEDP, right ventricular end-diastolic pressure; SBP, systolic blood pressure.

Tension Pneumothorax

The cascade of events resulting from pleural disruption is depicted in Figure 19. Air leakage into the pleural space, when combined with a one-way valve of egress into the pleural cavity, results in a tension pneumothorax. As this develops, intrathoracic pressure rises, resulting in decreased systemic venous return. Concomitantly, lung collapse causes hypoxemia and a precipitous rise in PVR. Right ventricular failure ensues, leading to interventricular septal shift. Impaired filling of both the right and left sides of the heart quickly results in cardiovascular compromise.

The cardinal signs of tension pneumothorax, cyanosis, hypotension, jugular venous distension, diminished breath sounds on the affected side, and tracheal shift, are thus easily explained by the pathophysiology of the disorder. Relief of the pressure can be achieved by the placement of a chest tube in the fifth intercostal space at the midaxillary line, or with an angiocatheter placed in the second intercostal space at the midclavicular line. This results in rapid clinical improvement. Whenever possible, the chest tube approach is preferred because it is not associated with internal mammary artery injury, and a chest tube will need

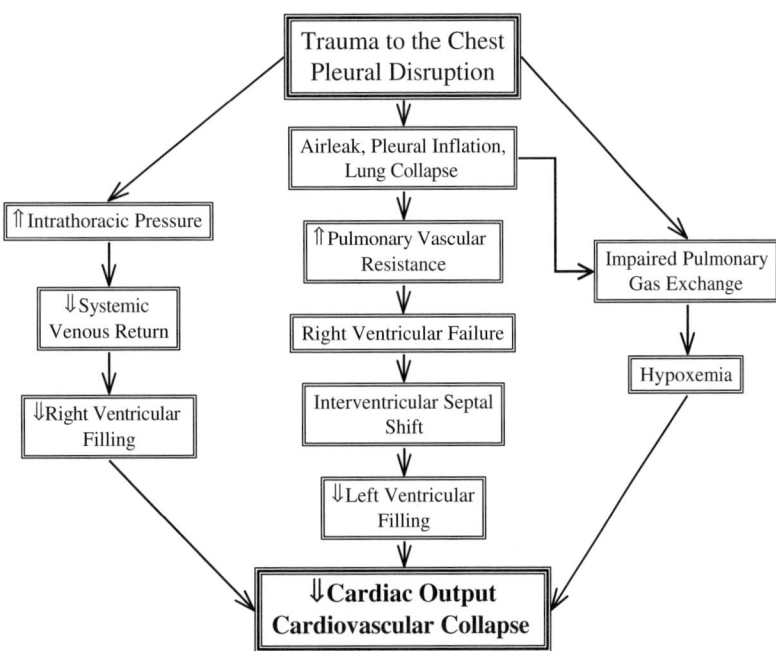

Figure 19 The cascade of events associated with tension pneumothorax.

to be placed anyway whenever a needle is inserted to decompress a tension pneumothorax.

Cardiac Contusion

Cardiac contusion usually results from blunt trauma or deceleration injury. The right ventricle, because of its anterior anatomic location, is the most commonly involved chamber. Direct injury to the myocardium may result in areas of electrical irritability, manifested as ventricular or atrial premature beats (39). ☞ **Conduction blockade is the most common mechanism of dysrhythmias in cardiac contusion patients (27). It results in reentrant dysrhythmias such as ventricular and atrial fibrillation (40,41), as well as heart block (42).** ☞ If extensive myocardial injury is present, cardiac failure or ventricular rupture may occur. Diagnosis can be made by measuring troponins, as well as by TEE. Treatment is mainly a supportive care and a dysrhythmia monitoring in a telemetry unit or the intensive care unit.

Head Trauma

Severe head trauma, with its associated cerebral edema, may result in increased intracranial pressure (ICP). When a severe increase in ICP occurs, bradycardia and systemic hypertension may ensue. The pathophysiologic mechanism for this is referred to as "Cushing's reflex." This is a vasoconstrictive response to cerebral ischemia, causing reflex bradycardia. The only successful treatment is the relief of the intracranial hypertension.

Head injury may also be associated with S-T and T wave ECG abnormalities, as well as myocardial dysfunction (43). These abnormalities appear to be unrelated to any cardiac pathology, indicating that the central nervous system control of electrical cardiac function is more complex than often appreciated.

EYE TO THE FUTURE

Transgenic research into cardiomyopathy involves the injection of adenylate cyclase genes into the cardiac muscle using viral vectors. The overexpression of adenylate cyclase in these animals shows improvement.

Mitochondrial regulation of oxygen consumption and energy metabolism is particularly pertinent in cardiac muscle. Indeed, the venous blood leaving myocardial tissue is the most desaturated of any vascular bed in the body for nonexercising patients. The mitochondrial story is recently just emerging and is a fascinating area of research.

Eukaryotic cells originally lacked the ability to undergo aerobic metabolism. These primordial eukaryotic cells were colonized by aerobic bacteria over a billion years ago. A symbiotic relationship developed, the bacteria evolved into mitochondria and the relationship became permanent. Structurally, mitochondria have four compartments: the outer membrane, the inner membrane, the intermembrane space, and the matrix (the region inside the inner membrane). They perform numerous tasks, such as pyruvate oxidation, the Krebs cycle, and metabolism of amino acids, fatty acids, and steroids, but the most crucial task is probably the generation of energy as ATP, by means of the electron transport chain and the oxidative phosphorylation system (the "respiratory chain").

Over the past 30 years there has been an explosion in technology for cardiovascular monitoring, and thus an exponential rise in knowledge of cardiovascular physiology. Techniques such as pulmonary artery catheterization and transesophageal echocardiography have become bedside procedures, thus revolutionizing our approach to cardiovascular problems. These technologies and improved understanding will continue to be applied to newer noninvasive techniques as well as improved therapies. Within the next 30 years, methods will be developed allowing complete assessment of the cardiovascular system with noninvasive tools.

Integrating such factors as pulse wave characteristics, echocardiographically derived Doppler flow attributes, heart sound characteristics, the timing of cardiovascular events, and advanced computerized analyses will allow such global assessments. These assessments, in turn, will themselves advance our understanding of cardiovascular function. Before long we will be narrating to our students, "Can you imagine, we used to put big catheters into the great veins and thread them into the heart…." The close relationship between cardiovascular physiology and hemodynamic diagnosis and treatment will continue to strengthen over time.

SUMMARY

Understanding the physiology of the cardiovascular system, as well as the pathophysiology of common traumatic disorders aids in the interpretation of physiologic data and choice of treatment modalities. Study of the physiologic basis of cardiac dysrhythmias and other acute pathological conditions facilitates their management, and guides future research. It is hoped that this chapter provides a framework for further study, as well a paradigm for the approach to the cardiovascular problems that critically ill patients present.

KEY POINTS

- ☞ Cardiac contraction is a complex three-dimensional event.
- ☞ The Frank-Starling mechanism causes enhanced myocardial performance when cardiac filling is increased.
- ☞ The healthy heart responds favorably to meet the demand of increased SVR, without exhibiting a decrease in output until the MAP is greater than 160 mmHg.
- ☞ Although vasodilation will augment cardiac output in the setting of high SVR, it may also decrease perfusion pressure to the needy tissue beds, including the coronary arteries.
- ☞ The pulmonary vascular system is a low-pressure, high-compliant network in health, with pressures approximately 1/10 systemic.
- ☞ The "Δ down" component of the systolic blood pressure variation with ventilation is quite sensitive in detecting hypovolemia.
- ☞ The heart and vasculature are under the constant influence of the autonomic nervous system. The resulting cardiac output and systemic blood pressure continuously reflect the intravascular blood volume and the relative parasympathetic and sympathetic "tone."
- ☞ When a myocardial energy deficit occurs, actin and myosin bridges fail to break, resulting in inability of the muscle to relax.

☞ Metabolic derangements resulting from abnormalities such as sepsis, systemic inflammatory response, hypovolemia, and diabetes can have devastating effects on the myocardium as well as other organs and tissues.

☞ The heart rate is by far the most significant factor in myocardial oxygen balance.

☞ In trauma and critical care management, a constant effort is made to balance the metabolic needs of the systemic tissues with the metabolic needs of the myocardium.

☞ Various electrolyte abnormalities, such as hypokalemia and hypomagnesemia, particularly when they occur together, as well as hypocalcemia increase the likelihood of cardiac dysrhythmias.

☞ Elderly patients and/or patients chronically receiving beta blockade may not mount a dramatic tachycardic response to hypovolemia or stress.

☞ Cardiac tamponade triggers the same sympathetic response as hypovolemia (tachycardia and vasoconstriction), but can usually be differentiated from hypovolemia by the presence of high filling pressures (or distended neck veins, in the absence of central monitoring).

☞ Conduction blockade is the most common mechanism of dysrhythmias in cardiac contusion patients, It results in reentrant dysrhythmias such as ventricular and atrial fibrillation, as well as heart block.

REFERENCES

1. Harvey W. Exercitatio Anatomica de Motu Cordis et Sanguinis in Amimalibus. Gryphon Editions, 1995.
2. Harvey W. William Harvey. In: Clendening L, ed. Sourcebook of Medical History. New York: Dover, Inc., 1942:152–169.
3. Simonson JS, Schiller NB. Descent of the base of the left ventricle: an echocardiographic index of left ventricular function. J Am Soc Echocardiogr 1989; 2:25–35.
4. Taber LA, Yang M, Podszus WW. Mechanics of ventricular torsion. J Biomech 1996; 29:745–752.
5. Gorman JH, 3rd, Gupta KB, Streicher JT, et al. Dynamic three-dimensional imaging of the mitral valve and left ventricle by rapid sonomicrometry array localization. J Thorac Cardiovasc Surg 1996; 112:712–726.
6. Guyton AC, Hall JE. Textbook of Medical Physiology. Philadelphia: W.B. Saunders Company, 2001:104.
7. Heineman FW, Kupriyanov VV, Marshall R, Fralix TA, Balaban RS. Myocardial oxygenation in the isolated working rabbit heart as a function of work. Am J Physiol 1992; 262:H255–H267.
8. Ino-oka E, Maruyama Y. Experimental study on vasodilator therapy and its clinical application. Jpn Circ J 1984; 48:373–379.
9. Taylor SH. Clinical pharmacotherapeutics of doxazosin. Am J Med 1989; 87:2S–11S.
10. Guyton AC, Hall JE. Textbook of Medical Physiology. Philadelphia: W.B. Saunders Company, 2001:216.
11. McGregor M. Current concepts: pulsus paradoxus. N Engl J Med 1979; 301:480–482.
12. Santoro IH, Neumann A, Carroll JD, Borow KM, Lang RM. Pulsus paradoxus: a definition revisited. J Am Soc Echocardiogr 1991; 4:408–412.
13. Abdalla IA, Murray RD, Awad HE, Stewart WJ, Thomas JD, Klein AL. Reversal of the pattern of respiratory variation of Doppler inflow velocities in constrictive pericarditis during mechanical ventilation. J Am Soc Echocardiogr 2000; 13:827–831.
14. Robotham JL, Cherry D, Mitzner W, Rabson JL, Lixfeld W, Bromberger-Barnea B. A re-evaluation of the hemodynamic consequences of intermittent positive pressure ventilation. Crit Care Med 1983; 11:783–793.
15. Tavernier B, Makhotine O, Lebuffe G, Dupont J, Scherpereel P. Systolic pressure variation as a guide to fluid therapy in patients with sepsis-induced hypotension. Anesthesiology 1998; 89:1313–1321.
16. Marik PE. The systolic blood pressure variation as an indicator of pulmonary capillary wedge pressure in ventilated patients. Anaesth Intensive Care 1993; 21:405–408.
17. Szold A, Pizov R, Segal E, Perel A. The effect of tidal volume and intravascular volume state on systolic pressure variation in ventilated dogs. Intensive Care Med 1989; 15:368–371.
18. Denault AY, Gasior TA, Gorcsan J, 3rd, Mandarino WA, Deneault LG, Pinsky MR. Determinants of aortic pressure variation during positive-pressure ventilation in man. Chest 1999; 116:176–186.
19. Mark JB. Atlas of Cardiovascular Monitoring. New York: Churchill Livingstone, 1998.
20. Baumgart D, Haude M, Gorge G, et al. Augmented alpha-adrenergic constriction of atherosclerotic human coronary arteries. Circulation 1999; 99:2090–2097.
21. Heusch G, Baumgart D, Camici P, et al. Alpha-adrenergic coronary vasoconstriction and myocardial ischemia in humans. Circulation 2000; 101:689–694.
22. Jalonen J, Halkola L, Kuttila K, et al. Effects of dexmedetomidine on coronary hemodynamics and myocardial oxygen balance. J Cardiothorac Vasc Anesth 1995; 9:519–524.
23. Guyton AC, Hall JE. Textbook of Medical Physiology. Philadelphia: W.B. Saunders Company, 2001:73–78.
24. Katz AM. Calcium channel diversity in the cardiovascular system. J Am Coll Cardiol 1996; 28:522–529.
25. Noma A. Ionic mechanisms of the cardiac pacemaker potential. Jpn Heart J 1996; 37:673–682.
26. Grant AO. Mechanisms of atrial fibrillation and action of drugs used in its management. Am J Cardiol 1998; 82:43N–49N.
27. Robert E, de La Coussaye JE, Aya AG, et al. Mechanisms of ventricular arrhythmias induced by myocardial contusion: a high-resolution mapping study in left ventricular rabbit heart. Anesthesiology 2000; 92:1132–1143.
28. Haissaguerre M, Shoda M, Jais P, et al. Mapping and ablation of idiopathic ventricular fibrillation. Circulation 2002; 106:962–967.
29. Johansson BW, Dziamski R. Malignant arrhythmias in acute myocardial infarction. Relationship to serum potassium and effect of selective and non-selective beta-blockade. Drugs 1984; 28(suppl 1):77–85.
30. Podrid PJ. Potassium and ventricular arrhythmias. Am J Cardiol 1990; 65:33E–44E, discussion 52E.
31. Singh RB, Singh VP, Bajpai HS. Refractory cardiac arrhythmia due to hypomagnesmia. Acta Cardiol 1975; 30:499–503.
32. Millane TA, Ward DE, Camm AJ. Is hypomagnesemia arrhythmogenic? Clin Cardiol 1992; 15:103–108.
33. Murros J, Luomanmaki K. A case of hypocalcemia, heart failure and exceptional repolarization disturbances. Acta Med Scand 1980; 208:133–136.
34. Schneider RR, Bahler A, Pincus J, Stimmel B. Asymptomatic idiopathic syndrome of prolonged Q-T interval in a 45-year-old woman. Ventricular tachyarrhythmias precipitated by hypokalemia and therapy with amitriptyline and prephenazine. Chest 1977; 71:210–213.
35. Collins KJ. Age-related changes in autonomic control: the use of beta blockers in the treatment of hypertension. Cardiovasc Drugs Ther 1991; 4(suppl 6):1257–1262.
36. Ismail S, Azam SI, Khan FA. Effect of age on haemodynamic response to tracheal intubation. A comparison of young, middle-aged and elderly patients. Anaesth Intensive Care 2002; 30:608–614.
37. Laitinen T, Hartikainen J, Vanninen E, Niskanen L, Geelen G, Lansimies E. Age and gender dependency of baroreflex sensitivity in healthy subjects. J Appl Physiol 1998; 84:576–583.
38. Olsen H, Vernersson E, Lanne T. Cardiovascular response to acute hypovolemia in relation to age. Implications for orthostasis and hemorrhage. Am J Physiol Heart Circ Physiol 2000; 278:H222–H232.

39. Ross P Jr, Degutis L, Baker CC. Cardiac contusion. The effect on operative management of the patient with trauma injuries. Arch Surg 1989; 124:506–507.

40. Vesterby A, Gregersen M. Atrial fibrillation resulting from cardiac trauma. Z Rechtsmed 1980; 85:153–157.

41. Crown LA, Hawkins W. Commotio cordis: clinical implications of blunt cardiac trauma. Am Fam Physician 1997; 55: 2467–2470.

42. Finn WF, Byrum JE. Fatal traumatic heart block as a result of apparently minor trauma. Ann Emerg Med 1988; 17:59–62.

43. Dujardin KS, McCully RB, Wijdicks EF, et al. Myocardial dysfunction associated with brain death: clinical, echocardio-graphic, and pathologic features. J Heart Lung Transplant 2001; 20:350–357.

44. Miller RD. Atlas of Anesthesia. Philadelphia: Churchill Livingstone, 1999.

45. Darovic DO. Hemodynamic Monitoring. Philadelphia: W.B. Saunders, 2002.

46. Guyton AC, Hall JE. Textbook of Medical Physiology. Philadelphia: W.B. Saunders, 2000.

47. Hansen JT, Koeppen BM. Netter's Atlas of Human Physiology. New Jersey: Icon Learning Systems, 2002.

48. Morgan GE, Mikhail MS, Murray MJ. Clinical Anesthesiology. 3rd ed. New York: McGraw-Hill, 2002.

4

Clinical Pharmacology Review

Doug Humber and Farivar Jahansouz

Department of Pharmacy, UC San Diego Medical Center, San Diego, California, U.S.A.

INTRODUCTION

Drug therapy is an essential component of critical-care management. The principles of clinical pharmacology outlined inthis chapter constitute the necessary knowledge for providing a rational approach to drug administration in critically ill patients. This chapter initially reviews the basic pharmacokinetic (PK) and pharmacodynamic (PD) principles of drug therapy. Subsequently, the focus changes to drug therapy in disease states which alter the PK and PD parameters. Therapeutic drug monitoring (TDM) is discussed as a means to adjust for these changes and to individualize drug regimens as required to provide optimal therapy in the intensive care unit (ICU).

Pharmacokinetics

The concept of PK modeling describes how administered drugs are handled in the body during health and critical illness and the subsequent plasma concentrations that result. This includes an understanding of route of administration, absorption, bioavailability, distribution, metabolism, and clearance, whereas PD modeling describes the pharmacological effect produced by any specific drug concentration in both healthy and diseased patients. The PK/PD concepts are depicted in Figure 1 (1).

Bioavailability

Bioavailability is defined as the fraction of a dose that reaches the systemic circulation. This fraction will vary depending on the route of administration, the chemical form of the drug (e.g., salt, ester), dosage form (e.g., extended-release vs. elixir), and the extent of "first-pass" elimination (when administered orally) (2).

Drugs administered as intravenous (IV) infusions have, by definition, 100% bioavailability. Administering a drug by the oral or rectal routes has variable bioavailability (1), as illustrated in Table 1. Two main processes are responsible for the bulk of this variability: incomplete absorption and first-pass metabolism. Incomplete absorption can be caused by a number of factors, including drug lipophilicity, drug hydrophilicity, the p-glycoprotein export pump system, and even bacterial degradation of the drug in the gut lumen (1). Enzymatic metabolism within the gut wall can also contribute to a reduced amount of drug reaching the circulation.

Enteral administration has the greatest number of factors affecting blood levels. After a drug has been absorbed across the gut wall, it is delivered to the liver by the hepatic portal system where it can undergo additional hepatic metabolism or biliary excretion. Removal of the drug by this process prior to reaching the systemic circulation is known as the first-pass effect. This effect can substantially decrease the amount of drug reaching the systemic circulation.

Some nonparenteral routes of administration can avoid or reduce the extent of first-pass metabolism (e.g., rectal, sublingual). In addition, parenteral routes (e.g., IV and transdermal preparations) also avoid the first-pass effect of the liver. The amount of drug that ultimately reaches the systemic circulation is calculated by multiplying the administered dose by the bioavailability factor (F) and the fraction of a dose that is active drug "salt form factor" (S) (Equation 1) (2).

$$\text{Amount reaching systemic circulation} = (S)(F)\text{dose} \quad (1)$$

Many drugs are administered as a salt form (e.g., erythromycin ethylsuccinate) and only a fraction of that salt would actually be the active drug.

Volume of Distribution

Once a medication reaches the systemic circulation, it is distributed in the body. The volume of distribution (V_d) is equal to the amount of drug administered (dose) divided by the concentration of the drug in the blood (Equation 2). The distribution of some drugs will be restricted to the vascular fluids and others may be distributed into fat, muscle, bone, or total body water.

$$V_d = \frac{\text{Amount of drug (dose)}}{\text{Concentration of drug}} \quad (2)$$

Factors that alter a drug's V_d include the lipophilicity, protein binding, and tissue binding (2,3). If a drug has extensive protein binding and little lipid solubility, the V_d is typically small (i.e., contained within the vascular compartment). In contrast, if a drug has a high degree of lipid solubility and tissue binding and low protein binding, then the V_d becomes very large. The V_d can also be altered by a number of pathological conditions. If the V_d changes, then the plasma concentration changes as well.

Perhaps the easiest way to conceptualize PK principles is to think of the body as one large compartment. However,

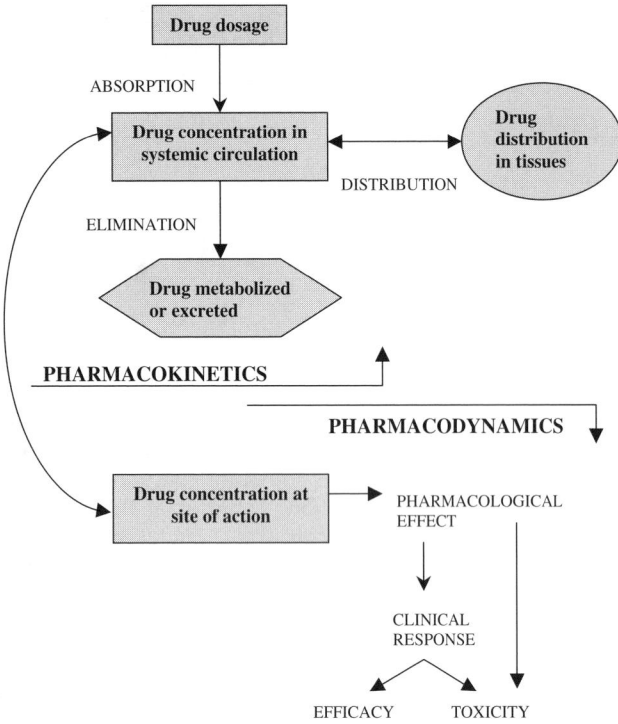

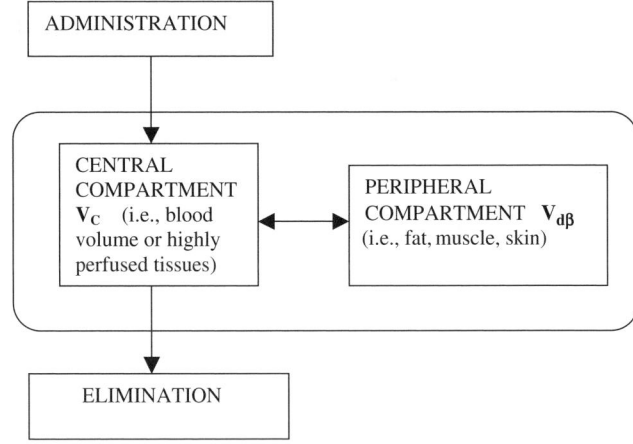

Figure 1　A schematic relationship between the concepts of pharmacokinetics (PK) (dose/concentration) and pharmacodynamics (PD) (concentration/effect). The key elements of pharmacokinetics include absorption, distribution, and elimination. The drug concentration at the site of pharmacological action links these two (PK and PD) concepts together. *Source*: Adapted from Ref. 1.

Figure 2　Schematic representation of a two-compartment pharmacokinetic model. Once the drug is administered and a percentage of it is absorbed (bioavailability), it will be distributed between all available compartments. Initially, the central compartment (V_c) will be exposed to the drug, and then the peripheral compartments ($V_{d\beta}$). During and after the distribution phase, elimination will occur. *Source*: Adapted from Ref. 3.

a multicompartment model is more appropriate when examining drug distribution, elimination, and movements between different parts of the body. Figure 2 represents a schematic of a two-compartment PK model where the drug is distributed between a central compartment (V_c) and a peripheral compartment ($V_{d\beta}$) (3).

Protein Binding

The plasma concentration that is reported by the laboratory represents protein-bound drug plus drug that is unbound.

Table 1　Routes of Administration and Bioavailability

Route	Bioavailability (%)	Comments
IV	100	Most rapid onset
IM	75 to ≤100	Increased volume of injection, may be painful
SC	75 to ≤100	Decreased volume of injection, may be painful
PO	5 to <100	Most convenient, first-pass effect may be large
PR	30 to <100	Less first-pass effect than oral
Inhalation	5 to <100	Often very rapid onset, no first pass effect; may cause bronchospasm
Transdermal	80 to ≤100	Slow absorption, no first-pass effect; convenience

Abbreviations: IM, intramuscularly; IV, intravenously; PO, by mouth; PR, per rectum; SC, subcutaneously.
Source: Adapted from Ref. 1.

☞ **The unbound ("free") drug molecule exerts the pharmacological effect by interacting with the cell receptor.** ☞ Two main plasma proteins bind drugs in the plasma: α_1-acid glycoprotein (basic drugs) and albumin (acidic and neutral drugs). This binding phenomenon is nonselective, meaning that other drugs with similar physiochemical properties can compete for binding sites. This competition can be concentration dependent or related to binding affinity with the plasma protein (2). For example, drugs A and B both bind to albumin but drug A has a higher binding affinity. Therefore, drug B may be displaced from the binding site yielding an increased "free" plasma concentration of drug B and therefore a greater pharmacological effect. The property of protein binding is of greatest concern for drugs that have a narrow therapeutic index (i.e., small range between subtherapeutic and toxic concentrations).

☞ **Protein-binding alterations occur in critically ill patients and must be considered in order to properly interpret measured drug concentrations and their predicted PD effects (4).** ☞ Certain physiological and disease states may alter the concentration of plasma proteins and therefore change the fraction of drug that is bound to these proteins. For example, nephrotic and cirrhotic patients commonly have low plasma albumin levels.

Trauma and burn patients also commonly suffer from low albumin levels following massive resuscitation. If these patients were to receive a drug, which is normally highly bound to albumin (e.g., phenytoin), then the fraction of drug that is unbound or free would be higher because fewer protein-binding sites are available to take it up. Accordingly, the PD effect would be greater than expected for the same measured drug concentration in a patient with normal albumin levels.

Clearance

Clearance (Cl) is defined as the volume of blood cleared of drug per unit of time. ☞ **The primary organs involved in clearance are the kidneys and the liver, but other organ systems (e.g., lungs) may be involved.** ☞ The total body clearance is the sum of the individual clearances as represented in Equation 3 (2,3).

$$Cl_{total} = Cl_{renal} + Cl_{liver} + Cl_{other} \quad (3)$$

Numerous factors affect drug Cl including plasma protein binding, extraction ratio, renal function, hepatic function, and cardiac output (Q). The Cl is reported in units of volume/time or if normalized to body weight, units of volume/body weight/time. If a patient is very large or small, but has normal organ function, there is an underlying assumption that the kidney and liver are proportionally large or small as well and therefore, clearance capabilities would be changed proportionately.

The extraction ratio is defined as the amount of drug that is removed after a single pass through the organ responsible for its clearance. It is proportional to the plasma or blood clearance of a drug and the plasma or blood flow to the eliminating organ. The impact of renal, hepatic, and cardiac failure on PK parameters will be discussed later.

Half-Life

The half-life ($t_{1/2}$) of a drug is the time it takes for the drug concentration in the body or plasma to be reduced by one-half. The half-life can be calculated as a function of the Cl and V_d (2).

$$t_{1/2} = \frac{0.693 \cdot V_d}{Cl} \quad (4)$$

The value of Cl/V_d is known as the elimination rate constant (K_d), so Equation 4 is often represented as shown in Equation 5:

$$t_{1/2} = \frac{0.693}{K_d} \quad (5)$$

In a similar fashion, the V_d can be calculated by combining the concepts derived in Equations 2–5, as shown in Equation 6.

$$V_d = \frac{Cl \cdot t_{1/2}}{0.693} \quad (6)$$

As the V_d and Cl change, the half-life changes also. In the simplest PK model (single compartment), the half-life is useful in determining an appropriate dosage interval as well as estimating the time it would take to eliminate the drug from the body. It takes five half-lives to reduce the concentration of a drug to about 3% of its original value once it has been discontinued.

It is also possible to estimate the time to reach steady state after the initiation or change of the maintenance dose. Steady state is defined as the state in which the amount of drug being administered in a given time period is equal to the amount eliminated in the same time period. In most clinical situations, it is appropriate to assume that steady state will be achieved after three to four half-lives have elapsed. However, many drugs display multiple compartment distribution and therefore equilibrate with each of the compartments at different rates. Half-lives reported in informational tables usually reflect the most clinically relevant half-life. For drugs administered intermittently, the clinical duration of action may be a more meaningful term (e.g., the time period that the drug concentration is within the clinically significant range).

Pharmacodynamics

The pharmacological response to a specific plasma drug concentration is defined as the PD effect of the drug. These effects result from the interaction of drugs with cellular macromolecules or receptors in the host organism. A number of factors can alter the PD response in critically ill patients. The pharmacological response to a drug is usually proportional to the unbound plasma concentration (i.e., PK properties). However, the specific PD response represents the interindividual variability in receptor binding and effect. Interindividual variations of responses to a given plasma drug concentration occur commonly. For example, the geriatric population is routinely more sensitive to the sedative effects of benzodiazepines than their younger counterparts (3). In addition, opioid-tolerant patients will require higher doses and blood levels to obtain adequate analgesia in the surgical intensive care unit (SICU).

In order for a drug to elicit a pharmacological response, it must be delivered and bound to the appropriate receptor. This drug–receptor complex can then evoke an effect. If the target site is heavily perfused (i.e., central circulation), then the pharmacological response is typically rapid. An example would be isoproterenol stimulation of the β_1-receptors in cardiac tissue resulting in tachycardia. Highly protein-bound drugs (e.g., phenytoin, valproic acid) may produce an increased pharmacological effect in the setting of hypoalbuminemia because only the free or unbound drug molecule binds to the target receptor. Many drugs also cause different pharmacological responses at different plasma drug concentrations. A classic example is the shift of pharmacological response with respect to α- and β-receptors which occurs as the dosage (and plasma concentration) of dopamine is increased.

ALTERATION OF PHARMACOKINETIC AND PHARMACODYNAMIC PARAMETERS IN THE CRITICALLY ILL

☞ **Multiple variables (PK and PD) affect the critically ill patient. Accordingly, multidisciplinary involvement and careful monitoring is required to optimize drug therapy.** ☞

A drug's PK parameters can be used to calculate an individualized drug regimen to assure optimal dosing. However, published PK parameters are usually determined in normal volunteers, and these values may not apply to critically ill patients. The clinician must therefore account for potential changes in these values based upon the disorders affecting their patients.

There are numerous reasons for alterations of PK and PD parameters in the critical-care setting. Organ failure, hyperdynamic states, disease-induced alterations in body physiology, acid–base disorders, and drug–drug interactions list some of the common confounders. Of these causes, organ failure is responsible for the majority of the changes in PK/PD parameters.

Organ Failure

Renal failure has an enormous impact on most drugs used in the ICU. Renal failure is easily detected because of the simplicity in recognizing "abnormal serum creatinine"; and changes in the urine output are easily detected in critically ill patients. ☞ **Glomerular filtration rate (GFR) is often estimated based on a patient's serum creatinine and ideal body weight. Since critically ill patients may have a decrease in** muscle mass, creatinine clearance (and GFR) can be overestimated. ☞

Liver function tests (LFTs) can indicate potential liver dysfunction (see Volume 2, Chapter 35); but, depending on the site of dysfunction, abnormal LFTs may or may not indicate an alteration in the PK or PD properties of a drug. Gastrointestinal (GI) changes can impact the bioavailability by altering the first-pass metabolism of enterally administered drugs. Cardiovascular dysfunction can cause hepatic congestion, which can decrease the drug metabolizing capacity of the liver. The following sections further discuss the failure of individual organ systems and their influence on the PK/PD parameters.

Renal

Many drugs depend at least in part on the kidneys for their excretion. Critically ill patients may already have or will develop renal failure during their course of stay in the ICU. Many medications can cause nephrotoxicity and renal insufficiency, and the clinician should assess whether medications are contributing to renal dysfunction (Table 2) (5,6). Renal dysfunction can alter both the V_d and ultimately the Cl of some drugs.

If renal excretion accounts for more than 30% of the total Cl of a drug, changes in renal function can have a significant impact on the PK of the drug. In drugs with a narrow therapeutic index, this change is much more important and alterations in renal clearance may necessitate dosage adjustment. Numerous sources of established guidelines for adjusting the drug dosages based on the degree of renal dysfunction exist (7). However, these guidelines are only first approximations to dose adjustments, and the physician must consider the patient's entire clinical picture and individualize the therapy. For drugs with a narrow therapeutic index, checking the serum drug level and performing a formal PK analysis is generally recommended.

☞ If renal dysfunction is severe enough to require dialysis, dosage adjustment is often required. ☞ Various types of dialysis require different dosage modifications. Intermittent hemodialysis is the most frequently employed modality outside of the SICU. Dosage adjustment guidelines for anuric patients on intermittent dialysis have been established for most drugs (7). A full or partial supplemental dose is recommended for some drugs that are cleared by hemodialysis.

Advances in continuous renal replacement therapy (CRRT) and the recognition that CRRT causes less perturbations to other organ systems have resulted in increased usage of this mode in unstable, critically ill patients. However, there are few well-established guidelines for dosage adjustments for many drugs that are given during CRRT. This is, in part, due to the fact that CRRT can be accomplished by several different modalities. Depending on the technique used, the dosage adjustments may be different. Continuous veno-venous hemodiafiltration (CVVHDF) has become a standard modality employed in most advanced ICUs.

Some drugs can be cleared by CVVHDF, and this clearance can be divided into three different processes (Table 3). Drugs can be cleared by diffusion (dialysis), convection (hemofiltration), and adsorption to the filter. The clearance by diffusion depends on the dialysate flow rate as well as on dialysate saturation (concentration of drug in dialysate divided by concentration of drug in plasma). This process depends on the molecular size, membrane pore size and its thickness, blood flow, and protein binding. During the convection process, as fluid (plasma water) gets filtered by hemofiltration, dissolved solutes (drugs) in the fluid are removed. This elimination depends on the drug's sieving

Table 2   Select Medications that Can Cause Renal Structural and Functional Changes

Acyclovir[c]	Hydralazine[d]
Aminoglycosides[a]	Indinavir[c]
Amphotericin B[a]	Intravenous immunoglobulin[a]
ACE inhibitors[b]	Lithium[e]
Angiotensin II	Mannitol[a]
receptor antagonists[b]	Methamphetamines[f]
Carboplatin[a]	Methicillin[e]
Cimetidine[g]	Mitomycin C[f]
Cisplatin[a]	NSAIDs[b,d,e]
Corticosteroids[g]	Radiographic contrast media[a]
Cyclosporine[e]	Sulfadiazine[c]
Cytokine therapy[d]	Triamterene[c]
Foscarnet[c]	Tricyclic antidepressants[c]
Gold[d]	Trimethoprim[g]

[a]Tubular epithelial cell damage.
[b]Hemodynamically mediated.
[c]Obstructive nephropathy.
[d]Glomerular disease.
[e]Tubulointerstitial disease.
[f]Renal vasculitis and thrombosis.
[g]Pseudo-renal failure.
Abbreviations: ACE, angiotensin-converting enzyme; NSAIDs, nonsteroidal anti-inflammatory drugs.
Source: Adapted from Refs. 5,6.

Table 3   Three Different Processes for Drug Clearance by Continuous Veno-venous Hemodiafiltration

Diffusion process (hemodialysis)
   Drugs pass through membrane from high concentration (blood) to lower concentration (dialysis)
   Process depends on
     Molecular weight
       Small and medium size drugs can easily pass through
       Larger (1000–5,000 dalton) drugs can pass through highly permeable membranes
     Protein binding
     Membrane pore size and thickness
     Blood flow and dialysate flow
     Concentration of unbound drug (only unbound drug can diffuse)
Convection process (hemofiltration)
   As fluid (plasma water) is removed, drugs dissolved in fluid are removed
   Process depends on
     Sieving coefficient
     Protein binding
     Filtration rate
Adsorption to filter
   Dependent upon type of filter used
     High flux (has large pore size leading to enhanced clearance of larger drugs)
     High efficiency (increased surface area leading to enhanced clearance of small solutes)

coefficient (the capacity of the drug to pass the membrane by convection) and the filtration rate. The sieving coefficient can be calculated directly by dividing the concentration of drug in the filtrate by the concentration of drug in the plasma. Drug removal via adsorption is not very well understood. Certain types of hemofilters (e.g., AN60S) are known to adsorb some drugs (e.g., aminoglycosides). This process is variable and can be a saturable process.

☞ **In general, the CVVHDF removal of small drugs depends on the diffusion and convection process, whereas removal of larger drugs depends mostly on convection and perhaps adsorption properties.** ☞ The total clearance of a drug is equal to CRRT clearance plus all other non-CRRT clearance. The non-CRRT clearance can be defined as the sum of hepatic, pulmonary, and other types of clearance plus any residual renal clearance.

A simple dosage adjustment guideline for CVVHDF (Fig. 3) has been developed (7 – 13). First, if the drug is normally cleared primarily via nonrenal routes, then it most likely does not have appreciable CRRT clearance (rare exceptions occur, e.g., phenobarbital). If the drug is cleared primarily by the renal route (more than one-third of the total clearance), then most likely there will be some degree of CRRT clearance. Second, if the drug has a narrow therapeutic index, the estimate of CRRT clearance must be accurately determined. In contrast, if it has a broad therapeutic index, the calculation of CRRT clearance can be estimated using clinical experience. Third, initial dosing for patients on CVVHDF should follow established guidelines tailored to the patient's clinical picture (7,8,14). Fourth, the patient's clinical course, as well as the CRRT parameters (blood flow rate, dialysis rate, ultrafiltrate rate, hemofilter), must be monitored closely. Fifth, significant changes in clinical status or CRRT parameters often require readjusting the dosage. For narrow therapeutic index drugs, the serum drug concentrations should be checked within the first 24 to 48 hours. Using the serum drug levels, PK analysis should be performed, and an individualized dosage can be developed. Finally, some inconsistencies exist with the CRRT drug clearance literature as there can often be more than one dosage recommendation for the same drug (15,16). The data may be derived from different modalities of CRRT in which CRRT parameters may have not been similar and the patient population may have been different. One must always account for the patient's residual renal function, and as the renal function improves, the possibility of improvement in renal clearance for some drugs exists.

If the renal function has not improved, but the patient is hemodynamically stable enough to tolerate intermittent dialysis, CRRT may be discontinued. In this case, the contribution of CRRT to the clearance of drugs is also stopped and dosage adjustments may be justified.

In summary, the CRRT clearance of a given drug is clinically important when it accounts for more than one-third of the total clearance. Drugs that are highly protein bound (e.g., phenytoin) or have large volumes of distribution (e.g., digoxin, cyclosporine) are not readily available for CRRT clearance. For narrow therapeutic index drugs, frequent monitoring of serum drug levels, clinical status, and CRRT parameters is essential.

Hepatic

☞ **Up to 54% of critically ill patients will develop some degree of liver dysfunction (17).** ☞ This can result from hypoperfusion due to decreased liver blood flow due to hypovolemia or cardiovascular dysfunction or can occur because of intrinsic changes such as altered hepatic microsomal enzyme activities associated with age, fever, stress, drug interactions, and hepatocellular damage. Both of these factors (hypoperfusion and intrinsic liver disease) can contribute to a decrease in hepatic drug metabolism (Table 4). Unlike renal dysfunction, which is relatively easy to quantify, the degree of liver dysfunction can be difficult to assess and the correlation with drug clearance is less consistent.

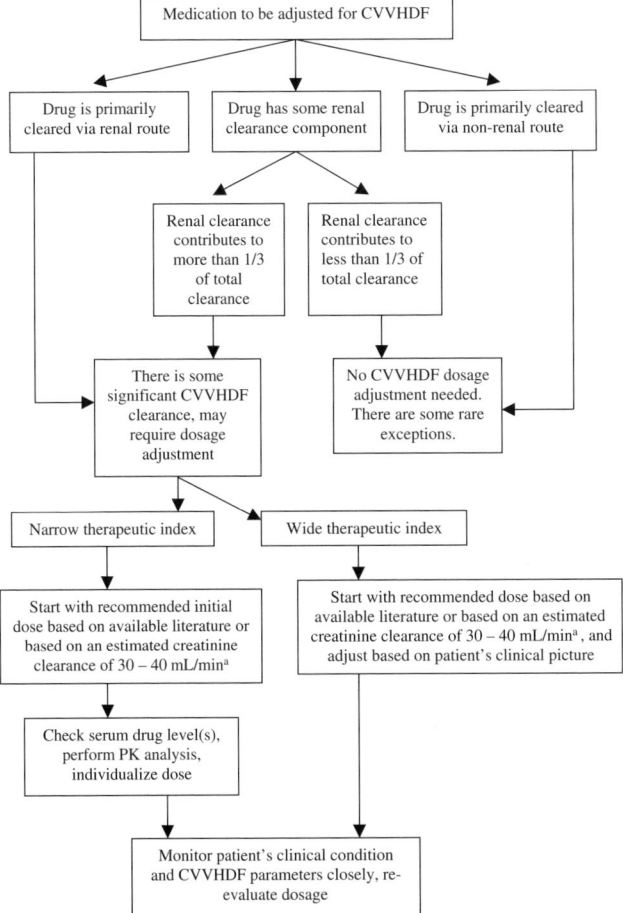

Figure 3 Decision tree for the management of drug dosing during continuous renal replacement therapy. ᵃEstimated creatinine clearance of 30–40 mL/min based on a CVVHDF combined clearance of 2000 mL/hr (dialysis + ultrafiltrate). *Abbreviations*: CVVHDF, continuous veno-venous hemodiafiltration, PK, pharmacokinetic.

Table 4 Factors that Can Decrease Hepatic Metabolism of Drugs in Critically Ill Patients

Hypoperfusion (decrease in hepatic blood flow)
   Hypovolemia
   Cardiovascular dysfunction
Intrinsic (altered hepatic enzyme activities)
   Age
   Fever
   Stress
   Systemic inflammatory response syndrome
   Hepatocellular damage
   Drug interactions

The liver is the site of metabolism for many drugs used in critically ill patients (4). In addition, some medications are hepatotoxic, especially if allowed to achieve high plasma concentrations, and can subsequently cause syndromes of hepatocellular necrosis, cholestasis, granulomas, fatty changes, or even chronic active hepatitis (Table 5) (18,19). Few well-established guidelines exist for adjusting medication dosages for hepatic dysfunction. One approach is to estimate the relevance of liver dysfunction by considering the contribution of liver metabolism to the total clearance of the drug. If this is more than 30%, then an empirical decrease in the drug dosage is often necessary in the setting of liver dysfunction.

A few specific drugs do have dosing recommendations based on the degree of hepatic dysfunction. For example, caspofungin, an IV antifungal agent, needs to be dose reduced based on the patient's Child–Pugh score (20). Metronidazole, a commonly prescribed antibiotic with anaerobic efficacy, carries a recommendation for a reduction in the dosage quantity or administration frequency depending on the clinical response and degree of hepatic dysfunction (20). The maintenance dose of sirolimus, an immunosuppressant, should be reduced by one-third for patients with mild to moderate hepatic impairment (20). Table 6 contains a select list of medications whose PK parameters may be affected by liver dysfunction and recommendations for dosage adjustments if available.

For drugs with a narrow therapeutic index, serum drug levels should be checked, PK analysis should be performed, and an individualized dose should be calculated. However, if the drug has a broad therapeutic index, the

Table 5   Select Medications that Can Cause Hepatotoxicity

Acetaminophen[a]	Haloperidol[b]	Phenobarbital[c]
Allopurinol[a]	Hydralazine[c,d]	Phenytoin[c,d]
Amiodarone[c,e]	Hydroxyurea[c]	Phenothiazines[b]
Ampicillin[a]	Ibuprofen[a]	Probenecid[a]
Azathioprine[c]	Indomethacin[a]	Procainamide[c,d]
Carbamazepine[a,b,d]	Isoniazid[a]	Propoxyphene[b]
Chlordiazepoxide[b]	Ketoconazole[a]	Propylthiouracil[c]
Chlorpropamide[b]	L-asparaginase[a,d]	Quinidine[c,d]
Clindamycin[a]	MAO inhibitors[a]	Ranitidine[c]
Cimetidine[c]	Methimazole[b]	Rifampin[a]
Contraceptives, oral[b]	Methotrexate[a,d]	Salicylates[a]
Corticosteroids[e]	Methyldopa[c,d,f]	Spironolactone[c]
Cyclophosphamide[c]	Metolazone[a,d]	Sulfonamides[c,d]
Dapsone[c]	Metronidazole[c]	Tetracyclines[a,e]
Diazepam[b]	Naproxen[c]	Thiazides[b]
Dicloxacillin[b]	Niacin[c]	Trazodone[a]
Diltiazem[d]	Nifedipine[c]	Tricyclic
Disopyramide[a]	Nitrofurantoin[c,d,f]	antidepressants[c]
Erythromycins[b]	Oxacillin[a,d]	Valproic acid[a,e]
Flurazepam[b]	Penicillin[c,d]	Verapamil[a]
Glyburide[a]	Phenazopyridine[a]	Warfarin[b]

[a]Hepatocellular necrosis.
[b]Cholestasis.
[c]Necrosis or cholestasis or both.
[d]Granulomas.
[e]Fatty change.
[f]Chronic active hepatitis.
Abbreviation: MAO, monoamine oxidase.
Source: Adapted from Refs. 18,19.

Table 6   Medications Whose Pharmacokinetic Parameters May Be Affected by Liver Dysfunction and Recommendations for Dosage Adjustment

Acyclovir[d,i]	Dobutamine[d,e,i]	Meropenem[d,i]
Amiodarone[a,d]	Dopamine[d,e,i]	Metronidazole[h]
Amphotericin B[d,i]	Enoxaparin[d,i]	Midazolam[b,d]
Azithromycin[d,i]	Epinephrine[d,e,i]	Milrinone[d,e,i]
Bumetanide[d,i]	Erythromycin[b,d]	Morphine[d,e]
Carbamazepine[b,d]	Esmolol[d,e,i]	Nafcillin[d,i]
Caspofungin[c]	Fentanyl[d,e,i]	Nitroprusside[d,e,i]
Cefazolin[d,i]	Fluconazole[d,i]	Norepinephrine[e]
Cefotaxime[d,i]	Foscarnet[d,i]	Oxacillin[d,i]
Cefotetan[d,i]	Furosemide[d,i]	Pancuronium[d,e,i]
Ceftazidime[d,i]	Haloperidol[d]	Penicillin[d,i]
Ceftriaxone[i]	Heparin[d,i]	Phenobarbital[a,d,f]
Cefuroxime[d,i]	Hydromorphone[d,e]	Phenytoin[d,e,f]
Ciprofloxacin[i]	Imipenem[d,i]	Procainamide[d,e,f]
Clarithromycin[d,i]	Itraconazole[d]	Dalfopristin-
Cyclosporine[b]	Levofloxacin[d,i,j]	Quinapristin[d,i]
Daltoparin[d,i]	Lidocaine[b,f]	Septra[d,i]
Dexmedetomidine[a,d,e]	Liposomal	Sirolimus[g,f]
Digoxin[d,f,i]	Amphotericin B[d,i]	Tacrolimus[b,f]
Diltiazem[b,e]	Lorazepam[a,b]	Valproic acid[f]
	Meperidine[d,e]	Vecuronium[d,e,i]

[a]Initial dose reduction recommended while monitoring for toxicity.
[b]Dose reductions may be needed.
[c]Dose reduction based on Child–Pugh score.
[d]No specific quantitative dose adjustment guidelines available; monitor closely.
[e]Dosage should be based upon clinical response.
[f]Dosage should be based upon serum level monitoring.
[g]Recommended to reduce maintenance dose by one-third in mild to moderate hepatic impairment.
[h]Daily dose may need to be reduced by 50% to 60% in severe hepatic disease.
[i]No dose adjustment needed with hepatic dysfunction alone.
[j]Avoid use in patients with active hepatic disease/impairment because of risk of severe hepatotoxicity.
Source: Adapted from Ref. 20.

patient's clinical picture and health care provider's assessment and experience can be used to guide an appropriate dosage. In either case, it is important to monitor the clinical course, therapeutic responses, and look for adverse effects.

In liver dysfunction, the effect of drug–drug interactions can be magnified. For example, if the hepatically cleared drug "A" can attenuate the metabolism of drug "B," and if the metabolism of drug "A" decreases as a result of liver dysfunction, not only can drug "A" accumulate and cause adverse effects, but also drug "B" could potentially accumulate and cause adverse effects. It may be difficult to evaluate whether decreased liver metabolism is due to liver dysfunction or decreased perfusion (21).

Drugs associated with increased elimination secondary to the first-pass phenomenon (described earlier) depend upon hepatic blood flow (22). If this blood flow is impaired, as in the setting of cirrhosis, portosystemic shunts are generated in order to bypass the liver. With this bypass, drugs that are normally subjected to a high degree of first-pass metabolism may have an increased bioavailability. Table 7 lists a select number of medications that undergo

Table 7 Medications with Marked First-Pass Removal

Aspirin	Metoprolol
Chlorpromazine	Morphine
Propoxyphene	Meperidine
Nitroglycerin	Prazosin
Hydralazine	Propranolol
Isoproterenol	Albuterol
Isosorbide dinitrate	Terbutaline
Labetalol	Verapamil
Lidocaine	

Source: Adapted from Ref. 23.

this first-pass phenomenon. ☞ **In critically ill patients with multiorgan failure, the net effect on drug metabolism is difficult to predict and must be carefully monitored.** ☞

Cardiovascular

Acute decompensated heart failure (ADHF) is characterized by low Q̇ and increased organ congestion. With the elevated right heart filling pressures and pulmonary hypertension seen with heart failure, renal, liver, and gut congestion may exist (23,24). With the associated low cardiac output state, perfusion to these organs is compromised as well. ☞ **ADHF can lead to an impairment of drug clearance and/or a reduction in the V_d by underperfusing organs responsible for metabolism or elimination (i.e., liver and kidneys) (23).** ☞ With changes in the clearance and volume of distribution, the half-life of a drug is usually affected. Medications that are titrated to effect (i.e., nitrates, diuretics, vasopressors) will be impacted to a lesser degree by the alteration of PK parameters.

Incomplete absorption of drugs from the GI tract can be related to the blood flow to the upper small bowel (primary site of drug absorption). If Q̇ is diminished, blood flow to the bowel is reduced and enteral absorption could be impaired. Congestion and gut edema have been implicated in the malabsorption of drugs (23). Other routes of drug administration may be affected by heart failure. Absorption of intramuscularly administered drugs is directly related to the blood flow to that muscle site. If Q̇ is reduced (as in cardiogenic shock or decompensated heart failure), absorption will be erratic and potentially impaired; therefore, intramuscular administration of drugs should be avoided unless no other administration options are available.

The main site of hepatic drug metabolism is the cytochrome P450 (CP450) enzyme system. This enzyme system is the rate-limiting step in drug metabolism, and decompensated heart failure can cause hepatic congestion, which may impair the metabolizing capacity of the P450 enzyme system (23). This impairment can lead to drug accumulation and potentially unwanted side effects.

Drugs that are eliminated from the body through the kidneys may accumulate during renal insufficiency. Decompensated heart failure and a low Q̇ state can lead to decreased renal perfusion and subsequent renal insufficiency. In this setting, modified administration regimens that decrease the dose or an increase in the dosing interval (or a combination of the two) should be employed. In particular, with ADHF and subsequent renal hypoperfusion, the renin–angiotensin system is stimulated to increase GFR. This process works independently of the effects on systemic blood pressure. In patients who have their angiotensin-converting enzyme (ACE) system inhibited, the decrease in

GFR can become more profound. This decrease in GFR can also contribute to drug toxicity (25).

One might incorrectly surmise that a drug's V_d would be increased in ADHF because of the commonly associated fluid retention. In fact, the excess fluid is generally restricted to the extravascular space and therefore is unable to directly participate in the distribution of drugs (23). The central volume in heart failure patients is actually reduced; therefore, the V_d of most drugs is reduced as well. Because the initial plasma concentration that results from a loading dose is dependent upon the V_d, an empiric reduction in the loading dose is often warranted to avoid toxic concentrations of narrow therapeutic index drugs (e.g., digoxin) (23).

The half-life of a drug is dependent upon the drug Cl and V_d (Equation 4). In ADHF, both of these parameters can be altered and therefore, drug elimination half-life may be altered. ☞ **Drugs with a narrow therapeutic index (i.e., digoxin, lidocaine, procainamide) require enhanced drug monitoring in patients with heart failure.** ☞

Endothelial (Burn)

Burn injury can cause marked changes in the PK and PD properties of some drugs (Table 8). Depending on the extent of the burn, the V_d, protein binding and Cl of some drugs can be altered. It is important to understand different phases of burn injury.

The acute phase (first 48 hours) of injury is characterized by fluid loss from the vascular system (26). This causes a drop in Q̇ and a decrease in tissue and organ perfusion. This phase is often managed with aggressive fluid resuscitation (e.g., hypertonic saline solutions), which can cause an increase in the V_d of some drugs, whereas the renal and hepatic hypoperfusion can decrease the Cl of some drugs.

The next phase begins immediately after the burn and may worsen 48 hours after the burn injury and consists of a hypermetabolic state. During this phase, the Q̇ is increased (provided the fluid repletion was adequate) as are kidney and liver blood flows (26). As a result, the Cl of some drugs (e.g., vancomycin) and neuromuscular blockade (NMB) agents is increased. Therefore, some dosage adjustments are needed to avoid subtherapeutic levels. This is most important for narrow therapeutic index drugs. Burn injuries can also cause hypoalbuminemia, increasing the free fraction of drugs that are normally highly bound to albumin (e.g., phenytoin). Consequently, there will be more

Table 8 Alteration of Pharmacokinetic Parameters After Massive Trauma or Burn Injury

Resuscitation phase (first 48 hrs)
↓ cardiac output
    ↓ renal perfusion (↓ renal clearance)
    ↓ hepatic perfusion (↓ hepatic clearance)
    ↑ volume of distribution
    ↑ intestinal permeability (changes in enteral absorption)
    ↓ albumin (changes in protein binding)
Hypermetabolic phase (after resuscitation phase)
↑ cardiac output
    ↑ renal perfusion (↑ renal clearance)
    ↑ hepatic perfusion (↑ hepatic clearance)
    ↓ albumin (changes in protein binding)
    ↑ α-1-acid glycoprotein (changes in protein binding)

unbound drug available to elicit its pharmacological action, increasing the potential for adverse effects. It may be necessary to calculate the total as well as free drug levels. Burn injury can also result in an increase in α-1-acid glycoprotein production (26). Drugs that are highly bound to this protein (e.g., carbamazepine) will have a lower amount of unbound (pharmacologically active) drug available. Therefore, the dosage of these drugs may need to be increased.

    ☞ **The clearance of some drugs during the hypermetabolic phase of burn injury may be increased.** ☞ The dosage of drugs with a narrow therapeutic index may require adjustment based on PK serum level analysis. For wide therapeutic index drugs, some empirical adjustments, based on available recommendations and the patient's clinical picture, can be used.

Central Nervous System

The PK and PD parameters of sedative and analgesics are altered in critically ill patients (27,28). The perception of pain can be affected by emotional and cognitive processes, as well as the physical restrictions of ICU patients. Sedative and analgesics are usually highly protein bound and depend on the liver for their metabolism. Change in protein binding, liver function, or perfusion can significantly impact therapeutic as well as adverse effects.

    In the setting of decreased liver and kidney perfusion, the clearance of these drugs is often reduced, necessitating significant decreases in dosage. Most of the commonly used sedatives and analgesic drugs used in the ICU exhibit multicompartment PK characteristics. With a typically prolonged course of exposure, they can accumulate. Critically ill patients may have an increased peak effect, faster onset of action, and a prolonged duration of action (27).

    Among the benzodiazepine class, lorazepam and midazolam are the most frequently used agents (29 − 32). Midazolam has a faster onset of action than lorazepam due to its increased lipophilicity and is metabolized to active compounds that are renally eliminated. Lorazepam has a longer duration of action; however, for prolonged use (continuous infusion over several days), lorazepam may be a better choice in critically ill patients because there are no active metabolites (29,30). Propofol, an IV anesthetic commonly used for ICU sedation, has a rapid onset and short duration of action. It does not appear to have major changes in its PK parameters in patients with renal and/or hepatic dysfunction (32).

    Many drugs that are commonly used in critically ill patients can cause QT interval prolongation, leading to possible ventricular dysrhythmias (e.g., Torsades de Pointes). Some antipsychotic medications (e.g., haloperidol, thioridazine, mesoridazine, chlorpromazine) and some other centrally acting drugs (e.g., droperidol and venlafaxine) are just a few drugs that carry a risk of prolonging the QT interval. Close monitoring of the electrocardiogram and attention to normal levels of magnesium and potassium are required when using these agents in critically ill patients with underlying conduction defects.

    The use of NMB drugs has been minimized in most modern ICUs. However, NMBs are still commonly employed for intubation and occasionally used during the treatment of patients with severe traumatic brain injury (TBI) and for acute respiratory distress syndrome (ARDS). The most common PK alteration for these NMB drugs in critically ill patients is related to changes in clearance.

Clearance is decreased by deterioration in renal, hepatic, cardiovascular, and endothelial systems (discussed earlier).

    Pancuronium is mostly cleared by the kidneys and any decrease in renal function or perfusion can result in its accumulation (30,33). Liver failure can cause a decrease in clearance of hepatically metabolized NMBs such as vecuronium because of an increase in their volume of distribution. Vecuronium is 85% cleared via the biliary route. Thus, any decrease in liver metabolism or perfusion can decrease its clearance (30). Cisatracurium relies on pH-dependent Hofmann elimination and nonspecific enzymatic ester hydrolysis for its clearance rather than the liver or kidney (34,35). ☞ **Cisatracurium is the ideal NMB drug for critically ill patients with liver and renal failure who require only a brief period of NMB.** ☞ Hypothermia and acidosis can slightly decrease the clearance of cisatracurium (36). However, this is rarely clinically significant. Important drug–drug interactions involving NMB drugs include corticosteroids, aminoglycosides, magnesium, and other agents that affect neuromuscular transmission can lead to the development of an acute myopathy in ICU patients (33).

Gastrointestinal

Critically ill patients often suffer altered GI motility (37). Changes in GI motility or changes in GI tract pH can affect the absorption and GI metabolism of some drugs. Postoperatively, patients can have hypoactive GI tracts secondary to the procedure or the use of opioid analgesics during the surgery or ICU stay. With some success, prokinetic agents have been used to improve gastric emptying and tolerability of enteral feeding (38,39). The effect of these prokinetic agents on drug absorption may not be easy to assess. Hyperactive GI motility is less frequently found in critically ill patients. This may be drug induced or result from the disease state. Often ICU patients are nutritionally supported with continuous enteral tube feedings which can interfere with the absorption of several drugs.

    In many ICU patients, it is standard practice to use protective agents to prevent the development of stress-induced gastritis (e.g., H_2-antagonists, proton pump inhibitors). Most of these agents cause an increase in gastric pH. This increase in pH can be detrimental to the absorption of some medications (e.g., itraconazole capsules) that require an acidic gastric environment for maximal absorption. Frequent presence of an ileus and decreased splanchnic perfusion may decrease the absorption of enterally administered drugs (40). Therefore, the IV route of administration is preferred in unstable ICU patients. However, this route of administration does have its inherent risks (infection) and costs. When GI absorption returns to a more reliable state, it is more desirable to give drugs by the GI route.

Respiratory

Respiratory failure does not generally have any direct impact on the PK or PD of a drug. However, indirectly it can cause changes in hepatic (hypoxemia) and renal (respiratory alkalosis or acidosis) clearance of some drugs (30). The pulmonary circulation also plays an important role in the metabolism of norepinephrine, angiotensin, and serotonin (40).

Muscle Disorders

Muscular disorders can be seen in critically ill patients. These can be associated with myopathy and neuromyopathy. In hemodynamically unstable patients the alteration in muscle perfusion can alter the intramuscular absorption of some drugs. The use of NMB drugs have the potential for causing or exacerbating neuropathy and myopathy, especially in patients with sepsis, poor glucose control, and those receiving steroids. Therefore, NMB drugs should be carefully monitored, used only when absolutely necessary (30), and discontinued as soon as possible (also see Volume 2, Chapter 6).

Hyperdynamic State

Some critically ill trauma patients experience an increased clearance of some drugs. For example, many patients with an extensive burn injury or closed head injury experience an early increase in metabolic rate. Therefore, for drugs with a narrow therapeutic range, it is important to monitor drug levels and perform PK studies early and repeatedly.

Acid–Base Disorders

☞ **Acidosis or alkalosis can change the protein binding of drugs (40).** ☞ However, the direct effects of acid–base disorders on PK and PD parameters of drugs in critically ill patients are not well studied. For highly protein-bound drugs, these changes are more profound. If there is an increase in the free fraction of drugs, the risks of adverse effects will be increased. In contrast, a decrease in the free fraction of a drug can lead to decreased therapeutic effect and potentially treatment failure. Changes in protein binding also can alter the V_d of drugs and consequently affect their Cl. Some drugs (e.g., cisatracurium) rely on pH-dependent Hofmann elimination and nonspecific enzymatic ester hydrolysis for their Cl (34). Acidosis causes a decrease in this clearance with a corresponding increased risk of accumulation. Respiratory acidosis can lead to a trapping of fentanyl within the central nervous system (CNS), prolonging and potentiating its effects (32). Alkalosis increases the lipophilicity of morphine and fentanyl, which can generate higher CNS levels during the initial distribution phase (32).

Drug Interactions

Mechanisms by which drugs can interact can be categorized into PK, PD, or combined interactions. PK interactions include those that alter absorption, distribution, metabolism, or excretion and are the most important. PD interactions include those that alter the effect of the drug on the body. Combined interactions are those that occur when two or more drugs are used together and increase the likelihood of combined toxicity (41).

Absorption

☞ **There are several ways by which the GI absorption of drugs may be affected,** ☞ such as the concurrent use of other drugs that (*i*) bind or chelate, (*ii*) have a large surface area for adsorption, (*iii*) alter gastric pH, (*iv*) alter GI motility, or (*v*) affect the GI transport proteins (41).

A classic example of binding and chelation involves the fluoroquinolone antibiotic class and the presence of divalent or trivalent cations commonly found in antacids, iron salts, dairy products, or continuous enteral feeding. It is recommended to not administer these cations enterally for two hours before or up to six hours after an oral dose of fluoroquinolone (42).

Activated charcoal is an example of a substance with a very large surface area available for drug adsorption and is commonly employed for reducing the absorption of toxic substances. Volume 1, Chapter 31 includes a discussion of the use of activated charcoal in treatments of poisonings.

Certain medications alter the pH of the stomach, and this can impact the degree of absorption. H2-antagonists (e.g., famotidine) or proton pump inhibitors (e.g., lansoprazole) can raise the gastric pH and alter the absorption of certain drugs. For example, itraconazole is an antifungal that requires an acidic environment in the stomach for optimal absorption. If the gastric pH is elevated, absorption can be impaired. Drugs that modify GI motility can also impact drug absorption (30).

Promotility agents (e.g., metoclopramide) can decrease intestinal transit time and therefore decrease the time a drug is in contact with absorptive surfaces in the GI tract. Inhibition of the GI transport proteins (e.g., PGP) can hinder the transluminal movement of drugs and ultimately the extent of absorption. It is important to understand the difference between rate and extent of absorption when discussing drug interactions. If the rate of absorption is reduced, it may not be clinically relevant but if the extent of absorption is reduced, there are usually clinical consequences.

Most modern ICUs support the early initiation of enteral nutrition. Some oral medications are not compatible with enteral nutrition, and knowledge of these interactions will help the clinician decide whether the enteral route of drug administration is desirable. Most drug interactions that occur with continuous feeding involve decreased or unpredictable absorption (43,44). Some common medications known to interact with continuous enteral nutrition are listed in Table 9. Medications with incompatibilities with tube feedings should not be mixed into the enteral formula. Rather, these should be administered separately, after evacuating the stomach contents, and subsequent tube feedings should be held one to two hours. Alternatively, different drugs, or route of administration can be selected.

Many commonly used medications in the critical care setting should not be crushed and administered via a feeding tube. In general, any product that is enteric coated or labeled as delayed-release, sustained-release, or extended-release should not be crushed (45). Always consult a pharmacist for alternatives.

Distribution

Drug interactions can alter drug distribution by two main mechanisms: (*i*) plasma protein binding competition and (*ii*) displacement from tissue-binding sites. When a drug competes with another drug for protein-binding sites, there is an increased concentration of free drug (i.e., unbound)

Table 9 Common Oral Medications that Interact with Continuous Enteral Nutrition

Carbamazepine (suspension)
Fluoroquinolones (e.g., ciprofloxacin, gatifloxacin)
Hydralazine
Levothyroxine sodium
Penicillin V potassium
Phenytoin sodium
Sucralfate
Theophylline
Warfarin

Source: Adapted from Ref. 45.

that is displaced into the plasma. This could increase the risk of adverse effects. If a drug were to be displaced from its tissue-binding site, then there would be a corresponding increase in the plasma concentration of the displaced drug; however, the clinical importance of this specific alteration is not clear (41).

Metabolism (Cytochrome P450 Enzyme System)

The CP450 isoenzymes are a group of heme-containing enzymes found primarily in the lipid bilayer of the endoplasmic reticulum of hepatocytes. They play a crucial role in the oxidative metabolism of exogenous (e.g., drugs) and endogenous substances (4,23,30,46,47). Other areas where these isoenzymes are found are the enterocytes of the small intestine and to a lesser extent in the kidneys, lungs, and brain. The way the isoenzymes are classified is based on family, subfamily, and individual gene (e.g., CP3A4). With the knowledge of individual substrates, inducers, and inhibitors of each isoenzyme, clinicians may be able to predict clinically important drug–drug interactions.

Differences do exist between patients, which include genetic polymorphism in the functional expression of some of the isoenzyme systems (e.g., CP2C9, CP2C19, and CP2D6) (47). This can lead to underexpression or overexpression of the enzyme system, which in turn can lead to adverse effects and/or therapeutic failures by either inhibiting or inducing metabolism. Other influences that can lead to variation in drug metabolism include age, nutrition, stress, hepatic disease, hormones, and other endogenous chemicals (48). The predominant enzyme systems responsible for most drug metabolism include CP3A4, CP2D6, CP1A2, and the CP2C subfamily.

Some drugs are metabolized by several isoenzyme systems, so it may be difficult to predict the magnitude of a drug–drug interaction if only one of the isoenzyme systems is being inhibited or induced. Also, some drugs may inhibit one isoenzyme system and be a substrate for another. For example, fluoxetine is an inhibitor of the CP3A4 enzyme, but it is metabolized by the CP2D6 enzyme system.

Inhibition of the CP450 system most often occurs as a result of competitive binding at the enzyme's active site (46). This inhibition is dependent on a few factors: binding affinity of both drugs, concentration of the substrate required for inhibition, and half-life of the inhibiting drug (46). Another important piece of information the clinician needs in order to interpret or predict drug–drug interactions is the onset and offset of enzyme inhibition. This is related to the half-life and time to steady state of the inhibiting drug. Classic examples would be cimetidine, which inhibits CP1A2 within 24 hours after a single dose, and amiodarone, which may take several months to inhibit CP3A4 because of its long half-life and considerable length of time to reach steady-state serum concentrations. Another common way by which inhibition may take place is noncompetitively, which results in inactivation of the enzyme by the inhibitor with normal substrate binding (46).

Enzyme induction is evidenced by an increase in hepatic blood flow or increased synthesis of the metabolizing CP450 enzymes (46). For example, enzyme-inducing anticonvulsants (e.g., phenobarbital) cause an increase in absolute liver size. Similar to enzyme inhibition, the effects of induction depend upon the precipitating drug's half-life. For example, rifampin has a relatively short

half-life and enzyme induction becomes apparent within 24 hours (46). Phenobarbital's half-life is much longer and therefore it may take 7 to 14 days before the effects of induction are seen (46). Once the causative drug is discontinued, the duration of induction depends on the half-life of the drug and the CP450 enzyme (half-life of one to six days). For example, once rifampin (half-life of three to five hours) has been discontinued, the duration or length of induction will be determined by the CP450 degradation time, not rifampin's presence in the body. Age, cirrhosis, and hepatitis may also impact the degree of induction.

With the knowledge of the CP450 enzyme systems and drugs that are known to be substrates, inducers, and inhibitors, health-care practitioners may be able to anticipate clinically important drug–drug interactions. This is most important for narrow therapeutic index drugs. Therefore, monitoring serum drug levels frequently and performing PK analysis to ensure appropriate drug regimens is essential. Lists of drugs commonly used in the ICU which are substrates, inducers, and inhibitors of various CP450 isoenzyme systems are readily available online and in pharmacology texts (46).

The following relevant examples illustrate how a health-care professional could utilize such information in predicting important drug–drug interactions. Example 1: a patient stable on warfarin with a therapeutic bleeding time gets initiated on amiodarone for atrial fibrillation. By identifying that both enantiomers of warfarin (R and S) are substrates of the CP450 enzyme system (CP3A4 and CP2C, respectively), one could predict that by adding an inhibitor of both isoenzyme subsystems (e.g., amiodarone) the bleeding time of the patient would probably rise and the chance of a clinically significant bleeding event would be elevated. Example 2: an intubated patient in the ICU is being sedated with midazolam by a continuous infusion. It was decided to treat his human immunodeficiency virus (HIV+) infection by initiating antiretroviral therapy, which included ritonavir. Noticing that ritonavir is an inhibitor of the CP3A4 isoenzyme subsystem and that midazolam is a substrate for that subsystem, the health-care practitioner may want to evaluate whether midazolam is the most appropriate choice of sedative in this particular patient.

↗ **Stimulation of the CP450 enzyme system in the liver and small intestine can lead to the increased metabolism of certain drugs; conversely, inhibition of this system can lead to elevated drug levels.** ↗

THERAPEUTIC DRUG MONITORING

TDM is a process of individualizing the dosage regimen of drugs with narrow therapeutic indices (a small range between its toxic plasma concentration and subtherapeutic plasma concentration). Using PK analysis, TDM includes continuous assessment of the therapeutic response and potential adverse effects and becomes more important in critically ill patients. Drugs can be divided into two general TDM categories: narrow therapeutic index agents and broad therapeutic index drugs. Here we will discuss some of the common drugs in the adult ICU that have a narrow therapeutic index. Because critically ill patients exhibit wide variable PK parameters, it is particularly important to monitor these drugs closely.

Antimicrobial Agents
Aminoglycosides

Aminoglycosides (e.g., gentamicin, tobramycin, amikacin) require TDM because of their narrow therapeutic index and risk for adverse effects (ototoxicity, nephrotoxicity). Critically ill patients often will display a larger V_d ($\sim$0.4 L/kg) than noncritically ill patients ($\sim$0.25 L/kg) (30,49,50). Many acutely ill patients will develop renal impairment and since the aminoglycosides are primarily excreted unchanged by glomerular filtration, frequent dosage adjustment based on PK analyses is necessary.

Within the past few years, once-daily dosing of aminoglycosides has gained popularity, and for good reason (49). Although aminoglycosides are themselves nephrotoxic, they remain a mainstay in the antimicrobial arsenal against aerobic gram-negative bacteria, as well as enterococcal and staphylococcal species (see Volume 2, Chapter 53).

The once-daily strategy is advantageous for a number of reasons. Aminoglycosides have concentration-dependent bactericidal activity, increasing the eradication of the organism(s) in the presence of higher serum drug concentrations. Once-daily therapy diminishes the ability of the organism to shut down the intracellular transport of the aminoglycoside (a form of resistance). This adaptive resistance occurs more frequently with multiple dose regimens. Aminoglycosides also possess a postantibiotic effect (PAE), a bacteriostatic environment after antibiotic exposure (the higher the aminoglycoside concentration, the longer the PAE). Most single-daily dose regimens (5–7 mg/kg/day) of gentamicin or tobramycin produce peak serum level concentrations approaching 15–20 mg/L and trough levels that are undetectable even in mild renal dysfunction.

Human studies have shown saturable uptake of aminoglycosides into the renal cortex (51). Therefore, the higher serum concentrations associated with once-daily administration does not predispose the patient to an increased risk of nephrotoxicity when compared with multiple daily dosing of aminoglycosides.

Vancomycin

Vancomycin is a bactericidal glycopeptide used for various gram-positive infections. It penetrates into most tissues well and is excreted almost entirely unchanged in the urine. Since compromised renal function is commonly seen in ICU patients, diligent monitoring of plasma levels is warranted. For intermittent hemodialysis patients, a dose of vancomycin (15 $\pm$ 5 mg/kg IV) every three to five days is common, whereas the same dose every 24 to 48 hours is common in those patients receiving CRRT. Since vancomycin primarily exhibits time-dependent killing, the routine monitoring of peak serum levels is generally not warranted unless an estimate of the patient's V_d is needed. Random or trough levels of vancomycin are generally sufficient to provide enough information to individualize a dosing regimen (30,52). For most indications, the goal vancomycin trough levels should be targeted between 5 and 15 mg/L. There are a few indications where clinicians might be more aggressive [e.g., methicillin-resistant *Staphylococcus aureus* (MRSA) bacteremia, endocarditis, meningitis, and osteomyelitis]. For these indications, the current trend is to target vancomycin trough levels of at least 10 mg/L (range 10–20 mg/L). For the treatment of MRSA-associated, ventilator-associated pneumonia, an even more aggressive dosing strategy is currently practiced to produce vancomycin trough levels approaching 15–20 mg/L. It is important to note

that vancomycin by itself infrequently causes nephrotoxicity. Only when it is administered in combination with other nephrotoxic agents (e.g., aminoglycosides) does the incidence of renal toxicity approach 30% (52).

Cotrimoxazole

Trimethoprim-sulfamethoxazole (TMP-SMX) is a combination antibiotic with a broad spectrum of activity against gram-positive and gram-negative organisms. There is a paucity of data that evaluates PK variables of TMP-SMX in critically ill patients. However, in hyperdynamic, acutely ill trauma patients [e.g., those with systemic inflammatory response syndrome (SIRS)], the half-life of SMX appears to be shorter and the V_d and Cl are larger (53). These data are in conflict with a study evaluating PK parameters of TMP-SMX in critically ill and noncritically ill AIDS patients where the V_d, Cl, and the half-life were similar between the two groups (54). Since there is potential for renal and bone marrow toxicity, monitoring of sulfonamide levels would be prudent in the critically ill patient, especially those patients with underlying renal dysfunction. A serum sulfonamide level of 50 to 150 mg/L is considered adequate for optimal therapy (30).

Miscellaneous Anti-infective Agents
Fluconazole and Itraconazole

Other agents that infrequently require TDM are the "azole" antifungal agents (e.g., fluconazole, itraconazole). Intact oral itraconazole capsules (not suspension) depend on the acidity of GI tract for absorption. It may be helpful to check an itraconazole level to assess oral absorption in those patients who are concomitantly taking gastric acid suppressing agents (e.g., H_2-antagonists and proton pump inhibitors) (55).

Ganciclovir

Ganciclovir is an antiviral agent used primarily for the treatment or prophylaxis of cytomegalovirus (CMV). It is highly nephrotoxic and can cause leukopenia and thrombocytopenia. The elimination of ganciclovir depends upon renal excretion, and therefore dose adjustments for impaired renal function is necessary in order to avoid adverse side effects (30). Guidelines for dosage adjustments for renal dysfunction exist (7). Occasionally, (especially patients on dialysis), it may be necessary to check the ganciclovir serum level and perform a PK analysis.

Cardiovascular Drugs
Digoxin

In critically ill patients, the most common use of digoxin is to control the heart rate in the setting of atrial fibrillation. The bioavailability of digoxin tablets is 50% to 90%. Although there is better bioavailability with the capsule formulation, the most common route of administration in the adult ICU is the IV route. Digoxin has a large V_d (about 7.3 L/kg) because of its extensive tissue binding (40,56).

However, in the setting of renal failure (estimated creatinine Cl <20 mL/min or those patients dependent on hemodialysis), the V_d is reduced. Loading and maintenance doses of digoxin will need to be adjusted accordingly for this reduction in V_d. Digoxin is not distributed into fat, and therefore the loading dose should be based on an estimate of ideal body weight (7). Digoxin has a long two-compartmental distribution phase, that explains the delay in its pharmacological action.

The sampling time of serum digoxin levels is important because serum digoxin levels drawn during the initial distribution phase may be falsely elevated. Therefore, it is important to wait at least four hours after an IV dose and six hours after an oral dose to check a serum digoxin level. Normally, 60% to 80% of digoxin is eliminated unchanged in the urine. Metabolism and biliary excretion contribute to nonrenal elimination.

The elimination half-life of digoxin is about one to two days in subjects with normal renal function and may be as long as five days in anuric patients. In critically ill patients with renal dysfunction, it is necessary to monitor digoxin serum levels closely and adjust the dosage as needed. The generally accepted therapeutic range of digoxin is 0.8–1.2 mcg/mL (for heart failure) and 0.8–2.0 mcg/mL (for atrial fibrillation). It is important to note that the immunoassays used to measure serum digoxin are not specific and may react with certain drug metabolites or endogenous digoxin-like substances (7,40), which could lead to a falsely elevated level.

Digoxin can interact with several drugs. Some of the most important digoxin–drug interactions involve the calcium channel blockers (e.g., diltiazem and verapamil) and amiodarone, both of which can increase the serum digoxin level significantly. Therefore, the dosage must be reduced and the digoxin level measured as needed.

Critically ill patients with electrolyte abnormalities (hypokalemia, hypomagnesemia, and hypercalcemia) are at higher risk of developing digoxin toxicity (ventricular arrhythmias, heart block, and other arrhythmias) (7,40). Close monitoring of serum electrolytes, renal function, and digoxin levels, performing PK analysis, and calculating an individualized dosage are highly recommended in ICU patients receiving digoxin.

Lidocaine

In critically ill patients, lidocaine is used to manage serious ventricular dysrhythmias. Because lidocaine has poor oral absorption, it is given initially by an IV bolus followed by a continuous IV infusion. Its V_d is about 1.3 L/kg (57). In ADHF, the V_d is decreased, whereas in chronic liver disease, it is increased (23). Lidocaine is mainly metabolized in the liver and its metabolites depend on renal clearance for their elimination. The usual elimination half-life of lidocaine is about 100 minutes, but in liver failure, the half-life may be prolonged. Frequent measurement of serum lidocaine levels is needed in critically ill patients with some degree of liver or heart failure. The therapeutic lidocaine level is 1–5 mg/L (57).

Procainamide

In critically ill patients, procainamide may be used in the treatment of ventricular and supraventricular dysrhythmias. It is usually used as continuous IV infusion in the ICU and switched to an oral form when appropriate. Oral bioavailability is about 75% to 100%, and it has a larger V_d than lidocaine (1.7–2.2 L/kg) (58). The therapeutic procainamide level is 4–8 mcg/mL, and although higher concentrations have been used in some patients, levels exceeding 8 mcg/mL have been associated with electrocardiographic changes (prolongation of the PR interval, QT, or QRS intervals) (59). The elimination half-life of procainamide is about three hours. It is metabolized in the liver to N-acetyl procainamide (NAPA), which is an active metabolite and is eliminated renally. In critically ill patients with some

degree of renal dysfunction, NAPA can accumulate and cause adverse effects. Therefore, close monitoring of serum procainamide and NAPA levels are needed.

Anticonvulsants

TBI patients often require treatment or prophylaxis for seizures. In these cases, the most commonly used agent is phenytoin. Carbamazepine, valproic acid, and phenobarbital may be used if phenytoin is ineffective or contraindicated.

Phenytoin

Phenytoin is the first-line agent for seizure prophylaxis following TBI. In the ICU, physical barriers or disease states can limit the appropriateness of administering medications enterally. Concurrent use of enteral feeding can further complicate the absorption of phenytoin; the intramuscular route is also unreliable and not recommended (60). The IV route is most commonly used in unstable, critically ill patients. Unlike the oral capsules, which are extended release, the injectable form of phenytoin is not and usually requires more than once-daily dosing.

Phenytoin is highly bound to albumin, and critically ill patients may have a significant degree of hypoalbuminemia, which results in an increased free fraction of phenytoin. There are formulas for adjusting the total phenytoin level that is usually reported by the laboratory in order to maintain a therapeutic-free level (60). However, the reliability of these equations is questionable; therefore, in critically ill patients, measurement of free and total phenytoin levels may be necessary.

Mainly metabolized in the liver, phenytoin is a low-extraction type drug; thus, changes in liver blood flow minimally affect its metabolism. However, induction or inhibition of liver microsomal enzymes will markedly affect the liver metabolism of phenytoin. This enzyme system is saturable, which explains the Michaelis–Menten elimination of phenytoin, that is, an increase in serum concentration of phenytoin beyond a certain point may not increase the rate of its clearance. So a small increase in dose can disproportionately increase the serum concentration and increase the risk of toxicity (60). The therapeutic range of serum phenytoin is 10–20 mg/L. The normal free fraction is about 10%, corresponding to a free plasma concentration of 1 to 2 mg/L.

In critically ill patients with oliguria and hypoalbuminemia, the free fraction of the drug can be increased; therefore, monitoring of both total and free serum phenytoin levels may be necessary. Following TBI, the rate of phenytoin metabolism may be increased (in the early hypermetabolic phase) and require an increased daily dosage. It is important to watch for changes in the rate of phenytoin metabolism in this subgroup. As the hypermetabolic state subsides, the rate of phenytoin metabolism may decrease substantially, and the dosage will have to be decreased.

Carbamazepine

Carbamazepine is usually the second-line anticonvulsant agent chosen in trauma patients. Carbamazepine is not available in an IV formulation and this limits its usefulness in the ICU setting. Oral bioavailability is about 75% but it may be variable and dissolution rate dependent (61). It is highly bound to α-1-acid glycoprotein, which can explain the increase in dosage requirement in some burn patients. It is mainly metabolized in the liver, and carbamazepine has the ability to induce its own metabolism. This self-induced metabolism usually starts after three to five days of therapy.

Frequent monitoring of carbamazepine serum concentrations in critically ill patients may be necessary. The therapeutic range is 4–12 mg/L (62). The adverse effects of carbamazepine include bone marrow suppression manifested by leukopenia and/or thrombocytopenia. It also can cause a hyponatremic hypo-osmolar condition similar to the syndrome of inappropriate antidiuretic hormone secretion (61).

Valproic Acid

Valproic acid is available in injectable form and this has increased its role in the ICU setting, usually as a second or third choice anticonvulsant in trauma patients. It is highly protein bound, mostly to albumin, and this binding appears to be saturable. The protein binding may actually decrease in TBI patients (61), so monitoring the free and total valproic acid levels may be necessary. Valproic acid is metabolized in the liver and because of its low extraction ratio, changes in liver perfusion usually do not alter its clearance. However, drugs that induce liver microsomal enzymes (e.g., phenytoin, phenobarbital, and carbamazepine) can increase valproic acid metabolism. Valproic acid itself is an inhibitor of liver enzymes and can affect the clearance of some drugs (63). The appropriate therapeutic range for valproic acid is not clear. It is thought that the minimum effective trough serum level for optimal seizure control is 50 mg/L (61) and the upper limit is probably about 120 mg/L. The most serious adverse effects are hepatotoxicity and thrombocytopenia.

Barbiturates

Barbiturates are not used as much in today's ICU as they historically have been used. Pentobarbital is occasionally used in TBI patients for control of resistant-increased intracranial pressure, and phenobarbital may be used as an anticonvulsant for other patients in the ICU. Phenobarbital is about 50% protein bound; however, in trauma and burn patients (especially those with uremia), the free fraction may be much higher (61). Hepatic enzymes oxidize phenobarbital, and changes in liver blood flow do not alter its clearance. It is a powerful inducer of liver enzymes, which can affect the metabolism of other hepatically metabolized drugs. The therapeutic range is 15–40 mg/L. The major adverse effects seen are those involving the CNS (e.g., drowsiness, lethargy, hangover).

Immunosuppressants

The immunosuppressant agent regiments used for both solid organ and bone marrow transplantations are usually metabolized in the liver and have drug interactions involving the CP450 enzyme system. In treating critically ill patients, clinicians must be familiar with these agents or seek the help of colleagues who are experts in this field. The interactions of immunosuppressants must be recognized and evaluated, and appropriate measures taken, if necessary.

Cyclosporine

Cyclosporine is a commonly used immunosuppressive agent alone and in combination with other immunosuppressive drugs. It is extensively metabolized in the liver to metabolites that depend on the biliary pathway for elimination. Cyclosporine is associated with a high degree of nephrotoxicity and has numerous drug–drug interactions (64). Cyclosporine levels must be monitored frequently because there is no practical PK model available for analysis. When evaluating cyclosporine levels, it is vital to consider the sample type (whole blood vs. plasma) and the technique used for measurement [(immunoassay vs. high performance liquid chromatography (HPLC)].

Different sample types and techniques used have different values. Therefore, care must be taken to assure that the desired serum level range is normalized for potential variables. The target immunosuppressant level is also highly variable and depends on the type of organ transplanted and the specific center that performed the transplant. Other variables that can help define the target level would include clinician experience, the clinical picture of the patient, the time after the transplant, past rejection history, adverse effects, and potential drug–drug interactions. Whenever a drug is added or discontinued, the effect on the cyclosporine level must be considered and the dosage should be reevaluated.

Cyclosporine can cause an increase in serum creatinine, which appears to be proportional to the cyclosporine level. Unless a decrease in the cyclosporine level is clinically indicated, there is no need for dosage adjustment for renal dysfunction or CRRT. With liver dysfunction, cyclosporine can accumulate resulting in an increased blood level. Cyclosporine can also increase the bilirubin level. Although this increase can be secondary to liver dysfunction, it is usually due to some degree of cholestasis. This is usually observed during initial cyclosporine therapy. After a few days, the bilirubin usually begins to decline; if not, the clinician should consider other causes including cyclosporine-induced hepatotoxicity. Drug interactions are extensive and can be divided into three types (Table 10) as those that can affect metabolism, bioavailability, or nephrotoxicity of cyclosporine.

Tacrolimus

Tacrolimus is an immunosuppressant similar to cyclosporine. It is extensively metabolized in the liver and can cause nephrotoxicity (64). Daily checking of the trough tacrolimus level is often necessary as the target range is quite variable. In addition, most of the previous discussion about cyclosporine also applies to tacrolimus. It is about 100 times more potent than cyclosporine on a weight basis; therefore, tacrolimus dosage and serum levels are about one-hundredth those of cyclosporine.

Sirolimus

Sirolimus is the newest immunosuppressive drug in the United States and its role is continually evolving. It is primarily used in combination with cyclosporine or tacrolimus to achieve an adequate level of global immunosuppression while minimizing the patient's exposure to the nephrotoxic immunosuppressants (e.g., cyclosporine and tacrolimus) (65). Many institutions strongly recommend monitoring sirolimus levels to avoid adverse effects, especially in critically ill patients. One of the serious unwanted effects of sirolimus is leukopenia (also see Volume 2, Chapter 57). More studies are needed to define an appropriate sirolimus level when it is used with cyclosporine- or tacrolimus-based immunosuppressive regimens. Investigators are studying sirolimus to determine whether it can be used without cyclosporine or tacrolimus. If so, the target level for various organ transplantations should be defined. Drug interactions with sirolimus are similar to those found with tacrolimus and cyclosporine (Table 10).

Table 10 Major Drug Interactions with Cyclosporine, Tacrolimus, and Sirolimus

Drugs that increase the absorption of cyclosporine (tacrolimus and sirolimus): grapefruit juice, metoclopramide, oral erythromycin, cyclosporine (increases sirolimus)
Drugs that affect the metabolism of cyclosporine (tacrolimus and sirolimus): drugs that increase metabolism: carbamazepine, phenobarbital, phenytoin, rifampin, St. John's wort
Drugs that decrease metabolism: allopurinol, amiodarone, androgens, azole antifungal agents (fluconazole, itraconazole, ketoconazole), bromocriptine, clarithromycin, erythromycin, diltiazem, nefazodone, nicardipine, nifedipine, oral contraceptives, sirolimus verapamil
Drugs that increase the nephrotoxicity of cyclosporine (tacrolimus): acyclovir, aminoglycosides, amphotericin B, foscarnet, ganciclovir, tacrolimus (cyclosporine), NSAIDs, vancomycin, and other nephrotoxic agents
Miscellaneous: digoxin (decrease clearance of digoxin by cyclosporine); neuromuscular blockers (prolonged neuromuscular blockage); HMG-CoA reductase inhibitors (increase risk of myopathy with cyclosporine); caspofungin (decreased tacrolimus and sirolimus levels, increased caspofungin level with cyclosporine)

Abbreviations: HMG-CoA, 3-hydroxy-3-methylglutaryl-Coenzyme A; NSAIDs, nonsteroidal anti-inflammatory drugs.

Miscellaneous (Mycophenolate and Azathioprine)

Azathioprine and mycophenolate belong to the antimetabolite class of immunosuppressive agents and are used in combination with corticosteroids and either cyclosporine or tacrolimus. The dosage ranges from 2 g/day up to 3 g/day and primarily depends on the type of organ transplanted. Azathioprine has an important drug–drug interaction with allopurinol. If used together, the dose of azathioprine should be reduced to avoid the accumulation of azathioprine's active metabolite (6-mercaptopurine). It is important to monitor for dose limiting adverse effects such as bone marrow suppression (neutropenia, pancytopenia), GI distress (nausea/vomiting, diarrhea, abdominal pain), and liver dysfunction (cholestasis, elevated hepatic enzymes).

DRUG-INDUCED FEVER

☞ Drug fever is defined as a febrile response to a drug without cutaneous manifestations and is estimated to occur in about 10% of hospitalized patients (66). ☞ The incidence may be higher in critically ill patients because they are on more medications. It may be difficult to recognize drug fever in ICU patients, as there are potentially multiple causes of fever (see Volume 2, Chapter 46). Although it usually occurs one to two weeks after a drug was started, it can occur at any time. This can lead to prolonged hospitalization and unnecessary tests. The most common cause of drug fever is a hypersensitivity reaction. Altered thermoregulatory mechanism, idiosyncratic reactions, and the pharmacological action of drugs can also be the cause of drug fever (66). Some common ICU drugs that are associated

with drug fever are listed in Volume 2, Chapter 46. Treatment of drug fever consists of discontinuation of the suspected offending medication.

DRUG-INDUCED RASH (TOXIC EPIDERMAL NECROLYSIS/ STEVENS–JOHNSON SYNDROME)

The most common adverse drug reactions (ADRs) are those involving the skin. They affect about 2% to 3% of hospitalized patients (67). Among those, only a small percentage are life threatening. Stevens–Johnson syndrome (SJS) is fatal in about 5% of patient cases and toxic epidermal necrolysis (TEN) in about 30% of patient cases (67). The clinical features and prognosis of these two diseases are different, yet they have similar histopathological findings and are caused by similar drugs. Some consider SJS to be a mild form of TEN.

If epidermal detachment is less than 10% of the total body surface area, it is classified as SJS. If it is greater than 30%, it is classified as TEN. If the affected area is between 10% and 30%, then it is considered an overlapped case of SJS–TEN. The incidence of SJS is 1.2 to 5 per million per year and for TEN 0.4 to 1.2 per million per year (67). Drugs that are associated with SJS and TEN and are commonly used in an adult ICU are listed in Table 11 (68).

Among drugs that can cause reactions, sulfonamides are the most frequent. Phenytoin, phenobarbital, and carbamazepine all can cause these severe cutaneous reactions. These three drugs have related chemical structures and are metabolized by similar pathways to reactive compounds. It is these reactive compounds that are thought to be immunogenic, causing the cutaneous reaction (69). Because of extensive skin detachment, the treatment is the same as for burn victims and requires a burn intensive care facility. The seriousness of these reactions and the lack of definitively

Table 11 Medications Associated with Stevens–Johnson Syndrome and/or Toxic Epidermal Necrolysis

Stevens–Johnson syndrome	Toxic epidermal necrolysis
Acetaminophen	Acetaminophen
Allopurinol	Allopurinol
Carbamazepine	Barbiturates
Cephalosporins	Carbamazepine
Cotrimoxazole	Chloramphenicol
Ibuprofen	Ibuprofen
Macrolides (e.g., erythromycin)	Imidazole antifungal agents (e.g., ketoconazole)
Penicillins	Indomethacin
Phenobarbital	Lamotrigine
Phenytoin	Macrolides
Propranolol	Penicillins
Quinolones	Phenytoin
Sulfadiazine	Quinine
Sulfonamides	Quinolones
Thiazides	Ranitidine
Valproic acid	Sulfonamides
	Sulindac
	Tetracyclines
	Valproic acid

Source: Adapted from Ref. 68.

effective treatment have produced a large body of literature on some effective and ineffective treatments (70).

As soon as the diagnosis of SJS/TEN has been made, the suspected agent(s) should be withdrawn. Early discontinuation of causative agents has been reported to improve the outcome (68,71). The principles of symptomatic treatments are the same as for burns, which include meticulous skin care, fluid replacement, nutritional support, and antimicrobial therapy (67). Plasmapheresis, immunosuppressive therapy, oral corticosteroids, human IV immunoglobulin, all have been used with varying degrees of success (70). Their role in the treatment of SJS and TEN remains to be established.

EYE TO THE FUTURE

Personalized medicine is a concept that describes patients receiving the most appropriate drugs with the most fitting dosage based on their genetic makeup (72). This concept appears to be gaining clarity as our knowledge regarding the human genome expands. Poor drug tolerability, adverse drug events, and therapeutic failure may be explained by genetic differences. Patients may express different alleles on genes that are responsible for creating certain drug-metabolizing enzymes (e.g., CP450 enzyme system, namely CP2C9, CP2C19, CP2D6). These differences may lead to diversity among patients' metabolic transformation of a particular medication, leading to individual variability in the efficacy and toxicity of drugs (73,74). It is important to remember that genetic polymorphisms do not always translate into phenotypic changes (75). The study of the genetic basis for individual drug response is called pharmacogenomics. Initially, pharmacogenomics focused on drug metabolism but has recently expanded to evaluate drug transporters that can influence the absorption, distribution, and excretion of medications as well as drug receptors (75).

Several examples of genetic differences in drug metabolism reside within the CP450 enzyme system. For example, approximately 8% to 10% of Caucasians are deficient in the isoform CP2D6, which represents the main metabolic pathway of drugs such as antidysrhythmic agents, β-adrenoreceptor blockers, tricyclic antidepressants, and certain opioids like codeine (76). For patients with this deficiency, β-adrenoreceptor blockade will be more pronounced and the effect of codeine will be much less because of the impaired production of the active metabolite, morphine. Another example of genetic polymorphism lies in the CP2C9 isoform and warfarin metabolism. Individuals expressing this mutation can only tolerate low doses of warfarin because their clearance is about 10% of those without the mutation (48).

Perhaps one of the more popular proteins that have recently been studied is PGP, that is involved in energy-dependent transport of drugs and their metabolites into urine, bile, and the intestinal lumen. PGP also plays a large role in regulating drug concentrations in the brain (e.g., digoxin, cyclosporine, and dexamethasone) (75). It is understood that individuals express PGP in differing amounts, contributing to the concept that genetic makeup plays a critical role in the PK of drugs.

Finally, there are genetic alterations in drug receptors which can result in a wide variation in drug effect. Some of these examples include the β2-adrenoreceptor and response to β2-agonists, the ACE and the renal protective effects of ACE inhibitors, and apolipoprotein E and the response to the HMG-CoA reductase inhibitors (77–81).

With the advent of genetic testing, pharmacogenomics may help health-care providers determine the most appropriate drug and dose for each patient. Until there is widespread availability of genetic testing (e.g., point-of-care), empiric, population-based treatment algorithms will probably remain the foundation of drug therapy. However, certain disease states may warrant a patient-specific genetic evaluation to identify the most effective treatment regimen and to minimize drug toxicity.

SUMMARY

Rational drug therapy is an essential part in the management of critically ill patients. Clinical pharmacology provides the necessary tools for an individualized approach to drug therapy, using PK and PD principles. With all of the variables that potentially can change in the critically ill patient, it is important to individualize drug therapy. This challenge can be minimized with multidisciplinary involvement and careful monitoring of the patient to prevent iatrogenic adverse reactions.

Organ failure is responsible for a majority of the alterations of PK and PD parameters in the critical-care setting. Renal dysfunction can alter the V_d and ultimately the Cl of some drugs. Liver dysfunction can be due to extrinsic causes such as decreased liver blood flow or as a result of some intrinsic changes such as altered hepatic microsomal enzyme activities. Both of these factors can contribute to a decrease in hepatic drug metabolism.

ADHF can lead to an impairment of drug Cl and/or a reduction in the V_d by underperfusing organs responsible for metabolism or elimination (i.e., liver and kidneys). PK changes are difficult to predict in heart failure and will assume importance with narrow therapeutic index drugs (i.e., digoxin, lidocaine, procainamide). Depending on the extent of the burn injury and time after the insult, the volume of distribution, protein binding, and Cl of some drugs can be altered.

In the setting of decreased liver and kidney perfusion, the clearances of sedatives and analgesic drugs are often reduced. Any change in their protein binding or changes in liver function may have a significant impact on their therapeutic or adverse effects. Changes in GI motility or changes in GI tract pH can affect the absorption and GI metabolism of some drugs. Often ICU patients are on tube feedings, which can interfere and lead to decreased or unpredictable absorption of many drugs.

There are several mechanisms by which drugs can interact, but most can be categorized into PK, PD, or combined interactions. PK interactions include those that alter absorption, distribution, metabolism, or excretion; PD interactions include those that alter the effect of the drug on the body. Stimulation of the CP450 enzyme system in the liver and small intestine can lead to an increased metabolism of certain drugs; conversely, inhibition of this system can lead to elevated drug levels. With the knowledge of the CP450 enzyme systems and drugs that are known to be substrates, inducers, and inhibitors, health-care practitioners may be able to anticipate clinically important drug interactions.

The critically ill patient's status can be dynamic and changes in bioavailability, V_d, protein binding, clearance, and half-life can generate suboptimal drug concentrations. There is great potential for diagnostic genetic tests to elucidate patient-specific polymorphisms, which will help the clinician develop a specific pharmacotherapeutic plan. Finally, it is important to frequently sample serum drug levels of narrow therapeutic index medications, in order to individualize therapy as much as possible.

KEY POINTS

- The unbound ("free") drug molecule exerts the pharmacological effect by interacting with the cellular receptor.
- Protein-binding alterations occur in critically ill patients and must be considered in order to properly interpret measured drug concentrations and their predicted PD effects.
- The primary organs involved in clearance are the kidneys and the liver but other organ systems (e.g., lungs) may be involved.
- Multiple variables (PK and PD) affect the critically ill patient. Accordingly, multidisciplinary involvement and careful monitoring is required to optimize drug therapy.
- GFR is often estimated based on a patient's serum creatinine and ideal body weight. Since critically ill patients may have a decrease in muscle mass, creatinine clearance (and GFR) can be overestimated.
- If renal dysfunction is severe enough to require dialysis, dosage adjustment is often required.
- In general, the CVVHDF removal of small drugs depends on the diffusion and convection process, whereas removal of larger drugs depends mostly on convection and perhaps adsorption properties.
- Up to 54% of critically ill patients will develop some degree of liver dysfunction (17).
- In critically ill patients with multiorgan failure, the net effect on drug metabolism is difficult to predict and must be carefully monitored.
- ADHF can lead to an impairment of drug clearance and/or a reduction in the V_d by underperfusing organs responsible for metabolism or elimination (i.e., liver and kidneys) (23).
- Drugs with a narrow therapeutic index (i.e., digoxin, lidocaine, procainamide) require enhanced drug monitoring in patients with heart failure.
- The clearance of some drugs during the hypermetabolic phase of burn injury may be increased.
- Cisatracurium is the ideal NMB drug for critically ill patients with liver and renal failure who require only a brief period of NMB.
- Acidosis or alkalosis can change the protein binding of drugs (40).
- There are several ways by which the GI absorption of drugs may be affected.
- Stimulation of the CP450 enzyme system in the liver and small intestine can lead to the increased metabolism of certain drugs; conversely, inhibition of this system can lead to elevated drug levels.
- Drug fever is defined as a febrile response to a drug without cutaneous manifestations and is estimated to occur in about 10% of hospitalized patients (66).

REFERENCES

1. Holford NHG. Pharmacokinetics & pharmacodynamics: rational dosing & the time course of action. In: Katzung BG, ed. Basic and Clinical Pharmacology. 8th ed. McGraw-Hill, 2001:35–50.
2. Winters ME. Basic Principles. Basic Clinical Pharmacokinetics. 3rd ed. Vancouver, WA: Applied Therapeutics, Inc., 1994:2–52.
3. Murray P, Corbridge T. Critical care pharmacology. In: Hall JB, Schmidt GA, Wood LD, eds. Principles of Critical Care. 2nd ed. New York: Mcgraw-Hill, 1998:1527–1550.
4. Mckindley DS, Hanes S, Boucher BA. Hepatic drug metabolism in critical illness. Pharmacotherapy 1998; 18(4):759–778.
5. Nolin TD, Abraham PA, Matzke GR. Drug-induced renal disease. In: DiPiro JT, Talbert RL, Yee GC, Matzke GR, Wells BG, Posey LM, eds. Pharmacotherapy: A Pathophysiologic Approach. 5th ed. New York: McGraw-Hill, 2002:889–910.
6. Henrich WL, Cronin RE. Drug-induced kidney disease. In: Schrier RW, Gambertoglio JG, eds. Handbook of Drug Therapy in Liver and Kidney Disease. 1st ed. Boston: Little, Brown and Company; 1991:257–271.
7. Aronoff GR, Berns JS, Brier ME, et al. Drug prescribing in renal failure, dosing guidelines for adults. 4th ed. Philadelphia: American College of Physician, 1998.
8. Gilbert DN, Moellering Jr RC, Sande MA. The Sanford Guide to Antimicrobial Therapy. 31st ed. Vienna: Antimicrobial Therapy, Inc., 2001.
9. Reetze-Bonorden P, Bohler J, Keller E. Drug Dosage in Patients during Continuous Renal Replacement Therapy. Clin Pharmacokinet 1993; 24(5):362–379.
10. Cockroft DW, Gault MH. Prediction of creatinine clearance from serum creatinine. Nephron 1976; 16:31–41.
11. Davies SP, Azadian BS, Kox WJ, et al. Pharmacokinetics of ciprofloxacin and vancomycin in patients with acute renal failure treated by continuous haemodialysis. Nephrol Dial Transplant 1992; 7:848–854.
12. Anon. Pharmacokinetic Dosage Guidelines for Adult Patients with Renal Impairment. UCSD Medical Center, Department of Pharmacy. 2001–2006.
13. Anon. Pharmacokinetic Dosing Guidelines for Adult Patients on CVVHDF. UCSD Medical Center, Department of Pharmacy. 2001.
14. Bugge JF. Pharmacokinetics and drug dosing adjustments during continuous venovenous hemofiltration or hemodiafiltration in critically ill patients. Acta Anaesthesiol Scand 2001; 45(8):929–934.
15. Giles LJ, Jennings AC, Thompson AH, et al. Pharmacokinetics of meropenem in intensive care unit patients receiving continuous hemofiltration or hemodiafiltration. Crit Care Med 2000; 28(3):632–637.
16. Verves TF, Van Dijk A, Vinks SA, et al. Pharmacokinetics and dosing regimen of meropenem in critically ill patients receiving continuous venovenous hemofiltration. Crit Care Med 2000; 28(10):3412–3416.
17. Hawker F. The critically ill patient with abnormal liver function tests. In: Park GR, ed. The Liver. London: WB Saunders Co Ltd, 1993:286–323.
18. Levine JS. Drug-induced liver disease. In: Schrier RW, Gambertoglio JG, eds. Handbook of Drug Therapy in Liver and Kidney Disease. 1st ed. Boston: Little, Brown and Company, 1991:242–256.
19. Lee WM. Drug-induced hepatotoxicity. N Engl J Med 2003; 349:474–485.
20. Anon. Clinical Pharmacology Online. URL: http://cpip.gsm.com.
21. Romac DR, Albertson TE. Drug interactions in the intensive care units. Clin Chest Med 1999; 20(2):385–399, ix.
22. Sherlock S. Disease of the Liver and Biliary System. 7th ed. Boston: Blackwell Scientific Publications, 1985:304–306.
23. Shammas FV, Dickstein K. Clinical pharmacokinetics of heart failure an updated review. Clin Pharmacokinet 1988; 15:94–113.
24. Johnson JA, Parker RB, Patterson JH. Heart failure. In: DiPiro JT, Talbert RL, Yee GC, et al., eds. Pharmacotherapy: A Pathophysiologic Approach. 5th ed. New York: McGraw-Hill, 2002:185–218.
25. Packer M, Lee WH, Kessler D. Preservation of glomerular filtration rate in human heart failure by activation of the renin-angiotensin system. Circulation 1986; 74:766–774.

26. Jaehde U, Sorgel F. Clinical pharmacokinetics in patients with burns. Clin Pharmacokinet 1995; 29(1):15–28.

27. Wagner BK, O'Hara DA. Pharmacokinetics and pharmacodynamics of sedatives and analgesics in the treatment of agitated critically ill patients. Clin Pharmacokinet 1997; 33(6):426–453.

28. Volles DF, Mcgory R. Pharmacokinetic considerations. Crit Care Clin 1999; 15(1):55–75.

29. Swart EL, van Schijndel RJ, van Loenen AC, Thijs LG. Continuous infusion of lorazepam versus midazolam in patients in the intensive care unit: sedation with lorazepam is easier to manage and is more cost-effective. Crit Care Med 1999; 27(8):1461–1465.

30. Power BM, Forbes AM, Heerden PV, Ilett KF. Pharmacokinetics of drugs used in critically ill adults. Clin Pharmacokinet 1998; 34(1):25–56.

31. American Society of Health-System Pharmacists. Clinical practice guidelines for the sustained use of sedatives and analgesics in critically ill adult. Am J Health-Sys Pharm 2002; 59:150–178.

32. Levine RL. Pharmacology of intravenous sedatives and opioids in critically ill patients. Crit Care Clin 1994; 10(4):709–731.

33. American Society of Health-System Pharmacists. Clinical practice guidelines for sustained neuromuscular blockade in the adult critically ill patient. Am J Health-Sys Pharm 2001; 59:179–195.

34. Topulos GP. Neuromuscular blockade in adult intensive care. New Horizons 1993; 1(3):447–462.

35. Miller RD, Katzung BG. Skeletal muscle relaxants. In: Katzung BG, ed. Basic and Clinical Pharmacology. 8th ed. New York: McGraw-Hill, 2001:446–462.

36. McManus MC. Neuromuscular blockers in surgery and intensive care, part 1. Am J Health-Sys 2001; 58:2287–2299.

37. Ritz MA, Fraser R, Tam W, Dent J. Impact and patterns of disturbed gastrointestinal function in critically ill patients. Am J Gastroenterol 2000; 95(11):3044–3052.

38. Chapman MJ, Fraser RJ, Kluger MT, Buist MD, De Nichilio DJ. Erythromycin improves gastric emptying in critically ill patients intolerant of nasogastric feeding. Crit Care Med 2000; 28(7):2657–2659.

39. MacLaren R, Kuhl DA, Gervasio JM, et al. Sequential single doses of cisapride, erythromycin, and metoclopramide in critically ill patients intolerant to enteral nutrition: a randomized placebo-controlled, cross over study. Crit Care Med 2000; 28(2):438–444.

40. Bodenham A, Shelly MP, Park GR. The altered pharmacokinetics and pharmacodynamics of drugs commonly used in critically ill patients. Clin Pharmacokinet 1988; 14:347–373.

41. Hansten PD. Appendix II: important drug interactions & their mechanisms. In: Katzung BG, ed. Basic and Clinical Pharmacology. 8th ed. New York: McGraw-Hill, 2001:1122–1133.

42. Schentag JJ, Scully BE. Quinolones. In: Yu VL, Merigan TC, Barriere SL, eds. Antimicrobial Therapy and Vaccines. Baltimore: Williams and Wilkins, 1999:875–901.

43. Mimoz O, Binter V, Jacolot A, et al. Pharmacokinetics and absolute bioavailability of ciprofloxacin administered through a nasogastric tube with continuous enteral feeding to critically ill patients. Intensive Care Med 1998; 24:1047–1051.

44. De Marie S, VandenBergh MFQ, Buijk SLCE, et al. Bioavailability of ciprofloxacin after multiple enteral and intravenous doses in ICU patients with severe gram-negative intra-abdominal infections. Intensive Care Med 1998; 24:343–346.

45. Engle KK, Hannawa TE. Techniques for administering oral medications to critical care patients receiving continuous enteral nutrition. Am J Health-Syst Pharm 1999; 56:1441–1444.

46. Michalets EL. Update: clinically significant cytochrome P-450 drug interactions. Pharmacotherapy 1998; 18(1):84–112.

47. Rautio A. Polymorphic CYP2A6 and its clinical and toxicological significance. Pharmacogenomics J 2003; 3(1):5–7.

48. Correia MA. Drug biotransformation. In: Katzung BG, ed. Basic and Clinical Pharmacology. 8th ed. New York: McGraw-Hill, 2001:51–63.

49. Nicolau DP, Freeman CD, Belliveau PP, et al. Experience with a once-daily aminoglycoside program administered to 2,184 adult patients. Antimicrob Agents Chemother 1995; 39: 650–655.

50. Winters ME. Aminoglycoside Antibiotics. Basic Clinical Pharmacokinetics. 3rd ed. Vancouver, WA: Applied Therapeutics, Inc., 1994:128–176.

51. De Broe ME, Verbist L, Verpooten GA. Influence on dosage schedule on renal cortical accumulation of amikacin and tobramycin in man. J Antimicrob Chemother 1991; 27(suppl C): 41–47.

52. Winters ME. Vancomycin. Basic Clinical Pharmacokinetics. 3rd ed. Vancouver, WA: Applied Therapeutics, Inc., 1994:474–499.

53. Hess MM, Boucher BA, Laizure SC, et al. Trimethoprim-sulfamethoxazole pharmacokinetics in trauma patients. Pharmacotherapy 1993; 13(6):602–606.

54. Chin TWF, Vandenbroucke A, Fong IW. Pharmacokinetics of trimethoprim-sulfamethoxazole in critically ill and non-critically ill AIDS patients. Antimicrob Agents Chemother 1995; 39(1):28–33.

55. Groll AH, Walsh TJ. Azoles: triazoles. In: Yu VL, Merigan TC, Barriere SL, eds. Antimicrobial Therapy and Vaccines. Baltimore: Williams and Wilkins, 1999:1158–1170.

56. Winters ME. Digoxin. Basic Clinical Pharmacokinetics. 3rd ed. Vancouver, WA: Applied Therapeutics, Inc., 1994:198–235.

57. Winters ME. Lidocaine. Basic Clinical Pharmacokinetics. 3rd ed. Vancouver, WA: Applied Therapeutics, Inc., 1994:242–56.

58. Bauman JL, Schoen MD. Arrhythmias. In: Dipiro JT, Talbert RL, Yee GC, et al, eds. Pharmacotherapy: A Pathophysiologic Approach, 5th ed. New York: McGraw-Hill, 2002:273–303.

59. Winters ME. Procainamide. Basic Clinical Pharmacokinetics. 3rd ed. Vancouver, WA: Applied Therapeutics, Inc., 1994:356–378.

60. Winters ME. Phenytoin. Basic Clinical Pharmacokinetics. 3rd ed. Vancouver, WA: Applied Therapeutics, Inc., 1994:312–348.

61. Gidal BE, Garnett WR, Graves N. Epilepsy. In: Dipiro JT, Talbert RL, Yee GC, et al. Pharmacotherapy: A Pathophysiologic Approach. 5th ed. New York: McGraw-Hill, 2002:1031–1059.

62. Winters ME. Carbamazepine. Basic Clinical Pharmacokinetics. 3rd ed. Vancouver, WA: Applied Therapeutics, Inc., 1994:177–184.

63. Winters ME. Valproic Acid. Basic Clinical Pharmacokinetics. 3rd ed. Vancouver, WA: Applied Therapeutics, Inc., 1994:463–473.

64. Burckart GJ, Venkataramanan R, Ptachcinski RJ. Overview of transplantation. In: Dipiro JT, Talbert RL, Yee GC, et al. Pharmacotherapy: A Pathophysiologic approach. 3rd ed. Connecticut: Appleton & Lange, 1997:129–147.

65. Johnson HJ, Heim-Duthoy KL. Renal transplantation. In: Dipiro JT, Talbert RL, Yee GC, et al. Pharmacotherapy: A Pathophysiologic Approach. 5th ed. McGraw-Hill, 2002:843–866.

66. Johnson DH, Cunha BA. Drug fever. Infect Dis Clin North Am 1996; 10(1):86–91.

67. Wolkenstein P, Revuz J. Drug-induced severe skin reactions: incidence, management and prevention. Drug Safety 1995; 13(1):56–68.

68. Elias SS, Patel NM, Cheigh NH. Drug-induced skin reactions. In: Dipiro JT, Talbert RL, Yee GC, et al. Pharmacotherapy: A Pathophysiologic Approach. 5th ed. McGraw-Hill, 2002:1705–1716.

69. Lott RS, McAuley JW. Seizure disorders. In: Young LY, Koda-Kimble MA, editors. Applied Therapeutics: The Clinical Use of Drugs. 7th ed. Philadephia: Lippincott Williams & Wilkins, 2001:52-1 to 52-41.

70. Stern RS. Improving the outcome of patients with toxic epidermal necrolysis and Stevens-Johnson syndrome [editorial]. Arch Dermatol 2000; 136:410–411.

71. Garcia-Doval I, LeCleach L, Bocquet H, Otero XL, Rojeau JC. Toxic epidermal necrolysis and Stevens-Johnson syndrome: does early withdrawal of causative drugs decrease the risk of death? Arch Dermatol 2000; 136:323–327.

72. Gurwitz D, Weizman A, Rehavi M. Education: teaching pharmacogenomics to prepare future physicians and researchers for personalized medicine. Trends Pharmacol Sci 2003; 24(3):122–125.

73. Severino G, Chillotti C, Stochino ME, Del Zompo M. Pharmacogenomics: state of the research and perspectives in clinical application. Neurol Sci 2003; 24:S146–S148.

74. Nicholls H. Improving drug response with pharmacogenomics. Drug Discov Today 2003; 8(7):281–282.

75. Evans WE. Pharmacogenomics: marshalling the human genome to individualise therapy. Gut 2003; 52(suppl 2):ii, 10–18.

76. Oates JA, Wilkinson GR. Principles of drug therapy. In: Fauci AS, Braunwald E, Isselbacher KJ, et al, eds. Harrison's Principles of Internal Medicine. 14th ed. McGraw-Hill, 1998:417–418.

77. Dishy V, Sofowora GG, Xie HG, et al. The effect of common polymorphisms of the beta2-adrenergic receptor on agonist-mediated vascular desensitization. N Engl J Med 2001; 14:1030–1035.

78. Liggett SB. Beta(2)-adrenergic receptor pharmacogenetics. Am J Respir Crit Care Med 2000; 161:S197–S201.

79. Lima JJ, Thomason DB, Mohamed MH, et al. Impact of genetic polymorphisms of the beta2-adrenergic receptor on albuterol bronchodilator pharmacodynamics. Clin Pharmacol Ther 1999; 5:519–525.

80. Nabel EG. Cardiovascular disease. N Engl J Med 2003; 349:60–72.

81. Jacobsen P, Rossing K, Rossing P, et al. Angiotensin converting enzyme gene polymorphism and ACE inhibition in diabetic nephropathy. Kidney Int 1998; 53:1002–1006.

5

Analgesia and Sedation for Trauma and Critical Care

Benjamin I. Atwater
Department of Anesthesiology, UC San Diego School of Medicine, San Diego, California, U.S.A.

Linda Pelinka
Department of Anesthesia and Critical Care, Lorenz Boehler Trauma Center, Vienna, Austria

Srdjan Nedeljkovic
Department of Anesthesiology and Critical Care Medicine, Brigham and Women's Hospital,
Harvard University School of Medicine, Boston, Massachusetts, U.S.A.

Agnes Ricard-Hibon
Department of Anesthesiology and Critical Care Medicine, Beaujon University Hospital, Clichy, France

INTRODUCTION

Pain is defined as an "unpleasant sensory or emotional experience associated with actual or potential tissue damage" (1). It is a complex phenomenon that combines strong emotional responses with ensuing physiological and psychological changes. Trauma patients often experience severe, and at times, poorly controlled pain (2). The administration of analgesics and sedatives is sometimes delayed or altogether avoided because of the concern that these drugs may produce hypotension, respiratory depression, or altered mental alertness (which could mask important diagnostic symptoms). ☞ **Without compromising cardiopulmonary status, judicious use of analgesics and sedatives can relieve pain, provide a state of emotional calm, and facilitate the diagnostic evaluation of trauma patients. ☞**

This chapter reviews the adverse effects of uncontrolled pain, and provides a clinical approach to analgesia and sedation for both acute trauma and critical care. The general approach utilizes the concept of the "analgesia and sedation pyramid" (Fig. 1), which emphasizes a graded hierarchy of treatment beginning with the removal of exacerbating factors and the baseline provision of a foundation of analgesia prior to administering any anxiolytic or sedative drugs. The pharmacology of the commonly employed analgesics and sedative drugs are extensively reviewed, and the assessment tools used in the evaluation of pain, sedation, and delirium are thoroughly surveyed.

Treatment guidelines are provided for the management of pain and anxiety in the prehospital period, in the trauma resuscitation suite (TRS), and surgical intensive care unit (SICU). Because delirium is an exceedingly common and difficult-to-treat condition in critical care, its evaluation, prevention, and treatment receives particular focus. In addition, sedation and analgesia guidelines for common trauma-related conditions are specifically reviewed. The "Eye to the Future" section provides a glimpse at a host of new analgesia and sedation therapies on the horizon.

ADVERSE EFFECTS OF UNCONTROLLED PAIN

Poorly controlled pain in trauma and burn patients can result in severe psychological trauma (3). When particularly severe or emotionally laden, painful experiences can culminate as post-traumatic stress disorder (PTSD), (see Volume 2, Chapter 65). Despite the high prevalence of psychological sequelae, these phenomena have only recently received the focus they merit.

The acute physiologic derangements resulting from uncontrolled pain have been more widely recognized. These include cardiovascular, pulmonary, and gastrointestinal (GI) effects. In addition, a link between the opioid receptors and the inflammatory response and coagulation system has been recently established.

☞ **PTSD affects up to 40% of major trauma patients (4,5).** ☞ Major trauma elicits a neurohumoral stress response manifested by the increased elaboration of catecholamines, antidiuretic hormone, cortisol, renin, angiotensin II, and aldosterone (6,7). Decreased insulin secretion, increased insulin resistance, proteinolysis, and glycogenolysis all contribute to hyperglycemia (with its own set of detrimental consequences). Physiological responses to the stress hormonal outflow include a hyperdynamic cardiovascular state, ileus, and urinary retention. The increased heart rate (HR), cardiac work, and O_2 consumption ($\dot{V}O_2$) can lead to a higher incidence of myocardial ischemia (8).

Poorly controlled pain in the chest wall or the upper abdomen impairs pulmonary function. Splinting and inability to cough lead to hypoventilation, atelectasis, hypoxemia, and elevated risk of pneumonia. Pulmonary function studies following these injuries show decreased tidal volumes, increased respiratory rate (RR), decreased functional residual capacity (FRC) and vital capacity, among other findings (9). Successful pain control can partially restore most of these processes, improving pulmonary function.

Coagulopathy commonly ensues after major injury (see Volume 2, Chapter 58), and opioid agonists have recently been shown to partially mitigate this disorder.

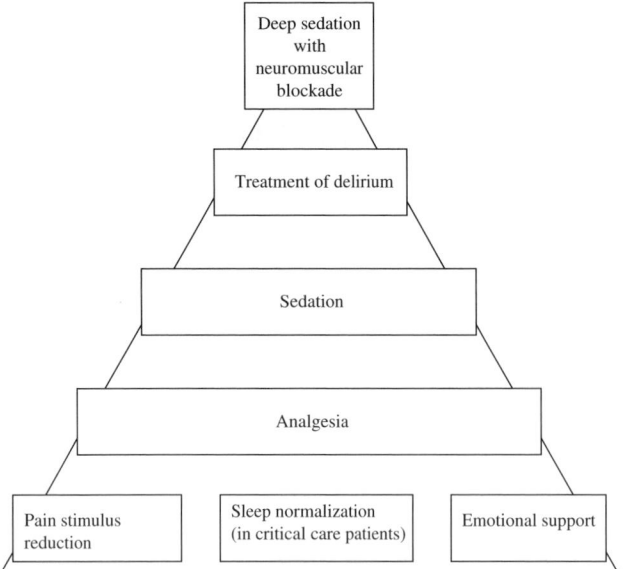

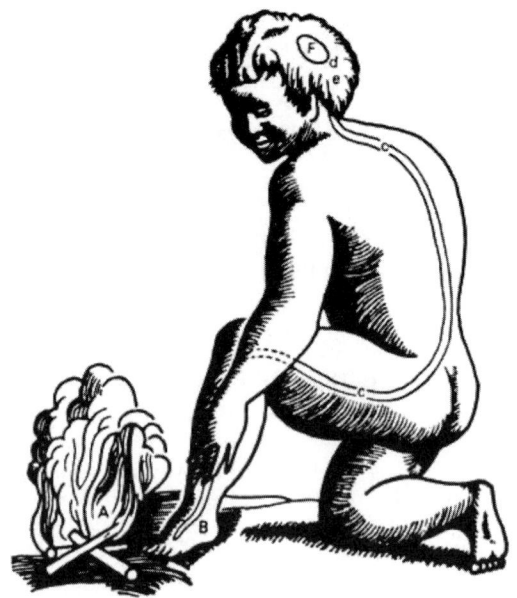

Figure 1 Analgesia and sedation pyramid. This figure graphically depicts the hierarchy of treatment with the most commonly employed drugs and techniques at the base of the pyramid, and the less often used drugs at the top. The base of the pyramid rests upon the three pillars of basic patient care techniques that, themselves, decrease the severity and emotional content of pain (emotional support, reduction of pain stimulus, and sleep normalization). Pain stimulus reduction techniques include splinting, immobilizing, and reducing fractures. Sleep normalization helps to decrease agitation and delirium; emotional support helps to decrease the secondary negative effects of pain. Considerations for analgesia consist of systemic administration and regional techniques. Emphasis with treatment begins on establishing adequate analgesia before ascending to anxiolysis (sedation treatment or to control delirium). Treatment of anxiety and agitation per se should be given after pain—an anxiety-provoking stimulus—has been addressed. Pharmacotherapy directed to treat delirium should be administered after delirium-inducing factors are mitigated. Neuromuscular blockade with deep sedation is reserved to the severely agitated or delirious patient unresponsive to a stepwise pharmacological approach.

Figure 2 Descartes' (1664) first conceptualized pain pathway. He writes: "If for example fire (**A**) comes near the foot (**B**), the minute particles of this fire, which as you know move with great velocity, have the power to set in motion the spot of the skin of the foot which they touch, and by this means pulling upon the delicate thread (**C**) which is attached to the spot of the skin, they open up at the same instant the pore (**D, E**) against which the delicate thread ends (**F**), just as by pulling at one end of a rope makes to strike at the same instant a bell which hangs at the other end." *Source*: From Refs. 15, 16.

Coagulation and inflammation are linked through numerous molecular pathways, including damaged endothelium, activated platelets, and the complexes of tissue factor, along with factors VIIa and Xa (10). In addition, G protein-coupled opioid receptors, expressed by T lymphocytes, neutrophils, monocytes, and macrophages have been found to modulate the inflammatory response (11) and (because coagulation and inflammation are linked) coagulaopathy (10). Opioid agonists have also been shown to reduce the inflammatory response by inhibiting the expression of proinflammatory cytokines (11,12).

GENERAL APPROACH: ANALGESIA AND SEDATION PYRAMID

☞ **Optimal pain management involves a stepwise, logical approach beginning with the elimination of obvious painful stimuli (e.g., fractures should be splinted), ascending to administration of analgesics prior to introducing sedatives or neuroleptic drugs; and, only in rare cases is**

deep sedation with neuromuscular blockade (NMB) required. ☞ This approach is summarized in the "Analgesia and Sedation Pyramid" (Fig. 1).

Initially, all patients should have their pain, discomfort, and anxiety treated by removal of exacerbating factors, reducing and splinting fractures, normalizing sleep, and becoming reintroduced to the environment (13,14). Next, analgesics are provided until the pain is adequately reduced. Dissipation of pain can by itself relieve anxiety and emotional distress. Only after adequate analgesia has been delivered, should antianxiety drugs be added.

Delirium can occur for numerous reasons, including the withdrawal or toxicity of psychoactive drugs, traumatic brain injury (TBI), and other causes of organic brain syndrome (OBS), including hypoxemia and organ dysfunction. Accordingly, delirium is treated medically only after considering all the precipitating factors and adjusting doses of all psychoactive drugs. Removing exacerbating factors and administering adequate analgesics, antianxiety drugs, and/ or delirium drugs almost always provides adequate analgesia, sedation, and the desired level of consciousness. However, when normally adequate doses of analgesia and sedation fail to control severe agitation, deep sedation and occasionally the use of NMB drugs may be required.

MECHANISMS OF PAIN
Neural Pathways

Over 300 years ago, René Descartes deduced that pain signals are transmitted from the periphery to the central nervous system (CNS) and interpreted in the brain. He hypothesized that the pain stimulus is analogous to pulling a string at the site of injury, while the other end of the string triggers an alarm bell inside the brain (Fig. 2) (15,16). Modern descriptions of pain pathways similarly refer to noxious stimuli that trigger signals from the periphery to the brain. However, in contrast to the model introduced by Descartes, the pain experience is now recognized as a dynamic process involving multiple humoral modulators and neurotransmitters, along with complex neural connectivity (Fig. 3).

Peripheral sensory nerve fibers that respond to noxious mechanical or chemical stimuli are known as primary nociceptors. These are typically thinly myelinated Aδ or unmyelinated C fibers with the cell bodies located within the dorsal root ganglia. As with other primary afferent nerves, these fibers form synapses with second order ascending neurons within the dorsal columns of the spinal cord. Important ascending nociceptive pathways contained within the spinal cord include the anterior spinothalamic, spinoreticular, and spinomesencephalic tracts along with the postsynaptic dorsal column fibers. Descending neural pathways in the spinal cord also play a role in pain modulation.

Details have recently emerged about the complexity of the cerebral nociceptive neuronal network. The ascending spinal tracts converge at the nuclei of the lateral and medial thalamus, which then project nerve fibers to the somatosensory cortex. This supratentorial neural network is primarily responsible for the sensory-discriminative aspects of the pain experience. The motivational component of pain is processed within the association cortex, involving the limbic system and the anterior cingulate gyrus (both integral structures involved in PTSD—see Volume 2, Chapter 65).

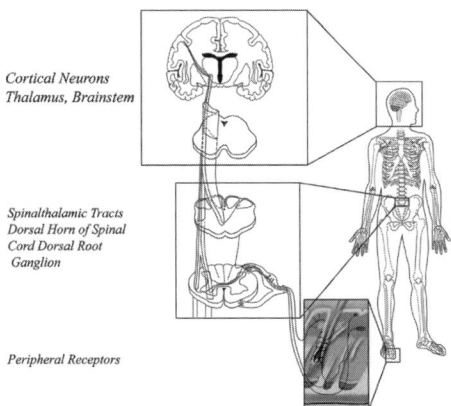

Sensory Nervous System
Pain Pathways

Cortical Neurons
Thalamus, Brainstem

Spinalthalamic Tracts
Dorsal Horn of Spinal
Cord Dorsal Root
Ganglion

Peripheral Receptors

Figure 3 Sensory pathway from skin to brain. Specialized axon terminals in skin transduce pain and sensory events for processing by first-order (peripheral) sensory neurons in the ipsilateral, segmental dorsal root ganglion, whose pseudo unipolar extension terminates in the dorsal horn (substantia gelatinosa) of the spinal cord. Additional processing occurs in deeper layers of the dorsal horn at the same and higher levels. Major sensory and pain pathways including the lateral and ventral spinothalamic tracts and medial lemniscus organize sensory fibers in their progression through the brainstem and thalamus before cerebral cortical termination. *Source*: Courtesy of Robert R. Myers, UCSD School of Medicine peripheral nerve research group.

Progression from Acute to Persistent Pain

The likelihood of developing chronic or persistent pain syndromes (pain that lasts longer than three months after injury despite the absence of ongoing trauma) is increased in patients who have inadequately managed pain in the immediate postinjury period (17). Sensitization of peripheral neurons takes place early after injury due to the release of inflammatory mediators such as H^+, K^+, prostaglandins, and bradykinin, as well as neuropeptides such as substance P and calcitonin gene-related peptide (CGRP). The sensitized peripheral nerves result in perception of pain in response to an innocuous stimulus (allodynia) and exaggerated pain response to a noxious stimulus (hyperalgesia).

Sustained stimulation of peripheral pain fibers can also lead to sensitization of the central neurons within the spinal cord. Following injury, persistent pain fiber stimulation activates *N*-methyl-D-aspartate (NMDA) receptors. This molecular change results in a facilitated pain state, now widely referred to as "wind-up." It can develop within several minutes after injury and is manifested by enhanced sensitivity to mechanical stimuli around the injured tissue. With healing, injury-related pain (including wind-up) usually resolves within a few days to several weeks. However, sometimes long-term changes in the peripheral or central nervous system take place leading to pain that persists long after the tissue has healed. Persistent pain due to the abnormal peripheral or central nerve conduction is referred to as neuropathic pain.

Preemptive Analgesia and Pain Reduction

Pre-emptive analgesia is a method of pain control aimed at reducing the initial intensity of pain, and thereby preventing the development of persistent or neuropathic pain syndromes (18). If transmission of the initial noxious stimulus is altogether prevented by the analgesics at the receptor sites, then the neuronal sensitization will be less likely to occur. In trauma, where significant secondary tissue injury occurs, very early postinjury analgesia can be preemptive if it improves pain control, reduces total analgesic requirements, and prevents progression to persistent pain.

☞ **The administration of analgesia at the earliest possible opportunity will likely have a beneficial effect on the long-term outcome of patients who sustain tissue injury from trauma or surgery.** ☞ This clinical consensus is supported by abundant experimental data; indeed, patients with initially poorly controlled pain are more prone to develop persistent pain than the patients who have received early satisfactory analgesia (17–19). However, contrary to this evidence and probably due to numerous confounding variables, some clinical studies of effectiveness of pre-emptive or early post-trauma analgesia in improving pain control and preventing persistent pain were inconclusive (20).

PHARMACOLOGY REVIEW

Because pain mechanisms are complex, analgesic pharmacotherapy often consists of several classes of drugs, each targeting a different neural pathway. Such an approach, known as multimodal analgesia, capitalizes upon analgesic synergy between various drugs while mitigating their deleterious side effects.

Nonsteroidal Anti-inflammatory Drugs/Cyclooxygenase Enzyme Inhibitors

Herbs containing nonsteroidal anti-inflammatory drugs (NSAIDs) were known by ancient Egyptians, and are referred to in the Ebers papyrus (21). In 1763, Edward Stone isolated salicin, the glycoside of salicylic acid, from the bark of a willow tree (*Salix alba*). Today NSAIDs are among the most commonly used medications worldwide. Although employed for centuries in the treatment of pain, fever, and inflammation, the molecular mechanism of NSAIDs was not elucidated until the 1970s by Vane et al. (22). It was then discovered that NSAIDs inhibit the enzyme cyclooxygenase (COX), and the subsequent formation of prostaglandin E (PGE). The predominant COX enzyme isoform, COX-1, is expressed constitutively in many tissues, including the kidneys, GI tract, platelets, and endothelium; whereas the COX-2 isoform is typically produced only following tissue injury. However, COX-2 is also expressed constitutively in some tissues, including the CNS, renal cortex, pancreas, and uterus.

Several well-known adverse effects, such as GI irritation, renal insufficiency, platelet inhibition, bronchospasm, and elevated liver enzyme levels, can complicate therapy with NSAIDs. Nonspecific inhibition of COX enzymes can cause platelet deactivation (irreversible with aspirin and indomethacin) (23), renal insufficiency, and GI mucosal erosion and perforation. COX-2 specific inhibitors are safer than nonspecific COX inhibitors, with respect to GI erosions and platelet inactivation (24,25). However, they retain the renal side effects seen with nonspecific COX inhibitors (26).

More recently, COX-2 enzyme inhibition has been shown to also retard angiogenesis and healing (27–29); however, these effects are probably mild. The ultimate decision for the use of NSAIDs and selective COX-2 inhibitors in trauma or critical care is based on the type and extent of injury (especially intracranial hemorrhagic lesions), and the presence of relative contraindications such as renal insufficiency or coagulopathy (including the concomitant use of anticoagulant or thrombolytic drugs), and so on.

Numerous NSAIDs are available as first-line analgesics for mild pain (Table 1). Among these, ketorolac is the only NSAID available in intravenous (IV) form in the United States. For this reason, and because of its relatively high analgesic efficacy, ketorolac is commonly selected for postoperative analgesia in trauma and critical care. Ketorolac inhibits platelet function; however, numerous studies were unable to define the risk of bleeding associated with this drug (30). Increase in bleeding time after administration of a high IV dose (60 mg) of ketorolac to healthy volunteers was shown to be mild and generally insignificant (31). Ketorolac can be administered IV or intramuscularly (IM) every six hours at 15- to 30-mg doses for five days. In trauma patients with massive tissue injury (especially in the CNS) and/or coagulopathy, ketorolac is contraindicated.

Acetaminophen (paracetamol) differs from typical NSAIDs in its mechanism of action and side effect profile. Its inhibition of prostaglandin synthesis appears to be limited to the CNS. Acetaminophen lacks anti-inflammatory activity in the peripheral tissues and, consequently, does not pose the same degree of bleeding risks as typical NSAIDs. However, at high doses acetaminophen (>100 mg/kg in adults or >150 mg/kg in children) can cause severe hepatotoxicity, and with chronic use has been shown to cause renal impairment (32,33).

Table 1 Nonsteroidal Anti-inflammatory Drugs Used for Analgesia

Generic drug (trade name)	Recommended dose
Aspirin	325–650 mg every 4 hr
Ibuprofen (Motrin®)	200–800 mg 3–4 times a day
Ketorolac (Toradol®)	Maximum duration of administration is 5 days
	IV/IM: 15–30 mg every 6 hrs, maximum dose is 60 mg/24 hrs in patients 65 yr or older
	Oral: 10 mg every 4–6 hrs not to exceed 40 mg/24 hrs (Note: IM dosing not recommended.)
Naproxen (Naprosyn®)	250–500 mg twice a day
Diclofenac (Voltaren®)	50–75 mg twice a day or 50 mg 3 times a day
Etodolac (Lodine®)	200–400 mg every 6–8 hrs
Flurbiprofen (Ansaid®)	200–300 mg daily divided 2 to 3 times a day
Indomethacin (Indocin®)	25–50 mg every 6–8 hrs
Ketoprofen (Orudis®)	25–50 mg every 6–8 hrs
Nabumetone (Relafen®)	1000–2000 mg daily or divided twice a day
Sulindac (Clinoril®)	150 mg twice a day

Abbreviations: IM, intramuscularly; IV, intravenously.

Paracetamol is available in IV and oral (PO) forms in Europe, whereas acetaminophen is only available in PO form in the United States. Side effects from short-term use of this medication are rare. However, liver toxicity following overdose can be lethal (see Volume 1, Chapter 31 and Volume 2, Chapter 36). Contraindications are limited to patients with severe hepatic disease and those allergic to the drug. Analgesia occurs approximately 30 minutes after IV administration of paracetamol (2 g over 15-minute infusion).

Local Anesthetics (Sodium Channel Blockers)

Structurally related to the prototype cocaine, local anesthetic drugs produce reversible block of voltage-gated sodium channels, thereby increasing the threshold required for electrical excitation of the neuron. These drugs can be applied topically, injected locally, IV, epidurally, intrathecally, and orally.

Lidocaine is available in the injectible form as well as in various topical formulations. This local anesthetic has relatively low levels of CNS and cardiovascular toxicity. The duration of action of subcutaneous (SQ) lidocaine can be prolonged by local vasoconstriction achieved by the addition of epinephrine. Lidocaine is also infused intravenously to treat ventricular dysrhythmias and has shown to be efficacious in the treatment of refractory pain in burn patients (34).

Bupivacaine is more potent, but has a slower onset than lidocaine. Its duration of action depends on vascular absorption at the site of injection and can persist for as long as 12 hours (more commonly three to six hours) with the peripheral nerve blocks and three hours with epidural or intrathecal blockade (more commonly 1.5–2 hours). Compared to other local anesthetics, bupivacaine exhibits greater sensory than motor blockade, and it is often used

Table 2 Maximum Doses of Local Anesthetics in 70-kg Patient

Drug	Commonly employed concentration (%)	Plain solution	Epinephrine-containing solution
Lidocaine	0.5–1.0	300 mg (4.5 mg/kg)	500 mg (7 mg/kg)
Bupivacaine	0.125–0.5	175 mg (3 mg/kg) per dose, 440 mg per 24 hrs	Not established
Ropivacaine	0.2–0.5	Dose of 770 mg/24 hrs has not been reported	Not established

for local infiltration and regional nerve blockade. Ropivacaine, structurally similar to bupivacaine, is slightly less potent, but is safer with respect to cardiotoxicity (35).

Systemically administered local anesthetics can be used to block sodium channels involved in pain transmission, and to decrease ventricular irritability (e.g., lidocaine infusion). However, when doses are too high (Table 2), sodium channels of inhibitory nerves located in the CNS can become blocked causing seizures; at higher plasma concentrations, myocardial tissue becomes irritable, causing dysrhythmias. The excitatory neurotoxic effects range from tremors and agitation to generalized seizures.

Myocardial toxicity can occur after administration of any local anesthetic, but it is most characteristically associated with the highly lipophilic agents (e.g., bupivacaine), which are characterized by "fast in, slow out" kinetics. Cardiac toxicity is manifested by depression of myocardial contractility, atrioventricular blocks, and ventricular dysrhythmias. In order to avoid neurotoxic and cardiovascular complications, local anesthetics are administered for regional and topical anesthesia incrementally at submaximal doses (Table 2). Inadvertent intravascular injections of local anesthetics are avoided by repeated aspiration through the needle.

⟟ **Local anesthetics do not work efficiently when injected in the vicinity of infected tissue.** ⟟ Local tissue acidemia occurs in the presence of cellulitis, abscess, and other forms of tissue infections. The impaired function of local anesthetics in infected tissues occurs because they are weak bases, and in aqueous solution, the relative concentration of neutral or ionized molecules is pH dependent. The neutral (nonionized) form of the local anesthetics preferentially permeates the cellular membrane of the neuron to its site of action at the sodium channel of the axon (Fig. 4). The fraction of neutral species decreases with a fall in tissue pH. Accordingly, their efficacy is diminished and onset of action is delayed in an acidic environment, where the polar (ionized) form predominates and is unable to traverse the nerve cell membrane.

Opioids
General Considerations
Opioids provide analgesia by stimulating $\mu - 1$ and κ opioid receptors. These receptors are distributed throughout the CNS particularly along the pain pathways and processing centers such as laminae I and II of the dorsal column of the spinal cord, spinal trigeminal nucleus, locus ceruleus, and periaqueductal gray. Opioid receptor activity results in the inhibition of the ascending pain pathways, and by activation of the descending inhibitory spinal pathways.

Specific Opioids
Morphine is a widely used opioid in treatment of acute pain. It conjugates in the liver to morphine-3-gluconoride (M3G) and morphine-6-gluconoride (M6G). M6G is a potent analgesic and probably contributes significantly to analgesia, particularly after prolonged morphine use. M3G, on the other hand, is neurotoxic and can result in hyperalgesia.

Following an IV administration, morphine provides peak analgesic and respiratory effects at 15 to 20 minutes with a clinical duration of two to three hours (Table 3).

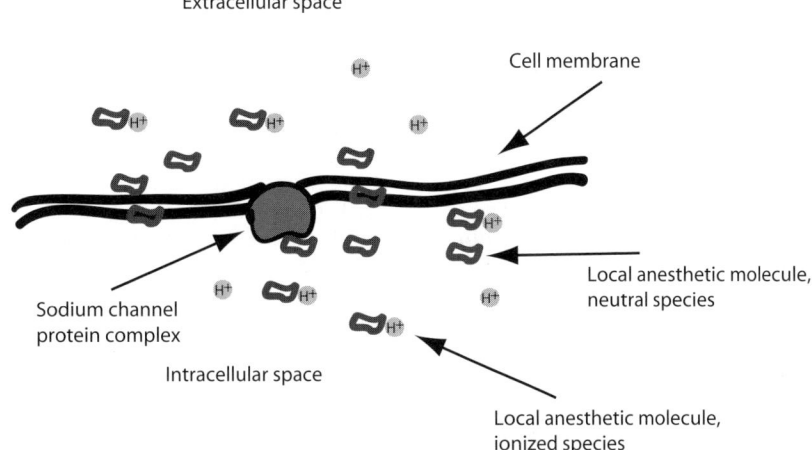

Extracellular space

Cell membrane

Sodium channel protein complex

Intracellular space

Local anesthetic molecule, neutral species

Local anesthetic molecule, ionized species

Figure 4 Schematic representation of ionized and neutral species of local anesthetic in the intracellular and extracellular media. The binding site of sodium channel receptor complex is located within the axon on the cytoplasm side of the cell membrane. Ionized (protonated) species of local anesthetics bind to the active site of the sodium channel protein complex, whereas neutral (deprotonated) local anesthetic species cross the cell membrane into the cytoplasm.

Table 3 Pharmacokinetic Properties (Onset, Peak, Effect, Clinical Duration, and Half-Life) After Single IV Bolus of Commonly Used Opioids

Drug/property	Onset (min)	Peak[a] (min)	Clinical duration of analgesia
Morphine	3–5	15–20	2–4 hr
Fentanyl	1	5	Low dose (25–150 μg): 30–45 min
			Moderate dose (150–500 μg): 45 min to 2 hr
			High dose (>500 μg): 2–4 hr
Hydromorphone	3–5	15–20	3–4 hr
Meperidine	3–5	15–20	2–4 hr

[a]Peak analgesia and respiratory depression effects tend to occur at the same time.

Peak analgesia with IM or SQ morphine is less predictable, but typically occurs after 45 to 90 minutes, with a clinical duration of three to four hours. Compared to the IV dose, a much smaller dose of morphine is required to produce analgesia with epidural administration, and up to 100 times less with intrathecal injection. The onset of analgesia following epidural administration of morphine is 30 minutes, with peak effect at two to three hours, and dose-dependent clinical duration of 4 to 18 hours. Intrathecal morphine bolus has an onset of around five minutes, and may provide analgesia for up to 24 hours. Bioavailability of PO morphine is 30%. Several formulations of PO morphine are able to provide sustained analgesia for up to 24 hours.

Fentanyl is a synthetic opioid structurally similar to meperidine. Peak analgesia following IV administration of this highly lipophilic drug is achieved within several minutes (Table 3). Fentanyl exhibits a two-phase pharmacokinetic profile. It is first taken up by the central compartments (lungs initially absorb 75% of IV fentanyl bolus). Fentanyl is then widely redistributed in body tissues (β-elimination), followed by a slow metabolism in the liver (β-elimination). Although the β-elimination half-life of fentanyl is slightly longer than that of morphine, its plasma concentration falls rapidly after a single small bolus (due to α-elimination), and its duration of analgesia is typically only 30 to 60 minutes following a small dose (50–100 μg), 60 to 90 minutes after moderate dose (150–250 μg), and two to four hours after larger doses (500–1000 μg).

Fentanyl is a potent opioid, and 100 μg of this drug is equianalgesic to 10 mg IV morphine. Because of its lipophilic properties and the propensity for redistribution, epidurally administered fentanyl provides analgesia at both the spinal level as well as at supraspinal CNS centers following systemic absorption and distribution. Fentanyl acts predominantly at the spinal level when administered as an epidural bolus, and at both spinal and supraspinal sites when continuously infused (36). In addition to the parenteral form, fentanyl is available as a sustained-release transdermal patch, and as a transmucosal lozenge applied to the buccal mucosa to treat breakthrough pain.

Other fentanyl derivatives are occasionally used in acute trauma and critical care. Alfentanil is an opioid that is approximately one-third as potent as fentanyl, and has a very short duration of action (15 to 25 minutes). In contrast to fentanyl, accumulation of alfentanil in the tissue is insignificant. The brief duration of action of alfentanil limits its use in acute post-traumatic pain except for very short-term procedural analgesia. Sufentanil is 5 to 10 times more potent than fentanyl. It causes approximately the same degree of respiratory depression and sedation as fentanyl at equipotent dosing.

Remifentanil is an opioid agonist with the most rapid onset (less than one minute) and the shortest duration of action of all clinically available opioids. It is metabolized via hydrolysis by tissue esterases; thus, its metabolism and elimination do not depend on hepatic or renal mechanisms. The blood concentration of remifentanil decreases by 50% after only three to six minutes, and its rapid elimination is independent of the duration of its administration. The dose range of IV infusion of remifentanil is 0.1–2 μg/kg/min. Rapid dissipation of analgesia and return of pain after remifentanil discontinuation precludes its routine use for acute trauma. However, intensivists and anesthesiologists experienced in its use can safely administer remifentanil for brief episodes of intense pain. Furthermore, as an IV infusion, remifentanil may be indicated in patients with multiple organ dysfunction syndrome (MODS), in whom unwanted prolonged analgesic and sedative effects might occur with the use of other drugs.

Hydromorphone is a semisynthetic morphine analog that can be administered PO, rectally (PR), IV, and epidurally. A 2-mg IV dose of this opioid is equipotent to 10 mg of IV morphine (Table 3). Following IV administration of hydromorphone, full analgesic and respiratory depressive effects are achieved within 15 minutes, lasting up to three to four hours (37). Hydromorphone is commonly used for epidural analgesia. Its water–lipid solubility properties lie between those of morphine and fentanyl; consequently, hydromorphone does not spread cephalad within the cerebrospinal fluid (CSF) as much as morphine, nor does it redistribute into the systemic circulation as much as fentanyl.

Meperidine is a synthetic opioid that is approximately one-tenth as potent as morphine. In patients with normal renal function, meperidine is injected IV or IM at incremental 12.5 to 75-mg doses to a maximum of 800 mg in 24 hours. Peak analgesia and respiratory depression occurs within 10 to 15 minutes following IV administration, with a clinical duration of two to three hours. Meperidine, as a member of the phenylpiperidine class, has strong local analgesic properties (38). It also exhibits activity at α_2-adrenoreceptors (39). Reported exacerbation of postoperative delirium and tachycardia are attributed to the anticholinergic properties of meperidine (40).

Meperidine has a neurotoxic metabolite, normeperidine. This renally excreted compound has a long elimination half-life and can induce myoclonus and seizures after repeated use, particularly in patients with renal impairment. Meperidine also interacts with monoamine oxidase inhibitors (MAOIs). This interaction can lead to accumulation of serotonin, resulting in hyperpyrexia (see Volume 1, Chapter 40 and Volume 2, Chapter 46), delirium, and seizures. Due to its severe side effects and potential complications, meperidine should be reserved for patients whose pain could not be adequately controlled with safer opioids.

Methadone is a synthetic opioid structurally unrelated to morphine. In addition to the opioid activity at the μ-receptors, methadone has an additional analgesic effect manifested through antagonism of NMDA receptors. Parenterally administered methadone is equipotent to IV morphine;

however, its pharmacokinetic profile is quite distinct. Typical onset of analgesia is 10 to 20 minutes following an IV bolus, and between 30 and 60 minutes after a PO dose.

Methadone bioavailability (41–99%) and elimination half-life (15 to 120 hours) can vary widely among patients (41). Furthermore, because of a rapid initial redistribution phase, and a long and unpredictable elimination phase, there is an apparent dissociation between the relatively short duration of analgesic properties (six to eight hours) and cumulative plasma concentration. Consequently, initial doses of this drug should be low, with gradual and infrequent (every three days) upward dose titration. Due to the diminished euphoric effects and low abuse potential, methadone is widely used to treat opioid addiction as a once-a-day dosing of approximately 30 mg. When used for analgesia, dosing is scheduled three to four times a day.

Naloxone is a semisynthetic opioid antagonist devoid of agonist activity. The competitive antagonism of opioid receptors is brief in duration, typically lasting less than 45 minutes. Therefore, repeated doses, or IV infusion, of naloxone are required to antagonize the effect of long-acting opioids. Onset of action is within one to two minutes after IV administration. Naloxone is primarily used to reverse opioid overdose. Administration of high dose (400 μg) of naloxone is recommended only in the situation of opioid-induced apnea accompanied by difficulty to maintain airway. Because of significant side effects, including pulmonary edema, prior practices of administering 2 mg of naloxone (equivalent to 5 ampules of naloxone each containing 400 μg) is no longer recommended as part of a routine prehospital or emergency department (ED) "coma cocktail." Instead, titration of opioid antagonism to effect is currently recommended, as dictated by the clinical circumstances.

Nalbuphine is a mixed opioid agonist/antagonist. It provides analgesia via κ receptor agonism, with analgesic potency equivalent to that of IV morphine. Nalbuphine is associated with opioid-specific side effects, including respiratory depression. Nalbuphine-produced analgesia, somnolence, and respiratory depression, are however, limited by a ceiling effect. Although nalbuphine is a potent analgesic, as a μ-receptor antagonist it reverses some of the opioid effects; it is accordingly used to treat opioid-induced pruritis, sedation, and respiratory depression.

Relative Potencies of Opioids

Clinicians are often faced with the need to change opioid regimens. Examples of such changes are conversion from the IV to PO route, and substitution of one opioid for another because of intolerable side effects.

When switching from one opioid to another in nonopioid-tolerant patients, equianalgesic doses are initially recommended. There is large variability in individual responses to different opioids; therefore, opioid equianalgesic conversion tables (Table 4) are used only as an approximate guide in establishing opioid therapy. In addition, it is generally recommended that only 75% of the calculated dose of the next opioid drug should be used in chronic pain patients, to account for the incomplete cross-tolerance effects. Particular caution should be exercised when the opioid regimen is changed to methadone, because of its long and unpredictable half-life.

Adverse Side Effects of Opioid Therapy

☞ **Among the side effects associated with opioids (Table 5), respiratory depression, loss of airway, and hypotension are**

Table 4 Equianalgesic Doses of Parenterally and Orally Administered Opioids

Drug	Intravenous (mg)	Oral equivalent (mg)
Morphine	10	30
Fentanyl	0.1	NA
Hydromorphone	2	7.5
Meperidine	100	300
Methadone	10	10–20
Oxycodone	NA	20

Abbreviation: NA, not available.

potentially the most dangerous. Indeed, fear of respiratory depression is a common cause of inadequate analgesia in critically ill patients. ☞ Opioids exhibit a dose-related increase in apneic threshold and CO_2 responsiveness (increasingly higher CO_2 partial pressure is required to stimulate spontaneous breathing). They also decrease the RR and, consequently, the $\dot{V}_E$. Longer-acting opioids such as morphine have slower onset and longer duration of respiratory depression than shorter-acting fentanyl. Opioid-induced respiratory depression can be mitigated by gradual titration. Monitoring of oxygen saturation, end-tidal CO_2, RR, and respiratory effort can provide accurate and continuous assessment of the respiratory status. ☞ **Pain stimulates the respiratory drive and counteracts the sedative effects of opioids. Consequently, patients on relatively high doses of opioids, who then undergo regional nerve blockade, can develop acute respiratory depression because of abrupt abolition of the afferent pain stimulus.** ☞

Decrease in GI motility and constipation develops in many patients treated with opioids. These patients are at increased risk of not tolerating enteral nutrition. In order to reduce this risk, it is prudent to administer bowel promotility agents early in critically ill patients who are receiving opioids and demonstrating decreased gut motility.

A progressive program involving a combination regimen, consisting of oral cellulose (e.g., Metamucil®) a softening agent (docusate), a cathartic (senna compounds), and an osmotic (lactulose, polyethylene glycol), is usually more effective than single-drug treatment. In refractory cases, patients require colonic lavage or oral bowel preparations. Severe GI stasis may respond to PO naloxone, starting at doses of 0.4–1.2 mg every four to six hours to induce bowel movement. Because of the risk of bowel perforation, PO naloxone is strictly contraindicated in patients with bowel obstruction. In addition, metoclopromide and/or erythromycin can be used as gastropropulsive drugs (both also contraindicated in the setting of bowel obstruction).

Opioid-induced nausea occurs in 10% to 40% of patients; however, it tends to abate gradually in most patients due to tolerance. Several mechanisms may be responsible for nausea, including delayed gastric emptying, vestibular sensitivity, and effects on the chemoreceptor trigger zone. Drugs effective for treating opioid-induced nausea include scopolamine, prochlorperazine, and serotonin receptor antagonists such as dolasetron or ondansetron, antihistimines, neuroleptic agents (haloperidol, chlorpromazine, and droperidol), benzodiazepines, and corticosteroids. Metoclopramide can treat nausea caused by delayed gastric emptying.

Sedation is a common opioid side effect that can be both beneficial and deleterious. The first step in reducing severity of this side effect is the discontinuation of any

Table 5 Opioid Receptor–Specific Analgesic Effects and Side Effects

Action or side effect	Receptor	Comments
Supraspinal analgesia	μ-1, κ	Cranial-level analgesia occurs with systemically administered opioids
Spinal analgesia	κ	Predominant-spinal level analgesia occurs with subarachnoid and epidural opioid administration
Respiratory depression	μ-2	Respiratory effects of opioids generally coincide with analgesic effects
Sympatholysis	μ-1, κ, σ	In patients with preexisting hypovolemia, opioids can precipitate severe decrease in blood pressure driven by sympatholysis
Sedation	μ-1, κ	Tolerance to sedative effects develops with time
Bradycardia	μ-1	Bradycardia is more prominent with fast-acting lipophilic opioids such as fentanyl
Miosis	κ	Tolerance to this effect develops with time
Constipation, intestinal motility retardation	μ-2	More common with systemic opioids than neuroaxial opioids
Pruritus	μ-2	Pruritis is more common with neuraxial than systemic opioids
Nausea and vomiting	μ-2	Nausea occurs in more than 30% of patients
Dysphoria, delirium, hallucinations	σ	Opioids contribute to development of delirium in intensive care
Euphoria, addiction, physical dependence	μ-2	Physical dependence is a normal physiologic response that develops over time

other CNS depressants and correction of coexisting metabolic problems. Subsequent steps include adjusting the opioid dose, rotating to a different opioid (42), or treating somnolence with psychostimulants such as methylphenidate or dextroamphetamine.

Modafinil (Provigil®) is a newer psychostimulant that was initially developed for treatment of narcolepsy; it is now also approved by the Food and Drug Administration (FDA) for reduction of daytime somnolence in shift workers. Modafinil reportedly has lesser abuse potential than traditional psychostimulant drugs, and may have a role in persistently somnolent critical care patients.

High-dose-opioid-induced myoclonus requires an immediate reduction in dose. Patients treated with opioids can develop tolerance, physical dependence, and addiction (discussed subsequently).

Sedative, Hypnotic, and Anxiolytic Drugs

Several classes of drugs are available for anxiolysis and sedation in trauma and critical care (Table 6). They include benzodiazepines, propofol, dexmedetomidine, and ketamine. Sedating properties of opioids are unpredictable

because of this property and respiratory depression, they are not used to primarily treat anxiety, agitation, or delirium. However, the early and adequate administration of opioid analgesia will often minimize the need for subsequent sedative administration. Benzodiazepines and propofol suppress respiration in a dose-related fashion. They also blunt and eventually lead to the obliteration of laryngeal airway protecting reflexes and pharyngeal muscle tone, thereby contributing to the risk of loss of airway and aspiration of gastric contents when heavily sedating doses are used. In contrast, dexmedetomidine does not depress respiration or airway reflexes and has other particular advantages as described subsequently.

Benzodiazepines

Midazolam is a potent, short-acting benzodiazepine used extensively as a sedative/anxiolytic in perioperative, acute trauma, and critical care settings. As with other benzodiazepines, midazolam increases the affinity for gamma amino butyric acid (GABA) receptor by changing the conformation of GABA$_A$ receptor complex. Onset of action following IV midazolam administration is within 1

Table 6 Pharmacology of Single-Dose Bolus of Sedatives, Hypnotics, and Neuroleptic Drugs

Drug	Typical dose IV	Onset time after IV bolus	Duration of action
Midazolam	1–2 mg	2–5 min	1–2 hr
Diazepam	1–5 mg	2–5 min	2–3 hr
Lorazepam	1–2 mg	20–30 min	3–4 hr
Propofol	50–100 mg	Less than 1 min	5–10 min
Dexmedetomide	Loading dose: 1 μg/kg for 10 min, followed by infusion: 0.2–0.7 μg/kg/hr	Less than 5 min	15–30 min
Ketamine	20–50 mg	Less than 1 min	15–45 min
Haloperidol	1–5 mg	5–10 min	4–8 hr
Ziprasidone	10–20 mg	30 min	3–5 hr

Typical initial doses are generally on the lower dose range, with titration upward as patient response warrants. These doses can cause apnea in elderly or hypovolemic patients and are suggested only for fully resuscitated patients requiring bolus dose of drug.
Abbreviation: IV, intravenously.

to 5 minutes. Sedation occurs 5 to 15 minutes after IM, and 10 to 30 minutes after PO administrations. It has an elimination half-life of one to five hours, and a clinical duration of action ranging from two to four hours depending upon dose and chronicity of use. Bioavailability of midazolam is approximately 35%. Typical adult IV anxiolytic dose is 0.5 to 2 mg; it may be repeated every five minutes until the desired level of sedation is delivered.

Lorazepam is an intermediate-acting benzodiazepine, and is available both IV and PO. Its half-life of 12 hours is intermediate between midazolam and diazepam. Despite the markedly longer half-life compared to midazolam, the clinical duration of action of lorazepam is only slightly longer (three to six hours). The durations of action of both midazolam and lorazepam are more predictable than that of diazepam (as described later). The onset of action following IV administration of lorazepam is, however, slower than that of midazolam or diazepam. Accordingly, lorazepam is less suitable for rapid treatment of titration and acute anxiety. Lorazepam does serve as an excellent drug for prolonged sedation (longer than 72 hours) in critically ill patients. It has no active metabolites, but the conjugated form (which is normally excreted in the urine) accumulates in patients with renal failure.

Diazepam is a longer-acting benzodiazepine than either midazolam or lorazepam. It can be administered IV, PO, or PR. In addition to its sedative and anxiolytic properties, diazepam is also used as an anticonvulsant and skeletal muscle antispasticity agent. Typical onset of action after an IV administration is one to five minutes. Diazepam has a half-life exceeding 30 hours; however, its clinical duration of action is only six hours. This discrepancy is presumed to be due to its extensive protein binding (98%). Diazepam is metabolized to active metabolite desmethyldiazepam, which accumulates in renal failure. Single-dose administration typically results in rapid onset as well as rapid dissipation of sedation. However, systemic absorption of diazepam even after a single IM dose can be slow and unpredictable. Repeated doses and continuous infusion cause accumulation of diazepam and its metabolites, resulting in delayed awakening.

Nonbenzodiazepine sedative-hypnotic drugs include zolpidem (Ambien®), zaleplon (Sonata®), and eszopiclone (Lunesta®). Although they are active at the GABA receptors, these drugs are chemically unrelated to classic benzodiazepines, and are less likely to produce residual sedation. After fast onset, the duration of action of zaleplon and zolpidem is approximately four hours and six to eight hours respectively.

Flumazenil is a specific benzodiazepine antagonist with strong affinity to the GABA receptors. It is useful in treating the respiratory depressant and sedative effects of benzodiazepines. In the absence of benzodiazepines, flumazenil is usually devoid of clinically significant intrinsic activity. However, it has been used to improve the mental state of critically ill patients with hepatic encephalopathy. The onset of action of IV flumazenil is less than one minute, with the peak effect in one to three minutes, and duration of action between 40 and 90 minutes. To reverse benzodiazepine-induced CNS depression, the typical initial adult dose of flumazenil is 0.2 mg; it may be repeated every minute to a total of 1 mg in five minutes. This titration sequence may be repeated at 20-minute intervals, up to a maximum of 3 mg/hr (43). ☞ **In long-term benzodiazepine users, and if given in too large of a dose (rather than titrated as recommended), flumazenil can precipitate seizures or** other withdrawal symptoms, including acute onset of severe anxiety, myoclonus, and tremors. ☞

Propofol

Propofol is a sedative-hypnotic agent not related to other anesthetics or sedatives. Within the CNS it exhibits agonist activity at the GABA$_A$ receptors by activating the chloride channels. In addition, propofol inhibits the NMDA subtype of glutamate receptors (44). It is administered IV as a series of bolus doses for procedural sedation, or more commonly in the SICU by continuous infusion. Injection of propofol is often associated with transient burning pain in the injection site veins. Pain is decreased if administered approximately five minutes after fentanyl 1–2 mg/kg, and/or after IV lidocaine is administered.

Following IV administration of general-anesthesia-induction dose (2 mg/kg), unconsciousness occurs within 20 to 40 seconds. The time to onset of sedation, which requires significantly smaller doses than for anesthesia, is one to five minutes. Sedation with propofol continues as long as the infusion provides adequate drug serum concentration. Emergence occurs approximately 10 minutes after administration of a single bolus dose, and awakening usually occurs in less than 30 minutes following cessation of infusions shorter than 72 hours in duration. Sedation with propofol typically requires infusion rates ranging from 25–150 µg/kg/min depending upon the patient's baseline level of consciousness, metabolism, and concomitant psychoactive drug administration.

Dexmedetomidine

Dexmedetomidine is a recently introduced selective α_2-adrenoceptor agonist that exerts centrally acting sedative, analgesic, and sympatholytic effects. Among the distinguishing properties of this sedative drug is the preservation of respiratory drive and protective airway reflexes.

Dexmedetomidine is clinically indicated for sedation of intubated trauma and critically ill patients in preparation for extubation, and in nonintubated patients requiring sedation. The relative absence of respiratory depression is unique to this drug, and allows for its continuation throughout the weaning process, including the first few hours to days after extubation. However, dexmedetomidine is more expensive than most of the other sedative drugs.

Dexmedetomidine is particularly beneficial in patients with obstructive sleep apnea (they tend to be more sensitive to the respiratory depressant properties of opioids and benzodiazepines than patients without the disorder). It is also particularly useful in those with alcohol or drug addiction (whose sedation is often difficult to titrate using propofol or benzodiazepines).

Dexmedetomidine is administered by an IV infusion. It is distributed to the tissues with an onset of action occurring within five minutes and a β-elimination half-life of six minutes. Recovery from the effects of dexmedetomidine is rapid (15 to 30 minutes) at normal sedative doses, although its terminal elimination half-life is in the order of two hours. Dexmedetomidine is commonly infused by first administering a loading bolus of 1 µg/kg over 10 minutes, followed by an initial infusion rates between 0.2 and 0.7 µg/kg/hr titrated to an effect. Chronic pain patients, alcoholics, and drug addicts frequently require much higher doses. The authors often employ doses ranging between 1 and 2 µg/kg/hr in patients with long-term sedative or opioid use, including those patients with a current history of chronic pain.

Hemodynamic changes are frequently observed during dexmedetomidine administration. A short-lived hypertensive response will occasionally occur during the initiation of dexmedetomidine infusion (especially during the bolus load). This effect is almost always followed by a decrease in blood pressure (BP) and HR. Patients with prominent vagal tone, such as young athletes, and those on β-blockers are particularly susceptible to severe bradycardia (treatable with vagolytic or sympathomimetic drugs) during dexmedetomidine infusion. Some of the side effects from dexmedetomidine can appear similar to those of opioids, with decreased HR, BP, and small pupils. However, in contrast to opioid administration, dexmedetomidine does not depress respiration.

Ketamine

Ketamine in doses of 2 mg/kg IV, 10 mg/kg IM, or 30 mg/kg PO serves as a sedative-hypnotic drug similar in structure and activity to phencyclidine (PCP). It produces profound analgesia even at subanesthetic doses. The analgesic and anesthetic effects of ketamine are achieved through several mechanisms. It inhibits cholinergic pathways and has strong sympathomimetic activity. Ketamine also noncompetitively inhibits NMDA receptors. Despite this theoretical neuroprotective property, ketamine also increases cerebral metabolic rate of oxygen ($CMRO_2$) and cerebral blood flow (CBF); thus, it has not been used in TBI patients for fear of increasing intracranial pressure (ICP).

In addition to contributing to analgesia, NMDA receptor blockade is responsible for psychosis-like side effects. Ketamine is particularly active within the limbic system and the cortex and thereby produces a feeling of dissociation from the environment. Its administration is typically followed by increased HR, BP (sympathomimetic effect), and muscle tone; a cataleptic state ensues with most patients, requiring only intermittent reassurances from the anesthesiologist. As this dissociative state occurs, horizontal nystagmus becomes evident.

The strong sympathetic activity is observed in most hemodynamically normal patients who have received ketamine. However, hypovolemic and other patients who are under physiologic stress, are often unable to mount strong adrenergic response, due to depletion of, and insensitivity to, already massively elaborated catecholamines and the direct myocardial effects will become predominant. ☞ **The hemodynamically unstable, hemorrhaging trauma patient is a classic example where ketamine predominantly exhibits cardiac depressant effects (45).** ☞

On the other hand, at therapeutic doses, ketamine offers several advantages, including preservation of pharyngeal and laryngeal reflexes and spontaneous respiration. Thus, in adequately resuscitated patients, ketamine is extremely useful and widely used by injection or infusion during painful procedures (e.g., wound debridement, or burn wound dressing changes). These beneficial properties make ketamine a good choice for use in austere military settings. Ketamine also possesses potent bronchodilator effects, and is particularly useful in the treatment of patients with bronchospasm. Ketamine also produces significant salivation and bronchorrhea; accordingly, small prophylactic doses of glycopyrrolate are recommended prior to its administration.

Neuroleptic Drugs

Several neuroleptic (antipsychotic) medications are available for the treatment of delirium. Haloperidol is arguably the most commonly used neuroleptic drug in the treatment of delirium and acute psychotic disorders in the trauma and critically ill patients. Its mechanism of action involves the blockade of postsynaptic dopamine-2 (D_2) receptors. Haloperidol has an FDA indication for PO and IM use. However, it is most commonly injected, a route of administration still without FDA approval. Onset of action after an IV dose of haloperidol occurs within 3 to 20 minutes, and the tranquilizing effect typically lasts two to four hours. Some mental status changes may, however, last as long as 12 hours.

Droperidol has long been used by anesthesiologists as both a neuroleptic drug and an antiemetic. The CNS properties of droperidol are similar to those of haloperidol; however, droperidol has a more pronounced α_1-adrenergic receptor blocking effect, which can exacerbate hypotension in hemodynamically unstable patients. Droperidol is also associated with prolongation of the QTc interval, with theoretically increased risk of serious ventricular dysrhythmias including Torsade de Pointes. Although the increased risk of cardiac dysrhythmias with droperidol has been recently widely publicized, many believe that this risk has been overemphasized in the literature (Volume 2, Chapter 20).

☞ **The slightly elevated risk of Torsade de Pointes associated with droperidol is also present with other antipsychotic drugs including haloperidol.** ☞

Ziprasidone, olanzapine, and risperidone represent newer atypical antipsychotic drugs. They tend to cause less sedation, fewer mental status changes, and extrapyramidal symptoms than the traditional neuroleptic drugs like haloperidol. The likelihood of developing tardive dyskinesia (TD) is reportedly reduced with the atypical compared to traditional neuroleptics. If PO administration of these drugs cannot be tolerated, then ziprasidone and olanzapine can be administered parenterally. Ziprasidone is administered IM to a total of 40 mg per 24 hours at 10-mg doses every two hours or 20-mg doses every four hours. Olanzapine is dosed at 5- to 10-mg IM every two hours to a maximum of two doses per 24 hours.

Skeletal Muscle Antispasticity Drugs

Muscle spasms contribute substantially to the pain due to injuries of spine and the extremities. For this reason, skeletal muscle antispasticity drugs play an important role in controlling acute postoperative and postinjury pain. These drugs are not related to NMB agents, which cause temporary skeletal muscle paralysis, and consequent complete apnea (Volume 2, Chapter 6). Drugs used for the purpose of relieving or preventing skeletal muscle spasms belong to various classes and include benzodiazepines (Table 7). Diazepam is the usual first-line drug for short-term spasticity; however, in presence of excessive somnolence or renal insufficiency, other drug categories, for example, cyclobenzaprine or baclofen, are typically used instead. Tizanadine, a newer antispasticity agent, also has analgesic properties through the activity at the central α_2-adrenergic receptors. Although muscle antispasticity drugs work by a variety of mechanisms, they all cause a certain degree of CNS depression manifested by drowsiness and sedation.

Other Analgesic Agents

Neuropathic pain conditions generally develop over time, yet there is mounting evidence that nerve sensitization and abnormal sensory nerve conduction originating at the initial time of trauma can serve to establish the pathologic neural pathways. Opioids are generally the most effective

Table 7 Antispasticity Drugs

Drug	Mechanism of action	Dosing	Common side effects
Diazepam	GABA agonist	5–10 mg IV or PO q6 hrs PRN	Sedation
Cyclobenzaprine (Flexeril®)	Unknown, centrally acting	5 mg PO TID, titrate to 10 mg PO TID	Sedation, dizziness
Baclofen	GABA_B agonist	5 mg PO TID, titrate to 80 mg a day	Sedation, delirium, urinary retention
Tizanidine (Zanaflex®)	Centrally acting α_2-adrenergic agonist	4–8 PO q6 hrs, maximum 36 mg per 24 hr	Dizziness, fatigue, dry mouth
Carispodol (Soma®)	Unknown, centrally acting	350 mg PO TID	Sedation, tremor, dizziness
Chlorzoxazone (Parafon Forte®, Paraflex®)	Unknown, appears to be sedation-related	250–500 mg PO TID to QID	Sedation, dizziness
Methocarbamol (Robaxin®)	Unknown, centrally acting	1–3 g IV/IM QD for 3 days; 1.5 g QID for 2–3 days	Sedation, dizziness
Orphenadrine (Norflex®)	Unknown, centrally acting, anticholinergic	60 mg IV/IM q12 hr; 100 mg PO q12 hr	Dry mouth and other anticholinergic effects

Abbreviations: GABA, gamma amino butyric acid; IV, intravenously; IM, intramuscularly; PO, orally; PRN, as needed; TID, three times a day; QD, once a day; QID, four times a day.

medications for systemic treatment of most categories of severe pain states. However, improved analgesia can be provided for some patients using adjuvant analgesics (anticonvulsants and antidepressant drugs) in concert with opioids.

Anticonvulsants constitute a class of several unrelated compounds that interfere with peripheral and central nerve conduction. Their mechanisms of action include sodium channel blockade, and modulation of calcium channels and GABA receptors. Gabapentin is a first-line anticonvulsant drug used in the treatment of neuropathic pain. Due to its pronounced sedative side effects, gabapentin is gradually titrated over one to two weeks from a single nightly dose of 300–900 mg three times a day. Pregabalin is a recently introduced anticonvulsant drug that also has received an FDA approval to treat several neuropathic pain states. It offers quicker onset of analgesia than gabapentin, with generally fewer side effects, and can be titrated to its maintenance dose of 300 mg per day in seven days (half the time of gabapentin).

The analgesic effects of tricyclic antidepressant (TCA) drugs probably result from sodium channel blockade and activity at the adrenergic α-receptors in the descending spinal pathways. Amitriptyline (Elavil®) is typically the first-line TCA employed in the treatment of neuropathic pain. It is usually administered at bedtime because of the profound sedative effects. If sedation is not desired, then other TCAs, such as nortriptyline or desipramine, can be used instead. The experience with selective serotonin reuptake inhibitors (SSRIs) for analgesia has been largely disappointing. In contrast, the new norepinephrine/serotonin reuptake inhibitor, duloxetine, is quite effective in treatment of neuropathic pain. Indeed, it has been approved by the FDA to treat diabetic peripheral neuropathy at a 60-mg-per-day dose.

Routes of Administration
Intravenous Route
Intermittent Bolus vs. Continuous Infusion
The IV route of administration is preferred for the initial titration of analgesic and sedative drugs in acute trauma and critically ill patients, since it is associated with the shortest onset time and the most predictable effect. Continuous IV infusion is advantageous in that it provides steady serum concentration of the drugs. However, continuous infusion can also result in the accumulation of the drug in the

tissues, and consequently delayed awakening. This requires vigilance and frequent reassessment of sedation and analgesia. Intermittent, demand-based, clinician-administered boluses are often helpful in avoiding excessive accumulation of the drug, but they can lead to undesirable peaks and troughs in the drug serum concentration (Fig. 5).

Patient-Controlled Analgesia
Because of relatively narrow therapeutic index of opioids, the concentration of the drugs tends to fluctuate widely between above and below the therapeutic level whenever administered as a bolus or on an "as needed" basis by the bedside nurse (Fig. 5). This often results in respiratory depression and oversedation alternating with poorly controlled pain. Whenever the patients are awake and cooperative, patient-controlled analgesia (PCA) can mitigate the problem of widely fluctuating drug serum concentrations. The use of PCA results in a decreased total opioid dosage during hospitalization and better pain control with smaller,

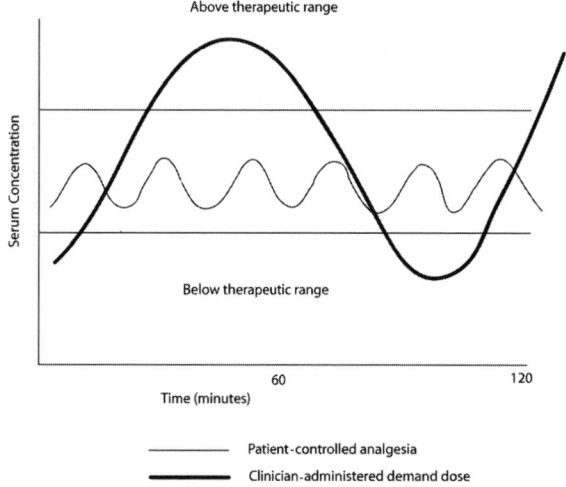

Figure 5 Serum concentrations of opioid analgesic delivered by patient-controlled analgesia (PCA) devices, versus clinician-administered doses. The serum concentration of opioid analgesics fluctuates within a narrower range in patients using PCA than patients receiving clinician-administered boluses only.

Table 8   Initial Intravenous Patient-Controlled Analgesia Schedule for Patients Who Are Not Opioid Tolerant

	Opioid drug and dose		
Modality	Morphine	Hydromorphone	Fentanyl
Continuous infusion (moderate pain)	None	None	None
Continuous infusion (severe pain)	1–1.5 mg/hr	0.2–0.4 mg/hr	0.005–0.01 mg/hr
Bolus dose (moderate pain)	1 mg	0.2 mg	0.01 mg
Bolus dose (severe pain)	1.5–2 mg	0.3–0.4 mg	0.015–0.02 mg
Lockout interval	8 min	8 min	8 min
Hourly clinician-activated dose	3 mg	0.6 mg	0.03 mg

For patients who are not opioid tolerant, continuous infusion is not recommended. The initial recommended dose may be incrementally increased to an effect. Moderate pain—fracture of lower or upper extremity. Severe pain—multiple rib fractures, large upper abdominal incision, or gunshot wound.

more frequent dosing. Typical IV PCA schedules for adult patients who are not tolerant to opioids are summarized in Table 8. Patients in a stable physiological and emotional state, who are awake and are able to operate the PCA button, are the most likely to benefit from IV PCA.

Intramuscular Injections
♂ Intermittent IM injections of drugs, although still widely practiced, are ill suited for analgesia and sedation in trauma and critical care. ♂ With IM injections, plasma concentrations can vary two-fold, and the time to peak concentration can vary three-fold in the same individual. In terms of interpatient variability, the maximum plasma concentration can differ five-fold, whereas the time to peak concentration can vary seven-fold (46). Furthermore, the patients must overcome the fear and unpleasantness of a needle puncture every time their trauma or surgical pain requires relief.

Enteral Administration
The GI tract provides unpredictable absorption of medications in hemodynamically unstable trauma and critically ill patients and those with impaired bowel function, such as ileus or bowel obstruction. However, patients with intact intestinal motility and the ability to tolerate enteral feeding are also capable of processing PO medications, and can generally receive analgesics and sedatives orally with predictable results. Some drugs, such as gradually released morphine and oxycodone, are absorbed systemically at a predictable rate only if the tablet or capsule is ingested intact. Ingestion of crushed tablets or opened capsules results in immediate, instead of gradual, systemic delivery of the drug and the risk of initial opioid overdose.

CLINICAL ASSESSMENT OF PAIN AND SEDATION

The clinical evaluation of pain is challenging, partly because of an inherently subjective nature of the pain experience. Emotional turmoil can exacerbate, while stoicism can diminish the outward expression of pain. Successful management of pain and emotional distress requires frequent assessments of pain, level of consciousness, and delirium. Several scoring systems have been developed for this purpose.

Pain Assessment Scores
The numeric rating scale (NRS) is an 11-point system widely used to assess acute pain in trauma and critical care. With this scale, the patients identify their pain level on a scale of zero (no pain) to 10 (the most severe pain imaginable). The NRS is a valid (47) and reliable (48) tool that is easy to administer and does not require any specialized tools or training.

The visual analog scale (VAS) represents another common pain assessment tool used in both clinical and research settings. The VAS pain score is obtained using a 100-mm ruler with "no pain" marked on the left, and "maximum pain" on the right ends. Patients slide the cursor along the ruler to a position that they believe reflects the intensity of their pain. Alternatively, the patients can report their pain by placing a mark along a 100-mm line drawn on a sheet of paper. Compared with the NRS, VAS ratings require greater attention and patient effort. It is therefore slightly less reliable than the NRS in acute trauma and critical care (48), but easier to use in awake, but nonverbal (e.g., intubated) patients.

Pain intensity in children and other individuals unable to respond to either the NRS or the VAS can be quantitatively assessed using scales showing a variety of facial expressions. These scales typically contain photographs or drawings of facial emotions ranging from laughing to crying (Fig. 6). These scales, usually displaying six to nine faces, are considered suitable for adults and children three years of age or older. Other nonverbal pain scores utilize behavioral and/or physiological parameters that reflect pain intensity. Such behavioral and physiologic variables as facial expression, activity, guarding, BP, RR, and pupil size can be scored (49). An inherent shortcoming of nonverbal pain scoring methods is the recognition that the behavioral and

Figure 6   Facial expression pain scale. This universal scale can be used with patients from all geographic areas of the globe and does not rely upon language. However, certain cultures (and individuals within any society) respond differently to the same level of pain. For instance, certain stoic patients may provide a facial score of 3–4, but may have pain only in the mild to discomforting range (2–4 of 10), yet have a hysterical component appearing like a 10 due to either their emotional make up or due to the stress they attribute to the event (see Volume 2, Chapter 65 for a review of acute stress disorders and posttraumatic stress disorder).

physiologic parameters associated with pain can also be exhibited in pain-free, but emotionally distressed or agitated patients. Distinguishing pain from agitation, delirium, or frank psychosis in these patients can be challenging.

Sedation Scoring Tools and Electric Brain Activity Monitoring

Nearly all sedative drugs result in varying degrees of respiratory depression; and, in higher doses, excessive sedation or delirium can occur. At the other extreme, inadequate sedation can result in physiologic stress and agitation leading to accidental self-extubation and the dislodgement of indwelling devices like intravascular catheters and feeding tubes (50,51). Frequent assessment of sedation is important for achieving and maintaining an optimal level of consciousness and avoiding the side effects of the drugs or the disruptive critical care environment.

Sedation Scores

Several sedation scoring systems are available for evaluating level of consciousness in trauma and critical care patients. Ramsay sedation score (RSS) is a semiquantitative scale based on the patient's response to the surroundings (Table 9) (52,53). This six-point scoring system describes the levels of consciousness ranging from the awake and agitated to an unconscious state with absent light glabellar tap response.

The Riker sedation agitation scale (SAS) evolved from the RSS and consists of seven points describing the states of sedation and agitation in terms of observed behavior of the patient, with calm and cooperative state located in the middle of the scale (Table 10) (54). SAS is highly correlated with the RSS in assessing sedation and agitation in the SICU. However, the SAS provides additional information by stratifying agitation into three separate categories (compared to only two in the RSS).

The Richmond agitation sedation scale (RASS) has further expanded the scoring possibilities and oriented the range of responses in a more intuitive format, offering improved validity and reliability compared to the RSS, SAS, and other scoring systems (55,56). ☞ **RASS is the first, and so far the only, sedation measuring tool that has been validated for its ability to detect changes in sedation over consecutive days in critical care (55).** ☞

Similar to other sedation scores, the RASS is designed to quantify the degree of sedation and agitation of the patient based on behavioral observation. In this scoring system, the patients who are alert and calm receive a balanced 0 score; others are assigned scores that deviate from the center in relation to their aberrancy with combative (score +4) at one extreme, and unarousable (score −5) at the other (Table 11).

Table 9 Ramsay Sedation Score

Awake levels	Patient description
1	Anxious, agitated, or restless
2	Cooperative, orientated, or tranquil
3	Responds to command only
4	Brisk response to a light glabellar tap
5	Sluggish response to a light glabellar tap
6	No response to a light glabellar tap

Table 10 Riker Sedation Agitation Scale

Score	Patient's state	Description of patient's behavior
7	Dangerous agitation	Pulls at endotracheal tube, tries to remove catheters, climbs over bedrail, strikes at staff, thrashes side to side
6	Very agitated	Does not calm despite frequent verbal reminding of limits, requires physical restraints, bites endotracheal tube
5	Agitated	Anxious or mildly agitated, attempts to sit up, calms down to verbal instructions
4	Calm and cooperative	Calm, awakens easily, follows commands
3	Sedated	Difficult to arouse, awakens to verbal stimuli or gentle shaking but drifts off again, follows simple commands
2	Very sedated	Arouses to physical stimuli, but does not communicate or follow commands, may move spontaneously
1	Unarousable	Minimal or no response to noxious stimuli, does not communicate or follow commands

Electric Brain Activity Monitoring

An established relationship exists between the electroencephalogram (EEG) and the effects of sedatives and anesthetics on the cerebral metabolic rate (57). In general, the observed decrease in EEG wave frequency is proportional to the lower neuronal firing rate produced by sedatives and anesthetics. However, interpretation of raw EEG wave patterns often requires considerable expertise. Furthermore, the unprocessed EEG signals do not always correlate well with drug-induced changes in neuronal activity except at very high doses.

Table 11 Richmond Agitation and Sedation Scale

Score	Descriptor	Characteristics
+4	Combative	Combative, violent, immediate danger to staff
+3	Very agitated	Pulls or removes tube(s) or catheter(s); aggressive
+2	Agitated	Frequent nonpurposeful movement, fights ventilator
+1	Restless	Anxious, apprehensive, but movements not aggressive or vigorous
0	Alert and calm	
−1	Drowsy	Not fully alert, but has sustained awakening to voice (eye opening and contact >10 sec)
−2	Lightly sedated	Briefly awakens to voice (eye opening and contact <10 sec)
−3	Moderately sedated	Movement or eye opening to voice (but no eye contact)
−4	Deeply sedated	No response to voice, but movement or eye opening to physical stimulation
−5	Unarousable	No response to voice or physical stimulation

In contrast to the raw EEG, analyzed processed EEG patterns, such as the 95% spectral edge frequency, appear to accurately reflect the degree of sedation (57). Proprietary tools, including the Bispectral Index Encephalographic analysis (BIS®) and patient state index (PSI®)<, are empirically derived methods of EEG processing with conversion to a linear analog scale. Neuronal activity in the fully awake brain is assigned a score of 100, and absence of activity is defined as a score of zero with both BIS and PSI systems (58,59). Patients are likely to respond to verbal commands when the BIS number is over 70, but not have any recall unless the BIS is >80 (Fig. 7). Patients are unlikely to respond to commands when the BIS values are <50 (60).

The ability of processed EEG methods (e.g., BIS or PSI) to assess the degree of sedation and awareness has been demonstrated in some (58–62), but not in other studies (63–65). Interpretation of BIS and PSI scores is complicated by the fact that similar levels of sedation that are brought about by different classes of drugs (opioids, benzodiazepines, or propofol) can result in different processed EEG scores (60). However, consistent and anesthetic-independent measurements of the states of awareness have been recently demonstrated (66).

The American Society of Anesthesiologists (ASA) has recently issued a Practice Advisory for Intraoperative Awareness and Brain Function Monitoring (67). This ASA advisory recommends against routine and universal use of electric brain activity monitors. It has, however, issued a consensus "that the decision to use a brain function monitor should be made on a case-by-case basis by the individual practitioner for selected patients (e.g., light anesthesia)." The ASA practice advisory did not make any specific recommendations concerning the use of electric brain activity monitors in the trauma or critical care settings. ☞ **Processed electric brain activity monitoring appears to correlate reasonably well with other sedation assessment methods such as the RASS (as described earlier); however, it remains unclear whether routine use of this technique improves the outcomes, and additional studies in acute trauma and critical care are needed.** ☞

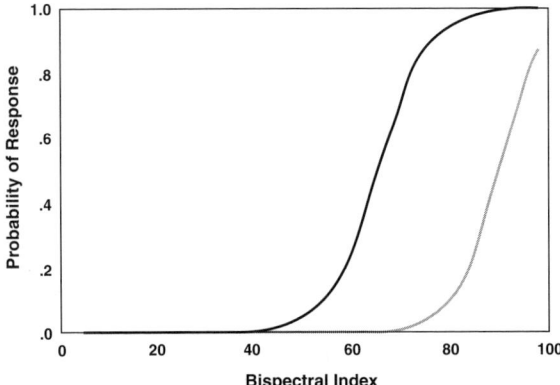

Figure 7   Relationship between BIS and probability of response to verbal command (*black line*) or ability to remember pictures or words (free recall test) (*shaded line*). Fractional probability of 1.0 = 100%. These relationships were determined using logistic regression analysis for volunteers receiving propofol, isoflurane, or midazolam. *Source*: From Ref. 60.

Assessment of Delirium

Delirium is manifested by the acute onset of an altered level of awareness or consciousness, inattention, lethargy or agitation, worsening of symptoms at night, and disorganized thinking. It can be precipitated by many factors, including primary cerebral diseases, such as cerebrovascular accident, seizure, mass lesions, and contusions. Other common factors that can cause or exacerbate delirium include medications or toxins, stessful environment and circumstances, alteration in sleep cycles, metabolic and endocrine disorders, and intracerebral infection (68).

☞ **Delirium in critical care is exceedingly common, with an estimated incidence between 60% and 80% (69–71).** ☞ Delirium is considered a psychiatric disorder with diagnositic criteria defined in the diagnostic and statistical manual of mental disorders (DSM-IV) (72). Delirium can appear as hypoactive (quiet), hyperactive, or mixed.

Patients with hyperactive delirium most commonly exhibit agitated and combative behavior. Administration of sedatives to patients in this state often results in a transition to hypoactive delirium (i.e., although the agitated behavior is apparently controlled, the patients continue to harbor disorganized thinking). Patients with hypoactive delirium appear withdrawn, lethargic, and apathetic. Mixed delirium describes the condition with fluctuating mental states between hyperactive and hypoactive.

Delirium invariably involves changes in consciousness, with the spectrum of states that include sedation or anxiety. Accordingly, evaluation of delirium is always entwined with assessment of sedation utilizing such tools as the RASS (as described earlier). In general, patients with hypervigilant altered level of consciousness (RASS = +4 to +1) are in need of evaluation for delirium. At the same time, presence of other conditions, such as dementia, psychogenic dissociative disorders, mania, and complex partial seizures, should be ruled out. Patients with RASS = −3 to −5 can also be suffering from an OBS causing a hypoactive form of delirium (or be oversedated with anxiolytic or antipsychotic drugs). Assessment and diagnosis of delirium on the basis of DSM-IV criteria requires extensive experience and knowledge of causes of OBS.

An additional diagnostic tool is available for characterization of delirium in patients with altered level of consciousness measured by RSS, SAS, or RASS. This tool, named CAM-ICU, is based on the confusion assessment method (CAM) scoring system (73). CAM-ICU allows rapid evaluation of delirium by clinicians who do not have extensive training in psychiatry. This test shows excellent validity and reliability when compared to determination of delirium using DSM-IV criteria (74). CAM-ICU evaluates delirium on the basis of four principal features: (*i*) acute or fluctuating mental status changes, (*ii*) inattention, (*iii*) disorganized thinking, and (*iv*) altered level of consciousness (Table 12). Delirium, according to CAM-ICU, is established when both features (*i*) and (*ii*), and either features (*iii*) or (*iv*) are positive.

ANALGESIA AND SEDATION FOR ACUTE TRAUMA

Pain and anxiety in trauma patients present a variety of challenges and circumstances. In some patients, extreme combative behavior, respiratory distress, inhalation burn injury, and neurological or mechanical loss of airway protection

Table 12 The Confusion Assessment Method for the Diagnosis of Delirium in the Intensive Care Unit (CAM-ICU)

Feature	Assessment variables
I. Acute onset of mental status changes or fluctuating course	Is there evidence of an acute change in mental status from the baseline?
	Did the (abnormal) behavior fluctuate during the past 24 hr, i.e., tend to come and go or increase and decrease in severity?
	Did the sedation scale (e.g., SAS or MAAS) or GCS fluctuate in the past 24 hr?
II. Inattention	Did the patient have difficulty focusing attention?
	Is there a reduced ability to maintain and shift attention?
	How does the patient score on the attention screening examination (ASE)?
III. Disorganized thinking	If the patient is already extubated from the ventilator, determine whether or not the patient's thinking is disorganized or incoherent, such as rambling or irrelevant conversation, unclear or illogical flow of ideas, or unpredictable switching from subject to subject
	For those still on the ventilator, can the patient answer simple, logical (yes/no) questions correctly?
IV. Altered level of consciousness [any level of consciousness other than alert (e.g., vigilant, lethargic, stupor, or coma)]	*Alert*: normal, fully aware of environment, interacts appropriately
	Vigilant: hyperalert
	Lethargic: drowsy but easily aroused, unaware of some elements in the environment
	Stupor: difficult to arouse, unaware of some or all elements in the environment, or not spontaneously interacting with the interviewer; becomes incompletely aware and inappropriately interactive when prodded strongly
	Coma: unarousable, unaware of all elements in the environment, with no spontaneous interaction or awareness of the interviewer

Patients are diagnosed with delirium if they have both features (I) and (II) and either feature (III) or (IV).

Abbreviations: SAS, sedation-analgesia scale; MAAS, motor activity assessment scale; GCS, Glasgow Coma Scale.
Source: From Refs. 51, 70.

dictate immediate intubation with relatively liberal analgesia and sedation. In other patients, the threat to safety or loss of airway is not immediate or severe; in these circumstances, analgesics and sedatives are administered gradually and judiciously. The discussion below reviews the analgesia and sedation considerations for trauma in the prehospital setting, during transport, and in the TRS.

Prehospital Considerations
General Approach and Recommendations
In general, pain in the field tends to be undertreated, and even in isolated limb injuries, only a minority (22%) of the patients receive analgesia before arriving in the hospital (75). Pain and anxiety should be treated as long as doing so does not interfere with patient's physiological status. Indeed, properly titrated analgesia can improve ventilatory and hemodynamic states, and facilitate patient evaluation. In all cases, IV analgesics and sedatives are withheld until IV access is established, O_2 is administered, pulse oximetry monitoring is applied, and the initial survey demonstrates that the patient is awake, alert, cooperative, and hemodynamically stable enough to tolerate medications.

Hemodynamic status is often deceptively stable immediately after the trauma; consequently, the ability to thoroughly assess the extent of injuries and blood loss in the field is limited. With this in mind, prehospital analgesia and sedation must be titrated gradually and with caution. In the presence of obvious major injuries, extensive blood loss, internal organ damage, or neurological compromise, analgesics should be withheld until the patient is transported to the hospital.

In patients meeting the above criteria for sedation and analgesia, opioids such as fentanyl (0.01–0.025 mg), morphine (1–3 mg), or hydromorphone (0.2–0.6 mg) can be administered IV at 5-minute (fentanyl) to 15-minute (morphine, hydromorphone) intervals. In initially stable patients, analgesia can be titrated to a RR of 12 to 15 breaths per minute and a reassuring blood pressure. Oxygen saturation and exhaled CO_2 (if available), should be continuously monitored.

Severe pain is a common cause of agitation following acute trauma. But so is hypovolemic shock. Accordingly, opioid administration must be titrated to a state of emotional calm without causing respiratory or hemodynamic compromise. Only if agitation persists after achieving adequate analgesia and continued cardiopulmonary stability, should sedatives such as midazolam be administered. Gradual titration of this drug should be limited to 0.5–1 mg every five minutes. Vital signs and the level of consciousness are frequently monitored, because the interpatient variability in the response to sedatives can be extreme and unpredictable, and coadministered benzodiazepines and opioids can have synergetic depressive hemodynamic and respiratory effects.

☞ **Nitrous oxide (N_2O) is not recommended in the acute trauma setting.** ☞ At therapeutic concentration it occupies substantial alveolar space, displacing O_2 and thus decreasing its partial pressure in arterial blood (PaO_2). In addition, N_2O causes rapid expansion of gas-filled spaces, such as pneumothorax or pneumocephalus (as described later).

N_2O does possess amnestic, hypnotic, and analgesic properties, and is thus favored by some prehospital practitioners. Indeed, analgesic properties of N_2O at a concentration of 20% to 25% are equivalent to 15-mg IV morphine dose (76). Because N_2O is used for analgesia and sedation during transport by some emergency medical systems in Europe (77–79), some treatment guidelines are provided. Most importantly, oxygen should always be administered first, and O_2 saturation monitoring should be established in all patients prior to initiating administration of N_2O. Secondly, oxygen must continue to be administered along with N_2O at all times, and N_2O fraction should never exceed 50% with 50% O_2.

N_2O can exacerbate pneumocephalus, pneumothorax, and pneumoperitoneum by the following mechanism. N_2O is carried in blood and rapidly accumulates in closed gas-filled spaces that are normally occupied with nitrogen. Because N_2O is 34 times more soluble in blood than nitrogen, it enters the gas-filled spaces faster than nitrogen can exit. Potentially catastrophic increase in pressure or volume in the gas-filled spaces ensues. For this reason, N_2O should not be used if injuries to the head, abdomen, or thoracic region are suspected.

Specific Prehospital Scenarios
Trapped Patient
Immediate extraction, stabilization, and transport of trapped patients are not always possible. While waiting for extrication from vehicles or structures, patients can be conscious and awake, and experience overwhelming anxiety in addition to severe pain. This experience can increase the risk of developing PTSD (see Volume 2, Chapter 65). Limited access to the trapped patient dictates extreme caution in pain and anxiety management. In addition to gentle reassurance, some pharmacologic treatment of pain and anxiety may be appropriate; however, drug administration should occur only after establishing an IV, administering oxygen, monitoring O_2 saturation with pulse oximetry, evaluating the ABCs, and confirming that the patient is not in an immediate risk of developing hypovolemic shock.

Because the threat of losing the airway is particularly dangerous in trapped patients, establishing physical access to the airway and administering supplemental O_2 are crucial prerequisites to analgesia administration. In these patients, severe pain and agitation can be treated with IV ketamine (0.1 mg/kg). These doses can be repeated every 5 to 10 minutes. Alternatively, repeated small IV doses of fentanyl (25–50 µg every three to five minutes) can be administered with particular attention to the preservation of wakefulness, adequate ventilation, absence of likely TBI, and reassuring hemodynamic status.

If adequate analgesia has been achieved but the patient develops agitation or becomes uncooperative, hypovolemia should be immediately assumed, and no additional analgesics or sedatives should be administered. Only after hemodynamic stability is assured, and agitation or anxiety continues, should midazolam be titrated IV in small (0.25–0.5 mg) doses every five minutes. Patients who become extremely uncooperative and hostile may require intubation and deeper sedation; these patients should be considered at high risk for TBI, and their pupil size and reactivity should be continuously monitored.

Long Transport
The treatment of pain, anxiety, and delirium in the injured trauma patient during transport (see Volume 1, Chapter 7) can be complicated particularly if the transit time is prolonged. One problem is that during transport by air, the partial pressure of oxygen is reduced in proportion to the decrease in ambient atmospheric pressure. At 5000 feet the atmospheric pressure is approximately 85%, and at 18,000 feet 50% of the pressure at sea level. In order to preserve oxygen supply, its fraction in the inhaled gas should be increased in proportion to the decrease in atmospheric pressure. Nitrous oxide is contraindicated in altitude because of the risk of expansion or increase in pressure in closed gas-filled cavities (as described earlier).

Because the extent of injuries in the majority of transported patients remains largely unknown, administration of opioid analgesics should be conservative. IV doses of fentanyl (0.01–0.025 mg), morphine (0.5–1.5 mg), or hydromorphone (0.1–0.3 mg) are administered at 15-minute intervals. Vital signs, including O_2 saturation and end-tidal CO_2 (if available), are continuously monitored.

As an alternative to systemic opioids, pain from injuries to upper and lower extremities can be treated with peripheral nerve blockade, provided that contraindications are not present (see Volume 1, Chapter 20). This is particularly important when the limb is anesthetized. Casts should be bivalved during transport to accommodate pressure changes, otherwise, the development of a compartment syndrome can go unnoticed.

Pharmacologic sedation is provided to agitated patients only after adequate analgesia has been achieved and intravascular volume has been shown to be adequate. For this purpose, IV midazolam can be titrated at 0.5- to 1-mg doses every three to five minutes, as the vital signs and level of consciousness are monitored.

Trauma Resuscitation Suite Considerations
General Approach and Recommendations
Analgesia and sedation guidelines for TRS are similar to those utilized in the prehospital setting. However, more monitoring and treatment resources are available in the TRS, and analgesics can be titrated to effect in a more controlled environment. Drugs are selected based upon the type of injury, severity, and location of pain along with the baseline mental and emotional status of the patient. Treatment choices include systemic analgesics, sedatives, and local and regional techniques.

In the TRS, as in the prehospital setting, analgesics and sedatives are withheld until oxygen is administered, functioning IV is placed, O_2 saturation is monitored, and the patient demonstrates cardiopulmonary stability after the initial ABCDEs of the primary survey.

Administration of analgesia and sedation in presence of isolated injuries of the extremities is usually relatively uncomplicated (80). Severe pain associated with such injuries is typically treated with IV fentanyl (0.01–0.05 mg), morphine (1–5 mg), or hydromorphone (0.2–1 mg) at intervals of 5 minutes (fentanyl) to 15 minutes (morphine and hydromorphone). Pain, vital signs, including oxygen saturation and end-tidal CO_2, are closely monitored during opioid titration. NSAIDs such as ketorolac or acetaminophen, and antispasticity agents (diazepam 5–10 mg IV or PO) can be used to augment opioid analgesia and reduce opioid requirements in otherwise stable patients with isolated extremity injuries.

Regional analgesia can be used to treat pain in the emergency. Techniques include neuroaxial (spinal and epidural) and peripheral nerve blockades (see Volume 1, Chapter 20 and Volume 2, Chapter 25). Neuroaxial administration of local anesthetics, in addition to providing analgesia, causes loss of sympathetic tone. This effect can result is severe cardiovascular compromise in trauma patients who depend on the sympathetic tone to maintain hemodynamic stability. For this reason, epidural and spinal analgesia are rarely used in the acute management of patients, except for those with isolated lower extremity injuries.

Specific Trauma Resuscitation Suite Scenarios
Procedural Analgesia
Analgesia and sedation are frequently required during invasive studies and minor procedures in the TRS. Procedures

Table 13 Analgesia and Sedation for Common Acute Trauma Procedures

Procedure	Local analgesia	Comments
Laceration repair	Yes	Local analgesia first, then systemic analgesia and sedation as needed
Fracture reduction	Yes[a]	Brief analgesia (+/−) sedation for severe transient pain
Dislocation	No	Brief sedation (to relax guarding muscle spasm, and to provide amnesia for severe transient pain) + minor postreduction analgesia
Chest tube placement	Yes	In hemodynamically unstable patients, only local anesthesia should be used. In others small doses of sedatives (+/−) analgesics are useful, but local anesthesia (at least 100 mg in 10 mL) is essential
Deep peritoneal lavage	Yes	Local analgesia is usually adequate in unstable patients. If fully stable (rare with this procedure), sedatives and analgesics are appropriate
Steinman pin placement	Yes	Local anesthesia does not cover the bone pain. Patients who are hemodynamically stable should receive analgesics +/− sedatives
Suprapubic catheter placement	Yes	Local anesthesia with supplemental sedatives and analgesics based upon patient status
Tongs/halo placement	Yes	Local anesthesia plus systemic analgesics +/− sedatives

[a]May use hematoma block (80)—especially for upper arm (distal radius fracture) reduction.

commonly performed in the ED and TRS are listed in Table 13, and include laceration repair and reduction of fractures and dislocations (81). Acute and transient pain exacerbation, which often accompanies such procedures, is optimally treated with short-acting analgesics or sedatives. The previously enumerated prerequisites for prehospital and TRS analgesia and sedation pertain to these patients as well, including the need for O_2 administration, functioning IV, and monitoring O_2 saturation, BP, echocardiogram (ECG), and RR. In addition, emergency airway management equipment must be available, and the patients must continue to be cooperative and stable.

Fentanyl and midazolam, with their rapid onsets and short durations of action, are commonly used for analgesia and sedation for minor procedures. In combination, these drugs provide a balance of analgesia and amnesia, with short-term sedation. During the titration of fentanyl and midazolam, the level of consciousness and vital signs, including oxygen saturation and end-tidal CO_2, are continuously monitored. In hemodynamically stable and awake patients, midazolam (0.5–1 mg) and fentanyl (0.025–0.05 mg) are administered at five-minute intervals. Although midazolam primarily treats anxiety and provides amnesia and fentanyl primarily treats pain, sedative and respiratory depressant effects of these drugs are synergistic. Furthermore, severe pain provoked by manipulation of injured tissue can rapidly dissipate following fracture or dislocation reduction. With abrupt reduction in the pain stimulus, patients who have received relatively large doses of sedatives and analgesics are at increased risk of losing control of airway, respiratory drive, and consciousness.

Propofol, with its short duration of action, quick onset, ease of titration, and relative safety, has also emerged as a commonly employed drug for procedural sedation. It is particularly suitable for procedures associated with severe, but short-lived pain, such as the reduction of a dislocated limb. However, in larger doses propofol can result in inadvertent unconsciousness, apnea and loss of airway reflexes, and hypotension. Adherence to the initially low and gradually increasing infusion rates is therefore important during propofol dose titration.

Typical initial infusion rate of propofol is 25 μg/kg/min. To achieve desired level of sedation, the infusion rate can be increased by 20% to 30% every five minutes. Propofol

can also be administered by intermittent 0.1–0.2 mg/kg boluses immediately prior to painful manipulation. Additional doses are typically injected at one- to five-minute intervals to the desired clinical effect.

As with other sedatives and analgesics, supplemental O_2 should be applied first, and vital signs be monitored, including oxygen saturation and end-tidal CO_2, and mental status (82). Throughout the procedure, the patients should be able to respond purposefully to verbal commands. Propofol and opioids, such as fentanyl, can be coadministered, however, propofol and opioid boluses should not be given simultaneously because of compounded risk of respiratory depression and excessive sedation (74).

Ketamine is another suitable procedural sedative-analgesic. It is commonly employed in the acute trauma due to rapid onset and dissipation of action, strong analgesic effect, sympathomimetic activity, bronchodilation, and preservation of laryngeal reflexes. Because of these beneficial physiological effects, which also support cardiopulmonary status and spontaneous ventilation, ketamine is frequently chosen in the military setting. However, because of other effects, particularly the unpleasant and emotionally disturbing dissociative mental state, ketamine is often supplemented with a benzodiazepine.

Ketamine can exhibit cardiovascular depressant effects in patients who are unable to mount additional sympathetic output, such as patients in hypovolemic shock (these patients should instead be promptly resuscitated, and may require intubation, positive pressure ventilation along with scopolamine for amnesia). Despite its unpredictable hemodynamic effects and contraindication in patients with TBI, ketamine remains a first-line drug for sedation and induction of anesthesia in the presence of severe bronchospasm, and in uncooperative patients without an IV access.

Combative Patient in the Trauma Resuscitation Suite
Evaluation and treatment of violent or combative patients can be uniquely challenging. Several factors can contribute to combative behavior in the acute trauma patient including TBI, hypoxia, hypovolemic shock, intoxication, psychiatric illness, and OBS from baseline organ failure. ✍ **Hypovolemic shock and/or TBI need to be immediately ruled out in all combative patients, because prompt and successful management of these problems can markedly improve outcomes.** ✍ Other

causes of combativeness that need to be considered include anxiety disorders precipitated by exposure to the confusing and chaotic environment of the TRS that are emotionally overwhelming to some patients.

Besides interfering with evaluation and treatment, combative patients are at risk of harming themselves and others. It is therefore essential for the treating clinicians to rapidly gain complete control of the patient. Some violent and completely uncooperative patients require deep sedation with induction of general anesthesia, with NMB and intubation. This measure is resorted to in circumstances where other means of analgesia and sedation are either ineffective or too risky, such as in patients with potential major organ compromise or tenuous airway.

Often agitated and combative patients identify severe pain as the main source of their distress. If these patients are not at risk of cardiovascular collapse or loss of airway, then their pain can, and should, be judiciously treated. The first choice for analgesia in severe pain (without concomitant TBI) is usually an opioid drug. Opioids are typically titrated to effect as a series of small sequential IV boluses of fentanyl (0.01–0.05 mg), morphine (1–5 mg), or hydromorphone (0.2–1 mg) every 5 minutes (fentanyl) or every 15 minutes (morphine and hydromorphone). Vital signs, especially RR and BP, and the level of consciousness are continuously monitored during opioid titration, with the endpoint being analgesia with a RR >10–12.

After achieving adequate opioid-based analgesia, midazolam can be administered to treat agitation. It is titrated in 0.5- to 1-mg doses every five minutes. Coadministered opioids and benzodiazepines can synergistically cause excessive respiratory depression and sedation (83).

Increasingly, dexmedetomidine (no intrinsic respiratory depression) is becoming the sedative of choice to supplement low-dose opioids in acute trauma patients. In those who require rapid recurrent evaluation of neurologic status, dexmedetomidine is particularly efficacious, because the sedative effect can continue without significant depression of mental acuity. In this setting dexmedetomidine is started as an infusion (without a bolus load) at 0.2–0.7 µg/kg/hr.

ANALGESIA AND SEDATION FOR CRITICAL CARE

Trauma patients in critical care exhibit diverse underlying pathologies, emotional states, pain levels, and analgesic and sedative dose requirements. The majority of these patients develop some degree of delirium during the intensive care unit (ICU) stay. Nonpharmacologic interventions, such as reduction of pain stimulus by repositioning, sleep normalization, verbal orientation and reassurance are the initial steps in treatment (Fig. 1).

Pharmacologic analgesia usually consists of opioids, whose doses are titrated and are empirically determined by clinical response. Titration of opioids should be rapidly completed with adequate serum drug levels achieved within 30 minutes of initiating therapy. Sedatives are introduced only after administering adequate analgesia and are likewise titrated to the desired effect. Deep sedation with muscle paralysis and mechanical ventilation may be initially required for some critical care patients.

Analgesia
Opioids remain the cornerstone of treatment for moderate to severe pain in critical care. The IV route of drug adminis-

tration is usually preferred since IM or SQ drug delivery can be painful and have unpredictable absorption rates. The latter problem is accentuated in critically ill patients, who can exhibit highly variable responses to opioids. In general, choice of an opioid for each patient depends on its potency, side effects, and ease of titration.

Fentanyl is often the first-line opioid analgesic in critical care. It provides rapid onset of analgesia and a relatively short clinical duration in small bolus doses, and is easily titratable by infusion. Fentanyl can be administered at 0.025- to 0.1-mg IV boluses every five minutes, or infused at an initial rate of 0.002–0.005 mg/kg/hr. The bolus doses and infusion rates can be gradually increased as needed to provide an adequate analgesic effect. Occasionally, opioid-tolerant patients may require fentanyl doses as high as 0.03 mg/kg/hr.

Morphine is also routinely used for analgesia in critical care. It can be gradually titrated with typical boluses of 1–5 mg every 15 minutes. After initial stabilization, morphine is generally infused IV at 3–10 mg/hr. Considerably higher doses and infusion rates may be required in opioid tolerant patients. Hydromorphone can be titrated to an analgesic effect with 0.2- to 1-mg IV doses every 10 to 15 minutes, or infused at 0.5–3 mg/hr.

Sedation for Treatment of Anxiety and Agitation
Assessment of the level of consciousness, including sedation and anxiety, is discussed earlier. Anxiety in the injured can arise from many causes, including pain, the circumstances, and sensory deprivation or overload. Treatment of pain often leads to dissipation of anxiety. Accordingly, sedatives should not be routinely administered until adequate analgesia has been delivered.

Because there is a continuum between light to deep levels of sedation, ultimately progressing to general anesthesia (84), the goals of sedation and its desired depth should be defined for each patient. This determination should be based on the nature and extent of injury, as well as the physiological and mental status of the patient. ☛ **Managing deeply sedated patients can be easier than those who are slightly sedated; however, deep sedation carries multiple risks, including delayed awakening, ventilator-associated pneumonia, postsedation delirium, muscle wasting, and pressure sores (85).** ☛ In most patients, the optimum level of sedation is achieved by titration to state of calm, or to comfortable but easily arousable states (e.g., RASS = 0). Deeper levels of sedation can be required when painful procedures are performed or to facilitate ventilatory support [i.e., patients with adult respiratory distress syndrome (ARDS) or TBI].

The sedative drug choice is generally guided by several factors, including the need for rapid awakening (e.g., to perform neurological exams) versus an anticipated prolonged sedation, without the need for awakenings. Other considerations include cost and the potential side effects. Drugs most commonly used for induction and maintenance of sedation are benzodiazepines, propofol, and dexmedetomidine.

Propofol with its rapid onset and short duration of action is well suited for short-term sedation in critical care, particularly in patients at risk for increased ICP, who may need frequent reversal sedation to conduct neurological exams.

Metabolism of propofol is minimally affected by hepatic and renal dysfunction, and its metabolites are inactive. Times of onset and levels of sedation with propofol and midazolam are similar, and after short-term sedation (less than 24 hours) propofol and midazolam exhibit similar times to awakening though they wake up from propofol faster and are more clear-headed (51,86–88). After sedation between 24 and 72 hours, the times to awakening with propofol (0.25–2.5 hours) are considerably shorter than with midazolam (2.8–30 hours). Similarly, sedation with propofol for longer than 72 hours provides significantly faster awakening and extubation than with midazolam (0.25–4 hours with propofol compared to 2.8–49 hours with midazolam) (51,89).

Because of its numerous side effects, propofol administration requires a high degree of vigilance. It causes respiratory depression, and reduces systemic vascular resistance and ionotropy. In some patients these effects result in significant systemic hypotension; whereas in others BP is relatively preserved. It is often impossible to predict the extent of hypotensive effect in the patient. Prolonged infusion of high-dose propofol increases serum triglycerides (51,90) and elevation of serum pancreatic enzymes (91,92). Lactic acidosis, bradycardia, and hyperlipidemia were reported in pediatric patients after 48-hour infusion of high-dose propofol (66 µg/kg/min) (as described later) (93). Prolonged infusion of even higher dose (>83 µg/kg/min) is associated with increased risk of cardiac dysrhythmias and arrest (94). Propofol is also relatively expensive and commonly causes pain in the peripheral vein during the injection. In consideration of all the benefits and risks associated with propofol, it is often the sedative of choice when rapid awakening or extubation are required (51).

Benzodiazepines remain the mainstay of sedative and anxiolytic therapy in chronically sedated critical care patients and those without acute TBI, primarily because they are relatively inexpensive and lack some side effects associated with propofol. Benzodiazepines, however, also possess several deleterious side effects. Although generally less severe than with propofol, respiratory and cardiovascular depression can occur even at moderate doses. Prolonged respiratory depression and delayed awakening are common after extended periods of benzodiazepine infusion. In order to mitigate delayed awakening and avoid excessive accumulation of the drug, level of consciousness should be frequently assessed and downward titration in the infusion rate should occur as tolerated.

An important practice consideration in this regard is the need to allow critical care patients to benefit from sleep that is not unnecessarily disrupted. One such approach allows the night shift nurse (19:00–07:00) to obtain a complete neurological exam of the patient at the beginning and end of shift, but limits evening awakenings to the bare minimum in otherwise stable patients. Pupils can be checked in sedated patients who are at risk for TBI on an hourly basis. Many of these patients will also have an ICP monitor in place during the early and most vulnerable stages of recovery. In these same patients, the day shift nurse tries to decrease the sedation to as low of a dose that is tolerated, (while analgesia is maintained), and efforts are made to increase the patient's orientation and interactions with treatments such as physical therapy, weaning from mechanical ventilation, and other activities.

Midazolam, with its strong amnestic properties and ease of titration, is one of the first-line benzodiazepines used in critical care and is particularly recommended for acute anxiolysis, rapid sedation, and infusion for less than two to three days (51). Indeed, it has largely replaced diazepam in critical care due to its shorter and more predictable duration of action. Time to awakening is less predictable after infusing midazolam for longer than three days,

particularly in patients who are obese, or with liver or renal insufficiency. Prolonged sedation in these patients is attributed to the accumulation of midazolam and its active metabolite, α-hydroxymidazolam.

Lorazepam has longer elimination half-life and slower onset than midazolam or diazepam (Table 6). It is, accordingly, less suitable for rapid titration of sedation because the responses to the dose changes are delayed. With prolonged high-dose infusion of lorazepam (over 18 mg/hr for longer than four weeks), its solvents (polyethylene glycol and propylene glycol) can be responsible for acute tubular necrosis (generally reversible), lactic acidosis, and hyperosmolar states (51). With this in mind, lorazepam is inexpensive and devoid of active metabolites. It offers predictable half-life and less variable time to awakening than even midazolam (51,95), and is a suitable choice for long-term (72 hours or longer) sedation at moderate doses (51).

Diazepam, similarly to midazolam, provides fast onset and is useful in acute sedation. Diazepam is, however, less suitable for continuous infusion or repeated boluses than midazolam or lorazepam because of gradual buildup of active metabolites with very long elimination half-life. In addition, diazepam can cause irritation of the veins and thrombophlebitis when injected peripherally. Because of unpredictable half-life of diazepam and its metabolites, it is not recommended for sedation in repeated doses or continuous infusion.

The benzodiazepine antagonist flumazenil is available, but not routinely used, in critical care for reversal of sedation after prolonged benzodiazepine administration. The duration of action of a single IV dose of flumazenil is approximately 30 minutes, and the reversal of benzodiazepine-induced sedation under these circumstances is likely to be short-lived. Several factors other than benzodiazepines could be responsible for prolonged sedation, and should always be considered prior to administration of flumazenil. Flumazenil at 0.5-mg doses can precipitate benzodiazepine withdrawal symptoms including seizures and increased cardiovascular oxygen demand (as described earlier). In patients who have received prolonged benzodiazepine infusion, residual sedation can be treated with short-term infusion of flumazenil (0.5 mg/hr) (96), instead of a single dose. However, only a single dose of flumazenil is recommended to test whether unexplained prolonged sedation is due to benzodiazepines (51).

Dexmedetomidine is increasingly utilized in critically ill patients whose sedation is difficult to manage with traditional (e.g., propofol or benzodiazepine) drugs. The pharmacologic properties of dexmedetomidine (described earlier) are distinct from those of other sedatives. **In therapeutic doses, dexmedetomidine does not suppress respiratory drive or airway reflexes, making it a very useful drug during weaning to extubation, particularly in cases where airway or breathing are subject to compromise (e.g., obesity, sleep apnea, and thoracic cage trauma).** Sedation produced by dexmedetomidine is characterized by a state of calm, in which patients are easily arousable to mild stimuli (97). Unlike propofol or benzodiazepines, dexmedetomidine is also an effective analgesic (98), whereas its hypnotic effects are insignificant (99).

Several prominent side effects require vigilance in administration of dexmedetomidine. Transient hypertension can initially occur especially when the loading dose is employed. Sympatholytic effects of dexmedetomidine result in often beneficial decrease in serum catecholamine levels (99). However, ensuing bradycardia and hypotension are also common.

Young and athletic patients with strong vagal tone are particularly susceptible to extreme bradycardia. These effects can be treated with vagolytic or sympathomimetic drugs.

With its unique pharmacologic properties, dexmedetomidine provides a balance of sedation, anxiolysis, and analgesia without respiratory drive suppression. In some patients dexmedetomidine is sufficient as a sole sedative-analgesic, and in other patients it is helpful in reducing the dose requirement of other sedatives and analgesics (36). Indeed, coadministration of dexmedetomidine with opioids decreases the opioid requirement and can produce optimal balance of analgesia and sedation (36). Similarly, combined infusion of propofol and dexmedetomidine produces a deeper sedation level than with dexmedetomidine alone, and decreases the dose requirement of propofol, thus mitigating its hypnotic and respiratory depressant effects.

Treatment of Delirium

Assessment of delirium is required in all critical care patients with an altered level of consciousness. The principal causes of delirium in the ICU includes: physical illness, infection, metabolic disorders, sleep deprivation, and psychoactive pharmacologic agents both resulting in a loss of frame of reference person, place, and time. Delirium is associated with increased morbidity and should be promptly treated and, if possible, prevented.

Preventive and nonpharmacological approaches to delirium include repeatedly reorienting the patients during the daytime and promoting sleep at night by reducing disruptive noise and light stimulation. Another important method for limiting delirium is by mobilizing patients as early as possible, and promoting physical and cognitive activities (71). Since opioids, sedatives, and other psychoactive drugs can exacerbate and even induce delirium; the ongoing analgesic and sedative doses are reviewed and, if possible, reduced.

If nonpharmacological measures and opioid and sedative dose reduction are not successful in treating delirium, then antipsychotic drugs, such as haloperidol, can be used. Haloperidol can be administered PO, IM, and IV (IV route, however, is not approved by the FDA) (as described earlier). Although compelling evidence is still emerging, there are numerous reports of successful use of newer atypical antipsychotic drugs—olanzapine, risperidone, and ziprasidone in treatment of delirium in critical care (100,101). These drugs cause less sedation, mental status changes, and extrapyramidal symptoms than traditional antipsychotics. Reportedly, the risk of developing tarditive dyskinesia with atypical antipsychotics is also reduced.

All antipsychotic medications active at the dopamine receptors carry the risk of inducing QTc interval prolongation and consequent ventricular arrhythmia. Patients with QTc >500 milli seconds, recent myocardial infarction, or uncompensated heart failure should be closely monitored if antipsychotic drugs are required. They should also receive concomitant magnesium infusion to a target serum magnesium ion concentration which is normal, or slightly above normal (typically 2–3 mg/dL). Tracking QTc changes with serial ECGs is necessary in all patients treated with antipsychotic drugs.

SPECIAL CONDITIONS IN TRAUMA AND CRITICAL CARE
Thoracic Trauma

Pain resulting from thoracic trauma, including chest wall contusions and rib fractures, severely restricts ventilatory efforts and efficiency. Systemic opioids can further depress ventilation in these patients. Without regional analgesia, some of these patients require deep sedation, intubation, and positive pressure ventilation. For patients who, because of significant pulmonary contusions or parenchymal injury, pneumonia, or polytrauma, are anticipated to require prolonged mechanical ventilation; systemic analgesia and sedation is fully appropriate.

However, in the awake patient with trauma limited to thoracic cage (i.e., multiple rib fractures) and no underlying pulmonary parenchymal injury, thoracic epidural analgesia is beneficial as it will allow earlier weaning, extubation, and mobilization of the patient. Regional techniques that have demonstrated better pain relief and safety than systemic analgesics include epidural and intrathecal analgesia, intercostal and paravertebral nerves blockade, and interpleural analgesia (102). The specifics of regional analgesia for chest injuries are further discussed in Volume 2, Chapter 25.

Regional analgesia techniques in the thoracic segments bear inherent risks of nerve injury, pneumothorax, uncontrolled bleeding, and infection. Risks and benefits of these techniques should be carefully weighed for each patient. **In general, thoracic regional analgesia should be considered in patients who are at risk of respiratory failure because of severe chest wall motion-related pain. Conversely, regional analgesia techniques should not be used in patients whose pain can be adequately controlled with systemic analgesics.**

Burns

Burn injury, discussed in Volume 1, Chapter 34 often results in severe pain, which is markedly exacerbated during dressing changes. Analgesia for burn injury almost universally includes opioids, typically fentanyl, morphine, or hydromorphone (103). At the time of dressing changes, the pain is usually treated with short- or ultrashort-acting fentanyl, sufentanil, or alfentanil. Ketamine, with its anesthetic and analgesic effect, sympathomimetic activity, and relative absence of respiratory depressive effects, is particularly suitable for short-duration analgesia during dressing changes in spontaneously ventilating, nonintubated patients.

Sedation and amnesia can be achieved with short-acting midazolam or propofol. **Titration of all sedatives and analgesics requires increased vigilance because protein-bound drugs often have increased bioavailability in the characteristically hypoalbuminemic burn patients (104).** These patients also have elevated metabolic rates and develop early tolerance to sedatives and analgesics, resulting in higher infusion rates and, consequently, increased risk of vasodilatation or myocardial depression. Regional analgesia is rarely used in burn injuries because of the infection risks. Adjuvant drugs such as antidepressants and anticonvulsants, as well as IV lidocaine infusion, can reduce pain and hyperalgesia (3,34).

Organ Dysfunction

The kidneys and liver are the primary organs of drug metabolism and excretion. Dysfunction of these organs inevitably results in significantly impaired drug and metabolite clearance. This usually results in markedly increased duration of action, enhanced pharmacological effect, and increased risk of dangerous side effects.

Accumulations of metabolic products of morphine and meperidine are particularly ominous. Renally excreted M3G is one of the main metabolic products of morphine.

Unlike M6G, it exhibits antianalgesic properties. It was also implicated in neurotoxic side effects, with resultant hyperalgesia, myoclonus, and seizures (as described earlier) (105). Clinically significant accumulation of morphine glucuronides have been clearly observed in patients with renal insufficiency (106). Accordingly, in these patients, morphine should be changed to opioids less affected by renal clearance (i.e., fentanyl or hydromorphone).

Meperidine is converted to a neurotoxic metabolite, normeperidine (as described earlier). It has long elimination half-life and can induce myoclonus and refractory generalized seizures. Meperidine should be used with caution even in patients with normal renal function, and completely avoided in all cases of renal insufficiency.

The effects of midazolam are enhanced in patients with hepatic or renal failure because of elevated unbound fraction of the drug (107). Furthermore, its plasma clearance is markedly decreased in patients with liver failure. Accumulation of renally excreted midazolam metabolites can result in prolonged sedation and coma (108). Even in healthy patients, midazolam tends to accumulate in the tissues, and after infusion longer than 48 to 72 hours, the time to awakening and extubation becomes prolonged and unpredictable (as described earlier).

Diazepam and its main active metabolite, desmethyldiazepam, tends to accumulate in all patients, resulting in prolonged and unpredictable sedation. In the presence of liver or kidney dysfunction, the ability to predict the effects and duration of action of diazepam is further diminished. For this reason, diazepam, which is rarely used in critical care, should never be used for sedation of patients with hepatic or renal insufficiency.

Use of propofol and fentanyl are generally the best choices of sedation and analgesia in patients with organ failure. Clearance of these short-acting drugs appears to be unaffected by hepatic or renal dysfunction, and their principal metabolic products are inactive. Clearance of dexmedetomidine, on the other hand, is impaired in the presence of liver and kidney dysfunction. Recent, yet unpublished studies have shown systemic hypertension and cerebral vasoconstriction at very high doses. Accordingly, dexmedetomidine must be used cautiously when organ dysfunction could significantly increase blood levels.

Drug Addiction, Dependence, and Tolerance

All opioid analgesics bear an inherent risk of developing tolerance, dependence, and addiction. ✐ **In the acute trauma and critically ill patients, presence or suspicion of opioid addiction should not preclude aggressive treatment of pain with opioids.** ✐ These behavioral and physiological manifestations of prolonged opioid use can be addressed and treated during recovery in the hospital or as an outpatient.

Physical dependence to opioids is defined by the development of an abstinence (withdrawal) syndrome when the opioid is discontinued. It is manifested by anxiety, irritability, chills, hot flashes, joint pain, lacrimation, rhinorrhea, diaphoresis, nausea and vomiting, abdominal cramps, diarrhea, and "flu-like" symptoms. Except for the patients who physiologically cannot tolerate a moderate increase in sympathetic outflow, opioid withdrawal symptoms are self-limiting and not life-threatening. Withdrawal symptoms can occur after as little as two weeks of opioid use. These symptoms appear 6 to 12 hours after discontinuing short-acting opioids. With long-acting opioids, the withdrawal symptoms are usually milder, and their onset is slower. To prevent these symptoms, opioids should never be discontinued abruptly, but tapered gradually. Clonidine, in topical or PO forms, is routinely administered to counteract the symptoms of opioid withdrawal. Similarly, dexmedetomidine has been recently used to facilitate discontinuation of opioids (109).

Opioid addiction, unrelated to drug dependence or tolerance, is characterized by an aberrant behavior and psychological dependence. Addicted patients crave, request, and consume opioids to satisfy the emotional urge. In the presence of severe acute pain, some patients may exhibit pseudoaddiction symptoms with behavioral patterns similar to that in addiction. In contrast to addicted patients, the pseudoaddicted patients revert to normal behavior once adequate analgesia is achieved, without developing symptoms of opioid intoxication, such as somnolence or slurred speech.

Opioid tolerance manifests as a gradually increased drug requirement to maintain the same level of analgesia. Tolerance has been shown to develop in laboratory animals as well as in patients who have undergone surgeries with even short-term courses of opioids. Younger patients tend to become opioid tolerant more rapidly than older adults. The development of tolerance to opioids should be expected in all critical care patients who receive these drugs for more than five to seven days. However, other causes for increased opioid requirement, such as progression of disease, infection, compartment syndrome, pressure ulcers, and so on, should always be considered first.

Dependence on benzodiazepines can also develop in critically ill patients after several weeks of continuous daily use. Unlike the opioid withdrawal, the abstinence symptoms after abrupt discontinuation of benzodiazepines can be life-threatening. Depending on the half-life of the benzodiazepine, the onset of symptoms usually occurs within one to two days. The symptoms can range from mild agitation to generalized seizures and include anxiety, increased HR and BP, diaphoresis, nausea and vomiting, and hallucinations. These symptoms are typically treated with administration of benzodiazepines, followed by a gradual taper.

Age-Related Considerations
Pediatric Patients

Children, including infants and neonates, are susceptible to the complications of the pain-induced stress response (79). Accordingly, adequate analgesia and sedation can suppress physiological responses to noxious stimuli, thereby improving postoperative recovery (110,111). Assessment of pain in children may be difficult, particularly in the critically ill. Physiological responses, parental interpretations, and facial expression interpretation scales can be helpful in assessing pain (as described earlier) (112).

Opioids such as fentanyl, morphine, and hydromorphone are usually the primary analgesics in treatment of moderate or severe pain in children. In addition to their analgesic properties, opioids can be even more effective than benzodiazepines for sedation of infants and neonates. Ketamine is used for sedation and analgesia in patients with bronchospasm or who are hemodynamically unstable. In patients with adequately controlled pain, sedation and amnesia can be achieved with bolus injection or continuous infusion of midazolam. Pentobarbital and other barbiturates can be effective, but benzodiazepines and opioids are usually more suitable to the provision of adequate sedation.

Chloral hydrate, a CNS depressant, is still available in PO and PR forms, but is rarely used because of serious side effects and toxicity (113). These include severe respiratory depression and low blood pressure, cardiac dysrhythmias, and liver damage.

Propofol is an effective sedative in children and can be safely used short-term for procedures and in critical care (114). However, safety of propofol for prolonged sedation in children remains undetermined. In addition to cardiovascular and respiratory depression, propofol use has been associated with numerous reports of rare but sometimes fatal "pediatric propofol infusion syndrome" (PRIS). This syndrome is the constellation of metabolic acidosis, cardiac and renal failure, and rhabdomyolysis. Although PRIS occurs primarily after prolonged (>48 hours) infusion of propofol, metabolic acidosis has been reported even after short periods of infusion (115). Exact mechanism of PRIS is unknown, but it may be related to the impairment of intracellular free fatty acid utilization (116). In children, doses of propofol exceeding 4 mg/kg/hr should generally be avoided. Experience with dexmedetomidine in children is still limited, but numerous reports describe successful sedation with this drug in pediatric critical care and anesthesia (109,117,118).

Elderly Patients

Although the age-related changes in the pharmacokinetic properties of drugs are not well defined, and can be gradual and unpredictable (119), the elderly often require reduced doses of sedatives and analgesics. Sedative effects of midazolam increase in intensity and duration with age. Indeed, it exhibits a twofold increase in the half-life between ages 20 and 80 (120). The elderly are also more susceptible than younger adults to the adverse side effects of benzodiazepines and often exhibit dizziness, confusion, hallucinations, hypothermia, urinary retention and constipation, and urinary or bowel incontinence (40,121). In general, it is prudent to use half or less the normal adult dose of the benzodiazepines in the elderly.

Propofol, in general, provides rapid recovery and relatively small propensity for accumulation or tolerance (122); however, in the elderly, clearance of this drug is decreased and its sedative effects are more pronounced. Consequently, the elderly generally require approximately one-half of the usual adult bolus doses or infusion rates of propofol.

In the elderly, fentanyl and related lipophilic opioids exhibit twofold potency with respect to analgesia and sedation, and their doses should be adjusted accordingly (123). Clearance of morphine and its active metabolites, M6G and M3G, decreases with age, resulting in increased apparent potency and risk of toxicity and overdose. Because of its slower metabolism, morphine is administered in smaller and less frequent doses in the elderly than in younger adults.

EYE TO THE FUTURE

The management of pain and anxiety in acute trauma and critical care is poised for a major transformation with the clinical introduction of a number of recently discovered agents, along with the continued developments of monitoring technologies, and refinements in the usage of existing drugs. Opioids, local anesthetics, and NSAIDs will likely retain a role in pain management of acute trauma and critical

care, whereas sedative/anxiolytic and antipsychotic drugs will see major changes. The balance between the increased cardiovascular risk and the benefit of prevention of GI bleeding will determine the future of selective COX-2 inhibitors, including the long-anticipated IV form.

Recently, a new variant of COX enzyme, COX-3, has been described (124). This isoenzyme modulates pain, inflammatory, and febrile response primarily by a central mechanism, and is a potential target of future COX-3-specific inhibitors. Indeed, some existing drugs, including acetaminophen, exert their analgesic effect primarily by their inhibition of the COX-3 enzyme.

Expanding knowledge and understanding of pain mechanisms provides the potential targets for new classes of analgesics. Such targets include NMDA receptor, calcium channels, tumor necrosis factor-α (TNF-α), spinal mitogen activated protein (MAP) kinase, and genes responsible for sodium channel synthesis. Compounds active at these sites are currently in various stages of development. Ziconitide, a calcium channel antagonist, has recently been introduced as a potent analgesic for intrathecal use. This peptide, derived from sea-snail venom, has shown strong analgesic effects in patients with refractory chronic pain.

Interestingly, erythropoietin, a compound involved in suppression of TNF-α synthesis, has shown promising analgesic effects in neuropathic pain, and its efficacy and safety are currently studied in animal models (125).

An isoform of spinal MAP kinase, p38β, is identified as an important mediator of pain processing and sensitization. Down-regulation of p38β in the spinal microglia was shown to prevent the development of hyperalgesia in rats who have received injection of formalin or intrathecal substance P (126). Such down-regulation of p38β has been demonstrated with intrathecal administration of minocycline, also resulting in blocking inflammation-induced hyperalgia (127). It appears that minocycline, an antibiotic, attenuates p38β as part of inhibition of microglia through a mechanism unrelated to its antibiotic activity.

A novel approach incorporating gene-related pain therapy has been recently described (128). This approach targets the synthesis of sensory nerve NaV1.8 sodium channels that are present in dorsal root ganglia and are implicated in pathogenesis of neuropathic and inflammatory pain. This in vitro study involved the synthesis of DNA fragments, designed to transcribe short hairpin RNA targeting synthesis the sodium channels. The DNA fragments were then incorporated in the recombinant lentoviruses. Infecting rat dorsal root ganglia cells expressing sodium channels with the lentoviruses resulted in a cessation of production of the sodium channel protein and its corresponding mRNA. Silencing sodium channel–producing DNA with internally transcribed RNA is conceptually attractive, particularly since the role of these sodium channels in mediating of neuropathic and inflammatory pain has already been established (129). Safety and efficacy of this technique in animals and humans is currently under investigation.

SUMMARY

Treating pain is compassionate, and a new impetus exists for meticulous and timely analgesia. If pain is treated early, immediate and long-term psychological and physiological postinjury complications can be reduced. Addressing analgesia is therefore imperative for all trauma and critically ill patients.

Management of pain and anxiety in the injured generally follows the path from the least to the more intensive and invasive approaches. In all situations, the treatment starts with reassurance, emotional support, and avoidance of pain-provoking stimuli. Pain is then treated with pharmacotherapy. Sedation should be added only after achieving an adequate foundation of analgesia (Fig. 1). Depending on the goals and desired results, sedation and treatment of delirium is a continuum ranging from mild sedation to a state of unconsciousness.

Most sedatives and opioids suppress respiratory drive, laryngeal reflexes, and hemodynamics. With vigilance and close attention to respiratory, neurologic, and cardiovascular parameters, administration of these drugs is performed by gradual titration. Peripheral or neuroaxial regional analgesic techniques are suitable for some acute trauma and critical care situations.

Children, the elderly, and those with substance abuse problems differ from the average adult patients in their responses to sedatives and analgesics. Like all humans, these patients exhibit severe stress response to injury and experience pain and anxiety.

Significant advances, both technical and conceptual, were made over the past several decades in the management of pain. However, to this day, opioids remain the mainstay of management of moderate to severe pain. It is becoming increasingly apparent that the pain signal is modulated in the periphery and within the CNS by multiple mechanisms. Some of these pain-modulating signaling molecules and receptors may in the future become targets for a new generation of analgesic drugs.

KEY POINTS

- Without compromising cardiopulmonary status, judicious use of analgesics and sedatives can relieve pain, provide a state of emotional calm, and facilitate the diagnostic evaluation of trauma patients.
- PTSD affects up to 40% of major trauma patients (4,5).
- Optimal pain management involves a stepwise logical approach beginning with the elimination of obvious painful stimuli (e.g., splinting fractures), ascending to administration of analgesics prior to introducing sedatives or neuroleptic drugs; and, only in rare cases is deep sedation with NMB required.
- There is a general consensus that administration of analgesia at the earliest possible opportunity will likely have beneficial effect on the long-term outcome of patients who sustain tissue injury from trauma or surgery.
- Local anesthetics do not work efficiently when injected in the vicinity of infected tissue.
- Among the side effects associated with opioids (Table 5), respiratory depression, loss of airway, and hypotension are potentially the most dangerous. Indeed, fear of respiratory depression is a common cause of inadequate analgesia in critically ill patients.
- Pain stimulates the respiratory drive and counteracts the sedative effects of opioids. Consequently, patients on relatively high doses of opioids, who then undergo regional nerve blockade, can develop acute respiratory depression because of abrupt abolition of the afferent pain stimulus.

- In long-term benzodiazepine users, and if given in too large of a dose (rather than titrated as recommended above), flumazenil can precipitate seizures or other withdrawal symptoms, including acute onset of severe anxiety, muscle jerks, and tremors.
- The hemodynamically unstable, hemorrhaging trauma patient is a classic example where ketamine predominantly exhibits cardiac-depressant effects (45).
- The slightly elevated risk of Torsade de Pointes associated with droperidol, is also present with other antipsychotic drugs including haloperidol.
- Intermittent IM injections of drugs, although still widely practiced, are ill suited for analgesia and sedation in trauma and critical care.
- RASS is the first and so far the only sedation measuring tool that has been validated for its ability to detect changes in sedation over consecutive days in critical care (55).
- Processed electric brain activity monitoring appear to correlate reasonably well with other sedation assessment methods such as the RASS; however, it remains unclear whether routine use of this technique improves the outcomes, and additional studies in acute trauma and critical care are needed.
- Delirium in critical care is exceedingly common, with an estimated incidence between 60% and 80% (69–71).
- Nitrous oxide (N_2O) is not recommended in the acute trauma setting.
- In ED and TRS, as in the prehospital setting, analgesics and sedatives are withheld until oxygen is administered, functioning IV is placed, O_2 saturation is monitored, and the patient demonstrates cardiopulmonary stability after the initial ABCDEs of the primary survey.
- Hypovolemic shock and/or TBI need to be immediately ruled out in all combative patients, because prompt and successful management of these problems can markedly improve outcomes.
- Managing deeply sedated patients can be easier than those who are slightly sedated; however, deep sedation carries multiple risks, including delayed awakening, ventilator-associated pneumonia, postsedation delirium, muscle wasting, and pressure sores (85).
- In therapeutic doses, dexmedetomidine does not suppress respiratory drive or airway reflexes, making it a very useful drug during weaning to extubation, particularly in cases where airway or breathing are subject to compromise (e.g., obesity, sleep apnea, and thoracic cage trauma).
- In general, thoracic regional analgesia should be considered in patients who are at risk of respiratory failure because of severe chest wall motion-related pain. Conversely, regional analgesia techniques should not be used in patients whose pain can be adequately controlled with systemic analgesics.
- Titration of all sedatives and analgesics requires increased vigilance because protein-bound drugs often have increased bioavailability in the characteristically hypoalbuminemic burn patients (104).
- In the acute trauma and critically ill patients, presence or suspicion of opioid addiction should not preclude aggressive treatment of pain with opioids.

REFERENCES

1. IASP Task Force on Taxonomy. Classification of Chronic Pain. In: Merskey H, Bogduk N, eds. Classification of Chronic

Pain: Descriptions of Chronic Pain Syndromes 2nd ed. Seattle: IASP Press; 1994:209–14.

2. Whipple J, Lewis K, Quebbeman E, et al. Analysis of pain management in critically ill patients. Pharmacotherapy 1995; 15(5):592–599.
3. Hedderich R, Ness T. Analgesia for trauma and burns. Crit Care Clin 1999; 15(1):167–184.
4. Holbrook T, Hoyt D, Stein M, Sieber W. Perceived threat to life predicts posttraumatic stress disorder after major trauma: risk factors and functional outcome. J Trauma 2001; 51(2):287–292.
5. Zatzick D, Kang S, Muller H, et al. Predicting posttraumatic distress in hospitalized trauma survivors with acute injuries. Am J Psychiatry 2002; 159(6):941–946.
6. Sedowofia K, Barclay C, Quaba A, et al. The systemic stress response to thermal injury in children. Clin Endocrinol (Oxf) 1998; 49(3):335–341.
7. Epstein J, Breslow M. The stress response of critical illness. Crit Care Clin 1999; 15(1):17–33.
8. Mangano D, Siliciano D, Hollenberg M, et al. Postoperative myocardial ischemia. Therapeutic trials using intensive analgesia following surgery. The Study of Perioperative Ischemia (SPI) Research Group. Anesthesiology 1992; 76(3):342–353.
9. Mackersie R, Karagianes T, Hoyt D, Davis J. Prospective evaluation of epidural and intravenous administration of fentanyl for pain control and restoration of ventilatory function following multiple rib fractures. J Trauma 1991; 31(4):443–449.
10. Strukova S. Blood coagulation-dependent inflammation. Coagulation-dependent inflammation and inflammation-dependent thrombosis. Front Biosci 2006; 11:59–80.
11. Rogers TJ, Peterson PK. Opioid G protein-coupled receptors: signals at the crossroads of inflammation. Trends Immunol 2003; 24(3):116–121.
12. McCarthy L, Wetzel M, Sliker J, et al. Opioids, opioid receptors, and the immune response. Drug Alcohol Depend 2001; 62(2):111–123.
13. De Witte J, Schoenmaekers B, Sessler D, Deloof T. The analgesic efficacy of tramadol is impaired by concurrent administration of ondansetron. Anesth Analg 2001; 92(5):1319–1321.
14. Dyson M. Intensive care unit psychosis, the therapeutic nurse-patient relationship and the influence of the intensive care setting: analyses of interrelating factors. J Clin Nursing 1999; 8(3):284–290.
15. Loeser JD, ed. Bonica's Management of Pain. 3rd ed. Philadelphia: Lippincott Williams & Wilkins, 2001.
16. Melzack R, Wall P. Pain mechanisms: a new theory. Science 1965; 150(699):971–979.
17. Muller H. Neuroplasticity and chronic pain. Anasthesiol Intensivmed Notfallmed Schmerzther 2000; 35(5):274–278.
18. Senturk M, Ozcan P, Talu G, et al. The effects of three different analgesia techniques on long-term postthoracotomy pain. Anesth Analg 2002; 94(1):11–15.
19. Bisgaard T, Rosenberg J, Kehlet H. From acute to chronic pain after laparoscopic cholecystectomy: a prospective follow-up analysis. Scand J Gastroenterol 2005; 40(11):1358–1364.
20. Møiniche S, Kehlet H, Dahl JB. A qualitative and quantitative systematic review of preemptive analgesia for postoperative pain relief: the role of timing of analgesia. Anesthesiology 2002; 96(3):725–741.
21. Vane J. The fight against rheumatism: from willow bark to COX-1 sparing drugs. J Physiol Pharmacol 2000; 51(4 pt 1): 573–586.
22. Ferreira S, Moncada S, Vane J. Prostaglandins and the mechanism of analgesia produced by aspirin-like drugs. 1973. Br J Pharmacol 1997; 120(4 suppl):401–412.
23. Loll P, Picot D, Garavito R. The structural basis of aspirin activity inferred from the crystal structure of inactivated prostaglandin H2 synthase. Nat Struct Biol 1995; 2(8):637–643.
24. Bombardier C, Laine L, Reicin A, Shapiro D, et al. Comparison of upper gastrointestinal toxicity of rofecoxib and naproxen in patients with rheumatoid arthritis. VIGOR Study Group. N Engl J Med 2000; 343(21):1520–1528.
25. Silverstein F, Faich G, Goldstein J, et al. Gastrointestinal toxicity with celecoxib vs nonsteroidal anti-inflammatory drugs for

osteoarthritis and rheumatoid arthritis: the CLASS study: a randomized controlled trial. Celecoxib Long-term Arthritis Safety Study. JAMA 2000; 284(10):1247–1255.
26. Schnitzer T. Cyclooxygenase-2—specific inhibitors: are they safe? Am J Med 2001; 110(1A):46S–49S.
27. Choy H, Milas L. Enhancing radiotherapy with cyclooxygenase-2 enzyme inhibitors: a rational advance? J Natl Cancer Inst 2003; 95(19):1440–1452.
28. Dormond O, Ruegg C. Regulation of endothelial cell integrin function and angiogenesis by COX-2, cAMP and Protein Kinase A. Thromb Haemost 2003; 90(4):577–585.
29. Perini R, Ma L, Wallace J. Mucosal repair and COX-2 inhibition. Curr Pharm Des 2003; 9(27):2207–2211.
30. Agrawal A, Gerson C, Seligman I, Dsida R. Postoperative hemorrhage after tonsillectomy: use of ketorolac tromethamine. Otolaryngol Head Neck Surg 1999; 120(3):335–9.
31. Singer A, Mynster C, McMahon B. The effect of IM ketorolac tromethamine on bleeding time: a prospective, interventional, controlled study. Am J Emerg Med 2003; 21(5):441–443.
32. Perneger T, Whelton P, Klag M. Risk of kidney failure associated with the use of acetaminophen, aspirin, and nonsteroidal antiinflammatory drugs. N Engl J Med 1994; 331(25):1675–1679.
33. Curhan G, Knight E, Rosner B, et al. Lifetime nonnarcotic analgesic use and decline in renal function in women. Arch Intern Med 2004; 164(14):1519–1524.
34. Jonsson A, Cassuto J, Hanson B. Inhibition of burn pain by intravenous lignocaine infusion. Lancet 1991; 338(8760): 151–152.
35. Heavner J. Cardiac toxicity of local anesthetics in the intact isolated heart model: a review. Reg Anesth Pain Med 2002; 27(6):545–555.
36. Ginosar Y, Riley ET, Angst MS. The site of action of epidural fentanyl in humans: the difference between infusion and bolus administration. Anesth Analg 2003; 97(5):1428–1438.
37. Hill H, Coda B, Tanaka A, Schaffer R. Multiple-dose evaluation of intravenous hydromorphone pharmacokinetics in normal human subjects. Anesth Analg 1991; 72(3):330–336.
38. Wagner LN, Eaton M, Sabnis S, Gingrich K. Meperidine and lidocaine block of recombinant voltage-dependent Na+ channels: evidence that meperidine is a local anesthetic. Anesthesiology 1999; 91(5):1481–1490.
39. Takada K, Clark D, Davies M, et al. Meperidine exerts agonist activity at the alpha(2B)-adrenoceptor subtype. Anesthesiology 2002; 96(6):1420–1426.
40. Marcantonio E, Juarez G, Goldman L, et al. The relationship of postoperative delirium with psychoactive medications. JAMA 1994; 272(19):1518–1522.
41. Ferrari A, Coccia C, Bertolini A, Sternieri E. Methadone—metabolism, pharmacokinetics and interactions. Pharmacol Res 2004; 50(6):551–559.
42. Quang-Cantagrel ND, Wallace MS, Magnuson SK. Opioid substitution to improve the effectiveness of chronic noncancer pain control: a chart review. Anasthesia and Analgesia 2000; 90: 933–937.
43. Hoffmann-La Roche Inc. ROMAZICON® (flumazenil) injection, complete product information.
44. Bansinath M, Shukla V, Turndorf H. Propofol modulates the effects of chemoconvulsants acting at the GABAergic, glycinergic, and glutamate receptor subtypes. Anesthesiology 1995; 83:809–815.
45. Weiskopf R, Bogetz M, Roizen M, Reid I. Cardiovascular and metabolic sequelae of inducing anesthesia with ketamine or thiopental in hypovolemic swine. Anesthesiology 1984; 60(3):214–219.
46. Stapleton J, Austin K, Mather L. Postoperative pain. Br Med J (Clin Res Ed) 1978; 2(6150):1499.
47. Bijur P, Latimer C, Gallagher E. Validation of a verbally administered numerical rating scale of acute pain for use in the emergency department. Acad Emerg Med 2003; 10(4):390–392.
48. Berthier F, Potel G, Leconte P, et al. Comparative study of methods of measuring acute pain intensity in an ED. Am J Emerg Med 1998; 16(2):132–136.

49. Odhner M, Wegman D, Freeland N, et al. Assessing pain control in nonverbal critically ill adults. Dimens Crit Care Nurs 2003; 22(6):260–267.

50. Fraser G, Riker R. Monitoring sedation, agitation, analgesia, and delirium in critically ill adult patients. Crit Care Clin 2001; 17(4):967–987.

51. Jacobi J, Fraser GL, Coursin DB, et al. Clinical practice guidelines for the sustained use of sedatives andanalgesics in the critically ill adult. Crit Care Med 2002; 30(1):119–141.

52. Avramon M, White P. Methods for monitoring the level of sedation. Crit Care Clin 1995; 11:803–826.

53. Ramsay M, Savege T, Simpson B, Goodwin R. Controlled sedation with alphaxalone-alphadolone. Br Med J 1974; 2:656–659.

54. Riker RR, Fraser GL. Prospective evaluation of the sedation-agitation scale for adult critically ill patients. Crit Care Med 1999; 27(7):1325–1329.

55. Ely E, Truman B, Shintani A, et al. Monitoring sedation status over time in ICU patients: reliability and validity of the Richmond Agitation-Sedation Scale (RASS). JAMA 2003; 289(22):2983–2991.

56. Sessler C, Gosnell M, Grap M, et al. The Richmond Agitation-Sedation Scale: validity and reliability in adult intensive care unit patients. Am J Respir Crit Care Med 2002; 166(10):1338–1344.

57. Alkire MT. Quantitative EEG correlations with brain glucose metabolic rate during anesthesia in volunteers. Anesthesiology 1998; 89(2):323–333.

58. Miner JR, Biros MH, Heegaard W, Plummer D. Bispectral electroencephalographic analysis of patients undergoing procedural sedation in the emergency department. Acad Emerg Med 2003; 10(6):638–643.

59. Schneider G, Heglmeier S, Schneider J, et al. Patient State Index (PSI) measures depth of sedation in intensive care patients. Intensive Care Med 2004; 30(2):213–216.

60. Glass P, Bloom M, Kearse L, et al. Bispectral analysis measures sedation and memory effects of propofol midazolam, isolurane, and alfentanil in healthy volunteers. Anesthesiology 1997; 86(4):836–847.

61. de Wit M, Epstein S. Administration of sedatives and level of sedation: comparative evaluation via the Sedation-Agitation Scale and the Bispectral Index. Am J Crit Care 2003; 12(4):343–348.

62. McDermott N, VanSickle T, Motas D, Friesen R. Validation of the bispectral index monitor during conscious and deep sedation in children. Anesth Analg 2003; 97(1):39–43.

63. Frenzel D, Greim C-A, Sommer C, et al. Is the bispectral index appropriate for monitoring the sedation level of mechanically ventilated surgical ICU patients? Intensive Care Med 2002; 28(2):178–183.

64. Gill M, Green S, Krauss B. A study of the Bispectral Index Monitor during procedural sedation and analgesia in the emergency department. Ann Emerg Med 2003; 41(2):234–241.

65. Nasraway SJ, Wu E, Kelleher R, et al. How reliable is the Bispectral Index in critically ill patients? A prospective, comparative, single-blinded observer study. Crit Care Med 2002; 30(7):1483–1487.

66. Prichep L, Gugino L, John E, et al. The Patient State Index as an indicator of the level of hypnosis under general anaesthesia. Br J Anaesth 2004; 92(3):393–399.

67. Apfelbaum J, Arens J, Cole D, et al. Practice Advisory for Intraoperative Awareness and Brain Function Monitoring . A Report by the American Society of Anesthesiologists Task Force on Intraoperative Awareness. American Society of Anesthesiologists Task Force on Intraoperative Awareness, Anesthesiology 2006; 104:847–864.

68. Lipowski Z. Delirium (acute confusional states). JAMA 1987; 258(13):1789–1792.

69. Trzepacz P, Breitbart W, Franklin J, et al. Practice guidelines: practice guideline for the treatment of patients with delirium. American Psychiatric Association. Am J Psychiatry 1999; 156(5 suppl):1–20.

70. Ely E, Margolin R, Francis J, et al. Evaluation of delirium in critically ill patients: validation of the confusion assessment method for the intensive care unit (CAM-ICU). Crit Care Med 2001; 29(7):1370–1379.

71. Inouye S, Bogardus S, Charpentier P, et al. A multicomponent intervention to prevent delirium in hospitalized older patients. N Engl J Med 1999; 340(9):669–676.

72. American Psychiatric Association. Diagnostic and statistical manual of mental disorders (DSM-IV). In: 4th ed. Washington, DC: American Psychiatric Association, 1994.

73. Inouye S, van Dyck C, Alessi C, et al. Clarifying confusion: the confusion assessment method. A new method for detection of delirium. Ann Intern Med 1990; 113(12):941–948.

74. Alpen M, Morse C. Managing the pain of traumatic injury. Crit Care Nurs Clin North Am 2001; 13(2):243–257.

75. McEachin C, McDermott J, Swor R. Few emergency medical services patients with lower-extremity fractures receive prehospital analgesia. Prehosp Emerg Care 2002; 6(4):406–410.

76. Chapman W, Arrowood J, Beecher H. The analgetic effects of low concentrations of nitrous oxide compared in man with morphine sulphate. J Clin Invest 1943; 22:871–875.

77. Baskett P. Nitrous oxide in prehospital care. Acta Anaesthesiol Scand 1994; 38:775–776.

78. Amey B, Ballinger J, Harrison E. Prehospital administration of nitrous oxide for control of pain. Ann Emerg Med 1981; 10:247–251.

79. Anand K, Ward-Platt M. Neonatal and pediatric stress responses to anesthesia and operation. Int Anesthesiol Clin 1988; 26(3):218–225.

80. Silka P, Roth M, Geiderman J. Patterns of analgesic use in trauma patients in the ED. Am J Emerg Med 2002; 20(4):298–302.

81. Miner J, Heegaard W, Plummer D. End-tidal carbon dioxide monitoring during procedural sedation. Acad Emerg Med 2002; 9(4):275–280.

82. American Society of Anesthesiologists Task Force on Sedation and Analgesia by Non-Anesthesiologists. Practice guidelines for sedation and analgesia by non-anesthesiologists, an updated report by the american society of anesthesiologists task force on sedation and analgesia by non-anesthesiologists. Anesthesiology 2002; 96(4):1004–1017.

83. Kissin I, Brown P, Bradley EJ, et al. Diazepam—morphine hypnotic synergism in rats. Anesthesiology 1989; 70(4):689–694.

84. Wilson W, Benumof J. Pathophysiology, evaluation, and treatment of a difficult airway. Anesth Clin North Am 1998; 16:29–75.

85. Park GR, Clarke S. Some is good and more is bad: getting the dose right in the critically ill. Eur J Anaesth 2001; 18(6):343.

86. Aitkenhead A, Pepperman M, Willatts S, et al. Comparison of propofol and midazolam for sedation in critically ill patients. Lancet 1989; 2(8665):704–709.

87. Higgins T, Yared J, Estafanous F, et al. Propofol versus midazolam for intensive care unit sedation after coronary artery bypass. Crit Care Med 1994; 22(9):1415–1423.

88. Ronan K, Gallagher T, George B, Hamby B. Comparison of propofol and midazolam for sedation in intensive care unit patients. Crit Care Med 1995; 23(2):286–293.

89. Hall R, Sandham D, Cardinal P, et al. Propofol vs midazolam for ICU sedation. A Canadian multicenter randomized trial. Chest 2001; 119(4):1151–1159.

90. Sanchez-Izquierdo-Riera J, Caballero-Cubedo R, Perez-Vela J, et al. Propofol versus midazolam: safety and efficacy for sedating the severe trauma patient. Anesth Analg 1998; 86(6):1219–1224.

91. Kumar A, Schwartz D, Lim K. Propofol-induced pancreatitis: recurrence of pancreatitis after rechallenge. Chest 1999; 115(4):1198–1199.

92. Possidente C, Rogers F, Osler T, Smith T. Elevated pancreatic enzymes after extended propofol therapy. Pharmacotherapy 1998; 18(3):653–655.

93. Bray R. Propofol infusion syndrome in children. Paediatr Anaesth 1998; 8(6):491–499.

94. Cremer O, Moons K, Bouman E, et al. Long-term propofol infusion and cardiac failure in adult head-injured patients. Lancet 2001; 357(9250):117–118.

95. Pohlman A, Simpson K, Hall J. Continuous intravenous infusions of lorazepam versus midazolam for sedation during mechanical ventilatory support: a prospective, randomized study. Crit Care Med 1994; 22:1241–1247.

96. Chern C, Chern T, Wang L, et al. Continuous flumazenil infusion in preventing complications arising from severe benzodiazepine intoxication. Am J Emerg Med 1998; 16(3):238–241.

97. Arbour RB, Ponzillo JJ. Appropriate utilization of intravenous sedatives and analgesics used in the care of the critically ill patient: Program sponsored By Medical Education Resources Inc. Med-Doc, Inc; 2002.

98. Jaakola M, Salonen M, Lehtinen R, Scheinin H. The analgesic action of dexmedetomidine—a novel alpha 2-adrenoceptor agonist—in healthy volunteers. Pain 1991; 46(3):281–285.

99. Ebert T, Hall J, Barney J, et al. The effects of increasing plasma concentrations of dexmedetomidine in humans. Anesthesiology 2000; 93(2):382–394.

100. Young C, Lujan E. Intravenous ziprasidone for treatment of delirium in the intensive care unit. Anesthesiology 2004; 101(3):794–795.

101. Schwartz TL, Masand PS. The role of atypical antipsychotics in the treatment of delirium. Psychosomatics 2002; 43:171–174.

102. Karmakar M, Ho A. Acute pain management of patients with multiple fractured ribs. J Trauma 2003; 54(3):615–625.

103. Choiniere M, Melzack R, Girard N, et al. Comparisons between patients' and nurses' assessment of pain and medication efficacy in severe burn injuries. Pain 1990; 40(2):143–152.

104. Bloedow D, Hansbrough J, Hardin T, Simons M. Postburn serum drug binding and serum protein concentrations. J Clin Pharmacol 1986; 26(2):147–151.

105. Andersen G, Christrup L, Sjogren P. Relationships among morphine metabolism, pain and side effects during long-term treatment: an update. J Pain Symptom Manage 2003; 25(1):74–91.

106. Pauli-Magnus C, Hofmann U, Mikus G, et al. Pharmacokinetics of morphine and its glucuronides following intravenous administration of morphine in patients undergoing continuous ambulatory peritoneal dialysis. Nephrol Dial Transplant 1999; 14(4):903–909.

107. Trouvin J, Farinotti R, Haberer J, et al. Pharmacokinetics of midazolam in anaesthetized cirrhotic patients. Br J Anaesth 1988; 60(7):762–767.

108. Bauer T, Ritz R, Haberthur C, et al. Prolonged sedation due to accumulation of conjugated metabolites of midazolam. Lancet 1995; 346(8968):145–147.

109. Finkel J, Johnson Y, Quezado Z. The use of dexmedetomidine to facilitate acute discontinuation of opioids after cardiac transplantation in children. Crit Care Med 2005; 33(9):2110–2112.

110. Anand K, Hickey P. Halothane-morphine compared with high-dose sufentanil for anesthesia and postoperative analgesia in neonatal cardiac surgery. N Engl J Med 1992; 326(1):1–9.

111. Anand K, Sippell W, Aynsley-Green A. Randomised trial of fentanyl anaesthesia in preterm babies undergoing surgery: effects on the stress response. Lancet 1987; 1(8524):62–66.

112. Grunau R, Craig K. Pain expression in neonates: facial action and cry. Pain 1987; 28(3):395–410.

113. Pershad J, Palmisano P, Nichols M. Chloral hydrate: the good and the bad. Pediatr Emerg Care 1999; 15(6):432–435.

114. Hertzog J, Campbell J, Dalton H, Hauser G. Propofol anesthesia for invasive procedures in ambulatory and hospitalized children: experience in the pediatric intensive care unit. Pediatrics 1999; 103(3):E30.

115. Koch M, De Backer D, Vincent J. Lactic acidosis: an early marker of propofol infusion syndrome? Intensive Care Med 2004; 30:522.

116. Vasile B, Rasulo F, Candiani A, Latronico N. The pathophysiology of propofol infusion syndrome: a simple name for a complex syndrome. Intensive Care Med 2003; 29(9):1417–1425.

117. Hammer G, Philip B, Schroeder A, et al. Prolonged infusion of dexmedetomidine for sedation following tracheal resection. Paediatr Anaesth 2005; 15(7):616–620.

118. Tobias J, Berkenbosch J. Sedation during mechanical ventilation in infants and children: dexmedetomidine versus midazolam. South Med J 2004; 97(5):451–455.

119. Crome P, Flanagan R. Pharmacokinetic studies in elderly people. Are they necessary? Clin Pharmacokinet 1994; 26(4):243–247.

120. Harper K, Collier P, Dundee J, et al. Age and nature of operation influence the pharmacokinetics of midazolam. Br J Anaesth 1985; 57(9):866–871.

121. Swift C. Prescribing in old age. Br Med J (Clin Res Ed) 1988; 296(6626):913–915.

122. Beller J, Pottecher T, Lugnier A, et al. Prolonged sedation with propofol in ICU patients: recovery and blood concentration changes during periodic interruptions in infusion. Br J Anaesth 1988; 61(5):583–588.

123. Shafer S. The pharmacology of anesthetic drugs in elderly patients. Anesthesiol Clin North America 2000; 18(1):1–29.

124. Chandrasekharan N, Dai H, Roos K, et al. COX-3, a cyclooxygenase-1 variant inhibited by acetaminophen and other analgesic/antipyretic drugs: cloning, structure, and expression. Proc Natl Acad Sci USA 2002; 99(21):13926–13931.

125. Campana W, Li X, Shubayev V, et al. Erythropoietin reduces Schwann cell TNF-alpha, Wallerian degeneration and pain-related behaviors after peripheral nerve injury. Eur J Neurosci 2006; 23(3):617–626.

126. Svensson C, Fitzsimmons B, Azizi S, et al. Spinal p38beta isoform mediates tissue injury-induced hyperalgesia and spinal sensitization. J Neurochem 2005; 92(6):1508–1520.

127. Hua X, Svensson C, Matsui T, et al. Intrathecal minocycline attenuates peripheral inflammation-induced hyperalgesia by inhibiting p38 MAPK in spinal microglia. Eur J Neurosci 2005; 22(10):2431–2440.

128. Mikami M, Yang J. Short hairpin RNA–mediated selective knockdown of NaV1.8 tetrodotoxin-resistant voltage-gated sodium channel in dorsal root ganglion neurons. Anesthesiology 2005; 103:828–836.

129. Laird J, Souslova V, Wood J, Cervero F. Deficits in visceral pain and referred hyperalgesia in NaV1.8 (SNS/ PN3)-null mice. J Neurosci 2002; 22:8352–8356.

130. Furia J, Alioto R, Marquardt J. The efficacy and safety of the hematoma block for fracture reduction in closed, isolated fractures. Orthopedics 1997; 20(5):423–426.

6

Neuromuscular Blockade for Trauma and Critical Care

Nitin Shah

Department of Anesthesiology and Critical Care, Long Beach VA Hospital, Long Beach, California, U.S.A.

INTRODUCTION

Neuromuscular blockade (NMB) use in trauma and critical care presents several unique challenges. First and foremost is its interference with the ability to repeatedly evaluate the neurological status of patients, both during initial resuscitation and later in the intensive care unit (ICU). Second, altered renal and hepatic function changes the pharmacokinetic and pharmacodynamic profiles of many NMB drugs. Third, some patients requiring prolonged administration of NMBs during their ICU stay, increase their risk of postparalytic syndrome. Fourth, critical illness polyneuropathy (CIP) and steroid-related myopathy are additional complications that may compound the issue of prolonged weakness. Finally, the emergent nature of severe traumatic injuries further complicate the situation (especially head trauma), as incomplete information about the patient's pre-injury neurological status or other underlying medical conditions, may be unavailable to guide the proper use of sedatives and NMBs (1–8).

In an ideal situation, appropriate sedation allows patients to remain in a calm, communicative state during their ICU stay, and illness does not become so severe that prolonged NMB use is required. However, the reality is different when one is dealing with head trauma and critically ill patients with multiple organ dysfunction syndrome (MODS). Treatable causes of agitation and confusion (e.g., meningitis or other systemic infections, hypoxia, pain, drug or alcohol withdrawal, and cerebral vascular events) should be investigated before sedation and high-dose analgesia is administered (9). Similarly, analgesia and sedation should be administered prior to the use of NMB drugs. Furthermore, paralyzed patients may be able to process external auditory and tactile stimuli since NMB drugs are devoid of sedative, amnestic, or analgesic activity. Hence, once hemodynamically stable, all patients receiving NMB drugs must receive sedative, amnestic, and analgesic drugs to prevent recall and discomfort (10–12).

This chapter will review the clinically relevant history, physiology, and pharmacology of the NMB drugs commonly employed in trauma and critical care. This review will also discuss reversal agents, interactions caused by various disease states and other drugs, as well as the specific indications for NMB use and monitoring techniques. Finally, the chapter reviews the complications of prolonged blockade, CIP, and steroid-related myopathy. The eye to the future focuses upon improving drugs and monitoring and limiting the complications.

HISTORY OF NEUROMUSCULAR BLOCKING DRUGS

As early as the 15th century, immediately following the explorations of Columbus, stories began to circulate through Europe of South American Indian tribes who used poisoned arrows. The preparation and use of the poisonous agent called curare (or Woorari), which probably meant "bird killer," was described by Peter Martyr, the royal chronicler for Spain following expeditions to Venezuela in a book entitled *De Orbe Novo* (13).

However, it was the noted geographer, Alexander von Humboldt (1807), who provided the first reliable eye witness accounts of the actual preparation of curare by South American natives. The concoction included the bark of *Strychnos toxifera* or *S. guianensis*, and especially *Chondrodendron tomentosum*. Other plant additives and, in some cases, venom from snakes or ants were also used depending upon the specific South American tribe making the curare (explaining the disparity in ingredients reported from various sources). The entire mixture was simmered in water for a couple days and condensed into a viscous resin. Dart tips were then dipped into the curare and fired through blowguns at small prey.

In 1811, Sir Benjamin Bodie discovered that during curare intoxication, the heart continues to beat even after breathing stops. By 1845, Claude Bernard had traced the action of curare to the neuromuscular junction (NMJ), by demonstrating that both neural conduction and direct muscular response were intact in the curarized frog. The work of Bernard and others led us to our current understanding of the structure and function of the NMJ. The nervous system innervates skeletal muscle to produce movement. Muscle depolarization results from a single action potential, which causes a brief contraction followed by relaxation. This response is called a muscle twitch (14).

However, curare's potential use as a medicinal agent was not realized until the 19th century. The first recorded clinical use of curare as a muscle relaxant during surgery occurred in Leipzig, Germany, in 1912, when a surgeon used it to facilitate abdominal closure (15). Curare was used by both American and English anesthetists in 1941–1943 with growing confidence and understanding about its dosing and side effects as it was beginning to be considered safe (16,17).

By 1946, one publication described a series of 1000 anesthetized patients where d-tubocurare (dTc) was used as a muscle relaxant (18). The authors of that publication described the intentional use of paralytic doses of dTc in conjunction with adjuvants to provide unconsciousness, analgesia, and relaxation (the components of a balanced anesthetic). However, a decade later, Beecher and Todd (19) report a sixfold increase in mortality of patients who had received an NMB. The increased mortality resulted from administering dTc to sicker patients and more widespread use by those who were less familiar with its pharmacology and reversal considerations. Additionally, the early anesthesiologists maintained spontaneous ventilation in their patients during curare anesthetics, further increasing the complexity of management and risk of complications.

During the last 60 years, a number of newer NMB drugs have been introduced to clinical practice. In addition, improved understanding of the prejunctional and postjunctional effects of drugs has helped explain some of the differences recognized between the benzylisoquinolinium and steroidal drugs, and explains the synergism produced when used together.

Better understanding of the limitations as well as the more sophisticated use of twitch monitors (e.g., post-tetanic fade, and double burst technologies) has increased safety. A supershort onset-drug (rapicuronium) has come and gone from clinical use due to its significant histamine release-related complications. Conversely, two long-acting drugs, doxacurnium (a benzylisoquinolinium) and pipercuronium (a steroidal drug), have come and gone due to complications related to their excessively long duration of action.

Another newer drug (rocuronium) has filled a particularly important niche in emergency trauma airway management; and another newer NMB drug (cisatracurium) has special properties of value in critically ill patients suffering from hepatic and renal failure requiring short term NMB in the ICU and OR. These and other clinically relevant NMB drugs are reviewed in subsequent sections of this chapter.

PHYSIOLOGY OF THE NEUROMUSCULAR JUNCTION

The nerve cell, together with the muscle fibers it innervates, is called the motor unit. The nerve impulse initiated in the nerve body travels along the axon to the nerve terminal, which synapses with somewhere between 15 and 1500 muscle fibers (depending upon the function). Muscles subserving fine movements, such as extraocular muscles, are richly innervated, with fewer muscle fibers per motor unit. Whereas, muscles such as the gastrocnemius, which do not require fine control, are less intensively innervated (i.e., large numbers of muscle fibers per motor unit) (20).

Neuromuscular Junction Anatomy

The NMJ consists of a motor nerve terminal (prejunctional side) and a motor endplate (postjunctional side), separated by a synaptic cleft (Fig. 1). The motor end plate is a uniquely chemosensitive and highly involuted area of muscle membrane located opposite the motor nerve terminal. A gap, or synaptic cleft (20–50 nm wide), separates the nerve terminal from the muscle fiber. ☞ **The neural signal is propagated along the axon electrically to the nerve terminal, but crossing the synapse requires the chemical messenger acetylcholine (ACh).** ☞ Electrical transmission then resumes in a second neuron or in a muscle fiber (in the case of neuromuscular transmission).

The Motor Nerve Terminal

The terminal portion of the motor axon is a specialized structure designed for the production and release of ACh (Fig. 2).

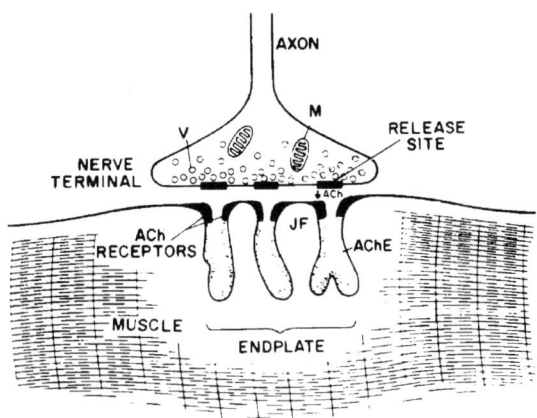

Figure 1 Neuromuscular junction anatomy. The nerve terminal is separated from the motor end plate by a synaptic cleft (or gap) approximately 20–50 nm wide. ACh is present in vesicles of the axon for release in response to nerve impulses. ACh diffuses across the synaptic cleft and binds to receptors concentrated on the JF of the skeletal muscle endplate. Acetylcholinesterase is present in the JF to facilitate rapid hydrolysis of ACh. *Abbreviations*: ACh, acetylcholine; AChE, acetylcholinesterase; JF, junctional folds; M, mitochondria; V, vesicles. *Source*: From Ref. 183.

The axon terminal contains subcellular structures involved with energy production, protein synthesis, as well as calcium binding and storage. It also synthesizes choline and acetate to form ACh. This reaction is catalyzed by the enzyme acetyltransferase. Choline is also recycled (as described below). ACh is the chemical messenger (a quaternary ammonium compound) for neural communication at several locations besides the NMJ, including some central nervous system pathways, the autonomic ganglia, all postganglionic parasympathetic nerve endings, and a few postganglionic sympathetic nerve endings (see Volume 2, Chapter 1) (21).

When an electrical impulse arrives at the nerve terminal of the NMJ, approximately 200 to 400 synaptic vesicles (SV) fuse with the nerve cell membrane after a calcium-calmodulin-mediated activation of the SV–SNARE complex triggers docking and priming. Soon after fusion, the ACh molecules are released into the synaptic cleft by exocytosis (Fig. 2). Calcium is required for the process and magnesium inhibits it. Each SV (or quanta) contains 5000 to 10,000 molecules of ACh, which diffuse across the synaptic cleft and bind with nicotinic ACh receptors (nAChRs) on the motor end plate of the muscle fiber, triggering a conformational change in the receptor allowing entry of sodium and the propagation of an action potential in the muscle.

In the absence of nerve stimulation, quanta are spontaneously released at random. These result in small depolarizations of the motor end plate known as miniature end-plate potentials (MEPPs). Although MEPPs can be recorded, they are not strong enough to allow any significant Na^+ entry and thus do not cause firing of the muscle cell.

Postjunctional Acetylcholine Receptor

Each nAChR is a protein complex made up of five subunits: two alpha, one beta, one gamma, and one delta (Fig. 3). These subunits form a transmembrane pore, as well as

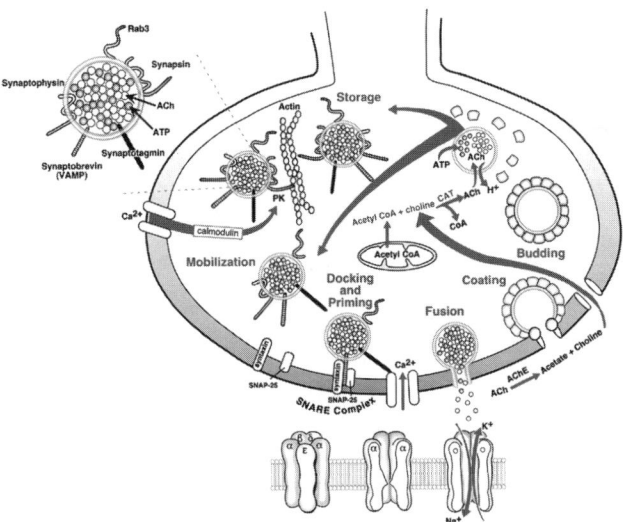

Figure 2 Motor nerve terminal. Schematic depiction of the synaptic vesicle exocytosis–endocytosis cycle. After an action potential and Ca^{2+} influx, phosphorylation of synapsin is activated by calcium-calmodulin activated protein kinases I and II. This results in the mobilization of synaptic vesicles (SVs) from the cytomatrix toward the plasma membrane. The formation of the complex is an essential step for the docking process. After fusion of SVs with the presynaptic plasma membrane, acetylcholine (ACh) is released into the synaptic cleft. Some of the released ACh molecules bind to the nicotinic ACh receptors on the postsynaptic membrane, while the rest is rapidly hydrolyzed by the acetyl-cholinesterase present in the synaptic cleft forming choline and acetate. Choline is recycled into the terminal by a high-affinity uptake system, making it available for the resynthesis of ACh. Exocytosis is followed by endocytosis in a process dependent on the formation of a clathrin coat and of action of dynamin. After recovering of SV membrane, the coated vesicle uncoats and another cycle starts again. *Source*: From Ref. 21.

binding sites for ACh NMB drugs. The M_2 transmembrane-spanning segment of each subunit lines the cation selective channel (Fig. 3) (21). The ACh binding sites are located on the $\alpha\delta$ and $\alpha\varepsilon$ subunits. In the absence of ACh the pore is closed. Simultaneous binding of two ACh molecules to a nAChR leads to a conformational change in the three dimensional shape of the subunits opening the pore (increased permeability to sodium). ☞ **If enough nAChR channels are opened (as occurs when 200–400 quanta of ACh are released into the synaptic cleft), the resultant change in transmembrane potential will exceed −50 mV, and an action potential will be propagated to the entire motor unit, resulting in muscular contraction (21).** ☞

The termination of normal, physiologic depolarization is caused by diffusion of free ACh from the cleft, unbinding of ACh from the receptor, and breakdown of the ACh molecule by fixed acetylcholinesterase (AChE) located in the invaginations of the motor end plate (Fig. 1). ACh is hydrolyzed by AChE to acetate and choline. The choline is reabsorbed into the nerve terminal, and in the presence of cholineacetyltransferanse (CAT) combines with acetyl-CoA (produced in the axon terminal mitochondria, via the Kreb's cycle) to reform ACh, which is then repackaged in vesicles (Fig. 2). The level of ACh falls below the threshold required for excitation before the end of the muscle's

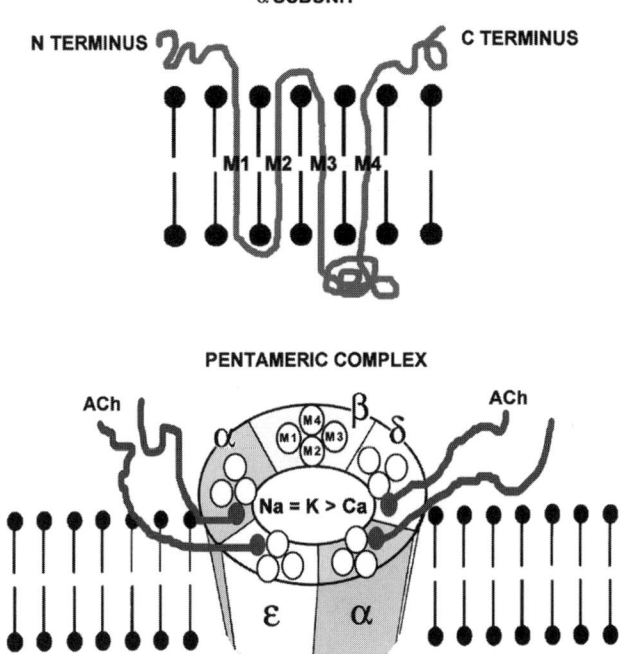

Figure 3 Subunit composition of the nicotinic acetylcholine receptor (nAChR) in the endplate surface of adult mammalian muscle. The adult AChR is an intrinsic membrane protein with five distinct subunits ($\alpha_2\beta\delta\varepsilon$). Each subunit contains four helical domains labeled M1 to M4. The M2 domain forms the channel pore. *Top*: A single α subunit (*gray*) with its N and C termini on the extracellular surface of the membrane lipid bilayer (*black*). Between the N and C termini, the α subunit forms four helices (M1, M2, M3, and M4) that span the membrane bilayer. *Bottom*: The pentameric structure of the nAChR of adult mammalian muscle. The N termini of two subunits cooperate to form two distinct binding pockets for acetylcholine. These pockets occur at the $\varepsilon-\alpha$ and the $\delta-\alpha$ subunit interface. The M2 membrane spanning domain of each subunit lines the ion channel. The doubly liganded ion channel has equal permeability to Na^+ and K^+; Ca^{2+} contributes approximately 2.5% to the total permeability. *Abbreviations*: Ach, acetylcholine; AChE, acetylcholinesterase; ATP, adenosine triphosphate; CAT, choline acetyltransferase; CoA, coenzyme A; PK, protein kinase. *Source*: From Ref. 21.

refractory period. Therefore, a single nerve action potential can elicit only one twitch (20,21).

CLINICAL PHARMACOLOGY OF NEUROMUSCULAR BLOCKADE DRUGS

The selection of NMB is based upon the clinical situation, the side effect profile, and cost. The clinical needs during the routine induction of anesthesia are different than during emergent intubation, and different still during maintenance of anesthesia—or during care in the ICU. For routine induction and intubation, a moderately rapid onset and brief duration of action are important NMB attributes, whereas in emergency intubation, an ultra rapidonset and minimal side effects are critical, while the duration of action is less important. This is true because in the emergency situation, waking the patient up and coming back another time

Table 1 Classification of Neuromuscular Blockade Drugs

Drug	Type of block	Duration	Structure
Succinylcholine	Depolarizing	Ultrashort	ACh-like
Atracurium	Nondepolarizing	Short	Benzylisoquinolinium
Cisatracurium	Nondepolarizing	Intermediate	Benzylisoquinolinium
Mivacurium	Nondepolarizing	Short	Benzylisoquinolinium
Doxacurium[a]	Nondepolarizing	Long	Benzylisoquinolinium
Pancuronium	Nondepolarizing	Long	Aminosteroid
Vecuromium	Nondepolarizing	Intermediate	Aminosteroid
Rocuronium	Nondepolarizing	Intermediate-long	Aminosteroid
Pipecuronium[a]	Nondepolarizing	Long	Aminosteroid

[a]No longer available clinically in United States.

to attempt intubation is almost never an option. For maintenance of NMB, facilitated paralysis (e.g., during anesthesia and in the ICU), reliability of duration, affordability and minimized side effects are the most important characteristics (22,23).

The NMB drugs can be classified in one of three common ways (Table 1): (*i*) according to the type of block produced (i.e., depolarizing vs. nondepolarizing), (*ii*) based upon the duration of action (i.e., ultrashort, short, intermediate, long), and (*iii*) in relation to the molecular structure (i.e., ACh-like, benzylisoquinolinium compound, or aminosteroid compound) (22–24). In this review, drugs will be organized into depolarizing (chiefly succinylcholine) and nondepolarizing (all the rest). The molecular structure does have certain clinical impacts, and will be referred to where appropriate (22).

Depolarizing Drugs (Succinylcholine)

The only depolarizing NMB drug in current clinical use is succinylcholine, which acts as an ACh analog binding to the nicotinic cholinergic receptors, initially causing depolarization. The blockade that ensues results from the slow hydrolysis of succinylcholine by AChE (relative to the rapid hydrolysis of ACh) and, consequently, repolarization is delayed until the succinylcholine is hydrolyzed. This results in a brief period of repetitive depolarizations of various motor units, often manifested by transient muscular fasiculations (25), particularly in the hands, feet, and face (26). This "fasciculation" phase is transient and followed by blockade of neuromuscular transmission and flaccid paralysis (25). Succinylcholine has a sufficiently rapid onset (45 to 60 seconds) to allow endotracheal intubation within 60 seconds and remains the NMB drug of choice for rapid-sequence induction (RSI), unless contraindicated due to its many known side effects (27).

Succinylcholine is administered in doses of 1–1.5 mg/kg intravenously. The duration of NMB due to succinylcholine is typically three to five minutes (28). However, some patients (who may be otherwise healthy or suffering from certain medical conditions in which plasma cholinesterase levels are depressed) can experience a prolonged duration of action. ☞ **Decreased quantity or quality of plasma cholinesterase results in a prolonged duration of NMB due to succinylcholine.** ☞ Pregnant patients, and those with impaired hepatic function, have depressed plasma levels of pseudocholinesterase; others may have congenitally abnormal pseudocholinesterase activity, both situations resulting in prolonged drug effect when succinlycholine is administered (Fig. 4) (18,28,29). These patients will have a prolonged

duration of action of other drugs dependent upon pseudocholinesterase for metabolism (e.g., mivicurium). Table 2 lists conditions that can cause decreased or increased activity of plasma cholinesterases.

In the ICU setting, succinylcholine is not used as a continuous infusion. Rather, it is utilized for rapid-sequence intubation (RSI) only, in order to achieve rapid paralysis and facilitate intubation of the airway in patients at increased risk for regurgitation of gastric contents. Succinylcholine has a number of cardiac side effects including sinus bradycardia, junctional rhythms, or even sinus arrest due to the concomitant binding to cardiac muscarinic receptors. These effects are more prominent in younger patients, and after administration of a second dose of the drug very soon (within minutes) after the first dose (21). The administration of succinylcholine ordinarily results in a small rise in serum K^+ concentration (0.5–1 mEq/L) because of muscle depolarization and potassium release.

☞ **In patients with denervated muscle, particularly following upper motor neuron injury or following muscle injury (burns, massive trauma), serum K^+ levels can increase by as much as 85% following succinylcholine administration (30), resulting in peaked T waves, widened QRS complexes, loss of P waves, and occasionally, ventricular fibrillation and cardiac arrest.** ☞ The therapy for succinylcholine-induced hyperkalemic ventricular fibrillation and arrest includes: (*i*) immediate institution of

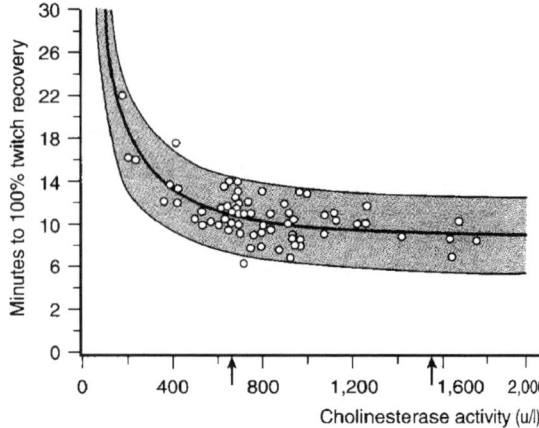

Figure 4 Correlation between the duration of succinylcholine neuromuscular blockade and butyrylcholinesterase activity. The normal range of activity lies between the arrows. *Source*: Modified From Ref. 184.

Table 2 Factors Affecting Plasma Cholinesterase Activity

Decreased activity of plasma cholinesterase	Increased activity of plasma cholinesterase
Inherited deficiency	Obesity, hyperlipidemia
Physiological variance: last trimester of pregnancy, newborns, infants	Essential hypertension Thyrotoxicosis Nephrosis
Acquired causes: liver diseases (acute hepatitis, hepatic metastasis), hyperpyrexia, myocardial infarction, acute infections, carcinomas, uremia, malnutrition, chronic debilitating diseases, burns, epilepsy	Asthma, alcoholism, schizophrenia
Iatrogenic causes: radiation therapy, anticancer therapy, MAO inhibitors, neostigmine, esmolol, organophosphorus insecticides	

Abbreviation: MAO, monaminoxidase.

cardiopulmonary resuscitation (CPR), (*ii*) administration of calcium chloride (to stabilize the membrane), (*iii*) alkalinization by hyperventilation and NaHCO$_3$ administration (to decrease the [K$^+$]), (*iv*) concomitant administration of glucose and insulin (to drive K$^+$ into cells), (*v*) β-agonist administration (to stimulate the Na$^+$/K$^+$ ATPase), (*vi*) Furosemide to promote diuresis and K$^+$ loss, and (*vii*) treatments using K$^+$ binding resins (e.g., kayexylate) administered via the GI tract are not efficacious acutely, but can help decrease serum [K$^+$] over time. CPR must continue until potassium levels have returned toward baseline. Cardioversion will not be effective until the serum [K$^+$] is decreased towards normal and the membrane stabilized by specific treatment (i.e., ionized calcium administration), all of which should occur concomitantly with CPR (Table 3).

The exaggerated potassium release seen with denervated, traumatized, or debilitated muscles is related to the proliferation of extrajunctional cholinergic receptors and the resultant increase in K$^+$ release following succinylcholine administration (31). Because of the delay between injury and receptor synthesis, patients can be given succinylcholine safely 72 hours after acute upper motor neuron injury, and/or 24 to 48 hours following major burns (32). The risk of potassium release has been shown to persist for as long as two years after injury in some cases, and should be presumed to be present in any patient with persistent denervation. Further discussions of succinylcholine-induced hyperkalemia resulting from neurologic injury and burns are found in Volume 1, Chapters 23 and 34, respectively.

Succincylcholine has a number of other side effects resulting in several relative contraindications for its use. A number of studies have shown increases in intracranial, intraocular, and intragastric pressure after administration of succinylcholine. It can also act as a trigger for malignant hyperthermia, and can cause myoglobinuria, trismus, and phase II block (a complex phenomenon resulting in NMJ dysfunction following prolonged exposure to depolarizing agents).

Nondepolarizing Drugs

Nondepolarizing NMB agents competitively inhibit the action of ACh at the NMJ through one of three mechanisms: (*i*) binding to nicotinic cholinergic receptors and preventing the conformational change that allows passage of sodium ions; (*ii*) physical obstruction of the channel, preventing passage of sodium; and (*iii*) presynaptic inhibition of ACh release (minimal clinical significance) (21). **The nondepolarizing agents are all derived from one of two chemical groups, benzylisoquoliniums and aminosteroids (Tables 1 and 4).** The benzylisoquolinium class of NMB drugs are characterized by the following main attributes: high potency, lack of vagolytic effect, propensity for histamine release (except for cisatricurium), and novel methods of degradation, for example, Hoffmann elimination (atricurium and cisatricurium) and enzyme-catalyzed ester hydrolysis (mivicurium). The oldest member of this class, dTc, also has a ganglion blockade effect, which may add to the hypotensive effect resulting from histamine release. Metocurine also has a

Table 3 Specific Therapy for Hyperkalemia

Drug	Dose/delivery	Rationale/comments
Calcium chloride	250–1000 mg IV push	Does not actually decrease [K$^+$]. Vitally important, however, and should be employed immediately to stabilize the myocardial membrane (separates the resting membrane potential from the threshold potential)
NaHCO$_3$	1–2 mEq/1 kg IV push	Alkalanization helps drive K$^+$ back into cells. Hyperventilation should also be employed, especially in the first 5–10 min
Epinephrine	0.1–0.2 mEq/kg/min IV drip	β-agonists increase the Na$^+$/K$^+$ ATPase which brings K$^+$ into cells, while moving Na$^+$ out
Lasix® (furosemide)	10–40 mg IV push	Lasix helps promote K$^+$ loss in the urine. Slow (takes minutes to hours to work)
Glucose and insulin	Administer 1 AmpD$_{50}$ and begin D$_{5W}$ drop; then administer 5 units of regular insulin	Insulin and glucose will drive K$^+$ into cells. The D$_{50}$ administration and D$_{5W}$ drop should be started prior to insulin administration, unless patient has a known blood glucose >150 at the time
Kayexalate® (sodium polystyrene sulfonate)	Depends upon starting [K$^+$]	Slowest (takes hours or days to work), only indicated if the patient's serum [K$^+$] was high prior to the succinylcholine administration

ganglion blockade effect, but weaker than dTc. Both DTc and metocurine are more precisely categorized as isoquinolinium drugs, and are no longer available in the United States. None of the benzylisoquinolinium drugs have a clinically significant ganglionic blockade effect.

Modifications of the steroidal nucleus of androstane resulted in potent synthetic NMBs, of which pancuronium was the first synthesized. Later, pipercuronium, vecuronium, rocuronium, and rapicuronium were synthesized. Renal excretion, elimination in the bile, and metabolism are all important characteristics of the steroidal NMBs. Uptake by the liver is more important for the intermediate-acting vecurunium and rocuronium, than for the longer-acting pancuronium and pipercuronium.

The onset of action of the nondepolarizing agents is dose dependent; as the dose is increased, the time to attain adequate intubating conditions is shortened (27). They produce a depression of evoked twitch amplitude, and they result in frequency-dependent suppression of neuromuscular transmission, which manifests either in tetanic fade or in train-of-four (TOF) fade (33). Metabolism of each nondepolarizing agent varies from drug to drug (34).

The use of muscle relaxants in ICU patients has increased significantly over the last 15 years, in large part because of their record of safe intraoperative use. However, it has become increasingly recognized that the long-term administration results in pharmacokinetics and side effect profiles are quite different from those found in the operating room (OR). A survey indicates that the NMB agents have been used in a variety of practices like bolus administration and continuous infusion with and without monitoring of degree of NMB (26). We will discuss the commonly used drugs in ICU in detail.

Rocuronium

Rocuronium is less potent than its predecessor steroidal NMBs but has a more rapid onset of action. ☞ **Rocuronium is mainly used as an NMB during RSI in patients with contraindications to succinylcholine [e.g., burns, upper motor neuron injury, chronic bedrest (>30 days), and history of malignant hyperthermia, etc.].** ☞ Rocuronium in a dose of 1.2 mg/Kg provides intubating conditions at 60 seconds, which are similar to that produced by succinylcholine (Table 4) (35).

Although it may cause mild vagolysis, it does not characteristically cause any significant hemodynamic perturbation. Rocuronium is hepatically metabolized and renally excreted. It is rarely used in ICU as a maintenance infusion NMB drug because of the availability of less expensive alternatives, for example, pancuronium and vecuronium. Closely related rapicuronium has the most rapid onset, but was never useful clinically in trauma or other RSI situations due to its propensity for significant histamine release and subsequent hypotension. Rapicuronium is no longer available clinically.

Vecuronium

Vecuronium is an intermediate-acting NMB drug, initially used during surgical anesthesia. Vecuronium has now come into widespread use in the ICU because of its negligible hemodynamic side effects and affordability, having become generic a decade ago. Vecuronium is an aminosteroid NMB drug produced by demethylation of the pancuronium molecule, with which it is roughly equipotent. Vecuronium undergoes spontaneous deacetylation in the liver to three metabolites with varying degrees of activity. ☞ **The main vecuronium metabolite, 3,17-dihydroxyvecuronium, has only 2% of the activity of the parent compound, whereas the 3-hydroxy derivative has 60% of the activity of the parent compound, and is excreted renally.** ☞ The half-life of vecuronium is moderately prolonged in both renal and hepatic failure. This effect is typically negligible after short-term use, but can become more significant with prolonged administration as in the ICU setting (36).

Pancuronium

Pancuronium is the first synthesized aminosteroid NMB drug with a 40-year history of clinical use. It is excreted primarily as an unchanged drug by the kidneys, although biliary excretion of unchanged drugs also occurs (13). Minimal metabolism in the liver produces an active 3-hydroxy metabolite with roughly one-half the activity of the parent compound. The 3-hydroxy metabolite is excreted equally in the kidney and bile. ☞ **Because pancuronium and its metabolites are mainly (70%) excreted in the urine, a prolonged duration**

Table 4 Infusion Dosing Recommendations for Intensive Care Unit and Routes of Elimination for Neuromuscular Blockade Agents

Structural classification	Relaxant	ETT bolus dose, mg/kg	ICU continuous infusion (usual range)	Routes of elimination
Depolarizing	Succinylcholine	1–2	—	Plasma cholinesterase
Nondepolarizing				
Benzylisoquinolinium	Mivacurium	0.15–0.25	4 mcg/kg/min (4–20)	Plasma cholinesterase
	Atracurium	0.3–0.5	11–13 mcg/kg/min (4.5–29.5) 3 mcg/kg/min (0.5–10.2)	Ester hydrolysis and Hoffmann elimination
	Cisatracurium	0.15–0.2	Not recommended	Hoffmann elimination
	Tubocurarine	0.25–0.5 every 2–3 hrs		Primarily renal, some biliary
Aminosteroid	Rocuronium	0.6 (elective) 1.2 (RSI)	10–12 mcg/kg/min (4–16)	Primarily hepatic, some renal
	Vecuronium	0.1	1 mcg/kg/min (0.8–1.2)	Biliary and hepatic; active metabolite (3-desacetyl)
	Pancuronium	0.03–0	1 mcg/kg/min (1–2)	Primarily renal, some biliary

Abbreviations: ETT, endotracheal tube/induction; ICU, intensive care unit; RSI, rapid sequence intubation/induction (when speed of onset is critical).

of action occurs in renal failure. ☞ Pancuronium has a vagolytic effect, which may cause tachycardia, and rarely mild hypertension (22,24). Pancuronium should be avoided in patients who cannot tolerate the vagolytic mediated increase in heart rate (e.g., severe coronary artery disease, severe aortic stenosis, severe mitral stenosis). Conversely, clinically significant bradycardia is occasionally seen after cessation of prolonged pancuronium infusion. For all other patients, especially the typical young, previously healthy trauma victim, the inexpensive pancuronium appears to be a suitable drug for prolonged NMB infusion in the ICU.

Atracurium

Atracurium is a short, acting benzylisoquinolinium NMB; this bis-quarternary nitrogen compound was designed to be independent of hepatic and renal elimination. Its metabolism (and offset) depends upon two mechanisms: the first is known as Hoffmann elimination, the nonenzymatic, chemical degradation of quarternary ammonium salts; the second, and probably more important, is the nonspecific ester hydrolysis occuring in plasma and tissue. Atracurium is relatively stable at pH 3.0 and 4°C, but becomes unstable when injected into the warm bloodstream. There are several metabolites of atracurium, one of which (laudanosine), has been shown to cause seizures in dogs when given in very high doses. Laudanosine is very unlikely to be of any significance in humans, as the atracurium dose given to the dogs was far higher than used clinically. Laudanosine does not have any muscle relaxant properties but it does have neuroexcitatory properties. Laudanosine is excreted by the kidneys and may accumulate in patients with renal failure. The accumulation of laudanosine in human subjects can theoretically result in excessive neural stimulation and seizures. However, despite two decades of clinical use, there has never been a single documented occurrence of atracurium-induced seizures in humans. Atracurium has essentially no effects on nicotinic autonomic receptors or muscarinic cardiac receptors. However, atracurium administration may lead to vasodilation and hypotension caused by histamine release, especially when it is administered rapidly and in large doses (24).

Cisatracurium

Cisatracurium is an intermediate-duration benzylisoquinolinium NMB drug. It is a sterioisomer of atracurium but is three times as potent per milligram, so less of the drug is required for an equivalent response. Cisatracurium, like atracurium, is rapidly inactivated in the plasma via Hoffmann degradation (nonenzymatic breakdown at normal body temperature and pH) and ester hydrolysis (24). ☞ **Because its elimination does not depend upon renal or hepatic function, cisatracurium is often used in patients with renal and hepatic dysfunction.** ☞ The amount of laudanosine released after prolonged infusion of cisatracurium is much less than that compared to atracurium. Cisatracurium does not cause histamine release, and therefore is not associated with the bronchospasm, hypotension, and tachycardia seen with atracurium (37–43). Patients requiring prolonged NMB infusion will not necessarily benefit from cisatracurium. However, patients with liver and/or renal disease, especially those who require a complete and prompt recovery, are likely to benefit from cisatracurium use.

Other Neuromuscular Blockade Drugs Seldom Used in Critical Care

A number of other NMB agents including mivacurium, doxacurium, and pipecuronium, have been used in the operative environment but have not come into widespread use in the ICU setting. Mivacurium is short acting but never became popular in the ICU setting, partly due to its propensity for histamine release. Mivacurium is rapidly hydralized by plasma cholinesterase (as occurs with succinylcholine), explaining its rather short duration of action in normal patients.

Mivacurium is useful for procedures such as bronchoscopies in intubated patients, when rapid return of neurological monitoring status is wanted. Doxacurium and pipecuroium were never used to any significant extent in the ICU due to their long durations of action. Both drugs have been taken off the market due to complications related to prolonged NMB. Table 4 provides a summary of the dose and routes of elimination of the NMB drugs commonly employed in trauma and critical care.

Pharmacokinetics and Pharmacodynamics

A useful way of distinguishing between pharmacodynamics and pharmacokinetics is that the former is what drugs do to patients; the latter is what patients do to drugs. Pharmacokinetics describes the time-dependent fate of a dosage of drug as it undergoes redistribution, metabolism and excretion. Because all NMBs are polar, highly ionized compounds and therefore very water soluble and fat insoluble, they have a small volume of distribution (mainly the extracellular fluid unless metabolized). The speed of onset of drug activity is best described as a function of dose and volume of distribution, whereas the offset depends on the method of elimination. The pharmacodynamics of NMBs are best described using a dose-response curve (Fig. 5) (24). This curve is determined at steady state (i.e., not during a period of drug administration or redistribution), and the effects of the drug are determined at several different doses. NMBs have a dose-response curve that is sigmoidal in

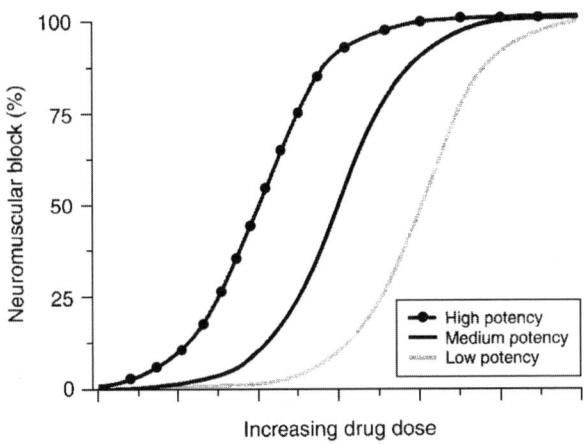

Figure 5 Schematic representation of a semilogarithmic plot of muscle relaxant dose versus neuromusucular block. A drug of high potency would be represented by doxacrium, one of medium potency by atracurium, and one of low potency by rocuronium. The graph illustrates that the relative potencies of the muscle relaxants span a range of approximately two orders of magnitude. *Source*: From Ref. 185.

shape, demonstrating a direct relationship between dose and response (24). Once the maximal effect is achieved (total paralysis), no further effect occurs at the NMJ regardless of the dose.

NEUROMUSCULAR BLOCKADE ANTAGONISTS

The muscle relaxant effects of nonodepolarizing NMB drugs can be reversed in one of two ways: (*i*) spontaneously, as the NMJ and plasma concentrations of the relaxant declines; or (*ii*) by pharmacologic reversal with AChE inhibitors (44).

Reversal agents function by raising the concentration of ACh at the NMJ. This can be achieved by either reducing the breakdown of ACh (e.g., AChE inhibitors), or by facilitating greater release of ACh at the nerve terminal (e.g., aminopyridines). This section focuses mainly on the effects of anticholinesterases drugs (AChE inhibitors) (24).

☞ AChE inhibitors produce their effects by binding to, and inhibiting the enzyme (AChE). The resulting increase in ACh in the synaptic cleft of the NMJ helps the ACh compete more favorably with NMB drugs for available ACh receptors. ☞ The reversal agents currently in use are neostigmine, pyridostigmine, and edrophonium. Neostigmine and pyridostigmine bind with AChE to form inert enzyme–substrate complexes (44). Edrophonium acts differently. It forms a reversible electrostatic bond with the enzyme (45,46). Table 5 lists the dosages and other key parameters of the three AChE inhibitors currently used in clinical practice.

However, AChE inhibitors should only be used when patients have at least 1 to 2 twitches on TOF, as elicited by the peripheral nerve stimulator (PNS) described below. In other words, some receptors must be free for ACh to work. With <1 twitch, the free ACh does not have an adequate number of unoccupied receptors to bind with to provide a return to normal muscle strength. The more intense the block (the less twitches present), the greater the dose of reversal drug needed. However, there is no advantage to giving more than 0.07 mg/kg of neostigmine (the appropriate dose if 1 to 2 twitches are present on TOF). If 3 to 4 twitches are present, neosigmine 0.04 mg/kg is suggested, or edrophonium 0.05 mg/kg.

An unpredictable response occurs at the NMJ to AChE inhibitors in the setting of a phase II block. Accordingly, reversal by AChE inhibitors is not recommended for this circumstance or for other causes of prolonged blockade following succinylcholine administration.

There is a limited role for AChE inhibitors in critical care; because, in contrast to the OR, there is rarely an urgent need to reverse NMB in the ICU. However, some situations may arise when AChE inhibitors are useful (41). Pyridostigmine is frequently used in myasthenia gravis patients; neostigmine

may be administered to patients with prolonged NMB, such as when the patient has only one twitch on PNS despite being many hours since the last NMB dose and a clinical benefit for early extubation is identified (i.e., following heart or lung transplantation).

Adverse effects commonly associated with the administration of AChE inhibitors include cardiac, gastrointestinal (GI), and respiratory effects, all of which are secondary to muscarinic stimulation. The cardiovascular effects are of greatest concern and include bradycardia, heart block, and cardiac arrest (24). Onset of bradycardia is rapid for edrophonium (45,46), slower for neostigmine (44), and slowest for pyridostigmine (47–49). GI side effects include increased salivary, gastric, and intestinal secretions and increased intestinal peristalsis (50). To prevent these side effects, anticholinergic agents such as atropine or glycopyrrolate are usually administered in conjuction with AChE inhibitors (44).

Atropine and gylcopyrrolate have muscarinic blocking effects but exert almost no activity on the nicotinic receptors (46). In general, atropine is coadministered with edrophonium, and glycopyrrolate is given with either neostigmine or pyridostigmine. Atropine's more rapid onset of action closely parallels that of edrophonium, while the less rapid onset of action of glycopyrrolate more closely matches the slower onset of neostigmine and pyridostigmine.

DISEASE STATE AND DRUG INTERACTIONS

Changes in disease processes (Table 6) alter drug requirements in the ICU patient (12,24). The diseases afflicting ICU patients may significantly impact NMB drug pharmacokinetics. The worsening condition of a patient leading to multiorgan system failure (including renal failure) may impact excretion of certain NMBs like pancuronium, and to a lesser degree vecuronium and rocuronium.

Table 6 Significant Disease State Electrolyte and Acid–Base Interactions with Neuromuscular Blockade Drugs

Potentiation of NMB	Neuromuscular diseases: myasthenia gravis, Eaton-Lambert syndrome
	Electrolyte disturbances: hypermagnesemia, hyponatrmeia, hypokalemia, hypocalcemia
	Acidosis (conditions that prolong metabolism): atypical plasma cholinesterase, renal disease, hepatic disease
Antagonism of NMB	Neuromuscular diseases: hemiparesis or paraparesis, demyelinating lesions, peripheral neuropathies
	Other: hypercalcemia, alkalosis, burn injury
Increased risk for cardiac arrhythmias or cardiac arrest with succinylcholine	Acute phase of injury following: major burns, multiple trauma, spinal cord injury, extensive denervation of skeletal muscle, upper motor neuron injury
	Other: hyperkalemia, digitalis toxicity

Abbreviation: NMB, neuromuscular blockade.

Table 5 Acetylcholinesterase Inhibitors

Agents	Dose (mg/kg)	Onset (min)	Duration (min)	Elimination
Edrophonium	0.5–1.0	0.5–1.0	50–73	70% renal, 30% hepatic
Neostigmine	0.025–0.075	3.0–7.0	70–82	50% renal, 50% hepatic
Pyridostigmine	0.1–0.3	4.0–12.0	123–137	75% renal, 25% hepatic

Table 7 Significant Drug Interactions with Neuromuscular Blockade Agents

Drug	Clinical effect	SUX	NDP	Management
Antidysrhythmics (e.g., quinidine, procainamide, lidocaine)	Enhanced NMB activity	+	+	Response should be monitored using lowest dose possible to achieve adequate blockade
Antibiotics (e.g., aminoglycosides, tetracyclines, polymyxins, clindamycin, piperacillin)	Potential for prolonged respiratory depression, excessive blockade	+	+	Observation for residual effects following NMB administration
Aprotinin (Trasylol®)	Enhanced NMB activity	+		Monitor with PNS, use lowest therapeutic dose
Azathioprine (various)	Reversal of NMB	+		Monitor effects of NMB agent and adjust dose as needed
Calcium channel blockers [nicardipine (various); verapamil (various)]	Enhanced NMB	+	+	Monitor effects of NMB agent and adjust dose as needed
Carbamazepine (various)	More rapid recovery time following NMB administration		+	Monitor patients for clinical response; may need higher/more frequent doses of NMB agent
Corticosteroids	Prolonged muscle weakness and myopathy		+	Minimize duration of coadministration; if prolonged concomitant use required, allow NMB-free periods to reduce total dose administered. Monitor with PNS, use lowest therapeutic dose
Digoxin (various)	Risk of cardiac arrhythmias	+	+	Noted specifically with succinylcholine and pancuronium; cardiac monitoring should be performed if used concomitantly
Fosphenytoin (Cerebyx®)	More rapid recovery time following NMB administration		+	Monitor patients for clinical response; may need higher/more frequent doses of NMB agent
Inhalation anesthetics	Enhanced NMB activity	+	+	When used concurrently, less NMB is required. Potentiation is greatest with enflurane and isoflurane
Lithium	Enhanced NMB activity		+	Monitor with PNS, use lowest therapeutic dose
Magnesium salts	Enhanced NMB activity	+	+	Monitor with PNS, use lowest therapeutic dose
Metoclopramide (various)	Enhanced NMB activity	+	+	Monitor with PNS, use lowest therapeutic dose
Oral contraceptives (when taken chronically)	Enhanced NMB activity	+	+	Monitor with PNS, use lowest therapeutic dose
Oxytocin (various)	Enhanced NMB activity		+	Monitor with PNS, use lowest therapeutic dose
Phenytoin (various)	More rapid recovery time following NMB administration		+	Monitor patients for clinical response; may need higher/more frequent doses of NMB agent
Tacrine (Cognex®)	Prolongation of NMB activity		+	Monitor with PNS, use lowest therapeutic dose
TCAs	Risk of ventricular arrhythmias		+	Documented in patients receiving chronic TCAs, who are anesthetized with halothane and administered pancuronium
Terbutaline (various)	Enhanced NMB activity		+	Monitor with PNS, use lowest therapeutic dose

Note: + indicates presence of interaction.
Abbreviations: NDP, nondepolarizing neuromuscular blockade drugs; NMB, neuromuscular blockade; PNS, peripheral nerve stimulator; SUX, succinylcholine; TCAs, tricyclic antidepressants.

Various electrolytes also have intrinsic effects on neuromuscular transmission also shown in Table 6.

Other drugs initiated or discontinued during the use of NMB drugs may have significant interaction with the duration of blockade (Table 7). Aminoglycoside antibiotics have synergistic actions with NMB drugs at the NMJ, and can influence both, the degree and duration of paralysis. They act by inhibition of presynaptic ACh release and depress postjunctional sensitivity (51). Anticonvulsants, conversely, can significantly increase the drug requirement for NMB drugs; phenytoin therapy has been shown to increase pancuronium requirements by 80% in neurosurgical patients (52).

The degree of paralysis should always be closely monitored to confirm adequacy of blockade. Monitoring may also help to recognize changes in organ function and NMB drug metabolism or excretion sooner than might be revealed by intermittent laboratory tests of organ function.

DOSING STRATEGIES

The NMB drugs can be administered by bolus technique as needed "pro re nata" (PRN), or via a regularly scheduled regimen, or via a continuous infusion. The PRN bolus techniques are only appropriate for patients who can tolerate intermittent movement in the ICU, without jeopardizing oxygenation, intracranial pressure (ICP) elevations, or life-sustaining therapy (e.g., intra-aortic balloon pump, etc.). Scheduled doses or infusions are best used in patients requiring constant paralysis. When tolerated, the intermittent lessening of the degree of NMB and occasional drug holiday may prevent or ameliorate the up regulation of ACh receptors seen with long-term blockade (53). Administration of NMB drug by infusion is convenient and minimizes the peak and valley effect typically seen with intermittent doses. However, if not monitored with PNS twitch monitoring, patients may receive an overdose of NMB drug. Drugs typically classified as shorter acting may be longer acting in the presence of organ failure because of the presence of active metabolites (36). Patients treated for long periods of time with NMB drugs often develop tolerance or resistance (54–56). Prolonged immobilization, by itself, results in muscle atrophy, enlargement of the ACh-sensitive area (31,57), receptor proliferation, and resistance to NMB drugs. There are a number of reports of neuropathy, myopathy, or abnormality of the NMJ in ICU patients treated with steroids and NMB drugs (58,59).

The appropriate dosing strategy varies from patient to patient, but it is clear that vigilance to prevent overdose, conservative use of paralytics, and prompt discontinuation when the drug is no longer necessary are essential. In critically ill patients, organ function, blood flow, and caregiving personnel change constantly. The risks inherent in paralyzing a patient (e.g., ventilator disconnection) are compounded by the duration of paralysis in the ICU.

INDICATIONS FOR NEUROMUSCULAR BLOCKADE DRUGS IN THE CRITICALLY ILL
Relative Requirements

The relative requirements for NMB drugs (as well as sedation, amnesia, and analgesia) depend upon the admitting condition, severity of disease, and the intensity of treatment (60,61). Some form of analgesia is usually required for patients who have suffered from trauma or have undergone surgery (see Volume 2, Chapter 5). Opiates provide the foundation as they are useful in relieving pain and provide some degree of anxiolysis. Benzodiazepines, propofol, or dexmeditomidine are useful drugs for minimizing anxiety and agitation. NMB drugs should only be employed when appropriate use of these drugs alone fails to provide safe nursing conditions in the ICU (Table 8). We are still searching

Table 8 Indications for Neuromuscular Blockade Drug Use in Critical Care

Indication	Comments
ETT placement or ETT change	Although intubation is best accomplished with complete paralysis, once the ETT tube is in place, there is no absolute need for continued NMB drug use.
Facilitate mechanical ventilation in ARDS patients	NMB drugs are never indicated to facilitate MV in normal patterns (adequate sedation and analgesia will accomplish this). However, in severe ARDS with stiff lungs and profound transpulmonary shunt, NMB drugs may be required to allow certain ventilatory techniques (i.e., prolonged I:E ratio) (also see Volume 2, Chapters 23, 24, 25, and 27).
Eliminate movement-related increased ICP in severe TBI	TBI patients with compliant cranial contents and normal ICP do not need, or benefit from, NMB drug use. However, very tight brains may have exacerbations in ICP associated with movement, coughing or bucking, and NMB drugs are appropriate, as long as maximum sedation and analgesia has already been employed (also see Volume 1, Chapter 23 and Volume 2, Chapters 1, 7, and 12).
Reduce $\dot{V}O_2$ and work of breathing in patient with shock	Temporary use of NMB drugs in this setting is acceptable. However, once the patient is resuscitated, NMB drugs should be halted, and sedatives should be titrated to effect.
Tetanus spasms	Tetanus spasms are painful, and are best treated with high-dose sedation and analgesics. However, supplementation with high NMB drugs while administering the antitoxin and penicillin is acceptable initial management.
Combative patients with severe injuries	Brief NMB drug use in this setting is appropriate as long as sedatives are also employed. Once life-threatening injuries are treated, or ruled out, paralysis should be discontinued and sedatives titrated to effect.
Following decompression of abdominal compartment syndrome or other surgical procedure where abdominal fascia is temporarily open	When patients are nursed in the ICU following procedures where the intra-abdominal contents are edematous, and the fascia is temporarily left open, NMB drugs are needed to maintain abdominal domain of the contents. However, after 3 to 5 days the fascia should be closed. If unable, then techniques not involving NMB drugs should be considered.
Abolish shivering; abolish status epilepticus; facilitation of hyperventilation	These are relatively nonsubstantiated reasons for NMB drugs. In the case of shivering, adequate sedation analgesia and warming is usually satisfactory. In status epilepticus, the patient should receive increasing doses of antiseizure medications, monitored by EEG (paralysis may dangerously mask seizure activity). Brief initial hyperventilation to control ICP prior to operative management is acceptable treatment. However, prophylactic, prolonged hyperventilation is associated with worse outcomes for TBI and not indicated (see Volume 1, Chapter 23 and Volume 2, Chapters 1, 12, and 14).

Abbreviations: ARDS, acute respiratory distress syndrome; EEG, electroencephalogram; ETT, endotracheal tube; ICP, intracranial pressure; ICU, intensive care unit; MV, mechanical ventilation; NMB, neuromuscular blockade; TBI, traumatic brain injury; $\dot{V}O_2$, oxygen consumption.

for better individual patient factors, which would indicate the requirements for different drugs. The studies published so far have tried to identify the needs for various combinations of drugs in ICU patients using three basic approaches (informed anecdotes, subjective impressions, and objective assessment).

Informed Anecdote

Informed anecdote is assessment of NMB needs on the basis of anecdotal experiences of medical and nursing personnel who have themselves been patients in an ICU before. Most commonly they reflect pain, anxiety, and disorientation. The use of NMB drugs causes particular concern. However, knowledge of the situation, diseases, and drugs might have influenced their fear and anxieties, causing bias.

Subjective Impressions

Subjective impressions are the recollections of the experiences of patients who have stayed in the ICU. Bion et al. (62), interviewed 60 patients after their discharge from a general ICU and found that the most common recollections were of physical therapy and of the presence of a urinary catheter (75% of patients recalled these), although these were not found to be particularly distressing by the majority of patients. Those who recalled having thirst, pain, or anxiety most commonly reported this to be an unpleasant experience.

Objective Assessment

Objective assessment occurs when the clinician uses a quantifiable bioassay to determine need and effect of NMB drugs. Objectively there are very few clinical tests available like the Glasgow Coma Scale, Visual Analog Scale for assessment of pain, and Ramsay Sedation Score for assessment of sedation. Rather, without a quantifiable bioassay, the only clinical endpoint is patient movement. Unfortunately, movement can be harmful in the few patient conditions that require NMBs [e.g., high ICP or severe acute respiratory distress syndrome (ARDS)]. PNSs, a form of bioassay, are used clinically to guide the titration of NMB drugs.

⚬ **Neuromuscular blocking drugs should never be administered without concomitant amnesics, sedatives, and/or analgesics.** ⚬ Patients too unstable to tolerate traditional analgesics or sedatives can receive scopolamine until stable. The administration of sedatives and analgesics also facilitates mechanical ventilation by improving patient comfort, suppressing cough-related bucking, and by minimizing responses to recurrent noxious stimuli such as suctioning (63).

Fentanyl, morphine, and dilaudid are the most commonly used parenteral narcotics. These drugs are potent respiratory depressants but have little direct effect on the cardiovascular system when administered as continuous infusions. These drugs do not increase Cerebral Metabloic Rate of Oxygen (CMRO$_2$), Cerebral Blood Flow (CBF), or Intracranial Pressure (ICP) when administered in conventional doses (see Volume 2, Chapter 5).

The past 25 years have witnessed a tremendous increase in the use of NMB agents in ICUs for a variety of interventions, paralleling advances in technology such as newer modes of mechanical ventilation. Along with the increased use of NMB agents have come reports about dangerous and costly complications including persistent paralysis (discussed below) (21,24,26,40,64–71). In addition, a disconcerting lack of knowledge about NMB agent therapy has been recognized (40,72–77).

Goal-Directed Indications

Goal-directed indications are those which dictate NMB use to achieve a specific goal (e.g., minimize perturbations in ICP). The most common indications for NMB drug use include those shown in Table 8 and discussed below. Intubation, control of ICP (Volume 2, Chapter 12), mechanical ventilation in ARDS patients (Volume 2, Chapters 24, 25, and 27), open abdominal fascia after damage control surgery (Volume 1, Chapter 21), release of abdominal compartment syndrome (Volume 2, Chapter 34), or control of hemodynamically unstable patients in shock, minimizes O$_2$ consumption (Volume 2, Chapter 18). Other indications are relative, and not necessarily based upon strong scientific principles (e.g., control of seizing or agitated patients), as these patients typically require sedation not more paralysis (78).

Although NMB drugs are occasionally required to help control ICP in patients with intracranial hypertension following traumatic brain injury (TBI), the routine use following TBI is not necessary (76). Chemical paralysis with minimal movement allowed (T1) (i.e., one twitch response out of four on a PNS) will mask neurologic deterioration that would normally be reflected in alteration of the motor examination. Pupillary changes, one of the few neurologic assessment tools available during NMB-induced paralysis, can indicate a cerebral event, but papillary function can also be altered by certain anticholinergic drugs used during resuscitation, including atropine and scopolamine (16). Prolonged absence of the motor examination is never optimal following TBI and should only be tolerated in cases of very high ICP requiring NMB and appropriate sedation (i.e., propofol) or barbiturates-induced coma.

The administration of NMB drugs to minimize airway pressures in patients with severe oxygenation and ventilation failure (e.g., ARDS) and those requiring ventilatory modes with prolonged Inspiratory : Expiratory (I:E) ratios, and hypercapnia, is well established. The goals of therapy here are to decrease peak inspiratory pressure and improve oxygenation (63).

The administration of NMBs to control movement of patients with severe hemodynamic instability and compromised oxygen delivery states may also be beneficial (20,24,79). In shock states, skeletal muscle activity (e.g., work of breathing), may utilize up to 24% of O$_2$ consumption (58). This increased metabolic demand may cause ischemia to vulnerable tissues. The administration of NMB agents may temporarily diminish the excess oxygen consumption (VO$_2$) allowing improved tissue oxygenation of at-risk tissue beds (e.g., myocardial emdothelium, or renal cortex) until medical intervention can intercede.

NMB drugs have occasionally been administered to control muscle rigidity in tetanus (80,81). Indeed, the contractures are painful and should be treated with NMB drugs. However, the mainstay of treatment is tetanus antitoxin (to neutralize unbound toxin), penicillin (to prevent further bacterial growth and toxin elaboration), and sedatives and analgesics to control anxiety and pain.

Occasionally, NMBs are used to facilitate a motionless state in patients with gaping and unstable surgical incisions (79). Vascular or reconstructive surgeons may request that a patient be immobile for 48 hours after a major flap reconstruction with tenuous vascular anastomosis. Similarly, the use of NMBs to immobilize severely agitated patients is not recommended. Indeed, given that sedatives and analgesics are titrated to effect, maximum doses of sedation and analgesics do not exist in intubated, mechanically ventilated patients.

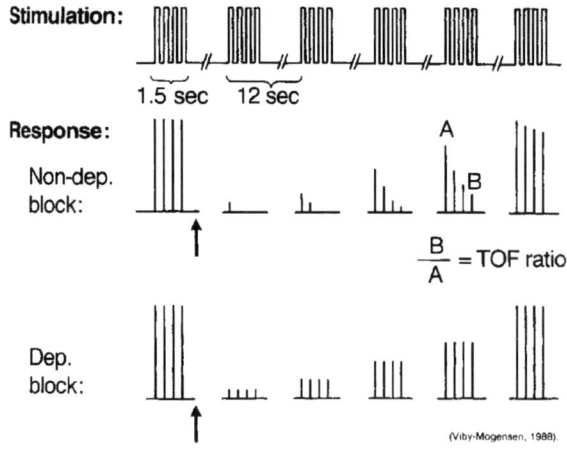

Figure 6 Pattern of electrical stimulation and evoked muscle responses to train-of-four (TOF) nerve stimulation before and after injection of nondepolarizing (Non-dep.) and depolarizing (Dep.) neuromuscular blocking drugs (*arrows*). *Source*: From Ref. 186. *Abbreviation*: TOF, train-of-four.

MONITORING OF NEUROMUSCULAR BLOCKADE

A combination of clinical oversight and a peripheral nerve stimulus monitoring (twitch monitoring) is recommended whenever patients are given NMB agents in an ICU. The goals of monitoring are to ensure adequate NMB effect during the therapeutic administration of the drug, and to verify full return of NMJ function after the drug is stopped. The clinical assessment of NMB drugs is dependent upon observation of muscle movement such as the ability to open the eyes, extend the tongue, or breathe spontaneously. ☞ **The most reliable single clinical measure of return of NMJ function is ability to head lift for five seconds or more.** ☞ However, this measurement requires patient cooperation and is influenced by sedatives and analgesics. When patients are capable of performing this task, they correlate with full return of TOF and absence of fade for five seconds. However, even with this full return of clinical function, as many as 50% of NMJ receptors may retain blockade. ☞ **The most objective measurement of the degree of blockade in noncooperative or sedated patients is obtained with the demonstration of sustained tetanus through the use of a PNS.** ☞ The PNS was first used to determine neuromuscular function during anesthesia in 1958 (82,83). Twitch monitoring with a PNS is the tool used to measure receptor occupancy. A supramaximal electrical stimulus (a stimulus sufficient to recruit all the motor units subserved by the stimulated nerve) is applied to a nerve and the motor response is measured. With depolarizing agents, the response to each stimulus in a series (a TOF successive stimuli, for example) is diminished equally. With nondepolarizing agents, on the other hand, each successive response is smaller than the previous one, demonstrating "fade" or fatigue (Fig. 6). The latter response is directly analogous to the response seen with myasthenia gravis, in which there is actual loss of ACh receptors, rather than pharmacologic blockade (21,24).

Technical Aspects of Peripheral Nerve Stimulator Monitoring

The PNS delivers electric current to the nerve through electrodes, which may be of three types: needle, ball, or pregelled.

Pregelled electrodes, the most commonly used, are self-adhering, comfortable, and noninvasive. However, the large surface area of the regular adult electrode may minimize current density and reduce the likelihood of attaining supramaximal stimulation (84). This potential problem may be eliminated with use of pediatric electrodes, which are smaller. The skin underneath the electrodes must be clean, dry, and hairless. For substantial edema or obesity, the ball electrode system is a good choice, allowing a precise location of the electrical stimulus. Needle electrodes are seldom used in patients with adequate skin coverage; because, although they provide excellent electrical conduction, they are uncomfortable and present risks for infection and nerve displacement (85). However, in burned patients and those with other exfoliative dermatological conditions, sterile disposable needle electrodes are commonly employed.

Several patterns of nerve stimulation are available, such as single twitch, tetanic stimulation, post-tetanic facilitation or potentiation, TOF, and doubleburst. Of these, TOF is the least painful and most frequently used in ICUs (86). The PNS should be able to deliver 50–60 mA at all frequencies. However, in lightly sedated patients lower current should be used. The frequency with which the PNS impulse is applied depends upon the technique of twitch monitoring employed. For example, single twitch 0.1–0.15 Hz, TOF is 2 Hz delivered every 0.5 seconds, and repeated every 10 seconds, tetanus is typically achieved with frequencies in the 50–100 Hz range.

Single Stimulus

The single twitch (aka single stimulus) mode involves one impulse with duration of 0.2 to 0.3 milliseconds. It may be repeated every 10 seconds and no sooner, to achieve optimum results, since more frequent stimulation may lead to ACh depletion, reduction of muscle twitch, and overestimation of blockade (82). A positive response to a single stimulus is not synonymous with absence of NMB. Muscle response is still present when 75% of the nicotonic receptors are occupied by the NMB agents (87). The muscle response disappears completely when 90% of the receptors have been occupied (85,88).

Train-of-Four Stimulation

The TOF method involves four electrical stimuli of 2 Hz delivered to a peripheral nerve at intervals of 0.5 seconds, repeatable every 10 seconds. Stimulation of the ulnar nerve with TOF evokes four twitches of the adductor pollicis muscle (83,89). The adductor pollicis muscle response is characterized by adduction of the thumb medially across the palm. In nondepolarizing block, the last thumb adduction of a TOF disappears first, and the first twitch disappears last. Blockade is quantified by counting the number of thumb adductions (90). Four twitches correlates with ≤75% receptor blockade. This level of blockade is clinically manifested by normal expiratory flow rate and vital capacity. Three twitches indicate a blockade of 80%; two, 85%; and one, 90%. When all four twitches are absent, 100% receptor occlusion is assumed to be present (82,83).

Tetanic Stimulation

Also called tetanus, this nerve stimulation test involves rapid impulses (30, 50, or 100 Hz) delivered to the nerve in which large amounts of ACh are synthesized, mobilized, and released. The frequencies most commonly used for

Table 9 Tests of Neuromuscular Junction Transmission and Reversal of Neuromuscular Blockade

Test	Acceptable value (results suggest normal clinical value)	% NMJ receptors occupied with NMB when acceptable value acheived	Comments
Single twitch	Qualitatively as strong as baseline	75–80	Uncomfortable, need to know twitch strength versus baseline. Insensitive as an indicator of recovery, but useful as a gauge of NMJ blockade depth.
TOF	No palpable fade	70–75	Still uncomfortable, but more sensitive as an indicator of recovery than single twitch is. Useful as a gauge of depth of block by counting the number of responses perceptible.
Sustained tetanus (50 Hz for 5 sec)	No palpable fade	70	Very uncomfortable, but reliable indicator of adequate recovery.
Double burst	No palpable fade	60–70	Uncomfortable, but more sensitive than TOF as an indicator of NMJ function. No perceptible fade indicates TOF recovery of at least 60%.
Sustained tetanus (100 Hz for 5 sec)	No palpable fade	50	Very painful—a "stress test." Lack of fade at 100 Hz is the most reliable indicator of NMJ recovery.
Tidal volume	At least 5 mL/kg	80	Insensitive as an indicator of NMJ recovery.
Vital capacity	At least 20 mL/kg	70	Requires patient cooperation, is not the best for determining clinical recovery of NMJ blockade.
Inspiratory force	At least −40 cm H_2O	50	Sometimes difficult to perform without endotracheal intubation, but reliable gauge of normal diaphragmatic function.
Head lift	Must be performed unaided with patient supine at 180° and sustained for 5 sec	50	Requires patient cooperation, but remains the gold standard test for determining clinical function (should be performed with patient in a completely supine position).
Hand grip	Sustained at a level qualitatively similar to pre-induction baseline	50	Only reliable if patient is awake and cooperative. Sustained strong grip is good gauge of normal function, but not of patient alertness or ability to protect the airway.
Sustained bite	Sustained jaw clench or tongue blade	50	Only reliable if patient is awake and cooperative. Often a poor measure of patient alertness or ability to protect airway.

Abbreviations: NMJ, neuromuscular junction; TOF, train-of-four.

this test (50–100 Hz) when delivered for five seconds, stresses the NMJ to the same extent as a maximal voluntary effort (82). At these higher frequencies, the duration of the refractory period is increased, fatigue of the end-plate occurs, and fade may be elicited due to the decreasing capacity of ACh to compete with the NMB drug at the postjunctional receptor (91). Tetanic stimulation may be repeated every one to two minutes to allow the end-plate to return to a steady state between stimuli (82). This test is a sensitive assessment of NMB (88,92). At 100 Hz for five seconds, fade develops when 50% of the receptors are blocked. Absence of fade is the best test using the PNS for assuring that the patient has enough ACh available at the NMJ to tolerate extubation of the trachea, and correlates with head lift for five seconds (Table 9). However, tetanus is painful and unacceptable to the nonsedated ICU patient (20,83).

Post-tetanic Facilitation or Potentiation

Mobilization and enhanced synthesis of ACh occur during and immediately after cessation of tetanic stimulation. There is an increase in the readily releasable fraction of ACh. This event is manifested in the stronger twitch response to the single stimulus test within three to five seconds after tetanic stimulation. This phenomenon, referred to as post-tetanic facilitation or potentiation (83–85,89), is seen only with nondepolarizing blockade (Fig. 7). This test is the best method for determining how soon a patient will likely begin to show a twitch in the absence of any detectable twitch with either TOF or tetanus by themselves.

Double-Burst Stimulation

Double-burst stimulation is a newer mode of electrical nerve stimulation developed with the specific aim of allowing manual (tactile) detection of small amounts of residual NMB under clinical conditions. It consists of two short bursts of 50-Hz tetanic stimulation separated by 750 milliseconds. The duration of each square wave impulse in the burst is 0.2 milliseconds. In the nonblocked NMJ, the response to double-burst stimulation over a peripheral nerve is two short muscle contractions of equal strength. In the partially blocked NMJ, the second response is weaker than the first (i.e., the response fades). Although useful and quantifiable for research purposes, this technique has not yet become popular in clinical use (83).

TOF stimulation is the most commonly employed method of peripheral nerve monitoring to assess the level of NMB, and is uncomfortable but not as painful as tetanus, and unlike single stimulus, the first twitch of a

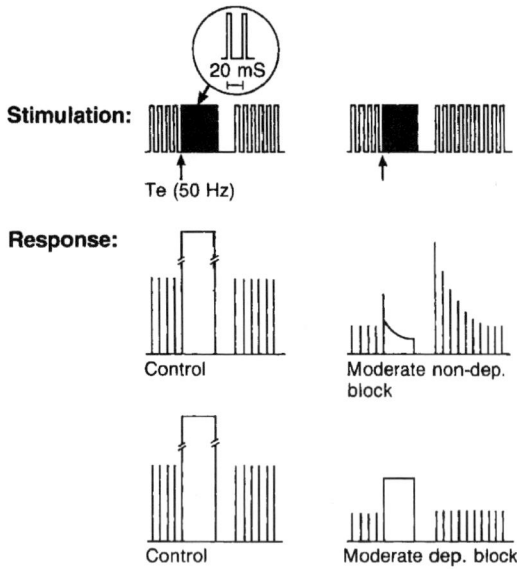

Figure 7 Pattern of stimulation and evoked muscle responses to tetanic nerve stimulation (50 Hz) for five seconds and post-tetanic stimulation (1.0 Hz) twitch. Stimulation was applied before injection of neuromuscular blocking drugs and during moderate nondepolarizing and depolarizing blocks. Note fade in the response to tetanic stimulation, plus post-tetanic facilitation of transmission during nondepolarizing blockade. During depolarizing blockade, the tetanic response is well sustained and no post-tetanic facilitation of transmission occurs. *Abbreviation*: Te, tetanic. *Source*: From Ref. 186.

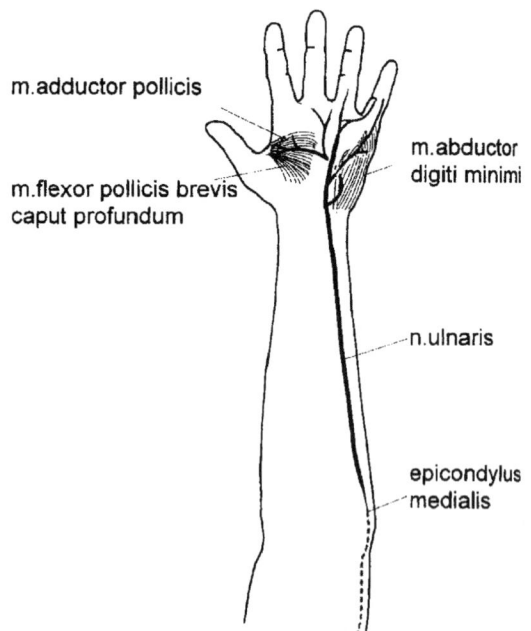

Figure 8 Ulnar nerve-innervated hand muscles suitable for monitoring of neuromuscular block. Stimulation of the nerve evokes contraction of the adductor pollicis muscle, which results in thumb adduction. Hence, the thumb is the recommended site for assessment of the mechanical twitch response. Other ulnar nerve-innervated hand muscles include the hypothenar (m. abductor digiti minimi) and the first dorsal interosseous (near the adductor pollicis, but on the dorsal side of the hand). *Abbreviations*: m, muscle; n, nerve. *Source*: From Ref. 187.

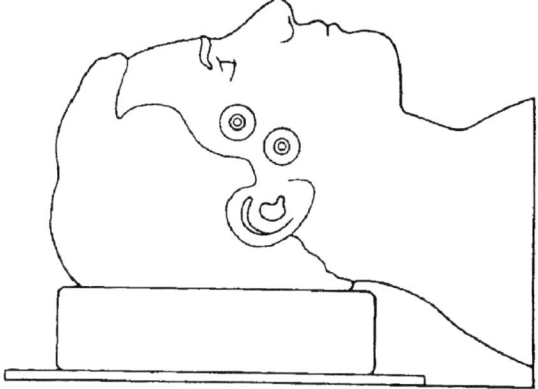

Figure 9 Positioning of stimulating electrodes over the facial nerve. The electrode nearest the eye is negative. *Source*: From Ref. 187.

TOF serves as a control for the fourth. Furthermore, in residual NMB, TOF is more sensitive than the single stimulus test (93). The degree of blockade that optimizes a patient's outcome depends upon the clinical circumstances, and thus, has not been scientifically determined (94). It is generally agreed that at least one or two of four (1/4–2/4) twitches should be maintained throughout therapy if clinically feasible (83,95–99).

Clinically, the most commonly used peripheral nerves for twitch monitoring are the ulnar (Fig. 8), and facial (Fig. 9). However, in some situations, other peripheral nerves (including the posterior fibial and peroneal nerves) are also employed. The ulnar nerve, which innervates the adductor pollicis muscle, is the most widely used for scientific quantification. The most accessible portion of the ulnar nerve is between the tendon of the flexor carpi ulnaris medially and the ulnar artery laterally, about 2–5 cm proximal from the flexor crease of the wrist (83). Electrodes must be placed along the nerve; improper placement increases resistance and reduces nerve stimulation. The electrodes should be rechecked for placement with each use (at least hourly) and they should be changed daily to assure adequate contact and that underlying skin is in good condition.

Current of stimulation—"submaximal" current is used to stimulate the nerve in ICU patients. This level of current is less than what is used during general anesthesia, which is typically "supramaximal" (and painful in awake or lightly anesthesized patients). Submaximal current is determined by identifying the least amount of current required for a positive evoked muscle response and then by increasing the current on the PNS by a one-number increment on the output dial. The typical PNS has a number range from 1 to 10, with 10 being maximum current (50–60 mA). Submaximal current usually correlates with numbers 4 through 6 on the current output dial (which relates approximately to 25 mA) (100).

Overestimation and Underestimation of Neuromuscular Blockade Using a Peripheral Nerve Stimulator

The degree of blockade may be overestimated when no muscle response is evoked, yet there are overt signs of muscle movement. Overestimation is usually due to improper technique, malfunction of the instrument, dead battery, increased resistance due to improper electrode placement, poor skin contact, or inadequate skin preparation. In case of difficulty, check connections, verify electrode placements, change the battery, ensure proper skin preparation, and increase output to maximal power (83,100,101). A completely blocked NMJ of the ulnar–adductor pollicis motor unit will result in an absence of twitch (thumb movement) when stimulating the ulnar nerve with the PNS. However, the muscle itself retains contractile function and will exhibit four thumb adductions to the TOF test if the muscle is directly stimulated by the electrical current (83). Hence, the level of blockade may be erroneously underestimated with improper direct muscle stimulation and the patient may receive an increased dose of the NMB agent. A similar effect can occur while monitoring with the facial nerve, if facial muscles are directly stimulated. Peripheral edema and obesity increase the distance between the nerve and electrodes, thus decreasing the amount of stimulus delivered to the nerve (101,102). Peripheral hypothermia causes impairment of neuromuscular transmission and may be a source of error in TOF evaluation (103,104). Sepsis or CIP may also affect nerve transmission and, theoretically, TOF monitoring (105).

Precautions While Using Peripheral Nerve Monitoring

Abnormal responses can occur in the presence of neuromuscular diseases, so an otherwise normal extremity should be used for TOF monitoring (106).

The frequency of TOF monitoring is dependent on whether the drug is actively titrated or is administered as an infusion (81,103). Testing has been advocated at least every four hours during active titration and every eight hours during maintenance infusion (81,103). Sensory alterations are experienced by chemically paralyzed patients who are inadequately sedated and those who do not receive any amnestic agents. This traumatic experience may be alleviated by frequent orientation, talking to patients before any procedure, and placing signs on the bedside to remind others about their unique needs (107).

Some people advocate discontinuing paralytics every so often (e.g., every 24 hours) to allow the NMJ to recover (20,108). The ability to do this will depend upon the patient's underlying condition.

Patients must be protected from the adverse effects of immobility (20,103,109). Changing body position every two hours and applying sequential compression stockings must be an integral part of their care. Passive range of motion exercises at regular intervals, as well as padding of elbows and bony prominences must be ensured. Low-dose anticoagulation may assist in the prevention of venous thrombosis. Because the ability to blink is absent, eyes should be lubricated and/or closed to prevent corneal drying and abrasions (81,103). To prevent aspiration, the head of the bed should be elevated, particularly during enteral feeding (unless spinal injury precautions don't allow).

PROLONGED MOTOR WEAKNESS FOLLOWING NEUROMUSCULAR BLOCKADE (AKA POSTPARALYTIC SYNDROME)

Postparalytic syndrome is also known as prolonged or persistent weakness after NMB drug use. The incidence of this complication is unknown, but a small prospective study estimated the risk for developing prolonged weakness as 5% to 10% if muscle relaxants had been used for more than 24 hours (110). Patients with severe asthma have also

been reported to develop myopathy (111), while several retrospective reports suggest that up to 70% of critically ill patients who share certain characteristics remain weak after prolonged administration of pancuronium or vecuronium (75,112–115). Although the majority of the cases reported in the literature are following the use of the more commonly employed aminosteroidal NMB drugs, there are case reports following the use of benzylisoquinoliniums as well (116).

☞ **The etiology of postparalytic syndrome is incompletely understood, but may result form injury mediated directly by the drug, its active metabolites, or by drug–drug or drug–disease state interactions.** ☞ Persistent NMB is most frequently associated with changes in pharmacokinetics secondary to renal or hepatic failure or to accumulation of active metabolites (117). All three metabolites of vecuronium (3-desacetylvecuronium, 17-desacetylvecuronium, and 3,17-desacetylvecuronium) have neuromuscular blocking properties. This has caused some to believe that atracurium or cisatracurium may be preferable in patients with renal and/or hepatic failure as they are metabolized spontaneously at body temperature and pH via Hoffmann elimination and also via hydrolysis by plasma esterase. Although their metabolite laudanosine may accumulate in patients with renal failure and/or hepatic failure (118), it does not have any muscle relaxant properties, and even after 71 days of infusion of atracurium the accumulation of laudanosine was minimal (119). The half-life of laudanosine is increased in patients with renal failure (120,121) and in animals with hepatic failure (122). Laudanosine is not eliminated by dialysis (123). Patients recovered faster after atracurium (105 minutes), compared to vecuronium (6 to 37 hours) in a study of ICU patients with renal impairment (36).

Intermittent dosage or continuous infusions of nondepolarizing relaxants can cause peripheral storage compartments to become saturated, resulting in decreased clearance of the drug (124–126). Prolonged weakness may also be caused by functional defects in the motor unit (nerve, muscle, or NMJ), that is, both myopathies and/or neuropathies may occur (131). Long-term use of NMB drugs in trauma patients is associated with other complications as well. For example, trauma patients are already at increased risk of infectious complications, and prolonged use of NMB drugs is characterized by significantly longer ICU stay, more frequent pneumonia, and a trend toward a higher rate of sepsis (8,127).

Additional factors contributing to prolonged duration of NMB include inadvertent overdosing (125), drug interactions (in particular with aminoglycosides and quinidine) (128–130), electrolyte abnormalities (e.g., hypermagnesemia, hypophosphatemia) acidosis (131–134), underlying muscular disorders (e.g., myasthenia gravis) (133–135), and hypothermia (136). Antibiotics and magnesium work on pre- and postsynaptic levels while several cardiovascular drugs (lidocaine, beta-blockers, calcium channel blockers, quinidine) influence ion transport at the NMJ and can potentiate NMB. Completeness of NMB must be monitored in these patients to guide the administration of drugs, to avoid overdoses, to maintain muscle activity, and to detect a chain of reactions among concomitant medications or pathophysiologic changes (137).

Neurologic examination of these patients often reveals paresis, or flaccid paralysis of distal and proximal muscles and the diaphragm in the presence of normal sensory function (117). Serum creatine kinase levels may be normal or increased up to 100-fold (115,138,139). Clinical examination may not be adequate for diagnosis and electrodiagnostic studies, and biopsies of muscles revealing degeneration of type I and II muscle fibers and nerves are often needed for accurate diagnosis of the cause of weakness in ICU patients. Electrophysiologic studies demonstrated reduced amplitude of motor-evoked responses and of compound action potentials, consistent with myopathy with unaltered sensory conduction (139,140). A general decrease in myofibrillar protein content, absence of myosin messenger RNA with very low thick-filament/thin-filament protein rations were also found (140). Histopathologic features include degenerative changes, fiber atrophy, evidence of regeneration with predominant involvement of the type I muscle fiber, and necrosis (141).

The complexities associated with pharmacological paralysis in critically ill patients warrants the comprehensive approach to care that multidisciplinary team members can provide (142). The weakness may persist from weeks to months. The management largely involves the same care that was given while patients were paralyzed. Regularly evaluate the patient for signs of recovery from NMBs. When patients can breathe on their own (i.e., weaned from mechanical ventilation—see Volume 2, Chapter 28), and are able to clear secretions and maintain some degree of pulmonary reserve, they can be discharged from the ICU.

CRITICAL ILLNESS POLYNEUROPATHY

✎ **CIP is acute axonal neuropathies involving both sensory and motor nerves, developing during critical illness, especially with sepsis or systemic inflammatory response syndrome (SIRS).** ✎ The severity of CIP can begin to remit spontaneously once the critical condition is under control (143). CIP was first reported by Bolton, Zochodne, and others in the 1980s (144). It is a sensory motor polyneuropathy as opposed to a myopathic polyneuropathy. The increased jitter in patients with CIP indicates that it is primarily an axonal neuropathy with a lesion of terminal motor axons (145). It is increasingly recognized, and occurs particularly in sicker, older patients with sepsis. Seventy percent of reported cases had sepsis during their stay in ICU (146–152). Other risk factors for the development of CIP include hyperosmolarity, parenteral nutrition, nondepolarizing NMBs, and neurologic failure (153). Investigators have speculated that the peripheral nerves are another organ system that is affected adversely by SIRS (see Volume 2, Chapter 63) (146,154). CIP can be seen in up to one-third of critically ill patients with SIRS (usually due to sepsis) (155). Disturbances in the microcirculation to peripheral nerves occur with sepsis and diabetes mellitus and can induce axonal hypoxia and degeneration. The local balance of leukocyte activities is of importance in the pathophysiology of muscle weakness in CIP and myopathy (156). Furthermore, the neurologic effects of SIRS are thought to be mediated by released mediators like cytokines and free radicals, affecting the microcirculation of the central and peripheral nervous system (157). The reduction in the risk of polyneuropathy with intensive insulin therapy (Volume 2, Chapter 60), regardless of the concomitant use of corticosteroids or aminoglycosides, suggests that hyperglycemia, insulin deficiency, or both contribute to axonal dysfunction and degeneration (146,158). The linear relation between blood glucose levels and the risk of polyneuropathy suggests that maintenance of the lowest possible level is necessary. The reduced need for mechanical ventilation in patients who received intensive insulin therapy is explained in part

by the reduced rate of critical-illness polyneuropathy, though a direct anabolic effect of insulin on respiratory muscles may also play a part (159).

The clinical picture of CIP is similar to that of the patient with an acute myopathy and may include delayed weaning from the respirator, muscle weakness, and prolonging of the mobilization phase. The onset is early, within 72 hours after onset of septic shock (160). CIP is an early feature of multiorgan dysfunction syndrome (142,140). Nerve conduction studies typically exhibit a reduction in amplitudes of compound muscle action potentials and sensory nerve action potentials (161). Abnormalities in phrenic nerve conductions also are observed frequently, and that may further contribute to delayed weaning from the ventilator in many patients (157,162). On needle electromyography (EMG) examination of the limb muscles and diaphragm, the most common finding is abnormal spontaneous activity (fibrillation potentials and positive sharp waves) (163). Biopsies of peripheral nerves reveal primary axonal degeneration of motor and sensory fibers. Inflammation of peripheral nerves is not observed in CIP; the absence of inflammation can help distinguish CIP from the Guillain-Barre syndrome. Muscle biopsies demonstrate denervation atrophy of proximal and distal muscles. Central chromatolysis of anterior horn cells and loss of dorsal root ganglion cells occur as the result of the peripheral nerve axonal changes (163,164). Because neuromuscular abnormalities seem to develop earlier than previously reported, EMG should be considered more frequently and earlier as a diagnostic test (165).

The specific course and long-term outcome of CIP remains unclear. The management of CIP is symptomatic, including the provision of adequate nutrition, sedation, analgesia, and amnesia, along with aggressive supportive care including long-term physical therapy and rehab (Volume 2, Chapter 66). Incomplete recovery within one to two years after the onset of disease occurs frequently in patients with CIP (166). If the underlying problem causing sepsis and/or SIRS can be treated successfully, full recovery from CIP can occur. This recovery often occurs in a matter of weeks in milder cases and in months in more severe cases (157). The longer the length of stay in the critical care unit, longer the duration of sepsis, and greater body weight loss were found to be significantly related with poor recovery (152). Mortality may be as high as 60% and relates to the medical rather than to the neurological condition (155). Advice to family and patients regarding long-term prognosis is related to the likely etiology of prolonged weakness (162).

CRITICAL ILLNESS–RELATED MYOPATHY

Several reports suggest that the prolonged weakness following NMB agent use in ICU patients has an association with concurrently administered corticosteroids. Sepsis has long been associated with muscle weakness. Critical illness–related muscle weakness delays recovery and often causes prolonged ventilator dependence (75,115,137,138,155,167–170). This entity may not necessarily be related to the provision of NMB drugs. However, both the administration of steroids and sepsis are likely implicated.

Steroid-Related Myopathy
Ramsay et al. proposed that critically ill patients have susceptible skeletal muscle that awaits a trigger to create the muscle damage. Ramsay et al. speculated that long-term and large-dose steroids prime the muscle in the ICU

patient, and the NMB agent might then trigger a cascade of severe muscle damage, reflected by increased serum creatine phosphokinase (CPK), and characterized microscopically as damage to the muscle cell proteins and gross muscle atrophy. The muscle membrane loses its ability to contract due to altered membrane sodium currents and loss of myosin thick filaments, resulting in profound and prolonged weakness (143,155,163). In a prospective study, Douglass et al. demonstrated elevated CPK in 19 of 25 patients who required mechanical ventilatory support for severe asthma and who received vecuronium for more than two days along with high-dose corticosteroids. Nine of the 25 patients developed a clinically apparent myopathy (114). Many other reports describe otherwise healthy asthmatic patients who remained quadriplegic days to weeks after simultaneous treatment with corticosteroids and NMB agents (114,115,138,168). In one instance after rapid tapering of systemic steroids, the patient quickly regained muscle strength, was extubated and sent for rehabilitation therapy (171). A recent case report shows that the metabolic alterations associated with hyperthyroidism may enhance the risk of developing critical illness myopathy after the administration of antibiotics, NMBs, and steroids in the ICU (171,172). Additional support for corticosteroid-induced muscular atrophy comes from animal studies. These studies have also shown that denervation increases the number of glucocorticosteroid receptors, which causes preferential depletion of myosin filaments and atrophy (164). ☛ **Corticosteroid-related myopathy primarily affects type 2 fibers; routine EMG most precisely evaluates type 1 fibers, and therefore its results can be equivocal or normal (163).** ☛ TOF monitoring was not employed in the studies published so far; although its use may be able to reduce the incidence of prolonged weakness, the assertion is speculative. While most reports of prolonged weakness involve the use of vecuronium and pancuronium, acute myopathy with atracurium and cisatracurium has also been reported (114,173–175).

Sepsis-Related Myopathy

Critical illness myopathy not related to steroids is also encountered in patients suffering from systemic inflammatory response syndrome (SIRS) and multiple organ failure (MOF). Muscle biopsy reveals fiber atrophy, internalized nuclei, rimmed vacuoles, fatty degeneration, fibrosis, and single fiber necrosis (176–178). Electrophoretic determination of the myosin/actin ratio is an alternate method for diagnosing critical illness myopathy (178).

In contrast to steroid-induced myopathy, the nonsteroid-involved version is not usually associated with elevated CPK. This entity is probably sepsis induced, and muscle force can be shown to be altered early in the course of sepsis. The pathology may be related to mitochondrial dysfunction and decreased ATP or increased concentration of reactive oxygen species (ROS) (179). Recently, Brealey et al. demonstrated that muscle biopsies obtained from septic patients had increased amounts of inducible nitric oxide synthase (iNOS) (180). This finding raised the concern that nitric oxide (NO) or other products of NO degradation (i.e., the highly toxic peroxynitrate molecule) might be the active factor. Wray et al. have introduced supporting data with the finding that the ubiquitin pathway is activated in the muscle of septic patients (181).

The ubiquitin pathway is responsible for degrading abnormal proteins in normal cells and may be causing unintended injury to skeletal muscle. Interestingly, ubiquitin is stimulated by peroxinitrate and other ROS and may also be involved in the pathway of corticosteroid induced muscle protein breakdown (182). Thus, the final common pathway for both sepsis-induced myopathy, and steroid-induced myopathy may be ROS-triggered activation of the ubiquitin pathway and resultant muscle protein degradation.

EYE TO THE FUTURE

The need for NMB use in critically ill patients is expected to increase over time since we care for increasingly sick and complex patients in the ICU. Our knowledge about complications of NMBs in this patient population also continues to increase. There is a need for an NMB drug that will be free from all the long-term side effects (prolonged motor weakness CIP, and steroid-related myopathy). Furthermore, the drug should also provide hemodynamic stability and ideally be void of harmful metabolites.

Improved capabilities for continuous monitoring of NMB will also be helpful. Currently available methods are increasingly being used, even though errors may occur in critically ill patients, especially in edematous or obese patients, and when the PNS is improperly utilized. Besides improved training, better techniques for evaluating the nerve, muscle and NMJ are needed. Recognition that some elements of CIP occur early in the ICU course of sepsis/SIRS should alert the clinician to avoid unnecessary NMB drug use and closely titrate serum glucose in these patients. Additionally, early use of EMG in this population might provide additional data on pathophysiology (though interrogation of type 2 fibers requires further enhancement and development of EMG technology).

SUMMARY

Several factors influence recovery after the use of NMB agents in ICU patients. These factors include concomitant drug use, length of therapy, end-organ function, primary disease process, and availability of neuromuscular monitoring devices. NMB drugs should be used only when their use is essential for optimal care. Clinicians need to be educated regarding the effects of NMB agents; in particular, they need to know that these agents are devoid of anxiolytic, amnestic, and analgesic properties. Prolongation of NMB carries the concomitant risk of prolonged ventilatory support, increased length of hospitalization, and higher associated costs.

Proposed methods to decrease the risk of prolonged blockade include peripheral nerve stimulation monitoring, periodic drug discontinuation, recognition of interacting drug therapy, and attention to electrolyte and acid–base management. Adjunctive therapies, such as early physical, occupational, and nutritional therapy, may also affect the length of blockade. Most importantly, patient-specific factors that may identify patients at risk for prolonged blockade, such as concomitant corticosteroid and/or aminoglycoside use, presence of renal and/or hepatic failure, should be assessed when deciding to use NMB agents.

The following is recommended if NMB agent use is indicated in the patient in ICU:

1. Never use an NMB unless absolutely required (Table 8).
2. Always administer an amnestic, analgesic and/or sedative agent before and throughout administration of an NMB agent.
3. Select NMB agent based on its pharmacokinetics, pharmacodynamics, and adverse-effect profile.
4. Carefully monitor the drug's effect by employing a PNS to prevent inadvertent overdosing. Intermittently discontinue the NMB agent to check for patient movement (and use this opportunity to revisit the need for NMB), whenever clinically feasible.
5. Recognize potential drug interactions and disease states that may potentiate or prolong the effects of the NMB agent.
6. Consider the cost of the agent, and also keep in mind the indirect costs of prolonged hospitalization secondary to prolonged NMB or persistent weakness.

KEY POINTS

☞ The neural signal is propagated along the axon electrically to the nerve terminal, but crossing the synapse requires the chemical messenger ACh.

☞ If enough nAChR channels are opened (as occurs when 200–400 quanta of ACh are released into the synaptic cleft), the resultant change in transmembrane potential will exceed −50 mV, and an action potential will be propagated to the entire motor unit, resulting in muscular contraction.

☞ Decreased quantity or quality of plasma cholinesterase results in a prolonged duration of NMB due to succinylcholine.

☞ In patients with denervated muscle (particularly following upper motor neuron injury) or following muscle injury (burns, massive trauma), serum K^+ levels can increase by as much as 85% following succinylcholine administration (30), resulting in peaked T waves, widened QRS complexes, loss of P waves, and occasionally ventricular fibrillation and cardiac arrest.

☞ The nondepolarizing agents are all derived from one of two chemical groups, benzylisoquinoliniums and aminosteroids (Tables 1 and 4).

☞ Rocuronium is mainly used as an NMB during RSI in patients with contraindications to succinylcholine [e.g., burns, upper motor neuron injury, chronic bedrest (>30 days), and history of malignant hyperthermia, etc.].

☞ The main vecuronium metabolite, 3,17-dihydroxyvecuronium, has only 2% of the activity of the parent compound, whereas the 3-hydroxy derivative has 60% of the activity of the parent compound and is excreted renally.

☞ Because pancuronium and its metabolites are mainly (70%) excreted in the urine, a prolonged duration of action occurs in renal failure.

☞ Because its elimination does not depend upon renal or hepatic function, cisatracurium is often used in patients with renal and hepatic dysfunction.

☞ AChE inhibitors produce their effects by binding to and inhibiting the enzyme (AChE). The resulting increase in ACh in the synaptic cleft of the NMJ helps the ACh compete more favorably with NMB drugs for available ACh receptors.

☞ Neuromuscular blocking drugs should never be administered without concomitant amnesics, sedatives, and/or analgesics.

☞ The most reliable single clinical measure of return of NMJ function is the ability to head lift for five seconds or more.

☞ The most objective measurement of the degree of blockade in noncooperative or sedated patients is obtained with the demonstration of sustained tetanus through the use of a PNS.

☞ The etiology of postparalytic syndrome is incompletely understood, but may result from injury mediated directly by the drug, its active metabolites, or by drug–drug or drug–disease state interactions.

☞ CIP is acute axonal neuropathies involving both sensory and motor nerves developing during critical illness, especially with sepsis or SIRS.

☞ Corticosteroid-related myopathy primarily affects type 2 fibers; routine EMG most precisely evaluates type 1 fibers, and therefore its results can be equivocal or normal.

REFERENCES

1. Aitkenhead AR, Pepplerman ML, Willatts SM, et al. Comparison of propofol and midazolam for sedation in critically ill patients. Lancet 1989; 23(2)iii:704–709.
2. Bullock R, Stewart L, Rafferty C, et al. Continuous monitoring of jugular bulb oxygen saturation and the effect of drugs on cerebral metabolism. Acta Neurochir 1993; S59:113–118.
3. Revelly JP, Chiolero R, Ravussin P. Use of benzodiazepines in neurosurgical resuscitation. Agressologie 1991; 32:387–390.
4. Chiolero RL, de Tribolet N. Sedatives and antagonists in the management of severely head-injured patients. Acta Neurochir Suppl 1992; 55:43–46.
5. Farling PA, Johnston JR, Coppel DL. Propofol infusion for sedation of patients with head injury in intensive care. Anaesthesia 1989; 44:222–226.
6. Hsiang JK, Chestnut RM, Crisp CB, et al. Early, routine paralysis for intracranial pressure control in severe head injury: is it necessary? Crit Care Med 1994; 22:1471–1476.
7. Prough DS, Joshi S. Does early neuromuscular blockade contribute to adverse outcome after head injury? Crit Care Med 1994; 22:1349–1350.
8. Petrozza PH. Is continuous neuromuscular blockade necessary in head-injured patients? J Neurosurg Anes 1994; 5:135.
9. Durbin CG. Sedation in the critically ill. New Horizons 1994; 2:64–74.
10. Loper KA, Butler S, Nessly M, et al. Paralyzed with pain: the need for education. Pain 1989; 37:315–317.
11. Coursin DB, Prielipp RC. Use of neuromuscular blocking drugs in the critically ill patients. Crit Care Clin 1995; 11: 957–981.
12. Prielipp RC, Coursin DB, Wood KE, Murray MJ. Complications associated with sedative and neuromuscular blocking drugs in critically ill patients. Crit Care Clin 1995; 11:983–1003.
13. Agoston S, Vermeer GA, Kersten UW, et al. The fate of pancuronium bromide in man. Acta Anaesthesiol Scand 1973; 17: 267–275.
14. Ford, E. Monitoring Neuromuscular blockade in the adult ICU. Monitoring Neuromuscular Blockade in the Adult ICU. Am J Crit Care 1995; 4(2):122–130.
15. Lawen A. Ueber die Verbindung der Lokalanasthesie mit der Narkose, Über hohe Extraduralanasthesie und epidurale Injektionen Anasthesia render Losungen bei tabischen Magenfrisen. Beitr Klin Chir 1912; 80:168–189.
16. Griffith H, Johnson GE. The use of curare in general anesthesia. Anesthesiology 1942; 3:418.
17. Cullen SC. The use of curare for improvement of abdominal relaxation during cyclopropane anesthesia: report on 131 cases. Surgery 1943; 14:216.

18. Gray TC, Halton J. A milestone in anesthesia? (d-tubocurarine chloride). Proc R Soc Med 1946; 39:400–410.

19. Beecher HK, Todd DP. A study of the deaths associated with anesthesia and surgery: based on a study of 599,548 anesthesias in ten institutions 1948–1952, inclusive. Ann Surg 1954; 140: 2–35.

20. Topulos G. Neuromuscular blockade in adult intensive care. New Horizons 1993; 1:447–462.

21. Naguib M, Flood P, Mc Ardle JJ, Benner HR. Advances in neurobiology of the neuromuscular junction: implications for the anesthesiologist. Anesthesiology 2002; 96(1):202–231.

22. Ramsey FM. Basic pharmacology of neuromuscular blocking agents. Anesthesiol Clin North Am 1993; 11:219–236.

23. Rathmell JP, Brooker RF, Prielipp RC, et al. Hemodynamic and pharmacodynamic comparison of doxacurium and pipecuronium with pancuronium during induction of cardiac anesthesia: does the benefit justify the cost? Anesth Analg 1993; 76:513–519.

24. Naguib M, Lien CA. Pharmacology of muscle relaxants and their antagonists. In: Miller RD, ed. Anesthesia. New York, NY: Churchill Livingstone, 2005.

25. Taylor P. Agents acting at the neuromuscular junction and autonomic ganglia. In: Gilman AG, Rall TW, Nies AS, Taylor P, eds. The Pharmacological Basis of Therapeutics. Elmsford, NY: Pergamon Press, 1990.

26. Prielipp RC, Coursin DB. Applied pharmacology of common neuromuscular blocking agents in critical care. New Horizons 1994; 2(1):34–47.

27. Donnelly AJ. Neuromuscular blocking agents. J Pharm Pract 1994; VII(1):22–23.

28. Foldes FF, Rendell-Baker L, Birch JH. Causes and prevention of prolonged apnea with succinylcholine. Anesth Analg 1956; 35:609.

29. Pantuck EJ, Pantuck CB. Cholinesterases and anticholinesterases. In: Katz RL, ed. muscle relaxants. Amsterdam: Excerpta Medica 1975:143.

30. Mazze RI, Escue HM, Houston JB. Hyperkalemia and cardiovascular collapse following administration of succinylcholine to the traumatized patient. Anesthesiology 1969; 31:540.

31. Gronert GA. Cardiac arrest after succinylcholine. Anesthesiology 2001; 194:523–529.

32. Kopriva C, Ratliff J, Fletcher JR, et al. Serum potassium changes after succinylcholine in patients with acute massive muscle trauma. Anesthesiology 1971; 43:246.

33. Isenstein DA, Venner DS, Duggan J. Neuromuscular blockade in the intensive care unit. Chest 1992; 102:1258–1266.

34. Lingle CH, Steinbach JH. Neuromuscular blocking agents. Int Anesthesiol Clin 1988; 26(4):288–301.

35. Magorian T, Flannery KB, Miller RD. Comparison of rocuronium, succinylcholine, and vecuronium for rapid-sequence induction of anesthesia in adult patients. Anesthesiology 1993; 80(6):1411–1412.

36. Segredo V, Caldwell JE, Matthay MA. Persistent paralysis in critically ill patients after long-term administration of vecuronium. N Engl J Med 1992; 327:524–528.

37. Ohlinger MJ, Rhoney DH. Neuromuscular blocking agents in the neurosurgical intensive care unit. Surg Neurol 1998; 49:217–221.

38. Prielipp RC, Coursin DB. Sedative and neuromuscular blocking drug use in critically ill patients with head injuries. New Horizons 1995; 3:346–368.

39. Kelly JS, MacGregor DA. Drugs acting at the cholineric receptor. In: Chernow B, ed. The Pharmacologic Approach to the Critically Ill Patient. Baltimore: Williams & Wilkins, 1994:534–547.

40. Gwinnutt CL, Eddleston JM, Edwards D, Pollard BJ. Concentrations of atracurium and laudanosine in cerebrospinal fluid and plasma in three intensive care patients. Br J Anaesth 1990; 65:829–832.

41. Yate PM, Flynn PJ, Arnold RW, et al. Clinical experience and plasma laudanosine concentrations during the infusion of atracurium in the intensive care unit. Br J Anaesth 1987; 59:211–217.

42. Donnelly AJ. A Review of Neuromuscular Blockers. New York, NY: Burroughs Wellcome, 1993.

43. Dickens, MD. Pharmacology of neuromuscular blockade: interactions and implications for concurrent drug therapies. Crit Care Nurs Q 1995; 18(2):1–12.

44. Bevan DR, Donati F, Kopman AF. Reversal of neuromuscular blockade. Anesthesiology 1992; 77:785–805.

45. Cronnelly R, Morris RB, Miller RD. Edrophonium: duration of action and atropine requirement in humans during halothane anesthesia. Anesthesiology 1982; 57:261–266.

46. Azar I, Pham AN, Karambelkar DJ, et al. The heart rate following edrophonium-atropine and edrophonium-glycopyrrolate mixtures. Anesthesiology 1983; 58:139–141.

47. Ravin MB. Pyridostigmine as an antagonist of d-tubocurarine-induced and pancuronium-induced neuromuscular blockade. Anesth Analg 1975; 54:317–321.

48. Samra SK, Pandit UA, Pandit SK, et al. Modification by halogenated anaesthetics of chronotropic responces during reversal of neuromuscular blockade. Can Anaesth Soc J 1983; 30:48–52.

49. Fogdall RP, Miller RD. Antagonism of d-tubocurarine- and pancuronium-induced neuromuscular blockade by pyridostigmine in man. Anesthesiology 1973; 39:504–509.

50. Olin BR, Hebel SK, eds. Drug Facts and Comparisons Loose-Leaf Drug Information Service. Philadelphia, PA: JB Lippincott, 1994.

51. Singh YN, Marshall JG, Harvey AL. Pre- and postjunctional blocking effects of aminogycoside, polymixin, tetracycline and lincosamide antibiotics. Br J Anaesth 1982; 54:1295–1306.

52. Chen J, Kim YD, Dubois M, et al. The increased requirement of pancuronium in neurosurgical patients receiving dilantin chronically. Anesthesiology 1983; 59:A288.

53. Hogue CW, Ward JM, Itani MS, et al. Tolerance and up-regulation of acetylcholine receptor follows chronic infusion of d-tubocurarine. J Appl Physiol 1992; 72:1326–1331.

54. Azar I, Kumar D, Betcher AM. Resistance to pancuronium in an asthmatic patient treated with aminophylline and steroids. Can Anaesth Soc J 1982; 29:280–282.

55. Callanan DL. Development of resistance to pancuronium in adult respiratory distress syndrome. Anesth Analg 1985: 64:1126–1128.

56. Coursin DB, Klasek K, Goelzer SL. Increased requirements for continuously infused vecuronium in critically ill patients. Anesth Analg 1989; 69:518–521.

57. Hogue SW Jr, Itani MS, Martyn JAJ. Resistance to d-tubocurarine in lower motor neuron injury is related to increased acetylcholine receptors at the neuromuscular junction. Anesthesiology 1990; 73:703–709.

58. Damon MJ, Carpenter S. Myopathy with thick filament (myosin) loss following prolonged paralysis with vecuronium during steroid therapy. Muscle Nerve 1991; 14:1131–1139.

59. Gorson KC, Ropper AH. Acute respiratory failure neuropathy: a variant of critical illness polyneuropathy. Crit Care Med 1993; 21:267–271.

60. Aitenhead AR. Analgesia and sedation in intensive care. Br J Anaesth 1969; 63:196–206.

61. Park SR, Gray PA. Infusions of analgesia, sedatives and muscle relaxants in patients who require intensive care. Anaesthesia 1989; 44:879–880.

62. Bion JF. Sedation and analgesia in the intensive care unit. Hospital Update 1988; 14:1272–1286.

63. Klessing HT, Geiger HJ, Murray MJ, et al. A national survey on the practice patterns of anesthesiologist intensivists in the use of muscle relaxants. Crit Care Med 1992; 20:1341–1345.

64. Halloran T. Use of sedation and neuromuscular paralysis during mechanical ventilation. Crit Care Nurs Clin North Am 1991; 3(4):651–657.

65. Buck ML, Reed MD. Use of nondepolarizing blocking agents in mechanically ventilated patients. Clin Pharmacol 1991; 10:32.

66. DeGarno BH, Dronen S. Pharmacology and clinical use of neuromuscular blocking agents. Ann Emerg Med 1983; 12:48.

67. Bevan DR, Donati F. Muscle relaxants. In: Barash PG, Cullen BF, Stoelting RK, eds. Clinical Anesthesia. Philadelphia, PA: JB Lippincott, 1992.

68. Jansen EC, Hansen PH. Objective measurement of succinyl-choline-induced fasciculations and the effect of pretreatment with pancuronium or gallamine. Anesthesiology 1979; 51:159–160.

69. Hunter JM. Neuromuscular blocking drugs in intensive therapy. Intensive Ther Clin Monit 1989; 3:1.

70. Bone RC, Sibblad WJ, Sprung CL. The ACCP-SCCM consensus conference on sepsis and organ failure. Chest 1992; 101:1481–1482, 1644–1653.

71. Davidson JE. Neuromuscular blockade: indications, peripheral nerve stimulation, and other concurrent interventions. New Horizons 1994; 2(1):75–84.

72. Coursin DB. Neuromuscular blockade: should patients be relaxed in the ICU? Chest 1992; 2(1):75–84.

73. Fiamengo SA, Savarese JJ. Use of muscle relaxants in intensive care units. Crit Care Med 1991; 19:1547–1559.

74. Hogue SW Jr, Ward JM, Itani MS, et al. Tolerance and upregulation of acetylcholine receptors following chronic infusion of d-tubocurarine. J Appl Physiol 1992; 72:1326–1331.

75. Gooch J, Suchytya M, Balbierz J, et al. Prolonged paralysis after treatment with neuromuscular junction blocking agents. Crit Care Med 1991; 19:1125–1131.

76. Werba A, Weinstabl C, Plainer B, et al. Vecuronium attenuates ICP increases during routine tracheobronchial suction. Anesth Analg 1990; 70:S430.

77. Kupfer Y, Okrent D, Twersky R, et al. Disuse atrophy in a ventilated patient with status asthmaticus receiving neuromuscular blockade. Crit Care Med 1987; 15:795–796.

78. Wheeler A. Sedation, analgesia, and paralysis in an intensive care unit. Chest 1993; 104:566–577.

79. Davidson J, Dattolo J, Goskowicz R, et al. Neuromuscular blockade: nursing interventions and case studies from infancy to adulthood. Crit Care Nurs Q 1993; 15:53–67.

80. Powles A, Ganta R. Use of vecuronium in the management of tetanus. Anesthesia 1985; 40:879–881.

81. Orko R, Rosenberg P, Himberg J. Intravenous infusion of midazolam, proporfol, and vecuronium in a patient with severe tetanus. Acta Anesthesiol Scand 1988; 32:590–592.

82. Hudes E, Lee L. clinical use of peripheral nerve stimulator in anesthesia. Can J Anesthesiology 1987; 4:525–534.

83. Viby-Mogensen J. Neuromuscular monitoring. In: Miller R, ed. Anesthesia, 6th ed. New York, NY: Churchill Livingstone, 2005:1551–1569.

84. Capan L, Satvanarayana T, Patel K. Assessment of neuromuscular blockade with surface electrodes. Anesth Analg 1981; 60:244–245.

85. Viby-Mogensen J. Clinical assessment of neuromuscular transmission. Br J Anesthesiol 1982; 54:209–223.

86. Tschida SJ, Hoey L, Mather D, et al. Train-of-four: to use or not to use. Pharmacotherapy 1995; 15(4):546–550.

87. Paton W, Waud D. The margin of safety of neuromuscular transmission. J Physiol 1967; 191:59–90.

88. Waud B, Waud D. The relation between tetanic fade and receptor occlusion in the presence of competitive neuromuscular block. Anesthesiology 1971; 35:456–464.

89. Ali H. Monitoring neuromuscular blockade. In: Rogers M, Tinker J, Covino B, Longnecker D, eds. Principles and Practice of Anesthesiology. St. Louis, MO: Mosby, 1993:827–845.

90. Lee C. TOF quantification of competitive neuromuscular blockade. Anesth Analg 1975; 54:639–643.

91. Stanec A, Heyduc J, Stanec G, et al. Tetanic fade and post tetanic tension in the absence of neuromuscular blocking agents in anesthetized man. Anesth Analg 1978; 57:102–107.

92. Gissen A, Katz R. Twitch, tetanus, and post tetanic potentiation as indices of nerve-muscle block in man. Anesthesiology 1969; 30:481–487.

93. Ali H, Savarese J. Monitoring of neuromuscular function. Anesthesiology 1976; 45:216–242.

94. Davidson J. Neuromuscular blockade: indications, peripheral nerve stimulation, and other concurrent interventions. New Horizons 1994; 2(1):75–83.

95. Hoyt J. Persistent paralysis in critically ill patients after the use of neuromuscular blocking agents. New Horizons 1994; 2(1):48–55.

96. Topulos G. Neuromuscular blockade in adult intensive care. New Horizons 1993; 1(3):447–460.

97. Agoston S, Seyr M, Khuenl-Brady K, et al. Use of neuromuscular blocking agents in the intensive care unit. Anesthesiol clin North Am 1993; 11(2):345–359.

98. Isenstein D, Venner D, Duggan J. Neuromuscular blockade in the intensive care unit. Chest 1992; 102:1258–1266.

99. Sgalio T. Monitoring the administration of neuromuscular blockade in critical care. Crit Care Nurs Q 1195; 18(2):41–59.

100. Davidson J. Neuromuscular blockade. Focus Crit Care 1991; 18:512–520.

101. Venner DS, Frazier WI, Isenstein DA. Neuromuscular blockade in the ICU (letter). Chest 1993; 104:1640–1641.

102. Casale LM, Siegel RE. Neuromuscular blockade in the ICU (letter). Chest 1993; 104:1639–1640.

103. Erikson LI, Lennmarken C, Jensen E, et al. Twitch tension and train-of-four ration during prolonged neuromusuclar monitoring at diefferent peripheral temperatures. Acta Anaesthesiol Scand 1991; 35:247–252.

104. Thornberry EA, Mazumdar B. The effect of changes in arm temperature on neuromuscular monitoring in the presence of atracurium blockade. Anaesthesia 1988; 43:447–449.

105. Bolton CF. The polyneuropathy of critical illness. J Intensive Care Med 1994; 9:132–138.

106. Azar I. Complications of neuromuscular blockers—interaction with concurrent diseases. Anesthesiol Clin North Am 1993; 11(2):409–443.

107. Parkeer M, Schubert W, Shelmer J, et al. perceptions of a critically ill patient experiencing therapeutic paralysis in an ICU. Crit Care Med 1984; 12:69–71.

108. Hansen-Flashen J, Brazinski S, Basile C, et al. Use of sedation drugs and neuromuscular blocking agents in patients requiring mechanical ventilation forrespiratory failure. JAMA 1991; 266:2870–2875.

109. Isestein D, Venner D, Dugan J. neuromuscular blockade in the intensive care unit. Chest 1992; 102:1258–1266.

110. Murray MJ, Strickland RA, Weiler C. The use of neuromuscular blocking drugs in the intensive care unit: a US perspective. Intensive Care Med 1993; 19:S40 – S44.

111. Douglass JA, Tuxen DV, Horne M, et al. Myopathy in severe asthma. Am Rev Respir Dis 1992; 146:517–519.

112. Hirano M, Ott B, Raps E, et al. Acute quadriplegic myopathy: a complication of treatment with steroids, neuromucular blocking agents, or both. Neurology 1992; 42:2082–2087.

113. Kupfer Y, Namba T, Kaldawi E, et al. Prolonged weakness after long-term infusion of vecuronium bromide. Ann Intern Med 1992; 117:484–486.

114. Op de Coul AA, Lambregts PC, Koeman J, et al. Neuromuscular complications in patients given pavulon (pancuronium bromide) during artificial ventilation. Clin Neurol Neurosurg 1985; 87:17–22.

115. Shee CD. Risk factors for hydrocortisone myopathy in acute severe asthma. Respir Med 1990; 84:229–233.

116. Davis NA, Rodgers JE, Gonzalez ER, et al. Prolonged weakness after cisatracurium infusion: a case report. Crit Care Med 1998; 26(7):1290–1292.

117. Lewis KS, Rothenberg DM. Neuromuscular blockade in the intensive care unit. Am J Health-Syst Pharm 1999; 56: 72–75.

118. Shah, NK. Management of Neuromuscular Blockers in Critically Ill patients. In 1st ISNAAC Conference, N. Delhi, 1999.

119. Peat SH, Peat SJ, Potter DR, Hunter JM. The prolonged use of atracurium in a patient with tetanus. Anaesthesia 1988; 43:962–963.

120. Fahey MR, Rupp SM, Cornfell C, et al. Effect of renal failure on laudanosine excretion in man. Br J Anaesth 1985; 57:1049–1051.

121. Parker CJR, Jones JE, Hunter JM. Disposition of infusions of atracurium and its metabolite laudanosine, in patients in renal and respiratory failure in an ITU. Br J Anaesth 1988; 61(5):531–540.

122. Pittet JF, Tassonyi E, Schopfer C, Monel DR, Menta G. Plasma concentrations of laudanosine, but not of atracurium, are increased during the anhepatic phase of orthotropic liver transplantation in pigs. Anesthesiology 1990; 72:145–152.

123. Shearer ES, O'Swliram EP, Hunter JM. Clearance of atracurium and laudanosine in the urine and by continuous venovenous haemofiltration. Br J Anaesth 1991; 67:569–573.

124. Henning RH, Houwertjes MC, Scaf AHJ, et al. Prolonged paralysis after long-term, high-dose infusion of pancuronium in anaesthetized cats. Br J Anaesth 1993; 71:393–397.

125. Vandenbrom, RHG, Wierda JM. Pancuronium bromide in the intensive care unit: a case of overdose. Anesthesiology 1998; 69:996–997.

126. Watling SM, Dasta JF, Seidl EC. Sedatives, analgesics, and paralytics in the ICU. Ann Pharmacother 1997; 31:148–153.

127. Pedersen T, Viby-Mogensen J, Ringsted C. Anaesthetic practice and postoperative pulmonary complications. Acta Anaesthesiol Scand 1992; 36:812–818.

128. Bevan DR, Donati F. Muscle relaxants. In: Barash P, Cullen B, Stoetling RK, eds. Clinical Anesthesia. Philadelphia, PA: Lippincott, 1992:481–508.

129. Dupuis JY, Martin R, Tetrault JP, et al. Atracurium and vecuronium interaction with gentamicin and tobramycin. Can J Anaesth 1989; 36:407–411.

130. Watling SM, Dasta JF. Prolonged paralysis in intensive care unit patients after the use of neuromuscular blocking agents: a review of the literature. Crit Care Med 1994; 22:884–893.

131. Sinatra RS, Philip BK, Naulty S, et al. Prolonged neuromuscular blockade with vecuronium in a patient treated with magnesium sulfate. Anesth Analg 1985; 64:1220–1222.

132. Wadon AJ, Dogra S, Anand S. Atracurium infusion in the intensive care unit. Br J Anaesth 1986; 68:64S–67S.

133. Buzello W, Noeledge G, Krieg N, et al. Vecuronium for muscle relaxation in patients with myasthenia gravis. Anesthesiology 1986; 64:1220–1222.

134. Ono K, Nagano O, Ohta Y, et al. Neuromuscular effects of respiratory and metabolic acid-base changes in vitro with and without nondepolarizing muscle relaxants. Anesthesiology 1990; 73:710–716.

135. Pollard B, Harper N, Doran B. Use of continuous prolonged administration of atracurium in the IRU to a patient with myasthenia gravis. Br J Anaesth 1989; 62:95–97.

136. Beaufort AM, Weirda JM, Belopavlovic M, et al. The influence of hypothermia (surface cooling) on the time-course of action and on the pharmacokinetics of rocuronium in humans. Eur J Anaesthesiol 1995; 12(suppl 11):95–106.

137. Lopez MP, Seiz A, Criado A. Prolonged muscle weakness associated with the administration of non-depolarizing neuromuscular blocking agents in critically ill patients. Revista Espanola de Anestesiologia y Reanimacion 2001; 48(8):375–383.

138. Griffin D, Fairman N, Coursin D, et al. Acute myopathy during treatment of status asthmaticus with coritcosteroids and steroidal muscle relaxants. Chest 1992; 102:510–514.

139. Zochodne DW, Ramsay DA, Viera S, et al. Acute necrotizing myopathy of intensive care: electrophysiological studies. Muscle Nerve 1994; 17:285–292.

140. Larsson L, Li X, Edstrom L, et al. Acute quadriplegia and loss of muscle myosin in patients treated with nondepolarizing neuromuscular blocking agents and corticosteroids: mechanisms at the cellular and molecular levels. Crit Care Med 2000; 28(1):34–45.

141. Wokke JHJ, Jennekens FGI, Van den Oord CJM, et al. Histological investigations of muscle atrophy and end plates with generalized weakness. J Neurol Sci 1988; 88:95–106.

142. Burry L, HoSang M, Hynes-Gay P. A review of neuromuscular blockade in the critically ill patient. Dynamics (Pembroke, Ont.) 2001; 12(3):28–33.

143. Hund E. Neurological complications of sepsis: critical illness polyneuropathy and myopathy. J Neurol 2001; 248(11):929–934.

144. Bolton CF. Neuromuscular complications of sepsis. Intensive Care Med 1993; (suppl 195): S58–S63.

145. Schwarz J, Planck J, Briegel J, Straube A. Single-fiber electromyography, nerve conduction studies, and conventional electromyography in patients with critical-illness polyneuropathy: evidence for a lesion of terminal motor axons. Muscle Nerve 1998; 20(6):696–701.

146. Bolton DF. Sepsis and the systemic inflammatory response syndrome: neuromuscular manifestations. Crit Care Med 1996; 24:1408–1416.

147. Dreijer B, Kledal S, Jennum PJ. Critical illness polyneuropathy—a neuromuscular complication in the intensive care patients. Ugeskrift for Laeger 2002; 164(43):5035–5036.

148. Bovan P, Blackburn W, Potter P. Critical illness polyneuropathy. AXON 2001; 22:25–29.

149. Khilnani GC, Bansal R, Malhotra OP, Bhatia M. Critical illness polyneuropathy: how often do we diagnose it? Indian J Chest Dis Allied Sci 2003; 45(3):209–213.

150. Motomura M. Critical illness polyneuropathy and myopathy. Rinsho Shinkeigaku—Clinical Neurology 2003; 43(11):802–804.

151. Leijten FSS, De Weerd AW, Poortvilet DCJ, De Ridder VA, Ulrich C, Harinck-De Weerd JE. Critical illness polyneuropathy in multiple organ dysfunction syndrome and weaning from the ventilator. Intensive Care Med 1996; 22(9):856–861.

152. de Seze M, Petit H, Wiart L, et al. Critical illness polyneuropathy. A 2-year follow-up study in 19 severe cases. Eur Neurol 2000; 43(2):61–69.

153. Garnacho-Montero J, Madrazo-Osuna J, Garcia-Garmendia JL, et al. Critical illness polyneuropathy: risk factors and clinical consequences. A cohort study in septic patients. Intensive Care Med 2001; 27(8):1288–1296.

154. Hund EF. Neuromuscular complications in the ICU: the spectrum of critical illness-related conditions causing muscular weakness and weaning failure. J Neurol Sci 1996; 136:10–16.

155. Bird SJ, Rich MM. Critical illness myopathy and polyneuropathy. Current Neurology & Neuroscience Reports 2002; 2(6):527–533.

156. De Letter MA, van Doorn PA, Savelkoul HF, et al. Critical illness polyneuropathy and myopathy (CIPNM): evidence for local immune activation by cytokine-expression in the muscle tissue. J Neuroimmunol 2000; 106(1–2):206–213.

157. van Mook WN, Hulsewe-Evers RP. Critical illness polyneuropathy. Curr Opin Crit Care 2002; 8(4):302–310.

158. Kane SL, Dasta JF. Clinical outcomes of critical illness polyneuropathy. Pharmacotherapy 2002; 22(3):373–379.

159. Murphy GS, Vender JS. Neuromuscular-blocking drugs. Crit Care Clin 2001; 17(4):925–942.

160. Tepper M, Rakic S, Haas JA, Woittiez AJ. Incidence and onset of critical illness polyneuropathy in patients with septic shock. Neth J Med 2000; 55(6):211–214.

161. Zifko UA, Zipko HT, Bolton CF. Clinical and electrophysiological findings in critical care illness polyneuropathy. J Neurol Sci 1998; 159:186–193.

162. Zochodne DW, Bolton CF, Wells GA, et al. Critical illness polyneuropathy: a complication of sepsis and multiple organ failure. Brain 1987; 110:819–842.

163. Ramsay DA, Zochodne DW, Robertson DM, et al. A syndrome of acute severe muscle necrosis in intensive care unit patients. J Neuropathol Exp Neurol 1998; 52:387–398.

164. Rouleau G, Karpati G, Carpenter S, et al. Glucocorticoid excess induces preferential depletion of myosin in denervated skeletal muscle fibers. Muscle Nerve 1987; 10:428–438.

165. Tennila A, Salmi T, Pettila V, Roine RO, Varpula T, Takkunen O. Early signs of critical illness polyneuropathy in ICU patients with systemic inflammatory response syndrome or sepsis. Intensive Care Med 2000; 26(9):1360–1363.

166. Zifko UA. Long-term outcome of critical illness polyneuropathy. Muscle Nerve 2000; 9(suppl):S49–S52.

167. Hirano M, Ott BR, Raps EC, et al. Acute quadriplegic myopathy: a complication of treatment with steroids, nondepolarizing blocking agents, or both. Neurology 1992; 42:2082–2087.

168. Williams RJ, O'Hehir RE, Czarney D, et al. Acute myopathy in severe acute asthma treated with intravenously administered corticosteroids. Am Rev Respir Dis 1998; 137:460–463.

169. Danon MJ, Carpenter S. Myopathy with thick filament loss following prolonged paralysis with vecuronium during steroid treatment. Muscle Nerve 1991; 14:131–139.

170. Al-Jumah MA, Awada AA, Al-Ayafi HA, Kojan SW, Al-Shirawi N. Neuromuscular paralysis in the intensive care unit. Saudi Med J 2004; 25(4):474–477.

171. Polsonetti BW, Joy SD, Laos LF. Steroid-induced myopathy in the ICU. Annals of Pharmacotherapy 2002; 36(11):1741–1744.

172. Riggs JE, Pandey HK, Schochet SS Jr. Critical illness myopathy associated with hyperthyroidism. Mil Med 2004; 169(1):71–72.

173. Hoey L, Joslin S, Nahum A, Vance-Bryan K. Prolonged neuromuscular blockade in two critically ill patients treated with atracurium. Pharmacotherapy 1995; 15(2):254–259.

174. Tousignanat CP, Bevan DR, Eisen AA, et al. Acute quadriparesis in an asthmatic treated with atracurium. Can J Anaesth 1995; 42:224–227.

175. Manthous CA, Chatila W. Prolonged weakness after the withdrawal of atracurium. Am J Respir Crit Care Med 1994; 130:1441–1443.

176. De Jonghe B, Sharshar T, Lefaucheur J, et al. Paresis acquired in the intensive care unit. A prospective multicenter study. JAMA 2002; 288:2859–2867.

177. Bednarik J, Lukas Z, Vondracek P. Critical illness polyneuromyopathy: the electrophysiological components of a complex entity. Intensive Care Med 2003; 29:1505–1514.

178. Stibler H, Edström L, Ahlbeck K, et al. Electrophoretic determination of the myosin/actin ratio in the diagnosis of critical illness myopathy. Intensive Care Med 2003; 29:1515–1527.

179. Brealey D, Brand M, Hargraves I, et al. Association between mitochondrial dysfunction and severity and outcome of septic shock. Lancet 2002; 360:219–223.

180. Brealey D, Rabuel C, Mebazza A, et al. iNOS expression and peroxynitrate production is associated with mitochondrial dysfunction in skeletal muscle of patients with severe sepsis. Intensive Care Med 2002; 28:517 (abstract).

181. Wray C, Mammen J, Hershko A, et al. Sepsis upregulates the gene expression of multiple ubiquitin ligases in skeletal muscle. Int J Biochem Cell Bio 2003; 35:698–705.

182. Sun X, Mammen J, Tian X. Sepsis induces the transcription of the glucocorticoid receptor in skeletal muscle cells. Clin Sci 2003; 105:383–391.

183. Stoelting RK, Miller RD. Muscle relaxants. In: Stoelting RK, Miller RD, eds. Basics of Anesthesia. 3rd ed. Philadelphia, PA: Churchill Livingstone, 1994:83–100.

184. Viby-Mogensen J. Correlation of succinylcholine duration of action with plasma cholinesterase activity in subjects with the genotypically normal enzyme. Anesthesiology 1980; 53:517–520.

185. Naguib M, Lien CA. Pharmacology of muscle relaxants and their antagonists. In: Miller RD, Fleisher LA, Johns RA, et al., eds. Miller's Anesthesia. 6th ed. Philadelphia, PA: Elsevier Churchill Livingstone, 2005:481–572.

186. Viby-Mogensen J. Neuromuscular monitoring. In: Miller RD, Fleisher LA, Johns RA, et al., eds. Miller's Anesthesia. 6th ed. Philadelphia, PA: Elsevier Churchill Livingstone, 2005: 1551–1569.

187. Kalli IS. Neuromuscular block monitoring. In: Kirby RR, Gravenstein N, Lobato EB, et al., eds. Clinical Anesthesia Practice. 2nd ed. Philadelphia, PA: W.B. Saunders Company, 2002:442–451.

7

Neurological Monitoring

Ahmed Fikry Attaallah

Department of Anesthesiology, West Virginia University, Morgantown, West Virginia, U.S.A.

W. Andrew Kofke

Department of Anesthesia, University of Pennsylvania Hospital, Philadelphia, Pennsylvania, U.S.A.

INTRODUCTION

This chapter reviews the equipment and techniques available for monitoring the brain and spinal cord for trauma and critical care. A detailed neurological examination is still the gold standard to evaluate brain and spinal cord function. Traditional examination includes assessment of the level of consciousness, pupillary response, motor function, sensory function, and cranial nerves (1). In many instances, such basic clinical neurological assessments guide surgical interventions and other important clinical decisions. However, sedatives, muscle relaxants, as well as existing neuropathology or acute trauma conditions may significantly impair the sensitivity or even the ability to perform a standard neurological examination.

A host of neurological monitoring devices have been developed as surrogates for the clinical neurological exam. The improved monitoring technology has made it possible to obtain real-time assessment of several parameters of central nervous system (CNS) function. However, not all aspects of CNS function can be monitored with the current technology. Furthermore, no monitoring modalities presently employed provide prospective prediction of deterioration in CNS function, or adequately warn of impending progression of injury. Nonetheless, monitoring provides useful information for evaluating the patient's current condition, recent progress, and need for therapy.

Research efforts continue to improve monitoring techniques in terms of predictive value, reliability, accuracy, and safety. The most important monitoring modalities in current clinical use are reviewed in this manuscript. The major focus of this chapter is in describing the technical aspects of these monitors and the indications for use. Because intracranial pressure (ICP) monitoring is so widely used clinically, we briefly review the basic anatomy and physiology underpinning the ICP volume relationship (elastance). We also provide high-quality figures showing the precise locations of the various ICP monitoring devices, anticipating that this additional review will improve the understanding and safety of ICP monitoring (also see Volume 2, Chapter 1). After reviewing the basic monitoring modalities, the chapter closes with a section dedicated to the monitoring modalities of the future (including cerebral microdialysis catheters and pupilometry).

INTRACRANIAL PRESSURE MONITORING
Anatomy and Physiology

Most neurosurgical catastrophes and much of the morbidity following traumatic brain injury (TBI) results from elevated ICP. Thus, a brief outline of the normal physiologic mechanisms that maintain the balance between pressure and volume inside the dural sac is useful to improve the understanding of the concepts underpinning ICP monitoring (2,3).

The normal adult produces approximately 500 mL of cerebrospinal fluid (CSF) in a 24-hour period. Approximately 150 mL is present in the intracranial space at any given time (see Volume 2, Chapter 1 for details of CSF production and removal). The intradural space consists of the intraspinal space plus the intracranial space. The total volume of this space in the adult is approximately 1700 mL, of which approximately 10% is spinal fluid, 10% blood volume, and 80% brain and spinal cord tissue. Because the spinal dural sac is not always fully distended, some increase in volume of the intradural space can be achieved at the expense of compression of the spinal epidural veins. Once the dural sac is fully distended, any further increase in volume of one component of the intracranial space must be offset by a decrease in volume of one of the other components. This concept is known by cerebral physiologists as the Monro-Kellie doctrine (summarized in Equation 1 later) (4,5).

The normal contents of the intracranial space are brain, blood, and CSF. When a formula is used to represent the intracranial volume–pressure relationships, a term is often included to represent the presence of any other intracranial mass (e.g., tumor or hematoma):

$$V_{csf} + V_{blood} + V_{brain} + V_{other} = V_{constant} \qquad (1)$$

Thus with a pathologic increase in one component, at least one of the others must decrease to maintain a constant volume. If the accommodating component volume decrease is equal to the volume added, then pressure does not change. The most effective and earliest compensation is displacement of CSF from the cranial space into the spinal space (compressing epidural veins), followed by reabsorption of CSF across the arachnoid villi (a less immediate accommodative process). As the ICP rises, the CSF production rate begins to decrease, further aiding compensation (this is a slower process). The second major volume compensation is the displacement of intracranial pial blood volume into the venous sinuses. Finally, the brain itself can be compressed to compensate for increases in volume. This is well exemplified by acute hydrocephalus, where the brain is compressed by the CSF resulting in ventricular enlargement, or in an acute epidural hematoma, when the brain is acutely compressed and distorted by the mass of the hematoma.

A diagrammatic summary of these principles is presented in Figure 1. The fundamental concept illustrated in the figure is that patients with the same ICP values may differ significantly in intracerebral compliance (i.e., ICP values taken in isolation can be quite misleading if they are not considered within the framework of compliance). Clinical factors affecting intracranial dynamics that should be considered when interpreting static ICP measurements include the intracranial pathology revealed in the computed tomography (CT) scan and/or witnessed in the operating room, the amount of therapy required to produce the present ICP value, and the sensitivity of the ICP reading to external stimuli (e.g., suctioning, turning, etc.).

The intracranial space is divided into a series of compartments by the foramen magnum and the folds of the dura, the falx, and the tentorium. The anterior fossa is separated from the middle fossa by the lesser wing of the sphenoid bone. The right half of the supratentorial space is separated from the left by the falx cerebri, and the supratentorial space is separated from the infratentorial space by the tentorium. Finally, the intracranial space becomes the intraspinal canal at the foramen magnum. Understanding

this compartmentalization is important because swelling or pressure increases in one compartment can result in distortion and displacement of brain into another compartment, with consequent tissue and vascular compression, resulting in brain dysfunction, damage, or death. These pathphysiogical mechanisms create the clinical brain herniation syndromes.

Normally, the CSF pressure is slightly lower than the cerebral venous pressure, but slightly higher than the central venous pressure. Because cerebral venous pressure is difficult to measure clinically, the ICP is used as a surrogate. The cerebral perfusion pressure (CPP) is defined as the difference between mean arterial pressure (MAP) and ICP (as shown in Equation 2).

$$CPP = MAP - ICP \qquad (2)$$

☞ **Any decrease in MAP or increase in ICP will result in a decrease in CPP.** ☞ Once the injured brain CPP falls below 50 to 60 mmHg, ischemia, compression, or herniation of the brain may occur (6–9). The interested reader may refer to Volume 1, Chapter 23 for a review of CPP within the context of TBI management.

Within the limits of autoregulation (CPP 50–150 mmHg) the cerebral vessels respond to decreased CPP by vasodilating, decreasing resistance to flow and thus maintaining the same cerebral blood flow (CBF), despite either a decline in arterial pressure or an increase in ICP. Below the limits of autoregulation, the CBF falls as the CPP is lowered. Cerebral metabolism is preserved to a CBF of about 50% of the normal level, after which some degree of cerebral ischemia begins. As blood flow falls below 25% of normal, irreversible damage begins. Thus, autoregulation is an additional brain protective mechanism against increased ICP. Unfortunately, autoregulation is not always preserved following TBI, and thus therapy is directed at maintaining normal or nearly normal ICP and MAP with the aim of preserving CBF (2,3,6–9).

It is also important to recognize that any obstruction to CSF drainage, such as jugular venous obstruction, increases in intrathoracic pressure (pneumothorax, excessive PEEP), which in turn can increase ICP just as an acute increase in brain edema or hemorrhage in the cranium. When the ICP increases above 20 mmHg, CPP may be impaired.

Continuous ICP monitoring has been used to guide the management of patients with head injury (Volume 1, Chapter 23 and Volume 2, Chapter 12), intracerebral hemorrhage (Volume 2, Chapter 14), and brain tumors. ICP monitoring is indicated in patients with severe head injury (GCS 3 to 8 after resuscitation) with nontrivial findings on CT scan. ICP monitoring is also appropriate in patients with severe head injury with a normal CT scan if two or more of the following features are noted at admission: age over 40 years, unilateral or bilateral motor posturing, and systolic blood pressure ≤90 mmHg (3). The relationship between uncontrolled ICP elevation and mortality has been firmly established in patients with head injury, and ICP monitoring is becoming a standard method of care for their management (3).

The common denominator for many neurosurgical catastrophes is elevated ICP, along with a resultant cerebral herniation, focal ischemia or globally elevated ICP, and diffused cerebral ischemia. As cerebral herniation progresses and the subarachnoid spaces are occluded, the transmission of pressure within the craniospinal axis is impeded, setting the stage for a larger increase in pressure for any given increase in volume [Fig. 1 and (Fig. 3 in Volume 1, Chapter 23)].

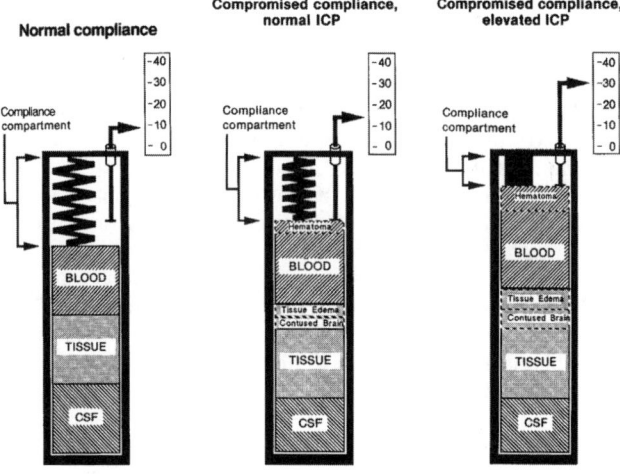

Figure 1 The interrelationship of compliance and ICP. In this figure, compliance is represented by the spring and ICP by the sliding indicator. The three components of the intracranial volume are shown as boxes (cerebrospinal fluid). The *left* shows the representation of the normal situation, in which compliance is maximal and ICP is within the normal range. The *center* shows the situation in which a postulated brain injury has resulted in an intracranial hematoma with contused and edematous brain. The resultant expansion of intracranial volume has used up the intracranial compliance (i.e., compressed the spring), but the ICP has not risen beyond the normal range. The *right* shows the situation in which the lesions have expanded further, expending the intracranial compliance and raising the ICP. It is important to note that in *left* and *center* figures the ICP is within the normal range despite critically different intracranial dynamics. *Abbreviations*: CSF, cerebrospinal fluid; ICP, intracranial pressure. *Source*: From Ref. 10.

The frequent waves of increased ICP may further abolish pressure autoregulation making the brain more prone to ischemia at the same CPP. A progressive loss of compensatory ability often follows an intracranial catastrophe, and an acute increase in volume that was tolerated (i.e., caused minimal increase in ICP) in the first few hours after the insult, may not be tolerated 24 hours later because of the exhaustion of the compensatory mechanisms (leading to dangerously elevated ICP). After TBI and cerebral aneurysm rupture, subarachnoid blood may clog the CSF reabsorption pathways (i.e., the arachnoid villi), further exacerbating ICP management.

Continuous ICP monitoring has been used to guide the management of patients with TBI and other causes of cerebral hypertension (e.g., intracerebral hemorrhage, large brain tumors, and hydrocephalus). The relationship between uncontrolled ICP elevation and fatality has been firmly established in TBI patients, and is the standard of care for the early management of severe closed head injury (GCS $\leq$ 8) (3,6–8). Although ICP monitoring does not measure neural function or recovery, its measurement does permit detection and prompt treatment of increased ICP (e.g., due to brain edema, hydrocephalus, or hemorrhage), which is known to impair neurological function (9). The techniques used to monitor ICP include ventricular catheters, subdural subarachnoid (Richmond) bolts, epidural transducers, and intraparenchymal fiberoptic devices (10).

Intracranial Pressure Monitoring Techniques

ICP monitoring can be performed with many different devices and requires knowledge of the indications, contraindications, and potential complications that may arise (Tables 1–3). Other than ventriculostomy, the remaining options for ICP monitoring do not provide the potential for CSF drainage in the management of ICP elevations. However, these other options (Richmond bolt, epidural

Table 2 Contraindications to Intracranial Pressure Monitoring

Contraindication	Rationale/comments
Coagulopathy	Ventricular catheterization should be avoided in thrombocytopenia (platelet count less than 100,000) or INR greater than 1.2. Other monitoring techniques are less risky; however, the patient should always have coagulopathy corrected prior to monitor placement
Immunosuppression	Patients with impaired immunologic status have an increased risk for infection creating a relative contraindication
Clinical irrelevance	Should not be used in patients with nonsurvivable prognosis

Note: International normalization ratio of the partial thromboplastin (PT) time (ratio of PT measured divided by the PT control).
Abbreviation: INR, international normalization ratio.

ICP monitors and intraparenchymal monitors) are associated with a decreased risk of intracerebral hemorrhage compared to ventriculostomy. Regardless of the ICP monitoring device employed, the ICP "number" should never be taken in isolation, and never substituted for a thorough neurological assessment, even when such examination is limited by coma or sedation.

Ventriculostomy

☛ **The intraventricular catheter, in addition to measuring ICP, allows therapeutic CSF drainage.** ☛ The intraventricular catheter is the gold standard method of

Table 1 Indications for Intracranial Pressure Monitoring

Indication	Criteria and rationale
Trauma	GCS $\leq$ 8 Inability to follow neurological exam from trauma or during necessary sedation or anesthesia
Intracranial hemorrhage	When expansion of hemorrhage would lead to surgical intervention, monitoring can provide immediate information. General ICP management
Intracranial neoplasm	Patients who develop brain swelling during operative resection or during closure, monitoring can be useful in the perioperative period
Post–AVM surgery	AVM resection leads to redistribution of blood flow and often postoperative edema requiring slow awakening from anesthesia and often postoperative sedation

Abbreviations: AVM, arterial venous malformation; GCS, Glasgow Coma Scale; ICP, intracranial pressure.

Table 3 Complications of Intracranial Pressure Monitoring

Complication	Rationale/comments
Infection	Placement of ICP monitors can lead to local wound infections, meningitis, ventriculitis, and brain abscess Risk of meningitis and ventriculitis greater with ventricular catheterization Unclear if routine replacement of devices prevents infection
Hemorrhage	Most morbid complication of monitor placement Can result from direct trauma (intracerebral or intraventricular) or overdrainage of CSF (subdural) Greatest risk with ventricular catheterization (1/70–100)
Measurement error	If devices are not placed and calibrated accurately, erroneous measurements may lead to inappropriate therapy or intervention

Abbreviations: CSF, cerebrospinal fluid; ICP, intracranial pressure.

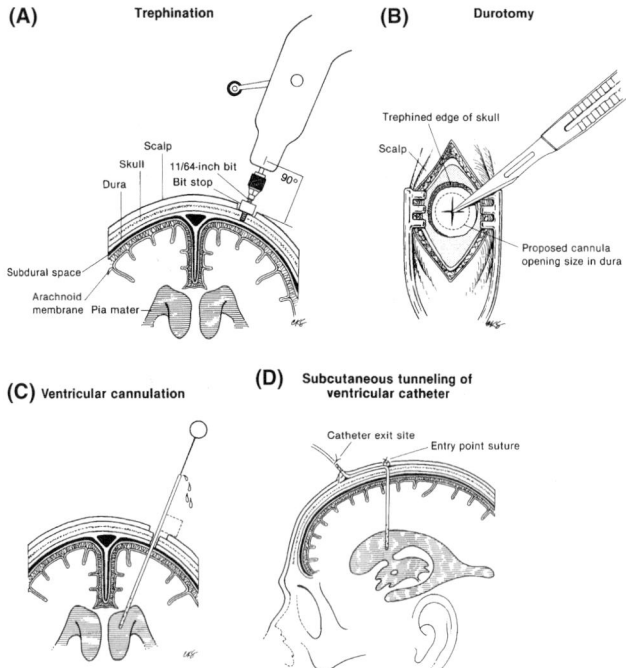

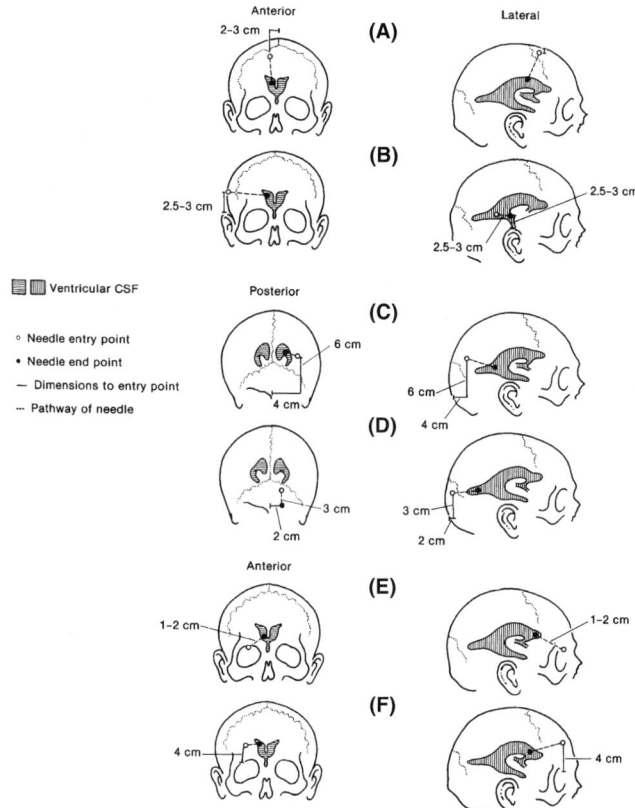

Figure 2 Ventirculostomy insertion technique including: trephination (**A**), durotomy (**B**), ventricular cannulation (**C**), and subcutaneous tunneling of catheter (**D**). Trephination (**A**) is accomplished with an 11/64-inch bit, care being taken not to lacerate the dura or plunge into the brain. Following trephination, the wound is thoroughly irrigated to remove all debris. A cruciate durotomy (**B**) is performed using a No. 11 blade. The size of the durotomy is limited so that the catheter will just pass through the opening, thereby avoiding a cerebrospinal fluid leak. Care is taken to avoid lacerating the underlying brain. The ventricle is cannulated (**C**) at no more than 5 cm from the dura, keeping the catheter at a right angle to the skull. The ventricular catheter is tunneled subcutaneously (**D**) external to the galea aponeurotica, and brought out through a separate exit wound, where it is well secured. *Source*: From Ref. 10.

monitoring ICP, which was first used in 1960 (11). A plastic catheter is introduced into the lateral ventricle and connected to an external transducer (Fig. 2). The intraventricular catheter measures ICP reliably, allows therapeutic CSF drainage, and is recommended for early ICP monitoring, following trauma in patients with anticipated ICP elevations (3,10). In the setting of trauma, ventricular size is often reduced subsequent to increased ICP, making the blind insertion of a ventricular catheter more difficult. If the ventricle cannot be cannulated by the third attempt, an alternative technique for ICP monitoring should be used, as the risk of complications increases with each passage.

Most neurosurgeons recommend using the frontal, parasagittal approach for the insertion site by employing Kocher's point (2–3 cm lateral to midline and just anterior to coronal suture). Other approaches do exist, however, the frontal approach offers good access to the frontal horn of the lateral ventricular system, minimizes the involvement of eloquent brain tissue during the passage of the catheter, and facilitates nursing care while the patient is supine in bed. Surgeon familiarity with whichever approach is chosen is paramount (Fig. 3). Some of the potential problems with ventriculostomies are occlusion and dampening,

Figure 3 Approaches for ventricular puncture. Six approaches for accessing the cerebral ventricles through trephines in the skull are shown in this figure. The ventricles are represented by the shaded areas, and the path of the ventricular cannula is shown as a dashed line. (**A**) Kocher's point: 2–3 cm from the midline, just anterior to the coronal suture. (**B**) Keen's point: 2.5–3 cm posterior and superior to the top of the ear. (**C**) Occipital parietal: 4 cm from the midline and 6 cm above the inion (external occipital protuberance). (**D**) Dandy's point: 2 cm from the midline and 3 cm above the inion. (**E**) Orbital: 1–2 cm behind the orbital rim. (**F**) Supraorbital: 4 cm above the orbital rim in the plane of the pupil. *Abbreviation*: CSF, cerebrospinal fluid. *Source*: From Ref. 10.

misplacement into important structures causing brain tissue damage, intracerebral hematoma, intraventricular hemorrhage and infection (12). The probability of clogging the ventricular catheter increases if it is left open in a collapsed ventricle, and it is not possible to monitor ICP with a ventriculostomy while it is left open to drain. In the setting of trauma we recommend one- to two-minute periods of drainage for ICPs >20 mmHg, with reclamping the catheter if no CSF is drained. This allows for CSF to build in the ventricle and the ICP measurements in the interim.

Richmond Bolt

The Richmond (subdural-subarachnoid) bolt usually consists of a certain type of hollow screw with its tip passing through the dura and thus projecting 1–2 mm below the inner table of the skull and gets seated adjacent to the arachnoid, covering the brain surface. If the bolt is seated to superficial position, there is a risk of dislodgement and/or loss of pressure (Fig. 4). If it is seated too deeply the brain

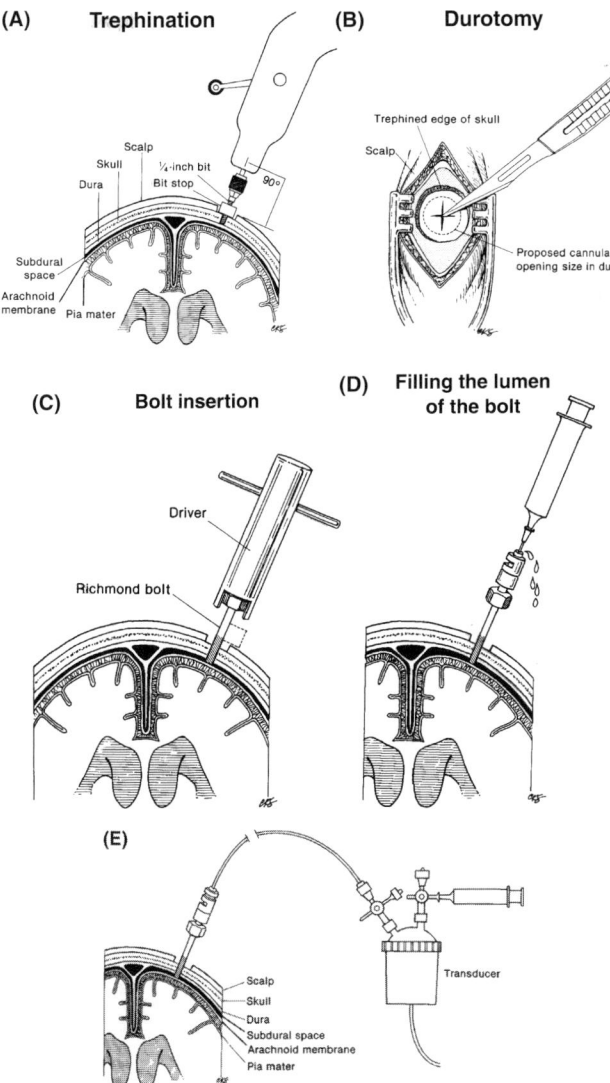

(A) Trephination   **(B) Durotomy**

(C) Bolt insertion   **(D) Filling the lumen of the bolt**

(E)

Figure 4 Richmond bolt trephination (**A**), durotomy (**B**), insertion (**C**), air evacuation (**D**), and completion (**E**). Trephination (**A**) is accomplished with a 1/4-inch bit, care being taken not to lacerate the dura or plunge into the brain. Following trephination, the wound is thoroughly irrigated to remove all debris. Durotomy (**B**) is performed in a cruciate fashion using a No. 11 blade. The two arms of the durotomy completely cross the orifice in the skull so that the resulting opening in the dura is of maximal size. Care is taken to leave the underlying arachnoid membrane intact. Insertion (**C**) is accomplished using the special driver; the bolt is screwed into the skull at right angle so that the tip projects 1–2 mm below the inner table. Air evacuation (**D**) is accomplished by gently filling the lumen of the bolt with nonbacteriostatic normal saline solution; continue until no air bubbles remain. The Richmond bolt monitoring system is completed when connected to the transducer as shown in (**E**). *Source*: From Ref. 10.

surface may be penetrated leading to herniation into the hollow screw and plugging up the system in the process.

The advantages of the Richmond bolt are its simple insertion technique and lack of brain tissue penetration. On the other hand, the bolt cannot be used to lower the ICP by CSF drainage, it can produce infection, epidural bleeding, and focal seizures. Furthermore, a blockage can occur in the

tubing, and the recording may get diminished or lost. Indeed, a significant shortcoming of the Richmond bolt is its tendency to become occluded with wound debris, dura and/or blood.

Epidural Intracranial Pressure Monitors

Two types of epidural ICP monitors have been developed. One uses a pressure sensitive membrane contacting the dura, and the other system uses a pressure sensitive pneumatic switch that deforms as the dura changes. Although the risk of infection to the brain is lower because of the extradural placement, there are several disadvantages, which include technically difficult placement, bleeding, difficult calibration after placement, and inability to conduct the drain of the CSF therapeutically.

Intraparenchymal Intracranial Pressure Monitors

✂ **Intraparenchymal devices, for example, Camino® ICP monitors (Camino Laboratories, San Diego, California, U.S.A.), use a catheter that is inserted within cortical gray matter, which allows direct measurement of brain tissue pressure.** ✂

A right frontal site is usually chosen for insertion and, because the intraventricular insertion (using Kocher's point) is not required, any cosmetic site in the lateral, frontal region can be used (Fig. 5A). After trephination, the barrel is threaded into the skull until it comes up against the plastic stop, leaving its distal tip 1 to 2 mm below the inner table of the skull (Fig. 5B). After creating a small hole in the dura, the fiberoptic sensor is zeroed and then inserted until the 5 cm mark is aligned with the top of the barrel, which typically places the distal end of the fiberoptic sensor 10 to 15 mm into the brain parenchyma (Fig. 5D). Newly developed intraparenchymal fiberoptic devices sense changes in the amount of light reflected off a pressure sensitive diaphragm that is located at the tip; and pressure can be displayed digitally on the device (Figs. 5E and 5G). Output cables can also be used to send data to a standard operating room (OR) or intensive care unit (ICU) monitor, allowing real time display of ICP waveforms (5,13,14).

In comparison to a ventriculostomy, Camino monitors are easier to insert and the intraparenchmal probe is of a small diameter, generally causing imperceptible neurologic injury. The advantages of this device are that infection is minimized, and that leaks and catheter occlusion are nonexistent. In addition, errors due to transducer malpositioning are minimized. The main disadvantage of this device is that it cannot be recalibrated after placement and drift may occur, necessitating the replacement of the fiberoptic probe under sterile conditions. The most significant limitation of the fiberoptic device is that it cannot be used for therapeutic CSF drainage (14).

In the setting of trauma, when the ICP is increased and the ventricles are compressed, only a small amount of CSF egress is seen during ventriculostomy placement. This occurs from collapse of the ventricle around the catheter, and if it is not recognized, the catheter may be withdrawn, and it will be impossible to recannulate the ventricle at that time. In this situation, the catheter should be left in place and an additional second monitor such as the Camino should be placed to monitor the ICP. When the intraventricular catheter begins to drain as CSF collects in the ventricle, one of the two monitors may then be removed depending upon the clinical situation.

Intracranial Pressure Waveforms

✂ **The normal ICP waveform is pulsatile and coincident with the cardiac cycle. However, the entire baseline rises**

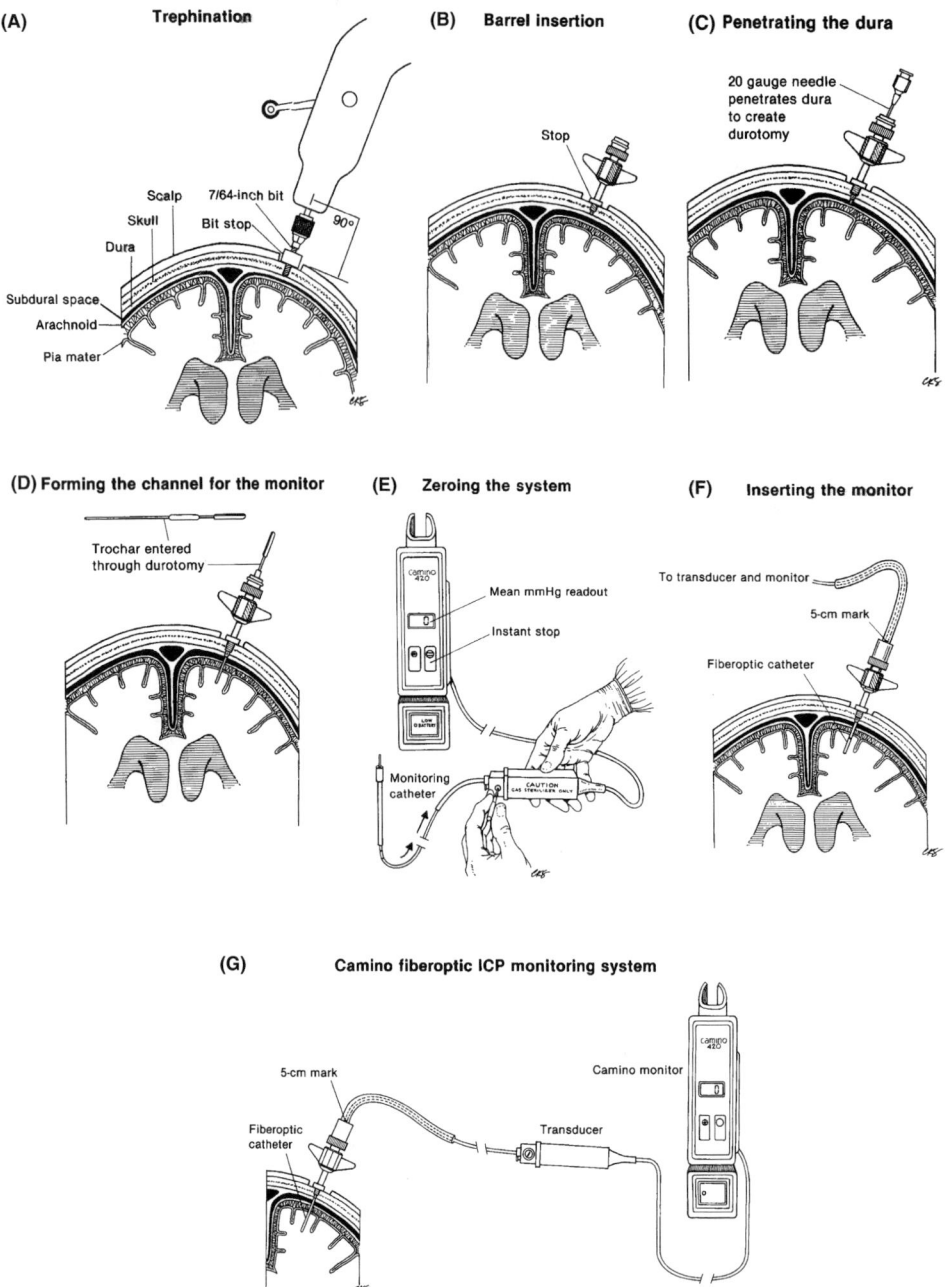

Figure 5   Insertion of the Camino fiberoptic intracranial pressure (ICP) monitoring system including trephination (**A**), barrel insertion (**B**), dural penetration (**C**), channel formation (**D**), zeroing (**E**), insertion (**F**), and completion (**G**). Trephination (**A**) is accomplished with a 7/64-inch bit, with care taken not to lacerate the dura or plunge into the brain. Following trephination, the wound is thoroughly irrigated to remove all debris. The barrel is screwed into the skull (**B**) until it comes up on the stop mounted on the device to control the depth of insertion. The dura is penetrated (**C**) with a 20-gauge needle passed only deep enough to create a small durotomy. Forming the channel for the monitor (**D**) is accompanied by passing the supplied trochar through the barrel and the durotomy as far as the trochar design allows. This forms a cavity for the monitor, which extends 15 mm beyond the tip of the barrel. Zeroing the system (**E**) must occur prior to insertion of the monitor. To accomplish this, the system is connected to the transducer and the small slotted knob is adjusted with the supplied screwdriver until the system is set to zero. Inserting the monitor (**F**) occurs after zeroing is accomplished. The monitor is passed through the barrel until the 5-cm mark is at the top. At this point, the catheter tip will project 13 mm beyond the tip of the barrel and will not touch the tip of the tissue cavity. The knurled knob is gently tightened to secure the fiberoptic catheter in place, and the collar is slid down over the top of the barrel, sealing the system. The complete Camino fiberoptic ICP monitoring system is shown in (**G**). *Source*: From Ref. 10.

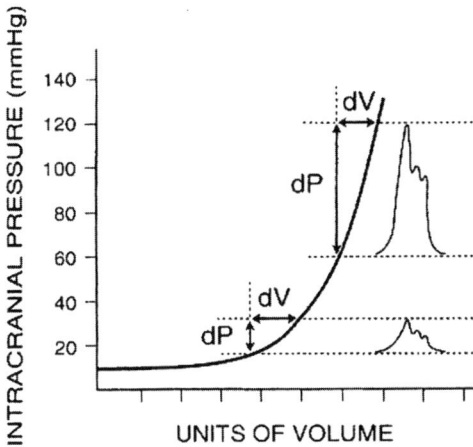

Figure 6 The intracranial pressure (ICP) volume (elastance) curve. Elastance is defined as the change (delta) in pressure (dP) for a unit change in volume (dV). The term elastance (dP/dV) is the inverse of compliance (dV/dP). The ICP waveform results from the arterial (and to a lesser extent venous) pressure waveforms occurring with the cardiac cycle, when the brain is compliant (low elastance), the dP/dV is small, whereas when the brain is noncompliant the elastance is large (i.e., the dP/dV is large), and the ICP waveforms have both a higher baseline, and a higher pulse pressure. *Source*: From Ref. 15.

and falls in concert with the respiratory cycle (as do all physiologic fluid waveforms). ☞ The normal fluctuations in the ICP waveform are characterized as having three pressure peaks (Fig. 6) (15). The initial, also the tallest peak (P_1) is due to the arterial pulsation transmitted to the brain parynchyma and CSF. The second peak (P_2) is termed as the tidal or rebound wave and reflects intracranial compliance. The third peak (P_3) is almost always lower than P_2, and is called the dicrotic wave representing venous pulsations that is transmitted to the brain. In the normal compliant brain the magnitude of pressure wave is small whereas, in tight brains the change in pressure with any change in volume (dP/dV) is large. Besides these characteristic three-peaked ICP waveforms, which occur with the cardiac cycle, additional changes to the entire baseline occur with alterations in intracranial compliance. Furthermore, changes in baseline occur with ventilation as follows: In the spontaneously breathing patient, inhalation decreases intrathoracic pressure and promotes venous drainage (lowering ICP). Whereas, exhalation leads to decreased venous outflow from the cranium causing increased ICP. The opposite is true with positive pressure ventilation. As ICP rises and cerebral compliance decreases (from any cause), the venous components disappear and the arterial pulses become more pronounced.

In 1960, Lundberg reported the results of direct ICP monitoring by means of ventriculostomy in 143 patients (11). In his report he outlined the pathophysiology and clinical significance of three pathologic ICP waveform patterns designated as "A" waves, "B" waves, and "C" waves.

Lundberg "A" waves, also known as plateau waves, are characterized by a steep ICP elevation to >50 mmHg lasting for two minutes to 20 minutes followed by an abrupt fall to initial ICP levels. Usually the new baseline is slightly higher after the "A" wave. These "A" waves recur with increasing frequency, duration, and amplitude and often occur with a simultaneous increase in mean arterial pressure. Lundberg recognized these waves as harbingers of impending uncontrollable ICP, probably resulting from an exhaustion of intracranial compliance and buffering capacity (Fig. 7A).

Lundberg "B" waves, also known as pressure pulses, are characterized by ICP elevations of 10 to 20 mm lasting between 30 seconds to two minutes. These waves are variations with types of periodic breathing and are more frequently seen with increased ICP and decreased intracranial compliance. Note the relationship is not entirely consistent and represents a qualitative finding during ICP elevations (Fig. 7B).

Lundberg "C" waves, reflecting Traube-Hering arterial waves, are characterized by variable ICP elevations with a frequency of four to eight per minute. They may represent preterminal state and are occasionally seen on top of plateau waves. Similar to "B" waves, they are suggestive but not pathognomonic of increased ICP (Fig. 7C) (11).

Currently the emphasis is on the early recognition and successful treatment of ICP elevations. Accordingly, the aforementioned Lundberg pathologic ("A", "B", and "C") pressure waves are infrequently seen. However, when they are seen in patients who are resistant to therapeutic interventions, they portend worse outcomes.

BRAIN ELECTRICAL ACTIVITY
Electroencephalogram

The electrical activity of the brain recorded by surface electroencephalogram (EEG) originates in the superficial layers of the cerebral cortex. Electrical activity of deep neurons adds to the complexity of surface signals. The analysis of EEG tracing primarily involves determination and evaluation of signal strength (amplitude) and pattern (frequency and morphology) (16,17). EEG is valuable in the investigation of intermittent or persistent brain dysfunction and remains essential in the evaluation of epilepsy. However, the role of EEG monitoring in trauma and critical care has been limited.

The classic EEG is recorded on up to 32 channels to improve sensitivity. The arrangement of electrodes is referred to as the "montage." Different montage patterns are designed to improve signal reception from the brain area of interest (16,17).

The different EEG patterns are characterized by their voltage, frequency, morphology, distribution, symmetry, persistence, and reactivity over the scalp. Brain electrical activity is commonly categorized according to its frequency: Delta, <4 Hz; theta, 4–8 Hz; alpha, 8–12 Hz; and beta, >12 Hz (Fig. 8). In 75% to 90% of the normal population, a dominant alpha range EEG is manifested, but this may be seen in only 28% to 50% of the elderly individuals. A dominant beta range is seen in 7% to 8%, whereas, 3% to 4% show dominant activity in the theta range. Only 1% has a mixed EEG without any classifiable dominant frequency (16,17).

Effect of Anesthetic Agents, Analgesics, and Sedatives on Electroencephalogram

In the normal brain, the induction of inhaled anesthetics initially decreases alpha activity and increases beta activity. As anesthesia deepens, EEG frequency decreases further until lower-frequency theta and delta moves predominate. Further increase in anesthetic depth will lead to burst suppression. At 2 MAC isoflurane, an electrical silence can be

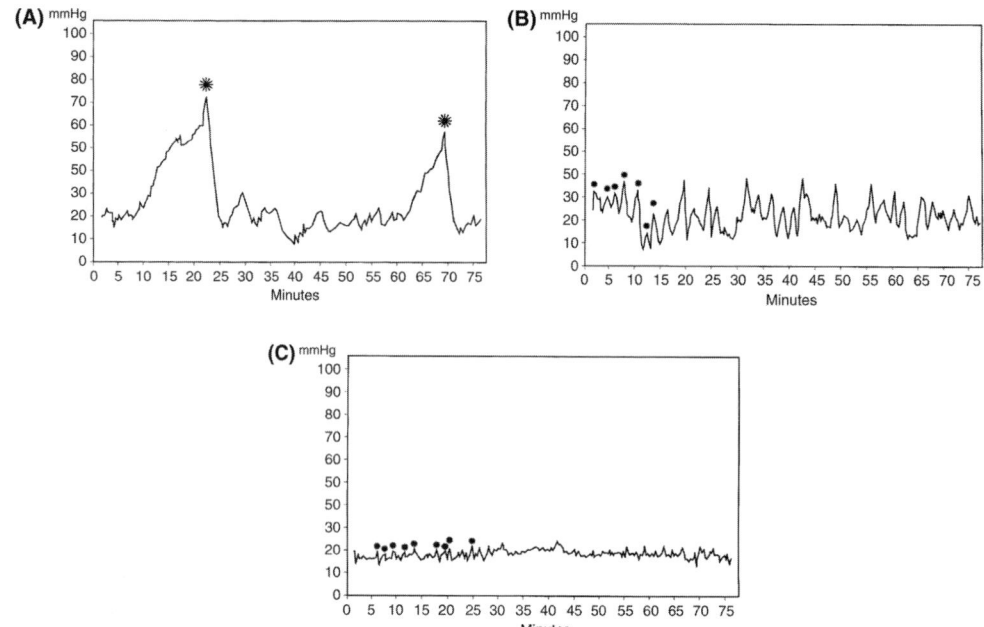

Figure 7 Lundberg's "A," "B," and "C" waves (respectively). Lundberg's "A" waves, also referred to as plateau waves (**A**), are actually intracranial pressure (ICP) waveform trends measured over 30 to 90 minutes. These ICP trends are characterized by a steep ramp up to pressures of nearly 50 to 80 mmHg, over a duration of 2 to 15 minutes. The peak ("A" wave) is followed by an abrupt fall to a new baseline slightly higher than that of the initial ICP waveform. Lundberg's "A" waveforms tend to recur at increasing frequencies, durations, and amplitudes with progressively higher baselines. Lundberg "A" waves reflect extreme compromise of intracranial compliance and are harbingers of uncontrollable ICP. Lundberg's "B" waves (**B**) are pressure pulses of 10–20 mmHg that occur at a frequency of 0.5 to 2 waves per minute. Lundberg's "B" waves illustrated in this figure are highlighted with asterisks. They usually occur in the setting of increased ICP and generally indicate decreased intracranial compliance, although in a less consistent manner than "A" waves. Lundberg's "C" waves (**C**) are ICP waveforms reflecting arterial Traube-Hering waves. They suggest diminished intracranial compliance in a qualitative fashion similar to "B" waves. "C" waves illustrated in this figure are highlighted with asterisks. *Source*: From Ref. 10.

noticed. These deep anesthetic charges are similar to hypothermia and brain death.

In lower doses, narcotics tend to increase the amplitude of alpha and beta frequencies. In higher doses, theta and delta bands develop, indicating sedation. Very high narcotic levels result in a steady decline in EEG frequency until delta predominates. Burst suppression does not occur with narcotics. At extremely high doses, seizure, like activity has been recorded in dogs and rodents (18) (also seen with high normeperidine levels in humans). However, in the absence of normeperidine, narcotics have not reproducibly caused convulsive seizures in humans (19,20). Although epileptiform activity (21) and temporal lobe activation (18) have been reported in humans, these changes are not analogous to seizures.

In low doses, benzodiazepines and barbiturates cause a decrease in the percentage of alpha waves, and an increase in the beta activity. At high doses, theta and delta activities predominate. In very high doses, they can cause periods of electrical silence interspersed with brief episodes of activity this pattern is termed burst suppression. The EEG verification of burst suppression is valuable when determining the dose that is required to induce and maintain barbiturate coma (22).

Etomidate and propofol administration alters EEG tracings in a fashion similar to barbiturates. In small doses (0.1 mg/kg) etomidate enhances interictal activity of seizure foci. However, the myoclonic activity sometimes seen with etomidate is not related to seizures. In higher

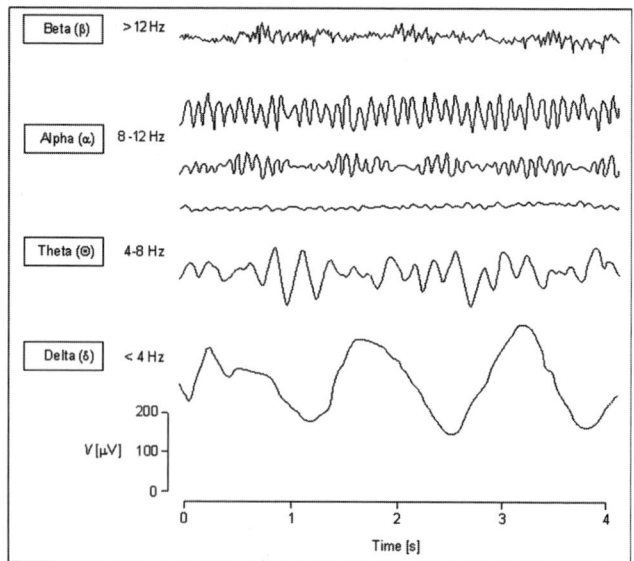

Figure 8 Electroencephalogram waves illustrated and labeled according to their classic frequency related distributions. Delta waves have frequencies <4 Hz but typically have higher amplitudes than beta or theta waves. Theta waves have frequencies between 8 and 12 Hz and typically have varying amplitude as shown. Beta waves have the highest frequencies (>12 Hz), but are low in amplitude. *Source*: From Ref. 150.

doses, etomidate causes EEG slowing and ultimately burst suppression. Propofol produces an increase in the alpha rhythm initially, followed by an increase in theta and delta activity, and finally (at very high doses) burst suppression (23). With regard to dexmedetomidine, human EEG data are not well characterized. However in the rat, dexmedetomidine causes progressive slowing of EEG with increasing doses of drug and some enhancements in amplitude (similar to the effects seen with opioids) (24).

Electroencephalogram Changes Resulting from Critical Care Events

In addition to the pharmacological effects, physiological changes can cause important EEG effects (25,26). It is essential that any EEG changes should be interpreted within the clinical context in which they are observed.

Carbon Dioxide, Oxygen, and Body Temperature

Hypocarbia causes slowing of the EEG and increased susceptibility to sedative/hypnotic drugs. Mild hypercarbia (5–20% above normal) causes decreased cerebral excitability and an increased seizure threshold. High level (30% above normal) results in increased cerebral excitability and epileptic activity. Very high levels (50% above normal) produce EEG depression (27).

Hyperoxia causes a low amplitude and fast frequency EEG pattern, characteristic of (but not essentially indicative of) cerebral excitation. Decreased brain oxygenation initially causes increased cerebral excitability. If hypoxia persists to cause anoxic death of enough brain cells, burst suppression or diffuse alpha pattern may emerge (both also seen in drug intoxication) (28). With brain and brainstem death EEG slows further, ultimately resulting in EEG silence (17,28).

Cerebral Blood Flow

✐ **The EEG has never been demonstrated to correlate with CBF except at very low levels.** ✐ Specifically, EEG changes begin to occur when CBF decreases <30% of normal (Fig. 9) (29). However, the EEG threshold for detection of ischemia in injured brain is unknown. Additionally, at the threshold of electrical failure, aerobic metabolism may still be occurring. Most clinical studies of EEG and CBF have occurred during carotid endarterectomy (30–32). Overall, neurological outcome is more dependent on the duration of anaerobic flow deficits than on the EEG changes, during the periods of low flow (29–32). Nonetheless, the EEG has certain value as a warning that CBF may be decreasing, thereby reaching a dangerous level.

Brain Death

Persistent EEG electrical silence is characteristic of, but not pathognomonic of brain death (33–35). However, barbiturate coma, metabolic dysfunction (e.g., hepatic encephalopathy), severe hypothermia (temperature <18°C), and other confounding factors may also produce cerebral electrical silence on EEG. Indeed, hypothermia causes progressive slowing of brain activity below 35°C. Complete EEG silence occurs with marked hypothermia (below 18°C) (36–39). ✐ **Because an EEG silence pattern is not specific for brain death, it should never be used exclusively to diagnose brain death, but rather only as a confirmatory test.** ✐ Particularly in the presence of any of these confounding factors, other confirming data (e.g., brain flow study) must be used to make the diagnosis of brain death (see Volume 2, Chapter 16).

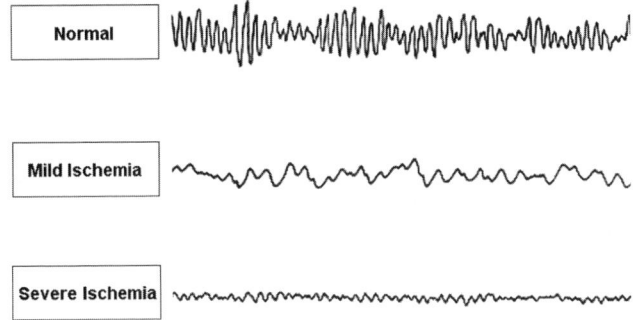

Figure 9 Detection of cerebral ischemia with electroencephalogram (EEG) monitoring. The normal adult brain has baseline EEG waveforms in the alpha range (8–12 Hz). With increasing ischemia the waveform slows some into the theta range (4–8 Hz), and the amplitude continues to diminish until electrical silence ultimately occurs (not shown). *Source*: From Ref. 151.

Processed Electroencephalogram Monitoring

Difficulty in using and interpreting the multichannel raw EEG stimulated the development of computerized processing of EEG data. The processed EEG generally does not employ many scalp electrodes to generate a satisfactory signal and typically uses adhesive contact electrodes that are easily replaceable. These electrodes have to be placed across the forehead. However, needles or standard cup electrodes can also be used.

Several signal processing techniques have been utilized; including compressed spectral array (CSA), power spectrum, zero cross, and a periodic analysis (40). The EEG signal is usually digitized, processed, and then graphically displayed. Advanced signal analyses such as source localization, quantitative EEG brain mapping, and high-resolution EEG are being developed, but their clinical applications are not yet fully defined (40).

✐ **The advantage of the processed EEG is that the real-time analysis can quickly interpreted with minimal training, resulting in a more rapid detection of clinical problems (e.g., ischemia, seizure), and institution of the treatment.** ✐

The processed EEG is potentially valuable in the ICU because it can be used to continuously monitor abnormal electrical activity and also the EEG effects of a given therapy, thus improving the titration of interventions in intensive care patients (40,41). For example, processed EEG monitoring can be used to assess and adjust sedation. Severe pain or discomfort increases EEG activity in the higher frequencies and increases the amplitude across all bands diffusely; while mildly sedated patients show decreased alpha and increased beta amplitude, and heavily sedated ones show decreased frequency and amplitudeacross all bands (40). Also, processed EEG may be useful for ischemia detection but sensitivity is decreased by electrode location and number of channels. Advanced signal analyses such as source localization, quantitative EEG brain mapping, and high-resolution EEG are being developed, but their clinical applications are not yet fully defined (26).

Bispectral Electroencephalogram Signal Processing and Monitoring

The bispectral index (BIS) is a complex EEG parameter composed by using statistical data analysis to identify the components of the EEG that were found to correlate with the clinical depth of sedation and amnesia with high accuracy and reproducibility (42). These data were normalized to a unitless scale from zero (no EEG activity) to 100 (awake). Its ability to measure these endpoints is thought to be significantly better than assessment by usual clinical signs alone (42). ☞ **Intraoperative experience shows that anesthetic drugs can be titrated to a specific quantitative endpoint (BIS monitor range of 50–60); to avoid recall, a level between 60 and 80 can be chosen if sedation and amnesia are the desired endpoints in the ICU (42–47).** ☞

Evoked Potentials

Nerve stimulation to evoke responses is used for monitoring the functional integrity of specific sensory and motor pathways. An evoked potential (EP) is an event gated sequential recording and averaging of multiple EEG traces in repetitive specified time epochs. Each EEG epoch is a reproducible EEG response to a specific stimulus that tests a certain neural pathway. EP technology has a specific nomenclature for waveform description: polarity (negative, positive), latency (msec), amplitude (mV), etc. (Fig. 10) (48).

☞ **Compromise of a neurological pathway is manifested as an increase in the latency, or a decrease in the amplitude of EPs, or both.** ☞ Various types of EPs have been used for many years in the OR. There is an increasing interest in the use of evoked potentials as monitors in ICUs (48,49). It has not yet achieved the anticipated widespread use due to technological complexity, required skills, relative patient discomfort, and signal deterioration with patient movement and/or use of sedatives (though etomidate tends to increase EPs). However, newer techniques may allow more robust signal monitors for the ICU, thus these neuro monitoring techniques will be reviewed here.

Brainstem Auditory Evoked Potentials

Brain stem auditory evoked potentials (BAEPs) are performed by the application of audible clicks to the ears by headphones or earplugs secured into one ear canal, while

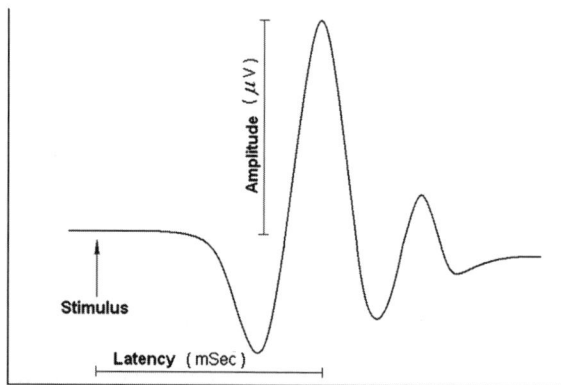

Figure 10 Evoked potential (EP) waveform. The latency is the duration in milliseconds (msec) between the stimulus and the EP waveform. The amplitude is typically recorded in microvolts (μV), but varies according to the type of EP. For example, somatosensory evoked potentials typically have amplitudes in the 1 to 3 μV range, whereas motor evoked potentials (MEPs) typically have amplitudes that range between 5 μV (neurogenic MEPs) and 25 μV (epidural MEPs), all the way up to 500 μV (myogenic MEPs).

white noise is used to mask the opposite ear (50). BAEPs are relatively resistant to drug effects. Benzodiazepines have been reported to have minimal effects, decreasing amplitude and increasing latency (51). However, no correlation between early latency BAEP and the presence of amnesia has been shown but there is probably a correlation with late latency BAEP (52). Analgesic opioids have no significant effects on amplitude or latency (53). Propofol may increase BAEPs latency minimally without changes in amplitude (54). In summary, drug-induced alterations to BAEPs are generally not very substantial. Thus BAEPs can be used to assess brainstem function in a patient treated with various CNS depressants in the ICU.

Visual Evoked Potentials

Visual evoked potentials (VEPs) are recorded by applying flashing lights to the eyes. In patients who are sedated or unconscious, the eyelids must be taped shut and the light is then applied through the closed lid or by light-emitting contact lenses applied under the lid. These patients present a challenge for recording VEPs because they cannot focus their eyes. Therefore, VEPs are technically difficult to obtain and questions have risen about their usefulness in monitoring. Also, VEPs are more sensitive than the other EP modalities, to the effects of different drugs further diminishing their usefulness in critical care (48).

Somatosensory Evoked Potentials

Somatosensory evoked potentials (SSEPs) electrodes usually are applied to the median, ulnar, peroneal, or tibial nerves (55). SSEPs are mainly used in the OR to monitor the spinal cord ascending pathways, functional integrity during spine surgery. SSEPs are also used to assess deep brain structures during some vascular neurosurgical procedures. SSEPs use in critical care is still not as common as a monitor. SSEPs are more sensitive to the effects of CNS depressant drugs than BAEPs (55). Benzodiazepines were reported to cause decreased amplitude and increase latency (56–58). Opioids have been reported to produce no effect or minimal increase in latencies and decrease in amplitude even in high doses (59–61). Propofol produces depression of SSEPs, but it still allows effective monitoring (62,63), whereas, etomidate increases SSEP amplitude (55).

Motor Evoked Potentials

Motor evoked potentials (MEPs) can be produced by direct (epidural) or indirect (transosseous) stimulation of the brain or spinal cord by either electrical or magnetic stimulation, causing contralateral peripheral nerve signals, electromyographic signals, or overt muscle contractions (64). MEPs are used to assess motor cortex, subcortical, and descending motor pathways. These are mainly used in the OR to monitor the spinal cord descending pathways, functional integrity during spine surgery. Further investigations with MEPs are needed to fully define their usefulness in critical care.

MEPs are extremely sensitive to depression by benzodiazepines, propofol, and inhaled anesthetic drugs (55). MEPs appear to be relatively unaffected by opioids and are less effected by etomidate (which actually enhances EPs) and dexmedetomidine (65,66). Neuromuscular blockade obviously affects the recorded electromyographic (EMG) response and must be carefully used (if used at all) to provide adequate monitoring conditions. Maintaining one or two twitches in a train of four can permit reliable MEP responses that has to be recorded (55,64). Due to the limitations of current technology, neither SSEPs nor MEPS are used in the ICU. However, both are used operatively (see Volume 1, Chapter 26).

Clinical Interpretation of Evoked Potential Changes in Context of Critical Care Events

The disease states commonly seen in the ICU produce EP changes due to ischemic insults and/or anatomic disruption of relevant neurological pathways. Compromise or injury of these pathways is manifest as an increase in the latency and/or a decrease in the amplitude of EP waveforms. It has been suggested that acute changes are more significant than gradual ones. Nonetheless, transient EP changes may occur without adverse effect (67). Also, in the ICU there may be considerable variability in the EP signals (related to temperature, PaO_2, $PaCO_2$, and artifacts related to nursing procedures) that make the interpretation of EP changes even more confusing.

Experimental reports of global cerebral ischemia describe monitoring of EPs to adequately reflect the integrity of CNS perfusion (68,69). Hypotension below levels of cerebral autoregulation produces progressive decreases in EP amplitudes until the waveform is completely lost (70). In addition, SSEPs have been noted to correlate with the severity of neurological deficits after cerebral ischemia (71,72). Persistence of SSEP waveforms, however, does not ensure the absence of infarction risk in nonmonitored areas. It has been shown that BAEPs are less sensitive than SSEPs to ischemia.

Several animal studies suggest that SSEPs can be used to detect focal ischemia (73,74). They have been used intraoperatively for that purpose (75), but up to date there have been few reports for EP use in the intensive care unit (76). In the ICU, EPs may find a role to monitor patients at risk of stroke (patients with transient ischemic attacks) or worsening of new strokes, to possibly assess the effects of peri-infarct edema, and in patients who already received thrombolytic therapy for probable recurrences (76).

Vasospasm can occur after subarachnoid hemorrhage and is characterized by increased blood velocity and decreased blood flow. SSEPs can be used to detect the onset of vasospasm (77,78). However, transcranial Dopplers (discussed later) are a better noninvasive monitor for vasospasm.

EPs are not yet developed to the degree that they can provide a prognosis of patients with head injuries. EPs are diminished in the setting of increased ICP (79,80). However, the minimal ICP required to begin altering EP signals is approximately 30 mmHg (81). Marked BAEPs changes occur with herniation (82). Thus, EPs lag behind other indicators such as IEP and Glasgow coma score in detecting danger or predicting the neurological outcome (83–85).

SSEPs can be used to monitor spinal cord integrity and may also be able to suggest prognosis after injury. Patients with spinal cord injury can experience ascent of the level of their deficit showing "spinal cord injury Potentials" (SCIPs) (55). SSEPs can be a useful device to detect progression of a deficit and instituting therapies to prevent or reverse this process (86). MEPs can be monitored in conjunction with SSEPs to evaluate the functional integrity of both motor and sensory pathways, although studies suggest that changes in only one modality are rare (55,87). EPs have not totally been studied in a controlled fashion for ICU monitoring of, spinal cord, and their utility remains to be studied.

Occasionally patients do not arouse quickly after lengthy neurosurgery even after procedures without expected anatomic neurological problem and an uneventful anesthesia. In this case, the routine postoperative neurological assessment cannot be performed in a satisfactory manner. In the setting of an unchanged brain CT, EPs may become useful in these unconscious patients to confirm the integrity of the central nervous system, until they regain consciousness (88,89).

Several reports document that EPs change with brain death, especially BAEP, which disappear in 80% of clinically brain dead subjects. Continuous BAEP monitoring may alert clinicians of the onset of brain death, sooner, and thus facilitate earlier decisions regarding organ donation (i.e., before hemodynamic instability ensues) (90–92). However, EPs cannot be used as a sole determinant of brain death. Accordingly, a change in EP is best used to trigger a review of patient status using other modalities.

CEREBRAL BLOOD FLOW
Transcranial Doppler Ultrasonography

✐ Transcranial Doppler (TCD) is a noninvasive method that uses sound waves for measuring CBF velocity. ✐ The waveform displayed is related to the velocity and flow direction of the blood and provides real-time, beat-to-beat information. TCD has been used in the ICU to detect cerebral vasospasm and determine its severity, following subarachnoid hemorrhage or aneurysm clipping (93–96). As a cerebral artery constricts, velocity of blood flow within the lumen increases to maintain blood flow. Mean velocity of the middle cerebral artery (MCA) blood flow over 120 cm/sec generally correlates with the presence of vasospasm by cerebral angiography (Fig. 11). TCD may also be helpful in monitoring head injured patients who go through three phases postinjury: hypoperfusion, hyperemia, and vasospasm (97,98).

Another important potential application of TCD is in stroke. TCD provides a reasonably accurate way to characterize the vascular system in ischemic stroke. Moreover, TCD can also detect cerebral emboli and provide information that can aid in making the needed therapeutic decisions. Embolic events are unpredictable, infrequent, and may or may not be symptomatic. Thus, TCD monitoring may be used in the future to detect, count, and measure the size of cerebral emboli (99–101).

TCD has also been used as a screening aid in the diagnosis of brain death. TCD in brain death shows a characteristic blood flow pattern with brief systolic inflow of blood followed by flow reversal in diastole (Fig. 12). Because the dead brain no longer has blood flowing to the parenchyma, the MCA takes a brief inflow of blood during systole and distends (but does not transmit blood further into the brain), and that blood then exits the MCA during diastole (flow reversal). TCD cannot be used as a sole determinant for brain death. Nonetheless, observation of normal TCD waveform, in some cases, can be used to rule out the diagnosis of brain death (102–105).

All intravenous anesthetics (except for ketamine) decrease CBF. Thiopental, propofol, and benzodiazepines tend to decrease cerebral flow velocity (CFV), while narcotics have little increase or no effect on CFV (106). It must be noted that many other physiological variables (e.g., temperature, hypoxia, hyper- or hypocarbia, hematocrit level, and

(A)
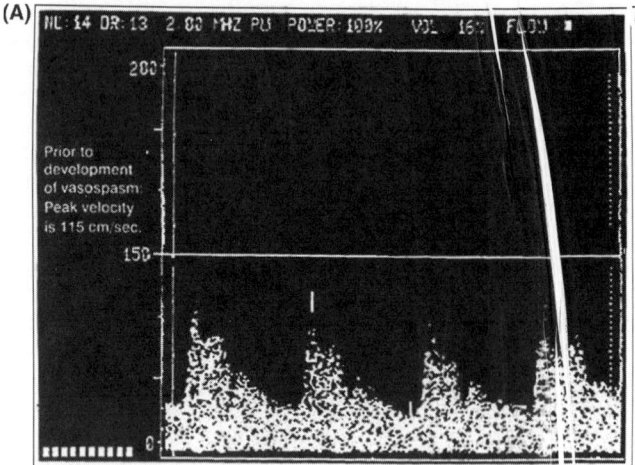

(B)
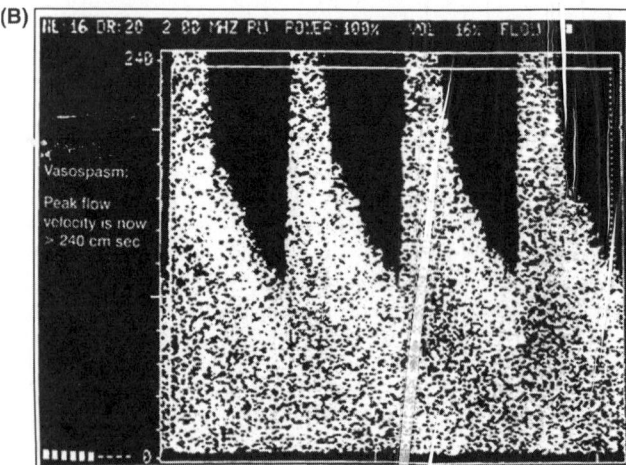

Figure 11   Transcranial Doppler (TCD) waves before (**A**) and after (**B**) the onset of cerebral vasospasm. Flow is shown on the X axis. Above zero is forward flow, and below zero is reverse flow. The top TCD profile (**A**) has a scale of 0 to 200 cm/sec with record flow peak velocity at 115 cm./sec. The bottom TCD profile (**B**), demonstrates vasospasm with peak velocities above scale (>240 cm/sec). *Source*: From Ref. 151.

atherosclerotic vascular disease) can also affect TCD values (106,107).

Laser Doppler Velocimetry/Flowmetry

The laser Doppler technique measures blood flow in the microvasculature. This technique depends on the Doppler principle where emitted light is scattered by moving red blood cells. As a consequence it is either reflected, or detected, or both after the wave frequency has changed. The Doppler frequency shift is processed to provide a blood flow measurement in the microvasculature. Scanning of tissues enables blood flow mapping, and color coded images of the blood flow can be displayed. The term commonly used to describe blood flow measured by the laser Doppler technique is "flux." Regions of interest can be defined and statistical data calculated and recorded. Assessments can be made using invasive procedures (needle fiber-optic probe) or noninvasive with skin probes on the forehead (108,109).

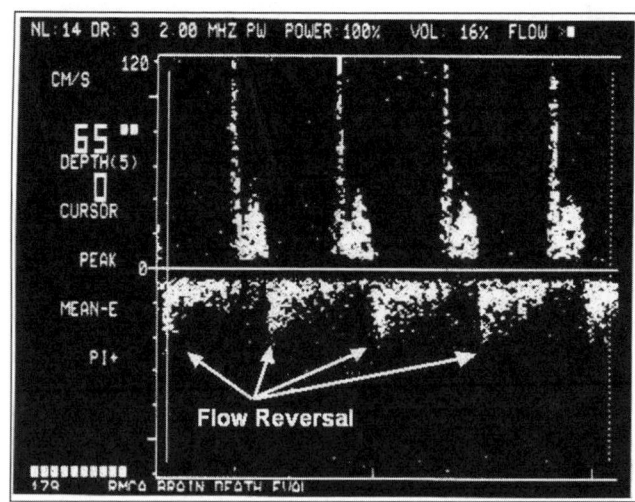

Figure 12   Reversal of transcranial Doppler (TCD) wave flow during diastole characterizing brain death. The top TCD profile shown has a scale of 0 to 120 cm/sec, above zero is forward flow, below zero is backward flow. During systole, a brief inflow of blood occurs in the middle cerebral artery (MCA), but due to the lack of forward flow beyond that point (due to brain death), the distended MCA expels its contained blood during diastole (flow reversal). *Source*: From Ref. 151.

Cerebral Angiography

The development of other noninvasive diagnostic modalities and the advancements in CT and magnetic resonance imaging (MRI) technology has diminished the use of angiography. Angiography uses X-ray imaging of the cerebral vessels after injection of a contrast medium via a catheter threaded into the carotid and/or vertebral arteries. Digital subtraction angiography (DSA) can show the vessels in isolation by subtraction of bone images, and portable units may soon find utility in the ICU (110). Potential risks are reaction to the contrast material, bleeding from puncture site and stroke by dislodged plaques or injury to cerebral vessels, followed by vasospasm or thrombosis (97,111).

Perfusion Computed Tomography (Helical Computed Tomography with Contrast Injection)

Continuous movement of the gantry of a CT scanner during ultrafast signal acquisition can create helical CT images. Overlapping the resulting two-dimensional (2-D) images creates virtual high-resolution, three-dimensional (3-D) images. Typical perfusion 3-D CTs have been carried out with intravenous bolus injection of contrast media. Helical CT scan can be extremely useful in the diagnosis of intracranial lesions and vascular abnormalities, but is not as important in most TBI patients (Fig. 14) (112–114).

Magnetic Resonance Angiography

The development of MRI has led to much of the progress in the diagnosis and management of neurological disorders (115). MRI is a form of tissue analysis in which magnetic field waves are applied and their resonance is analyzed to probe tissue characteristics. Magnetic resonance angiography (MRA) has also become a clinically useful tool; selective MRA provides information about the origin and direction of flow and circulation in collateral vessels, including the ability to visualize aneurysms and arterial venous malformations (AVMs) (Fig. 13) (115–117).

Xenon-Enhanced Computed Tomography

Improvements in CT technology using inhaled xenon as a radio-dense substance allowed acquiring three parameters describing the cerebral hemodynamics: regional cerebral blood volume (rCBV), blood mean transit time (MTT) through cerebral capillaries, and rCBF at multiple levels (Fig. 14 and 15) (118). It has also been used for many situations, these include: autoregulation assessment following trauma, outcome prediction, detection of vasospasm (and resultant regions of ischemia), and bedside titration of blood pressure and ventilation to CBF. In general it is an excellent method to detect and quantitate the blood flow (118–120).

Xenon-133 Clearance

The inert gas xenon-133 clearance technique relates the change in radiotracer activity over time (given intravenously or by inhalation) to blood flow. It is a valuable diagnostic and prognostic tool that allows bedside measurement of rCBF. Owing to xenon rapid clearance from the brain, multiple studies can be performed on the same day (121). Early post-traumatic findings are predictive of the outcome, whereas later measurements are correlated with functional recovery. Easily operated computerized systems are now available in which data are displayed as 2-D topographic brain maps (121). Stable xenon-enhanced CT (^{S}Xe/CT) uses a non radioactive stable xenon (131) and has been well validated as a measure for rCBF (122). However, ^{S}Xe/CT-induced rCBF activation may cause overestimation of actual rCBF in both TBI and subarachnoid hemorrhage (SAH) patients (122).

Positron Emission Tomography

Positron emission tomography (PET) is a complex method of brain imaging that requires a cyclotron to provide the positron emitting isotopes. PET provides 3-D images about cerebral metabolic rate, CBF, and oxygen extractions (quantitative and functional images) (123). Recent studies are showing high correlations with neuropsychological testing (124).

Single Photon Emission Computed Tomography

Single photon emission computed tomography (SPECT) technology uses a radionuclide to obtain 3-D images of its distribution with a gamma camera and CT techniques. The resultant images qualitatively reflect the regional blood flow and may be able to predict the likelihood of ischemia. Also, SPECT can differentiate neurological symptoms due to ischemia (hypoperfusion) from epilepsy (hyperperfusion) (125,126). SPECT is easily done but lacks the quantitative accuracy of PET and xenon-based techniques.

INTRACRANIAL OXYGEN SATURATION
Jugular Bulb Venous Oxygen Saturation

Jugular bulb venous oxygen saturation (SjvO$_2$) provides a measurement of the global balance between cerebral oxygen supply and demand. SjvO$_2$ can be measured by placing a fiberoptic catheter into the jugular bulb via the internal jugular vein retrograde. Assuming CMRO$_2$ to be constant, acute changes in CBF will be reflected by the SjvO$_2$. However, smaller focal areas of cerebral ischemia

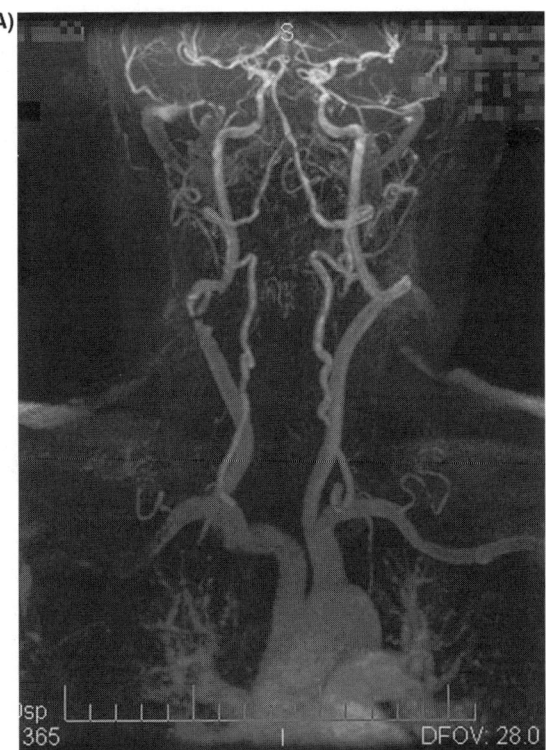
(A)

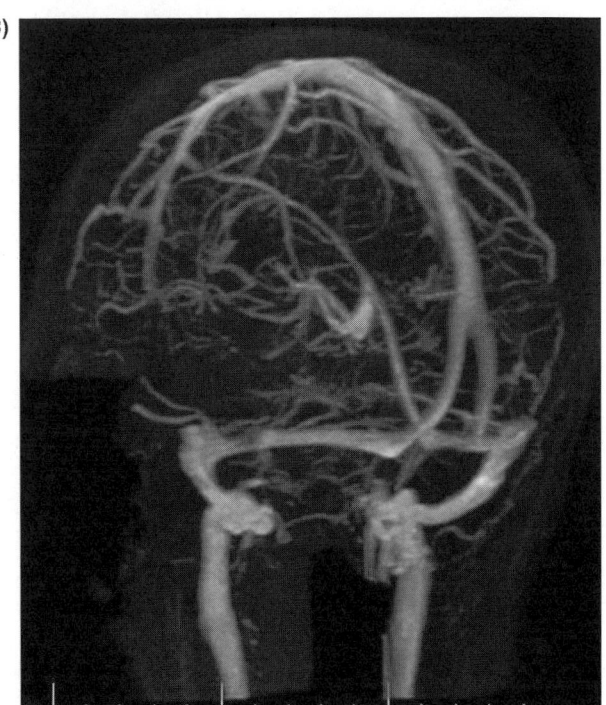
(B)

Figure 13 Magnetic resonance angiography (MRA) images of cerebral vessels. The arterial phase of the MRA image is shown in (**A**), whereas the venous phase is shown in (**B**). *Source*: From Ref. 152.

may go undetected with SjvO$_2$ monitoring (127–131). SjvO$_2$ measurements of below 50% are indicative of global cerebral ischemia. An increase in SjvO$_2$ above 85% implies either a rise in cerebral blood flow, shunting of blood away

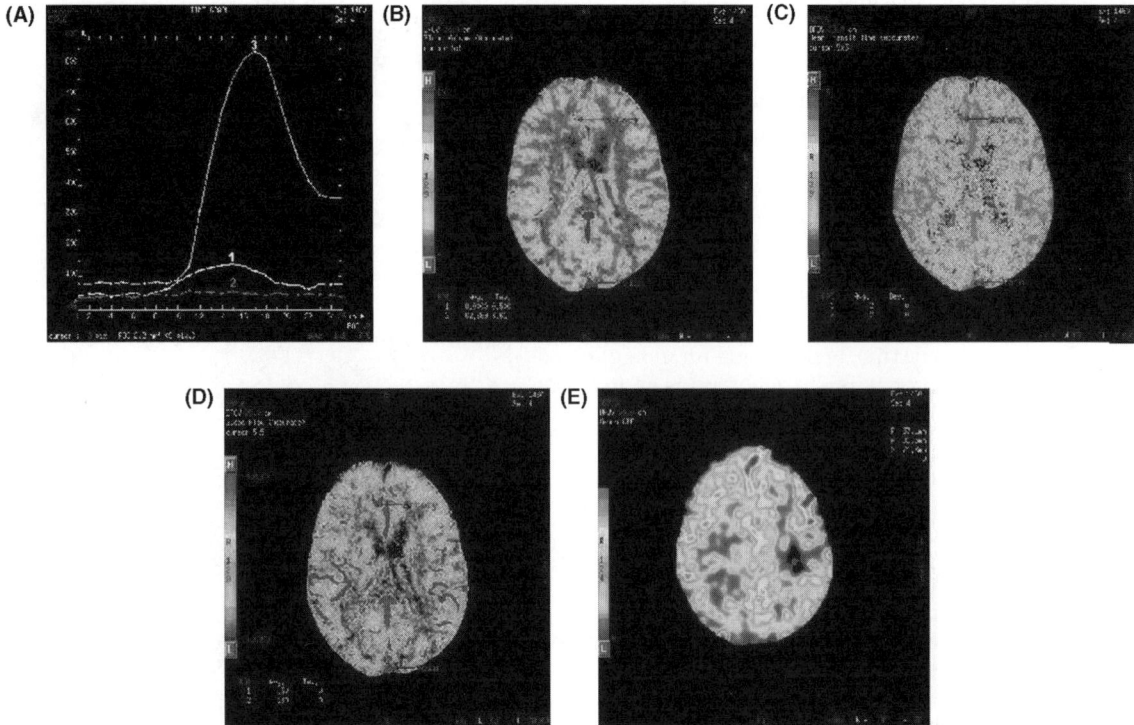

Figure 14   CT perfusional xenon enhanced computed tomography—normal brain. The output can be displayed as: (**A**) contrast media evolution in artery (curve 1), vein (curve 2), and cerebral parenchyma (curve 3); (**B**) regional cerebral blood volume; (**C**) regional cerebral mean transit time; (**D**) regional cerebral blood flow; and (**E**) xenon perfusion mapping. *Source*: From Ref. 153.

from neurons, or a decrease in cerebral metabolism as occurs in head injury, barbiturate coma, and impending brain death $SjvO_2$ monitoring is susceptible to artifacts caused by baseline drift of the catheter or by lodging of the sensor tip of the catheter against the wall of the vein.

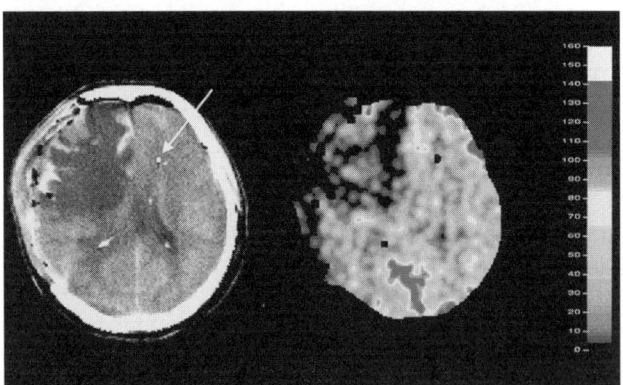

Figure 15   Xenon-enhanced computed tomography (CT)—traumatic brain injury. Xenon-enhanced CT blood flow study in a patient with severe head injury. *Left*, anatomic reference section [*arrow* indicates tip of regional cerebral blood flow (rCBF) probe]; *right*, corresponding rCBF (mL/100 g/min) image shows severe right hemispheric hypoperfusion (corresponding to the severe right-sided lesion seen on CT scan). *Source*: From Ref. 122.

Finally, areas of focal ischemia can occur with entirely normal $SjvO_2$ values (127–131).

Near Infrared Spectroscopy

Transcranial cerebral oximetry is a continuous, real-time, and noninvasive technique based on the measurement of infrared light wavelength's absorption by hemoglobin. It uses a near infrared light emitter and a dual receiver placed usually over the lateral forehead. HbO_2/Hb ratio is then determined. Interpretation principles afterwards are similar to those used with jugular bulb oxygen measuring (Fig. 16). Regional oxygen saturation (rSO_2) can thus be measured transcutaneously with near infrared spectroscopy (NIRS) to assess physiologic, pathologic, and therapeutic events. Absolute levels $<50\%$ or decrements $>10\%$ from baseline readings are thought to indicate cerebral hypoperfusion. The saturation values are representative only of the region beneath the sensor, and the presence of cerebral extravascular blood collections may interfere with the recordings or result in wrong values (132–134).

Brain Tissue PO_2 Probes

✍ **Microprobes can be inserted directly into the brain parenchyma to measure PO_2, PCO_2, pH, temperature, and many other variables, which indirectly indicate perfusion changes of that particular region of the brain (134).** ✍ One such monitor, the Neurotrend® Cerebral Tissue Monitoring System (Codman, Raynham, Massachusetts, U.S.A.) is commercially available, and has recently been shown to track declining brain pH and tissue PO_2 (Brain-$PtiO_2$) as brain PCO_2 and lactate (measured by microdialysis catheter—see later discussion in "Eye To The Future") increased in a feline model of fluid percussion injury (FPI) and secondary hypoxic injury (135). Insertion-related hemorrhagic and infectious complications are rare and the probes have little baseline drift (131).

Unfortunately, human studies in normal brain do not exist yet. Thus normal baseline and normal ischemic thresholds are not yet confirmed. However, decreasing human Brain-$PtiO_2$ values have correlated highly with outcome in patients with TBI (136,137). Brain tissue oxygen $PO_2 < 25$–30 mmHg is most likely an indication of impaired brain oxygenation (138). However, the anarobic threshold is probably in the range of an approximate Brain-$PtiO_2$ <20 mmHg (139).

EYE TO THE FUTURE

Recent technologies and improvement of monitoring techniques made it possible to have better, more accurate, and more user friendly equipment available for neurological monitoring in the ICU. However, most of the currently available monitors remain sensitive to interfering signals from other ICU equipment and patient movements, which causes frequent artifact recording. Improving monitor filters and sensitivity will allow better quality of signal detection and decrease both missed events and false alarms. As neurological monitors are becoming more popular every day, multimodal monitors will soon become available where different parameters can be detected simultaneously and displayed on a single monitor screen (140,141).

Pupillometry and microdialysis are two head-injury monitoring techniques on the horizon for clinical use. Quantitative pupillometry offers the possibility of measuring subtle changes in pupillary shape associated with intracranial volume expansion. Adding to the basic exam,

pupillometry aims to provide earlier and more sophisticated information about corresponding changes in brain elastance (dP/dV). A relationship exists between ICP higher than 20 mmHg and a reduction of constriction velocity of the pupil and a reduction of pupil size of less than 10% appears to be associated with increases in brain elastance (the inverse of compliance). Pupillometry is becoming a reliable technology capable of providing data on quantitative papillary function and further investigation is warranted to establish its clinical relevance and application (142).

Cerebral microdialysis catheters are a recently developed technology capable of directly measuring extracellular cerebral metabolites at the bedside (143). Microdialysis is a technique by which a fine tube is inserted into the brain that measures the concentration of chemicals in the extracellular space of the brain by mimicking the action of a blood capillary. Molecules that pass through the semipermeable membrane are collected into vials and the very small volumes are then analyzed.

Several substances can be studied, for example: energy metabolites (e.g., glucose, lactate, and pyruvate), excitatory amino acids (e.g., glutamate), and markers of cell damage (e.g., glycerol), and inflammatory substances (e.g., cytokines). In the setting of head injury reports have shown glutamate levels to increase, lactate to increase, and glucose and pyruvate levels to fall. Some studies have shown an alteration of chemical substances with the institution of therapy. Further investigation aims to detect changes in tissue chemistry at a stage when secondary brain damage can be prevented (143). Microdialysis catheters may be a useful monitor in the intensive care unit, especially in patients with head injury, epilepsy, stroke, and SAH (144–146).

Given evidence of prolonged neuromuscular blockade–induced myopathy, the use of peripheral nerve stimulators is recommended during neuromuscular blockade in the ICU (147). Nerve stimulators are an essential tool, especially during prolonged muscle relaxant infusions (148). Although specific monitors of neuromuscular junction health have not yet been developed, electrodiagnostictesting of neuromuscular disorders is continuing to evolve (149).

SUMMARY

The traditional means of clinically identifying neurological events is by conducting a periodic examination to detect neurologic deterioration. However, because of the high sensitivity of the brain to ischemia and anoxia, the reliance on intermittent examination may not immediately detect deterioration and therefore risks neurological damage to the patient.

Various neurological monitors are effective in detecting impending changes in brain electrical activity, cerebral ischemia, and anoxia, which make it possible that the onset of such neurological insult maybe detected earlier. It was proven that using these monitors in the ICU has dramatically improved the quality of patient care and outcomes.

Selection of the monitored parameter and modality depends on the clinical setting, diagnosis, and expected sequelae. However, frequent neurological examinations remain the gold standard of care.

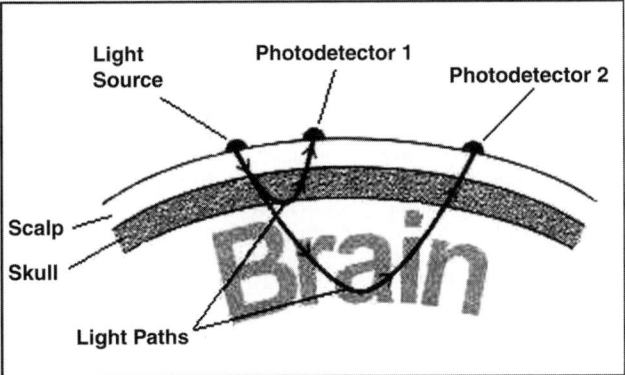

Figure 16 Schematic representation of near infrared spectroscopy (NIRS). The NIRS probe contains a light source and two photodetectors. Photodetector 1 detects infrared light absorption of scalp/extracranial blood and photodetector 2 detects infrared light absorption of both cerebral and extracranial blood. Cerebral oxygenation is calculated by subtracting absorption measured at detector 1 from that measured at detector 2. *Source*: From Ref. 151.

KEY POINTS

☞ The cerebral perfusion pressure (CPP) is equal to the difference between mean arterial pressure (MAP) and ICP (CPP = MAP − ICP). Accordingly, any decrease in MAP or increase in ICP will result in a decrease in CPP.

☞ The intraventricular catheter, in addition to measuring ICP, allows therapeutic CSF drainage.

☞ Intraparenchymal devices, for example, Camino® ICP monitors (Camino Laboratories, San Diego, California, U.S.A.), use a catheter that is inserted within cortical gray matter, which allows direct measurement of brain tissue pressure.

☞ The normal ICP waveform is pulsatile and coincident with the cardiac cycle. However, the entire baseline rises and falls in concert with the respiratory cycle (as do all physiologic fluid waveforms).

☞ The EEG has never been demonstrated to correlate with CBF except at very low levels.

☞ Because an EEG silence pattern is not specific for brain death, it should never be used exclusively to diagnose brain death.

☞ The advantage of the processed EEG is that the real-time analysis can be quickly interpreted with minimal training, resulting in a more rapid detection of clinical problems (e.g., ischemia, seizure), and institution of the treatment.

☞ Intraoperative experience shows that anesthetic drugs can be titrated to a specific quantitative endpoint (BIS monitor range of 50–60), to avoid recall; a level between 60 and 80 can be chosen if sedation and amnesia are the desired endpoints in the ICU.

☞ Compromise of a neurological pathway is manifested as an increase in the latency, or a decrease in the amplitude of EPs, or both.

☞ Transcranial Doppler (TCD) is a noninvasive method that uses sound waves for measuring CBF velocity.

☞ Jugular bulb venous oxygen saturation ($SjvO_2$) provides a measurement of the global balance between cerebral oxygen supply and demand.

☞ Microprobes can be inserted directly into the brain parenchyma to measure PO_2, PCO_2, pH, temperature, and many other variables, which indirectly indicate perfusion changes of that particular region of the brain.

REFERENCES

1. Haerer AF. Neurologic Examination. 5th ed. Philadelphia:JB Lippincott Co., 1992.
2. Lang EW, Chestnut RM. Intracranial pressure and cerebral perfusion pressure in severe head injury. New Horizons 1995; 3:400–408.
3. Brain Trauma Foundation. The American Association of Neurological Surgeons. Recommendations for Intracranial Pressure Monitoring trechnology. J Neurotrauma 2000; 17(6–7):497–506.
4. Monro A. Observations on the Structure and Function of the Nervous System. Edinburgh: Creech and Johnson, 1783.
5. Kellie G. On death from cold, and on congestions of the brain. An account of the appearance observed in the dissection of two of the three individuals presumed to have perished in the storm of 3rd and whose bodies were discovered in the vicinity of Leith on the morning of the 4th November 1821; with some reflections on the pathology of the brain. Trans Med Chir Soc (Edinburgh) 1824; 1:84–169.
6. Robertson CS, Valadka AB, Hannay HJ, et al. Prevention of secondary ischemic insults after severe head injury. Crit Care Med 1999; 27:2086–2095.
7. Brain Injury Foundation, American Association of Neurological Surgeons, Joint Section on Neurotrauma and Critical Care. Resuscitation of blood pressure and oxygenation. J Neurotrauma 2000; 17:471–8.
8. Procaccio F, Stocchetti N, Citerio G, et al. Guidelines for the treatment of adults with severe head trauma. J Neursurg Sci 2000; 44(1):11–18.
9. Juul J, Morris GF, Marshall SB, et al. Intracranial hypertension and cerebral perfusion pressure: influence on neurological deterioration and outcome in severe head injury. J Neurosurg 2000; 92:1–6.
10. Chestnut RM, Marshal LF. Intracranial pressure monitoring and cerebralspinal fluid drainage. In Benumof JL, ed. Clinical Procedures in Anesthesia and Intensive Care. Philadelphia, PA: Lippincott Williams & Wilkins Inc., 1992:695–724.
11. Lundberg N. Continuous recording and control of ventricular fluid pressure in neurosurgical practice. Acta Psych Neurol Scand 1960; 36(suppl):1–193.
12. Pfisterer W, Muhlbauer M, Czech T, et al. Early diagnosis of external ventricular drainage infection: results of a prospective study. J Neurol Neurosurg Psychiatry 2003; 74(7):929–932.
13. Martinez-Manas RM, Santamarta D, de Campos JM, et al. Camino intracranial pressure monitor: prospective study of accuracy and complications. J Neurol Neurosurg Psychiatry 2000; 69(1):82–86.
14. Poca MA, Sahuquillo J, Arribas M, et al. Fiberoptic intraparenchymal brain pressure monitoring with the Camino V420 monitor: reflections on our experience in 163 severely head-injured patients. J Neuotrauma 2002; 19(4):439–438.
15. Raksin PB, Alperin N, Sivaramakrishnan A, et al. Noninvasive intracranial compliance and pressure based on dynamic magnetic resonance imaging of blood flow and cerebrospinal fluid flow: reviews of principles, implementation, and other non-invasive approaches. Neurosurg Focus 2003; 14:1–8.
16. Schaul N. The fundamental neural mechanisms of electroencephalography. Electroencephalogr Clin Neurophysiol 1998; 106:101.
17. Niedermeyer E, Lopes da Silva F. Electroencephalography: Basic Principles, Clinical Applications, and Related Fields. 3rd ed. Baltimore: Williams and Wilkins, 1993.
18. Kofke WA, Attaallah AF, Kuwabara H, et al. Neuropathologic effects in rats and neurometabolic effects in humans of high-dose remifentanil. Anesth Analg 2002; 94:1229–1236.
19. Frenkle C, Kloos S, Ihmsen H, Rommelsheim K, Schuttler J. Rational ICU sedation on EEG monitoring and closed-loop dosing strategies. Anesthesiology 1992; A270.
20. Carlsson C, Smith DS, Keykhah MM. The effects of fentanyl on cerebral circulation and metabolism in rats. Anesthesiology 1994; 57:375–80.
21. Kearse LA Jr, Koski G, Husain MV, Philbin DM, McPeck K. Epileptiform activity during opioid anesthesia. Electroencephogr J Clin Neurophysiol 1993; 87:374–379.
22. Herkes GK, Wszolek ZK, Westmoreland BF, et al. Effects of midazolam on electroencephalograms of seriously ill patients. Mayo Clinic Proc 1992; 67:334–338.
23. Reddy RV, Moorthy SS, Mattice T, et al. An electroencephalographic comparison of effects of propofol and methohexital. Electroencephalogr Clin Neurophysiol 1992; 83:162–168.
24. Bol CJJG, Danhof M, Stanski DR, et al. Pharmakokinetic-pharmacodynamic characterization of the cardiovascular, hypnotic, EEG, and ventilatory response to Dexmedetomidine in the rat. Pharmacology 1997; 283(3):1051–1058.
25. Agarwal R, Gotman J, Flanagan D, Rosenblatt B. Automatic EEG analysis during long-term monitoring in the ICU. Electroencephalogr Clin Neurophysiol 1998; 17:44–58.
26. Claassen J. Continuous electroencephalographic monitoring in neurocritical care. Curr Neurol Neurosci Rep 2002; 2(6):534–40.
27. Kalkman CJ, Boezeman EH, Ribberink AA, et al. Influence of changes in arterial carbon dioxide tension on

electroencephalogram and posterior tibial nerve somatosensory cortical evoked potentials during alfentanil/nitrous oxide anesthesia. Anesthesiology 1991; 75:68–74.

28. Kraaier V, Van Huffelen AC, Weineke GH. Quantitative EEG changes due to hypobaric hypoxia in normal subjects. Electroencephalogr Clin Neurophysiol 1988; 69:303–312.

29. McGrail KM. Intraoperative use of electroencephalography as an assessment of cerebral blood flow. Neurosurg Clin N Am 1996; 7(4):685–692.

30. Lang W, Dinkel M. Cerebral ischemia during carotid clamping: diagnosis and prevention. Zentralbl Chir 2000; 125(3): 243–250.

31. Visser GH, Wieneke GH, van Huffelen AC. Carotid endarterectomy monitoring: patterns of spectral EEG changes due to carotid artery clamping. Clin Neurophysiol 1999; 110(2): 286–294.

32. Arnold M, Sturzenegger M, Schaffler L, Seiler RW. Continuous intraoperative monitoring of middle cerebral artery blood flow velocities and electroencephalography during carotid endarterectomy. A comparison of the two methods to detect cerebral ischemia. Stroke 1997; 28(7):1345–1350.

33. Korein J. Brain death. In: Cottrell JE, Turndorf H, eds. Anesthesia and Neurosurgery. St. Louis: Mosby-Year Book, 1986:293–351.

34. Paolin A, Manuali A, Di Paola F, et al. Reliability in diagnosis of brain death. Intensive Care Med 1995; 21(8):657–662.

35. Wijdicks EF. The diagnosis of brain death. N Engl J Med 2001; 19;344(16):1215–1221.

36. Levy WJ. Quantitative analysis of EEG changes during hypothermia. Anesthesiology 1984; 60:291–297.

37. Stecker MM, Cheung AT, Pochettino A, et al. Deep hypothermic circulatory arrest: I. Effects of cooling on electroencephalogram and evoked potentials. Ann Thorac Surg 2001; 71(1):14–21.

38. Kochs E. Electrophysiological monitoring and mild hypothermia. J Neurosurg Anesthesiol 1995; 7(3):222–228.

39. Rekand T, Sulg IA, Bjaertnes L, Jolin A. Neuromonitoring in hypothermia and in hypothermic hypoxia. Arctic Med Res 1991; 50(suppl 6):32–36.

40. Rampil IJ. A primer for EEG signal processing in anesthesia. Anesthesiology 1998; 89:980–1002.

41. Todd MM. EEGs, EEG processing, and the bispectral index. Anesthesiology 1998; 89:815–817.

42. Rosow C, Manberg PJ. Bispectral index monitoring. Anesthesiol Clin North America 2001; 19(4):947–966.

43. Johansen JW, Sebel PS. Development and clinical application of electroencephalographic bispectrum monitoring. Anesthesiology 2000; 93:1336–1344.

44. Deyne C, Struys M, Decruyenaere J, Creupelandt J, Hoste E, Colardyn F. Use of continuous bispectral EEG monitoring to assess depth of sedation in ICU patients. Intensive care medicine 1998; 24:1294–1298.

45. Simmons LE, Riker RR, Prato BS, Fraser GL. Assessing sedation during intensive care unit mechanical ventilation with the bispectral index and the Sedation-Agitation Scale. Crit Care Med 1999; 27:1499–1504.

46. Frenzel D, Greim CA, Sommer C, Bauerle K, Roewer N. Is the bispectral index appropriate for monitoring the sedation level of mechanically ventilated surgical ICU patients? Intensive Care Med 2002; 28:178–183.

47. Riess ML, Graefe UA, Goeters C, Van Aken H, Bone HG. Sedation assessment in critically ill patients with bispectral index. Eur J Anaesthesiol 2002; 19:18–22.

48. Chiappa KH. Evoked Potentials in Clinical Medicine. 3rd ed. New York: Lippincott, 1997.

49. Nuwer MR. Fundamentals of evoked potentials and common clinical applications today. Electroencephalogr Clin Neurophysiol 1998; 106:142.

50. Stockard, JJ, Pope-Stockard, JE, Sharbrough, FW. Brainstem auditory evoked potentials in neurology: Methodology, interpretation and clinical applications. In: Aminoff, M, ed. Electrodiagnosis in Clinical Neurology, 3rd ed. New York: Churchill-Livingstone, 1992:503.

51. Schwender D, Keller I, Klasing S, et al. Mid-latency auditory evoked potentials during induction of intravenous anesthesia using midazolam, diazepam and flunitrazepam. Anesth Intensivther Notf Med 1990; 25:383–390.

52. Samra SK, Bradshaw BG, Pandit SK, et al. The relation between lorazepam-induced auditory amnesia and auditory evoked potentials. Anesth Analg 1988; 67:526–533.

53. Schwender D, Keller I, Klasing S, et al. Middle-latency auditory-evoked potentials during high-dose opioid analgesia. Anaesthetist 1990; 39:299–305.

54. Chassard D, Joubaud A, Colson A, et al. Auditory evoked potentials during propofol anesthesia in man. Br J Anesth 1989; 62:522–526.

55. de Haan P, Kalkman CJ. Spinal cord monitoring: Somatosensory and motor evoked potentials. Anesthesiol Clin North America 2001; 19(4):923–945.

56. Banoub M. Pharmacologic and physiologic influences affecting sensory evoked potentials: implications for perioperative monitoring. Anesthesiology 2003; 99(3):716–737.

57. Koht A, Schutz W, Schmidt G, et al. Effects of etomidate, midazolam, and thiopental on median nerve somatosensory evoked potentials and the additive effects of fentanyl and nitrous oxide. Anesth Analg 1988; 67:435–441.

58. Young CC. Benzodiazepines in the intensive care unit. Crit Care Clin 2001; 17(4):843–862.

59. Loughnan BL, Sebel PS, Thomas D, et al. Evoked potentials following diazepam or fentanyl. Anesthesia 1987; 42:195–198.

60. Samra SK, Dy EA, Welch KB, Lovely LK, Graziano GP. Remifentanil- and fentanyl-based anesthesia for intraoperative monitoring of somatosensory evoked potentials. Anesth Analg 2001; 92(6):1510–1515.

61. Schubert A, Drummond JC, Peterson DO, et al. The effect of high-dose fentanyl on human median nerve somatosensory-evoked response. Can J Anesth 1987; 34:35–40.

62. Maurette P, Simeon F, Castagnera L, et al. Propofol anesthesia alters somatosensory evoked cortical potentials. Anesthesia 1988; 43(suppl):44–45.

63. Boisseau N, Madany M, Staccini P, et al. Comparison of the effects of sevoflurane and propofol on cortical somatosensory evoked potentials. Br J Anaesth 2002; 88(6):785–789.

64. Kalkman CJ, Drummond JC, Kennelly NA, et al. Intraoperative monitoring of tibialis anterior muscle motor evoked responses to transcranial electrical stimulation during partial neuromuscular blockade. Anesth Analg 1992; 75:584.

65. Kalkman CJ, Drummond JC, Ribberink AA, et al. Effects of propofol, etomidate, midazolam and fentanyl on motor evoked responses to transcranial electrical or magnetic stimulation in humans. Anesthesiology 1992; 76:502.

66. Thees C, Scheufler KM, Nadstawek J, et al. Influence of fentanyl, alfentanil, and sufentanil on motor evoked potentials. J Neurosurg Anesthesiol 1999; 11(2):112–118.

67. Nuwer MR. Electroencephalograms and evoked potentials: Monitoring cerebral function in the neurosurgical intensive care unit. Neurosurg Clin N Am 1994; 5(4):647–659.

68. Branston NM, Ladds A, Syrnon L, et al. Comparison of the effects of ischaemia on early components of the somatosensory evoked potential in brainstem, thalamus, and cerebral cortex. J Cereb Blood Flow Metab 1984; 4:68–81.

69. Kochs E, Schulte am Esch J. Somatosensory evoked responses during and after graded brain ischaemia in goats. Eur J Anaesthesiol 1991; 8(4):257–265.

70. Haghighi SS, Oro JJ. Effects of hypovolemic hypotensive shock on somatosensory and motor evoked potentials. Neurosurgery 1989; 24:246.

71. Karnaze D, Fisher M, Ahmadi J, et al. Short-latency somatosensory evoked potentials correlate with the severity of the neurological deficit and sensory abnormalities following cerebral ischemia. Electroencephalogr Clin Neurophysiol 1987; 67:147–150.

72. Madl C. Improved outcome prediction in unconscious cardiac arrest survivors with sensory evoked potentials compared with clinical assessment. Crit Care Med 2000; 28(3): 721–726.

73. Marinov M, Schmarov A, Natschev S, Stamenov B, Wassmann H. Reversible focal ischemia model in the rat: correlation of somatosensory evoked potentials and cortical neuronal injury. Neurol Res 1996; 18(1):73–82.

74. Minamide H, Onishi H, Yamashita J, Ikeda K. Reversibility of transient focal cerebral ischemia evaluated by somatosensory evoked potentials in cats. Surg Neurol 1994; 42(2):138–147.

75. Guerit JM, Witdoeckt C, de Tourtchaninoff M, et al. Somatosensory evoked potential monitoring in carotid surgery. I. Relationships between qualitative SEP alterations and intraoperative events. Electroencephalogr Clin Neurophysiol 1997; 104(6):459–469.

76. Jordan KG. Continuous EEG and evoked potential monitoring in the neuroscience intensive care unit. J Clin Neurophysiol 1993; 10(4):445–475.

77. Haralanov L, Klissurski M, Stamenova P. Functional methods for evaluation the occurrence of delayed ischemic deficit in patients with subarachnoid hemorrhage. Eur J Med Res 2001; 6(5):185–189.

78. Szabo S, Miko L, Novak L, Rozsa L, Szekely G Jr. Correlation between central somatosensory conduction time, blood flow velocity, and delayed cerebral ischemia after aneurysmal subarachnoid hemorrhage. Neurosurg Rev 1997; 20(3):188–195.

79. Moulton RJ, Brown JI, Konasiewicz SJ. Monitoring severe head injury: a comparison of EEG and somatosensory evoked potentials. Can J Neurol Sci 1998; 25(1):S7–S11.

80. Matsura S, Kuno M, Nakamura T. Intracranial pressure and auditory evoked responses of the cat. Acta Otolaryngol 1986; 102:12–19.

81. Kawahara N, Saski M, Mii K, et al. Reversibility of cerebral function assessed by somatosensory evoked potentials and its relation to intracranial pressure – report of six cases with sever head injury. Neurol Med Chir 1991; 31:264–271.

82. Krieger D, Jauss M, Schwarz S, Hacke W. Serial somatosensory and brainstem auditory evoked potentials in monitoring of acute supratentorial mass lesions. Crit Care Med 1995; 23(6):1123–1131.

83. Judson JA, Cant BR, Shaw NA. Early prediction of outcome from cerebral trauma by somatosensory evoked potentials. Crit Care Med 1990; 18:363–368.

84. Carter BG. Review of the use of somatosensory evoked potentials in the prediction of outcome after severe brain injury. Crit Care Med 2001; 29(1):178–186.

85. Pajeau AK. Somatosensory evoked potentials as predictors of outcome in patients with acute diffuse axonal injury. Crit Care Med 2001; 29(3):675–677.

86. Marsala M. Therapeutic window after spinal cord trauma is longer than after spinal cord ischemia. Anesthesiology 2000; 92(1):281.

87. Lips J. The role of transcranial motor evoked potentials in predicting neurologic and histopathologic outcome after experimental spinal cord ischemia. Anesthesiology, 2002; 97(1):183–191.

88. Robinson LR. Predictive value of somatosensory evoked potentials for awakening from coma. Crit Care Med 2003; 31(3): 960–967.

89. Young GB. Clinical neurophysiologic assessment of comatose patients. Crit Care Med 2003; 31(3):994.

90. Facco E, Casartelli-Liviero M, Munari M, et al. Short latency evoked potentials: new criteria for brain death? J Neurol Neurosurg Psychiat 1990; 53:351–353.

91. Lumente CB, Kramer M, von Tempelhoff W, et al. Brain stem auditory evoked potentials (BAEP) monitoring in brain death. Neurosurg Rev 1989; 12(suppl 1):317–321.

92. Facco E, Munari M, Gallo F, et al. Role of short latency evoked potentials in the diagnosis of brain death. Clin Neurophysiol 2002; 113(11):1855–1866.

93. Grosset DG, Straiton J, du Trevou M, Bullock R. Prediction of symptomatic vasospasm after subarachnoid hemorrhage by rapidly increasing transcranial Doppler velocity and cerebral blood flow changes. Stroke 1992; 23:674–679.

94. Grosset DG, Straiton J, McDonald I, et al. Use of transcranial Doppler sonography to predict development of a delayed ischemic deficit after subarachnoid hemorrhage. J Neurosurg 1993; 78:183–187.

95. Grosset DG, Straiton J, McDonald I, et al. Angiographic and Doppler diagnosis of cerebral artery vasospasm following subarachnoid hemorrhage. Br J Neurosurg 1993; 7:291–298.

96. Seckhar L, Wechsler LR, Yonas H, Luyckx K, Obrist W. Value of transcranial doppler examination in the diagnosis of cerebral vasospasm after subarachnoid hemorrhage. Neurosurgery 1988; 22:813–821.

97. Martin NA, Doberstein C, Zane C, Caron MJ, Thomas K, Becker DP. Postraumatic cerebraal arterial spasm: transcranial Doppler ultrasound, cerebral blood flow, and angiographic findings. J Neurosurg 1992; 77:575–583.

98. Martin NA, Parwardhan RV, Alexander MJ, et al. Characterization of cerebral hemodynamic phases following severe head trauma: hypoperfusion, hyperemia, and vasospasm. J Neurosurg 1997; 87:9–19.

99. Manno EM. Transcranial doppler ultrasonography in the neurocritical care unit. Crit Care Clinics 1997; 13:79–105.

100. Russell D. The detection of cerebral emboli using Doppler ultrasound. In: Newell DW, Aaslid R, ed. Transcranial Doppler. New York:Raven Press Ltd., 1992:207–213.

101. Spencer MP, Thomas GI, Nicholls SC, Sauvage LR. Detection of middle cerebral artery emboli during carotid endarterectomy using transcranial Doppler ultrasonography. Stroke 1990; 21:415–423.

102. Hassler W, Steinmetz H, Gawlowski J. Transcranial Doppler ultrasonography in raised intracranial pressure and in intracranial circulatory arrest. J Neurosurg 1988; 68:745–751.

103. Newell DW, Grady MS, Sirotta P, Winn HR. Evaluation of brain death using transcranial Doppler. Neurosurgery 1989; 24:500.

104. Petty GW, Mohr JP, Pedley TA, et al. The role of transcranial Doppler in confirming brain death: sensitivity, specificity, and suggestions for performance and interpretation. Neurology 1990; 40:300.

105. Cabrer C, Dominguez-Roldan JM, Manyalich M, et al. Persistence of intracranial diastolic flow in transcranial Doppler sonography exploration of patients in brain death. Transplant Proc 2003; 35(5):1642–1643.

106. Kofke WA. TCD in anesthesia. In: Babakian VL, Wechsler LR, ed. Transcranial Doppler Ultrasonography. St. Louis, MO: Mosby, 1993.

107. Steiger H-J, Aaslid R, Stoos R, et al. Transcranial doppler monitoring in head injury: relations between type of injury, flow velocities, and outcome. Neurosurgery 1994; 34:79–86.

108. Lam J, Hsiang J, Poon W. Monitoring of autoregulation using laser Doppler flowmetry in patients with head injury. J Neurosurg 1997; 86:438–445.

109. Kirkpatrick PJ, Smielewski P, Czosnyka M, Pickard JD. Continuous monitoring of cortical perfusion by laser Doppler flowmetry in ventilated patients with head injury. J Neurol Neurosurg Psychiatry 1994; 57(11):1382–1388.

110. Meguro K, Tsukada A, Matsumura A, Matsuki T, Nakada Y, Nose T. Portable digital subtraction angiography in the operating room and intensive care unit. Neurol Med Chir 1991; 31(12):768–772.

111. Suarez J. Symptomatic vasospasm diagnosis after subarachnoid hemorrhage: evaluation of transcranial Doppler ultrasound and cerebral angiography as related to compromised vascular distribution. Crit Care Med 2002; 30(6):1348–1355.

112. Koenig M, Klotz E, Luka B, et al. Perfusion CT of the brain: diagnostic approach for early detection of ischemic stroke. Radiology 1998; 209:85–93.

113. Rydberg J, Buckwalter KA, Caldemeyer KS, et al. Multi-section CT: Scanning techniques and clinical applications. Radiographics 2000; 20:1787–1806.

114. Mayer T, Hamann G, Baranczyk J, et al. Dynamic CT perfusion imaging of acute stroke. Am J of Neuroradiol 2000; 21: 1441–1449.

115. Leclerc X, Pruvo JP. Recent advances in magnetic resonance angiography of carotid and vertebral arteries. Curr Opin Neurol 2000; 13(1):75–82.

116. Kesava PP, Turski PA. MR Angiography of Vascular Malformations. Neuroimaging Clin N Am 1998; 8(2):349–370.

117. Bongartz GM, Boos M, Winter K, et al. Clinical utility of contrast-enhanced MR angiography. Eur Radiol 1997; 7(suppl 5):178–186.

118. Bouma G, Muizelaar J, Stringer W, Choi S, Fatouros P, Young H. Ultra-early evaluation of regional cerebral blood flow in severely head injured patients using xenon-enhanced computerized tomography. J Neurosurg 1992; 77:360–368.

119. Muizelaar JP, Fatouros PP, Schroder ML. A new method for quantitative regional cerebral blood volume measurements using computed tomography. Stroke 1997; 28(10):1998–2005.

120. Firlik KS, Firlik AD, Yonas H. Xenon-enhanced computed tomography in the management of cerebral vasospasm following aneurysmal subarachnoid hemorrhage. Keio J Med 2000; 49(suppl 1):A148–A150.

121. Obrist WD, Wilkinson WE. Regional cerebral blood flow measurement in humans by Xenon-133 clearance. Cerebrovasc Brain Metab 1990; 2:283–327.

122. Horn P, Vajkoczy P, Thome C, et al. Xenon-induced flow activation in patients with cerebral insult who undergo xenon-enhanced CT blood flow studies. AJNR 2001; 22:1543–1549.

123. Hoffman JM, Hanson MW, Coleman RE. Clinical positron emission tomography imaging. Radiological Clin of N Am 1993; 31(4):935–959.

124. Schneider F, Grodd W, Machulla HJ. Examination of psychological functions by functional imaging with positron emission tomography and magnetic resonance imaging. Nervenarzt 1996; 67(9):721–729.

125. Wiedmann KD, Wilson JTL, Wyper D. SPECT cerebral blood flow, MR imaging, and neuropsychological findings in traumatic head injury. Neuropsychology 1989; 3:267–281.

126. Cihangiroglu M, Ramsey RG, Dohrmann GJ. Brain injury: analysis of imaging modalities. Neurol Res 2002; 24(1):7–18.

127. Feldman Z. Monitoring of cerebral hemodynamics with jugular bulb catheters. Crit Care Clin 1997; 13:51–77.

128. Cruz J. The first decade of continuous monitoring of jugular bulb oxyhemoglobin saturation: Management strategies and clinical outcome. Crit Care Med 1998; 26:344–351.

129. Vigue B, Ract C, Benayed M, et al. Early SjvO$_2$ monitoring in patients with severe brain trauma. Intensive Care Med 1999; 25:445–451.

130. Schell RM. Cerebral monitoring: jugular venous oximetry. Anesth Analg 2000; 90(3):559–66.

131. Smythe PR, Samra SK. Monitors of cerebral oxygenation. Anesthesiol Clin North America 2002; 20(2):293–313.

132. Mancini DM, Bolinger L, Li K, et al. Validation of near-infrared spectroscopy in humans. J Appl Physiol 1994; 77:2740.

133. Kirkpatrick P, Smielewski P, Czosnyka M, et al. Near-infrared spectroscopy use in patients with severe head injury. J Neurosurg 1995; 83:963–970.

134. Samra SK, Dy EA, Welch K, et al. Evaluation of a cerebral oximeter as a monitor of cerebral ischemia during carotid endarterectomy. Anesthesiology 2000; 93:964–970.

135. Zauner A, Clausen T, Alves OL. Cerebral metabolism after fluid-percussion injury and hypoxia in a feline model. J Neurosurg 2002; 97(3):643–649.

136. Van Santbrink H, Maas A, Avezaat C. Continuous monitoring of partial pressure of brain tissue oxygen in patients with severe head injury. Neurosurgery 1996; 38(1):21–31.

137. Valadka AB, Gopinath SP, Contant CF, et al. Relationship of brain tissue PO$_2$ to outcome after severe head injury. Crit Care Med 1998; 26:1576–1581.

138. Kiening KL, Hartl R, Unterberg AW, et al. Brain tissue pO$_2$ monitoring in comatose patients: Implications for therapy. Neurol Res 1997; 19:233–240.

139. Zwienenburg M, Muizelaar JP. Cerebral perfusion and blood flow in neurotrauma. Neurol Res 2001; 23:167–174.

140. Czosnyka M, Kirkpatrick PJ, Pickard JD. Multimodal monitoring and assessment of cerebral haemodynamic reserve after severe head injury. Cerebrovasc Brain Metab Rev 1996; 8(4):273–295.

141. Kett-White R. Multi-modal monitoring of acute brain injury. Adv Tech Stand Neurosurg 2002; 27:87–134.

142. Taylor WR, Chen JW, Meltzer H, et al. Quantitative pupillometry, a new technology: normative data an preliminary observations in patients with acute head injury. J Neurosurg 2003; 98:205–213.

143. Sarrafzadeh AS, Kiening KL, Unternberg AW. Neuromonitoring: brain oxygenation and microdialysis. Curr Neurol Neurosci Rep 2003; 3(6):517–523.

144. Persson L, Hillered L. Chemical monitoring of neurosurgical intensive care patients using intracerebral microdialysis. J Neurosurg 1992; 76:72–80.

145. Unterberg AW, Sakowitz OW, Sarrafzadeh AS, et al. Role of bedside microdialysis in the diagnosis of cerebral vasospasm following aneurysmal subarachnoid hemorrhage. J Neurosurg 2001; 94:740–749.

146. Meixensberger J. Clinical cerebral microdialysis: brain metabolism and brain tissue oxygenation after acute brain injury. Neurol Res 2001; 23(8):801–806.

147. Raps EC, Bird SJ, Hansen-Flaschen J. Prolonged muscle weakness after neuromuscular blockade in the intensive care unit. Crit Care Clin 1994; 10(4):799–813.

148. Siverman DG, Brull SJ. Monitoring neuromuscular block. Anesthesiol Clin North America 1994; 12:237–260.

149. Barboi AC, Barkhaus PE. Electrodiagnostic testing in neuromuscular disorders. Neurol Clin 2004; 22:619–641.

150. Electroencephalography. In: Malmivuo J, Plonsey R, ed. Bioelectro-magnetism. New York, NY: Oxford University Press, 1995.

151. Mahla ME. Neurologic monitoring. In: Cucchiara, Black, Michenfelder, eds. Clinical Neuroanesthesia. 2nd ed. Amazon. Philadelphia, PA: Churchill Livingstone Inc., 1998.

152. Frab R. Magnetic resonance angiography. In: Toronto Brain Vascular Malformation Study Group. Website: http://brainavm.oci.utoronto.ca/malformations/content/MRA.html

153. Meuli R, Wintermark M. CT perfusion case study. In: GE Medical systems.

8

Respiratory Monitoring

Jonathan B. Cohen, Enrico M. Camporesi, and Hans W. Schweiger

Department of Anesthesiology and Critical Care, University of South Florida College of Medicine, Tampa, Florida, U.S.A.

INTRODUCTION

Monitoring of respiratory gases in critically ill patients is increasingly used, and with improved utilization and understanding come opportunities to improve outcomes. The widespread use of pulse oximetry in the late 1980s revolutionized anesthesia management and is responsible for saving countless lives. In the 1990s, this technology quickly spread outside the operating room (OR) to become a standard of care in the surgical intensive care unit (SICU) and the emergency department (ED). Carbon dioxide (CO_2) monitoring has long been used in anesthesia practice and is likewise becoming more commonly used in critical care areas outside of the OR. This chapter reviews the practical benefits of respiratory gas monitoring techniques that are commonly employed in the OR and are increasingly utilized in the trauma resuscitation suite (TRS) and in the SICU.

CARBON DIOXIDE MONITORING

The partial pressure of arterial CO_2 ($PaCO_2$) is commonly measured by arterial blood gas (ABG) sampling, but inhaled and exhaled CO_2 values provide additional clinically relevant information, and can also be monitored in the SICU. ☞ **Exhaled gas CO_2 concentrations provide physiologic information about both systemic perfusion and pulmonary function.** ☞ Monitoring of exhaled gas CO_2 can be accomplished by colorimetric, capnometric, or capnographic means. In colorimetric CO_2 monitoring, a disposable device, for example, Nellcor Easy Cap® II (Pleasanton, California, U.S.A.), is connected between the 15-mm airway adapter of the endotracheal tube (ETT) and the ventilator tubing. The presence of CO_2 in the exhaled gas causes a chemical reaction in the indicator device changing the color from a baseline purple to yellow. The Nellcor Easy Cap II is a commonly employed device for secondary confirmation of ETT placement in locations outside of the OR, where capnography may not be available (see Volume 1, Chapters 8 and 9). While colorimetric monitoring provides qualitative information, capnometric and capnographic monitoring devices provide more quantitative information. The numerical value of CO_2 measured is typically reported in mmHg. The end tidal CO_2 ($P_{ET}CO_2$) value is usually monitored in the OR, as this most closely reflects the $PaCO_2$. ☞ **The $P_{ET}CO_2$ provides information about four important issues: (*i*) the correct placement of the ETT, (*ii*) the ventilation status, (*iii*) the cardiac output ($\dot{Q}$), and (*iv*) the metabolic status of the patient.** ☞

Metabolic Status of the Patient

As the cellular byproduct of respiration, CO_2 blood levels mirror metabolic rate. When the rate of metabolism increases, the level of CO_2 produced ($\dot{V}CO_2$) also increases. A list of hypermetabolic disease processes commonly encountered in critically ill trauma patients are listed in Table 1. However, the $P_{ET}CO_2$ and the $PaCO_2$ can vary in response to a variety of conditions (described later).

Correct Placement of the Endotracheal Tube

Incorrect placement of an ETT leads to catastrophic results if it is not recognized immediately after it occurs. Historically, physical exam findings were used to confirm placement. Auscultation of the lungs is error prone, particularly in noisy environments such as the TRS of the ED, in an ambulance, or in a helicopter. Brunel et al. (1) found that 60% of main-stem intubations occurred despite the reported presence of equal breath sounds on examination. His group also found that cuff ballottement and referencing the markings on the ETT to the incisor line (as a measure of insertion depth) were not completely reliable (1).

Other clinical indicators of endotracheal versus esophageal intubation are likewise error prone. In one study condensation was observed in the ETT in more than 50% of patients intentionally intubated in the esophagus (2). White and Slovis (3) summarize the reliability of the clinical exam when they state that using physical exam alone as confirmation of correct ETT placement represents reliance on a "fool's gold standard."

☞ **The American Society of Anesthesiologists Difficult Airway (ASADA) guidelines, along with the Advanced Cardiac Life Support® (ACLS®) guidelines currently recommend secondary confirmation of ETT placement with exhaled CO_2 measurement or an esophageal detector device (EDD); as it has become increasingly recognized that physical exam alone is error prone.** ☞

Animal studies have indicated that recent ingestion of carbonated beverages may produce a false positive result (4). As a result, the manufacturer's recommendations for the Nellcor Easy Cap® II state that the colorimetric CO_2 detector color should be evaluated "after six full breaths"; the initial breaths being delivered to "wash out" any CO_2 artifact (5).

A concern with this technique is the potential delivery of six full breaths of gas to the esophagus and stomach, increasing the risk of aspiration. Capnometry, or better still capnography allows for more precise confirmation of tube placement, as long as the operator understands the workings and artifacts affecting these devices. If the putative ETT is actually incorrectly placed (e.g., in the esophagus), the exhaled CO_2 would decrease with each subsequent breath.

Table 1 Causes of Hypermetabolism

Postburn
Post-trauma
Post–CNS injury
Fever
Sepsis
Hyperthyroidism
Cocaine use
Methamphetamine use
Neuroleptic malignant syndrome
Malignant hyperthermia

The accuracy of either of these two modalities typically allows for a detection endpoint to occur before six full breaths have been delivered, provided the patient has adequate $\dot{Q}$. Silvestri et al. (6) found that in 153 patients, who received out-of-hospital intubation, no unrecognized misplaced intubations occurred in patients for whom paramedics used continuous $P_{ET}CO_2$ monitoring. Continuous monitoring can also alert the practitioner to accidental extubation of the patient, as ETT dislodgement is common during both out-of-hospital transport and intrahospital transport (7,8).

The major limitation of exhaled CO_2 monitoring is in patients with very low $\dot{Q}$, and those in complete cardiac arrest. If the time the patient has been without spontaneous circulation has been prolonged, lack of $P_{ET}CO_2$ may reflect an absence of pulmonary blood flow rather than incorrect tube placement. In this condition, an EDD is recommended (see Volume 1, Chapters 8 and 9).

Cardiac Output
The heart and the lungs are the only organs that receive 100% of $\dot{Q}$. ☞ **In patients with fixed ventilation/perfusion ($\dot{V}/\dot{Q}$) relationships in the lungs, and stable minute ventilation ($\dot{V}_E$), the $P_{ET}CO_2$ is proportional to $\dot{Q}$ (9)** ☞ Gudipati et al. (10) demonstrated that $P_{ET}CO_2$ during cardiopulmonary resuscitation (CPR) was predictive of animals that survived resuscitative efforts. The $P_{ET}CO_2$ also serves as a useful indicator of the return of spontaneous circulation after an arrest (11). The same group examined the effects of $P_{ET}CO_2$ on a controlled hemorrhage model in sheep, and documented a logarithmic relationship between $\dot{Q}$ and $P_{ET}CO_2$ (12).

Ventilation Status
The $P_{ET}CO_2$ levels usually provide an approximation of $PaCO_2$ levels. As such, they allow practitioners to rapidly determine if a patient is being hypoventilated, or more commonly hyperventilated. Aufderheide et al. (13) found that paramedics were consistently hyperventilating patients in cardiac arrest after they were intubated and that this was associated with poor outcomes. An important alternate explanation not considered by the authors that would perhaps better explain the increased mortality associated with low $P_{ET}CO_2$ was gross underresuscitation of intravascular volume. With either explanation, an excessively elevated $\dot{V}/\dot{Q}$ condition occurred, and this was most readily diagnosed with combined monitoring of capnography and $PaCO_2$ values.

Excessive and prolonged hyperventilation is also of concern in patients with traumatic brain injury (TBI) (Volume 1, Chapter 23). Although transient hyperventilation is an appropriate temporizing treatment in cases of impending herniation of brain tissue, its routine and prolonged use is no longer endorsed (14). Hyperventilation may cause

cerebral vasoconstriction and hypoxia to regions of the brain. There is evidence that paramedic-induced hyperventilation routinely occurs after head injury. Davis et al. (15,16) found that more than half of the patients studied had a $P_{ET}CO_2$ level of less than 25 mmHg. ☞ **A low $P_{ET}CO_2$ value in multi-trauma patients usually reflects insufficient $\dot{Q}$ (i.e., under resuscitation) and a resultant high ($\dot{V}/\dot{Q}$) as mentioned previously.** ☞ Accordingly, the study by Davis et al. (15) [as in the case of Aufderheide et al. (13)], may not necessarily have provided evidence of absolute hyperventilation (but rather, relative underresuscitation of intravascular volume).

Typically, the $P_{ET}CO_2$ value is slightly less than the concomitant $PaCO_2$. This $P_{ET}CO_2$–$PaCO_2$ gradient can be affected by a number of processes as summarized in Table 2. The use of capnometry to assist with tight ventilatory control during transport has been reported (17). However, the $P_{ET}CO_2$-$PaCO_2$ gradient needs to be established with an ABG to ensure that the $P_{ET}CO_2$ is truly reflecting the $\dot{V}_E$ [as would occur with stable alveolar dead space ($V_{D\ alveolar}$), $\dot{Q}$, and $\dot{V}CO_2$]. Otherwise, a decreasing $P_{ET}CO_2$ value is likely reflecting an increasing $\dot{V}/\dot{Q}$ condition, as occurs during exsanguination.

Waveform Analysis
If capnography is applied, analysis of the $P_{ET}CO_2$ waveform can be a useful tool. Figure 1 shows a normal waveform. Loss of the tracing altogether usually represents a circuit disconnect, kinked tubing, or extubation of the trachea. Gradually increasing levels of CO_2 in the $P_{ET}CO_2$ waveform may indicate ongoing gradual hypoventilation, hyperthermia, or increased metabolism. In contrast, gradually decreasing CO_2 levels may indicate hemorrhage in a patient with a fixed $\dot{V}_E$ and $\dot{V}CO_2$. Abrupt decreases in $P_{ET}CO_2$ often indicate cardiopulmonary arrest, pulmonary embolism, or sudden catastrophic blood loss (e.g., ruptured abdominal aortic aneurysm).

☞ **An exaggerated upstroke in segment C–D (also known as the plateau phase), as shown in Figure 2A, indicates an increase in airway resistance with associated $\dot{V}/\dot{Q}$ spread among the millions of alveoli.** ☞ Such an exaggerated slope to the plateau phase of the capnographic trace is often created by patients with reactive airways disease and

Table 2 Factors that Increase the End-Tidal Arterial CO_2 Gradient[a]

Low cardiac output states
Hypovolemia
Blood loss
"Third-space" fluid losses
Excessive diuresis
Excessive GI losses
Impaired contractility
Myocardial ischemia
Dilated cardiomyopathy
Valvular heart disease
Pulmonary embolism
Elevated alveolar pressure
Increased tidal volumes
Increased I:E ratios
Increased PEEP

[a]Note that all entities that cause an increase in the $P_{ET}CO_2$–$PaCO_2$ gradient are also factors that increase the alveolar dead space.
Abbreviation: PEEP, positive end expiratory pressure.

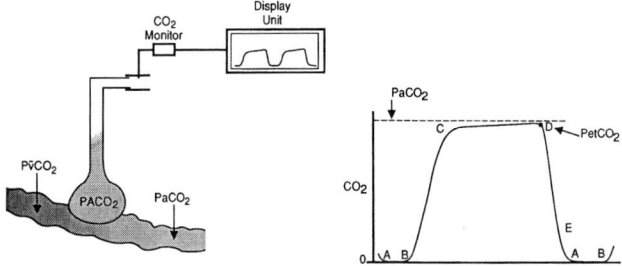

Figure 1 The essential elements of a normal capnogram. The left-sided drawing depicts the anatomic components monitored, and the apparatus involved in the capnographic display. The right-sided drawing shows a normal capnographic display. Segment A–B represents the zero baseline during early exhalation of CO_2-free gas from the anatomic dead space. Segment B–C represents mixed dead space and alveolar gas. The degree of slope in segment B–C represents the unevenness of the exhalation time constants of various lung segments (i.e., if all empty at the same time in a normal fashion, the upstroke is nearly vertical). Segment C–D represents alveolar plateau phase. D represents the end-tidal value. Segment D–E represents inhalation. *Source*: From Saidman LJ, Smith NT. Monitoring in Anesthesia, 3rd ed. Elsevier Science, p. 31, Fig. 22.

those with chronic obstructive pulmonary disease (COPD). However, an acute change in waveform during monitoring may represent mucous plugging, bronchospasm, or a partially kinked ETT. Changes in the shape of the capnographic waveform typically precede decreases in oxygenation, as would be detected by pulse oximetry monitoring; and thus capnography would potentially allow for earlier warning and intervention.

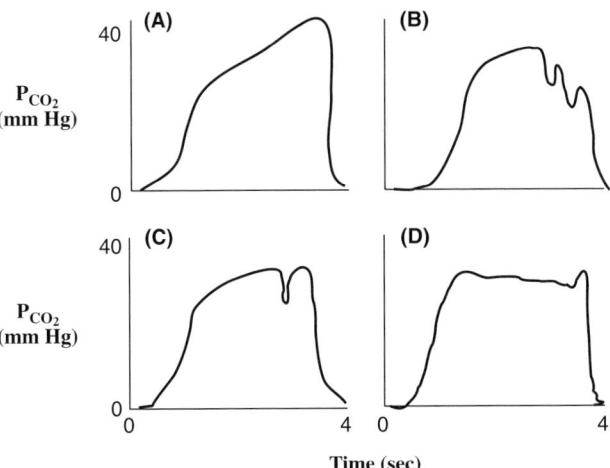

Figure 2 Common abnormalities seen in the alveolar plateau phase of the capnogram. (**A**) Increased slope of alveolar plateau. This waveform is consistent with increased airway resistance. The increasing slope of the plateau phase (segment C–D from Fig. 1) represents a gradient in CO_2 release from various alveoli as is commonly seen with bronchospasms or chronic obstructive pulmonary disease. (**B**) Cardiogenic oscillations. (**C**) Inspiratory effort during incomplete muscle relaxation during anesthesia. (**D**) Side-stream sampling tube leak. *Source*: Adapted from Ref. 60.

Prediction of Outcome in Trauma Patients

Several studies have examined $P_{ET}CO_2$ values and tried to extrapolate data on survivability after traumatic injury. As expected, Tyburski et al. (18) found the best survival rates in patients who had higher $P_{ET}CO_2$ levels and a lower $P_{ET}CO_2 - PaCO_2$, gradient at the end of emergency surgery. The same group followed these experiments with a study specifically examining the $P_{ET}CO_2–PaCO_2$ difference in over 500 patients. The average gradient of $P_{ET}CO_2–PaCO_2$ was less than 10 mmHg in all survivors at all times. The average gradient was greater than 10 mmHg in all nonsurvivors at all times (19). This difference also held true in patients who died more than 24 hours after surgery. Deakin et al. looked at prehospital $P_{ET}CO_2$ values as a predictor of mortality. He found that at 20 minutes after intubation, a $P_{ET}CO_2 < 3.25$ kPa (~24.4 mmHg) was associated with only a 5% survival rate to discharge rate (20). Aufderheide et al. showed that in cardiac arrest patients, the poor survival in hyperventilated patients may have been due to the decrease in cardiac preload, or may have been due to hypocarbia itself (which, in the authors' opinion, is the far less plausible explanation). As suggested earlier, whether or not the poor survival in trauma patients was a direct result of decreased $P_{ET}CO_2$, due to poor $\dot{Q}$ cardiac output and/or a decrease in cardiac preload against simple hyperventilation, as posited by the authors, remains unexplored.

Transcutaneous CO_2 (T_CCO_2) monitoring is a 20-year-old technology, which is enjoying a resurgence of interest. Heretofore, T_CCO_2 monitoring was largely utilized in the neonatal intensive care units (NICUs). Commercially available versions of T_CCO_2 measuring devices, such as the Novametrix $TCO_2M^®$ (Respironics, Inc., Murrysville, Pennsylvania, U.S.A.), combine the continuous measurement of T_CCO_2 and O_2. Studies are being conducted to determine its reliability of T_CCO_2 monitoring in adult SICU patients, and preliminary results look promising (21).

OXYGEN MONITORING

Oxygen serves as the substrate for aerobic metabolism. After entering the body via the lungs, O_2 travels down a partial pressure gradient from the atmosphere to its final site of action, the electron transport chain of mitochondria (Fig. 3). The O_2 levels can be monitored at key sites along the way, including the inspired gas, the alveolar gas (reflected in the end tidal O_2 concentration), the arterial blood, the mixed venous blood, and with transcutaneous sampling.

Inspired Gas and Alveolar Gas Monitoring

Monitoring the O_2 concentration of inspired gas is a necessity in anesthesia practice, and in other realms whenever the precise concentration of inhaled O_2 is important (i.e., whenever the potential for delivering a hypoxic gas mixture exists). ☞ **All mechanical ventilators in use in the SICU should also have the ability to measure and continuously display the fraction of inspired O_2 (F_IO_2).** ☞ This becomes of increasing importance when gas mixtures such as heliox, nitrous oxide (N_2O), and nitric oxide (NO) are administered (22). Monitoring the F_IO_2 of patients who are not intubated is problematic, as only an approximation can be made. Because the supplemental O_2 will blend with, and sometimes entrain, room air, the final F_IO_2 is related to numerous factors including the flow rate of O_2, the site of

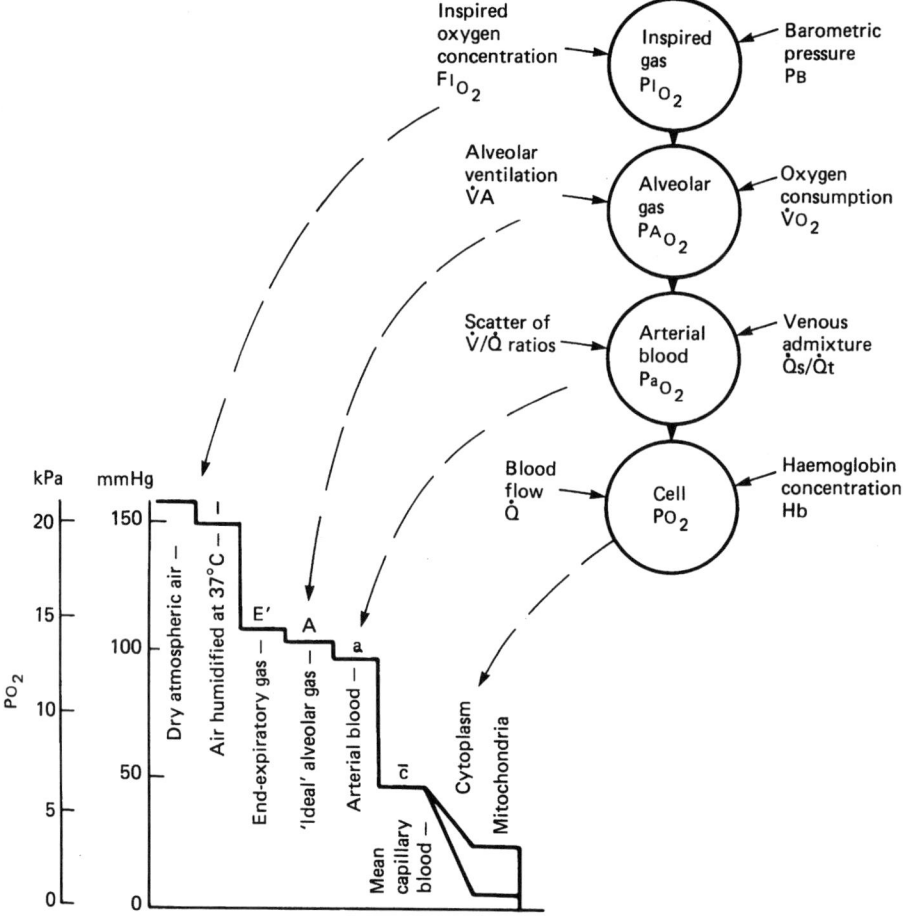

Figure 3 The oxygen cascade. The left side ("Y axis") shows the partial pressure of O_2 (PO_2) in both KPa and mmHg. Oxygen moves down a partial pressure gradient from dry atmospheric air (± 160 mmHg at sea level) to the mitochondria (± 3–20 mmHg), which is the site of utilization. On the right/top is a summary of the factors influencing oxygenation at different levels in the cascade. *Source*: From Ref. 61.

administration (i.e., nasal vs. oral), the devices used (i.e., simple mask vs. a nonrebreather), along with the $\dot{V}_E$ of the patient. The partial pressure of O_2 at the alveolus ($P_{A}O_2$) correlates directly with the F_IO_2, as shown in the alveolar air equation (Equation 1).

$$P_{A}O_2 = [F_IO_2 \cdot (P_B - P_{H2O})] - [PaCO_2/RQ] \quad (1)$$

Arterial Blood Gas Monitoring

Loading of the oxygen from the alveoli to the red blood cells (RBCs) within the pulmonary circulation is often impaired in critically ill patients. Monitoring this pulmonary transfer of O_2 is a factor that is of interest to many intensivists. The multiple inert gas elimination technique has been cited as the gold standard of oxygen transfer monitoring, but its use is cumbersome and not widely available except in research settings (23). One of the simplest methods of quantifying oxygen transfer is by determining the alveolar arterial partial pressure of O_2 [$P(A-a)O_2$] gradient, calculated as shown in Equation 2:

$$P(A-a)O_2 \text{ gradient} = P_{A}O_2 - PaO_2 \quad (2)$$

The $P(A-a)O_2$ gradient should be on the order of 7 to 14 mmHg for patients breathing room air. As a person ages, the normal PaO_2 decreases, and the $P(A-a)O_2$ gradient

conversely will increase. Breathing 100% oxygen (i.e., $F_IO_2 = 1.0$) also results in a discrepancy in the calculation of the $P(A-a)O_2$ gradient. These two factors taken into account, a elderly patient breathing at an F_IO_2 of 1.0 may have an $P(A-a)O_2$ gradient approaching 60 mmHg with healthy lungs. This example highlights one drawback to using the $P(A-a)O_2$ gradient. Following the $P(A-a)O_2$ gradient is most useful when examining trends. However, the F_IO_2 must remain approximately the same to accurately reflect the changes. Table 3 reviews common causes for $P(A-a)O_2$ gradient abnormalities.

Another method of estimating pulmonary oxygen transfer is the PaO_2/F_IO_2 (P/F) ratio. The normal P/F ratio is ≥ 500 mmHg; acute lung injury (ALI) is defined as a P/F ratio ≤ 300 mmHg, and the acute respiratory distress syndrome (ARDS) is defined as a P/F ratio ≤ 200 mmHg. Although its attraction is its simplicity, inaccuracies occur under a host of conditions seen in critically ill patients such as low oxygen extraction (24), COPD (25), and large intrapulmonary shunt (26).

☞ **Both right-to-left transpulmonary shunt ($\dot{Q}_s\dot{Q}_t$) and low $\dot{V}_A/\dot{Q}$ lung regions will contribute to an increase in the $P(A-a)O_2$ gradient.** ☞ The $P(A-a)O_2$ gradient does not readily distinguish between shunt (e.g., basilar atelectasis) and low $\dot{V}_A\dot{Q}$ (e.g., COPD) pathophysiology. Due to the sigmoid shape of the oxyhemoglobin dissociation curve, it

Table 3 Hypoxemia

Normal $P(A-a)O_2$ gradient	Increased $P(A-a)O_2$ gradient
$\downarrow PIO_2$	Right-to-left shunting
$\downarrow F_IO_2$	Transpulmonary
$\downarrow P_B$	Intracardiac
Hypoventilation	Diffusion defect
	Interstitial pulmonary
	fibrosis
	$\dot{V}/\dot{Q}$ mismatch

Abbreviations: $(A-a)O_2$ gradient, alveolar to arterial O_2 partial pressure gradient; PIO_2, $F_IO_2 \cdot P_B$; F_IO_2, fractional concentration of inhaled O_2; P_B, barometric pressure; $\dot{V}/\dot{Q}$; ventilation/perfusion; $\downarrow$, low.

is evident that any given $P(A-a)O_2$ gradient is more significant as the $P(A-a)O_2$ decreases and hemoglobin begins to desaturate. Accordingly, a more precise measure of oxygenation deficit may be the actual determination of right-to-left transpulmonary shunt or venous admixture.

Calculation of Right-to-Left Transpulmonary Shunt

In a simple two-compartment lung model (Fig. 4), consisting of a perfused and oxygen-ventilated lung compartment and a shunt lung compartment that is normally perfused but not ventilated, the pulmonary shunt ($\dot{Q}S$) fraction can be readily

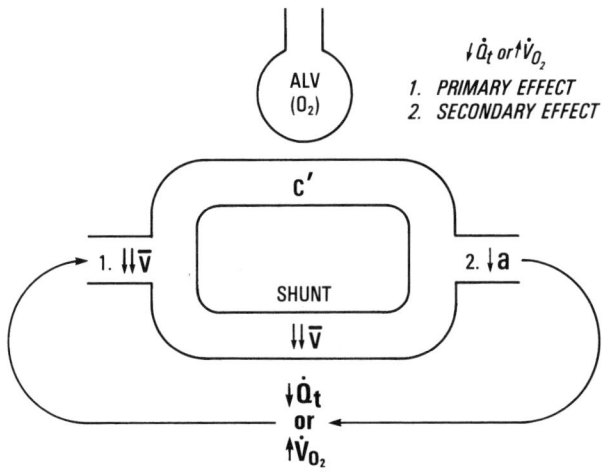

Figure 4 Two-compartment lung model. Mixed venous blood ($\bar{v}$) perfuses either ventilated alveolar (ALV O_2) capillaries and becomes oxygenated end-pulmonary capillary blood (c') or perfuses whatever true shunt pathways exist and remains the same in composition (desaturated). These two pathways must ultimately join together to form mixed arterial (a) blood. If the cardiac output ($\dot{Q}_T$) decreases and/or the O_2 consumption ($\dot{V}O_2$) increases, the tissues must extract more oxygen per unit volume of blood than under normal conditions. Thus, the primary effect of a decrease in $\dot{Q}_T$ or an increase in $\dot{V}O_2$ is a decrease in $\bar{v}O_2$ content. The $\bar{v}$ blood with a decreased O_2 content must flow through the shunt pathway as before (which may remain constant in size) and lower the arterial content of O_2. Thus, the secondary effect of a decrease in $\dot{Q}_T$ or an increase in $\dot{V}O_2$ is a decrease in arterial oxygen content. *Source*: Modified from Ref. 62.

derived by using the shunt equation (Equation 3)

$$\dot{Q}S/\dot{Q}T = (Cc'_{O_2} - Ca_{O_2})/(Cc'_{O_2} - C\bar{v}_{O_2}) \qquad (3)$$

where $\dot{Q}T$ is total cardiac output, Cc'_{O_2} is the end capillary O_2 content (C_{O_2}), which represents the blood leaving the normal lung unit, and is a valve that cannot be easily measured. The Cc'_{O_2} is assumed to be essentially the same as the PAO_2, and for calculation purposes, its value is derived by using the alveolar air equation (Equation 1), as this represents ideal oxygenation of arterial blood. The $C\bar{v}_{O_2}$ is the mixed venous C_{O_2}, and is measured in the blood aspirated from the distal [pulmonary artery (PA)] port of the Swan-Ganz catheter. The C_{O_2} for any sample of blood is calculated by using O_2 content equation (Equation 4).

$$C_{O_2} = [Hb] \times 1.34 \times Sat\ O_2 + 0.003 \times PO_2 \qquad (4)$$

Intuitively, the numerator of the shunt equation quantifies the oxygenation deficit (ideal oxygenation, Cc'_{O_2}, minus actual oxygenation, Ca_{O_2}), normalized by $\dot{Q}t$, which is estimated by the inverse of the denominator, that is, $1/(Cc'_{O_2} - C\bar{v}_{O_2})$. The term, $1/(Cc'_{O_2} - C\bar{v}_{O_2})$, closely approximates the expression, $1/(Ca_{O_2} - C\bar{v}_{O_2})$, which is proportional to $\dot{Q}_T$ during conditions of constant $\dot{V}O_2$, as given by rearrangement of the Fick equation (Equation 5).

$$\dot{Q}_T = \dot{V}O_2/(Ca_{O_2} - C\bar{v}_{O_2}) \qquad (5)$$

As the $\dot{Q}S/\dot{Q}T$ increases, the PaO_2 will decrease in a patient breathing the same F_IO_2. Thus, the ultimate PaO_2 depends also upon the F_IO_2 and the $\dot{Q}S/\dot{Q}T$, provided the other parameters remain stable. However, the greater the $\dot{Q}S/\dot{Q}T$ the less important is the F_IO_2 at determining the final PaO_2 (see Volume 2, Chapter 2). In addition, the Ca_{O_2} can be decreased by a decline in the $\dot{Q}T$ (at a constant $\dot{V}O_2$) and by an increased $\dot{V}O_2$ (for a constant $\dot{Q}T$). In either case (decreased $\dot{Q}T$ or increased $\dot{V}O_2$), along with a constant right-to-left shunt, the tissues must extract more O_2 from the blood per unit blood volume. Therefore, the $C\bar{v}_{O_2}$ must primarily decrease (Fig. 4). When the blood with lower $C\bar{v}_{O_2}$ passes through whatever shunt that exists in the lung and remains unchanged in its oxygen composition, it must inevitably mix with oxygenated end pulmonary capillary blood (c' flow) and secondarily decrease the Ca_{O_2} (Fig. 4). The pulmonary shunt fraction ($\dot{Q}S/\dot{Q}T$) is normally less than 5%. However, many conditions in trauma and critical care increase the $\dot{Q}S/\dot{Q}T$ including atelectasis, pneumonia, cardiogenic and noncardiogenic pulmonary edema, pneumothorax, hemothorax, and pulmonary contusion to name a few. Atelectasis is one of the most common problems that can dramatically increase $\dot{Q}S/\dot{Q}T$ in patients with otherwise normal lungs (Fig. 5).

If the lung is ventilated with an $F_IO_2 < 1.0$, then the oxygenation defects resulting from low $\dot{V}A/\dot{Q}$ units are added to it due to shunt regions. In this case, Equation 3 becomes an expression of the so-called venous admixture ($\dot{Q}_{VA}$). An attempt to discriminate between pulmonary shunt units ($\dot{V}A/\dot{Q} = 0$) and venous admixture units (low $\dot{V}A/\dot{Q}$) can be made by placing the patient on 100% O_2 ventilation. Then, the difference between the venous admixture fraction and the shunt fraction will estimate the amount of low $\dot{V}A/\dot{Q}$ units. However, this approach is limited because low $\dot{V}A/\dot{Q}$ lung units may collapse and

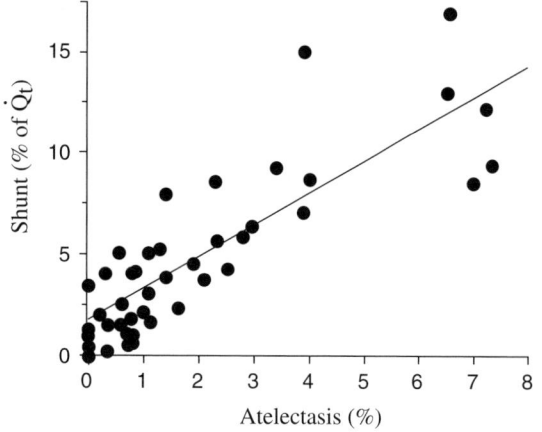

Figure 5 Association between shunt fraction and atelectasis in a normal subject. Atelectasis percentage data is derived from computed tomography scans taken through the caudal lung, just above the diaphragm, and right–left transpulmonary shunt $(\dot{Q}_s\dot{Q}_t)$ is calculated as a percent of the total cardiac output $(\dot{Q}_t)$ during anesthesia. In this study, there was a close correlation according to the equation: shunt = atelectatic area + 1.7 ($r = 0.1$, $P < 0.01$). *Source*: From Ref. 63.

convert themselves to shunt units during O_2 breathing (i.e., absorption atelectasis).

Venous admixture can be calculated if a PA catheter is in place, but requires numerous calculations. A simplified version of this equation was developed by Rasanen et al. (27) in 1988. These investigators termed this shunt approximation as the $\dot{V}/\dot{Q}$ index (Equation 6).

$$\dot{V}/\dot{Q} \text{ index} = \frac{1 - SaO_2}{1 - SvO_2} \qquad (6)$$

The $\dot{V}/\dot{Q}$ index ignores content calculations and substitutes only the saturations (assuming the pulmonary capillary saturation is 100%. Then the pulse oximeter saturation and mixed venous saturations and all that are required. The attractiveness of this equation is the ability to approximate shunt instantly from a continuous cardiac output PA catheter and a pulse oximeter. An example calculation is provided from a patient with a $SaO_2 = 90\%$ (or 0.9) and $SvO_2 = 60\%$ (or 0.6) the calculation would be as shown in Equation 7.

$$\dot{V}/\dot{Q} \text{ index} = \frac{1 - 0.9}{1 - 0.6} = \frac{0.1}{0.4} = 0.25 \qquad (7)$$

The 25% shunt calculated fails to reflect the severity of respiratory failure. Indeed, a $\dot{V}/\dot{Q}$ index of 0.25 for a patient breathing $F_IO_2 = 1.0$ is far worse than a $\dot{V}/\dot{Q}$ index of 0.25 for a patient breathing $F_IO_2 = 0.3$.

Complications with Arterial Blood Gas Measurement

An arterial puncture to obtain the sample may cause spasm, clot, hematoma, and distal ischemia, all of which need to be addressed immediately to prevent serious morbidity. The predictive value of the Allen's test in determining collateral flow to the palmar arch has been shown to be poor, and alternatives have been suggested (28). Care must be taken in those patients who are anticoagulated and those who have arterial occlusive diseases, such as Raynaud's disease.

If an arterial line is used, an adequate amount of dead space volume must be removed from the line before an accurate sample can be obtained.

A recent study suggests that discarding twice the dead space volume will ensure accurate blood gasses and electrolytes, while preventing unnecessary blood loss (29). Returning the dead space blood to the patient and using pediatric vials further diminishes the blood loss. Blood gases should be analyzed immediately after they are obtained to decrease the effects that metabolism and gas diffusion through the syringe have on the sample. The temperature of the patient may cause erroneous measurements. The solubility of oxygen increases as blood is cooled. By convention, blood gas analyzers are maintained at 37°C. In a hypothermic patient, the PaO_2 will be artificially elevated. Much debate has occurred over the years whether or not to correct for temperature. If the change in temperature is mild to moderate, it does not appear that temperature correction has any significant effect on therapy (30).

Complications with Pulse Oximetry Measurement

☞ Pulse oximetry relies on three principles: impedence plethysmography, absorption spectrophotometry, and the Beer-Lambert law. ☞ It distinguishes arterial blood from that of venous and capillary blood by relying on the fact that only arterial blood pulsates. All other sources of fluctuating light absorption are filtered out. Current pulse oximeters measure at two light wavelengths: 660 nm (red) and 940 nm (infrared). The effects of carbon monoxide (CO) on pulse oximetry have been studied in animals (31). Hemoglobin bound to CO (carboxyhemoglobin) absorbs light at 660 nm similarly to oxyhemoglobin, and at 940 nm it is virtually invisible to the photodetector. The result is that carboxyhemoglobin is spuriously detected by the pulse oximeter as oxyhemoglobin and the saturation levels of carboxyhemoglobin are artifactually elevated. Methemoglobin's effect on pulse oximetry has also been studied in animals (32). At both 660 nm and 940 nm, methemoglobin absorbs light equally. This corresponds to a saturation reading of 85% on a typical pulse oximeter calibration algorithm. Other causes of artifacts in pulse oximetry reading are listed in Table 4.

Despite the large number of artifacts affecting the pulse oximetry reading, it is an invaluable tool in reducing the occurrence of hypoxia in the TRS, the trauma OR, and the SICU. Patients with a high likelihood to have significant hemoglobin species other than oxy- and deoxyhemoglobin include inhalation burn victims (elevated carboxyhemoglobin) and those who have received benzocaine or prilocaine local anesthetics (elevated methemoglobin). These patients should have their O_2 saturation evaluated by a cooximeter

Table 4 Causes of Pulse Oximetry Artifact

Ambient lighting
Motion
Venous pulsations
Low perfusion: shock, low cardiac output
Malpositioned sensor
Hypothermia
Severe anemia
Dyes: methylene blue, indigo carmine, nail polish
Electrosurgical unit (Bovie) interference

with the ABG sample rather than the pulse oximeter, which will be erroneous.

Mixed Venous Oximetry

Mixed venous oximetry is an extension of pulse oximetry. Specially designed PA catheters emit light, which are reflected off of intact RBCs, down one set of fiberoptic cables. The light is carried by another set of fiberoptic cables to the photodetector. Mixed venous oxygen content is determined by the following formula:

$$SvO_2 = SaO_2 - [\dot{V}O_2/(\dot{Q} \times 1.36 \times Hgb)]$$

where $\dot{V}O_2$ is oxygen consumption, $\dot{Q}$ is cardiac output, and Hgb is hemoglobin concentration. From the formula, it is easy to see that a decrease in mixed venous oxygen saturation is caused by either a decrease in $\dot{Q}$ or a decrease in hemoglobin concentration, provided the oxygen consumption remains fixed. Causes of increased oxygen consumption that would decrease mixed venous saturation include sepsis, malignant hyperthermia, fever, and thyrotoxicosis. Continuous mixed venous saturation monitoring does not indicate to the practitioner the exact source of the disruption, but it does provide a finite list of them, which can be used in clinical assessment of the critically ill patient. The use of central venous saturation has gained attention as it does not require the placement of a PA catheter, but at least one recent study found lack of equivalence between these two methods (33). At the very least, the trends of central venous saturation and mixed venous saturation are interchangeable, and monitoring the trend may be of more clinical significance (34).

Tissue Oxygen Monitoring

Monitoring the oxygen at the tissues can either be noninvasive (cerebral oximetry, transcutaneous PO_2) or invasive. Transcutaneous PO_2 requires equipment maintenance, warmup time, and can result in skin burns. It has largely been replaced in the clinical setting by pulse oximetry. The data on cerebral oximetry is seemingly equivocal. Invasive tissue monitoring is fraught with complications and this provides information only about the tissue that the probe is located within.

Near Infrared Spectroscopy

A newer modality for cerebral ischemia monitoring is near infrared spectroscopy (NIRS). ✐ **NIRS is a technology designed to measure the adequacy of cerebral blood flow (CBF), but remains controversial because there is no universal agreement about normal values and the permissible degree of change.** ✐ The device utilizes infrared light of wavelengths 600–1300 nm to penetrate human tissue to a depth of several centimeters. Within the human brain this light is attenuated by the chromophores oxyhemoglobin, deoxyhemoglobin, and oxidized cytochrome aa3. Positioning a near infrared light source and a photodetector in a side-by-side configuration detects light attenuated and reflected in a parabolic path through the scalp, skull, and brain tissue (35). The standard probe placement of the NIRS devices is on the forehead, thus providing an estimation of tissue O_2 saturation in the vascular bed (primarily the venous component) of frontal lobes.

The most commonly utilized commercially available devices are the INVOS line of devices (Somanetics Corporation, Troy, Michigan, U.S.A.). Although the INVOS-3100

was introduced over a decade ago, and was utilized with minimal outcome data generated, questions arose regarding the validity of normal measurements and the meanings of abnormal numbers. The most notorious was the study by Schwartz et al. (36) who measured NIRS in 18 dead patients. They found that 6 of the 18 dead subjects (with obviously no cerebral blood flow) had values above the lowest values found in the healthy adults (or = 60%). Additionally, Lewis et al. (37) found poor correlation between NIRS and jugular venous saturation readings in head-injured patients. These findings raise serious concerns about the reliability of regional saturation (rSO_2) values obtained in adults by current generation NIRS monitoring devices.

The newest version of the INVOS line, the 5100B, provides an onscreen trend (graph) display, and is updated every 30 or 60 seconds (depending upon the settings). The generated data can be stored for one hour to 24 hours, and retrieved via supplied RS-232 port. The other widely used, commercially available device is the NIRO-300® (Hamamatsu Photonics K.K., Hamamatsu City, Japan). Although these devices are based upon the same principle, they both utilize different algorithms; however, studies generated on one device are not directly comparable with the other. Furthermore, currently no specific indications for these devices exist, and studies are still needed to correlate NIRS values with neurologic outcomes for various procedures (see "Eye to the Future" section).

Monitoring the Splanchnic System: Gastric Tonometry

Gastric tonometry uses the measurement of gastric intramucosal pH (pHim) as a method of determining the adequacy of oxygenation and perfusion of the splanchnic bed. Gastric pHim measurements are made to assess the adequacy of perfusion of the splanchnic circulation. The splachnic circulation may be particularly prone to injury as a consequence of hypoperfusion. Hypoperfusion-related tissue to the splanchnic circulation may allow intestinal bacteria and endotoxins to gain access to the systemic circulation (38). This so-called translocation of bacteria in hypoperfused patients may trigger the elaboration of several mediators of inflammation (interleukins, tumor necrosis factor, and activated white cells) that, in turn, contributes to the sepsis-like state of circulatory failure, which leads eventually to multiple organ failure (39). In an investigation in adult patients with acute circulatory failure, pHim was a highly predictive correlate of survival/nonsurvival, and its predictive accuracy was better than that of serum lactate determinations and greatly exceeded that of $\dot{D}CO_2$, $\dot{V}CO_2$, and cardiac index (39).

Because pHim requires steady-state conditions to establish baseline perfusion, it has been used more as an intensive care unit (ICU) management tool than as a monitor during initial resuscitation. Gastric pHim is calculated, using the Henderson-Hasselbach equation, from measurements of intragastric PCO_2 and arterial bicarbonate concentration. First, the intragastric PCO_2 is obtained via tonometry (using a small, saline-filled intragastric balloon). Next, the serum $[HCO_3^-]$ is measured, and the machine then calculates the pHim. At least one gastric tonometry device is available commercially (Tonocap; Instrumentarium Corp., Helsinki, Finland; and, Datex-Ohmeda). Gastric tonometry is discussed in greater detail in Volume 2, Chapter 10.

EYE TO THE FUTURE

As described earlier, T_CCO_2 and O_2 measurements are routinely used in pediatric ICUs in order to avoid serial arterial punctures; these technologies should likewise be utilized in adult units. A recent study involving COPD patients showed that T_CCO_2 values accurately reflected $PaCO_2$ values during mechanical ventilation in COPD patients (40). However, the accuracy of these data seem to be restricted to patients with $PaCO_2$ values of <56 mmHg (40).

Currently no reliable monitoring modality allows clinicians to assess the efficacy of CPR. As discussed earlier in this chapter, $P_{ET}CO_2$ provides an indication of the $\dot{Q}$ produced by chest compressions and can indicate return of spontaneous circulation. This fact is now also endorsed by the recent American Heart Association Guidelines for Cardiopulmonary Resuscitation (41). However, to accurately assess the $\dot{Q}$, one needs to evaluate the $P_{ET}CO_2$–$PaCO_2$ gradient. In the prehospital setting, ABG analysis may not be available. However, the T_CCO_2 values closely approximate the $PaCO_2$ and can likely be used as a surrogate, but this remains to be validated.

With regard to O_2 monitoring the future resides in increasing the ability to measure the saturation of various specific tissues, such as splanchnic and renal circulation (Volume 2, Chapter 10), cerebral (Volume 2, Chapter 7), etc. In terms of cerebral oximetry (introduced above), both the INVOS-5100® and the NIRO-300® are increasingly studied as indicators of CBF and cerebral tissue oxygenation. Although the data in TBI patients are mixed (37,42–47), these instruments have recently been used with some success in patients with cardiopulmonary bypass (CPB) (48–53), subarachnoid hemorrhage (54), and in carotid surgery (55,56).

Investigators are beginning to define threshold values for animals in various settings. Hagino et al. (53) studied pigs undergoing CPB, and were able to define a minimum safe flow rate during CPB in these animals using the NIRO-300®. Pigs were placed on CPB and cooled to various levels, and then run on various levels of low flow perfusion. Animals with an average tissue oxygenation index of less than 55% showed cerebral injury, whereas animals with an index of greater than 55% showed minimal or no evidence of injury (53).

The contribution of extracranial blood (57), and other artifacts continues to be a problem in some settings. In addition, comparisons between the various commercially available NIRS devices (e.g., NIRO-300 and the INVOS-5100) are only qualitative currently, as both manufacturers utilize different methodological approaches (including diodes with varying band widths and different algorithms to calculate saturations) (58). Once these concerns are addressed, the authors expect NIRS to become more widely employed in the near future, and ultimately begin to provide clinically useful in certain realms, such as CPB, carotid endartectomies, and certain neurosurgical procedures. Additional research is required before the role of NIRS in trauma and critical care can be defined.

SUMMARY

Monitoring gas exchange in patients who have undergone traumatic injury ranges from the simple, noninvasive monitoring to the more invasive and complex modalities. In the acutely decompensating patient, time to place a PA catheter is a luxury that is rarely afforded. Pulse oximetry

has gained acceptance as a universal monitor, since its introduction to the OR in the 1980s. Capnography which is well known to anesthesiologists, has yet to gain such widespread favor in the resuscitation area and the ICU. Despite the benefits of continuous $P_{ET}CO_2$ monitoring, one study found that in the centers that did have access to it, more than half "rarely" or "never" used it (59). It is perhaps the simplest and easiest-to-implement monitor that has yet to catch on. T_CCO_2 monitoring is in clinical use, but it cannot provide all of the useful information that is made available by capnography. Monitoring O_2 comprises testing the concentration of it at various points on its cascade from the atmosphere to the tissues. Currently, tissue oxygen monitoring is in its preliminary stage, and advances are eagerly anticipated.

KEY POINTS

- Exhaled gas CO_2 concentrations provide physiologic information about both systemic perfusion and pulmonary function.
- The $P_{ET}CO_2$ provides information about four important issues: (*i*) the correct placement of the ETT, (*ii*) the ventilation status, (*iii*) the cardiac output ($\dot{Q}$), and (*iv*) the metabolic status of the patient.
- The American Society of Anesthesiologists Difficult Airway (ASADA) guidelines, along with the ACLS® guidelines now recommend secondary confirmation of ETT placement with exhaled CO_2 measurement or an esophageal detector device (EDD) as it has become increasingly recognized that physical exam alone is error prone.
- In patients with fixed ventilation/perfusion ($\dot{V}/\dot{Q}$) relationships in the lungs, and stable minute ventilation ($\dot{V}_E$), the $P_{ET}CO_2$ is proportional to the $\dot{Q}$ (9).
- A low $P_{ET}CO_2$ value in multitrauma patients usually reflects insufficient $\dot{Q}$ (i.e., under resuscitation) and a resultant high ($\dot{V}/\dot{Q}$) as mentioned previously.
- An exaggerated upstroke in segment C–D (also known as the plateau phase), as shown in Figure 2A, indicates an increase in airway resistance with associated $\dot{V}/\dot{Q}$ spread among the millions of alveoli.
- All mechanical ventilators in use in the SICU should also have the ability to measure and continuously display the fraction of inspired O_2 (F_IO_2).
- Both right-to-left transpulmonary shunt ($\dot{Q}_s\dot{Q}_t$) and low $\dot{V}_A/\dot{Q}$ lung regions will contribute to an increase in the $P(A-a)O_2$ gradient.
- Pulse oximetry relies on three principles: impedence plethysmography, absorption spectrophotometry, and the Beer-Lambert law.
- NIRS is a technology designed to measure the adequacy of CBF, but remains controversial because there is no universal agreement about normal values and the permissible degree of change.

REFERENCES

1. Brunel W, Coleman DL, Schwartz DE, et al. Assessment of routine chest roentgenograms and the physical examination to confirm endotracheal tube position. Chest 1989; 96(5):1043–1045.
2. Andersen K, Hald A. Assessing the position of the endotracheal tube: the reliability of different methods. Anaesthesia 1989; 44:984–985.
3. White SJ, Slovis CM. Inadvertent esophageal intubation in the field: reliance on a fool's "gold standard." Acad Emerg Med 1997; 4(2):89–91.

4. Garnett AR, Gervin A. Capnographic waveforms in esophageal intubation: effect of carbonated beverages. Ann Emerg Med 1989; 18:387–390.
5. http://www.nellcor.com/_Catalog/PDF/Edu/CRT_B.f.00827v 1%20EasyCap%20Wall%20Ch.pdf. Last accessed November 22, 2005.
6. Silvestri S, Ralls GA, Krauss B. The effectiveness of out-of-hospital use of continuous end-tidal carbon dioxide monitoring on the rate of unrecognized misplaced intubation within a regional emergency medical services system. Ann Emerg Med 2005; 45(5):497–503.
7. Cummins RO, ed. ACLS Provider Manual Dallas: American Heart Association; 2001.
8. Christie JM, Dethlefsen M, Cane RD. Unplanned endotracheal extubation in the intensive care unit. J Clin Anesth 1996; 8:289–293.
9. Sullivan KJ, Kissoon N, Goodwin SR. End-tidal carbon dioxide monitoring in pediatric emergencies. Ped Emerg Care 2005; 21(5):327–335.
10. Gudipati CV, Weil MH, Bisera J, et al. Expired carbon dioxide: a non-invasive monitor of cardiopulmonary resuscitation. Circulation 1988; 77(1):234–239.
11. Garnet AR, Ornato JP, Gonzalez ER, Johnson EB. End-tidal carbon dioxide monitoring during cardiopulmonary resuscitation. JAMA 1987; 257(4):512–515.
12. Ornato JP, Garnett AR, Glauser FL. Relationship between cardiac output and the end-tidal carbon dioxide tension. Ann Emerg Med 1990; 19(10):1104–1106.
13. Aufderheide TP, Lurie KG. Death by hyperventilation: a common and life-threatening problem during cardiopulmonary resuscitation. Crit Care Med 2004; 32(9):S345–S351.
14. Stocchetti N, Maas AI, Chieregato A, van der Plas AA. Hyperventilation in head injury: a review. Chest 2005; 127(5):1812–1827.
15. Davis DP, Heister R, Poste JC. Ventilation patterns in patients with severe traumatic brain injury following paramedic rapid sequence intubation. Neurocrit Care 2005; 2(2):165–171.
16. Davis DP, Dunford JV, Poste JC, et al. The impact of hypoxia and hyperventilation on outcome after paramedic rapid sequence intubation of severely head-injured patients. J Trauma 2004; 57(1):1–8.
17. Palmon SC, Liu M, Moore LE, et al. Capnography facilitates tight control of ventilation during transport. Crit Care Med 1996; 24:608–611.
18. Tyburski JG, Collinge JD, Wilson RF, et al. End-tidal CO₂-derived values during emergency trauma surgery correlated with outcome: a prospective study. J Trauma 2002; 53(4):738–743.
19. Tyburski JG, Carlin AM, Harvery EH, et al. End-tidal CO₂-arterial CO₂ differences: a useful intraoperative mortality marker in trauma surgery. J Trauma 2003; 55(5):892–896.
20. Deakin CD, Sado DM, Coats TJ, Davies G. Prehospital end-tidal carbon dioxide concentration and outcome in major trauma. J Trauma 2004; 57(1):65–68.
21. Bendjelid K, Schutz N, Stotz M, et al. Transcutaneous PCO₂ monitoring in critically ill adults: clinical evaluation of a new sensor. Crit Care Med 2005; 33(10):2203–2206.
22. Brown MK, Willms DC. A laboratory evaluation of two mechanical ventilators in the presence of helium-oxygen mixtures. Respir Care 2005; 50(3):354–360.
23. D'Alonzo GE, Dantzker DR. Respiratory failure, mechanisms of abnormal gas exchange, and oxygen delivery. Med Clin North Am 1983; 67:557–571.
24. Pedersen T, Pederson P, Moller AM. Pulse oximetry for perioperative monitoring. Cochrane Database Syst Rev 2001; 2:CD 002013.
25. Morgan TJ, Venkatesh B. Monitoring oxygenation. In: Bersten AD, Soni N, Oh TE, eds. Oh's Intensive Care Manual. 5th ed. New York: Butterworth Heinemann, 2003: 95–106.
26. Nirmalan M, Willard T, Columb MO, Nightingale P. Effect of changes in arterial-mixed venous oxygen content difference on indices of pulmonary oxygen transfer in a model ARDS lung. Br J Anaesth 2001; 86:477–485.
27. Rasanen J, Downs JB, Malec DJ, et al. Real-time continuous estimation of gas exchange by dual oximetry. Intensive Care Med 1988; 14(2):118–122.
28. Barbeau GR, Arsenault F, Dugas L, et al. Evaluation of the ulno-palmar arterial arches with pulse oximetry and plethymography: comparison with the Allen's test in 1010 patients. Am Heart J 2004; 147(3):489–493.
29. Rickard CM, Couchman BA, Schmidt SJ, et al. A discard volume of twiche the deadspace ensures clinically accurate arterial blood gases and electrolytes and prevents unnecessary blood loss. Crit Care Med 2003; 31:1654–1658.
30. Durbin CG. Arterial blood gas analysis and monitoring. In: Lake CL, Hines RL, Blitt CD, eds. Clinical Monitoring. Philadelphia, PA: W.B. Saunders Company, 2001:335–353.
31. Barker SJ, Tremper KK. The effect of carbon monoxide inhalation on pulse oximeter signal detection. Anesthesiology 1987; 66:677–679.
32. Barker SJ, Tremper KK, Hyatt J, et al. Effects of methemoglobinemia on pulse oximetry and mixed venous oximetry. Anesthesiology 1989; 70:112–117.
33. Chawla LS, Zia H, Gutierrez G, et al. Lack of equivalence between central and mixed venous oxygen saturation. Chest 2004; 126(6):1891–1896.
34. Dueck MH, Klimek M, Appenrodt S, et al. Trends but not individual values of central venous oxygen saturation agree with mixed venous oxygen saturation during varying hemodynamic conditions. Anesthesiology 2005; 103(2):249–257.
35. Williams IM, Mortimer AJ, McCollum CN. Recent developments in cerebral monitoring—near-infrared light spectroscopy. An overview. Eur J Vasc Endovasc Surg 1996; 12(3):263–271.
36. Schwarz G, Litscher G, Kleinert R, et al. Cerebral oximetry in dead subjects. J Neurosurg Anesthesiol 1996; 8(3):189–193.
37. Lewis SB, Myburgh JA, Thornton EL, et al. Cerebral oxygenation monitoring by near-infrared spectroscopy is not clinically useful in patients with severe closed-head injury: a comparison with jugular venous bulb oximetry. Crit Care Med 1996; 24(8):334–338.
38. Lelli JL, Drongowski RA, Coran AG, Abrams GD. Hypoxia-induced bacterial translocation in the puppy. J Ped Surg 1992; 27:974–982.
39. Maynard N, Bihari D, Beale R, et al. Assessment of splanchnic oxygenation by gastric tonometry in patients with acute circulatory failure. JAMA 1993; 270:1203–1210.
40. Cuvelier A, Grigoriu B, Molano LC, et al. Limitations of transcutaneous carbon dioxide measurements for assessing long-term mechanical ventilation. Chest 2005; 127:1744–1748.
41. American Heart Association Guidelines for Cardiopulmonary Resuscitation and Emergency Cardiovascular Care. Part 7.4 Monitoring and Medications. Circulation 2005; 112:IV-78–IV-83.
42. Brawanski A, Faltermeier R, Rothoerl RD, Woertgen C. Comparison of near-infrared spectroscopy and tissue p(O₂) time series in patients after severe head injury and aneurysmal subarachnoid hemorrhage. J Cereb Blood Flow Metab 2002; 22:605–611.
43. Dunham CM, Sosnowski C, Porter JM, et al. Correlation of noninvasive cerebral oximertry with cerebral perfusion in the severe head injured patient: a pilot study. J Trauma 2002; 52(1):40–46.
44. Buchner K, Meixenberger J, Dings J, et al. Near-infared spectroscopy—not useful to monitor cerebral oxygenation after severe brain injury. Zentralbl Neurochir 2000; 61:69–73.
45. Macmillan CS, Andrews PJ. Cerebrovenous oxygen saturation monitoring; practical considerations and clinical relevance. Intensive Care Med 2000; 26:1028.
46. McLeod AD, Igielman F, Elwell C, et al. Measuring cerebral oxygenation during normobaric hyperoxia: a comparison of tissue microprobes, near-infared spectroscopy, and jugular venous oximetry in head injury. Anesth Analg 2003; 97:851–856.
47. Kirkpatric PJ, Smielewski P, Czonsnyka M, et al. Near-infared spectroscopy use in patients with head injury. J Neurosurg 1995; 83:963–970.

48. Reents W, Muellges W, Franke D, et al. Cerebral oxygen satur-
     ation assessed by near-infrared spectroscopy during coronary
     artery bypass grafting and early postoperative cognitive
     function. Ann Thorac Surg 2002; 74:109.
49. Janelle GM, Mnookin S, Gravenstein N, et al. Unilateral cerebral
     oxygen desaturation during emergent repair of a DeBakey type 1
     aortic dissection: Potential aversion of a major catastrophe.
     Anesthesiology 2002; 96:1263.
50. Kussman BD, Wypij D, DiNardo JA, et al. An Evaluation of bilat-
     eral monitoring of cerebral oxygen saturation during pediatric
     cardiac surgery. Anesth Analg 2005; 101:1294–1300.
51. Liebold A, Khosravi A, Westphal B, et al. Effect of closed mini-
     mized cardiopulmonary bypass on cerebral tissue oxygenation
     and microembolization. J. Thorac Cardiovasc Surg 2006;
     131(2):268–276.
52. Talpahewa SP, Lovell TA, Angelini GD, Ascione R. Effect of car-
     diopulmonary bypass on cortical cerebral oxygenation during
     coronary artery bypass grafting. Eur J Cardiothorac Surg
     2004; 26:676–681.
53. Hagino I, Anttila V, Zurakowski D, et al. Tissue oxygenation
     index is a useful monitor of histologic and neurologic
     outcome after cardiopulmonary bypass in piglets. J Thorac
     Cardiovasc Surg 2005; 130(2):384–392.
54. Springborg JB, Frederiksen HJ, Eskesen V, Olsen NV. Trends in
     monitoring patients with aneurysmal subarachnoid haemor-
     rhage. Br J Anaesth 2005; 94(3):259–270.
55. Samra SK, Dy EA, Welch K, et al. Evaluation of a cerebral oxi-
     meter as a monitor of cerebral ischemia during carotid endar-
     terectomy. Anesthesiology 2000; 93:964–970.
56. Beese U, Langer H, Lang W, et al. Comparioson of near-infared
     spectroscopy and somatosensory evoked potentials for the
     detection of cerebral ischemia during carotid endarterectomy.
     Stroke 1998; 29:2032.
57. Grubhofer G, Lassnigg A, Manlik F, et al. The contribution of
     extracranial blood oxygenation on near-infared spectroscopy
     during carotid thromboendarterectomy. Anesthesia 1997;
     52:116.
58. Thavasothy M, Broadhead M, Elwell C, et al. A comparison of
     cerebral oxygenation as measured by the NIRO 300 and the
     INVOS 5100 near-infrared spectrophotometers. Anaesthesia
     2002; 57(10):999–1006.
59. Deiorio NM. Continuous end-tidal carbon dioxide monitoring
     for confirmation of endotracheal tube placement is neither
     widely available nor consistently applied by emergency
     physicians. Emerg Med J 2005; 22(7):490–493.
60. Breen PH. Capnography: the science behind the lines. In:
     A.S.A. Annual Refresher Course Lectures. Park Ridge, IL:
     American Society of Anesthesiologists, 1994; 126:1–7.
61. Nunn JF. Applied Respiratory Physiology. 4 ed. London:
     Butterworth-Heinmann, 1993; 126:255.
62. Wilson WC, Benumof JL. Respiratory physiology and res-
     piratory function during anesthesia. In: Miller RD, ed.
     Anesthesia. 6th ed. New York: Churchill Livingstone,
     2005:701, chapter 17.
63. Gunnarsson L, Tokics L, Gustavsson H, et al. Influence of
     age on atelectasis formation and gas exchange impair-
     ment during general anesthesia. Br J Anaesth 1991;
     66:423–432.

9

Cardiovascular Monitoring

William C. Chiu

Department of Surgery, R Adams Cowley Shock-Trauma Center, Baltimore, Maryland, U.S.A.

INTRODUCTION

The clinical assessment and monitoring of the cardiovascular system is a fundamental necessity in severely injured and critically ill surgical patients to ensure optimal resuscitation and perfusion of organ systems. Traditional methods for cardiovascular evaluation were able to determine heart rate (HR), rhythm, and blood pressure using simple noninvasive means. The application of various invasive intravascular catheters then provided us with continuous pressure and flow measurements and was revolutionary to advanced hemodynamic monitoring. Now, current technological advances are returning to the development and perfection of noninvasive tools, with the hope that they will have the ability to acquire hemodynamic data with similar accuracy and reliability as invasive devices currently provide.

Many situations in critically ill trauma and surgical patients warrant monitoring of the heart and circulation. Guidelines from the American College of Cardiology (ACC)/American Heart Association (AHA) outline certain comorbid conditions that increase cardiac risk in surgical patients (Table 1) (1). Among these clinical predictors are ischemic coronary disease, congestive heart failure, significant dysrhythmias, and valvular heart disease. In the previously healthy patient, traumatic injury to the heart or aorta may require hemodynamic monitoring to ensure tissue oxygen delivery, while minimizing cardiac contractile force (2). Conversely, injuries to the central nervous system may require hemodynamic monitoring to facilitate resuscitation from neurogenic shock, and therapies to maintain cerebral and spinal cord perfusion pressure. Patients with significant blood loss from injury or surgery require monitoring to optimize resuscitation and determine response to therapy. In particular, geriatric blunt-trauma patients may have occult hypoperfusion, and are at risk for untreated shock (3). Finally, those patients developing overwhelming inflammatory response from trauma or sepsis require monitoring to limit organ system failure, and to guide supportive measures.

This chapter will provide a review of the tools in the intensivist's armamentarium to evaluate and monitor hemodynamics in the intensive care unit (ICU). These devices include electrocardiography, arterial pressure monitoring, central venous pressure (CVP) monitoring, pulmonary artery catheter (PAC) monitoring, and cardiac output monitoring. The focus of this chapter will be on the utilization of these devices and interpretation of the acquired data in the ICU. Further discussion on initial assessment of circulation and shock in the emergency room (see Volume 1, Chapter 12), preoperative evaluation and preparation (see Volume 1, Chapter 17), basic cardiovascular physiology (see Volume 2, Chapter 3), and management of cardiovascular problems in the ICU (see Volume 2, Chapters 17–22) can be found in other chapters of this book.

ELECTROCARDIOGRAPHY

Monitoring HR and rhythm has become a standard of care for patients admitted to the ICU. Einthoven first noted that the electrical activity of the heart produces electrical currents at the skin, giving rise to the development of surface electrocardiography. The electrocardiogram (ECG) depicts the electrical events of the heart, providing information on cardiac impulse morphology, HR, and abnormalities of these components. While a static 12-lead ECG may be comprehensive for the diagnosis of cardiac electrical abnormalities, continuous monitoring of one or two leads in the ICU allows the early detection of most HR changes, ischemic changes, transient abnormal beats, and dysrhythmias.

Heart Rate and Pulse Monitoring

Although the terms HR and pulse rate are commonly used interchangeably in clinical situations, there are subtle differences and implications that distinguish the two terms. The term HR, itself, may represent either the frequency of cardiac electrical activity or the frequency of cardiac contractions. The mechanical contraction results in ejection of blood into the aorta, which can be palpated in the arteries as a pulse. Natural coupling of electrical and mechanical cardiac events results in a condition where the pulse is equal to the electrically monitored HR. Certain conditions, such as pulseless electrical activity (PEA), are marked by a dissociation of electrical and mechanical events resulting in an electrical HR unequal to the mechanical HR.

Continuous ECG monitoring displays the electrical activity of the heart and is the best method for determining electrical HR, but does not always accurately reflect the mechanical HR (pulse). Since most modern telemetry monitors continuously display a computer-derived HR, it is critical that the clinician distinguish between cardiac electrical activity and artifacts. Inadequate electrode-skin contact or electrical interference within the monitoring equipment may produce artifacts resulting in an inaccurately derived HR. Patient motion or shivering may produce artifactual activity on the display. High-amplitude P or T waves may be incorrectly counted as QRS complexes by the telemetry computer, resulting in falsely elevated rates. In those patients with pacemakers, telemetry monitors may display the rate of pacemaker spikes. It is incumbent on the clinician

Table 1   Clinical Predictors of Cardiac Risk

Major clinical predictors
Unstable coronary syndromes
  Recent MI
  Unstable angina
Decompensated CHF
Significant dysrhythmias
  High-grade AV block
  Symptomatic dysrhythmias
  SVT
Severe valvular disease

Intermediate clinical predictors
Mild angina pectoris
Prior MI
Compensated or prior CHF
Diabetes mellitus

Minor clinical predictors
Advanced age
Abnormal ECG
Rhythm other than sinus
Low functional capacity
History of stroke
Uncontrolled systemic hypertension

Abbreviations: AV, atrioventricular; CHF, congestive heart failure; ECG, electrocardiogram; MI, myocardial infarction; SVT, supraventricular tachycardia.
Source: From Ref. 1.

to determine if electrical capture is present, and to evaluate whether there is a resultant mechanical contraction.

Accurate determination of mechanical HR, when necessary, may be assessed several ways: (*i*) observing the arterial pressure waveform of an intra-arterial catheter, (*ii*) observing ventricular contractions at echocardiography, or (*iii*) by observing change in pressures using a pulmonary artery catheter. Auscultation for cardiac sounds alone is often unreliable in the ICU, especially when HR is rapid and when there is excessive ambient noise. The most practical clinical estimate of mechanical HR is the pulse rate palpated at a peripheral arterial site.

The pulse rate typically equals the mechanical HR, except in conditions of irregular ventricular contractions such as ventricular fibrillation, conditions in which the contractile force is especially weak, or in association with perfusion deficit to the peripheral site. Pulse rate and rhythm information adds a valuable adjunct to complete evaluation of cardiac dysrhythmias. Accurate measurement of pulse rate depends on measuring pressure changes with an intra-arterial catheter, but may be estimated if a pulse oximeter is available. While palpation of peripheral pulse has similar shortcomings to auscultation of the heart in the ICU, it may be the most rapid method to assess pulse rate in those patients without other monitoring devices.

ECG lead II, displaying the electrical vector from the right arm electrode to the left leg electrode, is most commonly used for routine continuous monitoring. This lead best parallels the direction of forward electrical conduction, and results in the greatest P wave voltage of any surface lead configuration. The ability to rapidly detect and analyze P wave presence and regularity best facilitates evaluation of an abnormal rhythm. Placement of the limb electrodes is routinely adjusted proximal to the standard positions of the wrists and ankles, by placing arm electrodes over

the shoulders and leg electrodes over the lower torso (Fig. 1). This modification reduces electrical noise from extremity muscle contractions, while preserving the triangular cardiac axes.

Ischemia Monitoring

☞ **The precordial leads are the most sensitive for detecting myocardial ischemia in the operating room; this is presumably true in the ICU as well.** ☞ Indeed, London et al. studied a large cohort of patients with known coronary artery disease undergoing noncardiac, mainly vascular surgery and found that V_5 was most sensitive, detecting 75% of ischemic events (4). Simultaneously monitoring both leads, V_4 and V_5, increased sensitivity to 90%, whereas the standard II and V_5 array was only 80% sensitive. Because lead II is most sensitive for P wave evaluation and detects inferior wall ischemia, simultaneous monitoring of lead II and V_5 is recommended. The V_5 lead is classically placed over the left fifth intercostal space, in the anterior axillary line (also see Volume 2, Chapter 19).

ST Segment Depression

ECG changes suggestive of myocardial ischemia may occur with or without any associated clinical symptoms (e.g., chest pain, shortness of breath, dizziness, nausea) or signs (e.g., tachycardia, tachypnea, hypotension, or hypoxia). The recognition of acute ECG changes allows for the early detection and management of myocardial ischemia. ☞ **ST segment depression is the most common manifestation of subendocardial myocardial ischemia.** ☞ ST segment depression is commonly encountered during provocative ischemia studies (e.g., treadmill test), and clinically when perfusion pressure to a stenotic coronary artery drops below a critical threshold value (Fig. 2). The ST segment is that part of the ECG trace that immediately succeeds the QRS. The point at which it "takes off" from the QRS is called the J (junction) point. The position of the ST segment relative to baseline and its slope should be noted and monitored. Changes in the level of the ST segment are measured at the beginning of the ST segment (i.e., the "J" point), and are compared to the level of the isoelectric line, also known as the T-P segment. The standard criterion for diagnosing ischemia is ST segment depression of ≥ 0.10 mV or 1 mm (on a standard amplitude signal calibration of 1 mV $= 10$ mm), with a downsloping depression representing worse ischemia than a horizontal or upsloping segment (5).

ST Segment Elevation

☞ **Acute transmural myocardial ischemia, or infarction, results in acute ST segment elevation.** ☞ ST segment elevation of >1 mm from the J point is considered abnormal for women. However, ST segment elevation of 2 mm is the threshold for men. Indeed, 1 mm of ST segment elevation is normal for 90% of males, and the presence of prior myocardial infarction (MI) and other conditions must also be considered (6). In patients with Q waves, ST segment elevation may be related to wall motion abnormalities. In patients without Q waves, leads with ST segment elevation are very specific indicators of the location of ischemia. T wave inversions and new Q waves are suggestive of either recent or evolving MI. For more detailed information on the diagnosis and treatment of myocardial ischemia, the reader is referred to Volume 2, Chapter 19.

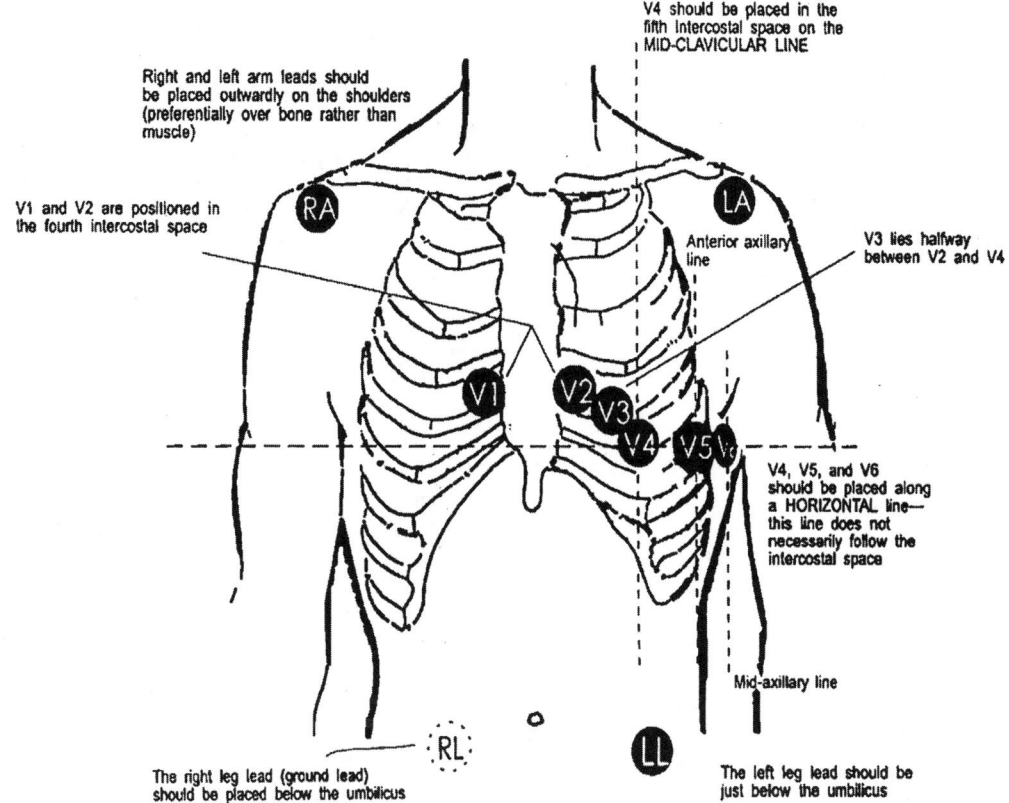

Figure 1 Recommendations for placement of 12-lead electrocardiogram electrodes. Electrodes are routinely adjusted proximal to the standard positions of the wrists and ankles by placing arm electrodes over the shoulders and leg electrodes over the lower torso for patients in the operating room, surgical intensive care unit, and during exercise testing. *Abbreviations*: RA, right arm; LA, left arm; RL, right leg; LL, left leg. *Source*: From Ref. 5.

Dysrhythmia Monitoring

Similar to monitoring for myocardial ischemia, continuous ECG monitoring in the ICU allows the early detection of changes in cardiac rhythm, or those dysrhythmias that are transient or episodic. The analysis of a dysrhythmia involves the delineation of three characteristics—anatomic origin, discharge sequence, and conduction sequence (7). After initially identifying the dysrhythmia as a bradycardia (ventricular rate <60) or a tachycardia (ventricular rate >100), the next priority in the analysis involves determining whether the origin of the electrical impulse is sinoatrial (SA), atrial, atrioventricular (AV), or ventricular. P waves

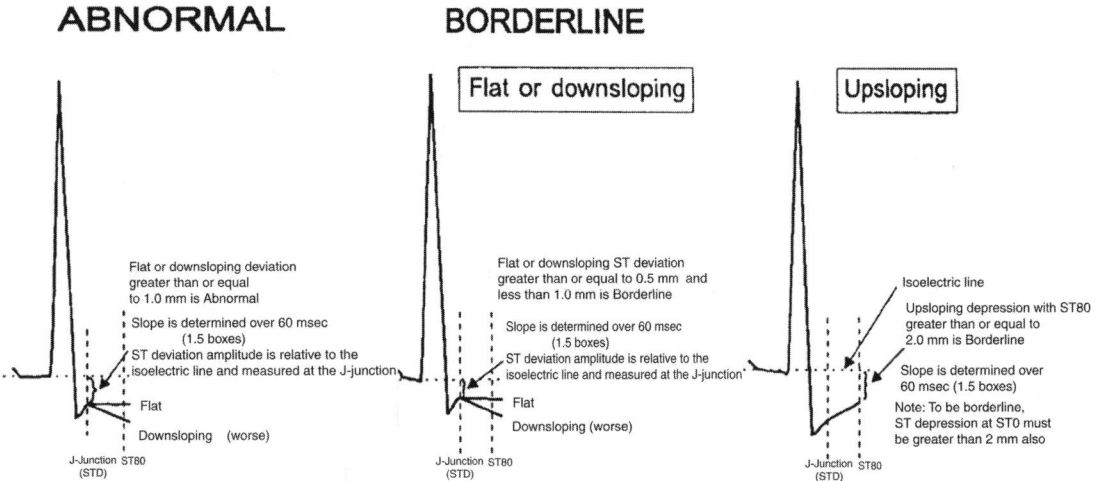

Figure 2 Abnormal and borderline ST segment depression criterion. ST depression is specific for ischemia when depressed greater than or equal to 1.0 mm, and flat or downsloping. The ST segment depression is borderline when ranging between 0.5 and 1.0 mm and flat or downsloping, or as much as 2.0 mm depressed but upsloping. *Source*: From Ref. 5.

Table 2 Common Dysrhythmias in the Intensive Care Unit

Supraventricular
Sinus tachycardia
Sinus bradycardia
Sinus arrest
Sick sinus syndrome
Sinus node re-entrant tachycardia
Atrial fibrillation
Atrial flutter
Multifocal atrial tachycardia
Ectopic atrial tachycardia
Atrial re-entrant tachycardia

Atrioventricular
Atrioventricular junctional rhythm
Accelerated atrioventricular junctional rhythm
Atrioventricular nodal re-entrant tachycardia
Wolff-Parkinson-White syndrome

Ventricular
Ventricular tachycardia
Ventricular flutter
Ventricular fibrillation

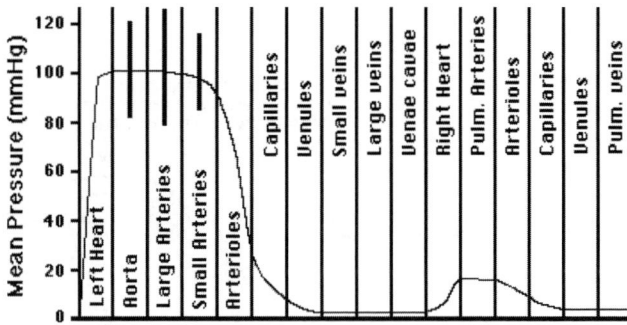

Figure 3 Mean arterial pressure throughout the normal circulation. Normal mean arterial blood pressure throughout the circulation is depicted by the continuous trace beginning in the left heart, and continuing through to the pulmonary veins. The systolic/diastolic pulse pressure is shown for the aorta, large arteries, and small arteries as a solid upright line, the top of which indicates the systolic pressure and the bottom of which indicates the diastolic pressure. *Source*: From Ref. 60.

suggesting SA node origin are best observed in lead II, while leads III, aV_F, and V_1 may be alternates. Lack of P waves or abnormal P wave morphology indicates an origin other than the SA node, and associated QRS complex widening may help localize the source to the AV junction or the ventricles.

A full ECG rhythm strip is critical in the analysis of dysrhythmias. Only with a rhythm strip can an adequate assessment be made, regarding whether the discharge sequence is normal sinus rhythm, atrial flutter, or atrial fibrillation, or whether some other ectopic or multifocal pattern exists. Conduction sequence analysis involves the determination of whether the electrical conduction pattern is normal, delayed, blocked, or aberrant. These identifying points facilitate appropriate treatment selection. Table 2 outlines the most common dysrhythmias encountered in surgical patients, and a more detailed discussion on the diagnosis and therapy of dysrhythmias can be found in Volume 2, Chapter 20.

ARTERIAL PRESSURE MONITORING
Physiology of Systemic Arterial Pressure

The function of the systemic arterial system is to distribute oxygenated blood to the capillary beds throughout the body, and to serve as a hydraulic filter and reservoir (8). Measurement of arterial blood pressure provides a quantitative assessment of the status of the hydraulic pressure head supplying the cardiovascular system. The mean arterial pressure (MAP) is the average blood pressure during the cardiac cycle. The MAP can be expressed by a cardiovascular equivalent of Ohm's law ($E = I \times R$; energy potential = current × resistance) as follows:

$$\dot{Q} \times SVR \qquad (1)$$

where $\dot{Q}$ is the cardiac output and SVR is the systemic vascular resistance. Thus, the blood pressure is dependent

upon the $\dot{Q}$ [HR × stroke volume (SV)] and the SVR:

$$\dot{Q} = HR \times SV \qquad (2)$$

The SV is dependent upon the preload, afterload, and contractility of the heart. The SVR is chiefly governed by the level of sympathetic stimulation. If SVR and HR are held constant, then the SV will correlate directly with the blood pressure. Indeed, Cullen found a correlation coefficient of 0.82 between changes in SV and systolic blood pressure (9).

☞ **The MAP is highest in the ascending aorta, and drops minimally until the peripheral arteriolar bed is reached (Fig. 3) (10).** ☞ Accordingly, in normal patients, the MAP measured in the larger arteries (radial, femoral, dorsalis pedis) will be an accurate measure of the MAP at the aorta. The pressure in the arterial system drives the flow of blood toward the arterioles and through the capillary system. Blood flow through the vast majority of the arterial system is fairly continuous (except for the proximal aorta), as only about 20% of the flow wave is pulsatile. The ascending aortic flow is quite pulsatile, with almost no flow occurring during diastole (except to the coronary arteries). Similarly, the arch of the aorta undergoes retrograde flow during diastole, as blood flows out the arch vessels from blood stored in the thoracic aorta. Blood flows out of the distal aorta at a relatively slow 0.5 m/sec during diastole, whereas the pulse pressure wave moves at about 10 m/sec (11). However, it is the arterial pressure wave that can be measured, and will be discussed further.

Arterial Pressure Waveform Characteristics

The arterial pressure waves are transformed as they proceed from the proximal aorta to the distal arteries (Fig. 4). These waveform changes include augmentation of the systolic component and attenuation of the diastolic component. These changes, along with dynamic response incompatibilities in the catheter-manometer system, are responsible for most disparities encountered between cuff pressures in the brachial artery and the invasively measured pressure in the radial artery (12).

The changing pattern in the arterial pressure waveform is chiefly due to the reflection of waves from the periphery.

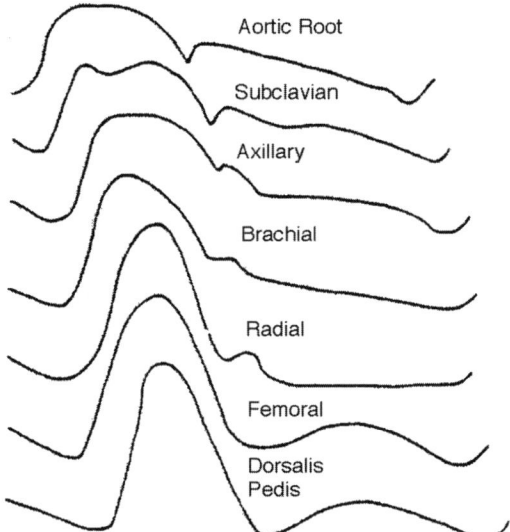

Figure 4 Changing pattern of arterial pressure waveforms from the aorta to the peripheral arteries. The contour of the arterial pressure waveform changes as the pressure wave moves from the proximal aorta to the periphery. The central aortic waveform is more rounded and has a definite dicrotic notch. The dorsalis pedis (and to a lesser degree the femoral) artery shows a delay in pulse transmission, a more rapid upstroke (dp/dt), and a slurring of the dicrotic notch. The systolic pressure increases and the diastolic pressure decreases as the pressure wave moves distally. However, the mean pressure remains the same. *Source*: From Ref. 61.

Just as waves are created in a still pool of water after an object is thrown into it, these waves reflect back after hitting the edge of the pool, producing a standing wave that adds to (or subtracts from) the incident wave. The artery-arteriole junction is thought to be the principal site of reflection. Additionally, branching points are sites of arterial waveform reflection and, finally, the tapering of arterial vessels as one proceeds toward the periphery acts to amplify waves, similar to how an ear trumpet amplifies sound waves (13).

Noninvasive Monitoring of Arterial Pressure

Arterial blood pressure can be measured noninvasively using indirect methods (including palpation, auscultation, and oscillometric technology) or invasively following direct arterial cannulation and pressure transduction. All of the noninvasive techniques of blood pressure determination utilize a Riva-Rocci cuff device. This apparatus involves the inflation of a pneumatic cuff (connected to a sphygmomanometer) that surrounds an extremity and occludes a peripheral artery to the point of no-flow. The physical changes that occur at the time of arterial occlusion and return of flow are sensed and correlated with an arterial blood pressure. Furthermore, the various noninvasive blood pressure measurement techniques actually interrogate different physical events. Thus, the blood pressure obtained is a function of the way in which it is measured. Additionally, there are many artifactual causes for blood pressure measurement problems with a noninvasive technique, which are not factors when monitoring the blood pressure directly (14). ✂ **In trauma situations and shock, the noninvasive automatic blood pressure devices often fail to work properly. In these situations, an invasive arterial line or manual techniques are preferred.** ✂

Table 3 Phases of Korotkoff Sounds

I.	First appearance of clear, repetitive, tapping sounds (systolic pressure)
II.	Sounds are softer and longer, with the quality of an intermittent murmur.
III.	Sounds again become crisper and louder.
IV.	Sounds are muffled, less distinct, and softer.
V.	Sounds disappear completely (diastolic pressure)

Manual Intermittent Techniques

A variety of methods for measuring blood pressure are available, ranging from basic manual intermittent techniques, to automated continuous technology. With only the means of a sphygmomanometer, systolic arterial blood pressure can be rapidly estimated by the Riva-Rocci technique, based on measuring the external pressure required to compress the brachial artery. This palpation method may be used when a stethoscope is not available. While palpating the radial arterial pulse, the cuff should be inflated to a level about 30 mmHg above the pressure, at which the pulse disappears. Pressure should then be released from the cuff slowly until the return of a regular palpable pulse, indicating a return of pulsatile blood flow. This pressure is the estimation of systolic arterial pressure.

With the assistance of a stethoscope, the auscultation method not only provides a more accurate systolic pressure, but also allows measurement of a diastolic arterial pressure. As the sphygmomanometer cuff pressure is slowly released, the return of pulsatile blood flow produces Korotkoff sounds. The AHA has published guidelines on the determination of blood pressure by sphygmomanometry, and has characterized five phases of Korotkoff sounds (Table 3) (15). The systolic arterial blood pressure corresponds to the pressure at which the sounds first appear at Phase I. The diastolic blood pressure corresponds to the pressure at which the sounds disappear at Phase V.

Automated Intermittent Devices

Noninvasive blood pressure monitoring has been automated to provide regular and repeated pressure measurements using oscillometry. This method is derived on the concept that as the occluding cuff is slowly deflated, the return of arterial pulsations results in a counterpressure onto the cuff. With continued cuff deflation and progressive increase in arterial pulsations, the oscillation amplitude increases. The definitions of systolic, diastolic, and mean arterial pressures vary somewhat with different device manufacturers. In general, the systolic pressure is determined to be the point of rapid increase in oscillation amplitude, while the mean pressure is determined to be the point of maximum oscillation amplitude. With some devices, diastolic pressure is taken to be the point of rapid decrease in oscillation amplitude [Dinamap (Critikon)], while with other manufacturers, the diastolic pressure is a derived value based on the systolic and mean pressure measurements.

Although the automated oscillometric blood pressure devices are quite accurate in normal patients, when the patients are hypotensive (systolic blood pressure less than 80 mmHg) they tend to overestimate blood pressure, compared to invasive monitoring (16). Furthermore, a recent study by Davis et al. demonstrated that automatic oscillometric blood pressure measurements were consistently higher in hypotensive patients (potentially providing a false sense of resuscitation adequacy) (17). Accordingly, automated devices are not recommended for field or hospital triage decisions.

Continuous Automated Technology

Newer methods of continuous noninvasive blood pressure measurement do exist, but these have not yet gained wide acceptance clinically. Photoplethysmography relies on infrared light transmission to monitor the volume of a finger. An inflatable cuff maintains the finger at a constant volume, and continuous arterial pressure is measured as the counter pressure required to maintain constant finger volume. One study performed in patients undergoing spinal anesthesia reported correlations of only approximately 0.72 to 0.79 between this technique [Finapres (Ohmeda)], and invasive indwelling radial artery catheter measurements, citing frequent unexplained large differences (18). Furthermore, it has been shown that measurements of pressure with this technique are very sensitive to malapplication of the finger cuff, contributing to errors and limiting the reliability of the device (19).

While photoplethysmography utilizes light transmission as the initial trigger to influence cuff counterpressure, the technique of arterial tonometry utilizes a surface pressure transducer applied onto the skin directly over an artery, to measure directly transmitted arterial pressure. This device generates a real-time continuous waveform and pressure measurement. A validation study of one of these devices (JENTOW) was performed, comparing it to intra-arterial catheter blood pressures in normotensive and hypertensive patients (20). The findings showed that tonometric pressures and waveforms correlated closely to the intra-arterial components. This reliability was limited in the conditions of rapid or large changes in blood pressure.

Invasive Monitoring of Arterial Pressure
History

The Reverend Stephen Hales became the first person to measure intra-arterial blood pressure when, in 1733, he cannulated the left crural artery of a horse (21). The resulting pressure column rose 8 feet, 3 inches (327 mmHg) and was noted to vary in height with the arterial pulse, and the baseline drifted in correlation to the horse's respiratory rate and level of pain. The first direct invasive blood pressure measurement in a human occurred in 1856, when the French physician Faivre cannulated the superficial femoral artery in the leg of an amputee. After McLean (22) discovered heparin in 1916, and the strain gauge was developed by Lambert and Wood (23) in 1947, the critical components necessary for widespread measurement of intra-arterial blood pressure were available. However, the routine measurement of intra-arterial blood pressure did not occur until the mid-1960s with the wide expansion of cardiothoracic and vascular surgery, and the description of the "catheter over the needle" cannulation technique by Barr in 1961 (24). Today, intra-arterial cannulation with continuous blood pressure transduction is considered the gold standard for arterial blood pressure monitoring by most clinicians. However, some maintain that the intra-arterial cannula must be calibrated with an indirect technique, such as "return to flow," prior to use (25,26).

Indications

Indications for intra-arterial blood pressure monitoring are listed in Table 4. These include "procedure related" indications (such as large fluid shifts, blood loss, or major vital organ surgery), and "patient related" conditions which require continuous arterial pressure monitoring irrespective of the surgical procedure. One of the most common indications for invasive monitoring of arterial pressure, is the need for continuous blood pressure data in a patient at risk of cardiovascular instability (27). There are indications for arterial cannulation for reasons other than arterial pressure monitoring as well, such as the need for frequent arterial blood gas sampling in patients with respiratory compromise.

Site Selection

Any peripheral artery can be used for catheterization. Sites commonly used include the radial, femoral, dorsalis pedis, brachial, and axillary arteries. In neonates, the umbilical artery is an excellent source of pressure monitoring and blood sample acquisition. The choice of site for arterial cannulation includes many factors. Typically, the radial artery of the nondominant hand is utilized. When this site is unsuitable, alternate sites are chosen based upon the following four criteria: (i) the artery should be large enough to accurately reflect systemic blood pressure, (ii) the chosen site should be free of cellulitis or nearby infected/devitalized tissue, (iii) there should be sufficient collateral flow to prevent distal ischemia, and (iv) the artery should be proximal to any anatomic aberrations (i.e., use the right arm for patients with aortic coarct or patent ductus arteriosis).

Certain disease states require particular attention to catheter placement site. The dorsalis pedis artery should be avoided in elderly patients, especially those with known peripheral vascular disease or diabetes mellitus.

Table 4 Indications for Invasive Intra-arterial Blood Pressure Monitoring

Procedure-related indications
Major procedures involving large fluid shifts and/or blood loss
Intrathoracic, intracardiac, intracranial procedures
Anticipated deliberate hypotension, hypothermia, hemodilution
Procedures with a high risk for spinal cord ischemia (thoracic aneurysm repair, aortic coarctation repair, scoliosis, and other spine surgery)
Liver, heart, and lung transplantation
Aortic X-clamp and other major vascular procedures

Patient-related indications
Significant coronary artery disease (unstable angina, recent MI)
Myocardial pump dysfunction (CHF, valvular HD, cardiomyopathy)
Shock (hypovolemic, cardiogenic, septic, neurogenic)
Significant cerebrovascular disease (internal carotid stenosis)
Patients with severe ascites
Significant pulmonary disease, COPD, pulmonary embolism, pulmonary hypertension, ARDS, pneumonia
Severe renal, acid–base, electrolyte, or metabolic disorders
Morbid obesity, massive burns, and other conditions where noninvasive monitoring is difficult

Abbreviations: ARDS, acute respiratory distress syndrome; CHF, congestive heart failure; COPD, chronic obstructive pulmonary disease; HD, heart disease; MI, myocardial infarction.

The superficial temporal artery, a branch of the external carotid artery, can be used as a vessel of last resort. This artery is tortuous and difficult to cannulate due to its proximity to the internal carotid artery; extreme care must be exercised during flushing. The radial, brachial, and dorsalis pedis arteries are contraindicated in patients with Raynaud's syndrome or Buerger's disease (thromboangiitis obliterans). In both of these conditions, cannulation of the femoral artery is indicated. These guidelines are especially important for Raynaud's syndrome, because environmental hypothermia is a known trigger for vasospasm.

Complications

The majority of complications after insertion of an arterial pressure-monitoring catheter are either mechanical or infectious. Thrombosis is the most common mechanical complication noted and partial or complete radial artery occlusion occurs in more than 25% of patients. Slogoff et al. (28) found that no ischemic damage or disability developed in any of their patients with catheter-associated radial artery occlusion, and most thromboses recannulate within two to four weeks after catheter removal.

Many investigators still recommend performing the modified Allen's test prior to cannulation of the radial artery, to assess adequacy of perfusion and collateral flow to the extremity (e.g., cold, ischemic digits are an absolute contraindication to cannulation of the vessel that supplies the digits). The modified Allen's test begins with compression of both the radial and ulnar arteries. Next, the patient's fist is clenched until it blanches. The patient's hand is then relaxed, and the pressure on the ulnar artery is released. If the patient's skin promptly becomes hyperemic, collateral ulnar flow is considered adequate for radial artery cannulation. The Allen's test, while recommended, has not been demonstrated to reduce the risk of digit ischemia (29), nor has an abnormal Allen's test been demonstrated to increase the risk of arterial cannulation. Indeed, Slogoff et al. cannulated the radial arteries in 16 patients with suboptimal ulnar flow assessed by the modified Allen's test, and none of these patients (0/16) had evidence of digital ischemia. ☞ **Although imperfect, if the Allen's test is markedly abnormal, and alternate sites are available, one of these other sites should be used.** ☞

When the radial artery is not available for cannulation, several other sites are available. One of the main concerns regarding the brachial artery is that few collaterals normally exist around this artery, so that a thrombotic or ischemic event may lead to morbidity. While this concept is valid anatomically, available evidence suggests that brachial artery cannulation is associated with an acceptable risk. Barnes et al. (30) reported their study on indwelling brachial artery cannulae and found no Doppler evidence of obstruction or vascular complications. Even with this information, it is generally recommended to use the axillary artery preferentially to the brachial artery, because of the abundant natural collateral blood supply.

After arterial cannulation, the tissues perfused by the artery should be routinely monitored for evidence of ischemic or thromboembolic events. Although permanent ischemic damage after arterial catheterization is uncommon, there have been rare reports of necrosis requiring amputation. Patients having certain risk factors deserve more careful surveillance for ischemic sequelae following catheterization (Table 5) (31). Any evidence of ischemia, infection, or embolic events should lead to immediate removal of the catheter.

Table 5 Predictors of Ischemic Risk for Radial Artery Catheterization

Proximal embolic source
Increased duration of cannulation
Long or large-caliber catheter
Hyperlipoproteinemia
Peripheral vascular disease
Low cardiac output
Vasoconstrictor agents
Female gender
Small wrist circumference

Another mechanical complication occasionally associated with arterial cannulation is pseudoaneurysm. A pseudoaneurysm is a persisting cavity that results from extravasation of blood from an injured vessel that is partially contained by surrounding tissues. It is thought that the technique of catheter insertion may predispose to pseudoaneurysm formation. If the posterior wall of the artery is punctured deliberately or unintentionally, or if multiple passes through the artery are attempted, then the risk of pseudoaneurysm is greater. These same factors increase the risk of arteriovenous fistula formation, where wounds to the artery and an adjacent vein persist. Smaller traumatic AV fistulae tend to close spontaneously, while larger fistulae may persist, because the venous outflow provides a path of least resistance for arterial inflow.

In consideration of femoral arterial cannulation, the clinician must always assess whether the patient may have a femoral arterial prosthesis. Patients with peripheral vascular disease often have previous femoral arterial reconstruction with a vascular graft. Puncture wounds through prosthetic material are at much higher risk for pseudoaneurysm formation. Upon removal of catheters from native arteries, endogenous arterial smooth muscle contraction facilitates closure of the wound, while this factor is absent in wounds to prosthetic grafts. Other predisposing factors for pseudoanaurysm formation seem to be prolonged cannulation and infection.

Embolization is a complication more frequently significant in femoral arterial cannulation. Flushing of catheters may result in thrombus or air emboli to distal regions. Less commonly, vessel instrumentation and catheterization alone may potentially cause atheromatous embolization from diseased femoral vessels. Routine pulse checks by palpation or Doppler sonography should be performed in those patients with indwelling femoral catheters.

Infection is the other main category of complications from arterial catheters. In cases of catheter-associated bacteremia and sepsis, the most common route of bacterial invasion is the insertion site, where organisms colonizing the catheter and skin have a portal of entry into the host. Strict aseptic insertion technique, catheter use, care, and dressing protocols help limit the incidence of infection. Unlike venous catheters, studies have shown that the risk of arterial catheter infections do not increase exponentially over time. Norwood et al. (32) performed a prospective study on prolonged arterial catheterization, and found that infection developed in less than 10% of radial and femoral sites used greater than 96 hours. It appears that arterial catheters may be left as long as skin colonization is well controlled and there is absence of systemic infection.

Systolic Pressure Variation

It has long been appreciated that large respiratory variation in the arterial pressure waveform correlates with hypovolemia. Perel (33) has developed a technique to better define the relative degree of volume depletion, using the systolic pressure variation (SPV) resulting from the dynamic response of the left ventricle to alterations in preload and afterload induced by mechanical ventilation. The SPV occurring during mechanical ventilation is divided into a delta up and a delta down component. When the delta down component exceeds a SPV of 10 mmHg (in patients ventilated at 10–15 cc/kg tidal volume), patients can generally be thought of as needing additional preload for the conditions (also see discussion on SPV in Volume 2, Chapter 3).

CVP and pulmonary artery wedge pressure (PAWP) are altered by both spontaneous and mechanical ventilation. The changes in these pressures, likewise, affect arterial blood pressure through changes in Q̇. Increased intrathoracic pressure during mechanical ventilation leads to increased right atrial pressure which decreases venous return to the right heart, while the left atrium and ventricle are being filled by blood which has been squeezed out of the pulmonary vascular system.

Similarly, there is an increase in the afterload on the right side of the heart due to increased airway pressure compressing the pulmonary artery (PA) vessels. In contrast, the left side of the heart has a relative decrease in afterload during positive pressure ventilation. This is because the increased pleural pressure is transmitted to the left ventricle and the thoracic aorta, and their pressure is transiently increased relative to the extrathoracic aorta. As exhalation occurs, these forces reverse. These changes in preload and afterload are most marked in the hypovolemic state and are reflected in the systolic arterial pressure variation (34).

CENTRAL VENOUS PRESSURE MONITORING

Indications

The CVP has long been used as an estimator of intravascular volume and a guide to fluid therapy in critically ill patients. The CVP gained popularity as a hemodynamic measure due to relatively simple catheter insertion and ease of interpretation. Some of the various indications for CVP monitoring include patients with the diagnosis of hemorrhage, trauma, sepsis, and cardiovascular dysfunction. Patients may benefit from CVP monitoring during the perioperative period, fluid resuscitation, or blood transfusion.

Site Selection

The three sites available for central venous catheterization are subclavian, jugular, and femoral. The internal jugular vein is probably the most commonly chosen site for placement of a central venous catheter, when the procedure is performed in the operating room. In this setting, the anesthesiologist typically has easiest access to the patient's head and neck. This site is associated with the least mechanical risk of insertion because inadvertent arterial puncture wounds can easily be compressed externally, and the possibility for pneumothorax is more remote.

Trauma patients having cervical collars, whether from spine injury or from an uncleared spine, pose a particular challenge for internal jugular venous access. Identification of surface landmarks is more difficult without the benefit of turning the head, and an assistant should immobilize the neck during the procedure. In those patients with tracheostomy, contamination of the catheter site and dressing is more likely with internal jugular vein catheters.

Outside the operating room, the subclavian vein is the favored site for central venous access. In those patients that are awake, an indwelling catheter on the chest wall is more comfortable than one in the relatively mobile neck. Trauma patients who already have a chest tube decompressing a pneumothorax do not have this associated risk factor during catheter insertion.

There are several situations that represent relative contraindications to subclavian venous catheterization. One of these is the coagulopathic or thrombocytopenic patient. Inadvertent arterial puncture wounds are more difficult to suppress with external compression, because the bony clavicle overlies the subclavian artery, and the pliable pleura and lung do not offer effective counterpressure. Patients who will not remain still for the procedure, such as the agitated uncooperative patient or the patient having active chest compressions during cardiopulmonary resuscitation, are poor candidates for subclavian venous catheter attempts because of the high risk for pneumothorax. However, subclavian lines are easier to maintain once in place in ICU patients, and less uncomfortable than neck lines for awake patients who are actively moving around. Accordingly, weighing the relative risks and benefits often results in placement of subclavian lines in patients who have some relative contraindications for the line.

ᗒ **In the acutely injured, or unstable, critically ill patient requiring central venous access, the femoral vein site is an excellent choice because of its relative ease of insertion.** ᗒ For prolonged CVP monitoring purposes, the femoral venous catheter is a less optimum choice than sites located above the waist (subclavian or internal jugular), because of increased risk of lower extremity deep venous thrombosis for femoral vein lines. Furthermore, the ideal catheter tip position for the assessment of preload is the atriocaval junction, near the right atrium. The usual central venous catheter inserted through the femoral vein will be remote from the atriocaval junction. While the pressure from a femoral venous catheter may be used to estimate CVP, it is important to recognize that factors concurrent in the abdomen and periphery may influence this pressure measurement. In those patients with an injured extremity, it is preferable to avoid catheterizing the respective femoral or subclavian vein. These injured extremities, typically, are burdened by hematoma and inflammatory edema and swelling. Optimal venous return from these injured extremities facilitates resolution of swelling and pain, limits the risk of elevated compartment pressures, and improves tissue perfusion and healing.

Interpretation

The CVP is measured as the pressure in the superior vena cava, an estimate of right atrial pressure. This pressure is an estimator of right atrial volume or cardiac preload. The normal range for CVP in critical care patients is 0–10 mmHg. The typical CVP waveform consists of three waves ("a," "c," and "v") and two descents ("x" and "y") (Fig. 5). While we use CVP to estimate the status of intravascular volume, the state of venous tone has an influence on the CVP. Rapid blood loss or fluid administration results in changes in CVP. A fluid challenge in a hypovolemic patient would result in an increase in CVP. The effect

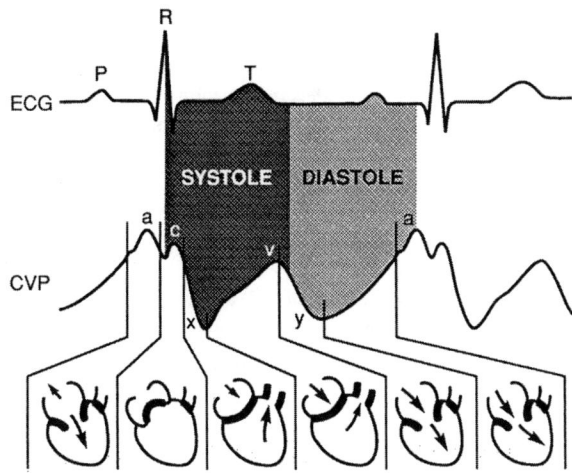

Figure 5 The cardiac cycle and the genesis of the a, c, and v waves. The a wave is caused by atrial contraction. The c wave is caused by bulging of the atrioventicular (AV) valve into the atrium during isovolemic ventricular contraction. The v wave is caused by passive venous filling of the atrium. The x descent results from ventricular decompression, following the opening of the ventricular outlet. The y descent results from draining the atrial blood into the ventricle, following the opening of the AV valve. The electrocardiogram trace serves as a useful marker to discern the components of the central venous pressure trace. *Abbreviations*: CVP, central venous pressure; ECG, electrocardiogram. *Source*: From Ref. 62.

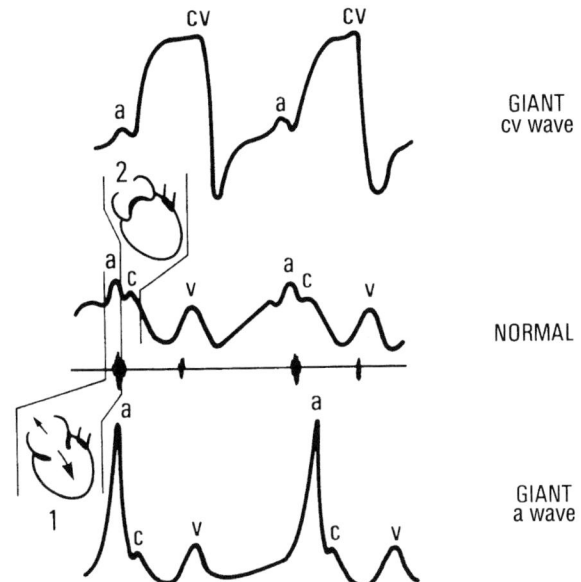

Figure 6 Giant cv waves and cannon (or Giant) a waves. Giant (or Cannon) a waves are caused by atrial contraction against a closed atrioventricular (AV) valve (as occurs with atrial ventricular dyssynchrony). Giant cv waves occur when the Giant c wave persists into the time when the v wave should be occurring, and are due to AV valve regurgitation. *Source*: From Ref. 62.

may be transient, in that venous compliance responds to these fluctuations in volume by adjusting venous tone. Elevation in CVP may represent hypervolemia, or impaired right ventricular function from congestive heart failure, or tricuspid valve regurgitation. The CVP may also be elevated in disease processes associated with pulmonary hypertension, such as pulmonary embolism, acute respiratory distress syndrome, or chronic obstructive pulmonary disease.

Effect of Mechanical Ventilation and PEEP
CVP measurements are affected by mechanical ventilation because of its effects on intrathoracic pressure. In the normally spontaneously ventilating patient, inspiration results in a negative intrathoracic pressure and resultant decrease in measured CVP. Expiration results in a positive intrathoracic pressure and a subsequent increase in measured CVP. These changes are considered normal respiratory variation of the CVP waveform. When patients are on positive pressure ventilation from a mechanical ventilator, the reverse effects are noted. Delivery of an inspiratory breath from a mechanical ventilator results in positive intrathoracic pressure and elevation in measured CVP, while the expiratory phase leads to a decrease in measured CVP.

It is recommended that serial CVP measurements be obtained at the same point of the respiratory cycle. In order to avoid the influence of intrathoracic pressure, CVP measurements are taken at end-exhalation in both spontaneously and mechanically ventilated patients. This is the point at which the intrathoracic pressure is most stable and least affected by ambient influences. When positive end-expiratory pressure (PEEP) is being administered, whether by the mechanical ventilator or by noninvasive means, the result is an increased intrathoracic pressure at end-expiration, and subsequent elevation in measured CVP.

Pathologic Central Venous Pressure Waveforms
Conditions of right heart flow pathology are manifested by changes in the normal CVP waveform (Fig. 5). The "a" wave, indicating the venous pressure during atrial contraction, is magnified in conditions of resistance to right atrial outflow. The classic giant or "cannon a" wave may be seen in situations where the atrium is contracting against a closed tricuspid valve (i.e., AV dyssynchrony or nodal rhythm) (Fig. 6). Less prominent "cannon a" waves are seen in situations with increased resistance to right atrial emptying (e.g., tricuspid stenosis). Other conditions in which the "a" wave is accentuated are right ventricular failure, pulmonary stenosis, and pulmonary hypertension. The "a" wave is absent during atrial fibrillation. In the condition of tricuspid regurgitation, the "c" and "v" waves are combined to form a large regurgitant CV wave, obliterating the normal "x" descent (Fig. 6).

PULMONARY ARTERY CATHETER MONITORING

Despite the controversy regarding its use, the PAC remains the ultimate invasive monitoring tool in the intensivist's armamentarium. Introduced into clinical practice in 1970, and initially used to diagnose patients with acute cardiac disease, the PAC allows us to directly measure three key parameters not available with any other invasive monitoring device: PAWP, Q̇, and mixed venous oxygen saturation. Acquisition and utilization of these measurements formulate the most fundamental indications for use of the PAC.

Indications

Previous studies have documented the unreliability of the CVP and right atrial pressure to accurately estimate left atrial pressure or left ventricular preload. Patients with isolated right- or left-sided heart failure, and those patients with altered systemic or pulmonary vascular resistance from shock or respiratory failure, may have discrepant right and left heart pressures. ☞ **The following clinical situations may benefit from monitoring with a PAC: cardiovascular dysfunction, MI, congestive heart failure, pulmonary hypertension, shock, geriatric patients, traumatic injury, sepsis, and respiratory failure.** ☞

Among the most common indications for PAC use is the hemodynamically unstable patient not responding predictably to conventional fluid resuscitation. The PAC may provide valuable hemodynamic data that will help evaluate the pathophysiology of the abnormality. Measurement of $\dot{Q}$ and calculation of SVR will help differentiate hypotension into hypovolemic shock, cardiogenic shock, or a form of distributive shock. The patient with respiratory failure requiring advancing ventilator support may benefit from a PAC. Measurement of the PAWP will allow the differentiation between cardiogenic and noncardiogenic pulmonary edema.

In addition to its diagnostic uses, the PAC is a valuable tool in guiding therapy in the critically ill. The PAWP may be used as a guide for fluid resuscitation as an estimate of left ventricular preload. Monitoring $\dot{Q}$ theoretically improves the appropriateness of inotropic therapy. Similarly, calculation of SVR using the PAC allows for improved titration of vasoactive agents. In those patients at risk for systemic inflammatory response syndrome, or sepsis and organ dysfunction, measurement of mixed venous oxygen saturation and calculation of oxygen transport variables may help determine presence of tissue ischemia, and guide resuscitation efforts.

There has been recent controversy regarding the utility and safety of PAC use. In 1996 Connors et al. (35) reported a multicenter observational study, showing that PAC use was associated with increased mortality and utilization of resources. This study stimulated intense debate, that even reached a point in which a moratorium on PAC use was recommended by the Food and Drug Administration (FDA), until a multicenter randomized clinical trial (RCT) could be performed. It was later realized that a study such as this would be too difficult to enroll patients and to practically complete, and the Connors study had several experimental design flaws.

The American Society of Anesthesiologists (ASA) established the Task Force on PACs in 1991 to determine the risk/benefits ratio for PAC use in settings encountered by anesthesiologists. The ASA guidelines (36) were adopted in 1992 and published in 1993. The ASA guidelines stated that the PAC should not be used routinely, but is likely beneficial when three high-risk variables intersected (patient, procedure, and clinical setting). The ASA guidelines also stated that the PAC will only prove beneficial when insertion and data interpretation are performed by competent individuals, and called for additional research.

Subsequently, in 1996, the Council of the Society of Critical Care Medicine (SCCM) hosted a consensus conference to examine important issues related to the PAC with representatives from the American Association of Critical-Care Nurses, the American College of Chest Physicians, the American College of Critical Care Medicine, the American Thoracic Society, the European Society of Intensive Care Medicine, and the SCCM in attendance (37). Among the consensus recommendations were that there was no basis for an FDA

Table 6 Indications for Pulmonary Artery Catheter Use in the Trauma Patient

To ascertain the status of underlying cardiovascular performance.
To direct therapy when noninvasive monitoring is inadequate or misleading.
To assess response to resuscitation.
To potentially decrease secondary injury when severe closed-head or acute spinal cord injuries are components of multisystem trauma.
To augment clinical decision making when major trauma is complicated by severe acute respiratory distress syndrome, progressive oliguria/anuria, myocardial injury, congestive heart failure, or major thermal injury.
To establish futility of care.

moratorium of PAC use and instead, that clinician knowledge about the use of the PAC and its complications should be improved (38).

In October 2003, the revised ASA guidelines were published, and the recommendations were essentially unchanged from those published a decade earlier (39). Also, in 2003, two large multicenter RCTs were completed with conflicting results. The first showed a slightly higher complication rate, and markedly higher incidence of pulmonary embolism in the group assigned to PACs (40). The other study by Richard et al. (41) demonstrated that PAC use is not associated with increased mortality or morbidity, as did a similar study by Rhodes et al. (42).

Accordingly, clinical decision making is still guiding the indications for PAC use. Table 6 lists the indications for PAC use in trauma patients, recommended by the SCCM consensus conference (albeit only supported by Level IV or V evidence).

Measurement of Cardiac Output
Thermomodification Technique

One of the most important capabilities of the PAC is the measurement of $\dot{Q}$. The PAC uses a thermodilution method for measuring $\dot{Q}$, with the injection of a bolus of cold solution. The technique is performed with the manual injection of 10 mL of a room temperature solution of 5% dextrose in water, into the right atrial port. The rate of blood flow determines the resultant temperature change, sensed by a thermistor at the tip of the catheter in the pulmonary artery. The device then calculates a $\dot{Q}$ by the integration of the change in temperature over time, where the area under the temperature-time curve is inversely proportional to the $\dot{Q}$.

Variability in $\dot{Q}$ measurement with the thermodilution technique may be either due to technical factors, or from physiologic causes (43). With repeated measurements, the injectate volume must be accurate and the injection administration speed must be consistent. The amount of fluid loaded into the syringe may vary simply from human error, or the volume may be altered when air becomes trapped within the catheter tubing. Any factors that may alter the injectate temperature may also affect the $\dot{Q}$ measurement. If the injection solution bag is changed between measurements, a significant difference in temperature may potentially occur between measurements.

Patients with tricuspid valve regurgitation have increased variability of $\dot{Q}$ measurement using the thermodilution technique. Some reports suggest an overestimation of $\dot{Q}$, based upon the concept that regurgitant blood flow warms the injectate more rapidly, resulting in a more rapid washout of temperature. Other reports point to the potential for a delay in flow of the injectate to the distal thermistor, resulting in an underestimation of $\dot{Q}$. Another physiologic source of $\dot{Q}$ variability arises in patients with dysrhythmias. One example is atrial fibrillation, where the actual $\dot{Q}$ may vary from beat to beat. Due to the great potential for variability, the possibility of artifactual signals and noise is also greater.

Fick Principle (Conservation of Mass)

While the PAC has allowed routine thermodilution $\dot{Q}$ measurement to be performed in the ICU, the Fick principle method remains the gold standard by which these methods are assessed. In the 1880s, Adolph Fick applied the law of conservation of mass to estimate $\dot{Q}$. The fundamental concept of Fick's principle is that the amount of oxygen exiting the heart equals the amount of oxygen entering the heart, plus or minus the amounts of oxygen added or removed from the heart, respectively. Thus, the $\dot{Q}$ equals the oxygen consumption ($\dot{V}O_2$) divided by the difference between arterial and venous oxygen concentrations ($CaO_2 - CvO_2$).

$$Q = \frac{VO_2}{CaO_2 - CvO_2} \qquad (3)$$

CaO_2 may be calculated by measuring hemoglobin concentration in blood and the oxygen saturation in arterial blood, and applying it to the following equation:

$$CaO_2(L/min) = Hb(g/dL) * SaO_2 * 1.36$$
$$(mL\ O_2/100\ mL\ blood) \qquad (4)$$

CvO_2 must be calculated from the oxygen saturation in mixed venous blood (SvO_2). The only practical site to obtain a sample with complete venous mixing of blood from throughout the body, is in the pulmonary artery. This sample is withdrawn from the pulmonary artery port at the tip of the PAC, and CvO_2 is calculated similarly to CaO_2:

$$CvO_2(L/min) = Hb\ (g/dL) * S\bar{v}O_2 * 1.36$$
$$(mL\ O_2/100\ mL\ blood) \qquad (5)$$

With the Fick principle, $\dot{V}O_2$ is calculated using indirect calorimetry results with a metabolic cart, measuring the differences in oxygen concentration between expired and inspired gas.

Measurement of $\dot{Q}$ further allows the assessment of the derived oxygen transport variables that are believed to estimate the body's overall state of tissue perfusion and oxidative metabolism (Table 7). Oxygen delivery ($\dot{D}O_2$) is calculated by the product of $\dot{Q}$ and CaO_2, while oxygen extraction is the ratio of $\dot{V}O_2$ to $\dot{D}O_2$:

$$\dot{D}O_2 = \dot{Q} * CaO_2 \qquad (6)$$

$$O_2\ extraction = \frac{\dot{V}O_2}{\dot{D}O_2} \qquad (7)$$

Low $\dot{D}O_2$ most often suggests inadequate $\dot{Q}$. Methods of improving $\dot{D}O_2$ include blood transfusion to increase [Hb] or inotropic support to increase $\dot{Q}$. SaO_2 is typically

Table 7 Derived Hemodynamic Variables from Pulmonary Artery Catheter Data

Cardiac index	$CI = \dot{Q}/BSA$
Stroke volume	$SV = \dot{Q}\ /\ HR$
Systemic vascular resistance	$SVR = (MAP - CVP) *$ $80/\dot{Q}$
Pulmonary vascular resistance	$PVR = (MPAP - PAWP)$ $* 80/\dot{Q}$
Arterial oxygen content	$CaO_2 = Hb * SaO_2 *$ $1.36 + (PaO_2 * 0.003)$
Mixed venous oxygen content	$CvO_2 = Hb * S\bar{v}O_2 *$ $1.36 + (PaO_2 * 0.003)$
Oxygen delivery	$\dot{D}O_2 = \dot{Q} * CaCO_2$
Oxygen consumption	$\dot{V}O_2 = \dot{Q} * (CaCO_2 -$ $CvO_2)$
Oxygen extraction	$O_2ext = \dot{V}O_2/\dot{D}O_2$

Abbreviations: BSA, body surface area; CVP, central venous pressure; Hb, hemoglobin; HR, heart rate; MAP, mean arterial pressure; MPAP, mean pulmonary artery pressure; $O_2ext = O_2$ extraction; PaO_2, partial pressure of O_2 in arterial blood; PAWP, pulmonary artery wedge pressure; SaO_2, O_2 saturation in blood; $S\bar{v}O_2 = O_2$, saturation in mixed venous blood; SVR, systemic vascular resistance; $\dot{Q}$, cardiac output.

near its maximum, where an increase would not result in significant change in $\dot{D}O_2$. Low $\dot{V}O_2$ may suggest inadequate tissue perfusion or oxygen metabolism. Tissue ischemia may result from inadequate supply of oxygen, or a maldistribution of microcirculatory perfusion to certain tissue regions. Decreased metabolism in critically ill patients may result from severe uncompensated shock states.

In those patients without a PAC, mixed venous blood is not available to assess oxygen transport dynamics. In an animal study of hypotensive hemorrhage, Scalea et al. (44) found that central venous oxygen saturation mirrored mixed venous oxygen saturation. In a subsequent study of trauma patients with evidence of hemorrhage, Scalea et al. (45) reported that central venous oxygen saturation, or the oxygen saturation of blood obtained from a central venous catheter, was a reliable and sensitive correlate of blood loss. They discovered that despite stable vital signs, the 39% of patients that had saturations under 65% had more serious injuries and required more transfusions.

Insertion Technique
Site Selection

The major sites for PAC insertion are similar to those of central venous access, with some special considerations. Ease of passage of the PAC into the pulmonary artery is influenced by the convolutions required for the catheter to reach its destination. The following sites are described in increasing level of technical difficulty. The most direct insertion route for the PAC is via the right internal jugular vein, where the PAC only requires one gentle curve to reach the right pulmonary artery. Access via the left subclavian vein also follows a generally smooth curve, but must traverse the left innominate vein to reach the superior vena cava. Access via the right subclavian vein requires the catheter to initially traverse the right innominate vein to reach the superior vena cava, then alter its curvature to enter the right atrium, in an S-shaped configuration. Finally, entry through the left internal jugular vein also requires an S-shaped configuration, with a greater travel distance.

Maneuvering through the left internal jugular vein to inno-minate vein curve is required, followed by an altered curve through the superior vena cava and right atrium. Femoral vein sites are acceptable alternatives, but are often more difficult to traverse into the right atrium. Fluoroscopic guidance may be necessary for those patients with unusual difficulty in placing the PAC.

Pulmonary Artery Catheter Advancement Considerations

After gaining central venous access via one of the above insertion points, the flushed and zeroed PAC is advanced, with the balloon deflated, to a distance of 12–15 cm (just past the introduction tip). At this point the flotation balloon is inflated, and the PAC is carefully advanced while simultaneously observing the pressure waveforms (Fig. 7), measured at the tip of the PAC. The initial CVP waveform leads to the right atrial pressure waveform,

which is not always easy to distinguish, depending on the sensitivity of the monitor settings. Upon reaching the right ventricle, there is an abrupt and obvious high spiking pressure waveform of 20–30 mmHg, representing the systolic right ventricular pressure, with a diastolic pressure that is unchanged from the CVP. This waveform leads to the pulmonary artery waveform with its characteristic step-up in diastolic pressure and a clear dicrotic notch. Finally, as the inflated balloon reaches a pulmonary arterial wedge, the waveform flattens as it loses its systolic and diastolic variation. After briefly observing the wedge waveform, the balloon should be deflated to confirm the reappearance of the pulmonary artery waveform.

☞ **Appropriate positioning of the PAC tip is critical to minimize risk for complications, and to achieve reliable data.** ☞ When the tip is in an appropriate position, a wedge waveform will be obtained with balloon inflation of 1.5 mL of air. If the wedge waveform does not appear, the catheter tip may need a slight advancement of several centimeters, with the balloon inflated, until the wedge reappears. If the wedge waveform is obtained with less than 1.5 mL, the catheter tip is probably in a small branch and should be withdrawn several centimeters, with the balloon deflated, followed by reinflation of the balloon and advancement back into a wedge position. After registering a wedge pressure, it is safest to pull the catheter back a few centimeters (with the balloon down), each time between readings to minimize the natural distal migration of the catheter.

Interpretation of PAC Waveforms and Pressures
Effect of Mechanical Ventilation

The PAWP, like the CVP, is best measured when there is the least influence from external transmural pressures, juxta-cardiac pressures, and intrathoracic pressures (46). This situation seems most closely approximated when the lungs return to their relaxed volume and state at end-expiration. In the spontaneously breathing patient, inspiration involves the development of a negative intrathoracic pressure that is transmitted through the pleura, lungs, alveoli, heart, and great vessels. In the mechanically ventilated patient, an increased intrathoracic pressure occurs with the positive pressure delivery of a breath. Still, in both spontaneously and mechanically ventilated patients, the chest returns to its most normal pressure configurations at end-expiration, and this is the most reliable for repeated measurements of intravascular pressure.

Effect of PEEP

PEEP may also influence the measurement of the PAWP. There are three physiologic lung zones, based upon the relationship between the pulmonary vascular and alveolar pressures (Fig. 8). In lung zones 1 and 2, the extent of alveolar pressure affects the pressure read by the PAC. The ideal position for the catheter tip is in lung zone 3, where the intravascular pressure always exceeds the alveolar pressure. In nonzone 3 situations, alveolar pressure may exceed intravascular pressure. The level of alveolar pressure and PEEP then affects measurement of PAWP.

Hemodynamic Profiles

Rational use of all the available data obtained from the PAC requires careful assessment of how individual data points fit into clinical scenarios. Hemodynamic profiles align several individual hemodynamic variables to fit into specified clinical patterns (Table 8). These specific patterns

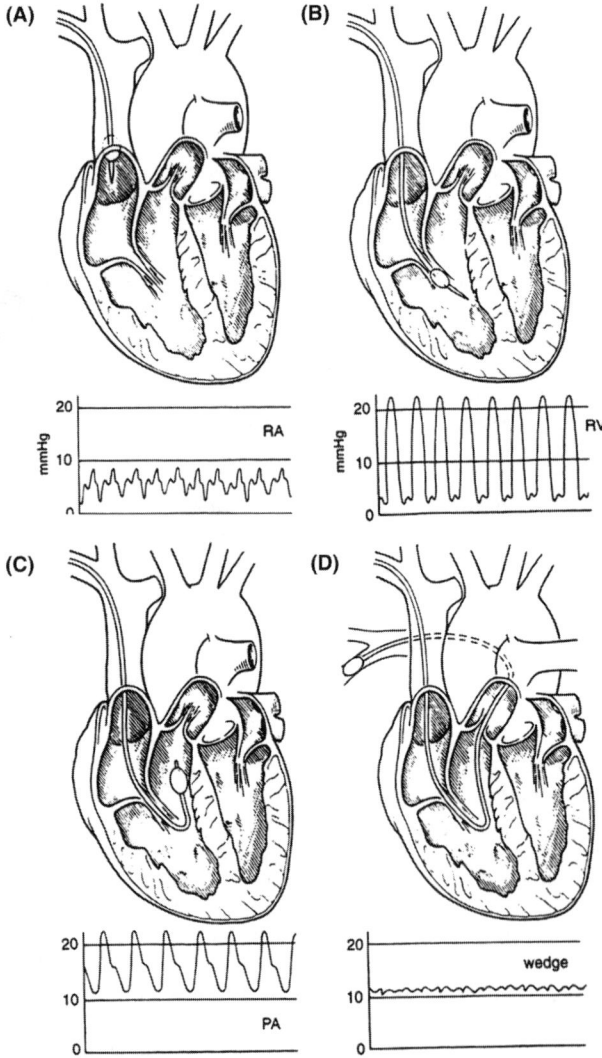

Figure 7 Advancement of the pulmonary artery catheter through the cardiac chambers and respective waveforms. (**A**) Pulmonary artery catheter (PAC) in right atrium. (**B**) PAC passing through tricuspid valve into the right ventricle. (**C**) PAC in the pulmonary artery (PA). (**D**) PAC in the distal PA in a wedge position. *Abbreviations*: RA, right atrium; RV, right ventricle. *Source*: From Ref. 63.

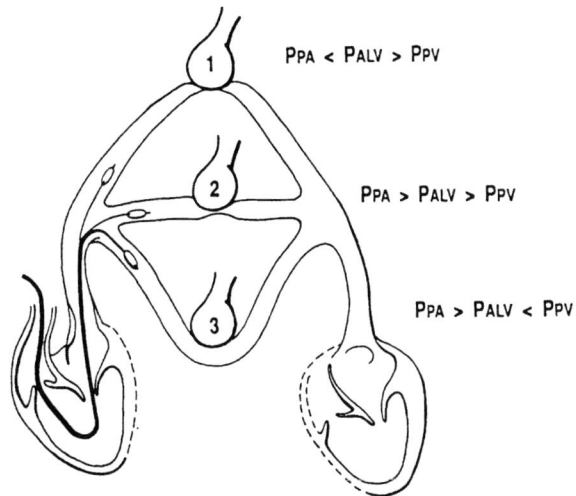

$P_{PA} < P_{ALV} > P_{PV}$

$P_{PA} > P_{ALV} > P_{PV}$

$P_{PA} > P_{ALV} < P_{PV}$

Figure 8 Physiologic lung "Zones of West." The zones are based upon alveolar–vascular pressure relationships. In either zone 1 or zone 2, P_{ALV} exceeds P_{PV}. During balloon occlusion of the pulmonary artery, wedge pressure reflects P_{PV} and left atrial pressure accurately only in zone 3. *Abbreviations*: P_{ALV}, alveolar pressure; P_{PA}, pulmonary arterial pressure; P_{PV}, pulmonary venous. *Source*: From Ref. 64.

are associated with certain appropriate therapeutic responses and subsequent prognoses (47). For example, a basic profile for acute hypovolemia would include low PAWP, low $\dot{Q}$, and high SVR.

CONTINUOUS CARDIAC OUTPUT MONITORING
Modified Pulmonary Artery Catheters
In response to increased monitoring needs in the ICU, technological advances have improved the utility of the PAC. Special catheters are now available that continuously monitor mixed venous oxygen saturation and/or cardiac output (48). In some ICUs, these modified catheters have become preferred.

Patients in whom oxygen transport variables are regularly followed require repeated blood draws for mixed venous oxygen analysis with the traditional PAC. In the Fick equation, the mixed venous oxygen saturation reflects the overall oxygen extraction, whereby a reduction in mixed venous oxygen saturation may suggest an uncompensated increase in oxygen consumption. Continuous mixed

Table 8 Hemodynamic Profiles Based on Three Variables

	PAWP	$\dot{Q}$	SVR
Hypovolemia	Low	Low	High
Fluid overload	High	High	Low
Septic shock	Low	High	Low
Left heart failure	High	Low	High
Pulmonary hypertension	Low	Low	Normal

Abbreviations: PAWP, pulmonary artery wedge pressure; $\dot{Q}$, cardiac output; SVR, systemic vascular resistance.

venous oximetry has given us the benefit of decreasing the labor of blood drawing required to measure mixed venous oxygen saturation, but an even greater advantage is that monitoring and therapeutic decisions can occur in real time, without the delay of laboratory processing of blood-work. The technology of continuous mixed venous oximetry uses fiberoptic bundles and an optical transducer in the tip of the catheter. As red blood cells flow past the catheter tip, a measurement of oxyhemoglobin relative to total hemo-globin is determined.

Another modification of the PAC that has gained some popularity in use is the continuous cardiac output ($\dot{Q}$ cont.) devices. The $\dot{Q}$ cont. PAC takes advantage of the thermodilution technique for measurement of $\dot{Q}$, but rather than injections of cold solution, it uses a heating filament on the catheter to deliver thermal pulses. The thermistor at the catheter tip senses the temperature change, and a computer-derived $\dot{Q}$ measurement is made. The $\dot{Q}$ displayed on the monitor is not truly continuous. Three- to six-minute periods of blood flow are analyzed to generate average $\dot{Q}$. Every 30 seconds, the $\dot{Q}$ is updated with these averages, thereby limiting extreme fluctuations that may occur with real-time measurements. ☞ **Several studies have since evaluated this $\dot{Q}$ cont. PAC was compared to bolus $\dot{Q}$ measurements in ICU patients, with the results showing that the $\dot{Q}$ cont. measurements compared favorably (49–51).** ☞

The technological advance in catheter capability is also associated with its own inherent drawbacks. Calibration of the measurements and troubleshooting dysfunctional catheters are occasional problems. Another potential pitfall lies in the reliability of the displayed measurements. Poor signal quality of the device may lead to inaccurate readings. Response to fluctuating readings may result in inappropriate therapy. Finally, the added cost of the modified catheters may be up to twice the cost of traditional PACs. While there is certainly time and labor saving with these options, the cost-efficiency of the devices must be assessed by the individual institutions using them.

One other PAC modification provides measurement of a hemodynamic variable that has yet to gain widespread acceptance in use. The right ventricular function catheter calculates the right ventricular end-diastolic volume index (RVEDVI) as the estimator of preload, and right ventricular ejection fraction as the estimator of contractility. The technology uses a thermodilution method, whereby the temperature changes between baseline and residual temperatures in successive heartbeats are computer analyzed to generate the ejection fraction. The SV and end-diastolic volume can be solved for (using an equation with a constant related to the specific gravity and heat capacity of blood) (52). A number of studies have attempted to assess the correlation between these measures and $\dot{Q}$. Martyn et al. (53) performed a study in acutely burned patients and reported that the RVEDVI is a better measure of right ventricular preload than CVP and PAWP. Subsequently, Chang et al. (54) reported a consecutive series of 46 trauma patients, who received volumetric PACs and required greater than 10 L of fluid in 24 hours. This study also concluded that the RVEDVI is a better predictor of preload than the PAWP in trauma patients during large-volume shock resuscitation, and promoted the idea that when the RVEDVI is 130 mL/m^2 or less, volume administration would increase the cardiac index. It still remains to be seen whether knowledge of right ventricular volumes and function and use of the volumetric PAC actually improve outcome.

Noninvasive Cardiac Output Monitoring Devices

☞ The esophageal Doppler monitor (EDM) is a relatively new advance in continuous Q̇ monitoring, and represents the most promising of noninvasive techniques (55). ☞ The Doppler method is based on the analysis of ultrasound waves to measure the velocity of blood flow. Doppler waveforms are analyzed to assess preload, afterload, and contractility. The EDM probe must be positioned to best visualize adjacent descending aortic blood flow through the esophageal wall. One of the drawbacks of this technique is that proper positioning is critical to achieving accurate results, and subsequent probe movement out of position is difficult to prevent. Studies have shown that this technique may better predict preload than either PAWP or CVP (56).

Thoracic electrical bioimpedance techniques are based on the concept that intrathoracic volume changes with each SV. An alternating current is applied by electrodes, whereby increased aortic flow during systole decreases the thoracic impedance. Q̇ is subsequently determined by computerized analysis of peak aortic flow, SV, and HR. Several different commercial devices are available, and at least one prospective study in 134 blunt-trauma patients concluded that bioimpedance Q̇ monitoring, as part of a multicomponent noninvasive system, approximated those of thermodilution methods shortly after admission (57). Conversely, a recent meta-analysis of 42 clinical studies instead found a wide variation of correlations between bioimpedance Q̇ and different invasive reference methods (58). Therefore, more work needs to be done on impedance cardiography before this technique can be recommended for clinical use in critically ill patients.

EYE TO THE FUTURE

The advent of invasive monitoring technology has been a significant factor in defining the role of the ICU and the intensivist in the care of critically ill patients, and the bulk of this chapter is devoted to the current invasive devices. We have recently seen that the minimally invasive movement is changing the approach to medical care. In critical care, there is a parallel movement to develop and refine noninvasive means to acquire cardiovascular and hemodynamic data. Some of the technologies discussed in this chapter are examples of this effort, applied clinically today.

Esophageal Doppler monitoring of continuous Q̇ is rapidly gaining interest, and clinical trials are actively investigating feasibility. Further improvement of probes is needed to limit the artifactual information and to more easily maintain proper positioning. Continued advances in ultrasonic probe technology and computer processing will provide higher level analytical information regarding ventricular volume and function. Contrast echocardiography and three-dimensional technology will certainly add additional anatomic and physiologic data (59). Photoplethysmography for continuous automated noninvasive arterial blood pressure monitoring using infrared light transmission, and arterial tonometry utilizing surface pressure transducers are undergoing clinical study and refinement, and may be applicable to clinical trials in the near future.

SUMMARY

Cardiovascular monitoring needs, in trauma and the critically ill, range from those patients needing just basic electrocardiography, to those patients that would benefit from intensive continuous assessment and oxygen transport evaluation. The level and extent of monitoring is dependent on the patient's injuries, comorbid diseases, current physiologic condition, and response to resuscitation and therapy. Arterial blood pressure, CVP, pulmonary artery pressures, CO, mixed venous oxygen saturation may now all be continuously monitored in those patients requiring advanced levels of care. The successful intensivist is one who clearly understands the technologies available, can appropriately analyze the data for accuracy and utility, and can integrate the findings with all the other relevant conditions and events in the patient, to formulate effective therapeutic strategies.

KEY POINTS

☞ The precordial leads are the most sensitive for detecting myocardial ischemia in the operating room; this is presumably true in the ICU as well.

☞ ST segment depression is the most common manifestation of subendocardial myocardial ischemia.

☞ Acute transmural myocardial ischemia, or infarction, results in acute ST segment elevation.

☞ The MAP is highest in the ascending aorta, and drops minimally until the peripheral arteriolar bed is reached.

☞ In trauma situations, and shock, the noninvasive automatic blood pressure devices often fail to work properly. In these situations, an invasive arterial line or manual techniques are preferred.

☞ Although imperfect, if the Allen's test is markedly abnormal, and alternate sites are available, one of these other sites should be used.

☞ In the acutely injured, or unstable, critically ill patient requiring central venous access, the femoral vein site is an excellent choice because of its relative ease of insertion.

☞ The following clinical situations may benefit from monitoring with a PAC: cardiovascular dysfunction, MI, congestive heart failure, pulmonary hypertension, shock, geriatric patients, traumatic injury, sepsis, and respiratory failure.

☞ Appropriate positioning of the PAC tip is critical to minimize risk for complications, and to achieve reliable data.

☞ Several studies have since evaluated this Q̇ cont. PAC compared to bolus Q̇ measurements in ICU patients, with the results showing that the Q̇ cont. measurements compared favorably.

☞ The esophageal Doppler monitor (EDM) is a relatively new advance in continuous Q̇ monitoring, and represents the most promising of noninvasive techniques.

REFERENCES

1. Eagle KA, Brundage BH, Chaitman BR, et al. Guidelines for perioperative cardiovascular evaluation for noncardiac surgery: Report of the American College of Cardiology/American Heart Association Task Force on Practice Guidelines [Committee on Perioperative Cardiovascular Evaluation for Noncardiac Surgery]. Circulation 1996; 93:1278–1317.
2. Fabian TC, Davis KA, Gavant ML, et al. Prospective study of blunt aortic injury: helical CT is diagnostic and antihypertensive therapy reduces rupture. Ann Surg 1998; 227:666–677.

3. Scalea TM, Simon HM, Duncan AO, et al. Geriatric blunt multiple trauma: Improved survival with early invasive monitoring. J Trauma 1990; 30:129–136.

4. London MJ, Hollenberg M, Wong M, et al. Intraoperative myocardial ischemia: localization by 12-lead ECG. Anesthesiology 1988; 69:233.

5. Fletcher GF, Balady GJ, Amsterdam EA, et al. Exercise standards for testing and training: a statement for healthcare professionals from the American Heart Association. Circulation 2001; 104:1694–1740.

6. Wang K, Asinger RW, Marriott HJL. ST-Elevation in conditions other than acute myocardial infarction. N Engl J Med 2003; 349:2128–2135.

7. Ferguson TB Jr, Cox JL. Cardiac rhythm disturbances. In: Barie PS, Shires GT, eds. Surgical Intensive Care. Boston: Little, Brown and Company, 1993:365–416.

8. Berne RM, Levy MN. The Arterial System, Cardiovascular Physiology. 4th ed. St. Louis: CV Mosby Co., 1981.

9. Cullen DJ. Interpretation of blood pressure measurements in anesthesia. Anesthesiology 1974; 40:6.

10. Guyton AC. Textbook of Medical Physiology. 8th ed. Philadelphia, PA: W.B. Saunders and Co., 1991.

11. Remington JW. Contour changes of the aortic pulse during propagation. Am J Physiol 1960; 199:331.

12. Bruner JM, Krenis LJ, Kunsman JM, et al. Comparison of direct and indirect methods of measuring arterial blood pressure, part III. Med Instrum 1981; 15:182.

13. Bedford RF. Invasive Blood Pressure Monitoring. Monitoring in Anesthesia and Critical Care Medicine. 2nd ed. New York: Churchill Livingstone, 1990.

14. Weinger MB, Scanlon TS, Miller L. A widely unappreciated cause of failure of an automatic noninvasive blood pressure monitor. J Clin Monit 1992; 8(4):291–294.

15. Perloff D, Grim C, Flack J, et al. Human blood pressure determination by sphygmomanometry. Circulation 1993; 88:2460–2470.

16. Gourdeau M, Martin R, Lamarche Y, et al. Oscillometry and direct blood pressure: a comparitive clinical study during deliberate hypotension. Can Anaesth Soc J 1986; 33:300–307.

17. Davis JW, Davis IC, Bennink LD, et al. Are automatic blood pressure measurements accurate in trauma patients? J Trauma 2003; 55:860–863.

18. Wilkes MP, Bennett A, Hall P, Lewis M, Clutton-Brock TH. Comparison of invasive and non-invasive measurement of continuous arterial pressure using the Finapres in patients undergoing spinal anaesthesia for lower segment caesarean section. Br J Anaesth 1994; 73:738–743.

19. Jones RD, Kornberg JP, Roulson CJ, Visram AR, Irwin MG. The Finapres 2300e finger cuff. The influence of cuff application on the accuracy of blood pressure measurement. Anaesthesia 1993; 48:611–615.

20. Sato T, Nishinaga M, Kawamoto A, Ozawa T, Takatsuji H. Accuracy of a continuous blood pressure monitor based on arterial tonometry. Hypertension 1993; 21:866–874.

21. Hales S. Statiskal essays: vegetable staticks, I(3):361. In: Innys W, Manby R, eds. London 1738. Cited in Geddes LA: The Direct and Indirect Measurement of Blood Pressure. Chicago: Yearbook Medical Publishers, 1970.

22. McLean J. The thromboplastic action of cephalin. Am J Physiol 1916; 41:250–257.

23. Lambert EH, Wood EH. The use of resistance wire strain gauge manometer to measure intra-arterial pressure. Proc Soc Exp Biol Med 1947; 64:186.

24. Barr PO. Percutaneous puncture of the radial artery with a multipurpose teflon catheter for indwelling use. Acta Physiol Scand 1961; 51:343.

25. Gardner RM. Hemodynamic monitoring: from catheter to display. Acute Care 1986; 12:3.

26. Gardner RM, Bond EL, Clark JS. Safety and efficacy of continuous flush systems for arterial and pulmonary artery catheters. Ann Thorac Surg 1977; 23:534.

27. Lodato RF. Arterial pressure monitoring. In: Tobin MJ, ed. Principles and Practice of Intensive Care Monitoring. New York: McGraw-Hill Companies, 1998:733–749.

28. Slogoff S, Keats AS, Arlund C. On the safety of radial artery cannulation. Anesthesiology 1983; 59:42–47.

29. Mangano DT, Hickey RF. Ischemic injury following uncomplicated radial artery catheterization. Anesth Analg 1979; 58:55–57.

30. Barnes RW, Foster EJ, Janssen GA, Boutros AR. Safety of brachial arterial catheters as monitors in the intensive care unit—prospective evaluation with the Doppler ultrasonic velocity detector. Anesthesiology 1976; 44:260–264.

31. Wilkins RG. Radial artery cannulation and ischaemic damage: a review. Anaesthesia 1985; 40:896–899.

32. Norwood SH, Cormier B, McMahon NG, Moss A, Moore V. Prospective study of catheter-related infection during prolonged arterial catheterization. Crit Care Med 1988; 16:836–839.

33. Perel A, Pizov R, Cotev S. Systolic blood pressure variation is a sensitive indicator of hypovolemia in ventilated dogs subjected to graded hemorrhage. Anesthesiology 1987; 67:498–502.

34. Pizov R, Ya'ari Y, Perel A. Systolic pressure variation is greater during hemorrhage than during sodium nitroprusside-induced hypotension in ventilated dogs. Anesth Analg 1988; 67:170–174.

35. Connors AF Jr, Speroff T, Dawson NV, et al. SUPPORT Investigators. The effectiveness of right heart catheterization in the initial care of critically ill patients. JAMA 1996; 276:916–918.

36. American Society of Anesthesiologists Task Force on Pulmonary Artery Catheterization: practice guidelines for pulmonary artery catheterization. Anesthesiology 1993; 78:380–394.

37. Pulmonary Artery Catheter Consensus Conference Participants. Pulmonary artery catheter consensus conference: consensus statement. Crit Care Med 1997; 25:910–925.

38. Kirton OC, Civetta JM. Do pulmonary artery catheters alter outcome in trauma patients? New Horiz 1997; 5:222–227.

39. American Society of Anesthesiologists Task Force on Pulmonary Artery Catheterization: practice guidelines for pulmonary artery catheterization: An updated report by the anesthesiology 2003; 99:988–1014.

40. Sandham JD, Hull RD, Brant RF, et al. A randomized, controlled trial of the use of pulmonary-artery catheters in high-risk surgical patients. N Engl J Med 2003; 348:5–14.

41. Richard C, Warszawski J, Anguel N, et al. Early use of the pulmonary artery catheter and outcomes in patients with shock and acute respiratory distress syndrome. JAMA 2003; 290:2713–2720.

42. Rhodes A, Cusack RJ, Newman PJ, Grounds RM, Bennett ED. A randomized, controlled trial of the pulmonary artery catheter in critically ill patients. Intensive Care Med 2002; 28:256–264.

43. Magder S. Cardiac output. In: Tobin MJ, ed. Principles and Practice of Intensive Care Monitoring. New York: McGraw-Hill Companies, 1998:797–810.

44. Scalea TM, Holman M, Fuortes M, et al. Central venous oxygen saturation: An early, accurate measurement of volume during hemorrhage. J Trauma 1988; 28:725–732.

45. Sclaea TM, Hartnett RW, Duncan AO, et al. Central venous oxygen saturation: A useful clinical tool in trauma patients. J Trauma 1990; 30:1539–1543.

46. Leatherman JW, Marini JJ. Pulmonary artery catheterization: interpretation of pressure recordings. In: Tobin MJ, ed. Principles and Practice of Intensive Care Monitoring. New York: McGraw-Hill Companies, 1998:821–837.

47. Pinsky MR. Hemodynamic profile interpretation. In: Tobin MJ, ed. Principles and Practice of Intensive Care Monitoring. New York: McGraw-Hill Companies, 1998:871–887.

48. Nelson LD. The new pulmonary artery catheters: continuous venous oximetry, right ventricular ejection fraction, and continuous cardiac output. New Horiz 1997; 5:251–258.

49. Burchell SA, Yu M, Takiguchi SA, Ohta RM, Myers SA. Evaluation of a continuous cardiac output and mixed venous oxygen saturation catheter in critically ill surgical patients. Crit Care Med 1997; 25:388–391.
50. Mihm FG, Gettinger A, Hanson CW III, et al. A multicenter evaluation of a new continuous cardiac output pulmonary artery catheter system. Crit Care Med 1998; 26:1346–1350.
51. Zollner C, Polasek J, Kilger E, et al. Evaluation of a new continuous thermodilution cardiac output monitor in cardiac surgical patients. Crit Care Med 1999; 27:293–298.
52. Cariou A, Laurent I, Dhainaut JF. Pulmonary artery catheterization: modified catheters. In: Tobin MJ, ed. Principles and Practice of Intensive Care Monitoring. New York: McGraw-Hill Companies, 1998:811–819.
53. Martyn JA, Snider MT, Farago LF, Burke JF. Thermodilution right ventricular volume: a novel and better predictor of volume replacement in acute thermal injury. J Trauma 1981; 21:619–626.
54. Chang MC, Blinman TA, Rutherford EJ, Nelson LD, Morris JA Jr. Preload assessment in trauma patients during large-volume shock resuscitation. Arch Surg 1996; 131:728–731.
55. Marik PE. Pulmonary artery catheterization and esophageal Doppler monitoring in the ICU. Chest 1999; 116:1085–1091.
56. Madan AK, UyBarreta VV, Aliabadi-Wahle S, et al. Esophageal Doppler ultrasound monitor versus pulmonary artery catheter in the hemodynamic management of critically ill surgical patients. J Trauma 1999; 46:607–612.
57. Velmahos GC, Wo CC, Demetriades D, et al. Invasive and non-invasive physiological monitoring of blunt trauma patients in the early period after emergency admission. Int Surg 1999; 84:354–360.
58. Woltjer HH, Bogaard HJ, de Vries PM. The technique of impedance cardiography. Eur Heart J 1997; 18:1396–1403.
59. Kohli-Seth R, Oropello JM. The future of bedside monitoring. Crit Care Clin 2000; 16:557–578.
60. Guyton AC, Hall JE. Textbook of Medical Physiology. 10th ed. Philadelphia: W.B. Saunders Company, 2000:145.
61. Bedford, RF. Invasive blood pressure monitoring. In: Blitt CD, ed. Monitoring in Anesthesia and Critical Care. New York: Churchill Liuingstone, 1985:505.
62. Benumof JL. Anesthesia for Thoracic Surgery. Philadelphia: W.B. Saunders Company, 1995:279.
63. Nakano KJM, Waxman K. Pulmonary artery catheterization. In: Shoemaker WC, Velmahos GC, Demetriades D, eds. Procedures and Monitoring for the Critically Ill. Philadelphia: W.B. Saunders Company, 2002:24.
64. O'Quin R, Marini JJ. Pulmonary artery occlusion pressure: Clinical physiology, measurement, and interpretation. Am Rev Respir Dis 1983; 128:322.

Splanchnic and Renal Monitoring

Eamon O'Reilly

Department of Surgery, Naval Medical Center San Diego, San Diego, California, U.S.A.

Eugenio Lujan

Department of Anesthesiology and Critical Care Medicine, Naval Medical Center San Diego, San Diego, California, U.S.A.

INTRODUCTION

Methods for monitoring resuscitation of patients in overt shock, as well as those with less obvious occult hypoperfused states, continues to be actively pursued. Along with research into shock states, increased standardization in definitions has been required. To this end, the American College of Surgeons Committee on Trauma (ACS-COT) defined shock as "an abnormality of the circulatory system that results in inadequate organ perfusion and tissue oxygenation" (1). The American College of Chest Physicians (ACCP) and the Society of Critical Care Medicine (SCCM) similarly established a Consensus Conference Committee, which defined shock associated with sepsis as "... hypotension [systolic blood pressure (SBP) <90 mmHg or reduction ≥40 mmHg from baseline] despite adequate fluid resuscitation, along with the perfusion abnormalities that may include, but are not limited to: (*i*) lactic acidosis, (*ii*) oliguria, or (*iii*) an acute alteration in mental status" (2).

These definitions and the inferred resuscitation endpoints are clinically relevant to goal-directed therapy for trauma (3,4) and sepsis respectively (5,6). Traditional endpoints of resuscitation include blood pressure (BP), pulse, urine output, and mentation. Invasive monitors of hemodynamic status include central venous pressure (CVP), indwelling arterial catheter and mean arterial pressure (MAP), and pulmonary artery occlusion pressure (PAOP). Invasively measured and derived variables, such as cardiac output (Q̇), mixed venous oxygen saturation, and central venous oxygen saturation, have also been widely utilized in the critical care settings as part of goal-directed therapy. Other markers of hypoperfusion include measuring serum lactate, base deficit (BD), and arterial pH.

The aforementioned global measures of resuscitation can be inaccurate and slow to change in the young or well-compensated patient (see Volume 1, Chapters 12 and 18) (7,8). In addition, these are nonspecific markers that reflect the overall patient status, and do not necessarily correlate with the specific well being of any particular vascular bed. Indeed, all of these parameters are incomplete predictors of resuscitation status (9).

Critically ill patients that are underresuscitated require prompt treatment to prevent further damage to their vital organs (see Volume 1, Chapter 12). Surrogate markers have been used for decades, in an attempt to assess the adequacy of circulation to end-organs and the end-points to resuscitation (see Volume 1, Chapter 18). 🗡 **The two organ systems most often initially impacted in** **the underresuscitated trauma patient are the kidneys and the gastrointestinal (GI) organs.** 🗡 Significant research efforts have been focused on developing techniques for measuring renal and splanchnic perfusion. Direct measurement is normally not available clinically, so surrogate markers have been studied as measures of resuscitation success.

This chapter will primarily focus on the intricacies and utility of the various monitoring modalities that reflect the adequacy of splanchnic and renal blood flow. In addition, some newer monitoring systems that correlate with splanchnic perfusion will be introduced.

SPLANCHNIC MONITORING

Due to the current limitations of global resuscitation markers, end-organ and tissue-specific markers of hypoperfusion continue to be sought. Splanchnic monitoring is one such area—examples include gastric tonometry and pH monitoring. Other measures that correlate, but are not direct measurements, include sublingual capnography, buccal tissue CO_2 monitoring, as well as biochemical markers of insult (e.g., abnormal increases in lactic acid), and other surrogates of splanchnic well-being (e.g., tolerance to enteral nutrition).

Anatomy and Pathophysiology
Splanchnic Circulation
The distribution of splanchnic blood flow is determined by well-known embryologic relationships (Table 1) (10). The abdominal foregut structures include the stomach, duodenum proximal to Wirsung's duct, liver, biliary drainage system, and pancreas. These structures are supplied by the celiac trunk via the common hepatic, left gastric, right gastric, and splenic arteries. Midgut structures encompass the bowel from the distal duodenum to the proximal two-thirds of the transverse colon, and are supplied by the superior mesenteric artery (SMA). The hindgut is composed of the remaining colon, rectum, and proximal anal canal. The inferior mesenteric artery (IMA) supplies these structures.

The renal blood supply is separate (individual right and left renal arteries, arising off the aorta between the SMA and IMA), but these vessels respond similarly to hypovolemia and hypotension (with relative hypoperfusion). Monitoring of renal perfusion and function is discussed below.

Table 1 Splanchnic and Renal Blood Supply

Artery (from aorta)	Major branch	Feeding artery	Organ perfused
Celiac	Common hepatic	Right and left hepatic	Liver (25% of flow, 50% O_2) The portal vein provides 75% of the hepatic inflow and 50% of the O_2
		Right hepatic	Gall bladder via cystic artery (branch of right hepatic)
		Gastroduodenal	First, second, and third part of duodenum, head of the pancreas
	Left gastric		Gastroesophageal junction
	Superior pancreatic		Midsection and tail of pancreas
	Splenic	Superior and inferior pancreatic	Midsection and tail of pancreas
		Short gastrics	Fundus of stomach
		Left gastroepiploic	Greater curvature of stomach (joins right gastroepiploic, which is the distal continuation of the gastroduodenal artery)
		Splenic	Spleen
Superior mesenteric	Inferior pancreaticoduodenal		Head of pancreas, and first and third part of duodenum
	Inferior pancreatic		Middle and tail of pancreas
	Superior mesenteric		Small intestine (including the fourth part of duodenum usually) to the proximal two-third of the transverse colon
Right and left renal arteries			Right and left kidneys
Inferior mesenteric	Left colic		Distal transverse and descending colon
	Sigmoid branches of IMA		Sigmoid colon
	Superior rectal branches of IMA		Rectum

Abbreviation: IMA, inferior mesenteric artery.

☞ **In the resting normovolemic patient, approximately 20% to 35% of the cardiac output is directed to the splanchnic circulation.** ☞ The tissues supplied by the splanchnic circulation have large metabolic compensatory abilities, in response to either increased or decreased demand, and these tissues can increase oxygen extraction upwards of 90%. During a sympathetic circulatory response to hypovolemic shock, blood is shunted to tissue beds most needed—heart, lungs, brain—and away from nonvital circulatory systems, such as the splanchnic circulation, via release of catecholamines and subsequent vasoconstriction (11,12). Nitric oxide (NO) is likely the most important regulator of splanchnic vascular tone at rest (11). The gut is susceptible to periods of hypoxemia, but due to the abundant collateralization of blood flow, and partly due to the countercurrent exchange of the vascular supply of the intestinal villi, ischemia is usually averted when hypotension periods are brief (11).

Pathological Consequences of Splanchnic Hypoperfusion

The splanchnic circulation is susceptible to episodes of hypoperfusion during shock. Due to the relatively low metabolic rate of the splanchnic organs (compared to heart and brain), these low perfusion states are generally well tolerated for brief periods. When periods of splanchnic hypoperfusion become prolonged ischemia and ultimately sepsis, the multiple organ dysfunction syndrome (MODS) can occur. The risk factors associated with splanchnic ischemia are listed in Table 2.

If splanchnic oxygen consumption is increased, as occurs in sepsis or other shock states, splanchnic hypoxemia can be exacerbated even if blood flow returns (13–16). ☞ **The pathogenesis of sepsis and MODS is multifactorial. The concept of a "leaky" gut barrier and translocation of bacteria (and cytokines) are likely the integral component.** ☞

During ischemic or low flow states in the viscera, proinflammatory cytokines are released. Tumor necrosis factor-α (TNF-α), interleukin-1, 6, 8, and interferon-γ lead to release of secondary inflammatory mediators such as NO and complement, all resulting in the upregulation of immune cell production and stimulation. Once activated, neutrophils adhere to endothelial cells, promoting cell permeability and occasionally injury. Endothelial and junctional damage leads to reductions in gut barrier function, and subsequent translocation of enteric bacteria, lipopolysaccharide, and endotoxin. This is thought to lead to the development of the systemic inflammatory response syndrome (SIRS), sepsis, and eventually MODS (Fig. 1) (16).

Gastric pH Monitoring
Physiological Tenets of Gastric pH Monitoring

Tonometry is the measurement of the partial pressure of a gas in a fluid or intravascular medium. ☞ **Gastric tonometry measures luminal CO_2 and mucosal CO_2 partial pressures (PCO_2), as they become equalized across a semipermeable membrane.** ☞

Most gastric tonometers utilize a saline-filled latex balloon (Fig. 2). CO_2 freely diffuses across the membrane,

Table 2 Risk Factors for Mesenteric Ischemia

Preexisting mesenteric disease	Chronic mesenteric ischemia
Systemic diseases associated with mesenteric disease	Coronary artery disease
	Acute or chronic heart failure
	Diabetes
	Hypertension
	Peripheral vascular disease
	Previous reconstruction for occlusive-stenotic arterial lesions
	Episodes of arterial embolism
	Congenital or acquired hemostatic disorders
	Oral contraceptives
	DVT or PE
Procedures associated with mesenteric ischemia	Trauma
	Abdominal surgery
	Cardiac surgery/CPB
Trauma-related risk factors	Hypotension/hypoperfusion
	SIRS/sepsis
	Vasopressor therapy
	Abdominal trauma
	Abdominal compartment syndrome
	Mechanical ventilation (with high PIP/PEEP)

Abbreviations: CPB, cardiopulmonary bypass; DVT, deep venous thrombosis; PE, pulmonary embolism; PEEP, positive end expiratory pressure; PIP, peak inspiratory pressure; SIRS, systemic inflammatory response syndrome.

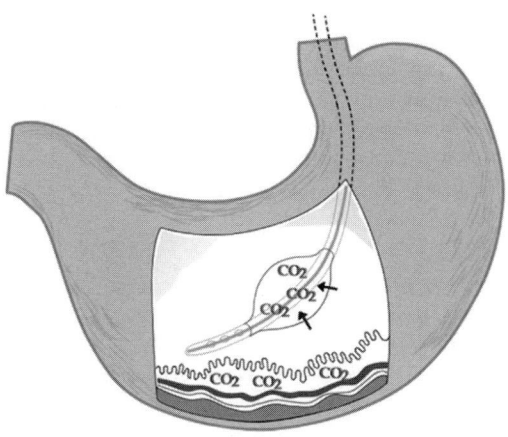

Figure 2 Gastric tonometry. Gastric mucosal CO_2 diffuses into the gastric tonometer balloon, and is measured using a blood gas analyzer. *Source*: Adapted from Ref. 16.

leading to equilibrium between the saline PCO_2 and the gastric mucosal PCO_2. The PCO_2 within the saline-filled balloon is used as a proxy for gastric mucosal CO_2, and is measured using a blood gas analyzer. Utilizing the Henderson-Hasselbach equation, and assuming that the partial pressure of stomach mucosa and arterial bicarbonate are equal, the intramucosal pH (pHi) can be calculated

(Table 3) (15). A decreased pHi is thought to reflect either an increased anaerobic metabolism or a low flow state, and thus ischemic states (15,16).

Two major assumptions enter into the calculation of pHi (15). First, the PCO_2 measured via gastric tonometry approximates the intramucosal PCO_2, because CO_2 freely diffuses in tissue. In animal studies, no difference has been found between luminal and mucosal CO_2 measurements (17). Second, intramucosal and arterial HCO_3^- measurements are the same. However, arterial HCO_3^- measurements are likely an overestimation of the mucosal HCO_3^- in decreased splanchnic flow states, due to the release of H^+ ions and subsequent buffering via bicarbonate (15). This may lead to altered measurements of pHi.

In the stomach and proximal duodenum, the assumption that mucosal and luminal PCO_2 equilibrates, may fail (15). Unlike the majority of the small and large bowel, the stomach actively secretes H^+ and the proximal duodenum

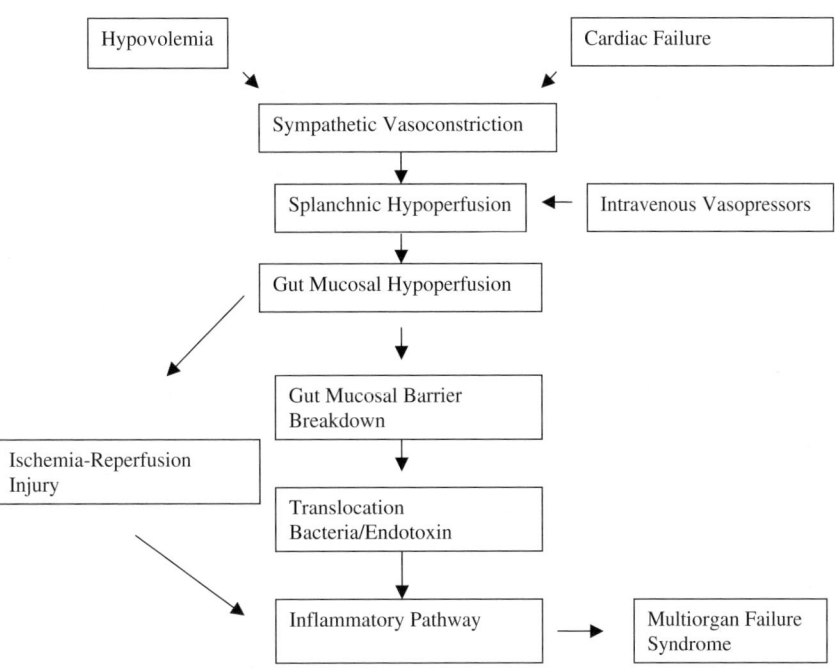

Figure 1 The gut hypothesis of sepsis and multiple organ dysfunction syndrome. *Source*: Adapted from Ref. 16.

Table 3 Physical Principles and Equations Used in Gastric Tonometry

Physical principle	Equation or relationship
Henderson-Hasselbach equation (adapted for pHi)	$pHi = 6.1 + \log 10\,[HCO_3^-]/[\alpha \cdot PCO_2]$ $\alpha = 0.03$ (solubility factor of CO_2 in plasma)
Bicarbonate buffer	$HCO_3^- + H^+ <-> H_2CO_3 <-> CO_2 + H_2O$

Abbreviation: pHi, intramucosal pH.

secretes HCO_3^-. Although the mucosal barrier in the stomach largely protects against the back diffusion of H^+, it does not completely do so. This back-diffused H^+ is buffered by bicarbonate in the mucosa, leading to the production of CO_2, and the reading of a falsely low pHi. Similarly, bicarbonate secreted by the duodenum may reflux into the stomach, buffering H^+, and artificially lowering the tonometrically measured PCO_2. Studies in animals have found that back diffusion of H^+ is not much of a confounding factor, whereas increased luminal CO_2 production is (18). It has been proposed that gastric H_2 blockers be utilized to decrease luminal H^+ and thus decrease error in tonometric PCO_2 measurements. In stable subjects, the measured variance between luminal PCO_2, luminal pH, and pHi were decreased when given an H_2 blocker, whereas when the same values were measured in a small study of critically ill patients on an H_2 blocker, no difference was found versus placebo (19,20).

Other physiological differences may affect the measured pHi (21). Differences in gastric mucosal temperature and arterial blood temperature may change the amount of gas dissolved in tissue or blood respectively. Also, the Haldane effect can increase the measured PCO_2 in the setting of increased oxygen consumption ($\dot{V}O_2$), without increased perfusion (16). Finally, the measured PCO_2 may be confounded by gastric H^+ secretion.

It has been suggested that the difference between gastric and arterial PCO_2 (the "PCO_2 gap") be utilized in order to eliminate the variables and confounding factors of gastric H^+ secretion. This idea of measuring this PCO_2 gap, and not the absolute marker pHi, is utilized in both resuscitation endpoints and in sublingual capnography. Recent expert consensus asserts that the PCO_2 gap is a more accurate reflection of gastric dysoxia (22). A normal PCO_2 gap is approximately less than 8 mmHg, whereas a normal intramucosal PCO_2 is less than 48 mmHg (22). Additional randomized controlled trials (RCTs) will be needed to settle this question.

Techniques of Gastric Tonometry
Conventional Gastric Tonometry
In most commercially available gastric tonometers, a saline solution is infused into a semipermeable balloon (composed of silicone or latex polymers) at the end of a nasogastric tube. Fundamental to the above physiology of tonometry, silicone is permeable to CO_2. The luminal and mucosal PCO_2 generally equilibrate in approximately 30 minutes, although equilibration times up to 90 minutes have been reported (13). The saline is drawn anaerobically from the saline-filled balloon, and PCO_2 is measured via standard blood-gas analysis. Once the PCO_2 equilibrates, this is used with an arterial bicarbonate measurement to determine pHi. Standard

values for pHi fall within two standard deviations of the norm as found in studies of H_2 blockers on stable subjects. Thus, it is generally accepted that a pHi < 7.32 represents mucosal acidosis (23). However, the type of saline solution and buffer composition used in the blood-gas analysis can skew results (24,25). Strict anaerobic conditions must be maintained, and saline is the preferred media over phosphate bicarbonate or succinylated gelatin solutions due to long equilibrium times (25).

Air-Semicontinuous Gastric Tonometry
In an effort to increase the reproducibility and accuracy of gastric tonometry and pHi monitoring, other methods such as air-semicontinuous tonometry are utilized to measure luminal PCO_2 (26,27). Air tonometry uses an air-filled CO_2 permeable balloon that rapidly equilibrates with luminal and mucosal PCO_2. This is directly measured in a semicontinuous manner, by an infrared sensor. While this too may under- or overestimate the PCO_2 depending on the blood gas machine and assumed equilibrium times, it has been found in animal studies to correlate well with gastric pHi monitoring and be more accurate in the in vitro laboratory (27,28,29). However, outcome data utilizing gastric air-semicontinuous tonometry is similar to traditional saline-filled balloon tonometry and, in fact, both are ubiquitous in research (30).

Outcome Studies
Numerous indications exist for gastric tonometry and pHi monitoring. It can be used in all critically ill patients in order to guide resuscitation and improve outcome in sepsis, cardiogenic, and hypovolemic shock (23). Most critically ill patients in the intensive care unit (ICU) have some method to monitor global monitors of ischemia. Gastric tonometry can be utilized as a regional corollary.

One of the earliest associations identified by gastric tonometry was that MODS rates are correlated with decreased pHi (31). Failure of the gut, liver, pancreas, lungs, and generalized sepsis have all been postulated to correlate with decreasing pHi (31). Outcome-driven critical care studies have found a correlation between optimization times for pHi guided resuscitation and survival; as a prognostic marker and independent predictor for mortality; as an independent predictor of MODS; and an association between decreased pHi and increased length of ICU stay (9,32–36). However, other studies have found that guiding resuscitation with pHi versus traditional resuscitation techniques does not yield improved outcomes in either overall survival or rates of MODS (37,38).

Other applications exist for gastric tonometry. In the preoperative setting, gastric pHi monitoring can be used to predict postoperative morbidity and mortality (39). Further, gastric pHi monitoring can guide vasoactive drug administration, particularly when norepinephrine or dopamine is used in conjunction with vasopressin for refractory shock (40,41). Physiologic doses of vasopressin (0.01–0.04 U/min) does not cause significant severe splanchnic vasoconstriction. However, higher doses can threaten gut perfusion. Gastric tonometry might evolve into a commonly employed monitor for preventing mesenteric ischemia during prolonged vasopressin use in the setting of refractory shock. However, due to the need for stable conditions in order to obtain baseline values and to monitor ongoing resuscitation efforts, gastric tonometry (in its current technological state) is not useful during the initial resuscitation efforts for the seriously injured trauma patient. With current technology, gastric tonometry is unlikely to provide additional useful information during the initial phase. However, technological advancements in stability calibration and equilibration time could result in early benefits to use.

Sublingual Capnography
Physiological Tenets of Sublingual Capnography
Due to the numerous limitations to gastric pHi monitoring utilizing PCO_2 as a surrogate marker, sublingual capnography surfaced as an alternative to directly monitoring tissue-perfusion. Although gastric tonometry measures tissue specific hypercapnia, other tissue, such as renal or brain tissue, have been suggested as sentinel markers for tissue hypoperfusion and shock states.

Unlike gastric monitoring, sublingual capnography is applied to a readily accessible site (42). This facilitates data gathered during initial resuscitation efforts in the trauma resuscitation suite (TRS) or in the trauma operating room (OR). In a fashion similar to gastric PCO_2 monitoring, the sublingual PCO_2 ($P_{SL}CO_2$) is measured against the arterial PCO_2 to define a $P_{SL}CO_2$ gap. Sublingual capnography does not necessarily reflect perfusion to the splanchnic circulation. Indeed, the sublingual mucosa is not perfused by the splanchnic circulation. However, the sublingual mucosal vascular bed shares similar characteristics with the splanchnic circulation, including a rich vascular supply and stimulatory parasympathetic innervation. Most importantly, several investigations have demonstrated that the $P_{SL}CO_2$ correlates closely with those values obtained in the stomach during low flow states (43–45).

Technique of Sublingual Capnography
Several sublingual capnographic measuring devices are commercially available. Studies reviewed here utilize either the MI-720 CO_2 electrode (Microelectrodes; Londonderry, New Hampshire, U.S.A.) or the Capnoprobe SL Monitoring System (Nellcor; Pleasanton, California, U.S.A.). The most popular device, the Capnoprobe SL, utilizes a specific CO_2-sensing optode consisting of a CO_2-permeable silicone bag with known buffer solution and a fluorescent dye solvent. This bag is attached to a light source that senses the wavelength changes of the fluorescent dye as it is acted upon by the pH of the solution. This is converted into a measurement of $P_{SL}CO_2$. It is imperative for measurement that the subject's mouth be closed around the monitor (42).

Outcome Studies
Studies on sublingual capnography were first conducted in animals, which found plausible reason to study sublingual CO_2 in humans due to correlations between rising $P_{SL}CO_2$ and systemic markers such as arterial lactate (43). Further, a head-to-head animal study comparing sublingual monitoring with gastric tonometry found similar monitoring characteristics and increases measured in both gastric intramucosal PCO_2 and $P_{SL}CO_2$ gap (44). Subsequently, the same investigators found that $P_{SL}CO_2$ values greater than 70 mmHg were predictive of hospital survival, and that $P_{SL}CO_2$ corrected in a more rapid manner than serum lactate (45). The $P_{SL}CO_2$ gap has also been found to correlate with gastric PCO_2 gap and lactate levels in critical care patients in circulatory or septic shock, and a small study has found that sublingual $P_{SL}CO_2$ gap is a better predictor of survival than lactic acid (46–48).

↗ A recent study has also found correlation between hemorrhage in penetrating trauma and rise in sublingual $P_{SL}CO_2$, coinciding with increasing in BD and lactate levels (49). ↗

Surrogate Measures of Splanchnic Well-Being
Lactic Acidosis
Lactic acidosis is a global marker of tissue hypoxia and is produced anaerobically from the substrate pyruvate. A normal plasma lactate level is less than 2.0–2.2 mmol/L; elevated levels correlate with oxygen delivery $\dot{D}O_2$ deficit and global under-resuscitation. Anaerobically produced lactate is generally independent of other metabolic processes (in comparison to other global hypoxia markers such as base deficit), although severe liver dysfunction can artificially prolong lactic acid levels (50). Outcome data has shown a correlation to lactate level normalization and mortality; development of acute respiratory distress syndrome; the SIRS and severe sepsis; and an increase in infection rates (51–55).

For the purposes of splanchnic monitoring, lactic acidosis is felt to be a generalized marker. Studies are mixed as to whether direct splanchnic monitoring (gastric tonometry), indirect splanchnic monitoring (sublingual capnography), or global markers of hypoperfusion are more sensitive guides to resuscitation. Early studies found gastric tonometry and pHi to better predict mortality and multiorgan system failure than traditional markers such as lactate levels and BD (9,35). The $P_{SL}CO_2$ was found, in one small study, to be a better predictor of mortality and a more sensitive marker than lactate levels (48). However, few RCTs exist comparing traditional endpoints with focused splanchnic monitoring. A recent small study, which randomized resuscitation in trauma patients to either "traditional" pHi markers (such as lactate) or gastric pH directed therapy, found no difference in outcomes (38).

Tolerance of Enteral Nutrition
↗ Tolerance of early enteral feeding has been shown to correlate with numerous markers, including decreasing bacterial translocation and morbidity from sepsis, overall mortality, the length of ICU stay, and cost of ICU admission (56). ↗ Although a majority of physicians begin enteral feeds within 48 hours of admission, less than half of patients started on enteral nutrition achieve tolerance to the feedings (56,57). Historically, tolerance of enteric feeding has been based on the concept of gastric residual volumes (GRVs). High GRVs are traditionally thought to correlate with poor outcomes, such as aspiration and pneumonia, or as a marker for intolerance of enteral nutrition (58). However, the definition of "high" by some (>150 mL in a 70-kg patient) is felt to be too low a threshold by most experienced intensivists. GRVs in this (150–200 mL) range are of little value in directing feedings due to: (i) lack of correlation with the measured value and adverse outcomes; and (ii) absence of standardization of GRV values. Using such low "acceptable" GRVs likely impedes the progression of feedings (58). The use of higher threshold GRVs (~450 mL in a 70-kg patient), along with the administration of promotility agents, and distal duodenum- or jejunal-placed feeding tubes, all correlate with increased tolerance of enteral nutrition (also see Volume 2, Chapter 32) (59,60). Due to conflicting opinions on the utilization of GVRs in the clinical setting, other methods for monitoring tolerance of enteral nutrition have been sought.

A few small studies have looked at tolerance of enteral nutrition and measuring Brix values, a measurement of the total amount of soluble solids in a solution. The Brix value is designed to help account for the amount of enteral formula versus gastric secretions and saliva contained in the GRV (61,62). The Brix value is obtained using a refractometer to assay the GRV aspirated from the patient. At best, these studies show the Brix value measurements as a clinical adjunct with GRV values, but have little clinical correlation to tolerance of enteral feedings or outcome.

Splanchnic monitoring via gastric tonometry or sublingual capnography may also serve as markers for tolerance to enteral nutrition. In theory, intolerance of enteral feedings can result from splanchnic hypoperfusion and, conversely, prolonged starvation could decrease splanchnic hypoperfusion. In cardiothoracic surgery patients, early enteral feedings did not show any effect on gastric tonometry measurements, potentially indicating tolerance of enteric feedings (although this was not an endpoint in the study) (63). Enteral feeding in burn patients has been shown via gastric tonometry to have beneficial effects on splanchnic circulation (64). In a small case study, a gastric pH less than 7.30 was found in all patients with nonocclusive bowel necrosis, one of the dreaded, but rare, complications of enteral feeds in the critically ill (65).

Stress Gastritis

Stress gastritis is associated with gastric mucosal ischemia (Volume 2, Chapter 30). A recurring paradigm of ischemia and reperfusion injury not only provides a plausible explanation for the development of stress gastritis (66,67), but also highlights the physiology and importance for other methods of splanchnic monitoring.

Mucosal ischemia (from various etiologies including occult hypoperfusion) interrupts gastric mucus production and has an overall negative effect on the gastroprotective prostaglandin (PG) and bicarbonate production. Further exacerbating the breakdown of the protective gastric mucus is reflux of bile salts into the gastric lumen in critically ill patients (67). The breakdown of gastric mucosa leads to subendothelial petechiae and small erosions from the acidic gastric contents. Ultimately, this may lead to frank ulceration (67).

Numerous risk factors, such as mechanical ventilation, coagulopathy, hypotension, sepsis, hepatic failure, renal failure, burns, and major trauma, may contribute to the development of mucosal ischemia and stress gastritis (67). All of these factors have specific physiological mechanisms, although two are particularly pertinent. Patients with critical illness often exhibit associated respiratory failure, and consequently require mechanical ventilation. The institution of mechanical ventilation can directly impair the splanchnic blood flow. Increased intrathoracic pressure and positive end expiratory pressures can decrease venous return and, thus, splanchnic perfusion (68).

The GI tract is susceptible to prolonged periods of decreased perfusion pressures. In addition to the increased risk of bacterial and cytokine translocation, the end result of gastric mucosal ischemia is stress gastritis. Medications that limit splanchnic perfusion also have the potential to cause mucosal ischemia and stress gastritis (67). Vasoactive agents, such as norepinephrine and vasopressin, can cause a decrease in splanchnic circulation, although correlations between these agents and stress gastritis are not as clear (69,70).

Prophylaxis against stress gastritis is recommended (Volume 2, Chapter 30), although the best choice is not readily apparent (71–73). Mechanical barriers, such as sucralfate, and pharmaceutical agents, such as H_2 blockers and proton pump inhibitors, are utilized. These agents have been shown to decrease the incidence of stress gastritis in the critical care setting, and subsequently decrease the utility of monitoring for stress gastritis as a marker for splanchnic ischemia and occult hypoperfusion—leading to the utility of gastric tonometry or sublingual capnography.

RENAL MONITORING
Introduction

Renal dysfunction and renal failure (Table 4) remain a serious complication in the critically ill trauma or postoperative patient (see Volume 2, Chapters 40–42). The trauma, burn, and the postoperative surgical patient have numerous risk factors that make them at high risk for the development of renal dysfunction (Table 5). Renal failure complicates the perioperative management of these patients. The onset of acute renal failure (ARF) portends a poor prognosis and a high association with mortality, sepsis, and MODS. The prevention of ARF lies in ensuring adequate resuscitation, preventing continued damage, minimizing the impact of coexisting disease, and minimizing the number of nephrotoxic drugs (Table 6).

As with other organ systems, renal function is intimately related to blood flow supplied by its arteries (renal artery). The detection of altered or diminished renal blood flow (RBF) is clinically difficult due to the limited available monitoring technologies. ☞ **Surrogate markers [urine output, serum creatinine, and glomerular filtration rates (GFRs—which is most commonly calculated from creatinine clearance (CL_{CR})] are routinely used to assess for clinically detectable alterations in RBF.** ☞ The most commonly employed tests and imaging studies used to evaluate renal perfusion and function are listed in Tables 7 and 8.

Anatomy and Physiology
Renal Circulation

Each kidney is supplied by a single renal artery arising from the aorta at the level of the intervertebral disc between L1 and L2 vertebrae. Each renal artery divides at the renal pelvis into 5 to 6 segmental arteries, which give rise to the interlobar arteries. At the division between the renal cortex and medulla, the interlobar arteries divide again into the arcurate arteries. Arcurate arteries then give rise to the interlobular arteries and the capsular perforating branches. Intelobular arteries directly supply each nephron through a

Table 4 Causes of Perioperative Renal Failure

Category	Description
Prerenal	Reversible increase in serum creatinine and blood urea. Results from a decreased renal perfusion, which leads to a decreased GFR
Postrenal	Caused by an obstruction of the urinary collection system by either intrinsic or extrinsic causes
Renal	The structures of the glomerulus, tubules, vessels, or interstitium are affected

Abbreviation: GFR, glomerular filtration rate.

Table 5 Risk Factors for Perioperative Acute Renal Failure

Risk factor category	Examples/comments
Preexisting renal insufficiency	The worse the preexisting renal insufficiency, the greater the risk
Systemic diseases associated with chronic renal failure	Coronary artery disease
	Congestive heart failure
	Diabetes
	Hypertension
	Liver failure, hepato-renal syndrome
	Peripheral vascular disease
	Polycystic kidney disease
	Scleroderma
	Systemic lupus erythematosus
	Rheumatoid arthritis
	Wegner's granulomatosis
Procedures associated with acute renal failure	Biliary surgery
	Burns
	Cardiac surgery
	Genitourinary surgery/obstetric surgery
	Transplant
	Trauma
	CAT scan
Trauma-related risk factors	Hypotension
	Hypovolemia
	Hypoperfusion
	Medication/antibiotics
	IV contrast
	Blood transfusion
	Rhabdomyolysis
	SIRS/sepsis
	Vasopressor therapy

Abbreviations: CAT, computerized axial tomography; IV, intravenous; SIRS, systemic inflammatory response syndrome.

single afferent arteriole (74). The microcirculation of the kidney is arranged into three separate blood flow zones, including that perfusing the cortex, the outer medulla, and the inner medulla (74).

Table 6 Medications Associated with Renal Failure

Nephrotoxic drug type	Examples/comments
IV radiocontrast	Nonionic less toxic than ionic
H_2 receptor antagonists	Cimetidine, rantidine, fomotidine
NSAIDs	Ibuprofen, Cox2 inhibitors, aspirin
Immunosuppressive drugs	Cyclosporin A, tacrolimus
Antibacterial drugs	Aminoglycosides, penicillins, sulfonamides, cephalosporins, vancomycin
Antifungal agents	Amphotericin B
Malignant chemotherapy drugs	Methotrexate, nitrosureas, cisplatin, asparginase,
Others	Acetaminophen, ACE inhibitors, allopurinol, IVIG, hydroxyethyl starch, antivirals, metoclopromide

Abbreviations: ACE, angiotensin-converting enzyme; Cox2, cyclo-oxygenase 2; IV, intravenous; IVIG, intravenous immunoglobulin; NSAIDs, nonsteroidal anti-inflammatory drugs.

Table 7 Commonly Used Tests and Studies in the Diagnosis of Acute Renal Failure

Category	Examples
Radiographic imaging	Ultrasound
	CT scan
	RUG
	Plain radiographs (KUB)
	IVP
	Angiography
Urine evaluation	Urine electrolytes
	Urine eosinophiles
	Urine analysis
	Urine culture
Tests of cardiac function	Cardiac echocardiography
	CVP
	Pulmonary capillary wedge pressure
	Left atrial pressure
Histological	Renal biopsy
	Autopsy

Abbreviations: CT, computed tomography; CVP, central venous pressure; IVP, intravenous pyelogram; KUB, kidneys, ureters, and bladder; RUG, retrograde urethrogram.

The blood flow through both kidneys constitutes approximately 20% to 25% of the total $\dot{Q}$, but can dramatically drop in patients that are hypovolemic or hypotensive. Approximately 80% of RBF supplies the cortical nephrons, whereas 10% to 15% supplies the juxtamedullary nephrons. Redistribution of RBF away from cortical nephrons, with short loops of Henle, to larger juxtamedullary nephrons with long loops, occurs during periods of stress and other times that are clinically relevant. Vasoactive hormones that regulate intrarenal blood flow originate from outside the kidney (vasopressin, norepinephrine, epinephrine), areas adjacent to the kidney (kinins, endothelins, adenosine), and from within the endothelium (NO, prostacyclin, endothelins) (74). Sympathetic nerve activation (75), angiotensin II (76), norepinephrine (76), and heart failure (77) have all been found to cause a redistribution of RBF away from the renal cortex and to the renal medulla. However,

Table 8 Physiologic Tests of Renal Tubular Function

Test	Prerenal	Renal (intrinsic)
U:P osmolality	>1.4:1	1:1
Urine osmolality	>500	<400
U:P creatinine	>50:1	<20:1
Urine Na level, mEq/L	<20	>40
FE_{Na}	<1	>3
CL_{CR}	15–20	<10
FE_{UA}	<35	>35
FE_{Li}	<15	>25
Urinary sediment	Normal, occasional hyaline, or finely granular casts	Renal tubular epithelial cells, granulars, and muddy brown granular casts

Abbreviations: CL_{CR}, creatinine clearance; FE_{Li}, fractional excretion of lithium; FE_{Na}, fractional excretion of sodium; FE_{UA}, fractional excretion of urea; P, plasma; U, urine.

not all vasopressors preferentially reduce cortical blood flow; vasopressin was recently found to preferentially reduce medullary blood flow in an animal model (76).

Contrast media is a major cause of hospital-acquired renal insufficiency. It has a heterogeneous effect on regional RBF, affecting outer medulla greater than the inner medulla or cortical blood flow (78). Iso-osmolar and high-osmolar contrast media, at normal and high doses, decrease outer medullary blood flow and place patients at significant risk for renal dysfunction (79).

The clinical significance of the redistribution of blood flow within the kidney can vary from situation to situation and patient to patient. Regardless of the stressor causing redistribution of RBF, it has been shown to be associated with sodium retention in both hypertensive and nonhypertensive patients. Initially, the redistribution of RBF serves to conserve sodium and free water. Prolonged periods of ischemia unleash a cascade of intrarenal mediators that potentially could lead to renal insufficiency and MODS. The role of NO and prostaglandin E_2 (PGE_2) in the prevention of this alteration in RBF is an ongoing area of research, but has shown promise in angiotensin II and norepinephrine dependent cortical constriction (80,81).

The kidney is the only organ in which oxygen consumption ($\dot{V}O_2$) is determined by RBF, this relationship seems to be maintained during periods of extreme stress (82–84). The rate of active transport of Na^+ best correlates with the $\dot{V}O_2$ (85,86). The simple relationship between $\dot{V}O_2$ and sodium transport best explains why the active transport of sodium decreases when RBF is diminished. ☞ **Renal physiology and pathophysiology are described by the relationships between RBF, renal $\dot{V}O_2$, O_2 extraction, and CL_{CR} in patients with normal and abnormal renal function (87).** ☞

Pathology of Renal Hypoperfusion

Trauma patients have multiple reasons for increased perioperative risk of renal failure (Table 5), including hypovolemia, hypotension, rhabdomyolysis, use of nephrotoxic agents (e.g., contrast, aminoglycosides, etc.). The risk increases further if they have associated intra-abdominal or renal trauma (e.g., renal contusion, lacerations, etc.). Trauma patients who are severely injured and have associated renal injury, have a much higher incidence of renal insufficiency and twice the mortality of those without renal injuries (88). In addition to direct renal trauma, secondary injury from conditions causing abdominal compartment syndrome (Volume 2, Chapter 34) are also important.

The renal circulation is extremely susceptible to periods of hypoperfusion. Prerenal causes account for 75% to 80% of the cases of perioperative dysfunction. Intrinsic causes account for 20% to 25% of the cases. The balance between renal $\dot{V}O_2$ and RBF tends to be maintained in states of shock or other shock states. However, with prolonged periods of renal hypoperfusion, ischemia and ultimately MODS can occur.

The role of the kidney in the propagation of SIRS and sepsis to MODS is incompletely understood. However, we do know that prolonged periods of reduced $\dot{D}O_2$ can lead to renal insufficiency. During periods of ischemia, the kidneys develop an O_2 debt and increase the release of vasoactive hormones, to include PGs, interleukins, and endothelin. Renal failure might supply a "second hit" in the development of sepsis, SIRS, and MODS in certain conditions (89).

Urine Output
Monitoring Urine Output

Serial measurements of urine output constitute the simplest form of RBF monitoring and assessment of renal function (see Volume 2, Chapter 40). Urine output is also one of the most commonly measured variables in the critically ill patient (90). However, resuscitation state, perioperative medications, and other interventions can alter the validity of this surrogate measure for RBF and renal function. ☞ **When evaluating a patient for alterations in urine output, the patient's medical history, medication use, type of surgery (or trauma), and relevant perioperative interventions must all be considered.** ☞

Urine output is an imperfect measure of renal function. Renal failure can occur in the setting of normal, elevated, or low urine output when confounders are present. That being said, urine formation is a sensitive marker of low flow states and prerenal causes of ARF. In the SICU, and especially in postsurgical and trauma patients, low urine output should be assumed to be prerenal until proven otherwise. Oliguria or low urine output, regardless of the setting, should prompt an evaluation of the patient and the correction of prerenal causes of renal dysfunction. Acute anuria suggests a mechanical or obstructive cause of renal failure, and the evaluation should be focused on the obstructive causes of renal failure in otherwise stable patients (e.g., kinked indwelling urine catheter).

However, in the setting of massive hemorrhage, oliguria and anuria reflect inadequate RBF due to insufficient intravascular volume repletion and/or inadequate renal perfusion pressure.

Oliguria is defined as urine output of 400 mL/day in a patient with previously normal kidneys. However, it is preferable to monitor urine output in the terms of hourly output, because prolonged periods of prerenal causes could lead to renal ischemia and acute tubular necrosis. Hence, oliguria has been traditionally defined as less than 0.5 mL/kg/hr. In critically ill, postoperative, or trauma patients, it should be expected that their trends of urine output should be greater than this value.

24-Hour Urine Output and Outcomes

Monitoring 24-hour urine output is useful in monitoring resuscitation, predicting the need for dialysis, and predicting mortality. Low urine output has been shown to be predictive of those patients requiring dialysis after cardiac surgery (91). It is predictive of those patients having higher mortality after myocardial infarction (92). Oliguric ARF was found to be an independent predictor for overall mortality in a subgroup of 348 patients with renal failure in the ICU (93).

Tubular Function
Creatinine and Creatinine Clearance

Creatinine is an end-product of skeletal muscle catabolism. Creatinine production is proportional to skeletal muscle mass, and is excreted solely by the kidneys. CL_{CR} measures the ability of the glomerulus to filter creatinine, and is the most reliable and widely used marker of GFR. Normal serum creatinine values range from 0.7 to 1.2 mg/dL. The formulas used to assess tubular function are listed in Table 9.

The most widely utilized formula to standardize GFR and renal function, according to age, is the Cockcroft-Gault equation: $CL_{CR} = [140 \ \text{age} \ \text{(yrs)}] \times \text{wt} \ \text{(kg)} \times 0.85$ (if

Table 9 Formulas Used to Assess Tubular Function

$CL_{CR} = (\text{creatinine})_U \times \text{urinary flow rate}/(\text{creatinine})_P$

$GFR = (140\text{-age})(\text{body weight in kg})/(\text{serum creatinine} \times 72)$

$FE_{Na} = (\text{urine sodium}/\text{serum sodium})/(\text{urine creatinine}/\text{serum creatinine}) \times 100\%$

$FE_{UA} = (\text{urine urea}/\text{serum urea})/(\text{urine creatinine}/\text{serum creatinine})$

Abbreviations: CL_{CR}, creatinine clearance; FE_{Na}, fractional excretion of sodium; FE_{UA}, fractional excretion of urea; GFR, glomerular filtration rate; P, plasma; U, urine.

female)$/72 \times$ [serum creatinine (mg/dL)] (94). Normal values range from 110 to 150 mL/min. Mild, moderate, and severe renal impairment have corresponding values of 40 to 60 mL/min, 20 to 40 mL/min, and less than 20 mL/min. Serial measurement of GFR is important for the early detection of renal dysfunction, determining the severity of renal impairment, and the need for further evaluation.

The CL_{CR} as a measure of GFR is commonly employed in the SICU for monitoring proper drug dosing and for the early detection of ARF. However, there is ongoing debate regarding the accuracy of these formulas for predicting CL_{CR} in critically ill patients. Wells et al. retrospectively evaluated 18 critically ill patients, nine without renal dysfunction, and nine with ARF. The investigators found statistically significant differences between measured CL_{CR} and the predicted values using the Cockcroft-Gault equation (94). Robert et al. assessed renal function utilizing inulin clearance, 30-minute CL_{CR}, 24-hour CL_{CR}, and the values estimated by the Cockcroft-Gault equation. They found that Cockcroft-Gault equation, using ideal body weight and the corrected serum creatinine concentration, was the best predictor of inulin clearance (95).

Furthermore, they found good correlation existed between inulin clearance and the Cockcroft-Gault equation, if the actual or ideal body weight and the actual or corrected serum creatinine were used in the calculation (95). Studies in trauma patients have shown that CL_{CR} can be used in those with stable renal function (96), and for the early detection of renal failure (97).

Fractional Excretion of Sodium

Fractional excretion of sodium (FE_{Na}) reflects tubular sodium reabsorption. FE_{Na} describes sodium clearance as a percentage of CL_{CR}. FE_{Na} less than 1% is seen in normal or hypovolemic patients. FE_{Na} above 3% indicates tubular damage or intrinsic causes of renal failure. Care must be taken when using FE_{Na} to evaluate for renal failure; medications are known to both raise and lower the FE_{Na}. Diuretics are the class of medications most notoriously known to alter the value and the usability of FE_{Na}. Both hydrochlothiazide and furosemide have been shown to increase the fraction of sodium excreted (98).

Fractional Excretion of Urea

Fractional excretion of urea (FE_{UA}) reflects the tubular reabsorption of urea. As with FE_{Na}, FE_{UA} describes urea clearance as a percentage of CL_{CR}. FE_{UA} less than 35% is seen in patients that are hypovolemic or prerenal. FE_{UA} above 35% indicates a normal, tubular damage or intrinsic causes of renal failure. In well-hydrated patients, the FE_{UA} is between 50% and 65% (99). Patients that have acute tubular necrosis (ATN) routinely have a FE_{UA} above 40%.

FE_{UA} may be a more sensitive and specific index than FE_{Na} in differentiating between prerenal-associated oliguria and ATN. **The FE_{UA} has a much higher positive predictive value in separating prerenal from ATN, 98% versus 89%.** It is especially useful in differentiating prerenal from intrinsic renal failure, after diuretics are used (100).

Urine-Concentrating Ability

The human body's ability to concentrate urine and maintain a normal serum osmolality is imperative. This is assessed by measuring urine osmolality, and comparing this value to the serum osmolality. Normal urine osmolality (U_{osm}) is 300 mOsm/kg (range 50–1200 mOsm/kg). Serum osmolality (278–298 mOsm/kg) should be measured in conjunction with urine osmolality. As serum tonicity increases, the release of antidiuretic hormone (ADH) increases, causing an increase in the reabsorption of free water and in the osmolality of urine. The opposite is true with a decrease in the serum tonicity; the decrease in ADH causes a decrease in the reabsorption of free water and in the osmolality of urine.

The most common times that clinicians will utilize these studies (S_{osm} and U_{osm}) is immediately postoperatively, ARF, and in the neurosurgical patient where diabetes insipidus (DI) results in a large quantity of dilute urine with increasing serum sodium and osmolality. The syndrome of inappropriate antidiuretic hormone (SIADH) can also occur in neurosurgical patients, and presents with a low quantity of concentrated urine, along with a concomitantly decreased serum sodium and osmolality (see Volume 2, Chapter 44).

Imaging in Genitourinary Conditions
Renal Ultrasound

The evaluation and workup of patients in acute, or acute on chronic, renal failure has traditionally focused on identifying the underlying etiology; prerenal, renal, or postrenal causes. Imaging techniques, especially ultrasound, can give an effective assistance in the differential diagnosis of ARF. **Imaging techniques can be used to exclude postrenal (obstruction) and prerenal (renal artery stenosis, low RBF) renal failure and confirm the diagnosis of intrinsic causes of renal failure.**

Color and pulse Doppler ultrasound are noninvasive tests that can be performed quickly and safely at the bedside. Color Doppler ultrasound has been utilized in diagnosing pyelonephritis (101), assessing RBF post-transplant (102,103), and differentiating between the causes of renal failure (104). However, many of the studies utilizing Doppler to assess for RBF have focused on renal transplant recipients.

Color Doppler (or duplex) ultrasound is commonly utilized in assessing patients with renal insufficiency and clearly has a role in the diagnosis of obstructive renal failure. Color Doppler has been increasingly utilized to assess for prerenal and renal causes of ATN as well. Izumi et al. evaluated 42 patients with ARF by Doppler ultrasound. Not only did they find that it was an effective tool to evaluate ARF caused by ATN, but also found it predictive of the recovery from ATN. However, its overuse in the initial diagnosis and management of ARF, especially in patients at low risk for obstructive renal failure, has been questioned (105).

Power Doppler ultrasound is a technique that has been in use since the mid-1990s, and is capable of detecting small-vessel, low-velocity flow (106,107). It has the ability to differentiate a wide spectrum of hypovascular renal pathologies. Renal hypoperfusion measured by power Doppler ultrasound has the ability to detect focal, multifocal, global, and cortical lesions (108). A recent animal study has found that image intensity of power Doppler ultrasound correlated well with invasively measured renal cortical blood flow (109). This technology has the greatest possibility to provide real-time measurement of renal perfusion during resuscitation of the injured and critically ill patient.

Computed Tomography

Computed tomography (CT) has primarily been used to evaluate renal injury following intra-abdominal and retro-peritoneal injuries sustained after blunt and penetrating trauma (110) (see Volume 1, Chapters 16, 27, and 28). Intrarenal blood flow derived from CT has been utilized in patients with renovascular disease (111), living kidney donors (112), and as an assessment prior to abdominal aortic aneurysm (113). In these studies, it was predominately utilized as a single occasion evaluation tool. Given the limitations of this technique and the advent of newer technologies that can be utilized continuously at the bedside, the role of CT in renal monitoring is obviously limited.

EYE TO THE FUTURE

The advent of newer technologies and biomarkers will allow for closer and more accurate monitoring of splanchnic and RBF. Many of the modalities described above represent techniques that require RCTs to better determine utility. Further, each of the techniques discussed is undergoing rapid technological improvements. Thus, the current notions of utility for various monitoring devices may change in the near future.

A relatively new perfusion monitoring tool that is on the clinical horizon is the buccal tissue CO_2 monitoring device (Fig. 3) (114). Increases in sublingual and buccal tissue PCO_2 (PCO_2 BU) have been shown to approximate those in the stomach and gut during low-flow states (115). At each of these sites, tissue PCO_2 was closely correlated with decreases in tissue blood flows (115–117).

Recently, Cammarata et al. (114) measured the PCO_2 BU in a rodent model of hemorrhagic shock. Rats were

bled over an interval of 30 minutes, in amounts estimated to be 25, 30, 35, or 40% of total blood volume. The PCO_2 BU was predictive of outcomes. Neither noninvasive end-tidal PCO_2, nor invasive aortic pressure measurements achieved such discrimination (114).

SUMMARY

Trauma patients commonly present hypotensive and hypovolemic. Optimal resuscitation requires early goal-directed therapy to prevent damage to organ systems and propagation of systemic inflammation. In addition to global measures, assessing perfusion adequacy for specific vascular beds (e.g., splanchnic and renal) are increasingly pursued, and newer technologies are becoming increasingly useful.

The splanchnic circulation is susceptible to prolonged periods of hypoperfusion. Markers used to assess adequacy of $\dot{D}O_2$ include gastric pH monitoring, sublingual capnography, lactic acidosis, tolerance of gastric feeds, and stress gastritis. The benefits and drawbacks of each of these methods for monitoring splanchnic circulation have been discussed.

The renal circulation has been established to preferentially shunt blood away from the cortex and supply the medulla. This places the kidney at high risk for ischemia and ATN, during periods of hypoperfusion as well. Markers used to assess RBF and renal dysfunction were described, including urine output, FE_{Na}, FE_{UA}, urine-concentrating ability, and imaging modalities.

Injuries to the splanchnic and renal systems likely play key roles in the propagation of SIRS to sepsis, septic shock, and ultimately MODS in the trauma patient. As we better understand the pathophysiology of trauma, SIRS, and MODS, the better we will understand the role played by splanchnic and renal hypoperfusion in the development of these conditions. By improving the circulation to these two organ systems and providing better ways to gauge and monitor that perfusion, we hope to improve the outcomes of patients who experience trauma.

KEY POINTS

- ☞ The two organ systems most often initially impacted in the underresuscitated trauma patient are the kidneys and GI organs.
- ☞ In the resting normovolemic patient, approximately 20% to 35% of the cardiac output is directed to the splanchnic circulation.
- ☞ The pathogenesis of sepsis and MODS is multifactorial. The concept of a "leaky" gut barrier and translocation of bacteria (and cytokines) are likely the integral component.
- ☞ Gastric tonometry measures luminal CO_2 and mucosal CO_2 partial pressures (PCO_2), as they become equalized across a semipermeable membrane.
- ☞ One of the earliest associations identified by gastric tonometry was that MODS rates are correlated with decreased pHi (31).
- ☞ Gastric tonometry might evolve into a commonly employed monitor for preventing mesenteric ischemia during prolonged vasopressin use in the setting of refractory shock.

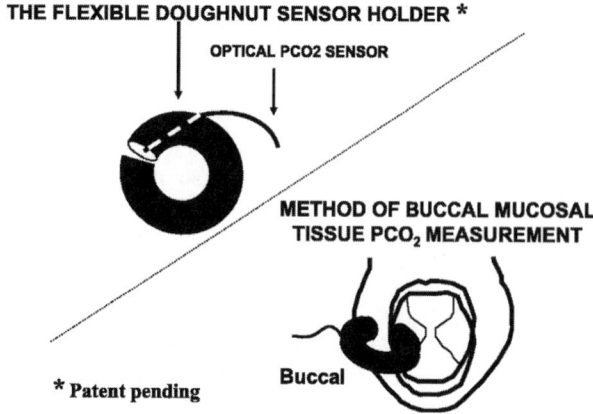

Figure 3 Buccal capnometry device (including positioning doughnut). A miniature CO_2 electrode (MI-720 CO_2 electrode; Microelectrodes, Londonderry, New Hampshire, U.S.A.), is positioned with the aid of a foam "doughnut." The doughnut helps maintain continuous contact with the mucosa without compromising local blood flow. *Source*: From Ref. 114.

☞ A recent study has also found correlation between hemorrhage in penetrating trauma and rise in sublingual $P_{SL}CO_2$, coinciding with increasing BD and lactate levels (49).

☞ Tolerance of early enteral feeding has been shown to correlate with numerous markers, including decreasing bacterial translocation and morbidity from sepsis, overall mortality, the length of ICU stay, and cost of ICU admission (56).

☞ The onset of acute renal failure (ARF) portends a poor prognosis and a high association with mortality, sepsis, and MODS.

☞ Surrogate markers [urine output, serum creatinine, and glomerular filtration rates (GFRs)—which is most commonly calculated from creatinine clearance (CL_{CR})] are routinely used to assess for clinically detectable alterations in RBF.

☞ Renal physiology and pathophysiology are described by the relationships between RBF, renal $\dot{V}O_2$, O_2 extraction, and CL_{CR} in patients with normal and abnormal renal function (87).

☞ Renal failure might supply a "second hit" in the development of sepsis, SIRS, and MODS in certain conditions (89).

☞ When evaluating a patient for alterations in urine output, the patient's medical history, medication use, type of surgery (or trauma), and relevant perioperative interventions must all be considered.

☞ Studies in trauma patients have shown that CL_{CR} can be used in those with stable renal function (96), and for the early detection of renal failure (97).

☞ The FE_{UA} has a much higher positive predictive value in separating prerenal from ATN, 98% versus 89%.

☞ Imaging techniques can be used to exclude postrenal (obstruction) and prerenal (renal artery stenosis, low RBF) renal failure and confirm the diagnosis of intrinsic causes of renal failure.

REFERENCES

1. American College of Surgeons, Committee on Trauma. Advanced Trauma Life Support. 7th Ed. Chicago, IL: American College of Surgeons, 2002:69–97.
2. Members of the American College of Chest Physicians/Society of Crit Care Med Consensus Conference Committee. American College of Chest Physicians/Society of Crit Care Med Consensus Conference: definitions for sepsis and organ failure and guidelines for the use of innovative therapies in sepsis. Crit Care Med 1992; 20:864–874.
3. Bilkovski RN, Rivers EP, Horst HM. Targeted resuscitation strategies after injury. Curr Opin Crit Care 2004; 10(6):529–538.
4. McKinley BA, Valdivia A, Moore FA. Goal-oriented shock resuscitation for major torso trauma: what are we learning? Curr Opin Crit Care 2003; 9(4):292–299.
5. Rivers E, Nguyen B, Havstad S, et al. Early goal-directed therapy in the treatment of severe sepsis and septic shock. N Engl J Med 2001; 345(19):1368–1377.
6. Dellinger RP, Carlet JM, Masur H, et al. Surviving Sepsis Campaign guidelines for management of severe sepsis and septic shock. Crit Care Med 2004; 32(3):858–873.
7. Abou-Khalil B, Scalea TM, Trooskin SZ, et al. Hemodynamic responses to shock in young trauma patients: need for invasive monitoring. Crit Care Med 1994; 22(4):633–639.
8. Dabrowski GP, Steinberg SM, Ferrara JJ, Flint LM. A critical assessment of endpoints of shock resuscitation. Surg Clin North Am 2000; 80(3):825–844.
9. Ivatury RR, Simon RJ, Islam S, et al. A prospective randomized study of end points of resuscitation after major trauma: global oxygen transport indices versus organ-specific gastric mucosal pH. J Am Coll Surg 1996; 183(2):145–154.
10. Moore KL, Persaud TVN. The Devloping Human: Clinically Oriented Embryology. 6th ed. Philadelphia, PA: W.B. Saunders Co., 1998.
11. Takala J. Determinants of splanchnic blood flow. Brit J Anaesthesia 1996; 77(1):50–58.
12. Jakob SM. Splanchnic blood flow in low-flowstates. Anesth Analg 2003; 96:1129–1138.
13. Hameed SM, Cohn SM. Gastric tonometry: the role of mucosal pH measurement in the management of trauma Chest 2003; 123(5 suppl):475S–481S.
14. Pastores SM, Katz DP, Kvetan V. Splanchnic ischemia and gut mucosal injury in sepsis and the multiple organ dysfunction syndrome. Am J Gastroenterol 1996; 91(9):1697–1710.
15. Gutierrez G, Brown SD. Gastric tonometry: a new monitoring modality in the intensive care unit. J Intens Care Med 1995; 10(1):34–44.
16. Ackland G, Grocott MP, Mythen MG. Understanding gastrointestinal perfusion in critical care: so near, and yet so far. Crit Care 2000; 4(5):269–281.
17. Cunningham JA, Cousar CD, Jaffin JH, Harmon JW. Extraluminal and intraluminal PCO2 levels in the ischemic intestines of rats. Curr Surg 1987; 44(3):229–232.
18. Fiddian-Green RG, Pittenger G, Whitehouse WM. Back diffusion of CO2 and its influence on the intramural pH in gastric mucosa. J Surg Res 1982; 33:39–48.
19. Heard SO, Helsmoortel CM, Kent JC, et al. Gastric tonometry in healthy volunteers: effect of ranitidine on calculated intramural pH. Crit Care Med 1991; 19(2):271–274.
20. Calvet X, Baigorri F, Duarte M, et al. Effect of ranitidine on gastric intramucosal pH in critically ill patients. Intensive Care Med 1998; 24(1):12–17.
21. Schlichtig R, Mehta N, Gayowski TJ. Tissue-arterial PCO2 difference is a better marker of ischemia than intramural pH (pHi) or arterial pH-pHi difference. J Crit Care 1996; 11:51–56.
22. Heard SO. Gastric tonometry: the hemodynamic monitor of choice (Pro). Chest 2003; 123(5 suppl):469S–474S.
23. Gutierrez G, Brown SD. Gastrointestinal tonometry: a monitor of regional dysoxia. New Horiz 1996; 4(4):413–419.
24. Kolkman JJ, Otte JA, Groeneveld AB. Gastrointestinal luminal PCO2 tonometry: an update on physiology, methodology, and clinical applications. Br J Anaesth 2000; 84(1):74–86.
25. Kolkman JJ, Zwarekant LJ, Boshuizen K, Groeneveld AB, Steverink PJ, Meuwissen SG. Type of solution and PCO2 measurement errors during tonometry. Intensive Care Med 1997; 23(6):658–663.
26. Groeneveld AJ. Tonometry of partial carbon dioxide tension in gastric mucosa: use of saline, buffer solutions, gastric juice or air. Crit Care 2000; 4(4):201–203.
27. Venkatesh B, Morgan J, Jones RD, Clague A. Validation of air as an equilibration medium in gastric tonometry: an in vitro evaluation of two techniques for measuring air PCO2. Anaesth Intensive Care 1998; 26(1):46–50.
28. Salzman AL, Strong KE, Wang H, et al. Intraluminal "balloonless" air tonometry: a new method for determination of gastrointestinal mucosal carbon dioxide tension. Crit Care Med 1994; 22(1):126–134.
29. Creteur J, De Backer D, Vincent JL. Monitoring gastric mucosal carbon dioxide pressure using gas tonometry: in vitro and in vivo validation studies. Anesthesiology 1997; 87:504–510.
30. Levy B, Gawalkiewicz P, Vallet B, et al. Gastric capnometry with air-automated tonometry predicts outcome in critically ill patients. Crit Care Med 2003; 31(2):474–480.
31. Fiddian-Green RG. Associations between intramucosal acidosis in the gut and organ failure. Crit Care Med 1993; 21(2 suppl):S103–S107.

32. Doglio GR, Pusajo JF, Egurrola MA, et al. Gastric mucosal pH as a prognostic index of mortality in critically ill patients. Crit Care Med 1991; 19(8):1037–1040.

33. Gutierrez G, Palizas F, Doglio G, et al. Gastric intramucosal pH as a therapeutic index of tissue oxygenation in critically ill patients. Lancet 1992; 339(8787):195–199.

34. Maynard N, Bihari D, Beale R, et al. Assessment of splanchnic oxygenation by gastric tonometry in patients with acute circulatory failure. JAMA 1993; 270(10):1203–1210.

35. Marik PE. Gastric intramucosal pH. A better predictor of multiorgan dysfunction syndrome and death than oxygen-derived variables in patients with sepsis. Chest 1993; 104(1):225–229.

36. Kirton OC, Windsor J, Wedderburn R, et al. Failure of splanchnic resuscitation in the acutely injured trauma patient correlates with multiple organ system failure and length of stay in the ICU. Chest 1998; 113(4):1064–1069.

37. Gomersall CD, Joynt GM, Freebairn RC, et al. Resuscitation of critically ill patients based on the results of gastric tonometry: a prospective, randomized, controlled trial. Crit Care Med 2000; 28(3):607–614.

38. Miami Trauma Clinical Trials Group. Splanchnic hypoperfusion-directed therapies in trauma: a prospective, randomized trial. Source American Surgeon 2005; 71(3):252–260.

39. Poeze M, Takala J, Greve JW, Ramsay G. Pre-operative tonometry is predictive for mortality and morbidity in high-risk surgical patients. Intensive Care Med 2000; 26(9): 1272–1281.

40. De Backer D, Creteur J, Silva E, Vincent JL. Effects of dopamine, norepinephrine, and epinephrine on the splanchnic circulation in septic shock: which is best? Crit Care Med 2003; 31(6): 1659–1667.

41. Dunser MW, Mayr AJ, Ulmer H, et al. Vasopressin in advanced vasodilatory shock: a prospective, randomized, controlled study. Circulation 2003; 107:2313–2319.

42. Maciel AT, Creteur J, Vincent JL. Tissue capnometry: does the answer lie under the tongue? Intensive Care Med 2004; 30(12):2157–2165.

43. Nakagawa Y, Weil MH, Tang W, et al. Sublingual capnometry for diagnosis and quantitation of circulatory shock. Am J Respir Crit Care Med 1998; 157(6 Pt 1):1838–1843.

44. Povoas HP, Weil MH, Tang W, et al. Comparisons between sublingual and gastric tonometry during hemorrhagic shock. Chest 2000; 118(4):1127–1132.

45. Weil MH, Nakagawa Y, Tang W, et al. Sublingual capnometry: a new noninvasive measurement for diagnosis and quantitation of severity of circulatory shock. Crit Care Med 1999; 27(7):1225–1229.

46. Marik PE. Sublingual capnography: a clinical validation study. Chest 2001; 120(3):923–927.

47. Rackow EC, O'Neil P, Astiz ME, Carpati CM. Sublingual capnometry and indexes of tissue perfusion in patients with circulatory failure. Chest 2001; 120(5):1633–1638.

48. Marik PE, Bankov A. Sublingual capnometry versus traditional markers of tissue oxygenation in critically ill patients. Crit Care Med 2003; 31(3):818–822.

49. Baron BJ, Sinert R, Zehtabchi S, et al. Diagnostic utility of sublingual PCO_2 for detecting hemorrhage in penetrating trauma patients. J Trauma 2004; 57(1):69–74.

50. Dasta JF, Brackett CC. Defining and achieving optimum therapeutic goals in critically ill patients. Pharmacotherapy. Review 1994; 14(6):678–688.

51. Husain FA, Martin MJ, Mullenix PS, Steele SR, Elliott DC. Serum lactate and base deficit as predictors of mortality and morbidity. Am J Surg 2003; 185(5):485–491.

52. McNelis J, Marini CP, Jurkiewicz A, et al. Prolonged lactate clearance is associated with increased mortality in the surgical intensive care unit. Am J Surg 2001; 182(5):481–485.

53. Kobayashi S, Gando S, Morimoto Y, et al. Serial measurement of arterial lactate concentrations as a prognostic indicator in relation to the incidence of disseminated intravascular coagulation in patients with systemic inflammatory response syndrome. Surg Today 2001; 31(10):853–859.

54. Rixen D, Siegel JH. Metabolic correlates of oxygen debt predict posttrauma early acute respiratory distress syndrome and the related cytokine response. J Trauma 2000; 49(3): 392–403.

55. Claridge JA, Crabtree TD, Pelletier SJ, et al . Persistent occult hypoperfusion is associated with a significant increase in infection rate and mortality in major trauma patients. J Trauma 2000; 48(1):8–14; discussion 14–15.

56. MacLaren R. Intolerance to intragastric enteral nutrition in critically ill patients: complications and management. Pharmacotherapy 2000; 20(12):1486–1498.

57. Heyland D, Cook DJ, Winder B, et al. Enteral nutrition in the critically ill patient: a prospective survey. Crit Care Med 1995; 23(6):1055–1060.

58. McClave SA, Snider HL. Clinical use of gastric residual volumes as a monitor for patients on enteral tube feeding. J Parenter Enteral Nutr 2002; 26(6 suppl):S43–S48.

59. Davies AR, Froomes PR, French CJ, et al. Randomized comparison of nasojejunal and nasogastric feeding in critically ill patients. Crit Care Med 2002; 30(3):586–590.

60. Booth CM, Heyland DK, Paterson WG. Gastrointestinal promotility drugs in the critical care setting: a systematic review of the evidence. Crit Care Med 2002; 30(7):1429–1435.

61. Chang WK, McClave SA, Lee MS, Chao YC. Monitoring bolus nasogastric tube feeding by the Brix value determination and residual volume measurement of gastric contents. J Parenter Enteral Nutr 2004; 28(2):105–112.

62. Chang WK, McClave SA, Chao YC. Continuous nasogastric tube feeding: monitoring by combined use of refractometry and traditional gastric residual volumes. Clin Nutr 2004; 23(1):105–112.

63. Revelly JP, Tappy L, Berger MM, et al. Early metabolic and splanchnic responses to enteral nutrition in postoperative cardiac surgery patients with circulatory compromise. Intensive Care Med 2001; 27(3):540–547.

64. Andel D, Kamolz LP, Donner A, et al. Impact of intraoperative duodenal feeding on the oxygen balance of the splanchnic region in severely burned patients. Burns 2005; 31(3):302–305.

65. Marvin RG, McKinley BA, McQuiggan M, et al. Nonocclusive bowel necrosis occurring in critically ill trauma patients receiving enteral nutrition manifests no reliable clinical signs for early detection. Am J Surg 2000; 179(1):7–12.

66. Spirt Mitchell J. Stress-related mucosal disease: risk factors and prophylactic therapy. Clin Ther 2004; 26(2):197–213.

67. Stollman N, Metz DC. Pathophysiology and prophylaxis of stress ulcer in intensive care unit patients. J Crit Care 2005; 20(1):35–45.

68. Mutlu GM, Mutlu EA, Factor P. GI complications in patients receiving mechanical ventilation. Chest 2001; 119(4):1222–1241.

69. Westphal M, Freise H, Kehrel BE, et al. Arginine vasopressin compromises gut mucosal microcirculation in septic rats. Crit Care Med 2004; 32(1):194–200.

70. van Haren FM, Rozendaal FW, van der Hoeven JG. The effect of vasopressin on gastric perfusion in catecholamine-dependent patients in septic shock. Chest 2003; 124(6):2256–2260.

71. Martindale RG. Contemporary strategies for the prevention of stress-related mucosal bleeding. Am J Health Syst Pharm 2005; 62:S11–S17.

72. Metz D. Preventing the gastrointestinal consequences of stress-related mucosal disease. Curr Med Res Opin 2005; 21(1):11–18.

73. Daley RJ, Rebuck JA, Welage LS, Rogers FB. Prevention of stress ulceration: current trends in critical care. Crit Care Med 2004; 32(10):2008–2013.

74. Pallone TL, Silldorff EP, Turner MR. Intrarenal blood flow: microvascular anatomy and the regulation of medullary perfusion. Clin Exp Pharmacol Physiol 1998; 25(6):383–392.

75. Leonard BL, Malpas SC, Denton KM, et al. Differential control of intrarenal blood flow during reflex increases in sympathetic nerve activity. Am J Physiol 2001; 280(1):R62–R68.

76. Evans RG, Correia AG, Weekes SR, Madden AC . Responses of regional kidney perfusion to vasoconstrictors in anaesthetized

rabbits: dependence on agent and renal artery pressure. Clin Exp Pharmacol Physiol 2000; 27(12):1007–1012.

77. Suehiro K, Shimizu J, Yi GH, et al. Selective renal vasodilation and active renal artery perfusion improve renal function in dogs with acute heart failure. J Pharm Exp Therap 2001; 298(3):1154–1160.

78. Lancelot E, Idee JM, Couturier V, et al. Influence of the viscosity of iodixanol on medullary and cortical blood flow in the rat kidney: a potential cause of nephrotoxicity. J Appl Toxicol 1999; 19(5):341–346.

79. Liss P, Nygren A, Hansell P. Hypoperfusion in the renal outer medulla after injection of contrast media in rats. Acta Radiol 1999; 40(5):521–527.

80. Tokuyama H, Hayashi K, Matsuda H, et al. Role of nitric oxide and prostaglandin E2 in acute renal hypoperfusion. Nephrology 2003; 8(2):65–71.

81. Rajapakse NW, Oliver JJ, Evans RG. Nitric oxide in responses of regional kidney blood flow to vasoactive agents in anesthetized rabbits. J Cardiovasc Pharmacol 2002; 40(2):210.

82. Flemming B, Seeliger E, Wronski T, et al. Oxygen and renal hemodynamics in the conscious rat. J Am Soc Nephrology 2000; 1(1):18–24.

83. Heemskerk AE, Huisman E, van Lambalgen AA, et al. Renal function and oxygen consumption during bacteraemia and endotoxaemia in rats. Nephrol Dial Transplant 1997; 12(8):1586–1594.

84. Weber A, Schwieger IM, Poinsot O, et al. Sequential changes in renal oxygen consumption and sodium transport during hyperdynamic sepsis in sheep. Am J Physiol 1992; 262(6 Pt 2):F965–F971.

85. Laycock SK, Vogel T, Forfia PR, et al. Role of nitric oxide in the control of renal oxygen consumption and the regulation of chemical work in the kidney. Circ Res 1998; 82(12):1263–1271.

86. Fleser A, Marshansky V, Duplain M, et al. Cross-talk between the Na(+)-K(+)-ATPase and the H(+)-ATPase in proximal tubules in suspension. Renal Physiology & Biochemistry 1995; 18(3):140–152.

87. Kurnik BR, Weisberg LS, Kurnik PB. Renal and systemic oxygen consumption in patients with normal and abnormal renal function. J Am Soc Nephrol 1992; 2(11):1617–1626.

88. McGonigal MD, Lucas CE, Ledgerwood AM. The effects of treatment of renal trauma on renal function. J Trauma 1987; 27(5):471–476.

89. Rotstein OD. Modeling the two-hit hypothesis for evaluating strategies to prevent organ injury after shock/resuscitation. J Trauma 2003; 54(5 suppl):S203–S206.

90. Fidler V, Nap R, Miranda DR. The effect of a managerial-based intervention on the occurrence of out-of-range-measurements and mortality in intensive care units. J Crit Care 2004; 19(3):130–134.

91. Lin CL, Pan KY, Hsu PY, et al. Preoperative 24-hour urine amount as an independent predictor of renal outcome in poor cardiac function patients after coronary artery bypass grafting. J Crit Care 2004; 19(2):92–98.

92. Lesage A, Ramakers M, Daubin C, et al. Complicated acute myocardial infarction requiring mechanical ventilation in the intensive care unit: prognostic factors of clinical outcome in a series of 157 patients. Crit Care Med 2004; 32(1):100–105.

93. de Mendonca A, Vincent JL, Suter PM, et al. Acute renal failure in the ICU: risk factors and outcome evaluated by the SOFA score. Intensive Care Med 2000; 26(7):915–921.

94. Wells M, Lipman J. Measurements of glomerular filtration in the intensive care unit are only a rough guide to renal function. So African J Surg 1997; 35(1):20–23.

95. Robert S, Zarowitz BJ, Peterson EL, Dumler F. Predictability of creatinine clearance estimates in critically ill patients. Crit Care Med 1993; 21(10):1487–1495.

96. Davis GA, Chandler MH. Comparison of creatinine clearance estimation methods in patients with trauma. Am J Health Syst Pharm 1996; 53(9):1028–1032.

97. Shin B, Mackenzie CF, Helrich M. Creatinine clearance of early detection of posttraumatic renal dysfunction. Anesthesiology 1986; 64(5):605–609.

98. Dussol B, Moussi-Frances J, Morange S, et al. A randomized trial of furosemide vs hydrochlorothiazide in patients with chronic renal failure and hypertension. Nephrol Dial Transplant 2005; 20(2):349–353.

99. Kaplan AA, Kohn OF. Fractional excretion of urea as a guide to renal dysfunction. Am J Nephrol 1992; 12(1–2):49–54.

100. Carvounis CP, Nisar S, Guro-Razuman S. Significance of the fractional excretion of urea in the differential diagnosis of acute renal failure. Kidney Int 2002; 62(6):2223–2229.

101. Eggli KD, Eggli D. Color Doppler sonography in pyelonephritis. Pediatr Radiol 1992; 22(6):422–425.

102. Tublin ME, Bude RO, Platt JF. The resistive index in renal Doppler sonography: where do we stand. Am J Radiology 2003; 180(4):885–892.

103. Baxter GM. Ultrasound of renal transplantation. Clin Radiol 2001; 56(10):802–818.

104. Izumi M, Sugiura T, Nakamura H, et al. Differential diagnosis of prerenal azotemia from acute tubular necrosis and prediction of recovery by Doppler ultrasound. Am J Kidney Diseases 2000; 35(4):713–719.

105. Keyserling HF, Fielding JR, Mittelstaedt CA. Renal sonography in the intensive care unit: when is it necessary? J Ultrasound in Medicine 2002; 21(5):517–520.

106. Helenon O, Correas JM, Chabriais J, et al. Renal vascular Doppler imaging: clinical benefits of power mode. Radiographics 1998; 18(6):1441–1454; discussion 1455–1457.

107. Martinoli C, Pretolesi F, Crespi G, et al. Power Doppler sonography: clinical applications. European J Radiology 1998; 27(suppl 2):S133–S140.

108. Clautice-Engle T, Jeffrey RB Jr. Renal hypoperfusion: value of power Doppler imaging. Am J Radiol 1997; 168(5):1227–1231.

109. Kuwa T, Cancio LC, Sondeen JL, et al. Evaluation of renal cortical perfusion by noninvasive power Doppler ultrasound during vascular occlusion and reperfusion. J Trauma 2004; 56(3):618–624.

110. Harris AC, Zwirewich CV, Lyburn ID, et al. CT findings in blunt renal trauma. Radiographics 2001; 21(spec no):S201–S214.

111. Lerman LO, Taler SJ, Textor SC, et al. Computed tomography-derived intrarenal blood flow in renovascular and essential hypertension. Kidney Int 1996; 49(3):846–854.

112. Patil UD, Ragavan A, Nadaraj, et al. Helical CT angiography in evaluation of live kidney donors. Nephrol Dial Transplant 2001; 16(9):1900–1904.

113. Blomley MJ, McBride A, Mohammedtagi S, et al. Functional renal perfusion imaging with colour mapping: is it a useful adjunct to spiral CT of in the assessment of abdominal aortic aneurysm (AAA)? Euro J Radiology 1999; 30(3):214–220.

114. Cammarata GAAM, Weil HM, Fries M, et al. Buccal capnometry to guide management of massive blood loss. J Appl Physiol 2006; 100:304–306.

115. Pellis T, Weil MH, Tang W, Sun S, Csapozi P, Castillo C. Increases in both buccal and sublingual PCO_2 reflect decreases in tissue blood flows during hemorrhagic shock. J Trauma 2005; 58:817–824.

116. Povoas HP, Weil MH, Tang W, et al. Decreases in mesenteric blood flow associated with increases in sublingual PCO_2 during hemorrhagic shock. Shock 2001; 15:398–402.

117. Jin X, Weil MH, Sun S, et al. Decreases in organ blood flows associated with increases in sublingual PCO_2 during hemorrhagic shock. J Appl Physiol 1998; 85:2360–2364.

11

Temperature Monitoring

Abdallah Kabbara
Department of Anesthesia, MetroHealth Medical Center, Cleveland, Ohio, U.S.A.

Charles E. Smith
Department of Anesthesiology, MetroHealth Medical Center, Case Western Reserve University, Cleveland, Ohio, U.S.A.

INTRODUCTION

Although fever has been recognized since antiquity as an accompaniment of illness (1), the ability to measure temperature clinically was developed only over the last 300 years (2–4). Temperature measurement continues to serve as a simple and direct method of tracking a patient's progress and recovery from disease (particularly infectious). Body temperature was not routinely measured during anesthesia until malignant hyperthermia was described in the mid-1960s (5). Over the years, the art of temperature measurement has evolved to incorporate new advances in technology. Like so many other areas of care, measuring a patient's temperature has become increasingly precise and efficient. Similarly, there is far better understanding of the ramifications and management of hypothermia and heat-related illnesses (Volume 1, Chapter 40), as well as the evaluation of fever (Volume 2, Chapter 46) following trauma and critical illness.

This chapter briefly reviews the history of thermometry extending back to the early Greeks, the rediscovery of their writings in the 1600s by Galileo, Sanctorio, et al., and subsequent developments. The "normal" temperature range was not established until 1868, by Wunderlich and his cadre of medical students (6,7); the major findings of this early research, along with the subsequent work on establishing the "normal temperature" is clearly presented. The mechanism of thermoregulation, heat loss, and the normal response to cold and heat are also reviewed. The importance of measuring temperature in trauma and critically ill patients is emphasized with examples of related complications. The pathophysiology of heat- and cold-related conditions is only briefly summarized here, as it is thoroughly covered in Volume 1, Chapter 40. The currently employed temperature measurement instrumentation, as well as the advantages and disadvantages of these devices for measuring temperature at various anatomic sites is thoroughly reviewed. In the "Eye to the Future" section, newer modes of temperature measurement are introduced. The evaluation of fever is the subject of Volume 2, Chapter 46 and not covered here.

HISTORY OF THERMOMETRY

The term "thermometer" is a compound word derived from the Greek *therme* (heat) and the Latin *metrum* (to measure). Early versions of this device were known as thermoscopes; the word scope is derived from the Greek *skopos*, (target, aim, or see).

The ancient Greeks knew that air could be expanded by heat, and in the second century BC, Philo of Byzantium (260–180 BC), a Greek engineer, constructed a crude thermoscope, as did Heron of Alexandria (250–150 BC) (2). A simple air-thermoscope traps air in a bulb so that applied heat expands and cold contracts it; the temperature variations are reflected in a rising or falling column of water in the tube connected to the bulb (Fig. 1) (3).

Galileo Galilei (1564–1642) has been credited with inventing the air/water thermoscope in 1593. However, he never claimed to have invented the device himself. Galileo most likely learned of the thermoscope from colleagues (described subsequently) and from reading Latin translations of Arabic documents that contained records of the aforementioned Greek engineer scholars Philo of Byzantium or Heron of Alexandria. It is likely that Giambattista della Porta (1535–1615), a wealthy Italian scholar, was the purveyor of such information. Della Porta, 31 years Galileo's senior, translated some of the Arabic records of Greek works into Latin, and initiated a scholarly society and convened meetings at his estate until these were closed down by the Inquisition. His book, "Natural Magic," (1558) described a Greek thermoscope (this was published 35 years prior to the time some claim that Galileo invented it).

The Italian physician-scientist Sanctorio Sanctorio of Padua (1561–1636), a colleague of both Galileo and della Porta, was the first to put a numerical scale on the instrument, thereby converting the thermoscope into the first thermometer (4). In his publication depicting medicine from Galen (Venice, 1612), Sanctorio acknowledges that he adapted his thermometer from one described by Heron of Alexandria.

In 1714, Daniel Gabriel Fahrenheit (1686–1736), a German physicist, invented the first mercury thermometer, which has now been in use for nearly 300 years. Fahrenheit discovered that mercury exhibits a more constant rate of expansion and a wider temperature range compared to the alcohol thermometer that he had invented a decade earlier (3).

Fahrenheit also devised a temperature scale to accompany his instrument. The coldest temperature he could reproducibly generate in his laboratory was an ice/salt mixture that Fahrenheit called "0°F"; on this scale the freezing point of pure water occurs at 32°F, and the boiling point is at 212°F (3).

In 1742, the Swedish astronomer and scientist, Anders Celsius (1701–1744), devised a centigrade scale using the mercury (Fahrenheit) thermometer. Initially he used 0° and 100° for the boiling point of water and the melting point of snow respectively (3). Later he reversed the numerical

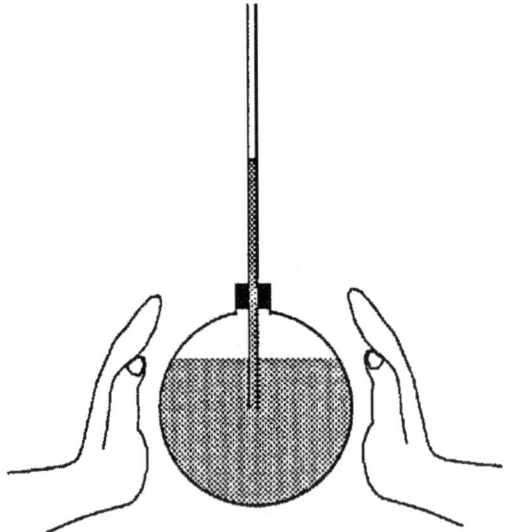

Figure 1 Simple air thermoscope. The initial design for the thermoscope was described by both Philo of Byzantium (260–180 B.C.) and Heron of Alexandria (250–150 B.C.). The illustration provided represents a modern-day depiction of the thermoscope described by these Greek inventors. A simple glass or thin metallic flask is partially filled with water and air, with an occluding stopper pierced by a glass tube. The heat derived from warming hands placed upon the sides of the flask warms the air and water, causing expansion of the gas forcing water up the thermoscope tube. This qualitative example of heat energy transfer was not useful for measuring temperatures until it became calibrated, as accomplished by Sanctorio (Fig. 2).

assignment so that 0°C represented the freezing point, and 100°C the boiling point. This revised centigrade scale gained widespread use. It was initially known simply as the centigrade scale until the term "Celsius" was adopted in 1948 by an international conference on weights and measures. The Celsius temperature scale is now part of the metric system of measurement (SI).

In 1848, the British physicist Lord William Thomson Kelvin (1824–1907) further developed the science of thermodynamics, but in order to do so, developed a new scale (in essence an expansion of the Celsius scale to a far more negative range) (3). Kelvin developed the concept of absolute zero, the temperature at which molecular energy stops (−273.15°C). Conversion factors have since been established to simplify calculations of temperature equivalences between the three commonly employed scales of Farenheit, Celsius and Kelvin (Table 1).

The early thermometers were at least a foot long and required 20 minutes to register a patient's temperature (3,7). In 1866, an English physician Sir Thomas Clifford

Table 1 Temperature Conversion Factors

From	To Fahrenheit	To Celsius	To Kelvin
°F	°F	(°F − 32) × 5/9	(°F − 32) × 5/9 + 273.15
°C	(°C × 9/5) + 32	°C	°C + 273.15
°K	(°K − 273.15) × 9/5 + 32	°K − 273.15	°K

Abbreviations: °C, Celsius; °F, Fahrenheit; °K, Kelvin.

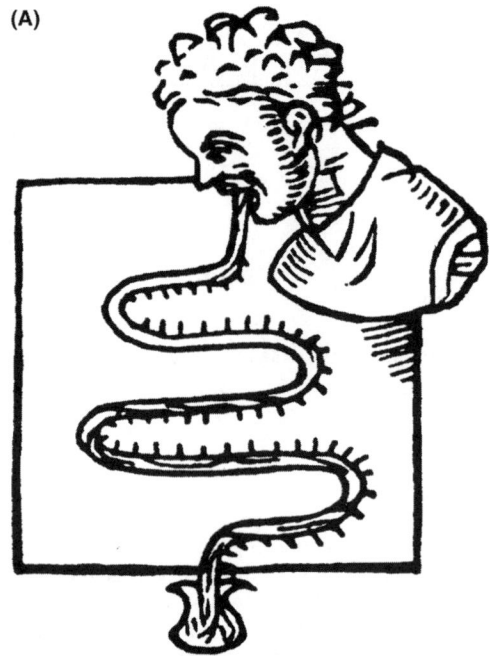

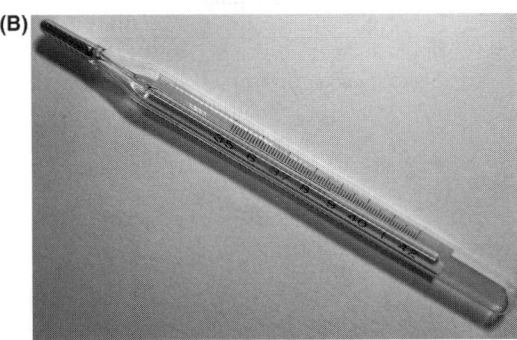

Figure 2 First thermometer—calibrated thermoscope. The first calibrated thermoscope (or thermometer) is credited to Sanctorio (1561–1636), who was driven to calibrate and measure all of the natural phenomena he observed. (**A**) is a wood cutting from the era, representing a stylistic depiction of the early Sanctorian thermometer. The hatch marks on the tube represent calibration lines. In (**B**) a modern-day mercury thermometer is shown.

Allbutt developed the shorter, modern mercury thermometer. Even the most recently developed glass mercury thermometers (Fig. 2) take time (2–3 minutes) to equilibrate with the patient's temperature; and prior to use, these thermometers need to be shaken so that the mercury is sequestered in the bulb at the start of temperature measurement.

In the 1980s, a series of newer technologies were developed for measuring temperature including electronic thermometers utilizing thermistors, for example, Diatec 500® (Diatec Inc., San Diego, California, U.S.A.). In 1984, David Phillips invented the infrared ear thermometer, for example, Braun Thermoscan® (Braun GmbH, Kronberg, Germany), or the ZT (ZyTemp, Hsin-Chu, Taiwan, China). These newer devices are described below in the section on current instrumentation.

ESTABLISHMENT OF NORMAL TEMPERATURE

The normal core temperature of 37°C was established by Professor Carl Reinhold August Wunderlich, the "father of

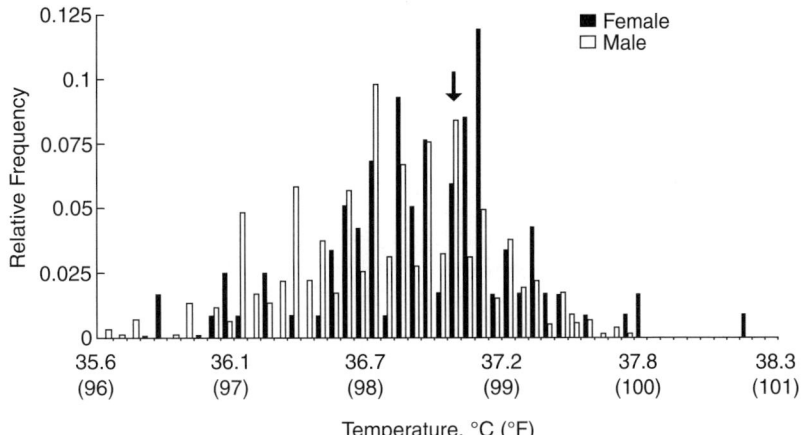

Figure 3 Frequency distribution of 700 baseline oral temperatures obtained during two consecutive days of observation in 148 healthy young male and female volunteers. *Arrow* indicates location of 37.0°C (98.6°F). *Source*: From Ref. 7.

prerounds," in the 1800s (6). Dr. Wunderlich instructed his medical students to measure the axillary temperature of the patients evaluated in the wards of St. James University Hospital, a large teaching hospital in Leipzig, Germany, until over one million temperature measurements were registered. Dr. Wunderlich was an early teacher of the pathologic basis of disease, and of empirical observation of patients. He was one of the first to write that fever is a symptom of disease, rather than a disease itself.

Macowiak (7), in 1996 repeated the study with a far smaller sample size, taking oral temperatures and essentially found the same results. In their sampling of 700 baseline oral temperatures from 148 young male and female volunteers, the mean temperature recorded was 36.8°C (Fig. 3). Macowiak et al. (7) claimed that their smaller, but more recent sampling demonstrated that the 37°C standard set by Wunderlich "should be abandoned." Perhaps a more enlightened interpretation of the Macowiak data is that oral temperatures are often slightly lower than true centrally obtained temperatures (e.g., via Swan-Ganz catheter); and that all individuals have their own thermoregulatory set point (TRSP) that is generally very near to 37°C.

✎ **Normal core temperature ranges between 36.5°C and 37.5°C, but may vary because of circadian rhythms and other factors.** ✎ The oral body temperature in a healthy

individual ranges between 35.6° and 38.2°C on average, which are slightly lower than core temperatures with a mean of 36.8°C [per Macowiak (7)]. Normal temperature also tends to increase slightly during the day from a nadir of 6:00 a.m. to a zenith at 4:00 to 6:00 p.m. (Fig. 4). Diurnal variation depends on activity throughout the day. Both gender and race are reflected in temperature difference with women having slightly higher normal temperatures than men, and black individuals having a trend toward higher temperatures compared to white subjects (7).

Persons working at night and sleeping during the day do not have the same changes in diurnal variation. When fever occurs, diurnal variation can also play a role accentuating or limiting fever, which generally reaches its peak in the evening. Accordingly, a very sick patient can have their temperature dip toward normal in the morning.

Young persons will have generally higher and more intense body temperature changes than older individuals. Body temperature may slightly or temporarily increase in a hot environment. Physical activity plays a role in increasing body temperature. During extreme effort, the increase may be very high. A marathon runner may have a core temperature increase to the 39–41°C range. Vasodilatation, hyperventilation and other compensatory mechanisms can slightly alter temperature.

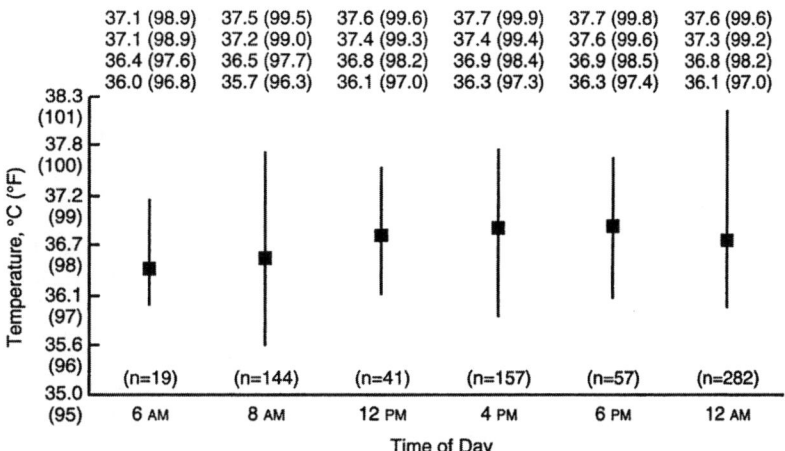

Figure 4 Diurnal variation of oral temperatures in 148 healthy young male and female volunteers. Mean (*solid squares*) oral temperatures and temperature ranges according to time of day. The four temperatures shown at each sample time are the 99th percentile (*top*), 95th percentile (*second from top*), mean (*second from bottom*), and 5th percentile (*bottom*) for each sample set. *Source*: From Ref. 7.

THERMOREGULATION
Hypothalamus

☞ **The hypothalamus is the center of thermoregulatory control.** ☞ Located at the base of the brain, the hypothalamus functions as the body's thermostat, and helps keep the core temperature constant at about 37°C by using physiological adjustments under its control (8). The hypothalamus monitors input from the central and peripheral heat sensors located throughout the body and relays information to various areas to raise or lower temperature by numerous mechanisms (vasodilation, vasoconstriction, and thermogenesis), to maintain the core temperature at the patient's TRSP, which is usually calibrated to a core temperature near 37°C. Close regulation of core temperature has evolved in organisms as a mechanism for optimizing enzymatic activities at the temperature of their best effect.

Mechanisms of Thermoregulation

The specific location of the thermoregulatory center within the hypothalamus is the preoptic area (anterior portion). This area receives input from peripheral thermoreceptors in the skin and mucous membranes and from central thermoreceptors, located in bone, spinal cord and brain, as well as the hypothalamus itself (Fig. 5) (8). The central core temperature is compared with the reference TRSP, which is the "normal" temperature for that individual. The hypothalamic thermostat works in conjunction with other hypothalamic, autonomic and higher nervous system thermoregulatory centers to maintain a constant core temperature by regulation of heat production and expenditure. When the hypothalamus senses a change in the core temperature, behavioral and physiologic mechanisms occur to oppose any deviation from the TRSP.

☞ **There are three components of the thermoregulatory system: (*i*) afferent input of temperature information; (*ii*) central processing of the information by the anterior**

hypothalamus; and (*iii*) efferent responses to control heat production and heat loss.** ☞

Numerous medications will alter the TRSP, and thus the ability to mount a normal thermoregulatory response. For example, nearly all sedatives and analgesics used in trauma, anesthesia, and critical care will alter the TRSP. This alteration in TRSP results in the requirement of a higher than normal core temperature to be registered before vasodilation occurs, and a lower than normal temperature to occur before vasoconstriction, shivering, and nonshivering thermogenesis mechanisms are invoked. Additional thermoregulatory dysfunction results following the administration of neuromuscular blockade (NMB) drugs and meperidine, which both inhibit shivering, whereas anticholinergics inhibit sweating.

Heat Production

Heat is produced by increasing the metabolic process in which energy is released in the form of heat. ☞ **The liver, heart, and skeletal muscle are the major heat generators, whereas the skin and respiratory system are the major organs responsible for heat loss.** ☞ Skeletal muscle, liver, splanchnic organs and the brain are the largest heat producers (8). Because of its weight, skeletal muscle plays an important role in heat production. Muscles are able to produce large amounts of heat in a short time period via several mechanisms including shivering and increased physical activity. During digestion, increased production of heat occurs in the gastrointestinal tract. Central nervous system regulation (chiefly at the hypothalamus) maintains optimal intensity of metabolism and regulates heat loss.

Nonshivering thermogenesis is mediated by brown fat and has an important function in increasing heat production in newborns and children. Brown fat is found between scapulas, on the neck, in the axilla, around the aorta, and the kidneys in children. It is a highly vascularized tissue, and has large mitochondria within its cells. Increased firing of the cold receptors leads to the release of norepinephrine from adrenergic nerve terminals, which in turn activates the enzyme lipase. Activated lipase splits the brown fat to glycerol and free fatty acids, and heat is released. Adults have very little brown fat.

Heat Loss

☞ **Heat is lost by radiation, conduction, evaporation, and convection (Table 2).** ☞ Radiation is the emission of electromagnetic energy in the infrared wavelengths (8–10). Conduction is the flow of heat energy from regions in contact between two objects: the warmer object transfers heat to the cooler object based upon the area in contact and the thermal conductivity of the objects. Air, sheets, and clothing have low thermal conductivity; water conducts heat 32× faster than air.

Evaporation is the heat loss to the atmosphere that occurs when water undergoes a change of phase (liquid to gaseous) following the discharge of aqueous fluid from an object by transfer of heat from skin (sweat), respiratory track (exhaled moist air), and exposed viscera in the operating room (OR). Each gram of water that vaporizes consumes 0.58 Kcal of heat (11). Sweating is mediated by postganglionic, cholinergic nerves. During intensive sweating, up to 1 L/hr of sweat can be formed with a heat elimination of 0.58 Kcal/g of evaporated sweat (or nearly 600 Kcal/hr).

When the humidity of the environment is higher, heat loss by sweating becomes less efficient. Yet, evaporation

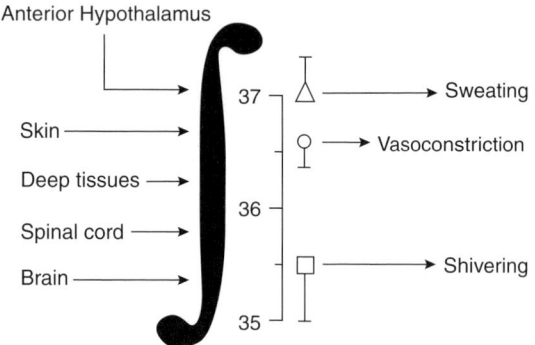

Figure 5 Thermoregulatory control system of the hypothalamus. The illustration shows the thermoregulatory control mechanisms utilized by the hypothalamic thermoregulatory control center. The left side of the image depicts the afferent input into the hypothalamus (including information from the hypothalamus itself, skin, deep tissues, spinal cord, and nonhypothalamic portions of the brain. The right side shows the temperature scale at which certain mechanisms of heat loss (e.g., sweating) and heat conservation (e.g., vasoconstriction and shivering) occur. No thermoregulatory responses are initiated when the core temperature is between these thresholds; these temperatures identify the interthreshold range, which in humans is usually only about 0.2°C. *Source*: From Ref. 72.

Table 2 Heat Loss Mechanisms

Mechanism of heat loss	Description (caloric loss example)
Radiation	Transmission of heat from exposed skin to surrounding objects (exposed patient: 50 Kcal/hr; draped and covered: 10 Kcal/hr)
Conduction	Transfer of heat due to direct contact of skin and viscera with colder objects Operating room table Spine backboard Skin-antiseptic solution Surrounding air Transfer of heat from patient's blood to colder intravenous fluids Crystalloid, 20°C, 16 Kcal/L Blood, 4°C, 30 Kcal/L
Convection	Removal of air warmed by skin or viscera Increases conductive heat loss by 10 Kcal/L
Evaporation	Transfer of heat from skin, respiratory tract, and viscera Skin and respiratory system: 12–16 Kcal/hr Exposed viscera and body cavities: up to 400 Kcal/hr Skin-antiseptic solutions: 6–8 Kcal/m
Redistribution	With redistribution of warm core blood to the periphery, heat is lost much faster via one of the above four mechanisms. Alcohol, as well as nearly all sedatives and analgesics used in anesthesia and critical care cause redistribution by altering the thermoregulatory set point. (e.g., first hour of anesthesia: 46 Kcal, next 2 hrs of anesthesia: 34 Kcal)

Note: It is estimated that for every 60–75 Kcal/hr heat loss in excess of heat production, a 1°C decrease in core temperature may occur (assumes 70-kg adult at 37°C). Note that the normal 60–75 Kcal/hr heat loss in an adult 70-kg patient is offset by 60–75 Kcal/hr metabolic heat production to maintain thermal steady state. If heat production is decreased (e.g., anesthesia, severe injury, medical diseases, extremes of age) greater decreases in core temperature may occur. All values are estimates only.
Source: Modified from Ref. 10.

(sweat and exhaled vapor) is an important mechanism, and the only one by which humans can eliminate heat into an environment exceeding core temperature (8). In addition to sweat, water vapor is lost during respiration. The volume of air, which is inhaled with each breath, is immediately humidified by the nasopharynx and lungs to full saturation. Some of this vapor is then exhaled, resulting in evaporative loss. At high altitudes, evaporative heat loss via the respiratory tract can rival sweat as a cooling factor.

Convection is the removal of air (warmed by the body) when blown away by a breeze or wind (i.e., the transfer of heat to an air current). Convection also describes the heat loss or gain when fluids are administered, or during cardiopulmonary bypass (CPB).

Countercurrent Heat Exchange (Vasoconstriction/Vasodilation)

Humans use a simple mechanism of countercurrent heat exchange to regulate blood flow through the skin and subcutaneous tissues. Distribution of heat occurs by blood

circulation. Heat goes from each cell to the surrounding liquid and afterwards to the circulated blood. The modulating factor of heat loss is the amount of blood that circulates through the body surface. The large blood flow through the subcutaneous area and the skin allows heat loss to the surrounding environment. When it is necessary to conserve heat, adrenergic stimuli cause reduction of blood flow through the skin, and the skin becomes an insulator (8,12).

Vasoconstriction allows the increased accumulation of central core heat, and vasodilation secures its quick loss. When vasodilation occurs in a cool environment (not normal, but does occur in sedated or anesthetized patients) a large flow of warm core blood will rapidly cool the core temperature. When vasodilation occurs in a warm environment heat loss is increased through the four aforementioned heat transfer mechanisms.

Pathophysiology of Temperature Change

Human life is only compatible within a narrow range of temperatures. If the core body temperature is increased above 42.2°C, irreversible damage occurs to the brain. Death occurs at core temperatures of ≥44°C due to protein denaturation. In humans, the temperature does not usually increase to levels above 41.1°C. Decreases in temperature to below 32.8°C is accompanied by confusion, and gradual loss of consciousness. If the decrease continues below 30°C, ventricular dysrhythmias may occur. At 28°C, there is a 50% decrease in cerebral metabolic requirement for oxygen (Table 3) (13).

Heat Balance

To maintain a constant body temperature, an individual must maintain a balance between the heat generated and the heat lost. Thus for temperature to be held constant and achieve thermal homeostasis, an individual must constantly vary many physiological and behavioral systems to maintain balance (14). This is achieved through integration of multiple systems (Table 4).

TEMPERATURE MONITORING RATIONALE

Humans require a nearly constant internal body temperature and when temperature deviates significantly from normal, metabolic function deteriorates and ultimately death can result. Trauma is a major condition where hypothermia (core temperature below 35°C) is common. The very young do not have fully developed thermoregulatory systems (14), and the elderly often have dysfunctional thermoregulation (15), hence both groups are more prone to hypothermia. Temperature should be monitored in all critically ill patients, particularly those with trauma and at the extremes of age.

Incidence and Risk Factors for Hypothermia in Trauma

In a study by Luna et al. (16), 23% of severely injured patients had core temperature <34°C with a range of 27–33.8°C. In a study of 71 patients with severe truncal injury and injury severity score (ISS) >25, 42% had core temperature <34°C, 23% <33°C, and 13% <32°C (17).

Multisystem trauma is the most common cause of hypothermia in patients requiring admission to the surgical intensive care unit (SICU) (18), and as many as 46% of injured patients leave the OR hypothermic (19). Fifty-seven percentage of trauma patients became hypothermic in the

Table 3 Physiologic Characteristics of the Three Stages of Hypothermia (Nonanesthetized, Nonintoxicated Patients)

Core temperature		
°C	°F	Characteristics
Mild		
37.6	99.6	Normal rectal temperature
37	98.6	Normal oral temperature
36	96.8	Increase in metabolic rate
35	95	Maximum shivering thermogenesis
34	93.2	Amnesia and dysarthria develop; maximum respiratory stimulation
33	91.4	Ataxia and apathy develop
Moderate		
32	89.6	Stupor; 25% ↓ in $\dot{V}O_2$, Osborne waves seen
31	87.8	Shivering thermogenesis extinguished
30	86	A-fib common, ↓HR and $\dot{Q}$; insulin ineffective
29	85.2	Progressive ↓ consciousness, pulse, and breathing; pupils dilated
28	82.4	V-fib susceptibility; 50% ↓ in VO_2 and HR
Severe		
27	80.6	Losing reflexes and voluntary motion
26	78.8	Major acid–base disturbances; no reflexes or response to pain
25	77	CBF 1/3 normal; $\dot{Q}$ 45% normal; pulmonary edema may develop
24	75.2	Significant hypotension
23	73.4	No corneal or oculocephalic reflexes
22	71.6	Maximum risk of V-fib; 75% ↓ in $\dot{V}O_2$
20	68	Lowest resumption of cardiac electro-mechanical activity
19	66.2	Flat electroencephalogram
18	64.4	Nerve and cardiac muscle silence
16	60.8	Lowest accidental hypothermia survival in an adult
15	59.2	Lowest accidental hypothermia survival in an infant
9	48.2	Lowest therapeutic hypothermia survival

Abbreviations: ↓, decrease; A-fib, atrial fibrillation; CBF, cerebral blood flow; HR, heart rate; $\dot{Q}$, cardiac output; V-fib, ventricular fibrillation; $\dot{V}O_2$, oxygen consumption.
Source: Modified from Ref. 13.

time interval between injury and completion of the initial surgical procedure.

☞ **Although hypothermia decreases the metabolic function of the body, and is neuroprotective, in traumatized individuals hypothermia most often results in deleterious effects such as coagulopathy, metabolic acidosis, and impaired immune response (8).** ☞ Injured patients in whom hypothermia develops have a higher mortality than do patients with a similar ISS who remain normothermic (17). Core rewarming increases the likelihood of successful trauma resuscitation (19). Hypothermia (<35°C) and acidosis (base deficit >12 mEq/L) were strong predictors of death in a retrospective review of exsanguinating trauma patients undergoing surgery (20).

Older data suggested that trauma alters thermoregulation, decreases heat production, and impairs shivering

Table 4 Integration of Behavioral and Autonomic Systems for Thermoregulation

System	Example
Behavioral	This is accomplished by adjusting clothing, modifying environmental temperature, assuming positions that oppose skin surfaces, voluntary movements, and timing of activities.
Autonomic	Vasodilation increases cutaneous blood flow and promotes either heat loss or heat gain depending on the environmental conditions.
	Vasoconstriction reduces peripheral flow. Cutaneous blood flow decreases to near zero in cold temperatures.
	Heart rate is often higher for any given core temperature during heating than during cooling, thus increasing heat transfer via the blood, decreasing rate of cooling and achieving optimal core temperature quicker.
	Piloerection increases insulation and slows heat exchange.
	Increased body fat. Fat conducts heat only one-third as fast as other tissues.
	Shivering is under central and peripheral control. Shivering increases heat production when the skin and/or body is cold.
	"Nonshivering" thermogenesis increases heat production without muscular activity. The principal heat producers are the liver, kidney, and brain via brown adipose tissue whose sole function is to produce heat in neonates.
	Evaporation, by increasing the amount of sweating.

(21,22). Impaired thermoregulation may transiently result from reduced cerebral and hypothalamic blood flow, constriction of hypothalamic blood vessels from release of endogenous substances such as norepinephrine, whereas, the major loss of hypothalamic thermoregulation results from alcohol and drug intoxication, and from direct traumatic brain injury (TBI) (8,10,13).

☞ **Risk factors that contribute to hypothermia include environmental exposure, alcohol and drug intoxication, intravenous (IV) infusion of room temperature fluid, transfusion of cold blood without warming, spinal cord injuries, head injury, shock, and associated medical conditions such as hypothyroidism and hypoglycemia (Table 5) (8,10,13).** ☞ Individuals at extremes of age are at greatest risk for accidental hypothermia (5,23). Exertional fatigue, sleep deprivation, and negative energy balance can also increase susceptibility to hypothermia (24).

Hypothermia-Associated Increased Mortality and Morbidity

Jurkovich et al. (17) demonstrated that survival, independent of injury severity, was dependent upon patient temperatures, such that core temperatures of 34°C, 33°C, and 32°C, correlated with mortality rates of 40%, 69% and 100%, respectively. In a retrospective review of 7045 patients admitted to a SICU, 661 (9.4%) had hypothermia with a mortality rate of 53% (18). ☞ **Trauma-associated hypothermia increases morbidity because of impaired cardiorespiratory**

Table 5 Risk Factors for Hypothermia

Mechanism	Examples
Impaired thermoregulation and decreased heat production	Alcohol
	Drugs: anesthetics, tricyclic antidepressants, phenothiazines, antipyretics, neuromuscular relaxants
	Head injury
	Spinal cord injury
	Severe injury and shock
	Extremes of age
	Autonomic nervous system dysfunction
	Medical disease: thyroid, adrenal, diabetes, malnutrition
	Bacterial toxins
Increased heat loss	Neonates
	Low ambient room temperature
	Burns
	Large blood loss
	Exposed abdominal and/or thoracic contents
	Combined general and neuraxial anesthesia
	Geriatrics
	Thin body type
	Low surface temperature of patient prior to trauma, intoxication, or anesthesia

Source: Modified from Ref. 10.

Table 6 Morbidity of Hypothermia in Trauma and Critical Care

System affected	Examples
Impaired cardiorespiratory function	Cardiac dysfunction
	Myocardial ischemia
	Cardiac dysrhythmias
	Peripheral vasoconstriction
	Decreased tissue oxygen delivery
	Increased oxygen consumption during rewarming
	Blunted response to catecholamines
	Increased blood viscosity
	Leftward shift of hemoglobin-oxygen dissociation curve
Coagulopathy	Decreased function of coagulation factors
	Decreased platelet function
Impaired hepatorenal function and decreased drug clearance	Decreased hepatic blood flow
	Decreased clearance of lactic acid
	Decreased hepatic metabolism of drugs
	Decreased renal blood flow
	Cold-induced diuresis
Altered immune response	Increased incidence of wound infection

Source: Modified from Ref. 56.

function, peripheral vasoconstriction, bleeding diathesis, metabolic acidosis, diminished hepatorenal function, and altered immune response (Table 6).

Cardiac Effects
Hypothermia exerts a negative inotropic effect on the myocardium, resulting in decreased left ventricular contractility (25), increased left ventricular ejection time, reduced early diastolic filling and total diastolic inflow time, and impaired peak velocity of left ventricular wall movement during systole and diastole (Table 6) (26). Hypothermia also impairs the inotropic effects of dopamine and norepinephrine.

Hypothermia is also associated with dysrhythmias. As the core temperature decreases, progressive bradycardia ensues. Below core temperatures of 30°C, ectopic atrial rhythms, atrial flutter, and atrial fibrillation commonly occur. Once the temperature decreases to 28°C, ventricular tachycardia and ventricular fibrillation are seen. Cardiac and neural tissues cease firing at a core temperature <15°C to 18°C (13). Even mild hypothermia can dramatically increase the incidence of morbid cardiac outcomes such as unstable angina, myocardial ischemia, and ventricular tachycardia in perioperative patients (27).

Vascular
Effects of hypothermia on the vasculature consists of peripheral vasoconstriction, increased blood viscosity (due to direct effect of hypothermia and cold-induced hemoconcentration), and the accumulation of metabolic acids in poorly perfused tissues (10). During rewarming, shivering can occur which will increase O_2 consumption ($\dot{V}O_2$), and potentially trigger myocardial ischemia in susceptible patients. In addition, the release of sequestered cold blood and acid metabolites from peripheral vascular beds following

re-warming can result in myocardial instability, even in patients without coronary artery disease.

Coagulopathy
Hypothermia leads to a bleeding diathesis due to impaired platelet function, inhibition of clotting enzymes, and altered kinetics of plasminogen activator inhibitors (e.g., alpha-2-antiplasmin). Mild hypothermia increases surgical blood loss and the need for blood transfusions (28,29). Core temperatures should be kept above 35°C because coagulopathy in trauma patients who required massive transfusion was predicted by temperature <34°C and progressive metabolic acidosis (30).

Respiratory
Moderate hypothermia decreases respiratory drive, and is associated with hypoventilation and the loss of protective airway reflexes (13). Hypothermia also inhibits hypoxic pulmonary vasoconstriction (HPV), increasing right-to-left transpulmonary shunt, and shifts the oxygen-hemoglobin saturation curve to the left. Pulmonary edema can occur at temperatures ≤28°C. Hypothermia also increases alveolar dead space.

Cellular Immune Response and Infection
Mild hypothermia increases the incidence of wound infection (31). It also impairs immune function, suppresses mitogen-induced activation of lymphocytes, and decreases production of interleukins-1β and interleukin-2. In addition, low tissue oxygen levels due to thermoregulatory vasoconstriction may be associated with impaired resistance to infection. Hypothermia tripled the incidence of surgical wound infection in one study (31), and had a relative risk of 6.3 in

another (32). Hypothermia also increases the risk of pneumonia in patients with closed head injuries (33).

Glucose and Electrolytes

Hypothermia can cause hypokalemia that can contribute to dysrhythmias and respiratory and cardiac insufficiency. Hyperglycemia commonly occurs at temperatures below 32°C due to decreased insulin production and utilization. Hyperglycemia can significantly aggravate neuronal ischemia.

Splanchnic and Renal Effects

Hepatic blood flow is decreased with hypothermia as is hepatocellular function. High-energy phosphates such as adenosine triphosphate are depleted in hypothermia, which may lead to organ failure (34). Hypothermia reduces the metabolism and activity of many anesthetics and other drugs, and also increases the solubility of many drugs in tissues. These effects all tend to result in delayed awakening and diminished organ function.

Due to the initial increased cardiac output (Q̇) and the mean arterial pressure, the renal perfusion pressures are increased. Accordingly, renal blood flow is increased leading to a "cold-induced" diuresis. However, glomerular filtration rates (GFR) are decreased and there is impaired renal tubular function. There is increased urinary loss of sodium, potassium, and water and a "cold-induced" diuresis. Despite increased urine output, renal clearance of water-soluble drugs is diminished as temperature drops further. Eventually, the Q̇ begins to fall due to decreased heart rate and contractility. However, the "cold-induced" diuresis persists as long as the heart continues to pump due to the persistent effect of these other factors.

General Anesthesia

☞**Hypothermia is common during general anesthesia because of impaired thermoregulation (Fig. 6), decreased heat production, and internal redistribution of body heat from the warmer core to the cooler peripheral tissue in the exposed patient (35,36).**☞

This is due to the alteration in the TRSP, which results from all anesthetic and sedative drugs. Most anesthetized patients will experience a drop in their core temperature of 1°C to 1.5°C in the absence of active warming measures. Patients may suffer additional hypothermic insults due to infusion of cold or inadequately warmed IV fluids as described during initial resuscitation (Fig. 6) (10,37).

Although malignant hyperthermia is a rare condition, the high mortality rate associated with this syndrome mandates routine core temperature monitoring in all anesthetic

$$\Delta\ MBT = (T_{fluid} - T_{patient})\ Sp_{fluid}/Weight \times Sp_{patient}$$

where

T_{fluid} = Outlet temperature of fluid delivered to the patient
$T_{patient}$ = Temperature of the patient, assumed to be 37°C
Sp_{fluid} = Specific heat of infused fluid, 1 Kcal/L/°C
$Sp_{patient}$ = Specific heat of the patient, 0.83 Kcal/L/°C

Figure 6   Change (Δ) in mean body temperature (MBT) as a function of administered intravenous fluid. Change in MBT is calculated in the figure. Note: Improvements in fluid warmer design together with set points of 42°C now allow the clinician to maintain thermal neutrality with respect to fluid management over a wide range of flow rates.

cases ≥30 minutes in duration. The use of effective warming technologies has now made it possible to overheat patients.

Regional Anesthesia

Core hypothermia can be nearly as common and severe during epidural and spinal anesthesia as during general anesthesia (38). With neuroaxial blockade, vasodilation below the level of the block can result in a core temperature drop due to both heat loss and redistribution. ☞ **Epidural and spinal anesthesia block afferent and efferent thermoregulatory responses and cause similar degrees of hypothermia as general anesthesia.** ☞

During regional anesthesia for trauma, core temperature should therefore be closely measured, especially in patients at highest risk to become hypothermic such as patients undergoing long extensive procedures in cold environments. Temperature monitoring is not usually required in otherwise healthy patients undergoing minor peripheral procedures <30 minutes in duration with local anesthetics (e.g., suture of finger laceration), because these drugs do not trigger malignant hyperthermia.

Deliberate Use of Hypothermia: In Cardiac and Neuro-anesthesia

A mainstay of neuroprotective therapy has been moderate systemic hypothermia (26). Mild to moderate hypothermia confers protection against tissue ischemia, especially during cardiac surgery and potentially during certain types of neurosurgery. Beneficial effects of hypothermia are thought to result from reduced metabolism and inhibition of deleterious effects of hypoxia such as free-radical reactions, excitotoxicity, and altered membrane permeability. Hypothermia increases the tolerance time for circulatory arrest and diminished blood flow during cardiopulmonary resuscitation. Improved neurologic outcome has been observed in cardiac surgery patients and in survivors of cardiac arrest treated with mild hypothermia (39). Hypothermia may prevent the initiation of some elements in the cascade of events that lead to cell death following trauma (13).

☞ **Mild hypothermia (1–2°C below normal) is neuroprotective, whereas mild hyperthermia (1–2°C above normal) may exacerbate cerebral ischemia.** ☞ Although hypothermia clearly has been shown to be neuroprotective, use of hypothermic CPB necessitates rewarming before discontinuation. Because most emboli occur during clamp removal and resumption of pulsatile flow when brain temperature may actually exceed 37°C, the brain may be even more susceptible to injury. Postoperative hyperthermia (37.2–39.3°C) is associated with worsened cognitive outcome after coronary surgery (40). Mild hyperthermia (1–2°C above normal) exacerbates the severity of cerebral ischemia (histopathological consequences, stroke severity, and mortality) by the following purported mechanisms: increased excitotoxic neurotransmitter release, increased free-radical production, increased intracellular acidosis, increased blood-brain barrier permeability, destabilized cytoskeleton, and abnormal modulation of protein kinase.

Hypothermia has long been touted as potentially beneficial for spinal cord ischemia and TBI (41,42). However, the clinical data is unclear. Two large prospective multicenter trials have failed to show improved neurologic outcome after therapeutic hypothermia for isolated TBI patients (43,44). Whereas, two others did show improvements for those having Glascow Coma Scale (GCS) values in the 5–8 range (see Volume 1, Chapter 40) (45,46). Accordingly, additional research is required.

External Factors Affecting Temperature Measurement

Body temperature can be altered by external factors, such as extremes of hot and cold weather, and by internal factors, such as circadian rhythms, infectious processes, and hormonal changes (Volume 1, Chapter 40). In addition, during extracorporeal circulation for cardiac and other surgeries, or as a result of malignant hyperthermia or damage to the hypothalamus, regulatory mechanisms may become ineffective in maintaining normal temperature, which causes hyperthermia or hypothermia.

The two most common factors influencing body temperature are age and gender. For example, when taken orally, adults' normal temperature ranges from 35.8°C to 37.4°C; elderly patients' temperatures will tend to be at the lower end of normal overall if taken correctly, lower still at the oral and axillary sites if tissue contact is inadequate. Children's temperatures normally range slightly higher (36.1–38°C) than adults. Women's temperatures can reach as high as 37.9°C during ovulation; men's generally stay in the range of 36.1–37.2°C (7).

THERMOMETER INSTRUMENTATION AVAILABLE

Electronic thermometers have largely replaced traditional mercury-in-glass thermometers; although these low-tech devices are still utilized in remote locations. The most common electronic thermometers utilize thermistors and thermocouples. Both devices are accurate for clinical use and sufficiently inexpensive to be widely available. Infrared tympanic membrane thermometers are also sufficiently accurate for clinical use.

A thermometer incorporated into an esophageal stethoscope is a simple and reliable method of measuring core temperature in tracheally intubated patients providing it is inserted deep enough (at least 5–10 cm past the carina).

During regional anesthesia or when patients are mask-ventilated, measurement of axillary, oral, or tympanic membrane temperatures at 15-minute intervals can be substituted for esophageal temperature monitoring.

TEMPERATURE MONITORING SITES

The core thermal compartment is composed of highly perfused tissues whose temperature is uniform and high compared with the rest of the body (Table 7). Core temperature is the most reliable thermal indicator of the body's condition. ☛ **The preferred technique of temperature monitoring is one that reflects core temperature such as distal esophageal, nasopharynx, pulmonary artery (PA), and tympanic membrane. Intermediate sites such as rectum, bladder, and mouth usually reflect core temperature.** ☛ Core temperature can be determined by measuring a single temperature adjacent to the distal esophagus, nasopharynx, PA, or tympanic membrane (8). Even during rapid thermal perturbations (e.g., CPB), these temperature monitoring sites remain reliable (47). Core temperature can be estimated with reasonable accuracy using oral, rectal, axillary, and

Table 7 Temperature Monitoring Sites

Core[a]	Intermediate
Pulmonary artery	Bladder
Distal esophagus	Rectal
Nasopharynx	Sublingual (mouth)
Tympanic membrane (ear)	Axilla
Jugular bulb	Skin surface (forehead better than extremity)[b]

[a]Core temperature monitoring sites are recommended.
[b]Skin surface temperature monitoring is the least reliable site.

bladder temperatures except during extreme thermal perturbations (48–50). Temperatures taken at more accessible sites such as the mouth, axilla, and rectum are clinically significant only in terms of how closely they correlate to core temperature. It should be noted that jugular bulb or cerebral temperatures may be higher than temperatures measured at other sites. In the SICU, patients' temperatures are monitored with PA catheters (if in place), or intermittently using tympanic membrane or electronic thermometers placed orally or rectally.

Temperature can be measured at numerous sites in the body. Consideration should be given to both reliability and accessibility. For example, the rectal site should not be used in patients undergoing hemorroidectomy. Some sites, primarily the mouth and axilla, are affected by environmental factors; less affected are the rectum and bladder, though they, too, can produce unreliable readings (51). ☛ **The most reliable core monitoring sites are the PA, distal esophagus, nasopharynx, and tympanic membrane (Table 7) (52).** ☛ These sites come closest to reflecting core temperature, which provides about 80% of thermal input to the hypothalamus, and are the best indicators of a deviation from homeostasis.

Core Sites
Esophagus
Distal esophageal thermometry is a highly accurate measure of core temperature. The distal esophagus is a useful site for core temperature measurement, especially in tracheally intubated patients (8). The esophageal stethoscope contains a thermistor and is also useful for monitoring heart and lung sounds (Fig. 7). Temperature readings are displayed on an electronic monitor (Fig. 8). Because of its proximity to the heart, a primary core temperature organ, the thermistor reacts quickly to changes, providing a fast and highly accurate reading (53). Placement is critical; if the probe containing the thermistor is not directly in front of the heart, readings are less reliable.

Esophageal probes should not be placed in patients with mediastinal traversing injuries due to the risk of esophageal trauma. Suction applied to a nasogastric tube will falsely lower the esophageal temperature. If the probe is not placed distally, temperature readings may be inaccurate. Temperature probes incorporated into esophageal stethoscopes must be positioned at the point of maximal heart sounds, or even more distally, to provide accurate readings.

Nasopharyngeal
Nasopharyngeal temperature probes usually correlate well with other centrally measured temperatures. Nasopharyngeal temperature exceeded tympanic temperature during

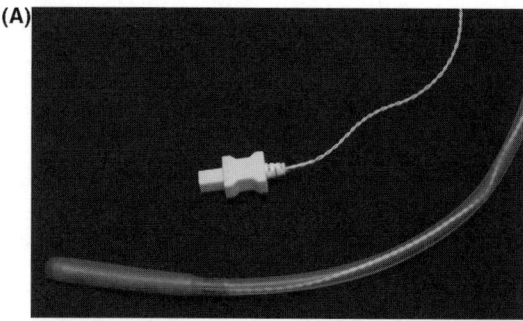

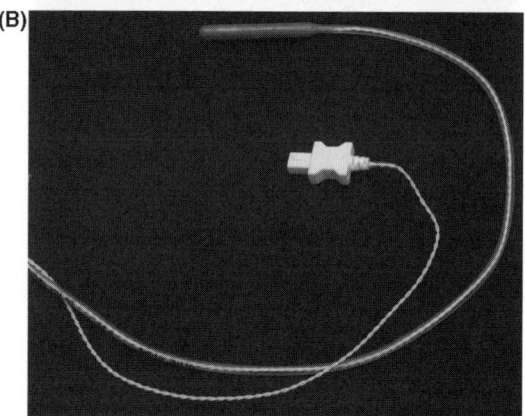

Figure 7 Distal esophageal (core) temperature is easily measured in tracheally intubated patients using an adult, 18 Fr (**A**), or pediatric, 9 Fr (**B**) esophageal stethoscope with thermocouple sensor. The esophageal stethoscope is positioned at the point of maximal heart sounds and temperature is continuously displayed on an electronic monitor. The temperature sensor in this device has an accuracy of $\pm 0.2°C$ over the range of $25–45°C$ (Series 400, Vitals Signs, Inc., Totowa, New Jersey, U.S.A.).

rewarming on CPB, which suggests that this site better reflects the brain temperature (54). When deep hypothermia is rapidly induced and reversed, temperature measurements made at standard monitoring sites may not reflect cerebral

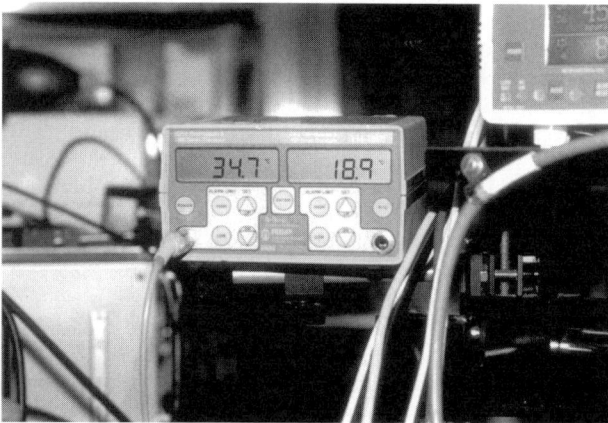

Figure 8 Two-channel electronic temperature monitor (Bi-Temp, Model TM-200D, Respiratory Support Products, Inc. SIMS, Irvine, California, U.S.A.). Core temperature is displayed on the *left* (34.7°C), and room temperature is displayed on the *right* (18.9°C). Low ambient operating room temperature, as seen in this example, is an important risk factor for intraoperative hypothermia in surgical patients.

temperature. Measurements from the nasopharynx, distal esophagus, tympanic membrane, and PA tend to match brain temperature best (8).

Problems with this site include the risk of nasopharyngeal bleeding. Temperatures may vary between different probe positions. This site is relatively contraindicated in patients with severe midface or basilar skull fractures with cribiform plate disruption.

Pulmonary Artery

To measure temperature in the PA, a catheter with a thermistor is placed in the PA during surgery or in critical care situations to monitor cardiac output and other hemodynamic parameters. ☞ **Because temperatures taken at the PA closely correlate with core temperature, many clinicians view this as the most accurate site for measuring body temperature in critical care; this site is far too invasive to use for temperature alone.** ☞ In any case, readings can be adversely affected by the temperature of the CPB fluids during cooling and re-warming, and by administration of cold or warm fluid directly into the right atrium, right ventricle or PA. The effect of cardiac output flush solution is generally transient and inconsequential.

Tympanic Membrane (Ear)

The ear canal—more specifically, the tympanic membrane— is just 1.4 inches (3.5 cm) from the hypothalamus, and can be readily monitored using an ear probe (Fig. 9). The temperature of the tympanic membrane is relatively well protected from the influence of ambient temperatures and is unaffected by respiration, eating, drinking, or smoking. Plus, of course, the ear has an equally usable twin on the other side of the head. ☞ **For these reasons, the tympanic membrane is a good noninvasive site to measure core body temperature in SICU and OR patients, but the probes are easily dislodged during patient movement and transport.** ☞

Although the tympanic membrane is perfused by the internal carotid artery, studies demonstrate that fanning the face decreases the temperature of the tympanic membrane but not the brain (55). Thus, tympanic membrane probes are not the best choice during initial resuscitation of a patient from the field. Sensor probes do not always abut the tympanum, and cerumen or dried blood in the auditory canal can result in a delayed response time. Tympanic membrane probes are contraindicated in patients with

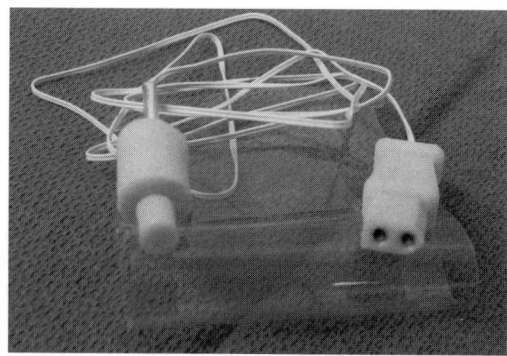

Figure 9 Tympanic membrane (TTS-400) temperature sensor. (Level-1, Rockland, Massachusetts, U.S.A.). The temperature probe is placed in close proximity to the tympanic membrane, and the external auditory meatus is covered with gauze and a piece of tape.

cerebrospinal fluid otorrhea and are easily dislodged during patient movement and transport. Measures may be inaccurate if the ears are cold or in the presence of otologic disease.

Intermediate Sites

☞ When body temperature is constant, intermediate sites such as sublingual, rectal, and urinary bladder are good estimates of core temperature (Figs. 10 and 11). When body temperature is rapidly changing (e.g., CPB, invasive rewarming, surgery), intermediate temperature sites are slower to change compared to core sites. ☞ Core temperature can be estimated with reasonable accuracy using oral, axillary, rectal, or bladder temperatures, except during extreme thermal perturbations. Rectal temperature is considered an intermediate temperature in deliberately cooled patients, and may not prove reliable during malignant hyperthermia episodes. During cardiac surgery, bladder temperature is similar or close to rectal temperature (and therefore intermediate) when urine flow is low, but similar or close to PA temperature (and thus core) when flow is high. Since bladder temperature is strongly influenced by urine flow, it may be difficult to interpret in these patients.

Mouth

Previously, the most common site for measuring temperature was the sublingual pocket under the tongue on either side of the frenulum. Normally, oral temperature is lower than core temperature by about 0.5°C. Correct placement of the thermometer is essential; dwell time is 15 to 45 seconds for electronic thermometers in the predictive mode, and three to five minutes for glass-mercury thermometers. The advantages of oral thermometry include accessibility, familiarity, and noninvasiveness. The disadvantages are chiefly related to inaccurate readings if the patient eats, drinks, smokes, or chews gum prior to the reading, fails to keep the thermometer properly placed under the tongue, breathes too fast (especially through the mouth), or talks.

Rectum

Rectal temperatures were long considered the "gold standard" for measuring core temperature, especially in children. Despite possible discomfort and embarrassment, the site has obvious advantages: It's easily accessible, requires an inexpensive thermometer, and provides an accurate reading when taken properly. What's more, it's usually quite close to core temperature—on average, it runs about 0.1°C higher.

Rectal thermometry does have some drawbacks (56). Because the rectum is a cavity, it can retain heat longer than other temperature sites. Rectal temperature normally correlates well with core temperature, but fails to increase rapidly during malignant hyperthermia crises and under other documented situations (51,56). When a patient's temperature is rising or falling rapidly, the temperature in the rectum can lag behind by as much as an hour. This may be because the rectum contains no thermoreceptors and thus is heated or cooled as an effect of hypothalamic control, rather than in response to it. Other possible causes of inaccurate rectal readings include heavy exercise of the large muscles in the buttocks and thighs, the insulating effect of fecal matter in the rectum, and heat produced by coliform bacteria.

(A)

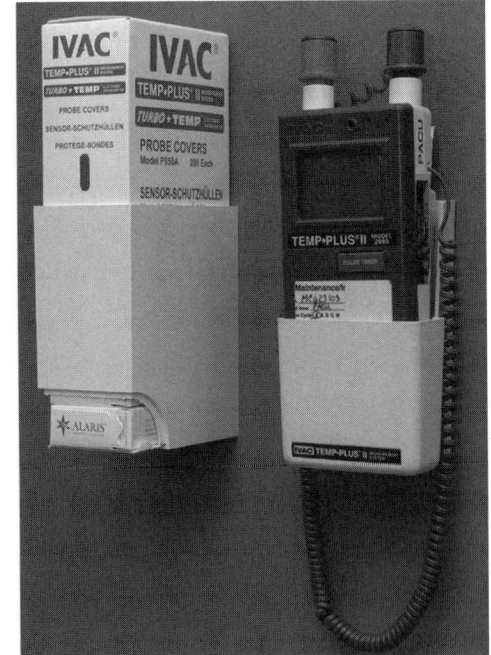

(B)

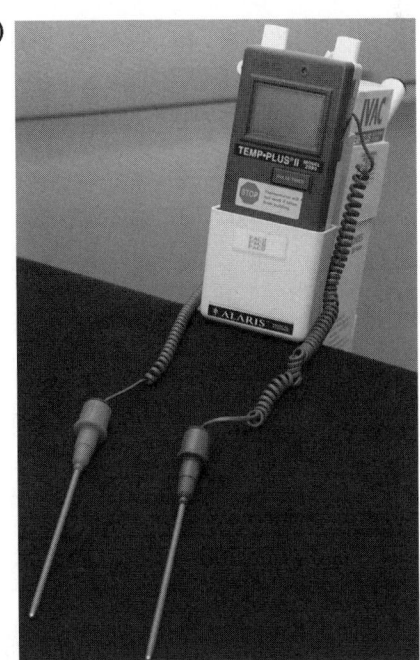

Figure 10 (**A**) and (**B**). An electronic thermometer can be used to accurately measure sublingual (*black probe*) or rectal (*gray probe*) temperatures (IVAC Temp Plus II, Model 2080, Alaris Medical, San Diego, California, U.S.A.).

To measure rectal temperature accurately—whether by electronic, glass-mercury, or single-use chemical thermometer—proper depth and dwell time are necessary. The proper depth for a rectal thermometer varies with the patient's age: for adults, it is 2 to 3 inches (5–7.5 cm); for children, 0.5 to 1.5 inches (1.25–3.75 cm); for neonates, 0.75 inch (1.9 cm). Proper dwell time is the same for all patients: 15 to 45 seconds for electronic thermometers in the predictive mode; three to five minutes otherwise.

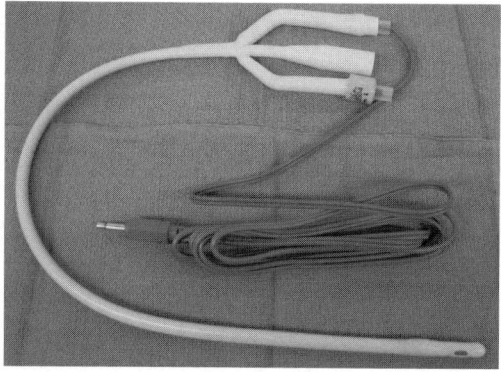

Figure 11 Bardex® Temperature-Sensing (400-Series) Foley catheter (C.R. Bard, Inc., Covington, Georgia, U.S.A.). This device is accurate to ±0.2°C.

Without proper depth and dwell time, rectal temperature readings will be inaccurate. Rectal probes can become lodged in fecal matter, which insulates them from the surrounding tissues.

Bladder

Bladder temperature is measured by an indwelling urinary catheter containing a thermistor (Fig. 11). High correlation exists between bladder and PA temperature. Drawbacks to bladder temperature monitoring include bladder irrigation, which, whether manual or continuous, will cause the thermistor to measure the temperature of the irrigant rather than of the urine. If the patient's urinary catheter does not have a thermistor attached, and most indwelling urinary catheters do not, it has to be changed to one that does. Finally, patients with hypothermia will show a slight lag in bladder temperature during rewarming.

Although bladder temperature sensors are convenient, they are influenced by urinary flow and consequently, may not provide a reliable measure of core temperature during shock with diminished urinary output or renal failure. Patients with urethral disruption require suprapubic placement of the urinary catheter (57). Open pelvic and lower abdominal trauma may falsely lower temperature readings

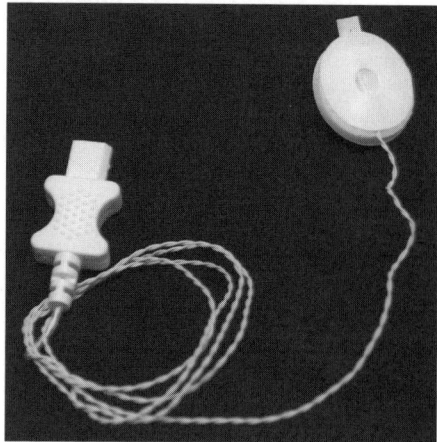

Figure 12 Skin surface temperature sensor with 400 series thermistor.

Table 8 Methods to Prevent and/or Treat Hypothermia

Method	Examples
Passive	a. Warm the room (e.g., 27–30°C)
	b. Warm blankets, insulating blankets, dry off wet skin
Active external	a. Forced air warming
	Intraoperative: rewarmed patients by 1–2°C/hr
	Postoperative: rewarmed patients at rate of 0.9°C/hr
	After cold water immersion: rewarmed at 2.4°C/hr°C
	Severe accidental hypothermia: rewarmed patients by 1.0–2.4°C/hr
	b. Circulating heated water mattress
	Most effective when placed on top of patient
	c. Radiant warmers
	Reduces shivering postoperatively regardless of effect on core temperature
Active internal	a. Heated humidified gases
	Insulates respiratory tract and prevents heat and moisture lost through breathing
	b. Warmed IV fluids
	Effective at preventing heat loss from IV fluid therapy
	2 L crystalloid at 20°C corresponds to 0.6°C decrease in core temperature in 70-kg adult
	2 L cold blood corresponds to 0.9°C decrease in core temperature in 70-kg adult
	c. Body cavity (e.g., peritoneal, mediastinal) lavage
	Rewarmed patients by 1–3°C/hr depending on flow and dwell time
	Problems with abdominal and thoracic trauma, adhesions, drainage, and flow
	d. Extracorporeal
	CAVR: rewarms by 1.3–2.2°C/hr. Does not require systemic heparinization
	CPB: most effective heat exchange device. Peserves organ blood flow and tissue oxygenation if mechanical cardiac activity is lost
	Requires systemic heparinization and cardiac perfusionist
	Hemodialysis: exchange cycle volumes of 200–250 mL/min are possible
	Venovenous rewarming: can achieve flows of 150–400 mL/min

Abbreviations: CAVR, continuous arteriovenous rewarming; CPB, cardiopulmonary bypass; IV, intravenous.
Source: Modified from Refs. 52 and 56.

from this site. Urinary flow may be negligible in the setting of shock or renal failure.

Axilla and Groin

When oral and rectal sites are inaccessible or inappropriate, the axilla or the groin may be used. Glass-mercury, electronic, or single-use chemical thermometers can be used in children at the axilla, but this site may not be reliable or accurate enough to use with adults. And, for both populations, it has

Table 9 Temperature Measuring Devices

Device	Pros	Cons
Glass mercury (oral, rectal, axillary)	Easy accessibility Familiarity Noninvasive	Long dwell time Inaccurate readings possible if patient is not cooperative Temperature read is lower than core temperature Breakable Requires disinfection between patients, or disposable covers
Infrared (tympanic membrane)	Noninvasive Close to the hypothalamus Can be used in either ear TM (but not ear canal) is protected from ambient temperatures Quick temperature acquisition	Current devices not continuous Measurement can be inaccurate in trauma due to blood, CSF, foreign body in ear canal Excessive cerumen interferes with temperature measurement
Thermister tipped ear probe (tympanic membrane)	Noninvasive Close to the hypothalamus Can be used in either ear TM (but not ear canal) is protected from ambient temperatures (positioning critical to reflect TM with this device)	Easily dislodged during movement or transport In setting of CSF otorrhea, other ear trauma, relatively contraindicated
Electronic thermocouple (oral, rectal, axillary)	Easy accessibility Familiarity Noninvasive Short dwell time compared to glass mercury	Inaccurate readings possible if patient is not cooperative Temperature read is usually lower than core temperature Requires disposable cover
Esophageal stethoscope—thermister (esophageal, nasopharyngeal)	Reflects core temperature Reacts quickly to changes Matches brain temperature (nasopharyngeal placement)	Critical placement Esophageal: must be distal to tracheal carina Nasopharyngeal: risk of nasal bleeding
PA catheter—thermister (CVP or PA locations)	Reflects core temperature Continuous measurement	Invasive Expensive
Indwelling urinary catheter—thermister	Convenient if requires catheter In stable patients, reflects core temperature	Influenced by urinary flow

Abbreviations: CSF, cerebrospinal fluid; CVP, central venous pressure; PA, pulmonary artery; TM, tympanic membrane.

inherent drawbacks: (*i*) skin contact with the thermometer must be maintained at the apex of the axilla for 8 to 11 minutes (using a glass-mercury thermometer); (*ii*) the resulting temperature reading must be adjusted because it can be 0.5°C to 1.2°C lower than core temperature; (*iii*) the temperature is less accurate in shock due to peripheral vasoconstriction.

Thermoregulatory vasoconstriction shunts blood away from the skin's surface, including the axilla (though less so than with distal extremities) during moderate hypothermia and prolongs thermal response times. During profound hypothermia, intense vasoconstriction redirects blood flow primarily to a very diminished central compartment. Thermal response time is altered by the volume of connective tissue and fat separating peripheral compartments from perfused vasculature.

For these reasons, axillary or groin temperatures are, at best, estimates and not always reliable enough to provide the basis for clinical intervention—except with neonates. Indeed, since neonates have a high rate of heat loss through their skin, the axilla and the groin are often preferred sites; in fact, for most neonates, the axillary site is standard. Because of the risk of perforation, the rectum is not used in neonates.

Peripheral Skin Sites

Adult temperature is rarely measured on the skin's surface, though this quick technique may help track a trend. At best, it provides a peripheral body temperature with measurements that can vary widely because of vasomotor activity and ambient temperatures (55). These drawbacks particularly apply when using single-use chemical thermometers to measure temperature at the forehead, a site constantly exposed to ambient temperatures. The skin provides approximately 20% of thermal input to the hypothalamus. A valid use of skin temperature is with incubated newborns. Electronic sensing elements (Fig. 12) attached to the skin provide a digital readout showing the trend of neonates' temperature and automatically maintain optimal environmental temperature in the incubator. Skin surface temperature is used in thermoregulatory research to determine mean body temperature, forearm to fingertip gradients and the degree of peripheral vasoconstriction or vasodilation.

Skin-surface temperatures are usually considerably lower than core temperature. However, in direct sun, the exposed skin temperature can be higher than core temperature. Skin-surface temperatures, when adjusted with an appropriate offset, can reflect core temperature reasonably well in stable patients located in protected enviroments

(53). However, skin temperatures do not reflect core temperature in resuscitation situations, and fail to reliably confirm the clinical signs of malignant hyperthermia (tachycardia and hypercarbia) in swine (58).

In a prospective comparison of esophageal, tympanic membrane, and forehead skin temperatures in adult surgical patients, there was a lack of precision between skin and distal esophageal temperatures with wide limits of agreement (55). Moreover, there was no relation between change in skin temperature and change in esophageal temperature. Accordingly forehead skin temperature should not be considered reliable, and sole reliance on this measurement can adversely affect patient care.

EYE TO THE FUTURE

Nonintended hypothermia in trauma victims is becoming a less common problem because of early recognition, accurate noninvasive body temperature monitoring, and thermally efficient devices that rapidly achieve desired body temperature (59). The lethal triad of hypothermia, acidosis, and coagulopathy will be easily controlled with interventions that restore organ perfusion, hemostasis, and tissue perfusion.

The role of therapeutic hypothermia in TBI patients will be further delineated in the next decade with increased focus upon the hypothermic intervention, duration of therapeutic hypothermia, and application of therapeutic hypothermia in carefully selected patients together with strict protocols and close monitoring to avoid complications such as hypovolemia, hypotension, and hyperglycemia (60–64).

A clear consensus will emerge as to which temperature monitoring site is best for trauma patients. Site of temperature monitoring will assume increased importance after head, spinal cord, and other injuries since central nervous system temperature may exhibit variability and discordance with respect to traditionally accepted core temperature measures.

SUMMARY

Body temperature is a vital sign which remains within a narrow range in normal patients. Body temperature is controlled by the hypothalamus, which integrates thermal information and coordinates increases in heat production such shivering and nonshivering thermogenesis, heat loss (sweating), and/or decreases in heat loss (vasoconstriction) in order to maintain thermal homeostasis (8).

Risk factors that contribute to hypothermia include environmental exposure, especially in the presence of impaired thermoregulation, extremes of age, spinal cord injury, TBI, shock, and administration of sedatives, analgesic, or anesthetic agents (65,66). Acute trauma patients should be warmed to maintain core temperatures >35.5°C (Table 8) (66). Standard methods available include warming the room to >28°C, forced air, inhalational gas warming (67,68), warming of IV fluids, and radiant heat (69,70).

Core temperature should be monitored in order to detect thermal disturbances and to maintain appropriate body temperature. Deliberate use of hypothermia is associated with improved neurologic outcome in cardiac and some forms of neuro-anesthesia, but has not been proven for isolated TBI with GCS 3–4, but may be useful in the young with GCS in the 5–8 range and elevated intracranial pressures. Hypothermia is associated with major morbidity

because of impaired cardiorespiratory function, peripheral vasoconstriction, bleeding diathesis, metabolic acidosis, diminished hepatorenal function, and altered immune response.

The preferred technique of temperature monitoring is one that reflects core temperature such as distal esophageal, nasopharynx, PA, and tympanic membrane (Table 9). Intermediate sites such as rectum, bladder, and mouth usually reflect core temperature. Brain temperature may exceed temperature measured elsewhere during hypothermia and subsequent rewarming.

KEY POINTS

- Normal core temperature ranges between 36.5°C and 37.5°C, but may vary because of circadian rhythms and other factors.
- The hypothalamus is the center of thermoregulatory control.
- There are three components of the thermoregulatory system: (*i*) afferent input of temperature information; (*ii*) central processing of the information by the anterior hypothalamus; and (*iii*) efferent responses to control heat production and heat loss.
- The liver, heart, and skeletal muscle are the major heat generators, whereas the skin and respiratory system are the major organs responsible for heat loss.
- Heat is lost by radiation, conduction, evaporation, and convection (Table 2).
- Although hypothermia decreases the metabolic function of the body, and is neuroprotective, in traumatized individuals hypothermia most often results in deleterious effects such as coagulopathy, metabolic acidosis, and impaired immune response (8).
- Risk factors that contribute to hypothermia include environmental exposure, alcohol and drug intoxication, IV infusion of room temperature fluid, transfusion of cold blood without warming, spinal cord injuries, head injury, shock, and associated medical conditions such as hypothyroidism and hypoglycemia (Table 5).
- Trauma-associated hypothermia increases morbidity because of impaired cardiorespiratory function, peripheral vasoconstriction, bleeding diathesis, metabolic acidosis, diminished hepatorenal function, and altered immune response (Table 6).
- Hypothermia is common during general anesthesia because of impaired thermoregulation (Fig. 6), decreased heat production, and internal redistribution of body heat from the warmer core to the cooler peripheral tissue in the exposed patient (35,36).
- Epidural and spinal anesthesia block afferent and efferent thermoregulatory responses and cause similar degrees of hypothermia as general anesthesia.
- Mild hypothermia (1–2°C below normal) is neuroprotective, whereas mild hyperthermia (1–2°C above normal) may exacerbate cerebral ischemia.
- A thermometer incorporated into an esophageal stethoscope is a simple and reliable method of measuring core temperature in tracheally intubated patients providing it is inserted deep enough (at least 5–10 cm past the carina).
- The preferred technique of temperature monitoring is one that reflects core temperature such as distal esophageal, nasopharynx, PA, and tympanic membrane.

Intermediate sites such as rectum, bladder, and mouth usually reflect core temperature.

☞ The most reliable core monitoring sites are the PA, distal esophagus, nasopharynx, and tympanic membrane.

☞ Because temperatures taken at the PA closely correlate with core temperature, many clinicians view this as the most accurate site for measuring body temperature in critical care; this site is far too invasive to use for temperature alone.

☞ For these reasons, the tympanic membrane is a good noninvasive site to measure core body temperature in SICU and OR patients, but the probes are easily dislodged during patient movement and transport.

☞ When body temperature is constant, intermediate sites such as sublingual, rectal, and urinary bladder are good estimates of core temperature (Figs. 10 and 11). When body temperature is rapidly changing (e.g., CPB, invasive rewarming, surgery), intermediate temperature sites are slower to change compared to core sites.

REFERENCES

1. Mackowiak PA. Concepts of fever. Arch Intern Med 1998; 158:1870–1881.
2. Berger RL, Clem TR, Harden VA, Mangum BW. Historical development and newer means of temperature measurements in biochemistry. Methods Biochem Anal 1984; 30:269–331.
3. Middleton WEK. A History of the Thermometer and Its Use in Meteorology. Baltimore: Johns Hopkins University Press, 1966.
4. Major RH. Sanctorio Sanctorio. Annals Med Hist 1938; 10:369–381.
5. Imrie MM, Hall GM. Body temperature and anesthesia. Br J Anesth 1990;64:346–354.
6. Wunderlich CD. Das Verhalten der Eiaenwarme in Krankenheiten. Leipzig, Germany: Otto Wigard, 1868.
7. Mackowiak PA, Wasserman SS, Levine MM. A critical appraisal of 98.6 degrees F, the upper limit of the normal body temperature, and other legacies of Carl Reinhold August Wunderlich. JAMA 1992; 268:1578–1580.
8. Sessler DI. Temperature monitoring. In: Miller RD, ed. Anesthesia. 6th ed. New York: Churchill Livingstone, 2005:1571–1597.
9. Morley-Foster PK. Unintentional hypothermia in the operating room. Can Anaesth Soc J 1986; 33:516–527.
10. Smith CE, Patel N. Hypothermia in adult trauma patients: anesthetic considerations. Part I. Etiology and pathophysiology. Am J Anesthesiol 1996; 23:283–290.
11. Hendrickx HHL, Trahey GE. Paradoxical inhibition of decreases in body temperature by use of heated and humidified gases. Anesth Analg 1982; 61:393–394.
12. Atkins E, Bodel P. Fever. N Engl J Med 1972; 286:27–34.
13. Danzl DF, Pozos RS. Accidental hypothermia. N Engl J Med 1994; 331:1756–1760.
14. Guyton, AC. Body temperature, temperature regulation and fever. In: Guyton AC, Hall JE (eds). Textbook of Medical Physiology. Philadelphia: W.B. Saunders Company, 1996:911–922.
15. Frankenfield D, Cooney RN, Smith JS, Rowe WA. Age-related differences in the metabolic response to injury. J Trauma 2000; 48(1):49–57.
16. Luna GK, Maier RV, Pavlin EG, et al. Incidence and effect of hypothermia in seriously injured patients. J Trauma 1987; 27:1014–1018.
17. Jurkovich GJ, Greiser WB, Luterman A, Curreri PW. Hypothermia in trauma victims: an ominous predictor of survival. J Trauma 1987; 27:1019–1024.
18. Rutherford EJ, Fusco MA, Nunn CR, et al. Hypothermia in critically ill trauma patients. Injury 1998; 29:605–608.
19. Gentilello LM, Jurkovich GJ, Stark MS, Hassantash SA, O'Keefe GE. Is hypothermia in the victim of major trauma protective or harmful? Ann Surg 1997; 226:439–449.
20. Krishna G, Sleigh JW, Rahman H. Physiological predictors of death in exsanguinating trauma patients undergoing conventional trauma surgery. Aust N Z J Surg 1998; 68:826–829.
21. Little RA, Stoner HB. Body temperature after accidental injury. Br J Surg 1981; 68:221–224.
22. Stoner HB, Marshall HW. Localization of the brain regions concerned in the inhibition of shivering by trauma. Br J Exp Pathol 1977; 58:50–56.
23. Hanania NA, Zimmerman JL. Accidental hypothermia. Crit Care Clinics 1999;15:235–249.
24. Young AJ, Castellani JW, O'Brien C, Shippee RL, Tikuisis P, Meyer LG. Exertional fatigue, sleep loss, and negative energy balance increase susceptibility to hypothermia. J Appl Physiol 1998; 85:1210–1217.
25. Tveita T, Ytrehus K, Myhre ESP, Hevroy O. Left ventricular dysfunction following rewarming from experimental hypothermia. J Appl Physiol 1998; 85:2135–2139.
26. Kuwagata Y, Oda J, Ninomiya N, Shiozaki T, Shimazu T, Sugimoto H. Changes in left ventricular performance in patients with severe head injury during and after mild hypothermia. J Trauma 1999; 47:666–672.
27. Frank SM, Fleisher LA, Breslow MJ, et al. Perioperative maintenance of normothermia reduces the incidence of morbid cardiac events: a randomized clinical trial. JAMA 1997; 227:1127–1134.
28. Schmied H, Kurz A, Sessler DI, et al. Mild hypothermia increases blood loss and transfusion requirements during total hip arthroplasy. Lancet 1996; 347:289–292.
29. Winkler M, Akça O, Birkenberg B, et al. Aggressive warming reduces blood loss during hip arthroplasty. Anesth Analg 2000; 91:978–984.
30. Cosgriff N, Moore EE, Sauaia A, Kenny-Moynihan M, Burch JM, Galloway B. Predicting life-threatening coagulopathy in the massively transfused trauma patient: hypothermia and acidoses revisited. J Trauma 1997; 42:857–861.
31. Kurz A, Sessler DI, Lenhardt R. Perioperative normothermia to reduce the incidence of surgical-wound infection and shorten hospitalization. N Engl J Med 1996; 334:1209–1215.
32. Flores-Maldonado A, Medina-Escobedo CE, Ríos-Rodríguez HM, Fernández-Domínguez R. Mild perioperative hypothermia and the risk of wound infection. Arch Med Res 2001; 32:227–223.
33. Gadkary CS, Alderson P, Signorini DF. Therapeutic hypothermia for head injury (Cochrane Review). Cochrane Database Syst Rev 2002; (1):CD001048.
34. Seekamp A, van Griensven M, Hildebrandt F, Wahlers T, Tscherne H. Adenosine-triphosphate in trauma-related and elective hypothermia. J Trauma 1999; 47:673–683.
35. Sessler DI, Sessler AM. Experimental determination of heat flow parameters during induction of general anesthesia. Anesthesiology 1998; 89:657–665.
36. Sessler DI. Consequences and treatment of perioperative hypothermia. Anesthesiol Clin North Am 1994; 12:425–456.
37. Patel N, Knapke DM, Smith CE, Napora TE, Pinchak AC, Hagen JF. Simulated clinical evaluation of conventional and newer fluid warming devices. Anesth Analg 1996; 82:517–524.
38. Sessler DI. Perianesthetic thermoregulation and heat balance in humans. FASEB J 1993; 7:638–644.
39. Bernard SA, Gray TW, Buist MD, et al. Treatment of comatose survivors of out-of-hospital cardiac arrest with induced hypothermia. N Engl J Med 2002; 346:557–563.
40. Grocott HP, Mackensen GB, Grigore AM, et al. Postoperative hyperthermia is associated with cognitive dysfunction after coronary artery bypass graft surgery. Stroke 2002; 33:537–541.
41. Mangano CM, Hill L, Cartwright CR, Hindman BJ. Cardiopulmonary bypass and the anesthesiologist. In: Kaplan JA, ed. Cardiac Anesthesia. 4th ed. Philadelphia: W.B. Saunders Co., 1999:1061–1110.

42. Kochanek PM, Safar P, Marion DW, et al. Therapeutic hypothermia after traumatic brain injury or hemorrhagic shock: from mild cooling to suspended animation. In: Smith CE, Grande CM, eds. Hypothermia in Trauma: Deliberate or Accidental. New York: XFP, 1998:17–20.

43. Shiozaki T, Hayakata T, Taneda M, et al. Mild Hypothermia Study Group in Japan. A multicenter prospective randomized controlled trial of the efficacy of mild hypothermia for severely head injured patients with low intracranial pressure. J Neurosurg 2001; 94:50–54.

44. Clifton GL, Miller ER, Choi SC, et al. Lack of effect of induction of hypothermia after acute brain injury. N Engl J Med 2001; 344:556–563.

45. Marion DW, Penrod LE, Kelsey SF, et al. Treatment of traumatic brain injury with moderate hypothermia. N Eng J Med 1997; 336:540–546.

46. Zhi D, Zhang S, Lin X. Study on therapeutic mechanism and clinical effect of mild hypothermia in patients with severe head injury. Surgical Neurology 2003; 29:381–385.

47. Stone JG, Yound WL, Smith CR, et al. Do temperature recorded at standard monitoring sites reflect actual brain temperature during deep hypothermia? Anesthesiology 1991; 75:A483.

48. Bissonnette B, Sessler DI, LaFlamme P. Intraoperative temperature monitoring sites in infants and children and the effect of inspired gas warming on esophageal temperature. Anesth Analg 1989; 69:192–196.

49. Cork RC, Vaughan RW, Humphrey LS. Precision and accuracy of intraoperative temperature monitoring. Anesth Analg 1983; 62:211–214.

50. Glosten B, Sessler DI, Faure EAM, Støen R, Thisted RA, Karl L. Central temperature changes are not perceived during epidural anesthesia. Anesthesiology 1992; 77:10–16.

51. Buck SH, Zaritsky AL. Occult core hyperthermia complicating cardiogenic shock. Pediatrics 1989; 83:782–784.

52. Benzinger M. Tympanic thermometry in surgery and anesthesia. JAMA 1969; 209:1207–1211.

53. Ikeda T, Sessler DI, Marder D, Xiong J. The influence of thermoregulatory vasomotion and ambient temperature variation on the accuracy of core-temperature estimates by cutaneous liquid-crystal thermometers. Anesthesiology 1997; 86:603–612.

54. Stone GJ, Young WL, Smith CR, et al. Do standard monitoring sites reflect true brain temperature when profound hypothermia is rapidly induced and reversed? Anesthesiology 1995; 82:344–351.

55. Patel N, Smith CE, Pinchak AC, Hagen JF. Comparison of esophageal, tympanic, and forehead skin temperatures in adult patients. J Clin Anesth 1996; 8:462–468.

56. Ash CJ, Cook JR, McMurry TA, Auner CR. The use of rectal temperature to monitor heat stroke. MO Med 1992; 89:283–288.

57. Smith CE. Trauma and hypothermia. Curr Anaesth Crit Care 2001; 12:87–95.

58. Iaizzo PA, Kehler CH, Zink RS, Belani KG, Sessler DI. Thermal response in acute porcine malignant hyperthermia. Anesth Analg 1996; 82:803–809.

59. Smith CE, Grande CM (ed.). Hypothermia in trauma: deliberate or accidental. Trauma Care 2004;14(2):45–91.

60. van Zanten AR, Polderman KH. Early induction of hypothermia: will sooner be better? Crit Care Med 2005; 33:1449–1452.

61. Nolan JP, Morley PT, Vanden Hoek TL, et al. Therapeutic hypothermia after cardiac arrest. Resuscitation 2003; 57:231–235.

62. Bernard SA, Buist M. Induced hypothermia in critical care medicine: a review. Crit Care Med 2003; 31:2041–2051.

63. Polderman KH. Application of therapeutic hypothermia in the ICU: opportunities and pitfalls of a promising treatment modality. Part 1: Indications and evidence. Intensive Care Med 2004; 30:556–575.

64. Polderman KH. Application of therapeutic hypothermia in the intensive care unit. Opportunities and pitfalls of a promising treatment modality-Part 2: Practical aspects and side effects. Intensive Care Med 2004; 30:757–769.

65. Smith CE, Yamat RA. Avoiding hypothermia in the trauma patient. Curr Opin Anaesthesiol 2000; 13:167–174.

66. Smith CE, Patel N. Hypothermia in adult trauma patients: anesthetic considerations. Part II. Prevention and treatment. Am J Anesthesiol 1997; 24:29–36.

67. Goheen MS, Ducharmme MB, Kenny GP, et al. Efficacy of forced-air and inhalation rewarming by using a human model for severe hypothermia. J Appl Physiol 1997; 83:1635–1640.

68. Steele MT, Nelson MJ, Sessler DI, et al. Forced air speeds rewarming in accidental hypothermia. Ann Emerg Med 1996; 27:479–484.

69. Smith CE, Kabbara A, Kramer RP, Gill I. A new IV fluid and blood warming system to prevent air embolism and compartment syndrome. Trauma Care 2001; 11(2):78–82.

70. Patel N, Smith CE, Pinchak AC. Comparison of fluid warmer performance during simulated clinical conditions. Can J Anaesth 1995; 42:636–642.

71. Lopez M, Sessler DI, Walter K, et al. Rate and gender dependence of the sweating, vasoconstriction, and shivering thresholds in humans. Anesthesiology 1994; 80:780–788.

72. Sessler DI. Perioperative hypothermia. N Engl J Med 1997; 336:1730–1737.

12

Traumatic Brain Injury: Critical Care Management

Anne J. Sutcliffe

Department of Anesthesia and Critical Care, Alexandra Hospital, Redditch, U.K.

INTRODUCTION

In the United States, the annual incidence of traumatic brain injury (TBI) is 1 per 1000 persons. Higher incidences are found in the age groups 15–24 years and 75 years or older (1). However, these data underestimate the true incidence of TBI because only patients dying before admission to the hospital and those admitted to the hospital are included. Prevalence estimates range from 2.5 to 6.5 million individuals living with the consequences of TBI.

Males are twice as likely to be affected as females, and there is a strong association of alcohol with TBI (1). Approximately half of TBIs are caused by motor vehicle, bicycle, and pedestrian-vehicle accidents. A further 10% of TBIs are caused by firearms and the incidence is increasing, 10% by nonfirearm assaults and 3% of total assaults are associated with sporting and recreational activities (1,2). TBIs are particularly associated with falls in the elderly and in the very young. Twenty-five percent of TBIs are due to nonaccidental mechanisms (1).

Mortality from TBI is falling and in 1992 was 19.3 per 1000 population per year (2). The decrease is accounted for by a decrease in deaths associated with blunt trauma. The incidence of deaths from penetrating injury due to firearms is increasing. This is important because most medical interventions for TBI are based on experimental evidence using a blunt trauma model. A different management approach may be more appropriate for penetrating injuries.

Acute care for TBI patients in the United States costs between $9 and $10 billion per year. The lifetime cost of care for a single person with severe TBI has recently been estimated at $1,857,000. This does not include loss of earnings or the cost of social services (1).

⚷ **The function of certain portions of damaged brain can be taken over by other areas, for example, the damaged brain is thought to exhibit a certain degree of neural plasticity.** ⚷ However, at present, little can be done to reverse the effects of primary brain injury. In the intensive care unit (ICU), management strategies are directed towards preventing and/or minimizing the damaging effects of secondary injury.

This chapter aims to describe the basics of primary brain injury and then address the critical care strategies employed to minimize secondary brain injury. The primary emphasis is on pharmacological interventions and maintenance of homeostasis in the intensive care setting. ⚷ **The goal of treatment for TBI is to reduce morbidity and improve outcome.** ⚷ New therapies are being actively investigated using animal models and some may prove successful in humans.

THE GOAL: TO FACILITATE A GOOD OUTCOME

Hospital-based research into outcome after TBI nearly always uses the Glasgow Outcome Scale (GOS) (3). However, TBI is a heterogeneous condition and the GOS conceals a huge variation in disabilities, consequently rehabilitation therapists often use alternative assessment tools that are more sensitive to these variations. Unfortunately, hospital outcome data are not routinely linked to rehabilitation outcome data. Copes et al. (4) have studied 375 patients linking the Major Trauma Outcome Study database and a national rehabilitation outcome database. These authors demonstrated correlations between the two databases' outcome measures, and, although the task of linking the databases is arduous, they recommend that hospital-based trauma registries should routinely include rehabilitation outcome data.

Defining a Good Neurological Outcome

For many patients, a good outcome appears to have been achieved but a follow-up study has shown that most patients have minimal physical disability at three months after mild or moderate TBI. However, 33% remain cognitively impaired at six months and 60% remain unemployed (5). High rates of depression, loneliness and psychomotor slowness can be demonstrated for up to 20 years after severe TBI (6). The consequences of TBI are summarized in Table 1.

Outcome measurement can be uni-dimensional or multifaceted: a specific function or functions are measured. Alternatively, surrogates such as employment status can be used. Sometimes, the patient's perception of the quality of a given outcome differs from that of his caretakers (7).

Duration Endpoints and Other Complexities of Outcome Measurements

⚷ **The full effects of the ICU management of head injury may not be apparent until years after rehabilitation is complete.** ⚷ Motor function improves to its best level relatively quickly, but cognitive function can improve for up to five years (8,9).

Table 2 compares the GOS and the Disability Rating Scale (DRS). These are two of the many outcome scales available. Different outcome scales survey different information, and thus predict different outcomes.

Glasgow Outcome Scale

The GOS is a simple classification. Possible outcomes are dead, vegetative, severely disabled, moderately disabled, or good recovery (3). The latter three categories depend on

Table 1 Consequences of Traumatic Brain Injury

Neurological consequence	Example-comments
Cognitive	Memory impairment
	Poor concentration
	Language difficulty
	Abnormal visual perception
	Difficulty with problem solving and abstract thought
	Impaired judgment and information processing
Functional	Hemiparesis
	Foot drop
Neuro-electrical	Seizures
	Sleep disorders
Behavioral	Verbal and physical aggression
	Altered sexual functioning
	Social disinhibition
	Depression
Social	Suicide
	Divorce
	Unemployment
	Economic strain
	Substance abuse

the patient's ability to live independently and their ability to return to work or school. The GOS is the most widely used outcome measure in head injury research. However, it is a global and relatively insensitive measure, precluding any description of the types of impairments that lead to the disability. The Glasgow Outcome Scale Extended (GOSE) was devised as a new outcome measure that retains the advantages of the existing GOS but allows comparison of patterns of recovery in different areas of function: behavioral, cognitive, and physical. Using a series of functional outcome measures, assessment of affective status, and neuropsychological tests as criteria, the validity of the GOSE generally exceeded the GOS, and the GOSE is more sensitive to change than the GOS (10).

Table 2 Comparison of Glasgow Outcome Scale and Disability Rating Scale as Outcome Scores

GOS score	Interpretation	DRS score	Interpretation
5	Good recovery	0	No TBI
		1	Mild TBI
		2–3	Partial TBI
4	Moderately disabled	4–6	Moderate TBI
		7–11	Moderately severe TBI
3	Severely disabled	12–16	Severe TBI
		17–21	Extremely severe TBI
2	Vegetative state	22–24	Vegetative state
		25–29	Extreme vegetative state
1	Dead		

Abbreviations: DRS, Disability Rating Scale; GOS, Glasgow Outcome Scale; TBI, traumatic brain injury.

Disability Rating Scale
The DRS was developed to describe the continuum of recovery and can be used by both acute and rehabilitation clinicians (11). Eye opening, communication ability, and motor response are measured in the same way as the Glasgow Coma Score. Feeding ability, toileting ability, grooming ability, level of functionality (physical and cognitive), and employability are also scored giving a total range of 0–29. Compared to the GOS with a range of 1–5, the DRS better describes the level of functioning from basic to complex.

Implications for Intensivists
Assessing the Evidence Base
Most studies of acute interventions for TBI measure mortality and gross morbidity either in ICU or in the hospital. Long-term improvements in outcome are not reported because insensitive measurement tools are used and recovery is often far from complete at the time of hospital discharge. This may explain why it has been impossible to prove that certain therapies that work in animals are helpful in humans.

Participating in a Multidisciplinary Approach to Care
Clinicians working in the ICU are aware that what they do has a significant impact on the patient's eventual outcome. However, there are therapies used by the rehabilitation team that are more effective if the TBI patient is discharged from an acute hospital without complications that restrict rehabilitative efforts. Earlier use of some rehabilitation therapies might speed up or improve the quality of recovery and are discussed in the section "Rehabilitation Begins in ICU."

Discussions with Relatives
Failure to appreciate that even minor TBI can cause significant morbidity can lead to misplaced optimism amongst patients and their families. It is important that relatives of those with severe TBI are given a realistic assessment of what the future might hold bearing in mind that it is impossible, even using magnetic resonance imaging (MRI), to predict with any certainty the outcome for an individual patient (12). However, families should be made aware that significant improvement can occur even after acute hospital discharge.

Mortality and Morbidity After Discharge Following TBI
Rehospitalization occurs in 23% of TBI patients in the first year after injury and declines to 17% at five years after injury (13). During the first year most readmissions are for elective reasons such as reconstructive surgery. By five years after injury, most admissions are related to seizures or psychiatric conditions. Mortality is also increased in the first five years after TBI. Most deaths are related to decreased mobility. The exception is death secondary to seizures (14).

PRIMARY BRAIN INJURY

Primary brain injury is caused directly by the initial impact, and this damage is generally referred to as the pathological state existing immediately following the trauma, whereas "secondary injury" refers to the destructive changes that evolve over time (hours to days) following the primary event. Direct injury can occur to the brain parenchyma, as well as to the skull, menengies, dura, or various blood

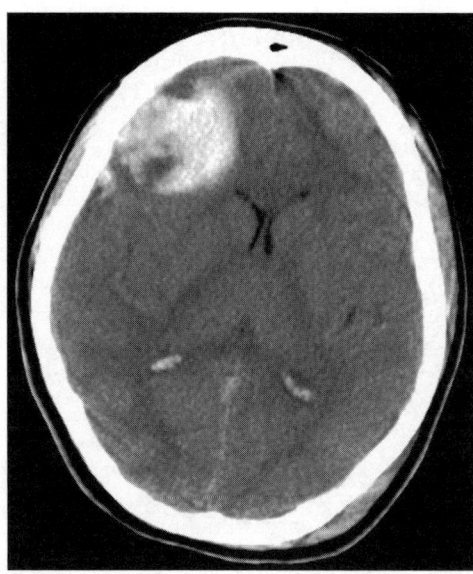

Figure 1 Computed tomograph of the brain showing an acute traumatic right frontal intracerebral contusion.

vessels, which result in space-occupying contusions or hematomas and consequent cell injury or death.

Parenchymal Tissue Damage

White and Grey Matter Injuries

Grey matter injury causes functional failure of neuronal cell bodies and synapses, whereas white matter injury causes abnormal axonal conduction. Head impact sets up pressure waves in the brain that can cause contusions on the crests of gyri that may extend into white matter (Fig. 1) (15). Shearing caused by angular acceleration of the head results in diffuse axonal injury (DAI). DAI is not always visible on early computed tomography (CT) scan but depending on its severity, the immediate effect can range from minimal cognitive changes to death. DAI can cause hemorrhage in the corpus callosum, diffuse cerebral swelling, subarachnoid hemorrhage (SAH), and hemorrhage around the third ventricle (16).

Anatomical Locations of Injury and Implications

Cortical contusion occurs under the site of impact but, because the brain is mobile within the skull, may also occur opposite the site of impact (contracoup injury). The majority of TBIs requiring ICU admission will be comatose, and a CT scan will have demonstrated areas of contusion and other abnormal features. Knowledge of the functions of various parts of the brain (Table 3) can enable an educated guess to be made on clinical evidence about the areas of likely damage. Furthermore, an understanding of the clinical signs associated with tentorial and or tonsillar herniation allows rapid intervention before radiological confirmation of the herniation (Table 4). For further information, readers are referred to a detailed text on correlative neuroanatomy (17).

Epidural Hematoma

Epidural hematomas (EDH) occur outside the dura and are also referred to as extradural hematomas. The incidence of EDH is between 5% and 15% (15). An EDH usually occurs

Table 3 Location-Based Guide to Brain Function

Location	Description	Function
Cortex	Dominant hemisphere	Speaking
		Reading
		Writing
		Calculating
	Nondominant hemisphere	Memory
		Drawing
		Copying
	Frontal lobes	Voluntary movement
		Emotion
		Motivation
		Social functioning
	Temporal lobes	Memory
		Receptive language
		Sequencing
		Musical awareness
	Parietal lobes	Sensation
		Hearing
		Spatial awareness
	Occipital lobes	Visual perception
Cerebellum		Muscle coordination
		Balance
Brainstem		Consciousness control
		Awareness
		Control of breathing
		Control of heart rate
		Control of blood pressure
		Control of temperature

after a skull fracture tears the middle meningeal artery. The hemorrhage, which has a smooth outline when visualized on CT scan, is usually located in the temporal or temporal-parietal region. Rupture of the sagittal or lateral sinus may also cause an EDH (Fig. 2).

Subdural Hematoma

The incidence of subdural hematoma (SDH) is 20% to 63% (15). An SDH occurs in isolation following rupture of

Table 4 Clinical Signs of Brainstem Herniation Based upon Type

Herniation type	Clinical signs of herniation
Sub-falcine	Usually none
Lateral tentorial	Pupil dilatation on ipsilateral side
	Loss of light reflex
	Ptosis
	Deterioration in conscious level
	Limb weakness on the contralateral side
Central tentorial	Pupils small, then moderately dilated
	Loss of light reflex
	Deterioration in conscious level
	Loss of upward gaze
	Diabetes insipidus
Tonsillar	Depression of conscious level
	Abnormal respiratory pattern, then apnea
	Neck stiffness

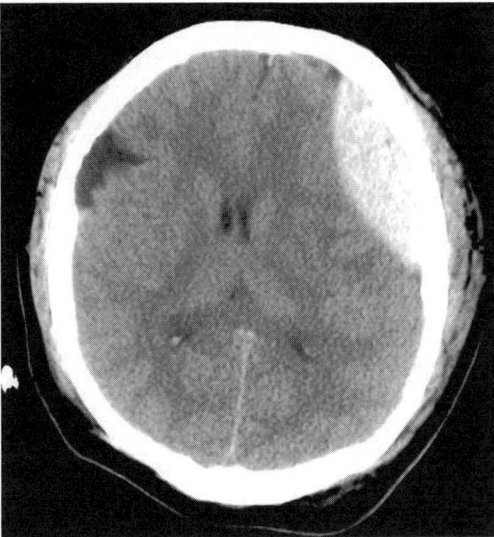

Figure 2 Computerized tomograph of the brain showing a left frontal epidural hematoma and mild left-to-right midline shift.

bridging veins (connecting the cortical surface to a venous sinus) (Figs. 3–5). Cerebral damage occurs because pressure from the clot causes ischemia. Frequently, there is underlying cerebral contusion particularly if the impact occurs over the frontal or temporal lobe. If the contusion is hemorrhagic, necrotic brain and blood escapes into the subdural space. This association of intracerebral and subdural hemorrhage is sometimes called a "burst lobe."

Intracerebral Hemorrhage

Closed head injury may also result in intraparenchymal hemorrhage, often referred to as hemorrhagic contusion (18). Seen as hyperdense areas within brain matter on

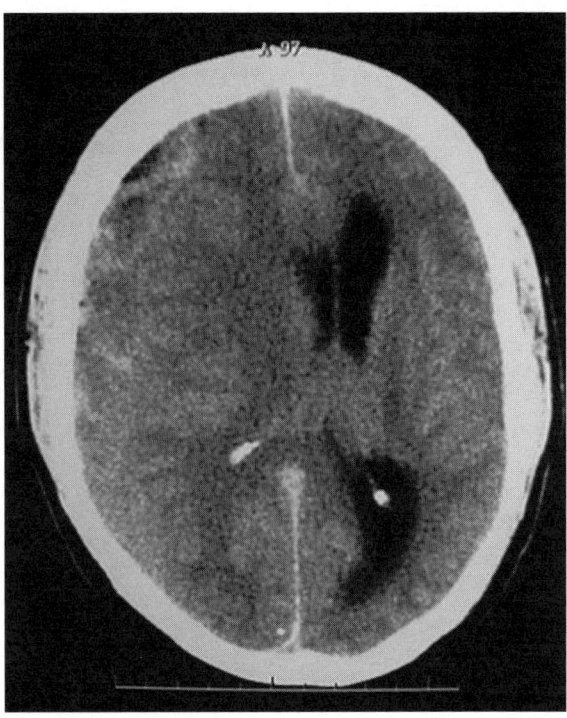

Figure 4 Computerized tomograph of the brain showing a right subacute subdural hematoma with significant right-to-left shift and effacement of the right ventricle (occipital horn). Note that the subacute hematoma (1–2 weeks) is nearly isodense with the density of the cerebral hemisphere.

CT imaging during the workup of head injury, these lesions most commonly occur in areas where sudden deceleration of the head causes the brain to impact bony intracranial surfaces in a coup or countercoup fashion.

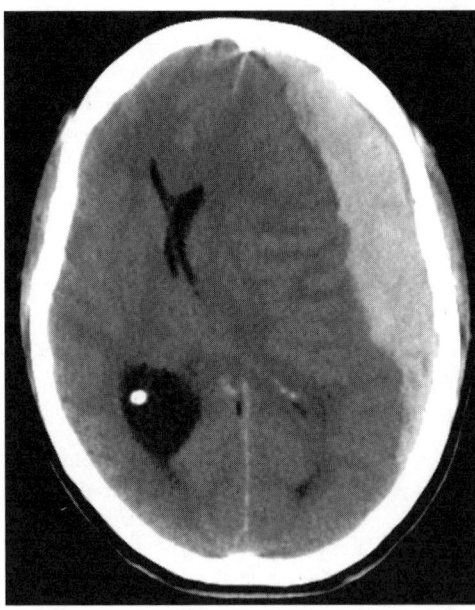

Figure 3 Computerized tomograph of the brain showing an acute left frontoparietal subdural hematoma with significant left-to-right midline shift.

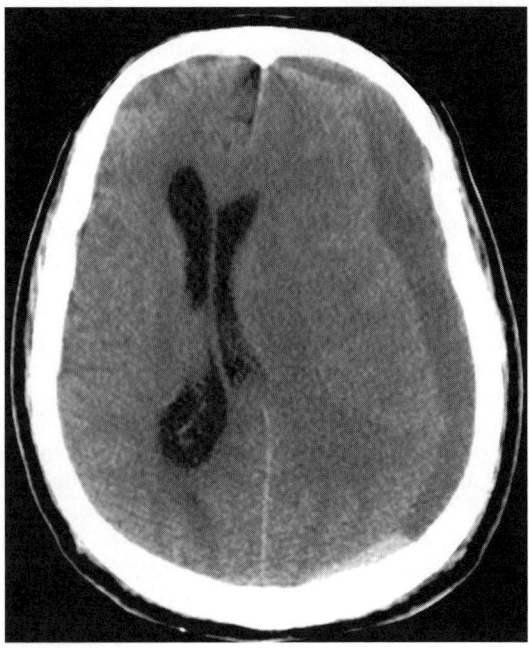

Figure 5 Computerized tomograph of the brain showing a left chronic subdural with significant left-to-right midline shift.

Surgical decompression is warranted if the mass effect threatens herniation and the temporal lobes in particular are housed in a region where uncal herniation can occur with smaller contusions (19). Chapter 14 more fully discusses the topics of intracerebral hemorrhage.

Subarachnoid Hemorrhage

SAH following head trauma is common and is associated with a poorer outcome (Fig. 6) (20). Animal experiments suggest that SAH causes an increase in intracranial pressure (ICP) and decrease in cerebral blood flow (CBF) independent of the effects of TBI (22). SAH also compromises the integrity of the blood-brain barrier. In some patients, SAH may be the primary cause of coma, secondarily leading to a motor vehicle accident or a fall which results in TBI. If this is suspected, following stabilization in the ICU, additional investigation is required to diagnose a possible cerebral aneurysm or arteriovenous malformation (also see Volume 2, Chapter 14).

Vascular Injury

Injury to the middle meningeal artery causing EDH is most common. Penetrating skull injuries can damage almost any vessel. Damage to the carotid artery by a blunt neck injury can mimic a severe head injury. The history and mechanism of the injury should alert the clinician to the possibility of this rare injury. Vertebral artery injuries also result from blunt neck trauma. These are diagnosed by CT angiography.

SECONDARY BRAIN INJURY

Secondary injury can result from pressure increases caused by hematomas and contusions, as they expand, as well as from the resultant edema, hyperemia, or release of inflammatory and cytotoxic mediators (as described below).

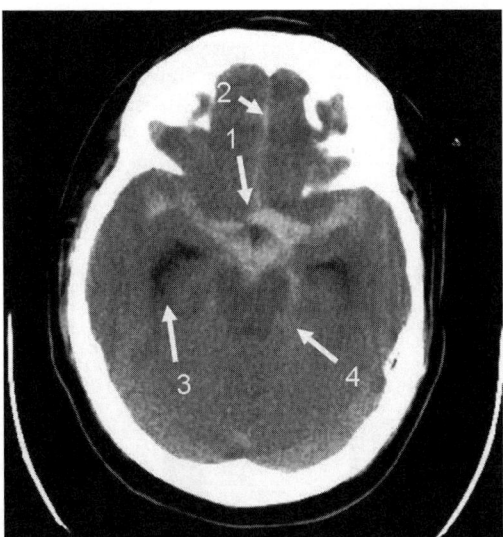

Figure 6   Computerized tomograph of the brain showing severe posttraumatic subarachnoid hemorrhage. Acute blood appears radiodense (white) on CT. The subarachnoid blood is seen in the suprasellar cistern (*arrow 1*), the interhemispheric cistern (*arrow 2*), temporal horn of the lateral ventricle (one of the radiological stigmata of hydrocephalus—*arrow 3*), and in the ambient cisterns around the midbrain (*arrow 4*).

Table 5   Causes of Secondary Brain Injury

Hypotension
Hypoxia
Herniation
Pyrexia
Seizures
Hyperglycemia
Hydrocephalus
Vasospasm
Cerebral infection
Reperfusion injury
Cytotoxic cellular edema
Vasogenic and hydrostatic interstitial edema

Edema can occur within the cell itself, as well as within the interstitial space (due to vasogenic and hydrostatic factors). Hypotension, hypoxia, and other non-physiologic conditions (e.g., hyperglycemia, hyperthermia, etc.), can cause or exacerbate secondary injury. ☞ **Secondary brain injuries (Table 5) are of particular interest because they are potentially preventable.** ☞

Cytotoxic Cellular Edema

Injured and dying neurons have disturbed ionic gradients that lead to swelling. Following mitochondrial swelling and failure of membranous ionic pumps, toxic factors are released that can cause further neuronal damage. These effects may be specific with respect to brain region and time (22). The mechanisms are complex and our understanding is far from complete. The cellular effects of TBI are commonly studied using rodents. A recent article shows that the method by which the animals are anesthetized can have an independent effect on mortality and calls into question the results of many earlier studies (23). Furthermore, it is not yet certain that different types of cellular injury, for example, DAI, contusion, hypoxic, are damaged by the same metabolic and biochemical mechanisms which include: anaerobic metabolism (producing lactate) glutamate toxicity, intracellular calcium influx, nitric oxide synthesis, and apoptosis (24–28).

These have been studied using specific antagonists of intracellular and cell membrane metabolic processes in cell culture and animal models. Unfortunately, although some experimental results are promising, they have not yet been successfully translated into neuroprotection in the clinical setting partly because most benefit occurs when the drug is applied prior to the initiation of trauma.

Interstitial Edema: Vasogenic and Hydrostatic

TBI causes an inflammatory response that involves cytokine production, chemokine release, inflammatory adhesion molecule upregulation and neutrophil recruitment (22). Macrophages from the circulation and microglia accumulate at the site of injury and release inflammatory mediators including tumor necrosis factor alpha (TNFα), and interleukin-6 (IL-6). These and other inflammatory mediators disrupt the tight junctions that normally exist between the cerebral capillary endothelial cells that form the blood-brain barrier. Leakage of protein-rich serous fluid from the capillaries causes vasogenic interstitial edema.

Hydrostatic interstitial edema occurs when there is a sudden increase in capillary transmural pressure. It may follow decompression of a mass lesion or occur in the presence of defective autoregulation. The fluid, which escapes into the interstitial space, unlike vasogenic edema, is low in protein.

Hyperemia

Animal experiments show that CBF increases immediately after injury, then decreases by up to 40% within a few minutes and returns to normal after approximately 24 hours (29). Hyperemia, defined as CBF in excess of metabolic demands, has been demonstrated in the hippocampus, and in the areas of brain close to the ischemic penumbra of injury (30). Usually hyperemia follows a period of increased ICP and/or reduced CBF. Its etiology is unexplained, but metabolic derangement, loss of vasomotor tone, or severe tissue acidosis are possible explanations.

Hypotension

⚡ **A systolic blood pressure of less than 90 mmHg occurring between the time of TBI and completion of resuscitation is associated with a 33% increase mortality (31).** ⚡ During the first 24 hours in ICU, the lowest recorded blood pressure is correlated with mortality (Fig. 7) (32). Systemic hypotension is particularly damaging in the setting of increased ICP and/or concomitant decreased systemic oxygenation (discussed subsequently).

Hypoxia

⚡ **An arterial oxygen tension (PaO$_2$) of less than 60 mmHg (8 kPa) occurring between the time of TBI and completion of resuscitation is also associated with an increase in morbidity and mortality but to a lesser extent than the effect of hypotension (31).** ⚡ An early hypoxic episode increases mortality by 6%. Hypoxia can be caused by airway obstruction or chest injury. Reduced cerebral blood flow, systemic hypotension or hypocapnic vasoconstriction may also cause cerebral hypoxia (Fig. 7). The effect of combined hypoxia and hypotension is synergistic and must be avoided (31).

Herniation

Brain herniation may be tentorial, subfalcine, or tonsillar. In general, the effect of herniation is compression of the adjacent brain, stretching or tearing of the blood vessels and ischemic damage (Table 4; Volume 2, Chapters 1 and 7).

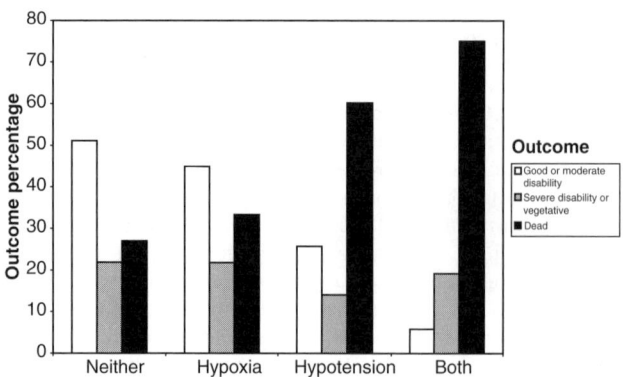

Figure 7 Bar graph demonstrating the relationship between hypoxia or hypotension or both hypoxia and hypotension and outcome following traumatic brain injury.

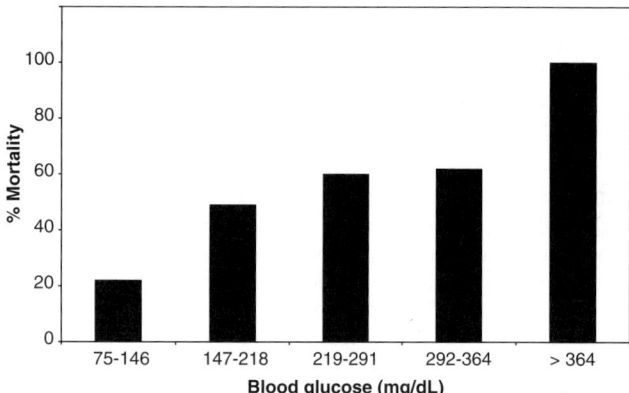

Figure 8 Bar graph demonstrating the relationship between highest measured blood glucose (mg/dL) in the first 24 hours in ICU and mortality. There is a 20% mortality for blood glucose in the normal range of 75–146 mg/dL (4.1–8 mmol/L). Moderately elevated glucose 147–218 mg/dL (8.1–12 mmol/L) is associated with more than twice the mortality. Blood glucose in the 219–291 mg/dL (12.1–16 mmol/L) range approaches 60% mortality. Patients with a blood glucose in the 292–364 mg/dL (16.1–20 mmol/L) range had slightly higher mortality than 60%. However, those patients with serum glucose measurements greater than 364 mg/dL (>20 mmol/L) had the highest mortality of all (approaching 100%).

Hyperglycemia

⚡ **The highest blood sugar occurring in the first 24 hours of ICU care is linearly correlated with mortality (Fig. 8) (32).** ⚡ It is not clear whether hyperglycemia is merely a manifestation of the stress response to injury or another secondary insult (also see Volume 2, Chapter 60) (33,34). It is interesting to observe that the correlation of blood glucose with mortality is closer than the inverse correlation between mean arterial pressure (MAP) with mortality (32). Furthermore, a high blood sugar combined with a MAP of 60 to 80 mmHg is associated with a poorer outcome than a low blood sugar and a MAP of less than 60 mmHg (Fig. 9) (32). In the cortical extracellular space, microdialysis has been used to

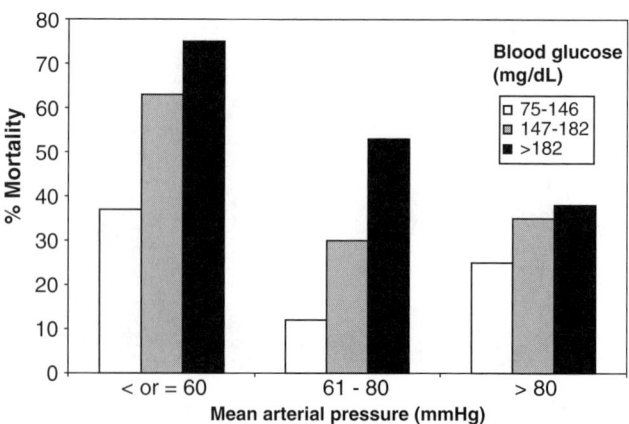

Figure 9 Bar graph demonstrating the relationship between highest blood glucose, lowest mean arterial pressure in the first 24 hours in ICU and mortality. *Key*: 75–146 mg/dL (4.1–8 mmol/L) = clear columns, 147–182 mg/dL (8.1–10 mmol/L) = grey columns, >182 mg/dL (>10 mmol/L) = solid columns.

show that lactate concentration is increased and glucose decreased indicating increased anaerobic glycolysis, which is associated with a poor outcome (24). The effects of delivering more glucose in the blood are debated. On the one hand, anaerobic metabolism is inefficient so additional glucose might provide fuel for more energy. On the other, increased energy production produces more lactate as a by-product, and lactate causes cellular damage.

Fever

The brain's metabolic rate alters in direct proportion to core temperature. Thus, a fever occurring in a patient with TBI will increase the oxygen requirement of cells that are already in an ischemic environment. Abundant animal data show moderate hypothermia to be protective (35). Conversely, hyperthermia increases mortality and morbidity by aggravating axonal and microvascular damage (36). ☞ **Although human outcome data is controversial, fever should be prevented in TBI patients.** ☞

Seizures

Within the first week after TBI, continuous electroencephalographic monitoring has shown that seizures occur in 20% of patients (37). Seizures cause intense local metabolic activity and can aggravate ischemic damage in affected areas of brain. Diagnosis can be difficult in the ventilated patient. Sedative drugs can mask typical tonic-clonic limb movements but twitching of the corner of the mouth is sometimes seen. An unprovoked episode of hypertension, tachycardia, increased ICP, and a small rise in core temperature is highly suggestive of undiagnosed seizures.

Hydrocephalus

Hydrocephalus is usually a late complication of TBI. The published incidence varies depending on whether the diagnosis is made on CT findings alone or whether combined clinical, physiologic, and imaging data are used (38). Distortion of the ventricular system by edema or intracerebral hemorrhage can obstruct cerebrospinal fluid (CSF) circulation. Alternatively a localized obstruction due to clot is common following SAH. In either event, the ventricles enlarge and ICP rises.

Vasospasm

Vasospasm occurs in 19% to 40% of patients following traumatic SAH and can contribute to brain ischemia from other causes (15). The pathogenesis of vasospasm is unclear, but it could be caused by blood or oxyhemoglobin binding with endothelial nitric oxide (the endogenous relaxant factor). Free radicals and inflammatory mediators have also been implicated. Transcranial Doppler ultrasonography is used for diagnosis. Reduced middle cerebral artery blood flow and increased pulsatility index are usual findings after severe TBI (39). These global changes must be differentiated from the more local increases in flow velocity associated with vasospasm.

Cerebral Infection

Meningitis may follow basal skull fractures, vault fractures, prolonged external ventricular drainage (EVD) or craniotomy. Meningitis can also cause hydrocephalus and a late deterioration in consciousness level. Post-traumatic brain abscess is rare and usually follows a penetrating injury, especially gunshot or shrapnel wounds.

Reperfusion Injury

Free-radical generation during reperfusion is facilitated by fresh oxygen carried by the recovering circulation and free iron derived from the breakdown of extravascular hemoglobin. Under normal circumstances, intracellular enzyme systems metabolize free radicals so that they do not cause damage. It is speculated that the influx of calcium that follows TBI inactivates these enzymes and allows an excess of free-radical species to cause significant endothelial damage. Although direct measurement of free radicals is impossible, indirect evidence suggests that there is an increase following TBI (40).

UNIFYING THE EFFECTS OF SECONDARY (AND SOME PRIMARY) INSULTS
Cerebral Metabolic Rate for Oxygen

Under normal conditions, the brain requires 3.5 mL oxygen per 100 g of brain tissue per minute. This accounts for 20% of total body oxygen consumption. Oxygen requirements increase if the patient is febrile or suffering seizures. In patients with severe TBI, global cerebral metabolic rate for oxygen ($CMRO_2$) may be decreased by one-third to one-half. It is thought that this reduction occurs in the energy expenditure component that governs cellular activation and that the brain's basal metabolic requirements are unchanged (41).

Cerebral Blood Flow, Cerebral Perfusion Pressure, and Autoregulation

Fifteen percent of the cardiac output is required to deliver the brain's oxygen requirements. In addition to a high basal oxygen utilization requirement, the brain has limited reserves of glucose, which must also be delivered by the cerebral circulation. Aerobic oxidation of glucose via the glycolytic and tricarboxylic acid pathways is essential for the production of high-energy phosphates. Most of the energy generated is used to maintain ionic gradients. In the intact brain, CBF closely matches $CMRO_2$. Anything that reduces $CMRO_2$, such as hypothermia or barbiturates, also reduces CBF. CBF is determined by the pressure difference across the cerebral circulation, known as cerebral perfusion pressure (CPP), and vascular resistance. MAP is easily measured but the measurement of mean cerebral venous pressure is more difficult. For convenience, mean cerebral venous pressure is usually equated to ICP. Hence:

$$CPP = MAP - ICP$$

The normal brain requires a constant blood flow, which is achieved by CBF autoregulation. Between a CPP of 50 and 150 mmHg, blood flow is controlled by alterations in the resistance of the arterioles and precapillary segments. Above and below these values, CBF is pressure dependent. In the injured brain, autoregulation is sometimes lost and CBF becomes pressure dependent over the entire CPP range. In this situation, the relationship between $CMRO_2$ and CBF can become uncoupled. ☞ **For the patient with TBI, a CPP of >60–70 mmHg is generally sufficient to maintain cerebral oxygenation (42).** ☞

Arterial carbon dioxide tension ($PaCO_2$) has a significant effect on CBF (3–6% change in CBF per mmHg change in $PaCO_2$) in the normal brain. Hypercarbia increases CBF and hypocarbia decreases it. This phenomenon is known as carbon dioxide reactivity and is caused by CO_2-mediated changes in hydrogen ion concentration. ✒ **Excessive hyperventilation of patients with TBI may cause ischemia if CO_2 reactivity is preserved.** ✒ However, those patients with moderate to severe TBI often have diminished or absent CO_2 reactivity.

Intracranial Pressure

Essentially, the skull is a semiclosed box of fixed volume (1600 mL). The contents of the skull are the brain representing 80% of the total intracranial volume, blood 12% and CSF 8%. Blood and CSF can be shifted away from the skull. This provides the total cerebral contents with some ICP buffering capacity. Reduced compliance implies increasing stiffness. Elasticity is the converse of compliance. Small, slow increases in the volume of the brain can be compensated for by a reduction in CSF volume and cerebral blood volume. Thus, normal ICP is maintained until elasticity is exhausted at which point pressure within the skull rises.

✒ **The interpretation of a given ICP measurement must be made in the light of the underlying pathology and the speed with which that pathology has occurred.** ✒ Cytotoxic cellular edema is initially compensated for by movement of CSF out of the skull into the subarachnoid space around the spinal cord. If, however, SAH has caused a blockage in the interventricular canals or the basal cisterns, CSF movement out of the skull is restricted, the total contents of the skull are less elastic and for the same amount of cerebral swelling, the rise in ICP will be greater. Although this description may be useful in clinical practice, it is important to realize that the relationships between intracranial blood, CSF, and brain volume with ICP are extremely complex and that greater understanding of these relationships may lead to improvements in the management of TBI (43). ✒ **Current evidence suggests that 20–25 mmHg is the upper threshold above which treatment to lower ICP should be started (42).** ✒

THE ROLE OF MONITORING IN THE MANAGEMENT OF TRAUMATIC BRAIN INJURY

Multimodal monitoring of the patient with TBI is discussed in detail in Volume 2, Chapter 7. The importance of adequate monitoring cannot be overemphasized. Many of the current treatments for TBI have never been proven in prospective, randomized trials. Furthermore, many of the monitoring techniques employed in the ICU setting are subject to inaccuracies and doubts about their benefit. However, their utilities in detecting the trends of therapy are valuable. A Canadian study has shown that although 98.1% of surgeons use ICP monitors for patients with severe TBI, only 20.4% have confidence that ICP monitoring improves outcome (44). If a treatment is administered with the expectation that it will cause a specific effect, monitoring is required to detect that effect. If the treatment is ineffective for the specific result required or fails to produce a reduction in mortality or morbidity, attention should be directed to inappropriate treatment not necessarily inappropriate monitoring. Vasopressor drugs may have a limited effect in the presence of hypovolemia, and mannitol may not reduce ICP in the presence of hyperemia. Monitoring should be used in conjunction with knowledge of the injury process, clinical examination, laboratory measurements, and imaging.

MANAGEMENT OF TBI IN THE INTENSIVE CARE UNIT
The Evolution of Intensive Care Unit Management for Traumatic Brain Injury

Much of the management of TBI is intuitive and preferred therapy varies between institutions and countries. Guidelines have been issued in the United States using published studies to make evidence-based recommendations and in Europe, based on consensus statements by experienced senior physicians (42,45). There is no doubt that neurosurgical ICU practice has changed in recent years (46,47). Whether this change has been brought about by the publication of guidelines, or in spite of them, is unclear. What is certain is that practice is not 100% uniform. However, overall, there are more common points of management in centers around the globe than divergent. In addition, the science behind our therapies is still in its infancy. Current specific management considerations for TBI are reviewed in the following section.

Specific Therapies of Importance in the Management of Traumatic Brain Injury
Oxygen

Postmortem studies of head-injured patients often show a high proportion of patients with secondary ischemia. It is hardly surprising, therefore, that most treatises on the management of TBI advise that oxygen be given to prevent hypoxia. ✒ **During the resuscitation phase it is recommended that PaO_2 be maintained above 60 mmHg (8 kPa) (42).** ✒ Hypoxic insults during intensive care also increase mortality (48). Nowhere is an upper limit of PaO_2 recommended. Consequently, it is not unusual to find ICU patients with TBI being managed with PaO_2 values well above the normal range.

This approach may not be as safe as is commonly supposed. High concentrations of oxygen are toxic to the lungs and can cause the acute respiratory distress syndrome (ARDS) (49). The role of oxygen free radicals in causing secondary brain damage has been described above. It seems sensible to suggest that sufficient supplemental oxygen be given to maintain PaO_2 within the normal range and that the dose should be titrated in the same way as for all other drugs and fluids.

Intravascular Repletion for Hypotension

During the early period after injury, hypotension is strongly associated with an increase in mortality suggesting that poor perfusion leads to reduced oxygen delivery to the brain with significant ischemic consequences. Hypotension in the ICU may be equally devastating. For patients whose only hypotensive episode occurred in ICU, 66% either died or remained in a vegetative state compared to 17% for those patients who never suffer a hypotensive episode (48). The target systolic blood pressure appears to be 90 mmHg or more (42).

In a small group of patients with severe TBI and significant extracranial injuries, aggressive fluid resuscitation is associated with remarkably good outcomes suggesting that archaic practices of fluid restriction (to reduce edema) is not only unnecessary but potentially harmful (51,52). A fluid deficit of only 594 mL has an adverse effect on outcome after isolated TBI (53). Animal studies suggest that resuscitation can be successfully completed using physiological saline, hypertonic saline, hetastarch or whole blood provided that adequate volumes are given. Hypertonic saline, however, appears to have the additional advantage of reducing ICP (53). It is important to remember that all hypertonic solutions exert their effect by increasing plasma osmotic pressure. Water is drawn first from the interstitial space and then from the cells. However, excessive use of hypertonic solutions can cause dangerous intracellular dehydration and increase mortality (54). Hypertonic saline should not be used for prolonged periods unless additional water is given in the form of other fluids.

Hypotension has many causes including vasodilator sedatives, ventilation, incomplete resuscitation prior to ICU admission, and continued blood loss from a known injury. The ICU doctor should always be alert to the possibility that there are other undiagnosed injuries causing occult bleeding. The chest and abdomen are common sites for such injuries. ☞ **The management of hypotension must include not only fluid replacement but also identification of the cause.** ☞

Ventilation, PaCO₂, and Effects of Intrathoracic Pressure

The patient with severe TBI requiring admission to ICU is typically comatose and at high risk of airway obstruction and pulmonary aspiration because airway reflexes are obtunded. Consequently, endotracheal intubation and mechanical ventilation will already have started or will be indicated shortly after ICU admission. At this time, ICP monitoring is very helpful. As expected venous return will be maximized if mean intrathoracic pressure is kept to the minimum required for adequate oxygenation and carbon dioxide removal. In theory, improving cerebral venous drainage will assist in the control of ICP by minimizing cerebral venous engorgement. This implies the use of head elevation, smaller tidal volumes, and proportionately increased respiratory rates. If TBI is associated with pulmonary contusion, positive end expiratory pressure (PEEP) may be used to aid alveolar recruitment. Also, postural drainage facilitates removal of secretions. The amount of PEEP or reversal of head elevation that can safely be used is variable. Their use should be guided by their effect on ICP. In theory, both of these interventions may raise ICP. In practice, their effect is very much dependant on individual patient variables. Accordingly, ICP monitoring is an invaluable aid to optimizing respiratory management. Positive pressure ventilation is often cited as a cause of hypotension. Hypotension is unlikely in euvolemic patients, when physiological (7–15 mL/kg) tidal volumes are used, and its occurrence should provoke further thought concerning the adequacy of fluid resuscitation.

For the patient with TBI, another important benefit of ventilation is the ability to control $PaCO_2$. For the majority of patients, $PaCO_2$ should be maintained in the low normal range. A $PaCO_2$ of between 30 and 35 mmHg (4–4.5 kPa) is recommended in the United Kingdom and between 35 and 40 mmHg (4.5–5 kPa) in the United States. Improved survival has been demonstrated for patients in whom $PaCO_2$ is maintained at 35 rather than 25 mmHg and local reductions in cerebral perfusion have been demonstrated when $PaCO_2$ is between 27 and 32 mmHg (55,56). Chronic hyperventilation should be avoided particularly in the early days after TBI (42). However, a brief period of hyperventilation is an appropriate option if there is an acute deterioration in neurological status (42). This allows time for other therapies such as increased sedation and mannitol to become effective and also allows time for diagnostic CT scanning and if appropriate, urgent surgical intervention to control raised ICP.

Monitoring of jugular bulb venous oxygen saturation (SjO_2) and arteriojugular venous oxygen content differences ($AVdO_2$) will facilitate the identification of hyperemia as a cause of raised ICP. An SjO_2 of more than 80% indicates that the brain is receiving more oxygen than it can extract. This may be because of high CBF and increased oxygen delivery, but can also occur if the brain has died and metabolic processes have ceased. In the presence of preserved CO_2 reactivity and hyperemia, temporary hyperventilation will reduce ICP and is generally considered safe provided that the SjO_2 does not fall below 55% and the $AVdO_2$ does not exceed 9%. Hyperventilation in excess of these values may cause cerebral ischemia. Recent research, however, shows that even in the presence of acceptable SjO_2, localized areas of ischemia are often present (56).

Sedation, Analgesia, Neuromuscular Blockade

Sedation and analgesia are essential components to the management of ventilated patients. They permit the patient to be comfortably settled on the ventilator. During unpleasant interventions, boluses obtund the hypertensive response. For the patient with TBI, the effects of sedatives and analgesics on ICP, CPP, CBF, CO_2 vasoreactivity and seizure activity must be considered and the beneficial effects balanced against detrimental effects. The choice of agent also depends upon whether it can be administered by infusion and its duration of action when the infusion is discontinued. Even opioids such as Morpline, when administered as a low dose infusion, will have minimal respiratory depression, sedation, pupillary constriction or unwanted cardiovascular effects (57). Short-acting drugs are preferred for patients where the ventilation period is expected to be brief or when brain death tests may need to be performed. In some centers, cost may also dictate the choice of drug, although it is important to remember that the cost of an expensive drug may be offset by reduced ICU costs brought about by a reduction in time to extubation. Minimal data exists upon which to base a recommendation that any particular drug is more or less beneficial to use in the TBI patient (58). Propofol (0.1–0.5 mg/hr) and midazolam (1–6 mg/hr) are equally successful for long-term sedation of critically ill patients (59). Propofol may, or may not, have a cost advantage because weaning is more rapid (59,60). Lorazepam (0.05 mg/kg, then 0.007 mg/kg/hr) has also been advocated as a safe, cost-effective sedative for critically ill trauma patients (61). Dexmedetomidine, a new α_2-agonist, is increasingly used in critically ill patients, and may become an ideal drug for patients recovering from TBI (62). If possible, evidence-based sedation guidelines should be followed (63).

In the past, nondepolarizing neuromuscular blockade (NMB) drugs were routinely given to prevent rises in ICP secondary to coughing on the endotracheal tube. With the advent of ICP monitoring, use of NMB has decreased and is now reserved for patients in whom persistently elevated ICP is difficult to control. NMB drugs are also frequently used during transport when movement may provoke coughing on the endotracheal tube and inceases in ICP, or accidental extubation. The choice of NMB drug depends on the side effects and the anticipated clinical duration of use, just as with sedatives and analgesics. Pancuronium, vecuronium, and cisatricurium are commonly used (58). Pancuronium can cause tachycardia and minimal hypertension that may or may not be desirable depending on the ICP, CPP, and CO_2 reactivity. Its main advantage is its long duration of action and low cost. A disadvantage is that excretion is dependant on normal renal function. Atracurium can cause histamine release and hence hypotension when administered as a bolus but cardiovascular stability is the rule when it is given by infusion. Cisatricurium does not cause histamine release (thus more stable hemodynamics), and does not depend upon renal or hepatic function for clearance. Cisatricurium is degraded spontaneously via Hoffman degradation, and is useful in patients with multiple organ dysfunction syndrome (MODS). Vecuronium causes minimal hemodynamic disturbances and is inexpensive, but its duration of action will be slightly prolonged in patients with liver disease. Guidelines are available for the prolonged use of NMB drugs in the general ICU population (also see Volume 2, Chapter 6) (64).

Head Elevation and Extracerebral Venous Drainage

It is traditional to nurse the head-injured patient with a 30° head up tilt. This usually reduces ICP by 1 or 2 mmHg. Hypovolemic patients may, however, become hypotensive causing a greater reduction in CPP. If CPP falls, the horizontal position should be used until blood pressure is restored by volume resuscitation or vasopressors.

There is no evidence that catheters sited in the internal jugular veins have an important effect on venous drainage. Placement of internal jugular catheters, however, can cause raised ICP, particularly if the head is turned and the patient is tilted head down. At many institutions, the placement of a subclavian catheter without causing a pneumothorax is the preferred method for skilled practitioners. In addition, tape used to secure the endotracheal tube should be sufficiently loose that engorgement of the jugular veins does not occur.

Surgery for Evacuation of Hematomas

The decision to evacuate hematomas is made by the neurosurgical team. Small hematomas may be observed but require regular CT assessment because they can enlarge. Any hematoma causing greater than 5 mm of midline shift or persistently raised ICP is usually removed urgently to minimize ischemic damage.

Ventriculostomy for External Ventricular Drainage

ICP can be reduced by the intermittent or continuous drainage of small volumes of CSF through a ventriculostomy. A ventriculostomy is a catheter inserted into one of the lateral ventricles (Fig. 10). Uncontrolled continuous drainage of CSF can lead to the complete collapse of the ventricles. A closed external ventricular drainage (EVD) system should always be used to reduce the risk of infection.

Osmotic Diuretics for Control of Cytotoxic and Vasogenic Edema

Used in single doses, all osmotic diuretics are reasonably safe. Potential risks of repeated doses are hypokalemia, hyperosmolarity possibly causing renal failure, subdural hematoma, congestive cardiac failure, and coagulopathy.

1. Mannitol is the most commonly used osmotic diuretic, and has been used for decades without randomized trials documenting its efficacy. However, a recent randomized trial has demonstrated clear benefit for the use of bolus doses of mannitol for patients with localizing signs in the emergency room (65). In the ICU, trials are needed to demonstrate benefit and an optimal dosing regime. Contrary to common belief, the osmotic effect of mannitol on the cells is probably the least important of its mechanisms of action. Its ability to reduce blood viscosity, increase the deformability of erythrocytes, and induce constriction of pial arterioles is most likely more important (66,67).

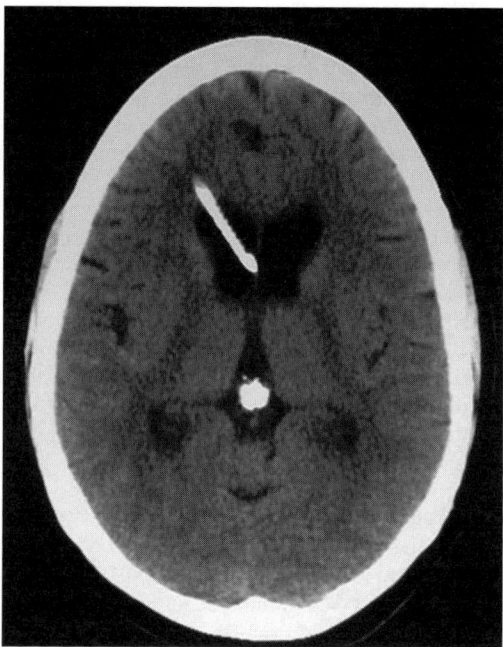

Figure 10 Computed tomograph of the brain showing the proper position and appearance of a ventriculostomy. The catheter is located in the frontal portion of the right lateral ventricle.

2. Hypertonic saline, from 3% to 23.4% has been used for ICP management; 7.5% saline as a single dose of 100 to 150 mL is commonly used for prehospital small volume resuscitation in Europe. Its use remains experimental in the United States. It reduces ICP but CBF is unaffected. This suggests that it works by an osmotic mechanism (68).

3. 23.4% saline has been used successfully for patients with refractory raised ICP who have failed to respond to mannitol (69). A single bolus of 30 mL given over 15 to 20 minutes through a central line did not alter the serum sodium concentration.

Loop Diuretics

Furosemide and other loop diuretics cause a diuresis and may reduce CSF formation. They may help to reduce ICP when used in conjunction with mannitol but are ineffective when used alone. Furthermore, both furosemide and mannitol may lead to hypotension, which requires volume repletion with physiological saline or colloid.

Steroids

The American standard is that steroids should not be used in the treatment of TBI (42). A more recent systematic review of randomized controlled trials concluded that "there remains considerable uncertainty over their effect" but this view has been challenged because exclusion of one of the trials changes the results to suggest that steroids do not have any benefit (70,71). Statistically, the systematic review could not rule out moderate harm from steroids (70). However, a significant increase in the incidence and severity of infectious complications has been noted in an observational study (72). Furthermore, dexamethasone can cause femoral and humeral head necrosis, and the non-steroid part of the methylprednisolone molecule causes anaphylaxis (73,74).

Vasopressors to Increase Cerebral Perfusion Pressure

Currently, a target CPP of >60 mmHg is recommended but some evidence suggests that this CPP may not be appropriate for all patients, particularly those who have preexisting hypertension (75,76). Vasopressors are used to increase CPP in euvolemic patients; adrenaline, noradrenaline, and dopamine are frequent choices. None have been specifically investigated with regard to outcome after TBI. The choice is typically made because of the personal preferences and/or biases of the ICU team. A more logical approach might be to monitor the circulation with a pulmonary artery flotation catheter and to choose a vasopressor after reviewing the findings. Pulmonary artery catheters can cause some morbidity and should not be used without an assessment of the risks and benefits.

Barbiturates

Barbiturates are thought to have several potentially useful mechanisms of action. These are altered vascular tone, suppression of metabolism, and free-radical scavenging. Regardless, the use of barbiturates is controversial. They may be helpful in reducing refractory raised ICP in salvageable, hemodynamically stable patients although there is no evidence that outcome is improved (42,77). Anaerobic metabolism is not always prevented even when electroencephalographic burst suppression is achieved (78).

Temperature Control Including Hypothermia

Pyrexia is associated with seizures, infection, an inflammatory response and thalamic injury. Depending on the cause, it is generally agreed that definitive treatment should be started and core temperature reduced to as near normal as possible. Paracetamol (acetaminophen) and surface cooling are simple, nonspecific methods that are easy to use.

Hypothermia reduces ICP but whether its use for the treatment of refractory raised ICP improves outcome is unproven (79). In the general population of blunt-trauma victims, hypothermia is an independent predictor of increased mortality (80). Despite numerous animal experiments suggesting that early hypothermia is protective in TBI, it has proved ineffective in the largest and most recent randomized human trial (81). The reasons for this disappointing finding are probably multifactorial but it has been shown that hypothermia below 35°C impairs cerebral oxygenation possibly because of a leftward shift of the oxygen dissociation curve (82). Other possible factors include prolonged time from injury to achieving hypothermia, the methods of cooling used, the difficulty of maintaining a constant temperature, and the duration of cooling (83).

Seizure Control

☞ **There is minimal evidence for the routine use of anticonvulsants to prevent seizures (84).** ☞ Phenytoin and sodium valproate are equally effective at treating seizures that do occur (85). Lamotrigine has not been tested for the prevention of early seizures but is of interest because it may also increase the speed of recovery from TBI (86). If anticonvulsants are used, they should be limited to the first week after head injury.

Decompressive Craniectomy

Decompressive craniectomy soon after TBI does not improve outcome (87). Some centers use decompressive craniectomy for refractory raised ICP but its benefit has not been tested in a controlled trial. Anecdotal evidence suggests that this procedure is useful when high doses of vasopressors are causing side effects and adequate perfusion pressure is becoming difficult to maintain (88). Until the bone flap is replaced, the brain is at greater than normal risk of injury particularly if the patient is confused or unstable while ambulatory. Furthermore, replacement of the bone flap is associated with the risks of postoperative EDH and significant infection. In the absence of clear evidence of benefit, the decision to proceed to decompressive craniectomy should be made after careful assessment of the risks and benefits for the individual patient.

Chest Physiotherapy and Endotracheal Suctioning

ICP and CPP increase with both these procedures. In the majority of patients, ICP falls to baseline values rapidly (89). If the patient has significant secretions, failure to provide physiotherapy and suction can result in consolidation and hypoxia, which may lead to ARDS. In order to reduce the intracerebral effects of suction and physiotherapy, many clinicians use preoxygenation and a bolus of sedative prior to the intervention.

Nimodipine to Control Vasospasm

Following nontraumatic SAH, the routine use of nimodipine has dramatically reduced the incidence of secondary ischemic damage due to vasospasm. Some favorable results have been obtained using nimodipine following traumatic SAH, yet its routine use in traumatic SAH is not universally accepted (90). Also see Volume 2, Chapter 14 for extensive discussion of nimodipine and other treatments for cerebral vasospasm following SAH.

Management of Hyperglycemia

In a study of 1548 surgical patients including 68 suffering from trauma or burns, intensive insulin therapy to control hyperglycemia reduced mortality by almost one-half (91). Patients with MODs and sepsis derived most benefit with significant reductions in the incidence of blood infections, acute renal failure, and polyneuropathy (also see Volume 2, Chapter 60). A reduction in red cell transfusion requirement and duration of mechanical ventilation were also observed. It is tempting to suggest that blood glucose should be maintained within the normal range because of the association of hyperglycemia with increased mortality following TBI particularly if the brain is ischemic. Although there are minimal standards for the management of hyperglycemia in TBI, it is clearly unacceptable to allow severe hyperglycemia to persist untreated. In the past, blood glucose was usually maintained between 125 and 175 mL/dL. However, with the newly recognized benefits of tight blood glucose with intensive insulin therapy, most units are now keeping the glucose in tighter range (e.g., 90–120 mg/dL).

Management by Standardized Protocol

☞ **A standardized protocol for the management of ICP appears to provide more consistent control (92).** ☞ Similarly, a standardized protocol for CPP management of patients admitted with a Glasgow Coma Scale (GCS) of less than 8 claimed a mortality rate better than any described previously. Only 31% of patients died or remained in a vegetative state (93). Another protocol designed to control both ICP and CPP also achieved a dead or vegetative rate of 30% but even better results were obtained when the therapy goal was cerebral extraction of oxygen. Use of this parameter permitted hyperventilation to be used for the treatment of hyperemia (94). A randomized study comparing a CBF targeted protocol against an ICP targeted protocol failed to show a significant difference in mortality between the groups. The most significant finding of the study was that both protocols prevented secondary ischemic insults (95).

In practice, equally good results are obtained by strict adherence to local protocols that may differ from each other in several ways. It has been suggested that this is because the use of a protocol implies exemplary critical care. The subtleties of management may be less important than the prevention of hypotension (96).

The Lund Protocol

There is evidence to support the belief that as much as 75% of brain swelling is due to cytotoxic edema and only 25% of increased brain bulk is due to vasogenic edema and hyperemia (97). The protocols discussed above share a common approach: treatment is designed to control cytotoxic and vasogenic edema with the primary intention of reducing ICP and increasing CPP, CBF, and hence cerebral oxygenation.

A completely different approach is used in Lund, Sweden. The two goals of therapy are prevention of cerebral hypoxia (by maintaining euvolemia) and control of vasogenic edema (by maintaining colloid osmotic pressure, reducing MAP, and constricting precapillary resistance vessels). The specifics of the Lund Management Protocol are summarized in Table 6. Of the 53 patients with severe TBI and ICP greater than 25 mmHg treated using the new Lund protocol, 8% died and 13% were left in a vegetative state or severely disabled (98). Like many other aspects of TBI management, the Lund protocol has not been tested in a randomized controlled trial. At present, all that can be concluded is that the results are impressive and have been replicated outside Lund (99). It may be that the Lund team has identified a key area where targeted intervention improves outcome. Alternatively, the Lund protocol may be yet another example of how exemplary ICU care combined with aggressive treatment of hypovolemia improves outcome.

ASSOCIATED ORGAN SYSTEM COMPLICATIONS FOLLOWING TRAUMATIC BRAIN INJURY
Neurogenic Pulmonary Edema

Neurogenic pulmonary edema is thought to be due to massive alpha-adrenergic discharge at the time of injury (100). A transient surge in left atrial and pulmonary artery occlusion pressure disrupts the alveolar-capillary membrane leading to massive fluid leakage into the lungs and airways. The clinical picture is similar to severe ARDS, and ideal respiratory management includes oxygen, ventilation with low tidal volumes of approximately 6 mL/kg, maximum peak airway pressures of 35 mmHg, PEEP of 5 to 10 mmHg, and an inverse inspiratory/expiratory ratio. The prone position also improves oxygenation in some patients. Clearly, some of these interventions may increase ICP or decrease CPP. Management should be individualized to each patient and compromises in the optimum management of both brain and lungs are often necessary. At its worst neurogenic pulmonary edema is so severe that the patient drowns in edema fluid. Even in the best institutions, adequate oxygenation cannot always be achieved. Accurate fluid management is crucial and a pulmonary artery flotation catheter can be very helpful to optimize cardiovascular parameters. Obviously fluid overload must be avoided but many of these patients become volume depleted as a result of the huge loss of proteinaceous fluid from the lungs.

Hypernatremia

Hypernatremia associated with TBI is usually a result of water depletion. Commonly, it is caused by the use of mannitol or diabetes insipidus.

Mannitol-induced hypernatremia is associated with excessive volumes of dilute urine that coincide with doses of mannitol. Treatment includes water replacement given via the enteral route or 5% dextrose given intravenously. Mannitol may also contribute to hypomagnesaemia and hypophosphatemia (101).

Diabetes insipidus should be suspected when the urine output is over 200 mL/hr for two consecutive hours and the serum sodium is rising. The diagnosis is confirmed if the urine osmolality is lower than plasma osmolality (also see Chapter 44). Desmopressin, 1–2 μg subcutaneously or intravenously, as single or repeated doses is the treatment of choice.

Table 6 The Lund Management Protocol

Goal	Target	Intervention
Reduce capillary hydrostatic pressure	CPP 60–70 mmHg (but 50 mmHg acceptable)	Metoprolol Clonidine Dihydroergotamine
Reduce cerebral blood volume	ICP < 25 mmHg	Thiopental Dihydroergotamine
Reduce stress response and cerebral energy metabolism	Adequate sedation and analgesia	Benzodiazepines Fentanyl Low-dose thiopental
Fluid balance and maintenance of colloid osmotic pressure	Hemoglobin 125–140 g/L Albumin 40 g/L Equal of slightly negative fluid balance	Albumin infusion Frusemide Blood Enteral nutrition
Intermittent CSF drainage	ICP < 25 mmHg	EVD

Abbreviation: EVD, external ventricular drainage.

Hyponatremia: SIADH vs. Cerebral Salt Wasting Syndrome

Hyponatremia is common in neurosurgical patients, and is often attributed to the syndrome of inappropriate secretion of antidiuretic hormone (SIADH). This syndrome is characterized by a urine osmolality which is greater than serum osmolality, and an elevated urinary sodium concentration (typically >20 mmol/L). Additionally, SIADH patients have normal or slightly elevated intravascular volume. Aggressive fluid restriction may be all that is needed to correct this syndrome.

It is important to distinguish between SIADH and the cerebral salt wasting syndrome, which also occurs commonly following TBI, because their treatments are divergent (102). Cerebral salt wasting syndrome occurs with concurrent water loss, and these patients are volume depleted. Careful assessment of trends in fluid and sodium balance combined with urine and serum osmolarity measurements usually provide the clues to the correct diagnosis. In cerebral salt wasting syndrome, there is an excess loss of sodium compared to changes in other parameters (osmolality may be increased with cerebral salt wasting syndrome). Treatment for SIADH is dramatically different from that for cerebral salt wasting syndrome. SIADH requires only fluid restriction, whereas cerebral salt wasting syndrome requires repletion of intravascular fluid as well as salt. Accordingly 3% saline is often administered for patients with cerebral salt wasting syndrome.

Hyponatremia when severe causes cerebral edema and seizures, thus treatment is required. However, hypertonic saline should be given slowly once the serum sodium is greater than 120 mmol/L. The reason for raising the serum sodium slowly is the association between rapid correction and central pontine myelinolysis (103). Accordingly, 3% saline is often given in addition to larger quantities of normal saline or albumin, until intravascular volume is replenished in the setting of cerebral salt wasting syndrome.

OTHER ASPECTS OF CRITICAL CARE FOR TRAUMATIC BRAIN INJURY PATIENTS
Enteral Nutrition

Patients with severe TBI are hypercatabolic and have reduced immune function (104). Early enteral feeding is essential to prevent malnutrition with attendant muscle wasting. Traditional wisdom had maintained that it is difficult to establish enteral nutrition early in head-injured patients because they have gastric stasis and/or intestinal ileus. However, early enteral feeding is successful in most patients. The benefits of jejunal versus gastric feeding have been studied, with the results showing that gastric feeding is successful in 97% of patients (105). Gastric feeding using a percutaneous endoscopic gastrostomy (PEG) starting on day 3 is also successful in 97% of patients (105). During the recovery phase, a PEG is helpful if the patient has dysphagia or diminished protective airway reflexes. Many centers believe that feeding via the gastric route using a nasogastric tube can and should be started shortly after admission, and is successful in the majority of patients. When enteral feeding is problematic, maxolon or low-dose erythromycin is used to encourage gastric emptying (106,107).

Acute Respiratory Distress Syndrome and Sepsis

ARDS is the most severe form of a spectrum of lung injury that occurs after injury and sepsis. In its less severe form, it is referred to as acute lung injury (ALI). ALI occurs in 20% of comatose TBI patients and is associated with the global severity of TBI rather than specific injury patterns (108). **TBI patients with ALI are almost three times more likely to die than patients with similar head injury severity but no ALI.**

ARDS causes more severe hypoxia than ALI. Numerous strategies have been suggested for the treatment of ALI/ARDS but although most of them increase PaO$_2$, none confer survival benefit (109,110). Over the years, however, mortality from ARDS has declined. The decline is probably due to better attention to fluid balance combined with lung-protective strategies. The patient with TBI and ARDS presents a particular challenge. Current treatment of ARDS includes reducing inspired oxygen concentration so that PaO$_2$ is maintained at around 60 mmHg (8 kPa) and adjustments to the ventilator so that tidal volumes and airway pressures are limited. These ventilator adjustments commonly cause hypercapnia. For the patient with TBI, relative hypoxia and absolute hypercapnia are undesirable with respect to brain recovery. Herein lies the challenge. Interventions must be tailored to each individual patient's physiological state, which will vary over time. It is helpful to maintain the PaO$_2$ at about 75 mmHg (10 kPa) and to manage PaCO$_2$ according to the ICP response.

Sepsis and multiorgan failure are common in critically ill patients, and patients with TBI are no exception. The use of prophylactic antibiotics is controversial except in the case of penetrating head injuries (111). Meticulous attention to infection control techniques will reduce the risk of infection.

Weaning and Extubation

There is little consensus regarding the best method of weaning patients with TBI from the ventilator. In addition to the normal respiratory parameters, the clinician should also be aware of the impact of weaning on ICP and CPP. For patients with uncomplicated TBI one method is to first reduce the respiratory rate so that PaCO$_2$ rises to at least 5 kPa. If ICP does not increase, paralysis is discontinued (if it is still being used). Lastly, sedation is reduced stepwise until either ICP rises or breathing commences. Assuming that ICP does not rise, the patient is weaned as rapidly as tolerated from synchronized intermittent mandatory ventilation to spontaneous ventilation with pressure support. As sedation is withdrawn, many relatively alert patients become hypertensive and ICP sometimes rises. At this point it is necessary for the clinician to decide whether hypertension and raised ICP will settle after extubation and whether the patient has sufficient airway control to manage following extubation. If it is thought that the patient will cope after extubation, weaning to independent breathing and extubation should proceed as quickly as possible watching for signs of clinical deterioration in the GCS. Commonly, the patient's GCS does not deteriorate despite the rise in ICP and extubation can be achieved uneventfully. In the event that the patient does not have adequate airway control and/or protective reflexes, a tracheostomy is indicated prior to a second attempt at weaning. TBI patients recovering from lower respiratory tract infection or ARDS usually require a tracheostomy to facilitate the weaning process.

Indications for Tracheostomy

In general tracheostomy is indicated to protect the lower airway, to aid weaning in the presence of copious secretions or muscle weakness, and as an aid to patient comfort. Predisposing factors indicating potential need for tracheostomy in patients with TBI include admission GCS of less than 8, injury severity score greater than 25 or ventilator days of more than 7 (112). Tracheostomy, whether performed percutaneously or by traditional surgical techniques, carries the risk of hypercarbia and sometimes hypoxia. For this reason, it is better to delay performing a tracheostomy until ICP is under control and the condition of the lungs has improved to a point where weaning is likely to be successful.

The Diagnosis and Treatment of Agitation Following Extubation

Agitation is a common problem following extubation of patients who have suffered a severe TBI. ☞ **It is essential to distinguish between agitation that results from the primary brain injury and agitation due to hypoxia, hypercarbia, or cerebral swelling; the latter are easily diagnosed by arterial blood gas analysis and the former by CT scan.** ☞

Whichever cause is identified, sedation and reintubation and ventilation for 24 hours are often the safest and most appropriate treatments. Sedatives such as benzodiazepines or haloperidol can be given but may reduce GCS to the point where there is a risk of airway compromise. Consequently, sedatives should be used with caution and frequent monitoring of GCS and airway status. Many head-injured patients suffer prolonged headache and simple analgesics sometimes reduce agitation. Physical restraint is an option but should only be used if this is believed to be in the patient's best interests and after discussion with members of the family.

REHABILITATION BEGINS IN THE INTENSIVE CARE UNIT

Most patients with severe TBI face a prolonged period of rehabilitation following discharge from acute hospital care. In the ICU, some rehabilitation techniques are appropriate. Even though dramatic improvements may not be achieved this early in the patient's care, an awareness of rehabilitation techniques and prevention of pressure sores and limb contractures can be important in facilitating eventual successful rehabilitation (see Volume 2, Chapter 66).

Appropriate Sensory Stimulation

Given that some aspects of recovery appear to be due to the recruitment of alternative neural pathways, sensory stimulation is commonly practiced in the ICU setting. Favorite music and frequent touching are encouraged. The evidence that these interventions make a real difference is sparse but involvement of family members comforts them at a time when they feel most helpless.

Spasticity and Contractures

Increased muscle tone is a common feature of severe TBI. Not only is this condition painful but also it can lead to permanent deformities of the limbs that can make subsequent mobilization difficult. Benzodiazepines, baclofen, dantrolene, and tinzandine (a clonidine analogue) have been recommended for the treatment of spasticity (113). All can cause sedation as a side effect. Consequently some specialized centers prefer to use botulinum toxin type A injected locally into affected muscles (113). Sometimes splints are used in addition or as an alternative to drug therapy. As with so many other aspects of head injury management, the long-term consequences of spasticity must be balanced against short-term side effects of drugs.

Heterotopic Ossification of Joints

Heterotopic ossification of joints occurs after severe head injury and can limit joint mobility. The diagnosis is likely if a joint becomes warm and swollen or the range of movement diminishes and is confirmed using plain radiography. Management is difficult and includes antiinflammatory drugs such as indomethacin, surgical removal of ectopic bone, physical therapy, and radiation treatment (114).

Management of Long Bone Fractures

Outcome following TBI with associated long bone fractures depends mainly on the severity of the TBI. Fracture management should be a secondary consideration in the immediate aftermath of injury. However, initial planning should anticipate full neurological recovery of the patient. Adequate resuscitation and control of ICP and CPP during anesthesia and surgery are of paramount importance (115). The treatment of fractures should be planned to facilitate nursing care and in the longer term, to ensure that mobilization is not hindered by limb deformities or nonunion of fractures.

DYING IN THE INTENSIVE CARE UNIT FROM A HEAD INJURY

All deaths following trauma are stressful for families and staff alike. Death from head injury can be particularly difficult because the external signs of injury may be minimal and the severity of the underlying injury may be difficult to comprehend (see Chapters 16 and 67–69).

Brain Death and Brainstem Death

Cultural, social, religious, and legal differences mean that the definition of death and hence the diagnosis of death differ between countries. Judaism, for example, requires that the patient's heartbeat and breathing cease before death can be certified. Some countries, such as the United Kingdom, require that the brainstem is dead for death to be legally diagnosed. Yet others require that the whole brain is dead before death can be declared. Consequently each country and/or state has its own criteria for the diagnosis of death after head injury, which is discussed in detail in Volume 2, Chapter 16.

Organ Donation After Traumatic Brain Injury

The diagnosis of brain death or brainstem death permits removal of organs for the purposes of transplantation while the heart is still beating and oxygenation of the tissues is maintained by means of mechanical ventilation. Although the grief of family members will be acute at the time of death, many relatives eventually take comfort from the knowledge that organ donation has taken place. One organ donor can save more than nine lives and improve the quality of life for many others. A complete review of the determination of brain death and management of the brain dead organ donor is proved in Volume 2, Chapter 16.

Communication with Family Members

The importance of sensitive and realistic communication with family members cannot be overemphasized. It is essential too that all members of the team communicate with one another so that confusing and contradictory information is not given. Death is much easier to accept if information is staged. Constant discussion with the family will ensure that deteriorations are communicated as they occur until the time that death becomes inevitable and the diagnosis is made. Preparation of the family for the death of the loved one is not only considerate but also facilitates the decision to proceed with organ donation (116,117).

Withhold or Withdrawal of Treatment

Not all head-injured patients die quickly as a result of brain death. Nevertheless, many injuries are ultimately not survivable, but death is delayed by the intensive support provided in an ICU. Current wisdom is that early intensive intervention is provided to all injured patients. When stabilization in the ICU has been achieved, the consequence of this approach is that ICU clinicians must, in conjunction with their neurosurgical colleagues, reassess the patient's potential for survival. For a few patients, the decision to withhold or withdraw active treatment is the inevitable consequence because further intervention is futile. The decision to withdraw treatment is based on experience and opinion and is emotionally difficult. Despite the risk of potential criticism from relatives, we owe it to our patients to ensure that inevitable death occurs in as dignified a manner as possible and with the minimum of medical intervention. This does not mean that routine nursing care and comfort sedation and analgesia should not be given. It does mean that prolonged ventilation and vasopressor support are inappropriate and should be discontinued.

UNCERTAINTIES IN THE MANAGEMENT OF TRAUMATIC BRAIN INJURY

The need for prolonged rehabilitation after TBI has already been alluded to and the consequences of TBI of all severities discussed. TBI also shortens the time to onset of Alzheimer's disease and increases the risk of suicide (118,119). No association has been found between TBI and the subsequent risk of primary brain tumors (120).

ICU management of TBI is targeted towards reducing secondary brain injury. In the future, antagonist cocktails that prevent the molecular cascades that occur shortly after injury will undoubtedly be developed. Because the molecular mechanisms of TBI are so complex and a balance between the protective and damaging effects of some of the cascades must be maintained, hopes that this will be an option in the near future are not realistic.

Many of the changes seen in the brain following TBI have been described in localized areas only. Currently, however, TBI management is restricted to global techniques in the hope that the damaged part of the brain will benefit. Some global therapies have the potential to damage normal brain. Hyperventilation, for example, is more effective in areas of brain that maintain the ability to autoregulate. Thus, excessive vasoconstriction will occur preferentially in areas of undamaged brain that could be rendered ischemic. Furthermore, blood flow may take the path of lesser resistance and be preferentially directed to damaged brain, thus causing local hyperemia. ☞ **All those who care for head-injured patients need to remember that the evidence for their management is strictly limited and that therapies considered acceptable today may be obsolete in the near future.** ☞ Not that many years ago, strict fluid restriction was recommended to reduce cerebral edema. It is now accepted that this treatment method may compromise circulating blood volume, increase viscosity, and reduce cerebral perfusion and blood flow (51).

There is a dearth of high quality evidence from randomized trials that the practitioner can refer to for guidance in the management of TBI. Clearly, there is a need to maintain CBF at a level sufficient to maintain the injured brain's global oxygen and glucose requirements. How this might be achieved is still debated.

EYE TO THE FUTURE

In the future, brain repair facilitated by nerve growth factors, tissue transplantation, and gene therapy may become available and would become the treatment of choice for TBI. Before that, it is likely that pharmacological interventions will be developed that either enhance natural protective mechanisms or that mitigate the damaging effects of the cascades activated by the release of toxic substances from dead and dying brain tissue. For example, intact female rats have a survival advantage over males and ovariectomized females (121). Progesterone given to male rats significantly reduces cerebral edema (122). Melatonin, a free-radical scavenger, is neuroprotective in mice (123). Cyclosporin A, which reduces mitochondrial membrane permeability and limits necrosis of cortical tissue, is neuroprotective in rats (124). These medications are already used and their safety profile is known, so with appropriate randomized controlled trials, they could be tested in humans relatively easily and rapidly. Also encouraging is the discovery of CNS 2103 in viper venom, which may lead to the development of brain-specific calcium antagonists (125). Ischemic preconditioning also significantly reduces contusion volume in rats, however, it is difficult to imagine how this might be used to protect humans (126).

Although there are many exciting developments that could become available in the next few years, we should not forget current possibilities. Hypothermia may yet prove to be helpful and despite evidence-based guidelines being available, clinical practice is still inconsistent (127). Although the search for new and better therapies must continue, it is probable that we could make further inroads into TBI mortality and morbidity if only we used existing therapies properly.

SUMMARY

☞ **The effects of a head injury are for life.** ☞ At present exemplary basic care is the best that can be offered. Adequate oxygenation and blood pressure are essential. Control of ICP by surgical means, gentle ventilation, control of $PaCO_2$, and the use of diuretics are standard therapies. Adequate sedation and analgesia are helpful in controlling ICP as well as a basic human right. Paralysis is sometimes needed. CPP should be maintained between 60 and 70 mmHg to facilitate cerebral oxygenation. Interventions to prevent secondary injury due to chemical mediators have been unsuccessful so far. Good nutrition is important. Prevention of fever, seizures, infection, and contractures can all contribute to an improved outcome. In the future, it may be possible to prevent secondary damage due to chemical mediators. An even more exciting development will be the facilitation of neuronal repair. In the meantime, it behooves us all to minimize secondary insults and to manage our patients guided by the best evidence available.

KEY POINTS

- The function of certain portions of damaged brain can be taken over by other areas, for example, the damaged brain is thought to exhibit a certain degree of neural plasticity.
- The goal of treatment for TBI is to reduce morbidity and improve outcome.
- The full effects of the ICU management of head injury may not be apparent until years after rehabilitation is complete.
- Rehospitalization occurs in 23% of TBI patients in the first year after injury and declines to 17% at five years after injury.
- Secondary brain injuries (Table 5) are of particular interest because they are potentially preventable.
- A systolic blood pressure of less than 90 mmHg occurring between the time of TBI and completion of resuscitation is associated with a 33% increase in mortality.
- An arterial oxygen tension (PaO_2) of less than 60 mmHg (8 kPa) occurring between the time of TBI and completion of resuscitation is also associated with an increase in morbidity and mortality but to a lesser extent than the effect of hypotension.
- The highest blood sugar occurring in the first 24 hours of ICU care is linearly correlated with mortality (Fig. 8).
- Although human outcome data is controversial, fever should be prevented in TBI patients.
- For the patient with TBI, a CPP of >60–70 mmHg is generally sufficient to maintain cerebral oxygenation.
- Excessive hyperventilation of patients with TBI may cause ischemia if CO_2 reactivity is preserved.
- The interpretation of a given ICP measurement must be made in the light of the underlying pathology and the speed with which that pathology has occurred.
- Current evidence suggests that 20–25 mmHg is the upper threshold above which treatment to lower ICP should be started.
- During the resuscitation phase it is recommended that PaO_2 be maintained above 60 mmHg (8 kPa).
- The management of hypotension must include not only fluid replacement but also identification of the cause.
- There is minimal evidence for the routine use of anticonvulsants to prevent seizures.
- A standardized protocol for the management of ICP appears to provide more consistent control.
- TBI patients with ALI are almost three times more likely to die than patients with similar head injury severity but no ALI.
- It is essential to distinguish between agitation that results from the primary brain injury and agitation due to hypoxia, hypercarbia, or cerebral swelling; the latter are easily diagnosed by arterial blood gas analysis and the former by CT scan.
- All those who care for head-injured patients need to remember that the evidence for their management is

strictly limited and that therapies considered acceptable today may be obsolete in the near future.
- The effects of a head injury are for life.

REFERENCES

1. 109 NIH Consensus Statement Online. Rehabilitation of persons with traumatic brain injury. 1998. Available at: http://consensus.nih.gov/1998/1998TraumaticBrainInjury109html.htm [Accessed-Nov. 8, 2006]; 16:1–41.
2. Sosin DM, Sniezek JE, Waxweiler RJ. Trends in death associated with traumatic brain injury, 1979 through 1992: Success and failure. JAMA 1995; 273:1778–1780.
3. Jennett B, Bond M. Assessment of outcome after severe brain damage. Lancet 1975; 1(7905): 480–484.
4. Copes WS, Stark MM, Lawnick MM, et al. Linking data from national trauma and rehabilitation registry. J Trauma 1996; 40:428–436.
5. Dombovy ML, Olek AC. Recovery and rehabilitation following traumatic brain injury. Brain Inj 1997; 11:305–318.
6. Hoofien D, Gilboa A, Vakil E, Donovick PJ. Traumatic brain injury (TBI) 10–20 years later: a comprehensive outcome study of psychiatric symptomatology, cognitive abilities and psychosocial functioning. Brain Inj 2001; 15:189–209.
7. Powell JM, Machamer JE, Temkin NR, Dikmen SS. Self-report of extent of recovery and barriers to recovery after traumatic brain injury: a longitudinal study. Arch Phys Med Rehabil 2001; 82:1025–1030.
8. Katz DI, Alexander MP, Klein RB. Recovery of arm function in patients with paresis after traumatic brain injury. Arch Phys Med Rehabil 1998; 79:488–493.
9. Millis SR, Rosenthal M, Novack TA, et al. Long-term neuropsychological outcome after traumatic brain injury. J Head Trauma Rehabil 2001; 16:343–355.
10. Levin HS, Boake C, Song J, et al. Validity and sensitivity to change of the extended Glasgow Outcome Scale in mild to moderate traumatic brain injury. J Neurotrauma 2001; 18(6):575–584.
11. Rappaport M, Hall KM, Hopkins K, Belleza T, Cope DN. Disability rating scale for severe head trauma: coma to community. Arch Phys Med Rehabil 1982; 63:118–123.
12. Azouvi P. Neuroimaging correlates of cognitive and functional outcome after traumatic brain injury. Curr Opin Neurol 2000; 13 Dec:665–669.
13. Marwitz JH, Cifu DX, Englander J, High WM. A multi-center analysis of rehospitalizations five years after brain injury. J Head Trauma Rehabil 2001; 16:307–317.
14. Shavelle RM, Strauss DJ, Whyte J, Day SM, Yu YL. Long-term causes of death after traumatic brain injury. Am J Phys Med Rehabil 2001; 80:510–516.
15. Cold GE, Dahl B. Topics in Neuroanaesthesia and Intensive Care. Berlin: Springer-Verlag, 2002.
16. Zimmerman RA, Bilaniuk LF, Generalli T. Computed tomography of shearing injuries in cortical white matter. Radiology 1978; 127:393–96
17. Waxman SG, deGroot J. Correlative Neuroanatomy. 22nd ed. Englewood Cliffs, New Jersey: Prentice Hall, 1995.
18. Hoff JT, Xi G. Brain edema from intracerebral hemorrhage. Acta Neurochir Suppl 2003; 86:11–15.
19. Miller MT, Pasquale M, Kurek S, et al. Initial head computed tomographic scan characteristics have a liner relationship with initial intracranial pressure after trauma. J Trauma 2004; 56(5):967–973.
20. Green KA, Jacobowitz R, Marciano FF, et al. Impact of traumatic subarachnoid hemorrhage on outcome in nonpenetrating head injury. Part 2: relationship to clinical course and outcome variables during acute hospitalization. J Trauma 1996; 41:964–971.
21. Jackowski A, Crockard A, Burnstock G, Russell RR, Kristek F. Time course of intracranial pathophysiological changes

following experimental subarachnoid haemorrhage in the rat. J Cereb Blood Flow Metab 1990; 10:835–849.

22. Sato M, Chang E, Igarashi T, Noble LJ. Neuronal injury and loss after traumatic brain injury: time course and regional variability. Brain Res 2001; 917:45–54.

23. Tecoult E, Mesenge C, Stutzmann JM, Plotkine M, Wahl F. Influence of anaesthesia protocol in experimental traumatic brain injury. J Neurosurg Anesthesiol 2000; 12:255–261.

24. Goodman JC, Valadka AB, Gopinath SP, Uzura M, Robertson CS. Extracellular lactate and glucose alterations in the brain after head injury measured by microdialysis. Crit Care Med 1999; 27:1965–1973.

25. Gong QZ, Phillips LL, Lyeth BG. Metabotropic glutamate receptor protein alterations after traumatic brain injury in rats. J Neurotrauma 1999; 16:893–902.

26. Weber JT, Rzigalinski BA, Willoughby KA, Moore SF, Ellis EF. Alterations in calcium mediated signal transduction after traumatic injury of cortical neurons. Cell Calcium 1999; 26:289–299.

27. Petrov T, Page AB, Owen CR, Rafols JA. Expression of the inducible nitric oxide synthetase in distinct cellular types after traumatic brain injury: an in situ hybridization and immunocytochemical study. Acta Neuropathol (Berl) 2000; 100:196–204.

28. Hutchinson JS, Derrane RE, Johnston DL, et al. Neuronal apoptosis inhibitory protein expression after traumatic brain injury in the mouse. J Neurotrauma 2001; 18:1333–1347.

29. Nilsson B, Nordström C-H. Experimental head injury in the rat. Rat 3: Cerebral blood flow and oxygen consumption after concussive impact acceleration. J Neurosurg 1997; 47: 262–273.

30. Bryan RM, Cherian L, Robertson C. Regional cerebral blood flow after controlled cortical impact injury in rats. Anesth Analg 1995; 80:687–695.

31. Chesnut RM, Marshall LF, Klauber MR, et al. The role of secondary brain injury in determinging outcome from severe head injury. J Trauma 1993; 34:216–222.

32. Walia S, Sutcliffe AJ. The relationship between blood glucose, mean arterial pressure and outcome after severe head injury. Injury 2002; 33(4):339–344..

33. Rovlias A, Kotsou S. The influence of hyperglycemia on neurological outcome in patients with severe head injury. Neurosurg 2000; 46:335–343.

34. Lam AM, Winn HR, Cullen BF, Sundling N. Hyperglycemia and neurological outcome in patients with head injury. J Neurosurg 1991; 75:545–551.

35. Chatzipanteli K, Alonso OF, Kraydieh S, Dietrich WD. Importance of posttraumatic hypothermia and hyperthermia on the inflammatory response after fluid percussion brain injury: biochemical and immunocytochemical studies. J Cereb Blood Flow Metab 2000; 20:531–542.

36. Dietrich WD, Alonso O, Halley M, Busto R. Delayed posttraumatic brain hyperthermia worsens outcome after fluid percussion brain injury: a light and electron microscopic study in rats. Neurosurgery 1996; 38:533–541.

37. Vespa PM, Nuwer MR, Nenov V, et al. Increased incidence and impact of nonconvulsive and convulsive seizures after traumatic brain injury as detected by continuous electroencephalographic monitoring. J Neurosurg 1999; 91:750–760.

38. Guyott LL, Michael DB. Post-traumatic hydrocephalus. Neurol Res 2000; 22:25–28.

39. Tan H, Feng H, Gao L, Huang G, Liao X. Outcome prediction in severe traumatic brain injury with transcranial Doppler ultrasonography. Chin J Traumatol 2001; 4:156–160.

40. Hall ED, Braughler JM. Central nervous system trauma and stroke. II. physiological and pharmacological evidence for involvement of oxygen radicals and lipid peroxidation. Free Radic Biol Med 1989; 6:303–313.

41. Robertson CS, Cormio M. Cerebral metabolic management. New Horizons 1995; 3:410–422.

42. Chesnut RM. Guidelines for the management of severe head injury: what we know and what we think we know. J Trauma 1997; 42:S19–S22.

43. Piper I. Intracranial pressure and elastance. In: Reilly P, Bullock R, eds. Head Injury: Pathophysiology and Management of Severe Closed Head Injury. London: Chapman and Hall, 1997.

44. Sahjpaul R, Girotti M. Intracranial pressure monitoring in severe traumatic brain injury—results of a Canadian survey. Can J Neurol Sci 2000; 27:143–147.

45. Maas AI, Dearden M, Teasdale GM, et al. (on behalf of the European Brain Injury Consortium) EBIC guidelines for the management of severe head injury in adults. Acta Neurochir (Wein) 1997; 139:286–294.

46. Marion DW, Spiegel TP. Changes in the management of severe traumatic brain injury: 1991–1997. Crit Care Med 2000; 28:16–18.

47. Wilkins IA, Menon DK, Matta BF. Management of comatose head-injured patients: are we getting any better? Anaesthesia 2001; 56:350–369.

48. Jones PA, Andrews PJ, Midgley S, et al. Measuring the burden of secondary insults in head-injured patients during intensive care. J Neurosurg Anesthesiol 1994; 6:4–14.

49. Kleen M, Messmer K. Toxicity of high PaO_2. Minerva Anestesiol 1999; 65:393–396.

50. Chesnut RM, Marshall SB, Piek J, et al. Early and late systemic hypotension as a frequent and fundamental source of cerebral ischemia following severe brain injury in the Traumatic Coma Data Bank. Acta Neurochir 1993; 59:121–125.

51. York J, Arrillaga A, Graham R, Miller R. Fluid resuscitation of patients with multiple injuries and severe closed head injury: experience with an aggressive fluid resuscitation strategy. J Trauma 2000; 48:376–380.

52. Clifton GL, Miller ER, Choi SC, Levin HS. Fluid thresholds and outcome from severe brain injury. Crit Care Med 2002; 30:739–745.

53. Qureshi AI, Suarez JI, Castro A, Bhardwaj A. Use of hypertonic saline/acetate infusion in treatment of cerebral edema in patients with head trauma: experience at a single center. J Trauma 1999; 47:659–665.

54. Huang PP, Stucky FS, Dimick AR, Treat RC, Bessey PQ, Rue LW. Hypertonic sodium resuscitation is associated with renal failure and death. Ann Surg 1995; 221:543–554.

55. Muizelaar JP, Marmarou A, Ward JD, et al. Adverse effects of prolonged hyperventilation in patients with severe head injury: a randomized clinical trial. J Neurosurg 1991; 75:731–739.

56. Imberti R Bellinzona G, Langer M. Cerebral tissue PO_2 and $SjvO_2$ changes during moderate hyperventilation in patients with severe traumatic brain injury. J Neurosurg 2002; 96:97–102.

57. Goldsack C, Scuplak SM, Smith M. A double-blind comparison of codeine and morphine for postoperative analgesia following intracranial surgery. Anaesthesia 1996; 51:1029–1032.

58. Ludbrook GL. Sedation and anaesthesia. In: Reilly P, Bullock R, eds. Head Injury: Pathophysiology and Management of Severe Closed Head Injury. London: Chapman and Hall, 1997.

59. Barrientos-Vega R, Sanchez-Soria MM, Morales-Garcia C, Robas-Gomez A, Cuena-Boy R, Ayensa-Rincon A. Prolonged sedation of critically ill patients with midazolam or propofol: impact on weaning and costs. Crit Care Med 1997; 25: 33–40.

60. Hall RI, Sandham D, Cardinal P, et al. Propofol vs midazolam for ICU sedation: a Canadian multicenter randomized trial. Chest 2001; 119:1151–1159.

61. McCollam JS, O'Neill MG, Norcross ED, Byrne TK, Reeves ST. Continuous infusions of lorazepam, midazolam and propofol for sedation of the critically ill surgery trauma patient: a prospective randomized comparison. Crit Care Med 1999; 27:2454–2458.

62. Kamibayashi T, Maze M. Clinical uses of α_2-adrenergic agonists. Anesthesiology 2000; 93:1345–1349.

63. Jacobi J, Fraser GL, Cousin DB, et al. Clinical practice guidelines for the sustained use of sedatives and analgesics in the critically ill adult. Crit Care Med 2002; 30:119–141.

64. Murray MJ, Cowen J, DeBlock H, et al. Clinical practice guidelines for sustained neuromuscular blockade in the adult critically ill patient. Crit Care Med 2002; 30:142–156.

65. Cruz J, Minoja G, Okuchi K. Improving clinical outcomes from acute subdural hematomas with emergency preoperative administration of high doses of mannitol: a randomized trial. Neurosurg 2001; 49:864–871.

66. Burke A, Quest DO, Chien S, Cerri C. The effect of mannitol on blood viscosity. J Neurosurg 1981; 55:550–553.

67. Muizelaar JP, Wei EP, Kontos HA, Becker DP. Mannitol causes compensatory cerebral vasoconstriction and vasodilation in response to blood viscosity changes. J Neurosurg 1983; 59:822–828.

68. Munar F, Ferrer AM, de Nadal M, et al. Cerebral hemodynamic effects of 7.2% hypertonic saline in patients with head injury and raised intracranial pressure. J Neurotrauma 2000; 17:41–51.

69. Suarez JI, Qureshi AI, Bhardwaj A, et al. Treatment of refractory intracranial hypertension with 23.4% saline. Crit Care Med 1998; 26:1118–1122.

70. Alderson P, Roberts I. Corticosteroids in acute traumatic brain injury: systematic review of randomised controlled trials. Br Med J 1997; 314:1855–1859.

71. Gregson B, Todd NV, Crawford D, et al. CRASH trial is based on problematic meta-analysis. Br Med J 1999; 319:578.

72. Demaria EJ, Reichman W, Kenney PR, Armitage JM, Gann DS. Septic complications of corticosteroid administration after central nervous system trauma. Ann Surg 1985; 202:248–252.

73. McCluskey J, Gutteridge DH. Avascular necrosis of bone after high doses of dexamethasone during neurosurgery. Br Med J 1982; 284:333–334.

74. Schonwald S. Methylprednisolone anaphylaxis. Am J Emerg Med 1999; 17:583–585.

75. Steiner LA, Czosnyka M, Pienchnik SK, et al. Continuous monitoring of cerebrovascular pressure reactivity allows determination of optimal cerebral perfusion pressure in patients with traumatic bran injury. Crit Care Med 2002; 30:733–738.

76. Bouma GJ, Muizelaar JP, Bandoh K, Marmarou A. Blood pressure and intracranial pressure-volume dynamics in severe head injury: relationship with cerebral blood flow. J Neurosurg 1992; 77:15–19.

77. Roberts I. Barbiturates for acute traumatic brain injury. Cochrane Database Syst Re 2000; CD000033.

78. Stover JF, Pleines UE, Morganti-Kossman MC, Stocker R, Kossman T. Thiopental attenuates energetic impairment but fails to normalize cerebrospinal fluid glutamate in brain-injured patients. Crit Care Med 1999; 27:1351–1357.

79. Vigue B, Ract C, Zlotine N, Leblanc PE, Sammi K, Bissonnette B. Relationship between intracranial pressure, mild hypothermia and temperature-corrected PaCO2 in patients with traumatic brain injury. Intensive Care Med 2000; 26:722–728.

80. Jurkovich GJ, Greisner WB, Luterman A, Curreri PW. Hypothermia in trauma victims: an ominous predictor of survival. J Trauma 1987; 27:1019–1024.

81. Clifton GL, Miller ER, Choi SC, et al. Lack of effect of induction of hypothermia after acute brain injury. N Engl J Med 2001; 344:556–563.

82. Gupta AK, Al-Rawi PG, Hutchinson PJ, Kirkpatrick PJ. Effect of hypothermia on brain tissue oxygenation in patients with severe head injury. Br J Anaesth 2002; 88:188–192.

83. Sutcliffe AJ. Hypothermia (or not) for head injury. Care Crit Ill 2001; 17:162–165.

84. Chadwick D. Seizures and epilepsy after traumatic brain injury. Lancet 2000; 355:334–336.

85. Temkin NR, Dikmen SS, Anderson GD, et al. Valproate therapy for the prevention of posttraumatic seizures: a randomized trial. J Neurosurg 1999; 91:593–600.

86. Snowalter PE, Kimmel DN. Stimulating consciousness and cognition following severe brain injury: a new potential clinical use for lamotrigine. Brain Inj 2000; 14:997–1001.

87. Munch E, Horn P, Schurer L, Piepgras A, Paul T, Schmiedek P. Management of severe traumatic brain injury by decompressive craniectomy. Neurosurgery 2000; 47:315–323.

88. Guerra WK, Gaab MR, Dietz H, Mueller JU, Piek J, Fritsch MJ. Surgical decompression for traumatic brain swelling: indications and results. J Neurosurg 1999; 90:187–196.

89. Kerr ME, Weber BB, Sereika SM, Darby J, Marion DW, Orndoff PA. Effect of endotracheal suctioning on cerebral oxygenation in traumatic brain-injured patients. Crit Care Med 1999; 27:2776–2781.

90. Harders A, Kakarieka A, Braakman R. German tSAH study group. Traumatic subarachnoid haemorrhage and its treatment with nimodipine. J Neurosurg 1996; 85:82–89.

91. Van den Berghe G, Wouters P, Weekers F, et al. Intensive insulin therapy in critically ill patients. N Engl J Med 2001; 345:1359–1367.

92. McKinley BA, Parmley CL, Tonneson AS. Standardized management of intracranial pressure: a preliminary clinical trial. J Trauma 1999; 46:271–279.

93. Rosner MJ, Rosner SD, Johnson AH. Cerebral perfusion pressure: management protocol and clinical results. J Neurosurg 1995; 83:949–962.

94. Cruz J. The first decade of continuous monitoring of jugular bulb oxyhemoglobin saturation: management stategies and clinical outcome. Crit Care Med 1998; 26:344–351.

95. Robertson CS, Valadka AB, Hannay HJ, et al. Prevention of secondary ischemic insults after severe head injury. Crit Care Med 1999; 27:2086–2095.

96. Chesnut RM. Avoidance of hypotension: conditio sine qua non of successful severe head-injury management. J Trauma 1997; 42:S4–S9.

97. Bullock R. Injury and cell function. In: Reilly P, Bullock R, eds. Head Injury: Pathophysiology and Management of Severe Closed Head Injury. London: Chapman and Hall, 1997.

98. Eker C, Asgeirsson B, Grande P-O, Schalen W, Nordstrom C-H. Improved outcome after severe head injury with a new therapy based on principles for brain volume regulation and preserved microcirculation. Crit Care Med 1998; 26:1881–1886.

99. Naredi S, Eden E, Zall S, Stephensen H, Rydenhag B. A standardized neurosurgical neurointensive therapy directed towards vasogenic edema after severe traumatic brain injury: clinical results. Intensive Care Med 1998; 24:446–451.

100. Wray NP, Nicotra MB. Pathogenesis of neurogenic pulmonary edema. Am Rev Resp Dis 1978; 118:783–786.

101. Polderman KH, Bloemers FW, Peerdeman SM, Girbes AR. Hypomagnesemia and hypophosphatemia at admission in patients with severe head injury. Crit Care Med 2000; 28:2022–2025.

102. Harrigan MR. Cerebral salt wasting syndrome. Crit Care Clinics 2001; 17(1):125–138.

103. Thomas PD. Fluid, electrolyte and metabolic management. In: Reilly P, Bullock R, eds. Head Injury: Pathophysiology and Management of Severe Closed Head Injury. London: Chapman and Hall, 1997.

104. Pepe JL, Barba CA. The metabolic response to acute traumatic brain injury and implications for nutritional support. J Head Trauma Rehabil 1999; 14:462–474.

105. Klodell CT, Carroll M, Carrillo EH, Spain DA. Routine intragastric feeding following traumatic brain injury is safe and well tolerated. Am J Surg 2000; 179:168–171.

106. Jackson MD, Davidoff G. Gastroparesis following traumatic brain injury and response to metoclopramide therapy. Arch Phys Med Rehabil 1989; 70:553–555.

107. Reignier J, Bensaid S, Perrin-Gachadoat D, Burdin M, Boiteau R, Tenaillon A. Erythromycin and early enteral nutrition in mechanically ventilated patients. Crit Care Med 2002; 30:1237–1241.

108. Bratton SL, Davis RL. Acute lung injury in isolated traumatic brain injury. Neurosurgery 1997; 40:707–712.

109. Kopp R, Kuhlen R, Max M, Rossaint R. Evidence-based medicine in the therapy of the acute respiratory distress syndrome. Intensive Care Med 2002; 28:244–255.

110. McIntyre RC, Pulido EJ, Bensard DD, Shames BD, Abraham E. Thirty years of clinical trials in acute respiratory distress syndrome. Crit Care Med 2000; 28:3314–3331.

111. Bayston R, de Louvois J, Brown EM, Johnston RA, Lees P, Pople IK. Use of antibiotics in penetrating craniocerebral injuries. Lancet 2000; 355:1813–1817.

112. Gurkin SA, Parikshak M, Kralovich KA, Horst HM, Agarwal V, Payne N. Indicators for tracheostomy in patients with traumatic brain injury. Am J Surg 2002; 68:324–328.

113. Anon. The management of spasticity. Drugs Therap Bull 2000; 38:44–46.

114. Sarafis KA, Karatzas GD, Yotis CL. Ankylosed hips caused by heterotopic ossification after traumatic brain injury: a difficult problem. J Trauma 1999; 46:104–109.

115. Townsend RN, Lheureau T, Protech J, Riemer B, Simon D. Timing of fracture repair in patients with severe brain injury (Glasgow Coma Score < 9). J Trauma 1998; 44:977–983.

116. Siminoff LA, Gordon N, Hewlett J, Arnold RM. Factors influencing families' consent for donation of solid organs for transplantation. JAMA 2001; 286:71–77.

117. Wendler D, Dickert N. The consent process for cadaveric organ procurement. JAMA 2001; 285:329–333.

118. Nemetz PN, Leibson C, Naessens JM, et al. Traumatic brain injury and the time to onset of Alzheimer's disease: a population based study. Am J Epidemiol 1999; 149:32–40.

119. Teasdale TW, Engberg AW. Suicide after traumatic brain injury: a population study. J Neurol Neurosurg Psychiatry 2001; 71:436–440.

120. Nygren C, Adami J, Ye W, et al. Primary brain tumors following traumatic brain injury—a population-based cohort study in Sweden. Cancer Causes Control 2001; 12:733–737.

121. Bramlett HM, Dietrich WD. Neuropathological protection after traumatic brain injury in intact female rats versus males or ovariectomized females. J Neurotrauma 2001; 18:891–900.

122. Wright DW, Bauer ME, Hoffman SW, Stein DG. Serum progesterone levels correlate with decreased cerebral edema after traumatic brain injury in rats. J Neurotrauma 2001; 18:901–909.

123. Mesenge C, Margaill I, Verrecchia C, Allix M, Boulu RG, Piotkine M. Protective effect of melatonin in a model of traumatic brain injury in mice. J Pineal Res 1998; 25:41–46.

124. Sullivan PG, Thompson M, Scheff SW. Continuous infusion of cyclosporin A postinjury significantly ameliorates cortical damage following traumatic brain injury. Exp Neurol 2000; 161:631–637.

125. McBurney RN, Daly D, Fischer JB, et al. New CNS-specific calcium antagonists. J Neurotrauma 1992; 9(suppl 2):S531–S543.

126. Perez-Pinzon MA, Alonso O, Kraydieh S, Dietrich WD. Induction of tolerance against traumatic brain injury by ischemic preconditioning. Neuroreport 1999; 10:2951–2954.

127. Thomas SH, Orf J, Wedel SK, Conn AK. Hyperventilation in traumatic brain injury patients: inconsistency between consensus guidelines and clinical practice. J Trauma 2002; 52:47–53.

13

Spinal Cord Injury: Critical Care Management

Christopher Junker and Lucia Palladino

Department of Anesthesiology and Critical Care Medicine, George Washington
University Hospital, Washington, D.C., U.S.A.

INTRODUCTION

Spinal cord injury (SCI) continues to be a devastating problem worldwide. In the United States alone, with more than 11,000 cases per year, SCI is a major cause of morbidity and mortality, especially in otherwise healthy young men (age 15–40) (1,2). The major causes of SCI are motor vehicle collisions accounting for 40% to 50%, falls (16%), and sports injuries (10–15%) (2). The cervical spine (C-spine) is involved in 55% of all SCIs (2–4).

Over the last decade, numerous major advances in our understanding of SCI pathophysiology have occurred. The possibility of beneficial treatment of acute injury with recovery of lost function and our improved ability to limit damage beyond the initial insult have begun to change the historically pessimistic attitude of physicians towards SCI (5,6).

The common assumption that patients who suffer SCI are inevitably unhappy following their injury is untrue. In one study of 128 patients with injuries at the C4 level or above, 64% of those who were ventilator dependent, 54% of those not dependent on a ventilator rated the quality of their lives as good or excellent, and more than 90% reported that they were glad to be alive (6). Old-fashioned approaches are characterized by words from the ancient Edwin Smith papyrus which declared: SCIs are "ailments not to be treated" (7). However, as new therapics promote neural regeneration in areas of the central nervous system (CNS) previously thought to be impossible, including the spinal cord, *these opinions will acquire* their appropriate status as merely historical footnotes. As new therapies promote neural regeneration in areas of the CNS previously thought to be impossible, including the spinal cord.

In this chapter, anatomic considerations and pathophysiology of SCI are reviewed. Only a brief mention is made of initial assessment and management considerations, as these topics are extensively covered in Volume 1, Chapters 15 and 26. This chapter reviews the critical care management and focuses upon the elimination of medical complications of SCI. By anticipating potential problems, the surgical intensive care unit (SICU) length of stay can be decreased, and emphasis can then be turned to rehabilitation.

ANATOMICAL CONSIDERATIONS
Skeletal Structure

The human vertebral column consists of 30 vertebrae: seven cervical, 12 thoracic, five lumbar, five sacral (fused), and the coccygeal bone. The cervical canal is typically wider at C1–C2 and tapers caudally through the thoracic vertebrae, widening again in the lumbar region. The impact on neurological function after trauma differs between cervical and thoracolumbar injuries, and is related to the change in spinal canal shape and diameter (8). The greatest degree of flexion and extension occurs at the atlanto-occipital junction, and the greatest rotatory capability takes place at the atlantoaxial joint. The bony elements of the spinal column articulate by intervertebral disks. Joint capsules and strong, elastic ligaments give the spine its unique combination of stability and flexibility.

Vascular Anatomy

The blood supply to the spinal cord is provided through paired anterior spinal arteries (branches off the vertebral arteries) that join to become the single anterior median spinal artery and supply the anterior two-thirds of the full length of the spinal cord. Paired posterior spinal arteries lie medial to the dorsal roots and supply the posterior one-third of the spinal cord. Collateral flow from radicular arteries emanating from the thoracic and abdominal aorta provides vital additional perfusion. The T4 to T8 region is most vulnerable to low flow because it is supplied mainly by a single thoracic radicular artery that branches off of the thoracic aorta at T7. The distribution from T9 to the sacrum is supplied mainly by a single left radicular artery at T11 called the artery of Adamkiewicz. ☞ **Because of the variable vascular anatomic distribution of the artery of Adamkiewicz, the upper thoracic portion of the spine has watershed zones that are extremely sensitive to ischemic and hypoxic insults.** ☞

PATHOPHYSIOLOGY OF SPINAL CORD INJURY AND THE BASIS OF PHARMACOLOGICAL INTERVENTION
Pathophysiology

Both experimental models and clinical observations reveal two overlapping phases of SCI regarded as primary and secondary injury (2,5,9–13). The primary injury is the direct, immediate, and irreversible mechanical injury of the spinal cord. Secondary injury is the subsequent destruction of neural elements caused by edema, ischemia, and compression from unstable fractures or bony elements impinging on the cord. SCI is the result of force applied directly to the cord or surrounding tissue.

The type of force applied influences the way in which the cord is injured. Traumatic distractional forces (flexion, extension, dislocation, rotation) cause stretching or shearing of the neural elements or the spinal vascular system. Compressive forces (edema, hematoma, or bone fragments within the spinal canal) cause crush injury and ischemia. Long-term mechanical instability leads to structural deformation (kyphosis, subluxation) and further neurological sequelae (10). The size of the spinal canal, the vascular distribution at the level of injury and its location relative to the conus medullaris are all important prognostic factors (8,10,14–16). Figure 1 gives a diagrammatic representation of the cascade of primary and secondary injury mechanisms.

Basis of Pharmacological Intervention

Current treatment of primary injury to the cord and supporting structures is limited to structural stabilization, maintaining mean arterial pressure (MAP), and limiting progression of the primary injury. Although recovery of function from primary injury to the cord through regeneration or grafting is still experimental, therapeutic interventions for secondary injury have a demonstrable, though limited, impact on

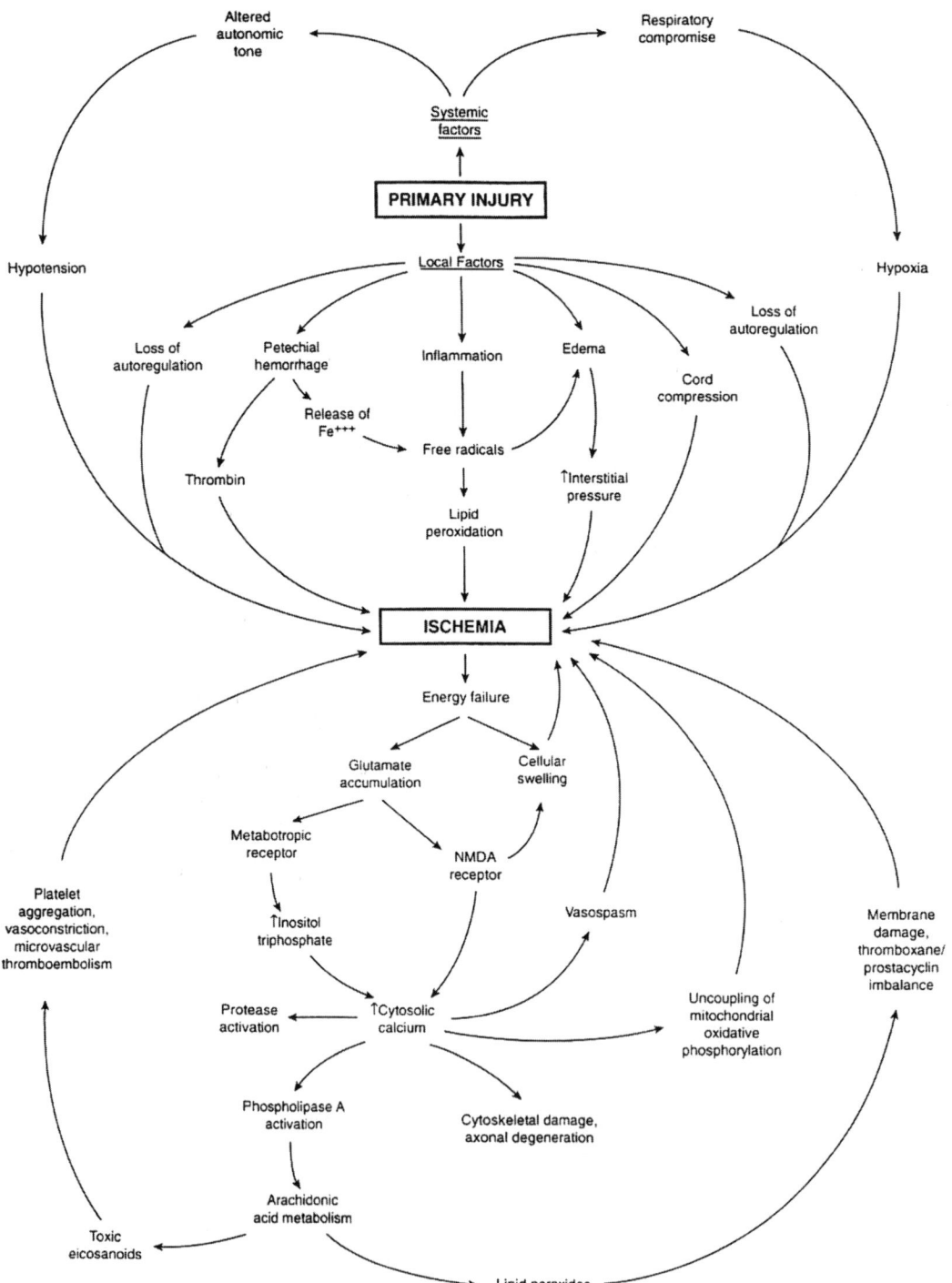

Figure 1 Schematic representation of key mechanisms, molecular species, and interrelations underlying the pathogenesis of acute spinal cord injury. Principal pathways of secondary injury that converge upon ischemia are emphasized and others have been omitted for simplicity. These pathogenetic determinants represent the logical targets for therapeutic modulation. *Abbreviation*: NMDA, *N*-methyl-D-aspartate. *Source*: From Ref. 5.

outcome (5,11). The primary insult to the spinal cord initiates the major determinants of secondary injury: vasospasm (13,17), axonal degeneration and demyelination, activation of the inflammatory response, intramedullary hemorrhage secondary to postcapillary venular rupture (18), disruption of the blood-cerebrospinal fluid barrier with edema formation as response to filtration of larger molecules, and water into the extracellular and interstitial space (18,19). Any of these secondary events can be exacerbated by hypotension, fever (20), and hypoxia. Hyperglycemia worsens neurological outcome in traumatic brain injury. Although its effect in SCI is less clear (21), meticulous control of glucose levels appears to be beneficial in other critically ill patients (22,23) and an insulin infusion protocol is recommended for any patient not easily controlled with a sliding scale insulin regimen.

Pharmacology for Specific Treatment of Spinal Cord Injury

The only agent supported by large human studies [i.e., National Acute Spinal Cord Injury Study (NASCIS) trials] and presently in widespread use is high-dose methylprednisolone (24–26) (Table 1). However, the results are controversial, and if therapy is not initiated within eight hours postinjury, the complications of treatment clearly outweigh the benefits. ☞ **The NASCIS trials supporting the use of methylprednisolone have been viewed as methodologically flawed, with the most encouraging results emerging only in posthoc analyses. Some prominent authors in the field of SCI have argued that 24-hour methylprednisolone should not be routinely used in SCI, and then only on a compassionate use basis (27).** ☞ The Spine Focus Panel offered this summary opinion, "Given the devastating impact of SCI and the evidence of a modest, beneficial effect of methylprednisolone, clinicians should consciously consider using this drug despite the well founded criticisms that have been directed against the NASCIS II and NASCIS III trials" (28). Despite the controversy, methylprednisolone remains a common treatment of SCI in the United States, and, if used, should be started as soon as a diagnosis is established.

Spinal cord ischemia results in lactic acid production due to anaerobic glycolysis, depletion of ATP, loss of cellular homeostasis and, finally, disruption of membrane function. The disruption of the ion pump compromises the membrane potentials and synaptic transmission. The pathological terminal membrane depolarization causes the release of excitatory amino acid (EAA) neurotransmitters, such as aspartate and glutamate, a phenomenon called excitotoxicity (5,11,29,30).

In experimental models of SCI, high extracellular levels of EAA appear within 15 minutes after the cord injury (5). These excitotoxins activate the N-methyl-D-aspartate (NMDA), nonNMDA receptors, and voltage-dependent Ca^{++} and Na^+ channels (2,5,11,31,32). As the energy-dependent ion pump loses the ability to maintain the concentration gradient between the intra- and extracellular space, the large influx of sodium and calcium into the cytosol leads to cellular swelling (2,31–33).

Increased calcium flux into the cells activates many Ca^{++}-dependent catabolic reactions that culminate in cellular necrosis and apoptosis (11,34–37). Phospholipase A_2 with generation of free fatty acid, synthesis of toxic eicosanoids, generation of free radicals (38), impairment of mitochondrial oxidative phosphorylation, and lytic enzymes activation (proteases, endonucleases) have all been linked to secondary neuronal injury.

Many of these observations suggest possible pharmacologic interventions to block or mitigate some of these effects, and in both animal models and human trials have shown promise, but none has yet proven a definitive convincing clinical success (Table 2).

INITIAL ASSESSMENT AND MANAGEMENT

☞ **All patients sustaining major trauma, a fall from greater than ten feet, MVC, or noticeable injuries to the head or neck should be thoroughly evaluated for evidence of SCI (12).** ☞ At the scene, the first goal is to protect the patient from further injury and provide resuscitation (39). Early stabilization of an SCI is imperative to prevent movement of the injured spine that can further neurological damage. The most effective way to stabilize the spine is with a rigid spine backboard and a cervical collar in combination with bilateral sandbags and supporting tape fixed across the forehead and secured to the spine board. If necessary, intubation in the field may be performed with manual inline traction and oral intubation (12,39,40). Airway management is discussed in Volume 1, Chapter 9. During the primary survey of the trauma patient, after airway, breathing, and circulation are assessed and stabilized, a brief neurological exam is performed. Once life-threatening problems are addressed, full neurological examination must be performed during the secondary survey. If, at any time during the primary or secondary survey, the neurological exam is suggestive of SCI, and high-dose methylprednisolone is part of the local treatment protocol, it should be started immediately for maximum potential benefit, even if the radiological examination is not complete (26,27,41–43).

There are several different systems for grading SCIs. These include: spinal cord injury severity scale (44,45), Sunnybrook cord injury scale (45), American Spinal Injury Association classification (46) (Fig. 2), and the Frankel classification (16), described in 1969 and still widely used. Grading systems facilitate the initial assessment, subsequent follow-up, and prognosis.

RADIOLOGIC DIAGNOSIS

Radiologic evaluation in SCI is used to assess alignment, detect ligamentous injuries or fractures, and visualize any compression of neural structures by soft tissue or bone fragments. The initial studies can be either plain radiographs or increasingly computed tomography (CT) scan. For cervical injury, the classic films include a lateral view of the C-spine followed by the anteroposterior, odontoid, and occasionally oblique views. A complete lateral view radiograph of the C-spine should include C7–T1 junction

Table 1 High-Dose Methylprednisolone Dosing for Acute Spinal Cord Injury

Time from injury	Loading dose	Infusion dose	Duration of infusion
1–3 hrs	30 mg/kg	5.4 mg/kg/hr	23 hrs
3–8 hrs	30 mg/kg	5.4 mg/kg/hr	48 hrs

Table 2 Agents Used to Block or Mitigate Secondary Neuronal Injury

Agent	Rationale	State of development	Note
Corticosteroids	Suppression of vasogenic edema Enhancement of spinal cord blood flow Stabilization of lysosomal membranes Inhibition of pituitary endorphin release Alteration of electrolyte concentrations in injured tissue Attenuation of the inflammatory response	Yes, some improvement in functional recovery, no change in level of care posthospital Multiple complications (especially with prolonged use) Additional studied needed	If started <3 hrs following injury should continue for 24 hrs If started between 4 and 8 hrs, must continue for 48 hrs If not started ≤8 hrs postinjury complications outweigh benefits
Gangliosides	Improve neuronal outgrowth, neural development and plasticity Increase synaptic transmission	Phase I trial showing motor improvement in lower extremities, Phase II in progress	May limit some effects of corticosteroids
Opiate antagonists	Antagonizes endogenous opioid peptides, which diminish micro-circulatory blood flow acting through the kappa subtype opioid receptor	Ineffective in NASCIS II by primary endpoints, reanalysis suggested functional improvement if given within 8 hrs	Dosing in NASCIS II was likely subtherapeutic
EAA receptor antagonists	NMDA receptor mediating excitotoxic neuronal damage have been found to be effective in both in vitro and in vivo models of cerebral ischemia, hypoglycemia, and trauma	A Phase III clinical trial of the NMDA receptor antagonist GK11 for acute SCI is currently under way	Most experimental models suggest that for brain lesions, window of effectiveness is narrow. In animal models of SCI within 15 min
Calcium channel blockers	Attenuation of vasospasm	Conflicting studies	No role at this time
Antioxidants and free-radical scavengers	Limit secondary damage after various types of CNS insults	Animal models	Primary protective effect only when administered before injury; possible role in surgical situations in which risk of injury exists

Abbreviations: CNS, central nervous system; EAA, excitatory amino acid; NASCIS, National Acute Spinal Cord Injury Study; NMDA, N-methyl-D-aspartate; SCI, spinal cord injury.

(12,47). Plain films of the spine are evaluated following the contour of four lines (Fig. 3) formed by the anterior margins of the vertebral body, the posterior vertebral margins, the anterior cortical margins of spinous process, and the tips of spinous process (47). The instability criteria include: widening of the interspinous process distance, translation of more than 3.5 mm, and segmental angulation more than 11° when compared to contiguous segments (48,49). Particularly important is the assessment of the posterior ligaments since three-column injury might necessitate an anterior and posterior stabilization procedure (16).

If the patient is conscious, without neurological deficit, has negative static images, yet complains of neck pain, flexion and extension views may be read to evaluate instability. Alternatively, the patient can be asked to rotate the head or the neck 45° in each direction (as per the Canadian C-spine Rule) (50). If the patient is able to do this, the chance of significant injury is exceedingly rare (50).

The stepwise approach to dynamic flexion and extension views exam includes the first film with the neck in extension position followed by the neutral position. If on comparison of the two views the alignment of the spine does not change, the flexion film may be taken. Ultimately,

if the alignment remains the same on flexion and extension, the spine is considered stable. If the patient exhibits any neurological deficit, dynamic images are contraindicated due to risk of causing further injury.

If the patient is unconscious and there is concern for SCI, further evaluation with CT (51) and/or magnetic resonance imaging (MRI) is indicated. Midsagittal T_1- and T_2-weighted images are considered the most reliable to assess spinal cord compression and/or contusion (Fig. 4) (49). MRI is particularly useful in situations where there is a discrepancy between the radiological images and the clinical neurological abnormalities or deterioration in the patient's neurological function. MRI is superior to CT in detecting cord hemorrhage or edema, hematoma, ligamentous disruption, and disc pathology. When MRI is unavailable or not feasible, CT myelography and two-dimensional reconstruction of the spinal CT are still useful.

Although angiography remains the standard for evaluation of vertebral artery injuries, noninvasive MR angiography is gaining acceptance (52). In addition, helical CT angiography is becoming increasingly capable of evaluating vascular injuries in the neck. CT scan, with three-dimensional reconstructions, remains superior to MRI in the evaluation of bony injuries (Figs. 5 and 6). Because of restrictions regarding ferrous materials in the area of the MRI

STANDARD NEUROLOGICAL CLASSIFICATION OF SPINAL CORD INJURY

MOTOR
KEY MUSCLES

	R	L	
C2			
C3			
C4			
C5			Elbow flexors
C6			Wrist extensors
C7			Elbow extensors
C8			Finger flexors (distal phalanx of middle finger)
T1			Finger abductors (little finger)

0 = total paralysis
1 = palpable or visible contraction
2 = active movement, gravity eliminated
3 = active movement, against gravity
4 = active movement, against some resistance
5 = active movement, against full resistance
NT = not testable

	R	L	
L2			Hip flexors
L3			Knee extensors
L4			Ankle dorsiflexors
L5			Long toe extensors
S1			Ankle plantar flexors

☐ Voluntary anal contraction (Yes/No)

TOTALS ☐ + ☐ = ☐ **MOTOR SCORE**
(MAXIMUM) (50) (50) (100)

LIGHT TOUCH / PIN PRICK

0 = absent
1 = impaired
2 = normal
NT = not testable

☐ Any anal sensation (Yes/No)

TOTALS { ☐ + ☐ → = ☐ } **PIN PRICK SCORE** (max: 112)
☐ ☐ = ☐ **LIGHT TOUCH SCORE** (max: 112)
(MAXIMUM) (56) (56) (56) (56)

SENSORY
KEY SENSORY POINTS

* Key Sensory Points

NEUROLOGICAL LEVEL The most caudal segment with normal function		R	L	**COMPLETE OR INCOMPLETE?** ☐ Incomplete = Any sensory or motor function in S4-S5	**ZONE OF PARTIAL PRESERVATION** Caudal extent of partially innervated segments		R	L
	SENSORY	☐	☐			SENSORY	☐	☐
	MOTOR	☐	☐	**ASIA IMPAIRMENT SCALE** ☐		MOTOR	☐	☐

This form may be copied freely but should not be altered without permission from the American Spinal Injury Association.   2000 Rev.

Figure 2 American Spinal Injury Association standard classification. *Source*: From Ref. 46.

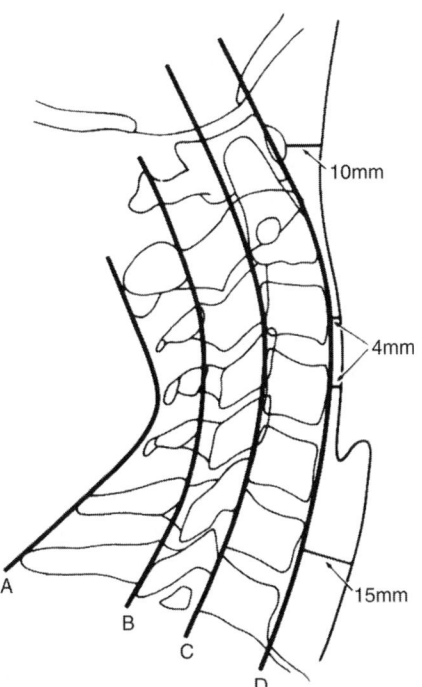

Figure 3 Representation of lateral radiograph of the cervical spine. This figure demonstrates the four imaginary lordotic lines that are formed by the anterior margins of the vertebral bodies (**A**), posterior vertebral margins (**B**), anterior cortical margins of the spinous process (**C**), and the tips of the spinous processes (**D**). Normal width of retropharyngeal soft tissue is also shown. *Source*: From Ref. 159.

scanner, many MRI suites are minimally equipped to monitor unstable or mechanically ventilated trauma patients, which is often a consideration in the early phases of critical care management.

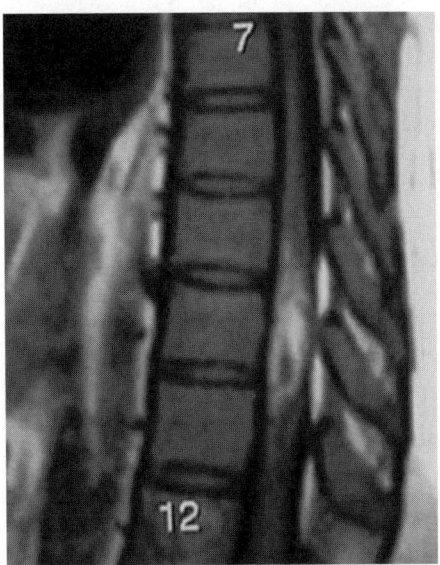

Figure 4 Magnetic resonance image of thoracic spine, sagittal T1WI, with midline spinal cord hyperintensity posterior to 10th thoracic vertebrae, consistent with spinal cord contusion.

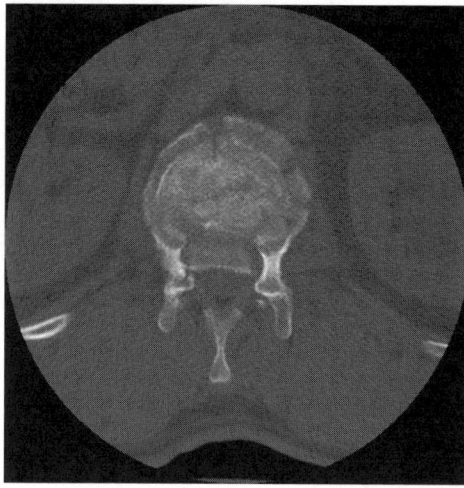

Figure 5 Computed tomography of lumbar spine, axial, with burst fracture of 1st lumbar vertebrae. Canal is 50% compromised from bony retropulsion.

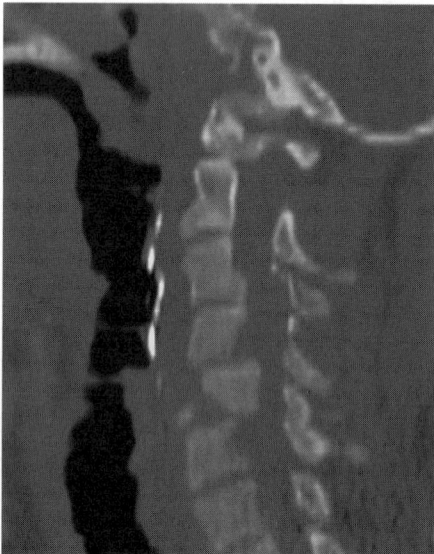

Figure 6 Computed tomography of cervical spine, sagittal 3-dimensional reconstructions, with fracture dislocation of 5th cervical vertebrae and significant canal compromise.

NONSURGICAL STABILIZATION

The goals of nonsurgical treatment are improvement or restoration of spinal alignment and decompression of neural elements with prevention of further injury. Stability is clinically confirmed by the ability of the spine to tolerate physiologic loads without additional neurological deficits, deformity, or pain. Spine fractures can be complicated, requiring evaluation of neurological status, biomechanical instability, and comorbidities, all of which influence the ultimate approach to management (12). However, many fractures are stable and require only limited restrictions, such as unilateral facet and small compression fractures.

An unstable fracture does not always necessitate operative reduction and fixation with hardware; it is important to remember that some unstable fractures may be treated with external immobilization and close clinical and radiographic follow-up. When a fracture warrants nonoperative stabilization, a vest or cuirass is fitted to the patient to limit movement of the spine and support the thorax and abdomen. However, if nonoperative therapy means prolonged bed rest, then operative intervention is almost always a better option when linked to early postoperative mobilization. The timing of intervention, surgical or nonsurgical, and its relation to neurological recovery remains controversial, and there is considerable variation in practice in the choice of surgical and nonsurgical methods of stabilization (12).

Currently, if indicated, traction to achieve realignment is applied as soon as possible after visualization of the injury on the imaging studies. Some experimental studies have reported reversal of neurological deficits if decompression is performed in six to eight hours from the time of injury (53), and clinical improvement of neurological deficits after cervical traction has been applied (54,55). The many traction devices fall into two basic design categories composed either of metal tongs or a halo ring apparatus attached to the head with screws and to a pulley system attached to a set of weights (47). The two essential components in cervical traction are the amount of weight and the direction of the applied force. The amount of applied weight depends on the location, type of injury, and the extent of subluxation (47). Excessive weight may cause overdistraction, exacerbating the injury directly or injuring vertebral arteries (12).

SPECIFIC SPINAL CORD INJURY SYNDROMES

☞ **Lesions in the spinal cord produce sensory and motor disturbances corresponding to the functions of the tracts that have been injured or transected.** ☞ Depending on the clinical exam, they are further categorized as incomplete or complete SCI (Table 3).

The segmental level of a lesion is indicated by the affected dermatomes and myotomes. The major descending motor tract is the crossed lateral corticospinal tract. This tract

Table 3 Neurological Conditions Associated with Partial or Complete Spinal Cord Injuries

Severity of injury	Associated neurological conditions
Complete spinal cord injury	Complete loss of voluntary movement, sphincter control, and sensation below the level of the injury
	No preservation of motor and sensory function more than three segments below the level of the injury
	The persistence of a complete spinal cord injury beyond 24 hrs indicates that no distal function will recover
	Hypotension, bradycardia, and priapism may also be present
Incomplete spinal cord injury	Central cord syndrome
	Anterior cord syndrome
	Brown-Sequard syndrome
	Posterior cord syndrome (very rare)

originates in the opposite hemisphere, crosses in the medulla, and ultimately descends in the lateral aspect of the spinal cord. Ascending sensory tracts include the uncrossed gracile and cuneate fasciculi (dorsal columns) and the crossed spinothalamic tract. The dorsal columns test provides proprioception/joint position sense as well as vibratory sensation; and the ascending crossed spinothalamic tract provides pain and temperature sensation.

There are several SCI syndromes with characteristic neurological deficits. Unilateral SCI causes Brown-Sequard syndrome that presents with ipsilateral loss of joint position sense, motor function deficits, contralateral pain, and temperature sensation deficits. The syndrome, rare in patients sustaining blunt trauma, was first described in victims with penetrating SCI (Table 4) (47,56).

The central spinal cord syndrome presents with severe upper extremity weakness with relative sparing of lower extremities. The degree of sensory deficit and the severity of bowel and bladder dysfunction are variable. This syndrome is often secondary to hyperextension of the neck and, most often, seen in the elderly population, in whom cervical spinal stenosis secondary to spondylosis is more common (47,57). The conus medullaris syndrome is secondary to lesions involving the thoraco-lumbar junction (T11–L1). Usually, the prognosis is more favorable if the lesion involves only the cauda equina. Patients affected by conus injury present with sexual and sphincter function loss.

The Wallenberg syndrome usually results from damage to a vertebral artery, often associated with forced flexion of the C-spine, but can also occur with cervical hyperextension and rotation. Typical findings are deficits of the ipsilateral cranial nerves (V, IX, X, XI), ipsilateral Horner syndrome, cerebellar ataxia, and contralateral impairment of pain and temperature perception. Atlanto-occipital injury should be considered in trauma patients with posterior occipital neck pain and a suboccipital hematoma upon physical exam (16).

Table 4 Syndromes Associated with Incomplete Spinal Cord Injuries

Syndrome	Definition and comments
Central cord syndrome	Most common type of incomplete spinal cord syndrome
	Disproportionately greater motor deficit in the upper extremities than lower, worst in hands
	Usually due to hyperextension injury
	Blunt trauma to forehead common
	Surgery often performed on a nonurgent basis
Anterior cord syndrome	Spinal artery syndrome
	Anterior cord compression causes cord infarct in the territory supplied by the anterior spinal artery
	Motor deficit and loss of pain and temperature sensation
	Preservation of proprioception and two-point discrimination (dissociated sensory loss)
Brown-Sequard syndrome	Spinal cord hemisection
	Usually due to penetrating trauma
	Ipsilateral loss of proprioception and motor function
	Contralateral loss of pain and temperature sensation

SYSTEMIC MANIFESTATIONS OF SPINAL CORD INJURY AND RELATED MANAGEMENT

Medical complications of SCI arise both from systemic effects of the cord injury itself and from prolonged immobilization secondary to paresis or paralysis. We will review the manifestations of each organ system and briefly discuss specific cord injury syndromes at the end of this section.

Cardiovascular
Spinal Shock
Spinal shock was first described by Hall more than 150 years ago, to distinguish it from arterial hypotension caused by hemorrhage or other cardiovascular problems. Spinal shock is defined as insufficient perfusion pressure to tissues, to maintain cellular function in concert with all phenomena surrounding physiologic or anatomic transection of the spinal cord that result in temporary loss or permanent depression of spinal reflex activity, below the level of the lesion (58). In animal models of SCI, spinal shock occurring in the acute setting differs from the one occurring with gradual compression of the spine, and the response varies with species (58,59). **Clinically, the term spinal shock refers to systemic hypotension due to a decrease in sympathetic fiber–mediated arterial and venous vascular resistance, along with venous pooling and loss of preload, with or without bradycardia.** Loss of the peripheral sympathetic vasomotor control occurs when SCI involves segments between T1 and L1 sympathetic innervations of the peripheral vasculature. Since the sympathetic innervation of the heart arises from T1 to T5, lesions involving the spine above T5, unopposed vagal stimulation especially from visceral stretch receptors can lead to severe bradycardia or asystole. With high thoracic lesions, hypotension can be especially severe and difficult to treat if the loss of chronotropic reflex inhibits the normal tachycardic response to decreased preload or peripheral vasodilation. Usually, symptoms resolve within days or weeks (58), but the patient may require intermittent doses of glycopyrrolate or atropine, external or temporary transvenous pacing, and invasive arterial pressure monitoring. Later, compression stockings and abdominal binders are useful to mitigate against orthostatic hypotension during rehabilitation.

Early Cardiovascular Resuscitation Following Spinal Cord Injury
The immediate end points for resuscitation in SCI are the same as with other major trauma: restoration of vital organ perfusion as evidenced by end organ function with adequate urine output, resolution of acidosis, and normal mental status off sedation.

Choice of Vasopressor Drugs
With impairment of normal cardiovascular reflexes, the selection of agents for blood pressure support should have both α- and β-adrenergic properties to cover both cardiac function and peripheral vascular tone. **Although phenylephrine, a nearly pure α-agonist, is commonly used in conjunction with volume in trauma resuscitation, for SCI we favor norepinephrine as a first choice, and if more β-adrenergic support is needed, epinephrine.**

Invasive Monitoring
Cord perfusion is crucial in the first 72 hours following injury, and even short periods of hypotension may have

severe consequences; all patients should receive an arterial line in the intensive care unit (ICU), and MAPs should not be allowed to fall below 60 to 70 mmHg. ☞ There is no outcome data to support the use of pulmonary artery catheterization in SCI, but recent studies of early goal-directed therapy in sepsis (60) and a meta-analysis supporting goal-directed hemodynamic management in acute critically ill patients (61) appear to support an aggressive approach to resuscitation using parameters beyond simple restoration of a normal blood pressure.

It appears likely that much of the benefit of resuscitation for limiting secondary damage to the spinal cord will occur early in the patient's course, including the first several hours of ICU management. Maintaining adequate perfusion to the injured cord is very important, and the combination of trauma and SCI can make assessment of volume status, arterial tone, and cardiac performance difficult, especially in elderly patients and those with coronary artery disease. Pulmonary artery catheterization can be helpful in guiding therapy in this setting (12,47,62).

With the combination of major trauma and the potentially confusing cardiovascular effects of SCI itself, we frequently place pulmonary artery catheters early in the resuscitation phase if cardiovascular stability without the use of vasopressors is not achieved quickly on admission to the ICU. Spinal cord perfusion pressure is defined as the difference between MAP and cerebrospinal fluid pressure. However, cerebrospinal fluid pressure is difficult to measure in the clinical setting, and spinal cord edema may increase flow resistance to tissues at risk, which makes the optimal MAP in the setting of SCI unknown. In one nonrandomized trial of goal-directed resuscitation and hemodynamic management by protocol, SCI patients were maintained at a MAP of 85 mmHg. The authors concluded, "Early and aggressive medical management (volume resuscitation and blood pressure augmentation) of patients with acute spinal cord injuries optimizes the potential for neurological recovery after sustaining trauma" (63). The selection of a MAP of 85 mmHg was essentially arbitrary. But some elevation of hemodynamic parameters above normal values is likely to prove useful, even if maintaining elevated parameters only decreases the incidence of hypotension by creating a margin of safety for the abrupt changes in blood pressure that is often seen in critical care settings.

Fluid Therapy for Spinal Cord Injury
The debate concerning fluids of choice for SCI resuscitation has produced a large volume of inconclusive literature. Hypotonic and glucose containing solutions have potential risks and offer no benefit during the initial resuscitation period. There is a trend toward improved outcomes using low-volume resuscitations with hypertonic saline and dextran for resuscitation in traumatic brain injury (64,65). Currently, the data is insufficient to recommend the routine use of hypertonic saline for resuscitation in SCI, however, its use should be considered in the setting of resuscitation when CNS edema amenable to osmotic therapy is present. Unlike mannitol, hypertonic saline does not need to be eliminated from the body to preserve its effect, thus it can serve both as an osmotic agent and a resuscitation fluid.

Autonomic Hyperreflexia
Spinally mediated sympathetic reflexes in segments distal to the injury typically start to reappear as early as three to six weeks after the injury, and these nerves are involved in autonomic dysreflexia. In the normal state, descending inhibitory

tracts that travel in the spinal cord moderate these reflexes, but in SCI patients with lesions above T6 the inhibitory pathways are disrupted leading to unopposed sympathetic discharge. These patients consequently experience episodes of massive, uncontrolled sympathetic discharge.

Often these responses are triggered by relatively minor autonomic stimuli, such as bladder distension 75% to 85% and fecal impaction 13% to 15% (66). Autonomic dysreflexia events can cause strokes, pulmonary edema, myocardial ischemia, and are occasionally fatal. ☞ **Somewhere between 19% to 70% of SCI patients have at least one episode of autonomic dysreflexia in their lifetime (67), and should always be anticipated when patients are scheduled for even small procedures, such as cystoscopy (68).** ☞

As SCI patients often have normal blood pressures in the 90/60 range, a rise to 150/95 mmHg, not necessarily alarming in another patient population, may represent an emergency in the SCI patient. Therefore, a heightened awareness of this phenomenon among nurses and physicians working with SCI patients is important. Treatment consists of sitting the patient up, if possible, to induce an orthostatic drop in blood pressure, removing the stimulus, and administration of rapid onset antihypertensives, primarily afterload reducers. Discontinuing any ongoing procedure, relieving bladder distension, or manually disimpacting stool will address the majority of cases. For blood pressure control hydralazine IV is an effective initial choice, moving to nitroprusside if blood pressure is not brought rapidly under control.

Pulmonary
☞ **Pulmonary complications, after the primary injury, are the largest cause of morbidity and mortality in SCI.** ☞ Pneumonia, aspiration, pulmonary embolism, airway complications, and neurogenic pulmonary edema are common in patients with SCI. Preexisting pulmonary conditions are exacerbated by SCI and most SCI patients will require mechanical ventilation at some time in their course.

Early Pulmonary Complications of Spinal Cord Injury
Aspiration and Ventilator-Associated Pneumonia
Ventilator-associated pneumonia (VAP) carries a high mortality rate (69), and the incidence increases by 1% to 3% per day of mechanical ventilation (70). Early mobilization, aggressive pulmonary toilet, and institution of the cough and breathing support are crucial in reducing the incidence of this complication. Accurate diagnosis and treatment of pneumonia is often difficult to make because the presence of fever, leukocytosis, pulmonary secretions, and an abnormal chest film are not uncommon findings in SCI patients without pneumonia. Initial, empiric therapy for VAP is based on the severity, the presence of coexisting illness, and length of hospital stay. Community-acquired *Streptococcus pneumonia* and *Hemophilus influenza* are the most common early pathogens. After a week, *Pseudomonas aeruginosa* or *Staphylococcus aureus* are more likely (62), and local antibiotic resistance patterns should be taken into consideration with increasing appearance of nosocomial organisms. Although some authors recommend the use of prophylactic antibiotics (71), most centers have not adopted this approach.

When aspiration of tube feeding or oral secretions is suspected, the use of antibiotics is controversial (72). We recommend antibiotic therapy for aspiration pneumonia for patients with persistent infiltrates >48 hours, suspicion of aspiration of bowel contents, or those who appear septic and are at risk for hemodynamic compromise. Supine body position has been identified as an independent risk factor for VAP (73), and SCI patients should be kept out of the supine position as soon as the stability of their injuries allows. Placement of the feeding tube past the pylorus or even past the ligament of Treitz has been advocated for aspiration prevention, however, current literature is equivocal regarding this approach and repeated attempts at post-pyloric placement often delay nutritional support (74).

Neurogenic Pulmonary Edema

Neurogenic pulmonary edema is an important complication occurring in some patients with SCI. Although there is some cardiac dysfunction associated with high cord level injuries, myocardial failure is not a significant component. In addition, there is no evidence for any direct nerve-mediated reflex. Rather, the mechanism appears to involve massive sympathetic activation triggered by the insult with associated marked systemic and pulmonary hypertension, leading to diffuse pulmonary capillary damage (62). Supportive care with close attention to fluid management to limit excessive hydrostatic pressures in the pulmonary circulation is the primary treatment.

Thromboembolic Complications

☞ **Acute SCI victims have the highest risk of developing deep venous thrombosis (DVT) among all hospitalized patients (75,76).** ☞ Venous stasis due to immobility and platelet and coagulation abnormalities occurring during the acute phase of injury are major factors contributing to DVT risk in SCI patients. Development of DVT and PE during the acute phase of SCI is both a cause of acute morbidity and mortality, and also contributes to long-term disability (77). The incidence of DVT is highest during the first three months postinjury (69,75,78–80), declining thereafter due to increased mobility during rehabilitation and resolution of the hypercoagulable state associated with acute injury (75,81). However, patients with SCI remain at risk for DVT and fatal PE in the rehabilitation phase as well (82). Accordingly, it is imperative that DVT prophylaxis should be instituted as soon as possible. Also see Volume 2, Chapter 56.

The ACCP consensus guidelines for antithrombotic therapy are based on several small, randomized trials of DVT prophylaxis in SCI patients (Table 5) (75). Low-molecular weight heparin (LMWH) is more effective than the combination of low-dose-unfractionated heparin, elastic stockings, and intermittent pneumatic compression. If there is evidence of perispinal hematoma, therapy with LMWH must be delayed for 24 to 72 hours and conversion to warfarin should be postponed at least for two weeks from the time of injury. Inferior vena cava (IVC) filter placement is recommended for protection against PE in patients with diagnosis of DVT who are not candidates for anticoagulation, documented failure of anticoagulation therapy, and patients in whom a PE would likely be fatal (83–85). However, despite the theoretical benefit, there are few controlled trials demonstrating the impact of IVC filters on recurrence rates and mortality from PE (86,87), and a large, retrospective study of over 8000 trauma patients (88) found no evidence to support prophylactic use of IVC filters. Only one randomized trial (89) suggested that the addition of IVC filter to standard anticoagulation showed short-term benefit in terms of decreased incidence of PE, but in the long term demonstrated a higher recurrence rate of DVT. Unfortunately, this study did

Table 5 American College of Chest Physicians Recommendations for Deep Venous Thrombus and Pulmonary Embolus Prophylaxis[a]

Risk group	Recommended prophylaxis
Intracranial neurosurgery	IPC device, with or without ES (grade 1A) LDUH or postoperative LMWH may be accepted alternatives (grade 2A) High-risk patients: ES or IPC device with LDUH or postoperative LMWH may be more effective than either prophylactic modality alone (grade 1B)
Trauma, with identifiable risk factor for thromboembolism	Prophylaxis with LMWH, as soon as considered safe (grade 1A); if delayed, or contraindicated because of bleeding concerns: initial use of ES or IPC device or both (grade 1C). If prophylaxis is suboptimal, offer screening of high-risk patients with duplex ultrasound (grade 1C). If proximal DVT is demonstrated and anticoagulation is contraindicated, IVC filter insertion (grade 1C+), but we do not recommend IVC filter insertion as primary prophylaxis (grade 1C)
Acute spinal cord injury	Prophylaxis with LMWH (grade 1B). We do not recommend LDUH, ES, and IPC as sole prophylaxis (grade 1C). ES and IPC may be offered in combination with LMWH or LDUH, or if early use of anticoagulants is contraindicated (grade 2B). In the rehabilitation phase, we recommend continued LMWH therapy or full-dose oral anticoagulation (both grade 1C).

[a]The Sixth Consensus Conference on Antithrombotic Therapy from the American College of Chest Physicians.
Abbreviations: DVT, deep venous thrombosis; ES, elastic stockings; IPC, intermittent pneumatic compression; IVC, inferior vena cava; LDUH, low-dose unfractionated heparin; LMWH, low-molecular-weight heparin.
Source: From Ref. 75.

not compare the efficacy of standard anticoagulation with IVC filter placement alone without any anticoagulation therapy. Morbidity and mortality from IVC filter placement are low (86), the most common complications being venous thrombosis at the insertion site and IVC obstruction. Filter migration and filter erosion through the IVC wall are rare, but can be catastrophic.

Chronic Pulmonary Complications of Spinal Cord Injury (Ventilator Weaning, Diaphragmatic Pacing, Chronic Ventilator Dependence)

The degree to which respiratory mechanics are affected depends on the level of the spinal injury and whether it is complete. Patients with injuries to lower thoracic cord or below typically have minimal changes in pulmonary function. Pulmonary mechanical dysfunction from SCI arises from decreased tidal volumes and minute ventilation and impaired cough with retained secretions (Table 6) (90).

Normal inhalation requires outward movement of the rib cage through contraction of the intercostal muscles with

Table 6 Comparison of Pulmonary Function in Patients with Cervical and Thoracic Spinal Cord Injury

Variable	C4 to C7	T3 to T12
FVC	52	69
FEV$_1$/FVC (%)	85	82
IC	71	—
ERV	21	64
TLC	70	82
FRC	86	86
RV	141	91
MVV	49	61
PI$_{max}$ (cmH$_2$O)	64	79
PE$_{max}$ (cmH$_2$O)	41	98

Note: Values expressed % predicates normal.
Abbreviations: ERV, expiratory reserve volume; FEV, forced expiratory volume in one second; FRC, functional residual capacity; FVC, forced vital capacity; IC, inspiratory capacity; MVV, maximal voluntary ventilation; PI, pressure inspiration; PE, equals pressure expiration; RV, residual volume; TLC, total lung capacity.
Source: From Ref. 90.

expansion of the lower rib cage. The intercostal muscles are required for chest expansion during inhalation (91). Paralysis of the intercostals and abdominal musculature impairs both expansion of the lungs and diaphragmatic stabilization, dramatically compromising vital capacity, deep breathing, and cough strength.

If the lesion is high enough to impair intercostal function, the diaphragm becomes the principal muscle of ventilation. In this setting, the rib cage often moves paradoxically inward during inhalation. On pulmonary function testing, SCI patients typically have decreased total lung, vital inspiratory capacities, and expiratory reserve volume, with increased residual volume. Patients with intact diaphragm function can maintain adequate minute ventilation through increased stimulation of their diaphragm. Table 7 shows the innervation of the respiratory muscles with the corresponding spinal cord level (92). ☞ **Diaphragmatic breathing is affected by body position. When supine, abdominal contents push the diaphragm up increasing excursion and tidal volume, but at the expense of functional residual capacity (FRC). When**

Table 7 Innervation of the Respiratory Muscles

Muscle group	Spinal cord level	Nerve(s)
Inspiratory muscles		
Diaphragm	C3 to C5	Phrenic
Parasternal intercostals	T1 to T7	Intercostal
Lateral external intercostals	T1 to T12	Intercostal
Intercostal	C4 to C8	
Sternocleidomastoid	XI, C1, C2	
Expiratory muscles		
Lateral internal intercostals	T1 to T12	Intercostal
Rectus abdominis	T7 to L1	Lumbar
External and internal obliques	T7 to L1	Lumbar
Transversus abdominis	T7 to L1	Lumbar

Source: From Ref. 43.

the patient is upright, FRC is preserved, but diaphragmatic "doming" and, thus, excursion is diminished. ☞ Patients with SCI below C5 often benefit from the use of an abdominal binder, which increases intra-abdominal pressure and thus helps the diaphragm start contraction in a more domed position. If the diaphragm is significantly weakened (i.e., injury level above C6), minute ventilation declines markedly when the patient is upright (93,94).

The phrenic nerve arises from the third to fifth cervical roots, so a complete C3 level or higher will cause near complete ventilatory muscle paralysis. High cervical injuries have the highest incidence of ventilation complications, are difficult to wean from mechanical ventilation (Volume 2, Chapter 28), and have the highest mortality when compared with other SCI injury levels (95–97). Injuries above C3 are at high risk for nosocomial pneumonia, and without recovery of some function, will require diaphragmatic pacing or chronic ventilatory support.

A diaphragmatic pacer delivers an electrical stimulus to the phrenic nerve, allowing some of these patients, who might otherwise require chronic mechanical support, to maintain adequate gas exchange. However, if the lesion affects the anterior horn cells of C3 to C4, Wallerian degeneration will impair propagation of electrical impulses in the phrenic nerves. Intercostal to phrenic nerve transfers with diaphragmatic pacing have shown promising improvements, and other surgical remedies are currently being developed in animal models.

Patients with SCI at levels C3 to C5 have variable loss of diaphragmatic strength, and often require mechanical ventilation during acute hospitalization, but permanent ventilatory support is usually unnecessary (98–100). Occasionally, the initial level of motor loss can be due to inflammation and edema of neural tissue that is not permanently injured and, in a high cervical lesion, even a small improvement of function as this resolves, allows recruitment of accessory ventilatory muscles. Retraining muscles that are deconditioned during the acute illness and the evolution from flaccid to spastic paralysis can also lead to improvement in respiratory function (98–103). ☞ **The use of abdominal thrusts or quad coughing, postural drainage, chest percussion, and effective pain management lower the incidence of pneumonia in these patients.** ☞

Lesions from levels C5 through C8 leave an intact diaphragm and the use of accessory muscles in the neck for inhalation, with exhalation primarily through the passive recoil of the chest wall and lungs. Injuries to the thoracic spinal cord have less impact on ventilatory muscle function, but have a higher incidence of associated chest trauma with pneumothorax, hemothorax, flail chest, and lung contusion, as well as damage to other thoracic structures (96,97).

Tracheostomy Decision Making in Spinal Cord Injury Patients

Decisions regarding chronic airway management are made based on the patient's overall condition, estimated duration of mechanical ventilation, type of injury, and any plans for surgical stabilization. For example, after anterior surgical stabilization for cervical SCI, a period of two weeks is usually required prior to tracheostomy to allow healing of tissue planes (62).

Tracheostomy results in greater comfort for the patient and diminished sedation requirements. Tracheostomy facilitates ventilator weaning, simplifies pulmonary toilet, decreases dead space (especially useful in patients with compromised minute ventilation), and may decrease the rate of pneumonia in trauma patients (104,105). The current consensus is to allow at least ten days for weaning attempts and performing the tracheostomies on patients who have been on the ventilator for more than 14 to 21 days (106,107).

However, these recommendations are for the general ventilated population, and if the likelihood of long-term mechanical ventilatory support is known with some degree of certainty based on the level of cord injury, the decision timing should be modified accordingly (108). The introduction of percutaneous tracheostomy in 1985 (109) has shortened the time to placing a chronic airway in some centers, and this technique has been used safely in patients with SCI, including patients with known cervical injury who cannot have their neck placed in extension (110).

Gastrointestinal System
Enteral Nutrition
☞ **Severe CNS injury causes a hypermetabolic response that peaks 5 to 12 days after injury and decreases to a level below pre-injury needs, depending on residual level of motor function.** ☞ Nutritional needs should be monitored and regularly reassessed because of the vulnerability of injured neural tissue to hyperglycemia and because overfeeding can impede weaning from mechanical ventilation, especially when pulmonary function is marginal. Most of the patients affected by SCI suffer from ileus due to autonomic dysfunction. A nasogastric or orogastric tube should be placed to avoid abdominal distension, and enteral feeding should be started as soon as it can be tolerated (see Volume 2, Chapter 32), which is often immediately.

Although the best enteral formulation for SCI patients is debatable, enteral feedings are preferred over parenteral nutrition to preserve intestinal function, minimize bacterial translocation, decrease complications of central venous catheters, and decrease ICU length of stay (111–121). In patients who are difficult to wean from the ventilator due to limited minute ventilation, a relatively high fat pulmonary formula can be used for nutrition which limits CO_2 production. The role of immunonutrition formulae, with arginine and omega3 polyunsaturated fatty acid versus the isocaloric isonitrogenous formulas in this ICU population is not established (122–124). Although gastric versus pyloric tube placement remains controversial, jejunal placement does reduce the incidence of abdominal distension, high gastric residuals, and vomiting compared with gastric placement (117). However, there is no increase in caloric administration or decrease in the incidence of nosocomial pneumonia (125–127).

Ulcer Prophylaxis
Stress ulcer prophylaxis should be instituted on admission (62,118,128), and some overlap between discontinuation of prophylaxis and successful enteral feeding are recommended, as the role of feeding in stress ulceration prevention is unclear in SCI patients (see Volume 2, Chapter 30) (125). The incidence of gastrointestinal (GI) bleeding in SCI patients peaks between postinjury days 4 to 10 (112,113). The pathogenesis of stress ulcer is not completely understood, increased destructive factors such as elevated levels of gastrin, bile, pepsin, acid, and diminished protective factors including prostaglandin production, mucous bicarbonate layer, and epithelial cell renewal have all been observed (125,129). Some authors (111,112) have postulated that unopposed vagal activity might predispose SCI victims to GI ulceration or hemorrhage.

A correlation exists between the level of injury and incidence of GI bleeding with cervical injuries that are at

highest risk. Patients with cervical and thoracic cord injury also have a higher incidence of pancreatitis, likely due to the predominant visceral parasympathetic tone. Accordingly, we check pancreatic enzymes as a part of nutritional monitoring. Simple antacids, H_2-antagonists, proton pump inhibitors (PPI), and sucralfate are all effective prophylactic agents for stress-related ulcer (114,115,129).

Some studies have shown that continuous infusion of a PPI or an H_2-antagonist is superior to both intermittent equivalent dosing or antacid and sucralfate (130,131), but whether this is true in the setting of CNS injury is unclear (132). Although early studies suggested that the use of pH-altering therapy increases the incidence of nosocomial pneumonia (130), a relatively recent large trial showed no significant difference (133). Currently, most centers use intermittent dosing of either an H_2-antagonist or a PPI as prophylaxis against stress gastritis (see Volume 2, Chapter 30).

Genitourinary System
Acutely, all SCI patients should be managed with a Foley catheter. As the patient enters the recovery phase, the indwelling Foley is replaced with an intermittent straight catheter regimen every four hours, provided that daily urine output is less than 2500 cc. If the use of a catheter is necessary, intermittent catheterization reduces the risk of infections [urinary tract infections (UTI), orchitis, epididymitis, urethritis, and periurethral abscess or fistula], as well as long-term complications such as calculi and bladder carcinoma (134,135). Condom catheters seem to carry the least risk of complicated UTI. In addition, recurrent UTI in patients using condom catheters should prompt examination for voiding problems (134,136). The incidence of UTI in catheterized patients can be reduced through education of patients and staff to use the appropriate technique, hand hygiene, use of closed drainage system (134,137), and use of silver alloy catheters (134,138). Topical antiseptic agents to the perineal area and the use of antiseptic solutions in drainage bags and bladder washout are not effective (134,136,137).

The clinical presentation of UTI in SCI patients is often problematic. Pyuria is commonly an irritative effect of the catheter on the urinary tract, and culture results are often polymicrobial. Bacteriuria in patients with indwelling catheter should be treated only if symptomatic (134,139), and treatment should be continued for 5 days, or 7 to 14 days for cases of reinfections and complicated UTI (134,136,140). Prophylactic antibiotics should not be used in patients with indwelling catheters, and the evidence is not clear enough to make a recommendation for patients using intermittent catheterization (3,141).

☞ **Chronic urinary tract dysfunction requiring catheter drainage and recurrent UTIs are a serious problem for patients with SCI.** ☞ In the past, urologic complications played a major role in SCI mortality (142,143), and renal insufficiency from ascending UTI is still one of the leading causes of morbidity in SCI patients (134,141). Incomplete voiding with large postvoiding residual (141,144), and outlet obstruction such as detrusor sphincter dyssynergia, high-pressure voiding, and vesicoureteral reflux are the well-recognized predisposing factors for UTI in patients with SCI (134).

Careful attention to bladder management also decreases the incidence of autonomic dysreflexia, often associated with UTI, bladder distention, and urogenital diagnostic testing (68,145,146). The diagnosis of possible structural and functional abnormalities is essential in order

Table 8   Neurosurgery, Trauma, and Acute Spinal Cord Injury

Risk group	Recommended prophylaxis
Intracranial neurosurgery	IPC device, with or without ES (grade 1A)
	LDUH or postoperative LMWH may be acceptable alternatives (grade 2A)
	High-risk patients: ES or IPC device with LDUH or postoperative LMWH may be more effective than either prophylactic modality alone (grade 1B)
Trauma, with identifiable risk factor for thromboembolism	Prophylaxis with LMWH, as soon as considered safe (grade 1A); if delayed, or contraindicated because of bleeding concerns: initial use of ES, or IPC device, or both (grade 1C)
	If prophylaxis is suboptimal, offer screening of high-risk patients with duplex ultrasound (grade 1C)
	If proximal DVT is demonstrated and anticoagulation is contraindicated, we recommend inferior vena cava (IVC) filter insertion (grade 1C+), but we do not recommend IVC filter insertion as primary prophylaxis (grade 1C)
Acute spinal cord injury	Prophylaxis with LMWH (grade 1B)
	We do not recommend LDUH, ES, and IPC as sole prophylaxis (grade 1C)
	ES and IPC may be offered in combination with LMWH or LDUH, or if early use of anticoagulants is contraindicated (grade 2B)
	In the rehabilitation phase, we recommend continued LMWH therapy, or full-dose oral anticoagulation (both grade 1C)

Abbreviations: DVT, deep venous thrombosis; ES, elastic stockings; IPC, intermittent pneumatic compression; LDVH, low-dose unfractionated heparin; LMWH, low-molecular-weight heparin.

to provide adequate care to SCI patients affected by UTI. Prior to transfer to rehabilitation phase, appropriate baseline urodynamic evaluation is recommended (141).

Cutaneous and Musculoskeletal Systems
Pressure Sores
Patients with SCI are particularly prone to develop pressure sores (decubitus ulcers). Pressure sores are potentially serious, putting patients at risk for osteomyelitis and septicemia, especially if they occur near the area of surgical intervention for spinal stabilization (147). Risk factors for pressure sores are immobility, nutritional status, fecal and urinary incontinence, and decreased sensory perception, all conditions commonly found in SCI patients. Table 8 summarizes the Braden scoring system for estimating risk of developing pressure sores.

Although pressure sores (decubitus ulcers) are often considered primarily a problem in long-term facilities, Figure 7 illustrates the findings of early development of pressure sores (Stage II or greater) in 18 of 183 SCI patients in a neuro-ICU over a three-month period (148). Establishing

a turning schedule with a recommended maximum duration time of two hours for any single position (as soon as conditions permit) is essential. Although still immobile, patients should be supported with pressure-reducing mattress materials, such as foam, static air, alternating air, gel, water, low air loss, or air-fluidized support surfaces (147), with proper alignment of extremities and cushioning devices between legs and ankles. Trapezes, transfer boards, and lift sheets should be employed to prevent mechanical injuries from friction and shearing forces during repositioning and transfer activities.

Contractures and Spasticity
Contractures and spasticity are problems that occur over time in SCI patients, but prevention begins in the ICU. Some patients may be able to undertake a partial active exercise regimen. But most will require either active assisted or passive movements to maintain full joint range, muscle length and extensibility and improve venous return. Shoulders, hands, hips, and ankles are at particular risk of contractures. Resting splints for the hands and feet should be employed in appropriate patients to maintain these joints in a neutral position. Spasticity is also a common cause of pressure sores. Spastic syndrome is characterized by exaggerated muscle tendon tap reflexes, increased muscle tone, and involuntary muscle contractions. Commonly used agents for spasticity include baclofen and diazepam with CNS action and dantrolene, which acts directly on skeletal muscles.

EYE TO THE FUTURE

For the short term, the most dramatic changes in the critical care of SCI will be in the improvements in critical care across the board. New developments in therapies for septic shock, protective ventilator strategies, reduced use of red cell transfusions, early renal replacement therapy, tight glucose control, to name a few examples, will dominate the improved care for all critically ill patients.

Longer term, ICU physicians will begin to introduce agents that reduce secondary SCI in incomplete lesions. Agents that either block endotoxicity or enhance cellular antiexcitotoxic activity may soon be available (149). There

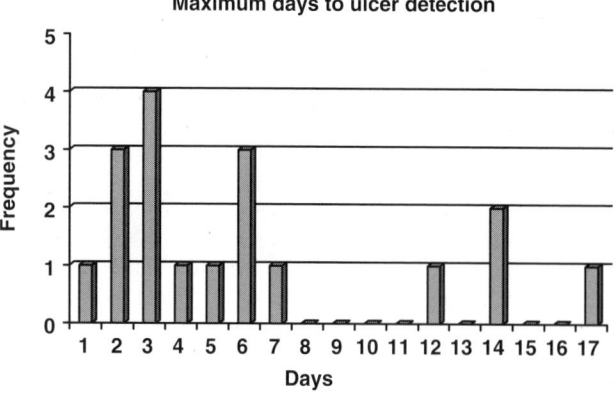

Figure 7   Maximum days to decubitus ulcer detection. This figure demonstrates the number of days that elapsed prior to decubitus ulcer formation in a group of spinal cord injured patients. *Source*: From Ref. 148.

is a very large research effort underway to understand apoptotic pathways and create medications targeted at interrupting or suppressing them (150). Control of apoptosis appears to be of central importance, and may be a precondition of regenerative strategies (151). Several other nonantioxidant approaches are under investigation for application with steroids: these include COX-2 inhibitors, inhibitors of calpain, and thyrotropine releasing hormone analogs (which act as opioid receptor antagonists).

When acute injury cannot be minimized and cell death occurs, the horizon of axonal regeneration research is increasingly showing promise. Regeneration avenues include neural growth factors (152); neural stem cell research (Fig. 8) (153,154); and the use of grafts, electrical stimulation, and physical therapy to induce neural plasticity (155).

Recently, human fetal spinal cord tissue has been cultured for neural stem cells and subsequently implanted into spinal cord injured primates (156). Eight weeks after transplantation, all animals were sacrificed and histological analysis revealed that not only did the human neural stem

cells survive, but they also differentiated into neurons, astrocytes, and oligodendrocytes. On a functional level, power and the spontaneous motor activity of the transplanted animals were significantly higher than those of sham-operated control animals (156). An important caveat for all of this research as it comes into human trials is the need for improvement in diagnostic testing to improve reliability of treatment protocol results (157).

SUMMARY

SCI represents a catastrophic event for the patient and his/her loved ones. The last decade has witnessed numerous significant improvements. Within the next five to ten years, further improvements are on the horizon. Pharmacological therapies are being developed to limit the extent of secondary injury, and soon thereafter we will likely see effective therapies for restoration of neurological function lost to primary spinal cord damage.

Recent research has shown that transplanted neural stem cells can repopulate damaged areas in the spinal cord. In addition, it is likely that the appropriate trophic factors will be discovered that will render the native spinal cord to transform into a growth permissive environment following SCI and allow regeneration of damaged neurons. In an effort to streamline research efforts and improve collaboration, a recent report from the Institute of Medicine states that the United States National Institutes of Health (NIH) and its subsidiary, the National Institute of Neurological Disorders and Stroke, should develop a centralized network to lead and organize diverse SCI research across the country (158).

In the meantime, meticulous critical care practices are proven to decrease morbidity and mortality in SCI patients and to hasten their readiness to enter rehabilitation. Aggressive rehabilitation should begin in the SICU (Volume 2, Chapter 66) and proceed on the ward, as well as following discharge. New techniques in early mobilization and training of transfers, self-cleansing, feeding, and dressing are also desperately needed. Significant additional funds need to be allocated in this arena as well in order to maximize the full potential for recovery, and return to productive lives following SCI.

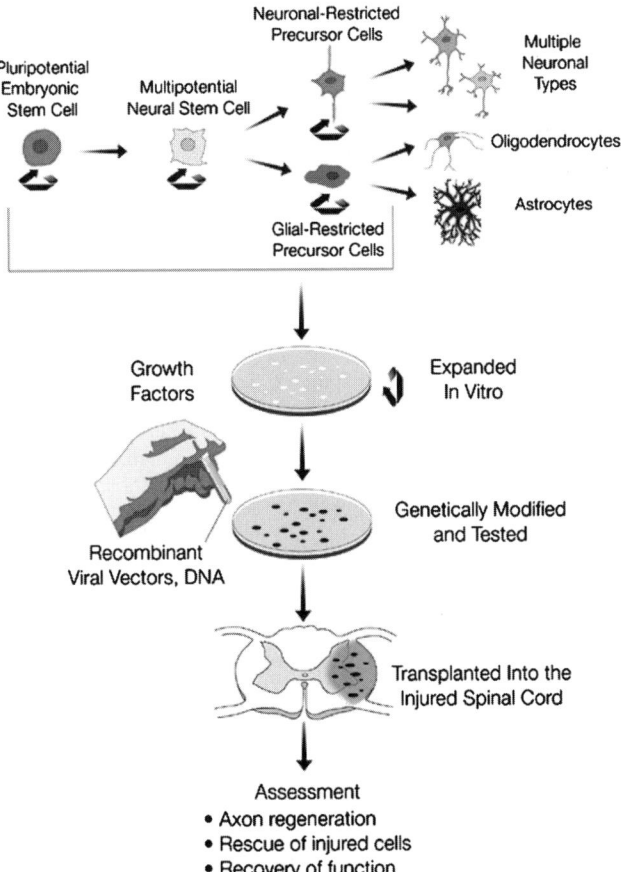

Figure 8 Process of transplanting neural stem cells (or their progeny mature cell types) into the spinal cord of injured patients. Multipotential neural stem cells have the ability to self-renew (*curved arrows*) and to generate all the mature cell types of the central nervous system—neurons, oligodendrocytes, and astrocytes. Neuronal-restricted precursor cells and glial-restricted precursor cells are more limited in their potential and ability to self-renew. These cells alone or in combination with ex vivo gene therapy are being evaluated for their potential to promote axon regeneration, rescue injured cells, and enhance functional recovery after spinal cord injury. *Source*: From Ref. 153.

KEY POINTS

- ☞ Because of the variable vascular anatomic distribution of the artery of Adamkiewicz, the upper thoracic portion of the spine has watershed zones that are extremely sensitive to ischemic and hypoxic insults.
- ☞ The NASCIS trials supporting the use of methylprednisolone have been viewed as methodologically flawed, with the most encouraging results emerging only in posthoc analyses. Some prominent authors in the field of SCI have argued that 24-hour methylprednisolone should not be routinely used in SCI, and then only on a compassionate use basis (27).
- ☞ All patients sustaining major trauma, a fall from greater than ten feet, MVC, or noticeable injuries to the head or neck should be thoroughly evaluated for evidence of SCI.
- ☞ Some experimental studies have reported reversal of neurological deficits if decompression is performed in six to eight hours from the time of injury (53), and

clinical improvement of neurological deficits after cervical traction has been applied (54,55).

✍ Lesions in the spinal cord produce sensory and motor disturbances corresponding to the functions of the tracts that have been injured or transected.

✍ Clinically, the term spinal shock refers to systemic hypotension due to a decrease in sympathetic fiber–mediated arterial and venous vascular resistance, along with venous pooling and loss of preload, with or without bradycardia.

✍ Although phenylephrine, a nearly pure α-agonist, is commonly used in conjunction with volume in trauma resuscitation, for SCI we favor norepinephrine as a first choice, and if more β-adrenergic support is needed, epinephrine.

✍ Cord perfusion is crucial in the first 72 hours following injury, and even short periods of hypotension may have severe consequences; all patients should receive an arterial line in the ICU, and MAPs should not be allowed to fall below 60 to 70 mmHg.

✍ Currently, the data is insufficient to recommend the routine use of hypertonic saline for resuscitation in SCI, however, its use should be considered in the setting of resuscitation when CNS edema amenable to osmotic therapy is present.

✍ Somewhere between 19% to 70% of SCI patients have at least one episode of autonomic dysreflexia in their lifetime (67), and should always be anticipated when patients are scheduled for even small procedures, such as cystoscopy (68).

✍ Pulmonary complications, after the primary injury, are the cause of morbidity and mortality in SCI.

✍ Acute SCI victims have the highest risk of developing DVT among all hospitalized patients (75,76).

✍ Diaphragmatic breathing is affected by body position. When supine, abdominal contents push the diaphragm up increasing excursion and tidal volume, but at the expense of FRC. When the patient is upright, FRC is preserved, but diaphragmatic "doming" and, thus, excursion is diminished.

✍ The use of abdominal thrusts or quad coughing, postural drainage, chest percussion, and effective pain management lower the incidence of pneumonia in SCI patients.

✍ Severe CNS injury causes a hypermetabolic response that peaks 5 to 12 days after injury, and decreases to a level below preinjury needs depending on residual level of motor function.

✍ Chronic urinary tract dysfunction requiring catheter drainage and recurrent UTIs are a serious problem for patients with SCI.

REFERENCES

1. Theodore N, Sonntag VK. Spinal surgery: the past century and the next. Neurosurgery 2000; 46(4):767–777.
2. Sekhon LH, Fehlings MG. Epidemiology, demographics, and pathophysiology of acute spinal cord injury. Spine 2001; 26(suppl 24):S2–S12.
3. Ditunno JF Jr, Formal CS. Chronic spinal cord injury. N Engl J Med 1994; 330(8):550–556.
4. De Vivo MJ, Richards JS, Stover SL, et al. Spinal cord injury. Rehabilitation adds life to years. West J Med 1991; 154(5):602–606.
5. Amar AP, Levy ML. Pathogenesis and pharmacological strategies for mitigating secondary damage in acute spinal cord injury. Neurosurgery 1999; 44(5):1027–1039.
6. Ross LF, Johnson DH, Bennahum D, et al. Life support for patients with cervical-level quadriplegia. N Engl J Med 1993; 329(9):663–664.
7. The Edwin Smith surgical papyrus. In: Wilkins RH, ed. Neurosurgical Classics. Chicago: American Association of Neurological Surgeons, 1992:1–5.
8. Vaccaro AR, Nachwalter RS, Klein GR, et al. The significance of thoracolumbar spinal canal size in spinal cord injury patients. Spine 2001; 26(4):371–376.
9. Chapman JR, Anderson PA. Thoracolumbar spine fractures with neurologic deficit. Orthop Clin North Am 1994; 25(4):595–612.
10. Tator CH. Spine-spinal cord relationships in spinal cord trauma. Clin Neurosurg 1983; 30:479–494.
11. Tymianski M, Tator CH. Normal and abnormal calcium homeostasis in neurons: a basis for the pathophysiology of traumatic and ischemic central nervous system injury. Neurosurgery 1996; 38(6):1176–1195.
12. Nockels RP. Nonoperative management of acute spinal cord injury. Spine 2001; 26(suppl 24):S31–S37.
13. Tator CH, Fehlings MG. Review of the secondary injury theory of acute spinal cord trauma with emphasis on vascular mechanisms. J Neurosurg 1991; 75(1):15–26.
14. Tator CH. Spinal cord syndromes with physiological and anatomical correlation. In: Arnold H. Menezes, Volker KH, eds. Principle of Spinal Injury, New York: McGraw-Hill, Health Professions Division, 1996:785–800.
15. Amar AP, Levy ML. Surgical controversies in the management of spinal cord injury. J Am Coll Surg 1999; 188(5):550–566.
16. An HS. Cervical spine trauma. Spine 1998; 23(24):2713–2729.
17. Anthes DL, Theriault E, Tator CH. Ultrastructural evidence for arteriolar vasospasm after spinal cord trauma. Neurosurgery 1996; 39(4):804–814.
18. Tator CH, Koyanagi I. Vascular mechanisms in the pathophysiology of human spinal cord injury. J Neurosurg 1997; 86(3):483–492.
19. Wagner FC Jr, Stewart WB. Effect of trauma dose on spinal cord edema. J Neurosurg 1981; 54(6):802–806.
20. Yu CG, Jagid J, Ruenes G, et al. Detrimental effects of systemic hyperthermia on locomotor function and histopathological outcome after traumatic spinal cord injury in the rat. Neurosurgery 2001; 49(1):152–158.
21. Sala F, Menna G, Bricolo A, et al. Role of glycemia in acute spinal cord injury. Data from a rat experimental model and clinical experience. Ann NY Acad Sci 1999; 890:133–154.
22. Van den Berghe G, Wouters P, Weekers F, et al. Intensive Insulin Therapy in Critically Ill Patients. N Engl J Med 2001; 345(19):1359–1367.
23. Van Den BG, Wouters PJ, Bouillon R, et al. Outcome benefit of intensive insulin therapy in the critically ill: Insulin dose versus glycemic control. Crit Care Med 2003; 31(2):359–366.
24. Bracken MB, Collins WF, Freeman DF, et al. Efficacy of methylprednisolone in acute spinal cord injury. JAMA 1984; 251(1):45–52.
25. Bracken MB, Shepard MJ, Collins WF, et al. A randomized, controlled trial of methylprednisolone or naloxone in the treatment of acute spinal-cord injury. Results of the Second National Acute Spinal Cord Injury Study. N Engl J Med 1990; 322(20):1405–1411.
26. Bracken MB, Shepard MJ, Holford TR, et al. Administration of methylprednisolone for 24 or 48 hours or tirilazad mesylate for 48 hours in the treatment of acute spinal cord injury. Results of the Third National Acute Spinal Cord Injury Randomized Controlled Trial. National Acute Spinal Cord Injury Study. JAMA 1997; 277(20):1597–1604.
27. Hurlbert RJ. The role of steroids in acute spinal injury: an evidence based analysis. Spine 2001; 26:39S–46S.
28. Fehlings MG. Editorial: Recommendations regarding the use of methylprednisolone in acute spinal injury: making sense out of the controversy. Spine 2001; 26(24S):S56–S57.
29. Shapiro S. Neurotransmission by neurons that use serotonin, noradrenaline, glutamate, glycine, and gamma-aminobutyric acid in the normal and injured spinal cord. Neurosurgery 1997; 40(1):168–176.

30. Lipton SA, Rosenberg PA. Excitatory amino acids as a final common pathway for neurologic disorders. N Engl J Med 1994; 330(9):613–622.

31. Fehlings MG, Sekhon LH. Acute interventions in spinal cord injury: what do we know, what should we do? Clin Neurosurg 2001; 48:226–242.

32. Agrawal SK, Fehlings MG. Role of NMDA and non-NMDA ionotropic glutamate receptors in traumatic spinal cord axonal injury. J Neurosci 1997; 17(3):1055–1063.

33. Agrawal SK, Fehlings MG. Mechanisms of secondary injury to spinal cord axons in vitro: role of Na+, Na(+)-K(+)-ATPase, the Na(+)-H+ exchanger, and the Na(+)-Ca2+ exchanger. J Neurosci 1996; 16(2):545–552.

34. Casha S, Yu WR, Fehlings MG. Oligodendroglial apoptosis occurs along degenerating axons and is associated with FAS and p75 expression following spinal cord injury in the rat. Neuroscience 2001; 103(1):203–218.

35. Lou J, Lenke LG, Ludwig FJ, et al. Apoptosis as a mechanism of neuronal cell death following acute experimental spinal cord injury. Spinal Cord 1998; 36(10):683–690.

36. Lu J, Ashwell KW, Waite P. Advances in secondary spinal cord injury: role of apoptosis. Spine 2000; 25(14):1859–1866.

37. Tymianski M, Charlton MP, Carlen PL, et al. Source specificity of early calcium neurotoxicity in cultured embryonic spinal neurons. J Neurosci 1993; 13(5):2085–2104.

38. Hall ED, Braughler JM. Free radicals in CNS injury. Res Publ Assoc Res Nerv Ment Dis 1993; 71:81–105.

39. American College of Surgeons. Advanced Tauma Life Support. Chicago: American College of Surgeons, 1995.

40. Lam AM. Spinal cord injury: management. Curr Opin Anesth 1992; 5:632–639.

41. Bracken MB. Treatment of acute spinal cord injury with methylprednisolone: results of a multicenter, randomized clinical trial. J Neurotrauma 1991; 8(suppl 1):S47–S50.

42. Bracken MB, Shepard MJ, Holford TR, et al. Methylprednisolone or tirilazad mesylate administration after acute spinal cord injury: 1-year follow up. Results of the third National Acute Spinal Cord Injury randomized controlled trial. J Neurosurg 1998; 89(5):699–706.

43. Bracken MB, Aldrich EF, Herr DL, et al. Clinical measurement, statistical analysis, and risk-benefit: controversies from trials of spinal injury. J Trauma 2000; 48(3):558–561.

44. Bracken MB, Webb SB Jr, Wagner FC. Classification of the severity of acute spinal cord injury: implications for management. Paraplegia 1978; 15(4):319–326.

45. Tator CH, Rowed DW, Schwartz TZ. Sunnybrook Cord Injury Scale for assessing neurological injury and neurological recovery. In: Tator CH, ed. Early Management of Spinal cord Injury. New York: Raven Press, 1982:7–24.

46. American Spinal Injury Association, http: www.asia-spinalinjury.org/. International Standards for Neurological Classification of SCI. ASIA. 2002.

47. Kaiser JA, Holland BA. Imaging of the cervical spine. Spine 1998; 23(24):2701–2712.

48. Rao SC, Fehlings MG. The optimal radiologic method for assessing spinal canal compromise and cord compression in patients with cervical spinal cord injury. Part I: An evidence-based analysis of the published literature. Spine 1999; 24(6):598–604.

49. Fehlings MG, Rao SC, Tator CH, et al. The optimal radiologic method for assessing spinal canal compromise and cord compression in patients with cervical spinal cord injury. Part II: Results of a multicenter study. Spine 1999; 24(6):605–613.

50. Stiell IG, Clement CM, McKnight RD, et al. The Canadian c-spine rule versus the NEXUS low-risk criteria in patients with trauma. N Engl J Med 2003; 349:2510–2518.

51. Schenarts PJ, Diaz J, Kaiser C, et al. Prospective comparison of admission computed tomographic scan and plain films of the upper cervical spine in trauma patients with altered mental status. J Trauma 2001; 51(4):663–668.

52. Giacobetti FB, Vaccaro AR, Bos-Giacobetti MA, et al. Vertebral artery occlusion associated with cervical spine trauma. A prospective analysis. Spine 1997; 22(2):188–192.

53. Delamarter RB, Sherman J, Carr JB. Pathophysiology of spinal cord injury. Recovery after immediate and delayed decompression. J Bone Joint Surg Am 1995; 77(7):1042–1049.

54. Grant GA, Mirza SK, Chapman JR, et al. Risk of early closed reduction in cervical spine subluxation injuries. J Neurosurg 1999; 90(suppl 1):13–18.

55. Brunette DD, Rockswold GL. Neurologic recovery following rapid spinal realignment for complete cervical spinal cord injury. J Trauma 1987; 27(4):445–447.

56. Schneider R. The syndrome of acute anterior spinal cord injury. J Neurosurg 1955; 12:95–122.

57. Schneider R. The syndrome of acute central spinal cord injury. J Neurosurg 1954; 11:546–577.

58. Atkinson PP, Atkinson JL. Spinal shock. Mayo Clin Proc 1996; 71(4):384–389.

59. Leis AA, Kronenberg MF, Stetkarova I, et al. Spinal motoneuron excitability after acute spinal cord injury in humans. Neurology 1996; 47(1):231–237.

60. Rivers E, Nguyen B, Havstad S, et al. Early goal-directed therapy in the treatment of severe sepsis and septic shock. N Engl J Med 2001; 345(19):1368–1377.

61. Kern JW, Shoemaker WC. Meta-analysis of hemodynamic optimization in high-risk patients. Crit Care Med 2002; 30(8):1686–1692.

62. Ball PA. Critical care of spinal cord injury. Spine 2001; 26(suppl 24):S27–S30.

63. Vale FL, Burns J, Jackson AB, et al. Combined medical and surgical treatment after acute spinal cord injury: results of a prospective pilot study to assess the merits of aggressive medical resuscitation and blood pressure management. J Neurosurg 1997; 87(2):239–246.

64. Vassar MJ, Fischer RP, O'Brien PE, et al. A multicenter trial for resuscitation of injured patients with 7.5% sodium chloride. The effect of added dextran 70. The Multicenter Group for the Study of Hypertonic Saline in Trauma Patients. Arch Surg 1993; 128(9):1003–1011.

65. Sheikh AA, Matsuoka T, Wisner DH. Cerebral effects of resuscitation with hypertonic saline and a new low- sodium hypertonic fluid in hemorrhagic shock and head injury. Crit Care Med 1996; 24(7):1226–1232.

66. Lindan R, Joiner E, Freehafer AA, et al. Incidence and clinical features of autonomic dysreflexia in patients with spinal cord injury. Paraplegia 1980; 18(5):285–292.

67. Blackmer J. Rehabilitation medicine: 1. Autonomic dysreflexia. CMAJ 2003; 169(9):931–935.

68. Naftchi NE, Richardson JS. Autonomic dysreflexia: pharmacological management of hypertensive crises in spinal cord injured patients. J Spinal Cord Med 1997; 20(3):355–360.

69. DeVivo MJ, Krause JS, Lammertse DP. Recent trends in mortality and causes of death among persons with spinal cord injury. Arch Phys Med Rehabil 1999; 80(11):1411–1419.

70. Craven DE. Epidemiology of ventilator-associated pneumonia. Chest 2000; 117(4, suppl 2):186S–187S.

71. D'Amico R, Pifferi S, Leonetti C, et al. Effectiveness of antibiotic prophylaxis in critically ill adult patients: systematic review of randomised controlled trials. BMJ 1998; 316(7140):1275–1285.

72. Marik PE. Aspiration pneumonitis and aspiration pneumonia. N Engl J Med 2001; 344(9):665–671.

73. Kollef MH. The prevention of ventilator-associated pneumonia. N Engl J Med 1999; 340(8):627–634.

74. Neumann DA, DeLegge MH. Gastric versus small-bowel tube feeding in the intensive care unit. Crit Care Med 2002; 30(7):1436–1438.

75. Geerts WH, Heit JA, Clagett GP, et al. Prevention of venous thromboembolism. Chest 2001; 119(suppl 1):132S–175S.

76. Prevention of thromboembolism in spinal cord injury. Consortium for Spinal Cord Medicine. J Spinal Cord Med 1997; 20(3):259–283.

77. McKinley WO, Jackson AB, Cardenas DD, et al. Long-term medical complications after traumatic spinal cord injury: a

regional model systems analysis. Arch Phys Med Rehabil 1999; 80(11):1402–1410.

78. Rossi EC, Green D, Rosen JS, et al. Sequential changes in factor VIII and platelets preceding deep vein thrombosis in patients with spinal cord injury. Br J Haematol 1980; 45(1):143–151.

79. Lamb GC, Tomski MA, Kaufman J, et al. Is chronic spinal cord injury associated with increased risk of venous thromboembolism? J Am Paraplegia Soc 1993; 16(3):153–156.

80. Merli GJ, Crabbe S, Paluzzi RG, et al. Etiology, incidence, and prevention of deep vein thrombosis in acute spinal cord injury. Arch Phys Med Rehabil 1993; 74(11):1199–1205.

81. Kim SW, Charalel JT, Park KW, et al. Prevalence of deep venous thrombosis in patients with chronic spinal cord injury. Arch Phys Med Rehabil 1994; 75(9):965–968.

82. Powell M, Kirshblum S, O'Connor KC. Duplex ultrasound screening for deep vein thrombosis in spinal cord injured patients at rehabilitation admission. Arch Phys Med Rehabil 1999; 80(9):1044–1046.

83. Pais SO, Tobin KD, Austin CB, et al. Percutaneous insertion of the Greenfield inferior vena cava filter: experience with ninety-six patients. J Vasc Surg 1988; 8(4):460–464.

84. Roehm JO Jr, Johnsrude IS, Barth MH, et al. The bird's nest inferior vena cava filter: progress report. Radiology 1988; 168(3):745–749.

85. Anderson FA Jr, Wheeler HB. Venous thromboembolism. Risk factors and prophylaxis. Clin Chest Med 1995; 16(2):235–251.

86. Becker DM, Philbrick JT, Selby JB. Inferior vena cava filters. Indications, safety, effectiveness. Arch Intern Med 1992; 152(10):1985–1994.

87. Streiff MB. Vena caval filters: a comprehensive review. Blood 2000; 95(12):3669–3677.

88. Maxwell RA, Chavarria-Aguilar M, Cockerham WT, et al. Routine prophylactic vena cava filtration is not indicated after acute spinal cord injury. J Trauma 2002; 52(5):902–906.

89. Decousus H, Leizorovicz A, Parent F, et al. A clinical trial of vena caval filters in the prevention of pulmonary embolism in patients with proximal deep-vein thrombosis. Prevention du Risque d'Embolie Pulmonaire par Interruption Cave Study Group. N Engl J Med 1998; 338(7):409–415.

90. Bennett DA, Bleck TP. Diagnosis and treatment of neuromuscular causes of acute respiratory failure. Clin Neuropharmacol 1988; 11(4):303–347.

91. Goldman JM, Rose LS, Morgan MD, et al. Measurement of abdominal wall compliance in normal subjects and tetraplegic patients. Thorax 1986; 41(7):513–518.

92. Aldrich TK, Rochester DF. The lungs and neuromuscular disease. In: Murray JR, Nadell J, eds. Textbook of Respiratory Medicine. Philadelphia: W.B. Saunders, 2002:2329–2356.

93. Bergofsky E. Mechanism for respiratory insufficiency after cervical cord injury. Ann Intern Med 1964; 61:435.

94. Danon J, Druz WS, Goldberg NB, et al. Function of the isolated paced diaphragm and the cervical accessory muscles in C1 quadriplegics. Am Rev Respir Dis 2002; 119:909.

95. DeVivo MJ, Stover SL, Black KJ. Prognostic factors for 12-year survival after spinal cord injury. Arch Phys Med Rehabil 1992; 73(2):156–162.

96. Jackson AB, Groomes TE. Incidence of respiratory complications following spinal cord injury. Arch Phys Med Rehabil 1994; 75(3):270–275.

97. Fishburn MJ, Marino RJ, Ditunno JF Jr. Atelectasis and pneumonia in acute spinal cord injury. Arch Phys Med Rehabil 1990; 71(3):197–200.

98. McMichan JC, Michel L, Westbrook PR. Pulmonary dysfunction following traumatic quadriplegia. Recognition, prevention, and treatment. JAMA 1980; 243(6):528–531.

99. Ledsome JR, Sharp JM. Pulmonary function in acute cervical cord injury. Am Rev Respir Dis 1981; 124(1):41–44.

100. Wicks AB, Menter RR. Long-term outlook in quadriplegic patients with initial ventilator dependency. Chest 1986; 90(3):406–410.

101. Axen K, Pineda H, Shunfenthal I, et al. Diaphragmatic function following cervical cord injury: neurally mediated improvement. Arch Phys Med Rehabil 1985; 66(4):219–222.

102. Haas F, Axen K, Pineda H, et al. Temporal pulmonary function changes in cervical cord injury. Arch Phys Med Rehabil 1985; 66(3):139–144.

103. Pichurko BM, McCool FD, Scanlon PD, et al. Factors related to respiratory function recovery following acute quadriplegia. Am Rev Respir Dis 1985; 131:A337.

104. Rodriguez JL, Steinberg SM, Luchetti FA, et al. Early tracheostomy for primary airway management in the surgical critical care setting. Surgery 1990; 108(4):655–659.

105. Gibbons KJ. Tracheostomy: timing is everything. Crit Care Med 2000; 28(5):1663–1664.

106. Heffner JE. Timing of tracheotomy in mechanically ventilated patients. Am Rev Respir Dis 1993; 147(3):768–771.

107. Plummer AL, Gracey DR. Consensus conference on artificial airways in patients receiving mechanical ventilation. Chest 1989; 96(1):178–180.

108. Harrop JS, Sharan AD, Scheid EH Jr, et al. Tracheostomy placement in patients with complete cervical spinal cord injuries: American Spinal Injury Association Grade A. J Neurosurg 2004; 100(suppl 1):20–23.

109. Ciaglia P, Firsching R, Syniec C. Elective percutaneous dilatational tracheostomy. A new simple bedside procedure; preliminary report. Chest 1985; 87(6):715–719.

110. Mayberry JC, Wu IC, Goldman RK, et al. Cervical spine clearance and neck extension during percutaneous tracheostomy in trauma patients. Crit Care Med 2000; 28(10):3436–3440.

111. Albert TJ, Levine MJ, Balderston RA, et al. Gastrointestinal complications in spinal cord injury. Spine 1991; 16(suppl 10):S522–S525.

112. Soderstrom CA, Ducker TB. Increased susceptibility of patients with cervical cord lesions to peptic gastrointestinal complications. J Trauma 1985; 25(11):1030–1038.

113. Gore RM, Mintzer RA, Calenoff L. Gastrointestinal complications of spinal cord injury. Spine 1981; 6(6):538–544.

114. Cook DJ, Laine LA, Guyatt GH, et al. Nosocomial pneumonia and the role of gastric pH. A meta-analysis. Chest 1991; 100(1):7–13.

115. Tryba M. Sucralfate versus antacids or H2-antagonists for stress ulcer prophylaxis: a meta-analysis on efficacy and pneumonia rate. Crit Care Med 1991; 19(7):942–949.

116. Guidelines for the use of parenteral and enteral nutrition in adult and pediatric patients. JPEN J Parenter Enteral Nutr 2002; 26(suppl 1):1SA–138SA.

117. Bistrian BR. Route of feeding in critically ill patients. Crit Care Med 2002; 30(2):489–490.

118. Round table conference on metabolic support of the critically ill patients—March 20–22, 1993. Intensive Care Med 1994; 20(4):298–299.

119. Jolliet P, Pichard C, Biolo G, et al. Enteral nutrition in intensive care patients: a practical approach. Working Group on Nutrition and Metabolism, ESICM. European Society of Intensive Care Medicine. Intensive Care Med 1998; 24(8):848–859.

120. Moore FA, Feliciano DV, Andrassy RJ, et al. Early enteral feeding, compared with parenteral, reduces postoperative septic complications. The results of a meta-analysis. Ann Surg 1992; 216(2):172–183.

121. Zaloga GP. Early enteral nutritional support improves outcome: hypothesis or fact? Crit Care Med 1999; 27(2):259–261.

122. Atkinson S, Sieffert E, Bihari D. A prospective, randomized, double-blind, controlled clinical trial of enteral immunonutrition in the critically ill. Guy's Hospital Intensive Care Group. Crit Care Med 1998; 26(7):1164–1172.

123. Galban C, Montejo JC, Mesejo A, et al. An immune-enhancing enteral diet reduces mortality rate and episodes of bacteremia in septic intensive care unit patients. Crit Care Med 2000; 28(3):643–648.

124. Beale RJ, Bryg DJ, Bihari DJ. Immunonutrition in the critically ill: a systematic review of clinical outcome. Crit Care Med 1999; 27(12):2799–2805.

125. Kearns PJ, Chin D, Mueller L, et al. The incidence of ventilator-associated pneumonia and success in nutrient delivery with gastric versus small intestinal feeding: a randomized clinical trial. Crit Care Med 2000; 28(6):1742–1746.

126. Kortbeek JB, Haigh PI, Doig C. Duodenal versus gastric feeding in ventilated blunt trauma patients: a randomized controlled trial. J Trauma 1999; 46(6):992–996.

127. Esparza J, Boivin MA, Hartshorne MF, et al. Equal aspiration rates in gastrically and transpylorically fed critically ill patients. Intensive Care Med 2001; 27(4):660–664.

128. Lu WY, Rhoney DH, Boling WB, et al. A review of stress ulcer prophylaxis in the neurosurgical intensive care unit. Neurosurgery 1997; 41(2):416–425.

129. Mutlu GM, Mutlu EA, Factor P. GI Complications in Patients Receiving Mechanical Ventilation. Chest 2001; 119(4):1222–1241.

130. Martin LF, Booth FV, Karlstadt RG, et al. Continuous intravenous cimetidine decreases stress-related upper gastrointestinal hemorrhage without promoting pneumonia. Crit Care Med 1993; 21(1):19–30.

131. Moore JG. Achieving pH control in the critically ill patient: the role of continuous infusion of H2-receptor antagonists. DICP 1990; 24(suppl 11):S28–S30.

132. Glavin GB. Role of the central nervous system in stress ulcers. Compr Ther 1991; 17(4):3–5.

133. Cook D, Guyatt G, Marshall J, et al. A comparison of sucralfate and ranitidine for the prevention of upper gastrointestinal bleeding in patients requiring mechanical ventilation. Canadian Critical Care Trials Group. N Engl J Med 1998; 338(12):791–797.

134. Biering-Sorensen F. Urinary tract infection in individuals with spinal cord lesion. Curr Opin Urol 2002; 12(1):45–49.

135. Cardenas DD, Mayo ME. Bacteriuria with fever after spinal cord injury. Arch Phys Med Rehabil 1987; 68(5 Pt 1):291–293.

136. Cardenas DD, Hooton TM. Urinary tract infection in persons with spinal cord injury. Arch Phys Med Rehabil 1995; 76(3):272–280.

137. Galloway A. Prevention of urinary tract infection in patients with spinal cord injury—a microbiological review. Spinal Cord 1997; 35(4):198–204.

138. Saint S, Elmore JG, Sullivan SD, et al. The efficacy of silver alloy-coated urinary catheters in preventing urinary tract infection: a meta-analysis. Am J Med 1998; 105(3):236–241.

139. Elden H, Hizmetli S, Nacitarhan V, et al. Relapsing significant bacteriuria: effect on urinary tract infection in patients with spinal cord injury. Arch Phys Med Rehabil 1997; 78(5):468–470.

140. Waites KB, Canupp KC, Chen Y, et al. Bacteremia after spinal cord injury in initial versus subsequent hospitalizations. J Spinal Cord Med 2001; 24(2):96–100.

141. Nygaard IE, Kreder KJ. Spine update. Urological management in patients with spinal cord injuries. Spine 1996; 21(1):128–132.

142. Hartkopp A, Bronnum-Hansen H, Seidenschnur AM, et al. Survival and cause of death after traumatic spinal cord injury. A long-term epidemiological survey from Denmark. Spinal Cord 1997; 35(2):76–85.

143. Selzman AA, Hampel N. Urologic complications of spinal cord injury. Urol Clin North Am 1993; 20(3):453–464.

144. Bors E, Comarr AE. Neurological urology physiology of micturition, its neurological disorders and sequelae. Baltimore: University Park Press, 1971:129–135.

145. Linsenmeyer TA, Campagnolo DI, Chou IH. Silent autonomic dysreflexia during voiding in men with spinal cord injuries. J Urol 1996; 155(2):519–522.

146. Linsenmeyer TA, Culkin D. APS recommendations for the urological evaluation of patients with spinal cord injury. J Spinal Cord Med 1999; 22(2):139–142.

147. Bates-Jensen BM. Quality indicators for prevention and management of pressure ulcers in vulnerable elders. Ann Intern Med 2001; 135(8 Pt 2):744–751.

148. Fife C, Otto G, Capsuto EG, et al. Incidence of pressure ulcers in a neurologic intensive care unit. Crit Care Med 2001; 29(2):283–290.

149. Mattson MP. Excitotoxic and excitoprotective mechanisms: abundant targets for the prevention and treatment of neurodegenerative disorders. Neuromolecular Med 2003; 3(2):65–94.

150. Kim DH, Vaccaro AR, Henderson FC, et al. Molecular biology of cervical myelopathy and spinal cord injury: role of oligodendrocyte apoptosis. Spine J 2003; 3(6):510–519.

151. Hains BC, Black JA, Waxman SG. Primary cortical motor neurons undergo apoptosis after axotomizing spinal cord injury. J Comp Neurol 2003; 462(3):328–341.

152. Blesch A, Tuszynski MH. Cellular GDNF delivery promotes growth of motor and dorsal column sensory axons after partial and complete spinal cord transections and induces remyelination. J Comp Neurol 2003; 467(3):403–417.

153. Han SSW, Fischer I. Neural Stem Cells and Gene Therapy: Prospects for Repairing the Injured Spinal Cord. JAMA 2000; 283:2300–2301.

154. Luque JM, Ribotta M. Neural stem cells and the quest for restorative neurology. Histol Histopathol 2004; 19(1):271–280.

155. Dobkin BH, Havton LA. Basic advances and new avenues in therapy of spinal cord injury. Annu Rev Med 2004; 55:255–282.

156. Iwanami A, Kaneko S, Nakamura N, et al. Transplantation of human neural stem cells for spinal cord injury in primates. J Neurosci Res 2005; 80:182–190.

157. Curt A, Schwab ME, Dietz V. Providing the clinical basis for new interventional therapies: refined diagnosis and assessment of recovery after spinal cord injury. Spinal Cord 2004; 42(1):1–6.

158. Hampton T. Spinal Cord Network. JAMA 2005; 293:2463.

159. Meyer PR Jr. Surgery of Spine Trauma. New York: Churchill Livingstone, 1989:210.

14

Management of Intracerebral Vascular Catastrophes

Rahul Jandial

Division of Neurosurgery, UC San Diego Medical Center, San Diego, and the Burnham
Institute for Medical Research, La Jolla, California, U.S.A.

Henry E. Aryan

Division of Neurosurgery, Department of Surgery, UC San Diego Medical Center, San Diego, California, U.S.A.

Samuel A. Hughes

Department of Neurosurgical Surgery, Oregon Health and Science University, Portland, Oregon, U.S.A.

Hoi Sang U

Division of Neurosurgery, Department of Surgery, UC San Diego Medical Center, San Diego, California, U.S.A.

INTRODUCTION

The management of vascular catastrophes in the brain requires both prompt diagnosis and treatment. It also requires a fundamental knowledge of the medical and surgical principles of neurological intensive care management of both operative and nonoperative cases. Often, the pathology comprising this arena is associated with high morbidity and mortality, underscoring the need for diligence and insight into the particulars of the neurological milieu.

Most neurological emergencies involve hemorrhage within the brain and/or other intracranial spaces, or ischemic insults to the central nervous system (CNS). Among intracranial hemorrhages, management of aneurysmal subarachnoid hemorrhage (SAH) is particularly demanding. Aside from operative or endovascular interventions, significant intensive care management is needed to treat the underlying pathologies and the associated complications. The principles of therapy aim to maintain adequate CNS blood flow to prevent cerebral ischemia, which threatens cell survival. In addition, treatment is focused upon preventing brain shift and herniation as a result of brain swelling. Intracerebral hemorrhage and ischemic cerebrovascular disease remain additional major sources of morbidity and mortality. Because of emerging therapies rapid evaluation is increasingly critical to their appropriate management. This chapter will focus on the pathophysiology, clinical presentation, and management of the aforementioned disease entities, as well as a brief discussion of traumatic cerebral aneurysms, venous sinus thrombosis, and carotid cavernous sinus fistulae.

SUBARACHNOID HEMORRHAGE

The major cause of nontraumatic SAH is aneurysmal rupture, which occurs in approximately 30,000 persons per year in the United States (1). ☞ **The mortality associated with the initial hemorrhage is around 20%.** ☞ Subsequently, the mortality is 30% within the first two weeks, and 45%

within the first month following the initial bleed. Among the survivors, as many as 50% suffer from significant neurological impairment (2,3). Most morbidity subsequent to SAH is due to complications from cerebral ischemia. This results from increased intracranial (ICP) pressure following the initial hemorrhage, and is exacerbated by rebleeding, vasospasm, and hydrocephalus. Nevertheless, outcomes following SAH have improved over the past 10 years as a result of improvements in the medical and surgical management of this disease (4).

Pathogenesis

☞ **Saccular aneurysms must be differentiated from traumatic, dissecting, mycotic, and/or tumor-associated aneurysms because the classification dictates management.** ☞ Saccular aneurysms arise at the sites in a blood vessel where the elastic component is either absent from birth or damaged by arteriosclerotic changes. A saccular outpouching eventually forms into an aneurysmal sac due to the constant impact of the blood stream (5). Aneurysms are also associated with systemic and familial diseases such as Marfan's syndrome, Ehlers-Danlos syndrome, fibromuscular dysplasia, polycystic disease, and coarctation of the aorta (6).

Presentation

The classical presentation of SAH is a sudden, severe headache, typically the worst in the life of the patient (often termed a thunder clap). This is often accompanied by neck pain, nausea and vomiting, photophobia, varying degrees of altered mental status, and even profound coma (7). The associated acute rise in intracranial pressure (ICP) may also produce subhyaloid hemorrhages. Up to 20% of patients experience a warning leak or sentinel hemorrhage prior to aneurysmal SAH. This is characterized by nuchal rigidity and/or meningismus lasting 24 to 48 hours. Unfortunately, a sentinel hemorrhage is misdiagnosed 20% to 40% of the time as another more benign disease such as migraine, cervical disease, or sinusitis (8,9). In order to minimize this, maintaining a high degree of suspicion for aneurysmal expansion or sentinel hemorrhage is imperative.

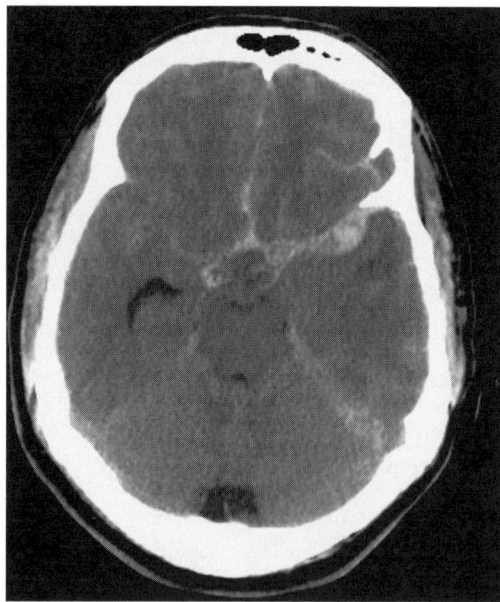

Figure 1 Head computed tomography (CT), noncontrast, with interhemispheric subarachnoid hemorrhage (between the frontal lobes along the left sylvian fissure). Also dilatation of the right temporal horn of the ventricle (one of the radiological hallmarks of hydrocephalus).

In addition to hemorrhage, aneurysmal expansion can cause neurological changes, allowing for the possibility of diagnosis prior to rupture. Depending on the location, the patient may have facial pain, papillary dilatation, ptosis, and/or visual field defects.

Diagnostic Evaluation

The diagnosis of SAH rests with identification of its classical clinical presentation. This should be confirmed with an emergent noncontrast computerized tomographic (CT) scan. The CT scan aids in detecting, localizing, and quantifying the SAH. It is successful 95% of the time in identifying SAH, when performed on the same day as the onset of symptoms (10) (Fig. 1). Additional information about cerebral edema and hydrocephalus is also provided by CT scan. In the setting of a sentinel hemorrhage from an aneurysm, a CT scan may be negative in up to 35% of patients (11). Patients presenting with a

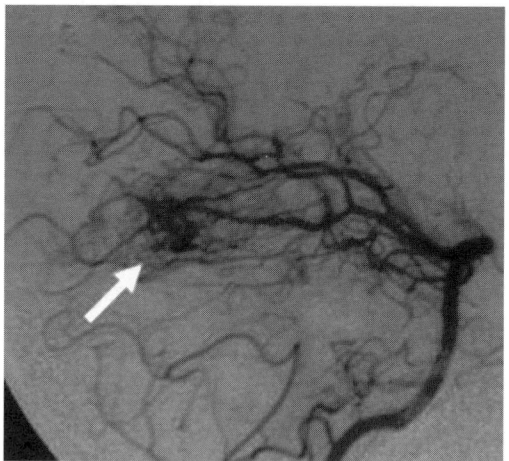

Figure 3 Cerebral angiogram, lateral projection, posterior circulation arterial venous malformation.

history which is suggestive of SAH, yet possessing a normal CT scan, warrant a lumbar puncture (first exclude intracranial mass lesion). This would consistently reveal elevated red blood cell counts in all tubes if SAH had indeed occurred. Lastly, a CT scan also reveals causes of SAH other than an aneurysm rupture. This includes pituitary apoplexy, which can mimic an aneurysm rupture clinically. The identification of a hemorrhagic pituitary adenoma can lead to prompt treatment with steroids to prevent a potentially lethal Addisonian crisis.

⚬ **Immediately following the documentation of SAH, attention is directed toward the identification of the responsible vascular abnormality, most commonly a ruptured aneurysm.** ⚬ The gold standard diagnostic examination is digital subtraction four-vessel cerebral angiography. This will identify an aneurysm in 95% of cases, and occasionally an arteriovenous malformation (AVM) (12) (Figs. 2 and 3). In addition, an angiogram will show details of the location, size and orientation of the aneurysm as well as demonstrate the presence or absence of vasospasm (Fig. 4). However, in 5% to 15% of the cases, the angiogram is negative. In this situation, the study should be repeated in two to three weeks and again in a few months, because an acute intraluminal thrombus may interfere with angiographic visualization (12,13).

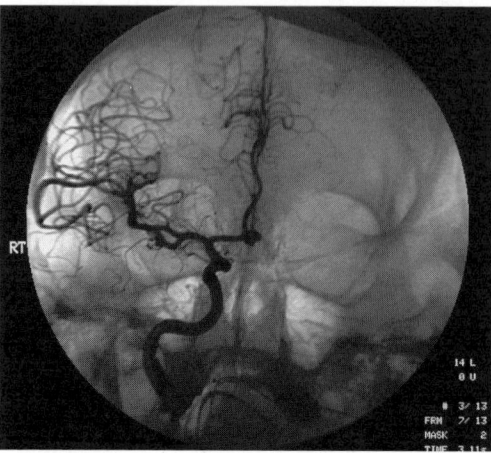

Figure 2 Cerebral angiogram, anterior–posterior projection, with anterior communicating artery aneurysm.

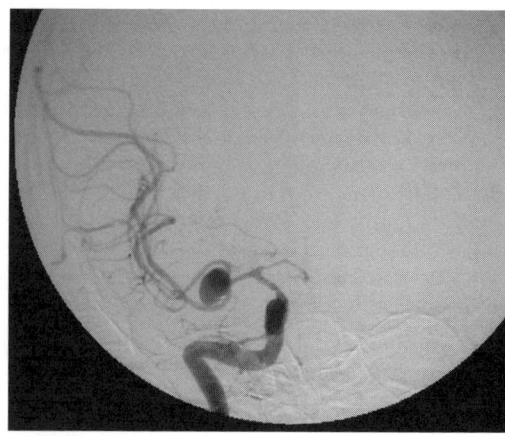

Figure 4 Cerebral angiogram, oblique projection, demonstrating the significant narrowing of vasculature beginning at the internal carotid artery and extending past the bifurcation in the middle cerebral vasculature, consistent with the angiographic diagnosis of vasospasm.

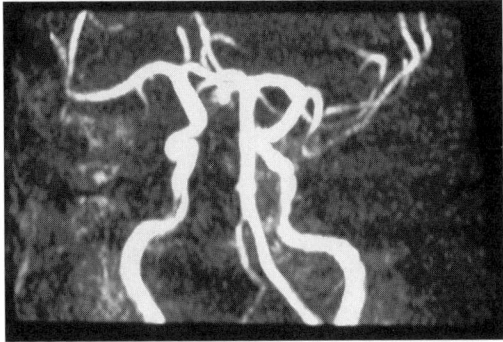

Figure 5 Magnetic resonance angiogram of the cerebral vasculature.

In addition to cerebral angiography for visualization of the cerebral vasculature, other noninvasive imaging modalities are available as well. Aneurysms can be demonstrated using magnetic resonance angiography (MRA); however, MRA has limited sensitivity in the detection of small (<5 mm) aneurysms (Fig. 5). On the other hand, CT angiography (CTA) is increasingly being employed for the assessment of the cerebral vasculature in the setting of SAH. This technique obtains images by contrast-enhanced, high-speed spiral CT. The axially acquired data are then reconstructed into three-dimensional angiographic images (14). The advantages of CTA include the rapidity with which images are obtained, its noninvasive nature, and its relative high sensitivity and specificity (15). However, aneurysms less than 3 mm still may escape detection. Additionally, extensive SAH may hinder the clear demonstration of an aneurysm. Finally, postoperative use of CTA is limited by scanning artifacts introduced by an aneurysm clip.

Clinical Grading

The clinical state of a patient presenting with SAH is highly predictive of the therapeutic outcome. A grading system has therefore been developed to document the severity of the patient's disease in order to guide therapy and prognostication. In 1968, Hunt and Hess developed a scale which has been useful in correlating the patient's clinical status and prognosis (Table 1) (16). Vasospasm, which is thought

Table 1 Hunt and Hess Grading Scale

Grade	Symptoms
I	Asymptomatic or minimal headache and slight nuchal rigidity
II	Moderate to severe headache, nuchal rigidity, no neurologic deficit other than a CN III palsy
III	Drowsiness, confusion, or mild focal deficit (e.g., any cranial nerve palsy other than CN III)
IV	Stupor, hemiparesis, possible early decerebrate rigidity
V	Deep coma, decerebrate rigidity, moribund appearance
Plus one	Serious systemic diseases, such as hypertension, diabetes, severe arteriosclerosis, chronic obstructive pulmonary disease, and severe vasospasm, result in placement of the patient in the next less-favorable category

Abbreviation: CN III, third cranial nerve.
Source: From Ref. 16.

Table 2 Fisher Grade

Grade	Blood on CT
1	No blood detected
2	Diffuse or vertical layers <1 mm thick
3	Localized clot and/or vertical layer greater than or equal to 1 mm
4	Intracerebral or intraventricular clot with diffuse or no subarachnoid blood

Abbreviation: CT, computed tomograph.
Source: From Ref. 17.

to be caused by subarachnoid blood and its breakdown products, is also responsible for marked morbidity and mortality. As a result, the Fisher grading system was developed to correlate the amount and distribution of subarachnoid blood on CT with the subsequent development of vasospasm (Table 2) (17). In both grading systems, a lower grade (smaller number) is correlated with a better prognosis.

Therapy

The initial goal in SAH management is stabilization of the neurologic and cardiopulmonary condition of the patient. Once this is accomplished, the necessary steps are taken to diagnose and treat the cause of the SAH. In the case of a ruptured aneurysm, the stabilization, workup, and operative therapy must be instituted expeditiously since rerupture usually occurs within the first 72 hours following SAH. The development of vasospasm may also occur within the first few days following SAH and tends to peak seven to eight days following the initial ictus. Depending on the grade of the SAH (Hunt/Hess and Fisher), the patient may need to be intubated for pulmonary support as well as to facilitate sedation. External ventricular drainage for the treatment of hydrocephalus may be needed. Once the diagnosis of a ruptured aneurysm is established by angiography, definitive treatment of the aneurysm may occur through surgical clipping or endovascular coiling. The algorithm for definitive treatment of aneurysmal SAH is changing rapidly (particularly the criteria for endovascular management).

Surgical Therapy

✄ Patients with a lower Hunt and Hess grade (Hunt and Hess grade I–III) should undergo an urgent craniotomy and surgical clipping of anatomically accessible aneurysms. ✄ The surgical treatment of higher-grade SAH patients (Hunt and Hess IV & V), who are less favorable operative candidates with a poorer prognosis, remains controversial.

✄ The goal of treatment is to secure the neck of the aneurysm by clipping, so that the common complications of SAH, such as rebleeding, vasospasm, and hydrocephalus can be eliminated or maximally treated (18,19). ✄ This is accomplished by a craniotomy through which the neck of the aneurysm is identified and excluded from the parent circulation by a clip (Fig. 6). The operative techniques may include temporary proximal arterial occlusion (20). Sometimes, aneurysms which are relatively inaccessible may need to be treated with proximal arterial ligation. In some of these cases, blood flow may need to be augmented with the aid of an extracranial to intracranial (carotid/vertebral) arterial bypass.

Endovascular Therapy

With the development of better fluoroscopy and catheters, endovascular techniques have become increasingly

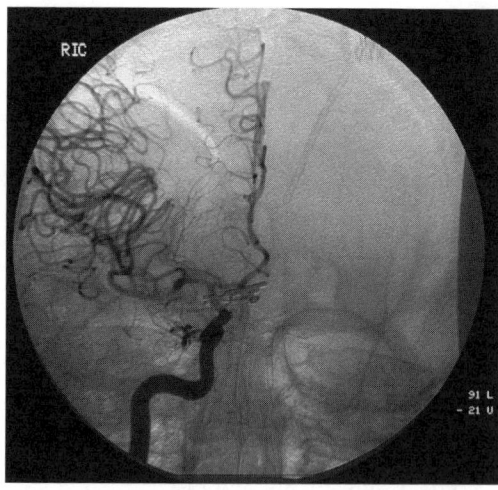

Figure 6 Cerebral angiogram, anterior–posterior projection, with anterior communicating artery aneurysm successfully clipped and excluded from the cerebral blood flow.

safe and effective in accessing the cerebral vasculature. Interventional neuroradiology has also become an indispensable adjunct in the management of cerebrovascular disease. A recent randomized International Subarachnoid Aneurysm Trial (ISAT) conducted in Europe, North America, and Australia, demonstrated better overall outcomes for those treated endovascularly. A total of 2143 patients were enrolled in 43 centers; the relative risk of death or significant disability at one year for patients treated with coils was 22.6% lower than those treated with surgical clipping (21).

☛ **Coil occlusion is indicated for the treatment of aneurysms which: (*i*) are difficult to clip surgically, (*ii*) occur in patients who are unsuitable for early surgery due to a poor SAH grade, and (*iii*) occur in patients who are medically unstable (22).** ☛ Detachable platinum-alloy microcoils are deployed through microcatheters into the aneurysm sac (23). The guidewire transmits a low positive direct electric current that detaches the coil from the stainless steel microcatheter. Coils "packed" into the aneurysm sac promote intra-aneurysmal electrothrombosis by attracting local blood components (Figs. 7 and 8) (22). In aneurysms which are treated with proximal parent artery ligation, endovascular balloon occlusion is also used. These include internal

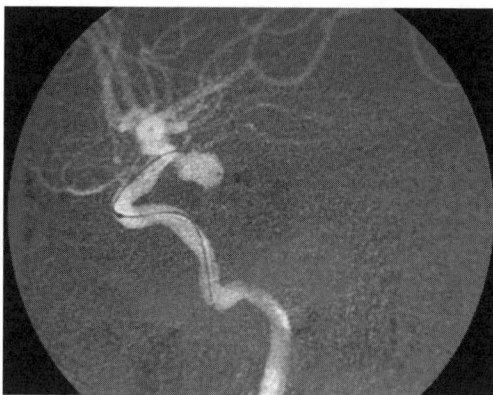

Figure 7 Cerebral angiogram with microcatheter seen in the internal carotid artery and entering the posterior communicating artery aneurysm.

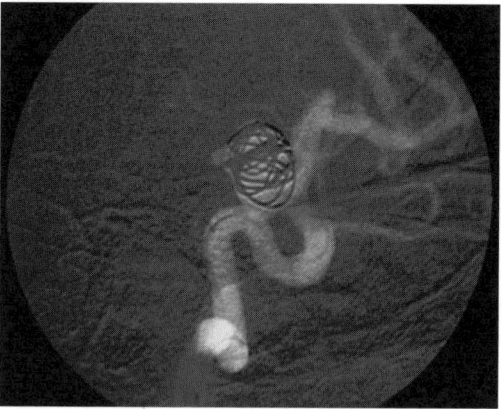

Figure 8 Cerebral angiogram with coils deployed within aneurysm.

carotid artery aneurysms in the cavernous sinus or selective vertebrobasilar aneurysms (24). Treatment of nonruptured aneurysms has not been studied prospectively. However, retrospective data tend to favor endovascular management at this time (25).

Vasospasm, diagnosed with angiography, can also be treated by endovascular interventions. Angioplasty can be used to increase luminal diameter and is indicated when calcium antagonist prophylaxis fails or when hypervolemic, hemodilutional, and hypertensive ("triple H") therapy is ineffective, or unsafe, in treating clinical vasospasm. A soft silicon balloon-tipped catheter is navigated into the affected cerebral vasculature and is inflated with 0.10 mL of saline to deliver 1–3 atm of pressure. This technique should not be employed when there is cerebral infarction or an unsecured aneurysm distal to the stenotic zone intended for angioplasty, as the postangioplasty increase in cerebral blood flow could precipitate a hemorrhage (26). Treatment of vasospasm also includes the perfusion of the stenotic segment with vasoactive drugs (e.g., papavarine). Repeated treatment is frequently necessary and effective.

Management of Subarachnoid Hemorrhage and Its Complications
Initial Management
Patients with SAH require intensive care management. All need to be closely monitored for potential medical, neurological, and surgical complications. Upon admission to the intensive care unit (ICU), patients are placed at bed rest with the head elevated to facilitate cerebral venous return. Measures are taken to prevent thrombophlebitis (with sequential pneumatic compression stockings), atelectasis and pneumonia (with good pulmonary toilet), and gastrointestinal ulceration (with the prophylactic use of H_2 antagonists and/or sulcrafate). External ventricular drainage of cerebrospinal fluid (CSF) may be necessary to treat acute hydrocephalus. All patients with an intraventricular hemorrhage should receive external ventricular drainage of CSF.

Systolic blood pressure should be maintained below 160 mmHg while the aneurysm is unsecured. Agents that are centrally sedating such as methyldopa should be avoided. Nausea and vomiting should be treated with agents that are not sedating as well (i.e., use odansatron rather than droperidol). Pain control should be addressed with minimal short-acting narcotics, without excessive sedation that may mask neurological (especially mental status) deterioration.

Neurological Consequences of Subarachnoid Hemorrhage

Rebleeding

After initial hemorrhage from a ruptured cerebral aneurysm, the greatest immediate concern is rehemorrhage of the unsecured aneurysm. In fact, the risk of rebleeding is greatest in the first 24 hours following SAH (1,3). Of untreated aneurysms, 20% rehemorrhage within two weeks, 50% rehemorrhage within one month, and by six months the risk stabilizes to approximately 2% to 3% per year (27,28). The consequences of rehemorrhage are devastating, with an overall mortality of 70% and accounting for 50% of all deaths occurring within 48 hours of the initial SAH (29,30). It is for these reasons that ruptured aneurysms should be treated early whenever feasible.

Vasospasm

Vasospasm is the constriction of arteries in the intracranial circulation in response to subarachnoid blood. A major complication that creates significant morbidity and mortality, vasospasm is noted angiographically in 70% of patients and leads to ischemic symptoms in 20% to 30% of patients (31). It may occur as early as the third day after the original SAH, with the incidence peaking between days 5 to 10 and remains a possible occurrence up to three weeks after the original hemorrhage (3). Ultimately, vasospasm leads to stroke or death in up to 15% of patients surviving the initial SAH (32).

Presentation and Diagnosis. During the pathological evaluation of vessels in vasospasm, intimal proliferation and medial necrosis is found. The amount of blood in the subarachnoid space and its location correlates directly with the likelihood of vasospasm and the vessels that are likely to be affected. The pathogenesis of vasospasm is unknown, but thought to result from the products of local erythrocyte degradation, and may be in part related to the sequestration of endothelial nitric oxide by the heme moiety of stroma-free hemoglobin.

The clinical presentation of vasospasm is variable and often progressive over a few hours, but can also occur suddenly. Symptoms may fluctuate ranging from a mild decrease in consciousness to focal neurological deficit from ischemic or infarcted brain, and even profound coma. The diagnosis is made when a delayed neurological deficit or deterioration occurs in a patient with SAH. Rehemorrhage and hydrocephalus must be excluded by urgent CT scan before attributing a delayed neurological deficit or deterioration to vasospasm. For definitive diagnosis of vasospasm, cerebral angiography should be performed. However, angiographic vasospasm is not always symptomatic. Since angiography carries a stroke risk of 1% to 2%, its utility as a screening or monitoring tool must be carefully considered (3,33).

The most commonly used bedside noninvasive monitoring technique to detect cerebral vasospasm is transcranial Doppler (TCD) ultrasonography (34). An inverse relationship between vessel caliber and flow velocity is predicted by the Bernoulli effect. Clinically, elevated TCD values and upward trends in TCD values are correlated with vasospasm, and guide the timing of noninvasive vasospasm treatment (35). This technique is also commonly used for monitoring poor-grade SAH patients in whom clinical signs of worsening neurological deterioration may be difficult to ascertain. Currently, xenon-13, single-photon emission computed tomography (SPECT), and positron emission tomography (PET) are being studied for their utility in directly measuring cerebral blood flow in vasospasm. Due to its noninvasive nature, TCD should be performed daily or every other day after aneurysmal SAH, reserving angiography for the diagnostic confirmation and therapeutic intervention of clinical vasospasm.

Management of Vasospasm. The goal of management is to minimize ischemic brain injury, especially from vasospasm. ✍ **The mainstay of therapy in the United States, once clinical vasospasm is suspected or confirmed, is nimodipine (to minimize vasospasm) and "triple-H" therapy; the three H's being hypervolemia, hypertension, and hemodilution.** ✍

A calcium channel antagonist such as nimodipine should be started upon admission to the ICU, since several studies with an oral nimodipine have demonstrated improved outcomes in SAH, particularly with poor-gradepatients (36,37). Fewer infarcts were noted, although there was no difference in the incidence or extent of angiographic vasospasm. Beneficial effects are most likely related to the calcium-blocking properties of these agents, which interfere with the ischemic cascade in marginally ischemic neurons (37). Calcium-channel blockers may also dilate leptomeningeal vessels, thereby improving collateral circulation to ischemic areas (38). Patients should be started on nimodipine 60 mg every four hours for 21 days, and if hypotension is encountered the dosage can be changed to 30 mg every two hours.

The other measure used to counteract the effects of vasospasm is triple-H therapy. The aim of triple-H therapy is to improve cerebral perfusion by raising systolic blood pressure and intravascular volume so as to optimize cardiac output. In the setting of SAH, circulating red blood cell volume is decreased, which predisposes patients to a higher incidence of delayed neurological deficit or deterioration from cerebral ischemia (39,40). Volume expansion, independent of effects on cerebral perfusion pressure, improves cerebral blood flow in patients with vasospasm (41). The critical factor in preventing or reducing cerebral ischemia may be the prevention of hypovolemia, rather than the creation of a hypervolemic state (42). Expanding the intravascular volume in patients with SAH also creates hemodilution. Hemodilution alone can improve both cerebral blood flow and oxygen delivery by decreasing blood flow viscosity (43). The use of hypertension in the treatment of vasospasm is based on the observation that cerebral autoregulation is lost with SAH. A direct correlation between mean arterial pressure and cerebral blood flow has also been demonstrated, and several studies have shown that such induced hypertension can reduce delayed neurological deficits from vasospasm in aneurysmal SAH (44,45). The combination of hypervolemia, hemodilution, and hypertension is now well accepted therapy for clinical vasospasm. The goal of intravascular volume expansion with isotonic crystalloid is to maintain a central venous pressure of 7–10 mmHg, and a hematocrit of 30% to 32%. Hypertension is induced in a stepwise fashion with volume and pressures, primarily beta agonists, to a systolic pressure of 160–200 mmHg until the neurological deficit or elevated TCD values improve (46). The use of triple-H therapy is not without risk, and should be instituted in the intensive care setting with a pulmonary artery catheter in place for continual cardiopulmonary assessment. This therapy has been associated with heart failure, pulmonary edema, and electrolyte disorders. Furthermore, induction of hypertension can lead to myocardial ischemia and infarction, intracranial hemorrhage, and rupture of unsecured aneurysms.

With the evolution of neuroendovascular techniques, another weapon in the armamentarium against vasospasm has been developed. Transluminal balloon angioplasty can be used to selectively dilate severely narrowed arteries. The ability to reverse clinical symptoms of vasospasm with this technique is related to how quickly after symptoms arise that angioplasty is performed. More significant improvement of symptoms is achieved when angioplasty is performed within 24 hours of neurological deterioration (47). In select patients, vasospasm refractory to medical therapy may be reversed in up to 98% of cases (48). Lastly, intra-arterial perfusion of vasoactive agents (e.g., papaverine) has also been used in treating vasospasm with varying degrees of success.

Hydrocephalus
Hydrocephalus may develop at different times after SAH. A large volume of blood in the subarachnoid space or in the ventricules can cause acute hydrocephalus due to obstruction of cerebrospinal drainage pathways. This may occur in up to 20% of patients and is more common in poor-grade patients since the degree of hemorrhage tends to be large in these patients (49). External ventricular drainage of CSF would be necessary to reduce ICP and to facilitate the removal of blood clots.

Hydrocephalus occurring in the subacute or late period after SAH is usually of the communicating type. The problem arises from decreased absorption of CSF by the arachnoid villi, caused by the products of blood degradation. These patients should be treated based on their clinical scenario. If there is ventriculomegaly and the patient is neurologically intact, then a period of observation and repeat CT scanning is warranted. However, if the patient has a neurological deficit or persistent headache, temporary CSF drainage and permanent CSF diversion with a ventriculoperitoneal or lumboperitoneal shunt may be needed. As many as 20% of patients with SAH will need permanent CSF diversion (50).

Seizures
Seizures occur in up to 25% of patients with aneurysmal SAH (51). Rebleeding or vasospasm can be exacerbated during the seizure episode. For this reason, anticonvulsants are used on a prophylactic basis for SAH patients in most American centers. Phenytoin is used for a two-week period and its use is extended to three months for witnessed seizure or postoperative intracranial hemorrhage. If fever, rash, or hepatotoxicity develops, phenytoin should be discontinued and a different anticonvulsant should be used (52).

Medical Consequences of Subarachnoid Hemorrhage
Cardiac Complications
Intracranial hemorrhage, particularly SAH, is associated with hypothalamic dysfunction and catecholamine release with unique cardiac complications. This adrenergic release causes prolonged myocardial contraction, decreased cardiac compliance, and is directly cardiotoxic. Sustained catecholamine release can eventually causes myofibrillar degeneration and necrosis (53). **Electrocardiogram (ECG) changes are common in patients with SAH, even in patients without prior history of cardiac disease.** Prominent U waves, inverted T waves, and minor elevation or depression of the ST segment can occur. Large upright T waves and prolonged QT intervals may also be encountered, and arrhythmias can occur in up to 30% of patients (54). Despite the aforementioned ECG changes in the setting of

SAH, permanent myocardial ischemia is relatively rare. The finding of pathologic Q waves warrants a diligent workup for myocardial infarction (55). Cardiac complications with SAH can be life threatening, and every patient should receive close cardiac monitoring, particularly during the first 48 hours after SAH when catecholamine release is greatest and during the institution of triple-H therapy.

Pulmonary Complications
After rebleeding, vasospasm, and hydrocephalus, morbidity following SAH can be attributable to pulmonary complications including pulmonary edema, pneumonia and/or pulmonary embolism. Pulmonary edema may be either neurogenic or cardiogenic in origin. The neurogenic pulmonary edema associated with SAH arises from induced alterations in pulmonary vascular permeability and results in edematous fluid with high protein content. Cardiogenic pulmonary edema is secondary to vascular congestion and results in edematous fluid with low protein content. This may be caused by primary cardiac failure or exuberant volume expansion in triple-H therapy, and underscores the need for using pulmonary artery catheters (56). Pneumonia occurs in 20% of SAH patients, usually from aspiration or prolonged mechanical ventilation. Timely intubation during neurological deterioration, vigilant pulmonary therapy, appropriate antibiotic management, and employment of tracheostomy are the basic principles guiding the management of pneumonia (57).

Thromboembolism
Thromboembolism poses a major concern in SAH patients who are frequently immobilized for long periods. These patients should receive intermittent pressure stockings. Anticoagulation is withheld until the aneurysm is secured. An established DVT in the setting of an unsecured aneurysm should be managed with an inferior vena caval filter. If anticoagulation is required, it is generally considered safe 48 hours after surgery.

ARTERIOVENOUS MALFORMATION
Pathogenesis
AVMs of the brain are congenital lesions of the vascular system. They begin to evolve between the fourth and eighth weeks of embryonic life, most likely from a defect in the development of the capillary system between the arteries and veins (58,59).

In a normally developed vascular system, cerebrovascular resistance, determined by the capillary system, prevents arterial blood from directly entering the veins. The capillary bed functions normally, allowing the developing brain access to nutrients from the blood. In the area of an AVM, however, this resistance bed does not exist and blood is shunted directly from the arterial into the venous system (Figs. 9 and 10). Since these anomalies arise during brain development, the part of the brain normally supplied by the absent capillary bed does not develop. Its function is subserved by surrounding cerebral components. For this reason, the patient may function normally and the AVM remains undetected. At the site where the AVM develops, a gliotic plane forms between the AVM and the surrounding brain. Lastly, the absence of the capillary bed also creates pathways which offer the least resistance to blood flow. These abnormal, low-resistance pathways

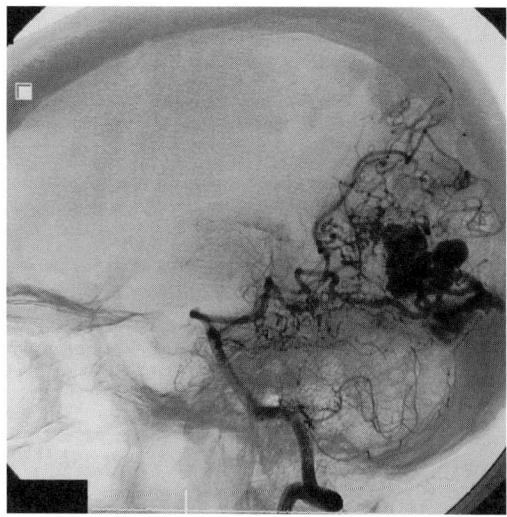

Figure 9 Cerebral angiogram, lateral projection, with occipital arterial venous malformation seen during the arterial phase.

gradually "capture" blood from the surrounding circulation and enlarge. The AVM eventually becomes a lesion comprised of abnormal channels of variable sizes. Aneurysms may also develop in this malformed vascular tree. AVMs may be extremely small and cryptic or so extensive as to involve an entire hemisphere. Because these vessels are malformed, under abnormal flow and pressure forces, they have a predilection to hemorrhage.

Presentation

☞ **AVMs are the leading cause of SAH in young people although they account for only 5% of SAH in adults (58,60).** ☞ AVMs may become symptomatic at any age. The most common presentation is an intracranial hemorrhage that occurs in up to 40% of the patients. This is more commonly seen in smaller AVMs. Seizure is also a presen-

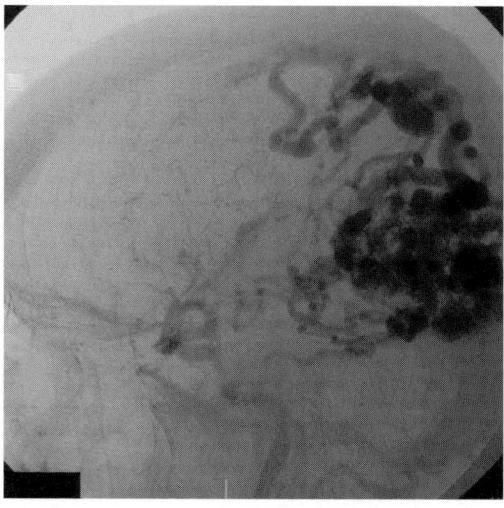

Figure 10 Cerebral angiogram, lateral projection, with occipital arterial venous malformation (AVM) seen during the venous phase; note the large dilated draining veins characteristic of an AVM.

tation of AVMs. This is presumed to arise from the gliotic plane between the AVM and the brain. Headache is the third symptom associated with an AVM. This is usually of a vascular pulsatile nature. In patients with large AVMs, progressive neurological deficits may develop, and this is thought to occur as blood is diverted from other areas of the brain to the malformation, causing progressive ischemia in those areas immediately surrounding the AVM. This diversion of blood is often referred to as steal.

The most threatening symptom of an AVM is hemorrhage. In those patients who did not present with a hemorrhage, the chance of a hemorrhage is 1% to 3% per year. On the other hand, AVMs which present with a hemorrhage, possess a hemorrhage risk of 3% to 5% per year. Since an AVM occurs mainly in younger individuals and the natural history in regard to hemorrhage for these patients is unfavorable, treatment is essential. In contrast to a mortality rate of 20% to 23% following rupture of an intracranial aneurysm, the initial mortality rate for a ruptured AVM is approximately 10% (58,60). The likelihood of surviving such a hemorrhage is, therefore, substantially higher than in a patient who suffers SAH from an aneurysm.

Diagnostic Evaluation

On CT scanning, a ruptured AVM assumes the appearance of an intracerebral hemorrhage. Blood can be intracerebral, intraventricular, subarachnoid, or some combination of the aforementioned. Calcifications may also be seen. Magnetic resonance (MR) imaging often shows signal voids as a result of traversing vessels and is more accurate at diagnosing AVM, particularly in the unruptured cases. The definitive diagnosis of an AVM is made using conventional cerebral angiography, which shows abnormal blood vessels and the classic early draining veins. In recent years CT angiography and MR angiography have been used increasingly in the diagnosis and evaluation of AVMs; however, therapy is offered only after establishing the diagnosis through a conventional cerebral angiogram (61).

Therapy

Therapy for AVMs has traditionally been operative. However, treatment of AVMs in critical areas (i.e., speech and motor centers) has been associated with marked morbidity and mortality. Therefore, alternative therapy is sought. Various forms of radiation have been tried and shown to be effective in selective situations (62–64). The limitation has been the size of the lesion. Focused radiation has particularly been effective in smaller AVMs. Gamma knife radiotherapy is now commonly used and can treat lesions up to 3.5 cm in diameter. The results, however, may not be evident for two years.

Concurrent developments of sophisticated flow-directed intravascular catheters and a variety of balloon occlusive devices, both stable and leaking, which allow the placement of glue into AVMs, have also contributed greatly to both the nonsurgical and surgical treatment of these lesions (65). Endovascular occlusion of AVMs can significantly reduce the size of the lesion facilitating operative resection, however, it is not used as the only treatment because of the risk of recanalization of the glued vessels.

Operative excision of small malformations, particularly those on the cortical surface, is usually straightforward (Table 3). Recent major improvements in surgical technique, as well as in nonsurgical methods such as radiographically guided embolization of such malformations,

Table 3 Spetzler–Martin Classification System

Characteristic	Points
Size	
<3 cm	1
3–6 cm	2
>6 cm	3
Eloquence	
No	0
Yes	1
Presence of deep drainage	
No	0
Yes	1
Total Score	1–5

Note: "Eloquence" denotes location in an anatomic location associates with higher brain functions e.g. speech, memory etc.
Source: From Ref. 65.

have made the large lesion somewhat less formidable than before. Nevertheless, large, deep-seated, or precariously located AVMs require a substantial amount of surgical expertise found only in a few centers with significant experience (60,66,67).

The intraoperative management of patients undergoing surgery for large AVMs is critical. Depending on the size and complexity of the AVM, surgery for removal may be done in either single or multiple stages. Staged excision is intended to allow for the gradual redistribution of blood from the AVM to the surrounding brain. Regardless of the staging, great care must be taken to successfully occlude all the vessels. Even small bleeders must be thoroughly coagulated because they may give rise to hemorrhage as the blood flow shifts from the malformation to other portions of the brain.

In the operative treatment of large, high-flow AVMs, catastrophic intraoperative as well as postoperative brain engorgement/hemorrhage can occur. The pathophysiology of such engorgement/hemorrhages lies in the redistribution of blood into vessels in the peri-AVM brain tissues that cannot accommodate the increased blood flow. Vasomotor paralysis ensues with resultant engorgement and hemorrhage. This bleeding, which has been called perfusion pressure breakthrough bleeding, is a major problem during operations on large and deep AVMs (68). Hemorrhage or malignant brain swelling can occur at a distance from the malformation in an area where the vasculature is normal, indicating that tremendous shifts in brain blood flow can occur in such patients. In such occurrences, reduction of cerebral blood flow through hypotension or the induction of barbiturate coma has been the most effective therapy.

Medical Intensive Care Unit Management

The combination of a large bed of recently divided and cauterized vascular elements and the risk of perfusion pressure breakthrough bleeding makes optimal postoperative management of patients undergoing resection of large AVMs very important. It is crucial that rapid increases in blood pressure during emergence from anesthesia be avoided. **Some large and deep AVMs are therefore rejected under deep barbiturate anesthesia. In such cases the goal of a smooth awakening is aided by the slow metabolism of pentobarbital.** If this is not the case, sedation must be maintained, often with propofol, to the extent of relaxing the patient without interfering with extubation. It is important for the anesthesiologist and surgeon to inform the patient thoroughly of the conditions under which he or she will emerge from anesthesia (ICU environment, endotracheal tube, etc.) prior to surgery (58). The blood pressure is frequently kept within very stringent limits (between 110 and 130 mmHg systolic). In the treatment of elevated blood pressure in the postoperative setting, sodium nitroprusside is generally avoided owing to its cerebral vasodilatory effects. Beta blockers such as labetalol are usually used, sometimes in very high dosages. In combination with sedation, these agents are usually sufficient to maintain stable cerebral perfusion dynamics during the critical postoperative period.

INTRACEREBRAL HEMORRHAGE

Pathogenesis

Spontaneous intracerebral hemorrhage accounts for as many as 25% of all strokes or up to 100,000 cases a year in the United States (69,70). Sudden intracerebral hemorrhage (ICH) is not always immediately catastrophic, although in many instances death occurs within minutes or hours. ICH is even more likely to result in death and major disability than SAH or ischemic stroke (71). Indeed, 35% to 52% are dead within one month; half of these dying within the first two days, and only 20% are able to live independently at six months (71).

Most hypertension-associated hemorrhagic strokes occur in the basal ganglia or the thalamus. An additional 10% occur in the cerebellar hemispheres, and a similar percentage in the brainstem (Table 4) (71). Occasionally, lobar hemorrhages (bleeding in a localized area of the brain near its outer surfaces) result from uncontrolled hypertension. However, amyloid angiopathy is the most common cause of lobar intracerebral hemorrhage in the elderly (Table 5).

Presentation

Hemorrhagic stroke classically presents as the sudden onset of a focal neurologic deficit that progresses over minutes to hours and is accompanied by severe headache, nausea, and vomiting. If the hemorrhage is large, there is often a rapid decline in the level of consciousness, and there is almost invariably an associated elevation in blood pressure. The clinical presentation is caused by a sudden and progressive expanding lesion that produces both a substantial shift of brain tissue and intracranial hypertension over a relatively short period.

Prognosis for patients suffering hemorrhagic stroke depends on age, location, size, and the rapidity with which the hemorrhage produces brain shift and distortion (72). In a recent Japanese study, 30-day mortality was 0% for cerebellar, 9% for thalamic, 11% for putaminal, 11% for lobar, 14% for caudate, and 53% for brainstem hemorrhage (73).

Table 4 Location of Intracerebral Hemorrhages

	%
Basal ganglia	50
Thalamus	15
Cerebral hemisphere	15
Cerebellum	10
Pons	10
Brainstem	3

Source: From Ref. 70.

Table 5 Common Causes of Intracerebral Hemorrhage

Hypertension	Most common cause
	Usually in the basal ganglia, thalamus or pons, but can occur anywhere
	Possibly secondary to microaneurysms in the lenticulostriates (supply putamen) and basilar pontine branches (supply pons)
Tumor	Tumors are highly vascular and some have a predilection for hemorrhage such as renal cell, choriocarcinoma, and melanoma
	Lung and breast cancer metastases are the most commonly found tumors, with hemorrhage due to a higher prevalence of these tumors
Amyloid angiopathy	Most common cause of hemorrhage in elderly patients who do not have hypertension
	Due to abnormal deposition of amyloid in the media of cerebral arteries
	Tends to be cortical and multifocal
AVM	Intracerebral hemorrhage is the most common presentation for an AVM
	Hemorrhage may extend to intraventricular space
Aneurysm	Usually cause subarachnoid hemorrhages but if abutting the parenchyma may have intracerebral component to hemorrhage
Stroke	Usually during reperfusion of an ischemic stroke (infarct), the injured area may hemorrhage from damaged vascular endothelium
Coagulopathy	Most commonly from anticoagulation treatment of cardiovascular or ischemic cerebrovascular disease with warfarin
	Also may be caused by thrombolytics
Infection	Fungal infections may have vascular invasion and consequent intracerebral hemorrhage
	Herpes virus may cause hemorrhage in the temporal lobes
Miscellaneous	Postoperative after carotid endarterectomy
	Leukemia
	Dural sinus thrombosis
	Substance abuse with cocaine or amphetamines resulting in vasospasm or arteritis

Abbreviation: AVM, arteriovenous malformation.
Source: From Ref. 72.

Outcome is directly related to the level of consciousness at the time the patient is first seen. A patient who has had a severe headache but is awake and stable at the time of hospitalization is likely to survive with optimum therapy, whereas the patient presenting in coma is likely to do poorly despite the most intense surgical and/or medical treatment.

Hemorrhages in the brainstem frequently result in a sudden loss of consciousness and death within a few hours or days. Patients with brainstem hemorrhages characteristically have disconjugate gaze, major disturbances of respiration, and dramatic swings in blood pressure with systemic arterial hypertension. In general, no specific therapy is currently available for such patients. Despite occasional reports of successful evacuation of brainstem hemorrhage, surgery should only be considered in very select cases (Table 6).

Table 6 Clinical Presentation of Intracerebral Hemorrhages Based on Location

Putamen	Contralateral hemiparesis or hemiplegia
	Altered level of consciousness if significant mass effect
Thalamus	Contralateral hemisensory loss
	If internal capsule is involved: hemiparesis
	If upper brainstem is involved: gaze and pupillary dysfunction
Frontal	Contralateral hemiparesis, usually of arm worse than leg
Parietal	Contralateral hemisensory loss and hemiparesis
Temporal	Dysphasia or aphasia if hemorrhage in dominant hemisphere
Occipital	Contralateral homonymous hemianopsia
Cerebellar	Ataxia
	If brainstem compression, then also decreased level of consciousness
	If obstructing fourth ventricle, acute hydrocephalus
Brainstem	Highly variable based on location; including but not limited to cranial nerve deficits, hemiplegia, hemisensory loss

Source: From Ref. 72.

Diagnostic Evaluation

CT scanning is the imaging test of choice in diagnosing intracerebral hemorrhage. Acute blood is hyperdense to surrounding brain and is readily identified on CT. Magnetic resonance (MR) imaging shows brain anatomy more clearly, but it can be difficult to identify acute hemorrhage on MR. In addition, the time it takes for an MR scan limits its practicality in the acute setting (Figs. 11–14).

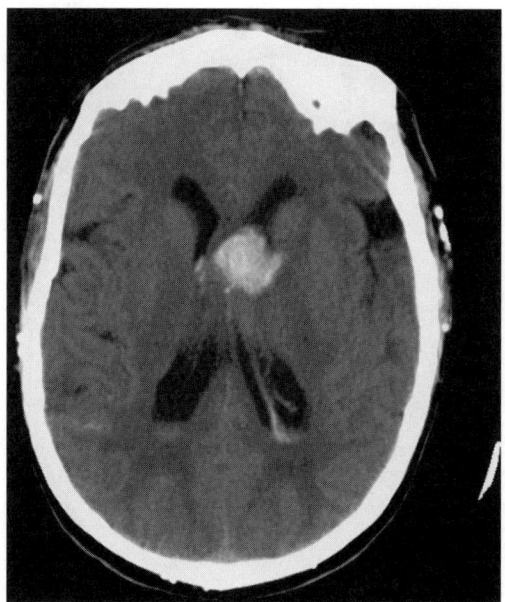

Figure 11 Head computed tomography, noncontrast, demonstrating a left thalamic hyperdensity consistent with acute intracerebral hemorrhage.

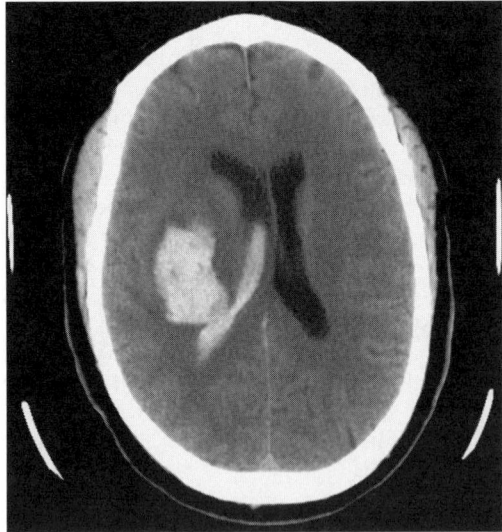

Figure 12 Head computed tomography, noncontrast, with right parietal hyperdensity consistent with acute intracerebral hemorrhage; note hemorrhage extends into right lateral ventricle.

Therapy

One of the major controversies regarding cerebrovascular disease is the treatment of hemorrhagic stroke. Japanese centers have been extremely aggressive in surgical intervention, in part perhaps because patients present earlier in Japan (74–76). In the United States there appears to be a much higher incidence of delay prior to hospitalization.

Morganstern et al. conducted a smalls single-center trial of surgical treatment for intracerebral hemorrhage (STICH) comparing standard craniotomy versus medical therapy. Entry criteria were supratentorial location of ICH, with volume $\geq 10 \, \mathrm{cm}^3$, and GCS between 5 and 15. Of the 34 patients entered, 17 were randomized to surgical therapy. The median time till surgery was 8.3 hours (range, 3.75–26.1 hours). The six-month mortality was 17.6% for the surgi-

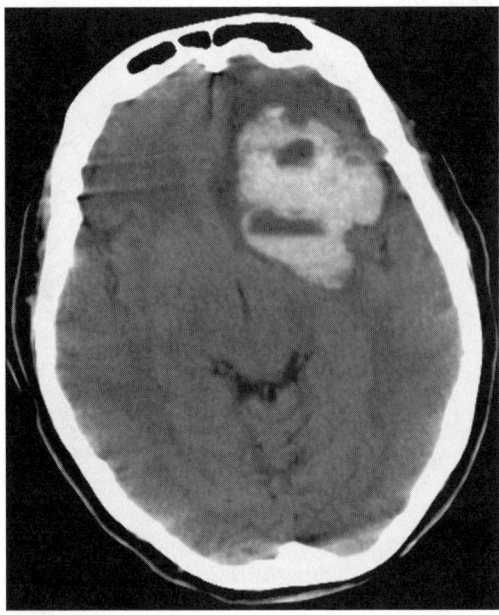

Figure 13 Head computed tomography, noncontrast, with left frontal hyperdensity consistent with intracerebral hemorrhage.

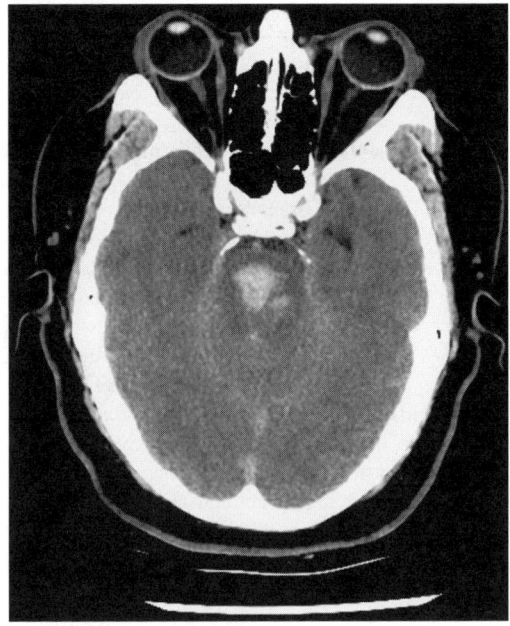

Figure 14 Head computed tomography, noncontrast, with pontine intracerebral hemorrhage.

cal group and 23.5% for the medical group ($P = \mathrm{NS}$). However, the surgical group had a greater number of hemorrhages located in an unfavorable location; only 1 of 17 patients (6%) had a lobar hemorrhage, whereas 7 of 17 (41%) of the medically treated patients had a lobar hemorrhage ($P = 0.04$).

In further pursuit of an answer to the debate of operative versus nonoperative management, a randomized international surgical trial for intracerebral hemorrhage (ISTICH) is now under way (77). In a recent update, Mendelow, the principal ISTICH investigator, reported on data collected from 985 patients at 107 centers (77). Unfortunately, the operation rates varied between 90% in Lithuania and 2% in Hungary (76). The disparity in operation rates could not be explained by differences in patient characteristics alone. This finding brings questions to the ultimate utility of this study, but also demonstrates the need for further trials given that current treatment for intracerebral hemorrhage appears to be at least partly governed by local custom. Since the treatment of patients with hemorrhagic stroke is still in flux, it is difficult to elaborate a specific set of rules regarding appropriate management.

As noted previously, patients who present awake will generally have a more favorable outcome and are less likely to require surgical intervention. It is the patient who presents with some impairment of consciousness, albeit mild, and then begins to deteriorate who presents the most difficulty (75,78,79). If the hemorrhage is large and located in a portion of the brain not involving the speech or motor systems, aggressive removal is frequently pursued with acceptable results. It appears that many nerve fiber tracts are separated and not destroyed by the intracerebral hemorrhage, particularly in younger patients, and that clot removal, if done through an appropriately placed small cortical incision, will often yield only a modest and relatively remediable neurological deficit. Lesions in the dominant hemisphere are mostly treated nonoperatively in the United States, especially when they are deep seated.

Historically, ICH bleeding was thought to be completed within a few minutes of onset, and the neurological deterioration resulting mainly from mass effect and cerebral edema. However, recent prospective data show that hematoma growth occurs in at least 38% of patients if scanned within three hours of onset, and that this expansion is highly correlated with neurological deterioration (80). On the basis of these observations, Mayer has hypothesized that ultra-early hemostatic therapy could reduce ultimate ICH volume and improve outcome (80). Mayer further hypothesized that recombinant factor VIIa (rFVIIa) was the most promising agent available as it promotes local hemostasis at sites of vascular injury in both coagulopathic and normal patients.

Mayer et al. presented the results of a recent phase IIb proof-of-concept study at the World Stroke Congress (Vancouver, California, June 26, 2004) (81). In that trial, rVIIa was shown to reduce the morbidity and mortality of ICH by about one-third of patients (81). Four hundred patients with ICH were randomized to one of four groups (rFVIIa at one of three doses vs. placebo). rFVIIa was administered at 40 mg/Kg, 80 mg/Kg, or 160 mg/Kg versus placebo within one hour of CT-demonstrated intracerebral hemorrhage (performed within three hours of onset of symptoms) in the trial. All three doses reduced the percentage increase in hematoma size (about 5 mL less blood on CT), with an attendant 35% reduction in mortality and morbidity (35). Therefore, treatment with rFVIIa holds promise in the nonoperative treatment of intracerebral hemorrhage. In addition to corroboration of this study with a definitive phase III study, similar trials will also need to be done in operative patients.

Medical Intensive Care Unit Management

Patients who are operated on for major intracranial hemorrhages require postoperative critical care management similar to that required for head injury. Frequently their decline is precipitous and the recovery period protracted. Respiratory care is particularly important in the early postoperative period.

Significant hypertension is frequent, and a modest attempt should be made to return the patient's blood pressure to premorbid levels. Systolic blood pressures under 200 mm Hg are usually tolerated in such individuals, and help prevent hematoma expansion. However, because the majority of these patients are more than 60 years of age and have had long-term hypertension with the attendant arterial changes, vigorous attempts to control the blood pressure may produce symptoms of cerebral ischemia and must be avoided (82–84). It is preferable to tolerate modest hypertension in such situations. After recovery, blood pressures can usually be lowered to a satisfactory range with oral medication.

The patient with hemorrhagic stroke is the stroke patient most often seen in the critical care unit. Owing to the sudden onset of neurological deficits in patients with hemorrhagic stroke, loss of consciousness and inadequate oxygen exchange are often encountered. Careful assessment of the patient's level of consciousness and neurological status provides valuable information about the stability of his or her intracranial compliance. A patient with a known intracerebral hemorrhage who deteriorates from lethargic to unresponsive needs immediate medical evaluation and intervention to control rising ICP (83,85,86).

There are a large number of patients who lie in an area of uncertainty with respect to management. These patients often have relatively large masses with intermediate shift of 3–6 mm and comparatively good clinical states. In these patients, there is a significant correlation between ICP and clinical status. Therefore, ICP monitoring can be quite useful in guiding management decision (78,79,83,84). If the ICP remains below 20 mmHg, the hemorrhage may be managed nonoperatively in the absence of other surgical indications. Conversely, ICP elevations above 30 mmHg indicate that deterioration is in progress and that surgical intervention should be promptly reconsidered.

ISCHEMIC CEREBROVASCULAR DISEASE

CVA is a focal neurological deficit of abrupt onset resulting from disturbance of the cerebral circulation and persisting more than 24 hours. Those deficits resolving within 24 hours are referred to as transient ischemic attacks (TIA). The incidence of CVA varies across ethnicities, rises exponentially with age, and is uniformly greater in men than in women. Furthermore, there is a recent increase in the annual incidence of stroke in the United States from 500,000 CVA in 1995 to roughly 750,000 events today (87,88). In total, the overall incidence for stroke has been estimated at 259 per 100,000 (age- and sex-adjusted for the 1995 U.S. population), and approximately 90% of patients undergoing CVA were hospitalized following the onset of symptoms.

The disturbance of the cerebral vasculature that results in focal neurologic deficit generally takes one of two forms. In one, the vasculature is affected by arteriosclerotic changes to produce vessel occlusion and subsequent focal ischemia in a condition referred to as ischemic stroke. In the other, the vasculature is disrupted to such a degree that intracranial bleeding results and a hemorrhagic stroke ensues. This following section will focus on the former form of cerebrovascular disease, ischemic stroke, which has been estimated to constitute roughly 85% of the cerebrovascular disease encountered in the clinical setting.

Pathophysiology

In order to sustain its normal level of function, the brain must maintain a highly active metabolic milieu. Although accounting for only 2% or so of overall body weight in the average adult, it receives roughly 20% of cardiac output at rest. Moreover, the brain is an obligate aerobe, highly dependent on the oxidative metabolism of glucose to meet its metabolic needs. Estimates of cerebral metabolic demands suggest that the average brain consumes roughly 50 mL of oxygen and 100 mg of glucose every minute. Consequently, the brain is exquisitely dependent on the maintenance of cerebral blood flow (CBF) for its continuing function. Mean CBF in the cortex has been estimated as roughly 50 mL/100 g/min. The cerebral vasculature maintains this value via autoregulation (vasodilation with lower pressures, and vasoconstriction in response to elevations in mean arterial pressure). Once the mean arterial pressure drops below the autoregulatory setpoint of around 50 mmHg, the cerebral blood flow drops down below the normal 50 mL/100 g/min. The brain has additional reserve mechanisms for lower flows, and is able to maintain brain oxygenation during a decrease in CBF to as low as 20 to 25 mL/100 g/min by increasing its oxygen extraction. Below that threshold, however, oxygen extraction fails and ischemic processes ensue that may progress to infarction.

☞ **Two distinct mechanisms by which CBF fails secondary to occlusion of the cerebral vasculature are**

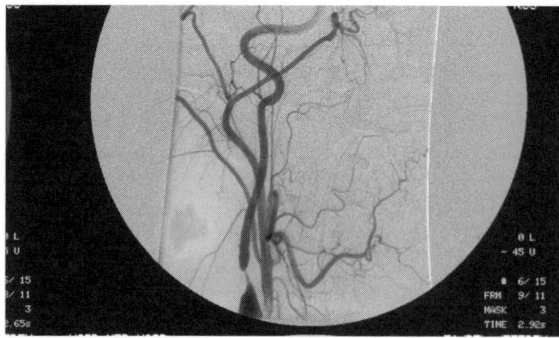

Figure 15 Carotid artery angiogram, with significant focal narrowing of the internal carotid artery just distal to the common carotid artery bifurcation.

generally recognized, one involving local thrombosis and the other embolism. ☞

Thrombosis of larger vessels (so-called atherothrombotic stroke) is rare and generally results from clotting initiated by debris originating from intracranial atherosclerotic plaques. This process may be slow in evolution and thus thrombotic stroke may take the form of so-called "stroke in progression," in which neurologic deficits progress over a few hours or days. Whether the progressive thrombosis occurs in a smaller vessel or a major vessel such as the internal carotid artery, heparin and thrombolytic therapy may arrest progression. Local thrombosis is also seen in small intracranial vessels (~30 to 100 μm in diameter) and results in so-called "lacunar strokes," in which a small volume of brain tissue supplied by an occluded end artery infarcts. In such cases, the most likely underlying pathology involves either lipohyalinosis or microatheroma and overlying thrombosis within the vascular lumen. Clinically, these insults may be asymptomatic or may produce a wide array of subcortical deficits.

Embolic stroke is classically differentiated from thrombotic stroke by the greater acuity of its onset and the maximal extent of its deficits at that time. The classical presentation is a transient alteration of mono-ocular vision called an amaurosis fugax or transient motor or speech dysfunction. Vessels in the middle cerebral artery distribution are the most commonly affected. A common source of emboli into the cerebral vasculature is an atherosclerotic plaque in a portion of the arterial tree proximal to the embolic destination. Such plaques, whether in the intracranial vasculature itself, along the course of the extracranial carotid artery (Fig. 15), or within the aortic arch, can generate thrombotic lesions that dislodge from the friable plaque and travel down arterial lumina of decreasing diameter until reaching a distal occluding point. Strokes of this sort are referred to as atherothromboembolic strokes. Another source of emboli is the heart itself. Strokes of this type, cardioembolic strokes, can involve a variety of emboli. Although most commonly consisting of red atrial thrombi as are generated in conditions such as atrial fibrillation, cardiogenic emboli may also consist of material such as infective elements from valvular lesions, necrotic endocardial tissue after acute myocardial infarct, and any of a number of entities from the venous system in the case of paradoxical emboli traversing a persistent foramen ovale. Embolic strokes have a higher risk of transforming into hemorrhagic strokes in which petechial or frank hemorrhage into the infarcted tissue follows the initial ischemic insult by hours or days (89).

Table 7 Differential Diagnosis of New, Sudden-Onset Neurological Deficit

Stroke/TIA
Postictal Todd's paralysis
Tumor
Migraine
Trauma: e.g., epidural hematoma, subdural hematoma
Infectious encephalopathy: e.g., abscess, encephalitis
Metabolic encephalopathy: e.g., hypoglycemia, drug toxicity, hepatic encephalopathy

Abbreviation: TIA, transient ischemic attacks.

Laboratory and Radiological Evaluation

The history of acute disease presentation in a patient with a new focal neurological deficit is exceedingly important in establishing a diagnosis of cerebrovascular disease. The physical examination identifies the extent of the patient's pathology. In atypical patients, intoxicant and medication history may be particularly relevant (Table 7). Even if the differential has been narrowed to CVA versus TIA, neither history nor physical can distinguish between ischemic and hemorrhagic causes. Accordingly, a noncontrast CT of the brain must be obtained immediately after presentation with a new focal neurological deficit. ☞ **Should the CVA prove to be of the ischemic variety (Fig. 16), immediate initiation of thrombolytic therapy should be considered (90).** ☞ If the CVA is of the hemorrhagic variety, thrombolytics and anticoagulants are contraindicated and clinical management should involve neurosurgical consultation. Ultimately, carotid Doppler ultrasound, MRI and MRA, and increasingly CT angiogram are useful in the workup of stroke (Figs. 17 and 18) (91–93).

The patient's vital signs will guide the evaluation of airway and respiratory management as well as the cardiovascular status, e.g., hypotension or hypertension. A

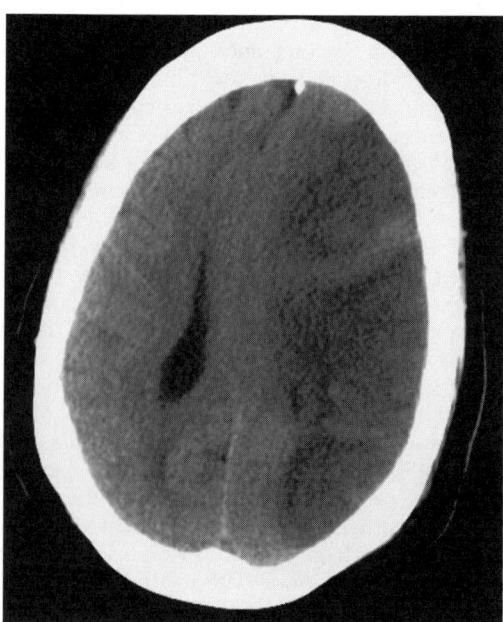

Figure 16 Head computed tomography, noncontrast, with left frontoparietal hypodensity consistent with left middle cerebral artery ischemic stroke.

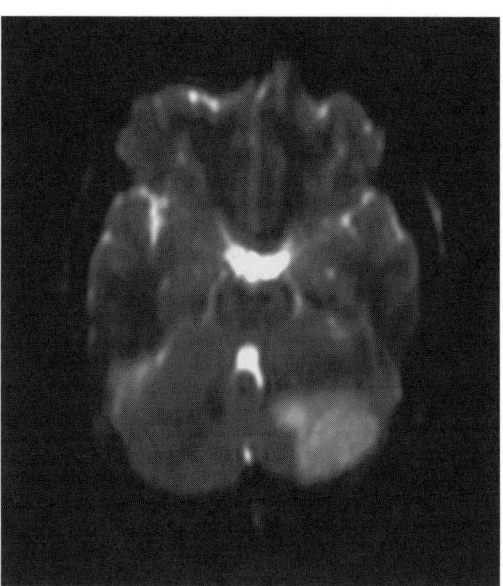

Figure 17 Magnetic resonance angiogram, diffusion weighted, with left cerebellar hyperintensity consistent with acute stroke.

complete blood count can suggest infectious causes of neurological deficit and diagnose polycythemia, thrombocytopenia, or thrombocytosis. A coagulation panel may detect hypo- or hypercoagulable states. Hypoglycemia will be detected by the metabolic panel, which also guides initial fluid resuscitation. A lipid panel may guide evaluation of the proximal arterial tree for atherosclerotic plaques, whereas an electrocardiogram may suggest (e.g., with a reading of atrial fibrillation) a cardiac source. A toxicology screen may suggest a triggering substance, but it will also guide initial management if the patient is prevented from gaining access to substances of chronic abuse when admitted. Finally, a chest radiograph will indicate whether or not the patient has suffered an aspiration incident (Tables 8 and 9).

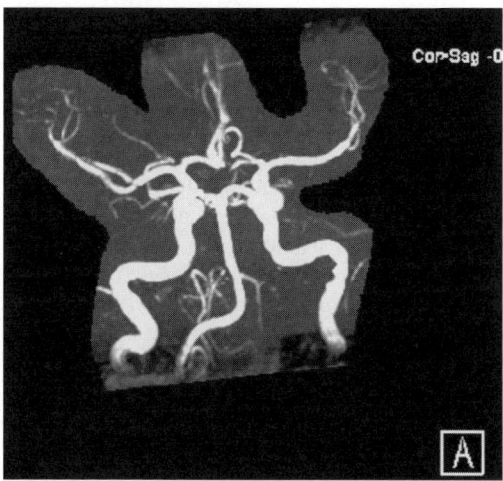

Figure 18 Magnetic resonance angiogram, with absent left vertebral artery and left posterior–inferior cerebellar artery causing the stroke in Fig. 17.

Table 8 Investigative Studies for Patients with Stroke or Transient Ischemic Attacks

Laboratory tests	Imaging studies
Complete blood count with platelet count	Chest roentgenogram
Metabolic panel (electrolytes, urea, glucose)	Electrocardiogram
Lipids	CT or MRI of head
Coagulation panel	
Toxin screen	

Abbreviations: CT, computed tomography; MRI, magnetic resonance image.

Management

Initial management of a patient who presents with a new, abrupt-onset neurological deficit goes hand in hand with assessment. Airway management, respiratory control, and cardiovascular status must be assessed and addressed prior to any further evaluation. Once the patient is sufficiently stable, neuroimaging must be obtained. A noncontrast head CT remains the imaging modality of choice in the setting of acute stroke for its rapidity, relatively low expense, and clarity in identifying new hemorrhage. When imaging indicates a hemorrhagic condition, appropriate measures should be immediately implemented (see above). If, however, CT reveals a normal or hypodense area consistent with acute ischemic stroke, the patient should be admitted to a level of care appropriate to disability and concomitant medical issues, and treatment should be initiated to reverse or reduce the amount of tissue undergoing ischemia and/or infarction. These treatments fall into five broad categories: (*i*) supportive care, (*ii*) thrombolytic therapy, (*iii*) anticoagulation, (*iv*) antiplatelet medication, and (*v*) neuroprotective measures.

Table 9 Uncommon Causes of Stroke

Disorder	Examples
Hypercoagulable states	Protein C deficiency
	Protein S deficiency
	Antithrombin III deficiency
	Antiphospholipid syndrome
	Factor V Leiden mutation
	Malignancy
	Polycythemia vera
	Systemic lupus erythematosus
	Nephrotic syndrome
	Inflammatory bowel disease
Fibromuscular dysplasia	Increased muscle and fibrous tissue in arterial wall of carotid and cerebral arteries
	Also affects kidneys, coronary arteries, mesenteric arteries, and iliac arteries
Vasculitis	Primary CNS vasculitis
	Systemic vasculitis (e.g., giant cell)
Cardiogenic syndrome	Atrial myxoma
	Marantic endocarditis
	Libman-Sacks endocarditis
	Mitral valve calcification

Supportive Care

The immediate goal of supportive care in patients suffering cerebral ischemia is optimization of cerebral perfusion to the at-risk periphery of the ischemic insult, the so-called "ischemic penumbra." Hypertension should be treated in the acute phase unless either cardiac risk factors are too great (in which case, rate reduction with the beta-1 antagonist esmolol is a first step) or malignant hypertension is developing. Hypotension should be addressed with intravenous fluids or vasopressor medications. Measures to facilitate prevention and treatment of common complications in debilitated patients such as pneumonia, urinary tract infections, or deep venous thrombosis formation are instituted. Fever is detrimental to neurons and should be treated aggressively with antipyretics. In the intermediate term, cerebral edema is a common sequela after ischemic insult (89). This effect peaks on roughly the second or third day after injury and persists for up to two weeks. In 5% to 10% of cases, edema is adequate to cause brain shifts leading to obtundation or coma. Care must be taken, therefore, to monitor progression of symptoms. Both medical and surgical management of ICP are instituted where adequate.

Thrombolytics, Anticoagulants, and Antiplatelet Drugs

Extensive study has been dedicated to the use of thrombolytic agents in acute ischemic cerebral infarct. Particular attention has been paid to recombinant tissue plasminogen activator (rtPA). Because of significant variations in study design, however, the precise effectiveness of intravenous thrombolytic agents for acute ischemic stroke remains unclear. The risk of intracranial hemorrhage is well established and appears to increase with increased size of infarct, increased duration of symptoms, and increased dose of rtPA administered (94). The drug is now approved for use in the United States and Canada within three hours of onset based on certain selection criteria (Table 10). Onset of symptoms is defined by either the moment symptoms

began or the last time the patient was observed at baseline. Consequently, patients "found down" or awakening with symptoms must have their onset of symptoms set at the last witnessed episode during which they were seen to be baseline (Table 11) (95). Studies are currently under way to evaluate the benefit of intra-arterial thrombolytic administration, but FDA approval has not yet been obtained.

The role of anticoagulation in the setting of acute ischemic stroke is unclear. Results from clinical trials do not support the use of heparinization for patients with atherothrombotic stroke of greater than 12 hours' duration. Heparin is widely used in the context of so-called "crescendo TIA," in which TIAs follow rapidly on one another with increasing frequency and severity. However, no definitive clinical evidence supports this practice. Since approximately 20% of patients with acute stroke show a continuing neurological decline over several hours to days, many physicians heparinize all patients with recent mild ischemic stroke to avoid this progression; some advise heparinization until demonstration of patency of all major carotid and intracranial vessels (96,97). In view of the 10% bleeding complication rate per week from heparinization, the value of this approach remains to be clarified.

Aspirin is the only antiplatelet agent demonstrated effective in prospective clinical trials for the treatment of acute ischemic stroke. These trials [international stroke trial (IST) and Chinese acute stroke trial (CAST)] show that the use of aspirin (150–300 mg) within 48 hours of the onset of symptoms is safe and produces a small, but definite net benefit in reducing both recurrence risk and mortality (98). For every 1000 patients given aspirin for acute ischemic stroke, roughly 9 patients will avoid death or nonfatal stroke recurrence in the early poststroke weeks and approximately 13 fewer will have died or been debilitated (98–101).

Table 10 Criteria for Recombinant Tissue Plasminogen Activator Eligibility in Setting of Acute Ischemic Cerebrovascular Accident

Indications	Contraindications
Clinical diagnosis of stroke	Sustained BP >185/110
Onset of symptoms less than three hours prior to rtPA administration	Platelets <100,000
	Hematocrit <25%
	Glucose <50 or >400
CT scan showing no hemorrhage or significant edema	Use of heparin within 48 hours and prolonged PTT, or elevated INR
Patient age at least 18 years	Rapidly improving symptoms
	Prior stroke or head injury within 3 mo
Consent by patient or surrogate	Prior intracranial hemorrhage
	Major surgery in preceding 14 days
	Minor stroke symptoms
	Gastrointestinal bleeding in last 21 days
	Recent myocardial infarction
	Coma or stupor

Abbreviations: BP, blood pressure; CT, computed tomography.

Table 11 Interventions Required for the Administration of Recombinant Tissue Plasminogen Activator for Acute Ischemic Cerebrovascular Accident

Intervention	Comments
Intravenous access	Two peripheral intravenous lines (arterial and central venous lines are to be avoided)
Bolus dose	Administer 0.9 mg/kg (to a maximum of 90 mg) intravenously as 10% total dose by bolus, followed by remainder of total dose over 1 hr
BP monitor	Continuous cuff manometer blood pressure monitoring, or arterial line (if patient debilitated)
Additional anticoagulants	No other antithrombotic treatment for 24 hr, no other anticoagulants
Reasons to halt therapy	Decline in neurologic status; Uncontrolled blood pressure
Additional treatment for neurological decline or uncontrolled BP requiring cessation of Rx	Administer cryoprecipitate; Reimage brain emergently; Avoid urethral catheterization or other elective invasive procedures for 2 or more hours

MISCELLANEOUS CEREBROVASCULAR LESIONS
Traumatic Aneurysms

Traumatic aneurysms comprise <1% of all intracranial aneurysms and are by definition false aneurysms (102). The aneurysm dome is formed by the surrounding cerebral structures and blood clot, subsequent to perforation of all layers of the vessel wall. This usually results from either penetrating head trauma or closed head injury. Penetrating trauma with gunshot wounds or actual penetration with a sharp object directly lacerates the vessel wall (103). The mechanisms behind the creation of traumatic aneurysms after closed head injury are less well understood, with the most widely accepted theories being either traction injury to the vessel wall or entrapment within a fracture. Traumatic aneurysms in closed head injury are usually accompanied by basal skull fractures (104).

☞ Any patient with significant SAH or intraventricular hemorrhage after penetrating head injury should be evaluated for a traumatic aneurysm. Also, dense subarachnoid blood after head trauma or delayed intracranial hemorrhage after head trauma should raise suspicion for traumatic aneurysm, and cerebral vessel evaluation with MRA or CT angiogram is essential. ☞ Traumatic aneurysms have a high rate of rupture and direct treatment is recommended. Internal carotid aneurysms at the skull base should undergo balloon trapping or embolization, and peripheral aneurysms should undergo endovascualr coiling or clipping (105).

Cerebral Venous Thrombosis

Intracranial venous thrombosis can develop rapidly with grave consequences. The thrombosis reduces venous outflow from the brain. The resultant venous engorgement causes white matter edema, which may cause cerebral venous infarction and intraparenchymal hemorrhage (106,107). This ultimately leads to elevated ICP, the severity of which will dictate neurological deterioration and clinical presentation. The patients usually have headache and nausea/vomiting, papilledema, blurred vision, seizures, and altered level of consciousness (108). The etiologies behind the development of cerebral venous thrombosis are many, but most include some element of hypercoagulable state, dehydration and/or trauma (Table 12).

The diagnosis is made with either a CT scan or MR study. Often the CT scan is performed first. The finding of hyperdense sinuses and veins and/or petechial intracerebral hemorrhages occurring bilaterally is highly suggestive of venous thrombosis (109). MRI with MR venogram is the mainstay of diagnosis. It is superior to CT in demonstrating both vascular and parenchymal changes and can differentiate an occluded sinus from its congenital absence (109,110).

Table 12 Etiologies of Cerebral Venous Thrombosis

Infection
Pregnancy
Dehydration
Ulcerative colitis
Diabetic ketoacidosis
Trauma
Iatrogentic
Hypercoagulable state

Source: From Ref. 99.

☞ The treatment of cerebral venous thrombosis should be aggressive, yet with the caution that interventions that counteract thrombosis tend to increase the risk of hemorrhage. ☞ The ICP should be monitored in the obtunded (GCS ≤8) patient. Hypertension should be controlled and any underlying abnormality that may have precipitated the event should be corrected. Also, the patient should be hydrated and treated with anticonvulsants. The mainstay of therapy is systemic heparin and conversion to Coumadin beyond the intensive care period. However, there is no consensus on the duration of these therapies (111,112). Even in the setting of intracranial hemorrhage, heparin remains the best treatment (113). If the patient continues to deteriorate, tPA systemically or locally injected into the clotted sinus can be attempted. Surgical or endovascular thrombectomy and surgical sinus reconstruction is rarely indicated due to the excessively high rates of rethrombosis (114).

Carotid Cavernous Sinus Fistulae

Carotid-cavernous sinus (CC) fistulae are rare vascular anomalies. They can arise spontaneously or result from maxillofacial and head trauma (60–80%) (115). The carotid artery courses through the cavernous sinus en route to its intradural distribution; subsequently perforations during this segment can lead to CC fistulae. The clinical features may include proptosis, chemosis (arteriolization of conjunctiva), bruit, ophthalmoplegia, visual deterioration, orbital pain and/or headache. Occasionally CC fistulae may present with SAH (115).

A bruit over the eye may be palpable or heard with a stethoscope, raising suspicion for a CC fistula, while the diagnostic procedure of choice is a cerebral angiogram. Because traumatic CC fistulae are high-flow vascular abnormalities and spontaneous closure is uncommon, intervention is indicated. The untreated patient may not deteriorate rapidly; the usual course is one of progressive visual loss from decreased retinal blood flow (116). Intolerable bruit and/or disfiguring proptosis may also progress.

Various approaches have been used to treat CC fistulae. The current treatment is occlusion of the fistula using a detachable balloon and/or coils with preservation of blood flow in the carotid artery. If this is technically unfeasible, two balloons may be placed on either side of the fistula to trap it, resulting in the deliberate sacrifice of the carotid artery. Test occlusion must be performed to establish patency of the circle of Willis, and the ability of the patient to tolerate loss of internal carotid artery flow to the distribution distal to the CC fistula (116,117).

EYE TO THE FUTURE

Expanding the horizon for improvement of therapeutic interventions in the arena of cerebrovascular disease is imperative given the morbidity and mortality associated with these disease entities. Future directions in the treatment of cerebrovascular diseases aim to correct the underlying pathologies and the deleterious ischemic effects they produce on the brain.

Tremendous improvements in endovascular occlusion of aneurysm and AVMs have recently occurred. Current investigations are exploring the use of even smaller microcatheters for the delivery of devices farther into the cerebrovasculature. Porous stents are being developed to provide a scaffold onto which wide-based aneurysms may be coil occluded without the risk of coil embolization (118–120).

Intracerebral hemorrhage management continues to be investigated. Thrombin is being studied as a major mediator of perihematoma edema. Accordingly, the use of antithrombin therapy for ICH management is being explored (121). Additionally, many patients requiring urgent neurosurgical intervention have coagulopathies. Standard use of blood products, including fresh-frozen plasma or cryoprecipitate to correct the coagulopathy, often leads to significant delays in treatment. Recombinant activated factor VII (rFVIIa) has recently been shown to reverse the coagulopathy in neurosurgical patients with intracerebral hemorrhage (ICH), intraventricular hemorrhage (IVH), hydrocephalus, diffuse cerebral edema, and epidural hematoma as early as 20 minutes after infusion (122). There were no procedural or operative complications, no postoperative hemorrhagic complications, and no thromboembolic complications observed with the use of rFVIIa in this group of patients (122). These experiences combined with the demonstrated 35% reduction in mortality and morbidity in hemopheliac patients with ICH treated with rFVIIa is likely to promote rFVIIa toward a mainstream treatment following ICH in the near future (80,81). More studies are currently required to provide dosing studies, and to review thrombotic complications in greater degree (122). Surgical approaches using early CT-guided clot aspiration and tPA for clot lysis remain possibilities as minimally invasive surgical approaches to intracerebral hematoma evacuation are developed (123,124).

Future directions in the management of acute cerebral ischemia focus on reperfusion and neuronal protection. Although intra-arterial thrombolysis was demonstrated to be effective in the prolyse in acute cerebral thromboembolism II (PROACT II) study, its use has been limited. Current investigations are exploring the use of both intravenous and intra-arterial thrombolysis as a sort of "bridging therapy" that may offer benefit over either alone in reestablishing blood flow.

A new, more potent form of tissue plasminogen activator t-PA, called TNKase™ (Tenecteplase), has recently been produced by Genetech (South San Francisco, California). TNKase™ is produced using recombinant DNA technology, and holds promise for accomplishing clot dissolution with fewer bleeding complications than t-PA. This new drug can be delivered faster as a single intravenous treatment rather than the prolonged infusion ordinarily needed to give t-PA. In the presence of fibrin, in vitro studies demonstrate that Tenecteplase conversion of plasminogen to plasmin is increased relative to its conversion in the absence of fibrin. This fibrin specificity (10 times more than normal t-PA) decreases systemic activation of plasminogen and the resulting degradation of circulating fibrinogen, and unwanted bleeding. A multicenter clinical trial is currently under way, with regional coordination occurring at two major university stroke centers, University of California, San Diego (UCSD) Medical Center, and the University of Virginia Health System in Charlottesville, VA. TNK is administered to patients who arrive at hospital emergency rooms with significant stroke three hours or less from symptom onset (personal communication from Patrick Lyden, M.D., UCSD Stroke Center director). The first phase of the study was completed in April 2004, and the results are in press; phase 2 (dosing regimen review) will begin in December 2004.

In the realm of neuronal protection, clinical administration of current pharmacological agents such as NMDA antagonists, calcium channel blockers, anti-inflammatory antibodies, and free-radical scavengers, have yet to demonstrate conclusive benefit in a large, prospective, randomized efficacy study (125,126). Nevertheless, animal models have demonstrated a beneficial effect using antioxidants to limit lipid peroxidation, an essential step in the pathogenesis of cerebral ischemia. Future research will continue to explore the molecular basis of cerebral ischemia and develop opportunities for the management of cerebral ischemia. This may include the use of neuronotrophic factors.

SUMMARY

Intracerebral vascular catastrophes have diverse etiologies but their effects on the brain share many common features. Management of ischemic insults is guided by many of the same basic principles of emergent neurosurgical intensive care. The patients receive basic cardiopulmonary support to protect the airway and maximize cerebral perfusion. Often this requires intubation and ICP management. Ultimately, ensuring adequate cerebral blood flow and neuronal preservation are the key goals of therapy.

Nontraumatic SAH is almost always secondary to aneurysmal hemorrhage and necessitates immediate intervention. Diagnostic evaluation for the possible aneurysm should be performed urgently with MRA or CT angiogram. Ultimately a cerebral four-vessel angiogram is necessary to plan exclusion of the aneurysm from the cerebral circulation with endovascular coils or surgical clipping. The clinician should maintain high suspicion for the complications that may arise, such as hydrocephalus and vasospasm.

Intracerebral hemorrhage, when in eloquent areas of the brain or large enough to cause significant mass effect, is a devastating event. Controversy exists regarding the timing and indications for operative evacuation, and is generally reserved for patients with acute mass effect and the possibility of a functional postoperative recovery. Ultra-early administration of rVIIa may soon become the standard of care for ICH management and viewed as the counterpart to thrombolytic treatment of acute ischemic stroke.

AVM hemorrhage may also present as an intracerebral hemorrhage, often with ventricular extension of the blood. Cerebral angiography is necessary for definition diagnosis and formulation of a treatment plan. In the nonemergent setting, most AVMs are treated with endovascular occlusion, stereotactic radiation and/or surgical resection. In large and deep AVMs, intraoperative challenges of hemostasis and potential cerebral edema/brain engorgement persist, and appropriate measures such as barbiturates may need to be instituted.

Ischemic cerebrovascular disease is associated with certain risk factors and may lead to fixed neurological deficit. Its management in the acute setting begins with a noncontrast CT of the head to exclude a hemorrhagic stroke, which would be a contraindication for rtPA. If certain inclusion criteria are met, rtPA is indicated. Subsequently, a workup for the particular etiology of the stroke is pursued to guide long-term management.

Future challenges include the selective elimination/correction of the underlying vascular pathologies, reestablishment/maintenance of adequate cerebral blood flow, and promotion of neuronal viability and function.

KEY POINTS

- The mortality associated with the initial hemorrhage is around 20%.

☞ Saccular aneurysms must be differentiated from traumatic, dissecting, mycotic and/or tumor-associated aneurysms because the classification dictates management.

☞ Immediately following documentation of SAH, attention is directed toward the identification of the responsible vascular abnormality, most commonly a ruptured aneurysm.

☞ Patients with a lower Hunt and Hess grade (Hunt and Hess grade I–III) should undergo an urgent craniotomy and surgical clipping of anatomically accessible (anterior circulation) aneurysms.

☞ The goal of treatment is to secure the neck of the aneurysm by clipping, so that the common complications of SAH, such as rebleeding, vasospasm, and hydrocephalus can be eliminated or maximally treated.

☞ Coil occlusion is indicated for the treatment of aneurysms which are: (*i*) difficult to clip surgically, (*ii*) occur in patients who are unsuitable for early surgery due to a poor SAH grade, and (*iii*) occur in patients who are medically unstable.

☞ Due to its noninvasive nature, TCD should be performed daily or every other day after aneurysmal SAH, reserving angiography for the diagnostic confirmation and therapeutic intervention of clinical vasospasm.

☞ The mainstay of therapy in the United States, once clinical vasospasm is suspected or confirmed, is nimodipine (to minimize vasospasm) and "triple-H" therapy; the three H's being hypervolemia, hypertension, and hemodilution.

☞ Electrocardiogram (ECG) changes are common in patients with SAH, even in patients without prior history of cardiac disease.

☞ After rebleeding, vasospasm, and hydrocephalus, morbidity following SAH can be attributable to pulmonary complications including pulmonary edema, pneumonia and/or pulmonary embolism.

☞ AVMs are the leading cause of SAH in young people although they account for only 5% of SAH in adults.

☞ Some large and deep AVMs are rejected under deep barbiturate anesthesia. In such cases the goal of a smooth awakening is aided by the slow metabolism of pentobarbital.

☞ Most hypertension-associated hemorrhagic strokes occur in the basal ganglia or the thalamus. An additional 10 percent occur in the cerebellar hemispheres and a similar percentage in the brainstem (Table 4).

☞ Two distinct mechanisms by which CBF fails secondary to occlusion of the cerebral vasculature are generally recognized. One involves local thrombosis and the other embolism.

☞ Should the CVA prove to be of the ischemic variety (Fig. 16), immediate initiation of thrombolytic therapy should be considered.

☞ Any patient with significant SAH or intraventricular hemorrhage after penetrating head injury should be evaluated for a traumatic aneurysm. Also, dense subarachnoid blood after head trauma or delayed intracranial hemorrhage after head trauma should raise suspicion for traumatic aneurysm, and cerebral vessel evaluation with MRA or CT angiogram is essential.

☞ The treatment of cerebral venous thrombosis should be aggressive, yet with the caution that interventions that counteract thrombosis tend to increase the risk of hemorrhage.

REFERENCES

1. Mayberg MR, Batjer HH, Dacey R, et al. Guidelines for the management of aneurysmal subarachnoid hemorrhage. Circulation 1994; 90(5):2592.
2. Broderick JP, Brott TG, Duldner JE, et al. Initial and recurrent bleeding are the major causes of death following subarachnoid hemorrhage. Stroke 1994; 25(7):1342.
3. Biller J, Geodersk JC, Adams HP. Management of aneurysmal subarachnoid hemorrhage. Stroke 1988; 19:1300.
4. Cesarini KG, Hardemark HG, Persson L. Improved survival after aneurismal subarachnoid hemorrhage; review of case management during a 12-year period. J Neurosurgery 1999/90(4):664.
5. Stebbens WE. Pathology of the cerebral blood vessels. St. Louis: Mosby-Yearbook Inc., 1972:351.
6. Heros RC, Kistler JP. Intracranial arterial aneurysm; an update. Stroke 1983; 14:628.
7. Fisher CM. Clinical syndromes in cerebral thrombosis, hypertensive hemorrhage, and ruptured saccular aneurysms. Clin Neurosurg 1975; 22:117.
8. Juvela S, Hillbom M, Numminen H, et al. Cigarette smoking and alcohol consumption as risk factors for aneurysmal subarachnoid hemorrhage. Stroke 1993; 24:639.
9. Jakobsson KE, Saveland H, Hillman J, et al. Warning leak and management outcome in aneurysmal subarachnoid hemorrhage. J Neurosurg 1996; 85:995.
10. Adams HP, Kassell NF, Torner JC, et al. Predicting cerebral ischemia after aneurysmal subarachnoid hemorrhage: influences of clinical condition, CT results, and antifibronolytic therapy. A report of the cooperative aneurysm study. Neurology 1987; 37(10):1586.
11. Leblanc R. The minor leak preceding subarachnoid hemorrhage. J Neurosurg 1987; 66:35.
12. Forster DM, Steiner L, Hakanson S, et al. The value of repeat pan-angiography in cases of unexplained subarachnoid hemorrhage. J Neurosurg 1987; 66(1):40.
13. West HH, Mani RI, Eisenberg RL. Normal cerebral anteriography in patients with spontaneous subarachnoid hemorrhage. Neurology 1972; 27:592.
14. Hsiang JNK, Liang EY, Lam HMK, et al. The role of computed tomographic angiography in the diagnosis of intracranial aneurysms and emergent aneurysm clipping. Neurosurgery 1996; 38:481.
15. Zouaoui A, Sahel M, Marro B, et al. Three-dimensional computed tomographic angiography in detection for cerebral aneurysms in acute subarachnoid hemorrhage. Neurosurgery 1997; 41(1):125.
16. Hunt WE, Hess RM. Surgical risk as related to time of intervention in the repair of intracranial aneurysms. J Neurosurg 1968; 28:14.
17. Fisher CM, Kistler JP, Davis JM. Relation of cerebral vasospasm to subarachnoid hemorrhage visualized by CT scanning. Neurosurgery 1980; 6(1):1.
18. Kassell NF, Torner JC, Haley EC, et al. The international cooperative study on the timing of aneurysm surgery. Part 1. Overall management results. J Neurosurg 1990; 73(1):18.
19. Sundt TM, Whisnant JP. Subarachnoid hemorrhage from intracranial aneurysm. N Engl J Med 978; 299:116.
20. Fox JL. Microsurgical exposure of intracranial aneurysms. J Microsurg 1979; 1:2.
21. Molyneux A, Kerr R, Stratton I, et al. International Subarachnoid Aneurysm Trial (ISAT) of neurosurgical clipping versus endovascular coiling in 2143 patients with ruptured intracranial aneurysms:a randomised trial. Lancet 2002; 360:1267–1274.
22. Weil SM, van Loveren HR, Tomisick TA, et al. Management of inoperable cerebral aneurysms by the navigational balloon technique. Neurosurgery 1987; 21:296.
23. Guglielmi G, Vinuela F, Sepetka I, et al. Electrothrombosis of saccular aneurysms via endovascular approach. J Neurosurg 1991; 75:1.

24. LeRoux PD, Elliott JP, Newell DW, et al. Prediction outcome in poor-grade patients with subarachnoid hemorrhage: a retrospective review of 159 aggressively managed cases. J Neurosurg 1996; 85:39.

25. Johnston SC, Wilson CB, Halbach VV, et al. Endovascular and surgical treatment of unruptured cerebral aneurysms: Comparison of risks. Ann Neurol 2000; 48:11–19.

26. Zubkov YN, Nififorov BM, Shustin VA. Balloon catheter technique for dilatation of constricted cerebral arteries after aneurysmal SAH. Acta Neurochir 1984; 70:65.

27. Higashida RT, Halbvach VV, Cahan LD, et al. Transluminal angioplasty for treatment of intracranial arterial vasospasm. J Neurosurg 1989; 71:648.

28. Kassell NF, Torner JC. Aneurysmal rebleeding: a preliminary report from the cooperative aneurysm study. Neurosurgery 1983; 13(5):479.

29. Winn HR, Richardson AE, O'Brien W, et al. The long-term prognosis in untreated cerebral aneurysms. Late morbidity and mortality. Ann Neurol 1978; 4(5):418.

30. Mayberg MR, Batjer HH, Dacey R, et al. Guidelines for the management of aneurysmal subarachnoid hemorrhage. Circulation 1994; 90(5):2592.

31. Kassell NF, Sasaki T, Colohan AR, et al. Cerebral vasospasm following aneurysmal subarachnoid hemorrhage. Stroke 1985; 16(4):562.

32. Mayberg MR. Cerebral vasospasm. Neurosurg Clin N Am 1998; 9(3):615.

33. Dion JE, Gates PC, Fox AJ, et al. Clinical events following neuroangiography: a prospective study. Stroke 1987; 18(6):997.

34. Asslid R, Huber P, Nornes H. Evaluation of cerbrovascular spasm with transcranial Doppler ultrasound. J Neurosurg 1984; 60(1):37.

35. Vora YY, Suarez-Almazor M, Steinke DE, et al. Role of transcranial Doppler monitoring in the diagnosis of cerebral vasospasm after suarachnoid hemorrhage. Neurosurgery 1999; 44(6):1237.

36. Allen GS, Ahn HS, Preziosi TJ, et al. Cerebral arterial spasm—a controlled trial of nimodipine in patients with aneurysmal subarachnoid hemorrhage. N Engl J Med 1983; 308(11):619.

37. Petruk KC, West M, Mohr G, et al. Nimodipine treatment in poor-grade aneurysm patients. Results of a multicenter double-blind placebo-controlled trial. J Neurosurg 1988; 68(4):505.

38. Solomon RA, Fink ME. Current strategies for the management of aneurysmal subarachnoid hemorrhage. Arch Neurol 1987; 311:432.

39. Kudo T, Suzuki S, Iwabuchi T. Importance of monitoring the circulating blood volume in patients with cerebral vasospasm after subarachnoid hemorrhage. Neurosurgery 1981; 9(5):514.

40. Solomon RA, Post KD, McMurtry JG. Depression of circulating blood volume in patients after subarachnoid hemorrhage: implications for management of symptomatic vasospasm. Neurosurgery 1988; 23(6):699.

41. McGillicuddy J, Knidt G, Giannotta S. Focal cerebral blood flow in cerebral vasospasm: the effect of intravascular volume expansion. Acta Neurol Scand Suppl 1979; 60:490.

42. Lennihan L, Mayer SA, Fink ME, et al. Effect of hypervolemic therapy on cerebral blood flow after subarachnoid hemorrhage: a randomized controlled trial. Stroke 2000; 31(2):383.

43. Wood JH, Simeone FA, Kron RE, et al. Experimental hypervolemic hemodilution: physiological correlations of cortical blood flow, cardiac output, and intracranial pressure with fresh blood viscosity and plasma volume. Neurosurgery 1984; 14(6):709.

44. Handa Y, Hayashi M, Takeuchi H, et al. Time course of impairment of cerebral autoregulation during chronic cerebral vasospasm after subarachnoid hemorrhage in primates. J Neurosurg 1992; 76(3):493.

45. Ostubo H, Takemae T, Inoue T, et al. Normovolaemic induced hypertension therapy for cerebral vasospasm after subarachnoid hemorrhage. Acta Neurochir 1990; 103(1–2):18.

46. Bailes JE, Spetzler RF, Hadley MN, et al. Management morbidity and mortality of poor-grade aneurysm patients. J Neurosurg 1990; 72(4):559.

47. Bejjani GK, Bank WO, Olan WJ, et al. The efficacy and safety of angioplasty for cerebral vasospasm after subarachnoid hemorrhage. Neurosurgery 1998; 42(5):979.

48. Brothers MF, Holgate RC. Intracranial angioplasty for treatment of vasospasm after subarachnoid hemorrhage: technique and modifications to improve branch access. Am J Neuroradiol 1990; 11(2):239.

49. Hasan D, Vermeulen M, Wijdicks EF, et al. Management problems in acute hydroephalus after subarachnoid hemorrhage. Stroke 1989; 20(6):747.

50. Vale FL, Bradley EL, Fisher WS III. The relationship of subarachnoid hemorrhage and the need for postoperative shunting. J Neurosurg 1997; 86(3):462.

51. Hart RG, Byer JA, Slaughter JR, et al. Occurrence implications of seizures in subarachnoid hemorrhage due to ruptured intracranial aneurysms. Neurosurgery 1981; 8(4):417.

52. Baker CJ, Prestigiacomo CJ, Solomon RA. Short-term perioperative anticonvulsant prophylaxis for the surgical treatment of low-risk patients with intracranial aneurysms. Neurosurgery 1995; 37(5):863.

53. Samuels MA. Neurogenic heart disease: a unifying hypothesis. Am J Cardio 1987; 60(18):15J.

54. Zarof JG, Rordorf GA, Newell JB, et al. Cardiac outcome in patients with subarachnoid hemorrhage and electrocardiographic abnormalities. Neurosurgery 1999; 44(1):34.

55. Hart GK, Humphrey L, Weiss J. Subarachnoid hemorrhage: cardiac complications. Crit Care Rep 1989; 1:88.

56. Simon RP. Neurogenic pulmonary edema. Neurol Clin 1993; 11(2):309.

57. Solenski MD, Haley EC Jr, Kassell NF, et al. medical complications of aneurysmal subarachnoid hemorrhage: a report of the multicenter, cooperative aneurysm study. Crit Care Med 1995; 23(6):1007.

58. Stein BM, Wolpert SM. Arteriovenous malformation of the brain. Current concepts and treatment. Arch Neurol 1980; 37:1–5.

59. Perret G, Nishioka H. Arteriovenous malformations: An analysis of 545 cases of craniocerebral arteriovenous malformations and fistulae reported of the cooperative study. J Neurosurg 1966; 25:467–490.

60. Yasargil M, Donaghy R. Microvascular surgery. Stuttgart: Geor Thieme Verlag, 1967.

61. Leblanc R, Meyer E, Zatorre R, Klein D, Evans A. Functional imaging of cerebral arteriovenous malformations with a comment on cortical reorganization. Neurosurg Focus 1996; 1(3):e4.

62. Pollock BE. Stereotactic radiosurgery for arteriovenous malformations. Neurosurg Clin N Am 1999; 10(2):281–290.

63. Steinberg GK, Chang SD, Levy RP, Marks MP, Frankel K, Marcellus M. Surgical resection of large incompletely treated intracranial arteriovenous malformations following stereotactic radiosurgery. J Neurosurg 1996; 84(6):920–928.

64. Pollock BE, Flickinger JC, Lunsford LD, Maitz A, Kondziolka D. Factors associated with successful arteriovenous malformation radiosurgery. Neurosurgery 1998; 42(6):1239–1244; discussion 1244–1247.

65. Taylor CL, Dutton K, Rappard G, Pride GL, Replogle R, Purdy PD, White J, Giller C, Kopitnik TA Jr, Samson DS. Complications of preoperative embolization of cerebral arteriovenous malformations. J Neurosurg 2004; 100(5):810–812.

66. Sisti MB, Kader A, Stein BM. Microsurgery for 67 intracranial arteriovenous malformations less than 3 cm in diameter. J Neurosurg 1993; 79(5):653–660.

67. Drake CG. Cerebral arteriovenous malformation. Consideration for and experience with surgical treatment in 166 cases. Clin Neurosurg 1979; 26:145–308.

68. Spetzer RF, Wilson CB, Weinstein P, et al. Normal perfusion pressure breakthrough theory. Clin Neurosurg 1974; 25:651–672.

69. Fisher CM. Hypertensive cerebral hemorrhage. Demonstration of the source of bleeding. J Neuropathol Exp Neurol 2003; 62(1):104–107.

70. Lammie GA. Hypertensive cerebral small vessel disease and stroke. Brain Pathol. 2002; 12(3):358–370.

71. Broderick JP, Adams HP, Barsan W, et al. Guidelines for the Management of Spontaneous Intracerebral Hemorrhage: A Statement for Healthcare Professionals From a Special Writing Group of the Stroke Council, American Heart Association. Stroke 1999; 30:905–915.

72. Ross DA, Olsen WL, Ross AM, Andrews BT, Pitts LH. Brain shift, level of consciousness, and restoration of consciousness in patients with acute intracranial hematoma. J Neurosurg 1989; 71(4):498–502.

73. Inagawa T, Ohbayashi N, Takechi A, et al. Primary Intracerebral Hemorrhage in Izumo City. Japan: Incidence Rates and Outcome in Relation to the Site of Hemorrhage. Neurosurgery 2003; 53:1283–1298.

74. Ohwaki K, Yano E, Nagashima H, Hirata M, Nakagomi T, Tamura A. Blood pressure management in acute intracerebral hemorrhage: relationship between elevated blood pressure and hematoma enlargement. Stroke 2004; 35(6):1364–1367.

75. Kazui S, Minematsu K, Yamamoto H, Sawada T, Yamaguchi T. Predisposing factors to enlargement of spontaneous intracerebral hematoma. Stroke 1997; 28(12):2370–2375.

76. Fujii Y, Takeuchi S, Sasaki O, Minakawa T, Tanaka R. Multivariate analysis of predictors of hematoma enlargement in spontaneous intracerebral hemorrhage. Stroke 1998; 29(6):1160–1166.

77. Mendelow AD. The International Surgical trial in intracerebral haemorrhage (I. S.T.I.C.H). Acta Neurochir Suppl 2003; 86:441–443.

78. Maira G, Anile C, Colosimo C, Rossi GF. Surgical treatment of primary supratentorial intracerebral hemorrhage in stuporous and comatose patients. Neurol Res 2002; 24(1):54–60.

79. Schwarz S, Jauss M, Krieger D, Dorfler A, Albert F, Hacke W. Haematoma evacuation does not improve outcome in spontaneous supratentorial intracerebral haemorrhage: a case-control study. Acta Neurochir (Wien) 1997; 139(10):897–903; discussion 903–904.

80. Mayer SA, et al. Ultra-early hemostatic therapy for intracerebral hemorrhage. Stroke 2002; 34:224–229.

81. Love R. Trial of haemophilia treatment for intracerebral haemorrhage. The Lancet 2004; 3:448.

82. Juvela S. Risk factors for impaired outcome after spontaneous intracerebral hemorrhage. Arch Neurol 1995; 52(12):1193–1200.

83. Garibi J, Bilbao G, Pomposo I, Hostalot C. Prognostic factors in a series of 185 consecutive spontaneous supratentorial intracerebral haematomas. Br J Neurosurg 2002; 16(4):355–361.

84. van Loon J, Van Calenbergh F, Goffin J, Plets C. Controversies in the management of spontaneous cerebellar hemorrhage. A consecutive series of 49 cases and review of the literature. Acta Neurochir (Wien) 1993; 122(3–4):187–193.

85. Schwarz S, Hafner K, Aschoff A, Schwab S. Incidence and prognostic significance of fever following intracerebral hemorrhage. Neurology 2000; 54(2):354–361.

86. Hemphill JC 3rd, Bonovich DC, Besmertis L, Manley GT, Johnston SC. The ICH score: a simple, reliable grading scale for intracerebral hemorrhage. Stroke 2001; 32(4):891–897.

87. Williams GR, Jiang JG, Matchar DB, et al. Incidence and occurrence of total (first-ever and recurrent) stroke. Stroke 1999; 30:2523.

88. Gorelick PB. TIA incidence and prevalence: the Stroke Belt perspective. Neurology 2004; 62(8 Suppl 6):S12.

89. Sacco RL. Risk factors for TIA and TIA as a risk factor for stroke. Neurology 2004; 62(8 Suppl 6):S7.

90. The ATLANTIS, ECASS, and NINDS rt-PA Study Group Investigators. Association of outcome with early stroke treatment: pooled analysis of ATLANTIS, ECASS, and NINDS rt-PA stroke trials. The Lancet 2004; 363:768–774.

91. Powers WJ, Zazulia AR. The use of positron emission tomography in cerebrovascular disease. Neuroimaging Clin N Am 2003; 13(4):741.

92. Schellinger PD. MRI-guided therapy in acute stroke. Expert Rev Cardovasc Ther 2002; 1(4):569.

93. Thijs VN. Imaging strategy for acute stroke therapy. JBR-BTR 2003; 86(6):350.

94. Gorter JW. Major bleeding during anticoagulation after cerebral ischemia. Patterns and risk factors. Stroke prevention in reversible ischemia trial (SPIRIT), European atrial fibrillation trial (EAFT) study groups. Neurology 1999; 53:1319.

95. Hacke W, Donnan G, Fieschi C, et al. Association of outcome with early stroke treatment: pooled analysis of ATLANTIS, ECASS, and NINDS rt-PA stroke trials. Lancet 2004; 363(9411):768.

96. Stahl JE, Furie KL, Gleason S, et al. Stroke: Effect of implementing an evaluation and treatment protocol compliant with NINDS recommendations. Radiology 2003; 228(3):659.

97. Albers GW. Advances in intravenous thrombolytic therapy for treatment of acute stroke. Neurology 2001; 59(5 Suppl 2):S77.

98. Chen ZM, Sandercock P, Pan HC, et al. Indications for early aspirin use in ischemic stroke: CAST and IST collaborative groups. Stroke 2000; 31(6):1240.

99. Albers GW. Antithrombotic and thrombolytic therapy for ischemic stroke. Fifth ACCP Consensus Conference on Antithrombotic Therapy. Chest 1998; 114:683S.

100. Rockson SG, Albers GW. Comparing the guidelines: anticoagulation therapy to optimize stroke prevention in patients with atrial fibrillation. J Am Coll Cardiol 2004; 43(6):929.

101. Meschia JF, Brott TG. New insights on thrombolytic treatment of acute ischemic stroke. Curr Neurol Neurosci Rep 2002; 1(1):19.

102. Parkinson D, West M. Traumatic intracranial aneurysms. J Neurosurg 1980; 52:11.

103. Kieck CF, de Villiers JC. Vascular lesions due to transcranial stab wounds. Neurosurgery 1984; 60:42.

104. Tureyen K. Traumatic intracranial aneurysm after blunt trauma. Br J Neurosurg 2001; 15(5):429.

105. Luo CB, Teng MM, Chang FC, et al. Endovascular management of traumatic cerebral aneuryms associated with traumatic carotid cavernous fistulas. Am J Neuroradiol 2004; 25(3):501.

106. Masuhr F, Mehraein S, Einhaupl K. Cerebral venous and sinus thrombosis. J Neurol 2004; 251(1):11.

107. Heller C, Heinecke A, Junker R, et al. Cerebral venous thrombosis in children; a multifactorial origin. Circulation 2003; 108(11):1362.

108. Ferrera PC, Pauze DR, Chan L. Sagittal sinus thrombosis after head injury. Am J Emergency Med 1998; 16:382.

109. Rao KCVG, Knipp HC, Wagner EJ. CT findings in cerebral sinus and venous thrombosis. Radiology 1981; 140:391.

110. Renowden S. Cerebral venous sinus thrombosis. Eur Radiol 2004; 14(2):215.

111. Gerszten PC, Welch WC, Spearman MP, et al. Isolated deep cerebral venous thrombosis treated by direct endovascular thrombolysis. Surg Neurol 1997; 48:261.

112. Levin SR, Twyman RE, Gilman S. The role of antigoagulation in cavernous sinus thrombosis. Neurology 1988; 38:517.

113. Einhaupl KM, Villringer A, Meister W, et al. Heparin treatment in sinus venous thrombosis. Lancet 1991; 338:597.

114. Horowitz M, Purdy P, Unwin H, et al. Treatment of dural sinus thrombosis using selective catheterization and urokinase. Ann Neurol 1995; 38:58.

115. Mostafa G, Sing RF, Matthews BD, et al. Traumatic carotid cavernous fistula. J Am Coll Surg 2002; 194(6):841.

116. Fattahi TT, Brandt MT, Jenkins WS, et al. Traumatic carotid-cavernous fistula: pathophysiology and treatment. J Craniofac Surg 2003; 14(2):240.

117. Coley SC, Pandya H, Hodgson TJ, et al. Endovascular trapping of traumatic carotid-cavernous fistulae. Am J Neuroradiol 2003; 24(9):1785.

118. Qureshi AL. Endovascular treatment of cerebrovascular diseases and intracranial neoplasms. Lancet 2004; 363(9411):804.

119. Doerfler A, Wanke I, Egelhof T, et al. Double-stent method: therapeutic alternative for small wide-necked aneurysms. J Neurosurg 2004; 100(1):150.

120. Howington JU, Hanel RA, Harrigan MR, et al. The Neuroform stent, the first microcather-delivered stent for use in the intracranial circulation. Neurosurgery 2004; 54(1):2.

121. Butcher KS, Baird T, MacGregor L, et al. Perihematomal edema in primary intracerebral hemorrhage is plasma derived. Stroke 2004; 4(2):223.

122. Park P, Fewel ME, Garton HJ, et al. Recombinant Activated Factor VII for the Rapid Correction of Coagulopathy in Nonhemophilic Neurosurgical Patients. Neurosurgery 2003; 53:34–39.

123. Collice M, D'Aliberti G, Talamonti G, et al. Surgery for intracerebral hemorrhage. Neurol Sci 2004; 25(Suppl 1):S10.

124. Marquardt G, Wolff R, Sager A, et al. Subacute stereotactic aspiration of hematomas within the basal ganglia reduces occurrence of complications in the course of hemorrhagic stroke in non-comatose patients. Cerebrovasc Dis 2003; 15(4):252.

125. DeGraba TJ, Pettigrew LC. Why do neuroprotective drugs work in animals but not humans? Neurol Clin 2000; 18:475.

126. Patel P. No magic bullets: the ephemeral nature of anesthetic mediated neuroprotection. Anesthesiology 2004; 100(5):1049.

15

Pediatric Neurological Trauma and Other Emergencies

Rukaiya K. Hamid

Department of Anesthesiology, UC Irvine Medical Center, Irvine, California, U.S.A.

Philippa Newfield

Department of Anesthesiology, UC San Francisco, Children's Hospital of San Francisco, San Francisco, California, U.S.A.

Michael L. Levy

Division of Neurosurgery, Department of Surgery, UC San Diego Medical Center, San Diego, California, U.S.A.

Rahul Jandial

Division of Neurosurgery, UC San Diego Medical Center, San Diego, and the Burnham Institute for Medical Research, La Jolla, California, U.S.A.

Peter J. Davis

Departments of Anesthesiology, Critical Care Medicine, and Pediatrics, Children's Hospital of Pittsburgh, Pittsburgh, Pennsylvania, U.S.A.

INTRODUCTION

Optimum management of pediatric neurosurgical emergencies requires the collaborative involvement by numerous specialties within a trauma center. This chapter describes the major pediatric neurosurgical conditions encountered, with an emphasis on the information that would aid trauma surgeons or critical care physicians in the management of such children. Other consulting specialties should also find this information germane when assisting in the management of pediatric neurosurgical patients.

Traumatic brain injury (TBI) is a significant cause of morbidity and mortality in children. This chapter emphasizes the injuries and pediatric management considerations that are dissimilar from those of adult trauma. Children engage in activities that can be associated with penetrating injuries; these lesions will also be explored. Traumatic birth injuries can lead to devastating effects that persist throughout life; accordingly, these are briefly reviewed. Trauma-related cerebral vascular lesions in children share significant overlap with those occurring in adults; hence, only the key points and the few pediatric-specific points will be discussed here. However, vascular lesions unique to children, such as vein of Galen aneurysms, which have classic clinical presentations, are reviewed in greater detail. Hydrocephalus, congenital or acquired, can present acutely and require emergent care as well. Pediatric tumors and infections are briefly discussed with an emphasis on the emergent issues. The chapter concludes with a discussion of pediatric intensive care unit (ICU) complications, and the "Eye to the Future" section reviews neuroprotective strategies and drugs that are currently under investigation.

PEDIATRIC-SPECIFIC INTRACRANIAL PRESSURE CONSIDERATIONS

Most neurosurgical catastrophes result from acute increases in intracranial pressure (ICP). The physiologic mechanisms that maintain the balance between pressure and volume inside the skull and dural sac were reviewed in Volume 2, Chapters 1 and 7, and are largely similar in adults and children (1,2). However, following trauma and other pathologic conditions, the manifestations of elevated ICP can be quite different in neonates and in children. This chapter provides an abbreviated review of ICP physiology, with a focus upon considerations that are specific to pediatric neurosurgical emergencies.

The contents of the intradural space are brain, brain stem, spinal cord, blood, and cerebral spinal fluid (CSF). ☞ **In an infant, with an open fontanel and open cranial sutures, small increases in the volume of intradural contents can be accommodated by separation of the sutures and distention of the fontanel.** ☞ This accommodation is generally achieved with a gradual increase in intradural volume. However, a sudden large increase in the intradural contents will only be minimally accommodated by distention of the dural sac and an open fontanel; under these circumstatnces, ICP will increase dramatically, as in adults.

The intradural space is divided into a series of compartments by the foramen magnum and the folds of the dura, the falx, and the tentorium. The compartments are important because increases in pressure in one compartment can result in distortion and displacement of brain into another compartment, with consequent tissue and vascular compression, ultimately resulting in brain dysfunction and herniation. The most frequent location for cerebral herniation is at the tentorial hiatus. Supratentorial pressure causes distortion and displacement of the mesial temporal lobe or lobes, forcing the parahippocampal gyrus through the tentorial notch (transtentorial herniation), thereby compressing the brain stem–perforating vessels, the posterior cerebral arteries, and the perforating vessels to the thalamus.

☞ **In children, hemiparesis occurs on the side ipsilateral to the herniation 50% of the time, whereas in adults hemiparesis is ipsilateral to the herniation 75% of the time.** ☞ Hemiparesis occurring on the same side as the intracranial lesion is due to the effect of brain stem itself shifting away from the mass and impinging upon Kernohan's notch of the tentorium, and is referred to as Kernohan's phenomenon. Why this occurs more often in children is unknown. But this finding can cause clinical confusion in pediatric neurosurgery, and must be quickly resolved with a neuroimaging study. Impending foramen magnum herniation can be heralded by complaints of headache and neck pain. The pain may initially be relieved by extension of the neck. As herniation progresses, the medulla oblongata is compressed with resulting elevation in ICP, systemic hypertension, and bradycardia (Cushing's triad), along with bradypnea, and finally apnea. In some cases, the onset of apnea may be preceded only by severe headache or neck pain with no other clinical signs.

A mass in the posterior fossa (common site for pediatric brain tumors) can occasionally cause herniation of the cerebellar vermis upward through the tentorial notch, with compression of the brain stem and posterior cerebral and thalamic perforating vessels. In children, this "upward herniation" is frequently precipitated by abrupt drainage of the lateral ventricles in the presence of a posterior fossa mass.

In addition to causing distortion and herniation of neural tissue and focal vascular compression, elevated ICP can affect general cerebral blood flow (CBF). As occurs in adults, the cerebral blood vessels of children exhibit autoregulation in response to changes in cerebral perfusion pressure (CPP). However, the range of autoregulation is different in children compared to that in adults. The CPP formula is provided below (where MAP is mean arterial pressure and ICP is intracranial pressure):

$$CPP = MAP - ICP$$

The cerebral vessels respond to a decrease in CPP by vasodilatation, decreasing resistance to flow and thus maintaining the same CBF despite either a decline in MAP or an increase in ICP. The exact limits of autoregulation are not known through the period of infancy and childhood but probably range between 35 and 40 mmHg at the lower end and is greater than 100 mmHg at the upper end. Below the limits of autoregulation, the CBF decreases as the CPP is lowered. Cerebral metabolism is preserved to a CBF of about 50% of normal, after which some degree of cerebral ischemia begins. As CBF decreases below 25% of normal, irreversible brain damage begins. Thus, autoregulation is a further brain-protective mechanism against increased ICP. Trauma in children often leaves autoregulation intact, whereas ischemia seems more likely to abolish autoregulation, making the CBF more sensitive to small changes in the CPP. ☞ **Unfortunately, the status of autoregulation is not known in the clinical setting, and thus therapy is directed at maintaining normal or nearly normal ICP and MAP in the hope that this will preserve CBF.** ☞ When the ICP is too high, or the MAP is too low, the CPP will be

inadequate to maintain CBF, and cerebral ischemia will result. The ultimate manifestation of this deficit is the cessation of CBF that results in brain death (2).

Before any surgical intervention, resuscitation of a child with a neurosurgical catastrophe addresses the usual concerns of airway patency, bleeding, and circulation. Specific therapy to lower the ICP (e.g., mannitol) depends on the severity and rapidity of the ICP elevation along with an evaluation of the degree of neurologic deterioration. The history is often the deciding factor, because absolute signs of intracranial hypertension are difficult in pediatrics, depending on the rate of increase in ICP. Papilledema is a sure sign of intracranial hypertension but is often absent because of the rapidity of the onset of symptoms or because the anatomy of the subarachnoid space in the optic nerve is such that papilledema does not occur. ☞ **Acute loss of consciousness after pediatric head trauma is less commonly the result of increased ICP unlike in adults. Accordingly, osmotic diuretics should not be routinely administered to children in coma after head trauma.** ☞

The most important initial issues to address in the child with TBI are the airway, breathing, and circulation (ABCs). When intracranial hypertension is suspected in a comatose child, endotracheal intubation is performed. Next, the immediate clinical presentation is addressed. Is the patient unconscious, seizing, posturing, exhibiting abnormal respiratory patterns, protecting his/her airway, displaying any focal neurologic deficits, or exhibiting any signs of high ICP? This information is quickly processed as a head computed tomography (CT) scan is being arranged. As the patient is being transported to CT, one can attain further details surrounding the injury. Indeed, from compiling the history and physical, one should have a pretty accurate prediction of what the head CT will reveal.

If a patient has a significantly large acute mass-occupying lesion, the child must be immediately rushed to the operating room for evacuation. If, on the other hand, there is no space-occupying lesion (just diffuse swelling), or a relatively small lesion, the patient may be initially managed nonoperatively in the ICU.

In the ICU, the head is maintained midline and (if the MAP is adequate and concomitant spinal trauma is ruled out), the head is elevated 30 degrees. The most important information in the brain-injured patient is the neurologic examination. ☞ **A reliable and reproducible neurologic examination is much more important than any number or value from an ICP monitor or ventriculostomy catheter.** ☞ If the child is at least able to localize the pain, the clinical neurologic examination is the best method of monitoring neurologic status. Close, hourly neurologic examinations should be able to detect any deterioration under these conditions. If the patient does not have a reliable examination either due to injury, intubation, or medications, ICP monitoring is required. However, an ICP monitor should only be placed after early resuscitation and verification that coagulation factors and platelets are adequate.

The preferred method of choice for ICP monitoring in children is with a ventriculostomy catheter (in infants the fontanel can be safely drained with a butterfly needle as needed). The ventriculostomy provides not only a reliable method of ICP monitoring, but also allows for efficacious treatment of high ICP pressures by drainage of CSF. There are certainly other means for treating high ICP, including hyperventilation, head elevation, sedation, mannitol, hypertonic saline, and so on. However, particularly in the setting of an acute closed head injury, the primary means of treating high ICP should always be CSF drainage. For this reason, ventriculostomy placement is the first method of choice for ICP monitoring (see Volume 2, Chapter 12, Fig. 10). If a ventriculostomy cannot be placed, then other means of ICP monitoring must be employed. The first 24 to 72 hours following a head injury are the most critical. If a ventriculostomy is present, one should be liberal in CSF drainage if the patient is exhibiting high ICP. In most instances, leaving the ventriculostomy open to drain at 15 cm of water pressure represents the optimum management. After allowing a few days for resolution of edema and secondary changes, the ventriculostomy should be weaned by slowly raising the drain reservoir height, then eventually clamping it. Some pediatric TBI patients will not be able to be weaned from ventricular drainage and will require placement of a ventriculoperitoneal (V-P) shunt (1–4).

CLOSED HEAD TRAUMA

Traumatic lesions that require surgical therapy in children are less common. They occur in 20% to 30% of children with a Glasgow Coma Scale (GCS) score ≤8. Traumatic unconsciousness is a neurologic emergency, and although it may be associated with elevated ICP, it most often requires rapid resuscitation rather than surgical intervention. ☞ **Lesions that may require immediate surgery are intracranial hematomas, compound depressed skull fractures, and penetrating trauma.** ☞ Post-traumatic subarachnoid hemorrhage (SAH), brain swelling, brain edema, arterial spasm, and focal strokes are all lesions not improved by surgery. Traumatic lesions that evolve over time and ultimately do require acute surgery include post-traumatic hydrocephalus, delayed intracranial hemorrhage, and ruptured traumatic aneurysm. Post-traumatic hydrocephalus can occur anytime up to one year after the injury, but most commonly requires a shunt in the first three months following the trauma. Delayed intracranial hemorrhage and ruptured traumatic aneurysm generally occur 7 to 14 days after injury.

Epidemiology

Injuries remain a leading cause of death for children over the age of one year in the United States. Pediatric trauma also results in an increased cost to society due to long-term disability (5,6). Nearly five million children sustain traumatic head injury in the United States each year, and about 200,000 of these children require hospitalization (7).

The mean age of pediatric trauma victims is between six and seven years with two-thirds of these being boys. Head injury is involved in as many as 80% of the children with multiple trauma. In 60% of these cases, head trauma is the most severe injury within the injury pattern and is the predominant factor that determines outcome. The most frequent combination of injuries is head trauma and an extremity fracture (8). The mortality of children related to trauma and head injury is second only to congenital diseases in the developing countries (9). Head injuries are responsible for 75% of all pediatric trauma hospital admissions and result in 70% of all trauma deaths in children (10). Children suffer TBI more frequently than any other age group (11,12). Head injuries account for up to 80% of fatal child abuse injuries at the youngest ages (13).

Mechanisms of Injury
Injuries from Falls

Falls represent the most common mechanism of injury in all pediatric age groups except for those less than one year of age. Child abuse is the most common cause of injury for those ≤1 year of age (14,15). Deaths in childhood can result from falls of less than 10 feet (16). Skull fracture is much less commonly associated with fatal head injury in children than in adults (16–18).

The mechanism of falling also differs according to age group. Younger children most often fall down stairs or out of windows. Prepubescent children tend to fall from a wide variety of places, with the majority occurring outside the home during play, whereas adolescents are reported to fall from much greater heights and sustain more severe injuries (19). The severity of the injuries resulting from falls varies according to the age of the child, the type of fall, and the height of the fall (16–21).

Although the incidence of possible complications is higher with increasing height of the fall, skull fractures and intracranial injuries can be sustained by children with falls of less than or equal to three feet (22–26).

Injuries Resulting from Vehicular Crash
Bicycle Collisions

Approximately 200,000 children and adolescents are injured and more than 600 die annually from bicycle-related trauma (5,27,28). Taken together, motor vehicle and bicycle collisions are the most common causes of head injury and death in children (29). It is the head injuries that cause most bicycle-related morbidity and mortality. More than half the deaths occur in children from 5 to 19 years of age (30,31). The use of bicycle helmets can prevent an estimated 85% of head injuries and 88% of brain injuries but many parents are unaware of the need for helmets, and children may be reluctant to use them (32,33). Helmet laws have resulted in a decreased number of head injuries in cyclists (34). A reduction in the risk of bicycle-related head injury among helmet wearers was demonstrated in cyclists of all ages in crashes, including crashes with automobiles (35). The principal injuries related to bicycle accidents include head trauma from road collisions, including compressive neuropathic injury (36–40).

Motor Vehicle Collisions

Motor vehicle–related trauma accounts for nearly half of all pediatric injuries and deaths (5,24). Proper use of seat restraints and lap-shoulder harnesses can prevent an estimated 65% to 75% of serious injuries and fatalities in passengers under four years of age, and 45% to 55% of all pediatric motor vehicle passenger injuries and deaths (41). Children and adolescents must be well secured in the car via a shoulder restraint and a lap belt. Although a 16-year-old boy sustained a common carotid artery and tracheal injury from a shoulder strap following a high-speed motor vehicle collision (MVC), most of these injuries occur with automated shoulder straps without a secured lap belt (42). Approximately 50% of adolescent motor vehicle fatalities involve alcohol (41), and a large proportion of all pediatric motor vehicle occupant deaths occur in vehicles operated by inebriated drivers (41).

Shaken Baby Syndrome and Other Forms of Child Abuse

Intentional injury is the most common cause of severe TBI in infants (43) and children less than one year of age (44,45). Additionally more child abuse deaths occur from head injuries than from any other form of trauma (46,47). Infants and toddlers who survive abusive head trauma often have serious neurologic sequelae (48–49). Intentional injuries, however, are more difficult to diagnose due to lack of accurate history and delay in presentation (50).

Utilizing the resources of the departments of health, social services, coroner, district attorney, and law enforcement, Wang et al. (49) documented that in Los Angeles County 54% of child abuse victims were under one year of age, and one-third of cases had a previous record of intervention by child-protective services. The cause of death in homicides was head trauma in 27% of the cases.

The most frequently inflicted form of infantile head injury results from the "shaken baby syndrome" (48). The classic description of abuse was documented by Kempe et al. (50) in 1962, as the "battered child syndrome" and later by Caffey (51), who coined the term "whiplash shaken baby syndrome." Briefly, the constellation of findings with "shaken baby syndrome" include subdural and subarachnoid hemorrhage, retinal hemorrhages, and traction-type metaphyseal fractures. This was based on evidence that angular (rotational) deceleration is associated with cerebral concussion and subdural hematoma (52). Furthermore, fewer than 2% of children with significant accidental head injuries have retinal hemorrhages. Blunt-force impact as well as vigorous shaking may play a role in the pathogenesis of these injuries (53,54).

Imaging Following Mild Alterations in Consciousness

Considerable controversy surrounds the appropriate evaluation of children with mild alterations in consciousness after closed head trauma (GCS score of 13–14). In a population-based, multicenter prospective study of all patients to whom Emergency Medical Services (EMS) responded over a 12-month period, 8488 patients in the pediatric age group (<15 years old) were transported by EMS for injuries. Of these, 209 had a documented field GCS score of 13 or 14. One hundred fifty-seven patients were taken to trauma centers and 135 (86%) received CT scans. Forty-three (27.4%) had an abnormal head CT scan, 30 (19.1%) had an intracranial hemorrhage, and five required a neurosurgical operative procedure for hematoma evacuation (55). Positive and negative predictive values of deteriorating mental status (0.500/0.844), loss of consciousness (0.173/0.809), skull fracture (0.483/0.875), and extracranial injuries (0.205/0.814) were poor predictors of intracranial hemorrhage. The incidence of intracranial injury in pediatric patients with mild alterations in consciousness in the field is significant. The great majority of these patients do not require operative intervention, but the implications of missing these hemorrhages can be significant for this subgroup of head-injured patients (55). ☞ **It is recommended that, because clinical criteria and skull X rays are poor predictors of intracranial hemorrhage, all children with a GCS score of 13 or 14 routinely have a screening noncontrast-enhanced CT scan.** ☞

Specific Pathologic Lesions
Intracerebral Hematoma

Most intracerebral hematomas occur with severe head trauma and often in association with diffuse axonal injury. They are encountered in 3% to 5% of postinjury CT scans in children who usually have a GCS score of <8. Many hematomas are in the deep white matter or basal ganglia, and it is rare that surgical evacuation is necessary or advisable. These children are at risk for elevated ICP and may require intense medical treatment to control brain swelling and edema. Large, more superficial hematomas are occasionally identified, and they may require surgical evacuation to control herniation and severely elevated ICP. Surgery, if necessary, should focus on evacuation of the hematoma, preserving as much brain tissue as possible. Acute cerebral contusions are relatively rare after pediatric head injury, and in general do not require surgical resection, primarily because of the need to remove brain that often can recover. In follow-up studies of children with moderate or severe head injuries, a high incidence of contusions has been identified (50%); the majority is in the frontal area, followed by the anterior temporal tip (55). Although some of these lesions were visible on the original CT scan, the majority was not. The latter are also clearly not surgical lesions and require no specific early intervention.

Epidural Hematoma

Epidural hematomas are usually of arterial origin, resulting from rupture of branches of the middle meningeal or posterior meningeal arteries. They are found in 6% to 8% of children who undergo CT scanning after head injury (see Volume 2, Chapter 12, Fig. 2). The children are almost equally divided into three groups, one-third never being unconscious, one-third being unconscious from the time of injury, and one-third demonstrating a lucid interval followed by unconsciousness. Early CT scanning to identify the lesion is important because the patient's outcome is closely correlated with the level of consciousness at the time of surgical evacuation and with the constellation of brain injuries present. In children younger than eight years of age, the epidural hematoma is more frequently situated in the parietal and temporal-parietal region rather than in the anterior temporal location typically observed in adults. Thus, blindly placing burr holes in children is rarely advisable. A CT scan should be obtained whenever possible to pinpoint the precise location of the lesion and to identify other intracranial lesions. However, if a child with a skull fracture is showing signs of rapid progression toward herniation, and if time does not permit a CT scan, surgery must be done emergently, with the center of the craniotomy located over the center of the fracture. Most epidural hematomas require surgical removal, but small lesions (especially frontal ones) in the presence of normal consciousness can often be treated nonoperatively.

Subdural Hematoma

Subdural hematomas are usually the result of tearing of the bridging cortical veins due to acceleration–deceleration injury or tearing of the cerebral cortex and cortical arteries following blunt trauma. The incidence varies from 5% to 30% in children hospitalized for head injury (see Volume 2, Chapter 12, Fig. 3). The highest frequency is in children younger than one year, and the cause is usually child abuse. In infants and toddlers, the lesions are usually small and bilateral and do not require surgery. Children with an open fontanel, and in extremis, can have their ICP lowered by withdrawing bloody fluid through the fontanel. The major problem with subdural hematoma is the underlying brain swelling. Thus treatment with ICP monitoring and medical management of the elevated ICP is essential.

Many of these lesions do not require surgery; rather, the emphasis is placed upon control of the brain swelling and ICP. In general, if the brain distortion is considerably more than the width of the subdural hematoma and the subdural hematoma is less than 1 cm, surgery is not performed; however, the indications for surgery vary with the condition of the individual child and the neurosurgeon's individual criteria for surgery in this setting.

Complex Depressed Skull Fractures

Compound depressed skull fractures are open wounds of the brain and require urgent surgical debridement as soon as the patient is stabilized and the associated cerebral edema minimized. These fractures are the most common reason for surgery after trauma in children. The aim of the surgery is to debride the brain of contamination including bone fragments, remove any associated hematomas, repair the dura to prevent cerebral herniation and CSF leakage, and reconstruct the skull either with the fragments present or with split cranial bone. It is usually possible to replace the fragments and avoid the need for a second reconstructive operation.

Cranial Burst Fractures in Infants

Cranial burst fracture is a unique type of head injury that occurs in infants (56). This lesion is characterized as a widely diastatic skull fracture associated with dural laceration and extrusion of cerebral tissue through the dural defect and outside the calvarium (but beneath the unbroken scalp). Prompt diagnosis and reduction of the cerebral hernia and repair of the dural tear prevents the sequelae of a "growing skull fracture." The diagnosis can be initially missed on skull X rays and even CT scans (Fig. 1) (56).

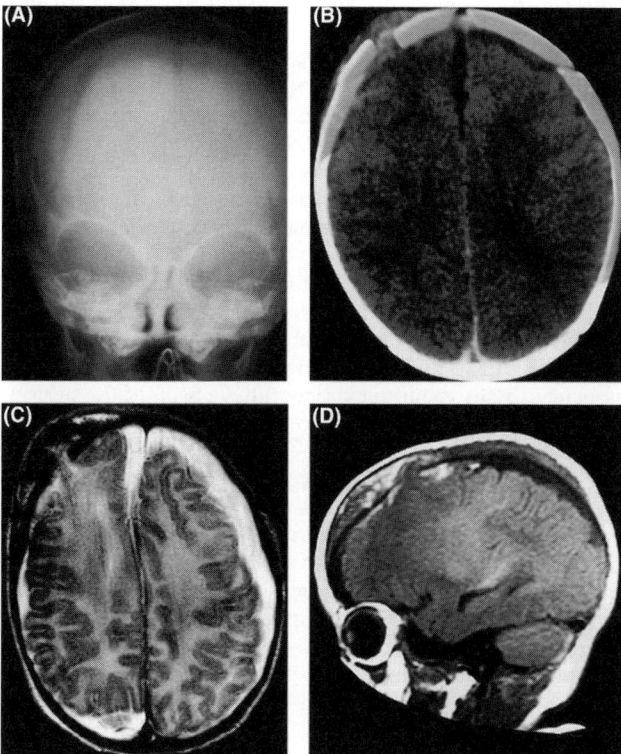

Figure 1 Cranial burst fracture. (**A**) Skull radiograph four hours after injury shows a widely diastatic right frontal skull fracture; (**B**) computed tomograph scan of acute cranial fracture four hours after injury shows hemorrhagic contusion beneath the fracture, overlying scalp swelling, and moderate eversion of fracture edges; (**C**) axial T2-weighted magnetic resonance (MR) image; and (**D**) sagittal T1-weighted MR image. Both (**C**) and (**D**) were taken 15 hours after injury and show acute transcalvarial brain herniation. Brain parenchyma is clearly differentiated from scalp soft tissue and hematoma. Note associated convexity and interhemispheric subdural hematoma and cortical contusions. *Source*: From Ref. 56.

Scalp swelling associated with cranial burst fracture can be misdiagnosed as a simple skull fracture with underlying subgaleal hematoma. Often the diagnosis is not made until weeks to years after the acute trauma, as this condition converts to a "growing skull fracture" (56).

Prompt treatment will likely increase neurologic outcomes, but acute neurologic imaging is the key to early delineation of the injury. Figure 1 elucidates one of the important pitfalls of using skull radiographs and CT alone, and also demonstrates the imaging characteristics seen on magnetic resonance imaging (MRI, the diagnostic modality of choice for cranial burst fractures).

PENETRATING TRAUMA

☞ **Most forms of penetrating cranial injury (PCI) require surgical exploration** ☞ (e.g., dog bites or dart injuries). Gunshot wounds of the head and other forms of PCI are increasingly common in children. The actual incidence is difficult to determine due to gaps in reporting, absence of a centralized database, and the presumption that—as in the adult population—a substantial number of victims die prior to arrival at emergency departments (57,58). The causes of PCI can be broadly categorized as follows: (*i*) accidental injury with sharp or semisharp objects, (*ii*) warfare, (*iii*) accidentally discharged firearms, (*iv*) suicide, and (*v*) homicides. Most PCIs require surgery to debride superficial bone fragments from the brain, remove intracranial hematomas, and repair the dura and cranium. The indications for surgery also depend upon an estimate of whether or not a child is likely to survive the injury.

By their very nature, children are prone to accidental injuries with common household and environmental objects. The literature has afforded scattered case reports of PCIs involving impalements with items such as pencils and chopsticks (59–62), broom handles, metal strips, plant branches, kitchen knives, dinner forks, wires, nails, spikes, scissors, and screwdrivers. Flying objects during automobile accidents have also been described as a cause of PCI (63–65). Low-velocity missiles such as arrows, and pellets accidentally discharged from pneumatic "toy" weapons would be included in this category as well (66,67). Lawn darts have been banned from retail sale in the United States due to the significant number of severe and fatal PCIs that occurred in young children; nonetheless, an estimated 10 to 15 million sets still remain in American households and will likely remain a significant mechanism of injury for years to come (68). A special consideration in the management of impalements is the frequent entrance through thin calvarial regions (such as the squamous temporal bone) or foramina or canals (such as the optic canal) with a high risk of vascular or cranial nerve damage, despite initial impressions that the injuries may be trivial. Accordingly, all these patients should receive prompt neurosurgical evaluation and brain CT scanning.

Prognostic Factors for Penetrating Head Injury

A discussion on outcomes in pediatric PCI is problematic, because most of the literature involves the adult population. The immediate and early mortality rates are high and the overall numbers are low enough that the generation of useful analyses and predictive models is difficult. As discussed above, it is reasonable to withhold aggressive care from the patient presenting with a GCS score of 3 and fixed pupils after initial resuscitative efforts. Furthermore, one recent series (69) found that no pediatric TBI patient with concomitant anoxic insult regained useful consciousness, implying that limited management is probably appropriate for this group. Conversely, patients with minimal initial neurologic impairments (i.e., GCS scores of 12–15) and limited parenchymal injuries generally make excellent functional recoveries, indicating that aggressive neurosurgical management is appropriate for all these patients.

The dilemma in neurosurgical management involves decision making in patients with moderate to severe injuries, and those with concomitant hypotensive and/or hypoxemic events. Most studies focus on closed head injuries; therefore, application to the PCI group must be done cautiously. Children with prolonged unconsciousness and vegetative states are more likely than adults to have protracted survivals; however, severe residual cognitive and motor deficits may occur (69–70). Children with milder injuries can be left with residual cognitive deficits, limitations in physical health, and behavioral problems. Although children generally fare better than adults with similar degrees of blunt TBI, Kaufman's analysis of PCI patients found similar incidences of functional disabilities, special educational needs, and extreme emotional lability (71). Other investigators have determined that cognitive recovery in moderately and severely injured children generally plateaus around the first postinjury year (72,73). For some patients with less severe injuries, the deleterious consequences on cognition, behavior, and psychosocial adjustment may not be fully realized until adulthood (74). One study found that only 23% of adults who sustained TBI in the preschool years were able to work, and only 36% lived independently at home (75). This correlated with the delayed development of cerebral atrophy and porencephalic cysts.

Surgical Approach to Penetrating Head Injury

A number of studies have concluded that it is unnecessary to reoperate for retained bone fragments and that it is often possible to temper the initial debridement in an effort to preserve additional cerebral tissue (60,61,76–78). Long-term follow-up in one series failed to document a significant difference between survivors with retained bone fragments (48%) and survivors without retained fragments with regard to epilepsy or central nervous system (CNS) infection (77). In a prospective series of 32 military patients with intracranial bone fragments who underwent debridement of the entry wound and dural closure, only one patient developed a subsequent CSF leak, seizure, and a CNS infection. No CSF leaks or infections were reported in the remaining 31 patients (76).

In summary, the current literature supports a conservative surgical approach. Surgical management begins with evacuation of mass lesions and debridement of necrotic tissue and bony fragments at entrance and exit sites. Only superficial or local bone fragments need be debrided. Deep parenchymal fragments and those not readily accessible should not be removed unless obviously grossly contaminated.

TRAUMATIC BIRTH INJURIES

The overall incidence of traumatic birth injuries has dramatically declined; however 2% to 5% of all neonates sustaining craniocerebral trauma die (79). Infants at an increased risk for birth injury include those born to primiparous women, those whose birth weight is greater than 3500 gm, and those who are born with forceps-assisted delivery. Furthermore, breech presentation and forceps or precipitous deliveries are significantly correlated with intracranial hemorrhage (80,81). Shoulder dystocia is associated with injury to the brachial plexus, as is prolonged pregnancy and macrosomia (82).

Although high-forceps deliveries have been abandoned in modern obstetrical care, mid-forceps deliveries have clear indications, such as fetal distress. A mid-forceps delivery involves the application of the instrument to a fetus whose biparietal diameter is somewhere between the pelvic inlet and the maternal labia in a vertex presentation. Mid-forceps deliveries have been associated with brachial plexus injury. When shoulder dystocia complicates a mid-pelvic delivery, the incidence of birth injury has been reported to be as high as 47%. Indeed, one recent review demonstrated that one-half of all brachial plexus injuries during delivery was attributed to mid-forceps extraction (83).

Vacuum cup extraction was introduced in an effort to reduce injury associated with forceps-assisted delivery. A pliable, soft cup is favored over the metal cup, which has been associated with a high incidence of scalp injuries and lacerations (84). Extraction by vacuum cup is associated with cephalohematoma (84) and has been associated with growing skull fractures (85); the overall incidence of complications from vacuum cup delivery is similar to that from forceps (86).

In addition, retinal hemorrhage appears to be higher with the vacuum cup method. This finding is assumed to represent exposure to sudden changes in ICP inherent in the vacuum extraction technique independent of the type of cup used (84). The significance of retinal hemorrhage in these neonates is unknown. Retinal hemorrhages have been reported with bloody CSF (82), but have not correlated with intracranial hemorrhage in other studies. Excluding an isolated report of SAH, intracranial hemorrhage has not been reported with vacuum cup extraction. Retinal hemorrhages associated with vacuum extraction have been of the peripheral type, and are thought to have no influence on the subsequent function of the eye (85–87).

It has been generally recognized that basic differences exist between the nature of tissue damage of craniocerebral trauma occurring in infants and that in children and adults (88). The scalp is subject to a considerable amount of stress and is frequently injured in the birth process. Exsanguination from a rapidly expanding subgaleal hemorrhage can occur and, as an isolated lesion, represents the most serious of superficial birth injuries. Extracranial cerebral compression may jeopardize the infant's life. Management consists of measures to correct hypovolemic shock and disseminated intravascular coagulation, as well as surgical intervention to control elevated ICP. Skull fractures are common but in general are not associated with underlying intracranial hemorrhage or pathology and require no treatment. The growing skull fracture and occipital osteodiastasis are exceptions.

Intracranial hemorrhage has many potential sources in the neonate with varying prognosis. Mass lesions require surgical management. All forms of intracranial hematomas are encountered in the neonatal period, but all are rare. Epidural hematomas occur in the supratentorial and infratentorial spaces and, if producing cerebral compression, require evacuation. Before any surgery is performed on a neonate, clotting studies must be performed and abnormalities corrected, if necessary. Subdural hematomas are a difficult problem to handle surgically, and if they are not large, efforts to control the ICP medically should usually be attempted before resorting to surgery. Most intracerebral hematomas in neonates are hemorrhagic infarctions or venous hemorrhages, and surgery is rarely indicated. The brain is 90% water, and hemostasis can be very difficult; the pia mater and cerebral vessels can be peeled off the brain by the operative suction devices, resulting in increased damage.

With the exception of scalp injury, trauma to the craniocerebrum and spine necessitates neurosurgical consultation and frequently surgical intervention. The brain of the newborn is not yet myelinated and is subject to shearing forces at junctional levels in a manner different from adult brain. In particular, cortical, subcortical, parenchymal-ventricular, interhemispheric–corpus callosum, and cerebral hemisphere–brain stem levels are at particular risk (14). Blunt head trauma in the newborn and infant produces tears in the cerebral white matter, parallel to the surface, and similar (microscopic) tears in the superficial cortical layers. When craniocerebral injury is of such a nature and severity as to produce the shearing forces, which result in intracranial mass lesions in the form of hematomas, the underlying brain damage is likely severe. In such a scenario, surgical evacuation of the clot may not alter the clinical outcome (88).

TRAUMATIC VASCULAR LESIONS

Cerebrovascular trauma includes a broad array of injuries both direct and indirect. Epidural hematoma and carotid-cavernous sinus fistula are two examples of the better-recognized sequelae of intracranial vascular disruption. Unfortunately, neither all vascular injuries associated with head trauma are as readily identifiable nor are they associated with definite treatment guidelines. Their management remains in evolution as medical, surgical, and endovascular options develop. Furthermore, many of the management strategies have arisen from the care of adults and will also be discussed in other chapters (Volume 1, Chapter 15 for initial evaluation of blunt cervical spine injuries and Volume 1, Chapter 24 for penetrating neck trauma).

Cervical Carotid Injury

Injury to the extracranial carotid and vertebral arteries is uncommon in pediatrics, but in adults represents one of the most common vascular injuries following neck trauma. Well over 90% of the major arterial trauma in the neck is caused by penetrating wounds (see Volume 1, Chapter 24) (89). Nonpenetrating traumatic lesions of the extracranial cerebral vasculature provide the most difficult diagnostic and management problems. The most important symptoms of carotid arterial injury are those of cerebral ischemia, including hemiparesis or hemisensory deficit with or without associated hemianopsia suggesting ischemia in the internal carotid territory. Symptoms may be fleeting as in transient ischemic attack (TIA), or more prolonged in their presentation. The neurologic deficit worsens and eventually becomes permanent. Also, the level of consciousness may be affected, but frequently the neurologic deficit is out of proportion to any reduction in the level of consciousness, in contradistinction to what would be expected solely as a result of the head injury.

Traumatically induced dissection of the internal carotid artery in the neck also occurs in association with head injury. As in thrombosis, the critical element is disruption of the intima. Aneurysms may also result from injury of the carotid artery in association with head trauma. The arterial wall is thinned and weakened, and the pulsatile column of blood produces an aneurysm in association with an area of dissection that is extensive enough to disrupt both the intima and adventitia. Turbulence may cause the aneurysm to enlarge and also provide for thrombus formation, which can subsequently embolize distally. Patients may complain of a pulsatile neck mass, dysphagia, or noise in the neck that may radiate into the head. Also, lower cranial nerve palsies including hoarseness or weakness of the tongue may occur in association with large aneurysms of the carotid artery (90).

Patients exhibiting signs or symptoms consistent with blunt cerebral vascular injury must undergo emergent diagnostic evaluation. Because a negative noninvasive study should not be accepted in this instance, the gold standard (four-vessel cervical arteriography) is the study of choice, but this is rapidly changing toward CT angiogram (CTA) and magnetic resonance angiogram (MRA) (Fig. 2).

⚬⁺ **The typical angiographic picture of trauma-induced occlusion of the cervical internal carotid artery is abrupt blockage of contrast flow approximately 1–3 cm above the bifurcation of the common carotid artery in the neck.** ⚬⁺ Although traumatic dissection can occur anywhere along the course of the internal carotid artery, it most frequently begins in the section of the artery adjacent to the C1 and C2 vertebra. Dissecting aneurysms may present as irregular enlargements of the contrast column in association with segmental narrowing of the cervical internal carotid artery. These aneurysms tend to become more localized and saccular in nature. Duplex scanning has well-documented limitations, which must be acknowledged if this test is used. Before exclusively embracing CTA or MRA, their limitations must also be acknowledged.

The treatment of patients with carotid thrombosis depends upon the stage at which it is diagnosed. Those with a completed stroke of more than 12 hours' duration or who present in a coma will most likely prove refractory to any type of treatment. ⚬⁺ **Patients with fluctuating neurologic symptoms in the face of an acutely occluded internal carotid artery may benefit from urgent exploration and thromboendarterectomy.** ⚬⁺ Prior to any thoughts

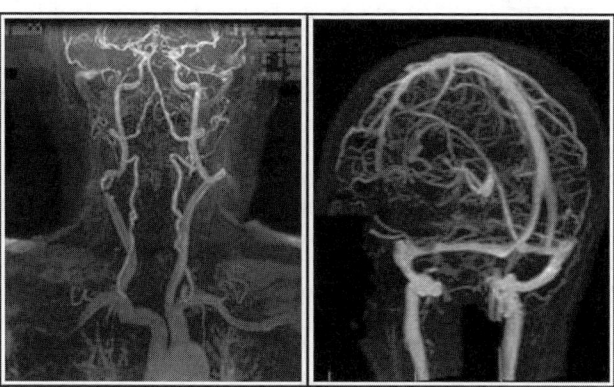

Figure 2 Magnetic resonance (MR) angiography. MR arteriogram (*left*) and MR venogram (*right*) revealing normal cervical and cerebral vasculature.

of surgical therapy, the patient who presents with an occluded carotid artery with or without ischemic neurologic deficits should be managed with attempts to increase cerebral perfusion. Hypotension resulting from associated injuries should be rapidly reversed with fluid therapy or pressor agents. In those few patients who are found to have a carotid occlusion in the absence of neurologic symptoms, a high circulating intravascular volume should be maintained in order to obviate any potential hypotensive episodes in the first few days following the injury. Those patients who have a mild to moderate neurologic deficit and who may or may not be candidates for surgical therapy, can benefit by trial of induced hypervolemia (91).

Therapeutic embolization of head and neck vascular injuries may be considered as an alternative to surgery particularly in lesions whose anatomic location makes them unsuitable for surgical treatment. Complications from therapeutic embolization, if carefully performed, are usually less than with surgery, and embolization can be performed in conjunction with the initial angiographic workup. Therapeutic embolization is preferably performed with preservation of parent arteries. When this is not possible, the involved carotid or vertebral arteries are occluded proximally by placing detachable balloons or coils. The safety of permanent arterial occlusion must be verified first by temporary test balloon occlusion, which provides information regarding the collateral blood flow.

Vertebral Artery Injuries

Injuries to the cervical portion of the vertebral artery occur infrequently. The relatively deep position of the vertebral artery in the neck associated with its protection by the foramina transversaria tends to reduce its vulnerability to both blunt and penetrating injuries. Further, the relative redundancy of the vertebral system makes injuries to one vertebral artery less likely to cause ischemic cerebrovascular symptoms. The majority of patients with vertebral artery injuries associated with head and neck trauma will present with the delayed onset of symptoms and signs of brain stem or cerebellar ischemia. Vertigo, blurred vision, ataxia, and dysarthria are common. In the setting of cervical vertebral artery trauma, neck ache, suboccipital pain, and headache are also frequent concomitants.

The classical Wallenberg syndrome as a result of trauma to the vertebral artery is also known to occur following minor head and neck injury (92). This consists of Horner's syndrome with decreased sensation to pain and temperature on the ipsilateral face and contralateral arm and leg in association with ataxia on the ipsilateral side. These symptoms may follow any traumatic incident that causes acute hyperextension or rotation of the cervical spine. Neurologic symptoms usually occur within 24 hours but may be delayed as long as a month after the trauma.

In some cases, associated neck movements serve to exacerbate the symptoms of ischemia. This clinical scenario should also alert the treating physician to a potential vertebral artery injury. Injuries to the cervical vertebral arteries most commonly result in thrombosis. However, intimal disruption, dissection, aneurysm formation, and fistula formation are also known to occur. Ischemia usually results from distal embolization but also may result from flow-restrictive lesions in dominant vertebral arteries.

As with carotid arterial injuries, treatment depends on the location and nature of the lesion as well as on any existing neurologic deficit. Total occlusion of the vertebral artery may not lead to ischemic symptoms because of a patent vertebral artery on the other side. In this instance, no further therapy is warranted. In those cases where vertebral thrombosis results in significant neurologic symptoms, attempts at thrombus removal or thromboendarterectomy of the vertebral artery have usually been unsuccessful (93). Supportive therapy with a trial of increased intravascular volume or mild hypertension may obviate some of the ischemic manifestations. Other injuries including traumatic narrowing, dissection, and mural hemorrhage with pseudoaneurysm formation are potential sources for distal embolization. In documented cases of embolization with mild or transient neurologic deficits, anticoagulation with heparin is recommended with consideration given to repair of the vessel. If angiography documents that the injured vessel is the dominant vertebra, reconstruction or repair using suitable graft material or possibly ligation or balloon occlusion with concomitant extracranial to intracranial bypass grafting can also be contemplated. In a situation where the nondominant vertebral artery is injured and is considered to be beyond repair, a successful trial of balloon occlusion under local anesthesia can be followed by permanent occlusion.

Intracranial Vascular Injury

Disruption of the intracranial vasculature is the rule rather than the exception with severe head injury. SAH due to loss of integrity of small pial vessels can be documented in the majority of fatal brain injuries. However, documentation of traumatic lesions in major branches of the circle of Willis or in dural venous sinuses is relatively uncommon in blunt head trauma.

☞ **The most common intracranial arterial structure to be occluded in blunt head injury is the internal carotid artery.** ☞ Although the majority of injuries to the internal carotid artery occur in its cervical portion, injury at the base of the skull, within the carotid canal, or at its cavernous segment have all been reported with some regularity (94). The patient is typically admitted comatose following an automobile accident. Within 24 hours the neurologic condition deteriorates further, and evidence of a hemiparesis tends to emerge, subsequent to infarction from internal carotid artery occlusion.

Occlusion of other major intracranial vessels has also been documented subsequent to head trauma. Evidence of ,injury to cerebral cortical branches may be seen, especially in relation to skull fractures. Findings may include branch occlusion, segmental narrowing, traumatic aneurysm formation, or slow flow in the cortical surface veins. A sharp angulation of a damaged cortical branch (Z deformity) is suggestive of entrapment of the vessel within the fracture line.

The mechanisms of middle cerebral artery thrombosis secondary to trauma are incompletely explained. The middle cerebral artery may become occluded indirectly secondary to injury to the internal carotid artery. Alternatively, the middle cerebral artery may be compressed by extracerebral or intracerebral hematomas. The management of traumatically induced middle cerebral artery occlusion remains empirical and relegated to supportive care. In the majority of those patients who survive and have follow-up angiography, the middle cerebral artery is again patent (95). In those cases where the artery does not recanalize or remain patent, the patient will progress to complete infarction of that vascular territory (Fig. 3).

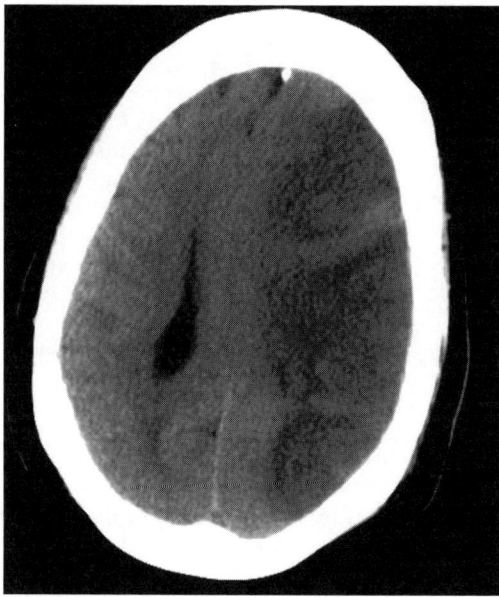

Figure 3 Computed tomography (CT) of the brain showing a left parietal hypodense area in the distribution of the left middle cerebral artery (MCA). This CT scan is consistent with infarct due to occlusion of the left MCA.

Basilar artery occlusion has also been noted secondary to head trauma (96). These patients invariably present with ischemic brain stem symptoms, and the majority of them do not survive. Basilar artery occlusion or stenosis can often be inferred from a carotid arteriogram that shows filling of the distal basilar artery through a posterior communicating artery. This observation should prompt complete examination of the vertebrobasilar circulation. Not infrequently, the basilar artery may be occluded due to associated injury to one or both vertebral arteries, which then act as a source of emboli. The majority of cases of basilar artery occlusion are documented at the time of autopsy; thus, no satisfactory treatment regimen has yet evolved.

Traumatic Aneurysms

Traumatically induced intracranial artery aneurysms are rare lesions. None of the intracranial aneurysms cataloged in the Cooperative Aneurysm Study was of traumatic origin. ♂ **The most common mode of presentation in symptomatic patients is that of delayed SAH following a head injury.** ♂ Typically, a decrease in the level of consciousness to the point of coma heralds the SAH. Further evaluation may reveal nuchal rigidity or complaints of a severe headache. Unless a high index of suspicion is maintained, the symptoms may be ascribed to an intracranial expanding process such as a hematoma or edema or possibly post-traumatic hydrocephalus. Other presenting symptoms include progressive deterioration following head trauma, most likely due to vasospasm following rupture of the aneurysm. Epistaxis or a delayed cranial nerve palsy following trauma may also give evidence of the presence of an internal carotid aneurysm near the skull base. Extracerebral hematomas following trivial head trauma and unexplained arterial bleeding during hematoma removal have all been reported as evidence of traumatically induced cerebral aneurysms (97).

Blunt head trauma is responsible for the majority of these lesions; however, penetrating lesions including bone fragments and missiles of various types including radio antennas, umbrella tips, bullets, knives, and surgical instruments are responsible for some of these cases.

The majority of traumatic cerebral aneurysms are located on branches of the middle cerebral artery. The next most common site is the internal carotid artery as it enters the skull. The pericallosal artery, most likely because of its proximity to the falx, is another important site for the occurrence of traumatically induced aneurysms. Angiographic hallmarks including delayed filling and emptying of the aneurysm, an irregular contour, the absence of a neck, and a peripheral location other than at a branching point tend to distinguish the traumatically induced aneurysm from that of the congenital or atherosclerotic forms. As with other types of intracranial aneurysm, management is directed toward avoiding recurrent hemorrhage, which is higher in traumatic aneurysms than in berry aneurysms. Aneurysm coiling or clipping should be pursued.

CONGENITAL VASCULAR ANOMALIES
Vein of Galen Aneurysm
♂ **Early high-output cardiac failure in neonates can occur with vascular shunting lesions in the cranium.** ♂ The most frequent cerebral vascular shunting lesion is the vein of Galen aneurysm, a misleading term. The vein of Galen aneurysm is actually an arteriovenous malformation (AVM) of the vessels that supply the choroid plexus of the third ventricle (98). It is different from most AVMs, which contain tangled webs of abnormal vessels. The vein of Galen aneurysm is a direct left-to-right shunting of branches of any or all of the following arteries into the vein of Galen: anterior cerebral, posterior lateral and medial choroidal, thalamic and hypothalamic perforators, posterior cerebral, anterior choroidal, and least likely the middle cerebral. The term aneurysm is also misleading: The aneurysm is of the internal cerebral veins or the vein of Galen itself and the straight sinus and is not arterial.

The vein of Galen aneurysm rarely bleeds in the first few months of life. Rather, the major clinical problem involves controlling secondary heart failure. This can often be accomplished by medical means. However, if medical management is insufficient, then selective embolization of particular arterial feeders with coils or balloons may help decrease the flow and attenuate the cardiac failure. Another option is embolization of the venous aneurysm via a transvenous route or directly through the torcula. Rarely is operative control of the feeder vessels successful in the first few days of life. If the heart failure can be initially controlled, and if after six weeks of age the failure should recur, then surgery to occlude the direct shunting arteries can usually be successfully accomplished. Interventional embolization of venous or arterial components represents a less dangerous option, although the risks of hemorrhage, pulmonary embolization by the coils, and myocardial ischemia remain concerns.

Other arteriovenous shunts that occur in neonates usually affect the dura mater, with or without cerebral involvement. Early treatment focuses on control of the heart failure with embolization if necessary. Early open surgery is rarely advisable because of the high risk of excessive blood loss.

Arteriovenous Malformations

AVMs are congenital anomalies of the vascular system and can occur anywhere in the cerebrum, brain stem, cerebellum, and spinal cord. Lesions in the spinal cord are rare in children. AVMs result in neurosurgical emergencies, as a result of rupture of usually venous components of the AVM and ensuing acute hemorrhage of blood at arterial pressure into the cerebral substance or the ventricular system (Fig. 4). In children, AVMs are four times more likely than aneurysms to be the cause of intracranial hemorrhage (99). The result is a sudden increase in ICP manifested clinically by the sudden onset of severe headache or sudden loss of consciousness. The signs and symptoms depend on the location of the hemorrhage and can include hemiparesis, aphasia, hemisensory loss, hemianopsia if the hemorrhage occurs in the supratentorial brain, or focal brain stem symptoms if the hemorrhage is in the posterior fossa. The only manifestation may be the acute onset of coma. The mortality from the first bleed has been reported to be as high as 24% in children (100). Standard resuscitation is followed by a CT scan to confirm the diagnosis of intraventricular or intraparenchymal hemorrhage. Treatment varies depending upon the clinical state of the patient. With signs of progressive herniation and impending death, acute evacuation of the hematoma may be necessary. Although obtaining an angiogram to identify the anatomy of the AVM is ideal, this is not always possible because of the rate of neurologic deterioration. The aim of surgery is to evacuate the clot, to decrease ICP, and to reverse any herniation. If an obvious AVM is encountered and is small, it may be possible to remove it. However, the safer course is to stop after evacuation of the clot. Arteriography can then be performed, followed subsequently by a second operation to resect the lesion.

Acute rebleeding from an AVM is rare, and urgent surgery therefore is not necessary to prevent a rebleed. If the blood is predominantly in the ventricle, an intraventricular catheter is required to monitor the ICP and provide for CSF drainage. Acutely, as little CSF as possible is drained to prevent the catheter becoming clogged by blood clot.

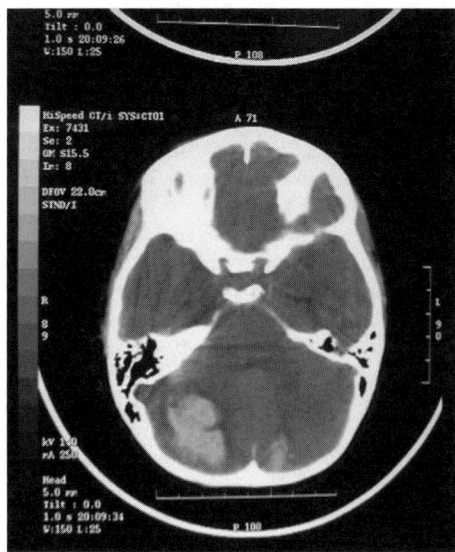

Figure 4   Computed tomograph of the brain showing a large right and small left cerebellar hemorrhage. Local mass effect on the fourth ventricle and absence of the perimesencephalic space is also noted; both findings are consistent with poor outcome.

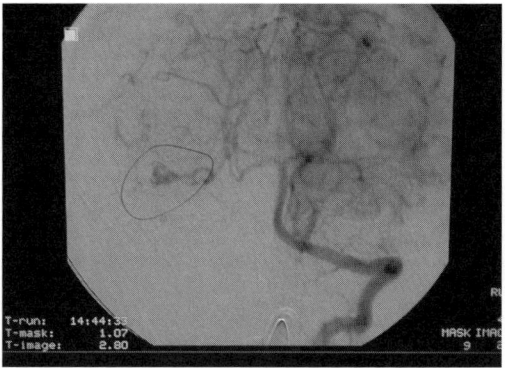

Figure 5   Vertebral arteriogram with an arteriovenous malformation nidus (*circled*).

The ICP is controlled by a combination of therapy. When a patient is stable and has recovered consciousness, arteriography (Fig. 5) and definitive therapy can be undertaken. When the clot is parenchymal, and the ICP and herniation can be controlled by medical means, it is advisable to postpone surgery until the clot has liquefied and the brain swelling and edema have subsided. This hiatus makes the surgery much safer and allows adequate investigation and therapeutic planning. Treatment is either surgery, embolization followed by surgery, or, for smaller deep lesions, focused radiation therapy. In a small percentage of cases, no obvious site of hemorrhage is identified. A repeat arteriogram some months later is required to be certain that a small lesion was not present but compressed by the acute hemorrhage. The rate of rebleeding from AVMs is 2% per year. In children in whom no lesion is identified, the rebleed rate is close to zero (101).

Aneurysms

As noted earlier, intracranial hemorrhage in children is less frequently a result of rupture of an aneurysm than that of an AVM (102). Aneurysms may be congenital or mycotic and may be found on the feeding arteries of an AVM. Aneurysms occur in the subarachnoid space, and thus SAH rather than intraparenchymal hemorrhage is the usual result of rupture. The signs and symptoms are typically sudden onset of unendurable headache followed by a stiff neck and photophobia and in about 50% of cases by coma. Diagnosis is made by the history and by a CT scan. The CT findings may appear normal or may show SAH. If the CT scan is normal while clinical suspicion for SAH remains high, the diagnosis can be made by lumbar puncture (seeking zanthochromic CSF).

Because aneurysms tend to rebleed in 24 to 48 hours, the next step in diagnosis is cerebral arteriography. MRI angiography is not adequate to visualize a small aneurysm (<5 mm). Although the most common location is at the bifurcation of the carotid, many aneurysms occur distally in children, and they are often gigantic (>2.5 cm). Mycotic aneurysms in particular occur on the distal branches of the cerebral vessels, and the rare post-traumatic aneurysm can occur on any vessel but is most frequently encountered on the anterior cerebral artery (102). Ruptured aneuryms are usually treated by angiographic coiling or by acute surgery to clip or trap the aneurysm. After rebleeding, the next major complication is cerebral ischemia, which usually results from cerebrovascular spasm (103). This is treated by volume expansion, calcium-channel blockers, and induced arterial hypertension as in adults (103,104). Because of the need for elevating the blood pressure to treat spasm, it is currently believed that early control (clipping or coiling) of the aneurysm makes this therapy to reverse or prevent ischemia safer. The use of free-radical scavengers is theoretically beneficial, but has not yet been shown to improve the outcome in patients with SAH. The grading of SAH in children is similar to the Hunt–Hess Classification used in adults (see Volume 2, Chapter 14, Table 1) (105).

Cavernous Angiomas and Venous Angiomas

Although both cavernous and venous angiomas can present with the acute onset of a new neurologic deficit and headache, it is rare that they require emergency surgery. Venous angiomas are most likely when the hematoma is in the posterior fossa, where brain stem compression can be sufficiently severe to require treatment by clot removal. In venous angiomas, the large draining vein should not be occluded because it is often the only venous drainage from a large area of the cerebellum (106,107).

The diagnosis is usually established on a noncontrast CT scan, which shows acute hemorrhage, and a contrast scan, which in the case of a cavernoma may demonstrate enhancement and in the case of a venous angioma shows the large vein and often its tributaries. Both cavernous and venous angiomas are well demonstrated on an MRI scan, which shows evidence of old hemorrhage and the surrounding edema. Cerebral arteriography usually shows no lesion in the case of the cavernous malformation and the caput of draining veins and the single large vein of the venous angioma. Acute hydrocephalus can occur as a result of posterior fossa hematoma and may require treatment with a ventriculostomy. The ventricle should be drained slowly, and the supratentorial pressure should be kept above 15 mm Hg in order to prevent upward herniation of the cerebellar vermis. This is true whenever a ventricular drain is required for relief of acute hydrocephalus secondary to a posterior fossa mass. Anticonvulsants are necessary if a patient presents with seizures, and corticosteroids are helpful to treat the cerebral edema that is often present. It is rare that severe intracranial hypertension is present. In most cases, definitive resection of the cavernous angioma is the treatment of choice once the hematoma and brain edema have subsided. The best treatment for venous angiomas often is to leave them alone unless repeated bleeding occurs, in which case a small AVM is often present and may be resected.

HYDROCEPHALUS

It is unusual for a newborn with hydrocephalus to present as a neurosurgical emergency. Because congenital hydrocephalus is a prenatal (i.e., chronic) condition, the brain accommodates and the sutures may be widely separated and the cranium may be significantly enlarged, accommodating the increased CSF volume without compression of neural structures (108). This also affords time to make an accurate diagnosis of the etiology of the hydrocephalus and to shunt the lesion electively. If signs such as apnea or bradycardia are present (representing increased ICP), the ventricle can be acutely tapped through the fontanel and the pressure relieved until an elective shunt is placed.

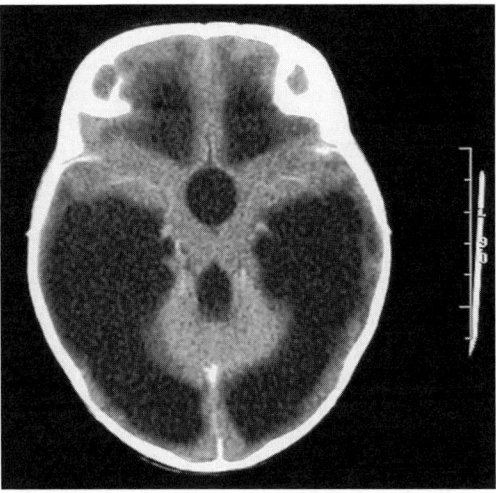

Figure 6 Computed tomograph of the brain showing massive bilateral ventriculomegaly subsequent to prolonged hydrocephalus.

Acute hydrocephalus due to congenital and acquired causes can present later in life, in a child with closed sutures (Fig. 6). In this case, rapid diagnosis and therapy may be required to prevent serious brain damage or death because the cranium cannot expand, and by the time a child presents for medical care, the compensatory mechanisms are usually exhausted. This also is true in children who have a CSF shunt in place and in whom a shunt malfunction has occurred. The difficulty with diagnosis in this group of patients is the lack of definitive signs that confirm the diagnosis. ☞ **The diagnosis of shunt malfunction or acute intracranial hypertension due to hydrocephalus is essentially based on the history and often confirmed by a neuroimaging study (CT or MRI), that shows ventricular dilatation.** ☞ In a small group of children with slit ventricle syndrome, the ventricles do not enlarge, or enlarge only minimally, in the presence of high ICPs and shunt dysfunction (109,110). In these children, it is important to compare their current scan with a previous scan; if none is available, act on the history and assume a shunt malfunction.

Because autoregulation of CBF is typically intact in a child presenting with acute hydrocephalus, the ICP waves that occur are often unassociated with any signs. The symptoms are of severe, episodic headache that may be associated with vomiting or visual disturbances. The pain may be located behind the eyes or in the back of the neck as a result of tonsillar herniation. The headache may be relieved by vomiting, because this triggers hyperventilation and thus a decrease in ICP that can abort the pressure wave. If a child is not having a wave of pressure at the time of the examination, he or she may appear perfectly normal, and even with a wave of high pressure there may be nothing to identify other than the pain of the headache, which is of course subjective to the patient.

The examination may reveal papilledema, but as mentioned earlier, the absence of papilledema does not rule out intracranial hypertension of a life-threatening degree. Decreased level of consciousness either accompanying the headache or continuously may occur as may a stiff neck due to tonsillar herniation, cranial nerve VI palsy due to diffuse ICP, or more rarely a cranial nerve III palsy. Visual acuity may be decreased as a result of chronic papilledema or optic atrophy. Changes in vital signs, such as bradycardia and hypertension, may occur but are often late manifestations, occurring at the time of brain stem decompensation, and cannot be relied upon as early indicators of increased ICP. Ventricular enlargement, as evidenced by CT imaging, can confirm the diagnosis of hydrocephalus.

When ICP elevation is suspected, it is preferable to avoid sedation in spontaneously breathing patients. If sedation is needed, it is best to give the minimum amount required and to recognize that sedation often leads to decreased ventilation, increased arterial partial pressure of carbon dioxide ($PaCO_2$), and further increased ICP. A plan to treat both hypoventilation (i.e., intubation or mask ventilation) and ICP should be in place before administering sedation. When hydrocephalus is present, urgent therapy is sometimes required to treat the increased ICP. Therapy ranges from acute administration of corticosteroids in those patients with a tumor and vasogenic edema, to ventriculostomy or an emergency shunt procedure in those with pathology unlikely to respond to steroids. In patients without a tumor or preexisting shunt, and in whom an acute or chronic CNS infectious process is not suspected, the ideal treatment is insertion of a shunt as an emergency procedure.

In children with a preexisting shunt, a radiographic shunt survey to evaluate the intactness and position of the shunt system is necessary in addition to the scan. If there is question about a shunt block, the shunt system can be tapped and the site of block identified as proximal or distal to the shunt reservoir. In children with the slit ventricle syndrome, when very little fluid is present in the ventricle and the ability to remove fluid is therefore limited, it is often better to test the proximal catheter by back-injecting contrast medium into the ventricle to establish the patency of the proximal shunt catheter. The distal end of the shunt can be checked by measuring the runoff pressure with a manometer. When the shunt is blocked proximal to the valve system such that CSF cannot be withdrawn, it is safer to revise the shunt immediately rather than to wait until the next day. If the shunt is blocked distal to the valve, adequate ventricular decompression can be attained by tapping the reservoir and removing CSF. In this setting, the shunt revision may be postponed until the next convenient opening in the operating schedule, and diamox and dexamethasone may be used to slow CSF production during the waiting period. Severe headaches need to be treated by further fluid withdrawal from the shunt and not treated with narcotics; if headaches persist, shunt revision is urgently required (109–111).

INFECTION

☞ **The most frequent setting in which an infectious process requires emergency neurosurgery is that of a brain abscess (111,112). The presentation is either with focal neurologic deficit or the signs of intracranial hypertension.** ☞ The aims of therapy are: (*i*) to obtain a specimen for culture and (*ii*) to evacuate any intracranial mass. CT scan usually identifies the lesion, and the therapy is increasingly often stereotactic drainage with or without leaving a catheter in situ for further drainage. It is rare that an attempt at abscess removal is performed as the primary procedure, unless the abscess is very large and superficially located in the brain. Even then, because of the surrounding edema, it

is generally preferable simply to drain the lesion, treat with antibiotics, and monitor with serial neuroimaging. Indeed, in many cases, craniotomy is never necessary and the abscess can be treated simply by antibiotics with or without repeated needle drainage.

The antibiotic selection depends upon the likely organisms (Volume 2, Chapter 53). For staphylococcus coverage, oxacillin is the first drug of choice unless the organism is methicillin-resistant, in which case vancomycin is used. Daptomycin or linazolid is used for vancomycin-resistant organisms. Ceftriaxone has excellent CSF penetration and is effective against most methicillin-sensitive gram-positive organisms. It also has activity against all gram-negative bacteria except for pseudomonas. If pseudomonas is present or suspected, ceftriaxone should be replaced by ceftazadime along with an aminoglycoside (e.g., amikacin). Metronidazole has excellent brain tissue penetration and is the drug of choice for anaerobic brain abscess. For fungal infections, seek infectious disease consultation and review Volume 2, Chapter 53.

Subdural and Epidural Empyema

Epidural empyema usually occurs with either severe air sinus infections or osteomyelitis of the skull (113). The mass effect is usually small, and acute drainage is only rarely necessary. In the frontal area, drainage of the frontal sinus often results in drainage of the epidural abscess.

Subdural empyema is a more catastrophic situation, with underlying pial and often cerebral inflammation, septic thrombophlebitis, and brain edema. In the past, this was always treated by urgent craniotomy and aspiration of the pus (114). Currently, with earlier diagnosis as a result of CT scan, burr hole aspiration for culture and immediate relief of mass effect is often all that is required, followed by antibiotics and corticosteroids. In children, the subdural empyema commonly recurs at different locations and may require repeated surgery, which may require extensive craniotomy if resolution is not achieved by medical management. Small lesions may require no surgery.

Meningitis

Bacterial meningitis is a medical emergency requiring antibiotic treatment. Because of vaccination programs, *Haemophilus influenzae* is less commonly seen in children. Currently, most common bacterial organisms carrying meningitis in children are *Meningococcus* and *Pneumococcus*, which can be treated with high-dose penicillin (115,116). Bacterial meningitis rarely requires acute neurosurgical management. However, acute hydrocephalus can occur with bacterial meningitis, and emergent placement of a ventricular drainage device may be necessary. This is most often the case in tuberculous meningitis but does also occur with the more common infectious organisms.

Shunt Infection

Most shunt infections do not require emergent shunt removal; rather they are treated by shunt culture and appropriate antibiotics. In children with an acute abdomen as a result of the shunt infection, emergency exteriorization of the abdominal end of the shunt may be required. Most commonly, the infecting organism is *Staphylococcus*, in which case the shunt will require elective removal and replacement. With other organisms, the shunt can often be saved (117).

NEOPLASMS

In only a few cases do pediatric brain tumors become neurosurgical catastrophes, but these must be rapidly identified and treated. These children are usually admitted with a history of headache, nausea, and vomiting, and are at risk of herniation while awaiting workup for a suspected gastrointestinal lesion. Others are admitted after a lesion is identified on CT or MRI scan, but the symptoms of increased ICP may be subtle, or initially ignored, resulting in clinical herniation and death. The problem is exactly as described in children with hydrocephalus, in whom autoregulation of CBF is intact and very high pressures can be tolerated without apparent clinical signs. Posterior fossa tumors often present this way when associated with hydrocephalus.

In 5% to 10% of cases of pediatric brain tumor, hemorrhage occurs into the tumor, producing acute deterioration that is no different from that related to other types of intracranial hemorrhage (118). Tumors in the supratentorial compartment are usually easier to diagnose because of accompanying local signs (e.g., hemiparesis, visual field defect) (Fig. 7). Rarely is an emergency operation necessary, but in the presence of progressive herniation, repeated ICP spikes and/or unconsciousness, rapid surgical debulking may be required. As noted previously, ventricular drainage in the presence of a large posterior fossa tumor can result in upward herniation; thus, resection of the tumor may be required at the time of insertion of the ventricular drain. In patients with less acute symptoms, corticosteroids usually bring about rapid clinical improvement, permitting surgery to be performed electively.

𝕠⚹ **Another presentation of tumor that requires emergency surgery is the rapid progression of visual loss.** 𝕠⚹ This may be due to local compression of the optic nerves, chiasm, or tracts by tumor, and can occur as a result of hemorrhage into such tumors as optic gliomas or pituitary tumors or can result simply from a tumor mass expansion, as in craniopharyngioma or meningioma. Such rapid visual loss that is the result of local compression is an indication for emergency surgical decompression. The other setting in which rapid visual loss can occur is the result of papilledema. In this setting, ventricular drainage or shunting plus steroids is usually chosen over emergency tumor resection in an effort to lower the ICP gradually and prevent the acute blindness that can occasionally occur after posterior fossa decompression. Rarely in children do tumors erode into adjacent structures, but epistaxis or bleeding from the ear occasionally is the first manifestation of a large skull base tumor. Although these rarely require acute neurosurgical intervention, if bleeding is severe or hard to control, CT or MRI scan may be necessary to make the diagnosis and acute embolization or vein ligation may be necessary to attain hemostasis.

SPINE

Spina Bifida

Spina bifida is derived from Latin, meaning "split spine." Spina bifida is a type of neural tube defect (NTD), which results in incomplete closure of one or more vertebral arches of the spine, and is often associated with malformation and/or malfunction of the spinal cord in the region of the lesion. Neurolation is the process whereby the neural plate is formed, and then closed dorsally to become the neural tube. Failure of this process results in an open NTD (119).

In the majority of cases, spina bifida is an isolated birth defect and can be minimized by the administration of folic acid 0.4 mg/day before conception and during the first three months of pregnancy. Alpha-fetoprotein (AFP) screening during the first 15 to 20 weeks of pregnancy can help identify mothers at risk for spina bifida, anencephaly, trisomy 21, and other anomalies.

Spina bifida occurs most commonly in the lumbar and sacral regions, and presents in the three major subtypes: oculta, cystica (myelomeningocele), and meningocele. Spina bifida oculta is the mildest form and does not require early surgical treatment. The skin completely covers the defect, and the spine can appear normal or have a tuft of hairs growing from it. There may or may not be a dimple over the defect. The posterior split in the vertebral arch is usually so small that the spinal cord does not protrude. However, mild sacral symptoms such as incontinence and some gait abnormalities are common.

Spina bifida cystica (myelomeningocele) is the most serious form. Failure of closure of the skin, muscle, bone, and spinal cord constitutes a myelomeningocele. These can occur at any level of the spinal canal but are most frequent in the lumbar area. These lesions frequently have disruption of the thin covering of arachnoid over the placode and leak CSF. There is no real emergency about closing these lesions, but in most pediatric neurosurgical centers they are closed within 24 to 48 hours after birth, assuming the neonate is otherwise stable (120). If closure is to be delayed more than a few hours, the lesions are covered with sterile saline-soaked sponges, and broad-spectrum antibiotics are begun.

𝕠⚹ **Closure of the open spinal NTD is undertaken within the first few days of life, in order to cease the leakage of CSF and cover the spinal cord with an intact epithelial barrier.** 𝕠⚹ If a marked kyphotic deformity is present,

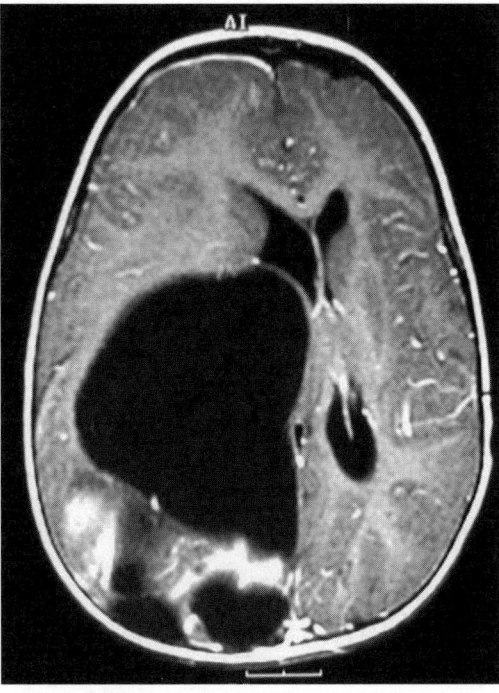

Figure 7 Magnetic resonance image with contrast revealing right parieto-occipital cystic mass/tumor with heterogeneous enhancing areas. Note significant mass effect and right-to-left midline shift.

this can be corrected at the time of closure with resection of one or more of the normal vertebral bodies. A CSF-diverting shunt may be placed concomitantly if hydrocephalus is already obvious. CNS deformities with the closed NTD are limited to the spinal cord and not associated with the Chiari II malformation and hydrocephalus. The prognosis for an infant at birth with a closed form of NTD is vastly better than one with an open NTD (121).

Meningoceles appear in 5% or less of open NTDs. Because meningoceles do not have exposed neural tissue and do not leak CSF, they can be closed electively. As the child grows, the neurologic deficit often progresses in an asymmetric fashion in lipomatous malformations, and operative intervention is advocated early in infancy to ameliorate further loss of neurologic function.

Congenital dermal sinuses are squamous epithelial lined tracts that occur in or very near the midline. These frequently go unnoticed until the patient presents with meningitis or an extra- or intradural abscess. *Staphylococcus aureus* is the most common infecting organism, although gram-negative bacteria are more frequently found in abscesses located at the low spinal region. Urgent operative intervention is required to drain these abscesses. If meningitis is present, surgical intervention should be briefly delayed until the patient receives a course of appropriate antibiotic therapy. It is often advisable to limit the procedure to drainage of purulent material, delaying the removal of the remaining tract or cyst capsule until the inflammation has subsided.

Diastematomyelia is a term used to describe the malformation in which the spinal cord is split into two hemicords. Neurologic abnormalities are similar to those found with lipomatous malformations. Treatment consists of an elective laminectomy at least one level above and below the area of deformity. Neuroenteric cysts may or may not be associated with other forms of closed NTD such as split cord malformations. The cysts slowly enlarge by the secretion of mucinous material, which leads to compression of the adjacent neural structures. The surgical approach is individualized, depending upon the extent of the associated malformations.

Arachnoid cysts may have either an intra- or extradural location, and the pathophysiology, clinical findings, and management are similar. The dominant symptom noted with arachnoid cysts of the thoracic region is progressive lower extremity weakness, often symmetrical, which can occasionally result in paralysis if not treated. MR is the initial imaging modality of choice. Treatment of symptomatic arachnoid cysts is surgical, because aspiration would provide only temporary relief. The prognosis for patients with these cysts is excellent and recovery dramatic if surgical treatment occurs before irreversible spinal cord damage has occurred.

Vascular Malformations

Vascular malformations of the spine are aneurysmal, arterial, arteriovenous, or venous, with the arteriovenous form being the most common (122). Spinal AVMs in children are difficult to treat surgically without causing additional damage to the spinal cord. The incidence of hemorrhage is over 50% in children, as opposed to only 10% in adults. Emergent decompression is indicated following hemorrhagic rupture.

Spine Neoplasms

It is exceedingly rare for intramedullary neoplasms of the spinal cord to be symptomatic at birth. In Von Hippel-Lindau disease (autosomal dominant neurocutaneous syndrome with variable penetrance), hemangioblastomas are found in the cerebellum, spinal cord, and medulla in decreasing order of frequency. Neurofibromatosis is associated with increased incidence of tumors of the entire nervous system and its coverings, including intramedullary spinal cord neoplasms (123). Intramedullary spinal cord metastases have also been found.

Intramedullary lipomas of the spinal cord are very rare congenital lesions that may first become manifest during rapid growth or excessive weight gain. If symptomatic, they can be surgically debulked; total removal is unnecessary and possibly hazardous (124).

In children, the most common extramedullary tumor is the result of seeding of the subarachnoid space from an intracranial neoplasm (such as primitive neuroectodermal tumor), which on occasion can be present at birth. Sometimes the spinal cord compression from subarachnoid seeding is the first manifestation of an intracranial tumor. Nerve sheath tumors and meningiomas are infrequently found in childhood. In children, the intra- and extradural (dumbbell) extension of a tumor is pathognomonic of a neurofibroma (125). Deformity of the spine may be the first manifestation of a neurofibroma but abnormal curvature in the spine in the absence of tumor is also common in neurofibromatosis. The diagnostic imaging modality of choice for spine tumors is MR, supplemented by CT and CT myelography if necessary. If an extramedullary tumor of the thoracic spinal cord is present, imaging of the entire CNS is advisable as multiple tumors are frequently found. Treatment is surgical removal of the tumor.

Neuroblastoma is the most common intra-abdominal malignancy of childhood. It may be manifest at birth with thoracic spinal cord compression secondary to extension of the tumor through neural foramina into the epidural space (126). Treatment is laminectomy for spinal cord decompression.

Failure of formation and segmentation of the vertebrae early in development can lead to clinical deformities that have neurologic sequelae. Spinal cord compression is most often seen in structural defects that produce kyphosis, as dorsal angulation of the spine is most likely to compromise the spinal canal (127).

Embryologic segmental maldevelopment can lead to hypoplastic or absent thoracic or lumbar vertebrae (128). The nerve roots adjacent to the bony deformity are either dysplastic or lacking in a condition referred to as segmental spinal dysgenesis. The neurologic deficit distal to the segmental dysgenesis can be partial or complete. The lower extremities are often deformed. The loss of neurologic function, if present, can occur secondary to rapidly increasing kyphosis from an unstable spine. Decompressive laminectomy in this situation would add to the lack of spinal stability. Thus, an anterior approach is advisable if necessary to decompress the spinal cord and stabilize the spinal column.

In achondroplasia, spinal cord compression can occur with development and growth. With aging, the stenosis can be further exacerbated by osteoarthritic spurs, disk degeneration, and kyphosis (129).

A severe form of kyphoscoliosis in the cervical and thoracic region is commonly seen in neurofibromatosis, regardless of the presence or absence of a neurofibroma. Such marked deformities, unless aggressively treated, can lead to paralysis secondary to spinal cord compression (130).

MISCELLANEOUS
Craniofacial Anomalies

Anomalies of the craniofacial skeleton can result in gruesome facial appearances including those involving amniotic band syndromes, facial clefts, cloverleaf skull appearance, and congenital absence of the nose or eyes. Children with severe Crouzon's, Apert's, or Pfeiffer's syndromes also appear dramatically abnormal, and a correct initial diagnosis often is not made. Despite their appearance, few of these children require emergency neurosurgery. The most common acute problem involves the airway, because choanal atresia or marked hypoplasia of the midface may interfere with ventilation (131). Endotracheal intubation can be very difficult, and a tracheostomy may occasionally be required to save a child's life. The globes of the eyes occasionally are completely dislocated out of the orbit, with closure of the lids posterior to the globe. This results in exposure and ischemia and requires treatment, first with lubricant and plastic wrap to keep the conjunctiva moist. Rarely is tarsorraphy adequate because of the degree of exorbitism, and early surgery with supraorbital rim advancement and tarsorraphy is occasionally the only way to obtain some coverage for the eyes. In general, craniofacial surgery for children with severe anomalies is delayed until after four months of age unless they show evidence of intracranial hypertension. It is almost impossible to correct any aspect of the facial anomaly before four months, even in the upper orbital area.

Encephaloceles

Encephaloceles occur at a rate of 1:10,000 live births in North America, and about 70% occur in the posterior region of the cranium and are either supratentorial or infratentorial (132). Despite presenting with a dramatic external appearance, most encephaloceles are not surgical emergencies. However, those with incomplete skin coverage, leaking CSF, or displaying visible brain tissue do require urgent closure (i.e., within 24 hours), provided the general condition of the neonate is otherwise stable. The exposed lesion is covered with sterile saline-soaked sponges, and broad-spectrum antibiotics are begun. CT or MRI scan or both are required to define the anatomy of the encephalocele and the intracranial brain.

Prognosis is best correlated with the size and anatomic appearance of the residual intracranial brain rather than with the size of the encephalocele. The herniated cerebral tissue is not normal and no effort is made to replace it within the cranial cavity; the abnormal tissue is removed, sparing the intracranial vasculature, and the dura closed. Hydrocephalus is common but usually does not need therapy in the first few days. With severe hydrocephalus, it is preferable to insert a shunt and decompress the brain before performing a definitive operation on the encephalocele. Anterior encephaloceles (in the nose or mouth), often in association with a cleft palate, can produce acute airway obstruction and feeding problems that require tracheostomy for emergency management of the airway. In such cases, it is advisable to postpone definitive surgery for as long as several months if possible to make the surgery safer.

Aplasia Cutis Congenita

Aplasia cutis congenita is an area of the skull where bone and skin fail to form, leaving exposed and occasionally slightly herniating dura, most commonly in the midline, associated with a suture or venous sinus. This is not an encephalocele and, because the dura is intact, often can be treated conservatively until a child is older, at which time surgery to rotate skin over the lesion is usually undertaken. Smaller lesions can be treated by immediate surgical closure of the skin.

Teratomas and Choristomas

Teratomas and choristomas are rare lesions, but they can present at birth as an emergency because of airway obstruction or feeding problems. The most common location is in the tongue or facies. These lesions are usually small at birth and grow rapidly in the first few days of life, yet they are rarely malignant. Tracheostomy and a feeding tube are often requited during the early life-threatening phase. Those that come to neurosurgical attention usually involve the intracranial space and exit from the cranium through the cranial nerve foramina, most frequently the trigeminal or superior or inferior orbital fissures, and present in the mouth and neck. These lesions can usually be completely removed in a single operation in the first few months of life, with cure of the lesions. It is unclear whether these should be categorized as congenital or neoplastic lesions, and in some cases true tumors are found.

PEDIATRIC INTENSIVE CARE UNIT COMPLICATIONS FOLLOWING CENTRAL NERVOUS SYSTEM TRAUMA
Hypotension

Marked worsening in outcome after TBI is associated with hypotension (133). The adverse effect of hypotension in head-injured children is as great as in head-injured adults. Children, in whom hypotension is present upon admission to the emergency department, suffer significantly higher mortality rates compared to those in children who are normotensive at the time of admission. The mechanism of the adverse effect of hypotension on outcome is thought to be decreased CPP (134,135).

Acute Lung Injury

Bratton and Davis used the Traumatic Coma Data Bank to study the incidence and negative prognostic sign of acute lung injury after isolated head trauma (136). Of the 100 patients in the study, the 20 who developed acute lung injury, most commonly in the form of neurogenic pulmonary edema, had more severe global brain injury: lower GCS scores, more frequent episodes of intracranial hypertension, and more ominous findings on the initial CT scan, and were almost three times more likely to die or survive in a persistent vegetative state.

Neuroinflammation

⚿ **There exists a neuroinflammatory response to TBI (137). This phenomenon contributes to the secondary injury that, along with the primary or biomechanical injury, is a major determinant of outcome.** ⚿ Whalen (138) noted elevated levels of interleukin-8 (IL-8) in the CSF of children in the first four to five days after head injury, which correlated directly with mortality. IL-8 might thus be a useful prognostic indicator of outcome in head-injured children.

Hypopituitarism

Hypopituitarism as a sequela of head trauma was first described by Escamilla and Lisser more than 50 years ago (139). Benvenga (140) reviewed a total of 367 cases of post head trauma hypopituitarism (PHTH) and pointed out that: (*i*) the head trauma could have been minor; (*ii*) the head trauma could have occurred several years before the onset of the hypopituitarism; and (*iii*) the patient could have forgotten about the head injury.

The epidemiology of PHTH indicates that the male-to-female ratio is five to one. In about 60% of cases, the head trauma had occurred when the patient was between the ages of 11 and 29. Although the majority of patients developed PHTH within one year after the trauma, 15% of patients were diagnosed five years or more after the accident.

EYE TO THE FUTURE

The horizon for pediatric neurosurgery is intertwined with the continual evolution of molecular biology, critical care medicine, and neuroimaging. Advances have been implemented such as neuroendoscopy and hyperosmolar therapy, and the future for molecular therapies remains promising.

Molecular Therapies

Historically, neoplasms such as medulloblastomas and other embroynal tumors have been classified by location, histology, and extent of surgical resection. More recently, molecular biologic studies have led to a new understanding of cell signaling pathways that promote tumor growth. Research continues to develop brain tumor therapies based on molecules that target growth factor receptors or downstream effectors. Also, molecular markers are being studied to validate outcome predictors and to stratify patients in standard and high-risk groups for clinical trials (141).

Whereas some cell damage occurs at the time of the traumatic event, much of the damage occurs between minutes and days after injury. This delayed injury process, known as secondary injury, is mediated by injury factors that, if identified, could be treated with "antifactors" that could prevent or at least attenuate the secondary injury process.

Four key mechanistic causes are associated with secondary damage from TBI. These include: (*i*) ischemic excitotoxicity, (*ii*) neuronal death cascades, (*iii*) cerebral swelling, and (*iv*) inflammation. Therapies have been aimed at all of these mechanisms.

Hypothermia

The therapeutic use of hypothermia in a patient with TBI was first described by Fay in 1943 (142). Because of the dearth of comparative studies during subsequent years, its therapeutic efficacy remained unestablished (143–145) despite the associated neuroprotection. Hypothermia can be utilized for neuroprotection. For every degree celsius (°C) decrease in body temperature, there is a 7% decrease in cerebral metabolic rate for oxygen ($CMRO_2$) (146). Moderate hypothermia to 32°C or 33°C for 24 hours, initiated soon after severe traumatic brain injury, significantly improved the outcome and decreased tissue injury in rats (147,148). However, moderate hypothermia for 24 hours following TBI in humans did not improve outcomes (149).

The specific putative beneficial effects of hypothermia include the reduction of cerebral ischemia, edema, and tissue injury, and the preservation of the blood-brain barrier (150). Hypothermia may mitigate secondary brain injury by suppressing the post-traumatic inflammatory response and by reducing the extracellular concentrations of excitatory neurotransmitters, particularly glutamate. Thus far, there are no studies documenting the routine use of hypothermia in the management of pediatric patients with head injury; however, a recent paper suggests that it is likely a safe therapeutic intervention for children after severe TBI up to 24 hours after injury. Although laboratory experimental research has shown beneficial effects of hypothermia in TBI, studies in humans (meta-analysis) have yielded conflicting results with respect to the risk of death and poor neurologic outcome (151–156). Part of the conflict arises from the fact that most studies have different speeds of induction of hypothermia. Neuroprotective measures may have limited time to be effective. The duration of hypothermia and the rate of rewarming, with the potential deleterious effects on ICP, were all different (149,151–159). Further studies are necessary and warranted to determine its effect on functional outcome and intracranial hypertension (160).

Hypertonic Saline

In pediatric patients, clinical experience with the use of hypertonic saline is still limited compared to use in adults. Hypertonic saline has been found to be helpful in the management of severe TBI in infants and children (161). Hypertonic saline decreases ICP by mechanisms similar to other hyperosmotic agents. Sodium has a low penetration of the blood-brain barrier. Saline restores normal cellular resting potential, cell volume, may inhibit inflammation, and lowers ICP. Hypertonic saline may have beneficial effects on excitatory neurotransmitters and the immune system (162,163). The major disadvantages of hypertonic saline include hypernatremia with consequent cellular dehydration and the development of central pontine myelinolysis and intracranial hemorrhage (164–170). Currently studies evaluating long-term neurologic outcome and the possible role of even more aggressive hyperosmolar therapy are needed (171). These studies should consider initiation of hypertonic saline as soon as feasibly possible, including the prehospital period (172).

New Intracranial Pressure Monitoring and Cerebrospinal Fluid Draining Techniques

Hydrocephalus treatment received great advancement with the application of endoscopic third ventriculostomy. Used in hydrocephalus where the point of obstruction is below the third ventricle (aqueduct and/or fouth ventricle), third ventriculostomy has obviated the need for ventricular shunting for certain etiologies and decreased the drainage dependence on shunts for other etiologies of hydrocephalus. Studies evaluating its efficacy in hydrocephalus from infection, hemorrhage, and other causes are currently under way. Given the many complications with shunting children, the role of third ventriculostomy will surely expand (173).

Magnesium Therapy

Work by McIntosh (1993) (174) revealed that a large number of intracellular metabolic processes implicated in TBI are regulated by magnesium (Mg^{2+}). These include energy metabolism, membrane stability, calcium-channel function, as well as protein and DNA synthesis (175,176). At the extracellular level, the ability of Mg^{2+} to block the *N*-methyl-D-aspartate channel is recognized as neuroprotective (177).

Several researchers have documented that TBI causes a reduction in the brain intracellular free Mg^{++} levels and that this is correlated with functional outcome (178). The possible beneficial role of Mg^{++} has been documented in a recent study that demonstrated a reduction in post-traumatic lesion size after treatment with Mg^{++} (179).

Magnesium therapy has been shown to reduce infarct size and volume, inhibit neuronal death, and attenuate motor impairment. Deficiencies in Mg^{++} can increase substance P release and induce a proinflammatory response. The proinflammatory responses accompanying TBI are also associated with a decrease in intracellular brain Mg^{++}. In animal studies, acute treatment with $MgSO_4$ attenuated the long-term hippocampal tissue loss after TBI, but did not affect the animal's learning (180–183). Although Mg^{++} has a tremendous beneficial potential in the treatment of TBI, it has not yet been studied in large randomized control trials in children.

SUMMARY

Severe head injuries are generally classified as a GCS score <8. By definition, a serious head injury is one in which the patient has a GCS score of 10 or less. A decrease in the GCS score by 3 following the initial examination, pupillary inequality greater than 1 mm, lateralized extremity weakness, a markedly depressed skull fracture, or an open fracture with evident brain or CSF leakage will require head CT scan. Approximately 50% of these patients will have an expanding intracranial clot and there is an overall 41% mortality, 26% good recovery, 16% moderate disability, and severe disability/vegetative state in 17%.

The usefulness of skull X rays was evaluated in a prospective study of 7035 patients with closed head injury. Patients with high risk for intracranial injury included those with a progressive decline or depression in level of consciousness, focal neurologic deficit, progressive headache and/or identified penetrating or depressed fracture. All were admitted for close in-house observation and underwent a CT of the head. Skull films were only helpful if penetrating injury was present.

The level of consciousness and arousability of the child is a key variable in assessing potential increases in ICP. The immediate examination includes the GCS score, pupillary, and motor function. All examinations should be performed promptly and sequentially with a final examination prior to discharge or admission. The contribution of intoxicants and hypotension must also be addressed. Clinical evidence of a basilar skull fracture includes CSF rhinorrhea or otorrhea, hemotympanum, blood in the external auditory meatus, subconjunctival hemorrhage, raccoon eyes, or a Battle's sign.

Pitfalls in the evaluation of patients following head injury include alternative causes for a blown pupil including direct ocular injury, vitreous hemorrhage, vitreal-retinal injury, and injury to the optic nerve. Monoparesis can result from brachial plexus injury and/or fracture. In addition, subgaleal hematomas can frequently mimic skull fractures on palpation. On examining children, evidence of a subhyaloid hemorrhage or full fontanel is usually assessed. The presence of a ventriculoperitoneal shunt and the potential for abuse are additional considerations that can modify the management of these children. As rules of thumb, all unconscious patients, all temporal skull fractures, all depressed and basilar fractures, and all serious head injuries undergo CT scanning. In multisystem trauma, low systemic blood pressure signifies depletion of blood volume until proven otherwise.

Once an injury has occurred, survival and good recovery mandate adequate initial assessment of the pediatric patient in the field with cardiovascular and mechanical stabilization, airway control, and either intravenous or intraosseous access for fluid resuscitation.

Innovative research efforts, aggressive injury prevention schemes focusing on the design of appropriately sized automotive and sports safety equipment (e.g., seatbelts, helmets), and intensified education of parents and caretakers in schools and playgrounds on the prevention of accidents and child abuse will all contribute to the reduction of head injuries in children.

KEY POINTS

- In an infant with an open fontanel and open cranial sutures, small increases in the volume of intradural contents can be accommodated by separation of the sutures and distention of the fontanel.
- In children, hemiparesis occurs on the side ipsilateral to the herniation 50% of the time, whereas in adults hemiparesis occurs ipsilateral to the herniation 75% of the time.
- Unfortunately, the status of autoregulation is not known in the clinical setting, and thus therapy is directed at maintaining normal or nearly normal ICP and MAP in the hope that this will preserve CBF.
- After pediatric head trauma, acute loss of consciousness is less commonly the result of increased ICP unlike in adults. Accordingly, there is no indication for routinely administering an osmotic diuretic to children in coma after head trauma.
- A reliable and reproducible neurologic examination is much more important than any number or value from an ICP monitor or ventriculostomy catheter.
- Lesions that may require immediate surgery are the intracranial hematomas, compound depressed skull fractures, and penetrating trauma.
- It is recommended that, because clinical criteria and skull X rays are poor predictors of intracranial hemorrhage, all children with a GCS score of 13 or 14 routinely have a screening noncontrast-enhanced CT scan.
- Most forms of penetrating cranial injury (PCI) require surgical exploration.
- The typical angiographic picture of trauma-induced occlusion of the cervical internal carotid artery is abrupt blockage of contrast flow approximately 1–3 cm above the bifurcation of the common carotid artery in the neck.
- Patients with fluctuating neurologic symptoms in the face of an acutely occluded internal carotid artery may benefit from urgent exploration and thromboendarterectomy.
- The most common intracranial arterial structure to be occluded in blunt head injury is the internal carotid artery.
- The most common mode of presentation of traumatic aneurysm in symptomatic patients is that of delayed SAH following a head injury.
- Early high-output cardiac failure in neonates can occur with vascular shunting lesions in the cranium.

✔ The diagnosis of shunt malfunction or acute intracranial hypertension due to hydrocephalus is essentially based on the history and often confirmed by a neuroimaging study (CT or MRI), that shows ventricular dilatation.

✔ The most frequent setting in which an infectious process requires emergency neurosurgery is that of a brain abscess (111,112). The presentation is either with focal neurologic deficit or the signs of intracranial hypertension.

✔ Another presentation of tumor that requires emergency surgery is the rapid progression of visual loss.

✔ Closure of the open spinal NTD is undertaken within the first few days of life, in order to cease the leakage of CSF and cover the spinal cord with an intact epithelial barrier.

✔ There exists a neuroinflammatory response to TBI (137). This phenomenon contributes to the secondary injury that, along with the primary or biomechanical injury, is a major determinant of outcome.

REFERENCES

1. Garton HJ, Piatt JH. Hydrocephalus: Pediatr Clin North Am 2004; 113(5):1375–1381.
2. Bruce DA. Pathophysiology of intracranial pressure. In: Asbury AK, McKhann GM, McDonald WI, eds. Diseases of the Nervous System. Vol. 2. Philadelphia: W.B. Saunders, 1986:1044–1062.
3. Rekate HL. Head injuries: management of primary injuries and prevention of secondary damage. A consensus conference on pediatric neurosurgery. Childs Nerv Syst 2001; 17(10):632–634.
4. Forbes ML, Kochanek PM, Adelson PD. Severe traumatic brain injury in children: critical care management. In: Albright AL, Pollack IF, Adelson PD, eds. Principles and Practice of Pediatric Neurosurgery. New York: Thieme, 1999:861–878.
5. Crawley-Coha T. Childhood injury: a status report. J Pediatr Nurs 2001; 16(5):371–374.
6. Guyer B, Ellers B. Childhood injuries in the United States: mortality, morbidity and cost. Am J Dis Child 1990; 144:649–562.
7. Dias MS. Traumatic brain and spinal cord injury. Pediatr Clin North Am 2004; 51(2):271–303.
8. Schmidt U, Frame SB, Nerlich ML, et al. On scene helicopter transport of patients with multiple injuries: comparison of a German and American system. J Trauma 1992; 33:548–555.
9. Feickert H-J, Drommer S, Heyer R. Severe head injury in children: Impact of risk factors on outcome. J Trauma 1999; 47(1):33–38.
10. Davis RJ, Fan Tait W, Dean JM, et al. Head and spinal cord injury. In: Rogers MC, ed. Text-Book of Pediatric Intensive Care. 2nd ed. Baltimore: Williams & Wilkins, 1992:805–857.
11. Aldelson PD, Kochanek PM. Head injury in children. J Child Neurol 1998; 13:2–15.
12. Diamond PT. Brain injury in the commonwealth of Virginia: an analysis of central registry data 1988–1993. Brain Injury 1996; 10:413–419.
13. Di Maio DJ, Di Maio VS. Forensic Pathology. 2nd ed. Boca Raton, FL: CRC Press, 1993:304.
14. Pierce MC, Bertocci GE, Berger R, et al. Injury biomechanics for aiding in the diagnosis of abusive head trauma. Neurosurg Clin N Am 2002; 13(2):155–168.
15. Baker SP, O'Neill B, Ginsberg MJ, et al. The Injury Fact Book. New York, NY: Oxford University Press, 1992:139.
16. Plunkett J. Fatal pediatric head injuries caused by short distance falls. Am J Forensic Med Pathol 2001; 22:1–12.
17. Reiber GD. Fatal falls in childhood. Am J Forensic Med Pathol 1993; 14:201–207.
18. Claydon SM. Fatal extradural hemorrhage following a fall from a baby bouncer. Pediatr Emerg Care 1996; 12:432–434.
19. Pillai S, Bethel CAI, Besner GE, et al. Fall injuries in the pediatric population: Safer and most cost-effective management. J Trauma 2000; 48(6):1048–1051.
20. Murray JA, Chen D, Velmahos GC, et al. Pediatric falls: is height a predictor of injury and outcome? Am Surg 2000; 66(9):863–865.
21. Musemache CA, Barthel M, Consentino C, et al. Pediatric falls from heights. J Trauma 1991; 31:1347–1349.
22. Williams RA. Injuries in infants and small children resulting from witnessed and corroborated free falls. J Trauma 1991; 31:1350–1352.
23. Chadwick DL, Chin S, Salerno C, et al. Death from falls in children: how far is fatal? J Trauma 1991; 31:1353–1355.
24. Gruskin K, Schutzman S. Head trauma in children younger than 2 years: Are there predictors for complications? Arch Pediatr Adolesc Med 1999; 153(1):15–20.
25. Ross SP, Cetta F. Are skull radiographs useful in the evaluation of asymptomatic infants following minor head injury? Pediatr Emerg Care 1992; 8:328–330.
26. Greenes DS, Schutzman SA. Infants with isolated skull fracture: what are their clinical characteristics, and do they require hospitalization? Ann Emerg Med 1997; 30:253–259.
27. DiGuiseppi CG, Rivera FP, Koepsell TD, et al. Bicycle helmet use by children: evaluation of a community-wide helmet campaign. JAMA 1989; 262:2256–2261.
28. Centers for disease control. Fatal injuries to children—United States. JAMA 1990; 264:952–953.
29. Luerssen TG. Head injuries in children. Neurosurg Clin N Am 1991; 2:399–410.
30. Maggi G, Aliberti F, Petrone G, et al. Extradural hematomas in children. J Neurosurg Sci 1998; 42:95–99.
31. Puranik S, Long J, Coffman S. Profile of pediatric bicycle injuries. South Med J 1998; 91:1033–1037.
32. Thompson RS, Rivara FP, Thompson DC. A case control study of the effectiveness of bicycle safety helmets. N Eng J Med 1989; 320:1362–1367.
33. DiGuiseppi CG, Rivara FP, Koepsell TD. Attitudes towards bicycle helmet ownership and use by school-age children. A J Dis Child 1990; 144:83–86.
34. Vulcan AP, Maxwell HC, Watson WL. Mandatory bicycle helmet use: experience in Victoria, Australia. World J Surg 1992; 16:389–397.
35. Thompson DC, Rivera FP, Thompson RS. Effectiveness of bicycle safety helmets in preventing head injuries: a case control study. JAMA 1996; 276:1968–1973.
36. Li G, Baker SP, Fowler C, et al. Factors related to the presence of head injury in bicycle-related pediatric trauma patients. J Trauma 1995; 38:871–875.
37. Cruz J, Minoja G, Mattioli C, et al. Severe acute brain trauma. In: Cruz J, ed. Neurologic and Neurosurgical Emergencies. Philadelphia: W.B. Saunders Co., 1998:405–436.
38. Weiss BD. Bycycle-related head injuries. Clin Sports Med 1994; 13(1):99–112.
39. Coffman S. Bicycle injuries and safety helmets in children. Orthop Nurs 2003; 22(1):9–15.
40. Depreitere B, Van Lierde C, Maene S, et al. Bicycle-related head injury: a study of 86 cases. Accid Anal Prev 2004; 36(4):649–654.
41. Margolis LH, Kotch J, Lacey JH. Children in alcohol-related motor vehicle crashes. Pediatrics 1986; 77:870–872.
42. McConnell EJ, Macbeth GA. Common carotid artery and tracheal injury from shoulder strap seat belt. Trauma 1997; 43(1):150–157.
43. Case M, Graham M, Handy TC, et al. Position paper on fatal abusive head injuries in infants and young children. Am J Forensic Med Pathol 2001; 22(2):112–122.
44. Osmond MH, Brennan-Barnes M, Shephard A. A 4-year review of severe pediatric trauma in Eastern Ontario: A descriptive analysis. J Trauma 2002; 52(1):8–12.
45. Vinchon M, Defoort-Dhellemmmes S, Desurmont M, et al. Accidental and nonaccidental head injuries in infants: a prospective study. J Neurosurg 2005; 102(4):380–384.

46. Wells RG, Vetter C, Laud P. Intracranial hemorrhage in children younger than 3 years: prediction on intent. Arch Pediatr Adolesc Med 2002; 156(3):252–257.

47. DiScala C, Sege R, Li G, et al. Child abuse and unintentional injuries: A 10 year prospective. Arch Pediatr Adolesc Med 2000; 154(1):16–22.

48. Duhaime AC, Christian CW, Rorke LB, et al. Current concepts: non-accidental head injury in infants—The "shaken-baby syndrome." N Eng J Med 1998; 338(25):1822–1829.

49. Wang MY, Griffith P, Tilton D, McComb JG, Levy M. 783 infant and child homicide from abuse in Los Angeles County. Neurosurgery 2000; 47(2):523.

50. Kempe CH, Silverman FN, Steele BF, et al. The battered-child syndrome. JAMA 1962; 181:17–24.

51. Caffey J. The whiplash shaken infant syndrome: manual shaking by the extremities with whiplash-induced intracranial and intraocular bleedings, linked with residual permanent brain damage and mental retardation. Pediatric 1974; 54:396–403.

52. Ommaya AK, Gennarelli TA. Cerebral concussion and traumatic unconsciousness: correlation of experimental and clinical observations on blunt head injuries. Brain 1974; 97:633–654.

53. Pierre-Kahn V, Roche O, Dureau P, et al. Opthalmologic findings in suspected child abuse victims with subdural hematomas. Ophthalmology 2003; 110(9):1718–1723.

54. Levine LM. Pediatric ocular trauma and shaken infant syndrome. Pediatr Clin North Am. 2003; 50(1):137–148.

55. Michael Y Wang, Pamela Griffith, Judy Sterling, Michael L Levy. A prospective population-based study of pediatric trauma patients with mild alterations in consciousness (Glasgow Coma Score of 13–14). Neurosurgery 2000; 46(5):1093–1099.

56. Ellis TS, Vezina LG, Donahue DJ. Acute identification of cranial burst fracture: Comparison between CT and MR imaging findings. Am J Neuroradiology 2000; 21:795–801.

57. Holmen CD, Sosnowski T, Latoszek KL, et al. Analysis of pre-hospital transport of head-injured patients after consolidation of neurosurgery resources. J Trauma 2002; 148(2):345–350.

58. Cooper A, DiScala C, Foltin G, et al. Prehospital endotracheal intubation for severe head injury in children: a reappraisal. Semin Pediatr Surg 2001; 10(1):3–6.

59. Kaufman HH. Civilian gunshot wounds to the head. Neurosurgery 1993; 32:962–964.

60. Ildan F, Bagdatoglu H, Boyar B, et al. The nonsurgical management of a penetrating orbitocranial injury reaching the brain stem. J Trauma 1994; 36:116–118.

61. Kasamo S, Asakura T, Kusumoto K, et al. Transorbital penetrating brain injury. No Shinkei Geka 1992; 20:433–438.

62. Oguz M, Aksungur EH, Altay M, et al. Orbitocranial penetration of a pencil: extraction under CT control. Euro J Radiology 1993; 17:85–87.

63. Al-Sebeih K, Karagiozov K, Jafar A. Penetrating craniofacial injury in a pediatric patient. J Craniofac Surg 2002; 13(2):303–307.

64. Domingo Z, Peter JC, De Villiers JC. Low-velocity penetrating craniocerebral injury in childhood. Pediatr Neurosurg 1994; 21:45–49.

65. LopezGonzalez A, Guiterrez Marin A, Alvarez Garijo JA, et al. Penetrating head injury in a pediatric patient caused by unusual object. Childs Nerv Syst 2005; 6:24–30.

66. Friedman D, Hammond J, Cardone J, et al. The air gun: toy or weapon? South Med J 1996; 89:475–478.

67. Medina M, Melcarne A, Ettorre F, et al. Clinical and neuroradiological correlations in a patient with a wandering retained air gun pellet in the brain. Surg Neurol 1992; 38:441–444.

68. Sotiropoulos SV, Jackson AJ, Tremblay GE, et al. Childhood lawn dart injuries. AJDC 1990; 144:980–982.

69. Kriel RL, Krach LE, Jones-Saeta C. Outcome of children with prolonged unconsciousness and vegetative states. Pediatr Neurol 1993; 9:362–368.

70. Haley SM, Graham RJ, Dumas HM. Outcome rating scales for pediatric head injury. J Intensive Care Med 2004; 19(4):205–219.

71. Kaufman HH, Levin HS, High WM Jr. Neurobehavioral outcome after gunshot wounds to the head in adult civilians and children. Neurosurgery 1985; 16:754–758.

72. Massagli TL, Jaffe KM, Fay GC, et al. Neurobehavioral sequelae of severe pediatric traumatic brain injury: a cohort study. Arch Phys Med Rehabil 1996; 77:223–231.

73. Jaffe KM, Polissar NL, Fay GC, et al. Recovery trends over three years following pediatric traumatic brain injury. Arch Phys Med Rehabil 1995; 76:17–26.

74. Corkin S, Rosen TJ, Sullivan EV, et al. Penetrating head injury in young adulthood exacerbates cognitive decline in later years. J Neurosci 1989; 9:3876–3883.

75. Koskiniemi M, Kyykka T, Nybo T, et al. Long-term outcome after severe brain injury in preschoolers is worse than expected. Arch Pediatr Adolesc Med 1995; 149:249–254.

76. George E, Dagi TF. Military penetrating craniocerebral injuries. Neurosurg Clin N Am 1995; 6:753–759.

77. Taha JM, Saba MI, Brown JA. Missile injuries to the brain treated by simple wound closure. Neurosurgery 1991; 29:380–383.

78. Singh P. Missile injuries of the brain: results of less aggressive surgery. Neuro India 2003; 51(2):215–219.

79. Zaidat O, Suarez JI. Intensive care management in the neurocritical care unit. In: Batjer HH, Loftus CM, eds. Textbook of Neurological Surgery: Principles and Practice. Philadelphia: Lippincott Williams & Wilkins, 2003:283–295.

80. Di Rocco C, Velardi F. Epidemiology and etiology of craniocerebral trauma in the first two years of life. In: Raimondi AJ, Choux M, Di Rocco CD, eds. Head Injuries in the Newborn and Infant. New York: Springer-Verlag, 1986:125–140.

81. Deulofeut R, Sola A, Lee B, et al. The impact of vaginal delivery in premature infants. Obstet Gynecol 2005; 105(3):525–531.

82. Hovind K. Traumatic birth injures. In: Raimondi AJ, Choux M, Di Rocco CD, eds. Head Injuries in the Newborn and Infant. New York: Springer-Verlag, 1986:87–109.

83. Al-Qattan MM. Obstetric brachial plexus palsy associated with breech delivery. Ann Plast Surg 2003; 51(3):257–264.

84. Johnson JH, Figueroa R, Garry D, et al. Immediate maternal and neonatal effects of forceps and vacuum-assisted deliveries. Obstet Gynecol 2004; 103(3):513–518.

85. Papaefthymiou F, Oberbauer R, Pendl G. Craniocerebral birth trauma caused by vacuum extraction: a case of growing skull fracture as a perinatal complication. Childs Nerv Syst 1996; 12:117–120.

86. McQuivey RW. Vacuum-assisted delivery: a review. J Matern Fetal Neonatal Med 2004; 16(3):171–180.

87. Croughan-Minihane MS, Petitti DB, Gordis L, Golditch I. Morbidity among breech infants according to method of delivery. Obstet Gynecol 1990; 75:821–825.

88. Bruce DA. Head injuries in the pediatric population. Curr Probl Pediatr 1990; 20:67–107.

89. Rommel O, Niedeggen A, Tegenthoff M, et al. Carotid and vertebral artery injury following severe head or cervical spine trauma. Cerebrovasc Dis 1999; 9(4):202–209.

90. Aleksic M, Heckenkamp J, Gawenda M, et al. Differentiated treatment of aneurysms of the extracranial carotid artery. J Cardiovasc Surg 2005; 46(1):19–23.

91. Turowski B, Zanella FE. Interventional neuroradiology of the head and neck. Neuroimaging Clin N Am 2003; 13(3):619–645.

92. Savitz SI, Caplan LR. Vertebrobasilar disease. N Engl J Med 2005; 352(25):2618–2626.

93. Norris JW, Beletsky V. Cervical arterial dissection. Adv Neurol 2003; 92:119–125.

94. Burke JP, Marion DW. Cerebral revascularization in trauma and carotid occlusion. Neurosurg Clin N Am 2001; 12(3):595–611.

95. Mobbs RJ, Chandran KN. Traumatic middle cerebral artery occlusion: case report and review of pathogenesis. Neurol India 2001; 49(2):158–161.

96. Sato S, Iida H, Hirayama H, et al. Traumatic basilar artery occlusion caused by a fracture of the clivus. Neurol Med Chir 2001; 41(11):541–544.

97. Uzan M, Cantasdemir M, Seckin MS, et al. Traumatic intracranial carotid tree aneurysms. Neurosurgery 1998; 43(6):1314–1320.

98. Jones BV, Ball WS, Tomsick TA, et al. Vein of Galen aneurismal malformation: diagnosis and treatment of 13 children with extended clinical follow-up. Am J Neuroradiol 2002; 13(12):1261–1264.

99. Brunelle F. Brain vascular malformations in the fetus: diagnosis and prognosis. Childs Nerv Syst 2003; 19(7–8):524–528.

100. Hoh Bl, Ogilvy CS, Butler WE, et al. Multimodality treatment of nongalenic arteriovenous malformation in pediatric patients. Neurosurgery 2000; 47(2):346–357.

101. Humphreys RP, Hoffman HJ, Drake JM, et al. Choices in the 1990s for the management of pediatric cerebral arteriovenous malformations. Pediatr Neurosurg 1996; 25(6):277–285.

102. Huang J, McGrit MJ, Gailloud P, et al. Intracranial aneurysms in the pediatric population: case series and literature review. Surg Neurol 2005; 63(5):424–433.

103. Wu CT, Wond CS, Yeh CC, et al. Treatment of cerebral vasospasm after subarachnoid hemorrhage: a review. Acata Anaesthesiol Taiwan 2004; 42(4):215–222.

104. Sert A, Aydin K, Pirgon O, et al. Arterial spasm following perimesencephalic nonaneurysmal subarachnoid hemorrhage in a pediatric patient. Pediatric Neurol 2005; 32(4):275–277.

105. Wijdicks EF, Kallmes DF, Manno EM, et al. Subarachnoid hemorrhage: neurointensive care. Mayo Clin Proc 2005; 80(4):550–559.

106. Buhl R, Hempelmann RG, Stark AM, et al. Therapeutical considerations in patients with intracranial venous angiomas. Eur J Neurol 2002; 9(2):165–169.

107. Masson C, Godefroy O, Leclerc X, et al. Cerebral venous infarction following thrombosis of the draining vein of a venous angioma. Cerebrovasc Dis 2000; 10(3):235–238.

108. Garton HJ, Piatt JH Jr. Hydrocehpalus. Pediatr Clin North Am 2004; 51(2):305–325.

109. Rekate HL. The slit ventricle syndrome: advances based on technology and understanding. Pediatr Neurosurg 2004; 40(6):259–263.

110. Virella AA, Galarza M, Masterman-Smith M, et al. Distal slit valve and clinically relevant CSF overdrainage in children with hydrocephalus. Childs Nerv Syst 2002; 18(1–2):15–18.

111. Ciurea AV, Stoica F, Vasilescu G, et al. Neurosurgical management of brain abscesses in children. Childs Nerv Syst 1999; 15(6–7):309–317.

112. Miyamoto RC, Miyamoto RT. Pediatric neurotology. Semin Pediatr Neurol 2003; 10(4):298–303.

113. Giannoni C, Sulek M, Friedman EM. Intracranial complications of sinusitis: a pediatric series. Am J Rhinol 1998; 12(3):173–178.

114. Bernaardini GL. Diagnosis and management of brain abscess and subdural empyema. Curr Neurol Neurosci Rep 2004; 4(6):448–456.

115. Kim KS. Pathogenesis of bacterial meningitis: from bacteraemia to neuronal injury. Nat Rev Neurosci 2003; 16(3):271–277.

116. Chavez-Bueno S, McCracken GH Jr. Bacterial meningitis in children. Pediatr Clin N Am 2005; 52(3):795–810.

117. Kaney PM, Sheehan JM. Reflections on shunt infection. Pediatr Neurosurg 2003; 39(6):285–290.

118. Laurent JP, Bruce DA, Schut L. Hemorrhagic brain tumors in pediatric patients. Childs Brain 1981; 8:263–266.

119. Stevenson KL. Chiari Type II malformation: past, present, and future. Neurosurg Focus 2004; 16(2):123–136.

120. Charney E, Weller S, Sutton IN, et al. Management of the newborn with myelo-meningocele: Time for a decision making process. Pediatrics 1985; 75:58–64.

121. Oakes WJ, Tubbs RS. Management of Chiari malformation and spinal dysraphism. Clin Neurosurg 2004; 51:48–52.

122. Aminoff MJ, Edwards MSB. Spinal arteriovenous malformations. In: Edwards MSB, Hoffman HJ, eds. Cerebral Vascular Disease in Children and Adolescents. Baltimore, MD: Williams and Wilkins, 1989:321–341.

123. Kumar R, Singh V. Intramedullary mass lesions of the spinal cord in children. Pediatr Neurosurg 2004; 40(1):16–22.

124. Lee M, Rezai AR, Abbott R, Coelho DH, Epstein FJ. Intramedullary spinal cord lipomas. J Neurosurg 1995; 82:394–400.

125. Parsa AT, Lee J, Parney IF, et al. Spinal cord and intradural-extraparenchymal spinal tumors: current best care practices and strategies. J Neurooncol 2004; 69 (1–3):291–318.

126. Asabe K, Handa N, Tamai Y, et al. A case of congenital intraspinal neuroblastoma. J Pediatr Surg 1997; 32(9):1371–1376.

127. Wiggins GC, Shaffrey CI, Abel MF, et al. Pediatric spinal deformities. Neursrg Focus 2003; 14(1):3–12.

128. Scott RM, Wolpert SM, Bartoshesky LE, et al. Segmental spinal dysgenesis. Neurosurg 1988; 22:739–744.

129. Misra SN, Morgan HW. Thoracolumbar spinal deformity in achondroplasia. Neurosurg Focus 2003; 14(1):4–13.

130. Tsirikos AI, Saifuddin A, Noordeen MH. Spinal deformity in neurofibromatosis: diagnosis and treatment. Eur Spine J 2005; 14(5):427–439.

131. Lo LJ, Chen YR. Airway obstruction in severe syndromic craniosynostosis. Ann Plast Surg 1999; 43(3):258–264.

132. Tubbs RS, Wellons JC, Oakes WJ. Occipital encephalocele, lipomeningomyelocele, and Chiari I malformation: case report and review of the literature. Childs Nerv Syst 2003; 19(1):50–53.

133. Chestnut RM. Avoidance of hypotension: conditio sine qua non of successful severe head injury management. J Trauma 1997; 42:S4–S9.

134. Bayir H, Kochanek PM, Clark RS. Traumatic brain injury in infants and children: mechanisms of secondary damage and treatment in the intensive care unit. Crit Care Clin 2003; 19(3):529–549.

135. Khoshyomn S, Tranmer BI. Diagnosis and management of pediatric closed head injury. Semin Pediatr Surg 2004; 13(2):80–86.

136. Bratton SL, Davis RL. Acute lung injury in isolated traumatic brain injury. Neurosurgery 1997; 40:707–712.

137. Bell MJ, Kochenek PM, Doughty LA, et al. Interleukin-6 and interleukin-10 in cerebrospinal fluid after severe traumatic brain injury in children. J Neurotrauma 1997; 14:451–457.

138. Whalen MJ, Carlos TM, Kochenek PM, et al. Interleukin 8 is increased in cerebrospinal fluid of children with severe head injury. Crit Care Med 2000; 28:929–934.

139. Escamilla RF, Lisser H. Simmonds Disease. J Clin Endocrinol 1942; 2:65–96.

140. Benvenga S, Campenni A, Ruggeri RM, Trimarchi F. Hypopituitarism secondary to head trauma. J Clin Endocrinol Metab 2000; 85:1353–1361.

141. Pomeroy SL, Sturla LM. Molecular biology of medulloblastoma therapy. Pediatr Neurosurg 2003; 39(6):299–304.

142. Fay T. Observation on generalized refrigeration in cases of severe cerebral trauma. Assoc Res Nerv Ment Dis Proc 1943; 24:611–619.

143. Sedzimir CB. Therapeutic hypothermia in cases of head injury. J Neurosurg 1959; 16:407–414.

144. Hendrick EB. The use of hypothermia in severe head injuries in childhood. Ann Surg 1959; 79:362–364.

145. Lazorthes G. Campan L. Hypothermia in the treatment of craniocerebral traumatism. J Neurosurg 1958; 15:162–167.

146. Rosomoff H, Holaday D. Cerebral blood flow and cerebral oxygen consumtion during hypothermia. Am J Physiol 1954; 179:85–88.

147. Busto R, Dietrich WD, Globus MT, et al. Small differences in intraischemic brain temperature critically determine the extent of ischemic neuronal injury. J Cereb Blood Flow Metab 1987; 7:729–738.

148. Smith SL, Hall ED. Mild pre- and posttraumatic hypothermia attenuates blood-brain barrier damage following controlled cortical impact injury in the rat. J Neurotrauma 1996; 13:1–9.

149. Marion D, Penrod L, Kelsey SF, et al. Treatment of traumatic brain injury with moderate hypothermia. N Eng J Med 1997; 336(8):540–546.

150. Pomeranz S, Safar P, Radovsky A, et al. The effect of resuscitative moderate hypothermia following epidural brain compression on cerebral damage in a canine outcome model. J Neurosurg 1993; 79:241–251.

151. Kochanek PM, Safar PJ. Therapeutic hypothermia for severe traumatic brain injury. JAMA 2003; 289:3007.

152. Henderson WR, Dhingra VK, Chittock DR, et al. Hypothermia in the management of traumatic brain injury. A systematic review and meta-analysis. Intensive Care Med 2003; 29:1637–1644.

153. Guha A. Management of traumatic brain injury: some current evidence and applications. Postgrad Med J 2004; 80:650–653.
154. Polderman KH, Ely EW, Badr AE, Birbes ARJ. Induced hypothermia in traumatic brain injury: considering the conflicting results of meta-analyses and moving forward. Intensive Care Med 2004; 30:1860–1864.
155. Henderson WR, Dhingra VK, Chittock DR, et al. Hypothermia in the management of traumatic brain injury. A systemic review and meta-analysis. Intensive Care Med 2004; 39:1637–1644.
156. McIntyre LA, Fergusson DA, Bebert PC, et al. Prolonged therapeutic hypothermia after traumatic brain injury in adults: a systemic review. JAMA 2003; 298:2992–2999.
157. Shiozaki T, Hayakata T, Taneda M, et al. A multicenter prospective randomized controlled trial of the efficacy of mild hypothermia for severely head injured patients with low intracranial pressure. Mild Hypothermia Study Group in Japan. J Neurosurg 2001; 94:50–54.
158. Polderman KH. Therapeutic hypothermia in the intensive care unit; problems, pitfalls and opportunities. I. Indications and evidence. Intensive Care Med 2004; 30:556–575.
159. Clifton GL, Miller ER, Choi SC, et al. Lack of effect of induction of hypothermia after acute brain injury. N Engl J Med 2001; 344:556–563.
160. Adelson PD, Ragheb J, Kanev P, et al. Phase II clinical trial of moderate hypothermia after severe traumatic brain injury in children. Neurosurgery 2005; 56(4):740–754.
161. Peterson B, Khanna S, Fisher B, et al. Prolonged hypernatremia controls elevated intracranial pressure in head-injured pediatric patients. Crit Care Med 2000; 28:1136–1143.
162. Munar F, Ferrer AM, deNadal M, et al. Cerebral hemodynamic effects of 72% hypertonic saline in patients with head injury and raised intracranial pressure. J Neurotrauma 2000; 17:41–51.
163. Dutton RP, McCunn M: Traumatic brain injury. Curr Opin Crit Care 2003; 9:503–509.
164. Worthley LI, Cooper DJ, Jones N. Treatment of resistant intracranial hypertension with hypertonic saline. Report of two cases. J Neurosurg 1988; 68:478–481.
165. Shackford SR, Bourguignon PR, Wald SL, et al. Hypertonic saline resuscitation of patients with head injury: a prospective, randomized clinical trial. J Trauma 1998; 44:50–58.
166. Fisher B, Thomas D, Peterson B. Hypertonic saline lowers raised intracranial pressure in children after head trauma. J Neurosurg Anesthesiol 1992; 4:4–10.
167. Simma B, Burger R, Falk M, et al. Aprospective, randomized, and controlled study of fluid management in children with sever head injury: lactated Ringer's solution versus hypertonic saline. Crit Care Med 1998; 26:1265–1270.
168. Hartle R, Ghajar J, Hochleuthner H, et al. Hypertonic/hyperoncotic saline reliably reduced ICP in severely head-injured patients with intracranial hypertension. Acta Neurochir Suppl (Wien) 1997; 70:126–129.
169. Sterns HR, Riggs JE, Schochet SS Jr. Osmotic demyelination syndrome following rapid correction of hyponatremia. N Engl J Med 1986; 314:1535–1541.
170. Finberg L, Luttrell E, Redd H. Pathogenesis of lesions in the nervous system in hypernatremic stats: II. Experimental studies of gross anatomic changes and alterations of chemical composition of the tissues. Pediatrics 1959; 23:46–66.
171. Carney NA, Chesnut R, Kochanek PM, et al. Use of hyperosmolar therapy in the management of severe pediatric traumatic brain injury. Pediatr Crit Care Med 2003; 4(3):S40–S44.
172. Cooper DJ, Myles PS, McKermott FT, et al. Prehospital hypertonic saline resuscitation of patient hypotension and severe traumatic brain injury. JAMA 2004; 291:1350–1357.
173. Smyth MD, Tubbs RS, Wellons JC, et al. Endoscopic third ventriculostomy for hydrocephalus secondary to central nervous system infection or intraventricular hemorrhage in children. Pediatr Neurosurg 2003; 39(5):258–263.
174. McIntosh TK. Novel pharmacological therapies in the treatment of experimental traumatic brain injury: A review. J Neurotrauma 1993; 10:215–261.
175. Vink R, Hu X, Bennett C, et al. Inhibition of neurogenic inflammation improves motor and cognitive outcome following diffuse traumatic brain injury. Rest Neurol Neurosci 2000; 16:164.
176. Biban C, Tassani V, Tonienello A, et al. The alterations in the energy linked properties induced in rat liver mitochondria by acetylsalicylate are prevented by cyclosporin A or Mg2+. Biochem Pharmacol 1995; 50:497–500.
177. Mayer ML, Westbrook GL, Gutherie PB. Voltage–dependent block by Mg^{2+} of NMDA responses in spinal cord neurons. Nature 1984; 309:261–63.
178. Heath DL, Vink R. Delayed therapy with magnesium up to 24 hours following traumatic brain injury improves motor outcome. J Neurosurg 1999; 90:504–509.
179. Heath DL, Vink R. Optimisation of magnesium therapy following severe diffuse axonal brain injury in rats. J Pharmacol Exp Ther 1999; 288:1311–1316.
180. McIntosh TK, Faden AI, Yamakami I, et al. Magnesium deficiency exacerbates and pretreatment improves outcome following traumatic brain injury in rats: 31P magnetic resonance spectroscopy and behavioral studies. J Neurotrauma 1988; 5:17–31.
181. Vink R, McIntosh TK, Demediuk P, et al. Decline in intracellular free Mg^{++} is associated with irreversible tissue injury after brain trauma. J Biol Chem 1988; 263:757–761.
182. Browne KD, Leoni MJ, Iwata A, et al. Acute treatment with $MgSO_4$ attenuates long-term hippocampal tissue loss after brain trauma in the rat. J Neurosci Res 2004; 77:878–883.
183. McKee JA, Brewer RP, Macy GE, et al. Analysis of the brain bioavailability of peripherally administered magnesium sulfate: A study in humans with acute brain injury undergoing prolonged induced hypermagnesemia. Crit Care Med 2005; 33:661–666.

16

Brain Death and Organ Donation

John K. Stene

Department of Anesthesiology, Penn State College of Medicine, Penn State University Hospital, Hershey, Pennsylvania, U.S.A.

Rahul Jandial

Division of Neurosurgery, UC San Diego Medical Center, San Diego, and the Burnham
Institute for Medical Research, La Jolla, California, U.S.A.

INTRODUCTION

Brain death is often perceived as the tragic end to the life of a loved one, and sometimes as a medical failure. However, the prospect of organ donation can refocus the grief emanating from an otherwise devastating event toward the greater good of extending the life of another patient who would otherwise also die. Indeed, the gift of organs provides tremendous benefits to the recipient, but also honors the departed patients, and assuages some of the grief experienced by the family and friends of the donor.

The concept of brain death is a relatively recent idea that began to emerge following advances in life support technology which occurred during the second half of the twentieth century (1,2). Classically, death had been defined as the cessation of respiration and heart beat. However, respiration can now be supported with mechanical ventilation, and cardiac function can be assisted both pharmacologically and mechanically well after the patient's brain has ceased viability. Despite science fiction stories, such as Robin Cook's *Coma* (3), the patient whose brain has died is incapable of recovery, and without special intervention typically succumbs to cardiac arrest within a week (2). Because several elements of the cardiovascular and endocrine system often become unstable following brain death, decisions regarding organ donation need to be made very soon after brain death is declared.

This chapter begins with a brief, partly historical survey of the medical advances, religious and philosophical principles involved in the conceptual evolution in the definition of brain death. Some religious and cultural objections to the definition of brain death remain, and these are discussed in greater detail in Volume 2, Chapter 68. After the historical review, the chapter focuses upon the main emphasis, which is diagnosis of brain death and the management of the brain dead organ donor. The diagnosis of brain death has clinical criteria (sufficient in the majority of cases) and confirmatory tests (occasionally required to expedite diagnoses) both of which are completely reviewed in this chapter. The management of the brain dead patient is divided between critical care considerations while awaiting organ procurement (section "ICU Management of the Brain Dead Organ Donor"), and operative management, which reviews both the anesthetic and surgical considerations for organ procurement (section "Operative Management During Organ Procurement"). Finally, this chapter provides a glimpse into the future with a sampling of ideas regarding a worldwide unification of brain death criteria, and search for earlier markers of brain death.

EVOLVING CONCEPT OF BRAIN DEATH
Advances in Organ Preservation and Transplantation

The concept that brain death is philosophically and ethically equivalent to the death of the person as a whole, developed very recently in response to prolonged futile maintenance of unrecoverable patients in intensive care units (ICUs) during the 1950s and 1960s. The nascent idea of brain death emerged as physicians and families grappled with the reality that medical technology had advanced beyond our philosophical constructs (see the section on philosophical evolution). Indeed, one half century ago medical science progressed to the degree that viable hearts, lungs (and other organs) could be maintained in patients long after blood flow to the brain had ceased and/or brain and brainstem neurons had become necrotic. One of the first clinical-pathological (and conceptual) descriptions of brain death was provided in France, when Mollaret and Goulon introduced the term *coma dépassé* (irreversible coma) in 1959 (4). In this report, 23 comatose patients are described, all with absent brainstem reflexes, documented apnea, and flat electroencephalograms (EEGs). The subsequent autopsy findings revealed necrotic brain and brainstem (4).

The concept of brain death also coincided with important advances in organ transplantation and an increased demand for organ donors. Pioneering trauma anesthesiologist, Henry K. Beecher, at Massachusetts General Hospital, chaired the Harvard University committee that defined the diagnosis and validity of brain death. ☞ **Beecher's white paper, published in JAMA in 1968, concentrated on limiting the use of ICUs to maintain futile life support for patients who had no chance of recovery secondary to death and necrosis of their entire brain (5).** ☞

Harvard University set out clinical and laboratory criteria required to declare a patient brain dead. These criteria (Table 1), which included lack of brainstem reflexes, unresponsiveness to noxious stimuli, and lack of spontaneous respiratory activity despite an elevated $PaCO_2$, were developed as safeguards to prevent withdrawal of life support from an otherwise viable patient in deep coma. Initially, these clinical criteria for brain death received rather slow acceptance among the medical community. Indeed, it took a decade before the uniform brain death act

Table 1 Original Harvard Criteria for Diagnosing Brain Death

Criteria	Clinical examination, testing results
Unreceptivity and unresponsivity	No response to intensely painful stimuli
No movements, and no breathing	No spontaneous movement observed by physicians during period of at least one hour, no effort to breathe when normocarbic and ventilator discontinued for three minutes
No reflexes	Fixed dilated pupils, no oculovestibular or oculocephalic reflex, no blinking, no postural activity (decerebrate), no swallowing, yawning, or vocalization, no corneal or pharyngeal reflexes
Flat EEG	Isoelectric at standard gains 50 μ V/5 mm for 10–20 min, also isoelectric at 25 μV/5 mm

Source: From Ref. 53.

legislation began to be prepared in 1979 by representatives of the medical community, the legal community, and state governments. The President's Commission for the Study of Ethical Problems in Medicine and Biomedical and Behavioral Research published the Uniform Determination of Death Act in 1981 (6). This act defined death as the irreversible cessation of circulatory and respiratory functions or irreversible cessation of brain and brainstem activities (1). The Uniform Determination of Death Act in the United States became a model for the 50 states to write legislation defining brain death. ☞ **Currently, the U.S. standard to declare brain death is to document the absence of brain and brainstem activity (7).** ☞

In 1995, the American Academy of Neurology (AAN) established practice parameters for the diagnosis of brain death (8). These guidelines represent a formalization of clinical practice incorporating the Harvard criteria. Follow-up studies have not identified any patient recovery subsequent to the strict application of these guidelines. In 2000, the Canadian Neurocritical Care Group published Guidelines for the Diagnosis of Brain Death, that closely mirror the AAN guidelines.

In 1971, brainstem death was shown to be the critical CNS lesion that when present was incompatible with unsupportive survival (9). Subsequently, the Medical Royal Colleges and their faculties published a statement in the United Kingdom that defined brain death as complete, irreversible loss of brainstem function (10). ☞ **The current U.K. standard for the diagnosis of brain death is complete and irreversible loss of brainstem function.** ☞

Although the medical community in both Europe and America has been proactive in developing the concept of brain death, the lay public continues to reveal confusion about the terminology and whether brain death means the person is irreversibly dead (11). A 1992 survey of over 6000 adults in the United States found that 21% believed it was possible for a brain dead person to recover and 16% were unsure (11). A similar survey of families of brain dead organ donors and nondonors performed in 1994 found similar levels of misunderstanding concerning brain death (12).

☞ **A patient who meets the clinical definition of brain death by either the U.S. or U.K. criteria is in essence dead as a person, as he/she will never recover sentient function.** ☞ Because cessation of cardiac activity usually proceeds relatively soon following the death of the brainstem, successful organ transplantation requires a reasonably brief duration between the declaration of brain death and the initiation of plans for organ procurement (12,13). Originally, the declaration of brain death required that two clinical examinations (both consistent with brain death) be conducted 24-hour apart. Two independent physicians are still required, but the 24 hours interval is no longer required in the United States. Experience has demonstrated that a rigorous clinical examination when properly performed clearly identifies patients with irreversible brain death. The purpose of the second examination is to confirm that the first examination was accurately performed. It is now considered ethical that the two examinations be performed within the same hour, because of the unstable homeostasis that develops soon after brain (and brainstem) death. However, because these patients are almost always receiving mechanical ventilation and have a spontaneously beating heart, the skin may be warm to the touch and the body could appear to be merely sleeping by family and others. The imperative that a patient meets the full criteria for brain death before organ procurement commences goes without saying (Table 2) (13–15).

Because experience demonstrates that a carefully performed clinical examination is fully sufficient to diagnose brain death, confirmatory laboratory tests are seldom needed (except for an arterial blood gas to document respiratory unresponsiveness to profound respiratory acidosis) (7,8). While EEG, angiography, transcranial Doppler, and radionuclide perfusion scans of the brain and brainstem are confirmatory of brain and brainstem death, they don't add any information to a properly performed clinical examination (8,13–15). However, these confirmatory studies can be useful when the etiology of a patient's profound coma is uncertain or when some elements of the clinical criteria cannot be determined (i.e., the patient denatures or becomes hemodynamically unstable during apnea testing).

International Variability in Definition

As mentioned above, in the United Kingdom, brain death is defined as "complete and irreversible loss of brainstem function" (7). In the United Kingdom, brain death is called "brain stem death" because a functioning brainstem is required to maintain life. Furthermore, a patient can suffer significant loss of cerebral cortex and maintain life through a functioning brainstem. Legally, the British physician only needs to document loss of brain stem function unlike the U.S. physician who must document brain (cerebral) and brainstem death.

As in America, the British public and medical community was initially relatively slow to accept the notion that brainstem death is equivalent to death of the patient. The U.K. criteria are observed by many of the previously colonized countries (including Australia and New Zealand), whereas Central and South American countries follow the U.S. criteria. Non-U.K. European countries, and those of the Middle East, Africa, Asia, and South Pacific have variable definitions (7). In Mainland China a specific legal definition of brain death does not yet exist, whereas Hong Kong follows the U.K. criteria. The brain death criteria in Japan have many unique features, and acceptance of

Table 2 American Academy of Neurology Practice Parameters for Determining Brain Death in Adults

Category	Criteria	Subcategory, explanation, comments
A	Prerequisite: document absence of exclusion criteria	Known reversible causes of coma or depressed brain function Complicating medical conditions Drug intoxication or poisoning Core temperature $\leq 32°C$
B_1	Coma or unresponsiveness	Lack of cerebral motor response (in any extremity) to pain by supraorbital pressur0e

B_2	Absence of brainstem reflexes	Pupils—midposition (5–7 mm) no response to bright light
		Ocular movement
		   No oculocephalic reflex (contraindicated with unstable c-spine)
		   No oculovestibular reflex (cold caloric)
		Facial sensation and facial motor response
		   No corneal reflex, no grimacing to deep pain
		   No jaw reflex
		Pharyngeal and tracheal reflexes (no gag or cough)

B_3	Apnea	Start with $PaCO_2 = 40$ and $PaO_2 \geq 200$
		Disconnect patient from ventilator
		Administer O_2 8–10 L/min via suction catheter with tip placed at
		   level of carina (optional)
		Observe closely for respiratory motion
		Measure $PaO_2/PaCO_2/pH$ at end of apnea trial (8–10 min)
		Reconnect the ventilator if respirations seen or hemodynamic instability occurs
		Positive result requires $PaCO_2$ to increase to ≥ 60 mmHg or by 20 mmHg
		   over baseline

C	Confirmatory tests (seldom required)	[99m]TcHM-PAO brain scan. "Hollow skull phenomenon" Angiography—no intracerebral filling at level of carotid bifurcation or circle of Willis EEG— no activity for 30 min[a] using minimal technical criteria for brain death TCD small systolic peaks and mediastolic flow or reverberating flow

To use table: (*i*) ensure all exclusion criteria in Catgeory A are absent, (*ii*) ensure that each criteria in B (first 3 points) are present, (*iii*) confirmatory tests only needed if unclear.

[a]Per minimal technical criteria for brain death.

Abbreviations: EEG, electroencephalography; TCD, transcranial Doppler ultransonography; [99m]TcHM-PAO, Technetium—99 m hexamethypropyleneamineoxine.
Source: From Ref. 8.

organ transplantation has been very slow because of religious and cultural difficulties with the concept of brain death (7). The variable worldwide definitions of brain death, and the associated cultural and religious considerations are discussed in greater detail in Volume 2, Chapter 68. Additionally, Wijdicks' review of international norms of brain death provides the best currently available survey of world wide practices for declaring brain death (Table 3) (7).

Religious and Legal Viewpoints

The various religious traditions have differing viewpoints on the concept of brain death. Most faith traditions consider the

Table 3 Worldwide Brain Death Laws

80 countries surveyed	Percent of countries
Laws concerning brain death	69
Guidelines concerning brain death	88
More than one physician required for declaration	50
Confirmatory laboratory testing required	40
Apnea testing with CO_2 target (50–60 mmHg)	59

Source: From Ref. 7.

time of death a medical diagnosis and accept a physician's diagnosis of death. Therefore, if the medical diagnosis is that brain death means the death of the patient, then the patient is dead and the soul has departed the body. However, a few religious groups still consider the cessation of breathing and heartbeat as a requirement for diagnosing death. State laws in the United States vary to accommodate such differences in religious views (7).

The legal community has been reluctant to define the precise nature of death (i.e., brain death was equivalent to the death of the whole person). Accordingly, most legal jurisdictions in the United States acknowledge that the diagnosis of death is a medical, not a legal issue (12). The Uniform Determination of Death Act serves as a template for most state legislation, and emphasizes that the person is dead when his brain and brainstem irreversibly cease function. However, it is left to the physician to declare when brain and brainstem death has occurred. Furthermore, the development of coma before the person meets the criteria of brain death is not synonymous with the time of death. The person is considered alive until all brain and brainstem activity cease.

Philosophical Evolution Continues

It is not surprising that philosophical disagreement about the concept of brain death continues, given the continuing debate about when life starts, and that the ancient quest for the source of the "mind" (sentient awareness) has only recently been resolved. The current philosophical understanding of brain death as equivalent to death of the sentient portion of the person, is the result of a journey several millennia in duration.

Hippocrates (460–377 BC) was convinced that consciousness derived from the brain, as evidenced in his writings: "men ought to know that from nothing else but the brain comes joys, delights, laughter and sports, and sorrows, grieves, despondency and lamentations" (16). Some contemporary Greek philosophers, for example, Plato (427–347 BC) published writings that placed the seat of thought in the brain [e.g., the Timaes (360 BC)] (17). However, other writings from Plato imply an extracorporeal source for the mind. Aristotle (384–322 BC.), the father of comparative biology, believed that the mind resided in the heart, and the function of the brain was to cool the heart. It is likely that Aristotle performed experiments on the brains of animals, and found it lacking sensation (17). The later Christian philosophers St. Augustine (354–430) and St. Thomas Aquinas (1225–1274) believed that the mind (or "soul") was separate from the body (18).

The early Greeks also theorized that all diseases shared a single cause: imbalance of the fluid portions of the body, specifically the four humors, yellow bile, black bile, blood and phlegm. This incorrect thinking paralyzed the advancement of philosophy, science and medicine, and is a major reason why physicians did not know the cause of a single important human disease until a little more than 150 years ago (19).

Galen (130–200) believed that the anatomical seat of the soul was the pineal gland. Unfortunately, Galen's dogma hopelessly hindered the advance of medical science and natural philosophy for 1300 years (17). Andreas Vesalius (1514–1564) believed the ventricles of the brain served as the seat of perception and cognition (17).

The pervasive belief at that time was that a "vital force" was responsible for life (an archaic philosophy now referred to as vitalism). Indeed, William Harvey (1578–1657) began his research in an effort to determine the precise location of where the vital spirits were brewed. He held the popular view that the blood was made in the liver, and that the heart and lungs made the vital spirits. He discovered the heart to be a muscular pump, and that the blood circulated (17).

Rene Descartes (1595–1650) believed that intellectual thought and reasoning is what makes humans unique among animal species; his famous "cognito ergo sum," literally, "I think, therefore I am," actually means I think, therefore I have a mind. However, this otherwise brilliant natural philosopher confused later scientific and philosophical thinking, with his dual substance view. Dualism contends that the mind's function of consciousness occurred via a process independently from the physical brain. The Cartesian model held that the mind and body were separate (18).

John Locke (1632–1704), founder of empiricism attacked the mind-body dichotomy of Descartes (18). The Scottish empiricist, David Hume (1711–1776), a central influence on Charles Darwin, discounted both mysticism and dualism. Although Hume was considered by contemporaries to be a skeptic and atheist, he became a leader of philosophical naturalism, a branch of philosophy which has evolved into neurophilosophy (18). Neurophilosophers believe that the brain is the seat of the mind, and that sound philosophy requires a strong understanding of neuroscience.

Joseph Priestley (1733–1804), naturalist, scientist, and philosopher, discovered oxygen, and that animals need it to survive. Priestley argued against spiritualism, in favor of materiality of the soul. The French philosopher and physician Cabanis (1757–1808) built upon Priestley's philosophy of materialism to forcefully state, for the first time since Hippocrates, that "the mind and the brain are one."

Giovanni Batista Morgagni (1682–1771) worked for 50 years to develop a compendium of clinical pathological correlations, in a book entitled "On the seats and causes of disease." Yet, the concept of living cells was still undiscovered. After Morgagni, Frenchman Xavier Bichat (1800) focused the origin of disease to the tissue level, and finally, Rudolph Virchow (1858) further refined it down to the cellular level. This set the stage for understanding neurological function on a cellular level.

The following scientists and philosophers discovered that the organized function of neurons within the brain are responsible for what we call the mind. Neurons were visualized for the first time by Purkinge (1837), and Santiago Ramon Y Cajal of Madrid (1852–1934), along with Camillo Golgi of Pavia (1843–1926) later won the Nobel Prize for describing the histologic anatomy of the brain and spinal cord.

Charles Bell (1774–1842), a Scottish surgeon, discovered that the ventral roots of the spinal cord contain only motor and the dorsal roots only sensory fibers. In so doing, he developed the foundation for neural organization within the CNS. Later, Johannes Muëller (1801–1858) of Berlin presented a unified theory of neurophysiology involving two cardinal principles (*i*) that the nervous system serves as an intermediary between the world and the mind, and (*ii*) the sensory nerve for vision is insensible to sound, as the nerve of audition is to light.

Paul Broca (1824–1880), the French physician, discovered that a lesion in the left frontal lobe was responsible for the pathology of a speechless, right hemiplegic patient. Finally, John Hughlings Jackson (1835–1911), an English Physician, provided the first general description of the functional organization of the nervous system. Discrete lesions of specific areas of the CNS have since been demonstrated to abolish the function attributed to it. However, death of the entire brain had never been observed in a patient with a pulse and warm skin until the modern development of ventilators.

Consciousness has reemerged as a topic in philosophical inquiry once again over the past three decades. Modern neurophilosophers such as Paul Churchland (20) are exploring the use of neural networks to help unlock the neurobiologic explanation of consciousness. Francis Crick and Christof Hoch are studying the visual system in an effort to find a universal clue to the mechanism of consciousness (21). All agree consciousness occurs in the brain, but there are likely discrete areas that are responsible for certain elements of consciousness and higher thought (including attention, reasoning, memory, etc.). For example, the area of the brain that governs free will may be located in Broadman's area 24 according to Crick (16). The future definition of brain death may relate to destruction or death of one of these vital structures.

DIAGNOSIS OF BRAIN DEATH
Clinical Determination of Brain Death
✍ **Brain death is diagnosed clinically with the establishment of three major criteria. First, the neurological injury**

Table 4 Confounding Agents/Conditions that Need to Be Excluded in Brain Death Testing

Agent/condition	Example
Pharmacologic	Anesthetics, paralytics, methaqualone, barbiturates, diazepam, bretylium, mecloqualone, amitrityline, meprobamate, trichloroethylene, alcohols, etc.
Metabolic	Hepatic encephalopathy
	Uremic encephalopathy
	Hyperosmolar coma
	Hypophosphatemia
Temperature	Hypothermia ?<32° Celsius
Vascular	Shock or hypotension
Infectious	Brain stem encephalitis
	Guillain–Barre syndrome

Source: From Refs. 8, 13, 15, and 47.

should be irreversible (1,13,15,22). Second, there is a loss of cerebral function. Third, there is a loss of brainstem function (13,15). ☞ Prior to establishing the clinical criteria for brain death, several potentially confounding factors must be eliminated (Table 4). For example, deep coma secondary to metabolic encephalopathy would not be compatible with the diagnosis of brain death, nor would lack of respiration solely due to a high spinal cord injury (23).

After brain death the pupils become fixed in midposition due to loss of parasympathetic and sympathetic input. Loss of cerebral or brainstem function due to cell death in this region of the CNS results in painful stimuli in absence of response. Any movement or other response that requires function of these structures is thus incompatible with brain death. For example, decerebrate and/or decorticate posturing usually correlates with severe TBI, but their presence demonstrates that the brain is not yet dead. ☞ Spinal reflexes, such as deep tendon reflexes and triple flexion responses, can be preserved following brain death. Release phenomena of the spinal cord are occasionally seen in the setting of brain death and do not exclude brain death; these include shivering, goose bumps, forced exhalation and some arm movements (13,14). ☞

Irreversible Etiology of Coma

Irreversibility is established when a structural disease or an irreversible metabolic cause (e.g., hypoxia, carbon monoxide poisoning) is known to have occurred to the patient resulting in brain cell death. At the same time, agents or conditions that confound the testing of brain death need to be excluded (Table 4). The patient must be documented as normothermic, free of reversible metabolic disturbances (e.g., renal failure, hepatic failure), CNS depressant drugs, or neuromuscular blocking agents. Therefore, it is imperative for the physician approaching a possibly brain dead patient to be fully aware of the patient's history of present illness, and the patient must also be screened for the presence of any drugs or conditions that mimic brain death (13). If any doubt exists, the observation period should be extended to 12 to 24 hours (two brain death examinations separated in time by 12 to 24 hours) (13,14). The role of confirmatory tests is discussed later in this section.

Loss of Cerebral Function

The loss of cerebral function can be found in some vegetative states; only when it occurs along with loss of brainstem function can a person be considered brain dead. In the setting of brain death, there should be no spontaneous movement, eye opening, breathing, or response to any auditory, visual, or painful stimuli. The painful stimuli should be applied to the face (preferably the supraorbital ridge) to rule out any spinal cord injury or spinal-mediated reflexive motor responses.

Loss of Brainstem Function

The brainstem houses the centers for arousal, respiratory drive, and the cranial nerve nuclei. Accordingly, its viability can be assessed with relevant clinical examinations (Table 2). Clinically, loss of brainstem function is verified by lack of: (*i*) pupillary reflex, (*ii*) corneal reflex, (*iii*) gag and cough, (*iv*) oculocephalic reflex (doll's eyes), (*v*) oculovestibular reflex (cold caloric), (*vi*) respiratory effort (apnea testing), and (*vii*) motor response. In practice, absence of cranial nerve reflexes is documented first and then apnea testing is performed. Confirmatory tests are not required when all of the above signs of brainstem function are clearly absent.

Absence of Brainstem Reflexes (Apart from Breathing)

Absence of pupillary reflex is demonstrated in the brain dead patient by pupils that are fixed (usually in mid position), and nonreactive to light (i.e., no change of pupil size, in either eye, after shining a strong light in each eye sequentially in a dark room). The pupillary reflex is mediated by cranial nerves II and III.

The lack of corneal reflex is documented in the brain dead patient when there is lack of eyelid movement after touching the cornea (not conjunctiva) with a cotton swab or tissue; the corneal reflex is mediated by cranial nerves V (afferent) and VII (efferent).

The absence of the gag reflex and cough reflex is documented in brain dead patients when there is a lack of retching or uvula movement after touching the back of the pharynx with a tongue depressor or after moving the endotracheal tube; the gag reflex is mediated by cranial nerves IX (afferent) and X (efferent). Additionally, there should be no coughing with deep tracheal irritation and suctioning; the cough reflex is mediated by cranial nerves IX and X.

The oculocephalic reflex ("doll's eyes" reflex) should be absent in brain dead patients. There should be no eye movement with brisk turning of the head from side to side. During this examination, the patient's head should be elevated 30° from the supine position in order to place the semicircular canals in the optimum orientation. This reflex is mediated by cranial nerves III, IV, and VI as well as the medial longitudinal fasciculus (MLF). Trauma patients with known or suspected cervical spine injuries should not have the "doll's eyes" reflex tested because the neck twisting might exacerbate neurologic injury. Instead, cervical spine injured patients should undergo the "cold caloric" test (below).

Brain dead patients should not exhibit any oculovestibular reflex ("cold caloric" reflex). There should be no eye movement with irrigation of each tympanic membrane sequentially with 50cc of ice water with the head of the patient 30° elevated from the supine position. Prior to performing this test the patient's external auditory meatus should be free of wax, and the tympanic membrane should be intact. This reflex is mediated by the cranial nerves III, IV, VI, and VIII as well as the MLF.

Brain dead patients also lack any motor response to pain or any other stimulatory input. There is no localization or withdrawal after painful stimuli, nor do they exhibit extensor or flexor posturing.

Apnea Testing (Documenting Absence of Respiratory Effort)
Prior to performing apnea testing, the following prerequisites are required: the core temperature needs to be $\geq 36.5°C$, the systolic pressure should be >90 mmHg, the patient should be euvolemic, the $PaCO_2$ should be normal or slightly above normal (i.e., ≥ 40 mmHg), and the PaO_2 should be supranormal (i.e., ≥ 200) to guard against desaturation during apnea. The arterial blood gas needs to be checked to establish baseline values prior to commencing apnea testing (24). The patient is preoxygenated with an F_iO_2 of 100%, preferably with an arterial line in place for rapid blood gas measurements, while adjusting ventilatory rate and volume to achieve a $PaCO_2$ of 40–45 mmHg. Next the patient is disconnected from the ventilator and humidified O_2 at 8–12 L/min is delivered via a cannula advanced 1–2 cm beyond the end of the endotracheal tube but still above the carina to facilitate apnea oxygenation (25). Pulse oximetry is used to detect oxygen desaturation, which usually does not occur when the above detailed oxygen supplementation maneuvers are employed. Usually after 8 to 10 minutes has elapsed the patient's $PaCO_2$ has typically increased above 60 mmHg, and an arterial bloodgas (ABG) is measured at this time for confirmation (26). The exact carbon dioxide level needed to ensure lack of respiratory drive is unknown, but a $PaCO_2$ of 60 mmHg is well accepted because higher partial pressures of CO_2 may begin to impart anesthetic effects and depress the respiratory centers in a positive feedback loop (13,15). The ventilator is reconnected after the 8–10 minute apnea event, if the patient is a candidate for organ donation. If there is no evidence of spontaneous respirations before reinstitution of mechanical ventilation in the presence of a $PaCO_2$ greater than 60 mm Hg or an increase of greater than 20 mmHg from the normal baseline value, the criteria for a positive apnea test are met. If the patient desaturates or becomes hemodynamically unstable during the apnea test, an ABG is immediately drawn and the patient is reconnected to the ventilator (27). Confirmatory tests are necessary for patients who do not achieve adequate levels of hypercarbia prior to becoming unstable.

Confirmatory Studies
☞ **Confirmatory tests are not necessary for the declaration of brain death in the vast majority of cases. They may be used in cases where the observation period needs to be shortened (unstable patient intended for organ donation), children younger than one, and when clinical brain death testing is confounded by certain agents and/or conditions (Table 5).** ☞

Confirmatory tests evaluate the loss of neuronal function or evaluate the cessation of intracranial blood flow (13,14). Neuronal function is best assessed with an electroencephalogram. The dead brain is no longer capable of maintaining cellular membrane potentials or electrical signals among cells, therefore, the EEG recorded from a dead brain is flat line with total electrical silence. The machine is set for minimal technical requirements for brain death and run for at least 30 minutes to document electrical

Table 5 Confirmatory Tests for Establishing Brain Death

Category or test	Specific test technique
Electrical neuronal activity	EEG
	Evoked potentials
Evaluation of intracranial blood flow	Nuclear medicine blood flow studies
	Four-vessel cerebral angiography
	Digital subtraction angiography
	Xenon-enhanced computed tomography
	Magnetic resonance angiography
	Transcranial Doppler study

silence. Measurements of evoked potentials have also been used but they are less widely used than EEG due to decreased specificity.

For the detection of intracranial blood flow, the four-vessel cerebral angiogram is the most sensitive and specific study. All other tests are less sensitive (digital subtraction angiography/venography, transcranial Doppler study), or indirect (CT, EEG). ☞ **Nuclear medicine cerebral blood flow studies are increasingly used as the confirmatory test, because the equipment can be brought to the ICU providing images with the presence or lack of radioactive tracer within the cranial vault (28) (Fig. 1).** ☞ Recent advances in positron emission tomography (PET) scanning using F-fluorodeoxyglucose to assess brain metabolism have introduced an alternative method for confirmation of brain death. However this test is not yet universally accepted (13). Other brain flow imaging techniques discussed in Volume 2, Chapter 7 may also be helpful.

Brain Death Determinations in Children
The assessment of brain death in children is performed using different guidelines than those for adults. For the purposes

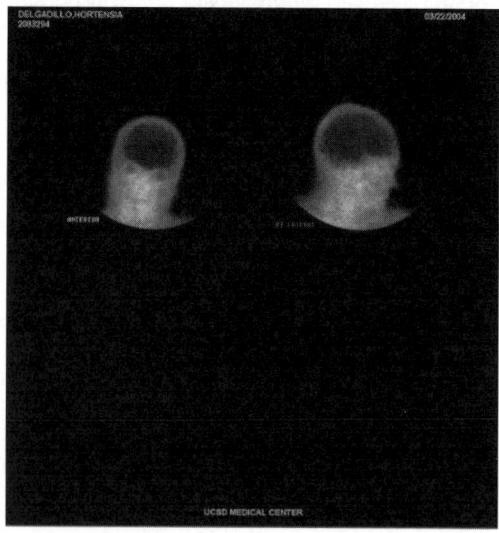

Figure 1 Nuclear cerebral blood flow study depicting lack of tracer in the intracranial circulation (supplied by the internal carotids and vertebral arteries) with preservation of tracer in the distribution of the external carotid arteries (face and scalp). The lack of tracer within the cranial vault is consistent with absence of intracranial blood flow.

Table 6 Brain Death Evaluation in Children

Evaluation element	Comments/specific details
History	Exclusion of reversible causes of coma (Table 4)
Clinical examination	Loss of consciousness, vocalization, and volitional activity
	Failed standard apnea test
	Absent brainstem function:
	Midposition or fully fixed and dilated pupils
	Absent spontaneous eye movements, oculocephalic, and oculovestivular reflexes
	Absent movement of lower cranial nerve musculature (pharynx, larynx, uvula, including gag or cough)
	Absent corneal, sucking, and rooting reflexes
	Flaccid tone and absent spontaneous or induced movements (excluding spinal cord reflexes)
	Findings should be consistent throughout entire examination observation period
Age-specific observation and retesting	7 days of age to 2 mo: two examinations and EEGs separated by 48 hr
	2 mo to 1 yr of age: two examinations and EEGs separated by at least 24 hrs or initial examination plus isoelectric EEG followed by nuclear medicine study confirming no cerebral blood flow
	>1 yr of age: two examinations at least 12 hrs apart, with EEG and cerebral nuclear medicine blood flow studies optional but recommended

Source: From Ref. 29.

of brain death documentation, the term child is applied to patients less than 7 to 12 years of age. After seven years of age most children can use abstract reasoning and communication skills. By 12 years of age, the differences with young adults are minimized. In younger children language, coping skills, and reasoning are less developed, and special clinical exam criteria are needed (29). Accordingly, a few changes in the clinical exam and retesting frequency are recommended (Table 6). These pediatric-specific principles are most useful for children less than seven years of age. ☞ **The criteria for assessing brain death in children incorporates the routine use of confirmatory tests as well as longer observation periods between examinations, as underscored by the variability of EEG and nuclear studies in newborns in comparison to the clinical exam (Table 6).** ☞

ORGAN DONATION
Balancing Sensitivity for the Grieving Family with the Need for Organ Donors

Most families have a better understanding of the organ donation process if the ICU staff entirely separates the declaration of brain death from discussions about organ donation. Thus, the determination of brain death is performed first

and presented to the family who are given time to digest the information (11,13,30). Before support is withdrawn, a request for organ donation is made by a representative of the Organ Procurement Organization (OPO). ☞ **Decoupling of the process of brain death declaration from the request for organ donation has resulted in an increase in next of kin authorizing organ donations (11,30,31).** ☞

Visceral organ transplantation is a relatively recent achievement with the first successful kidney transplant having occurred in 1954, from a twin living related donor, and the first successful cardiac transplantation in 1967 (1,2,6,33). Dramatic improvements in transplanted organ survival have occurred recent years due to advances in modern surgical techniques and immunosuppressive medications. Thus, a large backlog of patients with failing internal organs exists, all of whom are awaiting the donation of healthy organs. Advancements in immunosuppressive care and surgical techniques has improved both survival, following transplantation, and life style (34). Due to the expanding world population the number of patients awaiting transplantation has increased exponentially while available organs for donation has increased only linearly. On January 1, 2000, there were 71,380 patients in the United States on waiting lists for organ transplantation. For perspective on the availability of organs for transplantation, there were 64,579 transplant-eligible patients in 1998, and 21,197 received organ transplantation (personal communication—Gift of Life Organ Procurement Organization).

☞ **Several strategies have been developed to procure more organs for donation (27). These strategies include expanding the pool of acceptable donors, the use of living related donors, education of the public to the benevolence of organ donation, and use of non-heart-beating donors (33,35–38).** ☞

The trauma population provides a large pool of potential donors because serious head injury and subsequent brain death can frequently occur in an otherwise minimally injured patient. Experience with organ donation has demonstrated that donors who at one time were thought to be unsuitable can provide quality solid organs for transplantation (33,39). Table 7 lists the general requirements for live organ donations. Currently, organs are accepted from donors as old as 80, especially since many of the recipients are also elderly. The only two absolute contraindications for organ donation are systemic cancer and a disseminated viral infection such as rabies, HIV, or West Nile virus. Bacterial infections that are antibiotic sensitive are only relative contraindications.

Another technique to expand the pool of organ donors is the use of living related donors such as a sibling

Table 7 Requirements for Live Organ Donors

Competent—able to give consent
Willing to donate
Free of coercion
Medically suitable
Psychosocially suitable
Fully informed of risks and benefits as donor
Fully informed of risks and benefits to recipient
Benefits to both donor and recipient must outweigh risks of donation and transplantation

Source: From Ref. 35.

donating a kidney or lobar lung to a brother or sister or a parent donating part of his/her liver or lung to a child (33,36,37). Improved surgical techniques for obtaining organs from living related donors, such as laparoscopic nephrectomies should, increase the popularity of this technique by decreasing donors' morbidity. Improved recipient immunosuppression has allowed the potential donor pool to expand to those unrelated to the recipient, but with an emotional relationship such as a spouse (34). It is even possible for living donors to donate kidneys to strangers.

Public education of the desirability of postmortem organ donations has led to laws that present people with the opportunity to designate their wish to be an organ donor on their driver's license before they become critically ill. Permission must still be obtained from the next of kin in cases where the patients have expressed on their driver's license their desire to donate their organs.

Role of the Organ Procurement Organization

Public education about organ procurement has derived from studies conducted to determine what makes a family decide to donate or not donate their relatives' organs. These studies have revealed that decoupling the request for organ donation from the discussion of death (or brain death) with a relative increases the likelihood that families will agree to organ donation (11,30). Therefore, the medical staff discusses with the family the facts that the patient has suffered a devastating brain injury and will be tested for brain death. Later the ICU staff informs the family of the results of the brain death test. If the patient is declared brain dead, the relatives are provided time to grieve and accept their loss. After a brief period of mourning, a representative from the OPO approaches the family about the issue of organ donation. General principles of cadavaric organ donation are listed in Table 8. This process has been better accepted by families than a combined discussion of organ donation and possible brain death. Similarly, if a patient has irrecoverable brain damage, but is not brain dead and the family wishes to withdraw life support, the issue of non-heart-beating organ donation (NHBOD) should be introduced only after the decision to withdraw support is finalized (see below) (32).

Non-Heart-Beating Organ Donation (Special Case)

The NHBOD organ procurement protocol was designed to expand the pool of available organs for donation (35). In this (still controversial) scenario, a person with devastating, irrecoverable brain damage, but possessing a few residual brainstem reflexes (thus not brain dead), and whose family has decided to withdraw life support becomes an organ donor after support is withdrawn and the patient is declared

dead. Most commonly the patient is withdrawn from mechanical ventilatory support, and sedatives and analgesia are administered while the patient is allowed to die from respiratory and cardiac arrest. The sedatives and analgesics are administered to ensure that the patient does not suffer any more under the ethical principle of "double effect" (see Volume 2, Chapter 67). Double effect states that although sedatives and analgesics may hasten death as a secondary effect, their primary intent is to allow death to occur without pain, fear, anxiety; thus their administration is ethically moral.

The withdrawal of life support for NHBOD patients often takes place in the operating room (OR), but can occur in the ICU, or a room adjacent to the OR. After the cardiac death occurs the patient is transferred to the operating room for organ procurement. After the patient's heart stops, a suitable time period is allowed to pass (1–2 minutes of cardiac asystole) to ensure that the patient is indeed dead before transporting to the OR, and before the kidneys and/or liver are perfused with cold preservation fluid and removed (38).

Close monitoring of the actual support withdrawal and organ donation process at the University of Pittsburgh, in 15 NHBOD cases, demonstrated that no one's heart spontaneously restarted following more than one minute of circulatory cessation. Therefore, DeVita et al. recommend a two-minute wait following cessation of the circulation as documented by loss of the heart beat and pulse (40). This two-minute delay would ensure the patient's cardiopulmonary death, yet also minimize the warm ischemia time for donated kidneys and liver. This is an obviously important consideration, made even more salient when it is revealed that 45 minutes of warm ischemia time is the maximum tolerated by most solid organs, and at least one patient in the De Vita study took 33 minutes following extubation to become asystolic (i.e., likely had marginal organ perfusion for many of these 33 minutes prior to cardiac asystole).

Although initial organ transplantation was performed after the donors suffered cardiac arrest, this technique, which puts transplanted organs at risk for warm ischemic damage, has sparked medical and ethical debate about its propriety. Indeed, some in the medical community view NHBOD to be akin to euthanasia (38). Furthermore, the NHBOD technique is suitable only for donation of kidneys, livers, pancreas, and (occasionally) lungs.

Non-heart-beating organ donation is not euthanasia. Mechanical ventilation and intravenous hemodynamic support are withdrawn in NHBOD just as they would be in the ICU—while the patient receives sedatives and analgesics (but no neuromuscular blockade drugs), and no drugs with the specific intent of hastening death (i.e., no KCl solution) are administered, rather, patients are allowed to naturally expire. That the withdrawal often occurs in the operating room is the only difference. To avoid potential conflicts of interest, the anesthesiologist is usually tasked with declaring the patient dead before the transplant team begins organ procurement. If the patient's heart beat and respiration remain strong and he/she doesn't die within an hour, the organ procurement is canceled and the patient is returned to the ICU or to the floor for hospice-type care. Whether or not the patient is extubated after the termination of ventilator support is up to local hospital custom. Likewise, the use of intravenous opioids and sedatives as a comfort measure are also up to local hospital custom of withdrawing support for terminally ill patients (35,38). However, the

Table 8   General Principles of Cadavaric Organ Donation

Society benefits from promoting organ donation
Cadavaric donors of internal organs must be brain dead when organs are removed
Active euthanasia is absolutely prohibited
Policies and procedural protocols are completely open to the general public
Informed consent is required
Wishes of donors and their families are respected and honored

Source: From Ref. 50.

administration of sedatives and analgesics at withdrawal of life support from hopelessly ill patients at end of life is a well-established practice, and endorsed by medical ethicists as well as the authors (41). Heparin must be given in time to circulate through the solid organs to prevent post mortem coagulation from obstructing organ circulation. Many institutions also administer phentolamine to block vasoconstriction in the vital organs. Although phentolamine has the potential to cause systemic vasodilation, its use will result in better preservation of organs by preventing sympathetic nervous system vasoconstriction. Because, the systemic vasodilation effect of phentolamine may hasten death, phentolamine use is controversial (42). The survival of kidneys from non-heart–beating donors is comparable to kidneys from brain dead donors (43).

INTENSIVE CARE UNIT MANAGEMENT OF THE BRAIN DEAD ORGAN DONOR

Once an ICU patient has been identified as a potential organ donor and declared brain dead, management decisions are aimed at ensuring optimum survival of potential transplantable organs. ☞ **Optimal care of organ donors requires maintenance of organ perfusion, oxygen delivery, body temperature, and euvolemia with normal serum sodium values.** ☞ Boyd et al. suggest classifying organ donors according to their stability allowing clinicians to prioritize management (44). Stable patients can tolerate further ICU management while awaiting operating room time and the arrival of the transplant team (organ sharing, multiple procurements) without jeopardizing their organ function. Moderately stable patients that respond to vasopressors can be maintained in the ICU while the organ-tissue typing and recipient compatibility process occurs. However, moderately unstable patients with a poor response to therapy, and unstable patients who don't respond to corrective therapy need to proceed to the operating room with urgency, and in some case their organs offered for organ sharing during or after procurement. The only solid organs suitable for this emergent "crash" organ procurement process are for liver, kidney, and pancreas. The heart and lungs are much less tolerant of ischemia (maximum cold ischemia time 4–6 hours). Thus, crash organ procurement is not a viable procedure for heart or lung transplantation because the potential recipients must already be in the hospital and ready for the operating room at time of procurement, otherwise these organs will not be viable.

Recently declared "brain dead" donors occasionally undergo a brief period of medical optimization prior to organ procurement. ☞ **In these patients, simple volume resuscitation is adequate to achieve Phillips' Rule of Hundreds—systolic pressure >100 mmHg, PaO₂ >100 mmHg, and urine output >100 mL/hr (44).** ☞ Moderately stable patients are divided into two categories: those with a good response to volume loading and pressors to achieve Phillips' Rule of Hundreds and those with a transient response to volume loading and pressors. This second group often requires escalating pressor therapy to maintain systolic blood pressure. Finally, the grossly unstable patient never achieves Phillips' Rule of Hundreds and requires the greatest urgency to salvage transplantable organs (Table 9).

Table 9 Perioperative Management of the Multiorgan Donation

Step 1	Ensure that patient meets criteria for brain death or support withdrawal
Phillips' Rule of 100s	Systolic BP >100 mmHg PaO₂ > 100 mmHg urinary output >100 mL/hr
Cardiovascular	Maintain perfusion pressure through adequate hydration and inotropic/pressure support ot treat dysrrhythmias
Pulmonary	Maintain normal blood gases: PaO₂ 100–150 mmHg PaCO₂ 35–40 mmHg, pH 7.35–7.45 F₁O₂ ≤ 0.40 for heart-lungs donation
Endocrine	Treat diabetes insipidus—replace urine output and DDAVP or vasopressin titrate to urine output 2–3 mL/kg/hr
Hematology	Prevent anemia—maintain hematocrit near 30% Minimize coagulopathy

Abbreviations: BP, blood pressure; P$_a$O$_2$, partial pressure of oxygen in the arterial blood; P$_a$CO$_2$, partial pressure of carbon dioxide in arterial blood; FiO$_2$, fraction of inhaled oxygen; DDAVP, D-des-argenine-vasopressin (Desmopressin®).

Hemodynamic Management

Hypotension usually accompanies brain death when the vasomotor centers in the brainstem become impaired. Furthermore the hypotension is exacerbated by both the decreased cardiac output from diminished brainstem mediated inotropy, as well as the intra-vascular depletion resulting from diabetes insipidus (DI) (44,45). Patients should be monitored with an intra-arterial catheter and central venous pressure (CVP) catheter.

The first step toward improving blood pressure in the brain dead organ donor is to provide adequate volume resuscitation. Although transplantable kidneys perform very well when the donor is managed in the hypervolemic state causing a brisk diuresis, other transplantable organs (particularly heart and lungs) do not perform as well when obtained from a hypervolemic, edematous donor. Therefore, maintenance of a CVP in the 5–10 mmHg range and use of pressors/inotrops if the systolic pressure remains less than 100 mm Hg is recommended in heart and lung donor patients.

Volume loading should also lead to a urine output >100 mL/hr. If urine output is much greater than 100 mL/hr, intravenous fluid management must include replacement for urine output to keep CVP in the 5–10 mmHg range.

The decision to place a pulmonary artery catheter is usually based on the possibility of donation of a heart or lung for transplantation. The pulmonary artery catheter is optional for the management of a donor who is not going to donate heart or lungs. Additionally, the management of the stable and moderately stable patient is often facilitated by the information from a pulmonary artery catheter. End points of volume resuscitation are often more clearly achieved by following cardiac output and pulmonary artery pressure as well as CVP. The unstable donor who needs pressor and inotropic support as well as volume loading will be managed more optimally with a pulmonary artery catheter.

Ventilation Management and Infection Control

The brain dead organ donor has an obligatory dependence on mechanical ventilators for ventilation and gas exchange. The respiratory centers in the lower brainstem that normally integrate demand signals from blood pH, $PaCO_2$, and PaO_2 and match these signals with appropriate ventilatory response are dead and unresponsive. Therefore, the patient will not activate the respiratory muscles for ventilation in response to hypercarbia and hypoxia. Thus, the medical team caring for the organ donor must review the arterial blood gases and adjust the ventilator to optimize them.

Because the organs for potential donation require adequate oxygen delivery to maintain function, it is recommended to aim for a PaO_2 of 100 mmHg or greater. Controlled ventilation modes, either pressure control or volume control, are used on the ventilator because the donor is incapable of spontaneous ventilation. The F_IO_2 is adjusted to provide a PaO_2 >100 mmHg while ventilation is set to normalize $PaCO_2$. The brain dead donor has a lower metabolic rate and a reduced CO_2 production that needs to be cleared by ventilation to maintain $PaCO_2$.

Care must be exercised to prevent ventilator-induced lung injury for the potential lung donor. Thus, tidal volume should be kept in the 6–7 mL/kg range if lung compliance is low, whereas 10–15 mL/kg is acceptable if the compliance is normal. Additionally, the positive and expiratory pressure (PEEP) is kept at the minimum required to maintain the PaO_2 >100 mmHg or an $F_IO_2 \leq 0.4$ or less. These patients must continue to be turned and suctioned every two to four hours. Albuterol metered dose inhalers (MDI) are administered 2 to 4 puffs every four hours to minimize closure of small airways.

Endocrine Changes

Diabetes insipidus (DI) occurs very frequently in the brain dead donor secondary to infarction of the hypothalamus and pituitary. Loss of antidiuretic hormone (ADH) from the pituitary leads to inability of the kidney to concentrate the urine, thus the patient excretes copious dilute urine. The hallmarks of DI are urine output >4 mL/kg/hr, urine osmolality <300 mOsm/kg, with serum osmolality >310 mOsm/kg, serum sodium [Na] >145/meg/L, and a urine specific gravity <1.005. Treatment is with intravenous vasopressin for both blood pressure and urinary concentration or DDAVP to concentrate urinary solutes and conserve free water losses. Either drug is titrated to maintain urinary output at 2–3 mL/kg/hr (44,45).

Serum sodium also needs to be controlled because livers from donors with Na >155 have reduced graft survival. Extreme hyponatremia, which usually precedes the occurrence of brain death, must also be corrected before the patient is transferred to the operating room. Brain dead donors are also prone to develop profound hypokalemia, hypomagnesemia, and hypophosphatemia because of the high urinary output. These electrolyte abnormalities must be corrected prior to organ explantation in the operating room.

Other metabolic and endocrine abnormalities that must be corrected include hyperglycemia, thyroid insufficiency, and adrenal suppression. Hyperglycemia secondary to reduced insulin secretion or catecholamines and glucocorticoid administration is treated with intravenous insulin.

Brain dead donors often have depressed thyroid function similar to the "sick euthyroid" syndrome; it is controversial whether thyroid replacement is needed. Because T_3 levels are reduced by the "sick euthyroid" syndrome, the administration of thyroid replacement as a single dose of T_3 or T_4 is occasionally recommended.

The brain dead donor will have an impaired immune response; therefore, they must be managed with careful techniques to avoid seeding an infection in donor organs. Hyperthermia and fever is seldom a problem with the brain dead donor because hypothalamic temperature control centers are destroyed when the brainstem infarcts (i.e., these patients become poikilothermic) (44,45). These donors should be kept at 36°C to 37°C to optimize organ function before transplantation. If heated fluids and a warm room do not adequately maintain a normal body temperature, forced hot air warming (e.g., Bair Hugger®) may be required, but these are only recommended for temperature <36°C.

If the organ donor received enough dexamethasone to suppress adrenal function prior to brain death, he will need replacement therapy with hydrocortisone.

OPERATIVE MANAGEMENT DURING ORGAN PROCUREMENT

✐ **Management of the organ donor in the operating room (OR) is a continuation of the hemodynamic, temperature, and endocrine (diabetes insipidus) management of the organ donor in the ICU.** ✐ The goal of the donor procurement process is to recover viable organs with minimal warm ischemia time, hypotension, hypoxia, or surgical trauma. The procedure described below pertains to procurement from the brain dead organ donor only. Readers interested in a review of organ procurement considerations for the NHBOD are referred to the discussion by Von Norman (42).

General Considerations

Prior to transporting the brain dead donor to the OR, the anesthesiologist ensures that the patient meets appropriate criteria for brain death, has permission to be an organ donor, and that the consent stipulates which organs are to be procured. The stable patient can be managed on a more elective basis than the moderately unstable and unstable patient. Unstable patients must have priority of operating room space in order to procure viable organs for transplantation.

The operating room needs to be warm to prevent hypothermia, as the brain dead patient is poikilothermic, and regional cooling and perfusion of certain organs in situ, prior to perfusion of the heart and lungs, may cause premature hypothermia-induced dysrhythmias or arrest.

Phillips' Rule of 100s is the goal of cardiopulmonary management during the organ exposure phase of surgery prior to aortic cross clamping. Fluid management and pressors should be continued into the operating room to maintain blood pressure and urine output. The ventilator is adjusted to maintain PaO_2 greater than 100 mmHg. Frequently, anesthesiologists administer inhalational anesthesia and muscle relaxants to prevent Lazarus reflexes and occasional hypertension with surgical organ exposure (46–48).

Rationale for Organ Excision Sequence

The precise operative sequence depends upon the organs to be procured, and to some degree on the routine of the teams involved. However, certain general concepts are universally

Table 10 Donor Organ Excision Order and Cold Perfusion Solution Type, Amount, and Cannula Location

Standard excision order	Organ	Perfusion solution type (amount)	Cold perfusion cannula site
1	Heart	Cardioplegia (1–2 L)	Ascending aorta
2	Lungs	Pulmoplegia (3–6 L)	Pulmonary aorta
3	Liver	Viaspan™ᵃ (5–6 L)	Abdominal aorta and mesenteric vein
4	Pancreas	Viaspan™ᵃ (5–6 L)	Abdominal aorta
5	Kidneys	Viaspan™ᵃ (5–6 L)—if all abdominal organs procured (2 L)—if only kidneys procured	Abdominal aorta

ᵃBelzer's UW Solution.

followed (Table 10). The thoracic organs (heart and lungs) are less ischemia tolerant than the abdominal viscera (liver, pancreas, kidneys, small bowel), and are removed first when procured. Despite this, abdominal team will often start their part of the pre-excision visceral exposure and vessel cannulation prior to the thoracic team because the abdominal dissection takes longer. Both teams communicate with each other, and cold preservation fluids are never administered until after aortic cross clamp, which only occurs at a mutually agreed upon time in a special choreographed way (described below). This approach avoids premature or inadvertent cardiac arrest, which could damage the donor organs.

Technical Overview of Organ Procurement

The sequence provided below occurs when both the thoracic and abdominal teams begin operative exposure together. The donor patient is positioned on the OR table in the supine position, and the anesthesiologist assures all appropriate monitoring is applied and functioning optimally. Surgical skin preparation and draping commences with exposure of the entire anterior chest, abdomen, and both groins. The thoracic team makes a standard median sternotomy, then carries the incision down the midline to join the full-length midline abdominal incision created by the abdominal team (which carries down to the pubic symphasis).

Hemostasis is obtained while exposing the pericardium and great vessels. After pericardiotomy, the heart size and function is assessed, and the epicardial coronary arteries are grossly palpated for atherosclerotic plaques. Additionally, the heart is systematically inspected for any other abnormalities. Next, the lungs are inspected grossly for size and examined for any previously undiagnosed lesions or abnormalities. Once both the heart and lungs have passed the gross inspection, the ascending aorta is dissected and circumferentially freed of attachments, to the level of the left subclavian (in preparation for later placement of the thoracic aortic cross clamp). The superior vena cava (SVC) and inferior vena cava (IVC) have loosely placed circumferential vascular tapes with rubbershods for

later vascular control. The thoracic team may scrub out of the case for a brief respite while the abdominal team completes their, more time consuming, dissection.

The liver is exposed and freed from its ligamentous attachments to the diaphragm. The abdominal aorta above the celiac artery is encircled with loose ligature placed circumferentially, and rubbershods are placed for later. Next, the hepatic artery is identified, and the inferior mesenteric vein is cannulated with a tube and infused with normal saline to keep the vein open (Pre-Cool); later this line will be used to infuse cold perfusion fluid as part of the systemic cooling. The donor's kidneys are then dissected and renal arteries and veins are identified and vascular control is obtained (loose vascular tapes—with rubbershods as above). Similarly, other visceral organs to be transplanted are dissected out. Once this is done, the thoracic team returns, and the patient is systemically anticoagulated (typically 40,000 units heparin). Perfusion catheters are then inserted into the ascending aorta (which will soon be used to infuse 1–2 L of cold cardioplegia solution), and pulmonary artery (soon to be used to perfuse 3–6 L of cold pulmonoplegia solution). Cannulas are also placed in the abdominal vessels (which will soon receive 5–6 L) of cold Viaspan™ (Belzer's UW Solution) (Table 10). The typical placements for the two abdominal cannulas are the descending aorta (just below the previously placed loose ligature at the crus of the diaphragm) and the inferior mesenteric vein (which flows to the portal vein—this catheter was placed previously). Once all cold infusion catheters are properly placed, and all teams are ready, two aortic cross clamps are applied simultaneously. The first one is applied on the thoracic aorta; just proximal to the subclavian vein; and the other cross clamp is applied to the abdominal aorta, at the crus of the diaphragm. Immediately after aortic cross clamp, the cold preservation fluids are perfused through the previously situated cannulas, and the IVC is transected to vent the warm blood (some prefer to vent the IVC into the abdomen; some prefer to vent into a large, caliber drainage tube directly into the suction canister, diverting heat away from donor organs.

After all of the cardioplegia solution is infused in the heart (ascending aorta), and the pulmoplegia has perfused the lungs (via pulmonary artery), and the Viaspan™ (Belzer's UW Soln.) has perfused the visceral organs (via abdominal aorta and mesenteric vein), the organs are resected working from the top down (hearts, lungs, liver, pancreas, kidneys). After excision, some surgeons will administer additional cold flush to the excised organs on the back table (1–2 L of the appropriate fluid) prior to bagging for transport.

The heart is rinsed and examined for any valvular lesions or a patent foramen ovale (PFO); if present, the PFO is noted (for later repair at the recipient institution), and the heart is placed in a sterile plastic bag full of cold cardioplegia solution. This bag is placed within two other bags, and sealed, and then placed inside a bag of cold cardioplegia slush, placed in an ice chest and shipped to the recipient hospital (only 4–6 hours of ischemia time starting with x-clamp is allowed). Similarly, the perfused lungs are inspected again and placed inside a sterile plastic bag of cold pulmoplegia fluid, (triple bagged) and then placed inside a bag of cold pulmoplegia slush, and placed inside bags, and the organs are then placed in insulated labeled coolers for transport.

After the thoracic team has removed the heart and lungs, the abdominal team removes the organs located below the diaphragm. The common bile duct and hepatic artery are divided, and the freed liver is removed. Next, the ureters are dissected and divided, the aorta and vena cava on either side of the renal pedicles are transected, followed by enbloc nephrectomy. These organs are triple bagged in cold Viaspan™ (Belzer's UW Soln.) analogous to that described for the heart and lungs.

After the aorta is cross-clamped and organs perfused with their corresponding solutions, the ventilator is switched off and the anesthesiologist's role has concluded. During the entire procedure, the donor cadaver should be treated with dignity and respect, to honor ethical, religious, and cultural norms.

EYE TO THE FUTURE

Despite more than 30 years' experience with brain death as one criteria for determining death, some clinicians are still skeptical of the concepts (49,50). Thus, we are likely to see continued reevaluation of brain death criteria and refinement of the diagnosis. Additionally work needs to be done to educate the public that brain death is synonymous with death of the sentient portion of the individual, and that a declaration of brain death is synonymous with death of the patient even though some tissues (heart, lungs, liver, kidney, pancreas, bowel, skin) can be kept alive by artificial means. The medical profession also needs to emphasize to the public the difference between brain death and persistent vegetative state (51).

Alternatively, Truog and Robinson propose that society scrap the whole concept of brain death (47). They further propose that organ donation occur from patients who give informed consent to receive euthanasia under anesthesia while their vital organs are procured for recipients in organ failure. Society is unlikely to be persuaded by the arguments of Truog and Robinson, and it is unlikely that many anesthesiologists would agree to participate in the administration of such terminal anesthetics. Their arguments against brain death also fail to address the original need to acknowledge brain death: reduce the prolonged futile ICU management of patients who were already dead from permanent loss of brain function and infarction of most or all of their brain. A movement toward the simpler, yet equally valid, U.K. criteria of brainstem death would be a far more pragmatic remedy for the numerous confounding brain death definitions.

The search for chemical markers of brain death is probably at least a decade away. However, Dimopoulou et al. have recently identified a serum protein (S-100b), which is elevated in brain dead patients (52). These investigators found that the median S-100b level was higher in clinically brain dead patients than those patients who did not become brain dead ($p < 0.0001$). The S-100b protein has a high specificity for CNS lesions, is released in a time locked sequenced with injury, has a short half life, and does not have any significant age or gender variability. The presence of elevated S-100b in the serum indicates that both brain cell damage has occurred, and that there is increased permeability of the blood–brain barrier. Although far more additional work is required to determine the extents to which this protein can be used clinically, experimental results indicate that S-100b might be used in a fashion analogous to myocardial infarction markers (e.g., troponin), and when elevated, indicate the degree of brain injury (cell death) that has occurred. While the S-100b protein studies

are intriguing, they cannot be construed as a serological surrogate for the clinical determination of brain death.

Care of critically ill patients has revealed that death of various tissues or organs within the body occur as a complex temporal process, rather than as an instantaneous event for the entire body. This scientific fact has facilitated the philosophical and scientific concept of brain death. Skin cells, with their lower metabolic requirements, remain viable much longer than most other cells in the body, whereas neurons within the central nervous system are the least tolerant to ischemia, and some of these (i.e., hippocampal neurons) may be the least tolerant of all. In the critically ill TBI patient, supported by mechanical ventilation, death of the brain and brain stem may represent the first organs to die in a long succession of dying organs. With this current understanding and the ongoing research in neurophysiology and neurophilosophy, we may one day in the future evolve to a new definition of brain death; one where death of certain critical structures in the brain that are absolutely required for reasoning and understanding would be tantamount to brain death (16,18,20,21).

SUMMARY

Advances in life support techniques following World War II led to the appearance in intensive care units of patients who were unresponsive and totally dependent on ventilator support. When these patients succumbed to cardiac arrest, autopsy would reveal a liquefied brain, which was named "respirator brain." A Harvard University committee published a paper in JAMA that outlined the procedure to recognize that a critically ill patient's brain had died, thus rendering further care futile (5). This concept of brain death was used to effectively allow cessation of futile intensive care and coincided with the rapidly developing field of organ transplantation. Because it was recognized that death of the brain and brainstem was equivalent to death of the entire patient, it became permissible to procure solid organs from brain dead patients and minimize warm ischemic organ damage.

State laws have been updated to be consistent with guidelines of the Uniform Determination of Death Act, allowing physicians to declare a patient's death based on permanent cessation of brain and brain stem activity or permanent cessation of respiration and cardiac activity. The medical diagnosis of brain death requires: (i) brain damage consistent with permanent loss of brain function and lack of confounding metabolic or pharmacologic factors (not hypothermic, normal electrolytes, metabolism, metabolites, and no sedatives or neuromuscular blocking drugs), and (ii) total loss of responsiveness (spinal cord reflexes are allowed).

There continues to be an ever-increasing demand for organ donation from brain dead patients because of the advances in organ transplantation medicine has made it the treatment of choice for many types of organ failure. Strategies to increase the supply of donated organs include societal educational efforts to increase the percentage of brain dead patients who donate organs, expanding the pool of acceptable organs by accepting a wider age range of donors and less than perfect organs, increasing the use of live donors, and the use of non-heart–beating donors.

Although non-heart–beating donors or patients who died from cardiopulmonary arrest were the original cadavaric organ donors, this technique has fallen out of favor because the transplanted organs suffer longer warm ischemic times. Organs from brain dead donors that are procured while the heart is still beating have much shorter ischemic times. However, survival of kidney grafts from either procedure is comparable. Non-heart–beating donors are patients with extremely poor prognosis from brain injury who maintain some level of brainstem activity. Withdrawal of life support typically occurs in the operating room, and organ removal is delayed until the patient is declared dead (typically after 1–2 minutes of asystole).

The diagnosis and management of brain dead trauma patients is an important aspect of post-traumatic critical care to optimize the potential pool of organ donors and to prevent futile care of otherwise dead patients.

KEY POINTS

✐ Dr. Beecher's white paper, published in JAMA in 1968, concentrated on limiting the use of ICUs to maintain futile life support for patients who had no chance of recovery secondary to death and necrosis of their entire brain.

✐ Currently, the U.S. standard to declare brain death is to document the absence of brain and brain stem activity.

✐ The current U.K. standard for the diagnosis of brain death is complete and irreversible loss of brainstem function.

✐ A patient who meets the clinical definition of brain death by either the U.S. or U.K. criteria is in essence dead as a person, as he/she will never recover sentient function.

✐ Brain death is diagnosed clinically with the establishment of three major criteria. First, the neurological injury should be irreversible. Second, there is a loss of cerebral function. Third, there is a loss of brainstem function.

✐ Spinal reflexes, such as deep tendon reflexes and triple flexion responses, can be preserved and do not exclude brain death. Release phenomena of the spinal cord are occasionally seen in the setting of brain death and do not exclude brain death; these include shivering, goose bumps, forced exhalation, and some arm movements.

✐ Confirmatory tests are not necessary for the declaration of brain death in the vast majority of cases. They may be used in cases where the observation period needs to be shortened (unstable patient intended for organ donation), children younger than one, and when clinical brain death testing is confounded by certain agents and/or conditions.

✐ Nuclear medicine cerebral blood flow studies are increasingly used as the confirmatory test, because the equipment can be brought to the ICU providing images with the presence or lack of radioactive tracer within the cranial vault.

✐ The criteria for assessing brain death in children incorporates the routine use of confirmatory tests as well as a longer observation period between examinations, as underscored by the variability of EEG and nuclear studies in newborns in comparison to the clinical exam.

✐ Decoupling of the process of brain death declaration from the request for organ donation has resulted in an increase in next of kin authorizing organ donations.

✐ Several strategies have been developed to procure more organs for donation. These strategies include expanding the pool of acceptable donors, the use of living related donors, education of the public to the benevolence of organ donation, and, use of non-heart-beating donors.

✐ Optimal care of organ donors requires maintenance of organ perfusion, oxygen delivery, body temperature, and euvolemia with normal serum sodium values.

✐ In these patients, simple volume resuscitation is adequate to achieve Phillips' Rule of Hundreds—systolic pressure >100 mmHg, PaO_2 >100 mmHg, and urine output >100 mL/hr.

✐ Management of the organ donor in the OR is a continuation of the hemodynamic, temperature, and endocrine (diabetes insipidus) management of the organ donor in the ICU.

REFERENCES

1. Van Norman GA. A matter of life and death: what every anesthesiologist should know about the medical, legal, and ethical aspects of declaring brain death. Anesthesiology 1999; 91:275–287.
2. Jennett B, Gleave S, Wilson P. Brain death in three neurosurgical units. Brit Med J 1981; 282:533–539.
3. Cook R. Coma. Boston: Little, Brown. 1977.
4. Mollaret P, Goulon M: Le coma dépassé (mémoire préliminaire). Rev Neurol (Paris) 1959; 101:3–5.
5. Report of the Ad Hoc Committee of the Harvard Medical School to examine the definition of brain death. A definition of irreversible coma. JAMA 1968; 205:85–88.
6. Report of the Medical Consultants on the diagnosis of death to the President's commission for the study of ethical problems in medicine and biomedical behavioral research. Guidelines for the determination of brain death. JAMA 1981; 246:2184.
7. Wijdicks EFM. Brain death worldwide: accepted fact but no global consensus in diagnostic criteria. Neurology 2002; 58: 20–25.
8. American Academy of Neurology. Practice parameters for determining brain death in adults. Neurology 1995; 45:1012–1014.
9. Mohandas A, Chou SN. Brain death: a clinical and pathological study. J Neurosurg 1971; 35:211–218.
10. Diagnosis of brain death: statement issued by the honorary secretary of the conference of Medical Royal College and their Faculties in the United Kingdom on 11 October 1976. Brit Med J 1976; 2:1187–1188.
11. Franz HG, DeJong W, Wolfe SM, Nathan H, Payne D, Reitsma W, Beasley C. Explaining brain death: a critical feature of the donation process. J Transplant Coordination 1997; 7:14–21.
12. Plum F, Posner JB. The diagnosis of stupor and coma. 3rd edn. Philadelphia: F.A. Davis, 1980:313–324.
13. Wijdicks EFM. The diagnosis of brain death. N Engl J Med 2001; 344:1215–1221.
14. Wijdicks EFM. Neurology of critical illness. Philadelphia: F.A. Davis, 1995:323–337.
15. Beresford HR. Brain death. Neurologic Clinics 1999; 17: 295–306.
16. Crick Francis. The Astonishing Hypothisis: The Scientific Search for the Soul. New York: Simon and Schuster, 1994:317.
17. Singer C. A Short History of Anatomy and Physiology from the Greeks to Harvey. New York: Dover Publications, 1957.
18. Churchland PS. Brain-wise: Studies in neurophilosophy. Cambridge: MIT Press, 2002:471.
19. Major's Physical Diagnosis. An introduction to clinical process. 9th ed. Delp MT, Manning RT (ed), Philadelphia: W.B. Saunders, 1981.
20. Churchland PM. Matter and Consciousness—Revised Edition: A Contemporary Introduction to the Philosophy of Mind. Cambridge: MIT Press, 1988:181.
21. Hoch C. The Quest for Consciousness: A Neurobiological Approach. Englewood: Colorado Roberts and Co., 2004:429.

22. Rapenne T, Moreau D, Lenfant F, Boggio V, Cottin Y, Freysz M. Could heart rate variability analysis become an early predictor of imminent brain death? A pilot study. Anesth Analg 2000; 91:329–336.

23. Qureshi AI, Geocadin RG, Suarez JI, Ulatowski JA. Long-term outcome after medical reversal of transtentorial herniation in patients with supratentorial mass lesions. Crit Care Med 2000; 28:1556–1564.

24. Donselaar CV, Meerwaldt JD, Gijn JV. Apnea testing to confirm brain death in clinical practice. J Neurol Neurosur Psych 1986; 49:1071–1073.

25. Frumin J, Epstein RM, Cohen G. Apneic oxygenation in man. Anesthesiology 1959; 20:789–798.

26. Schafer JA, Caronna JJ. Duration of apnea needed to confirm brain death. Neurology 1978; 28:661–666.

27. Kuwagata Y, Sugimoto H, Yoshioka T, Sugimoto T. Hemodynamic response with passive neck flexion in brain death. Neurosurgery 1991; 29:239–241.

28. Harding JW, Chatterton BE. Outcomes of patients referred for confirmation of brain death by 99mTc-exametazime scintigraphy. Intensive Care Med 2003; 29:539–543.

29. Lynch J, Eldadah MK. Brain death criteria currently used by pediatric intensivists. Clin Pediatr 1992; 31:457–460.

30. Siminoff LA, Gordon N, Hewlett J, Arnold RM. Factors influencing families' consent for donation of solid organs for transplantation. JAMA 2001; 286:71–77.

31. Gortmaker SL, Beasley CL, Sheehy E, Lucas BA, Brigham LE, Grenvik A, Patterson RH, Garrison RN, McNamara P, Evanisko MJ. Improving the request process to increase family consent for organ donation. J Transplant Coordination 1998; 8:210–217.

32. Suthanthiran M, Strom TB. Renal transplantation. N Engl J Med 1994; 331:365–375.

33. Gridelli B, Remuzzi G. Strategies for making more organs available for transplantation. N Engl J Med 2000; 343:404–410.

34. Harlan DM, Kirk AD. The future of organ and tissue transplantation: can T-cell costimulatory pathway modifiers revolutionize the prevention of graft rejection? JAMA 1999; 282:1076–1082.

35. D'Alessandro AM, Hoffman RM, Belzer FO. Non-heart-beating donors: one response to the organ shortage. Transplantation Rev 1995; 9:168–176.

36. Benner P. Living organ donors: respecting the risks involved in the "gift of life." Am J Crit Care 2002; 11:266–268.

37. Live Organ Donor Consensus Group. Consensus statement on the live organ donor. JAMA 2000; 284:2919–2926.

38. Institute of Medicine. Non-heart-beating organ transplantation: medical and ethical issues in procurement. Washington, DC: National Academy Press, 1997.

39. Edwards J, Hasz R, Menendez J. Organ donors: your care is critical. RN 1997; 60(6):46–50.

40. DeVita MA, Snyder JV, Arnold RM, Siminoff LA. Observations of withdrawal of life-sustaining treatment from patients who became non-heart-beating organ donors. Crit Care Med 2000; 28:1709–1712.

41. Wilson WC, Smedira NG, Fink C, et al. Ordering and administration of sedatives and analgesics during the withholding and withdrawal of life support from critically ill patients. JAMA 1992; 267(7):949–953.

42. Van Norman G. Another matter of life and death: What every anesthesiologist should know about the ethical, legal, and policy implications of the non-heart beating cadaver organ donor. Anesthesiology 2003; 98(3):763–773.

43. Cho YW, Terasaki PI, Cecka JM, et al. Transplantation of kidneys from donors whose hearts have stopped beating. N Engl J Med 1998; 338:221–225.

44. Boyd GL, Phillips MG, Henry ML. Cadaver donor management. In: Phillips MG (ed), UNOS: Organ Procurement, Preservation and Distribution in Transplantation, 2nd ed. Richmond, VA, UNOS. 1996:81–98.

45. Robertson KM, Cook DR. Perioperative management of the multiorgan donor. Anesth Analg 1990; 70:546–556.

46. Wetzel RC, Setzer N, Stiff JL, Rogers MC. Hemodynamic responses in brain-dead organ patients. Anesth Analg 1985; 65:125–128.

47. Ropper AH. Unusual spontaneous movements in brain-dead patients. Neurology 1984; 34:1089–1092.

48. Saposnik G, Bueri JA, Maurino J, et al. Spontaneous and reflex movement in brain death. Neurology 2000; 54:221–223.

49. Truog RD, Robinson WM. Role of brain death and the dead-donor rule in the ethics of organ transplantation. Crit Care Med 2003; 31:2391–2396.

50. Doig CJ, Burgess E. Brain death: resolving inconsistencies in the ethical declaration of death. Can J Anesth 2003; 50:725–731.

51. Childs NL, Mercer WN. Late improvement in consciousness after post-traumatic vegetative state. N Engl J Med 1996; 334:24–25.

52. Dimopoulou I, Korfias S, Dafni U, et al. Protein S-100b serum levels in trauma-induced brain death. Neurology 2003; 60:947–951.

53. Henry Beecher. A definition of irreversible coma. JAMA 1968; 205:85–88.

17

Hemodynamic Management

Donnelle L. Crouse
Division of Trauma, Burns, and Critical Care, Department of Surgery, UC San Diego Medical Center, San Diego, California, U.S.A.

Martin Straznicky
Section of Cardiothoracic Anesthesia, Department of Anesthesiology, UC San Diego Medical Center, San Diego, California, U.S.A.

William C. Wilson
Department of Anesthesiology and Critical Care, UC San Diego Medical Center, San Diego, California, U.S.A.

INTRODUCTION

Optimum cardiovascular management of critically ill trauma patients often requires accepting hemodynamic indices that are reasonable rather than normal. When clinicians insist upon pushing the patient's hemodynamic system toward normal or even supranormal targets, iatrogenic complications can occur [1]

This chapter provides the trauma intensivist with a review of reasonable hemodynamic goals in hypertensive patients by surveying the normal cardiovascular indices during health, and explaining how these parameters are altered by trauma and critical illness [1–4]. This chapter also reviews the vasoactive drugs commonly used in trauma and critical care. A complete review of cardiovascular physiology is presented in Volume 2, Chapter 3 and cardiovascular monitoring in Chapter 9. Accordingly, these topics are only briefly reviewed here. The optimum management for both hypotension and significant hypertension is summarized for the most common etiologies. ☞ **Optimum hemodynamic management is based upon (*i*) the immediate cause of hypotension or hypertension, (*ii*) the presence of concomitant injuries, and (*iii*) the baseline medical conditions affecting the patient.** ☞

In the "Eye to the Future" section, we introduce some of the newer cardiovascular drugs as well as some diagnostic and monitoring tools that are on the horizon but not yet used in clinical practice.

NORMAL AND RATIONAL HEMODYNAMIC INDICES

Normal age-specific hemodynamic indices have been established for healthy patients. Following trauma and critical illness, the normal physiologic response is typified by abnormal hemodynamic indices. For example, massive hemorrhage leads to an increase in heart rate (HR), systemic vascular resistance (SVR), and contractility in compensation for the decreased intravascular volume (preload), blood pressure (BP), and cardiac output ($\dot{Q}$) [5–7]. For a brief period, these compensatory responses will help maintain $\dot{Q}$ and BP to the central circulation at the expense of an underperfused periphery. Sepsis results in an increased HR and decreased preload, but with an associated decrease in SVR and myocardial contractility. This results in a decreased BP despite an increased $\dot{Q}$.

Treatment of hemorrhage begins with control of bleeding and repletion of intravascular volume. Further decreases in BP in this setting can be potentially disastrous, as oxygen delivery ($\dot{D}O_2$) is already low. Likewise, the septic patient will likely require some additional intravascular volume, but the primary defect is sepsis-mediated vasodilation and myocardial depression. Accordingly, drainage of infected, necrotic tissue (as in necrotizing fasciitis) and immediate administration of appropriate antibiotics (Volume 2, Chapter 53) are equally important. Only after volume repletion, infection debridement, and appropriate antibiotics are instituted, should the inotropic support be initiated [8,9]. A summary of the normal hemodynamic parameters and the typical disease-related alterations in these variables is provided in Table 1.

Heart Rate

☞ **The HR should be maintained within a reasonable range in order to sustain adequate $\dot{Q}$ for tissue perfusion [10,11].** ☞ The normal resting adult HR ranges between 60 and 100 beats/min. Numerous physiologic perturbations (e.g., exercise, body temperature) and pathophysiologic insults (e.g., trauma, burns, and critical illness) result in variances in this "normal" range.

Although the relationship "$\dot{Q} = HR \times$ stroke volume (SV)" holds within the normal HR range, when HRs become excessively high, there begins to be an associated decrease in SV (i.e., decreased preload due to inadequate filling time). Accordingly, HRs above 120 should be discouraged in normal patients and rates above 90 should be prevented in patients with coronary artery disease (CAD).

Tachycardia is defined as a HR greater than 100 beats/min and is caused by mechanisms that increase the firing rate of the sinoatrial (SA) node (sinus tachycardia) and by atrial and ventricular dysrhythmias (Volume 2, Chapter 20). The most common causes of sinus tachycardia in the critical care setting result from conditions that increase sympathetic tone (e.g., hypovolemia, hypercarbia, hypoxemia, pain, fear, anxiety, etc.) and conditions that increase the metabolic rate (e.g., fever, thyroid storm, etc).

Trauma patients have several reasons why they may develop tachycardia, including hypovolemia from hemorrhage, pain, anxiety, and third spacing. Third spacing in the traumatized patient is a result of circulating cytokines causing leaky capillaries, as well as a result of decreased albumin from

Table 1 Normal Hemodynamic Parameters and the Direction of Alteration with Various Forms of Shock

	HR	MAP	PP	PACWP	Q̇	SVR	SVO$_2$	a-vdO$_2$	LAC
Normal	80	85	40	4–10	5	1200	75%	3–4	2–3
Hemorrhage	⇑⇑	⇓	⇓	⇓⇓	⇓	⇑⇑	⇓⇓	⇑	⇑⇑⇑
Sepsis	⇑	⇓	⇑⇓	⇓	⇑	⇓⇓	⇑	⇓	⇑
Cardiogenic	⇑	⇓	⇓	⇑	⇓	⇑	⇓	⇑	⇑⇑
Neurogenic	⇓	⇓	⇑⇓	⇓	⇓	⇓	⇑⇓	⇑⇓	⇑⇓

Abbreviations: HR, heart rate; LAC, lactate; MAP, mean arterial pressure; PP, pulse pressure; PACWP, pulmonary artery capillary wedge pressure; Q̇, cardiac output; SVR, systemic vascular resistance; SVO$_2$, mixed venous hemoglobin O$_2$ saturation; a-vdO$_2$, arterial–venous difference in O$_2$ saturation or content.

blood loss and crystalloid resuscitation. Additionally, hypoxemia from pulmonary contusion, pneumothorax or hemothorax, atelectasis, cardiac tamponade, myocardial contusion, sepsis, and pulmonary embolism may cause tachycardia (12). Trauma results in fever through numerous mechanisms including tissue injury, hematoma, subarachnoid blood, burns, and infection. ☞ **In a febrile patient, the basal metabolic rate increases approximately 8% per degree centigrade, which correlates with an increase in HR of approximately 18 beats/min (i.e., 10 beats/min for each degree Fahrenheit) (13,14).** ☞ Trauma patients may also develop tachycardia due to underlying medical conditions, such as thyrotoxicosis and withdrawal from alcohol or other psychotropic drugs.

Bradycardia is defined as a HR less than 60 beats/min and results from mechanisms that decrease the SA node firing rate (sinus bradycardia) as well as by pathology at the SA or atrial-ventricular (AV), node, leading to junctional or ventricular

bradydysrhythmias (Volume 2, Chapter 20). Following trauma, bradycardia can result from spinal cord injury that causes a decrease in the relative sympathetic tone (15). Brainstem ischemia, hypoxia, brainstem herniation (Cushing response), sick sinus syndrome, and myocardial ischemia (Volume 2, Chapter 19) are additional causes of bradycardia. Moderate to severe hypothermia (Volume 1, Chapter 40) is another important cause of bradycardia, as is opioid intoxication.

☞ **Some patients can manifest a form of bradycardia that is unresponsive to the elevated catecholamine state, associated with trauma or critical illness.** ☞ For example, patients taking beta-blockers, or occasionally young athletic patients with an exaggerated vagal tone, may not have the expected response to the elevated catecholamines during early shock following blunt or penetrating trauma (16). Some common causes and therapeutic options for the bradycardic patient are listed in Table 2.

Table 2 Bradycardia: Causes and Drug Options

Causes	Diagnosis	Treatment/comments
Increased vagal tone	Common in athletes and elderly/spinal cord injury	Only if symptomatic; atropine 0.5–1 mg
ETT at carina	Chest X ray	Reposition ETT
Large mucus plugs	Chest X ray	Suction or bronchoscopy
Gastric distention	Abdominal flat plate/chest X ray; hiccoughs	Nasogastric decompression
Overdistension of the bladder	Suprapubic pain/distended bladder	Bladder decompression via Foley catheter
Increased ICP	Cushing's reflex—bradycardia and hypertension with increased ICP	Decrease ICP
Hypothermia	Temperature ECG	Warm patient; treat underlying cause
Drug-induced (digitalis, beta blockers, calcium-channel blockers)	Electrolytes ECG digoxin level	Replace electrolytes; may need digibind, calcium chloride
Hypothyroidism	Thyroid function studies; electrolytes	Treat thyroid disorder
Sick sinus syndrome "tachy–brady syndrome"	ECG—intermittent sinus pauses	Pacemaker
Ischemic or hypertensive cardiomyopathy	ECG 2-D echo	If HR too low, may need nitroglycerin
First-degree AV block	ECG—pr interval >0.2 seconds	If symptomatic (e.g., hypotensive, syncope), treat with atropine 0.5–1 mg or glycopyrrolate 0.2 mg (longer acting)
Second-degree Mobitz Type I—Wenckebach	ECG—progressive prolongation of pr interval until beat is dropped	Treat if symptomatic with medications
Second-degree Mobitz Type II	ECG—regular dropping of ventricular beats	Treat with atropine or glycopyrrolate; if no response, infusion of dopamine, epinephrine, or isoproterenol until pacemaker can be inserted
Third-degree AV block	ECG—complete AV dissociation	Above medications; temporary pacemaker—transthoracic or transvenous, Permanent pacemaker
Inferior wall MI	ECG—cardiac enzymes	Fluid; treat MI

Abbreviations: AV, atrial-ventricular; ETT, endotrachial tube; ECG, electrocardiogram; ICP, intracranial pressure; MI, myocardial infarction.

Rhythm

Normal sinus rhythm is the ideal condition for both recently traumatized victims and those who are critically ill, because the atrial contraction preceding the ventricular contraction augments the left ventricular (LV) preload and coordination of myocardial mechanics. Several conditions following trauma (myocardial contusion, concomitant drug intoxication) and critical illness (ischemia, thyrotoxicosis, etc.) are associated with dysrhythmias and an impaired hemodynamic performance. Patients who have sustained a myocardial contusion after blunt trauma may present with sinus tachycardia or atrial and ventricular dysrhythmias, all of which can result in decreased myocardial performance.

✓ Elderly patients suffering from trauma or critical illness are prone to develop atrial fibrillation or supraventricular tachycardia, secondary to elevated catecholamines, baseline myocardial irritability, direct myocardial injury, or ischemia, all of which can impair pump function (17,18). ✓ These aberrations can eventually lead to inadequate perfusion of end organs and contribute to multiple organ failure. In order to maintain tissue perfusion, the astute physician maintains vigilance for, and is prepared to treat, these aberrations in the intensive care unit (ICU) setting.

Preload

Hemorrhage is the most common cause of decreased preload following acute trauma. When patients first present to the trauma bay, clinical signs are surveyed to assess preload. When the patient entering the trauma bay is pale, tachycardiac, and hypotensive, the patient is assumed to be in hemorrhagic shock and in need of intravascular volume. However, in less obvious situations, evaluation of the intravascular volume requires all the diagnostic tools and experience of a master clinician. ✓ Parameters measured by noninvasive means, such as HR, BP, urine output, skin color, turgor, and temperature, along with capillary refill, can be obtained quickly and reflect the patient's intravascular volume status prior to the placement of invasive monitors (19,20). ✓

The focused abdominal sonography for trauma (FAST) examination is designed to identify extra anatomic fluid within the peritoneal cavity. FAST can also be used to evaluate the intravascular volume status by estimating the size and function of the cardiac chambers. Although not as specific as transesophageal echocardiography (TEE), using FAST to perform a transthoracic echo (TTE) can yield gross measures of left ventricular (LV) volume and the presence or absence of cardiac tamponade. Later, central lines and pulmonary artery (PA) catheters can be inserted to assess intravascularly by measuring surrogates for pressure, including central venous pressure (CVP) or PA catheter wedge pressure. These invasive measures help to gauge the physiologic adequacy of the volume status, by determining the SV under similar conditions of contractility and afterload (i.e., construct a Starling curve, because SV = preload × contractility) (21–23). Additional specific monitoring techniques for the evaluation of intravascular volume are reviewed in Volume 2, Chapters 3, 9, and 21. Drugs (both endogenous and those discussed in this chapter) mainly affect the afterload and contractility and, to a somewhat lesser extent, the preload of the cardiovascular system.

Afterload

Afterload can be determined using Ohm's law (E = IR) as represented in the following estimates: PVR = [PA − left atrial pressure (LAP)]/Q̇ and SVR = (MAP − CVP)/Q̇. However, the clinician is warned that these measures are

not perfect. Indeed, Ohm's law refers to electricity or rigid pipes, and the blood vessels are not rigid structures. Additionally, one must account for the volume of blood that is pumped and pushed out of the way with each ejection of the heart. The true afterload is the sum of forces against which the LV must act to eject blood into the aorta.

✓ The measured SVR can be two to three times higher than normal following massive hemorrhage, due to catecholamine-mediated arteriolar constriction in compensation for the decreased intravascular volume. ✓ In this setting, the blood flow is shunted away from skin, muscle, splanchnic and renal circulation, with the majority of the dramatically diminished Q̇ directed centrally to the heart and brain via the large arteries. In this setting, increased alveolar dead space may cause V̇/Q̇ related hypoxemia (Volume 2, Chapter 2). Several abnormal patient conditions can complicate trauma resuscitation and SVR interpretation.

For example, patients with aortic stenosis (AS) or coronary artery disease (CAD) with left ventricular hypertrophy (LVH) typically have a higher than normal baseline SVR as a compensatory mechanism, to augment perfusion through the coronary arteries during diastole. Any reduction in afterload in these patients (as can occur with the administration of sedatives or analgesics), without first restoring the missing blood volume, will result in decreased coronary perfusion and likely cause myocardial ischemia. Conversely, cirrhotic patients will demonstrate a low baseline SVR because of arterio–venous (A–V) shunting. Patients suffering from septic conditions will also have a low SVR secondary to the systemic levels of circulating cytokines. Consequently, sepsis in a patient with coincident acute blood loss or baseline AS can unfavorably stress the myocardial supply/demand ratio and potentially cause myocardial ischemia.

Contractility

Myocardial contractility can be estimated by observing LV function with a TEE or by constructing Starling curves (via serial Q̇ measurements and a plot of SV vs. left ventricular end diastolic volume (LVEDV) or left ventricular end diastolic pressure (LVEDP)). Only when LVEDV and SVR are perfectly controlled can accurate determinations of contractility be made. Accordingly, clinical measures are never perfect.

In addition, drugs that increase both SV and afterload (e.g., norepinepherine) may not result in a measured increase in Q̇, partly because of the baroreceptor-mediated decrease in the HR and partly due to the elevated SVR. Drugs that increase contractility while decreasing afterload (e.g., dobutamine or milrinone) will likely demonstrate an increase in Q̇ (due to an increase in both SV and HR), but with a decrease in SVR and pulmonary vascular resistance (PVR).

When the myocardial perfusion is dependent upon the SVR for coronary artery perfusion (i.e., severe AS or CAD with significant LVH), ischemia can be precipitated when the afterload is reduced and result in decreased contractility and myocardial failure. However, a patient with a dilated cardiomyopathy and normal coronaries will likely benefit from a decreased SVR. A trauma patient who has been bleeding and requires intravascular volume may suffer profound hypotension following the administration of drugs with direct or indirect vasodilating effects, such as sedatives and analgesics. Drugs that increase afterload also tend to increase preload, and thus have countervailing effects on SV. Accordingly, monitoring multiple measures of these various parameters is the best way to keep track of the progress being made.

Adequacy of Perfusion (Oxygen Delivery = $\dot{D}O_2$)

☞ **Adequacy of perfusion to tissues is the most important endpoint of resuscitation.** ☞ Unfortunately, only global measures of oxygen delivery ($\dot{D}O_2$) are in wide clinical use (see Volume 1, Chapters 12 and 18, and Volume 2, Chapter 18). Global measures of $\dot{D}O_2$ tell only a part of the picture, $\dot{D}O_2 = O_2$ content $\times \dot{Q}$. Normal $\dot{Q} = 5$ L/min at rest in a 70-kg patient. The normal arterial O_2 content is 200 cc O_2/L, thus $\dot{D}O_2 = 1000$ cc O_2/min. Because a normal 70-kg patient will consume 250 cc O_2/min at rest, the mixed venous saturation at rest is normally approximately 75% in a healthy adult patient. Although the $\dot{D}O_2$ may be globally adequate, certain tissues may remain ischemic (24–26). Accordingly, specific measures of perfusion are required for each tissue bed of interest (this is an area of continued research).

When titrating therapy, the clinician has to anticipate variation in the patients' tissues needs. Exercising and febrile patients need higher $\dot{Q}$s, and certain disease states will be associated with supranormal $\dot{Q}$s [e.g., the systemic inflammatory response syndrome (SIRS)]. Conversely, other disease states are associated with low $\dot{Q}$s (e.g., hypothyroidism and hypothermia). Other conditions [e.g., congestive heart failure (CHF)] are associated with high preload, high SVR, and impaired pump function.

Clinically, the global adequacy of $\dot{D}O_2$ is determined by reviewing patient mentation, skin perfusion, BP, urinary output, base deficit, lactate, mixed venous saturation, and thermal dilution derived $\dot{Q}$ measurements.

OPTIMUM MANAGEMENT OF HYPOTENSION

Definitions and Causes of Hypotension in the Trauma ICU

Hypotension is the most common hemodynamic perturbation requiring immediate physician attention following trauma and critical illness. ☞ **When the mean arterial pressure (MAP) falls below 60 mmHg, organ perfusion to renal and splanchnic organs begins to fall. As the MAP dips below 50 mmHg, perfusion to brain and myocardium can become diminished.** ☞ In the setting of atherosclerotic disease, chronic hypertension, as well as in traumatic brain injury (TBI), cerebral ischemia may begin at higher MAPs, especially when the intracranial pressure (ICP) is elevated (27). Similarly, myocardial ischemia will occur at normally adequate MAPs when associated with severe tachycardia, anemia, or increased metabolic rate.

A normal MAP in a 70-kg adult varies with age and the degree of associated atherosclerotic disease, but typically ranges between 85 and 105 mmHg in healthy patients who are at rest. Patients who sustain trauma or critical illness often have tachycardia, and thus, those with coronary artery disease are at increased risk.

Although staying cognizant of the important concerns mentioned, it is sometimes necessary to accept lower MAPs in various conditions. For example, the patient with sepsis or SIRS may suffer from such a profound degree of vasodilation that administering drugs in high enough quantities to normalize MAP would potentially lead to additional complications, including renal insufficiency or decreased gut perfusion; thus compromises occasionally need to be accepted.

The most common cause of hypotension following trauma is hemorrhage. In the ICU, the most common causes are hypovolemia (due to numerous causes), vasodilation, and impaired cardiac output. Less commonly, bradycardia can be the culprit (Table 2).

Hypovolemia can result from hemorrhage, third spacing, increased intrathoracic pressure (tension pneumothorax, excessive PEEP, or high tidal volumes), excessive diuresis (e.g., iatrogenic, Lasix, mannitol), diabetes insipidus, hyperglycemia, alcohol or caffeine intoxication, excessive dialysis, evaporative losses following burns (Volume 1, Chapter 34), toxic epidermal necrolysis (TENS), and heat stroke. Anaphylaxis (Volume 1, Chapter 33) causes hypovolemia by two mechanisms, vasodilation and increased capillary permeability. Dysrhythmias (Volume 2, Chapter 20) can have an effect analogous to hypovolemia, by either not allowing enough LV filling time or due to loss of the atrial contraction, as occurs with a junctional rhythm. Pericardial tamponade is an important cause, which typically presents early following penetrating thoracic trauma, but can have a delayed and insidious presentation following blunt trauma and when resulting from numerous medical needs etiologies.

Decreased SVR, which leads to hypotension, occurs in various conditions such as sepsis (Volume 2, Chapter 47), spinal cord injury (Volume 2, Chapter 13), neuroaxial block (spinal or epidural anesthesia) with local anesthetics, after administration of systemic vasodilators (e.g., propofol for sedation, nimodipine to treat cerebral vasospasm, nitroglycerin to treat coronary artery spasm), and during SIRS (Volume 2, Chapter 63). SIRS is a common cause of hypotension in trauma and critical care, resulting from circulating inflammatory cytokines released following tissue injury from trauma, burns, infection, and pancreatitis (Volume 2, Chapter 39). Anaphylaxis (Volume 1, Chapter 33), also decreases SVR, as does cirrhosis and other etiologies of A–V shunting.

Another cause of hypotension in the critically ill patient is that of relative adrenal insufficiency (Volume 2, Chapter 62). ☞ **Any patient who is adequately fluid resuscitated and requiring vasopressor support, but remains unresponsive to these measures, may have adrenal insufficiency and may need steroid administration for improvement in vasomotor tone (28–33).** ☞ Relative adrenal insufficiency is common in patients with refractory septic shock, and moderate doses of steroids may restore cell sensitivity to vasopressors. A randomized, controlled trial performed in France demonstrated a significant survival benefit among patients receiving moderate-dose corticosteroid therapy in critically ill patients (34). A consyntropin (synthetic ACTH) stimulation test might help to diagnose this problem (Volume 2, Chapter 62). However, if adrenal insufficiency is suspected, and this test is not readily available, patients may benefit from empiric initiation of steroids without waiting for the results of this test.

Evaluation Principles

Bedside examination is initially employed in the evaluation of the hypotensive patient. Prior to a global exam of the patient (including evaluation of the skin, neck, cardiovascular system, pulmonary system, abdomen, extremities, and neurological systems), a careful survey of the patient's vital signs may offer some clues regarding the etiology of the hypotension. In addition to HR, BP, and respiratory rate, it is important to obtain information regarding the temperature, cardiac rhythm, skin color and temperature, oxygen saturation, and urine output.

TEE is the current gold standard for evaluating intravascular volume and can quickly diagnose most causes of hypotension because LV function and size are readily visualized, as is the presence or absence of tamponade (Volume 2, Chapter 21). However, TEE is not always immediately available in the ICU and may be contraindicated in patients with esophageal injury.

Accordingly, in addition to clinical examination parameters, an ECG, chest X ray, central lines (CVP, PA catheters), and TTE can assist in determining the cause of the hypotension (also see Volume 2, Chapter 9).

Management Goals Based upon Etiology and Other Conditions Present

☞ **The overall goal is to ensure adequate tissue perfusion by repletion of intravascular volume first. Vasoconstrictor or inotropic support drugs are generally best administered after intravascular repletion is assured. However, occasionally, both drug support and volume repletion must be employed concomitantly to maintain an adequate BP, until sufficient fluid repletion can be achieved.** ☞

Intravascular Volume Repletion

TEE is an excellent monitor for evaluating the efficacy of volume repletion. In the absence of TEE, intravascular pressure measurements (CVP, PACWP) are used as surrogates of intravascular volume status.

The choice of fluid for intravascular repletion depends upon several factors discussed at length in Volume 1, Chapter 11. In general, crystalloids are employed first. Colloids and blood products are added depending on the extent of hemorrhage and whether bleeding has been controlled or remains ongoing.

Vasopressor and Inotropic Drug Therapy

After ensuring adequate intravascular volume repletion, vasopressor therapy may be appropriate (e.g., when SVR is very low). Table 3 shows the dose range, receptor activity, predominant hemodynamic effects, and the complications for the most commonly employed vasopressor drugs. Note that some drugs, like norepinephrine and calcium chloride, have both inotropic and vasoconstrictor effects. Norepinephrine has recently been found to be less renal toxic than dopamine in euvolemic patients with sepsis (35–39).

Review of Vasopressors for Hypotension
Phenylephrine (Neo-Synephrine®)

Phenylephrine (Neo-Synephrine®) is commonly used in the treatment of hypotension due to hypovolemia, anaphylaxis,

or drug-induced vasodilation (40). This α_1-agonist causes arterial and venous vasoconstriction. It may cause a reflex decrease in HR. A loading dose is not required, and the drug is usually given as an infusion at 20–200 mcg/min titrating to effect in a 70-kg adult. It must be used with caution in patients with aortic insufficiency or mitral regurgitation. The drug usually decreases cardiac output as well as renal and splanchnic blood flow.

Phenylephrine is best infused via a central line, but can be initially administered using a peripheral IV. When a peripheral IV is used, it should be in concert with a carrier solution so as to prevent an unintentional bolus of a line containing pure phenylephrine. An arterial line should be used to monitor therapy and to titrate the infusion. The patient may also need a PA catheter to help guide therapy.

Norepinephrine (Levophed®)

☞ **Norepinephrine (Levophed®) can be used to increase BP in hypotensive patients who fail to respond to adequate volume resuscitation and other, less potent, vasopressors.** ☞ It is commonly employed in septic patients because it increases the BP and SVR without altering $\dot{Q}$ (38,39,41–44). Norepinephrine is an α- and β_1-agonist that causes arterial and venous vasoconstriction. It has minimal chronotropic effects and is typically infused at a rate of 0.05–40 mcg/kg/min. Norepinephrine causes vasoconstriction of the systemic, renal, and splanchnic beds. Complications include decreased renal perfusion in hypovolemic patients, peripheral vasoconstriction, and dysrhythmias. Norepinepherine can cause tissue necrosis following extravasation. The drug must be given through a central vein with careful monitoring of arterial pressure, perfusion, and renal function to prevent organ ischemia and excessive increases in ventricular afterload.

Arginine Vasopressin

Arginine vasopressin has been used for decades to treat esophageal variceal bleeding and diabetes insipidus. Recently, vasopressin has been shown to be useful in the treatment of refractory septic shock and during resuscitation from cardiac arrest (45–51).

The dose of vasopressin for treatment of diabetes insipidus is 2.5–10 U subcutaneously or intramuscularly three

Table 3 Vasopressors

Drug	Dose range	Receptor activity	Hemodynamic effects	Complications
Phenylephrine	20–200 mcg/min	α_1-agonist	↑ SVR ↑ MAP	Hypertension, bradycardia, myocardial ischemia, ⇓ renal perfusion
Norepinephrine	0.05–1.5 mcg/kg/min	Strong α_1-agoinst; moderate β-agonist	↑ Contractility ↑ SVR ↑ MAP	Peripheral vasoconstriction, arrhythmias, ⇓ renal perfusion, tissue necrosis with extravasation, hyperglycemia
Vasopressin	0.01–0.04 units/min	Neurohypophyseal peptide Vasoconstriction of vascular smooth muscle	Potent vasoconstrictor ↓ CO ↓ Renal perfusion	Mesenteric ischemia, ⇓ CBF, CNS disturbances, hyponatremia, metabolic acidosis, hypertension
Calcium chloride 10%[a]	Loading dose—90 mg 0.5–2 mg/hr adjusted to ionized calcium level	Stimulates the intracellular release of calcium from the sarcoplasmic reticulum	↑ SVR ↑ MAP ↑ Ionized concentration of calcium	Hypercalcemia, hypophosphatemia, ⇓ sensorium, arrhythmias, chemical burn if extravasates

[a] 1 ampule of 10% calcium chloride = 13.6 mEQ of calcium, 1 ampule of calcium gluconate = 4.65 mEQ calcium.
Abbreviations: CBF, cerebral blood flow; CNS, central nervous system; MAP, mean arterial pressure; SVR, systemic vascular resistance.

to four times a day. In the treatment of esophageal and gastric variceal bleeding, the dose is 20 U in 100 mL of normal saline given over 15 to 30 minutes or an infusion of 0.4 U/min intravenously. The recommended dose during Advanced Cardiac Life Support® (ACLS®) for refractory ventricular fibrillation is 40 U intravenously (52). Some investigators believe that vasopressin is superior to epinephrine in arrest situations (48). Although it is a weak vasopressor in normal subjects, the addition of vasopressin, infused at a fixed rate of 0.04 U/min, to norepinephrine is more effective in reversing late vasodilatory shock than norepinephrine infusion alone (41,53). ✍ **The use of vasopressin has also been shown to decrease the requirement for other vasopressors and is associated with a higher urine output and improved creatinine clearance (54,55).** ✍ Vasopressin is used with caution in patients with coronary artery disease. Complications include coronary and mesenteric ischemia, hyponatremia, pulmonary vasoconstriction, and skin necrosis from peripheral infusion. When using this agent as a vasopressor, it is preferably infused through a central line, and titrated based on invasive pressure monitoring (56).

Calcium Chloride

Calcium chloride is required for a wide variety of cellular functions. Ionized calcium is essential to the process of excitation–contraction coupling. When it is given exogenously, it stimulates the intracellular release of calcium from the sarcoplasmic reticulum. Indications for administration include ionized hypocalcemia, especially following rapid administration of citrate, containing blood products, or in continuous renal replacement therapy (CRRT). Calcium chloride is also recommended for the treatment of acute hyperkalemia, hypermagnesemia, and calcium-channel blocker overdose. Calcium administration can increase peripheral vascular tone and myocardial contractility, both serving to increase BP. Ionized calcium can also potentiate the peripheral vascular and inotropic effects of catecholamines.

The utility of calcium for the treatment of citrate intoxication is based upon the function of citrate. The citrate is used in blood products and with CRRT to bind calcium and inhibit clotting because Ca^{++} is needed in both the intrinsic and final common coagulation pathways. Exogenously administered citrate is rapidly cleared by the liver in normal healthy patients. However, when massive transfusion occurs, a concomitant massive quantity of citrate is coadministered and this can temporarily overwhelm the liver's ability to metabolize it, resulting in transient ionized hypocalcemia.

In severe liver disease, citrate is not metabolized and the citrate level in the blood will increase. When large quantities of citrate build up in the blood, free ionized Ca^{++} is diminished below the levels required to maintain vascular tone or myocardial contractility.

Calcium is given as a loading dose of 100 mg and then 1–5 mg/kg/hr, adjusted to the ionized calcium level. In the setting of massive blood product administration, or during the anhepatic stage of liver transplantation patients (where citrate is not being metabolized), much larger quantities of calcium are required. Calcium chloride has approximately three times the calcium bioavailability of the gluconate form. There are 13.6 mEQ of calcium in one 10-mL ampule of calcium chloride, whereas there are only 4.65 mEQ of calcium in one 10-mL ampule of calcium gluconate (57,58). Excessive calcium can precipitate or exacerbate digitalis toxicity, leading to dysrhythmias, and therefore

should be cautiously administered in patients taking digoxin. Calcium forms an insoluble precipitate if mixed with bicarbonate (calcium carbonate). Calcium chloride may sclerose peripheral veins and can produce a severe chemical burn if it infiltrates into the subcutaneous tissues. It is preferably infused through a central line to decrease the risk of peripheral vein injury.

Inotropes for Decreased Contractility Conditions

Perhaps the most commonly employed inotropic drug is dopamine. Though less potent than epinephrine, dopamine has a wide therapeutic range. Dopaminergic receptors are stimulated in the 2–3 mcg/kg/min range, whereas 5–10 mcg/kg/min stimulates beta-receptors, and >10 mcg/kg/min stimulates alpha-receptors. The dose ranges, receptor activities, predominant hemodynamic effects, as well as complications for the most commonly employed inotropic drugs are reviewed in Table 4.

Epinephrine

Epinephrine is an endogenous catecholamine with nonselective α- and β-adrenergic agonist effects. It is often used to treat hypotension and low $\dot{Q}$ following cardiopulmonary bypass (CPB), acute asthma, cardiac arrest, and anaphylaxis. Epinephrine is a third-line agent in the treatment of septic shock (after dopamine and norepinephrine) (59–62). Epinephrine at low dose (0.01–0.02 mcg/kg/min) stimulates predominantly β-receptors, and above 0.2–0.4 mcg/kg/min begins to have significant α-receptor agonist effects as well.

Low doses of epinephrine cause primarily β_1-adrenergic receptor agonist effects increasing inotropy and chronotropy, as well as β_2-adrenergic effects causing mild vasodilation; and the combined β_1 and β_2 effects increase $\dot{Q}$ and mildly increase MAP. High-dose epinephrine stimulates α_1 receptors causing vasoconstriction, and β_1 receptors increasing chronotropy and inotropy, producing a large increase in MAP. At high doses, the α_1 effects overwhelm the β_2 effects, causing an increased SVR. This, along with an increase in $\dot{Q}$ due to the concomitant β_1-adrenergic agonist effects-markedly elevate the MAP.

For the treatment of acute asthma, epinephrine is given as 0.3–0.5 mg of 1:100 dilution subcutaneously, repeated at 20-minute to four-hour intervals or one inhalation (metered dose) repeated in one to two minutes until symptoms abate. For emergency cardiac care, epinephrine is given at 0.5–1 mg (1:10,000) intravenously every three to five minutes to response. When used in the surgical intensive care unit (SICU) for inotropic support, it is infused at 0.01–0.4 mcg/kg/min. Complications include increased myocardial oxygen consumption with ischemia, dysrhythmias, hypertension, hyperglycemia, and decreased renal perfusion, especially in hypovolemic patients. Epinephrine should be administered through a central vein and monitored with an intra-arterial catheter.

Norepinephrine (Levophed®)

Norepinephrine is an endogenous catecholamine with potent α-adrenergic receptor agonist and moderate β_1-adrenergic agonist effects. It produces potent vasoconstriction with a less pronounced increase in cardiac output. A reflex bradycardia can occur in response to the increased SVR and MAP, so that the mild chronotropic effect is negated and the HR remains unchanged or even decreases slightly.

Table 4 Inotropes

Drug	Dose range	Receptor activity	Hemodynamic effects	Complications
Epinephrine	0.01–0.4 mcg/kg/min 0.5–1 mg (1:10,000) 0.3–0.5 mg SQ (1:1000)	Potent α_1-agonist Nonselective β- agonist	$\uparrow\uparrow$ Q̇ $\uparrow\uparrow$ Contractility $\uparrow$ HR $\uparrow\uparrow\uparrow$ Vasoconstriction (high dose) $\uparrow\uparrow$ Vasodilation (low dose) $\uparrow$ MAP Bronchodilation	$\Uparrow$ Myocardial consumption with ischemia; arrhythmia, hypertension, hyperglyce- mia, poor renal perfusion, local ulceration if infiltrated
Norepinephrine	0.05–1.5 mcg/kg/min	Potent α_1-agonist Moderate β_1-agonist	$\uparrow$ Contractility $\uparrow$ SVR $\uparrow$ MAP	Arrhythmias; peripheral vaso- constriction, tissue necrosis, hyperglycemia
Dopamine	1–3 mcg/kg/min 2–10 mcg/kg/min >10 mcg/kg/min	DA receptor β and DA α_1, β and DA	$\uparrow\uparrow$ Contractility $\uparrow$ HR Vasoconstriction $\uparrow$ SVR $\uparrow\uparrow\uparrow$ Renal blood flow $\uparrow\uparrow\uparrow$ Q̇	Arrhythmias; tachycardia, necrosis at injection site with extravasation
Dobutamine	2.5–20 mcg/kg/min	Potent β_1-agonist	$\uparrow\uparrow\uparrow$ Contractility $\uparrow$ HR $\uparrow\uparrow\uparrow$ Q̇ Peripheral vasodilator $\downarrow\downarrow$ SVR	Tachycardia, hypotension
Isoproterenol	0.01–0.1 mcg/kg/min	Potent β_1-and β_2- agonist	$\uparrow\uparrow\uparrow$ Contractility $\uparrow\uparrow\uparrow$ HR $\uparrow\uparrow\uparrow$ Vasodilation $\uparrow\uparrow\uparrow$ Q̇ Bronchodilator	Tachycardia, tachyarrhythmias, myocardial ischemia, flushing of the skin
Amrinone/ milrinone	Load 0.75 mg/kg over 3 minutes 2–15 mcg/kg/min Load 50 mcg/kg over 10 minutes 0.375–0.75 mcg/ kg/min	Inhibits phosphodiest erase $\Uparrow$ cAMP	$\uparrow\uparrow\uparrow$ Contractility; systemic and pulmonary vasodilation	Dose-related thrombocytopenia with amrinone, synergy with dobutamine, arrhythmia

Abbreviations: Q̇, dopaminergic; cAMP, cyclic adenosine monophosphate; HR, heart rate; MAP, mean arterial pressure; SVR, systemic vascular resistance; DA, cardiac output.

Norepinephrine is most commonly used in acute hypotensive states, especially to treat septic shock. Its major indication is to increase BP in hypotensive patients who fail to respond to adequate volume resuscitation and other, less potent, vasoconstrictors and inotropes. It causes systemic vasoconstriction and coronary artery vasodilation. Norepinephrine is inactivated by the pulmonary circulation, and thus does not cause an increase in PVR. Thus, it can be used in patients with PA hypertension (63,64).

Complications include dysrhythmias, hyperglycemia, and splanchnic vasoconstriction. When given to patients taking tricyclic antidepressants, norepinephrine can lead to a severe hypertension. As an inotrope, norepinephrine is infused at a rate of 0.05–1.5 mcg/kg/min, and titrated based on the arterial pressure. It is best given through a central vein to avoid tissue necrosis from extravasation. Careful monitoring of arterial pressure, perfusion, and renal function is necessary during infusions to prevent organ ischemia.

Dopamine

Dopamine has a variety of actions depending upon the dose administered. At doses of 1–3 mcg/kg/min, dopamine acts predominantly on D_1-receptors in the renal, mesenteric, cerebral, and coronary beds, resulting in selective vasodilation. It has been shown that this low-dose dopamine can increase urine output and renal blood flow (65–69). ☞ **Although low-dose dopamine increases renal blood**

flow, it does not ameliorate renal failure, and has not improved outcomes in nonoliguric patients recovering from acute tubular necrosis (ATN) (70,71). ☞ At 5–10 mcg/kg/min, the β_1-adrenergic effects of dopamine predominate. Dopamine at these doses will increase cardiac output by increasing SV and HR. The effect of dopamine on HR is variable at all dose ranges. At doses greater than 10 mcg/kg/min, the predominant effect of dopamine is to stimulate α_1-receptors. This dose will produce vasoconstriction and consequent increase in SVR. The vasoconstrictor effect of dopamine is weaker than that produced by norepinephrine. In some patients, doces greater than 3 mcg/kg/min result in dose-limiting dysrhythmias due to β_1-adrenergic receptor stimulation. Dopamine is most often used in hypotension due to sepsis, impaired cardiac function, and other combined vasodilated states. Once started, dopamine is titrated to a desired effect rather than a pharmacologic range. It is preferably administered through a central line and monitored with an intra-arterial catheter. Monitoring HR and rhythm, systemic and renal perfusion is also recommended. Dopamine has a mild increased effect on hypoxic pulmonary vasoconstriction but does not increase PVR and can be safely used in patients with pulmonary hypertension. Nausea, emesis, and tachyarrhythmias are the most common complications associated with dopamine infusion. Of note, patients on monoamine oxidase inhibitors (MAOI) can have exaggerated hypertensive effects following dopamine administration. Patients on MAOIs should only receive direct-acting drugs to increase BP (e.g., phenylephrine) and contractility (e.g., epinephrine).

If extravasation of the dopamine infusion occurs, tissue necrosis can develop if not treated by local injection of phentolamine (72–74).

Dobutamine

Dobutamine is a synthetic inotropic drug derived from isoproterenol, in an attempt to decrease the dysrhythmogenic and vasodilatory effects. Dobutamine has β_1-adrenergic receptor effects that increase $\dot{Q}$ and HR. It typically decreases both systemic and pulmonary vascular resistance because of minimal α_1- and moderate β_2-adrenergic receptor effects. Dobutamine is most frequently used in severe, medically refractory heart failure and cardiogenic shock. It is not routinely used in patients with sepsis or hypovolemic shock because it may exacerbate hypotension (72–80). Dobutamine is infused at a rate of 2.5–20 mcg/kg/min and is monitored by effect or cardiac parameters. Dysrhythmias and decreases in BP are the most frequent side effects.

Isoproterenol

Isoproterenol is a potent, nonselective β_1- and β_2-adrenergic receptor agonist with prominent chronotropic and vasodilator effects. The β_2 effects cause vasodilation and a decrease in MAP, and therefore isoproterenol has virtually no role in either the acute trauma or critical care setting. Isoproterenol can be used to treat pulmonary hypertension and right ventricular (RV) failure following heart transplantation, and in young patients without CAD. It can be used cautiously to treat hemodynamically significant bradycardia, but other choices are usually preferred (i.e., pacemakers, atropine, epinephrine, etc.).

Isoproterenol is avoided in patients with CAD because it can induce myocardial ischemia. Other complications are tachydysrhythmias and flushing of the skin. Isoproterenol is infused at a rate of 0.01–0.1 mcg/kg/min and is adjusted to produce the desired hemodynamic effect. Isoproterenol should never be used in patients without intra-arterial catheters, or in those with aortic stenosis, mitrial stenosis, hypertrophic left ventricles, CAD, or other disease states that will not tolerate combined hypotension and tachycardia.

Phosphodiesterase Inhibitors

Amrinone and milrinone inhibit phosphodiesterase, resulting in an increase in intracellular cyclic adenosine monophosphate cAMP. These are nonadrenergic drugs with inotropic and vasodilatory actions. These agents are most commonly used to treat patients with impaired cardiac function and heart failure refractory to β_2-agonists (81–83). Because these phosphodiesterase inhibitors cause systemic and pulmonary vasodilation, their role is limited in the trauma patient (84,85). Both drugs can cause dysrhythmias, and amrinone can also result in a dose-related thrombocytopenia (86,87).

Dopexamine

Dopexamine is a dopamine analog used intravenously in the treatment of heart failure and low $\dot{Q}$ states. It produces systemic vasodilation by stimulating β_2-adrenoceptors and peripheral dopamine receptors. It is a weak inotrope and has no α-adrenergic receptor activity. Dopexamine is given as an infusion ranging from 1 µg/kg/min to a maximum dose of 6 µg/kg/min. Although primarily used in heart failure, some studies have proposed its use in high-risk surgical and critically ill patients, because it preserves hepatosplanchnic and renal perfusion (88–92). This preservation of flow is thought to aid in the prevention of multiple organ dysfunction in critically ill patients. Dopexamine may also ameliorate the vasopressin-associated decrease in tissue oxygen in sepsis, thereby increasing the $\dot{Q}$ and $\dot{D}O_2$ in these patients (89). The most common complication associated with its use is tachyarrhythmias, which may be undesirable in the patient population subjected to its use.

OPTIMUM MANAGEMENT OF SIGNIFICANT HYPERTENSION
Definitions and Causes of Hypertension in the Trauma ICU

Most patients who present with hypertension in the ICU are baseline hypertensives who have stopped taking medications or who have a new medical problem that causes exacerbation of their normal conditions, for example, intracranial hemorrhage (ICH), aortic dissection, and cocaine or amphetamine intoxication.

In 2003, the Joint National Committee on Prevention, Detection, Evaluation, and Treatment of High Blood Pressure published their latest set of recommendations (JNC 7) on the diagnosis and treatment of hypertension (93–95) (Table 5). Hypertension is defined as a BP greater than 140/90. In contrast to JNC 6 (published in 1997), the new guidelines have only two stages of nonurgent or emergent hypertension. Unless there are compelling indications, stage 1 (140 to 159/90 to 99 mmHg) patients are recommended to receive

Table 5   Blood Pressure Classifications per Joint National Committee (JNC) 7 (2003)

BP classification	SBP (mmHg)	DBP (mmHg)	Comments (examples)
Normal	<120	and <80	In JNC 6 this was called optimal
Pre-HTN	120–139	or 80–89	In JNC 6 this was called normal or borderline
Stage 1 HTN	140–159	or 90–99	Thiazide diuretics first-line therapy
Stage 2 HTN	≥160	≥100	Thiazide + ACEI, or ARB, or BB, or CCB
HTN urgency	≥160	≥100	May have symptoms, but no evidence of end-organ failure (e.g., may have headache, but no ICH, encephalopathy, or seizure; e.g., may have shortness of breath, but not acute pulmonary edema)
HTN crisis	≥180	≥120	Evidence of impending or progressive target organ dysfunction (e.g., HTN encephalopathy, ICH, acute MI, acute LV failure with pulmonary edema, aortic dissection, eclampsia)

Abbreviations: ACEI, angiotensin-converting enzyme inhibitor; ARB, angiotensin receptor blocker; BB, β blocker; BP, blood pressure; CCB, calcium-channel blocker; DBP, diastolic blood pressure; HTN, hypertension; ICH, intracranial hemorrhage; JNC, Joint National Committee on Prevention, Detection, Evaluation, and Treatment of High Blood Pressure; LV, left ventricle; MI, myocardial infarction; SBP, systolic blood pressure.

thiazide diuretic therapy only, and stage 2 (>160/ > 100 mmHg) patients are treated with thiazide diuretics and a second drug such as an angiotensin-converting enzyme inhibitor, an angiotensin receptor blocker, a beta blocker, or a calcium-channel blocker.

The traumatologist and intensivist need to be aware of the pharmacology and side effects of these common drugs, because of their prevalence in the critically ill population and because they are used in the treatment of hypertensive crises. Hypertensive urgency is defined in JNC 7 as stage 2 hypertension plus symptoms, but no overt evidence of end-organ damage. Hypertensive crisis is defined by JNC 7 as BP greater than 180/120 mmHg and evidence of current or impending end-organ damage [(e.g., ICH, acute myocardial infarction (MI), acute LV failure with pulmonary edema, aortic dissection, pre-eclampsia)] (96,97).

Malignant hypertension (MHTN) is defined by the World Health Organization as severe hypertension with bilateral retinal hemorrhages and exudates. There is no defined level of systolic BP; however, the diastolic BP is usually greater than 120 to 130 mmHg (98–100).

Although the trauma intensivist must be cognizant of these definitions, common causes of hypertension may be present. Pain, fear, and anxiety are commonplace in the trauma ICU and need to be treated first. While evaluating and treating these common problems leading to hypertension, the intensivist must also search for the other life-threatening conditions. ☞ **In all scenarios, the goal of MHTN treatment is to prevent end-organ damage.** ☞

Evaluation Principles

Because the causes of hypertension in the ICU are numerous, bedside evaluation of the patient is imperative. It is most practical to obtain an assessment of pain, fear, and anxiety by examining the patient. By evaluating the patient at the bedside, the physician obtains a global assessment of the patient's condition and can begin treating the common problems of pain, fear, or anxiety. In examining the patient, the clinician can also rule in (or out) life-threatening conditions while surveying the patient for evidence of end-organ damage. Antihypertensive therapy can be started if there is no response to the other measures. However, it is important to avoid overcorrection because autoregulation is typically impaired, and hypotension can trigger hypoperfusion and organ ischemia.

During the bedside evaluation, a history of hypertension and medical treatment is sought. Hypertensive patients should be restarted on their antihypertensive medications as soon as it is safe to do so.

The physical exam provides clues to the cause and potential complications of hypertension. The head-to-toe examination focusses upon any obvious injuries that may cause pain and also evaluates the neurological status, checking for papilledema, assessing the HR and rhythm, and ruling out any occult injuries or causes.

Laboratory data should include a toxicology screen for cocaine, amphetamine, alcohol, and so on. Some withdrawal syndromes result in hypertension, including alcohol (e.g., delirium tremens) and abrupt cessation of clonidine. Serum chemistries and thyroid function studies help exclude renal vascular hypertension, thyroid storm, or hyperadrenalism. If the laboratory results and clinical evaluation does not return a clear etiology of the new-onset hypertension, it is important to rule out a pheochromocytoma (particularly when episodes of severe hypertension persistently recur) (101,102).

Imaging studies can define the cause of hypertension, such as in the setting of altered mental status. A CT scan of the head will help determine whether TBI or ICH is the culprit, while a CT scan of the abdomen and pelvis may lead to medical renal disease or an adrenal mass as the inciting factor.

Hypertension Management Goals Based upon Etiology

After ruling out pain, fear, or anxiety as the cause, it is important to treat the acutely hypertensive patient in order to prevent end-organ damage. Acutely, nitroprusside therapy is easily titrated, but beware of cyanide toxicity and exacerbation of tachycardia. If the patient is tachycardic, beta blockers are sometimes appropriate.

Peripheral Vasodilators
Nitroprusside
Nitroprusside is a direct vasodilator with rapid onset and elimination. Its use is indicated in the setting of hypertensive crisis, aortic dissection, or when rapid titration of vasodilatory effects is needed. The dose is 0.5–10 mcg/kg/min and the duration upon termination is three to five minutes. The dose is titrated to effect and to specific BP parameters. Monitoring with an indwelling arterial pressure line is a more accurate method of BP assessment when titrating the drug (Table 6).

Nitroprusside is contraindicated in the setting of acute TBI because of the cerebral vasodilatory effects that result in increased cerebral blood flow (CBF) and ICP (103).

Cyanide toxicity is the major concern with high dose (>8–10 mcg/kg/min) or prolonged therapy (e.g., >24 hours of dosages >2 mcg/kg/min) (104). Cyanide toxicity is particularly problematic in patients with thiosulfate deficiency (104). Other complications include metabolic acidosis, nausea, and coronary steal (103). Nitroprusside use is avoided in pregnant patients.

Nitroglycerin
Nitroglycerin is a venous and arterial dilator with a fast onset of action and a short duration. It is indicated in myocardial ischemia and postcoronary bypass. Its dose ranges from 0.1 to 10 mcg/kg/min and is titrated to symptomatic relief or desired effect. Because it increases CBF, it is relatively contraindicated in patients with TBI and elevated ICP. Complications of nitroglycerin infusion include headache, tachycardia, tolerance, and methemoglobinemia. Therapy is monitored based on desired effect. It is helpful to have an arterial line for more accurate BP control.

Hydralazine
Hydralazine is a direct arteriolar dilator. Its peak onset of action is 15 to 30 minutes, and its duration is two to four hours. Indications for hydralazine include pre-eclampsia and postoperative hypertension. Hydralazine can be given intravenously or intramuscularly. The intravenous dose is 10–20 mg, every 20 to 30 minutes as needed, and the intramuscular dose is 10–50 mg, every one to two hours as need. It is most commonly given in bolus doses without regularly scheduled times. Relative contraindications to use include patients with preexisting CAD, angina, or arrhythmias. Side effects include hypotension (especially when given more frequently than every 20–30 minutes IV). Tachycardia is common due to the vasodilator effects. Complications also include flushing, angina, and supraventricular tachycardia.

Table 6 Vasodilators

Drug	Dose	Action	Indications	Complications
Nitroprusside	0.25–10 mcg/kg/min	Direct vasodilation; rapid onset; rapid offset; onset: seconds. Duration: 3–5 minutes	Hypertensive crisis; aortic dissection, need for rapid titration of vasodilatory effects	Coronary steal; cyanide toxicity; metabolic acidosis; ⇑ ICP in TBI; nausea; avoid in pregnancy
Nitroglycerin	0.1–10 mcg/kg/min	Venous and arterial dilator Onset: 1–2 minutes. Duration: 5–10 min	Myocardial ischemia; post-coronary bypass	Headache; tachycardia tolerance; methemoglobinemia; ⇑ CBF
Nicardipine	5–15 mg/hr IV 10–50 mg IM	Ca^{2+} channel blocker onset: 3–5 minutes. Duration: 1–4 hours	CA vasodilator; prevents vasospasm	Tachycardia; hypotension
Hydralazine	10–20 mg IV 10–50 mg IM	Direct arteriolar dilation Onset: 15–30 minutes Duration: 2–4 hours	Eclampsia; postoperative hypertension	Tachycardia; SVT; flushing; angina; Lupus-like syndrome
Phentolamine	5–10 mg IV bolus every 15 minutes	α_1 blockade onset: 1–2 minutes. Duration: 3–10 minutes	Pheochromocytoma; recreational drugs; tyramine and MAOI ingestion; spinal cord dysreflexia	Tolerance; tachycardia vomiting; angina nausea
Diazoxide	Mini bolus 50–100 mg every 5 minutes up to 600 mg 7.5–30 mg/min	Direct arteriolar dilation Related to thiazides. Onset: 2–5 minutes. Duration: 4–12 hours	Causes ↑ CO, ↓ CBF, fluid retention; caution with Coumadin	Tachycardia; angina hyperglycemia; hyperuricemia; extrapyramidal symptoms
Fenoldopam	0.1 mcg/kg/min	Peripheral dopamine-1 agonist. Duration: 10 minutes.	Maintains or increases renal perfusion while it lowers BP	Contraindicated in patients with glaucoma

Abbreviations: BP, blood pressure; CBF, cerebral blood flow; CA, coronary artery; ICP, intracranial pressure; IM, intramuscular; MAOI, monoamine oxidase inhibitors; Q̇, cardiac ouput; SVT, supraventricular tachycardia; TBI, traumatic brain injury.

There is also a lupus-like syndrome that develops in as many as 10% of patients chronically using this drug. Therapy is monitored by desired effect.

Beta Blockers

Esmolol

Esmolol is a β_1-selective (i.e., cardioselective) adrenergic receptor blocking agent (Table 7). Its onset is immediate and has a clinical duration of 10 to 15 minutes after cessation of infusion. Esmolol is usually given as a loading dose of 500 mcg/kg/min over one minute, followed by an infusion rate of 50–100 mcg/kg/min. Indications for use include aortic

dissection and abdominal aortic aneurysm. Complications of esmolol included excessive bradycardia and rarely bronchospasm. It may prolong the effects of succinocholine and should be used with caution in patients with systolic cardiac dysfunction. It is easily titrated and is an appropriate drug to use when both a decrease in HR and BP are needed. Titration is based on BP measurements, preferably from an arterial line.

Metoprolol

Metoprolol is a selective β_1-adrenergic receptor blocking agent with a clinical duration of four to six hours. It is dosed intravenously in 5 mg increments, usually every six hours. The dose can be increased to a maximum of 10 mg

Table 7 β-Blockers

Drug	Dose	Action	Indications	Complications
Esmolol	Load 500 mcg/kg/min over 1 minute 10–300 mcg/kg/min	Selective β_1-blocker Onset: immediate Duration: 10–15 minutes	Aortic dissection; abdominal aortic aneurysm	Bradycardia; bronchospasm, may prolong effects of succinocholine; caution with systolic cardiac dysfunction
Metoprolol	5-mg increments	Selective β_1-blocker Duration: 3–4 hours	Myocardial infarction; hypertension; angina	Bradycardia
Labetolol	20-mg test dose 20–80 mg Q 10 minutes to total of 300 mg 0.5–2 mg/min	α_1 and nonselective β-blocker. Onset: 5–15 minutes. Duration: 2–12 hours	Eclampsia; spinal cord dysreflexia, intracranial process when nitroprusside not available	Bronchospasm; bradycardia

every six hours, or the frequency can be adjusted to every four hours or more frequently; with the physician at the bedside, 5 mg can be administered every 15 minutes for four doses. Once a stable IV dose is determined, metoprolol can be administered orally in doses of 25–200 mg twice daily. The maximum oral daily dose is approximately 450 mg in a 70-kg patient. The higher the dose, the less the cardioselective metoprolol becomes. It is indicated in myocardial infarction, hypertension, and angina. It is easily converted to an oral form once a regular dosing and effect has been established. Bradycardia is the main complication. Therapy is typically monitored based on increasing dosage, until the desired effect (control of BP and HR) is achieved or until important side effects occur.

Labetolol

Labetolol is a combined α_1-blocker and a nonselective β-adrenergic receptor blocker. Its peak onset of action is five minutes, with clinical duration of approximately six to eight hours. Indications include eclampsia, spinal cord dysreflexia, intracranial processes when nitroprusside is not available, and all situations where both a decrease in HR and a decrease in SVR are sought. Labetolol is administered intravenously in five-minute intervals starting with 5 mg aliquots, and increasing dose by 5–10 mg with each administration, until the desired effect is achieved or a complication occurs, up to a total of 300 mg in a 70-kg patient. Once the desired effect is achieved, the aggregate milligram dose required can be administered orally every eight hours to provide continued BP control. Additional IV doses can be administered as needed to supplement the baseline oral dose. It can also be given as an infusion of 0.5–2 mg/min; however, labetolol is not as easily titrated as esmolol, nitroprusside, or nitroglycerin because of the long duration of action.

Calcium-Channel Blockers

Calcium-channel blockers comprise two subclasses, dihydropyridines and nondihydropyridines, which are different with respect to vascular selectivity, negative inotropy, effect on cardiac impulse formation, and conduction. Both subclasses have efficacy as antihypertensive agents. However, several of these drugs have found certain niches. Diltiazam is commonly used for A–V nodal blockade and rate control of supraventricular tachycardias (Volume 2, Chapter 20), nimodipine is used for control of cerebral vasospasm following subarachnoid hemorrhage (SAH) (Volume 2, Chapter 14), and nicardipine is used for brief periods as an infusion in situations that were previously relegated to nitroprusside (discussed subsequently) (105).

Verapamil

Verapamil is calcium-channel blocker with an elimination half-life of four to five hours (Table 8). A loading dose of 5 to 10 mg over two to three minutes is given, and then it is infused at a rate of 5 mg/hour or 0.075–0.15 mg/kg/hr, and titrated to effect. Indications include angina, hypertension, hypertrophic cardiomyopathy, and supraventricular tachyarrhythmias (106). Hypotension, bradycardia, constipation, and AV block with beta blockers are some of the complications. Therapy is monitored based on desired effect, whether it is HR control, BP control, or chest pain control.

Nifedipine

Nifedipine is a calcium-channel blocker with an elimination half-life of three hours. Its use may be limited in the ICU setting because there is no intravenous dosing. It is given as a 10–20 mg orally or sublingually, with a maximum dose of 180 mg/day. Its indications include hypertension

Table 8 Calcium-Channel Blockers

Drug	Dose	Duration	Indications	Complications
Verapamil N	Load 5–10 mg over 2 to 3 minutes, 5 mg/hr (0.075 to 0.15 mg/kg/hr)	Elimination half-life: 4–5 hrs	Angina; hypertension, hypertrophic cardio-myopathy SVT	Hypotension, bradycardia, AV block with β-blockers[a] constipation
Nifedipine D	No IV dose 10–20 mg PO or SL Max 180 mg/day	Elimination half-life: 3 hrs	Angina, hypertension	Headache, hypotension reflex tachycardia
Diltiazem[b] N	Load 0.25 mg/kg over 2 minutes 5 to 15 mg/hr, max 360 mg/day	Elimination half-life: 2–5 hrs	Prevention of reinfarction angina, hypertension, rate control in atrial flutter/fibrillation	Hypotension, AV block with beta-blockers[a]
Nicardipine D	5–15 mg/hr	Onset: 3–5 minutes Duration: 1–4 hrs	Postoperative hypertension, prevention of vasospasm from SAH, angina, least potential cardiac contractility suppression	Long half-life, reflex tachy-cardia hypotension
Nimodipine N	60 mg PO every 4 hours		Prevention of vasospasms following SAH	

[a]Verapamil and diltiazam have significant A–V node blockade effect, thus useful in controlling the ventricular response to SVTs.
[b]Diltiazam has the least amount of vasodilation compared to A–V node blockade effect, thus is the best choice for infusion in critically ill patients with atrial fibrillation or flutter and hypotension.
Abbreviations: AV, artrial-ventricular D, dihydropyridine type; N, nondihydropyridine type; SVT, supraventricular tachycardia; PO, per oral; SAH, subarachnoid hemorrhage.

and angina. Complications are limited to headache, hypotension, and reflex tachycardia.

Diltiazem

Diltiazem is a calcium-channel blocker with an elimination half-life of two to five hours. It is given as a loading dose of 0.25 mg/kg over two minutes and then infused at 5 to 15 mg/hr. The maximum dose is 360 mg/day. Indications include prevention of reinfarction, angina, hypertension and, most commonly, rate control in atrial fibrillation or flutter. Hypotension is the main complication of this drug. Therapy is monitored based on desired effect.

Nicardipine

Nicardipine is a calcium-channel blocker with an onset of one to three minutes and duration of 15–40 minutes. Because of its relatively selective inhibition of vascular smooth muscle contraction along with its short half-life, some practitioners now use nicardipine in place of nitroprusside, especially in patients with evidence of cyanide toxicity or low endogenous thiosulfate levels (i.e., higher risk of cyanide toxicity).

Intravenous nicardipine was compared with nitroprusside in a randomized, multicenter trial, in 74 patients with hypertension (MAP ≥ 100 mmHg) following coronary artery bypass surgery (107). Nicardipine was administered as a 2.5- to 12.5-mg bolus followed by a 2- to 4-mg/hr infusion, and nitroprusside as a 0.5- to 6.0-mg/kg/min infusion. The aim was to reduce MAP to less than 90 mmHg within 50 minutes and maintain it stable at 85 ± 5 mmHg. Nicardipine was effective in 35 of 38 patients (92%), and nitroprusside in 29 of 36 (81%) (108). The decrease in MAP was not statistically different, but time until reaching the therapeutic endpoint was shorter with nicardipine ($P < 0.01$).

Nitroprusside was associated with greater increase in HR and decreases in mean PA, right atrial, and PACWP were more marked with $P < 0.01$ and $P < 0.05$, respectively, whereas nicardipine administration resulted in a greater elevation of $\dot{Q}$ and depression of SVR ($P < 0.01$ and $P < 0.05$, respectively). Patients on nicardipine had slightly more stable postreduction MAP and less need for drug titration with nicardipine. Interestingly, transfused blood volume was also lower with nicardipine (924 ± 644 mL) than nitroprusside (1306 ± 901 mL) ($P = 0.08$), despite similar postoperative blood losses.

Nicardipine is usually infused at 5–15 mg/hr. It is used in postoperative hypertension, the prevention of vasospasm from SAH, and angina. Nicardipine has the least potential cardiac contractility suppression of all calcium-channel blockers, but a long half-life. Complications include reflex tachycardia and hypotension. Therapy is titrated based on the drug's desired affect.

Nimodipine

Nimodipine is a calcium-channel blocker that only comes in oral form. It is usually given at 60 mg orally every four hours. The main indication for use is prevention of vasospasm following SAH. Nimodipine is a calcium-channel blocker that can alleviate vasospasm after SAH (see Volume 2, Chapter 14) (109). Intravenous nimodipine was recently used in two patients with primary thunderclap headache (TCH) after ischemia stroke had developed (110,111), with suggestive improvement. In addition, a small clinical series of nimodipine treatment in 11 consecutive patients with primary TCH showed some benefit in relieving vasospasm and headache. Similarly, intra-arterial nimodipine has been recently shown to reverse symptomatic vasospasm after SAH (112).

For the usual treatment of vasospasm following SAH, nimodipine is usually delivered in the oral form (the only available form until recently).

Angiotensin-Converting Enzyme Inhibitors

Enalaprilat is the only parenterally available ACE inhibitor, and thus the only drug of use for acute trauma or critical care related hypertensive crisis (113,114). The response to enalaprilat in variable and not predictable. The usual initial dose is 1.25 mg and is given every six hours. The maximum dose is 5 mg every six hours. The onset of action begins is 15 minutes but the peak effect may not be seen for four hours. The duration of action ranges from 12 to 24 hours. There are compelling indications for its use in heart failure, postmyocardial infarction, patients with high coronary disease risk, diabetes, chronic kidney disease, and for recurrent stroke prevention (Table 9). It is not used as a first-line agent for hypertension in the ICU setting. Typically, it is added as another agent to help control the hypertensive patient who needs a longer-acting drug, or in patients that are on oral forms of ACEIs at home. The main complication is hypotension. It is contraindicated in pregnancy.

SPECIAL CONSIDERATIONS
Coronary Artery Syndromes in the Trauma Patient

Suspicion of acute CAD in the critically ill trauma patient requires immediate attention and further diagnostic workup. This should include a 12-lead ECG to document progression of disease, an echocardiogram to evaluate function, and a consultation with the cardiology service. If the patient goes to Catheterization lab, the information contained in Table 10 will be obtained in order to assist in management.

Table 9   Compelling Indications for Antihypertensive Drugs Based upon Clinical Trials Reviewed in Joint National Committee 7

Compelling indication	Thiazide diuretic	BB	ACEI	ARB	CCB	Aldosterone antagonist
Heart failure	X	X	X	X		X
Post MI		X	X			X
High coronary disease risk	X	X	X		X	
Diabetes	X	X	X	X	X	
Chronic kidney disease			X	X		
Recurrent stroke prevention	X		X			

Abbreviations: ACEI, angiotensin-converting enzyme inhibitor; ARB, angiotensin receptor blocker; BB, β-blocker; CCB, calcium-channel blocker; MI, myocardial infarction.

Table 10 Ventricular Function Data Expected from the Catheterization Lab

Parameters evaluated on cath	Good	Impaired
RA, RV, PA, PACWP, LA, LV, AO contractility: EF, RVEDP, LVEDP wall motion abnormalities CA anatomy and description of lesions (>70% stenosis is significant)	EF > 0.55 LVEDP < 12 RVEDP <6 CI > 2.5	EF < 0.4 LVEDP > 18 RVEDP > 12 CI < 2.0

Abbreviations: AO, aorta; CA, coronary artery; CI, cardiac index; EF, ejection fraction; LA, left atrium; LV, left ventricle; LVEDP, left ventricular diastolic pressure; PA, pulmonary artery; PACWP, pulmonary capillary wedge pressure; RA, right atrium; RV, right ventricle; RVEDP, right ventricular and diastolic pressure.

Cardiac enzymes, including serial troponin, should be sent in addition to the other diagnostic studies. Therapy, such as aspirin, heparin, or platelet inhibitors, is essential in the management of acute cardiac ischemia. However, these therapies are contraindicated in the acutely traumatized patient with active CAD. Nitroglycerin may be considered in the trauma patient with acute CAD, but is harmful and essentially contraindicated in acute TBI with elevated ICP. Although the management is usually beta blockade if tolerated, following serial cardiac enzymes, supportive therapy, and watchful waiting, it is imperative to get the cardiology team involved early in these patients.

Once the information from the echocardiogram is obtained, there are certain hemodynamic goals to reach in the patient with cardiac ischemia. The echocardiogram will determine pump function, value function, intravascular volume, and rule out tamponade. The hemodynamic goals for the patient with myocardial ischemia may be at odds with the resuscitation requirement for hemorrhage. For instance, in the patient with myocardial ischemia, the goal is to decrease preload and increase the SVR. However, if the patient is traumatized and has ongoing hemorrhage, the goal is to increase the intravascular volume, which will start to normalize the SVR after fluid repletion (Table 11). As stated previously, some specific therapies for the CAD patient (e.g., heparin, aspirin, Plavix, etc.) are contraindicated in the trauma patient with active bleeding.

Valvular Heart Disease and Trauma/Critical Illness

The critically ill trauma patients with valvular heart disease may also create some management dilemmas. These patients may have specific hemodynamic requirements that may be contrary to the goals of resuscitation in hemorrhagic shock. Suspicion warrants immediate evaluation by the cardiology service, a 12-lead ECG, and an echocardiogram. Resuscitation considerations for patients with valvular heart disease are reviewed in Table 12. Managing these patients takes continuous communication with the

cardiology team, as well as constant reassessment of the hemodynamic goals.

EYE TO THE FUTURE

Developments in the cardiovascular management of critically ill patients continue to be made in diagnosis, monitoring, and support (mechanical and pharmacologic). Recent research indicates that early recognition and goal-directed therapy in septic patients improve outcomes (115,116). This concept of recognizing patients with sepsis syndromes early, so that aggressive therapy is instituted when patients arrive in the emergency department (ED), has led to a decrease in mortality from sepsis (117). Early goal-directed therapy in critically ill surgical patients has also led to better outcomes and a successful decrease in hospital stay (118,119).

Innovations in monitoring have also improved the care of the critically ill patient. Although invasive measures monitoring devices are still commonly employed, numerous noninvasive hemodynamic monitoring devices have become available that can provide accurate data in trauma and critically ill patients (120,121). These noninvasive devices can assess the adequacy of tissue perfusion and give hemodynamic parameters, such as cardiac index, without placing a Swan-Ganz catheter (122–124). A new form of inotropic drug is now being evaluated that may shorten the relaxation phase of the cardiac cycle and reduce filling pressures. These so-called "calcium sensitizers" provide better inotropic support in acute heart failure syndromes than the commonly employed inotropes (125,126).

Because the average age of the general population is increasing there are more elderly trauma and critically ill patients in our ICUs. The resuscitative efforts required to treat these elderly injured patients must now be more attuned to fluid overload, myocardial ischemia, or dysrhythmias, because the geriatric trauma patient is more prone to develop heart failure and inadequate tissue perfusion. The trauma intensivist needs to employ a wide array of strategies to ensure adequate tissue perfusion.

SUMMARY

The overriding management principles for the treatment of both the hypotensive and hypertensive conditions are firstly patient survival and secondly the prevention of end-organ damage. Although supranormal hemodynamic indices were at one time the goals of resuscitation, we now recognize that the side effects of attempting to achieve these supranormal values can cause ischemia, dysrhythmias, or be otherwise harmful.

The trauma intensivist now has a large armamentarium of diagnostic tools and therapeutic interventions to assist in

Table 11 Effects of Hemodynamic Parameters on Oxygen Supply and Demand of the Myocardium and Target Values for Patients with Coronary Artery Disease

Hemodynamic parameter	Effect on O₂ supply	Effect on M$_v$O$_2$	Target value
HR	⇓	⇑⇑	⇓⇓⇓
Dysrhythmia	⇓ – ⇓⇓⇓	⇑ – ⇑⇑	NSR
Preload	⇑	⇑⇑	⇓⇓
Afterload	⇑⇑	⇑	⇑⇑⇓
Contractility	⇑⇑	⇑⇑	⇑⇓

Abbreviations: HR, heart rate; NSR, normal sinus rhythm.

Table 12   Resuscitation Considerations for Patients with Valvular Heart Disease

	Aortic stenosis	Aortic insufficiency	Mitral stenosis	Mitral regurgitation
Pathophysiology	Concentric hypertrophy	Dilated LV volume overloaded	Dilated LA, ↑ PAP Empty and protected LV	Dilated LA and LV, volume overloaded
Hemodynamic goals	Hypertrophic LV requires high CA perfusion pressure (best assured by maintaining high SVR)	Stroke volume and ejection fraction maintained with preload reserve	May present with dyspnea, may be 2° to increased cardiac output (pregnancy or sepsis)	May underdiagnose LV failure because of regurgitant flow to LA despite severely decreased forward stroke volume
HR	⇓ ⇓	⇑	⇓ ⇓	⇑
Rhythm	SR[a]	–	Frequently in AS but NSR → AF = ↓	–
LV preload	↑	↑	↑	↑
SVR	⇑	↓	↔	⇓
PVR	↔	↔	↓ (These patients may have severe PA HTN)	↓
Contractility	↔ ↑	↔ ↑	↔	↔ ↑
RESUSC. pearls	Avoid myocardial depression, maintain CA perfusion pressure (↑ SVR, ↑ BP)	Minimize myocardial depression and keep the patient fast, full, and vasodilated	Avoid tachycardia (No Pavulon, inc. conduction through the AV node may dramatically inc. ventricular HR)	Isolated MR rare. Usually two papillary muscle dysfunction or RHD
	Be prepared to cardiovert if an arrhythmia occurs (CPR is futile)	A PAC is useful for measuring filling pressures and cardiac output	Don't decreases contractility. Inadequate sedation can precipitate extreme anxiety and tachycardia	MVP = most common cause of trivial isolated MR
	Treat hypotension with neo synephrine (etomidate = good induction choice)	Dobutamine is a reasonable supportive drug at induction	Consider esmolol to Rx tachycardia and hypotension	Maintain elevated HR, intervascular repletion and vasodilation (Have several ways to increase HR)

Note: Management of the patient with ischemic CAD is identical to that used for AS, except, the goal for the coronary artery patient should be to decrease the preload as hemodynamic improvement allows. Also note, for both AS and MS, CPR will be entirely ineffective, thus early cardioversion is required for the onset of V-fib, and very soon after the onset of atrial fib if medication does not quickly restore normal sinus rhythm.
[a]Maintaining SR is particularly critical in aortic stenosis.
Abbreviations: AV, atrial-ventricular; AI, aortic insufficiency; A-Fib, atrial fibrillation; BP, blood pressure; CA, coronary artery; CPR, cardiopulmonary resuscitation; CHF, congestive heart failure; Cong, congenital; HR, heart rate; HTN, hypertension; LA, left atrium; LV, left ventricle; MVP, mitral valve prolapse; mm, muscle; MR, mitral regurgitation; PA, pulmonary artery; PAC, pulmonary artery catheter; PAP, pulmonary artery pressure; PVR, pulmonary vascular resistance; RF, rheumatic fever; RHD, rheumatic heart disease; SBE, sub acute bacterial endocarditis; SVR, systemic vascular resistance.

resuscitative efforts. Therapy should be targeted to specific end points that provide adequate perfusion pressures and flows to critical organ beds. In order to monitor the success of therapy, the end points discussed in Volume 1, Chapters 12 and 18, and Volume 2, Chapter 18 should be reviewed.

In addition to understanding the hemodynamic goals of therapy, the clinician must be cognizant of side effects of the various drugs employed so that therapeutic goals can be obtained. As the patient population ages, more treatments are required on increasingly frail patients. Optimal management of these and other critically ill patients will likely be improved by early implementation of goal-directed therapy, where "reasonable" rather than "supranormal" resuscitation goals are targeted.

KEY POINTS

☞ Optimum hemodynamic management is based upon (*i*) the immediate cause of hypotension or hypertension, (*ii*) the presence of concomitant injuries, and (*iii*) the baseline medical conditions affecting the patient.

☞ The HR should be maintained within a reasonable range in order to sustain adequate Q̇ for tissue perfusion (10,11).

☞ In a febrile patient, the basal metabolic rate increases approximately 8% per degree centigrade, which correlates with an increase in HR of approximately 18 beats/min (i.e., 10 beats/min for each degree Fahrenheit) (13,14).

- Some patients can manifest bradycardia that is unresponsive to the elevated catecholamine state, associated with trauma or critical illness.

- Elderly patients suffering from trauma or critical illness are prone to develop atrial fibrillation or supraventricular tachycardia, secondary to elevated catecholamines, baseline myocardial irritability, direct myocardial injury, or ischemia, all of which can impair pump function (17,18).

- Parameters measured by noninvasive means, such as HR, BP, urine output, skin color, turgor and temperature, along with capillary refill, can be obtained quickly and reflect the patient's intravascular volume status prior to the placement of invasive monitors (19,20).

- The measured SVR can be two to three times higher than normal following massive hemorrhage, due to catecholamine-mediated arteriolar constriction in compensation for the decreased intravascular volume.

- Adequacy of perfusion to tissues is the most important end point of resuscitation.

- When the MAP falls below 60 mmHg, organ perfusion to renal and splanchnic organs begins to fall. As the MAP dips below 50 mmHg, perfusion to brain and myocardium can become diminished.

- Any patient who is adequately fluid resuscitated and requiring vasopressor support, but remains unresponsive to these measures, may have adrenal insufficiency and may need steroid administration for improvement in vasomotor tone (28–33).

- The overall goal is to ensure adequate tissue perfusion by repletion of intravascular volume first. Vasoconstrictor or inotropic support drugs are generally best administered after intravascular repletion is assured. However, occasionally, both drug support and volume repletion must be employed concomitantly to maintain an adequate blood pressure until sufficient fluid repletion can be achieved.

- Norepinephrine (Levophed®) can be used to increase BP in hypotensive patients who fail to respond to adequate volume resuscitation and other, less potent, vasopressors.

- The use of vasopressin has also been shown to decrease the requirement for other vasopressors and is associated with a higher urine output and improved creatinine clearance (54,55).

- Although low-dose dopamine increases renal blood flow, it does not ameliorate renal failure, and has not improved outcomes in nonoliguric patients recovering from ATN (70,71).

- The traumatologist and intensivist need to be aware of the pharmacology and side effects of these common drugs, because of their prevalence in the critically ill population and, more importantly, because they are used in the treatment of hypertensive crises.

- In all scenarios, the goal of MHTN treatment is to prevent end-organ damage.

REFERENCES

1. Kern JW, Shoemaker WC. Meta-analysis of hemodynamic optimization in high-risk patients. Crit Care Med 2002; 30(8):1686–1692.
2. Dasta JF, Brackett CC. Defining and achieving optimum therapeutic goals in critically ill patients. Pharmacotherapy 1994; 14(6):678–688.
3. Domsky MF, Wilson RF. Hemodynamic resuscitation. Crit Care Clin 1993; 9(4):715–726.
4. McGee S, Abernethy WB, Simel DL. The rational clinical examination. Is this patient hypovolemic? JAMA 1999; 281(11):1022–1029.
5. Gutierrez G, Reines HD, Wulf-Gutierrez ME. Clinical review hemorrhagic shock. Crit Care 2004; 8(5):373–381.
6. Chang MC, Martin RS, Scherer LA, Meredith JW. Improving ventricular–arterial coupling during resuscitation from shock: effects on cardiovascular function and systemic perfusion. J Trauma 2002; 53(4):679–685.
7. Drummond JC, Petrovitch CT. The massively bleeding patient. Anesthesiol Clin North Am 2001; 19(4):633–649.
8. Lee YT, Chou TD, Peng MY, Chang FY. Rapidly progressive necrotizing fasciitis caused by Staphylococcus aureus. J Microbiol Immunol Infect 2005; 38(5):361–364.
9. Young MH, Aronoff DM, Engleberg NC. Necrotizing fasciitis: pathogenesis and treatment. Expert Rev Anti Infect Ther. 2005; 3(2):279–294.
10. Kresh JY, Armour JA. The heart as a self-regulating system: integration of homeodynamic mechanisms. Technol Health Care 1997; 5(1–2):159–169.
11. McDonough KH, Giaimo M, Quinn M, Miller H. Intrinsic myocardial function in hemorrhagic shock. Shock 1999; 11(3):205–210.
12. Vincent JL, Prevention and therapy of multiple organ failure. World J Surg 1996; 20(4):465–470.
13. Roe CF. Temperature regulation and energy metabolism in surgical patients. Prog Surg 1973; 12:96–127.
14. Haight JS, Keatinge WR. Elevation in set point for body temperature regulation after prolonged exercise. J Physiol 1973; 229(1):77–85.
15. Fathizadeh P, Shoemaker WC, Wo CC, et al. Autonomic activity in trauma patients based on variability of HR and respiratory rate. Crit Care Med 2004; 32(6):1300–1305.
16. Vaz M, Sucharita S, Bharathi AV. HR and systolic blood pressure variability: the impact of thinness and aging in human male subjects. J Nutr Health Aging 2005; 9(5):341–345.
17. Hogue CW, J Creswell LL, Gutterman DD, et al. Epidemiology, mechanisms, and risks: American college of Chest Physicians guidelines for the prevention and management of postoperative atrial fibrillation after cardiac surgery. Chest 2005; 128(2):9S–16S.
18. Seguin P, Signouret T, Laviolle B, et al. Incidence and risk factors of atrial fibrillation in a surgical intensive care unit. Crit Care Med 2004; 32(3):722–726.
19. Bilkovski RN Rivers EP, Horst HM. Targeted resuscitation strategies after injury. Curr Opin Crit Care 2004; 10(6): 529–538.
20. Kaplan LJ, McPartland K, Santora TA, et al. Start with a subjective assessment of skin temperature to identify hypoperfusion in intensive care unit patients. J Trauma 2001; 50(4):620–627.
21. Asensio JA, Demetriades D, Berne TV, Shoemaker WC. Invasive and noninvasive monitoring for early recognition and treatment of shock in high-risk trauma and surgical patients. Surg Clin North Am 1996; 76(4):985–997.
22. Shoemaker WC, Appel PL, Kram HB. Hemodynamic and oxygen transport responses in survivors and nonsurvivors of high-risk surgery. Crit Care Med 1993; 21(7):977–990.
23. Jalonen J. Invasive haemodynamic monitoring: concepts and practical approaches. Ann Med 1997;29(4):313–318.
24. McKinley BA, Kozar RA, Cocanour CS, et al. Normal versus supranormal oxygen delivery goal in shock resuscitation: the response is the same. J Trauma 2002; 53(5):825–832.
25. Velmahos GC, Demetriades D, Shoemaker WC, et al. Endpoints of resuscitation of critically injured patients: normal or supranormal? A prospective randomized trial. Ann Surg 2000; 232(3):409–418.
26. Fleming A, Bishop M, Shoemaker W, et al. Prospective trial of supranormal values as goals of resuscitation in severe trauma. Arch Surg 1992; 127(10):1175–1179.

27. Stiefel MF, Tomita Y, Marmarou A. Secondary ischemia impairing the restoration of ion homeostasis following traumatic brain injury. J Neurosurg 2005; 103(4), 707–714.

28. Beeman BR, Veverka TJ, Lambert P, et al. Relative adrenal insufficiency among trauma patients in a community hospital. Curr Surg 2005; 62(6):633–637.

29. Thys F, Laterre PF. Hydrocortisone in septic shock: too much, too little, too soon? Crit Care Med 2005; 33(11):2683–2684.

30. Siraux V, De Backer D, Yalavatti G, et al. Relative adrenal insufficiency in patients with septic shock: comparison of low-dose and conventional corticotropin tests. Crit Care Med 2005; 33(11):2479–2486.

31. Chadda K, Annane D. The use of corticosteroids in severe sepsis and acute respiratory distress syndrome. Ann Med 2002; 34(7):582–589.

32. Rivers EP, Gaspari M, Saad GA. Adrenal insufficiency in high-risk surgical ICU patients. Chest 2001; 119:889–896.

33. Annane D, Bellissant E, Sebille V. Impaired pressor sensitivity to noradrenaline in septic shock patients with and without impaired adrenal function reserve. British J Clin Pharm 1998; 46:589–597.

34. Annane D, Sebille V, Charpentier C, et al. Effect of treatment with low doses of hydrocortisone and fludrocortisone on mortality in patients with septic shock. JAMA 2002; 288(7), 862–871.

35. Levy B, Dusang B, Annane D, et al. Cardiovascular response to dopamine and early prediction of outcome in septic shock: a prospective multiple-center study. Crit Care Med 2005; 33(10):2172–2177.

36. Guerin JP, Levraut J, Samat Long C, et al. Effects of dopamine and norepinephrine on systemic and hepatosplanchnic hemodynamics, oxygen exchange, and energy balance in vasoplegic septic patients. Shock 2005; 23(1):18–24.

37. Vincent JL, de Backer D. The International Sepsis Forum's controversies in sepsis: my initial vasopressor agent in septic shock is dopamine rather than norepinephrine. Crit Care 2003; 7(1):6–8.

38. Sharma VK, Dellinger RP. The International Sepsis Forum's controversies in sepsis: my initial vasopressor agent in septic shock is norepinephrine rather than dopamine. Crit Care 2003; 7(1):3–5.

39. Martin C, Papazian L, Perrin G, et al. Norepinephrine or dopamine for the treatment of hyperdynamic septic shock? Chest 1993; 103(6):1826–1831.

40. Mullner M, Urbanek B, Havel C, et al. Vasopressors for shock. Cochrane Database Syst Rev 2004; (3):CD003709.

41. Albanese J, Leone M, Delmas A, et al. Terlipressin or norepinephrine in hyperdynamic septic shock: a prospective, randomized study. Crit Care Med 2005; 33(9):1897–1902.

42. Beloeil H, Mazoit JX, Benhamou D, et al. Norepinephrine kinetics and dynamics in septic shock and trauma patients. BJA 2005; 95(6):782–788.

43. Marik PE, Mohedin M. The contrasting effects of dopamine and norephinephrine on systemic and splanchnic oxygen utilization in hyperdynamic sepsis. JAMA 1994; 272:1354–1357.

44. Morimatsu H, Singh K, Uchino S, et al. Early and exclusive use of norepinephrine in septic shock. Resuscitation 2004; 62(2):249–54.

45. Malay MB, Ashton RC Jr, Landry, DW, et al. Low-dose vasopressin in the treatment of vasodilatory septic shock. J. Trauma 1999;47(4):699–703; discussion 703.

46. Luckner G, Dunser MW, Jochberger S, et al. Arginine vasopressin in 316 patients with advanced vasodilatory shock. Crit Care Med 2005; 33(11):2659–2666.

47. Patel BM, Chittock DR, Russell JA, Walley KR. Beneficial effects of short-term vasopressin infusion during severe septic shock. Anesthesiology 2002; 96:576–582.

48. Buff DD. Vasopressin has cost and administration advantages over epinephrine in cardiac arrest. Arch Intern Med 2005; 165(14):1663.

49. Holmes CL, Walley KR. Vasopressin in the ICU. Curr Opin Crit Care 2004; 10(6):442–448.

50. Kam PC, Williams S, Yoong FF. Vasopressin and terlipressin: pharmacology and its clinical relevance. Anaesthesia 2004; 59(10):993–1001.

51. Abraldes JG, Bosch J. Medical management of variceal bleeding in patients with cirrhosis. Can J. Gastroenterol 2004; 18(2):109–113.

52. Koshman SL, Zed PJ, Abu Laban RB. Vasopressin in cardiac arrest. Ann Pharmacother 2005; 39(5):1687–1692.

53. Dunser MW, Mayr AJ, Ulmer H, et al. Arginine vasopressin in advanced vasodilatory shock: a prospective, randomized, controlled study. Circulation 2003; 107(18):2313–2319.

54. Lim TW, Lee S, Ng KS. Vasopressin effective in reversing catecholamine-resistant vasodilatory shock. Anaesth Intensive Care 2000; 28(3):313–317.

55. Leone M, Albanese J, Delmas A, et al. Terlipressin in catecholamine-resistant septic shock patients. Shock 2004; 22(4):314–319.

56. Dunser MW, Mayr AJ, Tur A, et al. Ischemic skin lesions as a complication of continuous vasopressin infusion in catecholamine-resistant vasodilatory shock: incidence and risk factors. Crit Care Med 2003; 31(5); 1394–1398.

57. Vincent JL, Bredas P, Jankowski S, et al. Correction of hypocalcaemia in the critically ill: what is the haemodynamic benefit? Intensive Care Med 1995; 21(10):838–841.

58. Drop LJ, Daniels AL, Hoaglin DC. Calcium chloride versus calcium gluconate: comparison of ionization and cardiovascular effects in children and dogs. Anesthesiology 1987; 66(4):465–470.

59. Levy B, Bollaert PE, Charpentier C, et al. Comparison of norepinephrine and dobutamine to epinephrine for hemodynamics, lactate metabolism, and gastric tonometric variables in septic shock: a prospective, randomized study. Intensive Care Med 1997; 23:282–287.

60. Di Giantomasso D, Bellomo R, May CN. The haemodynamic and metabolic effects of epinephrine in experimental hyperdynamic septic shock. Intensive Care Med 2005; 31(3): 454–462.

61. Beale RJ, Hollenberg SM, Vincent JL, et al. Vasopressor and inotropic support in septic shock: an evidence-based review. Crit Care Med 2004; 32(11):S455–S465.

62. Levy B. Bench-to-bedside review: is there a place for epinephrine in septic shock? Crit Care 2005; 9(6):561–565.

63. Jaillard S, Elbaz F, Bresson Just S, et al. Pulmonary vasodilator effects of norepinephrine during the development of chronic pulmonary hypertension in neonatal lambs. BJA 2004; 93(6):818–824.

64. Schindler MB, Hislop AA, Haworth SG. Postnatal changes in response to norepinephrine in the normal and pulmonary hypertensive lung. Am J Respir Crit Care Med 2004; 170(6):641–646.

65. Morelli A, Ricci Z, Bellomo R, et al. Prophylactic fenoldopam for renal protection in sepsis: a randomized, double-blind, placebo-controlled pilot trial. Crit Care Med 2005; 33(11):2451–2456.

66. Jones D, Bellomo R. Renal-dose dopamine: from hypothesis to paradigm to dogma to myth and, finally, superstition? J Intensive Care Med 2005; 20(4):199–211.

67. Di Giantomasso D, Morimatsu H, May CN, et al. Increasing renal blood flow: low-dose dopamine or medium-dose norepinephrine. Chest 2004; 125(6):2260–2267.

68. Gordon IL, Wesley R, Wong DH, et al. Effect of dopamine on renal blood flow and cardiac output. Arch Surg 1995; 130(8):864–868.

69. Duke GJ, Bersten AD. Dopamine and renal salvage in the critically ill patient. Anaesth Intensive Care 1992; 20(3):277–287.

70. Tumlin JA, Finkel KW, Murray PT, et al. Fenoldopam mesylate in early acute tubular necrosis: a randomized, double-blind, placebo-controlled clinical trial. Am J Kidney Dis 2005; 46(1):26–34.

71. Friedrich AD, Choi EK. Renal-dose dopamine: another nail in the coffin. Crit Care Med 2005; 33(6):1447–1448.

72. Subhani M, Sridhar S, DeCristofaro JD. Phentolamine use in a neonate for the prevention of dermal necrosis caused by dopamine: a case report. J. Perinatol 2001; 21(5):324–326.

73. Park JY, Kanzler M, Swette SM. Dopamine-associated symmetric peripheral gangrene. Arch Derm 1997;133(2): 247–249.

74. Boltax RS, Dineen JP, Scarpa FJ. Gangrene resulting from infiltrated dopamine solution. N Engl J Med 1977; 296(14):823.

75. Kerbaul F, Rondelet B, Motte S, et al. Effects of norepinephrine and dobutamine on pressure load-induced right ventricular failure. Crit Care Med 2004; 32(4):1035–1040.

76. Vincent JL, De Backer D. Inotrope/vasopressor support in sepsis-induced organ hypoperfusion. Semin Resp Crit Care Med 2001; 22(1):61–74.

77. Dellinger RP, Carlet JM, Masur H, et al. Surviving sepsis campaign guidelines for management of severe sepsis and septic shock. Crit Care Med 2004; 32(3):858–73. anesthesia. Anesthesiol 2004; 100(5):1188–1197.

78. Elatrous S, Nouira S, Besbes Ouanes, et al. Dobutamine in severe scorpion envenomation: effects on standard hemodynamics, right ventricular performance, and tissue oxygenation. Chest 1999; 116(3):748–753.

79. Huang L, Weil MH, Tang W, et al. Comparison between dobutamine and levosimendan for management of postresuscitation myocardial dysfunction. Crit Care Med 2005; 33(3): 487–491.

80. Feneck RO, Sherry KM, Withington PS, et al. Comparison of the hemodynamic effects of milrinone with dobutamine in patients after cardiac surgery. J Cardiothorac Vasc Anesth 2001; 15(3):306–315.

81. Iribe G, Yamada H, Matsunaga A, et al. Effects of the phosphodiesterase III inhibitors olprinone, milrinone, and amrinone on hepatosplanchnic oxygen metabolism. Crit Care Med 2000; 28(3):743–748.

82. Barton P, Garcia J, Kouatli A, et al. Hemodynamic effects of i.v. milrinone lactate in pediatric patients with septic shock. A prospective, double-blinded, randomized, placebo-controlled, interventional study. Chest 1996; 109(5):1302–1312.

83. Prielipp RC, MacGregor DA, Butterwoth JF, et al. Pharmacodynamics and pharmacokinetics of milrinone administration to increase oxygen delivery in critically ill patients. Chest 1996; 109(5):1291–301.

84. Taniguchi T, Shibata K, Saito S, et al. Pharmacokinetics of milrinone in patients with congestive heart failure during continuous venovenous hemofiltration. Intensive Care Med 2000; 26(8):1089–1093.

85. Scalea TM, Donovan R. Amrinone as an inotrope in managing hypermetabolic surgical stress. J. Trauma 1992; 32(3): 372–378.

86. Ross MP, Allen Webb EM, Pappas JB, et al. Amrinone-associated thrombocytopenia: pharmacokinetic analysis. Clin Pharm Ther 1993; 53(6):661–667.

87. Sadiq A, Tamura N, Yoshida M, et al. Possible contribution of acetylamrinone and its enhancing effects on platelet aggregation under shear stress conditions in the onset of thrombocytopenia in patients treated with amrinone. Thrombosis Res 2003; 111(6):357–361.

88. Renton MC, Snowden CP. Dopexamine and its role in the protection of hepatosplanchnic and renal perfusion in high-risk surgical and critically ill patients. BJA 2005; 94(4):459–467.

89. Westphal M, Sielenkamper AW, Van Aken H, et al. Dopexamine reverses the vasopressin-associated impairment in tissue oxygen supply but decreases systemic blood pressure in ovine endotoxemia. Anesth Analg 2004; 99(3):878–885.

90. Schilling T, Grundling M, Strang CM, Moritz KU, Siegmund W, Hachenberg T. Effects of dopexamine, dobutamine or dopamine on prolactin and thyreotropin serum concentrations in high-risk surgical patients. Intensive Care Med. 2004; 30(6):1127–1133.

91. Oberbeck R, Schmitz D, Schuler M, et al. Dopexamine and cellular immune functions during systemic inflammation. Immunobiology 2004; 208(5):429–438.

92. Hiltebrand LB, Krejci V, Sigurdsson GH. Effects of dopamine, dobutamine, and dopexamine on microcirculatory blood flow in the gastrointestinal tract during sepsis and anesthesia. Anesthesiology 2004; 100(5):1188–1197.

93. Chobanian AV, Bakris GL, Black HR, et al. and the National High Blood Pressure Education Program Coordinating Committee. The seventh report of the Joint National Committee on prevention, detection, evaluation, and treatment of high blood pressure: the JNC 7 report. JAMA 2003; 289: 2560–2572.

94. Wang Y, Wang QJ. The prevalence of prehypertension and hypertension among US adults according to the new joint national committee guidelines: new challenges of the old problem. Arch Intern Med 2004; 164(19):2126–2134.

95. Joint National Committee on Prevention, Detection, Evaluation, and Treatment of High Blood Pressure. The sixth report of the Joint National Committee on prevention, detection, evaluation, and treatment of high blood pressure. Arch Intern Med 1997; 157:2413–2446.

96. Reuler JB, Magarian GJ. Hypertensive emergencies and urgencies: definition, recognition, and management. J Gen Intern Med 1998; 3(1):64–74.

97. Vidaeff AC, Carroll MA, Ramin SM. Acute hypertensive emergencies in pregnancy. Crit Care Med 2005; 33(10), S307–S312.

98. Immink RV, van den Born BJ, van Montfrans GA, et al. Impaired cerebral autoregulation in patients with malignant hypertension. Circulation 2004; 110(15):2241–2245.

99. Fenves AZ, Ram CV. Drug treatment of hypertensive urgencies and emergencies. Semin Nephrol 2005; 25(4):272–280.

100. Vaughan CJ, Delanty N. Hypertensive emergencies. Lancet 2000; 356:411–417.

101. Manger WM, Eisenhofer G. Pheochromocytoma: diagnosis and management update. Curr Hypertens Rep 2004; 6(6): 477–484.

102. Rose JC, Mayer SA. Optimizing blood pressure in neurological emergencies. Neurocritical Care 2004; 1(3):287–299.

103. Curry SC, Arnold Capell P. Toxic effects of drugs used in the ICU. Nitroprusside, nitroglycerin, and angiotensin-converting enzyme inhibitors. Crit Care Clin 1991; 7(3):555–581.

104. Schulz V. Clinical pharmacokinetics of nitroprusside, cyanide, thiosulfate and thiocynate. Clin Pharmacokin 1984; 9:239–251.

105. Abernethy DR, Schwartz JB. Calcium-antagonist drug. N Engl J Med 1999; 341:1447–1457.

106. Pepine CJ, Handberg EM, Cooper DeHoff RM, et al. A calcium antagonist vs. a non-calcium antagonist hypertension treatment strategy for patients with coronary artery disease. The International Verapamil–Trandolapril Study (INVEST): a randomized controlled trial. JAMA 2003; 290(21):2805–2816.

107. David D, Dubois C, Loria Y. Comparison of nicardipine and sodium nitroprusside in the treatment of paroxysmal hypertension following aortocoronary bypass surgery. J Cardiothorac Vasc Anesth 1991; 5(4):357–361.

108. Lu SR, Liao YC, Fuh LJ, et al. Nimodipine for treatment of primary thunderclap headache. Neurology 2004; 62(8):1414–1416.

109. Feigin VL, Rinkel GJ, Algra A, et al. Calcium antagonists in patients with aneurysmal subarachnoid hemorrhage: a systematic review. Neurology 1998; 50:876–883.

110. Sturm JW, Macdonell RA. Recurrent thunderclap headache associated with reversible intracerebral vasospasm causing stroke. Cephalalgia 2000; 20:132–135.

111. Nowak DA, Rodiek SO, Henneken S, et al. Reversible segmental cerebral vasoconstriction (Call-Fleming syndrome): are calcium channel inhibitors a potential treatment option? Cephalalgia 2003; 23:218–222.

112. Firat MM, Gelebek V, Orer HS, et al. Selective intraarterial nimodipine treatment in an experimental subarachnoid hemorrhage model. Am J Neuroradiol 2005; 26:1357–1362.

113. Boldt J, Menges T, Wollbruck M, et al. Continuous i.v. administration of the angiotensin-converting enzyme inhibitor

enalaprilat in the critically ill: effects on regulators of circulatory homeostasis. J Cardiovasc Pharmacol 1995; 25(3):416–423.

114. Boldt J, Menges T, Wollbruck M, et al. Cardiopulmonary actions of intravenously administered enalaprilat in trauma patients. Crit Care Med 1994; 22(6):960–964.

115. Rivers E, Nguyen B, Havstad S, et al. Early goal-directed therapy in the treatment of severe sepsis and septic shock. N Engl J Med 2001; 345(19):1368–1377.

116. Rivers EP, McIntyre L, Morro DC, et al. Early and innovative interventions for severe sepsis and septic shock: taking advantage of a window of opportunity. CMAJ 2005; 173(9): 1054–1065.

117. Vincent JL, Abraham E, Annane D, et al. Reducing mortality in sepsis: new directions. Crit Care 2002; 6:S1–S18.

118. Pearse R, Dawson D, Fawcett J, et al. Early goal-directed therapy after major surgery reduces complications and duration of hospital stay. A randomised, controlled trial [ISRCTN38797445]. Crit Care 2005; 9(6):R687–R693.

119. Chapman M, Gattas D, Suntharalingam G. Why is early goal-directed therapy successful—is it the technology? Crit Care 2005; 9(4):307–308.

120. Velmahos GC, Wo CC, Demetriades D, et al. Early continuous noninvasive haemodynamic monitoring after severe blunt trauma. Injury 1999; 30(3):209–214.

121. Martin M, Brown C, Bayard D, et al. Continuous noninvasive monitoring of cardiac performance and tissue perfusion in pediatric trauma patients. J Pediatr Surg 2005; 40(12):1957–1963.

122. Reinhart K, Bloos F. The value of venous oximetry. Curr Opin Crit Care 2005; 11(3):259–263.

123. Marik PE. Regional carbon dioxide monitoring to assess the adequacy of tissue perfusion. Curr Opin Crit Care 2005; 11(3):245–251.

124. Cuschieri J, Rivers EP, Donnino MW, et al. Central venous–arterial carbon dioxide difference as an indicator of cardiac index. Intensive Care Med 2005; 31(6):818–822.

125. Follath F, Franco F, Cardoso JS. European experience on the practical use of levosimendan in patients with acute heart failure syndromes. Am J Cardiol 2005; 96(6A):80G–85G.

126. Mebazaa A, Barraud D, Welschbillig S. Randomized clinical trials with levosimendan. Am J Cardiol 2005; 96(6A):74G–79G.

18

Shock

James Gordon Cain

Department of Anesthesiology and Critical Care Medicine, University of Pittsburgh, Pittsburgh, Pennsylvania, U.S.A.

Jonathan B. Cohen

Department of Anesthesiology and Critical Care, University of South Florida College of Medicine, Tampa, Florida, U.S.A.

Erik B. Kistler

Department of Anesthesiology and Critical Care, UC San Diego Medical Center, San Diego, California, U.S.A.

Enrico M. Camporesi

Department of Anesthesiology and Critical Care, University of South Florida College of Medicine, Tampa, Florida, U.S.A.

INTRODUCTION

Shock was recognized by Hippocrates and his contemporaries as a "post-traumatic syndrome" occurring in those who had sustained major injuries. The origins of the word "shock" traces back to the French word *choc* meaning violent attack, and was first used by Le Dran in 1737 in his text, "A treatise on reflections drawn from practice on gunshot wounds" (1). The term "shock" entered into more common usage after Edwin Morris published his book "A practical treatise on shock after operations and injuries" in 1867 (2).

Prior to World War I, Cannon postulated a "toxic" theory, whereby shock was attributed to the effects of circulating toxins causing vasomotor pooling and loss of blood and fluids into the injured tissues (3). An alternative theory was presented by Dr. Alfred Blalock with his research on dogs, where he suggested that blood loss alone was responsible for the hypotension seen in traumatized animals. Blalock revolutionized the management of patients in hemorrhagic shock, and his enthusiasm for the transfusion of blood and blood products certainly saved numerous lives during World War II (4). It has become increasingly clear that both the volume loss and toxin production hypotheses are involved in various aspects of the current shock paradigm, and treatment today attempts to address both considerations.

In 1972, Hinshaw and Cox proposed a classification system for shock, which is among several currently utilized today. Their description is based largely on the cardiovascular characteristics seen with each type and includes hypovolemic, cardiogenic, obstructive, and distributive. The category of distributive shock is sometimes eschewed in favor of its constituent categories (septic, anaphylactic, neurogenic, and adrenal crisis) being listed separately. In addition, many investigators believe a fifth category should be added, which includes a "cellular" designation (Table 1) (5).

☞ **Shock is defined as inadequate perfusion of the tissue. This inadequacy can result from deficient oxygen delivery (D̄O₂), excessive utilization, or a combination of the two. In "cytotoxic" shock tissue, mitochondria are unable to utilize the O₂ delivered.** ☞

Hemorrhage and sepsis are common etiologies of shock, following central nervous system injury as the most common etiologies of death in trauma patients (6–9). Trauma patients are subject to a variety of shock etiologies, often progressing from one form to another. Neurohumoral mechanisms initially compensate for cardiovascular derangements and maintain vital organ perfusion, but compensatory mechanisms can ultimately become overwhelmed. When the perfusion of tissues with oxygenated blood falls below the basal state required to maintain cell viability, cellular injury, organ ischemia, multiple organ dysfunction, and death may ensue. Diagnosis and treatment of the underlying etiology is the foundation of shock treatment, and prompt initiation of therapy is vital to forestall adverse consequences.

☞ **Hypovolemic shock is caused by acute blood loss of greater than 30% of the circulating blood volume (class III/IV hemorrhage).** ☞ The severity of the hypovolemic shock is correlated with the degree of volume loss (Table 2) as well by the rapidity with which it occurs. Prolonged hypovolemic shock can proceed to irreversible shock with diffuse organ injury resulting in irreversible circulatory failure. Aggressive fluid resuscitation remains the mainstay of care. Cardiogenic shock is caused by primary myocardial dysfunction and inability to generate effective cardiac output (Q̇). Distributive shock is characterized by arterial and venous dilation with venous pooling. Its causes are numerous, including: bacterial sepsis and its byproducts, mediators of systemic inflammatory response syndrome (SIRS), anaphylactic and anaphylactoid reactions, neurogenic shock, and adrenal crisis. Obstructive shock results from mechanical impediment to blood flow; that is, obstruction of venous return and/or arterial outflow from the heart. Causes include tension pneumothorax, pericardial tamponade, pulmonary embolism (PE), excessive positive end expiratory pressure (PEEP), and abdominal compartment syndrome (ACS) (Volume 2, Chapter 34).

This chapter provides an overview of the pathophysiology, diagnosis, and management of various shock states, emphasizing those most commonly seen in trauma and critical care. Cellular shock etiologies are mentioned for completion,

Table 1 Classification of Shock and Common Etiologies

Categories	Common etiologies
Hypovolemic	External and occult hemorrhages, skin losses (severe burns), third spacing (pancreatitis, bowel obstruction, and prolonged abdominal surgery), gastrointestinal tract losses (vomiting, diarrhea), urinary tract losses
Cardiogenic	Acute myocardial infarction and its complications (e.g., acute mitral regurgitation, rupture of the interventricular septum, rupture of the free wall), myocarditis, end-stage cardiomyopathy, myocardical contusion, myocardial dysfunction after prolonged cardiopulmonary bypass, valvular heart disease, and hypertrophic obstructive cardiomyopathy
Obstructive	Cardiac tamponade, massive pulmonary embolism, tension pneumothorax, cor pulmonale, atrial myxoma, coarctation of aorta
Distributive	Septic shock, anaphylactic shock, neurogenic shock, adrenal crisis
Cellular[a]	Cyanide intoxication, carbon monoxide intoxication, iron intoxication

[a]Cellular shock results from processes that render the cell incapable of utilizing the O_2 which is delivered.

but not reviewed here. These conditions are thoroughly covered elsewhere (e.g., CN Toxicity in Volume 1, Chapter 34 and CO Toxicity in Volume 1, Chapters 31 and 34).

PATHOPHYSIOLOGY

The oxygen delivery ($\dot{D}O_2$) to tissues is related to the $\dot{Q}$ and arterial O_2 content (CaO_2) as seen in Equation 1. The $\dot{Q}$ component can be augmented by increasing either the stroke volume (SV) or the heart rate (HR) (Equation 2). The CaO_2 is derived from the hemoglobin concentration [Hgb] in g/dL, the amount of O_2 bound to the Hgb (generally, 1.34 mL O_2/g Hgb) multiplied by the SaO_2; and the amount of O_2 dissolved in the plasma ($0.003 \times PaO_2$) as per Equation 3.

$$\dot{D}O_2 = \dot{Q} \times CaO_2 \tag{1}$$

$$\dot{Q} = SV \times HR \tag{2}$$

$$CaO_2 = [Hgb] \times 1.34 \times SaO_2 + 0.003 \times PaO_2 \tag{3}$$

Stressful events affecting the body, for example, trauma, burns, sepsis, and so on, will increase O_2 demand (10). O_2 consumption ($\dot{V}O_2$) will usually increase to meet that demand so long as an adequate $\dot{D}O_2$ is being provided (11). If $\dot{D}O_2$ fails to increase adequately to meet the demands of the tissues, tissue ischemia develops and cell death and organ dysfunction may ensue (12). With studies supporting these relationships, it is easy to see why shock research initially became focused on maximizing $\dot{D}O_2$, either by increasing $\dot{Q}$ or CaO_2.

The targets for improving $\dot{D}O_2$ have been largely aimed at maximizing the $\dot{Q}$ after ensuring that hemoglobin concentration [Hgb] and saturation is adequate. Often the focus for increasing $\dot{Q}$ has been increasing the SV. Studies which demonstrate maximized $\dot{D}O_2$ have not, however, consistently shown improved survival (13,14).

In both hemorrhagic and septic shock, maximal $\dot{D}O_2$ has not consistently increased $\dot{V}O_2$. Therefore, two hypotheses emerged: (*i*) systemically adequate $\dot{D}O_2$ is not necessarily sufficient when measured at the tissue level (i.e., macrocirculation $\neq$ microcirculation); and (*ii*) cells in shock may be unable to utilize the O_2 being delivered.

Systemic $\dot{D}O_2$ Adequacy Does Not Ensure Sufficient Tissue Perfusion

✎ **Blood flow to organs is regulated by mechanisms that control systemic, regional, and local perfusion. Dysfunction can occur at any of these points.** ✎

Historically, clinicians have targeted the "macro"circulation, mainly because it was the only tissue bed that could be monitored. It is certainly easier to implement goal-directed therapy toward arterial blood flow than toward microcirculatory blood flow. Technological advances are

Table 2 Estimated Fluid and Blood Losses Based on Patient's Initial Presentation[a]

	Class I	Class II	Class III	Class IV
Blood loss (mL)	Up to 750	750–1500	1500–2000	>2000
Blood loss (% blood volume)	Up to 15%	15–30%	30–40%	>40%
Pulse rate	<100	>100	>120	>140
Blood pressure	Normal	Normal	Decreased	Decreased
Pulse pressure (mmHg)	Normal or increased	Decreased	Decreased	Decreased
Respiratory rate	14–20	20–30	30–40	>35
Urine output (mL/hr)	>30	20–30	5–15	Negligible
CNS/mental status	Slightly anxious	Mildly anxious	Anxious, confused	Confused, lethargic
Fluid replacement (3:1 rule)	Crystalloid	Crystalloid	Crystalloid and blood	Crystalloid and blood

[a]For a 70-kg man. The guidelines in this table are based on the 3:1 rule. This rule derives from the empiric observation that most patients in hemorrhagic shock require as much as 300 mL of electrolyte solution for each 100 mL of blood loss. Applied blindly, these guidelines can result in excessive or inadequate fluid administration. For example, a patient with a crush injury to the extremity may have hypotension out of proportion to their blood loss and require fluids in excess of the 3:1 guidelines. In contrast, a patient whose ongoing blood loss is being replaced by blood transfusion requires less than 3:1. The use of bolus therapy with careful monitoring of the patient's response can moderate these extremes.
Abbreviation: CNS, central nervous system.
Source: From Ref. 192.

increasingly allowing cellular perfusion to be evaluated, but these are still largely in the experimental phase and not yet validated in patient populations.

The microcirculation consists of vessels <300 μm in diameter. In excess of 10 billion capillaries supply nutrients and remove waste from cells in a normal 70-kg individual (15). Capillary PO_2 and Hgb saturation values are markedly decreased from arterial values at this level (15,16). In addition, the hematocrit in the microvasculature is decreased from arterial values and heterogeneously distributed leading to uneven $\dot{D}O_2$ at the tissue level (17).

The microcirculation is particularly vulnerable to dysfunction in diseased states (17). Hypovolemic shock is associated with decreased perfusion of muscle, skin, and the splanchnic circulation. Septic models have shown that a large number of capillaries are either not perfused or intermittently perfused in the shock state. Among the capillaries that are perfused, there exists a heterogeneity in blood flow (18,19). Failure of the microcirculation to function normally in the shock state has been attributed to a host of causes including acidosis (20), impaired nitric oxide (NO) (21), leukocyte activation and plugging, coagulation factor activation (22), and the elaboration of other inflammatory mediators (23,24).

Inability to Utilize Oxygen Hypothesis

☞ If $\dot{V}O_2$ cannot be increased after injury, even if adequate $\dot{D}O_2$ is assured, multiple organ dysfunction syndrome (MODS) may ensue and mortality is increased (12). ☞ Failure to accomplish effective oxidative metabolism, as measured by elevated lactate levels after injury, also predicts MODS (25).

The cytochrome *c* oxidase redox state has been used to reflect $\dot{D}O_2$ to the cells. When $\dot{D}O_2$ falls, the redox state moves toward reduction and when the $\dot{D}O_2$ is increased, the redox state is more oxidized (26). This relationship occurs in healthy cells, and hence the mitochondrial electron transport redox state is said to be "coupled" to $\dot{D}O_2$. If, for any reason, electron transport is inhibited proximal to the cytochrome *c* oxidase, the redox state will become relatively oxidized in the absence of increased O_2 availability. In this case, the mitochondrial electron transport redox state is said to be "decoupled" from $\dot{D}O_2$ (27), resulting in anomalous electron transport, the production of reactive oxygen species (ROS), and the potential for free radical–mediated damage (28). Trauma patients who subsequently develop MODS demonstrate decoupling in the setting of both normal or supranormal $\dot{D}O_2$ (28,29).

Evidence of decoupling has been seen in the brain (30), liver (28), and heart (28). Cardiac decoupling is particularly worrisome, as the heart is responsible for supplying itself and the rest of the body with the substrates for oxidative metabolism. Ischemia and reperfusion can produce organ injury by several mechanisms, including direct oxidative injury and the activation of NF-κB (31). It has been demonstrated that prolonged ischemia followed by reperfusion results in inhibition of mitochondrial oxidative metabolism enzyme systems (31). Free radical–mediated damage, resulting from ischemia and reperfusion, has been observed in every major organ predominantly from activated leukocytes (polymorphonuclear cells) in the vasculature, but also from intracellular processes such as mitochondrial dysfunction (32). These data infer that mitochondrial integrity or injury directly relates to cellular, and ultimately organ function in shock states.

Oxygen Extraction Ratio

☞ The normal 70-kg patient consumes approximately 250 mL O_2/min and has a $\dot{D}O_2$ = 1000 mL O_2/min. The $\dot{V}O_2/\dot{D}O_2$ is known as the extraction ratio (ER), which is normally about 25% (Fig. 1). ☞

As $\dot{V}O_2$ increases or $\dot{D}O_2$ falls, the ER will increase until a critical ER is achieved, generally thought to be approximately 60% to 70%. At this point anaerobic metabolism begins to predominate, and shock may become profound as tissues become ischemic. There is a family of $\dot{V}O_2/\dot{D}O_2$ curves, with each tissue/organ having its unique $\dot{V}O_2/\dot{D}O_2$ relationship, and values for maximum ER vary for each tissue, which will vary with stress and the disease state.

Current technology does not allow for determination of these organ-specific relationships in the critically ill patient, and inferences drawn from systemic oxygenation parameters may not be valid in different regional milieus.

One marker for hypoperfusion is compensatory increased oxygen extraction, demonstrated by decreased mixed venous oxygen saturation ($S\bar{v}O_2$) and increased difference between arterial oxygen saturation (SaO_2) and the $S\bar{v}O_2$ (Sa-vO_2). Generally, a $S\bar{v}O_2$ <50% is indicative of the shock state, as is a Sa-vO_2 >50%. Another marker for relative hypoperfusion is an increased O_2 ER, as can be seen in low delivery states, or high consumption conditions. However, certain disease processes (e.g., sepsis) may actually have an elevated $S\bar{v}O_2$ and a decreased O_2 ER due to

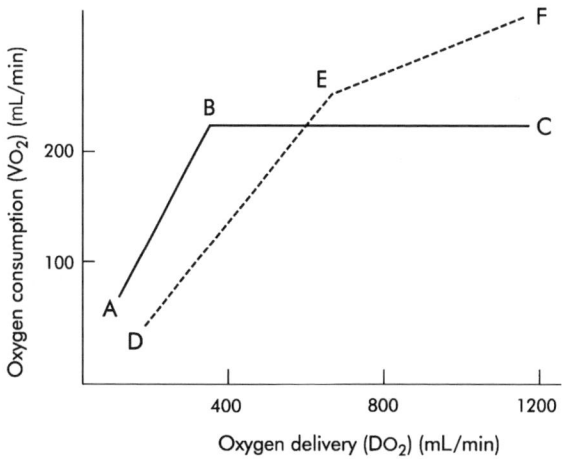

Figure 1 The normal relationship between $\dot{V}O_2$ and $\dot{D}O_2$ is illustrated by line ABC. The $\dot{V}O_2/\dot{D}O_2$ is known as the ER. As metabolic demand ($\dot{V}O_2$) increases or $\dot{D}O_2$ diminishes (C–B), the ER rises to maintain aerobic metabolism and consumption remains independent of $\dot{D}O_2$. However, at point B—called critical $\dot{D}O_2$ the maximum ER is reached. This is believed to be 60% to 70% and beyond this point any further increase in $\dot{V}O_2$ or decline in $\dot{D}O_2$ must lead to tissue hypoxia. In critical illness, particularly in sepsis, an altered global relationship is believed to exist (broken line DEF). The slope of maximum ER falls (DE vs. AB), reflecting the reduced ability of tissues to extract oxygen, and the relationship does not plateau as in the normal relationship. Hence consumption continues to increase (E–F) to "supranormal" levels of $\dot{D}O_2$, demonstrating so called "supply dependency" and the presence of a covert oxygen debt that would be relieved by further increasing $\dot{D}O_2$. *Abbreviation*: ER, extraction ratio. *Source*: From Ref. 191.

inability of the tissues to utilize the O_2 delivered. This probably reflects a mitochondrial O_2 utilization problem.

Stages of Shock
Compensated Shock
✿ The shock state has been described as evolving through stages. The first stage is typically called compensated shock. ✿ During this phase, compensatory mechanisms are successful at counteracting the hemodynamic perturbations of the shock state. The heart rate increases, the systemic vasculature constricts through autonomic involvement, and the renin–angiotensin–aldosterone (RAA) system shifts into a fluid retention mode (see Volume 2, Chapter 44). The decreased urine output in the early stages of the hypovolemic state represents renal compensation; later, renal failure (Volume 2, Chapter 40) can occur, as protective mechanisms are exhausted and cell injury begins to occur.

Local factors initially may compensate with rapid early changes mediated through endothelial stretch receptors, precipitating local bed vascular resistance changes. Additional mechanisms such as the release of CO_2, H^+, and NO cause further vascular dilatation, initially helping to preserve perfusion. These mechanisms are unable to fully compensate for extended periods of poor perfusion, and indeed, may exacerbate the perfusion deficit with vascular pooling.

In some patients, this compensated phase is short-lived. Either the total volume lost is too extensive (e.g., hemorrhagic shock), or the toxin load is too great (e.g., septic shock), and so on, or the patient is unable to fully compensate secondary to underlying medical conditions or advanced age. ✿ When compensation begins to fail, worsening circulatory changes and metabolic imbalances become manifest, and shock enters the second phase (uncompensated shock). ✿

Uncompensated Shock
The shock process progresses to the uncompensated stage when systemic blood pressure (BP) falls, and $\dot{D}O_2$ at the macrovascular level begins to suffer. At the same time, microvascular changes worsen as tissues become hypoxic. Ongoing uncompensated shock frequently precipitates a transition from aerobic to anaerobic metabolism in those vascular beds where $\dot{D}O_2$ becomes inadequate for tissue perfusion. Anaerobic metabolism (which occurs in the cytoplasm) is 19 times more energy-costly than aerobic metabolism (which occurs in the mitochondria). Intracellular adenosine biophosphate (ATP) is rapidly depleted and cellular repair systems become disrupted. Endoplasmic membranes swell, mitochondria distend (lack of ATP decreases ability to maintain membrane electrochemical gradients), and lysosomes are released. If shock continues to progress, the diminished end-organ perfusion is said to enter the "irreversible" stage of shock.

Irreversible Shock
✿ Irreversible shock is said to occur when cellular damage is so extensive that even if hemodynamics are restored, the degree of cell injury/death that has occurred (or will occur due to apoptotic mechanisms) cannot be sufficiently repaired to sustain life. ✿ Permanent cellular damage may ensue with lysosomal release and autolysis. Tissues with high metabolic demands and minimal energy reserves such as the brain, heart, and kidneys are particularly vulnerable to ischemia with hypotension.

The resulting cellular injury and death are responsible for the functional abnormalities affecting individual organs. Should cellular perfusion be restored, further injury may occur early in the reperfusion period due to generation of oxygen free radicals and other cytotoxic products. This cellular injury that occurs following the reestablishment of perfusion is referred to as reperfusion injury.

✿ The state of "irreversible" shock can result from numerous causes, but is particularly devastating following hypovolemia and hypotension due to hemorrhage. ✿ Patients suffering from hemorrhagic shock have usually lost at least 30% to 40% of their blood volume, and if replacement is not adequate, or too long of a duration occurs before the bleeding is controlled, hemodynamic instability can persist even after adequate volume resuscitation has occurred. As many as one-third of patients with massive hemorrhage (i.e., those who have lost greater than or equal to one blood volume within 24 hours) will die from this "irreversible" shock state (33). The study of these patients has been limited because the number of patients is small, and because of injury severity, these patients rarely have time for enrollment and randomization protocols (34).

The irreversible shock state is characterized by vasodilation, representing a failure of vascular smooth muscle regulation, endothelial dysfunction, and activation of white blood cells (WBCs) as well as other circulating cells (35). Initially, lactate was thought to be a prominent vasodilator; however, more recently, other vasodilating agents such as NO have been implicated (36). These vasodilating mechanisms overwhelm the normal compensatory vasoconstriction properties (that operate through elevated adrenergic tone) by at lease three mechanisms: (i) K_{ATP} channel activation, (ii) NO/cGMP overproduction, and (iii) vasopressin deficiency (37). An increase in exhaled NO concentration has been advocated as an early marker of a hypovolemic state (38). Currently, no analogous (noninvasive) assay exists to detect increased K_{ATP} or decreased vasopressin levels.

Neurohumoral Responses in Shock States
Neurohumoral responses to hypotension stimulate sympathetic discharge via carotid and aortic baroreceptors. The subsequent increase in adrenal release of epinephrine and norepinephrine enhances myocardial inotropy and chronotropy. In addition, the sympathetic-mediated increase in vascular tone temporarily increases BP during the compensated shock phase. Catecholamines, as well as stress hormones such as glucagon, aldosterone, adrenocorticotropic hormone (ACTH), and antidiuretic hormone (ADH) are secreted to maintain homeostasis during shock. Distal tubular sodium and water resorption are optimized to conserve intravascular volume. All of these factors combine to initially preserve hemodynamics.

The metabolic responses can be affected at both the neurohumoral and the local cellular level. Glucagon, epinephrine, and glucocorticocoids are part of the "fight or flight" response system leading to increased lipolysis and circulating glucose. Elevated levels of stress hormones promote muscle wasting, poor wound healing, loss of gastrointestinal (GI) mucosal integrity, and hypoalbuminemia. Inflammatory mediators, especially in conjunction with hypoxia, exacerbate proteolysis. Because all of these mediators are catabolic, it is not unusual for patients with chronic inflammatory (SIRS/sepsis) states to have difficulty in maintaining caloric balance, manifest inadequate wound healing, and suffer variable degrees of hemodynamic instability and difficulty in weaning from mechanical ventilation until the primary disorder is corrected.

EFFECT OF SHOCK ON ORGAN SYSTEMS

☞ **Hypoperfusion and inadequate $\dot{D}O_2$ to individual organ systems during shock can trigger a cascade of events that disrupt the function of these organs.** ☞ Systemic shock affects all organ systems, with earlier cellular damage and death seen in more rapidly metabolizing organs such as the brain, heart, lungs, kidneys, adrenals, and so on. Many circulating blood and humoral constituents also affect the GI tract, especially, the lining of the gut and the liver.

Central Nervous System

Central nervous system (CNS) dysfunction is often one of the first clinical signs reflecting from inadequate perfusion during shock states. This can be manifested as confusion or obtundation depending upon the severity of cerebral hypoperfusion, and/or the magnitude of circulating inflammatory mediators with CNS effects.

Although highly susceptible to hypoxemia and hypoperfusion, cerebral blood flow (CBF) is normally maintained at 50 mL/100 g brain tissue/minute as long as the mean arterial pressure (MAP) remains approximately between 50 and 150 mmHg. When MAP acutely moves outside this range, autoregulation of CBF may be compromised. Patients with chronic hypertension are more susceptible to cerebral hypoperfusion with relatively less significant hemodynamic perturbations than normal patients, due in part to a rightward shifted autoregulatory curve with subsequently lower hemodynamic reserve. Delirium and ultimately obtundation from inflammatory cytokines can occur during shock states even in the presence of normal CBF.

Profound hypotension may result in ventilatory and vasomotor collapse due to brainstem ischemia. Increased intracranial pressure (ICP), cerebral metabolic rate of O_2 consumption ($CMRO_2$), $PaCO_2$, and PaO_2 levels, as well as blood viscosity represent additional considerations affecting CBF and perfusion in trauma patients. Posterior pituitary ischemia or trauma can precipitate neurogenic diabetes insipidus (DI) initiated by the inhibition of ADH release by the posterior pituitary. The massive volume losses that accompany DI can dramatically exacerbate shock states occurring from any of the primary categories listed in Table 1.

Cardiovascular System

The cardiovascular system is greatly affected during shock states, both as a primary effector, and as a target of injury because of its extensive endothelial lining and contact with systemic inflammatory mediators. Sympathetic outflow provides mechanisms to initially maintain perfusion and resultant arteriolar constriction and increased HR are typical initial compensatory mechanisms seen with hypovolemic shock due to hemorrhage in trauma patients. Vascular tone is typically elevated in hypovolemic (early phase), cardiogenic, and obstructive shock whereas decreased in distributive shock states (Table 3).

Hypoperfusion and hypoxia may precipitate myocardial ischemia, decreased contractility, and dysrhythmias. Direct myocardial depression may also occur due to circulating mediators, such as in uncompensated hemorrhagic shock (e.g., following reperfusion and/or large-volume

Table 3 Shock Hemodynamics

	Hypovolemic	Distributive	Cardiogenic	Obstructive
HR	Increase	Increase	Variable	Increase
BP	Decrease	Decrease	Decrease	Decrease
CVP	Decrease	Decrease	Increase	Increase
P_{PA}	Decrease	Decrease	Increase	Increase
P_{PAO}	Decrease	Decrease	Increase	Increase/ no change
$\dot{Q}$	Decrease	Increase	Decrease	Decrease
SV	Decrease	Increase	Decrease	Decrease

Abbreviations: BP, blood pressure; CVP, central venous pressure; HR, heart rate; P_{PA}, pulmonary artery pressure; P_{PAO}, pulmonary artery occlusion pressure; $\dot{Q}$, cardiac output; SV, stroke volume.

blood product administration) and septic shock, particularly in the later stages (38). However, similar to the cerebral circulation, cardiac autoregulatory mechanisms normally maintain adequate perfusion to the coronary arteries between a MAP of 50 and 150 mmHg (39).

Patients with the underlying coronary artery disease or left ventricular (LV) hypertrophy (e.g., aortic stenosis), are particularly vulnerable to myocardial ischemia with shock. Myocardial ischemic risk is increased not just by diminished coronary arterial perfusion pressure resulting from hypotension, but also as a result of the compensatory tachycardiac response commonly occurring with hypotension.

Pulmonary System

Acute respiratory failure is another common finding seen early in the course of shock. Airway protection with intubation and mechanical ventilation support should be considered as an early intervention in the setting of significant shock. In addition to direct traumatic lung injury (e.g., pulmonary contusion), other factors (e.g., aspiration, drug intoxication, spinal cord injury, etc.) play a role in respiratory failure in the trauma patient.

☞ **Lung injury also results from circulating inflammatory mediators following reperfusion, or blood product transfusion in hemorrhagic shock, and from cellular injury following burns or massive blunt trauma, and bacterial toxins in septic shock.** ☞ Smooth muscle regulators such as thromboxane and certain prostaglandins may cause bronchospasm and acute pulmonary hypertension with subsequent ventilation/perfusion ($\dot{V}/\dot{Q}$) mismatch. These initial incidents often evolve into acute lung injury (ALI) and acute respiratory distress syndrome (ARDS). When ALI/ARDS develops following early injury, it often persists, contributing to critical illness and is a leading factor in delayed morbidity and mortality in trauma patients.

The P_aO_2 is monitored with arterial blood gas (ABG) measurement and pulse oximetry (see Volume 2, Chapter 2). Capnography is an increasingly appreciated monitor which is of significant value during resuscitation and subsequent management of trauma patients. Low expired end-tidal CO_2, in the setting of normal $\dot{V}_E$, correlates with low $\dot{Q}$, and/or increased alveolar dead space, as can occur in extremely hypovolemic patients (40). Continuous end-tidal CO_2 ($P_{ET}CO_2$) monitoring may aid in the determination of resuscitation of low $\dot{Q}$ states.

Renal System

The renal system is particularly vulnerable to the effects of shock. Shock stimulates compensatory mechanisms to maintain intravascular volume. One of the first clinical signs is oliguria and urinary concentration of solutes. Renal artery constriction and decreased glomerular filtration rate (GFR) occurs early in the shock state. Blood is redistributed from the cortex to the medulla in an attempt to conserve intravascular volume during hypovolemia. These events, mediated by circulating catecholamines, vasoconstrictor prostaglandins, and angiotensin predispose the renal cortex to ischemic injury. Shock patients with associated renal failure have a high mortality (41).

Ischemic injury to the kidney may result in acute tubular necrosis (ATN). Nephrotoxic agents (aminoglycosides or IV radiocontrast) further increase the risk for ATN. During the early phase of shock, patients may become oliguric or anuric. Other than optimizing hemodynamics to ensure adequate renal perfusion, no clear evidence exists that it is possible to alter the course of ATN through the use of such agents as diuretics to prevent tubular sludging or renal dopamine to enhance renal blood flow (RBF).

Gastrointestinal System

The GI system is particularly susceptible to hypoperfusion, and thus at risk for ischemia during shock states. Sympathetic stimulation during shock diverts blood flow from viscera to more "vital" organs such as the heart and brain. Gut mucosa can be compromised by splanchnic hypoperfusion, and damaged mucosa can then facilitate movement of toxic substances (e.g., proteolytically cleaved peptides, lipids) into the lymph and portal circulation. In addition, GI ulcers, GI hemorrhage, ileus, pancreatitis, and hepatic failure can also occur. Liver failure is an ominous sign given the significance of the liver's synthetic, metabolic, and clearance functions.

Splanchnic hypoperfusion results in a decrease in gastric intramucosal pH (pHi). Gastric pHi of less than 7.32 has been correlated with increased morbidity and mortality in shock patients (42). Measurement of gastric pHi may be useful in assisting with the estimation of disease severity (43). A 50% mortality has been demonstrated in critically ill patients with a pHi less than 7.32 obtained 24 hours after initial insult, compared with 11% mortality in those with pHi greater than 7.32 (44). Gastric intramucosal acidemia may be an early indicator of hypovolemia.

Hematological System

The hematologic system is widely affected in shock; in addition to anemia, WBC activation, platelet activation, and coagulopathies are commonly seen. Red blood cells, platelets, and coagulation factors can be diminished by both dilution and consumption. Consumption can result from disseminated intravascular coagulation (DIC), or more rarely, adverse drug reactions such as heparin-induced thrombocytopenia (HIT). Functional platelet dyscrasias can also occur without thrombocytopenia secondary to hypothermia, uremia, and sepsis. Blood products are commonly required in trauma patients with shock. The transfused blood products can themselves cause reactions that mimic or exacerbate shock.

HYPOVOLEMIC SHOCK

Hypovolemic shock often results from uncontrolled hemorrhage, and is the most common form of shock occurring in the acute trauma patient. External hemorrhage is usually easily detected following large lacerations, gunshot wounds, and open fractures, but these are not always easy to control. Thoracic and abdominal trauma are additional sources of blood loss that are usually apparent on chest radiograph and objective evaluation of the abdomen [e.g., focused abdominal sonography for trauma (FAST), computed tomography (CT) scanning, or diagnostic peritoneal lavage (DPL)]. However, concealed hemorrhage can be more problematic to diagnose. Common etiologies of concealed hemorrhage include long bone fractures, pelvic fractures, and other sources of retroperitoneal hemorrhage. Nonhemorrhagic hypovolemic shock can also result from diminished intravascular volume from etiologies other than hemorrhage. Causes of nonhemorrhagic hypovolemic shock include major burns, third space losses from crush injury, or major blunt trauma. Other sources include GI losses such as diarrhea and vomiting, and urinary losses such as DI or excess diuretics.

Pathophysiology

Hypovolemic shock is characterized by intravascular volume loss. The pathophysiology of hypovolemic shock can be revealed as a decrease in venous return, SV, $\dot{Q}$, BP, central venous pressure (CVP), pulmonary artery pressures, and pulmonary artery occlusion pressure. A compensatory increase in resorption of fluid into the capillaries decreases interstitial volume in an attempt to maintain intravascular volume. At some point, this compensatory mechanism may become inadequate and frank microcirculatory derangements (increases in capillary permeability, WBC plugging with no-reflow phenomenon, inflammatory mediator release, etc.) may occur.

Clinical Presentation

The patient's clinical presentation is dictated by the degree of hypovolemia along with comorbid conditions. The worse the premorbid state, the less the body tolerates the hypovolemia. The acutely volume-depleted patient has cool, moist, pallid, and/or cyanotic skin, especially at the extremities. Typical physical examination reveals diminished pulse pressure, rapid pulse, cold clammy integument, and flat neck veins. ☞ **Because of compensatory mechanisms, there may already be as much as 30% to 40% blood volume loss by the time hemodynamic changes occur (Table 2).** ☞ The greater the quantity and rate of volume loss, the greater the degree of shock sustained. Initial patient evaluation includes estimating blood volume deficit (Table 4), estimating rate of additional blood loss, completing a primary and secondary survey according to ATLS principles, evaluating cardiopulmonary reserve, and evaluating coexisting hepatic or renal dysfunction (45).

Table 4   Estimation of Blood Volume Deficit in Trauma

Unilateral hemothorax	1000–3000 mL
Hemoperitoneum with abdominal distension	2000–5000 mL
Full-thickness soft-tissue defect 5 cm^3	500 mL
Pelvic fracture	1500–2000 mL
Femur fracture	800–1200 mL
Tibia fracture	350–650 mL
Smaller fracture sites	100–500 mL

Management and Monitoring Priorities

☞ Major goals in resuscitation include controlling blood loss, repleting intravascular volume, and restoring adequate tissue $\dot{D}O_2$. ☞ Management and monitoring priorities in the acutely bleeding trauma patient target oxygenation and ventilation, BP measurement, electrocardiogram (ECG) monitoring, pulse oximetry, and capnography. The treating physician must establish or verify adequate intravenous (IV) access for infusion of normothermic fluids. Measurement of temperature, urine output, ABGs, hemoglobin, hematocrit, electrolytes, and parameters of coagulation is routine in severely injured patients. Arterial catheterization and monitoring is usually warranted once basic management priorities are fulfilled. Placement of invasive monitors (e.g., CVP, pulmonary artery catheter) and/or transesophageal echocardiography (TEE) may be considered, but should not delay definitive care.

A lag in restoration of normal organ perfusion may be present even after it appears the hemorrhagic shock patient has been adequately resuscitated (46). Despite recent suggestions that delayed fluid therapy may be preferable in isolated penetrating trauma, the current recommendation remains to optimize intravascular volume to prevent organ hypoperfusion. ATLS recommendations call for an initial bolus of 2000 mL crystalloid to determine hemodynamic response (Table 5).

Patients with higher preload, initially, after shock presentation maintain higher preload, demonstrate less intramucosal gastric acidemia, and have lower mortality (47). $\dot{Q}$, BP, and perfusion of oxygenated blood flow to vital organs are important determinants of outcome. A byproduct of massive volume resuscitation is tissue edema, in part, due to increased capillary permeability and perhaps decreased plasma oncotic pressure. Patients with comorbid cardiac dysfunction may be at risk for congestive heart failure (CHF) with even moderate volume overload. These patients may benefit from early placement of central monitoring to guide therapy.

Fluid Options

The choice of IV solutions for fluid resuscitation in all forms of shock remains controversial and is fully discussed in Volume 1, Chapter 11. Initial fluid resuscitation is most commonly performed with crystalloid solutions. Blood products are reserved for replacement of significant red blood cell loss, thrombocytopenia, or coagulopathies due to factor deficiency. Nonplasma colloids are generally used in low albumin states or when hypovolemia is so pervasive that crystalloid administration is not capable of resuscitating the patient.

Isotonic Crystalloids

Lactated Ringer's (LR) solution or isotonic 0.9% normal saline are given intravenously to replenish intravascular and interstitial volume (48). One-fourth to one-sixth of the isotonic fluids administered remains in the intravascular space. LR is a balanced electrolyte solution containing lactate, which is converted to bicarbonate by a functioning liver (49,50). This is useful in trauma patients with metabolic acidosis, as LR solution does not elevate circulating lactate levels in patients with a functioning liver (51). Because LR solution contains calcium, and can theoretically precipitate clotting when infused into blood products using citrate phosphate dextrose (CPD) as an anticoagulant, it should not be used with blood product. Rather, 0.9% normal saline is the solution of choice to dilute packed red blood cells. It is an acceptable alternative for fluid resuscitation; however, large volumes result in a hyperchloremic metabolic acidosis (Volume 2, Chapter 45), which may complicate patient care (49,52). Glucose solutions are avoided, as hyperglycemia may aggravate CNS injury (53,54).

Colloids

Colloids increase plasma volume to a larger degree than do crystalloids per unit volume infused, and remain intravascular for a longer period of time (55,56). However, several studies suggest worse outcomes in trauma patients receiving albumin (see Volume 1, Chapter 11). Trauma induces a state of inflammation which results in damaged endothelial integrity and altered microvascular permeability, promoting the extravasation of fluid and large molecules such as albumin into the interstitium (57), which may actually worsen interstitial edema (58).

Albumin is the least likely of the colloids to induce a coagulopathy, but both albumin and hetastarch can increase the risk of coagulopathy (59–62). In view of these concerns along with the expense of colloid compared to crystalloid, routine use of colloids in trauma patients appears unwarranted. Hetastarch doses greater than 1.5 L have been implicated in coagulopathy as a result of diminished factor VIII levels (63,64). Anaphylactoid reactions may also occur with colloid administration (65).

Hextend, a relatively new, physiologically balanced colloid plasma expander, does not appear to cause acidosis or coagulopathy following the infusion of up to 5 L in vivo and may be a promising colloid option (66). To date, no trauma outcome studies have been completed with Hextend.

Table 5 Responses to Initial Fluid Resuscitation[a]

	Rapid response	Transient response	No response
Vital signs	Return to normal	Transient improvement, recurrence of ↓ BP and ↑ HR	Remain abnormal
Estimated blood loss	Minimal (10–20%)	Moderate and ongoing (20–40%)	Severe (>40%)
Need for more crystalloid	Low	High	High
Need for blood	Low	Moderate to high	Immediate
Blood preparation	Type and cross-match	Type-specific	Emergency blood release
Need for operative intervention	Possibly	Likely	Highly likely
Early presence of surgeon useful	Yes	Yes	Yes

[a]2000 mL Ringer's lactate solution in adults, 20 mL/kg Ringer's lactate bolus in children.
Abbreviations: BP, blood pressure; HR, heart rate.
Source: From Ref. 192.

Hypertonic Saline

✤ Hypertonic fluids can provide rapid volume expansion, improved hemodynamics, lessen tissue edema, diminish inflammatory response, lower ICP, and decrease brain water when compared with isotonic solutions (67,68). ✤ Hypertonic solutions result in an osmotic translocation of extracellular and intracellular water. The intracellular half-life of hypertonic saline is similar to that of isotonic saline.

Despite the above described theoretical benefits, hypertonic saline has been associated with bleeding, hemodynamic deterioration, and increased mortality in some animal studies of uncontrolled hemorrhagic shock (69). A small study of septic patients demonstrated an improvement in cardiovascular parameters; however, patients receiving hypertonic saline had a higher incidence of bleeding, hemolysis, hypernatremia, and hyperchloremia (70). Hypertonic saline does not improve cerebral DO_2 after head injury and mild hemorrhage in animals (71). However, hypertonic saline combined with 6% hydroxyethyl starch may improve neurologic function and cerebral perfusion pressure (CPP) in patients with traumatic brain injury (TBI) (72). Such hypertonic fluid solution is currently used in Austria for resuscitation of all head-injured and major trauma patients in the field.

Blood Products

✤ Blood products should be reserved for patients who are hemorrhaging briskly, and in more stable patients who are requiring transfusion due to dangerously low levels of red blood cells, platelets, or other factors (see Volume 2, Chapter 59) (73). ✤ Blood products should not be transfused in stable patients for volume expansion without such deficiencies. Blood products are expensive, relatively scarce, and carry the risk for transmissible disease.

DO_2 is generally adequate with a hemoglobin of 7 g/dL in critically ill patients without underlying coronary artery disease (CAD) (see Volume 2, Chapters 54 and 59). A reasonable transfusion trigger in patients with significant CAD is a hemoglobin of 10 g/dL. Tissue oxygenation is maintained in otherwise healthy, normovolemic individuals, between hematocrits of 18% and 25% (74). Relatively restrictive transfusion triggers, maintaining hemoglobin between 7 and 9 g/dL, in critically ill patients appears to confer no added risk to organ function or survival compared with a liberal regimen trigger of 10 to 12 g/dL (75). The rate and magnitude of blood loss, degree of cardiopulmonary reserve, presence of atherosclerotic disease, and oxygen consumption should affect the transfusion trigger for red blood cells (73).

Actively bleeding patients with large volume blood loss in class III or IV (Table 2) shock, however, require immediate blood administration (76). Type O-negative, type-specific, typed and screened, or typed and cross-matched packed red blood cells are options. The initial choice of product depends upon the degree of hemodynamic stability and the acuity of the need for transfusion. Type O-negative red cells have no major antigens and may be given to patients with all blood types (76). Only 8% of the population have O-negative blood; therefore, O-positive red blood cells are frequently used. However, O-positive blood will predispose Rh-negative females of childbearing age to hemolytic disease of the newborn and should be avoided in this population if practicable.

If type O blood has been given in volumes of 50% to 75% of the patient's blood volume (e.g., approximately 10

units of red cells in an adult patient), it is prudent to continue to administer type O red cells if further transfusion is required. If possible, the use of type-specific red cells, requiring five to ten minutes in most institutions, is preferred over O-negative (77). Temporizing measures may sometimes be employed to gain the necessary time, as a full cross-match requires 45 minutes.

Post-traumatic bleeding is primarily due to surgical causes, hypothermia, and dilution. Additional coagulopathies may present due to preexisting defects or DIC (78). Correction of coagulopathies to forestall continued bleeding is essential in the care of hemorrhagic shock. Point-of-care testing and rapid reporting of coagulation test results should be used to guide decisions regarding administration of fresh frozen plasma (FFP), platelets, or cryoprecipitate (Table 6). Microvascular bleeding in this setting can be treated with FFP (79). Typically, 30% of coagulation factors, provided by two units of FFP (10–15 mL/kg), are required to achieve clinically adequate levels. Cryoprecipitate may be used to correct specific factor deficiencies. Dilutional thrombocytopenia, or a platelet count reduced to <50,000/μL, is a cause of hemorrhagic diathesis after transfusion of 1.5 to 2.0 blood volumes (80,81), corresponding to approximately 15 to 20 units of red cells in an adult trauma victim (82,83). Platelet transfusions are indicated in the presence of clinical bleeding and platelet count less than 75,000 to 100,000/μL. One unit of platelet (50 mL) increases the platelet count in an adult by 5000 to 10,000/mL.

Activated recombinant factor VII, although not approved by the FDA, is a relatively new approach to assist in the control of massive hemorrhage (84). A number

Table 6 Common Blood Components Used in Trauma

Blood component	Characteristics
Whole blood	RBC and plasma WBC and platelets not viable after 24-hr storage Labile clotting factors significantly decreased after 2 days of storage Hematocrit 35%
PRBC	PRBC with reduced plasma volume WBC, platelets, and coagulation factors as for whole blood Hematocrit 69%
Random-donor platelet concentrate	Platelets 5.5×10^{10} Some WBC (i.e., lymphocytes) 50 mL of plasma Few RBC Hematocrit <0.5%
Fresh frozen plasma	Plasma proteins All coagulation factors Complement
Cryoprecipitate	80 units of factor VIII Other plasma proteins Von Willebrand factor Factor XIII Fibrinogen (200 mg) Fibronectin

Abbreviations: PRBC, packed red blood cell; RBC, red blood cell; WBC, white blood cell.
Source: Adapted from Ref. 193.

of clinical and case reports indicate an improvement in hemostasis without the apparent activation of the coagulation cascade. Although no definitive dosing schedule has been determined, doses ranging from 40 to 221 µg/kg have been reported (85,86).

Hypothermia

☞ **Avoidance of hypothermia (Volume 1, Chapter 40) is another primary consideration in the resuscitation of hypovolemic trauma patients.** ☞ The patient's environment should be kept warm. Trauma patients often arrive to the hospital hypothermic. The subgroup of spinal cord injury (SCI) patients uniformly present with hypothermia. Detrimental effects of hypothermia include coagulopathies, cardiac dysrhythmias, and compromised immune function (87–89).

Standard coagulation tests are temperature corrected to 37°C and may not reflect hypothermia-induced coagulopathy (90–92). Hypothermia impairs coagulation due to decreased enzymatic rates and reduced platelet function. Hypothermia may also cause decreased myocardial contractility (93), cardiac dysrhythmias, and even cardiac arrest due to electromechanical dissociation, standstill, or ventricular fibrillation, particularly with core temperatures below 30°C. Citrate, lactate, and drug metabolism are impaired by hypothermia; increases in blood viscosity, impairment of red blood cell deformability, increases in intracellular potassium release, and a left-ward shift of the oxygen dissociation curve impairing oxygen offloading to tissues may also occur. One hundred percent mortality has been reported in trauma patients whose body temperature fell to 32°C (94), regardless of severity of injury, degree of hypotension, or fluid replacement.

Infusion of 4.3 L of room temperature crystalloid to a 70-kg trauma patient will result in a decrease of 1.5°C in core temperature (95,96). Similarly, infusion of 2.3 L of diluted red cells could result in a core temperature decrease between 1°C and 1.5°C. Thus, in addition to keeping the patient's environment warm, all fluids administered should be warmed.

The use of fluid-warming devices effective at delivering normothermic fluids to the patients at clinically relevant flow rates permit rewarming of hypothermic trauma patients; rewarming may be enhanced by an externally provided heat source such as a convective warming device (97). Fluid and blood resuscitation of the trauma patient is best accomplished with large-gauge IV catheters and effective fluid warmers with high thermal clearances (98). Countercurrent water and other fluid warmers using 42°C set points provide consistently warm fluid delivery, maintain thermal neutrality with respect to fluid, and do not damage red blood cells (97).

Pressors and Inotropes

☞ **Pressors and inotropes should be used only as temporizing measures in the setting of isolated hypovolemic shock.** ☞ Their use to maintain perfusion pressure within the range of autoregulation of the brain and the heart may occasionally be temporarily necessary while volume is being transfused. It must be recognized that such intervention will not necessarily provide adequate perfusion to other organs, and may worsen splanchnic and renal perfusion. In contrast to most pressors, vasopressin has shown potential in the early treatment of hemorrhagic shock without such compromise. The dosage for hemorrhagic shock is an initial bolus of 20 units followed by infusion of 0.2–0.4 units/min, increased up to 0.9 units/min as needed, per FDA guidelines. Vasopressin has an even greater role in the treatment of distributive shock (discussed further).

Calcium is also frequently required to restore hemodynamics in patients who have received large volumes of blood products. Packed red blood cells, FFP, and platelets are all stored in CPD with adenine or adsol at 4°C and may acutely decrease serum-ionized calcium levels (citrate-binding calcium) (99). Hypocalcemia decreases inotropy and vascular tone, and at severely decreased levels will exacerbate coagulopathy. Calcium administration is warranted during massive transfusion if large amounts of blood are transfused rapidly (50–100 mL/min) or if the patient is hypotensive and measured ionized calcium values are low. Ionized serum calcium typically normalizes when hemodynamic status is restored, so long as liver function remains intact.

CARDIOGENIC SHOCK

Cardiogenic shock is common, occurring in up to 25% of myocardial infarction patients in the United States. Cardiogenic shock is associated with an increased morbidity and mortality, approaching 60%. Cardiogenic shock can also be seen in such conditions as acute valvular dysfunction, dysrhythmia, or myocarditis. In trauma, myocardial contusion or coronary artery injury can also precipitate cardiogenic shock.

Pathophysiology

The pathophysiology of cardiogenic shock usually results from a decreased O_2 supply/demand ratio, and is characterized by a decrease in myocardial contractility. Consequently, SV, $\dot{Q}$, and ultimately BP are all diminished. The CVP, pulmonary artery (PA) pressure, and PA occlusion pressures are generally all increased as blood returns to the heart but is not subsequently pumped out efficiently. Heart rate is variable, but often is increased in order to compensate for decreased SV, in an effort to preserve $\dot{Q}$, and systemic vascular resistance (SVR) increases in order to preserve BP.

Among the more common etiologies of cardiogenic shock in trauma is myocardial contusion (100,101). Nonetheless, hemodynamic consequences precipitating shock from this etiology are not common. If myocardial failure occurs in the setting of blunt chest trauma, etiologies such as tamponade and cardiac rupture must be ruled out. Pulmonary artery catheter placement and/or optimally, TEE can discriminate between these diagnoses. Equilibration of pressures on pulmonary artery evaluation would indicate tamponade. TEE can quickly reveal or rule out tamponade, valvular dysfunction, contractility problems, and hypovolemia. The right ventricle (RV) is most frequently involved following blunt chest injury, demonstrating focal or general stunning.

Clinical Presentation

The clinical presentation of cardiogenic shock demonstrates hypoperfusion with peripheral vasoconstriction. Ejection fraction (EF) is decreased. Cold and mottled extremities, cyanosis, hypoxemia, altered sensorium, and decreased urine output are typical manifestations. Signs of elevated intravascular volume such as jugular venous distension, rales on chest examination, and an S3 gallop may be present. A new murmur may also be present. Invasive monitoring is generally diagnostic, with elevated CVPs along with diminished

Q̇ and SV. Chest X rays may demonstrate elevated pulmonary vascular volume with cephalization of vessels or frank pulmonary edema. TEE may demonstrate either global or segmental dysfunction with diminished EF or possibly an acute valvular defect. ECG may demonstrate ischemic signs such as ST-depression (subendocardial ischemia) or ST-elevation (transmyocardial ischemia).

In the case of myocardial contusion, it is rarely an isolated injury, and generally occurs in the setting of severe polytrauma. Abnormal ECGs and abnormal CK-MB and/or troponin values correlate with significant symptoms and the need for treatment, whereas normal ECGs and CK-MB and/or troponin values correlate with clinically insignificant complications. In patients with ECG abnormalities and/or echocardiographic abnormalities, cardiac troponin is not especially sensitive, nor specific for the diagnosis of myocardial contusion (102). Patients at risk for myocardial contusion who are younger than 55 years old, hemodynamically stable, without history of cardiac disease, and with a normal ECG have minimal likelihood for significant adverse events requiring subsequent intervention (103).

Monitoring and Management Priorities

Management of cardiogenic shock centers upon improving cardiac performance, improving cardiac output, maintaining sinus rhythm, and restoring effective organ perfusion. A variety of means may be employed, depending upon the etiology of the insult. Inotropic agents, arterial dilators, venodilators, appropriate sedation, and intra-aortic balloon counterpulsation (Volume 2, Chapter 22) may be indicated. Emergent definitive therapy such as emergent revascularization or valvular repair may be life-saving. Thrombolysis in the setting of acute myocardial infarction with cardiogenic shock has not been demonstrated to improve mortality.

Fluid Management

In the setting of cardiogenic shock, fluid administration must be judicious. These patients may be approaching the steep end of the Starling curve. Even moderate volume administration may place these patients at risk for CHF. Naturally, trauma patients with concomitant hypovolemia will require more aggressive fluid repletion. PA catheters and TEE monitoring can assist in guiding rational fluid therapy. For significant myocardial contusion, which is similar to other forms of RV failure, treatment requires adequate preload to maintain LV filling.

Inotropes

Inotropic agents should be considered early in cardiogenic shock. Inotropic agents improve myocardial contractility. Normal patients have a β_1- to β_2-myocardial receptor ratio of 80:20. Patients with a failing myocardium have a decreased absolute number of β_1-receptors along with a global diminished responsiveness to β-stimulation (104). Initial β-receptor down-regulation may occur within several hours of initial insult. With increased clinical severity of heart failure, there is greater reduction of β_1-receptors (105). This consideration must be entertained when choosing inotropic therapy for patients with myocardial dysfunction. Phosphodiesterase inhibitors do not rely on β-receptors, and may be helpful in cardiogenic shock. Phosphodiesterase inhibitors act primarily through inhibition of phosphodiesterase fraction III, found predominantly in cardiac muscle, increasing cyclic AMP and intracellular calcium to increase inotropy (see Volume 2, Chapter 17 for rational use of vasopressors in this population).

Vasodilators

Vasodilators can be considered in the treatment of severe cardiac dysfunction when SVR is very high. Decreasing SVR and preload decreases myocardial wall tension and cardiac work, thus improving the myocardial oxygen supply to demand ratio. However, in the setting of concomitant hypovolemic shock with compromised BP, isolated treatment with vasodilators is not beneficial, as it will further diminish coronary artery perfusion pressure, and simultaneously decrease perfusion pressure to other vital organs such as brain and kidneys. Rather simultaneous volume repletion and inotropic support is a superior initial management plan. As intravascular volume is repleted, the SVR will tend to decrease some. If ongoing cardiogenic shock keeps SVR high, despite adequate fluid repletion, then inotropes with vasodilatory side effects can be employed.

Inotropes such as dobutamine and phosphodiesterase inhibitors provide a component of vasodilation along with improved inotropy and are the most commonly utilized vasodilators in cardiogenic shock. In the postacute cardiogenic shock phase, primary vasodilator drugs such as angiotensin-converting enzyme (ACE) inhibitors, nitrates, along with rate-control drugs such as β-blockers have been shown to improve long-term outcomes.

Caution must also be exercised when instituting nitrates in patients with decreased preload, as nitrates can cause further intravascular depletion resulting in increased hypotension, with a compensatory response of increased HR (increasing the risk of ischemia). Rate-related ischemia is often best remedied by initially controlling HR, using a cardioselective β-blocker, such as esmolol 10–100 mg IV, titrated 10–20 mg per dose, and augmented by small doses of pressors such phenylephrine 40–80 µg IV during initiation of β-blocker therapy. As HR decreases, and MAP is maintained, ischemia often resolves. As ischemia resolves, myocardial performance typically improves. Systemic BP increases, organ perfusion improves, and the need for supplemental pressor support can be abated.

Ensuring Adequate Analgesia and Sedation

A cornerstone of patient care is providing adequate comfort, including both analgesia and anxiolysis (Volume 2, Chapter 5). Adherance to these precepts is particularly important in patients with cardiogenic shock. Indeed, these patients are uniquely prone to ischemia and dysrhythmias when pain and/or anxiety are inadequately treated. Reducing the hyperadrenergic state by effective analgesia reduces myocardial oxygen consumption by decreasing sympathetic discharge, decreasing vascular tone, and decreasing cardiac work.

Opioids are a reasonable first-line choice. Once adequate analgesia is provided, additional anxiolysis can be added, if required. Benzodiazepines are an appropriate choice in this setting. The synergistic effect of benzodiazepines with opioids must be kept in mind when initiating their use, both in terms of hemodynamics and respiratory depression. In general, the peak respiratory depressant effect of morphine occurs 15 to 20 minutes following an IV bolus.

An additional consideration for sedation are the newer α2-agonists such as dexmedetomidine. Dexmedetomidine offers analgesia and sedation with minimal respiratory-depressant properties. Dexmedetomidine also possesses potent sympatholytic properties, and directly produces both vasodilation and decreased HR.

Mechanical Assist Devices

Intra-aortic balloon pump (IABP) counterpulsation may be life-saving for patients in cardiogenic shock. The IABP was developed and entered into clinical practice 40 years ago (106,107), and improves survival in patients with severe or intractable cardiac shock (108) due to various forms of LV failure (Volume 2, Chapter 22). IABP is not a definitive therapy, but can be a bridge until definitive therapy can be initiated. Inflation of the IABP during diastole augments diastolic pressure improving coronary artery perfusion, whereas rapid deflation during systole decreases "afterload" and myocardial work.

Definitive Therapy

Definitive therapy, when appropriate, specifically addressing the underlying etiology of the cardiogenic shock should be instituted as soon as possible (Volume 2, Chapter 18). Thrombolysis for acute myocardial infarction is typically contraindicated in the setting of acute trauma. Alternative therapies such as percutaneous transluminal coronary angioplasty (PTCA) or surgery may also be contraindicated given the need for anticoagulation in such therapies. Surgical intervention, however, may be required as a life-saving measure in acute, traumatic valvular injury. Cardiac surgery and cardiology consultation should be obtained in such circumstances to access appropriate risk:benefit ratios.

DISTRIBUTIVE SHOCK STATES

Distributive shock states comprise a spectrum of disease processes with vasodilated hemodynamic profiles. The most commonly considered forms of distributive shock are septic shock, anaphylactic and anaphylactoid reactions, neurogenic shock, and adrenal crisis.

Septic shock, SIRS, and anaphylaxis are characterized by release of mediators that induce vasodilation, increase microvascular permeability, and affect capillary leakage of plasma proteins. Neurogenic shock refers to hypotension following spinal cord injury and is characterized by vascular dilation secondary to a diminished sympathetic outflow. Systemic hypotension secondary to vascular dilation is the hallmark in distributive shock. SV is often normal or elevated.

Septic Shock

Septic shock results of an infectious process (Volume 2, Chapter 47), cause an SIRS (Volume 2, Chapter 63) state. Because SIRS can result from either infectious or noninfectious etiologies (e.g., trauma, transfusions, pancreatitis) a wide differential should be initially considered. SIRS is characterized by tachycardia, tachypnea, hyperthermia (temperature >38.5°C) or hypothermia (temperature <36°C), leukocytosis (WBC >12,000/μL) or leukopenia (WBC <4,000/μL), or bandemia (elevation of immature WBC >10%). Should SIRS progress to involve failure of more than one organ system, it is termed MODS. Septic shock is characterized by hypotension not readily responsive to volume infusion, and dysfunction or failure of at least one organ system. It is the 13th leading cause of morbidity in the United States (109,110) with a mortality of more than 50%.

Bacteria, fungi, and rarely, viruses cause sepsis. Septic shock is a systemic inflammatory syndrome secondary to a suspected or documented infectious process accompanied by end-organ damage or refractory hypotension (111–113). Trauma and hemorrhage are the leading causes of noninfectious SIRS. Similar to sepsis, a neurohumoral cascade is initiated with major trauma or hemorrhage. Early changes are proinflammatory; inflammatory mediators such as cytokines are released and contribute to physiological changes of vascular dilation and impairment of intravascular integrity (i.e., leaky capillaries). Subsequent immunodepression may follow.

Pathophysiology

The pathophysiology of septic shock results from both direct action of microbial toxins and the body's response to the infection. Toxins such as endotoxin, peptidoglycan, and lipoteichoic acid (LTA) may trigger an inflammatory cascade. The body's response to these stimuli may be overzealous and precipitate SIRS, septic shock, and MODS. Cytokines and a host of other circulating inflammatory mediators are involved in the process. Among those cytokines implicated include tumor necrosis factor-α (TNF-α) and the interleukins. These cytokines mediate such systemic responses as hyperthermia, tachycardia, increased endothelial permeability, DIC, and shock. Systemic vasodilators include NO, prostacyclin, and prostaglandin E_2.

Clinical Presentation

The presentation of septic shock results from hypotension primarily from vasodilation, but also from intravascular hypovolemia secondary to extravasation of fluid into the interstitium. In addition, direct myocardial depressants may be present, impairing cardiac performance. Therefore, although septic shock is commonly considered as secondary to vasodilation, that is, distributive shock, it is apparent that components of hypovolemia and myocardial dysfunction are common. Components of obstructive shock, such as decreased venous return with either ACS or elevated ventilatory pressures, may also contribute to the overall condition. In this setting, multiple organ systems are impacted. The CNS may be affected directly with toxins causing obtundation, but may also be affected due to cerebral hypoperfusion during severe shock.

The cardiovascular system is affected in several ways. The vasculature dilates causing an effective intravascular hypovolemia. Additional intravascular hypovolemia occurs secondary to toxically mediated endothelial injury, resulting in extravasation of fluids into the interstitium. Furthermore, direct myocardial depression may occur (usually later in the course of disease). The overall hemodynamics of this setting are typically that of increased $\dot{Q}$, SV, HR, with decreased preload and SVR. TEE, early in the process, will demonstrate central hypovolemia with variable degrees of diminished myocardial performance.

The pulmonary system is also frequently affected in septic shock. The etiology of infection can be the lungs. However, even if the site of infection is distant from the lungs, pulmonary dysfunction is common. The body's entire circulation passes through the lungs, exposing the lungs to circulating toxins and mediators. Extravasation of fluids into the lung interstitium may cause significant declines in oxygenation due to increased diffusion gradients. Further injury may occur with the progression of ALI to ARDS.

Renal dysfunction is also prevalent, ranging from mild oliguria to frank ATN. Typically, the hypotension of septic shock and renal hypoperfusion is the precipitating event of the ATN; however, additional injury secondary to sepsis-related cytokines and nephrotoxic agents such as antibiotics (aminoglycosides) and radiocontrast agents can also occur.

The GI system may be involved in the pathogenesis of septic shock. Gram-negative sepsis is the most common etiology of septic shock. Sepsis from GI sources may also be a result of shock from other etiologies. During periods of significant hypotension, such as during traumatic hypovolemic shock, splanchnic blood supply and GI perfusion may be compromised. In this setting, mucosal integrity may be compromised with resulting systemic transfer of vasoactive peptides, lipids, and eventually the translocation of gut bacteria, resulting in sepsis.

The hematologic system also develops derangements. WBC count is typically elevated early in sepsis (predominantly neutrophils) but may decline to precipitously low levels in later stages of sepsis as immune function is compromised. Thrombocytopenia due to either the dilutional effects of volume resuscitation, consumption of platelets with DIC, or microvascular thromboses may occur. Bone marrow suppression may occur in critical illness or secondary to medications. Anemia requiring red blood cell transfusion may be required.

Management

Management of septic shock requires a multimodal approach. Care is not just focused upon the hypotension, but also must include treatment of the inciting infection (111,114,115). Appropriate antibiotic coverage should begin as soon as possible, with a goal of initiation of treatment within four to eight hours. Empiric broad-spectrum antibiotics may be a reasonable choice in the early period while definitive diagnosis and therapy is undertaken as reviewed in Volume 2, Chapter 53. Specific antimicrobial choices may be tailored to the suspected source of infection. Surgical management such as for bowel perforation or catheter placement for abscess drainage may be required. Additional care is supportive in nature, supporting the systems that may be affected by the septic shock. As in other forms of shock, initial therapy is aimed at maintaining adequate intravascular volume. Tissue oxygenation is dependent upon both supply and demand. During periods of excess inflammation, demand increases while supply must remain adequate to meet the increased demands.

Perhaps the best-known evidence-based publication for the treatment of sepsis and septic shock is the Surviving Sepsis Campaign Guidelines published in 2004 (116). Among the positive recommendations supported by at least one large randomized trial with clear-cut results is the use of "early, goal-directed therapy" (120). This method advocates aggressive optimization of hemodynamics and oxygen balance within six hours of diagnosis of septic shock.

The guidelines for sepsis and septic shock have been well articulated by the Surviving Sepsis Campaign. Recommendations were graded from A to E with category A representing evidence from two or more large randomized trials, and category E representing case series, uncontrolled studies, nonrandomized historical controls, or expert opinion. Here we review the findings of the Surviving Sepsis Campaign that were graded with an A or B (supported by at least one large randomized trial) (Table 7).

Volume resuscitation to replace fluids lost to leaky capillaries and decreased vascular tone is the cornerstone of therapy. Meta-analysis of sepsis patients shows no consistent benefit to crystalloid versus colloid use (117–119). In all forms of distributive shock, relative intravascular volume is depleted, whereas total body volume is usually elevated. It is common for infused volumes to exceed 5 L of crystalloid (120). An effective approach is to titrate volume until SV is maximized, typically at 100–150 cc/beat, while maintaining acceptable cardiac filling pressures, effectively defining the cardiac Starling curve.

Vasopressors are added when volume resuscitation is deemed adequate. They may also be used during early resuscitation to augment systemic BP while volume is being administered. Norepinephrine, phenylephrine, vasopressin, dopamine, and epinephrine are commonly used agents in the treatment of septic shock.

Vasopressors and Inotropes

Vasopressors are instituted in septic shock when volume resuscitation alone does not restore adequate BP and organ perfusion. Phenylephrine is often the first pressor chosen. As a direct-acting α-adrenergic agent, phenylephrine produces vasoconstriction without inotropic support. Phenylephrine has a rapid onset and a limited time of duration of less than 10 minutes following bolus. It may be given through a peripheral IV either in bolus or continuous infusion.

Norepinephrine is the pressor of choice in septic shock; it has both direct α and β sympathomimetic effects. Supplementation with norepinephrine will provide a greater Q̇ and SV for a given systemic BP than phenylephrine alone. Norepinephrine is a potent vasoconstrictor and should be infused via central access to lessen the risk of local ischemia, should peripheral extravasation occur. Recent studies demonstrate that norepinephrine may indeed be the drug of choice for patients with a low-tone state when used to support hemodynamics in patients with normal to elevated Q̇ (121). Models of distributive shock treated with norepinephrine have shown an increase in organ perfusion pressure along with an improvement of splanchnic, renal, and glomerular blood flow, and may be associated with better prognosis than either epinephrine or dopamine (122–124). While there has not been a controlled outcome study in humans, many distributive shock patient series demonstrate an increased GFR and urine output when norepinephrine is utilized (122), presuming that adequate volume resuscitation has been undertaken. Norepinephrine is also less likely to raise ICP than dopamine (125), and may be preferred in head trauma patients requiring vasopressor therapy with modest inotropy.

Dopamine, traditionally, has been the drug of choice for cardiovascular support in septic shock. Dopamine exerts various effects based upon the dose range. Doses in the range of 2–5 μg/kg/min have historically been used for as yet unproven "renal protective properties" (126), affecting predominantly the dopamine receptors located chiefly in the splanchnic circulation and renal beds. Doses in the 5–10 μg/kg/min range are used for inotropic effects as β-adrenergic effects come into play. Doses 10–20 mcg/kg/min are used for pressor effect as α-receptors become affected. The utility of dopamine as first-line pharmacotherapy has been questioned recently. Norepinephrine and vasopressin appear to offer improved outcomes in distributive shock when compared with dopamine. Dopamine is further limited by its propensity for tachydysrhythmias.

Table 7 Surviving Sepsis Campaign Guidelines

Category	Grade	Recommendation
Initial resuscitation	B	Resuscitation of a patient with severe sepsis or septic shock should begin at recognition. During the first 6 hrs, the following should be targeted: CVP 8–12 mmHg; MAP >65 mmHg; UOP >0.5 mL/kg/hr; SvO_2 >70%
	B	During the first 6 hrs, if SvO_2 of 70% is not achieved with a CVP of 8–12 mmHg, then transfusion of PRBCs to a hematocrit of 30% and/or a dobutamine infusion should be started to achieve this goal
Vasopressors	B	Low-dose dopamine should not be used for renal protection as part of the treatment of severe sepsis
Inotropic therapy	A	A strategy of increasing cardiac index to achieve an arbitrarily predefined elevated level is not recommended
Steroids	A	Doses of corticosteroids >300 mg hydrocortisone daily should not be used in severe sepsis or septic shock for the purpose of treating septic shock
rhAPC	B	rhAPC is recommended in patients at high risk of death (APACHE II ≥25, sepsis-induced multiple organ failure, septic shock, or sepsis-induced acute respiratory distress syndrome) and with no absolute contraindications related to bleeding risk or relative contraindication that outweighs the potential benefit
Blood product administration	B	Once tissue hypoperfusion has resolved and in the absence of extenuating circumstances, such as significant coronary artery disease, acute hemorrhage, or lactic acidosis, red blood cell transfusion should occur only when hemoglobin decreases to <7.0 g/dL to target a hemoglobin of 7.0–9.0 g/dL
	B	Erythropoietin is not recommended as a specific treatment of anemia associated with severe sepsis, but may be used when septic patients have other accepted reasons for administration of erythropoietin such as renal failure–induced compromise of red blood cell production
	B	Antithrombin administration is not recommended
Mechanical ventilation	B	High tidal volumes that are coupled with high plateau pressures should be avoided in ALI/ARDS. Tidal volumes should be 6 mL/kg and inspiratory plateau pressures should be <30 cmH₂O
	A	A weaning protocol should be in place and mechanically ventilated patients should undergo a spontaneous breathing trial to evaluate the ability to discontinue mechanical ventilation when they satisfy set criteria
Sedation, analgesia, and neuromuscular blockade	B	Protocols should be used when sedation of critically ill, mechanically ventilated patients is required
	B	Either intermittent bolus sedation or continuous infusion sedation to predetermined end-points with daily interruption/lightening of continuous infusion and retitration if necessary
Renal replacement	B	In acute renal failure, and in the absence of hemodynamic instability, continuous veno-venous hemofiltration and intermittent hemodiaysis are considered equivalent
DVT prophylaxis	A	Severe sepsis patients = low-dose unfractionated heparin or low-molecular–weight heparin; If contraindication to heparin = mechanical prophylaxis or intermittent compression device; High-risk patients = pharmacologic + mechanical therapy
Stress ulcer prophylaxis	A	Stress ulcer prophylaxis should be given to all patients with severe sepsis

Abbreviations: ALI, acute lung injury; APACHE II, Acute Physiology and Chronic Health Evaluation II; ARDS, acute respiratory distress syndrome; CVP, central venous pressure; MAP, mean arterial pressure; rhAPC, recombinant human activated protein C; UOP, urine output; DVT, deep venous thrombosis.
Source: From Ref. 116.

Care must be particularly exercised in this regard in patients at risk for heart rate-related ischemia. Dopamine also suppresses growth hormone, thyroid stimulating hormone, and prolactin. These additional detrimental effects in critically ill patients may induce immunosuppression and catabolism.

Epinephrine, similar to norepinephrine, is both a direct-acting α- and β-sympathomimetic. However, norepinephrine has been demonstrated to be superior to epinephrine in the treatment of septic shock, possibly partly related to its relatively greater α effects. Care must be taken in the use of epinephrine due to its propensity for significant tachycardia and dysrhythmias, which, in the setting of cardiac disease, can cause myocardial ischemia.

Vasopressin is becoming popular in the treatment of septic shock. Patients with septic shock refractory to volume infusion and standard pressor therapy have demonstrated restoration of adequate BP with the addition of small-dose vasopressin therapy. Septic shock patients have a relative vasopressin deficiency, and its exogenous administration can stabilize hemodynamics in advanced distributive shock (127–130). Septic shock patients require markedly smaller doses of vasopressin, in the range of 0.01 to 0.05 units/min, to improve BP (131). Vasopressin augments response to concomitant pressors, often allowing a reduction in other agents (132,133). Utilizing doses above 0.04 units/min in septic patients requires caution, as hemodynamics are not consistently improved in larger doses. Larger doses may compromise organ perfusion and contribute towards adverse events (134). A synthetic analog, terlipressin, has a longer half-life than vasopressin, and may be useful in potentially allowing intermittent dosing (135).

Inotropic support is frequently required given the myocardial depression secondary to the circulating toxins and mediators. Patients with supernormal physiology have been observed to have comparably improved outcomes. However, attempts to pharmacologically augment physiology to supernormal levels have not been shown to improve outcomes, and have indeed been shown to worsen outcomes. Pharmacological augmentation to normalize physiology is the current standard of care. Norepinephrine gives both vasoconstriction and moderate inotropy without significant tachycardia or dysrhythmias.

Corticosteroids

Steroids are sometimes utilized in septic shock patients in relatively modest dose replacement therapy to support hemodynamics. High doses of steroids (e.g., methylprednisolone 30 mg/kg) were given in the past for patients with septic shock, but were shown to have either no or detrimental effect on survival (136–139). A number of studies have explored the use of moderate steroid doses, in the range of steroid replacement therapy, and have shown improved outcomes (140–142). One effect may be to limit the systemic inflammatory response. Reduced HR, temperature, C-reactive protein, and phospholipase A_2 are noted (143).

Endogenous cortisol increases the pressor effect of catecholamines (Volume 2, Chapter 62). Cortisol increases β-adrenergic receptor cell density and synthesis by preventing desensitization (144,145), and its release from the pituitary is stimulated by stress and plays a role in homeostasis.

Half of the septic shock patients have relative adrenal suppression with serum cortisol levels less than 20 $\mu g/dL$ (146). Patients with pressor-dependent septic shock who are unresponsive to fluid resuscitation have a high likelihood of adrenal suppression. Those with an inadequate response to 0.25 mg cosyntropin (synthetic ACTH) stimulating test (147), that is, less than 9 $\mu g/dL$ increase over baseline serum cortisol level, had a 74% 28-day mortality when compared with 18% in those with positive response.

A follow-up randomized controlled outcome study showed 76% of patients with pressor-dependent septic shock unresponsive to volume replacement to have a nonresponsive cosyntropin stimulating test. In these nonresponders, patients who received steroid replacement therapy of 50 mg hydrocortisone as intravenous bolus every six hours along with 50 μg fludrocortisone orally, once per day had a 53% 28-day mortality versus 63% in the placebo group (148). The patients who had a positive response to the stimulation test showed a slight, nonsignificant trend towards increased mortality if given the above steroid replacement regimen.

Based on these findings, a reasonable approach in pressor-dependent septic shock patients nonresponsive to

volume replacement, given that roughly three-quarters of the patients will be nonresponders, is to perform a cosyntropin stimulation test, and then start low-dose steroid therapy. If there is a positive response to the test (i.e., appropriate increase of >18 $\mu g/dL$ plasma cortisol levels), discontinue steroids. If the patient is a nonresponder, continue steroid therapy for seven days.

In an analogous fashion, noninfectious inflammatory syndrome patients and posthemorrhagic patients with shock have been demonstrated to have a high incidence of adrenal cortical suppression with abnormal response to corticotropin stimulation test (149). In this group of patients, there was an increased requirement for norepinephrine support, both in the amount of drug administered and in the duration of treatment required (149). Nonetheless, it has not yet been demonstrated whether steroid replacement therapy, similar to that described earlier in the septic shock, will be efficacious in this patient population.

Activated Protein C

Despite the general lack of apparent efficacy targeting specific mediators and toxins, recombinant activated protein C (APC) has shown promise in the treatment of septic shock. Infection causes a procoagulant, antifibrinolytic, and inflammatory state. A variety of therapies have been explored for septic shock, including high-dose glucocorticoids (150,151), cytokine antagonists (152–162), bacterial modulators (163–165), anticoagulants (166,167), nonsteroidal anti-inflammatory agents (168), and NO inhibitors (169), which have all proven ineffectual or detrimental in patient studies.

On the other hand, APC appears to play a critical role in achieving regulation of thrombosis, fibrinolysis, and inflammation with subsequent improvement of survival in septic shock. Native APC reduces activated factor VIII and activated factor V leading to a reduction in thrombin formation with a decrease in fibrin clot formation. APC also reduces neutrophil activation and margination, plasminogen activating inhibitor, tissue factor, and monocyte activation by, as of yet, unknown mechanisms. In addition, APC deficiency is seen in 85% of severe sepsis patients (170). In a large randomized, placebo-controlled study, administration of recombinant APC showed a significant, overall reduction in mortality of 6.1% (171). A follow-up, open label trial dosed at 24 $\mu g/kg/hr$ for 96 hours showed similar results with even sicker patients (172). The sicker the patient, the more cost-effective the treatment with recombinant APC appears to be; the chief benefit of APC appears to be seen in patients with greater than one failing organ system (173). The major adverse event with APC is serious bleeding, with a small minority exhibiting fatal intracranial bleeding; this may be exacerbated in the pediatric population secondary to an immature blood–brain barrier. Nonetheless, the decreased mortality seen with APC is eight times less than the risk of a fatal bleed (in adults). It may soon be that all patients arriving in sepsis receive APC by protocol, as acute myocardial infarction and cerebral vascular accident patients today receive thrombolytic therapy.

Anaphylactic Shock

✪ **Anaphylaxis is an immunoglobulin E (IgE)-mediated allergic reaction, and requires an initial exposure with sensitization to an antigen with synthesis of IgE.** ✪ On re-exposure, the antigen binds to specific IgE antibodies bound to mast cells and basophils, and triggers the release of chemical mediators including histamine, tryptase, leuko-trienes, kinins, and prostaglandins (see Volume 1, Chapter 33).

These immunological mediators produce the systemic signs and symptoms of anaphylaxis. Common early symptoms are utricaria, edema, wheezing, excess airway secretions, vasodilation, and cardiovascular collapse. Anaphylaxis may be life-threatening, compromising both respiratory and cardiovascular systems, and be confused with etiologies such as sepsis, cardiogenic shock, and asthma. The most threatening manifestations of anaphylaxis are airway edema, bronchospasm, and shock. Anaphylactoid reactions are similar to anaphylaxis but not mediated by IgE and thus do not require a previous exposure. Anaphylactoid reactions are clinically indistinguishable from anaphylaxis and treated in the same fashion as anaphylaxis.

Inciting agents for anaphylaxis and anaphylactoid reactions may be environmental agents or medications. The temporal relationship to a triggering event often provides a clue. Bronchospasm and hematuria are consistent with the diagnosis. Elevated levels of serum histamine, tryptase, and IgE confirm the diagnosis. Common inciting environmental agents include latex products, hymenoptera (bee) stings, crotalid (snake) venom, and antivenom. Medications such as penicillins, cephalosporins, protamine, dextran, and radiocontrast agents are commonly noted to incite anaphylactic and anaphylactoid reactions. Immediately upon recognition of anaphylaxis or an anaphylactoid reaction, an attempt should be made to determine the inciting agent. The inciting agent should then be removed, for example, latex catheters, bee stingers, or medications.

The presentation of anaphylactic and anaphylactoid reactions has classic symptoms. Fifty percent of the deaths from anaphylaxis occur within the first hour. Seventy-five percent of the anaphylaxis deaths are from asphyxia, the remainder from circulatory collapse. Upper airway obstruction may occur from tongue and glottic edema. Bronchoconstriction may produce dyspnea, wheezing, air trapping, and acute respiratory collapse. Hypotension and tachycardia are typically present. Histamine is the most important mediator, affecting both H1 and H2 receptors. Vasodilation and vascular hyperpermeability ("leaky capillaries") cause hypotension. This marked hyperpermeability may occur rapidly, producing a fluid shift from the vascular to the extravascular space. Rapid, profound loss of intravascular volume may occur. Up to 50% of intravascular volume may be lost within 10 minutes (174). Secondary mediators are stimulated with an increase in serum catecholamines and a conversion of angiotensin I to angiotensin II (175,176). The $\dot{Q}$ and SV may be normal or increased, depending upon the patient's functional volume status and these compensatory mechanisms. Measurements of CVP, P_{PA}, and P_{PAO} are generally low. However, depending upon the effect of the toxic mediators upon the bronchial tree and pulmonary vasculature, the CVP and P_{PA} may be increased. Care must be taken not to interpret this as primary cardiac dysfunction.

Treatment of anaphylaxis and severe anaphylactoid reactions must be prompt and follow the ABCs (airway, breathing, and circulation) of patient management (177). Identify and remove the offending allergen. Supplemental O_2 and airway management take highest priority followed by administration of epinephrine and intravascular volume. Intubation prior to severe airway edema should be considered, both to ensure an adequate airway and also to enable positive pressure ventilation given the probability of significant bronchospasm. Aggressive volume resuscitation to correct the significant hypovolemia with infusion of 1000–2000 mL of crystalloid as an initial bolus to replete the intravascular volume, given the ongoing interstitial extravasation, is indicated.

Pharmacological therapy with epinephrine is the single most important specific therapy. Epinephrine is the ideal agent for the treatment of anaphylaxis and anaphylactoid reactions. Epinephrine increases vascular tone, increases cardiac output, stabilizes mast cells to prevent further deregulation, bronchodilates, and helps restore circulation. Initial dosing in early anaphylaxis is 100 µg IV bolus, followed by subsequent infusion. Alternatively, 300–500 µg should be administered intramuscularly (when an IV is not available). IM doses can be repeated several times at 10-minute intervals. Acute bronchospasm may be treated with 0.01 mg/kg IM epinephrine or SQ or, alternatively, with 0.5–0.1 µg/min IV. In the setting of fulminant cardiovascular collapse, continuous epinephrine infusions titrated to effect should be instituted. More severe or prolonged symptoms may be treated with 100–500 µg intravenous doses every five minutes as needed to maintain hemodynamic stability (177). Continue therapy with an IV infusion of 1–4 µg/min as necessary.

When administering epinephrine, the patient should be closely monitored. Cardiac ischemia and myocardial infarction have been reported in the use of epinephrine in anaphylactic shock. In the event of cardiac arrest, Advanced Cardiac Life Support® (ACLS®) protocol should be followed. Secondary treatment with corticosteroids and antihistamines inhibit further immune response. Antihistamines are particularly useful in the treatment of cutaneous symptoms. Since both H1 and H2 receptors are involved, both H1 and H2 blockers should be utilized. Diphenhydramine (25–50 mg) should be given either intramuscularly or intravenously along with 1 mg/kg of ranitidine intravenously, or 4 mg/kg of cimetidine intravenously. Corticosteroids may be considered, but do not have an immediate effect. However, corticosteroids may play a role in diminishing inflammatory respiratory reactions. Corticosteroids may be given IM, IV, or PO. Options include hydrocortisone 100 mg IV or prednisone 60 mg PO.

Neurogenic Shock

Neurogenic shock is caused by traumatic SCI. Neurogenic shock is characterized by an adrenergic deficiency characterized by vascular dilation and bradycardia. Higher SCI increases the incidence of significant bradydysrhythmias. If the SCI is above T1–T5 (level of the cardiac accelerator nerves), significant bradycardia, bradydysrhythmias, and even sinus arrest can occur.

The pathophysiology of neurogenic shock is hypotension due to loss of vasomotor tone. SCI ablates intrinsic sympathetic stimulus while allowing elevated or unopposed parasympathetic stimulus. Venous pooling occurs with decreased venous return and decreased cardiac output. Hypotension may ensue. Monitoring of BP, HR, and urinary output is necessary. Bradycardia may contribute to shock, and is a significant factor in post-SCI morbidity and mortality.

Neurogenic shock presents with significant vasodilation precipitating hypotension. The CVP, P_{PA}, P_{PAO} are all typically low, but depend upon the overall volume status. Bradycardia is often present if the injury is at or above the cardiac accelerator nerves (T1–T5). On physical examination, patients will have evidence of peripheral vasodilation, and may evidence signs of parasympathetic excess such as bradycardia, priaprism, diarrhea, and bronchospasm. Evidence of neurologic injury should be explored in trauma patients with shock symptoms. The etiology is generally clear; however, other types of shock such as hypovolemic shock must also be considered. Significant hypothermia is often present given inadequate temperature regulation.

Management of neurogenic shock begins with supportive measures. Airway management may be required should innervation of muscles of respiration be disrupted. Fluid resuscitation is necessary given the significant vascular dilation and pooling. Temperature control is critical, as these patients uniformly enter the hospital hypothermic due to their inability to autoregulate their temperatures secondary to peripheral vasodilation.

Early steroid loading with methylprednisolone (30 mg/kg loading dose followed by 5.4 mg/kg/hr × 24 hrs) may improve recovery in spinal cord injured patients for patients treated within four to six hours of the SCI. Pharmacological support is also at times necessary. The constellation of symptoms in neurogenic shock must be considered. In view of this, care must be exercised in using phenylephrine as the sole medication for restoration of vascular tone due to the potential to worsen bradycardia. Dopamine and epinephrine both offer vasoconstriction and increased chronotropy. If hypotension is severe, norepinephrine may be useful. For acute episodes of bradycardia, boluses of atropine or glycopyrrolate may be necessary. In SCI above the cardiac accelerator nerves, significant bradycardic events may be present.

Adrenal Crisis

Adrenal crisis (a.k.a. acute adrenal insufficiency or Addisonian crisis) is a medical emergency characterized by low serum cortisol and aldosterone with hypotension and tachycardia refractory to volume administration (Table 8). Prompt treatment with fluids, steroid replacement, and correction of metabolic derangements is necessary. A cosyntropin stimulation test (as described in the steroid treatment section for septic shock earlier) may still be utilized after a single dose of 2 mg of IV dexamethasone has been given (also see Volume 2, Chapter 62). Dexamethasone does not, however, offer mineral corticoid replacement. Therefore, in

primary adrenal failure, subsequent dosing with IV hydrocortisone 200 mg infusion over 24 hours should be initiated. Tapering of the initial large-dose steroids may be considered after resolution of the acute crisis, aiming for simple replacement doses.

OBSTRUCTIVE SHOCK

☞ Obstructive shock is due to mechanical impediment to blood flow; that is, obstruction of venous return and/or arterial outflow from the heart. ☞ Causes in trauma patients include PE, pericardial tamponade, ACS, increased intrathoracic pressure such as with tension pneumothorax, positive pressure ventilation and excessive PEEP (either iatrogenic or intrinsic). Obstructive shock is characterized by a diminished $\dot{Q}$ and SV, with increased HR, CVP, and intracardiac pressures. The CVP, P_{PA}, and P_{PAO} can all become elevated to similar values, which is termed as equalization of pressures.

Signs and symptoms common to all forms of obstructive shock include hypotension, tachycardia, respiratory distress, cyanosis, and jugular venous distension. Classical findings of pulsus paradoxus and Kussmaul's sign are also seen in forms of obstructive shock. Pulsus paradoxus is a greater than 10 mmHg decrease in systolic pressure during inspiration. Kussmaul's sign is an increase in venous pressure with inspiration during spontaneous ventilation.

Management of obstructive shock primarily focuses upon supportive care until diagnosis and definitive therapy such as decompression of tension pneumothorax, pericardiocentesis for pericardial tamponade, thrombolytic therapy for PE, or abdominal decompression for ACS are instituted. Supportive measures may include volume resuscitation and inotropic support. Volume therapy provides temporary support by improving intracardiac filling. Although the central pressures are elevated in obstructive shock, they are reflective of transmitted pressures rather than due to elevated intracardiac volumes. Inotropic support with dobutamine and phosphodiesterase inhibitors may also be considered while diagnosis is being accomplished. Pressors are not generally required, as peripheral vasoconstriction is typically present from sympathetic stimulation.

Pulmonary Embolism

PE is a common complication following deep venous thrombosis (DVT) formation after trauma. Virchow's triad of intimal damage, venous stasis, and a hypercoagulable state comprise the classically described conditions predisposing to thromboembolic disease (see Volume 2, Chapter 56), which exist in most trauma patients. Risk is reduced by utilization of both DVT prophylaxis and vena caval filter placement in patients unable to have anticoagulation. Mortality from PE increases in settings of significant comorbid disease, RV dysfunction, and age greater than 60 years. The risk of PE is further increased in TBI, SCI, pelvic fracture, and lower extremity fractures.

PE can present with classical symptoms of pleuritic chest pain and dyspnea (60–73% of the time). Apprehension is a common symptom as well, occurring in up to 60% of patients. Additional common symptoms include hemoptysis (20%), wheezing (9%), and palpitations (10%). However, syncope and sudden death may be the only signs at presentation. Examination is typically nonspecific. Tachypnea

Table 8 Common Causes of Adrenal Insufficiency

Primary	Secondary
Autoimmune adrenalitis	Sepsis
Acquired immunodeficiency syndrome (opportunistic infections)	Pituitary damage or dysfunction (tumors, metastasis, traumatic lesions, surgery, radiation)
Tuberculosis	Drugs
Metastatic carcinoma	Long-term glucocorticoids therapy
Systemic fungal infections	Interference with cortisol synthesis (etomidate, ketoconazole, aminoglutethimide)
Hemorrhage; necrosis or thrombosis of adrenal gland	Increased metabolism of cortisol (phenytoin, phenobarbital, rifampin)

Source: Adapted from Ref. 189.

(70%) is the most common finding, followed by crackles (50%) and tachycardia (30%).

Nonspecific ECG changes (50%) are common. The classically described pattern showing RV strain, right bundle branch block, and right axis deviation are present in less than one-third of the cases. Dysrhythmias, such as atrial fibrillation, premature ventricular contractions, and premature atrial contractions are present 5% of the time.

Radiographic imaging is helpful. Chest X rays are abnormal in 80% of patients. Parenchymal infiltrate (66%) is most common, followed by small effusions (50%), and atelectasis. The classic X-ray findings of Hampton's hump (a wedge-shaped pleural-based infiltrate) and Westermark's sign (prominent pulmonary artery with decreased pulmonary vascularity) are seen infrequently, but, if present, are strongly predictive of PE. Although $\dot{V}/\dot{Q}$ scans are often abnormal and useful in patients without other lung pathology, these are seldom useful in trauma patients due to the common presence of concomitant pulmonary infiltrates. Previously, pulmonary angiography represented the gold standard for diagnosis. ☞ **More recently, multidetector spiral CT angiography has emerged as the diagnostic imaging study of choice for pulmonary embolism (see Volume 2, Chapter 56).** ☞ Treatment is with systemic heparin, except for those with contraindications to anticoagulation (e.g., TBI) in whom placement of IVC filters is recommended.

Abdominal Compartment Syndrome

The ACS can result in refractory hypotension and ultimately obstructive shock in trauma patients (Volume 2, Chapter 34). Patients at risk are those with direct abdominal trauma, massive volume resuscitation, burns, intra- or retroperitoneal hemorrhage, along with those who have had gut ischemia, such as peritrauma episodes of significant hypotension.

The most common method to measure intra-abdominal pressures is to instill 100 cc of saline into the bladder, then transduce, and measure the bladder pressure. The syndrome may be classified as grade I, II, III, or IV based upon the pressure (Table 9). Elevated abdominal compartment pressure is transmitted to the vasculature and thorax. Its primary effects are seen upon the cardiac, pulmonary (decreased chest wall compliance), and renal systems. At pressures of 20 mmHg, effects are already seen in the kidney, with decreased renal perfusion and urine output. At pressures above 40 mmHg, renal perfusion is minimal, and urine output is usually absent. As intra-abdominal pressures rise, venous return decreases and afterload increases. Cardiac output decreases, pulmonary artery occlusion pressure rises, and hypotension may ensue. Typical symptoms include a distended tense abdomen, unexplained respiratory failure, decreasing blood pressure

Table 9 Intra-abdominal Compartment Syndrome

Grade	Intra-abdominal pressure (mmHg)	Recommended treatment
I	<15	Maintain normovolemia
II	16–25	Hypervolemic resuscitation
III	26–35	Decompression
IV	>35	Decompression and re-exploration

Source: Adapted from Ref. 190.

with increasing P_{PAO} and decreasing cardiac output, persistent gastric intraluminal acidosis, and oliguria (178).

Initial treatment is moderate fluid loading. If symptoms do not improve, or if the patient has grade III or IV pressures, consider surgical decompression as follows: pressures above 26 to 35 generally indicate that decompression is required. Those patients with compartment pressures >35 usually require decompression and consideration of re-exploration of abdomen if the prior surgery had occurred (179). Typically, symptoms quickly resolve after decompression. However, immediately after decompression, reperfusion syndrome is possible, with ensuing acute metabolic derangements, acidemia, and hypotension (see Volume 2, Chapter 34) (180).

Tension Pneumothorax

A tension pneumothorax is seen in trauma patients secondary to a variety of causes, including direct pulmonary trauma, placement of invasive monitoring, and positive pressure ventilation. Tachycardia is common along with an abnormal chest examination. Chest examination usually reveals hyporesonance to percussion along with diminished breath sounds on the affected side. Additional symptoms include agitation, arterial desaturation, air hunger, increasing peak airway pressures, hypotension with shock, and pulseless electrical activity. Chest radiograph or chest CT would confirm the diagnosis of pneumothorax. However, in the setting of likely pneumothorax with significant hemodynamic compromise, treatment should not be delayed to obtain imaging studies. Initial therapy may be placement of a 16- to 18-gauge angiocatheter in the second intercostal space in the mid-clavicular line. Definitive therapy with chest tube placement should follow.

Dynamic Hyperinflation

Dynamic hyperinflation, also known as auto-PEEP or intrinsic PEEP, occurs when a subsequent breath is initiated prior to complete exhalation of a prior breath. Auto-PEEP may be unrecognized by ventilator estimation due to frequent non-communication between some hyperinflated airways and site of airway measurement. Recognition of auto-PEEP is likely in the setting of failure to reach zero pressure at the end of exhalation. Dynamic hyperinflation may present with hemodynamic collapse due to decreased venous return and RV filling, increased RV afterload, and decreased LV compliance. When dynamic hyperinflation is suspected, the initial therapy should be to disconnect the patient from the ventilator, allowing the patient to fully exhale. Typically, hemodynamic effects readily resolve with such a trial. Should dynamic hyperinflation be confirmed, ventilator adjustments should be undertaken to administer bronchodilator therapy, and to ensure complete exhalation (i.e., decrease RR and increase exhalation time).

Cardiac Tamponade

Cardiac tamponade may be seen in trauma patients. The pericardium isolates the heart and great vessels from the mediastinum. It usually holds approximately 50 cc of fluid. While over the long-term, the pericardium can accommodate 2–3 L, in the acute setting, hemodynamic compromise should likely accumulate more than 200 cc of fluid in the pericardium. Pericardial injury is common with chest stab wounds. As pericardial pressure increases, intracardiac pressures equilibrate, and cardiac output is compromised. Pulsus paradoxus is seen. Percutaneous or surgical drainage is required to treat tamponade, should hemodynamics be significantly compromised.

EYE TO THE FUTURE

Experimental therapies targeting toxins and mediators of shock have been at the forefront of critical care research for some time. Trials utilizing dialysis in an effort to "wash" the blood of inflammatory mediators have not yet demonstrated benefit (see below). Similarly, antitoxin/antimediator antibodies have not yet proven efficacious. Work continues in this arena with hope that targeted therapy will one day provide a "magic bullet"; however, it is becoming increasingly clear that multimodal therapies offer the most reasonable approach for effective therapies in shock.

Orthogonal polarization spectral (OPS) imaging is a relatively new method of imaging the microcirculation, which may have some utility in the diagnosis and treatment of shock. De Backer et al. (181) used OPS to examine the microcirculation under the tongue in both healthy volunteers and in patients suffering from septic shock. They found that the proportion of perfused capillaries was significantly less in severely septic patients, and that this decrease in proportion of perfused capillaries correlated with the severity of the septic process. Sakr and associates (26) prospectively observed the microcirculation in another group of septic patients and correlated improvement in microvascular perfusion with survival, whereas most systemic hemodynamic and oxygenation variables did not differ between the survivors and the nonsurvivors. OPS is a fascinating new technology, which, when validated, may play a role in the understanding and possibly treatment of shock.

One of the new strategies emerging from the biotech sector is the marriage of rapid analysis of large numbers of data streams with biological problems of interest, including combinatorial analysis and computer-aided drug design. An illustrative example of diagnostic testing now in use includes gene (DNA microarrays) and protein chips as well as other "lab on a chip" devices, where trays are plated with large numbers of candidate molecule ligands for assay analysis. Increasing numbers of putative target molecule probes [e.g., known (heat) shock proteins or genetic precursors] can be put on chips, allowing simultaneous evaluation of large numbers of molecules, either manually or through artificial intelligence or neural network-type processing (182,183). At present, this kind of mass data analysis approach is limited by cost and understanding of shock pathophysiology, but may become clinically practical as design refinements occur.

Important strides are also being made in the treatment of shock. Although it has long been acknowledged that shock is a systemic phenomenon with global organ involvement, it has become increasingly clear that the nidus for MODS following shock may in fact be the gut (184). Proteolytic cleavage at the intestinal lumen is implicated in systemic shock, be it circulatory or septic in nature, and intraluminally-given protease inhibitors are efficacious in ameliorating the inflammatory response and subsequent mortality (185,186). Interventional techniques to block proteolytic enzymes in the gut may prove to be a valuable intervention against the initial shock process.

Alternatively, it may prove that either multipronged downstream approaches to modifying individual inflammatory mediators [oxygen free radicals including nitric oxide, prostaglandin derivatives and phospholipases, platelet activating factor, and other lipid mediators, TNF-α, high mobility group box 1 (HMGB1) as well as other cytokines, NF-κB and transcriptional factors, leukocytes, serine and metalloproteases, leukocyte integrins/selectins, protein activated receptors (PARs), lipopolysaccharides and Toll-like receptors (TLRs), the complement, coagulation, and kinin pathways, etc.] or inhibitors [heat shock proteins, nitric oxide, cytokines, growth factors (e.g., GM-CSF), erythropoietin, calcitonin, etc.] are efficacious. Thus far, all of the above candidate molecules have found some relevance in the preclinical arena but have not, in general, proven decisive in the clinical shock condition. This may be secondary to inadequate targeting, timing of intervention, or most importantly, the redundancy of the inflammatory response. As multiple therapies necessitate multiple toxicities and side effects, one method is to simply attempt to remove inflammatory mediators from the body (187). This assumes that mediators are circulating systemically (not merely locally diffusible molecules) and can be instrumented as an inflammatory "filter" that binds either nonspecifically or specifically via antigen–antibody complexing to mediators of interest. At present, prototype models are extracorporeal in the mode of continuous veno-venous hemodilution (CVVHD) (188). Their efficacy remains to be determined.

SUMMARY

The key to trauma care is a prompt recognition that the patient has sustained serious injury. Severely injured trauma patients may either present in shock or develop shock as a result of their injuries. Shock is a syndrome of hypotension and hypoperfusion with a broad variety of etiologies. Shock may progress from one hemodynamic classification to another. It is not unusual that a single patient may be treated for any and all of the four broad categories of shock: hypovolemic, cardiogenic, distributive, and obstructive during the peritrauma period. Diagnosis and treatment of shock's underlying etiology is always the foundation of shock treatment. Neurohumoral mechanisms initially maintain vital organ perfusion, yet cannot compensate long term. Aggressive intervention is warranted; without intervention, systemic ischemia with organ failure ensues.

Trauma patients have an array of etiologies of shock, with hypovolemic and distributive shock the most commonly seen. Hemorrhage and sepsis are among the most common specific etiologies of traumatic shock, following CNS injury as most common etiologies of death in trauma patients (7–9). Success in caring for the bleeding trauma patient and adherence to ATLS standards require rapid evaluation and treatment to ensure adequate tissue perfusion by skilled trauma personnel. Thermally efficient fluid warmers, effective transfusion services, and rapid availability of coagulation tests are practical aspects of trauma resuscitation that deserve priority. Preventing hypothermia, recognizing other complications of massive transfusions, as well as following trends in vital signs, urinary output, CVP, ABG analysis, and mixed venous blood gas analysis are critically important in managing patients with hemorrhagic shock.

Septic shock requires similar aggressive therapy. There is a growing belief that there may indeed be a "Golden Hour" in sepsis as well as trauma. Early, goal-directed therapy is rapidly becoming the gold standard in septic shock. Institution of appropriate antibiotics and optimization of hemodynamics through aggressive volume resuscitation and invasive monitoring, as early as in the emergency department, has been demonstrated to significantly improve outcomes.

Despite intensive research efforts in finding a magic bullet cure for shock, the foundations of management including airway, breathing, and circulation remain most vital in the care of the critically ill and injured trauma patient.

KEY POINTS

- Shock is defined as inadequate perfusion of the tissue. This inadequacy can result from deficient oxygen delivery ($\dot{D}O_2$), excessive utilization, or a combination of the two. In "cytotoxic" shock, tissue mitochondria are unable to utilize the O_2 delivered.
- Hypovolemic shock is caused by acute blood loss of >30% of the circulating blood volume (class III/IV hemorrhage).
- Blood flow to organs is regulated by mechanisms that control systemic, regional, and local perfusion. Dysfunction can occur at any of these points.
- If $\dot{V}O_2$ cannot be increased after injury, even if adequate $\dot{D}O_2$ is assured, MODS may ensue and mortality is increased (12).
- The normal 70-kg patient consumes approximately 250 mL O_2/min and has a $\dot{D}O_2 = 1000$ mL O_2/min. The $\dot{V}O_2/\dot{D}O_2$ is known as the ER, which is normally about 25% (Fig. 1).
- The shock state has been described as evolving through stages. The first stage is typically called compensated shock.
- When compensation begins to fail, worsening circulatory changes and metabolic imbalances become manifest, and shock enters the second phase (uncompensated shock).
- Irreversible shock is said to occur when cellular damage is so extensive that even if hemodynamics are restored, the degree of cell injury/death that has occurred (or will occur due to apoptotic mechanisms) cannot be sufficiently repaired to sustain life.
- The state of "irreversible" shock can result from numerous causes, but is particularly devastating following hypovolemia and hypotension due to hemorrhage.
- Hypoperfusion and inadequate $\dot{D}O_2$ to individual organ systems during shock can trigger a cascade of events that disrupt the function of these organs.
- Lung injury also results from circulating inflammatory mediators following reperfusion or blood product transfusion in hemorrhagic shock, and from cellular injury following burns or massive blunt trauma and bacterial toxins in septic shock.
- Because of compensatory mechanisms, there may already be as much as 30% to 40% blood volume loss by the time hemodynamic changes occur (Table 2).
- Major goals in resuscitation include controlling blood loss, repleting intravascular volume, and restoring adequate tissue $\dot{D}O_2$.
- Hypertonic fluids can provide rapid volume expansion, improved hemodynamics, lessen tissue edema, diminish inflammatory response, lower ICP, and decrease brain water compared with isotonic solutions.

- Blood products should be reserved for patients who are hemorrhaging briskly, and in more stable patients who are requiring transfusion due to dangerously low levels of red blood cells, platelets, or other factors (see Volume 2, Chapter 59).
- Avoidance of hypothermia (Volume 1, Chapter 40) is another primary consideration in the resuscitation of hypovolemic trauma patients.
- Pressors and inotropes should be used only as temporizing measures in the setting of isolated hypovolemic shock.
- Anaphylaxis is an IgE-mediated allergic reaction, and requires an initial exposure with sensitization to an antigen with synthesis of IgE.
- Obstructive shock is due to mechanical impediment to blood flow; that is, obstruction of venous return and/or arterial outflow from the heart.
- More recently, multidetector spiral CT angiography has emerged as the diagnostic imaging study of choice for pulmonary embolism (see Volume 2, Chapter 56).

REFERENCES

1. LeDran HF. A Treatise, or Reflections Drawn from Practice on Gun-Shot Wounds. London, 1737.
2. Morris EA. A Practicle Treatise on Shock After Operations and Injuries. Hardwicke, 1867.
3. Chambers NK, Buchman TG. Shock at the millennium. I. Walter B. Cannon and Alfred Blalock. Shock 2000; 13(6):497–504.
4. Sabiston, DC. The fundamental contributions of Alfred Blalock to the pathogenesis of shock. Archives of Surgery 1995; 130(7):736–737.
5. Hinshaw LB, Cox BG. The Fundamental Mechanisms of Shock. New York: Plenum Pub. Corp., 1972.
6. Pope A, French G, Longnecker D, eds. Fluid Resuscitation, State of the Science for Treating Combat Casualties and Civilian Injuries. National Academy Press, 1999.
7. Baker CC, Oppenheimer L, Stephens B, et al. Epidemiology of trauma deaths. Am J Surg 1980; 140:144–150.
8. Shackford SR, Mackersie RC, Holbrook TL, et al. The epidemiology of traumatic death. A population based analysis. Arch Surg 1993; 128:571–575.
9. Sauaia A, Moore FA, Moore E, et al. Epidemiology of trauma deaths: a reassessment. J Trauma 1995; 38:185–193.
10. Shoemaker WC, Appel PL, Kram HB, et al. Prospective trial of supranormal values of survivors as therapeutic goals in high-risk surgical patients. Chest 1988; 94(6):1176–1186.
11. Shoemaker WC, Appel PL, Kram HB. Role of oxygen debt in the development of organ failure, sepsis, and death in high-risk surgical patients. Chest 1992; 102:208–215.
12. Moore FA, Sauaia A, More EE, et al. Postinjury multiple organ failure: A bimodal phenomenon. J Trauma 1996; 40:501–510.
13. Hinds C, Waton D. Manipulating hemodynamics and oxygen transport in critically ill patients. N Engl J Med 1995; 333:1074–1075.
14. Gattinoni L, Brazzi L, Pelosi P, et al. A trial of goal-oriented hemodynamic therapy in critically ill patients. N Engl J Med 1995; 333:1025–1033.
15. Verdant C, De Backer D. How monitoring of the microcirculation may help us at the bedside. Current Opinion in Critical Care 2005; 11:240–244.
16. Tsai AG, Johnson PC, Intaglietta M. Oxygen gradients in the microcirculation. Physiol Rev 2003; 83:933–963.
17. Buwalda M, Ince C. Opening the microcirculation: can vasodilators be useful in sepsis? Intensive Care Med 2002; 28:1208–1217.

18. Drazenovic R, Samsel RW, Wylam ME, et al. Regulation of perfused capillary density in canine intestinal mucosa during endotoxemia. J Appl Physiol 1992; 72:259–265.

19. Dammers R, Wehrens XH, oude Egbrink MG, et al. Microcirculatory effects of experimental limb ischaemia-reperfusion. Br J Surg 2001; 88:816–824.

20. Cryer HM, Kaebrick H, Harris PD, et al. Effect of tissue acidosis on skeletal muscle microcirculatory responses to hemorrhagic shock in unanaesthetized rats. J Surg Res 1985; 39:59.

21. Bateman RM, Sharpe MD, Ellis CG. Bench-to-bedside review: microvascular dysfunction in sepsis-hemodynamics, oxygen transport, and nitric oxide. Crit Care 2003; 7:359–373.

22. Hoffman JN, Vollmar B, Laschke MW, et al. Microhemodynamic and cellular mechanisms of activated protein C action during endotoxemia. Crit Care Med 2004; 32:1011–1017.

23. Slotman GJ, Burchard KW, Williams JJ, et al. Interaction of prostaglandins in clinical sepsis and hypotension. Surgery 1986; 99:744.

24. Nakajima Y, Baudry N, Duranteau J, Vicaut E. Microcirculation in intestinal villi: a comparison between hemorrhagic and endotoxin shock. Am J Respir Crit Care Med 2001; 164:1526–1530.

25. Sauaia A, Moore FA, Moore EE, et al. Early predictors of post-injury multiple organ failure. Arch Surg 1994; 129:39–45.

26. Jobsis FF. Noninvasive infrared monitoring of cerebral and myocardial oxygen sufficiency and circulatory parameters. Science 1977; 198:1264–1267.

27. Cairns CB, Moore FA, Haenel JB, et al. Evidence for early supply independent mitochondrial dysfunction in patients developing multiple organ failure after trauma. J Trauma 1997; 42:532–536.

28. Hoch RC, Rodriguez R, Manning T, et al. Effects of accidental trauma on cytokine and endotoxin production. Crit Care Med 1993; 21:839–845.

29. Fink MP. Cytopathic hypoxia. Mitochondrial dysfunction as mechanism contributing to organ disfunction in sepsis. Crit Care Clin 2001; 17(1):219–37.

30. Veeramachaneni N, Ketcham E, Williams BT, et al. Oxidative metabolism does not recover with reperfusion following global cerebral ischemia. Acad Emerg Med 1997; 4:377–378.

31. Fink MP. Gastrointestinal mucosal injury in experimental models of shock, trauma, and sepsis. Crit Care Med 1991; 19:627–641.

32. Cairns CB. Rude unhinging of the machinery of life: metabolic approaches to hemorrhagic shock. Curr Opin Crit Care 2001; 7:437–443.

33. Hoyt DB, Bulger EM, Knudson MM, et al. Death in the operating room: an analysis of a multi-center experience. J Trauma 1994; 37:426–432.

34. Healey MA, Samphire J, Hoyt DB, et al. Irreversible shock is not irreversible: a new model of massive hemorrhage and resuscitation. J Trauma 2001; 50:826–834.

35. Robin JK, Oliver JA, Landry DW. Vasopressin deficiency in the syndrome of irreversible shock. J Trauma 2003; 54:S149–S154.

36. Thiemermann C, Szabo C, Mitchell JA, Vane JR. Vascular hyporeactivity to vasoconstrictor agents and hemodynamic decompensation in hemorrhagic shock is mediated by nitric oxide. Proc Natl Acad Sci 1993; 90:267–271.

37. Reilly JM, Cunnion RE, Burch-Whitman C, et al. A circulating myocardial depressant substance is associated with cardiac dysfunction and peripheral hypoperfusion (lactic acidemia) in patients with septic shock. Chest 1989; 95:1072.

38. Carlin RE, McGraw DJ, Camporesi EM, et al. Increased nitric oxide in exhaled gas is an early marker of hypovolemic states. J Surg Res 1997; 69:362–366.

39. Bond RF. Peripheral macro- and microcirculation. In: Schlag G, Redl H, eds. Pathophysiology of Shock, Sepsis and Organ Failure. Berlin: Springer-Verlag, 1993.

40. Weil MH, Bisera J, Trevino RP, Rackow EC. Cardiac output and end-tidal carbon dioxide. Crit Care Med 1985; 13:907–909.

41. Weinberger HD, Anderson RJ. Prevention of acute renal failure. J Crit Care 1991; 6:95.

42. Chang MC, Cheatham ML, Nelson LD, Rutherford EJ, Morris JA Jr. Gastric tonometry supplements information provided by systemic indicators of oxygen transport. J Trauma 1994; 37(3):488–494.

43. Roumen, RM, Vreugde JP, Goris RJ. Gastric tonometry in multiple trauma patients. J Trauma 1994; 36(3):313–316.

44. Kirton, OC, Windsor J, Wedderburn R, et al. Failure of splanchnic resuscitation in the acutely injured trauma patient correlates with multiple organ system failure and length of stay in the ICU. Chest 1998; 113(4):1064–9.

45. Stene J, Smith CE, Grande CM. Evaluation of the trauma patient. In: Longnecker DE, Tinker JH, Morgan GE, eds. Principles and Practice of Anesthesiology. 2nd ed. Philadelphia, PA: Mosby-Yearbook, 1997.

46. Wang P, Hauptman JG, Chaudry IH. Hemorrhage produces depression in microvascular blood flow which persists despite fluid resuscitation. Circ Shock 1990; 32:307.

47. Chang MC, Meredith JW. Cardiac preload, splanchnic perfusion, and their relationship during resuscitation in trauma patients. J Trauma 1997; 42(4):577–582.

48. Rackow EC, Falk JL, Fein IA, et al. Fluid resuscitation in circulatory shock: a comparison of the cardiorespiratory effects of albumin, hetastarch, and saline solutions in-patients with hypovolemic and septic shock. Crit Care Med 1983; 11:839.

49. Shires GT III, Shires GT. Fluid and electrolyte management of the surgical patient. In: Sabiston DC, ed. Textbook of Surgery: The Biological Basis of Modern Surgical Practices. 15th ed. Philadelphia, PA: W.B. Saunders Company, 1997:105.

50. Jurkovich GJ, Carrico J. Trauma: management of the acutely injured patient. In: Sabiston DC, ed. Textbook of Surgery: The Biological Basis of Modern Surgical Practices. 15th ed. Philadelphia, PA: W.B. Saunders Company, 1997:297.

51. Didwania A, Miller J, Kassel D, et al. Effect of intravenous lactated Ringer's solution infusion on the circulating lactate concentration: Part 3. Results of a prospective, randomized, double-blind, placebo-controlled trial. Crit Care Med 1997; 25(11):1851–1854.

52. Waters JH, Miller LR, Clack S, Kim JV. Cause of metabolic acidosis in prolonged surgery. Crit Care Med 1999; 27(10):2142–2146.

53. Lam AM, Winn HR, Cullen BF, et al. Hypoglycemia and neurological outcomes in patients with head injury. J Neurosurg 1991; 75:545.

54. Michaud LJ, Rivara FP, Longstreth WT, et al. Elevated initial blood glucose levels and poor outcome following severe brain injury in children. J Trauma 1991; 31:1356.

55. Alderson P, Schierhout G, Robers I, Bunn F. Colloids versus crystalloids for fluid resuscitation in critically ill patients. Cochrane Database Syst Rev 2000; (2):CD000567.

56. Choi PT, Yip G, Quinonez LG, Cook DJ. Crystalloids vs. colloids in fluid resuscitation: a systematic review. Crit Care Med 1999; 27(1):200–210.

57. Gosling P, Bascon JU, Zikria BA. Capillary leak, oedema and organ failure: breaking the triad. Crit Care Ill 1996; 12:191–197.

58. Weaver DW, Ledgerwood AM, Lucas CE, et al. Pulmonary effects of albumin resuscitation for severe hypovolemic shock. Arch Surg 1978; 113:387–392.

59. Jorgensen KA, Stofferson E. Heparin-like activity of albumin. Thrombus Res 1979; 16:573–578.

60. Dietrich G, Orth D, Haupt W, Kretschmer V. Primary hemostasis in hemodilution: infusion solutions. Infusionstherapie 1990; 17:214–216.

61. Tobias MD, Wambold D, Pilla MA, Greer F. Differential effects of serial hemodilution with hydroxyethyl starch, albumin, and 0.9% saline on whole blood coagulation. J Clin Anesth 1998; 9:366–371.

62. Jorgensen KA, Stofferson E. On the inhibitory effects of albumin on platelet aggregation. Thrombos Res 1980; 17:13–18.

63. Stogermuller B, Stark J, Willschke H, et al. The effect of hydroxyethyl starch 200 kD on platelet function. Anesth Analg 2000; 91:823–827.

64. Treib J, Haass A, Pindur G. Coagulation disorders caused by hydroxyethyl starch. Thromb Haemost 1997; 78(3):974–983.
65. Ring J, Messmer K. Incidence and severity of anaphylactoid reactions to colloid volume substitution. Lancet 1977; 1: 467–469.
66. Gan TJ, Bennett-Guerrero E, Phillips-Bute B, et al. Hextend, a physiologically balanced plasma expander for large volume use in major surgery: a randomized phase III clinical trial. Hextend Study Group. Anesth Analg 1999; 88(5):992–998.
67. Ducey JP, Mozingo DW, Lamiell JM, et al. A comparison of the cerebral and cardiovascular effects of complete resuscitation with isotonic and hypertonic saline, hetastarch, and whole blood following hemorrhage. J Trauma 1989; 29(11): 1510–1518.
68. Krausz MM. Controversies in shock research: hypertonic resuscitation—pros and cons. Shock 1995; 3(1):69–72.
69. Gross D, Landau EH, Klim B, et al. Quantitative measurement of bleeding following hypertonic saline administration in "uncontrolled" hemorrhagic shock. J Trauma 1989; 29:79.
70. Oliveira RP, Weiingartner R, Ribas EO, et al. Acute haemodynamic effects of a hypertonic saline/dextran solution in stable patients with severe sepsis. Intensive Care Med 2002; 28:1574–1581.
71. Dewitt DS, Prough DS, Deal DD, et al. Hypertonic saline does not improve cerebral oxygen delivery after head injury and mild hemorrhage in cats. Crit Care Med 1996; 24:109.
72. Hartl R, Ghajar J, Hochleuther H, Mauritz W. Treatment of refractory intracranial hypertension with repetitive hypertonic/hyperoncotic infusions. Zentrabl Chir 1997; 122:181–185.
73. ASA Task Force. Practice guidelines for blood component therapy. Anesthesiology 1996; 84:732.
74. Messmer K, Sunder-Plassman L, Jesch F, et al. Oxygen supply to the tissues during limited normovolemic hemodilution. Res Exp Med 1973; 159:152.
75. Herbert PC, Wells G, Blajchman MA, et al. A multicenter randomized, controlled clinical trial of transfusion requirements in critical care. Transfusion Requirements in Critical Care Investigators, Canadian Critical Care Trials Group. N Engl J Med 1999; 340:409–417.
76. Grande CM, Smith CE, Stene J. Anesthesia for trauma. In: Longnecker DE, Tinker JH, Morgan GE, eds. Principles and Practice of Anesthesiology. 2nd ed. Philadelphia, PA: Mosby-Yearbook, 1997.
77. Gervin AS, Fischer RP. Resuscitation of trauma patient with type-specific uncrossmatched blood. J Trauma 1984; 24:327.
78. Sohmer PR, Scott RL. Massive transfusion. Clin Lab Med 1982; 2:21.
79. Lucas CE, Ledgerwood AM, Saxe JM, Dombi G, Lucas WF. Plasma supplementation is beneficial for coagulation during severe hemorrhagic shock. Am J Surg 1996; 171(4):399–404.
80. Leslie SD, Toy PT. Laboratory hemostatic abnormalities in massively transfused patients given red blood cells and crystalloid. Am J Clin Path 1991; 96:770.
81. Valeri CR, Collins FB. Physiologic effects of 2,3-DPG_depleted red cells with high affinity for oxygen. J Appl Physiol 1971; 31:823.
82. Murray DJ, Pennell BJ, Weinstein SL, Olsen JD. Packed red cells in acute blood loss: dilutional coagulopathy as a cause of surgical bleeding. Anesth Analg 1995; 80:336.
83. Murray DJ, Olson J, Strauss R, Tinker JH. Coagulation changes during packed red cell replacement of major blood loss. Anesthesiology 1988; 69:839.
84. Dutton RP, Hess JR, Scalea TM. Recombinant factor VIIa for the control of hemorrhage: early experience in critically ill trauma patients. J Clin Anesth 2003; 15(3):184–188.
85. White B, et al. Successful use of recombinant FVIIa (NovoSeven) in the management of intractable post-surgical intraabdominal hemorrhage. Br J Haematol 1999; 107:677–678.
86. Martinowitz U, Kenet G, Segal E, et al. Recombinant activated factor VII for adjunctive hemorrhage control in trauma. J Trauma 2001; 51:431–438.
87. Smith CE, Patel N. Hypothermia in adult trauma patients: anesthetic considerations. Part II: Prevention and treatment. Amer J Anesthesiol 1997; 24:29.
88. Smith CE, Patel N. Hypothermia in adult trauma patients: anesthetic consideration. Part I: Etiology and pathophysiology. Am J Anesthesiol 1996; 23:283.
89. Sessler DI. Perianesthetic thermoregulation and heat balance in humans. FASEB J 1993; 7:638–644.
90. Valeri CR, Mac Gregor H, Cassidy G, et al. Effects of temperature on bleeding time and clotting in normal male and female volunteers. Crit Care Med 1995; 23:698.
91. Reed RL, Bracy AW, Hudson JD, et al. Hypothermia and blood coagulation: dissociation between enzyme activity and clotting factor levels. Circ Shock 1990; 32:141.
92. Reed RL, Johnston TD, Hudson JD, Fischer RP. The disparity between hypothermic coagulation and clotting studies. J Trauma 1992; 33:465.
93. Mizushima Y, Wang P, Cioffi WG, et al. Restoration of body temperature to normothermia during resuscitation following trauma-hemorrhage improves the depressed cardiovascular and hepatocellular functions. Arch Surg 2000; 135(2): 175–181.
94. Jurkovich GH, Greiser WR, Luterman A, et al. Hypothermia in trauma victims: an ominous predictor of survival. J Trauma 1987; 27:1019.
95. Mendlowitz M. The specific heat of human blood. Science 1948; 107:97.
96. Gentillo LM, Moujaes S. Treatment of hypothermia in trauma victims: thermodynamic considerations. J Intensive Care Med 1995; 10:5.
97. Patel N, Smith CE, Pinchak AC. Clinical comparison of blood warmer performance during simulated clinical conditions. Can J Anesth 1995; 42:636.
98. Scalea TM, Hartentt RW, Duncan AO, et al. Central venous oxygen saturation: a useful clinical tool in trauma patients. J Trauma 1990; 30:1539.
99. Kahn RC, Jasco HD, Carlon GC, et al. Massive blood replacement: correlation of ionized calcium, citrate, and hydrogen ion concentration. Anesth Analg 1979; 58:274.
100. Hossack KF, Moreno CA, Vanway CW, Burdick DC. Frequency of cardiac contusion in nonpenetrating chest injury. Am J Cardiol 1988; 61:392–394.
101. Pasquale M, Fabian TC. Practice management guidelines for trauma for the Eastern Association for the Surgery of Trauma. J Trauma 1998; 44:941–945.
102. Bertinchant JP, Polge A, Mohty D, et al. Evaluation of incidence, clinical significance, and prognostic value of circulating cardiac tropinin I and T elevation in hemodynamically stable patients with suspected myocardial contusion after blunt chest trauma. J Trauma 2000; 48:924.
103. Fildes JJ, Betlej TM, Manglano R, et al. Limiting cardiac evaluation in patients with suspected myocardial contusion complicating blunt chest injury. Am Surg 1995; 61:832.
104. Bristow MR, Ginsberg R, Umans V, et al. B_1 and B_2-adrenergic-receptor subpopulations in failing and nonfailing human ventricular myocardium: coupling of both receptor subtypes to muscle contraction and selective B_1 receptor downregulation in heart failure. Circ Res 1986; 59:297–309.
105. Englehardt S, Bohm M, Erdmann E, Lohse MJ. Analysis of beta-adrenergic receptor mRNA levels in human ventricular biopsy specimens by quantitative polymerase chain reactions: progressive reduction of beta₁-adrenergic receptor mRNA in heart failure. J Am Coll Cardiol 1996; 27:146–154.
106. Kantrowitz A, Tjonneland S, Freed PS, et al. Initial experience with intraaortic balloon pumping in cardiogenic shock. JAMA 1968; 203:113–118.
107. Moulopoulos SD, Topaz S, Kolff WJ. Diastolic balloon pumping (with carbon dioxide) in the aorta: mechanical assistance to the failing circulation. Am Heart J 1962; 63:669–775.
108. Moulopoulos SD, Stamatelopoulos S, Petroou P. Intraaortic balloon assistance in intractable cardiogenic shock. Eur Heart J 1986; 7:396–403.
109. Centers for disease control and prevention: increase in national hospital discharge survey rates for septicemia-United States, 1979–1987. JAMA 1990; 263:937.

110. Centers for Disease Control and Prevention, National Center for Health Statistics: mortality patterns-United States, 1990, Monthly Vital Statistics Report 1993; 41:5.

111. Matot I, Sprung CL. Definition of sepsis. Intensive Care Med 2001; 27:S2–S9.

112. Wheeler AP, Bernard GR. Treating patients with severe sepsis. N Engl J Med 1999; 340:207–214.

113. Bone RC, Balk RA, Cerra FB, et al. American College of Chest Physicians/Society of Critical Care Medicine consensus conference: definition for sepsis and organ failure and guidelines for the use of innovative therapies in sepsis. Chest 1992; 101:1644–1655.

114. Wheeler AP, Bernard GR. Treating patients with severe sepsis. N Engl J Med 1999; 340:207–214.

115. Bone RC, Balk RA, Cerra FB, et al. American College of Chest Physicians/Society of Critical Care Medicine consensus conference: definition for sepsis and organ failure and guidelines for the use of innovative therapies in sepsis. Chest 1992; 101:1644–1655.

116. Dellinger RP, Carlet JM, Masur H, et al. Surviving Sepsis Campaign guidelines for management of severe sepsis and septic shock. Crit Care Med 2004; 32(3):858–873.

117. Choi PTL, YIP G, Quinonez LG, Cook DJ. Crystalloids vs. colloids in fluid resuscitation: a systematic review. Crit Care Med 1999; 27:200–210.

118. Schierhout G, Roberts I. Fluid resuscitation with colloid or crystalloid solutions in critically ill patients. A systematic review of review of randomized trials. BMJ 1998; 316:961–964.

119. Finer S, Belloro R, Boyce N, et al. SAFE Study Investigators: A comparison of albumin and saline for fluid resuscitation in the intensive care unit. New Engl J Med 2004; 350:2247–2256.

120. Rivers E, Nguyen B, Havstad S, et al. Early goal directed therapy in the treatment of severe sepsis and septic shock. N Engl J Med 2001; 345:1368–1377.

121. Ruokonen E, Parviainen I, Uusaro A. Treatment of impaired perfusion in septic shock. Ann Med 2002; 34(7–8):590–597.

122. Bellomo R, Giantomasso DD. Noradrenaline and the kidneys: friends or foes? Crit Care 2001; 5(6):294–298.

123. Marik PE, Mohedin M. The contrasting effects of dopamine and norepinephrine on systemic and splanchnic oxygen utilization in hyperdynamic sepsis. JAMA 1994; 272:1354–1357.

124. Martin C, Viviand X, Leone M, et al. Effect of norepinephrine on the outcome of septic shock. Crit Care Med 2000; 28:2758–2765.

125. Ract C, Vigue B. Comparison of the cerebral effects of dopamine and norepinephrine in severely head injure patients. Intensive Care Med 2001; 27:101–106.

126. Bellomo R, Chapman M, Finfer S, Hickling Myburgh J. Low-dose dopamine in patients with early renal dysfunction: a placebo-controlled randomized trial. Lancet 2000; 356:2139–2143.

127. DW, Oliver JA. The pathogenesis of vasodilatory shock. N Engl J Med 2001; 345:588–595.

128. Chen P. Vasopressin: new uses in critical care. N Engl J Med 2001; 324:146–154.

129. Tsuneyoshi I, Yamada H, Kakihana Y, Nakamura M, Boyle WA III. Hemodynamic and metabolic effects of low-dose vasopressin in vasodilatory septic shock. Crit Care Med 2001; 29: 487–493.

130. Patel BM, Chittock DR, Russell JA, Walley KR. Beneficial effects of short-term vasopressin infusion during severe septic shock. Anesthesiology 2002; 96:576–582.

131. Landry DW, Levin HR, Gallant EM, et al. Vasopressin pressor hypersensitivity in vasodilatory septic shock. Crit Care Med 1997; 25:1279–1282.

132. Malay MB, Ashton RC Jr, Landry DW, Townsend RN. Low-dose vasopressin in the treatment of vasodilatory septic shock. J Trauma 1999; 47:699–703.

133. Dunser MW, Mayr AJ, Ulmer H, et al. The effects of vasopressin on systemic hemodynamics in catecholamine-resistant septic and postcardiotomy shock: a retrospective analysis. Anesth Analg 2001; 93:7–13.

134. Holmes CL, Walley KR, Chittock DR, Lehman T, Russell JA. The effects of vasopressin on hemodynamics and renal function on hemodynamics and renal function in severe septic shock: a case series. Intensive Care Med 2001; 27:1416–1421.

135. O'Brien A, Clapp L, Singer M. Terlipressin for norepinephrine-resistant septic shock. Lancet 2002; 359:1209–1210.

136. Bone RC, Fisher CJ Jr, Clemmer TP, et al. A controlled clinical trial of high-dose methyl prednisilone in the treatment of sever sepsis and septic shock. N Engl J Med 1987; 317:653–658.

137. The Veterans Administration Systemic Sepsis Cooperative Study Group. Effect of high-dose glucocorticoids therapy on mortality in patients with clinical signs of systemic sepsis. N Engl J Med 1987; 317:659–665.

138. Lefering R, Neugebauer EA. Steroid controversy in sepsis and septic shock: a meta-analysis. Crit Care Med 1995; 23:1294–1303.

139. Cronin L, Cook DJ, Carlet J, et al. Corticosteroid treatment for sepsis: a critical appraisal and meta-analysis of the literature. Crit Care Med 1999; 27:427–430.

140. Briegel J, Forst H, Haller M, et al. Stress doses of hydrocortisone to reverse hyperdynamic septic shock: a prospective, randomized, double-blind, single-center study. Crit Care Med 1999; 27:723–732.

141. Meduri GU, Kanangat S. Glucocorticoid treatment of sepsis and acute respiratory distress syndrome: time for a reappraisal. Crit Care Med 1998; 26:630–633.

142. Bollaert PE. Stress doses of glucocorticoids in catecholamine dependency: a new therapy for a new syndrome. Intensive Care Med 2000; 26:3–5.

143. Briegel J, Kellermann W, Forst H, et al. Low-dose hydrocortisone infusion attenuates the systemic inflammatory response syndrome. Clin Investig 1994; 72:782–787.

144. Saito T, Fuse, A Gallagher ET, et al. The effect of methylprednisilone on myocardial beta-adrenergic receptors and cardiovascular function in shock patients. Shock 1996; 5241–5246.

145. Saito T, Takanashi M, Gallagher, et al. Corticosteroid effect on early beta-adrenergic down-regulation during circulatory shock: hemodynamic study and beta-adrenergic receptor assay. Intensive Care Med 1995; 21:204–210.

146. Schein RM, Sprung CL, Marcial E, et al. Plasma cortisol levels in patients with septic shock. Crit Care Med 1990; 18:259–263.

147. Annane D, Sebille, Troche G, et al. A 3-level prognostic classification of septic shock based on cortisol levels and cortisol response to corticotropin. JAMA 2000; 283:1038–1045.

148. Annane D, Sebille V, Charpentier C, et al. Effect of treatment with low dose of hydrocortisone and fludrocortisone on mortality in patients with septic shock. JAMA 2002; 288:862–871.

149. Hoen S, Asehnoune K, Brailly-Tabard S, et al. Cortisol response to corticotropin stimulation in trauma patients: influence of hemorrhagic shock. Anesthesiology 2002; 97(4):807–813.

150. Bone RC, Fisher CJ, Clemmer TP, Slotman GJ, et al. A controlled clinical trial of high-dose methylprednisone in the treatment of severe sepsis and septic shock. N Engl J Med 1987; 317:653–658.

151. Cronin L, Cook DJ, Carlet J, et al. Corticosteroid treatment for sepsis: a critical appraisal and meta-analysis of the literature. Crit Care Med 1999; 27:427–430.

152. Fisher CJJ, Agosti, Opal SM, et al. Treatment of septic shock with the tumor necrosis factor receptor: Fc fusion protein. N Engl J Med 1996; 334:699–709.

153. Abraham E, Laterre PF, Garbino J, et al. Lenercept (p55 tumor necrosis factor receptor fusion protein) in severe sepsis and early septic shock: a randomized, double-blind, placebo-controlled, multi-center phase III trial with 1342 patients. Crit Care Med 2001; 29:503–510.

154. Cohen J, Carlet J. INTERSEPT: an international multicenter, placebo-controlled trial of monoclonal antibody to human tumor necrosis factor alpha in patients with sepsis. Crit Care Med 1996; 24:1431–1440.

155. Opal SM, Fisher CJJ, Dhainault JF, et al. Confirmatory interleukin-1 receptor antagonist trial in severe sepsis: a phase III randomized, double-blind, placebo-controlled, multi-center trial. Crit Care Med 1997; 25:1115–24.

156. Dhainault JF, Tenaillon A, Le Tulzo Y. Platelet-activating factor receptor antagonist BN 52021 in the treatment of severe sepsis: a randomized, double-blind, placebo-controlled, multicenter clinical trial. Crit Care Med 1994; 22:1720–1728.

157. Fisher CJJ, Dhainault JF, Opal SM, et al. Recombinant human interleukin 1 receptor antagonist in treatment of patients with sepsis syndrome: results from a randomized, double-blind, placebo-controlled trial. JAMA 1994; 271:1836–1843.

158. Reinhart K, Menges T, Gardlund B, et al. Randomized, placebo-controlled trial of the anti-tumor necrosis factor antibody fragment afelimimab in hyperinflammatory response during severe sepsis: the Ramses study. Crit Care Med 2001; 29:765–769.

159. Abraham E, Anzueto A, Guitierrez G, et al. Double blind randomized controlled trial of monoclonal antibody to human tumor necrosis factor in treatment of septic shock. Lancet 1998; 351:929–933.

160. Abraham E, Wondering R, Silverman H, et al. Efficacy and safety of monoclonal antibody to human tumor necrosis alpha in patients with sepsis syndrome: a randomized, controlled, double-blind, multicenter clinical trial. JAMA 1995; 273:934–941.

161. Abraham E, Glauser M, Butler T, et al. p55 Tumor necrosis factor receptor fusion protein in the treatment of patients with severe sepsis and septic shock: a randomized controlled multicenter trial. JAMA 1997; 277:1531–1538.

162. Fisher CJJ, Slotman GJ, Opal SM, et al. Initial evaluation of human recombinant interleukin-1 receptor antagonist in the treatment of sepsis syndrome: a randomized, open-label, placebo-controlled multicenter trial. Crit Care Med 1994; 22:12–21.

163. Ziegler EJ, Fisher CH, Sprung CL, Straube RC, Sadoff JC, Foulke GE. Treatment of gram-negative bacteremia and septic shock with HA-1A human monoclonal antibody against endotoxins: a randomized, double-blind, placebo-controlled trial. N Engl J Med 1991; 324:429–436.

164. Bone RC, Balk RA, Fein AM, et al. A second large controlled clinical study of E5, a monoclonal antibody to endotoxins: results of a prospective, multicenter, randomized controlled trial. Crit Care Med 1995; 23:994–1006.

165. McCloskey RV, Straube RC, Sanders C, Smith SM, Smith CR. Treatment of septic shock with human monoclonal antibody to endotoxins: results of a prospective, multicenter, randomized, controlled trial. Ann Intern Med 1994; 121:1–5.

166. Bernard GR, Vincent JL, Laterre PF, et al. Efficacy and safety of recombinant human activated protein C for severe sepsis. N Engl J Med 2001; 344:699–709.

167. Abraham E, Reinhart K, Svoboda P, et al. Assessment of the safety of recombinant tissue factor pathway inhibitor in patients with severe sepsis: a multicenter, randomized, placebo-controlled, single-blind, dose escalation study. Crit Care Med 2001; 29:2081–2089.

168. Bernard GR, Wheeler AP, Russell JA, et al. The effects of ibuprofen on the physiology and survival of patients with sepsis: the ibuprofen study group. New Engl J Med 1997:912.

169. Nasraway SA. Sepsis research: we must change course. Crit Care Med 1999; 27:427–430.

170. Fisher CJ Jr, Yan SB. Protein C levels as a prognostic indicator of outcome in sepsis and related diseases. Crit Care Med 2000; 28(9 suppl):S49–S56.

171. Bernard GR, Vincent JL, Laterre PF, et al. Efficacy and safety of recombinant human activated protein C for severe sepsis. N Engl J Med 2001; 344:699–709.

172. Bernard GR, Margolis B, Shanies H, et al. Efficacy and safety of drotecogin alpha (activated) in the treatment of adult patients with severe sepsis: report from a single-arm open-label trial in the United States. Chest 2002; 1229(suppl 4):50S.

173. Mannis BJ, Lee H, Doig CJ, Johnson D, Donaldson C. An economic evaluation of activated protein C treatment for severe sepsis. N Engl J Med 2002; 347:993–1000.

174. Fisher M. Clinical observations on the Pathophysiology and implications for treatment. In: Vincent JL, ed. Update in Intensive Care and Emergency Medicine. New York: Springer-Verlag, 1989:309–316.

175. Fahmy NR. Hemodynamics, plasma histamine and catecholamine concentrations during anaphylactoid reaction to morphine. Anesthesiology 1981 55:329–331.

176. Hanashiro PK, Weil MH. Anaphylactic shock in man: report of two cases with detailed hemodynamic and metabolic studies. Arch Int Med 1967:119–129.

177. Levy JH, Levi R. Diagnosis and treatment of anaphylactic/anaphylactoid reactions. In: Assem E-SK, ed. Allergic Reactions to Anaesthetics. Clinical and Basic Aspects. Monogr Allergy. Vol. 30. Basel, Karger, 1992:130–144.

178. Stassen NA, Luken JK, Dixon MS, et al. Abdominal compartment syndrome. Scand J Surg 2002; 91:104–108.

179. Berger P, Nijsten MW, Paling JC, Zwaveling JH. The abdominal compartment syndrome: a complication with many faces. Neth J Med 2001; 58(5):197–203.

180. Eddy V, Nunn C, Morris JA Jr. Abdominal compartment syndrome. The Nashville experience. Surg Clin North Am 1997; 77:801–812.

181. De Backer D, Creteur J, Preiser JC, et al. Microvascular blood flow is altered in patients with sepsis. Am J Respir Crit Care Med 2002; 166:98–104.

182. Grigoryev DN, Finigan JH, Hassoun P, Garcia JG. Science review: searching for gene candidates in acute lung injury. Crit Care 2004; 8(6):440–447.

183. Kingsmore SF. Multiplexed protein measurement: technologies and applications of protein and antibody arrays. Nat Rev Drug Discov 2006; 5(4):310–320.

184. Senthil M, Brown M, Xu DZ, et al. Gut-lymph hypothesis of systemic inflammatory response syndrome/multiple-organ dysfunction syndrome: validating studies in a porcine model. J Trauma 2006; 60(5):958–965.

185. Acosta JA, Hoyt DB, Schmid-Schonbein GW, et al. Intralumenal pancreatic serine protease activity, mucosal permeability, and shock: a review. Shock 2006; 26(1):3–9.

186. Schmid-Schonbein GW, Hugli TE. A new hypothesis for microvascular inflammation in shock and multiorgan failure: self-digestion by pancreatic enzymes. Microcirculation 2005; 12(1):71–82.

187. Taniguchi T, Hirai F, Takemoto Y, et al. A novel adsorbent of circulating bacterial toxins and cytokines: the effect of direct hemoperfusion with CTR column for the treatment of experimental endotoxemia. Crit Care Med. 2006; 34(3):800–806.

188. Kellum JA, Song M, Venkataraman R. Hemoadsorption removes tumor necrosis factor, interleukin-6, and interleukin-10, reduces nuclear factor-kappaB DNA binding, and improves short-term survival in lethal endotoxemia. Crit Care Med 2004; 32(3):801–805.

189. Lamberts SW, Bruining HA, de Jong FH. Corticosteroid therapy in severe illness. N Engl J Med 1997; 337:1285–1292.

190. Meldrum DR, Moore FA, Moore EE, et al. Prospective characterization and selective management of abdominal compartment syndrome. Am J Surg 1997; 174:667–672.

191. Leach RM, Treacher DF. The pulmonary physician in critical care: 2. Oxygen delivery and consumption in the critically ill. Thorax 2002; 57:170–177.

192. Advanced Trauma Life Support for Doctors. Student Course Manual 7th Edition. American College of Surgeons Committee on trauma, Chicago, IL: American College of Surgeons, 2004.

193. Boral LI, Henry JB. Transfusion medicine. In: Henry JB, ed. Clinical Diagnosis and Management by Laboratory Methods. 19th ed. Philadelphia, PA: W.B. Saunders Company, 1996:804–805.

19

Myocardial Ischemia

Steven L. Orebaugh

Department of Anesthesiology, University of Pittsburgh Medical Center, Pittsburgh, Pennsylvania, U.S.A.

EPIDEMIOLOGY OF CORONARY ARTERY DISEASE

Myocardial ischemia results from an abrupt decrease in the myocardial oxygen supply/demand relationship. This may result from rupture of pre-existing atherosclerotic plaque or an acute increase in demand in a patient with significant pre-existing coronary artery disease (CAD) (1). In the trauma setting, coronary vasospasm and coronary emboli may occur, along with direct trauma to the heart, resulting in ischemia in the absence of known pre-existing coronary disease (2). However hypoperfusion of myocardium supplied by coronary arteries with pre-existing lesions is the predominant ischemic mechanism. Additionally, coronary spasm, in response to a variety of stimuli, plays a variable role in the development of myocardial ischemic episodes when superimposed upon CAD (3).

An epidemic of cardiovascular diseases exists, with atherosclerosis as the chief among them (4). By far, the most common cause of overall mortality in the United States is CAD, which is responsible for one in five deaths (5). More than 1.1 million myocardial infarctions (MIs) occur annually in the United States, with a significant male predominance (as with trauma). Sudden cardiac death (SCD) is responsible for 250,000 premature deaths each year in the United States, and in over half of these patients, there was no pre-existing knowledge or symptoms of CAD (6).

Obstructive CAD is manifested in a variety of ways. It is useful to envision a continuum, based on the severity of signs and symptoms, which is influenced by the degree of coronary obstruction, the stability of atherosclerotic plaques, activation levels of the platelet and fibrin systems, coronary arterial spasm, and systemic and local inflammatory factors (7). Patients with CAD are often asymptomatic (8). When symptoms of the disease exist, they may manifest as stable angina (SA) pectoris, unstable angina (UA), nonST-segment elevation MI (NSTEMI), and transmural or ST-segment elevation MI (STEMI). In addition, CAD may present as SCD (1). Further complexity is added by the realization that myocardial ischemia is often clinically silent. Indeed, 17% of all MIs occur without symptoms, and another 17% are unrecognized due to atypical symptoms (8).

✍ **The presence of CAD significantly increases the risk of morbidity and mortality to any acutely injured patient.** ✍ The incidence of CAD in trauma patients ranges from 0.3% (9) to as high as 15% (10). Mortality rates in trauma patients with pre-existing CAD have been reported to be as high as 11.2% (10) and 18.4% (9) compared with a mortality of only 2.6% (10) and 3.2% (9) in corresponding cohorts without CAD. Given the high prevalence

of asymptomatic ischemic heart disease (6), many trauma patients with CAD at the time of injury may be undiagnosed.

Although several cases of direct traumatic coronary occlusion have been reported in trauma patients (11), the most common cause of myocardial ischemia in the trauma patient with CAD is hypoperfusion due to hemorrhagic shock. While young patients without CAD can tolerate a low flow state for brief periods, patients with critical coronary artery lesions will develop immediate myocardial ischemia, further exacerbating the shock state, and complicating the resuscitation.

In one retrospective study at a busy tertiary trauma center, only five cases of post-traumatic MI occurred over a 10-year period (12). Only one of these patients had chest pain, but all five developed heart failure. However, the expectation is that prospective studies would reveal more patients. Indeed, about 4% of trauma patients (and a large percentage of elderly) have pre-existing ischemic heart disease, which confers a higher mortality rate after trauma (13).

This chapter will review the considerations for CAD for the general population, and then discuss the specific issues related to the trauma patient. Many of the first-line treatments for acute coronary syndromes (ACS) in the nontrauma setting are relatively contraindicated following trauma (e.g., anticoagulation or antiplatelet drugs in setting of bleeding, nitrates in the setting of hypovolemia, or closed head injury, and beta blockers in the setting of hemorrhagic shock). Accordingly, many aspects of management for CAD in the trauma victim are complicated and different.

PATHOPHYSIOLOGY OF MYOCARDIAL ISCHEMIA
Atherosclerosis of the Coronary Arteries

As the majority of cases of myocardial ischemia result from atherosclerosis of the coronary arteries, it is important to review the pathogenesis of this process. Focal changes of the vessel wall of middle-sized and large arteries lead to a softening of the intima and a hardening around it from a combination of lipid accumulation, smooth muscle cell proliferation, and immune cell activation (14). The epicardial coronary arteries, aorta, iliofemoral, and carotid arteries appear to be most susceptible to this process.

Atherogenesis begins with endothelial cell dysfunction at susceptible sites, including increased permeability to lipoproteins, accumulation of leukocytes, and other processes related to thrombosis, fibrosis, and neovascularization (15). "Fatty streaks," asymptomatic collections of lipid-laden macrophages or "foam cells," are the initial lesions of atherosclerosis and can be seen in the fetuses of hypercholes-terolemic women, as well as in normal adolescents (16). The grossly apparent streaks may regress if serum cholesterol is lowered, or progress to symptomatic atherosclerotic plaques. The activation of macrophages and T-cells is an important contributor to the progression of these lesions, perhaps allowing progression to full-fledged atherosclerotic plaques (17). ☞ **Atheromatous lesions progress in association with known risk factors for CAD, such as hypertension, and the influx of inflammatory cells.** ☞

Risk factors for CAD, such as hypertension, diabetes, smoking, advanced age, and elevated cholesterol levels, are associated with endothelial dysfunction (17). Further, intimal thickening, resulting from mechanical influences on the vessel wall, tends to develop at areas frequently affected by atherosclerotic lesions. This focal adaptive thickening of the intima in association with endothelial dysfunction seems to predispose the development of atherosclerosis at these sites (18).

When the foam cells of a fatty streak begin to release lipid into the vessel wall, or when lipoproteins from the serum become trapped within the lesion, the streak begins to mature into a atherosclerotic plaque. Concomitant patholo-gic changes include proliferation of connective tissue, denuded areas of intima with platelet adhesion, and neo-vascularization at the base of the plaque (19). Additional inflammatory cells then migrate into the lesion, resulting in further progression (Table 1). An advanced plaque contains cellular debris, apoptic cells, connective tissue cells, and free cholesterol crystals. This is very rich in tissue factor (Fig. 1) (7).

Atherosclerotic Plaque Vulnerability to Rupture

Some atherosclerotic lesions are vulnerable to rupture or fissuring, which results in superimposed thrombosis of varying degrees. Thrombotic occlusion of the coronary lumen, whether subtotal or complete, is the basis for the majority of ACS (Fig. 2) (20,21). ☞ **Atheromatous plaque may be vulnerable to rupture, with resultant coronary artery thrombosis and occlusion, despite a relatively modest baseline impingement of the coronary lumen.** ☞ Plaques which are rich in lipid, especially those with greater degrees of inflammation and with thin fibrous "caps" are most susceptible to rupture (22). These are termed "vulnerable plaques." Surprisingly, the size of a plaque tells little about its vulnerability to rupture (23). Lesions which rupture and cause ACS show greater degrees of inflammation than other plaques (Fig. 3) (24). A

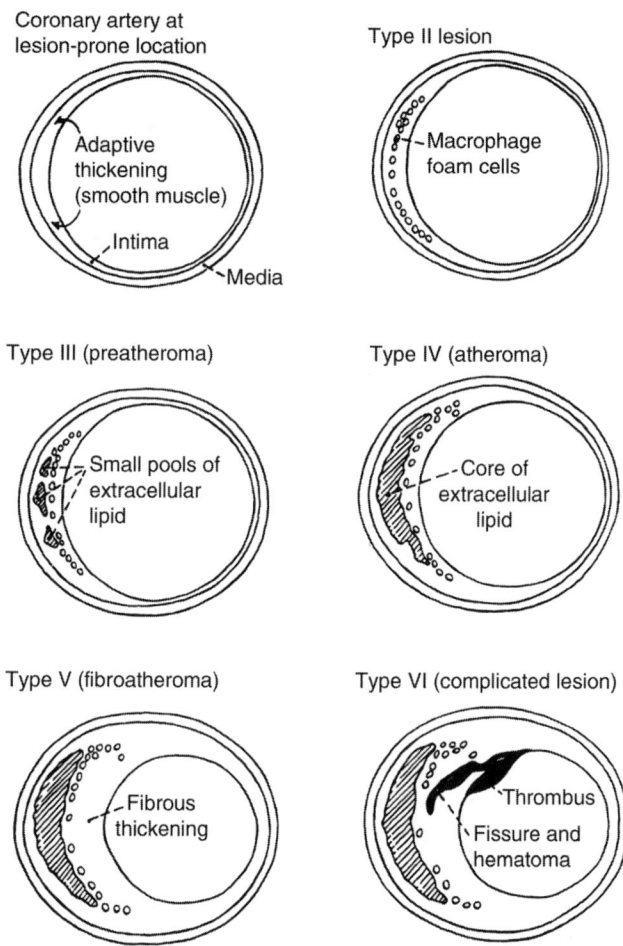

Figure 1   Progression of atheromatous lesions in a coronary artery using the American Heart Association classification. Adaptive smooth muscle thickening constitutes a type I lesion; type II lesions require the infiltration of macrophage foam cells; type III lesions are characterized by small pools of extracellular lipid; type IV lesions contain a large core of coalesced lipid; fibrous thickening of the intema (so called fibroatheroma) characterizes the type V lesion; and type VI lesion involves intimal fissures with thrombus formation. *Source*: From Ref. 15.

role for infectious agents in atherosclerosis has been suggested but is not well elucidated (25).

Vulnerable, advanced plaques rupture with great fre-quency, and most of these episodes are asymptomatic. However, such lesions are subject to worsening inflam-mation and rapid progression (26). Plaque rupture may lead to formation of a small mural thrombus, which seals the lesion; or of a more substantial thrombus, which pro-duces UA or MI. Both platelet adhesion and the deposition of fibrin are important components of the dynamic thrombo-sis, which complicates plaque rupture (27).

Rupture of a plaque may also be followed by hemor-rhage into the atheroma, thereby encroaching on the lumen of the vessel. In addition, the rupture may also be followed by a coronary vasospasm. Such lesions may either cause chest pain, or other anginal equivalents, or may remain clini-cally silent. Obstruction of the lumen is often dynamic, with a fluctuating impediment to distal blood flow (20,21).

While unstable, ruptured plaques are usually evident on coronary angiography, the majority of atherosclerotic

Table 1   The Pathologic Characteristics of an Atheromatous Plaque

General characteristics	High vulnerability characteristics
Intimal thickening	↑ inflammation
Accumulation	(e.g., ↑ CRP)
of lipid-laden macrophages	Rich in lipid
(foam cells)	↑ IL-18
Proliferation of connective tissue	Exuberant neo-
Neovascularization at base of	vascularization
lesion	Small "cap"
Fibrous "cap" on lumen	↑ greater degrees of
surface of lesion	inflammation

Abbreviations: CRP, C-reactive protein; IL-18, interleukin-18.

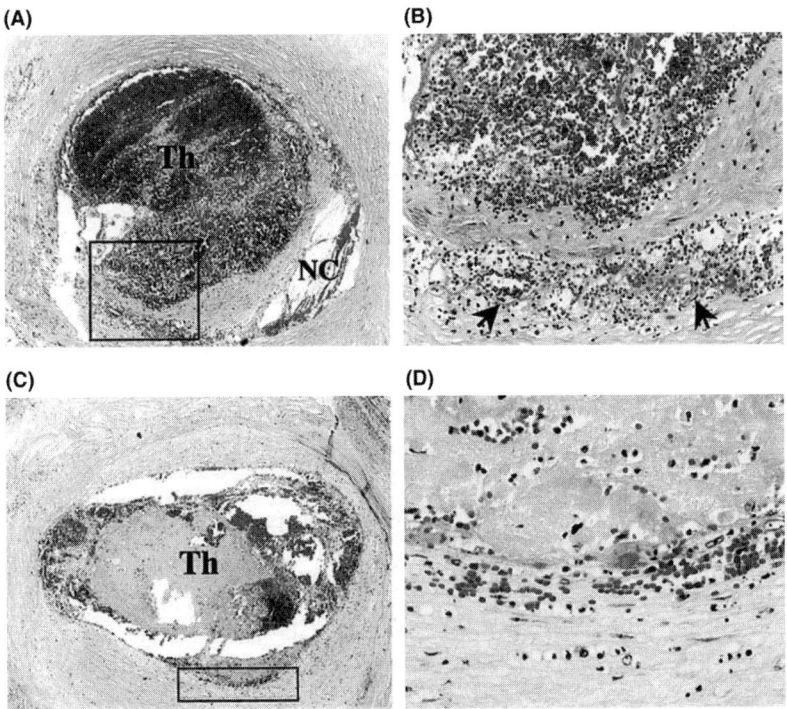

Figure 2 Coronary artery lesions showing areas of rupture and erosion. (**A**) Coronary section with plaque rupture containing a luminal thrombus, disrupted thin fibrous cap, and underlying necrotic core. (**B**) A high-power view of the region outlined by the box in (**A**), showing macrophage infiltration of the thin fibrous cap (*arrows*). (**C**) Section proximal to rupture site (**A**) showing the propagated thrombus over a lesion resembling plaque erosion. (**D**) A high-power view of the region outlined by the box in (**C**) showing a smooth muscle cell—and proteoglycan-rich plaque. Without serial sectioning, the rupture site may not have been identified. This case exemplifies the histological diversity of some lesions that confound the diagnosis underlying the patient's demise. *Abbreviations*: NC, necrotic core; Th, thrombus. *Source*: From Ref. 18.

plaques do not cause significant lumen narrowing and are thus not apparent during cardiac catheterization (28,29). Furthermore, regions of vessel wall affected by atheromas often undergo remodeling, which preserves the integrity of the vessel lumen.

    ☞ **Coronary angiography does not identify all high-risk lesions, because neither the size of the plaque nor the degree of stenosis correlates with its vulnerability to rupture (23).** ☞ Most MIs result from lesions that are not angiographically significant (7). Coronary calcification identified by electron beam computed tomography (CT) reflects the overall burden of atherosclerosis, although calcium-containing plaques may actually be more stable than lesions without calcium (30,31).

The Ischemic Continuum

CAD may present as a continuum of clinical ischemic manifestations ranging from stable angina to STEMI (see box below).

> **Box 1.** The Ischemic Continuum
> stable angina → UA → NSTEMI → STEMI

    Atherosclerosis remains silent until the coronary lumen is reduced to the degree that blood flow is insufficient to meet the metabolic needs of the myocardium, typically when more than 70% of the cross-sectional area of the artery is obstructed. Such compromise classically produces a stable angina pattern, wherein the metabolic demand exceeds the oxygen delivery only during exertion, producing chest discomfort or other symptoms. When stable angina occurs, reductions in metabolic demand result in restoration of the balance of oxygen supply and myocyte demand. Symptoms generally resolve at this point, and no myocardial damage occurs (32).

    Patients with stable angina generally complain of exercise-induced (or emotionally induced) chest discomfort, but are symptom free at rest. Anginal "equivalents" include jaw or neck pain, shoulder or arm pain, and shortness of breath. Rest alone suffices to ameliorate the symptoms in these patients. The physiologic perturbations associated with major trauma (hypotension, tachycardia) as well as the supratentorial component (stress, pain, fear, and anxiety) can escalate a previously stable patient toward the right side of the ischemic continuum (Box 1), leading to myocardial ischemia or infarction.

    More severe coronary obstruction gives rise to the ACS, including UA, NSTEMI, and STEMI (Table 2). ☞ **Instability and rupture of nonocclusive plaque leads to most episodes of ACS, because the subsequent exposure of reactive elements within the lesion leads to unpredictable degrees of thrombosis at the vascular luminal site (33).** ☞ Platelet adhesion occurs, following the luminal exposure of thrombin inducing constituents, and fibrin deposition is initiated. The extent of resultant thrombosis is related to local vessel wall abnormalities, rheologic characteristics of blood, and systemic factors, as originally described by Virchow (34). The thrombus which arises may occlude the coronary lumen embolize small particles downstream, or promote coronary vasospasm through the release of

PLAQUE HETEROGENEITY

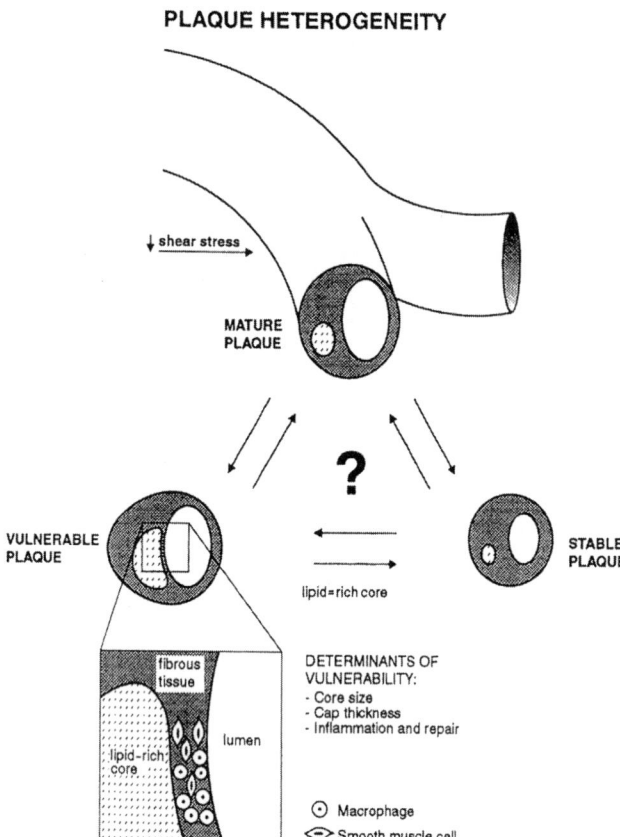

Figure 3 Range of plaque heterogeneity, determinants of rupture vulnerability (core size, cap thickness, inflammation, and repair), and the transformation from mature plaque to vulnerable plaque. *Source*: From Ref. 19.

vasoactive substances (35). Therapeutic maneuvers in ACS are leveled at these causes of compromised perfusion.

Table 2 Pathophysiology of the Coronary Syndromes

Coronary syndrome	Pathophysiologic derangements
Stable angina pectoris during demand	Narrowing of coronary lumen, reduced blood supply, ischemia resolves with rest, no cellular injury
Unstable angina myocardial	Plaque disruption, dynamic coronary thrombosis, ischemia, limited cellular injury
NSTEMI myocardial ischemia	Plaque disruption, dynamic coronary thrombosis, greater degree of ischemia, some cell death
STEMI throughout the territory	Occlusive coronary thrombosis, ischemia
Death	Served by the affected coronary, transmural cell

Abbreviations: NSTEMI, nonST-segment elevation myocardial infarction; STEMI, ST-segment elevation myocardial infarction.

Autopsy evidence reveals that plaque rupture or fissuring occurs frequently in atherosclerotic lesions, but most of these undergo remodeling and heal without deleterious consequences to the patient (36,37). It appears that widespread activation of inflammatory biomolecules results in frequent plaque disruption in those with CAD. Only a small minority of these occurrences result in ACS (3). Certain inflammatory markers, such as C-reactive protein, may predict adverse outcome in such patients (38,39).

A wide range (in terms of size and thrombus content) of coronary lesions occurs in UA. Necropsy typically shows disrupted plaques with intralumenal thrombus, and some degree of preserved lumen patency. Most plaques which cause UA contain thrombus, implying disruption, while most other plaques in patients with stable angina do not contain any thrombus. In milder cases of UA, repeated episodes of vasospasm occurring at sites of lumen narrowing may be part of the underlying cause (7,40–42).

Intravascular ultrasound confirms that many "stable" coronary plaques are angiographically invisible due to arterial remodeling. Thus, angiography accurately demonstrates anatomic stenosis, but is an imperfect test for predicting the likelihood of future plaque rupture and consequent MI locations. Indeed, high grade (more than 50%) stenosis is responsible for less than one-third of MI (22). These lesions may progress to complete occlusion, but this tends to occur over years, and usually does not lead to acute MI due to the development of collateral coronary blood flow (43). The precise morphology of disrupted plaques leading to MI cannot currently be determined in vivo (7).

☞ STEMI is caused by complete occlusion of a coronary artery, with simultaneous myocyte death in the territory supplied by that vessel (44). NSTEMI results from small areas of infarction of differing ages, probably caused by repeated episodes of transient occlusion, platelet emboli, or both (7,45). ☞ In addition, it appears that SCD may be related to plaque rupture and thrombosis as well (33,46). Fifty percent to 70% of cases of CAD-related SCD are due to coronary thrombi (47).

TRAUMA RELATED CAUSES OF MYOCARDIAL ISCHEMIA
Direct Mechanisms of Cardiac Injury
Myocardial Contusion

Direct trauma to the heart may cause a variety of disturbances of cardiac structure and function, depending on whether the mechanism is blunt or penetrating (Table 3). ☞ Myocardial ischemia is often clinically silent in the trauma patient. ☞ Myocardial ischemia and infarction may be caused by cardiac trauma, blunt or penetrating, even in the absence of atherosclerosis of the coronary arteries. Such episodes are relatively infrequent, but require suspicion on the part of the examining physician. Numerous conditions in the trauma patient may mask myocardial injury or distract the examiner, including altered mental status (from head injury or intoxication), as well as coexisting painful fractures or soft-tissue injury.

Myocardial contusion is more common than coronary artery obstruction-related ischemia, after blunt chest trauma; and most of these cases arise from motor vehicle accidents (MVA). The mechanism of cardiac injury in this setting involves severe compressive forces delivered to the thorax.

Table 3 Injuries Sustained Following Direct Cardiac Trauma (Blunt and Penetrating)

Blunt trauma	Penetrating trauma
Myocardial contusion	Myocardial laceration
Coronary dissection	Coronary laceration
Coronary thrombosis	Arteriovenous fistula
Coronary injury with delayed aneurysm formation	Coronary injury with aneurysm
Pericardial tamponade (may be delayed)	Pericardial tamponade (after acute presentation)
Posttraumatic pericarditis	Valvular or papillary muscle laceration
Valve or papillary muscle disruption	Foreign body retention embolism

Histopathologically, cardiac contusion is marked by hemorrhage into the myocardium, disruption of myofibrils, and followed by inflammatory cell infiltrates (48). Chest pain may be identical to that of myocardial ischemia, or may appear to be due to injury to the chest wall (49).

Myocardial contusion should be suspected in all patients with significant blunt chest trauma. No laboratory test has proven completely accurate in confirming the diagnosis. Cardiac enzyme determination [creatine kinase (CK)] suffers from a lack of specificity, as it is frequently liberated by major trauma to skeletal muscle in multitrauma patients. The cardiac troponins are far more specific for injury to the myocardium (47,50,51). Nevertheless, the ability of these biomarkers to predict complications in the blunt chest trauma patient is poor (52). Electrocardiographic (ECG) abnormalities which may occur with myocardial contusion include tachycardia, nonspecific ST-segment and T-wave abnormalities, and supraventricular or ventricular tachydysrhythmias. None of these findings is very specific for contusion, as they occur with numerous other conditions (53). However, patients with normal troponins and a normal ECG are very unlikely to have significant myocardial contusion (52). Gated scintigraphy has also proven useful in the diagnosis of myocardial contusion (52).

Echocardiography, both transesophageal (TEE) and transthoracic (TTE), has proven to be a more useful immediate diagnostic tool in the patient with suspected myocardial contusion, and is especially useful in those with structural abnormalities resulting from trauma, such as papillary muscle injury (54). However, even when wall motion abnormalities appear on echocardiogram after blunt chest trauma, there is a low likelihood of complications that require intervention (48).

✔ **Most myocardial contusions require no specific therapy (other than monitoring), and these patients usually have an excellent prognosis.** ✔ Therapy for cardiac contusion is largely symptomatic and supportive. Only 2% to 4.5% of patients with myocardial contusion from blunt chest trauma require treatment of complications (55). Unlike ACS, there is no obstructing coronary lesion or thrombus at which to direct the therapy. Patients are generally monitored for early treatment of significant dysrhythmias, and if severe left ventricular dysfunction exists, concomitant coronary artery thrombosis or spasm should be ruled out, and inotropic agents may be useful (48). Patients with atrial or ventricular dysrhythmias should be monitored with continuous ECG for at least 24 hours following trauma.

Significant dysrhythmia, or hypotensive episodes, or both warrant an echocardiographic exam. Large contusions may result in prolonged or permanent left ventricular compromise, with the patient experiencing intermittent bouts of congestive heart failure (CHF). Patients who develop left ventricular aneurysms may benefit from surgical repair (56). However, the vast majority of patients with myocardial contusion do well and do not have long-term sequelae or ventricular dysfunction (57).

Blunt Coronary Artery Injury

Coronary thrombosis secondary to blunt chest trauma is rare. Such cases appear to be due to intimal tears of the coronary arteries with dissection and subsequent thrombosis. These thrombi will result in MI unless either spontaneous thrombolysis or emergent invasive therapy intervenes to rapidly re-establish blood flow (Fig. 4) (58). ✔ **Blunt chest injury may produce injury to the right coronary artery (RCA) or left anterior descending (LAD) artery. These injuries often involve dissections resulting in MI, especially when the LAD coronary artery is injured.** ✔ Most case reports involve the LAD and RCAs, with the circumflex (CIRC) rarely becoming injured (58–60).

Electrocardiography, cardiac enzymes and troponins, and echocardiography may all prove useful in making the diagnosis of MI in blunt chest trauma. Each of these modalities provides greater specificity for the diagnosis of coronary artery injury than for the diagnosis of myocardial contusion. ST-segment elevation, reflecting a current of transmural injury, is common in this situation (58,59,61,62). Both creatine kinase MB isoenzyme (CKMB) and cardiac troponins will be elevated, reflecting infarcting myocardium, and the echocardiography will reflect wall motion abnormalities in the ischemic territory.

When coronary dissection with thrombotic occlusion is suspected, the patient should undergo coronary angiography if the clinical condition permits. Intracoronary thrombolysis has been described in the management of one such patient but severely injured patients may develop life-threatening hemorrhage from this intervention (60). Both percutaneous transluminal coronary angioplasty (PTCA) and coronary stenting have been successfully utilized in these patients to emergently re-establish coronary blood flow (58,59,62). Ventricular septal defect, coronary aneurysm, or ventricular aneurysm mandate surgical intervention (58).

Penetrating Cardiac Trauma

Penetrating cardiac trauma commonly results from injury by sharp instruments or missiles. Mortality from these injuries is greater than 50% (63). As with myocardial contusion, the right side of the heart is injured more frequently than the left due to its orientation within the thorax (64). Coronary lacerations constitute only 5% of these injuries, and are usually sufficiently distal in the artery to minimize the degree of resultant myocardial injury (65).

Chest radiography, ECG, and echocardiography are utilized in the diagnosis of complications from penetrating chest trauma. When the patient has signs of life in the field or the emergency department, but becomes acutely unstable or experiences cardiac arrest, immediate resuscitative thoracotomy (Volume 1, Chapter 13) for presumed pericardial tamponade may be life saving (65). Surgical repair of any cardiac laceration is required after resuscitation.

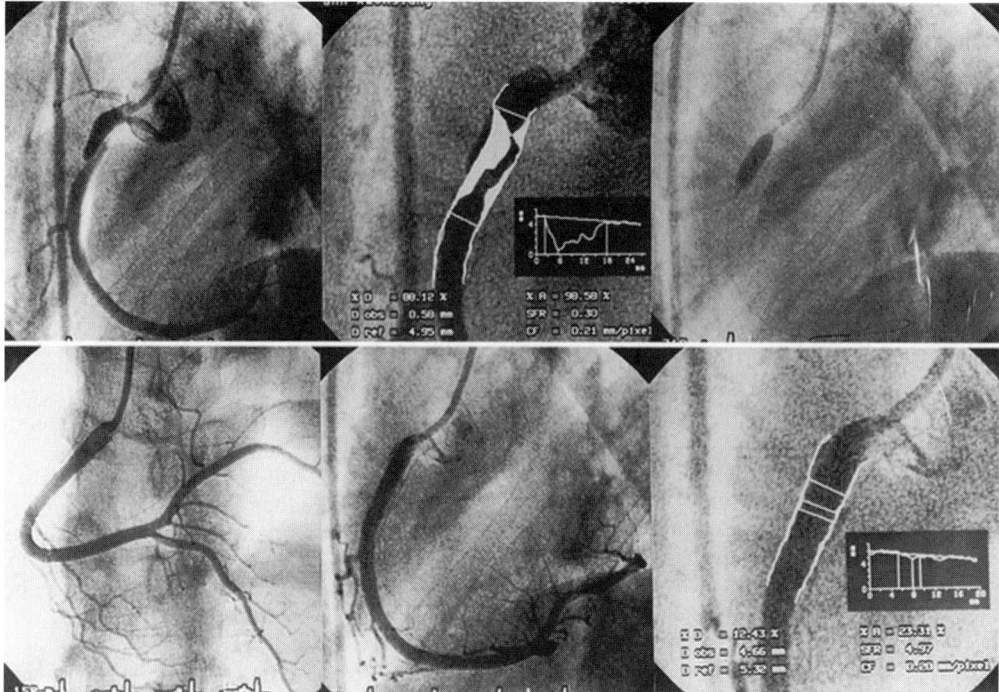

Figure 4 Angiogram showing a right coronary artery dissection (*upper left* and *middle*) following blunt chest trauma. After percutaneous transluminal coronary angioplasty and stenting (*upper right* and *lower*). The patient's ischemic symptoms improved after this procedure and was doing well after the one-year follow up. *Source*: From Ref. 58.

Another potential complication of penetrating chest trauma is arterial air embolism, which may produce myocardial ischemia or infarction. ☞ **Arterial air embolism, a complication of penetrating chest trauma, may be rapidly fatal and requires early suspicion and familiarity to diagnose the condition and effectively intervene.** ☞ This is typically the result of pulmonary laceration, with positive pressure ventilation favoring entrainment of air into open pulmonary veins (66). Subsequent embolization to the arterial tree and various arterial capillary beds follows, with resultant ischemia. Patients may present with typical manifestations of penetrating lung trauma, only to rapidly deteriorate when positive pressure ventilation is initiated (67). Management includes reducing airway pressures, ventilating with 100% oxygen, appropriate inotropic support, and immediate thoracotomy to clamp the hilum of the involved lung, thereby excluding the source of air embolization (68).

Indirect Mechanisms of Cardiac Injury

The indirect stressors of hypotension and hypoperfusion probably trigger the majority of ischemic episodes occurring during the resuscitation phase of trauma patients with pre-existing CAD. However, many ischemic episodes occur two to three days or more following trauma and surgery (69,70). Inflammation also plays a seminal role in the progression and rupture vulnerability of atherosclerotic plaque. Multiple trauma leads to the release of inflammatory biomolecules and initiation of inflammatory cascades in animals and humans (71), but the relationship of these factors to plaque progression or instability after trauma is not well established.

The primary cause of death to trauma patients outside of the immediate period of injury is multiple organ system failure. This appears to result from widespread inflammatory changes in the organ systems that are affected, more often out of proportion to the degree of insult (72). Complement activation, release of anaphylotoxins, as well as activation of both the coagulation and fibrinolytic systems often accompany major trauma. Each of these cascades can activate granulocytes. Adverse neutrophil-endothelium interaction occurs, leading to local microvascular dysfunction, dysregulation of blood flow, intravascular coagulation, and ischemic injury superimposed on toxic injury from oxidants and other products of activated neutrophils (73). A systemic inflammatory response syndrome (SIRS) often follows, which, when unregulated, causes further release of cytokines and prolonged activation of inflammatory cells, causing end-organ injury (also see Volume 2, Chapter 63) (72–77). Higher cytokine levels correlate with increased mortality rates in these patients (78,79).

Systemic inflammation is likewise deleterious in CAD. Various markers of inflammatory activation, such as C-reactive protein (CRP) and circulating leukocyte levels, have been linked to the progression of atherosclerotic plaques (80,81). Loss of smooth muscle cells in the fibrous caps of plaques has been suggested to result from cytokine production by activated leukocytes (82,83). This loss of smooth muscle cells predisposes a plaque to rupture. It is possible that circulating inflammatory molecules in trauma may adversely affect smooth muscle cells in pre-existing plaque, predisposing these patients to plaque rupture and increasing the likelihood of ACS.

☞ **Systemic inflammation and adverse physical conditions (common accompaniments of major trauma) probably predispose the existing atheromatous plaques toward instability, followed by their rupture.** ☞ Shear forces may be exaggerated due to trauma, and labile vital signs in such patients can result in altered coronary dynamics, leading to plaque fissuring or rupture. Adrenergic stimulation, a concomitant of multiple trauma, may play a role as well (80). Lastly, the determinants of clotting and clot stability can be dramatically altered by systemic trauma, with ill-defined effects on the process of coronary thrombus formation.

Major surgical procedures, much like multisystem trauma, can initiate a widespread inflammatory response, which, when unchecked, can have deleterious consequences. Incision, tissue dissection, vessel ligation, and cauterization may all result in cellular injury, release of tissue factor and cytokines, and initiation of the coagulation and fibrinolytic cascades (84,85). A SIRS may result, with progression to multiple organ system failure (73).

Both surgery and multiple trauma provide favorable conditions for the development of acute instability in atherosclerotic plaques. Each of these processes has been shown to release tissue factor and other inflammatory biomolecules, activate the thrombotic and fibrinolytic systems, and activate platelets and leukocytes, thus predisposing to small-vessel dysfunction and widespread tissue injury. Epidemiologic and pathophysiologic studies of myocardial ischemia and infarction in the trauma patient are scarce, but much work has been done to elucidate the nature and mechanisms of myocardial ischemia in surgical patients during the perioperative period.

As is the case with ACS outside of these settings, vulnerable atheromatous plaques put the patient at risk for plaque rupture, fissuring, or denudation with subsequent coronary thrombosis, followed by UA, MI, or spontaneous clot dissolution with re-establishment of coronary flow. A variety of historical factors and laboratory abnormalities have been established to qualify the likelihood of perioperative cardiac morbidity (Table 4). Those placing patients at high risk include recent MI with ongoing ischemia, active CHF, uncontrolled dysrhythmias, UA, or severe valvular disease (86). A large area of ischemic myocardium or ischemia in multiple different coronary territories on preoperative radionuclide perfusion studies or stress echocardiography also portends high risk (69). Intermediate degrees of risk are suggested by stable angina, diabetes mellitus, history of CHF, and more modest degrees of ischemia on perfusion/functional testing (69,86). Poor exercise capacity also helps

stratify risk of cardiac disease and the need for preoperative testing.

The invasiveness and immediacy of surgery are also important variables, with major vascular surgery carrying one of the highest risk profiles (70). Intraoperative factors are also closely tied to the risk of perioperative cardiac morbidity. Hypotension and tachycardia, particularly when they occur in tandem, are important contributors to myocardial ischemia and adverse cardiac sequalae (87). This may be related to increased myocardial oxygen demand, decreased oxygen delivery, shear stress on vulnerable plaques, or a combination of these.

Intraoperative ST-segment depression, and ischemic ECG changes in the immediate postoperative period are associated with postoperative MI (88). Segmental wall motion abnormalities evident on intraoperative TEE are more sensitive to ischemia than ST-segment analysis, but are not necessarily more predictive of outcomes (89). ☞ **Continuous electrocardiographic ST-segment evaluation provides the most practical means of monitoring for intraoperative myocardial ischemia.** ☞

The postoperative period is just as important as the intraoperative period, perhaps more so, in the genesis of perioperative cardiac morbidity (PCM). Up to 90% of perioperative MIs occur in the first 72 hours postoperatively, with very few actually occurring in the operating suite (69,87). It is likely that systemic inflammatory mediators, liberated by surgical trauma, place patients at risk of plaque rupture and thrombosis throughout the perioperative period. ☞ **The risk of myocardial ischemia in the perioperative period is higher postoperatively than intraoperatively.** ☞

DIAGNOSIS OF MYOCARDIAL ISCHEMIA FOLLOWING TRAUMA
Clinical Diagnosis

In stable angina pectoris, ischemia is typically manifested by chest pain, which may be dull, heavy, squeezing, or merely a sensation of pressure. Discomfort may be felt in the precordial or substernal region, or in the neck, jaw, arm, or shoulder. It is often difficult for the patient to precisely localize the pain (32). In the case of stable angina, symptoms occur with exertion or after exertion, and generally resolve within a few minutes of ceasing the activity.

In some patients, pain is not sensed, but anginal "equivalents" are experienced during ischemia. These include shortness of breath and vague chest heaviness (90). Ischemic episodes occur with no symptoms at all, in many patients, with ischemia detectable only by ambulatory ECG (91). The extreme variability among patients in symptoms experienced during myocardial ischemia makes the diagnosis challenging, and explains why significant numbers of patients are discharged inappropriately from emergency departments when experiencing MI (92).

Angina is considered unstable when (*i*) anginal symptoms occur at rest, or (*ii*) with increasing frequency, with levels of activity that were previously well tolerated, or (*iii*) becomes refractory to previously effective therapy (93). This intensifying symptomatology portends a poor prognosis. Like stable angina, many episodes of UA occur without producing symptoms or with atypical symptoms (91). ☞ **UA and NSTEMI are commonly indistinguishable on clinical grounds, manifesting as rest angina. They are, therefore, approached in a similar diagnostic and therapeutic fashion.** ☞ Unlike stable angina, in which atherosclerotic plaque produces limitations of blood flow in the

Table 4 Major Risk Factors for Perioperative Cardiac Morbidity

Risk factors	Clinical examples
Historical	Recent MI with ongoing ischemic symptoms
	Active CHF
	Unstable angina
	Severe valve dysfunction
Surgical	Emergency surgery
	Major vascular (aortic) or peripheral vascular surgery
	Abdominal or thoracic surgery with large blood or fluid losses
Intraoperative	Prolonged tachycardia and/or hypotension
	ST-segment depression on ECG monitoring
Postoperative	ST-segment depression on ECG monitoring
	Prolonged tachycardia

Abbreviations: CHF, congestive heart failure; ECG, electrocardiogram; MI, myocardial infarction.

face of increased myocardial demand, UA and NSTEMI are caused by occlusive coronary thrombus at the site of a ruptured or denuded plaque. Arterial occlusion is probably intermittent, fluctuating with propagation and lysis of the clot, coronary vasospasm, mechanical disruption of the obstruction, and distal platelet emboli (94). In NSTEMI, symptoms are likely to prevail for a longer period of time before relief, implying a greater period of ischemia and cellular injury, detectable by chemical markers.

In STEMI, the signs and symptoms of classic MI are more likely to be manifest. These include unrelenting chest pain or pressure, dyspnea, and visceral symptoms such as diaphoresis and nausea (95). Hemodynamic instability, such as tachycardia and hypotension, are common, as are dysrhythmias. Chest pain in STEMI is frequently refractory to nitrate therapy, and often requires opioids or effective reperfusion to ameliorate its severity.

Despite the classic descriptors of anginal or ischemic pain, up to 90% of perioperative ischemic episodes are asymptomatic (70), and the majority of such events, after major trauma, appear to be clinically silent (12). ☞ **The diagnosis of myocardial ischemia is difficult to make on clinical grounds, especially in the trauma patient, who may have altered pain response for a variety of reasons, such as distracting injury, analgesic medications, or CNS injury.** ☞

Electrocardiographic Diagnosis

Historical and physical examination data are notoriously unreliable in diagnosing myocardial ischemia, following severe trauma or major surgery, making laboratory data (especially ECG and troponin values) essential. Electrocardiographic evidence of ischemia includes ST-segment depression, T-wave inversion, or both, in the territory of a particular coronary artery (96). In the operating room (OR), and potentially in the intensive care unit (ICU), continuous computer analysis of ST-segments improves the sensitivity of ECG for detecting ischemic episodes (88). For patients at high risk, ambulatory ECG can be utilized to document and quantify the number and duration of ischemic episodes (97). The number and duration of such episodes predicts the risk of PCM.

The diagnosis of MI by ECG criteria must be made rapidly for effective institution of therapy to commence. The changes on ECG reflect numerous processes in the myocardium so that coronary thrombi can be manifest in a number of different patterns, varying with artery length and size, location of the thrombus, degree of necrosis, collateral circulation, and cardiac orientation in the thorax (98). The time honored terms used to locate an MI include anterior, inferior, and lateral, corresponding to occlusion of the LAD, RCA, and CIRC arteries, respectively. Some authors maintain that the appropriate anatomic correlate of these occlusions should actually be anterior, lateral, and posterior (99).

ST-segment elevations permit the most rapid recognition of MI, though sensitivity of ECG for MI is only fair. ☞ **Classic ECG criteria for MI are only about 50% sensitive.** ☞ The standard criteria for diagnosis of acute STEMI is to have the ST-segment elevation greater than 1 mm in at least one lead (anterior or inferior), and ST-segment elevation greater than 2 mm in at least one anterior lead. This combination produces a sensitivity of 56% and specificity of 94% for MI (100). ST-segment depression in uninvolved areas of the myocardium as reflected on the ECG may reflect "reciprocal" forces. The position of the

ST-segment elevation in the precordial leads helps to identify the position of LAD occlusion as proximal or distal. Elevation in leads I and aVL predicts occlusion of the first diagonal branch of the LAD (98,101).

Inferior MI is classically manifested by ST-segment elevation in leads II, III, and aVF, 80% to 90% of which represent RCA occlusions. The other 10% to 20% represents CIRC occlusion, depending upon the patient's anatomy (102). ☞ **MI may manifest with ST-segment depression rather than elevation.** ☞ It will often be accompanied by ST-segment depression in the lead aVL (103). ST-segment elevations in V_5 or V_6 accompanying the pattern of inferior MI indicate posterolateral myocardial injury (104).

Unfortunately, the variable territory served by the CIRC and the placement of ECG leads renders occlusion of this artery difficult to diagnose. Only half of the occlusions are manifest as ST-segment elevation, most often in II, III, and aVF (105). When an inferior infarction pattern is accompanied by ST-segment depression in the precordial leads, posterior myocardial wall injury is likely (106–109), implicating the CIRC rather than the RCA as the infarct artery. To further elucidate injury to the posterior wall of the LV, leads V_7 through V_9 can be placed. These leads are placed in the same horizontal plane as V_6, on the posterior thorax, and will show ST-segment elevation in posterior wall injury (102,105). They are much more sensitive and specific for posterior MI related to CIRC occlusion than the standard precordial leads (104).

Infarctions of the interventricular septum usually manifest as ST-segment elevation in leads V_3 and V_4 (110). Occlusion of the left main coronary produces a combination of ST-segment elevation in aVR and ST-segment depression inferiorly in lead II, with lateral depression in leads I and V_4–V_6 (110). Infarction of the right ventricle often accompanies inferior MI and manifests on ECG as ST-segment elevation in V_1 and in the right precordial leads, especially V_4R (111).

Many patients with acute MI do not have ST-segment elevations despite coronary occlusion. ST-segment depression is sometimes the only manifestation evident on the ECG. Depressions of 4 mm or more (except in aVR) are highly specific for acute MI, though not very sensitive (112). Diffuse precordial ST-segment depression, if maximal in leads V_4–V_6, suggests LAD occlusion. When this depression is maximal in V_2–V_3, CIRC involvement is more likely (113). When such depression is evident in the inferior leads and across the precordium, left main coronary or triple vessel disease is probably present (98).

An ECG monitor that can simultaneously display two channels is optimal for ischemia monitoring of high-risk patients in the OR and the ICU. Lead II is superior for monitoring the cardiac rhythm because of the clarity and size of the P wave. However, the precordial leads are the most sensitive for detecting significant myocardial ischemia. Indeed, London et al. (114) studied a large cohort of patients with known CAD undergoing noncardiac, mainly vascular surgery using continuous 12-lead ECG monitoring, and found that V_5 was most sensitive, detecting 75% of ischemic events. Simultaneously, monitoring both leads V_4 and V_5 increased sensitivity to 90%, whereas the standard II and V_5 array was only 80% sensitive (Fig. 5). However, lead II and concomitant V_5 monitoring is recommended, because lead II is most sensitive for P-wave evaluation and detects inferior wall ischemia (geographically separated from, and perfused by a different coronary artery than the V_5 area). The V_5 lead is usually placed over the left fifth intercostal

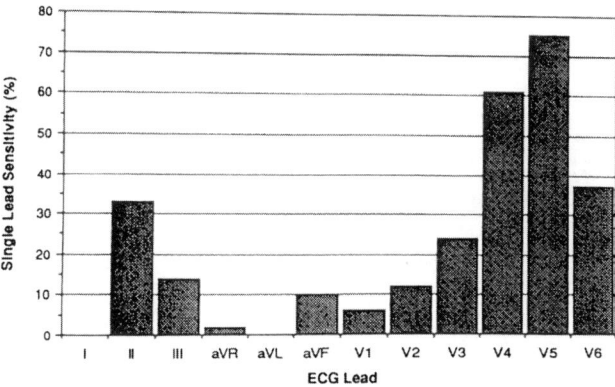

Figure 5 Single-lead sensitivity for detection of myocardial ischemia during noncardiac surgery. *Abbreviation*: ECG, electrocardiogram. *Source*: From Ref. 114.

space just lateral to the mid-clavicular line. However, we frequently need to modify this location to accommodate surgical management in the OR and chest wall dressings following trauma in the ICU.

Conduction defects, such as bundle branch blocks, can make the diagnosis of MI more difficult, because repolarization abnormalities commonly accompany these disorders. However, the right bundle branch block (BBB) does not usually obscure the ECG evidence of MI (115). The left BBB presents more difficulty to the physician. Criteria have been proposed to distinguish new myocardial injury patterns in the left BBB (116), but the clinical utility of these criteria remains controversial (117). ⚐ **Symptoms of acute myocardial ischemia, combined with new ECG manifestations of left bundle branch block, together are sufficient to diagnose acute MI.** ⚐ Strong clinical evidence of myocardial ischemia

in association with a new left BBB is an indication for thrombolytic therapy or percutaneous coronary interventions (118).

A number of conditions may mimic acute MI or ischemia on ECG, and must be considered in the differential diagnosis. These include electrolyte abnormalities, acute pericarditis, acute pulmonary thromboembolism, thoracic aortic dissection, ventricular aneurysms, left ventricular hypertrophy and left BBB, hypothermia, and early repolarization patterns (98). Electronic permanent pacemakers may obscure the diagnosis of acute MI. ST-segment elevation of more than 0.5 mV in leads with negative QRS complexes have high specificity for acute MI, though these changes only occur in about half of the cases (119).

A significant proportion of patients with MI do not have the expected ECG changes described. ⚐ **Ten percent of patients with acute MI have a normal ECG on presentation (92).** ⚐ In one analysis of diagnostic modalities for acute cardiac ischemia, the sensitivity of prehospital ECG for acute myocardial ischemia was 76% (120). Thus, the diagnosis of acute myocardial ischemia or infarction may depend upon clinical suspicion and other laboratory data, as well as the ECG.

Biochemical Testing

Several biochemical tests are available to assist in the diagnosis of myocyte injury. These include creatine kinase (CK) and the MB fraction of CK, cardiac troponins I and T (cTnI and cTnT), and myoglobin (Table 5). These biomarkers have been primarily evaluated for the diagnosis of MI and not for myocardial ischemia. When infarction occurs, cellular proteins and enzymes are released into the bloodstream in time dependent fashion. This is less likely in the setting of ischemia without infarction.

CK is an enzyme found in myocytes, of which several subunits exist. The subunit most specific to cardiac

Table 5 Biochemical Markers of Cardiac Injury

Marker	Hours til elevated	Peak elevation	Duration of elevation	Sensitivity, specificity, and comments
AST	8–12	1–2 days	3–6 days	Low sensitivity and specificity elevated with skeletal trauma and liver injury.
LDH	8–12	2–3 days	7–10 days	Low sensitivity and specificity elevated with skeletal trauma and liver injury.
CK	4–6	12–36 hrs	3–4 days	Low sensitivity and specificity elevated with skeletal trauma and liver injury.
CKMB	4–6	12–24 hrs	2–3 days	99% sensitive, 90–95% specific in absence of skeletal injury. Skeletal muscle has trace amounts of CKMB, thus limiting usefulness following trauma and surgery.
Myoglobin	2–3	6–12 hrs	24–48 hrs	Heme protein located in both skeletal and cardiac muscle. Nonspecific in setting of trauma or surgery. However, very sensitive, and an early marker.
HFABP	2–3	8–10	18–30	HFABP not widely available clinically yet, may emerge as useful measure of infarct size.
Troponins (T and I)	4–6	12–24 hrs	7–10 days	99–100% sensitive, 85–96% specific, increased specificity compared to others in the setting of trauma and surgery.

Note: Troponin T and I are isoforms of troponin.
Abbreviations: AST, aspartate transaminase; CK, creatine kinase; CKMB, creatine kinase MB isoenzyme; HFABP, heart fatty acid binding protein; LDH, lactate dehydrogenase.

myocytes is the MB subunit, though it appears in variable degrees in skeletal muscle as well. CK is reported in units of total enzyme activity, while CKMB is reported in units, or concentration, or as a percentage of total CK. Since CK and its MB subunit also appear in skeletal muscle, they may be elevated in circumstances which cause skeletal muscle injury, such as trauma, vigorous exercise, rhabdomyolysis, heat illness, and inflammatory conditions. These markers become detectable in serum four hours after myocyte injury, and peak levels occur at 12 to 24 hours (110,111), returning to normal at 24 to 36 hours. ✐ **In acute MI, serial determination for CKMB is more sensitive for the diagnosis than a single determination at presentation.** ✐ In a recent meta-analysis of studies conducted to evaluate the accuracy of CKMB in the diagnosis of acute MI, sensitivity of serial testing ranged from 68% to 90%, if samples were drawn at presentation and three or four hours later. However, sensitivity improved to nearly 100% in studies in which serial testing was performed at six hours or more after presentation (114). Specificities ranged from 90% to 96%, depending on whether the assay was drawn at presentation or serially thereafter.

Myoglobin is the best early indicator of myocardial ischemia in patients who have not sustained trauma or surgery. Indeed, it is detectable in serum at two to four hours after infarction, providing improved early sensitivity compared to CKMB (110). Sensitivity is improved for myoglobin as symptom duration increases, as with CKMB. The sensitivity of myoglobin for MI at presentation varies from 43% to 55% and specificity from 82% to 94% (114). When drawn serially, the sensitivity of myoglobin determinations improves to about 90%. However, myoglobin is also released from injured skeletal muscle myocytes. Accordingly, myoglobin is a useless marker of myocardial injury in the trauma or postsurgical patient.

Troponins are another type of protein released from cardiac myocytes during cellular injury. cTnI and cTnT are highly specific for myocardial injury, as they differ in significant ways from their skeletal muscle counterparts (121). Thus troponin assays are more specific for cardiac injury, and help to differentiate this condition from elevated CKMB due to skeletal muscle trauma (49–51). Troponin measurement is an essential feature of diagnosing MI or injury after surgical or accidental trauma (122).

Cardiac troponins appear in the serum four to six hours after myocyte injury. ✐ **Cardiac troponins are often released during myocardial ischemia, even without infarction.** ✐ The peak activity occurs at about 12 hours, but these markers remain elevated for around 3 to 10 days (123). Unlike CKMB or myoglobin, the cardiac troponins are also released during some episodes of UA, providing useful diagnostic and prognostic information that are not available from other biomarkers (3). In diagnosing acute MI, serial assays of cTnI and cTnT yielded a sensitivity of 90% to 100%, with a specificity that ranges from 85% to 96% (114). Because troponins are specific for the heart, they are, by far, the best measure of myocardial ischemia and infarction in trauma patients.

In summation, individual biomarkers drawn at the time of patient presentation for possible myocardial ischemia are not very sensitive, but their specificity is quite good, generally greater than 85%. When these markers are drawn serially over several hours after presentation, sensitivity is increased from less than 50% to over 80%. ✐ **Cardiac troponins are more useful than CKMB to diagnose MI in the multiple trauma patient, as they are more**

specific for cardiac muscle injury. ✐ In the future, markers of systemic inflammation, such as CRP and fibrinogen, may provide important diagnostic and prognostic information for those suffering from myocardial ischemia without infarction (124).

Imaging Modalities and Stress Testing

The imperfect sensitivity of biochemical testing for acute MI is troublesome, but serial testing markedly improves this sensitivity. On the other hand, the sensitivity of biomarkers for acute myocardial ischemia without infarction, as in UA, is poor. In such circumstance noninvasive testing is frequently utilized to support (or exclude) the diagnosis. These testing modalities, which include rest and stress echocardiography, and radionuclide perfusion studies, are particularly valuable in patients with suspicious symptoms or findings who have normal biochemical testing and normal ECG, or nonspecific ECG abnormalities only (Table 6) (125).

Both TTE and TEE can be used to detect acute ischemia or prior infarction. In addition, Doppler color flow analysis can provide evidence of valvular dysfunction. Information about global cardiac function and abnormal anatomy or pathology can be obtained from these tests. Evidence of ischemia includes reduced contractility and segmental wall motion abnormalities. However, differentiation of prior infarction and current ischemic wall motion abnormalities is difficult. Resting echocardiography in the emergency department to evaluate low to moderate risk patients has shown sensitivity of 81% to 97% for cardiac ischemia (125,126). Exercise echocardiography or dobutamine stress echocardiography may improve upon the specificity of this test, which is reported to be between 43% and 83% for acute myocardial ischemia (127). TEE has proven to be extremely sensitive for intraoperative monitoring of ischemia (88).

Technetium-99m Sestamibi scanning utilizes radionuclide distribution to image myocardial blood flow, and is useful to demonstrate areas of reduced perfusion. This study has been shown to have high sensitivity for the diagnosis of ischemia in patients presenting with chest pain, ranging from 91% to 100%, with a range of specificity for MI between 49% and 84%. The sensitivity of this technique for acute myocardial ischemia, without infarction, is also quite good (126).

Exercise stress electrocardiography is less complex, less expensive, and less dependent upon operator expertise than the studies described previously. ✐**Imaging modalities or stress testing may be utilized to improve the accuracy of the diagnosis of myocardial ischemia or**

Table 6 Diagnostic Modalities for the Detection of Myocardial Ischemia and Infarction

Echocardiography
Exercise echocardiography
Dobutamine echocardiography
Transesophageal echocardiography (intraoperative)
Technicium-99m Sestamibi scanning (with adenosine or persantine)
Exercise electrocardiography
Computed ST-segment analysis during ECG monitoring
Ambulatory (Holter) ECG monitoring

Abbreviation: ECG, electrocardiogram.

infarction in patients with equivocal or nonspecific ECG and biochemical testing. ☞ Reported sensitivities vary widely, from 29% to 90%, while specificity ranges from 50% to 99% (128,129).

Detecting Intraoperative Myocardial Ischemia

Detection of intraoperative myocardial ischemia and ischemia in the ICU are more or less limited by logistical considerations. As noted earlier, TEE is highly sensitive in this regard. However, this technology is both very expensive and operator dependent. Computed ST-segment analysis of continuous ECG, utilizing two leads, has a high degree of sensitivity and reasonable specificity for detection of ischemia in the OR (88). Typically, leads II and V$_5$ are monitored (Fig. 5) (114). However, controversy exists as to which of the precordial leads is most sensitive (130). Ambulatory ECG is useful for detection of ischemia in the postoperative period, during which around 90% of episodes of myocardial ischemia are without symptoms (70).

In summary, the clinical diagnosis of myocardial ischemia and MI is unreliable. Electrocardiography is rapidly obtainable, inexpensive, noninvasive, and relatively accurate. However, some patients with MI have a normal ECG and others have a nonspecific tracing. NSTEMI is often indistinguishable from ischemia without infarction on ECG. For this reason, biochemical testing with CKMB isoenzymes, or cardiac troponins, or both markedly improves the diagnosis of MI. When the diagnosis remains uncertain, or when it is essential to exclude mechanical complications of infarction, imaging modalities such as echocardiography, gated scintigraphy, and radionuclide perfusion scanning are of value.

THERAPY FOR MYOCARDIAL ISCHEMIA AND INFARCTION

The therapy for myocardial ischemia has substantially changed in the past decade. More emphasis is placed upon early re-establishment of coronary flow in the catheterization lab when such therapy is available, and medical therapy is more effective ever since the introduction of several new classes of drugs. It is convenient to discuss therapeutic interventions with respect to the ischemic continuum.

Stable Angina Pectoris

Stable angina (SA) pectoris may occur during exertion or stress, and therefore may occur in the perioperative period or after trauma. However, angina or evidence of ischemia in hospitalized patients will usually be considered UA, since the patients are generally at rest. The therapy of SA involves coronary vasodilation, preload reduction, reduction of myocardial oxygen demand, and prevention of platelet aggregation (Table 7) (131). ☞ **Nitrates, calcium-channel blockers, and beta- blockers, along with platelet inhibition,**

Table 7 Therapy of Stable Angina Pectoris

Nitrates (oral, sublingual, topical)
Calcium channel blockers
Beta-receptor blockers
Aspirin
Revascularization

are the mainstays of medical management of stable angina. ☞

Nitroglycerine, whether sublingual or topical, is the time-honored method of providing selective coronary vasodilation, while at the same time reducing preload, wall tension, and therefore myocardial oxygen demand (132). Typically, sublingual nitroglycerine is utilized by the patient or physician for acute therapy of angina attacks, while more prolonged therapy is delivered via slow-release oral formulations or topical patches. The latter seem most efficacious when they are incorporated into a regimen, which includes a daily nitrate-free period (133).

Both calcium-channel blocking agents and beta-blocking drugs are utilized in SA to reduce myocardial oxygen demand. Calcium-channel blocking agents may also contribute to coronary vasodilation. Both these drug classes also have antihypertensive properties, thus reducing the afterload as well as contractility (131).

Aspirin is beneficial in SA, as it is in all of the ACS (134). By preventing platelet aggregation, which serves as the nidus for obstructing thrombosis, aspirin reduces the likelihood of MI and death in this population (135). Revascularization procedures, such as PTCA, coronary stenting, and coronary artery bypass grafting (CABG), are utilized selectively to reduce symptoms, improve quality of life, and increase life expectancy.

Unstable Angina and Non-ST-Elevation Myocardial Infarction

In UA/NSTEMI, which are often indistinguishable at presentation, management is conducted with immediate attention to reducing ischemia, preventing further platelet aggregation, preventing fibrin deposition and, in some cases, re-establishing coronary patency by invasive means (Table 8) (124). Therapy of ischemia generally includes sublingual or intravenous nitroglycerine, although evidence for its efficacy is only fair. Supplemental oxygen is necessary if the patient is hypoxic, and morphine sulfate should be instituted if ischemic signs and symptoms are not relieved with nitrates (136). ☞ **Antiplatelet and antithrombotic agents assume increasing importance in the therapy of UA and NSTEMI.** ☞

Beta-receptor blockade is effective in ACS (136). Patients should receive a first dose intravenously if evidence of ischemia persists after the aforementioned interventions, and orally within 15 minutes thereafter (137). If beta-blockade cannot be tolerated due to adverse effects, a nondiydropyridine calcium-channel blocking agent should be used instead (136). For persistent hypertension despite beta-receptor blockade and nitrate administration, an angiotensin-converting enzyme (ACE) inhibitor should be initiated, especially in patients with CHF or diabetes.

Because of the central role of intracoronary thrombus in causing ACS, antiplatelet and anticoagulation therapies are essential components of the management strategy in this population. Aspirin is the primary antiplatelet agent used, and should be started immediately and continued indefinitely (136). Anticoagulation should be acutely instituted in these patients, with either intravenous unfractionated heparin or low-molecular–weight heparin (138). Several studies have established improved outcomes in ACS when enoxaparin, a low-molecular–weight heparin, was compared to unfractionated heparin (124). In addition, the American College of Cardiology recommends the addition of a glycoprotein IIbIIIa receptor antagonist to the

Table 8   Management of Myocardial Ischemia and Infarction

Goal	Drug or treatment	Comments
Ameliorate ischemia	Oxygen Nitrates (if not contraindicated by increased ICP) Morphine sulfate Beta-receptor blockade	Add ACE inhibitor within first 24 hrs for MI with ST-segment elevation
Prevent further platelet aggregation	Aspirin	In nontrauma setting may add glycoprotein IIb/IIIa inhibitor
Prevent further fibrin deposition	Intravenous unfractionated heparin, or Subcutaneous low-molecular–weight heparin	Anticoagulation with heparin contraindicated immediately following head injury, and in patients with trauma- or hemorrhage-related coagulopathy
Re-establish coronary patency	Percutaneous coronary intervention (especially if not a candidate for thrombolytics) Emergent coronary artery bypass grafting (when appropriate)	Thrombolysis (tissue plasminogen activator) in nontrauma patient Both PTCA and off-pump CABG have been successfully accomplished in selected trauma patients (see text for explanation)

Abbreviations: ACE, angiotensin converting enzyme; CABG, coronary artery bypass grafting; ICP, intracranial pressure; MI, myocardial infarction; PTCA, percutaneous transluminal coronary angioplasty.

aforesaid measures in patients who have continuing evidence of ischemia, hypotension or bradycardia, new bundle branch block, or markedly elevated biochemical markers of cardiac myocyte injury (124,136,138,139). These agents, which block platelet receptors permitting aggregation and progression of thrombus formation, are also indicated in patients in whom percutaneous coronary intervention (PCI) is to be conducted within the ensuing 24-hour period (138).

Opinions differ as to the necessity of early PCI, as opposed to a conservative strategy of medical management with deferred coronary arteriography, pending further clinical events or symptoms. ☛ **Certain subsets of patients with UA/NSTEMI benefit from early percutaneous coronary intervention.** ☛ Patients who appear to benefit from early PCI include those with high-risk profiles, such as recurrent rest angina, CHF, hemodynamic instability, sustained ventricular tachycardia, and prior CABG or PCI (136).

Indications for coronary revascularization in patients with ACS are similar to those for patients with chronic SA, depending upon coronary anatomy, life expectancy, ventricular function, functional capacity, severity of symptoms, and degree of myocardium at risk. The objective of such revascularization is to improve functional capacity, prevent progression of disease, relieve symptoms, and alter the prognosis. CABG is generally recommended for those with left main coronary disease, three vessel disease, and two vessel disease with significant LAD disease or with ischemia on noninvasive testing (135). Those with normal LV function and suitable multivessel CHD are generally treated with PCI.

ST-Elevation Myocardial Infarction

Acute STEMI, also referred to as transmural or Q-wave MI, represents the most damaging of the ACS, with the greatest extent of cell death and the highest rate of early complications. However, prognosis of this entity has dramatically improved in the last two decades, with the introduction of effective thrombolytic drugs and establishment of the effi-

cacy of several other classes of medications, ushering in the modern era of active management of MI.

Historically important therapies, such as oxygen, nitrates, and morphine sulfate, have become ancillary interventions to the main focus of therapy, which is re-establishment of patency of the infarct-related artery (140). ☛ **Re-establishing early patency of the infarct-related artery is key to limiting damage in STEMI.** ☛ As in UA/NSTEMI, management of thrombosis is carried out with multiple classes of drugs, which act by distinctly different mechanisms. Antiplatelet agents, anticoagulants, and fibrinolytic agents all play an essential role in the therapy of STEMI (141). Numerous studies have shown that re-establishment of patency of the infarct-related vessel improves inhospital and long-term survival (140).

Nearly three decades ago, randomized trials established that aspirin significantly reduced mortality in STEMI (142). Subsequent mega-trials investigated the efficacy of thrombolytic agents, demonstrating a reduction in mortality from approximately 15% to 7% (143). Tissue plasminogen activator (tPA) and its derivatives have become the favored agents for reperfusion in the United States, but controversy exists over whether or not these expensive agents are actually more efficacious or safer than streptokinase. Nevertheless, these large, randomized trials established that earlier intervention with thrombolytic agents in STEMI resulted in greater preservation of myocardium with reduced early and late adverse effects. Optimum benefit occurs when thrombolytics are administered within six hours of symptoms, although some benefit may be derived up to 12 hours later (140).

Criteria for thrombolysis include ST-segment elevation of greater than 1 mm in at least two contiguous limb leads or more than 2 mm in at least two contiguous precordial leads. The left BBB and permanent pacemakers may obscure this diagnosis, although diagnostic criteria have been proposed to detect acute MI, even under these circumstances (116).

Several adjunctive agents have proven beneficial in MI when used in conjunction with thrombolytics. Heparin is administered to prevent coagulation, and intravenous unfractionated heparin is most commonly used in this setting (141). Aspirin is of established benefit, as noted earlier. Beta-receptor blockade is initiated early in the course of STEMI, if there are no contraindications, and continued thereafter, with a reduction in early and long-term mortality (144). ACE inhibitors, usually begun in the first 24 hours after presentation, also reduce postinfarction mortality, probably due to alterations of adverse neurohumoral influences on the myocardium, along with a favorable effect on ventricular remodeling (145). Nitroglycerine, useful for symptomatic improvement, has not been clearly shown to improve the outcome.

ᵒ⁴ **Percutaneous coronary intervention is evolving as the preferred therapy in STEMI, when available.** ᵒ⁴ Up to two-thirds of patients with STEMI are not candidates for thrombolysis, due to contraindications to these agents, while PCI is almost always applicable, if available (146). Several randomized trials have been conducted which provide evidence that percutaneous coronary intervention is as efficacious as thrombolysis, or even more so, in the management of STEMI (147,148). Patients undergoing primary percutaneous coronary intervention appear to have improved infarct-related artery patency and a lower rate of intracranial hemorrhage compared to patients receiving thrombolytics (146). A meta-analysis of 10 studies, evaluating primary percutaneous coronary intervention compared to thrombolysis for STEMI, concluded that percutaneous coronary intervention confers a 34% reduction in mortality along with reduced nonfatal MI and hemorrhagic stroke rates (149).

Unfortunately, recurrent ischemia occurs before hospital discharge in around 10% to 15% of patients who receive angioplasty. Placement of coronary stents has been found to be safe and practical at the time of primary PCI in STEMI, with a reduction in the rate of restenosis. Glycoprotein IIbIIIa inhibiting agents are efficacious in reducing restenosis in this setting as well, and are recommended as cotherapy for all patients receiving percutaneous coronary intervention (150). Percutaneous coronary intervention has been most effective for those older than 65 years of age, those with prior CABG, and for those patients with CHF or cardiogenic shock in association with STEMI (146).

Myocardial Ischemia in the Multiple Trauma Patient

The treatment of MI in trauma is complicated by the likelihood of hemorrhagic complications in this population with many of the agents that are used to manage ACS. Thrombolysis is absolutely contraindicated in patients with major trauma, active bleeding, or surgery within the prior 10-day period, most of which apply to the hospitalized, injured patient (12). ᵒ⁴ **Since thrombolysis is not feasible in the trauma patient, percutaneous coronary intervention is an important alternative for therapy of MI.** ᵒ⁴ Even heparin may cause significant hemorrhage in the traumatized or postoperative patient, and its use must, therefore, be carefully balanced against the risk of complications. Management of ischemia and MI may well be confined to aspirin, nitrates [except in the setting of closed head injury with elevated intracranial pressure (ICP)], beta-blockers (may not be tolerated in acute shock state), and ACE inhibitors in this setting, along with the usual management of complications, such as CHF.

Some authors recommend early invasive monitoring for elderly trauma patients who have evidence of shock on presentation, or a high injury severity score, maintaining that this allows improved titration of oxygen delivery and

thus reduces organ injury and post-traumatic mortality (151,152). For patients with hemodynamic instability due to myocardial ischemia or infarction after major trauma, or who have persistent evidence of ischemia despite supportive therapy as outlined earlier, percutaneous coronary intervention is appropriate to re-establish coronary blood flow.

Prophylaxis Against Myocardial Ischemia

Perioperative beta-blockade is associated with a significant reduction in ischemic episodes (153,154). One validated method entails postoperative titration of esmolol to a heart rate (HR) of 20% less than that which was determined preoperatively as the individual's ischemic threshold HR (153). The benefit of esmolol is its β_1 selectivity, titratability, and short clinical duration. Most clinicians titrate beta-blockade to a HR of 60 beats per minute (153–155). As HR slows, myocardial oxygen demand decreases (less contractions per unit time) and supply increases (diastolic time increases, especially as HR falls below 70) because most of the coronary blood flow occurs during diastole, especially for the left ventricle. Indeed, diastolic time increases 15% when HR decreases from 70 to 50 beats per minute (156). With few contraindications (Table 9), beta-blockers are recommended for most high risk patients for prophylaxis against perioperative MI (PMI) undergoing major surgery (153,155). Poldermans reported a striking reduction in cardiac complications within 30 days postoperatively (3.4% vs. 34%) (153). In a placebo-controlled, double-blind study of 200 men with or at risk for CAD, Mangano (155) found a perioperative atenolol regimen that was associated with a reduction in two year mortality.

The ACC/AHA Perioperative Practice guidelines limits specific recommendations for beta-blockade use to patients with inducible ischemia (157). In this high-risk population, beta-blockers should be started days to weeks before surgery, and titrated to a resting HR from 50 to 60 beats/min preoperatively. No specific recommendations are made for lower-risk patients, or for intraoperative or postoperative therapy (157).

A recent review by London et al. (158) provides a thorough overview of the known and theoretical benefits and hazards of perioperative beta-blockade. They also recommend that the ACC/AHA guidelines be followed until the results from several recently launched, large-scale trials provide more substantial data. This paper, and the accompanying editorial by Kertai (159) triggered a flurry of correspondence regarding the relative merits of perioperative beta-blockade (160–162). The ongoing Perioperative Ischemic Evaluation (POISE) trial is currently enrolling patients in six countries, and will evaluate the effectiveness

Table 9 Contraindications to Beta-Blockade

Absolute	Relative (strong)	Relative (weak)
Acute broncho-spasm following treatment	Strong Hx of bronchospastic disease	Epidural or spinal anesthetic
Third-degree heart block	SBP < 100 mmHg (after treatment with Neosynephrine)	Fluid shifts anticipated
Starting HR < 55 bpm	Current exam or lab evidence of CHF	Hypovolemia Concurrent antihypertensives

Abbreviations: CHF, congestive heart failure; HR, heart rate; Hx, history; SBP, systolic blood pressure.

of perioperative beta-blockade in 10,000 moderate to high risk patients undergoing noncardiac surgery (160,161).

When beta-blockers are contraindicated (Table 9), calcium channel blockers or α_2 agonists (clonidine, or dexmedetomidine) may be better tolerated. Although nitroglycerin is effective in treating ischemia, it is not effective prophylactically. Nicardipine has been found to be more useful in reducing ischemia after coronary artery bypass (perhaps helping to decrease spasm) (163). Although dexmedetomidine caused a 20% reduction in blood pressure in both vascular surgery patients and healthy volunteers (treatable with phenylephrine), it was associated with fewer ST ischemic changes than placebo (164). The level of ischemia reduction and sedation appears to be similar to that found with clonidine, but future studies will delineate clinical situations for which each drug is indicated.

PROGNOSIS

The prognosis for the patient with post-traumatic MI is less favorable than for patients who infarct outside of this setting. In one study, the mortality rate was 20% for patients with MI after trauma, as compared to an approximate 7% mortality rate for STEMI in the first 30 days after infarction (12). The elderly suffer higher rates of mortality after trauma than patients under 55 years of age, largely due to multisystem organ failure (MSOF) and sepsis (165). Ischemic heart disease, along with several other pre-existing conditions, significantly increases the post-traumatic mortality rate (13). Among 326 multitrauma patients older than 60 years, Tornetta (166) found that MI, along with acute respiratory distress syndrome (ARDS) and sepsis, was a major predictor of mortality. He reported 62% mortality in those sustaining MI in this retrospective investigation.

EYE TO THE FUTURE

In the future, ongoing investigation into the underlying causes of atherosclerosis, including the role of systemic inflammatory influences and infectious agents, may permit more effective intervention in the early stages of this disorder. In particular, elucidation of inflammatory cascades in trauma and their role in influencing plaque vulnerability and ACS, will be of importance to the development of therapies which block this response to injury.

Research will continue into the epidemiology and therapy of MI in the setting of trauma and in the perioperative period, especially with regard to the safety of anticoagulation and antiplatelet agents, and the utility of percutaneous coronary therapy. As the nature of anticoagulant therapy is refined, more specific inhibitors of the particular steps in the coagulation cascade, such as factor Xa, may permit effective prevention of thrombosis, with less likelihood of systemic bleeding (34).

Recently, Le Manach et al. (167) have introduced a new approach to reduction of perioperative cardiac morbidity through the use of monitoring troponin I (cTnI). They studied 1152 consecutive patients undergoing abdominal infrarenal aortic surgery and measured cTnI release. One group did not have any abnormal elevations, and a second group had only mild increases of cTnI. However, two groups demonstrated increases of cTnI consistent with a

PMI. One of these "ischemic groups" demonstrated acute (<24 hours) increases of cTnI above threshold, and the other demonstrated prolonged low levels of cTnI release, followed by a delayed (>24 hours) increase of cTnI. The authors suggest that these two different ischemic patterns represent two distinct pathophysiologies: (i) acute coronary occlusion for early morbidity and (ii) prolonged myocardial ischemia for late events. They also suggest that early anti-ischemic treatment should occur in patients with elevated cTnI levels (prior to the development of irreversible necrosis).

The role of early percutaneous coronary intervention in trauma patients is currently under investigation. At the time of this writing, only seven cases have been reported describing the use of PCI to relieve acute CA occlusions, following blunt chest trauma (58,134,137,168–170), and only one case of concomitant PCI during repair of penetrating trauma (gunshot wound to the chest) (171). Temporary anticoagulation was used, with complete reversal at the end of the procedure to facilitate this last case. Furthermore, the development of specialized tools for off-pump coronary revascularization (e.g., shunts and coronary suturing devices) have already provided new techniques for the treatment of traumatic coronary artery lesions (172). These reports are illustrative of the multisystem approach required for successful treatment of these life-threatening injuries, and a great deal of work still needs to be done in this area.

Lastly, existing imaging technologies are being used in innovative ways to facilitate the diagnosis of myocardial and coronary artery injury in chest trauma. These include application of MRI (173) and intracoronary echocardiography (174).

SUMMARY

Myocardial ischemia and infarction due to atherosclerosis are most likely to affect the geriatric trauma population, which is predisposed to poor outcomes due to this and a variety of other underlying diseases. Hypoperfusion of pre-existing coronary artery lesions is the dominant cause of ischemia in this population. Direct cardiac trauma with left ventricular dysfunction or infarction due to coronary artery thrombosis or laceration is less common but may affect any age group following chest trauma. Detection of myocardial ischemia in traumatized patients involves several subtle differences compared to the nontrauma population. Furthermore, the reliance on diagnostic laboratory testing is greater due to the inability of seriously injured patients to communicate their chest pain or distinguish it from that due to chest wall trauma. As one moves along the ischemic continuum from stable angina to STEMI, there is greater therapeutic emphasis on platelet inhibition, antithrombotic agents, and direct attempts to disrupt clot in the infarct related artery with fibrinolysis or PCI.

The management of suspected myocardial ischemia and infarction in trauma is complicated by the propensity of these patients to bleed with anticoagulation and the contraindication to thrombolytic administration in this population. Additionally, the use of nitroglycerine and other nitrates is relatively contraindicated in the setting of severe traumatic brain injury and elevated ICP. Anticoagulation must be carefully weighed against its hazards, as must use of antiplatelet agents. A greater reliance on percutaneous angioplasty and stent placement in this population in the setting of severe myocardial ischemia or MI should reduce morbidity, though only case reports exist to support this therapeutic strategy.

KEY POINTS

- The presence of CAD significantly increases the risk of morbidity and mortality to any acutely injured patient.
- Atheromatous lesions progress in association with known risk factors for CAD, such as hypertension and the influx of inflammatory cells.
- Atheromatous plaque may be vulnerable to rupture, with resultant coronary artery thrombosis and occlusion, despite a relatively modest baseline impingement of the coronary lumen.
- Coronary angiography does not identify all high-risk lesions, because neither the size of the plaque nor the degree of stenosis correlates with its vulnerability to rupture.
- Instability and rupture of nonocclusive plaque leads to most episodes of ACS, because the subsequent exposure of reactive elements within the lesion leads to unpredictable degrees of thrombosis at the vascular luminal site.
- STEMI is caused by complete occlusion of a coronary artery, with simultaneous myocyte death in the territory supplied by that vessel (44). NSTEMI results from small areas of infarction of differing ages, probably caused by repeated episodes of transient occlusion, platelet emboli, or both.
- Myocardial ischemia is often clinically silent in the trauma patient.
- Most myocardial contusions require no specific therapy (other than monitoring), and these patients usually have an excellent prognosis.
- Blunt chest injury may produce injury to the RCA or LAD. These injuries often involve dissections resulting in MI, especially when the LAD coronary artery is injured.
- Arterial air embolism, a complication of penetrating chest trauma, may be rapidly fatal and requires early suspicion and familiarity to diagnose the condition and effectively intervene.
- Systemic inflammation and adverse physical conditions (common accompaniments of major trauma), likely predispose existing atheromatous plaques to instability and rupture.
- Continuous electrocardiographic ST-segment evaluation provides the most practical means of monitoring for intraoperative myocardial ischemia.
- The risk of myocardial ischemia in the perioperative period is higher postoperatively than intraoperatively.
- UA and NSTEMI are commonly indistinguishable on clinical grounds, manifesting as rest angina. They are therefore approached in a similar diagnostic and therapeutic fashion.
- The diagnosis of myocardial ischemia is difficult to make on clinical grounds, especially in the trauma patient, who may have altered pain response for a variety of reasons, such as distracting injury, analgesic medications, or CNS injury.
- Classic ECG criteria for MI are only about 50% sensitive.
- MI may manifest with ST-segment depression rather than elevation.
- Symptoms of acute myocardial ischemia, combined with new ECG manifestations of left bundle branch block, together are sufficient to diagnose acute MI.
- Ten percent of patients with acute MI have a normal ECG on presentation.
- In acute MI, serial determination for CKMB is much more sensitive for the diagnosis than a single determination at presentation.
- Cardiac troponins are often released during myocardial ischemia, even without infarction.
- Cardiac troponins are more useful than CKMB to diagnose MI in the multiple trauma patient, as they are more specific for cardiac muscle injury.
- Imaging modalities or stress testing may be utilized to improve the accuracy of the diagnosis of myocardial ischemia or infarction in patients with equivocal or nonspecific ECG and biochemical testing.
- Nitrates, calcium-channel blockers and beta-blockers, along with platelet inhibition, are the mainstays of medical management of stable angina.
- Antiplatelet and antithrombotic agents assume increasing importance in the therapy of UA and NSTEMI.
- Certain subsets of patients with UA/NSTEMI benefit from early percutaneous coronary intervention.
- Re-establishing early patency of the infarct-related artery is the most important factor for limiting damage in STEMI.
- Percutaneous coronary intervention is evolving as the preferred therapy in STEMI, when available.
- Since thrombolysis is not feasible in the trauma patient, percutaneous coronary intervention is an important alternative for therapy of MI.

REFERENCES

1. Large GA. Contemporary management of acute coronary syndrome. Postgrad Med J 2005; 81:217–222.
2. Tun A, Khan IA. Myocardial infarction with normal coronary arteries: the pathologic and clinical perspectives. Angiology 2001; 52:299–304.
3. Crossman D. Acute coronary syndromes. Clin Med 2001; 1:206–213.
4. Lloyd-Jones DM, Larson MG, Beiser A, et al. Lifetime risk of developing coronary heart disease. Lancet 1999; 353:89–92.
5. National Center for Health Statistics. Fast Stats A–Z Heart Disease. www.edu.gov.risks/fastats/heart.htm.
6. Rogot E, Sorlie PD, Johnson NJ, et al. Second data book: a study of 1.3 million persons: by demographic, social and economic factors: 1979–1985 follow up: US National Longitudinal Mortality Study. US Dept of Health and Human Services, National Institutes of Health, pub no. 92-3297;1992.
7. Davies MJ. The pathophysiology of acute coronary syndromes. Heart 2000; 83:361–366.
8. Kannel WB. Clinical misconceptions dispelled by epidemiologic research. Circulation 1995; 92:3350–3360.
9. MacKenzie EJ, Morris JA Jr, Edelstein SL. Effect of pre-existing disease on length of hospital stay in trauma patients. J Trauma 1989; 29:757–765.
10. Wilson RF. Trauma in patients with pre-existing cardiac disease. Crit Care Clin 1994; 10:461–506.
11. Neiman J, Hui WK. Postermedial papillary muscle rupture as a result of right coronary artery occlusion after blunt chest injury. Am Heart J 1992; 123:1694–1699.
12. Moosikasuwan JB, Thomas JM, Buchman TG. Myocaridal infarction as a complication of injury. J Am Coll Surg 2000; 190:665–670.

13. MacKenzie EJ, Morris JA, Edelstein SL. Effect of pre-existing disease on the length of hospital stay in trauma patients. J Trauma 1989; 29:757–765.
14. Davies MJ. Atlas of Coronary Artery Disease. Philadelphia, PA: Lippincott-Raven, 1998.
15. Stary HC, Chandler AB, Dinsmore RE, et al. A definition of advanced types of atherosclerosis: A report from the "Committee on Vascular Lesions of the Council on Ateriosclerosis," American Heart Association. Circulation 1995; 92:1355–1374.
16. Napoli C, Glass CK, Witztum JL, et al. Influence of maternal hypercholesterolemia during pregnancy on progression of early atherosclerotic lesions in childhood: fate of Early Lesions in Children Study. Lancet 1999; 354:1234–1241.
17. Biegelsen ES, Loscalzo J. Endothelial function and atherosclerosis. Coron Art Dis 1999; 10:241–256.
18. Virmani R, Kolodgie FD, Burke AP, et al. lessons from sudden coronary death: a comprehensive morphological classification scheme for atherosclerotic lesions. Arterioscler Thromb Vasc Biol 2000; 20(5):1262–1275.
19. Falk E, Fuster V. Atherogenesis and its determinants. In: Fuster V, Alexander RW, O'Rourke RA, et al., eds. Hurst's The Heart. 10th ed., New York: McGraw Hill Medical Publishing, 2001:1072–1073.
20. Fuster V, Badimon L, Badimon J, et al. The pathogenesis of coronary artery disease and the acute coronary syndromes. NEJM 1992; 326:242–250.
21. Fuster V, Fayad ZA, Badimon JJ. Acute coronary syndromes: biology. Lancet 1999; 353(suppl II):5–9.
22. Falk E, Shah PK, Fuster V. Coronary plaque disruption. Circulation 1995; 92:657–671.
23. Mann JM, Davies MJ. Vulnerable plaque: retention of characteristics to degree of stenosis in human coronary arteries. Circulation 1996; 94:928–931.
24. Moreno PR, Falk E, Palacios IF, et al. Macrophage infiltration in acute coronary syndromes: Implications for plaque rupture. Circulation 1994; 90:775–778.
25. Libby P, Egan D, Skarlatos S. Roles of infectious agents in atherosclerosis. Circulation 1997; 96:4095–4103.
26. Mann J, Davies MJ. Mechanisms of progression in native coronary artery disease: role of healed plaque disruption. Heart 1999; 82:265–268.
27. Falk E, Fuster V, Shah PK. Interrelationship between atherosclerosis and thrombosis. In: Verstroete M, Fuster V, Topol EJ, eds. Cardiovascular Thrombosis: Thrombocardiology and Thromboneurology. Philadelphia, PA: Lipincott-Raven, 1998:45.
28. Ge J, Erbel R, Gerber T, et al. Intravascular ultrasound imaging of angiographically normal coronary arteries: a prospective study in vivo. Br Heart J 1994; 71:572–578.
29. Roberts WC. Diffuse extent of coronary atherosclerosis in fatal coronary artery disease. Am J Cardiol 1990; 65:2F–6F.
30. Sangiorgi G, Rumberger JA, Severson A, et al. Arterial calcification and not lumen stenosis is highly correlated with atherosclerotic plaque burden in humans. J Am Coll Cardiol 1998; 31:126–133.
31. Mintz GS, Pichard AD, Popma JJ, et al. Determinants and correlates of target lesion calcium in coronary artery disease. J Am Coll Cardiol 1997; 29:268–274.
32. Davies SW. Clinical presentation and diagnosis of coronary artery disease: stable angina. Br Med Bull 2001; 59:17–27.
33. Burke AP, Farb A, Malcom GT, et al. Coronary risk factors and plaque morphology in men with coronary artery disease who died suddenly. NEJM 1997; 336:1276–1282.
34. Rauch U, Osende JI, Fuster V, et al. Thrombus formation on atherosclerotic plaques: Pathogenesis and clinical consequences. Ann Intern Med 2001;134:224–238.
35. Willerson JT, Golino P, Eidt J, et al. Specific platelet mediators and unstable coronary artery lesions. Circulation 1989; 80:198–205.
36. Davies MJ, Thomas A. Thrombosis and acute coronary artery lesions in sudden cardiac ischemic death. NEJM 1984; 310:1137–1140.
37. Goldstein JA, Demetriou D, Grimes CL, et al. Multiple complex coronary plaques in patients with acute myocardial infarction. NEJM 2000; 343:915–922.
38. Haverkate F, Thompson SG, Pyke SDM, et al. Production of C-reactive protein and risk of coronary events in stable and unstable angina. Lancet 1997; 349:462–466.
39. Koenig W, Sund M, Frohlich M, et al. C-reactive protein, a sensitive marker of inflammation, predicts future risk of coronary heart disease in initially healthy middle-aged men. Circulation 1999; 99:237–242.
40. Braunwald E. Unstable angina. An etiologic approach to management. Circulation 1998; 98:2219–2222.
41. Ambrose J, Winters S, Stern A, et al. Angiographic morphology and the pathogenesis of unstable angina. J Am coll Cardiol 1985; 5:609–616.
42. Mann J, Koski J, Pereira W, et al. Histologic patterns of atherosclerotic plaque in unstable angina patients vary according to clinical presentation. Heart 1998; 80:19–22.
43. Glagov S, Weisenberd BA, Zarins, et al. Compensatory enlargement of human atherosclerotic coronary arteries. NEJM 1987; 316:1371–1375.
44. DeWood M, Spores J, Notske R, et al. Prevalence of total coronary occlusion during the early hours of transmural myocardial infarction. NEJM 1980; 303:897–902.
45. Ambrose JA, Weinrauch M. Thrombosis in ischemic heart disease. Arch Int Med 1996; 156:1382–1394.
46. Gutstein ED, Fuster V. Pathophysiology and clinical significance of atherosclerotic plaque. Cardiovasc Res 1999; 41: 323–333.
47. Swaanenburg JC, Klaase JM, DeJongste MJ, et al. Troponin I, Troponin T, CKMB activity and CKMB mass as markers for the detection of myocardial contusion in patients who experienced chest trauma. Clin Chim Acta 1998; 272:171–181.
48. Symbas PN. Traumatic heart disease. In: Fuster V, Alexander RW, O'Rourke RA, eds. The Heart. 10th ed. New York: McGraw-Hill, 2001:2219–2226.
49. Kissane RW. Traumatic heart diseases, especially myocardial contusion. Postgrad Med 1954; 15:114–119.
50. Chapelle JP. Cardiac troponin I and T: recent players in the field of myocardial markers. Clin Chem Lab Med 1999; 37: 11–20.
51. Ruppert M, Van Hee R. Creatinine-kinase MB determination in non-cardiac trauma: its difference with cardiac infarction and its restricted use in trauma situations. Eur J Emerg Med 2001; 8:177–179.
52. Rosen CL, Wolfe RE. Blunt chest trauma. In: Ferrera PC, Coluciello SA, Marx JA, et al., eds. Trauma Management. St. Louis: Mosby, 2001:232–258.
53. Snow N, Richardson JD, Flynt LM Jr. Myocardial contusion: implications for the patient with multiple traumatic injuries. Surgery 1982; 92:744–750.
54. Shapiro NG, Yanofsky SO, Trapp I, et al. Cardiovascular evaluation in thoracic blunt trauma using transesophageal echocardiography. J Trauma 1991; 131:835–839.
55. Maenza RL, Seaburg D, D'Amico F. A meta-analysis of blunt cardiac trauma. Am J Emerg Med 1996; 14:237–241.
56. Singh R, Nolan JP, Schrank JP. Traumatic left ventricular aneurysm: two cases with normal coronary angiography. JAMA 1975; 234:412–414.
57. Sturaitis M. Lack of significant long-term sequelae following myocardial contusion. Arch Int Med 1986; 146:1765–1769.
58. Lee TB, Lee W-Z. Blunt chest injury with traumatic dissection of right coronary artery. J Trauma 2002; 53(3):617.
59. Maram JL, Booth DC, Sapin PM. Acute myocardial infarction caused by blunt chest trauma: Successful therapy by direct coronary angiography. Am Heart J 1996; 132:1275–1277.
60. Atalar E, Acl T, Aytemir K, et al. Acute anterior myocardial infarction following a mild nonpenetrating chest trauma. Angiology 2001; 52:279–282.
61. Banzo I, Montero A, Uriarte I, et al. Coronary artery occlusion and myocardial infarction. Clin Nuc Med 1999; 24:94–96.

62. Thorban S, Ungeheuer A, Blasini R, et al. Emergent interventional transcatheter revascularization in acute right coronary artery dissection after blunt chest trauma. J Trauma 1997; 43:365–367.

63. Kaplan AJ, Norcross ED, Crawford FA, et al. Predictors of mortality in penetrating cardiac injury. Am Surg 1993; 59: 338–344.

64. Brown J, Grover FL. Trauma to the heart. Chest Surg Clin North Am 1997; 7:325–341.

65. Powell DW, Moore EE, Cothren CC, et al. Is emergency department resuscitative thoracotomy futile care for the critically injured patient requiring prehospital cardiopulmonary resuscitation? J Am Coll Surg 2004; 199(2):211–215.

66. Thomas AN, Stephens BG. Air embolism: a cause of morbidity and death after penetrating chest trauma. J Trauma 1974; 14:633–637.

67. Estrera AS, Pass LJ, Platt MR. Systemic arterial air embolism in penetrating lung injury. Ann Thor Surg 1990; 50:257–261.

68. Yee ES, Verrier ED, Thomas AN. Management of air embolism in blunt and penetrating chest trauma. Thorac Cardiovasc Surg 1983; 85:661–668.

69. Mangano D. Assessment of the patient with cardiac disease: an anesthesiologist's paradigm. Anesthesiology 1999; 91: 1521–1529.

70. Mangano D. Assessment of risk for cardiac and noncardiac surgical procedures. Anesth Clin North Am 1991; 9:521–551.

71. Michie HR, Wilmore DW. Sepsis, signals, and surgical sequelae. Arch Surg 1990; 125:531–536.

72. Baue AE. Predicting outcome in injured patients and its relationship to circulating cytokines. Shock 1995; 4:39–40.

73. Lee C, Marill K, Carter W, et al. A current concept of trauma-induced multiorgan failure. Ann Emerg Med 2001; 38:170–176.

74. Sauaia A, Moore FA, Moore EE, et al. Early risk factors for post-injury multiple organ failure. World J Surg 1996; 20:392–400.

75. Gullo A, Berlot G. Ingredients of organ dysfunction or failure. World J Surg 1996; 20:430–436.

76. Guirao X, Lowry SF. Biologic control of injury and inflammation. World J Surg 1996; 20:437–446.

77. Saadia R, Schein M. Multiple organ failure: how valid is the "two hit" model? J Accid Emerg Med 1999; 16:163–167.

78. Roumen R, Redl H, Schlag G, et al. Inflammatory mediators in relation to the development of multiple organ failure in patients with severe blunt trauma. Crit Care Med 1995; 23:474–480.

79. Pape HC, Remmers D, Grotz M, et al. Reticuloendothelial system activity and organ failure in patients with multipe injury. Arch Surg 1999; 134:421–427.

80. Robbie L, Libby P. Inflammation and atherothrombosis. Ann NY Acad Sci 2001; 947:167–180.

81. Koenig W. Inflammation and coronary heart disease: An overview. Cardiol Rev 2001; 9:31–35.

82. Geng Y-J, Wu Q, Muszynski M, et al. Apoptosis of vascular smooth muscle cells induced by in-vitro stimulation with interferon-gamma, TNF-alpha and interleukin-1-beta. Arterioscler Thromb Vasc Biol 1996; 16:19–27.

83. Geng Y-J, Libby P. Evidence for apoptosis in advanced human atheroma. Am J Pathol 1995; 147:251–266.

84. Pape HC, Schmidt RE, Rice J, et al. Biochemical changes after trauma and skeletal surgery of the lower extremity: quantification of the operative burden. Crit Care Med 2000; 28: 3441–3448.

85. Roumen RM, Hendrijks T, Ven der Ven-Jonge K, et al. Cytokine patterns in patients after major vascular surgery, hemorrhagic shock, and severe blunt trauma. Ann Surg 1993; 218:769–776.

86. Eagle K, Brundage B, Chaitman B, et al. Guidelines for perioperative cardiovascular evaluation of noncardiac surgery: a report of the AHA/ACC Task Force on the assessment of diagnostic and therapeutic cardiovascular procedures. Circulation 1996; 93:1278–1317.

87. Tuman K. Perioperative cardiovascular risk: assessment and management. Anesth J Analg 2001; 92(3S):106–112.

88. Fleischer L, Weiskopf RB. Real-time intraoperative monitoring of myocardial ischemia in noncardiac surgery. Anesthesiology 2000; 92:1183–1188.

89. Eisenberg MJ, London MJ, Leung JM, et al. Monitoring for myocardial ischemia during noncardiac surgery: a technology assessment of transesophageal echocardiography and 12-lead electrocardiography. JAMA 1992; 268:210–216.

90. Paraskas JA. Approach to the patient with chest pain. In: Rippe JM, Irwin RS, Alpert JS, et al. eds. Intensive Care Medicine. 2nd ed. Boston: Little, Brown and Company, 1991:359–364.

91. Amsterdam EA, Marschiske R, Laslett LJ, et al. Symptomatic and silent myocardial ischemia during exercise testing in coronary artery disease. Am J Cardiol 1986; 58:43B.

92. Pope JH, Aufderheide TP, Selker HP, et al. Missed diagnosis of acute cardiac ischemia in the emergency department. NEJM 2000; 342:1163–1170.

93. Theroux P, Fuster V. Acute coronary syndromes: unstable angina and non-ST segment elevation myocardial infarction. Circulation 1998; 97:1195–1206.

94. Reeder GS. Contemporary diagnosis and management of unstable angina. Mayo Clin Proc 2000; 75:953–957.

95. Panju AA, Hemmelgam BR, Guyatt GH, et al. Is this patient having a myocardial infarction? JAMA 1998; 280:1256–1260.

96. Jesse RL, Kontos MC. Evaluation of chest pain in the emergency department. Curr Prob Cardiol 1997; 22:149–162.

97. Mangano DT, Browner WS, Hollengerg M, et al. Association of perioperative myocardial ischemia with cardiac morbidity and mortality in men undergoing noncardiac surgery. NEJM 1990; 323:1781–1788.

98. Sgarbossa EB, Birnbaum Y, Parillo J. Electrocardiographic diagnosis of acute myocardial infarction. Am Heart J 2000; 141:507–517.

99. Parker AB, Waller BF, Gering LE. Usefulness of the 12-lead EKG in detection of myocardial infarction. Clin Cardiol 1996; 19:141–148.

100. Menown IB, MacKenzie G, Adgey AA. Optimizing the initial 12-lead EKG diagnosis of acute myocardial infarction. Eur Heart J 2000; 21:275–283.

101. Tamura A, Katooka H, Mikuriya Y, et al. Inferior ST-segment depression as a useful marker of identifying proximal left anterior descending coronary artery occlusion during acute myocardial infarction. Eur Heart J 1995; 16:1795–1799.

102. Braat SH, Brugada P, Den Dulk K, et al. Value of lead V4R for recognition of the infarct coronary artery in acute inferior myocardial infarction. Am J Cardiol 1984; 53:1538–1541.

103. Hasdai D, Birnbaum Y, Herz I, et al. ST-segment depression in lateral limb leads in inferior wall acute myocardial infarction. Eur Heart J 1995; 16:1549–1553.

104. Assali AR, Sclarovsky, Herz I, et al. Comparison of patients with inferior wall myocardial infarction with, versus without, ST-segment elevation in leads V5 and V6. Am J Cardiol 1998; 81:81–83.

105. Matetzky S, Freimark D, Chocuraqui P, et al. Significance of ST-segment elevations in posterior chest leads in patients with acute inferior myocardial infarction. J Am Coll Cardiol 1998; 31:506–511.

106. Porter A, Vatui M, Adler Y, et al. Are there differences among patients with inferior acute myocardial infarction with ST-segment depression in leads V2 and V3 and positive versus negative T waves in these leads on admission? Cardiol 1998; 90:295–298.

107. Boden WE, Bough EW, Korr KS, et al. Inferoseptal myocardial infarction: another cause of precordial ST-segment depression in transmural inferior wall MI? Am J Cardiol 1984; 54: 1216–1223.

108. Gorgels APM, Vos MA, Mulleneers R, et al. Value of the EKG in diagnosing the number of severely narrowed coronary arteries in rest angina pectoris. Am J Cardiol 1993; 72:999–1003.

109. Lopez-Sendon J, Coma-Canella I, Alcasena S, et al. EKG findings in acute right ventricular infarction. J Am Coll Cardiol 1985; 6:1273–1279.

110. Zimmerman J, Fromm R, Meyer D, et al. Diagnostic marker cooperative study for the diagnosis of myocardial infarction. Circulation 1999; 99:1671–1681.

111. Balk E, Ioannidis JPA, Salem D, et al. Accuracy of biomarkers for the diagnosis of acute cardiac ischemia in the emergency department: a meta-analysis. Ann Emerg Med 2001; 37: 479–494.

112. Lee HS, Cross SJ, Rawles JM, et al. Patients with suspected myocardial infarction who present with ST-segment depression. Lancet 1993; 342:1204–1207.

113. O'Keefe JH, Sayed-Taha K, Gibson W, et al. Do patients with left circumflex coronary artery-related acute myocardial infarction without ST-segment elevation benefit from reperfusion? Am J Cardiol 1995; 75:718–720.

114. London M, Hollenberg M, Wong M, et al. Intraoperative myocardial ischemia: localization by continuous 12 lead electrocardiography. Anesthesiology 1988; 69:237.

115. Eriksson P, Gunnarsson G, Dellborg M. Diagnosis of acute myocardial infarction in patients with chronic right bundle branch block using standard 12-lead electrocardiogram compared with dynamic vector cardiography. Cardiol 1998; 90:58–62.

116. Sgarbossa EB, Pinski SL, Barbagelata A, et al. Electrocardiographic diagnosis of evolving acute myocardial infarction in the presence of left bundle branch block. NEJM 1996; 334:481–487.

117. Kontos M, McQueen RH, Jesse RL, et al. Can myocardial infarction be rapidly identified in emergency department patients who have left bundle branch block? Ann Emerg Med 2001; 37:431–438.

118. Ryan TJ, Anderson JL, Antman EM, et al. ACC/AHA Guidelines for management of patients with acute myocardial infaraction: report of the AHA/ACC Task Force on Practice Guidelines. J Am Coll Cardiol 1996; 28:1328–1428.

119. Sgarbossa EB, Pinski SL, Crates KB, et al. Electrocardiographic diagnosis of acute myocardial infarction in the presence of ventricular paced rhythm. Am J Cardiol 1996; 77:423–424.

120. Lau J, Ioannidis JPA, Balk EM, et al. Diagnosing acute cardiac ischemia in the emergency department: a systematic review of the accuracy and clinical effect of current technologies. Ann Emerg Med 2001; 37:453–460.

121. Mair J, Genser N, Morandell D, et al. Cardiac troponin I in the diagnosis of myocardial injury and infarction. Clinica Chemica Acta 1996; 245:19–38.

122. Benoit MO, Paris M, Silleran J, et al. Cardiac troponin I. Its contribution to the diagnosis of perioperative myocardial infarction and various complications of cardiac surgery. Crit Care Med 2001; 29:1880–1886.

123. Adams J III. Impact of troponin on the evaluation and therapy of patients with acute coronary syndromes. Curr Opin Cardiol 1999; 14:310–313.

124. O'Rourke RA, Gochman JS, Cohen NF, et al. New approaches to the diagnosis and management of unstable angina and non-ST segment elevation myocardial infarction. Arch Int Med 2001; 161:674–682.

125. Garber AM, Solomon NA. Cost-effectiveness of alternative test strategies for the diagnosis of coronary artery disease. Ann Intern Med 1999; 130:719–725.

126. Ioaniddis JPA, Salem D, Chew P, et al. Accuracy of imaging technologies in the diagnosis of acute cardiac ischemia in the emergency department: A meta-analysis. Ann Emerg Med 2001; 37:471–477.

127. Trippi JA, Lee Ks, Kopp G, et al. Dobutamine stress tele-echocardiography for evaluation of emergency department patients with chest pain. J Am Coll Cardiol 1997; 30:627–632.

128. Gibler WB, Runyon JP, Levy RC, et al. A rapid diagnosis and treatment center for patients with chest pain in the emergency department. Ann Emerg Med 1995; 25:1–8.

129. Zalenski RJ, McCarren M, Roberts R, et al. An evaluation of a chest pain diagnostic protocol to exclude cardiac ischemia in the emergency department. Arch Intern Med 1997; 157:1085–1091.

130. Landesberg G, Mosseri M, Yehuda W, et al. Perioperative myocardial ischemia and infarction. Anesthesiology 2002; 96:264–270.

131. Thadani U. Treatment of stable angina. Curr Opin Cardiol 1999; 14:349–358.

132. Thadani U. Role of nitrates in angina pectoris. Am J Cardiol 1992; 70:43B–53B.

133. Thadani U. Current management of chronic stable angina. J Cardiovasc Pharmacol Ther 2004; 9 suppl 1:511–529.

134. Sigmund M, Nase-Huppmeier S, Uebis R, Hanrath P. Emergency PTCA for coronary artery occlusion after blunt chest trauma. Am Heart J 1990; 119:1408–1410.

135. Ridker PM, Marlon JE, Gaziano M, et al. Low dose aspirin therapy for chronic stable angina- a randomized, placebo-controlled trial. Ann Intern Med 1991; 114:835–839.

136. Braunwald E, Antman EM, Beasley JW, et al. American College of Cardiology/ American Heart Association guidelines for management of patients with unstable angina and nonST-elevation myocardial infarction: executive summary and recommendations. Circulation 2000; 102:1193–1209.

137. Calvo Orbe L, Garcia Gallego F, Sobrino N, et al. Acute myocardial infarction after blunt chest trauma in young people: need for prompt intervention. Cathet Cardiovasc Diagn 1991; 24:182–185.

138. Reeder G. Contemporary diagnosis and management of unstable angina. Mayo Clin Proc 2000; 75:953–957.

139. Gibler WB, Wilcox RG, Bode C, et al. Prospective use of glycoprotein IIb IIIa inhibitors in the emergency department setting. Ann Emerg Med 1998; 32:712–722.

140. Ryan TJ, Antman EM, Brooks NH, et al. 1999 update: ACC/AHA guidelines for the management of patients with acute myocardial infarction: a report of the ACC/AHA Task Force on Practice Guidelines. J Am Coll Cardiol 1999; 34:890–911.

141. Ryan TJ, Melduni RM. Highlights of the latest ACC/AHA guidelines for management of patients with acute myocardial infarction. Cardiol Rev 2002; 10:35–43.

142. ISIS-2 Collaborative Group. Randomized trial of intravenous streptokinase, oral aspirin, both or neither among 17,181 cases of suspected acute myocardial infarction: ISIS-2. Lancet 1988; 2:349–360.

143. GUSTO Angiography Investigators. The effects of tissue plasminogen activator, streptokinase, or both on coronary artery patency, ventricular function and survival after acute myocardial infarction. NEJM 1993; 329:1615–1622.

144. Hennekens CH, Albert CM, Godried SL, et al. Adjunctive drug therapy of acute myocardial infarction-evidence from clinical trials. NEJM 1996; 335:1660–1667.

145. ACE Inhibitor Myocardial Infarct Collaborative Group. Indications for ACE inhibitors in the early therapy of acute myocardial infarction. Circulation 1998; 97:2202–2209.

146. DeGeare VS, Dangus G, Stone GW, et al. Interventional protocols in acute myocardial infarction. Am Heart J 2001; 141: 15–25.

147. GUSTO-IIb Angiography Substudy Investigators. A clinical trial comparing primary coronary angioplasty with tissue plaminogen activator for acute myocardial infarction. NEJM 1997; 336:1521–1528.

148. Zijlstra F, DeBoer MJ, Hoomtje JCA. A comparison of immediate percutaneous translumenal coronary angioplasty with intravenous streptokinase in acute myocardial infarction. NEJM 1993; 328:680–684.

149. Weaver WD, Simes RJ, Betriu A, et al. Comparison of primary coronary angioplasty and intravenous streptokinase therapy for acute myocardial infarction: a quantitative review. JAMA 1997; 278:2093–2098.

150. Colombo A, Briguori C. Primary stenting and glycoprotein IIb IIIa inhibitors in acute myocardial infarction. Am Heart J 1999; 138:S153–S157.

151. Santora TA, Schinco MA, Troskin SZ. Management of trauma in the elderly patient. Surg Clin North Am 1994; 74:163–186.

152. Scalea TM, Simon HM, Duncan AO, et al. Geriatric blunt multitrauma: improved survival with early invasive monitoring. J Trauma 1990; 30:129–136.

153. Poldermans D, Boersma E, Bax J, et al. The effect of bisoprolol on perioperative mortality and myocardial infarction in high-risk patients undergoing vascular surgery. N Engl J Med 1999; 341:1789–1794.

154. Urban MK, Markowitz SM, Gordon MA, et al. Postoperative prophylactic administration of beta-adrenergic blockers in patients at risk for myocardial ischemia. Anesth Analg 2000; 90:1257–1261.

155. Mangano D, Layug E, Wallace A, et al. Effect of atenolol on mortality and cardiovascular morbidity after noncardiac surgery. N Engl J Med 1996; 335:1713–1720.

156. Boudoulas H, Rittgers S, Lewis R, et al. Changes in diastolic time with various pharmacologic agents. Circulation 1979; 60:164–169.

157. Eagle KA, Berger PB, Calkins H, et al. ACC/AHA guideline update for perioperative cardiovascular evaluation for noncardiac surgery-executive summary: a report of the American College of Cardiology/American Heart Association Task Force on Practice Guidelines (Committee to update the 1996 Guidelines on Perioperative Cardiovascular Evaluation for Noncardiac Surgery). J Am Coll Cardiol 2002; 39:542–553.

158. London MJ, Zaugg M, Schaub MC, et al. Perioperative beta-adrenergic receptor blockade: physiologic foundations and clinical controversies. Anesthesiology 2004; 100:170–175.

159. Kertai MD, Bax JJ, Klein J, et al. Is there any reason to withhold beta blockers from high-risk patients with coronary artery disease during surgery? Anesthiology 2004; 100:4–7.

160. Kate L, Deveraux PJ. A large trial is vital to prove perioperative beta-blockade effectiveness and safety before widespread use. Anesthesiology 2004; 101(3):803.

161. London MJ, Zaugg M, Schaub MC, et al. A large trial is vital to prove perioperative beta-blockade effectiveness and safety before widespread use. Anesthesiology 2004; 101(3): 804–805.

162. Kertai MD, Bax JJ, Klein J, et al. A large trial is vital to prove perioperative beta-blockade effectiveness and safety before widespread use. Anesthesiology 2004; 101(3):805–806.

163. Apostolidou I, Skubas N, Bakola A, et al. Effects of nicardipine and nitroglycerin on perioperative myocardial ischemia in patients undergoing coronary artery bypass surgery. Semin Thorac Cardiovasc Surg 1999; 11:77–83.

164. Talke P, Li J, Jain U, et al. Effects of perioperative dexmedetomidine infusion in patients undergoing vascular surgery. Anesthesiology 1995; 82:620–633.

165. Schwab CW, Kauder DR. Trauma in the geriatric patient. Arch Surg 1992; 127:701–706.

166. Tornetta III P, Mostafavi H, Riina J, et al. Morbidity and mortality in elderly trauma patients. J Trauma 1999; 46:702–706.

167. Le Manach Y, Perel A, Coriat P, et al. Early and delayed myocardial infarction after abdominal aortic surgery. Anesthesiology 2005; 102:885–891.

168. Bokelman TA, Rahko PS, Meany BT, Fausch MD. Traumatic occlusion of the right coronary artery resulting in cardiogenic shock successfully treated with primary angioplasty. Am Heart J 1996; 131:411–413.

169. Marcum JL, Booth DC, Sapin PM. Acute myocardial infarction caused by blunt chest trauma: successful treatment by direct coronary angioplasty. Am Heart J 1996; 132:1275–1277.

170. Thorban S, Ungeheuer A, Blasini R, Siewert JR. Emergent interventional transcatheter revascularization in acute right coronary artery dissection after blunt chest trauma. J Trauma 1997; 43:365–367.

171. O'Neill PA, Sinert RH, Sian KU, et al. Percutaneous transluminal coronary angioplasty in a patient with myocardial infarction after penetrating trauma. J Trauma 2003; 54(5): 1000–1005.

172. Fedalen PA, Bard MR, Piacentino V III, et al. Intraluminal shunt placement and off-pump coronary revascularization for coronary artery stab wound. J Trauma 2001; 50(1):133.

173. Southam S, Jutila C, Ketai L. Contrast-enhanced cardiac MRI in blunt chest trauma: differentiating cardiac contusion from acute peritraumatic myocardial infarction. J Thor Imaging 2006; 21:176–178.

174. Moreno R, Perez del Todo J, Nieto M, et al. Primary stenting in acute myocardial infarction secondary to right coronary artery dissection following blunt chest trauma. Usefulness of intracoronary ultasound. Int J Cardiol 2005; 103:209–211.

20

Dysrhythmia: Diagnosis and Management

Janice Bitetti

Department of Anesthesiology and Critical Care Medicine, George Washington University Hospital, Washington, D.C., U.S.A.

Sung Lee

Division of Cardiology, Department of Medicine, George Washington University Hospital, Washington, D.C., U.S.A.

INTRODUCTION

Dysrhythmias are commonly seen in the electrocardiogram (ECG) of patients suffering from trauma and critical illness. Some dysrhythmias result as exacerbations of underlying rhythm disorders. Most are due to the changes in the autonomic nervous system and electrolyte levels that often occur in the critically ill. Dysrhythmias in the trauma patient also result from ischemia, direct mechanical injury to the heart (e.g., myocardial contusion), or occur secondary to drugs or toxins. A review of normal electrophysiologic function will precede the discussion of the dysrhythmias most frequently encountered in trauma and critical illness.

NORMAL SINUS RHYTHM

The conduction system of the heart comprises specialized cardiac myocytes. These myocytes spontaneously depolarize at their own intrinsic frequency. The normal sinus rhythm originates from sinus node cells located at the junction of the superior vena cava and right atrium (see Volume 2, Chapter 3, Fig. 13) and has spontaneous depolarization frequencies ranging from 60 to 100 beats per minute (bpm). The normal ECG reveals upright P waves in the inferior leads (I, II, and aVF) and lateral leads (I and aVL) and all of the V leads except for V1, where the P wave is biphasic. The P wave is normally inverted in aVR. Figure 1 shows a normal sinus rhythm in leads II and V5. The commonly measured intervals are shown in Figure 2. Alterations in these intervals will have both diagnostic and prognostic implications as described in this text.

The sinus node is richly innervated with both sympathetic and parasympathetic nerves. As a result, the heart rate is closely regulated by the autonomic nervous system. An increase in sympathetic tone, as often occurs in critically ill patients due to pain, fear, anxiety, hypovolemia, or withdrawal from opiates or alcohol, increases sinus rate. An increase in parasympathetic (vagal) tone or a decrease in sympathetic tone (as occurs with spinal shock) will decrease the sinus node-firing rate.

BRADYCARDIA

Bradycardia is defined as a heart rate less than 60 bpm. However, bradycardia is not necessarily pathologic and needs to be interpreted in the light of the clinical setting.

A heart rate of 60 bpm or less may be appropriate for a patient at rest or sleeping. However, the same heart rate would be inappropriately low for a critically ill patient with fever and hypotension. Because the cardiac output is a product of heart rate and stroke volume, bradycardia leads to a decrease in cardiac output that can result in decreased tissue perfusion. Pathologic bradycardia, therefore, can be better defined as a heart rate that is too slow to meet the metabolic demand. The causes of pathologic bradycardia can be divided into two categories: sinus node dysfunction and heart block.

Sinus Node Dysfunction

Failure of the sinus node to generate a cardiac impulse can result in sinus bradycardia, sinus pauses, or sinus arrest. Sinus node dysfunction can be due to either intrinsic structural abnormality of the sinus node or to extrinsic factors that affect the normally functioning sinus node. The most common cause of intrinsic sinus node dysfunction is idiopathic and is thought to be due to diffuse fibrosis of atrial tissue (including cardiac conduction fibers). Intrinsic sinus node dysfunction is most commonly seen in elderly patients and in patients with atrial tachydysrhythmias. Extrinsic factors that affect the sinus node are common (Table 1). Extrinsic factors that cause sinus node dysfunction do not cause structural changes in the sinus node and thus can be reversed once the offending factors are removed. The most common extrinsic causes of sinus node dysfunction include high vagal tone and sinus node-depressant drugs. High vagal tone can be seen in critically ill patients during endotracheal suctioning, in association with inferior wall myocardial infarction (MI) and with cervical spinal cord injury that results in unopposed vagal effect on the heart. Drugs such as beta-receptor blockers and calcium-channel blockers are common extrinsic drug-related causes of sinus node dysfunction. Nondrug-related extrinsic causes of sinus node dysfunction include hypothyroidism, increased intracranial pressure (ICP), and hypothermia. One of the important manifestations of sinus node dysfunction is tachycardia–bradycardia syndrome in which termination of an atrial tachydysrhythmia is followed by a sinus pause.

⊄ **Bradycardia per se does not require specific treatment as long as it does not cause symptoms of hemodynamic compromise.** ⊄ Symptoms related to sinus node dysfunction are often nonspecific and are difficult to identify. The first step in the treatment of sinus node dysfunction should be removal of extrinsic factors such as sinus

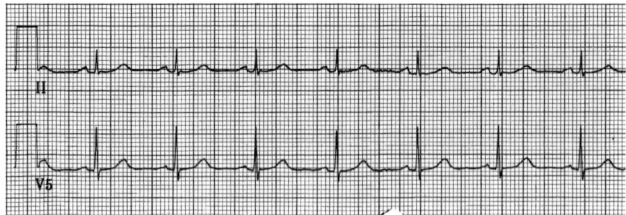

Figure 1 Normal sinus rhythm obtained from an otherwise healthy 67-year-old male. The P waves are upright in leads II and V5. Heart rate: 76 bpm, PR interval: 148 msec, QRS duration: 76 msec, QT/QT$_C$: 370/416 msec.

node-depressant drugs. Catecholaminergic drugs, such as isoproterenol and epinephrine, and vagolytic agents, such as atropine or glycopyrrolate, can acutely increase sinus rate and can be used if urgent intervention for bradycardia is needed. If bradycardia causes symptoms and is resistant to pharmacologic therapy, or if there is concern that the heart rate may decline further, a temporary transcutaneous pacemaker can be placed on the surface of the patient. Esophageal stethoscopes with pacing capabilities have also been used successfully. If one needs prolonged heart rate support, a transvenous temporary pacemaker, or a permanent pacemaker, is required.

Abnormal Atrio-ventricular Conduction

Atrio-ventricular (AV) block occurs when there is a delay or failure of the atrial impulse to conduct to the ventricles. Abnormal AV conduction can occur at the level of the AV

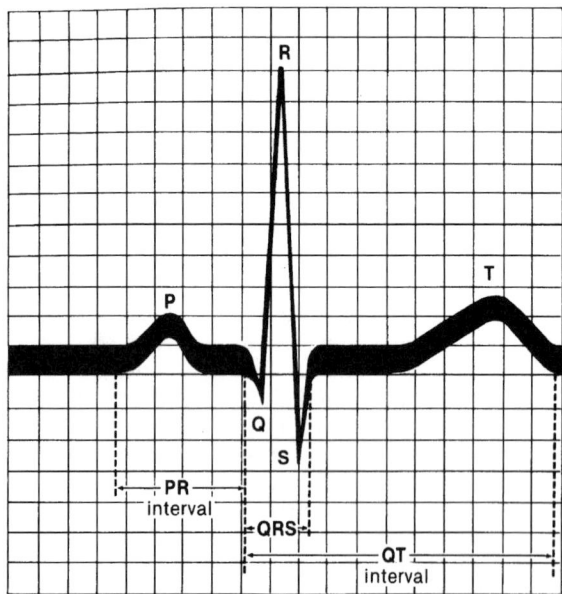

Figure 2 Commonly measured intervals on the electrocardiographic trace. The normal PR interval duration ranges between 0.12 and 0.2 seconds (120–200 msec). The QRS interval normally ranges from 0.05 to 0.12 seconds (50–120 msec). The normal QT interval varies with heart rate, age, and sex. In general, the QT interval should be less than half the preceding RR interval. However, when the heart rate is ≤65 bpm the normal heart rate corrected QT interval (QT$_C$) is even lower. When the QT$_C$ becomes >500 msec there is increased risk of torsades de pointes and V-fib.

Table 1 Extrinsic Causes of Sinus Node Dysfunction Resulting in Bradycardia

Drugs	Beta-receptor blockers
	Calcium-channel blockers
	Digitalis
	Antidysrhythmic drugs
High vagal tone	Inferior wall myocardial infarction
	Endotracheal suctioning
	Carotid massage
Increased ICP	Bradycardia associated with hypertension
	Mechanism of this "Cushing response" is not completely understood
	Traditionally, the hypertensive component is believed to result from brainstem ischemia
	Could result from activation of intracranial baroreceptors, or loss of supratentorial inhibition of brainstem vasomotor centers
	Bradycardia can be direct effect, or reflexic (of brainstem ischemia)
Hypothyroidism	Decreased inotropy and chronotropy
Apnea	Initially HR is increased due to increased sympathetic tone. Later, perhaps due to brainstem ischemia, bradycardia results
Hypothermia	Decreased sinus rate, and decreased PR interval, and decreased contractility ultimately. Osborn waves are seen just prior to V-fib (see Volume 1, Chapter 40, and Volume 2, Chapter 11)

Abbreviations: HR, heart rate; ICP, intracranial pressure; V-fib, ventricular fibrillation.

node or below in the bundle of His or beyond. Identification of the level of block is important because it determines the treatment strategy. Conduction block at the level of the AV node is usually due to abnormal vagal tone or to medications and does not usually require permanent intervention. However, an AV block below the level of the AV node represents damage to the conduction system and requires a permanent pacemaker.

AV block can be classified into first-degree AV block, second-degree AV block, high-degree AV block, and third-degree AV block or complete heart block. First-degree AV block is characterized by prolongation of the PR interval to more than 200 msec. In general, first-degree AV block does not cause any significant hemodynamic compromise and does not need intervention. Second-degree AV block can be classified into type I and type II. Type I, or Wenckebach AV block, is characterized by gradual prolongation of the PR interval, eventually leading to a P wave that does not conduct, resulting in the absence of a QRS complex (Fig. 3A). The level of block for type I second-degree AV block is in the AV node and is most commonly due to high vagal tone or to medications that produce block at the AV nodal level such as beta-blockers, nondihydropyridine calcium-channel blockers, and digoxin. One must inquire specifically about eye drops containing beta-blockers because they can have significant systemic absorption and can cause bradycardia and AV block. Type II AV block is characterized by a sudden drop in a QRS complex without gradual prolongation of the PR interval and represents more extensive disease in the conduction system (Fig. 3B). In general, type I second-degree AV block is associated

(A)

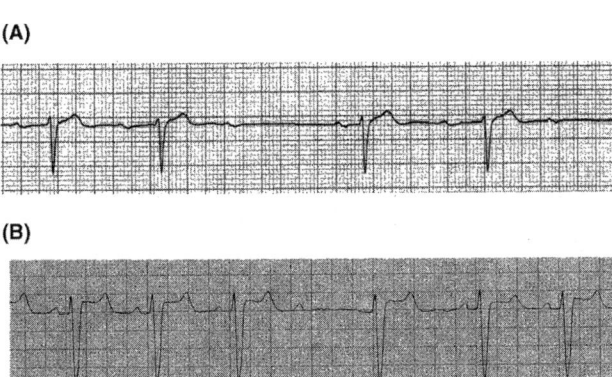

(B)

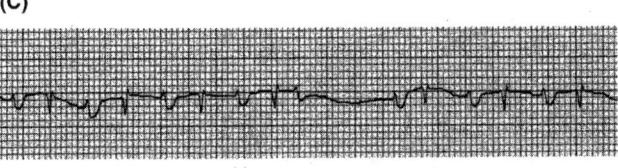

(C)

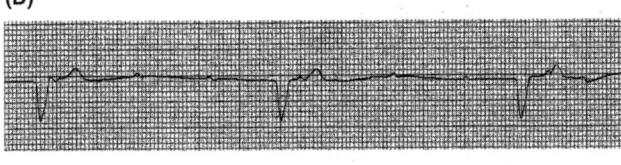

(D)

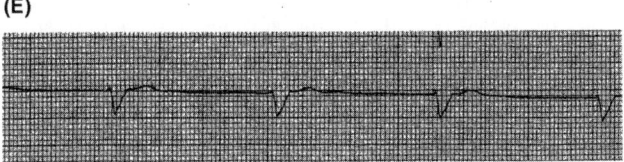

(E)

Figure 3 (**A**) Type I second-degree AV block. There is a gradual prolongation of the PR interval prior to a nonconducted P wave. (**B**) Type II second-degree heart block. The PR interval is fixed prior to a nonconducted P wave. (**C**) Late coupled premature atrial contraction mimicking type II second-degree AV block. The fifth P wave is premature and has a P-wave morphology that is slightly different from other P waves. (**D**) Complete heart block with ventricular escape. (**E**) A-fib with complete heart block. The ventricular rate is slow and regular.

with narrow QRS complex escape beats, because these arise from the AV node. Type II AV block is associated with wide QRS complex escape beats, which arise from the ventricle. Late coupled premature atrial contractions (PACs) that do not result in ventricular contraction can be confused with second-degree AV block. Therefore, the P-wave morphologies prior to AV block need to be carefully scrutinized (Fig. 3C). Complete heart block or third-degree heart block is due to complete blockade of AV conduction. Complete heart block at the level of the AV node usually results in a junctional escape rhythm with narrow QRS complexes and a heart rate of approximately 50 bpm. Junctional rhythm is relatively stable and prolonged asystole is uncommon. Complete heart block occurring below the level of the AV node results in a slow ventricular escape rhythm with wide QRS complexes, typically at a rate less than 40 bpm (Fig. 3D). A ventricular escape rhythm is an unstable rhythm and may suddenly disappear, resulting in prolonged asystolic period. When there is a slow, regular ventricular rhythm in the setting of underlying atrial fibrillation (A-fib), complete heart block should be suspected (Fig. 3E).

Slow ventricular rates from heart block will result in a decreased left ventricular end diastolic volume (LVEDV) due to the lack of atrial contraction at end diastole. The subsequent decrease in cardiac output may be significant enough to result in inadequate tissue perfusion. Patients with heart block and moderate hypertension may maintain what appears to be an adequate blood pressure, but truly have occult inadequate tissue perfusion, which is evidenced by prerenal azotemia, hepatocelluar injury, and congestive heart failure. In addition, complete heart block with a slow ventricular escape rate can be associated with bradycardia-dependent torsades de pointes. Therefore, patients with evidence of inadequate tissue perfusion should be promptly treated.

☞ **Heart block at the level of the AV node usually does not require invasive therapy and only requires withdrawal of the offending agents, such as beta-blockers and calcium-channel blockers.** ☞ Sometimes, infusion of a beta-agonist such as isoproterenol, or temporary pacing with either a transvenous or a transcutaneous pacemaker, can be used to support the heart rate until the medications are metabolized or excreted. A permanent pacemaker is almost never needed. However, heart block below the level of the AV node often causes more significant symptoms and requires a permanent pacemaker (Table 2).

Table 2 Atrio-ventricular Blocks Categorized by Degree, and by Anatomic Location Relative to the AV Node, Along with Common Symptoms and Treatment

Degree of block	Level of block	Symptoms	Treatment
First-degree AV block	Proximal	No	None
(prolonged PR interval)	Distal	No	None
Second-degree AV block	Proximal	No	None
(intermittent block)		Yes	Removal of offending factors, temporary pacemaker
	Distal	No	Permanent pacemaker
		Yes	Permanent pacemaker
Third-degree AV block	Proximal	No	None
(no conduction of atrial		Yes	Temporary pacemaker
impulses to the ventricles)	Distal	No	Permanent pacemaker
		Yes	Permanent pacemaker

Abbreviation: AV, atrio-ventricular.

TACHYDYSRHYTHMIAS
Sinus Tachycardia

Sinus tachycardia is defined as a heart rate more than 100 bpm. The morphology of the P wave is similar to that in the baseline sinus rhythm, with positive P-wave deflections in leads I, II, III, aVF, and aVL. ☞ **Sinus tachycardia usually has a gradual onset and termination.** ☞ Sinus tachycardia in critical care settings is an appropriate physiologic response to stresses such as fever, hypovolemia, hypotension, pulmonary embolism, congestive heart failure, respiratory distress, and thyrotoxicosis. Drugs such as dobutamine, epinephrine, caffeine, and alcohol can also cause sinus tachycardia. In patients with unexplained sinus tachycardia, a vigilant search for its cause should be made. Pulmonary embolism, in particular, should be considered as a possible cause in a chronically ill patient in the critical care setting.

In general, sinus tachycardia does not require specific interventions to correct the heart rate itself, and treatment should be directed at addressing the underlying cause of the sinus tachycardia and removing any offending agents. However, beta-blockers such as esmolol and metoprolol, and calcium-channel blockers such as diltiazem and verapamil, can be used to slow the ventricular rate in patients in whom tachycardia might be harmful (e.g., myocardial ischemia, aortic stenosis, mitral sentosis, etc.). In the trauma intensive care unit (ICU) setting, sinus tachycardia often means the patient requires additional intravascular repletion, is hypoxemic or febrile, or suffering from pain and anxiety requiring opioid analgesics or other sedatives. Even when the problem is mainly anxiety or pain driven, adequacy of oxygenation, ventilation, fluid repletion, and systemic perfusion must be assured.

Atrial Tachydysrhythmias

Atrial tachydysrhythmias include A-fib, atrial flutter, atrial tachycardia, and multifocal atrial tachycardia (MAT). Frequent symptoms associated with atrial tachydysrhythmias include a sensation of the heart racing, palpitations, dizziness, syncope, fatigue, shortness of breath, and chest pain. These symptoms are usually due to a rapid ventricular rate, which decreases cardiac output because of inadequate ventricular filling time.

A-fib is the most common sustained tachydysrhythmia and is frequently seen in critically ill and elderly patients. The cause of new-onset A-fib in ICU patients is not always obvious, although it is almost always related to elevated catecholamine levels associated with physiologic or pathophysiologic stress. Treatable causes of A-fib, such as thyrotoxicosis and pulmonary embolism, should always be sought.

The heart with A-fib is characterized by disorganized atrial depolarizations, with an irregularly irregular ventricular contraction rate. The fibrillating atria resembles a "bag of worms" when directly visualized or examined with transesophageal echocardiography (TEE). The ECG reveals baseline undulations without discernable P waves, and an irregularly irregular QRS with A-fib. The disorganized atrial depolarizations range between 300 and 500 depolarizations per minute and the ventricular rate in untreated patients varies from 100 to 180 bpm.

Atrial flutter is commonly seen in ICU patients, others with high catecholamine levels, and those with structural heart disease. Typically, the atrial rate is regular and ranges from 260 to 300 bpm, and the corresponding ventricular rate is 130–150 bpm due to a 2:1 AV block. Thus,

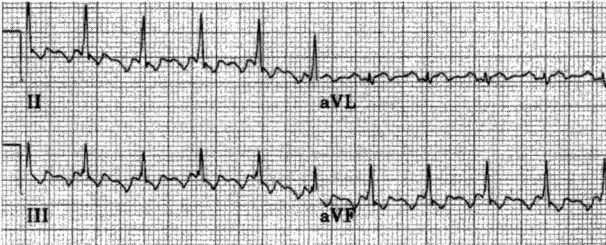

Figure 4   Typical atrial flutter with sawtooth flutter waves in the inferior leads.

atrial flutter should be considered as the most likely rhythm when a patient develops an acute narrow complex tachycardia with a ventricular rate near 140 bpm. The ECG classically reveals a sawtooth pattern in the inferior leads and narrow positive flutter waves in leads II, III, and aVF (Fig. 4).

Ectopic atrial tachycardia (EAT) is most commonly due to an automatic focus and is usually seen in patients with chronic lung disease and digitalis toxicity. The automatic focus of atrial tachycardia is enhanced by catecholamines. Similar to sinus tachycardia, EAT typically has a gradual onset and termination. The ECG reveals an atrial rate of 120–250 bpm with a P-wave morphology that is different than that seen in sinus rhythm.

MAT is also commonly seen in patients with severe lung disease, especially in the setting of increased atrial stretch (i.e., volume overload) and in high catecholamine states. The atrial rate is, in general, 120–180 bpm. The ECG reveals multiple P-wave morphologies. Patients with MAT are usually elderly and often have prolonged ICU stays due to their pulmonary disease and comorbid conditions (see Volume 1, Chapter 37). Of the atrial tachydysrhythmias, MAT is one of the most difficult to treat, partly due to the triggering pathophysiology (long-standing pulmonary disease and atrial stretch).

Acute treatment of atrial tachydysrhythmias includes ventricular rate control, as well as acute conversion to and maintenance of sinus rhythm (Table 3). For ventricular rate control, agents that block AV nodal conduction, such as calcium-channel blockers, beta-blockers, or digoxin, can be used in hemodynamically stable patients. Repletion of potassium and magnesium is universally beneficial. Digoxin, once the foundation of therapy, is no longer recommended as the initial or stand-alone treatment when other (less toxic) AV node-blocking agents are available. In hemodynamically unstable patients, synchronized direct current (DC) cardioversion should be employed before rate-controlling drugs are administered.

☞ **Acute conversion of atrial tachydysrhythmias to sinus rhythm can be accomplished either by synchronized DC cardioversion or by administration of antidysrhythmic agents.** ☞ Hemodynamically unstable atrial tachydysrhythmias should be treated promptly with synchronized DC cardioversion. Atrial flutter requires less energy than A-fib to convert to sinus rhythm. Antidysrhythmic drugs can be used to convert atrial tachydysrhythmias and to maintain sinus rhythm in hemodynamically stable atrial tachydysrhythmias. Antidysrhythmic drugs will be discussed in more detail in a subsequent section.

Inadequate atrial contraction associated with A-fib and atrial flutter can result in thrombus formation in the atria, which may lead to systemic thromboembolism. The

Table 3 Atrial Tachydysrhythmias: Diagnosis and Treatment

Atrial rhythm disorder	Heart rate (atrial/ ventricular)	P waves	Treatment
Sinus tachycardia	100–180/100–180	Same as sinus rhythm	Treat underlying illness Beta-blocker, if symptomatic
Ectopic atrial tachycardia	120–250/variable	Different from sinus	Rate control with AV-blocking agents Rhythm control with antidysrhythmic drugs
Multifocal atrial tachycardia	100–140/100–140	Multiple P-wave morphologies	Rate control with AV-blocking agents Rhythm control with antidysrhythmic drugs
Atrial flutter	250–300/150 if untreated	Sawtooth in leads II, III, and aVF	Adenosine Rate control with AV-blocking agents
Atrial fibrillation	300–400/120–180 if untreated	No discernable P waves	Rhythm control with antidysrhythmic drugs Anticoagulation, if more than 48 hrs

Note: In most situations, normalizing $[Mg^{2+}]$ and $[K^+]$ and decreasing catecholamine levels will increase the ability to maintain normal sinus rhythms.
Abbreviations: AV, atrio-ventricular; VF, ventricular fibrillation.

risk of thromboembolism increases after A-fib or flutter is sustained for more than 48 hours. Therefore, cardioversion should be performed within 48 hours from the onset of A-fib or flutter to minimize the risk of embolization that can occur following cardioversion as the atria return to normal contraction. Beyond 48 hours, patients should receive a TEE to rule out mural thrombi, and be considered for anticoagulation prior to electric cardioversion.

Atrio-ventricular Node-Mediated Dysrhythmias

The most common AV node-mediated tachycardias are the AV nodal re-entrant tachycardia (AVNRT) and the AV re-entry tachycardia (AVRT) shown schematically (Fig. 5). In patients with AVNRT, there are two inputs into the AV node, a slow pathway and a fast pathway. During the AVNRT, the electrical impulse propagates antegrade through the slow pathway and then retrograde through the fast pathway (Fig. 5A). The ECG reveals a narrow complex tachycardia with no discernable P wave, or retrograde conducted P waves that are visualized at the terminal portion of the QRS complexes (referred to as a pseudo r-prime). In AVRT tachycardias (Fig. 5B), the AV node is used for antegrade conduction and the accessory pathway is used for retrograde conduction; this larger circuit is sometimes referred to as macrorecurrent. The P waves in AVRT will be retrograde conducted and seen between the QRS and the T wave (Fig. 5B).

ơ⁴ **Treatment of AV node-mediated tachycardias (AVNRT and AVRT) can be accomplished by administering drugs that increase the refractory period of the AV node. These drugs include calcium-channel blockers, beta-blockers, digoxin, and adenosine.** ơ⁴ In patients without hypotension, vagal maneuvers (e.g., carotid massage) are often sufficient to terminate these dysrhythmias. However, in the setting of hypotension, the judicious administration of phenylephrine in 0.1 mg increments may terminate the dysrhythmia on its own or increase the pressure enough to allow the patient to tolerate the administration of a calcium-channel blocker or adenosine. A diagnostic test as well as therapeutic dysrhythmia conversion can be performed simultaneously by giving an intravenous bolus of 6–12 mg of adenosine. Because adenosine is rapidly degraded in the blood stream, it should be given through a large bore (preferably central) intravenous line followed by a bolus flush of intravenous fluids. Intravenous verapamil (2–10 mg) or diltiazem (10–20 mg) can also be used for acute termination of AVNRT or AVRT. Because both of these calcium-channel blockers can cause some systemic vasodilation and hypotension, calcium chloride can be administered concomitantly in (250 mg) aliquots without inhibiting the calcium-channel blockade effect at the AV node. Digoxin is too slow acting, and should not be used emergently to control AVNRT or AVRT, but digoxin is typically added to further increase tone at the AV node. Maintenance and prevention can be accomplished with either intravenous or oral calcium-channel blockers or beta-blockers.

Accessory-Pathway Mediated Tachycardia (Wolf-Parkinson-White Syndrome)

Wolf-Parkinson-White (WPW) syndrome is due to antegrade conduction down an accessory pathway linking the atrium and the ventricle. As a result, activation of ventricular depolarization is fused between the activation occurring through the normal AV nodal pathway and that occurring through the accessory pathway (a process referred to as pre-excitation). The resulting ECG trace reveals a characteristic "delta wave" type widening of the QRS, which is relegated to the basal portion of the ascending limb of the QRS complex. WPW affects about two to three out of 1000 people in the general population. Accessory-mediated tachycardias include orthodromic AVRT (retrograde conduction through the accessory pathway) and WPW atrial dysrhythmias (antegrade conduction down the accessory pathway) with a variable degree of pre-excitation and delta wave formation. Orthodromic AVRT uses the AV node–His bundle as the antegrade limb, and the accessory pathway for the retrograde limb during the tachycardia. Therefore, the ventricular activation pattern is normal and the QRS complex is narrow. Antidromic AVRT (e.g., WPW) uses the accessory pathway as the antegrade limb and the AV node–His bundle as the retrograde limb. When the ventricular activation is purely through the accessory pathway, the ECG reveals a wide complex tachycardia that can be difficult to differentiate from ventricular tachycardia (VT).

AVRT, like AVNRT, requires the AV node as the critical limb for re-entry. Therefore, agents that slow conduction in the AV node can terminate and prevent both of these dysrhythmias. Acutely, AVRT can be terminated with an intravenous bolus of either adenosine (6–12 mg) or a

(A)   **AVNRT**

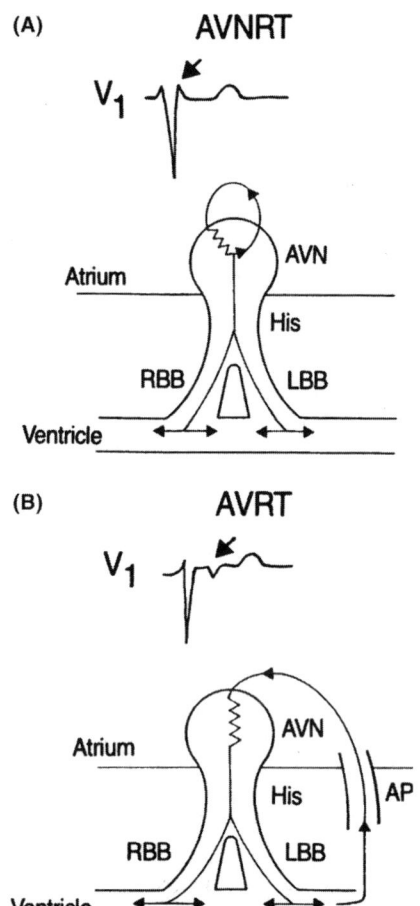

(B)   **AVRT**

Figure 5 Schematic of AV node re-entry tachycardia (AVNRT) and AV re-entry tachycardia (AVRT). (**A**) V₁ lead showing the typical electrocardiographic trace of AVNRT, along with a schematic of the re-entrant circuit. There is relatively slow anterograde conduction over the AV node with nearly simultaneous activity of the atrium and ventricle. This leads to P-wave activity within or at the end of the QRS complex. The arrow points to a pseudo r-prime in V₁, which represents P-wave activity during tachycardia. (**B**) In AVRT, the tachycardia circuit is macro re-entrant. Anterograde conduction occurs over the AV node–His Purkinje system to activate the ventricle. Retrograde conduction proceeds from the ventricle over the accessory pathway to activate the atrium. There is a requisite amount of time necessary from ventricular activation to atrial activation. This usually allows sufficient time for P-wave activity to be noted in the early ST segment (*arrow* in V₁). *Abbreviations*: AVN, atrial-ventricular node; AP, accessory pathway; LBB, left bundle branch; RBB, right bundle branch. *Source*: From Ref. 77.

calcium-channel blocker such as diltiazem (10–20 mg) or verapamil (2–10 mg) (Table 4). Oral calcium-channel blockers or beta-blockers can be used on a regular dosing schedule to prevent recurrence.

Patients with WPW syndrome also commonly have atrial tachydysrhythmias such as A-fib requiring particular caution during termination. Because the accessory pathway can allow more rapid conduction than the AV node, the ventricular rate during atrial tachydysrhythmias is often quite rapid. Ventricular activation during atrial tachydysrhythmias is fused between activation through the

AV node–His bundle and the accessory pathway. Therefore, an ECG during A-fib in patients with WPW syndrome reveals a wide complex tachycardia that is irregularly irregular (Fig. 6).

☞ **Acute treatment of pre-excited A-fib should be targeted at slowing conduction in the accessory pathway rather than in the AV node. Pre-excited A-fib can be treated acutely with cardioversion (if patient is hemodynamically unstable) or adenosine, intravenous procainamide, ibutilide (1,2), or amiodarone (3).** ☞ One should avoid AV node-blocking agents (e.g., digoxin, calcium-channel blockers, or beta-blockers) in pre-excitation AVRT (WPW), because these may facilitate more rapid conduction through the accessory pathway and result in hemodynamic compromise. Chronic treatment of WPW syndrome includes radiofrequency ablation (RFA) or chronic administration of the above-mentioned antidysrhythmic drugs.

Differential Diagnosis of Narrow Complex Tachycardias

Accurate diagnosis of a narrow complex tachycardia in the acute care setting is important, because the treatment options depend on accurate recognition and diagnosis of the tachycardia (Table 5). The first step is to determine whether the rhythm is regular or irregular. Irregular rhythms include A-fib, MAT, and sinus tachycardia with frequent PACs. Regular narrow complex rhythms include EAT, atrial flutter, AVNRT, or AVRT.

The ventricular rate is sometimes helpful. With a ventricular rate of 140–150 bpm, the most likely diagnosis is atrial flutter with 2:1 block. AVNRT or AVRT have ventricular rates of 160–240 bpm.

The onset and termination of the supraventricular tachycardia (SVT) are also helpful. Atrial tachycardia tends to have a warm-up period with a slight increase in heart rate as the tachycardia warms up. AVNRT and AVRT have relatively fixed heart rates.

When determining the type of SVT, one must evaluate the presence and morphology of the P waves. The best leads in which to look for P waves are leads II and V1. Subtle changes in the ST-T waves may allow detection of P waves. With an EAT, P waves are usually seen at the terminal portion of the T waves or after the T waves. With an AVNRT, retrograde P waves are usually not visible, because they are buried within the QRS complex or are disguised as an R′ in the V1 lead. With an AVRT, retrograde P waves can be seen in the ST segments.

Administration of adenosine can be used not only to acutely terminate the rhythm, but also as a diagnostic tool. A bolus injection of adenosine (6–18 mg) will result in termination of AV node-mediated re-entrant tachycardias including AVNRT and AVRT. A bolus injection of adenosine in atrial tachycardias, such as atrial flutter and EAT, will result in increased AV block and may allow visualization of P waves or flutter waves when the rhythm returns, helping to make an accurate diagnosis.

Ventricular Tachydysrhythmias
Accelerated Idioventricular Rhythm

An accelerated idioventricular rhythm (AIVR) is a dysrhythmia of ventricular origin that is slower than 120 bpm, and is most commonly seen in patients with recent myocardial injury. In general, it does not cause hemodynamic compromise and does not require treatment.

Table 4 Atrio-ventricular Node and Accessory Pathway–Mediated Tachycardias: Diagnosis and Treatment

Rhythm disorder	Heart rate	P wave	Treament

AVNRT	150–250	Retrograde P wave in the QRS or at the terminal portion of the QRS	AV-blocking agents
			  Adenosine (A)
			  Beta-blockers (A, C)
			  Calcium-channel blockers (A, C)
			  Digoxin (C)

AVRT	150–250	Retrograde P wave in ST segment	AV-blocking agents
			  Adenosine (A)
			  Beta-blockers (A, C)
			  Calcium-channel blockers (A, C)
			Antidysrhythmics
			  Class IA, IC, and III (C)
			RF ablation
			Cardioversion adenosine

Atrial fibrillation with WPW	150–300	Irregularly irregular wide complex QRS. No discernable P waves	Antidysrhythmics RF ablation Class IA (A, C), IC (C), and III (A, C)

Abbreviations: A, acute treatment; AV, atrio-ventricular; AVNRT, AV nodal re-entrant tachycardia; AVRT, AV re-entrant tachycardia (uses accessory pathway rather than the AV node); C, chronic treatment; RF, radiofrequency; WPW, Wolf-Parkinson-White syndrome.

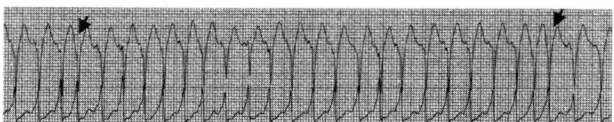

Figure 6 Pre-excited atrial fibrillation. There are slight irregularities in the RR interval (*arrows*).

Nonsustained Ventricular Tachycardia

VT is commonly seen in critically ill patients. Nonsustained VT does not always cause symptoms, but does require prompt evaluation because it may proceed to sustained VT or ventricular fibrillation (V-fib). In evaluating patients with nonsustained VT, one needs to assess left ventricular (LV) function and search for underlying coronary artery disease, and determine if it is multifocal or unifocal.

Nonsustained VT in patients with preserved LV function and without myocardial ischemia has a good prognosis and does not require further evaluation or treatment. In addition, nonsustained VT is seen frequently in patients with nonischemic dilated cardiomyopathy and usually does not require further evaluation or treatment. However, nonsustained VT in patients with ischemic cardiomyopathy and an LV ejection fraction (EF) less than 40% requires an electrophysiologic test to further assess the risk of sudden cardiac death (4,5).

⚓ Of the nonsustained VTs, nonsustained polymorphic VTs with a rapid ventricular rate require special attention, because these unstable dysrhythmias are very likely to progress to V-fib. ⚓ Nonsustained polymorphic VTs are most commonly associated with active myocardial ischemia or a prolonged QT interval. Recognition of nonsustained VT due to QT prolongation (Fig. 7) is particularly important, because administration of antidysrhythmic agents such as amiodarone would further prolong the QT interval, slow the heart rate, and increase the likelihood of causing a sustained polymorphic VT that could progress to V-fib.

Table 5 Differentiation of Narrow Complex Tachycardias

Regular vs. irregular	Irregular	Atrial fibrillation, multifocal atrial tachycardia, sinus tachycardia with PACs
	Regular	EAT, atrial flutter, AVNRT, AVRT
Rate	140 – 150 bpm	Atrial flutter
	160–240 bpm	EAT, AVNRT, AVRT
Onset/termination	Sudden	Atrial flutter, AVNRT, AVRT
	Gradual warm up	Sinus tachycardia, EAT
P waves	Not seen or at the terminal portion of QRS complex	AVNRT
	Seen on the ST segment	AVRT
	Sawtooth pattern	Atrial flutter
Response to adenosine	Increased AV block	EAT, atrial flutter
	Termination	AVNRT, AVRT

Abbreviations: AV, atrio-ventricular; AVNRT, AV nodal re-entrant tachycardia; AVRT, AV re-entrant tachycardias; EAT, ectopic atrial tachycardia; PACs, premature atrial contractions.

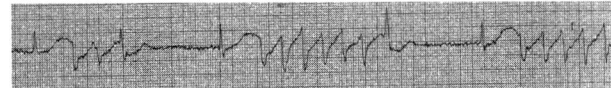

Figure 7 Nonsustained torsades de pointes in a patient taking sotalol. Note the prolonged QT interval and a large T wave from which nonsustained ventricular tachycardia starts.

Nonsustained polymorphic VT with QT prolongation should be treated promptly with intravenous magnesium, correction of underlying electrolyte disturbances, and withdrawal of offending drugs. Judicious doses of phenylephrine 0.05–0.1 mg bolus or phenylephrine infusion (25–75 µg/min) may be required to maintain blood pressure in patients with this rhythm. If the nonsustained polymorphic VT continues despite the above measures, a transvenous temporary pacemaker can be placed to overdrive suppress the nonsustained VT.

Sustained Ventricular Tachycardia

Sustained VT can be divided into monomorphic VT and polymorphic VT. The ECG reveals a wide complex tachycardia. Differentiation of VT from SVT with aberration will be discussed in a later section. Monomorphic VT is most commonly seen in patients with underlying heart disease including previous MI and cardiomyopathy (Fig. 8).

Sustained VT is occasionally seen in patients with a structurally normal heart. In patients with normal hearts, VT often arises from either the right ventricular (RV) outflow tract or the LV septum. Sustained VT originating in the RV outflow tract has tall upright R waves in the inferior leads (leads II, II, and avF) and has a left bundle branch block (LBBB) pattern. Sustained VT originating in the LV septal area has a right bundle branch block (RBBB) pattern and normal or left axis deviation. The unique feature of these VTs in patients with normal hearts is that they behave more like SVTs and respond well either to calcium-channel blockers or to beta-blockers, sedatives, and analgesics. This is not surprising, given the typical trigger is a high catecholamine state (secondary to pain, fear, anxiety, or underresuscitation).

Sustained polymorphic VTs are divided into those with and without QT prolongation. Polymorphic VT with QT prolongation is called torsades de pointes, which is characterized by QRS complexes that alternately widen and narrow continuously as the electrophysiologic axis of the heart changes "twists around a point." The underlying mechanism for QT prolongation is abnormal and prolonged repolarization of the ventricles. As a result, the T wave becomes abnormal and the QT duration becomes prolonged to an interval greater than the upper limit of the normal corrected QT duration (QT_c) of 440 msec.

There are primary (or congenital) and acquired long QT syndromes. Primary long QT syndrome is a familial disorder. The acquired long QT syndrome is most commonly caused by

(*i*) drugs such as quinidine, procainamide, sotalol, amiodarone, tricyclic antidepressants, antihistamines, and quinolone antibiotics; and (*ii*) electrolyte disorders such as hypokalemia and especially hypomagnesemia. Other causes of QT prolongation are discussed below. Torsades de pointes due to acquired QT prolongation is more likely to occur in the setting of bradycardia (bradycardia-dependent) or it can follow long pauses (pause-dependent). Prolonged QT interval (and frequent PVCs due to the prolonged QT interval) should be promptly treated, so that polymorphic VT does not progress to V-fib, and the subsequent need for cardiac resuscitation can be prevented.

Acute treatment of sustained unifocal (monomorphic) VT depends on whether or not hemodynamic decompensation is associated. ☞ **Hemodynamically unstable VT should be treated promptly with DC electrical cardioversion.** ☞ Monomorphic VT can be treated using a synchronized low-energy shock. However, when the rate of VT is too rapid, synchronization may not work well, may delay treatment, may accelerate VT, or may convert VT to V-fib. When a nonsynchronized shock is given for rapid VT or fibrillation, the output should be high enough to depolarize enough myocardium to terminate VT. In general, the minimum output for a nonsynchronized shock should be 120 J with a biphasic defibrillator and 200 J with a monophasic defibrillator. If V-fib results, reshock with 300 J to convert to sinus rhythm, increasing to 360 J, if subsequent shocks are needed. Closed chest cardiopulmonary resuscitation (CPR) should always be started if cardioversion is not immediately available in the case of V-fib or hemodynamic unstable VT (without a pulse or pressure). Following termination of the VT, an antidysrhythmic agent such as amiodarone should be started to prevent recurrent VT while the causes of the VT are sought after. ☞ **Hemodynamically stable VT can be treated with a pharmacologic agent. The first line of treatment is intravenous amiodarone or procainamide (6).** ☞

Sustained polymorphic VT, in general, causes hemodynamic decompensation and requires prompt nonsynchronized DC cardioversion. Again, the output should be high enough to depolarize enough myocardium to terminate VT. Following termination of VT, the QT interval should be determined to rule out torsades de pointes. If the QT interval is not prolonged, an antidysrhythmic agent can be started. However, if the QT interval is prolonged, a magnesium infusion should be started, any underlying electrolyte disturbances should be corrected, and offending drugs should be withdrawn.

Similar to the atria in A-fib, the appearance of the entire heart during V-fib resembles a "bag of worms." There is no significant ejection out of a ventricle during V-fib. Low-amplitude fibrillatory waves are seen on ECG. Accordingly, treatment of V-fib is immediate CPR until a defibrillator is available; then immediate cardioversion should proceed with 300 J escalating to 360 J.

Differential Diagnosis of Wide Complex Tachycardias

The diagnosis of wide complex tachycardia is often difficult to make. However, accurate diagnosis of wide complex tachycardia is important for prompt and appropriate initial treatment and subsequent management. The differential diagnosis of wide complex tachycardias includes VT, SVT with aberration, SVT with underlying bundle branch block (BBB) or conduction delay, and SVT with ventricular depolarization through an accessory pathway. Several criteria have been developed to distinguish among wide

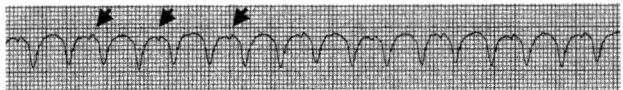

Figure 8 Sustained monomorphic ventricular tachycardia. Note the retrograde P wave seen after every other QRS complex (*arrows*).

complex tachycardias. Factors to be considered include presenting symptoms, past medical history, and the ECG.

Presenting symptoms are not always reliable in deciding whether a wide complex tachycardia is VT or SVT with aberration. Although SVT tends to be more hemodynamically stable, sustained VT does not necessarily cause hemodynamic instability. One should not assume that if a patient is alert and hemodynamically stable, the wide complex tachycardia must be an SVT; the misdiagnosis of VT as SVT, and the treatment as such, may lead to catastrophic consequences.

Past medical history is important in differentiating VT from SVT with aberration (7). In patients with a history of previous heart disease, such as previous MI, heart failure, and congenital heart disease, a wide complex tachycardia is more likely to be VT than SVT and should be presumed to be VT unless one can be sure that it is an SVT with aberration. ☞ **The ECG is quite useful in distinguishing VT from SVT with aberration.** ☞

Ventricular rate is not a useful differentiation between VT and SVT because there is significant overlap between the two. However, AV dissociation, capture beats, and fusion beats are all associated with VT. Right superior axis, that is, −90° to −180°, is more likely to be VT than SVT. Additionally, the wider the QRS complex, the more likely the dysrhythmia is VT rather than SVT. A QRS duration longer than 140 msec with an RBBB morphology and a QRS duration more than 160 msec with an LBBB morphology, are more likely to be VT than SVT. Finally, QRS morphology is useful. In general, SVT with aberration leads to a more typical BBB pattern than VT, whether it is an RBBB or an LBBB pattern, whereas VT usually has a BBB pattern that is bizarre and atypical. The following features of the QRS morphology favor diagnosis of VT: (*i*) concordance of the precordial leads, that is, the QRS complex in the precordial leads are either all negative or all positive; (*ii*) presence of Q waves; and (*iii*) an RS interval longer than 100 msec. These criteria are useful in distinguishing VT from SVT with aberration. However, for most clinicians, distinguishing VT from SVT with aberration and remembering all the criteria is difficult. The more important determination is the patient's hemodynamic status. If the patient is stable, abundant time is available to measure RS intervals, and so on. If the patient is unstable, cardioversion is indicated. ☞ **The criteria for distinguishing VT from SVT include: (*i*) VT is more common than SVT with aberration, especially in patients with structural heart disease, (*ii*) SVT with aberration usually has a typical BBB pattern, (*iii*) when in doubt, treat wide complex tachycardias as VT, and (*iv*) obtain as much electrocardiographic documentation as possible including a 12-lead ECG and rhythm strips of the tachycardia's onset and termination.** ☞

ANTIDYSRHYTHMIC DRUG SELECTION

Many dysrhythmias are triggered by reversible factors such as ischemia, stress, electrolyte imbalance, systemic illness, and drugs. Antidysrhythmic drugs themselves can cause as well as treat dysrhythmias. In a broad sense, the agents that are used to treat underlying illness can be considered to be antidysrhythmic agents. However, in this section, we will focus more on the drugs that are classically classified as antidysrhythmic due to their electrophysiologic effects on the heart (Table 6). Despite some shortcomings, the Vaughn-Williams drug classification system is a useful way of classifying antidysrhythmic agents. Class I drugs affect sodium channels and thus depress the phase 0 (Fig. 9) of the action potential and slow conduction. This group of drugs is further subdivided into A, B, and C depending on their potency and their effect on repolarization. Subclass A has modest effects on the sodium channel, but prolongs repolarization. Subclass B has weak sodium channel-blocking action and has no effect on repolarization. Subclass C is the most potent sodium-channel blocker and has minimal or no effect on repolarization. Class II drugs are those that block beta-receptors. Class III antidysrhythmic drugs are those that prolong repolarization. Class IV drugs are those that block the calcium channel. All antidysrhythmic drugs have undesirable side effects, including the propensity to cause some dysrhythmias. For example, class IA and III drugs can prolong repolarization and cause polymorphic VT (torsades de pointes). Class IC drugs, especially in patients with underlying coronary artery disease, can cause sustained VT. Class II and IV drugs can cause heart block and bradycardia. Class I and III drugs can delay conduction in the His-Purkinje system, especially in patients with underlying conduction system disease, and may cause distal AV block with a very slow or no ventricular escape. Therefore, initiation of antidysrhythmic agents in patients with underlying LBBB or RBBB should be done cautiously.

Class IA drugs include quinidine, procainamide, and disopyramide. Because the class IA drugs affect the atria, AV node, and ventricles, class IA drugs work well for both atrial and ventricular dysrhythmias. It is particularly important to follow QT intervals in patients receiving class IA drugs due to their potential for causing QT prolongation resulting in torsades de pointes. Prolongation of the rate-corrected QT interval (QTc) is idiosyncratic and can occur with the first dose of class IA drugs. In general, drugs should be stopped if the QTc prolongs by 25% or beyond 550 msec.

Class IB drugs include lidocaine, mexiletine, and tocainamide. These drugs are useful in the treatment of ventricular dysrhythmias, but not in the treatment of atrial dysrhythmias. Class IB drugs have sodium channel-blocking effects with minimal QT interval prolongation.

Class IC agents include flecainide, moricizine, and propafenone. These drugs are also sodium-channel blockers but have minimal effects on repolarization. Class IC drugs are particularly useful in both converting and preventing the recurrence of atrial dysrhythmias. Although these drugs also work well for ventricular tachydysrhythmias, they are only employed when all other drugs and RFA are inadequate in patients with structural heart disease, particularly those with coronary artery disease (8). Intravenous forms of these drugs are not available in the United States.

Class III drugs prolong repolarization and affect the sinus node, AV node, atrial tissue, and ventricular tissue. They work well for atrial and ventricular dysrhythmias. Similar to class IA drugs, class III drugs also prolong the QT interval. The QTc interval should be carefully monitored and the drugs discontinued if the QTc interval is prolonged by 25% or beyond 550 msec.

Beta-blockers (class II) and calcium-channel blockers (class IV) drugs have their primary effect on the sinus node and AV node. These drugs are useful for ventricular rate control in atrial tachydysrhythmias, or to treat and prevent tachycardias involving the AV node. Like the class II and IV drugs, adenosine and digoxin affect the AV node, and are

Table 6 Intravenous Antidysrhythmia Drugs of Use in Trauma and Critical Care Patients

IV drugs	Class	Route elimination	Half-life	Doses	Indication
Adenosine	Other	RBC and EC	<10 sec	6–18 mg IV bolus followed by a bolus of flush	Termination of AV node-mediated tachycardia; diagnosis of SVT
Digoxin	Other	Renal	30–50 hrs	0.5 mg IV and then 0.25 mg × 2 over the next 4–8 hrs	Ventricular rate control in patients with LV dysfunction and CHF
Procainamide	IA	Both	6–8 hrs	500 − 1000 mg IV (max 50 mg/min) and then 1–4 mg/min Follow levels	Termination/prevention of atrial dysrhythmias
Lidocaine	IB	Hepatic	1–4 hrs	50–100 mg IV and then 1–4 mg/min	VT due to myocardial ischemia/infarct
Flecanide	IC	Hepatic, 75% Renal, 25%	7–24 hrs	50–100 mg PO BID	SVT (including A-fib/flutter ventricular rhythms only if refractory to other drugs and RFA)
Esmolol	II	RBC	9 min	0.5 mg/kg over 1 min and then 0.05–0.2 mg/kg/min	Termination and prevention of AVNRT and AVRT; ventricular rate control in atrial dysrhythmias
Propranolol	II	Hepatic	1–6 hrs	0.1–1.0 mg q3 min; maximum 10 mg	Termination and prevention of AVNRT and AVRT; ventricular rate control in atrial dysrhythmias
Amiodarone	III	Hepatic	3–15 wks	150 mg over 10 min followed by 1 mg/min for 6 hrs and then 0.5 mg/min	Atrial fibrillation; hemodynamically stable VTs
				300 mg IV push followed by 1 mg/min for incessant VT/V-fib Maximum daily dose of 2 g	Hemodynamically unstable VT and V-fib
Ibutilide	III	Mostly liver	6 hr	1 mg over 10 min and may repeat × 1 in 10 min	Acute termination of atrial dysrhythmias
Diltiazem	IV	Hepatic	3–5 hrs	10–20 mg IV	Termination and prevention of AVNRT and AVRT; ventricular rate control in atrial dysrhythmias
Verapamil	IV	Hepatic	3–7 hrs	5–10 mg IV	Termination and prevention of AVNRT and AVRT; ventricular rate control in atrial dysrhythmias

Abbreviations: AV, atrio-ventricular; AVNRT, AV nodal re-entrant tachycardia; AVRT, AV re-entrant tachycardia; CHF, congestive heart failure; EC, endothelial cells; IV, intravenous; LV, left ventricle; PO, per os; BID, twice a day; RBC, red blood cells; RFA, radiofrequency ablation; SVT, supraventricular tachycardia; V-fib, ventricular fibrillation; VTs, ventricular tachycardias.

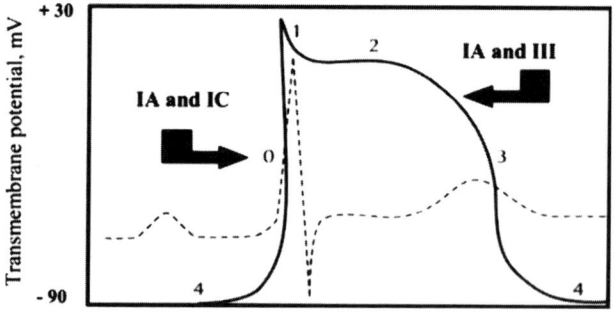

Figure 9 Ventricular muscle transmembrane potential (*solid line*) with superimposed ECG. Phase 4 is the resting membrane potential; phase 0 is the rapid depolarization phase (fast sodium channels open, making the inside of the cell less negative). Phase 1 is when the slower calcium channels open. During phase 2, the potassium channels open. During phase 3 (repolarization), the sodium is pumped back out, the potassium is pumped back inside the cell, and resting membrane potential is restored. Vaughn-Williams class IA and class IC drugs block the fast sodium channels and decrease phase 0. Class IA and class III drugs prolong repolarization reflected in a prolonged QT interval and increased risk of torsades de pointes.

used for ventricular rate control in atrial tachydysrhythmias, or to treat and prevent tachycardias involving the AV node.

PACING AND NONPHARMACOLOGIC INTERVENTIONS
Transcutaneous Pacing
☞ Transcutaneous pacing can be a useful adjunctive therapy in patients who require urgent heart rate support for symptomatic bradycardia. ☞ It can serve as a bridge to transvenous pacing, or be sufficient by itself for those patients whose risk of symptomatic bradycardia is too low to warrant a transvenous pacemaker. The major advantage of transcutaneous pacing is that it is noninvasive, and can be applied quickly by staff members who have no expertise in the insertion of transvenous pacemakers. However, transcutaneous pacing is less reliable and can cause significant discomfort in awake patients. As a result, long-term use is never indicated. During temporary use (in the operating room or ICU), patients should be anesthetized or at least sedated. When using transcutaneous pacing, it is imperative to ensure that each pacing output results in a ventricular capture. Watching only the ECG rhythm strip can be

misleading, because the high-energy output required for transcutaneous pacing may mask the QRS complex on the cardiac monitor. Therefore, a measure of stroke volume must be used to assess the ventricular response to each delivery of the electrical impulse. This is best done by following the arterial pulse in the invasive arterial line. In the absence of an arterial line, this is done by simply checking for a palpable pulse, or by assuring that each pulse-oximeter wave corresponds with a pacing output event.

Temporary Transvenous Pacing

✍ **A transvenous pacemaker is needed in patients with symptomatic bradycardia, whether it is due to sinus node dysfunction or to AV block.** ✍ In general, a single-chamber ventricular pacemaker is adequate for the majority of patients.

There are two types of transvenous pacing catheters: a soft, balloon-tipped catheter, and a stiffer, nonballoon-tipped catheter. In general, a balloon-tipped catheter is preferable. However, during CPR in which there is inadequate cardiac output to direct the balloon into the RV, a stiffer catheter may be more successful. These stiffer catheters are best manipulated under fluoroscopic guidance.

Venous access can be obtained through the left subclavian, right internal jugular, or femoral veins. Placement of a transvenous catheter through the femoral vein requires fluoroscopic guidance.

Once venous access is obtained, a catheter can be placed in the RV using the guidance of intracardiac ECG. A precordial "V" lead is attached to the distal electrode of the catheter with the other four leads attached in standard position. As the catheter tip enters the right atrium, there is a sharp deflection corresponding to the surface P wave. As the catheter tip approaches the tricuspid valve, both the atrial and ventricular deflections can be seen. Once there is only a ventricular signal, the balloon is deflated and the catheter advanced until ST elevation is demonstrated on the monitor (Fig. 10). The distal electrode is attached to the negative pole and the proximal electrode to the positive pole ("proximal" for "positive"). The location of the catheter tip can be determined by the morphology of the paced QRS complex. An apical location of the catheter will give deep negative QRS complexes in leads II, III, and aVF, and a location in the outflow tract will give positive QRS complexes in the same leads.

Once the catheter is positioned, the pacing and sensing thresholds should be determined. The pacing threshold is the lowest amount of energy required to depolarize the ventricle. The pacing threshold is determined by setting the pacing frequency to a rate greater than the intrinsic pulse and then gradually decreasing the pacing output current until there is loss of ventricular capture. The usual ventricular pacing threshold is about 1 mA. The sensing threshold is the amplitude of depolarization or QRS complex detected by the pacemaker. The sensing threshold can be tested by setting the pacing frequency to a level below the intrinsic heart rate and then gradually decreasing the sensing setting on the pacemaker or increasing the millivolt setting. When the sensing is lost and the pacemaker starts pacing, the sensing setting is increased or the millivolt setting is decreased until every QRS complex is appropriately sensed. The maximum millivolt setting at which every QRS complex is sensed is the sensing threshold. One should try to obtain a ventricular sensing threshold of above 5 mV. The pacing and sensing threshold should be

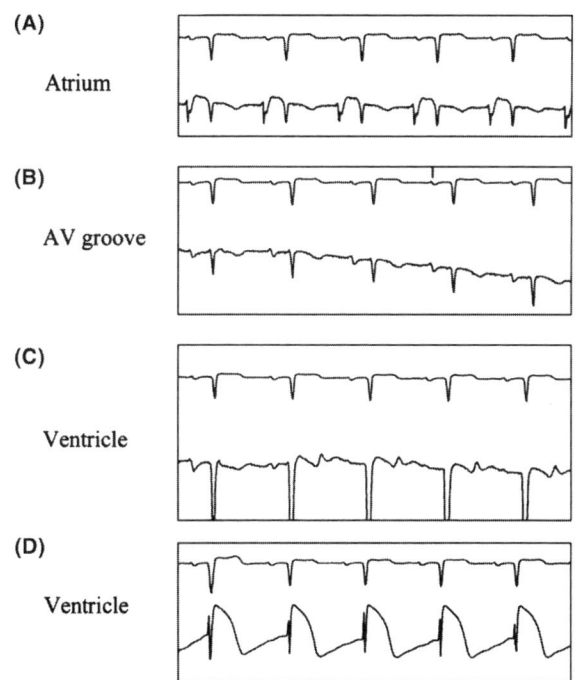

Figure 10 (A–C) Intracardiac electrograms recorded as the pacing wire is advanced from the right atrium, the atrio-ventricular (AV) groove, the right ventricle and then in contact with the ventricular wall. Note ST elevation when the pacing lead comes in contact with the ventricular wall (**D**).

checked daily to ensure proper functioning of the pacemaker.

Once the pacing and sensing thresholds have been determined, a temporary pacemaker can be programmed. In general, the ventricular output is set at 10–20 mA and the sensitivity at 1–2 mV.

Cardioversion Therapy

Transthoracic DC cardioversion is an effective and rapid means to restore normal heart rhythms in patients with tachydysrhythmias. ✍ **When a tachyarrhythmia causes hemodynamic instability, urgent DC cardioversion is recommended.** ✍ The energy should be high enough to effectively terminate the tachyarrhythmia. The biphasic mode is more efficient at an equivalent energy dose. The mean energy for successful cardioversion of A-fib is 200 J with a monophasic waveform and 120 J with a biphasic waveform (9). For cardioversion of A-fib, electrode patches should be placed in an anterior and posterior location rather than anteriorly and apically. Conversion of atrial flutter usually requires less joules (and should be synchronized), whereas version of V-fib requires at least 300 J.

TRAUMA CONDITIONS ASSOCIATED WITH DYSRHYTHMIAS
Myocardial Contusion
Predisposing Mechanisms
Myocardial contusion refers to damage occurring to the myocardium from blunt trauma. The classic setting is a decelerational injury where an individual is moving forward, the chest strikes an immobile or slower object, and the heart is compressed within the thorax. Motor

vehicle accidents or falls from a significant height are common causes of decelerational injuries. However, any mechanical motion that generates stress on the heart or any direct transfer of energy to the heart can result in tissue damage and contusion (10).

It is estimated that anywhere from 16% to 76% of patients who suffer blunt trauma to the chest sustain a myocardial contusion. The huge variation in incidence is due to major differences in the method of defining contusion (11). Also see Volume 1, Chapter 25, and Volume 2, Chapters 19 and 25.

Associated Injuries

A contusion caused by a deceleration injury is often accompanied by other injuries including aortic disruption, coronary or valvular disruption, pulmonary contusion and hemorrhage, and flail chest and tracheobronchial injuries. Patients who sustain more than one of these serious associated injuries often do not survive during transport to the hospital. If they do, the mortality with coexisting chest injuries is high, up to 67% in one series (12). Other less serious injuries, such as sternal fracture, are also associated with myocardial contusions, and when present should increase the awareness that a myocardial contusion may be present (13,14).

Pathology

The pathology of contusion includes hemorrhage, edema and multiple foci of myocyte necrosis, and cellular fragmentation that can result in reduced blood flow and function. Contraction bands, seen in areas of necrosis, may result from ischemia-reperfusion and ionic abnormalities. The RV and septum are most commonly injured because of their location in the anterior portion of the thorax. Histologic lesions are similar to those observed after severe ischemic stress (15). The myocyte damage can result in a decreased contractile force and can affect the coronary vascular bed.

The Diagnosis of Myocardial Contusion

It is known that mechanical injury to the heart can cause abnormalities of conduction, rhythm, and mechanical performance. Identifying the patients likely to have such complications, in order to monitor and treat them accordingly, is very difficult. Depending on diagnostic criteria, between 0% and 76% of patients with blunt chest trauma have a myocardial contusion (11). Because cardiac contusion may be complicated by lethal dysrhythmias, selecting the proper patients for monitoring is important (Table 7).

Contusion is, in essence, a pathological diagnosis, but because most cases of contusion are best diagnosed prior to reaching autopsy, clinical signs and symptoms are sought that would suggest injury. The various criteria for diagnosis include a predisposing mechanism of trauma, ECG abnormalities, cardiac enzyme elevation, and an abnormal echocardiogram.

Electrocardiogram Abnormalities

Many studies have used any abnormality of ECG in the setting of a mechanical force to the chest as diagnostic of contusion. The most common findings are sinus tachycardia and extrasystoles. Frequent conduction abnormalities are RBBB, AV blocks, and A-fib. VT and V-fib are less commonly seen on ECG but are the most feared complications and are the impetus for monitoring patients with contusion. The anterior RV is more often affected by contusion than the more protected LV, so the classic leads do not always detect injury.

Table 7 Diagnostic Criteria for Myocardial Contusion

Diagnostic criterion		Example
I	Predisposing mechanism	Blunt chest trauma
IIa	ECG dysrhythmias and other abnormalities	PACs, PVCs, sinus tachycardia, extrasystoles, right bundle branch block, atrial fibrillation, ventricular tachycardia, ventricular fibrillation
IIb	Elevated troponin	All other markers (CPK, MB) are nonspecific in the setting of trauma or major surgery
IIc	Abnormal echocardiogram (transesophageal or transthoracic)	Abnormal wall function (hypokinesis, dyskinesis, and akinesis) in the injured area (typically right ventricle)
IId	Contusion of heart directly visualized	Thoracotomy autopsy

Note: To make the diagnosis of myocardial contusion, there must be a category I criterion and at least one of the four category II criteria. The more category II criteria present, the higher the diagnostic accuracy.
Abbreviations: CPK, creatine phosphokinase; ECG, electrocardiogram; MB, the CPK isoform predominantly found in cardiac muscle; PACs, premature atrial contractions; PVCs, premature ventricular contractions.

Many patients with contusion may not have any ECG abnormalities on presentation, and concern has been raised that this criterion may eliminate too many patients who need observation. In one study, abnormal ECGs were present in 50% of patients with blunt trauma; the positive predictive value for needing some form of cardiac therapy was 28% with a 95% negative predictive value. In conjunction with troponin I, ECG had a 62% positive predictive value and 100% negative predictive value for blunt cardiac trauma victims requiring cardiac therapy (16). In another study, the presence of ECG abnormalities was 100% sensitive for those needing antidysrhythmic drugs or defibrillation (17). ☞ **Some authors suggest that a normal ECG three hours after minor cardiac trauma can exclude those who might develop cardiac complications (Table 7) (18).** ☞

Cardiac Enzymes

Creatine phosphokinase (CPK) isoenzymes: CPK and CPK-MB (the CPK isoform predominantly found in cardiac muscle) are frequently elevated in trauma patients, and thus, should not be used for diagnosing contusion. Even the MB isoform is released in patients with rhabdomyolysis; it accounts for 1% of CPK activity in skeletal muscle.

Troponin: Troponin T and I are released after both MI and contusion. Troponin I is exclusive to the myocardium and is superior to CPK-MB in diagnosing contusion. Troponin T may have some cross-reactivity with skeletal muscle, but depending on the assay, it too can be useful in detecting myocardial injury (11). Both troponins become positive four to eight hours after injury and peak 24 hours after injury. In animals, troponin I is a marker of anatomic and functional consequences of contusion and correlates well with extent of contusion (10,15,19). ☞ **Troponins are neither 100%**

specific nor sensitive; small injuries with undetectable troponin could lead to dysrhythmias; conversely hemorrhage and shock may lead to troponin release without contusion (10). ✐ In one study, troponin I had a positive predictive value of 48% and negative predictive value of 93% when detecting patients requiring cardiac therapy (16). Another study showed only a 23% sensitivity, a positive predictive value of 77% and negative predictive value of only 75% (11). However, differences in the definition of contusion account for much of the variability in studies of contusion.

If ECG and troponins suggest a MI, then angiography should be considered to detect coronary injuries, especially in young patients. As the population ages, the possibility of concurrent MI in the trauma victim will increase.

Echocardiography
✐ TEE is preferable to transthoracic echocardiography in evaluating trauma patients except for viewing the pericardium (20). It is superior to helical computed tomography (CT) in detecting contusions (21). Unfortunately, the RV is more difficult than the LV to visualize, and the RV is more frequently involved in contusions. ✐ A study of 117 patients with blunt chest trauma showed that 42% had echocardiographic evidence of contusion: RV dysfunction in 32%, LV dysfunction in 15%, and both in 5%. A review of 50 records of patients who suffered sternal fracture and who had echocardiograms revealed that 22% of echocardiograms showed a pericardial effusion, which in no case was associated with other abnormal clinical findings. The authors concluded that a pericardial effusion on echo after trauma is not suggestive of contusion or other injuries (22).

Complications of Contusion
✐ Myocardial contusion is associated with dysrhythmias and functional impairment, especially of the ventricle. ✐ It is also associated with an increased risk of hypotension, dysrhythmias, and arrest in the perioperative period (10). The incidence of complications is highest in the period immediately after injury. Most patients who survive admission to the hospital have a favorable prognosis (11).

Dysrhythmias
Dysrhythmias are important complications because they are insidious, difficult to predict, and occur with increasing frequency when greater myocardial injury has occurred, as quantified by troponin levels (Fig. 11) (23). They can occur even after minor contusions and may be worsened by the metabolic and hemodynamic consequences of other injuries or heart failure. VT and V-fib are the most dangerous. Animal models show that the degree of arrhythmogenesis is related to the increasing kinetic energy of the blow. A blow leads to shortened and dispersed ventricular refractory periods with re-entrant VTs developing around an electrically silent area or a line of fixed conduction block. Almost all contusion-related dysrhythmias are re-entrant (Table 7) (24) (see section on treatment of "Ventricular Tachydysrhythmias").

Following myocardial contusion, A-fib has been noted in 2% to 15% of patients (11). In one series of 312 patients, A-fib was the most significant marker of outcome (25). It is usually treated with antidysrhythmics including cardiac glycosides, but direct cardioversion can be effective as well (26) (see section on treatment of "Atrial Tachydysrhythmias"). Intraoperative dysrhythmias were seen in 6% of patients who had had a myocardial contusion as well as intraopera-

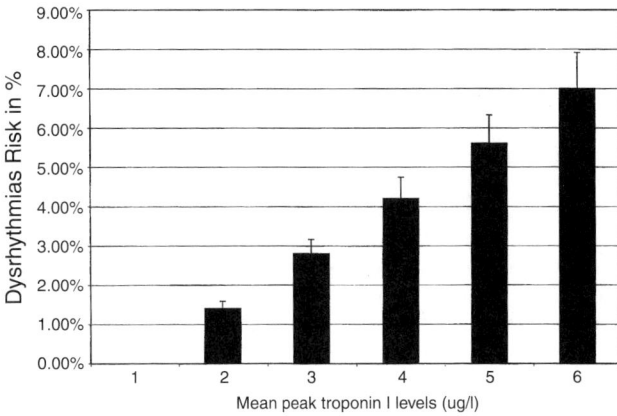

Figure 11 Cardiac troponin I (cTnI) levels increase linearly with the risk of dysrhythmias following myocardial contusion. When the cTnI level is less than 1.0, the risk of dysrhythmia is negligible. *Source*: From Ref. 23.

tive hypotension in 16% (27). ✐ **Risk factors for perioperative mortality associated with contusion are old age, A-fib, and aortic rupture (14).** ✐

Functional Impairment
The RV is commonly involved in contusion, and echocardiography may show impairment of function. Although cardiogenic shock is rarely observed with myocardial contusion, the RV impairment can become significant in patients with pulmonary hypertension or acute respiratory distress syndrome (ARDS). In animal models, there is decreased ventricular compliance after myocardial contusion and shock and early decreases in LV maximal change in pressure over time (dp/dt max) (15).

Therapy for Myocardial Contusion
There is no single therapy that prevents the complications of a myocardial contusion. The presence of RV dysfunction mandates careful preload, manipulation of mechanical ventilation to minimize airway pressures, and attention to other causes of increased RV afterload. Monitoring for dysrhythmias is important, and predisposition to malignant dysrhythmias must be considered when administering any treatment.

Head Trauma and Myocardial Effects
Head trauma, subarachnoid hemorrhage, and other causes of increased ICP can lead to indirect lesions of the heart. It is postulated that increases in sympathetic activity with catecholamine release can lead to myocardial beta-receptor desensitization, coronary vasoconstriction, and myocyte damage (10,24). The elevated catecholamine state should be considered when treating any dysrhythmias (see section "Sinus Tachycardia"). In addition, the prolonged QT syndrome can occur in any head injury, which raises ICP.

Thoracic Blast Injuries/Pulmonary Contusions
Blast injuries result from the direct effect of changes in atmospheric pressure. In addition, injuries can occur from objects accelerated by the blast or from the body itself being propelled by the blast energy. The role of myocardial contusions as a cause of dysrhythmias has been discussed above. Pulmonary

contusions are discussed in Volume 1, Chapter 25, and Volume 2, Chapter 25; however, the dysrhythmogenic blast effect is described here.

The high-energy release of an explosion leads to blast waves that can be propelled faster than the speed of sound. Primary injuries from the blast waves usually occur in gas-containing organs, including the chest. The pulmonary contusions that result are associated with bradycardia and hypotension unrelated to hemorrhage. Animal studies suggest that severe hypotension is not related to myocardial injury but to vagal nerve–mediated bradycardia and cardiogenic shock without compensatory vasoconstriction (28,29). Pulmonary C-fiber stimulation activates a vagal nerve reflex with bradycardia, peripheral vasodilation, and apnea, followed by rapid respirations. Bilateral vagotomy resolves these reflexes in an animal model (28,29). Treatment in patients is supportive, including administration of anticholinergic drugs (atropine and glycopyrollate) and beta-agonists.

Commotio Cordis

Commotio cordis is Latin for "cardiac concussion," and refers to a blunt precordial chest impact that results in dysrhythmias and sudden death without evidence of heart injury at autopsy. Commotio cordis is separate from myocardial contusion because no actual heart damage occurs in the former, and the lethal dysrhythmias are thought to result from a purely electrical phenomenon. Commotio cordis commonly results from low-energy impacts, usually during sporting activities (e.g., baseball impact to anterior chest), where cardiac arrest likely results from ventricle fibrillation or from complete heart block (1). When the timing of a precordial impact occurs precisely within 1/100 of a second period before the peak of the T wave, these minor traumas will reliably result in ventricular fibrillation (30,31). Occasionally, impacts outside of this period result in unsustained polymorphic VT or transient complete heart block if delivered during the QRS complex (30,31).

DRUG INTOXICATIONS AND ASSOCIATED DYSRHYTHMIAS
Cocaine

Cocaine is a powerful sympathomimetic drug; popular for the energized, euphoric state it produces. The most common associated medical problem is chest pain. Cocaine use is also associated with cardiac ischemia and infarction, hypertension, dysrhythmias, sudden death, thrombosis, myocarditis, and cerebrovascular events (32–34).

Cocaine-Induced Cardiovascular Toxicity: Overview

The cardiovascular complications of cocaine are ascribed to its inhibition of norepinephrine reuptake and stimulation of central sympathetic outflow, raising circulating catecholamines up to fivefold (35). The initial effect of cocaine on the cardiovascular system is vagotonic, followed by increased sympathetic stimulation (36). The blood pressure–raising effect of cocaine should normally be offset by a baroreceptor response lowering central sympathetic outflow—cocaine may offset this by directly increasing central sympathetic outflow to the heart leading to tachycardia and increased contractility. It is postulated that patients with conditions that impair baroreflex responses (such as heart failure, long-standing hypertension, or chronic cocaine abuse) may have exaggerated hypertensive responses to cocaine (37). An additional effect of cocaine is

its class I antidysrhythmic properties, which can impair cardiac conduction.

Cocaine-Induced Ischemia

Cocaine-related ischemia can be caused by two mechanisms: (*i*) increased oxygen demand from an elevated heart rate and blood pressure; or (*ii*) decreased flow from vasospasm, coronary constriction, platelet aggregation, or thrombosis (33,38). Long-term use of cocaine is associated with premature atherosclerotic disease. Short- and long-term use are associated with an early coronary vasodilation that is followed by a transient decrease in coronary artery caliber, probably through alpha-adrenergic mechanisms. This constriction is most pronounced in diseased coronaries (33). Some of the vasospasm associated with cocaine may be due to endothelin-1 release that may sensitize the vasculature to vasoconstrictor stimuli (38). Cocaine use is also associated with intravascular thrombosis and platelet activation, predisposing to ischemia and infarction. Smoking exacerbates some of the effects of cocaine. The ECG in cocaine-induced chest pain may be difficult to interpret. J-point and ST-segment elevation due to early repolarization or LV hypertrophy can interfere with the diagnosis of ischemia.

Cocaine-Induced Hypertension

Hypertension and hypertensive crises result from the direct effects of impaired norepinephrine uptake as well as from the enhanced sympathetic outflow. Conversely, hypotension can occur from a state of relative catechol depletion, from paradoxical suppression of the central nervous system (CNS), from ischemia, or from a direct toxic effect on the myocardium.

Cocaine-Induced Dysrhythmias

Dysrhythmias associated with cocaine are diverse and are often associated with other cardiovascular disturbances such as hypertension, hypotension, or MI. It is reported that in 4% to 14% of patients with cocaine-induced MI, ventricular dysrhythmias will occur, with death in less than 2%.

There are many mechanisms whereby cocaine can facilitate dysrhythmias. It has sodium channel-blocking properties, its sympathomimetic effects lower the threshold for fibrillation, and it increases intracellular calcium that can result in afterdepolarizations and triggered dysrhythmias. However, the increased metabolic demands associated with the tachycardia and hypertension of an acute intoxication also predispose the myocardium to dysrhythmias. In the setting of abnormal myocardium, these can be particularly worrisome. Cocaine can produce ventricular dysrhythmias and fibrillation in the setting of ischemia. Long-term cocaine use leads to left ventricular hypertrophy (LVH) that predisposes to ventricular dysrhythmias.

There is evidence that differences in calcium channels may partly explain different sensitivities to cocaine-induced dysrhythmias including AV conduction block and sinus arrest (39). In studies of cocaine toxicity in animals, calcium-channel antagonists prevent malignant dysrhythmias and protect against MI.

Treatment of Cocaine-Induced Ischemia and Dysrhythmias
🖋 **Benzodiazepines and nitroglycerin (NTG) are the first-line agents for patients with cocaine-induced ischemia (40).**
🖋 Benzodiazepines should be administered first as

they protect the brain against many of the ravages of acute cocaine intoxications and also decrease any CNS-mediated manifestations. Both NTG and verapamil reverse cocaine-induced hypertension and vasoconstriction. However, calcium-channel blockers may exacerbate the CNS toxicity of cocaine. Thus, all cocaine-toxic patients should receive benzodiazepine therapy. Furthermore, NTG and calcium-channel blockers should be given only after benzodiazepines have been used to stabilize the CNS (Table 8) (36). Phentolamine has also been shown to reverse cocaine-induced coronary constriction and is considered third-line therapy after benzodiazepine and NTG (32).

☞ **Because beta-blockers exacerbate this constriction, they should be avoided in patients with cocaine use.** ☞ Labetalol is likewise not indicated because the beta-antagonist effects outweigh the alpha-blocking effects. Sodium bicarbonate has been shown to reduce the cocaine-induced widening of the QRS complex and to reduce the incidence of associated VT. The use of benzodizepines is considered first-line therapy, because they attenuate the cardiac and CNS toxicity of cocaine in animal studies (36). The use of aspirin is encouraged on a theoretical basis.

Lidocaine use in cocaine-induced dysrhythmias is controversial because, like cocaine, it is a sodium-channel blocker and could be prodysrhythmic in combination with cocaine. Limited studies suggest that lidocaine is probably safe several hours after cocaine use. Sodium bicarbonate is safe to use immediately following cocaine use and it reverses cocaine-induced QRS prolongation (36). The proposed guidelines from the Toxicologic Oriented ACLS for treatment of cocaine-induced VT/V-fib are sodium bicarbonate and lidocaine and the avoidance of epinephrine and non-selective beta-blockers (40).

Amphetamines

Amphetamines, like cocaine, are sympathomimetic agents. Also like cocaine, the cardiovascular complications from amphetamines can include vasoconstriction, unpredictable blood pressure effects, dysrhythmias, and ischemia (35). The amphetamine class includes amphetamine, metamphetamine, and the popular drug, ecstasy. Ecstasy (3,4-methylenedioxymethamphetamine or "MDMA") is a variant of metamphetamine but also has some of the properties of mescaline (41).

An abundance of evidence suggests that MDMA acts by increasing release of the monoamine neurotransmitters, noradrenaline, and to a lesser extent dopamine and by inhibiting the reuptake of serotonin (41). The increase in noradrenaline is responsible for the cardiac effects; the most common arrhythmia is sinus tachycardia, but sudden death has also been reported. MDMA has a plasma half-life of appproximately eight hours with some active metabolites, so effects may be seen well after the original ingestion (see section on treatment of "Sinus Tachycardia").

Ma Huang and the Ephedra Alkaloids

Ma huang, also known as ephedra, is one of the Chinese herbs belonging to the ephedra alkaloid class. It is a non-catecholamine sympathomimetic agent, which leads to release of endogenous catecholamines and directly stimulates alpha- and beta-receptors (41–43). Excess intake is associated with ischemia, hypertension, stroke, cardiomyopathy, and sudden death in the absence of structural heart disease (42). Dysrhythmias are similar to those induced by commercially available ephedrine and include VT (see section "Ventricular Tachydysrhythmias").

Alcohol

Light to moderate intake of alcohol has been associated with improvements in cardiac risk. Moderate drinking appears to lower the risk of stroke, peripheral vascular disease, and perhaps type 2 diabetes (44). Heavier alcohol consumption (>3 drinks per day) increases the risk of hypertension, dysrhythmias, and hemorrhagic stroke. Chronic heavy alcohol use can be damaging to the heart and is associated with LV hypertrophy, mild systolic or diastolic dysfunction, and occasional biventricular dilatation, resembling a dilated cardiomyopathy (45). Early stages are often asymptomatic and associated with diastolic dysfunction; later symptomatic stages show systolic dysfunction as well (46). Dysrhythmias and other symptoms associated with alcoholic cardiomyopathy are similar to those of other dilated cardiomyopathies (46). ☞ **Acute effects of alcohol intoxication include paroxysmal A-fib, or "holiday heart," which can be seen in healthy patients with structurally normal hearts (Table 3) (46–48).** ☞ In animals, acute alcohol can raise cardiac troponin-T levels, decrease systolic blood pressure, and increase heart rate (49). ☞ **Chronic heavy consumption causes an increase in catecholamine release and is associated with poor contractility, mitochondrial dysfunction, and ventricular dysrhythmias (49–51).** ☞

Table 8 Pharmacotherapy for Cocaine-Induced Ischemia and Dysrhythmias

Priority	Drug	Rational/comments
First line	Benzodiazepines	Most patients with myocardial ischemia while toxic on cocaine have central nervous system effects that will only be controlled with benzodiazepines. Thus, midazolam should be administered first, followed by ativan.
	Nitroglycerin	Whenever myocardial ischemia is the predominant presenting symptom, nitroglycerin is indicated for direct coronary artery dilation.
Second line	Magnesium sulfate	Useful for the management of both atrial and ventricular tachydysrhythmias, including SVT and VT and torsades de pointes.
Third line	Consider sodium bicarbonate	Recommended in cases of severe acidosis (pH < 7.0, and/or rhadidomyolysis, or wide complex dysrhythmias). High-dose cocaine causes type I sodium channel blockade in the myocardium, which can be partially reversed with alkalinization.

Abbreviations: SVT, supraventricular tachycardia; VT, ventricular tachycardia.

Tricyclic Antidepressant Toxicity
Diagnosis

𝔯 Tricyclic antidepressants are a leading cause of morbidity and mortality due to drug intoxication in the United States. Initial ECG changes include widening of the QRS interval to >100 msec, an R-wave amplitude of >3 mm in aVR, and abnormalities in the terminal 40-msec QRS axis (T40-msec) (an axis between 120° and 270° rotation). These abnormalities on the presenting ECG are reported to predict seizures and dysrhythmias. 𝔯 In addition, it has been shown that the degree of QRS widening and T40-msec axis changes and the duration of their abnormality correlate with the likelihood of developing seizures and dysrhythmias. However, there is huge variability in the resolution of these changes and clinical improvement can occur despite persistence of ECG changes in some patients (51). Tricyclic antidepressants can behave like class IA antidysrhythmics and can prolong the QT interval as well (see section "Antidysrhythmic Drug Selection").

Treatment

𝔯 Alkalinization is considered standard treatment for conduction delays or dysrhythmias associated with tricyclic toxicity. 𝔯 The goal is a systemic pH of 7.5 to 7.55; boluses are preferable to constant infusion (40). The beneficial effects of sodium bicarbonate are due to alkalosis and hypertonic sodium. Some have used hypertonic saline to treat tricyclic overdoses, but the experience with saline is not as extensive as with sodium bicarbonate (40). 𝔯 If dysrhythmias are resistant to sodium bicarbonate, then lidocaine is considered the drug of choice. 𝔯 Procainamide is contraindicated due to its class IA properties that are shared by the tricyclics (40). Whom to monitor and how long are difficult questions. Some authors recommend that patients with an abnormal QRS or T40-msec axis should be admitted and monitored for 24 hours with serial ECGs to determine worsening; patients who improve clinically and whose ECGs improve can be discharged from the ICU after that period (51).

Theophylline Toxicity

Theophylline toxicity used to be very common; its incidence has somewhat decreased as beta-agonists, inhaled steroids, and other modalities have become pre-eminent in the treatment of asthma. 𝔯 Theophylline has a narrow therapeutic window and so overdose is not uncommon. The serious complications are hypotension, dysrhythmias, seizures, and death (52). Peak serum concentrations are helpful in predicting toxicity, but chronic users may be toxic at lower serum concentrations. 𝔯 In chronic users, age is a major predictor of toxicity (53).

Dysrhythmias Associated with Theophylline Toxicity

Theophylline has direct effects on membrane depolarization; in addition, it antagonizes endogenous adenosine and has sympathomimetic effects (53). Dysrhythmias associated with theophylline toxicity are most commonly sinus tachycardia; other minor dysrhythmias include ventricular premature contractions, SVTs, and PACs. Major toxicity is associated with SVT, A-fib or flutter with rapid ventricular conduction, and VT.

Treatment of Theophylline-Associated Dysrhythmias

𝔯 Treatment of dysrhythmias should be supportive and accompanied by treatment of the overdose: multiple doses of activated charcoal or hemoperfusion for those at highest risk, cardiorespiratory support, and correction of electrolyte abnormalities. 𝔯 Predictors of toxicity depend on whether the theophylline use is chronic or acute; chronic users are at greater risk of toxicity and the peak serum level is less predictive of toxicity in this group of patients (52). In acute theophylline intoxication, peak serum levels of >110 mg/L predict a 50% chance of major toxicity. In chronic intoxication, serious side effects can occur at lower peak levels, and age is a better predictor of poor outcomes. Many will dialyze theophylline at lower levels: >60 mg/L for chronic ingestion or >80 mg/L with acute ingestion (54).

Other Drugs of Abuse Associated with Dysrhythmias

Lighter fluid, glue, and other volatile hydrocarbons (e.g., toluene, gasoline, solvents, spray paint, and nail polish) are commonly abused by adolescents, and are commonly associated with cardiac dysrhythmias as well as neurotoxic effects. Cardiac dysrhythmias are the main cause of sudden death, and initial as well as prolonged use can lead to hypoxia, seizures, and fatal dysrhythmias (55). Sympathetic activation can lead to tachydysrhythmias and myocardial sensitization (35). Suppression of cardiac conduction or sinus node activity may also be seen (see subsections "Sinus Node Dysfunction" and "Abnormal Atrio-Ventricular Conduction").

Tetrahydrocannabinol (THC), the active ingredient in marijuana, can also cause dysrhythmias in susceptible individuals. Low doses of marijuana can increase sympathetic tone, whereas higher doses lead to bradycardia and hypotension from increased parasympathetic tone.

Drugs and Conditions Associated with QT Prolongation and Torsades de Pointes
Mechanisms Underlying Torsades de Pointes

Torsades de pointes is a polymorphic VT in which the axis of the QRS complex appears to twist around an isoelectric zero point. Torsades de pointes is triggered by early afterdepolarizations, and most commonly occurs in the setting of QT prolongation. Early afterdepolarizations are depolarizing potentials that develop because of failure of normal repolarization. They are referred to as "triggered" because they only occur in the presence of a preceding action potential. They are due to an imbalance in repolarizing currents due to reduced net outward current or enhanced net inward current. This can lead to oscillation of membrane potential, which can conduct to the ventricular myocardium and lead to tachydysrhythmias. Slowed outward potassium currents, enhanced inward calcium currents, or slowed inactivation of inward sodium currents can prolong the QT interval (56,57).

A number of clinical conditions are associated with QTc prolongation (Table 9). Foremost among these are acquired etiologies, including conditions that increase catecholamines, decrease potassium and magnesium (e.g., excessive diuretics), and drugs. Prolonged QT intervals are an important side effect of several antidysrhythmic drugs including class III and some class IA agents (Table 10).

A number of other drugs (Table 10) commonly used in critically ill patients have also been shown to prolong the QTc. There are variations in susceptibility to drug-induced

Table 9 Clinical Conditions Associated with QT Prolongation and Torsades de Pointes

Condition type	Example
Acquired	Drugs (Table 10) causing QT prolongation
	Long pauses or bradycardia
	Short-long-short RR interval sequence
	Adrenergic stimulation
	Hypokalemia, hypomagnesemia, hypocalcemia
	Ischemia, hypoxia, stroke, subarachnoid hemorrhage, HIV, autonomic neuropathy
Hereditary syndrome	Sympathetic activation

torsades de pointes. Some patients have torsades de pointes without a markedly prolonged QT interval suggesting that other modulating factors must exist besides prolongation of the action potential. These modulating factors may include adrenergic stimulation, low heart rate, hypokalemia, ischemia, or hypoxia (57).

Droperidol, Ondansetron, and Food and Drug Administration Black Box Warning

On December 5, 2001, the Food and Drug Administration (FDA) issued a black box warning regarding the use of droperidol because of concerns that droperidol leads to QT prolongation and may increase the risk of torsades. However, many anesthesiologists immediately expressed concerns that the FDA had overreacted, given droperidol's long track record of safety in the treatment of postoperative nausea and vomiting (PONV) (58). To further underscore this reality, Habib et al. (59) used the Freedom of Information Act to gain access to the 273 cases reported to the FDA between November 1, 1997, and January 2, 2002, upon which the FDA based their warning. Their survey of those 273 cases revealed that the vast majority had no direct connection between the administration of droperidol and QT prolongation or torsades (59).

Using a square-root model to simulate the expected prolongation of the QTc interval that would be produced by droperidol 0.625–1.25 mg IV, Paul White's group found that small "antiemetic" doses of droperidol (1.25 mg) would be unlikely to produce clinically significant proarrhythmogenic effects in the perioperative period. Indeed, their calculations predicted QTc prolongation of up to only 18 ± 3 msec (60).

The degree of QTc prolongation and the risk of developing ventricular dysrhythmias following droperidol administration was recently studied by a Charbit et al. (61) in a PONV treatment study, and by White et al. (62) in a perioperative prophylayxsis model. Charbit et al. compared QTc prolongation in patients receiving either 0.75 mg droperidol or 4 mg ondansetron for the treatment of PONV symptoms experienced in the postanesthesia care unit after surgery. The observed mean maximal prolongation in QTc were 17 ± 9 msec for droperidol and 20 ± 13 msec for ondansetron (Fig. 12) (61). These QTc prolongations were similar to those reported by White et al. (62) who demonstrated 15 ± 40, and 22 ± 41 msec for placebo, 0.625 mg droperidol, and 1.25 mg droperidol, respectively. White

Table 10 Antidysrhythmia Drugs Strongly Associated with QT Prolongation and Torsades de Pointes

Classification	Drugs
Class IA Antidysrhythmics (torsades occurs at low-normal doses)	Quinidine
	Procainamide
	Disopyramide
Class III Antidysrhythmics (High doses are typically required to cause Torsades)	Sotalol
	Ibutilide
	Azimilide
	Dofetilide
	Amiodarone (rarely leads to torsades)
Antifungal	Itraconazole
	Ketaconazole
Antihistamine	Terfenadine
	Astemizole
Antioxidant–antiinflammatory	Probucol
Antiparasitic	Chloroquine
	Pentamidine
Antipsychotic/antidepressant	Haloperiodl
	Tricyclic antidepressants
Antiviral	Amantadine
	Indinavir
	Ritonavir
Gastro propulsive	Cisapride
Immunosuppressant	Tacrolimus
Local anesthetic	Cocaine
Natural-occurring poison	Arsenic trioxide[a]
Neuroleptic-tranquilizer	Droperidol[b]
	Phenothiazines
Vasodilator and smooth muscle relaxant	Papaverine

[a]Encountered in contaminated ground water and as an industrial poisoning.
[b]Droperidol received a black box warning by the Food and Drug Administration (FDA) which was most likely not warranted (see text for explaination).
Source: From Ref. 44.

et al. (62) further demonstrated that the droperidol QT prolongations were not different from those achieved with saline placebo, and that other anesthetic drugs (including inhaled vapors) cause modest QT prolongation themselves. An accompanying editorial to the Charbit et al. and White et al. studies provides additional perspective about the general safety of droperidol, despite the clinically insignificant QT prolongation (63).

Treatment of Torsades de Pointes

☞ The mainstay of treatment for torsades de pointes is intravenous magnesium (2 g bolus over two to three minutes, then IV infusion at 2–4 mg/min with second 2 g bolus if necessary), potassium (if K is low), temporary cardiac pacing (at rates of 90–110 to prevent short-term recurrence), and correction of electrolyte imbalance. ☞ Rarely, an isoproterenol infusion to keep the heart rate at >90 is required. Isoproterenol should not be used in congenital forms of prolonged QT syndrome or in patients with ischemia, because beta-stimulation classically exacerbates hereditary long QT syndromes.

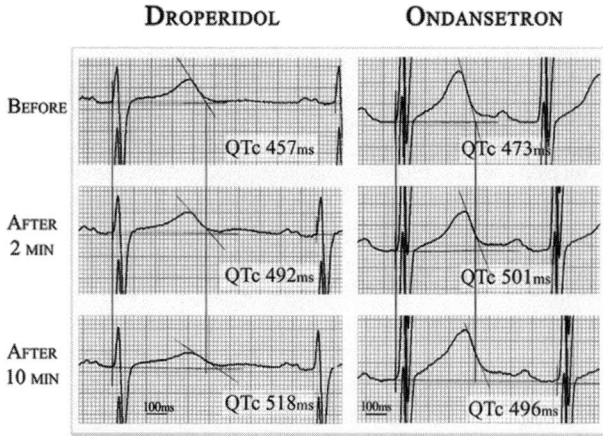

DROPERIDOL   ONDANSETRON

BEFORE   QTc 457ms   QTc 473ms

AFTER
2 MIN   QTc 492ms   QTc 501ms

AFTER
10 MIN   100ms QTc 518ms 100ms QTc 496ms

Figure 12   Electrocardiogram (ECG) recordings in two representative subjects who received 0.75 mg droperidol (female, *left*) or 4 mg of ondansetron (male, *right*) to treat postoperative nausea and vomiting. Upper ECGs were obtained immediately before antiemetic administration, and the recordings performed after 2 and 10 minutes are shown below. The same chest lead is shown for each patient. Note the flattened T wave occurring after droperidol and changes in T-wave morphology after ondansetron. Recordings of ECGs conducted at a paper speed of 50 mm/sec and an amplitude of 20 mm/mV. *Source*: From Ref. 61.

Table 11   Potassium-Related Electrophysiologic Changes Predicted in the Electrocardiogram

Plasma potassium	ECG changes
Hyperkalemia	Decrease T-wave amplitude
	ST-segment depression
	Presence U wave
	Other findings (especially with low Mg^{2+}):
	Prolonged QT
	Extrasystoles
	VT, torsades de pointes, V-fib
Hypokalemia	Early changes:
	Peaked T waves (best seen in leads II, III, and V2–4)
	Later changes:
	P wave widens/flattens
	PR segment lengthens
	P waves disappear
	Terminal changes:
	QRS widens
	QRS merges with T wave: Sine wave pattern degrades to ventricular fibrillation

Abbreviations: ECG, electrocardiogram; V-fib, ventricular fibrillation; VT, ventricular tachycardia.

ELECTROLYTE IMBALANCE–ASSOCIATED DYSRHYTHMIAS
Hypokalemia

Hypokalemia is a risk factor for dysrhythmias including conduction abnormalities and ventricular fibrillation. Potassium is the predominant intracellular cation and is important in the maintenance of the resting membrane potential. Disruption of the potassium gradient can lead to impaired cellular function and dysrhythmias. Hypokalemia increases the transmembrane potential, impairing conduction, enhancing automaticity, and leading to afterdepolarizations. The classic ECG changes of hypokalemia are a low-amplitude T wave associated with a "U" wave and are usually only seen at potassium levels <2.7 mmol/L (Table 11) (64).

In trauma patients, hypokalemia is usually due to catecholamines and the stress response, diuretics, or nasogastric drainage. Hypokalemia is exacerbated by sympathomimetic drugs.

Mild hypokalemia (3–3.5 mmol/L) is usually asymptomatic. More severe hypokalemia (2.5–3.0 mmol/L) may lead to symptoms of malaise, weakness, and constipation; symptoms correlate with the rapidity of the decrease in potassium (67). Severe hypokalemia is associated with rhabdomyolysis and renal magnesium wasting. Conduction abnormalities are unusual in patients without underlying heart disease, even with severe hypokalemia. At potassium levels below 2.5 mmol/L, ventricular extrasystoles may be seen, as well as paroxysmal atrial tachycardia, MAT, A-fib, or flutter (64,65). Severe hypokalemia can increase the likelihood of ventricular dysrhythmias including VT and V-fib (68).

In patients with ischemia, heart failure, or LVH, mild to moderate hypokalemia can lead to dysrhythmias. The prolonged repolarization associated with hypokalemia can lead to torsades de pointes in susceptible patients, especially in those with concurrent hypomagnesemia. In hypertensive patients, potassium depletion associated with diuretic use has been correlated with the presence of ventricular dysrhythmias (69). In the absence of sodium restriction, hypokalemia can lead to increased systolic and diastolic blood pressure, presumably from urinary sodium retention. Hypokalemia may cause resistance to antidysrhythmic drugs (70).

☞ **The treatment of hypokalemia is potassium supplementation, intravenously if dysrhythmias are present. The rate of infusion should be no more than 20 mmol/hr and the ECG should be monitored.** ☞ Glucose-containing solutions should be avoided in the treatment of hypokalemia (71). Glucose can lower potassium levels in patients with initially normal potassium levels as well as in those with hypokalemia. This is presumably due to the stimulation of insulin, which drives potassium into cells and lowers serum potassium levels. Studies and case reports have shown decreases in serum potassium, the appearance of life-threatening cardiac dysrhythmias, and worsening muscle weakness during the infusion of potassium with glucose for the treatment of hypokalemia (Table 12). In addition to potassium, magnesium should be repleted because hypomagnesemia is often coexistent and can impair repletion of potassium.

Hyperkalemia

In trauma patients, hyperkalemia may be due to renal failure or rhabdomyolysis (following burns, crush injuries, or compartment syndromes). Transient elevations in potassium may also be seen following the use of succinylcholine or as a result of acute acidosis.

Hyperkalemia reduces the transmembrane potential, which results in a shortened action potential, increased conduction, and lessened automaticity. In extreme cases, it can lead to very prolonged cardiac conduction manifesting as

Table 12 Treatment of Abnormalities in Plasma Potassium Concentration

Treatment of hypokalemia	Treatment of hyperkalemia
Potassium: IV not >20 mm	Calcium IV
Monitor the ECG	Sodium bicarbonate IV
Proceed with extreme care if abnormal renal function	Insulin 10 units regular IV
Avoid glucose-containing solutions	Dextrose 50% ampule IV
Replete magnesium	β-agonist
	Diuretic

Abbreviations: ECG, electrocardiogram; IV, intravenously.

peaked T waves on ECG followed by QRS prolongation appearing as sine wave activity (Table 11) (72). This must be treated emergently.

✍ **Acute treatment of hyperkalemia consists of membrane stabilization with calcium and transcellular shifting of potassium facilitated by insulin, glucose, bicarbonate, and beta-agonists.** ✍ Removal of potassium takes longer to accomplish and can be done with dialysis for severe cases, loop diuretics, fluodrocortisone, or cation exchange resins (Table 12).

Hypomagnesemia

Hypomagnesemia is a common condition associated with trauma and critical care. Hypomagnesemia is caused by decreased intestinal absorption or increased excretion through the kidneys. Renal excretion is enhanced by osmotic diuresis, as seen in hyperglycemia, or by drugs such as ethanol, aminoglycosides, or cisplatinum (73). Hypomagnesemia leads to irritable membranes in both nervous and cardiac conduction tissues. Hypomagnesemia, like hypokalemia and hypocalcemia, can lead to prolongation of the action potential and triggered afterdepolarizations, which may lead to torsades de pointes.

✍ **Treatment of hypomagnesemia is repletion of magnesium. This may be done by a single 2-g bolus of magnesium over two to three minutes followed by an infusion of 2–4-mg/min in severe cases.** ✍ The usual total deficit is 1–2 mEq/kg of body weight; twice this amount must be administered to account for renal excretion of the repleted cation. This can be repleted more slowly by giving 49 mEq IV over three to six hours and repeating every 12 hours as necessary (73).

Hypermagnesemia

Increased magnesium lowers the transmembrane potential, stabilizes the membrane, and lessens automaticity and afterdepolarizations. It can occasionally cause slowed AV conduction and ventricular conduction. In general, the arrhythmogenic risk of low magnesium is much greater than that of elevated magnesium levels, and hypermagnesemia is not usually associated with clinical dysrhythmias (72). At the neuromuscular junction, the action of magnesium is antagonized by calcium.

Treatment of pre-eclampsia with magnesium leads to marked maternal hypercalciuria, decreased serum calcium and ionized calcium, and an increase in parathyroid hormone in response. However, clinically significant hypocalcemia in either mother or fetus is unusual (74). ✍ **If hyper-**

magnesemia is symptomatic and causing CNS depression, administration of calcium is appropriate. ✍ Calcium can be given as 10 cc of 10% calcium gluconate diluted in 50–100cc of D5W and repeated, depending on calcium levels (73).

Further treatment, though rarely required, consists of renal excretion of magnesium, which can usually be accomplished with fluid administration and furosemide. Dialysis is necessary in symptomatic patients with renal failure.

Hypocalcemia

Hypocalcemia, although less important in triggering dysrhythmias than hypokalemia and hypomagnesemia, is nevertheless a factor in prolonged action potential duration and triggered afterpotentials. The ionized calcium should be checked to determine if arrhythmogenic hypocalcemia is present; total calcium may be misleading if albumin levels are abnormal. Hypocalcemia can contribute to susceptibility to torsades de pointes. It can also mask digitalis toxicity. The ECG in hypocalcemia shows prolongation of the QTc interval.

Risk factors for hypocalcemia include renal failure, alkalosis, gastrointestinal bleeding, pancreatitis, and large volume transfusions of blood products due to the presence of the anticoagulant citrate-phosphate-dextrose (CPD) (73). Another important source of hypokalemia in critical care is renal replacement therapies, which commonly utilize citrate anticoagulant. Postoperative patients at risk for hypocalcemia include those following parathyroid adenoma resection (Volume 2, Chapter 61).

Symptoms of hypocalcemia include tetany, tingling, paresthesias, and in severe cases, seizures. ✍ **The treatment of hypocalcemia is IV repletion of calcium, which can be accomplished by either 10% calcium gluconate (93 mg of calcium per 10 cc) or 10% calcium chloride (272 mg of calcium per 10 cc) (73).** ✍ Both agents should be diluted to prevent venous irritation. In patients with possible digitalis toxicity, calcium should be given slowly with ECG monitoring, because it can enhance the effects of digitalis.

Hypercalcemia

✍ **Excess extracellular calcium rarely leads to dysrhythmias.** ✍ Excess intracellular calcium, from catecholamines, ischemia, or digoxin, for example, may lead to dysrhythmias but these rhythms are not treated by lowering extracellular calcium. The ECG in hypercalcemia is characterized by prolongation of the PR interval, widened QRS, and shortening of the QT interval, followed by prolongation of the T wave (which may then normalize the QT interval) (74). The enhanced myocardial contractility associated with hypercalcemia can rarely result in midsystolic arrest.

Hypercalcemia is treated by saline hydration and loop diuretics to enhance renal excretion of calcium. Calcitonin and biphosponates can be used if saline hydration is inadequate. Octreotide does not lower plasma calcium; its use is only in prevention of stones.

Hyponatremia and Hypernatremia

Hyponatremia and hypernatremia, while requiring correction due to CNS effects, are not associated with particular dysrhythmias. The diagnostic significance and treatment of these, and other, electrolyte disorders are discussed in Volume 2, Chapter 44.

EYE TO THE FUTURE

Many of the recent advances in dysrhythmia management have occurred in the area of catheter-based ablation and device-based therapy. Catheter-guided RFA therapy has become the treatment of choice for various SVTs including accessory pathway-mediated tachycardia, AVNRT, EAT, and atrial flutter. More recently, there have been significant advances in our understanding of A-fib, and catheter-based ablation of A-fib is still time-consuming but increasingly successful. It appears that the posterior wall of the left atrium near the pulmonary veins is a key area in the initiation of A-fib. Catheter-based ablation targeted to this area appears very promising, with a high success rate and a low complication rate (75,76). If these early findings can be reproduced, catheter-based ablation of A-fib may become a more routine procedure.

Device-based therapy of dysrhythmias is another area of rapid development. It has been shown that automatic implantable cardiac defibrillators (AICDs) are more effective than antidysrhythmic drugs in treating VT and V-fib (4,5). Furthermore, indications for AICD implantation are expanding and an increasing number of patients are eligible for an AICD device. It has also become more common to see these devices in critically ill patients. Understanding and management of these devices by critical care providers will be important.

Most of the dysrhythmias seen in critical care settings such as paroxysmal SVT, A-fib, atrial flutter, and VT respond well to currently available antidysrhythmic therapies. However, the need still remains: (*i*) to deliver therapies that are more effective with fewer side effects and (*ii*) to identify patients who are more likely to develop dysrhythmias. Development of therapies with higher efficacy with few or no side effects is the goal of new therapeutic approaches. One of the major drawbacks of the currently available antidysrhythmic agents is their effect on other organs. Delivery of drugs to the target tissues by either local delivery or targeted delivery systems may lessen the systemic complications. One example of this approach is delivery of antidysrhythmic agents to the pericardial space to obtain high myocardial concentration without significant systemic concentration. In addition, there are drugs in development for atrial dysrhythmias that are specific to atrial tissue and thus avoid potential ventricular prodysrhythmias.

Another area of future advancement will be in targeting patients at high risk for dysrhythmias through genetic testing. For example, electrolyte disturbances such as hypokalemia and hypomagnesemia and the usage of QT-prolonging medications are common in the critical care setting. Unfortunately, QT prolongation and torsades de pointes are not uncommon in trauma and critical care. Although only a small fraction of trauma patients develop acute MI (Volume 2, Chapter 19), many develop dysrhythmias. Along with improved monitoring techniques, identification of these susceptible patients using noninvasive markers, or with genetic testing, may facilitate management of these patients and may become feasible in the near future.

SUMMARY

Dysrhythmias are commonly associated with critical illness and trauma. Bradyarrhythmias should be treated only when symptomatic. At such time, placement of an external or transvenous pacemaker (depending on the availability of devices and personnel) can be life-saving. Atrial and ventricular tachydysrhythmias can often be distinguished from each other by past medical history as well as by distinguishing features on the ECG. Treatment of hemodynamically stable atrial and ventricular dysrhythmias can be accomplished with medical therapy. Atrial and ventricular dysrhythmias in unstable patients must be treated promptly with electrical cardioversion or pacing.

Many mechanisms of trauma, such as decelerating injuries, blunt trauma to the chest, blast injuries, and head trauma can cause myocardial contusions complicated by dysrhythmias. Careful diagnosis and monitoring are essential to the care of these patients.

Overdoses of medications and other substances are commonly seen in emergency departments and associated with acute trauma, and can lead to critical illness and dysrhythmias. Treatment of these overdoses and dysrhythmias is tailored to the substance ingested; for example, tricyclic overdoses are treated with alkalinization, and then lidocaine if dysrhythmias persist. Cocaine overdoses are treated with benzodiazepines as first-line therapy along with NTG; beta-blockers are avoided in this setting.

Other common causes of dysrhythmias in critical illness and trauma are related to electrolyte disturbances. Hypokalemia and hypomagnesemia are the most common and are treated with prompt IV replacement. Hyperkalemia can be life-threatening and should be treated emergently if ECG changes are detected. Because potassium is painful when administered to peripheral veins, it should be given via central line or via a peripherally inserted central catheter (PICC) line whenever possible.

KEY POINTS

- Bradycardia per se does not require specific treatment as long as it does not cause symptoms of hemodynamic compromise.
- Heart block at the level of the AV node usually does not require invasive therapy and only requires withdrawal of the offending agents, such as beta-blockers and calcium-channel blockers.
- Sinus tachycardia usually has a gradual onset and termination.
- Acute conversion of atrial tachydysrhythmias to sinus rhythm can be accomplished either by synchronized DC cardioversion or by administration of antidysrhythmic agents.
- Treatment of AV node-mediated tachycardias (AVNRT and AVRT) can be accomplished by administering drugs that increase the refractory period of the AV node. These drugs include calcium-channel blockers, beta-blockers, digoxin, and adenosine.
- Acute treatment of pre-excited A-fib should be targeted at slowing conduction in the accessory pathway rather than in the AV node. Pre-excited A-fib can be treated acutely with cardioversion (if patient is hemodynamically unstable) or adenosine, intravenous procainamide, ibutilide (1,2), or amiodarone (3).
- Of the nonsustained VTs, nonsustained polymorphic VTs with a rapid ventricular rate require special attention, because these unstable dysrhythmias are very likely to progress to V-fib.
- Hemodynamically unstable VT should be treated promptly with DC electrical cardioversion.

- Hemodynamically stable VT can be treated with a pharmacologic agent. The first line of treatment is intravenous amiodarone or procainamide.
- The ECG is quite useful in distinguishing VT from SVT with aberration.
- The criteria for distinguishing VT from SVT include: (*i*) VT is more common than SVT with aberration, especially in patients with structural heart disease, (*ii*) SVT with aberration usually has a typical BBB pattern, (*iii*) when in doubt, treat wide complex tachycardias as VT, and (*iv*) obtain as much electrocardiographic documentation as possible including a 12-lead ECG and rhythm strips of the tachycardia's onset and termination.
- Transcutaneous pacing can be a useful adjunctive therapy in patients who require urgent heart rate support for symptomatic bradycardia.
- A transvenous pacemaker is needed in patients with symptomatic bradycardia, whether it is due to sinus node dysfunction or to AV block.
- When a tachyarrhythmia causes hemodynamic instability, urgent DC cardioversion is recommended.
- Some authors suggest that a normal ECG three hours after minor cardiac trauma can exclude those who might develop cardiac complications.
- Troponins are neither 100% specific nor sensitive; small injuries with undetectable troponin could lead to dysrhythmias; conversely hemorrhage and shock may lead to troponin release without contusion.
- TEE is preferable to transthoracic echocardiography in evaluating trauma patients except for viewing the pericardium. It is superior to helical computed tomography (CT) in detecting contusions. Unfortunately, the RV is more difficult than the LV to visualize, and the RV is more frequently involved in contusions.
- Myocardial contusion is associated with dysrhythmias and functional impairment, especially of the ventricle.
- Risk factors for perioperative mortality associated with contusion are old age, A-fib, and aortic rupture.
- Benzodiazepines and nitroglycerin (NTG) are the first-line agents for patients with cocaine-induced ischemia.
- Because beta-blockers exacerbate this constriction, they should be avoided in patients with cocaine use.
- Acute effects of alcohol intoxication include paroxysmal A-fib or "holiday heart," which can be seen in healthy patients with structurally normal hearts.
- Chronic heavy consumption causes an increase in catecholamine release and is associated with poor contractility, mitochondrial dysfunction, and ventricular dysrhythmias.
- Tricyclic antidepressants are a leading cause of morbidity and mortality due to drug poisoning in the United States. Initial ECG changes include widening of the QRS interval to >100 msec, an R-wave amplitude of >3 mm in aVR, and abnormalities in the terminal 40-msec QRS axis (T40-msec) (an axis between 120° and 270° rotation). These abnormalities on the presenting ECG are reported to predict seizures and dysrhythmias.
- Alkalinization is considered standard treatment for conduction delays or dysrhythmias associated with tricyclic toxicity.
- If dysrhythmias are resistant to sodium bicarbonate, then lidocaine is considered the drug of choice.

- Theophylline has a narrow therapeutic window and so overdose is not uncommon. The serious complications are hypotension, dysrhythmias, seizures, and death (54). Peak serum concentrations are helpful in predicting toxicity, but chronic users may be toxic at lower serum concentrations.
- Treatment of dysrhythmias should be supportive and accompanied by treatment of the overdose: multiple doses of activated charcoal or hemoperfusion for those at highest risk, cardiorespiratory support, and correction of electrolyte abnormalities.
- The mainstay of treatment for torsades de pointes is intravenous magnesium (2-g bolus over two to three minutes, then IV infusion at 2–4 mg/min with second 2-g bolus if necessary), potassium (if K is low), temporary cardiac pacing (at rates of 90–110 to prevent short-term recurrence), and correction of electrolyte imbalance.
- The treatment of hypokalemia is potassium supplementation, intravenously if dysrhythmias are present. The rate of infusion should be no more than 20 mmol/hr and the ECG should be monitored.
- Acute treatment of hyperkalemia consists of membrane stabilization with calcium and transcellular shifting of potassium facilitated by insulin, glucose, bicarbonate, and beta-agonists.
- Treatment of hypomagnesemia is repletion of magnesium. This may be done by a single 2-g bolus of magnesium over two to three minutes followed by an infusion of 2–4 mg/min in severe cases.
- If hypermagnesemia is symptomatic and causing CNS depression, administration of calcium is appropriate.
- The treatment of hypocalcemia is IV repletion of calcium, which can be accomplished by either 10% calcium gluconate (93 mg of calcium per 10 cc) or 10% calcium chloride (272 mg of calcium per 10 cc).
- Excess extracellular calcium rarely leads to dysrhythmias.

REFERENCES

1. Glatter KA, Dorostkar PC, Yang Y, et al. Electrophysiological effects of ibutilide in patients with accessory pathways. Circulation 2001; 104(16):1933–1939.
2. Varriale P, Sedighi A, Mirzaietehrane M. Ibutilide for termination of atrial fibrillation in the Wolff-Parkinson-White syndrome. Pacing Clin Electrophysiol 1999; 22(8):1267–1269.
3. Fuster V, Ryden LE, Asinger RW, et al. Guidelines for the management of patients with atrial fibrillation. A report of the American College of Cardiology/American Heart Association and the European Society of Cardiology ACC/AHA/ESC. Eur Heart J 2001; 22(20):1852–1923.
4. Buxton AE, Lee KL, Fisher JD, et al. Multicenter Unsustained Tachycardia Trial investigators: a randomized study of the prevention of sudden death in patients with coronary artery disease. N Eng J Med 1999; 341:1882–1890.
5. Moss AJ, Hall WJ, Cannom DS, et al. Improved survival with an implanted defibrillator in patients with coronary disease at high risk for ventricular arrhythmias. N Eng J Med 1996; 335:1933–1940.
6. Guidelines 2000 for Cardiopulmonary Resuscitation and Emergency Cardiovascular Care. Part 6: section 1: Introduction to ACLS 2000: overview of recommended changes in ACLS from the guidelines 2000 conference. The American Heart Association in collaboration with the International Liaison Committee on Resuscitation. Circulation 2000; 102(8 suppl):I86–189.

7. Baerman JM, Morady F, DiCarlo LA, et al. Differentiation of ventricular tachycardia from SVT with aberration. Ann Intern Med 1987; 106:807–814.

8. Echt DS, Liebson PR, Mitchell LB, et al. Mortality and morbidity in patients receiving encainide, flecainide or placebo: the cardiac arrhythmia suppression trial. N Eng J Med 1991; 324:781–788.

9. Page RL, Kerber RE, Russell JK, et al. Biphasic versus monophasic shock waveform for conversion of atrial fibrillation: the results of an international randomized, double-blind multicenter trial. J Am Coll Cardiol 2002; 39(12):1956–1963.

10. Orliaguet G, Ferjani M, Riou B. The heart in blunt trauma. Anesthesiology 2001; 95(2):544–548.

11. Bertinchant JP, Polge A, Mohty D, et al. Evaluation of incidence, clinical significance, and prognostic value of circulating cardiac troponin I and T elevation in hemodynamically stable patients with suspected myocardial contusion after blunt chest trauma. J Trauma 2000; 48(5):924–931.

12. Swan KG, Swan BC, Swan KG. Decelerational thoracic injury. J Trauma 2001; 51(5):970–974.

13. Martin M, Mullenix P, Rhee, et al. Troponin increases in the critically injured patient: mechanical trauma or physiologic stress? J Trauma 2005; 59(5):1086–1091.

14. Wojcik JB, Morgan AS. Sternal fractures: the natural history. Ann Emerg Med 1988; 17:912–914.

15. Okubo N, Hombrouck C, Fornes P, et al. Cardiac Troponin I and Myocardial Contusion in the Rabbit. Anesthesiology 2000; 93(3):811–817.

16. Salim A, Velmahos GC, Jindal A, et al. Clinically significant blunt cardiac trauma: role of serum troponin levels combined with electrocardiographic findings. J Trauma 2001; 50(2):237–243.

17. Healey MA, Brown R, Fleiszer D. Blunt cardiac injury: is the diagnosis necessary? J Trauma 1990; 30:137–146.

18. Wisner DH, Reed WH, Riddick RS. Suspected myocardial contusion: triage and indication for monitoring. Ann Surg 1990; 212:82–86.

19. Bertinchant JP, Robert E, Polge A, et al. Release kinetics of cardiac troponin I and cardiac troponin T in effluents from isolated perfused rabbit hearts after graded experimental myocardial contusion. J Trauma 1999; 47(3):474–480.

20. Garcia-Fernandez MA, Lopez-Perez JM, Perez-Castellano N, et al. Role of transesophageal echocardiography in the assessment of patients with blunt chest trauma: correlation of echocardiographic findings with the electrocardiogram and creatine kinase monoclonal antibody measurements. Am Heart J 1998; 135(3):476–481.

21. Vignon P, Boncoeur MP, Francois B, et al. Comparison of multiplane transesophageal echocardiography and contrast-enhanced helical CT in the diagnosis of blunt traumatic cardiovascular injuries. Anesthesiology 2001; 94(4):615–622.

22. Wiener Y, Achildiev B, Karni T, et al. Echocardiogram in sternal fracture. Am J Emerg Med 2001; 19(5):403–405.

23. Rajan GP, Zellweger R. Cardiac troponin I as a predictor of arrithymia and ventricular dysfunction in trauma patients with myocardial contusion. J Trauma 2004; 57(4):801–808.

24. Robert E, de La Coussaye JE, Aya AGM, et al. Mechanisms of ventricular arrhythmias induced by myocardial contusion. Anesthesiology 2000; 92:1132–1143.

25. Van Wijngaarden MH, Karmy-Jones R, Talwar MK, et al. Blunt cardiac injury: a 10 year institutional review. Injury 1997; 28:51–55.

26. Ellis DY, Hutchinson NP. Synchronized direct current cardioversion of atrial fibrillation after blunt chest trauma. J Trauma—Injury Infection & Critical Care 2000; 49(2): 342–344.

27. Baum VC. The patient with cardiac trauma. J Cardiothorac Vasc Anesth 2000; 14:71–81.

28. Wightman JM, Gladish SL. Explosions and blast injuries. Annals of Emergency Medicine 2001; 37(6):664–678.

29. Irwin RJ, Lerner MR, Bealer JF, et al. Shock after blast wave injury is caused by a vagally mediated reflex. J Trauma—Injury Infection & Critical Care 1999; 47(1):105–110.

30. Curfman GD. Fatal impact—concussion of the heart. N Engl J Med 1998; 338(25):1841–1843.

31. Link MS, Wang PJ, Pandian NG, et al. An experimental model of sudden death due to low-energy chest-wall impact (commotio cordis). N Engl J Med 1998; 338(25):1805–1811.

32. Lange RA, Hillis LD. Medical progress: cardiovascular complications of cocaine use. N Engl J Med 2001; 345(5): 351–358.

33. Benzaquen BS, Cohen V, Eisenberg MJ. Effects of cocaine on the coronary arteries. Am Heart J 2001; 142(3):402–410.

34. Curtis BM, O'Keefe JHL. Autonomic tone as a cardiovascular risk factor: the dangers of chronic fight or flight. Mayo Clin Proc 2002; 77(1):45–54.

35. Ghuran A, van der Wieken LR, Nolan J. Cardiovascular complications of recreational drugs: are an important cause of morbidity and mortality. BMJ 2001; 323(7311):464–466.

36. Hollander JE. Current concepts: the management of cocaine-associated myocardial ischemia. N Engl J Med 1995; 333(19):1267–1272.

37. Tuncel M, Wang Z, Arbique D, et al. Mechanism of the blood pressure-raising effect of cocaine in humans. Circulation 2002; 105(9):1054–1059.

38. Wilbert-Lampen U, Seliger C, Zilker T, et al. Cocaine increases the endothelial release of immunoreactive endothelin and its concentrations in human plasma and urine: reversal by coincubation with sigma-receptor antagonists. Circulation 1998; 98(5):385–390.

39. Shi B, Heavner JE, Wang MJ, et al. Calcium channel blockade differentially modifies sensitivity to cocaine-induced arrhythmias in two genetically-selected strains of rats. Circulation 1997; 96(8 suppl):293-I.

40. Albertson TE, Dawson A, de Latorre F, et al. TOX-ACLS: toxicologic-oriented advanced cardiac life support. Ann Emerg Med 2001; 37(4 suppl):S78–S90.

41. Kalant H. The pharmacology and toxicology of "ecstasy" (MDMA) and related drugs. Can Med Assoc J 2001; 165(7):917–928.

42. Samenuk D, Link MS, Homoud MK, et al. Adverse cardiovascular events temporally associated with ma huang, an herbal source of ephedrine. Mayo Clin Proc 2002; 77(1):12–16.

43. Ang-Lee MK, Moss J, Yuan CS. Herbal medicines and perioperative care. JAMA 2001; 286(2):208–216.

44. Klatsky AL. Should patients with heart disease drink alcohol? JAMA 2001; 285(15):2004–2006.

45. Kajander OA, Kupari M, Laippala P, et al. Dose dependent but non-linear effects of alcohol on the left and right ventricle. Heart 2001; 86(4):417–423.

46. Piano MR. Alcoholic cardiomyopathy: incidence, clinical characteristics, and pathophysiology. Chest 2002; 121(5):1638–1650.

47. Prystowsky EN, Benson DW Jr, Fuster V, et al. Management of patients with atrial fibrillation: a statement for healthcare professionals from the subcommittee on electrocardiography and electrophysiology, American Heart Association. Circulation 1996; 93(6):1262–1277.

48. Thornton JR. Atrial fibrillation in healthy non-alcoholic people after an alcoholic binge. Lancet 1984; II:1013–1015.

49. Patel VB, Ajamal R, Sherwood RA, et al. Cardioprotective effect of propranolol from alcolol-induced heart muscle damage as assessed by plasma cardiac troponin-t. Alcoholism: Clin & Exp Res 2001; 25(6):882–889.

50. Fenton RA, Chung ES. Chronic ethanol enhances adenosine antiadrenergic actions in the isolated rat heart. Alcoholism: Clin & Exp Res 2001; 25(7):968–975.

51. Liebelt EL, Ulrich A, Francis PD, et al. Serial electrocardiogram changes in acute tricyclic antidepressant overdoses. Crit Care Med 1997; 25(10):1721–1726.

52. Shannon M. Predictors of major toxicity after theophylline overdose. Ann Int Med 1993; 119(12):1161–1167.

53. Raggi P. Therapeutic theophylline levels and adverse cardiac events. Ann Int Med 1994; 120(10):891.

54. Zimmerman, JL. Drug overdoses. 16th Comprehensive update and board review. Crit Care Med. April 2002.

55. Bruner AB, Fishman M. Adolescents and illicit drug use. JAMA 1998; 280(7):597–598.
56. Khan IA. Clinical and therapeutic aspects of congenital and acquired long QT syndrome. Am J Med 2002; 112(1):58–66.
57. Tan HL, Hou CJY, Lauer MR, et al. Electrophysiologic mechanisms of the long QT interval syndromes and torsade de pointes. Ann Int Med 1995; 122(9):701–714.
58. White PF. Droperidol: a cost-effective antiemetic for over thirty years (editorial). Anesth Analg 2002; 95:789–790.
59. Habib AS, Gan TJ. Food and Drug administration black box warning on the perioperative use of droperidol: a review of the cases. Anesth Analg 2003; 96:1377–1379.
60. Zhang Y, Luo Z, White PF. A model for evaluating droperidol's effect on the median QTc interval. Anesth Analg 2004; 98:1330–1335.
61. Charbit B, Albaladejo P, Funck-Brentano C. Prolongation of QTc interval after postoperative nausea and vomiting treatment by droperidol or ondansetron. Anesthesiology 2005; 102(6):1094–1100.
62. White PF, Song D, Abrao J, et al. Effect of Low-dose droperidol on the QT interval during and after general anesthesia: a placebo-controlled study. Anesthesiology 2005; 102(6):1101–1105.
63. Scuderi PE. You (still) can't disprove the existence of dragons. Anesthesiology 2005; 102(6):1081–1082.
64. Slovis C, Jenkins R. Conditions not primarily affecting the heart. BMJ 2002; 324(7349):1320–1323.
65. Agarwal A, Wingo CS. Treatment of hypokalemia. N Eng J Med 1999; 340(2):154–155.
66. Gennari FJ. Current concepts: hypokalemia. N Eng J Med 1998; 339(7):451–458.
67. Christians KK, Wu B, Quebbeman EJ, et al. Postoperative atrial fibrillation in noncardiothoracic surgical patients. Am J Surg 2001; 182(6):713–715.
68. Hayakawa M, Sugimoto S, Matsubara I, et al. Ventricular fibrillation after pseudo-Bartter's syndrome. Ann Emerg Med 2002; 39(2);205–206.
69. He FJ, MacGregor G. A beneficial effects of potassium. Brit Med J 2001; 323(7311):497–501.
70. Wong KC. Hypokalemia and dysrhythmias. J Cardiothorac Anesth 1989; (5):529–531.
71. Gennari JF. Treatment of hypokalemia. N Eng J Med 1999; 340(2):154–155.
72. Ramaswamy K, Hamdan MH. Ischemia, metabolic disturbances, and arrhythmogenesis: mechanisms and management. Crit Care Med 2000; 28(10 suppl):N151–N157.
73. Rippe JM, et al. Intensive Care Medicine. 3rd ed. Little, Brown and Company, 1996.
74. Cruikshank DP, Chan GM, Doerrfeld D. Alterations in vitamin D and calcium metabolism with magnesium sulfate treatment of preeclampsia. Am J Ob & Gyn 1993; 168(4):1170–1177.
75. Pappone C. Mortality, morbidity, and quality of life after circumferential pulmonary vein ablation for atrial fibrillation: outcomes from a controlled nonrandomized long-term study. J Am Coll Cardiol 2003; 42(2):185–197.
76. Chen MS. Pulmonary vein isolation for the treatment of atrial fibrillation in patients with impaired systolic function. J Am Coll Cardiol 2004; 43(6):1004–1917.
77. Prystowsky EN. Supraventricular arrhythmias. In: Messerli FH, ed. Cardiovascular Drug Therapy. Philadelphia, PA: W.B. Saunders CO. 1990:1207–1285.

21

Transesophageal Echocardiography for Trauma and Critical Care

Peter Mair

Department of Anesthesia and Intensive Care Medicine, Division of Cardiovascular Anesthesia,
University of Innsbruck School of Medicine, Innsbruck, Austria

Daniel P. Vezina

Division of Cardiovascular Anesthesiology, Department of Anesthesiology, and the Division of Cardiology, Department of Medicine,
University of Utah School of Medicine, and the VA Medical Center, Salt Lake City, Utah, U.S.A.

Ramon Sanchez

Sections of Cardiothoracic Anesthesia and Liver Transplantation, Department of Anesthesiology,
UC San Diego Medical Center, San Diego, California, U.S.A.

INTRODUCTION

The use of transesophageal echocardiography (TEE) has expanded tremendously since its introduction into clinical use in the mid-1970s. TEE is used daily in the echocardiography laboratory, the operating rooms, and also the surgical intensive care unit (SICU). Its usefulness derives from its high capacity for both diagnosis and monitoring. Ultrasound studies are considered noninvasive procedures when performed from the thoracic surface (transthoracic tomographic views) and minimally invasive when performed from the esophagus (transesophageal tomographic views).

This chapter reviews the basic physical principles of ultrasound and echocardiography, echoanatomy, and a practical approach to performing an abbreviated trauma TEE examination when time is limited. Assessment of preload, afterload, contractility, and diastolic dysfunction will be reviewed. This is followed by a discussion of common valvular heart lesions and the general approach to the trauma patient. Clinically oriented discussions regarding the usefulness of TEE in the management of trauma patients in the operating room, SICU, and use of TEE as an emergency "rescue diagnostic tool" in the hemodynamically unstable patient are also provided.

A task force formed by the American Heart Association (AHA), the American College of Cardiology (ACC), and the American Society of Echocardiography (ASE) published guidelines in 1997 for clinical application of TEE (1) (Table 1). Class 1 indications are conditions for which there is scientific evidence and/or general agreement that the procedure is useful and effective. Class 2a indications are those of which there is conflicting evidence and/or divergence of opinion about usefulness, but the final assessment weighs in favor of its use. Class 2b indications are still useful but with less well established evidence or opinion. In SICU and trauma clinical scenarios, Class 1 indications for TEE include the evaluation of acute and life-threatening hemodynamic disturbances, evaluation of heart structure for possible endocarditis, guidance for placement of intracardiac devices, and drainage of pericardial effusion. Class 2a indications include the monitoring for myocardial ischemia, diagnosis of myocardial infarction, and evaluation

for a cadiac source of emboli (atheromatous disease, intracardiac thrombus/tumor, and intracardiac shunt). Finally, class 2b indications are related to diagnosis of post-traumatic cardiac lesions and acute aortic dissection.

PHYSICS AND PRINCIPLES
Physics of Ultrasound

Sound waves are defined as mechanical vibrations that create rarefaction and compression of any medium through which they travel. The human ear can analyze sound waves with frequencies ranging from 20 Hz to 20 KHz. Ultrasound frequencies used for echocardiography are above this level, ranging between 1 and 20 MHz. Sound waves can be characterized by amplitude (dB), frequency (Hz), wavelength (mm), and velocity (m/sec). Increasing transducer frequency will give better resolution but less depth of penetration due to tissue absorption. For example, a 3.5 MHz TEE transducer (low frequency) will have decreased image resolution, but will be able to assess a structure far away from the probe [i.e., the apex of a large dilated left ventricle (LV) at a depth of 16–18 cm]. In contrast, a 7.5-MHz transducer (high frequency) will give excellent spatial resolution of a near structure, but depth of penetration will be diminished.

Ultrasound emitted by a transducer has a known frequency and a defined constant velocity within the medium through which it passes (1540 m/sec in soft tissue). This relationship between frequency, velocity, and wavelength is used to acquire appropriate data regarding cardiac structure and function. TEE utilizes two different technologies: structural imaging (A-Mode, M-mode, B-Mode, and 2D) and Doppler.

Structural Imaging: Two-Dimensional Echocardiography

The structural imaging process relies on the fact that a transducer will emit a signal at a known frequency, ranging from 2.5 to 7.5 MHz, and a known constant velocity, 1540 m/sec. After emission of the sound wave, the transducer becomes a receptor and waits for the signal to be reflected back by the structures along its pathway. Because the propagation velocity of the ultrasound is constant, the distance

Table 1 Indications for Transesophageal Echocardiography in the Operating Room or Surgical Intensive Care Unit (ASA Practice Guidelines)

Indication	Examples
Class 1	Acute, persistent and life-threatening hemodynamic instability
	Unstable ICU patients with suspected valve disease or thromboembolic problems
	Patients with suspected aortic dissection/aneurysm/ disruption who need immediate evaluation
Class 2	Monitoring for myocardial ischemia, myocardial infarction
	Patients with increased risk for hemodynamic disturbances in the perioperative setting
	Patients with intracardiac foreign bodies
	Intraoperative detection of air emboli in patients at risk
	Suspected cardiac trauma
Class 3	Intraoperative monitoring for emboli during orthopaedic procedures
	Intraoperative assessment of repair of thoracic aortic injury
	Perioperative evaluation of pleuro-pulmonary diseases
	Monitoring placement of central venous or pulmonary artery catheters

Note: Class 1, frequently useful in improving clinical outcome; class 2, perhaps useful with less clear influence on clinical outcome; class 3, controversial indication with unclear influence on clinical outcome
Abbreviations: ASA, American Society of Anesthesiologists; ICU, intensive care unit.
Source: From Ref. 4.

between the transducer and the reflected structure will be determined by the time it takes for the initial signal to emit and return to the transducer. The same signal will also have defined amplitude, which is related to the reflective characteristics of the structures met. The processing component of the echo machine can display this information in various ways. The earliest echo systems displayed the data by A-mode (amplitude vs. depth) on an oscilloscope screen. With increasingly powerful processing systems, the same data can be presented by M-mode (motion) where the different returned signals are presented on a gray-scale display over time on the horizontal axis. The temporal aspect of M-mode is useful for analyzing highly mobile structures, but is limited in its ability to provide information about the relationship between multiple structures. The M-mode gives data about only a thin cut of the cardiac structure (single scan line). The B-mode (brightness), also called two-dimension (20) imaging, is the ultimate way to display the same data by dots on a screen monitor. The position of the dot on the screen is related to the calculated distance between the transducer and the structure represented. The brightness of the dot is related to the amplitude of the returning signal. With a high-capacity processing system, multiple scan lines can be analyzed quickly to produce a moving image with adequate temporal resolution. This is how 2D images of moving cardiac structures are produced in echocardiography. The reflection which occurs at the interface between two tissues and the intensity of the reflected signal will be related to the acoustic impedance between those tissues. Since ultrasound does not travel well through air, it is essential to have an adequate medium between the transducer and the tissue, such as a water-soluble jelly. In order to obtain optimal 2D images, the angle between the transducer and the imaged structure should be as close to 90° as possible in order to minimize refraction and artifact formation (the angle of incidence of the transmitted ultrasound wave equals the angle of reflection).

Doppler Echocardiography

The second physical principle used in cardiac ultrasound imaging is the "Doppler effect," defined as the apparent change in frequency observed when the source and observer are in motion relative to each other. For echocardiography, the Doppler shift is the difference between the initial known frequency and the backscattered signal returned from moving blood cells. **From the Doppler shift, the velocity of the moving blood cells can be calculated.** Ideally, the ultrasound beam should be parallel to blood flow with the scattered signal moving directly towards or away from the transducer. Keeping the crossing angle to less than 20° will limit error in blood flow velocity measurements.

The returning backscattered signal from the moving blood cells is composed of several different frequencies, which are analyzed by a fast Fourier transformation before being displayed using spectral analysis. Spectral analysis displays time on the horizontal axis and velocity on the longitudinal axis. The Doppler shifts indicating that the moving red cells are coming toward the transducer will appear above the baseline, whereas those traveling away from the transducer will appear below the baseline. Doppler echocardiography is commonly used to measure blood flow velocities in cardiac chambers, across valves, and in great vessels. These measured velocities are helpful for both diagnostic and monitoring applications. **The modified Bernoulli equation can be used to transform velocities obtained by TEE into pressure units.**

$$P = 4v^2$$

where P = peak pressure gradient (mmHg) and v = peak velocity (m/sec) of flow across the valve. Data for this equation are usually obtained using continuous wave (CW) Doppler echo (described subsequently).

There are three types of Doppler echocardiography modalities: CW, pulsed wave (PW), and color Doppler. The use of CW Doppler necessitates two different crystals in the transducer. One is used for emitting ultrasound continuously and the other for receiving the returned signal. The CW Doppler will be able to measure all the velocities along a scanning line, but is unable to differentiate the exact location of the maximum velocity along that line (range ambiguity). The PW Doppler is different in that it uses one crystal that alternates between emitting and receiving. A sampling area for velocity measurement is determined by the echocardiographer, along a scanning line. The Doppler shift will correspond to the velocity measured at the sampling volume. The PWD signals must be sampled twice in order to get an accurate determination of the wavelength. This limits its ability to measure high velocities. The major limitation of PWD is that it can only measure a limited range of velocities without ambiguity in the speed or direction. Velocities outside the limits of the spectral display (the Nyquist limit) will "wrap around" and falsely appear as a reversal of flow (aliasing).

The color Doppler is a variation of PW Doppler. Simply explained, a larger sampling area for velocity measurements is analyzed and presented as color-coded images superimposed on 2D images instead of a spectral display. ✍ **By convention, the velocities going away from the transducer are coded in shades of blue, whereas velocities coming toward the transducer are coded in shades of red (BART: Blue Away, Red Towards).** ✍ In clinical practice, color Doppler is used to get a semi-quantitative evaluation of velocities in cardiac chambers and valves. Precise quantification is done using either CW or PW Doppler. Color Doppler has the same intrinsic limit for maximum velocity measurement (Nyquist limit) as PW Doppler. When the measured velocities in the mapping area of color Doppler are above the Nyquist limit, they appear as an aliasing signal, depicted as a sudden reverse in color. For example, when evaluating normal mitral valve (MV) inflow during diastole using color Doppler, blue color would appear in the left atrium (LA) because blood flow is going away from the probe at low velocity. If red color suddenly appeared during diastole near the valve, the velocities measured at that point are above the Nyquist limit of the color Doppler setting, suggestive of mitral stenosis.

In summary, echocardiography is done with ultrasound using two different modalities: 2D showing live motion images of the heart and great vessels in a gray scale, and Doppler echocardiography measuring blood velocity in cardiac chambers, valves, and orifices.

TRANSESOPHAGEAL ECHOCARDIOGRAPHY ANATOMY
Nomenclature
In 1999, the ASE and the Society of Cardiovascular Anesthesiologists (SCA) published a landmark paper with guidelines for performing a comprehensive perioperative multiplane TEE (2). This publication describes in detail the 20 cross-sectional views of a comprehensive TEE examination (Fig. 1). An experienced echocardiographer can perform

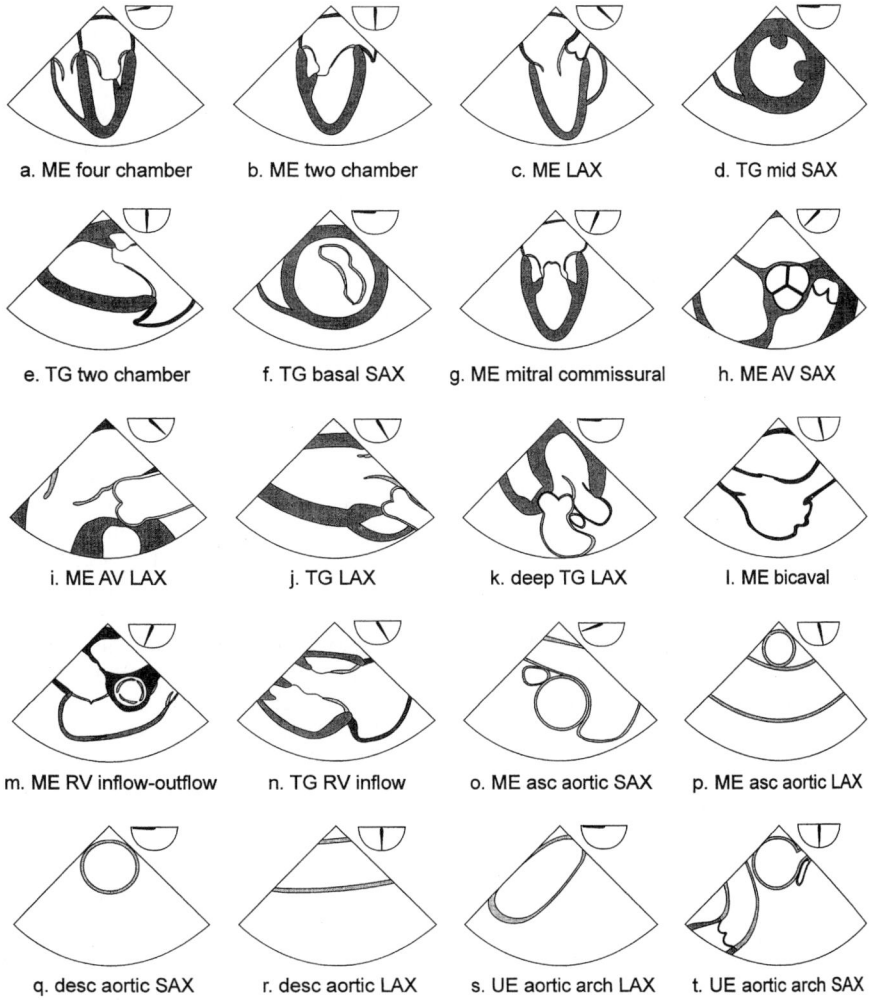

a. ME four chamber   b. ME two chamber   c. ME LAX   d. TG mid SAX

e. TG two chamber   f. TG basal SAX   g. ME mitral commissural   h. ME AV SAX

i. ME AV LAX   j. TG LAX   k. deep TG LAX   l. ME bicaval

m. ME RV inflow-outflow   n. TG RV inflow   o. ME asc aortic SAX   p. ME asc aortic LAX

q. desc aortic SAX   r. desc aortic LAX   s. UE aortic arch LAX   t. UE aortic arch SAX

Figure 1 The ASE/SCA 20-view exam. Transesophageal echocardiography cross-sections in a comprehensive examination. Twenty standard cross-sections and their abbreviated names are depicted by the line drawings. Probe manipulations required to produce each of the cross-sections are described in the text. *Abbreviations*: ME, mid-esophageal; ME LAX, mid-esophageal long-axis view; TG mid SAX, transgastric mid-short-axis view; TG basal SAX, transgastric basal short axis view; ME AV SAX, mid-esophageal aortic valve short-axis view; ME AV LAX, mid-esophageal aortic valve long-axis view; TG LAX, transgastric long-axis view; ME RV inflow–outflow, mid-esophageal right ventricle inflow–outflow; TG RV inflow, transgastric right ventricle inflow; ME asc aortic SAX, mid-esophageal ascending aortic short-axis view; ME asc aortic LAX, mid-esophageal ascending aortic long-axis view; desc aortic SAX, descending aorta short-axis view; desc aortic LAX, descending aorta long-axis view; UE aortic arch LAX, upper esophageal aortic long-axis view; UE aortic arch SAX, upper esophageal aortic short-axis view. *Source*: From Ref. 2.

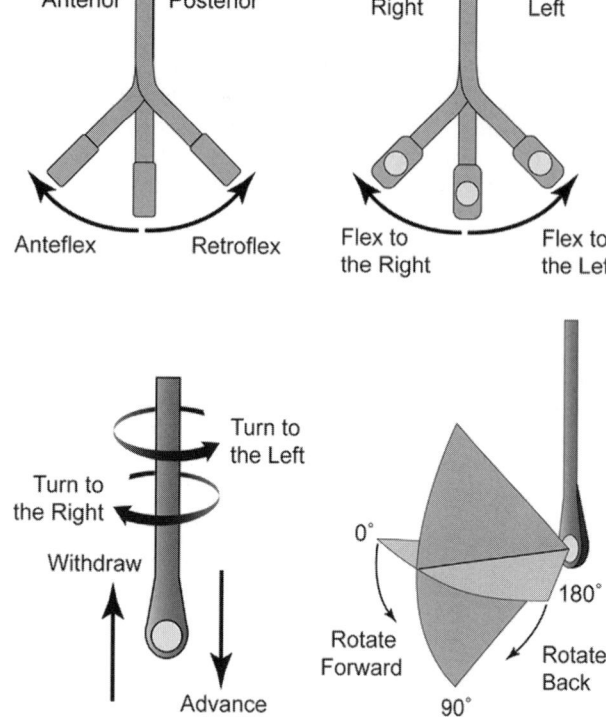

Figure 2 Terminology used for transesophageal echocardiography probe and transducer manipulations.

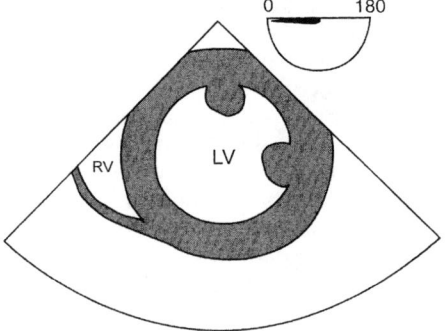

Figure 3 Transgastric mid-short-axis (TG mid SAX) view. *Abbreviations*: LV, left ventricle; RV, right ventricle.

this exam in less than 10 minutes; however, for those less experienced, a complete exam can be time consuming and overwhelming. In this chapter, a concise and practical approach to the trauma patient will be presented, followed by a completion of the 20-view exam.

The modern multiplane TEE probe consists of a central flexible shaft with a controllable distal portion (last 10 cm). The transducer is embedded into the tip of the flexible shaft and mounted on an electric motor that permits rotation for multiplane imaging. With the patient supine and the TEE imaging structures in front of it, the terminology is always in reference to the heart. Superior is toward the head, inferior toward the feet, posterior toward the spine, anterior toward the sternum, and right and left being the patient's right and left sides, respectively. The probe itself can be advanced inferiorly, withdrawn superiorly, and rotated right and left (Fig. 2). The tip of the probe can be anteflexed or retroflexed with the large rotating knob. It can also be flexed left and right with the smaller knob. The internal transducer (multiplane) can be rotated forward (0–180° clockwise) or backward (180–0° counterclockwise) by another control on the handle. The depth of the scanning area and the multiplane angle should always be adjusted to have the screen show only the structures being evaluated. In general, cross sections of structures seen at multiplane angles below 45° are called short axis and those above 45° are called long axis.

Abbreviated Trauma Transesophageal Echocardiography Examination

✤ **The abbreviated trauma examination includes 12 of the 20 cross sections of the ASE/SCA comprehensive examination.** ✤ The goal of this approach will be to identify

trauma-related injuries and evaluate the causes of hemodynamic instability. Additional views can be used for further evaluation if felt necessary by the echocardiographer.

The first view obtained is the transgastric mid-short axis (TG mid SAX) (Fig. 3). The authors would recommend starting with this view as one can rapidly diagnose many causes of hemodynamic instability. This view is obtained by advancing the probe past the esophagus and into the stomach, followed by anteflexion. The multiplane angle is generally best placed between 0° and 30°. Once the LV is seen in the center of the image, the probe is advanced or withdrawn slightly until both the anterolateral and posteromedial papillary muscles are shown equally. This will indicate that the probe is at the mid-level of the LV. Volume status, global and regional LV contractile function, right ventricular (RV) function, and evidence of pericardial effusion can all be evaluated with this highly versatile cross section.

The next view obtained is the mid-esophageal four-chamber view (ME 4 Chamber) (Fig. 4). From the TG mid-SAX view, the probe is withdrawn into the mid-esophagus with the multiplane angle at 0°. The tip of the probe often has to be slightly retroflexed in order to reduce apical fore-shortening. This cross section shows the four chambers [right atrium (RA), RV, LA, and LV], as well as the MV and tricuspid valves (TV). The free wall of the RV is shown on the left, the septum is located in the middle, and the lateral wall of the LV appears on the right. With this view, chamber size and global contractile function can be examined. Regional wall motion of the septum and lateral wall of the LV at the basal, mid, and apical levels can be evaluated. The color Doppler can be used to evaluate the MV and TV for stenosis or regurgitation.

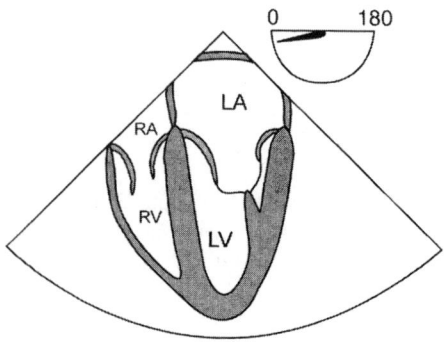

Figure 4 Mid-esophageal four-chamber (ME 4 Chamber) view. *Abbreviations*: LV, left ventricle; RV, right ventricle; LA, left atrium; RA, right atrium.

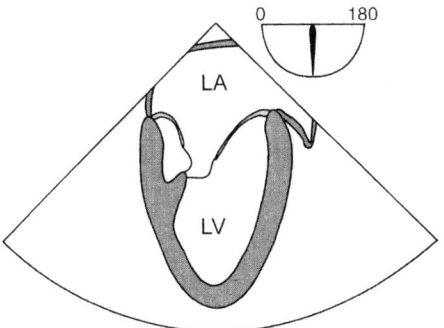

Figure 5 Mid-esophageal two-chamber (ME 2 Chamber) view. *Abbreviations*: LA, left atrium; LV, left ventricle.

Keeping the LV in the middle of the screen and rotating the multiplane forward to about 90° will give the mid-esophageal two-chamber view (ME 2 Chamber) (Fig. 5). The LA is seen at the top of the figure with the MV and LV below. The anterior LV wall on the right side of the figure and the inferior wall on the left side can be evaluated for regional contractile function. The LA appendage can also be visualized as a part of the LA covering the upper part of the anterior wall of the LV. Chamber size, LV contractile function, MV abnormalities, and thrombus in the LA appendage can be studied in this view. Color Doppler can be used to further study the MV, if necessary.

From the ME 2 Chamber view, the multiplane is then rotated to approximately 130° to obtain the mid-esophageal long-axis view (ME LAX) (Fig. 6). This view shows the anteroseptal wall on the right side facing the posterior wall on the left, which can be evaluated for regional contractile function. The LV outflow tract (LVOT) and the aortic valve (AV) in long axis are above the anteroseptal wall.

From the ME LAX view, rotating the multiplane back to 0° will give the ME 4 Chamber. Withdrawing the probe until the cusps of the AV are seen, and then turning the multiplane angle to approximately 30° will give the mid-esophageal AV short axis (ME AV SAX) (Fig. 7). The coaptation of the three aortic cusps (which resemble a Mercedes Benz sign) should be visualized in this view. The optimal depth is between 8 and 10 cm. The main focus of this cross section is to evaluate the AV structure and function. A nonquantitative estimation of LV stroke volume and cardiac output can be done, based on the extent of AV opening and the heart rate.

From the ME AV SAX view (approximately 30°), rotating the multiplane angle to approximately 115° will give the

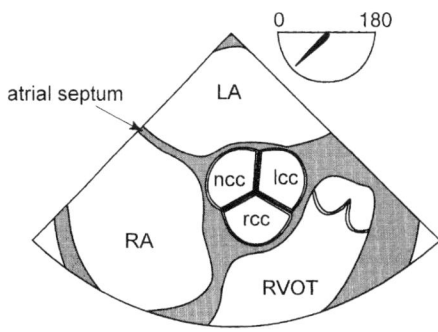

Figure 7 Mid-esophageal aortic valve short-axis (ME AV SAX) view. *Abbreviations*: LA, left atrium; RA, right atrium; RVOT, right ventricular outflow tract.

mid-esophageal AV long-axis view (ME AV LAX) (Fig. 8). The AV is now seen in long axis in the middle with the LA shown above, the proximal ascending aorta on the right, and the LVOT below and to the left. The optimal multiplane angle is found when one visualizes the coaptation point between the right coronary cusp on the bottom of the figure and either the noncoronary or left coronary cusp in the middle of the aortic root. This view is optimal for color Doppler studies of the AV to look for aortic regurgitation (Nyquist limit above 50 cm/sec). This view is also useful for evaluation of AV structure and function as well as its relationship with the MV. A small part of the ascending aorta is also seen, along with the sino-tubular junction, the sinuses of Valsava, and the aortic annulus. An aortic dissection flap may be seen in the proximal ascending aorta if present.

The remaining views of the abbreviated trauma exam include important views of the aorta and pulmonary artery (PA). The descending aortic short-axis view (desc. aortic SAX) (Fig. 9) is obtained by placing the probe deep in the stomach and turning the probe to the left so that the ultrasound beam is pointing posterior. Depth is decreased to 6–8 cm. The probe can be withdrawn until the entire descending aorta has been visualized from its distal to proximal end. If the aorta is tortuous, the probe may be turned left or right to keep the image centered. At any level of the descending aorta, the multiplane angle can be rotated to 90° to image the aorta in long axis to obtain the descending aortic long-axis view (desc. aortic LAX) (Fig. 10). From the desc. aortic SAX view, the probe can be withdrawn into the upper esophagus until the aorta arches to the left side of the figure. This is the upper esophageal aortic arch long-axis view (UE aortic arch LAX) (Fig. 11). From this view, the

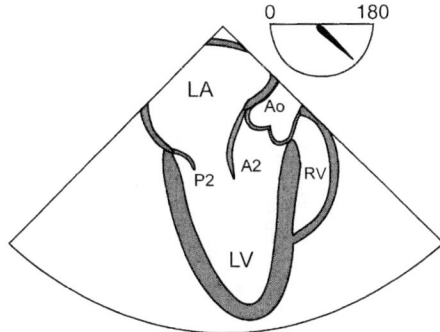

Figure 6 Mid-esophageal long-axis (ME LAX) view. *Abbreviations*: Ao, aorta; LA, left atrium; LV, left ventricle; RV, right ventricle.

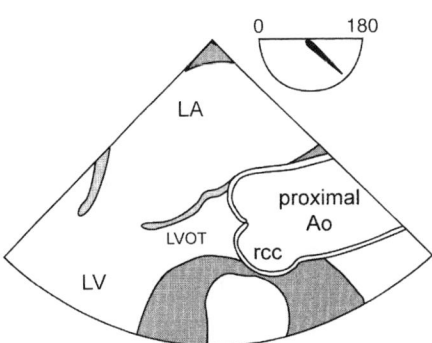

Figure 8 Mid-esophageal aortic valve long-axis (ME AV LAX) view. *Abbreviations*: Ao, aorta; LA, left atrium; LV, left ventricle; LVOT, LV outflow tract.

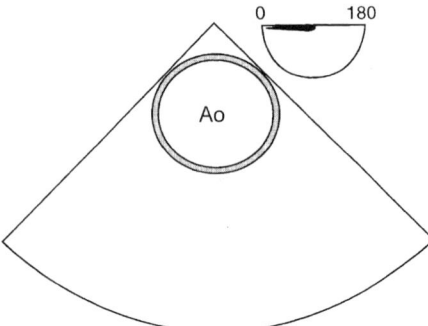

Figure 9   Descending aorta short-axis (desc aortic SAX) view. *Abbreviation*: Ao, aorta.

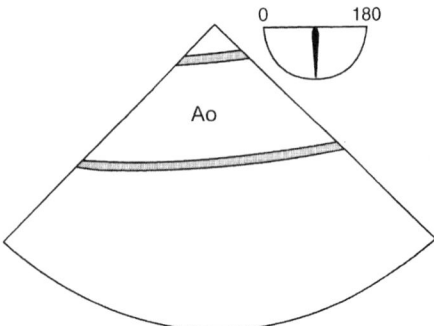

Figure 10   Descending aorta long-axis (desc aortic LAX) view. *Abbreviation*: Ao, aorta.

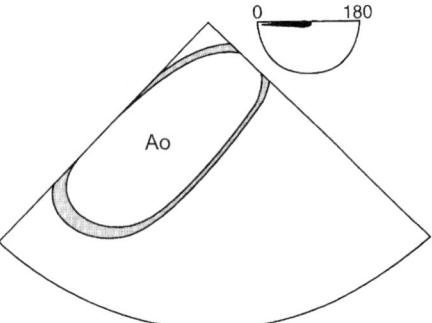

Figure 11   Upper esophageal aortic long-axis (UE aortic arch LAX) view. *Abbreviation*: Ao, aorta.

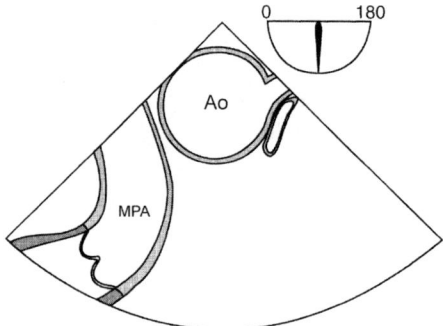

Figure 12   Upper esophageal aortic short-axis (UE aortic arch SAX) view. *Abbreviations*: Ao, aorta; MPA, main pulmonary artery.

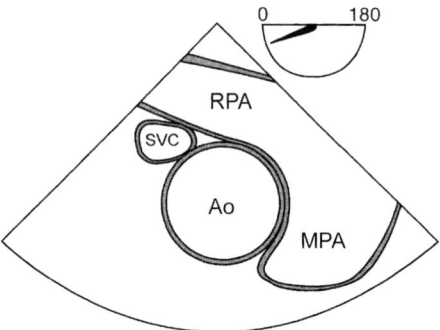

Figure 13   Mid-esophageal ascending aortic short-axis (ME asc aortic SAX) view. *Abbreviations*: Ao, aorta; RPA, right pulmonary artery; MPA, main pulmonary artery; SVC, superior vena cava.

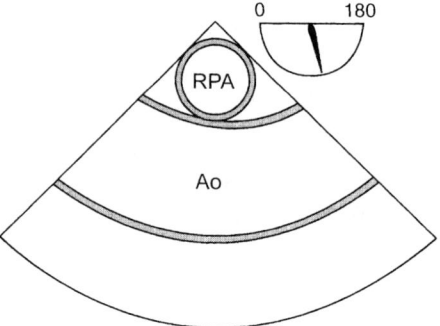

Figure 14
Mid-esophageal ascending aortic long-axis (ME asc aortic LAX) view. *Abbreviations*: Ao, aorta; RPA, right pulmonary artery.

transducer is rotated 90° until the distal arch is seen in short axis [upper esophageal aortic arch short-axis view (UE aortic arch SAX)] (Fig. 12). In this view, the takeoff of the left sub-clavian artery can be seen in the upper right of the figure. These aortic views can be used to examine the proximal ascending aorta, the distal portion of the aortic arch, and the entire descending thoracic aorta for evidence of dissection, aneurysm, and atheromatous plaque. However, the distal ascending aorta and proximal arch cannot be examined because of the interposition of the air-filled trachea and left bronchus. The desc. aortic SAX view is also useful to visualize fluid in the pleural space. The last view of the abbreviated trauma exam is the mid-esophageal ascending aortic short-axis view (ME asc. aortic SAX) (Fig. 13). This view is obtained from the ME 4 Chamber view by rotating the multiplane to about 40° and withdrawing the probe, until a short-axis view of the proximal ascending aorta and a long-axis view

of the main and right PA are seen. The superior vena cava (SVC) is seen in its location between the right PA and the aorta. This view can be useful for Doppler studies across the PA and evaluation for a proximal pulmonary embolus (PE). The mid-esophageal ascending aortic long-axis view (ME asc. aortic LAX) (Fig. 14) provides additional information about the ascending aorta, and is obtained by rotating the multiplane 90° from the previous image. The authors believe that these 12 views are the most important and are sufficient for the initial brief evaluation of the acute trauma patient.

Exam Completion

In hemodynamically stable patients, as well as in previously unstable trauma patients, a complete examination should

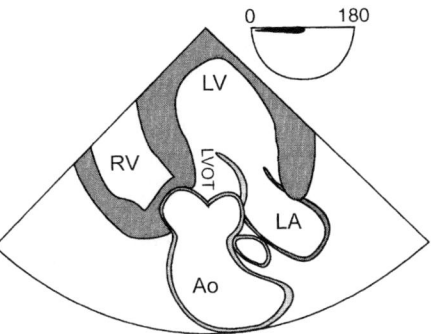

Figure 15 Deep transgastric long-axis (deep TG LAX) view. *Abbreviations*: LV, left ventricle; RV, right ventricle; LA, left atrium; Ao, aorta; LVOT, LV outflow tract.

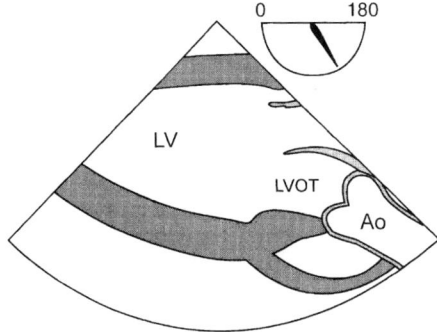

Figure 17 Transgastric long-axis (TG LAX) view. *Abbreviations*: Ao, aorta; LV, left ventricle; LVOT, LV outflow tract.

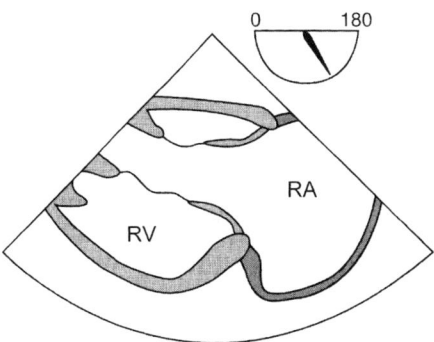

Figure 18 Transgastric right ventricle inflow (TG RV inflow) view. *Abbreviations*: RA, right atrium; RV, right ventricle.

be performed as soon as time permits. To complete the ASE/SCA comprehensive 20-view exam, eight additional views are necessary. The deep transgastric view (deep TG LAX) (Fig. 15) is obtained by advancing the probe to approximately 45–50 cm, followed by anteflexion, left flexion, and a multiplane angle of 0°. The CW and PW Doppler can be used across the AV and the LVOT to evaluate for aortic stenosis and for calculating a left-sided cardiac output. The transgastric two chamber view (TG 2 chamber) (Fig. 16) is obtained by rotating the multiplane to about 90° from the TG mid-SAX view. Evaluation of wall motion of the anterior and inferior wall as well as the apex can be performed. The MV and subvalvular structures can also be seen. Rotating the multiplane angle forward to between 90° and 120° and turning the probe slightly to the right from the previous view will give the transgastric long-axis view (TG LAX) (Fig. 17). With this view, Doppler studies can be performed across the AV and LVOT. The transgastric RV inflow view (TG RV inflow) (Fig. 18) is obtained by turning the probe to the right from a TG mid-SAX view until the RV is in the center, then rotating the multiplane to about 90°. This view is useful for evaluating RV function and TV anatomy. The transgastric basal short-axis view (TG basal SAX) (Fig. 19) view is obtained by withdrawing the probe slightly from the TG mid-SAX view until the MV is seen. This view is useful for evaluating the MV as well as wall motion of all the basal segments of the LV. The ME mitral commissural view (ME mitral commissural) (Fig. 20) can be found by decreasing the multiplane angle to about 60° from the ME 2 Chamber view. This view is useful for further evaluation of MV anatomy. Portions of the posterior and anterior leaflets

can be closely studied. From the ME AV SAX view, the multiplane is rotated to 80° and turned to the left to obtain the mid-esophageal right ventricular inflow-outflow view (ME RV inflow–outflow) (Fig. 21) to show the TV and pulmonic valve. The RV inferior free wall is seen on the left, and the right ventricular outflow tract (RVOT) is seen on the right. This view is valuable in the assessment of RV function, tricuspid and pulmonary regurgitation. The last view, mid-esophageal bicaval view (ME bicaval) (Fig. 22) is obtained by turning the probe to the patient's right from the ME AV LAX view and rotating the multiplane to approximately 110°. Here, the RA is seen at the bottom with the LA above and the intra-atrial septum between. This view may be useful to look for a patent foramen ovale, evidence of pericardial tamponade, and assist with line placement.

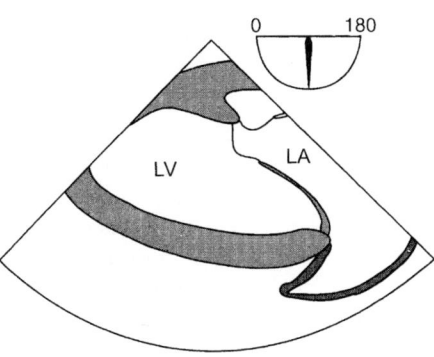

Figure 16 Transgastric two-chamber (TG two chamber) view. *Abbreviations*: LA, left atrium; LV, left ventricle.

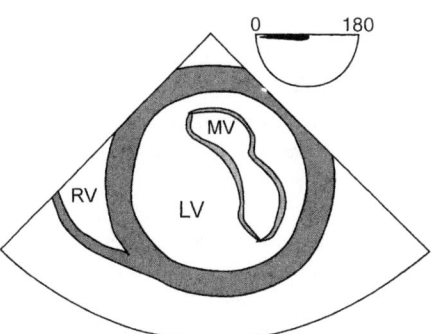

Figure 19 Transgastric basal short-axis (TG basal SAX) view. *Abbreviations*: LV, left ventricle; MV, mitral valve; RV, right ventricle.

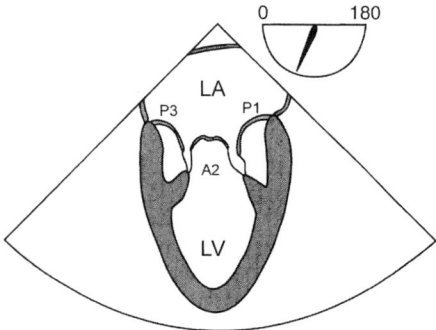

Figure 20 Mid-esophageal mitral commissural (ME mitral commissural) view. *Abbreviations*: LA, left atrium; LV, left ventricle.

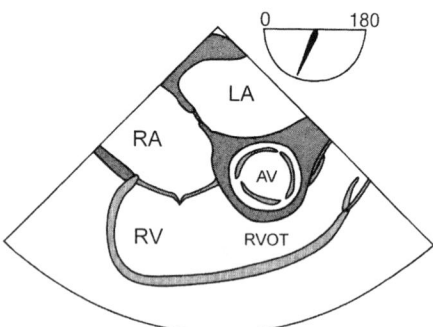

Figure 21 Mid-esophageal right ventricle inflow–outflow (ME RV inflow–outflow) view. *Abbreviations*: AV, aortic valve; LA, left atrium; RA, right atrium; RV, right ventricle.

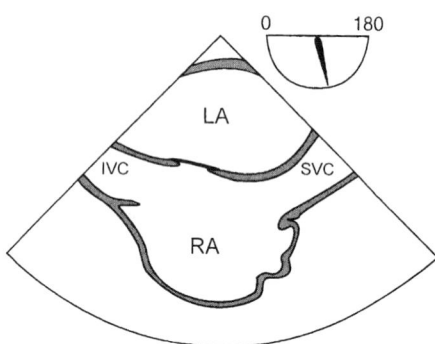

Figure 22 Mid-esophageal bicaval (ME bicaval) view. *Abbreviations*: LA, left atrium; RA, right atrium; IVC, inferior vena cava; SVC, superior vena cava.

ASSESSMENT OF PRELOAD, AFTERLOAD, AND MYOCARDIAL FUNCTION
Left Ventricular Preload Evaluation
Right Heart Filling Pressures vs. Transesophageal Echocardiography

Heart muscle fibers need a particular baseline stretch (preload) to produce optimal fiber shortening. Consequently, the heart depends on an adequate end-diastolic volume to produce optimal stroke volume. Even with normal myocardial contractility the heart cannot produce normal stroke volume and cardiac output if end-diastolic volume, and thus muscle fiber baseline stretch are reduced. In clinical practice, myocardial preload is typically assessed indirectly, using pressure measurements in the RA [central venous

pressure (CVP) or pulmonary circulation—pulmonary artery capillary occlusion pressure (PACOP)].

There is a rather close correlation between PACOP or even CVP and LV end-diastolic volume (LVEDV) in most patients with normal LV function and normal pulmonary vascular resistance (PVR). Consequently, indirect assessment using pressure measurements may often be sufficient to guide volume therapy. However, in several subgroups of patients, indirect assessment of end-diastolic volume by pressure measurements becomes less reliable, because of poor correlation between PACOP and LV end-diastolic volume (3–6). Loss of correlation between pressure and volume measurements is typically found in patients in whom pressure measurements do not represent transmural filling pressure (e.g., high intrathoracic pressure, high PEEP), and in patients in whom higher filling pressures are needed to maintain end-diastolic volume because of an impaired ability of myocardial muscle fibers to relax (diastolic dysfunction) (4) (Table 2).

The improved ability of TEE in preload assessment was initially described for cardiac surgical patients (5–7), but is now also well documented and widely accepted for emergency patients or unstable patients in the SICU (8–11). Preload assessment is among the most common indications for a TEE examination in the SICU, and a TEE examination should always be added to filling pressure measurements if there is any doubt about adequacy of preload (9,11,12). However, echocardiographic preload assessment has a few limitations, particularly in patients with diastolic dysfunction and pre-existing cardiac disease (8). In these patients it is not possible to define a clear threshold for LV end diastolic area (EDA), below which there is no volume recruitable increase in LV function (8). In these instances, it is often helpful to repeatedly assess EDA, fractional area shortening and filling pressure during volume administration, and not to base the decision on a single TEE exam. It has also been suggested that adding PW Doppler data of transmitral (ventricular filling) and pulmonary venous blood flow (atrial filling) may further improve echocardiographic preload assessment. However, these parameters are markedly influenced by heart rate, rhythm, afterload, and other physiologic parameters that are poorly defined and constantly changing in SICU patients. Therefore, PW Doppler estimation of preload is of limited clinical usefulness.

Practical Approach
↺ Normally, the TG mid-SAX view is used to assess RV and LV myocardial preload. ↺ In the transgastric short-axis

Table 2 Common Clinical Scenarios with Poor Correlation Between Pulmonary Artery Capillary Occlusion Pressure and Left Ventricular End-Diastolic Volume

Cause	Example
Elevated intrathoracic pressure	Ventilation with markedly increased I:E ratios
	Ventilation with high PEEP values
Elevated abdominal pressure	Retroperitoneal hematoma
	Abdominal compartment syndrome
Diastolic dysfunction	Sepsis
	High-dose catecholamine therapy
	Hypertrophic myocardium

Abbreviation: PEEP, positive end expiratory pressure.

Table 3 Echocardiographic Findings Associated with Reduced Left Ventricular Preload (Hypovolemia)

End-systolic papillary muscle contact and loss of LV lumen (TG SAX view)
LV end-diastolic area <5.5 cm^2/m^2 body surface area
Reduced LV end-diastolic area compared to baseline measurement
Increased fractional area shortening with decreased LV end-diastolic area

Abbreviations: LV, left ventricle; TG SAX, transgastric short-axis view.

view, the TEE beam can be easily directed to precisely traverse both papillary muscles, thereby producing a consistent and highly reproducible echocardiographic view. In contrast, it is often impossible to direct the TEE beam to exit through the apex of the heart in the four-chamber view, thereby typically underestimating end-diastolic volume. One can trace the area of the LV along the endocardial border at end diastole and see changes in EDA with volume loading. Echocardiographic indicators of reduced LV preload are listed in Table 3, the systolic papillary muscle attachment (kissing papillary muscle phenomenon) being the most obvious, consistent, and clinically useful. In the trauma and critical care setting, repeated evaluation of LV function and EDA before and after volume loading can add to the echocardiographic diagnosis of reduced LV preload (8,10).

Left Ventricular Afterload Estimation

Using volume determinations and measurements of myocardial thickness, LV afterload can be assessed by calculating LV wall stress. In lesions where forward stroke volume does not equal total stroke volume [e.g., mitral insufficiency, ventricular septal defect (VSD)], LV wall stress may be a better way to assess LV afterload when compared to systemic vascular resistance (SVR), calculated from PA catheter data (13). Wall stress may be a better predictor of clinical outcome (e.g., myocardial ischemia) when compared to SVR (13). However, due to the complexity of the method and multiple confounding factors, LV wall stress has never gained widespread acceptance in clinical practice. Echocardiographic findings in a state with isolated low SVR show a vigorously contracting ventricle and a reduced end systolic area (ESA) similar to hypovolemia. However, the EDA is normal. In uncertain cases or when dealing with a mixed picture, information from a PA catheter can be useful.

Global and Regional Left Ventricular Function Evaluation

TEE enables direct visualization of both global and regional LV function. Semi-quantitative assessment of global LV function is possible with basic knowledge in TEE, and in general is sufficient to solve most clinical problems. Detection and assessment of regional LV function is often subtle and should be done only by an experienced echocardiographer. The midpapillary region of the heart generates 80% of LV stroke volume and all three major branches of the coronary circulation (left anterior descending, circumflex, and right coronary) contribute to blood supply of this region (Fig. 23) (3,14). Consequently, the TG mid-SAX view (Fig. 3) is the imaging plane of choice to quickly assess LV function in the unstable patient or to continuously monitor LV function in the operating room.

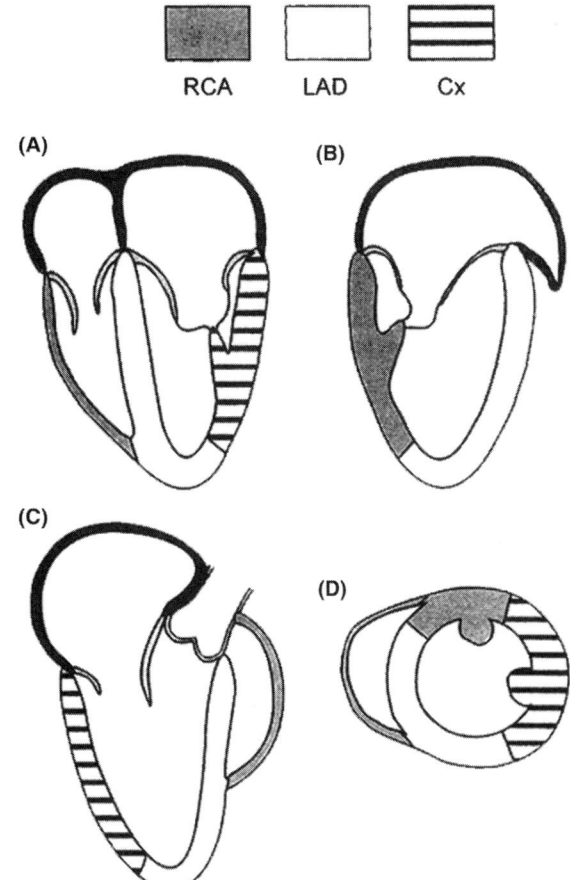

Figure 23 Coronary artery perfusion territories. Typical regions of myocardium perfused by each of the three major coronary arteries to the left ventricle. Other patterns exist because of normal anatomic variations or coronary disease with collateral flow. Mid-esophageal 4 Chamber (**A**), 2 Chamber (**B**), long-axis (**C**), and transgastric mid-short-axis views (**D**). *Abbreviations*: RCA, right coronary artery; LAD, left anterior descending (coronary artery); Cx, circumflex artery.

Global Systolic Left Ventricular Function

☞ The evaluation of global LV function in the ICU and emergency patient is typically done semi-quantitatively, describing global LV function as hyperdynamic, normal, moderately impaired, or severely impaired. ☞ Semi-quantitative assessment of LV function has several advantages. It does not direct attention away from the important task of resuscitating the patient and allows complicated calculations to be done with the echo software. In addition, it does not give the impression of highly accurate values, which takes more time to perform. One must realize that semi-quantitative assessment relies on using a single diameter to assess three-dimensional LV ejection. Impaired LV function is often the consequence of coronary artery disease, which may be associated with significant regional wall motion abnormalities. The calculation of LV function using diameter or area measurements in a single plane in the presence of regional wall motion abnormalities may therefore be less accurate. Fractional area change (FAC) is the proportional area change during systole, and provides a rapid and reliable index of global LV systolic function. The TG mid-SAX view (Fig. 3) is used, and areas are derived by freezing and tracing the endocardial borders during systole (ESA) and diastole (EDA). The papillary muscles should be excluded from the trace.

$$FAC = EDA - ESA/EDA \times 100$$

The normal range of FAC is from 36% to 64%. In the presence of wall motion abnormalities, FAC overestimates the true ejection fraction (EF). Using two orthogonal echocardiographic views, ME 4 Chamber (Fig. 4) and ME 2 Chamber (Fig. 5), EF can be calculated using the modified Simpson's formula. This method is the most accurate in the presence of regional wall motion abnormalities.

Although sufficient for clinical practice, all parameters of global LV function mentioned earlier are preload and afterload dependent and therefore have their limitations in describing myocardial contractility. Echocardiographic parameters, such as length of pre-ejection period, end-systolic pressure–volume relationship, circumferential fiber shortening rate, and end-systolic stress/end-systolic area relationship, have all been evaluated in clinical or experimental studies as less pre- and afterload–dependent indices to describe myocardial contractility.

Cardiac output measurements can be done with TEE using 2D echocardiographic measurements alone or more commonly, adding transmitral or aortic Doppler flow velocity data. Difficulties in obtaining a proper Doppler signal (angle) and a number of assumptions when calculating the orifice of flow (errors in diameter measurements are squared) cause significant variability and miscalculations. In addition, repeated cardiac output determinations are necessary in most SICU patients, making PA catheter the preferred option to determine cardiac output. Computer software has become commercially available for continuous echocardiographic LV function monitoring. It automatically detects end-diastolic and end-systolic LV endocardial borders and does a beat-by-beat calculation of fractional area shortening. This technique has many pitfalls and problems and is rarely used in clinical practice.

Echocardiographic Evaluation of Diastolic Function

Diastolic dysfunction has become increasingly more recognized as an important reason for cardiac dysfunction and morbidity in SICU patients, in particular in those with septic syndrome or high-dose inotropic support. The causes of diastolic dysfunction include abnormal reuptake of calcium, myocardial ischemia, hypertension, aortic stenosis, and hypertrophic cardiomyopathy. Several echocardiographic parameters to characterize and assess diastolic dysfunction are available, based on Doppler flow measurements of transmitral and pulmonary venous blood flow. The 2D echocardiographic findings associated with LV diastolic dysfunction include increased myocardial thickness, reduced end-diastolic volume despite high filling pressures, and a typical interrupted biphasic pattern of diastolic filling (instead of the smooth continuous pattern of normal diastolic filling). Doppler echocardiography is used to characterize diastolic dysfunction more in detail (4). The PW Doppler signal at the tips of the atrioventricular valves (ventricular inflow) is typically biphasic with a larger E-wave (early ventricular filling) and a smaller A-wave (atrial systole) with the normal E to A ratio being 2:1 (Fig. 24). In patients with diastolic dysfunction, the contribution of atrial contraction to diastolic filling becomes more important, and the ratio between E- and A-wave is

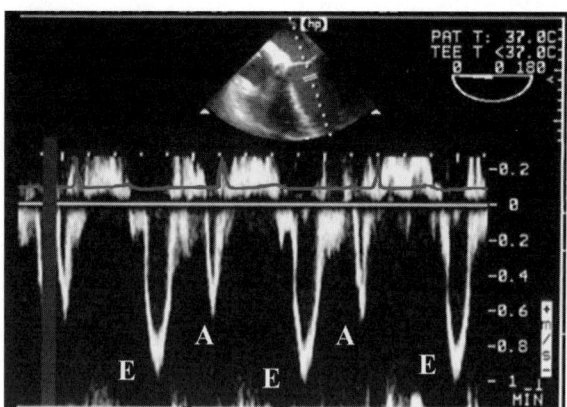

Figure 24 Pulse wave Doppler flow characteristics at the tips of mitral valve leaflets (left ventricular inflow), mid-esophageal 4 Chamber view. Normal biphasic pattern of the signal with a larger E-wave (diastolic ventricular filling), and a smaller A-wave (atrial contraction).

altered (maximum velocity, velocity time integral, acceleration and deceleration, duration of E/A-wave). To reduce the confounding influence of LA pressure and compliance on LV filling, PW Doppler signals at the tips of the atrioventricular valves are often combined with the PW Doppler flow profiles in the left upper pulmonary vein (atrial inflow). Mitral annular Doppler tissue imaging and color M-mode transmitral propogation velocity are relatively preload, insensitive measures of LV diastolic dysfunction. However, it should be noted that the sensitivity and specificity of Doppler echo findings used to characterize diastolic dysfunction in the unstable SICU patient is limited, and they should be interpreted very cautiously.

Regional Left Ventricular Function

Monitoring of regional LV function to detect intraoperative myocardial ischemia was one of the first indications for the perioperative use of TEE by anesthesiologists. Standard ECG and PA catheter monitoring detect less than 50% of all intraoperative ischemic events (3,15). Considering the therapeutic and prognostic significance of myocardial ischemia in the increasing number of older perioperative and post-traumatic patients, a sensitive tool to detect myocardial ischemia is undoubtedly of significant clinical importance.

Regional wall motion is characterized by a systolic inward motion (endocardial movement) and systolic wall thickening (Fig. 25). Regional wall motion may be classified as normal, hypokinetic, akinetic, or dyskinetic. Endocardial movement is easier to assess when compared to myocardial thickening (Table 4). Assessment of myocardial thickening is significantly improved with M-mode echocardiography, in particular with the less experienced investigator. A reduction in myocardial blood flow of about 20% will create hypokinesis, and the segment will become akinetic with a reduction in blood flow of more than 90% (16). For a rapid initial assessment of regional wall motion in emergency situations, the TG mid-SAX view is chosen (Fig. 26). All three major branches of the coronary circulation are represented in this echocardiographic plane. The mid-esophageal views (ME 4 Chamber, ME 2 Chamber, and ME LA) supplement the TG mid-SAX view (especially when difficult to obtain), providing a more thorough evaluation

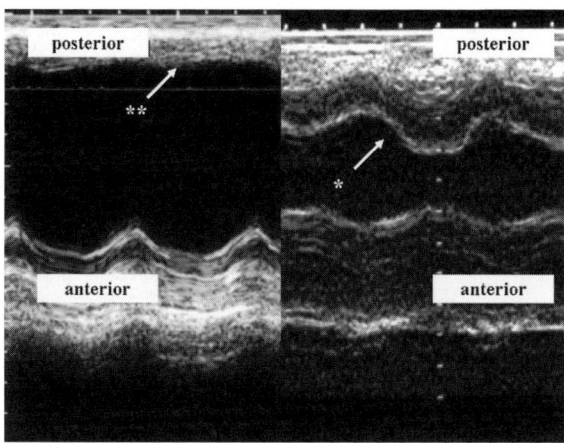

Figure 25 Impaired (*left*) and normal (*right*) regional left ventricular wall motion, transgastric short-axis view, M-Mode. *Note:* Normal pattern of contractility with systolic thickening and inward motion. Akinetic myocardial segment with loss of systolic thickening and inward motion (of the posterior wall).

of the basal, mid and apical levels of the LV (Fig. 26). For a comprehensive echocardiographic evaluation of regional LV function, the 16-segment model endorsed by the ASE is recommended (14).

☞ **The single most important cause of regional wall motion abnormality is myocardial ischemia.** ☞ Other causes of wall motion abnormalities include myocardial hematoma, myocardial contusion, intraventricular conduction abnormalities (left anterior hemiblock or pacemaker stimulation), myocardial stunning, intracoronary air, hypovolemia, and mitral stenosis. Loss of active thickening of the myocardium is an earlier (seconds) and more sensitive sign of interrupted myocardial blood flow compared to ST-T segment alterations (minutes) or increases in PACOP (low sensitivity and specificity) (3,11). However, TEE assessment of regional wall motion abnormalities has some limitations, in particular with the less experienced investigator. Oblique echocardiographic views can mimic (foreshortening) or miss (pseudo thickening) even significant, extensive regional wall motion abnormalities.

Right Ventricular Function

Compared to evaluation of global LV function, echocardiographic assessment of global and regional RV function is complicated by the nongeometric, asymmetric, crescent shape of this chamber, making quantitative measurements less reliable. Thus, RV size and function is best assessed in a qualitative manner (17). Standard views in which to evaluate RV size and function are IG mid-SAX, ME 4

Table 4 Contraction Patterns of Normal and Altered Regional Left Ventricular Function

Contractility	Radial shortening	Thickening
Normal	More than 30%	>30%
Hypokinetic	10–30%	10–30%
Akinetic	None	None
Dyskinetic	Systolic radial widening	Systolic thinning

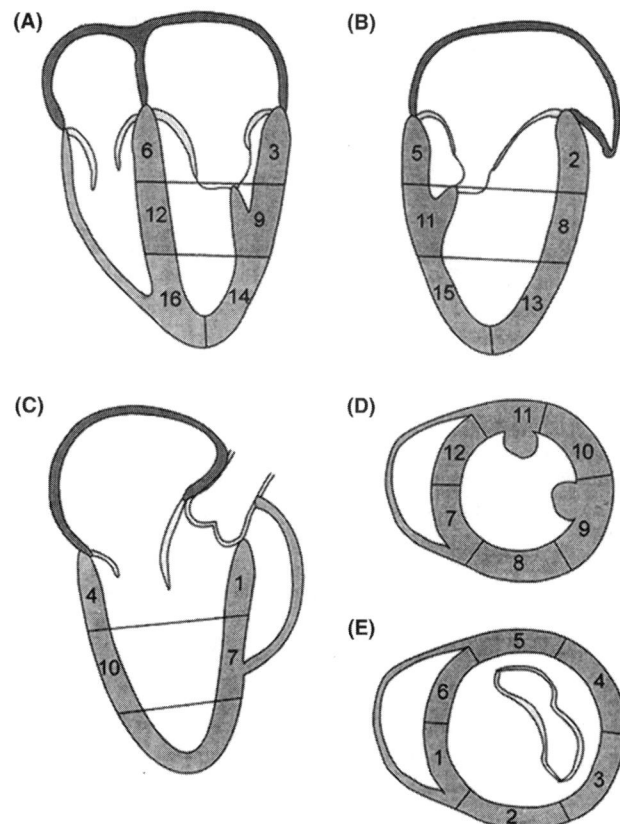

Figure 26 Sixteen-segment model of the left ventricle. (**A**) Four-Chamber view shows the three septal and three lateral segments. (**B**). Two-Chamber view shows the three anterior and three inferior segments. (**C**) Long-axis view shows the two anteroseptal and two posterior or inferolateral segments. (**D**) Mid-short-axis view shows all six segments at the midlevel. (**E**) Basal short-axis view shows all six segments at basal level. Basal segments—1, basal anteroseptal; 2, basal anterior; 3, basal lateral; 4, basal posterior (inferolateral); 5, basal inferior; and 6, basal septal. Mid-segments—7, mid-anteroseptal; 8, mid-anterior; 9, mid-lateral; 10, mid-posterior (inferolateral); 11, mid-inferior; and 12, mid-septal. Apical segments—13, apical anterior; 14, apical lateral; 15, apical inferior; and 16, apical septal.

Chamber, TG RV inflow, and the ME RV inflow–outflow views (Table 5).

The RV consists of an RV free wall and a septal wall, which it shares with the LV. The RV free wall can be divided into basal, mid, and apical segments corresponding to the adjacent LV segments in the ME 4 Chamber view. Normal RV thickness is less than half of the LV and measures <5 mm at end diastole. Right ventricular hypertrophy (RVH) is present when RV wall thickness exceeds 6 mm. In patients with RVH, a prominent trabeculae pattern is often seen, especially at the apex.

In the ME 4 Chamber view, normal RV appearance is triangular compared to the elliptical LV, and its length extends for only about two-thirds the length of the LV. The apex in this view is formed by only the LV, and the end diastolic cross-sectional area of the RV is less than 60% of the LV area. When RV area exceeds LV area, severe RV enlargement is present. As the RV dilates, its shape changes from triangular to round. When the cardiac apex is formed by the RV rather than the LV, the RV is dilated. Because of the

Table 5 Echocardiographic Parameters that Describe Right Ventricular Function

Parameter	Normal	Pathological
RV shape	Semilunar	Round, dilated
RV size	<2/3 LV size	<LV size, moderate enlargement
		>LV size, severe enlargement
RV free wall thickness	<6 mm	<10 mm, moderate hypertrophy
		>10 mm, severe hypertrophy
RV free wall motion	Normal	Hypokinetic, moderate dysfunction
		Akinetic, severe dysfunction
Septal motion	Contraction with LV	Paradoxical contraction with RV
		Diastolic leftward shift

Abbreviations: LV, left ventricle; RV, right ventricle.

complex geometry and contraction pattern of the RV, regional wall motion can be difficult to assess. In general, akinesia or dyskinesia of the RV free wall needs to be present for wall motion abnormality to be definitively diagnosed.

Normally, the ventricular septum functions as part of the LV and maintains a convex curvature toward the RV throughout the cardiac cycle. As the RV dilates or hypertrophies, the septum flattens. When RV mass exceeds LV mass, paradoxical septal motion appears (inward movement toward LV in diastole). With RV volume overload (atrial septal defect, tricuspid regurgitation, and pulmonic regurgitation) septal distortion is maximal at end diastole, corresponding with timing of peak diastolic overfilling of the RV. During systole, the end-diastolic septal flattening reverses, and there is paradoxical systolic septal motion toward the RV cavity. In RV pressure overload, maximal septal distortion is at end systole and early diastole, corresponding to the time of peak systolic afterload of the RV.

ASSESSMENT OF VALVULAR FUNCTION

Quantitative detailed assessment of valvular dysfunction necessitates advanced knowledge in echocardiography, valvular anatomy, and cardiology. It should be done only after a comprehensive echocardiographic examination, including multiple 2D planes and various PW and CW Doppler calculations. There are a number of possible pitfalls when assessing the hemodynamic significance of a valvular lesion, and only specially trained cardiologists and cardiovascular anesthesiologists should do advanced echocardiographic evaluation of valvular lesions. However, an abbreviated 2D and semi-quantitative color Doppler examination of the valves must be done in the case of hemodynamically unstable or septic patients. This preliminary qualitative echocardiographic valve assessment can be done with a basic level of education in echocardiography, and allows one to exclude significant valvular pathology and reliably detect common valvular lesions relevant for the trauma or critically ill patient in the SICU: vegetations in patients with endocarditis, acute valvular regurgitation after trauma, myocardial infarction, septic valve destruction, and acute aortic insufficiency (AI) in patients with type A aortic dissection.

Mitral Valve Evaluation

The MV can be easily examined with TEE. The MV structures include the annulus, leaflets, chordae tendinae,

papillary muscles, myocardium, and the fibrous skeleton of the heart. The MV annulus is described as a saddle-shaped, three-dimensional ellipsoid with a high, more basal short axis (seen in the ME LAX view), and a lower, more apical long axis (seen in the ME commissural view). The MV is bileaflet with an anterior and posterior cusp (Fig. 27). The larger anterior cusp covers approximately two-thirds of the area of the mitral annulus and one-third of the circumference. The smaller posterior cusp covers approximately one-third of the area of the mitral annulus and about two-thirds of the circumference. The valve leaflets join at the anterolateral and posteromedial commissures. The posterior leaflet is divided into three scallops (P1, P2, and P3: Carpentier classification) with corresponding adjacent anterior valve segments (A1, A2, and A3).

The anterolateral and posteromedial papillary muscles attach to the MV via the chordae tendinae with both muscles

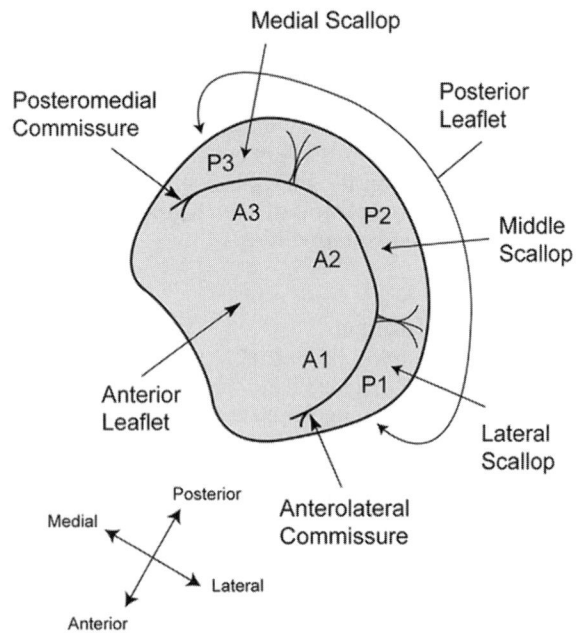

Figure 27 Mitral valve anatomy: transgastric basal short-axis view. The valvular tissue can be divided into two commissural regions: anterolateral and posteromedial. There are two leaflet areas: anterior and posterior. Clefts along the free margin of the posterior leaflet identify the individual scallops as P1, P2, and P3. The anterior leaflet has less clearly defined segments, designated A1, A2, and A3.

attaching to both valve leaflets. TEE examination consists of four mid-esophageal views (ME 4 chamber, ME commissural, ME 2 Chamber, and ME LAX) and two transgastric views (TG basal SAX and TG 2 Chamber). Using the mid-esophageal views one can closely look at all segments of the MV (Fig. 27). The systematic evaluation of the MV is depicted in Figure 28.

♂ Color flow Doppler serves as an important screening tool in the mid-esophageal views to detect evidence of mitral regurgitation (MR). ♂ Secondary effects of MR include dilation of the LA or LV. If MR is detected, a more thorough evaluation can be done with transmitral and pulmonary venous PW Doppler studies. The causes of MR can be divided into abnormalities of the valve leaflets, mitral annulus, chordae tendinae, and papillary muscles.

Mitral stenosis is now a rare finding, as the occurrence of rheumatic heart disease has decreased with the use of antibiotics. Features of mitral stenosis seen on TEE exam include restricted movement of the valve leaflets, commissural fusion, and calcification of the valvular and subvalvular structures. Left atrial dilatation with a normal or more typically small empty LV may also be seen. Additional valuable information can be obtained by using CW Doppler studies.

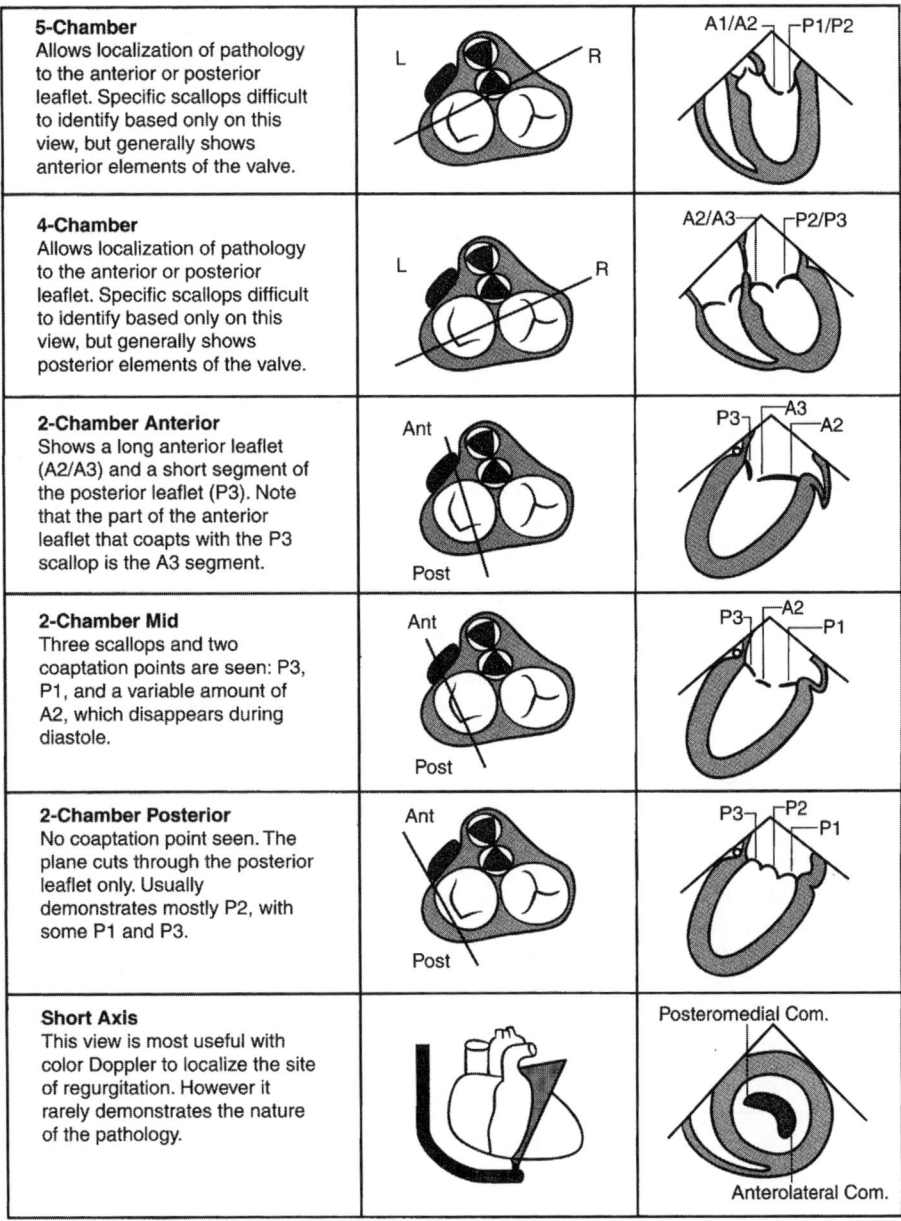

Figure 28 Systematic examination of the mitral valve. In this examination, the mitral valve is viewed in multiple cross-sections to delineate leaflet anatomy. The "5-Chamber" cross-section is accomplished by withdrawing the probe slightly from the standard 4-Chamber cross-section, until the left ventricular outflow track is in view. The center column shows the planes of the different cross-sections as viewed from directly above the base of the heart. The 2-Chamber "anterior," "mid," and "posterior" cross-sections are variations of the standard 2-Chamber cross-section and are accomplished by turning the probe from the patient's right to left. P1, P2, and P3 refer to the three scallops of the posterior mitral leaflet, and A1, A2, and A3 refer to the juxtaposed segments of the anterior mitral leaflet. The right column shows the leaflet segments seen in the corresponding cross-section. *Source*: From Ref. 49.

Aortic Valve Evaluation

High-resolution images of the AV can easily be obtained with TEE because of its close proximity to the esophagus. The AV consists of three cusps (right, left, and noncoronary) with three outpouchings called the sinuses of Valsalva. Normal AV area ranges from 2–4 cm². TEE examination includes the ME aortic short axis, ME LAX, TGLAX, and deep TGLAX views.

The most frequent cause of aortic stenosis is calcific degeneration associated with aging. Other causes include rheumatic disease, congenital bicuspid or unicuspid valve, subaortic and supravalvular stenosis. In the ME AV SAX view, findings may include fusion of the commissures, calcification, and restricted valve movement. Planimetry can be used to estimate valve area, but in the presence of calcifications. Doppler studies across the valve in the deep transgastric view give a better estimate of valve area. In the ME AV LAX view restricted valve movement, calcifications- and doming of the valve leaflets may also be seen.

AI can be caused by problems of the aortic cusps or by problems with the ascending aorta. Valvular problems include endocarditis, traumatic injury, rheumatic and myxomatous changes, and congenital abnormalities. Conditions affecting the ascending aorta include aortic dissection (from blunt trauma or hypertension), chronic hypertension, Marfan's syndrome, cystic medial necrosis, and aneurysm. The 2D echocardiography using the aortic views can be used to look for structural abnormalities of the AV, such as vegetations, abscess formation, failure of aortic cusps to coapt properly, thickening of aortic cusps, dilatation of the aortic annulus, and presence of a bicuspid valve. Dilatation of the LV occurs from chronic volume overload, and may also be noted. Color Doppler using the ME AV SAX view can help localize the site of regurgitation. Color Doppler of the AV long-axis view can be used to screen for and quantify AI. Using the ratio of jet width to LVOT has been used to quantify the severity of AI (<0.25: 1+, 0.25–0.46: 2+, 0.47–0.64: 3+, and >0.64: 4+).

Endocarditis

Suspected infective endocarditis is a common indication for a TEE examination in medical ICU patients (18–20). TEE is superior to transthoracic echocardiography (TTE) for the diagnosis of smaller vegetations and/or complications of endocarditis (Fig. 29). This TEE examination frequently leads to significant changes in the patient's clinical management (18–24). ☞ **The classic echocardiographic features of infective endocarditis are vegetations: shaggy, irregular, highly mobile echo-dense structures located on the low-pressure side of a valve leaflet.** ☞ On occasion, the

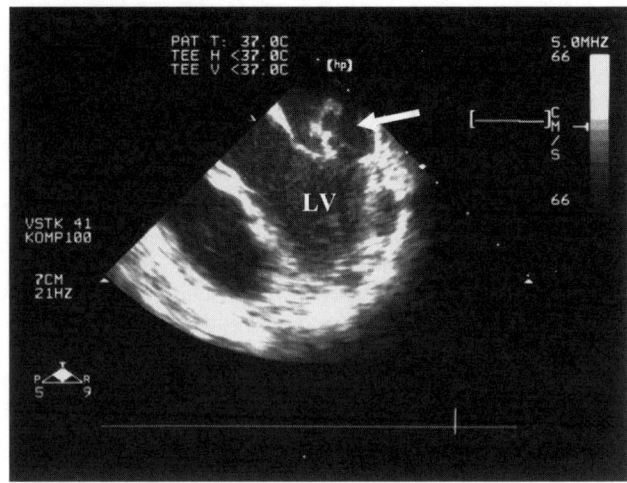

Figure 29 Infective endocarditis with highly mobile vegetation (*arrow*) on the anterior mitral valve leaflet. *Abbreviation*: LV, left ventricle.

vegetation will appear to be attached to an intracardiac foreign body, such as a central venous catheter or a pacemaker lead. The length of the vegetation (>15 mm) and the mobility (highly mobile, small basis) seem to predict probability of embolism. Consequently, besides complications (leaflet perforation, abscesses, valve destruction, and fistulas), length and mobility of the vegetation should be considered when discussing a possible surgical intervention. Diagnostic sensitivity and specificity of TEE for infective endocarditis is high (>90%) (1,3,15,22). However, pre-existing valve pathology (myxomatous degeneration, annular calcifications) can make the diagnosis less reliable. Only repeated examinations documenting progression or regression of the echo densities establish a definite diagnosis. Acute endocarditis remains a clinical diagnosis and requires positive blood cultures. The 2D examination should also focus on leaflet thickening or calcifications, reduced systolic valve opening with doming of leaflets (in mitral stenosis typically combined with LA enlargement and spontaneous echo contrast), structural lesions causing acute valvular regurgitation (aortic cusps prolapse into LVOT, MV leaflet prolapse into LA, leaflet perforation, ruptured chordae tendinae or papillary muscle), and mitral or tricuspid annular dilatation.

Color Doppler interrogation in multiple cross sections allows a good semi-quantitative assessment of the hemodynamic significance of a regurgitant lesion using length,

Table 6 Color Doppler Classification of the Severity of Mitral and Aortic Valve Regurgitation

Severity	Mitral regurgitation extension of regurgitant jet in LA	Aortic regurgitation extension regurgitant jet in LVOT
Trivial, grade 1	Mitral annulus area only	25% LVOT diameter
Mild, grade 2	1/3 LA height	25–45% LVOT diameter
Moderate, grade 3[a]	2/3 LA height	45–60% LVOT diameter
Severe, grade 4[a]	Roof of LA or pulmonary veins	60% LVOT diameter

[a]Any mitral regurgitant jet with a width more than 5.5 mm at the origin (vena contract) and any aortic regurgitant jet exceeding the tip of the anterior mitral valve leaflet should be considered hemodynamically significant. Note that an equivalent classification of regurgitant jets in the right atrium may be used to stage tricuspid regurgitation.
Abbreviations: LA, left atrium; LVOT, left ventricle outflow tract.

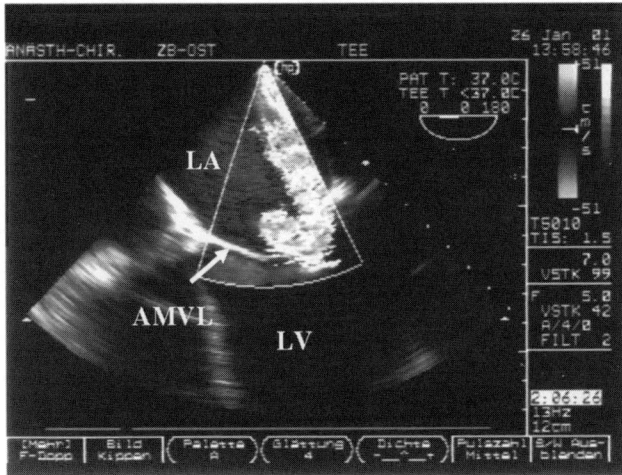

Figure 30 Mitral valve regurgitation, grade IV, mid-esophageal 4-Chamber view, color Doppler. Eccentric jet, along the posterior MV leaflet reaching the roof of the LA. *Abbreviations*: LV, left ventricle; LA, left atrium; AMVL, anterior mitral valve leaflet.

diameter, and area of the regurgitant jet (Table 6; Fig. 30). Previously unknown stenotic lesions are a rather uncommon echocardiographic finding in ICU patients evaluated with TEE and should always be assessed by a cardiologist, as should any suspected pathology in patients with valve prosthesis.

ACUTE TRAUMA EVALUATION

TEE is an important tool for the evaluation of the heart, great vessels, and surrounding tissues in the trauma patient. It is useful following both penetrating and blunt chest traumatic injuries. The following section will first discuss the clinical usefulness of TEE in trauma patients, followed by a description of the main differential diagnosis of lesions found in that population. Limitations and safety issues of TEE in trauma patients will also be discussed.

A retrospective study published by Mollod and Felner (25) in patients with either penetrating or blunt chest trauma, showed that 15 of 16 patients had significant abnormal findings, resulting in new surgical or medical management of the lesions. In a landmark prospective study on the systematic use of TEE on patients with multiples injuries, Catoire et al. (26) studied 70 patients: group 1 (patients in whom the initial clinical evaluation supported the need for further evaluation), and group 2 (patients without symptoms of thoracic or mediastinal injury). Use of the TEE yielded new diagnoses in 70% of trauma patients in group 1, but only in 33% of those in group 2. They concluded that TEE is of utmost importance in patients with multiple injuries, with or without clinical evidence of thoracic or mediastinal injuries. Another prospective study with 34 consecutive blunt chest traumas revealed that 65% of the patients had clinically relevant TEE findings, ranging from myocardial contusions to valvular ruptures (27). Karalis et al. (28) compared TTE with TEE in a prospective study of 105 patients with severe blunt chest traumas. TEE appeared to be more sensitive than TTE, especially for aortic lesions.

However, compared to newer multidetector CT scans, TEE is supplementary (see Volume 1, Chapter 25). TEE misses significant injuries in the arch and in branch

vessels, which are seen on newer multidetector CT scans, and lacks the ability to provide comprehensive information about other thoracic structures. On the basis of available literature, TEE is an adjunct diagnostic modality evaluation of the multiply injured patient. Its greatest asset is in the realm of continuous intraoperative monitoring of myocardial function, filling states, and assessment of hemodynamic instability. ☞ **The use of TEE in the acute trauma patient is only indicated in patients without esophageal injury, and after intubation of the trachea has been achieved.** ☞

Practical Approach

Most of the information necessary for an accurate assessment of the heart and surrounding vascular structures on a trauma patient can be obtained with the abbreviated TEE examination described earlier (section "Abbreviated Trauma Transesophageal Echocardiography"). In addition, the proximal ascending aorta, distal arch, and the descending aorta views must be evaluated for a complete assessment. PW and color Doppler can be used to characterize aortic flow and velocity. In aortic dissection, the presence or absence of flow in one lumen is very helpful to identify the true and false lumen. Laminar versus the turbulent characteristic of the flow pattern can be used for a better understanding of the anatomy of the lesion. It is crucial to begin the examination with a differential diagnosis in mind. Common traumatic injuries include myocardial contusion, pericardial effusion with or without tamponade physiology, valvular rupture, traumatic shunts and fistulas, thrombus, aortic trauma, and hypovolemia. Aortic dissection, myocardial contusion, and surgically correctable lesions will be discussed elsewhere in more detail.

Pericardial Diseases: Effusion, Hematoma, and Tamponade

☞ **Echocardiography is the diagnostic tool of choice to detect and evaluate pericardial effusion and tamponade (29).** ☞ Pericardial tamponade is an important diagnostic consideration in patients presenting with tachycardia, low cardiac output, and high filling pressures. Theoretically, pericardial tamponade can be differentiated from myocardial failure by pulsus paradoxus. However, in clinical practice, echocardiography leads to the diagnosis. Pericardial effusion and hematoma are characteristically echo-free spaces between the epicardium and the pericardium, and are detectable and diagnosed with sensitivity and a specificity of almost 100% (Fig. 31). Quantification has been tried, but in clinical practice semi-quantitative description of the amount of pericardial effusion is more common. Pericardial thrombus from coagulated blood is difficult to detect, as the echo density is almost the same as that in myocardium (Fig. 32). Coagulated blood in the pericardium is often found in atypical locations and restricted to a small area (Fig. 33). Therefore, diagnosis of shock secondary to pericardial tamponade by thrombus may be very tricky and should be done only by an experienced echocardiographer. Whether pericardial effusion is of any hemodynamic relevance can be judged by certain echocardiographic findings (Table 7), but if there is any doubt, decision for emergency pericardiocentesis should be based predominately on hemodynamics. The most important echocardiographic indicator of hemodynamic significance is the systolic inward shift of the RA (Fig. 34). The most specific finding is diastolic collapse of the RV wall. Diastolic collapse of the RV indicates that the pericardial pressure exceeds the intramural pressure and is

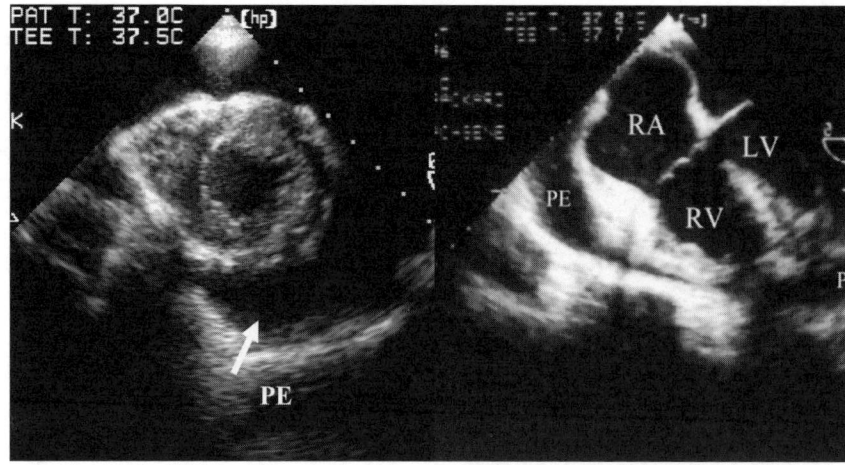

Figure 31   Pericardial effusion. (*Left*) A transgastric mid-short-axis view demonstrating pericardial effusion (PE) surrounding heart. (*Right*) A mid-esophageal four-chamber view demonstrating fluid PE within the pericardial sac impinging upon the right atrium and ventricle. *Abbreviations*: RA, right atrium; RV, right ventricle; LV, left ventricle; PE, pericardial effusion.

consequently a rather late indicator of tamponade in case of RV pressure overload (e.g., pulmonary hypertension). The amount of effusion present is also a poor indicator of the hemodynamic relevance. Small amounts of blood (60–80 mL) accumulating within minutes may cause shock, whereas large amounts of effusion accumulating over weeks may be well tolerated.

Aortic Trauma

Approximately 80% of patients who sustain traumatic aortic injury (TAI) die at the accident site (30). For the remaining 20% that reach the hospital alive, an expeditious and precise evaluation of their injuries is conducted as described in Volume 1, Chapters 8 and 14. Computed tomography (CT) technology has become the dominant imaging modality for providing definitive diagnosis of blunt TAI (see Volume 1, Chapter 25). Aortography is used where new-generation

CT is not available, and in the further evaluation of aortic branch vessel injuries that are ambiguously visualized on thoracic CT. TEE also can be used in the early diagnosis of aortic injuries (aortic wall hematoma, intimal flap, and disruption), and is useful in the setting of critically ill trauma victims because it can be performed in the operating room, SICU, or the trauma resuscitation unit. However, the TEE is manly adjunctive to multidetector CT angiography in terms of initial evaluation.

In order to understand the images seen with TEE during the aorta evaluation, a brief review of the aortic anatomy and history is useful. The aorta is formed by three main layers of tissue, from the inside lumen to the outside. There is the intima, a regular, smooth and thin layer of endothelial cells; the media, which is a thicker muscular layer; and the adventitia, a stronger and more fibrotic layer of tissue. Current TEE probes provide sufficient spatial resolution to differentiate between the intima, media

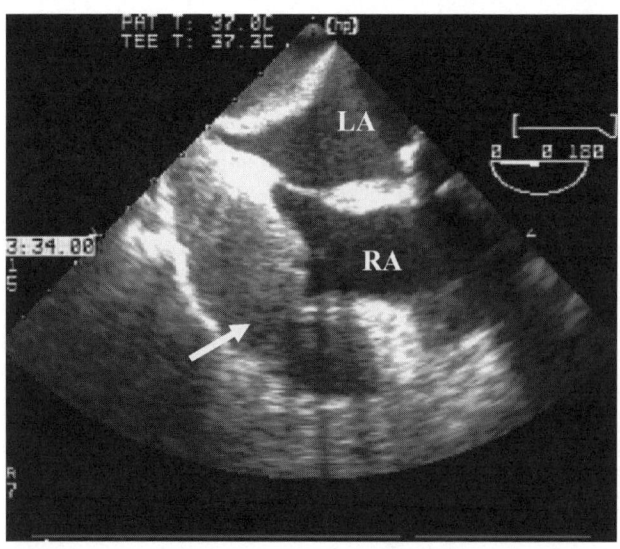

Figure 32   Pericardial thrombus—mid-esophageal bicaval (ME bicaval) view. *Arrow* denotes pericardial thrombus. There is increased echodensity of the thrombus compared to blood. *Abbreviations*: LA, left atrium; RA, right atrium.

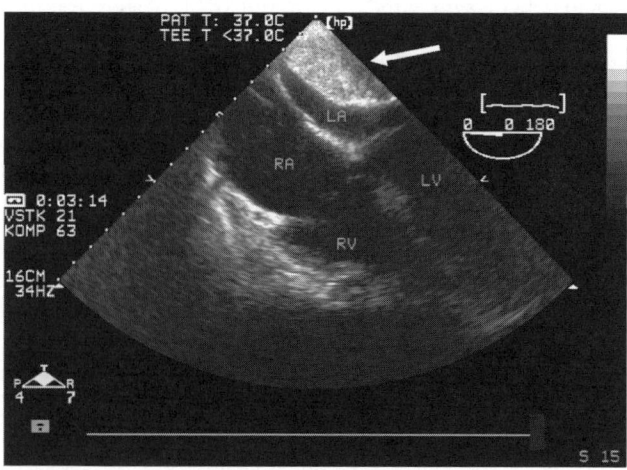

Figure 33   Atypical locations of coagulated blood—mid-esophageal 4 Chamber view—demonstrates left atrium compression from pericardial thrombus. *Abbreviations*: LA, left atrium; RA, right atrium; LV, left ventricle; RV, right ventricle.

Table 7 Echocardiographic Signs of Pericardial Tamponade

Moderate to large pericardial effusion

RV collapse during diastole

RA collapse during systole

LA collapse during systole

LV collapse during diastole

Decreased LV filling with inspiration and decreased transmitral E-wave velocity with inspiration[a]

Increased RA and RV filling with inspiration and increased tricuspid E-wave velocity with inspiration[a]

---

[a]Assumes spontaneously breathing patient.

Abbreviations: LV, left ventricle; RV, right ventricle; RA, right atrium; LA, left atrium.

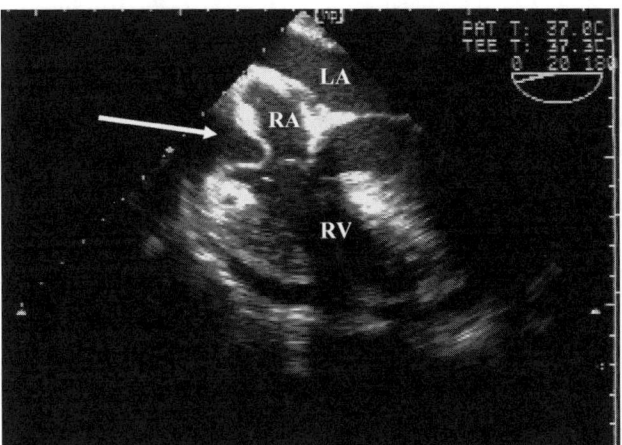

Figure 34 Systolic inward shift of right atrium (RA)—ME 4 Chamber view showing tamponade with inward indentation of the RA. *Abbreviations*: LA, left atrium; RA, right atrium; RV, right ventricle.

and adventitia, based on their thickness and differing echogenicities. Accordingly, a variety of traumatic aortic injuries have been described, depending on reference consulted (30,31). Traumatic aortic injuries include intimal tears, either localized or with extension creating a traumatic aortic dissection, aortic ruptures, and intramural and mural hematomas. In more than 90% of the cases, the initial tear occurs at the aortic isthmus, defined as the aortic segment between the left subclavian and the first intercostal arteries.

Abrupt decelerations have a maximal impact at this location because the aorta is relatively immobile (attached by the ligamentum arteriosum) compared to the more freely mobile arch. Lesions can also be found in the arch vessels and in the descending thoracic aorta at the level of the diaphragm.

Although aortography had long been considered the gold standard for aortic evaluation, this modality presents significant limitations in its ability to diagnose intimal lesions without dissection and intramural hematoma. CT angiography using high-resolution multidetector devices is now emerging as the gold standard. The sensitivity and specificity of both TEE and spiral CT angiography are clearly above 95%, when compared to surgical or post-mortem diagnosis (32). In 1993, Nienaber et al. (33) compared TEE, CT scan, and MRI for their diagnostic ability for aortic dissection on 110 patients. The sensitivity and specificity of MRI proved to be slightly superior to TEE and CT scan. However, MRI accessibility for the unstable patient is somewhat limited, and that represents a significant problem for the trauma population. Panco et al. showed that TEE was not only very accurate in the establishment of the appropriate diagnosis, but provided other crucial information, such as presence and localization of intraluminal thrombus, function of the AV, possible retrograde coronary dissections with LV contractile dysfunction, and hemodynamically significant pericardial effusions. TEE has also been proven to be highly valuable for follow-up evaluation of the initial pathology (34).

Intimal Tears

☞ Localized intimal tears appear as small (1–2 mm), thin, mobile, echo-dense intraluminal appendages of the aortic walls. ☞ The media and adventitia are intact, and no turbulent intra-aortic flow is visualized when color Doppler mapping studies are done over the aortic wall. The aortic contour is also preserved. Vignon et al. (31) showed in their 1995 study that the conservative management of localized tears was appropriate, and that no surgical intervention was needed. At the other end of the spectrum, it is possible that an intimal tear can be large enough to create an entry point for the blood stream and create a separation between the intima and the media. This will result in the creation of an intraluminal intimal flap (Fig. 35). These lesions are called traumatic aortic dissections. The intimal flap is usually thin (2.2 ±0.7 mm), highly mobile, and travels parallel to the isthmus wall. The short-axis view of the aortic lumen will usually present two lumens of different sizes. The difference between the true and the false lumen is

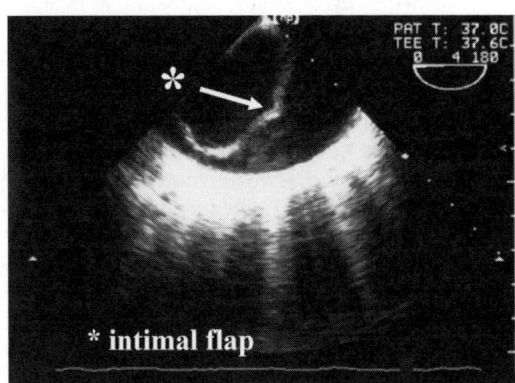

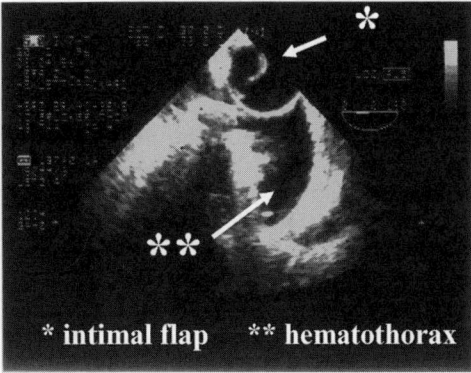

Figure 35 Aortic tear. Both images are descending aortic short-axis views (*left*). The descending aorta is visualized and the intimal flap (*) is shown (*right*). The aortic dissection with intimal flap (*), as well as the accompanying hemothorax (**) are shown.

made by evaluating the systolic flow expansion of the true lumen. Interestingly, the true lumen is very often the smaller one. Finally, the aortic contour is usually symmetrically enlarged (31). The management of traumatic aortic dissection is usually medical, if limited to the descending aorta and if no organ perfusion appears to be compromized. This is supported by the natural history of these lesions: the false lumen will most likely thrombose and a clot can be seen on follow-up studies.

Aortic Ruptures

Aortic ruptures, also called traumatic aortic disruptions, occur when the lesions involve the entire intimal and medial layers, with the adventitia usually intact. Appropriately, these lesions are also called subadventitial ruptures. An aortic rupture will present with a thick, relatively immobile medial flap (4.2 ± 0.8 mm) traveling perpendicular to the aortic isthmus and traversing the entire aortic lumen (31). Two lumens can be seen in the short-axis views, but they are usually about the same size and have even flows, with Doppler evaluation. The aortic contour will also appear irregularly enlarged. Because those patients may die suddenly secondary to a rupture of the adventitial layer, they should be managed surgically as soon as possible. TEE can help the trauma physician distinguish between an intimal tear with dissection and an aortic rupture. This difference is of crucial importance, because of their different management strategies.

Intramural Hematoma

Aortic trauma can also result in rupture of the vasa vasorum, resulting in an intramural hematoma. TEE examination shows no intimal flap and an intact intima. The aortic wall appears to have a crescent or circular increased wall thickness. Intramural hematoma involving the ascending aorta typically measure 7 ± 2 mm, whereas descending aorta hematoma measure 15 ± 6 mm. The intima is still smooth with no apparent rupture. The wall hematoma may also contain a hypoechoic area, representing small pockets of blood inside the wall. There is no communication between the thickened wall and the vessel lumen when evaluated by Doppler echocardiography. The natural history of intramural hematoma is such that 60% of patients will progress to rupture or dissection within a one-year follow-up. Nienaber et al. (35) clearly demonstrated that intramural hematoma are part of the spectrum of aortic dissection with flap and should clinically be managed the same way.

Myocardial Contusion

Myocardial contusion is characterized by direct myocardial injury or cell death of a variable portion (width and thickness) of the heart muscle. Clinically, this diagnosis can be made by EGG changes, cardiac enzyme elevation, nuclear studies, or echocardiographic evaluation (see also Volume 1, Chapter 25).

The classic echocardiographic myocardial contusion will be defined by the presence of new segmental wall motion abnormalities, often associated with a reduced global contractile function and an anterior pericardial effusion. Because most of the myocardial trauma is related to the rapid deceleration and contact between the heart and the sternum, the most anterior myocardial structures (RV free wall and anterior wall of the LV) are more commonly involved. The ME RV inflow–outflow view, the ME 4 Chamber view, and the ME 2 Chamber views are most useful for evaluation of the relevant structures. In addition, the TG mid-SAX view can help identify anterior pericardial effusions. New wall motion abnormalities are present in areas where there is enough myocardium to be damaged and will usually appear to be more echogenic compared to other segments. This precision is important because the patient may have significant baseline wall motion abnormalities.

One important point related to the early diagnosis of myocardial contusion is to identify the diagnostic modality that will be more powerful in predicting serious complications. In a large meta-analysis including more than 4000 patients of both retrospective and prospective studies, Maenza et al. (36) showed that EGG abnormalities and high rise in CPK-MB enzymes were the best ways to identify patients who will develop complications related to myocardial contusion. Only a few recent TEE studies were included in this meta-analysis. A more recent study published in 2001 by Wiener et al. (37) compared the usefulness of TEE to the CPK-MB, in 50 patients. Even though the study was limited, TEE was shown to be a better diagnostic tool compared to the use of cardiac enzymes alone, for the diagnosis of more serious myocardial contusions, including those with significant pericardial effusions and severe wall motion abnormalities.

Surgically Correctable Lesions

Significant chest trauma, either blunt or penetrating, can cause structural damage to the heart. Most frequently involved are one or both atrioventricular valves. The TV and MV can have either a valve laceration or rupture of a supporting structure (chordae tendinae, papillary muscle), resulting in hemodynamically significant regurgitant lesions (38–41). Traumatic fistulas between the sinuses of Valsalva and the main PA or the aorta have also been described (25). Penetrating trauma can cause pericardial lesions and potentially myocardial tear with pseudoaneurysm formation or VSD. In all these cases, TEE permits prompt diagnosis and aggressive intervention leading to successful surgical repair of complex cardiac traumatic lesions. The abbreviated TEE examination described earlier can help the clinician to establish or rule out the presence of those diagnoses, even during the early evaluation period.

Other Diagnoses

Wall thrombus secondary to severe hypokinetic or akinetic wall segments can develop quickly after trauma and represent a serious threat for either pulmonary or systemic emboli (38). The thrombi are usually adjacent to the less contractile myocardial segments and will appear as an echo-dense (brighter) signal with an apparent increase in wall thickness protruding inside the chamber cavity. Mobile thrombus may indicate impending embolization.

Limitations of TEE for Trauma Evaluation

Like any other diagnostic modality, TEE has limitations that must be considered when evaluating the trauma patient. Of great initial importance is the recognition that TEE is contraindicated in the setting of known or likely esophageal injury (31). The next important consideration is that the trauma patient is at high risk for pulmonary aspiration. Thus, TEE should only be employed in those patients who are already tracheally intubated (i.e., the airway is protected).

The acoustic shadow created by the trachea and left bronchus make it difficult, if not impossible, to visualize the distal part of the ascending aorta and proximal arch.

Fortunately, isolated lesions of these areas are extremely rare, and when injuries are present, they typically extend beyond this "blind spot," becoming accessible for evaluation by TEE. Another potential pitfall is the misdiagnosis of artifacts for real lesions. For example, reverberation artifact from a PA catheter or side lobes artifact from atherosclerotic plaque can be mistaken for aortic dissection, particularly in the proximal ascending aorta. It must be kept in mind that a real pathologic finding will be seen consistently in multiple imaging planes and not only in one specific view. One must also keep in mind that TEE is not the perfect tool to evaluate the LV apex. TTE can complete the initial TEE examination if nothing convincing is seen with TEE.

ECHOCARDIOGRAPHY IN THE SURGICAL INTENSIVE CARE UNIT

Studies conclusively demonstrating that diagnostic information yielded by a TEE exam can reduce morbidity or mortality in particular clinical scenarios are completely missing (3). Training and availability of TEE vary markedly between institutions, and often TEE is not used only because the equipment or an experienced echocardiographer is not available. Consequently, indications for a TEE examination in the SICU vary tremendously among institutions. An increasing number of retrospective studies have demonstrated increasing benefit of TEE on patient management in the ICU. About 20% to 40% of all TEE examinations in the ICU yield new unexpected information with therapeutic consequences (Table 8) regardless of whether surgical, general, or medical ICUs are studied (18–24). The most common cardiocirculatory problems evaluated with TEE were hemodynamic instability, monitoring of LV filling, monitoring of global RV or LV function, suspected valvular lesions, and endocarditis in septic patients (Table 1).

TEE vs. Transthoracic Echocardiography

Although the focused abdominal sonography for trauma (FAST) is now a standard portion of the initial evaluation of the trauma patient as described in Volume 1, Chapters 8, 16, and 27, the surface or TTE can also be used in selected patients in the ICU. The diagnostic sensitivity and specificity of TTE is often limited in surgical, post-traumatic, or ventilated patients. Inability to adequately position the patient, positive-pressure ventilation, hematoma, subcutaneous emphysema, wounds, surgical incisions, chest tubes, and dressings all limit the possible windows for a comprehensive

transthoracic examination and often result in poor imaging quality (20). In about 25% to 50% of all ICU patients investigated with both TTE and TEE, only TEE revealed important diagnostic information. This new information changed the diagnosis or treatment prescribed by TTE in 15% of patients (19,22). Furthermore, TEE was more specific and sensitive when compared to TTE in certain clinical scenarios involving suspected endocarditis and evaluation of valvular dysfunction (Table 9). Therefore, TEE is often preferred to TTE for post-traumatic or postsurgical patients in the ICU requiring evaluation of cardiothoracic structures.

TEE vs. Pulmonary Artery Catheter

The PA catheter has served as the gold standard for the advanced hemodynamic monitoring of unstable critically ill patients over the last several decades. No prospective clinical study has evaluated if or when semi-invasive monitoring with TEE should replace PA catheterization. In clinical practice, TEE has replaced PA catheterization in some institutions. In a significant number of patients, TEE yields important additional diagnostic information and a complete evaluation of an unstable patient is probably optimized if the PA catheter data and TEE are used together (5,7,9,11). Both techniques have their particular advantages and limitations (Table 10); hence, these modalities should be considered to be complementary. TEE yields anatomic information that cannot be obtained with a PA catheter (valvular dysfunction, septal rupture, pericardial tamponade, and end-diastolic LV dimension) and provides a fast answer to most questions that a clinician may have concerning a hemodynamically unstable patient. The major advantage of a PA catheter is the easy and reliable determination of cardiac output, stroke volume, filling pressures, and mixed venous oxygen saturation. TEE allows estimation of systolic PA pressure in the presence of tricuspid regurgitation; however, a detailed characterization of pulmonary vascular pathology (e.g., pulmonary arterial resistance) is only possible with PA catheter. Stroke volume calculations are possible with TEE, but can be quite cumbersome in clinical practice.

Contraindications and Complications of TEE for Critical Care

☞ **There are few contraindications for a TEE examination, most of them related to a pre-existing oropharyngeal or esophageal pathology.** ☞ Some of these contraindications (i.e., esophageal varices, penetrating

Table 8 Impact of New Diagnostic Information from Transesophageal Echocardiography

Patient type/number	Total impact[a] (%)	Major impact[b] (%)	Reference
Cardiovascular $n = 51$	59	24	18
40% Septic $n = 69$	25	17	24
16% Multitrauma $n = 111$	37	9	19
Unstable $n = 61$	28	20	20
Medical/surgical $n = 108$	42	—	21
TEE after TTE $n = 61$	33	20	22
OR and ICU $n = 214$	40	9	23

[a]Any new diagnostic information obtained with echocardiography.
[b]New diagnostic information with major impact on medical or surgical management.
Abbreviations: TEE, transesophageal echocardiography; TTE, transthoracic echocardiography; OR, operating room; ICU, intensive care unit.

Table 9 Cardiac Pathologies Where Transesophageal Echocardiography Has Improved Sensitivity and Specificity Compared with Transthoracic Echocardiography

---

Poor image quality in transthoracic examination

Evaluation of valvular lesions

Evaluate/exclude intracardiac shunt

Suspected endocarditis

Evaluation of mitral or aortic valve prosthesis

Aortic dissection, aortic rupture

Evaluation of left atrial pathology (e.g., left atrial appendage thrombus)

Search for cardiac source of emboli

---

chest trauma without prior esophagoscopy) may be considered relative in the case of life threatening hemodynamic instability (Table 11).

Most experts consider TEE a safe technique with a low complication rate, which has been well documented for sedated and nonintubated cardiac patients (Table 12). Frequency and type of complication may be different in anesthetized, intubated patients in the ICU; however, data are almost completely missing. Theoretically, pressure or thermal lesions may occur during prolonged probe insertion. Therefore, the probe should be left in the esophagus only for a few hours. Transient bacteremia is another theoretical consideration, which is considered trivial by most experts. Prophylactic antibiotics are not generally used. In smaller children, esophageal probes may cause airway compromise. Mortality associated with TEE has been solely secondary to esophageal perforation in patients with unidentified pre-existing esophageal pathologies.

RESCUE TRANSESOPHAGEAL ECHOCARDIOGRAPHY FOR THE HEMODYNAMICALLY UNSTABLE PATIENT

Sudden, unexpected hemodynamic instability is the most common indication for a TEE examination in the ICU (18–22). ☞ **TEE examinations in patients with acute hemodynamic disturbances result in a major therapeutic impact (surgical or medical) in over 50% of patients examined (10,19,21).** ☞ According to the ASA practice guidelines, (3)

acute and persistent life-threatening hemodynamic instability is a class 1 indication for a perioperative TEE investigation in noncardiac surgical patients. Although there are only few clinical studies prospectively or independently evaluating the diagnostic efficiency of TEE in patients with hemodynamic instability, those who regularly use the TEE to diagnose unstable patients in the SICU are well aware of the benefits. TEE is a minimally invasive bedside test and can avoid potentially dangerous transport of unstable patients within the hospital (e.g., to the radiology department for CT scan or angiography). Compared to the invasive evaluation of right heart catheterization, diagnostic information is typically available more rapidly with TEE. In addition, TEE yields information about anatomical lesions and blood flow abnormalities that cannot be obtained with alternative diagnostic tests in clinical practice (e.g., traumatic MV insufficiency, post infarct VSD).

Practical Approach

In patients with acute hemodynamic instability, there are five echocardiographic parameters that should be evaluated as rapidly as possible: (*i*) preload of the RV and LV, (*ii*) global and regional myocardial function, (*iii*) acute valvular dysfunction, and (*iv*) cardiac, and (*v*) extracardiac anatomical or structural lesions that may be responsible for shock. The time necessary to evaluate these parameters may vary, but the establishment of a diagnosis is possible within a few minutes. A basic, abbreviated trauma TEE exam (see section "Abbreviated Trauma Transesophageal Echocardiography") rather than a comprehensive echocardiographic evaluation is often most appropriate, especially when cardiopulmonary arrest is imminent. Abnormal LV preload and myocardial dysfunction are important diagnostic possibilities (Table 13). Common anatomical or structural lesions amenable to immediate echocardiographic diagnosis in patients with sudden, unexpected hemodynamic instability include (*i*) pericardial effusion hematoma, (*ii*) valvular dysfunction, (*iii*) myocardial infarction with or without ventricular septal rupture/free wall rupture, (*iv*) aortic rupture, aortic dissection, (*v*) LVOT obstruction, SAM phenomenon, and (*vi*) pulmonary embolism direct embolus visualization not always possible (Table 14). Diagnostic sensitivity and specificity for these anatomical and structural lesions vary to some degree but are in general high enough to establish diagnosis and initiate emergency therapeutic interventions.

Table 10 Advantages and Limitations of Using Transeosphageal Echocardiography vs. a Pulmonary Artery Catheter in Critically Ill Patients

Parameter	TEE	PA catheter
Left and right ventricular	Direct	Indirect
End-diastolic volume (preload)	+++	++
Cardiac output	+(+)	+++
Pulmonary circulation	+(+)	+++
Anatomical information	+++	None
Abnormal blood flow, shunts	+++	+
Pericardial tamponade	+++	Indirect signs
Valvular dysfunction	+++	Indirect signs
Observer dependency	Significant	Moderate
Complications	<0.1%	1–5%

Note: +++, optimal information, diagnostic and monitoring method of choice; ++, often adequate information, significant limitations in particular patients; +, limited clinical usefulness.

Abbreviations: PA, Pulmonary artery; TEE, transesophageal echocardiography.

Table 11 Contraindications to a Transesophageal Echocardiography Examination in Acutely Injured Patients

Trauma to the oropharynx or esophagus
Unprotected airway
Recent esophageal or gastric surgery
Tumor of the esophagus or esophageal stenosis
Pathology of the oropharynx (Zenker diverticulum)
Unstable cervical spine injury[a]
Penetrating chest/neck trauma before esophagoscopy[a]
Esophageal varices more than grade II[a]
History of unclear dysphagia[a]

[a]May be used if patient is in acute life-threatening condition and diagnostic information from TEE is considered essential for patient management.

Table 12 Transesophageal Echocardiography Examination: Incidence of Complications

Complications	Incidence (%)
Hypoxia	~0.5
Hypo-, hypertension	~0.5
Dysphagia, bleeding	~0.5
Dysrhythmias	~0.2
Laryngospasm	~0.1
Esophageal perforation	0.02
Death	0.01

Source: From Ref. 51.

In the rare cases where TEE is not diagnostic, it still provides valuable information about the exclusion of the most frequent clinical entities causing hemodynamic compromise.

Echocardiographic Features of Common Acute Problems
Hypovolemia

The advantages of TEE include not only a rapid and minimally invasive diagnostic approach, but also an increased sensitivity in the detection of reduced LV preload in emergency situations. (5,9,11,19). To assess RV and LV preload, the TG mid-SAX view is the imaging plane of choice. There are typical 2D echocardiographic findings indicating hypovolemia (Table 3), the systolic papillary muscle attachment (kissing papillary muscles) being the most obvious, consistent and useful in clinical practice (Fig. 36A,B). The clinical usefulness of 2D echo is sometimes limited by the significant variations in the LV end-diastolic area representing

normovolemia. Both systolic papillary muscle attachment (e.g., in patients with LV hypertrophy) and a LV end-diastolic area more than 5.5 cm^2/m^2 body surface area (e.g., patients with pre-existing dilated cardiomyopathy) may represent normal LV preload in particular patients.

Myocardial Ischemia, Infarction, and Left Ventricular Failure

TEE enables a direct visualization of both global and regional LV and RV function. Semi-quantitative assessment of myocardial function is sufficient in emergency situations and allows a rational diagnostic approach (Figs. 37 and 38). ☞ **A particular advantage of echocardiography in the unstable patient is its ability to promptly diagnose structural complications.** ☞ Structural abnormalities seen by TEE in patients with acute myocardial infarction include aneurysm, papillary muscle rupture with MV insufficiency, ventricular septal rupture, pericardial effusion, and LV free wall rupture.

Tamponade

Myocardial tamponade can occur acutely following penetrating trauma to the heart, or chronically following blunt trauma. Tamponade can also occur postoperatively following surgery on the heart where the pericardium is open but clot and blood are contained in the anterior or posterior mediastinum resulting in tamponade physiology (Table 7).

Pulmonary Embolism

The echocardiographic diagnosis of PE (Fig. 39) is based on the signs of RV pressure overload (hypokinetic, dilated RV with leftward shift of the interventricular septum) and in more than half of the patients by the direct visualization of embolic material (Fig. 39) in the RA or central pulmonary circulation (Table 14). TEE is more sensitive in cases with significant pulmonary hypertension, where at least 30% of the pulmonary vessels are obstructed by embolic material. However, TEE is more specific (i.e., if seen less on diagnostic), but not as sensitive as spiral CT (i.e., may have significant distal emboli not seen at all with TEE).

Echocardiographic signs of RV pressure overload are detected in 80% to 90% of patients with PE and hemodynamic instability (42,43). In patients with acute cor pulmonale based on clinical findings or TTE, TEE can identify pulmonary emboli with high sensitivity and specificity (42–46) Therefore, in many institutions TEE is considered the diagnostic tool of choice for unstable patients with suspected PE, as it not only allows diagnosis with high sensitivity, but also allows exclusion of diseases mimicking PE, such as myocardial infarction, aortic dissection, or

Table 13 Common Echocardiographic Findings and Underlying Cardiac Pathologies in Patients with Unexpected Prolonged Hemodynamic Instability and Abnormal Preload or Myocardial Contractility

Clinical condition	TEE findings
Reduced LV preload (hypovolemia)	Systolic papillary muscle contact and reduced RV EDA Consider pulmonary hypertension if RV EDA increased!
Reduced global myocardial function (left or biventricular contractile failure)	Increased RV and LV EDA Moderate to severely reduced FAC (consider myocardial ischemia or myocardial infarction when regional wall motion abnormalities are present!)
Regional myocardial dysfunction (myocardial infarction)	Regional wall motion abnormalities with normal/increased LV EDA and moderate to severely reduced FAC

Abbreviations: EDA, end diastolic area; FAC, fractional area of contraction; LV, left ventricle; RV, right ventricle; TEE, transesophageal echocardiography.

Table 14 Echocardiographic Findings in Patients with Pulmonary Embolism

Finding	Frequency
Dilated, hypokinetic right ventricle[a]	85%
Leftward shift of ventricular septum	70%
Dilated pulmonary artery[b]	70%
Signs of right ventricular failure	≤50%
Right atrial enlargement	
Leftward shift atrial septum	
Tricuspidal valve regurgitation	
Direct emboli visualization	≥50%[c]
Right atrium	Rarely
Pulmonary artery, right pulmonary artery	Common

[a]Typically combined with hyperdynamic left ventricle with end-systolic papillary muscle contact.
[b]Compared to aortic diameter in basal short-axis view.
[c]In case of severe pulmonary embolism with significant hemodynamic compromise.
Source: From Ref. 25.

pericardial tamponade. Echocardiography is not as useful for patients with suspected PE and stable hemodynamics; rather, a spiral CT scan is superior. It should be noted that detection of embolic material in the central pulmonary circulation by TEE is limited by inability to image the left main PA. Therefore, TEE can never be used to definitely exclude the uncommon scenario of central PE limited to the left PA. Without direct embolus visualization, echocardiographic

signs of PE may be mimicked by RV infarction and RV pressure overload secondary to respiratory insufficiency.

Aortic Dissection

Aortic dissection (Fig. 39) is another possible reason for acute hemodynamic instability, where TEE has significant diagnostic abilities not only in the emergent but also in the elective evaluation of the patient. Diagnostic sensitivity and specificity ranges from 88% to 100% and 77% to 100%, respectively (3,47,48). Diagnostic sensitivity and specificity of TEE was initially comparable to CT scan or angiography (48). However, with the newer multidetector CT scans, TEE plays a secondary and supplemental role (see also Volume 1, Chapter 25). ☞ **Although TEE has a definite role in the diagnosis of aortic dissection, an important diagnostic pitfall occurs when the dissection is restricted to the proximal part of the ascending aorta (extraordinarily rare).** ☞ Many institutions use the simplified Stanford classification to grade aortic dissection, as it allows one to differentiate two distinct risk groups with a different therapeutic approach (Table 15) (Fig. 40). The echocardiographic characteristics of aortic dissection include a true (extension with systole) and a false lumen, divided by an intimal flap (highly mobile echo-dense structure in the aortic lumen). In most cases, TEE can clearly define the extent of the dissection (type A or B), the intimal tear (Doppler) and diagnose possible complications, such as pericardial effusion/tamponade, pleural effusion, coronary artery involvement (type A) and AV insufficiency (type A).

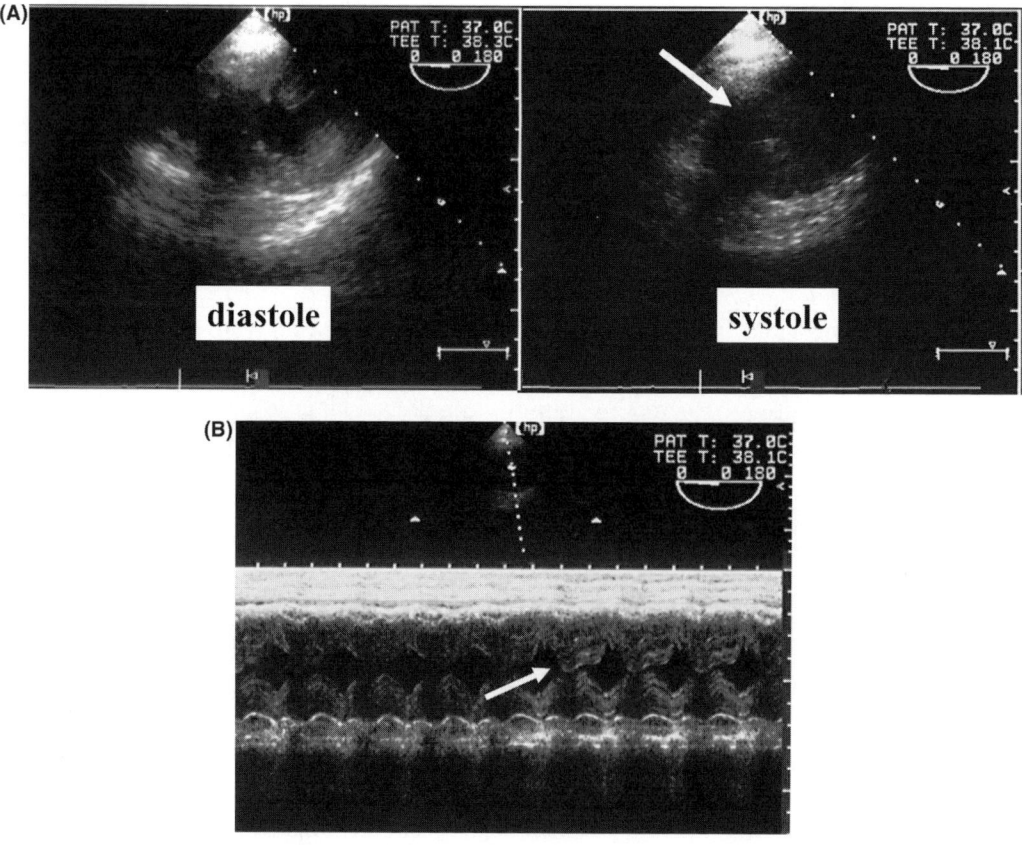

Figure 36 The "kissing papillary muscle phenomenon." Transgastric short-axis view, 2D echo (**A**), and M-Mode (**B**). *Arrow* indicates end systolic papillary muscle contact (**B**) and loss of left ventricular volume.

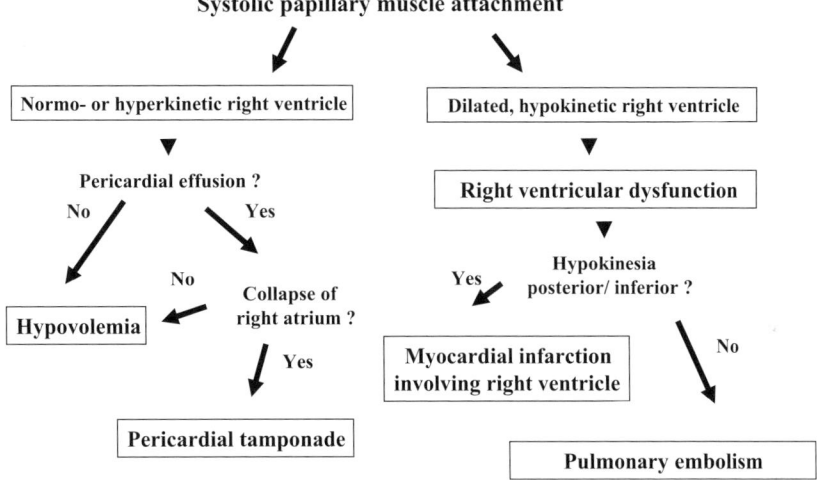

Figure 37 Diagnostic considerations in the hemodynamically unstable patient with the echocardiographic finding of systolic papillary muscle attachment (kissing papillary muscle phenomenon).

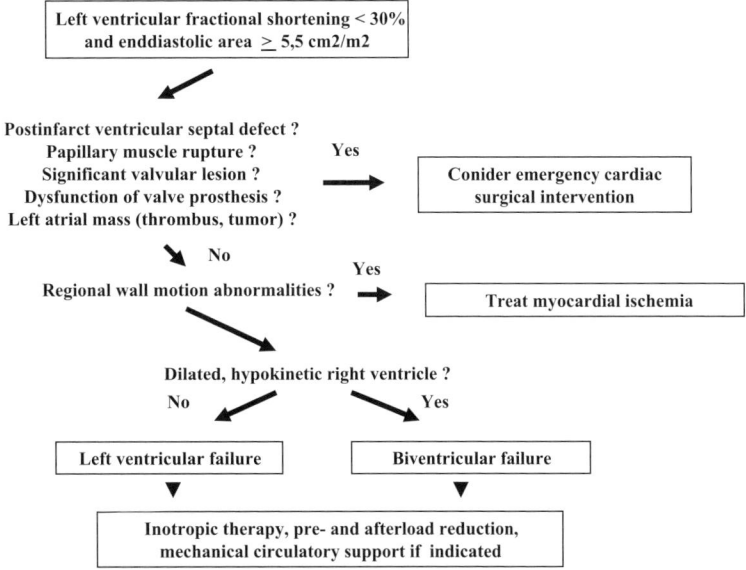

Figure 38 Diagnostic considerations based on transesophageal echocardiography findings in the emergency patient with reduced left ventricular function.

EYE TO THE FUTURE

The field of echocardiography has evolved quickly in the last decade. The introduction of multiplane TEE probes has dramatically changed our perspective on the heart structures. More changes will come in the next decade. Echocardiography is a very dynamic area of medicine with a substantial amount of research conducted every year. Myocardial echo contrast and 3D echocardiography are probably the two most exciting technologies of the future.

Echo contrast agents have been used for research purposes for about 10 years and are now commonly used for clinical applications. These intravenous agents contain microbubbles (4–8 μ in diameter) that possess a high reflective capacity. When present in the cardiac chambers, it raises the impedance between the blood and the tissue and improves the quality of the signal returned to the ultrasound system. The clinical result is an improvement in the echocardiographic viewed endocardial borders, which allows for

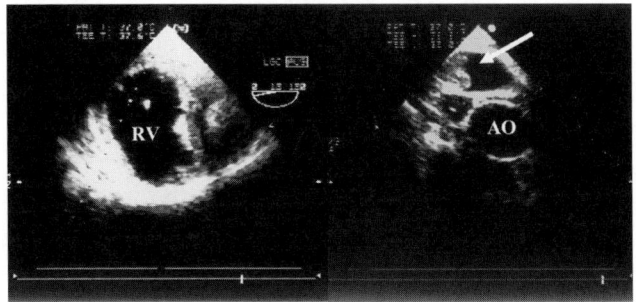

Figure 39 Pulmonary embolism. (*Left*) A transgastric mid-short-axis view demonstrating a distended right ventricle and a small left ventricle. (*Right*) A mid-esophageal ascending aortic short-axis view showing the pulmonary embolus in the right pulmonary artery (*arrow*). *Abbreviations*: AO, aorta; RV, right ventricle.

Table 15   Standford Classification of Aortic Dissection

	Stanford type A	Stanford type B
Aortic segments involved	Involves ascending aorta	Restricted to descending aorta
Frequency	More common	Less common
Mortality without surgery	More than 90%	About 40%
Therapeutic approach	Surgical intervention	More conservative[a]

[a]Surgical intervention in selected cases and in case of complications (ischemic, bleeding).

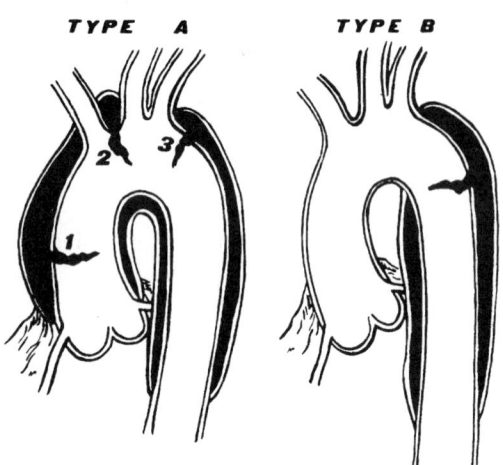

Figure 40   Stanford classification of aortic dissections based upon the presence or absence of involvement of the ascending aorta. The primary intimal tear in type A dissections can be in the ascending aorta (1), arch (2), or descending aorta (3). The intimal tear is usually distal to the left subclavian artery in a type B dissection. *Source*: From Ref. 50.

improved evaluation of global and segmental contractile function of the heart. Some agents are composed of bubbles small enough to enter the myocardial microcirculation. With adequate circulation, the myocardium should appear to be very echo-dense (brighter) because of the presence of the contrast agent. If significant coronary stenosis is present, the contrast agent should not be able to reach the myocardium and no echo-dense signal would come from that specific area. Clinically, it could help the clinician to identify noninvasively the myocardial perfusion and be able to distinguish coronary artery disease from stunned or contused myocardium related to trauma.

With the spectacular evolution of computer processing systems, it is becoming increasingly possible to analyze huge amounts of information in a very short period of time. This represents the basic requirement for 3D echocardiography. As stated in the introduction, one of the main challenges of echocardiography is to use several 2D planes to recreate a 3D composite of the heart structure. By letting computers integrate this information and display it in a 3D representation, echocardiography in the next generation will be much more intuitive and easier to analyze.

SUMMARY

TEE will likely play an increasing role in the evaluation of the trauma patient. The main indications for TEE, in the context of this chapter, are assessment of the hemodynamically unstable patient, evaluation of valvular

pathologies, diagnosis of blunt cardiac injury and myocardial ischemia, and assessment of traumatic aortic lesions.

Echocardiography is supported by two different applications: 2D imaging and Doppler echo. The 2D echo presents a real-time image of the heart, based on the time it takes for the ultrasound to travel back and forth between the transducer and the imaged structure. Doppler echo measures the velocity of blood flow in the chambers or across the valves. Color Doppler represents an easy way to display the measured velocities superimposed on the 2D image. Using the modified Bernoulli equation, measured velocities can be transformed to pressure units, and echo becomes a non-invasive tool to estimate intracardiac pressures.

The abbreviated trauma TEE examination consists of 12 imaging planes aimed at diagnosing causes of hemodynamic instability and traumatic lesions. With experience, the abbreviated TEE exam can be done in less than five minutes and can provide an excellent assessment of heart and great vessel structures and function.

TEE adds important diagnostic information to the hemodynamic evaluation of the patient in the operating room and in the ICU. It enables direct visualization of both global and regional ventricular function. In addition, it improves preload assessment, especially in patients in whom the right heart filling pressures do not correlate well with LV end diastolic volume.

A TEE examination should include a 2D as well as semi-quantitative color Doppler evaluation of valve function to detect endocarditis and traumatic or septic valve destruction.

Although indications for a TEE examination vary markedly between institutions, studies consistently demonstrate that 20% to 40% of all TEE exams in the ICU yield new, important diagnostic information. A complete hemodynamic evaluation of the unstable patient is greatly facilitated by the immediate availability of TEE.

According to the ASA, TEE evaluation of patients with acute, persistent, and life-threatening hemodynamic instability will improve clinical outcome. TEE has proven to be invaluable in diagnosing and treating pericardial tamponade and other causes of acute myocardial dysfunction.

KEY POINTS

- From the Doppler shift, the velocity of the moving blood cells can be calculated.
- The modified Bernoulli equation can be used to transform velocities obtained by TEE into pressure units .
- By convention, the velocities going away from the transducer are coded in shades of blue, whereas velocities coming toward the transducer are coded in shades of red (BART: Blue Away, Red Towards).
- The abbreviated trauma examination includes 12 of the 20 cross sections of the ASE/SCA comprehensive examination.

- Normally, the TG mid-SAX view is used to assess RV and LV myocardial preload.
- Evaluation of global LV function in the ICU and emergency patient is typically done semi-quantitatively, describing global LV function as hyperdynamic, normal, moderately impaired, or severely impaired.
- Regional wall motion may be classified as normal, hypokinetic, akinetic, or dyskinetic.
- The single most important cause of regional wall motion abnormality is myocardial ischemia.
- Color flow Doppler serves as an important screening tool in the mid-esophageal views to detect evidence of MR.
- The classic echocardiographic features of infective endocarditis are vegetations: shaggy, irregular, highly mobile echo-dense structures located on the low-pressure side of a valve leaflet.
- The use of TEE in the acute trauma patient is only indicated in patients without esophageal injury, and after intubation of the trachea has been achieved.
- Echocardiography is the diagnostic tool of choice to detect and evaluate pericardial effusion and tamponade (29).
- Localized intimal tears appear as small (1–2 mm), thin, mobile, echo-dense intraluminal appendages of the aortic walls.
- There are few contraindications for a TEE examination, most of them related to a pre-existing oropharyngeal or esophageal pathology.
- TEE examinations in patients with acute hemodynamic disturbances result in a major therapeutic impact (surgical or medical) in over 50% of patients examined (9,19,21).
- A particular advantage of echocardiography in the unstable patient is its ability to promptly diagnose structural complications.
- Although TEE has a definite role in diagnosis of aortic dissection, an important diagnostic pitfall occurs when the dissection is restricted to the proximal part of the ascending aorta (extraordinarily rare).

REFERENCES

1. Cheitlin MD, Alpert JS, Armstrong WF, et al. ACC/AHA guidelines for the clinical application of echocardiography: a report of the American College of Cardiology/ American Heart Association Task Force on practice guidelines (Committee on Clinical Application of Echocardiography). Developed in collaboration with the American Society of Echocardiography. Circulation 1997; 95:1686–1744.
2. Shanewise JS, Cheung AT, Aronson S, et al. ASE/SCA guidelines for performing a comprehensive intraoperative multiplane transesophageal echocardiography examination: recommendations of the American Society of Echocardiography Council for Intraoperative Echocardiography and the Society of Cardiovascular Anesthesiologists Task Force for Certification in Perioperative Transesophageal Echocardiography. Anesth Analg 1999; 89: 870–884.
3. Thys DM, Abol M, Bullen B, et al. Task force on perioperative transesophageal echocardiography of the American Society of Anesthesiologists and the Society of Cardiovascular Anesthesiologists. Practice guidelines for perioperative transesophageal echocardiography. Anesthesiology 1996; 84:986–1006.
4. Oh JK, Seward JB. Assessment of diastolic function. In: Oh JK, Steward JB, Tajik AJ, eds. The Echo Manual. Philadelphia: Lippincot Williams & Wilkins, 1999: 45–58.
5. Reichert CL, Visser CA, Koolen JJ, et al. Transesophageal echocardiography in hypotensive patients after cardiac operations. J Thorac Cardiovasc Surg 1992; 104:321–326.
6. Rich DL, Konstadt SN, Nejat M, Abrams HP, Bucek J. Intraoperative transesophageal echocardiography for the detection of cardiac preload changes induced by transfusion and phlebotomy in pediatric patients. Anesthesiology 1993; 79:10–15.
7. Benjamin E, Griffin K, Leibowitz AB. Goal directed transesophageal echocardiography performed by intensivists to assess left ventricular function: comparison with pulmonary artery catheterization. J Cardiothorac Vasc Anesth 1998; 12:10–15.
8. Tousignant CP, Walsh F, Mazer CD. The use of transesophageal echocardiography for preload assessment in critically ill patients. Anesth Analg 2000; 90:351–355.
9. Voga G, Krivec B. Echocardiography in the intensive care unit. Curr Opin Crypt Care 2000; 6:207–213.
10. Loubieres Y, Vieillard-Baron A, Beauchet A, Fourme T, Page B, Jardin F. Echocardiographic evaluation of left ventricular function in critically ill patients. dynamic loading challenge using medical antishock trousers. Chest 2000; 118:1718–1723.
11. Fontes ML, Bellows W, Ngo L, Mangano DT. Assessment of ventricular function in critically ill patients: limitations of pulmonary artery catheterization. J Cardiothoracic Vasc Anesth 1999; 13:521–527.
12. Swenson JD, Bull D, Stringham J. Subjective assessment of left ventricular preload using transesophageal echocardiography: corresponding pulmonary artery occlusion pressure. J Cardiothoracic Vasc Anesth 2001; 15:580–583.
13. Lang RM, Borow KM, Neumann A, Janzen D. Systemic vascular resistance: an unreliable index of left ventricular afterload. Circulation 1986; 74:1114 –1123.
14. Schiller NB et al. Recommendations for quantitation of the left ventricle by two-dimensional echocardiography. American Society of Echocardiography Committee on Standards, Subcommittee on Quantitation of two-dimensional echocardiograms. J Am Soc Echo 1989; 2:358–367.
15. Cahalan MK. Transesophageal echocardiography. In: Miller RD, ed. Anesthesia. 5th ed. Philadelphia, PA: Elsevier 2000:1207–229.
16. Vatner SF. Correlation between acute reductions in myocardial blood flow and function in conscious dogs. Circ Res 1980; 47:201–207.
17. Feigenbaum H. Echocardiographic evaluation of cardiac chambers. In: Feigenbaum H, ed. Echocardiography. Philadelphia: Lippincott Williams & Wilkins, 1994:134–181.
18. Oh Jk, Seward JB, Khandheria BK, et al. Transesophageal echocardiography in critically ill patients. Am J Cardio 1990; 66:1492–1495.
19. Vignon P, Mentec H, Terre S, Gastinne H, Gueret P, Lemaire F. Diagnostic accuracy and therapeutic impact of transthoracic and transesophageal echocardiography in mechanically ventilated patients in the ICU. Chest 1994; 106:1829–1834.
20. Heidenreich PA, Stainback RF, Redberg RF, Schiller NB, Cohen NH, Foster E. Transesophageal echocardiography predicts mortality in critically ill patients with unexplained hypotension. J Am Coll Cardio 1995; 26:152–158.
21. Poelaert TJ, Trouerbach J, De Buyzere M, Everaert J, Colardyn FA. Evaluation of transesophageal echocardiography as a diagnostic and therapeutic aid in a critical care setting. Chest 1995; 107:774–779.
22. Slama MA, Novara A, Van de Putte P, et al. Diagnostic and therapeutic implications of transesophageal echocardiography in medical ICU patients with unexplained shock, hypoxemia, or suspected endocarditis. Intensive Care Med 1996; 22: 916–922.
23. Denault AY, Couture P, Mkenty S, et al. Perioperative use of transesophageal echocardiography by anesthesiologists: impact in non-cardiac surgery and the intensive care unit. Can J Anesth. 2002; 49:287–293.
24. Foster E, Schiller N.B. The role of transesophageal echocardiography in critical care: UCSF experience. J Am Soc Echo 1992; 5:368–374.
25. Mollod M, Felner JM. Transesophageal echocardiography in the evaluation of cardiothoracic trauma. Am Heart J 1996; 132 (4):841–849.

26. Catoire P, Orliaguet G. Liu N, et al. Systematic transesophageal echocardiography for detection of mediastinal lesions in patients with multiple injuries. J Trauma 1995; 38:96–102.

27. Sousa RC, Garcia-Fernandez- MA, Moreno M, et al. Value of TEE in the assessment of blunt chest trauma: correlation with EKG, heart enzymes and TEE. Rev Port Cardiol 1994; 13:833–843.

28. Karalis DG, Victor MF, Davis GA, et al. The role of echocardiography in blunt chest trauma: a transthoracic and transesophageal echocardiography study. J Trauma 1994; 36:53–58.

29. Feibenbaum H. Pericardial disease. In: Feigenbaum H, ed. Echocardiography. Williams & Wilkins, Philadelphia: Lippincott 1994:556–589.

30. Parmley LF, Mattingly TW, Manion WC, Jahnke EJ. Nonpenetrating traumatic injury of the aorta. Circulation 1958; 17:1086–1101.

31. Vignon P, Gueret P, Vedrinne JM, et al. Circulation 1995; 92:2959–68.

32. Wintermark M, Wicky S, Schnyder P. Imaging of acute traumatic injuries of the thoracic aorta. Euro Radiol 2002; 12:431–442.

33. Nienaber CA, von Kodolitsch Y, Nicolas, et al. The diagnosis of thoracic aortic dissection by noninvasive imaging procedures. N Engl J Med 1993; 328:1–9.

34. Penco M, Paparoni S, Dagianti A, et al. Usefulness of transesophageal echocardiography in the assessment of aortic dissection. Am J Cardio 2000; 86(4A):53G–56G.

35. Nienaber CA, von Kodolitsch Y, Peterson B, et al. Intramural hemorrhage of the thoracic aorta. Circulation 1995; 92:1465–1472.

36. Maenza RL, Seaberg D, D'Amico F. A meta-analysis of blunt cardiac trauma: ending myocardial confusion. Am J Emerg Med 1996; 14:237–241.

37. Wiener Y, Achildiev B, Karni T, Halevi A. Echocardiogram in sternal fracture. Am J Emerg Med 2001; 19:403–405.

38. Sold M, Silber R, Hopp H, Meesmann M, Ertl G. A successful procedure in mitral rupture accompanied by the rupture of the papillary muscle and the chordae tendinae following multiple injuries and blunt thoracic trauma. Anaesthesist 1989; 38:262–265.

39. RuDusky BM, Cimochowski G. Traumatic tricuspid insufficiency—a case report. Angiology 2002; 53:229–233.

40. Pelligrini RV, Copeland CE, DiMarco RF, et al. Blunt rupture of both atrio-ventricular valves. Ann Thorac Surg 1986; 42:471–472.

41. Ruvolo G, Fattouch K, Speziale G, Macrina F, Tonelli E, Marino B. Left ventricular thrombosis after blunt chest trauma. J Cardiovasc Surg 2001; 42:211–212.

42. Wittlich N, Erbel R, Eichler A, Detection of central pulmonary artery thromboemboli by transesophageal echocardiography in patients with severe pulmonary embolism. J Am Soc Echo 1992; 5:515–524.

43. Vieillard-Baron A, Quanadli SD, Antakly Y, et al. Transesophageal echocardiography for the diagnosis of pulmonary embolism with acute cor pulmonale : a comparison with radiological procedures. Intensive Care Med 1998; 24:429–433.

44. Steiner P, Lund GK, Debatin JF, et al. Acute pulmonary embolism: value of transthoracic and transesophageal echocardiography in comparison with helical CT. Am J Roentgenol 1996; 167:931–936.

45. Pruszczyk P, Torbicki A, Pacho R, et al. Noninvasive diagnosis of suspected severe pulmonary embolism: transesophageal echocardiography vs. spiral CT. Chest 1997; 112:722–728.

46. Pruszczyk P, Torbicki A, Kuch-Wocial A, Szulc M, Pacho R. Diagnostic value of transesophageal echocardiography in suspected hemodynamically significant pulmonary embolism. Heart 2001; 85:628–634.

47. Erbel R, Alfonso F, Boileau C, et al. For the task force on aortic dissection of the European Society of Cardiology. Diagnosis and management of aortic dissection. Eur Heart J 2001; 22:1642–1681.

48. Nienaber CA, Kodolitsch Y, Nicolas V, et al. The diagnosis of thoracic aortic dissection by non-invasive imaging procedures. New Engl J Med 1993; 328:1–9.

49. Lambert AS, Miller JP, Foster E, et al. Improved evaluation of the location and mechanism of mitral valve regurgitation with a systematic transesophageal echocardiograpy examination. Anesth Analg 1999; 88:1205–1212.

50. Miller DC, Stinson EB, Oyer PE, et al. Operative treatment of aortic dissections. J Thorac Cardiovasc Surg 1979; 78:365.

51. Daniel WG, et al. Safety of TEE: a multicenter survey of 10,419 examinations. Circulation 1991; 83:817–821.

22

Cardiopulmonary Mechanical Assist Devices

Marc E. Stone

Department of Anesthesiology, Mount Sinai School of Medicine, New York, New York, U.S.A.

Sacha Salzberg

Department of Cardiothoracic Surgery, Mount Sinai School of Medicine, New York, New York, U.S.A.

Douglas N. Mellinger

Division of Cardiothoracic Surgery, Department of Surgery, UC San Diego Medical Center, San Diego, California, U.S.A.

William C. Wilson

Department of Anesthesiology and Critical Care, UC San Diego Medical Center, San Diego, California, U.S.A.

INTRODUCTION

Mechanical cardiopulmonary assist devices have been infrequently employed following trauma, mainly due to concerns of anticoagulation and exacerbation of bleeding from injuries. In addition, solitary injury to the heart requiring use of only an intra-aortic balloon pump (IABP), right ventricular assist device (RVAD), or left ventricular assist device (LVAD) is also rare. More common in trauma is the need for combined therapy with extracorporeal life support (ECLS) due to bilateral pulmonary contusions and concomitant right and/or left ventricular failure (1). Although still rarely used in support of the acute trauma patient, a few case reports from specialized centers have demonstrated successful results using these support modalities (discussed below).

More commonly, cardiac surgical patients often require short durations of IABP use or RVAD/LVAD support, whereas ischemic injury recovers following infarction and/or surgery. Finally, a large number of critically ill patients who are admitted to surgical intensive care units (SICUs) with end-stage cardiomyopathies require long-term cardiopulmonary support as a bridge to heart transplantation, a bridge to recovery, or as final "destination therapy." All of these devices are undergoing dramatic advances and are increasingly employed in SICU patients.

This chapter reviews the state-of-the art mechanical cardiopulmonary assist devices that can be of use in SICU patients following cardiac surgery, trauma, or chronic heart disease. Although many trauma and critically ill patients will not be candidates for these therapies, this field of medicine is rapidly evolving. Accordingly, all clinically active intensivists must be aware of the available technologies, because the indications for these devices continue to broaden.

The chapter begins with a review of standard IABP indications and use, followed by an introduction to a new implantable IABP device. Next, the basics of RVADs, LVADs, and biventricular assist devices (BiVADs) are provided, focusing on short-term use (i.e., bridge to recovery of native myocardial tissue). The current status of long-term ventricular assist devices (VADs) are presented as a bridge to transplantation, as well as a permanent solution (i.e., destination therapy). The common complications associated with VADs are reviewed, and the pulsatility considerations in VAD design are also discussed.

Next, the role of ECLS, including veno-arterial support with extracorporeal membrane oxygenation (ECMO), for trauma and critically ill patients and pump failure is summarized. The use of veno-veno circuits (where only oxygenation is impaired and pump function is adequate) is contrasted with the veno-arterial ECMO systems (which are required if pump function is also impaired). The "Eye to the Future" section reviews the recent innovations in miniaturization of these devices.

INTRA-AORTIC BALLOON PUMP

☞ **The IABP is a percutaneously inserted device, which provides intra-aortic counterpulsation.** ☞ Thus, it does not truly pump blood systemically, but rather augments diastolic pressure (and coronary arterial blood flow) and decreases the afterload of the left ventricle (LV) immediately prior to systole [improving LV ejection fraction (EF)]. In contrast to the VADs and the total artificial heart (TAH), the IABP requires a pumping heart to work (the pump may be failing, but must have some baseline function). In situations where the LV function is nonexistent or so diminished that meaningful ejection is absent, IABP is often insufficient, and an evaluation for VAD may be required.

Insertion Principles

Initially, IABP devices were inserted via a femoral artery (FA) cut down (2). However, since 1979, percutaneous placement of the IABP has been achieved via the FA, using a modified Seldinger technique (3). The IABP device is approximately 70 cm long and the balloon is positioned in the descending aorta, just distal to the left subclavian artery takeoff (Fig. 1). Positioning can be verified in the operating room (OR) or SICU using transesophageal echocardiography (TEE), or via chest radiography.

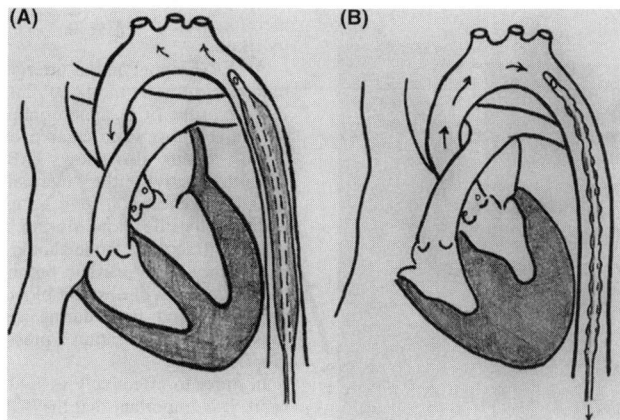

Figure 1 Intra-aortic balloon counterpulsation increases cardiac output and coronary and cerebral perfusion, and decreases ventricular workload by inflating (**A**) and deflating (**B**) during cardiac diastole (aortic valve closure) to displace blood to peripheral vessels.

Inflation/Deflation Physiology

The IABP balloon is rapidly inflated and deflated by a pneumatic system that shuttles helium through an electronically controlled solenoid valve between the IABP console and the balloon (4). The inflation–deflation sequence is timed to the cardiac cycle by sensing the "R" of the electrocardiogram (ECG) rhythm or the diastolic notch (or other features) of the arterial pressure waveform. The IABP inflates during diastole (Figs. 1A and 2) and deflates just prior to systole (Figs. 1B and 2).

The inflation period provides diastolic augmentation, which can significantly increase intra-aortic diastolic blood pressure. This diastolic inflation increases the retrograde flow from the aorta into the coronary arteries and the great vessels and, to a much lesser degree, helps speed along the blood distal to the balloon down the descending aorta.

Deflation occurs immediately prior to systolic ejection, thus causing a vacuum-like effect in the aorta, decreasing the afterload of the LV, and enhancing LV EF. Deflation occurs during the PR interval of the ECG waveform, and the exact

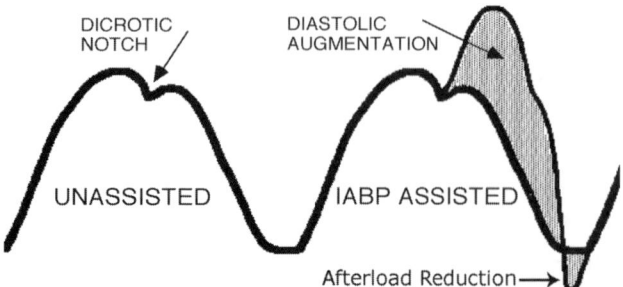

Figure 2 Arterial pressure waveform in the unassisted (*left*) and intra-aortic balloon pump (IABP) assisted condition (*right*). The balloon inflates during diastole following a trigger signal from the T-wave of the electrocardiogram or the diastolic notch on the A-line trace. This diastolic inflation increases the flow into the coronary arteries and the great vessels, and to a much lesser degree, helps speed along the blood distal to the balloon. Deflation causes afterload reduction.

Table 1 Intra-aortic Balloon Pump Inflation/Deflation Errors

Error	Physiologic effects
Early inflation (inflation prior to dicrotic notch)	Potential premature closure of aortic valve
	Potential increase in LVEDV and LVEDP or PCWP
	Increased left ventricular wal stress or afterload
	Aortic regurgitation
	Increased $M\dot{V}O_2$ demand
Late inflation (inflation after the dicrotic notch)	Suboptimal diastolic augmentation
	Suboptimal coronary artery perfusion
Early deflation (deflation prior to end diastole)	Suboptimal coronary perfusion
	Potential for retrograde coronary and carotid blood flow
	Angina may occur as a result of retrograde coronary blood flow
	Suboptimal afterload reduction
	Increased $M\dot{V}O_2$ demand
Late deflation (deflation after end diastole)	Afterload reduction is essentially absent
	Increased $M\dot{V}O_2$ consumption, due to the left ventricle ejecting against a greater resistance and a prolonged isovolumetric contraction phase
	IABP may impede left ventricular ejection and increase the afterload.

Abbreviations: IABP, intra-aortic balloon pump; LVEDP, left ventricular end diastolic pressure; LVEDV, left ventricular end diastolic volume; $M\dot{V}O_2$, myocardial oxygen consumption; PCWP, pulmonary artery capillary wedge pressure.

timing can be easily adjusted using controls on the IABP console.

Timing of inflation and deflation is critical, as errors (Table 1) can increase myocardial oxygen consumption ($M\dot{V}O_2$), and decrease coronary artery perfusion. If inflation is too early or deflation too late, ventricular afterload is actually increased. If inflation is too late or deflation too early, then the diastolic augmentation is less robust. Initial settings generally require some adjustment by the bedside clinician while viewing the nonaugmented versus augmented arterial blood pressure (BP) waveforms that are generated with manipulations of the inflation and deflation times. Anticoagulation with heparin is utilized to maintain an activated clotting time (ACT) between 180 and 200 seconds.

Indications and Contraindications

The IABP should be considered for use in patients who have LV dysfunction, but still have some ejection, and in whom short-term recovery is expected (Table 2). In those with coronary artery disease, or a hypertrophic LV myocardium (as occurs with aortic stenosis or long-term hypertension), the diastolic augmentation may be the most important component supplied by the IABP. Whereas those in congestive heart failure from a weak and dilated cardiomyopathy, may benefit most from the afterload reduction properties provided by the IABP. In both cases, the expectation is that the IABP will help improve the perfusion and function of

Table 2 Indications and Contraindications for Intra-aortic Balloon Pump

Indications for IABP
Cardiogenic shock
Acute cardiac instability following PTCA misadventure
Unstable angina
Preheart transplant/post failed transplant
Myocardial contusion following blunt abdominal trauma
Inability to wean from CPB
Acute mechanical deterioration (VSD, MR)

Contraindications of IABP
Aortic valve insufficiency
Acute aortic trauma
Severe aorto-illiac atherosclerotic disease
Irreversible myocardial disease in a nontransplant candidate

Abbreviations: CPB, cardiopulmonary bypass; IABP, intra-aortic balloon pump; MR, mitral regurgitation; PTCA, percutaneous transluminal coronary artery angioplasty; VSD, ventricular septal defect.

the LV and that, over time, intrinsic function is expected to recover.

Absolute contraindications of IABP are relatively few; mainly aortic insufficiency and/or recent aortic injury (Table 2). Relative contraindications include severe athero-sclerotic aorto-illiac disease, an irreversible LV failure in a patient who is not a candidate for an implantable device or transplant.

As patients recover from LV failure, the IABP can be weaned off, initially transitioning from 1:1 to 1:2, then 1:3, and 1:4 or less, and finally off IABP augmentation. If the LV dysfunction worsens while on IABP, considerations for placement of a VAD may need to be contemplated.

Long-Term Implantable Intra-aortic Balloon Pump (Kantrowitz CardioVad™)

Recently, an implantable IABP has been introduced, the "Kantrowitz CardioVad" (LVAD Technology, Detroit, Michigan, U.S.A.) (Fig. 3). This electrically powered, pneumatically driven device functions in a manner similar to a standard IABP, but is permanently anastomosed in a side-to-side fashion to an oval-shaped window in the descending thoracic aorta. A textured polyurethane surface subsequently develops a nonthrombogenic psuedointima, which maintains contact with the blood. Inflation and deflation of the device are triggered automatically from the electrical activity of the heart.

Like the IABP, the CardioVad provides diastolic augmentation of coronary perfusion pressures and systolic unloading of the failing ventricle, but this device retracts from the aortic lumen during systolic deflation. The result is that cardiac output ($\dot{Q}$) can reportedly be increased by around 40% with the CardioVad (depending on the after-load) (5), in comparison to the 20% to 25% augmentation of forward $\dot{Q}$ achievable with the conventional IABP (6,7). In addition, as there is an ostensibly nonthrombogenic surface in contact with the blood, anticoagulation is not required, and the device can be turned on and off at will by the patient without increasing the risk for thromboembolic events. Thus, this new device is characterized as "non-obligatory."

The initial clinical experience with the CardioVad in nontransplant-eligible patients with end-stage cardiac failure (5), demonstrated that it can be implanted with

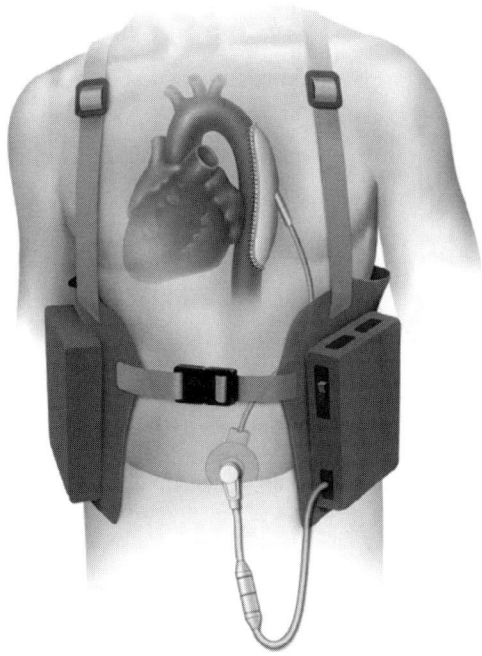

Figure 3 The Kantrowitz CardioVad™. As described in the text, the device is surgically anastomosed in a side-to-side fashion to an oval window cut from the proximal descending aorta. Because the balloon retracts fully during deflation, an increased forward augmentation of stroke volume is realized, compared to the conventional IABP. System control and pneumatic power are delivered to the device through a unique "percutaneous" cable. The modular design of this mechanism makes it more like a phone jack than a percutaneous cable. The internal aspect of the "jack" is coated with the recipient's fibroblasts to potentially decrease the incidence of infection at the site. *Source*: Courtesy of LVAD Technology, Inc.

very low perioperative morbidity and mortality, and the degree of support obtained was sufficient to reverse heart failure, improve end-organ dysfunction, and remove inotrope dependency. By 30 days, investigators observed significant increases in cardiac index, and significant decreases in right atrium (RA) pressures, pulmonary artery capillary wedge pressure, blood urea nitrogen (BUN), and creatinine. No significant differences were found in platelet counts.

Recent modifications to the CardioVad™ have decreased device length and improved forward stroke volume to 60 mL (Dr. Valluvan Jeevanandam, personal communication). A feasibility trial is now in progress, testing the CardioVad in patients with compensated heart failure, who are on intermittent or continuous inotropic therapy. Pilot and pivotal trials are planned.

VENTRICULAR ASSIST DEVICES

Several Food and Drug Administration (FDA)-approved VADs are available to support the circulation in patients with ventricular failure refractory to maximal pharmacologic interventions and/or IABPs. Circulatory support with these devices is generally accomplished by placing cannulas in the heart and great vessels, so as to divert blood from the failing side of the heart to a pump, which then returns the diverted blood to the arterial circulation immediately downstream of the failing ventricle.

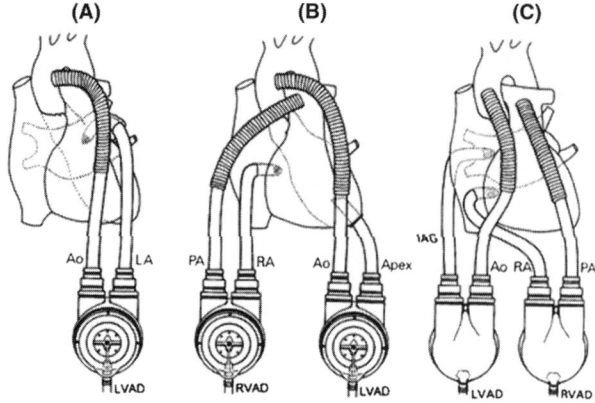

Figure 4 The Thoratec® Ventricular Assist Device and cannulation approaches for univentricular left heart support (**A**) and biventricular support (**B** and **C**). Although the Thoratec device is depicted, this figure illustrates commonly used cannulation strategies for all currently available ventricular assist devices. As described in the text, cannulas are placed in the heart and great vessels to divert blood returning to the failing side of the heart to the pump. The blood collected in the ventricular assist device blood chamber is then ejected into the arterial circulation, immediately downstream of the failing ventricle. *Abbreviations*: AO, aorta; Apex, left ventricular apex; IAG, cannula inserted via the interatrial groove and directed towards the LA roof; LA, left atrial appendage; LVAD, left ventricular assist device; PA, pulmonary artery; RA, right atrium; RVAD, right ventricular assist device. *Source*: Courtesy of Thoratec Corporation.

These devices are becoming increasingly used in patients with bleeding risks (e.g., trauma patients), due to the heparin-bonded circuits that obviate the need for full systemic heparinization and the consequent bleeding complications.

As depicted in Figure 4, for LV support, blood is continuously drained as it returns to the left side of the heart from the left atrium (LA) or the LV, and is then pumped into the ascending aorta. For RV support, venous return to the right side of the heart is continuously drained from the RA or RV, and pumped into the main pulmonary artery (PA). The diverted blood not only provides the stroke volume, which will be pumped forward as the output from the supported side of the heart, but by unloading (decompressing) the failing ventricle, wall tension is markedly decreased. This dramatically reduces myocardial oxygen demand in the failing ventricle, which potentially facilitates myocardial recovery.

Short-Term Ventricular Assist Device Support Overview

Acute ventricular failure can result from a variety of insults, including ischemia (e.g., acute myocardial infarction (AMI) or stunned myocardium during cardiotomy), acute and/or chronic pressure and volume overloads (e.g., severe acute valvular dysfunction), and inflammatory processes (e.g., acute viral myocarditis).

In the trauma setting, myocardial contusion and ventricular failure generally affect the RV to a greater extent than the LV. This is because the RV is directly underneath the anterior thorax and is more often contused following blunt trauma to the anterior chest. However, heretofore RVADs have rarely been employed following acute

trauma. Rather, in cases of severe chest trauma, combined pulmonary contusions and concomitant heart failure can call for the use of ECMO to support both the injured heart and lungs (discussed subsequently).

In cases where acute LV dysfunction is the primary problem, regardless of the etiology, counterpulsation therapy with an IABP (Fig. 1) can often provide sufficient short-term LV "assistance" to allow hemodynamic stabilization, preventing cardiogenic shock. (Note use of the IABP is contraindicated in cases of acute aortic injury or aortic regurgitation). ☞ **When maximal pharmacologic interventions and an IABP fail to restore hemodynamic stability, extracorporeal support may be required to re-establish and maintain systemic perfusion, and to prevent the catastrophic sequelae of cardiogenic shock.** ☞ Currently approved VADs include:

- The Abiomed BVS5000® (Abiomed, Danvers, Massachusetts, U.S.A.; Fig. 5)
- The AB5000 ventricle® (Abiomed, Danvers, Massachusetts, U.S.A.; Fig. 6)
- The Thoratec® VAS (Thoratec Laboratories, Pleasanton, California, U.S.A.; Fig. 7)
- Standard centrifugal pumps (several manufacturers; Fig. 8) (8)

All of the devices listed above are paracorporeal (the pump heads reside outside the body), and can provide left (LVAD), right (RVAD), or biventricular (BiVAD) support. With the exception of centrifugal pumps (which provide continuous flow), these devices provide pneumatically driven pulsatile outflow. Anticoagulation during short-term

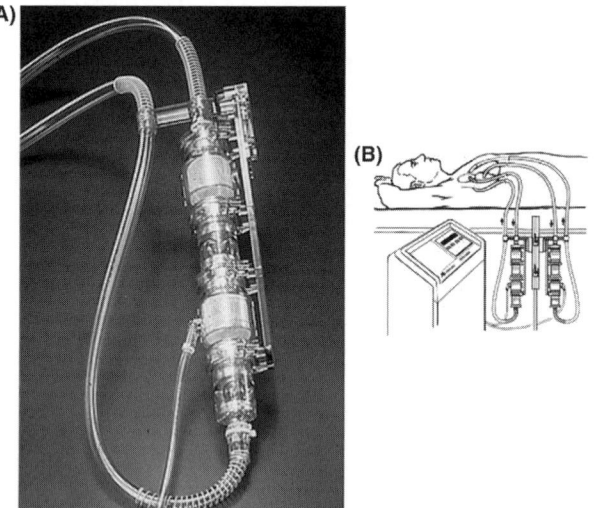

Figure 5 The Abiomed BVS5000®. Since FDA approval as a bridge-to-recovery in 1992, the BVS5000 has been used to support more than 6000 patients, in over 500 U.S. centers. The device is available in more than 85% of adult cardiac transplant centers and more than 85% of all cardiac surgery teaching institutions. (**A**) The BVS5000 blood pump. (**B**) The BVS5000 system controller and pole-mounted blood pumps. The typical configuration for biventricular support with the BVS5000. Pumps are kept mounted on a pole at the bedside. The height of the pumps can be adjusted to optimize gravity-drainage filling and pneumatically accomplished ejection. *Source*: From Ref. 9; courtesy of ABIOMED.

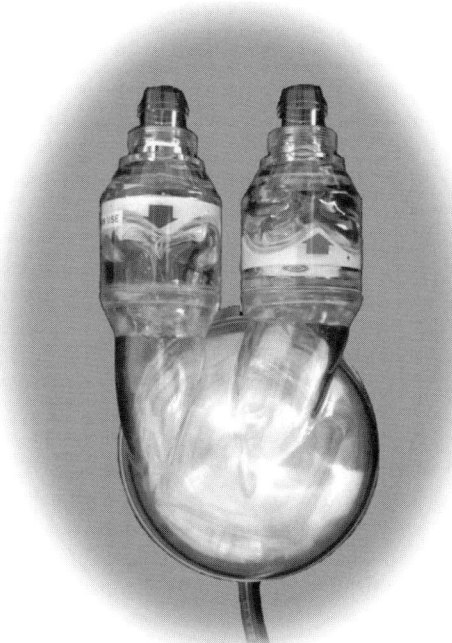

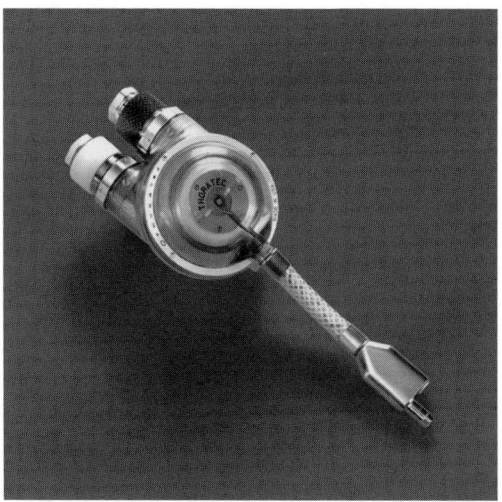

Figure 6 The AB5000® ventricle. The pump head, pictured here, is connected to the heart and great vessels by cannulas tunneled through the skin of the upper abdomen (Fig. 1). The drive-line emerging from the left of the device alternately provides vacuum to assist filling and compressed air to accomplish ejection. According to the Abiomed worldwide voluntary registry, since FDA approval in October 2003, the AB5000 ventricle has been used to support more than 88 patients, in more than 35 U.S. centers. The longest duration of support was 149 days, with an average duration of support of 15 days; 22% of those supported were transitioned from BVS5000 pumps. *Source*: From Ref. 10; courtesy of ABIOMED.

Figure 7 The Thoratec® VAS. Although it was originally introduced in 1976, and FDA-approved as a bridge to transplantation in 1994, the Thoratec VAS was not FDA-approved for postcardiotomy support until 1998. Since then, Thoratec reports the use of its device to bridge more than 806 patients to recovery. The maximum reported duration of support was 340 days, with a mean duration of 19 days. As depicted, the inflow and outflow cannulas are connected to the heart and great vessels by cannulas tunneled through the skin of the upper abdomen. The drive-line (lower right of the device) alternately provides vacuum to assist filling and compressed air to accomplish ejection. *Source*: From Ref. 8; courtesy of Thoratec Corporation.

support is generally maintained with heparin to a minimum ACT of 180 to 200 seconds. It should also be noted that none of these devices by themselves can provide oxygenation or removal of waste from the blood. They simply act as pumps to maintain effective output from the failing side of the heart (Fig. 8A). However, oxygenators can be inserted between the pump heads and the systemic arterial cannula site, in situations requiring ECMO support (e.g., Fig. 8B).

Myocardial recovery may be rapid or slow. If short-term support cannot be weaned, consideration for chronic circulatory support devices must be made. The rates of successful weaning from short-term circulatory support have improved over the last decade, from the previously dismal past. Abiomed, for example, recently reported that experienced centers, with well-defined protocols for patient selection and timing of intervention, are achieving

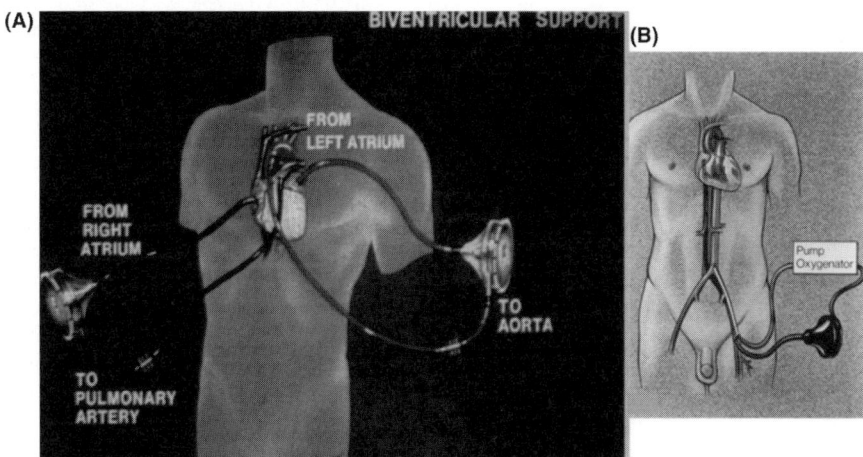

Figure 8 Potential cannulation strategies for circulatory support with centrifugal pumps. (**A**) Cannulations of the heart and great vessels (Fig. 1). The large controllers that power the pump heads are not shown. (**B**) Percutaneous femoral cannulations.

ventricle survival approaching 50% in the postcardiotomy cardiogenic shock population using the BVS5000 and AB5000 VADS (9,10). When used to support the circulation following an AMI, the survival of patients is reported to be 42% with the AB5000 ventricle (mean number of days supported = 25.4) and 27% with the BVS5000 (mean number of days supported = 5.2) (11).

☛ **The importance of prompt intervention to restore adequate systemic perfusion, and careful patient selection for prolonged treatment cannot be understated, if expectations are for successful bridge to recovery with a VAD.** ☚
Clearly, any patient who is unlikely to survive, regardless of the re-establishment of effective systemic perfusion, should not even be considered for VAD support. When the myocardial injury is deemed to be of the variety that is likely to recover and the clinical assessment is otherwise favorable, VAD support may be considered. However, one cannot wait until there is profound cardiogenic shock, with significant injury to the lungs, kidneys, liver, brain, and splanchnic beds, to initiate mechanical circulatory assistance, because experience has shown that the patient is unlikely to survive (12). Factors influencing outcome with the Abiomed BVS5000 device are shown in Table 3. It is likely, however, that such principles apply to virtually every bridge-to-recovery support device. A variety of important considerations and relative contraindications to mechanical circulatory assistance that must be duly considered, prior to implantation of a VAD are provided in Table 4.

☛ **If the myocardium does not recover after a period of short-term support, then a decision must be made as to whether the patient is an acceptable transplant candidate.** ☚
If so, their support may be maintained until a donor heart becomes available (device permitting), or their VAD may be switched to a device capable of providing long-term support, as a bridge to transplantation. If the patient is not transplant eligible, he must either be evaluated for permanent implantation of an approved VAD as "destination therapy" (discussed below), or the difficult decision must be made to terminate support.

Table 3 Factors Influencing Outcomes with the Abiomed BVS5000®

Good outcomes occur when
  Support is commenced to correct marginal hemodynamics within 30–45 min of attempted pharmacologic treatment (with or without an IABP)
  The time between the first attempt to wean from CPB and BVS implant is <6 hr
  The BVS implant occurs as part of the initial operation
  Due consideration is given to whether the patient requires uni- or biventricular support; and
  Hemostasis is assured before leaving the operating room

Poor outcomes occur when
  Signs of other end-organ failure are present
  The patient is >75 yr old; and
  The patient is brought back to the operating room for implantation after a period of time

Abbreviations: BVS, ABIOMED BVS5000 left ventricle assist device; CPB, cardiopulmonary bypass; IABP, intra-aortic balloon pump.

Table 4 Considerations Before Initiation of Rescue Mechanical Circulatory Assistance with a Ventricular Assist Device

Patient is not a transplant candidate (though VAD use may allow improvements in clinical status that may improve transplant eligibility)
Presence of prosthetic valves (increased risk of thromboembolic complications)
Significant aortic regurgitation (decreased effective forward flow from an LVAD and failure of LV decompression that will encourage myocardial recovery. Aortic valve must be repaired or replaced before engaging LVAD support)
Congenital heart disease (certain forms may preclude conventional VAD support. Ironically, extracorporeal membrane oxygenation may be the only hope for some patients with CHD)
Patent foramen ovale (must be recognized and closed before engaging VAD support with currently available LVADs)
Prior cardiac surgery (reoperative sternotomy may predispose to significant perioperative bleeding. Femoral cannulations can potentially be used to ensure rapid restoration of adequate systemic perfusion, whereas careful mediastinal dissection proceeds)
Small body surface area (outflow from the many currently available devices may be too high for patients with BSA < 1.5 m². Possibly can use the Thoratec® VAS for small adults or centrifugal pumps for pediatric patients)
Presence of advanced systemic disease (comorbidities, such as severe COPD, malignancy, end-stage renal or hepatic disease, overwhelming sepsis, progressive neurological disorder, etc., may make meaningful recovery unlikely)

Note: This is a nonexhaustive list of anatomical issues and other patient factors that either make urgent ventricular assist device placement or use difficult, make the patient more likely to have major complications, or make meaningful recovery unlikely. Some of the issues on this list are easily resolved as long as they are recognized, but must be considered nonetheless.
Abbreviations: CHD, congenital heart disease; COPD, chronic obstructive pulmonary disease; LV, left ventricle, LVAD, left ventricular assist device.

Recent Innovations in Short-Term Ventricular Assist Device Support

Approximately 7% to 10% of patients with AMI develop cardiogenic shock, and this remains the leading cause of mortality in this population (13–15). As discussed above (Table 3), a key determinant of the overall success of bridge-to-recovery is the rapidity with which the failing ventricle can be decompressed, and resumption of adequate systemic perfusion assured. One of the recognized limitations of the currently available devices, which can serve as a bridge-to-recovery following an AMI, is that they must be implanted in a cardiac OR, often utilizing cardiopulmonary bypass (CPB). Even assuming the immediate availability of the OR, the device, and the necessary surgical, anesthesia, perfusion, and nursing personnel, delays are inevitable. A likely factor contributing to the low success rates of previous bridge-to-recovery studies was a delay in treatment due to the need to coordinate these various resources prior to transport and VAD implantation. During this interval, the failing ventricle is likely to be pressure and volume overloaded, while the renal, splanchnic, and peripheral tissue beds are underperfused.

The ability to deploy a rescue device rapidly, at the first diagnosis of acute ventricular insufficiency in the emergency department, the cardiac catheterization laboratory, or the SICU, without the need for sternotomy and CPB would potentially have great impact on not only immediate, but ultimate patient survival. In addition, some complications of CPB, such as perioperative bleeding and the sequelae of the systemic inflammatory response, would be minimized. Once immediate survival is assured, such a device can conceivably be changed later, to another capable of providing a longer term of support. It was considerations such as these that drove the development of several new and innovative short-term assist devices.

The TandemHeart® pVAD™

Extracorporeal centrifugal pumps have long been used to provide mechanical circulatory assistance via both intrathoracic (Fig. 8A) and percutaneous femoral (Fig. 8B) cannulation strategies (16). Although standard intrathoracic cannulations require sternotomy in the OR, percutaneous femoral arterial and venous cannulations can be performed in many locations outside the OR setting. The downside of femoral venous cannulation, however, is that ventricular decompression is usually inadequate to substantially reduce MV̇O₂.

The TandemHeart pVAD (percutaneous ventricular assist device; Cardiac Assist, Inc., Pittsburgh, Pennsylvania, U.S.A.; Fig. 9) utilizes a full-sized centrifugal pump and an innovative cannulation strategy that does result in significant decompression of the failing LV. In addition, a percutaneous, Seldinger-type, cannula deployment system enables rapid cannula placement to assure rapid resumption of systemic perfusion.

With this device, a 21 French venous inflow cannula is percutaneously advanced retrograde from the femoral vein, through the RA, and across the interatrial septum into the LA (Fig. 9). Continuous, nonpulsatile outflow from the centrifugal device (strapped to the patient's leg) is directed into the FA. LA to FA flows of 2.5–5 L/min can be generated by pump speeds in the range of 4500–7500 RPM, to encourage resolution of cardiogenic shock. Heparinization to an ACT of 180–200 seconds is used during support.

Reportedly, the TandemHeart has been implanted in more than 100 patients as a bridge-to-recovery, following acute MI-induced cardiogenic shock. A review by Thiele et al. (17), reports the results of TandemHeart use in 18 consecutive patients with cardiogenic shock following AMI. Fifty-six percent of the patients in their series survived, and were successfully weaned from support. The TandemHeart has also been successfully employed as a bridge-to-recovery following cardiotomy with failure to wean from CPB (18), and as a margin of safety in high-risk patients undergoing percutaneous coronary interventions with stenting (19–21). Although a theoretical downside to cannulation of the FA for device outflow is retrograde arterial perfusion through the potentially diseased aorta of a patient with atherosclerosis, cerebral embolism has not been reported as a significant problem. The TandemHeart already holds a CE mark (Conformité Européene) in Europe. FDA approval of this device in the United States is pending.

Hemopump®

Miniaturized continuous flow devices that employ a longitudinal "Archimedes Screw"-like impeller have also been used in the past as a "bridge-to-immediate survival." In the late 1980s and early 1990s, the Hemopump (Nimbus Medical, Inc., Rancho Cordova, California, U.S.A.; Fig. 10) was implanted in patients in cardiogenic shock, in

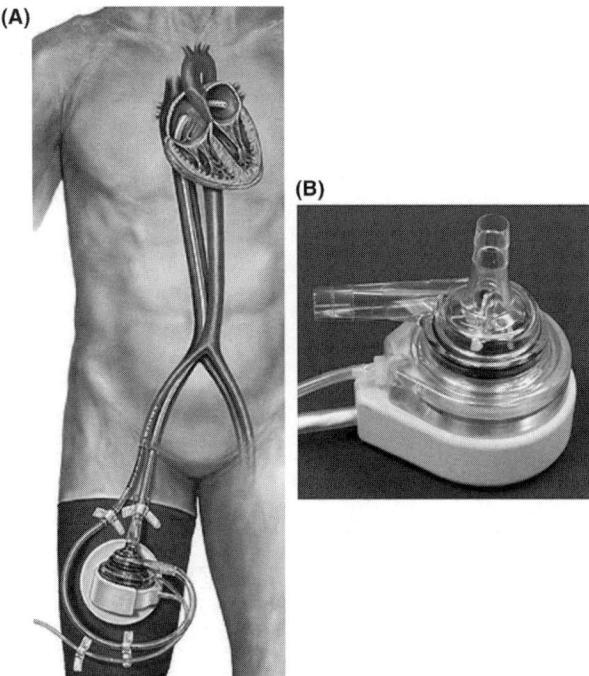

Figure 9 The TandemHeart® pVAD™. (**A**) As described in the text, the femoral artery and vein are percutaneously cannulated. The venous cannula is advanced across the interatrial septum into the left atrium. Outflow from the device is directed into the femoral artery. (**B**) A close-up of the centrifugal mechanism. *Source:* Courtesy of Cardiac Assist, Inc.

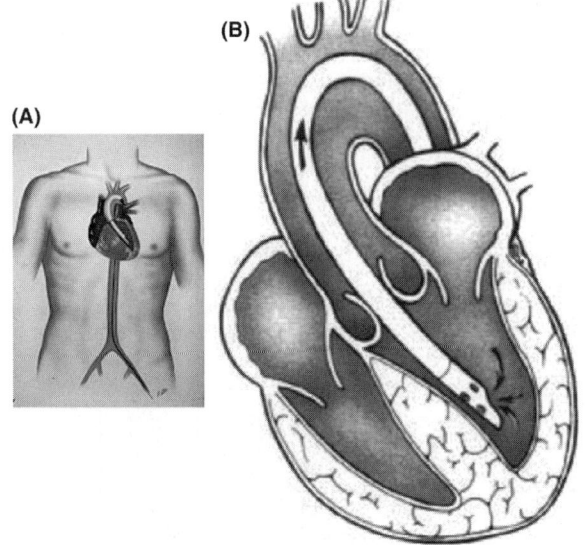

Figure 10 The Hemopump®. (**A**) As described in the text, the Hemopump was inserted via surgical cut-down into the femoral artery, and advanced retrograde up the aorta and across the aortic valve into the left ventricle (LV). Blood was impelled from the LV to the ascending aorta. (**B**) A close-up of the Hemopump. The arrows indicate the direction of blood flow.

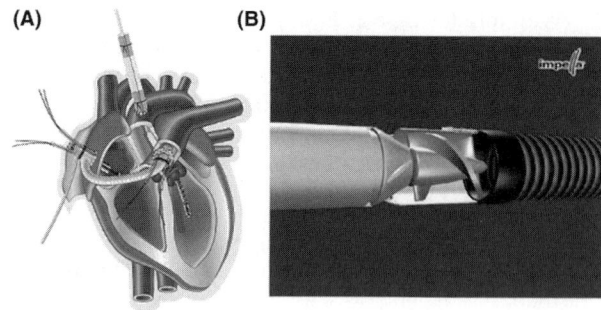

(A)   **(B)**

Figure 11 The Impella®. (**A**) Biventricular support with the Impella. The left ventricle (LV) is supported here by surgical placement of the microaxial catheter into the LV retrograde from the ascending aorta. The right ventricle is supported here by surgical cannulation of the right atrium, with the output directed into the main pulmonary artery. (**B**) A cutaway view reveals the impeller design of the Impella device. *Source*: Courtesy of ABIOMED.

FDA-approved clinical trials. This axial flow device was surgically introduced into the FA and advanced retrograde under fluoroscopic guidance, up the aorta and across the aortic valve into the LV. A high-speed impeller inside the device casing drew blood from the LV, and propelled it into the ascending aorta at a maximum of approximately 3.5–4 L/min. Reportedly, decompression of the failing LV was adequate to decrease myocardial oxygen demand (22), and the observed improvements of cardiac output, mixed venous oxygen saturation, pulmonary capillary wedge pressure, and splanchnic blood flows were found to be superior to that with IABP counterpulsation therapy (23–25). However, actual clinical results were modest at best with this device [survival around 32% at 30 days (26)], and failure of device insertion occurred in nearly 25% of patients (27). The high cost of conducting clinical trials eventually forced the abandonment of the Hemopump, but it did serve to show that an intraventricular axial flow device could be successfully employed to provide mechanical circulatory support.

Impella®

The Impella Pump System (Abiomed Inc., Danvers, Massachusetts, U.S.A.) (28) is a new, catheter-based, axial flow device that can be used to support the left, right, or both ventricles (Fig. 11). Depending on the location and status of the patient, the device can be deployed surgically or percutaneously. The Impella system may also be of use in high-risk patients undergoing off-pump coronary artery bypass grafting (CABG) surgery or difficult percutaneous coronary interventions. A mechanical or severely calcified aortic valve contraindicates the use of the Impella for LV support. Significant aortic insufficiency may also represent a relative contraindication.

A recent review of an initial clinical experience with the Impella in patients with cardiogenic shock reports significantly increased cardiac outputs, decreased pulmonary capillary wedge pressures, and decreased lactate levels by six hours of support (29). Sixty-eight percent of the patients were successfully weaned from support, though only 38% survived. Among the observed complications were clinically significant hemolysis in 38% of the patients and one instance of pump displacement. The Impella system was recently acquired by Abiomed, and clinical trials intended to establish its efficacy as a bridge-to-recovery are ongoing.

Long-Term Ventricular Assist Device Support
Bridge-to-Transplantation

Critically ill patients with chronic, progressive ventricular failure due to cardiomyopathy can often be temporized with medications, and occasionally with biventricular pacing. But for those who progress to end-stage ventricular failure, the HeartMate® LVAD (Thoratec Corporation, Woburn, Massachusetts, U.S.A.; Fig. 12) and the Novacor® LVAD (WorldHeart Corporation, Ottawa, Canada; Fig. 13) are the devices most often used as a bridge-to-transplantation in the United States. The original pneumatically powered HeartMate device was FDA-approved in 1994, and the Novacor in 1998. Both are used as LVADs only, draining blood from the LV apex to a large pump head implanted in the preperitoneal space of the abdomen, and returning blood to the ascending aorta (Figs. 4, 12, and 13). Both devices produce pulsatile flow by mechanical compression of a blood chamber, and both devices require a

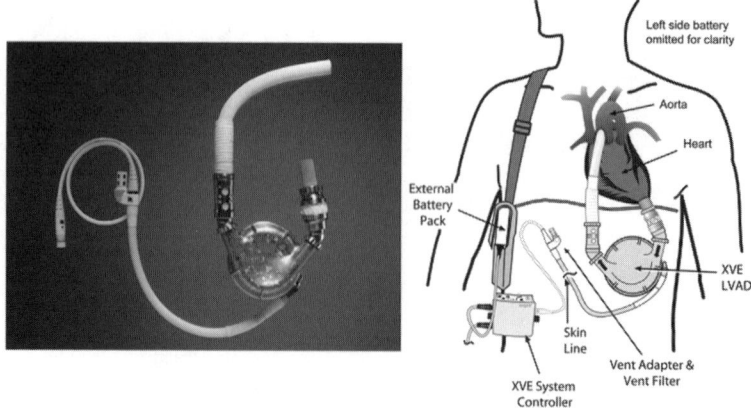

Figure 12 The HeartMate® XVE LVAD. Blood is drained from the left ventricle apex to the pump and ejected into the ascending aorta. The pump head is completely implanted in the preperitoneal space of the abdomen. The current model requires that a cable from the device be tunneled through the abdominal wall to connect to the external system controller and power supply. *Source*: Courtesy of Thoratec Corporation.

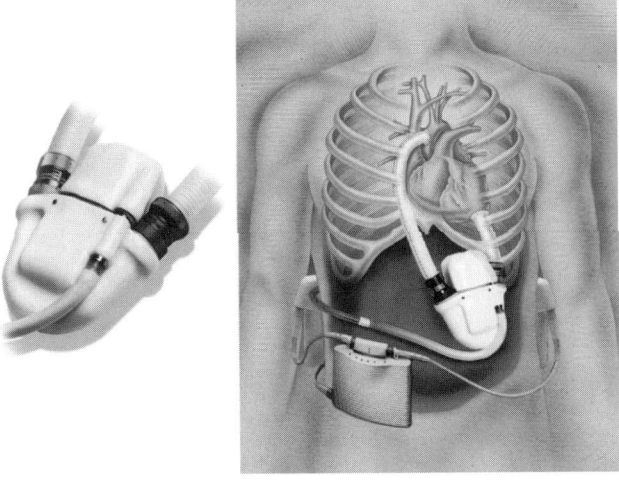

Figure 13 The Novacor® LVAD. Blood is drained from the left ventricle apex to the pump and ejected into the ascending aorta. The pump head is completely implanted in the preperitoneal space of the abdomen. The current model requires that a cable from the device be tunneled through the abdominal wall to connect to the external system controller and power supply. *Source*: Courtesy of WorldHeart, Inc.

percutaneous cable to connect the implanted device to an external power source and system controller.

Since FDA approval in 1995, patients with biventricular failure are most often bridged to transplantation with the Thoratec VAD (Fig. 7). Available statistics from their respective manufacturers indicate that more than 1300 patients have been implanted with the Novacor, more than 4100 with the HeartMate, and more than 1700 with the Thoratec worldwide. Recently reported rates of successful

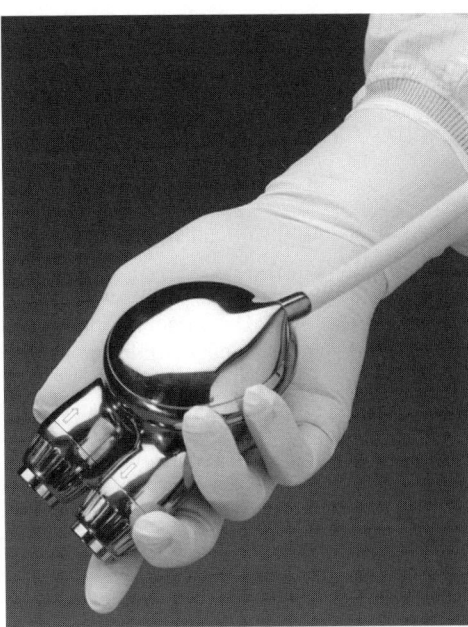

Figure 14 The implantable ventricular assist device (IVAD). Titanium clad pump IVAD. *Source*: Courtesy of Thoratec Corporation.

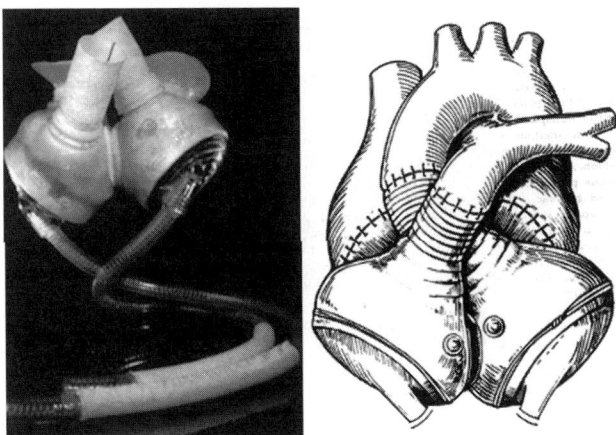

Figure 15 The CardioWest™ TAH. As described in the text, the failed native heart is removed and the CardioWest TAH is implanted orthotopically, anastomosed to cuffs of native atria and the great vessels. *Source*: Courtesy of SynCardia Systems.

bridging-to-transplantation with these devices are in the range of 51–78% (30–33).

Thoratec has recently introduced a titanium-clad implantable version of their Thoratec pump: the IVAD® (implantable ventricular assist device; Thoratec Corporation, Woburn, Massachusetts, U.S.A.; Fig. 14). Currently, the IVAD is the only FDA-approved implantable device that can provide biventricular assistance. According to the manufacturer, as of September 2003, 30 patients with advanced heart failure have been supported with the IVAD as a bridge-to-transplantation or for postcardiotomy ventricular failure, in Europe and the United States. Sixty-eight percent were successfully treated through transplantation or ventricular recovery, with many of these patients discharged to their homes through the use of the TLC-II Portable VAD Driver. At the time of this writing, no published reports of IVAD use in patients have appeared in the peer-reviewed, indexed literature.

The CardioWest™ TAH (Total Artificial Heart; SynCardia Systems, Tucson, Arizona, U.S.A.; Fig. 15) is also currently available, in select centers in the United States, Canada, and France, as a bridge-to-transplantation for patients with biventricular failure. This device is a pneumatically powered biventricular pump that is implanted orthotopically (the native heart is removed and replaced by this device). Since 1993, approximately 225 of these devices have been implanted clinically (34). The reported rate of successful bridge-to-transplantation with this device is in the order of 79% (35). When compared to devices like the HeartMate and the Novacor, a major potential disadvantage of the CardioWest device as a bridge-to-transplantation is a lack of portability, significantly limiting potential for physical rehabilitation and outpatient use, though a smaller and more portable driver is reportedly in development. Another potential disadvantage to a device of this type is that the native heart must be excised, significantly limiting therapeutic options if device failure occurs or infection develops.

Permanent Support (Destination Therapy)
↗ **Only one out of every 2273 patients with end-stage heart failure is likely to receive a heart transplant.** ↗

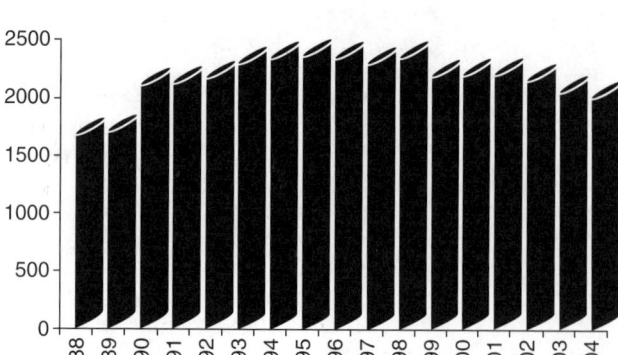

Figure 16   The number of adult cardiac transplants performed in the United States, 1998–2004. *Source*: From Ref. 39.

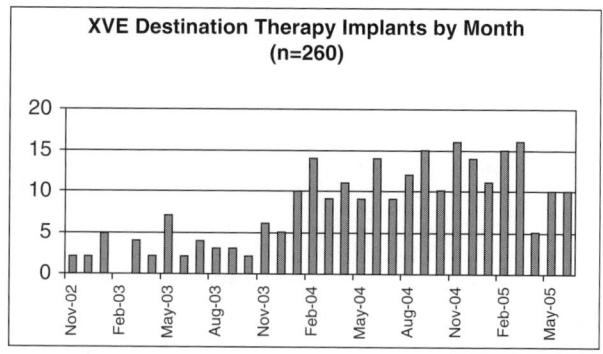

Figure 17   Patient accrual for destination therapy with the HeartMate® XVE by month and year. *Source*: From Ref. 41.

Permanent replacement of the failing heart has always been the major driving force behind research and development in the field of mechanical circulatory assistance. Of the estimated 5,000,000 patients currently living with heart failure in the United States (36), it is estimated that only between 40,000 (37) and 100,000 (38) could potentially meet transplant criteria. Furthermore, transplantation may not be a feasible option for the vast majority of heart failure patients, because there are only around 2200 donor organs available annually in the United States (Fig. 16) (39). In addition, many heart failure patients are ineligible to receive a transplant because of advanced age and comorbidities.

The REMATCH trial (Randomized Evaluation of Mechanical Assistance for the Treatment of Congestive Heart failure, completed June 2001) demonstrated that the use of an LVAD (the HeartMate VE) was not only an effective tool to treat patients with advanced heart failure, but resulted in more than twice the survival rate and an improved quality of life, in comparison to optimal medical management (40–42). This was especially the case if the patient was less than 60 years old (Table 5). Thus, for the vast majority of patients with end-stage cardiac disease, it would appear that intentionally permanent implantation of a mechanical assist device may be the best option available, if they are to survive. Based on the results of REMATCH, the FDA approved the HeartMate in November 2002 for transplant-ineligible patients as "destination therapy"; in essence, permanent implantation of a VAD is their "final destination." By November 2002, improvements to the HeartMate device resulted in the HeartMate XVE, and it is this device that has been implanted for destination therapy patients.

According to the manufacturer, as of May 2005, 260 patients have been implanted with the HeartMate XVE as Destination therapy. The statistics presented in Figure 17 (41) indicate that patient accrual for destination therapy started out slowly, but has steadily increased with time, reflecting a growing acceptance of this management strategy by cardiologists and patients with end-stage heart failure.

Thus far, destination therapy with the HeartMate XVE has been associated with fewer observed adverse events and a better survival rate than reported in the REMATCH trial (42). The authors' conclusion was that improved outcomes likely reflect improvements in the HeartMate XVE device (compared to the HeartMate VE used in REMATCH), and increased experience with patient management.

The INTrEPID trial (Investigation of NonTransplant-Eligible Patients who are Inotrope Dependent) was recently conducted to establish the ability of the Novacor LVAS to provide destination therapy, but the FDA failed to approve the Novacor for this indication based on the INTrEPID data. The RELIANT trial (Randomized Evaluation of the Novacor LVAS In A NonTransplant Population) currently randomizes patients to receive either the Novacor LVAS or the HeartMate XVE LVAS as a bridge to transplantation. The purpose of this trial is to demonstrate that use of the Novacor LVAS is superior to optimal medical therapy, by demonstrating equivalence to HeartMate XVE LVAS, which has already been approved for destination therapy.

Complications Associated with Ventricular Assist Device Support

☞ **Despite the impressive rates of successful short- and long-term support with VADs, infection, thromboembolic complications, and mechanical problems remain major issues to be overcome.** ☞

Table 5   Summarized Results of the REMATCH Trial

	HeartMate®	Medical therapy
1 yr survival (age <60)	52% (74%)	25% (33%)
2 yr survival	23%	8%
Median survival	408 days	150 days

Note: REMATCH stands for Randomized Evaluation of Mechanical Assistance for the Treatment of Congestive Heart failure.
Source: From Ref. 42.

Table 6   Summarized Rates of Infectious Complications from a Large Series of Long-Term Support at a Single Center in Germany

	Novacor®	HeartMate®	Thoratec®
Driveline infection	26%	18%	2%
Pocket infection	11%	24%	NA
Systemic sepsis	24%	11%	26%

Abbreviation: NA, not applicable.
Source: From Ref. 30.

Infection

Infections associated with currently available devices tend to be more common with long-term devices, and often occur along the percutaneous components and in the device pocket. Although infections within the devices themselves are rare, sepsis is not uncommon. A recent large series, reviewing bridge-to-transplantation with the HeartMate in the United States, reported that 45% of patients developed "infection," with 72% of the observed infections at the exit site of the percutaneous driveline (32). Table 6 summarizes the rates of infectious complications from a recent large series of long-term support in Germany (30). Thus, the presence of percutaneous components appears to be an important predisposing factor to infectious complications.

Thromboses

For short-term devices, heparin therapy is usually utilized to maintain an ACT of 180 to 200 seconds. If the ACT is allowed to drift lower for a significant time, thrombosis can form in the rotor heads and/or circuits, requiring replacement. Thromboembolic complications remain a major problem with all of these devices. A recent review of 228 patients on long-term support with the Thoratec, Novacor, and HeartMate as a bridge to transplantation reported cerebral embolism in 24%, 39%, and 16%, respectively, despite adherence to recommended anticoagulation protocols (30). The HeartMate has a blood chamber composed of sintered titanium microspheres, to encourage the ingrowth of a neointima. Once the neointima is developed, formal anticoagulation with warfarin is generally considered to be unnecessary, though some centers maintain their patients on antiplatelet therapy during support. By comparison, the Novacor has a blood chamber made of smooth polyurethane which is thrombogenic, and mandates anticoagulation with warfarin. The international normalized ratio (INR) is generally maintained at 2.5 to 3.5 times normal, during support with a Novacor. Anticoagulation during long-term Thoratec support is with warfarin (INR 2.5–3 times normal), though antiplatelet agents are often prescribed as well.

Mechanical Problems and Device Durability

Short-term support devices rarely have problems of durability, however, the long-term devices do have a finite life span. On July 26, 2005, WorldHeart (the manufacturer of the Novacor LVAS) proudly announced that a Novacor recipient from the INTrEPID trial has entered his fifth year of support. However, despite such encouraging results, it is not currently known for how long available "long-term" devices like the HeartMate and the Novacor can function. Destination therapy ideally refers to at least 10 to 15 years of support, and experience has shown that the Novacor and the HeartMate have a limited lifespan. Although they may be able to sustain a patient for a few years, these devices were intended as temporary bridges-to-transplantation; they were neither designed nor engineered with permanent use in mind.

Based on anecdotal and published worldwide in vivo experience to date, a reasonable estimate of the average lifespan of a single Novacor device is in the order of three and a half to four years, and that of a single HeartMate VE device is around two years (though the HeartMate XVE that is currently available may have an increased longevity). Results of in vitro testing of these devices (43–45) by their respective manufacturers reveals that the "reliability" of the HeartMate VE at two months and one year is reportedly 93.5% and

84.7%. In contrast, that of the Novacor is greater than 99.9% at both of these timepoints. Additionally, the reported "reliability" of the Novacor at two years and three years is 98.3% and 85.9%, respectively. Unfortunately, information about the reliability of the HeartMate at these later timepoints is not available.

In addition to issues of overall longevity, a recent large series of LVAD support for bridge-to-transplantation reported that 9% of patients supported by a HeartMate experienced mechanical problems with their device (compared to no mechanical problems observed with the Novacor) (30). Although only 1% of HeartMate-supported patients in a large multicenter series in the United States experienced "mechanical failure," there were 435 "confirmed device malfunctions" of one sort or another in the 280 supported patients, and 9% of the supported patients needed to use "backup components" because of "cable or controller malfunction" or "pump stoppage" (32).

Importance of Pulsatility in Ventricular Assist Device Design

Pulsatility has always been considered a desirable characteristic of VAD design, due to the ability of pulsatile flow to maintain "normal" physiology. However, creating 5–6 L/min of pulsatile flow creates several physical engineering conundrums: (*i*) The blood chamber must be of sufficient size to allow a physiologically meaningful stroke volume. Because there is an upper limit to the possible number of pump strokes per minute, a fairly large device is required, which tends to exclude small adults and pediatric patients. (*ii*) To facilitate the requisite pumping action, artificial unidirectional valves are required to prevent retrograde flow during pump systole. The presence of these valves (as well as the potentially thrombogenic blood contacting surfaces and the potential for periods of stasis during the pulsatile pump cycle) mandates anticoagulation. (*iii*) Although the pump heads of the Novacor and the HeartMate are implantable, they currently require connection to an external controller and power source. The presence of percutaneous lines, connecting the external components to the implanted pump, greatly increases the potential for infection. High rates of infection, with requisite antibiotic treatment, and repeated trips to the OR for incision and drainage of driveline abscesses certainly impair a patient's quality of life, and makes systems with percutaneous components less attractive as a long-term, permanent management strategy for heart failure. (*iv*) Durable, reliable pumping action requires some fairly complex engineering, which (by definition) is always going to be less than maximally efficient (and unquestionably more intrinsically expensive) than some simpler device. Current diaphragm type pumps like the Novacor and HeartMate require pusher plates, with struts, springs, bearings, and servo-mechanisms. All these moving parts are subject to wear and tear, and ultimate mechanical failure (usually, it's the bearings that wear out first).

Biomechanical engineers have designed a variety of continuous flow devices, with an eye toward providing solutions to the above mentioned problems. (*i*) From a mechanical standpoint, continuous flow devices are simple, consume less power, and are generally more durable because there is essentially only one moving part (the impeller). (*ii*) Since the flow is continuous, artificial unidirectional valves are not required and stasis is minimized, decreasing the need for formal anticoagulation. (*iii*) There is a potential for less hemolysis with the newly designed continuous flow devices, than with pulsatile flow (46). (*iv*) These devices can be miniaturized and produce a wide range of flow rates, making them suitable for adult or pediatric use.

However, the physiologic consequences of long-term, continuous, nonpulsatile flow continue to raise concern. ☞ **Pulsatile flow has long been felt to be superior to continuous flow, in terms of its ability to maintain normal homeostasis and physiology.** ☞ It has been demonstrated that nonpulsatile flow initially causes: (*i*) stagnation in capillary beds, leading to tissue edema and increased arteriovenous shunting, resulting in decreased oxygen extraction and impaired lactate clearance (47); (*ii*) redistribution of intrarenal and intrahepatic blood flow, resulting in renal and hepatic insufficiency (48,49); (*iii*) impairment of carotid baroreceptor function, resulting in increased mean arterial pressure (MAP) and systemic vascular resistance (50); (*iv*) adverse alterations of catecholamines, prostaglandins, and cytokine levels (49); (*v*) electrolyte imbalance, fluid overload, and anemia (51,52).

☞ **More recent studies conducted over the last decade have demonstrated that humans and animals can adapt to nonpulsatile flow, so long as that flow is maintained at somewhat supranormal levels (46).** ☞ If one maintains at least 20% or 30% higher flows than generally utilized for pulsatile support, the abnormal physiology tends to correct itself. Although pulsatile flow does appear to better maintain physiologic homeostasis and allows more efficient oxygen metabolism at lower flow rates (especially in elderly patients with noncompliant blood vessels), many of the differences appear to be attenuated as the rate of nonpulsatile flow increases on a mL/kg/min basis, with no demonstrable differences as nonpulsatile flow rates approach 100 mL/kg/min (7 L/min for a 70-kg person) (39). As a conventional point of reference, the typical flow rates employed during the routine conduct of nonpulsatile CPB are in the range of 50–60 mL/kg/min. This information, along with technological advances over the last two decades in the areas of miniaturization technology, computer chips, and biocompatible materials, have allowed for the design and development of the axial flow VADs and miniaturized, implantable centrifugal pumps, now in human clinical trials.

A final major desirable feature of the VAD of the future is total implantability; there should be no percutaneous components (cables, conduits, or wires) to encourage infection. With the development of the so-called "TET coil" (TET stands for transcutaneous energy transmission), one can deliver power and programming across the skin without skin puncture. One no longer needs cables, wires, or conduits crossing the skin. Basically, two sophisticated induction coils are aligned (one external, one internal), and energy is transduced across the skin. In addition to energy to power the device, programming information and functional interrogation can be relayed via the TET coils.

EXTRACORPOREAL MEMBRANE OXYGENATION AND CO$_2$ REMOVAL

The use of ECLS in trauma and critical care is a relatively recent event. Indeed, ECMO was first employed in a trauma patient in 1972, when conventional therapeutic modalities were exhausted in a patient with respiratory failure. One of the major reasons why ECMO has not been widely used for respiratory failure in trauma patients is the common contraindication to systemic heparinization that

results in the presence of concomitant injuries to brain, liver, and other organs. Another reason for the initial reluctance to use ECMO in trauma and critical care resulted from the initial prospective controlled trial, using ECMO in patients with severe acute respiratory distress syndrome (ARDS) by Zapol et al. (53), which demonstrated extremely high mortalities in both the ECMO (91%) and control (91%) groups. This experience resulted in minimal utilization of ECMO, even in severe, refractory cases. However, many criticized this study, because the ECMO was started very late in the course, and because lung protection ventilation strategies were not employed.

In 1979, Gattinoni et al. (54) provided far better results in patients who were started on veno-venous extracorporeal oxygenation and CO$_2$ removal (ECCO$_2$R) early in the progression of their disease. Because this strategy utilized a veno-venous system to manage severe respiratory failure, no arterial pressure support was provided to the patients. This technique involved the extrathoracic cannulation of both the internal jugular (IJ) vein and the femoral vein, using cutdown. Blood was drained from the common femoral vein (both proximally and distally) and the distal IJ vein, and then was returned to the proximal IJ vein (54). This cannulation system was later improved to a percutaneous system (55).

Later, Alan Morris (56) performed a prospective, controlled, computer-randomized study, comparing standard ventilation therapy (using pressure control) to ECCO$_2$R, and did not demonstrate any survival benefit from the ECCO$_2$R.

Despite the results from these early prospective studies, there are more recent retrospective, uncontrolled, prospective, and anecdotal reports of the successful use of ECMO in severe, refractory ARDS, including those with trauma. Lewandowski et al. (57), in a prospective, noncontrolled trial, demonstrated a 55% survival in patients treated with ECMO utilizing a clinical algorithm. Kolla et al. (58), retrospectively reviewed 100 patients that were treated with ECMO between 1990 and 1996, and found a 54% survival rate in ARDS patients with severe hypoxia.

☞ **Michaels et al. (59) retrospectively reviewed the results of ECMO in trauma patients, and found 50% mortality and documented a 59% nonlethal bleeding complication rate.** ☞ Most publications in trauma patients have consisted of case reports involving combined RV failure, LV hypokinesis, and respiratory failure (60,61). Despite significant additional trauma including splenic and liver injuries (61), and even a ruptured thoracic aorta (62), ECLS has been successfully employed without significant bleeding complications, and with excellent clinical results (50–62).

The current ECLS technique recommended for isolated respiratory failure is veno-veno cannulation, using a percutaneously placed arterial CPB cannula (Bio-Medicus; Eden Prairie, Minnesota, U.S.A.) placed in the right IJ vein (advanced to the mid-RA) and either femoral vein (advanced to the common iliac vein), as per the technique used by Pranikoff et al. (63). Using the percutaneously placed bio-medicus cannulas, Prannikoff et al., were able to achieve flows ranging between 22.4 and 127.8 mL/kg/min, with cannulas ranging from 19–23 F (Table 7). In these patients, a jugulo-femoral bypass direction is used preferentially over a femoro-jugular bypass, because the right IJ access to the RA allows for use of a short, low-resistance cannula, and drainage is better. In patients with respiratory failure along with concomitant pump failure, a form of mechanical cardiopulmonary support is also required, and an

Table 7 Characteristics of Bio-Medicus Cannulas

Cannula size	Length, cm	M-number	Expected flow at 100 cm H$_2$O gradient, L/min
17 F	25	3.05	2.4
	50	3.4	1.8
19 F	25	2.8	3.8
	50	3.15	2.3
21 F	25	2.6	5.0
	50	2.9	3.5
23 F	25	2.4	6.5
	50	2.65	4.8
25 F	50	2.55	5.5
27 F	50	2.4	6.5
29 F	50	2.3	7.0

Note: The "M-number" is an experimentally derived resistive factor that describes this pressure/flow relationship, and it allows for the estimation of flow for any specific cannula, given a defined pressure change across the circuit.

oxygenator that returns blood to the arterial circulation (i.e., ECMO) is optimal.

In trauma patients, femoral vein to common FA cannulation has been successfully used (61), as has the RA to ascending aorta cannulation technique (60). Those with the most experience in trauma patients all emphasize the importance of aggressive resuscitation and early employment of ECLS technology (1,59,63,64). However, these patients should be systematically evaluated for appropriateness of utilizing all forms of extracorporeal support.

EYE TO THE FUTURE

☞ **Rotary continuous flow pumps represent the next generation of VAD technology, and can employ an axial or centrifugal design.** ☞ Although axial flow devices can be smaller and often consume less power, they typically require much higher rotational speeds to generate clinically relevant blood flow, compared to centrifugal devices, which (despite miniaturization) tend to be larger, heavier, and are sensitive to changes in afterload. A potential advantage of centrifugal devices, however, is that they can generate higher pressures at lower flow rates, due to a typically larger forward displacement volume.

As all of the new devices described below are still in human clinical trials at the time of this writing, details of patient outcomes and information about specific complications with the various devices are limited to a handful of publications in the indexed literature. Moreover, the majority of available publications report results of relatively early clinical experiences with the new devices, some of which have been modified/improved as a result of information obtained in the course of their trials. Thus, one must bear in mind that a given device may eventually prove better suited to certain indications and clinical situations than another, and that the ultimate success (or failure) of a given device will only be revealed with the passage of time, and increased experience with that device. It should also be noted that many more devices have been designed and tested than are discussed below. Those

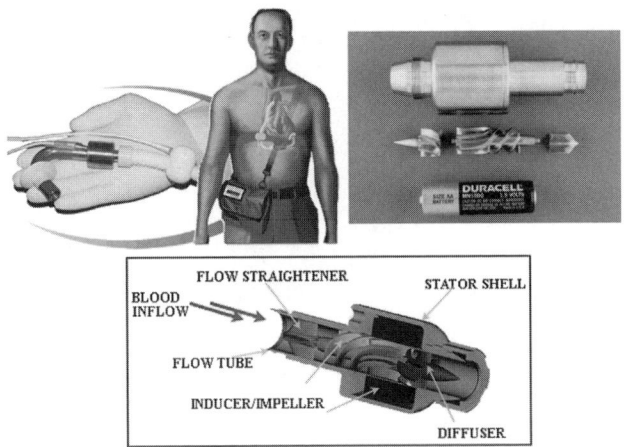

Figure 18 The MicroMed DeBakey VAD®. *Top left*: As described in the text, the DeBakey VAD is used as a left ventricular assist device, drawing blood from the left ventricle apex and returning it to the ascending aorta. A percutaneous cable providing power and system control exits the skin at the right lower abdomen. *Top right*: As a size comparison, the device and impeller can be seen with a standard AA battery. *Bottom*: A cutaway view of the device. *Source*: Courtesy of Micromed Technologies, Inc.

presented here are key devices, about which there is information published in peer-reviewed, indexed literature.

The Axial Flow Pumps
MicroMed DeBakey VAD®
In the mid-1980s, a fortuitous collaboration between Drs. DeBakey and Noon (65), and engineers from the NASA Johnson Space Center in Houston, resulted in the development of one of the first axial-flow LVADs. This device eventually became the LVAD we know today as the MicroMed DeBakey VAD (MicroMed Technologies, Houston, Texas, U.S.A.; Fig. 18), now in human clinical trials. As depicted in Figure 18, the 75 mm long × 25 mm in diameter device is used as an LVAD, positioned between the left ventricular apex and the ascending aorta; 10,000 rpm will produce 5–6 L/min flow at a pressure of 100 mmHg, and consumes less than 10 W of power.

According to the manufacturer, more than 330 patients have already been implanted with the DeBakey VAD at 14 centers, in seven countries. European and U.S. clinical trials of the device as a bridge to transplantation began in November 1998 and June 2000, respectively. A CE mark in Europe was awarded in May 2001. Also in 2001, the device was modified with the addition of a Carmeda® heparin coating of the blood-contacting surfaces (which has subsequently been removed). A further miniaturized version of the DeBakey VAD (the DeBakey VAD Child heart pump) received FDA Humanitarian Device Exemption (HDE) approval in March 2004, and successfully served as a bridge to transplantation in a 14 year old with congenital heart disease, from September to November 2004.

Though the device is still the subject of human clinical trials, a few investigators have published the details of their early experiences with the DeBakey VAD (66–68). Despite overall survival of 50% or more in these trials, reported impressions of the device have varied (based apparently on complications encountered).

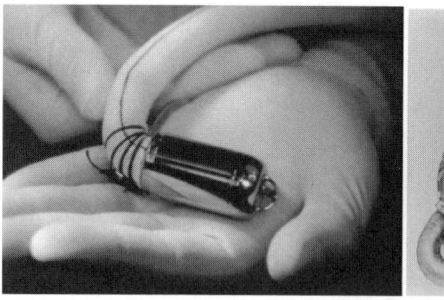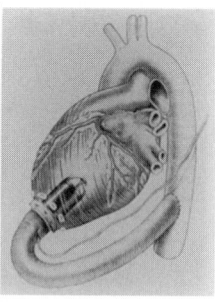

Figure 19   Jarvik 2000 Flowmaker®. This axial flow pump was formerly known as the Jarvik 2000 LVAS. *Left*: the size of the device can be seen compared to a surgeon's hand. *Right*: The Flowmaker is implanted in the left ventricle apex with outflow directed into the descending thoracic aorta. The cable providing power and system control can be seen emerging from the device, and heading craniad to emerge from the skin at the base of the skull (see text for details). *Source*: Courtesy of Texas Heart Institute, 2000.

The DELTA™ trial (Destination Evaluation of Long Term Assist) currently randomizes transplant-ineligible patients with end-stage failure to receive either the DeBakey VAD or the HeartMate XVE LVAS as destination therapy. Up to 360 patients, at 30 clinical sites, will be enrolled in a 2:1 randomization scheme (DeBakey VAD:-HeartMate), under the supervision of the International Center for Health Outcomes and Innovation Research (InCHOIR). The first DELTA patient was implanted with a DeBakey VAD at California Pacific Medical Center in November 2004.

The Flowmaker® (the Device Formerly Known as the Jarvik 2000 LVAD)

The Flowmaker (Jarvik Heart, Inc., New York, New York, U.S.A.; Fig. 19) is an electrically powered, miniaturized axial flow pump, now in human clinical trials in the United States and Europe. The entire device weighs 85 grams and measures 2.5 cm in diameter × 5.5 cm long. It has typically been described by the media as "the size of a C-cell battery." All blood-contacting surfaces are composed of smooth titanium. A number of surgical approaches have been used to implant the device, including midline sternotomy, left thoracotomy, and subcostal incision. As depicted in Figure 19, the device is implanted in the left ventricular apex, and outflow from the device can be directed into the descending thoracic aorta or ascending aorta, depending on the surgical approach. Anticoagulation is recommended when the outflow is to the descending aorta, to prevent stasis and potential thrombosis in the aortic root. The current version of the Flowmaker uses a percutaneous cable to provide power and system control (though a totally implantable configuration with a TET coil is under development). The cable exits the skin of the abdomen with devices implanted as a bridge to transplantation, but when the device is implanted for permanent use (destination therapy), the cable is tunneled craniad (through the pleura and across the neck), to exit the skin at the base of the skull just behind the left mastoid process. Apparently, the vascularity of the skin in this area permits a very low incidence of infection in this site.

When physiologic conditions are optimal, impeller rotation at 8000–12000 rpm can produce flows on the order 6–7 L/min (69) to assist native ventricular ejection. Increasing pump speed has been demonstrated to have direct effects on hemodynamic indices, in direct relation to the level of ventricular unloading. Increasing impeller rotation from 8000 to 12,000 rpm results in linear increases in MAP and cardiac index, and linear decreases in pulmonary capillary wedge pressure and the amount of time the aortic valve stays open in systole. Impeller speeds greater than 12,000 rpm reportedly produce complete unloading of the LV, with a resultant pulse pressure less than 20 mmHg (70).

As mentioned above, the various new devices will undoubtedly declare themselves as best suited to specific clinical scenarios and certain patient populations, once experience has demonstrated their individual strengths and weaknesses. This already appears to be the case with the Flowmaker. According to a recent publication by Dr. Frazier (71), the main goal of this device is to "partially reduce the LV size and end-diastolic pressure," as this may allow reverse remodeling of the failing LV. Thus, patients likely to benefit most from the Flowmaker are those who require "true left ventricular assistance," and not "total capture of the LV output." Further, that the use of the Flowmaker "may be justified in severely impaired class III and IV (but not preterminal) patients."

Human clinical trials of this device as a bridge-to-transplantation in the United States, began at the Texas Heart Institute (THI) in April 2000. In 2002, the FDA gave permission for patients to be discharged to home with an implanted Flowmaker. A recent review (71) reports that, as of 2004, 35 patients have received the device as a bridge-to-transplantation, in four U.S. clinical centers (29 were implanted at the THI). Three were discharged home to await their new heart. Eighteen patients were successfully bridged to transplantation, and 12 died during support. The average duration of support was 67 days. One patient had his Flowmaker explanted and exchanged for an approved pulsatile device, and four patients remained supported.

European clinical trials began shortly after the U.S. trials, and are evaluating the Flowmaker for both destination therapy and as a bridge to transplantation. As of 2004, 17 patients had been implanted (14 permanent implants and three bridges) in five clinical centers. Ten patients have reportedly been discharged home in the European trials (71). There have, thus far, been no reported device failures nor episodes of significant hemolysis. One European patient has reportedly been supported by the Flowmaker for longer than four and a half years (72).

RV failure is known to occur in up to 30% of LVAD supported patients (73,74), due to alterations in RV geometry resulting in increased RV compliance and decreased RV contractility, in the presence of increased RV preload (75). Feasibility studies using the Flowmaker for biventricular support (in calves) yielded favorable results (76). Although the LVAD was implanted in the LV, the RVAD was implanted in the RA (through the same left thoracotomy incision). Further study is required to assess the efficacy of biventricular support with the Flowmaker in humans with biventricular heart failure.

HeartMate II®

The HeartMate II LVAS (Thoratec Corporation, Pleasanton, California, U.S.A.; Fig. 20) is an axial flow pump that

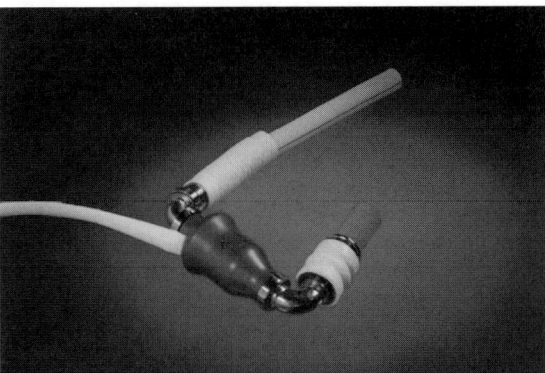

Figure 20 The HeartMate II®. The HeartMate II is implanted in a configuration similar to that shown for the DeBakey VAD (video clip 1) and many other axial flow devices now in clinical trials. Blood is drawn from the left ventricle apex to the device and impelled into the ascending aorta. *Source*: Courtesy of Thoratec Corporation.

evolved from the original Hemopump. At 7 cm long, it occupies approximately one-eighth the volume of the pulsatile HeartMate® I, but can generate the same output. Using the battery analogy mentioned earlier, this device is about the size of a D-cell battery. Impeller speeds range from 6000–15,000 rpm with a 10 L/min maximum output. A microprocessor-controlled algorithm adjusts pump speed to meet the changing flow demands of the body. Like the pulsatile HeartMate I, some of the blood-contacting surfaces are lined with sintered titanium microspheres to encourage neoendothelialization. The impeller is made of smooth titanium. Inflow and outflow cannulations of the left ventricular apex and the ascending aorta are similar to that of the Heart-Mate (and most of the other devices). Although a totally implanted configuration with a TET coil is under development, the current system requires a percutaneous driveline that exits the skin of the right lower abdomen.

The first human implant was performed at the Sheba Medical Center in Israel, in July 2001 (77), but the specific results have not been made publicly available. It is known, however, that the initial European clinical trial was terminated early, due to thrombus formation at the inlet and outlet of the device. Since that time, the device has been redesigned (the positions of textured surfaces have been altered), and is now being implanted in a U.S. clinical trial. The redesigned HeartMate® II was recently implanted in an 18-year-old male with severe heart failure (idiopathic cardiomyopathy) and multisystem organ dysfunction, as a bridge-to-transplantation (78). For this patient, 8600 rpm produces approximately 4.4 L/min of flow, during which he still has native ventricular ejection (echocardiographically demonstrated by aortic valve opening). During exercise, his pump speed adjusts up to 9000 rpm (approximately 5.3 L/min of flow). There has been no significant hemolysis observed, and he has been supported for longer than six months with a New York Heart Association (NYHA) class I status (maintained on warfarin anticoagulation).

The Berlin Heart INCOR® and the MagneVad®—Magnetically Levitated, Bearingless Axial Flow Pumps

All the axial flow pumps discussed above utilize bearings at the two ends of their impeller. Thrombus formation at the sites of these bearings has been a problem with several of

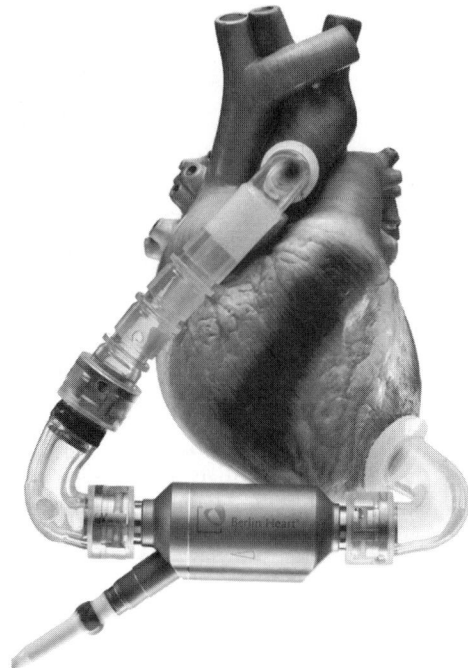

Figure 21 The Berlin Heart INCOR®. Like the majority of the new axial flow VADs, the INCOR draws blood from the left ventricle apex and returns it to the ascending aorta. However, unlike all the other devices, the impeller is magnetically levitated. Without bearings, the durability of the device is likely to be very long, and the potential for thrombosis is markedly diminished. *Source*: Courtesy of Berlin Heart.

the new axial flow devices (67,68). As discussed above, the HeartMate II had to be redesigned after thrombus formation was detected at the inlet and outlet stators, in the initial human implantation experience. The Berlin Heart INCOR® (Berlin Heart AG, Berlin, Germany; Fig. 21) and the Magnevad (Gold Medical Technologies, Inc, Valhalla, New York, U.S.A.; Fig. 22) are innovative axial flow devices, with non-contacting magnetic bearings. Theoretically, this should eliminate the potential for thrombus formation at the points of impeller-bearing contact. Additionally, without points of contact, the durability of such a device is likely to be very long, because there are no contacting moving parts to wear out.

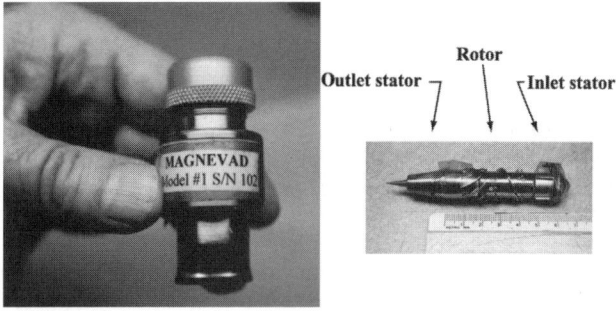

Figure 22 The Magnevad®. Like the Berlin Heart INCOR, the Magnevad is a bearingless, magnetically levitated axial flow device, now under development in the United States. *Source*: Courtesy of Gold Medical Technologies, Inc.

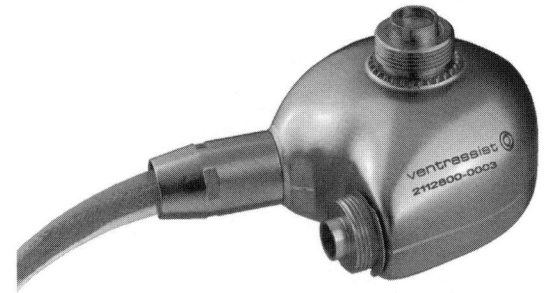

Figure 23 The VentrAssist™ LVAS. *Source*: Courtesy of Ventracor, Ltd.

The INCOR is a very successful axial flow device that has been implanted in more than 200 patients in Europe since June 2002. According to the manufacturer, 12,000 rpm produces 7 L/min of flow against a pressure of 150 mmHg, and consumes 8.5 W of power. The efficiency of the magnetically levitated rotor is reportedly greater than 90%. The INCOR received a European CE mark in 2003. According to press releases from Berlin Heart, as of July 2005, the longest duration of support is more than 1000 days. The average duration of support has been 167 days, with 24 patients supported for more than one year, and four for longer than two years. Twenty-five patients have been successfully discharged to home during support. As discussed above, the advantage of magnetic levitation of the impeller (without bearings) is a minimization of thrombotic risk. Presentations by Berlin Heart at the 2003 ASAIO conference in Washington, DC, indicated that thrombus formation had not been observed in patients (79). The Magnevad is still under development in animal trials, and has not yet been implanted in humans.

Centrifugal Continuous Flow Pumps
VentrAssist™

The VentrAssist LVAS (Ventracor Ltd., Sydney, Australia; Fig. 23) is a hydrodynamically suspended, electromagnetically driven, miniaturized centrifugal blood pump that provides continuous flow of up to 10 L/min at 3000 rpm (80). It weighs just 298 grams (10 oz) and measures 60 mm (2.5 inches) in diameter, making it suitable for both children and adults. This new device was primarily designed for destination therapy, but has been successfully used as a bridge-to-transplantation, and has also shown promise as a bridge-to-recovery.

According to the manufacturer, the VentrAssist has now been implanted in more than 30 patients in Australia, New Zealand, and Europe as part of a CE mark trial. Although press releases have been extremely positive and it is known that several VentrAssist patients have been successfully discharged to home, no specific information about the device recipients, complications, or durations of support, has been published as of the time of this writing. The first implant in the United States was performed on July 18, 2005, at the University of Maryland Medical Center in Baltimore, as part of a feasibility study intended to establish an application for FDA approval. This U.S. feasibility trial will enroll 10 patients, in up to five hospitals across the country, and is managed by the InCHOIR.

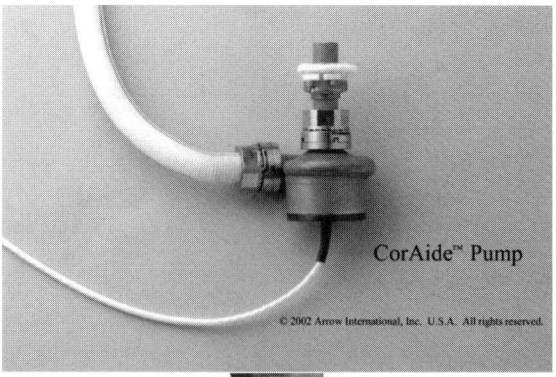

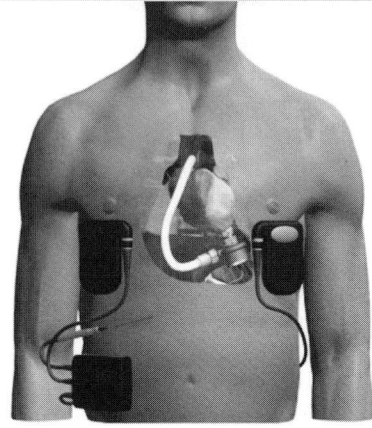

Figure 24 The CorAide™ Pump. *Top*: The device. The percutaneous cable which delivers power and system control can be seen emerging from the bottom, and the outflow cannula can be seen emerging from the side of the device. *Bottom*: The configuration of the implanted CorAide is demonstrated. *Source*: Courtesy of Arrow International.

CorAide™

The CorAide LVAS (Arrow International, Inc, Reading, Pennsylvania, U.S.A.; Fig. 24) is a magnetically and hydrodynamically suspended miniaturized centrifugal blood pump that provides continuous flow of 2–8 L/min. Weighing just 293 grams with a forward displacement of 84 mL, flows of 3–5 L/min have been achieved with this device, at pump speeds around 2700 rpm, consuming just 4 watts of power (81). This new device was developed by Arrow International and the Cleveland Clinic Foundation, and, according to the manufacturer, can serve as a potential bridge-to-recovery, a bridge-to-transplantation, or can provide long-term cardiac support.

The CorAide is currently in a European clinical trial to assess its safety and performance. According to the manufacturer, the first implant took place in Germany in May 2003, in a 65-year-old male, as a bridge-to-transplantation. Though the implantation was reportedly uneventful, high levels of hemolysis were noted by postoperative day 3. The CorAide was explanted and replaced by a different support device to bridge the patient to transplantation. As a result, the clinical trial was temporarily put on hold. There have now been five patients implanted with the CorAide, since the trial was resumed in February 2005, and "all patients are recovering as expected" (Carl Botterbusch, personal communication). No specific information about these patients is available in the peer-reviewed, indexed literature at the time of this writing.

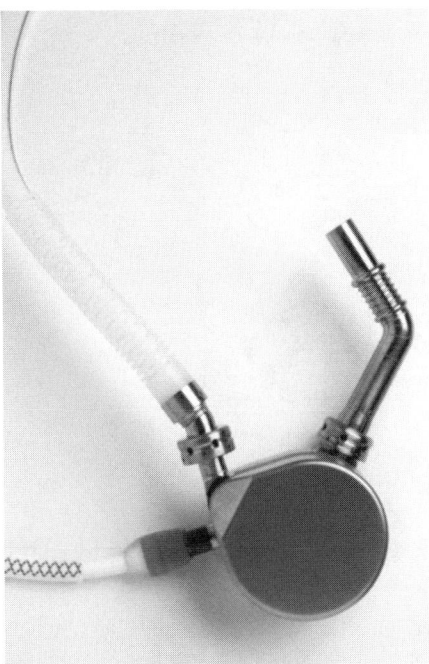

Figure 25 The Terumo Duraheart®. *Source*: Courtesy of Terumo Heart, Inc.

Duraheart®

The Terumo Duraheart (Terumo Cardiovascular Systems Corporation, Ann Arbor, Michigan, U.S.A.; Fig. 25) is an implantable centrifugal device with a magnetically levitated impeller, but its inner surfaces are heparin bonded, eliminating the need for anticoagulation during support. Compared to the VentrAssist and the CorAide, the Duraheart is larger (72 mm diameter, 45 mm height), heavier (540 g), and has a significantly bigger forward displacement volume (180 mL). A pump speed of 2600 rpm can produce flows of 10 L/min (82).

A European clinical trial of the Duraheart began in January 2004. According to a very recently published review, as of August 2004, 10 patients have been implanted. Reportedly, three patients "met the primary endpoint" of the trial (evaluating the safety and performance of the Duraheart), four were able to be discharged, and one underwent transplantation after 138 days of support. The outcome of the remaining patients is unknown, but it is reported that "there were no cerebrovascular accidents, deaths, or infections," and that the longest support duration was 170 days (82).

The NEDO Projects

From 1995 to 2004, the NEDO projects (New Energy and Industrial Technology Development Organization) encompassed a number of mechanical circulatory support devices (MCSD) in development at Japanese universities, hospitals, national research institutes, and private companies. The Terumo Duraheart described above was one such project. Another of the NEDO projects focused on a pivot-bearing-supported centrifugal flow pump that could be used for uni- or biventricular support, and could be configured in different ways, depending on the needs of the patient. Currently called the Miwatec/Baylor® biventricular MCSD (Miwatec Co., Ltd., Hokkaido, Japan; Fig. 26), this multipurpose miniaturized centrifugal device produces 5 L/min of flow at rotational pump speeds under 2000 rpm, and

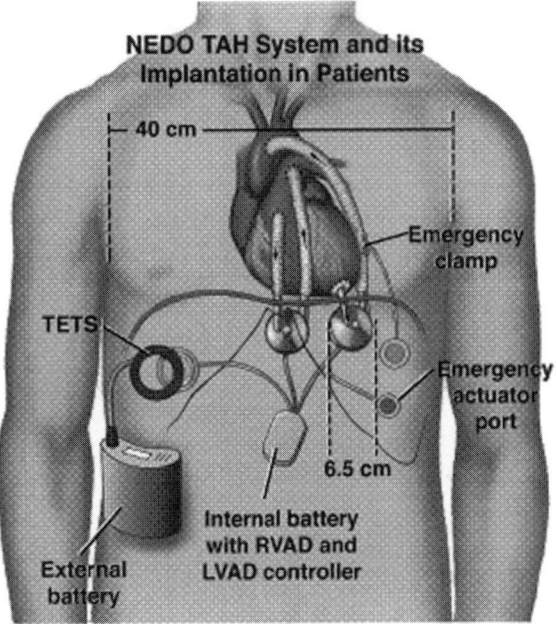

Figure 26 The Miwatec/Baylor® Device. As discussed in the text, this miniaturized centrifugal pump is intended to be multipurpose, and can be configured to suit the needs of the individual patient. Specifically, the miniaturized centrifugal devices can be paracorporeal (like a Thoratec) for short-term assistance (bridge to recovery), implanted in the preperitoneal space for long-term assistance (bridge to transplantation), or permanent (destination therapy). *Abbreviations*: LVAD, left ventricular assist device; RVAD, right ventricular assist device; TET, transcutaneous energy transmission. *Source*: From Ref. 82.

consumes around 7 watts of power (82). Reportedly, clinical trials are planned for the United States and Europe in the near future.

The HeartMate III®

The HeartMate III (Thoratec Corporation, Woburn, Massachusetts, U.S.A.; Fig. 27) is a miniaturized centrifugal flow device with a magnetically levitated impeller. The device occupies approximately one-third the volume of the HeartMate I, but reportedly can produce flows of 7 L/min at a pressure of 135 mmHg, at just under 5000 rpm. The device

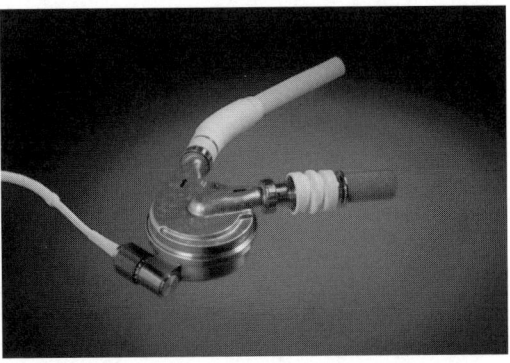

Figure 27 The HeartMate III®. The HeartMate III is implanted in a manner similar to most of the other new continuous flow devices, drawing blood from the left ventricle apex and returning it to the ascending aorta.

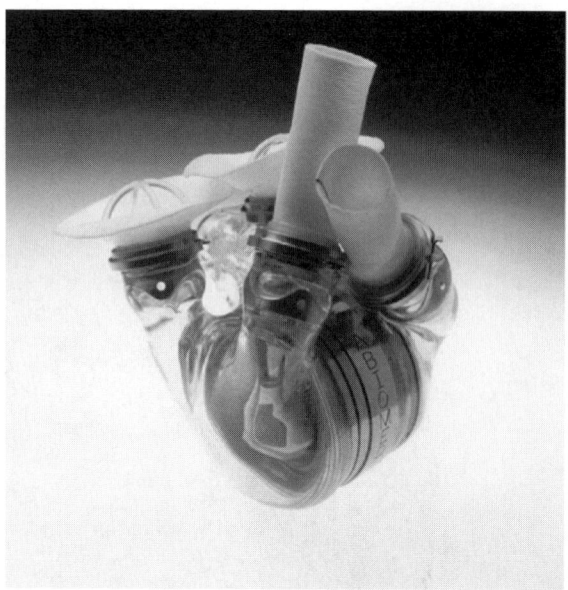
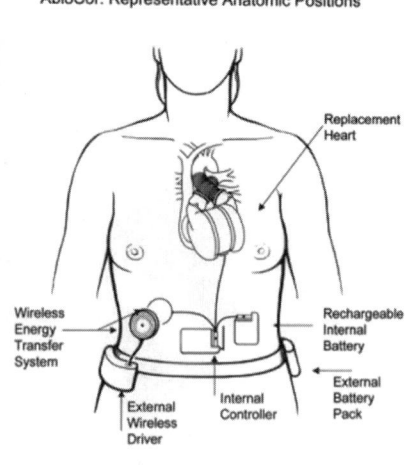
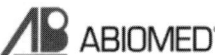

Figure 28 The AbioCor™ Implantable Replacement Heart. *Left*: The device as it appeared at the beginning of the feasibility study. Note the struts on the atrial inflow appendages. These struts were removed from subsequent implantations during the feasibility study, once they were identified as a likely location of thrombus formation. *Right*: The appearance of an implanted AbioCor with components labeled.

will use a totally implanted configuration, with power transfer and system control via a TET coil. Sophisticated control algorithms will allow device responsiveness to physiologic demand, and alternating rotational speeds will allow for some pulsatility. This device is not yet in human clinical trials. A recent feasibility study using the HeartMate III for biventricular support (in sheep) yielded favorable results (72). Further study is required to assess the efficacy of biventricular support with the HeartMate III, in humans with biventricular heart failure.

New Innovations in Total Artificial Heart Technology

The AbioCor™ Implantable Replacement Heart (Abiomed, Danvers, Massachusetts, U.S.A.; Fig. 28) represents a major advance in artificial heart technology, because it is electrically powered and truly, totally implantable. Unlike the pneumatically driven TAHs of the past (83–85) and the CardioWest device available today, the AbioCor is motor driven, so a percutaneous source of compressed air is not required. Additionally, TET is used to supply the motor-driven hydraulic pumping of the artificial ventricles with power and system control.

As depicted in Figure 28, the failed, native heart is removed, and this device is implanted orthotopically, directly anastomosed to cuffs of native atrial tissue and the great vessels. The AbioCor weighs around two pounds, and consists of two ventricular pumps, each with SV 60 mL. Instead of compressed air, ejection from the artificial ventricles is hydraulically effected by a high-efficiency centrifugal pump, which operates unidirectionally, whereas a cylindrical rotary valve alternates the direction of hydraulic fluid flow between right and left pumping chambers. A microprocessor controller allows device output to be responsive to physiologic demand. Overall, the AbioCor can reportedly produce pulsatile flows in the range of 4–8 L/min. Because the device produces pulsatile flow, there are four artificial trileaflet valves to prevent retrograde flow

during pump systole, mandating formal anticoagulation with Coumadin.

A clinical feasibility study for the AbioCor was approved in January 2001, for up to 15 patients. The purpose of this study was to assess the safety and probable benefit of the AbioCor, as a potential therapy for those patients with biventricular failure whose therapeutic options had otherwise been exhausted, and had a high probability of dying within 30 days. Fourteen patients were implanted with the AbioCor, at six clinical centers. Although all 14 have now expired, device performance was truly impressive, with one patient supported for more than a year. Figure 29 shows the length of AbioCor support of the initial 14 implantees. Of the 14 patients enrolled in the feasibility study, two died in the OR, 10 did not leave the hospital (except for day passes for four patients), one was discharged to a nearby hotel, and one was discharged home (86).

As might be expected in any study population with significant comorbidities, complications were frequently

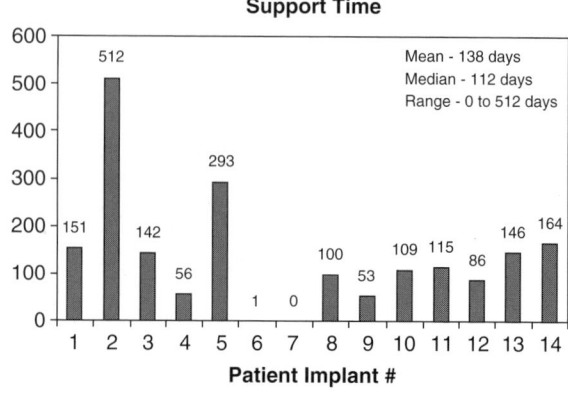

Figure 29 Length of support of the initial 14 implantees with the AbioCor™ Implantable Replacement Heart. *Source*: From Ref. 86.

encountered. Details of the AbioCor experience with the first seven human implants was recently published (87). Thromboembolic complications were a big problem initially, but the ostensible source of the thrombi was identified fairly early as the struts on the atrial inflow appendages (Fig. 28), and these were removed prior to subsequent implants. Other encountered complications were not so unusual for any cardiac surgical population requiring mechanical circulatory assistance, and included perioperative bleeding, respiratory failure, transient renal and/or hepatic insufficiency, and multisystem organ failure. One patient reportedly died of a severe aprotinin reaction in the OR. Interestingly, one of the two patients who were ultimately discharged to home, survived multiple episodes of aspiration requiring tracheostomy and an episode of neuroleptic malignant syndrome.

Results from the initial implants were submitted to the FDA in September 2004, for marketing approval under a HDE. Under the HDE application, up to 4000 patients a year who are not eligible for a heart transplant would have the potential to be eligible for an AbioCor. On June 23, 2005, the FDA ultimately denied the application, citing concerns about patient inclusion criteria and device labeling, potential benefit versus risk of the device, anticoagulation protocols, and quality-of-life versus quantity-of-life issues. The complete transcript of the FDA Medical Devices Advisory Committee Circulatory System Devices Panel Meeting can be viewed online (88).

Abiomed has acquired the rights to the Penn State TAH, and have now introduced the AbioCor II (Fig. 30). This device incorporates the best technologies of both the AbioCor and the Penn State heart. The AbioCor II is 35% smaller than the original AbioCor (potentially implantable in more of the adult population), and has been designed with the goal of five-year reliability. This device is currently being evaluated in preclinical animal studies. Abiomed reportedly intends to submit for an Investigational Device Exemption in 2006, in order to begin clinical trials, with a goal of seeking premarket approval by 2008.

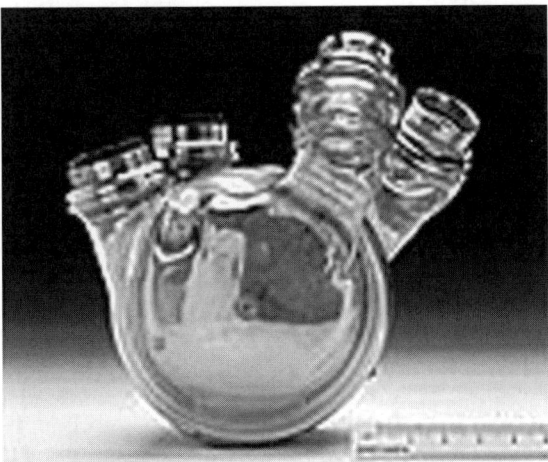

Figure 30 The AbioCor™ II. The AbioCor II combines the best technologies of the AbioCor I and the Penn State total artificial heart, in an implantable replacement heart that is 35% smaller than the AbioCor I.

SUMMARY

Cardiopulmonary mechanical assist devices represent powerful assets in our armamentarium against acute and chronic cardiopulmonary failure. In the case of pure cardiac failure, LV support is most commonly required, and the initial short-term assistance is generally provided with an IABP. An LVAD is required when combined inotropic and IABP utilization results in inadequate Q̇ and perfusion pressures. The most common cause of RV failure is LV failure. However, occasionally a temporary RVAD is employed for acute RV dysfunction, following ischemia related to coronary artery disease or following a heart transplantation. When biventricular dysfunction is present, a BiVAD is employed.

Whether used as a bridge-to-recovery, a bridge-to-transplantation, or as permanent "destination therapy," outcomes have been increasingly encouraging as experience has grown, and the various components comprising these devices continue to be improved.

In the case of respiratory failure not responding to conventional mechanical ventilator therapy, utilization of ECLS devices have resulted in improved outcomes. For those without pump failure, veno-venous ($ECCO_2R$) technologies are adequate. Whereas, when both cardiac and respiratory failure are present together, a veno-arterial (ECMO) type of ECLS is required. Due to the recent improvements in membrane technologies, and because of heparin bonding to ECLS circuits, systemic heparinization is no longer required. Rather, ACTs in the 180 to 200 seconds range are adequate to prevent thromboembolic complications. Thus, these devices are suitable for acute trauma patients, providing brain injuries are absent or of a nonhemorrhagic type.

Miniaturization and newer pump technologies are being studied as the next generation of VAD. Innovative new devices promise increased device longevity, with fewer complications and an improved quality of life for patients who would otherwise succumb to heart failure.

KEY POINTS

- The IABP is a percutaneously inserted device, which provides intra-aortic counterpulsation.
- When maximal pharmacologic interventions and an IABP fail to restore hemodynamic stability, extracorporeal support may be required to re-establish and maintain systemic perfusion, and to prevent the catastrophic sequelae of cardiogenic shock.
- The importance of prompt intervention to restore adequate systemic perfusion, and careful patient selection for prolonged treatment cannot be understated, if expectations are for successful bridge to recovery with a VAD.
- If the myocardium does not recover after a period of short-term support, then a decision must be made as to whether the patient is an acceptable transplant candidate.
- Only one out of every 2273 patients with end-stage heart failure is likely to receive a heart transplant.
- Despite the impressive rates of successful short- and long-term support with VADs, infection, thromboembolic complications, and mechanical problems remain major issues to be overcome.
- Pulsatile flow has long been felt to be superior to continuous flow, in terms of its ability to maintain normal homeostasis and physiology.

- More recent studies conducted over the last decade have demonstrated that humans and animals can adapt to nonpulsatile flow, so long as that flow is maintained at somewhat supranormal levels (46).

- Michaels et al. (59), retrospectively reviewed the results of ECMO in trauma patients, and found 50% mortality and documented a 59% nonlethal bleeding complication rate.

- Rotary continuous flow pumps represent the next generation of VAD technology, and can employ an axial or centrifugal design.

REFERENCES

1. Michaels AJ. Management of posttraumatic respiratory failure. Crit Care Clin 2004; 20:83–99.
2. Kantrowitz A, Tjonneland S, Freed PS, et al. Initial clinical experience with intra-aorta balloon pumping in cardiogenic shock. JAMA 1968; 203: 113–118.
3. Bregman D, Casarella WJ. Percutaneous intraaortic balloon pumping: Initial clinical experiences. Ann Thorac Surg 1981; 29:153.
4. Aguirre FV, Kern MJ, Bach R, et al. Intraaortic balloon pump support during high-risk coronary angioplasty. Cardiology 1994; 84(3):175–86.
5. Jeevanandam V, Jayakar D, Anderson A, et al. Circulatory assistance with a permanent implantable IABP: initial human experience. Circ 2002; 106(suppl 1):I183– I188.
6. Maccioli G, Lucas W, Norfleet E. The intra-aortic balloon pump: a review. J Cardiothorac Anesth 1988; 2:365–373.
7. Dietl CA, Berkheimer MD, Woods EL, et al. Efficacy and cost effectiveness of pre-operative IABP in patients with ejection fraction of 0.25 or less. Ann Thorac Surg 1996; 62:401–408.
8. Cumulative data from the Thoratec Voluntary Worldwide Registry, November 2004. www.thoratec.com/medical-professionals/pdf/Thoratec_VAD_Clinical_Results_112004.pdf
9. www.abiomed.com/clinical_information/BVS5000_Update.cfm
10. www.abiomed.com/clinical_information/AB5000_Update.cfm
11. www.abiomed.com/clinical_information/physician_videos. cfm, Data presented in video lecture from Dr. Ralph de la Torre: AMI Patients and Mechanical Support.
12. BVS5000 Bi-ventricular Support Training Manual, Abiomed, Inc. Danvers, MA, July 1997.
13. Goldberg RJ, Samad NA, Yarzebski J, et al. Temporal trends in cardiogenic shock complicating acute myocardial infarction. N Engl J Med 1999; 340:1162–1168.
14. Holmes DR Jr, Bates ER, Kleiman NS, et al. Contemporary reperfusion therapy for cardiogenic shock: the GUSTO-I trial experience. The GUSTO-I investigators. Global utilization of streptokinase and tissue plasminogen activator for occluded coronary arteries. J Am Coll Cardiol 1995; 26:668–674.
15. Mueller HS. Role of intra-aortic counterpulsation in cardiogenic shock and acute myocardial infarction. Cardiol 1994; 84:168.
16. Noon GP, Ball JW, Short HD. Bio-medicus centrifugal ventricular support for postcardiotomy cardiac failure: a review of 129 cases. Ann Thorac Surg 1996; 61:291–295.
17. Thiele H, Lauer B, Hambrecht R, et al. Reversal of cardiogenic shock by percutaneous left atrial-to-femoral arterial bypass assistance. Circ 2001; 104:2917–2922.
18. Pitsis A, Dardas P, Nikoloudakis N, et al. Temporary assist device for postcardiotomy cardiac failure. Ann Thorac Surg 2004; 77:1431–1433.
19. Aragon J, Lee MS, Kar B, et al. Percutaneous left ventricular assist device: "tandemheart" for high-risk coronary intervention. Catheter Cardiovasc Interv 2005; 65(3):346–352.
20. Vranckx P, Foley DP, de Feijter PJ, et al. Clinical introduction of the TandemHeart as a percutaneous left ventricular assist device for circulatory support during high-risk percutaneous coronary intervention. Int J Cardiovasc intervent 2003; 5(1):35–39.
21. Kar B, Butkevich A, Civitello AB, et al. Hemodynamic support with a percutaneous left ventricular assist device during stenting of an unprotected left main coronary artery. Tex Heart Inst J 2004; 31(1):84–86.
22. Merighe ME, Smalling RW, Cassidy D, et al. Effect of the hemopump left ventricular assist device on regional myocardial perfusion and function: reduction of ischemia during coronary occlusion. Circ 1989; 80:158–166.
23. Baldwin RT, Radovancevic B, Matsuwaka R, et al. Peripheral organ perfusion augmentation during left ventricular failure. A controlled bovine comparison between the intraaortic balloon pump and the hemopump. Tex Heart Inst J 1993; 20:275–280.
24. Phillips SJ, Barker L, Balentine B, et al. Hemopump support for the failing heart. ASAIO Trans 1990; 36:M629–M632.
25. Deeb GM, Bolling SF, Nicklas J, et al. Clinical experience with the nimbus pump. ASAIO Trans 1990; 36:M632–M636.
26. Sweeney MS. The hemopump in 1997: a clinical, political, and marketing evolution. Ann Thorac Surg 1999; 68:761–763.
27. Burnett CM, Vega JD, Radovancevic B, et al. Improved survival after hemopump insertion in patients experiencing postcardiotomy cardiogenic shock during cardiopulmonary bypass. ASAIO Trans 1990; 36:M626–M629.
28. www.abiomed.com/clinical_information/physician_videos. cfm, Data presented in video lecture from Dr. Donald S. Baim. The Future Role of Short-Term Support Devices.
29. Meyns B, Dens J, Sergeant P, et al. Initial experiences with the impella device in patients with cardiogenic shock. Thorac Cardiovasc Surg 2003; 51:312–317.
30. Minami K, El-Banayosy A, Sezai A, et al. Morbidity and outcome after mechanical support using Thoratec, Novacor®, and HeartMate for bridging to heart transplantation. Artif Organs 2000; 24(6):421–426.
31. Robbins RC, Kown MH, Portner PM, et al. The totally implantable Novacor® left ventricular assist system. Ann Thorac Surg 2001; 71:S162– S165.
32. Frazier OH, Rose EA, Oz MC, et al. Multicenter clinical evaluation of the HeartMate vented electric left ventricular assist system in patients awaiting heart transplantation. J Thorac Cardiovasc Surg 2001; 122:1186–1195.
33. Pasque MK, Rogers JA. Adverse events in the use of HeartMate vented electric and Novacor® left ventricular assist devices: comparing apples and oranges. J Thorac Cardiovasc Surg 2002; 124:1063–1067.
34. Copeland JG, Arabia FA, Smith RG, et al. Mechanical assist device; my choice: the CardioWest total artificial heart. Transplant Proc 2000; 32:1523–1524.
35. Copeland JG, Smith RG, Arabia FA, et al. Cardiac replacement with a total artificial heart as a bridge to transplantation. NEJM 2004; 351(9):859–867.
36. American Heart Association. Heart Disease and Stroke Statistics—2005 Update. Dallas, Texas: American Heart Association, 2005.
37. Song X, Throckmorton AL, Untaroiu A, et al. Axial flow blood pumps. ASAIO J 2003; 49:355–364.
38. Westaby S, Narula J. Preface: surgical options in heart failure. Surg Clin N Am 2004; 84:xv–xix.
39. Data source: Organ Procurement and Transplant Network (OPTN) data, accessed 7/25/05.
40. Rose EA, Gelijns AC, Moskowitz AJ, et al. Long-term use of a left ventricular assist device for end-stage heart failure. NEJM 2001; 345(20):1435–1443.
41. Data source: personal communication from Ed Burke, Thoratec Corporation.
42. Long JW, Kfoury AG, Slaughter MS, et al. Long term destination therapy with the HeartMate XVE left ventricular assist device: Improved outcomes since the REMATCH study. Congest Heart Fail 2005; 11(3):133–138.
43. HeartMate Sutures Not Applied Vented Electric (SNAP-VE) Left Ventricular Assist System (LVAS): directions for use.

Thoratec Corporation, Pleasanton, CA. Document 29123, revision B; April 25, 2001, p. 1–66.

44. Physician's Manual Novacor® LVAS. Baxter Healthcare Corporation, Novacor® Division, Technical Support Department, Deerfield (IL). Document GCP 9 105–1097, revision B; 1998, p. 1.1 –16.2.

45. Lee J, Miller PJ, Chen H, et al. Reliability model from the in-vitro durability Tests of a left ventricular assist system. ASAIO J 1999; 45:595–601.

46. Allen GS, Murray KD, Olsen DB. The importance of pulsatile and nonpulsatile flow in the design of blood pumps. Artif Org 1997; 21(8):922–928.

47. Mavroudis C. To pulse or not to pulse. Ann Thorac Surg 1978; 25(3):259–271.

48. Sezai A, Shiono M, Orime Y, et al. Major organ function under mechanical support: Comparative studies of pulsatile and non-pulsatile circulation. Artif Org 1999; 23(3):280–285.

49. Orime Y, Shiono M, Hata H, et al. Cytokine and endothelial damage in pulsatile and nonpulsatile cardiopulmonary bypass. Artif Org 1999; 23(6):508–512.

50. Shomura Y, Tanaka K, Takabayashi S, et al. Arterial baroreceptor afferent activity in nonpulsatile systemic circulation. Artif Org 1998; 22(12):1056–1063.

51. Golding L, Murakami G, Harasaki H, et al. Chronic nonpulsatile flow. ASAIO Trans 1982; 28:81–89.

52. Golding L. Centrifugal pumps. In: Unger F, ed. Assisted Circulation 2. Berlin: Springer Verlag, 1984.

53. Zapol WM, Snider MT, Hill JD, et al. Extracorporeal membrane oxygenation in severe acute respiratory failure? A randomized study. JAMA 1979; 242:2193–2196.

54. Gattinoni L, Kolobow T, Damia G. Extracorporeal carbon dioxide removal (ECCO₂R): a new form of respiratory assistance. Int J Artif Organs 1979; 2:183–185.

55. Gattinoni, L, Pesenti, A, Mascheroni, D, et al. Low-frequency positive-pressure ventilation with extracorporeal CO_2 removal in severe acute respiratory failure. JAMA 1986; 256:881–886.

56. Morris AH, Wallace CJ, Menlove RL, et al. Randomized clinical trial of pressure-controlled inverse ratio ventilation and extracorporeal CO_2 removal for adult respiratory distress syndrome. AM J Respir Crit Care Med 1994; 149:295–305.

57. Lewandowski K, Rossaint R, Pappert D, et al. High rate in 122 ARDS patients managed according to a clinical algorithm including extracorporeal membrane oxygenation. Intensive Care Med 1997; 23:819–835.

58. Kolla S, Awad SS, Rich PB, Schreiner RJ, Hirschl RB, Bartlett RH. Extracorporeal life support for 100 adult patients with severe respiratory failure. Ann Surg 1997; 226:544–564.

59. Michaels AJ, Schriener RJ, Kolla S, et al. Extracorporeal life support in pulmonary failure after trauma. J Trauma 1999; 46:638–645.

60. Sasadeusz KJ, Long WB, Kemalyan N, et al. Successful treatment of a patient with multiple injuries using extracorporeal membrane oxygenation and inhaled nitric oxide. J Trauma 2000; 49:1126–1128.

61. Masiakos PT, Hirsch EF, Millham FH. Management of severe combined pulmonary and myocardial contusion with extracorporeal membrane oxygenation. J Trauma 2003; 54:1012–1015.

62. Masroor S, Tehrani H, Pham S, et al. Extracorporeal life support in pulmonary failure after traumatic rupture of the thoracic aorta: A case report. J Trauma 2004; 57:389–391.

63. Pranikoff T, Hirschl RB, Remenapp R, et al. Venovenous extracorporeal life support via percutaneous cannulation in 94 patients. Chest 1999; 115:818–822.

64. Bartlett RH, Roloff DW, Custer JR, et al. Extracorporeal life support: the University of Michigan experience. JAMA 2000; 283(7):904–908.

65. DeBakey ME, Noon GP, Teitel ER. The rotary blood pump: lessons learned and future directions. Artif Org 2004; 28(10):865–868.

66. Salzberg S, Lachat M, Zünd G, et al. Left ventricular assist device as bridge to heart transplantation—lessons learned with the Micromed DeBakey Axial blood flow pump. Eur J Cardiothorac Surg 2003; 24:113–118.

67. Jurmann MJ, Weng Y, Drews T, et al. Permanent mechanical circulatory support in patients of advanced age. Eur J Cardiothorac Surg 2003; 25:610–618.

68. Noon GP, Morley DL, Irwin S, et al. Clinical experience with the Micromed DeBakey ventricular assist device. Ann Thor Surg 2001; 71:S133–S138.

69. Frazier OH, Myers TJ, Gregoric ID, et al. Initial clinical experience with the Jarvik 2000 implantable axial-flow left ventricular assist system. Circ 2002; 105:2855–2860.

70. Frazier OH, Meyers TJ, Jarvik RK, et al. Research and development of an implantable axial-flow left ventricular assist device: The Jarvik 2000 heart. Ann Thorac Surg 2001; 71:S125– S132.

71. Frazier OH, Shah NA, Myers TJ, et al. Use of the Flowmaker (Jarvik 2000) left ventricular assist device for destination therapy and bridging to transplantation. Cardiol 2004; 101:111–116.

72. Frazier OH, Tuzun E, Cohn W, et al. Total heart replacement with dual centrifugal ventricular assist devices. ASAIO J 2005; 51:224–229.

73. Fukumachi K, McCarthy PM, Smedira NG, et al. Preoperative risk factors for right ventricular failure after implantable left ventricular assist device insertion. Ann Thorac Surg 1999; 68:2181–2184.

74. Elbeery JR, Owen CH, Savitt MA, et al. Effects of the left ventricular assist device on right ventricular function. J Thorac Cardiovasc Surg 1990; 99:809–816.

75. Santamore WP, Gray LA Jr. Left ventricular contributions to right ventricular systolic function during LVAD support. Ann Thorac Surg 1996; 61:350–356.

76. Radovancevic B, Gregoric ID, Tamex D, et al. Biventricular support with the Jarvik 2000 axial flow pump: A feasibility study. ASAIO J 2003; 49:604–607.

77. Griffith BP, Kormos RL, Borovetz HS, et al. Hearmate II left ventricular assist system: From concept to first clinical use. Ann Thor Surg 2001; 71:S116– S120.

78. Frazier OH, Delgado RM III, Kar B, et al. First clinical use of the redesigned HeartMate II left ventricular assist system in the United States. Tex Heart Inst J 2004; 31:157–159.

79. Goldowsky M. Magnevad—The world's smallest magnetic bearing turbo pump. Artif Org 2004; 28(10):945–952.

80. James NL, van der Meer AL, Edwards GA, et al. Implantation of the VentrAssist implantable rotary blood pump in sheep. ASAIO J 2003; 49(4):454–458.

81. Doi K, Golding LAR, Massiekko AL, et al. Preclinical readiness testing of the arrow international CorAide left ventricular assist system. Ann Thorac Surg 2004; 77;2103–2110.

82. Takatani S, Matsuda H, Hanatani A, et al. Mechanical circulatory support devices (MCSD) in Japan: current status and future directions. J Artif Org 2005; 8:13–27.

83. Cooley DA, Liotta D, Hallman GL, et al. Orthotopic cardiac prosthesis for two staged cardiac replacement. Am J Cardiol 1969; 24(5):723–30.

84. Cooley DA, Akutsu T, Norman JC, et al. Total Artificial Heart in Two-Staged Cardiac Transplantation. Tex Heart Inst J 1981; 8:305–319.

85. DeVries WL, Anderson JL, Joyce LD, et al. Clinical use of the total artificial heart. NEJM 1984; 310:273–8.

86. FDA Questions for Circulatory System Devices Panel, June 23, 2005, H040006Abiomed AbioCor Implantable Replace/ ment Heart; www.fda.gov/ohrms/dockets/ac/05/questions/ 2005-4149q2_01_Abiomed%20Panel%20Questions-draft%20final.doc

87. Dowling RD, Gray JA Jr, Etoch SW, et al. Initial experience with the Abiocor implantable replacement heart system. J Thorac Cardiovasc Surg 2004; 127(1):131–141.

88. www.fda.gov/ohrms/dockets/ac/05/transcripts/2005-4149t2.htm

23

Acute Respiratory Failure: Initial Diagnosis and Management

Michael J. Yanakakis

Department of Anesthesia and Perioperative Care, UC San Francisco Medical Center, San Francisco, California, U.S.A.

Michael A. Gropper

Department of Anesthesia and Critical Care Medicine, UC San Francisco Medical Center, and the UCSF Cardiovascular Research Institute, San Francisco, California, U.S.A.

William C. Wilson

Department of Anesthesiology and Critical Care, UC San Diego Medical Center, San Diego, California, U.S.A.

INTRODUCTION

Respiratory failure is one of the most common reasons for admission to the intensive care unit (ICU) following trauma or critical illness, and remains a leading cause of morbidity and mortality. This chapter reviews the pathophysiology of acute respiratory failure (ARF), and provides a practical approach to diagnosis and therapeutic management. This review is complementary to the material covered in Volume 2, Chapter 24, which surveys the acute respiratory distress syndrome (ARDS).

Apart from the application of life-support measures during management of ARF, the initial emphasis involves an intense search for the primary etiology of respiratory failure. The important principles of early and accurate diagnosis are emphasized throughout this text. Early diagnosis (in the first hours or days of disease) increases the likelihood that appropriate specific therapy will be applied, and decreases the likelihood that the patient will progress from ARF to full-blown ARDS.

Pulmonary embolus (PE) is an important and common source of ARF following trauma and critical illness. Because the problem of deep venous thrombosis (DVT) and consequent PE is so pervasive in patients suffering from trauma, burns, and critical illness, an entire chapter has been dedicated to the subject (Volume 2, Chapter 56). Accordingly, PE is only briefly reviewed here.

This chapter does provide an important survey of infectious causes of pneumonia, because almost all ICU patients with ARF will either begin with an infectious etiology, or become secondarily infected. In addition to reviewing the organisms commonly associated with respiratory infections, practical strategies to minimize nosocomial infections are provided. This chapter is also complementary to Volume 2, Chapter 48, which reviews ventilator-associated pneumonia (VAP), and focuses more closely on the organisms that cause VAP. Therefore, this chapter surveys all of the clinically relevant organisms causing respiratory failure.

Finally, this chapter provides only an abbreviated summary of management principles for patients with ARF, because Volume 2, Chapters 24 to 29 in this volume cover these topics in exquisite detail.

DEFINITIONS AND EPIDEMIOLOGY
Consensus Definitions

The presence of persistent hypoxemia (with or without hypercapnia) is clearly evidence of respiratory system failure. However, a universally accepted definition of ARF does not yet exist. In contrast, definitions for acute lung injury (ALI) and ARDS have been agreed upon by the American-European Consensus Conference, and are summarized in Table 1 (1). Additionally, the American College of Chest Physician (ACCP)/Society of Critical Care Medicine (SCCM) consensus statement on sepsis syndrome defines respiratory failure as a respiratory rate >20 breaths/min or $PaCO_2$ <32 mm Hg, or the need for mechanical ventilation to treat an acute respiratory process (2). The ACCP/SCCM definition of respiratory failure does not specifically account for hypercapneic respiratory failure. Because the most important consideration in assessing the need for mechanical ventilatory support is the overall clinical condition of the patient, any complete definition of ARF should include criteria for ALI, along with a measure of overall patient status.

Respiratory failure can be classified as oxygenation failure (hypoxemic), ventilation failure (hypercapneic), or both (combined). Differentiation between these conditions can be made on the basis of the arterial blood gas (Table 2).

 ☞ **Arterial blood gas (ABG) analysis is the single most important laboratory test for defining the severity of ARF. In addition to quantifying the severity, ABG analysis assists in differentiating the cause of ARF, and is useful in decision making regarding intubation and mechanical ventilation.** ☞

Age should be considered when quantifying the degree of hypoxemia appropriate for patients, when breathing room air. A physiologic increase in the alveolar to arterial (A-a) oxygen gradient occurs during aging, with a gradient as high as 30 mmHg at age 80 (3). This gradient will be exacerbated when higher inspired oxygen concentrations are used, as there is a normal increase in A-a gradient of 5–7 mmHg with every 10% increase in inspired oxygen concentration (4).

If the patient has not improved with the administration of supplemental oxygen, or if the work of breathing (WOB) is excessive, or the patient's debilitated state does not allow him to perform the required WOB, the patient should be

Table 1   American–European Consensus Conference Definitions of Acute Lung Injury and Acute Respiratory Distress Syndrome

Acute lung injury	Acute respiratory distress syndrome
Acute onset of respiratory failure	Acute onset of respiratory failure
Bilateral infiltrates on chest radiograph	Bilateral infiltrates on chest radiograph
No evidence of left atrial hypertension (PAOP[a] < 18 mmHg)	No evidence of left atrial hypertension (PAOP < 18 mmHg)
$PaO_2/FiO_2 < 300$ mmHg	$PaO_2/FiO_2 < 200$ mmHg

[a]Although classically, pulmonary artery occlusion pressure (PAOP) should be < 18 to make the diagnosis of noncardiogenic pulmonary edema, occasionally noncardiogenic etiologies will occur with PAOP ≥ 18. *Abbreviations*: PaO_2/FiO_2, ratio of partial pressure of oxygen in arterial blood to the fraction of inhaled oxygen; PAOP, pulmonary artery occlusion pressure. *Source*: From Ref. 1.

transported to the ICU for more aggressive interventions and closer monitoring. Most importantly, the clinician needs to vigorously pursue the inciting cause of respiratory failure, rather than merely provide supportive care in the form of endotracheal intubation and mechanical ventilation. Importantly, the clues to the etiology are usually most apparent during the initial hours of respiratory failure, and may become lost after 24 to 48 hours of ventilatory support. Furthermore, recent clinical trials suggest that early intervention in the form of antibiotics and fluid resuscitation may decrease mortality from respiratory failure, so identifying the precipitating cause will suggest the most effective therapy (5,6).

Epidemiology

In a recent European study, the incidence of ARF was 78 patients per 100,000/yr, with an overall 90-day mortality of 41% (7). In addition, the lung is often the primary source for sepsis syndrome in patients presenting with ARF (8). The common need for mechanical ventilation, and the costs and complications associated with this intervention, make this patient population responsible for a significant component of health care expenditures.

ARF is the leading cause of admission to the ICU in most settings. Using the definition of a PaO_2/FiO_2 200 and the need for mechanical ventilatory support, Vincent (9) estimated that 34% of all ICU admissions were for ARF that progressed to ARDS, and that those patients had a mortality of 34% versus a mortality of 16% for patients admitted for other diagnoses. Arroliga et al. (10), identified the incidence of ARDS at 15 cases/100,000/yr in Ohio. As ARDS is only a subset of all patients with ARF, the overall incidence of ARF would be expected to be much higher. Clearly, ARF, along with sepsis syndrome, are leading causes of both ICU admission and morbidity and mortality. Volume 2, Chapter 24 discusses the pathophysiology and progression from ALI to ARDS that results, when any one of a multitude of disorders becomes severe enough to disrupt the alveolar epithelial capillary barrier.

PATHOPHYSIOLOGY OF ACUTE RESPIRATORY FAILURE
Acute Hypoxemic Respiratory Failure: Gas Exchange Dysfunction

Hypoxemia is defined as inadequate blood oxygenation, and should be conceptually differentiated from hypoxia, which indicates deficient oxygen concentration anywhere (inside or outside the body), but typically means low PO_2 in the tissues. Acute hypoxemic respiratory failure is present when the partial pressure of oxygen in arterial blood (PaO_2) is less than 60 mmHg, in the setting of low or normal arterial partial pressure of carbon dioxide ($PaCO_2$). The presence of tissue hypoxia leads to anaerobic cellular metabolism, and if the tissue PO_2 remains too low for too long, cell death will occur. Hypoxemia in ARF can result from a number of conditions, listed in Table 3. Each of these pathologic processes leading to hypoxemia will be considered separately. However, the critically ill patient with respiratory failure often presents with a combination of these processes coexisting. Additionally, others begin after the initial event, and all conditions may contribute to the degree of hypoxemia experienced by the patient.

Table 2   Classification of Respiratory Failure by Arterial Blood Gas Analysis

Classification	Acute hypoxemic	Hypercapneic (ventilatory failure)	Combined (periop, posttrauma)
$P_{(A-a)}O_2$	↑	→	↑
PaO_2	↓	↓[a]	↓
$PaCO_2$	Initially ↓ Later, may ↑	↑	Initially maybe ↑, →, or ↓ Later ↓
Examples	Pulmonary edema pneumonia	CNS depression Neuromuscular weakness Airflow obstruction	Postchest trauma or post-op with pain and atelectasis
Comments	Any condition causing mixed venous blood to traverse nonventilated lung units results in right-to-left transpulmonary shunt. When severe, acute hypoxemic respiratory failure results	In ventilatory failure, gas exchange abnormalities result from decreased alveolar ventilation, resulting in hypercapnea and proportional hypoxia	Combined respiratory failure is common following trauma and postop. Lower lung volume due to splinting from pain leads to atelectasis, smoking history, fluid resuscitation, and leaky capillaries (burns, SIRS, sepsis, etc.) all contribute further

[a]PaO_2 often becomes normal with ↑ FIO_2 in pure hypoventilatory (hypercapneic) respiratory failure.
Abbreviations: ↓, decreased; ↑, increased; →, normal; CNS, central nervous system; $PaCO_2$, partial pressure of carbon dioxide in the arterial blood; PaO_2, partial pressure of oxygen in the arterial blood; $P_{(A-a)}O_2$, alveolar-to-arterial oxygen gradient; SIRS, systemic inflammatory response syndrome.

Table 3 Five Pathophysiologic Processes that Cause Acute Hypoxemic (Low PaO_2) Respiratory Failure

Process	P(A-a)O₂	Response to 100% O₂	PaCO₂	Clinical examples
Low PIO_2	Normal	↑↑ PaO_2	Normal	Elevation (e.g., Denver, Mexico City) low FIO_2 (e.g., plumbing or tank hook-up error)
Hypoventilation	Normal	↑↑ PaO_2	↑↑	Opiate overdose Myasthenia Gravis Guillian-Barre syndrome
$\dot{V}_A/\dot{Q}$ mismatch	↑↑	↑↑ PaO_2	Normal	Segmental atelextasis (low $\dot{V}_A/\dot{Q}$) or sub segmental pulmonary emboli (high $\dot{V}_A/\dot{Q}$)
Shunt ($\dot{Q}_s/\dot{Q}_t$)	↑↑	No improvement	Normal	Noncardiogenic pulmonary edema (2° aspiration, sepsis, SIRS, etc.)
Diffusion limit	↑↑	↑↑ PaO_2	Normal	Pulmonary edema and associated interstitial edema

Note: $PIO_2 = FIO_2 (P_B - P_{H_2O})$.

Abbreviations: ↑↑, increased; FIO_2, fractional concentration of inspired oxygen; P_B, barometric pressure; $P_{H_2}O$, partial pressure of water; $PaCO_2$, partial pressure of carbon dioxide in the arterial blood; PaO_2, partial pressure of oxygen in the arterial blood; $P_{(A-a)}O_2$, alveolar-to-arterial oxygen gradient; SIRS, systemic inflammatory response syndrome (see Volume 2, Chapter 63); $\dot{V}_A/\dot{Q}$, alveolar ventilation to perfusion ratio.

Oxygen Consumption and Delivery

In order to fully evaluate the adequacy of tissue oxygenation, the concepts of oxygen delivery ($\dot{D}O_2$) and oxygen consumption ($\dot{V}O_2$) will be briefly reviewed. The factors contributing to the value of $\dot{D}O_2$ are oxygen content (CaO_2) and cardiac output ($\dot{Q}$), as shown in Equation 1:

$$\dot{D}O_2 = CaO_2 \times \dot{Q} \qquad (1)$$

where CaO_2 is the arterial oxygen content (expressed in mLO_2/dL blood) and $\dot{Q}$ the cardiac output (expressed as L blood/min). The CaO_2 can be calculated by simultaneously measuring an ABG and hemoglobin (Hb) concentration in a patient, as shown in Equation 2.

$$CaO_2 = [Hb] \times 1.34 \times Sat_{arterial} + 0.003 \times PaO_2 \qquad (2)$$

Using Equation 2, a patient with an Hb = 15, and 100% saturation of arterial Hb with O_2 has a calculated $CaO_2 = 20$ mL O_2/dL blood = 200 mL O_2/L blood. Some O_2 is also dissolved in plasma ($0.003 \times PaO_2$), the amount of which is generally negligible. However, in low O_2 saturation conditions, where patients are supported with high FIO_2, and especially at higher barometric pressures (i.e., at sea level or in a hyperbaric chamber), the dissolved O_2 component can become more significant.

The $\dot{Q}$ is most often measured using the thermodilution method, via a pulmonary artery (PA) catheter. The normal resting $\dot{Q}$ for a 70-kg patient is approximately 5 L blood/min. Thus, the normal $\dot{D}O_2$ for a 70-kg patient is 1000 mL O_2/min (5 L blood/min × 200 mL O_2/L blood).

The $\dot{V}O_2$ can be determined for various vascular beds or organs. However, if not otherwise stated, the $\dot{V}O_2$ represents the total amount of O_2 consumed by all tissues in the body and is expressed as $mL/O_2/min$.

The $\dot{V}O_2$ can be determined clinically in two ways, either by indirect calorimetry, where actual oxygen uptake is measured (subtraction of expired from inspired volume of oxygen), or by use of the Fick mass balance equation (Equation 3):

$$\dot{V}O_2 = \dot{Q} \times (Ca_{O2} - Cv_{O2}) \qquad (3)$$

where Ca_{O_2} is calculated using Equation 2 and using the saturation of the arterial blood (obtained from the ABG),

and the Cv_{O_2} is also calculated by using Equation 2, but uses the venous O_2 saturation taken from the mixed venous blood gas (obtained with a PA catheter). The Fick method does not take into account oxygen consumed by the lungs. Normally, lung tissue oxygen extraction is negligible. However, in the setting of ALI, pulmonary oxygen consumption may be significantly increased. Thus, the Fick method may be prone to inaccuracy compared to indirect calorimetry, in the setting of ALI (11). The normal value for $\dot{V}O_2$ is about 250 mL/min for a 70-kg patient, or about 3 to 4 mL/kg/min. The $\dot{V}O_2$ varies in concert with the metabolic needs of the body, and may be increased by fever or the systemic inflammatory response syndrome (SIRS), as described in Volume 2, Chapter 63.

Ventilation–Perfusion Abnormalities

Ventilation and perfusion ($\dot{V}/\dot{Q}$) are normally well matched (see Volume 2, Chapter 2). However, when hypoxic pulmonary vasoconstriction (HPV) is blunted, underventilated areas of the lung are overperfused, resulting in hypoxemia. Conversely, when certain areas of the lung are underperfused (as occurs in pulmonary embolism), areas of high $\dot{V}/\dot{Q}$ (and alveolar dead space) result. The oxygen content of these high $\dot{V}/\dot{Q}$ regions is elevated, and the CO_2 content is lower than normal. Following a PE, blood will also be forced to increase flow to nonobstructed low $\dot{V}/\dot{Q}$ regions. Because the very low oxygen content of the now overperfused (low $\dot{V}/\dot{Q}$) lung units cannot be sufficiently compensated by the higher oxygen content of the underperfused (high $\dot{V}/\dot{Q}$) lung units, the aggregate mixing of the blood results in hypoxemia. Furthermore, pulmonary emboli release factors into the pulmonary circulation that increase the right-to-left transpulmonary shunt (discussed subsequently), further impairing oxygenation.

A number of factors influence alveolar dead space, including age, posture, and body size (12). Significant abnormalities in alveolar dead space result from a number of pathologic conditions occurring in trauma and critical care. The processes that increase the alveolar dead space include all conditions that increase ventilation beyond the concomitant pulmonary perfusion, as occurs when excessive tidal volume or positive end expiratory pressure (PEEP) is employed; as well as when impaired cardiac output occurs, due to hypovolemia (common in trauma), pump failure (myocardial ischemia, tamponade), and so on. Alveolar dead space is also increased by pulmonary embolism (Volume 2, Chapter 56). Additionally, situations that impair HPV (e.g., inhaled anesthetics and other pulmonary vasodilators) will increase alveolar dead space. The anatomic dead space is defined as the volume of gas in the conducting airways. The alveolar dead space and anatomic dead space combined yields the physiologic dead space. The physiologic dead space can be measured by determining the dead space to tidal volume ratio using the Bohr equation (Equation 4):

$$V_D/V_T = Pa\ CO_2 - P_{ET}CO_2/PaCO_2 \qquad (4)$$

where V_D/V_T represents the dead space to tidal volume ratio, $PaCO_2$ is the partial pressure of carbon dioxide in arterial blood, and $P_{ET}CO_2$ is the partial pressure of carbon dioxide in a mixed-expired gas sample.

The most common clinical scenarios leading to ventilation-perfusion mismatching include blood loss following trauma or during surgery, and in the nonoperative setting, exacerbations of chronic obstructive pulmonary disease (COPD), pneumonia, and atelectasis. Many drugs will blunt the ability of the pulmonary circulation to respond appropriately to hypoxia by vasoconstriction. These drugs are commonly used in the ICU, and include nitrates, inotropes, inhaled anesthetics, and calcium-channel blockers (13).

σ⁺ **Many of the drugs used in the ICU have vasodilator properties and can worsen oxygenation by blunting HPV and exacerbating $\dot{V}/\dot{Q}$ mismatching.** σ⁺

Right-to-Left Transpulmonary Shunt

Right-to-left transpulmonary shunting, sometimes referred to as venous admixture, refers to alveoli that are perfused but not ventilated, resulting in the effluent of nonoxygenated blood from these lung units, and ultimate mixing of oxygenated and nonoxygenated blood, decreasing the Pa_{O_2}. The normal healthy person has less than 5% transpulmonary shunt. This normal shunted blood results from two sources: (i) the anatomic shunt of blood that empties directly to the left atrium or left ventricle (LV); and (ii) a very small amount of normal, transpulmonary shunting (blood that flows through the lungs in the normal pathways, past alveolar units that are not exposed to gas exchange). The anatomic shunts that are present in all normal patients include the thebesian veins and the bronchial circulation, both of which empty their deoxygenated blood directly into the left side of the heart. Intracardiac shunts are pathologic, and not considered part of the normal right-to-left transpulmonary shunt. When pathologic intracardiac shunts are present, they can contribute large quantities of deoxygenated blood to the left side of the heart, resulting in profound hypoxemia. The foramen ovale is physiologically closed in most normal adults; however, it remains probe patent in as many as 30% of adult patients. The probe-patent foramen ovale may open in the setting of elevated right atrial pressures, as can occur in secondary RV failure (i.e., due to pulmonary artery hypertension—as occurs in numerous disease states such as advanced ARDS). Other pathologic anatomic shunts include pleural-based arteriovenous shunts seen in patients with hepatic cirrhosis—so-called hepato-pulmonary syndrome—reviewed below (also see Volume 2, Chapters 36 and 37). σ⁺ **The most common causes of right-to-left transpulmonary shunting in ICU patients are direct pulmonary pathologic entities, such as pneumonia, atelectasis, and noncardiogenic pulmonary edema.** σ⁺ Each of these entities causes blood flow to bypass gas-exchanging portions of the lung.

The degree of shunt can be calculated using the shunt equation (Equation 5):

$$\frac{\dot{Q}s}{\dot{Q}t} = \frac{C_{CO_2} - Ca_{O_2}}{C_{CO_2} - Cv_{O_2}} \qquad (5)$$

where $\dot{Q}s/\dot{Q}t$ is the shunt blood flow expressed as a fraction of total blood flow, Cc_{O_2} the calculated alveolar capillary blood content, CaO_2 the measured oxygen content of arterial blood, and CvO_2 the measured oxygen content of mixed venous blood. Although some intensivists will calculate the $\dot{Q}s/\dot{Q}t$ using the above shunt equation, a clinically useful estimate can be made using the shortcut suggested by Pierson (14). Providing the patient is on an FiO_2 of 1.0, and the PaO_2 is 150 mmHg or more, there is approximately 5% shunt for every 100 mmHg the PaO_2 is below 700 (14).

The degree of right-to-left transpulmonary shunt is also reflected in the PaO_2/FiO_2 (or "P/F") ratio (normally approximately 500) (15,16). Using the alveolar air equation (Equation 6), one can calculate the expected P_AO_2 and, as first proposed by Bendixen, calculate the alveolar-to-arterial PO_2 difference $[P(A-a)O_2]$ (17). In the absence of any significant right-to-left transpulmonary shunt, the PaO_2 (measured with an ABG) will be essentially the same as the P_AO_2, calculated from the alveolar air equation (Equation 6).

$$P_AO_2 = [(P_B - P_{H_2}O) \cdot F_IO_2] - \left[\frac{PaCO_2}{RQ}\right] \qquad (6)$$

The alveolar air equation predicts that the P_AO_2 will be decreased when there is: (i) a decrease in either the barometric pressure, or the F_IO_2, or (ii) an increase in the $PaCO_2$. The PaO_2/F_IO_2 ratio can be used to roughly, and quickly, determine the degree of right-left transpulmonary shunt. When the PaO_2/F_IO_2 is <300, the threshold for ALI is achieved, whereas a PaO_2/F_IO_2 <200 meets the criteria for ARDS (Table 1).

Although shunt units will not be affected by the administration of 100% oxygen, hypoxemia from $\dot{Q}s/\dot{Q}t$ mismatching will be improved. In clinical practice, patients often have a combination of both shunt and $\dot{V}/\dot{Q}$ mismatch. Thus, oxygen should always be administered to the hypoxemic patient regardless of the putitive mechanism.

Diffusion Impairment

Impairment of oxygen diffusion into alveolar capillaries may occur with infiltration of the alveolar airspaces. This occurs most commonly with pulmonary edema, either cardiogenic or noncardiogenic. The increased diffusion distance for oxygen may result in incomplete oxygenation of venous blood, especially when diffusion impairment exists in combination with high $\dot{Q}$ and/or anemia. It is unclear what the clinical significance of diffusion impairment is, as other mechanisms, such as ventilation-perfusion mismatching and right-to-left transpulmonary shunting, are likely more significant causes of hypoxemia.

Decreased Mixed Venous Oxygen Content

Decreased CVO_2 rarely exists as an isolated entity, but commonly occurs in concert with other causes of hypoxemia such as anemia, low cardiac output, and increased systemic oxygen consumption (i.e., fever). If venous blood is not fully oxygenated during passage through the lungs, then unsaturated blood enters the arterial circulation. Treatment of low mixed venous oxygen content is based upon the etiology.

In the setting of anemia (Volume 2, Chapter 54), treatment consists of transfusion, and in the setting of low $\dot{Q}$, inotropes are used, whereas in the case of fever, antipyretic therapy may be indicated. Sedatives may be administered to critically ill patients to decrease the $\dot{V}O_2$. Paralytic agents by themselves should not be employed for this purpose. Considerable controversy exists regarding the precise goals of DO_2 in critically ill patients (see Volume 2, Chapter 17).

Alveolar Hypoventilation

The alveolar air equation (Equation 6) predicts a decrease in P_AO_2 if there is an increase in $PaCO_2$ (as occurs with hypoventilation). So, even if alveolar uptake of O_2 is normal and DO_2 is normal, the patient may ultimately become hypoxic, because the increase in partial pressure of CO_2 in the alveoli leaves less space for O_2.

The CO_2 concentration in the alveoli increases during alveolar hypoventilation. Accordingly, the alveolar partial pressure of oxygen and other gases must fall. In the absence of supplemental oxygenation, hypoxemia will occur. The most common clinical scenario for alveolar hypoventilation is decreased respiratory drive from opiate administration, although patients with neuromuscular or central nervous system (CNS) disorders can develop the same complication. In trauma patients, drugs, CNS disorders, and mechanical ventilatory problems (e.g., pneumothorax) can all occur simultaneously.

The oxygenation defect seen with alveolar hypoventilation may be overcome by increasing the F_IO_2, thereby increasing the diffusion gradient for oxygen into the alveolar capillaries. The most common clinical entities associated with acute hypoxemic respiratory failure are listed in Table 4.

Acute Hypercapneic Respiratory Failure: Ventilation Dysfunction

Failure of the ventilatory system results in hypercapnea and respiratory acidosis, and in the absence of supplemental oxygen, hypoxemia. Ventilatory failure can result from CNS injury or dysfunction, with consequent alterations in respiratory drive, as well as from respiratory musculature weakness as in patients with Guillin-Barré syndrome, or due to increased WOB, as occurs in severe bronchospasm or decreased C_L or increased V_D (e.g., PE), or patients with COPD. A review of the medical history, physical examination, chest radiograph (CXR), and blood gas analysis can usually identify the etiology of the ventilatory failure. In the case of neuromuscular disease, electromyography (EMG) testing or consultation by a neurologist may be required to differentiate between neuronal, muscular, or neuromuscular junction (NMJ) dysfunction. Acute hypercapneic respiratory failure can be identified when the ABG reveals a $PaCO_2$ greater than 50 mmHg. Each of these systems will be examined independently.

Carbon Dioxide Production and Clearance

Carbon dioxide is produced as an end product of cellular metabolism, with a normal steady-state production of approximately 200 mL/min in a 70-kg patient. If alveolar ventilation is inadequate to eliminate the total CO_2 produced, then hypercapnea and respiratory acidosis will ensue. Therefore, in the steady state, $\dot{V}CO_2$ can be defined as the product of alveolar ventilation and arterial $PaCO_2$,

as shown in Equation 7.

$$P_ACO_2 \approx PaCO_2 = \frac{\dot{V}CO_2}{\dot{V}_A} \qquad (7)$$

The alveolar PCO_2 (P_ACO_2) varies during the ventilatory cycle. P_ACO_2 falls at the commencement of inhalation, and rises during exhalation. The end tidal P_ACO_2 is nearly equal to the $PaCO_2$, whereas the exhaled PCO_2 (measures is $P_{ET}CO_2$) is slightly lower; the greater the alveolar dead space, the greater the difference between the $P_{ET}CO_2$ and the $PaCO_2$.

An increase in $PaCO_2$ must be due to either an increase in production or a decrease in elimination, with decreased elimination due to either a decreased minute ventilation or increased dead space ventilation (or both). Increased CO_2 production may result from fever or overfeeding, both of which should be corrected in patients with severe ARF. Diagnosis of increased CO_2 production can be made with indirect calorimetry. Adjustment of enteral or parenteral nutrition, or treatment of fever, can be further monitored with indirect calorimetry to follow the expected decrease CO_2 production.

Ventilatory Mechanics

A number of factors will contribute to abnormalities in ventilatory mechanics, including decreased lung or chest wall C_L, increased intra-abdominal pressure, and neuromuscular dysfunction. Pure ventilatory failure will manifest itself by hypercapnea. Having an intubated patient perform a spontaneous breathing trial provides information regarding the patient's ability to do their WOB. However, a high RSBI (i.e., RR/Vt >100) does not specifiy whether the WOB is too high, or if the patient is too weak. Accordingly, the evaluation of mechanical failure seeks pulmonary mechanic data that isolate the variables of interest. The maximum inspiratory pressure (P_{IMAX}) is another weaning parameter (pulmonary mechanic) that reflects the patient's strength. The P_{IMAX} is obtained by occluding the endotracheal tube (ETT) with a negative pressure measuring device (see Volume 2, Chapter 28). The P_{IMAX} may vary with age and gender, but normal healthy individuals can usually generate negative pressures less negative than -80 to $-100\,cmH_2O$ (18). Having a patient perform a vital capacity (VC) breath will also identify mechanical abnormalities related to respiratory muscle weakness, but this measurement is also dependent upon the lung and chest wall compliance. In mechanically ventilated patients, measurement of peak inspiratory pressure, plateau pressure, and dynamic hyperinflation or intrinsic positive end-expiratory pressure (PEEP) further characterize the mechanical abnormalities associated with ARF.

Work of Breathing

In normal circumstances, the WOB is very small, representing less than 2% of the basal metabolic rate. Under pathologic conditions, however, when respiratory system compliance decreases and/or airway resistance increases, the WOB can be substantial, utilizing a larger portion of the oxygen delivery. In patients with ARF, minute ventilation demands are high because of increased dead-space fraction (e.g., PE), or cause airflow obstruction (e.g., kinked ETT or copious secretions). With further increases in airflow obstruction, the WOB is markedly elevated because of active expiratory

Table 4 Pathophysiology and Diagnostic Clues Associated with Common Clinical Conditions Causing Acute Respiratory Failure

Clinical condition	Physiologic abnormality	Diagnostic clues
Acute bacterial pneumonia	$\Uparrow$'d $\dot{Q}_S/\dot{Q}_T$, ($\Downarrow$'d PaO_2), fever ($\Uparrow$'d $\dot{V}CO_2$), $\Downarrow$'d C_L, and $\Uparrow$'d R_{AW} all cause $\Uparrow$ WOB	Fever, WBC (left shift), infiltrate on CXR, purulent sputum
Viral and atypical (*Mycoplasma, Legionella*) pneumonias	S/A	WBC not very elevated, more monocytes, diffuse alveolar pattern on CXR, sputum normal
Fungal pneumonia	S/A	Immunosuppressed patient, cavitary lesions on CXR
Asthma	Broncho constriction and mucus plugging of airways, $\Uparrow$'d $\dot{V}/\dot{Q}$, $\Uparrow$'d R_{AW} all cause $\Uparrow$ WOB	Wheezing, $\Uparrow$'d expiratory phase, CXR: flat diaphragms, and $\Uparrow$'d A-P diameter; use of accessory muscles
COPD	S/A, plus bronchitis and or emphysema: ($\Downarrow$'d DLCO)	S/A, often $\Uparrow$'d serum $[HCO_3^-]$ due to chronic hypercarbia
Upper airway obstruction	$\Uparrow$'d R_{AW}, $\Uparrow$'d $PaCO_2$	Stridor (heard in neck), snoring
Aspiration	Epithelial injury: R → L shunting, ($\Downarrow$'d PaO_2), $\Uparrow$'d lung H_2O: $\Downarrow$'d C_L, bronchial injury: $\Uparrow$'d R_{AW}: $\Uparrow$ WOB	CXR infiltrate classically in superior segments of lower lobes (especially right side)
Pulmonary embolism	$\Uparrow$'d V_D/V_T, $\Uparrow$'d $\dot{V}_E$, $\Uparrow$'d $\dot{V}/\dot{Q}$, $\Uparrow$'d $\dot{Q}_S/\dot{Q}_T$	Hx DVT, Hx trauma, abrupt $\Uparrow$'d dyspnea after position change
Myocardial failure	$\Uparrow$'d $\dot{Q}_S/\dot{Q}_T$ (cardiogenic pulmonary edema)	$\Downarrow$'d $\dot{Q}$, $\Uparrow$'d atrial pressures, ECG changes
Neuromuscular disorders	$\Downarrow$'d $\dot{V}_E$—due to $\Downarrow$'d NMJ function	$\Downarrow$'d twitch and $\Downarrow$'d muscle strength Tensilon improves (if myasthenia G)
Chest wall trauma	$\Downarrow$'d $\dot{V}_E$—due to pain induced splinting	Rib fractures, $\Downarrow$'d V_T, $\Downarrow$'d MIF
Pulmonary contusion	$\Uparrow$'d $\dot{Q}_S/\dot{Q}_T$ (noncardiogenic pulmonary edema)	Lung contusion on CXR or CT
Hemo-pneumothorax	$\Uparrow$'d $\dot{Q}_S/\dot{Q}_T$ (lung collapse 2° blood or air)	Hemo-pneumothorax on CXR/CT
Fluid overload	$\Uparrow$'d $\dot{Q}_S/\dot{Q}_T$ (hydrostatic pulmonary edema)	$\Uparrow$ $\Uparrow$ Fluid resuscitation, $\Uparrow$'d atrial pressures, $\Downarrow$'d Albumin ú
Fat embolism	$\Uparrow$'d $\dot{Q}_S/\dot{Q}_T$ (noncardiogenic pulmonary edema)	Hx proximal long bone Fx
Near-drowning	$\Uparrow$'d $\dot{Q}_S/\dot{Q}_T$ (noncardiogenic pulmonary edema)	Trauma involving water
Burns	$\Uparrow$'d $\dot{Q}_S/\dot{Q}_T$ (noncardiogenic pulmonary edema)	$\Uparrow$ BSA Burn, or inhaled smoke
Head injury	$\Uparrow$'d $\dot{Q}_S/\dot{Q}_T$ (neurogenic pulmonary edema)	Especially with SAH
Renal failure	$\Uparrow$'d $\dot{Q}_S/\dot{Q}_T$ (hydrostatic and noncardiogenic pulmonary edema), $\Downarrow$'d C_L, $\Uparrow$ WOB	left atrial pressures, $\Downarrow$'d albumin, ± LV dysfunction
Pancreatitis	$\Uparrow$'d $\dot{Q}_S/\dot{Q}_T$ (noncardiogenic pulmonary edema)	$\Uparrow$ amylase, $\Uparrow$ lipase, $\Uparrow$ inflammation
Liver failure	$\Uparrow$'d $\dot{Q}_S/\dot{Q}_T$ (noncardiogenic pulmonary edema)	$\Uparrow$ LFTs, $\Downarrow$'d albumin, edema, ± porto-pulmonary syndrome
Sepsis/SIRS	$\Uparrow$'d $\dot{Q}_S/\dot{Q}_T$ (noncardiogenic pulmonary edema)	$\Uparrow$ inflammation (multiple etiologies)

Abbreviations: $\Uparrow$, increase; $\Downarrow$, decrease; BSA, body surface area; BUN, blood urea nitrogen; C_L, compliance; CO_2, CO_2 production; Cr, creatinine; CT, computed tomography; CXR, chest radiograph; DLCO, diffusion capacity; DVT, deep venous thrombosis; ECG, electrocardiogram; Fx, fracture; Hx, history of; LV, left ventricle; MIF, maximum inspiratory force; NMJ, neuromuscular junction; $PaCO_2$, partial pressure of CO_2 in arterial blood; PaO_2, partial pressure of oxygen in arterial blood; $\dot{Q}$, cardiac output; $\dot{Q}_S/\dot{Q}_T$, shunt flow/cardiac output (in this context same as right-to-left transpulmonary shunt); R_{AW}, airway resistance; S/A, same as above; SAH, subarachnoid hemorrhage; $\dot{V}_E$, minute ventilation; V_T, tidal volume; $\dot{V}/\dot{Q}$, ventilation/perfusion ratio; V_D/V_T, dead space to tidal volume ratio; WBC, white blood cell count; WOB, work of breathing.

efforts. This increased demand will often lead to ventilatory failure, as respiratory and accessory muscles fatigue. The WOB can be measured with esophageal manometry, and the workload partitioned between the patient and the mechanical ventilator. The precise WOB threshold that should be done by the patient is not well understood. A more detailed discussion of ventilatory mechanics and the WOB, in terms of normal pulmonary physiology and weaning parameters are found in Volume 2, Chapters 2 and 28, respectively.

Neural Control of Breathing

Respiratory drive originates in the medulla and triggers inspiratory efforts. In rare cases, patients may have primary alveolar hypoventilation, usually secondary to other disease processes. The most common associated illnesses are obesity, with obesity hypoventilation syndrome, and chronic poliomyelitis. Far more common is respiratory depression secondary to the use of opiates or benzodiazepines. Patients in the ICU are particularly prone to disorders of the NMJ, so-called "critical illness polyneuropathy" (Volume 2, Chapter 6). This is a syndrome that may be present 50% to 70% of the time in mechanically ventilated patients with sepsis (19). Critical illness polyneuropathy is characterized by polyneuropathy-induced muscular weakness and difficulty weaning from mechanical ventilation. Diagnosis may be made by EMG. Other myopathies may result from steroid use (20), and in particular, from the combination of steroids and neuromuscular blocking drugs in acute asthmatics (21). Patients proving difficult to wean from mechanical ventilation should be evaluated for myopathy or other neurologic dysfunction.

CLINICAL PRESENTATION OF ACUTE RESPIRATORY FAILURE
Diagnostic Approach to Acute Respiratory Failure

The importance of determining the etiology of ARF cannot be overstated. Often, the clues regarding the etiology are fleeting, and may only be available at the bedside immediately prior to intubation. These clues (Table 4) must be actively sought out, gathered, and chronicled by the physician called to intubate the patient, prior to transfer to the ICU. Examples of clues that should be sought, and will be missed if not reported by the intubating physician, include the presence of: (*i*) vomit in a patient's oropharynx passing below cords, involving the trachea and bronchi; (*ii*) ST segment depression during the ARF event, which resolves following intubation and mechanical ventilation; (*iii*) pulmonary edema fluid prior to intubation and the administration of PEEP; 4) stridor; etc. Accordingly, the diagnostic approach to ARF starts with a focused medical history, and physical examination at the bedside.

History

Because of critical illness, a patient's complete medical history cannot always be fully obtained. Clinical clues to the history of present illness (relevant to ARF) are invaluable, as mentioned above. Regarding the past medical history, it is useful to ascertain whether the patient has any underlying lung pathology such as COPD or asthma, whether the patient has a history of tobacco use, or whether s/he has had any recurrent problems such as congestive heart failure (CHF), pneumonia, or bronchitis. Knowledge of underlying pulmonary or cardiac conditions may influence the clinician's decision to move directly to endotracheal intubation, or to temporize with noninvasive positive pressure ventilation (NIPPV). A patient who was doing well prior to moving or getting out of bed, who abruptly develops respiratory failure, shows no signs of aspiration, and has clear lungs provides a good history and physical for an acute PE. Historical factors may also influence the choice of induction agents for endotracheal intubation, and may further guide the selection of a particular mode of mechanical ventilatory support, impact the level of PEEP, tidal volume setting, or initial setting of I:E ratio. Finally, knowledge of pulmonary function testing and baseline oxygenation and ventilation (via ABG evaluation) can help establish acceptable weaning parameters when respiratory status begins to improve.

Physical Examination

Physical examination of the patient with respiratory failure begins with chest observation of respiratory rate and pattern (including use of accessory muscles or pardoxic breathing), auscultation of breath sounds and any evidence of stridor, and blood pressure measurement. Although this valuable diagnostic information is being obtained, it is essential that the "ABCs" of resuscitation are being employed, by assuring a patent airway, and treating with supplemental oxygen. Examination may reveal surgical scars, indicating prior surgery, such as a thoracotomy or prior tracheotomy. Barrel-chested patients, for instance, are more likely to have COPD. The presence of subcutaneous emphysema is highly suggestive of pneumomediastinum, and tracheal deviation may indicate tension pneumothorax.

Ausculatation of breath sounds may reveal a variety of diffuse or specific findings, which may help to diagnose an underlying condition or the cause of ARF. Close observation of the patient's respiratory pattern can provide valuable information: Is the chest moving paradoxically? Does the patient appear to be breathing with diaphragmatic, or more with accessory, musculature? Is there equal excursion of both sides of the chest? Is there dullness (effusion, acteletasis, pneumonia), or hyperresonance (pneumothorax, blebs) in any areas of the lungs? Heart rate and blood pressure measurement are essential.

A patient with an acute exacerbation of COPD or reactive airway disease may have low systolic blood pressure, resulting from dynamic hyperinflation, increased intrathoracic pressure and consequent decreased venous return to right atrium, increased afterload of the right ventricle (RV) and consequent decreased LV filling and stroke volume. Patients may be diaphoretic or confused, and patients with hypercapnea may exhibit somnolence, seizures, or myoclonic jerks.

Arterial Blood Gas Analysis

Initial assessment of a patient with ARF is facilitated by obtaining focused laboratory data; especially pulse oximetry, CXR, ECG, and ABG. Only with an ABG can quantitative determinations about the severity of the ARF be made. These determinations include calculation of shunt fraction ($\dot{Q}s/\dot{Q}t$), P_aO_2/F_IO_2, and alveolar dead space ventilation. Analysis of the ABG and serum electrolyte panel can provide additional clues that may facilitate the diagnosis and management of these patients. Elevated $PaCO_2$ in the presence of a high serum bicarbonate level suggests chronic CO_2 retention. The Henderson-Hasselbach equation may be used to estimate the patient's baseline degree of CO_2 retention. The PaO_2 will be essential in assessing those patients who are receiving supplemental oxygen, and for whom the institution of NIPPV or endotracheal intubation may be imminent. Furthermore, the PaO_2 may serve to provide the only accurate measure of oxygenation for those patients whose decreased peripheral perfusion limits the use of pulse oximetry.

Oximetry and Capnometry

In patients with ARF, the decision to proceed to endotracheal intubation may be made on the basis of physical examination and oximetry, particularly if the patient is in distress and there is no time to obtain an arterial blood gas. Most patients require oxygen saturation greater than 90%, particularly in the setting of critical illness. Oximetry provides a rapid, reliable assessment of oxygenation in critically ill patients, and is the standard of care for continuous monitoring in both the ICU and operating room (OR). However, oximetry is prone to errors; for example, carbon monoxide poisoning may show falsely high oxygen saturation, whereas patients with methemoglobinemia will present with a pulse oximeter saturation of 85%, regardless of the true oxygen saturation as determined by co-oximetry (see Volume 2, Chapter 8). The reason for these errors with pulse oximetry is that only the two species oxy-Hb and Hb are measured by these devices. Accordingly, the initial blood gas assessment of the patient with ARF should include co-oximetry, which will characterize the various hemoglobin species present (including oxy-Hb, Hb, met-Hb, and carboxy-Hb).

σ **Many commonly used drugs can cause methemoglobinemia, which will worsen hypoxemia and acidosis. These drugs include dapsone, local anesthetics (benzocaine and prilocaine), commonly used nitrates (nitroprusside, nitroglycerin), and sulfonamides. Diagnosis may be made with co-oximetry that measures various hemoglobin species. Treatment is with methylene blue.** σ

Capnometry allows measurement of end-tidal CO_2 ($PetCO_2$). In normal subjects, the $PetCO_2$ is usually 3–5 mmHg less than the arterial PCO_2. Patients with COPD, and those with respiratory failure, have an increased dead space fraction, and the $PetCO_2$-$PaCO_2$ gradient will be much larger. However, capnometry is extremely useful in a number of settings; for continuous respiratory monitoring, and importantly, for documenting intratracheal placement of the ETT during intubation. Capnometry also allows detection of expiratory flow obstruction, as the expiratory curve will fail to reach a plateau, suggesting delayed release from alveoli with long exhalation time constants.

Radiographic Evaluation

Chest radiography is an essential component in the diagnostic work up of ARF; it can substantially narrow the differential and sharpen the focus in developing a treatment plan. A clinical diagnosis of pneumonia, for example, is supported by the presence of an infiltrative process on the radiograph. Chest radiography will also help to diagnose underlying pathology that may be linked directly or indirectly to the ARF, such as an enlarged cardiac silhouette or the presence of apical scarring in a patient with a history of mycobacterial disease. The presence of an increased anterior-posterior diameter, flattened diaphragms, and hyperinflation are common findings associated with COPD. The presence of pulmonary interstitial emphysema can alert the clinician to a potential imminent pneumothorax. Pulmonary interstitial emphysema can appear as perivascular halos, pneumatoceles, intraseptal air collections, and linear streaks of air radiating from the hila, parenchymal cysts, and subpleural air collections. However, most pneumothoraces are not diagnosed until an apicolateral visceral pleural line is detected. Reliance on this presentation will result in the underdiagnosis of pneumothorax in critically ill patients. Subpulmonic pneumothorax can be detected by visualizing a "deep sulcus" sign, as well as by hyperlucency of the superior abdominal area. Anteromedial pneumothorax may be diagnosed by the presence of a mediastinal border outlined by pleural air or by a linear air density along that border. Many patients with ARF are unable to be positioned upright, thereby making the detection of pneumothorax more difficult with chest radiography. Tracheal deviation with contralateral displacement of the heart and mediastinal structures, as well as ipsilateral lung collapse, may provide essential clues of a potentially life-threatening tension pneumothorax.

Differentiation of cardiogenic versus noncardiogenic pulmonary edema can be difficult. The presence of Kerley-B lines represent interstitial edema, and their presence, along with evidence of vascular cephalization, suggests the presence of cardiogenic pulmonary edema. However, even experienced clinicians may be unable to determine the cause of edema in the supine ICU patient (22). Likewise, the severity of pulmonary infiltration does not always correlate with the severity of respiratory failure.

An entirely normal appearing CXR (other than slight decreased pulmonary arterial markings), in a patient with acute onset respiratory failure, is suggestive of an acute PE. Chest radiography will not always provide the clinician with specific clues that will lead to a clear diagnosis, but it can rule out many of the common etiologies of ARF, allowing the clinician to narrow the likely list of causes.

Sputum Evaluation

Sputum evaluation is an essential component of the diagnosis of both community-acquired and nosocomial pneumonias. Both culture and Gram stain can provide important diagnostic therapeutic information. The Gram stain can be more reliable than sputum culture for diagnosing pneumonia, whereas the culture helps define antimicrobial resistance. Indeed, if an organism is cultured from sputum, but not shown as a predominant species in the Gram stain, it often represents colonization of the tracheo-bronchial tree. The Gram stain is an excellent tool for determining the focus of early antibiotic therapy. The sensitivity and specificity of sputum culture depends on criteria used for a definition of positivity and negativity. There is a very hazy evidence base defining the efficacy of sputum culturing, and is often most useful in the identification of unusual infectious causes of respiratory failure, and in identifying antibiotic resistance of certain organisms. It should be kept in mind that even in the setting of bacterial pneumonia, sputum culture is positive less than 50% of the time (23).

Clinical Entities Associated with Acute Respiratory Failure
Airway and Airflow Disorders

Airflow disorders are frequently life-threatening, with the most common processes being asthma and exacerbations of COPD (Table 4). Both disease entities are common, with more than 17 million individuals having asthma in the United States (24). Physical examination may demonstrate expiratory wheezing, which may decrease in intensity as the patient fatigues. Other physical examination findings associated with both asthma and COPD include a prolonged expiratory phase and accessory muscle use. ARF with airflow limitation is usually hypercapneic, so ABG sampling is essential. The use of oximetry may be misleading, as these patients usually oxygenate well, even with impending ARF.

Asthma

Asthma is an inflammatory process characterized by both bronchoconstriction and mucus plugging of small airways. A number of precipitating factors may trigger an asthma exacerbation, including upper respiratory infections, pneumonia, inhaled irritants, and allergens (25,26). σ **Patients with acute asthma exacerbations are normally hypertensive because of catechol release. Those that are normotensive or hypotensive and tachycardic may have elevated intrathoracic pressure impeding venous return, and are at increased risk for cardiopulmonary arrest during endotracheal intubation.** σ Although an asthma attack is usually easy to identify on physical examination, measurement of fraction of exhaled volume in the first second (FEV_1) and forced vital capacity (FVC) can be used to track the severity of illness.

Patients develop ARF from asthma exacerbations when expiratory flow obstruction progresses to the point where accessory muscles fail, resulting in hypercapnea and acidosis. Wheezing may be inspiratory and/or expiratory. Other physical examination findings can include pulsus paradoxus. A rising $PaCO_2$ in the setting of maximal noninvasive therapy is a worrisome sign, and is suggestive that the patient may require intubation and mechanical ventilation. Particularly worrisome is the presence of hypotension, which suggests high intrathoracic pressure and decreased venous return; these patients are at particularly high risk for hypotension and/or cardiac arrest during endotracheal intubation and with positive pressure ventilation (27,28). Mechanical ventilation management includes a prolonged exhalation phase, slow respiratory rate, low tidal volume, and intravascular bolus of fluid, while waiting for medical therapy (e.g., inhaled β-agonists, etc.) to work.

Radiographic findings in asthma may be unimpressive, but a CXR should be obtained to rule out pneumothorax, to identify a pneumonic process, and to evaluate the degree of pulmonary hyperinflation or diaphragmatic flattening. Laboratory testing should be done, as intensive bronchodilator therapy may result in life-threatening hypokalemia. Creatine phosphokinase levels may be elevated from respiratory muscle fatigue (29). Arterial blood gases should be obtained to assess the severity of acidosis and hypoxemia, and to help decide the need for intubation and/or ICU admission. Acidosis is often multifactorial, with a major respiratory component and a variable metabolic contribution (depending upon the systemic perfusion) (30).

Initial therapy begins with inhaled β-agonists, and consideration given to the addition of inhaled anticholinergic therapy with ipratroprium bromide (31). However, in pure asthma, ipratroprium bromide provides minimal additional benefit beyond that caused by the inhaled β-agonist. Additionally, because asthma is an inflammatory disorder, early, aggressive treatment with corticosteroids is essential. The recommended dosing is intravenous methylprednisolone, 120–180 mg/day, divided in three or four doses, for at least 48 hours (25). Theophylline, a phosphodiesterase inhibitor, is preferable to placebo, but has more toxicity than β-agonist and steroid therapy, and does not provide additional benefit to those drugs once they have been instituted (32).

Acute COPD Exacerbations

Patients with COPD often develop respiratory failure, as a result of exacerbation of their chronic bronchitis and/or emphysema. It can be particularly difficult to define ARF in this patient population, as the severity of their baseline pulmonary function is highly variable. Many patients are on chronic oxygen therapy, and others have varying degress of carbon dioxide retention. COPD is a common disease, affecting as many as 16 million Americans (33). Clinical presentation usually includes dyspnea, cough, and sputum production. Wheezing may be variably present, and accessory muscle use is common. Patients may have a history of upper respiratory infection, and sputum should be obtained for Gram stain and culture. The precipitating factors for COPD exacerbation include infection, medication noncompliance, and environmental exposures (34). Admission labs revealing an elevated $[HCO_3^-]$ may provide clues that the patient is a chronic CO_2 retainer (Table 4).

Like asthmatics, patients with COPD are also faced with impaired expiratory flow of gases. However, these patients may also experience these limitations at baseline.

It is useful to follow these patients with periodic evaluations of their $PaCO_2$, FEV_1, and FEV_1/FVC. If a significant component of emphysema is present, diffusing capacity (DLCO) should be measured in order to assess diffusing capacity. The COPD patient not only exhales against a markedly elevated resistance, but also breathes with a higher residual volume, making the WOB more difficult to accomplish, with increased reliance on accessory muscles. Dynamic hyperinflation results in increased intrinsic PEEP, which further limits alveolar ventilation. Areas of hyperinflation impair blood flow and give rise to an increasing dead space fraction, making the elimination of a given quantity of carbon dioxide dependent on a larger minute ventilation. Although exacerbations are characterized primarily by hypercapnea, hypoxemia is often present in those breathing room air, because of alveolar hypoventilation and poor ventilation/perfusion matching (35). With exacerbations, the patient can no longer maintain the required WOB, and endotracheal intubation with mechanical ventilatory support may become necessary.

Management of COPD exacerbations starts with supplemental oxygen. Many of the clinical signs and symptoms may be treated with oxygen alone, as ventilation/perfusion matching and pulmonary hypertension will both respond favorably (36). Oxygen therapy should not be withheld because of concern about blunting the hypoxic drive to breathe, rather it should be titrated to keep oxygen saturation at least 90% (37,38). As with acute asthmatics, corticosteroid therapy is essential, and should be supplemented with inhaled β-agonists. However, these patients (in contrast to younger asthmatics) will further benefit from inhaled ipatroprium bromide (Atrovent®) therapy. Ipatroprium bromide is an anticholinergic drug, which does not cause tachycardia. Ipatroprium bromide is administered as an inhaler, by itself, or along with albuterol as combination therapy (Combi-vent®). Severely bronchospastic patients should receive 125 mg methylprednisolone intravenously, every six hours, for three days, followed by an oral prednisone taper (39). Inhaled corticosteroids are useful for chronic therapy, but may not be efficacious without intravenous methylpredinisolone for acute exacerbations.

COPD and Upper Airway Obstruction

Upper airway obstruction may result in ARF, either directly through interference with oxygenation and ventilation, or indirectly by causing negative pressure pulmonary edema. Patients usually present with stridor, and careful auscultation may help identify the anatomic site of obstruction: inspiratory stridor is generally associated with an extrathoracic obstruction, whereas expiratory stridor is associated with intrathoracic obstruction (Table 4). High-pitched stridor is usually glottic in origin. There are numerous causes of airway obstruction, including trauma, infection, tumor, angioedema, foreign body aspiration, and vocal cord dysfunction.

☞ **Inspiratory stridor is usually due to an extrathoracic obstruction (supraglottic or periglottic) and expiratory stridor is usually due to an intrathoracic process.** ☞ Physical examination can help determine the cause of stridor.

After initial resuscitation, radiographic evaluation is essential, and may be done with chest and lateral neck radiography, but may require computerized tomography or magnetic resonance imaging (40). Arterial blood gases should be obtained to assess the severity of hypercapnea and oxygenation deficit. Patients with trauma-induced neck injuries and stridor should go directly to the OR for airway evaluation and management. ☞ **The key principles** of airway management for stridor are: (*i*) maintain spontaneous ventilation, (*ii*) avoid blind intubation techniques (may convert partial obstruction into complete obstruction), (*iii>*) awake fiberoptic intubation is often the best diagnostic tool and method of airway intubation, and (*iv>*) equipment and personnel capable of performing a surgical airway must be present until the airway is secured. ♂ All patients presenting with airway obstruction should be admitted to the ICU for observation, if surgical intervention is not planned. A carefully designed plan for emergent airway access needs to be in place, with appropriate equipment and personnel immediately available.

Aspiration of Gastric Contents

Aspiration pneumonia occurs when gastric contents enter the lung. Injury can result from three major factors: (*i*) epithelial burn from the low pH of gastric juice, (*ii*) obstruction from particulate matter, and (*iii*) infection from oropharyngeal bacteria. The aspiration injury that occurs also predisposes the lung to secondary infection. Patients at risk for aspiration pneumonia include those with diminished pharyngeal reflexes, and those with a decreased level of consciousness. Critically ill patients are at risk because of the presence of gastroparesis, resulting in high gastric volume. Early enteral nutrition, when tolerated (defined as residuals < 400 cc), does not increase the risk of this complication.

Diagnosis may be difficult, as CXR may initially appear grossly normal. Diagnostic testing is controversial, as transtracheal aspiration may primarily identify colonizing flora, rather than organisms causing pneumonia. Sputum culture or blood culture will identify organisms in only a small percentage of patients, whereas protected brush specimens also have low sensitivity (41). CXR may eventually show infiltrate in the superior segment of the right lower lobe (Table 4). However, diffuse bilateral infiltrates may develop as the lung injury progresses. Care is primarily supportive, with empiric antibiotic therapy used only in immunocompromised patients, or in those having rapid deterioration. Focused therapy can be started when specific organisms are identified by bronchoalveolar lavage (BAL) Gram stain, or a predominant organism is cultured from BAL, sputum, or blood.

Thromboembolism

Venous thromboembolism is a ubiquitous and difficult problem in all trauma and critically ill patients, and is covered in greater detail in Volume 2, Chapter 56. Prophylaxis is essential, but still imperfect. The most worrisome complication is PE. The occurrence of PE in a spontaneously ventilating patient is usually associated with significant tachypnea and moderate hypoxemia, associated with an acute increase in alveolar dead space and shunting without a concomitant new lung infiltration (Table 4). Patients who are weak and debilitated may not be able to do the requisite increased WOB to overcome the increased alveolar dead space, and may become hypercapnic. Similarly, patients entirely dependent upon the mechanical ventilator for breathing will have an acute decrease in $P_{ET}CO_2$, and a consequent increase in $PaCO_2$ due to the increased alveolar dead space following PE (providing the minute ventilation is maintained stable). Hypoxia also occurs in all of these scenarios; partly due to the redistribution of pulmonary blood flow to low $\dot{V}/\dot{Q}$ and shunt regions, and partly due to the vasogenic factors released from the embolus increasing alveolar capillary leak (e.g., histamine, bradykinin, etc). This hypoxemia can be

further exacerbated in the settling of alveolar hypoventilation, in the absence of supplemental oxygen therapy.

All trauma and ICU patients require thromboprophylaxis, guidelines for which have recently been published by the American College of Chest Physicians (Volume 2, Chapter 56) (42). The source of emboli are multiple and generally involve the lower extremities and pelvic veins, but also include the upper extremity venous system, particularly in patients with central venous catheterization. Diagnosis of pulmonary embolism relies on a high index of suspicion, and is confirmed with objective testing including spiral computed tomography or angiography. Respiratory failure from thromboembolism is usually hypoxemic, with ventilation-perfusion mismatching and increased alveolar dead space as a result of vascular obstruction.

Immediate treatment with heparinization (unless contraindicated) will prevent further clot formation, and although it has no intrinsic fibrinolytic effect, will provide clot dissolution results at the end of one week, similar to that provided by thrombolytic therapy, with far less side effects. When heparin is contraindicated, high-risk patients should receive inferior vena caval filters (Volume 2, Chapter 56).

Collagen-Vascular Pulmonary (Autoimmune) Disease

Patients may develop ARF from parenchymal abnormalities, due to aspiration (discussed earlier), infectious pneumonias (discussed subsequently), neoplasm (not reviewed here), and collagen-vascular disease-related conditions described in this section. Patients with pulmonary fibrosis are particularly susceptible to these conditions. It is increasingly recognized that collagen vascular diseases result from autoimmune disorders (see Volume 2, Chapter 52).

These patients most commonly present with dyspnea and cough. Chest radiography may be normal, or may demonstrate reticular densities. These abnormalities may make it difficult to document a pulmonary infection. Indeed, infection may be the precipitating factor for ARF in patients with underlying pulmonary fibrosis. Many of these patients are on chronic steroid therapy, and may require stress-dose supplementation if they develop ARF.

Goodpasture's syndrome and Wegner's glomerulotosis are common causes of patients presenting with alveolar hemorrhage (43). These are both pulmonary-renal autoimmune syndromes associated with substantial morbidity and mortality. The pathophysiology includes antibodies against basement membrane proteins in the lung and kidney, resulting in both respiratory and renal failure. Patients will require immunosuppressive therapy, usually with both corticosteroids and an antiproliferative agent like cyclophosphamide (44). Hemodialysis is commonly required, and may be combined with plasma exchange. Presentation of ARF secondary to systemic lupus erytematosus (SLE) may be similar to that seen in Goodpasture's, but alveolar hemorrhage is less common (45). As in Goodpasture's disease, infection should be vigorously pursued and treated in patients with SLE.

Cardiovascular Failure

Effective management of ARF requires knowledge of the underlying processes. Unraveling these processes can be complicated, as when trying to differentiate between cardiogenic and noncardiogenic pulmonary edema (Table 4). Both, ventricular systolic and diastolic dysfunction can give rise to ARF, as can valvular abnormalities such as severe mitral valve insufficiency (46). Clinical differentiation can be made on the basis of history and physical examination, but most patients will require echocardiography or PA catheterization to make a definitive diagnosis. Supplemental oxygen therapy should be implemented initially before any other intervention. Not only will this help with hypoxemia, it may directly treat ischemic cardiac dysfunction that is giving rise to the ARF. If pulmonary edema fluid can be obtained, then measurement of the edema fluid protein/plasma protein ratio can identify an exudative (sepsis or ALI) versus transudative (left atrial hypertension or CHF) cause for the pulmonary edema (47). Diastolic dysfunction, whether in combination with myocardial ischemia or secondary to systemic hypertension, may also cause ARF secondary to pulmonary edema.

Noninvasive positive pressure ventilation should only be considered if the underlying process causing the respiratory failure has resolved, and if there is no evidence of active cardiac ischemia. In patients with ongoing ischemia, endotracheal intubation and mechanical ventilation should be used. Many of the patients who present with ARF in this setting respond well to pharmacologic therapy, such as diuretics and afterload reducing agents. Although several studies have shown a benefit with NIPPV in the setting of ARF, few have indicated a clear benefit when the etiology of the ARF is clearly cardiac. The use of NIPPV may be comforting for the patient with pulmonary edema secondary to CHF, and may help to unload the LV while improving oxygenation. But the clinician should consider endotracheal intubation if there is no improvement after several hours of pharmacologic interventions, if there is any evidence of cardiac ischemia, or if the patient's WOB becomes too great (see Volume 2, Chapter 27).

Neuromuscular Disorders

Although there are multiple neurologic disease processes that cause ARF, several occur much more commonly in the ICU setting. The end result for most of these processes, such as myasthenia gravis or the Guillain-Barré syndrome, is respiratory muscle weakness (48).

Myasthenia gravis is a disorder of the NMJ, which can present as ARF. The disease is caused by circulating antibodies that target the junctional acetylcholine receptors. The result can be marked inhibition of muscle contraction. Although the extraocular muscles, eyelid levators, and other head and neck musculature are most typically affected, respiratory muscles can fatigue, whereas sensation and reflexes are normal. Weakness and fatigability of the diaphragm and chest wall musculature is most commonly invoked as the etiology of ARF, but bulbar symptoms can be responsible as well. The P_{IMAX} and VC can both be utilized to assess respiratory muscle strength (48). Given the fluctuating weakness and fatigability characterized by this disease, it can be difficult to interpret the P_{IMAX} and VC.

Once the diagnosis of mysthemia gravis is suggested, confirmation should be sought with a "Tension test." Edrophonium hydrochloride (Tensilon®) is a rapid-onset, short-acting cholinesterase inhibitor (Table 4). Myasthenic weakness typically resolves dramatically within one minute of intravenous administration, and improved strength (including P_{IMAX} and VC) will persist for at least 10 minutes after the administration of 5–10 mg. Cholinergic side effects (gastrointestinal hyperactivity, bradycardia, cardiac dysrhythmias, diaphoresis, etc.) can occur. Accordingly, patients should be monitored with ECG, and intubation and resuscitation equipment must be available. Once the diagnosis of myasthenia gravis is made, a neurological consultation should be obtained, and the patient may be started on pyridostigmine, a longer-acting oral anticholinesterase. Definitive therapy may include plasmapharesis, corticosteroids, and a thymectomy. Failure to inspire with normal tidal volume breaths leads to increased areas of atelectasis and $\dot{V}/\dot{Q}$ mismatch, which then results in hypoxemia. If tidal volume breaths are excessively low, then hypercapnea ensues, and the patient will become distressed. In the minority of patients, myasthenic exacerbations will require mechanical ventilatory support. Given that the time course of the exacerbation is uncertain, most patients require intubation. This intervention also provides airway protection for more generalized weakness that may involve upper airway muscles. Intubation, if required, is best accomplished without the use of neuromuscular blocker drugs. These severe exacerbations that require mechanical ventilatory support are most commonly caused by infection. The administration of neuromuscular blockers in the surgical setting cholinergic crisis, and poor compliance with medications represent other situations that further inhibit NMJ function.

Other diseases of the NMJ that can result in ARF are the Eaton-Lambert syndrome and botulism. Both of these entities are rarely seen, compared to myasthenia gravis. As opposed to myasthenia, which usually presents in females in the third decade of life, the Eaton-Lambert syndrome is more commonly seen in elderly men with small cell bronchogenic carcinoma (49). Botulism occurs when the neurotoxin produced by the anaerobic, gram-positive, sporulating bacterium, *Clostridium botulinum*, binds irreversibly to the presynaptic terminal, resulting in inhibition of acetylcholine release. Because the bulbar musculature is affected first, most patients present with diplopia and dysphagia. Most patients' symptoms will progress to descending weakness or frank paralysis of the skeletal musculature that can cause profound respiratory failure. As with myasthenia, patients will often require urgent endotracheal intubation, both for the ability to provide adequate positive pressure ventilation, as well as to provide airway protection in the setting of bulbar muscle weakness. Again, following the MIF and VC will be helpful for the clinician in assessing the progression of disease.

The Guillain-Barré syndrome is a disease of the peripheral neurons, and results from a nonspecific infectious etiology. The disease, which is also referred to as acute postinfectious polyneuropathy, is commonly encountered in the critical care setting. The pathophysiology of the disease involves demyelination of the peripheral and autonomic nervous systems, which is believed to be caused by a hypersensitivity reaction within several weeks of an upper respiratory tract or gastrointestinal tract infection. The disease is characterized by progressive weakness that is most commonly symmetric. Despite the fact that not all patients with the Guillain-Barré develop ARF, patients should be monitored closely. Should there be evidence of declining respiratory (VC) or bulbar muscle strength (poor handling of secretions or a weak cough or gag), patients should be admitted to the ICU for closer monitoring.

Trauma-Related Etiologies of Acute Respiratory Failure
Chest Trauma
Chest Wall Injury

Patients presenting with chest trauma may have multiple etiologies of ARF (also see Volume 2, Chapter 25). Initial failure may be due to hypoventilation, such as that seen with multiple rib fractures. Flail chest is defined as multiple fractures occurring in two or more places, in three or more adjacent ribs, which results in paradoxical chest wall movement. The flail segment results in pendelluft, where ventilation passes between the normal and abnormal thoraces. Disarticulation and fractures of ribs cause low tidal volume breathing and splinting, with resulting hypercapnea (Table 4). Diagnosis may be made by CXR or chest computed tomography (CT) scan. ☞ **Thoracic epidural anesthesia can improve respiratory function in patients with rib injuries.** ☞ Management of chest wall injuries is primarily supportive, with pain management paramount. Epidural anesthesia has been demonstrated to improve respiratory function, and should be considered for patients with flail chest (50). Pain management should be instituted prior to the institution of mechanical ventilation, as this intervention alone may be adequate for treatment. Patients with chest trauma are at risk for other thoracic injuries, including diaphragmatic disruption. A high index of suspicion is required to identify diaphragmatic rupture, which may be hidden by herniation of the liver through the right side of the diaphragm.

Pulmonary Contusion

Pulmonary contusion commonly results from chest trauma. This injury is characterized by hypoxemia, and may result in a clinical picture indistinguishable from ARDS. The pathophysiology of this injury is from alveolar-capillary disruption. Contusion may also occur as a result of intraoperative injury, particularly with lung retraction during thoracic aortic surgery. Diagnosis is made by a constellation of clinical findings, including hypoxemia and the presence of diffuse infiltrates on CXR. The injury may be exacerbated by excessive fluid resuscitation, as the normal safety factors for the prevention of pulmonary edema have been disrupted (51).

Pneumothorax and Hemothorax

Chest trauma may cause disruption of small or large airways or blood vessels, resulting in pnemothorax or hemothorax. Although more common with penetrating trauma, pneumothorax may result from blunt trauma and airway disruption. Both of these conditions may be immediately life-threatening. Mechanical ventilation may also cause barotrauma-induced pneumothorax. Whatever the cause of pneumo or hemothorax, the result is the same: increased pleural pressure that impedes venous return and decreases ventricular filling and ejection fraction. If the injury leads to tension pneumothorax or hemothorax, then cardiovascular collapse will result. To diagnose pneumothorax, CXR and physical examination with auscultation of the chest are essential, and should be components of initial evaluation of the trauma patient. A high index of suspicion is required, especially for unsuspected hypotension, in the setting of mechanical ventilation. CXR of the supine patient may show a deep sulcus sign, representing air in the costophrenic sulcus. In hemothorax, partial or complete opacification of the thorax will be seen. Treatment should not be delayed, and tube thoracostomy should be performed. For small pneumothoraces, observation or catheter aspiration may be sufficient, however, in larger pneumothoraces, hydrothoraces, and particularly hemothoraces, placement of a larger tube is required to assure drainage. These procedures are particularly urgent in a patient receiving mechanical ventilation. For example, Steier et al. (52) showed that delay of treatment for more than 30 minutes, of patients

with pneumothorax from mechanical ventilation, was associated with a mortality rate of greater than 30%. When thoracostomy was done sooner, mortality rate was 7%.

Fluid Overload

Trauma patients are particularly prone to volume overload during resuscitation. One of the most important consequences of fluid overload is hydrostatic pulmonary edema (Table 4). Early placement of a central venous catheter may help guide fluid resuscitation and minimize this complication. PA catheters do not appear to be superior in preventing this complication in normal, young, previously healthy trauma patients (53). Other conditions that predispose trauma patients to pulmonary edema include inflammatory mediator release from shock, and tissue injury from transfusion of blood and blood products. Diagnosis of fluid overload pulmonary edema must be differentiated from ARDS. This will be determined by identifying the presence of left atrial hypertension, usually associated with right atrial hypertension, recognized on the central venous pressure (46). Many patients may have a combination of syndromes, with increased vascular permeability, followed by increased hydrostatic pressure from overresuscitation. Chest radiography usually shows bilateral pulmonary edema, but is not specific for the etiology of the edema (22). Treatment consists of supportive care with oxygen, diuretic administration (only after intravascular volume adequacy is established) and, if necessary, mechanical ventilation. In the setting of renal failure, emergent hemodialysis may be required.

Fat Embolism

Fat embolism syndrome may cause respiratory failure in trauma and orthopedic patients. It is clinically indistinguishable from ARDS. This syndrome is most commonly associated with long bone and pelvic fractures, where fat from the bone marrow enters the circulation, causing inflammatory injury to the lung and a noncardiogenic pulmonary edema picture (Table 4). The reaction may be triggered by thromboplastin with complement and coagulation system activation, and activation of leukocytes. The embolization is microscopic and difficult to diagnose; essentially a diagnosis of exclusion. Clinical manifestations include neurologic changes, hypoxemia and, rarely, right heart failure. Skin manifestations include petechiae, found in 50% to 60% of patients. Treatment includes routine care of patients with ARDS, with the caveat that the long bone fractures must be stabilized surgically. Steroids after the onset of the syndrome are controversial, with at least one study showing efficacy of methylprednisolone 7.5 mg/kg/6 hrs for 12 doses for prevention, but not treatment (54).

Near-Drowning

Near-drowning (Volume 1, Chapter 35) is often a catastrophic event that is associated with high morbidity (i.e., anoxic encephalopathy) and mortality. Most victims do not aspirate large quantities of water, and aspirated water is usually reabsorbed rapidly. Most complications occur as a result of hypoxia and delayed-onset pulmonary edema. Associated pathology includes spinal cord injury, myocardial infarction, and seizures. Patients may develop late-onset cerebral edema as well. Seawater drowning results in the introduction of hypertonic water into the alveolar space, where it draws additional liquid across the alveolar epithelium from the capillaries. Cardiac output may be impeded from the increase in pulmonary vascular resistance caused by

Table 5 Orlowski Score

Points	Factor
1	Age 3 or older
1	Submersion time greater than 5 min
1	No resuscitation attempts for at least 10 min after rescue
1	Coma on admission to emergency department
1	Arterial blood pH ≤ 7.10

Note: One point is given for each category, and score ≤ 3 is associated with 90% intact recovery; if >3, then 5% intact recovery.

alveolar compression. Fresh water does not draw additional water into the alveolar space, but the hypotonic liquid denatures surfactant and other alveolar proteins, causing atelectasis, shunting, and hypoxemia. The ultimate clinical syndrome that results is similar, whether the drowning is in fresh or seawater.

Initial resuscitation is no different than that of any trauma patient, with establishment of an airway and supplemental oxygen administration paramount. In awake, cooperative patients, NIPPV may be effective. Prognostication of outcome is reflected by the Orlowski score (Table 5) (55). An Orlowski score ≤ 3 is associated with a 90% chance of recovery (55).

Burns
Burn injury is a complex form of trauma that may result in ARF due to inhalation injury or due to tissue destruction and fluid third space from the thermal injury itself (Table 4). Burn injury is covered in great detail in Volume 1, Chapter 34. The severity of inhalation injury depends on both the type and concentration of inhaled material, and where they are deposited in the lungs. Exposure to smoke in an enclosed space may result in lung injury, with severity ranging from mild to fatal. Thermal injury is usually limited to the upper airway, as the alveolar liquid layer and high blood flow rapidly dissipate high temperatures. Both thermal injury and particles may initiate an inflammatory process that results in ARDS. Full manifestation of the severity of injury may not be evident for hours, so these patients require close observation and ICU admission. Clinical presentation includes wheezing, stridor, dyspnea, and tachypnea. Physical examination of the oropharynx and nares may reveal burns or soot. Whenever there is suspicion of an inhalational injury, patients should have their airways evaluated with fiberoptic bronchoscopy, and endotracheal intubation should be undertaken immediately, before swelling causes asphyxiation. Carboxyhemoglobin levels can be measured, but are not necessarily prognostic. Treatment is supportive, with the same considerations as for those patients with ARDS. Steroids should be avoided initially, as no clinical trials have demonstrated clear efficacy, and they may increase infectious complications. Similarly, empiric antibiotic therapy has no demonstrated efficacy.

Other Injuries Promoting or Worsening Acute Respiratory Failure
Head Injury
Patients with traumatic head injury are at high risk for respiratory failure (Volume 1, Chapter 23 and Volume 2, Chapter 12). These patients may develop respiratory failure as a result of multiple factors, including aspiration pneumonitis, neurogenic pulmonary edema, or increased vascular permeability, from the

release of vasoactive substances from the injured brain; this is more common in the setting of subarachnoid hemorrhage (Table 4). Patients with head injury may also develop respiratory failure from altered mental status, with resulting hypercapnea. Neurogenic pulmonary edema is a complex phenomenon, which results from specific brainstem injuries, and likely is caused by a combination of increased vascular permeability and elevated pulmonary hydrostatic pressures (56). Patients with head injury often require endotracheal intubation for airway protection, and initially have no primary cause of respiratory failure, but are at particularly high risk of ventilator-associated pneumonia (57).

Renal Failure
Renal failure may contribute to ARF through multiple routes (Volume 2, Chapter 41). Most commonly, acute renal failure leads to fluid overload that causes hydrostatic pulmonary edema (Table 4). Additionally, failure to clear acid results in acidemia, creating a large minute ventilation burden, and retained products of metabolism lead to leaky capillaries (noncardiogenic pulmonary edema). Critically ill patients may not be able to sustain the elevated minute ventilation required to compensate for the metabolic acidosis, and respiratory failure results. Alkalinization of the blood may be appropriate in the setting of a renal tubular acidosis, where there is bicarbonate loss into the urine. Other metabolic functions of the kidney, including failure of toxin clearance, may contribute to altered mental status and subsequent ARF. Electrolyte abnormalities may contribute to respiratory muscle weakness, and should be corrected to optimize respiratory function. A recent study of critically ill patients with acute renal failure suggests that intensive hemodialysis can decrease multiple organ failure and mortality (58).

Pancreatitis
Pancreatic injury and pancreatitis create a systemic inflammatory response similar to sepsis syndrome, which often results in ALI (Volume 2, Chapter 39). Release of cytokines and proteases into the circulation injures endothelial cells, causing increased pulmonary vascular permeability and pulmonary edema. The consequences of these abnormalities are not significantly different from the consequences of severe sepsis syndrome. ARDS appears commonly in patients with pancreatitis, and usually requires mechanical ventilation (59). Electrolyte abnormalities and hyperglycemia may contribute to the ARF seen with acute pancreatitis.

Hepatic Injury
Traumatic liver injury shock and drug intoxications may result in fulminant hepatic failure, leading to multiple organ dysfunction and ARF (Volume 2, Chapter 36). Release of vasoactive substances into the circulation creates a syndrome similar to that seen with sepsis, but with higher mortality. Hypoxemia may be seen due to intrahepatic and intrapulmonary shunting, and can be refractory (Table 4).

The hepatopulmonary syndrome is characterized by the clinical triad of advanced chronic liver disease, pulmonary vascular dilatations, and reduced arterial oxygenation (i.e., increased A-a gradient) in the absence of intrinsic cardiopulmonary disease. This syndrome is common in patients with liver cirrhosis or portal hypertension (60). The pathophysiology includes arteriovenous shunting in the lung, predominantly in the bases, and are equivalent to "spider angiomata" in the lung. Echocardiography will reveal a positive bubble study with intravenous agitated saline (61).

Increasing the FIO$_2$ improves oxygenation, but because shunting is not the only problem, there is also a combination of $\dot{V}/\dot{Q}$ mismatching and diffusion abnormalities.

Although permanent cure has only been achieved following liver transplantation, the role of nitric oxide (NO) was suggested in 2002, when methylene blue was found to transiently improve oxygenation in patients with hepatopulmonary syndrome (62). Recently, the role of TNF-α has been implicated, with the demonstration that pentoxifillin improves oxygenation (63). The interactions of NO, endothelin, and TNF-α have been summarized in a recent editorial by Dinh-Xuan and Naeije (64). ARDS develops in approximately 30% of these patients, and the hepatopulmonary syndrome is associated with sepsis.

COMMUNITY-ACQUIRED PNEUMONIAS CAUSING ACUTE RESPIRATORY FAILURE

Patients admitted to the ICU frequently have pre-existing respiratory infections (65). Because community-acquired pneumonia (CAP) may progress to ARF, recognition and appropriate treatment of this entity is essential. Many trauma patients will have signs and symptoms of CAP prior to their traumatic injuries, so CAP must be included in the differential diagnosis of ARF in the trauma patient. The emergence of antibiotic resistance makes careful analysis and antibiotic selection more important than ever. The recommendations in this chapter are consistent with those recommended by the American Thoracic Society for both community-acquired pneumonias (66) and hospital-acquired pneumonias (67).

Chronic illness is the largest single risk factor for CAP. Diseases of the respiratory tract, especially COPD, predispose patients to pneumonia. Other coexisting illnesses, which should raise the index of suspicion for CAP, include diabetes, renal failure, malignancy, AIDS, and chronic cardiac disease. Use of either alcohol or tobacco similarly inhibits defense mechanisms and predisposes to CAP.

Diagnosis of CAP relies on the physical examination, CXR, Gram stain sputum culture, and blood count. Patients requiring ICU admission should also have an arterial blood gas and two sets of blood cultures obtained. The presence of a number of factors predict those patients with increased risk of death: coexisting illness, shock, WBC $<4 \times 10^9$/L or $>30 \times 10^9$/L, coexisting acute renal failure, anemia, pH <7.35. These factors should be taken into consideration when determining if the patient requires ICU admission. Therapy should initially be empiric and broad, with antibiotic coverage narrowed once the organism and sensitivities are known. As in nosocomial infections, current knowledge of the community antibiogram should guide antibiotic selection (Table 6).

Bacterial Pneumonias (Community Acquired)
Streptococcus pneumoniae *(Pneumococcus)*
Pneumococcus (*Streptococcus pneumoniae*) is the most commonly identified pathogen, comprising 30% to 60% of isolates in patients requiring hospitalization. The Centers for Disease Control (CDC) estimates that *S. pneumoniae* causes 40,000 deaths and 500,000 cases of pneumonia annually in the United States (68). Pneumococcal pneumonia is characterized by high fever, rigors, productive cough, dyspnea, tachypnea, pleural pain, and meningitis. *S. pneumoniae* causes approxi-

mately 20% of all bacterial meningitis, and bacteremia occurs in 25% to 30% of patients with pneumococcal pneumonia. When bacteremia occurs, it is associated with higher mortality. Diagnosis is made by Gram stain, where the organisms appear as gram-positive, lancet-shaped diplococci. Definitive identification must be made either by bacterial culture or counter immunoelectropheresis. Antibiotic sensitivities should be obtained, as resistance is common. Treatment of sensitive *S. pneumoniae* is with penicillin, ampicillin, or amoxicillin. However, the increasing prevalence of resistant organisms (up to 40% of isolates are resistant) mandates that empiric therapy for high-risk patients admitted to the ICU include an intravenous b-lactam *plus* an intravenous macrolide (e.g., azithromycin), or an antipneumococcal fluoroquinolone alone. Lower risk patients can be treated with either azithromycin or an antipneumococcal fluoroquinolone. Patients who have undergone splenectomy are at particularly high risk of infection with this organism, and must be immunized prior to discharge.

Hemophilus influenzae
Hemophilus influenzae is most commonly present as the type b serotype (Hib). Hib is responsible for 3% to 10% of all CAP. Children and infants are at particulary high risk for infection with Hib, which usually presents with coryza and pleural effusions; and most adults present with bronchopneumonia. Presumptive diagnosis is made with Gram stain, which shows small, gram-negative coccobacilli, and definitive diagnosis by culture. About 30% of *H. influenzae* strains produce β-lactamase, and are resistant to ampicillin. Thus, preferred treatment is trimethoprim-sulfamethoxazole. Fluoroquinolones and azithromycin are also active.

Staphylococcus aureus
Staphylococcus aureus accounts for about 2% of CAP. High-risk groups include the elderly, intravenous drug users, and those with preceding viral infections. *S. aureus* pneumonia is characterized by signs and symptoms similar to those already described for pneumococcal pneumonia. *S. aureus* is particularly prone to causing abscesses and infections on prosthetic devices. Diagnosis is made by examination of sputum, blood cultures, or empyema fluid, which reveals gram-positive cocci. Differentiation from *S. epidermidis* and *S. saprophyticus* is made by the coagulase test. *S. aureus* produces a number of toxins, including toxic shock syndrome toxin, epidermolysin, and enterotoxin, all of which may cause clinically important, and often lethal, clinical syndromes. The clinical course of patients with *S. aureus* is also characterized by empyema formation, which requires tube thoracostomy. This organism is particularly adept at developing antibiotic resistance, with methicillin-resistant *S. aureus* increasingly present in the community. Treatment of *S. aureus* pneumonia in patients requiring ICU admission consists of an intravenous β-lactam (cefotaxime or ceftriaxone), *plus* either an intravenous macrolide (azithromycin) or intravenous fluoroquinolone. If methicillin resistance is present, the organism should be considered resistant to all β-lactam antibiotics, and should be treated with vancomycin. Linezolid, although only bacteriostatic, is effective against methacillin-resistant *S. aureus*, and in two double-blind studies, showed lower mortality than vancomycin for VAP (69). The 2005 American Thoracic Society/Infectious Disease Society of America guidelines for hospital-acquired pneumonias suggest it may be preferred, due to its higher penetration of epithelial lining fluid (67). In the case of vancomycin-resistant *S. aureus* (VRSA) pneumonia, Linazolid is clearly the drug of

Table 6 Organisms that Cause Acute Respiratory Failure Requiring Ventilatory Support

Type	Organism (Gram stain)	Presentation, diagnostic factors, other comments	Drug treatment
CAP	*Streptococcus pneumoniae*, aka: Pneumoccus (Gm Pos diplococcus—lancet shaped)	S&S: Fever, rigors, coughs, dyspnea, (meningitis may occur): increased risk following splenectomy. Causes 30–60% of CAP	Ampicillin (if sensitive), resistant organisms require azithromycin, or fluoroquinolone
CAP	*Staphylococcus aureus* (Gm Pos cocci—grapelike clusters)	S&S: Similar to pneumococcus, propensity to form abscesses and infect prosthetic devices. Common in IVDA.	Ancef or ceftriaxone (if sensitive). For MRSA, vancomycin is required[a]
CAP	*Hemophilus influenzae* (Gm Neg coccobacilli)	Presenting S&S: (adults) bronchopneumonia, (kids) coryza and pleural effusions	TMP-SMX or ciprofloxacin
CAP	*Klebsiella penumoniae* (Gm Neg bacilli)	Presenting S&S: Bronchopneumonia, ↑ risk in alcoholics and elderly. "Current jelly" sputum with Gm Neg bacilli	Ceftriaxone, extended spectrum penicillin[b], ciprofloxacin
CAP/NOS	*Acinetobacter* (Gm Neg bacilli)	S&S similar to *Klebsiella*, common nosocomial pneumonia source. Increasingly resistant organisms (i.e., ESBLs)	Ceftriaxone, extended spectrum penicillin[b], ciprofloxacin[c]
NOS	*Pseudomonas aeruginosa* (Gm Neg rods)	Fever, chills dyspnea, productive cough, purulent sputum, CXR diffuse patchy infiltrates, common in burn patients. Also, increasing ESBLs	Ceftazidime[d] and ciprofloxacin or ceftriaxone, antipseudomonal penicillin[b], and aminoglycoside[c]
NOS	*Enterobacter* spp. (Gm Neg rods)	Can present like *Pseudomonas*, or have primarily tracheo-bronchitis. Increasingly resistant organism (i.e., ESBLs)	Ceftriaxone and ciprofloxacin[c]
NOS	*Serratia marcasens* (Gm Neg bacilli)	Increased risk in immunocompromised, and following prolonged IV catheterization. Increasing ESBLs	Ceftriaxone or ciprofloxacin[c]
ASP	All above organisms plus mouth anaerobes	Fever, cough, and purulent sputum. Classic CXR: infiltrate superior segments of lower lobes (particularly right)	Acute aspiration may not need Rx. However, fever and purulent sputum, rx: ciprofloxacin and clindamycin
ATYP	*Mycoplasma pneumoniae* (scant bacteria on Gram stain)	Interstitial pneumonia, bronchitis, culture takes 10 days. Diagnosis by culture. Treatment only necessary if severe	Erythromycin, tetracycline, or azithromycin
ATYP	*Legionella penumophylia* (scant bacteria on Gram stain)	Headache, fevers, malaise, patchy alveolar infiltrates. Diagnosis by serology or urine antigen, or DFA	Erythromycin ↑ dose 2–3 wk, or azithromycin for 2–3 wk
ATYP	*Chlamydia pneumoniae* (scant bacteria on Gram stain)	Fever, malaise, pharyngitis, pneumonia Diagnosis requires embryonic cell culture or DFA	Erythromycin or tetracycline 3–4 wk
ATYP	Q-fever *Coxiella burnettii* (scant bacteria on Gram stain)	Exposure to farm animals (especially sheep). Fever, chills, HA, myalgias. Diagnosis is by blood culture or serology	Tetracycline, doxycycline
ATYP	Pneumocystis Carinii (scant bacteria on Gram stain)	Fever, nonproductive cough, interstitial diffuse infiltrates on CXR immunocompromised host (especially cell mediated). Diagnosis by sputum silver stain	TMP-sulfa, pentamidine
VIRAL	Influenza A and B, RSV, CMV, VZV (scant bacteria on Gram stain)	Low WBC, few bacteria on sputum, need viral cultures or serology for diagnosis—herpetic tracheobronchitis may be suggested by bronchoscopic appearance—confirmed with viral culture	Acyclovir for—herpes tracheobronchitis or varicella, Ganciclovir for CMV, intravenous IgG and Interferon may help in some
FUNGI	Cryptococcus (massive, round, Gm Pos)	Almost never causes ARF in immunocompetent individuals. AIDS patients may develop ARF. Dx BAL or serology: cryptococcal polysaccharide capsular antigen	Fluconazole (mild disease), For advanced disease: ampho B or voriconazole

(Continued)

Table 6 Organisms that Cause Acute Respiratory Failure Requiring Ventilatory Support (*Continued*)

Type	Organism (Gram stain)	Presentation, diagnostic factors, other comments	Drug treatment
FUNGI	Coccidioidiomycosis (scant bacteria on Gram stain)	Fever, cough (productive, sometimes blood) pleuritis—CXR may show cavitary lesion. Hx—contact with fossils or digging in San Joaquin Valley. Diagnosis by serology	Fluconazole (mild disease), For advanced disease: ampho B or voriconazole
FUNGI	Histoplasmosis (scant bacteria on Gram stain)	S&S S/A Cocci, but Hx exposure to Mississippi River Valley. Diagnosis by serology and by urine antigens (may have retinal involvement)	Fluconazole (mild disease), For advanced disease: ampho B or voriconazole
FUNGI	Blastomycosis (scant bacteria on Gram stain)	S&S S/A Cocci, but Hx exposure to Mississippi or Ohio River Valleys	Fluconazole (mild disease), For advanced disease: ampho B or voriconazole
FUNGI	Aspergillosis (scant bacteria on Gram stain)	Fever, cough, usually fatal respiratory failure, ↑ risk in immunocompromised (s/p BMTxP)	Ampho B or voriconazole or caspofungin
TB	Mycobacterium (acid-fast bacilli) Ziel Neilson Stain (MTD) auramine	↑ risk with foreign birth on travel, immuno-compromised heatlth (epidemic in HIV infected patients). Recent PCR (MTD) test allows more rapid diagnosis	Multiple drug resistance increasing (see Volume 2, Chapter 53 and consult ID)
WMD	Anthrax aka *Bacillis anthracis* (very large Gm Pos Rods) Large cells with square ends	Inhalational anthrax almost entirely due to weaponized preparation, or occupational exposure, fever, chills, sweats, dyspnea, ↑ WBC, ↑ liver transaminases	Ciprofloxacin or doxycycline

Note: *Candida* is a cause of disseminated disease, but very rarely causes acute respiratory failure.
Also note: Daptomycin is contraindicated in pneumonia. It is inactivated by surfactant. Linezolid should be used for vancomycin resistant organisms causing pneumonia.
[a]Linezolid, though only bactereostatic, is effective against MRSA, and has greater epithelial lining penetration than vancomycin.
[b]Extended spectrum (antipseudomaonal) penicillins include pipercillin and mezlocillin.
[c]Extended spectrum beta lactamases (ESBLs) are increasingly prevelant, and require one of the two following carbapenems: imipenem or meropenem (ertapenem lacks activity against *Pseudomonas* or *Acinetobacter*).
[d]Although ceftazidime is effective against all of the gram-negative organisms, we recommending reserving it for known pseudomonal infections.
Abbreviations: Ampho B, Amphotericin B; ATYP, atypical pneumonia; CAP, community-acquired pneumonia; DFA, direct fluorescent antibody; ESBLs, extended spectrum beta lactamases; FUNGAL, fungal pneumonia; Gm Neg, gram-negative organism; Gm Pos, gram-positive organism; IVDA, intravenous drug abuse; NOS, nosocomial pneumonia; MRSA, methacillin resistant staph aureus; TB, tuberculosis; WMD, weapons of mass destruction; S&S, signs and symptoms.

choice. Daptomycin is contraindicated in the treatment of pneumonia. Although daptomycin has excellent cidal effects against VRSA, in other tissues, it is inactivated by surfactant. In addition to Linazolid, Tigecycline (a derivative of tetracycline) has activity against VRSA. Tigecycline has no activity against *Pseudomonas*, but has recently (June 2005) been approved by the FDA for skin structure infections, and will likely become useful in the treatment of resistant nonpseudamonal pneumonia.

Klebsiella pneumoniae

Klebsiella pneumonia is the most important community-acquired gram-negative pathogen. Mortality can be as high as 50%, even with antibiotic treatment. Patients with CAP due to *Klebsiella pneumoniae* typically present with bronchopneumonia. This organism is more frequently associated with the elderly, alcohol use, nosocomial pneumonia, and neutropenic patients. Diagnosis is made by the presence of "currant jelly" sputum, which on Gram stain shows numerous gram-negative bacilli. False-positive cultures due to other organisms that colonize the airways are common. For definitive diagnosis, culture from other sources, such as blood or pleural fluid, should be obtained.

Treatment consists of a cephalosporin (e.g., ceftriaxone), antipseudomonal penicillin, or fluoroquinolone. Each of these drugs can be given alone, or in combination with an aminoglycoside. Aminoglycosides should not be used alone. Another class of antibiotics that can be combined with an aminoglycoside to combat *K. pneumoniae* is the monobactams (e.g., aztreonam).

Acinetobacter

Acinetobacter is a gram-negative bacillus, which tends to cause respiratory disease in patients with diminished host defense. Although more commonly associated with nosocomial pneumonias, it is also a significant community-acquired pathogen, and thus listed here. The clinical presentation is similar to that described for *K. pneumoniae*. Diagnosis is, similarly, difficult because of the presence of colonizing organisms. Attempts should be made to isolate the organism from the blood or other fluids. Treatment of *Acinetobacter* pneumonia consists of a cephalosporin (e.g., ceftriaxone), antipseudomonal penicillin, or fluoroquinolone. Each of these drugs can be given alone, or in combination with an aminoglycoside. Aminoglycosides should not be used alone. Other drugs that can be combined with an aminoglycoside are a monobactam. β-lactams are frequently associated with treatment failure, or relapse, when used against *Acinetobacter*. Additionally, a marked increase in drug resistance due to extended spectrum beta lactamases (ESBLs), produced by gram-negative pathogens, has begun to plague many hospitals and ICUs, and are particularly expressed in *Acinetobacter, Enterobacter* spp., *Serratia marcasens*, and *Pseudomonas* spp. When ESBLs are causative of pneumonia, one of the two following carbapenems should be used: imipenem or meropenem (ertapenem lacks activity against *Pseudomonas* and *Acinetobacter*).

Aspiration Pneumonitis Coinciding with Hospital Admission

Patients with aspiration pneumonitis from community-acquired organisms present with a bacterial infection of the lower airways. The most common pathogens are anaerobic bacteria that normally colonize the oropharynx. Unlike aspiration pneumonia from chemical pneumonitis, bacterial infection is more insidious. Clinical presentation is with fever, cough, and purulent sputum. CXR most commonly shows infiltration in the superior segments of lower lobes, which drain dependently (posterior) in supine patients. This is particularly common on the right, possibly due to the straighter right mainstem bronchus. Posterior segments of upper lobes may also be involved, depending on the patient's position at the time of aspiration. Anaerobic infection may lead to abscess formation or empyema, which may be visible on the CXR. Diagnosis may be difficult, as expectorated sputum will be contaminated with upper airway flora. The preferred specimen source is a transtracheal aspirate (in nonintubated patients), and BAL or protected bronchoscopic specimen in intubated patients. Additionally, pleural fluid (in presence of effusion/empyema) infections frequently include multiple organisms, particularly *S. aureus*, in addition to mouth anaerobes. For the anaerobic infection, clindamycin is usually effective. For sicker patients, an aminoglycoside or fluoroquinolone, combined with a third-generation cephalosporin or extended-spectrum penicillin is effective.

Atypical Pneumonias (Community Acquired)
Mycoplasma pneumoniae

Mycoplasma infection is the most common cause of CAP in the younger age group from 5 to 35, and is often spread in epidemic form. This organism has the ability to adhere to, and destroy, ciliated epithelial cells. This characteristic results in a clinical syndrome of interstitial pneumonitis, bronchitis, and bronchiolitis. Patients initially present with symptoms of influenza, with pharyngitis, cough, and malaise. Sputum may be mucopurulent or blood-tinged. Disease progresses gradually, and most patients recover uneventfully; however, some may progress to respiratory failure. Diagnosis is difficult, as isolation from sputum culture may take up to 10 days. Gram stain shows few bacteria. Chest X ray is characterized by a patchy, infiltrative pattern, rather than dense consolidation. Treatment is often not required, and if deemed necessary, should be with erythromycin, tetracycline, or azithromycin.

Legionella pneumophila

Pneumonia from *Legionella pneumophila* is normally a limited flu-like illness. Legionnaires' disease is the more commonly recognized form, and is characterized by a more severe pneumonia, and occasionally, soft-tissue infections. Legionnaires' disease accounts for approximately 5% of CAPs that lead to hospitalization. Patients at risk for this disorder include those that smoke, use alcohol, and are immunosuppressed, especially with steroids. There is a greater prevalence in males than females. Signs and symptoms of Legionnaires'disease include headache, fever, and myalgias initially, which then progress to a nonproductive cough and high fever. CXR is notable for patchy lobar or alveolar infiltrates. Pleural effusions and abscesses may be seen. Diagnosis may be obtained by serology, urine antigen measurement, or direct fluorescent antibody (DFA) staining. Treatment consists of high-dose erythromycin (1 g IV every 6 hours). Alternatives include a fluoroquinolone or azithromycin. Treatment should be continued for two to three weeks because of the risk of relapse. In spite of treatment, mortality may be as high as 15%, especially in immunosuppressed patients (80).

Chlamydia pneumoniae

Chlamydia pneumoniae can be isolated in 5% to 10% of patients with CAP. Clinical presentation of *C. pneumoniae* pneumonia is similar to other atypical pneumonias, particularly that of *M. pneumoniae*. Patients present with fever, malaise, pharyngitis, bronchitis, and variably productive sputum. Risk factors are not known, except for advanced age. Diagnosis of *C. pneumoniae* pneumonia is difficult, as it requires embryonic cell culture or DFA. More often, diagnosis is made clinically in a patient who has not responded to β-lactam antibiotics. Treatment should be with tetracycline or erythromycin, and continued for two to three weeks.

Q-Fever

Q-fever is the acute illness caused by *Coxiella burnettii*. This organism is normally associated with farm animals, particularly sheep, and an exposure history is essential. Almost all cases are those of occupational exposure, which occurs by inhalation. Signs and symptoms include high fever, chills, headache, and myalgias. Nonproductive cough is variably present. Many patients also develop hepatitis. Lobar pneumonia may occur, and the chest radiographic pattern is similar to other atypical pneumonias. Diagnosis must be made by clinical history of exposure, and may also be documented by blood culture or serology. Treatment is with tetracycline, doxycycline, or chloramphenicol (third tier due to toxicity).

Pneumocystis carinii

Pneumonia due to *P. carinii* is most frequently associated with immunocompromised patients, especially those with defects in cell-mediated immunity, including AIDS. Susceptibility to *P. carinii* pneumonia in AIDS patients is dependent on their T-cell function, which becomes inadequate when CD4 cells are below 150–200/μL. Symptoms of *P. carinii* pneumonia include dyspnea, fever, and nonproductive cough. CXR may show diffuse infiltrates, but is not reliable. Patients may be profoundly hypoxemic, causing dyspnea. Diagnosis is made with sputum silver staining, which may be induced or obtained bronchoscopically. Bronchoscopy is much more reliable for diagnosis, and bronchoalveolar lavage specimens should be obtained in intubated patients and considered in others that can tolerate the procedure. Treatment consists of trimethoprim-sulfamethoxazole at 20 mg/kg/day, IV for 21 days. In patients with severe hypoxemia, corticosteroids have been demonstrated to decrease hypoxemia and duration of mechanical ventilation (70). Noninfected AIDS patients with CD4 counts <200/mm^3 should receive prophylaxis with trimethoprim-sulfamethoxazole.

Common Viral Pneumonias

Influenza A and B: In adults, the most common viral pneumonias result from influenza infection. In elderly or debilitated patients, parainfluenza, respiratory syncitial virus, cytomegalovirus (CMV), and varicella-zoster may be pathogens. The vast majority of these infections are self-limited, but patients with inadequate immune responses may develop a full-blown pneumonia. Most of these infections start as bronchitis or bronchiolitis, and then progress to pneumonia. Herpes tracheo bronchitis is commonly seen in critically ill trauma patients. Clinical diagnosis is suggested by hemorrhagic bronchial lesions seen during bronchoscopy. Viral cultures confirm the diagnosis, but acyclovir therapy can be started immediately after seeing the lesions, and continued (or stopped) on the basis of cultures.

Identification of viral pneumonia is important, as many patients will progress to a bacterial pneumonia, and present with constitutive symptoms including headache, malaise, and myalgias. CXR usually shows an interstitial pattern, rather than focal infiltrates. Laboratory findings often include a low WBC count. Diagnosis may be difficult, with sputum examination showing few bacteria. Demonstration of a rash, in conjuction with the respiratory illness, may be helpful. Only serologies or viral culture can establish a definite diagnosis. Treatment is usually supportive, but acyclovir for herpes or varicella infections, ganciclovir for CMV infections, or intravenous immune globulin have been used.

Severe Acute Respiratory Syndrome

Severe acute respiratory syndrome (SARS) is an acute form of viral respiratory illness that became recognized as a global infectious disease threat in March 2003, when the World Health Organization was called in to help evaluate and contain the epidemic. First appearing in Foshan, in the Guangdong province of southern China in November 2002, SARS became the first new serious contagious illness to emerge in the 21st century, with almost 800 people killed, and nearly 8100 suffering serious illness in 2003 alone. Outbreaks in 30 countries threw public health systems into chaos and disrupted international travel (71).

The spread of SARS illustrates how quickly infection can proliferate in the modern, mobile, global economy. Conversely, the rapid discovery of the infectious agent, as well as the containment of the epidemic and elucidation of the pathophysiologic patterns associated with SARS, illustrates the sophistication of modern epidemiological and infectious disease research capabilities (72). Indeed, in April 2003 (approximately one month after the epidemic was identified), Peiris et al. (73) had isolated the SARS-associated coronavirus (SARS-CoV). In less than one month after that, Marra et al. (74) had already sequenced the SARS-CoV genome. In November 2003, one year after the initial outbreak, Li et al. (75) had discovered the critical role of the angiotensin-converting enzyme 2 (ACE2) as a functional receptor for the SARS-CoV. The subsequent research into the role of the ACE2 receptor (and its possible role in ARF of other etiologies) is discussed in the "Eye to the Future" section (76,77). Here, the clinical characteristics of SARS will be briefly reviewed.

Etiology

SARS is caused by a previously unrecognized coronavirus, called (SARS-CoV) (72). It is believed that the SARS-CoV jumped species from a palm civet to humans and exploited opportunities provided by crowded living conditions and the warm, humid climate in southern China, evolving into a virus that is now readily transmissible between humans via respiratory secretion droplets. Hospitals and international travel provided the "amplifiers" that facilitated the initially local outbreak to rapidly achieve global dimensions (72).

Epidemiology

The primary method of SARS infection is by close person-to-person contact. SARS-CoV is transmitted most readily by respiratory droplets. When respiratory secretions from the cough or sneeze of an infected person are propelled a short distance (generally up to three feet) through the air, droplets are deposited on the mucous membranes of the mouth, nose, or eyes of nearby persons. The virus can also spread when a person touches a surface or object contaminated with infectious droplets, and then touches his or her mouth, nose, or eye(s). In addition, it is possible that SARS-CoV might be spread more broadly through the air (airborne spread) (72).

Signs and Symptoms

The illness usually begins with a high fever (>38.0°C). The fever is sometimes associated with chills or other symptoms, including headache, malaise, and body aches. Some people also experience mild respiratory symptoms at the outset. However, in contrast to most respiratory viruses, minimal upper respiratory symptoms are initially present following SARS-CoV infection. Diarrhea is seen in 10% to 20% of patients. After two to seven days, SARS patients may develop a dry, nonproductive cough that usually progresses to a viral pneumonia, with variable degrees of right-to-left transpulmonary shunt. In 10% to 20% of patients, mechanical ventilation is required.

Incubation Period and Contagious Duration

The SARS-CoV has a long incubation period for a respiratory virus: typically four to seven days and, occasionally, as long as 14 days. The illness has a relatively insidious onset, upper respiratory tract symptoms are uncommon, and lower respiratory tract symptoms worsen slowly, but steadily, during the first 10 to 15 days (78). Persons with SARS are most likely to be contagious only when they have symptoms, such as fever or cough. Patients are most contagious during the second week of illness, when their viral loads and respiratory symptoms are most severe. However, as a precaution against spreading the disease, the CDC recommends that persons with SARS limit their interactions outside of the home for an additional 10 days after the fever has dissipated and their respiratory symptoms have resolved.

Pathology and Laboratory Testing

On gross examination, the typical lung infected with SARS virus will demonstrate diffuse hemorrhage on the lung surface (79). Several laboratory tests can now be used to detect SARS-CoV. A reverse-transcription polymerase chain reaction test can detect SARS-CoV in clinical specimens such as blood, stool, and nasal secretions. Serologic testing also can be performed to detect SARS-CoV antibodies, produced after infection. Finally, viral culture has been used to detect SARS-CoV.

Prognosis and Treatment

The prognosis of this infection is fair, provided that the patient is in good health and within the younger age group. But death occurs in 3% to 12% of cases. A poorer prognosis is found in those with coexisting conditions such as diabetes mellitus, renal failure, and other chronic medical conditions.

Treatment remains mainly supportive. All patients suspected of SARS infection should be admitted to the hospital, and isolated to prevent further spread of disease. The CDC recommends that patients with SARS receive the same treatment that would be used for a patient with any serious community-acquired atypical pneumonia (e.g., macrolide antibiotic), as this condition is commonly confused with SARS infection. SARS-CoV is being tested against various antiviral drugs; so far no specific antiviral remedy has been identified. Riboviron has specifically been found to be noneffective (72). Monoclonal antibodies from memory B-cells have recently been shown to neutralize SARS-CoV, but research is ongoing (72).

Fungal Pneumonias

Fungal pneumonia may be primary, or may result from superinfection of a pre-existing bacterial or viral infection. These pneumonias are seen primarily in immunocompromised hosts, but patients on suppressive antibacterial therapy are at risk as well. These infections may be complicated by hypersensitivity pneumonitis and the formation of cavitary lesions. There are geographic considerations in fungal pneumonias; *Coccidioides immitis* causes coccidiomycosis, primarily in the Southwest of the United States and the central valley of California.

Coccidioidiomycosis

Infection with *C. immitis* is endemic to the western United States. Infection occurs with inhalation of spores, which transform into spherules at body temperature. Although usually self-limited, impaired hosts may develop invasive pneumonia. Patients develop a granulomatous pneumonia characterized by fever, pleuritis, cough, and production of sputum, which may be bloody. Cavitary lesions may form, which can be life-threatening if they erode into the pulmonary vasculature. Diagnosis of coccidiomycosis is made by culture of sputum or pleural fluid. Occasionally, the spherules can be seen with staining. Complement fixation or immunoassay testing may also demonstrate elevated titers. Treatment choice depends on the severity of infection. For milder infections, fluconazole or itraconazole are adequate, but in invasive infections, amphotericin, posiconazole, voriconazole, or caspofungin should be administered (81). In patients with concomitant meningitis, intrathecal therapy may be required.

Histoplasmosis

Infection with *Histoplasma capsulatum* occurs globally, and in the United States, most frequently is seen in the Mississippi River Valley. *H. capsulatum* occurs naturally as a mold, but when inhaled and warmed to body temperature, transforms into yeast cells. Patients with chronic exposure, and immunocompromised hosts are those at highest risk of infection. Acute primary histoplasmosis is characterized by fever, cough, and malaise, and may cause acute pneumonia.

Progression of infection may result in disseminated infection, and in the lung may cause cavitary lesions. Diagnosis may be made by culture of sputum or biopsy samples, and occasionally, staining of the blood buffy coat will demonstrate organisms. Acute primary infection is usually self-limited, but invasive infection should be treated with amphotericin or voriconazole (82).

Aspergillosis

Aspergillus sp. are ubiquitous molds that become pathogenic in immunocompromised hosts. Exposure occurs by inhalation of conidia, and invasion may occur in the setting of immunosuppression. Bone marrow transplant patients, in particular, are susceptible to invasive infections, which may be life-threatening. Symptoms range from mild fever and cough, to fatal, progressive respiratory failure. Diagnosis is complicated by the fact that these organisms are ubiquitous, so the presence of *Aspergillus* sp. in sputum or other cultures may merely represent environmental contamination. Bronchial washings are preferred over sputum, and tissue diagnosis may be required. Because of the risk of biopsy in mechanically ventilated patients, empiric therapy may be required in patients with suspected infection. Treatment is with amphotericin B, and pulmonary infection may be more effectively treated using liposome-encapsulated amphotericin. Voriconazole has recently been approved for invasive fungal infections, and may eventually replace amphotericin due to less renal toxicity.

Mycobacterial Pneumonia

Chronic infection with mycobacteria may develop into mycobacterial pneumonia. The commonly identified organisms causing tuberculosis (TB) include *M. tuberculosis*, *M. bovis*, and *M. afrocanum*. Most patients at risk include the elderly, immunocompromised patients, and recently have appeared as an epidemic in those with HIV infection. More worrisome has been the emergence of multiple, drug-resistant organisms. Active TB may occur as a new infection, or reactivation of a chronic pulmonary infection. Awareness of the possibility of TB is essential, both for optimal patient care and to prevent exposure of health care workers and others, via inhalation of aerosol. Primary infection may result in a dormant phase, where organisms may persist a lifetime. Reactivation usually occurs as a result of an immunosuppressive insult.

Symptoms of pulmonary TB include cough, fever, and variably productive sputum. There may be associated lymphadenopathy. Diagnosis is often suspected by CXR, which may show apical scarring. If the patient is immunocompetent, skin testing may be done. Pulmonary TB is usually diagnosed by the demonstration of acid-fast bacilli on a sputum smear, and then confirmed by culture. This process may take many days, however. More recently, polymerase chain reaction testing has allowed much more rapid diagnosis. Treatment requires a full course of therapy, with at least two drugs, to prevent the emergence of resistance (see Volume 2, Chapter 53). Additional drugs may be required, depending on the risk group and degree of immunosuppression; an infectious disease consultation should be obtained by those who do not routinely treat this disease.

Anthrax

Bacillis anthracis is the causative agent of anthrax, a weaponized version of which has recently been used as a biological agent of terror (83). Early recognition of anthrax infection by health care workers is essential for early intervention, to prevent widespread exposure. Anthrax is normally pathogenic for herd animals, including cattle and deer, and vegetative bacteria have poor survival outside their hosts. Spores are hardier, and they may survive for decades. Weaponization occurs when the spores are treated, so they become more readily dispersed and inhaled. Inhalational anthrax occurs following inhalation of the spores, which then germinate. Symptoms include fever, chills, sweats, nausea, dyspnea, and chest discomfort. Physical findings include fever, tachycardia and, rarely, hypotension. Laboratory findings are largely nonspecific, with elevated WBC count and transaminases most common. CXR is usually abnormal, with mediastinal widening a fairly specific finding. Infiltrates and hemorrhagic pleural effusions are common. Chest CT may show mediastinal lymphadenopathy (responsible for the mediastinal widening seen on CXR) and pleural effusions which, when sampled, are usually bloody. The presence of a markedly widened mediastinum, in a formerly healthy patient with severe respiratory illness, should be suspicious for inhalational anthrax. Because of the rarity of this disease, diagnosis may be difficult, but therapy should be initiated while the diagnosis is pursued. *B. anthracis* is a gram-positive, encapsulated, nonhemolytic, penicillin-sensitive, spore-forming bacillus, which may be visible on peripheral blood smear. Most public health facilities now have reference laboratories in place to assist with rapid identification.

Therapy should be initiated with doxycycline or ciprofloxacin, although penicillin is usually effective and is approved by the FDA. The recommended initial dosing for adults, with clinically evident inhalational anthrax, is ciprofloxacin 400 mg administered intravenously every 12 hours (84). The use of dual initial therapy (ciprofloxacin plus penicillin) may be considered, in view of the frequent and rapid development of complicating meningitis, and the clinical experience of cerebrospinal-fluid penetration with high-dose intravenous penicillin (84). More complete recommendations for special groups, such as pregnant women, immunosuppressed patients, and children, are available elsewhere (84).

Prompt notification of public health authorities is essential, as infection control, postexposure prophylaxis, and decontamination are required to prevent widespread loss of life.

NOSOCOMIAL PNEUMONIAS CAUSING ACUTE RESPIRATORY FAILURE

The ICU is associated with a greatly increased risk of nosocomial infection, with rates three to five times greater than that seen for patients who are not admitted to the ICU (85). These infections are associated with substantial morbidity and mortality, in addition to cost. Prevention of these infections is clearly the most effective therapy, and a strong evidence base exists that demonstrates the cost-effectiveness of such measures. Nosocomial pneumonia is most often associated with intubated patients who develop VAP. This subject is covered in detail in Volume 2, Chapter 48. Antibiotic resistance develops in the ICU as a result of exposure of organisms to broad-spectrum antibiotics. One strategy that may limit this selection pressure is the use of antibiotic rotation (86,87). In addition to *Acinetobacter* (discussed

above), the following microorganisms are commonly associated with nosocomial pneumonia.

Nosocomial Organisms
Pseudomonas aeruginosa

P. aeruginosa respiratory infections occur almost entirely in patients who are immunocompromised. Patients with chronic lung disease and CHF are particularly susceptible. Along with *S. aureus*, it is the most common cause of VAP. Pneumonia occurs as a result of aspiration of *P. aeruginosa* from the oropharynx, which becomes colonized during the course of hospitalization. *P. aeruginosa* pneumonia is associated with high morbidity and mortality, in part because of the propensity of *P. aeruginosa* to cross the alveolar epithelium and cause bacteremia (88). The clinical presentation of *P. aeruginosa* pneumonia includes chills, fever, severe dyspnea, productive cough with purulent sputum, and cyanosis. CXR may reveal focal or diffuse infiltrates. Bacteremia is common, so blood cultures should be obtained in addition to sputum culture or bronchoalveolar lavage. Because of the increasing prevalence of resistant organisms, double coverage (e.g., ciprofloxacin and ceftazidime combined) is recommended in critically ill patients. Because combined, the critically ill patients are at risk for renal insufficiency, aminoglycosides are reserved for second-line therapy, in combination with a fluoroquinolone or an antipseudomonal penicillin.

Enterobacter spp.

Enterobacter spp. is a common cause of nosocomial pneumonia, and like *P. aeruginosa*, causes lung infection via aspiration of colonizing oropharyngeal organisms. The lung may also be infected by the intravenous route, as a result of central venous catheter infections, which are frequently caused by *Enterobacter* spp. These organisms tend to colonize patients who have been treated with antibiotics, and therefore are abundant in the ICU. Most are resistant to first-, second-, and frequently third-generation cephalosporins. Blood cultures are rarely positive, so surveillance sputum cultures should be obtained, when possible. More aggressive pursuit of VAP is discussed in Volume 2, Chapter 48. Treatment of *Enterobacter* pneumonia consists of a second-generation cephalosporin, a nonpseudomonal third-generation cephalosporin (e.g., ceftriaxone), or ciprofloxacin. When ESBLs are produced by resistant *Enterobacter*-causing pneumonia, imipenem or meropenem should be used.

Serratia marcasens

Serratia is a frequent cause of nosocomial infections, of both the urinary and respiratory tract. These infections are rare outside the ICU, as they are commonly associated with catheters and other foreign bodies. Antibiotic resistance is common, especially with monotherapy using cephalosporins. The combination of ceftriaxone and an aminoglycoside is recommended for serious infections requiring prolonged therapy. When ESBLs are produced by resistant *S. marcasens* causing pneumonia, imipenem or meropenem should be used.

Factors Predisposing to Nosocomial Pneumonias

Nosocomial pneumonia is the second most common hospital-acquired infection after urinary tract infection (85). Although the majority of nosocomial pneumonias occur in nonintubated patients, the risk of pneumonia is up to 20 times greater in intubated patients (87). Other common risk factors include age, decreased level of consciousness, the presence of a nasogastric tube, postsurgical patients, and recent bronchoscopy (89).

A number of strategies have been examined, in an effort to decrease risk of nosocomial pneumonia. Clearly, the most effective is prevention or prophylaxis. The implementation of ventilator weaning protocols that decrease the duration of mechanical ventilation, will decrease risk. VAP is discussed in detail in Volume 2, Chapter 48. Other preventive measures include aggressive infection control policies, such as hand washing, postpyloric nasogastric feeding, and appropriate antibiotic usage. Inadequate treatment of VAP may also contribute to increased prevalence of nosocomial pneumonia; if initial broad-spectrum therapy is ineffective, then treatment should be de-escalated (90). More innovative concepts like zinc-coated ETTs show promise, but await definitive clinical trials.

> ☞ **Decreasing duration of mechanical ventilation, through the use of weaning protocols, can reduce the incidence of VAP.** ☞

SUMMARY OF CARE FOR THE PATIENT WITH ACUTE RESPIRATORY FAILURE
Respiratory Insufficiency Criteria for Intensive Care Unit Admission
Triage of patients with ARF to the ICU focuses initially upon severity of the ARF. However, in patients with moderate disease, not in itself requiring ICU admission, additional factors that must be evaluated include coexisting illness in the patient, anticipated difficulty of intubation, clinical course, and availability of monitoring and nursing. Patients requiring high-flow supplemental oxygen for hypoxemia, or those requiring noninvasive ventilatory support, require close monitoring if they are not physically admitted to the ICU.

Patients with progressive pneumonia or sepsis syndrome should be evaluated for admission to the ICU earlier rather than later, as hypoxemia, hypercapnea, and acidosis may develop rapidly in patients who do not have intact compensatory mechanisms. The Society of Critical Care Medicine has established guidelines for ICU admission, discharge, and triage (65). Table 7 describes the two major respiratory criteria (oxygenation and ventilation abnormalities) that should be considered for ICU admission. Other considerations include the availability of qualified nursing or respiratory care personnel (e.g., patient in need of frequent suctioning, encouragement to cough, deep breath, etc.).

Intubation and Mechanical Ventilation Criteria
The decision to intubate the trachea and implement mechanical ventilation is multifactorial, and may be determined by the degree of hypoxemia, hypercapnea, respiratory distress, stridor, or altered mental status. NIPPV has been demonstrated to be efficacious in a number of settings, particularly in exacerbations of COPD. However, noninvasive ventilation should only be employed in situations where the respiratory insufficiency is expected to be transient. This is seldom the case in trauma. The various modes of mechanical ventilation are fully described in Volume 2, Chapter 27.

Table 7 Criteria for Intensive Care Unit Admission: Emphasis on ARF, Postoperative, Post-Trauma Conditions

Priority	ICU admission criteria	Respiratory related examples
1A	Critically ill, unstable patients in need of intensive R_x or monitoring that cannot be provided outside of the ICU.	ARF requiring MV. Shock requiring MV and continuous vasoactive drug infusions, etc.
1B	Postoperative or post-trauma patients requiring MV, and monitoring or R_x for shock or HD instability.	S/P polytrauma, S/P TBI, S/P thoracic or major vascular surgery, S/P liver transplant, S/P major abdominal surgery, S/P surgery in critically ill patient.
2	Patients requiring intensive monitoring and may potentially need immediate intervention.	S/P neck or thoracic injuries, who are initially oxygenating and ventilating adequately. New onset pneumonia in patient with chronic comorbid condition(s).
3A	Unstable critically ill patients with a reduced likelihood of recovery because of underlying disease or nature of their acute illness.	End stage liver disease with acute severe TBI, disseminated malignancy or AIDS with major (>30% BSA) burn.
3B	Patients that might benefit from ICU to relieve acute illness, however, have set forth limits on therapeutic efforts (e.g., no intubation or CPR).	Metastatic malignancy complicated by infection, or pneumonia in patient with living will, or advanced directive that prohibits aggressive life-saving therapy.
4A	Patients not ill enough to significantly benefit from ICU care.	S/P uncomplicated peripheral vascular surgery; hemodynamically stable DKA, mild CHF, etc.
4B	Patients with terminal and irreversible illness facing imminent death (i.e., ICU therapy is considered futile). Patients with decision-making capacity (or a living will or advanced directive) that prohibits intensive care who receive comfort care only.	Brain death or severe irreversible brain injury (however, these patients may be suitable organ donors; if so they advance to priority 1 or 2). Irreversible multiorgan system failure. Patients with decision-making capacity (or a living will/advanced directive) that prohibits ICU and/or invasive monitoring or ETT.

Abbreviations: AIDS, acquired immunodeficiency syndrome; ARF, acute respiratory failure; BSA, body surface area; CHF, congestive heart failure; CPR, cardiopulmonary bypass; DKA, diabetic ketoacidosis; ETT, endotracheal tube; HD, hemodynamic; ICU, intensive care unit; MV, mechanical ventilation; R_x, treatment; S/P, status post; TBI, traumatic brain injury.
Source: From Ref. 65.

Patients who continue to be hypercapneic, acidotic, or hypoxemic despite noninvasive measures should have their trachea intubated and be started on mechanical ventilation. This decision may be influenced by both the rate of disease progression, as well as the need for interventional and/or diagnostic procedures. For example, if it is deemed necessary to place a central venous catheter, many patients with tenuous respiratory status are unable to tolerate lying supine (much less in the Trendellenberg position), due to decreased functional residual capacity, and may require intubation to facilitate line placement or more complex procedures. Likewise, patients who must undergo diagnostic procedures like magnetic resonance imaging or CT scanning (where monitoring of respiratory status is compromised), or in need of cerebral angiography (where sedation and absence of movement is critical) should be intubated to protect against respiratory failure, gastric aspiration, or complications of the procedure.

Finally, patients with stridor, or airway exams that indicate intubation is likely to be difficult, should have their tracheas intubated earlier, under controlled, semi-elective conditions, rather than later, under less controlled emergent conditions. In many cases, maintaining spontaneous ventilation, and intubating the trachea using an awake-intubation technique (e.g., fiberoptic bronchoscopy) represents the optimum approach when stridor is present, or difficult intubation is anticipated (see Volume 1, Chapter 9).

EYE TO THE FUTURE

The management of patients with respiratory failure has improved exponentially over the last decade. The future holds promising therapies, which include improved diagnostic equipment, which will allow real-time measurement of arterial blood gases, which in concert with therapist-driven weaning protocols may allow faster weaning from mechanical ventilation. As respiratory failure is often a byproduct of other disease processes, such as sepsis (Volume 2, Chapter 47) and pancreatitis (Volume 2, Chapter 39), specific therapies for those diseases, currently evolving, will have a positive impact on ARF as well. Exciting new work into the molecular mechanisms of cellular regulation, immunology (Volume 2, Chapter 52), and microbial-host interactions is beginning to elucidate the fundamental mechanisms underlying the sources of some etiologies of respiratory failure. These research pursuits will yield new therapeutic tools, some of which may become available soon.

Researchers now believe that the ACE2 receptor involved in SARS has broad applicability in the pathogenesis and treatment of numerous etiologies of pulmonary edema, beyond infection with SARS-CoV. The SARS-CoV requires ACE2 to gain entry into cells (75). However, once the virus enters the cell, the expression of ACE2 is downregulated, and the subsequent paucity of ACE2 expression appears to be the mechanism that promotes respiratory failure. Insight garnered from this research has suggested methods for treating humans infected with SARS-CoV, by administrating ACE2 to reverse the often deadly condition (77,91). ACE2 administration may also help alleviate pulmonary edema from other sources.

The ACE2 receptor is required for the SARS-CoV to infect cells and replicate itself. Using tissue culture, researchers have demonstrated that, in the presence of cells expressing ACE2, SARS-CoV replicate to levels 100,000 times greater than when incubated with cells not expressing ACE2. Furthermore, compounds that inhibit ACE2 in humans decrease SARS-CoV viral replication.

The "Spike," or S proteins on SARS-CoV, are used like a hook to grab onto ACE2; this binding enables cell membranes to fuse together, a process that is critical for a virus to enter a cell (92). The unexpected secondary relationship of SARS-CoV infection and ACE2 receptors was discovered by Kuba et al. (77), who found that infections with SARS-CoV result in ACE2 downregulation, also through binding of SARS-CoV Spike protein to ACE2.

The role of ACE2 as a protector against pulmonary edema was first demonstrated when lab mice were infected with the SARS corona virus, and it was noticed that the resulting drop in ACE2 was associated with the mice lungs filling with fluid, triggering acute pulmonary edema-mediated respiratory failure. Armed with their new knowledge, the researchers theorized that if a lack of ACE2 causes respiratory failure, then restoring it should halt the process. They injected the mice with bioengineered ACE2, which, as they predicted, shut down the SARS-induced pulmonary edema (77).

Recent data in a small cohort of individuals with SARS suggested that an insertion/deletion ACE polymorphism that affects ACE function correlates with disease severity, underscoring the relevance of these findings in humans (93). Indeed, Marshal et al. demonstrated that ACE plays a likely role in the pathogenesis of ARDS (perhaps via effects on pulmonary vascular tone/permeability, epithelial cell survival, and fibroblast activation). They noted that 47% of the variance in plasma ACE activity is accounted for by the ACE insertion/deletion polymorphism, and that the D allele is associated with higher activity. Accordingly, they hypothesized that the D allele might be associated with ARDS. In their study, they demonstrated that the DD genotype was markedly increased in the patients with ARDS, compared to other ICU patients ($p = 0.00008$), coronary artery bypass graft patients ($p = 0.0009$), and general population ($p = 0.00004$) control groups, and was significantly associated with mortality in the ARDS group ($p < 0.02$), suggesting a potential role for renin-angiotensin systems in the pathogenesis of ARDS and, for the first time, implicating genetic factors in the development and progression of ARDS (94).

The aggregate analysis of this exciting aforementioned new research, regarding the molecular mechanisms of SARS-mediated infection and pulmonary edema (involving the renin-angiotensin system), has now suggested a broader role of ACE2 in lung failure and ARDS of multiple etiologies. Recombinant ACE2 protein might, therefore, not only serve as a treatment to block spreading of SARS-CoV, modulation of the renin-angiotensin system could also be used to protect individuals infected with other viruses (such as strains of avian influenza A), and other disease processes (such as pancreatitis-mediated noncardiogenic pulmonary edema), from developing acute severe lung failure and ARDS (77). Numerous additional examples of ongoing research into the molecular mechanisms of disease, and also the genetic predisposition (relating to the expression, or nonexpression of permissive or protective proteins) will continue to provide bright new avenues for treatment of respiratory failure in the future.

SUMMARY

ARF continues to be the most common reason for admission to the ICU for both nontrauma and trauma patients.

Table 8 Categorization of Common Sources of Respiratory Failure Based upon the Primary Physiologic Abnormality (Oxygenation or Ventilation)

Oxygenation problem	Ventilation problem
Direct pulmonary dysfunction	Airway obstruction
Pneumonia	Stridor
Atelectasis	Excessive snoring
Pulmonary contusion	
Noncardiogenic	Excessive WOB
pulmonary edema	Low compliance
(ALI/ARDS)	$\Uparrow\Uparrow$ Airway resistance
Sepsis, SIRS	$\Uparrow$'d V_D/V_T
$\Uparrow\Uparrow$ Nonthoracic trauma	CO_2 production
Fat emboli	Inability to do the WOB
Burns	Generalized weakness
Pancreatitis	Critical illness
$\Downarrow \ni \delta$ albumin[a]	polyneuropathy
Cirrhosis	Steroid myopathy
Acute renal failure	
Cardiogenic pulmonary	Lung mechanical problem
edema	($\Downarrow$'d ventilatory drive
Left heart failure	or strength)
Ischemia	Opiate overdose
Mitral valve disease	Brainstem injury
Viral cardiomyopathy	Spinal cord injury
Hydrostatic pulmonary edema	($\Downarrow$'d NMJ function)
Neurogenic pulmonary edema	Myasthenia gravis
NPPE	Botulism

[a]Hypoalbuminemia can result from massive blood loss and resuscitation with crystalloid, nephrosis, cirrhosis, malnutrition, excessive catabolism, etc.

Abbreviations: $\Downarrow$, decrease; $\Uparrow$, increase; ALI, acute lung injury; ARDS, acute respiratory distress syndrome; NMJ, neuromuscular junction; NPPE, negative pressure pulmonary edema; SIRS, systemic inflammatory distress syndrome; V_D/V_T, dead space to tidal volume ratio; WOB, work of breathing.

The specific diagnosis can often be categorized as primarily a problem of oxygenation or ventilation (Table 8). The precise etiology of the respiratory failure should be aggressively sought after, beginning when patients are first evaluated in the ICU, or immediately prior to transfer. Although culture data will generally take at least 48 hours, often the clues explaining the cause of respiratory failure become irretrievable 12 to 24 hours after presentation, forcing treatment to remain empirical and suboptimal for much longer durations. Even though oxygenation and ventilation problems are often coinvolved, one form is often predominant initially, and reflects the inciting insult. It is extremely important to search for the initial trigger of respiratory failure, because it has both prognostic and therapeutic implications.

ARF can result from problems directly related to the lungs, aspiration, pulmonary emboli pneumonia, and blunt chest trauma (e.g., pulmonary contusion). However, many critically ill patients develop ARF after primary pathology in another organ system (e.g., renal failure, liver failure) or a generalized condition causing systemic inflammation (sepsis, pancreatitis, trauma, burn). Because their etiologies are covered in other chapters, this chapter has focused upon primary problems affecting the lungs and causing ARF.

The SARS-CoV Spike protein-mediated ACE2 down-regulation contributes to the severity of pulmonary edema, and explains how this family member of the normally relatively harmless coronaviruses has evolved into a lethal virus. Furthermore, the significance of the discovery of the molecular nature behind the pulmonary edema component of SARS-CoV extends beyond SARS itself. Indeed, understanding the role of ACE2 in pulmonary edema has suggested a possible means of preventing lung failure from numerous other forms of ARF and ARDS, including sepsis, anthrax, and avian flu (the agent that, many infectious disease experts believe, will launch the next flu pandemic) (95).

Finally, a more sobering thought is the continuing emergence of antibiotic resistance in the ICU. Aggressive infection control, limitation of excessive antibiotic usage and, possibly, devices like antimicrobial-coated ETTs may help stem the tide.

KEY POINTS

☞ Arterial blood gas (ABG) analysis is the single most important laboratory test for defining the severity of ARF. In addition to quantifying the severity, ABG analysis assists in differentiating the cause of ARF, and is useful in decision making regarding intubation and mechanical ventilation.

☞ Many of the drugs used in the ICU have vasodilator properties and can worsen oxygenation by blunting HPV and exacerbating $\dot{V}/\dot{Q}$ mismatching.

☞ The most common causes of right-to-left transpulmonary shunting in ICU patients are direct pulmonary pathologic entities, such as pneumonia, atelectasis, and noncardiogenic pulmonary edema.

☞ Many commonly used drugs can cause methemoglobinemia, which will worsen hypoxemia and acidosis. These drugs include dapsone, local anesthetics (benzocaine and prilocaine), commonly used nitrates (nitroprusside, nitroglycerin), and sulfonamides. Diagnosis may be made with co-oximetry that measures various hemoglobin species. Treatment is with methylene blue.

☞ Patients with acute asthma exacerbations are normally hypertensive because of catechol release. Those that are normotensive or hypotensive and tachycardic may have elevated intrathoracic pressure impeding venous return, and are at increased risk for cardiopulmonary arrest during endotracheal intubation.

☞ Inspiratory stridor is usually due to an extrathoracic obstruction (supraglottic or periglottic), and expiratory stridor is usually due to an intrathoracic process.

☞ The key principles of airway management for stridor are: (*i*) maintain spontaneous ventilation, (*ii*) avoid blind intubation techniques (may convert partial obstruction into complete obstruction), (*iii*) awake fiberoptic intubation is often the best diagnostic tool and method of airway intubation, and (*iv*) equipment and personnel capable of performing a surgical airway must be present until the airway is secured.

☞ Thoracic epidural anesthesia can improve respiratory function in patients with rib injuries.

☞ Decreasing duration of mechanical ventilation, through the use of weaning protocols, can reduce the incidence of VAP.

REFERENCES

1. Bernard GR, Artigas A, Brigham KL, et al. The American-European Consensus Conference on ARDS. Definitions, mechanisms, relevant outcomes, and clinical trial coordination. Am J Respir Crit Care Med 1994; 149:818–824.

2. Bone RC, Balk RA, Cerra FB, et al. Definitions for sepsis and organ failure and guidelines for the use of innovative therapies in sepsis. The ACCP/SCCM Consensus Conference Committee. American College of Chest Physicians/Society of Critical Care Medicine. Chest 1992; 101:1644–1655.

3. Marshall BE, Wyche MQ, Jr. Hypoxemia during and after anesthesia. Anesthesiology 1972; 37:178–209.

4. Lumb A. Nunn's Applied Respiratory Physiology. Oxford, UK: Butterworth, 2000.

5. Rivers E, Nguyen B, Havstad S, et al. Early goal-directed therapy in the treatment of severe sepsis and septic shock. N Engl J Med 2001; 345:1368–1377.

6. Kollef MH. Optimizing antibiotic therapy in the intensive care unit setting. Crit Care 2001; 5:189–195.

7. Luhr OR, Antonsen K, Karlsson M, et al. Incidence and mortality after acute respiratory failure and acute respiratory distress syndrome in Sweden, Denmark, and Iceland. The ARF Study Group. Am J Respir Crit Care Med 1999; 159:1849–1861.

8. Bochud PY, Glauser MP, Calandra T. Antibiotics in sepsis. Intensive Care Med 2001; 27:S33–48.

9. Vincent JL, Akca S, De Mendonca A, et al. The epidemiology of acute respiratory failure in critically ill patients. Chest 2002; 121:1602–1609.

10. Arroliga AC, Ghamra ZW, Perez Trepichio A, et al. Incidence of ARDS in an adult population of northeast Ohio. Chest 2002; 121:1972–1976.

11. Nunn JF. Pulmonary oxygen consumption. Intensive Care Med 1996; 22:275–276.

12. Harris EA, Hunter ME, Seelye ER, Vedder M, Whitlock RM. Prediction of the physiological dead-space in resting normal subjects. Clin Sci Mol Med 1973; 45:375–386.

13. Eisenkraft JB. Effects of anaesthetics on the pulmonary circulation. Br J Anaesth 1990; 65:63–78.

14. Pierson DJ. Weaning from mechanical ventilation in acute repsiratory failure: concepts, indications, and techniques. Respir Care 1983; 28(5):646–662.

15. Lecky JM, Ominsky AJ. Postoperative respiratory management. Chest 1972; 62:505–575.

16. Gilbert R, Keighley JF. The arterial/alveolar oxygen tension ratio. An index of gas exchange applicable to varying inspired oxygen concentrations. Am Rev Respir Dis 1974; 109:142–145.

17. Bendixen HH, Egbert LD, Hedley-Whyte J, Laver MB, Pontoppidan H. Respiratory Care. St. Louis: CV Mosby, 1965:149–150.

18. Bruschi C, Cerveri I, Zoia MC, et al. Reference values of maximal respiratory mouth pressures: a population-based study. Am Rev Respir Dis 1992; 146:790–793.

19. Witt NJ, Zochodne DW, Bolton CF, et al. Peripheral nerve function in sepsis and multiple organ failure. Chest 1991; 99:176–184.

20. Decramer M, de Bock V, Dom R. Functional and histologic picture of steroid-induced myopathy in chronic obstructive pulmonary disease. Am J Respir Crit Care Med 1996; 153:1958–1964.

21. Segredo V, Caldwell JE, Matthay MA, Sharma ML, Gruenke LD, Miller RD. Persistent paralysis in critically ill patients after long-term administration of vecuronium. N Engl J Med 1992; 327:524–528.

22. Aberle DR, Wiener-Kronish JP, Webb WR, Matthay MA. Hydrostatic versus increased permeability pulmonary edema: diagnosis based on radiographic criteria in critically ill patients. Radiology 1988; 168:73–79.

23. Levy M, Dromer F, Brion N, Leturdu F, Carbon C. Community-acquired pneumonia. Importance of initial noninvasive bacteriologic and radiographic investigations. Chest 1988; 93: 43–48.

24. Hartert TV, Peebles RS Jr. Epidemiology of asthma: the year in review. Curr Opin Pulm Med 2000; 6:4–9.

25. Georgitis JW. The 1997 Asthma Management Guidelines and therapeutic issues relating to the treatment of asthma. National Heart, Lung, and Blood Institute. Chest 1999; 115:210–217.

26. Lee TH. Precipitating factors of asthma. Br Med Bull 1992; 48:169–178.

27. Zimmerman JL, Dellinger RP, Shah AN, Taylor RW. Endotracheal intubation and mechanical ventilation in severe asthma. Crit Care Med 1993; 21:1727–1730.

28. Papiris S, Kotanidou A, Malagari K, Roussos C. Clinical review: severe asthma. Crit Care 2002; 6:30–44.

29. Burki NK, Diamond L. Serum creatine phosphokinase activity in asthma. Am Rev Respir Dis 1977; 116:327–331.

30. Appel D, Rubenstein R, Schrager K, Williams MH Jr. Lactic acidosis in severe asthma. Am J Med 1983; 75:580–584.

31. Karpel JP, Schacter EN, Fanta C, et al. A comparison of ipratropium and albuterol vs albuterol alone for the treatment of acute asthma. Chest 1996; 110:611–616.

32. Littenberg B. Aminophylline treatment in severe, acute asthma. A meta-analysis. JAMA 1988; 259:1678–1684.

33. NHLBI. Strategies in preserving lung health and preventing COPD and associated diseases. The National Lung Health Education Program (NLHEP). Chest 1998; 113:123S–163S.

34. McHardy VU, Inglis JM, Calder MA, et al. A study of infective and other factors in exacerbations of chronic bronchitis. Br J Dis Chest 1980; 74:228–238.

35. Barbera JA, Roca J, Ferrer A, et al. Mechanisms of worsening gas exchange during acute exacerbations of chronic obstructive pulmonary disease. Eur Respir J 1997; 10:1285–1291.

36. Hunt JM, Copland J, McDonald CF, et al. Cardiopulmonary response to oxygen therapy in hypoxaemic chronic airflow obstruction. Thorax 1989; 44:930–936.

37. Aubier M, Murciano D, Fournier M, et al. Central respiratory drive in acute respiratory failure of patients with chronic obstructive pulmonary disease. Am Rev Respir Dis 1980; 122:191–199.

38. Agusti AG, Carrera M, Barbe F, Munoz A, Togores B. Oxygen therapy during exacerbations of chronic obstructive pulmonary disease. Eur Respir J 1999; 14:934–939.

39. Niewoehner DE, Erbland ML, Deupree RH, et al. Effect of systemic glucocorticoids on exacerbations of chronic obstructive pulmonary disease. Department of Veterans Affairs Cooperative Study Group. N Engl J Med 1999; 340:1941–1947.

40. Loevner LA. Anatomic and functional lesions resulting in partial or complete upper airway obstruction. Semin Roentgenol 2001; 36:12–20.

41. Marik PE. Aspiration pneumonitis and aspiration pneumonia. N Engl J Med 2001; 344:665–671.

42. Hirsh J, Dalen J, Guyatt G. The sixth (2000) ACCP guidelines for antithrombotic therapy for prevention and treatment of thrombosis. American College of Chest Physicians. Chest 2001; 119:1S–2S.

43. Young KR Jr. Pulmonary-renal syndromes. Clin Chest Med 1989; 10:655–675.

44. Salama AD, Levy JB, Lightstone L, Pusey CD. Goodpasture's disease. Lancet 2001; 358:917–920.

45. Prakash UB. Respiratory complications in mixed connective tissue disease. Clin Chest Med 1998; 19:733–746.

46. Gropper MA, Wiener-Kronish JP, Hashimoto S. Acute cardiogenic pulmonary edema. Clin Chest Med 1994; 15:501–515.

47. Matthay MA, Folkesson HG, Clerici C. Lung epithelial fluid transport and the resolution of pulmonary edema. Physiol Rev 2002; 82:569–600.

48. Bella I, Chad DA. Neuromuscular disorders and acute respiratory failure. Neurol Clin 1998; 16:391–417.

49. Oh SJ, Dwyer DS, Bradley RJ. Overlap myasthenic syndrome: combined myasthenia gravis and Eaton-Lambert syndrome. Neurology 1987; 37:1411–1414.

50. Cicala RS, Voeller GR, Fox T, et al. Epidural analgesia in thoracic trauma: effects of lumbar morphine and thoracic bupivacaine on pulmonary function. Crit Care Med 1990; 18:229–231.

51. Fulton RL, Peter ET. Physiologic effects of fluid therapy after pulmonary contusion. Am J Surg 1973; 126:773–777.

52. Steier M, Ching N, Roberts EB, Nealon TF Jr. Pneumothorax complicating continuous ventilatory support. J Thorac Cardiovasc Surg 1974; 67:17–23.

53. Polanczyk CA, Rohde LE, Goldman L, et al. Right heart catheterization and cardiac complications in patients undergoing noncardiac surgery: an observational study. JAMA 2001; 286:309–314.

54. Byrick RJ, Mullen JB, Wong PY, Wigglesworth D, Kay JC. Corticosteroids do not inhibit acute pulmonary response to fat embolism. Can J Anaesth 1990; 37:S130.

55. Orlowski JP, Szpilman D. Drowning. Rescue, resuscitation, and reanimation. Pediatr Clin North Am 2001; 48:627–646.

56. Simon RP. Neurogenic pulmonary edema. Neurol Clin 1993; 11:309–323.

57. Ewig S, Torres A, El-Ebiary M, et al. Bacterial colonization patterns in mechanically ventilated patients with traumatic and medical head injury. Incidence, risk factors, and association with ventilator-associated pneumonia. Am J Respir Crit Care Med 1999; 159:188–198.

58. Schiffl H, Lang SM, Fischer R. Daily hemodialysis and the outcome of acute renal failure. N Engl J Med 2002; 346:305–310.

59. Banerjee AK, Haggie SJ, Jones RB, Basran GS. Respiratory failure in acute pancreatitis. Postgrad Med J 1995; 71:327–330.

60. Naeije R. Hepatopulmonary syndrome and portopulmonary hypertension. Swiss Med Wkly 2003; 133:163–169.

61. Krowka MJ, Tajik JA, Dickenson RE, et al. Intrapulmonary vascular dilations in Liver transplant candidates. Screening by two-dimensional contrast enhanced echocardiography. Chest 1990; 97:1165–1170.

62. Rolla G, Bucca C, Brussino L. Methylene Blue in the Hepatopulmonary Syndrome. N Engl J Med 1994; 331:1098.

63. Sztrymf B, Rabiller A, Nunes H, et al. Prevention of hepatopulmonary syndrome and hyperdynamic state by pentoxifylline in cirrhotic rats. Eur Respir J 2004; 23:752–758.

64. Dinh-Xuan AT, Naeije R. The hepatopulmonary syndrome: NO way out? Eur Respir J 2004; 23:661–662.

65. Guidelines for intensive care unit admission, discharge, and triage. Task Force of the American College of Critical Care Medicine, Society of Critical Care Medicine. Crit Care Med 1999; 27:633–638.

66. Niederman MS, Bass JB Jr, Campbell GD, et al. Guidelines for the initial management of adults with community-acquired pneumonia: diagnosis, assessment of severity, and initial antimicrobial therapy. American Thoracic Society. Medical Section of the American Lung Association. Am Rev Respir Dis 1993; 148:1418–1426.

67. ATS/IDSA. Guidelines for the management of adults with hospital-acquired, ventilator-associated, and healthcare-associated pneumonia. Am J Resp Crit Care Med 2005; 171:388–416.

68. Robinson KA, Baughman W, Rothrock G, et al. Epidemiology of invasive Streptococcus pneumoniae infections in the United States, 1995–1998: Opportunities for prevention in the conjugate vaccine era. JAMA 2001; 285:1729–1735.

69. Wunderink RG, Rello J, Cammarata SK, et al. Linezolid vs Vancomycin: analysis of two double-blind studies of patients with methicillin-resistant Staphylococcus aureus nosocomial pneumonia. Chest 2003; 124:1789–1797.

70. Gagnon S, Boota AM, Fischl MA, et al. Corticosteroids as adjunctive therapy for severe Pneumocystis carinii pneumonia in the acquired immunodeficiency syndrome. A double-blind, placebo-controlled trial. N Engl J Med 1990; 323:1444–1450.

71. Drazen JM. SARS-looking back over the first 100 days. N Engl J Med 2003; 349:319–320.

72. Peiris JSM, Guan Y, Yuen KY. Severe acute respiratory syndrome. Nat Med 2004; 10:S88–S97.

73. Peiris JSM, Lai ST, Poon LLM, et al. Coronavirus as a possible cause of severe acute respiratory syndrome. Lancet 2003; 361:1319–1325.

74. Marra MA, Jones SJ, Astell CR, et al. The genome sequence of the SARS-associated coronavirus. Science 2003; 300:1399–1404.

75. Li W, Moore MJ, Vasilieva N, et al. Angiotensin-converting enzyme 2 is a functional receptor for the SARS coronavirus. Nature 2003; 426:450–454.

76. Nicholls J, Peiris M. Good ACE, bad ACE do battle in lung injury, SARS. Nat Med 2005; 11:821–822.

77. Kuba K, Imai Y, Rao S, et al. A crucial role of angiotensin converting enzyme 2 (ACE2) in SARS coronavirus-induced lung injury. Nature Medicine 2005; 11:875–879.

78. Low DE, McGeer A. SARS-One Year Later. N Engl J Med 2003; 349:2381–2382.

79. Lang ZW, Zhang LJ, Zhang SJ, et al. A clinicopathological study of three cases of severe acute respiratory syndrome (SARS). Pathology 2003; 35(6):526–531.

80. Traggiai E, Becker S, Subbarao K, et al. An efficient method to make human monoclonal antibodies from memory B cells: potent neutralization of SARS coronavirus. Nat Med 2004; 10:871–875 .

81. Galgiani JN, Catanzaro A, Cloud GA, et al. Comparison of oral fluconazole and itraconazole for progressive, nonmeningeal coccidioidomycosis. A randomized, double-blind trial. Mycoses Study Group. Ann Intern Med 2000; 133:676–686.

82. Goldman M, Johnson PC, Sarosi GA. Fungal pneumonias: The endemic mycoses. Clin Chest Med 1999; 20(3):507–519.

83. Inglesby TV, O'Toole T, Henderson DA, et al. Anthrax as a biological weapon, 2002: updated recommendations for management. JAMA 2002; 287:2236–2252.

84. Swartz MN: Recognition and management of anthrax—an update. N Engl J Med 2001; 345:1621–1626.

85. Craven DE, De Rosa FG, Thornton D. Nosocomial pneumonia: emerging concepts in diagnosis, management, and prophylaxis. Curr Opin Crit Care 2002; 8:421–429.

86. Raymond DP, Pelletier SJ, Crabtree TD, et al. Impact of a rotating empiric antibiotic schedule on infectious mortality in an intensive care unit. Crit Care Med 2001; 29:1101–1108.

87. Chastre J, Fagon JY. Ventilator-associated pneumonia. Am J Respir Crit Care Med 2002; 165:867–903.

88. Savel RH, Yao EC, Gropper MA. Protective effects of low tidal volume ventilation in a rabbit model of Pseudomonas aeruginosa-induced acute lung injury. Crit Care Med 2001; 29:392–398.

89. Joshi N, Localio AR, Hamory BH. A predictive risk index for nosocomial pneumonia in the intensive care unit. Am J Med 1992; 93:135–142.

90. Hoffken G, Niederman MS. Nosocomial pneumonia: the importance of a de-escalating strategy for antibiotic treatment of pneumonia in the ICU. Chest 2002; 122:2183–2196.

91. Li W, Zhang C, Sui J, et al. Receptor and viral determinants of SARS-coronavirus adaptation to human ACE2. The EMBO J 2005; 24:1634–1643.

92. Holmes KV. SARS-associated coronavirus. N Engl J Med 2003; 348:1948–1951.

93. Itoyama S, Keidio N, Quy T, et al. ACE1 polymorphism and progression of SARS. Biochem. Biophys. Res. Commun. 2004; 323:1124–1129.

94. Marshall RP, Webb S, Bellingan GJ, et al. Angiotensin converting enzyme insertion/deletion polymorphism is associated with susceptibility and outcome in acute respiratory distress syndrome. Am J Respir Crit Care Med 2002; 166: 646–650.

95. Monto AS. The threat of an avian influenza pandemic. N Engl J Med 2005; 352:323–325.

24

The Acute Respiratory Distress Syndrome

Paul A. Campbell and Benoit Misset

Department of Medicine and Anesthesiology, UC San Francisco Medical Center, San Francisco, California, U.S.A.

Jeanine P. Wiener-Kronish and Michael A. Matthay

Departments of Medicine, Anesthesia, and Critical Care Medicine, UC San Francisco Medical Center, and the UCSF Cardiovascular Research Institute, San Francisco, California, U.S.A.

DEFINITIONS AND EPIDEMIOLOGY

Definitions

Formally recognized over four decades ago (1), acute lung injury and the acute respiratory distress syndrome (ALI/ARDS), are defined by descriptive physiologic and clinical criteria set forth by the American-European Consensus Conference (AECC) of 1994 (Table 1) (2). Three primary features define ALI/ARDS; a profound oxygenation defect (right-to-left transpulmonary shunt), impaired carbon dioxide excretion, and the presence of noncardiogenic pulmonary edema. The oxygenation defect is characterized by the partial pressure of oxygen in the arterial blood (PaO_2)/fraction of inspired oxygen (FiO_2) ratio (P/F ratio). When the P/F ratio is <300, the criteria for ALI is met, whereas if <200, the ARDS threshold is achieved. The AECC definitions for ALI and ARDS build upon the experience of the lung injury severity score introduced by Murray et al. (3). That scoring system combines the magnitude of physiologic impairment (severity of oxygenation defect, required level of positive end-expiratory pressure, and decreased respiratory compliance) along with the degree of alveolar consolidation on the chest radiograph (3). Several studies have compared the diagnostic accuracy between these criteria concluding statistical agreement (4). The intent of the simplified definition is to characterize a syndrome without reference to a specific etiology (5).

Epidemiology

An accurate incidence of ALI/ARDS has been difficult to determine. Several epidemiological studies using the AECC definition suggest an incidence of 12.6 to 18.9 cases per 100,000 population per year (6). However, new data recently generated in King's County, Washington, demonstrated the incidence may be as high as 75 cases per 100,000, or approximately 200,000 cases per year in the United States (7). Previous studies that did not apply the AECC criteria described lower estimates, ranging from 1.5 to 17.9 cases per 100,000 population per year (8).

Associated Clinical Disorders, Risk Factors, and Mortality

♂ Both ALI and ARDS, can result from a multitude of disorders (Table 2) with the common thread being injury to the epithelial capillary barrier of lung alveoli. ♂ This injury can result from direct injury, or indirectly through local or systemic inflammation. The most common associations from prospective studies are sepsis syndrome accounting for 40%, aspiration and pneumonia combining for 40%, as well as trauma, and multiple transfusions (9). ♂ **Because of the frequency of associated septic conditions, infectious foci must be actively pursued and treated in ARDS patients (10).** ♂

Several independent predictors of mortality have been reported including comorbid states and age >65 (Table 3) (8). The patient's immunological status (particularly neutrophil function) is an important determinant of ALI/ARDS severity. Patients suffering from chronic alcoholism are more susceptible to lung injury, likely a result of deranged neutrophil activation (11). Conversely, diabetics with impaired neutrophil function from hyperglycemia may be protected from lung injury, but are more likely to succumb to sepsis syndrome (12).

Interestingly, the only pulmonary-specific physiologic predictor of mortality appears to be a bedside measure of pulmonary dead-space fraction (13). Patients with diminished alveolar fluid clearance, determined by sequential samples of pulmonary edema fluid, also have a higher mortality (14).

Estimates over the past several decades for the overall mortality rate of ALI/ARDS patients range from 30% to 60% (10). Most deaths seem to be a consequence of multiorgan dysfunction rather than primary pulmonary failure. Fortunately, more recent calculations suggest a decreasing mortality trend, approximately 35% to 40% (7).

PATHOPHYSIOLOGY

Regardless of the etiology of ALI/ARDS, the extravasation of protein-rich fluid into the alveolar space leads to pathologic, radiographic, and clinical changes that can be delineated into acute, subacute, and chronic phases (Table 4).

Acute Exudative Phase

♂ **The acute exudative phase is a consequence of widespread protein-rich alveolar edema.** ♂ In the initial hours, the permeability edema has a high alveolar to plasma protein ratio (16). Findings on bronchoalveolar lavage and

Table 1 Criteria for Acute Lung Injury and Acute Respiratory Distress Syndrome

Acute onset
$PaO_2/FiO_2 \leq 300$ mmHg (ALI)
  $PaO_2/FiO_2 \leq 200$ mmHg (ARDS)
Bilateral pulmonary infiltrates on anterior-posterior chest radiograph
Absence of left arterial hypertension (PCWP < 18 mmHg when measured)

Abbreviations: ALI, acute lung injury; ARDS, acute respiratory distress syndrome; FiO₂, fraction of inspired oxygen; PaO₂, partial pressure of oxygen in the arterial blood; PCWP, pulmonary artery capillary wedge pressure.

lung biopsy include diffuse alveolar damage with cellular infiltration by neutrophils, macrophages and erythrocytes, alveolar-epithelial disruption, and hyaline membrane deposition (17).

Radiographically, nonspecific findings predominate with bilateral infiltrates that may not be symmetrical and may be associated with pleural effusions (Fig. 1) (18). Computed tomography may further reveal a bilateral heterogeneous alveolar filling without enlargement of pulmonary vessels. It tends to occur in dependent lung zones with associated consolidation and atelectasis (19).

☞ **Alveolar flooding results in significant transpulmonary shunting and ventilation-perfusion ($\dot{V}/\dot{Q}$) imbalance causing profound hypoxemia that is refractory to supplemental oxygen.** ☞ A reduction in static lung compliance, the tidal volume divided by the plateau pressure minus the level of positive end-expiratory pressure (PEEP), leads to an increase in the work of breathing. Hypoxemia may worsen with increasing metabolic demand (e.g., fever, and high work of breathing) decreased oxygen delivery (e.g., anemia, impaired cardiac output), or derangement in acid-base status (20). The initiation of mechanical ventilation attempts to reverse the hypoxemia due to alveolar flooding and increased work of breathing by providing assisted ventilation with PEEP and supplemental oxygen. However, the oxygen delivery can be further decreased with positive pressure ventilation due to impairment of cardiac output. Accordingly, ARDS patients with impaired cardiac output often require some degree of inotropic support.

Table 2 Clinical Disorders Associated with the Development of Acute Lung Injury and Acute Respiratory Distress Syndrome

Direct lung injury	Indirect lung injury
Pneumonia	Sepsis
Aspiration of gastric contents	Severe trauma with shock and multiple transfusions
Pulmonary contusion	Cardiopulmonary bypass
Fat emboli	Drug overdose
Near-drowning	Acute pancreatitis
Inhalational injury	Transfusions of blood products
Reperfusion pulmonary edema after lung transplantation or pulmonary embolectomy	Reperfusion of ischemic gut and extremities

Table 3 Predictors of Increased Mortality in Acute Lung Injury and Acute Respiratory Distress Syndrome (Based on Epidemiologic Studies)

Risk factor	Examples
Severe, nonpulmonary systemic disease	Liver dysfunction/cirrhosis
	Sepsis
	Nonpulmonary organ dysfunction
	HIV infection
	Active malignancy
	Chronic alcoholism
	Renal failure
Pulmonary factors	Increased alveolar dead space
	Prolonged, decreased pulmonary compliance
Age-related factors	>65
Miscellaneous poor predictors	Organ transplantation
	APACHE II >25

Table 4 Stages of Acute Lung Injury and Acute Respiratory Distress Syndrome

Stage	Pathophysiology/clinical presentation	Pathogenesis
Acute exudative	Onset—hours to days Hypoxemia—intra-pulmonary shunting and ventilation perfusion imbalance Static lung compliance worsening Increasing dead space Bilateral pulmonary edema on the chest radiograph	Disruption of alveolar-capillary unit from: Primary injury Secondary injury such as inflammatory and procoagulant mechanism Protein-rich alveolar edema accumulating secondary to inflammatory and procoagulant mechanism
Subacute fibrosing alveolitis	Onset—hours to weeks Hypoxemia—as above plus diffusion defect Pulmonary hypertension with right ventricular failure Susceptibility to ventilator-associated pneumonia Reticulation and distortion of bronchovascular markings and baro-trauma on the chest radiograph	Interstitial and air space fibrosis from: Mesenchymal cellular infiltrate Disorganized collagen deposition
Chronic resolution	Onset—hours to months Hypoxemia improved Lung compliance improved Persistent restrictive defects and diffusion abnormalities by pulmonary function testing Long-term neuro-muscular deficits and diminished quality of life	Resolution of alveolar edema through: Regenerated alveolar-capillary integrity Apoptosis of inflammatory cells

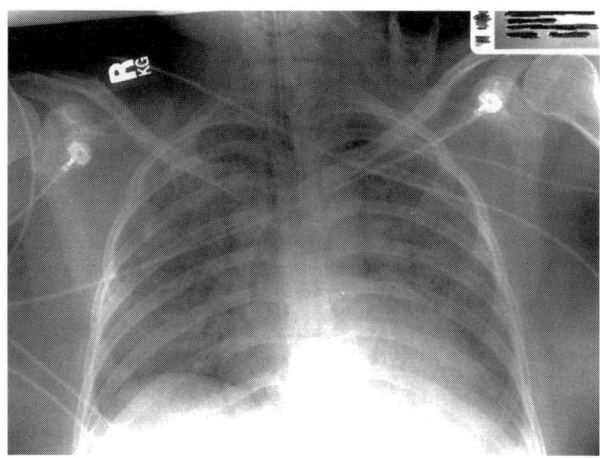

Figure 1 The anterior–posterior chest radiograph shows bilateral patchy alveolar infiltrates consistent with noncardiogenic pulmonary edema. This patient has acute respiratory distress syndrome from gram-negative sepsis due to a perforated duodenal ulcer. *Note*: There is an endotracheal tube in place to deliver positive pressure ventilation.

Concomitant abnormalities in pulmonary blood flow lead to mismatched ventilation–perfusion. This physiologic dead space is the component of wasted ventilation that impairs the excretion of carbon dioxide and may cause hypercapnia. As mentioned previously, increased dead-space ventilation early in the disease course is predictive of mortality (13). Interestingly, the recent therapeutic shift towards permissive hypercapnia is not associated with worse outcome (21).

Subacute Fibrosing Alveolitis Phase
☞ **Some patients recover from the acute insult without sequelae, however, some progress to a subacute fibrosing alveolitis phase.** ☞ This phase is characterized by fibrotic alteration of the interstitium and air spaces of the lung and chronic inflammatory cell infiltrate (14). The evolving fibrosis is evident on the chest radiograph as linear opacities (18). Likewise, computed tomography demonstrates interstitial reticulation and distortion of bronchovascular markings (19). Dependent lung zone barotrauma, in the form of pneumothorax and other air leaks, is anticipated in approximately 5% to 10% of patients. Surprisingly, there is not an increase in mortality associated with barotraumas (22).

Gas exchange abnormalities persist; hypoxemia, from the ongoing transpulmonary shunt and ventilation-perfusion imbalance as well as hypercapnia, from increased alveolar dead-space ventilation (20). In severe cases, the obliteration of the pulmonary capillary bed can lead to worsening pulmonary compliance, pulmonary hypertension, and ultimately right ventricular failure (23).

The clinical course of ALI/ARDS is frequently complicated by nosocomial infections, particularly ventilator- associated pneumonia (VAP). Estimates of ALI/ARDS patients suffering VAP have been as high as 60% (24). The increased risk is partly due to the consequences of endotracheal intubation and mechanical ventilation. These include the microbial colonization of the lungs and changes in alveolar epithelial integrity (25). Endotracheal tubes facilitate bacterial entry and limit physical clearance of organisms. Once established, these flora alter the innate response to infection by reducing surfactant protein secretion that is critical in the process of

clearance, and by increasing the quantity of proinflammatory cytokines (26). In the setting of VAP, specific attributable mortality increases, particularly with the presence of *Pseudomonas* and *Acinetobacter* species (27).

Chronic Resolution Phase
Gradual resolution, typically weeks after the insult, is heralded with improving oxygenation and lung compliance, as slow radiographic resolution occurs. ☞ **Postextubation pulmonary function testing among ALI/ARDS survivors shows restrictive impairments and diffusion abnormalities.** ☞ At 6 to 12 months, lung volume and spirometric measurements normalize, however, diffusion derangements persist (28). This is accompanied by a low health-related quality of life not entirely explained by changes in pulmonary function. Some of the postrecovery sequalae of ARDS (including prolonged or chronic weakness and fatigue), result from critical illness neuromuscular disease (see Volume 2, Chapter 6) (29). Neuro-psychological deficits, another consequence of critical illness, are an additional burden to survivors (6).

PATHOGENESIS
Mechanisms of Lung Injury
The alveolar-capillary unit is composed of the alveolar epithelium, lined with type I and II pneumocytes, and the microvascular endothelium. The acute exudative phase of ALI/ARDS is a result of a compromised vascular and epithelial barrier allowing an influx of protein-rich edema fluid into the air space.

The pathogenesis of the alveolar edema depends on both inflammatory and coagulation-dependent mechanisms. Inflammatory mediators may be generated focally or systemically depending on the initial insult (Table 2). ☞ **The release of inflammatory mediators into the systemic circulation amplifies the injury to both nonpulmonary organs as well as the lung itself, a process referred to as innate immunity (30).** ☞ Severe alveolar epithelial injury results in disorganized collagen deposition and imbalanced apoptosis, subacute fibrosing alveolitis. Ultimately, resolution and removal of alveolar edema and cellular debris requires the restoration of the alveolar-capillary unit that actively transports fluid, electrolytes, and proteins.

Direct Lung Injury
A large number of direct or indirect injuries to the alveolar capillary-epithelial barrier can lead to ALI/ARDS (Table 2). The most important direct exposure injuries include bacteria, aspiration, and trauma (mechanical at smoke inhalation). These more common etiologies are described in greater length here.

Bacterial Pneumonia
Direct exposure of the epithelial–endothelial barrier to bacteria increases permeability influx while decreasing active fluid transport across the alveolar epithelial membrane. ☞ **The bacteria-causing pneumonia (particularly those associated with ALI/ARDS) possess a variety of virulence factors disruptive to alveolar epithelial cells.** ☞ The capsule surrounding *Streptococcus pneumoniae*, *Haemophilus influenzae*, and *Klebsiella pneumoniae* is designed to protect bacteria against phagocytosis (31). *Staphylococcus aureus* produces extracellular and cell wall–associated proteases (32). Gram-positive bacteria have a surface-associated adhesion molecule,

lipoteichoic acid, whereas the gram-negative bacteria express lipopolysaccharides, both potent stimuli of the host defense (33). Further, animal models with *Pseudomonas aeruginosa* demonstrate some bacterial products, including phospholipase C and exoenzyme S, which injure the epithelial barrier and impair the resolution of alveolar edema. Similarly, influenza virus alters epithelial ion transport with the enzymatic activity of phospholipase C and protein kinase C, also known to disrupt these sodium channels (34).

Aspiration

Similar disruption of the lung barrier is noted with aspiration of gastric contents. ☞ **The severity of alveolar epithelial injury following gastric aspiration is a consequ-ence of both the volume and acidity of the aspirate.** ☞ Quantities as small as 30 mL in an adult with a pH less than 2.5 are adequate to induce ALI (35). ALI/ARDS animal studies routinely use a standard protocol with hydrochloric acid solutions. There is a biphasic lung injury. First, the direct caustic effect injures the barrier integrity, becoming evident in minutes. Hours later, a systemic response may develop (36). The sterility of gastric contents under normal conditions likely explains the findings that only one-third of those aspirating develop clinical symptoms. Even fewer patients progress to ALI/ARDS (37).

Trauma and Burns

Patients exposed to direct thoracic trauma will develop variable degrees of pulmonary contusions (disruptions of alveolar-capillary barrier in all areas of contusion), lacerations, etc. This direct injury may occur concomitantly with other direct lung insults (e.g., aspiration, smoke inhalation, etc.). Later, in the course of their illness, these patients may be exposed to additional direct injuries (e.g., bacterial colonization and ventilator-associated pneumonia) as well as a multitude of indirect insults (e.g., sepsis, hemorrhagic shock, and fluid overload) discussed below. The magnitude of the direct lung injury is related to the impact of the trauma, but also to the condition of the lung prior to the injury. Patients with low serum albumin, liver disease, coagulopathy, or sepsis, prior to the direct injury, suffer more severe ALI/ARDS for similar degrees of trauma. In the case of burn trauma, patients may suffer direct lung injury from smoke inhalation, as well as secondary lung injury from the systemic manifestations of thermal injury (see Volume 1, Chapter 34). The special pulmonary considerations related to lung trauma are discussed in far greater detail in Volume 2, Chapter 25.

Indirect Lung Injury

Sepsis

In both pulmonary and extrapulmonary infections, the initial response to a localized infection is a systemic release of endotoxins or exotoxins, inducing macrophages to generate inflammatory cytokines, termed innate immunity. The occurrence of ARDS in sepsis is a marker of an exaggerated inflammatory response that overwhelms the capacity of the immune system to balance between pro- and anti-inflammatory factors (also see Volume 2, Chapter 47 on Sepsis and Volume 2, Chapter 63 on SIRS).

Early on, alveolar macrophages, the first line of cellular defense, generate inflammatory cytokines [tissue necrosis factor-alpha (TNF-α), interleukin 1-beta (IL-1β), interleukin-6 (IL-6), and chemokines similar to interleukin-8 (IL-8)] as well as consuming, processing, and presenting foreign elements (38). This initial response activates and attracts polymorphonuclear neutrophils (PMNs) to the site of infection or

injury. Additionally, there is a systemic response through the stimulation of blood monocytes (releasing and transcribing more cytokines, growth factors, and chemokines) and endothelial cells (activating the coagulation cascade). Growth factors, such as granulocyte colony-stimulating factor, augment the production of neutrophils, whereas chemokines attract them to the peripheral organs (39).

Once activated, the PMNs, the second cellular line, express integrins that act as mediators for sequestration on small capillaries, for adhesion to endothelial cells and for migration across barriers (39). At the same time, the endothelium is stimulated to express surface receptors for adhesion of PMNs that will cross the alveolar-capillary membrane. These PMNs can release toxic products including reactive oxygen species and proteolytic enzymes that can increase endothelial permeability and alveolar epithelial damage (40). In the presence of bacteria or other foreign organisms, the PMNs assist macrophages in the process of phagocytosis and antigen presentation.

The third cell line of immunity involved in the acute response is the type II pneumocyte. These cells produce cytokines, complement growth factors, plus they express adhesion molecules and secrete several surfactant proteins (41). Some of the surfactant proteins participate in the recognition of nonself patterns, such as the gram-positive lipoteichoic acid molecule and opsonize for antigen presentation (42). Injury to the pneumocytes may be the result of PMNs producing proteolytic enzymes and reactive oxygen species in the alveoli, resulting in worse alveolar-capillary permeability and impairing edema fluid removal (43).

Endothelial cells stimulated by TNF-α and IL-1β, activate coagulation. The trigger is the expression of tissue factor (TF), a transmembrane cell surface receptor similar to a cytokine receptor. Concurrently, the endothelial cell-bound pool of TF pathway inhibitor is depleted. This leads to the formation of thrombin and fibrin clot. The procoagulant thrombin is also capable of stimulating inflammatory pathways and further suppressing the endogenous fibrinolytic system (43). These same activated endothelial cells release platelet-activating factor leading to platelet aggregation (44). The combination of systemic inflammatory cytokines and thrombin can impair the endogenous fibrinolytic pathway resulting in obstruction, injury to small capillaries, tissue hypoxia, and alveolar injury. The compromised epithelial barrier facilitates alveolar flooding.

Hemorrhagic Shock

Massive hemorrhage impacts distal alveolar fluid clearance. With acute blood loss of greater than 30% blood volume, there is a sharp rise in plasma epinephrine leading to a doubling of alveolar fluid clearance. Similar to early sepsis, elevated epinephrine levels upregulate the epithelial fluid transport capacity. However, prolongation of either the hemorrhagic or septic shock state results in the inability to up-regulate alveolar fluid clearance, despite an intact epithelial barrier. This process probably requires both neutrophils and macrophages that trigger a systemic cascade that alters adrenergic activity and increases the release of oxidant radicals. Expression of nitric oxide synthase leads to the release of nitric oxide, further impairing the function of sodium channels and alveolar fluid transport. The mechanisms may explain part of the susceptibility to alveolar flooding after major trauma (34). Additionally, circulatory inflammatory cytokines (either released from the trauma that caused the blood loss or from blood and blood products during transfusion) can cause pulmonary capillaries to begin leaking fluid.

Massive alveolar and interstitial edema may also result from the administration of large quantities of resuscitation fluids. Also, patients who start out with low serum albumen or liver disease are more prone to ALI. Finally, patients may manifest secondary injury following massive trauma or burns due to the circulating inflammatory cytokines (see Volume 1, Chapter 34 and Volume 2, Chapter 63).

Resolution Phase
Fluid Clearance
For alveolar edema to be actively reabsorbed several factors must be overcome. Reversal of hypoxia is required. There appears to be a hypoxia-induced decrease in alveolar fluid clearance caused in part by fewer sodium transport proteins being inserted into the alveolar epithelial membranes (45). Also, mechanical ventilation–induced stretch injury in type I epithelial cells must be minimized. Lower tidal volumes are protective to both epithelial and endothelial cells and allow faster alveolar fluid clearance (46).

Another significant factor in the resolution of alveolar edema is the active ion transport of sodium and chloride from the alveoli to the interstitium. This is both catecholamine-dependent and independent. Water fluxes passively via aquaporins, epithelial water channels (47). Fluid clearance may be apparent within hours of the acute phase onset and directly correlates with improved survival and shorter duration of mechanical ventilation. Impairment of alveolar fluid clearance defined as rates of less than 14% per hour, correlate with worse outcome in ALI/ARDS patients (Fig. 2) (14).

Protein Clearance
In severe alveolar epithelial injury, repair of the barrier does not occur normally. The alveoli are filled with mesenchymal cells and their by-products, collagen precursors, as well as hyaline membranes and cellular debris. Within the first week, a fibrotic process stimulated in part by IL-1β is well under way (48).

Effective removal of these insoluble proteins by the epithelial cells occurs by endocytosis and transcytosis (49). This process limits the extent of hyaline membrane composition and fibrous tissue networking. Soluble proteins diffuse between epithelial cells. Meanwhile, previously

activated PMNs and other inflammatory cells appear to undergo programmed cell death, apoptosis (50). Overactivation of the apoptotic cascade may contribute to on-going leakage of proteins, whereas inadequate apoptosis may impair removal of activated cells (51).

Remodeling
The type II pneumocyte is the progenitor for re-epithelialization of denuded alveoli. Proliferation and differentiation into type I cells restores the epithelial integrity, a process that is controlled, in part, by keratinocyte and other growth factors (52).

EVIDENCE-BASED TREATMENT

The mainstay of treatment is to stabilize the respiratory failure using mechanical ventilation, search aggressively for and treat reversible etiologies, and administer supportive care (41). Approaches to therapies have followed the theories regarding the pathogenesis of lung injury.

Mechanical Ventilation and Gas Exchange Mechanisms
Mechanical ventilation in patients suffering from ALI/ARDS has evolved over the past decade. ☞ **Since the early 1990s, consensus statements began recommending lower tidal volume ventilation and airway pressures allowing for permissive hypercapnia and hypoxemia (53).** ☞ The strategy was based on growing awareness of ventilator-induced lung injury, probably a consequence of cyclic opening and closing of atelectatic lung zones that trigger an inflammatory cascade (54). This therapeutic approach was definitively supported by the publication of the National Institutes of Health (NIH)/National Heart Lung and Blood Institute (NHLBI) ARDS Network Ventilation Protocol (Table 5) (21). The study compared ventilation with lower tidal volumes (6 mL/kg predicted body weight and plateau pressures <30 cm H_2O) to traditional tidal volumes (12 mL/kg

Table 5 National Institutes of Health/National Heart Lung and Blood Institute Acute Respiratory Distress Syndrome (ARDS) Network Lower Tidal Volume Ventilation for Acute Lung Injury/ARDS Protocol Summary

Variables	Protocol
Ventilator mode	Volume assist-control
Tidal volume	<6 mL/kg predicted body weight
Plateau pressure	<30 cm H_2O
Ventilation set rate/pH goal	6–35/min, adjusted to achieve arterial pH > 7.30 if possible
Inspiratory flow, I:E	Adjust flow to achieve I:E ratio of 1.1–1.3
Oxygenation goal	55 mm Hg < PaO_2 or 88% < SpO_2
F_iO_2/PEEP (mmHg) combinations	0.3/5, 0.4/5, 0.4/8, 0.5/8, 0.5/10, 0.6/10, 0.7/10, 0.7/12, 0.7/14, 0.8/14, 0.9/14, 0.9/16, 0.9/18, 1.0/18, 1.0/22, 1.0/24
Discontinuation	Attempts to wean by pressure support required when F_iO_2/PEEP < 0.4/8

Abbreviations: F_iO_2, fraction of inspired oxygen; I:E, inhalation to exhalation ratio; PaO_2, partial pressure of oxygen in the arterial blood; PEEP, positive end-expiratory pressure.

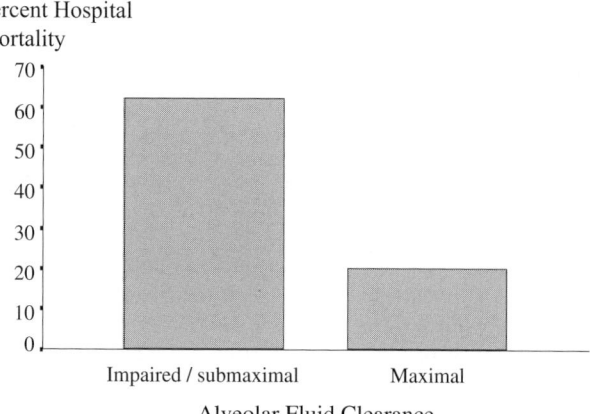

Percent Hospital Mortality

Alveolar Fluid Clearance

Figure 2 Percent hospital mortality versus alveolar fluid clearance in patients with acute lung injury and acute respiratory distress syndrome. Maximal clearance >14%/hr; impaired/submaximal <14%/hr.

and pressures <50 cm H_2O). ☞ **The critical finding of the NIH/NHLBI study was a 22% reduction in mortality using the lung protective strategy, regardless of the clinical etiology (55).** ☞ The number of patients needed to be treated with this strategy, to prevent one death from ARDS, was 12.5 patients (21). The strategy was effective in patients with different clinical risk factors for ALI/ARDS (55).

The relationship of F_IO_2 to oxygen-induced lung injury is not clearly understood. A F_IO_2 <0.6 has been considered safe (56). PEEP may allow for lower F_IO_2 levels by increasing functional residual capacity and reducing trans-pulmonary shunt (57). However, excessive PEEP may worsen cardiac output, increase pulmonary hypertension, and increase alveolar dead space. Correction of oxygenation deficits usually require a balance of F_IO_2 and PEEP. The protocol above, adjusts the F_IO_2 and PEEP by using a sliding scale (Table 5) (58). A follow-up trial by the ARDS Network reported that higher levels of PEEP did not have an additional value in reducing mortality, although this subsequent trial reported a further decrease in mortality to 27% with the 6 mL/kg low tidal volume strategy (Table 5) (59).

Despite maximal F_IO_2 and PEEP, patients may suffer refractory hypoxemia. Definitive trials have explored both extracorporeal membrane oxygenation (ECMO) and extracorporeal carbon dioxide removal ($EC_{CO_2}R$) to counter the seemingly irreversible gas exchange (60,61). ECMO optimizes oxygenation through extrinsic circulation, whereas $EC_{CO_2}R$ normalizes $PaCO_2$ via filtration, thereby decreasing the amount of ventilator support and subsequent associated lung injury. Neither technique has demonstrated improvements, beyond standard mechanical ventilation and supportive care, in the adult trauma population.

Reversal of Underlying Etiology
Infectious Foci
Identifying and reversing an underlying cause may reduce mortality. Particular attention should focus on infection that is responsive to antibiotics and/or surgical intervention as well as the prevention of nosocomial infection (41). Empiric antibiotics should be based on hospital antimicrobial sensitivities.

Activated Protein C
☞ **Patients suffering from severe sepsis and ALI/ARDS should be considered for the administration of recombinant human activated protein C.** ☞ Activated Protein C is an inhibitor of both the procoagulant and the inflammatory cascades that reduces absolute mortality by 6.1% in severe sepsis (62). The Food and Drug Administration (FDA) performed a subgroup analysis of the original trial. It indicates that the greatest benefit is observed in patients with Acute Physiology and Chronic Health Evaluation II scores >25 (63). Recommended activated protein C dosing is a 24 mcg/kg/hr infusion for 96 hours.

Insulin Therapy
Intensive insulin therapy (blood glucose kept between 80–110 mg/dL by exogenous insulin infusion) has been shown to improve outcomes in critically ill surgical patients and in some medical patients when admitted to the ICU beyond three days (64). Optimal blood glucose levels and most at risk patient populations are still being determined (64). Also see Volume 2, Chapter 60 for an expanded discussion of this topic.

Supportive Care
Hemodynamics
Hemodynamic management remains a controversial issue. Current recommendations are to restore intravascular volume to achieve euvolemia and reverse hypotension. This can be approximated by a central venous pressure of 6–12 mmHg or pulmonary capillary wedge pressure of 6–14 mmHg in patients with normal hearts and relatively mild ALI. However, patients with severe ARDS and/or pulmonary hypertension may require higher filling pressures to achieve appropriate cardiac outputs and systemic pressures [especially if higher levels of PEEP or inversed inhalation to exhalation (I:E) ratios are employed]. Accordingly, titrating filling pressures to a more physiologic endpoint, for example, stroke volume of at least 1 mL/kg, is pursued. Vasopressors are added to maintain a mean arterial pressure greater than 60 mmHg or higher. The attainment of supranormal oxygen delivery does not provide an outcome benefit (65). Instead, the clinician is guided by clinical indexes of organ perfusion (65). Currently, the NIH ARDS Clinical Trials Network is completing a large multicenter trial of 1000 patients, to evaluate a conservative versus a liberal fluid strategy guided by either a central venous or pulmonary artery catheter measurements in ALI/ARDS patients.

Nutrition
An additional important supportive measure is early enteral nutrition using standard nutritional formulations. Using the patient's own gastrointestinal system for caloric and nutrient administration serves the dual purpose of preserving the gut barrier (an implicated source of ARDS when impaired) and allowing for nutrition to be delivered without the infection risks of total parental nutrition (see Volume 2, Chapters 47 and 49). When enteral feeding is contraindicated (e.g., small bowel obstruction), critically ill patients should receive nutrition parenterally. Nutritional goals should balance the metabolic demand and the prevention of nutrient deficiencies with complications of delivery mode and overfeeding (66). Metabolic charts can be used to measure oxygen consumption and CO_2 production and can help guide caloric needs (see Volume 2, Chapter 31).

Pharmaceutical Interventions
Inhaled Nitric Oxide
Nitric oxide, a potent, short-acting pulmonary vasodilator, can be delivered directly to the pulmonary vasculature by inhalation with resultant reduction in pulmonary vascular resistance and improved oxygenation. Improved oxygenation occurs when the blood vessels associated with well-ventilated alveolar are vasoditated by the inhaled nitric oxide (INO). However, the pulmonary vasoditation dose of INO (20–60 ppm) is much higher than the dose recommended for improving $\dot{V}/\dot{Q}$ mismatch (<1 ppm). When higher concentrations of INO are employed, not only the vessels associated with the well-ventilated alveoli are dilated, but so too are the adjacent blood vessels (some of which are poorly ventilated), causing $\dot{V}/\dot{Q}$ mismatch and oxygenation impairment. Furthermore, INO has no clinical mortality benefit nor does it seem to reduce the duration of mechanical ventilation (67). Thus, INO is no longer widely used for ARDS but, rather, is used in rare individual cases.

Surfactant
Supplemental treatment with surfactant for ALI/ARDS has been driven by the successful application in neonatal

pulmonary failure. Surfactant reduces wall stress across the alveoli, thereby reducing potential stretch injury. To date, however, replacement strategies with aerosolized exogenous surfactant have only resulted in transient clinical benefits in ALI/ARDS (68,69). However, as part of a multimodal therapeutic regimen, surfactant may have some merit, but these studies are yet to be performed.

Glucocorticoids

Recognition of the inflammatory nature of ALI/ARDS has prompted interest in glucocorticoid therapy. There has been no convincing outcome benefit in early nor late course ALI/ARDS (70). A recently completed NHLBI, ARDS Network randomized clinical trial showed no mortality benefit in patients treated with glucocorticoid (71).

Antioxidants

Intrinsic antioxidants or oxygen free-radical scavengers play a role in mediating endothelial injury caused by reactive oxygen species. Scavengers interrupt parts of the neutrophil-mediated inflammatory cascade. Encouraging results in phase II clinical trials utilizing procysteine, one such scavenger, have been tempered by a placebo-controlled trial failing to show significant benefit (41).

Conservative Fluid Management

A recent randomized clinical trial demonstrated a significant increase in ventilator-free days with a fluid conservative versus a fluid liberal strategy for patients with acute lung injury. After patients had been treated so that they were no longer in shock (did not require vasopressors for 12 hours), they were randomized to a fluid liberal or fluid conservative strategy. The fluid conservative strategy, which included fluid restriction and diuretic therapy to reduce pulmonary vascular pressures, was successful in improving oxygenation, reducing airway pressures, and decreasing the duration of positive pressure ventilation (72).

β2-Adrenergic Agonists

More recently, there is interest in pharmaceutical strategies that accelerate removal of pulmonary edema (73). In the intact epithelial barrier, β2-agonists can stimulate the resolution of edema and surfactant secretion. When given prophylactically, salmeterol, a long-acting β2-agonist, reduces high-altitude pulmonary edema (74). Clinical trial will be done to test the value of this therapy in ALI/ARDS by The ARDS Network.

EYE TO THE FUTURE
Targeting Epithelial Growth Factors

Ultimately, effective lung function depends on the reconstruction of the alveolar unit. Growth factors modulate alveolar epithelial function and enhance its repair; in particular, keratinocyte and hepatocyte growth factors. These growth factors serve as mitogens of type II alveolar epithelial cells. Coupled with this cellular proliferation is improved alveolar fluid clearance (75). Intratracheally administered, these growth factors decrease the severity of injury in animal models challenged with caustic agents. Clinical trials are anticipated.

β2-Adrenergic Agonist

As already discussed, β2-adrenergic agonist therapy may be effective as a treatment to enhance the resolution of alveolar edema and to decrease lung endothelial injury (37,73,76). Clinical trials are needed to test this possibility.

Applied Genomics in Screening and Therapeutics

Predicting an individual patient's susceptibility to certain microorganisms or their clinical response to medications, particularly antibiotics, is now a major research focus. The completion of the Human Genome Project has modified the fundamental paradigm of a "reaction" to illness, to "screening, predicting, and preventing" illness. This paradigm includes the critically ill. The future intensivist may have the ability to identify patients who have an unchecked inflammatory cascade in response to an infectious organism like *Pseudomonas* and host DNA-sequence variations to choose the most efficacious anti-*Pseudomonal* therapy (77,78). A recent NHLBI conference summarized several future directions that are needed to advance basic and clinical research in ALI/ARDS (79).

SUMMARY

The simplified definition of ALI/ARDS (Table 1), has allowed for considerable progress in understanding the epidemiology of ALI/ARDS as well as conducting clinical trials. Advances in delineating the pathogenesis have revealed new leads into the potential role of targeted therapies that interrupt or redirect the procoagulant and inflammatory cascades, such as activated protein C, insulin, and glucocorticoids. However, reversal of the underlying infectious process and institution of supportive care measures remain paramount.

Finally and most importantly, there is now a lung-protective ventilator strategy using low tidal volumes, which reduces mortality (Table 5). These combined efforts are a direct result of the creation of and support from, the NIH ARDS Network (21). Forthcoming trials hope to clarify optimal volume status, the role of invasive monitoring, and therapies that target the repair of the alveolar unit and the resolution of pulmonary edema in lung injury.

KEY POINTS

- Both ALI and ARDS can result from a multitude of disorders (Table 2) with the common thread being injury to the epithelial capillary barrier of lung alveoli.
- Because of the frequency of associated septic conditions, infectious foci must be actively pursued and treated in ARDS patients.
- The acute exudative phase is a consequence of widespread protein-rich alveolar edema.
- Alveolar flooding results in significant transpulmonary shunting and ventilation-perfusion ($\dot{V}/\dot{Q}$) imbalance causing profound hypoxemia that is refractory to supplemental oxygen.
- Some patients recover from the acute insult without sequelae; however, most progress to a subacute fibrosing alveolitis phase.
- Postextubation pulmonary function testing among ALI/ARDS survivors shows restrictive impairments and diffusion abnormalities.

☛ The release of inflammatory mediators into the systemic circulation amplifies the injury to both nonpulmonary organs as well as the lung itself, a process referred to as innate immunity.

☛ The bacteria-causing pneumonia (particularly those associated with ALI/ARDS) possess a variety of virulence factors disruptive to alveolar epithelial cells.

☛ The severity of alveolar epithelial injury following gastric aspiration is a consequence of both the volume and acidity of the aspirate.

☛ Since the early 1990s, consensus statements began recommending lower tidal volume ventilation and airway pressures allowing for permissive hypercapnia and hypoxemia.

☛ The critical finding of the NIH/NHLBI study was a 22% reduction in mortality using the lung protective strategy, regardless of the clinical etiology.

☛ Patients suffering from severe sepsis and ALI/ARDS should be considered for the administration of recombinant human activated protein C.

☛ There does appear to be a survival benefit of one in seven when steroids are used as an adjuvant in hypotensive septic patients suffering from "relative" adrenal insufficiency.

REFERENCES

1. Ashbaugh DG, Bigelow DB, Petty TL, et al. Acute respiratory distress in adults. Lancet 1967; ii:319–323.
2. Bernard GR, Artigas A, Brigham K, et al. The American-European consensus conference on ARDS. Am J Respir Crit Care Med 1994; 149:818–824.
3. Murray JF, Matthay MA, Luce JM, et al. An expanded definition of the adult respiratory distress syndrome. Am Rev Respir Dis 1988; 138:720–723.
4. Meade MO, Guyatt GH, Cook RJ, et al. Agreement between alternative classifications of acute respiratory distress syndrome. Am J Respir Crit Care Med 2001; 163:490–493.
5. Abraham E, Matthay MA, Dinarello CA, et al. Consensus conference definitions for sepsis, septic shock, acute lung injury, and acute respiratory distress syndrome: time for reevaluation. Crit Care Med 2000; 28:232–235.
6. Hudson LD, Steinberg KP. Epidemiology of acute lung injury and ARDS. Chest 1999; 116:74S–82S.
7. Rubenfeld G, Caldwell E, Peabody E, et al. Incidence and outcomes of acute lung injury. N Engl J Med 2005; 353:1685–1693.
8. Atabai K, Matthay MA. Acute lung injury and the acute respiratory distress syndrome: definitions and epidemiology. Thorax 2002; 57:452–458.
9. Doyle RL, Szaflarski N, Modin GW, et al. Identification of patients with acute lung injury predictors of mortality. Am J Respir Crit Care Med 1995; 152:1818–1824.
10. Bell RC, Coalson JJ, Smith JD, et al. Multiple organ system failure and infection in adult respiratory distress syndrome. Ann Intern Med 1983; 99:293–298.
11. Moss M, Bucher B, Moore FA, et al. The role of chronic alcohol abuse in the development of acute respiratory distress syndrome in adults. JAMA 1996; 275:50–54.
12. Moss M, Guidot DM, Steinberg KP, et al. Diabetic patients have a decreased incidence of acute respiratory distress syndrome. Crit Care Med 2000; 28:2187–2192.
13. Nuckton TJ, Alonso JA, Kallet RH, et al. Pulmonary dead-space fraction as a risk factor for death in acute respiratory distress syndrome. N Engl J Med 2002; 346:1281–1286.
14. Ware LB, Matthay MA. Alveolar fluid clearance is impaired in the majority of patients with acute lung injury and the acute respiratory distress syndrome. Am J Respir Crit Care Med 2001; 163:1376–1383.
15. Abel SJC, Finney SJ, Brett SJ, et al. Reduced mortality in association with the acute respiratory distress syndrome. Thorax 1998; 53:292–294.
16. Matthay MA. Pathophysiology of pulmonary edma. Clin Chest Med 1985; 6:301–314.
17. Bachofen M, Weibel ER. Alterations of the gas exchange apparatus in adult respiratory insufficiency associated with septicemia. Am Rev Respir Dis 1977; 116:589–615.
18. Aberle DR, Wiener-Kronish JP, Webb WR, Matthay MA. Hydrostatic versus increased permeability pulmonary edema: diagnosis based on radiographic criteria in critically ill patients. Radiology 1988; 168:73–79.
19. Goodman LR. Congestive heart failure and adult respiratory distress syndrome: new insights using computed tomography. Radiol Clin North Am 1996; 34:33–46.
20. Dantzker DR. Gas exchange in the adult respiratory distress syndrome. Clin Chest Med 1982; 3:57–67.
21. http://www.ardsnet.org, ARDS Network: Ventilation with low tidal volumes as compared with traditional tidal volumes for acute lung injury and the acute respiratory distress syndrome. N Engl J Med 2000; 342:1301–1308.
22. Weg JG, Anzueto A, Balk RA, et al. The relation of pneumothorax and other air leaks to mortality in the acute respiratory distress syndrome. N Engl J Med 1998; 338:341–346.
23. Matthay MA, Broaddus VC. Fluid and hemodynamic management in acute lung injury. Semin Respir Crit Care Med 1994; 15:271–288.
24. Markowicz P, Wolff M, Djedaini K, et al. Multicenter prospective study of ventilator-associated pneumonia during acute respiratory distress syndrome. Incidence, prognosis, and risk factors. ARDS Study Group. Am J Respir Crit Care Med 2000; 161:1942–1948.
25. George DL, Falk PS, Wunderink RG, et al. Epidemiology of ventilator-acquired pneumonia based on protected bronchoscopic sampling. Am J Respir Crit Care Med 1998; 157:1839–1847.
26. Martin TR. Recognition of bacterial endotoxin in the lungs. Am J Respir Cell Mol Biol 2000; 23:128–132.
27. Chastre J, Fagon JY. Ventilator-associated pneumonia. Am J Respir Crit Care Med 2002; 165:867–903.
28. Herridge MS, Cheung AM, Tansey CM, et al. One-year outcome in survivors of the acute respiratory distress syndrome. N Engl J Med 2003; 348:683–693.
29. Angus DC, Musthafa AA, Clermont G, et al. Quality-adjusted survival in the first year after the acute respiratory distress syndrome. Am J Respir Crit Care Med 2001; 163:1389–1394.
30. Kurahashi K, Kajikawa O, Sawa T, et al. Pathogenesis of septic shock in pseudomonas aeruginosa pneumonia. J Clin Invest 1999; 104:743–750.
31. Lindberg AA. Polyosides (encapsulated bacteria). C R Acad Sci III 1999; 322:925–932.
32. Chan PF, Foster SJ. Role of SarA in virulence determinant production and environmental signal transduction in Staphylococcus aureus. J Bacteriol 1998; 80:6232–6241.
33. Ginsberg I. Role of lipoteichoic acid in infection and inflammation. Lancet Infect Dis 2002; 2:171–179.
34. Matthay MA, Folkesson HG, Clerici C. Lung epithelial fluid transport and the resolution of pulmonary edema. Physiol Rev 2002; 82:569–600.
35. Marik PE. Aspiration pneumonitis and aspiration pneumonia. N Engl J Med 2001; 344:665–670.
36. Kennedy TP, Johnson KJ, Kunkel RG, et al. Acute acid aspiration lung injury in the rat: biphasic pathogenesis. Anesth Analg 1989; 69:87–92.
37. Warner MA, Warner ME, Weber JG. Clinical significance of pulmonary aspiration during the perioperative period. Anesthesiology 1993; 78:56–62.
38. Parrillo JE. Pathogenetic mechanisms of septic shock. N Engl J Med 1993; 328:1471–1477.
39. Doerschuk CM. Mechanisms of leukocyte sequestration in inflamed lungs. Microcirculation 2001; 8:71–88.

40. Lee WL, Downey GP. Neutrophil activation and acute lung injury. Curr Opin Crit Care 2001; 7:1–7.
41. Ware LB, Matthay MA. The acute respiratory distress syndrome. N Engl J Med 2000; 342:1334–1349.
42. Ginsberg I. Role of lipoteichoic acid in infection and inflammation. Lancet Infect Dis 2002; 2:171–179.
43. Gunther A, Mosavi P, Heinemann S, et al. Alveolar fibrin formation caused by enhanced pro-coagulant and depressed fibrinolytic capacities in severe pneumonia. Comparison with the acute respiratory distress syndrome. Am J Respir Crit Care Med 2000; 161:454–462.
44. Zimmerman GA, McIntyre TM, Prescott SM, et al. The platelet-activating factor signaling system and its regulators in syndromes of inflammation and thrombosis. Crit Care Med 2002; 30:S294–S301.
45. Planes C, Blot-Chabaud M, Matthay MA, Couette S, Uchida T, Clerici C. Hypoxia and beta 2-agonists regulate cell surface expression of the epithelial sodium channel in native alveolar epithelial cells. J Biol Chem 2002; 277(49):47318–47324.
46. Frank JA, Gutierrez JA, Jones KD, et al. Low tidal volume reduces epithelial and endothelial injury in acid-injured rat lungs. Am J Respir Crit Care Med 2002; 165:242–249.
47. Matthay MA, Folkesson HG, Verkman AS. Salt and water transport across alveolar and distal airway epithelia in the adult lung. Am J Physiol 1996; 270:L487–L503.
48. Martinet Y, Menard O, Vaillant P, et al. Cytokines in human lung fibrosis. Arch Toxicol Suppl 1996; 18:127–139.
49. Folkesson HG, Matthay MA, Westrom BR, et al. Alveolar epithelial clearance of protein. J Appl Physiol 1996; 80:1431–1435.
50. Matute-Bello G, Liles WC, Radella F II, et al. Neutrophil apoptosis in the acute respiratory distress syndrome. Am J Respir Crit Care Med 1997; 156:1969–1977.
51. Albertine KH, Soulier MF, Wang Z, et al. Fas and Fas ligand are up-regulated in pulmonary edema fluid and lung tissue of patients with acute lung injury and the acute respiratory distress syndrome. Am J Pathol 2002; 161:1783–1796.
52. Folkesson HG, Nitenberg G, Oliver BL, et al. Upregulation of alveolar epithelial fluid transport after sub-acute lung injury in rats from bleomycin. Am J Physiol 1998; 275:L478–L490.
53. Esteban A, Anzueto A, Alia I, et al. How is mechanical ventilation employed in the intensive care unit? Am J Respir Crit Care Med 2000; 161:1450–1458.
54. Dreyfuss D, Soler P, Basset G, et al. High inflation pressure pulmonary edema: respective effects of high airway pressure, high tidal volume, and positive end-expiratory pressure. Am Rev Respir Dis 1988; 137:1159–1164.
55. Eisner MD, Thompson T, Hudson LD, et al. Efficacy of low tidal volume ventilation in patients with different clinical risk factors for acute lung injury and the acute respiratory distress syndrome. Am J Respir Crit Care Med 2001; 164:231–236.
56. Albert RK. Least PEEP: primum non nocere [editorial]. Chest 1985; 87:2–4.
57. Falke KJ, Pontoppidan H, Kumar A, et al. Ventilation with end-expiratory pressure in acute lung disease. J Clin Invest 1972; 51:2315–2323.
58. Brower RG, Ware LB, Berthiaume Y, et al. Treatment of ARDS. Chest 2001; 120:1347–1367.
59. ARDS Clinical Trials Network. Higher versus lower positive end-expiratory pressures in patients with the acute respiratory distress syndrome. N Engl J Med 2004; 351(4):327–336.
60. Zapol WM, Snider MT, Hill JD, et al. Extracorporeal membrane oxygenation in severe acute respiratory distress failure. A randomized prospective study. JAMA 1979; 242:2193–2196.
61. Morris AH, Wallace CJ, Menlove RL, et al. Randomized clinical trial of pressure-controlled inverse ratio ventilation and extra-corporeal CO_2 removal for adult respiratory distress syndrome. Am J Respir Crit Care Med 1994; 149:295–305.
62. Bernard GR, Vincent J-L, Laterre P-F, et al., for the Recombinant Human Activated Protein C Worldwide Evaluation in Severe Sepsis (PROWESS) Study Group. Efficacy and safety of recombinant human activated protein C for severe sepsis. N Engl J Med 2001; 344:699–709.
63. Manns BJ, Lee H, Doig CJ, et al. An economic evaluation of activated protein C treatment for severe sepsis. N Engl J Med 2002; 347:993–1000.
64. Van den Berg G, Wilmer A, Hermans G, et al. Intensive insulin therapy in the medical ICU. N Engl J Med 2006; 354:449–461.
65. Hayes MA, Timmins AC, Yau EHS, et al. Elevation of systemic oxygen delivery in the treatment of critically ill patients. N Engl J Med 1994; 330:1717–1722.
66. Cerra FB, Benitez MR, Blackburn GL, et al. Applied nutrition in ICU patients, a consensus statement of the american college of chest physicians. Chest 1997; 111:769–778.
67. Payen D, Vallet B, Genoa Group. Results of the French prospective multicentric randomized double-blind placebo-controlled trial on inhaled nitric oxide in ARDS. Intensive Care Med 1999; 25(suppl):S166 [abstract].
68. Anzueto A, Baughman RP, Guntupalli KK, et al. Aerosolized surfactant in adults with sepsis-induced acute respiratory distress syndrome. N Engl J Med 1996; 334:1417–1421.
69. Spragg RG, Lewis JF, Walmrath HD, et al. Effect of recombinant surfactant protein C-based surfactant on the acute respiratory distress syndrome. N Engl J Med 2004; 351(9):884–892.
70. Luce JM, Montogomery AB, Marks JD, et al. Ineffectiveness of high-dose methylprednisolone in preventing parenchymal lung injury and improving mortality in patients with septic shock. Am Rev Respir Dis 1988; 136:62–68.
71. ARDS Network. Efficacy and safety of corticosteroids for persistent acute respiratory distress syndrome. N Engl J Med 2006; 354:1671–1684.
72. ARDS Network. Comparison of two fluid-management strategies in acute lung injury. N Engl J Med 2006; 354:2564–2575.
73. Berthiaume Y, Lesur O, Dagenais A. Treatment of adult respiratory distress syndrome: plea for the rescue therapy of alveolar epithelium. Thorax 1999; 54:150–160.
74. Sartori C, Allemann Y, Duplain H, Salmeterol for the prevention of high-altitude pulmonary edema. N Engl J Med 2002; 346:1631–1636.
75. Wang Y, Folkesson HG, Jayr C, Ware LB, Matthay MA. Alveolar epithelial fluid transport can be simultaneously upregulated by both KGF and beta-agonist therapy. J Appl Physiol 1999; 87:1852–1860.
76. McAuley DF, Frank JA, Fang X, Matthay MA. Clinically relevant concentrations of beta2-adrenergic agonists stimulate maximal cyclic adenosine monophosphate-dependent airspace fluid clearance and decrease pulmonary edema in experimental acid-induced lung injury. Crit Care Med 2004; 32(7):1470–1476.
77. Khoury MJ, McCabe LL, McCabe ERB. Population screening in the age of genomic medicine. N Engl J Med 2003; 348:50–58.
78. Weinshilboum R. Inheritance and drug response. N Engl J Med 2003; 348:529–537.
79. Matthay MA, Zimmerman GA, Esmon C, et al. Future research directions in acute lung injury: summary of a National Heart, Lung, and Blood Institute working group. Am J Respir Crit Care Med 2003; 167(7):1027–1035.

25

Critical Care Considerations Following Chest Trauma

Judith C. F. Hwang
Department of Anesthesiology, UC Davis Medical Center, Sacramento, California, U.S.A.

Eric R. Amador and Leland H. Hanowell
Department of Anesthesia, Stanford University Medical Center, Stanford, California, U.S.A.

INTRODUCTION

Injuries to the chest are often serious, resulting in significant morbidity and prolonged stays in the intensive care unit (ICU). Several reasons account for the serious and debilitating nature of these injuries. First, trauma significant enough to injure internal organs, protected by the semirigid bony thorax, is typically quite severe. Second, the organs contained within the thoracic cavity (i.e., heart and lungs) are required for survival, and when these vital structures are injured, the flow of oxygenated blood to the systemic tissues is impaired. Third, although small, solitary stab wounds may damage only a single organ or structure within the thoracic cavity (e.g., intercostal artery, lobe of lung, etc.), blunt trauma and high-velocity missile injuries may destroy or injure large quantities of intrathoracic tissue and adjacent organ systems.

The acute resuscitative management and intraoperative care of thoracic wounds is discussed in Volume 1, Chapter 25, whereas this chapter provides an overview of the special ICU management considerations related to chest injuries. This review begins with a survey of the common mechanisms of lung and thoracic trauma, including both direct injury (see the section on direct trauma to the thorax) as well as indirect lung injury (see the section on, lung injury resulting from trauma-associated conditions). The acute lung injury and adult respiratory distress syndrome section briefly reviews the pathophysiology of acute lung injury (ALI) and the adult respiratory distress syndrome (ARDS) as these entities relate to trauma and trauma-associated pulmonary conditions. The mechanical ventilation considerations section provides a brief summary of mechanical ventilation considerations for thoracic trauma, and special analgesic techniques for thoracic trauma are surveyed in the acute lung injury and adult respiratory distress syndrome section. The chapter concludes with an eye to the future section that previews methods of pulmonary diagnosis, monitoring, and support.

DIRECT TRAUMA TO THE THORAX

Direct injuries to the lungs or thoracic structures may result from penetrating or blunt trauma. Major life-threatening injuries should be diagnosed and treated during the primary survey (Table 1). Although other critical injuries that are not immediately life-threatening are evaluated and treated during the secondary survey, there are multiple mechanisms for chest injury yielding pathophysiology unique to the particular injury, and requiring injury-specific interventions. The etiology of chest injury also bears upon the prognosis for successful resuscitation, intensive care management, and eventual recovery. For example, cardiopulmonary arrest in the field after blunt chest trauma has a much worse prognosis for recovery than transient arrest following a penetrating injury (1).

Penetrating Trauma

Penetrating chest trauma is increasingly common as urban unrest and regional conflicts escalate. These injuries may be temporized in the field and must be definitively managed in a trauma facility (Volume 1, Chapter 25). Penetrating chest trauma should always be considered a potentially lethal injury. However, if appropriately managed, even some victims arriving in profound shock can be rescued. ☞ **The most common etiologies of shock from penetrating chest injury include tension pneumothorax, massive hemothorax, cardiac wounds, and cardiac tamponade.** ☞

Stab wounds to the chest may present anywhere in the continuum between solitary peripheral injury to the chest wall, or lung injury requiring only a chest tube, versus severe hemorrhagic shock and death from injury to a great vessel, or one of the abovementioned common etiologies. These individual injuries are briefly discussed later in this chapter and more fully covered in Volume 1, Chapter 25. Stab wounds and other low-velocity penetrating chest injuries may injure only the internal mammary artery, or intercostal artery, and classically present with a slightly delayed onset of hemorrhagic shock. Resuscitative thoracotomy (Volume 1, Chapter 13) is indicated for patients presenting in extremis, or arrest following penetrating trauma.

Gunshot wounds (GSWs) and shrapnel injuries have a combination of blunt and penetrating trauma components, with a wide area of adjacent tissue at risk. ☞ **The magnitude of destruction resulting from the secondary shock wave occurring with high-velocity GSWs and shrapnel injuries may not be initially apparent.** ☞ Accordingly, GSWs and shrapnel injuries require sequential monitoring for progression of injury, and complete evaluation of all organs and tissues in proximity of the GSW or shrapnel injury. These injuries often require prolonged periods of mechanical ventilation and supportive care in the ICU. Specific injuries are discussed below.

Table 1   Thoracic Injuries that Should Be Detected During the Primary and Secondary Surveys

Injury category	Specific injury
Immediate threat to life— should be detected in primary survey	Airway obstruction
	Tension pneumothorax
	Open pneumothorax
	Flail chest
	Massive hemothorax
	Cardiac tamponade
Critical injuries— generally identified during secondary survey	Simple pneumothorax
	Hemothorax
	Pulmonary contusion
	Tracheobronchial disruption
	Myocardial contusion
	Aortic laceration
	Diaphragmatic rupture
	Wounds transversing the mediastinum

Source: Adapted from Ref. 201.

Blunt Trauma
Pulmonary Contusion

Pulmonary contusion accompanies deceleration injuries, blast wounds, crush injuries, and blows to the chest. It is often associated with bony trauma to the chest involving rib, scapula, thoracic spine and/or clavicle fracture. Contusion-induced lung dysfunction can be accompanied by bronchial or vascular disruption in the chest. Hemothorax due to chest wall or lung bleeding can compound the pulmonary dysfunction and also contribute to hemodynamic compromise in the chest trauma patient.

Lobar collapse and atelectasis frequently accompany pulmonary contusion. Atelectasis and collapse occur when aspirated secretions become inspissated in the airway. Aspiration is more common, following a lapse in consciousness. Additionally, secretions become increasingly difficult to clear from the airway in patients with an impaired ability to take deep breaths and cough (due to pain or flail chest). Impaired ventilation after lung contusion, particularly in those with chest wall fracture, can ultimately lead to respiratory failure. The respiratory failure results from decreased lung and chest wall compliance to increased right-to-left transpulmonary shunt (see below).

Compliance (C) is defined as volume/pressure, and is usually expressed in liters (or milliliters) per centimeter of water, that is, the volume of air moved by each centimeter of water pressure applied. The total respiratory compliance (C_T) may be diminished either via alterations in the chest wall compliance (C_{CW}), for example, in the patient with massive chest wall edema or eschar due to burn, or due to alterations in compliance of the lung (C_L) itself. However, the values are not merely additive. Rather, compliance is analogous to electrical capacitance. Accordingly, total compliance is calculated in a similar fashion to total capacitance for capacitors in series (the individual reciprocals are added to obtain the reciprocal of the total value), thus:

$$\frac{1}{C_T} = \frac{1}{C_L} + \frac{1}{C_{CW}}$$

Gastric distention associated with thoracoabdominal trauma may further impair pulmonary compliance, if severe and untreated. Gastroparesis can be treated with gastropropulsive drugs (i.e., erythromycin or metoclopromide) and by minimizing systemic opiates. Gastric distension is managed by nasogastric (NG) tube placement and intermittent gastric suction.

Hypoxemia and frank respiratory failure require airway instrumentation and mechanical ventilation. Bronchoscopy may be required to alleviate airway obstruction from inspissated secretions and blood. Additionally, bronchoscopy is required to assess for evidence of tracheal or bronchial disruption. After thoracic injury, an increase in right-to-left transpulmonary shunt occurs due to abnormalities of lung parenchyma from pulmonary contusion, atelectasis, pulmonary edema, or ARDS. This is reflected by a widening of the alveolar-arterial oxygen gradient. The factors affecting shunt fraction are reviewed in Volume 2, Chapter 2.

Dead-space ventilation may be markedly increased as well after thoracic injury, such as when pain after chest wall injury yields a state of rapid and shallow respiration, or when hypotension results in an increase in the extent to which alveoli are ventilated but not perfused. The factors increasing dead-space ventilation are further reviewed in Volume 2, Chapter 2.

Thoracostomy tube drainage is commonly required to eliminate collections of air, fluid, or blood from the chest cavity. Ideally, these procedures are done under strict sterile precautions; however, because of the emergency nature of such interventions, bacteria may enter the chest cavity resulting in the later development of empyema (Figs. 1 and 2). In our experience, empyema is rare following emergency thoracostomy. However, rarely, when infection and true empyema do develop, or the viscous fluids and coagulated blood in the chest do not drain well via thoracostomy tubes, open or thoracoscopic removal of these contents may be required.

Primary blast injury is a common mechanism of injury in urban warfare. Naturally, these patients are at high risk for

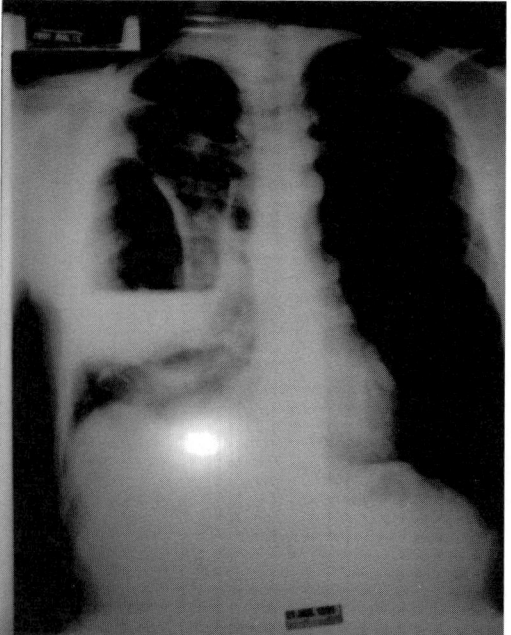

Figure 1   Radiographic appearance of empyema of the right chest.

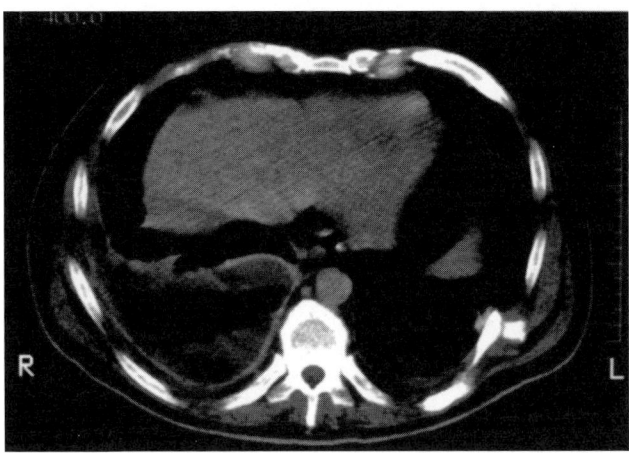

Figure 2 Computed tomograph demonstrating empyema in the right chest.

pulmonary contusion. Blast lung injury occurs under circumstances of contained explosions, for example, those occurring on civilian buses, when explosive materials are detonated in an enclosed space.

Thoracoabdominal injuries and common associated injuries, especially ear drum perforation, are the result of high amplitude air pressure waves as great as 5 atm exerted for several seconds (2). In addition, abdominal blast wounds can be associated with bowel perforation.

Rib Fractures/Flail Chest

Rib fractures are problematic for several reasons. First, rib fractures are painful, particularly with movement. This leads to "splinting," the process whereby the patient (both voluntarily and involuntarily) limits movement of the fracture site during position changes and respiratory effort. ☞ **Atelectasis will develop as a result of splinting of the chest and will compound the shunt attributable to lung contusion itself.** ☞ Lobar collapse may also occur, resulting in severe hypoxia and a radiographic picture of unilateral or bilateral volume loss in the area of the lobar collapse.

Pain is stressful and leads to sleep deprivation if untreated. Hypoxemia will become exacerbated when confusional states develop, particularly in patients who are not receiving adequate analgesia (becoming increasingly fatigued and sleep deprived). Therefore, it is imperative that the pain cycle be interrupted by intervention. Such intervention may be simply the administration of oral or intravenous analgesics in the most minor of injuries. However, parenterally administered sedatives and analgesics may occasionally contribute to confusional states. Accordingly, thoracic epidural analgesia (or another form of regional analgesia) is recommended for solitary chest wall injuries in hemodynamically stable patients with a normal coagulation system. When regional analgesia is initiated the first few hours following admission to the trauma center, the cascade of splinting, atelectasis, hypoxemia, and respiratory failure can be markedly diminished (see later discussion on analgesia, in the analgesia for thoracic trauma section, as well as Volume 2, Chapter 5).

A "flail segment" is generally defined as three or more ribs broken in two or more places. Some clinicians consider a "flail chest," as any mechanical chest dysfunction resulting from thoracic trauma where the patient is unable to ventilate adequately due to that injury, even in the absence of a true flail segment. Additionally, a flail segment can be missed upon admission to the trauma center, as a weak or "splinting" patient may not be capable of generating sufficient inspiratory forces to cause an inward and paradoxical movement of the chest in the area of the contiguous rib fractures. The extent of the underlying lung contusion in flail injury is probably the most import aspect of the lung dysfunction under these circumstances. It must therefore be understood that even with perfect analgesia, patients with flail chest will almost invariably progress to respiratory failure. Furthermore, when the pulmonary contusion itself is severe, the consequent right-to-left transpulmonary shunt worsens and respiratory failure will ensue (see Volume 2, Chapter 24).

When respiratory insufficiency due to flail chest and/or significant pulmonary contusion is present, intubation and mechanical ventilation are warranted. Indeed, an older study by Sankaran and Wilson (3) found that early intubation in these patients resulted in only 6% mortality, whereas delayed intubation (waiting until the patient developed clinical evidence of hypoxia or hypercapnea) led to >50% mortality. Although modern techniques may provide lower mortalities today, early intubation and mechanical ventilation remain as a cornerstone of therapy.

Analgesia is another critical element in the management of these patients. Mechanically ventilated patients do not benefit from regional anesthesia to the same degree as nonintubated patients. Accordingly, intravenous analgesia and sedation is initially more appropriate in these mechanically ventilated patients.

Hemothorax and Pneumothorax

Pneumothorax can result from blunt trauma due to compression of the air-filled alveoli and airways, as well as from puncture following rib fractures. Hemothorax due to chest wall or lung bleeding can compound pulmonary dysfunction and contribute to hemodynamic compromise in the chest trauma patient. Both hemothorax and pneumothorax can be diagnosed by clinical and radiological methods (Volume 1, Chapters 8 and 25). Typically, these injuries are diagnosed and treated during the primary survey (Volume 1, Chapter 8). However, they may have a delayed presentation in the operating room (OR) or ICU, with abrupt hypotension or by a sudden increase in peak inspiratory pressures and concomitant decreased breath sounds in the affected hemithorax. These clinical findings are often associated with subcutaneous emphysema (pneumothorax) and/or decreased hematocrit (hemothorax). However, they also present occultly, with subtle changes in vital signs, and the only clinical clue being decreased breath sounds on the affected side.

Specific Intrathoracic Injuries
Airway Injury (Trachea and Bronchi)

Airway injury may result from blunt trauma or penetration from a knife, GSW, or a piece of shrapnel, causing injury to the larynx, trachea, bronchi, or more distal airway. ☞ **Bronchoscopy is an essential part of the evaluation of the victim of thoracic or neck trauma whenever there is a suspicion of airway disruption.** ☞ The author, Hanowell, has diagnosed airway injury or disruption by fiberoptic bronchoscopy on numerous occasions, and has even had to remove a bullet from the mainstem bronchus of a GSW victim via the use of bronchoscopy. Airway disruption may be heralded by finding of subcutaneous emphysema and/or an unusual or persistent pneumothorax accompanied by an obvious air leak after placement of a thoracostomy tube (so-called broncho-pleural fistula). The majority of tracheo-bronchial lesions associated with blunt trauma occur in the intrathoracic portion of the major airways within a few centimeters of the carina (4). Surgical correction is required, and failure to promptly diagnose such injuries can lead to grave pulmonary complications or death.

Blunt thoracic trauma may also be associated with disruption of the smaller airways and pulmonary veins, leading to an alveolar-pulmonary venous communication that is associated with air embolism to the left heart. At the time of thoracotomy for major trauma, the first sign of this may be the surgeons' observation of air in the coronary arteries. ☞ **When left heart air embolism is recognized, the team must prevent further entry of air into the left heart. The first maneuver is isolation of the injured lung via one-lung ventilation (1LV).** ☞ Placement of a double lumen tube (DLT) is one way to accomplish 1LV, but should be done by a skilled anesthesiologist, with precision and speed, augmented by bronchoscopic positioning. Alternatively, intubated patients in respiratory failure may not tolerate changing to a DLT (presence of airway swelling, cardiopulmonary instability). In these cases, advancing a bronchial blocker through an existing endotracheal tube and into the injured bronchus with fiberoptic bronchoscopy is the method of choice (5). Use of the Arndt bronchial blocker has made this procedure far less cumbersome (5). For a complete review of lung separation techniques, including the use of DLTs and various bronchial blockers, the reader is referred to the review by Wilson et al. (5). When a bronchial blocker is not available, a lifesaving maneuver may entail simply directing the existing single lumen tube into the mainstem bronchus of the uninvolved lung with the aid of bronchoscopy. In the case of the need for left lung isolation, the anesthesiologist can even attempt at blindly advancing the single lumen tube into the right mainstem. However, positioning and verification with a fiberoptic bronchoscopic technique is always recommended. Definitive treatment is surgical with bronchial repair or exclusion of the injured lung. Initial surgical, control may involve cross-clamping the involved bronchus to prevent further ingress of air from the alveoli into the pulmonary venous system (Table 2).

Table 2 Clinical Features of Air Embolism in Thoracic Trauma

Clinical feature	Description/comments
Predisposing conditions and presentation	Lung laceration, airway disruption
	Hypotension (R/O tamponade, pneumothorax, hemorrhage)
	Onset of hypotension during mechanical ventilation
Diagnosis	Air visualized in coronary arteries/fundi
	Air bubble seen in heart on TEE
Treatment	Close the fistula connecting lung bronchi to vasculature
	Avoid nitrous oxide when air embolism suspected
	Administer pure oxygen: favors elimination of nitrogen
Sequelae of air embolism	Cerebrovascular air embolism and stroke
	Coronary air embolism and coronary insufficiency

Abbreviations: R/O, rule out; TEE, transesophageal echocardiogram.

Esophageal Injuries

Esophageal injuries are extremely lethal, particularly those resulting from high-velocity missiles and those associated with any delay in diagnosis. Understanding esophageal anatomy explains much of the morbidity associated with these injuries. ☞ **Early evaluation and prompt management are the most critical factors in optimum outcomes following esophageal injury.** ☞ Because of the high morbidity and relative rarity of injuries, some debate continues regarding the best techniques and algorithms for evaluation and management. However, none debate the need for early, prompt diagnosis and treatment.

Anatomy

The adult esophagus is approximately 25 cm in length, extending from the cricopharyngeus muscle in the neck to the fundus of the stomach. The esophagus descends in the midline of the neck, behind the membranous portion of the trachea, continues downward through the esophageal hiatus of the diaphragm, and enters the stomach. Three anatomic areas of narrowing occur in the esophagus: (*i*) at the level of the cricoid cartilage (pharyngoesophageal sphincter), (*ii*) in the mid-thorax, from compression of the aortic knob and the left mainstem bronchus, and (*iii*) at the esophageal hiatus of the diaphragm (gastroesophageal junction).

The musculature of the pharynx and upper third of the esophagus is the skeletal type, the remainder being smooth muscle. The muscular alignment is similar to the rest of the gastrointestinal tract (inner circular and outer longitudinal). The entire esophagus lies in a loose areolar tissue bed, which communicates with the entire mediastinum. Accordingly, any contaminated spillage is highly likely to develop into mediastinitis.

The arterial supply to the esophagus is consistent, but quite segmental, with little collateralization. The upper portion is supplied by branches of the inferior thyroid arteries. The thoracic portion is supplied by both branches of the bronchial arteries and esophageal segmental arteries (emanating directly from the aorta). Occasionally, intercostal arteries contribute. The diaphragmatic and abdominal portions of the esophagus are nourished by branches of the left gastric artery. The venous drainage is quite variable and complex. The most important veins are those draining the inferior portion. These empty into the coronary vein, a tributary of the portal vein. This connection results as esophageal varices in cirrhotic patients.

Clinical Presentation

The vast majority of esophageal injuries result from penetrating trauma and caustic ingestion. When blunt traumatic esophageal injuries occur, they are located almost exclusively in the neck. Classical signs of esophageal injury include pain, fever, and crepitus, but these become increasingly predominant when diagnosis is delayed. Hamman's sign, mediastinal crunching, may be present in thoracic esophageal injuries. Some signs are more prominent in particular regions of the esophagus (e.g., dyspnea and vomiting are common in thoracic esophageal injuries, but rare in cervical esophageal injuries). Additionally, the mechanism of trauma affects the prevalence of clinical signs (present in only 50% of patients following stab wounds, and nearly 100% of patients following GSWs) (6). Because these signs and symptoms are nonspecific, a high degree of suspicion must accompany any injury with proximity to the esophagus.

Radiographic and Endoscopic Evaluation

Plain films of the neck or chest are abnormal in 80% of perforations, but are nonspecific. Contrast studies are needed with specificities ranging between 94% and 100% (6). Endoscopy does pose a risk of worsening injury (e.g., converting a trivial perforation into a frank perforation with contamination). However, combining esophagoscopy (in experienced hands) with contrast esophography, improves diagnostic accuracy, with some series reporting no missed injuries (7).

Operative Management

Care of the commonly associated injuries to the major airways and vasculature naturally take, precedence. However, because delayed treatment results in far worse outcomes, diagnosis and treatment of esophageal injuries must occur as soon as the patient's condition allows. Indeed, the rate of esophageal anastomotic leak and esophagocutaneous fistula rose from 20%, when treatment occurred within 12 hours of injury, to 100% when treatment was delayed beyond 24 hours (8).

A complete review of operative techniques for esophageal repair is beyond the scope of this chapter. However, the following general considerations should be reviewed. For stab wounds, primary repair may follow irrigation and debridement, whereas following high-velocity GSWs or shrapnel injuries, a portion of the esophagus may need to be resected. A closed suction (i.e., Jackson Pratt) drainage device is usually employed, and perioperative antibiotics with efficacy against mouth and skin flora should be initiated immediately following diagnosis. In the presence of combined esophageal and tracheal injuries, it is advisable to interpose one of the strap muscles to decrease the delayed fistula rate.

Postoperative Management and Nutrition

Some advocate placing a NG tube to decompress the esophagus, relying on total parental nutrition (TPN). Others advocate early enteral feeding through the NG tube. The duration of NG tube insertion (for those advocating TPN) is as variable as the number of surgeons performing the procedure. Analgesia is often problematic, especially for thoracic esophageal repairs, and pain should be aggressively treated. However, excessive postoperative pain in the face of fever and leukocytosis should warn of an esophageal leak.

Cardiac Injuries

Thoracic trauma victims must be evaluated for cardiac injuries whenever wounds have proximity to the heart. Discovery may require echocardiographic and electrocardiographic, radiographic and/or biochemical findings depending upon the mechanism of injury.

In the case of suspected cardiac contusion, guidelines that define the extent to which victims are appropriately evaluated and monitored, are based upon the overall severity and likelihood of injury. In minor trauma, a normal electrocardiogram and transthoracic echocardiogram will generally be adequate to screen for significant injury. When these tests are negative, no further specific measures are indicated. In the patient with more severe injuries and high suspicion of myocardial contusion, the use of electrocardiography (ECG), troponin I measurements, and transesophageal echocardiography (TEE) are indicated (9). Patients with positive findings on these tests are at increased risk of serious dysrhythmias, and deserve a higher level of monitoring to include at least ECG telemetry. Perioperative

evidence of myocardial contusion is also important in planning anesthesia and surgery for the multiple trauma victim.

Assessment of structural abnormalities of the heart and pericardial effusion (blood) and possible early or frank cardiac tamponade, can be quickly evaluated with transthoracic echocardiography (TTE) as part of the FAST exam (Volume 1, Chapters 14, 16, and 25). However, TEE is preferable to TTE whenever structural lesions or valve abnormalities are to be evaluated.

Great Vessel Injuries

Chest trauma may entail injury to any vessel in the thorax or contiguous areas including the neck or abdomen. Tears of the thoracic aorta occur after sudden deceleration injury and constitutes one of the most common and important injuries following blunt thoracic trauma. The most common site of aortic injury is adjacent to the ligamentum arteriosum, where the thoracic aorta is fixed and most subject to the shearing forces of sudden deceleration. However, thoracic aortic rupture or dissection may occur at other sites as well.

Diagnosis should be considered in the presence of shoulder harness marks on the patient, or a steering wheel imprint in unrestrained drivers. Pulses in the left upper or lower extremities may be diminished compared to the right upper extremity, but this is not universally present. The diagnosis of thoracic aortic rupture should also be considered when any of the following findings are noted on chest radiography: first or second rib fractures, a wide mediastinum, blurring of the aortic knob, left hemothorax, downward deflection of the left mainstem bronchus, or a rightward-shifted trachea or NG tube.

Evaluation of the aorta and arch structures should proceed following suspicion of injury with computerized tomography or aortogram. The TEE can also demonstrate aortic defects, and given that TEE is extremely useful in diagnosing multiple cardiac lesions associated with blunt thoracic trauma, the concomitant evaluation of the aorta is warranted in all of these patients. However, certain areas in the aorta are poorly visualized via TEE; thus it is an imperfect screening tool. Cinnella et al. (10) believe the TEE should be considered as a first-line evaluation tool to evaluate aortic injury following blunt trauma, but they acknowledge that randomized trials are lacking.

The current standard is spiral computed tomographic (CT) imaging for aortic injury, and some still prefer arteriography for aortic branch lesions (11). The rapid development in CT scanning technology has resulted in dramatic improvement in anatomic clarity in recent years. When one includes three-dimensional reconstructions for aortic lesions and injuries to the great vessels, it is difficult to beat CT angiography, though this continues to be a rapidly changing area.

Due to the propensity of aortic tears to progress to rupture in a large percentage of nonoperated patients, treatment of thoracic aortic rupture has traditionally involved urgent replacement with a synthetic aortic conduit. However, endovascular approaches are increasingly being utilized with success (especially in patients with concomitant injuries) (12). Some patients require delayed operative management due to contraindications to blood pressure perturbations and/or systemic heparinization (e.g., intracranial hemorrhage/hematoma), or the need to manage other higher-priority lesions (e.g., exploratory laparatomy for hemorrhage, or evacuation of intracerebral hematoma). For patients requiring delayed management, beta blockade associated with significant opioid analgesia, sedation, and judicious vasodilator therapy should be a main pillar of critical care management.

Patients without contraindications to immediate treatment generally go to the OR as soon as the surgical and anesthetic teams are assembled, and the patient has been resuscitated and fully worked up for intercurrent injuries. Aortic tears at or distal to the left subclavian artery may be treated by short-term clamping and resection of the damaged aortic tissue, with repair utilizing a short segment of Dacron tube graft with or without heparin or shunts (Fig. 3A–C). When clamp time is ≤30 minutes, paraplegia rates are <7% (comparable to bypass rates). For these patients, a left lateral thoracotomy and DLT are utilized, and require close communication and cooperation between the surgeon and anesthesiologist to optimally manage these cases (see below—anesthetic management). Several commonly employed adjuncts for descending thoracic tear repair include atriofemoral bypass (Fig. 3B), and passive proximal to distal aortic shunts (Fig. 3C). More proximal aortic tears involving the ascending aorta or arch will require full heparinization and cardiopulmonary bypass. The anesthetic

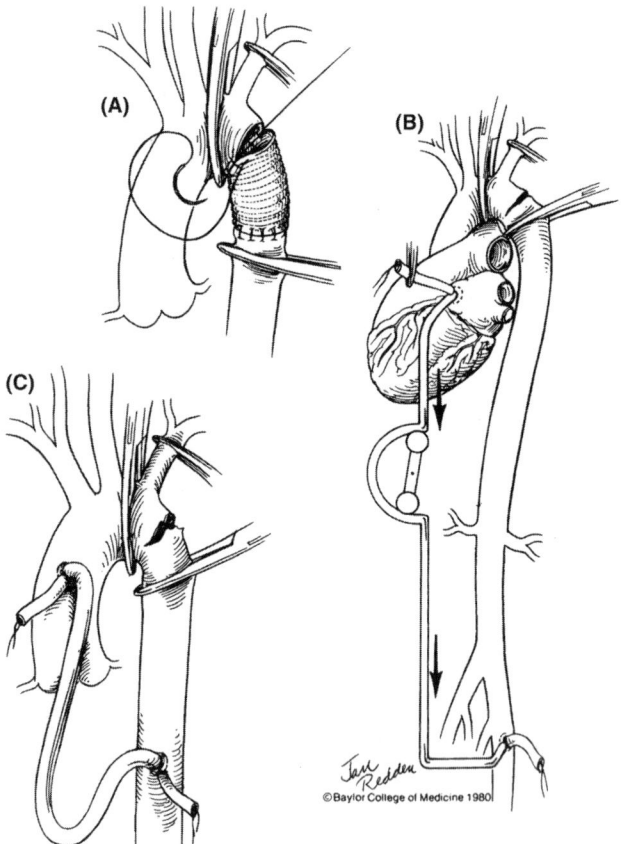

Figure 3 Techniques used for repair of blunt injuries to the descending thoracic aorta. (**A**) Clamp and sew technique (sometimes accomplished without heparinization or shunting). (**B**) Atriofemoral (partial) bypass, provides perfusion to the spinal cord and structures below the level of the aortic clamp, and diverts some blood away from the native heart, thus decreasing the stress on the left ventricle and possibility of very elevated ascending aortic blood pressure (requires heparinization). (**C**) Passive shunt bypass (Gott shunt), requires a small amount of heparinization. *Source*: Courtesy of Baylor College of Medicine.

management for these cases is similar to that utilized for repair of aortic aneurysms or dissections in these areas (and is beyond the scope of this chapter). The interested reader is referred to standard cardiothoracic anesthesia textbooks for further information.

Anesthetic management for repair of distal aortic tear includes the attainment of adequate intravenous access, volume infusion for associated hemorrhage, and placement of central venous access. Optimally, two arterial lines are placed, one in the right radial artery to reflect proximal aortic and cerebral blood flow pressures, and one in either femoral artery to reflect distal pressures and spinal cord perfusion pressures. The other femoral arterial area is prepped into the field in case needed during the operation (e.g., atrial femoral bypass). In the absence of an associated esophageal or cervical spine injury, TEE is an extremely useful monitor, reflecting ventricular preload and contractility, and can often be used to help determine the extent of aortic tear.

Blood pressure control with beta-blockers, opioids, and vasodilators can be employed preoperatively in hypertensive patients to decrease the incidence of further injury or frank rupture. Induction of anesthesia without triggering hypertension and tachycardia is essential to avoid further shearing of the aorta. However, many of these patients present in hemorrhagic shock from their other injuries and require massive volume resuscitation. Accordingly, avoiding myocardial depressants and or vasodilators in the hemorrhagic shock patient is equally mandatory.

A DLT or bronchial-blocking device is used to isolate the lungs and to facilitate surgical exposure to the left chest. A lumbar cerebral spinal fluid (CSF) drain can occasionally be placed even in the trauma setting if the patient is sufficiently stable. The goal of CSF drainage is to decrease retrograde pressure on the spinal cord and limit neurological sequela resulting from the sacrifice of any aortic branches to the spinal cord. This measure may be precluded by the emergency nature of these surgeries and instability of the severely injured patient. Mannitol infusion may be utilized for suprarenal clamping to promote urinary flow and as an antioxidant so as to avert acute tubular necrosis. Prior to aortic cross-clamping, vasodilators and beta-blocker infusion can be utilized to attenuate the rise in blood pressure associated with this surgical manipulation.

Prior to aortic unclamping, appropriate volume loading by monitoring central venous pressure, pulmonary artery occlusion pressure, and/or left ventricular cavity dimension by TEE is essential to avoid hypotension. Additionally, vasodilation therapy should be weaned off. Heparinization and various circulatory bypass techniques may be utilized to assure continued perfusion to the vital organs and spinal cord during vascular repair. As patients undergoing surgical repair of the thoracic aorta require left thoracotomy, appropriate measures to postoperatively manage pain are necessary (see later discussion).

After exsanguinations, paraplegia is the most dreaded and significant complication. Paraplegia results from insufficient perfusion of the anterior spinal cord. In a large meta-analysis of 1742 patients, Von Oppell (13) found that 2.9% of patients with thoracic aortic injuries had already developed paraplegia preoperatively. Postoperative paraplegia was found in 19.3% of clamp/repair patients, 6.1% of bypassed patients, 11.1% of passive shunt patients, and in 2.3% of active shunted patients (13). He also reported that full heparinization in patients with multiple injuries yielded a higher mortality compared to no heparin.

Renal failure and/or mesenteric ischemia may also complicate the postoperative course of these patients.

Traumatic Asphyxia

Traumatic asphyxia is a rare condition which results from massive increased intrathoracic and venacaval pressure due to a thoracic crush injury in the presence of a closed glottis. The syndrome was first described by D'Angers in 1837 (14). Retrograde flow of blood through valveless veins of the head and neck results in swelling and petechiae or cyanotic discoloration of the face and neck. Neurological manifestations frequently include transient loss of consciousness, but rarely involve focal neurological deficits or cord syndromes, unless additional injuries are present (15).

No specific lung injuries may occur from traumatic asphyxia, rather, neurological impairment is the concern. Although the patient may appear moribund upon initial presentation, emergent airway management and supportive care can result in remarkable improvement in patient status in the first 48 hours, providing the duration of asphyxia is brief and the associated injuries are not severe.

Initial Management of the Patient in Extremis

The primary survey, reviewed in Volume 1, Chapter 8, should identify most life-threatening injuries (Table 1), and these must all be promptly treated. Immediate recognition and treatment of the thoracic trauma patient in extremis (impending death) provides the best chance for survival. Some thoracic trauma patients, particularly those following penetrating trauma, will require an emergency department resuscitative thoracotomy for survival. However, most are initially managed with a thoracostomy tube, and later (if bleeding persists) may require urgent thoracotomy.

Resuscitative Thoracotomy

The term "resuscitative thoracotomy" is used to mean a thoracotomy performed on a patient in extremis, typically outside the OR (in the emergency department or resuscitation bay). However, many of these patients are sent directly to a prepared trauma OR (Volume 1, Chapter 5). Thus, from a nomenclature perspective, the physical location of the thoracotomy is not as important as the reason and timing. The concept underlying a resuscitative thoracotomy (Volume 1, Chapter 13) is to improve perfusion to both cerebral and coronary circulation by performing open cardiac massage and cross-clamping of the descending aorta. Additional benefits of resuscitative thoracotomy include control of intrathoracic bleeding, release of pericardial tamponade, control of the pulmonary hilum to minimize bleeding, and air leaks.

Rhee et al. (16) have recently reviewed the combined data from 24 previously published series. This study confirmed the importance of mechanisms of injury, location of injury, and signs of life during transport (and upon arrival), on predicting survival (Table 3). Although the overall survival rate was only 7.4%, normal neurological function at discharge was observed in 92.4% of these surviving patients (16). An important factor that correlated with survival was successful tracheal intubation in the field. A complete review of resuscitative thoracotomy is provided in Volume 1, Chapter 13, and interested readers are referred there for additional information.

Thoracostomy Tube Alone vs. Urgent Thoracotomy

The decision to place a thoracostomy tube for hemothorax versus urgent operative thoracotomy is a fundamental

Table 3 Survival Factors for Patients Following Resuscitative Thoracotomy

Survival factor	Specific category and survival (%)
Mechanism of injury	Blunt trauma (1.4)
	Gunshot wound (4.3)
	Stab wound (16.8)
Location of major injury	Multiple major injuries (0.7)
	Abdominal (4.5)
	Thoracic (10.7)
	Cardiac (19.4)
Signs of life	Absent in the field (1.2)
	Present during transport (8.9)
	Absent on arrival (2.6)
	Present on arrival (11.5)

Source: Adapted From Ref. 16.

determination that needs to be made in every thoracic trauma patient who presents with hemodynamically unstable hemothorax. The current Advanced Trauma Life Support® (ATLS®) guidelines call for urgent operative thoracotomy to control bleeding and allow full lung expansion when the initial chest tube output exceeds 1500 mL of blood, or when the hourly output exceeds 250 mL for three consecutive hours (though we do not believe anyone should wait this long). Other indications for urgent and nonurgent thoracotomy following trauma are provided in Table 4. The surgical approach for urgent thoracotomy is beyond the scope of this chapter, and is found in standard surgical texts.

LUNG INJURY RESULTING FROM TRAUMA-ASSOCIATED CONDITIONS

In addition to direct wounding of the heart, lung, and chest wall, secondary injuries can afflict the trauma patient due to multiple associated conditions including aspiration, burns, inhalation injury, near-drowning, fat embolization, pulmonary embolization, and acute respiratory distress syndrome (ARDS). Each of these injuries increase morbidity and have their own special considerations for managing the thoracic trauma patient, and will be discussed below.

Aspiration of Gastric Contents

Trauma patients may aspirate blood or gastric contents before, during, or immediately after their injury. Aspiration during airway management is also common and problematic. The rate of aspiration after urgent intubation ranges from less than 1% in the OR under controlled circumstances, to almost 40% in other circumstances (17–21). Patients at risk for aspiration include those with a full stomach, a history of reflux, a decreased level of consciousness, depressed laryngeal reflexes, morbid obesity, emergency abdominal surgery following alcohol consumption, or in the presence of pain or stress (18). Trauma victims often have one or more of these risk factors.

Prevention

☞ **The proper use of cricoid pressure (Sellick's maneuver) may help prevent regurgitation of gastric contents into the trachea during intubation (22).** ☞ However, no studies

Table 4 Indications for Urgent and Nonurgent Thoracotomy

Indications for urgent thoracotomy	Cardiac tamponade
	Acute hemodynamic deterioration
	Initial chest tube output >1500 mL
	Ongoing chest tube output > 250 mL/hr for >3 hr
	Vascular injury at the thoracic outlet
	Traumatic thoracotomy (loss of chest-wall substance)
	Massive air leak from the chest tube
	Known or suspected tracheal or bronchial injury
	Esophageal injury
	Great vessel injury
	Mediastinal traverse with a penetrating object
	Significant missile embolism to the heart or pulmonary artery
	Transcardiac placement of inferior venal caval shunt for hepatic vascular wounds
Indications for nonurgent thoracotomy	Nonevacuated clotted hemothorax
	Chronic traumatic diaphragmatic hernia
	Traumatic cardiac septal or valvular lesions
	Chronic traumatic thoracic aortic pseudoaneurysms
	Nonclosing thoracic duct fistula
	Chronic (or neglected) post-traumatic empyema
	Traumatic lung abscess
	Missed tracheal or bronchial injury
	Tracheoesophageal fistula
	Innominate artery/tracheal fistula (often urgent)
	Traumatic arterial venous fistula (often urgent)

have confirmed the effectiveness of cricoid pressure in reducing aspiration and its associated morbidity and mortality. Another strategy to minimize the risk of aspiration is inserting a nasogastric tube (NGT) into the patient, prior to induction, to reduce the volume of gastric contents (orogastric tubes are placed in patients with maxillofacial trauma). Many of these same practitioners will remove the NGT, after emptying the stomach, to decrease the incidence of gastroesophageal reflux (23,24). However, others prefer leaving the NGT in place, using the rationale that it may help drain residual gastric contents (25). If the NGT is left in place, Salem et al. (26) have shown that the NGT does not impair the efficacy of cricoid pressure. However, the effect of the NGT on laryngoscopic view and ease of intubation has not been studied. Accordingly, patients with anticipated difficult intubation (see Volume 1, Chapter 9) should be intubated without the NGT in place. The use of histamine-2 receptor antagonists has been shown to decrease gastric volume and acidity; this option may rarely be implemented effectively in the trauma patient who is presented for urgent or emergent surgery (27). Additionally, metoclopramide may be administered to promote gastric emptying (as long as there is no bowel obstruction).

Diagnosis and Management

Up to 40% of patients who aspirate during intubation may subsequently developed a clinical pneumonitis (16,19). When aspiration-induced pneumonitis does occur, it is more often associated with greater than 0.4 mL/kg of gastric contents and a gastric content pH of 2.5 or less (16,19). Of those patients who do develop aspiration pneumonitis, about half may require mechanical ventilation (16,19). The patients who develop aspiration pneumonitis often have symptoms of wheezing or coughing, decreased oxygen saturation, or abnormalities on chest roentograms, within two hours of aspiration (19). Patients who suffer an aspiration should have bronchial suctioning performed, especially if the aspirate contains particulate matter. Corticosteroids do not appear to be beneficial when given prophylactically. Similarly, antibiotics should not be given unless the aspirate is grossly contaminated (e.g., patient with upper gastrointestinal obstruction), or the patient has been institutionalized for more than 72 hours, or after a sputum culture returns positive with specific organisms (28,29).

However, aspiration of gastric contents can account for up to 20% of ARDS patients (30,31). Aspiration is one of the most common conditions associated with the development of ARDS. Therefore, patients symptomatic after aspiration should be carefully monitored for progressive respiratory failure, because the mortality rate increases up to 50% (16,19).

Burns and Inhalation Injury
Incidence and Etiology

Although it is less common for a trauma patient to also have sustained a thermal injury (32), up to 7% of patients who suffer burns have concomitant nonthermal injuries (32–34). Burn victims suffer concomitant inhalation injury up to 35% of the time (35,36). Inhalation injury should be suspected in patients who have a history of smoke or flame exposure in a closed space, a history of loss of consciousness, facial burns, carbonaceous particles in their nares, carbonaceous sputum, or a carboxyhemoglobin level greater than 10% (36). However, even when the burn patient does not have an inhalation injury, respiratory complications occur in 18% to 33% of all burn patients (36). When a burn patient has an inhalation injury, there is a significant increase in respiratory complications and mortality can be as high as 77% (35–39). Interestingly, Hollingsed (36) found that burn patients with an inhalation injury but no additional respiratory complications (e.g., pneumonia) had no higher mortality than those without an inhalation injury. Instead, Hollingsed noted that burn patients who develop respiratory failure have a higher mortality rate (27–50%) than those without pulmonary failure (0–3%), regardless of the history of inhalation injury. There is, nonetheless, a propensity for respiratory failure to develop in those who have suffered inhalation injury (see Volume 1, Chapter 34).

Pathophysiology and Treatment

Inhalation injury can occur in several forms and affect different portions of the airway. The most obvious consequence of inhalation injury is hypoxemia and its attendant complication of ischemia. Hypoxemia should be immediately treated with a high-inspired concentration of oxygen. Patients may also develop severe tissue edema of the oropharyngeal and laryngeal areas, secondary to direct thermal injury (40,41). Since the edema may take over 12 hours to develop, patients suspected of having an inhalation injury should be closely monitored (42). These patients often benefit from early intubation and mechanical support until the edema resolves.

The various components found in smoke may cause carbon monoxide or cyanide toxicity, as well as a chemical pneumonitis marked by sloughing of the mucosa and plugging of the airways (41). Patients suffering from carbon monoxide or cyanide poisoning may present with metabolic acidosis and neurological symptoms progressing from headache and confusion to hallucinations and coma (42,43). ☞ **The treatment of carbon monoxide toxicity involves the use of a high-inspired concentration of oxygen.** ☞ Depending on the severity of the carbon monoxide poisoning, the patient may require intubation or, if available, hyperbaric oxygen treatment (also see Volume 1 Chapter 34 and Chapter 73 in this Volume). In addition to mechanical ventilation and circulatory support, the patient with cyanide toxicity may benefit from the intravenous administration of sodium thiosulfate or sodium nitrite to bind the cyanide molecules. Patients with a chemical pneumonitis require ventilatory support with vigorous pulmonary toilet to minimize the risk of secondary complications such as pneumonia. Prophylactic antibiotics and corticosteroids should be avoided (44). However, appropriate antibiotics should be initiated when an infection is identified by Gram stain and culture data.

Trauma patients who sustain a thermal injury may also have pulmonary complications aside from inhalation injury. The burn itself may result in the formation of a thick eschar circumferentially around the thorax, which may impede chest wall excursion until the patient undergoes escharotomy. The fluid resuscitation needed for burns with inhalation injury are about twice those needed for thermal injury without inhalation injury, but this additional fluid requirement has rarely been associated with the development of pulmonary edema (45). Inhalation injury itself is not associated with a large accumulation of extravascular lung water, though this too varies (45,46). Finally, the development of sepsis in a burn patient may also be accompanied by the development of increasing lung water (47,48).

Fat Embolism Syndrome

Fat embolism is defined as the presence of fat droplets in the circulation, usually after a major trauma or long-bone fracture (49,50). The fat embolism syndrome results in a constellation of clinical signs and symptoms, including tachypnea, hypoxemia, tachycardia, petechial rash, thrombocytopenia, fever, and deteriorating neurological status, associated with fat globules in the circulation (49–51). Diagnosis of fat embolism syndrome is made by exclusion of other etiologies, given the nonspecific nature of many of the signs and symptoms. Although fat embolism is very common, with over 90% of patients suffering from a long-bone fracture found to have some degree of fat embolism, the fat embolism syndrome is much less common with an incidence ranging from 0.5% to 19% (49–55).

Pathophysiology

The clinical course of fat embolism syndrome proceeds in one of two variants: a fulminant form and a progressive form. The severe form begins within 12 hours of injury is associated with significant neurological deficits and cardiovascular compromise, and has a higher mortality rate compared to the progressive form that presents 24 to 72 hours after injury, and has a wide range in severity of signs and symptoms (54–57).

The precise mechanism by which the fat enters the systemic circulation remains unclear. There is evidence that fractures as well as repair of fractures with reamed intramedullary nails, increase the intramedullary pressure with resultant fat embolization (58,59). The fat may enter the systemic circulation either through the venous drainage of the femur, via a shunt between the arterial and venous systems in bone, or through the pulmonary capillaries (50,58).

Once in the circulation, fat may cause hypoxia and respiratory compromise by either mechanically occluding pulmonary capillaries or by participation in a biochemical chain of events related to the presence of fat in the pulmonary vasculature. The latter includes the possibilities that lipase converts the fat into free fatty acids that subsequently cause vasculitis and alveolar damage; fat provides a surface for the activated platelets to adhere and coagulation to occur; and fat enhances the inflammatory process triggered by trauma (50,58–61).

Fat embolism syndrome can occur without respiratory effects, however, it is more commonly associated with hypoxemia (49). Fat embolism syndrome may also be associated with severe respiratory failure accompanied by chest radiographs demonstrating bilateral diffuse infiltrates indistinguishable from ARDS. In these patients with ARDS, the mortality of fat embolism syndrome is about 10% (49,62).

Treatment

Randomized studies treating fat embolism syndrome with corticosteroids have had limited success with improving the respiratory effects (62–66). In one study, up to 45% of patients suffering from fat embolism syndrome required ventilatory support either due to severe hypoxemia or significant central nervous system depression (49). The same study documented 96% of patients as having some degree of hypoxia. Given the prevalence of respiratory involvement, patients with fat embolism syndrome should be closely monitored for hypoxemia and supported with mechanical ventilation as medically indicated.

Thromboembolism and Pulmonary Embolism
Incidence and Etiology

Deep venous thrombosis (DVT) and pulmonary embolism (PE) are major factors of morbidity and mortality in trauma patients (see Volume 2, Chapter 56). DVT occurs in 6% to 80% of trauma patients (67–71), whereas PE occurs in 0.3% to 2.3% of trauma patients (69,72–76). DVTs may result in morbidity, due either to recurrent DVTs or to the development of post-thrombotic syndrome. Although DVTs may recur in trauma patients, the risk of recurrence is significantly less than in patients who develop DVTs secondary to inherited coagulation disorders and malignancy (77). Post-thrombotic syndrome occurs in approximately 30% of patients with DVT and is characterized by leg pain, pretibial edema, induration of the skin, hyperpigmentation, venous ectasia, and ulceration that occur within the first two years after acute DVT (77,78). Although fatal PE occurs rarely in trauma patients, PEs (fatal and subclinical) occur in up to 50% of patients with DVTs (79,80). Equally concerning is the fact that despite a PE mortality rate between 20% and 50% (72,80,81), up to 70% of patients who die of PE are not clinically suspected of having suffered a PE (82–84). ☞ **For patients who survive the first 24 hours after traumatic injury, PE is the third leading cause of death (76).** ☞

Patients at risk for DVT and for PE include those who have sustained direct venous trauma, a spinal cord injury, severe head injury, pelvic fracture, fracture of the lower extremities, or severe trauma with subsequent shock or multiple transfusions (67,70,72,74). These conditions result in varying combinations of prolonged immobilization, stasis, endothelial damage, and hypercoagulability. Consequently, these patients may develop DVTs that can then embolize.

Diagnosis

Patients with DVTs are frequently asymptomatic until they suffer a fatal PE. Consequently, clinical findings, such as a swollen and painful leg, palpable cord, and erythema, are unreliable for the diagnosis of DVT (70,75,80). Similarly, PE can be difficult to diagnose clinically because the symptoms and signs of pleuritic chest pain, dyspnea, tachypnea, and hemoptysis are nonspecific (80,85). A high index of suspicion for PE should be maintained in any trauma patient who subsequently develops dyspnea, hypoxemia, and respiratory failure without obvious pulmonary pathology. PEs can occur in trauma victims as early as within the first 24 hours after injury or as late as two weeks after trauma (75,86).

The most common methods used to detect the development of DVTs include contrast venography, impedance plethysmography, and duplex ultrasound (80,85). Although venography is considered the gold standard for diagnosing DVT, its use is limited by its invasiveness and cost. Impedance plethysmography and duplex ultrasound have the advantage of being noninvasive in nature, however, they require trained personnel to perform and can be limited by technical difficulties (67). Of these two methods, duplex ultrasound is considered to be superior to impedance plethysmography in detecting DVT (80,85). Knudson et al. (67) found that serial duplex ultrasound venous examinations of trauma patients serve as an ideal noninvasive surveillance method for patients deemed to be at risk for developing DVTs. However, routine surveillance has not been proven to reduce the incidence of PE and is more costly than DVT prophylaxis (76,87). Techniques used to diagnose PE include pulmonary angiography, ventilation-perfusion ($\dot{V}/\dot{Q}$) lung scan, and spiral CT angiography (85).

☞ **Pulmonary angiography had been the gold standard for diagnosing PE. As with contrast venography, pulmonary angiography is limited by its invasiveness and cost. Spiral CT is emerging as the new gold standard. However, some patterns of PEs such as distal small vessel disease are better seen by angiography, whereas others are better seen by CT (85).** ☞

The $\dot{V}/\dot{Q}$ lung scan was evaluated in the landmark Prospective Investigation of Pulmonary Embolism Diagnosis (PIOPED) study, and determined to be useful in diagnosing PE primarily when the $\dot{V}/\dot{Q}$ scan was considered to be of high probability and correlated with a high clinical suspicion of PE (88). At the same time, the $\dot{V}/\dot{Q}$ scan was also noted to be useful in excluding the diagnosis of PE when the $\dot{V}/\dot{Q}$ scan was of low probability and associated with a low clinical suspicion of PE (88). Overall, the $\dot{V}/\dot{Q}$ scan is diagnostic in 30% to 50% of the patients (88). Consequently, spiral CT angiography is increasingly viewed as the best technique to diagnose PE. Early studies suggest that spiral CT angiography is more accurate than $\dot{V}/\dot{Q}$ scan and less invasive and expensive than pulmonary angiography (85,89). However, spiral CT angiography is limited when evaluating for PE in the subsegmental arteries (85). Hopefully, an ongoing PIOPED II study to evaluate spiral CT angiography will provide more definitive answers (90).

Treatment

The primary treatment for thromboembolism and PE remains prophylactic anticoagulation in patients identified as being at risk for developing DVT. Numerous studies have demonstrated the effectiveness of early prophylactic anticoagulation in decreasing the incidence of DVT (69,91,92). According to the American College of Chest Physicians recommendations, trauma patients should be started on prophylactic low-molecular-weight heparin (LMWH) if they have no contraindications, such as active hemorrhage, intracranial hematoma, partial spinal cord injury, uncorrected coagulopathy, and development of major complications related to heparin (76,93). Prophylactic treatments in order of decreasing efficacy are LMWH, such as dalteparin and Lovenox, fixed low-dose unfractionated heparin, and low-dose warfarin at fixed dose or titrated to increase the prothrombin time by 1.5 to 3 seconds (94). If LMWH is contraindicated, the patient should be placed on a mechanical treatment such as sequential pneumatic compression devices (SCD) (76). Potential problems with SCD include limited use in patients with lower extremity trauma requiring dressings, casts, or traction (67,68,95). In these patients, an SCD can be placed on an upper extremity.

Prophylactic inferior vena cava (IVC) filters are often employed in trauma patients who meet the following three conditions: (*i*) are at high risk for DVT and PE, (*ii*) are not candidates for anticoagulation, and (*iii*) for whom SCDs are either not feasible or considered insufficient prophylaxis. Conflicting studies exist regarding the efficacy of prophylactic IVC filters in preventing PE in high-risk trauma patients (72,73,87,93,96–98). However, most authors agree that when IVC filters are placed prophylactically, it should occur early in the patient's hospital course (72,93,97). Less controversial is the use of IVC filters in trauma patients who have already developed DVTs and who also have contraindications to anticoagulation, or who have suffered a PE despite standard DVT prophylaxis (76,93). IVC filters, however, do not guarantee the prevention of future PEs (76,93). Therefore, the efficacy of prophylactic IVC filters must be weighed against potential complications associated with IVC filters including migration of the filter, IVC occlusion, new DVT or propagation of previous DVT, venous insufficiency, and erosion of filter into adjacent viscera (93,96,98,99). The interested reader is referred to Volume 2, Chapter 56 for further review of DVT management.

Neurogenic Pulmonary Edema
Incidence and Etiology

Neurogenic pulmonary edema (NPE) may develop in patients following traumatic brain injury (TBI), or a subarachnoid hemorrhage (100,101). The true incidence of NPE is unknown (102–105), although one study suggests it may be as high as 50% of patients with severe TBI (106). Similarly, the overall mortality rate of NPE is difficult to define, with rates from 9.5% to over 90% found in the literature (103,105,107).

The pathophysiology of NPE remains unclear. One animal study suggests that the brainstem may be the neuroeffector site responsible for a massive sympathetic discharge (108). However, several other specific areas in the medulla, including the area postrema, Area A1 (a cluster of adrenergic receptors) of the ventrolateral medulla, the medial reticular nucleus, and the nucleus tractus solitarius are also possible sites (109–111). As a result of the massive outflow of sympathetic activity, the patient undergoes systemic and pulmonary vasoconstriction, hypertension, ventricular wall stress, and damage to endothelial cells (101,104,109,110,112).

Diagnosis

The patient with NPE presents with tachypnea, hypoxemia, tachycardia, hypertension, and frothy sputum. The signs and symptoms may appear within minutes to hours of the central nervous system injury, or develop gradually over the course of several days (112,113). Although the patient has pulmonary edema, the pulmonary capillary wedge pressure is usually low (112). Accordingly, NPE is a subset of noncardiogenic pulmonary edema. The chest X ray demonstrates diffuse patchy alveolar infiltrates, similar to those seen in patients with ARDS in the majority of patients (105).

Treatment

Fortunately, NPE is frequently a self-limited process (105,109,113). The patients require ventilatory support with positive end-expiratory pressure (PEEP) to prevent hypoxemia until the NPE resolves, which can be as quickly as within several hours of instituting mechanical ventilation (112). Some recent studies suggest that the use of dobutamine may be useful in resolving NPE in those patients with left ventricular dysfunction (114,115).

Fluid Overload
Incidence and Etiology

The true incidence of fluid overload in trauma patients is difficult to determine. One retrospective review of patients sustaining thoracic trauma had 2.6% rate of pulmonary edema in 187 patients (116), whereas a prospective review of pulmonary complications in trauma patients showed a 0.2% incidence of pulmonary edema in the 3289 patients analyzed (117). Pulmonary edema can be defined as the presence of clinical or radiographic findings that responds to fluid restriction or diuresis (117).

The etiology of fluid overload is related to the trauma patients receiving significant crystalloid resuscitation as well as massive transfusion to treat hemorrhagic shock. At the same time, respiratory failure due to fluid overload may be partially attributed to pulmonary contusions sustained at the time of injury, new onset or exacerbation of pre-existing cardiac failure, and the development of sepsis (118).

Pathophysiology

The pathophysiology of fluid overload remains controversial. Pulmonary edema may be the result of increased pulmonary capillary permeability, which can occur due to trauma itself (118,119), due to hemorrhagic shock (118), or due to the development of sepsis (118,120). However, several studies show that despite an increase in pulmonary microvascular permeability, pulmonary edema has not consistently occurred (121,122). Fluid overload may occur in some trauma patients, because they have a decreased compliance in the interstitial compartment that is exacerbated by decreased renal perfusion (123). The third and most popular theory is that pulmonary edema develops because massive fluid resuscitation, particularly with crystalloid solutions, results in a decrease in the plasma colloid oncotic pressure, with subsequent movement of fluid from the intravascular space to the interstitial compartment (124–126).

Once again, several studies dispute this idea (118,127–131). However, this theory has been critical to the still unresolved issue of whether colloid solutions are better than crystalloid solutions when massive fluid resuscitation is required in patients. Multiple studies suggest that colloids do not significantly improve pulmonary function or decrease the incidence of pulmonary edema when compared to crystalloids (128,132,133). In fact, several studies and reviews suggest that colloids may actually worsen pulmonary function and survival in trauma patients (129,132,134,135). More rigorous, randomized clinical trials, however, are still needed to better understand the phenomenon of fluid overload, and the role played by crystalloids and colloids.

Near-Drowning
Definition, Incidence, and Etiology

Near-drowning is reviewed in detail in Volume 1, Chapter 35, and has been defined by Modell (136) as "survival, at least temporarily, after suffocation by submersion in water." The exact incidence of near-drowning can only be estimated from data regarding drownings, but is at least double the incidence of drowning (137,138). According to the World Health Organization, at least 450,000 people drown annually world wide (139). However, since not all drownings are reported, this figure is undoubtedly an underestimation (140,141). Less than 10% of drowning accidents occur in salt water (141).

Drownings, and thus also near-drownings, are associated with a variety of causes including swimming, cramps while swimming, the consumption of alcohol and drugs near bodies of water, epilepsy or cardiac attacks while in the water, lapse of supervision around bodies of water, the use of hyperventilation to increase the duration of underwater swimming, and the immersion syndrome (141–145). The immersion syndrome occurs when a person is suddenly exposed to water 5°C less than body temperature and develops arrhythmias and syncope (144). Drownings can also be associated with boating accidents, car-in-water accidents, diving accidents, and suicide.

Pathophysiology

When drowning, victims may or may not have initially aspirated water (145). Regardless, the person experiences laryngospasm severe enough to cause not only panic but also hypoxemia. As hypoxia eases the laryngospasm, the victim swallows as well as aspirates water (144). Contrary to previous theories, the impact of the aspirated water on the respiratory system is more a function of the volume rather than the composition of fluid (144). The aspirated fluid, whether salt or fresh water, destroys surfactant resulting in decreased pulmonary compliance and the development of alveolitis and noncardiogenic pulmonary edema (141,144). All of these developments interfere with normal alveolar-capillary gas exchange, increase intrapulmonary shunting, and subsequently worsen the near-drowning victim's hypoxemia (146). Increasing hypoxia leads to high pulmonary vascular resistance, compromised cardiac function, and systemic hypotension despite severe peripheral vasoconstriction (144). Eventually, the near-drowning victim develops both metabolic and respiratory acidosis. Although rare, the aspirated water may cause electrolyte disturbances, hemolysis, and subsequent arrhythmias (144,147–149).

Management

Immediately upon rescuing a drowning victim, pulmonary resuscitation should be promptly begun without first attempting to drain the aspirated water from the lungs (e.g., using the Heimlich maneuver) (150). Restoration of oxygenation and ventilation is the key to convert a drowning victim to a near-drowning survivor (142). If the water is fresh water, it will rapidly be absorbed into the vascular system (151,152). If the water is seawater, pulmonary edema fluid will be exuded into the alveolar spaces (143,144,149). The priority should be to re-establish oxygenation and ventilation, with or without mechanical support. The near-drowning victim's pulmonary status may be further complicated by emesis and aspiration of gastric contents (153). Treatment for aspiration should be judiciously begun only when infection is suspected and cultures are pending, unless the near-drowning victim is known to have aspirated grossly contaminated water (142,154).

Although the near-drowning victim's initial chest X ray on admission to the hospital may be normal, it does not necessarily correlate with the patient's arterial oxygen concentration or pulmonary artery to inspired oxygen concentration ratio (147). More importantly, a later radiograph may reflect the pulmonary edema that can develop up to 12 hours after the drowning accident (144,155). The pulmonary edema that occurs may be the result of the process described above or the onset of either NPE or ARDS (156). Regardless, the patient often requires mechanical ventilatory support to ensure adequate oxygenation and that ventilation is maintained. (For greater specifics regarding the respiratory management of the patient with NPE or ARDS, please see the corresponding sections.) The use of steroids has not been shown to be of benefit (147).

The near-drowning patient's pulmonary status may be further compromised by the development of cardiac failure. Cardiac dysfunction occurs as the severe hypoxemia experienced during drowning produces increased pulmonary vascular resistance that decreases the cardiac output and increases central venous pressure (157,158). Subsequently, the patient develops cardiogenic pulmonary edema in addition to the ongoing pulmonary edema secondary to drowning (159). These patients may benefit from either increased intravascular volume or dobutamine to improve cardiac function and oxygen delivery (160). The use of furosemide, however, is strongly discouraged (144).

Although not addressed in detail here, there are other potential medical concerns to be considered when treating a near-drowning victim. These include hypothermia due to exposure in the water and cerebral edema secondary to cerebral hypoxia; both should be individually addressed (141,142,144). For additional study on near-drowning, the reader is referred to Volume 1, Chapter 35.

ACUTE LUNG INJURY AND ARDS

✔ **ALI can result from all of the lesions that progress to the ARDS (also see Volume 2, Chapters 23 and 24).** ✔

Indeed, ALI, by recent definition, merely means that the PaO_2/F_IO_2 is <300, whereas ARDS has a PaO_2/F_IO_2 <200 (161). Typically, ALI begins with an injury to both components of the alveolar-capillary barrier: the alveolar epithelium and the pulmonary capillary. The loss of alveolar epithelium has multiple effects (162). First, the increased permeability of the alveolar epithelium permits the development of alveolar edema. Next, the impaired fluid and ion transport inhibits the normal reabsorption of fluid and, further, enhances the development of alveolar edema. Finally, decreased surfactant production and turnover further compromises the gas exchange function of the alveoli. Surfactant diminution results in increased surface tension of alveoli that are still open, causing them to collapse and develop atelectasis.

Simultaneously, an increase in pulmonary vascular permeability leads to an influx of protein-rich edema into the alveoli (163–166). Hence, this phase of the injury process is known as the exudative phase. Besides proteins, the alveolar edema fluid also contains a high concentration of neutrophils (167). Studies of neutrophils show that their activation causes lung injury and their depletion can prevent or reduce injury (168,169). However, ARDS can develop in neutropenic patients (170). Recent work has focused on preventing adhesion of neutrophils to endothelial and epithelial cells, in an effort to decrease their migration from the vascular lumen and slow their injurious interaction with epithelium (171). The exact role of neutrophils remains unclear, however, they do participate in the pulmonary inflammatory process (162,172).

The combination of alveolar edema and surfactant dysfunction increases intrapulmonary shunting, increases dead-space ventilation, and decreases lung compliance. Shunting can increase to 25% to 50% of cardiac output and present as severe refractory hypoxemia (173). Increased dead-space ventilation results from the rapid shallow breathing, even when the alveoli are relatively normal. The decrease in lung compliance is due to increased lung water edema and a reduction in the aeratable lung volume to 20% to 30% of normal (174). CT studies of the lungs of patients diagnosed with ARDS show localization of densities to dependent areas, correlating with loss of gas volume rather than edema (174). As ARDS progresses from the exudative to the proliferative and, finally, the fibrotic phase, the decrease in lung compliance begins to result from a change in the intrinsic elastic properties of lung tissue.

For many of these complications, ARDS is the final common pathway. ✔ **ARDS-inciting events may be associated with primary injuries to the lung, such as aspiration, pneumonia, pulmonary contusions, near-drowning, and toxic inhalation (160,161). On the other hand, the initiating event may be an extrapulmonary illness that injures the lungs through activation of systemic inflammation response syndrome.** ✔ Examples of indirect causes of ARDS include sepsis, shock, multiple emergency transfusions, major multiple fractures, pancreatitis, burns, cardiopulmonary bypass, and disseminated intravascular coagulation (161,162). Seventy to eighty percent of ARDS is accounted for by sepsis, aspiration, and trauma (163,164). The onset of ARDS varies with approximately 80% of patients developing ARDS within 48 hours after an inciting event, 90% of patients developing ARDS in the first 72 hours, and the remaining patients developing ARDS over the next several days (164,165). Mortality ranges from 10% to 90%, with average mortality slightly greater than 50%. Death is primarily due to multiorgan dysfunction syndrome and sepsis, rather than pulmonary failure or hypoxia.

Ashbaugh (166), first described ARDS in 1967 as an acute onset of severe respiratory distress with cyanosis refractory to oxygen therapy, decreased lung compliance, and diffuse infiltrates on chest radiograph. In 1994, the American-European Consensus Conference on ARDS simplified the definition to improve the determination of incidence and mortality and their response to interventional strategies. ALI is defined as "a syndrome of inflammation and increased permeability that is associated with a constellation of clinical, radiologic, and physiologic abnormalities that cannot be explained by, but may coexist with, left atrial or pulmonary capillary hypertension" (161). ARDS is reserved for the most severe form of ALI. The defining criteria for both include acute onset, chest X rays consistent with bilateral infiltrates, pulmonary artery occlusion pressure of less than 19 mm Hg or no clinical evidence of congestive heart failure, and a low PaO_2/FiO_2 ratio. The cut-off for ALI is a PaO_2/FiO_2 ratio of less than 300, whereas that for ARDS is less than 200 (161).

MECHANICAL VENTILATION CONSIDERATIONS

Mechanical ventilation for trauma and critical care is reviewed extensively in Volume 2, Chapter 27. ARDS-affected lungs can be further traumatized by mechanical ventilation when a high fraction of inspired oxygen (FiO_2) is used, plateau pressures exceed 30–40 cm H_2O causing barotrauma, and high tidal volumes are used resulting in volutrauma (175). ⚔ **Current ventilation management for ARDS involves an open lung technique with tidal volumes in the 6 cc/kg range and enough PEEP to keep alveoli open at end exhalation.** ⚔

Maintaining the PEEP at a level that keeps alveoli open allows ventilation to occur above the lower inflection point on the P/V curve (see Volume 2, Chapter 27). Similarly, by keeping the tidal volume less than 7 cc/kg, the ventilation is typically occurring below the upper inflection point on the P/V curve. This is the so-called "lung protective strategy."

Best PEEP

Best PEEP decreases or abolishes the lower inflection point to prevent cyclic alveolar collapse and recruitment, whereas minimizing overdistension of alveoli already open (176). At the same time, best PEEP permits decreases in the FiO_2 and minimally affects the cardiac performance of a patient with adequate intravascular volume. Gattinoni (177) demonstrated on computed tomography that PEEP has an immediate effect on lung densities by acting as a counterforce to hydrostatic pressure. The effect of PEEP, therefore, reopens dependent alveoli and reduces the amount of nonaerated tissue. His studies show that the maximal amount of PEEP should not exceed ventral to dorsal height of lung in centimeters when applied in the supine patient (178).

Small Tidal Volumes

Amato (179) defines the open lung approach as the use of (*i*) PEEP above the lower inflection point of the pressure-volume curve, (*ii*) tidal volumes <6 mL/kg, (*iii*)) static peak pressures <40 cm H_2O, (*iv*) permissive hypercapnia, and (*v*) stepwise use of pressure-limited modes. Their study shows that using the open lung approach improved lung compliance, increased PaO_2/FiO_2 and decreased shunt, decreased periods of high FiO_2 use and resulted in faster weaning from the ventilator. Unfortunately, Amato was unable to demonstrate any significant difference in mortality. A study by the National Institutes of Health (NIH) ARDS Network also supports the use of small tidal volumes, which were associated with a decreased plasma concentration of IL-6, an increased number of early extuba-

tions, an increase in ventilator-free days, and decreased mortality (180). This study reinforces earlier research demonstrating ventilator-associated lung injury (181–183). A more recent trial by the NIH ARDS Network corroborates the results of the earlier work and suggests that small tidal volumes should be used in patients with ALI or ARDS, regardless of its etiology (184).

Prone Position

Having the patient in prone position can improve oxygenation and decrease shunt without deleterious effects on hemodynamics. The beneficial effects of prone position include: changes of chest wall compliance, changes in gravitational ventilation/perfusion distribution, changes in regional diaphragmatic motion, improvement of postural drainage of bronchial secretions, and compliance of thoracoabdominal cage decreased. Prone position may cause gas to be distributed toward the ventral, dependent portion of the lung resulting in a more homogeneous regional inflation and improved oxygenation.

Perfusion of the lung continues to be greater in the dorsal area than the ventral area, even after the patient has been in the prone position for a prolonged period of time (185). The beneficial effect of the prone position does not immediately disappear on return to the supine position.

Partial Liquid Ventilation

Partial liquid ventilation involves filling the functional residual capacity volume with perfluorocarbons (PFC) in combination with conventional mechanical ventilation (186). The PFC acts as the carrier for oxygen and carbon dioxide. PFC improves gas exchange by decreasing surface tension and thus increasing compliance, promoting recruitment of previously collapsed dependent lung regions, facilitating the use of lower ventilator pressures to achieve desired tidal volumes, and facilitating removal of airway secretions (185,187). Recruitment also occurs by physical distension by a noncompressible fluid. PFC preferentially re-expands gravity-dependent dorsal alveoli and simultaneously redirects blood flow toward the nondependent lung. Recruitment of alveoli improves ventilation/perfusion matching and, thus, decreases intrapulmonary shunting. Studies are under way to evaluate the efficacy of this treatment modality. The reader is referred to Volume 2, Chapter 27 for further study.

ANALGESIA FOR THORACIC TRAUMA

Patients with thoracic trauma are at significant risk of respiratory morbidity and mortality (188). Respiratory failure and/or pneumonia can be prevented with aggressive respiratory care; however, this is limited by the adequacy of pain control (188,189). Pain from rib fractures due to blunt thoracic trauma can severely limit patient mobilization, deep breathing, and cough. First-line pain management predominantly consists of a patient-controlled analgesia (PCA) deliverance of parenteral opioids, with or without other adjuncts such as nonsteroidal anti-inflammatory drugs (NSAIDS). Unfortunately, systemic analgesics may be ineffective, or result in oversedation and a decrease in the cough reflex (190). Patients who are failing first-line (systemic analgesic) therapy or who are at high risk for respiratory failure can derive benefit from several different regional anesthetic techniques (Fig. 4) available for the treatment of thoracic pain.

Although invasive, regional blocks tend to be more effective than systemic opioids and produce less systemic side effects. However, the current literature does not support the application of any particular method of analgesia for all circumstances, for patients with multiple fractured ribs (191). Rather, the data supports having superbly trained trauma anesthesiologists and surgeons that understand the strengths and weaknesses of the various analgesic techniques (191). In this setting, the clinician can weigh the risks and benefits and individualize the pain management based on the clinical setting and the extent of trauma.

The following regional analgesic options should be considered along with systemic opioids: epidural analgesia, thoracic paravertebral block, intercostal nerve block, and interpleural analgesia. These have all been used effectively, and will be reviewed sequentially next.

Epidural

Thoracic epidural analgesia is a commonly employed mode of pain management for thoracic trauma. The use of a thoracic epidural analgesia has been shown to decrease the amount of opiate utilized, increase tidal volumes, and improve negative inspiratory force (191–193). When started within 24 hours of admission, thoracic epidural analgesia with bupivacaine and fentanyl have been shown to provide superior analgesia than intravenous PCA morphine (188).

Several forms of epidural analgesia have been used and are acceptable for the treatment of thoracic trauma. Debate continues concerning the level of placement (lumbar vs thoracic) and the ideal epidural solution (opiate vs local anesthetic or combination). However, the general consensus is that a combined (opiate and local anesthesia) technique tends to be optimal by providing superior analgesia with fewer side effects (188). Although technically more difficult, a thoracic epidural with a local anesthetic/opiate mixture is superior, especially if using a local anesthetic-based technique. If a lumbar epidural catheter is placed, an opiate without local anesthetic should be used for pain management. The addition of patient-controlled epidural analgesia, along with continuous epidural drug infusions, has further increased the effectiveness of this technique. Thoracic epidural is considered by many to be the most effective of the regional techniques available to treat thoracic trauma (194). However, several known complications of thoracic epidural need to be considered (188). Epidural analgesia is contraindicated in patients with significant ongoing hemorrhage, abnormalities in coagulation factors, thrombocytopnia, or hypotension for any reason, systemic infection, and neurological trauma (i.e., spinal cord damage). The most common side effect of epidural analgesia is hypotension

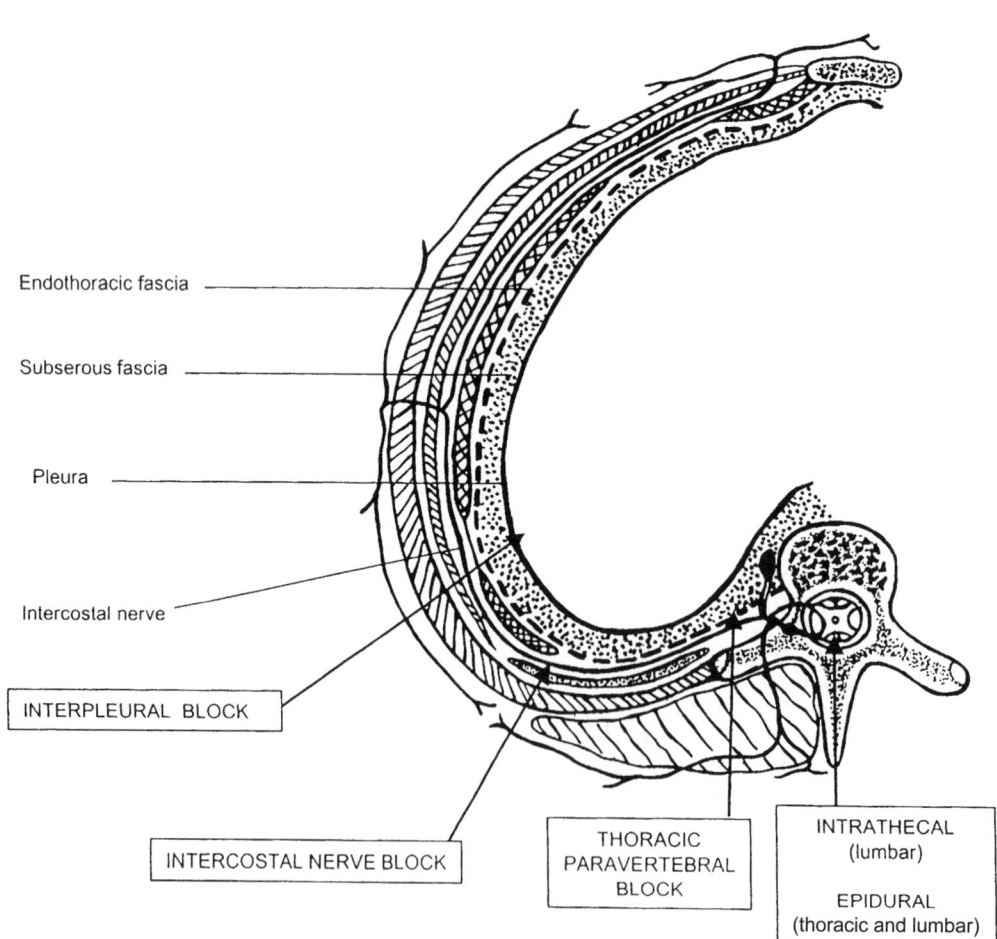

Endothoracic fascia

Subserous fascia

Pleura

Intercostal nerve

INTERPLEURAL BLOCK

INTERCOSTAL NERVE BLOCK

THORACIC PARAVERTEBRAL BLOCK

INTRATHECAL (lumbar)

EPIDURAL (thoracic and lumbar)

Figure 4   Regional analgesic techniques available for patients with thoracic trauma (including rib fractures). The figure shows the basic anatomy including the intercostal nerve, pleura, muscle, and fascial layers, as well as the anatomic target location for each of the regional techniques. *Source*: From Ref. 191.

that usually responds to volume infusion. There is also always the rare risk of epidural hematoma or abscess.

☞ **Placement of an epidural catheter in the trauma victim, especially at the thoracic level, takes significant expertise and should only be performed by an appropriately trained anesthesiologist.** ☞ Furthermore, management should be conducted by an established and dedicated pain management team.

Trauma patients who have suffered unilateral chest trauma, with or without neurological compromise, are good candidates for pain management with thoracic paravertebral block. This regional technique should be performed by an appropriately trained anesthesiologist. Several variations of this technique can be utilized in the thoracic trauma patient. A continuous catheter can be placed or a "single-shot" can be performed. Advantages over an epidural technique include not interfering with neurological examinations, a decreased incidence of hypotension, and coagulopathy is only a relative contraindication (195). Risks of this technique include pneumothorax, vascular puncture, hypotension and, occasionally, epidural spread resulting in pulmonary compromise.

Intercostal Block

Easy to perform and not requiring an anesthesiologist, the intercostal nerve block is a popular technique for management of trauma localized to the seventh rib and below. Performance of this block on higher ribs is problematic due to interference from the scapula. Due to the dual innervation of ribs, the inner space above and below each rib must be injected. The block can be repeated as often as needed but one study found that 89% of patients required only two interventions and subsequently did well with systemic opiates (196). The predominant risk of this technique is pneumothorax, which is roughly 1.5% per block. This technique is most appropriate for patients with isolated lower rib fractures who do not suffer from other injuries. Catheter placement has been described and is successful, especially if the catheters are actually intentionally placed extrapleural as described by Haenel et al. (190). Increased spread is achieved and additional levels can be covered by a single catheter placed in this manner.

Intrapleural Block

Extremely easy to perform and only limited by local anesthetic toxicity secondary to absorption, interpleural analgesia can be utilized if the previously described regional techniques cannot be performed. Unfortunately, the efficacy of this technique is suspect, and certainly is not as effective as the aforementioned ones (197,198).

EYE TO THE FUTURE

The future management of thoracic trauma will integrate methods to enhance delivery of care via use of mobile systems, incorporate newer technology and pharmacological agents, and strive for less invasive surgical and monitoring techniques. There continues to be a need for solutions for common trauma-related complications. For example, there is a need for enhanced methods for protection of the spinal cord in circumstances of direct cord injury, as well as prevention of anterior spinal cord injury occurring during surgical repair of thoracic aortic rupture and/or

dissection. Additionally, newer methods of airway management, with the utilization of bronchial-blocking devices and enhanced bronchoscopic imaging, will be welcome advances in perioperative management of thoracic trauma. Echocardiographic assessment of hemodynamics can permit a less invasive alternative to pulmonary artery catheterization. More effective technology and miniaturization of TEE devices could enhance diagnosis of injury and perioperative hemodynamic monitoring of the thoracic trauma victim. The development of safe and effective blood substitutes will be important as the risk of blood-borne pathogens lingers. Recombinant blood factors may enhance the treatment of coagulopathy and provide solutions for trauma-related coagulopathies. For example, recombinant factor VIIa has treated bleeding refractory to other interventions, and there is now experimental and early clinical evidence that these recombinant factors can be effective in the treatment of trauma-related hemorrhage (199). Thoracoscopic diagnosis and repair of injury is more prevalent in trauma care. Analgesic methods, though good, are not yet optimal. New strategies of mechanical ventilation and sedation during ICU care are necessary. Triage and field management of casualties may save more lives as more prompt care requires training of individuals in immediate proximity to the trauma scene, to utilize portable systems of resuscitation and trauma care. Endovascular management of thoracic aortic injury is now becoming available clinically (200).

SUMMARY

Thoracic trauma is a common problem in both urban trauma and military conflicts. Optimal management requires early diagnosis and prompt treatment of life-threatening injury (hemothorax, pneumothorax, pericardial tamponade, etc.). Besides treatment of the primary injury, outcome is improved when secondary injury (e.g., aspiration, fluid overload, etc.) is prevented or minimized. When feasible, the use of thoracoscopic technology speeds recovery, because additional trauma and pain is minimized. Lung-protective ventilation strategies allow for oxygenation and ventilation without causing exacerbation of the existing lung injury.

Analgesia must be optimized to facilitate early return to spontaneous ventilation and minimize splinting-related atelectasis and pneumonia. Patients capable of breathing on their own, despite extensive rib or chest-wall trauma, are optionally managed with thoracic epidural analgesia. Those requiring prolonged mechanical ventilation can receive intravenous opiates during the most painful period (first two to four days following injury).

Optimum care of the thoracic trauma patient requires a unifying management approach which includes the above concepts. By so doing, the significant morbidity and prolonged ICU stays common so those injuries can be minimized.

KEY POINTS

☞ The most common etiologies of shock penetrating chest injury include tension pneumothorax, massive hemothorax, cardiac wounds, and cardiac tamponade.

☞ The magnitude of destruction resulting from the secondary shock wave occurring with high-velocity GSWs and shrapnel injuries may not be initially apparent.

☞ Atelectasis will develop as a result of splinting of the chest and will compound the shunt attributable to lung contusion itself.

☞ Bronchoscopy is an essential part of the evaluation of the victim of thoracic or neck trauma whenever there is a suspicion of airway disruption.

☞ When left heart air embolism is recognized, the team must prevent further entry of air into the left heart. The first maneuver is isolation of the injured lung via one-lung ventilation (1LV).

☞ Early evaluation and prompt management are the most critical factors in optimum outcomes following esophageal injury.

☞ Assessment of structural abnormalities of the heart and pericardial effusion (blood) and possible early or frank cardiac tamponade, can be quickly evaluated with TTE as part of the FAST exam (Volume 1, Chapters 14, 16, and 25). However, TEE is preferable to TTE whenever structural lesions or valve abnormalities are to be evaluated.

☞ The proper use of cricoid pressure (Sellick's maneuver) may help prevent regurgitation of gastric contents into the trachea during intubation (22).

☞ The treatment of carbon monoxide toxicity involves the use of a high-inspired concentration of oxygen.

☞ For patients who survive the first 24 hours after traumatic injury, PE is the third leading cause of death (76).

☞ Pulmonary angiography had been the gold standard for diagnosing PE. As with contrast venography, pulmonary angiography is limited by its invasiveness and cost. Spiral CT is emerging as the new gold standard. However, some patterns of PEs, such as distal small vessel disease, are better seen by angiography, whereas others are better seen by CT (85).

☞ Acute lung injury (ALI) can result from all of the lesions that progress to the ARDS (also see Volume 2, Chapters 23 and 24).

☞ ARDS-inciting events may be associated with primary injuries to the lung, such as aspiration, pneumonia, pulmonary contusions, near-drowning, and toxic inhalation (160,161). On the other hand, the initiating event may be an extrapulmonary illness that injures the lungs through activation of systemic inflammation response syndrome.

☞ Current ventilation management for ARDS involves an open lung technique with tidal volumes in the 6 cc/kg range and enough PEEP to keep alveoli open at end exhalation.

☞ Placement of an epidural catheter in the trauma victim, especially at the thoracic level, takes significant expertise and should only be performed by an appropriately trained anesthesiologist.

REFERENCES

1. Martin SK, Shatney CH, Sherck JP, et al. Blunt trauma patients with prehospital pulseless electrical activity (PEA): poor ending assured. J Trauma 2002; 53(5):876–880.
2. Katz E, Ofek B, Adler J, Abramowitz HB, Krausz MM. Primary blast injury after a bomb explosion in a civilian bus. Ann Surg 1989; 209(4):484–488.
3. Sankaran S, Wilson RF. Factors affecting prognosis in patients with flail chest. J Thorac Cardiovasc Surg 1970; 60(3):402–410.
4. Orliaguet G, Mustapha F, Riou B. The heart in blunt trauma. Anesth 2001; 95:544–548.
5. Wilson WC, Benumof JL. Anesthesia for thoracic surgery. In: Miller RD, ed. Anesthesia. 6th ed. Philadelphia: Churchill Livingston, 2005.
6. Weigelt JA, Thai ER, Snyder WH, et al. Diagnosis of penetrating cervical esophageal injuries. Am J Surg 1987; 154:619–628.
7. Richardson JD, Tobin GR. Closure of esophageal defects with muscle flaps. Arch Surg 1994; 129:541.
8. Armstrong WB, Detar TR, Stanley RB. Diagnosis and management of external penetrating cervical esophageal injuries. Ann Otorhinolaryngeal 1994; 103:863.
9. Garcia-Fernandez MA, Lopez-Perez JM, Perez-Castellano N, et al. Role of transesophageal echocardiography in the assessment of patients with blunt chest trauma: correlation of echocardiographic findings with the electrocardiogram and creatinine kinease monoclonal antibody measurements. Am Heart J 1998; 135:476–481.
10. Cinnella G, Dambrosio M, Brienza N, et al. Transesophageal echocardiography for diagnosis of traumatic aortic injury: an appraisal of the evidence. J Trauma 2004; 57(6):1246–1255.
11. Melton SM, Kerby JD, McGiffin D, et al. The evolution of chest computed tomography for the definitive diagnosis of blunt aortic injury: a single-center experience. J Trauma 2004; 56(2):243–250.
12. Zager JS, Ohki T, Simon JE, et al. Endovascular repair of a traumatic pseudoaneurysm of the thoracic aorta in a patient with concomitant intracranial and intra-abdominal injuries. J Trauma 2003; 55(4):778.
13. Von Oppell UO, Dunne TT, De Greeot MK, et al. Traumatic aortic rupture: Twenty-year meta analysis of mortality and risk of paraplegia. Ann Thorac Surg 1994; 58:585–593.
14. D'Angers O. Relation medicale des evenements survenus au Champs-de- Mars le 14 juin, 1837. Ann d'Hyg 1837; 18:485.
15. Jongewaard WR, Cogbill TH, Landercasper J. Neurological consequences of traumatic asphyxia. J Trauma 1992; 32:28.
16. Rhee PM, Acosta J, Bridgeman A, et al. Survival after emergency department thoracotomy: review of published data from the past 25 years. J Am Col Surg 2000; 190:288–298.
17. Olsson GL, Hallen B, Hambreus-Jonzos K. Aspiration during anaesthesia: a computer-aided study of 185,358 anaesthetics. Acta Anaesthesiol Scand 1986; 30:84–92.
18. Oswalt JL, Hedges JR, Soifer BE, Lowe DK. Analysis of trauma intubations. Am J Emerg Med 1992; 10:511–514.
19. Warner MA, Warner ME, Weber JB. Clinical significance of pulmonary aspiration during the perioperative period. Anesthesiology 1993; 78:56–62.
20. Lockey DJ, Coats T, Parr MJA. Aspiration in severe trauma: a prospective study. Anaesthesia 1999; 54:1097–1109.
21. Thibodoeau LG, Vedile VP, Bartfield JM. Incidence of aspiration after urgent intubation. Am J Emerg Med 1997; 15: 562–565.
22. Fanning GL. The efficacy of cricoid pressure in preventing regurgitation of gastric contents. Anesthesiology 1970; 32:553–555.
23. Manning G, McGreal G, Winter DC, Kirwan WO, Redmond HP. Nasogastric intubation causes gastro-oesophageal reflux in patients undergoing elective laparotomy. Br J Surg 2000; 87:637.
24. Ferrer M, Bauer TT, Torres A, Hernandez D, Piera C. Effect of nasogastric tube size on gastroesophageal reflux and microaspiration in intubated patients. Ann Intern Med 1999; 130: 991–994.
25. Ng A, G Smith. Gastroesophageal reflux and aspiration of gastric contents in anesthetic practice. Anesth Analg 2001; 93:494–513.
26. Salem MR, Joseph NJ, Heyman HJ, Belani B, Paulissian R, Ferrara TP. Cricoid compression is effective in obliterating the esophageal lumen in the presence of a nasogastric tube. Anesthesiology 1985; 63:443–446.
27. Escolano F, Sierra P, Ortiz JC, Cabrera JC, Castano J. The efficacy and optimum time of administration of ranitidine in the prevention of the acid aspiration syndrome. Anaesthesia 1996; 51:182–184.

28. Barlett JG, Gorbach SL, Finegold SM. The bacteriology of aspiration pneumonia. Am J Med 1974; 56:202–207.

29. Zorab JSM. Pulmonary aspiration. Br Med J 1984; 288:1631–1632.

30. Zilberberg M, Epstein SK. Acute lung injury in the medical ICU: Comorbid conditions, age, etiology, and hospital outcome. Am J Respir Crit Care Med 1998; 157:1159–1164.

31. Valta P, Ususaro A, Nunes S, Ruokonen E, Takala J. Acute respiratory distress syndrome: Frequency, clinical course, and costs of care. Crit Care Med 1999; 27:2367–2374.

32. Brandt CP, Yowler, CJ, Fratianne RB. Burns with multiple trauma. Am Surg 2002; 68:240–244.

33. Dougherty W, Waxman K. The complexities of managing severe burns with associated trauma. Surg Clin North Am 1996; 76:923–958.

34. Purdue G, Hunt J. Multiple trauma and the burn patient. Am J Surg 1989; 158:536–538.

35. Shirani KZ, Pruitt BA Jr, Mason AD Jr. The influence of inhalation injury and pneumonia on burn mortality. Ann Surg 1987; 205:82–87.

36. Hollingsed TC, Saffle JR, Barton RG, Craft WB, Morris SE. Etiology and consequences of respiratory failure in thermally injured patients. American J of Surgery 1993; 166:592–597.

37. Blinn DL, Slater H, Goldfarb W. Inhalation injury with burns: a lethal combination. J Emerg Med 1988; 6:471–473.

38. Thompson PB, Herndon DN, Traber DL, Abston S. Effect on mortality of inhalation injury. J Trauma 1986; 26:163–165.

39. Darling GE, Keresteci MA, Ibanez D, Pugash RA, Peters WJ, Neligan PC. Pulmonary complications in inhalation injuries with associated cutaneous burn. J Trauma 1996; 40:83–89.

40. Cahalane M, Demling RH. Early respiratory abnormalities from smoke inhalation. JAMA 1984; 251:771–773.

41. Peitzman AB, Shires GT 3rd, Teixidor HS, Curreri PW, Shires GT. Smoke inhalation injury: evaluation of radiographic manifestations and pulmonary dysfunction. J Trauma 1989; 29:232–1239.

42. Zikria BA, Weston GC, Chodoff M, Ferrer JM. Smoke and carbon monoxide poisoning in fire victims. J Trauma 1972; 12:641–645.

43. Jones J., McMullen MJ, Dougherty J. Toxic smoke inhalation: Cyanide poisoning in fire victims. Am J Emerg Med 1987; 5:317–321.

44. Demling RH, Chen C. Pulmonary function in the burn patient. Semin Nephrol 1993; 13:371–381.

45. Tasaki O, Dubick MA, Goodwin CW, Pruitt B. Effects of burns on inhalation injury in sheep: a 5-day study. J Trauma 2002; 52(2):351–358.

46. Peitzman AB, Shires GT 3rd, Corbett WA, Curreri PW, Shires GT. Measurement of lung water in inhalation injury. Surgery 1981; 90:305–312.

47. Chrysopoulo MT, Barrow RE, Muller M, Rubin S, Barrow LN, Herndon DN. Chest radiographic appearances in severely burned adults. A comparison of early radiographic and extravascular lung thermal volume changes. J Burn Care Rehabil 2001; 22:104–110.

48. Tranbaugh RF, Lewis FR, Christensen JM, Elings VB. Lung water changes after thermal injury: the effects of crystalloid resuscitation and sepsis. Ann Surg 1980; 192:479–490.

49. Bulger EM, Smith DG, Maier RV, Jurkovich GJ. Fat embolism syndrome. Arch Surg 1997; 132:435–439.

50. Mellor A, Soni N. Fat embolism. Anaesthesia 2001; 56:145–154.

51. Batra P. The fat embolism syndrome. J Thorac Imaging 1987; 2:12–17.

52. Gitin TA, Seidel T, Cera PJ, Glidewell OJ, Smith JL. Pulmonary microvascular fat: the significance? Crit Care Med 1993; 21:673–677.

53. Williams AG Jr, Mettler FA Jr, Christie JH, Gordon RD. Fat embolism syndrome. Clin Nucl Med 1986; 11:495–497.

54. Eddy A, Rice C, Carrico C. Fat embolism syndrome: monitoring and management. J Crit Illness 198; 2:24–37.

55. Fabian T, Hoots A, Stanford D, Patterson CR, Mangiante EC. Fat embolism syndrome: prospective evaluation in 92 fracture patients. Crit Care Med 1990; 18:42–46.

56. Pell AC, Hughes D, Keating J, Christie J, Busuttil A, Sutherland GR. Brief report: fulminating fat embolism syndrome caused by paradoxical embolism through a patent foramen ovale. NEJM 1993; 329:926–929.

57. Sevitt S. The significance and pathology of fat embolism. Ann Clin Res 1977; 9:173–180.

58. Giannoudis PV, Pape HC, Cohen AP, Krettek C, Smith RM. Review: Systemic effects of femoral nailing. Clin Orthop 2002; 404:378–386.

59. Robinson CM. Current concepts of respiratory insufficiency syndromes after fracture. J Bone Joint Surg(Br) 2001; 83-B:781–791.

60. Peltier L. Fat embolism: a current concept. Clin Orthop 1969; 66:241–253.

61. Muller C, Rahn BA, Pfister U, Meinig RP. The incidence, pathogenesis, diagnosis, and treatment of fat embolism. Orthopaedic Review 1994; 23:107–117.

62. Schonfeld SA, Ploysongsang Y, DiLision R, et al. Fat embolism prophylaxis with corticosteroids. Ann Intern Med 1983; 99:433–438.

63. Lindeque BG, Schoeman HS, Dommisse GF, Boeyens MC, Vlok AL. Fat embolism and the fat embolism syndrome. A double-blind therapeutic study. J Bone Joint Surg (Br) 1987; 69:128–131.

64. Kallenbach J, Lewis M, Zaltzman M, Feldman C, Orford A, Zwi S. 'Low-dose' corticosteroid prophylaxis against fat embolism. J Trauma 1987; 27:1173–1176.

65. Shier MR, Wilson RF, James RE, Riddle J, Mammen EF, Pedersen HE. Fat embolism prophylaxis: a study of four treatment modalities. J Trauma 1977; 17:621–629.

66. Byrick RJ, Mullen JB, Wong PY, Kay JC, Wigglesworth D, Doran RJ. Prostanoid production and pulmonary hypertension after fat embolism are not modified by methylprednisone. Can J Anaesth 1991; 38:660–667.

67. Knudson MM, Lewis FR, Clinton A, Atkinson K, Megerman J. Prevention of venous thromboembolism in trauma patients. J Trauma 1994; 37:480–487.

68. Shackford SR, Davis JW, Hollingsworth-Fridlund P, Brewer NS, Hoyt DB, Mackersie RC. Venous thromboembolism in patients with major trauma. Am J Surg 1990; 159:365–369.

69. Dennis JW, Menawat S, Von Thron J, et al. Efficacy of deep venous thrombosis prophylaxis in trauma patients and identification of high-risk groups. J Trauma 1993; 35:132–138.

70. Geerts WH, Code KI, Jay RM, Chen E, Szalai JP. A prospective study of venous thromboembolism after major trauma. N Engl J Med 1994; 331:1601–1606.

71. Kudsk KA, Fabian TC, Baum S, Gold RE, Mangiante E, Voeller G. Silent deep vein thrombosis in immobilized multiple trauma patients. Am J Surg 1989; 158:515–519.

72. Tuttle-Newhall JE, Rutledge R, Hultman CS, Fakhry SM. Statewide, population-based, time series analysis of the frequency and outcome of pulmonary embolism in 318,554 trauma patients. J Trauma 1997; 42:90–99.

73. Winchell RJ, Hoyt DB, Walsh JC, Simons RK, Eastman AB. Risk factors associated with pulmonary embolism despite routine prophylaxis: implications for improved protection. J Trauma 1994; 37:600–606.

74. Rogers FB, Shackford SR, Ricci MA, Wilson JT, Parsons S. Routine prophylactic vena cava filter insertion in severely injured trauma patients decreases the incidence of pulmonary embolism. J Am Coll Surg 1995; 180:640–647.

75. O'Malley KF, Ross SER. Pulmonary embolism in major trauma patients. J Trauma 1990; 30:748–750.

76. Geerts WH, Heit JA, Clagett GP, et al. Prevention of venous thromboembolism. Chest 2001; 119:132S–175S.

77. Prandoni P, Villalta S, Bagatella P, et al. The clinical course of deep-vein thrombosis: a prospective long-term follow-up of 528 symptomatic patients. Haematologica 1997; 423–428.

78. Franzeck UK, Schalch I, Jager KA, Grimm ES, Bollinger A. Prospective 12-year follow-up study of clinical and hemodynamic sequelae after deep vein thrombosis in low-risk patients (Zurich Study). Circulation 1996; 93:74–79.

79. Prandoni P, Lensing AW, Cogo A, et al. The long-term clinical course of acute deep venous thrombosis. Ann Intern Med 1996; 125:1–7.

80. Baker WF. Diagnosis of deep venous thrombosis and pulmonary embolism. Med Clin North Am 1998; 82:459–476.

81. National Institutes of Health Consensus development Conference Statement: Prevention of venous thrombosis and pulmonary embolism. JAMA 1986; 256: 744–749.

82. Ryu JH, Olson EJ, Pellikka PA. Clinical recognition of pulmonary embolism. Mayo Clin Proc 1998; 73:873–879.

83. Morgenthaler TI, Ryu JH. Clinical characteristics of fatal pulmonary embolism in a referral hospital. Mayo Clin Proc 1995; 70:417–424.

84. Landefeld CS, Chren MM, Myers A, Geller R, Robbins S, Goldman L. Diagnostic yield of the autopsy in a university hospital and a community hospital. N Engl J Med 1988; 318:1249–1254.

85. Ryu JH, Swensen SJ, Olson EJ, Pellikka PA. Diagnosis of pulmonary embolism with use of computed tomographic angiography. Mayo Clin Proc 2001; 76:59–65.

86. Owings JT, Kraut E, Battistella F, Cornelius JT, O'Malley R. Timing of the occurrence of pulmonary embolism in trauma patients. Arch Surg 1997; 132:862–867.

87. Spain DA, Richardson JD, Polk HC Jr, Bergamini TM, Wilson MA, Miller FB. Venous thromboembolism in the high-risk trauma patient: do risks justify aggressive screening and prophylaxis? J Trauma 1997; 42:463–469.

88. Value of the ventilation/perfusion scan in acute pulmonary embolism. Results of the prospective investigation of pulmonary embolism diagnosis (PIOPED). The PIOPED Investigators. JAMA 1990; 263:2753–2759.

89. Lorut C, Ghossains M, Horellou MH, Achkar A, Fretault J, Laaban JP. A noninvasive diagnostic strategy including spiral computed tomography in patients with suspected pulmonary embolism. Am J Respir Crit Care Med 2000; 162:1413–1418.

90. Gottschalk A, Stein PD, Goodman LR, Sostman HD. Overview of prospective investigation of pulmonary diagnosis II. Seminar Nucl Med 2002; 32:173–182.

91. Geerts WH, Jay RM, Code KI, et al. A comparison of low-dose heparin with low-molecular-weight heparin as prophylaxis against venous thromboembolism after major trauma. N Engl J Med 1996; 335:701–707.

92. Prevention of venous thromboembolism. International consensus statement (guideline according to scientific evidence). Int Angiol 1997; 16:3–38.

93. McMurtry AL, Owings JT, Anderson JT, Battistella FD, Gosselin R. Increased use of prophylactic vena cava filters in trauma patients failed to decrease overall incidence of pulmonary embolism. J Am Coll Surg 1999; 189:314–320.

94. Bick RL, Haas S. Thromboprophylaxis and thrombosis in medical, surgical, trauma, and obstetric/gynecologic patients. Hematol Oncol Clin North Am 2003; 17:217–258.

95. Gersin K, Grindlinger GA, Lee V, Dennis RC, Wedel SK, Cachecho R. The efficacy of sequential compression devices in multiple trauma patients with severe head injury. J Trauma 1994; 37:205–208.

96. Rodriguez JL, Lopez JM, Proctor MC, et al. Early placement of prophylactic vena caval filters in injured patients at high risk for pulmonary embolism. J Trauma 1996; 40:797–802.

97. Carlin AM, Tyburski JG, Wilson RF, Steffes C. Prophylactic and therapeutic inferior vena cava filters to prevent pulmonary emboli in trauma patients. Arch Surg 2002; 137:521–527.

98. Decousus H, Leizorovicz A, Parent F, et al. A clinical trial of vena caval filters in the prevention of pulmonary embolism in patients with proximal deep vein thrombosis. N Engl J Med 1998; 338:199–205.

99. Rogers FB, Strindberg G, Shackford SR, et al. Five-year follow-up of prophylactic vena cava filters in high-risk trauma patients. Arch Surg 1998; 133:406–411.

100. Pender ES, Pollack CV Jr. Neurogenic pulmonary edema: case reports and review. J Emerg Med 1993; 11:207–211.

101. Fahy BG, Sivaraman V. Current concepts in neurocritical care. Anesthesiol Clin North America 2002; 20:441–462.

102. Yabumoto M, Kuriyama T, Iwamoto M, Kinoshita T. Neurogenic pulmonary edema associated with ruptured intracranial aneurysm: case report. Neurosurgery 1986; 19:300–304.

103. Colice GL, Matthay MA, Bass E, Matthay RA. Neurogenic pulmonary edema. Am Rev Respir Dis 1984; 130:941–948.

104. Ell SR. Neurogenic pulmonary edema: a review of the literature and a perspective. Invest Radiol 1991; 26:499–506.

105. Fontes RB, Aguiar PH, Zanetti MV, Andrade F, Mandel M, Teixeira MJ. Acute neurogenic pulmonary edema: case reports and literature review. J Neurosurg Anesthesiol 2003; 15:144–150.

106. Rogers FB, Shackford SR, Trevisani GT, Davis JW, Mackersie RC, Hoyt DB. Neurogenic pulmonary edema in fatal and nonfatal head injuries. J Trauma 1995; 39:860–866.

107. Casey WF. Neurogenic pulmonary oedema. Anaesthesia 1983; 38:985–988.

108. Chen HI. Hemodynamic mechanisms of neurogenic pulmonary edema. Biol Signals 1995; 4:186–192.

109. Colice GL. Neurogenic pulmonary edema. Clin Chest Med 1985; 6:473–389.

110. Simon RP. Neurogenic pulmonary edema. Neurol Clin 1993; 11:309–323.

111. Inobe JJ, Mori T, Ueyama H, Kumamoto T, Tsuda T. Neurogenic pulmonary edema induced by primary medullary hemorrhage: a case report. J Neurol Sci 2000; 172:73–76.

112. Wijdicks EFM, Borel CO. Respiratory management in acute neurologic illness. Neurology 1998; 50:11–20.

113. Wiercisiewski DR, McDeavitt JT. Pulmonary complications in traumatic brain injury. J Head Trauma Rehabil 1998; 13:28–35.

114. Deehan SC, Grant IS. Haemodynamic changes in neurogenic pulmonary oedema: effect of dobutamine. Intensive Care Med 1996; 22:672–676.

115. Knudsen F, Jensen HP, Petersen PL. Neurogenic pulmonary edema: treatment with dobutamine. Neurosurgery 1991; 29:269–270.

116. Segers P, Van Schil P, Jorens Ph, Van Den Brande F. Thoracic trauma: an analysis of 187 patients. Acta Cir Belg 2001; 101:277–282.

117. Hoyt DB, Simons RK, Winchell RJ, et al. A risk analysis of pulmonary complications following major trauma. J Trauma 1993; 35:524–531.

118. Tranbaugh RF, Elings VB, Christensen J, Lewis FR. Determinants of pulmonary interstitial fluid accumulation after trauma. J Trauma 1982; 22:820–825.

119. Sturm JA, Wisner DH, Oestern HG, Kant CJ, Tscherne H, Creutzig H. Increased lung capillary permeability after trauma: a prospective clinical study. J Trauma 1986; 26:409–418.

120. Pietra GG, Ruttner JR, Wust W, Glinz W. The lung after trauma and shock: fine structure of the alveolar capillary barrier in 23 autopsies. J Trauma 1981; 21:454–462.

121. Holcroft JW, Trunkey DD. Extravascular lung water following hemorrhagic shock in the baboon: comparison between resuscitation with Ringer's lactate and plasmanate. Ann Surg 1974; 180:408–417.

122. Northrup WF, Humphrey EW. The effect of hemorrhagic shock on pulmonary vascular permeability to proteins. Surgery 1978; 83:264–273.

123. Lucas CE, Ledgerwood AM, Shier MR, Bradley VE. The renal factor in the post-traumatic "fluid overload" syndrome. J Trauma 1977; 17:667–676.

124. Weil MH, Henning RJ, Puri VK. Colloid oncotic pressure: clinical significance. Crit Care Med 1979; 7:113–116.

125. Rackow EC, Fein IA, Leppo J. Colloid oncotic pressure as a prognostic indicator of pulmonary edema and mortality in the critically ill. Chest 1977; 72:709–713.

126. Rackow EC, Falk JL, Fein IA, et al. Fluid resuscitation in circulatory shock: a comparison of the cardiorespiratory effects of albumin, hetastarch, and saline solutions in patients with hypovolemic and septic shock. Crit Care Med 1983; 11:839–850.

127. Virgilio RW, Rice CL, Smith DE, et al. Crystalloid vs. colloid resuscitation: is one better? Surgery 1979; 85:129–139.

128. Shires GT 3rd, Peitzman AB, Albert SA, et al. Response of extravascular lung water to intraoperative fluids. Ann Surg 1983; 197:515–518.

129. Goodwin CW, Dorethy J, Lam V, Pruitt BA Jr. Randomized trial of efficacy of crystalloid and colloid resuscitation on hemodynamic response and lung water following thermal injury. Ann Surg 1983; 197:520–529.

130. Gallagher TJ, Banner MJ, Barnes PA. Large volume crystalloid resuscitation does not increase extravascular lung water. Anesth Analg 1985; 64:323–326.

131. Choi PT, Yip G, Quinonez LG, Cook DJ. Crystalloids vs. colloids in fluid resuscitation. Crit Care Med 1999; 27:200–210.

132. Lowe RJ, Moss GS, Jilek J, Levine HD. Crystalloid vs colloid in the etiology of pulmonary failure after trauma: a randomized trial in man. Surgery 1977; 81:676–683.

133. Moss GS, Lowe RJ, Jilek J, Levine HD. Colloid vs crystalloid in the resuscitation of hemorrhagic shock: a controlled clinical trial. Surgery 1981; 89:434–438.

134. Schierhout G, Roberts I. Fluid resuscitation with colloid or crystalloid solutions in critically ill patients: a systematic review of randomized trials. BMH 1998; 316:961–964.

135. Cochrane Injuries Group Albumin Reviewers. Human albumin administration in critically ill patients: a systematic review of randomized controlled trials. BMJ 1998; 317:235–240.

136. Modell JH. Drown vs near drown: a discussion of definitions. Crit Care Med 1981; 9:351–352.

137. Lindholm P, Steensberg J. Epidemiology of unintentional drowning and near drowning in Denmark in 1995. Inj Prev 2000; 6:29–31.

138. Gonzalez-Rothi RJ. Near-drowning: consensus and controversies in pulmonary and cerebral resuscitation. Heart Lung 1987; 16:474–482.

139. Krug E (ed) for the World Health Organization. Injury: A Leading Cause of the Global Garden of Disease. Geneva, Switzerland: WHO, 1999.

140. Langley JD, Chaimera DJ. Coding the circumstances of injury: ICD-10 a step forward or backwards? Inj Prev 1999; 5:247–253.

141. DeNicola LK, Falk JL, Swanson ME, Gayle NO, Kissoon N. Submersion injuries in children and adults. Crit Care Clin 1997; 13:477–502.

142. Bierens JJ, Knape JT, Gelissen HP. Drowning. Curr Opin Crit Care 2002; 8:578–586.

143. Weinstein MD, Krieger BP. Near-drowning: epidemiology, pathophysiology, and initial treatment. J Emerg Med 1996; 14:461–467.

144. Orlowski JP, Szpilman D. Drowning: rescue, resuscitation, and reanimation. Pediatr Clin North Am 2001; 48:627–646.

145. Modell JH. Drowning without aspiration: is this an appropriate diagnosis? J Forensic Sci 1999; 44:1119–1123.

146. Modell JH, Moya F, Williams HD, Weibley TC. Changes in blood gases and A-a DO$_2$ during near-drowning. Anesthesiology 1968; 29:456–465.

147. Modell JH. Clinical course of 91 consecutive near-drowning victims. Chest 1976; 70:231–238.

148. Modell JH. Serum electrolyte changes in near-drowning victims. JAMA 1985; 253:253–257.

149. Cohen DS, Matthay MA, Cogan MG, Murray JF. Pulmonary edema associated with alt water near-drowning: new insights. Am Rev Respir Dis 1992; 146:794–796.

150. Rosen P, Soto M, Harley J. The use of Heimlich maneuver in near-drowning: Institute of Medicine Report. J Emerg Med 1995; 13:397–405.

151. Conn AW, Barker GA. Fresh water drowning and near-drowning—an update. Can J Anaesth 1984; 31:S38.

152. Modell JH. Drowning. N Engl J Med 1993; 328:253–256.

153. Smyrnios NA, Irwin RS. Current concepts in the pathophysiology and management of near-drowning. J Intensive Care Med 1991; 6:26–35.

154. Oakes DD, Sherck JP, Maloney JR, Charter AC 3rd. Prognosis and management of victims of near-drowning. J Trauma 1982; 22:544–549.

155. Ornato JP. The resuscitation of near-drowning victims. JAMA 1986; 256:75–77.

156. Rumbak MJ. The etiology of pulmonary edema in fresh water near-drowning. Am J Emerg Med 1996; 14:176–179.

157. Hildebrand CA, Hartmann AG, Arcinue EL, Gomez RJ, Bing RJ. Cardiac performance in pediatric near-drowning. Crit Care Med 1988; 16:331–335.

158. Orlowski JP, Abulleil MM, Phillips JM. The hemodynamic and cardiovascular effects of near-drowning in hypotonic, isotonic, or hypertonic solutions. Ann Emerg Med 1989; 18:1044–1049.

159. Tabeling BB, Model JH. Fluid administration increases oxygen delivery during continuous positive ventilation after fresh water near-drowning. Crit Care Med 1983; 11:693–696.

160. Luce JM. Acute lung injury and acute respiratory distress syndrome. Crit Care Med 1998; 26:369–376.

161. Bernard GR, Artigas A, Brigham KL, et al. The American-European consensus conference on ARDS: Definitions, mechanisms, relevant outcomes and clinical trial coordination. Am J Respir Crit Care Med 1994; 149:818–824.

162. Ware LB, Matthay MA. The acute respiratory distress syndrome. NEJM 2000; 342:1334–1349.

163. Pepe PE, Potkin RT, Reus DH, Hudson LD, Carrico CJ. Clinical predictors of the adult respiratory distress syndrome. Am J Surg 1982; 144:124–130.

164. Hudson LD, Milberg JA, Anardi D, et al. Clinical risks for development of the acute respiratory distress syndrome. Am J Respir Crit Care Med 1995; 151:293–201.

165. Fowler AA, Hamman RF, Good JT, et al. Adult respiratory distress syndrome: risk with common predispositions. Ann Inter med 1983; 98:593–597.

166. Ashbaugh DG, Bigelow DB, Petty TL, Levine BE. Acute respiratory distress in adults. Lancet 1967; 2:319–323.

167. Pittet JF, MacKersie RC, Martin TR, Matthay MA. Biological markers of acute lung injury: prognostic and pathogenetic significance. Am J Respir Crit Care Med 1997; 155:1187–1205.

168. Zimmerman GA, Renzetti AD, Hill HR. Functional and metabolic activity of granulocytes from patients with adult respiratory distress syndrome: evidence for activated neutrophils in the pulmonary circulation. Am Rev Respir Dis 1983; 127:290–300.

169. Heflin AC, Brigham KL. Prevention by granulocyte depletion of increased vascular permeability of sheep lung following endotoxemia. J Clin Invest 1981; 68:1253–1260.

170. Laufe MD, Simon RH, Flint A, Keller JB. Adult respiratory distress syndrome in neutropenic patients. Am J Med 1986; 80:1022–1026.

171. Bevilacqua MP. Endothelial-leukocyte adhesion molecules. Ann rev Immunol 1993; 11:767–804.

172. Gropper M, Wiener-Kronish JP. The adult respiratory distress syndrome: diagnosis, pathophysiology, and treatment. In: Hanowell LH, Junod FL, ed. Pulmonary Care of the Surgical Patient. Mount Kisco, NY: Futura Publishing Company, Inc., 1994:139–182.

173. Dantzker DR, Brook CJ, Dehart P, et al. Ventilation-perfusion distribution in the adult respiratory distress syndrome. Am Rev Respir Dis 1979; 120:1039–1052.

174. Pelosi P, Crotti S, Brazzi L, Gattinoni L. Computed tomography in adult respiratory distress syndrome: what has it taught us? Eur Respir J 1996; 9:1055–1062.

175. Artigas A, Bernard GR, Carlet J, et al. The American-European Consensus Conference on ARDS. Part 2: Ventilatory, Pharmacologic, supportive therapy, study design strategies, and issues related to recovery and remodeling. Am J Respir Crit Care Med 1998; 157:1332–1347.

176. Gattinoni L, Pesenti A, Avalli L, Rossi, F, Bombino M. Pressure-volume curve of total respiratory system in acute respiratory failure. Computed tomographic scan study. Am Rev Respir Dis 1987; 136:730–738.

177. Gattinoni L, Pesenti A, Bombino M, et al. Relationships between lung computed tomographic density, gas exchange, and PEEP in acute respiratory failure. Anesthesiology 1988; 69:812–814.

178. Gattinoni L, D'Andrea L, Pelosi P, et al. Regional effects and mechanism of positive end-expiratory pressure in early adult respiratory distress syndrome. JAMA 1993; 269:2122–2127.

179. Amato MB, Barbas CS, Medeiros DM, et al. Beneficial effects of the "open lung approach" with low distending pressures in acute respiratory distress syndrome: a prospective randomized study on mechanical ventilation. Am J Respir Crit Care Med 1995; 152:1835–1846.

180. Ventilation with lower tidal volumes as compared with traditional tidal volumes for acute lung injury and the acute respiratory distress syndrome. The Acute Respiratory Distress Syndrome Network. NEJM. 2000; 342:1301–1308.

181. Tremblay L, Valenza F, Ribeiro SP, et al. Injurious ventilatory strategies increase cytokines and c-fos m-RNA expression in an isolated rat lung model. J Clin Invest 1997; 99:944–952.

182. Chiumello D, Pristine G, Slutsky AS. Mechanical ventilation affects local and systemic cytokines in an animal model of acute respiratory distress syndrome. Am J Respir Crit Care Med 1999; 160:109–116.

183. Ranieri VM, Suter PM, Tortorella C, et al. Effect of mechanical ventilation on inflammatory mediators in patients with acute respiratory distress syndrome. JAMA 1999; 282:54–61.

184. Eisner MD, Thompson T, Hudson LD, et al. Acute Respiratory Distress Syndrome Network. Efficacy of low tidal volume ventilation in patients with different clinical risk factors for acute lung injury and the acute respiratory distress syndrome. Am J Respir Crit Care Med 2001; 164:231–236.

185. Lamm WJ, Graham MM, Albert RK. Mechanism by which the prone position improves oxygenation in acute lung injury. Am J Respir Crit Care Med 1994; 150:184–193.

186. Greenspan JS, Wolfson MR, Shaffer TH. Liquid ventilation: clinical experiences. Biomed Instrum Technol 1999; 33:253–259.

187. Davies MW. Annotation: liquid ventilation. J Paediatr Child Health 1999; 35:434–437.

188. Wu CL, Jani ND, Perkins FM, Barquist E. Thoracic epidural analgesia versus intravenous patient-controlled analgesia for the treatment of rib fracture pain after motor vehicle crash. J Trauma 1999; 47(3):564–567.

189. Rodriguez JL. Pneumonia: incidence, risk factors, and outcome in injured patients. J Trauma 1991; 31:907.

190. Haenel JB, Moore FA, Moore EE, et al. Extrapleural bupivacaine for amelioration of multiple rib fracture pain. J Trauma 1995; 38(1):22–27.

191. Karmakar MK, Ho AM-H. Acute pain management of patients with multiple fractured ribs. J Trauma 2003; 54(3):615–625.

192. Worthy LI. Thoracic epidural in the management of chest trauma. A study of 161 cases. Intensive Care Med 1985; 1:312.

193. Cicala RS, Voeller GR, Fox T, et al. Epidural analgesia in thoracic trauma: Effects of lumbar morphine and thoracic bupivacaine on pulmonary function. J Trauma 1990; 18:229.

194. MacKersie RC, Karagianes TG, Hoyt DB, et al. Prospective evaluation of epidural and intravenous administration of fentanyl for pain control and restoration of ventilatory function following multiple rib fractures. J Trauma 1991; 31:443.

195. Karmakar MK, Chui PT, Joynt GM, Ho AM. Thoracic paravertebral block for management of pain associated with multiple fractured ribs in patients with concomitant lumbar spinal trauma. Reg Anes Pain Med 2001; 26(2):169–173.

196. Shanti CM, Carlin AM, Tyburski JG. Incidence of pneumothorax from intercostals nerve block for analgesia in rib fractures. J Trauma 2001; 51(3):536–539.

197. Luchette FA, Radafshar SM, Kaiser R, Flynn W, Hassett JM. Prospective evaluation of epidural versus intrapleural catheters for analgesia in chest wall trauma. J Trauma 1994; 36(6):865–869.

198. Schneider RF. Lack of efficacy of interpleural bupivacaine for postoperative analgesia following thoracotomy. Chest 1993; 103:414.

199. Jeroukhimov I, Jewelewicz D, Zaias J, et al. Early injection of high-dose recombinant factor VIIa decreases blood loss and prolongs time from injury to death in experimental liver injury. J Trauma 2002; 53(6):1053–1057.

200. Kuriwoto Y, Morishita K, Kawaharda N, et al. The first case report of stent-grafting for blunted extended aortic dissection. J Trauma 2002; 53:571–573.

201. ATLS guidelines. 6th ed. Chicago, IL: American College of Surgeons, 1997.

26

Respiratory Care

William T. Peruzzi and Kenneth D. Candido

Department of Anesthesiology, Northwestern University Medical School, and Department of Respiratory Care,
Northwestern Memorial Hospital, Chicago, Illinois, U.S.A.

INTRODUCTION

Trauma and critically ill patients routinely require respiratory care ranging from supplemental oxygen administration to lung separation and unilateral or independent lung ventilation. Respiratory support encompasses a wide range of prophylactic, therapeutic, and diagnostic interventions, including airway mucus clearance, increasing lung volumes, improving oxygenation, and recruiting collateral airway units. Expectorants, mucolytics, mucokinetics, and modifiers of airway water transport may each have a role in the management of these patients. Anti-inflammatory agents, anticholinergics, and some macrolide antibiotics may prove to be mainstays in the care and treatment of certain cases.

Airway management is one of the foundations of resuscitation from trauma of all types, and may pose a formidable challenge for the caregiver called upon to urgently stabilize such patients. A variety of complications may develop following the securing of the airway and the implementation of respiratory care, necessitating prolonged vigilance and a high degree of skill to minimize the potentially severe morbidity associated with these scenarios. One of the goals of respiratory care is to maximize the quantity of oxygen (O_2) arriving at the sites of intracellular utilization.

This chapter concerns itself with the optimization of O_2 delivery (DO_2) and carbon dioxide (CO_2) elimination, as therapeutic goals in the management of trauma patients. The application of the correct respiratory care modality at the appropriate time will often result in a favorable outcome with minimization of the inherent risks. Inappropriate or delayed application of the necessary respiratory care modality may result in serious clinical morbidity and the need for more extensive supportive measures at a later time.

DISORDERS OF OXYGENATION

By definition, hypoxemia is an abnormally low PO_2 in arterial blood (PaO_2). Hypoxia exists when oxygen tension at the cellular level is inadequate for cellular function (tissue oxygen deprivation). Distinguishing the terms is important because each may exist without the other. Pulmonary conditions associated with hypoxemia may be routinely associated with trauma and include hypoventilation, diffusion impairment, shunt, and ventilation-perfusion inequalities. Blood-related conditions including anemia and carbon monoxide (CO) intoxication, among others can

be seen in trauma patients. Tissue factors associated with hypoxemia, notably cyanide toxicity, are rarely associated with general trauma, yet can occur in structural fires, and must be considered in any presentation of hypoxemia that is unresponsive to supplemental oxygen administration—because all the previously mentioned factors do, indeed, respond in some measure to supplemental oxygen.

The alveolar oxygen tension (P_AO_2) is determined by a balance between the rate of removal of O_2 by the blood and the rate of replenishment of O_2 from alveolar ventilation. The O_2 removal is a function of the metabolic demands of tissues, which may be quite high as a result of endogenously or exogenously administered catecholamines in the trauma patient. Hypoventilation is said to occur when abnormally low alveolar ventilation causes a rise in PCO_2 and a fall in PO_2. Trauma patients intoxicated with opioids, barbiturates, or ethanol are at risk for developing hypoxemia from hypoventilation. Similarly, victims of trauma to the chest wall, or those in whom the respiratory muscles are paralyzed as a result of a central nervous system injury, can also suffer hypoventilation. As PO_2 falls, PCO_2 rises in hypoventilation, and this relationship is expressed by the alveolar gas equation:

$$P_AO_2 = P_IO_2 - \frac{P_ACO_2 + F}{RQ}$$

where P_AO_2 is the alveolar oxygen tension, P_IO_2 the partial pressure of humidified oxygen, $P_IO_2 = F_IO_2 ([P_B - P_{H2O}])$, F_IO_2 the inspired oxygen concentration, P_ACO_2 the alveolar CO_2 tension, RQ the respiratory quotient (CO_2 production/ O_2 consumption) (typically 200/250 mL/min, or 0.8), and F is a small correction factor (typically = 2 mmHg).

Similarly, the relationship between alveolar ventilation and PCO_2 demonstrates why hypoventilation increases alveolar (and arterial) PCO_2:

$$PCO_2 = \frac{\dot{V}CO_2 \times K}{\dot{V}_A}$$

where PCO_2 is the arterial CO_2, $\dot{V}CO_2$ the CO_2 production, $\dot{V}_A$ the alveolar ventilation, and K is a constant.

Diffusion impairment is another factor potentially associated with hypoxemia in trauma. Under ideal conditions, the PO_2 difference between alveolar gas and end-capillary blood resulting from incomplete diffusion is exceedingly small, yet this difference may become larger during stressful states such as trauma, or if the blood-gas barrier becomes thickened, or if an oxygen-poor admixture is administered to a patient. Although this mechanism of hypoxemia may not be routinely present in the trauma patient, it remains a practical concern in respiratory care, because it may be one presentation of the patient who manifests low oxygen tension in the face of normal PCO_2. This type of insult is typically responsive to the administration of supplemental oxygen.

The P_AO_2 results from a dynamic equilibrium between oxygen delivery to the alveolus and oxygen extraction from the alveolus. Oxygen delivery to the alveolus is a function of the minute ventilation ($\dot{V}_E$) and the inspired oxygen fraction (F_IO_2), whereas oxygen extraction from the alveolus is a function of the de-oxygenation status of blood presented to the alveolus ($SVO_2 \times Hgb = CVO_2$) and the capillary blood flow (Q_C). If the factors governing oxygen extraction remain static, a decrease in alveolar ventilation or F_IO_2 will result in less oxygen delivery to the alveolus. Since the alveolar contents of nitrogen and water vapor remain essentially unchanged, the P_AO_2 must decrease; therefore, the capillary blood will equilibrate with a lower P_AO_2.

If factors determining alveolar oxygen delivery remain constant, a decrease in pulmonary artery oxygen content (CVO_2) or an increase in capillary blood flow, will result in more oxygen extraction from the alveolus. There are three major reasons for mixed venous blood to have decreased oxygen content. First, an increase in metabolic rate increases oxygen consumption ($\dot{V}O_2$). If there is no increase in perfusion, the tissues will extract more oxygen from each deciliter of blood and thereby decrease the venous blood oxygen content. Second, decreased oxygen delivery at a constant $\dot{V}O_2$ requires that the tissues extract more oxygen from each deciliter of blood, thereby decreasing the venous blood oxygen content. Third, a decreased arterial oxygen content will result in a lower venous oxygen content after the normal extraction of oxygen by the tissues. A compensatory mechanism for all three scenarios is an increase in cardiac output ($\dot{Q}$). The above presentation expresses the gas-exchange factors that are traditionally referred to as the ventilation-perfusion ($\dot{V}/\dot{Q}$) relationship. Low $\dot{V}/\dot{Q}$ refers to perfusion in excess of ventilation, leading to a decreased alveolar oxygen tension and hypoxemia. It is important to recognize that changes in F_IO_2 and S_VO_2 can change the alveolar PO_2 without changing the $\dot{V}/\dot{Q}$ relationship. Therefore, arterial oxygenation deficits must be considered beyond the scope of $\dot{V}/\dot{Q}$ relationships.

Anatomic right-to-left shunting is defined as blood that goes from the right side to the left side of the heart without traversing pulmonary capillaries. Capillary shunting is defined as blood that goes from the right side to the left side of the heart by traversing pulmonary capillaries that are adjacent to unventilated alveoli. In both circumstances, right heart blood enters the left heart without an increase in O_2 content. This phenomenon is traditionally referred to as zero $\dot{V}/\dot{Q}$, or true shunting, because the blood does not interact with alveolar gas.

Shunting and hypoxemia are not synonymous terms, nor do they have linear relationships. The hypoxemic effect of any shunt will depend both on the size of the shunt and on the oxygenation status of the blood that is shunted. A small shunt in a patient with a low SvO_2 may have profound hypoxemic effects, whereas a large shunt in patients with a high SvO_2 may cause only mild hypoxemia.

Oxygen diffusion defects, due to edema fluid or fibrous tissue between the alveolar epithelium and the capillary epithelium, can impose a significant impediment to O_2 diffusion and inhibit equilibration between pulmonary capillary and alveolar O_2 tensions. This impaired O_2 exchange is worsened as blood transit time decreases (blood traverses the lung more rapidly). Arterial hypoxemia secondary to diffusion defects is not common in trauma but is responsive to an increase in P_AO_2.

$\dot{V}/\dot{Q}$ mismatch, not infrequently, occurs in trauma and can result from retained bronchial secretions, bronchospasm, obstructive endobronchial lesions, chronic obstructive pulmonary disease, pulmonary edema, or other pulmonary pathology. The hallmark of hypoxemia due to $\dot{V}/\dot{Q}$ mismatch is that it is responsive to oxygen therapy. In order to determine O_2 responsiveness, an appropriate oxygen challenge must be given (1). If, at sea level, the F_IO_2 is increased by 0.2 (i.e., from 0.2 to 0.4, or 0.3 to 0.5), the PAO_2 of all ventilated alveoli should increase by 90–100 mmHg. Subsequently, the PAO_2 will increase by significantly more than 10 mmHg if less than 15% true right-to-left shunt is present; however, it will increase by significantly less than 10 mm Hg if greater than 30% true shunt exists.

True right-to-left shunt can result from several different pathological conditions—intracardiac shunt; alveolar collapse, as occurs in acute lung injury (ALI); pulmonary consolidation associated with lung infections; segmental or lobar lung collapse due to retained secretions or other lung pathology; pulmonary arterial-venous malformations or pulmonary-capillary dilatation, as is sometimes seen in liver disease; and large vascular lung tumors. Oxygen therapy has limited effect on blood traversing true shunt units. The reason for this is that, regardless of the F_IO_2 or P_AO_2, O_2 transfer cannot occur when blood does not come into contact with functional alveolar units. Therefore, true shunt pathology is refractory to O_2 therapy. Functional alveolar units may be impaired or destroyed by penetrating chest wall trauma, among other causes. For several types of pathology resulting in true shunt, there is little or no available therapy; antibiotics or surgical interventions may help other types of true shunt–producing disease. The type of lung pathology that is the most responsive to therapy is that involving diffuse or focal lung collapse. Segmental or lobar lung collapse can often be reversed with appropriate bronchial hygiene or removal of the source of obstruction.

Diffuse alveolar collapse often results from destabilization of the alveolar architecture due to disruption of the surfactant layer and alveolar epithelial damage associated with ALI (2,3). This type of pathology is responsive to positive end expiratory pressure (PEEP) (4). PEEP levels of 5 to 10 cm H_2O will increase alveolar size and redistribute interstitial lung water from the interstitial regions between the alveolar epithelium and pulmonary-capillary endothelium to the peribronchial and hilar regions of the lung (5,6). PEEP levels >15 cm H_2O no longer increase alveolar size; rather, these levels of PEEP "recruit" nonfunctional and collapsed alveoli to expanded and functional alveolar units (7).

☞ **The three major reasons for mixed venous blood to have low O_2 content include: (*i*) metabolic rate; (*ii*) ↓ O_2 delivery; and (*iii*) ↓ arterial O_2 content.** ☞

OXYGEN ADMINISTRATION

In order to understand the indications for O_2 therapy, the physiologic responses to hypoxemia and hypoxia must be appreciated. First, there is an increase in minute ventilation that increases alveolar ventilation and the work of breathing. Second, there is an increase in $\dot{Q}$, which maintains DO_2 in the face of a decreased arterial O_2 content, but increases the stress placed on the cardiovascular system. Therefore, the goals of oxygen therapy are to improve arterial O_2 content and subsequently decrease the work of breathing and myocardial stress.

Oxygen Content
ơ⁺ **The primary determinants of oxygen content are the Hgb concentration and the degree of Hgb saturation.** ơ⁺

Oxygen content is determined by the concentration of Hgb in the blood, the percentage of the Hgb that is saturated with oxygen, the maximal amount of oxygen that can be bound to Hgb (constant of 1.34 mL O_2g Hgb), and the amount of O_2 dissolved in the plasma (0.003 mL O_2mm Hg). Thus,

$$CaO_2 = [Hgb] \times [SaO_2] \times [1.34] + [PaO_2] \times [0.003]$$

Obviously, the primary determinants of O_2 content are the Hgb concentration (g/dL) and the degree of Hgb saturation (expressed as a decimal). At atmospheric pressure, the amount of O_2 dissolved in the plasma ([PaO_2][0.003]) is usually negligible. The value of 1.34 mL/g Hgb represents the amount of O_2 that can be bound to Hgb contained within the red blood cell membrane; a value of 1.39 mL/g Hgb is sometimes used and represents the amount of O_2 that can be bound by stroma-free Hgb, which occurs when cells are lysed during co-oximetry measurements (8).

Oxygen Delivery Systems
There are three basic types of gas delivery systems: rebreathing systems, nonrebreathing systems, and partial rebreathing systems. Rebreathing systems collect exhaled gases into a reservoir on the expiratory limb of the system, which contains a CO_2 absorber (permitting the re-entry of expiratory gases into the inspiratory gas flow without rebreathing of CO_2). This system is used primarily for the delivery of anesthetic gases in order to conserve expensive volatile anesthetics. Such systems have little or no use in current critical care settings.

A partial rebreathing system is one in which the initial portion of the expired gases, consisting mainly of gas from the anatomical dead space, is expired into a reservoir, whereas the latter portions of the expiratory gases are vented in the atmosphere through one-way valves. The expiratory gases from the anatomic dead space contain very little CO_2 and, therefore, can be rebreathed without significant consequences. The reservoir also receives fresh inspiratory gas flow; thus, the patient breathes both expiratory gas containing little CO_2 and fresh inspiratory gas.

Most oxygen-delivery systems are nonrebreathing systems in that all expiratory gases are vented in such a fashion that exhaled CO_2 is not rebreathed during subsequent breaths. This is often accomplished with one-way valves to prevent mixing of inspired and expired gases.

ơ⁺ **Nonrebreathing systems are divided into high-flow (fixed performance) and low-flow (variable performance) systems.** ơ⁺ A high-flow system means that the inspiratory gas flow rate delivered to the system is sufficient to meet the peak inspiratory-flow demands of the patient. Thus, all inspiratory gas is supplied by the O_2-delivery system and the F_IO_2 is both known and stable. In order to accomplish this, the inspiratory gas flows must be three to four times the measured minute ventilation (9). The use of high-flow O_2-delivery systems is indicated whenever there is a need

Table 1 Low-Flow Oxygen-Delivery Devices, Flow Rates, and F_IO_2

Low flow system	Oxygen flow rates (L)	F_IO_2
Nasal cannula	1	0.24
	2	0.28
	3	0.32
	4	0.36
	5	0.40
	6	0.44
Simple facemask	5–6	0.40
	6–7	0.50
	7–8	0.60
Partial rebreathing mask	6	0.60
	7	0.70
	8	0.80
	9	0.80+
	10	0.80+
Nonrebreathing mask	10	0.80+
	−15	0.90+

Note: Predicted F_IO_2 values for low-flow systems assume a normal and stable pattern of ventilation.
Source: From Ref. 95.

for a consistent and predictable F_IO_2, especially in patients with unstable ventilatory patterns.

Conversely, a low-flow system delivers a fixed amount of O_2 to the patient, and entrainment of room air is necessary in order to meet the patient's peak inspiratory-flow rates. In this setting, the F_IO_2 is variable and unpredictable if the patient has an abnormal or changing pattern of ventilation. If the patient has a stable, normal pattern of ventilation, however, low-flow O_2-delivery systems can deliver a relatively predictable and consistent F_IO_2 (Table 1).

It must be understood that use of a low-flow O_2-delivery system does not imply delivery of low O_2 concentrations. For example, it is possible to calculate the F_IO_2 for a low-flow system, such as a nasal cannula, if certain assumptions are made as follows: (*i*) the anatomic reservoir (nose, nasopharynx, and oropharynx) is approximately 50 mL or one-third of the anatomic dead space (150 mL); (*ii*) the O_2 flow rate is 6 L/min (100 mL/sec) via the nasal cannula; (*iii*) the patient's respiratory rate of 20 breaths/min results in a one-second inspiratory phase and a two-second expiratory phase; and (*iv*) there is negligible gas flow during the terminal 0.5 seconds of the expiratory phase, thus allowing the anatomic reservoir to completely fill with O_2. Using the above assumptions, the F_IO_2 can be calculated for variable tidal volumes (V_T) (Table 2). This variability in F_IO_2 at 6 L/min of O_2 flow clearly demonstrates the effects of a changing ventilatory pattern on F_IO_2. In general, the larger the V_T or the faster the respiratory rate, the lower the F_IO_2; the smaller the V_T or lower the respiratory rate, the higher the F_IO_2. With a stable, unchanging ventilatory pattern and O_2 flow rate, low-flow systems can deliver a relatively consistent F_IO_2.

Low-Flow Systems
Low-flow O_2 devices are the most commonly employed O_2-delivery systems because of their simplicity, ease of use, familiarity, low cost, and patient acceptance. In most clinical situations, low-flow systems are acceptable and even preferable.

Table 2 Variability in F_IO_2 with Low-Flow O_2-Delivery Systems and Variable Patterns of Ventilation

	$V_T = 500$ cc	$V_T = 250$ cc
Anatomic reservoir	50 cc O_2	50 cc O_2
Inspiratory phase (1 sec)	100 cc O_2	100 cc O_2
Entrained room air	350 cc	100 cc
O_2 from entrained room air (21% oxygen)	70 cc O_2	20 cc O_2
Total volume O_2/V_t	220 cc/500 cc	170 cc/250 cc
F_IO_2	0.44	0.68

Source: From Ref. 96.

Nasal Cannula

The nasal cannula is the most frequently used O_2-delivery device because of its simplicity and comfort. To be effective, the patient's nasal passages must be patent in order to allow filling of the anatomic reservoir; however, the patient does not need to breathe through the nose. Oxygen will be entrained from the anatomic reservoir even in the presence of mouth breathing. If the O_2 flow rate exceeds 4 L/min, the gases should be humidified to prevent drying of the nasal mucosa. Flow rates greater than 6 L/min will not increase the F_IO_2 significantly above 0.44, and are often poorly tolerated by the patient.

Simple Facemask

A simple facemask consists of a mask with two side ports. The mask provides an additional 100–200 mL oxygen reservoir and will provide a higher F_IO_2 than will a nasal cannula. The open ports in the sides of the mask allow entrainment of room air and venting of exhaled gases. ☞ **A minimum flow of at least 5 L/min is necessary to prevent CO_2 accumulation and rebreathing during facemask-assisted breathing.** ☞ Flow rates greater than 8 L/min will not increase the F_IO_2 significantly above 0.6.

Partial Rebreathing Mask

A partial rebreathing mask (Fig. 1) is similar in construction to the simple facemask, but it also incorporates a 600–1000 mL reservoir bag into which fresh gas flows. The first one-third of the patient's exhaled gas fills the reservoir bag. Because this gas is primarily from the anatomic dead space, it contains very little CO_2. With the next breath, the patient inhales a mixture of the exhaled gas and fresh gas. If the fresh gas flows are equal to or greater than 8 L/min and the reservoir bag remains inflated throughout the entire respiratory cycle, adequate CO_2 evacuation and the highest possible F_IO_2 should occur. The rebreathing capacity of this system allows some degree of O_2 conservation that may be useful while transporting patients with portable O_2 supplies.

Tracheostomy Collars

Tracheostomy collars are primarily used to deliver humidity to patients with artificial airways. Oxygen may be delivered with these devices, but, similar to other low-flow systems, the F_IO_2 is unpredictable, inconsistent, and depends upon the ventilatory pattern.

High-Flow Systems

Although high-flow systems are more complex, more labor intensive to initiate and maintain, and more expensive,

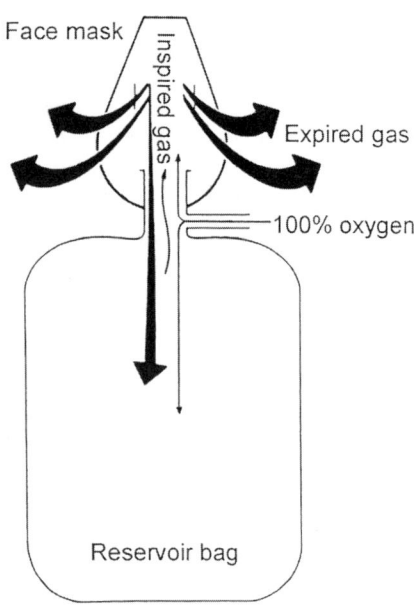

Figure 1 Air flow during inspiration and expiration through a partial rebreathing mask. Note the first part of the exhaled gas from the anatomic dead space enters the respiratory bag to be inspired with the next breath. *Source*: From Ref. 93.

clinical situations in which it is important to deliver a precise F_IO_2 require their use.

Venturi Masks

These masks entrain air using the Bernoulli principle and constant pressure-jet mixing (10). This physical phenomenon is based on a rapid velocity of gas (e.g., O_2) moving through a restricted orifice (Fig. 2). This movement produces viscous shearing forces, which create a subatmospheric pressure gradient downstream relative to the surrounding gases. This pressure gradient causes room air to be entrained until the pressures are equalized. In this manner, flows high enough to meet the patient's peak-inspiratory demands can be generated. As the desired F_IO_2 increases, the air-to-O_2-entrainment ratio decreases with a net reduction in total gas flow. Therefore, the probability of the patient's needs exceeding the total flow capabilities of the device increases with higher F_IO_2 settings. Occlusion of or impingement on the exhalation ports of the mask can cause backpressure and can alter gas flow ("Venturi stall"). In addition, the O_2-injector port can become clogged, especially with water droplets. Therefore, aerosol devices should not be used with Venturi masks; if humidity is necessary, a vapor-type humidifier should be used. There are two basic types of Venturi systems: (*i*) a fixed-F_IO_2 model, which requires specific color-coded inspiratory attachments with labeled jets that produce a known F_IO_2 with a given flow, and (*ii*) a variable-F_IO_2 model, which has graded adjustments of the air-entrainment port that can be set to allow variation in delivered F_IO_2.

Nonrebreathing Masks

A nonrebreathing mask (Fig. 3) is similar to a partial rebreathing mask, but with the addition of three unidirectional valves. Two of the valves are located on opposite sides of the mask. They permit venting of exhaled gas and prevent entrainment of room air. The remaining

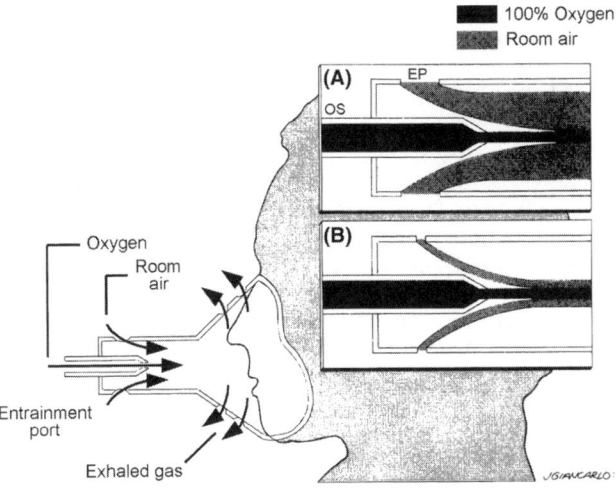

100% Oxygen
Room air

Figure 2 Principle of an air-entrainment device. Pressurized O_2 is forced through a constricted orifice; the increased gas velocity distal to the orifice creates a shearing effect that causes room air to be entrained through the entrainment ports. The high flow of gas fills the mask; holes allow both exhaled and delivered gases to escape. Insets (**A**) and (**B**) illustrate that the size of the entrainment ports (EP) determines the amount of room air to be entrained; OS is the O_2 source. Large ports (**A**) result in relatively low F_IO_2; small ports (**B**) result in relatively higher F_IO_2. For any size EP, the F_IO_2 is stable; however, the total gas flow will vary with the pressurized O_2 flow (see text). *Source*: From Ref. 94.

unidirectional valve is located between the mask and the reservoir bag, and prevents exhaled gases from entering the fresh-gas reservoir. As with the partial rebreathing mask, the reservoir bag should be inflated throughout the entire ventilatory cycle in order to ensure adequate CO_2 clearance from the system and the highest possible F_IO_2.

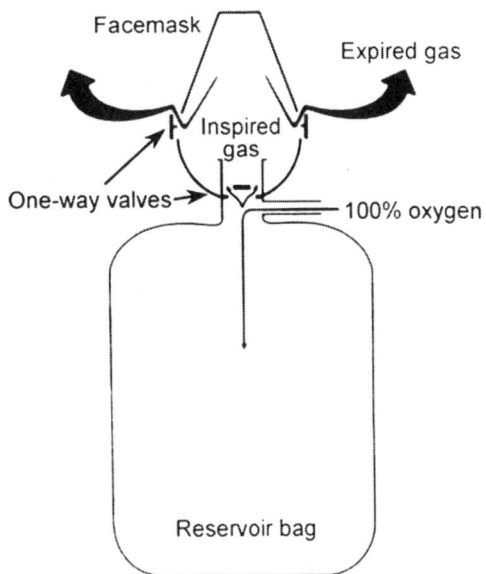

Figure 3 Air flow during inspiration and expiration through a nonrebreathing mask. Note that all expired gas exits through one-way valves on the sides of the mask and is precluded from entering the reservoir bag by an additional one-way valve. *Source*: From Ref. 93.

To avoid air entrainment around the mask and dilution of the delivered F_IO_2, masks should fit snugly on the face, but excessive pressure should be avoided. If the mask is fitted properly, the reservoir bag should respond to the patient's inspiratory efforts. Unfortunately, if fresh-gas flows and the volume of the reservoir bag are insufficient to meet inspiratory demands, the patient could be compromised. Therefore, masks may be fitted with a spring-loaded tension valve that will open and allow entrainment of room air as needed, to meet inspiratory demands. If such a valve is not present, another option is to remove one of the unidirectional valves that prevent room air entrainment. If the total ventilatory needs of the patient are met by the nonrebreathing system, the system then functions as a high-flow system. If room air entrainment occurs, then a low-flow system is operating.

Aerosol Mask and T-Piece

An F_IO_2 greater than 0.40 with a high-flow system is best provided with a large-volume nebulizer and wide-bore tubing. Aerosol masks, in conjunction with air-entrainment nebulizers or air/O_2 blenders, can deliver a consistent and predictable F_IO_2 regardless of the patient's ventilatory pattern. A T-piece is used in place of an aerosol mask for patients with an endotracheal or tracheostomy tube. An air-entrainment nebulizer can deliver an F_IO_2 of 0.35 to 1.0, produce an aerosol, and generate flow rates of 14–16 L/min. As with Venturi masks, a higher F_IO_2 results in less room air entrainment and lower flow rates. Should a greater total flow be required, two nebulizers can feed a single mask and increase total flow. In addition, large diameter corrugated tubing can be placed on one or both exhalation holes on a standard facemask to serve as O_2 reservoirs, and further decrease the chance of entraining room air. Air/oxygen blenders can deliver a consistent F_IO_2 in the range of 0.21 to 1.0, with flows up to 100 L/min. These devices are usually used in conjunction with humidifiers Oxygen therapy should never be withheld from a patient with respiratory failure for fear of respiratory drive suppression.

COMPLICATIONS OF OXYGEN THERAPY
Suppression of Respiratory Drive

When patients who retain CO_2 receive O_2 therapy, they may exhibit a depression in their respiratory drive. The resultant decrease in minute ventilation produces an increase in the $PaCO_2$, CO_2 narcosis, and further depression of the respiratory drive. Oxygen should be administered with caution to patients who retain CO_2. More recent studies indicate that the increase in $PaCO_2$ is often due to an increase in VD/V_T with O_2 therapy, rather than a decrease in respiratory drive. Oxygen therapy should never be withheld from a patient with respiratory failure for fear of respiratory drive suppression.

Oxygen Absorption Atelectasis

Absorption atelectasis occurs when high alveolar O_2 concentrations cause alveolar collapse. Normally, nitrogen, which is at equilibrium with the blood, remains within the alveoli and "splints" alveoli open. When a high F_IO_2 is administered, nitrogen is "washed out" of the alveoli, and the alveoli are filled primarily with oxygen. In areas of the lung with reduced $\dot{V}/\dot{Q}$ ratios, O_2 will be absorbed into the blood faster than ventilation can replace it. The alveoli then become progressively smaller until they reach the critical volume at which surface-tension forces cause alveolar collapse. This phenomenon is precipitated primarily by the

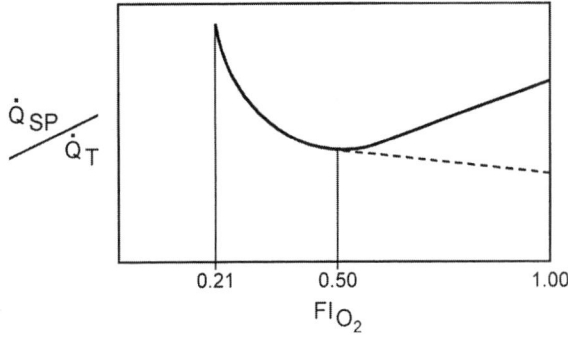

Figure 4 The general relationship between intrapulmonary shunt fractions ($\dot{Q}_{SP}/\dot{Q}_T$) and increasing inspired O_2 concentration (F_IO_2). The shunt fraction diminishes as the F_IO_2 is increased from 0.21 (room air) towards 0.50. This diminution is readily attributed to the decreasing hypoxemic effect of low ventilation perfusion ($\dot{V}/\dot{Q}$) as the alveolar PO_2 increases. As the F_IO_2 is increased from 0.50 toward 1.0, the shunt fraction increases. Broken line depicts what would be anticipated if all low $\dot{V}/\dot{Q}$ alveoli remained open as the F_IO_2 increased. The observed increase in shunt fraction must be attributed to increased zero $\dot{V}/\dot{Q}$. *Source*: From Ref. 95.

administration of an F_IO_2 greater than 0.5 and is illustrated in Figure 4.

Oxygen Toxicity

A high F_IO_2 can be injurious to the lungs. The mechanism of O_2 toxicity is related to production of O_2 free radicals such as superoxide anions (O_2^-), hydroxyl radicals (OH), hydrogen peroxide (H_2O_2), and singlet oxygen ($1O_2$). These radicals affect cell functions by inactivating sulfhydryl enzymes, interfering with DNA synthesis, and disrupting the integrity of cell membranes. During periods of lung-tissue hyperoxia, the normal oxygen-radical-scavenging mechanisms are overwhelmed, and toxicity results (11). The F_IO_2 at which oxygen toxicity becomes important is controversial and variable depending upon animal species, degree of underlying lung injury, ambient barometric pressure, and duration of exposure. ☞ **In general, it is best to avoid exposure to an F_IO_2 of 0.5 or greater for more than 24 hours.** ☞

AIRWAY CLEARANCE TECHNIQUES

Bronchial hygiene is useful and effective when the patient is carefully evaluated, the goals of therapy are clearly defined, and the appropriate modalities are applied. Normal respiratory secretions include mucus, surfactant, and periciliary fluid. Airway mucus is a secretory product of goblet cells and submucosal glands. It is a nonhomogeneous, adhesive, viscoelastic gel composed of water, carbohydrates, proteins, and lipids. In health, the mucus gel is primarily composed of a three-dimensional tangled polymer network of mucus glycoproteins or mucin.

Airway mucus is moved by three basic mechanisms: slug flow, which describes how airflow may push forward a mucus plug obstructing an airway; annular flow, describing mucus moving along the walls of an airway by expiratory air flow or cilia; and mist flow, describing aerosolized mucus that is exhaled as suspended droplets (12). Mucus transportation can be affected by traumatic lung injury

or damage to the oropharynx or nasopharynx. ☞ **Disruption of normal secretion or mucociliary clearance impairs pulmonary function and lung defenses, and predisposes the individual to infection.** ☞

Extensive ciliary damage and mucus hypersecretion render the individual dependent upon airflow-assisted mucus clearance mechanisms such as cough, to maintain airway hygiene (13). Likewise, acute and chronic airway inflammation may lead to ciliary dysfunction and sloughing of the ciliary epithelium, effectively disrupting the "mucociliary elevator" system of mucus clearance. Because the trauma patient may have an impaired cough mechanism due to central or peripheral abnormalities, they may need assistance in mobilizing and expelling retained airway secretions.

Prophylactic vs. Therapeutic

Prophylactic bronchial hygiene therapy is administered to trauma patients who are essentially free of acute pulmonary pathology, with the intent of preventing inadequate bronchial hygiene. Therapeutic bronchial hygiene therapy is aimed at the reversal of pre-existing inadequate bronchial hygiene, specifically, the mobilization of retained mucus and secretions, and the reinflation of atelectatic lung regions.

Humidification

☞ **Humidification of inhaled gases is required to maintain normal respiratory epithelial function.** ☞ Air inspired through the nose is warmed and nearly 90% humidified by the time it passes through the pharynx. The administration of dry O_2 lowers the water content of the inspired air, and the use of artificial airways bypasses the nasopharynx and oropharynx where the humidification of gases primarily takes place. If adequate humidification of inspired gases is not provided before the gas enters the trachea, the deficit of humidity is provided by moisture from the mucus blanket of the tracheobronchial tree. Thus, both O_2 administration and the use of artificial airways can increase the demands on the lung to humidify inspired gases. If humidification of inspired gases is not appropriately addressed, drying of the tracheobronchial tree, ciliary dysfunction, impairment of mucus transport, inflammation and necrosis of the ciliated pulmonary epithelium, retention of dried secretions, atelectasis, bacterial infiltration of the pulmonary mucosa, and pneumonia may occur. To prevent these complications, a humidifier or nebulizer should be used to increase the water content of inspired gases. Humidification can be accomplished by passing gas over heated water (heated pass-over humidifier); by fractionating gas into tiny bubbles as gas passes through water (bubble humidifiers); by allowing gas to pass through a chamber that contains a heated, water-saturated wick (heated-wick humidifier); or by vaporizing water and selectively allowing the vapor to mix with the inspired gases (vapor-phase humidifier).

A nebulizer increases the water content of the inspired gas by generating aerosols (small droplets of particulate water) of uniform size, which become incorporated into the delivered gas stream and then evaporate into the inspired gas as it is warmed in the respiratory tract. There are two basic types of nebulizers. Pneumatic nebulizers operate from a pressurized-gas source and are either jet or hydronomic; electric nebulizers are powered by an electrical source and are referred to as "ultrasonic." There are several varieties of the above nebulizers, which are more dependent on design differences than on the power source.

Incentive Spirometry

☞ **The incentive spirometer is an effective and inexpensive prophylactic and therapeutic bronchial hygiene tool.** ☞ This device provides a visual goal or "incentive" for the patient to achieve and sustain a maximal inspiratory effort. When performed on an hourly basis, this modality provides optimal lung inflation, distribution of ventilation, and improved cough. Thus, atelectasis and the retention of bronchial secretions are minimized. Incentive spirometry can also be helpful in the diagnosis of acute pulmonary pathology, in which a sudden decrease in a patient's ability to perform at a previously established level may herald the onset of severe atelectasis, pneumonia, or other pulmonary pathology. For incentive spirometry to be effective, the patient must be cooperative, motivated, and well instructed in the technique (by the respiratory therapist, nurse, or physician); the patient should be able to obtain a vital capacity greater than 15 mL/kg or an inspiratory capacity greater than 12 mL/kg; and the patient should not be tachypneic or receiving a high F_IO_2.

Chest Physical Therapy

Chest physical therapy (CPT) techniques can be classified into those that promote bronchial hygiene, improve breathing efficiency, or promote physical reconditioning. The CPT techniques considered here will be those concerned with bronchial hygiene. Chronic mucus hypersecretion is associated with a high mortality and a rapid decline in pulmonary function (14,15). In asthma, secretions may worsen $\dot{V}/\dot{Q}$ mismatch, and result in more severe or life-threatening exacerbations (16,17). For these reasons, CPT is a valuable tool in combating pulmonary morbidity in trauma patients.

Postural Drainage

Postural drainage is a technique that uses different body positions to facilitate gravitational drainage of mucus from various lung segments (Fig. 5). Although gravity is not a primary mechanism for normal secretion clearance, it plays a major role in depth and pattern of ventilation, perfusion, and lymphatic drainage (18). Postural drainage improves mobilization of secretions, but requires a considerable investment of time. ☞ **The key elements of postural drainage are posture, time, breathing, and cough.** ☞ Although postural drainage may be the gold standard to which all other bronchial hygiene techniques are compared, it has limited applicability in victims of trauma except for those who have excessive sputum production, and in spinal cord injured, and/or spine/thoracic trauma where both mobilization and cough are diminished. This is because the viscosity of the normal mucus blanket is such that it does not typically flow into gravity-dependent terminal airways (18). On the other hand, diseases that are amenable to postural drainage therapy include cystic fibrosis, bronchiectasis, COPD, acute atelectasis, and lung abscess, among others.

In hospitalized trauma patients, the basilar lung regions can often benefit from postural drainage, because most hospital bed positions do not permit adequate drainage of these segments. The patient should be positioned so that the affected lung segments are superior to the carina, with each position maintained for 3 to 15 minutes (18). Simply turning the patient may be a primary technique for lung expansion and for matching ventilation with perfusion. When performing postural drainage in unilateral lung disease, the healthier lung should be initially placed down to improve oxygenation and to follow with drainage of the contralateral lung. The reason for this is that

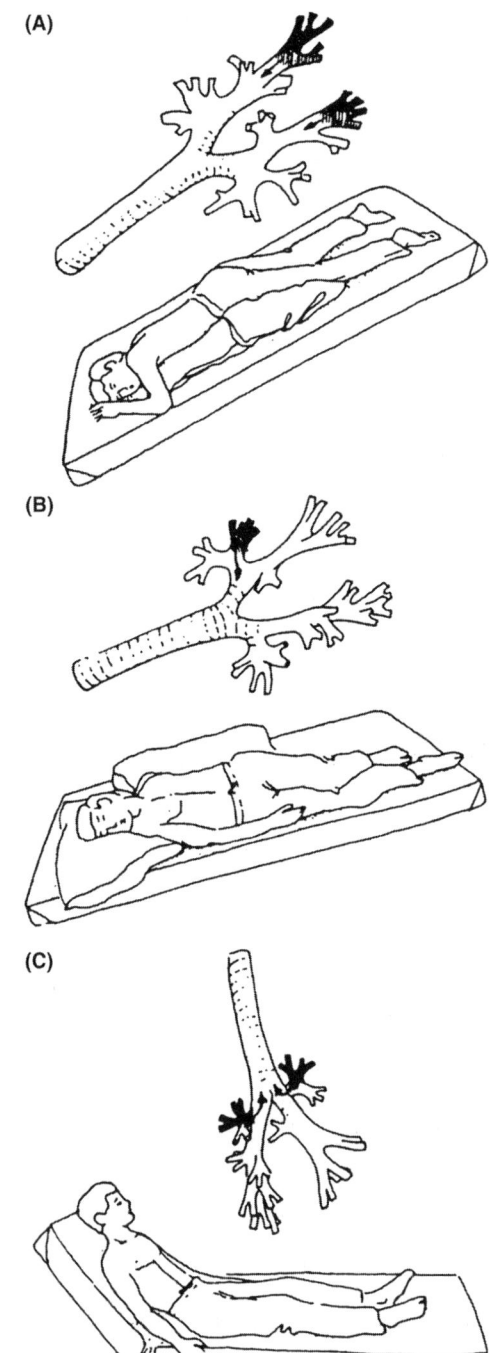

Figure 5 Common postural drainage positions for **(A)** posterior basilar segments; **(B)** middle lobe and lingual; **(C)** apical segments of upper lobes. *Source*: From Ref. 93.

crosscontamination of the nondiseased lung is always a possibility.

It is also important to avoid inappropriate positioning during postural drainage. Patients with increased intracranial pressure (ICP) or congestive heart failure (CHF) may not tolerate head-down positioning to facilitate drainage of the basilar lung segments. Shifting of abdominal and thoracic contents with gravity in the Trendelenburg position may be deleterious for patients at risk for aspiration with uncontrolled airways, distended abdomens, or recent esophageal injury. Also, it is important to avoid direct pressure on sites of injury, operations, or burns. The technique has been associated with hypoxemia, bronchospasm, acute hypotension, increased ICP, pulmonary hemorrhage, pain, vomiting, and aspiration (18).

Percussion and Vibration

☞ **Percussion assists secretion mobilization by loosening adherent secretions and centralizing them for more effective expectoration or easier suctioning.** ☞ External manipulation of the thorax, in the form of percussion and vibration, is used to facilitate the process of postural drainage. Theoretically, percussion assists secretion mobilization by shaking secretions loose, like "shaking ketchup from a bottle" (18). The goal of therapy is to intermittently apply kinetic energy to the chest wall and lung, to loosen and mobilize secretions that adhere to bronchial walls and improve airflow-dependent clearance by moving secretions from the periphery of the lung to more proximal airways, where greater secretion depth and higher expiratory air flow can improve expectoration. Mucus transport by expiratory air flow (including cough) is the primary transport mechanism in patients with pulmonary diseases when mucociliary transport is damaged (19).

Chest percussion is accomplished by rhythmically striking the thorax with cupped hands or a mechanical device placed directly over the lung segment to be drained. Percussion and vibration should be cautiously considered for trauma patients suffering burns, open wounds, skin infections, recent skin grafts, subcutaneous emphysema, recently placed pacemakers, or recent injection of local anesthetic through continuous-infusion epidural catheters. Mechanical percussion devices are available and have some theoretic advantages in that they apply vibratory or percussive forces in a more consistent, uniform fashion, and they are not subject to fatigue. Clinically, however, there is no demonstrable advantage between the two approaches (20).

Vibration normally follows percussion and involves the application of a fine tremorous action that is manually performed by pressing in the direction of the ribs and soft tissue of the chest. Chest vibration is accomplished by placing the hands on the chest wall and generating a rapid vibratory motion in the arms (from the shoulders), and gently compressing the chest wall in the direction that the ribs normally move during exhalation (21–23). Vibrations should be delivered over the draining area during the patient's expiration for optimal effect.

Overall, percussion and vibration appear to be relatively ineffective, and do not seem to add to the effectiveness of the combination of coughing, breathing exercises, and postural drainage—whereas forced expiratory technique, even without postural drainage, enhances tracheobronchial clearance (18).

Indications and Contraindications

Indications for the use of CPT are the inability or reluctance of a patient to change body position (i.e., during mechanical ventilation or in paralyzed patients); the presence of segmental atelectasis; physical evidence of retained secretions; and the presence of diseases, such as cystic fibrosis, bronchiectasis, or cavitating lung disease, that result in increased mucus production.

Contraindications to the use of CPT include situations in which proper positioning cannot be safely accomplished, when a patient's injuries would preclude appropriate percussion or vibratory maneuvers, or when pre-existing disease processes could be exacerbated during the procedure (23). Specifically, contraindications to the Trendelenburg position include increased ICP; recent neurosurgical procedures; unclipped cerebral-artery aneurysms; uncontrolled hypertension; pulmonary edema associated with CHF; abdominal distension; increased risk for gastroesophageal reflux or aspiration (e.g., esophageal operations, altered airway-protective reflexes, or decreased mental status); ongoing epidural opioid or anesthetic infusions; and recent eye surgery. The reverse-Trendelenburg position is contraindicated for use in patients with hypotension or other hemodynamic instability.

External manipulation of the thorax, such as percussion and vibration, is contraindicated in patients with subcutaneous emphysema; a recent skin graft or myocutaneous flap procedures on the thorax; thermal injuries, open wounds or skin infections of the thorax; flail chest or fractures, osteomyelitis, or osteoporosis of the ribs; soft-tissue injuries to the thorax or complaints of chest-wall pain due to other causes; temporary transvenous pacemakers or recently inserted permanent pacemakers; suspected pulmonary tuberculosis, pulmonary embolism, pulmonary contusions, or a bronchopleural fistula; large pleural effusions or an undrained empyema; increased ICP or other unstable intracranial pathology; unstable spine injuries or recent spine operation; active hemorrhage with hemodynamic instability; severe or uncontrolled coagulopathies; and confused or combative patients who do not tolerate physical manipulation.

Another hazard associated with CPT is the development of hypoxemia during the procedure. In many cases, hypoxemia can be treated by initiating oxygen therapy or increasing the oxygen concentrations during CPT. The decision to use CPT requires that the physician assess potential benefits versus potential risks and limitations. Therapy should be provided for no longer than is necessary to obtain the desired therapeutic results.

ALTERNATIVE AIRWAY-CLEARANCE TECHNIQUES

In addition to the traditional CPT techniques, alternative airway-clearance methods, such as positive-expiratory-pressure (PEP) therapy, forced-expiratory technique, autogenic drainage (AD), and high-frequency oscillation (HFO), have recently gained support in the literature and are widely used in Europe (21,24–26). These techniques either serve as replacement for the traditional CPT or are used in conjunction with CPT to remove retained secretions and promote aerosol deposition. These techniques focus on controlled breathing and modified coughing techniques, but patients require significant training before they can adequately master the various maneuvers. Patients who actively participate in alternative airway-clearance methods are usually those with long-standing pulmonary processes, such as cystic fibrosis patients who can cooperate and tolerate the maneuvers. ☞ **Trauma patients in the intensive care unit (ICU) or those with long-term pulmonary complications, such as spinal cord injury, severe ARDS, etc., may also be good candidates for treatment with alternative airway-clearance methods.** ☞

HFO of the air column in the conducting airways is designed to facilitate secretion removal in select individuals. A variety of devices are available that generate HFO by applying forces either at the airway opening or across the chest wall (27). HFO reduces the viscosity of sputum, potentially influencing its clearance by a cough. HFO may also increase the volume of air distal to airways partially obstructed with mucus.

Devices used to administer HFO include the Flutter valve (VarioRaw SA, Scandipharm, Birmingham, Alabama, U.S.A.), which is shaped like a pipe with a steel ball in a "bowl" that is loosely covered by a perforated cap. The weight of the ball serves as an expiratory positive airway pressure (EPAP) device, creating a pressure of approximately 10 cm H_2O. The shape of the bowl permits the ball to repeatedly move on or off the bowl in a flutter movement, thereby generating oscillations at about 15 Hz (range: 2–32 Hz). The proposed mechanism of action includes a shearing of mucus from the airway wall by oscillatory forces, preventing early airway closure by stabilizing the airways with EPAP. This facilitates the cephalad flow of mucus. Oscillations may decrease mucus viscoelasticity at frequencies and amplitudes achievable with the Flutter device (27).

A pneumatic device called the Percussionator is used to provide intrapulmonary percussive ventilation (IPV). IPV treats diffused patchy atelectasis, enhances mobilization and clearance of secretions, and delivers nebulized medications and wetting agents to the distal airways (27). Patients using this device breathe through a mouthpiece delivering a high flow of "mini-bursts" at rates of >200 Hz. Impaction pressures of 25–40 PSI are delivered with a frequency between 100 to 225 percussive cycles/min.

High-frequency chest wall compression is designed to increase tracheal mucus clearance and improve ventilation by reducing viscoelastic and cohesive properties of mucus. The vest (Advanced Respiratory, St. Paul, Minnesota, U.S.A.) is a device originally designed to promote secretion clearance and, more recently, for sputum induction (27). It is intended for self-administered therapy and consists of a large-volume variable-frequency air-pulse delivery system attached to a nonstretching, inflatable vest worn by the patient over the entire torso. The patient uses a foot pedal to control pressure pulses, during expiration or the entire respiratory cycle. Pulse frequency is adjustable from 5 to 25 Hz, with pressure in the vest ranging from 28 to 39 mmHg.

The Hayak Oscillator is an electrically powered, microprocessor-controlled, noninvasive oscillator ventilator, which applies negative and positive pressures to the chest wall to deliver noninvasive oscillation to the lungs. Frequency range, inspiratory–expiratory ratios, and inspiratory pressures may be adjusted.

Intermittent Positive Pressure Breathing

Intermittent positive pressure breathing (IPPB) is the application of inspiratory positive pressure to the airway in order to provide a significantly larger tidal volume than the patient can produce spontaneously. IPPB should not be confused with positive-pressure ventilation delivered with a mechanical ventilator, which is intended to provide ventilatory support. It should also not be confused with IPV, a therapeutic technique of CPT that utilizes a pneumatic device called the Percussionator. IPPB is most useful in disease states in which the patient's depth of breathing is limited. This type of therapy is very expensive; therefore, for this mode of therapy to be indicated, the patient's vital capacity should be less than 15 mL/kg and the IPPB treatment should augment this volume by at least 100%. In addition, some end point should be planned for the

therapy. The use of IPPB should be limited to those patients with severely compromised respiratory reserves who are suffering an acute illness, or an exacerbation of a chronic condition that causes a temporary deterioration in their overall respiratory state. Patients with more severe and chronic ventilatory-reserve limitations will often require a chronic artificial airway (i.e., tracheostomy) in order to maintain consistent bronchial hygiene.

Suctioning

Removal of bronchial secretions via suction catheters is a commonly employed bronchial-hygiene technique. Performed appropriately, this procedure is safe and effective. Performed without appropriate caution, it can result in significant complications or death. Airway suctioning can be accomplished safely in patients with artificial airways (endotracheal or tracheostomy tubes) in place. In these circumstances, the patient should be ventilated with a manual resuscitation bag and a high F_IO_2. This "preoxygenation/denitrogenation" will minimize the hypoxemia that is induced by removing the patient from an O_2 source and applying suction to the airways. A sterile suction catheter should then be placed into the airway and advanced, without the application of vacuum, beyond the tip of the artificial airway until the catheter can no longer be easily advanced. The catheter should then be withdrawn slightly before suction is applied. Suctioning is then accomplished by the intermittent application of vacuum and the gradual withdrawal of the catheter in a rotating fashion. The duration of the entire procedure should not exceed 20 seconds. Following the completion of suctioning, the patient should be manually ventilated with an O_2-enriched atmosphere to ensure adequate lung re-expansion and oxygenation. The patient should be monitored for signs of distress, bronchospasm, hemodynamic instability, or dysrhythmias throughout the entire procedure.

In the mechanically ventilated patient whose condition creates concerns of infection, either to the patient or to the healthcare professional who is rendering care, a closed-system suction catheter may be of benefit (28). Unlike open-system suction catheters, the closed-system suction catheters can be reused and physically incorporated into the patient's ventilator circuit at the connection between the ventilator circuit and the artificial airway. This closed-system suction catheter can also be used when any disconnection from mechanical ventilation or intermittent discontinuation of high levels or PEEP may result in pulmonary compromise.

In the closed system, the catheter itself is shrouded in a protective sleeve that allows the versatility of advancing or retracting the catheter in the patient's airway without interrupting mechanical ventilation. Although preoxygenation is not as critical with closed-system suctioning, it should still be used. Hypoxemia is best avoided by temporarily increasing the F_IO_2 to 100% shortly before and during any suction maneuver. When fully retracted, the closed-system suction catheter does not create airway interference or obstruction and can be left in line for extended periods of time, usually 24 to 48 hours, or as determined by an institution's infection-control policy.

Suctioning of the tracheobronchial tree without an artificial airway in place (i.e., nasotracheal suctioning) is practiced in many centers but carries several risks. Because the patient cannot be manually ventilated and "preoxygenated" before the procedure, hypoxemia and hemodynamically significant arrhythmias can occur (29,30). In addition, passing the suction catheter through the vocal cords can result in laryngospasm or vocal-cord injury with subsequent airway obstruction. In many patients who have impaired but reasonable ventilatory reserves, this technique is often carried out without significant problems. However, patients with extremely marginal ventilatory reserves are at the greatest risk for the aforementioned complications.

Suctioning of the tracheobronchial tree should only be undertaken when appropriately indicated. The primary indication is the presence of bronchial secretions that can be identified visually or on auscultation. Rising airway pressures in mechanically ventilated patients may also indicate the presence of retained bronchial secretions. Mucosal irritation, trauma, and bleeding can be precipitated by frequent and aggressive suctioning in the absence of bronchial secretions. Routine suctioning of the airway is, however, required in intubated patients including adults, and especially in neonates, where small airways can be acutely obstructed by a small accumulation of secretions.

Bronchoscopy

☛ **Therapeutic bronchoscopy is indicated for clearance of secretions or when atelectasis persists despite aggressive bronchial-hygiene maneuvers, or for retrieval of aspirated foreign bodies.** ☚

Bronchoscopy can be used for both diagnostic and therapeutic purposes in various clinical settings. In the trauma critical care setting, the indications for bronchoscopy tend to be focused on diagnosing infections, removing retained secretions or foreign bodies, and assessing and controlling hemoptysis. In the ICU, bronchoscopy is often performed on patients undergoing mechanical ventilatory support and necessitates a different approach than that taken with awake, stable, spontaneously ventilating patients. Observations of the patient during bronchoscopy are essential and should be delegated to personnel other than the bronchoscopist or the immediate assistant. It is often best to have a respiratory therapist to provide manual ventilation during the procedure and also monitor the patient for adverse physiological effects. Introduction of a bronchoscope into the airways of a mechanically ventilated patient will often result in increased airway pressures, interference with distribution of ventilation, and inhibition of ventilator function. Manual ventilation of the patient by a respiratory therapist during bronchoscopy can be useful, because the therapist can instantly feel changes in airway resistance, alter the pattern of ventilation to compensate for the problem, inform the bronchoscopist that a problem exists, and assist with maneuvers that will alleviate the compromising situation before a deterioration in the patient's condition can occur.

There are several relative contraindications to bronchoscopy, but no absolute contraindications exist. The decision to perform the procedure must be based upon the balance of potential risks and benefits. Considerations that should be taken into account include: (*i*) the hemodynamic stability of the patient; (*ii*) the patient's respiratory status, including oxygenation, ventilation, PEEP level, airway pressures, etc.; (*iii*) the presence of coagulopathies and the potential for their correction or amelioration before the procedure; and (*iv*) the patient's mental status. Bronchoscopy may be life-saving in the presence of these factors, and should never be omitted if determined to be indicated for emergency clearance of the airway.

Therapeutic bronchoscopy is indicated for clearance of secretions when radiographic studies show evidence of segmental or lobar atelectasis, and the patient's clinical condition requires urgent intervention or when atelectasis is persistent despite aggressive bronchial-hygiene maneuvers (i.e., postural drainage, percussion, and vibration), and is likely to result in detrimental sequelae such as pneumonia or lung abscess. In such circumstances, inspissated bronchial secretions may not be effectively mobilized by any means other than direct visualization, lavage, and manual removal. Therapeutic bronchoscopy is also useful in the retrieval of aspirated foreign bodies. Such foreign bodies may range from particulate food material, which may not be evident on chest radiographs, to any number of inanimate objects. The degree of difficulty encountered with the location and removal of a foreign body depends upon several factors, such as its size, consistency, location, and the duration of time it has been in the bronchial tree. Various foreign-body-retrieval tools (Fig. 6) are designed to be passed through the suction channel of the bronchoscope and grasp or snare objects of various size, shape, and consistency.

The localization and control of bleeding in the airways is one of the most difficult challenges in bronchoscopy for several reasons. Depending upon the severity of the bleeding, visualization is often difficult. One of the risks of bronchoscopy is mucosal injury and its associated additional hemorrhage. Once located, the source of bleeding may not be amenable to control via bronchoscopic techniques. Despite all of these problems, bronchoscopy can be important in obtaining information that is useful in the planning of procedures necessary to further diagnose and control sites of pulmonary hemorrhage, such as localizing the bleeding to a specific lung, lobe, or segment for more rapid angiographic

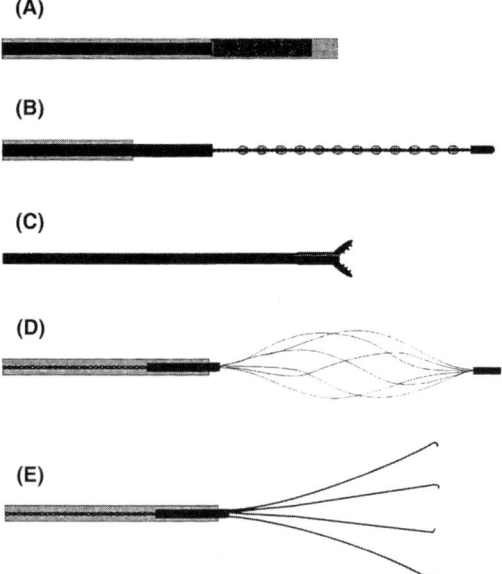

Figure 6 (**A**) Protected bronchial microbiology brush in the retracted position with the protective diaphragm in place. (**B**) Protected bronchial microbiology brush in the extended sampling position before retraction into the protective sleeve. (**C**) Foreign-body-retrieval forceps with "teeth." (**D**) Retrieval basket for grasping irregularly shaped or difficult-to-grasp objects from the bronchial tree. (**E**) Retrieval device for grasping large, soft objects from the bronchial tree.

location and intervention. Bronchoscopy is also useful in diagnosis and treatment of retained clots in the airway (31) and for stent placement needed to alleviate bronchial obstruction due to tumor or collapse (32).

In the critical care setting, diagnostic bronchoscopy is useful for the detection and characterization of bacterial and opportunistic lung infections. However, the use of bronchoscopy for the diagnosis of nosocomial pneumonia, especially ventilator-associated pneumonia, is controversial. The methods by which cultures are obtained, the use of quantitative or semiquantitative culture techniques, the threshold of bacterial growth necessary for the diagnosis of pneumonia versus colonization, and the other factors that are most useful in differentiating bacterial colonization from pneumonia in different patient populations, are all debated (33–35).

There are several reasons to perform bronchoscopy for the diagnosis of lung infections. Cultures of endotracheal aspirates may not yield results consistent with the pathologic organism because of oropharyngeal contamination or tracheal colonization. The use of clinical (fever, leukocytosis, and purulent secretions) and radiologic (focal infiltrates) criteria for differentiation of pneumonia from airway colonization is generally limited, especially in intubated patients (33–35). Microbiologic specimens obtained from localized areas of the lung, especially if they include samples of alveolar contents, provide more specific information regarding the pathologic process (36); however, sensitivity and specificity for the diagnosis of pneumonia can be influenced greatly by the type of pathology present, the bronchoscopic technique, and interpretive thresholds (33,37).

Bronchoscopy permits the direct visualization of the airways so that anatomic abnormalities, such as tumors or aberrant bronchial anatomy which can predispose the patient to developing airway obstruction and infection, can be detected. Occasionally, it is important to obtain tissue samples via transbronchial biopsy in order to further elucidate the pathologic process when culture results alone are insufficient.

The diagnosis of lung infections can be accomplished with various bronchoscopic techniques, including protected bronchial brushing, bronchoalveolar lavage (BAL) (protected or unprotected), or transbronchial biopsy. Each of these methods has indications and limitations, which must be considered when planning diagnostic procedures. Protected bronchial brushing is useful for the diagnosis of bacterial pneumonia, because this technique permits the avoidance of contaminated upper-airway secretions and more select sampling of the region of lung of interest. This technique has limitations because the potential for contamination with upper-airway secretions continues, but it is much more likely that positive cultures from the area of the lung in question will be representative of the pathologic process.

The type of protected brush and the methods used to obtain samples will vary, but it is primarily the ability to obtain quantitative cultures (38) that justifies the risks and expense of this procedure. This technique allows the retrieval of 0.001–0.01 mL of lung secretions (39). The level of bacterial growth used to diagnose a ventilator-associated pneumonia with protected bronchial brushing is generally accepted as >10^3 colony-forming units (cfu)/mL (40).

BAL also permits sampling from a specific region of lung and has several added advantages compared to protected bronchial brushing. BAL samples a large area of the distal airways and alveoli, is appropriate for all types of

microbiological diagnoses [bacterial, fungal, *Pneumocystis carinii* (PCP), etc.], and provides a sample volume that is adequate for a large number of tests (35).

BAL can be performed either in a nonprotected or a protected manner. The nonprotected technique involves isolating the bronchus of interest from the remainder of the tracheobronchial tree, by wedging the tip of the bronchoscope into an airway lumen and lavaging with a large-volume (approximately 120–200 mL in 5–10 aliquots) of nonbacteriostatic saline.

One may expect to obtain a return of less than 50% of the lavage fluid that will contain approximately 1 mL of actual lung secretions (35). The first lavage sample is likely to be contaminated with central-airway secretions and is often discarded or treated as bronchial washings (41). ✍ **Protected BAL has been developed to decrease the potential contamination of the lavage fluid with secretions contained within the lumen of the bronchoscope.** ✍ This technique uses a protected transbronchoscopic balloon-tipped catheter to lavage from the level of third-generation bronchi following expulsion of the protective polyethylene-glycol diaphragm and occlusion of the bronchi with the air-filled balloon (42).

When using BAL, the level of bacterial growth accepted as being consistent with a ventilator-associated pneumonia is 10^4 cfu/mL because of dilution of the alveolar secretions (33,40). Some clinicians would use a higher diagnostic threshold (10^5 cfu/mL) with nonprotected BAL, because of the increased chance of sample contamination, and would accept the fact that this threshold will increase the specificity but decrease the sensitivity of the test.

The use of "blind" (nonbronchoscopic), nonprotected BAL in order to monitor and diagnose ventilator-associated pneumonia in trauma patients has been advocated (43). Although this use may be generally appropriate and cost-effective for pneumonia surveillance in this group of patients, the results may be misleading in patients with chronic lung disease or who are immunocompromised. Thus, the patient population must be considered carefully when diagnostic bronchoscopic techniques are chosen.

A special nonbronchoscopic catheter for BAL has been developed and proven to be useful in the diagnosis of PCP (44). This device is also useful in circumstances, such as mechanical ventilation with high PEEP when the risks of bronchoscopy are considered to be too high; however, bleeding and pneumothorax can occur with the use of this device. The use of transbronchial biopsy in the critical care setting is most often not necessary and is frequently contraindicated, especially for patients who are being treated with positive-pressure ventilation.

Bronchoscopy remains a valuable diagnostic tool-in these clinical settings: (*i*) immunocompromised patients (i.e., HIV infected and organ transplant patients), (*ii*) ventilator-associated pneumonia, and (*iii*) severe persistent community- or hospital-acquired pneumonia. Fiberoptic bron- choscopy is especially useful in the diagnosis of atypical pneumonia (i.e., cytomegalovirus, *Mycobacterium tuberculosis*, *Pneumocystis carinii*) (37). Again, risks and benefits must be weighed before choosing the diagnostic technique.

The administration of antibiotic therapy before obtaining bronchoscopic bacterial cultures has been shown both to decrease sensitivity (likely due to inhibition of growth) and to decrease specificity (probability due to increased airway colonization) (35). Obviously, the preferred method is to obtain culture samples before instituting antibiotic therapy, but if antibiotics have already been administered, the only recourse is to interpret the culture results accordingly. When lidocaine is used during bronchoscopy from which bacterial cultures are to be obtained, the lidocaine may inhibit the growth of some microorganisms (45), but this finding has not been noted with lidocaine used in nebulization (35,36).

AEROSOL THERAPY

An aerosol is a suspension of fine particles of a liquid in a gas. Aerosols have three basic applications in respiratory care: as an aid to bronchial hygiene, to humidify inspiratory gases, and to deliver medications. When dealing with medical aerosols for inhalation, particle size should be 5 mm or less in order for gravitational effects to be sufficiently small to permit deposition in the pulmonary tree (46).

Bland Aerosol Therapy

When used as an aid to bronchial hygiene, water is one of the most important physically active agents. Aerosol therapy can be useful in the hydration of dried, retained secretions and the restoration and maintenance of the mucus blanket. This hydration, in conjunction with appropriate cough mechanisms and other bronchial-hygiene techniques, will permit the mobilization of retained secretions. Care must be taken, however, because bland (i.e., without medication) aerosols used for these purposes can result in the patient's clinical deterioration due to either increased airway resistance (bronchospasm) or swelling and expansion of dried secretions (47). These detrimental effects may be ameliorated by the administration of a bronchodilator or the use of techniques to mobilize the expanding secretions. Although bland-aerosol therapy is widely used, evidence to support the utility of such therapy is not available (46,48). Generally, it appears that there is a need to reassess the clinical utility of this modality.

The major indication for nebulized saline, either hypotonic or hypertonic, is for induction of sputum specimens. The administration of high-volume aerosolized saline for 30 minutes via a continuous ultrasonic aerosol is appropriate to achieve sputum induction, provided the patient has a strong effective cough and there is sputum in the airways that can be mobilized and expectorated.

Obtaining sputum specimens for the diagnosis of PCP in immunocompromised individuals requires a special procedure. The diagnosis is confirmed by visualization of the organisms in samples of sputum, BAL fluid, or lung tissue obtained on biopsy. Sputum samples should be obtained after the patients have brushed their teeth and rinsed their mouths. The patient inhales an ultrasonic mobilization of 3% sodium chloride through his or her mouth to promote a vigorous cough and produce a sample containing alveolar cells and contents. With this technique, the diagnosis can be obtained in 50% to 80% of patients with PCP due to the acquired immunodeficiency syndrome (AIDS) (49–51). This diagnostic yield may be decreasing in light of current inhaled and systemic antibiotic prophylaxis of PCP.

Complications associated with ultrasonically nebulized aerosols include wheezing or bronchospasm, infection, overhydration, and patient discomfort. Other individuals in the room may be exposed to droplet nuclei of *M. tuberculosis* or other airborne infections produced as a consequence of coughing particularly during sputum induction. The use of sputum induction for diagnostic purposes is only effective

if the patient has a productive cough and is able to produce a "deep specimen" that is not contaminated. Success in obtaining quality sputum specimens is best accomplished early in the morning after the patient has been supine for several hours. In the presence of an effective cough and adequate hydration, which is possible after using an ultrasonic nebulizer for 30 minutes, a patient should, in most cases, successfully mobilize any retained secretions to the level where an adequate specimen can be expectorated, collected, and sent to the laboratory for analysis.

Aerosolized Medications

The airway mucosa responds to infection and inflammation in several ways. These include goblet cell and submucosal gland hyperplasia and hypertrophy, with resultant mucus hypersecretion. Mucoactive medications either increase the ability to expectorate sputum or decrease mucus hypersecretion. The delivery of medications for the reversal and prevention of bronchoconstriction is an important application of aerosol therapy. PEP and aerosol therapy done simultaneously, either by hand-held nebulizer or metered-dose inhaler (MDI) can improve the response to bronchodilators (52). Table 3 provides data on the most commonly used aerosolized pharmacologic agents.

These medications include β-agonists, anticholinergic agents, and anti inflammatory agents. The β-agonists and anticholinergic agents act primarily by enhancing bronchodilation through increases in intracellular cyclic adenosine monophosphate levels or decreases in intracellular cyclic guanosine monophosphate levels. The use of anti-inflammatory agents has gained popularity in the treatment of bronchospastic disorders because the disease process has been demonstrated to be of an inflammatory nature.

When delivered in aerosolized form, antibiotic medications, such as pentamidine isethionate and amphotericin B, have been found to be effective for the prophylaxis and treatment of opportunistic pulmonary infections, such as PCP and pulmonary aspergillosis (53–56). Nebulized pentamidine decreases the frequency, severity, and occurrence of PCP in patients with AIDS (57). Pentamidine aerosolization should generate particles with a mass median aerodynamic diameter (MMAD) of less than 3.0 μm in order to ensure adequate penetration to the lung parenchyma and to minimize the irritation associated with deposition in the airways. The currently recommended dosage regimen is 300 mg, administered via an ultrasonic nebulizer (Fisoneb®) or a jet-type nebulizer (Respigard II ®) every month (57,58).

Invasive pulmonary fungal infections are significant problems in immunocompromised patients, especially those undergoing bone marrow transplantation during their neutropenic stages. Aerosolization and inhalation of amphotericin B has been investigated as a method to provide prophylaxis against pulmonary fungal infections while minimizing the adverse side effects of the drug (55,59). Aerosolized amphotericin appears to be well tolerated and has minimal systemic absorption (54,60); however, well-controlled outcome data are not available. Aerosolized antibiotic therapy for infections associated with cystic fibrosis has also been explored, but found to be of equivocal efficacy (61).

Ribavirin has been recommended for the treatment of respiratory syncytial virus (RSV) in children, especially those with congenital heart disease, immunnodeficiency, or bronchopulmonary dysplasia (61). This drug has also been used in certain immunocompromised adults;

Table 3 Aerosolized Bronchodilators and Antiasthmatic Drugs

Drug	Method	Adult dosages[a]	Frequency action (hr)	Duration of effects	Intended effect (side effect)	Mechanism
Sympathomimetics						
Albuterol 0.5% (Ventolin®, Proventil®)	MDI[b]	2 puffs (90 μg/puff)	q4-6h or qid	≤6	Bronchodilation	β_2-agonist, increase in cAMP
	Nebulized	2.5-5.0 mg in 4 mL				
Isoetharine hydrochloride 1% (Bronkosol®)	Nebulized	0.25-0.50 mL in 4.0 mL	q2-4h	1.5-3.0	Bronchodilation (tachycardia)	β_2-agonist, increase in cAMP
	MDI[b]	2 puffs (10 mg/puff)				
Isoproterenol 0.5% (Isoprel®)	Nebulized	0.25-0.50 mL in 3.5 mL	q2-4h	1.5-2.0	Bronchodilation (tachycardia, vasodilation, flushing)	Prototype β-agonist; significant β_1 side effects
Metaproterenol sulfate 5% (Alupent®)	Nebulized	0.3 mL in 4.0 mL	q4-6h or qid	≤5	Bronchodilation	β_2-agonist, increase in cAMP
	MDI	2 puffs (0.655 mg/puff)				
	Rotocaps®b	1-2 capsules (200 μg/cap)				
Racemic epinephrine 2.25%	Nebulized	0.5 mL in 3.5 mL	q1h, prn	≤1	Mucosal decongestion	Weak β_2 agonist and mild a mucosal vasoconstrictor
Terbutaline 0.1% (Brethane®, Bricanyl®)	Nebulized	2-5 mg in 2-5 mL	q4-6h	4-6	Bronchodilation	β_2-agonist
Anticholinergic drugs						
Atropine sulfate 2% or 5%	Nebulized	0.025 mg/kg up to 2.5 mg in 2-5 mL	q6-8h	4-6	Bronchodilation	Cholinergic blocker, decreases cGMP
Ipratropium bromide 0.02% (Atrovent®)	MDI	2 puffs (18 μg/puff)	q4h or qid	3-4	Bronchodilation	Cholinergic blocker, decreases cGMP
	Nebulized	0.5 mg in 2.5 mL	tid or qid			
Antiallergy agents						
Beclomethasone acetonide (Vanceril®, Beclovent®)	MDI	2 puffs (42 μg/puff)	q6h or qid	6	Anti-inflammatory	Anti-inflammatory; inhibit leukocyte migration; potentiate effects of β-agonists
Cromolyn sodium (Intel®)	Nebulized	20 mg in 2-4 mL	q6h or qid	6	Stabilization of mast cell membranes	Suppression of mast cell response to Ag-ab reactions; used prophylactically
	MDI	2-4 puffs (800 μg/puff)				
	Spinhaler®b	1 capsule (20 μg/cap)				
Dexamethasone sodium phosphate (Decadron®)	Nebulized	1 mg in 2.5 mL	q6h	6	Anti-inflammatory	Anti-inflammatory; inhibit leukocyte migration; potentiate effects of β-agonists
Flunisolide (Aerobid®)	MDI[b]	2-4 puffs (250 μg/puff)	bid		Anti-inflammatory	Anti-inflammatory; inhibit leukocyte migration; potentiate effects of β-agonists
Triamcinolone (Azmacort®)	MDI[b]	2 puffs (100 μg/puff) 4 puffs (100 μg/puff)	tid-qid bid		Anti-inflammatory	Anti-inflammatory; inhibit leukocyte migration; potentiate effects of β-agonists

[a]Dosages may vary. References to specific drug inserts are recommended.
[b]Rotocaps and Spinhaler = inhaled powder.
Abbreviations: Ag-ab, antigen-antibody; cAMP, cyclic adenosine monophosphate; cGMP, cyclic guanosine monophosphate; MDI, metered dose inhaler.

however, because of the high expense of treatment and the rarity of severe RSV infections in adults, the diagnosis of RSV infection should be confirmed with rapid laboratory testing before commencing therapy.

The U.S. FDA has recommended the "Small Particle Aerosol Generator" (SPAG) for aerosolization of ribavirin for the treatment of RSV in children, but SPAG may also be used for adults if such therapy is deemed appropriate. The SPAG system will generate particles with a MMAD of less than 1.5 mm. The delivery of bronchodilators and antibiotics, and the use of aerosolization, are being investigated as means by which to deliver other drugs, such as insulin (62), that otherwise require chronic parenteral administration.

Unfortunately, a high incidence of bronchospastic reactions is associated with the administration of aerosolized antibiotics and other medications. These reactions necessitate either pretreatment or concurrent treatment with an aerosolized β-agonist. In addition, these agents potentially have toxic effects for healthcare-delivery personnel who are administering the treatments; therefore, appropriate exhaust, scavenging, or filtering systems should be used during administration of the treatments.

Small-Volume Nebulizers, Metered-Dose and Dry-Powder Inhalers

The delivery of medications via small-volume nebulizers (SVN) has historically been the standard for aerosol-medication delivery. Small and relatively easy to use, the SVN does require a gas source that can produce a flow of 5–10 mL/min. Optimal gas-source flow settings and specific design characteristics of a particular SVN are variables that determine aerosol particle size. As such, this method of drug delivery is expensive and potentially inefficient (63) and requires a significant time commitment on the part of the respiratory therapist.

Recent variations in the SVN design that incorporate a reservoir bag to collect and suspend aerosol particles of desired therapeutic size, and the addition of a PEP valve to promote better aerosol deposition, have been engineered to improve SVN efficiency. Advocates of these design changes suggest that the result is better aerosol-particle size, less systemic absorption of medication, and more medication targeted and deposited to the airways; however, no published clinical studies have supported this claim.

A functional alternative to the SVN is the MDI. The MDI is a device that permits the patient to rapidly self-administer an inhaled drug. The delivery of drug to the lower airways, with appropriate use of the MDI, has been demonstrated to be approximately 10% of the total dose and is comparable to that attained with the SVN (64–66). However, in contrast to the SVN, with which 66% of the drug is deposited in the apparatus and 2% is deposited in the mouth and stomach, MDI administration results in only 5% to 10% of drug deposition in the apparatus, with 80% deposited in the mouth and stomach (64,67). This factor carries implications pertaining to local side effects and tissue toxicity (i.e., oral thrush associated with inhaled-steroid use) (64).

☞ **In terms of clinical effects, no differences between MDI and SVN therapy have been found for peak expiratory-flow rates or severity of symptoms in stable patients treated with either modality (68).** ☞ In addition to having clinical efficacy equal to that of SVN devices, administering bronchodilator therapy with MDI devices requires less manpower and offers significant cost savings to the hospital (69).

Studies suggest that there can be a substantial benefit from the increased use of MDI with spacer and a percentage of patients can replace SVN with MDI using a spacer device (70,48,49,71). The effective use of an MDI requires that the patient meet certain clinical criteria. The patient must be able to appropriately position and actuate the device, inspire deeply, and coordinate the inspiratory effort with the device actuation.

In order to ensure efficacious use, a successful coordination of efforts is necessary, which requires appropriate instruction, training, and practice (72). Problems with proper technique are especially pronounced with patients who are either young or elderly (73). In order to ameliorate some of the problems associated with MDI use, "spacer devices" have been developed (74). A spacer effectively acts as a reservoir into which the drug is discharged by attaching and actuating the MDI device (Fig. 7). The use of spacer eliminates the need for significant coordination of hand, mouth, and breathing functions and improves delivery of the drug to the airways.

A breath-activated variation to the MDI is the Autohaler®. This device addresses concerns related to particle deposition and coordination issues inherent to the use of conventional MDI devices (75). Objectively comparing the conventional MDI devices and the Autohaler is difficult, because the Autohaler is limited to use with one drug (pirbuterol acetate) in the United States. As do conventional MDI devices, the Autohaler uses chlorofluorocarbons (CFC) as a propellant, a factor that is of environmental concern and strictly regulated by the government. A comparison of therapy with an MDI-spacer system versus SVN treatments indicated that a greater spirometric response was initially obtained with SVN, but this response

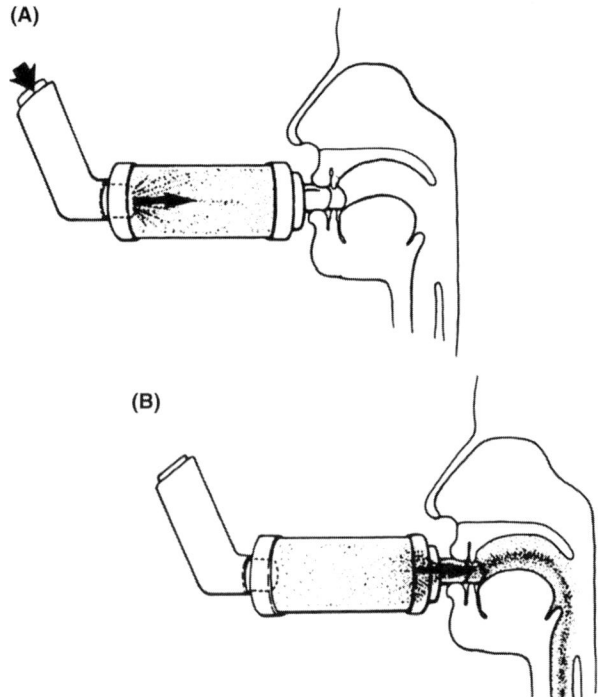

Figure 7 Illustration of a spacer with a metered-dose inhaler (MDI). (**A**) Demonstrates the aerosol suspension dispersing equally in the gas volume within the spacer following ejection from the MDI. (**B**) The patient takes a deep, slow inhalation of the medication. *Source*: From Ref. 93.

equalized over time to hospitalization (76). A study comparing MDI versus SVN delivery of albuterol in mechanically ventilated patients indicated equal clinical responses in both groups (77). In light of such information, it is reasonably clear that SVN administration of bronchodilators should be reserved for those patients who are unstable or otherwise incapable of using an MDI device. Patients can be assigned to MDI-spacer therapy if they meet the following criteria (78):

1. Respiratory rate <25 breaths/min.
2. Ability to breath-hold for 5 seconds or more.
3. Vital capacity >15 mL/kg.
4. Ability to understand verbal and visual instructions.
5. Appropriate hand-mouth-inspiratory coordination.
6. Peak expiratory flow rates of 150 mL/min for females and 200 mL/min for males.

Patients should be instructed in MDI-spacer use by a properly trained respiratory therapist. Before patients completely switch to this device, their technique should be evaluated, and additional training should be given if necessary.

Delivery of bronchodilators to patients undergoing mechanical ventilation can be effective but is also problematic. The use of an SVN to deliver bronchodilation during mechanical ventilation can result in bacterial contamination of the ventilator circuit, alteration in the delivered V_T, increased work of breathing during patient-initiated modes of ventilation, and damage to flow-measurement devices incorporated into some ventilator circuits (79). In addition, administration of aerosols via an endotracheal tube will reduce penetration to the lower airways (80). MDIs, in conjunction with mechanical ventilatory supports, have been evaluated for use in delivery of bronchodilators and have been shown to be comparable to SVN delivery systems—without the associated problems (79).

The use of MDI devices with spacers has undergone nonclinical bench testing with evidence of increased aerosol delivery; however, trials to document an improvement in clinical response are not yet available (73). Improved aerosol delivery can also be accomplished by adapting a nozzle-extension system to the MDI and extending the nozzle tip beyond the end of the endotracheal tube (81,82). Again, clinical studies to support the improved efficiency of this method of aerosol delivery are lacking, and the results of animal studies indicate that tracheal epithelial injury may occur when this system is used (73,83).

Another method of inspired-drug delivery is the dry-powder inhaler (DPI). DPIs create aerosols by drawing air through an aliquot of dry powder. The powder contains either micronized (<5 μm in diameter) drug particles bound into loose aggregates or micronized drug particles that are loosely bound to large (>30 μm in diameter) lactose or glucose particles (1). Patients using a DPI must be able to generate an inspiratory flow rate of greater than 30 to 60 L/min to be effective, and DPIs are not recommended for patients in acute bronchoconstriction or for children under the age of six years. DPIs are recommended for prophylactic and maintenance therapy because of the inspiratory flow requirements (84). These devices have two major advantages over SVN or MDI devices: they are activated by the patient's inspiratory effort and, therefore, do not require a high degree of hand-mouth-inspiratory-effort coordination, and they do not use fluorocarbon propellants.

This drug-delivery method appears to have equal efficacy compared to MDI and SVN delivery systems (64). The use of these devices may increase as the concern for environmental protection results in the elimination or severe restriction of CFC propellants (46). Although patients can find DPIs more convenient and easier to use than MDIs, one report suggests that as many as 25% of patients may use DPIs improperly (46). Clinicians must understand the required technique involved with DPIs and provide the necessary instruction and periodic review of technique, for patients to receive the benefits of medication delivery utilizing a DPI (47,48,70).

CONTINUOUS POSITIVE AIRWAY PRESSURE

Positive airway pressure has been used since the 1930s to improve oxygenation, increase lung volumes, and reduce venous return. More recently, continuous positive airway pressure (CPAP) has been identified as an effective method of splinting airways during expiration, improving collateral ventilation, increasing response to inhaled bronchodilators, and aiding secretion clearance in patients with various lung disorders. CPAP bronchial hygiene techniques may be effective alternatives to CPT for expanding lungs and mobilizing secretions (52). CPAP therapy may be more effective than spirometry and IPPB in the management of postoperative atelectasis (86). CPAP is the application of positive airway pressure during both inspiration and expiration, during spontaneous breathing. A typical continuous-flow CPAP system includes a medium-volume, high-compliance reservoir bag (5–10 L) and maintains system flow in excess of the patient's peak inspiratory flow demands (Fig. 8). Characteristically, system-continuous flows are maintained at 60–90 L/min. The adequacy of continuous flow is evaluated by observing gas continuously exiting from the system, even during peak inspiratory-flow periods. A system-pressure manometer and, ideally, an O_2 analyzer should be included in all CPAP circuits. A threshold resistor is located on the expiratory limb of the pressurized circuit. Finally, a pressure pop-off valve is included in all systems to prevent excessive pressure (such as occurs with system obstruction or when the patient coughs with a high-flow resistance or PEEP device) from building up in the system. With all circuits, some fluctuations in system pressure are noted, with the acceptable range being about ±2 cm H_2O. Fluctuations of greater magnitude during inspiration may be corrected by increasing system flow, increasing the size of the circuit reservoir, or increasing the flow and the size of the reservoir. Changes in baseline pressures during exhalation are primarily affected by the flow-resistance properties of the PEEP device.

CPAP, applied by full-face mask or nasal mask, has been used for respiratory support in patients with various types of pulmonary pathology, ranging from CHF to obstructive sleep apnea. The primary respiratory effects of CPAP are that it increases functional residual capacity; improves distribution of ventilation, lung compliance, and oxygenation; and decreases work of breathing. CPAP applied with a nasal mask is more comfortable, often better tolerated, and allows the patient to communicate more effectively than does CPAP applied with a full-face mask. Additionally, should vomiting occur, nasal-mask CPAP does not present an obstacle to airway clearance. However, in severely hypoxemic patients, nasal CPAP may not permit a seal sufficient to sustain the airway pressure necessary to maintain oxygenation. Conditions in the trauma patient, such as sinusitis, ear infection, epistaxis, or recent facial, oral or skull injury, should be individually

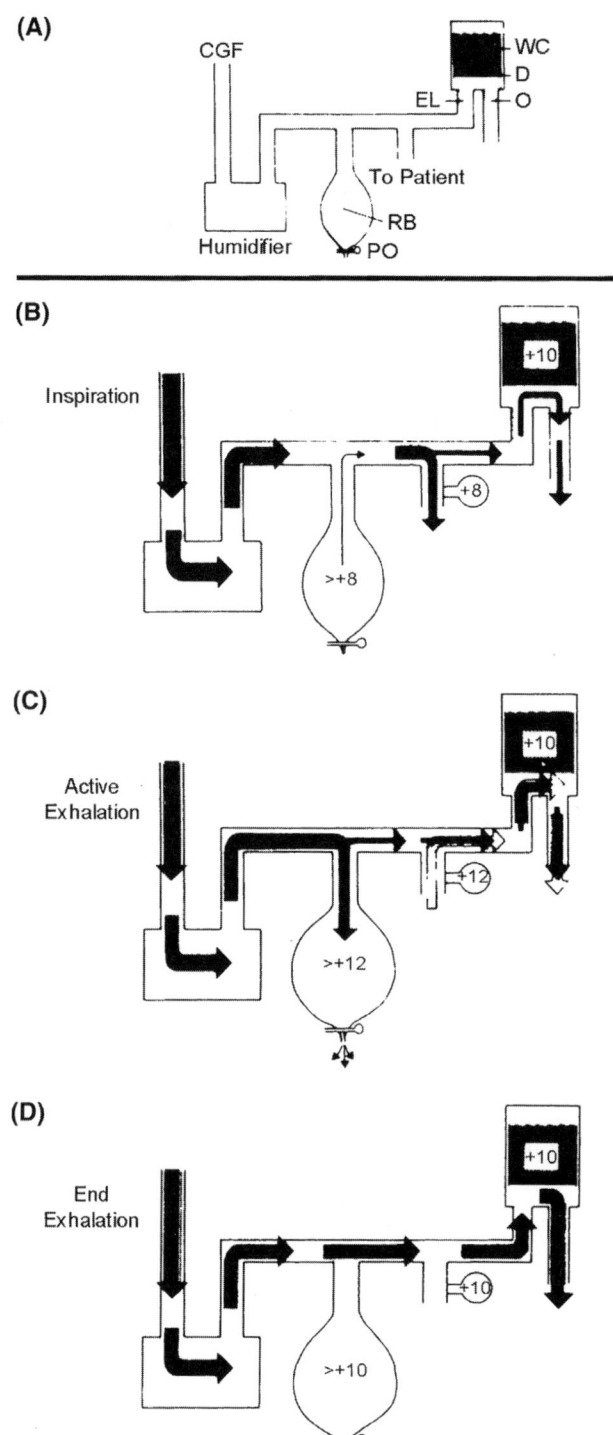

Figure 8 (**A**) Schematic representation of a continous positive airway pressure device. The continuous gas flow must be great enough to force some gas to continuously enter the reservoir bag except during peak inspiratory flow. Through adjustment of the pop-off mechanism, the pressure in the bag is maintained equal to or greater than the threshold pressure. Thus, gas will always flow through the outlet port of the PEEP device. Note that the patient's airway pressure fluctuates no more than ± 2 cm H_2O of the threshold pressure. (**B**) Inspiration: most of the gas flow will enter the patient's airway without added impedance, whereas the remainder of the gas flows through the outlet port of the PEEP device. Note that at the moment of the patient's peak inspiratory flow, there may be a small amount of gas entering the patient from the reservoir bag. (**C**) Active exhalation: airway pressure is greater than threshold, causing more of the continuous gas flow to enter the reservoir bag. The increased expiratory flow may create increased pressure if the PEEP device has orificial resistor properties and thus increases the work of breathing. (**D**) End exhalation: the continuous gas flow and reservoir bag maintain the circuit pressure at the threshold pressure. *Abbreviations*: CGF, continuous gas flow source; D, diaphragm of the PEEP device; EL, exhalation line of the patient circuit; OP, outlet port of the PEEP device; PEEP, post end expiratory pressure; PO, pop-off mechanism, which is an open nipple with an adjustable clamp; RB, elastic reservoir bag; WC, water column determining the threshold pressure of 10 cm H_2O. *Source*: From Ref. 93.

evaluated prior to considering a decision to initiate this therapy. Those with hemoptysis or unresolved pneumothorax are not candidates for this treatment modality (52).

Biphasic-airway-pressure (BiPAP) therapy is effectively the combination of CPAP with pressure-support augmentation of spontaneous inspiration. This method permits mechanical support of spontaneous ventilatory efforts without the need for intubation. This method of "noninvasive" ventilatory support has been demonstrated to be efficacious in patients demonstrating hypoxemia, hypercapnia, or hypercapnia and hypoxemia due to COPD, CHF, ARDS, and PCP (86–88). Although pressure injury to the nose has been reported with the use of biphasic airway pressure, the potential complications of gastric distention and aspiration do not appear to be significant. Of course, this mode of ventilatory support would not be appropriate for patients with a compromised ability for airway protection or glottic pathology (i.e., supraglottitis, thermal injury, or laryngeal edema). Additionally, patients must be observed carefully to ensure that the device does not become displaced and that spontaneous ventilation continues.

☞ BiPAP therapy combines CPAP with a pressure-support augmentation of spontaneous inspiration. ☜

EYE TO THE FUTURE

Impaired mucus clearance or mucus hypersecretion have potentially grave consequences for the individual. Aside from discomfort and dyspnea, excess mucus in the airway may lead to airway obstruction, atelectasis, infection, bronchiectasis, and other pulmonary morbidity (83). Concepts regarding airway secretion clearance are continuing to evolve. Included in any discussion of these evolving techniques is ultra-low-frequency airway oscillation, also known as the Insufflator/Exsufflator. This device, admittedly not newly developed, may be uniquely suited to assist in airway clearance in trauma victims, as well as in those individuals who have neuromuscular weakness and other infirmities. It may prove to be a valuable adjunctive measure when added to postural drainage and lung expansion therapy. Other new modalities include AD, active cycle of breathing technique, PEP methods, high-frequency airway oscillation (flutter), high-frequency chest-wall oscillation (The Vest), and IPV. Patient motivation and understanding of the disease process may greatly affect outcomes when utilizing devices such as these. The greatest challenge may be in educating our patients in the relative risk-benefit and alternative paradigms of care available to them.

SUMMARY

The practice of respiratory care has always been integral to the practice of critical care medicine. The advancements of technology and medical science have made this role even more important but, also more complex and difficult. These advancements require appropriate training and understanding of the equipment now used to deliver state-of-the-art respiratory care. Also, the complexity of patients requiring critical care necessitates the inclusion of individuals capable of making complicated clinical assessments and decisions. The complexity of this situation will only increase as medical science advances. Therefore, the training and capabilities of respiratory care practitioners must advance to keep pace with these changes.

KEY POINTS

- ☞ The three major reasons for mixed venous blood to have low O_2 content include: (*i*) metabolic rate; (*ii*) ↓ O_2 delivery; and (*iii*) ↓ arterial O_2 content.
- ☞ The primary determinants of oxygen content are the Hgb concentration and the degree of Hgb saturation.
- ☞ Nonrebreathing systems are divided into high-flow (fixed performance) and low-flow (variable performance) systems.
- ☞ Flow rates greater than 6 L/min will not increase the F_IO_2 significantly above 0.44 and are often poorly tolerated by the patient.
- ☞ A minimum flow of at least 5 L/min is necessary to prevent CO_2 accumulation and rebreathing during facemask-assisted breathing.
- ☞ In general, it is best to avoid exposure to an F_IO_2 of 0.5 or greater for more than 24 hours.
- ☞ Disruption of normal secretion or mucociliary clearance impairs pulmonary function and lung defenses, and predisposes the individual to infection.
- ☞ Humidification of inhaled gases is required to maintain normal respiratory epithelial function.
- ☞ The incentive spirometer is an effective and inexpensive prophylactic and therapeutic bronchial hygiene tool.
- ☞ The key elements of postural drainage are posture, time, breathing, and cough.
- ☞ Percussion assists secretion mobilization by loosening adherent secretions, and centralizing them for more effective expectoration or easier suctioning.
- ☞ Trauma patients in the ICU or those with long-term pulmonary complications, such as spinal cord injury, severe ARDS, etc., may also be good candidates for treatment with alternative airway-clearance methods.
- ☞ Therapeutic bronchoscopy is indicated for clearance of secretions or when atelectasis persists despite aggressive bronchial-hygiene maneuvers, or for retrieval of aspirated foreign bodies.
- ☞ Protected BAL has been developed to decrease the potential contamination of the lavage fluid with secretions contained within the lumen of the bronchoscope.
- ☞ In terms of clinical effects, no differences between MDI and SVN therapy have been found for peak expiratory-flow rates or severity of symptoms in stable patients treated with either modality (68).
- ☞ BiPAP therapy combines CPAP with a pressure-support augmentation of spontaneous inspiration.

REFERENCES

1. Shapiro BA, Kacmarek RM, Cane RD, Peruzzi WT, Hauptman D. Limitations of oxygen therapy. In: Shapiro BA, Kacmarek RM, Cane RD, Peruzzi WT, Hauptman D, eds. Clinical Application of Respiratory Care. 4th ed. St. Louis: Mosby Year Book, 1991:135–150.
2. Solliday NH, Shapiro BA, Gracey DR. Adult respiratory distress syndrome. Clinical conference in pulmonary disease from Northwestern University-McGaw Medical Center, Chicago, IL. Chest 1976; 69:207–213.
3. Lamy M, Fallat RJ, Koeniger E, et al. Pathologic features and mechanisms of hypoxemia in adult respiratory distress syndrome. Am Rev Respir Dis 1976; 114:267–284.
4. Shapiro BA, Cane RD, Harrison RA. Positive end-expiratory pressure in acute lung injury. Chest 1983; 558–563.

5. Shapiro BA, Cane RD. Metabolic malfunction of the lung: non-cardiogenic edema and adult respiratory distress syndrome. Surg Ann 1981; 13:271–298.

6. Miller WC, Rice DL, Unger KM, Bradley BL. Effect of PEEP on lung water content in experimental noncardiogenic pulmonary edema. Crit Care Med 1981; 9:7–9.

7. Shapiro BA, Cane RD, Harrison RA. Positive end-expiratory pressure therapy in adults with special reference to acute lung injury: a review of the literature and suggested clinical correlations. Crit Care Med 1984; 12:127–141.

8. Shapiro BA, Peruzzi WT, Templin R. Arterial Oxygenation. In: Clinical Application of Blood Gases, 5 Ed. St. Louis: Mosby Year Book, 1994: 33–53.

9. Schacter EN, Littner MR, Luddy P, Beck GJ. Monitoring of oxygen delivery systems in clinical practice. Crit Care Med 1980; 8:405–409.

10. Scacci R. Air entrainment masks: jet mixing is how they work; the Bernoulli and Venturi Principles are how they don't. Respir Care 1979; 24:928–931.

11. Deneke SM, Fanberg BL. Normobaric oxygen toxicity of the lung. N Engl J Med 1980; 303:76–86.

12. Lapin CD. Airway physiology, autogenic drainage, and active cycle of breathing. Respir Care 2002; 47(7):778–785.

13. Mengr BKR. Physiology of airway mucus clearance. Respir Care 2002; 47(7):761.

14. Lange P, Nyboe J, Appleyard M, et al. Relation of ventilatory impairment and of chronic mucus hypersecretion to mortality from obstructive lung disease and from all causes. Thorax 1990; 45(8):579–585.

15. Vestbo J, Prescott E, Lange P. Association of chronic mucus hypersecretion with FEV$_1$ decline and chronic obstructive pulmonary disease mortality. Copenhagen City Heart Study Group. Am J Respir Crit Care Med 1996; 153(5): 1530–1535.

16. Maxwell GM. The problem of mucus plugging in children with asthma. J Asthma 1985; 22(3):131–137.

17. Aikawa T, Shimura S, Sasaki H, et al. Marked goblet cell hyperplasia with mucus accumulation in the airways of patients who died of severe acute asthma attack. Chest 1992; 101(4):916–921.

18. Fink JB. Positioning versus postural drainage. Respir Care 2002; 47(7):769–777.

19. Kim CS, Rodriguez CR, Eldridge MA, Sackner MA. Criteria for mucus transport in the airways by two-phase gas-liquid flow mechanism. J Appl Phsiol 1986; 60(3):901–907.

20. Maxwell M, Redmond A. Comparative trial of manual and mechanical percussion technique with gravity-assisted bronchial drainage in patients with cystic fibrosis. Arch Dis Child 1979; 54:542–544.

21. Hardy AK. A review of airway clearance: New techniques, indications, and recommendations. Respir Care 1994; 39: 440–452.

22. Shapiro BA, Kacmarek RM, Cane RD, Peruzzi WT, Hauptman D. Applying and evaluating bronchial hygiene therapy. In: Shapiro BA, Kacmarek RM, Cane RM, Peruzzi WT, Hauptman D, eds. Clinical Application of Respiratory Care, 4th ed. St. Louis: Mosby Year Book, 1991:85–108.

23. AARC clinical practice guideline: Postural drainage therapy. Respir Care 1991; 36:1418–1426.

24. Lieberman JA, Cohen NH. Evaluation of a fixed orifice device for the delivery of positive expiratory pressure to non-intubated patients. Anesthesiology 1992; 77:A587.

25. Mahlmeister M, Fink J, Hoffman G, Fifer L. Positive-expiratory-pressure mask therapy: theoretical and practical considerations and a review of the literature. Respir Care 1991; 36:1218–1229.

26. Van Hengstum M, Festen J, Beurskens C, Hankel M, Beckman F, Corstens F. Effect of positive expiratory pressure mask physiotherapy (PEP) versus forced expiration technique (FET/PD) on regional lung clearance in chronic bronchitis. Eur Respir J 1991; 4:651–654.

27. Fink JB, Mahlmeister MJ. High-frequency oscillation of the airway and chest wall. Respir Care 2002; 47(7):797–807.

28. Sloan HE. Vagus nerve in cardiac arrest; effect of hypercapnia, hypoxia and asphyxia on reflex inhibition of heart. Surg Gynecol Obstet 1950; 91:257–264.

29. Crimlisk JT, Paris R, McGonagle EG, Calcutt JA, Farber HW. The closed tracheal suction system: implications for critical care nursing. Dim Crit Care Nurs 1994; 13:292–300.

30. Shim C, Fine N, Fernandez R, Williams MH Jr. Cardiac arrhythmias resulting from tracheal suctioning. Ann Intern Med 1969; 71:1149–1153.

31. Arney KL, Judson MA, Sahn SA. Airway obstruction arising from blood clot: three reports and a review of the literature. Chest 1999; 115(1):293–300.

32. Hautmann H, Bauer M, Pfeifer KJ, Huber RM: Flexible bronchoscopy: a safe method for metal stent implantation in bronchial disease. Ann Thoracic Surg 2000; 69(2):398–401.

33. Bonten MJM, Gaillard CA, Wouters EFM, van Teil FH, Stobberingh EE, van der Geest S. Problems in diagnosing nosocomial pneumonia in mechanically ventilated patients: a review. Crit Care Med 1994; 22:1683–1691.

34. Garrard CS, A'Court CD. The diagnosis of pneumonia in the critically ill. Chest 1995; 108:17S–25S.

35. Baselski VS, Wunderink RG. Bronchoscopic diagnosis of pneumonia. Clin Microbiol Rev 1994; 7:533–558.

36. Cook DJ, Fitzgerald JM, Guyatt GH. Evaluation of the protected brush catheter and bronchoalveolar lavage in the diagnosis of nosocomial pneumonia. J Inten Care Med 1991; 6:196–205.

37. Emad A: Bronchoalveolar lavage: a useful method for diagnosis of some pulmonary disorders. Respir Care 1997; 42(8): 765–790.

38. Pollack HM, Hawkins EL, Bonner JR, Sparkman T, Mass JB. Diagnosis of bacterial pulmonary infections with quantitative protected catheter cultures obtained during bronchoscopy. J Clin Microbiol 1983; 17:255–259.

39. Wimberley N, Faling LJ, Bartlett JG. A fiberoptic bronchoscopy technique to obtain uncontaminated lower airway secretions for bacterial culture. Am Rev Respir Dis 1979; 119:337–343.

40. Baselski VS, Robinson MK, Pifer LW, Woods DR. The standardization of criteria for processing and interpreting laboratory specimens with suspected ventilator-associated pneumonia. Chest 1992; 102:571S–579S.

41. Davis GS, Giancola MS, Costanza MC, Low RB. Analyses of sequential bronchoalveolar lavage samples from healthy human volunteers. Am Rev Respir Dis 1982; 126:611–616.

42. Meduri GU, Geals DH, Maijub AG, Baseleski V. Protected bronchoalveolar lavage. A new bronchoscopic technique to retrieve uncontaminated distal airway secretions. Am Rev Respir Dis 1991; 143:855–864.

43. Pugin J, Auckenthaler R, Mili N, Janssens JP, Lew PD, Suter PM. Diagnosis of ventilatory-associated pneumonia by bacteriologic analysis of bronchoscopic and nonbronchoscopic "blind" bronchoalveolar lavage fluid. Am Rev Respir Dis 1991; 143:1121–1129.

44. Bustamante EA, Levy H. Sputum induction compared with bronchoalveolar lavage by Ballard catheter to diagnose Pneumocystis carinii pneumonia. Chest 1994; 105:816–822.

45. Wimberley N, Willey S, Sullivan N, Bartlett JC. Antibacterial properties of lidocaine. Chest 1979; 6:37–40.

46. Aerosol consensus statement. Consensus conference of aerosol delivery. Chest 1991; 100:1106–1109.

47. Kuo CD, Lin SE, Wang JH. Aerosol, humidity and oxygenation. Chest 1991; 99:1352–1356.

48. Ward JJ, Helmholz HF Jr. Applied humidity and aerosol therapy. In: Burton GG, Hodgkin JE, Ward JJ, eds. Respiratory Care: A Guide to Clinical Practice. 3rd ed. Philadelphia: JB Lippincott Co., 1991:355–396.

49. Bigby TD, Margolskee D, Curtis JL, et al. The usefulness of induced sputum in the diagnosis of Pneumocystis carinii pneumonia in patients with the acquired immunodeficiency syndrome. Am Rev Respir Des 1986; 133:515–518.

50. Kovacs JA, Ng VL, Masur H, et al. Diagnosis of Pneumocystis carinii pneumonia: improved detection in sputum

with use of monoclonal antibodies. N Engl J Med 1988; 318: 589–593.

51. Masur H, Gill VJ, Ognibene FP, Shelhamer J, Godwin C, Kovacs JA. Diagnosis of Pneumocystis pneumonia by induced sputum technique in patients without the acquired immunodeficiency syndrome. Ann Intern Med 1988; 109:755–756.

52. Fink JB. Positive pressure techniques for airway clearance. Respir Care 2002; 47(7):786–796.

53. Leoung GS, Hopewell PC. Pneumocystis carinii pneumonia: Therapy and prophylaxis. In: Cohen PT, Sande MA, Volberding PA, eds. The AIDS Knowledge Base. 2nd ed. Vol. 6. 1994:17–26.

54. Myers SE, Devine SM, Topper RL, et al. A pilot study of prophylactic aerosolized amphotericin B in patients at risk for prolonged neutropenia. Leuk Lymphoma 1992; 8:229–233.

55. Hertenstein B, Kern WV, Schmeiser T, et al. Low incidence of invasive fungal infections after bone marrow transplantation in patients receiving amphotericin B inhalations during neutropenia. Ann Hematol 1994; 68:21–26.

56. Niki Y, Bernard EM, Edwards FF, Schmitt HJ, Yu B, Armstrong D. Model of recurrent pulmonary aspergillosis in rats. J Clin Microbiol 1991; 29:1317–1322.

57. Hardy WD. Prophylaxis of AIDS-related opportunistic infections (Ols). Current status and future strategies. AIDS Clin Rev 1991; 145–180.

58. Newman SP, Simonds AK. Aerosol therapy in AIDS. Lung 1990; suppl:685–691.

59. Schmitt HJ. New methods of delivery of amphotericin B. Clin Infect Dis 1993; 17(suppl 2):S501–S506.

60. Beyer J, Barzen G, Risse G, et al. Aerosol amphotericin B for prevention of invasive pulmonary aspergillosis. Antimicrob Agents Chemother 1993; 37:1367–1369.

61. Ziment I. Drugs used in respiratory therapy. In: Burton GG, Hodgkin JE, Ward JJ, eds. Respiratory Care: A Guide to Clinical Practice. 3rd ed. Philadelphia: JB Lippincott Co., 1991:411–448.

62. Laube BL, Georgopoulos A, Adams GK III. Preliminary study of the efficacy of insulin aerosol delivered by oral inhalation in diabetic patients. JAMA 1993; 269:2106–2109.

63. Newman SP. Aerosol deposition considerations in inhalation therapy. Chest 1985; 88:152S–160S.

64. Kacmaret RM, Hess D. The interface between patient and aerosol generator. Respir Care 1991; 36:952–976.

65. Newman SP, Pavia D, Moren F, Sheahan NF, Clarke SW. Deposition of pressurized aerosols in the human respiratory tract. Thorax 1981; 36:52–55.

66. Spiro SG, Singh CA, Tolfree SE, Partridge MR, Short MD. Direct labeling of ipratropium bromide aerosol and its deposition pattern in normal subjects and patients with chronic bronchitis. Thorax 1984; 39:432–435.

67. Lewis RA, Fleming JS. Fractional deposition from a jet nebulizer: How it differs from a metered dose inhaler. Brit J Dis Chest 1985; 79:361–367.

68. Jenkins SC, Heaton RW, Fulton TH, Moxham J. Comparison for domiciliary nebulized salbutamol and salbutamol from a metered-dose inhaler in stable chronic airflow limitation. Chest 1987; 91:804–807.

69. Bowton DL, Goldsmith WM, Haponik EF. Substitution of metered-dose inhalers for hand-held nebulizers. Success and cost savings in a large, acute-care hospital. Chest 1992; 101:305–308.

70. Hess D. The open forum: reflections on unanswered questions about aerosol therapy delivery techniques (Editorial). Respir Care 1988; 33:19–20.

71. Camargo CA, Kenney PA. Assessing costs of aerosol therapy. Respir Care 2000; 45(6):756–763.

72. Roberts RJ, Robinson JD, Doering, PL, Dallman JJ, Steeves RA. A comparison of various types of patient instruction in the proper administration of metered inhalers. Drug Intell Clin Pharm 1982; 16:53–59.

73. Armitage JM, Williams SJ. Inhaler technique in the elderly. Age Ageing 1988; 17:275–278.

74. Sackner MA, Kim CS. Recent advances in the management of obstructive airways disease. Auxiliary MDI aerosol delivery systems. Chest 1985; 88:161S–170S.

75. Chapman KR, Lover L, Brubaker H. A comparison of breath-activated and conventional metered-dose inhaler inhalation techniques in elderly subjects. Chest 1993; 104:1332–1337.

76. Morley TF, Marozsan E, Zappasodi SJ, Gordon R, Greisback R, Giudice JC. Comparison of beta-adrenergic agents delivered by nebulizer versus metered dose inhaler with InspirEase in hospitalized asthmatic patients. Chest 1988; 94:1205–1210.

77. Gay PC, Patel HG, Nelson SN, Gilles B, Hubmayr RD. Metered dose inhalers for bronchodilator delivery in intubated, mechanically ventilated patients. Chest 1991; 9:66–71.

78. Leiner GC, Abramowitz S, Small MJ, et al. Expiratory peak flow rate standard values for normal subjects. Use as a clinical test of ventilatory function. Am Rev Respir Dis 1963; 88:644–651.

79. Hess D. Inhaled bronchodilators during mechanical ventilation: delivery techniques, evaluation of response, and cost-effectiveness. Respiratory Care 1994; 39:105–122.

80. Ahrens RC, Ries RA, Popendorf W, Wiese JA. The delivery of therapeutic aerosols through endotracheal tubes. Pediatr Pulmonol 1986; 1:19–26.

81. Niven RW, Kacmarek RM, Brain JD, Peterfreund RA. Small bore nozzle extensions to improve the delivery efficiency of drugs from metered dose inhalers: laboratory evaluation. Am Rev Respir Dis 1993; 146:1590–1594.

82. Taylor RH, Lerman J, Chambers C, Dolovich M. Dosing efficiency and particle-size characteristics of pressurized metered-dose inhaler aerosols in narrow catheters. Chest 1993; 103:920–924.

83. Spahr-Schopfer IA, Lerman J, Cutz E, Dolovich M. Airway mucosal damage induced by high dose aerosol in rabbits (abstract). Am Rev Respir Dis 1992; 145:A364.

84. Fink JB. Aerosol device selection: evidence to practice. Respir Care 2000; 45(7):874–885.

85. Paul WL, Downs JB. Postoperative atelectasis: intermittent positive pressure breathing, incentive spirometry, and face-mask positive end-expiratory pressure. Arch Surg 1981; 116(7): 861–863.

86. Meduri GU, Conoscenti CC, Menashe P, Nair S. Noninvasive face mask ventilation in patients with acute respiratory failure. Chest 1989; 95:865–870.

87. Brochard L, Isabey D, Piquet J, et al. Reversal of acute exacerbations of chronic obstructive lung disease by inspiratory assistance with a face mask. N Engl J Med 1990; 323:1523–1530.

88. Pennock BE, Kaplan PD, Carlin BW, et al. Pressure support ventilation with a simplified ventilatory support system administered with a nasal mask in patients with respiratory failure. Chest 1991; 100:1371–1376.

89. Weber K, Milligan S. Therapist-driven protocols: The state-of-the-art (conference report). Respir Care 1994; 39:746–756.

90. Hart SK, Dubbs W, Gil A, Myers-Judy M. The effects of therapist-evaluation of orders and interaction with physicians on the appropriateness of respiratory care. Respir Care 1989; 34:185–190.

91. Shapiro BA, Cane RD, Peterson J, Weber D. Authoritative medical direction can assure cost-beneficial bronchial hygiene therapy. Chest 1988; 93:1038–1042.

92. Fink JB. Bronchial hygiene and lung expansion. In: Fink JB, Hunt J, eds. Clinical Practice of Respiratory Care. Philadelphia: Raven-Lippincott, 1999.

93. Shapiro BA, Kacmarek RM, Cane RD, Peruzzi WT, Hauptman D. Clinical Application of Respiratory Care. 4th ed. St. Louis: Mosby Year Book, 1991:127.

94. Burton GG, Hodgkin JE, Ward JJ. Respiratory Care. 3rd ed. Philadelphia: JB Lippincott Co., 1991.

95. Sharpiro BA, Peruzzi WT, Templin R. Clinical Application of Blood Gases. 5th ed. St. Louis: Mosby Year Book, 1994.

96. Vender JS, Spiess BD. Post Anesthesia Care. Phliladelphia: W.B. Saunders Co., 1992.

27

Mechanical Ventilation

William C. Wilson and Anushirvan Minokadeh
Department of Anesthesiology and Critical Care, UC San Diego Medical Center, San Diego, California, U.S.A.

Richard Ford
Department of Respiratory Care, UC San Diego Medical Center, San Diego, California, U.S.A.

Tobias Moeller-Bertram
Section of Pain Management, Department of Anesthesiology, UC San Diego Medical Center, and
VA Medical Center, San Diego, California, U.S.A.

INTRODUCTION

The ability to provide mechanical ventilation (MV) is the cornerstone of critical care medicine. More than 50 years of clinical experience with MV has shaped current understanding of the four fundamental relationships involved in an MV breath (time, pressure, volume, and flow). These factors affect more than merely MV, as manipulation of these values will affect both oxygenation and CO_2 elimination, but also affects patient comfort, secondary lung injury, ventilator-associated pneumonia (VAP), and hemodynamic stability.

Despite the one half century of experience with MV, controversy exists regarding many aspects [e.g., benefit of high-frequency ventilation (HFV), inverse ratio, pressure control ventilation, proning, permissive hypercapnia, etc.]. The controversy results from the paucity of randomized controlled trials (RCTs) investigating MV, the variety of patients and disease processes requiring MV, the plethora of ventilators and modes available, as well as the confusing and inconsistent terminology.

HISTORY

Although the scientific basis of oxidative metabolism was not established until the 1900s, ancient Egyptian, Chinese, and Greek medical papyri provide evidence that physicians in early civilizations understood the need for air to move into the airway to sustain life. Indeed, an engraving of the tracheostomy procedure was chiseled into Egyptian tablets dating back to 3600 B.C. (1). The earliest known textual references to tracheostomy are found in the *Rigveda*, a sacred Hindu book, published around 2000 B.C. (1). Hippocrates (460–370 B.C.) is quoted in his corpus to have said: "Whoever wishes to investigate medicine properly, should consider the pulsations of veins and breathing of the lungs according to age, harmonious and inharmonious, signs of disease more than health, for breath too is nutrient." Furthermore, in his "Treatise on Air," Hippocrates may have provided the first written description of endotracheal intubation when he instructed that: "One should introduce a cannula into the trachea along the jawbone so that air can be drawn into the lungs" (2).

Aristotle (384–322 B.C.) demonstrated the essential requirement of fresh air for the maintenance of life when he showed that animals placed in airtight boxes perished. Although his deduction on the cause of death (that the animals died due to their inability to cool themselves) was incorrect, he established that fresh air was required to sustain life. The first written account of mouth-to-mouth resuscitation is attributed to the prophet Elisha in the Old Testament (~800 B.C.), though the mechanism of resuscitation was attributed to divine intervention.

Galen (130–200), surgeon to the gladiators of Pergamos and later physician to the emperor Marcus Aurelius, performed vivisection and understood the role of the airway as a conduit to move air into the lungs, as evidenced in his writings: "If you take a dead animal and blow air through its larynx (using a reed), you will fill its bronchi and watch its lungs attain the greatest dimension" (3). However, Galen incorrectly deduced, and others were wrongly taught for over 1500 years that the function of the lungs was to cool the heart.

Andreas Vesalius (1514–1564) published an anatomically correct sequel to Galen's writings, in his opus "De Humani Corporis Fabrica, 1543" in which an ornate wood cutting depicts a group of cherubs performing a tracheostomy on a sow. Vesalius is credited with popularizing the notion that resuscitation is possible when he introduced a reed into a dying animal's trachea and through the intermittent application of positive pressure ventilation, successfully restored its heartbeat (4). In *Fabrica*, he wrote: "But that life may be restored to the animal, an opening must be attempted in the trunk of the trachea, into which a tube of reed or cane should be put; you will then blow into this, so that the lung may rise again and take air."

In 1530, Paracelsus (1493–1541) experimented with lung function using a fire bellows connected to a tube inserted in a patient's mouth as a ventilation device (4). Interestingly, William Harvey (1578–1657) solved the riddle of the circulation, but never went on to clearly speculate on the importance of respiration. Harvey did, however, cite references from Galen and others that addressed respiration in the incomplete and inaccurate fashion that was understood at the time.

Robert Hooke (1635–1703) became interested in establishing the cause of death that results when the thorax is opened to atmospheric air (5). He experimented with dogs and found that he was able to sustain an animal's life by using a fire bellows connected to an opening in the trachea. Hooke presented his results to the Royal Society of England in 1667. However, his technique would not be applied to human surgery until nearly two centuries later (5).

In 1744, John Fothergill of England reported a successful incident of mouth-to-mouth resuscitation. In 1767, the Dutch formed the "Society for the Rescue of Drowned Persons" later known as the "Human Society" (also see Volume 1, Chapter 1). One of the more progressive techniques was to keep the victim warm, give mouth-to-mouth breathing, and compress the chest and stomach to assist exhalation (4). Although there was no apparent focus or intention to increase inhalation, these maneuvers did have this effect.

In 1775, John Hunter of London developed a double bellows system for resuscitation: one for blowing air in and the second for drawing the "bad air" out. He also recommended the use of finger pressure over the larynx to help prevent gastric inflation with air. This maneuver predated the description attributed to Sellick (6) by 200 years. This technique was adapted for patient use by the Royal Humane Society in 1782.

In 1911, Dräger designed an artificial breathing device that fire and police units used for resuscitation. The Dräger "Pulmotor" held the head of the victim in the head-tilt position. Pressure by the operator on the cricoid cartilage (as described by John Hunter) helped prevent gastric inflation (4).

From the mid-1800s to the early 1900s, an incredible number of ventilator assist devices were invented that applied negative pressure (pressure below ambient) around the body (7). Cuirass is a French word, which was used to describe the part of a suit of armor that covered the front of the chest. It has also come to mean a type of negative pressure ventilator that covers the anterior thorax and sometimes the abdomen as well. In Austria, Hungary, and the United States, Ignez von Hauke (1874), Rodolf Eisenmenger (1901), and Alexander Graham Bell (1882), respectively, constructed various early models of chest cuirass-negative pressure ventilators. The first really successful negative pressure ventilator was designed in 1928 by Engineer Philip Drinker, physiologist Louis Agassiz Shaw, and Dr. Charles F. McKhann at the Department of Ventilation, Illumination, and Physiology of the Harvard Medical School (8).

The use of endotracheal intubation and MV in the operating room (OR) was used sparingly after the introduction by Jackson, but accelerated after 1934 when Gudel (9) popularized the use of a cuffed endotracheal tube (ETT) (see Volume 1, Chapter 1) and controlled ventilation during anesthesia, facilitating operations on the upper abdomen and also making possible open chest thoracic procedures. But the skills of anesthesiologists in providing positive pressure ventilation via tracheostomy or translaryngeal intubation were virtually unknown outside the walls of the OR. The tank respirator ("iron lung") or cuirass respirator were the only ventilators available for use on patients with respiratory failure due to polio. Other patients with respiratory failure severe enough to require intubation and MV simply did not survive.

The Copenhagen polio epidemic of 1952 provided the setting for the union for the expertise of anesthesiologists (with their knowledge of cardiopulmonary physiology) and the need for widespread MV. This need served as the birth of the specialty of critical care medicine.

From August to December of 1952, over 2200 patients with the documented diagnosis of polio (345 with respiratory failure) were admitted to the Blegdam Infectious Disease Hospital in Copenhagen. At the beginning of the epidemic, only one tank respirator and six cuirass respirators were available at this hospital. After 27 of the first 31 patients with respiratory failure died, Dr. H.C.A. Lassen (chief physician of Blegdam Hospital) asked an anesthesiologist, Dr. Bjorn Ibsen, for consultation to determine whether positive pressure ventilation used during anesthesia might be of benefit (10).

Almost overnight, the management of choice for polio became tracheostomy with cuffed ETT and manual ventilation using an anesthesia bag and a to-and-fro system fitted with a CO_2 absorber. At the height of the epidemic, the medical schools in Copenhagen were closed and up to 250 medical students took daily shifts to hand ventilate the tracheotomized polio victims. At the end of the epidemic, valved systems without CO_2 absorbers were employed and a number of manufacturers modified their OR ventilator machines (previously only used in surgery) for use as long-term positive pressure ventilators.

Several North American anesthesiologists visited Denmark during the epidemic and news of the Copenhagen experience spread rapidly. It was soon recognized that the techniques used to treat the polio victims could be applied to respiratory failure due to other ailments (drug overdose, tetanus, myasthenia gravis, etc.). This recognition led to the opening of the first respiratory intensive care units (ICUs). Subsequently, surgical intensive care units (SICUs) developed as a natural progression for patients who were ventilated postoperatively in the recovery room. Ventilating patients outside of the OR for prolonged periods, for other processes began as well (e.g., pulmonary contusions, various traumatic injuries) which caused a paradigm shift in thinking. All of these factors served as the impetus to create the first respiratory ICUs.

The founding fathers of critical care medicine in North America were these same anesthesiologists who spread the lessons learned from the Copenhagen experience, and who were attending in large teaching programs. Indeed, several well-known anesthesiologist-intensivists opened the first ICUs in North America including Safer (11) in Baltimore, Fairley (12) in Toronto (later at San Francisco General Hospital and Stanford), and Pontoppidan and Bendixen (13) at Massachussets General Hospital, then at UCSD (later at Columbia).

Dr. Bendixen was recruited to UCSD in 1969 to run the newly established department of anesthesiology. He in turn was responsible for the recruitment of pulmonary physiologists Eric Wahrenbrock, Jonathan Benumof, along with past editor of *Anesthesiology*, Larry Saidman, to the department of anesthesiology at UCSD.

These pioneering respiratory physiologists collaborated with others at UCSD, such as John B. West and Peter D. Wagner, to shape the thinking about both the research and the teaching of pulmonary physiology for decades to come. Since then, many leaders in pulmonary physiology, airway management, and MV have contributed new ventilator modes and strategies for patient care. These investigators continue to push the threshold of knowledge forward. The fruit of their labors are reviewed in this chapter.

INDICATIONS FOR MECHANICAL VENTILATION

Indications for MV are distinct from indications for intubation (see Volume 2, Chapter 9). The two most basic

Table 1 Indications for Mechanical Ventilation

Hypoxic respiratory failure	Hypercapnic respiratory failure
Low F$_I$O$_2$ (i.e., high altitude)	Spinal injury, denervation injury (i.e., spinal cord transection, phrenic nerve injury)
Hypoventilation (i.e., flail chest, opioids)	Respiratory center depressants (i.e., opioids, anesthetics, CNS injury)
$\dot{V}_A/\dot{Q}_t$ mismatch (i.e., hypovolemia, hyperinflation)	Neuromuscular disease (i.e., myasthenia gravis)
Shunt R → L ($\dot{Q}_s/\dot{Q}_t$) (i.e., pneumothorax, pulmonary contusion)	Myopathy (i.e., critical illness myopathy)
Diffusion abnormality (i.e., ARDS, pulmonary edema)	Pleural cavity (i.e., hemothorax, pleural effusion)
Anemia (i.e., hemorrhage)	Abdominal compression (i.e., ascites, surgical packing)
Low cardiac output (i.e., ischemia, tamponade)	COPD (i.e., COPD exacerbation, status asthmaticus)
Histocytic hypoxia (i.e., cyanide poisoning)	Chest wall (i.e., flail chest, splinting)

Abbreviations: ARDS, acute respiratory distress syndrome; CNS, central nervous system; COPD, chronic obstructive pulmonary disease; F$_I$O$_2$, fraction of inhaled gas due to oxygen; $\dot{Q}_s/\dot{Q}_t$, transpulmonary shunt/total cardiac output; R → L, right to left.

indications for MV include (*i*) conditions where the patient is unable to oxygenate the blood without a very high F$_I$O$_2$ and/or elevated continuous positive airway pressure (CPAP), and (*ii*) conditions where the patient is unable to do the work of breathing without MV (Table 1) (11–14).

VENTILATOR TYPES

☞ **Ventilators can be categorized into two major types: (*i*) negative pressure, and (*ii*) positive pressure ventilators.** ☞ This section reviews the differences between positive and negative pressure ventilators.

Negative Pressure

Negative pressure ventilators, such as the "iron lung" or the chest cuirass, were known since the turn of the last century. The operational mechanism of negative pressure ventilators involves the development of negative extrathoracic pressure, which expands the chest wall and in so doing, initiates flow of gas into the lungs. Exhalation occurs when the pressure inside the iron lung increases, transmitting positive pressure to the external chest and abdomen.

This technology is suitable for patients who are unable to breathe due to skeletal muscle paralysis or weakness, but possess otherwise normal lung parenchyma and function. In this situation, when the lung parenchyma and airways are essentially normal and chest wall compliance is normal, iron lung ventilation is satisfactory. However, negative pressure ventilation has the following disadvantages compared to positive pressure ventilation: (*i*) airway protection

relies solely on the patient's reflexes; (*ii*) when the lungs and chest wall are noncompliant, massive pressures are required to promote airflow; (*iii*) in the iron lung and the cuirass, there is impaired access to the patient for hygiene, examination, or resuscitation purposes.

Despite these distinct disadvantages, negative pressure ventilation via the iron lung continues to be a successful ventilation modality for patients with poliomyelitis and less commonly for chronic obstructive pulmonary disease (COPD) patients (14,15).

The cuirass functions in a fashion similar to the iron lung, but is physically less bulky and more portable. Negative pressure ventilation using a body cuirass is uncommon today. However, this mode of ventilation has been successfully used in the OR, where the airway is part of the surgical field, as occurs during bronchoscopies (16,17). Negative pressure ventilators became aggressively developed and widely distributed to support polio victims during the pandemics of the 1940s and 1950s.

Positive Pressure

Although negative pressure devices (described earlier) were the first widely applied apparatus for MV, their limitations along with progress in anesthetic techniques led to the development of improved airway and ventilatory control in the OR, the recovery room, and into modern SICUs. Instrumental in this progress was the introduction of the laryngoscope in 1913 by Jackson and, in 1943, Gudel (9) introduced the cuffed ETT. These tubes featured a high pressure–low volume cuff, which caused tracheal mucosal ischemic problems during long-term placement. Cuffs with a higher volume and low pressure (high compliance) replaced the original tubes in the 1970s. Nonetheless, these devices ushered in the use of positive pressure ventilators (described in the remainder of this chapter).

Intubation of the trachea can be accomplished using a variety of routes and techniques as described in Volume 1, Chapter 9. The standard intubation in the OR or ICU consists of an ETT, inserted into the trachea via the mouth or nose. Other possibilities include percutaneous cricothyroidotomy or tracheotomy, mainly used in emergency situations or for prolonged intubations.

Placement of a cuffed ETT protects the airway from major aspirations, although ETT cuffs do not reliably prevent subglottic fluid from passing to the tracheobronchial tree. Microaspiration, which occurs along the longitudinal folds within the wall of an inflated cuff, is directly linked to VAP (18). A recent study showed a reduced incidence of aspiration when the cuff was lubricated with gel (19). In a small number of tracheostomy patients, the protection lasted for a mean duration of 42 hours (19).

Once a cuffed tube seals the trachea, a closed system is made of the lungs, breathing circuit, and the ventilator. In this situation, it is possible to apply positive airway pressures to the airway without inflating the stomach. Changes in flow and/or pressure generated by the patient can be easily detected by the ventilator sensors in such a closed system.

FOUR PHASES OF MECHANICAL VENTILATION

☞ **Mechanically ventilated breaths can be divided into four distinct phases to best understand the changes that occur in pressure, flow, and volume of the inhaled and** exhaled gases. ☞ The terminology used in this chapter is that most consistently used in clinical medicine today, initially adopted at a 1992 consensus conference on MV (Fig. 1) (20).

Phase 1 (trigger phase) is defined as the changeover from exhalation to inhalation, and phase 2 (inhalation phase) is the period when gas flows into the lungs increasing both alveolar pressure and lung volume. Phase 3 (cycle phase) is the changeover from inhalation to exhalation, and phase 4 (exhalation phase) extends between phase 3 until the next breath occurs. In most modes of MV, gas exits the lungs passively during phase 4. Understanding these four phases and how they are manipulated is fundamental to comprehending the mechanisms used in modern ventilations. Each of these phases will be further characterized below using a pressure versus time graphic, useful in describing these four phases (Fig. 1).

Phase 1, "Trigger Phase" (Changeover from Exhalation to Inhalation)

☞ The "trigger phase" refers to a point in time (P1 in Fig. 1) when the ventilator initiates the positive pressure breath (changes over from exhalation to inhalation). ☞ The mechanism used by the ventilator to trigger a machine-generated

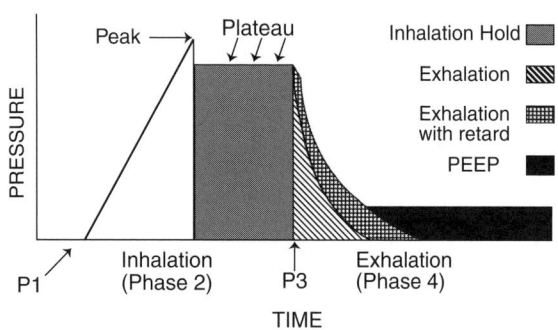

Figure 1 Phases of mechanical ventilation. Phase 1 (P1) "trigger phase" is the changeover from exhalation to inhalation. The trigger phase is just a point in time (P1) when the machine initiates the positive pressure breath. The jargon used to describe the trigger phase also commonly referred to as the "mode of ventilation" [i.e., synchronized intermittent mandatory ventilation (SIMV), assist- controlled, etc.]. The ventilator can be triggered by the patient in the SIMV or assist controlled mode, whereas the breath is triggered by a timer circuit in the controlled mode or during the machine-initiated portions of the assist control and SIMV breaths. The variable that triggers the ventilator to deliver a patient initiated breath include: (*i*) a sensed pressure drop in the system (pressure sensitivity) or (*ii*) a sensed change in flow (flow-by sensitivity), whereas machine-triggered breaths are initiated by a timer. Phase 2 is the "inhalation phase." This is the period of time extending between the initiation of inhalation to the start of exhalation (i.e., between P1 and P3). During the inhalation phase, most ventilators will control either flow (volume-controlled) or pressure (pressure-controlled). Phase 3 (P3) "cycle phase" is the changeover from inhalation to exhalation. In short, how the ventilator decides to end the breath and cycle into exhalation. The cycle phase is just a point in time (P3). This changeover can be pressure cycled, time cycled, volume cycled, or flow cycled. Phase 4 is the "exhalation phase," is generally passive but can be influenced by positive end-expiratory pressure (PEEP) or by the placement of a retarding mechanism.

breath can either be patient triggered (where the ventilator senses a negative inspiratory pressure or flow profile) or time triggered (where the ventilator delivers breaths at a rate set by the clinician). Ventilator terms that describe the trigger phase of the mechanical ventilatory cycle include: (*i*) controlled mechanical ventilation (CMV), (*ii*) assist control (A/C), (*iii*) synchronized intermittent mandatory ventilation (SIMV), and so on. These conventional modes of triggering MV are shown diagrammatically in Figure 2, and are discussed in detail below.

Controlled Mechanical Ventilation

When inhalation is triggered by a computer-generated signal from a respiratory rate timing mechanism, it is referred to as CMV (Fig. 3). This is the trigger methodology used on most OR ventilators. ICU ventilators with

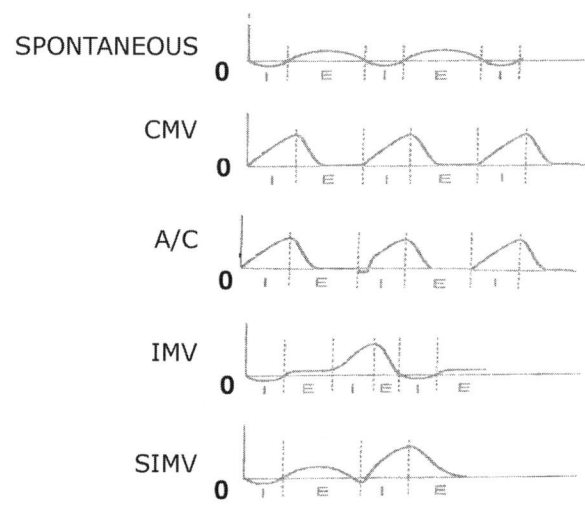

Figure 2 The conventional modes of mechanical ventilation (MV) are shown in this figure with a series of pressure versus time graphs. Note that with spontaneous ventilation, airway pressure is negative during inhalation and positive during exhalation, whereas in the controlled mechanical ventilation (CMV) mode, airway pressure is positive during inhalation and exhalation, beginning and ending at zero (also see Fig. 3). The patient will only receive the set number of breaths in the CMV mode, and cannot trigger additional breaths. If positive end expiratory pressure were applied, the end-exhalation pressure would be positive in each of these modes. In the assist control (A/C) mode of MV, the machine provides a certain number of positive pressure breaths (number set by the clinician); however, the patient can trigger the ventilator to provide additional breaths by making a negative inspiratory pressure effort. In the intermittent mandatory ventilation (IMV) mode the machine will provide a certain number of positive pressure breaths (number set by the clinician). However, in contrast to A/C, if the patient cares to take any additional breaths s/he must do all the work of breathing. In the standard (non-synchronized) IMV mode, the ventilator can trigger a machine breath when the patient does not want one, and cause ventilator-patient dyssynchrony. In the synchronized IMV mode (SIMV), the machine-delivered breaths are synchronized with the patient's intrinsic ventilatory efforts, thus markedly minimizing patient-ventilator dyssynchrony.

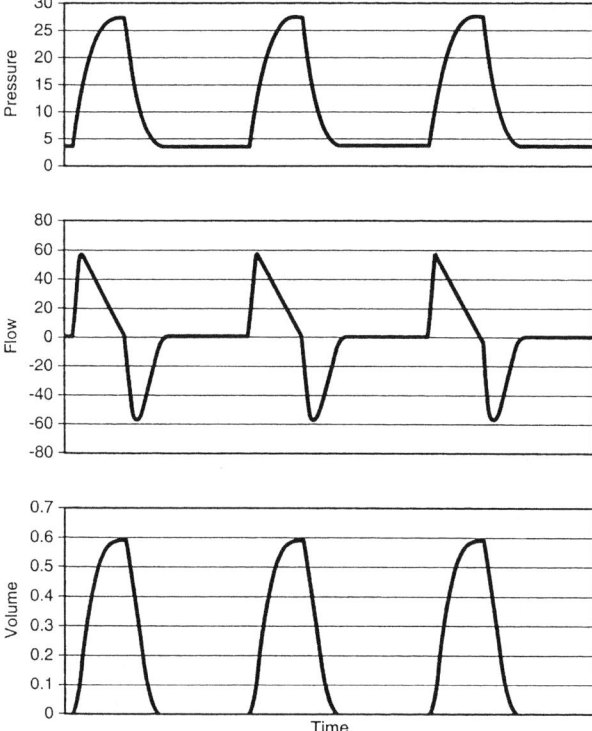

Figure 3 Controlled mechanical ventilation (CMV). Pressure, flow, and volume versus time during volume-controlled CMV mode. *Source*: From Ref. 150, p. 58.

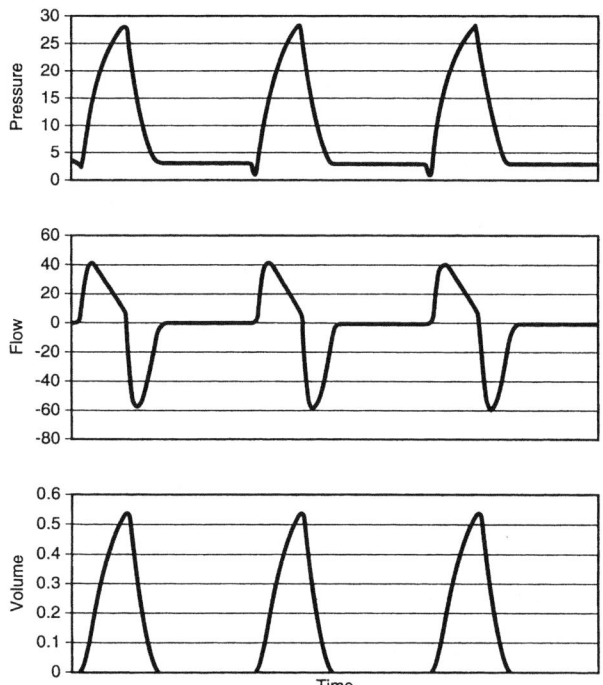

Figure 4 Assist control ventilation (A/C). Pressure, flow, and volume versus time during volume-controlled AC ventilation. *Source*: From Ref. 150, p. 60.

automatic timing mechanisms, called controllers, can also trigger the inhalation phase on the ventilator. In the control mode, the patient will receive the set rate of mandatory positive pressure breaths, regardless of his/her own respiratory efforts. This feature is satisfactory for deeply sedated or anesthetized patients and essential in caring for patients without any ventilatory drive of their own. However, patients capable of triggering some breaths on their own can become extremely agitated if maintained on CMV mode. This is because in the pure CMV mode, patients are "locked out" of initiating inhalation. However, the true CMV mode as described here is only available on older ICU ventilators and on anesthesia machines. No modern-day ICU ventilators are solely controllers, hence, all currently produced ventilators have escape mechanisms so that patients can receive some ventilatory support in response to their efforts.

Assist Control
Ventilator devices that trigger a machine delivered breath in response to patient-initiated ventilatory efforts are called assistors. In the A/C mode, the patient may initiate a machine-delivered breath as frequently as he/she would like, merely by making minimal ventilatory effort which is immediately sensed by the machine as a negative inspiratory pressure or flow change (depending upon the trigger sensing mode employed) (Fig. 4). The A/C mode allows the patient to increase their minute ventilation by triggering additional breaths at a rate higher than set. However, if the patient on the A/C mode becomes heavily sedated or anesthetized and does not trigger any breaths of her/his own, s/he will only receive the baseline number of breaths set by the rate control. In this situation, A/C is

indistinguishable from the CMV mode. Later, when the patient recovers from deep sedation or anesthesia and begins to seek additional breaths, full machine-delivered breaths can be triggered by the patient's efforts, when ventilated using the A/C mode.

Synchronized Intermittent Mandatory Ventilation
The intermittent mandatory ventilation (IMV) mode was initially developed as a weaning tool. In the IMV mode, the patient will receive a preset number of machine-delivered breaths but is allowed unrestricted ability for spontaneous breathing (although with increased work, as the patient does not get any assistance for the spontaneous breaths taken above the background set rate). The rudimentary IMV mode is problematic because the machine can deliver a controlled breath just after the patient has taken thier own spontaneous, nonassisted breath. Thus, stacking of breaths can occur resulting in barotrauma/volutrauma and patient distress from patient-ventilator dyssynchrony.

Because of these considerations, SIMV was developed (Fig. 5). The SIMV mode allows the ventilator to sense when the patient takes a non-machine-aided breath and will space the preset machine-assisted breaths so as not to stack breaths. If the patient on SIMV becomes sedated or anesthetized, then s/he will only receive the number of breaths programmed into the machine. However, once the patient begins to take additional breaths, they must perform all of the work required to achieve the supplemental breaths. The baseline pressure waveforms generated when patients fail to trigger additional SIMV or A/C breaths are indistinguishable from those occurring with the CMV mode.

Phase 2, "Inhalation Phase"
↗ The inhalation phase is characterized as that period of time when gas is flowing into the lungs, as well as that time when

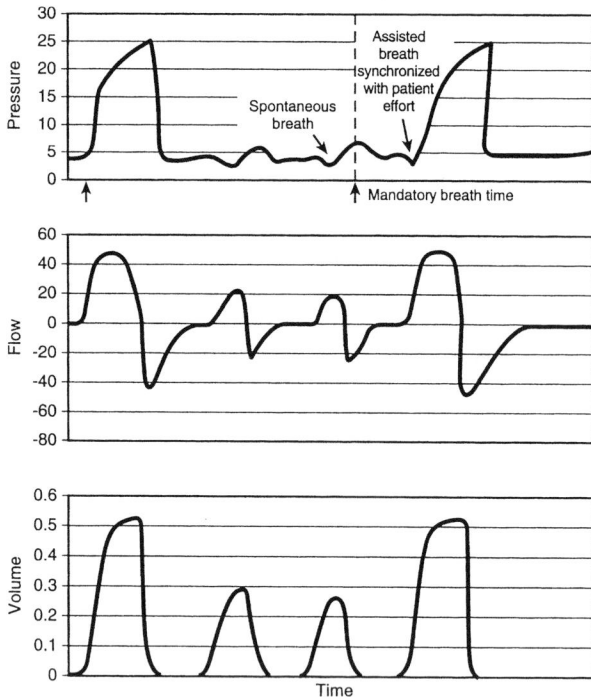

Figure 5 Synchronized intermittent mandatory ventilation (SIMV). Pressure, volume, and flow versus time waveforms during SIMV ventilation. The first breath is a machine time-triggered breath. At the *second arrow*, the patient is exhaling after a spontaneous breath. At this time, the mandatory (assisted) breath is synchronized with the patient's spontaneous exhalation. The *bottom arrow* indicates the mandatory breath time based on set respiratory frequency. *Source*: From Ref. 150, p. 63.

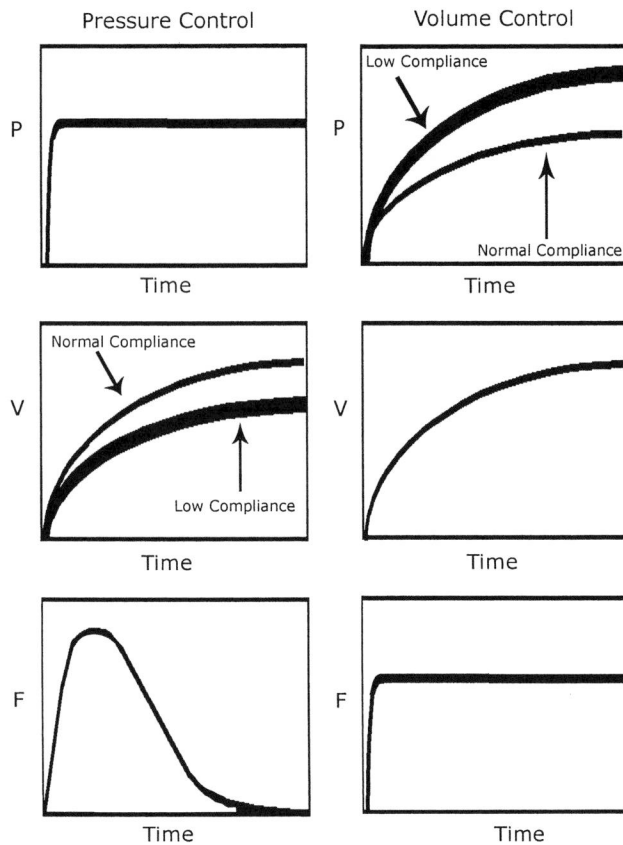

Figure 6 Pressure control and volume control ventilation differences, showing the pressure, volume, and flow versus time waveform profiles. *Abbreviations*: F, flow; P, pressure; V, volume.

already delivered gas remains in the lungs (i.e., until the ventilator cycles into exhilaration). ↗ As gas flows into the lungs, ventilators use one of two basic mechanisms to control the physical characteristics of pressure, flow, and volume (volume control and pressure control). These two major types of control systems characterize the active (gas flow) portion of the inhalation phase. The differences between volume control and pressure control are shown graphically in Figure 6 and are summarized in Table 2.

Volume Control (Set Volume with Constant Flow Generation)

The volume set/flow-controlled ventilators maintain a constant preset volume with every machine-delivered breath, whereas the flow rate is constant, and the pressure required to attain this volume will increase until the preset volume is delivered (Fig. 6, right side panel). The advantage of a volume set/flow-controlled ventilator is that a constant volume will be delivered with each machine-generated breath regardless of changing airway resistance or

Table 2 Volume Control Versus Pressure Control Breaths

Variable	Volume control breath	Pressure control breath
Tidal volume	Set by clinician; remains constant	Variable with changes in patient effort and respiratory system impedance
Peak inspiratory pressure	Variable with changes in patient effort and respiratory system impedance	Set by clinician; remains constant
Inspiratory time	Set directly or as a function of respiratory frequency and inspiratory flow settings	Set by clinician; remains constant
Inspiratory flow	Set directly or as a function of respiratory frequency and inspiratory flow settings	Variable with changes in patient effort and respiratory system impedance
Inspiratory flow waveform	Set by clinician; remains constant; can use constant, sine, or decelerating flow waveform	Variable with changes in patient effort and respiratory system impedance; flow waveform always decelerating

compliance (as can occur in a patient with bronchospasm, a kinked ETT, the acute development of a pneumothorax, or decreased pulmonary compliance). This is why most ventilators in current usage are volume set/flow-controlled ventilators. Of course, if the set high-pressure limit is reached during the delivery of a volume set flow-controlled breath, inhalation will terminate on some ventilators and the set volume will not be delivered. If undetected, this could result in under-ventilation, however, alarms should alert the clinicians of this occurrence so that the problem can be rectified.

Volume control is often considered the conventional mode of controlling the pressure, volume, and flow of gas during the inhalation phase. It is also somewhat of a misnomer as it is really the flow that is controlled, whereas the volume is fixed. The advantage of the volume control mode is that tidal volume remains stable with changes in compliance or resistance. The disadvantage is that increased peak inhalation pressure occurs as lungs become less compliant or airway resistance increases. The newer variants of volume control provide options for variable flow profiles during the inhalation phase, but Figure 6 describes the classic waveform patterns.

Pressure Control (Constant Pressure)

Pressure control is a mode of controlling the inhalation phase so that pressure remains stable (square wave) throughout inhalation. Typically, flow occurs as a decelerating wave in this mode (Fig. 6, left side panel). The overriding attractive feature in this mode of inhalation control is the fact that pressure remains constant throughout. The downside is that as compliance decreases or resistance increases, the tidal volume delivered to the patient will decrease.

Pressure-controlled ventilators have the pressure maintained at a preset level. Thus, the volume delivered varies depending on the resistance and compliance characteristics of the patient's lungs (Fig. 6). Accordingly, hypoventilation can occur. Therefore, if CO_2 elimination is a major concern, pressure control may not be the optimal choice. If on the other hand, limiting the pressure applied to the airways and alveoli is of particular interest, this ventilator mode guarantees control. This may be the case in lung diseases like acute respiratory distress syndrome (ARDS), where the lung involvement is heterogeneous with the risk of damaging healthy areas.

In addition, patient-ventilator synchrony can be achieved easier with pressure control compared to the volume control mode (21). Another small study showed that pressure control ventilation tends to require a lower work of breathing than the volume control mode (22).

Phase 3, "Cycle" (Changeover from Inhalation to Exhalation)

☞ The cycle phase represents the changeover from inhalation to exhalation. ☞ The ventilator can cycle into exhalation via a number of mechanisms (pressure, time, volume or flow). Pressure-cycled ventilators terminate inhalation when a preset pressure is reached in the ventilator circuit, regardless of what tidal volume has been delivered. This is the way the old-fashioned intermittent positive pressure breathing (IPPB) ventilators used to work; and, because of this variable volume delivery, it is a rarely used mode today. In contrast, time-cycled ventilators will continue in the inhalation phase for a preset time interval. Most commonly, a set volume is delivered, then a passive inhalation hold period will occur

until the preset time elapses, at which time the ventilator cycles into exhalation. The time until exhalation in this mode is dependent upon respiratory rate and the set I:E ratio. This is the method of cycling used in the pressure-controlled, inverse ratio mode of ventilation, and on OR ventilators.

☞ **Volume-cycled ventilators terminate inhalation after a preselected volume has been delivered to the patient.** ☞ Volume-cycled ventilators are most commonly employed for phase 3. However, decreased patient's lung or chest wall compliance or increased airway resistance will decrease the amount of volume delivered to the patient's airways. Flow-cycled ventilators terminate inhalation when a preselected flow is reached (this is the method of cycling used in the pressure support mode of MV).

Phase 4, "Exhalation Phase"

☞ **The exhalation phase is the time period when the previously inhaled gas is exhausted, and is generally passive (i.e., occurs by natural recoil if elastic forces in lung and in chest wall).** ☞ However, early prototypes of positive pressure ventilators applied a negative pressure (suction) during exhalation called negative end-exhalation pressure. This feature has been abandoned on all modern ventilators due to the propensity to decrease functional residual capacity (FRC), cause atelectasis, and increase right-to-left transpulmonary shunt. Modern day oscillator ventilators actually provide a "to and fro" function during ventilation. However, this occurs on top of a standing wave of pressure.

Positive End Expiratory Pressure

Whenever the pressure in the airways at end-exhalation is greater than ambient, this is referred to as positive end expiratory pressure (PEEP). The application of PEEP increases the FRC—the lung volume at end-exhalation during normal tidal breathing. Increasing FRC recruits alveoli during inhalation and prevents closure of airways at end-exhalation thus increasing the number of lung units participating in gas exchange. Prevention of airway closure and recruitment of alveoli improves the ventilation-perfusion relationships, reverses atelectasis, and thus decreases right-to-left transpulmonary shunt (23–26). ☞ **Although the application of PEEP will decrease shunt, it can also increase alveolar dead space, particularly in West's zone 1 regions.** ☞ West's zone 1 is the portion of the lung in which the intra-alveolar pressure exceeds the arterial pressure ($P_A > P_a$); these are high $\dot{V}/\dot{Q}$ regions. Furthermore, the application of PEEP can reduce cardiac output ($\dot{Q}$) (27). This can occur through several mechanisms including a decrease in venous return (28,29), an increase in pulmonary vascular resistance (30), right ventricular dysfunction (30), leftward displacement of the intraventricular septum (31), and decreased transmural ventricular filling pressures.

Through these mechanisms, the application of excessive PEEP can actually worsen the delivery of oxygen ($\dot{D}O_2$) to the body tissues, since $\dot{Q}$ is a major determinant:

$$\dot{D}O_2 = \dot{Q} \times 1.34 \, [Hb] \times SaO_2 + 0.003 \times PaO_2$$

The net effect of PEEP on $\dot{D}O_2$ depends on the relative changes on both the increase in SaO_2 and the decrease in $\dot{Q}$.

The end point of PEEP application should be the lowest level of PEEP that allows an adequate PaO_2 with an F_1O_2 of 0.5 or less. Some have called this the "best PEEP"

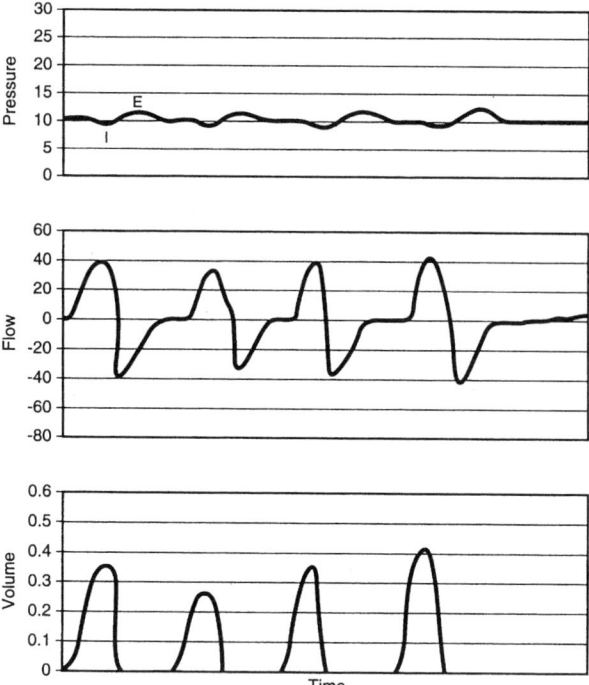

Figure 7 Continuous positive airway pressure (CPAP). Pressure, flow, and volume versus time during CPAP. *Abbreviations*: E, exhalation; I, inhalation. *Source*: From Ref. 150, p. 69.

(32). An "adequate PaO_2" is approximately 60 mm of mercury. A PaO_2 of 60 mmHg is just above the steep part of the oxyhemoglobin dissociation curve. In other words, an increase in PaO_2 will not correlate with an improvement in $\dot{D}O_2$, when the mechanisms used to increase the PaO_2 decrease $\dot{Q}$ too much. Also, the ideal level of PEEP should cause the least amount of hemodynamic change when increasing oxygenation. Therefore, $\dot{Q}$ and $\dot{D}O_2$ should be monitored when high (>10 cm H_2O) PEEP levels are used.

Continuous Positive Airway Pressure

In continuous positive airway pressure (CPAP) breathing both the inspiratory and expiratory limbs of the ventilator are pressurized to a set level (frequently 5 cm H_2O) (Fig. 7) (33). The patient provides all of the ventilatory work. The mean airway pressure (mPaw) is increased but, if effective, the work of breathing can be less and oxygenation improved because of recruitment of previously atelectatic alveoli. For the temporary prevention of upper airway closure at night in patients with obstructive sleep apnea, CPAP delivered via nasal mask is widely used.

Bilevel Positive Airway Pressure

Bilevel positive airway pressure (BiPAP) ventilatory support system is used in spontaneously breathing patients (34). As the name bilevel implies, two different levels of pressure flow, inspiratory and expiratory positive airway pressure (IPAP and EPAP), can be chosen to support the patient's ventilation. The upper (inspiratory) and lower (expiratory) pressures are set by the clinician. The gradient between the EPAP and IPAP levels determines the degree of tidal volume augmentation, or pressure support. The patient determines the time that the higher and lower airway

pressures are applied by their spontaneous respiratory cycle. BiPAP can be administered noninvasively utilizing various types of masks; however, some devises are also approved for use with intubated patients (34,35).

SUPPORT MODES
Pressure Support

Pressure support ventilation is a pressure-triggered and flow-cycled mode of ventilatory support. The trigger mechanism of pressure support ventilation is similar to the A/C mode because both trigger on when a negative pressure (or decreased flow in some models) is sensed. The inhalation phase is similar to pressure control (square wave pressure, decelerating flow). However, the method of cycling into exhalation is unique for pressure support (using flow rate to determine exhalation point).

In pressure support ventilation, flow is delivered to the patient until the inspiratory flow decreases below a preset value (such as 25% below the peak inspiratory flow). Thus, the delivered tidal volume will depend on the resistance and compliance of the lungs and chest wall.

The inspiratory pressure is maintained by a computer-controlled servomechanism in the ventilator that continually adjusts the inspiratory flow to maintain the desired pressure. Therefore, there is a square wave pressure and decelerating flow pattern with each machine-delivered breath. Most of the newer ICU ventilators are capable of providing the pressure support mode of ventilation. ☞ **Pressure support ventilation can be used as the sole method of ventilation or, more frequently, as a method to support weaning.** ☞

As the level of pressure support is decreased, more patient effort is required to maintain the minute ventilation. This makes pressure support ventilation a suitable ventilation setting for weaning from MV (36). With pressure support weaning, the level of pressure support is decreased as tolerated by the patient. Pressure support has shown to be well tolerated in COPD patients (37,38), and can be used as a noninvasive method in these patients (e.g.) BiPAP (39).

Volume Support

As pressure support provides a constant level of positive pressure during the inhalation phase of every spontaneous breath, volume support provides variable levels of positive pressure for a constant, preset tidal volume (40). Using a closed-loop control system, ventilators adapt the level of inspiratory pressure support required to deliver the volume, despite changes in the patient's inspiratory effort or the compliance and resistance characteristics of the lungs. The triggering mechanism is the same as pressure support (pressure-triggered), but phase 3 occurs once the inspiratory flow decreases to 5% of the peak flow. Volume support is thought to be a potential automated ventilator weaning approach (41).

VENTILATOR-INDUCED LUNG INJURY
Evidence for Ventilator-Induced Lung Injury

Positive pressure ventilation was first linked to damage of the lung, in as early as the 1940s, where a study by Macklin and Macklin (42) showed interstitial emphysema of lungs and the mediastinum, which the authors linked to alveolar rupture caused by critically high-pressure gradient between alveolus and surrounding interstitium.

In 1974, Webb and Tierney (43) first showed positive pressure-induced lung damage in the form of edema, hyaline membrane formation, and hemorrhage, similar to the findings in ARDS. Other studies demonstrated complications like bacterial translocation from the respiratory tract (44) or an increase in circulating cytokines (45) from positive pressure ventilation in ARDS patients.

Other mechanisms found to cause lung damage and possibly contribute to ventilator-induced lung injury (VILI) include surfactant depletion and ventilation at low-end-expiratory lung volumes (46).

VOLUTRAUMA VS. BAROTRAUMA CONTROVERSY
Evidence for Barotrauma

For lung pathologies caused by the presence of extra-alveolar air in abnormal locations like pneumothorax, pneumomediastinum, pneumopericardium, pulmonary interstitial air, pneumatoceles, and venous air emboli, both terms barotrauma and volutrauma can be found in the literature. These complications affect 4% to 15% of all mechanically ventilated patients, however, more common in patients with ARDS, status asthmaticus, and aspiration pneumonia (47). Several studies looked for whether the predominant factor for VILI was excessive volume or pressure (48,49).

A relationship between high peak inspiratory pressures (PIP) and barotrauma has been suggested by findings in some studies (49–51), whereas others found poor correlation (52–54). There are also studies that found an inverse relationship between PIP and barotrauma, showing a lower incidence of barotrauma in the study groups with higher PIP (55–57). A similar controversy can be found in reviewing the literature for correlations of PEEP and barotrauma (54,55,58). The role of PEEP in lung protective ventilation strategies will be reviewed later.

☞ **One explanation for the confounding relationship between PIP and barotrauma is that the actual pressure applied at the alveolus is lower than that measured at the ventilator tubing, and it is the pressure distending the alveolus that is most injurious.** ☞

Evidence for Volutrauma

Abundant animal and human data now exists supporting the concept of volutrauma (59–61). Studies in dogs, rabbits (60), and rats (61) showed induction of volutrauma by high inflation pressures during MV. This could be prevented by drastically reducing the lung compliance by strapping or banding of the thorax and/or the abdomen.

The amount of lung distension is dependent on the transalveolar pressure rather than airway pressure. Transalveolar pressure is the difference between airway pressure and intrapleural pressure. For a normal pleural pressure (0 mmHg), depending on the moment in the respiratory cycle, the transpulmonary pressure needed to achieve vital lung capacity is around 35–40 mmHg.

Thus for patients with normal compliant lungs, the pressure limit during MV should be set at 35–40 mmHg to avoid volutrauma. Higher alveolar pressures may not cause volutrauma in situations where there is reduced chest wall or abdominal compliance, resulting in transpulmonary pressures below potential harmful values (62).

LUNG PROTECTIVE VENTILATION STRATEGY: DEFINED
Different Approaches

After it was established that MV could prolong or cause lung injury, a significant effort has been expended in searching out ventilation strategies that minimize stress on the lung.

Variations of PIP, PEEP levels, tidal volumes (VTs), and the use of HFV and inverse I:E ratio ventilation are several of the most commonly employed strategies that have been examined to determine their impact on VILI. Most of these studies use acute lung injury (ALI)/ARDS models or patients, since these pathologies are most prone to lung injury. In these syndromes, the lung is affected in a patchy, heterogeneous matter, leaving some areas densely consolidated, and others virtually normal. This leads to decreased surfactant function, diffuse atelectasis and alveolar consolidation and flooding (63).

Traditionally, the goal of MV had been to keep the $PaCO_2$ in a physiologic normal range and to apply adequate oxygenation using tidal volumes of 10–15 mL/kg to achieve this. In lungs with pathologies like ARDS, this often results in very high PIP. The recognition that this ventilation regimen can injure the already damaged lung further, led to an approach of using reduced tidal volumes and a pressure limit.

Hickling and Henderson (64) showed that the use of a tidal volume of 5 mL/kg and a PIP of less than 30 cm H_2O was associated with a reduced mortality rate among subjects with ARDS. Three large multicenter, randomized clinical trials followed, and failed to show a decrease in mortality by using low tidal volumes in the study group compared to a group with traditional higher tidal volumes (62,65,66).

National Institutes of Health–National Heart, Blood, and Lung Institute Study: First Investigation to Show Decreased Mortality with a Mode of Ventilation

☞ **The first trial showing a decrease in mortality for a low tidal volume strategy compared with traditional, higher tidal volumes was conducted by the National Institutes of Health–National Heart, Blood, and Lung Institute ARDS Network Study (67).** ☞ In this multicenter, randomized clinical trial, a total of 861 patients were assigned to either a starting tidal volume of 12 mL/kg predicted body weight (traditional) or 6 mL/kg (low tidal volume group). Ventilation had to be established no later than 36 hours after ALI criteria were met. Adjustments to lower tidal volumes were made in both groups if needed to avoid excessive end inspiratory plateau pressures.

The mortality rate in the traditional tidal volume group was 40% compared with only 31% in the low tidal volume group. The low tidal volume group had statistically significant more ventilator-free days and more days without nonpulmonary organ failures. Explanation as to why this study could demonstrate an outcome difference, where previous studies failed, may include the larger study population. Another reason could be the larger differences in tidal volume between groups as compared to some of the previous studies.

Open Lung Approach

In addition to high tidal volumes and lung stretch causing VILI, ventilator patterns promoting increased amounts of atelectasis have been shown to be harmful. Mechanical forces that occur in small bronchioles and alveoli that repeatedly

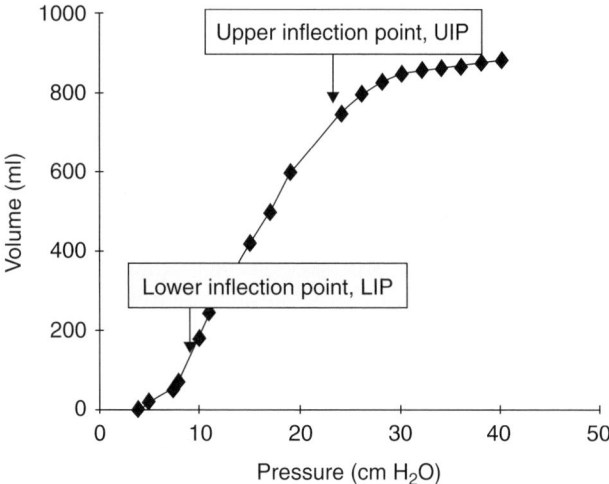

Figure 8   Static pressure–volume curve. The lower inflection point defines optimal PEEP level, whereas the upper inflection point defines the maximal lung inflation pressure (end inhalation pressure). *Abbreviations*: LIP, lower inflection point; UIP, upper inflection point. *Source*: From Ref. 151.

snap open and close may play a role in the development of the injury (68). In addition, the region between normal and atelectatic lung may be affected by physical stress (68).

  ⚲ **In the open lung approach, the patient is ventilated between the upper and lower inflection points on the pressure–volume curve.** ⚲ Pressure–volume (P–V), aka "elastance" curves, can be useful in determining the optimal PEEP that prevents atelectasis at end-expiration and does not cause overdistension (Fig. 8) (69). The term "lower inflection point" describes the point on the lower portion of the P–V curve where the flat slope becomes more steep (first knee in the curve). The upper inflection point marks the point where the steep curve becomes flat again (second knee in the curve). The optimal ventilation would theoretically lie in-between those two points in order to avoid atelectasis and overdistension. Studies by Amato et al. (70,71) suggest beneficial outcomes in ARDS patients who were ventilated with a PEEP above the lower inflection point.

  This approach in determining the optimum amount of PEEP has some limitations: First, the P–V curve represents the combined elastance of both lung and chest wall (72). Second, not every static P–V curve shows a clearly distinguished inflection points (69). Also, a single point on the P–V curve does not represent the global events throughout the lung. The determination of a P–V curve is labor intensive and several studies have demonstrated the wide variability in measuring and reporting the upper and lower inflection points.

  Furthermore, the P–V curve shows hysteresis: at each level of airway pressure, volume is greater during deflation than during inflation. Hysteresis can be accounted for by the differences in surface tension and pressures of small bronchioles and alveoli during inflation and deflation (73). So, after initial opening of a lung unit, lower pressures are needed to maintain ventilation. This phenomenon has led to the newly developed interest in intermittent recruitment maneuvers. Overall, it seems that there is no straightforward answer to the question of the ideal amount of PEEP. However, most experienced intensivists agree that the best PEEP is the least PEEP required to maintain an "open lung" strategy during ventilatory support.

NEWER MODES: AIMED AT LUNG PROTECTIVE VENTILATION
Airway Pressure Release Ventilation
Airway pressure release ventilation (APRV) is a newer mode of ventilatory support, which combines CPAP with a release valve on the expiratory limb that can open at end-exhalation. The patient is breathing spontaneously during APRV and this modality can be used either invasively or noninvasively. The putative advantage of this mode of ventilation is less positive pressure transmitted to the cardiovascular system. ARDS patients showed improved cardiopulmonary function and oxygenation in spontaneous breathing patients receiving APRV, compared to similar patients on standard MV (74–76). The benefit may result from improved recruitment of nonventilated lung units. Improved oxygenation with APRV was again shown recently in an animal study on pigs with induced lung injury (77).

Time-Cycled, Pressure-Controlled Inverse Ratio Ventilation
Time-cycled, pressure-controlled inverse ratio ventilation (TCPCIRV), is a mode of MV used for patients with ARDS (78–80). This ventilatory mode was developed to counteract three major pathologic findings associated with ARDS: (*i*) decreased compliance (C_L), (*ii*) increased transpulmonary shunt ($\dot{Q}_s/\dot{Q}_t$), and (*iii*) the inhomogeneous (i.e., diffuse, but scattered) alveolar involvement associated with ARDS. By controlling the pressure and increasing the I:E ratio, gas flows into the lungs in a more physiologic way, decreasing barotrauma previously prevalent with ventilation of lungs with low C_L. Increasing the I:E ratio keeps alveoli open longer to participate in gas exchange longer, thus decreasing the $\dot{Q}_s/\dot{Q}_t$. Because of the heterogeneity of the lung injury associated with ARDS, some long inhalation time-constant alveoli do not expand when conventional I:E ratios are employed. By increasing the I:E ratio, the long inhalation time-constant alveoli (that would otherwise be atelectatic) are able to contribute to gas exchange. Since ARDS lungs are extremely stiff, they empty quickly, and the shorter exhalation time is generally well tolerated. When conventional ventilation with PEEP is used, the normal, compliant lung units may become overdistended, leading to $\dot{V}/\dot{Q}$ inequality with worsening gas exchange.

  ⚲ **In severe ARDS, the concept of applying PEEP preferentially to the diseased lung units is hypothesized to improve gas exchange.** ⚲ By prolonging inspiratory time (inverse of the usual I:E ratio), the expiratory flow time is decreased, and with extreme inverse I:E, exhalation flow does not complete before the next delivered breath occurs. This results in alveolar gas trapping or "intrinsic" (auto) PEEP. Because the diseased alveolar units are the slowest to empty, the intrinsic PEEP will mainly be present in these units, that is, the normal units will have already emptied. This "selective" PEEP is hypothesized to improve $\dot{V}/\dot{Q}$ matching (i.e., decreased shunt and dead space), resulting in improved oxygenation and CO_2 elimination. However, if too much intrinsic PEEP is used, alveolar dead space can increase just as it can when too much extrinsic PEEP is used. The initial setup for TCPCIRV is shown in Table 3.

  ⚲ **Because of improved gas exchange with TCPCIRV, one can generally ventilate and oxygenate patients at lower peak airway pressures.** ⚲ The risk of barotrauma is then theoretically reduced. However, because inspiration is prolonged, mPaw increases. Hence, significant decreases in $\dot{Q}$ can occur, especially in hypovolemic patients, as has been described by Perel (81). Thus, all patients treated with

Table 3 Initial Setup for Time-Cycled, Pressure-Controlled, Inverse Ratio Ventilation

Step	Parameter	Comments
1	F_IO_2	Temporarily increases F_IO_2 to 1.0 (may be there already), then wean down as tolerated. Same as during previous mode
2	Set PEEP	Maintain at value used during conventional MV
3	Inspiratory pressure	Start with inspiratory pressure = peak pressure during volume controlled breath—set PEEP (e.g., if patient is receiving 10 of PEEP and peak pressure is 45–50, initial inspiratory pressure should be 35–40 with PEEP at 10 cm H_2O)
4	RR	Generally not adjusted during TCPCIRV. Usually an initial rate of 15–25 is common
5	I:E ratio	The normal I:E ratio is 1:2. Increasing the I:E ratio increases the time alveoli are pressurized and the time for oxygen to diffuse across the alveolar epithelium
6	Inspiratory time	Determined by the I:E ratio. If the patient is set on a RR = 20 and an I:E ratio of 1:1, then a 1.5 sec inhalation time and a 1.5 sec exhalation time results

Note: The effects of TCPCIRV on $PaCO_2$ and $\dot{D}O_2$ are less predictable than the effects on PaO_2 (see text). Accordingly, frequent monitoring of blood gases and $\dot{D}O_2$ is necessary.
Abbreviations: F_IO_2, fraction of inhaled gas due to oxygen; MV, mechanical ventilation; PEEP, positive end-expiratory pressure; RR, respiratory rate; TCPCIRV, time-cycled, pressure-controlled, inverse ratio ventilation.

TCPCIRV should have invasive arterial pressure monitoring (and when unstable either a TEE or pulmonary artery catheter). In addition, high levels of sedation and (usually supplemental) paralysis are required to effectively ventilate patients in this mode. Although TCPCIRV is a beneficial mode for ventilating ARDS, guidelines for initiating TCPCIRV in less severe forms of ARF are less well defined and further studies are needed.

High-Frequency Ventilation
✎ HFV has several variants defined in the literature, but in general terms describes a form of MV utilizing high ventilatory rates and low tidal volumes (82). ✎ The V_T used in HFV is usually at, near, or below the anatomic dead space volume; accordingly, gas exchange occurs by bulk flow, coaxial flow, pendelluft, Taylor dispersion, or facilitated molecular diffusion (83). The Food and Drug Administration (FDA) considers HFV to occur when the rate of ventilation is >150 breaths/min.

Because HFV uses much smaller tidal volumes and lower peak inspiratory airway pressures than conventional ventilation, it possesses many of the attributes required for lung protective ventilation of ARDS patients. Its main clinical use has been for neonatal patients with respiratory failure (84,85). Indeed, HFV has only been shown to be superior to

conventional ventilation for pediatric respiratory distress syndrome (RDS). HFV can be categorized into five separate types by using criteria of ventilation rate and type of gas delivery mechanism.

High-Frequency Positive Pressure Ventilation
High-frequency positive pressure ventilation (HFPPV) utilizes conventional positive-pressure ventilators with low compliance circuits set at high rates and small tidal volumes. The V_T is usually in the range of 3–4 mL/kg with a set frequency of 60 to 120 breaths/min (1–2 Hz). HFPPV does not meet the FDA threshold for HFV because the rates are typically <150.

High-Frequency Jet Ventilation
In high-frequency jet ventilation (HFJV), a high-velocity pulse of gas is delivered into the lungs through a narrow cannula (usually within the lumen of a conventional ETT). The respiratory frequency typically ranges from 1.5 to 10 Hz. Originally developed in the 1970s, HFJV results in delivery of V_T smaller than the V_D (2–5 mL/kg). The consequent minimized tidal movement of the operative field led to its use in the OR for patients undergoing thoracic surgery (e.g., bronchopleural fistula repair) and for surgery on the upper airway (e.g., trachea, carina, and mainstem bronchus) (86). Today HFJV is mainly used in pediatrics and flow is delivered via a specially made triple-lumen ETT (National Catheter Corporation). Ventilators designed specifically for HFJV include the Bunnell Life Pulse (Bunnell, Inc., Salt Lake City, Utah, U.S.A.). Under most conditions, gas entrainment occurs around the jet, increasing the V_T by a physical process termed jet mixing.

High-Frequency Flow Interruption
High-frequency flow interruption (HFFI) is similar to HFJV, achieving frequencies as high as 15 Hz. This is the HFV apparatus invented by Emerson, which uses interrupted bulk gas flow using a ball moving back and forth across a nozzle. The ball alternates between obstructing the output flow and allowing the flow. The HFFI device can be used as a bulk flow device connected to an ETT or with a jet catheter in the airway when a high-pressure source is intermittently interrupted. This technology is not widely used clinically.

High-Frequency Oscillatory Ventilator
Utilizing an oscillator (piston pump) to create rapidly changing positive and negative pressure fluctuations is called high-frequency oscillatory ventilation (HFOV). High frequencies of 5–50 Hz are commonly used with this modality. HFOV aims to maintain an open lung volume by the application of a stable mPaw. The F_IO_2 and the mPaw are the main determinants of oxygenation during HFOV, whereas the effectiveness of ventilation (CO_2 elimination) is dependent upon the magnitude of pressure fluctuations and the set frequency.

The role of HFOV in treatment of neonates with RDS is well established (84,85). In early case studies (86,87) and later in clinical trials (88–90), HFOV was used as a rescue therapy for adults with severe ARDS not responding to conventional MV (91). HFOV improved oxygenation best when used in combination with recruitment maneuvers (92,93).

A recent review by Derdak (94) using HFOV in adult ARDS patients suggests it may benefit patients who require both a high F_IO_2 (>0.6) and high mPaw (≥20 cm

H_2O). Whether HFOV actually reduces mortality compared to other ventilation modes that also increase with mPaw (e.g., TCPCIRV) and its role outside of the rescue and/or research setting remains to be determined in future RCTs (95–97).

High-Frequency Percussive Ventilation
High-frequency percussive ventilation (HFPV) is a recent ventilatory mode, which combines conventional cycles with high-frequency percussions. HFPV was initially instituted as salvage therapy after acute respiratory failure following smoke inhalation injury achieving in each case a dramatic improvement of oxygenation, $PaCO_2$, and ventilatory pressures.

Complications of HFV common to all five basic modes include pneumothorax, drying of the airways, and airway injury including necrotizing tracheobronchitis. In addition, significant potential for air trapping and auto-PEEP exists [especially in the elderly COPD population, and other patients with reactive airways disease (RAD)]. Therefore, monitoring of airway pressure is extremely important in high-frequency ventilation.

The use of any or all of the five major types of HFV for the treatment of ARDS is still unproven in adults. However, many of the attributes of HFV seem ideal for adult ARDS, since the principles of lung-protective ventilation, including an open lung strategy with low tidal volume, peak pressure limitation, maintenance of an adequate end-expiratory lung volume, and the use of the low F_IO_2. However, large RCTs comparing HFV to conventional protective ventilation are still needed to prove HFV as effective, or more effective than conventional ventilation.

Liquid Ventilation
The use of perfluorocarbons as a respiratory medium was used as early as the 1960s (98). These colorless fluids have a greater density, lower surface tension, and higher solubilities for oxygen and CO_2, than water. This mode of ventilation in the form of total liquid ventilation (complete filling of the lung with liquid requiring a special ventilator) or partial liquid ventilation (usually to functional residual capacity using a conventional ventilator), has been successfully used in pediatric and adult patients (99–104). The results so far suggest that it is safe and efficacious in improving gas exchange by recruitment of dependent, atelectatic alveoli (liquid PEEP) and minimizing lung injury by requiring lower ventilator pressures and improving lung compliance in regions of lung injury. Disadvantages include the inability to assess lung parenchyma by chest radiography, because the liquid-filled lungs appear "white" on the chest film. Also, minimal data exists describing possible long-term toxicity. Results from ongoing and future studies will determine its adaptation into clinical practice.

Permissive Hypercapnia
Minimizing overdistension of the diseased lung and reducing the risk of stretch injury have become predominant goals in ventilating patients with lung disease like ARDS (105,106). This usually necessitates the use of small tidal volumes and lower minute ventilations to keep maximal transpulmonary pressures low. The resulting low minute ventilation often leads to hypoventilation with increased $PaCO_2$ and respiratory acidosis. Willingness to tolerate this respiratory acidosis is referred to as permissive hypercapnia

(105,106). Most patients can tolerate pH values in the range of 7.1 to 7.2 (106). Deep sedation is often required to decrease the respiratory drive caused by the hypercarbia. The role of $NaHCO_3$ as a buffering agent is controversial. High doses are required at low pH, and this may lead to paradoxical intracellular acidosis and increased intracellular CO_2 production. The clinician should also carefully consider potential harmful effects of permissive hypercapnia like central nervous system depression, increased intracranial pressure (ICP), dysrhythmias, myocardial ischemia or myocardial depression, and pulmonary hypertension.

Prone Ventilation
Placing ventilated patients with ARDS in the prone position to improve oxygenation was initially used in the early 1970s (107), and has been shown to improve oxygenation in patients with severe ALI/ARDS (108,109). The reason for underutilization of this ventilation technique is related to the special nursing and technical requirements, and the increased risk of dislodging the ETT and other important lines during the repositioning.

The improved oxygenation in the prone position is thought to be at least partially due to: (*i*) improved $\dot{V}/\dot{Q}$ matching by redistribution of perfusion to the better ventilated lung areas; (*ii*) better clearance of secretions by gravity; (*iii*) increased FRC; and (*iv*) a favorable change in regional diaphragm motion (110).

A large multicenter, randomized trial confirmed the improved oxygenation in the prone group but did not show a significant difference in outcome (111). Criticism of this study (112) included the short time spent in the prone position (at least six hours). It has been shown that the benefit from the proning increases with time spent in the prone position (113).

Inhaled Nitric Oxide
Since the endogenous vasodilator, endothelium derived relaxing factor, has been identified as nitric oxide (NO), it is not surprising that inhaled NO selectively vasodilates the pulmonary vasculature and has been used for patients with ARDS (114).

☞ **The potential benefit of inhaled NO in ARDS patients lies in improving the shunt fraction in the diseased lung.** ☞ Since it only dilates vessels in areas of ventilated alveoli, it diverts blood flow to these alveoli. The effects are kept local by its very short half-life and rapid inactivation. Although improved oxygenation with NO has been observed, prospective trials in ARDS showed no improved long-term outcome (115–118). As of this publication, FDA has only approved NO for the treatment of neonatal hypoxemia.

These results have led to the controversy about its use. Further studies need to show favorable outcome to prove it as a beneficial adjunct in the treatment of severe lung injury before its recommended routine use.

Noninvasive Positive-Pressure Ventilation
Noninvasive positive-pressure ventilation (NIPPV) has been shown to be beneficial in settings where the patient is not intubated, but needs ventilatory support. NIPPV is a technique in which the ventilator is connected to the patient via a tightly fitting facemask, potentially avoiding complications from endotracheal intubation (i.e., VAP). But NIPPV has its own disadvantages, including potential air leaks from suboptimal mask fit, pressure-induced skin

damage where the mask and face contact, and intolerable discomfort. Furthermore, patients should be sufficiently oriented, committed, able to handle their secretions, and capable of working with the NIPPV system.

Successful use of NIPPV in decreasing the need for endotracheal intubation has been shown to be the case in patients with acute respiratory failure (119), cardiogenic pulmonary edema (120), as well as in patients with acute hypercapnic respiratory failure from COPD (121,122). However, this technique has minimal application during the initial resuscitation and MV phase of critically injured trauma and burn patients.

WRITING VENTILATOR ORDERS

Initial ventilator orders should include the mode of ventilation (usually A/C or SIMV), the set tidal volume calculated based on the patient's weight, the backup set respiratory rate, the F_IO_2, and the amount of PEEP desired. Ventilator parameters typically determined by the respiratory therapist include the inhalation waveform, the I:E ratio (generally 1:2), trigger sensitivity, peak inhalation flow (usually 70–110 L/min is adequate), pressure limit, and P–V alarms. However, the responsible physician must understand the ramifications of improperly setting any of these variables. Furthermore, whenever TCPCIRV is used, the responsible physician should also order I:E ratio, and discuss the plan of care with the respiratory therapist.

Rarely used ventilatory settings include the use of an inflation hold, expiratory retard, and/or sigh. Indeed, most modern ventilators no longer have these capabilities. The reason these lung recruitment functions are no longer used is because in awake patients these maneuvers are uncomfortable and distressful.

The choice of ventilatory mode is based on the physician preference, but typically A/C offers the advantage of decreasing work of breathing and allows patients with respiratory muscle weakness to increase ventilation without performing the work of breathing on their own. With A/C, there is a theoretical increased risk for respiratory alkalosis because with each patient effort, a full machine-delivered breath results. The IMV mode offers the advantage of lower mPaw (since patient-initiated breaths are negative pressure breaths) allowing the patient to perform a greater portion of their work of breathing (if desired). However, the increased work of breathing with the IMV mode is often excessive in patients in severe respiratory failure.

The initial V_T can be calculated based on the patient's lean body weight, typically between 10 to 12 mL/kg in young healthy patients without lung injury. It is recommended that patients with a low FRC (such as those with ARDS) receive V_T ranging from 5–7 mL/kg with supplemental PEEP to keep the exhalation volume above the lower inflection point of the P–V curve. In addition, patients with a high FRC, resulting from bronchospasm (such as a patient with COPD or asthma) should also be ventilated with a smaller tidal volume in the range of 5–7 mL/kg in order to avoid hyper inflation, or any further increase in intrinsic PEEP.

The respiratory rate is set to assure an adequate $\dot{V}_E$ and to avoid respiratory acidosis or alkalosis. In a normal patient with normal lungs, an arterial carbon dioxide tension ($PaCO_2$) of 40 mm of mercury is usually achieved with an initial rate of 8 to 12 breaths/min.

The initial fractional inspired oxygen concentration (F_IO_2) should be 1.0 in order to document a level of right to-left shunt (by measuring the alveolar to arterial oxygen tension difference) and at the same time, minimize the risk of hypoxemia during transport and the initial ventilator set-up period in the ICU. Administration of 100% oxygen for a short period of time (i.e., <4 hours) is nontoxic. Later, based upon arterial blood gases, the F_IO_2 should be decreased by titrating the PEEP up. The goal should be to decrease the F_IO_2 into the nontoxic (<0.5) range as soon as possible.

The amount of PEEP initially set for most patients without elevated ICP should be 5 cm water, as this is thought to be physiologic and should decrease the incidence of atelectasis by increasing FRC. However, in the case of severe hypoxemia, the PEEP may need to be increased to as high as 15–20 cm H_2O pressure. The goal should be to use the least amount of PEEP possible, although still allowing the F_IO_2 to be 0.5 or less and obtain a $PaO_2 \geq 60$ mmHg.

COMPLICATIONS OF MECHANICAL VENTILATION

Complications of MV can be classified into those that cause an increase in airway pressure and those that cause a decrease in airway pressure (Table 4). Differentiation of peak versus plateau pressures can further differentiate the source of certain high-pressure problems. For instance, if the patient has a very high PIP but only a modest plateau airway pressure, an increase in airway resistance should be suspected. An increase in airway resistance may result from increased secretions, too small of an ETT, or bronchospasm.

☞ **When the patient seems to be "fighting the ventilator," an appropriate first diagnostic and therapeutic step is to separate the patient from the ventilator and hand-ventilate the patient with 100% oxygen.** ☞ Separating the patient from the ventilator assures that the ETT is properly placed and functioning in the patient and that the patient him/herself is not the problem. While the patient is receiving hand-generated bag/mask ventilation, attention can be turned to the ventilator to correct problems.

Complications of Prolonged Tracheal Intubation
There are also complications that arise simply as a result of endotracheal intubation. Although this review does not specifically address intubation, it is extremely uncommon

Table 4 Complications of Mechanical Ventilation

High pressure	Low pressure
Kinked ETT	Tube disconnect
ETT migration (mainstem)	Extubation
Increased secretions	Air leak around the cuff
Tension pneumothorax	Balloon rupture
Light anesthesia	TE fistula
Worsening of lung disease	BP fistula (early)
Fighting the vent	
Intrinsic ("auto") PEEP	

Abbreviations: BP, broncho-pleural; ETT, endotracheal tube; PEEP, positive end expiratory pressure; TE, tracheo-esophageal.

Table 5 Complications of Tracheal Intubation

During intubation
  Trauma to the C-spine, nose, teeth, lips,
  tongue, oropharynx, larynx, and trachea
  Aspiration (blood, tooth, gastric contents, etc.)
  Esophageal intubation
  Endobronchial intubation
  Hemodynamic instability
  Hypnotic drugs: myocardial depression, vasodilation
  Relative hypovolemia: decreased venous return
  Loss of sympathetic tone: hyperventilation (CO_2 elimination),
    administration of sedatives
  Exaggerated ANS reflexes
    Sympathetic (hypertension, tachycardia, myocardial
      ischemia)
    Vagal (hypotension, bradycardia, cardiac arrest)
Endotracheal tube in place
  Bronchospasm
  Tracheomalacia
  Tracheal perforation (by cuff, by tip of tube)
  Inadequate removal of secretions (possible ETT obstruction)
  Trauma to areas of contact (exacerbated by patient
    movement)
  Excessive inflation of cuff causing tube lumen narrowing
  Ruptured cuff causing air leak or aspiration
During extubation
  Trauma to the glottis by inflated cuff
  Aspiration of supraendotracheal tube cuff secretions
  Laryngospasm
  Respiratory obstruction by immediate edema of any part of
    the airway previously in contact with the endotracheal tube
After extubation
  Sore throat, dysphagia
  Aphonia
  Paralysis of the hypoglossal and/or lingual nerves
  Vocal cord paralysis
  Ulceration, inflammation, infection, edema of any part of the
    airway previously in contact with the endotracheal tube
  Laryngeal granulomas and polyps
  Laryngeal membranes and webs
  Tracheal stenosis

Abbreviations: ANS, autonomic nervous system; C-spine, cervical spine; ETT, endotracheal tube.

that we perform MV without concomitant endotracheal intubation (Table 5). For an expanded discussion of the complications of endotracheal intubation and tracheostomy, see the review by Stauffer et al. (123).

Pathologic Airway Injury

The presence of an ETT in the larynx causes characteristic pathology. The incidence of laryngeal complications after prolonged intubation is between 4% and 13%. The earliest of these changes are nonspecific hyperemia and edema due to mucosal irritation. Edema within the submucosa in the subglottis at the level of the cricoid may increase slowly, leading to delayed airway obstruction hours after the removal of the ETT.

As the tube remains in place, ulceration occurs with varying degrees of granulation tissue formation. The most susceptible site to irritation from the ETT is in the posterior larynx, especially the mucosa overlying the vocal processes of the arytenoids (124).

Subglottic stenosis, which is more easily recognized, may be coexistent with posterior glottic stenosis. Prolonged intubation is the most common cause of subglottic stenosis in both adults and children. By definition, subglottic stenosis is a narrowing of the subglottic space above the inferior margin of the cricoid cartilage and below the level of the glottis.

True vocal cord paralysis may occur as a result of endotracheal intubation. The paralysis is most commonly unilateral, but bilateral paralysis with airway obstruction has been reported. Brandwein et al. (125) examined the course of the anterior branch of the recurrent laryngeal nerve and discovered it to be vulnerable to compression between the inflated cuff of the ETT, the lateral projection of the abducted arytenoid, and the thyroid cartilage. Injury to the recurrent laryngeal nerve most commonly results in the cord lying in the paramedian position. Occasionally, true vocal cord edema persists long after extubation.

Obstruction of the Endotracheal Tube

Due to the plastic nature of the ETT, bending can occur at any time. Kinking can lead to hypoventilation and high peak airway pressures. The ventilator alarm should alert the clinician to a sudden increase in ventilator circuit resistance. Appropriate vigilance must be taken to avoid this occurrence.

Adequate pulmonary toilet and clearance of secretions is difficult in the mechanically ventilated patient. Secretions can be due to an inflammatory process (i.e., pneumonia, tracheitis) or mobilization of third space fluids. Nevertheless, the need for airway suctioning and pulmonary toilet should be assessed on a regular basis and achieved by in-line suctioning to minimize the risk of contamination. Mucous plugs can cause airway obstruction as severe as segmental and lobar collapse. Also, bronchospasm can occur in the patient with reactive airway disease.

Complications Related to Endotracheal Tube Securement

Once the position of the ETT is confirmed, there are multiple methods to prevent movement of the ETT. Tape, umbilical tape, and cloth Velcro contraptions have been used to maintain the position at the level of the vermilion border of the lips. Unfortunately, complications can arise from the mere securing of the ETT. Patients with sensitive skin and tape allergies can develop rashes or skin ulcers. The tape adhesive can be compromised by virtue of moist secretions and sweat, which can result in ETT migration and potential extubation. Umbilical tape that wraps around the neck of the patient can occlude the venous outflow and cause facial plethora. Special care must be taken to prevent such catastrophes associated with securing the ETT.

Complications Related to Breach of Airway Protection
Atelectasis and Impaired Clearance of Secretions

Atelectasis is a major contributor to postoperative respiratory failure in critically ill trauma patients, especially following thoracic and high abdominal trauma. Lung collapse secondary to decreased respiratory muscle tone, cephalad displacement of the diaphragm, compression of lung tissue, and splinting, all contribute to a reduction of FRC (126). Postoperative persistence of atelectasis often results secondary to postoperative pain, decreased cough, inability to clear secretions, and inability to take deep breaths; all of which can be improved with adequate analgesia (126).

Ventilator-Associated Pneumonia

VAP is the most frequent ICU-acquired infection among patients receiving MV. VAP is defined as an inflammation of the lung parenchyma caused by infectious agents occurring >48 hours after the time MV was started. Cook et al. (127) found, in a larger series of 1014 mechanically ventilated patients, that the cumulative risk of VAP was 3% per day up to day 5, 2% per day up to day 10, and 1% per day thereafter. The attributable mortality for VAP has been reported to be as high as 33% to 55% (128). Independent predictors, in decreasing order, were a primary admitting diagnosis of burn, trauma, central nervous system disease, respiratory disease, cardiac disease, and witnessed aspiration (127–129).

Sources of infection for VAP include inoculation by healthcare workers, aspiration of oropharyngeal pathogens around the ETT cuff, and invasive respiratory devices (129). Many preventive strategies have been prescribed, such as hand washing, semi-recumbency, ventilator device care, subglottic suctioning, noninvasive ventilation, and intensive insulin therapy. Treatment is focused at early recognition, broad-spectrum antibiotics, antibiotic de-escalation at three to five days, and curtailing therapy duration to eight days if there is clinical improvement (130).

Barotrauma/Volutrauma

Barotrauma refers to complications of MV, such as pneumothorax, pneumomediastinum, and other forms of extra-alveolar air (131–134). It became clear in the 1990s that the production of high pressures is not the only reason for formation of extraalveolar air (135). However, controversy continues regarding the term barotrauma, because it implies that injury is related only to pressure. Other investigators will use volutrauma to denote that lung injury associated with positive pressure is from high distending volumes rather than high pressures. Evidence is increasing that volume, not pressure alone, causes overdistension and is associated with iatrogenic lung injury (136–137). Thus, the term VILI (described earlier) is now used when referring to lung injury that can result from either barotrauma or volutrauma (138).

Types of conditions that predispose to barotrauma include: high PIPs, bullous lung disease such as may occur with emphysema, high levels of PEEP, high tidal volumes, aspiration of gastric acid, and ARDS. The result of this overdistension can be pneumothorax, pneumomediastinum, subcutaneous emphysema, systemic air embolism, and bronchopleural fistula. Ways of reducing the likelihood of alveolar rupture during MV include: setting smaller tidal volumes, decreasing tidal volume when high PEEP is used, maintaining alveolar pressures below 30 cm H_2O, omitting use of sigh breaths with high tidal volumes, monitoring for auto-PEEP when present, and considering permissive hypercapnia and lung-protective ventilation strategies when necessary (139).

EYE TO THE FUTURE

Today's ventilators are primarily microprocessor driven. As rapid as there are advances in information technology, so too will advances be made in the features and capabilities of tomorrow's ventilator devices. As with information systems and other electronics, ventilators continue to be smaller, incorporate expanded capabilities, and process and display information better and faster as time progresses.

Closed-Loop Ventilation

We have discussed the breath-delivery phases of MV and several modes of ventilation that are available. Closed-loop ventilation is now possible with the ability of technology to rapidly sense and respond to patient-generated variables. In its simplest form, Auto-Flow (Drager Medical, Telford, Pennsylvania, U.S.A.) and Volume Control Plus (Puritan Bennett, Tyco Healthcare, Pleasanton, California, U.S.A.) represent forms of closed-loop ventilation in which there is automatic next breath changes in pressure using tidal volume as the feedback control, with the objective of keeping tidal volume constant. Manufacturer's engineering teams continue to devise more sophisticated methods to provide closed-loop ventilation to improve the responsiveness of breath delivery to patients needs. However, there is no uniformity regarding how manufacturers name or classify these new modes. This leads to confusion among caregivers, and training programs have become more focused on understanding manufacturer-specific vocabulary. Closed-loop systems do provide for pressure support, volume targeted pressure control, mandatory minute ventilation, and other modes commonly found on ICU ventilators.

Manufacturers are quickly responding to gain a clinical advantage by partnering with clinicians to develop new modes of closed-loop ventilation. Adaptive support ventilation (ASV) is designed to titrate ventilator output on a breath-to-breath basis. The level of support is determined by the mechanical characteristics of the patient and their own breathing efforts. Based on ideal body weight and the % minute ventilation control, a target minute ventilation is determined. By delivering a series of "test breaths" the ventilator measures respiratory system compliance, airway resistance, and intrinsic PEEP. From those measures and the % minute volume setting, the ventilator will determine the target breath rate and tidal volume. Campbell et al. (140) evaluated ASV and determined that the ventilator would self-adjust to achieve a lower PIP, lower V_T, and higher rate than clinician-selected settings, but was associated with an improved efficiency of ventilation and reduction in dead space when compared to conventional ventilation.

Proportional assist ventilation (PAV) is not currently available in the United States and remains limited to investigational use. PAV is a form of closed-loop ventilation designed to increase or decrease airway pressure in proportion to the patient's effort (141). PAV is an intrabreath, positive feedback controller that amplifies airway pressure proportional to inspiratory flow and volume (142). Puritan Bennett (Puritan Bennett, Tyco Healthcare, Pleasanton, California, U.S.A.) will be the first manufacturer to release PAV in the United States. The feature will be incorporated in their 840 series ventilator in which the clinician sets the % support, tube size and type, an expiratory sensitivity, the high and low tidal volume limits, and the ventilator— and on every 4 to 10 breaths the ventilator will measure resistance, compliance, flow, and volume every five milliseconds. Studies have validated the feasibility of PAV in a variety of patient conditions (143–145).

Closed-loop advances include the use of occlusion pressure measures to control the level of pressure support (146,147), the use of end tidal CO_2 to control the level of pressure support (148), and the concept of neurally-adjusted ventilator assist using diaphragm electrical activity to trigger the ventilator (149).

Decision-Making Algorithms

Although technology advances continue to arm the clinician with new options for ensuring that MV and breath delivery meet the needs of the patients, decisions about the selection of these modes and changes in clinician set parameters will remain important.

Monitoring systems will continue to evolve so that ventilator information is displayed in ways that the clinician can configure, that allows storage of selected information, that allows breath-to-breath comparisons of measured parameters to assess the effectiveness of MV.

Nearly all modern-day ICU ventilators allow connectivity with information systems so that clinicians can spend less time charting, and data is integrated and stored. Point of care access to such information will assist future clinicians in making critical decisions about the patient's plan of care.

With the increasing number of monitored and derived parameters, clinicians will also need new tools to assist in making safe and appropriate changes in the patient's ventilator care plan. Decision-based algorithms are being investigated and incorporated in new technology. The ability to preconfigure facility-specific algorithms to target initial settings, adjust those settings based on user-selected inputs, and to manage the liberation from MV are incorporated in emerging technology.

SUMMARY

A strong understanding of the ventilator is paramount when taking care of the critically ill patient. Because so many machines are made for the same purpose, the stratification of phases of ventilation enhances one's understanding of the ventilator. Choosing the appropriate mode of ventilation depends on the patient's clinical situation. The vast majority of patients in the SICU are appropriately placed on volume control ventilation. However, in the patient with severe respiratory failure, multiple lung protective modes should be used to minimize the risk of barotrauma/volutrauma and other forms of secondary lung injury.

Knowledge of the complications surrounding the procedures involved with MV is very important. Placement of an ETT and delivering positive pressure to the critically ill patient is not a benign process. In the future, newer modes will be available to further improve morbidity and mortality associated with MV by minimizing the risk of secondary lung injury.

KEY POINTS

- Ventilators can be categorized into two major types: (*i*) negative pressure and (*ii*) positive pressure ventilators.
- Mechanically ventilated breaths should be divided into four distinct phases to best understand the changes that occur in pressure, flow, and volume of the inhaled and exhaled gases.

- The "trigger phase" refers to a point in time (P1 in Fig. 1) when the ventilator initiates the positive pressure breath (changes over from exhalation to inhalation).
- The inhalation phase is characterized as that period of time when gas is flowing into the lungs, as well as that time when already delivered gas remains in the lungs (i.e., until the ventilator cycles into exhalation).
- The cycle phase represents the changeover from inhalation to exhalation.
- Volume-cycled ventilators terminate inhalation after a preselected volume has been delivered to the patient.
- The exhalation phase is the time period when the previously inhaled gas is exhausted, and is generally passive (i.e., occurs by natural recoil if elastic forces in lung and in chest wall).
- Although the application of PEEP will decrease shunt, it can also increase alveolar dead space, particularly in West's zone 1 regions.
- Pressure support ventilation can be used as the sole method of ventilation or, more frequently, as a method to support weaning.
- One explanation for the confounding relationship between PIP and barotrauma is that the actual pressure applied at the alveolus is lower than that measured at the ventilator tubing, and it is the pressure distending the alveolus that is most injurious.
- The first trial showing a decrease in mortality for a low tidal volume strategy compared with traditional, higher tidal volumes was conducted by the National Institutes of Health—National Heart, Blood, and Lung Institute ARDS Network Study (67).
- In the open lung approach, the patient is ventilated between the upper and lower inflection points on the pressure–volume curve.
- In severe ARDS, the concept of applying PEEP preferentially to the diseased lung units is hypothesized to improve gas exchange.
- Because of improved gas exchange with TCPCIRV, one can generally ventilate and oxygenate patients at lower peak airway pressures.
- HFV has several variants defined in the literature, but in general terms describes a form of MV utilizing high ventilatory rates and low tidal volumes (82).
- The potential benefit of inhaled NO in ARDS patients lies in improving the shunt fraction in the diseased lung.
- When the patient seems to be "fighting the ventilator," an appropriate first diagnostic and therapeutic step is to separate the patient from the ventilator and hand-ventilate the patient with 100% oxygen.

REFERENCES

1. Stock CR. What is past is prologue: A short history of the development of the tracheostomy. Ear Nose Throat J 1987; 66(4):166–169.
2. Comroe JH. Retrospectroscope: Insights Into Medical Discovery. Menlo Park: Von Gehr Press, 1977.
3. Stoller JK. The history of intubation, tracheostomy and airway appliances. Respir Care 1999; 44(6):595–603.
4. Mørch ET. History of mechanical ventilation. In: Kirby RR, Smith RA, DeSautels DA, et al., eds. Mechanical Ventilation. New York: Churchill Livingstone, 1985.
5. Hook R. An account of an experiment made by M. Hook, of preserving animals alive by blowing through their lungs with bellows. Philos Trans 1667; 2:539–540.

6. Sellick BA. Cricoid pressure to control regurgitation of stomach contents during induction of anaesthesia. Lancet 1961; 2: 404–406.
7. Emerson JH. The Evolution of the "Iron Lung." Cambridge, MA: JH Emerson, 1978.
8. Drinker PA, McKhann CF. The iron lung: first practical means of respiratory support. JAMA 1986; 255(11):1476.
9. Gudel AE, Treweek DN. Ether apnoeas. Anesth Analg 1934; 13:263–264.
10. Snider GL. Historical perspective on mechanical ventilation: from simple life support system to ethical dilemma. Am Rev Respir Dis 1989; 140:S2–S7.
11. Safer P, DeKornfield TJ, Pearson JW, Redding JS. The intensive care unit; a three year experience at Baltimore City Hospitals. Anaesthesia 1961; 16:275–84.
12. Fairley HB. The Toronto General Hospital Respiratory Unit. Anaesthesia 1961; 16:267–274.
13. Bendixen HH, Egbert LD, Hedley-Whyte J, Laver MB, Pontoppidan H. Respiratory Care. Vol. 4. St Louis: Mosby, 1965.
14. Corrado A, De Paola E, Gorini M, et al. Intermittent negative pressure ventilation in the treatment of hypoxic hypercapnic coma in chronic respiratory insufficiency. Thorax 1996; 51:1077–1082.
15. Corrado A, Gorini M, Ginanni R, et al. Negative pressure ventilation versus conventional mechanical ventilation in the treatment of acute respiratory failure in COPD patients. Eur Respir J 1998; 12:519–525.
16. Natalini G, Cavaliere S, Seramondi V, et al. Negative pressure ventilation versus external high-frequency oscillation during rigid bronchoscopy. Chest 2000; 118:18.
17. Natalini G, Vitacca M, Cavaliere S, et al. Negative pressure ventilation versus spontaneous assisted ventilation during rigid bronchoscopy. Acta Anaesthesiol Scand 1998; 42:1063.
18. Seegobin RD, Van Hasselt GL. Aspiration beyond endotracheal cuffs. Can Anaesth Soc J 1986; 33:273–279.
19. Young PJ, Basson C, Hamilton D, Ridley SA. Prevention of tracheal aspiration using the pressure-limited tracheal tube cuff. Anaesthesia 1999; 54:559–563.
20. American Association for Respiratory Care. Consensus statement on the essentials of mechanical ventilators—1992. Respir Care 1992; 37(9):1000–1008.
21. MacIntyre NR, McConnell R, Cheng K-C G, Sane A. Patient-ventilator flow dyssynchrony: flow-limited versus pressure-limited breaths. Crit Care Med 1997; 25:1671–1677.
22. Cinnella G, Conti G, Lofaso F, et al. Effects of assisted ventilation on the work of breathing: volume controlled versus pressure controlled ventilation. Am J Respir Crit Care Med 1996; 1: 1025–1033.
23. Kumar A, Falke KJ, Geffin B, et al. Ventilation with end-expiratory pressure in acute lung disease. N Engl Med 1970; 283:1430–1436.
24. McIntyre RW, Laws AK, Ramachandran PR. Positive expiratory pressure plateau: improved gas exchange during mechanical ventilation. Canad Anaesth Soc J 1969; 16:477–486.
25. Shapiro BA, Cane RD, Harrison RA. Positive end-expiratory pressure in acute lung injury. Chest 1983; 83:558–563.
26. Weisman IM, Rinaldo JE, Rogers RM. Positive end-expiratory pressure in adult respiratory failure. N Engl J Med 1982; 307:1381–1384.
27. Cournand A, Motley HL, Werko L, et al. Physiological studies of the effects of intermittent positive-pressure breathing on cardiac output in man. Am J Physiol 1998; 152: 162–174.
28. Qvist J, Pontoppidan H, Wilson RS, et al. Hemodynamic responses to mechanical ventilation with PEEP: the effect of hypervolemia. Anesthesiology 1975; 42:45–55.
29. Fewell JE, Abendschein DR, Carlson CJ, et al. Mechanism of decreased right and left ventricular end-diastolic volumes during continuous positive-pressure ventilation in dogs. Circ Res 1980; 47:467–472.
30. Henning RJ. Effects of positive end-expiratory pressure on the right ventricle. J Appl Physiol 1986; 61:819–826.
31. Scharf SM, Brown R, Saunders N, et al. Changes in canine left ventricular size and configuration with positive end-expiratory pressure. Circ Res 1979; 44:672–678.
32. Sutur PM, Fairley HB, Isenberg MD. Optimum end-expiratory airway pressure in patients with acute pulmonary failure. N Engl J Med 1975; 292:284–289.
33. Schlobohm RM, Falltrick RT, Quan SF, Katz JA. Lung volumes, mechanics, and oxygenation during spontaneous positive-pressureventilation: the advantage of CPAP over EPAP. Anesthesiology 1981; 55:416–422.
34. Rappard S, Hickey J. Just the Berries. Use of CPAP and BiPAP in acute respiratory failure. Can Fam Physician 2001; 47:269–270.
35. Henzler D, Dembinski R, Bensberg, et al. Ventilation with biphasic positive airway pressure in experimental lung injury: influence of transpulmonary pressure on gas exchange and haemodynamics. Intensive Care Med 2004; 30:935–994.
36. Brochard L, Rauss A, Benito S, et al. Comparison of three methods of gradual withdrawal from ventilatory support during weaning from mechanical ventilation. Am J Respir Crit Care Med 1994; 150:896–903.
37. Keilty SEF, Ponte J, Fleming TA, et al. Effect of inspiratory pressure support on exercise tolerance and breathlessness in patients with severe stable chronic obstructive pulmonary disease. Thorax 1994; 49:990–994.
38. Maltais F, Seissman H, Gottfried SB. Pressure support reduces inspiratory effort and dyspnea during exercise in chronic airflow obstruction. Am J Respir Crit Care Med 1995; 151:1027–1033.
39. Meecham Jones DJ, Paul EA, Jones PW. Nasal pressure support ventilation plus oxygen compared with oxygen therapy along in hypercapnic COPD. Am J Respir Crit Care Med 1995; 152:538–544.
40. Sottiaux TM. Patient-ventilator interactions during volume support ventilation: asynchrony and tidal volume instability: a report of three cases. Respir Care 2001; 46(3):255–262.
41. Pilbeam SP. Mechanical Ventilation: Physiological and Clinical Applications. St. Louis: Mosby, 1998:201–203.
42. Macklin MI, Macklin CC. Malignant interstitial emphysema of the lungs and mediastinum as important occult complications in many respiratory diseases and other conditions: interpretation of clinical literature in light of laboratory experiments. Medicine 1944; 23:281.
43. Webb HH, Tierney DF. Experimental pulmonary edema due to intermittent positive pressure ventilation with high inflation pressures: protection by positive end-expiratory pressure. Am Rev Respir Dis 1974; 110:556–565.
44. Nahum A, Hoyt J, Schmitz et al. Effect of mechanical ventilation strategy on dissemination of intratracheally instilled *Escherichia coil* in dogs. Crit Care Med 1997; (10):1733–1743.
45. Chiumello D, Pristine G, Slutsky AS, et al. Mechanical ventilation affects local and systemic cytokines in an animal model of acute respiratory distress syndrome. Am J Respir Crit Care Med 1999; 160:109–116.
46. Tasker V, John J, Evander E, et al. Surfactant dysfunction makes lungs vulnerable to repetitive collapse and reexpansion. Am J Respir Crit Care Med 1997; 155:313–320.
47. De Latorre F, Tomasa A, Klamburg J, et al. Incidence of pneumothorax and pneumomediastinum in patients with aspiration pneumonia requiring ventilatory support. Chest 1977; 72:141–144.
48. Gammon RB, Shin MS, Buchalter SE. Pulmonary barotrauma in mechanical ventilation. Chest 1992; 102:568–572.
49. Peterson GW, Baier H. Incidence of pulmonary barotraumas in a medical ICU. Crit Care Med 1983; 11:67–69.
50. Kumar A, Pontopiddan H, Falke KJ, et al. Pulmonary barotraumas during mechanical ventilation. Crit Care Med 1973; 1:181–186.
51. Woodring JH. Pulmonary interstitial emphysema in the adult respiratory distress syndrome. Crit Care Med 1985; 13: 786–791.
52. Rohlfing BM, Webb WR, Schlobolm RM. Ventilator-related extra-alveolar air in adults. Radiology 1976; 121:25–31.

53. Leatherman J, Ravenscroft SA, Iber C, et al. High peak inflation pressures do not predict barotraumas during mechanical ventilation of status asthmaticus. Am Rev Repir Dis 1989; 139:A154.

54. Weg JG, Anzueto A, Balk RA, et al. The relation of pneumothorax and other air leaks to mortality in acute respiratory distress syndrome. N Engl J Med 1998; 338:341–346.

55. Mathru M, Rao TLK, Venus B. Ventilator-induced barotraumas in controlled mechanical ventilation versus intermittent mandatory ventilation. Crit Care Med 1983; 11:359–361.

56. Clevenger FW, Acosta JA, Osler TM, et al. Barotrauma associated with high-frequency jet ventilation for hypoxic salvage. Arch Surg 1990; 125:1542–1545.

57. Tharratt RS, Allen RP, Albertson TE. Pressure-controlled inverse-ratio ventilation in acute respiratory distress syndrome. Chest 1988; 94:755–762.

58. Gammon RB, Shin MS, Groves RH Jr, et al. Clinical risk factors for pulmonary barotrauma: a multivariate analysis. Am J Respir Crit Care Med 1995; 152:1235–1240.

59. Polak B, Adams H. Traumatic air embolism in submarine escape training. US Naval Med Bull 1932; 30:165–177.

60. Hernandez LA, Peevy KJ, Moise AA, et al. Chest wall restriction limits high pressure-induced lung injury in rabbits. J Appl Physiol 1989; 66:2364–2368.

61. Dreyfuss D, Basset G, Soler P, et al. Intermittent positive pressure hyperventilation with high inflation pressures produces pulmonary microvascular injury in rats. Am Rev Respir Dis 1985; 132:880–884.

62. Stewart TE, Meade MO, Cook DJ, et al. Evaluation of a ventilation strategy to prevent barotraumas in patients at high risk for acute respiratory distress syndrome. N Engl J Med 1998; 338:355–361.

63. Gattinoni L, Pesenti A, Avalli L, et al. Pressure–volume curve of total respiratory system in acute respiratory failure: Computed tomographic scan study. Am Rev Respir Dis 1987; 136:730–736.

64. Hickling KG, Henderson SJ, Jackson R. Low mortality associated with low volume pressure limited ventilation with permissive hypercapnia in severe adult respiratory distress syndrome. Intensive Care Med 1990; 16:372–377.

65. Brochard L, Roudot-Thoraval F, Roupie E, et al. Tidal volume reduction for prevention of ventilator-induced lung injury in acute respiratory distress syndrome. The Multicenter Trial Group on Tidal Volume reduction in ARDS. Am J Respir Crit Care Med 1998; 158:1831–1838.

66. Brower RG, Shanholtz CB, Fessler HE, et al. Prospective, randomized, controlled clinical trial comparing traditional versus reduced tidal volume ventilation in acute respiratory distress syndrome patients. Crit Care Med 1999; 27:1492–1498.

67. Acute Respiratory Distress Syndrome Network. Ventilation with lower tidal volumes as compared with traditional tidal volumes for acute lung injury and the acute respiratory distress syndrome. N Engl J Med 2000; 342:1301–1308.

68. Muscedere JG, Mullen JBM, Gan K, et al. Tidal ventilation at low airway pressures can augment lung injury. Am J Respir Crit Care Med 1994; 149:1327–1334.

69. Matamis D, Lemaire F, Hart A, et al. Total respiratory pressure–volume curves in the adult respiratory syndrome. Chest 1984; 86:58–66.

70. Amato MBP, Barbas CSV, Medeiros DN, et al. Beneficial effects of the "open lung approach" with low distending pressures in acute respiratory distress syndrome. Am J Respir Crit Care Med 1995; 152:1835–1846.

71. Amato MBP, Barbas CSV, Medeiros DM, et al. Effect of a protective-ventilation strategy on mortality in the acute respiratory distress syndrome. N Engl J Med 1998; 338:347–354.

72. Mergoni M, Martelli A, Volpi A, et al. Impact of positive end-expiratory pressure on chest wall and lung pressure–volume curve in acute respiratory failure. Am J Respir Crit Care Med 1997; 156:846–854.

73. Gaver DP, Samsel RW, Solway J. Effects of surface tension and viscosity on airway reopening. J Appl Physiol 1990; 69:74–85.

74. Putensen C, Zech S, Wrigge H, et al. Long-term effects of spontaneous breathing during ventilatory support in patients with acute lung injury. Am J Respir Crit Care Med 2001; 164:43–49.

75. Sydow M, Burchardi H, Ephraim E, Zielmann S. Long-term effects of two different ventilatory modes on oxygenation in acute lung injury: comparison of airway pressure release ventilation and volume controlled inverse ratio ventilation. Am J Respir Crit Care Med 1994; 149:1550–1556.

76. Putensen C, Mutz NJ, Putensen-Himmer G, Zinserling J. Spontaneous breathing during ventilatory support improves ventilation-perfusion distributions in patients with acute respiratory distress syndrome. Am J Respir Crit Care Med 1999; 159:1241–1248.

77. Wrigge H. Spontaneous breathing improves lung aeration in oleic acid-induced lung injury. Anesthesiology 2003; 99(2):376–384.

78. Wang S-H, Wei T-S. The outcome of early pressure-controlled inverse ratio ventilation on patients with severe acute respiratory distress syndrome in surgical intensive care unit. Am J Surg 2002; 183(2)151–155.

79. Gurevitch MJ, Dyke JV, Young ES, et al. Improved oxygenation and lower peak airway pressure in severe adult respiratory distress syndrome: treatment with inverse ratio ventilation. Chest 1986; 89:211–213.

80. Manthous CA, Schmidt GA. Inverse ratio ventilation in ARDS: improved oxygenation without autoPEEP. Chest 1993; 103:953.

81. Perel A, Minokovich L, Presiman S, et al. Assessing fluid-responsiveness by a standardized ventilatory maneuver: the respiratory systolic variation test. Anesth Analg 2005; 100(4):942–945.

82. Sjostrand Ulf. High-frequency positive-pressure ventilation (HFPPV): a review. Crit Care Med 1980; 8:345–364.

83. Chang HK. Mechanisms of gas transport during high frequency ventilation. J Appl Physiol 1984; 56:553–563.

84. Abbasi S, Bhutani VK, Spitzer AR, et al. Pulmonary mechanics in preterm neonates with respiratory failure treated with high-frequency oscillatory ventilation compared with conventional mechanical ventilation. Pediatrics 1991; 87:487.

85. Clark RH, Gertsmann DR, Null DM, et al. Prospective randomized comparison of high-frequency oscillatory and conventional ventilation in respiratory distress syndrome. Pediatrics 1992; 89:5.

86. Benumof JL (ed.). High-frequency and high-flow apneic ventilation during thoracic surgery. In: Anesthesia for Thoracic Surgery. Philadelphia: W.B. Saunders, 1987:288.

87. Clark RH, Yoder BA, Sell MS. Prospective, randomized comparison of high-frequency oscillation and conventional ventilation in candidates for extracorporeal membrane oxygenation. J Pediatr 1994; 124:447–454.

88. Gerstmann DR, Minton SD, Stoddard RA, et al. The Provo multicenter early high-frequency oscillatory ventilation trial: Improved pulmonary and clinical outcome in respiratory distress syndrome. Pediatrics 1996; 98:1044–1057.

89. Plavka R, Kopecky P, Sebron V, et al. A prospective randomized comparison of conventional mechanical ventilation and very early high frequency oscillatory ventilation in extremely premature newborns with respiratory distress syndrome. Intensive Care Med 1999; 25:68–75.

90. Chiche JD, Boukef R, Laurent I, et al. High frequency oscillatory ventilation (HFOV) improves oxygenation in patients with severe ARDS. Am J Respir Crit Care Med 2000; 161:A48.

91. Claridge JA, Hostetter RG, Lowson SM, et al. High-frequency oscillatory ventilation can be effective as rescue therapy for refractory acute lung dysfunction. Am Surg 1999; 65:1092–1096.

92. Fort P, Farmer C, Westerman J, et al. High-frequency oscillatory ventilation for adult respiratory distress syndrome—a pilot study. Critical Care Med 1997; 25:937–947.

93. Mehta S, Lapinsky SE, Hallett DC, et al. A prospective trial of high frequency oscillatory ventilation in adults with acute respiratory distress syndrome. Crit Care Med 2001; 29(7):1360–1369.

94. Derdak S, Mehta S, Stewart T, et al. High frequency oscillatory ventilation for acute respiratory distress syndrome: a randomized, controlled trial. Am J Respir Crit Care Med 2002; 166: 801–808.

95. Ferguson ND, Kacmarek RM, Mehta S, et al. Safety and efficacy of high frequency oscillatory ventilation (HFOV) and recruitment maneuvers (RMS) in early severe ARDS. Am J Respir Crit Care Med 2001; 163:A767.

96. Froese AP. High-frequency oscillatory ventilation for adult respiratory distress syndrome: let's get it right this time! J Crit Care Med 1997; 25:906–908.

97. Derdak S. High-frequency oscillatory ventilation for acute respiratory distress syndrome in adult patients. Crit Care Med 2003; 31(4):S317–S323.

98. Clark LC, Gollan F. Survival of mammals breathing organic liquids equilibrated with oxygen at atmospheric pressure. Science 1966; 152:1755.

99. Greenspan JS, Wolfson MR, Rubenstein SD, et al. Liquid ventilation of human preterm neonates. J Pediatr 1990; 117:106.

100. Gauger PG, Pranikoff T, Schreiner RJ, et al. Initial experience with partial liquid ventilation in pediatric patients with the acute respiratory distress syndrome. J Crit Care Med 1996; 24:16.

101. Hirschl RB, Pranikoff T, Wise C, et al. Initial experience with partial liquid ventilation in adult patients with the acute respiratory distress syndrome. JAMA 1996; 275:383–389.

102. Spitzer AR, Lipsky CL. Partial liquid ventilation with perflubron in premature infants with severe respiratory distress syndrome. Clin Pediatr (Phila) 1997; 36:181–182.

103. Leach CL, Greenspan JS, Rubenstein SD, et al. Partial liquid ventilation with perflubron in premature infants with severe respiratory distress syndrome. The LiquiVent Study Group. N Engl J Med 1996; 335:761–767.

104. Hirschl RB, Croce M, Wiedemann H, et al. Prospective, randomized, controlled pilot study of partial liquid ventilation in adult acute respiratory distress syndrome. Am J Respir Crit Care Med 2002; 165:781–787.

105. Hickling KG, Walsh J, Henderson S, et al. Low mortality rate in adult respiratory distress syndrome using low-volume, pressure-limited ventilation with permissive hypercapnia: A prospective study. Crit Care Med 1994; 22:1568–1578.

106. Fiehl F, Perret C. Permissive hypercapnia—How permissive should we be? Am J Respir Crit Care Med 1994; 150:1722–1737.

107. Douglas W, Rehder K, Beynen RM, et al. Improved oxygenation in patients with acute respiratory failure: the prone position. Am J Respir Crit Care Med 1977; 115:559–566.

108. Albert RK. The prone position in acute respiratory distress syndrome: Where we are, and where do we go from here? Crit Care Med 1997; 25:1453–1454.

109. Chatte G, Sab JM, Dubois JM, et al. Prone position in mechanically ventilated patients with severe acute respiratory failure. Am J Respir Crit Care Med 1997; 155:473–478.

110. Lamm WJ, Graham MM, Albert RK. Mechanism by which the prone position improves oxygenation in acute lung injury. Am J Respir Crit Care Med 1994; 150:184–193.

111. Gattinoni L, Tognoni G, Pesenti A, et al. Effect of prone positioning on the survival of patients with acute respiratory failure. N Engl J Med 2001; 345:568–573.

112. Meade M. Prone positioning for acute respiratory failure improved shortterm oxygenation but not survival. Evid Based Nurs 2002; 5:52–62.

113. McAuley DF. What is the optimal duration of ventilation in the prone position in acute lung injury and acute respiratory distress syndrome? Intensive Care Med 2002; 28(4):414–418.

114. Roissant R, Falke KJ, Lopez F, et al. Inhaled nitric oxide for the adult respiratory distress syndrome. N Engl J Med 1993; 328:399–405.

115. Michael JR, Barton RG, Saffle JR, et al. Inhaled nitric oxide versus conventional therapy: effect on oxygenation in ARDS. Am J Respir Crit Care Med 1998; 157:1372–1380.

116. Troncy E, Collet JP, Shapiro S, et al. Inhaled nitric oxide in acute respiratory distress syndrome: a pilot randomized controlled study. Am J Respir Crit Care Med 1998; 157:1483–1488.

117. Dellinger RP, Zimmerman JL, Taylor RW, et al. Effects of inhaled nitric oxide in patients with acute respiratory distress syndrome: results of a randomized phase II trial. Crit Care Med 1998; 26:15–23.

118. Lundin S, Mang H, Smithies M, et al. Inhalation of nitric oxide in acute lung injury: Results of a European multicenter study. Intensive Care Med 1999; 25:911–919.

119. Antonelli M, Conti G, Rocco M, et al. A comparison of noninvasive positive-pressure ventilation and conventional mechanical ventilation in patients with acute respiratory failure. N Engl J Med 1998; 339:429–435.

120. Lin M, Yang Y-F, Chiang H-T, et al. Reappraisal of continuous positive airway pressure therapy in acute cardiogenic pulmonary edema. Chest 1995; 107:1379–1386.

121. Vitacca M, Rubini F, Foglio K, et al. Noninvasive modalities of positive-pressure ventilation improve the outcome of acute exacerbations in COLD patients. Intensive Care Med 1993; 19:450–455.

122. Miro AM, Shivaram U, Hertig I. Continuous positive airway pressure in COPD patients in acute hypercapnic respiratory failure. Chest 1993; 103:266–268.

123. Stautfer JL, Olson DE, Petty TL. Complications and consequences of endotracheal intubation and tracheostomy. A prospective stuy of 150 critically ill adult patients. Am J Med 1981; 20(1):65–76.

124. Benjamin B. Laryngeal trauma from intubation: endoscopic evaluation and classification. In: Cummings CW, et al., ed. Otolaryngology-Head & Neck Surgery. 3rd ed. St. Louis: Mosby, 1998:2013–2035.

125. Brandwein M, Abramson AL, Shikowitz MJ. Bilateral vocal cord paralysis following endotracheal intubation. Arch Otolaryngol Head Neck Surg 1986;112:877–882.

126. Karmakar MK, Ho AM-H. Acute pain management of patients with multiple fractured ribs. J Trauma 2003; 54(3):615–625.

127. Cook DJ, Walter SD, Cook RJ, et al. Incidence of and risk factors for ventilator-associated pneumonia in critically ill patients. Ann Intern Med 1998; 129:433–440.

128. Heyland DK, Cook DJ, Griffith L, et al. The attributable morbidity and mortality of ventilator-associated pneumonia in the critically ill patient. Am J Respir Crit Care Med 1999; 159: 1249–1256.

129. American Thoracic Society. Guidelines for the management of adults with hospital-acquired, ventilator-associated, and healthcare-associated pneumonia. Am J Respir Crit Care Med 2005; 171:388–416.

130. Shorr AF, Kollef MH. Ventilator-associated pneumonia: insights from recent clinical trials. Chest 2005;128:583–591.

131. Cullen DJ, Caldera DL. The incidence of ventilator-induced pulmonary barotraumas in critically ill patients. Anesthesiology 1979; 50:185–190.

132. Downs JB, Chapman RL. Treatment of bronchopleural fistula during continuous positive pressure ventilation. Chest 1976; 63:363–366.

133. Lewis FR Jr, Blaisdell FW, Schlobohm RM. Incidence and outcome of post-traumatic respiratory failure. Arch Surg 1977; 112:436–443.

134. Rohlfing BM, Webb WR, Schlobohm RM, Ventilator-related extra-alveolar air in adults. Radiology 1976; 121:25–31.

135. Chao DC, Scheinhorn DJ. Barotrauma vs volutrauma. Chest 1996; 109(4):1127–1128.

136. Kolobow T. Volutrauma, barotrauma, and ventilator-induced lung injury: lessons learned from the animal research laboratory. Crit Care Med 2004; 32(9):1817–1824.

137. Gajic O, Dara SI, Mendez JL, et al. Ventilator-associated lung injury in patients without acute lung injury at the onset of mechanical ventilation. 2004; 32(9):1817–1824.

138. Pierson DJ. Barotrauma and bronchopleural fistula. In: Tobin MJ, ed. Principles and Practice of Mechanical Ventilation. New York: McGraw-Hill, 2006:945–946.

139. Pilbeam SP. Mechanical Ventilation: Physiological and Clinical Applications. St. Louis: Mosby, 1998:150.

140. Campbell RS, Sinamban RP, Johanningman JA, et al. Clinical evaluation of a new closed loop ventilation mode: adaptive support ventilation. Respir Care 1998; 43(10):856.

141. Thompson JD. Computerized control of mechanical ventilation: closing the loop. Respir Care 1987; 32(6):440–444; discussion 444–446.

142. Branson RD, Johanningman JA, Campbell RS, Davis K. Closed loop mechanical ventilation. Respir Care 2002; 47(4):427.

143. Younes M, Puddy A, Roberts D, et al. Proportional assist ventilation: results of an initial clinical trial. Am Rev Respir Dis 1992; 145(1):121–129.

144. Youmes M. Patient-ventilator interaction with pressure-assisted modalities of ventilatory support. Semin Respir Med 1993; 14:299–322.

145. Ambrosino N, Vitacca M, Polese G, et al. Short-term effects of nasal proportional assist ventilation in patients with chronic hypercapnic respiratory insufficiency. Eur Respir J 1997; 10(12):2829–2834.

146. Iotti G, Braschi A. Closed-loop support of ventilatory workload: the Po.1 controller. Respir Care Clin N Am 2001; 7(3):441–464.

147. Iotti G, Brunner JX, Braschi A, et al. Closed-loop control of airway occlusion pressure at 0.1 second (Po.1) applied to pressure support ventilation: algorithm and application in intubated patients. Crit Care Med 1996; 24(5):771–779.

148. Dojat M, Brochard L, Lemaire F, Harf A. A knowledge based system for assisted ventilation of patients in intensive care units. Int J Clin Monit Comput 1992; 9(24):239–250.

149. Sinderby C, Navalesi P, Beck J, et al. Neural control of mechanical ventilation in respiratory failure. Nat Med 1999; 5(12):1433–1436.

150. Macintyre NR, Branson, RD. Mechanical Ventilation. Philadelphia, PA: W.B. Saunders Company. 2001:58,60,63,69.

151. Macnaughton, PD. New ventilators for the ICU: usefulness of lung performance reporting. Br J Anaesth 2006; 97:57–63.

28

Weaning from Mechanical Ventilation

Ulrike B. Eisenmann, Anushirvan Minokadeh, and William C. Wilson

Department of Anesthesiology and Critical Care, UC San Diego Medical Center, San Diego, California, U.S.A.

INTRODUCTION

Weaning from mechanical ventilation describes the process of progressively reducing mechanical ventilatory support until the patient is entirely capable of performing the work of breathing (WOB) on his/her own. Severely injured and critically ill patients are increasingly dependent upon mechanical ventilation for their survival, and their subsequent weaning from ventilatory support has become increasingly complex. These conditions have evolved from our improved resuscitation capabilities, the increasing complexity of surgical corrective procedures, and the increased baseline comorbidities associated with our aging population (1–7).

The art and science of weaning from mechanical ventilation has continued to evolve since the widespread use of mechanical ventilators for intensive care began in the late 1960s (8,9). Optimization of the weaning process is aimed at diminishing the time on the ventilator, and reducing the adverse complications associated with prolonged mechanical ventilation. Some authors object to the term "weaning" (10–13). Accordingly, Hall and Wood (10) introduced and promoted the term "liberating" from mechanical ventilation. In more recent publications, the term "discontinuing" from mechanical ventilation is increasingly used (14). This chapter will review the important concepts and use the terms weaning, liberating, and discontinuing from mechanical ventilation, interchangeably.

In the simplest terms, ventilatory dependence occurs whenever the WOB exceeds the patient's ability to perform that work. However, there are a host of other factors that may intervene and prolong ventilatory dependence in addition to the simple WOB supply/demand relationship (15–18). The section "Weaning Sequence: Seven-Step Pathway to Extubation" provides an overview of the seven goals that must be achieved to accomplish successful weaning from mechanical ventilation and safe extubation. This section serves as an in-depth overview of the entire process, whereas the subsequent sections review the data supporting the seven-step approach. All major recommendations in this chapter are in concert with the recent American College of Chest Physicians (ACCP)/American Association for Respiratory Care (AARC)/Society of Critical Care Medicine (SCCM) evidence-based guidelines for weaning and discontinuing ventilatory support (18).

WEANING SEQUENCE: SEVEN-STEP PATHWAY TO EXTUBATION

🗡 **The weaning sequence should proceed along a logical stepwise evaluation pathway.** 🗡 The successful achievement of each goal in the pathway leads to the next step in the sequence (Table 1). The first step in the weaning process begins when the clinician judges that the patient's condition has improved, and the underlying disease process (requiring mechanical ventilation) is improving or has resolved (Table 1). The second step is to verify that the patient is free of any intercurrent conditions that might complicate weaning.

Once these first two goals are achieved, the clinician ensures that the patient can oxygenate adequately, defined as being capable of maintaining PaO_2 >60 mmHg on an $FIO_2 \leq 0.4$ with ≤ 5 to 8 cm positive end expiratory pressure (PEEP) (step 3). The fourth and fifth steps (or weaning goals) are the verification that the patient does not have an excessive WOB and that he/she is capable of performing that work. Once these thresholds are met (as demonstrated by various weaning parameters), the clinician must verify that the patient is able to protect his/her airway (step 6). Finally, prior to extubation, a determination is made regarding whether extubation, and possibly reintubation, will be easy or difficult (step 7). If reintubation is expected to be difficult, the trachea should be extubated over an airway exchange catheter (AEC), and/or with a fiberoptic bronchoscope (FOB). Patients with tracheostomies in place need not achieve goals 6 and 7 prior to advancing to tracheostomy collar. Furthermore, many neurologically impaired patients will not be capable of achieving step 6; and some pathologic processes causing tracheal stenosis (or airway swelling) obviate safe breathing through their natural airway. Whenever steps 6 and 7 cannot be safely accomplished, a tracheostomy should be considered.

🗡 **Clinicians should closely review the contributors to respiratory failure at the moment the patient is intubated, and commence optimization of all anticipated impediments to weaning from the beginning.** 🗡 The details of this seven-step process and the weaning goals required to proceed down the pathway from full ventilatory support to weaning and extubation are reviewed below.

Improvement in Primary Disease Process Requiring Ventilatory Support

Without resolving or significantly improving the original disease process that triggered the need for mechanical ventilatory support, it is illogical to expect successful liberation from mechanical ventilation. Assessing the degree to which the patient has improved and adequately reversed the process that required mechanical ventilation involves the interpretation of weaning parameters discussed in this chapter, and an overall application of the art and science of medicine reviewed in other chapters of this textbook.

Table 1   Weaning from Mechanical Ventilation Goals

Weaning goal	Pathophysiologic process requiring normalization	Demonstrated by
1	Reversal/recovery from primary disease causing ARF	Determined by appropriate evaluation
2	Absence of acute processes that may impede weaning	
	Afebrile	Temperature $\leq 38°C$
	Stable hemodynamics	HR and MAP within 20% of baseline with no or minimal vasoactive agents
	Stable metabolism and electrolytes	Laboratory data
3	Oxygenation adequacy demonstrated	$F_IO_2 \leq 0.4$
		PEEP ≤ 5–8 cmH$_2$O
		PaO$_2 \geq 60$ mmHg
		PaO$_2$/F$_I$O$_2 > 150$–200
4	WOB not excessive	$\dot{V}_E < 12$ L/min (70-kg patient)
		$V_D/V_T < 0.6$
		$C_L > 30$ mL/cmH$_2$O
		Absence of wheezing or prolonged exhalation time
5[a]	Demonstrated ability to perform the required WOB	RR < 25 min^{-1} during SBT
		$V_T > 5$ cm^3/kg during SBT
		RSBI < 100 during SBT
		$P_{IMAX} > 25$ cmH$_2$O
		$P_{0.1}$
		$P_{0.1}/P_{IMAX}$
6	Verify patient's ability to protect airway	Awake and following commands
		Intact gag reflex, vigorous cough, empty stomach (relative requirement)
7	Ensure reintubation not anticipated to be difficult	History, exam of airway
		If reintubation is likely difficult, should be extubated with AEC and only after evaluation with FOB

[a]Patients with existing tracheostomies need only to achieve above to goal 5 prior to advancing to a tracheostomy collar. However, the tracheotomy site should be evaluated for maturity, and the ease of tracheostomy recannalization (in the event of cannula dislodgment) should be evaluated.

Abbreviations: AEC, airway exchange catheter; ARF, acute respiratory failure; C_L, compliance; F$_I$O$_2$, inspired fraction of oxygen; FOB, fiber-optic bronchoscope; HR, heart rate; MAP, mean arterial pressure; PaO$_2$, arterial oxygen tension; PEEP, positive end-expiratory pressure; RSBI, rapid shallow breathing index (RR/V_T expressed in Liters); P_{IMAX}, maximum inspiratory pressure; $P_{0.1}$, mouth occlusion pressure; $P_{0.1}/P_{IMAX}$, ratio of mouth occlusion pressure to maximum inspiratory pressure; RR, respiratory rate; SBT, spontaneous breathing trial; V_D/V_t, deadspace to tidal volume ratio; $\dot{V}_E$, minute ventilation; V_T, tidal volume; WOB, work of breathing.

Determining the patient's level of recovery from respiratory failure (Volume 2, Chapter 26) and fitness for weaning requires insight into the underlying process that required mechanical ventilation. Recovery from respiratory failure, resulting from a primary pulmonary event, is generally easier to gauge because only one organ system is involved. Evaluating recovery from respiratory failure that occurred secondary to dysfunction of another organ (e.g., renal failure), or as sequelae of sepsis (Volume 2, Chapter 47), multiple trauma, or the systemic inflammatory response syndrome (Volume 2, Chapter 63), requires both an evaluation of the pulmonary system and a review of the injured organs that initiated the event (14). When multiple organs are injured, the weaning sequence is even more complicated than when failure of only one organ initiated respiratory failure (15–17). In severely ill patients, the duration of weaning may extend for weeks or even months after the primary insult, as multiple systems and the lungs recover.

Absence of Intercurrent Processes that Impede Weaning

Although the patient may have substantially recovered from the primary disease that required mechanical ventilatory support, the physician must also ensure the absence of intercurrent disease processes (e.g., renal failure, or congestive heart failure) that may complicate the primary injury, and doom the weaning process. Similarly, acute disease states that increase the WOB (e.g., sepsis, fever, etc.) or decrease the patient's ability to do that work (e.g., chronic bed rest, muscle wasting, critical illness polyneuropathy, steroid myopathy, malnutrition, etc.) must be addressed and treated prior to expecting any significant progress in weaning. Finally, the patient should be optimized from a respiratory care perspective, receiving nutrition, hemodynamically stable (defined as in a stable rhythm—preferably sinus, and off or on minimal doses of vasoactive drips), as per weaning goal 2 in Table 1.

Adequacy of Oxygenation Demonstrated

☞ The patient is not ready to proceed with weaning until he/she can maintain adequate oxygen saturation, both at rest and with modest exertion (i.e., during weaning). ☞ The generally accepted oxygenation threshold required to safely commence weaning is the demonstrated ability to maintain PaO$_2$/FIO$_2 \geq 150$ to 200; or a PaO$_2 \geq 60$ mmHg (i.e., $> 90\%$ saturation) on an FiO$_2 \leq 0.4$ with a minimal (< 5–8 cmH$_2$O) of PEEP.

The acceptable oxygenation threshold listed in Table 1 (step 3) is far below the normal resting oxygen status of healthy patients. Indeed, normal individuals maintain a PaO$_2$ ranging between 100 and 70 mmHg when breathing room air and not receiving exogenous PEEP. However, because of the immense physiologic reserve within the normal mammalian oxygen delivery system (Volume 2, Chapter 2), these lower oxygenation threshold criteria will generally allow for the provision of adequate oxygenation to tissues during the weaning process. This subnormal threshold of the PaO$_2$/FiO$_2$ ratio is also adequate for supplying tissue oxygenation following extubation, and provides latitude for minor setbacks (e.g., transient atelectasis or fever).

Work of Breathing Is Not Excessive

☞ When the WOB is excessive (Fig. 1), even young and otherwise healthy patients can develop respiratory failure. ☞ Accordingly, an assessment of the WOB must demonstrate that it is not too excessive prior to commencing the weaning process (Table 1, goal 4).

Numerous weaning parameters and clinical measures have been used. These will be thoroughly reviewed in the

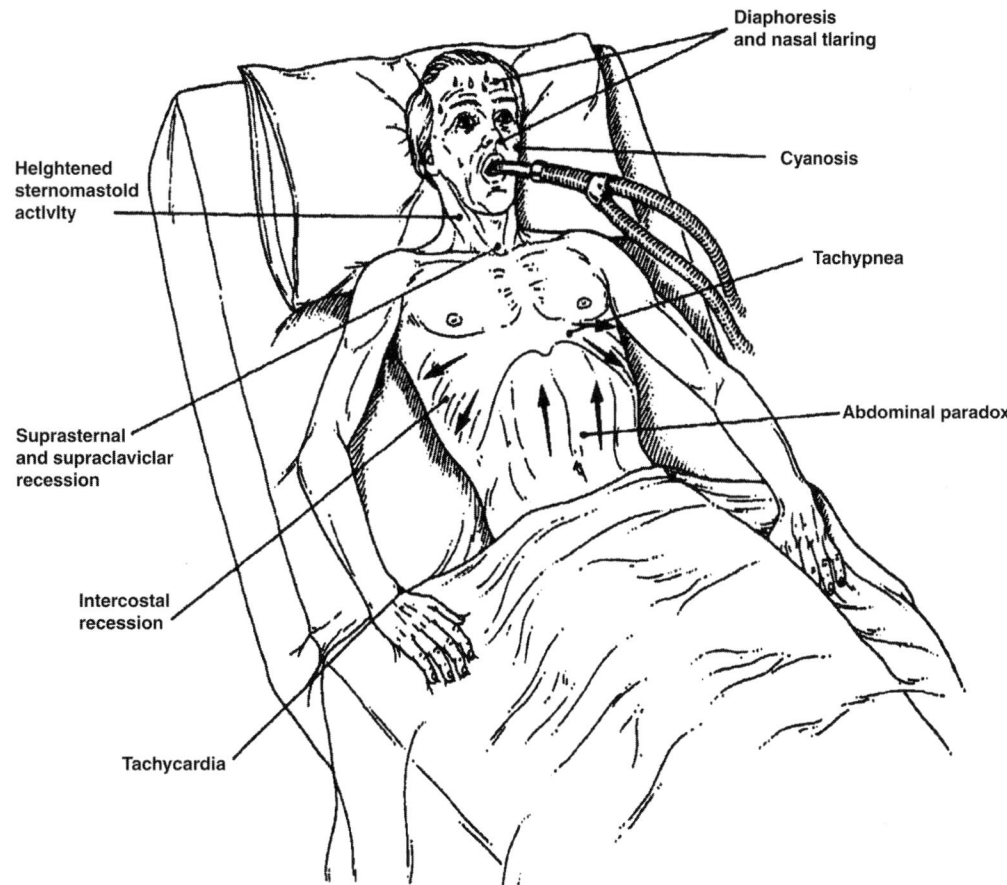

Figure 1 Patient in respiratory distress. Clinical signs include tachypnea (with a rapid shallow breathing pattern), increased accessory muscle (sternocleidomastoid and strap muscle) activity, diaphoresis, nasal flaring, abdominal paradox (especially when spinal cord injury or flail chest present), and when severe, cyanosis may develop (especially when supplemental oxygen is insufficient). *Source*: From Ref. 222.

following section. However, it is useful at this point to identify some of the weaning parameters that specifically assess the WOB [e.g., minute ventilation ($\dot{V}_E$), the dead space to the tidal volume ratio (V_D/V_T), compliance (C_L), airway resistance (R_{AW}), etc.].

To increase the predictive power of weaning parameters, multiple factors should be evaluated (discussed further subsequently). One way to conceptually combine the clinically important parameters reflecting the WOB into a single formula is with the WOB equation:

$$\frac{\dot{V}_E \times R_{AW}}{C_L} = \text{WOB} \qquad (1)$$

The three components of the WOB equation ($\dot{V}_E$, R_{AW}, and C_L) have been defined above. The factors that contribute to altering these fundamental measures of the WOB will be discussed subsequently. The $\dot{V}_E$ for a normal 70-kg patient is approximately 6 L/min. When $\dot{V}_E$ is ≤ 12 L/min, and there are minimal additional coincident factors known to increase the WOB (e.g., wheezing, chest wall stiffness, etc.), patients with normal strength should be considered weanable. The normal V_D/V_T is approximately 0.3; when it is ≥ 0.6, patients are seldom weanable due to the excessive WOB. The $\dot{V}_E$ is comprised of both alveolar ventilation ($\dot{V}_A$) and dead space ventilation ($\dot{V}_D$). Accordingly, the V_D/V_T does not need to be specifically measured unless the $\dot{V}_E$ is extremely elevated especially in the absence of

fever, obvious hypermetabolism, or overfeeding (Volume 2, Chapter 31). R_{AW} is normally negligible. However, patients with reactive airway disease, COPD, bronchitis, or a current cold will have an increased R_{AW} reflected in the clinical exam as wheezing. Similarly, kinks in the ET, or inspissated secretions on the endotracheal tube (ETT) may increase the R_{AW}. Ventilated patients demonstrating a large increase in the peak airway pressure compared to the plateau pressure on volume control ventilation reflect significantly increased R_{AW}. Those ventilated on the pressure control mode will show a decreased in tidal volume at any set inhalation pressure when the R_{AW} is elevated. The clinical exam should reveal the absence of bronchospasm or wheezing indicating R_{AW} is negligible, prior to commencing a trial of weaning.

The C_L is defined as a change in volume divided by a change in pressure (typically expressed as mL air/cmH$_2$O). The normal C_L is >80 mL/cmH$_2$O; however, following trauma, resuscitation, and critical care, C_L is often decreased (especially in the setting of lung injury). The lower the C_L, the greater the WOB. When the C_L is <30 mL/cmH$_2$O, the WOB is often too great to allow weaning from mechanical ventilation unless the patient is also very fit.

Ability to Perform the Work of Breathing Demonstrated

Once the patient's WOB has been evaluated and determined to be "reasonable" (i.e., not so high that weaning is impractical), the next goal is to determine if the patient can perform the required work (Table 1, weaning goal 5). The easiest way to assess this is by having the patient perform a spontaneous breathing trial (SBT). For example, place the patient on a T-piece or on a continuous positive airway pressure (CPAP) of 5 cmH$_2$O, without or with minimal (i.e., 5 cmH$_2$O) of pressure support, and assess if he/she can do the WOB.

The most clinically useful (and predictive) weaning parameter used at the beginning and end of an SBT is the rapid shallow breathing index (RSBI), defined as the respiratory rate (RR) (expressed in breaths/min) divided by the tidal volume (V_T) (expressed in liters) (9,13,18). Other weaning parameters have less predictive power, but are still instructive in determining why a patient may have a high RSBI during an SBT. Some of the more commonly employed weaning parameters are the maximum inspiratory pressure (P_{IMAX}), also known as the maximum inspiratory force (MIF), both are typically expressed as negative cmH$_2$O pressure; the vital capacity (VC), expressed either as mL or L; and the maximal voluntary ventilation (MVV) previously known as the maximal breathing capacity. The MVV is determined by asking the patient to perform their maximal $\dot{V}_E$ for 12 to 30 seconds. The threshold goal is achieved if the patient can breathe twice their baseline $\dot{V}_E$ for the entire 12- to 30-second duration. Patients able to accomplish this MVV goal demonstrate that they possess significant cardiopulmonary reserve, and are more likely to tolerate weaning.

Airway Protection Intact and Reintubation Difficulties Fully Evaluated

After the patient meets all of the criteria for weaning from mechanical ventilation (Table 1, goals 1–5), the clinician must verify that the patient can safely have their trachea extubated by fulfilling goal 6 (demonstrating ability to protect their airway) and goal 7 (verification that reintubation is not anticipated to be difficult). If the patient has a pre-existing tracheostomy, then after fulfillment of goal 5, the patient may advance to tracheal collar. Conversely, if the patients cannot fulfill goals 6 and 7, a tracheotomy is often warranted (discussed in the tracheostomy section).

The ability to protect one's airway (Table 1, goal 6) is demonstrated by verifying: (*i*) the patient is awake and follows commands and (*ii*) that the patient has an intact gag and cough [sensory limb of the reflex is mediated by cranial nerve (CN) IX, and motor response is mediated by CN X]. As an additional margin of safety, it is best to ensure that the patient has an essentially empty stomach at the time of extubation (in case reintubation is required). For example, tube feeds should be held two to six hours prior to extubation. Patients at high risk for aspiration (i.e., those with altered mental status) should have tube feeds held the full six hours prior to extubation. Note that high gastric outputs (≥ 1500 cm^3/day) from a nasogastric or orogastric tube represent a relative contraindication to extubation (Table 1, goal 6), because the relative gastric outlet obstruction increases the patient's risk of regurgitation and aspiration, and is a sign that pathological processes are not fully resolved.

The final hurdle to be cleared, prior to extubation of the trachea, is determining if the airway would be difficult to reintubate urgently. For example, if the patient was a difficult intubation preop, or has a halo in place for cervical immobilization postop, he/she would be considered difficult to reintubate using conventional means (i.e., direct laryngoscopy). When the airway is anticipated to be difficult to

reintubate, extubation should occur over an AEC as described in greater detail in "The Patient is Weaned, Can the Trachea Be Safely Extubated?" and more fully in Volume 2, Chapter 29. Additionally, in situations where airway swelling has been problematic (e.g., following neck surgery/trauma), the vocal cords and supraglottic structures should be evaluated with an FOB prior to and during extubation.

WEANING PARAMETERS: WHICH ARE PREDICTIVE?

Weaning parameters are bedside tests developed to assess the patient's readiness to be weaned from mechanical ventilation. **Some weaning parameters reflect the WOB that must be performed by the patient (e.g., $\dot{V}_E$, C_L, R_{AW}), whereas others reflect the patient's ability to perform that work (e.g., MIF, VC, RSBI).** When properly performed and interpreted, weaning parameters help in the decision-making process to liberate the patient from the ventilator (15). Since the introduction of artificial ventilation, weaning parameters have been developed and modified. The early parameters included simple measures of ventilation status, such as RR and V_T (while breathing spontaneously), as well as the VC and MIF (16,17). Over the last 40 years, more than 60 weaning parameters have been evaluated (18,19).

When clinical researchers investigate the statistical relationship between weaning parameter results and the success of weaning, the data for each weaning parameter threshold can be plotted in a 2 × 2 table (Table 2). Chi-square analysis can be applied to the data in order to assess the statistical significance of the association between the weaning parameter and the success or failure of weaning. It is also useful to express the data in ways that are clinically relevant in order to communicate the results in a consistent manner. In this regard, the definitions summarized in Table 2 have been developed.

A true positive is a patient who achieves a positive result on the weaning parameter (at some threshold set by the researcher), and successfully weans from mechanical ventilation. A false positive is a patient who achieves a positive result on the weaning parameter (at a given threshold), but does not successfully wean. A true negative is a patient who fails to achieve the threshold weaning parameter value, and also fails to wean from mechanical ventilation. A false negative is a patient who fails to achieve the threshold weaning parameter value, but actually does successfully wean.

Table 2 Comparing Weaning Parameter Results with Success of Weaning Using a 2 × 2 Table

		Weaning	
		Success	Failure
Weaning	Positive	True positive	False positive
parameter result	Negative	False negative	True negative

Sensitivity = True Positives/(True Positives + False Negatives).
Specificity = True Negatives/(False Positives + True Negatives).
Positive Predictive Value = True Positives/(True Positives + False Positives).
Negative Predictive Value = True Negatives/(True Negatives + False Negatives).
Accuracy = (True Positives + True Negatives)/(True Positives + False Positives + True Negatives + False Negatives).

Sensitivity is the probability that a weaning parameter test is positive given that the person actually weans successfully. Sensitivity is also known as the true positive rate. Specificity is the probability that a weaning parameter test is negative given that the person fails to wean from mechanical ventilation. Specificity is also known as the true negative rate (Table 2).

The positive predictive value is the probability that a person successfully weans given a positive weaning parameter result is achieved at some threshold. The negative predictive value is the probability that a person fails weaning given a negative weaning parameter result is achieved. Accuracy, the most important statistical measure, reflects the combined positive and negative predictive values (Table 2).

When reviewing clinical trials that purport to compare various weaning parameters with the success of weaning, only those studies that provide a 2 × 2 table of the data should be trusted. The remainder (unfortunately most studies) are less useful in terms of providing meaningful data that can be compared with your own practice, or with other studies. A review of the clinically employed weaning parameters is provided in the following sections.

No Weaning Parameter Is Perfect—Most Are Useful

None of the clinically available weaning parameters are perfect; they all have their drawbacks. However, most are useful in clinical practice, and they tend to be complementary (Table 3) (20–62). The best weaning parameters are those that are easy to measure, can be obtained at the bedside, and have the greatest predictive power (63).

Unfortunately, no single weaning parameter test yields 100% accuracy. The reason for the imperfect predictive power of weaning parameters is that: (*i*) numerous factors are involved in ventilatory dependence (steps 1–5, Table 1), (*ii*) no single weaning parameter reflects all these factors, and (*iii*) clinicians have often already considered the weaning parameter results prior to selecting patients for trials of weaning (9,18).

Weaning parameters should only be used as supportive tests to bolster the clinical appraisal, and should never be used as a substitute for clinical judgment (64). If the clinical picture does not support the weaning parameter data reported by respiratory therapists (RTs), then either the data is flawed or the clinical picture has changed from when the weaning parameters were obtained. In this setting, it is best to carefully reassess the situation, and either obtain the parameters oneself, or ask the RT to obtain them while the clinician is present at the bedside. Finally, if the clinician habitually relies on only one weaning parameter to decide likelihood of weaning success, errors will inevitably occur. It is far better to obtain several weaning parameters to improve the overall predictive power. It is also important to clearly understand the data being obtained; some weaning parameters reflect an increased WOB, whereas others demonstrate a decreased ability to do that work (as explained earlier).

Survey of Traditional Weaning Parameters

This section reviews all the commonly employed weaning parameters from the perspective of both "normal" and

Table 3 Commonly Used Weaning Parameters

Parameter	Typical threshold required	Element evaluated
SaO_2 on $F_IO_2 = 0.4$	>90%	Oxygenation
PaO_2/F_IO_2	>300–350 mmHg	Oxygenation
$\dot{Q}_s/\dot{Q}_t$	<20%	Oxygenation (as reflected in right-to-left transpulmonary shunt)
$\dot{V}_E$	≤12 L/min (70 kg)	Demand component of WOB
C_L	>40 mL/cmH$_2$O	Demand component of WOB
R_{AW}	Absence of bronchospasm Minimal P_{PK} vs. P_{PL} difference	Demand component of WOB
V_D/V_T	<0.6	Demand component of WOB
MIF or P_{IMAX}	≤−20 cmH$_2$O (if thin with compliant lung)[a] ≤−35 if the C_L is decreased	Strength
VC	≥15 mL/kg	Strength/C_L
$P_{0.1}$	≤−5 cmH$_2$O	Strength of respiratory fitness
$P_{0.1}/P_{IMAX}$	<0.09 (see text for details)	Strength and respiratory fitness
RR	≤35 breaths/min	Ability to tolerate the WOB
V_T	≥5 mL/kg	A measure of strength/C_L, and ability to tolerate the WOB
RSBI	RR (breaths/min)/V_T (L) ≤100	Ability to perform the WOB
CROP	>13 (incorporates multiple factors)	Oxygenation and WOB
MVV	>2 × $\dot{V}_E$ for 12–30 sec	Measure of ventilatory reserve
$\dot{V}_E$ recov time	<3–5 min	Measure of ventilatory reserve

[a]The MIF is a negative number; the more negative the number the stronger the patient.

Abbreviations: C_L, compliance; CROP, index composed of C_L; F_IO_2, inspired fraction of oxygen; MIF, maximal inspiration force; MVV, maximum voluntary ventilation; PaO$_2$, arterial oxygen tension; $P_{0.1}$, mouth occlusion pressure (maximum inspiratory pressure 0.1 sec after airway occlusion); $P_{0.1}/P_{IMAX}$, ratio of $P_{0.1}$ to P_{IMAX}; P_{IMAX}, maximal inspiratory pressure; $\dot{Q}_s/\dot{Q}_t$, right-to-left transpulmonary shunt; R_{AW}, airway resistance; RR, respiratory rate; RSBI, rapid shallow breathing index (RR/V_T expressed in Liters); SaO$_2$, oxygen saturation; VC, vital capacity; V_D, dead space; $\dot{V}_E$, minute ventilation; V_T, tidal volume; WOB, work of breathing.

"acceptable" values; recognizing that "acceptable" values almost always reflect a level of function far below "normal." The first parameter most often assessed clinically is the RR. A normal, healthy, nonintubated 70-kg adult at rest has an RR of 12 to 14 breaths/min. However, the general acceptable threshold for a patient weaning from mechanical ventilation is an RR of 30 to 35 (9,18). This upper limit of 30 to 35 is a threshold that makes sense for otherwise healthy adults, but will have variable predictive power in other patient populations. Indeed, stable, nonintubated patients with pulmonary fibrosis (a restrictive lung disease) often have a baseline RR in the 20 to 30 range. A patient without any previous underlying lung disease presenting with a resting RR above 30 likely represents acute respiratory failure (14). The RR is also age dependent; a newborn's normal RR ranges from 30 to 40, and rates above 60 to 80 are required to represent respiratory failure in this population (65). Similarly, temporarily hypermetabolic patients will have an expected increased $\dot{V}_E$ (66,67).

The RR can be normalized to some degree by adding the patient's V_T, as occurs with the RSBI (RR/V_T in liters). When the RSBI is <50 at the end of a two-hour SBT, patients are almost always capable of being weaned from the ventilator. When the RSBI is >100 to 105, they often are incapable of being liberated from mechanical ventilation (but what about the patients with RSBI in between?). Many weaning trials have used an RSBI threshold of 100 to 105, and thus do not have perfect predictive power (9,18). If the predictive threshold were decreased to the 50 to 65 range for the RSBI, then the positive predictive value would increase dramatically, but the negative predictive value would suffer (i.e., many patients who could actually tolerate weaning would still be receiving mechanical ventilation). Conversely, increasing the RSBI threshold to some number >105 would increase the negative predictive value (i.e., few patients with higher indices would tolerate extubation), but the positive predictive value would be lower (i.e., many patients with RSBI just below the 105 threshold would fail to tolerate extubation).

The MIF, also known as the maximum inspiratory pressure (P_{IMAX}), or negative inspiratory force, has been evaluated as a weaning parameter in many studies with variable predictive results (68–71). A healthy female can create an MIF of at least $-90\,cmH_2O$, a male can generate less than $-120\,cmH_2O$. Various clinical trials use different thresholds from $-15\,cmH_2O$ to $-50\,cmH_2O$ depending upon the average C_L and WOB of the study population.

Accordingly, simple comparisons between studies are challenging. One study demonstrated an accuracy of 66% for medical and cardiac intensive care patients capable of achieving a P_{IMAX} less negative than $-20\,cmH_2O$ (38). A 71% accuracy was achieved in a multidisciplinary intensive care unit (ICU) (including trauma and surgical patients) but required a P_{IMAX} of less than $-50\,cmH_2O$ (72).

The maximum negative pressure in the first 0.1 second ($P_{0.1}$), with a threshold of $<-5\,cmH_2O$ is listed with an accuracy of 88%, specificity of 91%, and negative predictive value of 96% for multidisciplinary patients. However, this measurement is not readily available in most modern ICUs today (72).

The VC is determined in most ICUs before extubation with a commonly accepted threshold of 10–15 mL/kg. A healthy person generates a VC of approximately 70 mL/kg (5000 mL for a 70-kg adult). Accordingly, the minimum acceptable VC for weaning is far below the "normal" value achievable in healthy patients. The lower 10–5 mL/kg "threshold" value is often acceptable because of the

enormous reserve in the mammalian respiratory system. The 10–15 mL/kg VC target (like all weaning parameter thresholds) is a relative number, only adequate if the patient is not debilitated in areas other than those reflected in this one weaning predictor. Inability to generate the minimum acceptable VC can result from (*i*) a very noncompliant thorax or lungs and (*ii*) significant respiratory to muscle weakness. In either case, successful discontinuation from mechanical support is unlikely, and obtaining other weaning parameters (e.g., MIF, C_L) will help explain the etiology problem.

A V_T of 6–8 mL/kg is required to maintain sufficient ventilation in a normal, spontaneously breathing patient. In ICU patients recovering from trauma and critical illness, breathing spontaneously (T-piece or C-PAP), a reasonable threshold is 4–6 mL/kg. Naturally, the RR will need to increase in patients with lower than normal V_T in order to maintain the $\dot{V}_E$ required to exhale the normal CO_2 produced.

Note that this V_T threshold is not as predictive when one is interrogating the muscle strength, and relative reversal from neuromuscular blockade drugs; in this setting, V_T measurements are not nearly as predictive as measuring the VC or evaluating a five-second head lift in a patient (Chapter 48).

Minute ventilation ($\dot{V}_E$) is one of the most commonly used weaning parameters, because it is easily obtainable with today's ventilators and serves as a gross measure of respiratory status. However, when taken in isolation, without clinical correlation, $\dot{V}_E$ will not be as predictive (64). It is influenced by numerous clinical conditions like body weight, age (65), postoperative hypermetabolic state (66), and nutrition (67). The $\dot{V}_E$ is, therefore, listed with a wide range of acceptable upper limits (10–15 L/min), and corresponding accuracies are lower than those resulting from other weaning parameters (62% for $\dot{V}_E \leq 10$ L/min) (38).

The ratio of mouth occlusion pressure in the first 0.1 second to maximum inspiratory pressure ($P_{0.1}/P_{IMAX}$) is a very accurate weaning parameter, in the setting of close experimental observations (Fig. 2). A $P_{0.1}/P_{IMAX}$ ratio below 0.09 predicted successful extubation with a very high accuracy in one study (72). The authors explained these results based on ventilatory pattern changes being different in health and disease. Patients with imminent respiratory failure tend to take quick shallow breaths, as if gasping for air, which is reflected by a $P_{0.1}/P_{IMAX}$ ratio of >0.09. This test detected successful weaning in a group of multidisciplinary critical care patients with an accuracy of 98%, PPV of 100%, and NPV of 92% (73).

Greater accuracy occurs when more than one weaning parameter is used to predict success. A formal approach by Yang and Tobin to further combine indices resulted in the index composed of C_L, RR, oxygenation, and pressure (CROP) index (73). This acronym integrates dynamic compliance C, respiratory rate R, oxygenation (P_aO_2/P_AO_2), and maximum inspiratory pressure P_{IMAX}. The higher the CROP index, the higher the likelihood of successful weaning (73).

The Rapid Shallow Breathing Index May Be the Single Most Useful Weaning Parameter

☞ The RSBI is the most widely used weaning parameter, because it is easy to obtain, predictive, and illustrative; patients failing to wean develop a breathing pattern characterized by small tidal volumes and increased RRs. ☞ In clinical practice, an RSBI of >100 usually predicts

Predictive Accuracy of
Weaning Parameters

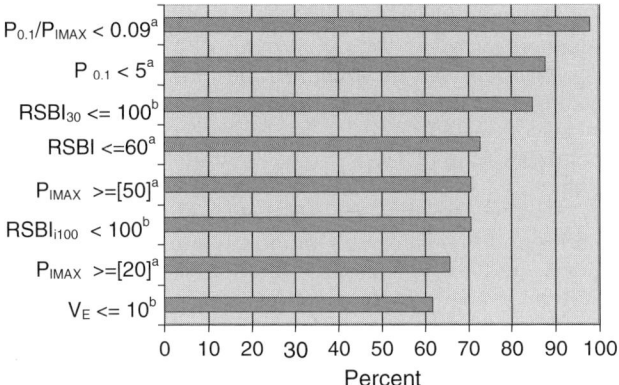

Figure 2 Predictive accuracy of weaning parameters: from highest accuracy (*top*) to lowest accuracy (*bottom*) in percent. *Abbreviations*: $P_{0.1}/P_{IMAX}^{a}$, mouth occlusion pressure to maximum inspiratory pressure; $P_{0.1}^{a}$, mouth occlusion pressure (cmH$_2$O); $RSBI_{30}^{b}$, RSBI after 30 minutes breathing begin; $RSBI^{a}$, rapid shallow breathing index (breaths/min/L); $P_{IMAX}50^{a}$, maximum inspiratory pressure >50 cmH$_2$O; $RSBI_i 100^{b}$, initial RSBI <100; $P_{IMAX}20^{a}$, maximum inspiratory pressure >20 cmH$_2$O; $\dot{V}_E^{b}$, minute ventilation (cmH$_2$O). *Source*: [a]Multidisciplinary patient group (72). [b]M/CICU patient group (38).

failure, and when this threshold was used the accuracy of predicting a weaning success was only 71% in MICU/CCU patients (38,74). A better prediction results when the RSBI is evaluated after 30 minutes of CPAP breathing ($RSBI_{30}$), using a threshold of 100; the $RSBI_{30}$ results in an accuracy of 85% in the same patient group. If the threshold were lowered to the 50 to 65 range, the RSBI would predict nearly 100% of patients that could be safely weaned to extubation, but (as discussed earlier) would result in far too many patients remaining ventilated who could tolerate weaning to extubation despite having RSBI >65.

The RSBI only scored higher than the $P_{0.1}/P_{IMAX}$ for the negative predictive value in medical/cardiac ICU patients (73,75). However, as we have discussed above, some of the differences in predictive power result from the threshold values chosen. If the experimentally derived statistical significance were the only important factor for predicting weaning success, then the arcane and cumbersome to measure $P_{0.1}/P_{IMAX}$ ratio would be widely utilized (in some studies, the $P_{0.1}/P_{IMAX}$ accuracy approaches 98–100%). However, the practical clinical realities require ease of use and reproducibility.

The RSBI is easy to obtain, and its use provides additional information beyond a calculated number (i.e., a description of the patient's ventilatory status during SBT). Accordingly, the RSBI should be considered the single most useful weaning parameter. However, the threshold number used will determine the predictive power. A patient could have an RSBI of less than 100, the commonly used threshold, and still not be ready for extubation (other factors must always be considered). An RSBI less than 50 almost always successfully predicts a patient's ability to be weaned to extubation. The threshold value chosen by the clinician will markedly alter the predictive power of any given weaning parameter.

Evaluating weaning parameters obtained by the RT results in an incomplete interpretation of data available from the patient. The clinician should be physically present at the bedside during at least part of any SBT that is being used to determine a patient's fitness for weaning to extubation. The absence or presence of signs and symptoms of respiratory distress communicated through facial expressions, restlessness, perspiration, or hemodynamic changes all serve to supplement the weaning parameter data (in this case the RSBI), and helps the clinician determine the patient's likelihood of tolerating weaning (Fig. 1) (75,76).

Greatest Success Occurs When Multiple Parameters Are Combined with Clinical Judgment

Any of the single weaning parameters used in isolation will result in many errors in management. Accordingly, multiple parameters should be used (according to Bayes's theorem). Furthermore, when the decision to remove an ETT from a patient recovering from respiratory failure is complicated, clinical judgment that incorporates all aspects of the patient's condition and progress is required. The acquisition and interpretation of multiple weaning parameters provide the supplemental information needed by the clinician to formulate the weaning decision-making process (64,77).

WEANING STRATEGIES: WHICH ONE IS BEST?

There are nearly as many weaning strategies as there are intensivists (8–13). Patients, who are not sick, rarely require weaning evaluation and may not need any special strategies (Table 4). However, patients who are debilitated

Table 4 Strategies Employed to Facilitate Weaning

Weaning strategy	How accomplished/ comments	Likelihood of expediting weaning success
SBT	Patient placed on a T-piece or CPAP, ± supplementation with PSV and evaluated for 30–120 min; optimum duration of SBT varies with patient condition	Generally considered to be as good as any other weaning strategy
SIMV	Stepwise reduction in SIMV set rate until a set rate of 2 is achieved; SIMV set rate usually decreased 2–4 breaths/ min every 12 hr	Generally considered the slowest strategy of weaning
PSV	Stepwise reduction in driving pressure until a threshold of <5– 8 cmH$_2$O is achieved; the driving pressure is usually decreased every 2–4 breaths/min every 12 hr	In some patients, PSV may facilitate weaning

Abbreviations: CPAP, continuous positive airway pressure; PSV, pressure support ventilation; SBT, spontaneous breathing trial; SIMV, synchronized intermittent mandatory ventilation.

and recovering from critical illness often need some time to both decrease their WOB (through healing) and to increase their strength (through exercise) (4). The WOB is increased following trauma and critical illness secondary to decreased C_L of the lungs and chest wall, increased V_D/V_T, and increased R_{AW}.

Spontaneous Breathing Trial

During an SBT, the physician evaluates the patient's ability to breathe on his or her own (i.e., spontaneously) (78). To accomplish this, the patient is placed either on a T-piece or on the CPAP mode, typically set at 5 cmH$_2$O PEEP, and supplemented with 5–10 cmH$_2$O pressure support (Table 4) (79,80). The term "T-piece" stems from its shape. One arm of the T-shaped piece connects to the ETT, one arm connects to the fresh gas flow, and the third arm serves as the exhalation limb of the apparatus. The exhalation tubing should be at least 25 cm long to prevent entrainment of room air, and the fresh gas flow should equal at least twice the patient's spontaneous minute ventilation to eliminate rebreathing.

Although the patient performs the SBT, the RR, ventilatory pattern, and breathing efforts are closely monitored along with the SpO$_2$, pulse rate, and blood pressure. RRs of 25 to 35 per minute are considered acceptable as long as the rate remains stable, the patient appears comfortable, and there is no deterioration in other parameters.

Most SBTs are now performed using the CPAP mode with the patient still connected to the ventilator apparatus. Advantages of this setup include the collection of more complete and continuous monitoring of many parameters, including tidal volume, RR, and minute ventilation, as well as ease of transition from baseline ventilatory support to the SBT.

☞ **Resistance created by the ETT, ventilator tubing, and circuit valves can be overcome by the addition of a minimal amount (i.e., 5 cmH$_2$O) of pressure support.** ☜ Insufficient pressure support will result in increased WOB due to the high resistance of the relatively narrow ETTs (79,80). Too much pressure support augments the patient's spontaneous volumes and will cause a false-positive result during the SBT. The formula for determining airway resistance experienced by a patient on mechanical ventilation is shown in the airway resistance equation:

$$R_{AW} = \frac{P_{PK} - P_{PL}}{V_{INSP}} \qquad (2)$$

where R_{AW} is the airway resistance, P_{PK} the peak inspiratory pressure, P_{PL} the plateau pressure, and V_{INSP} the inspiratory flow rate delivered with the breath. However, the R_{AW} equation includes the resistance of the entire system (ETT, trachea, bronchi, distal airways, etc.). The pressure support level required to counterbalance the resistive workload imposed by a narrow ETT varies widely (3–14 cmH$_2$O) and cannot be easily measured noninvasively (79).

Historically, SBTs have been performed when the patient was deemed ready to be separated from ventilatory support (78). They can also be used as an intermittent assessment of the progress made in a patient's recovery from respiratory failure (78,81,82). Esteban et al. (82,83) showed that SBTs alternated with the assist control ventilation mode led to faster weaning when compared with pressure support ventilation (PSV) or synchronized intermittent mandatory ventilation (SIMV) weaning. Interestingly, there was no difference in time to extubation whether SBTs were performed only once a day or multiple times per day. As both weaning methods were equally fast, the advantage of using only one SBT per day derived from saving time and human resources.

The optimal duration of the SBT for predicting weaning success is unclear because no large randomized, controlled trials (RCTs) exist. The Spanish Lung Failure Collaborative Group (83) reported a 30-minute trial to be just as effective as a two-hour trial in predicting weaning outcome (84). However, in debilitated patients who need to build muscles and ventilatory endurance, two to three SBTs per day of gradually increasing duration is more likely to result in strength training (RCTs are needed to verify). Some ICUs refer to these SBT exercise periods as "sprints" invoking the sports analogy, and a connotation that training of muscle strength and endurance is occurring.

Ultimately, the benefits of a regimented weaning strategy derived not just from the training of the respiratory muscles, but also from the organized process of exercise and progress monitoring (leading to earlier recognition of patients who are ready to be discontinued from mechanical ventilation) (84).

Synchronized Intermittent Mandatory Ventilation Weaning

The SIMV mode of MV was described in Chapter 69. In SIMV weaning, the goal is a step-by-step reduction in mechanical support, promoting the patient's own ventilatory efforts (and strength), by sequentially decreasing the number of machine delivered breaths (Table 4). The initial set rate is progressively decreased until a rate of 2 to 4 breaths/min is achieved. The stepwise decrease in SIMV set rate typically occurs at intervals of 2 to 4 breaths/min every 12 hours, as tolerated and monitored by various parameters (i.e., the RSBI). The patient is evaluated at each level of ventilatory support, both clinically and with the use of weaning parameters, and laboratory data (i.e., arterial blood gas). The patient is considered successfully weaned and ready to evaluate for extubation if he/she is tolerating an SIMV rate of ≤2 to 4 breaths/min for at least 120 minutes. Note that Brochard et al. (85) and Esteban et al. (82) used an SIMV endpoint of 4 to 5 breaths/min for their definition of success (Tables 4 and 5). Some investigations require 24 hours of tolerating ≤4 breaths/min SIMV before meeting the weaning criteria for success (85). Pressure support (5 cmH$_2$O) may be added to overcome the resistance created by the ventilator tubing and valves in the circuit during the spontaneous breaths.

One of the disadvantages of both SIMV weaning and T-piece weaning is the absence of automatic adjustments for changes in a patient's ventilatory demands (i.e., there is no compensation if the patient's minute ventilation declines). This implies that the patient cannot be left unattended during SIMV (or T-piece) weaning. SIMV weaning was initially promoted to prevent the patient from "fighting" the ventilator, decreasing the need for sedation, and reducing the likelihood of weaning fatigue. So far, no study has proven any of these claims or shown superiority of SIMV weaning over any other modes (82,85–87).

Pressure Support Ventilation Weaning

As previewed above, PSV augments a spontaneous breath through a set amount of positive pressure, usually 5–20 cmH$_2$O during inspiration. The PSV mode is a ventilation package, which is pressure triggered and flow cycled. In addition, the pressure, flow, and volume profiles mimic the pressure control mode during the inhalation flow period (PSV is fully described in Volume 2, Chapter 27) (88–91).

Weaning with PSV usually begins by titrating the pressure support so that the patient starts with a reasonable RSBI (i.e., between 50 and 100), and is accomplished by reducing the pressure support gradually in 2–4 cmH$_2$O decrements every 12 hours (Table 4) (82,85). Weaning is generally considered successful if the patient is tolerating a pressure support level of <5–8 cmH$_2$O for ≥30 to 120 minutes, confirmed by adequate weaning parameters and blood gases at the end of the SBT. In a prospective, randomized controlled study, Brochard et al. (85) demonstrated PSV weaning to be faster and more successful than T-piece or SIMV weaning. However, Esteban et al. (82) failed to demonstrate any particular advantage of PSV weaning. A comparison of the Brochard and Esteban studies is provided in Table 5. Some patients tend to tolerate PSV weaning well, and for these individuals it remains a viable weaning methodology.

Weaning Strategy Hybrids

Most intensivists currently use hybrids of the above weaning strategies (92). For example, regardless of which weaning plan is followed (once or twice a day SBTs, SIMV, or PSV), PSV is often added to compensate for the extra WOB caused by the R_{AW} of the ETT during spontaneous ventilatory efforts.

Microprocessors have increased the variety of ventilation modes available both during ventilatory support and weaning from respiratory failure (Volume 2, Chapter 27) (93,94). For example, airway pressure release ventilation

(APRV) has been developed for augmentation of alveolar ventilation (95). Modes have also been developed to adapt to a patient's change in respiratory support, like pressure-assisted ventilation (PAV) (96), automatic tube compensation (ATC) (97–103), adaptive support ventilation (ASV) (104–106), and adaptive lung ventilation (ALV) (107).

Modes purely used for ventilation of ARDS patients, such as time cycled pressure control inverse ratio ventilation (TCPCIRV), have been developed. These advanced modes add another layer of complexity to weaning because they require a transition from this aggressive level of support back to conventional mechanical ventilation before classical weaning can commence. To tolerate the TCPCIRV mode, patients require a deep level of sedation and usually neuromuscular blockade, underscoring the complexity of weaning from the TCPCIRV mode. Other options to modify oxygenation and ventilation in ARDS patients are numerous, and are fully reviewed in Volume 2, Chapter 27 (108–111).

Summarizing Weaning Mode Trials

Three commonly applied modes of weaning a patient from ventilatory support have emerged: the SBT, where either CPAP or T-piece is utilized; SIMV; and pressure support (PSV) weaning. All three modes employ a stepwise reduction in ventilatory support as described above. Similarly, all three modes can be referred to as "sprints" when used to exercise debilitated, difficult-to-wean patients.

The literature offers hundreds of studies focusing on weaning, however, none have been conducted with sufficient power to provide a definitive answer. Only a few studies have been designed well enough to begin answering

Table 5 Comparison of Brochard and Esteban Trials that Examined Pressure Supported Ventilation vs. Synchronized Intermittent Mandatory Ventilation vs. Spontaneous Breathing Trial Strategies of Weaning

	Brochard et al. (85)	Esteban et al. (82)
Number of patients screened	456	546
Number of patients randomized	109	130
Duration of MV before randomization	14 days	9 days
Starting condition	PSV—titrates to RR = 20–30 SIMV—half of AC rate T-piece 5–60 min as tolerated	PSV—titrates to RR ≤25 SIMV—half of AC rate T-piece as tolerated
Protocol	PSV: ↓ by 2–4 cmH$_2$O, twice a day SIMV: ↓ by 2–4 breaths/min, twice a day T-piece: progressively increase to 2 hr	PSV: ↓ by 2–4 cmH$_2$O, twice a day SIMV: ↓ by 2–4 breaths/min, twice a day T-piece (once): as tolerated up to 2 hr T-piece (multiple): T-piece or CPAP 5 cmH$_2$O as tolerated multiple times per day (up to 2 hr per trial)
Criteria for success	PSV: 8 cmH$_2$O for 24 hr SIMV: 4 breaths/min for 24 hr T-piece: 2 hr (1–3 times/24 hr)	PSV: 5 cmH$_2$O for 2 hr SIMV: 5 breaths/min for 2 hr T-piece: 2 hr (once/24 hr)
Definition of failure	Unweaned at 21 days	Unweaned at 14 days
Results	PSV decreased percentage of patients with weaning failure (23% vs. T-piece 43%, SIMV 42%) Shorter mean duration of weaning with PSV (5.7 days) compared with pooled T-piece and SIMV patients (9.3 days)	Weaning failure: once daily T-piece (29%), multiple daily T-piece (18%), PSV (38%), SIMV (31%) Shorter mean duration of weaning with T-piece, once (3 days) and T-piece (3 days) compared with PSV (4 days) and SIMV (5 days)

Abbreviations: AC, assist control; CPAP, continuous positive airway pressure; MV, mechanical ventilation; PSV, pressure-supported ventilation; RR, respiratory rate; SIMV, synchronized intermittent mandatory ventilation.

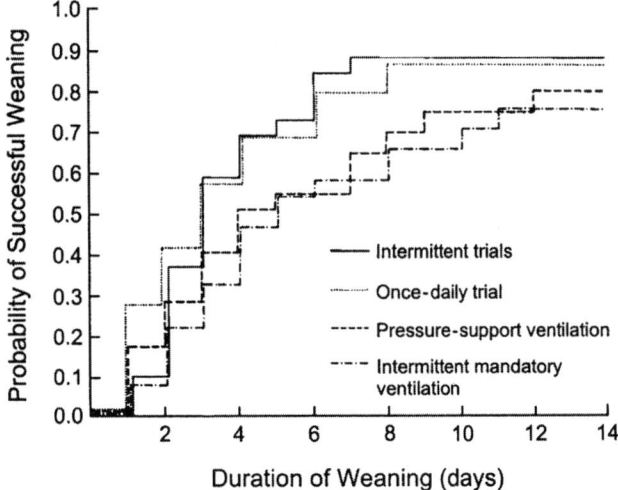

Figure 3 Kaplan–Meier curves of the probability of successful weaning with intermittent mandatory ventilation, pressure support ventilation, intermittent trials of spontaneous breathing, and once-daily trial of spontaneous breathing. Demonstrating once-daily trials at least as good as any other modality. *y*-axis: probability of successful weaning; *x*-axis: duration of weaning (days). *Source*: From Ref. 82.

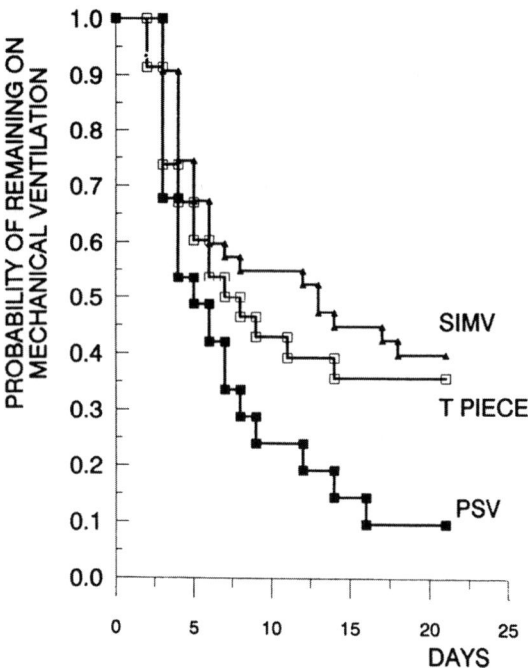

Figure 4 Probability of remaining on mechanical ventilation in previously ventilator-dependent patients based upon the method of weaning. In this study, weaning was more rapid using a PSV weaning mode than for T-piece or SIMV weaning. See text for details. *y*-axis: probability of remaining on mechanical ventilation; *x*-axis: duration of weaning (days). *Abbreviations*: PSV, pressure support ventilation; SIMV, synchronized intermittent ventilation. *Source*: From Ref. 85.

some of the questions about what constitutes the most effective means of weaning (82,85,86,112,113). None of the three most commonly employed weaning modes has been consistently identified to be superior to the others (114,115). Esteban et al.'s (82) study showed the two-hour SBT using a T-piece to be at least as good, if not superior, to both PSV and SIMV (Fig. 3). In Brochard et al.'s study (85), PSV was marginally superior (Fig. 4), but as reviewed in Table 5, Brochard et al.'s protocol was more favorable to PSV than Esteban et al.'s (82,85). In both these widely referenced studies, SIMV weaning was shown to be the slowest method (8,87,116,117).

☞ **Most experienced intensivists recognize that no single mode of weaning is best for all patients in all circumstances.** ☞ Rather, the most critical elements of weaning are the repeated evaluation of the ventilator-dependent patient by both the respiratory therapist and the physician in charge; this is sometimes facilitated by protocols (118).

Patients with the need for prolonged ventilatory support may further benefit from specialized weaning facilities once they have recovered from their critical illness (119–125). In these centers, more attention can be paid to incorporating occupational and physical therapy into respiratory rehabilitation (126,127), than is possible in the acute care–centered (and more expensive) critical care unit environment (79,113,128,129). The weaning success rate ranges from 50% to 68%. It is highest within the first three months of institution of mechanical ventilation. In recent years, improved weaning techniques have accomplished separation from the ventilator in patients who were previously considered lifelong ventilator dependent, and the success rates for long-term weaning are continuing to improve (130–134).

Given that many chronic ventilator-dependent patients may have been near ventilator dependence due to poor cardiopulmonary fitness, even prior to sustaining their injury, an additional tool for improving pulmonary rehabilitation is cardiovascular fitness training.

Weaning Protocols

An organized approach (i.e., weaning protocol) helps ensure that an organized and systematic approach is followed (118). Weaning protocols also increase the frequency and uniformity with which the patient's status is evaluated, helping to more quickly sort out the patients who are ready to be discontinued from mechanical ventilation.

The main benefit of weaning protocols is the consistent and systematic approach to weaning (135–143). When protocols are utilized, patients can be liberated from the ventilator faster (112,118). Protocols in the form of an algorithm can be followed by the RTs and/or nurses without the requirement for continuous physician presence (refer to UCSD Weaning Protocol, Fig. 5). However, review of the overall ventilatory status of the patient by the supervising physician remains indispensable in difficult-to-wean patients; and bedside presence of the clinician during SBTs provides important data that supplement weaning parameters. By employing a standardized regimen, unnecessary and potentially detrimental variations in weaning approaches are reduced and patients are extubated earlier than controls (84,105,106,108,109,144–154). Decreasing the duration of mechanical ventilation results in a reduction of adverse events secondary to mechanical ventilation and in shortening of ICU and hospital length of stay, and has been shown to improve the overall outcome (108,117,118,122,155). Earlier extubation has also been shown to decrease laryngeal damage from the ETT, and decrease the incidence of self-extubation, volutrauma/barotrauma, ventilator-associated pneumonia, ventilator-associated lung injury,

UCSD VENTILATOR **S.T.E.E.R.** WEANING PROTOCOL

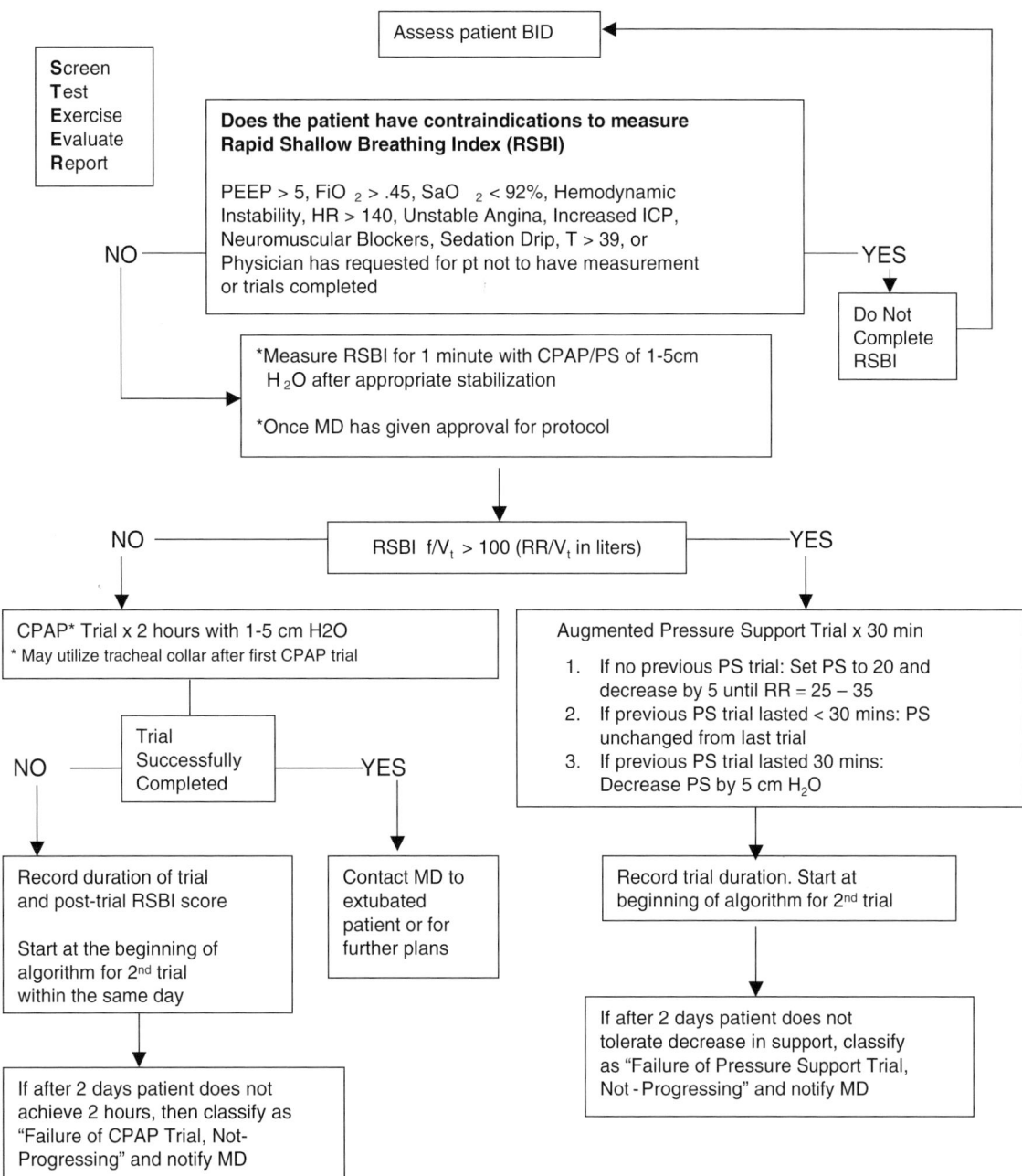

Figure 5 UCSD weaning protocol. *Abbreviations*: BID, twice a day; CPAP, continuous positive airway pressure (cmH$_2$O); F$_i$O$_2$, fraction of inspired oxygen; HR, heart rate (beats/min); MD, medical doctor; PEEP, positive end expiratory pressure (cmH$_2$O); PS, pressure support (cmH$_2$O); RSBI, rapid shallow breathing index [Respiratory rate/tidal volume (expressed in liters)]; STEER is an abbreviation for Screen, Test, Exercise, Evaluate, Report; *T*, temperature (°C).

cardiac compromise, patient discomfort, and respiratory muscle dysfunction (84,156).

☞ **The benefits of weaning protocols derived partly from the more frequent evaluations of respiratory status, decreasing delays caused by the false assumption that the patient is not yet weanable.** ☞ Protocols are thought to provide closer attention to the patient's respiratory status and decreased distraction from other sick patients. Part of this success is also attributable to a learning effect and

refining of management skills. If an organized weaning approach is already in place, less benefit occurs following implementation of a protocol (139,149,157). So far, mortality has not been shown to change by any specific weaning strategy, and weaning failures generally occur at similar rates in both protocol and control groups (136,137). However, an overall significant reduction of financial costs has been demonstrated using numerous protocol-driven weaning systems (84,105, 143,144,157).

UCSD Weaning Protocol

The weaning protocol employed at UCSD (Fig. 5) has been developed through the work of several critical care practitioners over two decades. Patients are divided into two groups: (*i*) those that are expected to undergo an uncomplicated weaning to extubation (i.e., no focused weaning maneuvers required) and (*ii*) those that require a controlled weaning program. In the "uncomplicated weaning" group, the patient to be extubated fulfills steps 1 to 5 in Table 1, and is required to be awake, alert, with minimal WOB, is not expected to have difficulty controlling his/her airway, and not expected to have a difficult reintubation (i.e., also fulfills steps 6 and 7 in Table 1). The patient is placed on CPAP or T-piece, and providing that the weaning parameters are acceptable (RR ≤25, RSBI <100) and that oxygenation and ventilation are satisfactory (confirmed by arterial blood gas analysis), the trachea is extubated.

The "controlled weaning" group patient fulfills all criteria of the "uncomplicated" patient but must prove that he/she can do the WOB for a prolonged period of time. These patients, who are recovering from critical illness, frequently require strength and endurance training. They are placed on our "STEER" protocol: S for screen, T for test, E for exercise, E for evaluate, and R for report (Fig. 5). If the initial RSBI is <100, the patient undergoes a two-hour CPAP trial, and if completed successfully is deemed ready for extubation (i.e., ready to be evaluated for goals 6 and 7, Table 1). If the patient becomes fatigued—RR of more than 30 and/or tidal volume decrease by 50 cm^3 (or more than 10% below baseline) he/she is rested, but may undergo a second trial later the same day, if there is an observed likely reversible reason to explain why the patient did not tolerate the first SBT (e.g., fever spike).

If the initial RSBI is >100, pressure support is increased to allow a CPAP trial for 30 minutes; if tolerated the pressure support is then gradually decreased. The patient is rested until a second trial later that same day if a CPAP trial is not possible, or a decrease of pressure support is not tolerated.

Tracheostomy

Surgical airway techniques have been described for more than 5000 years (158) but the debate regarding indications in the critically ill patient has been most intense over the last 50 years. Some authors believe that early tracheostomy (within one to seven days) is associated with a reduction in duration of mechanical ventilation and shorter ICU and hospital stays when compared with translaryngeal endotracheal intubation and late (eight or more days after admission) tracheostomy (101,113,130,131). This is controversial because others cannot demonstrate any significant difference in duration of ventilatory support, ICU length of stay, frequency of pneumonia, or death in either early (3–5 days), or late (10–14 days) tracheostomy groups (132,159,160). In one study, about half of the patients underwent postextubation laryngoscopy: vocal cord ulceration and subglottic inflammation were more often present in the continued intubation group, but the difference was not significant (159). None of these patients demonstrated evidence of late vocal cord or laryngeal stenosis during the follow-up visit. Although there is a significant improvement in PaO$_2$/FiO$_2$ ratios within 24 hours, there is only negligible change in V_D/V_T, if the patient remains hooked up to the ventilator tubing following a tracheostomy (73,161). However, V_D/V_T is decreased following tracheostomy when comparing

T-piece to tracheal collar. Additionally, there is a decreased WOB following tracheostomy compared to an ETT (162). In an RCT with burn patients, 26% of the conventional therapy group (continued endotracheal intubation with tracheostomy performed on postburn day 14 if necessary) were successfully extubated on postburn day 14 compared to only one patient of the early tracheostomy group (159). The authors attributed this partly to the ease of initiating or discontinuing mechanical ventilation with a tracheostomy in place decreased the rate of early tracheostomy decannulation. Additionally, the early tracheostomy group had larger full thickness burns than did the control group (159). Other benefits attributed to tracheostomy that have not been proven, but are generally accepted, include increased patient comfort, improved oral hygiene, easier airway suctioning, and greater options for oral communication.

THE DIFFICULT-TO-WEAN PATIENT

Extubation failures and prolonged mechanical ventilation fall into the category of the difficult-to-wean patient. Most affected are elderly and COPD patients (10,163). Reinstitution of ventilatory support within 24 to 72 hours of planned ETT removal occurs in 2% to 25% of extubated patients (164,165). Failures are associated with higher incidence of hospital mortality, longer ICU and hospital stay, prolonged duration of mechanical ventilation, higher hospital costs, and increased need for tracheostomy (122,128,166,167).

Inadequacies in pulmonary gas exchange, increased WOB, and physical debility are the most common causes for failure to wean (79). If extubation fails or the patient is extubated but at risk for being reintubated, noninvasive positive pressure ventilation (NIPPV) is an alternative that can be applied successfully (Volume 2, Chapter 27) (2,106,151,168–185). However, NIPPV should not be expected to be successful if the reason for weaning failure is stridor and/or airway obstruction or any process with rapidly worsening respiratory failure. In contrast, NIPPV is particularly useful for the treatment of asthma, COPD, and cardiogenic edema, and brief episodes of hypercarbic or hypoxemic acute respiratory failure (185,186). Conversely, NIPPV is rarely successful in avoiding intubation in trauma and postsurgical surgical patients, partly because the underlying disease etiology is generally of greater severity and not quickly reversible (176,179,185).

☞ **Dysfunction of other (nonpulmonary) organ systems can also prolong weaning. Treating functional organ failures can help to turn a difficult-to-wean patient into one who can be successfully weaned.** ☞ The following survey of ventilation-associated organ system dysfunctions should be reviewed in each patient with prolonged weaning (Table 6).

Central Nervous System (Neurological and Psychiatric) Considerations

Numerous neurologic conditions contribute to weaning difficulty (187,188). Traumatic brain injuries can impair the patient's wakefulness and ability to protect their airway; brainstem injuries can impair the respiratory drive as well as the gag and cough. Injuries to the phrenic nerve (from high cervical spine trauma) (189) and/or paralysis of thoracic cage muscles (high and low cervical spine trauma) can all impair the patient's strength, prolong

Table 6 Special Considerations in the Difficult-to-Wean Patient: An Organ Systems Approach

Organ system	Common problems and solutions
CNS	Psychiatric/psychological: prolonged stress, fear and anxiety can lead to an acute disaster, which untreated may advance to PTSD; sleep deprivation and drug withdrawal are common problems (see text for solutions); excessive sedation and inadequate sedation can both prolong weaning, SCI can decrease the ability to do the WOB, TBI can alter the drive to breath and ability to protect the airway
Respiratory care	Secretion management and treatment of bronchospasm are frequent respiratory care problems that prolong weaning; ETTs can become kinked, or narrowed with inspissated secretions leading to significantly elevated WOB due to increased R_{AW}; positioning during the SBT can alter success; obese patients benefit from reverse Trendelenberg, SCI at C5–7 benefit from an abdominal binder (see text for explanation)
Cardiovascular	Myocardial ischemia may occur when there is an increased WOB, and or when the loading conditions on the heart change during the SBT; monitoring of ECG and evaluation with echo before and during an SBT can be diagnostic
GI/nutrition	Numerous GI and nutritional ailments can prolong weaning; severe malnutrition and excessive feeding syndromes are two ends of a spectrum that can impact weaning
Renal (electrolytes, etc.)	Fluid overload, as occurs with ARF, and deficiency in PO_4^{2-}, or Ca^{2+}, or K^+ can cause weakness, whereas excess Mg^{2+} also cause weakness, deficiency of Mg^{2+}/K^+ are associated with dysrhythmias
ID	Fever, sepsis, and inadequately treated pneumonias or abscess, all contribute to respiratory failure
Hematological	Anemia in an already debilitated patient can increase cardiac work and lead to increase BMR and ischemia
Endocrinological	Hypothyroidism and adrenal suppression both decrease MAP and ability to do the WOB, hyperthyroidism increases WOB

Abbreviations: ATN, acute tubular necrosis; BMR, basal metabolic rate; CNS, central nervous system; ECG, electrocardiogram; ETTs, endotracheal tubes; MAP, mean arterial blood pressure; PTSD, posttraumatic stress disorder; R_{AW}, airway resistance; SBT, spontaneous breathing trial; SCI, spinal cord injury; TBI, traumatic brain injury; WOB, work of breathing.

weaning, and, in some cases, result in lifelong ventilator dependence (188).

Psychiatric issues also commonly contribute to the difficult-to-wean situation. Fear of respiratory failure and

death can hinder progress in some patients; this is particularly common in patients with underlying pulmonary disease and a history of prior ventilator dependence. One of the more common causes of prolonged weaning is the inappropriate titration of sedative drugs (7,190,191). Excessive sedation causes the patient to become obtunded. Inadequate drugs/doses promote increased pain, fear, anxiety, and psychosis during weaning. Delirium is present in the majority of ICU patients requiring mechanical ventilation, and its presence correlates with a prolonged duration of intubation and weaning (191).

Many institutions use relatively short-acting benzodiazepines (e.g., midazolam, lorazepam) or propofol for sedation. Newer sedatives such as the alpha-2 agonist dexmedetomidine provide excellent sedation and decrease analgesic requirements (192–197). Dexmedetomidine also maintains the respiratory drive despite the central depressant and sedative effects (Volume 2, Chapter 5). Daily evaluation and interruption of sedation have also been shown to accelerate the weaning process (198).

However, patients who are severely agitated and suffering from delirium often benefit from holoperidol. Many severely agitated patients are withdrawing from drugs, and most are extremely sleep deprived, as a result of the noisy ICU environment. Ensuring adequate sleep at night and increasing environmental stimulation during the daytime are beneficial goals. Evening efforts to promote sleep include placing less acutely ill weaning patients further away from noisy ICU doors and the main nursing desk to minimize sleep interruption from ambient noise. Newer specific benzodiazepine drugs such as zaleplon (Sonata®) or zolpidem (Ambien®) are increasingly used sleep medicines. Additionally, playing soothing music may have a positive biofeedback benefit.

Daytime stimulation is promoted by keeping the lights on and/or window shades open during the day, and reorienting patients to large clocks and calendars placed on the wall in clear view of the patient. Providing aggressive physical and occupational therapy, as well as other daytime activities also increases the environmental stimulation and daytime wakefulness of these patients. Some find the use of a bedside fan can help the patient endure SBTs. The psychological effect of cool air on the face during an SBT is analogous to jogging in a gentle cool breeze (vs. jogging on a stifling hot, humid windless day). Clinically depressed or psychotic patients should receive a psychiatric consultation and be restarted on their preinjury psychiatric medications. Review of the above neurological-, psychological-, and sedation-related causes of failure to wean comprises the first step in evaluating the difficult-to-wean patient (190,191).

Optimize Respiratory Care

Secretion management is another, often overlooked, source of weaning failure. Although the patient may be able to oxygenate and ventilate, they may not be optimized from a respiratory care perspective. First and foremost, the clinician must ensure the absence of bronchospasm. Bronchospasm occurring in an otherwise ready to wean patient should be treated with albuterol (if COPD is prominent, ipatroprium bromide should be added), and if steroid dependent, a short course of intravenous steroids in addition to aerosolized steroids should be employed.

Airway secretions are normally cleared by the tracheobronchial mucocilliary system. This system is impaired in the intubated patient. In chronically intubated patients, these stagnant pools of secretions become colonized or infected with nosocomial flora, producing an increased bacterial load in the secretions. The inability to maintain sufficient pulmonary toilet (excess respiratory secretions, inadequate cough) combined with impaired respiratory muscle capacity results in weaning failures and the need to reinstitute mechanical ventilation.

Aggressive physical therapy, including chest vibrations and pulmonary drainage, in combination with bronchodilators, frequent incentive spirometry, deep coughing, repeated suctioning, and abdominal binders (when appropriate), are all important measures for satisfactory weaning.

The ETT internal diameter (i.d.) should be evaluated in difficult-to-wean patients. A reduction in the i.d. of the ETT increases R_{AW} inversely to the fourth power of the radius. Kinks, retained secretions, and foreign bodies adherent inside the lumen of an otherwise adequately sized EET can similarly increase the WOB.

Inspiratory muscle fatigue and atrophy are common causes of failure to tolerate weaning (199–204). The use of inspiratory muscle strength training is gaining more recognition as a method to combat these changes (187,188,205–207). The proposed benefits of inspiratory training include: (*i*) the effect of improving the inspiratory muscle strength (206,207), (*ii*) standardization, (*iii*) routine use of beneficial breathing patterns, and (*iv*) other (not defined) training effects (205–207).

Patient positioning during SBTs can have a significant impact on ventilatory mechanics and weaning success. The upright position can decrease airway resistance compared with the supine position and results in increased lung volume and FRC (especially in obese patients). Most importantly, the increased FRC also protects against atelectasis and the consequent right-to-left transpulmonary shunting. Sitting a patient up in bed will achieve this goal, if their body habitus is thin. However, morbidly obese patients often need to be placed in the reverse Trendelenberg position to improve FRC. Indeed, placing morbidly obese patients in the sitting position may increase abdominal pressure and upward excursion of the diaphragm decreasing FRC.

In contrast to patients with a normally functioning thoracic cage, the supine position or slight Trendelenberg position results in superior pulmonary function (as documented by MIF and VC) in quadriplegic patients with diaphragm-sparing cervical spine injuries (i.e., C5–6, C6–7, C7–T1). These patients ventilate almost solely by the functioning diaphragm (along with a minor contribution from strap muscles). In these patients, the intercostal muscles and entire thoracic bucket handle ventilatory system is paralyzed (and paradoxically involutes during inhalation). By placing these patients supine or in slight Trendelenberg position, the diaphragm starts in the more optimized domed position (due to cephalad displacement by the weight of the abdominal contents), and has a greater excursion during diaphragmatic contraction, than occurs in the upright position. Most patients do not enjoy breathing in the reverse Trendelenberg position; accordingly, an abdominal binder can be placed and provide the same benefit (increasing abdominal pressure–mediated doming of the diaphragm prior to contraction).

Cardiovascular Issues

Ongoing cardiac dysrhythmias, myocardial ischemia, or other cardiovascular causes of hemodynamic instability can render weaning difficult (208–215). Up to 35% of chronically ventilator-dependent patients show evidence of myocardial ischemia, which is associated with failure to discontinue mechanical ventilation (210,211). Cardiac dysfunction needs to be diagnosed and treated early, in order to maximize the likelihood of weaning success. A large variety of cardiac abnormalities can lead to weaning failure. However, myocardial ischemia is the most important cardiovascular impediment to weaning (210). Using continuous ECG monitoring, Chatila et al. (211) demonstrated myocardial ischemia in 6% of all weaning patients during SBTs. Lemaire et al. (213) first noted that intrathoracic pressure changes in patients with COPD changed markedly during the transition from positive pressure ventilation to spontaneous breathing, and that these alterations affected the cardiac loading conditions. Large, negative intrathoracic pressure swings increase both left ventricular preload and afterload. The consequent decrease in LVEF observed in COPD patients can be offset by the administration of PSV, further demonstrating the importance of heart–lung interactions during weaning (214). Patients demonstrating signs of myocardial ischemia during weaning should receive a cardiac consultation, an echocardiogram, and an examination of their coronary artery anatomy. Those with critical coronary artery lesions should be considered for treatment.

Gastrointestinal and Nutritional Impediments to Weaning

Although any acute gastrointestinal process (e.g., small bowel obstruction, perforated viscus) will prolong weaning, these processes are normally recognized promptly, and are uncommon causes of failure to wean. Rather, malnourishment and abnormalities in essential vitamins and nutrients represent the gastrointestinal conditions that more commonly postpone weaning from mechanical ventilation. Preexisting malnourishment and debility, compounded by the delayed start of nutritional support, can prolong weaning due to muscle weakness and easy fatigability. Conversely, feeding the patient a diet too high in carbohydrates can increase the respiratory quotient (RQ), defined as $\dot{V}CO_2/\dot{V}O_2$. Worse still is the massive overfeeding of calories, which results in fat synthesis and an extremely increased RQ. The reader is referred to Volume 2, Chapter 31 for a review of the clinically relevant metabolic and nutritional assessment measures.

Genitourinary Considerations

Abnormalities in fluid status and acid–base balance (controlled mainly by the lungs and kidneys) can complicate weaning. In order to compensate for acidosis (e.g., renal failure), the respiratory drive to ventilate CO_2 off is increased; this will lead to higher-a-minute-ventilation (increasing the WOB) and making weaning more difficult. Conversely, metabolic alkalosis will decrease the brainstem-mediated drive to breath causing hypercarbia, and in the absence of increased F_IO_2 results in hypoxemia (Volume 2, Chapter 2). In-hospital metabolic alkalosis is most commonly due to contraction alkalosis, from aggressive diuretic therapy and/or H^+-loss secondary to continuous gastric suctioning. A decrease in minute ventilation can eventually lead to hypoxemia and persistent respiratory failure. Correction of electrolyte abnormalities [calcium, magnesium, phosphate (216,217), potassium (218–220)] and other vitamin and trace elements are likewise essential.

Renal failure almost always leads to respiratory failure when not treated. Early correction of fluid overload electrolyte and uremic toxin abnormalities increases the likelihood of weaning success. A complete normalization of acid–base status may not be possible, except with continuous renal replacement modalities (Volume 2, Chapter 43). Unstable ICU patients with renal failure may not become weanable until these aggressive therapies are instituted.

Infectious Disease Impediments to Weaning

Infectious conditions increase the WOB by increasing the metabolic rate (e.g., fever), increasing lung water due to capillary leak, and decreasing lung compliance. Accordingly, weaning failure can sometimes serve as the first hint of an ongoing or new infectious process. In ventilator-dependent patients, the lung is generally colonized and a common source of pneumonia and/or tracheobronchitis. Careful examination of all other potential sources (e.g., wound sites, invasive catheter sites, all body surface cavities, and fluids) is appropriate in any weaning patient showing evidence of infection (fever, leukocytosis, fluid retention, hyperglycemia, etc.). Appropriate antibiotic selection is guided by the clinical picture, Gram stain, and culture results (Volume 2, Chapter 53).

Hematological Considerations

Abnormal hematological conditions can impair weaning and recovery from respiratory failure in a number of ways. Anemia can contribute to ischemia of multiple organs and increase the work of both the heart and lungs in compensation for the decreased O_2-carrying capacity of the blood (211). The decreased O_2 content can also lead to generalized weakness and early fatigability of the muscles (including the diaphragm). Blood transfusion is indicated if ischemia or impaired DO_2 is prolonging weaning. Iron and erythropoietin are indicated in debilitated, chronically ill patients with anemia of chronic disease.

Thrombocytosis and immobility increase the risk of deep venous thrombosis (DVT) and subsequent pulmonary emboli. All critically ill trauma patients should receive DVT prophylaxis (as reviewed in Volume 2, Chapter 56).

Endocrine Issues

Endocrine dysfunction can impair the ability to wean. The most relevant endocrinological conditions include hyperthyroidism, hypothyroidism, and adrenal suppression. Hyperthyroidism increases the metabolic rate, CO_2 production, and, consequently, the WOB, whereas hypothyroidism decreases the mental and physical condition, decreasing the patient's ability to do the WOB. Adrenal suppression decreases the patient's stamina and impairs the cardiovascular system. These entities are discussed in greater detail in Volume 2, Chapters 61 and 62.

SPECIAL CONSIDERATIONS RELATED TO THORAX TRAUMA
Direct Lung Injury

Pulmonary contusion and lung lacerations are the most pertinent direct lung injuries occurring following trauma and are fully discussed in depth in Volume 1, Chapters 25, and Volume 2, Chapters 23–25. Accordingly, only the key points affecting weaning will be outlined in the section. The contused lung is prone to shunting from alveolar damage and atelectasis, resulting in hypoxemia and increased alveolar dead space, all of which can impair weaning and result in increased WOB.

Indirect Lung Injury

Fluid resuscitation complicates weaning following trauma. Loss of colloid oncotic pressure and consequent increased third spacing of fluid increase the diffusion distance for the oxygen molecule, resulting in increased V/Q-mismatching, shunt, and dramatically increased WOB.

Release of inflammatory mediators from sepsis and from systemic response to severe injury (Chapter 105) further exacerbates the noncardiogenic pulmonary edema. This condition impairs oxygenation through V/Q-mismatching and leads to increased WOB and a possible difficult-to-wean situation.

Mechanical Issues
Flail Chest

A flail segment is defined as two or more ribs broken in two or more places, whereas a flail chest is a chest which does not function for any number of reasons (Volume 2, Chapter 25 discusses these entities in detail); pain can lead to splinting, whereas mechanical dysfunction can lead to paradoxical breathing. Both are worsened by hemo- or pneumothorax. The overall net result is a reduction in minute ventilation. Furthermore, the perfusion in the flail segment continues; however, the expansion of the lung decreases resulting in regional shunting. A patient with a flail chest typically compensates by increasing his RR and by decreasing his tidal volume rendering weaning from a respirator challenging.

Pneumothorax and Hemothorax

Both pneumothorax and hemothorax are discussed in Chapter 25 of both volumes. These lesions are both acutely treated with chest tubes. Prior to initiating weaning, the patient should be free of any acute process.

Spinal Cord Injury

Site, mechanism of injury, and clinical findings of secondary spinal cord injury determine whether a patient is at risk for respiratory failure and/or in need for airway protection. Severe spinal cord injuries with lesions around vertebral body C3 and higher lead, almost always, to long-term respiratory failure and in cases of C4–5 lesions to long-term respiratory insufficiency (phrenic nerve arises from spinal nerve roots C3–5).

THE PATIENT IS WEANED—CAN THE TRACHEA BE SAFELY EXTUBATED?
Does the Patient Have an Intact Gag and Cough?

Once oxygenation and ventilation have been normalized and the patient is deemed ready to be liberated from the ventilator, the next question is whether the patient has a sufficient gag reflex, and is able to protect his/her airway. Without a gag reflex, extubation is contraindicated (Table 1, step 6). The next important question is whether the patient has a strong enough cough to bring up secretions and clear the airway from obstructing substances. **Only after verifying that the patient has a normal vigorous gag and cough mechanism should the clinician advance to the step of considering ETT removal.**

Does the Patient Have a Difficult Airway?

A history of difficult intubation, or an examination that concludes the airway will be difficult to reintubate

(i.e., presence of a halo), requires a planned extubation sequence usually involving fiberoptic bronchoscopy and or an AEC. ☞ If placing an ETT is known to be difficult, helpful tools as described in the ASA Difficult Airway Algorithm (Volume 1, Chapter 9) should be at the bedside and a person comfortable with the application of these tools present. It is prudent to have a surgeon—capable of doing an emergency tracheostomy— aware of a planned "difficult" extubation and standing by. To minimize the chance of serious complications, it is most reasonable to extubate these patients only if successful extubation and discontinuation from mechanical support is highly likely.

Strategies for Extubating the Difficult Airway

The first step is to keep the patient NPO following the usual NPO guidelines by the American Society of Anesthesiology in order to decrease the risk of aspiration. Please see also the ASA Difficult Airway Algorithm for options to extubate a patient safely. It is not a particular technique but one's familiarity with the technique that decides safety and success.

A good first choice is the use of a tube exchanger: a long (>50 cm) rigid plastic tubing which is placed through the in situ ETT allowing the ETT to slide over it. Ideally, the patient is appropriately informed, well prepared, and compliant. The ETT is removed carefully: close observation for respiratory sufficiency is obligatory. The tube exchanger is removed if the patient is breathing comfortably.

If later on the patient fails extubation, it is critical to maintain spontaneous ventilation until an ETT can be placed successfully (e.g., via fiberoptic bronchoscopy). If the patient becomes obtunded, he/she might tolerate an LMA through which an ETT can be placed, preferably with fiberoptic guidance (221).

EYE TO THE FUTURE

Ongoing research will help us to improve outcomes and promote more successful recovery from respiratory failure. One such new approach, by Martinez et al. (62), plots $\dot{V}_E$ recovery time after a two-hour SBT. In this introductory study, $\dot{V}_E$ recovery time outperformed RR (cut off = 38 breaths/min) and RSBI (cut off = 105 breaths/min/L) (62). Unfortunately, the number of patients evaluated in the Martinez et al. study was small, as was the number of patients requiring prolonged mechanical ventilation. Although the results are encouraging, the threshold for discrimination between weaning success and failure is not robust enough as a single measure of weaning.

Newer sedative drugs that do not inhibit ventilatory drive (e.g., dexmedetomidine) are proving potent adjuncts to standard practices in the difficult-to-wean patients.

In the future, more sophisticated ventilators will help us to determine the earliest and safest time to discontinue mechanical ventilation by integrating and extrapolating numerous weaning parameters.

Finally, "step-down" weaning units are likely to play a more prominent role in acute patient care. These units would accept chronically ventilatordependent patients who have recovered from their acute disease processes but have become debilitated and ventilator dependent. Most of these patients would already have had a tracheostomy performed, and failed weaning for a significant period of time.

SUMMARY

Weaning remains a major challenge for patients recovering from respiratory failure. Employing the seven-step approach reviewed in Table 1 ensures that patients are capable of tolerating weaning (steps 1–5), patients are evaluated for ability to protect their airway once extubated (step 6), and the likelihood that reintubation will be difficult (step 7).

The search continues to find the single weaning parameter that best predicts success, but currently the RSBI provides the best indicator. Nearly all patients with RSBI <50 are capable of breathing on their own, whereas those with RSBI >100 are unlikely to tolerate weaning and require strength training, or further improvement in their overall condition. Patients with RSBI in the middle of these two extremes require additional data to make the correct weaning decision. One newer weaning parameter that may provide such data is the $\dot{V}_E$ recovery time (62). No particular weaning strategy (SBT, SIMV, PSV, etc.) has proven superior to others. In difficult-to-wean patients, efforts are spent in reviewing each organ system and optimizing these, as the patient recovers from the primary disease. Additionally, strength and endurance training are thought to be beneficial, especially in debilitated patients. The optimum methodology and duration of sprinting regimens are the subject of ongoing research.

KEY POINTS

- ☞ The weaning sequence should proceed along a logical stepwise evaluation pathway.
- ☞ Clinicians should closely review the contributors to respiratory failure at the moment the patient is intubated, and commence optimization of all anticipated impediments to weaning from the beginning.
- ☞ The patient is not ready to proceed with weaning until he/she can maintain adequate oxygen saturation, both at rest and with modest exertion (i.e., during weaning).
- ☞ When the WOB is excessive (Fig. 1), even young and otherwise healthy patients can develop respiratory failure.
- ☞ Some weaning parameters reflect the WOB that must be performed by the patient (e.g., $\dot{V}_E$, C_L, R_{AW}), whereas others reflect the patient's ability to perform that work (e.g., MIF, VC, RSBI).
- ☞ The RSBI is the most widely used weaning parameter, because it is easy to obtain, predictive, and illustrative; patients failing to wean develop a breathing pattern characterized by small tidal volumes and increased RRs.
- ☞ Resistance created by the ETT, ventilator tubing, and circuit valves can be overcome by the addition of a minimal amount (i.e., 5 cmH$_2$O) of pressure support.
- ☞ Most experienced intensivists recognize that no single mode of weaning is best for all patients in all circumstances.
- ☞ The benefits of weaning protocols derived partly from the more frequent evaluations of respiratory status, decreasing delays caused by the false assumption that the patient is not yet weanable.
- ☞ Dysfunction of other (nonpulmonary) organ systems can also prolong weaning. Treating functional organ failures can help to turn a difficult-to-wean patient into one who can be successfully weaned.
- ☞ Only after verifying that the patient has a normal vigorous gag and cough mechanism should the clinician advance to the step of considering ETT removal.

✍ A history of difficult intubation, or an examination that concludes the airway will be difficult to reintubate (i.e., presence of a halo), requires a planned extubation sequence usually involving fiberoptic bronchoscopy and or an AEC.

REFERENCES

1. Afessa B, Hogans L, Murphy R. Predicting 3-day and 7-day outcomes of weaning from mechanical ventilation. Chest 1999; 116(2):456–461.
2. Esteban A, Anzueto A, Alia I, et al. How is mechanical ventilation employed in the intensive care unit: an international utilization review. Am J Respir Crit Care Med 2000; 161(5):1450–1458.
3. Sevransky JE, Haponi EF. Respiratory failure in elderly patients. Clin Geriatr Med 2003; 19(1):205–224.
4. Ely EW, Wheeler AP, Thompson BT, et al. Recovery rate and prognosis in older persons who develop acute lung injury and the acute respiratory distress syndrome. Ann Intern Med 2002; 136(1):25–36.
5. Epstein CD, El-Mokadem N, Peerless JR. Weaning older patients from long-term mechanical ventilation: a pilot study. Am J Crit Care 2002; 11(4):369–377.
6. Esteban A, Anzueto A, Frutos-Vivar F, et al. Outcome of older patients receiving mechanical ventilation. Intensive Care Med 2004; 30(4):639–646.
7. Criswell DS, Shanley RA, Betters JJ, et al. Cumulative effects of aging and mechanical ventilation on in vitro diaphragm function. Chest 2003; 124(6):2302–2308.
8. Papadakos PJ, MacIntyre NR, Tobin MJ. Weaning from mechanical ventilation. Controversies Crit Care 1996; 2(4):1–6.
9. Meade M, Guyatt G, Griffith L, et al. Introduction to a series of systematic reviews of weaning from mechanical ventilation. Chest 2001; 120(suppl 6):396S–399S.
10. Hall JB, Wood LD. Liberation of the patient from mechanical ventilation. J Am Med Assoc 1987; 257(12):1621–1628.
11. Manthous CA, Schmidt GA, Hall JB. Liberation from mechanical ventilation: a decade of progress. Chest 1998; 114(3):886–901.
12. Manthous CA. The anarchy of weaning techniques. Chest 2002; 121(6):1738–1739.
13. Truwitt JD. Viewpoints to liberation from mechanical ventilation. Chest 2003; 123(6):1779–1780.
14. Ware LB, Matthay MA. The acute respiratory distress syndrome. N Engl J Med 2000; 342:1334–1339.
15. Sapijaszko MJ, Brant R, Sandham D, et al. Nonrespiratory predictor of mechanical ventilation dependency in intensive care unit patients. Crit Care Med 1996; 24(4):601–607.
16. Sahn SA, Lakshminarayan S. Bedside criteria for discontinuation of mechanical ventilation. Chest 1973; 63(6):1002–1005.
17. Pierson DJ. Weaning from mechanical ventilation in acute respiratory failure: concepts, indications, and techniques. Respir Care 1983; 28(5):646–662.
18. MacIntyre NR, Cook DJ, Ely EW, et al. Collective Task Force (ACCP, AARC, SCCM): evidence-based guidelines for weaning and discontinuing ventilatory support. Chest 2001; 120(6):375S–395S.
19. Yang KL. Reproducibility of weaning parameters: a need for standardization. Chest 1992; 102(6):1829–1832.
20. Bach JR, Manthous CA, Schmidt GA, et al. Liberation from mechanical ventilation. Chest 1999; 115:1217.
21. Esteban A, Alia I. Clinical management of weaning from mechanical ventilation. Intensive Care Med 1998; 24(10):999–1008.
22. Tobin MJ. Weaning patients from mechanical ventilation using gastric pH. Ann Intern Med 1994; 120(5):439.
23. Yang KL. Inspiratory pressure/maximal inspiratory pressure ratio: a predictive index of weaning outcome. Intensive Care Med 1993; 19(4):204–208.
24. Mohsenifar Z, Hay A, Hay J, et al. Gastric intramural pH as a predictor of success or failure in weaning patients from mechanical ventilation. Ann Intern Med 1993; 119(8):794–798.
25. Rochester DF. Weaning patients from mechanical ventilation using gastric pH. Ann Intern Med 1994; 120(5):438–439.
26. Burns SM, Burns JE, Truwit JD. Comparison of five clinical weaning indices. Am J Crit Care 1994; 3(5):342–352.
27. Bach JR, Saporito LR. Criteria for extubation and tracheostomy tube removal for patients with ventilatory failure: a different approach to weaning. Chest 1996; 110(6):1566–1571.
28. Gluck EH. Predicting eventual success or failure to wean in patients receiving long-term mechanical ventilation. Chest 1996; 110(4):1018–1024.
29. Jacob B, Chatila W, Manthous CA. The unassisted respiratory rate/tidal volume ratio accurately predicts weaning outcome in postoperative patients. Crit Care Med 1997; 25(2):253–257.
30. O'Keefe GE, Hawkins K, Boynton J, et al. Indicators of fatigue and of prolonged weaning from mechanical ventilation in surgical patients. World J Surg 2001; 25(1):98–103.
31. Montgomery AB, Holle RHO, Neagley SR, et al. Prediction of successful ventilator weaning using airway occlusion pressure and hypercapnic challenge. Chest 1987; 91(4):496–499.
32. Stroetz RW, Hubmayr RD. Tidal volume maintenance during weaning with pressure support. Am J Respir Crit Care Med 1995; 152(3):1034–1040.
33. Jacob B, Amoateng-Adjepong Y, Rasakulasuriar S, et al. Preoperative pulmonary function tests do not predict outcome after coronary artery bypass. Conn Med 1997; 61(6):327–332.
34. Epstein SK. Etiology of extubation failure and the predictive value of the rapid shallow breathing index. Am J Respir Crit Care Med 1995; 152(2):545–549.
35. Patel RG, Petrini MF, Norman JR. Strategies for maximizing your chances for weaning success: limitations—and advantages—of common predictive indices. J Crit Illn 1995; 10(6):411–413, 417–418, 421–423.
36. Scheinhorn DJ, Hassenpflug M, Artinian BM, et al. Predictors of weaning after 6 weeks of mechanical ventilation. Chest 1995; 107(2):500–505.
37. Yende S, Wunderink R. Validity of scoring systems to predict risk of prolonged mechanical ventilation after coronary artery bypass graft surgery. Chest 2002; 122:239–244.
38. Chatila W, Jacob B, Guaglionone D, et al. The unassisted respiratory rate–tidal volume ratio accurately predicts weaning outcome. Am J Med 1996; 1010(1):61–67.
39. Manczur TI, Greenough A, Pryor D, et al. Comparison of predictors of extubation from mechanical ventilation in children. Pediatr Crit Care Med 2000; 1(1):28–32.
40. Krieger BP, Ershowsky PF, Becker DA, et al. Evaluation of conventional criteria for predicting successful weaning from mechanical ventilatory support in elderly patients. Crit Care Med 1989; 17(9):858–861.
41. Marini JJ. What derived variables should be monitored during mechanical ventilation? Respir Care 1992; 37(9):1097–1107.
42. Krieger BP, Chediak A, Gazeroglu HB, et al. Variability of the breathing pattern before and after extubation. Chest 1988; 93(4):767–771.
43. Whelan J, Simpson SQ, Levy H. Unplanned extubation: predictors of successful termination of mechanical ventilatory support. Chest 1994; 105(6):1808–1812.
44. Zeggwagh AA, Abouqal R, Madani N, et al. Weaning from mechanical ventilation: a model for extubation. Intensive Care Med 1999; 25(10):1077–1083.
45. Venkataraman ST, Khan N, Brown A. Validation of predictors of extubation success and failure in mechanically ventilated infants and children. Crit Care Med 2002; 28(8):2991–2996.
46. Smina M, Salam A, Khamiees M, et al. Cough peak flows and extubation outcomes. Chest 2003; 124:262–268.

47. Vassilakopoulos T, Zakynthinos S, Roussos C. The tension–time index and the frequency/tidal volume ratio are the major pathophysiologic determinants of weaning failure and success. Am J Respir Crit Care Med 1998; 158:378–385.

48. Clochesy JM, Daly BJ, Montenegro HD. Weaning chronically critically ill adults from mechanical ventilatory support: a descriptive study. Am J Crit Care 1995; 4(2):93–99.

49. Capdevila X, Perrigault PF, Ramonatxo M, et al. Changes in breathing pattern and respiratory muscle performance parameters during difficult weaning. Crit Care Med 1998; 26(1):79–87.

50. Moody LE, Lowry L, Yarandi H, Voss A. Psychophysiologic predictors of weaning from mechanical ventilation in chronic bronchitis and emphysema. Clin Nurs Res 1997; 6(4):311–330.

51. Johannigman JA, Davis K Jr, Campbell RS, et al. Use of the rapid/shallow-breathing index as an indicator of patient work of breathing during pressure support ventilation. Surgery 1997; 122(4):737–741.

52. Dojat M, Harf A, Touchard D, et al. Evaluation of a knowledge-based system providing ventilatory management and decision for extubation. Am J Respir Crit Care Med 1996; 153(3):997–1004.

53. Khamiees M, Raju P, DeGirolamo A, et al. Predictors of extubation outcome in patients who have successfully completed a spontaneous breathing trial. Chest 2001; 120:1262–1270.

54. Ashutosh K, Lee H, Mohan CK, et al. Prediction criteria for successful weaning from respiratory support: statistical and connectionist analyses. Crit Care Med 1992; 20(9):1295–1301.

55. Shoults D, Clarke TA, Benumonf JL, Mannino FL. Maximum inspiratory force in predicting successful neonate tracheal extubation. Crit Care Med 1979; 7(11):485–486.

56. Belani KG, Gilmour IJ. Maximum inspiratory force. Crit Care Med 1980; 8(9):528–529.

57. Jaeschke RZ, Meade MO, Guyatt GH, et al. How to use diagnostic test articles in the intensive care unit: diagnosing weanability using F/Vt. Crit Care Med 1997; 25(9):1514–1521.

58. Miwa K, Mitsuoka M, Takamori S, et al. Continuous monitoring of oxygen consumption in patients undergoing weaning from mechanical ventilation. Respiration 2003; 70(6):623–630.

59. Hendra KP, Bonis PA, Joyce-Brady M. Development and prospective validation of a mode for predicting weaning in chronic ventilator dependent patients. BMC Pulm Med 2003; 3(1):3.

60. Conti G, Montini L, Pennisi MA, et al. A prospective, blinded evaluation of indexes proposed to predict weaning from mechanical ventilation. Intensive Care Med 2004; 30(5):830–836.

61. Bien MY, Hseu SS, Yien HW, et al. Breathing pattern variability: a weaning predictor in postoperative patients recovering from systemic inflammatory response syndrome. Intensive Care Med 2004; 30(2):241–247.

62. Martinez A, Seymour C, Nam M. Minute ventilation recovery time: a predictor of extubation outcome. Chest 2003; 123(4):1214–1221.

63. Soo Hoo GW, Park L. Variations in the measurement of weaning parameters: survey of respiratory therapists. Chest 2002; 121(6):1947–1955.

64. Leitch EA, Moran JL, Grealy B. Weaning and extubation in the intensive care unit: clinical or index-driven approach? Intensive Care Med 1996; 22(8):752–759.

65. Gillespie LM, White SD, Sinha SK, Donn SM. Usefulness of the minute ventilation test in predicting successful extubation in newborn infants: a randomized controlled trial. J Perinatol 2003; 23(3):205–207.

66. Tulla H, Takala J, Alhava E, et al. Hypermetabolism after coronary artery bypass. J Thorac Cardiovasc Surg 1991; 101(4):598–600.

67. Laaban JP, Lemaire F, Baron JF, et al. Influence of caloric intake on the respiratory mode during mandatory minute volume ventilation. Chest 1985; 87(1):67–72.

68. Caruso P, Friedrich C, Denari SD, et al. The unidirectional valve is the best method to determine maximal inspiratory pressure during weaning. Chest 1999; 115(4):1096–1101.

69. Bruton A. A pilot study to investigate any relationship between sustained maximal inspiratory pressure and extubation outcome. Heart Lung 2002; 31(2):141–149.

70. Chen JY. Maximum inspiratory pressure: a neonatal criterion for weaning from mechanical ventilation. Gaoxiong Yi Xue Ke Xue Zhi 1992; 8(10):535–541.

71. Fernandez R, Raurich JM, Mut T, et al. Extubation failure: diagnostic value of occlusion pressure (P0.1) and P0.1-derived parameters. Intensive Care Med 2004; 30(2):234–240.

72. Capdevila XJ, Perrigault PF, Perey PJ, et al. Occlusion pressure and its ratio to maximum inspiratory pressure are useful predictors for successful extubation following T-piece weaning trial. Chest 1995; 108(2):482–489.

73. Yang KL, Tobin MJ. A prospective study of indexes predicting the outcome of trials of weaning from mechanical ventilation. N Engl J Med 1991; 324:1445–1450.

74. Tobin MJ, Perez W, Guenther SM, et al. The pattern of breathing during successful and unsuccessful trials of weaning from mechanical ventilation. Am Rev Respir Dis 1986; 134:1111–1118.

75. Lee KH, Hui KP, Chan TB, et al. Rapid shallow breathing (frequency–tidal volume ratio) did not predict extubation outcome. Chest 1994; 105(2):540–543.

76. Tobin MJ, Jubran A, Hines E Jr. Pathophysiology of failure to wean from mechanical ventilation. Schweiz Med Wochenschr 1994; 147(47):2139–2145.

77. Epstein SK. Weaning parameters. Respir Care Clin N Am 2000; 6(2):253–301.

78. El-Khatib M, Jamaleddine G, Soubra R, Muallem M. Pattern of spontaneous breathing: potential marker for weaning outcome: spontaneous breathing pattern and weaning from mechanical ventilation. Intensive Care Med 2001; 27(1):52–58.

79. Brochard L, Rual F, Lorino H, et al. Inspiratory pressure support compensates for the additional work of breathing caused by the endotracheal tube. Anesthesiology 1991; 75:739–745.

80. Perrigault PFO, Pouzeratte YH, Jaber S, et al. Changes in occlusion pressure (P0.1) and breathing pattern during pressure support ventilation. Thorax 1999; 54:119–123.

81. Frutos-Vivar F, Esteban A. When to wean from a ventilator: an evidence-based strategy. Cleve Clin J Med 2003; 70(5):389, 392–393, 397.

82. Esteban A, Frutos F, Tobin MJ, et al. A comparison of four methods of weaning patients from mechanical ventilation. N Engl J Med 1995; 332:345–350.

83. Esteban A, Alia I, Tobin MJ, et al. Effect of spontaneous breathing trial duration on outcome of attempts to discontinue mechanical ventilation: Spanish lung failure collaborative group. Am J Respir Crit Care Med 1999; 159(2):512–518.

84. Ely EW, Baker AM, Dunagan DP, et al. Effect on the duration of mechanical ventilation of identifying patients capable of breathing spontaneously. N Engl J Med 1996; 335(25):1864–1869.

85. Brochard L, Rauss A, Benito S, et al. Comparison of three methods of gradual withdrawal from ventilatory support during weaning from mechanical ventilation. Am J Respir Crit Care Med 1994; 150:896–903.

86. Tomlinson JR, Miller KS, Lorch DG, et al. A prospective comparison of IMV and T-piece weaning from mechanical ventilation. Chest 1989; 96(2):348–352.

87. Dries DJ. Weaning from mechanical ventilation. J Trauma 1997; 43(2):372–384.

88. Putensen C, Hering R, Wrigge H. Controlled versus assisted mechanical ventilation. Curr Opin Crit Care 2002; 8(1):51–57.

89. Putensen C, Zech S, Wrigge H, et al. Long-term effects of spontaneous breathing during ventilatory support in patients with acute lung injury. Am J Respir Crit Care Med 2001; 164:43–49.

90. MacIntyre NR. Respiratory function during pressure support ventilation. Chest 1986; 89(5):677–683.

91. Koksal GM, Sayilgan C, Sen O, Oz H. The effects of different weaning modes on the endocrine stress response. Crit Care 2004; 8(1):R31–R34.

92. Kuhlen R, Rossaint R. The role of spontaneous breathing during mechanical ventilation. Respir Care 2002; 47(3):296–307.

93. Lessard MR, Brochard LJ. Weaning from ventilatory support. Clin Chest Med 1996; 17(3):475–489.

94. Strickland JH Jr, Hasson JH. A computer-controlled ventilator weaning system. Chest 1991; 100(4):1096–1099.

95. Rasanen J, Cane RD, Downs JB, et al. Airway pressure release ventilation during acute lung injury: a prospective multicenter trial. Crit Care Med 1991; 19(10):1234–1241.

96. Shen HN, Lin LY, Chen KY, et al. Changes of heart rate variability during ventilator weaning. Chest 2003; 123(4): 1222–1228.

97. Guttmann J, Berhnard H, Mols G, et al. Respiratory comfort of automatic tube compensation and inspiratory pressure support in conscious humans. Intensive Care Med 1997; 23(11):1119–1124.

98. Cohen JD, Shapiro M, Grozovski E, Singer P. Automatic tube compensation-assisted respiratory rate to tidal volume ratio improves the prediction of weaning outcome. Chest 2002; 122:980–984.

99. Haberthur C, Mols G, Elsasser S, et al. Extubation after breathing trials with automatic tube compensation, T-tube, or pressure support ventilation. Acta Anaesthesiol Scand 2002; 46(8):973–979.

100. Guttmann J, Haberthur C, Mols G, Lichtwarck-Aschoff M. Automatic tube compensation (ATC). Minerva Anesthesiol 2002; 68(5):369–377.

101. Maeda Y, Fujino Y, Uchiayama A, et al. Does the tube-compensation function of two modern mechanical ventilators provide effective work of breathing relief? Crit Care 2003; 7(5):R92–R97.

102. Kuhlen R, Max M, Dembinski R, et al. Breathing pattern and workload during automatic tube compensation, pressure support and T-piece trials in weaning patients. Eur J Anaesthesiol 2003; 20(1):10–16.

103. Knight DJ, Moppett IK, Hardman JG. Breathing pattern and workload during automatic tube compensation, pressure support and T-piece trials in weaning patients. Eur J Anaesthesiol 2003; 20(11):932–933.

104. Cassina T, Chiolero R, Mauri R, Revelly JP. Clinical experience with adaptive support ventilation for fast-track cardiac surgery. J Cardiothorac Vasc Anesth 2003; 17(5):571–575.

105. Petter AH, Chiolero RL, Cassina T, et al. Automatic "respirator/weaning" with adaptive support ventilation: the effect on duration of endotracheal intubation and patient management. Anesth Analg 2003; 97(6):1743–1750.

106. Brunner JX, Iotti GA. Adaptive support ventilation (ASV). Minerva Anesthesiol 2002; 68(5):365–368.

107. Linton DM, Potgieter PD, Davis S, et al. Automatic weaning from mechanical ventilation using an adaptive lung ventilation controller. Chest 1994; 106(6):1843–1850.

108. Cook D, Meade M, Guyatt G, et al. Trials of miscellaneous interventions to wean from mechanical ventilation. Chest 2001; 120(S6):S438–S444.

109. Gatti G, Cardu G, Bentini C, et al. Weaning from ventilator after cardiac operation using the Ciaglia percutaneous tracheostomy. Eur J Cardiothorac Surg 2004; 25(4):541–547.

110. Gross D, Shenkman Z, Bleiberg B, et al. Ginseng improves pulmonary functions and exercise capacity in patients with COPD. Monaldi Arch Chest Dis 2002; 57(5–6):242–246.

111. Holliday JE, Lippmann M. Reduction in ventilatory response to CO_2 with relaxation feedback during CO_2 rebreathing for ventilator patients. Chest 2003; 124(4):1500–1511.

112. Grap MJ, Strickland D, Tromey L, et al. Collaborative practice: development, implementation, and evaluation of a weaning protocol for patients receiving mechanical ventilation. Am J Crit Care 2003; 12(5):454–460.

113. Rodriguez JL, Steinberg SM, Luchetti FA, et al. Early tracheostomy for primary airway management in the surgical critical care setting. Surgery 1990; 108(4):655–659.

114. Vitacca M, Vianello A, Colombo D, et al. Comparison of two methods for weaning patients with chronic obstructive pulmonary disease requiring mechanical ventilation for more than 15 days. Am J Respir Crit Care Med 2001; 164(2):225–230.

115. Tobin MJ. Current concepts: mechanical ventilation. N Engl J Med 1994; 30(15):1056–1061.

116. Schachter EN, Tucker D, Beck GJ. Does intermittent mandatory ventilation accelerate weaning? J Am Med Assoc 1981; 246(11):1210–1214.

117. Hess D. Ventilator modes used in weaning. Chest 2001; 120(suppl 6):474S–476S.

118. Stoller JK, Mascha EJ, Kester L, Haney D. Randomized controlled trial of physician-directed versus respiratory therapy consult service-directed respiratory care to adult non-ICU inpatients. Am J Respir Crit Care Med 1998; 158(4):1068–1075.

119. Scheinhorn DJ, Artinian BM, Catlin JL. Weaning from prolonged mechanical ventilation: the experience at a regional weaning center. Chest 1994; 105(2):534–539.

120. Scheinhorn DJ, Chao C, Hassenpflug MS, Gracey DR. Post-ICU weaning from mechanical ventilation: the role of long-term facilities. Chest 2001; 120(suppl 6):482S–484S.

121. Schonhofer B, Euteneuer S, Nava S, et al. Survival of mechanically ventilated patients admitted to a specialised weaning centre. Intensive Care Med 2002; 28(7):908–916.

122. Stoller JK, Xu M, Mascha E, Rice R. Long-term outcomes for patients discharged from long-term hospital-based weaning unit. Chest 2003; 124(5):1892–1899.

123. Ceriana P, Delmastro M, Rampulla C, Nava S. Demographics and clinical outcomes of patients admitted to a respiratory intensive care unit located in a rehabilitation center. Respir Care 2003; 48(7):670–676.

124. Scheinhorn DJ, Chao DC, Stearn-Hassenpflug M, et al. Post-ICU mechanical ventilation: treatment of 1123 patients at a regional weaning center. Chest 1997; 111(6):1654–1659.

125. Nevins ML, Epstein SK. Weaning from prolonged mechanical ventilation. Clin Chest Med 2001; 22(1):13–33.

126. Ntoumenopoulos G, Presneill JJ, McElholum M, Cade JF. Chest physiotherapy for the prevention of ventilator-associated pneumonia. Intensive Care Med 2002; 28:850–856.

127. Martin AD, Davenport PD, Franceschi AC, Harman E. Use of inspiratory muscle strength training to facilitate ventilator weaning: a series of 10 consecutive patients. Chest 2002; 12(1):192–196.

128. Epstein SK, Ciubotaru RL, Wong JB. Effect of failed extubation on the outcome of mechanical ventilation. Chest 1997; 112(1):186–192.

129. Sprague SS, Hopkins PD. Use of inspiratory strength training to wean six patients who were ventilator-dependent. Phys Ther 2003; 83(2):171–181.

130. Harrop JS, Sharan AD, Scheid EH Jr, et al. Tracheostomy placement in patients with complex cervical spinal cord injuries: American spinal injury association grade A. J Neurosurg 2004; 10(suppl 1):20–23.

131. Heffner JE. Tracheotomy application and timing. Clin Chest Med 2003; 24(3):389–398.

132. Sugerman HJ, Wolfe L, Pasquale MD, et al. Multicenter, randomized, prospective trial of early tracheostomy. J Trauma 1997; 43(5):741–747.

133. Modawal A, Candadai NP, Mandell KM, et al. Weaning success among ventilator-dependent patients in a rehabilitation facility. Arch Phys Med Rehabil 2002; 83(2):154–157.

134. Lindsay ME, Bijwadia JS, Schauer WW, Rozich JD. Shifting care of chronic ventilator-dependent patients from the intensive care unit to the nursing home. Jt Comm J Qual Saf 2004; 30(5):257–265.

135. Horst HM, Mouro D, Hall-Jenssens RA, Pamukov N. Decrease in ventilation time with a standardized weaning process. Arch Surg 1998; 133:483–489.

136. Kollef MH, Shapiro SD, Silver P, et al. A randomized, controlled trial of protocol-directed versus physician-directed weaning from mechanical ventilation. Crit Care Med 1997; 25(4):567–574.

137. Price AM. Nurse-led weaning from mechanical ventilation: where's the evidence? Intensive Crit Care Nurs 2001; 17(3):167–176.

138. Kollef MH, Horst HM, Prang L, Brock WA. Reducing the duration of mechanical ventilation: three examples of change in the intensive care unit. New Horiz 1998; 6(1):52–60.

139. Henneman E, Dracup K, Ganz T, et al. Effect of a collaborative weaning plan on patient outcome in the critical care setting. Crit Care Med 2001; 29(2):297–303.

140. Ely EW, Meade MO, Haponik EF, et al. Mechanical ventilator weaning protocols driven by nonphysician health-care professionals: evidence-based clinical practice guidelines. Chest 2001; 120(suppl 6):454S–463S.

141. Pierson DJ. The future of respiratory care. Respir Care 2001; 46(7):705–718.

142. Walsh TS, Dodds S, McArdle F. Evaluation of simple criteria to predict successful weaning from mechanical ventilation in intensive care patients. Br J Anaesth 2004; 92(6):793–799.

143. Ely EW, Baker AM, Evans GW, Haponik EF. The prognostic significance of passing a daily screen of weaning parameters. Intensive Care Med 1999; 25(6):581–587.

144. Henneman E, Dracup K, Ganz T, et al. Using a collaborative weaning plan to decrease duration of mechanical ventilation and length of stay in the intensive care unit for patients receiving long-term ventilation. Am J Crit Care 2002; 11(2):132–140.

145. Duane TM, Riblet JL, Golay D, et al. Protocol-driven ventilator management in a trauma intensive care unit population. Arch Surg 2002; 137:1223–1227.

146. Marelich GP, Murin S, Battistella F, et al. Protocol weaning of mechanical ventilation in medical and surgical patients by respiratory care practitioners and nurses: effect on weaning time and incidence of ventilator-associated pneumonia. Chest 2000; 118(2):459–467.

147. Saura P, Blanch L, Mestre J, et al. Clinical consequences of the implementation of a weaning protocol. Intensive Care Med 1996; 22(10):1052–1056.

148. Meade M, Guyatt G, Cook D, et al. Predicting success in weaning from mechanical ventilation. Chest 2001; 120:400S–424S.

149. Ibrahim EH, Kollef MH. Using protocols to improve the outcomes of mechanically ventilated patients: focus on weaning and sedation. Crit Care Clin 2001; 17(4):989–1001.

150. Auriant I, Jallot A, Herve P, et al. Noninvasive ventilation reduces mortality in acute respiratory failure following lung resection. Am J Respir Crit Care Med 2001; 164(7):1231–1235.

151. Elliott MW, Confalonieri M, Nava S. Where to perform noninvasive ventilation? Eur Respir J 2002; 19(6):1159–1166.

152. Smyrnios NA, Connolly A, Wilson MM, et al. Effects of a multifaceted, multidisciplinary, hospital-wide quality improvement program on weaning from mechanical ventilation. Crit Care Med 2002; 30(6):1224–1230.

153. Hill NS. Following protocol: weaning difficult-to-wean patients with chronic obstructive pulmonary disease. Am J Respir Crit Care Med 2001; 164(2):186–187.

154. Ely EW. The utlity of weaning protocols to expedite liberation from mechanical ventilation. Respir Care Clin N Am 2000; 6(2):3019–3030.

155. Slutsky AS, Ranieri VM. Mechanical ventilation: lessons from the ARDSNet trial. Respir Res 2000; 1(2):73–77.

156. MacIntyre NR. Issues in ventilator weaning. Chest 1999; 115:1215–1216.

157. Krishnan JA, Moore D, Robeson C, et al. A prospective, controlled trial of a protocol-based strategy to discontinue mechanical ventilation. Am J Respir Crit Care Med 2004; 169(6):673–678.

158. Pryor JP, Reilly PM, Shapiro MB. Surgical airway management in the intensive care unit. Crit Care Clin 2000; 16(3):473–488.

159. Saffle JR, Morris SE, Edelman L. Early tracheostomy does not improve outcome in burn patients. J Burn Care Rehabil 2002; 23(6):431–438.

160. Heffner JE. The role of tracheostomy in weaning. Chest 2001; 120:4778–4815.

161. Mohr AM, Rutherford EJ, Cairns BA, Boysen PG. The role of dead space ventilation in predicting outcome of successful weaning from mechanical ventilation. J Trauma 2001; 512(5):843–848.

162. Diehl JL, El Atrows S, Touchard D, et al. Changes in the work of breathing induced by tracheostomy in ventilation-dependent patients. Am J Respir Crit Care Med 1999; 159:383–388.

163. Kupfer Y, Tessler S. Weaning the difficult patient: the evolution from art to science. Chest 2001; 119:7–9.

164. Epstein SK. Predicting extubation failure. Chest 2001; 120:1061–1063.

165. Rothaar RC, Epstein SK. Extubation failure: magnitude of the problem, impact on outcomes, and prevention. Curr Opin Crit Care 2003; 9(1):59–66.

166. Epstein SK, Ciubotaru RL. Independent effects of etiology of failure and time to reintubation on outcome for patients failing extubation. Am J Respir Crit Care Med 1998; 158(2):489–493.

167. De Jonghe B, Bastuji-Garin S, Sharshar T, et al. Does ICU-acquired paresis lengthen weaning from mechanical ventilation? Intensive Care Med 2004; 30:1117–1121.

168. Aberegg SK. Noninvasive ventilation and weaning. Am J Respir Crit Care Med 2004; 169(7):882.

169. Tulaimat A, Mokhlesi B. Noninvasive ventilation for persistent weaning failure. Am J Respir Crit Care Med 2004; 169(9):1073–1074.

170. Burns KE, Meade MO. Noninvasive ventilation reduces duration of mechanical ventilation and ICU stay more than conventional weaning. ACP J Club 2004; 140(2):35.

171. Welte T. Noninvasive ventilation in the intensive care unit—is it still negligible? Wien Klin Wochenschr 2003; 115(3–4):89–98.

172. Ferrer M, Esquinas A, Arancibia F, et al. Noninvasive ventilation during persistent weaning failure: a randomized controlled trial. Am J Respir Crit Care Med 2003; 168(1):70–76.

173. Giacomini M, Iapichino G, Cigada M, et al. Short-term noninvasive pressure support ventilation prevents ICU admittance in patients with acute cardiogenic pulmonary edema. Chest 2003; 123(6):2057–2061.

174. Burns KE, Adhikari NK, Meade MO. Non-invasive positive pressure ventilation as a weaning strategy for intubated adults with respiratory failure. Cochrane Database Syst Rev 2003; (4):CD004127.

175. Baudouin S, Blumenthal S, Cooper B, et al. Non-invasive ventilation in acute respiratory failure. Thorax 2002; 57: 192–211.

176. Nava S, Ceriana P. Causes of failure of noninvasive mechanical ventilation. Respir Care 2004; 49(3):295–303.

177. Meduri GU, Turner RE, Abou-Shala N, et al. Noninvasive positive pressure ventilation via face mask. Chest 1996; 109:179–193.

178. Janssens JP, Derivaz S, Breitenstein E, et al. Changing patterns in long-term noninvasive ventilation: a 7-year prospective study in the Geneva Lake area. Chest 2004; 123(1):67–79.

179. Smailies ST. Non-invasive positive pressure ventilation in burns. Burns 2002; 28(8):795–801.

180. Conti G, Antonelli M, Navalesi P, et al. Noninvasive vs conventional mechanical ventilation in patients with chronic obstructive pulmonary disease after failure of medical treatment in the ward: a randomized trial. Intensive Care Med 2002; 28(12):1701–1707.

181. Chadda K, Annane D, Hart N, et al. Cardiac and respiratory effects of continuous positive airway pressure and noninvasive ventilation in acute cardiac pulmonary edema. Crit Care Med 2002; 30(11):2457–2461.

182. Van de Louw A, Brocas E, Boiteau R, et al. Esophageal perforation associated with noninvasive ventilation: a case report. Chest 2002; 122(5):1857–1858.

183. Thys F, Roeseler J, Reynaert M, et al. Noninvasive ventilation for acute respiratory failure: a prospective randomised placebo-controlled trial. Eur Respir J 2002; 20(3):545–555.

184. Ferrer M, Bernadich O, Nava S, Torres A. Noninvasive ventilation after intubation and mechanical ventilation. Eur Respir J 2002; 19(5):959–965.

185. American Thoracic Society, European Respiratory Society, European Society of Intensive Care Medicine, Societe de Reanimation de Langue Francaise. International Consensus Conferences in Intensive Care Medicine: Noninvasive Positive Pressure Ventilation in Acute Respiratory Failure. Am J Respir Crit Care Med 2001; 163(1):283–291.

186. Keenan SP, Powers C, McCormack DG, Block G. Noninvasive positive-pressure ventilation for postextubation respiratory distress: a randomized controlled trial. J Am Med Assoc 2002; 287(24):3238–3244.

187. Lerman RM, Weiss MS. Progressive resistive exercise in weaning high quadriplegics from the ventilator. Paraplegia 1987; 25(2):130–135.

188. Gutierrez CJ, Harrow J, Haines F. Using an evidence-based protocol to guide rehabilitation and weaning of ventilator-dependent cervical spinal cord injury patients. J Rehabil Res Dev 2003; 40(5, suppl 2):99–100.

189. Williams O, Greenough A, Mustfa N, et al. Extubation failure due to phrenic nerve injury. Arch Dis Child Fetal Neonatal Ed 2003; 8(1):F72–F73.

190. MacIntyre NR. Psychological factors in weaning from mechanical ventilatory support. Respir Care 1995; 40(3):277–281.

191. Ely EW, Margolin R, Francis J, et al. Evaluation of delerium in critically ill patients: validation of the confusion assessment method for the intensive care unit (CAM-ICU). Crit Care Med 2001; 29:1370–1379.

192. Herr DL, Sum-Ping ST, England M. ICU sedation after coronary artery bypass graft surgery: dexmedetomidine-based versus propofol-based sedation regimens. J Cardiothorac Vasc Anesth 2003; 17(5):576–584.

193. Groeben H, Mitzner W, Brown RH. Effects of the alpha 2-adrenoceptor agonist dexmedetomidine on bronchoconstriction in dog. Anesthesiology 2004; 100(2):359–363.

194. Takrouri MS, Seraj MA, Channa AB, et al. Dexmedetomidine in intensive care unit: a study hemodynamic changes. Middle East J Anesthesiol 2002; 16(6):587–595.

195. Tritsch AE, Welte M, von Homeyer P, et al. Bispectral index-guided sedation with dexmedetomidine in intensive care: a prospective randomized, double blind, placebo-controlled phase II study. Crit Care Med 2002; 30(5):1007–1014.

196. Venn RM, Hell J, Grounds RM. Respiratory effects of dexmedetomidine in the surgical patient requiring intensive care. Crit Care 2000; 4(5):302–308.

197. Multz AS. Prolonged dexmedetomidine infusion as an adjunct in treating sedation-induced withdrawal. Anesth Analg 2003; 96(4):1054–1055.

198. Kress JP, Pohlman AS, O'Connor MF, Hall JB. Daily interruption of sedative infusions in critically ill patients undergoing mechanical ventilation. N Engl J Med 2000; 342(20):121–127.

199. Laghi F, Cattapan SE, Jubran A, et al. Is weaning failure caused by low-frequency fatigue of the diaphragm? Am J Respir Crit Care Med 2003; 167(2):120–127.

200. Shanely RA, Coombes JS, Zergergolu AM, et al. Short-duration mechanical ventilation enhances diaphragmatic fatigue resistance but impairs for production. Chest 2003; 123(1): 195–201.

201. Bernard N, Matecki S, Py G, et al. Effects of prolonged mechanical ventilation on respiratory muscle ultrastructure and mitochondrial respiration in rabbits. Intensive Care Med 2003; 29(1):111–118.

202. Gayan-Ramirez G, de Paepe K, Cadot P, Decramer M. Detrimental effects of short-term mechanical ventilation on diaphragm function and IGF-ImR in rats. Intensive Care Med 2003; 29(5):825–833.

203. Vassilakopoulos T, Zakynhinos S, Rousssos C. Respiratory muscles and weaning failure. Eur Respir J 1996; 9(11):2283–2400.

204. Anzueto A, Andrade FH, Maxwell LC, et al. Diaphragmatic function after resistive breathing in vitamin E-deficient rats. J Appl Physiol 1993; 74(1):267–271.

205. Gosselink R, Kovacs L, Ketelaer P, et al. Respiratory muscle weakness and respiratory muscle training in severely disabled multiple sclerosis patients. Arch Phys Med Rehabil 2000; 81(6):747–751.

206. Sturdy G, Hillman D, Green D, et al. Feasibility of high-intensity, interval-based respiratory muscle training in COPD. Chest 2003; 123(1):142–150.

207. Romer LM, McConnell AK. Specificity and reversibility of inspiratory muscle training. Med Sci Sorts Exerc 2003; 35(2):237–244.

208. Weinberger SE, Weiss JW. Weaning from ventilatory support. N Engl J Med 1995; 332(6):388–389.

209. Nayak AK, Aggarwal K, Flaker GC. Minute ventilation-sensor driven pacemaker related difficulty in weaning from mechanical ventilation: a case report. Mo Med 2001; 98(5): 181–183.

210. Hurford WE, Favorito F. Association of myocardial ischemia with failure to wean from mechanical ventilation. Crit Care Med 1995; 23(9):1475–1480.

211. Chatila W, Ani S, Guaglianone, et al. Cardiac ischemia during weaning from mechanical ventilation. Chest 1996; 109(6):1577–1583.

212. Legras A, Dequin PF, Hazouard E, et al. Right-to-left interatrial shunt in ARDS: dramatic improvement in prone position. Intensive Care Med 1999; 25(4):412–414.

213. Lemaire F, Teboul JL, Cinotti L, et al. Acute left ventricular dysfunction during unsuccessful weaning from mechanical ventilation. Anesthesiology 1988; 69:171–179.

214. Richard C, Teboul JL, Archambaud F, et al. Left ventricular pulmonary disease. Intensive Care Med 1994; 20:181–186.

215. Smith-Blair NJ, Pierce JD, Clancy RL. The effect of dobutamine infusion on fractional diaphragm thickening and diaphragm blood flow during fatigue. Heart Lung 2003; 32(2):111–120.

216. Agusti AG, Torres A, Estopa R, Agustividal A. Hypophosphatemia as a cause of failed weaning: the importance of metabolic factors. Crit Care Med 1984; 12(2):142–143.

217. Varsano S, Shapiro M, Taragan R, Bruderman I. Hypophosphatemia as a reversible case of refractory ventilatory failure. Crit Care Med 1983; 11(11):908–909.

218. Peltz S, Hashmi S. Severe hypokalemia and ventilator-dependent generalized paralysis. NY State J Med 1991; 91(1):32–33.

219. Chandrashekar R, Claxton AR. Acute respiratory failure secondary to severe hypokalaemia. Anaesthesia 2000; 55(12):1221–1222.

220. Davies RG, Gemmell L. Severe hypokalaemia causing acute respiratory failure. Anaesthesia 2001; 56(7):694–695.

221. Glaisyer HR, Pary M, Lee J, et al. The laryngeal mask airway as an adjunct to extubation on the intensive care unit. Anaesthesia 1996; 51(12):1187–1188.

222. Tobin MJ, Jubran A, Hines E Jr. Pathophysiology of failure to wean from mechanical ventilation. Schweiz Med Wochenschr 1994; 124(47): 2139–2145.

29

Extubation of the Difficult Airway and Endotracheal Tube Change in the Surgical Intensive Care Unit

Ahmed Elrefai

Department of Anesthesiology, INOVA Fairfax Hospital, Falls Church, Virginia, U.S.A.

Michael Berrigan

Department of Anesthesiology and Critical Care Medicine, George Washington University Hospital, Washington, D.C., U.S.A.

INTRODUCTION

☞ **Extubation of a known difficult airway and especially planned endotracheal tube (ETT) change in a critically ill patient should be approached with a similar degree of concern and preparation as that given to initial intubation.** ☞ That is, the patient should be evaluated for difficulty of reintubation due to known anatomic or pathologic airway conditions. In addition, the likelihood of difficulty maintaining cardiopulmonary function during the reintubation interval must be incorporated into the airway plan of patients dependent upon high levels of ventilatory support. Similarly, perturbations in intracranial pressure (ICP) in patients with decreased intracranial compliance must be considered in trauma patients requiring ETT change. The basic aphorism "Never take out that which you can not put back in" should be followed when the tube is critical to the patient's survival.

The incidence of tracheal reintubation in the surgical intensive care unit (SICU) setting has been reported as 4% in a study of 700 consecutive extubations (1). It should be noted that a very low incidence of reintubation may not necessarily be a good thing. It might indicate excessively conservative management and an unnecessarily prolonged course of mechanical ventilation (MV) in many patients. The reintubation rates reported in the postanesthesia care unit are much lower, less than 0.2% (2,3). In the intensive care unit (ICU), self-extubation, either deliberate or accidental, accounts for slightly more than 10% of all extubations (4). After controlling for comorbidities and severity of illness, the need for reintubation has been shown to be an independent predictor of mortality (5). Although this higher mortality was associated with nonairway problems, rather than with complications of the reintubation itself, in a medical ICU (6), numerous airway-related mishaps are involved in the morbidity of reintubation, especially in the SICU where postextubation stridor can result from numerous complications of resuscitation, primary disease, trauma, or burns.

Practice guidelines for management of the difficult airway developed by the American Society of Anesthesiologists (ASA) in 1993, and updated in 2003, recommend that airway practitioners should have a "Preformed strategy for extubation of the difficult airway" (7,8). The recommended components of the preformed extubation strategy are listed in Table 1 (7).

This chapter reviews the risk factors for difficult extubation in critically ill patients, or ETT change, along with other criteria that should be evaluated prior to extubation. Next the value of airway exchange catheters (AECs) and fiberoptic bronchoscopes (FOBs) during ETT change or removal is surveyed. Guidelines for the use of other adjunct devices and rescue maneuvers are also provided. This chapter should be reviewed along with Volume 1, Chapter 9, and Volume 2, Chapter 28.

EXTUBATION/REINTUBATION CONSIDERATIONS/ RISK FACTORS

Some extubations in the ICU are inherently more risky than others. For example, patients with a history of difficult intubation, and those who have undergone a procedure or developed a condition that makes reintubation more challenging are considered "difficult intubation" patients. Others with risk factors for surgical-airway difficulty (e.g., radiation therapy or tissue swelling) represent risks in terms of backup procedures. In addition, those with physiologic risk factors [e.g., requirement for high F_IO_2, positive end expiratory pressure (PEEP), inability to do the work of breathing (WOB) or clear secretions] will not likely tolerate ETT removal for long. Likewise, those with unstable ICP or hemodynamic status, and those pharmacological risk factors all require specific preparation and treatment (Table 2).

Although the presence of an indwelling ETT implies previous intubation success, the ease with which the ETT was placed is not necessarily obvious. Consequently, it is important to determine the circumstances (ease or difficulty) with which the previous intubation occurred. The medical record is helpful in this regard if the documentation was well done. However, there are many instances when this information will not be available.

Intubation History

Any mention of a difficult intubation during prior airway manipulations requires further investigation and clarification. If the patient came from the operative suite, a record of the intubation should be chronicled in the anesthesia record. When difficult intubation is mentioned, it is

Table 1   The Preformulated Extubation Strategy

A consideration of the relative merits of awake extubation versus
  extubation
An evaluation for general clinical factors that may produce an
  adverse impact on ventilation after the patient has been
  extubated
The formulation of an airway management plan that can be
  implemented if the patient is not able to maintain adequate
  ventilation after extubation
A consideration of the short-term use of an AEC that can serve as a
  guide for expedited reintubation; this type of device is usually
  inserted through the lumen of the tracheal tube and into the
  trachea before the tracheal tube is removed; the device may be
  rigid to facilitate intubation and/or hollow to facilitate
  ventilation

Abbreviation: AEC, airway exchange catheter.

important to note the circumstances surrounding the intubation and the technique(s) used. Among the variables to be noted are whether or not the patient was easily ventilated by mask, the position of the patient, the specifics of the equipment used, the number of attempts required, and which member of the health-care team (novice vs. senior airway expert) performed the intubation.

Physical Examination of the Airway

Physical evaluation techniques for determining the ease or difficulty of intubation are improving in precision. A

Table 2   Causes of Difficult Extubation/Reintubation

Causes	Mechanism	Examples
Difficult reintubation/ventilation	Anatomic	I-IG, OPV, MS, H&N ROM
	Pathologic	Trauma, fluid, angioedema
	Mechanical	Halo, fused spine, IMF
Will not tolerate extubation for long (i.e., patients are not weaned, but need an ETT change)	Impaired oxygenation	↑ PEEP, ↑ F_IO_2
	↑'d WOB	↑R_{AW}, ↑ PIPs, ↑ $\dot{V}_E$, ↑ CO_2, ↑ V_D
	↓'d ability to WOB	↑RSBI, or ↓ MIF
	Other systemic or neurologic conditions	Shock—numerous etiologies (Volume 2, Chapter 18) ↑'d ICP

Abbreviations: CO_2, carbon dioxide; F_IO_2, fraction of inhaled O_2; H&N, head and neck; ICP, intracranial pressure; I-IG, inter-incisor gap; IMF, intermaxillary fixation; MIF, maximum inspiratory force; MS, mandibular space; OPV, oral-pharyngeal view; PEEP, positive end expiratory pressure; PIPs, peak inspiratory pressure; ↑ R_{AW}, airway resistance; ROM, range of motion; RSBI, rapid shallow breathing index; WOB, work of breathing; ↑, high; ↓'d, decreased; ↑'d, increased; $\dot{V}_E$, minute ventilation; V_D, dead space; ↓, low.

formal 11-step airway evaluation as outlined in Volume 1, Chapter 9 should be performed in all patients prior to intubation, and prior to elective ETT change in the ICU. There is a high predictive value in addressing measurements such as the thyromental distance (TMD), mouth opening, and neck extension (9). The Mallampati test, which involves visual inspection of the pharynx, is less precise in the intubated patient. However, a receding chin (short TMD), a pronounced dental overbite, a short, thick neck, a highly arched palate, and a small mouth can all be appreciated by physical exam. All have been associated with a difficult tracheal intubation. The reader is referred to Volume 1, Chapter 9 for complete guidelines on the 11-step airway examination. In addition, those patients whose neck movement is restricted by pathology or by external restraint such as a cervical collar or rigid halo device represent additional hazards likely due to technical difficulties in intubating the trachea.

Postsurgical/Trauma Considerations

☞ A critical airway consideration in the posttrauma or critically ill surgical patient is the likelihood of periglottic swelling or pathology that could lead to postextubation stridor and possible inability to intubate or ventilate the patient. ☞

Risk factors for postextubation stridor include: airway edema due to massive resuscitation and/or hypoalbuminemia, high levels of circulating inflammatory mediators due to sepsis/systemic inflammatory response syndrome, direct neck trauma, or burns (especially to neck and face). In addition, prolonged intubation can cause ulcers to develop on the vocal cords, or cysts to form, which can obstruct the airway following extubation. Another important consideration is recurrent laryngeal nerve injury, which will cause unopposed adduction of the vocal cord involved, and consequent stridor.

Techniques for Predicting Postextubation Stridor

☞ In the case of patients at high risk for postextubation stridor, a formal evaluation for periglottic swelling should be performed prior to attempts at extubation or ETT exchange. Options for evaluation of airway swelling include: (*i*) cuff-leak test, (*ii*) FOB evaluation, and (*iii*) imaging studies. ☞

Cuff-Leak Test

The cuff-leak test has been used in a variety of ways over the years, with varying degrees of success. Potgieter and Hammond (10) described a qualitative cuff-leak test performed by deflation of the ETT cuff, digital occlusion of the tube, and an assessment of air movement around the tube. They evaluated this in 10 patients who had previously had required intubation for upper-airway obstruction due to edema. They did not describe the extubation of patients without a cuff-leak or the implications of leaving the tube in place until a cuff-leak develops. The authors also failed to emphasize the difference in evaluation success rates when flow is characterized during exhalation versus inhalation. When clear flow occurs during exhalation only (where there is less propensity for airway closure), but not during inhalation (where collapse is more likely to occur due to dynamic resistive changes), then the predictive power of extubation success is likely to be lower than in situations where clear airflow is heard around the obstructed ETT during both inhalation and exhalation. Kemper et al. (11) confirmed Potgieter's observation in a pediatric burn and trauma unit, concluding that the absence of a cuff leak was the best predictor of the need for reintubation or tracheostomy.

Fisher and Raper (12) observed that all 60 patients with a cuff leak were successfully extubated, but two patients extubated without a cuff leak required reintubation, and five patients who repeatedly failed the test required tracheostomy. They subsequently studied 10 patients without a cuff leak; only three of whom required reintubation or tracheostomy, whereas the majority tolerated extubation despite "failing" the cuff-leak test.

Owing to the generally poor positive predictive value (true positive tests divided by total positive tests) of the qualitative cuff-leak test (with a "positive test" defined as absent airflow around the obstructed ETT with the cuff down) (12,13), techniques for quantitating the cuff-leak test were developed. Indeed, investigators can now quantify the degree of leak around an indwelling ETT, with the cuff deflated, in mechanically ventilated patients. The leak volume in these studies is quantified by measuring the difference in exhaled tidal volume before and after cuff deflation occurs while patients continue to receive positive pressure ventilation.

In the two largest studies of this type to date, the cuff-leak test was not found to be predictive. Engoren (14) studied 524 patients, defining failure as those with <110 mL leak-volume, the study yielded a positive predictive value of zero. Kriner et al. (15) performed a quantitative cuff test on 464 patients who had been intubated an average of 5 ± 4 days in a medical–surgical ICU, a failed cuff-leak test in this study was defined as ≤110 mL, or ≤15.5% of exhaled volume before cell deflation. These authors conclude that the cuff-leak test is an unreliable indicator of postextubation stridor. A large part of the variability relates to the many factors (besides the cross-sectional area around the ETT that contributes to the degree of leak, e.g., the respiratory mechanics, the inspiratory flow, pressure, and I:E ratio) (16).

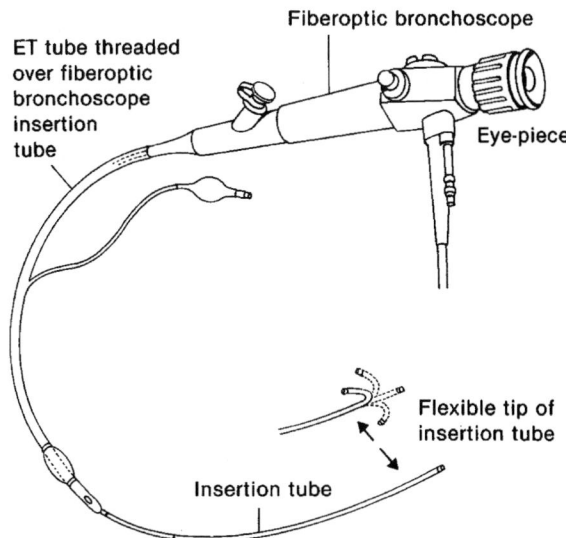

Figure 1 Fiberoptic bronchoscope (FOB). FOB is integral to the evaluation of periglottic swelling often responsible for postextubation stridor. The FOB is also useful in facilitating reintubation of the difficult airway.

Fiberoptic Bronchoscopy Evaluation

☛ **In situations where the patient is at high risk for postextubation stridor, additional specific evaluation with FOB (Fig. 1) is warranted.** ☛ The FOB can be used to suction debris from the airway and improve the immediate postextubation ventilatory status. It can also be used to evaluate the airway for anatomic and pathologic evidence of airway swelling that will increase the risk of postextubation stridor. The use of the FOB for airway manipulations is fully reviewed in Volume 1, Chapter 9.

The patient should be placed on 100% O_2, and be topicalized with local anesthetics delivered above the glottis (including in the nasal and oral passages), as well as through the ETT to anesthetize the tracheal and bronchial mucosa. The patient should also receive any necessary systemic analgesia and sedation as required to tolerate the procedure. Besides small doses of opioid titrated to a respiration rate (RR) ≥12, sedation can be titrated as needed, but should not be so excessive as to obtund the patient. Sedation choices range from low doses of benzodiazepine or propofol, to dexmedetomidine, a newer α_2 agonist that does not depress respiration, but does decrease opioid requirements. The primary side effect of dexmedetomidine is hypotension due to its activation of the α_2-adrenergic receptor (17). It is dosed intravenously and maintained via intravenous infusion. Currently, dexmedetomidine is approved for up to 24 hours of use; however, there are several reports of longer use in the ICU without complications (18).

Reassuring findings during airway evaluation by FOB include: (*i*) ability to clearly visualize the vocal cords around the indwelling ETT, (*ii*) absence of significant supraglottic swelling (that might progress following removal of the ETT), (*iii*) visualization of room between the anterior commissure of the vocal cords and the ETT (i.e., should be able to pass the FOB alongside the ETT and enter the trachea), (*iv*) confirmation that the airway passages (trachea and main bronchi) are patent, without massive retained secretions or bronchial plugs, and (*v*) verification that the posterior membrane of the trachea stays expanded during inhalation (rather than involuting and causing a subglottic form of postextubation stridor). Although these above mentioned findings are reassuring, their predictive power has yet to be confirmed in prospective, randomized, controlled trials (RCTs).

Imaging Studies

All available imaging data should be evaluated prior to extubation or elective ETT change in patients with likely anatomic or pathologic airway problems that could contribute to postextubation stridor. Although this recommendation constitutes common wisdom, there have not been any prospective RCTs investigating the predictive power of computed tomography or magnetic resonance imaging findings and the likelihood of postextubation stridor.

A recent development in this area has been the introduction of laryngeal ultrasound (US) (19). Laryngeal US is less invasive than FOB. The laryngeal US probe is placed on the skin of the anterior neck at the level of the cricothyroid membrane. Using this technique, Ding et al. demonstrated that laryngeal US was capable of evaluating the vocal cords, laryngeal morphology, and the ease of airflow through the vocal cords. The air column width during cuff deflation appeared to be a potential predictor of postextubation stridor; however, because it was a pilot study, it was not powered enough to provide definitive data.

ET tube threaded over fiberoptic bronchoscope insertion tube

Fiberoptic bronchoscope

Eye-piece

Flexible tip of insertion tube

Insertion tube

Evaluating Ease of Performing Surgical Airway

☞ In the case where airway management is difficult and both conventional and adjunct procedures (described subsequently) all fail, then a surgical airway should be performed. ☞ In fact, in some patients, a surgical airway will be the best first option for definitive airway exchange in the ICU. For example, converting the ETT to a tracheostomy would be warranted in the patient with respiratory failure who requires an ETT change due to balloon cuff rupture, but is expected to have a very difficult reintubation, or has documented tight-swelling around the indwelling ETT. In these cases, going to the operating room and performing a formal tracheostomy under a controlled setting is a safer choice than risking an ETT change in the ICU.

Regardless of planned surgical airway, or if the surgical option is relegated as a "Plan B," an evaluation of the anatomic structure in the neck should be undertaken to determine the ease of performing a surgical airway. In addition, the ability to flex and extend the neck should be determined. Finally, the cricothyroid membrane should be palpated and marked on the neck (in case of need), and a surgical airway kit should be at the bedside, along with a trained surgeon capable of performing the procedure. In the very highest risk cases of all, the neck should even be prepped and draped and the head extended so that an emergency surgical airway could be more easily conducted if needed.

Other Factors

There are other conditions associated with the inability to safely exchange an ETT or tolerate extubation which do not directly involve upper-airway swelling, or impairment of pulmonary status. There are numerous physiologic risk factors which predispose a patient toward altered mental status, perhaps respiratory insufficiency and systemic inflammation (Volume 2, Chapter 63). In addition, poor planning or absence of qualified airway experts or assistance can be detrimental. It has been estimated that as much as 62% of reintubations are the result of an error of judgment/problem recognition (20). Other contributing factors included high unit activity, difficult patient habitus, and lack of patient cooperation. ☞ When considering ETT change or extubation, decisions must be made on an individual basis with evaluation of the entire clinical picture considered rather than focusing upon a single event or parameter. ☞ Patient secretions are often overlooked; adequate suctioning of the oropharynx should be performed prior to any attempt at extubation or ETT exchange. An antisialogogue may be useful in this regard.

EXTUBATION IN THE INTENSIVE CARE UNIT

In preparing a patient for extubation in the ICU, all the points discussed in "Extubation/Reintubation Considerations/Risk Factors" should be considered. Several additional observations and laboratory studies should be considered to determine the patient's overall fitness for weaning, but above all, sound clinical judgment is required. Prior to attempting ETT removal or exchange, the checklist provided in Table 3 should be followed.

In terms of weaning criteria, the seven-step approach to weaning detailed in Table 1 of Volume 2, Chapter 28 should be used. It is required that the patient has adequate affirmative responses to all seven parameters prior to safe extubation

Table 3 Criteria Checklist Prior to Extubation/Tube Change

Criteria	Examples/comments
Fulfills all weaning criteria	Necessary if extubation is planned (seven-step approach according to Volume 2, Chapter 28)
Successful "cuff-leak test"	No leak = ↑'d risk of stridor
Pre-extubation FOB exam	Evaluate periglottic anatomy when no leak on cuff-leak test, and other high-risk patients
Extubate over appropriately sized AEC	Use whenever in doubt about airway caliber adequacy for extubation, and when reintubation expected to be difficult
Assistance tools available	The following tools are useful: O_2, suction, RDL, FOB (pre-ensleeved), LMA, Combitube, TTJV, surgeon

Abbreviations: AEC, airway exchange catheter; FOB, fiberoptic bronchoscope; LMA, laryngeal mask airway; O_2, oxygen; RDL, rigid direct laryngoscopy; TTJV, transtracheal jet ventilation; ↑'d, increased.

in the SICU. The seven requirements are: (*i*) the patient has recovered from or improved sufficiently from the primary disease process that necessitated intubation and MV; (*ii*) there is no intercurrent condition that will require continued MV (e.g., renal failure, liver failure, neuromuscular weakness, etc.); (*iii*) the patient is able to maintain adequate oxygenation with reduced FiO_2 ($PaO_2 > 90$ mmHg on $FiO_2 \leq 0.4$ with PEEP ≤ 8); (*iv*) the WOB is not high (i.e., the $\dot{V}_E$ is not excessive, the airway resistance is not elevated, and the compliance is not too low); (*v*) the patient must be able to do the WOB [i.e., the maximum inspiratory force (MIF) and vital capacity are high, and the rapid shallow breathing index (RSBI) is low (<50 is excellent, <100 may be adequate)]; (*vi*) the patient is awake, cooperative, and has intact airway reflexes (e.g., gag and cough); and (*vii*) the patient does not have a reason for difficult reintubation if he/she fails extubation. If reintubation is expected to be difficult, the patient should initially be extubated over an AEC.

☞ In terms of weaning parameters, the RSBI is probably the single best indicator for determining the patient's ability to perform the required WOB. ☞ The RSBI is defined as the RR divided by the tidal volume in liters achieved while breathing spontaneously. Those patients with an RSBI >100 generally cannot tolerate extubation (21,22).

No one set of criteria or parameters will be able to predict the success of extubation with certainty. The following criteria are a list of guidelines which may be employed in evaluating the patient for a potential extubation.

ENDOTRACHEAL TUBE EXCHANGE

Although extubation ultimately remains the goal for every patient on MV, ETT exchange may be required until the patient has improved enough to fulfill the seven criteria for weaning. Indications for ETT exchange include damaged ETT, exchange of a specialized ETT (e.g., double-lumen ETT), and exchange of ETT size to allow for bronchoscopy (Table 4). In addition, if an excessively small ETT is in place, optimal ventilator settings may not be achieved due

Table 4 Indications for Endotracheal Tube (ETT) Exchange

Damaged ETT
Exchange of a specialized ETT (e.g., double-lumen tube)
ETT exchange to allow for bronchoscopy
Exchange of a small ETT for a larger one to aid in positive pressure
  ventilation

to the resistance encountered due to the small internal diameter of the ETT.

To determine the feasibility of safe ETT exchange, all elements discussed in "Extubation/Reintubation Considerations/Risk Factors" should be considered. In addition, an FOB examination should be performed and the FOB should be available for the management of the difficult airway (23). The other methods mentioned in Table 5 are used less frequently depending upon experience and familiarity.

Direct Laryngoscopy—Simple Endotracheal Tube Exchange

☞ **Direct laryngoscopy is the most common and simplest method for establishing airway access and appropriate when reintubation is not expected to be difficult (Fig. 2).** ☞ As with all procedures, experienced personnel should perform direct laryngoscopy. It is the procedure of choice for simple and uncomplicated ETT exchange, as would be anticipated in patients with known easy airway and without swelling which could cause postextubation stridor. However, the critically ill patient is seldom simple and uncomplicated. The postsurgical and physiologic changes in the airway that develop in the ICU patient may make direct laryngoscopy more difficult. Any attempts to perform direct laryngoscopy should be done carefully, and numerous attempts will be harmful to the patient. If the airway structures are in any way obscure, another method of airway access should be considered so that edema and hemorrhage will not complicate the picture further. These alternative methods are considered subsequently.

Airway Exchange Catheters

AECs are devices designed to allow the exchange of one ETT for another without losing access to the airway (Fig. 3). The AEC can also be used to administer O_2 and to detect O_2 (Table 6). These are especially useful when the airway was difficult or is expected to be difficult to reestablish. These AECs have been used safely for the extubation of patients

Table 5 Commonly Used Devices for Endotracheal Tube Exchange

Direct laryngoscopy
ETT exchangers
FOB
LMA—to facilitate FOB
Airway intubating mask—to facilitate FOB
Intubating LMA—only when airway obstruction or injury is absent
Lighted stylette
Wu scope
Bullard scope

Abbreviations: ETT, endotracheal tube; FOB, fiberoptic bronchoscope; LMA, laryngeal mask airway.

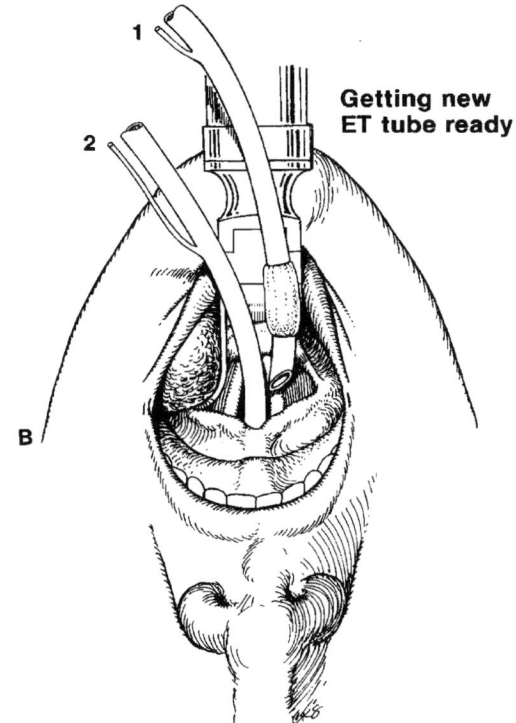

Getting new ET tube ready

Figure 2 Use of direct laryngoscopy for endotracheal tube (ETT) change. Changing an ETT with direct laryngoscopy is appropriate in patients without expected airway difficulty. However, other techniques, involving use of an airway exchange catheter and/or a fiberoptic bronchoscope are recommended for difficult airways. *Note*: "1" refers to new ETT and "2" refers to malfunctioning ETT.

with a known difficult airway for two decades. In a study of 40 patients with a known difficult airway who were extubated using the AEC, four required reintubation; all were accomplished successfully using the AEC (24).

The most frequent indication for the use of an AEC is a damaged ETT, or the need for a different sized or specialized ETT. In addition to use as a stylette, or guide for reintubation, AECs can also be used as a backup, left in the trachea following extubation for minutes to hours. The hollow lumen can be used for insufflating oxygen or to sample CO_2. These catheters are specially designed to facilitate their use. The features include: (*i*) measurement markings allowing the determination of the catheter length relative to that of the ETT. (*ii*) Distal openings and a standard 15-mm adapter which allow for ventilation using a ventilator circuit or ambu bag during the exchange or as a bridge between ETTs. (*iii*) These are available in different sizes and lengths to accommodate differing ETT inner diameters and lengths (Table 7).

Risks

☞ **The risks involved in using AECs include loss of the established airway and damage to the airway from the device.** ☞
The loss of the airway may result from kinking or flexing the AEC while withdrawing the damaged ETT. The use of a small amount of water-based lubricant may help protect against this. AEC has a blunt tip, however, there remains the risk of penetrating a bronchus or creating a clinically significant mucosal tear while using this device. It is

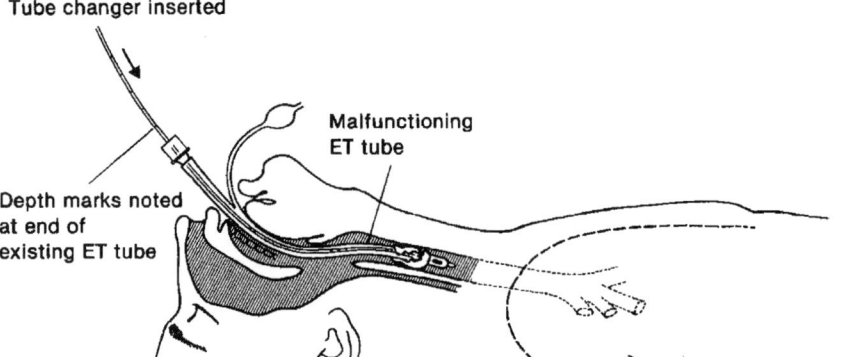

Figure 3 Use of airway exchange catheter (AEC) for endotracheal tube change. An AEC can be used as a stylette to guide reintubation, as well as a conduit for providing O_2 and/or measuring CO_2 during airway manipulations.

recommended that the tip of the AEC remain 2–3 cm above the carina in order to avoid the more sensitive areas of lung architecture.

Technique

The process for exchanging an ETT over AEC is relatively intuitive. There are a few points which should be emphasized so that patient safety is maintained throughout the procedure. Whenever possible, the original ETT position should be determined by FOB. If this is not done, the equipment should be immediately available. All standard airway equipment should be immediately on hand as well (laryngoscope with multiple blades, ETT sizes, and stylettes).

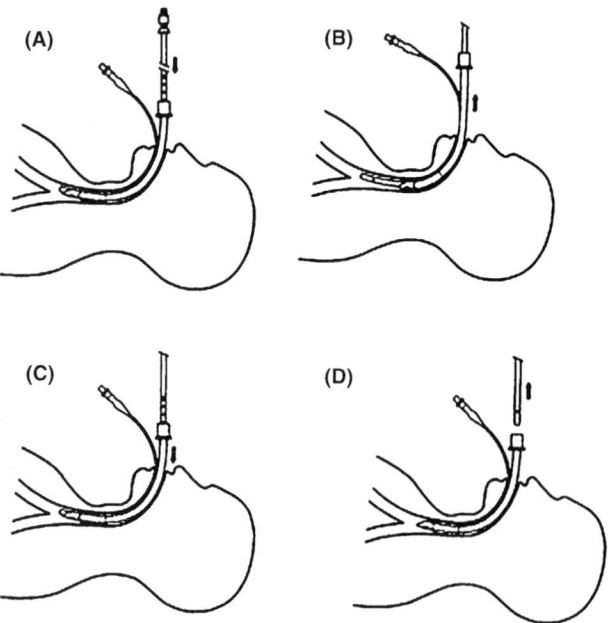

Figure 4 Technique for airway exchange catheter-assisted endotracheal tube (ETT) exchange. (**A**) The AEC is placed down the indwelling ETT. (**B**) Removal of the ETT tube over the AEC while keeping position of the AEC unchanged. (**C**) Placement of the new ETT over the AEC. (**D**) Removal of the AEC while firmly securing placement of the new ETT.

The method for confirming ETT position should be determined in advance. Capnography, whenever available, should be used. Waiting for an AP chest film is inadequate management.

Even seasoned experts of AEC use should refamiliarize themself with the AEC and the ventilation adapters. The AEC should be lubricated prior to use. The AEC is placed into the ETT, and the depth is noted against a landmark such as the level of the upper incisors. If possible, the AEC should be confirmed to be in the trachea by capnography. Once confirmed, the cuff balloon is deflated on the ETT and the ETT is removed without moving the AEC. The new ETT is then threaded over the indwelling AEC and advanced into the appropriate depth. The cuff balloon is inflated on the new ETT, and the AEC is removed. Confirmation of proper ETT position (Fig. 5) should be accomplished by capnography and/or by FOB.

☞ **If excessive resistance is encountered while removing the ETT, the withdrawal should be halted while the apparatus is reexamined.** ☞ Providing the ETT is still within the trachea, the AEC can be removed, and an FOB inserted to investigate. If the AEC and the ETT get stuck together, both may need to be removed completely and an alternative method of airway access may need to be attempted. Having an FOB pre-ensleeved with an ETT for emergency use can be useful at this time. Bag-mask ventilation may need to be employed between the time of ETT removal and the reestablishment of the ETT. If the patient remains hemodynamically stable with good oxygenation and adequate ventilation, several attempts to complete a

Table 6 Airway Exchange Catheter[a] Uses

Use	Example/comments
Stylet	To facilitate reintubation
Administer O_2	Insufflation; manual or jet ventilation
Measure: $P_{ET}CO_2$	In both SV and MV patients; ensures gas exchange throughout the ETT change procedure

[a]AECs are long, small ID, hollow, or semi rigid tubes.
Abbreviations: ETT, endotracheal tube; ID, internal diameter; MV, mechanical ventilation; O_2, oxygen; $P_{ET}CO_2$, end-tidal pressure of carbon dioxide; SV, spontaneously ventilating.

Table 7 Airway Exchange Catheter: Common Manufacturers and Sizes

	3.0 ID ETT	4.0 ID ETT	5.0 ID ETT	7.0 ID ETT	DLT
Cook (Bloomington, Ind.)	2.7 ED (45 cm)	3.7 ED (83 cm)	4.7 ED (83 cm)	6.3 ED (83 cm)	Yes
Sheridan (Argyle, NY)	2.0 ED (56 cm)	3.3 ED (81 cm)	4.8 ED (81 cm)	5.8 ED (81 cm)	Yes (Jettex = 100 cm)
CardioMed (Gromley, Ont., Canada)	—	—	4.0 ED (65 cm)	→	No

Abbreviations: AECs, airway exchange catheter; DLT, double lumen endotracheal tube; ED, external diameter; ETT, endotracheal tube; ID, internal diameter.

smooth transition can be attempted. In less stable patients, use of an airway-intubating mask, or laryngeal mask airway (LMA) can provide ventilation, while intubation is achieved using the FOB (as explained subsequently).

Fiberoptic Intubation

☞ **FOB-assisted techniques are useful for cases of suspected or confirmed difficult airway and as an adjunct to use of the AEC.** ☞ It is also useful for confirmation of ETT placement. In addition, airway obstructions, particularly those below the vocal cords, can be evaluated and treated with FOB, as can airway blockages due to secretions and plugs.

In patients who have known or suspected pathology involving the airway, extubation using the FOB is indicated. There are several techniques used for ETT exchange using the bronchoscope. The FOB (with pre-ensleeved ETT) can be inserted into the oropharynx alongside the in situ ETT and passed down to the carina if there is sufficient room in the trachea. The ETT can be slid over the FOB into position using it as a stylette guide. Sometimes using concomitant direct laryngoscopy can help facilitate ETT passage in appropriately sedated or anesthetized patients. Alternatively, the old ETT can be removed after the FOB is in

place, and before inserting the new ETT passed over the FOB into position.

Another possibility is passing an AEC down the existing ETT and slowly backing both the old ETT out, then intubating the trachea with a "pre-ensleeved" FOB alongside the AEC. The technique carries a slightly higher risk than using the AEC as a guide for both removal of the old ETT and insertion of the new ETT because the airway is insecure for a short period of time and the field of view through the bronchoscope may change rapidly.

It is recommended that a full bronchoscope examination occurs prior to the planned extubation in high-risk patients. This allows for the adequate sedation of the patient reducing the stress of airway manipulation or loss of the airway in an uncooperative patient. Information obtained from this inspection will better prepare the health-care team to have any emergency equipment or personnel available should the patient deteriorate acutely following extubation.

Laryngeal Mask Airway and Intubating Laryngeal Mask Airway Devices

The LMA was developed by Dr. Archie Brain in 1981. It became commercially available in Europe in the late 1980s. As its inception, the LMA has gained wide acceptance as a tool for airway management. Its role in the difficult airway algorithm was established in the 1990s, and was incorporated into the emergency limb of the American Society of Anesthesiology Difficult Airway (DA) Algorithm in 1993. The LMA has more recently been inserted into the main limb of the "revised" ASA DA algorithm in 2003. It can be a useful device in the ICU setting as well.

Several types of LMA products are available, although the basic design principle is same throughout. The teardrop shape of the LMA conforms to the oropharynx to create a seal in the soft tissues directly above the airway. When positioned properly, it effectively removes the upper-airway soft-tissue obstruction to the trachea allowing for easy ventilation.

☞ **The LMA can be a life-saving measure, as it can provide ventilation, and serves as a guide to FOB-assisted intubation.** ☞ It does not by itself, however, deliver a definitive airway. Patients with the LMA device are still susceptible to aspiration. In addition, the LMA can become dislodged at any time and these patients must be closely monitored.

There is a specially designed intubating LMA, also known as the Fastrach™, which has a larger aperture facing the vocal cords, which allows for blind passage of the ETT (Fig. 6) (25). This device is not recommended in situations where blind manipulation could convert a partial airway obstruction into a complete airway obstruction. For example, in all cases of stridor or airway injury, a technique using visualization through an FOB is far safer. Whenever intubating patients through a preexisting LMA, a longer ETT is optimal (26).

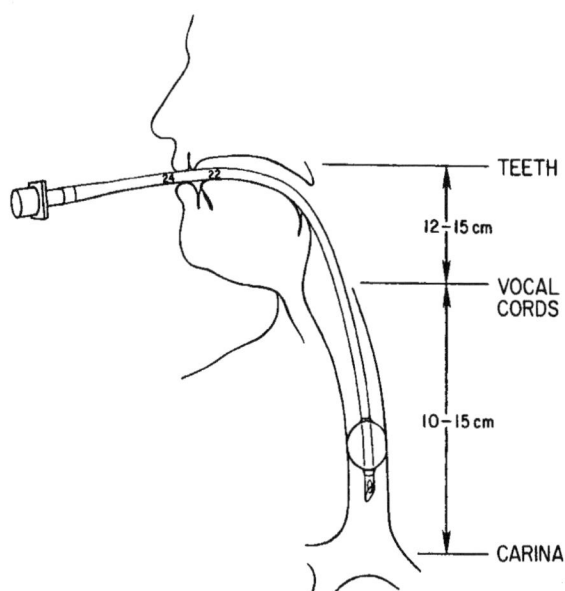

Figure 5 Endotracheal tube depth of insertion. The figure shows standard distances from key anatomic landmarks. When using an airway exchange catheter (AEC), it should not be positioned below the carina, especially if used to provide jet ventilation. To protect against barotrauma, place AEC no deeper than 26 cm from upper incisors, and use <25 psi pressure if using jet ventilation.

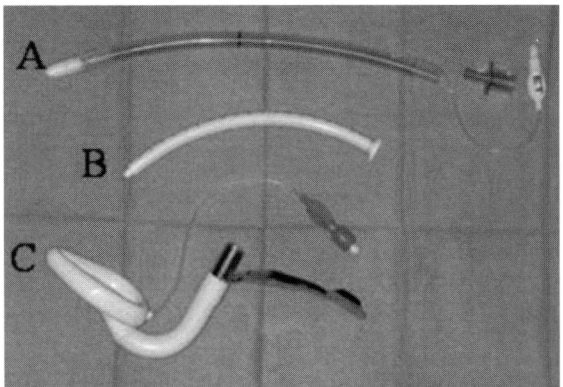

Figure 6   The intubating laryngeal mask airway (LMA) or LMA Fastrach™. (**A**) The ETT with removable 15-mm adapter for passage down the lumen of the LMA device. (**B**) The stabilizing rod which holds the position of the ETT while the intubating LMA device is withdrawn. (**C**) The LMA Fastrach™ device.

The LMA is ideally used in a spontaneously breathing patient. MV is possible, although the pressures generated by the ventilator should not exceed 20 mmHg (the pressure at which the lower esophageal sphincter opens) so that insufflation of the stomach can be avoided. Ventilation may be required in this manner as a "bridging" measure while the airway is secured.

One advantage of using a properly placed LMA as a guide for FOB-assisted intubation is the ability to deliver an elevated FiO_2 in a patient who may be in respiratory failure. Volume 1, Chapter 9 provides additional insight into the uses of the LMA. Briefly, placement of the LMA occurs as follows.

Lighted Stylette

A lighted stylette may be useful as an emergency backup for intubating patients whose vocal cords may not be visualized under direct laryngoscopy (Fig. 7). The stylette has a light source at the tip which can be appreciated through the soft tissues of the neck and airway. It is very simple to use and one can become rapidly proficient in performing ETT intubation using this technique (27). It is very important to dim the ambient light surrounding the patient while using this device because success is dependent upon visualizing the light source through the soft tissues of the neck and upper

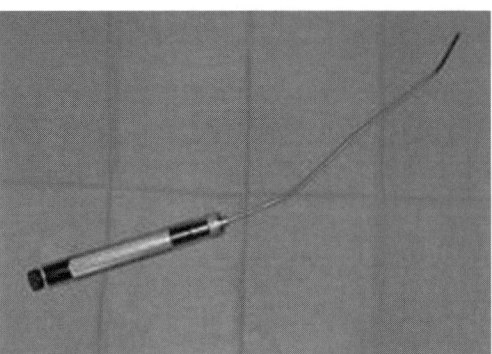

Figure 7   The lighted stylette. The light at the tip transilluminates the cartilage and soft tissues of the trachea and the neck.

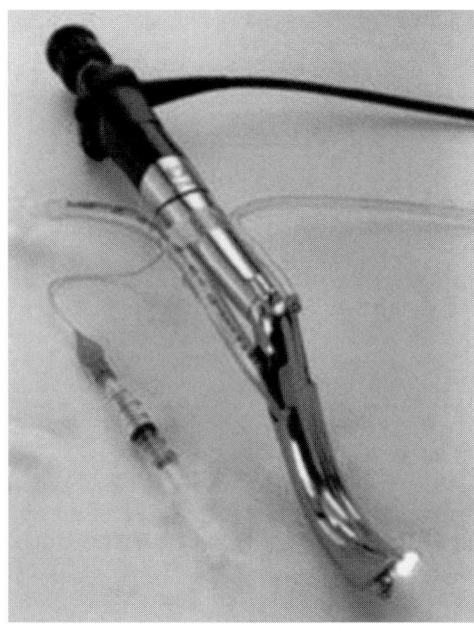

Figure 8   The Wu scope. This scope has specific positions for placement of the endotracheal tube (ETT) and the fiber-optic scope which is used to guide the suction catheter and ETT past the vocal cords and into the tracheal lumen.

neck, making this tool less useful in emergency trauma situations where lighting can be diminished.

Wu Scope

The Wu Scope is a specially designed device: a tubular laryngoscope blade. A fiberoptic light source is passed down the tubular blade, illuminating the tip (Fig. 8). An ETT is passed though the Wu Scope and placed under direct visualization. The device requires some practice to become proficient. However, the Wu Scope offers the advantage of allowing laryngoscopy without neck extension and jaw lift while allowing direct visualization of the vocal cords.

ETT exchange using the Wu Scope has been described and may be used as a backup device in a patient with a difficult airway (28). The tubular design of the Wu Scope provides an avenue for the ETT to bypass the soft tissue of the oropharynx. When using the Wu Scope, the vocal cords should be identified, and a soft flexible device such as a flexible suction catheter should be passed down through the ETT and through the vocal cords. This serves as a soft guide over which the ETT is passed into the trachea under direct vision.

Bullard Scope

The Bullard Scope is another laryngoscope which may be used for ETT exchange in the same manner as the Wu Scope. The laryngoscope blade is flat and the ETT sits over a contoured stylette attached to the blade. The Bullard Scope uses a standard laryngoscopy handle, and when attached it illuminates a light source at the tip of the blade. The eyepiece of the scope is located near the handle, and the lens is located at the tip of the blade adjacent to the light source. Placement of the Bullard Scope should be done carefully to avoid iatrogenic trauma to the mouth and teeth. Once the view of the vocal cords has been obtained, the old ETT should be removed carefully and the new one passed under visualization through the Bullard Scope.

Surgical Airway

Both tracheostomy and cricothyroidectomy provide definitive airway options. In elective situations, the tracheostomy is preferred, whereas the cricothyroidectomy is more rapidly established and therefore favored in an emergency. In some patients, converting an existing ETT airway to a tracheostomy is the best first choice for ETT exchange. The cricothyroidectomy is relegated to situations where the airway cannot be established using the above mentioned standard measures. These techniques are described in greater detail in Volume 1, Chapter 9.

EYE TO THE FUTURE

New advances for facilitating extubation of the difficult airway and ETT exchange in high-risk patients are anticipated to occur in the realms of diagnosis, monitoring, and management. No single laboratory test or imaging study can yet definitively predict airway difficulty, or ability to tolerate extubation. Research advances are anticipated in airway imaging, and in staging airway swelling by FOB exam. Accurate prediction of safe extubation and ETT exchange is facilitated by sound judgment that considers the patient's condition and all of the possible tools available for diagnosis, monitoring, and facilitation of the difficult airway.

SUMMARY

Extubation and ETT exchange have not received the same emphasis in literature as intubation and definitive airway management. The extubation or ETT exchange of the patient with a difficult airway presents a unique problem affecting critically ill trauma patients with potentially rapid and severe complications. It is important to note that any patient can develop a difficult airway depending upon their physical status and operative care. Extubation and ETT exchange can most safely be performed by physicians with up-to-date knowledge of the tools available, training and experience in their use, and sound clinical judgment in their use, along with preparations, attention to detail, and adequate help when they are employed.

KEY POINTS

- Extubation of a known difficult airway and especially planned ETT change in a critically ill patient should be approached with a similar degree of concern and preparation as that given to initial intubation.
- A critical airway consideration in the posttrauma or critically ill surgical patient is the likelihood of periglottic swelling or pathology that could lead to postextubation stridor and possible inability to intubate or ventilate the patient.
- In the case of patients at high risk for postextubation stridor, a formal evaluation for periglottic swelling should be performed prior to attempts at extubation or ETT exchange. Options for evaluation of airway

swelling include: (*i*) cuff-leak test, (*ii*) FOB evaluation, and (*iii*) imaging studies.
- In situations where the patient is at high risk for postextubation stridor, additional specific evaluation with FOB (Fig. 1) is warranted.
- In the case where airway management is difficult and both conventional and adjunct procedures (described subsequently) all fail, then a surgical airway should be performed.
- When considering ETT change or extubation, decisions must be made on an individual basis with evaluation of the entire clinical picture considered rather than focusing upon a single event or parameter.
- In terms of weaning parameters, the RSBI is probably the single best indicator for determining the patient's ability to perform the required WOB.
- Direct laryngoscopy is the most common and simplest method for establishing airway access and appropriate when reintubation is not expected to be difficult (Fig. 2).
- The risks involved in using AECs include loss of the established airway and damage to the airway from the device.
- If excessive resistance is encountered while removing the ETT, the withdrawal should be halted while the apparatus is reexamined.
- FOB-assisted techniques are useful for cases of suspected or confirmed difficult airway and as an adjunct to use of the AEC.
- The LMA can be a life-saving measure, as it can provide ventilation, and serves as a guide to FOB-assisted intubation.

REFERENCES

1. Demling RH, Read T, Lind LJ, et al. Incidence and morbidity of extubation failure in surgical intensive care patients. Crit Care Med 1988; 16:573.
2. Rose DK, Cohen MM, Wigglesworth DF. Critical respiratory events in the postanesthesia care unit. Anesthesiology 1994; 81:410–418.
3. Mathew JP, Rosenbaum SH, O'Connor T, et al. Emergency tracheal intubation in the postanesthesia care unit: physician error or patient disease. Anesth Anal 1990; 71:691–697.
4. Vassal T, Anh NG, Gabillet JM, et al. Prospective evaluation of self-extubation in a medical intensive care unit. Intensive Care Med 1993; 19:340.
5. Epstein SK, Ciubotaru RL, Wong JB. Effect of failed extubation on the outcome of mechanical ventilation. Chest 1997; 112: 186–192.
6. Daley BJ, Garcia-Perez F, Ross SE. Reintubation as an outcome predictor in trauma patients. Chest 1996; 110(6):1577–1580.
7. Practice Guidelines for Management of the Difficult Airway: a report by the American Society of Anesthesiologists Task Force on management of the difficult airway. Anesthesiology 1993; 78(3):597–602.
8. Practice Guidelines for Management of the Difficult Airway: an updated report by the American Society of Anesthesiologists Task Force on management of the difficult airway. Anesthesiology 2003; 98(5):1269–1277.
9. Turkan S, Ates Y, Cuhruk H, Tekdemir I. Should we reevaluate the variables for predicting the difficult airway in anesthesiology? Anesth Analg 2002; 94(5):1340–1344.
10. Potgieter PD, Hammond JMJ. "Cuff" test for safe extubation following laryngeal edema. Crit Care Med 1988; 16:818.
11. Kemper KJ, Benson MS, Bishop MJ. Predictors of postextubation stridor in pediatric trauma patients. Crit Care Med 1991; 19:352.

12. Fisher MM, Raper RF. The "cuff-leak" test for extubation. Anaesthesia 1992; 47(1):10–12.

13. Marik P. The cuff-leak test as a predictor of postextubation stridor: a prospective study. Respir Care 1996; 41(6):509–511.

14. Engoren M. Evaluation of the cuff-leak test in a cardiac surgery population. Chest 1999; 116(4):1029–1031.

15. Kriner EJ, Shafazan S, Colice GL. The endotracheal tube cuff-leak test as a predictor for postextubation stridor. Respir Care 2005; 50(12):1632–1638.

16. Prinianakis G, Alexopoulou C, Mamidakis E, et al. Determinants of the cuff-leak test: a physiological study. Crit Care 2005; 9:R24–R31.

17. Gehlbach BK, Kress JP. Sedation in the intensive care unit. Curr Opin Crit Care 2002; 8(4):290–298.

18. Ebert T, Maze M. Dexmedetomidine: another arrow for the clinician's quiver. Anesthesiology 2004; 101(3):568–570.

19. Ding L-W, Wang H.-C, Wu H.-D, et al. Laryngeal ultrasound: a useful method in predicting post-extubation stridor: a pilot study. Eur Respir J 2006; 27:384–338.

20. Beckmann, Ursula, Gillies, Donna MRN. Factors associated with reintubation in intensive care*: an analysis of causes and outcomes. Chest 2001; 120(2):538–542.

21. Morgan GE, Mikhail MS, Murray MJ. Clinical Anesthesiology. 3rd ed. 2002:967.

22. Miller, Kirk A, Harkin, Christopher P, Bailey, Peter L. Postoperative tracheal extubation. Anesth Analg 1995; 80(1):149–172.

23. Rosenblatt, William H, Wagner, et al. Practice patterns in managing the difficult airway by anesthesiologists in the United States. Anesth Analg 1998; 87(1):153–157.

24. Loudermilk, Eric P, Hartmannsgruber, et al. A prospective study of the safety of tracheal extubation using a pediatric airway exchange catheter for patients with a known difficult airway. Chest 1997; 111(6):1660–1665.

25. Stix, Michael S, Borromeo, et al. A modified intubating laryngeal mask for endotracheal tube exchange. Anesth Analg 2000; 91(4):1021–1023.

26. Benumof, Jonathan L. Laryngeal mask airway and the ASA difficult airway algorithm. Anesthesiology 1996; 84(3):686–699.

27. Fisher QA, Tunkel DE. Lightwand intubation of infants and children. J Clin Anesth 1997; 9(4):275–279.

28. Andrews SR, Norcross SD, Mabey MF, Siegel JB. The Wu Scope technique for endotracheal tube exchange. Anesthesiology 1999; 90(3):929–930.

30

Gastrointestinal Prophylaxis

Jeffrey S. Upperman

Division of Pediatric Surgery, Department of Surgery, University of Southern California School of Medicine, Children's Hospital Los Angeles, Los Angeles, California, U.S.A.

Faisal Qureshi and Henri R. Ford

Department of Surgery, University of Southern California School of Medicine, Children's Hospital Los Angeles, Los Angeles, California, U.S.A.

INTRODUCTION: STRESS ULCERS

☞ **Stress ulcers are common in critically ill patients, but clinically important bleeding occurs in only 5% or less of these patients. Mortality in this small group of patients can be as high as 50%.** ☞ Stress-induced gastritis and ulcers have been reported to occur in 75% to 100% of patients admitted to critical care units (1). These lesions are associated with major trauma, surgical procedures, shock, sepsis, hemorrhage, coagulopathy, hepatic, renal, and pulmonary failure (2). Stress ulcers occurring in severely burned patients are called Curling's ulcers, while those associated with central nervous system (CNS) diseases are referred to as Cushing's ulcers (3,4). Curling's ulcers are merely a form of stress ulcer, whereas they appear to be a unique entity that behaves more like peptic ulcers. ☞ **Stress ulcers are found in the proximal stomach and are usually multiple, superficial, and diffuse. Deeper lesions can lead to major hemorrhage.** ☞

The pathogenesis of peptic ulcers appears to be different from that of common stress ulcers. For example, common ("non-Cushing") stress ulcers usually occur in the proximal stomach, whereas peptic ulcer lesions usually develop in the gastric antrum and in the duodenum. In addition, common "non-Cushing" stress ulcers are typically superficial and more numerous than peptic ulcer lesions. The shallow, diffuse stress ulcers typically result in clinically occult or mild bleeding. However, deeper ulcerated lesions can occur and lead to significant gross hemorrhage.

Occult bleeding is exemplified by a patient with guaiac positive gastric aspirate or stool sample. Overt bleeding can present as hematemesis, hematochezia, or melena with or without hemodynamic instability. Clinically significant hemorrhage is characterized by overt bleeding with signs and symptoms of hemodynamic instability requiring aggressive resuscitation, often with blood transfusion. Although only a small proportion (1–6%) of patients with stress gastritis develops clinically significant bleeding, the mortality rate among this subset of patients approaches 50% (5–7).

Therefore, the prevention and effective management of these ulcers constitute a major clinical imperative in critically ill patients. Not surprisingly, in recent years, there has been rapid proliferation of a variety of therapeutic agents designed to combat or prevent stress ulcers in critically ill patients. These drugs include: sucralfate, histamine type-2 receptor antagonists (H_2RAs), proton pump inhibitors (PPIs), prostaglandins (PGs) (e.g., misoprostol), and antacids among others. Early enteral nutrition (Volume 2, Chapter 32) is another important protective factor against stress ulcer formation.

This chapter reviews the pathogenesis of stress gastritis including the protective role of normal mucosal blood flow and the injurious effects of H^+ ions following ischemia and reperfusion. The protective barriers provided by mucus production and bicarbonate secretion are discussed, along with conditions that disrupt these factors and promote epithelial injury. Endogenous PGs and nitric oxide (NO) are produced by the luminal epithelium and their protective roles are also elaborated upon. The benefits of normal gut motility and nutrition comprise some of the other known, protective factors, and these are identified. This chapter also reviews the pathologic appearance and risk factors for stress ulcer formation. The rationale for various ulcer prophylactic agents and their specific mechanisms of action are then described. Finally, the complications of gastrointestinal prophylaxis and the management principles for gastrointestinal (GI) bleeding are reviewed, along with the patient populations at greatest risk [those with coagulopathes, requiring mechanical ventilation, and severe trauma (especially CNS injury)].

PATHOPHYSIOLOGY

The pathogenesis of stress gastritis and ulceration is multifactorial; however, splanchnic hypoperfusion, mucosal injury, and low pH are probably the most important risk factors. The presence of amino acids in the stomach stimulates gastrin release by the G cells in the gastric antrum. Gastrin and pituitary adenylate cyclase-activating polypeptide trigger histamine release (8,9). Histamine and calcium in turn promote acid release by the parietal cells. Although acid production plays a central role in the development of gastric mucosal injury, a low pH alone not sufficient to induce stress ulcer formation (10–13). Increased acid production only partially explains why critically ill patients are at risk for gastric mucosal ulceration. In fact, acid production is sometimes diminished in this group of patients (13).

Compromised mucosal barrier function, which is often associated with critical illness (e.g., sepsis, shock, hemorrhage), is also operative. Indeed, relatively small

Table 1 Pathophysiologic Factors that Are Involved in the Development of Stress Ulcers

Protective	Deleterious
Mucosal blood flow	Acid secretion
Mucus production	Hypotension
CGRP	Reperfusion
Bicarbonate secretion	Reactive oxygen species
Intact epithelia	α- and β-adrenoreceptor agonists
Nitric oxide	Nitric oxide
Prostaglandins	Pylori
Intact gastric and intestinal motility	Reflux of bile salts
Adequate nutritional status	
Epidermal growth factor	

Abbreviation: CGRP, calcitonin gene-related peptide.

amounts of acid can lead to significant mucosal injury and the subsequent development of stress gastritis in this setting. The physiological function in the stomach and proximal small intestine are known to be impaired during critical illnesses (14,15). For example, mucosal blood flow is reduced, gastric emptying is impaired, and acid production is deranged (16,17). The small bowel exhibits decreased motility and mucosal perfusion (14,16). The combination of these derangements leads to an unfavorable balance between protective and deleterious factors resulting in mucosal injury (Table 1).

Mucosal Blood Flow, Ischemia, and Reperfusion Injury

Mucosal blood flow plays an essential role in maintaining mucosal homeostasis and when impaired gastritis and ulceration are common (18). Mucosal blood flow is dependent on total gastric blood flow and microcirculatory perfusion. These are important in maintaining the mucosal barrier. The microcirculation provides epithelial cells with the necessary nutrients and oxygen for generating the ATP that is essential for maintenance of normal homeostasis. In addition, the microcirculation transports deleterious protons and other agents that traverse the epithelial barrier away from the mucosa and brings them into the interstitial fluid. Therefore, gastric and mucosal blood flow prevents epithelial injury by tightly regulating the local pH. In addition, the microcirculation supports the repair of injured epithelium by removing harmful reactive oxygen species from the local microenvironment.

☞ **Decreases in blood flow to the gastric epithelium, whether as a result of globally diminished circulating blood volume or reduced microcirculatory blood flow, leads to impairment of the epithelial defense mechanisms.** ☞

Critically ill patients may have low blood pressure resulting in diminished gastric blood flow. Shock leads to a drop in gastric mucosal blood flow secondary to a decrease in circulating blood volume, vasodilatation or local vasoconstriction (19). Consequently, in shock states the normal oxygen and nutrient supply to the epithelial lining of the stomach is compromised resulting in decreased cellular ATP (18). Experimental animal data suggest that in shock states, gastric blood flow may be intact while the microcirculation is impaired (20). Diminution in microcirculatory blood flow can give rise to shunting in the local environment, thereby reducing the gastric mucosa's ability to counter the damage caused by hydrogen ions. A disruption in blood flow results in anaerobic metabolism and the buildup of oxygen-free radicals, leading to lipid peroxidation and

damage to mucosal cells (21,22). Additional experiments have shown the relationship between blood flow and the development of gastric and duodenal injury (23). Even if adequate blood flow is restored, secondary reperfusion injury may occur as a result of oxidative stress (24–27).

Another mechanism that can lead to gastric mucosal injury is the inhibition of the gastric hyperemic response to acid back diffusion. It is thought that under normal conditions, gastric mucosal blood flow increases when the mucosa is acidified. This defense mechanism is mediated by the release of the vasodilator calcitonin gene-related peptide (CGRP) from capsaicin-sensitive nerve fibers (28). Endogenous and exogenous α- and β-adrenoreceptor agonists can block the release of the transmitter and suppress the gastric mucosal vasodilator response. Critically ill patients often have increased levels of endogenous catecholamines which can block the release of CGRP. In addition, therapeutic agents such as dobutamine are often used in critically ill patients to improve cardiac output and regional perfusion; the global hemodynamic improvement afforded by such agents may paradoxically result in local gastric mucosal hypoperfusion leading to epithelial damage (29).

Mucus Production and Bicarbonate Secretion

The gastric mucosa is covered by a tightly adherent thin layer of mucus that functions as the first line of defense against stress-related injury. This physical mucus barrier is composed of a glycoprotein matrix and bicarbonate that prevents the direct contact of pepsin and hydrogen ions with the gastric mucosa. Ischemia, fasting states, and steroids can change the composition of the mucus layer by reducing the level of glycoprotein and allowing hydrogen ions access to the mucosa (30,31). Shock states lead to a diminution of ATP, which in turn leads to reduced secretion of mucus and bicarbonate (32). Additionally, as reperfusion occurs, reactive oxygen species are generated which further destroy the mucus layer disrupting its protective properties (21,33).

Intact Epithelium

The epithelium of the stomach forms another effective defense mechanism. Any condition that leads to tissue hypoxia such as shock, sepsis, and trauma can disrupt the normal cell turnover and proliferation rate. DNA, RNA, and protein synthesis rates are diminished during periods of stress, starvation, and catabolism. Mucosal injury is further exacerbated by the resultant cellular acidosis, release of proteases, and phospholipases. The normal proliferation/apoptotic balance is altered as mucosal injury progresses with increasing cell necrosis and initiation of the inflammatory cascade. This cascade may exacerbate the inciting event and contribute to the development of multiorgan failure that is seen in critically ill patients.

Prostaglandins and Nitric Oxide

Prostaglandins normally play a protective role in maintaining an intact gastric mucosal barrier. They increase mucosal blood flow and stimulate the production of mucus and bicarbonate to protect the mucosa against acid-induced injury. Prostaglandins also attenuate the vasoconstrictive effects of angiotensin II in shock states (34). Both prostaglandin E-2 (PGE_2) and prostaglandin I-2 (PGI_2) are present in the gastric mucosa and protect against the deleterious effects of substances such as nonsteroidal anti-inflammatory drugs (NSAIDs), aspirin, and alcohol (35–37).

NO is a potent local vasodilator that appears to play a protective role in gastric mucosal barrier function. The constitutive isoform of NO synthase is present throughout the gastrointestinal tract. Physiologic levels of NO support the defense mechanisms of the gastric mucosa by maintaining gastric mucosal perfusion. In addition, NO downregulates neutrophil and platelet activation, thus attenuating the inflammatory response. Under hypoxic conditions, the inducible form of NO synthase (iNOS) is upregulated, leading to sustained overproduction of NO. Paradoxically, while physiological (i.e., low) levels of NO contribute to normal mucosal homeostasis, pathological (high) levels of NO can trigger an inflammatory response in the gastric mucosa (related to excess free-radical production) resulting in gastric mucosal damage and cell death (38).

Gastrointestinal Motility and Nutritional Status

Up to 50% of critically ill patients develop gastrointestinal dysmotility (15). This dysmotility may be a result of local or central factors. The failure of the migrating motor complex, which is responsible for gastroduodenal peristalsis, to originate in the stomach leads not only to local hypokinesis but also to small bowel dysmotility (14). These motility disturbances may be further exacerbated by the use of pharmaceutical agents such as dopamine in the critically ill by reducing antral contractions and increasing duodenal contractions (39). The resulting reluctance to feed these patients may lead to an increased risk of developing stress gastritis.

Nutritionally depleted patients are at risk for stress gastritis. Inadequate protein levels may lead to gastrointestinal mucosal edema, which in turn leads to malabsorption. Protein malabsorption triggers a cycle where absorption of amino acids and peptides is limited resulting in increased mucosal edema (Volume 2, Chapter 32).

OTHER FACTORS

Other pathophysiologic factors that contribute to stress gastritis include bile reflux, *Helicobacter pylori*, and epidermal growth factor (EGF) deficiency. Bile reflux is a consequence of gastric and proximal small bowel dysmotility. Bile reflux can injure the gastric mucosa and contribute to stress gastritis (40).

While *H. pylori* has been linked to peptic ulcer disease, its role in the pathogenesis of stress gastritis is not clear. Elevated levels of anti–*H. pylori* immunoglobulin A are associated with increased risk of bleeding secondary to stress gastritis in critically ill patients. In contrast, patients with peptic ulcer disease have elevated anti–*H. pylori* IgG levels. In stress gastritis, patients have colonization of both the body and antrum of the stomach, but in peptic ulcer disease the body and antrum have significantly less *H. pylori* infestation. The difference in microbial exposure between the two ulcer conditions may determine the divergence in virulence and inflammatory response observed between the two conditions (41).

EGF is produced by the salivary glands. Evidence suggests that EGF is necessary not only to maintain an intact intestinal epithelial lining, but also for effective repair of the damaged gastric mucosa (42,43). EGF is important for gastric mucosal restitution and for the maintenance of intracellular pH in mucosal epithelia, which is largely regulated by various isoforms of Na^+/H^+ exchangers (NHEs) throughout the gastrointestinal tract (44). EGF is known to stimulate the expression and function of NHEs (43,45).

Pathogenesis of CNS-Related Stress Ulcers

The pathogenesis of stress gastritis secondary to CNS injury or illness differs from stress gastritis related to other forms of trauma and critical illnesses. CNS-related ulcers are commonly referred to as Cushing's ulcers. Patients with CNS injuries develop increased gastric acid secretion in response to autonomic dysregulation originating in the hypothalamus (46–48). In experimental conditions, direct vagal nerve stimulation leads to gastric acid hypersecretion (49). Cushing's ulcers are similar to peptic ulcers. They are single and deeper than lesions that are traditionally associated with stress gastritis. Thus, Cushing's ulcers are more prone to perforation.

An important clinical note is that patients on high-dose steroids are also at increased risk. Furthermore, patients with spinal cord injuries may not present with typical signs of peritonitis (due to skeletal muscle paralysis) despite a frank perforated duodenal ulcer. Accordingly, vigilance is required in this patient population.

Pathophysiology Summary

In summary, hydrogen ions are necessary for the development of stress ulcers. But stress ulcers do not occur without the disruption of basal mucosal defense mechanisms. Acidotic critically ill patients have inadequate mucosal blood flow and an impaired ability to neutralize hydrogen ions. In addition, microcirculatory hypoperfusion diminishes mucus, bicarbonate, and PG production. This impairment in epithelial protective mechanisms allows the mucosa to become damaged. Restitution and regeneration are inhibited in the face of inadequate nutrition, reduced proteins, diminished ATP, PGs, and EGF. The injured mucosa is unable to protect itself against deleterious factors such as hydrogen ions, bile, and oxygen-free radicals. Even when adequate blood flow is reestablished, reperfusion can initially accentuate the mucosal injury by producing reactive oxygen and nitrogen species that exacerbate the inflammatory response. CNS-related stress ulcers (Cushing's ulcers) are related to elevated hydrogen ion levels (like common stress ulcers), but they are usually singular, deep, and prone to perforation.

☞ Hydrogen ions play a central role in the development of stress ulcers. However, stress ulcers do not develop under normal circumstances because mucosal epithelial damage is limited by protective mechanisms including adequate blood flow, normal mucus production, buffering by bicarbonate secretion, mucosal PGs, and NO, as well as epithelial repair facilitated by EGF. ☞

PATHOLOGICAL APPEARANCE

The gross and microscopic appearance of stress gastritis is time dependent. In the first 24 hours, stress gastritis ulcers are diffuse and shallow, and accompanied by focal hemorrhage. Histologically, stress gastritis ulcers have a leukocytic infiltrate. After 24 to 72 hours, tissue reactions occur; the ulcers lose their erythematous appearance and develop coagulation necrosis, cell infiltration, and hemorrhage with extension into the deeper mucosal layers. Extension into the submucosa leads to bleeding. If the patient's clinical condition improves, these ulcers will heal.

☞ Stress ulcers appear differently at various stages of development, and lesions of dissimilar morphological stages can be seen in the same patient. ☞

Table 2 Risk Factors in the Development of Stress Ulcers in Adult and Pediatric Patients

Adult	Pediatric
Mechanical ventilation (>48 hr)	Coagulopathy
Coagulopathy (platelets <50,000; INR >2.5; PT >2 control)	Surgery (>3 hr)
Major surgery	Trauma
Head or multiple trauma	Burns (>13% BSA)
Burn injury (>30% BSA)	Pneumonia
Sepsis	Pediatric Risk of Mortality Score >10
Shock	
Multisystem organ failure	
Steroid therapy	
Solid organ transplantation	
Prolonged intensive care unit stay	
History of ulcer disease or gastro-intestinal bleeding	

Abbreviations: BSA, body surface area; INR, international normalized ratio; PT, prothrombin time.

RISK FACTORS

Several clinical states are associated with the development of stress gastritis (2). Coagulopathy (platelets <50,000; INR >2.5, PT >2 control) and respiratory failure (mechanical ventilation > 48 hr) are the two most important clinical factors related to clinically significant bleeding from stress gastritis (2). Additional high-risk groups include patients who have had recent major surgery, head or multiple trauma, burn injury (>30%), sepsis, shock, multiorgan system failure, steroid therapy, solid organ transplantation, or prolonged intensive care unit stay (50).

Despite physiologic differences between adults and children, pediatric patients are also at risk for the development of stress gastritis (51,52). In the pediatric population, coagulopathy, shock, surgery greater than three hours, burns [>13% body surface area (BSA)], trauma, pneumonia, and Pediatric Risk of Mortality Score greater than 10 are considered important risk factors for the development of stress gastritis ulcers (Table 2) (53–56).

♂ **Respiratory failure and coagulopathy are the two most important factors associated with the development of stress ulcers.** ♂

CLINICAL SIGNS AND SYMPTOMS

Stress gastritis ulcers are generally asymptomatic in the early stages and do not manifest overt bleeding. As stress becomes prolonged or more severe, bleeding is often detected. Categorizing ulcer-associated hemorrhages is crucial for patient care and clinical research endeavors. Ulcer-associated bleeding is categorized into three types: (*i*) hemodynamically stable patients with superficial diffuse ulcers and guaiac-positive gastric aspirate or stool samples have occult bleeding. Occult bleeding is the most common type of stress gastritis–related hemorrhage. Most lesions are not very deep and do not erode into any large vessels; (*ii*) hemodynamically stable patients with overt bleeding may have hematemesis, hematchezia, or melena but it is generally not clinically significant; gastric aspirates contain gross blood or coffee-ground material; (*iii*) hemodynamically unstable patients with clinically significant bleeding are those demonstrating cardiovascular and hematological signs associated with overt bleeding. These signs include: (*i*) >20 mmHg decrease in the resting systolic blood pressure (SBP); (*ii*) an orthostatic decrease of >10 mmHg in SBP; >20 bpm increase in heart rate; >2 g/dL drop in hemoglobin concentration (2). Bleeding classification assists clinicians and researchers in stratifying patients at risk for bleeding and determining appropriate therapeutic regimens (Table 3).

♂ **Patients with stress ulcers are usually asymptomatic. Those patients who do bleed can have occult or overt bleeding, with or without hemodynamic instability.** ♂

GI PROPHYLAXIS RATIONALE AND GOALS

The key to stress gastritis prophylaxis is selecting high-risk patients and treating them early. Several risk factors are associated with stress gastritis and due to the identification of these factors and institution of prophylaxis measures, few patients develop clinically significant bleeding now. Improvements in resuscitation, early enteral nutrition, and basic supportive care help sustain "at-risk" patients who are susceptible to stress gastritis. Hydrogen ions play a pivotal role in the pathogenesis of stress gastritis. Therefore, the inhibition of acid secretion is the central target in ulcer prophylaxis. Several drugs reduce gastric pH including antacids, H$_2$RAs, and PPIs.

Stress ulcer prophylaxis is an important therapeutic maneuver in the critical care setting. The most significant consequence from stress-induced ulcers is hemorrhage. Mechanical ventilation and coagulopathy are the only independent risk factors connected to clinically relevant bleeding. Gastric acid production is central to the development of stress-induced ulcers; hence, inhibition of acid production is the main goal in preventing stress gastritis. Clinical trials demonstrate that keeping gastric pH above 3.5 can prevent mucosal injury (57). The following section will review the

Table 3 Bleeding States Associated with Stress Ulcers

Type	Occult bleeding	Overt bleeding	Clinically significant bleeding
Hemodynamic stability	Stable	Stable	Unstable
Type of ulcer	Superficial	Deep	Erosion into vessel
Clinical signs/symptoms	Guaiac-positive gastric aspirate or stool sample	Hematemesis, melena, gross blood in gastric aspirate or coffee-ground material	↓ SBP >20 mmHg; ↑ Heart rate >20 bpm; ↓ orthostatic SBP 20 mmHg; ↓ Hemoglobin 2 g/dL

Abbreviation: SBP, systolic blood pressure.

therapeutic strategies commonly used to prevent the development of stress gastritis.

Ulcer prophylaxis is designed to raise the intragastric pH to >4.0. A pH <4.0 does not inactivate pepsin and permits fibrinolysis. Once upper gastrointestinal bleeding starts, intragastric pH >4.0, but <6.0 may be inadequate to prevent recurrent bleeding. During overt bleeding, a pH of >6.0 should be achieved to prevent the breakdown of blood clots and the spread of bleeding (58–60). Under acidic conditions, platelets do not aggregate and gastric mucosa does not heal (58,61). The next section will deal with the options available for stress ulcer prophylaxis.

✧ As hydrogen ions play a central role in stress ulcer development, raising gastric pH is necessary for prevention of stress gastritis. Maintaining gastric pH >4.0 will prophylax against stress ulcer formation, but once bleeding starts, a pH greater than 6.0 is required to prevent rebleeding. ✧

ULCER PROPHYLAXIS OPTIONS

Drugs/treatments used for stress ulcer prophylaxis can be broadly classified into cytoprotective agents (e.g., sucralfate, misoprostol, and enteral nutrition) and acid reducers (e.g., H$_2$RAs, PPIs, and antacids). Each of these commonly employed drugs and treatments will be reviewed.

Sucralfate
Background and Mechanism of Action
Sucralfate is an orally administered basic aluminum salt of sulfated sucrose. It is a nonabsorbable agent that exerts its cytoprotective effects by binding to the gastric mucosa and forming a gel-like barrier that allows mucosal healing beneath the protective gel-like layer. In acidic environments, the aluminum and sulfate disassociate into ions. The highly polar sulfide anions bind to cations such as mucins and exposed proteins serving to coat mucosal defects.

Although its mechanism of action is not entirely known, some theorize that sucralfate acts as a physical barrier to acid-induced damage or stimulates local PG synthesis (62). Other reports suggest that sucralfate downregulates endothelin 1 expression, binds to bile salts, inhibits pepsin, and increases bicarbonate excretion (62–64).

Efficacy vs. Complication Profile
Various meta-analyses examined the difference in efficacy between sucralfate and H$_2$RAs or antacids and placebo. These analyses revealed disparate conclusions. Messori et al. did not show any difference in efficacy between sucralfate and H$_2$RAs as compared to placebo (65). A meta-analysis by Cook et al. suggested that sucralfate and H$_2$RAs were comparable in preventing clinically overt bleeding. Interestingly, sucralfate administration correlated with a reduction in mortality (61). A prospective randomized trial revealed that the H$_2$RA, ranitidine, was more efficacious than sucralfate in preventing clinically important bleeding, but there was no difference in length of stay or mortality (66). These studies suggest that sucralfate is equivalent to H$_2$RAs in preventing overt bleeding from stress gastritis.

The sucralfate complication profile is low. One potential risk is nosocomial pneumonia. As sucralfate is delivered via a nasogastric tube directly into the stomach, the gastroesophageal junction is stented open, thus permitting aspiration of stomach contents into the lung. However, sucralfate does not alter stomach flora, a process that is linked to nosocomial pneumonia. Nonetheless, controversy persists regarding the role of sucralfate therapy in the development of nosocomial pneumonia when compared to antacids or H$_2$RAs.

Additional complications include aluminum absorption (only 3–5% absorbed) in patients with renal failure. Aluminum binds to the phosphate which prevents absorption. Therefore, aluminum absorption can cause hypophosphatemia even in patients with normal renal function. Constipation and drug interactions (fluroquindones, phentoin, and warfarin) can occur in some patients. Bezoar formation has been reported with the use of sucralfate in pediatric patients (67). Sucralfate is on the Food and Drug Administration (FDA) "Class B" agent (safe to use during pregnancy).

Although readily available, sucralfate is not FDA approved for use as prophylaxis against stress gastritis. Sucralfate is generally underused, partly due to its four-times-a-day dosing compared to once-daily dosing for PPIs. Another problem with sucralfate is its disrupting effect on viewing the gastric mucosa using endoscopy.

✧ Sucralfate works by binding to the stomach lining and thus has to be introduced directly into the stomach. It is efficacious in preventing stress ulcers, with a low complication profile, but has not been shown to improve outcome. ✧

H$_2$ Receptor Antagonists
Background and Mechanism of Action
Histamine binds to the histamine receptor-2 on parietal cells and stimulates the production and release of hydrochloric acid. In the late 1970s, cimetidine, a prototypical H$_2$RA, was introduced as the treatment for peptic ulcer disease. Since the introduction of H$_2$RAs, they have been a mainstay in acid-suppressing treatment.

H$_2$RAs block the histamine receptor and subsequently reduce hydrogen ion production levels. H$_2$RAs have limitations as global hydrogen ion production regulators as histamine does not completely activate all intramural hydrogen production.

Efficacy vs. Complication Profile
Approximately 70% to 80% of duodenal ulcers and 55% to 65% of gastric ulcers are healed by H$_2$RAs after four to six weeks of therapy. Based on the early successes in preventing the progression of peptic ulcer disease, clinicians began to investigate the efficacy of H$_2$RAs in controlling acute upper gastrointestinal bleeding. Little data support the use of H$_2$RAs in abrogating bleeding complications of peptic ulcer disease (68,69). In a meta-analysis by Collins et al., they collated and analyzed 27 randomized prospective trials with approximately 2500 total patients who were treated with H$_2$RAs. The data suggest that H$_2$RAs limited rebleeding in patients after endoscopic control of upper GI bleeding. Walt et al. tested this hypothesis by examining the ability of famotidine to limit upper GI bleeding in patients with peptic ulcer disease; however, they found no improvement over placebo controls (69).

Complications and side effects related to H$_2$RA are significant. In some cases, raising intraluminal pH makes gastric mucosa susceptible to injury by lowering the intracellular pH. Some investigators propose that stress ulceration may be related to intramural pH and not to intraluminal pH (70). H$_2$RAs are associated with tachyphylaxis, diarrhea, headache, mental status changes, hyperprolactinemia (cimetidine), rashes, vomiting, and drowsiness. In pediatric patients, there is a higher incidence of thrombocytopenia as compared to adults with the use of cimetidine (71).

Other medications that rely on an acidic environment for absorption must be used with caution in all drugs that increase gastric pH. Ampicillin and ketoconazole both have lower serum concentrations and bioavailability in this setting. Additionally, some H_2RAs (cimetadine more than ranitidine) inhibit the cytochrome P450 (CYP450) system. Famotidine and nizatidine do not affect the CYP450 enzyme.

Furthermore, H_2RA use is associated with nosocomial infection for several reasons: (*i*) H_2RAs alter the composition of the gastric microbial flora and lead to selection of more virulent microbes; (*ii*) critically ill patients are at higher risk of aspiration; and (*iii*) aspiration is followed by the onset of nosocomial pneumonia (72). But some believe that the role of H_2RAs in nosocomial infection is overstated. The risk of nosocomial pneumonia has not been validated in the meta-analysis by Messori et al. or by the randomized control study by Cook et al. (65,66). Some evidence suggests that H_2RAs lose their inhibitory effect on acid secretion over time (73,74). H_2RA tachyphylaxis and the association with nosocomial pneumonia have led to a reduction in H_2RA use as the mainstay in controlling stress-related gastritis and its most significant consequence, upper GI bleeding.

Cimetidine, ranitidine, famotidine, and nizatidine are widely available in the United States. Only cimetidine is FDA approved for the prevention of bleeding in critically ill patients as a continuous intravenous infusion. The oral H_2RAs are limited by malabsorption.

☞ **H_2RAs work by blocking histamine receptors on parietal cells. They are efficacious in raising pH, but they are associated with nosocomial pneumonia and tachyphylaxis. Survival benefit has not been demonstrated with H_2RAs.** ☞

Proton Pump Inhibitors
Background and Mechanism of Action
The goal of PPIs is to provide substantial, long-lasting elevation in gastric pH. PPIs are the most potent acid-suppressing agents available. The first PPI, omeprazole, was made clinically available in an oral formulation in 1989. Recently, intravenous PPIs were introduced and added to the therapeutic armamentarium for the prevention of stress ulcers. Pantoprazole, introduced in 2001 in the U.S. market, is the first intravenous PPI used in the United States.

The hydrogen (H^+)/potassium (K^+) ATPase pump exchanges H^+ ions for K^+ ions in parietal cells leading to the production of extracellular hydrochloric acid. PPIs directly block the H^+/K^+ ATPase proton pump in parietal cells. PPIs bind to cysteine residues in the transmembrane domains of the adenosine triphosphatase enzyme. The bound enzyme is unable to produce acid. Most PPIs are delivered enterally, absorbed beyond the pylorus and then transported in the blood stream to the parietal cells. PPIs are activated in an acidic environment and therefore only inhibit actively secreting proton pumps. PPIs bind irreversibly to the proton pump enzyme; and the inhibitory effects can only be overcome by the de novo production of a new proton pump enzyme. New proton pumps are synthesized every 72 hours.

Efficacy vs. Complication Profile
PPIs maintain higher gastric pH than H_2RAs (74). PPIs decrease the rate of duodenal ulcers by 80% to 100%, and the formation of gastric ulcers by 70%. However, no study

has definitively demonstrated the efficacy of PPIs in stress ulceration protection (75–77).

PPIs are metabolized through the CYP450 system and sulfate conjugation in the liver. PPIs appear to have minimal interactions with other medications, which make them particularly useful in the critical care setting. Nonspecific adverse events associated with the use of PPIs include vomiting, diarrhea, constipation, and rashes. Tachyphylaxis has not been documented with PPIs.

Originally PPIs were only available as enteral agents. PPIs are acid labile and therefore they are enteric coated to protect against gastric inactivation. The use of oral PPIs in the critical care setting is limited because many patients do not have postpyloric feeding tubes. The introduction of intravenous PPIs in the United States has permitted their use in critically ill patients at the highest risk of developing stress ulcers.

☞ **PPIs work by irreversibly binding the proton pump, thereby preventing release of hydrogen ions. Efficacious in raising gastric pH, their role in preventing stress ulcers is not defined. Most PPIs are available in oral form, although intravenous agents are now available.** ☞

Antacids
Antacids are no longer considered the mainstay in stress gastritis prophylaxis. Antacids are efficacious in preventing stress-related mucosal damage. But frequent enteral dosing and side effects limit their use in most settings. Side effects include hypermagnesemia, hypophosphatemia, intestinal distension, diarrhea, constipation, bezoar formation, and nosocomial pneumonia (78–90). Antacids are FDA approved for the prevention of stress-related mucosal disease.

☞ **Antacids are efficacious but difficult to use in critically ill patients.** ☞

Misoprostol
Misoprostol is a PG analog that inhibits gastric acid secretion, and may improve muscosal blood flow. The anti-secretory activity is less potent than that provided by the H_2RAs or PPIs. Misoprostol is the only FDA-approved PG analog that has shown benefit in the prevention of peptic ulcer disease. Although PGs are important in preventing acid-related mucosal injury under physiological conditions, and peptic ulcers due to NSAIDs, the use of synthetic PG analogues has not yet been shown to be efficacious in preventing stress gastritis or stress-related bleeding.

Enteral Nutrition
Enteral nutrition is ineffective in preventing stress gastritis. The inconsistency attributed to enteral feeding may be due to the inability of enteral feeds to consistently raise gastric pH (81). In addition, the mode of delivering enteral feedings is not resolved. Some clinicians prefer prepyloric feedings while others favor postpyloric feeding. Enteral feeds may play an important role in reducing the incidence of stress gastritis by helping to maintain positive nitrogen balance.

COMPLICATIONS OF GASTROINTESTINAL PROPHYLAXIS

Specific complications related to the different agents have been discussed in detail in the aforementioned section. Interactions between prophylactic agents and other medications are not uncommon and should be monitored. Agents that increase gastric pH promote bacterial overgrowth in the stomach and nosocomial pneumonia. Studies are discordant in their results. Some studies find an increase in nosocomial pneumonia in antacid- or H2RAs-treated patients compared to sucralfate-treated patients (82,83), while other studies find no difference among these agents (60,84,85). In a randomized trial involving 1200 patients comparing sucralfate and ranitidine no statistical difference between the groups was seen with regard to the development of nosocomial pneumonia, although there was an overall lower incidence in the sucralfate group (66). Environmental factors such as the use of nasogastric tubes that stent open the lower esophageal sphincter and allow reflux of gastric contents into the upper airway complicate the analyses. The issue of increased nosocomial pneumonia associated with prophylactic agents is unresolved but with current data the differences between medications seems small.

☞ Nosocomial pneumonia is a theoretic complication with all agents that raise gastric pH; however, the incidence of this complication is very low. ☜

MANAGEMENT OF ACUTE BLEEDING ASSOCIATED WITH STRESS GASTRITIS

Critically ill patients who bleed from stress ulcers are initially managed with standard resuscitation ATLS protocols. The principles involve the ABCs of resuscitation including airway protection and hemodynamic stabilization. Intravenous PPIs should be started promptly. A nasogastric tube is placed into the stomach and the stomach is lavaged until clear. Serial hematocrit measurements are monitored. Endoscopy is performed as necessary, and all high-risk lesions in the stomach should be treated with injection of epinephrine and thermocoagulation.

Gastric pH measurements should be monitored, and a pH >6 is targeted in order to prevent rebleeding (57). PPIs have been shown to be effective in preventing recurrent bleeding after successful endoscopic therapy (86,87).

OVERALL STRATEGY FOR GI PROPHYLAXIS

Based on the pathophysiology of stress ulcer formation, one of the most important maneuvers in preventing the development of stress gastritis in critically ill patients is to increase mucosal blood flow and subsequent oxygen delivery. Therapies directed at achieving this objective reduce the overall progression of stress gastritis and its major sequelae, clinically overt bleeding.

Stress gastritis prophylaxis is strongly recommended in coagulopathic patients, and all those who are anticipated to require mechanical ventilation for greater than 48 hours. Ulcer prophylaxis is also recommended in patients with at least two of the following risk factors: anticipated ICU stay more than one week; occult bleeding of any duration; sepsis; and steroids use (250 mg/day hydrocortisone or equivalent). In addition, patients with CNS injury, >10% BSA burn or a history of ulcer disease or gastrointestinal bleeding should be placed on prophylactic medication (88).

The best agent for prophylaxis is not clear. Sucralfate and H2RAs have similar efficacy but H2RAs are easier to use and a reasonable first-line therapy. If famotidine has been used in the past without success, sucralfate may be used. Although PPIs are more effective than H2RAs in raising intragastric pH, their efficacy in preventing stress gastritis is not markedly different. However, PPIs may be most beneficial when the prevention of recurrent bleeding is necessary after endoscopic therapy; monitoring gastric pH has not been documented to be beneficial in stress ulcer prophylaxis. However, pH monitoring (to maintain pH >6.0) is likely valuable after successful endoscopic management of stress gastritis–related bleeding. Figure 1 outlines the prophylaxis algorithm and management of stress ulcer bleeding.

EYE TO THE FUTURE

It has not been clearly demonstrated which agent is most efficacious in the prevention of stress ulcers. Current options include sucralfate, misoprostol, H2RAs, or PPIs. As only one intravenous PPI is currently approved for use in the United States, experience is limited and comparisons with H2RAs are continuing. Furthermore, whether any of these agents will actually prevent clinically important bleeding and reduce mortality may be ultimately more relevant.

Investigation into the etiology, prevention and treatment of stress ulcers continues to progress. The subsequent discussion reviews some of these new investigations in the clinical management of stress gastritis, including diagnostic technologies and novel mediator manipulation.

Diagnostic Screening for High-Risk Patients

The identification of patients at risk for developing stress gastritis continues to be an elusive target. Although several risk factors (burns, trauma, CNS catastrophes) have been identified and analyzed as outlined in the section "Risk Factors," modern pharmacogenetic-based strategies may offer customized patient-specific data that pinpoint the risk in other populations, and may influence appropriate drug and dosage targets for previously identified high-risk patients. For example, gene microarray and proteomic analyses may reveal the pertinent gene and protein variations in critically ill patients most likely to suffer from stress gastritis. Furthermore, these approaches may identify a set of genes or proteins that predict positive therapeutic responses or the potential for deleterious drug side effects. This knowledge would provide the clinician and pharmacist with a detailed report of what drug or drug combination may be most efficacious.

Novel Candidate Mediators

Some postulate that the increasing levels of proapoptotic proteins lead to gastric injury and therefore, antiapoptosis therapy could potentially attenuate the development of stress gastritis. For instance, apoptosis-modulating proteins (e.g., Bcl-2 family members or Fas/FasL) may play a role in stress ulcer pathogenesis. Zhonghua et al. studied bcl-2 (an antiapoptotic protein), Bax (a proapoptotic protein), and Fas/Fas ligand (proapoptotic proteins) in a rat model of stress-induced ulceration (89–95). They found that in rats immersed in water and restrained, decreased bcl-2 and increased Bax levels correlated with apoptosis but Fas/FasL protein levels did not correlate with stress ulcer injury.

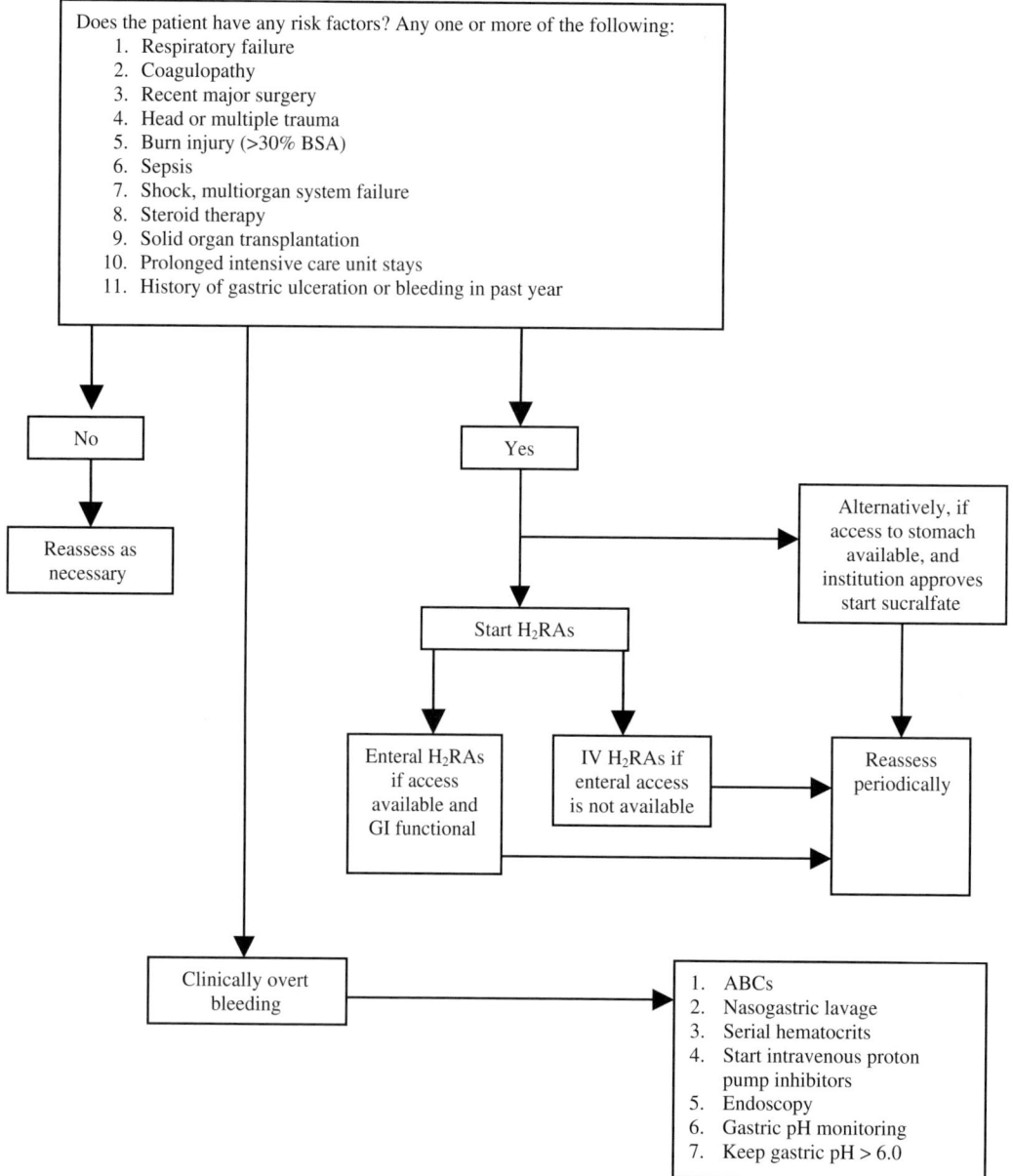

Figure 1 Prophylaxis and management of stress ulcers bleeding. *Abbreviations*: BSA, body surface area; H₂RAs, histamine type-2 receptor antagonists; ABCs, airway, breathing, and circulation.

Therefore, increasing bcl-2 and decreasing Bax expression may play a crucial role in abrogating stress ulcer pathogenesis. Another protein that could reduce the development of stress gastritis is heat shock protein 70 (hsp70). Shichijo et al. have shown that spontaneously hypertensive rats with increased levels of hsp70 are protected against water stress and restraint-induced gastritis (96). The authors propose that hsp70 protects against ulceration by increasing mucosal blood flow. Therapies directed at increasing hsp70 levels could also lead to decreases in stress gastritis.

Novel Therapeutics Nearing Clinical Trials

Several modalities are on the horizon that hold promise for reducing the formation of stress-induced gastritis by blocking the effects of reactive oxygen species. Ohta et al. determined that injecting stressed rats with superoxide

dismutase and catalase attenuated the formation of stress-related gastric ulcers (97). In addition, Bulbuller et al. demonstrated that intragastric L-tryptophan reduces the mucosal damage in immobilized rats as compared to controls by an alternative antioxidant mechanism (90). Hormonal strategies have been tested in a number of laboratories and these approaches may also augment our current armamentarium of antiulcer therapy. Bombesin and candesartan, the angiotensin II AT1 receptor antagonist, prevent hemorrhagic and cold-induced stress ulcers in rats. Bombesin is thought to work via a cholecystokinin receptor mechanism while candesartan works by a combination of gastric blood flow protection, decreased sympathoadrenal activation, and anti-inflammatory effects while maintaining the protective glucocorticoid effects and PGE-2 release (89,98). All of these therapeutic measures remain largely experimental and human testing is still required.

Nontraditional antiulcer therapeutics may also provide clues to the pathogenesis and treatment. Recently, two studies report the use of herbal remedies for the treatment of gastric ulcers. Shirwaikar et al. examined the effects of the ethanol extract of *Ageratum conyzoides* in preventing cold restraint stress ulcer in rats and found that it reduces the ulcer size and number mediated possibly by its antioxidant activity, Ca^{2+} channel blocking and antiserotogenic properties (99). In another report, Sairam et al. demonstrated the protective activity of *Asparagus racemosus* against cold restraint stress-induced gastric ulcers (100). They showed significant protection against acute gastric ulcer formation and an increase in mucosal defensive factors such as mucus secretion, cellular mucus, and the life span of cells. *A. racemosus* had little or no effect on the production of offensive factors like acid and pepsin.

SUMMARY

All critically ill patients are at risk to develop stress-related gastric mucosal disease. A small number of patients go on to develop clinically significant bleeding. The need for prophylactic therapy in these patients is particularly important in the group of patients who are at highest risk: those with coagulopathy and/or in respiratory failure requiring mechanical ventilation. Current data demonstrate that sucralfate and H2RAs are comparable in preventing stress gastritis, but the impact that this has on stress gastritis–related bleeding and mortality is less clear. Maximizing hemodynamic management combined with PPIs may be the best method to reduce mortality and bleeding (and rebleeding) from stress gastritis in the highest-risk patients.

Finally, while future work in stress gastritis is necessary, it is also very critical to determine the most efficacious management algorithm in patients at risk for stress gastritis. Current options include H2RAs, PPIs, sucralfate, misoprostol, and antacid therapy. The least manpower is used on H2RAs, PPIs, however, the side effects of increased gram-negative organisms and other side effects must be weighed against the use of other agents. The ability of H2RAs or PPIs to prevent clinically important bleeding and reduce mortality may be ultimately more relevant but this comparison remains untested. Additionally studies designed to compare the efficacies of the H2RAs and PPIs in various high-risk populations are also required. Finally, several new and novel modulators may be on the horizon of stress ulcer prophylaxis and treatment following trauma and critically illness.

KEY POINTS

- Stress ulcers are common in critically ill patients, but clinically important bleeding occurs in only 5% or less of these patients. Mortality in this small group of patients can be as high as 50%.
- Stress ulcers are found in the proximal stomach and are usually multiple, superficial, and diffuse. Deeper lesions can lead to major hemorrhage.
- Decreases in blood flow to the gastric epithelium, whether as a result of globally diminished circulating blood volume or reduced microcirculatory blood flow, leads to impairment of the epithelial defense mechanisms.
- Hydrogen ions play a central role in the development of stress ulcers. However, stress ulcers do not develop under normal circumstances because mucosal epithelial damage is limited by protective mechanisms including adequate blood flow, normal mucus production, buffering by bicarbonate secretion, mucosal PGs, and NO, as well as epithelial repair facilitated by EGF.
- Stress ulcers appear differently at various stages of development and lesions of dissimilar morphological stages can be seen in the same patient.
- Respiratory failure and coagulopathy are the two most important factors associated with the development of stress ulcers.
- Patients with stress ulcers are usually asymptomatic. Those patients who do bleed can have occult or overt bleeding, with or without hemodynamic instability.
- As hydrogen ions play a central role in stress ulcer development, raising gastric pH is necessary for prevention of stress gastritis. Maintaining gastric pH >4.0 will prophylax against stress ulcer formation, but once bleeding starts, a pH >6.0 is required to prevent rebleeding.
- Sucralfate works by binding to the stomach lining and thus has to be introduced directly into the stomach. It is efficacious in preventing stress ulcers, with a low complication profile, but has not been shown to improve outcome.
- H2RAs work by blocking histamine receptors on parietal cells. They are efficacious in raising pH, but they are associated with nosocomial pneumonia and tachyphylaxis. Survival benefit has not been demonstrated with H2RAs.
- PPIs work by irreversibly binding the proton pump, thereby preventing release of hydrogen ions. Efficacious in raising gastric pH, their role in preventing stress ulcers is not defined. Most PPIs are available in oral form, although intravenous agents are now available.
- Antacids are efficacious but difficult to use in critically ill patients.
- Nosocomial pneumonia is a theoretic complication with all agents that raise gastric pH; however, the incidence of this complication is very low.

REFERENCES

1. Fennerty MB. Pathophysiology of the upper gastrointestinal tract in the critically ill patient: rationale for the therapeutic benefits of acid suppression. Crit Care Med 2002; 30:S351–S355.
2. Cook DJ, Fuller HD, Guyatt GH, et al. Risk factors for gastrointestinal bleeding in critically ill patients. Canadian Critical Care Trials Group. N Engl J Med 1994; 330:377–381.
3. Lamb FS, Silva YJ, Walt AJ. Thomas Blizard Curling—the man and the ulcer. Surgery 1971; 69:646–649.
4. Alexander E Jr. Harvey Cushing. J Neurosurg 1996; 84:1077.
5. Zandstra DF, Stoutenbeek CP. The virtual absence of stress-ulceration related bleeding in ICU patients receiving prolonged mechanical ventilation without any prophylaxis: a prospective cohort study. Intensive Care Med 1994; 20:335–340.
6. Peura DA, Johnson LF. Cimetidine for prevention and treatment of gastroduodenal mucosal lesions in patients in an intensive care unit. Ann Intern Med 1985; 103:173–177.
7. Pinilla JC, Oleniuk FH, Reed D, et al. Does antacid prophylaxis prevent upper gastrointestinal bleeding in critically ill patients? Crit Care Med 1985; 13:646–650.

8. Zeng N, Athmann C, Kang T, et al. PACAP type I receptor activation regulates ECL cells and gastric acid secretion. J Clin Invest 1999; 104:1383–1391.

9. Pisegna JR, Wank SA. Molecular cloning and functional expression of the pituitary adenylate cyclase-activating polypeptide type I receptor. Proc Natl Acad Sci USA 1993; 90:6345–6349.

10. Miller TA. Mechanisms of stress-related mucosal damage. Am J Med 1987; 83:8–14.

11. Kivilaakso E, Barzilai A, Schiessel R, et al. Ulceration of isolated amphibian gastric mucosa. Gastroenterology 1979; 77:31–37.

12. Moody FG, Aldrete JS. Hydrogen permeability of canine gastric secretory epithelium during formation of acute superficial erosions. Surgery 1971; 70:154–160.

13. Stremple JF, Molot MD, McNamara JJ, et al. Posttraumatic gastric bleeding: prospective gastric secretion composition. Arch Surg 1972; 105:177–185.

14. Dive A, Moulart M, Jonard P, et al. Gastroduodenal motility in mechanically ventilated critically ill patients: a manometric study. Crit Care Med 1994; 22:441–447.

15. Ritz MA, Fraser R, Tam W, Dent J. Impacts and patterns of disturbed gastrointestinal function in critically ill patients. Am J Gastroenterol 2000; 95:3044–3052.

16. Reilly PM, Wilkins KB, Fuh KC, et al. The mesenteric hemodynamic response to circulatory shock: an overview. Shock 2001; 15:329–343.

17. Heyland DK, Tougas G, King D, Cook DJ. Impaired gastric emptying in mechanically ventilated, critically ill patients. Intensive Care Med 1996; 22:1339–1344.

18. Cheung LY, Ashley SW. Gastric blood flow and mucosal defense mechanisms. Clin Invest Med 1987; 10:201–208.

19. Bulkley GB, Oshima A, Bailey RW, Horn SD. Control of gastric vascular resistance in cardiogenic shock. Surgery 1985; 98:213–223.

20. Payne JG, Bowen JC. Hypoxia of canine gastric mucosa caused by Escherichia coli sepsis and prevented with methylprednisolone therapy. Gastroenterology 1981; 80:84–93.

21. Perry MA, Wadhwa S, Parks DA, et al. Role of oxygen radicals in ischemia-induced lesions in the cat stomach. Gastroenterology 1986; 90:362–367.

22. Reilly PM, Schiller HJ, Bulkley GB. Pharmacologic approach to tissue injury mediated by free radicals and other reactive oxygen metabolites. Am J Surg 1991; 161:488–503.

23. Leung FW, Itoh M, Hirabayashi K, Guth PH. Role of blood flow in gastric and duodenal mucosal injury in the rat. Gastroenterology 1985; 88:281–289.

24. Yasue N, Guth PH. Role of exogenous acid and retransfusion in hemorrhagic shock-induced gastric lesions in the rat. Gastroenterology 1988; 94:1135–1143.

25. Itoh M, Guth PH. Role of oxygen-derived free radicals in hemorrhagic shock-induced gastric lesions in the rat. Gastroenterology 1985; 88:1162–1167.

26. Das D, Bandyopadhyay D, Bhattacharjee M, Banerjee RK. Hydroxyl radical is the major causative factor in stress-induced gastric ulceration. Free Radic Biol Med 1997; 23:8–18.

27. Kayabali M, Hazar H, Gursoy MA, Bulut T. Free oxygen radicals in restraint-induced stress gastritis in the rat. Surg Today 1994; 24:530–533.

28. Li DS, Raybould HE, Quintero E, Guth PH. Calcitonin generelated peptide mediates the gastric hyperemic response to acid back-diffusion. Gastroenterology 1992; 102:1124–1128.

29. Holzer P, Painsipp E. Differential effects of clonidine, dopamine, dobutamine, and dopexamine on basal and acid-stimulated mucosal blood flow in the rat stomach. Crit Care Med 2001; 29:335–343.

30. Cheung LY, Chang N. The role of gastric mucosal blood flow and H^+ back-diffusion in the pathogenesis of acute gastric erosions. J Surg Res 1977; 22:357–361.

31. Gordon MJ, Skillman JJ, Zervas NT, Silen W. Divergent nature of gastric mucosal permeability and gastric acid secretion in sick patients with general surgical and neurosurgical disease. Ann Surg 1973; 178:285–294.

32. Menguy R. Role of gastric mucosal energy metabolism in the etiology of stress ulceration. World J Surg 1981; 5:175–180.

33. Smith SM, Grisham MB, Manci EA, et al. Gastric mucosal injury in the rat. Role of iron and xanthine oxidase. Gastroenterology 1987; 92:950–956.

34. Wood JG, Yan ZY, Cheung LY. Role of prostaglandins in angiotensin II-induced gastric vasoconstriction. Am J Physiol 1994; 267:G173–G179.

35. Peskar BM, Maricic N. Role of prostaglandins in gastroprotection. Dig Dis Sci 1998; 43:23S–29S.

36. Konturek PK, Brzozowski T, Konturek SJ, Dembinski A. Role of epidermal growth factor, prostaglandin, and sulfhydryls in stress-induced gastric lesions. Gastroenterology 1990; 99:1607–1615.

37. Zinner MJ, Rypins EB, Martin LR, et al. Misoprostol versus antacid titration for preventing stress ulcers in postoperative surgical ICU patients. Ann Surg 1989; 210:590–595.

38. Nishida K, Ohta Y, Ishiguro I. Changes in nitric oxide production with lesion development in the gastric mucosa of rats with water immersion restraint stress. Res Commun Mol Pathol Pharmacol 1998; 100:201–212.

39. Dive A, Foret F, Jamart J, et al. Effect of dopamine on gastrointestinal motility during critical illness. Intensive Care Med 2000; 26:901–907.

40. Ritchie WP Jr. Role of bile acid reflux in acute hemorrhagic gastritis. World J Surg 1981; 5:189–198.

41. Ellison RT, Perez-Perez G, Welsh CH, et al. Risk factors for upper gastrointestinal bleeding in intensive care unit patients: role of Helicobacter pylori. Federal Hyperimmune Immunoglobulin Therapy Study Group. Crit Care Med 1996; 24:1974–1981.

42. Basson M, Modlin I, Madri J. Human enterocyte (Caco-2) migration is modulated in vitro by extracellular matrix composition and epidermal growth factor. J Clin Invest 1992; 90:15–23.

43. Yanaka A, Suzuki H, Shibahara T, et al. EGF promotes gastric mucosal restitution by activating $Na(+)/H(+)$ exchange of epithelial cells. Am J Physiol Gastrointest Liver Physiol 2002; 282:G866–G876.

44. Furukawa O, Matsui H, Suzuki N, Okabe S. Epidermal growth factor protects rat epithelial cells against acid-induced damage through the activation of Na^+/H^+ exchangers. J Pharmacol Exp Ther 1999; 288:620–626.

45. Xu H, Collins JF, Bai L, et al. Epidermal growth factor regulation of rat NHE2 gene expression. Am J Physiol Cell Physiol 2001; 281:C504–C513.

46. French JD, Porter RW, von Amerongen FK, Raney RB. Gastrointestinal hemorrhage and ulceration associated with intracranial lesions: a clinical and experimental study. Surgery 1952; 32:395–407.

47. Feldman S, Birnbaum D, Behar A. Gastric secretions and acute gastroduodenal lesions following hypothalamic and preoptic stimulation: an experimental study in cats. Arch Neurol 1961; 4:308–317.

48. Cushing H. Peptic ulcers and the interbrain. Surg Gynecol Obstet 1932; 55:1–34.

49. Norton L, Fuchs E, Eiseman B. Gastric secretory response to pressure on vagal nuclei. Am J Surg 1972; 123:13–18.

50. Fisher RL, Pipkin GA, Wood JR. Stress-related mucosal disease. Pathophysiology, prevention, and treatment. Crit Care Clin 1995; 11:323–345.

51. Kuusela AL, Ruuska T, Karikoski R, et al. A randomized, controlled study of prophylactic ranitidine in preventing stress-induced gastric mucosal lesions in neonatal intensive care unit patients. Crit Care Med 1997; 25:346–351.

52. Sevitt S. Duodenal and gastric ulceration after burning. Br J Surg 1967; 54:32–41.

53. Lacroix J, Infante-Rivard C, Gauthier M, et al. Upper gastrointestinal tract bleeding acquired in a pediatric intensive care unit: prophylaxis trial with cimetidine. J Pediatr 1986; 108:1015–1018.

54. Lacroix J, Nadeau D, Laberge S, et al. Frequency of upper gastrointestinal bleeding in a pediatric intensive care unit. Crit Care Med 1992; 20:35–42.

55. Cochran EB, Phelps SJ, Tolley EA, Stidham GL. Prevalence of, and risk factors for, upper gastrointestinal tract bleeding in critically ill pediatric patients. Crit Care Med 1992; 20:1519–1523.

56. Bruck HM, Pruitt BA Jr. Curling's ulcer in children: a 12-year review of 63 cases. J Trauma Injury Infect Crit Care 1972; 12:490–496.

57. Vorder Bruegge WF, Peura DA. Stress-related mucosal damage: review of drug therapy. J Clin Gastroenterol 1990; 12(suppl 2):S35–S40.

58. Brunner G, Luna P, Hartmann M, Wurst W. Optimizing the intragastric pH as a supportive therapy in upper GI bleeding. Yale J Biol Med 1996; 69:225–231.

59. Brunner G, Luna P, Thiesemann C. Drugs for pH control in upper gastrointestinal bleeding. Aliment Pharmacol Ther 1995; 9(suppl 1):47–50.

60. Labenz J, Peitz U, Leusing C, et al. Efficacy of primed infusions with high dose ranitidine and omeprazole to maintain high intragastric pH in patients with peptic ulcer bleeding: a prospective randomised controlled study. Gut 1997; 40:36–41.

61. Cook DJ, Reeve BK, Guyatt GH, et al. Stress ulcer prophylaxis in critically ill patients. Resolving discordant meta-analyses. J Am Med Assoc 1996; 275:308–314.

62. McCarthy DM. Sucralfate. N Engl J Med 1991; 325:1017–1025.

63. Lipsett P, Gadacz TR. Bile salt binding by maalox, sucralfate, and meciadanol: in vitro and clinical comparisons. J Surg Res 1989; 47:403–406.

64. Slomiany BL, Piotrowski J, Slomiany A. Role of interleukin-4 in down-regulation of endothelin-1 during gastric ulcer healing: effect of sucralfate. J Physiol Pharmacol 2000; 51:69–83.

65. Messori A, Trippoli S, Vaiani M, et al. Bleeding and pneumonia in intensive care patients given ranitidine and sucralfate for prevention of stress ulcer: meta-analysis of randomised controlled trials. Br Med J 2000; 321:1103–1106.

66. Cook D, Guyatt G, Marshall J, et al. A comparison of sucralfate and ranitidine for the prevention of upper gastrointestinal bleeding in patients requiring mechanical ventilation. Canadian Critical Care Trials Group. N Engl J Med 1998; 338:791–797.

67. Algozzine GJ, Hill G, Scoggins WG, Marr MA. Sucralfate bezoar. N Engl J Med 1983; 309:1387.

68. Barer D, Ogilvie A, Henry D, et al. Cimetidine and tranexamic acid in the treatment of acute upper-gastrointestinal-tract bleeding. N Engl J Med 1983; 308:1571–1575.

69. Walt RP, Cottrell J, Mann SG, Freemantle NP, Langman MJ. Continuous intravenous famotidine for haemorrhage from peptic ulcer. Lancet 1992; 340:1058–1062.

70. Fiddian-Green RG, McGough E, Pittenger G, Rothman E. Predictive value of intramural pH and other risk factors for massive bleeding from stress ulceration. Gastroenterology 1983; 85:613–620.

71. Agarwal AK, Saili A, Pandey KK, et al. Role of cimetidine in prevention and treatment of stress induced gastric bleeding in neonates. Ind Pediatr 1990; 27:465–469.

72. Garvey BM, McCambley JA, Tuxen DV. Effects of gastric alkalization on bacterial colonization in critically ill patients. Crit Care Med 1989; 17:211–216.

73. Merki HS, Wilder-Smith CH. Do continuous infusions of omeprazole and ranitidine retain their effect with prolonged dosing? Gastroenterology 1994; 106:60–64.

74. Netzer P, Gaia C, Sandoz M, et al. Effect of repeated injection and continuous infusion of omeprazole and ranitidine on intragastric pH over 72 hours. Am J Gastroenterol 1999; 94:351–357.

75. Lasky MR, Metzler MH, Phillips JO. A prospective study of omeprazole suspension to prevent clinically significant gastrointestinal bleeding from stress ulcers in mechanically ventilated trauma patients. J Trauma Injury Infect Crit Care 1998; 44:527–533.

76. Phillips JO, Metzler MH, Palmieri MT, et al. A prospective study of simplified omeprazole suspension for the prophylaxis of stress-related mucosal damage. Crit Care Med 1996; 24:1793–1800.

77. Levy MJ, Seelig CB, Robinson NJ, Ranney JE. Comparison of omeprazole and ranitidine for stress ulcer prophylaxis. Dig Dis Sci 1997; 42:1255–1259.

78. Kaplan M, Ozeri Y, Agranat A, Brisk R, Eylath U. Antacid bezoar in a premature infant. Am J Perinatol 1995; 12:98–99.

79. Grosfeld JL, Schreiner RL, Franken EA, et al. The changing pattern of gastrointestinal bezoars in infants and children. Surgery 1980; 88:425–432.

80. Thomason MH, Payseur ES, Hakenewerth AM, et al. Nosocomial pneumonia in ventilated trauma patients during stress ulcer prophylaxis with sucralfate, antacid, and ranitidine. J Trauma 1996; 41:503–508.

81. Spilker CA, Hinthorn DR, Pingleton SK. Intermittent enteral feeding in mechanically ventilated patients. The effect on gastric pH and gastric cultures. Chest 1996; 110:243–248.

82. Tryba M. Sucralfate versus antacids or H2-antagonists for stress ulcer prophylaxis: a meta-analysis on efficacy and pneumonia rate. Crit Care Med 1991; 19:942–949.

83. Tryba M. Prophylaxis of stress ulcer bleeding. A meta-analysis. J Clin Gastroenterol 1991; 13(suppl 2):S44–S55.

84. Cook DJ, Reeve BK, Scholes LC. Histamine-2-receptor antagonists and antacids in the critically ill population: stress ulceration versus nosocomial pneumonia. Infect Control Hosp Epidemiol 1994; 15:437–442.

85. Cook DJ, Laine LA, Guyatt GH, Raffin TA. Nosocomial pneumonia and the role of gastric pH. A meta-analysis. Chest 1991; 100:7–13.

86. Lau JY, Sung JJ, Lee KK, et al. Effect of intravenous omeprazole on recurrent bleeding after endoscopic treatment of bleeding peptic ulcers. N Engl J Med 2000; 343:310–316.

87. Lin HJ, Lo WC, Lee FY, et al. A prospective randomized comparative trial showing that omeprazole prevents rebleeding in patients with bleeding peptic ulcer after successful endoscopic therapy. Arch Intern Med 1998; 158:54–58.

88. ASHP Therapeutic Guidelines on Stress Ulcer Prophylaxis. ASHP Commission on Therapeutics and approved by the ASHP Board of Directors on November 14, 1998. Am J Health Syst Pharm 1999; 56:347–379.

89. Bregonzio C, Armando I, Ando H, et al. Anti-inflammatory effects of angiotensin II AT1 receptor antagonism prevent stress-induced gastric injury. Am J Physiol Gastrointest Liver Physiol 2003; 285:G414–G423.

90. Bulbuller N, Akkus MA, Ilhan YS, et al. The effects of L-tryptophan and pentoxiphylline on stress ulcer. Ulus Travma Derg 2003; 9:90–95.

91. Deeb D, Xu YX, Jiang H, et al. Curcumin (diferuloyl-methane) enhances tumor necrosis factor-related apoptosis-inducing ligand-induced apoptosis in LNCaP prostate cancer cells. Mol Cancer Ther 2003; 2:95–103.

92. Ferrero E, Belloni D, Contini P, et al. Transendothelial migration leads to protection from starvation-induced apoptosis in $CD34^{+}CD14^{+}$ circulating precursors: evidence for PECAM-1 involvement through Akt/PKB activation. Blood 2003; 101:186–193.

93. Ikeda M, Yoshikawa H, Liu J, et al. Apoptosis-inducing protein derived from hepatocyte selectively induces apoptosis in lymphocytes. Immunology 2003; 108:116–122.

94. Kudsk KA. Effect of route and type of nutrition on intestine-derived inflammatory responses. Am J Surg 2003; 185:16–21.

95. Takahashi M, Ota S, Shimada T, et al. Hepatocyte growth factor is the most potent endogenous stimulant of rabbit gastric epithelial cell proliferation and migration in primary culture. J Clin Invest 1995; 95:1994–2003.

96. Shichijo K, Ihara M, Matsuu M, et al. Overexpression of heat shock protein 70 in stomach of stress-induced gastric ulcer-resistant rats. Dig Dis Sci 2003; 48:340–348.

97. Ohta Y, Nishida K. Protective effect of coadministered superoxide dismutase and catalase against stress-induced gastric mucosal lesions. Clin Exp Pharmacol Physiol 2003; 30:545–550.

98. Unluer EE, Denizbasi A, Ozyazgan S, Akkan AG. Role of bombesin and cholecystokinin receptors in gastric injury induced by hemorrhagic shock in the rat. Pharmacology 2003; 68:74–80.

99. Shirwaikar A, Bhilegaonkar PM, Malini S, Sharath Kumar J. The gastroprotective activity of the ethanol extract of *Ageratum conyzoides*. J Ethnopharmacol 2003; 86:117–121.

100. Sairam K, Priyambada S, Aryya NC, Goel RK. Gastroduodenal ulcer protective activity of *Asparagus racemosus*: an experimental, biochemical and histological study. J Ethnopharmacol 2003; 86:1–10.

31

Nutritional and Metabolic Evaluation and Monitoring

Eugene Golts
Department of Surgery, UC San Diego Medical Center, San Diego, California, U.S.A.

Jua Choi
Department of Nutrition, UC San Diego Medical Center, San Diego, California, U.S.A.

William C. Wilson
Department of Anesthesiology and Critical Care, UC San Diego Medical Center, San Diego, California, U.S.A.

Samme Fuchs
Department of Nutrition, UC San Diego Medical Center, San Diego, California, U.S.A.

Niren Angle
Department of Surgery, UC San Diego Medical Center, San Diego, California, U.S.A.

INTRODUCTION

The administration of enteral or parenteral nutrition constitutes one of the pillars of modern critical care, as nutritional status directly affects morbidity and mortality (1,2). Nutritional needs vary in response to metabolic changes, age, sex, growth periods, stress (i.e., trauma, disease, pregnancy, etc.), and physical condition. During critical illness, retention of sodium and water, along with loss of lean body mass from immobility and hypermetabolism, is related with the risk of multiorgan dysfunction syndrome, infection, and healing difficulties. Furthermore, these inflammatory changes can confound the monitoring of factors usually used in nutritional assessment.

The phenomenon of hypermetabolism was first described over 70 years ago in a landmark paper by Cuthbertson (3). More recently, hypermetabolism is recognized to occur in most critically ill patients, when in the catabolic state due to inflammatory mediators from severe trauma, burns, and disease states such as sepsis or the systemic inflammatory response syndrome (SIRS). This results in a rapid loss of total body mass, mainly from muscles. Early identification of high-risk patients and efficacious monitoring of nutritional support can reduce postoperative complications and decrease surgical intensive care unit (SICU) length of stay.

Nutritional assessment tools should be easy to use, reliable, reproducible, and inexpensive. Furthermore, these tools should be continuously available, and minimally perturbed by conditions associated with the underlying illness. ✒ **No gold standard in nutritional assessment currently exists.** ✒ All the tools mentioned in this chapter fulfill certain criteria but are lacking in other aspects.

This chapter reviews the nutritional and metabolic assessment tools commonly employed in critically ill trauma and burn patients. The nutritional assessment parameters that should be initially evaluated are first reviewed in the chapter, including pertinent information that should be sought in a carefully taken history and physical (H&P).

In addition, the anthropometric measurements commonly determined by registered dietitians, are surveyed along with laboratory values, predictive equations, and indirect calorimetry. The principal determinants of nitrogen balance and the continuous measurement of caloric expenditures are also provided. The chapter finishes with a survey of the pitfalls of nutritional assessment and the eye to the future.

INITIAL ASSESSMENT
History and Physical

The initial nutritional assessment is focused on determining the baseline nutritional state through information gleaned in the H&P exam, including a review of the patient's medical, surgical, social, and drug history, along with the review of systems.

The history as related to nutritional assessment should at minimum include the following: age, sex, and history of present illness (including duration of the disease process and of the state of malnutrition prior to seeking medical care). Any history of gastrointestinal (GI) symptoms should be elucidated, including changes in appetite, eating, or bowel patterns that would suggest alteration in the patient's absorption and/or metabolism (e.g., diarrhea, constipation, and steatorrhea).

Patients who have been vomiting for days with or without gastric outlet obstruction will have struggled with maintaining adequate caloric intake and electrolyte balance. Patients with drug addiction, alcoholism, or psychiatric disorders or malignancy often have anorexia and rarely meet their bodies' metabolic demands. Patients should also be screened for the presence of systemic diseases (e.g., liver, renal, congestive heart failure, or diabetes), and metabolic disorders. Similarly, patients with pretrauma symptoms of malabsorption (i.e., symptomatic Crohn's disease with progressive weight loss) are likely to be malnourished despite reporting seemingly adequate caloric intake.

Use of appropriate nutrition supplementation and providing adequate macro- and micronutrients will help maintain or improve nutritional status during hospitalization.

Previously hospitalized patients, those who are institutionalized, or transferred from another facility will need to provide a list of current medications.

Diuretics decrease the amount of body water and therefore affect body composition studies. Some medications such as propofol are lipid based, and their administration in itself provides patients with caloric intake that needs to be included into evaluations and later calculations of total caloric intake. Steroid use induces hyperglycemia which requires close monitoring and control via carbohydrate controlled diets and effective insulin therapy. Calories from dextrose-containing intravenous fluid and alcohol drips should also be accounted for.

The review of systems relevant to nutritional status includes: (*i*) history of recent weight change (particularly involuntary weight loss of 20% over two to six months or 10% over one month), (*ii*) difficulty in chewing/swallowing (dependence on thickened liquids and mechanically altered diets), (*iii*) emesis, nausea, and change in appetite, and (*iv*) bowel habits (presence of diarrhea or constipation for more than three days).

The nutritional history should be aimed at screening for individuals who are at risk of having protein-calorie malnutrition as well as identifying individuals with potential macro- and micronutrient deficiencies (Table 1). Hence, a nutrition support care plan should be established with

Table 1 Physical Examination Findings Consistent with Malnutrition

Physical examination	Deficiency/interpretation
General appearance	
Weight loss, decreased muscle mass, decreased subcutaneous fat	Protein/calorie malnutrition (<90% IBW), severe malnutrition (<70% IBW)
Skin	
Xerosis (dryness)	Essential fatty acids
Dermatitis	Vitamin C
Easy bruising	Vitamin K
Perifollicular hemorrhages	Vitamin C
Poor wound healing	Protein and zinc
Nails	
Koilonychia	Iron
Spoon-shaped, transverse ridging	Protein
Head, eyes, ears, nose, throat (HEENT)	
Hair	
Pigment changes, alopecia, easily pluckable without pain, flag spin (transverse depigmentation of hair)	Protein
Eyes	
Conjunctival pallor	Iron
Bitot's spot (triangular, shiny, gray spots on conjunctiva)	Vitamin A
Opthalmoplegia	Thiamine, phosphorus
Impaired night vision	Vitamin A
Nose	
Nasolabial seborrhea	Vitamin A, zinc, fatty acids, riboflavin, pyridoxine
Mouth/throat	
Glossitis	Riboflavin, niacin, vitamin B12
Cheilosis	Pyridoxine, folate
Angular stomatitis	
Swollen, bleeding, retracted gums	Vitamin C
GI	
Diarrhea	Zinc, niacin
Extremities	
Edema	Protein
Muscle wasting	Protein
Osteoporosis/osteomalacia	Calcium, vitamin D
Neurologic system	
Disorientation, confabulation	Niacin, phosphorus
Impaired cerebellar functioning	Thiamine
Peripheral neuropathy	Thiamine, pyridoxine, vitamin E
Impaired vibratory/position sense	Vitamin B12

Abbreviation: IBW, ideal body weight.
Source: From Ref. 105.

Table 2 Severity of Weight Loss as Percent of Weight Loss over Time

Time	Significant weight loss (%)	Severe weight loss (%)
1 wk	1–2	>2
1 mo	5	>5
3 mo	7.5	>7.5
6 mo	10	>10

Values charted are for percent weight change: % weight change = (usual weight − actual weight) × 100/usual weight.
Source: From Ref. 7.

goals to prevent starvation-induced complications, to improve clinical outcomes, and to correct existing metabolic or nutritional deficiencies that arise from a disease or treatment. For example, trauma patients admitted with alcohol dependence develop water-soluble vitamin (e.g., thiamine) deficiencies, and those on prolonged courses of broad-spectrum antibiotics will develop vitamin K malabsorption and depletion of healthy gut flora.

The most important element of the careful nutritional history is the presence or absence of recent weight change. This parameter has been evaluated extensively and is linked to mortality in several trials (4–6). Blackburn et al. (7) provide the clinician with the guidelines for the determination of the severity of the weight change (Table 2).

Part of the history includes the patient's current injuries. In particular, injuries or burns to the arms or bilateral upper extremity fractures should be noted. These patients can easily become malnourished because physical limitations prevent them from cutting their food and/or transferring it to their mouth. The nutrition support care plan should include an order that an individual is directed to assist them with eating. Another source of malnutrition is repeated periods of fasting prior to anesthesia for surgical procedures. Again, a review of all injuries will predict how many surgeries may be required. Thus, in addition to planning practical measures such as ensuring that the time of surgery is predictable so that the fasting period is minimized, caloric intake can be calculated to compensate for these periods.

The physical characteristics reflecting nutritional status include the baseline muscle mass, body fat, and subjectively the quality of hair and skin. Presence of stomatitis, friable gingival mucosa, easily pluckable hair, dermatological changes, and poor dentition may be associated with nutritional and vitamin deficiencies.

The abbreviated H&P performed during the primary and secondary surveys as per the Advanced Trauma Life Support® (ATLS®) paradigm should be supplemented with a complete H&P as part of the tertiary survey (Volume 1, Chapter 42).

Subjective Global Assessment Method

Several formal assessment tools have been designed to help organize nutrition-oriented H&P data into a format that facilitates the analysis. Among these, the Subjective Global Assessment (SGA) is the most widely used (Fig. 1) (8,9). The SGA summarizes weight change, dietary intake, GI symptoms, functional impairment, and physical examination. Both long- and short-term weight changes are assessed, and the severity of the weight change in the last six months is expressed as the percentages (A = <5%; B = 5–10%; C = >10%).

Symptoms of nausea, emesis, diarrhea, and anorexia are noted. These GI symptoms should be present almost daily for one to two weeks preceding the assessment to be considered significant. The degree and duration of the functional impairment related to nutritional intake is recorded. Finally, four observations derived from the physical examination are evaluated (loss of subcutaneous fat, muscle wasting, edema, and ascites). Once the assessment is complete, the patient is graded as well nourished, mildly or severely malnourished.

In general, the patient with significant weight loss, poor intake, severe nausea, emesis or anorexia, is bedridden, and has evidence of fat and muscle wasting would be considered severely malnourished. In contrast, the patient with no weight loss, no decrease in dietary intake, no nausea or anorexia, appropriate functional status, and no signs of muscle or fat wasting would be deemed well nourished. The method is only semiquantitative, and absolute numbers are not used. Rather, the tool serves more as a score card where trends are revealed. For example, even significant weight loss over the last six months is not a strong indicator of severe malnutrition, when offset by the recent (previous two weeks) trend toward weight gain in the setting of minimal or no stress (10).

The SGA has been found to be an inexpensive, quick, and reliable tool for the initial screening of patients who are malnourished (11,12). In the recent evaluation of 100 surgical patients, SGA was found to be a highly sensitive (100%) and specific (69%) tool for the identification of malnutrition (13). Despite its partly subjective and semiquantitative nature, it possesses good interobserver correlation (9,14). The SGA has also been found to be a sensitive and specific assessment tool in the pediatric surgical subgroup of patients (15). As such, ☞ **SGA is a valuable tool in the initial screening for malnutrition in the majority of the situations where the information regarding the status of the patient prior to admission is readily available.** ☞

Anthropometric Measurements

Anthropometry describes quantitative measurements in patients that assist in the evaluation of nutritional status. Anthropometrics were first used in the nineteenth century as an element of forensic science. Anthropometric measurements are the oldest and most studied ways to assess the nutritional status of patients. These are generally rapid, inexpensive, and noninvasive methods for assessing nutritional status. Although operator- and technique-related errors do occur, when performed consistently with adherence to the stringent set of rules, anthropometric measurements provide a solid basis not only for the initial assessment, but also allow for the ongoing monitoring nutritional status.

The most basic anthropometric measurements are the height and weight, which are obtained on admission. Weight should be measured daily to facilitate detection of changes in fluid status and to globally monitor nutritional trends. Both absolute weight and weight change over time could be used as predictors of outcome for the patients.

☞ **Weight loss is expected during hospitalization, and nutrition therapy goal should include maintaining ≥90% admit or usual weight.** ☞ Losses of 40% or more of admit weight is often fatal due to the substantial loss of lean body mass (16). Clinicians should be aware that weight loss, although occurring, may not be apparent in critically ill patients who develop tissue edema secondary to SIRS. Only when the edema resolves, will true weight loss

Risk Factor	Subcategories	SGA SCORE A	B	C
Weight Change	Total weight loss over last 6 months: ____ kg.			
Over the past 6 Months	A. No weight gain, no change, or mild (<5%) weight loss			
	B. Moderate weight loss (5- 10 %)			
	C. Severe weight loss (> 10%)			
In the past 2 weeks	A. Weight is increasing			
	B. No change in weight			
	C. Weight is decreasing			
Dietary Intake				
Change in Dietary Intake	A. No change or slight change for short duration			
	B. Intake borderline and decreasing; intake poor and increasing; intake poor, no change based on prior intake			
	C. Intake poor and decreasing			
Duration and degree of change	A. Less than 2 weeks, little or no change			
	B. More than 2 weeks, mild to moderate suboptimal diet			
	C. Unable to eat or starvation			
Presence of GI Symptoms				
	A. Few or no symptoms intermittently			
	B. Some symptoms for >2 weeks; severe symptoms that are improving			
	C. Symptoms daily or frequently >2 weeks			
Functional Status				
	A. No impairment in strength, stamina and full functional capacity; mild-moderate loss and improving			
	B. Mild to moderate loss of strength, stamina / some loss of daily activity or severe loss but now improving			
	C. Severe loss of function, stamina and strength			
Metabolic Demand				
	A. No stress			
	B. Low or moderate stress			
	C. High stress			
Physical Examination				
Subcutaneous loss of fat	A. Little or no loss			
	B. Mild-moderate in all areas; severe loss in some areas			
	C. Severe loss in most areas			
Muscle wasting	A. Little or no loss			
	B. Mild to moderate in all areas; severe loss in some areas			
	C. Severe loss in most areas			
Edema	A. Little or no edema			
	B. Mild to moderate edema			
	C. Severe edema			
Ascites	A. No ascites or only on imaging			
	B. Mild to moderate ascites or improving clinically			
	C. Severe ascites or progressive ascites Overall SGA score A or B or C			

Figure 1 SGA scoring sheet. SGA is a mainly subjective means of assessing the nutritional status. SGA classifies the patient as: A—well-nourished, B—moderately malnourished, and C—severely malnourished. The clinician rates each parameter as A, B, or C. If there are no more B or C ratings, the patient is more likely to be malnourished. If the ratings are on the left-hand side, the patient is likely to be well nourished. *Abbreviation*: SGA, subjective global assessment. *Source*: From Ref. 10.

become apparent by which time protein losses may be significant.

The pioneering paper by Studley (16) published in 1936 was the first to link outcome to the weight loss in patients undergoing surgery for peptic ulcer disease. He noticed that those with the most rapid weight loss had worse outcomes than the patients whose weight remained stable. Hill and Jonathan (17) have categorized the degree of weight loss with functional abnormalities. Weight loss of <10% of body weight is not associated with functional abnormalities, whereas weight loss of 10% to 20% is accompanied by functional abnormalities, with weight loss of >20% being most indicative of malnutrition, and multiple functional abnormalities are detectable in virtually all patients (17).

Patient's admission weight can be used as a determinant of nutritional status. The Hamwi "rule of thumb" calculation is one of the most commonly used methods to determine ideal body weight (IBW):
Men: 106 lb for the first 5 ft, then 6 lb for every inch over 5 ft.
Women: 100 lb for the first 5 ft, then 5 lb for every inch over 5 ft.

An acceptable body weight is ±10% of their ideal weight for all frame sizes.

Another standard available for estimation of IBW is the 1983 Metropolitan Life Height and Weight Table and the NHANES I (1971–1974)/NHANES II (1976–1980)

Table 3 Ideal Body Weight Ranges

IBW (%)	Classification
<70	Severely underweight
70–80	Moderately underweight
80–90	Mildly underweight
90–119	Healthy
120–134	Overweight
135–149	Obese
>150	Morbidly obese

Abbreviation: IBW, ideal body weight.

nutrition surveys (18,19). The tables provide clinicians one of the earliest examples of the anthropometric measurements used as the predictors of life expectancy and mortality (Table 3), however, it is not commonly used in the clinical setting.

It is important to note that comparing the patient's current weight to usual body weight is usually more useful than comparing current weight to an ideal weight. Body mass index (BMI) has been used as the measurement that correctly captures the relationship between the height and the weight, and is somewhat independent of height. BMI of 14 to 15 kg/m^2 is associated with significant mortality (20,21). BMI of less than 20 was found to be highly sensitive in elderly patients, or patients with cancer, but not in cirrhotic patients with tense ascites, cardiovascular, and neurological patients (22).

A study of lung transplant patients from the University of Toronto demonstrated that BMI <17 kg/m^2 or >25 kg/m^2 increased the risk of dying within 90 days posttransplant (23). However, not all literature supports the use of BMI as a sensitive indicator of malnutrition. In a prospective study of 640 hospitalized patients, four different widely available and locally accepted nutritional assessment methods were compared. BMI was shown to be the least sensitive method of the four (refer Table 4 for BMI classifications) (24).

Anthropometric measurements of fat stores are inexpensive, simple, and effective means of estimating the size of the largest energy-rich component of the human body. These measurements require only the skin fold caliper and measuring tape to perform. However, the amount of fat in the healthy subjects varies widely. For example, very little fat is sufficient in an athlete who is able to maintain his energy intake from food and has large muscle mass. The same amount of fat is insufficient in the critically ill patient who struggles with infection and stress from major abdominal surgery or trauma with little or no energy intake.

Table 4 Interpretation of Body Mass Index for Males and Females

BMI interpretation	Males	Females
Lean	<18.5	<19.5
Normal	18.5–23.5	19.5–24.5
Excess weight	>23.5–29.5	>24.5–29.5
Obese	>29.5	>29.5

Abbreviation: BMI, body mass index.

In order to assess total body fat stores, both skin fold thickness and the estimation of the limb fat area are the methods focused on the single measurement. Skin fold thickness can be measured over the biceps, triceps, thigh, or calf. Alternatively, subscapular or suprailiac skin folds can be used. Skin fold measurements are preferably done in the standing position (which partially limits their use for critically ill trauma patients).

In a study of 1561 patients admitted to the hospital emergently, mid-upper arm circumference was found to be a better predictor of the poor outcome than BMI (25). Similarly, mid-thigh circumference was found to be a statistically significant predictor of mortality in 142 patients with chronic obstructive pulmonary disease (COPD) (26). Not all studies, however, fall on the side of anthropometric measurements being reliable in the clinical settings. In the study of 158 consecutive medical admissions, mid-arm circumference was found to have poor validity in evaluation of malnutrition (27). Therefore, care should be exercised in using these measurements as the stand-alone methods for the evaluation of nutritional status.

Laboratory Values
Nitrogen Balance
Evaluation of the nitrogen balance is one of the oldest methods to estimate protein needs and adequacy of nutritional status. This method is based on the fact that protein is the only constituent in the human body composed of nitrogen. Therefore, by comparing protein intake and nitrogen waste, conclusions can be made regarding the nutritional balance of nitrogen and hence overall nutrition. Proper evaluation of the nitrogen balance involves total urea nitrogen (TUN) measurement of all the waste including urine, feces, nails, hair lost, etc. over the course of several days. Many facilities, however, do not have the equipment to determine TUN. Instead, they obtain a urinary urea nitrogen (UUN) value and estimate the other losses. It has been proposed that up to seven days are required to reflect the adaptation to the dietary change (28). However, the most dramatic drop in the urinary nitrogen excretion occurs in response to the deficiency in protein intake occurring in the first three days (29).

From the clinically relevant standpoint, it is acceptable to approximate the losses by measuring the UUN content over the course of 24 hours and compare it to the protein/nitrogen intake over the same period. The most common conversion factor for dietary protein is 6.25 g protein for every gram of nitrogen. Heymsfield et al. (30), for example, consider that total daily nitrogen excretion is urea nitrogen plus 1.5–2.0 g for most hospitalized patients. Other estimates, however, place the amount of nonurinary nitrogen losses at approximately 4 g/day.

Nitrogen balance = nitrogen intake − nitrogen losses.
Nitrogen intake = protein intake/6.25 (or appropriate conversion factor for nutrition regimen).

Nitrogen losses equal to 4 g is a commonly used factor to estimate nitrogen losses from the GI tract, in addition to UUN.

The goal is to be in +2 nitrogen balance. To estimate protein requirements based on a UUN value:

Estimated protein needs = [UUN+4 (insensible loss)+2 (for positive N balance)] × 6.25.

It should be pointed out that the 4 g/day allowance for the nonurinary nitrogen losses from fecal matter and skin is

Table 5 Approximate Values of Nitrogen Loss in Normal and Catabolic States

24 hrs urinary nitrogen loss (g)	24 hrs nonurinary nitrogen losses (g)	Level of metabolism
<6	4	Normal
6–12	4	Mild catabolism
12–18	4	Moderate catabolism
>18	4	Severe catabolism

only applicable in the situations when the patient's major source of excretion is urine. In the cases of renal failure (BUN >50 mg/dL or urine output <500 mL/day), severe diarrhea, lymphatic leak, or exudative drainage from the body (i.e., burns, high-volume fistula output, multiple decubitus ulcers, surgical drains, chyelothorax, etc.) nitrogen losses can be very substantially higher, and should be considered in any calculations of the nitrogen balance. In 1987, Waxman et al. (31) attempted to quantify protein losses through severe burns by deriving the formula: (g) = 1.2 × body surface area (m²) × % burn.

Critically ill patients are usually in a heightened state of catabolism. In this condition, patients often lose 16–20 g of nitrogen per day (up to 24 g/day in some cases) as opposed to nonstressed individuals who lose only 10–12 g/day. The classification of the degree of catabolism based on the nitrogen excretion in the urine is summarized in Table 5.

The degree of catabolism following trauma, burns, and critical illness is notoriously difficult to control. Nutritional supplementation by any route may blunt, but will never completely reverse the catabolic state of the patient (32,33). ✍ **The goal for nutritional support is to minimize the degree of catabolism and to maintain the patient in the normal to only mildly catabolic state throughout the acute phase of illness.** ✍ The protein intake for the critically ill patient should be tailored to this goal.

Hepatic Transport Proteins

Several proteins produced by the liver have been used to estimate the nutritional status of the patient. The most commonly used proteins are albumin, prealbumin, transferrin, and retinol-binding protein (RBP) (Table 6). Of these, albumin has been studied most extensively. Serum albumin concentration represents the balance between the hepatic synthesis and albumin degradation and clearance from the body. Approximately two-thirds of the albumin reside in the extravascular compartment (34). The half-life of albumin is approximately 21 days. Several well-designed studies demonstrated the correlation of low serum albumin and increased rate of complications (35–37).

For example, a study of 54,215 patients undergoing major noncardiac surgery in the VA system demonstrated that compared with the patients whose albumin levels was 46 g/L, the patients with the albumin levels of 21 g/L and above had increase in mortality from less than 1% to 29% and increase in morbidity rates from 10% to 65% (38). The levels of albumin drop in response to malnutrition. The drop, however, is offset by the shift of the albumin from the extravascular pool and by decreased degradation. Fol-

lowing trauma, sepsis, or after major surgery, the levels of albumin usually decrease precipitously. The mechanisms responsible are decreased hepatic synthesis, increased degradation, and hemodilution due to fluid resuscitation (39–41). Despite above mentioned confounding factors, albumin remains one of the easiest and most well studied parameters for the long-term assessment of the nutritional status of the patients.

However, due to its relatively long half-life (21 days), albumin is not a good indicator of the acute changes in the nutritional status. Accordingly, other proteins are used for the assessment of nutritional status and monitoring of nutritional progress in critical care. Transferrin has a half-life of approximately eight days. It therefore would seem to be better suited for the evaluation of acute changes in metabolism and nutritional status. However, transferrin concentration varies widely in healthy subjects. Furthermore, as this protein is part of the hepatic acute-phase response (APR), its concentration is elevated in both anemia and infection.

The preferred protein parameter for assessing nutritional status in critically ill patients is prealbumin. This protein has rapid turnover with a half-life of approximately 72 hours. As such, its levels fall and rise as nutrition status deteriorates and improves, respectively (42). In burn patients, the initial drop in prealbumin reaches maximum decline on postburn days six to eight (42). In a study of more than 1600 patients on maintenance hemodialysis therapy, prealbumin was inversely related to mortality, with a relative risk reduction of 6% per 1 mg/dL increase in prealbumin (43). Prealbumin levels are elevated in renal failure due to decreased excretion and long-term steroid therapy and lowered in liver failure due to decreased synthesis. Acceptable prealbumin levels for patients with renal failure, receiving hemodialysis, and on steroids are ≥30 mg/dL (44). The presence of these conditions as well as the acute response phase should be considered when making interpretations of prealbumin level.

Acute-Phase Proteins

Despite adequate nutritional support, prealbumin levels may not rise at goal improvement rate of 0.5–1 mg/dL/day. Drawing a C-reactive protein (CRP) level may be helpful to confirm decreased constitutive protein (i.e., albumin, prealbumin, RBP, and transferrin) synthesis. ✍ **During critical illness, the liver reprioritizes protein synthesis to acute-phase proteins (i.e., CRP, alpha$_1$-acid glycoprotein, alpha$_1$-protease inhibitor, fibrinogen, and haptoglobulin) instead of constitutive proteins (i.e., albumin, prealbumin, and RBP) (45), hence an inverse relationship between CRP and prealbumin levels develops.** ✍

A prompt increase in prealbumin may be seen when CRP levels fall below 10–15 mg/dL. If prealbumin levels do not rise, the nutrition support regimen should be reevaluated (refer to Table 7 for more information). The body's response to physical and psychological stress is called the APR and occurs during strenuous exercise, childbirth, burn, trauma, tissue ischemia, surgical operation, and allergic reactions. Clinical symptoms of APR include increased heart rate, fever, hemodynamic instability, altered level of consciousness and/or anorexia in addition to changes in body mineral stores, hormone levels, coagulation factors, blood cellular components, and plasma proteins. During APR, 30% of total body protein synthesis is dedi-

Table 6   Hepatic Transport Proteins

Serum protein	Clinical significance	Half-life (days)	Function	Causes of increased values	Causes of decreased values
Albumin	2.8–3.5 g/dL (mild depletion)	14–20	Carrier protein, maintenance of plasma oncotic pressure	Dehydration	Blood loss associated with trauma and surgery, fluid repletion during resuscitation, liver disease, infection, nephrotic syndrome, overhydration, malabsorption
	2.1–2.7 g/dL (moderate depletion) <2.1 g/dL (severe depletion)				
Transferrin	150–200 mg/dL (mild depletion) 100–150 mg/dL (moderate depletion) <100 mg/dL (severe depletion)	8–10	Carrier protein for iron	Pregnancy, hepatitis, iron deficiency, dehydration, chronic blood loss	Chronic infection, acute catabolic states, nephritic syndrome, increased iron stores, liver damage, overhydration, malnutrition
Prealbumin	10–15 mg/dL (mild depletion)	2–3	Carrier protein for RBP, transport protein for thyroxine	Chronic renal failure, steroid use	Acute catabolic states, past surgery, altered energy and nitrogen balance, liver disease, infection, dialysis
	5–10 mg/dL (moderate depletion) <5 mg/dL (severe depletion)				
RBP	Neglects acute changes in protein malnutrition; normal range of 2.7–7.60 mg/dL	0.5	Transports retinol	Renal failure, pregnancy	Vitamin A deficiency, acute catabolic states, past surgery, liver disease

Abbreviation: RBP, retinol binding protein.
Source: From Ref. 106.

cated to the production of acute-phase proteins—mainly CRP with a half-life of approximately 48 to 72 hours (Table 7) (46).

RBP has a small body pool and very short half-life (<12 hours). Like prealbumin, its concentration responds rapidly to variations in the energy intake and protein intake. Both prealbumin and RBP are therefore suited for the evaluation of the changes in the nutritional status with the limitations aforementioned.

Triglyceride Levels

Another important nutrition laboratory marker is serum triglyceride levels. Patients who are receiving propofol (Diprivan®) for sedation are receiving approximately 1.1 kcal/mL, which may add up to a significant source of fat calories. When greater than 1 g/kg/day or 0.1 g/kg/hr of lipid are infused, hepatic fat clearance may be compromised leading to elevated triglycerides. It is recommended to check triglyceride levels weekly for a goal of ≤400 mg/dL.

If elevated triglyceride levels continue, changing to a fat-free sedative (i.e., dexmetodomidine), is recommended. If elevated triglycerides continue after the halt of parenteral intralipid infusion or propofol, an evaluation for carnitine deficiency should be initiated.

Patients receiving parenteral intralipids with elevated triglycerides (>400 mg/dL) should have intralipids checked five hours after the lipid infusion is stopped. If levels continue to be elevated, approximately 500 mL of 10% intralipids or 250 mL of 20% intralipids should be provided over 8 to 10 hours, three times a week (47). Five hundred milliliters of 20% intralipid may also be given once per week. ☛ **Essential fatty acid deficiency arises one to three weeks after fat-free parenteral nutrition is initiated.** ☛ Propofol and parenteral intralipids should be used with caution because they are mainly composed of soybean oil or omega-six fatty acids, which have been shown to be immunosuppressive.

In a study done by Mayer et al. (48) on 10 critically ill patients with septic shock randomly receiving either n-6

Table 7 Nutritional Assessment Parameters

Parameters	Significance	Goals
Prealbumin	Half-life 2–3 days Synthesized by: liver Filtered by: kidneys Mild depletion: 10–18 Elevated values: steroid use and renal failure Decreased values: stress, infection, and critical illness or elevated CRP	When nutrition support initiated, goal improvement is 1 mg/dL/day Normal: >18 Moderate: 5–10 Severe: <5 Renal failure or steroids: ≥30 (44)
APP	Opsonins: CRP, protein protease inhibitors: alpha₁-protease inhibitor, hemostatic agents: fibrinogen, transporters: haptoglobulin Alpha₁-acid glycoprotein (45) Levels ≤48–72 hr postinjury When APP levels elevated, prealbumin levels decrease	CRP levels goal Baseline normal: <3 CRP level during bacterial infection: 30–35 Viral infection: <20 Posttrauma: 20–35 (107)
24 hr—UUN	Formula to estimated protein needed to achieve 0 N balance: (24 hr UUN + four for skin and fecal losses) = Y Y × 6.25 g protein/1 g N = g protein Waxman formula: (g) = 1.2 × BSA (m²) × % burn	Positive N balance 2–4 g Values inaccurate when: BUN >50 mg/dL urine output <500 mL/dL, multiple wounds/burns/large fistula and surgical output, dialysis
Triglycerides	To assess tolerance of TPN intralipids or fat containing sedative (i.e., propofol); to determine if hepatic fat clearance is optimal	Acceptable level: <400 mg/dL; if levels are higher, hold fats for 5 hrs and recheck; if levels remain elevated, infuse 250 mL TPN intralipids weekly to prevent EFAD; if levels are elevated, check for carnitine deficiency
Dry weight	To monitor losses of lean body mass; however, values may fluctuate with fluids, different scale use, dialysis, and burns; used to calculate calorie, protein, and fluid needs	Prevent loss of ≥10% admit or dry weight Losing ≥40% admit or dry weight is generally fatal (due to loss of substantial lean body mass)
Visual assessment, GI losses	Monitoring for symptoms of macro- and micronutrient deficiency, lean body mass wasting, edema, etc. GI losses may cause electrolyte imbalances (i.e., NG/OG fluids, ileostomy/rectal output, surgical drains)	Provide adequate MVI and mineral supplementation and electrolyte repletion to prevent deficiencies which may arise from long-term nutrition support or present illness
Indirect calorimetry	Gold standard to determine energy expenditure RQ: $\dot{V}CO_2/\dot{V}O_2$ Requires skilled personnel to interpret data Patient must be in the supine position either with continuous nutrition support or measurement taken 2 hrs postmeal	Caution when interpreting data RQ <0.7 oxidation of alcohol, ketones, carbohydrate synthesis, measurement problem 0.70–0.75 mostly lipid oxidation, possible starvation >1.00 lipogenesis, primarily carbohydrate oxidation, hyperventilation, measurement problem

Abbreviations: APP, acute-phase proteins; BSA, body surface area; BUN, blood urea nitrogen; $\dot{V}CO_2$, CO_2 production; $\dot{V}O_2$, O_2 consumption; EFAD, essential fatty acid deficiency; MVI, multivitamins; N, nitrogen; NG, nasogastric; RQ, respiratory quotient; TPN, total parenteral nutrition; UUN, urine urea nitrogen.

or n-3 lipid emulsion as parenteral nutrition for 10 days, CRP concentration and leukocyte count were increased in the n-6 group and decreased in the n-3 group—but the difference was not statistically significant. The same authors showed that n-3-enriched parenteral lipid emulsions may improve immunocompetence and inflammation in critically ill patients with sepsis (49). The FDA has not approved the use of omega-3 parenteral emulsions till now despite wide use in Europe.

Despite the reasonable biochemical basis for the use of protein levels for the evaluation of the nutritional status and multiple studies which validated this approach, some have found a discrepancy between anthropometry and use of nutritional markers for the assessment of nutritional status (50). ☞ **Clinicians, therefore, are advised to exercise some degree of caution while using the biochemical markers exclusively for the nutritional assessment.** ☞

Predictive Equations for Determining Caloric Requirements

The accurate estimation of the energy requirements allows intensivists to avoid the dangers of overfeeding critically ill patients while providing enough calories to combat malnutrition. Adequate nutrition is used to reduce the rate of complications and to decrease the hospital stay (51,52). It is also important in attenuating APR in critical illness (53,54).

The energy requirements of the individual are composed of resting metabolic rate, thermogenic response to food, and physical activity. Of these, the resting energy expenditure (REE) is the largest contributor to the total energy expenditure (TEE).

In 1919, Harris and Benedict (55) published their landmark study on the prediction of the basal metabolic rate in healthy individuals.

Box 1. Harris–Benedict Equations

Male: REE $= 66 + 13.7$ (weight in kg) $+ 5$ (height in cm) $- 6.8$ (age in years)
Female: REE $= 665 + 9.6$ (weight in kg) $+ 1.8$ (height in cm) $- 4.7$ (age in years)

Since then, the Harris–Benedict equations have been used to predict energy requirements in diverse groups of patients. These equations, however, were derived from the measurements of healthy subjects. Together with the realization that nutrition plays a crucial role in the care of critically ill patients came the attempts to use the equations to estimate the energy requirements of the critically ill patients. Through decades, these equations remained the standard for the assessment of the energy requirements. Their validity has been challenged recently (56,57). Multiple coefficients have been used to adjust the equations to evaluate the patients under various degrees of stress (Table 8) (58).

Other equations have been developed to improve accuracy over these original ones. Of these, the equations designed by Owen et al. (59) and the World Health Organization (WHO) have been shown to be more accurate.

Box 2. Owen et al. (60) Estimation of Caloric Requirements

Men EE $= [879 = 10.20 \times$ weight (kg)$] \times 4.184$
Women EE $= [795 + 7.18 \times$ weight (kg)$] \times 4.184$

Table 8 Injury Correction Factors for Different Surgical Insults

Injury correction factor	Clinical situation
1.3	Nonstressed, nutritionally sound patient
1.4	For minimal stress (elective surgery, cancer, minimal trauma)
1.5	Moderate stress (orthopedic surgery, major musculoskeletal trauma)
1.6	Severe stress (major trauma, sepsis)
1.7	Extreme stress (severe closed head injury, ARDS, sepsis)
2.1	Major burn

Abbreviation: ARDS, acute respiratory distress syndrome.
Source: From Ref. 50.

Box 3. WHO Estimation of Caloric Requirements (61)

Men 18 to 30 years old EE $= 64.4 \times$ weight (kg) $- 113.0 \times$ height (m) $+ 3000$
30 to 60 years old EE $= 19.2 \times$ weight (kg) $= 66.9 \times$ height (m) $+ 3769$
Women 18 to 30 years old EE $= 55.6 \times$ weight (kg) $+ 1397.4 \times$ height (m) $+ 146$
30 to 60 years old EE $= 36.4 \times$ weight (kg) $- 104.6 \times$ height (m) $+ 3619$

Another useful set of equations was developed by Ireton-Jones et al. (63). Unlike the other sets, these equations are designed to be used specifically for critically ill patients from the outset without the need for the correction factors.

Box 4. Ireton–Jones Equations

Spontaneously breathing patients: EEE $= 629 - 11A + 25W - 609O$
Ventilator-dependent patients: EEE $= 1784 - 11A + 5W + 244G + 239T + 804B$
EEE $=$ estimated energy expenditure, A $=$ age (years), W $=$ weight (kg), O $=$ presence of obesity ($>30\%$ IBW; $0 =$ absent, $1 =$ present), G $=$ gender (1—male, 0—female), T $=$ diagnosis of trauma (0—absent, 1—present), B $=$ diagnosis of burn (0—absent, 1—present)

These equations have been validated in several studies (64,65).

Lastly, a simple but commonly used energy expenditure equation is to calculate calorie and protein range based on weight in kilograms. Ranges of 20–35 kcal/kg would be appropriate for trauma, critical illness, and mild to severe stress. Estimating energy needs for obese patients ($>135\%$ IBW) brings a challenge. The use of the Ireton-Jones et al. (62) equation has closely estimated indirect calorimetry results. However, 11–14 kcal/kg of actual body weight per day and 1.5–2.1 g protein/kg IBW per day would be an appropriate initial range to meet energy needs of the critically ill obese patient (66). For trauma and critical care patients, providing protein of at least 1–1.2 g protein/kg initially for one to two weeks is adequate (67). Providing greater than 1.5 g protein/kg does not further reduce nitrogen losses (68). Azotemia may result when protein of more than 2 g protein/kg is provided (69) (refer to Table 9 for kcal, protein, and fluid guidelines).

Determination of kcal, fluid, and protein needs weight should be adjusted for patients with multiple amputations to prevent overfeeding or underfeeding. Table 10 provides adjustment information. For example, when calculating the IBW of a 5 ft 5 in. tall, 70-kg male with a below-knee amputation (BKA), using the Hamwi method IBW is 62 kg but when adjusted for BKA the patient's IBW would be: 62 kg—62 (7.1% for BKA) $= 57.5$ kg. Therefore, the patient would be 122% of IBW—slightly overweight.

☞ **The Harris–Benedict equations remain the standard, and most widely used equation for the estimation of the energy expenditures.** ☞ It is worth noting that the equipment used by Harris and Benedict consisted of the humidified breathing circuit in which $\dot{V}CO_2$ was trapped and weighted. The $\dot{V}O_2$ was determined by the amount of O_2 injected into the circuit (70). The formulas, therefore, have been designed on the same principle as indirect calorimetry.

Table 9 General Guidelines for Estimating Calorie, Protein, and Fluid Needs

Degree of metabolic stress	Total kcal/kg/day	Grams protein/kg/day	Fluid
Mild to moderate stress	25–30	0.8–1.5	1–1.5 mL/kcal for maintenance unless
Severe stress	30–35	1.5–2	restricted; additional free water indicated
Standard ICU	20–25	1.2–2	in absence of IVF in all tube fed patients
Obese (BMI > 27)	11–14 of actual weight	1.5–2.1 IBW	unless restricted
Burn	BEE × 1.2–1.5	2–2.5	
Trauma	20–35	1.2–2	

Abbreviations: BMI, body mass index, BEE, basal energy expenditure; ICU, intensive care unit; IBW, ideal body weight; IVF, intravenous fluids.
Source: From Ref. 66.

Indirect Calorimetry

Two types of calorimetry have been employed for the calculation of the energy expenditure. Direct calorimetry measures heat produced by the subject, as a direct measure of energy expenditure. This method is plagued by high cost and complicated engineering. Alternatively, indirect calorimetry has emerged as the viable method for the estimation of the REE. It is based on the measurements of $\dot{V}O_2$ and the $\dot{V}CO_2$ by the subjects. From these data, the energy expenditure is estimated. The equation used for the calculation of the energy expenditure is called the Weir equation:

$$EE = [\dot{V}O_2 \ (3.941) + \dot{V}CO_2 \ (1.11)] \times 1440 \ \text{min/day}$$

(71). In more general terms, the Weir equation assumes the following form:

$$EE = [(K_1 \times VO_2) + (K_2 \times VCO_2) \times 1.44 - (K_3 \times UN)] \quad (1)$$

where K_1, K_2, and K_3 are the constants. Various sources report different numbers for the K_{1-3} with the range for K_1 being 3.58 to 5.5, K_2 1.10 to 1.7, and K_3 1.44 to 3.44 (72–74). For the sake of simplicity, the urinary nitrogen measure can be omitted, as its contribution to the overall caloric expenditure is minimal. As a matter of fact, it has been shown that 100% error in the calculation of the nitrogen contribution would result in less than 4% error in the overall energy expenditure calculation (75).

Metabolic monitoring using indirect calorimetry has the advantage over formulas to account for variables that are difficult to measure such as energy expended from pain, physical therapy, sepsis, or respiratory complications. To perform the measurements, the equipment should be capable of measuring basic spirometry as well as performing the measurements of the partial pressures of gases in the inhaled and exhaled gas mixtures (76). The machines currently available measure and calculate the REE (intermittent

Table 10 Adjusting Weight for Amputation

Body parts	Adjustment (%)
Hand	0.8
Forearm and hand	3.1
Entire arm	6.5
Foot	1.8
Lower leg and foot	7.1
Above knee	11
Entire leg	16

Source: From Ref. 107.

monitor), which is slightly higher than the basic energy expenditure and lower than the TEE (continuous monitor). Nonetheless, indirect calorimetry has been shown to accurately approximate the caloric requirements (56,73,77–78). As defined in the review written by Brandi et al. (73), indirect calorimetry plays the role in the assessment of the patients who fail to respond adequately to traditional nutritional therapy. It is currently considered by many that **indirect calorimetry is the standard technique in the clinical armamentarium against which all other methods of nutritional assessment should be measured.** Some of the limitations of using a metabolic monitor include chest tubes with pulmonary air leaks, air leak past the tracheal cuff, or requirement of >80% FiO_2 (79,80)

Respiratory quotient (RQ) is defined as the ratio of $\dot{V}CO_2$ produced to $\dot{V}O_2$ consumed ($\dot{V}CO_2/\dot{V}O_2$). RQ above 1.0 is suggestive of overfeeding and of lipogenesis. Likewise the values of RQ below 0.85 suggest underfeeding and continued use of endogenous fat stores (Table 10). In the study of 263 patients from 30 kindred (long-term ventilator weaning) hospitals demonstrated the RQ measurement of more than 1.0 to be 85.1% specific but only 38.5% sensitive in detecting patients being overfed. Likewise, an RQ measurement of less than 0.85 was shown to be 72.2% specific and 55.8% sensitive for the detection of underfeeding. **Based on these numbers, it is hard to use the RQ as the monitoring tool or as assessment tool for the determination of the adequacy of nutritional regimen (81).**

RQ, however, can be used for the validation of the indirect calorimetry measurements with RQ values outside the physiologic range resulting from problems with the quantity or quality of nutritional intake, as well as from problems with the testing process.

MONITORING METABOLIC DEMANDS/NUTRITIONAL SUPPLY
Nitrogen Balance

Nitrogen balance, which requires 24-hour urine collection, is necessary to assess the net protein delivery. The goal of nutritional support is to achieve the positive nitrogen balance of 2–4 g/day in critically ill patients (as described earlier).

The context in which nitrogen balance is discussed here is as a measure of metabolic demand. The 2–4 g/day goal might not be obtainable in the patients in the acute phase of the critical illness (82–84). In the study of eight patients in septic shock, Streat et al. (84) found a significant degree of loss of the lean body mass despite aggressive nutritional regimen. In another study of the 20 medical patients in multiorgan system failure, the researchers have found that neither hypercaloric nor isocaloric nutritional support prevented protein catabolism; in contrast, they enhanced the metabolic burden (83).

Nonetheless, continuous monitoring of the nitrogen balance allows clinicians to tailor the diet regimens to offset the effects of the catabolic state of the acute illness (85). Nitrogen balance should be calculated weekly for critically ill patients and others at risk for malnutrition by the screening methods described elsewhere in this chapter.

Measurement of Continuous Caloric Expenditure

As discussed previously, indirect calorimetry has emerged as the robust tool for the management of the challenging patients with severe trauma and sepsis. The continuous metabolic measurements during the 24-hour period eliminate the theoretical problems with the errors in assessment of the metabolic needs caused by circadian rhythms, intermittent feedings, and stress of the treatments. Continuous indirect calorimetry is laborious and expensive as it ties the machine to the particular patient for the duration of the measurement. In the past, metabolic cart or a tent was used for the determination of the energy expenditure. This technique implied intermittent assessment, or, in other words, the "snapshot" picture of the energy expenditure. Recently, research has focused on the accuracy of intermittent indirect calorimetry as a tool for the determination of the energy expenditure (86–90). In the study by Smyrnios et al. (86), 30-minute indirect calorimetry measurements between 11 P.M. and 3 P.M. were found to predict energy expenditure acceptably well for clinical use. Similarly, van Lanschot et al. (89) concluded that acceptable accuracy can be achieved with two 15-minute measurements in a 24-hour period. It appears that there is sufficient evidence to recommend short-period measurements as a viable way to estimate 24-hour energy expenditure.

PITFALLS IN NUTRITIONAL SYSTEMS EVALUATION

The acute response to injury alters metabolism dramatically (91). Most of the baseline tables need modifications for critical illness. In patients with multiple trauma or severe sepsis, there is less correlation between the levels of IGF-1, prealbumin, and transferrin and the change in the total body protein, making these markers less useful for following changes in protein stores early in the course of critical illness (91). Anthropometrics are easy to perform on the patients in the upright position. However, trauma patients, especially in the critical care settings, usually have major limitations in mobility rendering anthropometric measurements difficult to perform and sometimes unreliable.

Nutritional history preceding the accident or onset of critical illness is sometimes unobtainable by the changes in the patient's mental status. SGA discussed earlier in this chapter has been used fairly extensively to recognize nutritional problems in patients (9,14,92,93). It has been shown to be the accurate predictor of malnutrition in the geriatric population (14,93) and in acute renal failure patients (94) specifically.

The SGA depends on careful collection of the information by trained observers. In at least one study, SGA failed to distinguish between the levels of malnutrition in the dialysis patients. In comparison with the total body nitrogen, the authors concluded that SGA is not a reliable predictor of degree of malnutrition (95).

Indirect calorimetry use is best reserved for the monitoring of the change in metabolic demands of severely injured or sickest patients when other methods fail to help in achievement of adequate nutritional status.

EYE TO THE FUTURE

Several body composition testing techniques have been suggested to be more accurate than currently employed methods. Among these are nuclear magnetic resonance, dual-energy X-ray absorptiometry (96,97), whole body conductance/impedance (98–101), neutron activation (102), air displacement plethysmograph (103), and hydrodensitometry (99,104). These methods are currently very expensive and difficult to implement on a broad scale. However, if the current trends in the search for a more precise tool continue, some of these new techniques might gain more popularity and, therefore, would become more suitable for the bedside applications.

SUMMARY

This chapter provides an overview of the armamentarium readily available to the interested clinicians in the majority of large trauma centers and SICU. The tools described have all been successfully employed in the nutritional assessment of the critically ill and injured patients. However, as it has been pointed out previously, all of the methods described here possess certain limitations. Despite great advances in the field of nutrition over the recent decades, the search for the cheap, easy to use, and reliable nutrition assessment tool continues. ☞ **At present there remains no viable substitution to the continuous and relentless attention to multiple small details of the patient's progress for the accurate assessment and monitoring of the nutritional status.** ☞

KEY POINTS

☞ No gold standard in nutritional assessment currently exists.

☞ SGA is a valuable tool in the initial screening for malnutrition in the majority of the situations where the information regarding the status of the patient prior to admission is readily available.

☞ Weight loss is expected during hospitalization, and nutrition therapy goal should include maintaining ≥90% admit or usual weight.

☞ The goal for nutritional support is to minimize the degree of catabolism and to maintain the patient in the normal to only mildly catabolic state throughout the acute phase of illness.

☞ During critical illness, the liver reprioritizes protein synthesis to acute-phase proteins (i.e., CRP, alpha$_1$-acid glycoprotein, alpha$_1$-protease inhibitor, fibrinogen, and haptoglobulin) instead of constitutive proteins (i.e., albumin, prealbumin, and RBP) (45), hence an inverse relationship between CRP and prealbumin levels develops.

☞ Essential fatty acid deficiency arises one to three weeks after fat-free parenteral nutrition is initiated.

☞ Clinicians, therefore, are advised to exercise some degree of caution while using the biochemical markers exclusively for the nutritional assessment.

☞ The Harris–Benedict equations remain the standard, and most widely used equations for the estimation of the energy expenditures.

☞ Indirect calorimetry is the standard technique in the clinical armamentarium against which all other methods of nutritional assessment should be measured.

☞ Based on these numbers, it is hard to use the RQ as the monitoring tool or as assessment tool for the determination of the adequacy of nutritional regimen (81).

☞ At present, there remains no viable substitution to the continuous and relentless attention to multiple small details of the patient's progress for the accurate assessment and monitoring of the nutritional status.

REFERENCES

1. Sungurtekin H, Sungurtekin U, Balci C, Zencir M, Erdem E. The influence of nutritional status on complications after major intraabdominal surgery. J Am Coll Nutr 2004; 23(3):227–232.
2. Dannhauser A, Van Zyl JM, Nel CJ. Preoperative nutritional status and prognostic nutritional index in patients with benign disease undergoing abdominal operations—part II. J Am Coll Nutr 1995; 14(1):91–98.
3. Cuthbertson DP. Further observations on the disturbance of metabolism caused by injury, with particular reference to the dietary requirements of fracture cases. Br J Surg 1936; 23:505.
4. Stanley KE. Prognostic factors for survival in patients with inoperable lung cancer. J Natl Cancer Inst 1980; 65(1):25–32.
5. Dewys WD, Begg C, Lavin PT, et al. Prognostic effect of weight loss prior to chemotherapy in cancer patients: Eastern Cooperative Oncology Group. Am J Med 1980; 69(4):491–497.
6. Keller HH, Ostbye T. Body mass index (BMI), BMI change and mortality in community-dwelling seniors without dementia. J Nutr Health Aging 2005; 9(5):316–320.
7. Blackburn GL, Bistrian BR, Maini BS, Schlamm HT, Smith MF. Nutritional and metabolic assessment of the hospitalized patient. J Parenter Enteral Nutr 1977; 1(1):11–22.
8. Duerksen DR. Teaching medical students the subjective global assessment. Nutrition 2002; 18(4):313–315.
9. Detsky AS, McLaughlin JR, Baker JP, et al. What is subjective global assessment of nutritional status? J Parenter Enteral Nutr 1987; 11(1):8–13.
10. Kozar RA, McQuiggan MM, Moore FA. Trauma. In: Cresci G, ed. Nutrition Support for the Critically Ill Patient: A Guide to Practice. Florida: Taylor & Francis, 2005:452.
11. Martinez Olmos MA, Martinez Vazquez MJ, Martinez-Puga Lopez E, del Campo Perez V. Nutritional status study of inpatients in hospitals of Galicia. Eur J Clin Nutr 2005; 59(8):938–946.
12. Sungurtekin H, Sungurtekin U, Hanci V, Erdem E. Comparison of two nutrition assessment techniques in hospitalized patients. Nutrition 2004; 20(5):428–432.
13. Mourao F, Amado D, Ravasco P, Vidal PM, Camilo ME. Nutritional risk and status assessment in surgical patients: a challenge amidst plenty. Nutr Hosp 2004; 19(2):83–88.
14. Ek AC, Unosson M, Larsson J, Ganowiak W, Bjurulf P. Interrater variability and validity in subjective nutritional assessment of elderly patients. Scand J Caring Sci 1996; 10(3):163–168.
15. Rojratsirikul C, Sangkhathat S, Patrapinyokul S. Application of subjective global assessment as a screening tool for malnutrition in pediatric surgical patients. J Med Assoc Thai 2004; 87(8):939–946.
16. Studley HO. Percentage of weight loss: a basic indicator of surgical risk in patients with chronic peptic ulcer, 1936. Nutr Hosp 2001; 16(4):141–143; discussion 0–1.
17. Hill GL. Jonathan E. Rhoads Lecture: body composition research: implications for the practice of clinical nutrition. J Parenter Enteral Nutr 1992; 16(3):197–218.
18. Wilber JA. Build and blood pressure study a review. Proc Annu Meet Med Sect Am Counc Life Insur 1980; 37–43.
19. Build Study: Society of Actuaries and Association of Life Insurance Medical Directors of America Recording and statistical Corporation; 1980.
20. Jeejeebhoy KN. Nutritional assessment. Gastroenterol Clin North Am 1998; 27(2):347–369.
21. Rapp-Kesek D, Stahle E, Karlsson TT. Body mass index and albumin in the preoperative evaluation of cardiac surgery patients. Clin Nutr 2004; 23(6):1398–1404.
22. Campillo B, Paillaud E, Uzan I, et al. Value of body mass index in the detection of severe malnutrition: influence of the pathology and changes in anthropometric parameters. Clin Nutr 2004; 23(4):551–559.
23. Madill J, Gutierrez C, Grossman J, et al. Nutritional assessment of the lung transplant patient: body mass index as a predictor of 90-day mortality following transplantation. J Heart Lung Transplant 2001; 20(3):288–296.
24. Galvan O, Joannidis M, Widschwendter A, et al. Comparison of different scoring methods for assessing the nutritional status of hospitalised patients. Wien Klin Wochenschr 2004; 116(17–18):596–602.
25. Powell-Tuck J, Hennessy EM. A comparison of mid-upper arm circumference, body mass index and weight loss as indices of undernutrition in acutely hospitalized patients. Clin Nutr 2003; 22(3):307–312.
26. Marquis K, Debigare R, Lacasse Y, et al. Mid-thigh muscle cross-sectional area is a better predictor of mortality than body mass index in patients with chronic obstructive pulmonary disease. Am J Respir Crit Care Med 2002; 166(6): 809–813.
27. Burden ST, Stoppard E, Shaffer J, Makin A, Todd C. Can we use mid-upper arm anthropometry to detect malnutrition in medical inpatients? A validation study. J Hum Nutr Diet 2005; 18(4):287–294.
28. Matthews D. Proteins and amino acids. In: Shils ME, Olson J, Shike M, Ross AC, eds. Modern Nutrition in Health and Disease. 9th ed. Philadelphia: Williams & Wilkins, 1999: 11–48.
29. Scrimshaw NS, Hussein MA, Murray E, Rand WM, Young VR. Protein requirements of man: variations in obligatory urinary and fecal nitrogen losses in young men. J Nutr 1972; 102(12):1595–1604.
30. Heymsfield SB, Tighe A, Wang ZM. Nutritional assessment by anthropometric and biochemical methods. In: Shils ME, Olsen JA, Shike M, eds. Modern Nutrition in Health and Disease. 8 ed. Philadelphia: Lea & Febiger, 1994:812–841.
31. Waxman K, Rebello T, Pinderski L, et al. Protein loss across burn wounds. J Trauma 1987; 27:136–140.
32. Wilmore DW. Catabolic illness: strategies for enhancing recovery. N Engl J Med 1991; 325(10):695–702.
33. Lowry SF. Modulating the metabolic response to injury and infection. Proc Nutr Soc 1992; 51(2):267–277.
34. Jeejeebhoy KN. Cause of hypoalbuminaemia in patients with gastrointestinal and cardiac disease. Lancet 1962; 1: 343–348.
35. Reinhardt GF, Myscofski JW, Wilkens DB, Dobrin PB, Mangan JE Jr., Stannard RT. Incidence and mortality of hypoalbuminemic patients in hospitalized veterans. J Parenter Enteral Nutr 1980; 4(4):357–359.
36. Apelgren KN, Rombeau JL, Twomey PL, Miller RA. Comparison of nutritional indices and outcome in critically ill patients. Crit Care Med 1982; 10(5):305–307.
37. Anderson CF, Wochos DN. The utility of serum albumin values in the nutritional assessment of hospitalized patients. Mayo Clin Proc 1982; 57(3):181–184.
38. Gibbs J, Cull W, Henderson W, Daley J, Hur K, Khuri SF. Preoperative serum albumin level as a predictor of operative mortality and morbidity: results from the National VA Surgical Risk Study. Arch Surg 1999; 134(1):36–42.
39. Lopez-Hellin J, Baena-Fustegueras JA, Schwartz-Riera S, Garcia-Arumi E. Usefulness of short-lived proteins as

nutritional indicators surgical patients. Clin Nutr 2002; 21(2): 119–125.

40. Fleck A, Raines G, Hawker F, et al. Increased vascular permeability: a major cause of hypoalbuminaemia in disease and injury. Lancet 1985; 1(8432):781–784.

41. Brugler L, Stankovic A, Bernstein L, Scott F, O'Sullivan-Maillet J. The role of visceral protein markers in protein calorie malnutrition. Clin Chem Lab Med 2002; 40(12):1360–1369.

42. Cynober L, Prugnaud O, et al. Serum transthyretin levels in patients with burn injury. Surgery 1991; 109:640–644.

43. Chertow GM, Ackert K, Lew NL, Lazarus JM, Lowrie EG. Prealbumin is as important as albumin in the nutritional assessment of hemodialysis patients. Kidney Int 2000; 58(6): 2512–2517.

44. Duggan A, Huffman FG. Validation of serum transthyretin (prealbumin) as a nutritional parameter in hemodialysis patient. J Ren Nutr 1998; 8(3): 142–149.

45. Fuhrman MP, Charney P, Mueller CM. Hepatic proteins and nutrition assessment. J Am Diet Assoc 2004; 104:1258–1264.

46. Preston T, Slater C, McMillan DC, et al. Fibrinogen synthesis is elevated in fasting cancer patients with an acute phase response. J Nutr 1998; 128:1355.

47. Seidner DL, Mascioli EA, Istfan NW, et al. Effets of long-chain triglyceride emulsions on reticuloendothelial system function in humans. J Parenter Enteral Nutr 1989; 13:614–619.

48. Mayer K, Fegbeutel C, Hattar K, et al. Omega-3 vs. omega-6 lipid emulsions exert differential influence on neutrophils in septic shock patients: impact on plasma fatty acids and lipid mediator generation. Intensive Care Med 2003; 29:1472–1481.

49. Mayer K, Gokorsch S, Fegbeutal C, et al. Parenteral nutrition with fish oil modulates cytokine response in patients with sepsis. Am J Respir Crit Care Med 2003; 167:1321–1328.

50. Lemonnier D, Acher S, Boukaiba N, et al. Discrepancy between anthropometry and biochemistry in the assessment of the nutritional status of the elderly. Eur J Clin Nutr 1991; 45(6): 281–286.

51. McClave SA, Snider HL, Spain DA. Preoperative issues in clinical nutrition. Chest 1999; 115(suppl 5): 64S–70S.

52. Heyland DK. Nutritional support in the critically ill patients: a critical review of the evidence. Crit Care Clin 1998; 14(3): 423–440.

53. Windsor AC, Kanwar S, Li AG, et al. Compared with parenteral nutrition, enteral feeding attenuates the acute phase response and improves disease severity in acute pancreatitis. Gut 1998; 42(3):431–435.

54. Moore FA, Feliciano DV, Andrassy RJ, et al. Early enteral feeding, compared with parenteral, reduces postoperative septic complications: the results of a meta-analysis. Ann Surg 1992; 216(2):172–183.

55. Harris JA, Benedict FG. A biometric study of basal metabolism in men. Carnegie Institute of Washington, 1919.

56. Weissman C, Kemper M, Askanazi J, Hyman AI, Kinney JM. Resting metabolic rate of the critically ill patient: measured versus predicted. Anesthesiology 1986; 64(6):673–679.

57. Foster GD, Wadden TA, Mullen JL, et al. Resting energy expenditure, body composition, and excess weight in the obese. Metabolism 1988; 37(5):467–472.

58. Donaldson-Andersen J, Fitzsimmons L. Metabolic requirements of the critically ill, mechanically ventillated trauma patient: measured versus predicted energy expenditure. Nutr Clin Pract 1998; 13(1):25–31.

59. Owen OE, Holup JL, D'Alessio DA, et al. A reappraisal of the caloric requirements of men. Am J Clin Nutr 1987; 46(6): 875–885.

60. Owen OE, Kavle E, Owen RS, et al. A reappraisal of caloric requirements in healthy women. Am J Clin Nutr 1986; 44(1):1–19.

61. Energy and protein requirements. Report of a joint FAO/ WHO/UNU Expert Consultation. World Health Organ Tech Rep Ser 1985; 724:1–206.

62. Ireton-Jones CS, Turner WW Jr, Liepa GU, Baxter CR. Equations for the estimation of energy expenditures in patients with burns with special reference to ventilatory status. J Burn Care Rehabil 1992; 13(3):330–333.

63. Ireton-Jones C, Jones J, McClave S, Spain D. Metabolic requirements of the critically ill mechanically ventilated trauma patient: measured versus predicted energy expenditure. Nutr Clin Pract 1998; 13(1):141–145.

64. Amato P, Keating KP, Quercia RA, Karbonic J. Formulaic methods of estimating calorie requirements in mechanically ventilated obese patients: a reappraisal. Nutr Clin Pract 1995; 10(6):229–232.

65. Gagliardi E, Brathwaite L, Ross S. Predicting energy expenditure in trauma patients: validation of the Ireton–Jones equation (abstract). J Parenter Enteral Nutr 1995; 19(suppl):22S.

66. Elamin E. Nutritional care of the obese intensive care unit patient. Curr Opin Crit Care 2005; 11:300–303.

67. Ishibashi N, Plank LD, Sando K, Hill GL. Optimal protei requirements during the first two weeks after the onset of critical illness. Crit Care Med 1998; 26:1529–1535.

68. Larsson J, Lennmarken C, Martensson J, Sandstedt S, Vinnars E. Nitrogen requirements in severely injured patients. Br J Surg 1990; 77:413–416.

69. Gault MH, Dixon ME, Doyle M, Cohen WM. Hypernatremia, azotemia, and dehydration due to high protein tube feeding. Ann Intern Med 1968; 68:778–791.

70. Garrel D, Jobin N, de Longe L. Should we still use the Harris and Benedict equations? Nutr Clin Pract 1996; 11(3):99–103.

71. Weir JB. New methods for calculating metabolic rate with special reference to protein metabolism. J Physiol 1949; 109(1–2):1–9.

72. Headley JM. Indirect calorimetry: a trend toward continuous metabolic assessment. AACN Clin Issues 2003; 14(2):155–167; quiz 266.

73. Brandi LS, Bertolini R, Calafa M. Indirect calorimetry in critically ill patients: clinical applications and practical advice. Nutrition 1997; 13(4):349–358.

74. Flancbaum L, Choban PS, Sambucco S, Verducci J, Burge JC. Comparison of indirect calorimetry, the Fick method, and prediction equations in estimating the energy requirements of critically ill patients. Am J Clin Nutr 1999; 69(3):461–466.

75. Bursztein S, Saphar P, Singer P, Elwyn DH. A mathematical analysis of indirect calorimetry measurements in acutely ill patients. Am J Clin Nutr 1989; 50(2):227–230.

76. McClave SA, McClain CJ, Snider HL. Should indirect calorimetry be used as part of nutritional assessment? J Clin Gastroenterol 2001; 33(1):14–19.

77. McClave SA, Spain DA, Skolnick JL, et al. Is achievement of steady state required when performing indirect calorimetry? J Parenter Enteral Nutr 1999; 23:S8.

78. Daly JM, Heymsfield SB, Head CA, et al. Human energy requirements: overestimation by widely used prediction equation. Am J Clin Nutr 1985; 42(6):1170–1174.

79. Branson RD. The measurement of energy expenditure; instrumentation, practical considerations, and clinical application. Respir Care 1990; 35(7):640–659.

80. Weissman C, Kemper M. Metabolic measurements in the critically ill. Crit Care Clin 1995; 11(1):169–197.

81. McClave SA, Lowen CC, Kleber MJ, McConnell JW, Jung LY, Goldsmith LJ. Clinical use of the respiratory quotient obtained from indirect calorimetry. J Parenter Enteral Nutr 2003; 27(1):21–26.

82. Streat SJ, Plank LD, Hill GL. Overview of modern management of patients with critical injury and severe sepsis. World J Surg 2000; 24(6):655–663.

83. Muller TF, Muller A, Bachem MG, Lange H. Immediate metabolic effects of different nutritional regimens in critically ill medical patients. Intensive Care Med 1995; 21(7): 561–566.

84. Streat SJ, Beddoe AH, Hill GL. Aggressive nutritional support does not prevent protein loss despite fat gain in septic intensive care patients. J Trauma 1987; 27(3):262–266.

85. Wolfe RR, Goodenough RD, Burke JF, Wolfe MH. Response of protein and urea kinetics in burn patients to different levels of protein intake. Ann Surg 1983; 197(2):163–171.

86. Smyrnios NA, Curley FJ, Shaker KG. Accuracy of 30-minute indirect calorimetry studies in predicting 24-hour energy

expenditure in mechanically ventilated, critically ill patients. J Parenter Enteral Nutr 1997; 21(3):168–174.

87. Damask MC, Askanazi J, Weissman C, Elwyn DH, Kinney JM. Artifacts in measurement of resting energy expenditure. Crit Care Med 1983; 11(9):750–752.

88. Mann S, Westenskow DR, Houtchens BA. Measured and predicted caloric expenditure in the acutely ill. Crit Care Med 1985; 13(3):173–177.

89. van Lanschot JJ, Feenstra BW, Vermeij CG, Bruining HA. Accuracy of intermittent metabolic gas exchange recordings extrapolated for diurnal variation. Crit Care Med 1988; 16(8):737–742.

90. van Lanschot JJ, Feenstra BW, Vermeij CG, Bruining HA. Calculation versus measurement of total energy expenditure. Crit Care Med 1986; 14(11):981–985.

91. Clark MA, Hentzen BT, Plank LD, Hill GI. Sequential changes in insulin-like growth factor 1, plasma proteins, and total body protein in severe sepsis and multiple injury. J Parenter Enteral Nutr 1996; 20(5):363–370.

92. Detsky AS, Smalley PS, Chang J. The rational clinical examination. Is this patient malnourished? J Am Med Assoc 1994; 271(1):54–58.

93. Persson MD, Brismar KE, Katzarski KS, Nordenstrom J, Cederholm TE. Nutritional status using mini nutritional assessment and subjective global assessment predict mortality in geriatric patients. J Am Geriatr Soc 2002; 50(12):1996–2002.

94. Fiaccadori E, Lombardi M, Leonardi S, Rotelli CF, Tortorella G, Borghetti A. Prevalence and clinical outcome associated with preexisting malnutrition in acute renal failure: a prospective cohort study. J Am Soc Nephrol 1999; 10(3):581–593.

95. Cooper BA, Bartlett LH, Aslani A, Allen BJ, Ibels LS, Pollock CA. Validity of subjective global assessment as a nutritional marker in end-stage renal disease. Am J Kidney Dis 2002; 40(1):126–132.

96. Kohrt WM. Preliminary evidence that DEXA provides an accurate assessment of body composition. J Appl Physiol 1998; 84(1):372–377.

97. Tataranni PA, Ravussin E. Use of dual-energy X-ray absorptiometry in obese individuals. Am J Clin Nutr 1995; 62(4):730–734.

98. Barbosa-Silva MC, Barros AJ, Wang J, Heymsfield SB, Pierson RN Jr. Bioelectrical impedance analysis: population reference values for phase angle by age and sex. Am J Clin Nutr 2005; 82(1):49–52.

99. Brodie D, Moscrip V, Hutcheon R. Body composition measurement: a review of hydrodensitometry, anthropometry, and impedance methods. Nutrition 1998; 14(3):296–310.

100. Dumler F, Kilates C. Use of bioelectrical impedance techniques for monitoring nutritional status in patients on maintenance dialysis. J Ren Nutr 2000; 10(3):116–124.

101. Pichard C, Kyle UG, Morabia A, Perrier A, Vermeulen B, Unger P. Nutritional assessment: lean body mass depletion at hospital admission is associated with an increased length of stay. Am J Clin Nutr 2004; 79(4):613–618.

102. Silva AM, Shen W, Wang Z, et al. Three-compartment model: critical evaluation based on neutron activation analysis. Am J Physiol Endocrinol Metab 2004; 287(5):E962–E969.

103. Dewit O, Fuller NJ, Fewtrell MS, Elia M, Wells JC. Whole body air displacement plethysmography compared with hydrodensitometry for body composition analysis. Arch Dis Child 2000; 82(2):159–164.

104. Demerath EW, Guo SS, Chumlea WC, Towne B, Roche AF, Siervogel RM. Comparison of percent body fat estimates using air displacement plethysmography and hydrodensitometry in adults and children. Int J Obes Relat Metab Disord 2002; 26(3):389–397.

105. Halsted CH. Malnutrition and nutritional assessment. In: Braunwald E, Fauci AS, Kasper DL, Hauser SL, Longo DL, Jameson JL, eds. Harrison's Principles of Internal Medicine. 15th ed. New York: McGraw-Hill, 2001:455–461.

106. Gottschlich MM, Matarese LE, Shronts EP (eds). Nutrition Support Dietetics Core Curriculum. 2nd ed. Silver Springs, MD: American Society for Parenteral and Enteral Nutrition, 1993:41–52.

107. Osterkamp LK. Current perspective on assessment of human body proportions of relevance to amputees. J Am Diet Assoc 1995; 95:215–218.

32

Enteral Nutrition

Cristina Guerra

Department of Trauma and Critical Care Surgery, Alamogordo, New Mexico, U.S.A.

Joseph F. Rappold

Division of Trauma and Critical Care, Department of Surgery, Naval Medical Center San Diego,
San Diego, California, U.S.A.

Jua Choi

Department of Nutrition, UC San Diego Medical Center, San Diego, California, U.S.A.

INTRODUCTION

Nutritional depletion is associated with malnutrition, increased morbidity—including delayed wound healing—increased lengths of hospital stay, and increased mortality (1). Malnutrition is common in hospitalized trauma patients with an incidence of 30% to 55% (2). Nutrition provides vital cell substrates, antioxidants, vitamins, and minerals required for recovery from illness (3). The two current mainstays of nutritional therapy are enteral and parenteral, with most investigators agreeing that the enteral route should be utilized when at all feasible (2–6).

Anatomically, enteral nutritional support requires a functional gut, a minimum of 100 cm of jejunum and 150 cm of ileum, and some colon, preferably with an intact ileocecal valve (7). Physiologically, the gut must receive adequate splanchnic blood flow and be free of obstruction, infection, ileus, or major mucosal injury. The earlier feeding resumes after resuscitation from trauma or burns, the more likely these conditions will be met.

The benefits of enteral nutrition include the maintenance of gut microflora and decreased bacterial translocation leading to enhanced immune function (2). Increasing gastric blood flow protects the gastric mucosa (4) and assists in maintaining mucosal barrier integrity (2), which results in decreased stress ulceration in critically ill and ventilated patients. Enteral nutrition is associated with decreased catabolic response to injury and improved wound healing (4). Utilization of enteral nutrition is associated with lower cost and fewer major complications than that of parenteral feeding (2). Also, it appears to improve survival in patients with severe injuries, acute pancreatitis, inflammatory bowel disease, and posthepatic transplantation (5). An outcome study by Adams et al. (2) demonstrated a significant reduction in septic morbidity in patients receiving enteral feeds against those on total parenteral nutrition (TPN).

It has become increasingly established that enteral feeding is generally well tolerated in critical illness, including following trauma and surgery. ✐ **In situations where full enteral nutrition is not tolerated, as little as 20% of overall nutrient calories administered to the gut can be sufficient to show benefits as opposed to TPN alone (5).** ✐

TRAUMA AND CRITICAL ILLNESS CONSIDERATIONS

Body stores will be adequate to provide nutrients during short periods of moderate stress without compromising physiologic functions or altering resistance to infection, or impairing wound healing. However, the greater the physiologic stress and the worse the baseline nutritional status, the shorter the duration of starvation tolerated before these complications begin to occur. ✐ **Patients most likely to benefit from nutritional support are those with baseline malnutrition in whom a protracted period of starvation would otherwise occur (8).** ✐ By definition, patients categorized as malnourished have lost greater than 10% of their ideal body weight (9). Enteral nutrition should be considered in healthy uninjured patients who have been without nutrition for three to five days and whose disease process is anticipated to last more than ten days (10). In previously well-nourished persons with short (<1 week) anticipated duration of fasting, it is difficult to demonstrate improvement in outcome with nutrition support (8). The Eastern Association for the Surgery of Trauma (EAST) practice management guidelines for nutritional support provide helpful recommendations on when, what, and where to feed various types of trauma injuries, which include head injury, spinal cord injury, postgastrointestinal surgery, and pancreatitis, based on 28 clinical studies between 1976 and 2000 (Table 1).

Post-Trauma

Multisystem trauma results in a hypermetabolic state resulting in an energy expenditure of 120% to 140% of basal levels (11). Generally speaking, the higher the injury severity score (ISS), the greater the hypermetabolic state. Without provision of exogenous substrates, amino acids are leached from endogenous protein stores including skeletal muscle and visceral structural elements. The resultant acute protein malnutrition is associated with cardiac, pulmonary, hepatic, gastrointestinal (GI), and immunologic dysfunctions. Late infectious complications can prolong the hypermetabolic or hypercatabolic state, eventually resulting in multiple-organ failure (12). ✐ **Early enteral feeding should be instituted in all severely injured trauma patients (ISS > 17) without contraindications.** ✐

Table 1 EAST Practice Nutrition Support Management Guidelines[a]

Diagnosis	Head injury	Abdominal injury	Spinal cord injury	Post-GI surgery	Pancreatitis
When to feed	As soon as possible	Immediately after patient is resuscitated	Within 72 hr of admission	Within hours after surgery if feasible	Immediately
What to feed	Immune-enhanced or high-protein formulas	Immune-enhanced or high-protein formulas	Immune-enhanced or high-protein formulas	Immune-enhanced or high-protein formulas	High nitrogen elemental formula
Where to feed	Stomach if feasible, if not tolerated in 48 hrs feed distally	Stomach if feasible, distally if undergoing laparatomy for injury	Stomach if feasible	Stomach if feasible, distally if not	Distally, preferably past the ligament of Treitz
Calorie needs	30 kcal/kg; 25 kcal/kg if pharmacologically paralyzed	25–30 kcal/kg	20–22 kcal/kg for quadriplegia; 22–24 kcal/kg for paraplegia	25–30 kcal/kg	25–35 kcal/kg
Protein needs	1.5–2 g/kg	1.5–2 g/kg	1–1.5 g/kg	1–1.5 g/kg	1–1.5 g/kg

[a]EAST = Eastern Association for the Surgery of Trauma.

Though trauma victims are generally young, well nourished, and free of pre-existing comorbid diseases, long-term catabolism can have detrimental effects. Biffl et al. (12) evaluated the effect of early nutritional support on patients with major torso trauma. They found early feeding to be feasible in this population, and that enteral nutrition resulted in higher total lymphocyte counts, cumulative positive nitrogen balance, and a lower rate of septic complications versus patients receiving TPN (12). Intensive study has been performed to determine the optimal route of nutrition to prevent the breakdown of lean muscle. In 1986, Moore and Jones compared enteral and parenteral feeding in patients who underwent laparotomy for severe abdominal trauma. Though nutritional parameters and overall complications were not different between groups, septic morbidity was higher in the parenteral group (11).

Kudsk et al. (13) also reported a decreased rate of septic complications including pneumonia, intra-abdominal abscess, and line sepsis in enterally fed patients with severe abdominal trauma. Furthermore, the sicker patients' abdominal trauma index [(ATI) ≥ 24, ISS ≥ 20, transfusions = 20 units, and reoperation] had significantly fewer infections when enterally fed (13). In addition, enteral feeding produced greater increases in constitutive proteins and greater decreases in acute-phase proteins after severe trauma (13).

The current EAST guidelines (Fig. 1) recommend that patients with blunt and penetrating abdominal injuries be fed enterally because of the lower incidence of septic complications compared with parenterally fed patients (11). As trauma patients are hypermetabolic, depletion of nutrient stores proceeds more rapidly in the case of total starvation than it does in healthy patients. So, the consequences of starvation evolve more rapidly in stressed, catabolic patients than in healthy individuals. Because of this, nutritional support in a severely injured patient should be achieved no later than the seventh day, whether by enteral or parenteral means, or by a combination of the two (Fig. 1). Over time, the dose of parenteral nutrition can be incrementally decreased as GI function returns (11).

Burn Injury

The goal in burn patients is to initiate enteral nutrition within six hours of presentation to prevent body weight loss of more than 10% of their baseline status (14). When a person sustains a burn, healing of the wound consumes large quantities of energy (14), resulting in elevation of the basal metabolic rate and doubling of the resting energy expenditure (REE) (15). The burn-related hypermetabolism results from elevation in catabolic hormones, cortisol, and catecholamines as well as from a decrease in the normal endogenous activity of the anabolic agents (14). This intense metabolic demand causes loss of body fat stores as well as loss of visceral and structural protein mass. In addition, burn injury predisposes to immunosuppression, delayed wound healing, and generalized muscle weakness, all of which prolong rehabilitation (15). In severely malnourished states, lean body mass loss of more than 40% correlates with imminent mortality, whereas limiting weight loss to less than 10% of baseline state is associated with better outcomes (14). Finally, the length of time and severity of the hypermetabolic and catabolic responses persist for over a year following the initial burn injury (14).

Severely burned children receiving a protein supplemented enteral diet demonstrated a higher survival rate

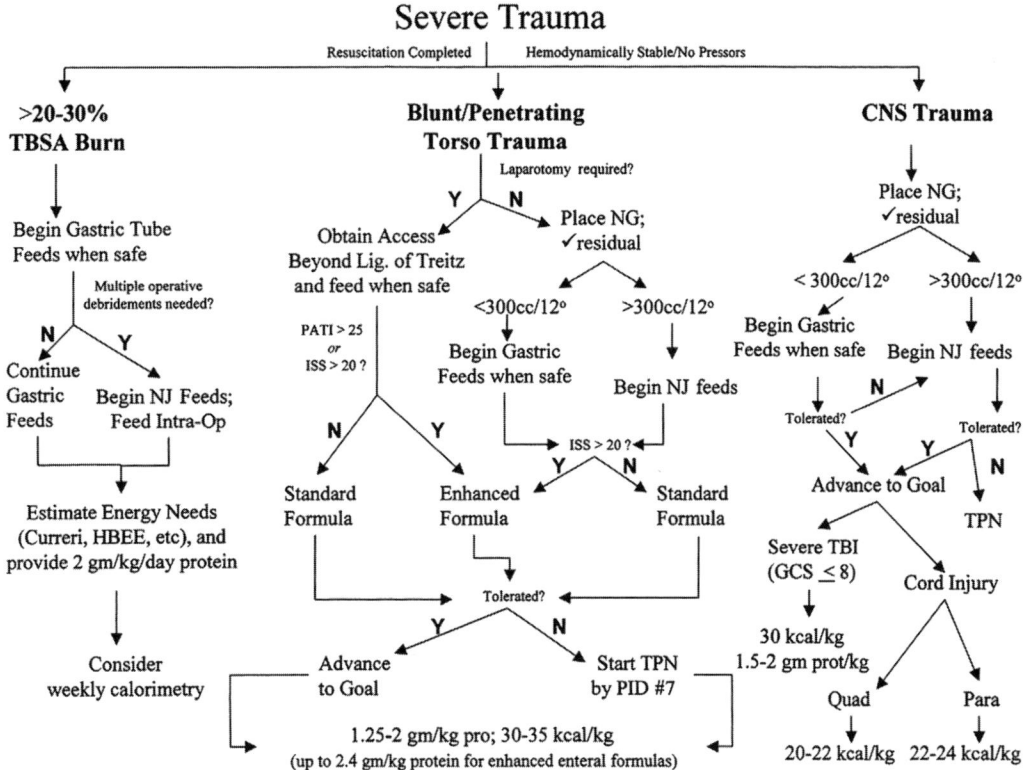

Figure 1 One proposed algorithm for feeding trauma and burn patients. *Abbreviations*: NJ, naso-jejunal; PID, post-injury day. *Source*: From Ref. 11.

and lower sepsis rate than those on a normal enteral diet (13). Based on studies such as these, it is not surprising that the American Society of Parenteral and Enteral Nutrition (ASPEN) Guidelines of 2002 recommend administering adequate amounts of calories and increased protein following burns (16).

The ASPEN Guidelines of 2002 also recommend enteral over parenteral nutrition (16). Studies in burn patients have shown that enteral nutrition provides superior nutritional support through maintenance of gut mucosal integrity, prevention of increased secretion of catabolic hormones (14), and higher survival rates (13). Though there is concern over inadequate splanchnic blood flow to support the use of the gut in the early postburn period, the immediate use of high calorie enteral feeding during the postburn shock phase has a positive effect on splanchnic perfusion. Conversely, the use of supplemental parenteral nutrition in burned patients leads to a significantly decreased survival rate (14). Intraoperative enteral feeding not only is well tolerated in burn patients but also leads to more successful attainment of calorie and protein goals in those requiring frequent burn wound debridements (11).

Critically ill, anuric ventilated patients on continuous renal replacement therapy (CRRT) have also been shown to have better outcomes with enteral compound to parenteral nutrition ($P = Q 04$) (17). The REE tended to be higher than predicted, and the use of a metabolic cart was found to be particularly useful in ensuring adequate energy provision (17), as is common in many burn patients (13–15).

Traumatic Brain Injury
Patients with traumatic brain injury (TBI) are hypermetabolic and catabolic similar to trauma patients. Numerous studies

have been performed to investigate the effect of TBI on nutritional need. On average, caloric expenditure following TBI averages 140% of normal REE (18). The increased REE is due to elevated oxygen consumption ($\dot{V}O_2$) caused by increased elaboration of stress hormone. Other factors increasing the metabolic demand include hyperventilation, fever, seizures, and posturing when present. Patients with decerebrate or decorticate posturing have demonstrated elevations in energy expenditure of 200% to 250% of the predicted value. TBI patients with elevated intracranial pressures (ICPs) refractory to standard therapy benefit from pharmacologic manipulation. High-dose barbiturates used to induce pharmacologic coma can decrease REE by as much as 40% below predicted levels. Other common pharmacologic interventions, such as neuromuscular blockade, reduce energy expenditure by 42% below predicted energy expenditure (11). So, patients requiring pharmacologic sedation or coma have a lower caloric expenditure of 100% to 120% of the predicted value (18).

☞ **To prevent devastating losses of nutrient stores and improve patient outcome, nutritional supplementation should begin no later than 72 hours following TBI (18).** ☞ Nitrogen loss of 0.2 g/kg/day occurs in TBI patients, which is two to three times higher than normal fasting nitrogen loss. After seven days without nutritional supplementation this rate of nitrogen loss can decrease lean body mass by 10% (18). During the first two weeks after injury, REE rises regardless of the patient's clinical course. Undernutrition during this two-week interval can result in up to 30% weight loss and increased mortality rate. Although steroids are a contributing factor for hyperglycemia in the TBI patient, no difference has been observed in the nutritional status of these patients who do or do not receive these drugs (19).

Spinal Cord Injury

Nutritional supplementation is associated with decreased mortality and disability in patients who have sustained a spinal cord injury (SCI) (20). Though there is no study showing a benefit of enteral versus parenteral nutrition in SCI patients, enteral nutrition is preferred due to decreased cost and lower rate of complications (11).

After the initial period of increased REE, SCI patients exhibit a decrease in energy expenditure. During this acute period, nitrogen excretion is increased, which may be due to muscle denervation and atrophy in the muscle segments distal to the injury. Within four weeks of an SCI, patients can lose up to 10% to 20% of their body weight, 85% of which is from loss of lean body mass. This loss is extremely difficult to correct even with aggressive nutritional replacement. Finally, the enforced immobility and nutritional compromise increase the patient's risk of infections, respiratory, wound, and urinary, thereby increasing ventilatory time, antibiotic administration, hospital length of stay, and recovery (20).

✍ **After the acute SCI phase, there is a period of reduced REE in proportion to the amount of paralyzed muscle mass.** ✍ So, the higher the lesion, the lower the REE measurement; for example quadriplegics require 55% to 90% of predicted REE and paraplegic patients require 80% to 90% (11). Although it is imperative to recognize the hypometabolic response in SCI patients to avoid the adverse effects of overfeeding, the precise time window when the hypermetabolic response gives way to the hypometabolic state is often complicated by intercurrent medial problems (e.g., pneumonia), which themselves increase the REE. Accordingly a metabolic cart is useful in these patients when their caloric needs are not obvious on the basis of normal nutritional markers (e.g., prealbumin levels) (Volume 2, Chapter 31).

Pancreatitis

Acute pancreatitis begins with a localized inflammatory process within the pancreas. However, with severe forms of the disease, extensive surrounding tissue destruction can occur. This results in profound systemic, metabolic derangements due to release of hydrolytic enzymes, toxins, and cytokines (21). The resulting condition is one characterized as hypermetabolic, hyperdynamic, systemic inflammatory response syndrome (SIRS), which leads to a highly catabolic stress state (22). The consequent rapid consumption of nutrient stores is characterized as a negative nitrogen balance condition. The REE increases by 77% to 139% of predicted value due to the hypermetabolic state. Catabolism and proteolysis of skeletal muscle increases by as much as 80% and nitrogen loss increases as much as 20–40 g/day. Gluconeogenesis increases, and glucose clearance and oxidation diminish, leading to glucose intolerance. Finally, development of hypocalcemia is common due to saponification, hypoalbuminemia, hypomagnesemia, increased calcitonin release, and decreased parathyroid hormone secretion (21).

Historically, the standard of care has involved gut rest and utilization of TPN for nutritional supplementation (22). Recent studies have shown that enteral feeding is safe and well tolerated in severe acute pancreatitis (23), with the caveat that pancreatic stimulation be avoided (24). Animal studies have shown that the site of GI feeding determines whether the pancreas is stimulated (22). With this in mind, current recommendations include placement of an enteral feeding tube distal to the ligament of Treitz (24) as jejunal

feeding results in a negligible increase in pancreatic exocrine secretion of enzymes and bicarbonate, and volume (22).

A recent meta-analysis by Marik and Zaloga (22) showed that patients who received enteral nutrition had lower rates of pneumonia, pancreatic and abdominal abscess, as well as wound and blood stream infections, than those receiving parenteral nutrition. In addition, enterally fed patients had a lower requirement for surgical intervention and shorter length of hospital stay (23,24).

Severe ileus preventing enteral feeding is common in the early stages of disease; most patients tolerate continuous low-volume nasojejunal (N-J) infusion. ✍ **Enteral feeding by an N-J tube or percutaneous jejunostomy has largely replaced TPN in the management of patients with pancreatitis (24).** ✍

More recently, a randomized study by Eatock et al. (25) compared elemental tube feeds administered via nasogastric (N-G) and N-J routes in patients with severe acute pancreatitis. The results indicated that N-G feeding was safe when an elemental diet formula was used with little difference in pain, analgesic requirements, serum C-reactive protein (CRP) concentrations, and clinical outcome (25). So, patients with severe acute pancreatitis without ileus may tolerate N-G administration of semielemental low-fat feeding. This would be favored, as the placement of N-G tubes is far easier and more cost-effective (23). Thus, patients with moderate to severe pancreatitis (Ranson's score >3) should be considered for enteral nutrition. Patients with mild pancreatitis normally resume oral intake within 48 hours, thereby negating the benefit of enteral nutrition.

Systemic Inflammatory Response Syndrome

SIRS, as well as sepsis and multiple organ dysfunction syndrome (MODS) (Volume 2, Chapter 63), are all associated with an increased REE and nutritional stress. These conditions represent a spectrum of illnesses with increasing severity of catabolism and increasing associated mortalities (26).

✍ **Patients with SIRS with or without MODS have elevated total caloric requirements, increased net protein catabolism, and increased micronutrient requirements (27).** ✍ The REE increases to at least 55% above predicted levels (28), so caloric requirements may need to be increased by 10% to 20%. The increased net protein catabolism necessitates an increase in protein administration. In general, nitrogen retention is promoted with 1.5–2.0 g/kg/day of protein (amino acids). In addition, hyperglycemia and triglyceride intolerance are common. Hyperglycemia, even in the absence of diabetes mellitus, is frequently present and requires tight control (27).

Surgery/Peritonitis

Patients undergoing surgery face many metabolic and physiologic challenges that compromise nutrition. Postoperative nausea, emesis, pain, anorexia, catabolism, infection, and wound healing tax the patient's nutritional reserves. Poor nutritional status in postoperative patients compromises organ and immune function, as well as muscle strength, and puts the patients at an increased risk for the development of infectious complications. In addition, delayed wound healing leads to prolonged recovery time. All of these factors contribute to increased length of hospital stay, readmission rates, and health-care costs (Fig. 2) (29).

Patients with peritonitis were historically treated with bowel rest and gastric decompression until return of normal GI function. Recent studies of surgical patients including those with peritonitis refute this early thinking (30). In an

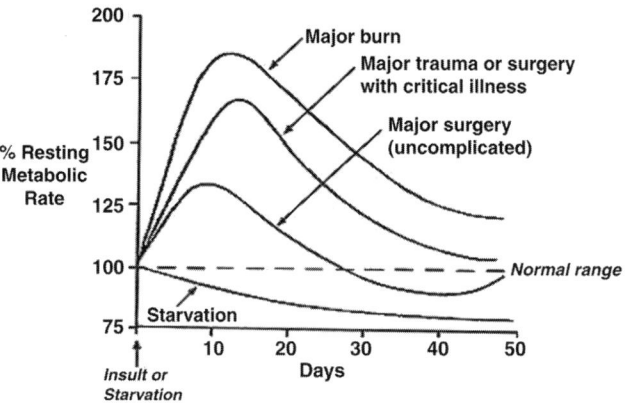

Figure 2 Variability of the metabolic rate depending on the level of injury. *Source*: From Ref. 77.

analysis of patients with generalized peritonitis, the GI tract recovers its tone and function within 48 hours (30). Early enteral nutrition not only is tolerated in these patients but also results in improved weight gain, nitrogen balance, and serum albumin (30). ☞ **Gut perforation after repair generally remains secure and is not necessarily put at risk of leakage by enteral nutrition started at 48 hours after surgery (30).** ☞

Malignancy

There is no evidence to support routine use of preoperative enteral nutrition in well-nourished patients undergoing chemotherapy or surgery for cancer; but it is indicated in malnourished patients with a functional GI tract who are unable to ingest sufficient nutrients orally (31). By virtue of their location, upper aero digestive tract tumors can profoundly impair swallowing and cause dysphagia (32). Patients with cancer of the head and neck are predisposed to malnutrition due to pre-existing alcohol and tobacco use. It is estimated that up to 57% of patients with cancer of the head and neck have significant weight loss prior to beginning treatment (31). In addition, therapies to treat these tumors, including surgery, radiation, and chemotherapy, will adversely affect nutritional status (31) and even when successful may further impair swallowing function (33). So, most patients with advanced malignancies will have compromised nutritional status at the initial medical evaluation (32).

Though the complications from the tumor or therapies prevent oral intake, the remaining GI tract is usually functional and enteral nutrition can be administered via a feeding tube. In addition, numerous studies have shown the importance of maintaining the patient's nutritional status during the treatment of these tumors (33). In a prospective study of patients with esophageal cancer undergoing chemoradiation, enteral nutrition effectively prevented weight loss during therapy. Patients who are better nourished have been found to have fewer complications and improved survival (33). ☞ **For malnourished patients undergoing resection of their tumor, 7 to 10 days of preoperative enteral nutrition support is associated with a 10% reduction in morbidity and improved quality of life (31).** ☞

Finally, when a severe, acute insult is superimposed on the underlying debilitating effects of cancer, malnutrition is almost unavoidable. It is no surprise that malnutrition is almost universally present in cancer patients requiring admission to a surgical intensive care unit (SICU). Enteral feeding is superior to TPN and can prevent or reverse host tissue wasting, broaden the spectrum of clinical options, and possibly improve clinical outcome (31).

Contraindications

The only absolute contraindication to enteral nutrition associates with intestinal obstruction, perforation, ischemia, and major ileus. Other contraindications include patients with intractable vomiting, severe diarrhea, circulatory shock, and GI hemorrhage. Large-volume (500 mL/day) enterocutaneous fistulas represent relative contraindications that can sometimes tolerate elemental diets and/or tubes that both administer nutrients and control fistula drainage.

Finally, though a patient may qualify for nutritional supplementation, it is imperative both to consider the patient's wishes (29) and to determine whether enteral nutrition is appropriate for patients whose prognosis does not warrant aggressive nutritional support due to futility of the disease process (8) (Volume 2, Chapter 67).

INITIATION AND ADVANCEMENT OF ENTERNAL NUTRITION
Early vs. Late

Historically, delayed institution of feeding was preferred due to the prevalence of gastroparesis and lack of bowel sounds in critically ill, injured, and postoperative patients, both of which were thought to indicate an increased risk of tube feeding intolerance. However, it is now known that small-bowel function, including the ability to absorb nutrients, remains intact despite critical illness, gastroparesis, and lack of bowel sounds. Finally, it has been popularly propagated that patients can easily tolerate five to seven days of starvation without clinical detriment. However, it is now recognized that critically ill trauma and burn patients (as aforementioned) are hypermetabolic following injury and are at increased risk of secondary complications (including infections and wound breakdown) if nutrition is withheld even for a couple of days following injury (11–16).

Tube Feed Advancement

Tolerance of enteral nutrition advancement is partly dependent upon the formula administered and the route of administration. When feeding gastrically, the osmolality can be higher than when feeding into the jejunum. But because of gastric atony in numerous situations, advancement may be slower than when fed distally. Gastric tube feeding should be initiated at a rate of 10–20 mL/hr of volume via a pump in critically ill patients. After four hours of feeding, enteral administration is temporarily held and the gastric contents aspirated to evaluate the residual gastric volume (RGV). If the RGV is less than 400–500 mL, the tube feeding should be considered to be tolerated and can be advanced after readministrating the aspirated volume. Advancement occurs with 10–20 mL increments every two to four hours until the goal rate is attained. The implementation of tube feed advancement can be successfully increased more rapidly in many patients to more rapidly attain the goal rate (5).

When small-bowel feeding occurs, the volume should be increased first using a hypo-osmotic solution followed by advancement of the osmolality. Administration of solutions composed of greater than 300–400 mOsm is not tolerated and can result in diarrhea. The authors have found that the jejunum can tolerate up to 110 mL/hr of iso-osmotic enteral formula with minimal GI distress. As previously discussed, the presence of bowel sounds and the passage of flatus or stool are not necessary for initiation of tube feeding (27).

Though full feeding can usually be achieved within one to three days, many patients remain underfed despite receiving enteral feeding (1). Reasons include slow tube feed advancement, feeding interruption due to surgery, procedures, and patient transport. When patients have tolerated enteral nutrition well for several days, intermittent bolus supplementation can often be tolerated to make up for the lost nutrition due to procedural interruptions.

Continuous vs. Bolus Feeding

Continuous feeding involves administering the total daily nutritional volume in equal hourly increments. Proponents note less abdominal distention and regurgitation due to the lower total stomach volume, and is generally the optimal method to initiate tube feedings.

Bolus or intermittent feeding involves dividing the total volume for 24 hours into equal portions to be administered as four to six separate feedings given over approximately an hour each. Adequate free water flushes should also be provided to meet hydration needs and prevent clogging of feeding tube. The benefits of this approach include increased patient mobility and freedom. As such, bolus feeding is more appropriate for ambulatory (rather than critically ill) patients. Some patients may note early satiety, nausea, or emesis, which can be resolved by administering the bolus over a longer duration (32). Intermittent feeding is also believed to decrease gastric pH between feedings, causing bacterial destruction and a decreased risk of pneumonia after aspiration of regurgitated gastric contents.

A prospective, randomized study of 41 mechanically ventilated patients was performed to compare intermittent gastric feeding, continuous gastric feeding, continuous jejunal feedings, and the risk of aspiration by Metheny et al. (34). Though they noted some variability in gastric pH, there was no difference in the rate of aspiration (34). The most important factor in determining which patients best qualify for intermittent versus continuous feeding is the route of administration. As noted earlier, the small bowel will not tolerate large volumes, so bolus feeds are not recommended and continuous feeding is preferred. If the patient is receiving intragastric feeds then it is possible to achieve nutritional goals with either intermittent or continuous feeding (32). However, bolus feeding should only be considered in patients that have already demonstrated the ability to tolerate continuous feeds for several days.

Transitional Feeding

When patients are transitioning from parenteral to enteral nutrition the physician should provide clear weaning procedures to the nurses. There is no set formula on how to wean parenteral nutrition and increase enteral goal rate. However, with parenteral nutrition, trophic feeding of 10–20 mL/hr should be initiated when GI function is stable. If the patient is able to tolerate trophic feeding based on presence of residuals (<400 mL), discontinuing parenteral intralipids would be the first action. Precise weaning would be achieved if nutrient calculation is conducted by the physician or the clinical dietitian; however, as this is a time-consuming process, equations such as increasing

enteral rate and decreasing TPN rate every two to four hours to sum the enteral goal rate have been helpful. When patients are ready for oral intake, a swallowing evaluation should be ordered to assess for thin liquid tolerance.

ROUTES OF ADMINISTRATION

☞ The route of enteral nutrition administration is influenced by the patient's clinical prognosis, anticipated duration of feeding, gut patency, motility and anatomy, and risk of aspiration (32). ☞ Though there are many forms of access for enteral feeding, they all result in placement of the nutrient load into either the stomach or small bowel.

Normal Physiology of the Stomach and the Small Intestine

When selecting the appropriate route for feeding, it is necessary to consider the normal function of the location selected. The stomach neutralizes and dilutes osmotic loads. So, when a hyperosmotic fluid enters the stomach, gastric motility is inhibited to allow time for gastric secretion to convert the hyperosmotic fluid to an iso-osmotic fluid. Once the fluid is adequately diluted, it can be transferred via the pylorus into the duodenum.

The small bowel, unlike the stomach, is unable to tolerate large osmotic loads. The small intestine is the primary area for nutrient absorption. Products of protein digestion, such as dipeptides, oligopeptides, and single amino acids, are completely absorbed in the first 120 cm of jejunum. Carbohydrates are absorbed high in the jejunum. Though simple sugars are preferred, more complex carbohydrates are absorbed after additional enzymatic cleavage. Fat is the most difficult nutrient to absorb, as it is dependent upon proper release and mixing of bile and pancreatic enzymes (5).

Short-Term Access

Options for short-term access involve placement of a tube via either the nose or the mouth with location of the distal tip into the stomach for gastric feeds or into the duodenum or jejunum for postpyloric feeding (2). Regardless of the location chosen, it should be utilized for short-term access of no more than two to four weeks, after which placement of a long-term device [e.g., percutaneous endoscopic gastrostomy (PEG)] should be considered (1).

Larger, 16- or 18-French diameter N-G tubes are satisfactory for short-term use as they are less likely to clog and allow for assessment of GI tolerance via checking gastric residuals (5). Unfortunately, these tubes have been known to increase the risk of sinusitis, nasopharyngeal ulceration, nasal septum necrosis, nasal ala necrosis, otitis, hoarseness, and vocal cord paralysis (1), and can be uncomfortable for the conscious patient (2).

Smaller-diameter (Dobhoff® and Kaofeed®) feeding tubes are constructed with a weighted tip and an insertion stylet to facilitate placement (32). These tubes allow short-term access but due to the small diameter more easily clog and do not easily allow evaluation of gastric residuals as they collapse when aspirating through them. The primary benefit is greater patient satisfaction and decreased risk of sinusitis (5). It is appropriate to initiate tube feeding with the larger-bore feeding tube and convert to a smaller-bore N-G tube once it has been proven that the patient will tolerate gastric feeding. In addition, once the GI tract becomes functional, it is possible to attempt feeding orally with an N-G/N-J tube in place (35). Oroenteric tubes, unlike nasoenteric tubes, involve tube insertion via the mouth. These tubes are useful in sedated and intubated patients, but commonly stimulate the gag reflex in conscious patients (2).

Naso/oroenteric feeding requires tube passage via the nose or mouth with placement distal to the pylorus. Standard-length feeding tubes (e.g., Dobhoff and Kaofeed) are placed with the distal tip in the duodenum, whereas the longer (Stayput®) tubes allow placement of the distal tip into the jejunum (5). Methods to assist placement include use of weighted tubes, administration of prokinetic agents (i.e., metroclopramide, erythromycin salts) before inserting the tube, and finally fluoroscopic or endoscopic placement (1). Some studies have demonstrated that small-bowel feeding allows the goal rate to be obtained more rapidly, although these results have not been consistent (36).

If an aggressive advancement protocol is utilized, naso/orogastrically fed patients receive equivalent amounts of enteral nutrition as those fed in the duodenum. The only groups with potential benefit from postpyloric feeding are those with gastroparesis and gastric atony (35), gastric outlet obstruction, and possibly those with pancreatitis (21–25) and those at high risk of pulmonary aspiration due to elevated gastric residuals (e.g., TBI patients) (37). Although some investigators have found that jejunal feeding leads to earlier achievement of daily caloric goal compared with patients fed intragastrically, overall rates are similar in those who can tolerate gastric feeds (38).

The primary drawback is the difficulty in positioning the feeding tube postpylorically and frequent proximal tube migration. Therefore, these tubes must be monitored radiographically to avoid gastric feeding, aspiration, and possible pneumonia in high-risk patients. Other disadvantages of these small-bowel feeding tubes include increased cost and risk of occlusion (36). To decrease the risk of complication, tube position should be confirmed by air insufflation and auscultation of the epigastrium, or aspiration of gastric contents. Radiologic confirmation is the most accurate test to assess feeding tube placement (35).

All of the above tubes are associated with potential complications. Esophageal and gastric erosions (5), esophageal stricture, and esophagitis occur due to mucosal irritation by repetitive contact with the feeding tube. Pneumothorax and intrapulmonary feeding (35) can occur when the tip of a metal-weighted feeding tube enters the trachea and punctures the lung. Patients at the highest risk have a depressed cough reflex due to sedation or coma. Some feeding tubes, e.g., Stayput, contain an indwelling, removable metal stylet to facilitate tube placement. Malposition of the tube and stylet can cause esophageal perforation and pneumothorax (5).

Tube occlusion occurs frequently due to inspissated feedings, pulverized medications (7), and inadequate flushing (35). This is prevented by flushing the tube with 15–20 mL of fluid (13) every six hours (35) before and after the instillation of medications (13), avoiding administration of pill fragments or thick medications, and conversion of medications to a liquid form when possible (7). Once a tube is clogged, flushing with warm water, carbonated beverages, acidic juices, proteolytic enzymes, and meat tenderizer may clear the obstruction. Although cleaning the tube with a guidewire is often mentioned, it should be avoided as there is a risk of tube perforation (13). Finally, the most common complication is the removal of the feeding tube by the patient (35).

Intragastric feeding tubes are associated with gastroesophageal reflux and pulmonary aspiration. Possible causes include high residual gastric volumes (RGVs) (5) and incomplete closure of the lower esophageal sphincter due to stenting by the feeding tube (2). Occurrence of aspiration and subsequent pulmonary infection can be minimized by elevating the head of the bed (>30°), radiographic confirmation of feeding tube placement, utilization of feeding protocols, and monitoring RGVs. Generally, RGVs less than or equal to 500 mL are tolerated in adults, whereas larger residual volumes are correlated with increased risk of reflux into the esophagus. The use of RGVs is not a reliable marker to predict aspiration in the critically ill patient (39). As aforementioned, occlusion of the nasal passages with large-bore tubes increases the risk of sinusitis (Fig. 5).

Long-Term Access

◢ **Patients who require long-term, that is, more than two to four weeks, enteral nutrition require permanent access for feeding.** ◢ Options include gastrostomy, jejunostomy, or a combination of both, which can be placed via percutaneous or transabdominal approaches (35).

Gastrostomy

The first option is intragastric feeding with a gastrostomy. This can be performed surgically or percutaneously (i.e., PEG). For this route to be successful, the patient must tolerate gastric feeding. Patients with gastroparesis, multiple episodes of aspiration, esophageal obstruction, wired jaw, multiple previous laparotomies, and gastric malignancy are not candidates for this procedure (40). Due to the risk of aspiration with intragastric feeding, it is recommended that feeds be discontinued one to two hours preoperatively with low continuous naso- or orogastric suction (2).

Jejunostomy

An alternative to gastrostomy is jejunostomy placement, which is appropriate for patients at high risk of aspiration or with abnormal gastric function (35). A jejunostomy requires formation of a stoma between a loop of proximal jejunum and the skin, which can be accomplished surgically or percutaneously. Thus, nutrients are administered directly into the upper small intestine while bypassing or resting the proximal GI tract. Indications for jejunostomy placement include gastric outlet obstruction, gastroparesis, nonfunctioning gastrojejunostomy, anastomic leak or stricture after esophagectomy, and aspiration (31). Regardless of the approach, jejunostomy placement allows prompt attainment of caloric goals. Though the complications of jejunostomy placement are very few, they include intraperitoneal leak, bowel obstruction, wound infection, fistula formation, and aspiration pneumonitis (41).

Combined Gastrojejunostomy Tube Placement

The final option is placement of a gastrojejunostomy (G-J) tube. This can be performed surgically or percutaneously. A G-J tube provides access for concomitant continuous jejunal feeding as well as gastric decompression with the gastrostomy. This route allows feeding tolerance in patients with gastric paresis and does not need to be discontinued for operative intervention. A disadvantage of these tubes is tube migration proximally into the stomach, which then requires endoscopic repositioning. This tube was proposed to reduce reflux and aspiration; however, studies have found a higher rate of tube dysfunction, 50% to 85%, and no reduction in the risk of aspiration (32).

TECHNIQUES FOR PLACING PERCUTANEOUS FEEDING TUBES
Open Surgical Technique

The open surgical gastrostomy was first performed in 1876, by Vernueuil with later modifications in technique by Witzel, Janway, and Stamm. Although rarely done following trauma surgery, it can be performed during laparotomy or as a separate procedure. Open surgical gastrostomies are mostly indicated in patients with esophageal disease including atresia, stricture, or malignancy, as well as cancer and neuromuscular dysphagia. Relative contraindications include primary gastric disease, abnormal gastric or duodenal emptying, and significant esophageal reflux (35).

The Stamm gastrostomy is the most common surgical gastrostomy performed. It involves creating two incisions in the anterior abdominal wall. One is placed midline to access the intra-abdominal contents, and the other is placed over the stomach for the gastrostomy tube (Fig. 3A). The gastrostomy is passed through the anterior abdominal wall and inserted into the stomach via a gastrotomy, an incision in the stomach (Fig. 3B). The feeding tube is secured by balloon inflation and an inner purse-string suture (Fig. 3C). After the feeding tube is passed through the anterior abdominal wall (Fig. 3D), a second purse-string suture is utilized to reinforce the gastric opening and anchor the anterior gastric wall to the anterior abdominal wall (42) (Fig. 3E).

An alternative to surgical gastrostomy is a surgical jejunostomy. Contraindications include Crohn's disease and ascites (35). A jejunostomy can be created by performing a subserosal, "Witzel" tunnel, or with a needle catheter jejunostomy. In the Witzel procedure, an opening is created in the jejunum for feeding tube insertion. The bowel is then plicated to cover the feeding tube with the external surface of the jejunum and attached to the undersurface of the anterior abdominal wall.

The needle catheter jejunostomy is performed by passing a 16-gauge polyvinyl catheter through the antimesenteric border of the jejunum, 15 cm distal to the ligament of Trietz (32). The opposite end of the jejunal feeding tube is passed through the abdominal wall distant from the laparotomy incision (35). A rare complication of needle jejunostomy feeding is bowel necrosis, occurring with an incidence of 0.15% to 0.29% (41).

Complications for both the surgical gastrostomy and jejunostomy include local irritation, hemorrhage, skin excoriations, wound infection, wound dehiscence, and intraperitoneal leakage (35).

Laparoscopic Feeding Tube Placement

General anesthesia is not necessarily required for this procedure. A prospective randomized study by Duh et al. (43) compared the use of general anesthesia versus local anesthesia for the placement of laparoscopic feeding tube placement, demonstrating that the use of intravenous sedation and local injection at the trocar sites allowed adequate relaxation of the abdominal musculature and adequate pain and anxiety control to safely accomplish the procedure. In these cases, pneumoperitoneum is typically decreased to 6–8 mmHg from the standard 15 mmHg, thus decreasing patient discomfort without compromising intra-abdominal visualization (43).

This procedure is most useful in patients with total or incomplete obstruction of the hypopharynx or esophagus.

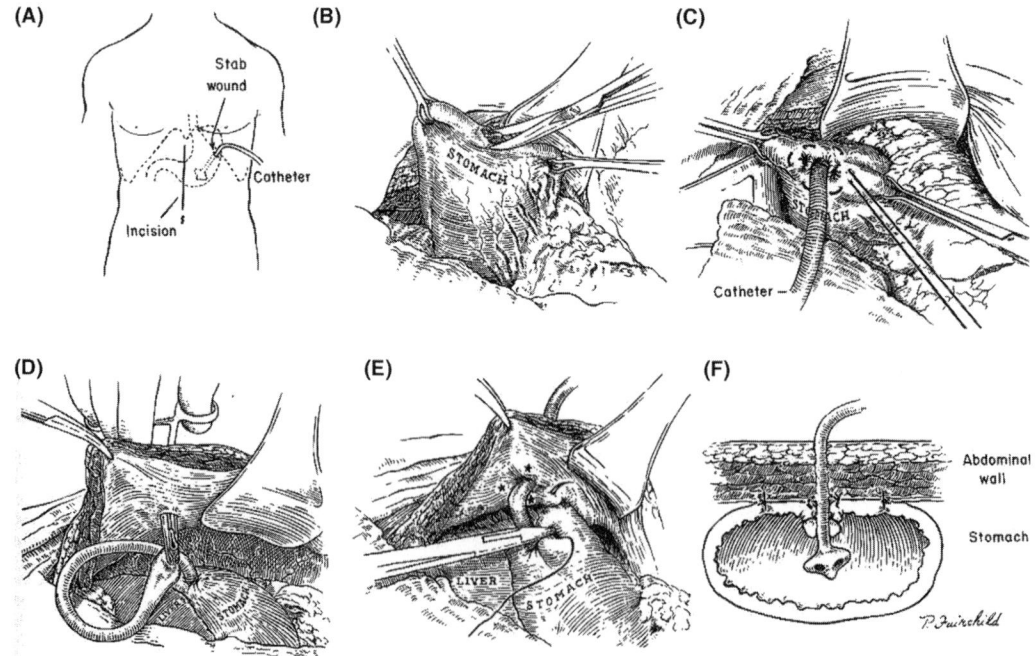

Figure 3 (**A**) Small incision is made in the midline. (**B**) Grasp midanterior gastric wall with babcock forceps and a small incision made in the stomach wall. (**C**) Gastrostomy tube inserted into the stomach and held in place with a purse-string suture. A second purse-string suture is placed around the gastrostomy tube. (**D**) Stab wound made in left midrectus region over the stomach for passage of the gastrostomy tube. (**E**) Stomach wall is anchored to the peritoneum with the second purse-string suture. (**F**) Side view after gastrostomy procedure is complete. *Source*: From Ref. 78.

The procedure utilizes port placement and insufflation of the abdomen to visualize the intra-abdominal contents. A site for gastrostomy placement is chosen and must easily reach the abdominal wall without tension. The stomach is fixed in four sites with sutures to both elevate and stabilize the organ (Fig. 4A). A needle with a catheter is inserted into the stomach and the needle removed. The Seldinger technique is utilized to insert the feeding tube (Fig. 4B). The gastrostomy is inserted and held in place with T-fasteners (Fig. 4C) (44).

Percutaneous Techniques

The percutaneous approach was first described in 1979 by Gauderer (38) and has widely replaced surgical gastrostomies due to the inherent safety and rapidity of the procedure (2). This procedure can be performed by multiple specialists in the GI suite, or at the bedside in the SICU or a step-down unit. A percutaneous gastrostomy utilizes a single exit wound and can be performed with local anesthesia and light sedation or general anesthesia. Combined, these differences result in a significantly lower cost than that of surgical gastrostomy. Enteral feeds can be instituted within 24 hours after gastrostomy placement as opposed to waiting for bowel sounds two to three days postsurgical gastrostomy (38). Both percutaneous gastrostomy and jejunostomy placement can be performed with an endoscope or laparoscope, or radiologically.

However, true percutaneous jejunostomies carry a high rate of complications including dislodgement, occlusion, bowel obstruction, and small-bowel ischemia (5).

Endoscopic

PEG is preferred to surgical gastrostomy due to increased safety, increased cost-effectiveness, decreased procedure-related mortality (2%), and complication rate (35). Endoscopic

gastrostomy involves placing an endoscope through the mouth into the stomach (Fig. 5A). Once the stomach is insufflated, the endoscope is manipulated to view the anterior wall of the stomach. An assistant locates the area of endoscopic illumination on the abdominal wall (Fig. 5B) and inserts a needle with catheter at this site. Once the needle is removed, a guidewire is passed into the stomach via the catheter and grasped by the endoscopic snare (Fig. 5C). The guidewire and endoscope are removed to allow the PEG tube to be attached to the guidewire. The assistant pulls the extra-abdominal portion of the guidewire to move the gastrostomy through the mouth into the stomach until the tube portion of the gastrostomy passes through the abdominal wall (Fig. 5D). The extra-abdominal portion of the gastrostomy is cut to attach to a feeding port. Movement of the gastrostomy is inhibited by a plastic bolster on the extra-abdominal side, along with a bell or diaphragm placed against the gastric mucosa (Fig. 5E). This causes the stomach to become adherent to the inner wall of the abdomen. A variation of endoscopic gastrostomy placement includes the push. This procedure is relatively contraindicated in morbidly obese patients, as gastric transillumination

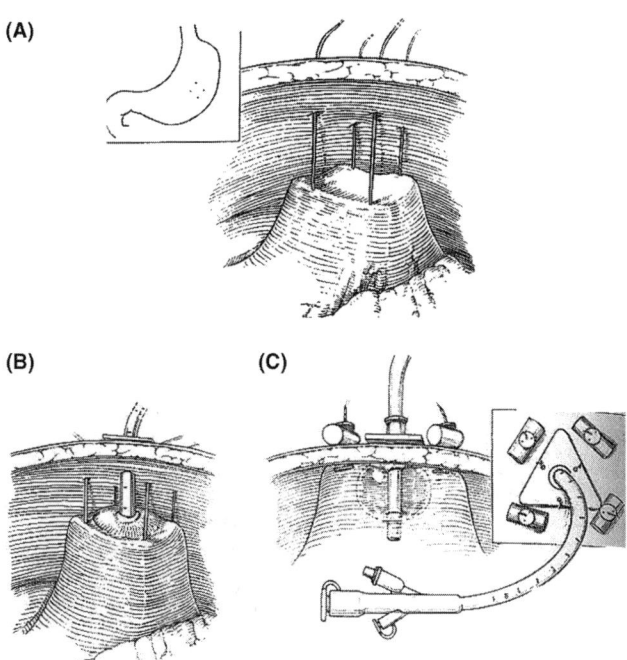

Figure 4 (**A**) Four sutures are placed to elevate and stabilize the anterior gastric wall. (**B**) The needle catheter complex is inserted into the anterior gastric wall. (**C**) The feeding tube has been inserted and the balloon inflated. Finally, the sutures are tightened with T-fasteners to maintain approximation of the gastric wall and the peritoneum. *Source*: From Ref. 44.

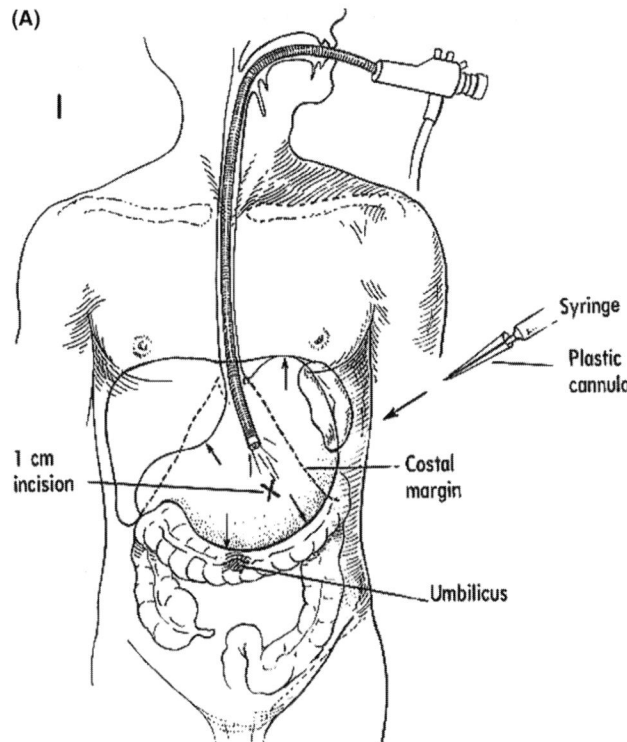

Figure 5 (*Continued on next page*) (**A**) The endoscope is placed into the stomach and the stomach insufflated. (**B**) Once the endoscope is in the stomach, the stomach is insufflated with air and the endoscope positioned to transilluminate through the stomach. (**C**) The needle and catheter are passed through the abdominal wall into the stomach. The needle is removed and the guidewire inserted into the stomach via the catheter. The guidewire is grasped by the endoscopic snare. (**D**) The endoscope, snare, and guidewire are pulled out via the mouth. The guidewire is attached to the PEG tube and pulled back through the mouth into the stomach by putting traction on the guidewire. (**E**) The PEG is pulled through the stomach and anterior abdominal wall. The guidewire is cut and the PEG held in place by the bolster and diaphragm. *Abbreviation*: PEG, percutaneous endoscopic gastrostomy. *Source*: From Ref. 79.

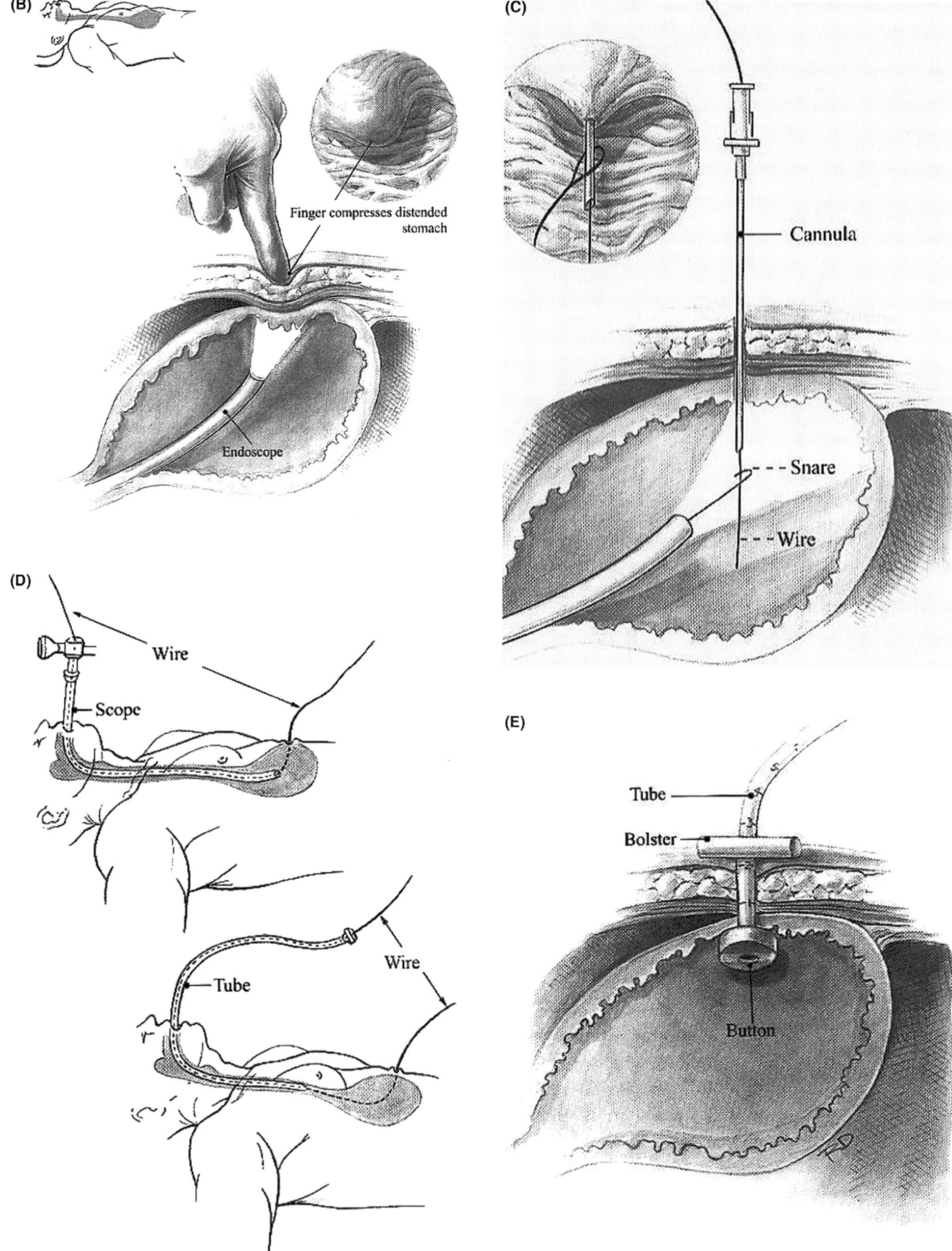

Figure 5 (*Continued from previous page*)

is often not possible. So, there is an increased risk of inappropriate placement and injury to intra-abdominal structures (32). Other contraindications include occluding pharyngeal or esophageal tumors, ascites, peritoneal dialysis, and coagulopathy (35). Endoscopic percutaneous jejunostomy requires placement of an extension through an existing gastrostomy tube creating a G-J tube (5). These have limited usefulness due to the difficulty with insertion and common proximal migration into the stomach (35).

Interventional Radiologic

Interventional radiologically placed feeding tubes are becoming increasingly used in patients who are difficult to treat endoscopically. Patients who benefit most from this approach are morbidly obese, require gastric decompression (5), have ascites, require peritoneal dialysis (35), or have an esophageal obstruction or other anatomic features inhibiting oral endoscopic entry (32).

Radiographic placement can be performed using one of two methods. In the first, the stomach is inflated with air via the N-G tube to allow fluoroscopic visualization of the gas-filled viscous (45). The stomach is then stabilized with two or three gastropexy T-fasteners placed around the intended puncture site. A small incision is then made in the center of the gastropexy fasteners (46) and the stomach punctured with an 18-gauge needle aimed at the greater curvature. A stiff guidewire is passed through the needle and looped into the stomach. The percutaneous tract is serially dilated and a locking loop pigtail catheter or an inflatable balloon catheter (12–28 French) is inserted. A T-fastener is utilized to anchor the gastric wall to the anterior abdominal wall, thereby promoting adherence and preventing leakage of gastric contents into the peritoneal cavity. Once the tube is secured to the abdominal wall with either an in-built fixation device or suture (45), the tube may be used after 24 hours. The sutures and T-fasteners can be removed after two weeks.

The second option mimics the procedure for PEG placement. After the stomach is insufflated, a small incision is created in the skin and the stomach punctured with a single T-fastener. Once the stomach is stabilized, the stomach is punctured and a guidewire inserted and advanced toward the G-E junction. The guidewire exits via the mouth and attached to the gastrostomy mushroom catheter. The gastropexy fastener is cut and the mushroom catheter pulled through the mouth to exit via the stomach and anterior abdominal wall. It should be noted that the pigtail catheter has shorter patency rates and a higher likelihood of dislodgement, peritonitis, and wound infection. So, if the esophagus is patent, the mushroom catheter appears to be the superior method (46).

Radiographic jejunostomy placement with fluoroscopic guidance involves opacification of the small bowel with iodinated contrast medium. A loop of jejunum near the anterior abdominal wall is visualized fluoroscopically and punctured with a fine needle (20–22 gauge) for passage of a stiff guidewire into the distal jejunum. The jejunum is affixed to the abdominal wall by T-fasteners and a locking pigtail catheter is inserted into the distal jejunum. Problems of this technique include difficulty in puncturing the jejunum, because it tends to be pushed away from an approaching needle. Jejunal puncture can be facilitated by the use of a target such as a snare or a catheter which has been passed perorally into the jejunum to the site of puncture. The target is easily visualized fluoroscopically to aid percutaneous jejunal catheterization. A second problem is the difficulty of obtaining appropriate antegrade positioning in the distal jejunum if the guidewire is passed retrogradely in the jejunum after the initial puncture (47).

Radiographic G-J placement requires insufflation and puncture of the stomach. Next, an angled-tip catheter is manipulated through the pylorus into the duodenum and jejunum. An extra stiff guidewire is passed through the catheter into the jejunum and the tract through the abdominal wall dilated. Finally, a percutaneous G-J tube is inserted so that the tip is in the proximal jejunum (47).

The technical success of radiographically placed gastrostomies and G-J tubes is close to 100% in most series. This procedure may not be possible in patients with previous partial gastrectomy and large left lobe of the liver and in patients in whom it is unable to separate the stomach and transverse colon (47). In addition, extreme caution must be exercised in patients with portal hypertension, as puncture of gastric varices can result in hemorrhage (45). Major complications such as peritonitis from leakage into the abdomen, puncture of the transverse colon, and puncture of the transverse colon occur in 1% to 6% of cases. Minor complications occur in 3% to 12% of cases and are due to tube occlusion or dislodgement (47).

Complications

Major complications of gastrostomy placement include gastric perforation, bleeding, peritonitis, subcutaneous abscess, necrotizing fasciitis, ileus, and aspiration. Hemorrhage is due to injury to an abdominal wall blood vessel, erosion caused by pressure from the gastrostomy bolster on the anterior wall of the stomach, ulcers caused by balloon gastrostomy placement in the posterior gastric wall, and duodenal ulcer (48).

Minor complications include wound infection, tube removal, and pneumoperitoneum. A recent meta-analysis of seven published studies established that a single intravenous dose of a broad-spectrum antibiotic was effective in reducing the incidence of peristomal wound infections (32). Inadvertent tube removal by the patient is a frequent occurrence. Though prevention is not always possible, attempts can be made by covering the gastrostomy with a dressing or abdominal binder and covering the hands of an agitated patient with mitts or restraints (48). Minor complications are usually not life threatening and merely require tube replacement or exit site care and do not require surgical intervention (47).

Tube-related complications include small-bowel obstruction, obstruction of bile flow at the ampulla of vater, cologastric and colocutaneous fistulas, acute gastric dilation, and retrograde migration of the gastrostomy tube into the abdominal wall or sinus tract. Perforation of the colon or cologastric fistula is a rare but potentially catastrophic complication. If the colon lies between the stomach and the anterior abdominal wall, gastrostomy placement perforates the colon. Initially patients may be asymptomatic. Once symptoms develop, they range in severity from perigastrostomy drainage to sepsis with fever, hemodynamic instability, abdominal tenderness, rebound, and leukocytosis.

In addition, peritonitis and intra-abdominal abscess can develop from enteral feeds leaking into the abdomen. Diagnosis is especially difficult in an unconscious patient in whom symptoms may be masked. So, it is imperative to have a high index of suspicion (48).

An alternate presentation occurs when the gastrostomy tube migrates into the colon via the gastrocolic fistula. Huang described a patient who within minutes of PEG feeding developed sudden, transient diarrhea composed of undigested tube feed formula. Patients may deposit fecal material in the PEG tube or may present with foul-smelling eructations or feculent vomiting resulting from retrograde passage of fecal material from the colon into the stomach via the gastrocolic fistula.

Diagnosis necessitates performance of a contrast study by either the gastrostomy tube or per rectum. Urgent operative repair is indicated in patients with peritonitis (49). In patients with peritonitis, correction methods include exploratory laparotomy, resection of the through-and-through colonic injury, irrigation of the abdomen, and closure with a colostomy or primary anastomosis (48). As most patients do not have peritonitis, the gastrostomy can be removed without the need for operative intervention. The residual tract to the skin closes within several days. If a new feeding tube is required, another gastrostomy can be placed. These complications can be minimized by ensuring a well-defined transillumination site before insertion of the needle (35,49).

ENTERAL FORMULA OPTIONS

Nutritional requirements are affected by size, age, and energy expenditure of the patient. Nutritional requirement can be calculated using the Harris–Benedict formulas (see Volume 2, Chapter 31). In a healthy patient, protein requirement is 0.8 g/kg/day, but due to the hypermetabolism associated with critical illness, protein requirements are increased to $1.5-2$ g/kg/day. The goal is to provide adequate amounts of protein to maintain a positive nitrogen balance (10). However, protein delivery of more than 2.5 g/kg is not recommended as it can cause azotemia and exacerbate metabolic acidosis in critically ill patients. Carbohydrates provide 50% to 80% of nonprotein calories (50). Carbohydrates act to prevent protein gluconeogenesis for glucose-dependent tissues, such as bone marrow, erythrocytes, and brain tissue, as well as prevent ketogenesis (29). The remaining nonprotein calories are derived from fat. A minimum of 2% to 4% of calories from linoleic acid is necessary to prevent essential fatty acid deficiency. Multivitamins, such as vitamins A, B, C, and E, and trace elements, such as zinc, chromium, and selenium, are provided as well (50).

Obesity is the most common chronic disease in the United States and the incidence is continuing to increase. Over 50% of adults are overweight [body mass index (BMI)] 25 to 29; 15% are obese (BMI 30–34); 5% are seriously obese (BMI 35–40); and 3% are morbidly obese (BMI >40). As with any other patient, for a patient who suffers from a catabolic illness such as trauma, burn, or sepsis, nutritional support must be instituted expeditiously. Starvation is not an appropriate strategy as it results in loss of lean body mass (1). When determining the calorie needs of an obese patient it is imperative to utilize ideal body weight and not actual body weight (10). Some institutions have begun to implement hypocaloric regimens for critically ill obese patients. Hypocaloric nutritional supplementation has allowed a positive nitrogen balance to be obtained. This may occur due to utilization of endogenous fat stores for energy. In a recent study of obese patients admitted to surgical or trauma ICUs, patients receiving hypocaloric

nutrition had shorter ICU stay, fewer days with antibiotic therapy, and fewer ventilator days (29).

When selecting a formula, one must consider the patient's nutrient intake, GI function, existence of comorbid diseases, as well as organ function. Appropriate selection can be daunting as there are over 100 varieties and brands of tube feeds available for use (51). The types and use of tube feeds can be divided into general categories, which include standard, elemental, immune modulating, and disease-specific formulas.

Standard Formulas

♂ **Standard formulas are the most widely utilized form of enteral nutrition. They are designed for patients with normal or near-normal GI function.** ♂ Due to adequate GI function, the nitrogen source can be provided by whole protein. The carbohydrates are composed of partial enzyme hydrolysates of starch. Due to the number of lactose-intolerant patients and the prevalence of transient acquired lactase deficiency in critically ill patients, most formulas do not include lactose as a carbohydrate source (5). The lipid source is either composed of long-chain triacylglycerols or medium-chain triacylglycerols. These formulas provide an energy source as well as fluid, fiber, trace elements, and vitamins (51).

Elemental Formulas

♂ **Elemental formulas were created to provide a complete set of nutrients in a form that required little or no digestion; thus, it could be utilized in patients with a dysfunctional GI tract (52).** ♂ For example, patients with short bowel syndrome or diseased bowel have difficulty tolerating complex diets. When presented with complex nutrients, inadequate luminal hydrolysis and brush border membrane hydrolysis lead to decreased ability to break down the nutrients to their most basic form (51). The few nutrients that are successfully processed are inadequately absorbed due to the markedly decreased area for absorption. In short, the inadequate amalgamation leads to malnutrition (5).

To facilitate maximal absorption, the nutrients are provided in their most basic form. Proteins consist of small peptides of two to three amino acid residues in chains. The carbohydrates consist of maltodextrins, a heterogenous mixture of glucose polymers with more than 10 glucose molecules. As many of these patients suffer from steatorrhea, the lipids in elemental formulas consist of either long-chain fatty acids or medium-length fatty acids. Formulas with long-chain fatty acids use linoleic acid in the hope of preventing essential fatty acid deficiency. Unlike long-chain fatty acids, medium-chain fatty acids are less complex, allowing increased absorption (51).

Of great concern are the fluid and electrolyte losses in patients with diseases of malabsorption. Patients with end jejunostomies and/or resection of the ileum and large intestine are at the highest risk for loss of large quantities of sodium, potassium, magnesium, and zinc. Though sodium absorption is promoted by luminal carbohydrate, bicarbonate, and amino acids, passive secretion down a concentration gradient overwhelms the active transcellular absorption. Ingestion of low-sodium products results in net sodium losses. So it is recommended that these formulas contain sodium concentrations between 80 and 90 mmol/L (51).

Immune Modulating Formulas

Immune-modulating formulas were created in an attempt to modify the impaired immune status of critically ill patients, which increases the risk of the development of infectious complications (53), SIRS, and MODS (54). Nutritional deficits produce atrophy and impaired function of lymphoid organs, leading to an increased risk of infection. Excessive nutrition, especially large quantities of fat intake (especially ω-6 fatty acids), can cause immunosuppression as well (9). For this reason, extensive research has been invested to determine formula components which would facilitate modification of the disease-induced immune dysfunction. To date supplements studied include arginine, glutamine, nucleotides, and ω-3-fatty acids (5).

Arginine

Arginine is a nonessential amino acid which modulates the immune system by promoting normal T-cell proliferation and function (53), enhancing delayed type hypersensitivity and lymphocyte blastogenesis as well as stimulating macrophages and natural killer cell function (9). In addition, it is a substrate for several enzymes and is the sole precursor for the production of nitric oxide (NO). Under normal conditions, arginine is not required for normal growth and development. In humans, de novo synthesis from citrulline provides adequate levels of arginine. In periods of stress induced by trauma or severe sepsis, arginine is depleted from the plasma and may become essential. A potential drawback of supplementation with arginine is increased production of NO, which has been hypothesized to have a potentially detrimental vasodilatory effect in septic shock. A decreased level of NO metabolites has been found in the plasma of trauma patients (53). So it has been hypothesized that arginine-mediated NO production might lead to an exacerbation of vasodilation in septic patients (53). Other studies indicate arginine supplementation can improve nitrogen balance (29) and aid in wound healing (5).

Glutamine

Glutamine is an oxidative fuel for rapidly replicating cells, including GI mucosal cells, hepatocytes, lymphocytes, and macrophages. It also serves as a nitrogen shuttle among organs (9), and as a substrate for gluconeogenesis (29). It is also a precursor of the antioxidant glutathione (9), nucleic acids, nucleotides, amino acids, and protein (55). Though glutamine is typically considered nonessential, during stressed states glutamine levels decline as consumption exceeds synthesis (29). An exogenous source of glutamine is necessary to avoid catabolism and muscle glutamine depletion (9). Human studies have shown that glutamine attenuates gut atrophy in the fasting state, maintains ATP levels in oxidant injured cells, and preserves immune cellularity of the gut in prolonged parenteral feeding. In addition, a systematic review of randomized controlled trials in adult surgical or critically ill patients suggests that glutamine supplementation may reduce infectious complications, duration of hospital stay, and possibly mortality (55). However, glutamine supplementation has also been associated with elevated levels of liver enzymes (29).

Nucleotides

The purine (adenine, guanine) and pyrimidine (thymidine, uracil) nucleotides are precursors for DNA and RNA (11). Purines and pyrimidines are synthesized by the liver from amino acids. Reduction in dietary nucleotides results in suppression of cellular immune responses via inability of T cells to undergo blastogenesis (10). Administration of nucleotides appears to be essential for cell energetics (adenosine triphosphate) and may also play a role as physiologic mediators (cyclic adenosine monophosphate). Administration of these agents promotes natural killer cell cytotoxicity and enhances resistance to infection (11). Finally, they may also increase the disease-free duration of cancer patients undergoing treatment (56).

Fatty Acids

Dietary lipids are essential components of all living cells and aid formation of the bilipid structure of cell membranes, are sources of energy, and are precursors to numerous biologically active compounds (57). Linoleic acid, ω-6 fatty acid, is metabolized to arachidonic acid. This is further metabolized to eicosanoid prostanoids responsible for inflammation and increased immunosuppression and leukotrienes. Whereas, α-linoleic acid, ω-3 fatty acid, is a precursor of eicosapentaenoic acid which leads to prostanoids and leukotrienes, which have anti-inflammatory and immune-enhancing properties. In addition, ω-3 fatty acids have been shown to inhibit the formation of ω-6 fatty acid products, thereby blocking their immunosuppressive effects (51). The eicosanoids alter cytokine production and intracellular signaling. As an example, prostaglandin E_2 (PGE$_2$) significantly increases intracellular cAMP levels and prevents the increase in intracellular calcium that is an early event in T-cell activation. Both PGE1 and PGE2 are potent inhibitors of interleukin-2 (IL-2) and IL-2 receptor production, and they modulate protein kinase C (PKC) activation. In contrast, leukotriene (LT) B4 enhances the generation of IFNg and IL-2 (57).

Humans can synthesize all the lipids necessary for health except ω-3 and ω-6 long-chain fatty acids. Both of these essential fatty acids are found in common dietary substances, such as canola oil, soybean oil, and fish oil (57). For this reason, ω-3 fatty acids are being studied in immunonutrition to evaluate their ability to act as substrate for the synthesis of immune-modulating prostanoids and leukotrienes (9). To date, ω-3 fatty acid supplementation has been shown to improve survival after burn injury, reduce postinjury infectious complications, and diminish immunosuppression secondary to transfusion.

Initial results indicated that immune-modulating formulas could decrease infection rates and length of stay. A multicenter prospective randomized clinical trial with administration of immune-modulating formula for 7 to 10 days showed reduced rates of infection and wound complications and shorter hospital stays for critically ill patients. Another multicenter trial with trauma patients revealed significantly fewer intra-abdominal abscesses and less multiple organ failure (8). More recent studies dispute these findings.

Nonetheless, the immune-enhancing diet summit of 2000 recommended administration of immune-enhancing diets to patients with blunt and penetrating torso trauma especially when the ISS is greater than or equal to 18, or the ATI is greater than or equal to 20. In addition, administration of immune-enhancing diets was also recommended for patients with Glasgow coma score less than 8, patients with 30% or greater third-degree burns, and ventilator-dependent nonseptic patients. It is not recommended in septic patients, as two studies demonstrated increased mortality in septic patients receiving immune-modulating diets (16).

Disease-Specific Formulas

When a patient presents to the intensive care unit critically ill, pre-existing diseases must be accounted for, as they can affect the care of the patient and may worsen during the course of illness. In cases where there were no pre-existing diseases, patients may develop pulmonary, hepatic, and renal dysfunction due to their disease process. For this reason, research has been performed to determine the effects, if any, of disease-specific enteral formulas.

Pulmonary Formulas

Most patients with isolated respiratory failure will receive adequate nutrition with the application of standard enteral formulas. Overfeeding (with a high ratio of calories from carbohydrates or a total excess of calories) results in excessive CO_2 production and an increased work of breathing which results in difficulty weaning. This should be considered in patients receiving nutritional support with difficulty weaning from the mechanical ventilator, and a metabolic cart evaluation can be helpful (Volume 2, Chapter 31) (27).

Pulmonary formulas are composed of high fat (50%) and diminished levels of carbohydrates to reduce CO_2 production. In preclinical studies, tailored pulmonary formulas reduced pulmonary neutrophil accumulation and inflammatory cytokines and improved cardiopulmonary hemodynamics and gas exchange. This disease-specific pulmonary formulation contains eicosapentaenoic acid, α-linolenic acid (which modify production of proinflammatory cytokines), and antioxidants (vitamin E, vitamin C, and beta-carotene), and is a calorically dense formula, suitable, in particular, for fluid-restricted patients with ARDS (8).

Hepatic Formulas

The normal functioning liver has many complex functions. Hepatic Kupfer cells engulf and detoxify intestinal bacteria and endotoxins. It also clears activated inflammatory mediators such as leukotrienes and cytokines. When liver function is impaired, inflammatory mediators are incompletely filtered, contributing to increased caloric expenditure, protein catabolism, hyperinsulinemia, hyperglucagonemia, and ultimately malnutrition. Depending on disease severity, patients present with hyperbilirubinemia, coagulopathy, vasodilation, and alterations in mental status (58). In addition, patients with liver failure have increased losses of potassium, magnesium, and zinc (27). As long as the patient is not at risk of developing encephalopathy, a standard or elemental formula is appropriate.

Hepatic encephalopathy can occur in both patients with and without pre-existing liver disease. Acute hepatic encephalopathy most commonly occurs in patients without pre-existing hepatic disease due to fulminant viral or toxic hepatitis. Patients with pre-existing liver disease can develop acute episodic hepatic encephalopathy due to excessive intake of proteins, from an upper GI bleed, or from other precipitating conditions, such as spontaneous bacterial peritonitis (or other form of sepsis). Possible theories to explain the occurrence of encephalopathy include inability of the liver to clear gut-derived substances, such as ammonia and gamma-aminobutyric acid, due to portosystemic shunting or severe hepatocellular failure, as well as altered amino acid metabolism, which results in creation of false neurotransmitters.

Normally aromatic amino acids (AAAs), such as phenylalanine, tyrosine, and tryptophan, are produced in the gut during digestion and cleared by the liver. With hepatic dysfunction, branch chain amino acid (BCAA) levels decrease while AAA levels increase. The reduction in the plasma BCAA/AAA ratio favors brain uptake of aromatics because they compete for transport across the blood–brain barrier leading to an influx of false neurotransmitters (58). So patients with liver failure and risk of encephalopathy should receive formulas containing high concentrations of BCAAs (27), and low concentrations of methionine, AAA, phenylalanine, tyrosine, and tryptophan are indicated (51). BCAA, leucine, isoleucine, and valine are essential amino acids required for protein synthesis (27). Infusion of BCAAs corrects the imbalance between AAAs and BCAAs in plasma and the central nervous system that contribute to mental disturbances (8). These modified formulas permit greater protein intake without inducing encephalopathy unlike standard protein formulas (58), which lead to improved nitrogen balance (8).

Regardless of the risk of encephalopathy, the nonprotein energy content is predominantly carbohydrate rather than lipid, as many patients have cholestatic jaundice and are unable to assimilate long-chain triacylglycerols. In elemental formulas, 5% of the energy content is linoleic acid to prevent central fatty acid deficiency. The sodium content is low as most patients have high total body sodium content due to underlying hyperaldosteronism (51). In addition, patients with ascites benefit from fluid restriction (27).

Renal Formulas

Renal failure is characterized as fluid intolerance and elevated plasma levels of potassium, magnesium, and phosphate. Frequent monitoring of these electrolytes is required and the amounts administered reduced to maintain appropriate plasma levels. In the ICU, patients may require continuous renal replacement therapy (CRRT) (which tends to decrease phosphate levels), and the use of high-protein or standard formula to provide up to 2.5 g/kg/day is recommended, as a large percentage of protein is lost through the filtration process (59).

Patients with end-stage renal disease commonly have malnutrition and muscle catabolism, resulting in muscle wasting and fatigue. Blood levels of essential amino acids, especially BCAAs, are lower in patients than in control subjects with the same protein intake (56). In chronic renal failure, large protein and volume loads must be avoided. For this reason, enteral formulas have been created which consist of higher total calories (1.5–2 cal/mL) in a smaller total volume. These formulas provide the calories with increased proportions of fat and less protein (e.g., Nepro, Nutrirenal, Novasource Renal) (5). The protein dose of 0.5–0.8 g/kg/day is associated with preservation of renal function (27). Finally, maintaining an arterial blood pH of 7.35 is associated with reduced net catabolism.

Acute renal failure (ARF) occurs most commonly in the setting of shock, trauma, sepsis, or multiple organ failure. It is characterized by excessive protein catabolism and negative nitrogen balance. This is most likely due to the toxic effects of high metabolic byproduct concentration, altered levels of catabolic hormones, circulating cytokines and serum proteases, insulin resistance, metabolic acidosis, and inadequate supply of nutritional substrates.

Mitigation of the hypermetabolic state can be accomplished by controlling infection, optimizing oxygen transport, and providing adequate metabolic and nutritional support. If unsuccessful, the generalized nutritional deficiency can progress to MODS (60).

Similar to patients with chronic renal failure, those with ARF have a high prevalence of malnutrition which increases the likelihood of in-hospital complications and death (61). Unlike patients with chronic renal failure, there is no demonstrable advantage to limitation of protein load in patients with acute renal insufficiency (27), in fact, prolonged delivery of protein-restricted diets can lead to increased skeletal muscle protein breakdown (13). Protein intake should be between 1.2 and 1.5 g/kg/day in patients with ARF to maintain a neutral nitrogen balance (61).

For patients with both chronic and acute renal failure, dialysis therapy further complicates nutritional supplementation. Adjustment of glucose administration is often needed in patients receiving peritoneal dialysis, which contains a significant amount of glucose, thereby increasing the risk of hyperglycemia. In addition, peritoneal dialysis, hemodialysis, and hemodilution remove considerable amounts of amino acids (27). The study by Scheinkestel et al. (17) evaluated the effect of improved nitrogen balance on the outcome in critically ill patients on CRRT. They found that nitrogen balance was inversely proportional to REE, that is, higher levels of stress cause an increase in REE, which results in decreased nitrogen balance. In addition, nitrogen balance correlates with both hospital and intensive care unit outcomes. So, patients with positive nitrogen balance were more likely to survive, and every 1-g/day increase in nitrogen balance correlated with a 21% increased probability of survival (17).

The Kidney Disease Outcome Quality Initiative recommends protein intake in maintenance dialysis patients who are acutely ill to be at least 1.2 g/kg/day for hemodialysis and 1.3 g/kg/day for peritoneal dialysis. Due to the highly catabolic state associated with critical illness, patients with sepsis or CRRT may have greater protein requirements. This is supported by the fact that during CRRT 10% to 15% of amino acids are lost in the dialysate (60). In the critically ill patients, a positive nitrogen balance is attained with a protein ingestion of 2 g/kg/day or more (17).

Oral Dietary Supplements

Canned liquid meal replacement beverages are widely available commercially. ✐ **The oral dietary supplements are true supplements, that is, they are not nutritionally complete. The use of these products is as an additional, highly concentrated nutritional source for individuals who are unable to ingest adequate nutrients with a standard oral diet (1).** ✐ Unlike tube feed formulas, these products must be palatable for patient tolerance. In general, they are packaged in 200–250 mL containers as a liquid, and a few are produced in semisolid or solid form. The products are composed of whole proteins, and nonprotein calories are derived from carbohydrates and long-chain triacylglycerols. They usually lack fiber, lactose, and gluten, making them safe for those who are lactose intolerant and have celiac sprue (51).

Use of Probiotics and Functional Fibers

Probiotics are live microorganisms (e.g., *Lactobacillus* species, *Bifidobacterium* species, and normal GI yeasts) that can be administered with enteral nutrition to restore the intestinal microflora balance, which is often disturbed in critically ill trauma patients. Some desirable properties resulting from probiotic strains when they colonize the human intestine include resistance to acid and bile, production of antimicrobial substances, and antagonism against pathogenic bacteria. Probiotics also produce nutrients and antioxidants,

participate in growth regulation, reduce endotoxins, and activate mucosa-associated lymphoid tissues (MALT) (62).

Probiotic effects on humoral processes include stimulating IgA and NO, inhibiting IgE, and modulating cytokines (62). On the cellular level, probiotics stimulate macrophage function, natural killer cell activity, growth, regeneration, and apoptosis (62). Putative clinical effects include decreased incidence and severity of sepsis in ICU and major surgery patients, decreased duration or prevention of diarrhea, *Clostridium difficile* infections, and decreased septic manifestations in pancreatitis.

Prebiotics or dietary fibers (i.e., fructooligosaccharides, glycomannans, insulin, algal fibers, and pectin) have been supplemented into a variety of enteral nutrition solutions to help control diarrhea and maintain fluid absorption in the colon. A recent prospective multicenter study evaluated the effects of a high-protein formula enriched with artinine, fiber, and antioxidants compared with a standard high-protein formula for early enteral nutrition in 200 critically ill patients. The supplemented group had a lower incidence of catheter-related sepsis than the control group (63).

The combined use of probiotics with prebiotics has been recently coined "synbiotics." The beneficial effects of synbiotics have been studied in arteriosclerosis, Crohn's disease, chronic liver disease, acute pancreatitis, abdominal surgery, liver transplantation, the ICU, and ulcerative colitis (64).

For the critically ill patients, the stress, extensive medication treatment, antibiotic variety, all contribute to the depletion of invaluable gut flora and the overabundance of pathogenic harmful bacteria. Synbiotics in the twenty-first century may become the main foundation for the nutrition therapy of the sickest patients.

Though these specialty products are available, they are markedly more expensive than standard formulas. Therefore, clinicians should be challenged to evaluate both the appropriate macronutrients and micronutrients as well as to justify the additional cost in relation to the patient's outcome (29).

TUBE FEED INTOLERANCE

The enteric nervous system consists of GI neurons that can function independently of the central nervous system to control motility, exocrine and endocrine secretion, and gut microcirculation. The enteric nervous system communicates with the CNS via sympathetic and parasympathetic afferent and efferent neurons. Normally when a food bolus enters the small intestine, serotonin is released due to mucosal stimulation or mechanical distention of the gut lumen, which triggers activity of intrinsic afferent neurons. Above the site of intraluminal stimulus, ascending cholinergic interneurons relay the signal to excitatory motor neurons that contain acetylcholine and substance P. This results in contraction of the circular muscle layer above the stimulus. At the same time, descending cholinergic interneurons activate inhibitory motor neurons that contain NO, vasoactive intestinal polypeptide, and adenosine triphosphate, causing relaxation below the stimulus. The resultant forces propel the bolus in an antegrade direction also called peristalsis (65).

Disruption of this complex process (i.e., inadequate mucosal stimulation, altered neurotransmitter production, inhibitors to neurotransmission) can result in diminished gut motility. Acute gastric and intestinal ileus can also result from selective suppression of excitatory motor reflexes via sympathetic nerves or sustained intrinsic inhibitory neural overactivity. Dopamine-2 receptors in the gut decrease gastric emptying and intestinal motility. Increased production of NO due to activation of the nonneuronal inducible NO synthase or decreased production of motilin may result in ileus. Other putative causes include use of continuous liquid enteral feeding (which decreases mucosal stimulation) and decreased production of adenosine triphosphate, or substance P (65).

Though many critically ill patients suffer from tube feed intolerance (5), or gastroparesis, the exact cause is often unknown. Numerous etiological agents have been shown to depress gastric motor activity, including pain, anxiety, recent abdominal surgery, peritonitis, sepsis, pancreatitis, diabetes mellitus/hyperglycemia, head injury, increased intracranial pressure, burn injury, and medications (beta agonists, anticholinergic agents, dopamine, and opioids). Gastroparesis leads to increased gastric residuals and predisposes the patient to gastroesophageal reflux, emesis, and aspiration. Also, it impairs absorption of drugs and nutrients administered into the stomach (66). So, the required nutritional demands of the patient cannot be met, leading to inadequate protein and calorie administration (5).

It is important to note that although gastric residuals are measured to determine tube feed tolerance, this correlation has yet to be validated. It is thought that high gastric residuals (>500 mL) correlate with tube feed intolerance and increased risk of aspiration. Low residuals of less than 100 mL should indicate a low risk of aspiration. Though GRVs are frequently associated with comorbidities such as vasopressor use, sedation, sepsis, and emesis, GRVs alone have little independent clinical utility. A prospective study by McClave and associates showed no relationship between GRVs and risk of aspiration or regurgitation as well as no association between aspiration or regurgitation and pneumonia. Of note, there was no difference in regurgitation or aspiration and pneumonia in patients with gastric residual cutoffs of 200 or 400 mL (39). As there is no consensus on the safe or normal GRV utilized, the higher value (400–500 mL) to determine tube feed tolerance can be used safely.

The least labor-intensive adjustments to promote GI motility include control of pain, anxiety, and blood sugar levels (66), and adjusting the level of the head of the bed (67). In the management of the polytrauma or postoperation surgical patient, opioid administration is often required. If opioids are thought to impair gastric motility, the use of dilaudid (less gastroparesis) should be considered with supplemental sedation using dexmedetomidine (on α-2 agonist with opioid sparing properties). ☞ **When these adjustments fail to alleviate gastroparesis, institution of promotility agents, metoclopramide and erythromycin, can be utilized.** ☞

Promotility Drugs

Metoclopramide is a well-known prokinetic medication with an unclear mechanism of action. Studies have shown that it facilitates the release of acetylcholine from gut cholinergic neurons, antagonizes the inhibitory effects of dopamine on GI motility, and has a direct effect on lower esophageal smooth muscle. In high concentrations, it blocks 5-hydroxytryptamine (5-HT) receptors in the upper GI tract. Finally, it enhances antropyloroduodenal coordination and propagation of duodenal contractions (66). Through these physiologic effects, metoclopramide facilitates peristalsis and

gastric emptying (68), as well as esophageal and small intestine promotility (13). It has been proven effective in diabetic patients with gastroparesis as well as critically ill patients (65). Metaclopramide is administered IV, as a tablet, or syrup (13).

In a normal patient, the enterochromaffin cells of the proximal small intestine produce a 22-amino acid peptide called motilin. Motilin binds motilin receptors found on cholinergic nerves. Motilin receptor activation causes release of acetylcholine, which acts on cholinergic pathways in the enteric nervous system to mediate motility.

In the esophagus, motilin increases lower esophageal sphincter tone and esophageal peristalsis to assist propulsion and avoid reflux. It is thought that motilin release is inhibited in critically ill patients and results in gastroparesis. Erythromycin, a macrolide antibiotic, affects gastric motility by activating the motilin receptors in the gut. Erythromycin has been found to improve gastric emptying in patients with diabetic gastroparesis, vagotomy, chronic intestinal pseudo-obstruction, and denervated whole stomach after esophageal resection.

Chapman and colleagues investigated the effect of erythromycin in critically ill patients with depressed gastric emptying. They assessed gastric residuals to determine the effect of erythromycin on gastric emptying in 20 mechanically ventilated patients being given enteral nutrition.

Erythromycin significantly diminished gastric residuals, presumably by increasing gastric emptying. Enteral feeding was subsequently successful in 90% of the erythromycin patients versus 50% of the control patients (65). Erythromycin can be administered IV, IM, or orally. The optimum dose has not been clearly established, but 250 mg IV every six hours is commonly utilized (36). Patients in the ICU will occasionally have large gastric residuals regardless of receiving metoclopramide. The addition of erythromycin frequently improves gastric emptying in these patients (65). Though there are no studies supporting it, there is concern that erythromycin therapy in critically ill patients may alter native bacterial flora, increase the risk of infection, and promote antibiotic resistance, especially to *Streptococcus pneumoniae* (69). Also, there is concern that erythromycin may increase the risk of cardiac dysrhythmias (36).

Postpyloric Feeding

A final option involves institution of postpyloric feeding. Spontaneous duodenal passage of weighted feeding tubes occurs in approximately 95% of general ward surgical patients, but only in 61% of critically ill patients (68). Manipulation of the tube into the duodenum or jejunum can be enhanced in some patients with metoclopramide, but predicting which patients will be assisted is difficult (68). Erythromycin is a second option for pharmacologic manipulation of feeding tubes. Three adult studies have shown that erythromycin facilitates passage of feeding tubes in both healthy and critically ill patients (65). The highest success rates for feeding tube placement involve the use of endoscopy, which is an expensive solution. Another option utilizes feeding tube manipulation with fluoroscopic guidance (also expensive). Recent modifications in tube feed catheters involve the addition of flaps to facilitate placement into the jejunum by allowing peristalsis to gently drag the catheter into the small bowel. This tube is promoted as allowing rapid bedside placement by clinicians without the additional cost of endoscopy or fluoroscopy (36).

Although distal tubes allow feeding in the small bowel in patients who do not tolerate gastric feeding, studies do not show a reduction in the incidence of aspiration between those fed postpylorically and those fed intragastrically (68).

In a recent study comparing the efficacy of gastric feeding supplemented with prokinetic agents to distal small-bowel feeding tubes, it has been demonstrated that gastric feeding with erythromycin (200 mg intravenously every eight hours) was equivalent to distal feeding both in terms of meeting nutritional goals and in overall clinical outcomes (36).

Prone Positioning Considerations

Some critically ill patients with ARDS will require prone positioning during mechanical ventilation. There is an increased risk of regurgitation in this position compared with the supine position with 30° of head of bed elevation. Enteral nutrition should be stopped at least two hours before proning to prevent aspiration pneumonia, vomiting, and GI distress. According to a 71-patient, prospective, comparative study, enteral nutrition during the prone position was poorly tolerated, and postpyloric feeding tube placement with promotility agents was recommended for optimal enteral feeding tolerance (70). Tube feeding goal rate adjustments should be made in order to provide adequate calories and protein for patients during the nonprone portion of the SICU care.

COMPLICATIONS OF ENTERAL NUTRITION
Aspiration and Pneumonia

All critically ill tube-fed patients are at risk of tube feed aspiration due to altered level of consciousness, abnormal gastric motility, emesis, and reflux. Decreased level of consciousness is due to patient sedation from iatrogenically administered medications, alcohol, and drug ingestion. In addition, a GCS less than 9 is a significant risk factor for aspiration and pneumonia. Patients with decreased level of consciousness have a depression of upper airway reflexes (cough and gag) and a reduction of lower esophageal sphincter pressure. Absence of these safeguards for airway protection allows accumulated oropharyngeal secretions and regurgitated gastric contents to be aspirated into the lungs. For critically ill patients requiring mechanical ventilation, cuffed endotracheal tubes were designed to seal the lower airway and prevent the entry of materials from the upper airway. Unfortunately they often fail to provide a consistent barrier against aspirated materials (34).

Decreased gastric motility is a frequent problem in critically ill patients because of underlying disease or injury. Dive et al. utilized manometry to compare gastroduodenal motility in 12 critically ill, mechanically ventilated patients with that in 12 healthy control volunteers. The frequency of contractions was significantly decreased in the critically ill group, and more importantly the loss of peristaltic activity was greater in the stomach than in the duodenum. Factors that decrease GI motility include neurologic impairment with elevated ICP and medications.

For example, propofol is a visceral smooth muscle relaxant. In healthy persons the effect is insignificant, but it may contribute to delayed gastric emptying in patients receiving other medications that slow gastric motility. Low-dose dopamine slows gastroduodenal motility in mechanically ventilated, critically ill patients. Opioids can delay gastric emptying, through both central and peripheral mechanisms. The enteral administration of opioid antagonists has been suggested as a possible method to improve gastric emptying and decrease the frequency of aspiration in mechanically ventilated patients receiving opioid analgesia.

When gastric motility is moderately or seriously impaired, feedings accumulate in the stomach along with gastric secretions and predispose patients to reflux and aspiration. Another risk factor is recurrent episodes of emesis; in these patients tube feedings should be held or reduced and antiemetic medications administered (34). Aspiration can result from refluxed tube feedings or oropharyngeal secretions that are unrelated to feedings (32). Pulmonary aspiration of tube feed can result in hypoxia and/or pneumonia (67).

To determine whether tube feeds are contaminating the lungs, the color of respiratory secretions can be assessed after adding several drops of blue food coloring to the feeding formula. However, one study showed that the sensitivity of blue dye for the detection of aspiration was only 15%, and a study in animals determined that the sensitivity of blue dye detection of aspiration decreased after multiple aspiration events. However, the FDA in a public health bulletin in 2003 noted an association between the use of blue dye in enteral feedings and discoloration of body fluids and skin as well as serious metabolic complications including death. The FDA suggested that patients at risk for increased intestinal permeability, including those with sepsis, burns, trauma, shock, surgical interventions, renal failure, celiac sprue, and inflammatory bowel disease, appear to have an increased risk of absorbing blue dye from tinted enteral feedings.

An alternative for detecting tube feed aspiration is the use of glucose oxidase reagent strips. Proponents believe glucose strips are safer and more accurate than blue dye. Drawbacks of glucose strips include the possibility of false positives in the presence of blood in tracheobronchial aspirates and the possibility of false negatives in patients receiving low-glucose enteral feeding. In addition, glucose reagent strips were not designed to test for pulmonary aspirate, cost more than blue dye, and may require certification before clinicians can integrate them into care (71).

When trauma or surgery causes significantly delayed GI motility, small-bowel function usually returns before gastric or colonic activity. Also, small-bowel activity may be less adversely affected than either gastric or colonic function in acute medical conditions such as pancreatitis. So if gastric motility is significantly slowed, small-bowel feedings are preferred (34). Though small-bowel feeding is thought to decrease the risk of aspiration, it has not been proven in studies (32). Studies have revealed that feeding the duodenum or jejunum results in stimulation of gastric secretions and duodenogastric reflux. So utilizing a postpyloric feeding tube to insert feeds and a separate nasogastric tube (NGT) to aspirate gastric contents or a combination gastrojejunostomy tube may be the safest option. Finally, if bolus or intermittent gastric feedings are not tolerated, continuous feedings may be better tolerated. There are no studies that demonstrate a reduced rate of aspiration with administration of continuous feeding, yet this is more commonly used in critically ill patients.

Continuous subglottic suction appears to help prevent or delay the development of nosocomial pneumonia in mechanically ventilated patients by removing pooled secretions that may leak around the endotracheal tube cuff. A sleep study suggested that continuous aspiration of subglottic secretions could decrease bacterial colonization of the respiratory tract, but may also result in mucosal damage at the level of the suction port (34).

Bacterial Contamination

Microbial contamination of enteral feeds is associated with pneumonia (35), diarrhea (72), and sepsis. Anderson et al. compared locally prepared, manipulated, and nonmanipulated formulas and the development of diarrhea. As would be expected, the locally prepared and manipulated formulas contained a significantly higher number of organisms than the nonmanipulated formulas. The risk of contamination in manipulated or reconstituted tube feeding has been supported in numerous studies. Manipulated formulas have a 30% to 60% risk of preadministration contamination, whereas Okuma et al. (72) found sterile ready-to-use formulas have a 2% risk. Okuma et al. (72) studied liquid ready-to-use enteral feeds and found 10 of 48 postadministration samples were contaminated. Though there were a high number of contaminated samples, only two patients developed diarrhea (72).

Due to the high morbidity and mortality due to infection in the critically ill, recommendations have been created to decrease the risk of bacterial contamination in tube feeds. Use of a closed enteral nutrition delivery system, where the tube feed is prepackaged with a tube for administration, may carry the lowest risk of contamination (72).

Diarrhea

GI side effects of tube feeding include nausea and vomiting, abdominal pain, and diarrhea (32). Diarrhea is the most common complication, with a rate of 30% to 50% of critically ill patients receiving tube feedings being affected (72). As diarrhea results in ongoing GI protein, electrolyte, fluid losses, and malabsorption, control is mandatory. Numerous causes of diarrhea exist and include medications (promotility agents, antibiotics, sorbitol-containing elixirs/suspensions), hyperosmolar formulas, prolonged bowel rest, severe hypoproteinemia, infection, and increased dietary fat (10). Additional causes include infected diets, lactose intolerance, ingestion of laxatives, and hypoalbuminemia (51).

The most rapid intervention involves a review of medications, and all prokinetic agents should be discontinued (73). A common pharmacologic cause of diarrhea in tube-fed patients is administration of large doses of nonabsorbable carbohydrate such as sorbitol (32). Sorbitol is a component of common medicinal elixirs, such as acetaminophen, theophylline, and cimetidine, to improve palatability and results in osmotic shifts and diarrhea (7). Finally, the combination of antibiotics and infection is responsible for three-quarters of the cases of diarrhea (13). Antibiotic use can lead to proliferation of *C. difficile* and development of pseudomembranous colitis. In a normal patient, short-chained fatty acids (SCFAs) have multiple functions. In the colon, they enhance water and electrolyte absorption, increase colonocyte proliferation and metabolic energy production, enhance blood flow, stimulate the autonomic nervous system, and increase GI hormone production (51). When *C. difficile* occurs, it blocks the conversion of carbohydrates to SCFAs, causing diarrhea development (32). ☞ **It is mandatory that clostridial infection as the cause of diarrhea be eliminated, as pharmacologic manipulation of gut motility in an infected patient can result in severe toxicity.** ☞

Once infectious causes of diarrhea have been eliminated, enteral formula, concentration, and rate of administration can be altered. If the diarrhea persists, trials of

antidiarrheal agents such as diphenoxylate or loperamide are justified in an effort to maintain adequate delivery of nutrients (32). In some cases, administration of opiates may be necessary. They act by slowing intestinal motility, but are contraindicated in patients with infectious diarrhea, or they may lead to prolonged retention of the toxins. Only in the most severe cases will discontinuation of enteral feeding and temporary administration of parenteral nutrition be necessary (10).

Overfeeding/Hyperglycemia

Though catabolic patients require higher levels of nutritional supplementation, care must be taken to avoid overfeeding. When this occurs, the high-carbohydrate diet leads to accumulation of increased fat mass without changes in lean body mass. In addition, the overfed patient commonly suffers from hyperglycemia, which leads to an increased insulin requirement. Hyperglycemia has also been associated with a negative influence on the outcome of septic and critically ill patients. Detrimental effects of hyperglycemia include a predisposition to severe infections, MODS, and death. In addition, the elevated plasma levels of glucose impair immune function by altering macrophage cytokine productions, diminishing lymphocyte proliferation, and depressing intracellular bactericidal activity of leucocytes. So, preventing hyperglycemia results in improved immune response and wound healing (14). In addition, recent studies have revealed reduction in mortality rate of critically ill patients treated aggressively with insulin (Volume 2, Chapter 60) (10).

It is important to note that overfeeding is associated with inability to wean patients from mechanical ventilation. Administration of excessive carbohydrate loads (>500 g/day or >50% total calories from carbohydrate) results in overproduction of CO_2. When ability to excrete CO_2 by the lungs is overwhelmed, hypercapnia results (10). Therefore, ensuring adequate but not excessive feeding is mandatory.

Small-Bowel Necrosis

A dreaded yet rare complication of both gastric and small bowel feedings is nonocclusive small-bowel necrosis (34). To date, nonocclusive bowel necrosis has been reported in 0.3% of critically ill patients who are given tube feedings. Bowel necrosis is hypothesized to be due to a combination of factors which cause ischemia, or compromised blood flow to the bowel. Factors include hypotension and the use of vasoconstrictive medications. The body responds by shunting the blood flow from the small intestine to maintain cerebral and cardiac perfusion. In general, the remaining blood flow to the bowel is adequate to maintain perfusion in the resting state (32). Addition of an iatrogenic stressor, which increases the metabolic demand of the intestine, increases the flow necessary to provide adequate bowel perfusion. Ischemia is induced which, if uncorrected with fluid resuscitation and discontinuation of tube feeding, may result in necrosis (41).

Patients with ischemia commonly have abdominal pain and tenderness, but it is difficult to detect as many of the patients at risk are typically sedated and mechanically ventilated. Furthermore, both enteral feed intolerance and paralytic ileus are common in this group of patients (74). So, any critically ill patient who experiences abdominal distention, pain (34), tachycardia, temperature elevation (13), and possibly increasing GRVs while receiving either continuous gastric or small-bowel feedings must be evaluated for tube feed necrosis. The use of gastric tonometry may be useful for detecting nonocclusive small-bowel necrosis; for example, low mucosal pH (<7.30) measurements were detected in three patients who demonstrated this condition during enteral feeding advancement. If there is concern of tube feed necrosis, enteral feeding should be immediately discontinued. If the ischemia progresses, the patient may continue to deteriorate and show signs of hypotension and septic shock with fever, tachycardia, and abnormal white blood cell count. Emergent surgical intervention often is mandated (34).

A study by Desai et al. found ischemic intestinal pathology to be a common autopsy finding in patients with large burns, being present in more than 50% of those patients who succumb to their injury, although it was clinically identified in less than 1%. In addition, the mortality rate associated with ischemic enterocolitis is extremely high (60–69%) (74). So, a high index of suspicion is mandatory for this unusual complication.

Refeeding Syndrome

Refeeding syndrome is a common condition in previously malnourished patients, where aggressive nutritional supplementation increases the basal metabolic rate with the use of glucose as the primary energy source. As minerals shift intracellularly, the serum levels fall precipitously (35). The resulting hypophosphotemia, hypokalemia, thiamine deficiency, and hypomagnesemia (50) lead to cardiorespiratory and neurologic dysfunction. Patients develop congestive heart failure, respiratory failure, lethargy, confusion, coma, convulsions, and death (35). Patients most at risk have a history of anorexia, chronic alcoholism (50), chronic malnutrition, prolonged fast, or intravenous hydration only (35). In addition, increased insulin levels result in an antinaturetic effect and fluid retention. The sudden expansion of extracellular fluid leads to cardiac decompensation. On the other hand, the dextrose load can result in hyperglycemia, osmotic diuresis, and dehydration (1). So, it is imperative to closely monitor electrolyte and glucose serum levels so as to diagnose and treat refeeding syndrome rapidly.

NUTRITIONAL MONITORING

Once nutritional supplementation is instituted, it is mandatory to evaluate the adequacy of the supplementation. Many of the common markers of nutritional deficiency such as weight loss and anthropometric measurements are not useful in trauma patients due to massive fluid shifts.

Of the laboratory values currently available clinically to assess nutritional status, albumin, transferrin, and prealbumin are the most common. In addition, collecting a 24-hour urine urea nitrogen, indirect calorimetry, estimating nutritional needs via energy formulas, and monitoring overall improvement in medical condition help determine if the nutritional care plan is appropriate and effective (refer to Volume 2, Chapter 31 for additional information on nutritional monitoring).

EYE TO THE FUTURE

Though the ideal enteral feeding formula has yet to be identified, it is clear from research over the last 20 years that the gut is the preferred method with which to restore nutritional integrity in both trauma and critically ill patients. The importance of various strains of fibers and beneficial bacteria or synbiotics continues to peak interest in hopes to help fight infection and nutrient absorption. Astaxanthin, a reddish-orange carotenoid pigment, has been studied in animal models and shown to have antioxidative and anti-inflammatory effects, bringing promise to human health (75).

Increased interest in polyphenol and its antioxidant capacity, especially Curcumin, has brought promise to the treatment of atherosclerosis, cancer, diabetes, respiratory, liver, pancreatic, gastric, and intestinal diseases when supplemented in the oral diet (76). Synbiotic therapy also brings promise to improving nutrient absorption for the critically ill patients.

Future research will concentrate on improved modes of delivery and attempts at identifying immune-enhancing substances that can prevent the deleterious effects of nutritional depletion and starvation.

SUMMARY

Due to the prevalence of pre-existing malnutrition and the risk of developing malnutrition in critically ill patients, it is imperative to consider early nutritional supplementation. When the patient's GI tract is functional, the enteral route is preferred. Again, the route of administration and the formula used should take into account the patient's clinical state, anticipated duration of feeding, gut patency, and risk of aspiration. Care must be taken to minimize the interruption of nutritional administration, and efficacy of nutritional supplementation should be determined with weekly measurements of metabolic parameters.

KEY POINTS

- In situations where full enteral nutrition is not tolerated, as little as 20% of overall nutrient calories administered to the gut can be sufficient to show benefits as opposed to TPN alone (5).
- Patients most likely to benefit from nutritional support are those with baseline malnutrition in whom a protracted period of starvation would otherwise occur (8).
- Early enteral feeding should be instituted in all severely injured trauma patients (ISS > 17) without contraindications.
- The current EAST guidelines (Fig. 1) recommend that patients with blunt and penetrating abdominal injuries be fed enterally because of the lower incidence of septic complications compared with parenterally fed patients (11).
- The goal in burn patients is to initiate enteral nutrition within six hours of presentation to prevent body weight loss of more than 10% of their baseline status (14).
- To prevent devastating losses of nutrient stores and improve patient outcome, nutritional supplementation should begin no later than 72 hours following TBI (18).

✄ After the acute SCI phase, there is a period of reduced REE in proportion to the amount of paralyzed muscle mass.

✄ Enteral feeding by an N-J tube or percutaneous jejunostomy has largely replaced TPN in the management of patients with pancreatitis (24).

✄ Patients with SIRS with or without MODS have elevated total caloric requirements, increased net protein catabolism, and increased micronutrient requirements (27).

✄ Gut perforation after repair generally remains secure and is not necessarily put at risk of leakage by enteral nutrition started at 48 hours after surgery (30).

✄ For malnourished patients undergoing resection of their tumor, 7 to 10 days of preoperative enteral nutrition support is associated with a 10% reduction in morbidity and improved quality of life (31).

✄ The route of enteral nutrition administration is influenced by the patient's clinical prognosis, anticipated duration of feeding, gut patency, motility and anatomy, and risk of aspiration (32).

✄ Patients who require long-term, that is, more than two to four weeks, enteral nutrition require permanent access for feeding.

✄ Standard formulas are the most widely utilized form of enteral nutrition. They are designed for patients with normal or near-normal GI function.

✄ Elemental formulas were created to provide a complete set of nutrients in a form that required little or no digestion; thus, it could be utilized in patients with a dysfunctional GI tract (52).

✄ The oral dietary supplements are true supplements, that is, they are not nutritionally complete. The use of these products is as an additional, highly concentrated nutritional source for individuals who are unable to ingest adequate nutrients with a standard oral diet (1).

✄ When these adjustments fail to alleviate gastroparesis, institution of promotility agents, metoclopramide and erythromycin, can be utilized.

✄ It is mandatory that clostridial infection, as the cause of diarrhea be eliminated, as pharmacologic manipulation of gut motility in an infected patient can result in severe toxicity.

REFERENCES

1. August D, Teitelbaum D, Albina J, et al. Guidelines for the use of parenteral and enteral nutrition in adult and pediatric patients. J Parenter Enteral Nutr 2002; 26:1–137.
2. Adams G, Guest D, Ciraulo D, et al. Maximizing tolerance of enteral nutrition in severely injured trauma patients: a comparison of enteral feedings by means of percutaneous endoscopic gastrostomy versus percutaneous endoscopic gastrojejunostomy. J Trauma 2000; 48:459–465.
3. Marik PE, Zaloga GP. Early enteral nutrition in acutely ill patients: a systemic review. Crit Care Med 2001; 29:2264–2270.
4. Doherty W, Winter B. Prokinetic agents in critical care. Crit Care 2003; 7:206–208.
5. Tawa NE, Maykel JA, Fischer JE. Metabolism in surgical patients. In: Townsend CM, Beauchamp RD, Evers BM, eds. Sabiston Textbook of Surgery. 17th ed. Elsevier Saunders, 2004:137–182.
6. Roy S, Rigal M, Doit C, et al. Bacterial contamination of enteral nutrition in a paediatric hospital. J Hosp Infection 2005; 59: 311–316.
7. Nisim A, Allins A. Enteral nutrition support. Nutrition 2005; 21:109–112.
8. Chan S, McCowen K, Blackburn G. Nutrition management in the ICU. Chest 1999; 115:145S–148S.
9. Slone S. Nutritional support of the critically ill and injured patient. Crit Care Clin 2004; 20:135–157.
10. Rolandelli RH, Gupta D, Wilmore DW. Nutritional support. In: Souba WW, Fink MP, Jurkovich GJ, eds. American College of Surgeons ACS Surgery Principles and Practice. WebMD, Inc., 2004:1444–1465.
11. Jacobs D, Kudsk K, et al. For the EAST Practice Management Workshop. Practice management guidelines for nutritional support of the trauma patient. J Trauma 2004; 57:660–679.
12. Biffl W, Moore EE, Haenel JB. Nutrition support of the trauma patient. Nutrition 2002; 18:960–965.
13. Kudsk KA, Sacks GS, Brown RO. Nutritional support. In: Moore EE, Feliciano DV, Mattox KL, eds. Trauma. 5th ed. McGraw-Hill, 2004:1351–1381.
14. Andel H, Kamolz LP, Horauf K, Zimpfer M. Nutrition and anabolic agents in burned patients. Burns 2003; 29: 592–595.
15. Peck MD, Kessler M, Cairns BA, et al. Early enteral nutrition does not decrease hypermetabolism associated with burn injury. J Trauma 2004; 57:1143–1149.
16. Wernerman J. Guidelines for nutritional support in intensive care unit patients: A critical analysis. Curr Opin Clin Nutr Metab Care 2005; 8:171–175.
17. Scheinkestel CD, Kar L, Marshall K, et al. Prospective randomized trial to assess caloric and protein needs of critically ill, anuric, ventilated patients requiring continuous renal replacement therapy. Nutrition 2003; 19:909–916.
18. Robertson C. Critical care management of TBI. In: Marshall L, Grady M, Winn H, eds. Youmans Neurological Surgery. 5th ed. Saunders, 2004:5103–5144.
19. Brain Trauma Foundation. Management and Prognosis of Severe TBI. Brain Trauma Foundation, 2000:143–158.
20. Dvorak M, Noonan V, Belanger L, et al. Early versus late enteral feeding in patients with acute cervical spinal cord injury: a pilot study. Spine 2004; 29:E175–E180.
21. Abou-Assi S, O'Keefe S. Nutrition support during acute pancreatitis. Nutrition 2002; 18:938–943.
22. Marik PE, Zaloga GP. Meta-analysis of parenteral nutrition versus enteral nutrition in patients with acute pancreatitis. Br Med J 2004; 328:1407.
23. Raimondo M, Scolapio J. Editorial—What route to feed patients with severe acute pancreatitis: vein, jejunum, or stomach? Am J Gastroenterol 2005; 2:440–441.
24. Mitchell RMS, Byrne MF, Baillie J. Pancreatitis. Lancet 2003; 361:1447–1455.
25. Eatock FC, Chong P, Menezes N, et al. A randomized study of early nasogastric versus nasojejunal feeding in severe acute pancreatitis. Am J Gastroenterol 2005; 100:432–439.
26. Balk RA. Pathogenesis and management of multiple organ dysfunction or failure in severe sepsis and septic shock. Clin Crit Care 2000; 16:337–350.
27. Cerra F, Benitez M, Blackburn G. Applied nutrition in ICU patients: a consensus statement of the American College of Chest Physicians. Chest 1997; 111:769–778.
28. Hill G. Implications of critical illness, injury, and sepsis on lean body mass and nutritional needs. Nutrition 1998; 14: 557–558.
29. Huckleberry Y. Nutritional support and the surgical patient. Am J Health Syst Pharm 2004; 61:671–682.
30. Malhotra A, Manthur AK, Gupta S. Early enteral nutrition after surgical treatment of gut perforations: a prospective randomized study. J Postgrad Med 2004; 50:102–106.
31. Schattner M. Enteral nutritional support of the patient with cancer: route and role. J Clin Gastroent 2003; 36:297–302.
32. Klein S, Rubin DC. Enteral and parenteral nutrition. In: Feldman, ed. Sleisenger and Fordtran's Gastrointestinal and Liver Disease. 7th ed. Elsevier, 2002:287–293.
33. Ahmed K, Samant S, Vieira F. Gastrostomy tubes in patients with advanced head and neck cancer. Laryngoscope 2005; 115:44–47.

34. Metheny N, Schallom M, Edwards S. Effect of gastrointestinal motility and feeding tube site on aspiration risk in critically ill patients: a review. Heart and lung. J Acute Crit Care 2004; 33:131–145.

35. Pearce CB, Duncan HD. Enteral feeding. Nasogastric, nasojejunal, percutaneous endoscopic gastrostomy, or jejunostomy: its indications and limitations. Postgrad Med J 2002; 78:198–204.

36. Davies A, Bellomo R. Establishment of enteral nutrition: prokinetic agents and small bowel feeding tubes. Curr Opin Crit Care 2004; 10:156–161.

37. Boivin M, Levy H. Gastric feeding with erythromycin is equivalent to transpyloric feeding in the critically ill. Crit Care Med 2001; 10:1916–1919.

38. Marik PE, Zaloga GP. Gastric vs. post-pyloric feeding: a systematic review. Crit Care 2003; 7(3):R45–R51.

39. McClave SA, Lukan JK, Stefates JA, et al. Poor validity of residual volumes as a marker for risk of aspiration in critically ill patients. Crit Care Med 2005; 33(2):449–450.

40. Dwyer K, Watts D, Thurber J, Benoit R, Fakhry S. Percutaneous endoscopic gastrostomy: the preferred method of elective feeding tube placement in trauma patients. J Trauma 2002; 51:26–31.

41. Munshi I, Steingrub J, Wolpert L. Small bowel necrosis associated with early postoperative jejunal tube feeding in a trauma patient. J Trauma 2000; 49:163–165.

42. Khatri V, Asensio J. Operative Surgery Manual. 1st ed. Elsevier, 2003:123.

43. Duh Q, Senokozlieff-englehart A, Choe Y, et al. Laparoscopic gastrostomy and jejunostomy. Safety and cost with local vs. general anesthesia. Arch Surg 1999; 134:151–154.

44. Crawford DL. Laparoscopic gastric surgery. In: Cameron JL, ed. Current Surgical Therapy. 8th ed. Elsevier Mosby, 2004: 1224–1226.

45. Ozman M, Akhan O. Percutaneous radiologic gastrostomy. Euro J Rad 2002; 43:186–195.

46. Funaki B, Zaleski G, Lorenz J. Radiologic gastrostomy placement: pigtail versus mushroom retained catheters. Am J Roentgenol 2000; 175:375–379.

47. Grainger R, Allison D, Adam A, et al., eds. Grainger and Allison's Diagnostic Radiology: a Textbook of Medical Imaging. 4th ed. Churchill Livingstone, 2001.

48. Guloglu R, Taviloglu K, Alimoglu O. Case report: colon injury following percutaneous endoscopic gastrostomy tube insertion. J Laparoendosc Adv Surg Tech 2003; 13:69–72.

49. Huang S, Levine M, Raper S. Case report: gastrocolic fistula with migration of feeding tube into transverse colon as a complication of percutaneous endoscopic gastrostomy. Am J Roentgenol 2005; 184:S65–S66.

50. Minard G. Nutrition/metabolism in the trauma patient. In: Peitzman AB, Rhodes M, Schwab CW, Yealy DM, Fabian TC, eds. The Trauma Manual. 2nd ed. Lippincott Williams & Wilkins, 2002:420–427.

51. Silk DBA. Formulation of enteral diets. Nutrition 1999; 15: 626–632.

52. Gardner M, Earl S, Wood D. Elemental diets in the repair of small intestinal damage. Nutrition 1997; 13:755–759.

53. Tsuei BJ, Bernard AC, Barksdale AR, et al. Supplemental enteral arginine is metabolized to ornithine in injured patients. J Surg Res 2005; 123:17–24.

54. Weimann A, Bastian L, Bischoff W, et al. Influence of arginine, omega-3 fatty acids and nucleotide-supplemented enteral support on systemic inflammatory response syndrome and multiple organ failure in patients after severe trauma. Nutrition 1998; 14:165–172.

55. Tubman TRJ, Thompson SW, McGuire W. Glutamine supplementation to prevent morbidity and mortality in preterm infants. Cochrane Database Systematic Reviews 2005; CD001457.

56. Lin E, Kotani J, Lowry S. Nutritional modulation of immunity and the inflammatory response. Nutrition 1998; 14:545–550.

57. Alexander J. Immunonutrition: the role of ω-3 fatty acids. Nutrition 1998; 14:627–633.

58. Mizock B. Nutritional support in hepatic encephalopathy. Nutrition 1999; 15:220–228.

59. Scheinkestal CD, Kar L, Marshall K, et al. Prospective randomized trial to assess caloric and protein needs of critically ill patients with acute renal failure. J Parenter Enteral Nutr 1996; 20:56.

60. Herselman M. Protein and energy requirements in patients with acute renal failure on continuous renal replacement therapy. Nutrition 2003; 19:813–815.

61. Lefrance J, Leblanc M. Metabolic, electrolytes, and nutritional concerns in the critically ill. Crit Care Clin 2005; 21:318–322.

62. Bengmark S. Gut microbial ecology in critical illness: is there a role for prebiotics, probiotics, and synbiotics? Curr Opin Crit Care 2002; 8:145–151.

63. Caparros T, Lopez J, Grau T. Early enteral nutrition in critically ill patients with a high-protein diet enriched with arginine, fiber, and antioxidants compared with a standard high-protein diet: the effect on nosocomial infections and outcome. J Parenter Enteral Nutr 2001; 25:299–308.

64. Bengmark S, Martindale R. Prebiotics and synbiotics in clinical medicine. Nutr Clin Pract 2005; 20:244–261.

65. Zaloga GP, Marik P. Promotility agents in the intensive care unit. Crit Care Med 2000; 28:2657–2658.

66. Jooste CA, Mustoe J, Collee G. Metaclopromide improves gastric motility in critically ill patients. Intensive Care Med 1999; 25:464–468.

67. Zaloga GP. The myth of the gastric residual volume. Crit Care Med 2005; 33:449–450.

68. Heiselman DE, Hofer T, Vidovich RR. Enteral feeding tube placement success with intravenous metoclopramide administration in ICU patients. Chest 1995; 107:1686–1688.

69. Berne J, Norwood S, McAuley C, et al. Erythromycin reduces delayed gastric emptying in critically ill trauma patients: a randomized, controlled trial. J Trauma 2002; 53:422–425.

70. Reignier J, Thenos-Jost N, Fiancette M, et al. Early enteral nutrition in mechanically ventilated patients in the prone position. Crit Care Med 2004; 32(1):94–99.

71. Klein L. Is blue dye safe as a method of detection for pulmonary aspiration? J Am Dietetic Assoc 2004; 104:1651–1652.

72. Okuma T, Nakamura M, Totake H, Fukunaga Y. Microbial contamination of enteral feeding formulas and diarrhea. Nutrition 2000; 16:719–722.

73. Mechanick J, Brett E. Nutritional support of the chronically critically ill patient. Crit Care Clin 2002; 18:597–618.

74. Wilson MD, Dziewulski P. Severe gastrointestinal haemorrhage and ischaemic necrosis of the small bowel in a child with 70% full-thickness burns: a case report. Burns 2001; 27:763–766.

75. Hussein G, Sanakawa U, Goto H, et al. Astaxanthin, a carotenoid with potential in human health and nutrition. J Nat Prod 2006; 69(3):443–449.

76. Bengmark S. Curcumin, an atoxic antioxidant and natural NFκB, cyclooxygenase-2, lipooxygenase, and inducible nitric oxide synthase inhibitor: a shield against acute and chronic diseases. J Parenter Enteral Nutr 2006; 30:45–51.

77. Demling RH, Desanti L. Complications of acute weight loss due to stress response injury. Curr Opin Crit Care 1996; 2:482–491.

78. Zollinger RM, eds. Atlas of Surgical Operations. 7th ed. McGraw-Hill, 1993:30–31.

79. Brasel K, Weigelt JA. Intensive care unit. In: Thal ER, Weigelt JA, Carrico CJ, eds. Operative Trauma Management. 2nd ed. McGraw-Hill, 2002:458–471.

80. Lutornski DM, Gora ML, Wright SM, Martin JE. Sorbitol content of selected oral liquids. Ann Pharmacother 1993; 27:269.

33

Parenteral Nutrition

Grant V. Bochicchio and Shelley Nehman
Department of Surgery, University of Maryland School of Medicine, Baltimore, Maryland, U.S.A.

Jua Choi
Department of Nutrition, UC San Diego Medical Center, San Diego, California, U.S.A.

INTRODUCTION

The concept and implementation of parenteral nutrition (PN) began nearly a century ago. In 1912, Fohn and Denis (1) reported that protein hydrolysis led to gut absorption. These findings fostered the idea that the gut could be bypassed to provide nutrition, and inspired Henriques and Anderson (2), in 1913, to administer hydrolyzed protein intravenously in an animal study. PN was actively investigated following that study. A significant breakthrough occurred in 1925 when Seibert (3) discovered that pyrogens, elicited from bacteria, were responsible for the fever and chills associated with the infusion of intravenous (IV) substances. In 1939, Elman and Weiner (4) reported on the first successful use of total parenteral nutrition (TPN) in man. However, TPN did not become widely accepted until 1967 when Dudrick et al. (5) at the University of Pennsylvania demonstrated that normal growth and development could occur solely with the administration of TPN [without any enteral nutrition (EN) at all].

TPN became the predominant route of nutrition administration in the 1970s, because it was widely available, and could be used regardless of the patient's gastrointestinal (GI) function. In the 1980s, however, several unique advantages of EN became more apparent, including the benefit of direct nourishment of the gut endothelium by enteral amino acids such as glutamine, the first-pass effect of EN through the liver, decreased nitrogen losses compared to TPN, less glucose intolerance, and so on. Furthermore, data began to emerge demonstrating a survival advantage with EN in certain trauma conditions (especially the burn patient; see Volume 1, Chapter 34), as well as a decrease in complication rates (e.g., line sepsis; see Volume 2, Chapter 49). According to a meta-analysis of prospective, randomized clinical trials among 27 studies, TPN is associated with a higher rate of infection than EN in both malnourished and nonmalnourished patients (6). PN is expensive because of cost of admixture, placing venous access, laboratory monitoring, and costs to treat complications (7). Protection against gut atrophy, preservation of gut flora, and improved immunocompetence became even greater positive attributes of EN, and in the early 1990s the trend had reverted back toward using EN whenever possible (Volume 2, Chapter 32).

Although the enteral route remains the favored portal for nutritional administration to critically ill patients, TPN is still required for patients who cannot be fed enterally. This chapter reviews the indications for PN, the routes of administration, and nutritional requirements in terms of macronutrients (protein, carbohydrate, and fat) and micronutrients (vitamins, trace elements, and electrolytes). Next, the clinical applications of PN are discussed in terms of initiation, maintenance, and withdrawal. The complications of PN are then reviewed, followed by a brief summary of nutrient monitoring considerations for patients receiving PN (Volume 2, Chapter 31). Special disease states that are common in critical illness (e.g., diabetes, renal failure, and liver failure) are also reviewed in terms of their effect on TPN. In the section "Eye to the Future," current areas of research are discussed.

INDICATIONS

EN (Volume 2, Chapter 32) represents the preferred route of nutrition administration when the gut is functional and can be used, whereas TPN remains the mainstay of nutritional support whenever EN is contraindicated (Table 1), or gut function is impaired either due to injury or ileus (from surgical manipulation, infection, or medications, especially opiates) (Table 2). In these settings, TPN should be considered after three to four days of starvation in previously healthy critically ill patients. In previously ill, malnourished, or severely injured patients with a nonfunctioning GI tract or no enteral feeding access, TPN should be considered earlier in their care, that is, immediately postresuscitation when prolonged critical care is anticipated. For example, patients who suffer from small-bowel obstruction or malabsorptive capacity such as inflammatory bowel disease or short gut syndrome, and are expected to be nil per os (NPO) for greater than seven days should be considered for TPN as soon as possible.

In a large study, TPN was only shown to benefit severely malnourished patients, whereas TPN was associated with a worse risk benefit ratio in previously healthy patients (i.e., complications including infections were greater than nutritional benefits) (8). Thus, the risks of TPN (line-related infections, hyperglycemia, refeeding syndrome, hepatic dysfunction) must be weighed against the presumed harm of a short-term (three to seven days) fasting.

ROUTES OF ADMINISTRATION

Vein location, macronutrient concentration, and volume capacity of the patient need to be carefully reviewed before

Table 1   Indications for Total Parenteral Nutrition

TPN indication	Issue and relative importance	Exceptions—recommendations
SBO	Distended bowel	Rest gut—no exception
Ischemic colon	May not tolerate feeding	Rest gut—until POD#1 surgical revision or with improvement
Pancreatitis	Feeding causes pancreatic enzymes to be elaborated	Recent data support trophic enteral feeding, some believe full EN is indicated providing the tube is in the jejunum
Short gut syndrome	Inability to absorb nutrients	Need jejunum to absorb water, need distal ileum to absorb vitamin B12, lack of colon, not as devastating as lack of small bowel?
Pancreatitis (now controversial)	Feeding causes pancreatic enzymes to be elaborated	Recent data supports trophic enteral feeding, some believe full EN is indicated providing the tube is in the jejunum

The authors believe that the above total parenteral nutrition (TPN) indications encompass the major clinical situations where enteral nutrition is contraindicated. Whenever the gut can be used, the authors recommend providing enteral nutrition (EN) rather than administering TPN.
Abbreviations: EN, enteral nutrition; POD, postoperative day; SBO, small bowel obstruction.

the initiation of PN. Central vessels are able to handle higher macronutrient concentrations compared with peripheral vessels without the risk of thrombophlebitis or vessel damage (9). True peripheral veins can tolerate no more than 900 mOsm/L. Concentrations of calcium ≤5 mEq/L and potassium ≤40 mEq/L should be used whenever possible, and the infusion of lipids to decrease osmolarity (10). ☞ **As TPN solutions are hyperosmolar, a large-diameter vein with adequate flow rate is required to allow for rapid dilution of TPN products within the vessel.** ☞ Common peripheral PN (PPN) solutions contain no more than 10% dextrose and 4% amino acids for safe administration. Full calorie and protein needs can only be met when a patient is able to tolerate larger volumes of dilute (compared with centrally administered) PN. Peripheral veins can be used to administer isotonic fat emulsions and hypocaloric dextrose solutions (i.e., <10% dextrose). However, their use is limited to merely preventing starvation adaptation and minimizing nitrogen loss, because they cannot accommodate the high osmolar load needed to provide calories and nutrients required for TPN. Accordingly, the authors recommend that TPN be administered through either a standard central line or a peripherally inserted central catheter line.

Owing to the anatomical location of the large veins where central lines are placed, complications such as pneumothorax, arterial cannulation, and air embolism can occur. In addition, catheter-associated sepsis can be a potentially lethal complication of this procedure in combination with TPN use. Therefore, experienced personnel utilizing proper sterile technique are recommended for placement of central lines for PN.

Practical Considerations Regarding IV Site Selection

The technical details of central vein insertion are reviewed in Volume 1, Chapter 10 and infectious considerations are provided in Volume 2, Chapter 49; these topics are beyond the scope of this chapter, but certain practical considerations warrant inclusion here.

☞ **The preferred site of central venous catheter placement for PN is the subclavian vein.** ☞ This route is most comfortable for the patient, following insertion, and is less easily

Table 2   Reasons Why Physicians May Halt Enteral Nutrition

Reason to halt Enteral Nutrition	Cause	Treatment
High residuals 7 cm³/kg (after 4–5 hr of tube feeding)	Gastric atony, small bowel obstruction, ileus, rate of feeding too fast	Rule out obstruction (rectal exam, KUB and lateral decub or upright abdominal film); if no obstruction, resume feeding, at slower rate; if high residuals occur second time, provide a brief period of bowel rest (4–24 hr), then resume enteral feeding; also, attempt to reduce opiates, and add or increase reglan or cisapride
Vomiting	All above, plus hypotension, improper tube placement, TF osmolality too high, medications coadministered, critical illness	Same as above, except rest till patient no longer vomiting; also, consider antiemetics, including odansatron
Diarrhea	Sorbitol elixirs, intolerance of medications (e.g., antibiotics), bacterial infection (e.g., *Closridium difficile*)	Omit offending agents, provide bulk, treat infection (e.g., *C. difficile* Rx with Flagyl or oral vancomycin)
Constipation	Opiates, dehydration, lack of fiber	Limit opiates (e.g., switch to nonsteroidal antiinfilamatory drugs), hydrate, suppositories, fiber

Abbreviations: KUB, kidneys, ureter, bladder; TF, tube feeds.

dislodged as compared with the internal jugular route. Furthermore, the subclavian site has the lowest infection rate of the common central line access locations (Volume 2, Chapter 49). When the subclavian site is unavailable, the internal jugular (uncomfortable) or the femoral vein (increased risk of lower extremity deep vein thrombosis and limitation of mobility) may be used.

If a pulmonary artery (PA) catheter is placed, some recommend against infusing through the distal PA port, with the concern that this may lead to pulmonary infiltrates. However, there are no published data to support this assertion. Consequently, PN can be instilled through any of the ports not being used for other drugs (typically the right atrium or right ventricle infusion ports, but even the PA distal port can be used for short durations when needed).

Skin Site Preparation and Maintenance

The skin site should be scrubbed with a chlorhexidine preparation and permitted to dry for at least 30 seconds prior to catheter insertion. Surgical caps, mask, sterile gown, and gloves are mandatory. In addition to the site drape provided in the kit, a sterile full body sheet should be draped across the patient in order to minimize contamination.

After the catheter is inserted and sutured in place, the skin should be thoroughly washed with a saline-soaked gauze and dried with a clean sterile gauze to eliminate any residual blood—which can become a nidus for infection. Next, a clear adhesive dressing should be placed over the venepuncture and catheter suture sites, in order to further decrease the infection rate (11). A postprocedure chest radiograph is obtained to confirm placement and assure proper anatomical location. Dressings should be sterilely changed daily.

The catheter should be used solely for PN, to minimize the possibility of contaminating an entry port to the catheter. The catheter should be routinely changed per standard protocols (Volume 2, Chapter 49).

ENERGY, FLUID, AND MACRONUTRIENT REQUIREMENTS

Energy Requirements

There are several methods that can be used to determine energy expenditure (Volume 2, Chapter 31). ☞ **Indirect calorimetry is considered as the golden standard for the measurement of metabolic rate and substrate utilization.** ☞ The measurement of inspired oxygen (O_2) and expired carbon dioxide (CO_2) are used to calculate resting energy expenditure and respiratory quotient (RQ). The RQ is the ratio of CO_2 production ($\dot{V}CO_2$) and O_2 consumption ($\dot{V}O_2$), and reflects the net substrate utilization of carbohydrate, protein, and fat. The goal of normal RQ in parenteral nutrition and TPN is to obtain mixed fuel utilization, which is demonstrated by an RQ of approximately 0.8, within the range 0.85–0.95 (7). A low RQ ≤ 0.7 indicates fat oxidation, and a high RQ (>1.0) indicates lipogenesis, which occurs with excess total calorie or carbohydrate administration (12). However, the low specificity and sensitivity of RQ may be an unreliable tool in the assessment of under- or overfeeding the critically ill patient (13).

Limitations to indirect calorimetry include inaccuracies in the measurement of gas exchange, cost, and availability of the apparatus. When indirect calorimetry is not available, the use of predictive equations is necessary to determine energy requirements.

The Harris–Benedict equation is commonly used to estimate basal energy expenditure (BEE) (14). Developed in 1919, the equation was derived from indirect calorimetry measurement of healthy men and women:

$$\text{Men:} \quad \text{BEE} = 66 + 13.8(\text{wt in kg}) + 5(\text{ht in cm}) - 6.8(\text{age})$$
$$\text{Women:} \quad \text{BEE} = 655 + 9.6(\text{wt in kg})$$
$$+ 1.8(\text{ht in cm}) - 4.7(\text{age})$$

Activity and stress factors, which add to the BEE, have also been studied (15). The overaddition of these factors may cause an overestimation of energy requirements and overfeeding (16). Therefore, hypermetabolism and nutrition requirements in critically ill patients should be carefully scrutinized, with the goal of providing adequate calories, but not overfeeding.

In general, the increases observed in metabolic rate are reported to be 110% to 120% in elective surgery and medical patients, 135% to 150% in trauma, and 150% to 170% in burns and sepsis (17–22). Comparisons between the Harris–Benedict equation and measured energy expenditure have demonstrated that these formulas only provide a good first approximation, and that actual measurements (e.g., indirect calorimetry) are required to provide conclusive caloric requirements and expenditure data. Other methods may be used to determine the adequacy of nutrition (see subsequently, and Volume 2, Chapter 31).

General recommendations for most acutely ill patients are to provide a range of 25 to 30 nonprotein calories per kilogram per day (23,24), and 1.25–2 g protein per kilogram per day (25). The caloric requirements should be individualized with respect to the degree of stress and/or sepsis, organ failure, percentage of ideal body weight (IBW) or BMI, age, pharmacological therapy, and presence of quadri- or paraplegia. IBW may be derived by using the Hamwi method. For men: 106 lb (for first 5 ft) + 6lb (for each additional inch past 5 ft). For women: 100 lb (for first 5 ft) + 5 lb (for each additional inch past 5 ft). For example, the IBW for a 6-ft 1-in male would be 106 lb + 6(13 in) = 178 lb. IBW $<90\%$ is considered underweight, $>125\%$ overweight, $>130\%$ obese, and $>150\%$ morbidly obese. The calories should be provided in the form of protein, carbohydrate, and fat as described subsequently.

Fluid Requirements

The fluid management in PN depends upon the hydration status of the patient. Solutions may be concentrated or volume expanded as necessary. In the acute care setting, supplemental IV fluids can be provided in case of dehydration or resuscitation. In terms of baseline fluid requirements, administering the equivalent milliliter of fluid as the patient's calculated basal caloric requirements generally provides the appropriate hydration (e.g., approximately 30 mL/kg/day in a 70-kg patient equals about 2.1 L of TPN solution per day).

Generally TPN orders should be written twice daily, so that changes in electrolytes or acid base status can be addressed on an every 12-hour basis, without wasting too much of the costly TPN solution. Additional fluid requirements are supplemented via additional IV fluid. In the hemodynamically stable patient, this is administered as one-half normal saline. In hemodynamically unstable patients, larger fluid volumes with higher sodium-containing formulations are utilized.

Macronutrients

Protein

☞ **The provision of adequate protein as an energy source is necessary for proper utilization of amino acids.**

Table 3   Water and Nutrient Requirements for Total Parenteral Nutrition

Water/nutrient	Per kg basis	Average amount for 70-kg patient over 24 hr
Water	4 cm^3/kg/hr (first 10 kg)	960 cm^3
	2 cm^3/kg/hr (second 10 kg)	480 cm^3
	1 cm^3/kg/hr (subsequent kg)	1200 cm^3 2640 mL/24 hr
Carbohydrate (D$_{20}$)	4–6 g/kg/min (GIR); D$_{20}$ = 200 g glucose L	2 mg/kg/min GIR
Protein	0.8–1 g/kg/day—healthy	56–70 g/day
	1–1.2 g/kg/day—mild stress	70–84 g/day
	1.2–1.5 g/kg/day—moderate stress (i.e., dialysis, trauma)	84–105 g/day
	1.5–2 g/kg/day—severe stress (i.e., CVVHD/HDF, burns)	105–140 g/day
Fat (240 mL/day, 20% intralipid)	<1 g/kg/day or <0.1 g/kg/hr	0.8 g/kg/day or 0.03 g/kg/hr

Abbreviations: CVVHD, continuous veno-venous hemodiafiltration; GIR, glucose infusion rate; HDF, hemodialysis filtration.

Healthy adults require 0.8–1.0 g of protein per kilogram per day (26).

The role of protein administration in critical illness is to decrease muscle catabolism, aid wound healing, and support/enhance immune function. Recommendations for hospitalized patients vary with disease state (Table 3). Critically ill patients without renal or hepatic dysfunction generally require ~1.5 g of protein per kilogram per day (27–29). Patients with protein-losing medical conditions such as burns, large wounds, or high, output GI fistulas may require additional protein of up to 2.0 g of protein per kilogram per day.

Patients with chronic renal failure should have their protein restricted to 0.6–0.8 g/kg/day (30). In patients who are dependent on hemodialysis or peritoneal dialysis, protein requirement may be increased from 1.2 to 1.3 g/kg/day (31,32). Patients who receive renal replacement therapy (CRRT, CVVHD, or CVVHDF) have daily protein requirements of up to 2.5 g/kg/day in order to achieve nitrogen balance due to the hypercatabolic nature of acute renal failure and protein losses during filtration (33).

In hepatic disease, protein restriction is not recommended (in the absence of encephalopathy) due to the prevalence of catabolism and malnutrition. **In acute hepatic encephalopathy, a temporary restriction of protein to 0.8 g/kg/day may be warranted (34,35).** Furthermore, patients with hepatic encephalopathy have an impaired ability to metabolize aromatic amino acids (AAAs) and may have a depressed concentration of branched chain amino acids (BCAAs). Accordingly, BCAAs should be used rather than AAAs in the case of chronic hepatic encephalopathy unresponsive to protein restriction and pharmacotherapy. BCAAs by themselves, as a specific treatment for hepatic encephalopathy, have not been shown to decrease mortality (36–39).

Currently, parenteral protein is provided as crystalline amino acids. This formulation does not promote microbial growth and has improved nitrogen balance when compared to previously used casein solutions (40). The amino acid profile is based on the recommendations of the World Health Organization (WHO) for adequate essential amino acid (EAA) proportions (41). The concentration of the solutions ranges from 2.25% to 15%. Generally, 1 g of protein provides four calories in PN solutions.

There are several modified amino acid profiles that are available for certain diseases or conditions. In renal failure, it was hypothesized that if only EAAs were provided it would result in improved urea recycling and conversion to nonessential amino acids. Studies have challenged the theory of urea recycling and have demonstrated that synthesis of all amino acids is not accomplished (42–44). Several studies have not shown improvement in renal function, catabolism, or mortality when parenteral EAAs are provided (44–47).

In sepsis and injury, exogenous BCAAs may improve protein synthesis as they are used preferentially by skeletal muscles when plasma levels are depressed. Several studies on parenteral BCAAs in critical illness have yielded varying results. Some have shown improved protein synthesis, however, mortality was not improved (48–51). The use of parenteral BCAAs is therefore controversial.

Glutamine is a conditional EAA during hypercatabolic states, such as stress, trauma, or burns (52,53). Glutamine is involved in protein synthesis, transport, and supports rapidly dividing cells such as lymphocytes and enterocytes. Glutamine is absent from commercially available parenteral feeding formulas because it is unstable, and is degraded to the toxic pyroglutamic acid when stored in aqueous solution. In experimental protocols, glutamine has been added successfully to the PN solution, and is available for parenteral use in Europe as a dipeptide. In parenteral solutions, glutamine has recently been shown to be stable, and dipeptides have been included in PN (54,55). Glutamine in EN has been shown to stimulate the gut luminal mucosa, however, in the parenteral form this has not been shown.

Several recent studies regarding parenteral supplementation of L-glutamine or L-alanyl-L-glutamine in critical illness have shown improved nitrogen balance, decreased length of stay, decreased infection, and in some studies, reduced mortality (56–63). However, not all studies have been able to replicate these results (64). The level of glutamine supplementation varied and thus the role of parenteral glutamine remains controversial.

Glutamine is absent from commercially available parenteral formulas because of its aforementioned instability and degradation to pyroglutamic acid (toxic in aqueous solution). However, parenteral glutamine is mainly useful for gut luminal nutrition when administered enterally; hence, its absence from parenteral formulas is not considered problematic. In protocol settings, glutamine may be added to parenteral solutions. Further research and development is required to consider glutamine as part of a commercially mandatory supplement in PN solution.

Carbohydrate

Within 24 hours of metabolic stress, glycogen stores in the liver and skeletal muscle are depleted. The body converts skeletal muscle protein (primarily glutamine and alanine) to glucose via gluconeogenesis to meet basal metabolic demand. The minimum requirement of glucose is 100–150 g/day to fuel the brain, renal medulla, and white and red blood cells (65). The maximum glucose utilization rate in critical illness is 5–7 mg/kg/min (66,67). ☞ **Providing carbohydrate in excess can lead to hyperglycemia, hypertriglyceridemia, and an increased RQ (>1.0).** ☞

The primary purpose of parenteral carbohydrate is to provide an energy source. The parenteral carbohydrate approved and commonly used in the United States is glucose. Parenteral glucose solutions are in the form of dextrose monohydrate, which is available in concentrations of 2.5% to 70%. A 5% dextrose solution contains 5 g/100 cm^3 or 50 g/L. ☞ **Most TPN regimens utilize ≤25% dextrose (D$_{25}$) and most PPN regimens utilize ≤10% dextrose (D$_{10}$) for safe osmolarity infusion.** ☞ One gram of dextrose provides 3.4 calories. Thus, 1 L of D$_{25}$ provides 250 g or 850 calories, and most 70-kg patients would receive about 2 L of this solution at a glucose infusion rate of 2.5 mg/kg/min (Table 3). Owing to the high osmolarity of parenteral dextrose, concentrations >10% require infusion through a central line. Other forms of carbohydrate have been studied, including fructose (68), sorbitol (which is converted to fructose), xylitol (69,70), and glycerol in traumatized patients (71,72). Alternate carbohydrate sources are not available in the United States.

Fat

Lipids in parenteral solutions provide calories and prevent essential fatty acid deficiency (EFAD). EFAD can develop in three weeks of fat-free PN. ☞ **Providing approximately 2% to 4% of total calories as linoleic acid can prevent the occurrence of EFAD (73,74).** ☞ The use of topical vegetable oils to prevent EFAD is controversial (75–78). Additional topics relating to EFAD are discussed subsequently.

The type of parenteral lipid available in the United States is composed of long-chain triglycerides (LCTs). There have been studies suggesting LCTs impair the immune system, specifically the reticuloendothelial system (RES) (79). Current recommendations are to limit lipids to 1 g/kg/day or <0.1 g/kg/hr (Table 3). Alternatively, patients can receive 25% to 30% total calories as lipids as a result of concern over the impact of immune suppression in hospitalized patients (80,81).

In the United States, parenteral lipids contain soybean and/or safflower oil, egg yolk phospholipid, and glycerol emulsifiers. The concentrations available are 10%, 20%, and 30%, with the latter available only in total nutrient admixtures. The 10% emulsion contains 1.1 calories per mL, the 20% contains 2 calories per mL, and the 30% contains 3 calories per mLl.

Owing to the impairment of the RES with LCTs, investigations into alternative lipid sources are ongoing. The "structured lipids" commonly studied are a mix of LCT and medium-chain triglycerides (82,83). Structured lipids are not commercially available in the United States. The outcomes reported are improved liver function tests, no increase in low-density lipoprotein:high-density lipoprotein cholesterol ratio, and correction of fatty acid pattern imbalance. Additional alternatives to LCTs are omega-3 fatty acids (84) and short-chain fatty acids (85).

The maximum infusion time of intralipids for 2-in-1 PN solutions should be limited to less than 12 hours as recommended by the Centers for Disease Control, due to reports of gram-negative sepsis associated with IV fat emulsions infusing for periods >12 hours (86). However, intralipids composed in TNA or 3-in-1 mixtures have decreased the risk of bacterial growth because of the low pH environment (87).

MICRONUTRIENT REQUIREMENTS
Electrolytes

Electrolytes are added to PN for maintenance or repletion. The quantity will vary depending on the clinical condition of the patient and prescribed medications. Electrolytes provided in PN are sodium, potassium, magnesium, chloride, lactate, and phosphorus. Sodium and potassium can be provided as acetate or chloride if an acid–base imbalance exists. In situations where the patient is noted to have a hyperchloremic metabolic acidosis (e.g., large diarrhea output, fistulas, or renal tubular acidosis, or iatrogenic), then acetate should be provided in larger quantity than chloride. Typically, calcium is provided as gluconate, and magnesium is provided as sulfate due to improved solubility and compatibility (88). Phosphorus may be provided as the sodium or potassium salt.

Guidelines for the quantity of electrolytes to be provided in parenteral solutions vary (Table 4). Generally, the following range of electrolytes are recommended per liter: sodium 100–150 mEq, potassium 60–120 mEq, magnesium 8–24 mEq, calcium 9–22 mEq, and phosphorus 15–30 mEq (89). A sum of less than 40 mEq/L should be used for calcium and phosphorus to prevent precipitation. Management of electrolytes should be assessed with clinical judgment. Medical situations such as renal failure, cardiac issues, hydration status, and intestinal losses should be considered.

Vitamins

The current recommendation for the vitamin solutions for PN is from the Nutrition Advisory Group of the American Medical Association (AMA) in 1975 (Table 5) (90). The recommendations were created to prevent clinically significant deficiency or toxicity. Most multivitamin preparations are formulated to meet the recommendations. The multivitamin preparation (MVI-12) was studied and found to provide adequate amounts of vitamins except for ascorbic acid in a few of the subjects (91). There has been concern over the possibility of increased vitamin requirements in critically ill or injured patients. Individual vitamin preparations are available, if needed. Parenteral multivitamin preparations are being reformulated to include vitamin K; however, currently vitamin K should be added to the parenteral solution weekly.

Trace Elements

The most commonly supplemented trace elements are zinc, chromium, manganese, selenium, and copper, based in part on 1977 AMA recommendations (Table 6) (92). Other elements may be additionally supplemented, if needed. There are commercially available trace element preparations for PN. Molybdenum is not routinely supplemented; however, there is one single case of deficiency in a patient on long-term PN (93).

Table 4   Electrolyte and Mineral Requirements for Total Parenteral Nutrition

Electrolyte	Recommended daily intake (adults)	Effects of serum deficiency	Effects of serum excess
Sodium	100–150 meq	Generalized edema, confusion, hypotension, irritability, lethargy, seizures	Decreased skin turgor, mild irritability in some cases, elevated BUN and hematocrit
Potassium	60–120 meq	Cardiac dysrhythmias (U-waves), multiple irritable dysrhythmias	Cardiac dysrhythmias (peaked T-waves), may not be able to resuscitate without calcium chloride
Chloride/acetate	100–150 meq to maintain acid/base balance	Seen in contraction alkalosis	Non-gap metabolic acidosis
Bicarbonate	Not added to PN: precipitates with calcium and magnesium; changes pH with solution	Metabolic acidosis	Metabolic alkalosis
Calcium	10–15 meq	Parasthesias, irritability, tetany, ventricular arrhythmias	Confusion, dehydration, muscle weakness, nausea, vomiting, coma
Phosphorus	400–900 mg	Muscle weakness, (muscle injury when severe), red blood cell rigidity, leftward shift in the Oxy-Hbg curve (increased O_2 affinity for oxygen and decreased release at tissues)	Parasthesias, flaccid paralysis, mental confusion, hypertension, cardiac arrythmias, soft-tissue calcification with prolonged elevated levels
Magnesium	120–240 mg	Cardiac dysrhythmias, neurological irritability (including seizures), neuromuscular irritability (including tetany)	Respiratory paralysis, hypotension, premature ventricular contractions, lethargy, cardiac arrest, coma, liver dysfunction

Abbreviations: BUN, blood urea nitrogen; Hbg, hemoglobin; PN, parenteral nutrition.

In patients with hepatic dysfunction, withholding manganese and copper may be warranted as they are excreted in bile (94–99). Iron has not been included in trace element preparations due to the potential for anaphylactic reaction. If a patient is on long-term PN and NPO, small amounts of iron dextran may be added to parenteral solutions containing amino acids and dextrose (100). There are conflicting reports on the compatibility of iron with lipid-containing parenteral solutions (101,102).

IMPLEMENTATION OF PARENTERAL NUTRITION
Initiation
Before initiation of PN, abnormal electrolytes must be corrected. Once electrolytes are within normal limits, there are a variety of ways to initiate PN. Important factors to consider are the patient's ability to tolerate fluid volume, glucose intolerance, and renal function (i.e., electrolyte status). If fluid tolerance is not known, initiation of PN with 1000 mL of fluid may be prudent. For patients without known diabetes or glucose intolerance, dextrose may be started at 200 g. If diabetes or glucose intolerance is a concern, dextrose may be restricted to 100–150 g and sliding scale regular insulin ordered with blood glucose monitored every four to six hours (67,103). ✍ **Regular insulin may then be added to the parenteral solution at one-half to two-thirds the previous day's total sliding scale insulin coverage.** ✍ As the dextrose is increased to goal, the insulin requirements will increase. If a patient is unstable, septic or otherwise physiologically stressed [common in the surgical intensive care unit (SICU) setting], a separate insulin infusion line will better

control glucose due to fluctuations from changes in clinical status. The goal range of blood glucose in the hospital setting has been recently studied (Volume 2, Chapter 60), and tighter glucose control has been observed to improve outcomes, and shown decreased rates of infection, ventilator days, renal failure, length of stay, and mortality (104–106). Current recommended goals in critically ill patients are glucose levels between 80 and 110 mg/dL (Volume 2, Chapter 60).

Amino acids may be given at goal on the first day of PN if renal function is normal, and the patient is hemodynamically stable. Lipids may also be given on the first day if serum triglycerides are less than 400 mg/dL and remain at this level after lipids are infused (107).

Advancement and Maintenance
The limits to advancing PN are hyperglycemia and fluid tolerance. If these factors are controlled, PN may be advanced on the second day. If hyperglycemia persists, the dextrose content may be increased to goal in increments as insulin is increased.

Cyclic Feeding Strategies
Cycling PN may be beneficial in stable patients on long-term support. In addition to allowing a patient time-off of an infusion pump at home, cycling can also decrease hepatic complications (108). The potential benefit is derived from mimicking the physiologic fast and feed states. Cycling usually occurs gradually over a two- to three-day period to monitor tolerance to fluid volume and glucose load (109). Patients with impaired renal, cardiac, or hepatic function may not tolerate the rapid volume infusion. Depending

Table 5 Vitamin Requirements for Total Parenteral Nutrition

Vitamin	Recommended daily Intake	Effects of serum deficiency
A	4500 IU	Infections/sepsis
Thiamine (B1)	5 mg	Wernicke's encephalopathy and Korsakoff's psychosis acidosis, inability to metabolize nutrients via Kreb cycle
Pyridoxine (B6)	6 mg	Neuropathy, dermatitis, irritability
B12	3 µg	Megaloblastic anemia, glossitis
C	50 mg	Scurvy
D	400 IU	Ricketts but exposure to sunlight recommended rather than IV vitamin D which causes bone pain and fractures
E	15 IU	Increased oxidants, and dermatitis
K	Up to 10 mg/day	Decreased vitamin K-dependent coagulation factors: II, VII, IX, X, and decreased anticoagulation factors: protein C, protein S
Folic acid	400 µg	Neuropathy, glossitis
Niacin	15 mg	Delerium, confusion, dermatitis pelagra: dark red erethema of exposed skin, cracked skin, stomatitis, diarrhea
Riboflavin	1.8 mg	Glossitis, cheilosis, pruritis, anogenital inflammation
Pantothinic acid	15 mg	Listlessness, fatigue, irritability, restlessness, malaise, sleep disturbances, nausea, abdominal cramps, vomiting, diarrhea, neuromuscular disturbances, hypoglycemia, increased insulin sensitivity
Biotin	60 µg	Anorexia, pallor, glossitis, nausea, vomiting, depression, lethargy, muscle pain, hair loss, erythematous seborrheic dermatitis, elevated bile pigments/cholesterol

Abbreviation: IV, intravenous.

on patient tolerance, PN can be cycled down to 12 hours, a one-hour taper up and down with either 50 mL or one-half of the goal infusion rate is recommended. Patients with diabetes or glucose intolerance will require slow down (at least a two-hour taper) to prevent hypoglycemia.

COMPLICATIONS
Refeeding Syndrome
Refeeding syndrome may occur in malnourished or underfed patients. Hospitalized patients at risk of refeeding syndrome are those who have sustained significant recent weight loss, been kept NPO for greater than 7 to 10 days, as well as those with chronic medical conditions, or alcoholism (110,111). **Refeeding syndrome is characterized by hypophosphatemia, hypomagnesemia, hypokalemia, and hyperinsulinemia.** Hypophosphatemia is the most frequently observed. Refeeding syndrome is the result of the body shifting from utilizing stored fat to

Table 6 Trace Element Requirements for Total Parenteral Nutrition

Trace element	Recommended daily intake	Effects of deficiency
Zinc	2–4 mg/L (catabolic)	Dermatitis, alopecia, impaired wound healing, impaired immune function, psychiatric disturbances, gonadal atrophy
	12.2 mg/L (small bowel losses)	17.7 mg/L (ileostomy or rectal losses)
Copper	300–500 µg	Anemia, demineralization of bone, vascular aneurysms
Iron	0.5–1.5 mg/day in fat-free PN in the form of iron dextran	Anemia
Selenium	50–100 µg	Cardiomyopathy, myositis, arthritis, hair, and nail changes
Chromium	10–15 µg	Glucose intolerance, peripheral neuropathy, hyperlipidemia
Manganese	2–5 mg	Bleeding disorders, impaired wound healing
Molybdenum	10–50 µg	Amino acid intolerance

Abbreviation: PN, parenteral nutrition.

carbohydrate as the primary energy source. As a result, insulin levels increase and as the body shifts to anabolism, electrolytes are consumed via intracellular pathways (112). Thiamine deficiency may contribute to the effects of refeeding syndrome. Fluid retention occurs due to hypoalbuminemia, elevated sodium levels, and carbohydrate metabolism (113,114). Signs and symptoms of refeeding syndrome may include lethargy, weakness, edema, respiratory depression, and cardiac dysrhythmias.

Reducing the occurrence of refeeding syndrome should be considered in patients at risk of developing symptoms. It is ideal to correct electrolyte imbalances prior to initiating nutritional support. Patients with a history of alcoholism should receive vitamin repletion including supplemental thiamine (115). The patient's actual weight should be used in determining calorie and protein requirements. In addition, energy goals for PN should be achieved over the course of several days. When PN is initiated, additional phosphorus, magnesium, and potassium may be added to the solution. During advancement of PN, electrolytes, fluid volume status, and the general condition of the patient should be monitored closely.

Glycemic Control
Difficulty in managing glucose levels is frequently encountered during PN. Critical illness and stress may compound the problem. Hypoglycemia and, more frequently, hyperglycemia can occur.

Hyperglycemia is a common complication of PN. The causes include stress, insulin resistance or diabetes, steroids, infection, organ failure, and high dextrose concentrations. ☞ **Morbidity and mortality are affected by untreated or poorly treated hyperglycemia (Volume 2, Chapter 60), therefore controlling glucose is a priority (104–106).** ☞ If a patient is a known diabetic, or has elevated glucose values prior to initiation of PN, sliding scale regular insulin and blood glucose monitoring should be started. If a patient has normal glucose values, monitoring blood glucose changes for the first three days of PN may be prudent. The use of insulin drips in the ICU or monitored setting may be beneficial in achieving tight control.

Hypoglycemia is a complication of PN when exogenous insulin is provided in excess of need. Symptoms include dizziness, impaired vision, diaphoresis, headache, and confusion. If a patient has labile glucose values, an insulin drip may improve glucose control. When insulin is added to the parenteral solution, caution should be used in determining the quantity. Insulin adsorbs to glass bottles, polyvinyl chloride bags, and tubing used for PN infusion and therefore, insulin requirements may be increased and bring a challenge to excellent blood sugar control (116). Insulin availability may be increased when a combination of MVIs and trace elements are present in the PN solution (117). Changes in medical condition or medications, such as resolution of an infection or tapering of steroids, should be monitored. Whenever PN is discontinued or cycled, insulin infusion should be likewise turned down. Tapering the PN solution for one to two hours may prevent rebound hypoglycemia. When unplanned interruptions in PN infusion occur, administering a dextrose-containing IV fluid such as dextrose 10% at the same rate for up to four hours may prevent hypoglycemia from abrupt termination of the high dextrose infusion.

Essential Fatty Acid Deficiency

The occurrence of EFAD with PN in the United States is primarily the result of allergic reactions to IV lipids, or in patients with a contraindication for lipids for several weeks both resulting in lipid-free solutions. In hospitalized, stressed patients, reports of EFAD occurred in one to three weeks (75,76). In stable patients, EFAD may occur within one month (78). The symptoms include dermatitis, alopecia, poor wound healing, increased platelet aggregation, increased capillary fragility, and hepatic dysfunction (118).

Providing 2% to 4% total calories as fat prevents EFAD. There are reports of using topical vegetable oils to correct EFAD, however the results varied (75–78). If EFAD is suspected as a result of lipid-free PN for >1 month, assessing fatty acid status should be completed. A sensitive diagnostic indicator is the triene:tetraene ratio (119). A ratio above 0.4 indicates EFAD.

Hepatic Dysfunction

The hepatic dysfunction that develops during PN is multifactorial, contributes to morbidity, and it is not well understood. With long-term PN, in particular, there exists a pattern of hepatic dysfunction and potentially hepatic failure. Laboratory abnormalities develop in succession, initially with aspartate animotransferase, then alkaline phosphatase (AP), and finally with bilirubin (120). Malnourished patients reveal an early rise in AP in addition to cholestasis (121). The incidence of laboratory abnormalities varies from 25% to 100% (122). Both intrahepatic and extrahepatic

abnormalities and complications may occur. Generally, the pathophysiology is reversible after the discontinuation of PN. When long-term PN is given with a modest amount of macronutrients and a minimal amount of fat emulsions, abnormal liver enzymes are common, but severe liver dysfunction is unusual (123).

The most common and earliest intrahepatic complication from PN in adults is steatosis (124). Steatosis can occur as early as five to seven days after the initiation of PN with elevation of liver enzymes with in the first three weeks. The causes may include EFAD, choline deficiency, carnitine deficiency, glutamine deficiency, bacterial translocation, and excessive caloric or carbohydrate provision.

The development of cholestasis is more common in infants than adults. Cholestasis generally follows steatosis if PN is not discontinued. Other risk factors for cholestasis include sepsis, EFAD, particular amino acid deficiencies, and length of time on PN. The pathogenesis in adults is unknown.

Although treatment for hepatic dysfunction remains under investigation, there are proposed options for reducing the risk and potentially reversing steatosis and cholestasis. Cycling PN may improve laboratory values and resolve hepatomegaly (108). Providing PN over a shorter duration of time allows for the conversion to fat oxidation, which promotes lipid mobilization and transport (125–127). The addition of a lipid emulsion to PN in place of carbohydrates has decreased the incidence of hepatic dysfunction (128), and it allows one to avoid excessive caloric or dextrose loads. Modifying the amino acid content to include taurine may be beneficial, especially in pediatric PN (129–131). Supplementing PN with choline (132,133), glutamine (134,135), and/or carnitine (136) have been proposed as treatment options for hepatic steatosis. Choline may be mandatory for the synthesis of lipoproteins used in triglyceride transport from the liver to peripheral locations (137). Glutamine may minimize hepatic fat uptake and increase alanine flow through the portal route, thereby promoting ideal hepatic metabolism. Carnitine supplementation (1 g/day for home PN patients) has not shown improvement in steatosis although carnitine deficiency has been proposed as a possible cause of steatosis (136). Of course any amount of enteral feeding, if possible, may decrease hepatic dysfunction (138).

Micronutrient Deficiencies

Once PN tolerance of macronutrients is established, the daily focus of management shifts to electrolyte balance, and potential deficiencies of electrolytes, vitamins, and minerals. In critical illness, deficiencies may occur due to GI losses, organ dysfunction, surgery, injury, and certain medications. Increased need for zinc due to GI losses should be considered (Table 6) (12). In long-term PN, there have been reports of vitamin and mineral deficiencies. This became apparent during the nationwide multivitamin shortage when several cases of thiamine deficiency and death were reported (139,140). In addition, reports of selenium deficiency due to long-term, selenium-free PN were documented (141,142). Clinical judgment and laboratory values should be used to prevent or treat potential deficiencies in patients who are at risk.

NUTRITION MONITORING

When initiating PN support, the patient's baseline nutritional status should be evaluated, and the ongoing nutritional adequacy must be monitored and assured. Volume 2, Chapter 31 covers this topic in greater detail, but it will be briefly discussed here in general terms. A simple and relatively inexpensive way to evaluate nutritional status is to measure serum proteins. The most common proteins that are measured include albumin (half-life = 21 days), transferrin (half-life = 8–9 days), and prealbumin (half-life = 2–3 days) (143).

The most accurate reflection of a critically ill patient's current nutritional state is obtained from the prealbumin level. Of course, multiple factors can impact on the concentration of these proteins including resuscitation, hemoglobin level, and degree of liver failure. Accordingly, following the trend of these proteins in addition to the absolute value is most beneficial. It is optimal to institute standard protocols for obtaining monitoring of nutritional status; for example, every Monday and Thursday, so that the level of progress can be assessed. If the albumin, transferrin, and prealbumin levels have increased, this represents a positive trend and the nutritional plan should be maintained. If the trend is negative or improvement continues at a slow rate, one must reassess the nutritional needs in order to determine an alternative plan to reverse the negative trend. In addition to prealbumin levels, triglyceride levels and liver function enzymes should be monitored on a weekly basis. Triglyceride levels of <250 mg/dL after four hours and <400 mg/dL after continuous infusion are acceptable (144). If levels remain elevated, providing intralipids of 250 mL two to three times weekly to prevent EFAD is appropriate. An increased trend of liver function enzymes may suggest the need for cycling PN, decreasing macronutrient concentrations, and minimizing trace elements to zinc, chromium, and selenium (see subsequently for more information).

SPECIAL DISEASE STATES AND PARENTERAL NUTRITION

Disease processes such as diabetes, renal failure, and hepatic failure present special concerns and considerations for PN. Tailoring the parenteral prescription for each individual is vital when meeting nutrient needs.

Diabetes Mellitus

Diabetes mellitus (DM), one of the most common but devastating metabolic diseases, affects more than 16 million Americans. Diabetes is marked by abnormal glucose metabolism, insulin deficiency, and/or irregular insulin response which cause short- and long-term consequences that include hyperglyceridemia, hyperlipidemia, obesity, heart disease, retinopathy, nephropathy, and vascular damage. Appropriate glucose control is imperative for patients with DM due to risk for catheter infection, wound healing, and mortality. Conservative action may be taken when formulating macronutrient composition. ☞ **Maximum glucose infusion rate for nondiabetic patients may be 4–6 mg/kg/min.** ☞ This rate allows peripheral glucose uptake to be maximized and hepatic glucose production to be minimized (66). As mentioned earlier, dextrose in the initial PN infusion may be limited to 100–150 g (103). Once glucose levels are stable and less than 200 mg/dL, dextrose content may be increased by 50–75 g/day. Close attention and adjustments should also be made for outside sources of dextrose (i.e., dextrose intravenous piggybacks and dextrose absorbed from dialysate). In addition, lipid infusion of less than or equal to 30% of nonprotein calories is safe and may decrease exogenous insulin requirements.

Sliding scale insulin is adequate for stable floor patients on PN if blood glucose levels are >140 mg/dL, and one-third to one-half of the previous day's sliding scale insulin dose may be subsequently added to the parenteral bag. For critically ill DM patients, intensive insulin therapy managed with an insulin drip is usually the best choice to achieve glucose between 80 and 110 mg/dL, hence decreasing risk of sepsis, condensing antibiotic therapy, decreasing mechanical ventilation dependence, reducing endogenous glucose production, and further preventing lean body catabolism (106,145). Improved glucose tolerance has been reported in populations with chromium deficiency receiving chromium-supplemented PN solutions. Thus, strong clinical suspicion should accompany any decision to supplement above currently recommended levels (146).

Renal Failure

Renal failure rapidly causes nutritional imbalances, thereby shifting a patient to a hypercatabolic state. Hypercatabolism in patients with renal failure may be due to inadequate use of nutrients, increased production of catabolic factors, drug therapy, protein losses via dialysis membrane, and toxic-related symptoms such as nausea, vomiting, and anorexia. Renal failure patients in the ICU challenge the entire health team because these patients are in negative nitrogen balance, and the presence of infection intensifies their underlying malnutrition (147,148). PN may be indicated for the renal failure patients who do not tolerate enteral support. Nutrition therapy varies with both the presence of dialysis and type of dialysis [i.e., hemodialysis (HD), CVVHD, peritoneal dialysis (PD)]. Benefits of commercially available renal parenteral formulations have been controversial because patients with renal failure are highly variable based on their renal function, hypermetabolism, and hypercatabolism (45,47,149). ☞ **Despite the increased need for macro- and micronutrients, supplementing trace minerals in the parenteral solution for patients with renal failure must be carefully evaluated.** ☞ Moreover, trace mineral excretion is minimal in CVVHD (150).

Hepatic Failure

Hepatic failure results in a number of different metabolic dysfunctions, such as the ability to metabolize ammonia into urea thereby triggering hepatic encephalopathy. The specific etiological factors related to HD that result in hepatic failure have not been clearly identified; however, they may be associated with increased dietary protein intake, GI bleeding, infections, electrolyte imbalances, surgical procedures, and drugs (151,152). PN support is appropriate for hepatic failure patients who cannot receive enteral support due to active GI hemorrhage or small-bowel obstruction. Central PN is preferred over peripheral because less volume is required to provide adequate calories and protein. According to Plauth et al. (153), parenteral amino acids are less likely to precipitate encephalopathy, however, most patients will accept standard tube-feeding formulas (refer to Volume 2, Chapter 32). Abnormal amino acid profiles have been present under conditions of hepatic encephalopathy: AAA (i.e., tyrosine, tryptophan, and phenylalanine) levels are elevated, whereas BCAA (i.e., isoleucine, valine, and leucine) levels are depressed. Significant liver dysfunction may be seen in patients with a molar ratio of BCAA: AAA of 1.4:2.0 and those encephalopathic patients with a ratio ≤1.0 (144). Five of the nine randomized controlled studies reviewed in a meta-analysis by Naylor et al.

(39) showed significant improvement in mental recovery from acute encephalopathy with parenteral BCAA formulation and a significant decrease in mortality. However, due to mortality differences and short-term follow-up time among trials, the authors concluded that using parenteral BCAA over standard therapy is not suggested. ☞ **Most hepatic encephalopathy patients suffer from protein-calorie malnutrition and have been supported with standard solutions under careful awareness of protein intake.** ☞ HepatAmine® (B. Braun, Irvine, California, U.S.A.) is the only modified amino acid solution that contains high amounts of BCAA versus AAA and should be reserved for patients who have refractory HE. Strict criteria should be implemented to prevent the inappropriate use of hepatic parenteral formula which is more costly than standard solutions. As with renal failure, trace element supplementation (especially copper and manganese) should be minimized to prevent hepatic toxicity.

EYE TO THE FUTURE

In future research, two areas of focus that are particularly interesting include the use of PN as an enteral growth stimulant and as a cancer-inhibitory factor. Glucagon-like peptide-2 (GLP-2) is an intestinal trophic enteroendocrine peptide that is associated with intestinal adaptation following resection. Martin et al. (154) demonstrated that GLP-2 alone in PN, without enteral feeding, stimulated indices of intestinal adaptation in an animal study. Further studies are warranted to establish the mechanisms of action and therapeutic potential of GLP-2 in animal studies prior to the initiation of human studies.

Jordan et al. examined the effects of a fish oil (FO)-based lipid emulsion rich in omega-3 fatty acids, which is used in humans as a component of PN, on the growth of the colon cancer cell line Caco-2. The authors concluded that FO has a potent antiproliferative effect on Caco-2 cells, at least in part due to a decrease in the progression of the cell cycle and the induction of apoptosis. The combination of FO with 5-fluorouracil resulted in an additive growth inhibitory effect (155).

Dipeptide glutamine and alanyl-glutamine parenteral supplementation helped improve nutrition status (weight, plasma proteins, urinary accumulated creatinine, and nitrogen retention) in rats and may be a helpful supplementation in critically ill patients with moderate or severe stress (156). PN support has been shown to preserve body protein composition for patients with severe acute pancreatitis who are unable to meet nutritional needs solely on EN (157). Patients suffering from severe GI diseases and with irreversible intestinal failure have been supported with long-term PN. Small-bowel transplantation, in addition to development of immunosuppressant medication, has been a life-saving procedure for those who can no longer be maintained on PN.

The growth of digestive disease and intestinal rehabilitation centers in collaboration with new techniques and phenomena such as gut trophic factors, natural additives, small-bowel transplantation, restorative surgery, and PN have helped the specific patient population receive the safest and physiologically appropriate treatment while improving quality of life.

SUMMARY

Over the past 100 years, there has been significant advancement in the field of nutrition, in which PN has clearly been one of the most significant. Indirect calorimetry has become the golden standard for energy assessment and nutritional requirements. However, serum proteins still play a major role in the daily clinical practice of nutrition providers. Although there are complications of PN, the benefits clearly outweigh them for patients that cannot tolerate enteral feeds.

Continuing nutrition assessment and monitoring should be practiced in order to potentially wean patients from PN support and begin trophic enteral or oral feeds (Volume 2, Chapters 31 and 32). The three macronutrients of PN, such as carbohydrates, proteins, and fats, should be individualized based on the patient's medical condition and adjusted regularly. Vitamins and minerals should be supplemented and reviewed for appropriateness in order to prevent deficiency, toxicity, and help meet metabolic needs. Lastly, the best PN prescription may be accomplished by proactive efforts made by each health-care team player.

KEY POINTS

- As TPN solutions are hyperosmolar, a large-diameter vein with adequate flow rate is required to allow for rapid dilution of TPN products within the vessel.
- The preferred site of central venous catheter placement for PN is the subclavian vein.
- Indirect calorimetry is considered as the golden standard for the measurement of metabolic rate and substrate utilization.
- The provision of adequate protein as an energy source is necessary for proper utilization of amino acids. Healthy adults require 0.8–1.0 g of protein per kilogram per day (26).
- In acute hepatic encephalopathy, a temporary restriction of protein to 0.8 g/kg/day may be warranted (34,35).
- Glutamine is a conditional EAA during hypercatabolic states, such as stress, trauma, or burns (52,53).
- Providing carbohydrate in excess can lead to hyperglycemia, hypertriglyceridemia, and an increased RQ (>1.0).
- Most TPN regimens utilize ≤25% dextrose (D_{25}), and most PPN regimens utilize ≤10% dextrose (D_{10}) for safe osmolarity infusion.
- Providing approximately 2% to 4% of total calories as linoleic acid can prevent the occurrence of EFAD (73,74).
- Regular insulin may then be added to the parenteral solution at one-half to two-thirds the previous day's total sliding scale insulin coverage.
- Refeeding syndrome is characterized by hypophosphatemia, hypomagnesemia, hypokalemia, and hyperinsulinemia.
- Morbidity and mortality are affected by untreated or poorly treated hyperglycemia (Volume 2, Chapter 60), therefore controlling glucose is a priority (104–106).
- Maximum glucose infusion rate for nondiabetic patients may be 4–6 mg/kg/min.
- Despite the increased need for macro- and micronutrients, supplementing trace minerals in the parenteral solution for patients with renal failure must be carefully evaluated.
- Most hepatic encephalopathy patients suffer from protein-calorie malnutrition and have been supported with standard solutions under careful awareness of protein intake.

REFERENCES

1. Fohn O, Denis W. Protein metabolism from the standpoint of blood and tissue analysis: absorption from the large intestine. J Biol Chem 1912–1913; 12:253.
2. Henriques V, Andersen AC. Uber parenterale Ernahrung durch intravenose Injektion. Zeit Physiol Chem 1913; 88: 357–678.
3. Seibert FF. Fever producing substances found in some distilled water. Am J Physiol 1923–1924; 67:90.
4. Elman R, Weiner DO. Intravenous alimentation with special reference to protein (amino-acid) metabolism. J Am Med Assoc 1939; 112:796.
5. Dudrick SJ, Wilmore DW, Vars HM. Long-term total parenteral nutrition with growth in puppies and positive nitrogen balance in patients. Surg Forum 1967; 18:356.
6. Braunschweig, Carol L. Enteral compared with parenteral nutrition: a meta-analysis. Am J Clin Nutr 2001; 74:534–542.
7. Mirtallo F. Introduction to parenteral nutrition. In: Gottschlich M, ed. The Science and Practice of Nutrition Support. Kendal Hunt Publishing 2001:211–224.
8. The Veteran Affairs Total Parenteral Nutrition Cooperative Study Group. Perioperative nutrition in surgical patients. N Engl J Med 1991; 325(8):525–532.
9. Dickerson RN, Brown RO, White KG. Parenteral nutrition solutions. In: Rombeau JL, Caldwell MD, eds. Parenteral Nutrition. 2nd ed. Philadelphia: WB Saunders, 1993:310–333.
10. Isaacs JW, Millikan WJ, Stackhouse J, et al. Parenteral nutrition of adults with a 900 milliosmolar solution via peripheral veins. Am J Clin Nutr 1977; 30:552–559.
11. Conly JM, Grieves K, Peters B. A prospective, randomized study comparing transparent and dry gauze dressings for central venous catheters. J Infect Dis 1989; 159(2):310–319.
12. Wolman SL, Anderson GH, Marliss EB, Jeejeebhoy KN. Zinc in total parenteral nutrition: requirements and metabolic effects. Gastroenterology 1979; 76:458–467.
13. McClave SA, Lowen CC, Kleber MJ, McConnell JW, Jung LY, Goldsmith LJ. Clinical use of the respiratory quotient obtained from indirect calorimetry. J Parenter Enter Nutr 2003; 27:21–26.
14. Harris JA, Benedict FG. Biometric Studies of Basal Metabolism in Man. Publication No. 270. Washington, DC: Carnegie Institution of Washington, 1919.
15. Long CL, Schaffel N, Geiger JW, et al. Metabolic response to injury and illness: estimation of energy and protein needs from indirect calorimetry and nitrogen balance. J Parenter Enter Nutr 1979; 3:815–818.
16. Frankenfield D. Energy dynamics. In: Matarese LE, Gottschlich MM, eds. Contemporary Nutrition Support Practice: A Clinical Guide. Philadelphia: WB Saunders, 1998:79–95.
17. Frankenfield DC, Wiles CE, Bagley S, Siegel JH. Relationships between resting and total energy expenditure in injured and septic patients. Crit Care Med 1994; 22:1796–1804.
18. Weissman C, Kemper M, Danask MC, et al. Effect of routine intensive care interactions on metabolic rate. Chest 1984; 86:815–818.
19. Fredrix EW, Soesters PB, von Meyenfeldt MF, et al. Resting energy expenditure in cancer patients before and after gastrointestinal surgery. J Parenter Enter Nutr 1991; 15:604–607.
20. Mann S, Westenshkow DR, Houtchens BA. Measured and predicted caloric expenditure in the acutely ill. Crit Care Med 1985; 13:173–177.
21. Boulanger BR, Nayman R, McClean RF, et al. What are the clinical determinants of early energy expenditure in critically injured adults? J Trauma 1994; 37:969–974.
22. Kreymann G, Grosser S, Buggisch P, et al. Oxygen consumption and resting metabolic rate in sepsis, sepsis syndrome, and septic shock. Crit Care Med 1993; 21:1012–1019.
23. Hunter DC, Jaksik T, Lewis D, et al. Resting energy expenditure in the critically ill: estimations versus measurement. Br J Surg 1998; 75:875–878.
24. National Advisory Group on Standards and Practice Guidelines for Parenteral Nutrition. Special Report: safe practices for parenteral nutrition formulations. J Parenter Enter Nutr 1998; 22:49–66.
25. Jacobs DG, Jacobs DO, Kudsk KA, et al. Practice management guidelines for nutritional support of the trauma patient. J Truama 2004; 57:660–679.
26. National Research Council. Recommended Daily Allowances. 10th ed. Washington, DC: National Academy Press, 1989:3.
27. Cerra FB, Blackburn G, Hirsh J, et al. The effect of stress level, amino acid formula, and nitrogen dose on nitrogen retention in traumatic and septic stress. Ann Surg 1987; 205:282–287.
28. Shaw JF, Wild bore M, Wolfe RR. Whole body protein kinetics in severely septic patients: the response to glucose infusion and total parenteral nutrition. Ann Surg 1987; 205:288–294.
29. Shaw JF, Wolfe RR. Whole body protein kinetics in patients with early and advanced gastrointestinal cancer: the response to glucose infusion and total parenteral nutrition. Surgery 1988; 103:148–155.
30. K/DOQI, National Kidney Foundation. Clinical practice guidelines for nutrition in chronic renal failure. Am J Kidney Dis 2000; 35:S1–S140.
31. Ikizler TA, Flankoll PF, Parker RA, et al. Amino acid and albumin losses during hemodialysis. Kidney Int 1994; 46:830–837.
32. Blumenkrantz MJ, Gahl GM, Kopple JD, et al. Protein losses during peritoneal dialysis. Kidney Int 1981; 19:593–602.
33. Scheinkestel CD, et al. Prospective randomized trial to assess caloric and protein needs of critically ill patients with acute renal failure. J Parenter Enter Nutr 1996; 20:56.
34. Nompleggi DJ, Bonkovsky HL. Nutritional supplementation in chronic liver disease: an analytical review. Hepatology 1994; 19:518–533.
35. Mullen KD, Weber FL. Role of nutrition in hepatic encephalopathy. Semin Liver Dis 1991; 11:292–304.
36. Erikkson LS, Conn HO. Branched-chain amino acids in the management of hepatic encephalopathy: an analysis of variants. Hepatology 1989; 10:228–246.
37. Rossi-Fanelli F, Riggio O, Cangiano C, et al. Branched-chain amino acids vs lactulose in the treatment of hepatic coma: a controlled study. Dig Dis Sci 1982; 27:929–935.
38. Wahren J, Denis J, Desurmont P, et al. Is intravenous administration of branched chain amino acids effective in the treatment of hepatic encephalopathy? A multicenter study. Hepatology 1983; 3:475–480.
39. Naylor CD, O'Rourke K, Detsky AS, Baker JP. Parenteral nutrition with branched-chain amino acids in hepatic encephalopathy: a meta-analysis. Gastroenterology 1989; 97:1003–1042.
40. Goldmann EA, Martin WT, Worthington JW. Growth of bacteria and fungi in total parenteral nutrition solutions. Am J Surg 1973; 126:314–318.
41. WHO (World Health Organization): Energy and protein requirements: Report of a joint FAO/WHO/UNU expert consultation. Technical Report Series 724. WHO: Geneva, 1985.
42. Ell S, Fynn M, Richards P, Halliday D. Metabolic studies with keto acid diets. Am J Clin Nutr 1978; 31:1776–1783.
43. Long C, Jeevanandam M, Kinney JM. Metabolism and recycling of urea in man. Am J Clin Nutr 1978; 31:1367–1382.
44. Richards P. Nutritional potential of nitrogen recycling in man. Am J Clin Nutr 1972; 25:615–625.
45. Feinstein EI, Blumenkrantz MJ, Healy M, et al. Clinical and metabolic responses to parenteral nutrition in acute renal failure: a controlled, double-blind study. Medicine 1981; 60:124–137.
46. Feinstein EI, Kopple JD, Silberman H, Massry SG. Total parenteral nutrition with high or low nitrogen intakes in patients with acute renal failure. Kidney Int 1983; 26:319–323.
47. Mirtallo JM, Schneider PJ, Mavko K, et al. A comparison of essential and general amino acid infusions in the nutritional support of patients with compromised renal function. J Parenter Enter Nutr 1982; 6:109–113.
48. Bower RH, Muggia-Sullam M, Vallgren S, et al. Branched-chain amino acid-enriched solutions in the septic patient: a randomized, prospective trial. Ann Surg 1986; 203:13–20.
49. Chiarla C, Siegel J, Kidd S, et al. Inhibition of posttraumatic septic proteolysis and ureagenesis and stimulation of hepatic acute-phase protein production by branched-chain amino acid TPN. J Trauma 1988; 28:1145–1172.

50. Kuhl DA, Brown RO, Vehe KL, et al. Use of selected visceral protein measurements in the comparison of branched-chain amino acids with standard amino acids in parenteral nutrition in injured patients. Surgery 1990; 107:503–510.

51. von Meyenfeldt MF, Soeters PB, Vente JP, et al. Effect of branched chain amino acid enrichment of total parenteral nutrition of nitrogen sparing and clinical outcome of sepsis and trauma: a prospective randomized double blind trial. Br J Surg 1990; 77:924–929.

52. Lacey JM, Wilmore DW. Is glutamine a conditionally essential amino acid? Nutr Rev 1990; 48:297–309.

53. Souba WW, Smith RJ, Wilmore DW. Glutamine metabolism by the intestinal tract. J Parenter Enter Nutr 1985; 9:608–617.

54. Hornsby-Lewis L, Shike M, Brown P, et al. L-Glutamine supplementation in home total parenteral nutrition patients: stability, safety, and effects on intestinal absorption. J Parenter Enter Nutr 1994; 18:268–273.

55. Lowe DK, Benefell K, Smith RJ, et al. Safety of glutamine-enriched parenteral nutrient solutions in humans. Am J Clin Nutr 1990; 52:1101–1106.

56. Stehle P, Zander J, Mertes N, et al. Effect of parenteral gluta-mine peptide supplements on muscle glutamine loss and nitro-gen balance after major surgery. Lancet 1898; 1:231–233.

57. Hammarqvist F, Wernerman J, Ali R, et al. Addition of gluta-mine to total parenteral nutrition after elective abdominal surgery spares free glutamine in muscle, counteracts the fall in muscle protein synthesis, and improves nitrogen balance. Ann Surg 1989; 209:455–461.

58. Ziegler TR, Young LS, Benfell K, et al. Clinical and metabolic efficacy of glutamine-supplemented parenteral nutrition after bone marrow transplantation: a randomized, double-blind controlled study. Ann Intern Med 1992; 116:821–828.

59. Morlion BJ, Stehle P, Wachtler P, et al. Total parenteral nutrition with glutamine dipeptide after major abdominal surgery: a randomized, double-blind, controlled study. Ann Surg 1998; 227:302–308.

60. Mertes N, Schulzki C, Goeters C, et al. Cost containment through L-alanyl-L-glutamine supplemented total parenteral nutrition after major abdominal surgery: a prospective ran-domized double-blind controlled study. Clin Nutr 2000; 19:395–401.

61. Jian ZM, Cao JD, Zhu XG, et al. The impact of alanyl-glutamine on clinical safety, nitrogen balance, intestinal permeability, and clinical outcome in postoperative patients: a randomized, double-blind, controlled study of 120 patients. J Parenter Enter Nutr 1999; 23:S62–S66.

62. Griffiths RD, Jones J, Palmer MD. Six-month outcome of criti-cally ill patients given glutamine-supplemented parenteral nutrition. Nutrition 1997; 13:295–302.

63. Goeters CG, Wenn A, Mertes N, et al. Parenteral L-alanyl-L-glutamine improves 6-month outcome in critically ill patients. Crit Care Med 2002; 30:2032–2037.

64. Powell-Tuck J, Jamieson CP, Bettany GEA, et al. A double blind randomized, controlled trial of glutamine supplementation in parenteral nutrition. Gut 1999; 45:82–88.

65. McMahon MM. Glucose vs. lipid as a calorie source. In: Pro-ceedings of the ASPEN 19th Clinical Congress, Miami, January 15–18, 1995. Silver Spring, MD: American Society for Parenteral and Enteral Nutrition, 1995.

66. Wolfe RR, O'Donnell TF Jr, Stone MD, et al. Investigation of factors determining the optimal glucose infusion rate in total parenteral nutrition. Metabolism 1980; 29:892–900.

67. Michael SR, Sabo CE. Management of the diabetic patient receiving nutritional support. Nutr Clin Pract 1989; 4:179–183.

68. Fryburg DA, Gelfand RA. Is exogenous fructose metabolism truly insulin independent? J Parenter Enter Nutr 1990; 14:535–537.

69. Georgieff M, Moldawer LL, Bistrian BR, Blackburn GL. Xylitol, an energy source for intravenous nutrition after trauma. J Parenter Enter Nutr 1985; 9:199–209.

70. Karlstad MD, DeMichele SJ, Bistrian BR, Blackburn GL. Effect of total parenteral nutrition with xylitol on protein and energy metabolism in thermally injured rats. J Parenter Enter Nutr 1991; 15:445–449.

71. Singer P, Bursztein S, Kirvels O, et al. Hypercaloric glycerol in injured patients. Surgery 1992; 112:509–514.

72. Waxman K, Day AT, Stellin GP, et al. Safety and efficacy of glycerol and amino acids in combination with lipid emulsion for peripheral parenteral nutrition support. J Parenter Enter Nutr 1992; 16:374–378.

73. Barr LH, Dunn GD, Brennan MF. Essential fatty acid deficiency during total parenteral nutrition. Ann Surg 1981; 193:304–311.

74. McCarthy MC. Nutritional support in the critically ill surgical patient. Surg Clin North Am 1991; 71:831–841.

75. McCarthy MC, Turner WW, Whatley K, Cottam GL. Topical corn oil in the management of essential fatty acid deficiency. Crit Care Med 1983; 11:373–375.

76. Sacks GS, Brown RO, Collier P, Kudsk KA. Failure of topical vegetable oils to prevent essential fatty acid deficiency in a critically ill patient receiving long-term parenteral nutrition. J Parenter Enter Nutr 1994; 18:274–277.

77. Clemans GW, Yamanaka W, Flournoy N, et al. Plasma fatty acid patterns of bone marrow transplant patients primarily supported by fat-free parenteral nutrition. J Parenter Enter Nutr 1981; 5:221–225.

78. Miller DG, Williams SK, Palombo JD, et al. Cutaneous appli-cation of safflower oil in preventing essential fatty acid deficiency in patients on home parenteral nutrition. Am J Clin Nutr 1987; 46:419–423.

79. Kinsella JE, Lokesh B. Dietary lipids, eicosanoids and the immune system. Crit Care Med 1990; 18:S94–S113.

80. Siedner DL, Mascioli EA, Istfan MW, et al. Effects of long-chain triglyceride emulsions on reticulothelial system function in humans. J Parenter Enter Nutr 1989; 13:614–619.

81. Jensen GL, Mascioli EA, Seidner DL, et al. Parenteral infusion of long- and medium-chain triglycerides and reticulothelial system function in man. J Parenter Enter Nutr 1990; 14:467–471.

82. Hyltander A, Sandstrom R, Lundholm K. Metabolic effects of structured triglycerides in humans. Nutr Clin Pract 1995; 10:91–97.

83. Baldermann H, Wicklmayr M, Rett K, et al. Changes of hepatic morphology during parenteral nutrition with lipid emulsions containing LCT or MCT/LCT quantified by ultrasound. J Parenter Enter Nutr 1991; 15:601–603.

84. Morlion BJ, Torwesten E, Lessire H, et al. The effect of parent-eral fish oil on leukocyte membrane fatty acid composition and leukotriene-synthesizing capacity in patients with postopera-tive trauma. Metabolism 1996; 45:1208–1213.

85. Tappenden KA, Thomson AB, Wild GE, McBurney MI. Short-chain fatty acid-supplemented total parenteral nutrition enhances functional adaptation to intestinal resection in rats. Gastroenterology 1997; 112:792–802.

86. Brown DH, Simkover RA, Maximum hang times for i.v. fat emulsions. Am J Hosp Pharm 1987; 44:282.

87. Gilbert M, Gallagher SC, Eads M, Elmore MF. Microbial growth patterns in a total parenteral nutrition formulation containing lipid emulsion. J Parenter Enter Nutr 1986; 10:494.

88. Henry RS, Jurgens RW, Sturgeons R, Athanikar AN. Compat-ibility of calcium chloride and calcium gluconate with sodium phosphate in a mixed TPN solution. Am J Hosp Pharm 1980; 37:673–674.

89. Matarese LE, ed. Nutrition Support Handbook, Cleveland: Cleveland Clinic Foundation, Departments of General Surgery and Hospital Pharmacy, 1997:52.

90. Nutrition Advisory Group. Guidelines for essential trace elements preparations for parenteral use. A statement by the Nutrition Advisory Group. American Medical Association. JPEN 1979; 3(4):263–267.

91. Shils ME, Baker H, Frank O. Blood vitamin levels of long-term adult home total parenteral nutrition patients: the efficacy of the AMA-FDA parenteral multivitamin formulation. J Parenter Enter Nutr 1985; 9:179–188.

92. American Medical Association Department of Foods and Nutrition. Guidelines for essential trace element preparations for parenteral use. J Am Med Assoc 1979; 241:2051–2054.
93. Fleming CR. Trace element metabolism in adult patients requiring total parenteral nutrition. Am J Clin Nutr 1989; 49:573–579.
94. Hambidge KM, Sokol RJ, Fidanza SJ, et al. Plasma manganese concentrations in infants and children receiving parenteral nutrition. J Parenter Enter Nutr 1898; 13:168–171.
95. Mehta R, Reilly JJ. Manganese levels in jaundiced long-term total parenteral nutrition patient: potentiation of haloperidol toxicity? J Parenter Enter Nutr 1990; 14:428–430.
96. Ejima A, Imamura T, Nakamura S, et al. Manganese intoxication during total parenteral nutrition. Lancet 1992; 339:426.
97. Taylor S, Manara AR. Manganese toxicity in a patient with cholestasis receiving total parenteral nutrition. Anaesthesia 1994; 49:1013.
98. Fredstrom S, Rogosheske J, Gupta P, Burns LJ. Extrapyramidal symptoms in a BMT recipient with hyperintense basal ganglia and elevated manganese levels. Bone Marrow Transplant 1995; 15:989–992.
99. Albina JE, Melnik G. Fluid, electrolytes and body composition. In: Rombeau JL, Caldwell MD, eds. Clinical Nutrition: Parenteral Nutrition. 2nd ed. Philadelphia: WB Saunders, 1993: 132–149.
100. Kwong KW, Tsallas G. Dilute iron dextran formulation for addition to parenteral nutrient solutions. Am J Hosp Pharm 1990; 47:1745–1746.
101. Vaughan LM, Small C, Plunkett V. Incompatibility of iron dextran and total nutrient admixture. Am J Hosp Pharm 1990; 47:1745–1746.
102. Tu YH, Knox NL, Biringer JM, et al. Compatibility of iron dextran with total nutrient admixture. Am J Hosp Pharm 1992; 49:2233–2235.
103. McMahon M, Manji N, Driscoll DF, Bistrian BR. Parenteral nutrition in patients with diabetes mellitus: theoretical and practical considerations. J Parenter Enter Nutr 1989; 13(5):545–553.
104. Finney SJ, Zekveld C, Elia A, Evans TW. Glucose control and mortality in critically ill patients. J Am Med Assoc 2003; 290:2041–2047.
105. Van den Berghe G, Wouters PJ, Bouillon R, et al. Outcome benefit of intensive insulin therapy in the critically ill: insulin dose versus glycemic control. Crit Care Med 2003; 31:359–366.
106. Van den Berghe G, Wouters P, Weekers F, et al. Intensive insulin therapy in the critically ill patients. N Engl J Med 2001; 345:1359–1367.
107. Adamkin DH, Gelke KN, Andrews BF. Fat emulsions and hypertriglyceridemia. J Parenter Enter Nutr 1984; 8:563–567.
108. Maini B, Blackburn GL, Bistrian BR, et al. Cyclic hyperalimentation: an optimal technique for preservation of visceral protein. J Surg Res 1976; 20:515–525.
109. Bennett KM, Rosen GH. Cyclic total parenteral nutrition. Nutr Clin Pract 1990; 5:163–165.
110. Solomon SM, Kirby DF. The refeeding syndrome: a review. J Parenter Enter Nutr 1990; 14:90–97.
111. Brooks M, Melnik G. The refeeding syndrome: an approach to understanding its complications and preventing its occurrence. Pharmacotherapy 1995; 15:713–726.
112. Jolly AF, Blank R. Refeeding syndrome. In: Zaloga GP, ed. Nutrition in Critical Care. St. Louis: Mosby, 1994:765–782.
113. McClave SA, Short AF, Mattingly DB, Fitzgerald PD. Total parenteral nutrition: conquering the complexities. Postgrad Med 1990; 88:235–248.
114. Apovian CM, McMahon MM, Bistrian BR. Guidelines for refeeding the marasmic patient. Crit Care Med 1990; 18:1030–1033.
115. Gloria L, Cravo M, Camilo ME, et al. Nutritional deficiencies in chronic alcoholics: relation to dietary intake and alcohol consumption. Am J Gastroenterol 1997; 92:485–489.
116. Weber SS, Wood WA, Jackson EA. Availability of insulin from parenteral nutrient solutions. Am J Hosp Pharm 1977; 34(4): 353–357.
117. Christianson MA, Schartz MW, Suzuki N. Determinants of insulin availability in parenteral nutrition solutions. J Parenter Enter Nutr 2006; 30:6–9.
118. Stegink LD, Freeman JB, Wispe J, Connor WE. Absence of the biochemical symptoms of essential fatty acid deficiency in surgical patients undergoing protein sparing therapy. Am J Clin Nutr 1977; 30:388–393.
119. Holman RT. Essential fatty acid deficiency. In: Holman RT, ed. Progress in the Chemistry of Fats and Other Lipids. Vol. 9, Part 2. New York: Pergamon Press, 1971:275–348.
120. Tayek JA, Bistrian B, Sheard NF, et al. Abnormal liver function in malnourished patients receiving total parenteral nutrition: a prospective randomized study. J Am Coll Nutr 1990; 9:76–83.
121. Leaseburge LA, Winn NJ, Schloerb PR. Liver test alterations with total parenteral nutrition and nutritional status. J Parenter Enteral Nutr 1992; 16:348–352.
122. Clarke PJ, Ball MJ, Kettlewell MGW. Liver function tests in patients receiving parenteral nutrition. J Parenter Enter Nutr 1991; 15:54–59.
123. Salvino R, Ghanta R, Seidner DL. Liver failure is uncommon in adults receiving long-term parenteral nutrition. J Parenter Enter Nutr 2006; 30:202–208.
124. Quigley EMM, Marsh MN, Shaffer JL, Markin RS. Hepatobiliary complications of total parenteral nutrition. Gastroenterology 1993; 104:286–301.
125. Just B, Messing B, Darmaun D, et al. Comparison of substrate utilization by indirect calorimetry during cyclic and continuous total parenteral nutrition. Am J Clin Nutr 1990; 51:107–111.
126. Lerebours E, Rimbert A, Hecketsweiler B, et al. Comparison of the effects of continuous and cyclic nocturnal parenteral nutrition on energy expenditure and protein metabolism. J Parenter Enter Nutr 1988; 12:360–364.
127. Messing B, Pontal PJ, Bernier JJ. Metabolic study during cyclic total parenteral nutrition in adult patients with and without corticosteroid-induced hypercatabolism: comparison with standard total parenteral nutrition. J Parenter Enter Nutr 1983; 7:21–25.
128. Buchmiller CE, Kleinman-Wexler RL, Ephgrave KS, et al. Liver dysfunction and energy source: results of a randomized clinical trial. J Parenter Enter Nutr 1993; 17:301–306.
129. Belli DC, Roy CC, Fournier LA, et al. The effect of taurine on the cholestatic potential of sulfated lithocholate and its conjugates. Liver 1991; 11:162–169.
130. Guertin F, Roy CC, Lepage G, et al. Effect of taurine on total parenteral nutrition-associated cholestasis. J Parenter Enter Nutr 1991; 15:247–251.
131. Dorvil NP, Yousef IM, Tuchweber B, et al. Taurine prevents cholestasis induced by lithocholic acid sulfate in guinea pigs. Am J Clin Nutr 1983; 37:221–232.
132. Buchman AL, Dubin M, Jenden D, et al. Lecithin increases plasma free choline and decreases hepatic steatosis in long-term total parenteral nutrition patients. Gastroenterology 1992; 102:1363–1370.
133. Buchman AL, Dubin MD, Moukarzel AA, et al. Choline deficiency: a cause of hepatic steatosis during parenteral nutrition that can be reversed with intravenous choline supplementation. Hepatology 1995; 22:1399–1403.
134. Li SJ, Nussbaum MS, McFadden DW, et al. Addition of L-glutamine to total parenteral nutrition and its effects on portal insulin and glucagons and the development of hepatic steatosis in rats. J Surg Res 1990; 48:421–426.
135. Grant JP, Snyder PJ. Use of L-glutamine in total parenteral nutrition. J Surg Res 1988; 44:506–513.
136. Bowyer BA, Miles JM, Haymond MW, Fleming CR. L-Carnitine therapy in home parenteral nutrition patients with abnormal liver tests and low plasma carnitine concentrations. Gastroenterology 1988; 94:434–438.
137. Shronts EP. Essential nature of choline with implication for total parenteral nutrition. J Am Diet Assoc 1997; 97:639–649.
138. Zamir O, Nussbaum MS, Bhadra S, et al. Effect of enteral feeding on hepatic steatosis induced by total parenteral nutrition. J Parenter Enter Nutr 1994; 18:20–25.

139. Oriot D, Wood C, Gottesman R, Huault G. Severe lactic acidosis related to thiamine deficiency. J Parenter Enter Nutr 1991; 15:105–109.

140. Barrett TG, Forsyth JM, Nathavitharana KA, Booth IW. Potentially lethal thiamine deficiency complicating parenteral nutrition in children. Lancet 1993; 341:901.

141. Lane HW, Lotspeich CA, Moore CE, et al. The effect of selenium supplementation on selenium status of patients receiving chronic total parenteral nutrition. J Parenter Enter Nutr 1987; 11:177–182.

142. Cohen HJ, Brown MR, Hamilton D, et al. Glutathione peroxidase and selenium deficiency in patients receiving home parenteral nutrition: time course for development of deficiency and repletion of enzyme activity in plasma and blood cells. Am J Clin Nutr 1989; 49:132–139.

143. Schlictig T, Ayres S. Nutritional Support of the Critically Ill. Chicago: Year Book Medical Publishers, 1988:78–79.

144. Guidelines for the use of parenteral and enteral nutrition in adult and pediatric patients. J Parenter Enteral Nutr 1993; 17(4):1SA–52SA.

145. Thorell A, Rooyackers O, Myrenfors P, et al. Intensive insulin treatment in critically ill trauma patients normalizes glucose by reducing endogenous production. J Clin Endocrinol Metab 2004; 89(11):5382–5386.

146. Anderson RA, Polansky M, Bryden NA, Canary J. Supplemental chromium effects on glucose, insulin, glucagons, and urinary chromium losses in subjects consuming controlled low chromium diets. Am J Clin Nutr 1991; 54(5): 909–916.

147. Butler B. Nutritional management of catabolic renal failure requiring renal replacement therapy. Am Nephrol Nurses Assoc 1991; 3(18):247–259.

148. Wolk R, Swartz R. Nutritional support of patients with acute renal failure. Nutr Support Serv 1986; 2(6):38–46.

149. Freund HR, Atamian S, Fischer JE. Comparative study of parenteral nutrition in renal failure using essential and nonessential amino acid containing solution. Surg Gynecol Obstet 1980; 151:652.

150. Pasko DA, Btaiche IF, Jain JC, Mueller BA. Trace element clearance in critically ill patients treated with continuous venovenous hemodiafiltration (CVVHDF). Blood Purif 2006; 24:247–273.

151. Sherlock S, Dooley J. Hepatic encephalopathy. In: Schiff ER, Sorrell MF, Maddrey WC, eds. Schiff's Diseases of the Liver. Vol. 1, 8th ed. Philadelphia: Lippincott-Raven, 1999:545–581.

152. Sherlock S, Dooley J. Hepaic encephalopathy. In: Sherlock S, Dooley J, eds. Diseases of the Liver and Biliary System. 10 ed. Oxford: Blackwell, 1997:87–102.

153. Plauth M, Roske AE, Romaniuk P, et al. Post-feeding hyperammonemia in patients with transjugular intrahepatic portosystemic shunt and liver cirrhosis: role of small intestinal ammonia release and route o nutrient administration. Gut 2000; 46(6):849–855.

154. Martin GR, Wallace LE, Sigalet DL. Glucagon-like peptide-2 induces intestinal adaptation in parenterally fed rats with short bowel syndrome. Am J Physiol Gastrointest Liver Physiol 2004; 286(6):G964–972.

155. Joradan A, Stein J. Effect of an omega-3 fatty acid containing lipid emulsion alone and in combination with 5-fluorouracil (5-FU) on growth of the colon cancer cell line Caco-2. Eur J Nutr 2003; 42(6):324–331.

156. Ortiz de Urbina JJ, Jorquera F, Culebras JM. Effects of parenteral nutrition supplemented with alanyl-glutamine on nutrition status in rats. J Parenter Enteral Nutr 2005; 29: 262–265.

157. Chandrasegaram MD, Plank, KD, Windsor JA. The impact of parenteral nutrition on the body composition of patients with acute pancreatitis. J Parenter Enteral Nutr 2005; 29:65–73.

34

Abdominal Compartment Syndrome

Devashish J. Anjaria

Division of Trauma, Burns, and Critical Care, Department of Surgery, UC San Diego Medical Center, San Diego, California, U.S.A.

David B. Hoyt

Department of Surgery, UC Irvine Medical Center, Irvine, California, U.S.A.

HISTORY AND INTRODUCTION

Compartment syndrome is defined as a "condition in which increased pressure in a confined anatomical space adversely affects the circulation and threatens the function and viability of the tissues therein" (1). Compartment syndromes have been traditionally described to occur within the closed fascial spaces of the extremities. However, in the past 20 years the term has been appropriately extended to include the abdomen. Although the term abdominal compartment syndrome (ACS) was first used by Kron et al. (2) in 1984, the pathophysiology of elevated intra-abdominal pressure (IAP) has been recognized for nearly a century. This review of ACS represents an organizational summation of the factors that have been recognized over that duration to cause critically elevated IAP causing morbidity and mortality.

In 1876, Wendt (3) described the reduction of urinary blood flow which occurs in response to elevated IAP (4). Emerson (5) was the first to describe the cardiovascular derangements associated with elevated IAP in 1911. Although intra-abdominal hypertension (IAH) was shown to increase mortality in animal models by the late nineteenth century, it was the fashioning of a rudimentary ventilatory support device that allowed Emerson to do his work (6). Since that time, the effects of elevated IAP on nearly every organ system have been described. The classic presentation remains the "high-risk" patient with decreasing urinary output and increasing peak inspiratory pressures.

In the late 1940s and early 1950s, pediatric surgeons attempting to repair omphaloceles and gastroschisis discovered that although primary repair was possible, there was a high mortality rate, and these neonates usually died of acute respiratory failure (7,8). These were the first descriptions of ACS in children. By the late 1960s, the need for a staged reduction of abdominal contents was described by Allen and Wrenn (9) with the creation of plastic silos or chimneys, which allowed for temporary abdominal closure (TAC) until the loss of abdominal domain could be overcome. This is the basis for modern decompressive laparotomies with TAC.

With the evolution of laparoscopy in the 1970s, the cardiovascular effects of elevated IAP on patients was increasingly recognized, observed, and further characterized in animal models (10–12). In 1984, with this foundation already laid, Kron coined the term, ACS. In addition, he described an easy, reproducible method for measurement of IAP, and the successful treatment of ACS with decompressive laparotomy (2). After this report, there has been a plethora of literature describing and characterizing the etiology, diagnosis, and pathophysiology of ACS.

ETIOLOGY

With improved understanding and recognition of ACS, the reported etiologies have become increasingly varied (Table 1). ☛ **Because of the numerous etiologies, a high index of suspicion is required to consider the diagnosis of ACS.** ☛ Despite the disparate etiologies, a simple unifying classification scheme has been developed. The initial classifier is the rapidity with which the process develops (acute or chronic). In the acute setting, IAH/ACS is further subclassified as a primary abdominal process (1° ACS), or secondary to accumulation of "third space" fluid; as occurs with massive resuscitation secondary to capillary leak without a primary abdominal process (2° ACS). Regardless of the etiology, if the diagnosis of acute ACS is made, prompt treatment must be undertaken to minimize the morbidity and mortality associated with this condition. Because of this, the recognition and increasing incidence of acute ACS have paralleled the evolution of damage control surgery (Volume 1, Chapter 21) first described in 1983 by Stone et al. (13). Individuals with chronic IAH have had time for the abdomen to accommodate and therefore are usually compensated; however, this baseline IAH may become exacerbated in the setting of acute illness.

Acute Intra-abdominal Hypertension

A rapid rise in IAP, over hours, which does not allow for accommodation by the abdominal wall results in acute IAH. With progressively increasing IAP, patients have the physiological consequences of IAH which cause progression to ACS. A grading system has been proposed and prospectively evaluated by Meldrum et al. (14) as shown in Table 2. Although this is useful in considering IAH as mild, moderate, or severe, the absolute cutoffs used in creation of the grading scale are somewhat arbitrary. The transition from IAH to ACS is a continuum which is dependent upon many factors including the etiology of the IAH, medical condition of the patient, and the physiological response to the IAH. The exact incidence of ACS in all patients is not known given the wide variety of etiologies. A prospective study reviewing all trauma patients admitted to the intensive care unit (ICU) at the University of Miami

Table 1 Etiologies of Intra-abdominal Hypertension

Timing and categorization	Etiology
Acute primary	
Intraperitoneal origin	Intraperitoneal hemorrhage (137)
	Blunt hepatic trauma (127)
	Bowel obstruction (138)
	Ileus (139)
	Acute gastric dilation (46)
	Pneumoperitoneum (38)
	Abdominal packing (140)
	Abscess (141)
	Ascites (125)
	Visceral edema (137)
	Mesenteric revascularization (142)
	Transplant kidney (143)
Retroperitoneal origin	Pancreatitis (133)
	Pelvic or retroperitoneal hemorrhage (134)
	Contained abdominal aortic aneurysm rupture (107,135)
	Abscess (136)
Abdominal wall	Rectus sheath hematoma (144,145)
	Burn eschar (146)
	MAST trousers (147)
	Repair of large hernia with loss of domain (140)
	Repair of gastroschisis or omphalocele (148)
	Laparotomy closure under extreme tension
Acute secondary	Burns (19)
	Significant nonabdominal trauma (20,149)
Chronic	Obesity (29,150)
	Ascites (122)
	Pregnancy (151)
	Large abdominal tumors (121)
	Peritoneal dialysis (152)

Abbreviation: MAST, military anti-shock trousers.

found that of 706 patients, 15 (2%) developed IAH. Of these 15, six patients (40%) progressed to ACS with derangement of physiologic parameters, reversed by abdominal decompression (15). A patient with initially mild IAH (grade I) can rapidly progress into severe (grades III and IV) ACS; therefore, in the high-risk patient frequent re-evaluation is indicated. Given the morbid consequences of IAH and ACS, it is better to treat more aggressively if in doubt.

Table 2 Treatment of Intra-abdominal Hypertension/Abdominal Compartment Syndrome Based on Grade

Grade	Bladder pressure (mmHg)	Recommended treatment
I	10–15	Maintain normovolemia
II	16–25	Hypervolemic resuscitation
III	26–35	Decompression
IV	>35	Decompression and re-exploration

Source: From Ref. 14.

Primary

As the name suggests, primary ACS is an acute process with an intra-abdominal etiology. The majority of patients seen with ACS will fall into this category. In the trauma setting, hemorrhage (intra-abdominal, retroperitoneal, or pelvic) is the most common etiology. In the severely injured, this sets the stage for shock with massive resuscitation of crystalloid and blood products, which in turn leads to acidosis, hypothermia, and coagulopathy, also known as the "triarchy of death." This is the setting in which trauma surgeons developed the concept of damage control surgery, as these patients are at very high risk of developing ACS. The abdomens of these patients are often edematous and unable to be closed without developing IAH; in this setting TAC should be employed. Indeed, every patient requiring an abbreviated or damage control laparotomy must be considered at increased risk of developing ACS. In a study examining patients who underwent damage control surgery, 37% subsequently developed ACS requiring decompression (16). This is significantly greater than the 2% incidence in all trauma patients admitted to the University of Miami ICU (15). This disparity underscores the reason why many consider the need for damage control surgery and the likelihood of developing of ACS linked. A prospective study examining the risk factors for developing ACS following trauma found that shock requiring significant crystalloid resuscitation, acidosis, hypothermia, and anemia were all independent predictors of primary ACS (Table 3) (17). Similarly, another study found that a protocol for supranormal resuscitation which required administration of larger quantities of crystalloid and blood products resulted in a higher than conventional resuscitation, and an increased incidence of IAH and ACS (18).

In the general surgery patient, a multitude of etiologies can lead to the development of ACS. Devastating intra-abdominal catastrophes are the most common cause (e.g., ruptured aortic aneurysm, significant intra-abdominal infection/peritonitis, severe pancreatitis, bowel obstruction). Similar to the trauma patient, many of these can be predicted at the primary laparotomy with the observation of visceral edema, and an abdomen that would be difficult to close, necessitating TAC. As in the trauma patient, when initial closure in a high-risk patient is possible, diligent re-evaluation is required to avoid missing the development of ACS.

Secondary

Although occurring less frequently, ACS is also seen in the absence of abdominal trauma or pathology and is referred to as secondary ACS. A very common setting is the patient with significant extra-abdominal trauma or burns, requiring significant volumes of crystalloid and blood resuscitation, resulting in visceral and retroperitoneal edema and ascites (19,20). Studies examining this subgroup of acute ACS patients reveal that treatment with decompression reversed the immediate physiological consequences of IAH (21). However, Maxwell et al. (22) found the overall incidence of secondary ACS was 0.5% (6 in 1216 surgical ICU patients) with an overall mortality of 67%. While examined for mortality based on etiology, there was 38% mortality for trauma patients and 100% mortality for nontrauma patients with the development of secondary ACS (21). However, centers which use supranormal resuscitation [goal to maintain oxygen delivery index ($\dot{D}O_2I$) $\geq$600 mL/min m^2] have shown that this results in a significantly increased incidence of IAH and ACS (18,23). This is because to achieve supranormal

Table 3 Independent Predictors of Abdominal Compartment Syndrome in Trauma Patients During Initial Emergency Department Resuscitation and Subsequent 24 Hours in the Intensive Care Unit

ACS category	Emergency department		Intensive care unit	
	Independent predictor	Odds ratio	Independent predictor	Odds ratio
All ACS	Crystalloid $\geq$ 3 L	23	$GAP_{CO_2} \geq 16$	>999.9
	SBP <86	4.9	Crystalloid $\geq$ 7.5 L	166.2
			UO $\leq$ 150 mL	89.8
			Hb $\leq$ 8 g/dL	252.5
			CI $\leq$ 2.6 L/min/m^2	12.5
1° ACS	To OR $\leq$ 75 min	102.7	$GAP_{CO_2} \geq 16$	54.3
	Crystalloid $\geq$ 3 L	69.8	Temperature $\leq$ 34°C	22.9
			Hb $\leq$ 8 g/dL	206.1
			BD $\geq$ 12 meq/L	3.5
2° ACS	Crystalloid $\geq$ 3 L	15.8	$GAP_{CO_2} \geq 16$	>999.9
	No urgent surgery	0.3	Crystalloid $\geq$ 7.5 L	38.7
	PRBC $\geq$ 3 units	5.6	UO $\leq$ 150 mL	64.1

Abbreviations: ACS, abdominal compartment syndrome; BD, base deficit; Hb, hemoglobin; CI, cardiac index; GAP_{CO_2}, gastric regional carbon dioxide; OR, operating room; UO, urine output; PRBC, packed red blood cell; SBP, systolic blood pressure.
Source: From Ref. 17.

resuscitation, significantly greater volumes of crystalloid and blood resuscitation are required. In another study, independent predictors of secondary ACS were found to include significant crystalloid or blood requirement and shock, as measured by gastric tonometry (Table 3) (17).

Chronic

With the increasing awareness of the effects and multifactorial prevalence of IAH, it was recognized that chronic conditions could produce IAH and in the proper setting ACS. Examples of conditions that can cause chronic IAH include morbid obesity, ascites, large abdominal tumors, peritoneal dialysis, and pregnancy. Chronic conditions result in slow increases in IAP which are compensated by increasing compliance of the abdominal wall (24). Therefore, these patients usually do not experience the acute deterioration seen with ACS. Despite this, chronic IAH is not benign, as some of the morbidity associated with these conditions is secondary to IAH. For example, some of the ventilatory dysfunction as well as pseudotumor cerebri seen in patients with morbid obesity have been linked to chronic elevation of IAP (25–27). Most importantly, some of these morbidities can be ameliorated by successful therapy (e.g., surgical treatment of morbid obesity, delivery of fetus) (6,28,29).

DIAGNOSIS
Clinical Features

Depending on the clinical scenario, the onset and presentation of IAH and ACS can range from insidious to expected. This means that diagnosis of ACS often requires a high index of suspicion, because if missed, the consequences can be disastrous, priming the patient for multiple organ failure or even death. Therefore, it would be beneficial to predict which patient is at a higher risk for the development of ACS. McNelis et al. (30) looked at a cohort of surgical ICU patients who developed ACS and found that using multivariate analysis only 24-hour fluid balance and an elevated peak airway pressure were correlated with the development of ACS. The elevated peak airway pressure is usually a side

effect and not the primary cause of ACS. However, a high peak airway pressure can contribute to IAH. A predictive equation was created to estimate the risk of ACS based upon the 24-hour fluid balance, $P = 1/(1 + e^{-z})$, where $z = -6.7291 + 0.005$ (net 24-hr fluid balance). Looking at trauma patients, as they are at the highest risk of developing ACS, factors as early as three hours postinjury can predict the development of ACS (17). Independent predictors of ACS are listed in Table 3. Markers indicating a need for significant crystalloid resuscitation, hypoperfusion, and need for urgent/emergent surgery (more likely to be damage control) are seen as independent risk factors for the development of ACS.

In a patient with IAH progressing to ACS, the first signs are decreasing urinary output, respiratory failure, and decreased lung compliance, reflected as an elevation in peak airway pressure. However, even with this clinical suspicion, physical examination has a minimal role in the diagnosis of IAP or ACS, as studies looking at physical examination have shown poor sensitivities and specificities. Looking prospectively at abdominal girth, there is a poor correlation ($R^2 = 0.12$) between abdominal girth and IAP (31). This is because there can be significant increase in IAP without significant changes in girth. Palpation of the abdomen has also been shown to have a sensitivity of 40% in diagnosing ACS (32,33). Therefore, when the possibility of IAH or ACS exists, "if you don't measure IAP you cannot make a diagnosis of IAH or ACS" (34).

Measurement of Intra-abdominal Pressure

☞ **Because of the limitations of clinical examination in diagnosing ACS, measurement of IAP is essential to making the diagnosis.** ☞ The abdomen is normally a compliant cavity with minimal pressure. Although overdistended, the compliance decreases and the abdomen becomes a fixed compartment which is relatively noncompressible. The contents of the abdomen can be considered fluid and therefore is subject to Pascal's law (34). Therefore, IAP can be measured in almost every part of the abdomen, resulting in the myriad of techniques described for IAP measurement. Normally, IAP is equal to atmospheric or subatmospheric pressure with spontaneous respiration (6,35). In a study examining hospitalized patients with indwelling bladder catheters, the mean IAP was 6.5 mmHg, with a range of 0.2–16.2 mmHg (35). With positive pressure ventilation, IAP is nearly equal to end expiratory pressure with positive end expiratory pressure (PEEP) (36).

Direct Intra-abdominal Catheter Placement

Earlier experiments used either a metal cannula/wide-bore needle or catheter directly inserted into the peritoneal cavity connected to a pressure transducer for measurement of IAP (12,37). The only modern application of direct IAP measurement is that of real-time IAP measurement during laparoscopic surgery (38). The direct measures of IAP were largely abandoned in the mid-1980s, and replaced by indirect techniques once IAP measurements began to be obtained frequently for clinical purposes and used as a criterion for abdominal decompression (2).

Inferior Vena Cava Pressure

A central venous catheter placed via the femoral route can be used to measure pressure in the inferior vena cava. This pressure has good correlation with IAP measured either by direct measurement or urinary bladder pressure (39,40). This method carries the risks of central venous catheters including thrombosis and infection. However to date, no human studies have validated its use prospectively in the setting of ACS.

Gastric Pressure

Intragastric pressure can be used as a measure of IAP. A nasogastric or gastrostomy tube is placed and the stomach instilled with 50–100 mL of water. The proximal end is held perpendicular to the floor or attached to a pressure transducer with the mid-axillary line being used as the zero point (41). Alternatively, a balloon catheter can be placed on the tip of a nasogastric tube with measurement of the balloon pressure as a surrogate to IAP still using the mid-axillary line as a zero point (42). Human studies show correlation between gastric pressure and urinary bladder pressure. No large series have validated the use of this technique in the setting of a patient with suspected ACS. However, this may be a valid alternative for measurement of IAP in patients with bladder trauma in whom bladder distension may be contraindicated.

Urinary Bladder Pressure

✐ **Despite the variety of methods described for measurement of IAP, the gold standard continues to be urinary bladder pressure.** ✐ Originally described by Kron et al. (2), the urinary bladder pressure technique requires a supine patient with an indwelling Foley catheter (Fig. 1). After complete drainage of urine, the bladder is instilled with 50–100 mL of sterile saline to form a continuous column of fluid (without distending the bladder which might cause detrussor spasm). The tubing of the drainage bag is clamped and a 16-gauge needle is inserted through the aspiration port while connected to a pressure transducer or water manometer. The zero reference for the transducer is the pubis symphysis. Many variations on this original technique have been described to eliminate the need for a needle or repeated breaks of the sterile urinary drainage system; however, the basic principle of using a column of fluid to conduct intravesicular pressure which correlates to IAP

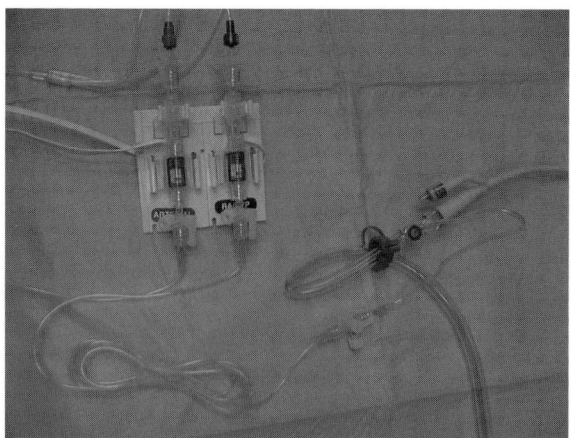

Figure 1   Setup for measurement of urinary bladder pressure.

has not changed (43–46). Critics of this method cite the potential errors from using a fluid-filled transduction system, loss of accurate urinary output measurement, and the risks of infection by breaking a sterile system (34). Despite this, urinary bladder pressure has become the gold standard due to its relative ease of measurement, minimal invasiveness, reproducibility, and the wealth of literature validating its use.

Other Measurements of Intra-abdominal Pressure

Literature describes the use of fluid balloons or open catheters with slow continuous flow for transduction of rectal or uterine pressures as a surrogate for measuring IAP (34,40,47,48). These are more difficult with no validation in the ICU setting and therefore have no clinical implications at this time. Work has also been done to evaluate microchip-tipped catheters as a source of continuous real-time IAP measurement which could be introduced by any of the above mentioned routes (49). Although this may be promising in the future, currently these catheters are expensive, not readily available, and have not been validated for use in the clinical arena.

PATHOPHYSIOLOGY

The physiological consequences of IAH and ACS are almost as numerous as the etiologies which cause it. ✐ **Renal dysfunction is the most common presentation, however the morbidity of ACS is not limited to intra-abdominal organs, and has the potential to effect nearly every major system.** ✐ The pathophysiological implications of IAH/ACS on the most commonly impaired organ systems are summarized in Figure 2 (50). ✐ **Most of the pathophysiologic effects of ACS are reversible, making early diagnosis and prompt treatment imperative.** ✐

Renal

The classical effect of IAH/ACS on the renal system is oliguria progressing to anuria with increasing IAP (39,51,52). ✐ **An IAP of 15–20 mmHg may result in oliguria, while IAP greater than 30 mmHg can lead to anuria.** ✐ The mechanism of renal dysfunction is multifactorial. ACS results in cardiovascular derangements including decreased cardiac output (Q̇) (as discussed subsequently), decreased renal arterial

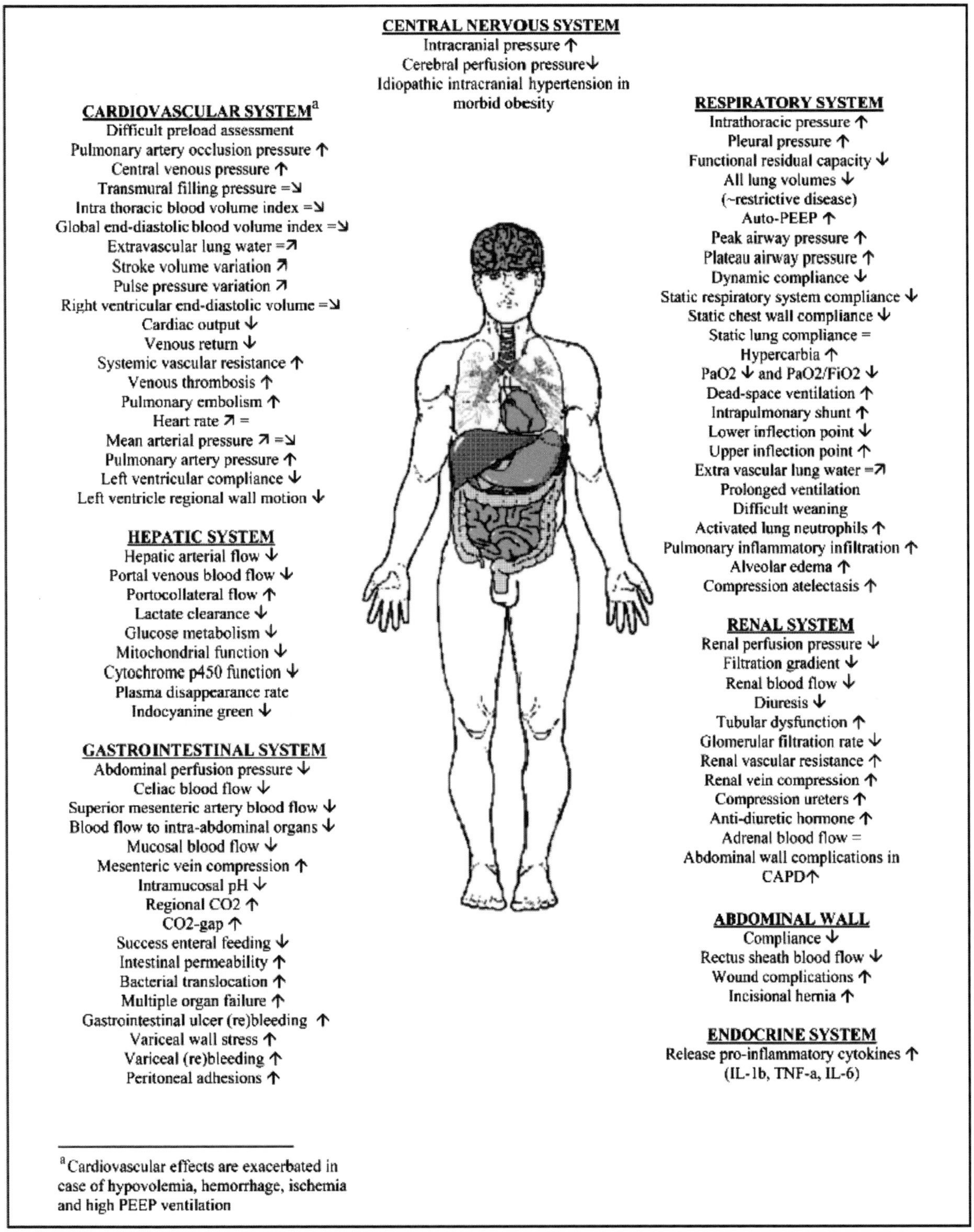

CENTRAL NERVOUS SYSTEM
Intracranial pressure ↑
Cerebral perfusion pressure ↓
Idiopathic intracranial hypertension in morbid obesity

CARDIOVASCULAR SYSTEM[a]
Difficult preload assessment
Pulmonary artery occlusion pressure ↑
Central venous pressure ↑
Transmural filling pressure =↘
Intra thoracic blood volume index =↘
Global end-diastolic blood volume index =↘
Extravascular lung water =↗
Stroke volume variation ↗
Pulse pressure variation ↗
Right ventricular end-diastolic volume =↘
Cardiac output ↓
Venous return ↓
Systemic vascular resistance ↑
Venous thrombosis ↑
Pulmonary embolism ↑
Heart rate ↗ =
Mean arterial pressure ↗ =↘
Pulmonary artery pressure ↑
Left ventricular compliance ↓
Left ventricle regional wall motion ↓

HEPATIC SYSTEM
Hepatic arterial flow ↓
Portal venous blood flow ↓
Portocollateral flow ↑
Lactate clearance ↓
Glucose metabolism ↓
Mitochondrial function ↓
Cytochrome p450 function ↓
Plasma disappearance rate
Indocyanine green ↓

GASTROINTESTINAL SYSTEM
Abdominal perfusion pressure ↓
Celiac blood flow ↓
Superior mesenteric artery blood flow ↓
Blood flow to intra-abdominal organs ↓
Mucosal blood flow ↓
Mesenteric vein compression ↑
Intramucosal pH ↓
Regional CO2 ↑
CO2-gap ↑
Success enteral feeding ↓
Intestinal permeability ↑
Bacterial translocation ↑
Multiple organ failure ↑
Gastrointestinal ulcer (re)bleeding ↑
Variceal wall stress ↑
Variceal (re)bleeding ↑
Peritoneal adhesions ↑

RESPIRATORY SYSTEM
Intrathoracic pressure ↑
Pleural pressure ↑
Functional residual capacity ↓
All lung volumes ↓
(~restrictive disease)
Auto-PEEP ↑
Peak airway pressure ↑
Plateau airway pressure ↑
Dynamic compliance ↓
Static respiratory system compliance ↓
Static chest wall compliance ↓
Static lung compliance =
Hypercarbia ↑
PaO2 ↓ and PaO2/FiO2 ↓
Dead-space ventilation ↑
Intrapulmonary shunt ↑
Lower inflection point ↓
Upper inflection point ↑
Extra vascular lung water =↗
Prolonged ventilation
Difficult weaning
Activated lung neutrophils ↑
Pulmonary inflammatory infiltration ↑
Alveolar edema ↑
Compression atelectasis ↑

RENAL SYSTEM
Renal perfusion pressure ↓
Filtration gradient ↓
Renal blood flow ↓
Diuresis ↓
Tubular dysfunction ↑
Glomerular filtration rate ↓
Renal vascular resistance ↑
Renal vein compression ↑
Compression ureters ↑
Anti-diuretic hormone ↑
Adrenal blood flow =
Abdominal wall complications in CAPD ↑

ABDOMINAL WALL
Compliance ↓
Rectus sheath blood flow ↓
Wound complications ↑
Incisional hernia ↑

ENDOCRINE SYSTEM
Release pro-inflammatory cytokines ↑
(IL-1b, TNF-a, IL-6)

[a] Cardiovascular effects are exacerbated in case of hypovolemia, hemorrhage, ischemia and high PEEP ventilation

Figure 2 Pathophysiology of end-organ dysfunction secondary to intra-abdominal hypertension. *Abbreviations*: CAPD, long term ambulatory peritoneal dialysis; IL, interleukin; PEEP, positive end-expiratory pressure; TNF-α, tumor necrosis factor α. *Source*: From Ref. 50.

flow, increased renal vascular resistance, decreased glomerular filtration, and compression of the renal vein (51,53,54). All these factors contribute to the pathophysiology because maintenance of a normal or supranormal Q with resuscitation in the face of IAH, renal dysfunction persists, and only corrects after abdominal decompression (39). In addition, the decreased glomerular filtration secondary to arterial, venous, and direct parenchymal compression results in the elaboration of antidiuretic hormone, rennin, and aldosterone. This compensatory endocrine response further contributes to the clinical renal dysfunction in ACS (55). Compression of the ureter has been ruled out as a potential etiology as stenting of the ureters has not improved renal function (39,56).

Pulmonary

☞ **The pulmonary dysfunction resulting from IAH is secondary to elevation of bilateral hemidiaphragms in response to the pressure (57).** ☞ This results in secondary compression atelectasis, creating a potential for pulmonary infections and barotrauma. However, more importantly, this results in a reduction in the pulmonary compliance with increasing peak inspiratory pressures seen in patients with volume control ventilation (58). This also results in a reduction of the functional residual capacity, total lung capacity, and residual volume (25,59). Similarly, patients receiving pressure control ventilation will have smaller tidal volumes generated by the same driving pressure. Studies have shown that the overall decreased compliance of the respiratory system is due primarily to decreased compliance of the thoracic cavity and not due to a change in the compliance of the lung itself (60). These changes manifest as hypoventilation, ventilation-perfusion mismatch, and eventual hypercarbia hypoxia (43,57,59). This also causes increased vascular resistance (61).

The elevated IAP results in a direct elevation of intrathoracic pressure (62). To counteract the effects, increased ventilatory pressures and specifically increased PEEP are required, exacerbating the increased intrathoracic pressures caused by the IAH (63). This can result in falsely elevated central venous pressure (CVP) and pulmonary capillary wedge pressures (PCWPs), parameters used for patient management, including determination of the onset of acute respiratory distress syndrome (ARDS). This pathophysiology complicates the standard treatment of ARDS which requires lung-protective strategies including decreased tidal volumes, and limiting peak and plateau inspiratory pressures (64). In patients with elevated intrathoracic pressures secondary to IAH, accurate determination of central pressures becomes increasingly difficult and therefore some have suggested subtracting the IAP from the inspiratory pressure as a better judge of therapy (50). All these effects are effectively treated with abdominal decompression.

Cardiovascular

☞ **The primary cardiovascular derangement seen secondary to IAH is reduction of CO (36,39,59,62,65–67).** ☞ Multiple etiologies factor into this end result (including decreased preload and contractility with concomitant increased systemic and pulmonary vascular resistance). First, increased IAP causes decreased blood flow in the inferior vena cava and retroperitoneal veins (68,69). This decrease in flow can be seen with IAP of 15 mmHg but continues to decreases with increasing IAP. The area of maximal resistance to caval flow is at the IVC just below the diaphragm. It has been hypothesized that this is secondary to the transition between the high-pressure abdomen and the low-pressure thoracic cavity, as well as possible mechanical stretching of the diaphragmatic crura with protrusion secondary to IAH (68). This is attenuated by decreased venous return from the lower extremities secondary to IAH (70). This decreased venous outflow from the lower extremities can be overcome with the use of intermittent pneumatic compression devices during laparoscopic cholecystectomy (71). In addition, the secondarily increased intrathoracic pressure (i.e., elevated

diaphragms as described aforementioned) result in decreased flow in both the inferior and superior vena cava, thereby causing decreased cardiac preload.

The elevated intrathoracic pressures also result in decreasing ventricular compliance and stroke volume (59,72). At mild elevations of IAP, the heart is able to compensate with increasing rate (73). However, with increasing pressures, there is a concomitant increase in pulmonary vascular resistance (as discussed previously) as well as systemic vascular resistance (69). The exact etiology for the increased systemic vascular resistance is unclear, but it is likely the result of sympathetic stimulation resulting from the relatively low effective circulating blood volume. However, others have also postulated that it is secondary to direct arterial compression (as well as compression of many of the capillary beds) resulting from the increased intra-abdominal and intrathoracic pressures. In addition, IAH results in increased intracranial pressures (ICPs) (see subsequently), which cause the release of vasoconstricting agents such as vasopressin and catecholamines from the central nervous system in order to maintain cerebral perfusion pressure (CPP) by increasing systemic vascular resistance (74). The net result of this decreased preload, decreased cardiac compliance, and increased afterload is a marked reduction in $\dot{Q}$ seen with increasing IAP, eventually leading to cardiovascular collapse as described by Emerson almost a century ago (4).

In the face of significantly increased IAP, false elevation of CVP and PCWP measurements are seen (57,59,62). When this is taken in context with decreased stroke volume and $\dot{Q}$, the clinical picture can resemble cardiac failure. However, the setting of increased inspiratory pressures and increased IAP measurements, the diagnosis of ACS can be surmised. Confirmation of intraventricular volume status and contractility is easily achieved with the use of transesophageal echocardiography.

In the early stages of IAH/ACS, the cardiovascular derangements can be overcome with fluid resuscitation, in contrast to congestive heart failure which can be exacerbated by this therapy (6). In a porcine model of IAH, intravascular volume depletion was seen secondary to prolonged (24-hour) IAH despite elevated CVP (75). Some authors have suggested using volumetric Swan-Ganz catheters to help guide resuscitation in this setting, as all pressure measurements are altered (76). All of these derangements are reversed with treatment of the elevated IAP.

Hepatic

☞ **Diminished hepatic arterial, portal venous, and microcirculatory blood flow have all been associated with IAH (77).** ☞ When anesthetized pigs had IAP increased to 20 mmHg, despite constant $\dot{Q}$ and mean arterial pressure, hepatic arterial flow was decreased by 55%, portal vein flow was decreased by 35%, and hepatic microcirculatory flow was decreased 29% compared to controls. Similar decreases in hepatic microcirculatory flow have been seen in patients undergoing laparoscopic cholecystectomy (78). Trauma patients may be at increased risk secondary to the alterations in visceral and portal blood flow occurring during shock (4). Although it is theorized that this in addition to the ischemia-reperfusion injury seen in treated ACS, results in a secondary decrease in hepatic function, commonly referred to as "shock" liver, detailed studies on the effects of ACS on hepatic dysfunction have not been published.

Splanchnic

Similar to effects seen on the liver, kidney, and the inferior vena cava, the predominant effect of elevated IAP is that of decreased splanchnic perfusion. Splanchnic hypoperfusion can be seen with IAP as low as 15 mmHg, with case reports of intestinal ischemia requiring operative intervention after elective laparoscopy maintaining 15 mmHg pneumoperitoneum (79). This is a rare occurrence and has been hypothesized to require pre-existing vascular compromise to have this outcome. However, mesenteric arterial, intestinal mucosal, and portal venous blood flows have shown to be decreased with elevation of IAP. This can be measured in the clinical setting with gastric tonometry indicating decreased perfusion to the stomach, which has been described by many authors (80–83). One study showed that the decrease in gastric perfusion as inferred by gastric pHi was decreased earlier than the traditional signs of ACS (oliguria, increased peak inspiratory pressures) (84). This decreased gastrointestinal perfusion occurs independent of a decreased $\dot{Q}$ as it can be shown to occur even when $\dot{Q}$ is held constant (85). This is a factor to be considered in deliberating the creation of gastrointestinal anastomoses in patients at high risk of developing IAH and secondary complications of the anastomosis.

Elevated IAP has also been shown to increase portal venous pressure (77). This may be a contributing factor in the pathophysiology of esophageal varices in patients with liver failure. Increasing IAP by 10 mmHg resulted in an increase in variceal pressure, radius, volume, and wall tension. Therefore, the elevated IAP that many cirrhotics have secondary to ascites may be a causative factor in the development of variceal hemorrhage (86).

In animal models, there has been suggestion of increased incidence of bacterial translocation in rats as a result of IAH (87). However, this finding has not been reproduced in a larger porcine model (88). In addition, the decreased splanchnic perfusion and reperfusion injury has been shown to result in the production of cytokines from the gut (89). These may play a role in the development of septic complications and or subsequent systemic inflammatory response syndrome (SIRS) and multiple organ failure (Volume 2, Chapter 63).

Central Nervous System

Although ACS does not cause central nervous system failure, there is a strong relationship between IAH and increased ICP with secondary reduction in CPP shown both in animal models (90–93) as well as humans (92,94). The proposed mechanism for this is the elevated intrathoracic pressures, which result from the IAH, mediated elevation of the diaphragms. The increased intrathoracic pressures, in turn, increase the jugular venous pressure and ICP. This is demonstrated in a porcine model when the effects of IAH on ICP are completely ameliorated by a sternotomy, thereby releasing increased intrathoracic pressure (91).

In humans, Citerio et al. (92) showed that inducing IAH by placing 15-L water bags on the abdomen of patients with moderate-to-severe head injury, a significant increase in intracranial and internal jugular pressures resulted. Patients with clinical ACS and elevated ICP have had correction of ICP with decompressive laparotomy (94). Therefore, monitoring of IAP is recommended in patients with neurotrauma and abdominal injury or reason to suspect IAH, with consideration to decompression in refractory elevation of ICP (95). In addition, chronic IAH associated with morbid obesity has been implicated in intracranial hypertension and even the development of pseudotumor cerebri (28,94,96). In these cases, weight loss by bariatric surgery results in improvement in the chronic intracranial hypertension (28,94,96).

Abdominal Wall

Increased IAP causes hypoperfusion of the abdominal wall secondary to a direct compressive effect. In a porcine model, Diebel et al. (97) showed decreased abdominal wall perfusion at all levels of IAH despite maintenance of constant $\dot{Q}$ and blood pressure. This results in localized ischemia and reperfusion. This has been implied in the high rate of abdominal wound complications (infection, hernia, and dehiscence) in this population. In addition, similar increase in abdominal wall complications have been seen in patients with stable peritoneal dialysis with increased rates of leaks and hernias with increased IAP being an independent risk factor (98).

Multiple Organ Dysfunction Syndrome

Studies have shown that ACS is an independent predictor for multiple organ dysfunction syndrome (MODS) and that prevention of ACS can decrease the incidence of MODS (17,99,100). In addition to the direct pressure-related effects of IAH on these organs, the process of ACS has been shown to prime the immune system as a result of activating neutrophils and increasing the elaboration of cytokines (89,101). This can set the stage for SIRS and subsequent MODS (Volume 2, Chapter 63) (100,101). In a porcine model, a modest elevation of IAP to 15 mmHg for only 24 hours has been shown to result in MODS (102). ⚔ **The priming of the immune system and the resultant enhanced inflammatory response may predispose patients with ACS to MODS even after abdominal decompression.** ⚔ This may relate to ACS being one of the hits in the two-hit theory of multiple organ failure (99). Because of this, prevention of ACS is paramount in the treatment of the high-risk patient.

TREATMENT

These diverse affects of ACS, although potentially life-threatening, can be abrogated with early recognition and appropriate treatment. Depending on the clinical scenario, the appropriate treatment strategy may entail resuscitation, minimally invasive decompression, surgical decompression, and the use of TAC as an initial potential preventative measure.

Prevention

An ounce of prevention is worth a pound of cure. This is as true for ACS as it is for a compartment syndrome of the extremity. Similar to the patient with a significant vascular injury or long-bone fracture who should receive a prophylactic fasciotomy, a patient at high risk of developing IAH or ACS at the time of laparotomy, as is often seen in trauma patients requiring damage control surgery, it is best not to close the abdomen, but instead to treat with a prophylactic "open abdomen," or TAC. This is the cornerstone of "damage control" trauma surgery. The classic presentation is the patient with severe injuries who is becoming hypothermic, coagulopathic, and acidotic, and requiring massive resuscitation. Paradoxically, the fluid repletion needed to bring the patient back from the so-called "death spiral," is the very thing that makes these patients at greatest risk for developing ACS (99,103). Therefore, damage control (Volume 1, Chapter 21) aims to abbreviate definitive control and usually incorporates a TAC both as prophylaxis for ACS as well as lessening operative time and allowing for more prompt return to the ICU for resuscitation.

Numerous TAC techniques have been described in the literature including towel clip closure, Bogota bag, mesh closure, and vacuum packs (104,105). The specific TAC used is less important than to understand and feel comfortable with at least one of these methods for surgeons who may potentially treat patients at risk for or with ACS. ☞ **When used in appropriately selected patients, the use of TAC can be effective in preventing the development of ACS (106).** ☞ Although level I data for improved survival is not available, case–control studies have shown that patients treated at initial laparotomy for potential ACS have a lower incidence of multiple organ failure and lower mortality as compared to those who develop ACS and require a second decompressive laparotomy (107,108). ☞ **When abdominal swelling continues following TAC, it is still possible to develop ACS despite the theoretical "open abdomen"; therefore, in the setting of a patient with significant risk for developing ACS, regular IAP measurements should still be obtained (109).** ☞

Resuscitation

Although decompressive laparotomy is the gold standard for the treatment of patients with ACS, the exact IAP at which that is indicated is less clear. A grading system for IAH/ACS was proposed and prospectively evaluated by Meldrum et al. (14), and this is shown in Table 2. Grade I IAH usually requires no intervention and has subsequently been shown to be within the upper range of IAPs measured in "normal" hospitalized patients. Patients with grade II IAH may respond to hypervolemic resuscitation. Depending on the etiology in a given patient, this may be sufficient with careful observation and repeated measurement to track the trends of the IAP. However, as previously discussed, supranormal resuscitation can lead to visceral and retroperitoneal edema, thereby worsening IAH. In a study of trauma patients matched for severity of illness, the patients who progressed toward ACS did not respond to fluid loading and did not demonstrate a significant increase in $\dot{Q}$ to crystalloid/colloid boluses (110). The conclusion of this study was that fluid resuscitation could not overcome impending ACS, much as fluid resuscitation, by itself, will not overcome cardiac tamponade. Other authors have argued that given the poor sensitivity of IAP to predict ACS, that a surrogate marker of abdominal perfusion pressure (APP), which is equal to IAP minus mean arterial pressure, be used to drive resuscitation. The argument being that APP is a measure of overall abdominal perfusion and therefore a better indicator of the end effects of IAH. They recommend that APP be maintained greater than 50 mmHg and that if this is not possible, decompressive laparotomy be performed (111). However, although this may be a useful guide, APP has not been validated in multiple trials. Therefore, the overall clinical picture (oliguria, increased peak inspiratory pressure, worsening of acidosis) and trends in the IAP should guide therapy rather than relying upon any single absolute number. There is a suggestion that abdominal muscular tone may play a role in elevating IAP, and therefore case report exists of the treatment of ACS with

neuromuscular blockade with resulting decreased IAP preventing the need in that patient for decompressive laparotomy (112). If in doubt, err toward decompressive laparotomy as it is the only therapy for all of the pathological consequences of elevated IAP.

Abdominal Decompression
Considerations Prior to Laparotomy

☞ **The mainstay of treatment of suspected or confirmed ACS is laparotomy with abdominal decompression and TAC.** ☞ Realizing that this may result in an initial drop in systemic and pulmonary vascular resistance as well as venous pooling prior to decompressing the abdomen, the patient's intravascular volume should be restored and metabolic perturbations corrected (acidosis, hypothermia, coagulopathy) prior to decompression if at all possible. However, decompression should not be delayed if this is not easily achieved (65). Fluid resuscitation should be continued after decompression as an ischemia-reperfusion washout syndrome can occur with the possibility of instability, dysrhythmias, or cardiac arrest. Cases of asystole have been reported with an incidence as high as 12% in some series (113). Because of this, the authors recommend having a cardiac arrest cart at the bedside prior to undertaking decompression in patients with advanced (grade IV) ACS.

☞ **During mesenteric reperfusion immediately following abdominal decompression, a washout of the products of anaerobic metabolism occurs, and can lead to significant hypotension (113).** ☞ Because of this, preparation for abdominal decompression involves maneuvers similar to those taken immediately prior to aortic cross-clamp removal after aneurysm repair: (*i*) large-bore intravenous access; (*ii*) warm intravenous fluids infusing prior to decompression with availability of a rapid infuser; (*iii*) dopamine or other vasopressors prepared and in line (only to be used when intravascular volume replacement is inadequate to treat the hypotension resulting from reperfusion product-mediated venous pooling and decreased vascular resistance); (*iv*) prepare to compensate for the washout of lactate (and CO_2) from the gut and lower extremities by temporarily increasing the overall minute ventilation; (*v*) because acidosis is anticipated, sodium bicarbonate should be immediately available if needed; (*vi*) calcium chloride 250–500 mg should be prophylactically administered immediately following decompression to protect against myocardial irritability from potassium washout during reperfusion, as well as to bolster the transient hypocalcemia associated with sodium bicarbonate administration. Morris et al. (114) recommend 2 L of normal saline, with 50 g mannitol and 50 meq sodium bicarbonate per liter intravenous fluids prior to decompression.

Fortunately, with abdominal decompression there is a sudden increase in pulmonary compliance with a resultant increase in tidal volume delivered to the patient. Although beneficial to blow-off CO_2 in the severely debilitated patients with anticipated acid washout, this can eventually result in respiratory alkalosis after the acute decompression, and should be adjusted as needed, after stabilization.

The other consideration prior to decompression is whether the ACS is secondary to or associated with significant hemorrhage. The importance of this is determining the ideal location for abdominal decompression. Patients with full ACS are difficult to ventilate and unstable, making bedside ICU decompression an attractive option. However, recognizing that a significant portion of these patients will have significant hemorrhage especially in the trauma setting, if the patient is stable for transport, decompression should be undertaken in the operating room. If the patient is unstable, bedside decompression can be performed, with operating room standby. If significant hemorrhage is encountered, temporary hemostasis is achieved with packing and following stability the patient is transported to the operating theater for definitive surgical hemostasis.

Temporary Abdominal Closure

Once a decompressive laparotomy is performed, the question as to the ideal TAC arises. There is a wide variety of TAC described in the literature and a complete review of these is beyond the scope of this discussion. In brief, the goal is to open the fascia, releasing pressure, and allowing the intra-abdominal volume to expand into the new space, while still providing coverage of the bowel and abdominal contents preventing desiccation. The original TAC was the towel clip closure of the skin, however, this still limits the amount that the intra-abdominal compartment can expand and is therefore rarely used in cases of ACS (Fig. 3) today (115). ✍ **One of the easiest methods of achieving TAC is using the Bogota bag technique, a variation of the silos created by pediatric surgeons in the treatment of gastroschisis and omphaloceles.** ✍ First described by Londoni while he was a chief resident in Bogota, Colombia, this involves suturing a sterile plastic 3-L urologic irrigation bag to either the fascia or skin to allow visualization of the bowel as well as ample volume for the intra-abdominal contents to expand (Fig. 4) (116).

Recently, the vacuum pack closure has also gained popularity in which a polypropylene sheet is tucked into the abdomen on top of which a towel is tucked into the

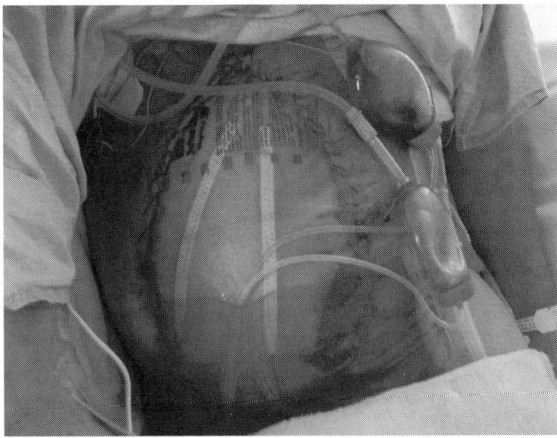

Figure 4 The "Bogota bag" method of temporary abdominal closure. A urological irrigation fluid bag is sutured to the skin and external drains are placed for control and quantification of leaking fluid or hemorrhage.

abdomen. This is covered with drains and sealed with plastic adhesive drape. The drains are then placed to continuous suction, allowing for an easily created TAC (117). A variety of commercial TAC devices are now available, including Velcro, zippers, vacuum-assisted devices, and others, but availability and experience with these are still institution dependent (118,119). The important point is that the surgeon is to be familiar and experienced with at least one of these techniques if the need for TAC arises. In the case of a patient with a TAC who develops ACS, abdominal reexploration with a wider/looser TAC is required (109).

Once a TAC or "open abdomen" is created, the goal is to correct the factors causing the ACS and closure of the abdomen. This requires correction of the initial disease process (coagulopathy, acidosis, etc.), and usually mobilization of visceral and abdominal wall edema to facilitate closure. Of note, all the open abdomen techniques result in colonization of the skin and open wound, and therefore if fascial closure is possible, the skin should be left open because of the high rate of wound complications if closed. If this is not possible in a single operation, staged procedures may be needed with gradual approximation of the abdominal fascia. In some patients, fascial closure is impossible, necessitating closure with absorbable mesh with eventual skin graft to create a controlled ventral hernia (Figs. 5 and 6). These patients will eventually require abdominal wall reconstruction six months to a year after all the inflammation has resolved and the intra-abdominal adhesions are remodeling (120).

Percutaneous/Laparoscopy

Although the gold standard for the treatment of ACS is decompressive laparotomy, in selected circumstances a less invasive method may be adequate. The most common circumstance in which a percutaneous approach may be a viable option is that of ACS secondary to ascites or a large loculated fluid collection (121,122). In cases of ascites secondary to hepatic failure, this is the preferred method as a laparotomy carries a risk of a persistent ascites leak. In addition, there are reports of using percutaneous decompression in cases of 2° ACS with significant ascites in burn patients and trauma patients, although there is some data to suggest that this is less effective in patients with >80% total body surface area

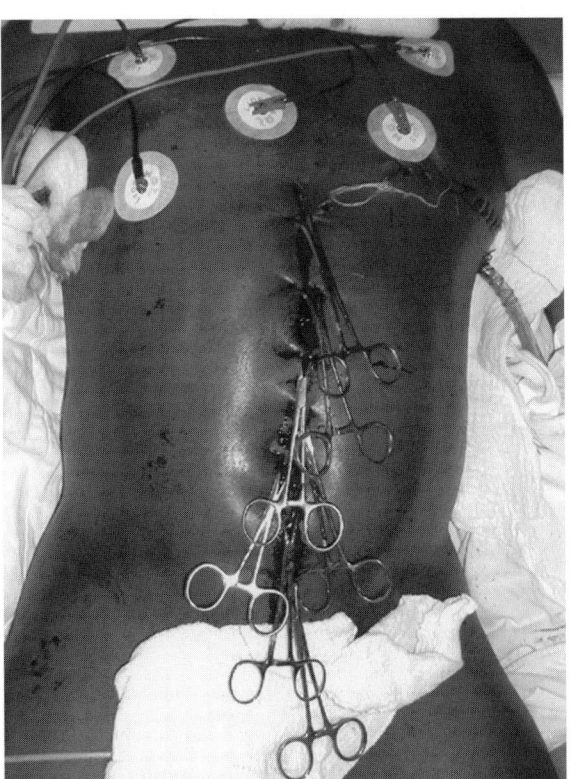

Figure 3 Towel clip closure of the abdomen. As the skin is still approximated, the increase in abdominal domain is modest.

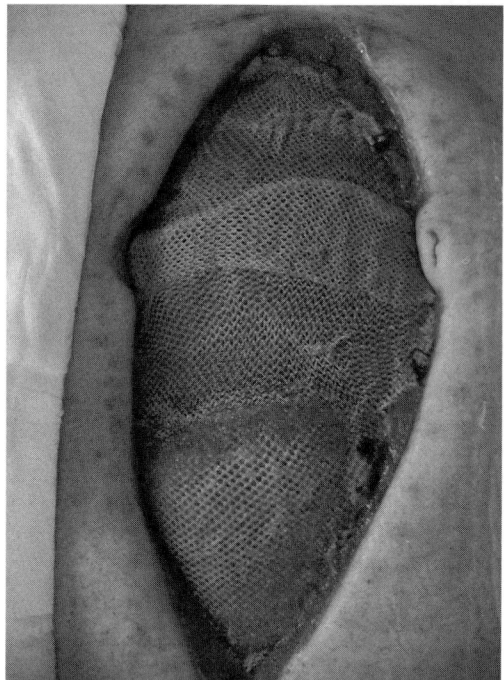

Figure 5 In cases where primary closure of the fascia is not possible at reoperation, temporary abdominal closure is accomplished using an absorbable mesh fascial closure. This allows coverage and the formation of granulation tissue to occur over the bowel and omentum.

(TBSA) burns (123–125). Even in the setting of secondary ACS secondary to burn, the frequency of being able to treat with percutaneous techniques is limited. In a retrospective review of 1014 consecutive burn patients, 10 developed ACS requiring surgical interventions, only two cases (both with isolated ascites) were amenable to percutaneous drainage (19). Case reports also exist of the use of laparoscopy or percutaneous drainage for the treatment of ACS secondary to blunt hepatic trauma (126,127). This should only be used in cases of isolated injury where ACS is secondary to hemoperitoneum

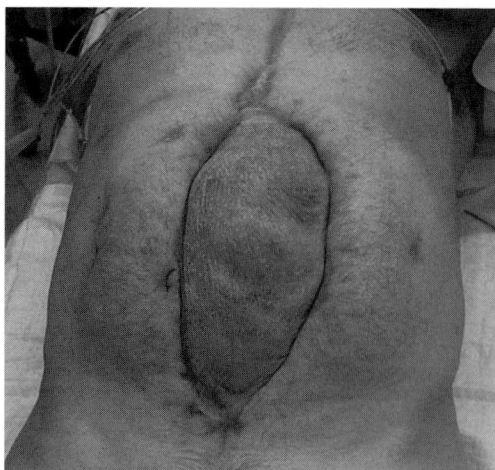

Figure 6 Once adequate granulation has occurred with an absorbable mesh closure, the mesh is removed and the abdomen is "closed" with a split thickness skin graft to create a controlled ventral hernia.

without edematous bowel from resuscitation; and therefore application of this technique is limited. If one of these minimally invasive methods fails to correct the IAH, then decompressive laparotomy should naturally be performed.

EYE TO THE FUTURE

In the future, real-time IAP measurement may be possible using microchip-tipped catheters allowing earlier diagnosis and treatment of IAH or impending ACS in high-risk patients rather than intermittent bladder pressure (34). The future of ACS therapy will be in prevention rather than treatment. Once ACS has occurred, significant mortality results, and therefore the optimal goal will be prevention by better predictive models and prophylactic decompressive celiotomy before the onset. In addition, improved resuscitative techniques and modalities (i.e., synthetic blood substitutes) may reduce the amount of crystalloid needed and therefore the incidence of ACS (128,129). Once ACS has set in, work in animal models using pharmacological therapy with either octreotide or vasopressin is showing potential for being able to attenuate the effects of the ischemia/reperfusion after abdominal decompression, and therefore potentially decreasing the incidence of MODS and mortality (130,131). Finally, improvements in the management of open abdomens may result in fewer patients requiring a planned ventral hernia and delayed abdominal reconstructions (132).

SUMMARY

IAH and ACS are relatively common phenomena with a wide range of etiologies. Given the often subtle and insidious onset, and the potentially grave consequence when the diagnosis/treatment is delayed or missed, a high index of suspicion is required. If the possibility of IAH is entertained, IAP must be measured, as objective measurement is the only method to diagnose or rule out ACS. The result of IAH is seen most readily in the renal and respiratory systems, however, almost every organ system can be affected. In trauma or other patients at high risk for developing ACS on the basis of perioperative findings, the best treatment is the use of a TAC to decrease the incidence (if not completely prevent) the development of ACS. If ACS develops, prompt treatment with decompression will afford the best therapy with resolution of cardiovascular, pulmonary, and renal derangements, although the stage may be set for subsequent multiple organ failure.

KEY POINTS

- ☞ Because of the numerous etiologies, a high index of suspicion is required to consider the diagnosis of ACS.
- ☞ Because of the limitations of clinical examination in diagnosing ACS, measurement of IAP is essential to making the diagnosis.
- ☞ Despite the variety of methods described for measurement of IAP, the gold standard continues to be urinary bladder pressure.
- ☞ Renal dysfunction is the most common presentation, however, the morbidity of ACS is not limited to intra-abdominal organs, and has the potential to effect nearly every major system.

☞ Most of the pathophysiologic effects of ACS are reversible, making early diagnosis and prompt treatment imperative.

☞ An IAP of 15–20 mmHg may result in oliguria, while IAP greater than 30 mmHg can lead to anuria.

☞ The pulmonary dysfunction resulting from IAH is secondary to elevation of bilateral hemidiaphragms in response to the pressure (57).

☞ The primary cardiovascular derangement seen secondary to IAH is reduction of $\dot{Q}$.

☞ Diminished hepatic arterial, portal venous, and microcirculatory blood flow have all been associated with IAH.

☞ The priming of the immune system and the resultant enhanced inflammatory response may predispose patients with ACS to MODS even after abdominal decompression.

☞ When used in appropriately selected patients, the use of TAC can be effective in preventing the development of ACS.

☞ When abdominal swelling continues following TAC, it is still possible to develop ACS despite the theoretical "open abdomen"; therefore, in the setting of a patient with significant risk for developing ACS, regular IAP measurements should still be obtained.

☞ The mainstay of treatment of suspected or confirmed ACS is laparotomy with abdominal decompression and TAC.

☞ During mesenteric reperfusion immediately following abdominal decompression, a washout of the products of anaerobic metabolism occurs, and can lead to significant hypotension (113).

☞ One of the easiest methods of achieving TAC is using the Bogota bag technique, a variation of the silos created by pediatric surgeons in the treatment of gastroschisis and omphaloceles.

REFERENCES

1. Stedman's Medical Dictionary. 26th ed. Baltimore: Williams & Wilkins, 1995.
2. Kron IL, Harman PK, Nolan SP. The measurement of intra-abdominal pressure as a criterion for abdominal re-exploration. Ann Surg 1984; 199:28–30.
3. Wendt EC. Über den Einflus des intraabdominellen Druckes auf die Absonderungsgeschwindigkeit des Harnes. Arch Heilkunde 1876; 17:527–546.
4. Wittmann DH, Iskander GA. The compartment syndrome of the abdominal cavity: a state of the art review. J Intensive Care Med 2000; 15:201–220.
5. Emerson H. Intra-abdominal pressures. Arch Intern Med 1911; 7:754–784.
6. Saggi BH, Sugerman HJ, Ivatury RR, Bloomfield GL. Acute abdominal compartment syndrome in the critically ill. J Intensive Care Med 1999; 14:207–219.
7. Gross R. A new method for surgical treatment of large omphaloceles. Surgery 1948; 24:277–292.
8. Moore TC, Stokes GE. Gastroschisis. Surgery 1953; 33:112–115.
9. Allen RG, Wrenn EL Jr. Silon as a sac in the treatment of omphalocele and gastroschisis. J Pediatr Surg 1969; 4:3–8.
10. Kleinhaus S, Sammartano R, Boley SJ. Effects of laparoscopy on mesenteric blood-flow. Arch Surg 1978; 113:867–869.
11. Ivankovich AD, Miletich DJ, Albrecht RF, Heyman HJ, Bonnet RF. Cardiovascular effects of intraperitoneal insufflation with carbon-dioxide and nitrous-oxide in dog. Anesthesiology 1975; 42:281–287.
12. Diamant M, Benumof JL, Saidman LJ. Hemodynamics of increased intra-abdominal pressure—interaction with hypovolemia and halothane anesthesia. Anesthesiology 1978; 48:23–27.
13. Stone HH, Strom PR, Mullins RJ. Management of the major coagulopathy with onset during laparotomy. Ann Surg 1983; 197:532–535.
14. Meldrum DR, Moore FA, Moore EE, et al. Prospective characterization and selective management of the abdominal compartment syndrome. Am J Surg 1997; 174:667–672.
15. Hong JJ, Cohn SM, Perez JM, et al. Prospective study of the incidence and outcome of intra-abdominal hypertension and the abdominal compartment syndrome. Br J Surg 2002; 89:591–596.
16. Raeburn CD, Moore EE, Biffl WL, et al. The abdominal compartment syndrome is a morbid complication of postinjury damage control surgery. Am J Surg 2001; 182:542–546.
17. Balogh Z, McKinley BA, Holcomb JB, et al. Both primary and secondary abdominal compartment syndrome can be predicted early and are harbingers of multiple organ failure. J Trauma 2003; 54:848–859.
18. Balogh Z, McKinley BA, Cocanour CS, et al. Supranormal trauma resuscitation causes more cases of abdominal compartment syndrome. Arch Surg 2003; 138:637–642.
19. Hobson KG, Young KM, Ciraulo A, Palmieri TL, Greenhalgh DG. Release of abdominal compartment syndrome improves survival in patients with burn injury. J Trauma 2002; 53:1129–1133.
20. Kopelman T, Harris C, Miller R, Arrillaga A. Abdominal compartment syndrome in patients with isolated extraperitoneal injuries. J Trauma 2000; 49:744–747.
21. Biffl WL, Moore EE, Burch JM, et al. Secondary abdominal compartment syndrome is a highly lethal event. Am J Surg 2001; 182:645–648.
22. Maxwell RA, Fabian TC, Croce MA, Davis KA. Secondary abdominal compartment syndrome: an underappreciated manifestation of severe hemorrhagic shock. J Trauma 1999; 47:995–999.
23. Balogh Z, McKinley BA, Cocanour CS, et al. Secondary abdominal compartment syndrome is an elusive early complication of traumatic shock resuscitation. Am J Surg 2002; 184:538–543.
24. Mutoh T, Lamm WJE, Embree LJ, Hildebrandt J, Albert RK. Abdominal distension alters regional pleural pressures and chest-wall mechanics in pigs in vivo. J Appl Phys 1991; 70:2611–2618.
25. Sugerman HJ. Pulmonary-function in morbid-obesity. Gastroenterol Clin North Am 1987; 16:225–237.
26. Sugerman HJ. Ventilation and obesity. Int J Obes 1995; 19:686.
27. Sugerman HJ, Felton WL, Sismanis A, et al. Gastric surgery for pseudotumor cerebri associated with severe obesity. Ann Surg 1999; 229:634–642.
28. Sugerman HJ, Felton WL, Salvant JB, Sismanis A, Kellum JM. Effects of surgically induced weight-loss on idiopathic intracranial hypertension in morbid-obesity. Neurology 1995; 45:1655–1659.
29. Sugerman HJ. Effects of increased intra-abdominal pressure in severe obesity. Surg Clin North Am 2001; 81:1063–1075.
30. McNelis J, Marini CP, Jurkiewicz A, et al. Predictive factors associated with the development of abdominal compartment syndrome in the surgical intensive care unit. Arch Surg 2002; 137:133–136.
31. Van Mieghem N, Verbrugghe W, Daelemans R, Lins R, Malbrain M. Can abdominal perimeter be used as an accurate estimation of intra-abdominal pressure? Crit Care 2003; 7(suppl 2): S90.
32. Kirkpatrick AW, Brenneman FD, McLean RF, Rapanos T, Boulanger BR. Is clinical examination an accurate indicator of raised intra-abdominal pressure in critically injured patients? Can J Surg 2000; 43:207–211.
33. Sugrue M, Bauman A, Jones F, et al. Clinical examination is an inaccurate predictor of intraabdominal pressure. World J Surg 2002; 26:1428–1431.

34. Malbrain ML. Different techniques to measure intra-abdominal pressure (IAP): time for a critical re-appraisal. Intensive Care Med 2004; 30:357–371.

35. Sanchez NC, Tenofsky PL, Dort JM, et al. What is normal intra-abdominal pressure? Am Surg 2001; 67:243–248.

36. Moffa SM, Quinn JV, Slotman GJ. Hemodynamic-effects of carbon-dioxide pneumoperitoneum during mechanical ventilation and positive end-expiratory pressure. J Trauma 1993; 35:613–618.

37. Richardson JD, Trinkle JK. Hemodynamic and respiratory alterations with increased intra-abdominal pressure. J Surg Res 1976; 20:401–404.

38. Safran DB, Orlando R. Physiological-effects of pneumoperitoneum. Am J Surg 1994; 167:281–286.

39. Harman PK, Kron IL, McLachlan HD, Freedlender AE, Nolan SP. Elevated intra-abdominal pressure and renal function. Ann Surg 1982; 196:594–597.

40. Lacey SR, Bruce J, Brooks SP, et al. The relative merits of various methods of indirect measurement of intraabdominal pressure as a guide to closure of abdominal wall defects. J Pediatr Surg 1987; 22:1207–1211.

41. Collee GG, Lomax DM, Ferguson C, Hanson GC. Bedside measurement of intra-abdominal pressure (IAP) via an indwelling naso-gastric tube: clinical validation of the technique. Intensive Care Med 1993; 19:478–480.

42. Sugrue M, Buist MD, Lee A, Sanchez DJ, Hillman KM. Intra-abdominal pressure measurement using a modified nasogastric tube: description and validation of a new technique. Intensive Care Med 1994; 20:588–590.

43. Iberti TJ, Kelly KM, Gentili DR, Hirsch S, Benjamin E. A simple technique to accurately determine intra-abdominal pressure. Crit Care Med 1987; 15:1140–1142.

44. Iberti TJ, Lieber CE, Benjamin E. Determination of intra-abdominal pressure using a transurethral bladder catheter: clinical validation of the technique. Anesthesiology 1989; 70:47–50.

45. Cheatham ML, Safcsak K. Intraabdominal pressure: a revised method for measurement. J Am Coll Surg 1998; 186:368–369.

46. De Keulenaer BL, De Backer A, Schepens DR, et al. Abdominal compartment syndrome related to noninvasive ventilation. Intensive Care Med 2003; 29:1177–1181.

47. Shafik A, El Sharkawy A, Sharaf WM. Direct measurement of intra-abdominal pressure in various conditions. Eur J Surg 1997; 163:883–887.

48. Dowdle M. Evaluating a new intrauterine pressure catheter. J Reprod Med 1997; 42:506–513.

49. Schachtrupp A, Tons C, Fackeldey V, et al. Evaluation of two novel methods for the direct and continuous measurement of the intra-abdominal pressure in a porcine model. Intensive Care Med 2003; 29:1605–1608.

50. Malbrain ML. Is it wise not to think about intraabdominal hypertension in the ICU? Curr Opin Crit Care 2004; 10: 132–145.

51. Kirsch AJ, Hensle TW, Chang DT, et al. Renal effects of CO_2 insufflation: oliguria and acute renal dysfunction in a rat pneumoperitoneum model. Urology 1994; 43:453–459.

52. Platell C, Hall J, Dobb G. Impaired renal function due to raised intraabdominal pressure. Intensive Care Med 1990; 16: 328–329.

53. Chiu AW, Azadzoi KM, Hatzichristou DG, et al. Effects of intra-abdominal pressure on renal tissue perfusion during laparoscopy. J Endourol 1994; 8:99–103.

54. Jacques T, Lee R. Improvement of renal function after relief of raised intra-abdominal pressure due to traumatic retroperitoneal haematoma. Anaesth Intensive Care 1988; 16:478–482.

55. Bloomfield GL, Blocher CR, Fakhry IF, Sica DA, Sugerman HJ. Elevated intra-abdominal pressure increases plasma renin activity and aldosterone levels. J Trauma 1997; 42:997–1004.

56. Celoria G, Steingrub J, Dawson JA, Teres D. Oliguria from high intra-abdominal pressure secondary to ovarian mass. Crit Care Med 1987; 15:78–79.

57. Cullen DJ, Coyle JP, Teplick R, Long MC. Cardiovascular, pulmonary, and renal effects of massively increased intra-abdominal pressure in critically ill patients. Crit Care Med 1989; 17:118–121.

58. Nguyen NT, Anderson JT, Budd M, et al. Effects of pneumoperitoneum on intraoperative pulmonary mechanics and gas exchange during laparoscopic gastric bypass. Surg Endosc 2004; 18:64–71.

59. Ridings PC, Bloomfield GL, Blocher CR, Sugerman HJ. Cardiopulmonary effects of raised intra-abdominal pressure before and after intravascular volume expansion. J Trauma 1995; 39:1071–1075.

60. Malbrain ML, Deeren D, Nieuwendijk R, et al. Partitioning of respiratory mechanics in intra-abdominal hypertension. Intensive Care Med 2003; 29(suppl 1):S85.

61. Barnes GE, Laine GA, Giam PY, Smith EE, Granger HJ. Cardiovascular responses to elevation of intra-abdominal hydrostatic pressure. Am J Physiol 1985; 248:R208–R213.

62. Quintel M, Pelosi P, Caironi P, et al. An increase of abdominal pressure increases pulmonary edema in oleic acid-induced lung injury. Am J Respir Crit Care Med 2004; 169:534–541.

63. Suwanvanichkij V, Curtis JR. The use of high positive end-expiratory pressure for respiratory failure in abdominal compartment syndrome. Respir Care 2004; 49:286–290.

64. The Acute Respiratory Distress Syndrome Network. Ventilation with lower tidal volumes as compared with traditional tidal volumes for acute lung injury and the acute respiratory distress syndrome. N Engl J Med 2000; 342:1301–1308.

65. Shelly MP, Robinson AA, Hesford JW, Park GR. Haemodynamic effects following surgical release of increased intra-abdominal pressure. Br J Anaesth 1987; 59:800–805.

66. McDermott JP, Regan MC, Page R, et al. Cardiorespiratory effects of laparoscopy with and without gas insufflation. Arch Surg 1995; 130:984–988.

67. Windberger U, Siegl H, Ferguson JG, et al. Hemodynamic effects of prolonged abdominal insufflation for laparoscopic procedures. Gastrointest Endosc 1995; 41:121–129.

68. Rubinson RM, Vasko JS, Doppman JL, Morrow AG. Inferior vena caval obstruction from increased intra-abdominal pressure: experimental hemodynamic and angiographic observations. Arch Surg 1967; 94:766–770.

69. Kashtan J, Green JF, Parsons EQ, Holcroft JW. Hemodynamic effect of increased abdominal pressure. J Surg Res 1981; 30:249–255.

70. Beebe DS, McNevin MP, Crain JM, et al. Evidence of venous stasis after abdominal insufflation for laparoscopic cholecystectomy. Surg Gynecol Obstet 1993; 176:443–447.

71. Christen Y, Reymond MA, Vogel JJ, et al. Hemodynamic effects of intermittent pneumatic compression of the lower limbs during laparoscopic cholecystectomy. Am J Surg 1995; 170:395–398.

72. Robotham JL, Wise RA, Bromberger-Barnea B. Effects of changes in abdominal pressure on left ventricular performance and regional blood flow. Crit Care Med 1985; 13:803–809.

73. Ho HS, Gunther RA, Wolfe BM. Intraperitoneal carbon dioxide insufflation and cardiopulmonary functions: laparoscopic cholecystectomy in pigs. Arch Surg 1992; 127:928–932.

74. Rosin D, Rosenthal RJ. Adverse hemodynamic effects of intraabdominal pressure is it all in the head? Int J Surg Investig 2001; 2:335–345.

75. Schachtrupp A, Graf J, Tons C, et al. Intravascular volume depletion in a 24-hour porcine model of intra-abdominal hypertension. J Trauma 2003; 55:734–740.

76. Durham R, Neunaber K, Vogler G, Shapiro M, Mazuski J. Right ventricular end-diastolic volume as a measure of preload. J Trauma 1995; 39:218–223.

77. Diebel LN, Wilson RF, Dulchavsky SA, Saxe J. Effect of increased intra-abdominal pressure on hepatic arterial, portal venous, and hepatic microcirculatory blood flow. J Trauma 1992; 33:279–282.

78. Eleftheriadis E, Kotzampassi K, Botsios D, et al. Splanchnic ischemia during laparoscopic cholecystectomy. Surg Endosc 1996; 10:324–326.

79. Hasson HM, Galanopoulos C, Langerman A. Ischemic necrosis of small bowel following laparoscopic surgery. JSLS 2004; 8:159–163.

80. Engum SA, Kogon B, Jensen E, et al. Gastric tonometry and direct intraabdominal pressure monitoring in abdominal compartment syndrome. J Pediatr Surg 2002; 37:214–218.

81. Balogh Z, McKinley BA, Moore FA. Gastric tonometry is an early independent predictor of abdominal compartment syndrome. Shock 2004; 21:101.

82. Chang MC, Miller PR, D'Agostino R, Meredith JW. Effects of abdominal decompression on cardiopulmonary function and visceral perfusion in patients with intra-abdominal hypertension. J Trauma 1998; 44:440–445.

83. Schwarte LA, Scheeren TW, Lorenz C, De Bruyne F, Fournell A. Moderate increase in intraabdominal pressure attenuates gastric mucosal oxygen saturation in patients undergoing laparoscopy. Anesthesiology 2004; 100:1081–1087.

84. Ivatury RR, Porter JM, Simon RJ, et al. Intra-abdominal hypertension after life-threatening penetrating abdominal trauma: prophylaxis, incidence, and clinical relevance to gastric mucosal pH and abdominal compartment syndrome. J Trauma 1998; 44:1016–1021.

85. Diebel LN, Dulchavsky SA, Wilson RF. Effect of increased intra-abdominal pressure on mesenteric arterial and intestinal mucosal blood flow. J Trauma 1992; 33:45–48.

86. Luca A, Cirera I, Garcia-Pagan JC, et al. Hemodynamic effects of acute changes in intra-abdominal pressure in patients with cirrhosis. Gastroenterology 1993; 104:222–227.

87. Eleftheriadis E, Kotzampassi K, Papanotas K, Heliadis N, Sarris K. Gut ischemia, oxidative stress, and bacterial translocation in elevated abdominal pressure in rats. World J Surg 1996; 20:11–16.

88. Doty JM, Oda J, Ivatury RR, et al. The effects of hemodynamic shock and increased intra-abdominal pressure on bacterial translocation. J Trauma 2002; 52:13–17.

89. Oda J, Ivatury RR, Blocher CR, Malhotra AJ, Sugerman HJ. Amplified cytokine response and lung injury by sequential hemorrhagic shock and abdominal compartment syndrome in a laboratory model of ischemia-reperfusion. J Trauma 2002; 52:625–631.

90. Bloomfield GL, Ridings PC, Blocher CR, Marmarou A, Sugerman HJ. Effects of increased intra-abdominal pressure upon intracranial and cerebral perfusion pressure before and after volume expansion. J Trauma 1996; 40:936–941.

91. Bloomfield GL, Ridings PC, Blocher CR, Marmarou A, Sugerman HJ. A proposed relationship between increased intraabdominal, intrathoracic, and intracranial pressure. Crit Care Med 1997; 25:496–503.

92. Citerio G, Vascotto E, Villa F, Celotti S, Pesenti A. Induced abdominal compartment syndrome increases intracranial pressure in neurotrauma patients: a prospective study. Crit Care Med 2001; 29:1466–1471.

93. Josephs LG, Este-McDonald JR, Birkett DH, Hirsch EF. Diagnostic laparoscopy increases intracranial pressure. J Trauma 1994; 36:815–818.

94. Bloomfield GL, Dalton JM, Sugerman HJ, et al. Treatment of increasing intracranial pressure secondary to the acute abdominal compartment syndrome in a patient with combined abdominal and head trauma. J Trauma 1995; 39:1168–1170.

95. Morken J, West MA. Abdominal compartment syndrome in the intensive care unit. Curr Opin Crit Care 2001; 7:268–274.

96. Sugerman HJ, DeMaria EJ, Felton WL, Nakatsuka M, Sismanis A. Increased intra-abdominal pressure and cardiac filling pressures in obesity-associated pseudotumor cerebri. Neurology 1997; 49:507–511.

97. Diebel L, Saxe J, Dulchavsky S. Effect of intra-abdominal pressure on abdominal wall blood flow. Am Surg 1992; 58:573–575.

98. del Peso G, Bajo MA, Costero O, et al. Risk factors for abdominal wall complications in peritoneal dialysis patients. Perit Dial Int 2003; 23:249–254.

99. Balogh Z, McKinley BA, Cox CS Jr., et al. Abdominal compartment syndrome: the cause or effect of postinjury multiple organ failure. Shock 2003; 20:483–492.

100. Rezende-Neto JB, Moore EE, Melo de Andrade MV, et al. Systemic inflammatory response secondary to abdominal compartment syndrome: stage for multiple organ failure. J Trauma 2002; 53:1121–1128.

101. Rezende-Neto JB, Moore EE, Masuno T, et al. The abdominal compartment syndrome as a second insult during systemic neutrophil priming provokes multiple organ injury. Shock 2003; 20:303–308.

102. Schachtrupp A, Toens C, Hoer J, et al. A 24-h pneumoperitoneum leads to multiple organ impairment in a porcine model. J Surg Res 2002; 106:37–45.

103. Moore EE. Staged laparotomy for the hypothermia, acidosis, and coagulopathy syndrome. Am J Surg 1996; 172:405–410.

104. Losanoff JE, Richman BW, Jones JW. Temporary abdominal coverage and abdominal compartment syndrome. Arch Surg 2003; 138:565–566.

105. Navsaria PH, Bunting M, Omoshoro-Jones J, Nicol AJ, Kahn D. Temporary closure of open abdominal wounds by the modified sandwich-vacuum pack technique. Br J Surg 2003; 90:718–722.

106. Mayberry JC, Mullins RJ, Crass RA, Trunkey DD. Prevention of abdominal compartment syndrome by absorbable mesh prosthesis closure. Arch Surg 1997; 132:957–961.

107. Rasmussen TE, Hallett JW Jr., Noel AA, et al. Early abdominal closure with mesh reduces multiple organ failure after ruptured abdominal aortic aneurysm repair: guidelines from a 10-year case-control study. J Vasc Surg 2002; 35:246–253.

108. Offner PJ, de Souza AL, Moore EE, et al. Avoidance of abdominal compartment syndrome in damage-control laparotomy after trauma. Arch Surg 2001; 136:676–681.

109. Gracias VH, Braslow B, Johnson J, et al. Abdominal compartment syndrome in the open abdomen. Arch Surg 2002; 137:1298–1300.

110. Balogh Z, McKinley BA, Cocanour CS, et al. Patients with impending abdominal compartment syndrome do not respond to early volume loading. Am J Surg 2003; 186:602–607.

111. Cheatham ML, White MW, Sagraves SG, Johnson JL, Block EF. Abdominal perfusion pressure: a superior parameter in the assessment of intra-abdominal hypertension. J Trauma 2000; 49:621–626.

112. De Waele JJ, Benoit D, Hoste E, Colardyn F. A role for muscle relaxation in patients with abdominal compartment syndrome? Intensive Care Med 2003; 29:332.

113. Eddy V, Nunn C, Morris JA Jr. Abdominal compartment syndrome: the Nashville experience. Surg Clin North Am 1997; 77:801–812.

114. Morris JA Jr., Eddy VA, Blinman TA, Rutherford EJ, Sharp KW. The staged celiotomy for trauma. Issues in unpacking and reconstruction. Ann Surg 1993; 217:576–584.

115. Burch JM, Ortiz VB, Richardson RJ, et al. Abbreviated laparotomy and planned reoperation for critically injured patients. Ann Surg 1992; 215:476–483.

116. Burch JM, Moore EE, Moore FA, Franciose R. The abdominal compartment syndrome. Surg Clin North Am 1996; 76:833–842.

117. Barker DE, Kaufman HJ, Smith LA, et al. Vacuum pack technique of temporary abdominal closure: a 7-year experience with 112 patients. J Trauma 2000; 48:201–206.

118. Wittmann DH, Aprahamian C, Bergstein JM, et al. A burr-like device to facilitate temporary abdominal closure in planned multiple laparotomies. Eur J Surg 1993; 159:75–79.

119. Losanoff JE, Richman BW, Jones JW. Temporary abdominal coverage and reclosure of the open abdomen: frequently asked questions. J Am Coll Surg 2002; 195:105–115.

120. Jernigan TW, Fabian TC, Croce MA, et al. Staged management of giant abdominal wall defects: acute and long-term results. Ann Surg 2003; 238:349–355.

121. Oray-Schrom P, St. Martin D, Bartelloni P, Amoateng-Adjepong Y. Giant nonpancreatic pseudocyst causing acute anuria. J Clin Gastroenterol 2002; 34:160–163.

122. Savino JA, Cerabona T, Agarwal N, Byrne D. Manipulation of ascitic fluid pressure in cirrhotics to optimize hemodynamic and renal-function. Ann Surg 1988; 208:504–511.

123. Corcos AC, Sherman HF. Percutaneous treatment of secondary abdominal compartment syndrome. J Trauma 2001; 51:1062–1064.

124. Latenser BA, Kowal-Vern A, Kimball D, Chakrin A, Dujovny N. A pilot study comparing percutaneous decompression with decompressive laparotomy for acute abdominal compartment syndrome in thermal injury. J Burn Care Rehabil 2002; 23:190–195.

125. Mayberry JC, Welker KJ, Goldman RK, Mullins RJ. Mechanism of acute ascites formation after trauma resuscitation. Arch Surg 2003; 138:773–776.

126. Chen RJ, Fang JF, Lin BC, Kao JL. Laparoscopic decompression of abdominal compartment syndrome after blunt hepatic trauma. Surg Endosc 2000; 14:966–967.

127. Yang EY, Marder SR, Hastings G, Knudson MM. The abdominal compartment syndrome complicating nonoperative management of major blunt liver injuries: recognition and treatment using multimodality therapy. J Trauma 2002; 52:982–986.

128. Shafi S, Kauder DR. Fluid resuscitation and blood replacement in patients with polytrauma. Clin Orthop 2004; 37–42.

129. Gould SA, Moore EE, Hoyt DB, et al. The life-sustaining capacity of human polymerized hemoglobin when red cells might be unavailable. J Am Coll Surg 2002; 195:445–452.

130. Kacmaz A, Polat A, User Y, et al. Octreotide: a new approach to the management of acute abdominal hypertension. Peptides 2003; 24:1381–1386.

131. Kacmaz A, Polat A, User Y, et al. Octreotide improves reperfusion-induced oxidative injury in acute abdominal hypertension in rats. J Gastrointest Surg 2004; 8:113–119.

132. Miller PR, Meredith JW, Johnson JC, Chang MC. Prospective evaluation of vacuum-assisted fascial closure after open abdomen—planned ventral hernia rate is substantially reduced. Ann Surg 2004; 239:608–614.

133. Gecelter G, Fahoum B, Gardezi S, Schein M. Abdominal compartment syndrome in severe acute pancreatitis: an indication for a decompressing laparotomy? Dig Surg 2002; 19:402–404.

134. Hessmann M, Rommens P. Bilateral uretheral obstruction and renal failure caused by massive retroperitoneal hematoma: is there a pelvic compartment syndrome analogous to abdominal compartment syndrome? J Orthop Trauma 1998; 12:553–557.

135. Oelschlager BK, Boyle EM Jr., Johansen K, Meissner MH. Delayed abdominal closure in the management of ruptured abdominal aortic aneurysms. Am J Surg 1997; 173:411–415.

136. Wittmann DH. Operative and nonoperative therapy of intraabdominal infections. Infection 1998; 26:335–341.

137. Ertel W, Oberholzer A, Platz A, Stocker R, Trentz O. Incidence and clinical pattern of the abdominal compartment syndrome after "damage-control" laparotomy in 311 patients with severe abdominal and/or pelvic trauma. Crit Care Med 2000; 28:1747–1753.

138. Blevins DV, Khanduja KS. Abdominal compartment syndrome with massive lower-extremity edema caused by colonic obstruction and distention. Am Surg 2001; 67:451–453.

139. Madl C, Druml W. Gastrointestinal disorders of the critically ill: systemic consequences of ileus. Best Pract Res Clin Gastroenterol 2003; 17:445–456.

140. de Cleva R, Silva FP, Zilberstein B, Machado DJ. Acute renal failure due to abdominal compartment syndrome: report on four cases and literature review. Rev Hosp Clin Fac Med Sao Paulo 2001; 56:123–130.

141. Krivoruchko IA, Boiko VV, Seidametov RR, Andreeshchev SA. Re-laparotomy and damage control during surgical treatment of postoperative intra-abdominal purulent-septic complications. Klin Khir 2004; (1):5–8.

142. Sullivan KM, Battey PM, Miller JS, McKinnon WM, Skardasis GM. Abdominal compartment syndrome after mesenteric revascularization. J Vasc Surg 2001; 34:559–561.

143. Wiebe S, Kellenberger CJ, Khoury A, Miller SF. Early Doppler changes in a renal transplant patient secondary to abdominal compartment syndrome. Pediatr Radiol 2004; 34:432–434.

144. O'Mara MS, Semins H, Hathaway D, Caushaj PF. Abdominal compartment syndrome as a consequence of rectus sheath hematoma. Am Surg 2003; 69:975–977.

145. Yamamoto S, Sato Y, Takeishi T, et al. Liver transplantation in an endostage cirrhosis patient with abdominal compartment syndrome following a spontaneous rectus sheath hematoma. J Gastroenterol Hepatol 2004; 19:118–119.

146. Tsoutsos D, Rodopoulou S, Keramidas E, et al. Early escharotomy as a measure to reduce intraabdominal hypertension in full-thickness burns of the thoracic and abdominal area. World J Surg 2003; 27:1323–1328.

147. Cheatham ML. Intra-abdominal hypertension and abdominal compartment syndrome. New Horizons 1999; 7:96–115.

148. Kidd JN Jr., Jackson RJ, Smith SD, Wagner CW. Evolution of staged versus primary closure of gastroschisis. Ann Surg 2003; 237:759–764.

149. Bar-El Y, Kertzman V, Klein Y. The abdominal compartment syndrome as a consequence of penetrating heart injury. J Card Surg 2003; 18:312–314.

150. Sugerman HJ. Increased intra-abdominal pressure in obesity. Int J Obes 1998; 22:1138.

151. Eddy VA, Key SP, Morris JA Jr. Abdominal compartment syndrome: etiology, detection, and management. J Tenn Med Assoc 1994; 87:55–57.

152. Ali SZ, Freeman BD, Coopersmith CM. Abdominal compartment syndrome in a patient resulting from pneumothorax. Intensive Care Med 2003; 29:1614.

35

Liver Dysfunction in the Previously Well Patient

Joel R. Peerless

Department of Surgical Critical Care, MetroHealth Medical Center, Case Western Reserve University, Cleveland, Ohio, U.S.A.

INTRODUCTION

The hepatobiliary system plays a major role in energy metabolism, bilirubin metabolism, coagulation, digestion, and the immune response. The liver receives a large portion of the cardiac output and, as such, critically ill patients with any combination of trauma, hemodynamic instability, and sepsis are subject to hepatic dysfunction. Most critically ill patients are administered multiple medications which may affect hepatic function, and hepatic dysfunction may require alterations in drug dosing. Knowledge of the etiologies of hepatic dysfunction, hepatic function in disease states, and alterations in drug metabolism in the critically ill patient will aid the clinician in the generalized support of the critically ill patient with hepatic dysfunction.

OVERVIEW OF NORMAL HEPATIC ANATOMY
Hepatic Anatomy and Blood Supply

The liver weighs approximately 1500 g, is enclosed within a fibrous sheath (Glisson's capsule), and is located in the right upper quadrant of the abdomen. The upper border of the liver lies approximately at the level of the nipples. The lower border corresponds to the costal cartilage of the right ninth and left eighth ribs.

The liver receives approximately 25% of the total cardiac output. The blood supply to the liver is situated to process, modify, and detoxify nutrients and metabolic fuels from the intestinal lumen (1). Blood supply to the liver is derived from two sources, the portal vein and the hepatic artery. Blood in the portal vein drains blood from the digestive tract between the proximal stomach to the upper rectum, spleen, pancreas, and gall bladder (2,3). The portal vein accounts for 75% of the total hepatic blood flow (1–4).

The common hepatic artery is one of three major branches of the celiac axis, and provides branches to the gall bladder via the cystic arteries (2,3). Although the hepatic artery accounts for only 25% of hepatic blood flow, it provides 50% of the oxygen requirements to the hepatocytes, and hepatic arterial flow may become predominant in a cirrhotic liver with decreased portal vein perfusion (2,3). Hepatic collateral circulation can be dilated in cases of cirrhosis or thrombosis of portal or hepatic veins. The most common sites of increased collateral portal circulation are the submucosal vessels of the esophagus and stomach (Fig. 1).

Hepatic Microcirculation

Hepatocytes are polyhedral cells with a central spherical nucleus, arranged in plates one cell in thickness with blood-filled sinusoids on each side of the plates (2,3). Hepatocytes comprise 65% of the cells in the liver, have specialized oxidative activities, and are spatially arranged to achieve these functions (2,3).

The liver is classically divided into lobules (1–2 mm hexagons) oriented around a central vein (the terminal hepatic vein) which drains into the hepatic vein. At every other apex of the hexagonal lobule is a portal triad, which includes a bile duct, a branch of the hepatic artery, and a branch of the portal vein. The portal venous blood and the hepatic arterial blood mix and bathe the hepatocytes via sinusoids.

Sinusoids are the major site for blood-flow regulation, hepatic capacitance, and solute exchange between blood and hepatocyte (4). The flow of mixed portal vein blood and hepatic arterial blood is in the opposite direction of the bile formation. The hepatic sinusoids eventually empty into the terminal hepatic venule. Hepatic sinusoids are fenestrated with scanty subendothelial stromal material, permitting passage of large macromolecules (2,3). Sinusoids bridge the gap between terminal portal venules (inflow) and hepatic venules (outflow) (2–4). This low-pressure system results in a constant, sluggish blood flow through the sinusoids (2,3).

The three-dimensional organization of the functional liver anatomy can be further described by the Acinar model, in which hepatocytes surround a terminal central hepatic vein which forms the pericentral zone (Fig. 2) (2,3). Pericentral hepatocytes differ from the hepatocytes that surround the central vein in synthetic capabilities, enzymes, and susceptibility to liver injury (Fig. 3) (2,3). Hepatocytes that are further away from the portal blood supply are more prone to hypoxic effects of ischemia and react differently to toxin exposure. ✐ **The geographic position of hepatocytes and their exposure to gradients of nutrients and waste products leads to location-related variations in susceptibility to ischemia and drug toxicity (2).** ✐

Biliary System

Bile drains from each hepatic segment through bile canaliculi, to small hepatic ducts, to right and left hepatic ducts, which eventually form a common hepatic duct (Fig. 4). The common hepatic duct joins with the cystic duct to form the common bile duct (CBD) emptying into the duodenum via the ampulla of Vater. The function of the gall bladder is to concentrate and store bile during fasting; and

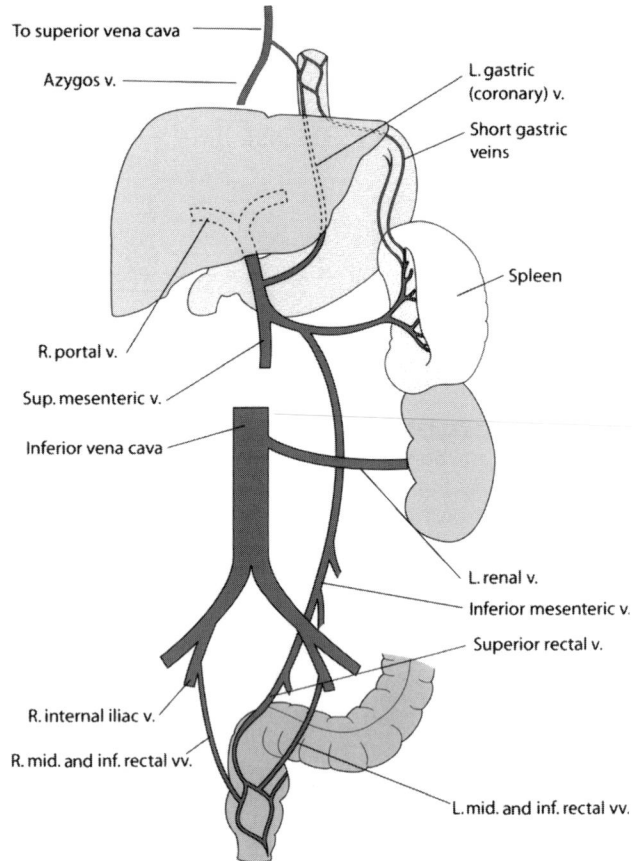

Figure 1   Diagram of the portal circulation. The most important sites for the potential development of portosystemic collateral vessels involve the areas where systemic veins join the portal system. (*i*) Esophageal submucosal veins, supplied by the left gastric vein and draining into the superior vena cava through the azygos vein. (*ii*) Paraumbilical veins, supplied by the umbilical portion of the left portal vein and draining into abdominal wall veins near the umbilicus (not shown). These veins may form a caput medusa at the umbilicus. (*iii*) Rectal submucosal veins, supplied by the inferior mesenteric vein through the superior rectal vein and draining into the internal iliac veins through the middle rectal veins. (*iv*) Splenorenal shunts: created spontaneously or surgically. (*v*) Short gastric veins communicate with the esophageal plexus. *Source*: From Ref. 84.

having a volume of 30–70 mL may add this stored bile following a large fatty meal (1).

NORMAL HEPATIC FUNCTION
Energy Metabolism
Carbohydrate Metabolism

The liver is responsible for maintenance of normal glucose levels through regulation of glycogenolysis and gluconeogenesis (5). In the fed state, glucose is stored as glycogen or converted to fatty acids that are then stored in adipose tissue (5). Hepatic glycogen is the main storage site for glucose-dependent organs [brain, red blood cells (RBCs), retina, and renal medulla] (1). The normal liver has a 24- to 48-hour supply of glycogen. Alcoholics and malnourished patients have little or no stored glycogen and are more

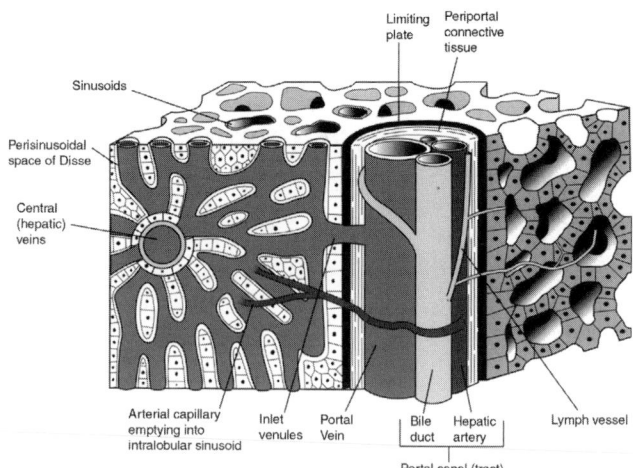

Figure 2   Three-dimensional architectural drawing of the normal human liver. The major components of the portal tract (or canal) include a branch of the portal vein, a hepatic arteriole, a bile duct, and some lymphatics (not shown). Also shown in the figure are cholangioles that carry bile from the canaliculi to the bile duct (listed as lymphatic). The hepatic arterial blood empties into the interlobular sinusoids mixing with the portal venous blood which enters the sinusoids via inlet venules. This nutrient-rich blood eventually empties into the central hepatic veins. The perisinusoidal space of Disse separates the sinusoidal blood from the hepatocytes. The hepatocytes empty their bile on the opposite side of their cells into the bile canaliculi. *Source*: From Ref. 85.

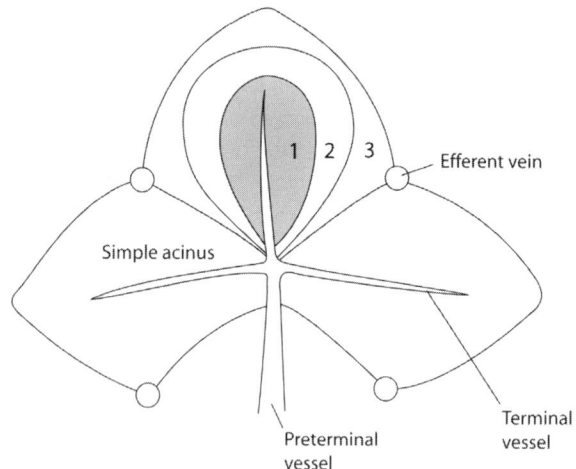

Figure 3   The complex acinar structure as conceived by Rappaport. The preterminal vessel is the proximal portion of the mixed hepatic arterial and portal venous sinusoidal blood, and the terminal portion is the distal end. The terminal hepatic venule is labeled as efferent vein. The margins of the shaded zones represent planes of equal blood pressure (isobars), oxygen content, or other characteristics. Periportal tissue (zone 1) receives blood that is higher in oxygen content than perivenular (zone 3) tissue. The acinus is bulb shaped, and the classic lobule is composed of several wedge-shaped portions, (called primary lobule, not indicated). The hepatic microcirculatory subunit is the smallest functional unit in which there is the potential for countercurrent flow. *Source*: From Ref. 85.

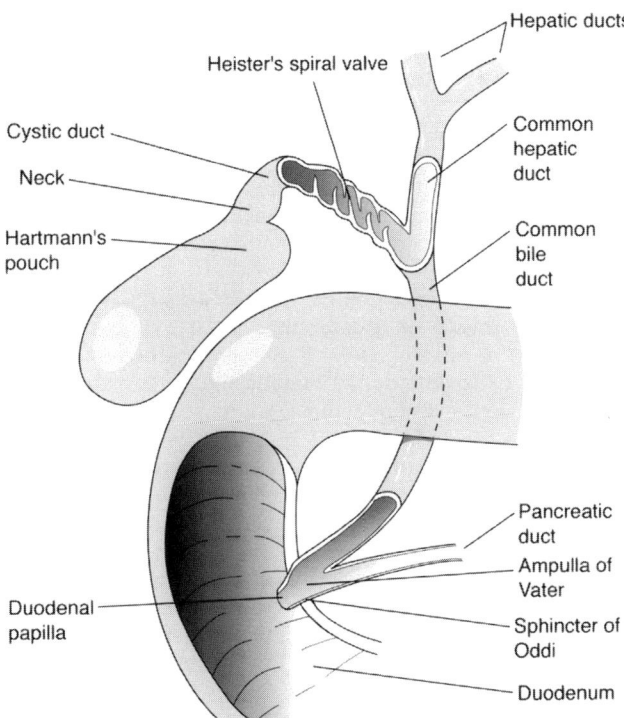

Figure 4 Gallbladder and biliary system. The right and left hepatic ducts coalesce to form the common hepatic duct which can empty into the CBD or into the cystic duct for storage in the gallbladder for later use. The CBD joins the pancreatic duct at the ampulla of Vater and empties into the duodenum via the duodenal papilla. This anatomy explains why the passage of gall stones can either cause obstruction of the CBD and result in dilation of intrahepatic ducts (causing cholestatic jaundice), or obstruct pancreatic exocrine function resulting in gall stone pancreatitis. When the stone is only obstructing the cystic duct (simple cholelithiasis), the patient may complain of pain, and could later develop secondary infection related to the obstruction, but will not necessarily have an elevation of either bilirubin levels or pancreatic enzymes. *Abbreviation*: CBD, common bile duct. *Source*: From Ref. 85.

prone to hypoglycemia. Insulin stimulates the formation of glycogen and inhibits gluconeogenesis (5). Glycogenolysis and gluconeogenesis are stimulated by glucagon and epinephrine. Precursors for glucose formation are lactate, pyruvate, and amino acids (1,2).

Lipid Metabolism

The liver plays a central role in fatty acid metabolism (1). Oxidation of fatty acids to carbon dioxide and water yields the highest production of adenosine triphosphate (1). In the fed state, the liver esterifies fatty acids to triglycerides and other esters, which provide energy for the liver. In the fasting state, fatty acid synthesis is inhibited. Obesity, diabetes mellitus, corticosteroid therapy, and ethanol ingestion can result in fatty liver, an excess accumulation of triglyceride. Alcoholic ketosis occurs secondary to ethanol or acetaldehyde-mediated impairment of fatty acid oxidation (5).

Amino Acid and Protein Metabolism

The liver is the major site for the synthesis of proteins involved in coagulation, transport, and acute phase reactants. Plasma protein synthesis accounts for 80% of all hepatic protein synthesis, and is regulated by multiple factors, including availability of nutritional components, genetic determinants, drugs, toxins, as well as the presence of inflammatory or catabolic states (5). ☞ **Acute hepatic disease will have a greater effect on proteins with rapid turnover (i.e., coagulation factors) than those that turn over more slowly, such as albumin (5).** ☜

Bilirubin Metabolism

Almost 70% of bilirubin is derived from the heme moiety of hemoglobin from erythrocytes sequestered in the spleen, liver, and bone marrow. The remaining bilirubin results from the breakdown of nonhemoglobin protein, cytochrome P-450, in the liver. Unconjugated bilirubin is water insoluble, highly bound to albumin, and not excreted in the urine. Following transport to the liver, carrier proteins mediate passage through large fenestrations in the cells of the sinusoidal lining and contact the hepatocyte plasma membrane. Bilirubin is conjugated with glucuronic acid, becoming water soluble, and secreted into the bile canaliculus. Serum bilirubin is normally at least 70% conjugated (Fig. 5) (4–8).

Bile Formation

Bile is composed of conjugated bile acids, cholesterol, phospholipids, and protein. In the initial formation of bile, bile acids and bilirubin are taken up at the sinusoidal membrane (4). Bile is formed at a rate of 0.42 mL/min (4). Eighty percent of bile is secreted by hepatocytes and 20% by the bile duct epithelial cells (4). Inhibition of the sphincter of Oddi by cholecystokinin stimulates expulsion of preformed bile into the duodenum (1,4).

The formation of bile is a high-energy expenditure process. To conserve energy and maintain the large stores of bile required for digestive purposes, an enterohepatic circulation recirculates bile 6 to 15 times per day (4). Active secretion of bile salts across the canalicular membrane is the primary metabolic pump of the enterohepatic circulation (4). Malfunction of the enterohepatic circulation leads to a decreased bile acid pool, which predisposes to gall stone formation (4).

Vitamin Metabolism

The liver is vital to the uptake, storage, and mobilization of many vitamins. Bile salts are required for absorption of the fat-soluble vitamins A, D, E, and K. Vitamin D conversion to 25-hydroxycalciferol, the first step of vitamin D activation, occurs in the liver (4). Vitamin K is essential for the activation of the coagulation factors II, VII, IX, and X (4).

BIOCHEMICAL EVALUTION OF HEPATIC DYSFUNCTION

The liver is one of the most frequently damaged organs in the body, but also has one of the greatest regenerative capacities, and has enormous functional reserve. Only 10% of hepatic parenchyma is required for normal liver function. Thus, evidence of liver injury does not necessarily mean that hepatic dysfunction is occurring.

The most common method of assessing hepatic health is to obtain a measure of liver function tests (LFTs). The common LFTs include hepatic enzymes called bilirubin. When liver injury occurs, hepatic enzymes leak into the circulation, and bilirubin levels increase. An additional

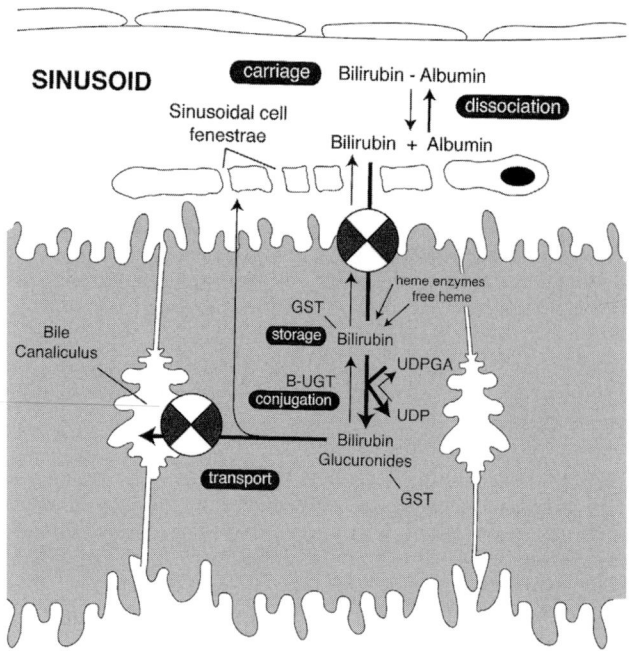

SINUSOID

Figure 5 Schematic diagram summarizing the structural and biochemical pathways involved in bilirubin metabolism. During its carriage in the plasma, bilirubin is strongly, but reversibly bound to albumin. In hepatic sinusoids, this complex comes in direct contact with the basolateral domain of the hepatocyte plasma membrane through fenestrae of the specialized hepatic endothelial cells. At the hepatocyte surface, dissociation of the albumin-bilirubin complex occurs, and bilirubin enters hepatocytes by a specific uptake mechanism. A fraction of the bilirubin is also derived from catabolism of hepatocellular heme proteins. Storage within the hepatocyte is accomplished by binding of bilirubin to a group of cytosolic proteins, glutathione-S-transferases (GSTs) (also termed ligandin or Y-protein). Binding to these proteins keeps bilirubin in solution and inhibits its efflux from the cell, thereby increasing the net uptake. Conjugation of bilirubin in the endoplasmic reticulum is catalyzed by bilirubin-UDP-glucuronosyltransferase, forming bilirubin monoglucuronide and diglucuronide. Both conjugates may bind to GSTs in the cytosol. Conjugation is obligatory for efficient transport across the bile canaliculus. This process is normally rate-limiting in bilirubin throughput, and is shared by other organic anions, but not bile salts. *Source*: From Ref. 85.

measure of liver function is provided by assessing the synthetic function of the liver (e.g., albumin, prealbumin, and coagulation factors). These various methods of evaluating liver injury and viability with biochemical measurements will be reviewed in the following sections.

Hepatic Enzymes
Aminotransferases
The aminotransferases, aspartate aminotransferase (AST, formerly serum glutamic oxaloacetic transaminase), and alanine aminotransferase (ALT, formerly serum glutamic pyruvic transaminase) measure liver injury (Table 1). While ALT is relatively specific to the liver, AST is found in the liver as well as skeletal and cardiac muscle, kidney, brain, pancreas, and blood (7). Absolute elevations of AST and ALT reflect leakage from damaged liver cells (7), as well as the early phase of acute biliary obstruction (8).

The level of elevation of aminotransferases may be an indication of the etiology of hepatic dysfunction. ALT and AST levels less than 300 IU/L are seen in alcoholic hepatitis and biliary obstruction. Patients with advanced cirrhosis may have normal or near normal levels of aminotransferases (7).

Mild to moderate elevations of aminotransferases (250–1000 IU/L) are seen with viral infection, drug-induced hepatitis, nonsteroidal antiinflammatory agents, cocaine, modest hepatic inflammation, steatosis, drugs, alcohol, chronic viral hepatitis, and cirrhosis (7). ☞ **Aminotransferase levels of greater than 1000 IU/L are almost always due to hepatocellular injury, and can be seen with drug- and or toxin-induced hepatic injury, ischemic liver injury, and acute viral hepatitis (7).** ☞

The level of elevation of aminotransferases correlates poorly with the extent of necrosis, and is not predictive of outcome (7,8). Aminotransferase levels may fall during the course of massive hepatic necrosis, and a rapid fall in enzyme levels in combination with a rising bilirubin and prolonged prothrombin time may portend a poor prognosis (7,8).

☞ **In most hepatic injuries, the ratio of AST to ALT is usually 1:1; however, ratios of 2:1 or greater are common in alcoholic hepatitis.** ☞ A high AST to ALT ratio in the absence of alcohol abuse may represent cirrhosis (7).

Alkaline Phosphatase
Alkaline phosphatase (AP) is present mostly in liver and bone. Hepatic AP is present in the hepatocyte plasma membrane and the lumen of the bile duct epithelium (7). Elevations of AP are secondary to increased synthesis and release of enzyme into the circulation (7). Hepatocyte plasma membranes are solubilized by bile acids, which are retained in settings of cholestasis. The retention of bile acids facilitates the release of AP, thus the rise of AP after acute biliary obstruction (7). Because elevations of AP require synthesis of new enzymes, AP may not increase for one to two days after biliary obstruction (7). The half-life of AP is approximately one week, thus levels may remain elevated for days to weeks after resolution of biliary obstruction (8).

Levels of AP of 3 to 10 times normal are seen in both intrahepatic and extrahepatic obstruction of bile flow. Slight to moderate increases in AP may be seen in hepatitis and cirrhosis. Higher levels may be seen with infiltrative hepatic disorders secondary to intrahepatic bile duct compression (7,8). Severe bacterial infection is also associated with an isolated rise in AP (7).

Lactate Dehydrogenase
Elevations of lactate dehydrogenase (LDH) are seen in many different tissue injuries, including skeletal and cardiac muscle, hemolysis, stroke, and renal infarct. LDH is especially high in ischemic hepatitis. A sustained elevation of LDH with AP is indicative of malignant infiltration of the liver (7).

Gamma-Glutamyl Transpeptidase
Gamma-glutamyl transpeptidase (GGTP) is present in many tissues, but not in bone, and thus may be useful in confirming hepatic elevations of AP (7,8). GGTP is inducible by alcohol, and thus may be useful in detecting alcohol abuse. GGTP is also elevated in biliary obstruction, but is not as sensitive for obstruction as 5′-nucleotidase (NT).

Table 1 Biochemical Liver Function Tests

Test/basis of abnormality	Normal range	Level of elevation	Extrahepatic sources
Aminotransferases/leakage from damaged tissue	AST 10–40 U/L	Modest—many types of hepatic disease	ALT—relatively specific for hepatocellular necrosis
	ALT 10–55 U/L	Marked—hepatitis (ischemic, viral, toxic)	AST—skeletal and cardiac muscle; kidney, brain, pancreas, RBCs
		Levels <300 U/L with AST:ALT ratio >2:1—alcoholic hepatitis, cirrhosis	
AP/Overproduction and leakage into serum	45–115 U/L	Modest—many types of hepatic disease Marked—extra and intrahepatic cholestasis, diffuse infiltrating disease (tumor); occasional alcoholic hepatitis	Bone growth or disease (tumor, fracture, Paget's disease); placenta, intestine, tumors
Gammaglutamyl transpeptidase/overproduction and leakage into serum	0–30 U/L	Same as AP Induced by ethanol, drugs GGTP:AP ratio >2.5 suggestive of alcoholic liver disease	Kidney, spleen, pancreas, heart, lung, brain
5′NT/overproduction and leakage into serum	0–11 U/L	Same as AP	Relatively specific for liver disease
Bilirubin/decreased hepatic clearance	0–1.0 mg/dL 0–17 μmol/L	Modest—many types of hepatic disease Marked—extra and intrahepatic cholestasis; alcoholic, drug-induced or viral hepatitis	Increased breakdown of hemoglobin
Prothrombin time/decreased synthetic activity	10.9–12.5 sec	Acute or chronic liver failure (unresponsive to vitamin K) Biliary obstruction (responsive to vitamin K)	Vitamin K deficiency (malabsorption, malnutrition, antibiotics); consumptive coagulopathy
Albumin/decreased synthetic activity; increased catabolism	4.0–6.0 g/dL	Chronic liver failure	Decreased in nephrotic syndrome, protein losing enteropathy, vascular leak, malnutrition, malignancy, inflammatory states

Abbreviations: AST, aspartate aminotransferase; ALT, alanine aminotransferase; RBC, red blood cells; GGTP, gamma-glutamyl transpeptidase; AP, alkaline phosphatase; 5′NT, 5′-nucleotidase.
Source: From Ref. 1, p. 1127.

5′-Nucleotidase

5′-NT is present in small quantities in numerous organs, but is only present in high concentrations in liver tissue (7,8). The enzyme is located in the hepatocyte sinusoidal and canalicular bile membranes and may reflect bile obstruction (7,8). Because 5′-NT is predominantly located in or near the bile canalicular membrane, its elevation is more specific for biliary obstruction than either AP or GGTP, both of which are diffusely distributed throughout the liver.

Bilirubin

Normal Serum Bilirubin Levels (in Health)

Bilirubin results from the metabolism of the porphyrin ring component of heme-containing proteins (chiefly hemoglobin and myoglobin). Bilirubin exists in the blood in two forms, conjugated (water soluble) and unconjugated (water insoluble, bound to albumin). Most clinical labs use the Van den Bergh assay to determine the conjugated "direct" reacting component (reacts prior to addition of alcohol) and the total bilirubin (the amount that reacts after the addition of alcohol). The indirect amount is the total minus the direct, and correlates with the unconjugated portion. ☞ **Normally, the total bilirubin is less than 1 mg/dL, and at least 70% is conjugated (direct reacting).** ☞ The rate-limiting step in bilirubin metabolism is not conjugation (a property which remains intact even with severe liver disease). Rather, transport of conjugated bilirubin into the bile canaliculi is the rate limiting step, explaining why elevated bilirubin is seen in all forms of acute liver disease including that due to ischemia and shock liver.

Causes of Hyperbilirubinemia (Jaundice)
Overproduction of Bilirubin
In the trauma patient, the administration of multiple blood transfusions may result in a bilirubin load that overwhelms the conjugation and excretory capacity of the liver (9,10). In an effort to rotate stocks of packed RBCs, those first released from the blood bank are usually the oldest ones on the shelf. These older, more fragile RBCs lyse quickly within the reticuloendothelial system, and the resultant increase in unconjugated bilirubin is analogous to any other source of hemolytic anemia. The normal rate of bilirubin production is approximately 250–300 mg/day, an amount equal to a 500 mL transfusion of RBCs.

Resorption of hematomas is another common cause of unconjugated hyperbilirubinemia, in patients with major trauma or those undergoing major aortic procedures (7,10). Drug-induced or immune-mediated hemolysis, mechanical damage to RBCs (mechanical heart valves), or hemoglobinopathies (sickle cell anemia) may also result in overproduction of bilirubin (7,9,10). The inability to respond to an increased bilirubin load is accentuated with underlying liver disease or acute ischemic injury (9).

Acute Hepatocellular Injury
Acute hepatocellular injury may occur secondary to hypoperfusion, ischemia, iatrogenic injury to blood vessels of the liver, following toxic exposure (acetaminophen, Amanita phalloides) and to many classes of medications (10). Conjugated hyperbilirubinemia results from impaired hepatic excretion and regurgitation of bilirubin from hepatocytes into the serum. However, in the setting of "ischemic hepatitis" or "shock liver," the predominant picture is hepatocellular necrosis, with extremely high enzyme elevations.

Cholestasis
Cholestasis describes any disturbance of the bile secretory process (extrahepatic or intrahepatic). Extrahepatic refers to an obstructor at the bile duct level. Obstruction may occur from cholelithiasis, inflammatory processes, or extraluminal compression (11,12). Intrahepatic cholestasis is more common than extrahepatic in the trauma and critical care setting. Intrahepatic cholestasis is sometimes referred to as benign postoperative jaundice, and may be secondary to prolonged hypotension and multiple blood transfusions among other causes. Intrahepatic inflammatory disorders such as sepsis, primary biliary cirrhosis, infiltrative or granulomatous disease, drug toxicity, and viral or alcoholic hepatitis may result in cholestasis (11,12).

Serum bilirubin can be elevated as high as 40 mg/dL in cholestasis (10). AP levels are elevated; however, aminotransferase levels, prothrombin time, and albumin levels are not initially altered in pure cholestasis. Although this process is usually self-limited, patients can progress to sepsis and multiorgan failure (10). In prolonged cholestasis, the delta fraction of circulating conjugated bilirubin is tightly bound to albumin, and may account for the prolonged resolution of bilirubin when other parameters are improving (7).

Tests of Hepatic Synthetic Function
Albumin and Prealbumin
Albumin is the predominant serum binding protein with a half-life of approximately three weeks (2,8). Production is 100–200 mg/kg/day, and is influenced by nutritional state, the presence of systemic disease, toxins, liver disease, and thyroid and glucocorticoid hormones (8). Albumin

levels reflect hepatic synthesis and volume of distribution, and may decrease with nephrotic syndrome, protein-losing enteropathy, severe burns, traumatic blood loss, peritoneal losses, exfoliative dermatitis, and gastrointestinal bleeding (2,8) Thus, the albumin concentration is limited as an acute indicator of liver disease severity (8). Prealbumin has a half-life of three to four days. However, a low prealbumin level is not specific for hepatic disease. Indeed, malnutrition in a patient with a normal liver will result in decreased prealbumin.

Prothrombin Time
The prothrombin time measures the rate of conversion of prothrombin to thrombin, and reflects the activity of factors II, VII, IX, and X, the factors involved in the extrinsic coagulation pathway (7). Elevations of prothrombin time occur with vitamin K deficiency, warfarin, disseminated intravascular coagulation (DIC), acute and chronic liver disease, and chronic cholestasis with fat malabsorption (7). ☞ **The coagulation factors have a short half-life, especially factor VII (five to seven hours); thus prothrombin time is a useful indicator of hepatic synthetic function providing vitamin K levels are normal (4,8).** ☞

ETIOLOGY OF LIVER DYSFUNCTION IN THE TRAUMA/ INTENSIVE CARE UNIT PATIENT
Ischemic Hepatitis
Etiology and Pathogenesis
Trauma and Shock
Ischemic hepatitis, or "shock liver," refers to acute circulatory failure of the liver in the setting of trauma, major surgery, and critical illness (13–17). Liver cell necrosis occurs secondary to prolonged cellular hypoxia, due to arterial hypotension, hypoxemia, or passive venous congestion (16). Hypotension is the most important factor contributing to post-traumatic liver dysfunction and jaundice (13,17). Hypotension may be secondary to, or accompanied by, hypovolemia, hypoxemia, prolonged surgery, and anemia with the requirement for massive transfusion (13). Multiple etiologies are usually present in such situations.

Patients with ischemic hepatitis may present clinically with jaundice, encephalopathy, hepatomegaly, or acholic stools (13). Marked elevations of aminotransferases and LDH are common, with lesser elevations of AP (two to three times normal) and bilirubin (5–20 mg/dL) (14–16). Prothrombin time may be elevated two to three seconds (14). Elevations in LFTs occur within the first 12 to 24 hours, peak within one week of the inciting event, and resolve to normal in 7 to 10 days (Fig. 6) (15,16).

Ischemic Hepatitis in Cardiac and Medical Patients
Cardiogenic ischemic hepatitis occurs in the setting of overt cardiogenic shock or in heart failure patients with an acute decline in cardiac function (18–22). Elevations of serum ALT, AST (usually 10–20 times normal values) and bilirubin occur, as well as prolongation of prothrombin time. Abnormal values decrease by 50% within 72 hours.

Congestive liver fibrosis and congestive cirrhosis (cardiac cirrhosis) occur secondary to elevated venous pressure, hypoxia or hepatocellular necrosis, with varying degrees of fibrosis in different regions of the liver (18). The diagnosis is suggested by the triad of right heart failure,

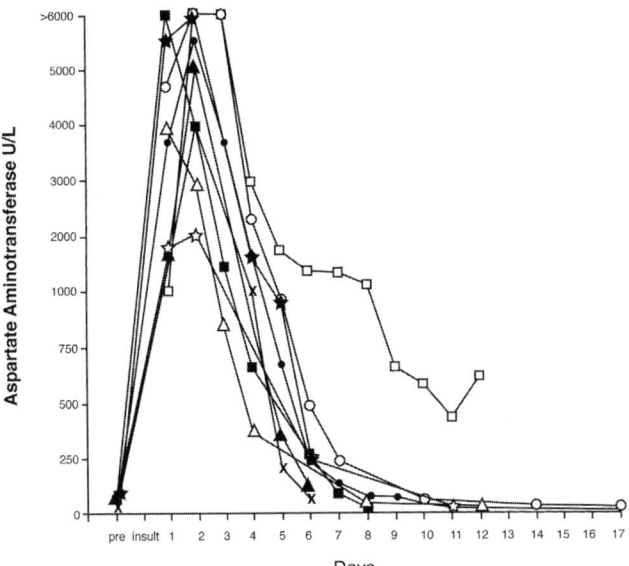

Figure 6 The course of aspartate aminotransferase (AST) elevation and normalization in ischemic hepatitis. Each of nine individual patients is represented by a separate symbol. All but one had AST values sore above 2000 U/L by postinsult day 3 (most reaching above 4–6000 U/L). All but one had values return to normal by day 10, with most demonstrating values below 250 U/L by day 7. *Source*: From Ref. 15.

hepatomegaly, and ascites with high protein content. Aminotransferases, AP, bilirubin, and albumin levels are usually initially normal (18).

Pathology and Pathophysiology

The hepatic arterial buffer response (HABR) is a compensation mechanism by which hepatic arterial dilation compensates for inadequate portal blood flow (19,22). Hepatic oxygen consumption is maintained due to the higher oxygen saturation of hepatic arterial blood (22). Following injury, splanchnic blood flow decreases as splanchnic vascular resistance is increased. Hepatic oxygen consumption may be maintained by an increase in oxygen extraction, which may actually exceed oxygen extraction in other areas of the body (17). Although the HABR is maintained early in hemorrhage, as blood loss exceeds 30%, splanchnic vasoconstriction becomes significant, and hepatic oxygen supply decreases (22).

Patients with acute circulatory failure secondary to organic heart disease demonstrate both hepatic hypoperfusion and hepatic venous congestion, which may further predispose the liver to ischemic injury (22). ☞ **Ischemic hepatitis is associated pathologically with centrilobular necrosis. This is described histologically as necrosis to hepatocytes surrounding the central vein (furthest away from the nutrients supply) and hence, most susceptible to ischemic damage (16).** ☞ The reticular framework of the lobule is preserved, however, and allows for regeneration after recovery of the hypoperfusion (16).

Biochemical Liver Tests in the Differential Diagnosis of Ischemic Hepatitis

Many other conditions that cause abnormalities of liver function may be present in the critically ill patient. These include viral hepatitis, sepsis, intravascular hemolysis, and venous congestion. The time course and level of hepatic enzyme increases suggest an ischemic etiology. In benign postoperative cholestasis, bilirubin and AST levels will be lower and AP levels higher than in ischemic hepatitis. LDH levels may be useful in differentiating ischemic from viral hepatitis, as only a moderate rise in LDH occurs in viral hepatitis (16). Viral hepatitis has a longer time course than ischemic hepatitis (viral titers are required to make that diagnosis).

Treatment

Treatment of ischemic hepatitis is entirely supportive, including resuscitation, antibiotic treatment of infection and sepsis, control of gastrointestinal bleeding, nutritional support, and adjustment of medications for hepatic dysfunction (13,18). Mortality is increased when ischemic hepatitis occurs in patients with pre-existing chronic liver disease (16).

Hepatic Response to Infection and Sepsis
Hepatic Blood Flow and Oxygen Consumption

There is conflicting evidence related to hepatic blood flow in sepsis (Volume 2, Chapters 47 and 63). Several studies have demonstrated decreased hepatic blood flow secondary to mesenteric vasoconstriction, or to the hypovolemia and cardiac dysfunction that occurs with sepsis (22–24). Hepatic hypoperfusion may occur in the absence of hypotension, and may persist despite fluid resuscitation (25). In addition, there may be alterations in the regional distribution of hepatic blood flow that may lead to areas with decreased oxygen utilization (22). In some models of sepsis, there has been speculation that hepatic hyperperfusion may occur due to increased cardiac output and decreased systemic vascular resistance (25,26). In these models, hepatic hypoxia is postulated to occur from increased flow of desaturated portal blood (25).

Oxygen consumption is increased in sepsis. Increased splanchnic uptake of lactate, amino acids and free fatty acids, and concomitant increased splanchnic glucose output has been demonstrated after endotoxin bolus in humans (27). Because of increased amino acid and lactate concentrations, gluconeogenesis and glucose uptake are upregulated. The mismatch of hepatic blood flow and metabolic demand is a major etiology of sepsis-induced hepatic dysfunction (22–29).

Hepatic Cellular Response to Bacteremia and Endotoxemia

The hepatic cellular response to sepsis involves Kupffer cells, hepatocytes, and sinusoidal endothelial cells (24,30,31). The majority of the body's reticuloendothelial system surface area is contained within the liver, primarily the macrophage Kupffer cells that line the sinusoidal vascular network (24,30,31). The Kupffer cells scavenge and filter bacteria and endotoxins from portal vein blood, preventing them from entering the systemic circulation. Kupffer cells also limit the systemic inflammatory response by scavenging inflammatory mediators and cytokines (24,30). Spillover of bacterial, endotoxin, and inflammatory mediators leads to activation of the coagulation, kallikrein, and complement cascades, leading to generalized microvascular injury, the systemic inflammatory response syndrome, and when severe, irreversible shock and multiple organ dysfunction syndrome (Volume 2, Chapter 63) (24).

Hepatic Mediator Production and Secondary Cellular Dysfunction

Kupffer cells produce and release mediators such as proinflammatory cytokines such as tumor necrosis factor-alpha (TNF-α), and interleukins-6 (IL-6), as well as nitric oxide, reactive oxygen products, and granulocyte colony stimulating factors (24,30,31).

Secondary hepatic dysfunction occurs in Kupffer cells as a result of tissue factor–induced fibrin deposition and microcirculatory disturbances, with resultant hepatocyte and endothelial cell injury. Endotoxin and TNF may induce cellular dysfunction, even without microcirculatory changes (24). Consumption of fibronectin as a result of reticuloendothelial system phagocytosis of particulate material may impair reticuloendothelial system efficiency (30). Mediators of reperfusion injury may cause additional injury to endothelial and parenchymal cells following resuscitation (21).

Effects of Infection and Sepsis on the Immune Response and Coagulation

Hepatocytes have receptors for endotoxin, cytokines, inflammatory mediators, and vasoactive substances (24). Hepatocytes demonstrate increased synthesis and release of coagulation factors, complement and antiproteolytic enzymes (24). Acute-phase proteins such as C reactive protein, alpha-one antitrypsin, fibrinogen, and prothrombin are also increased. There is an overall procoagulant response secondary to enhanced inhibition of protein C, lower protein S, decreased synthesis of protein C and antithrombin III, increased tissue factor, and enhanced inhibition of fibrinolysis (24).

Lactate and the Liver

While lactate production increases in settings of hypoperfusion, the presence of lactate in sepsis may represent the hypermetabolism that is stimulated by inflammatory mediators. The liver is both a source of lactate as well as the primary organ responsible for lactate clearance. Hepatic production of lactate is based on the presence of macrophages in the liver, increased hepatic neutrophil sequestration, and endotoxin-induced glucose uptake and synthesis of free radicals in hepatic phagocytes (32). Lactate metabolism by the normal liver usually results in negative lactate balance. However, lactate balance can be positive in the presence of underlying hepatic dysfunction or sepsis-induced hepatic dysfunction due to increased lactate production. ☞ **The major source of hyperlactatemia in sepsis results from dysfunctional clearance of lactate by the liver (31,32).** ☞

Sepsis and Cholestasis

Intrahepatic cholestasis is the most common finding in bacteremic patients with jaundice (12,31,33). There are a number of mechanisms by which sepsis results in cholestasis. Bile flow and biliary excretion are reduced after exposure to endotoxin. Endotoxemia impairs the transport of organic anions at the sinusoidal and canalicular membranes. Endotoxin and proinflammatory cytokines may also lead to increased neutrophil migration and adhesion, resulting in hepatocyte injury and portal tract inflammation (12,30). It is likely that both decreased hepatic perfusion and decreased urinary excretion of conjugated bilirubin play a role.

Biochemical Liver Tests in the Hepatic Response to Infection and Sepsis

In sepsis, LFTs commonly demonstrate intrahepatic cholestasis (12,30,34). Elevations of serum bilirubin occur in a high percentage of septic patients (34–36). Although peak serum bilirubin usually is in the 5–10 mg/dL range, mostly conjugated, levels may reach as high as 40 mg/dL. Often, there are only modest elevations of aminotransferases (34–37). The level of elevation of serum bilirubin and serum enzymes are often discrepant (33,35,36). AP is elevated one to three times normal, and rarely 5 to 10 times normal (34–37).

The differential diagnosis of sepsis-induced cholestasis includes gall stone disease, sludge, acute acalculous cholecystitis (AAC), drug-induce hepatitis, hemolysis, and cholestasis or jaundice associated with total parenteral nutrition (TPN) (30). Sepsis should be considered when fever and jaundice occur without aminotransferase elevations or evidence of primary hepatic or biliary tract disease. Although the level of bilirubin is not always predictive of outcome, persistent hyperbilirubinemia portends a poor prognosis (34–37).

PHARMACOLOGY AND HEPATIC DYSFUNCTION
Hepatic Biotransformation
Pathways of Drug Elimination

Three phases of drug elimination are accomplished by the liver. Phase I involves alteration of the parent molecule by oxidation, reduction, and hydrolysis. Phase II includes conjugation of a drug or metabolite with small, endogenous molecules such as glucuronic acid, glutathione acetate or glutathione sulfate, making the products water soluble, allowing excretion into the bile or urine. Conjugation usually detoxifies active metabolites. Phase III involves excretion of the parent compound or metabolite from the hepatocyte (37–40). Any or all of these three steps may be involved in drug elimination (37–40).

Cytochrome P-450 System

The cytochrome P-450 proteins (P-450) are responsible for most phase I reactions (37–40). In the reaction cycle, oxygen is bound and reduced, resulting in activated oxygen, which is incorporated in lipophilic substrates (drugs, toxins, fatty acids, and steroid hormones) (37–41). Chemically reactive intermediates (e.g., free radicals) are formed and reduced. There are more than 20 P-450 isozymes in the liver (37,41). Patient variation in drug metabolism is due to polymorphisms in the genes coding for P-450 (Volume 2, Chapter 4) (38). There are decreased P-450 levels in severe liver disease, with resultant decrease in drug clearance (38).

Enzyme induction is the synthesis of new enzyme proteins secondary to exposure of the P-450 system to lipophilic substances. Enzyme induction occurs with medications such as isoniazid, phenytoin, rifampicin, and St. John's wort, as well as commonly used agents such as alcohol, tobacco, and cannabis. Enzyme induction affects the metabolism of other drugs, as well as drug–drug interactions (37).

Mechanisms of Drug Toxicity
Intrinsic (Direct) Hepatotoxicity

Toxic hepatic injury occurs with agents that damage liver cells of all exposed patients (intrinsic toxicity) (Table 2).

Table 2 Mechanisms of Drug-Induced Liver Disease

Mechanism	Direct/indirect physiochemical destruction	Idiosyncratic toxicity	
		Aberrant metabolism leading to toxic metabolite	Hypersensitivity (drug allergy) reaction immune-mediated
Examples	Acetaminophen	Isoniazid Ketoconazole Troglitazone	Halothane Phenytoin Carbamazepine Valproate Sulfonamides
Clinical features	Fulminant (acute hepatitis)	Elevated LFTs, acute hepatitis, jaundice	Fever, rash, eosinophilia, arthralgias accompany hepatitis
Risk of injury	Very high (predictable)	Low (unpredictable)	Low (unpredictable)
Latency	Hours (acute)	Weeks-months (variable)	1–5 wk (fixed)
Dose dependency	Yes	No	No
Morphologic injury pattern	Usually necrosis	Broad spectrum	Broad spectrum, granulomas
Positive response to rechallenge	No	Possibly, delayed	Expected, prompt
Animal models	Yes	No	No

Abbreviation: LFTs, liver Function tests.
Source: From Ref. 43.

Intrinsic hepatotoxins cause predictable liver injury, either from the drug itself (as with Amanita phalloides mushroom, chloroform, and carbon tetrachloride) or from a toxic metabolite of the agent (as with acetaminophen toxicity), and are usually not related to host factors (Volume 1, Chapter 31). Most toxic hepatic injury results from the actions of active metabolites of the drug (37,41,42). Electrophilic radicals, the probable mechanism for injury from acetaminophen and isoniazid, bind to molecules of cell membranes and lead to necrosis (41). Most cases of acute drug-induced liver disease occur within days of a direct hepatotoxin (37,41).

Idiosyncratic Toxicity
The majority of drugs associated with drug-induced liver disease are idiosyncratic hepatotoxins (37,38,40). Unstable drug metabolites may bind to cellular proteins or macromolecules that cause a direct toxic effect on hepatocytes (38,40). Idiosyncratic agents may be due to aberrant metabolism of the drug to a toxic intermediate that induces liver injury in the susceptible patient, or may be immunologic in nature (37,38,40–42).

Metabolic Idiosyncracy
Metabolic idiosyncracy is the susceptibility of agents to formation of intrinsic toxins, resulting in hepatic cellular injury. These reactions usually result from genetic or acquired differences in drug metabolism (37,40,42). Agents associated with metabolic idiosyncracy include isoniazid, fluconazole, troglitazone, fluoxitene, paroxitene, and trazodone.

Immunoallergic or Hypersensitivity Reactions
Immunoallergic or hypersensitivity reactions involve the covalent binding of the drug to enzymes, forming adducts, which can serve as immune targets (40). Adducts can induce the formation of antibodies or induce direct cytolytic T-cell responses (40). The pattern of liver disease can be hepatitic, cholestatic, or mixed (38,40,42). This reaction

occurs after a predictable sensitization period, usually one to five weeks (42). Rash, fever, and eosinophilia may accompany immunoallergic reactions.

Immunoallergic reactions have been reported with sulfonamides and anticonvulsants (37,40). Rare cases have occurred from barbiturates, beta-blocking agents, calcium-channel blockers, nifedipine, verapamil, diltiazem, and gastric acid suppression drugs such as cimetidine, ranitidine, and famotidine (37).

Targets of Cellular Injury
Drug-induced hepatic injury can be classified by clinical, histologic or laboratory features, and depends on the area of the hepatobiliary tree that is injured. Covalent binding of a drug to intracellular proteins may occur and migrate to the cell surface, resulting in cell lysis. Enzyme-drug adducts can migrate to the cell surface and serve as targets for cytolytic T-cells or cytokines. Disruption of the actin filaments near the canaliculus, or interruptions of transport proteins that affect bile flow, may result in cholestasis. Interruption of transport pumps may prevent excretion of bilirubin and other compounds. Drugs may activate apoptotic pathways via TNF-α. Others may affect fatty acid oxidation and respiratory chain enzymes, leading to lactic acidosis and reactive oxygen species. Triglyceride accumulation within cells leads to steatohepatitis (aforementioned) (40). Many drugs cause a spectrum of features, however, and some produce mixed disorders (37).

Presentations of Hepatic Injury
Hepatic Adaptation
Hepatic adaptation refers to alterations in hepatic function without significant liver injury. Patients are frequently asymptomatic (42). Drugs commonly involved include phenytoin, warfarin, and the statin class of cholesterol-lowering agents (37,42). Rash, eosinophilia, and fever are uncommon (37).

Hepatocellular Necrosis

Acute hepatocellular necrosis is characterized by marked elevations in ALT and AST (8–100 times normal), with normal or minimally elevated AP (<3 times normal) (41,43). Serum bilirubin levels always increase, but the degree of elevation is quite variable. Patients with drug-induced hepatocellular necrosis may progress to fulminant hepatic failure, which carries a poor prognosis (41,43).

Steatosis and Steatohepatitis

Steatosis is fatty liver, whereas steatohepatitis is fatty liver with inflammation of the hepatic cells. Steatosis is typically divided into two types, microvesicular (owing to mitochondrial problems), and macrovesicular (hepatic export/import and manufacturing abnormality). Steatosis can progress to steatohepatitis, fibrosis, and cirrhosis. Steatohepatitis may present with jaundice and elevations of aminotransferases, but levels are typically less than those seen with hepatocellular necrosis (41,42).

Cholestatic Liver Injury

Drugs associated with cholestatic liver injury presumably result from immunologic activities against the bile ducts. The predominant histologic features are portal inflammation and biliary injury (38).

Cholestatic liver injury may present with anorexia, malaise, fatigue, jaundice, dark urine, and pruritis (37,38,40,42,43). Elevations of AP, GGTP, and 5′NT may indicate bile duct injury (37,43). There are modestly elevated aminotransferases and conjugated hyperbilirubinemia (37,41,42). The ratio of ALT to AP is <2:1 in cholestasis (37). ☞ **Drug-induced cholestatic injury has a better prognosis than hepatocellular injury, but may become fatal if the drug is continued after appearance of symptoms (40,41).** ☜

Common Drugs Associated with Hepatoxicity in the Trauma/Intensive Care Unit Patient
Antibiotics

Acute hepatic necrosis and liver failure may occur with isoniazid, rifampin, ketoconazole, and oxacillin (43,44). Sulfonamides are associated with hepatitis, especially in combination agents, such as sulfamethoxazole/trimethoprim (37). Fatalities have occurred with trovafloxacin (44). Ceftriaxone and linezolid have been associated with hyperbilirubinemia (44). Cholestasis may occur with erythromycin, trovafloxacin, sulfonamides, angiotensin converting enzyme (ACE) inhibitors, and tricyclics (37,44). Tetracycline hepatotoxicity is dose related (44). Many of the antiretroviral agents prescribed to HIV-positive patients are also associated with hepatotoxicity (37).

Acetaminophen

Acetaminophen overdosage is well known to cause liver failure. Liver toxicity is common with acetaminophen doses of 15 g or more, but doses as low as 6–10 g can also be toxic. Glutathione binds with acetaminophen metabolites, and acetaminophen overdose causes the amount of metabolite to exceed the amount of glutathione. Due to cytochrome induction, there are higher levels of a toxic quinone metabolite (37,43). Hepatic injury occurs at about 48 hours after ingestion. Elevations of AST and ALT to greater than 10,000 U/L can be seen (43). A characteristic feature is a large increase in AST compared with ALT (41). Acetaminophen

toxicity results in higher levels of aminotransferases than in viral hepatitis (40). Centrilobular necrosis and hepatic failure result.

Acetaminophen toxicity is exacerbated in patients with regular intake of alcohol, and therapeutic doses of acetaminophen in alcohol users can lead to severe toxicity (45). This enhanced reaction may be secondary to induction of cytochrome P-450 by ethanol, depletion of glutathione, alcohol-induced malnutrition, and the fasting state (45,46). Enhanced P-450 activity also occurs with isoniazid, rifampin, anticonvulsants, and zidovudine, and increases acetaminophen toxicity (43).

Acetylcysteine causes a repletion of glutathione (41), and can ameliorate liver injury if administered within 12 to 24 hours (37,41). Later administration of acetylcysteine can still reduce the mortality of hepatotoxicity (37). Some patients may require hepatic transplantation (47).

Aspirin

Aspirin (ASA) injury is dose–dependent, at 4 to 6 g/day or with blood levels of 25 mg/dL (37,43). ALT levels rise. Recovery is usually rapid following prompt discontinuation of the drug without occurrence of chronic liver disease (37). ASA has been identified in inducing Reye's syndrome in febrile children (37).

Amiodarone

Hepatotoxicity from the antidysrhythmic agent, amiodarone, has been described (37,48,49). The most common abnormality is a mild elevation of serum AST and ALT levels in 15% to 80% of patients. Acute liver failure occurs in 0.6% of patients. Most changes resolve spontaneously without discontinuation of the agent. Fatalities from liver dysfunction are rare (37,48).

The most typical lesion is steatohepatitis (37). Progression of the disease may occur even with discontinuation of the agents. Chronic liver disease may occur with prolonged use of amiodarone. Clinical presentation includes fatigue, nausea, vomiting, malaise, weight loss, ascites, hepatomegaly, jaundice, and bruising (37). Use of oral amiodarone may be safe in some patients who demonstrate acute hepatitis with the parenteral form of this agent (49).

Anticonvulsants

Carbamazepine, phenytoin, and phenobarbital have been associated with cytotoxic hepatic injury (37,38,50,51). These reactions occur with intermediate (usually one to eight weeks) or long latency (up to 12 months) after exposure, and may occur with rash, fever, eosinophilia, and lymphadenopathy (37,38,41–43). Aminotransferase levels are high (38), and fulminant hepatic failure may result (50). Effects may not be seen until after the drug is discontinued, or may be nonspecific; thus the drug is not discontinued. Diagnosis is made by a rechallenge of the agent. The incidence is 1/3000 exposures (43). Valproic acid is associated with severe hepatotoxicity, but usually in young children (37).

Drugs of Abuse

Phencyclidine, cocaine, angel dust, and 3,4 methylenedioxymethamphetamine (MDMA) (ecstasy) have been associated with hepatic injury. Associated hyperthermia, rhabdomyolysis, respiratory, and renal failure may occur. Cocaine-induced liver injury is usually secondary to hypoxia, hypotension, and hyperthermia (37).

Anesthesia-Induced Hepatotoxicity (Exceedingly Rare)

General anesthetics are not common sources of hepatitis. However, fulminant hepatic failure, secondary to immune-mediated toxicity, occurs very rarely. The oxidative metabolism of halothane by cytochrome P-450, to trifluoroacetyl chloride, leads to trifluoroacetylation of specific proteins which idiosyncratically act as antigens in the immune response. It is thought that patients who develop halothane hepatitis either produce unusually large amounts of hepatotoxic metabolites or have an idiosyncratic immunologic response that initiates the hepatic damage (52). An allergic etiology is suggested by the occurrence after repeated exposure in certain patients, and the occurrence of fever, rash, and eosinophilia (52). Halothane hepatitis is exceedingly rare and is a diagnosis of exclusion. Treatment is entirely supportive (38,52). Enflurane, isoflurane, and desflurane undergo less oxidation, and are thus associated with fewer cases of hepatotoxicity. There has not yet been any reported association between sevoflurane and hepatotoxicity (52).

Clinical Aspects of Drug-Induced Hepatic Disease

The trauma/intensive care unit (ICU) patient may have numerous factors that influence the effects of drugs on the liver, such as age, previous excessive use of alcohol, poor nutritional status, and shock (37). In addition, the recognition of drug-induced liver disease in the surgical and trauma patient is complicated by the effects of surgery, trauma and hemodynamic instability on hepatic function, underlying medical conditions which impact on liver function, and the large number of medications which are used in the critically ill patient.

A drug reaction should be considered in any critically ill patient with hepatic dysfunction. Eliminating other causes of liver disease is essential. Temporal associations with new agents, and improvement after drug cessation, may aid in the diagnosis (40). If the offending agent is discontinued, acute hepatocellular injury is reversible and heals without sequelae (43).

Dechallenge and rechallenge may be used, but puts the patient at risk for severe injury (40,42). Findings on liver biopsy that suggest drug-induced hepatotoxicity include eosinophils in an inflammatory infiltrate, granulomatous hepatitis, hepatitis-like hepatocellular injury, cholestatic hepatitis, severe acute injury with zonal, and submassive or massive hepatic necrosis (42).

There is little effective treatment for drug-induced hepatotoxicity (37). Prevention, detection, and discontinuation of any possible hepatotoxic agents are critical (37). There is no data that corticosteroids are useful in immunoallergic reactions (40). Mortality may approach 10% in cases of hepatocellular necrosis or toxic steatosis. Agents that produce cholestatic injury rarely produce fatalities (43). ☞ **The presence of jaundice worsens the prognosis in hepatocellular injury. Patients with coagulopathy or with encephalopathy may be candidates for hepatic transplantation (40).** ☞

Alterations in Drug Dosing in the Trauma/Intensive Care Unit Patient with Hepatic Dysfunction
Hepatic Drug Metabolism

Hepatic clearance depends primarily on hepatic blood flow, enzyme activity and, to a lesser extent, protein binding. The effects of changes in hepatic blood flow and enzyme activity are synergistic, not additive. When drug clearance is reduced, drugs can reach a higher steady-state concentration. Drugs with a high hepatic extraction rapidly undergo biotransformation and biliary excretion, and are sensitive to changes in hepatic blood flow. Thus, conditions associated with hepatic hypoperfusion, such as hemorrhagic shock, sepsis, application of positive end-expiratory pressure, and use of alpha-adrenergic agents, may prolong the metabolism of such agents (39).

Drugs with a low hepatic extraction are sensitive to variations of the activity of drug-metabolizing enzymes, and not to hepatic blood flow changes. Hepatic enzyme activity is an important factor in metabolism of drugs with low hepatic extraction, and may be altered in the absence of liver injury. Oxidative metabolism of drugs is primarily catalyzed by enzymes of the P-450 system, some of which are more susceptible to liver disease than others. Binding of drugs to albumin and alpha-1 acid glycoprotein is affected in critical illness, and thus drugs that are highly protein bound may have altered metabolism (39).

Analgesics

The liver is responsible for the metabolism of many analgesic agents. Morphine metabolism is dependent on liver blood flow. Prolonged clearance can occur in severe cirrhosis and septic shock. The metabolite morphine-6-glucronide can have a prolonged duration of action, especially in patients with renal failure or insufficiency (53).

Fentanyl is more highly lipid soluble, with increased volume of distribution and longer limitation half-life than morphine. Fentanyl is metabolized to inactive metabolites, which are eliminated by the kidney. Metabolism is affected by liver blood flow, thus decreased hepatic perfusion can affect clearance (53).

Meperidine is metabolized in the liver to normeperidine, and is renally excreted. Central nervous system toxicity limits its use in ICU patients with renal failure (53).

Hydromorphone is metabolized in the liver to hydromorphone-3-glucronide. This metabolite may accumulate in renal failure and cause central nervous system toxicity. Metabolism is dependent on hepatic blood flow.

Sedatives

Diazepam is highly lipid soluble and protein bound. The drug is metabolized to the active compound, desmethyldiazepam, which has a long half-life (100–200 hours) and is eliminated by the kidney. Diazepam metabolites are converted by oxidation, which undergo conjugation before elimination. The elimination half-life is thus prolonged in patients with liver disease (54).

Lorazepam is five to six times more potent than diazepam, and is 90% protein bound. It is metabolized to inactive products by hepatic glucuronidation, and thus there are fewer drug interactions than with other benzodiazepines. The half-life of 10 to 20 hours is prolonged in liver disease. Lorazepam clearance has shown variability, depending on the underlying trauma mechanism, increased after head and thermal injury, decreased after spinal cord injury (39).

Midazolam is 95% protein bound and three to four times more potent than diazepam. It is metabolized by hepatic microsomal oxidation (5). Midazolam has a prolonged clearance and half-life with severe liver disease (54).

Propofol has the largest volume of distribution of any sedative, with rapid return to consciousness after discontinuation. Although metabolized by the liver, propofol recovery is not affected by liver disease (55).

Muscle Relaxants

The effects of vecuronium, pancuronium, mivacurium, rocuronium, and *d*-tubocurarine are prolonged in patients with liver disease (56). A metabolite of vecuronium, 3-desacetylvecuronium, has muscle relaxant properties, and prolonged muscle relaxation can occur in renal failure (56).

Miscellaneous Agents

Agents used in the ICU, which are also affected by liver disease, include metoclopramide and ondansetron. Cirrhosis can markedly affect the metabolism of the proton pump inhibitors lansoprazole, pantoprazole, and omeprazole. Patients with cirrhosis may have decreased sensitivity to loop diuretics.

✄ **Although clearance of many drugs has been shown to be diminished after trauma, phenytoin and lorazepam clearance are normally increased after head trauma (39).** ✄

SELECTED CLINICAL ISSUES IN LIVER DYSFUNCTION IN THE TRAUMA/SURGICAL PATIENT
Total Parenteral Nutrition and Hepatic Function
Steatosis

Steatosis (fatty liver), the most common hepatic abnormality in adult patients receiving TPN, is reversible and benign providing additional insults do not occur, and duration is short (57,58). Onset is usually one to four weeks after initiation of TPN. Hepatic function tests reveal mild-to-moderate elevation of aminotransferases, and less pronounced elevations of serum AP and bilirubin (57). However, long-term steatosis may progress to steatohepatitis, fibrosis, and cirrhosis (57,58). Excessive calories from carbohydrates can stimulate insulin-induced lipogenesis, essential fatty acid deficiency, and choline deficiency (58). Reducing the calories of TPN solutions, cycling of TPN, and choline supplementation have been shown to reduce hepatic steatosis (58).

Cholestasis

Long-term TPN is a risk factor for cholestasis (57,58). A mechanism in adults may relate to inadequate stimulation of cholecystokinin release, with resultant bile stasis in the gall bladder. Intestinal stasis may lead to small intestinal bacterial overgrowth, which results in transformation of chenodoxycholate to lithocholate. Lithocholate has been shown in animals to impair bile flow and induce cholestasis (57). Lack of enteral nutrition may lead to intestinal hypoplasia, which increases lithocholate absorption and promotion of bacterial translocation across the gastrointestinal tract. Treatment options include the use of metronidazole to suppress bacterial overgrowth, and ursodeoxycholic acid to improve the fluidity of the bile (58). Cholestasis can lead to calculous gall bladder disease. Sludge is present in all patients after six weeks of TPN. Acalculous cholecystitis can occur in a small percentage of patients on long-term TPN (57,58).

Acalculous Cholecystitis
Definition and Incidence

AAC is an acute inflammation of the gall bladder that occurs in the absence of gallstones (9,16,59,60). AAC occurs in the setting of trauma, burns, major intra-abdominal surgery, and sepsis, often in patients who require mechanical ventilation, hemodynamic support, and multiple blood transfusions or TPN (9,16,59). As opposed to the equal incidence of calculous cholecystitis in men and women, the incidence of the acalculous form of cholecystitis is more common in men and in children (9,59).

Etiology and Pathogenesis

The pathogenesis of ACC is multifactorial, and includes bile stasis, infection, and ischemia. Prolonged fasting can lead to bile stasis secondary to reduced gallbladder emptying, and volume depletion may result in concentration of bile (9,59,61). Hypoperfusion secondary to sepsis, the use of vasoactive agents, and splanchnic vasoconstriction, combined with an increased metabolic requirement of the gall bladder epithelium, can result in ischemia of the gall bladder (9,16,59,60). Increased intraluminal pressure from inspissated bile can further exacerbate gall bladder ischemia (9,16,60). Mechanical ventilation may contribute to biliary stasis and decreased portal blood flow when continuous positive air way pressure (CPAP) is applied for prolonged periods or high levels (62). Multiple arterial occlusions are present histologically (63), and gangrene is present in 50% of the cases (9).

Clinical Manifestations and Diagnosis

The clinical presentation of AAC is usually nonspecific, and requires a high index of suspicion. Any combination of fever, leukocytosis, elevated hepatic function tests, and hyperbilirubinemia may be present. Patients may be septic, yet this may be a cause or a result of AAC. Perforation may occur in 10% to 20% (9,16,59).

Abdominal findings may be absent or difficult to ascertain in this patient population secondary to critical illness, endotracheal intubation, use of narcotics and sedatives, and the presence of previous abdominal pathology (9).

Ultrasound is the diagnostic test of choice. Findings are nonspecific, and may include a thickened gall bladder wall, gall bladder distention, biliary sludge, pericholecystic fluid, and a sonographic halo around the gall bladder without gallstones (9,59,64). Hepatic scintigraphy has a high incidence of false negative and false positive results. Prolonged fasting with decreased bile production and absence of gall bladder contraction, narcotic-induced contraction of the sphincter of Oddi, and biliary stasis secondary to TPN leads to nonvisualization of the gall bladder (64,65). CT has not been shown to be more accurate, and requires transport from the ICU, thus limiting its utility in diagnosing AAC (61,65).

Treatment

Cholecystectomy should be performed, but carries a high rate of complications and mortality. Thus, percutaneous cholecystostomy may be an option in an unstable critically ill patient. Percutaneous drainage has been shown to be effective as both a diagnostic and treatment modality in critically ill patients (66,67). The cholecystostomy tube is left in place for three weeks so a tract can form.

Antibiotic therapy should be directed against the common bacterial isolates, including *Escherichia coli*, *Klebsiella*, and *Enterococcus faecalis* (59). In patients with previous antibiotic therapy, resistant bacteria may be encountered. Pseudomonas, staphylococci, enterobacter, and anaerobic organisms may be recovered in such patients (59). However, patients with documented AAC may have negative bile cultures (64,66,68).

Coagulopathy Associated with Liver Failure
Etiologies of Coagulopathy
The liver is the site of synthesis of all the major coagulation factors except for factor VIII and vWF. In addition, antithrombotic factors protein C and protein S are synthesized by the liver. Antithrombin is produced in the liver, and can be decreased in patients with acute hepatic failure and cirrhosis. Decreased platelet counts are common in liver disease, but rarely result in bleeding (69).

The prothrombin time depends on prothrombin and the clotting factors synthesized in the liver, factors II (fibrinogen), V, VII, and IX (6,69). Vitamin K, a fat-soluble vitamin found in many foods and produced by intestinal bacteria, is required for many of these factors, and may be deficient in cases of malnutrition and malabsorption. Deficiency of vitamin K may occur in cases of biliary obstruction, cholestasis, and with antibiotic suppression of intestinal bacteria (2,6,70).

Coagulopathy can occur in cases of hepatic necrosis. Etiologies include increased tissue factor activity, decreased clearance of activated factors, and decreased synthesis of inhibitors (69). Patients with liver disease may demonstrate a reduction of coagulation factors and a quantitative or qualitative platelet defect.

DIC may be difficult to differentiate from bleeding secondary to advanced hepatic disease. DIC results from unopposed thrombin generation and action resulting from endothelial or tissue injury (69).

Clinical bleeding is unusual in toxic hepatitis, unless the hepatitis becomes fulminant or hepatic failure occurs (69). Coagulation factor deficiencies, especially factor VII, may occur. Hyperfibrinolysis can occur in patients with liver disease in whom there is increased reduction of physiologic inhibitors alpha 2-antiplasmin and PAI-1 combined with decreased clearance of activated factors (70).

Coagulopathy Evaluation and Management
Coagulopathy is multifactorial in the patient with liver dysfunction. The plasma half-life of most coagulation factors is short, and thus prothrombin time is helpful in following the course of acute liver failure. When prolonged prothrombin time is secondary to vitamin K deficiency, administration of vitamin K will decrease prothrombin time by 30% within 24 hours (8). Vitamin K can be administered as a single dose

of 10 mg IV, at a rate of 1 mg/min (69). Intramuscular injection is not recommended in cases of coagulopathy (69). **In cases of parenchymal liver disease, there may be minimal or absent response to vitamin K.**

Evaluation of Hepatic Dysfunction in the Trauma/Intensive Care Unit Patient
The etiology of post-traumatic and postoperative jaundice is often multifactorial. Critically ill patients have experienced any combination of hemodynamic instability, infection and/or sepsis, multiple blood transfusions, and have been exposed to potentially hepatotoxic medications.

Evaluation of Biochemical Liver Function Tests
The initial step in the investigation of jaundice is to identify the pattern of biochemical LFTs. Jaundice may be classified on the basis of etiology, pathophysiology, or time course of appearance of jaundice. Evaluations based on pathophysiology would differentiate between increased pigment load, hepatic parenchymal disease, or intrahepatic or extrahepatic cholestasis (Table 3).

Unconjugated hyperbilirubinemia suggests hemolysis, resorption of hematomas or, less likely, inherited defects of conjugations (e.g., Gilbert's syndrome).

Patients who are critically ill usually have an element of hepatocellular dysfunction, and bilirubin is predominantly conjugated. Unconjugated bilirubin is always bound to albumin and is not filtered by the kidney (except in protenuria states). Accordingly, bilirubin in the urine is conjugated and indicates hepatobiliary disease (6) in the absence of protenuria.

Hepatocellular injury is characterized by elevations in direct bilirubin and amino-transferases, with only modest elevations of AP. A rise in conjugated bilirubin without an increase in AP suggests alcohol, drugs, viral hepatitis, or inherited disorders of bilirubin excretion (Dubin Johnson, Rotor's syndrome) (6). Cholestasis is identified by jaundice with bilirubin levels 2–10 mg/dL, a mild to moderate rise in AP, and smaller elevations in aminotransferases. Clinical evidence of encephalopathy does not occur.

Ischemic hepatitis and drug-induced liver disease are usually associated with higher levels of aminotransferases. Sepsis, extrahepatic biliary obstruction, calculus cholecystitis, and TPN should be considered.

Table 3 General Patterns of Biochemical Liver Tests

Test	Hepatocellular necrosis			Biliary obstruction		Hepatic infiltration
Causative agent	Toxin/ischemia Viral	Alcohol		Complete	Partial	
Examples	Acetaminophen, shock liver	Hepatitis A or B		Pancreatic carcinoma	Hilar tumor	Primary or metastatic carcinoma, TB, sarcoid, amyloidosis
Amino-transferases	50–100	5–50	2–5	1–5	1–5	1–3
AP	1–3	1–3	1–10	2–20	2–10	1–20
Bilirubin	1–5	1–30	1–30	1–30	1–5	1–5; often normal
Prothrombin time	Prolonged and unresponsive to vitamin K in severe liver disease			Often prolonged and responsive to vitamin K		Usually normal
Albumin	Decreased in subacute or chronic disease			Usually normal; decreased in advanced disease		Usually normal

Abbreviation: AP, alkaline phosphatase.
Source: From Ref. 1.

Measurements of conjugated and unconjugated bilirubin are of limited utility in distinguishing between intrinsic liver disease and biliary obstruction (6,8). Isolated marked elevations of AP with conjugated hyperbilirubinemia, is consistent with partial biliary obstruction and hepatic infiltration. Both GGTP and AP are typically elevated in cholestasis; the combination of an elevated AP and normal GGTP suggests that the AP is from bone (8). An isolated elevation of GGTP may result from certain drugs (8). In prolonged homeostasis, the delta fraction of circulating conjugated bilirubin is tightly bound to albumin, and may account for the prolonged resolution of bilirubin when other parameters are improving (6).

Unrecognized pre-existing liver diseases, including viral hepatitis, alcoholic hepatitis, and cirrhosis, are possible in the trauma population, and may contribute to hepatic dysfunction.

Timing of hepatic dysfunction is important. ☞ **While ischemic hepatitis has a short latent period and characteristic biochemical pattern, drug-induced liver disease may occur further into the patient's hospital course.** ☜

Diagnostic Imaging

Ultrasound or computed tomography can reveal the presence of dilated ducts. If dilated ducts are present, endoscopic retrograde cholangiopancreatography (ERCP) can be performed (10). The advantage of ultrasound is that it is noninvasive and portable. No contrast agents are required. However, bowel gas may obscure visualization. Abdominal CT is also noninvasive, and has a higher resolution than ultrasound. However, the patient requires transport, and only calcified gallstones may be visualized. Contrast may be contraindicated in the patient with hypovolemia or renal dysfunction. ERCP provides direct imaging of the bile ducts and periampullary region. This test is technically difficult in the critically ill patient. Percutaneous cholangiography provides direct imaging of the bile ducts, but interpretation may be difficult with nondilated intrahepatic ducts (8).

Management Goals of the Trauma/Intensive Care Unit Patient with Hepatic Dysfunction

Many trauma and ICU patients have abnormalities of biochemical LFTs with evidence of hepatic dysfunction. Prolonged elevations in biochemical LFTs may only reflect the severity of the patient's underlying condition, rather than intrinsic hepatic dysfunction. Most critically ill patients are at risk for intrahepatic cholestasis, which may persist as long as the patient remains critically ill. It is essential to continually review medications for possible drug-induced hepatic disease. Stabilization of the patient's hemodynamic status is essential in preserving hepatic blood flow. Metabolic and coagulation abnormalities should be treated as they arise. Medication doses should be adjusted for changes in hepatic function.

EYE TO THE FUTURE
Evaluation of Hepatic Function in Critical Illness and Injury

Patients who are critically ill or injured are at risk for multiple organ dysfunction, including hepatic failure. However, abnormal tests of hepatic function are often nonspecific and reflect multiple mechanisms of hepatic injury. Two

studies may prove to be useful in the early detection of disorders of hepatic function.

Indocyanine Green Clearance as an Evaluation of Hepatic Injury

In an attempt to investigate hepatic perfusion, indocyanine green clearance was measured in patients with sepsis, and showed that indocyanine green elimination failed to increase in survivors. Measurement of indocyanine green clearance may be able to identify reversible liver injury early in the course of septic shock, and may predict patients with a poor outcome (71).

Cytochrome P-450 Activity as a Monitor for Liver Dysfunction in Trauma Patients

Alterations in CYP activity can be evaluated by measuring metabolism of medications specific for CYP isoforms. The metabolism of medications that test different CYP isoforms were administered following resuscitation, stabilization and initial treatment of a group of critically injured adult patients. The metabolizing capacity of the some of the CYP isoforms were found to be altered compared with control subjects, and several of these alterations correlated with measures of organ dysfunction and illness severity (72).

Improving Hepatosplanchnic Perfusion in Sepsis
N-Acetylcysteine (NAC)

The properties of NAC which make it a potentially useful agent in sepsis have been reviewed, including its antioxidant properties, modulation of the activity of inducible nitric oxide synthase, decreased formation of proninflammatory cytokines, and inhibition of neutrophil activation (73). Animal studies have shown positive effects of NAC on hepatosplanchnic perfusion (75), and clinical trials have demonstrated increased liver blood flow and function (74–76). However, other studies in human subjects have shown deleterious effects on cardiac and respiratory function (73). Further studies will be required to assess the utility of NAC on hepatic function and other organ systems in sepsis.

Fenoldopam and Dopexamine

Studies using fenoldopam, a dopamine-1 receptor agonist, and dopexamine, an inotoropic agent have shown conflicting results in improving hepatosplanchnic perfusion (22,77,78).

Bioartificial Support

Bioartificial hepatic support has been in development since the 1950s. Extracorporeal liver perfusion, transplantation of hepatocytes, and hybrid liver support devices are among the modalities being studied (80–83). Meta-analysis has shown conflicting results in the effect of bioartificial liver support on mortality in acute-on-chronic liver failure and in hepatic encephalopathy (82). A prospective, randomized, multicenter controlled trial of the Hepatassist liver support system, an extracorporeal porcine hepatocyte-based BAL, has demonstrated improved survival in patients with fulminant and subfulminant hepatic failure (83). (Also see Volume 2, Chapter 38.)

SUMMARY

Trauma and critical illness may affect all aspects of hepatic function, including energy, bilirubin and vitamin metabolism, biliary function, and production of plasma proteins and coagulation factors. The trauma/ICU patient is at risk for hepatic ischemia secondary to hepatic hypoperfusion from hypotension and anemia. The liver of the septic, critically ill patient is subject to hypoperfusion and mismatch of oxygen delivery and consumption. Sepsis can result in Kupffer cell spillover of bacteria and inflammatory mediators, hepatic mediator production with secondary hepatocellular dysfunction, and a procoagulant response.

Jaundice is commonly seen in the critically ill patient, and may be secondary to bilirubin overload, hepatocellular dysfunction, or cholestasis. Elevations of aminotransferases reflect hepatocellular damage. Intrahepatic cholestasis is common in patients with sepsis. The level of elevation of serum bilirubin and serum enzymes are often discrepant. Persistent hyperbilirubinemia portends a poor prognosis.

Hepatic injury can occur from direct injury by intrinsic hepatotoxins, causing predictable hepatic injury, or from idiosyncratic reactions related to aberrant metabolism or immunoallergic reactions against drugs or their metabolites. Although drugs may affect hepatic function tests without significant liver injury, hepatocellular necrosis, steatosis, or cholestasis may occur. Drug effect must be considered in any critically ill patient with hepatic dysfunction.

Hepatic dysfunction may affect the pharmacokinetics and pharmacodynamics of many drugs. Analgesics, sedatives, and muscle relaxants may have prolonged metabolism in patients with hepatic dysfunction.

Identifying the pattern of biochemical LFTs is the initial step in investigating hepatic dysfunction in the critically ill patient's. Timing of hepatic dysfunction in relation to the patient course of illness may help differentiate etiologies of hepatic dysfunction. Measurements of conjugated and unconjugated hyperbilirubinemia are of limited value in distinguishing between intrinsic liver disease and biliary obstruction. Sepsis, extrahepatic biliary obstruction, acalculous cholecystitis, TPN, and drug effect should be considered as etiologies for hepatic dysfunction in critically ill patients.

KEY POINTS

- The geographic position of hepatocytes and their exposure to gradients of nutrients and waste products leads to location-related variations in susceptibility to ischemia and drug toxicity (2).
- Acute hepatic disease will have a greater effect on proteins with rapid turnover (i.e., coagulation factors) than those that turn over more slowly, such as albumin (5).
- Aminotransferase levels of greater than 1000 IU/L are almost always due to hepatocellular injury, and can be seen with drug- or toxin-induced hepatic injury, ischemic liver injury, and acute viral hepatitis (7).
- In most hepatic injuries, the ratio of AST to ALT is usually 1:1; however, ratios of 2:1 or greater are common in alcoholic hepatitis.
- Normally, the total bilirubin is less than 1 mg/dL, and at least 70% is conjugated (direct reacting).
- The coagulation factors have a short half-life, especially factor VII (five to seven hours); thus prothrombin time is a useful indicator of hepatic synthetic function providing vitamin K levels are normal (4,8).
- Ischemic hepatitis is associated pathologically with centrilobular necrosis. This is described histologically as necrosis to hepatocytes surrounding the central vein

(furthest away from the nutrients supply) and hence, most susceptible to ischemic damage (16).
- The major source of hyperlactatemia in sepsis results from henobarbital clearance of lactate by the liver (32,33).
- Drug-induced cholestatic injury has a better prognosis than hepatocellular injury, but may become fatal if the drug is continued after appearance of symptoms (40,41).
- The presence of jaundice worsens the prognosis in hepatocellular injury.
- Although clearance of many drugs has been shown to be diminished after trauma, phenytoin and lorazepam clearance are normally increased after head trauma (39).
- In cases of parenchymal liver disease, there may be minimal or absent response to vitamin K.
- While ischemic hepatitis has a short latent period and characteristic biochemical pattern, drug-induced liver disease may occur further into the patient's hospital course.

REFERENCES

1. Stolz A. Liver physiology and metabolic function. In: Feldman H, Friedman L, Sleisenger M, eds. Sleisenger and Fordtran's Gastrointestinal and Liver Disease. 7th ed. Elsevier Science, 2002:1202–1223.
2. Wanless IR. Physioanatomic considerations. In: Schiff ER, Sorrell MF, Maddrey WC, eds. Schiff's Diseases of the Liver. 8th ed. Philadelphia: Lippincott–Raven Publishers, 1999:3–33.
3. Wanless IR. Anatomy, histology, embryology, and developmental anomalies of the liver. In: Feldman H, Friedman L, Sleisenger M, eds. Sleisenger and Fordtran's Gastrointestinal and Liver Disease. 7th ed. Elsevier Science, 2002:1197–1200.
4. Meyers WC, Ricciardi R. Liver: function. In: Townsend C, ed. Sabiston Textbook of Surgery. 16th ed. Philadelphia, PA: W.B. Saunders Company, 2001:1005–1012.
5. Weisiger RA. Hepatic metabolism in liver disease. In: Goldman L, ed. Cecil's Textbook of Medicine. 21st ed. W.B. Saunders Company, 2000:768–770.
6. Weisiger RA. Laboratory tests in liver disease and approach to the patient with abnormal tests. In: Goldman S, ed. Cecil' Textbook of Medicine. 21st ed. W.B. Saunders Company, 2000:775–779.
7. Davern TJ, Scharschmidt BF. Biochemical liver tests. In: Feldman H, Friedman L, Sleisenger M, eds. Sleisenger and Fordtran's Gastrointestinal and Liver Disease. 7th ed. Elsevier Science, 2002:1112–1122.
8. Scharschmidt BF. Bilirubin metabolism, hyperbilirubinemia, and approach to the jaundiced patient. In: Goldman S, ed. Cecil' Textbook of Medicine. 21st ed. W.B. Saunders Company, 2000:770–775.
9. Molina EG, Reddy KR. Postoperative jaundice. Clin Liver Dis 1999; 3:477–488.
10. Nyber LM, Pockros PJ. Postoperative jaundice. In: Schiff ER, Sorrell MF, Maddrey WC, eds. Schiff's Diseases of the Liver. 8th ed. Philadelphia, PA: Lippincott–Raven Publishers, 1999:599–605.
11. Kullak-Ublick GA, Meier PJ. Mechanisms of cholestasis. Clin Liver Dis 2000; 4:357–385.
12. Moseley RH. Sepsis and cholestasis. Clin Liver Dis 1999; 3:465–475.
13. Orlinsky M, Shoemaker W, Reis ED, Kerstein MD. Current controversies in shock and resuscitation. Surg Clin North Am 2001; 81:1217–1262.
14. Schafer DF, Sorrell MF. Vascular diseases of the liver. In: Feldman H, Friedman L, Sleisenger M, eds. Sleisenger and Fordtran's Gastrointestinal and Liver Disease. 7th ed. Elsevier Science, 2002:1370–1374.

15. Gitlin N, Serio KM. Ischemic hepatitis: widening horizons. Am J Gastroenterol 1992; 87:831–836.

16. Sheth SG, LaMont JT. Gastrointestinal problems in the chronically critically ill patient. Clin Chest Med 2001; 22:135–147.

17. Gottlieb ME, Sarfeh IJ, Stratton H, Goldman ML, Newell JC, Shah DM. Hepatic perfusion and splanchnic oxygen consumption in patients postinjury. J Trauma 1983; 23:836–843.

18. Naschitz JE, Slobodin GS, Lewis RJ, Zuckerman E, Yeshurun D. Heart diseases affecting the liver and liver diseases affecting the heart. Am Heart J 2000; 140:111–120.

19. Giallourakis CC, Rosenberg PM, Friedman LS. The liver in heart failure. Clin Liver Dis 2002; 6:947–967.

20. Fuchs S, Bogomolski YV, Paltiel O, Ackerman Z. Ischemic hepatitis: clinical and laboratory observations in 34 patients. J Clin Gastroenterol 1998; 26:183–186.

21. Nouel O, Henrion J, Bernuau J, Degott C, Rueff B, Benhamou JP. Fulminant hepatic failure due to transient circulatory failure in patients with chronic heart disease. Dig Dis Sci 1980; 25:49–52.

22. Jakob SM. Splanchnic blood flow in low-flow states. Anesth Analg 2003; 96:1129–1138.

23. Navaratnam RL, Morris SE, Traber DL, Flynn J, et al. Endotoxin (LPS) increases mesenteric vascular resistance (MVR) and bacterial translocation. J Trauma 1990; 30:1104–1113.

24. Dhainaut JF, Marin N, Mignon A, Vinsonneau C. Hepatic response to sepsis: interaction between coagulation and inflammatory processes. Crit Care Med 2001; 29:S42–S47.

25. Wang P, Zheng F, Ayala A, Chaudry IH. Hepatocellular dysfunction persists during early sepsis despite increased volume of crystalloid resuscitation. J Trauma 1992; 32:389–397.

26. Dahn MS, Lange P, Wilson RF, et al. Hepatic blood flow and splanchnic oxygen consumption measurements in clinical sepsis. Surgery 1990; 107:295–301.

27. Maynard ND, Bihari DJ, Dalton RN, et al. Liver function and splanchnic ischemia in critically ill patients. Chest 1997; 111:180–187.

28. Fong YM, Marano MA, Moldawer LL, Wei H, et al. The acute splanchnic and peripheral tissue metabolic response to endotoxin in humans. J Clin Invest 1990; 85:1896–1904.

29. Matuschak GM, Rinaldo JE. Organ interactions in the adult respiratory distress syndrome during sepsis: role of the liver in host disease. Chest 1988; 94:400–406.

30. Szabo G, Romics L, Frendl G. Liver in sepsis and systemic inflammatory response syndrome. Clin Liver Dis 2002; 6:1045–1066.

31. Mizock B. The hepatosplanchnic area and hyperlactatemia: a tale of two lactates. Crit Care Med 2001; 29:447–449.

32. DeBacker D, Creteur J, Silva E, Vincent JL. The hepatosplanchnic area is not a common source of lactate in patients with severe sepsis. Crit Care Med 2001; 29:256–261.

33. Thiele DL. Hepatic manifestations of systemic disease and other disorders of the liver. In: Feldman, ed. Sleisenger and Fordtran's Gastrointestinal and Liver disease. 7th ed. 1612–1617.

34. Miller DJ, Keeton GR, Webber BL, et al. Jaundice in severe bacterial infection. Gastroenterology 1976; 71:94–97.

35. Franson TR, Heirholzer WJ, LaBrecque DR. Frequency and characteristics of hyperbilirubinemia associated with bacteremia. Rev Infect Dis 1985; 7:1–9.

36. Franson, TR, LaBrecque DR. Buggy BP, et al. Serial bilirubin determinations as a prognostic marker in clinical infections. Am J Med Sci 1989; 297:149–152.

37. Farrell GC. Liver disease caused by drugs, anesthetics and toxins. In: Feldman, ed. Sleisenger and Fordtran's Gastrointestinal and Liver Disease. 7th ed. 2002:1403–1447.

38. Liu ZL, Kaplowitz N. Immune-mediated drug-induced liver disease. Clin Liver Dis 2002; 6:73–96.

39. McKindley DS, Hanes S, Boucher BA. Hepatic drug metabolism in critical illness. Pharmacotherapy 1998; 18:759–778.

40. Lee WM. Drug-Induced hepatotoxicity. New Engl J Med 2003; 349:474–485.

41. Zimmerman HJ, Ishak KG. General aspects of drug-induced liver disease. Gastroenterol Clin North Am 1995; 24:739–757.

42. Goodman ZD. Drug hepatotoxicity. Clin Liver Dis 2002; 6:381–397.

43. Lewis JH. Drug-Induced liver disease. Med Clin North Am 2000; 84:1275–1311.

44. Cunha BA. Antibiotic side effects. Med Clin North Am. 2001; 85:149–185.

45. Zimmerman HJ, Maddrey WC. Acetaminophen (Paracetamol) hepatotoxicity with regular intake of alcohol: analysis of instances of therapeutic misadventure. Hepatology 1995; 22:767–773.

46. Whitcomb DC, Block GD. Association of acetaminophen hepatotoxicity with fasting and ethanol use. J Am Med Assoc 1994; 272:1845.

47. Bailey B, Amre DK, Gaudreault P. Fulminant hepatic failure secondary to acetaminophen poisoning: a systematic review and meta-analysis of prognostic criteria determining the need for liver transplantation. Crit Care Med 2003; 31:299–305.

48. Lewis JH, Ranard RC, Caruso A, et al. Amiodarone hepatotoxicity: prevalence and clinicopathologic correlations among 104 patients. Hepatology 1989; 9:679–685.

49. Gregory SA, Webster JB, Chapman GD. Acute hepatitis induced by parenteral amiodarone. Am J Med 2002; 113:254–255.

50. Knowles SR, Shapiro LE, Shear NH. Anticonvulsant hypersensitivity syndrome: incidence, prevention and management. Drug Saf 1999; 21:489–501.

51. Schlienger RG, Shear NH. Antiepileptic drug hypersensitivity syndrome. Epilepsia 1998; 39(suppl 7):S3–S7.

52. Badem JM, Rice SA. Metabolism and toxicity of inhaled anesthetics. In: Miller, ed. Anesthesia. 5th ed. Churchill Livingstone, Inc., 2000:157–160.

53. Volles DF, McGory R. Perspectives in pain management: pharmacokinetic considerations. Crit Care Clin 1999; 15:55–75.

54. Young CC, Prelipp RC. Benzodiazepines in the intensive care unit. Crit Care Clin 2001; 17:843–862.

55. Angelini G. Ketzler JT. Coursin DB. Use of propofol and other nonbenzodiazepine sedatives in the intensive care unit. Crit Care Clin 2001; 17:863–880.

56. Murphy GS, Vender JS. Neuromuscular blocking drugs: use and misuse in the intensive care unit. Crit Care Clin 2001; 17:925–942.

57. Sandhu IS, Jarvis C, Everson GT. Total parenteral nutrition and cholestasis. Clin Liver Dis 1999; 3:489–508.

58. Chung C, Buchman AL. Postoperative jaundice and total parenteral nutrition-associated hepatic dysfunction. Clin Liver Dis 2002, 6:1067–1084.

59. Barie PS, Fischer E. Acute acalculous cholecystitis. J Am Coll Surg 1995; 180:232–244.

60. Mutlu GM, Mutlu EA, Factor P. GI complications in patients receiving mechanical ventilation. Chest 2001; 119:1222–1241.

61. Brugge WR, Brand DL, Atkins, HL, Lane BP, Abel WG. Gallbladder dyskinesia in chronic acalculous cholecystitis. Dig Dis Sci 1986; 31:461–467.

62. Johnson EE, Headley-Whyte J. Continuous positive pressure ventilation and choledochoduodenal flow resistance. J Appl Physiol 1975; 39:937–942.

63. Warren BL. Small vessel occlusion in acute acalculous cholecystitis. Surgery 1992; 111:163–168.

64. Mirvis ST, Vainright JR, Nelson AW, et al. The diagnosis of acute acalculous cholecystitis: a comparison of sonography, scintigraphy, and CT. AJR 1986; 147:1171–1175.

65. Boland G, Lee MJ, Mueller PR. Acute cholecystitis in the intensive care unit. New Horiz 1993; 2:246–260.

66. Boland GW, Lee MJ, Leung J, Mueller PR. Percutaneous cholecystostomy in critically ill patients: early response and final outcome in 82 patients. AJR 1994; 163:339–342.

67. Melin MM, Sarr MG, Bender CE, van Heerden JA. Percutaneous cholecystostomy: a valuable technique in high-risk patients with presumed acute cholecystitis. Br J Surg 1995; 82:1274–1277.

68. McGahan JP, Lindfors KK. Acute cholecystitis: diagnostic accuracy of percutaneous aspiration of the gall bladder. Radiology 1988; 167:669–671.

69. Rutherford CJ, Frenkel EP. Hemostatic disorders in liver disease. In: Schiff ER, Sorrell MF, Maddrey WC, eds. Schiff's Diseases of the Liver. 8th ed. Lippincott–Raven Publishers, 1999:583–595.

70. McKenna R. Abnormal coagulation in the postoperative period contributing to excessive bleeding. Med Clin North Am 2001; 85: 1277–1310.

71. Kimura S, Yoshioka T, Shibuya M, et al. Indocyanine green elimination rate detects hepatocellular dysfunction early in septic shock and correlates with survival. Crit Care Med 2001; 29:1159–1163.

72. Harbrecht BG, Frye RF, Senati MS, et al. Cytochrome P-450 activity is differentially altered in severely injured patients. Crit Care Med 2005; 33:541–546.

73. Vassilev D, Hauser B, Bracht H, et al. Systemic, pulmonary and hepatosplanchnic effects of N-acetylcysteine during long-term porcine endotoxemia. Crit Care Med 2004; 32:525–532.

74. Rank N, Michel C, Haertel C, et al. N-acetylcysteine increases liver blood flow and improves liver function in septic shock patients: results of a prospective, randomized, double blind study. Crit Care Med 2000; 28:3799–3807.

75. Devlin J, Ellis A, McPeake J, et al. N-acetylcysteine improves indocyanine green extraction and oxygen transport during hepatic dysfunction. Crit Care Med 1997; 25:236–242.

76. Hein OV, Ohring R, Schlling A, et al. N-acetylcysteine decreases lactate signal intensities in liver tissue and improves liver function in septic shock patients, as shown by magnetic resonance spectroscopy: extended case report. Crit Care 2004; 8:R66–71.

77. Renton MC, Snowden CP. Dopexamine and its role in the protection of hepatosplanchnic and renal perfusion in high-risk surgical and critically ill patients. Br J Anaesth 2005; 94:459–467.

78. Morelli A, Rocco M, Conti G, et al. Effects of short term fenoldopam infusion on gastric mucosal blood flow in septic shock. Anesthesiology 2004; 101:576–582.

79. Maguire PJ, Stevens C, Humes HD. Bioartificial organ support for hepatic, renal, and hematologic failure. Crit Care Clin 2000; 16:681–694.

80. Sechser A, Osorio J, Freise C, Osorio RW. Artificial liver support devices for fulminant liver failure. Clin Liver Dis 2001; 5:415–430.

81. Kjaergard LL, Jianping L, Als-Nielsen B, Cluud C. Artificial and bioartificial support systems for acute and acute-on-chronic liver failure. JAMA 2003; 289:217–222.

82. Liu JP, Gludd LL, Als-Nielsen B, et al. Artificial and bioartificial support systems for liver failure. Cochrane Database Syst Rev 2004; CD003628.

83. Demetriou AA, Brown RS, Busuttil RW, et al. Prospective, randomized, multicenter, controlled trial of a bioartificial liver in treating acute liver failure. Ann Surg 2004; 239:660–670.

84. Feldman. Sleisenger & Fordtran's Gastrointestinal and Liver Disease, 6th ed. W.B. Saunders Company, 2002:3–33.

85. Sherlock & Dooley. Diseases of the Liver and Biliary System, 10th ed. Blackwell Science, 1997:7.

36

Acute Fulminant Hepatic Failure

Brian McGrath

Department of Anesthesiology and Critical Care Medicine, George Washington University School of Medicine,
Washington, D.C., U.S.A.

Shobana Chandrasekar

Department of Anesthesiology, Baylor College of Medicine, Houston, Texas, U.S.A.

Rhonda K. Martin and Tarek Hassanein

Division of Hepatology and Liver Transplantation, Department of Medicine, UC San Diego Medical Center,
San Diego, California, U.S.A.

INTRODUCTION

Acute fulminant hepatic failure (FHF) is the abrupt onset of hepatocyte dysfunction, typically associated with massive necrosis of the liver, resulting in hepatic encephalopathy and multiple organ system dysfunction (MODS). It is a devastating condition associated with mortality rates as high as 80% in the absence of liver transplantation (1,2). Affected patients are often previously healthy, and thus without the typical stigmata of chronic liver disease or cirrhosis (Volume 2, Chapter 37), prior to illness.

Care is mainly supportive, however, a small number of important etiologies have specific treatments that will limit disease if begun early, and the full course of therapy is completed (e.g., N-acetylcysteine for acetaminophen toxicity). In addition, newer methods of extracorporeal support are being investigated to temporarily serve the function of the liver while it recovers. However, liver transplantation remains the only long-term life-saving therapy when hepatic failure is severe. Indeed, emergent liver transplantation has improved survival significantly for those eligible for the procedure, and FHF now accounts for 6% of adult liver transplants in the United States (3).

This chapter reviews the various etiologies of FHF, then discusses the diagnosis, classification, and prognosis. Next, the associated nonliver organ dysfunction syndromes are reviewed with a focus on both the pathophysiology and current management principles. Specific sections reviewing extracorporeal hepatic support and liver transplantation are also provided. The "Eye to the Future" section summarizes some of the new discoveries in diagnosis, monitoring, and management of liver failure currently on the horizon.

ETIOLOGIES OF ACUTE FULMINANT HEPATIC FAILURE

A variety of causes can trigger acute FHF including infection, toxic ingestion, drug reactions, malignancy, veno-occlusive disease, and ischemia, among others (Table 1). Drug toxicity, idiosyncratic drug reactions, and viral infections produce the majority of cases of FHF. Recent data

indicate that acetaminophen toxicity has become the leading cause of FHF in the United States. This is an example of drug-induced liver injury that results from a direct hepatotoxic agent acting in a dose-dependent manner (4,5). Acetaminophen-induced liver failure typically results from intentional overdose; although significant toxicity can occur unintentionally with therapeutic doses of the drug in chronic ethanol abusers and those exposed to other enzyme-inducing medications such as phenytoin or isoniazid (6,7).

The majority of drugs that produce liver failure do so in an unpredictable, dose-independent pattern through a variety of mechanisms including immune-mediated allergic reactions and the production of toxic metabolites. Phenytoin and halothane represent examples of compounds that can produce such idiosyncratic drug reactions. There are multiple viruses capable of producing severe liver injury. The incidence of viral etiologies varies geographically with hepatitis B virus (HBV) being most common in the United States and other Western countries (5). Liver failure resulting from chronic hepatitis C virus (HCV) is also one of the most common causes of end-stage liver disease requiring liver transplant; however, it is an uncommon cause of FHF in Western countries.

☞ **A rapid diagnosis and identification of the etiologic agent increases the likelihood that specific therapy will be beneficial in the treatment of FHF.** ☞ Determining the etiology is particularly important in cases of acetaminophen toxicity as early treatment with N-acetylcysteine can be lifesaving. The same is true for other toxic exposures that may benefit from temporary support by extracorporeal blood cleansing technologies (Volume 2, Chapter 38).

DIAGNOSIS, CLASSIFICATION, AND PROGNOSIS

The diagnosis of FHF is based on the clinical findings of jaundice and encephalopathy with associated laboratory abnormalities such as elevated aminotransferases, bilirubin, ammonia, coagulopathy, and/or hypoglycemia. Histology is helpful in determining etiology in some circumstances, but the use of liver biopsy is limited by the risks imposed by coexisting coagulopathy.

Table 1   Etiology of Fulminant Hepatic Failure

Type	Toxic agent
Infectious	Viral hepatitis: HAV, HBV, HCV[a], HDV, HEV, HSV$_1$, HSV$_6$, EBV, CMV
	Bacterial toxin: *Bacillus cereus, Leptospirosis*
Drug toxicity	Direct
	Acetaminophen
	Alcohol
	Idiosyncratic
	Isoniazid
	Halothane
	Phenytoin
	Statins
	Sulfonamides
	Many others reported
Toxins	Amanita phalloides
	Organic solvents, for example, carbon tetrachloride
	Phosphorous
	Many others reported
Vascular/hemodynamic	Budd–Chiari syndrome
	Congestive heart failure
	Shock/ischemia
Infiltrative disease	Lymphoma
	Leukemia
	Metastatic carcinoma
Other	Acute fatty liver of pregnancy
	Wilson's disease
	Reye's syndrome
	Hyperthermia
	Autoimmune hepatitis

[a]HCV is virtually unheard of as a cause of FHF in Western countries, but has been occasionally reported to cause FHF in Asia.
Abbreviations: CMV, cytomegalovirus; EBV, Epstein–Barr virus; HAV, hepatitis A virus; HBV, hepatitis B virus; HCV, hepatitis C virus; HDV, hepatitis D virus; HEV, hepatitis E virus; HSV$_1$, herpes simplex virus type 1; HSV$_6$, herpes simplex virus type 6.

Classification systems for FHF denote subdivisions based on the interval from the onset of jaundice to encephalopathy, a defining characteristic of FHF (Table 2). A short jaundice to encephalopathy interval has been correlated with a better outcome in some series (8,9). Other factors associated with survival include age, etiology, coagulation factors, pH, bilirubin, renal function, grade of hepatic encephalopathy, and neurologic status.

Table 2   Classification Systems of Fulminant Hepatic Failure

Number of stages	Classification	Jaundice–encephalopathy interval (wk)
2	FHF	≤2
	Sub-FHF	2–12
3	Hyper-ALF	1
	Acute liver failure	1–4
	Subacute liver failure	5–12

Abbreviations: ALF, acute liver failure; FHF, fulminant hepatic failure.
Source: From Refs. 8, 9.

Table 3   King's College Criteria for Nonsurvival in Fulminant Hepatic Failure

Acetaminophen etiology
  Arterial pH <7.30 (with adequate volume resuscitation)
  or arterial serum lactate level >3 mmol/L (6 mg%)
  or association with any of the following:
    INR >6.5 (PT >100 sec)
    Serum creatinine level >3.4 mg%
    Hepatic encephalopathy of grade 3 or 4
Non-acetaminophen etiology
INR >6.5 or any three of the following:
  Age <10 or >40 yr
  Interval between jaundice and encephalopathy >7 days
  Etiology of "drug-induced" or sero-negative hepatitis
  INR >3.5 (PT >50 sec)
  Total bilirubin >17.5 mg/dL

Abbreviations: INR, international normalization ratio; PT, prothrombin time.
Source: From Ref. 10.

☛ **Accurate assessment of severity and prognosis in FHF is particularly important for identifying those patients requiring liver transplantation.** ☛ Several schemes have been proposed to aid in transplant decision making, and the King's College Hospital criteria are perhaps the best known and most widely used (10). The influence of acetaminophen as the cause of FHF is particularly important in this evaluation system (Table 3).

SUPPORTIVE CARE TARGETING ASSOCIATED ORGAN SYSTEM DYSFUNCTION

FHF exerts its effects on multiple organ systems in the body through loss of the synthetic, metabolic, and immune-protective functions of the liver (Table 4). Herniation from intractable intracranial hypertension and sepsis with MODS remain important causes of death.

Central Nervous System
☛ **Hepatic encephalopathy is a defining feature of fulminant liver failure.** ☛ The reversible metabolic encephalopathy that accompanies FHF manifests a broad range of neuropsychiatric abnormalities. Encephalopathy related to FHF is more complex than that associated with chronic liver disease in part because of elevations in intracranial pressure (ICP) and the neurologic sequelae of MODS that accompany FHF.

The severity of hepatic encephalopathy is traditionally classified into four stages (Table 5) (11). Behavioral changes in hepatic encephalopathy range from subtle personality disturbances to profound coma (stage IV). Motor changes include hypertonia and hyperreflexia in earlier stages and hypotonia and loss of deep tendon reflexes with progression. Asterixis, the classic "liver flap," may be seen in early stages.

Pathophysiology
The pathogenesis of encephalopathy in FHF is complex, multifactorial and includes cerebral edema as well as the effects of accumulating gut-derived encephalopathic substances that

Table 4 Organ Dysfunction in Fulminant Hepatic Failure

Organ	Dysfunction	Treatment/comments
CNS	Hepatic encephalopathy	Lactulose, neomycin (or rifaxamine), aromatic amino acid, and protein restriction
	Cerebral edema, elevated ICP	Minimize (ammonia), elevate HOB, avoid hypotension, hypercarbia and hypoxia; ICP monitoring does not improve survival
Cardiovascular	Hyperdynamic circulation, vasodilation, hypovolemia, dysrhythmias, sepsis, septic shock, MODS	Fluid resuscitation (if hypovolemic) with invasive monitoring (if unstable) systemic vasopressor support if needed
Respiratory	Hyperventilation, aspiration, pneumonia, ARDS	Intubation, mechanical ventilation with PEEP
Metabolic	Hypoglycemia, metabolic acidosis, hypokalemia, hypomagnesemia	Glucose drip (if ↓ [glu]). Repletion of electrolytes feedings with low aromatic amino acid diet
Renal	ATN, functional renal failure (hepatorenal syndrome)	Maintenance of hemodynamics to preserve renal perfusion, avoid nephrotoxic drugs and infection; CVVHD if dialysis is needed
Hematologic	Coagulopathy, depletion of clotting factors, thrombocytopenia, platelet dysfunction, accelerated fibrinolysis, DIC, bleeding/anemia	Repletion of coagulation factors, treatment of infection, TEG monitoring may be useful, especially during OLT
GI bleed	Worsens organ failure and hypovolemia	H₂RA or PPI
ID/immune	Impaired phagocyte function	Surveillance for infection, prompt treatment of infections; there is a role for prophylactic antibiotics
	Bacterial and fungal infections are easily acquired leading to sepsis and MODS	

Abbreviations: ARDS, acute respiratory distress syndrome; ATN, acute tubular necrosis; CNS, central nervous system; CVVHD, continuous venovenous hemodialysis; DIC, disseminated intravascular coagulation; H₂RA, histamine 2 receptor agonist; HOB, head of bed; ICP, intracranial pressure; MODS, multiple organ dysfunction syndrome; OLT, orthotopic liver transplant; PEEP, positive end expiratory pressure; PPI, proton pump inhibitor; ↓, decreased; [glu], plasma glucose concentration; TEG, thromboelastogram;

are normally cleared by the liver. Ammonia is often implicated, and most patients will have elevated blood levels of this substance that crosses the blood–brain barrier (12). The role of ammonia in the pathophysiology of hepatic encephalopathy has been unclear in the literature, as plasma levels correlate poorly with severity, and many of the clinical and neurophysiologic disturbances induced by ammonia in other settings are not characteristic of hepatic encephalopathy (13,14). However, ammonia may exert some of its effects in FHF by potentiating gamma aminobutyric acid (GABA)-mediated neuronal depression and contributing to cerebral edema via increased conversion of glutamate to glutamine (15). Furthermore, arterial plasma ammonia levels have been shown to correlate with cerebral herniation (16).

Table 5 Hepatic Encephalopathy

Grade	Neurologic status
I	Mild confusion, euphoria, depression, slowing of mental tasks, slurred speech, irritability, abnormal sleep pattern
II	Drowsiness, lethargy, gross deficits in mental tasks, personality change, inappropriate behavior, disorientation
III	Somnolent, unable to perform mental tasks, persistent disorientation to time and/or place, amnesia, incoherent speech, profound confusion, agitation
IV	Coma with or without response to painful stimuli

Source: From Ref. 2.

Many other substances have been proposed as causative agents in hepatic encephalopathy. For example, increased concentrations of mercaptans, fatty acids, phenol, tryptophan, octopamine, phenylethanolamine, and taurine have been found in increased concentrations in the setting of liver failure. The role, if any, for these substances in the pathogenesis of FHF-induced encephalopathy has not been well established (17).

GABA activity is believed to be very important in the pathogenesis of hepatic encephalopathy. Increased GABA activity in FHF has been demonstrated secondary to increased synaptic availability and increased synthesis (18). Increased concentrations of endogenous benzodiazepine receptor agonists have been found in the brain and plasma of patients with hepatic encephalopathy, and benzodiazepine receptor antagonists such as flumazanil provide transient improvement in clinical and electrophysiologic abnormalities in some patients (19,20). As noted above, ammonia may enhance GABA-receptor activity as well.

Many factors can exacerbate the neurologic dysfunction associated with hepatic encephalopathy. Use of central nervous system (CNS) depressants such as benzodiazepines for sedation can worsen the encephalopathic state, presumably via GABA-receptor activity. Gastrointestinal (GI) bleeding and excess protein loads present more substrate to the gut for the production of encephalopathic substances. Alkalosis further promotes the movement of ammonia into the brain. Sepsis, electrolyte abnormalities, and hypoglycemia are also common in FHF and impart additional neurologic dysfunction.

Cerebral edema is the most prominent feature of FHF, occurring in up to 80% of patients with stage IV encephalopathy (21). Elevated ICP distinguishes encephalopathy in FHF from that associated with chronic liver disease, and a short jaundice to encephalopathy interval is associated with a greater risk of cerebral edema. Uncontrolled ICP produces ischemic neurologic injury as well as the potential for herniation, a common event in nonsurvivors (22). Clinical signs of intracranial hypertension in encephalopathic patients may be difficult to detect. Computed tomography (CT) is useful in detecting abnormalities such as intracranial hemorrhage but unreliable in diagnosing elevated ICP (23). ✍ **Because of the potential for complications, ICP monitoring remains controversial in managing patients with stage III and IV encephalopathies.** ✍ Although it is important for optimizing patient's management, ICP monitoring via an epidural transducer is associated with fewer complications, whereas an intracranial transducer offers a higher fidelity and more reliable signal (24). Techniques to control serum ammonia levels may be beneficial, because arterial ammonia levels >200 μmol/L have been shown to predict cerebral herniation within 24 hours after the development of stage III/IV encephalopathy (Fig. 1).

Measurements of cerebral blood flow (CBF) vary widely in patients with FHF-induced encephalopathy (25). As encephalopathy worsens, uncoupling of cerebral metabolism and CBF develops. Autoregulation to blood pressure is lost, rendering CBF more passively pressure-dependent and the brain more sensitive to hypotension (26). An absolute hyperemia develops in some and has been correlated with worsening edema and mortality (27).

Cerebral oxygen utilization and CBF can be inferred from jugular venous oximetry monitoring which is a more practical bedside technique than measurement of regional CBF. Increases in arterial-jugular venous oxygen (AjVdO$_2$) content difference imply low CBF and cerebral ischemia when oxygen utilization is constant. The assumption that cerebral oxygen consumption is constant in FHF may not be correct in all cases, however (25). A narrowed AjVdO$_2$ correlates with relative or absolute hyperemia. CBF has also been measured noninvasively with transcranial Doppler, although the utility of this technique has not been established relative to the use of jugular venous oximetry (28).

Electroencephalogram monitoring is useful in more severe cases, as subclinical seizure activity has been identified in FHF patients with advanced encephalopathy. It is also essential in managing patients who require barbiturate coma for control of intracranial hypertension (29).

Management

✍ **The most important aspect of treatment for encephalopathy in FHF is control or elimination of factors known to increase ICP and cerebral edema.** ✍ Maintaining an adequate cerebral perfusion pressure (CPP), the difference between mean arterial pressure (MAP) and ICP, is critical to preventing ischemia. A CPP less than 50 mmHg has been associated with poor outcome after hepatic transplantation, and values of 50 to 60 mmHg have been advocated as therapeutic targets (30–32). Efforts to improve CPP include reducing elevated ICP as well as increasing blood pressure with vasoconstrictors and/or inotropes. Maintaining adequate intravascular volume is important in maintaining cardiac output and MAP, but the optimum fluid regimen to use in patients with hepatic encephalopathy is unknown. Unnecessary free water is avoided, as it will exacerbate cerebral edema.

Although CPP improvement results from both ICP reduction and MAP augmentation, control of ICP also prevents herniation. Osmotherapy with mannitol is effective in reducing ICP in many patients, while corticosteroids have not been found to be helpful (33). Barbiturates are used to reduce refractory intracranial hypertension, however, hypotension from barbiturate-induced vasodilation and myocardial depression can compromise CPP. Therefore, aggressive hemodynamic monitoring and support may be necessary. Clinical neurologic examination is lost with barbiturate coma, and the drug effects can persist for a prolonged period of time in the face of impaired hepatic metabolism.

✍ **Hypothermia has emerged as an integral supportive maneuver in the care of FHF patients.** ✍ Hypothermia has been used in other settings of intracranial hypertension (32–34°C) and mild hypothermia has been shown to reduce cerebral edema in animal models of FHF (34,35). Techniques employed to achieve hypothermia include use of cooling blankets, reducing room temperature, and reducing ventilator circuit temperature settings. Reductions in ICP with commensurate improvement in CPP have been reported in patients with liver failure treated with hypothermia although prospective outcome data are lacking (34,35).

A head-up position has been advocated by some to decrease ICP, although the optimal head position has not been established as CPP may actually be compromised despite the reduction in ICP. Phenytoin reduces subclinical

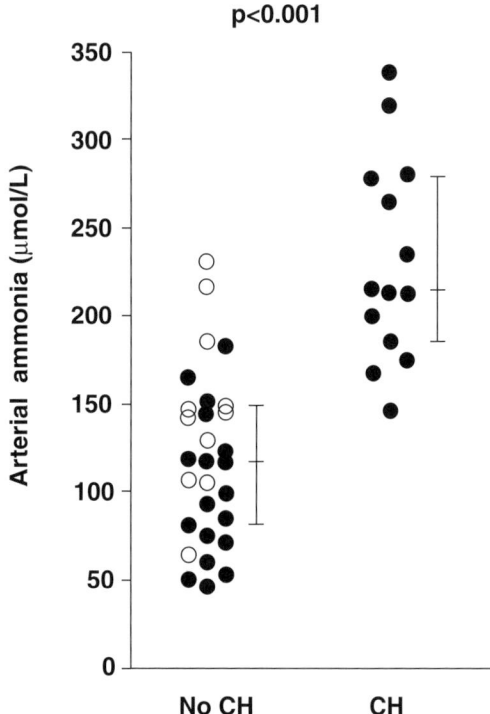

p<0.001

Figure 1 Arterial plasma ammonia concentration in 30 patients with acute liver failure (ALF) who did not develop cerebral herniation (No CH), and 14 patients who died from cerebral herniation (CH). *Left side:* open circles indicate patients who underwent liver transplantation; full circles indicate patients who died from other reasons. *Source:* From Ref. 16.

seizure activity as well as cerebral edema in some patients (29). Monitoring of phenytoin levels if used is warranted given the potential for alterations in hepatic metabolism and plasma protein levels in FHF.

Airway control and mechanical ventilation are required in comatose patients, and neuromuscular blockade can be necessary to prevent coughing and ventilator bucking with consequent increases in ICP and to protect the airways in patients considered for liver transplantation. Routine hyperventilation should be avoided as it may further reduce CBF in brain areas that are already marginally perfused. Lowering the $PaCO_2$ should be reserved for the subset of patients with hyperemia as identified by jugular venous saturation or CBF measurement.

Lactulose is commonly used to treat encephalopathy in patients with chronic liver disease. It is not clear whether there is any benefit in acute liver failure (ALF). However, ammonia exerts neurotoxicity via accumulation of glutamine within astrocytes (Fig. 2), and this rapid increase in astrocyte osmolarity triggers cerebral edema and cerebral hyperemia via unknown mechanisms (36).

The benzodiazepine receptor antagonist flumazenil has been shown to improve clinical and electrophysiological derangement in a significant proportion of patients with encephalopathy in both FHF and chronic liver disease (37). Unfortunately, the effects are transient (consistent with the drug's pharmacokinetics) and there is no improvement in prognosis.

Supportive measures also include correction/prevention of hypoxemia, hypoglycemia, and electrolyte abnormalities. N-Acetylcysteine improved oxygen transport in some studies of liver failure independent of its effects on acetaminophen metabolism and is used by some in FHF of any cause (31). The beneficial effect of N-acetylcysteine on oxygen transport has been challenged, and is currently under investigation in a multicenter clinical trial (38).

Cardiovascular

☞ **Circulatory abnormalities in liver failure include a decreased effective intravascular volume, vasodilation, and a hyperdynamic circulation.** ☞ The decreased effective intravascular volume results from altered intake (particularly in encephalopathic patients), bleeding, and

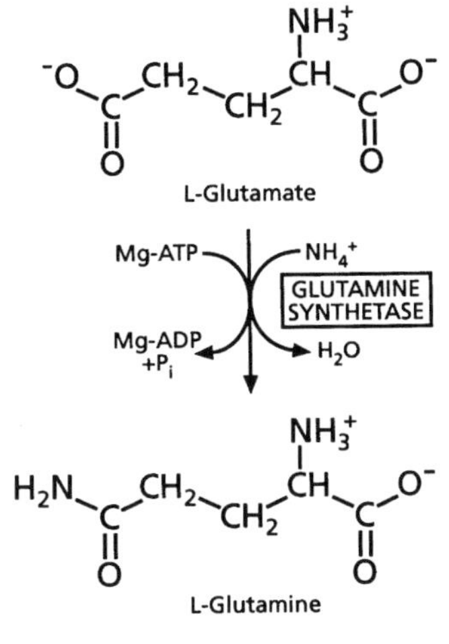

Figure 2 Astrocytic incorporation of ammonium into L-glutamine as first step for development of cell swelling, cerebral edema, and hyperemia. *Source*: From Ref. 36.

venodilation and third space of fluid due to circulating inflammatory mediators, hyponatremia, and later hypoalbuminemia. Systemic arteriolar dilation and afterload reduction contribute to the supranormal cardiac index in FHF. Supervening sepsis will exacerbate this vasodilated, hyperdynamic, state. Additionally, barbiturate therapy, if used for intracranial hypertension produces myocardial depression, vasodilation, and hypotension. Dysrhythmias occur frequently in FHF and include ventricular ectopy, A–V block, and atrial fibrillation (39).

Pathophysiology

The pathophysiology of the cardiovascular changes in FHF is unknown. The decreased systemic vascular resistance (SVR) was first reported in 1953 by Kowalski and Abelmann (40). Since then, it has been documented that systemic shunts open up and that much of the increased cardiac output is circulating in muscle and skin, rather than through the liver. However, investigators have yet to determine if these shunts are opened up because of a substance that is elaborated by the injured liver, or by some substance that is not being cleared by the injured liver, or by the absence of some factor which is normally produced by a well-functioning liver.

Following liver transplantation, the shunts will close down and the SVR will subsequently normalize. In many patients, the increased cardiac output and decreased SVR has little deleterious impact. However, in the elderly, or those with severe coronary artery disease, the hyperdynamic circulatory state can trigger myocardial ischemia or low perfusion-related renal failure.

Management

☞ **Hemodynamic management in ALF is aimed at providing adequate cerebral perfusion in the setting of intracranial hypertension, avoiding hemodynamically mediated deterioration in hepatic function, and preventing multiple organ failure.** ☞ Continuous intra-arterial blood pressure monitoring identifies hypotension quickly while facilitating blood gas analysis and calculation of parameters such as CPP. Pulmonary artery catheterization (PAC), while controversial, can help guide fluid and vasoactive drug therapy via preload assessment and cardiac output measurement when patients are unstable, and particularly when the cardiovascular parameters are confusing. However, there is no role for the PAC in routine management of stable patients with liver failure.

☞ **Maintaining intravascular volume and therefore cardiac preload is essential to preserve cardiac output and oxygen delivery.** ☞ In contrast, overly zealous fluid therapy risks exacerbation of cerebral edema, hepatic congestion, and worsening pulmonary edema in patients with acute respiratory distress syndrome (ARDS). Fluid choice is controversial and there is no clear evidence supporting the use of colloid over crystalloid solutions, although, as noted previously, excess free water should be avoided when cerebral edema is present. Red blood cell transfusion is indicated in bleeding and anemic patients and represents the ideal volume expander in such settings. A target hematocrit of 30% is advisable given the ongoing risks for multiple organ ischemia by providing a reasonable balance between oxygen carrying capacity and peripheral oxygen delivery.

☞ **Hypotension not responding to fluid therapy should be treated with vasoactive drug infusion.** ☞ Norepinephrine is being used more often as it combines potent inotropy with vasoconstriction. Many other vasoactive drug and drug combinations have been used, however. The endpoints for resuscitation include maintenance of adequate CPP in patients with elevated ICP, restoration/maintenance of renal function, and relief of lactic acidosis. The practice of resuscitation to target values of oxygen delivery and consumption has been called into question in other settings and a role, if any, in FHF has not been established. Correction of electrolyte abnormalities, for example, hypokalemia and hypomagnesemia, may ameliorate cardiac dysrhythmias.

Respiratory

Severe encephalopathic patients are at risk for pulmonary aspiration and upper airway obstruction. Respiratory alkalosis is often present early secondary to central hyperventilation, which can increase ammonia. Hypercapnic respiratory failure is more likely in later stages of hepatic encephalopathy.

Pathophysiology

σ⁴ **Gas exchange abnormalities in FHF result from transpulmonary shunting, and in some cases aspiration pneumonia, atelectasis, acute lung injury, or hepatopulmonary syndrome.** σ⁴ Patients with intracranial hypertension will be particularly sensitive to episodes of hypoxemia. The ARDS occurs in a significant number of patients and produces hypoxemia and reduced compliance (Volume 2, Chapter 24) (41). Ventilatory therapy in ARDS, particularly high PEEP levels, can exacerbate intracranial hypertension.

Management

Endotracheal intubation for airway protection and patency will be necessary for comatose patients and those with intracranial hypertension who require mechanical ventilation while receiving paralytics, barbiturates, or hyperventilation therapy. Hypoxemia will exacerbate cerebral ischemia and should be treated aggressively with supplemental oxygen and ventilatory support. Mechanical ventilation has the potential to adversely affect hepatic function, particularly when high levels of positive end-expiratory pressure (PEEP) are used which impede hepatic venous drainage. High PEEP levels may also adversely affect ICP. Such patients should receive close ICP monitoring as ventilatory support is titrated.

Coagulation System
Pathophysiology

Coagulopathy in acute hepatic failure results from a variety of causes. Loss of hepatic synthesis of the major plasma clotting factors is a prime reason. Levels of factors I, II, V, VII, IX, and X are reduced, ultimately leading to a prolonged prothrombin time (PT), and consequent elevated international normalization ratio (INR). Indeed, the PT serves as an important diagnostic and prognostic role. Platelet counts are reduced as is platelet function (42). Plasminogen, protein C, and protein S levels are reduced with evidence of disseminated intravascular coagulation (DIC) in many. Simultaneously, accelerated fibrinolysis is present, further contributing to the risk of hemorrhage (43).

Management

σ⁴ **Correction of coagulation and platelet abnormalities is necessary in bleeding patients and those undergoing invasive procedures such as ICP monitor placement or** surgery. σ⁴ Routine correction of clotting factor deficiencies with fresh frozen plasma (FFP) and/or factor VII infusion is unnecessary and concern has been raised regarding the subsequent loss of the PT as a prognostic sign (36). Vitamin K should be administered, as biliary absorption of this clotting cofactor may be impaired. Prophylaxis with H_2 antagonists can reduce the risk of GI bleeding.

Renal

Acute renal failure occurs in FHF with an incidence ranging from 30% to 70% and is associated with poor outcome particularly in those with severe encephalopathy (44–46). A variety of etiologies can contribute to renal failure singularly or as collective insults. Chief among these are prerenal states, hepatorenal syndrome, and toxin-induced acute tubular necrosis (ATN).

Pathophysiology

Renal dysfunction in the setting of FHF is often multifactorial in origin but prerenal factors are implicated in the majority of cases. σ⁴ **Potentially reversible hepatorenal syndrome occurs in a significant proportion of FHF patients with renal dysfunction.** σ⁴ The hepatorenal syndrome is associated with the same laboratory findings as the prerenal state, for example, elevated blood urea nitrogen/Cr ratio, and low fractional excretion of sodium (FeNa), that is, typically <1.0. In contrast to the prerenal state, patients with hepatorenal syndrome will not improve their renal function following the restitution of intravascular volume alone. Rather, the hepatorenal state will only resolve if the liver injury recovers, or following liver transplantation. Hypovolemia and vasodilation are often present in patients with FHF. This state is often exacerbated by secondary sepsis, leading to further reductions in renal blood flow which can progress to ATN.

Renal injury can also result from a toxic ingestion that is the primary cause of liver failure (e.g., acetaminophen toxicity). Furthermore, numerous nephrotoxic drugs, such as aminoglycosides, and radiocontrast are utilized in the care of FHF patients, and can contribute to renal injury.

Management

Prevention of acute renal failure is a major goal of the critical care management of patients with liver failure, and close monitoring of urine output via an indwelling bladder catheter is warranted. Cardiovascular resuscitation with fluids, prior to institution of supplemental vasoconstrictors and inotropes, is the best way to prevent acute renal failure. Furthermore, this therapy should be guided by hemodynamic monitoring data aimed at maintaining normal renal blood flow and perfusion pressure.

Nephrotoxic drugs such as aminoglycosides and nonsteroidal antiinflammatory drugs should be avoided whenever possible. N-acetylcysteine therapy for acetaminophen-induced FHF has been reported to reduce the incidence and severity of renal failure (47).

Patients who develop ATN often require some type of renal replacement therapy. Intermittent hemodialysis produces significant reductions in blood pressure and ICP elevations in the setting of FHF encephalopathy. Continuous renal replacement therapy (typically venovenous hemodialysis) is a better option than intermittent hemodialysis in patients with elevated (or potentially elevated) ICP because of the reduced risk of hypotension and ICP spikes (Volume 2, Chapter 43) (48).

Metabolic

☞ **Patients with ALF develop multiple metabolic and electrolyte abnormalities including hypoglycemia, hypokalemia, hypomagnesemia, hypophosphatemia, and metabolic acidosis.** ☞

Pathophysiology

Hypoglycemia occurs frequently as a result of impaired gluconeogenesis, persistent insulin effects, and decreased glycogenolysis. Neurologic dysfunction induced by low blood glucose can exacerbate or be confused with hepatic encephalopathy.

Metabolic acidosis is a poor prognostic factor in ALF. Lactate accumulation results from impaired hepatic metabolism as well as increased production by the liver and peripheral tissues. Uncorrected hemodynamic derangement and persistent hypoperfusion will exacerbate lactate production (49,50).

Management

Frequent monitoring of blood glucose is necessary in FHF patients. Hypoglycemia is treated aggressively with intravenous 50% dextrose solution by bolus followed by continuous glucose infusions. Ten percent dextrose infusions are used commonly, whereas some patients may require more concentrated glucose solutions. Phosphate levels may dramatically decrease, following the administration of large volumes or high concentrations of dextrose solutions.

Improvement in lactic acidosis will follow adequate hemodynamic resuscitation, control of secondary sepsis, and improved liver function. Treatment of low pH levels with bicarbonate is only recommended when severe and associated with hyponatremia. Potassium and magnesium repletions are required to treat and prevent cardiac dysrhythmias.

Infectious Disease

Sepsis is an ever-present risk in FHF that can be difficult to recognize. Serious infection contributes to the development of hyperdynamic shock, multiorgan failure, and death.

Pathophysiology

Susceptibility to infection is increased due to poor phagocyte function, low complement levels, and invasive therapies (51). *Staphylococcus* and *Candida* species have become increasingly important causative organisms (52).

Management

A high index of suspicion is necessary to detect and treat new infections. Whenever possible, therapeutic antibiotic choice should be based on culture results and sensitivities. Some centers advocate the use of prophylactic parenteral antibiotics for all FHF patients. Enteral decontamination does not appear to add additional protection (31).

SPECIFIC DRUG THERAPY

Treatment and support strategies targeted directly at the liver in acute hepatic failure include prevention or attenuation of toxic liver injury with resuscitative drugs (e.g., for acetaminophen toxicity, antiviral, etc.) and extracorporeal substitution of hepatocyte function (following section).

Acetaminophen Toxicity

Overdosage of acetaminophen should be treated with gastric lavage and activated charcoal within two hours of ingestion, the period of GI absorption. N-acetylcysteine is indicated in any case of known or suspected acetaminophen toxicity. Oxidation of acetaminophen by the cytochrome P-450 enzyme system produces N-acetyl-p-benzoquinoeimine (NAPQI), a highly reactive compound which binds to intracellular hepatocyte proteins producing injury and subsequent necrosis (53). N-acetylcysteine prevents or attenuates hepatocyte injury by serving as a glutathione source and substitute to which NAPQI binds producing nontoxic metabolites. Institution of therapy may be beneficial as late as 24 hours after ingestion (54). N-acetylcysteine is currently available in the United States as an oral or intravenous form, which is the preferred way of treatment. For oral use, it is given as a loading dose of 140 mg/kg, which is followed by 70 mg/kg maintenance doses at four-hour intervals. The duration of treatment is somewhat controversial. Food and Drug Administration (FDA) guidelines prescribe 17 doses of oral N-acetylcysteine given at four-hour intervals following the loading dose, however, shorter duration protocols using the intravenous form is preferred.

Antiviral Therapy

Specific antiviral treatment markedly improves survival of herpetic hepatitis in immunocompetent patients. In a study of 93 patients, without antiviral therapy survival was only 11% with vidarabine, survival improved to 38% and with acyclovir survival was 57% (55). More recent results demonstrate approximately 40% survival rate (55). Patients with hepatitis caused by herpes virus may benefit from acyclovir therapy. Likewise, patients with cytomegalovirus (CMV) may benefit from gancyclovir.

There are four FDA approved treatments for hepatitis B infection in the United States, interferon alpha-2b, which is contraindicated in cases with HBV-FHF, lamivudine, adefovir dipivoxil, and entecavir (56). In cases of acute exacerbation or flare of hepatitis B, these drugs are the choice for therapy; however, in patients on long-time lamivudine who develop a flare, other drugs such as adefovir are probably better, as the flare likely represents a lamivudine-resistant mutation in the virus (57).

Hepatitis C is an uncommon cause of fulminant hepatitis, but a recent report demonstrated improved survival with a combined treatment of alpha interferon and ribavirin (58).

Mushroom Toxin Support

The numerous syndromes associated with mushroom poisonings, along with their associated diagnostic and management principles, have recently been reviewed (Volume 1, Chapter 31) (59). Amanita mushroom poisoning has been treated with penicillin, which displaces amatoxin from protein-binding sites and may inhibit penetration into hepatocytes. Silibinin, which inhibits toxin binding, has also been used in amanita poisoning (60).

Combined treatment with silibinin and N-acetylcysteine appears to be more effective than other medical treatments in amatoxin poisoning (61). As a bridge to transplantation, and occasionally as a successful therapy in its own right, extracorporeal liver-cleansing techniques are beginning to show promise following mushroom intoxication as well as following other hepatic injuries (Volume 2, Chapter 38) (62,63).

Other Specific Therapies

Autoimmune hepatitis has been treated with prednisone and azathioprine for over 30 years. However, there are a variety of types of autoimmune hepatitis, and more specific therapies are on the horizon (64). Each specific autoimmune disease has a specific regulatory dysfunction that can be targeted (65).

Galactosemia and fructosemia are etiologies of FHF, which are treated with dietary elimination. Hereditary tyrosinemia type I is treated with dietary elimination and 2-(2-nitro-4-trifluoromethylbenzoyl)-1,3-cyclohexanedione.

EXTRACORPOREAL SUPPORT

A variety of techniques have been used in patients with ALF to temporarily replace hepatic function while awaiting spontaneous recovery or liver transplantation. Plasmapheresis decreases plasma concentrations of substances such as bilirubin, aminotransferases, and ammonia (66). In combination with plasma exchange, plasmapheresis can correct coagulation abnormalities and has been associated with improved survival in noncontrolled studies (67). Charcoal hemoperfusion and hemodiafiltration with charcoal or an albumin adsorbent circuit, the so-called "molecular absorbent recirculating system" have also demonstrated improvement in various clinical and biochemical parameters (Volume 2, Chapter 38) (68).

Bioartificial livers incorporate hepatocyte cells in a synthetic framework through which whole blood, plasma, or a dialysate are perfused via an extracorporeal circuit. The hepatocytes used in these devices are derived from human hepatoblastoma cells [extracorporeal liver-assist device (ELAD)] or porcine livers ("Bioartificial Liver"). Improvement in mental status with the ELAD has been reported, however, a randomized, controlled trial did not show reduced mortality (69). Similarly, the bioartificial device has been associated with improved neurologic function, but improved survival has yet to be demonstrated (Volume 2, Chapter 38).

Extracorporeal perfusion of both human and porcine livers has been undertaken with improvement in encephalopathy and prolonged survival in small numbers of patients (70).

LIVER TRANSPLANTATION

Liver transplantation offers the best hope for survival for patients with FHF. Given the limited availability of human donors, replacement of liver tissue has also been undertaken by implantation of hepatocytes, auxiliary liver transplantation, and xenotransplantation; techniques which have not had the success of allotransplantation.

Transplantation Types and Nomenclature
Hepatocyte Transplantation

Implantation of hepatocytes into the splenic bed has been carried out in a limited number of patients, and decreased ammonia levels, improved neurologic function, and a slight mortality advantage over controls have been described (71). Randomized trials have not been performed to date, however.

Xenotransplantation

Transplantation of animal livers has been performed as a bridge to human organ transplant in a very small number

of patients. Baboon, chimpanzee, and pig livers have been implanted with variable success including reports of graft function as long as 70 days (72). Rejection of the xenograft remains a significant problem along with concerns about transmission of infectious agents.

Allotransplantation

Allotransplantation denotes a species-to-species transplant, in this usage human-to-human. Liver transplantation with a human allograft has significantly reduced the mortality for patients with liver failure. Although survival following transplantation for patients with FHF is less than in other settings, one-year survival rates of 60% to 70% in FHF have been achieved (73). Patients with liver failure from acetaminophen fare somewhat better than those with FHF from other causes.

When the diseased liver is totally removed, and the transplanted allograft is positioned in the location of the native liver, it is referred to as an orthotopic liver transplant (OLT). OLT is the most commonly employed liver transplant. Heterotopic grafts refer to situations where the native diseased liver is left in place (because it might recover) and the transplanted liver is placed in another location (e.g., below the native liver) in the abdomen, and all connections are shared.

The shortage of donor organs remains the biggest hurdle to OLT. In response to the shortage of cadaveric donors, transplant centers have begun using "higher-risk" donor livers such as those from non-heart-beating donors (NHBDs) or with ABO incompatibility or from older donors or donors with fatty liver. Split-liver grafts from a single donor and living-donor transplantation are also being used (31).

Auxiliary transplantation allows the native liver to remain in place with the hope of eventual recovery and discontinuation of immunosuppressive therapy. While reported survival rates for the partial technique are similar to OLT, complications are more frequent with auxiliary transplantation (74). Although acute cellular rejection is a complication that is associated with a longer hospital stay, it rarely occurs in a severe form with the current immunosuppression protocols.

Perioperative Considerations for OLT in Acute Liver Failure Patients

Liver transplantation is the second most common transplant surgery, accounting for 21% of all organ transplants in the United States (75). In the period from 1997 to 2001, acute hepatic necrosis accounted for 9% of cadaveric liver transplants (76,77). In the last 20 years, emergency liver transplantation has emerged as the most beneficial therapeutic intervention for patients with ALF (78). Most of these are OLTs. Living donor transplants have increased since 1999. Management considerations for living donors will not be included in this discussion.

Recipient Selection

Accurate prediction of successful transplantation is an important goal in patient selection due to a small organ donor pool, lack of proven alternatives to transplantation, and lifelong complications secondary to immunosuppression (79).

The commonly used King's College Hospital critera are the most utilized, and studies evaluating these criteria have shown positive predictive values ranging from 70% to 100% in predicting outcome as compared to other prognostic scoring systems (80,81). In a recent meta-analysis, various prognostic criteria (Table 3) were compared in ALF patients (82). This included King's College Hospital criteria, elevated serum creatinine, encephalopathy, PT elevations, decreased factor V levels, the acute physiology and chronic health evaluation II scores, and Gc-globulin (vitamin D-binding protein, a liver-derived component of the actin scavenging system). The analysis indicated that King's College Hospital criteria and pH <7.3 alone were both fairly specific in predicting a poor outcome. Other proposed prognostic criteria include: (i) the severity of systemic inflammatory sepsis syndrome, (ii) alpha feto protein (AFP) levels, (iii) ratios of factors VIII and V, (iv) liver histology, (v) CT scanning of liver, (vi) cytokine levels, (vii) serum phosphate levels, and (viii) adrenal insufficiency. Further research is needed to determine the validity of each of these aforementioned prognostic variables.

Potentially helpful indicators of poor prognosis include: (i) based on etiology: drug injury, acute hepatitis B and autoimmune hepatitis, mushroom poisoning, Wilson's disease, Budd, Chiari syndrome (hepatic vein thrombosis), and grades III and IV encephalopathy on admission; (ii) based on King's College criteria (Table 3); (iii) model for end-stage liver disease (MELD) score (a logarithmic grading system based upon serum bilirubin, creatinine, and INR), introduced by the United Network for Organ Sharing in 2002 to prioritize organ allocation (83). MELD is an objective measurement that unlike the Child–Pugh scoring system, was not influenced by subjective assessments like hepatic encephalopathy. The MELD score has become a widely used tool for recipient selection and organ allocation but despite its objectivity and reliability, more studies regarding short-term and long-term outcomes are needed; (iv) the U.S. ALF group criteria is also predictive of mortality and categorizes the presence of three values: stage 3 or 4 hepatic encephalopathy, serum creatinine ≥2.0; and INR ≥3.0. ALF patients with zero criteria have 4% mortality; 1 factor = 15% mortality; 2 factors = 50% mortality; and all 3 factors = 80% mortality (84).

In summary, currently available prognostic scoring systems do not perfectly determine recipient selection or predict outcome for liver transplantation; however, they are useful when combined with clinical judgment, and factored in with donor selection.

Donor Selection
Standard criteria for donor selection initially excluded advanced age, obesity (body mass index >30), donor hypernatremia (serum sodium >155 meq/L), prolonged intensive care unit stay, large doses of vasopressor requirement, positive hepatic serologies, and the use of NHBDs.

However, over the last 20 years there is a growing disparity between demand and supply of organs. The expanded criteria for donors or marginal donors now include older livers, organs from the opposite gender, grafts with steatosis (obesity, alcohol use, diabetes), NHBDs, HCV-positive liver grafts, hepatitis B core antibody-positive grafts, donor hypernatremia, split liver grafts from deceased donors, and prolonged cold ischemia time (85). Marginal grafts have shown poorer immediate graft function, but careful matching of donors and recipients with these grafts has shown promising results in some centers.

Preoperative Preparation
All patients with clinical or laboratory evidence of severe acute hepatitis should have the coagulation status evaluated and alterations in mental status closely monitored. If the diagnosis of liver failure is established, transfer to the ICU facilitates optimum management, and in a center with a liver transplant program preparation for OLT. Exposure to viral infections, drugs or toxins, and history of chronic liver disease and alcohol intake is determined and all medications and supplements the patient used are reviewed.

A detailed history from the patient or the family and a physical examination is performed. The physical examination includes an assessment of neurologic status, the presence of jaundice, and stigmata of acute and/or chronic liver disease, right upper quadrant tenderness and palpable mass, ascites, edema, and congestive heart failure.

Laboratory examination consists of routine chemistries, complete blood counts, renal function tests, arterial blood gas measurements, blood typing and cross-matching, drug screens, viral hepatitis serologies, AFP levels, tests for Wilson's disease, autoimmune antibodies, HIV testing, and a pregnancy test in females. Plasma ammonia levels, lactate levels, and a liver biopsy via the transjugular route may also be indicated in certain clinical situations.

All the above is done to determine a precise etiology to help guide further management decisions. Once the etiology is determined, specific therapies should be initiated. A key factor for improving survival is early contact with a transplant center for transfer of patients.

Therapy
Apart from focused therapy for the specific etiology, general supportive management should continue. Attention to fluid balance is of primary importance. Hemodynamic status should be monitored and treatment of infection should be carried out promptly. Metabolic parameters should be evaluated and GI prophylaxis for bleeding provided.

Management of Raised Intracranial Pressure
In early stages of FHF, sedation should be avoided. Nonabsorbable disaccharides (e.g., lactulose) and antibiotics may be used, keeping in mind the possibility of bowel distention. If evidence of intracranial hypertension is present, the head should be elevated 30° and mannitol infusion is given. Patients progressing into grade III or IV hepatic encephalopathy should have airway protection and ICP monitoring established, particularly if they are considered for liver transplantation. Prompt treatment of seizures with benzodiazepines is recommended. Short-acting barbiturates and hyperventilation are temporary measures and are used only for short-term management of severe intracranial hypertension. Moderate hypothermia has been effective in reversing cerebral edema in some patients and is currently the subject of a clinical trial (34).

Infection Screening and Antibiotic Prophylaxis
Patients with FHF are vulnerable to bacterial or fungal sepsis. This may preclude transplantation; hence periodic surveillance cultures should be performed and treated accordingly. Prophylactic antibiotics and antifungals have not been shown to improve overall outcomes.

Coagulopathy
Patients are at increased risk for bleeding complications due to decreased synthesis and increased consumption of clotting factors. In preparation for liver transplant, use of FFP, vitamin K, platelet transfusions, and recombinant factor VII has been administered with temporary correction of coagulopathy. There are no reliable predictors of perioperative bleeding. It is known that patients who require more

perioperative transfusions are associated with lower graft and patient survival rates. This may be due to increased proinflammatory cytokine release, which worsens bleeding and worsens graft and patient survival.

The effort taken to temporarily normalize the coagulation status immediately prior to transplantation is generally worthwhile. Indeed all three phases of OLT are associated with metabolic and hemorrhagic derangements that can worsen any pre-existing coagulopathy. ☞ **Sudden massive blood loss can occur intraoperatively and this in conjunction with baseline hyperfibrinolysis, coagulation factor deficiencies, and thrombocytopenia results in the need for massive blood and blood product transfusions with that have potentially severe consequences.** ☞ Use of thromboelastogram (TEG) intraoperatively (Volume 1, Chapter 17) has been shown to decrease transfusion requirements during OLT surgery.

Intravascular Volume Status

The high cardiac output, low SVR caused by a hyperdynamic circulation causes hypotension which may require inotropes and vasoactive drugs. Supportive therapy with fluid resuscitation and attempt to maintain intravascular volume is paramount. Monitoring should include an arterial blood pressure and pulmonary artery catheter to help guide fluid management perioperatively. Systemic vasopressor support with epinephrine, norepinephrine, or dopamine is preferred.

Intraoperative Management
Monitoring

Invasive monitoring devices include a radial or femoral arterial line placed prior to induction. A pulmonary artery catheter is used routinely for perioperative fluid and hemodynamic management and for monitoring PA pressures. A transesophageal echocardiography (TEE) lead is placed for monitoring left ventricular filling, detection of air emboli during reperfusion, and assessing global left ventricular function. TEE is increasingly being used without reports of variceal bleeding after insertion.

Venous access is obtained with two 9-French introducers centrally. At UCSD, a rapid infuser circuit incorporating a cardiotomy reservoir, roller pump, heat exchanger, and safety features for monitoring air embolism and occlusion is set up by a cardiovascular perfusionist. Use of the rapid infusion device allows rapid administration of warmed blood and fluids through large-bore central lines. Usual rates of transfusion are 200 cm³/min, but more rapid rates up to 1000 cm³/min can be administered.

The volume of infusion is guided by blood pressure, CVP, PA, and TEE. The composition of fluid replaced is determined by Hct, platelet count, PT/PTT, and TEG, as evaluated by the anesthesiologist.

Veno-venous Bypass

Venovenous bypass is used by some surgeons during liver transplantation to provide hemodynamic stability, decrease splanchnic congestion, improve renal perfusion, and decrease metabolic acidosis when the vena cava is clamped. Venous return from the femoral circuit and portal circulation is returned to the internal jugular/subclavian/axillary veins. In our center, percutaneous venovenous bypass lines are placed by the anesthesiologist prior to incision. A 17-French cannula is placed in the internal jugular vein and can be used for both bypass and for rapid infusion. Problems

with venovenous bypass include air embolism, thromboembolism, and inadvertent decannulation.

Factor VII

Recombinant factor VIIa seems to enhance local hemostasis by a local thrombin burst effect. Recombinant factor VIIa might have the potential to be an effective hemostatic measure in patients undergoing liver transplantation (86). This impression is based on clinical data from a limited number of case histories and small clinical trials. A recent study in patients undergoing hepatectomy showed that rfactor VIIa (rFVIIa) did not result in a statistically significant reduction in either the number of patients transfused or the volume of blood products administered (87).

Clinical trials are ongoing to determine the safety and efficacy of rFVIIa in patients undergoing OLT surgery, but no conclusive information has been obtained yet (Volume 2, Chapters 58–59) (88).

Thromboelastogram

In FHF patients receiving transplantation, pre-existing coagulopathy is often present secondary to decreased synthesis of coagulation factors and platelets, increased utilization of these, and decreased platelet function. During transplantation, this is complicated by fibrinolysis due to reduced clearance of activators of coagulation and after reperfusion of the grafted liver. A heparin-like effect is observed in one-third of patients following transplantation, and intraoperative changes in blood coagulation and TEG monitoring are also observed during liver transplantation.

Heparin used during venovenous bypass, heparin present in the grafted organ, and persisting fibrinolysis from poor graft function all may contribute to severe bleeding after reperfusion if the newly grafted liver is functioning poorly. TEG gives a global evaluation of clotting function and helps in assessing response to administration of corrective factors such as cryoprecipitate, platelets, or protamine (89,90). The TEG is also useful in detecting a prothrombotic state, as some patients are at a risk for hepatic arterial thrombosis after liver transplantation.

Anesthetic Drugs

Anesthetic induction incorporates a rapid sequence technique after three to five minutes of preoxygenation due to the increased risk of aspiration secondary to abdominal distension from ascites. Fentanyl is the opioid of choice and is useful to blunt the sympathetic response. Midazolam with its minimal hemodynamic effects is useful for amnesia. A balanced anesthetic technique is used in most centers, and volatile agents like isoflurane are used in low concentrations to minimize hypotension in patients with FHF. Isoflurane preserves splanchnic blood flow and is the preferred agent. Cisatracurium because of its organ-independent elimination, is used for neuromuscular blockade.

Antifibrinolytics

Reperfusion can trigger severe fibrinolysis, which requires cryoprecipitate and possibly antifibrinolytics. Earlier studies did not show any advantage to the use of prophylactic antifibrinolytics, but a European multicenter study showed decreased transfusion requirements with aprotonin and no thrombotic events in the aprotonin group (91).

Table 6 Stages of Liver Transplantation

Preanhepatic (stage of dissection)	Anhepatic (stage of no liver)	Postanhepatic (stage of reperfusion)
Surgical incision to cross-clamp PV, HA, IVC	Occlusion of vascular flow to perfusion of grafted liver	Perfusion of new liver to completion of biliary reconstruction and closure of surgical incision
Blood loss	Hemodynamic changes due to clamping and then unclamping IVC	Hypotension
Hypoglycemia	Splanchnic congestion	Acidosis
Hypocalcemia	Decreased renal perfusion	Hypothermia
Coagulopathy	Hypocalcemia	Hyperkalemia
		Blood loss

Abbreviations: HA, hepatic artery; IVC, inferior vena cava; PV, portal vein.

Stages of Liver Transplant Surgery

Preanhepatic Stage (Phase of Dissection)
The preanhepatic stage begins with surgical incision and ends with cross-clamp of portal vein, supra- and infrahepatic parts of the inferior vena cava, and hepatic artery (Table 6). Dissection and mobilization of the liver along with pre-existing coagulopathy result in blood loss and hypovolemia. Transfusions of blood and blood products are administered based on hematocrit, coagulation profile, platelet count, and TEG.

Metabolic parameters are monitored and treated. Citrate intoxication in the absence of hepatic function causes hypocalcemia from infusion of blood products. Hypoglycemia in acute hepatic failure and hyperkalemia secondary to renal dysfunction worsened by massive blood transfusion all need to be frequently monitored and corrected. Hypothermia should be avoided and hourly urine output monitored closely.

Anhepatic Stage
This begins with occlusion of vascular inflow and ends with perfusion of the grafted new liver. Hemodynamic changes dominate this stage when vena caval cross-clamping causes significant decreases in venous return, splanchnic congestion, metabolic acidosis, and decreased renal perfusion pressure.

Hemodynamic stability is maintained by administration of blood and blood products and correction of coagulopathy. This is important as the combined effect of absent clotting factors and fibrinolysis due to the unopposed action of tissue plasminogen activator can cause severe coagulopathy in this stage.

Neohepatic Stage (Reperfusion Stage)
Reperfusion of the new liver through the portal vein begins the neohepatic stage and is associated with hypotension, hyperkalemia, acidosis, and hypothermia. One-third of patients experience profound hypotension after reperfusion. This can be due to metabolic abnormalities, vasodilatation, emboli (air or thrombotic), hypothermia, arrhythmias, or myocardial dysfunction (92,93). Some risk factors for this include suboptimal grafts and prolonged graft cold ischemia time. Hepatic artery followed by biliary tree anastomosis is done following portal vein anastomosis. Improvement in acidosis, decreasing requirements for calcium, improvement of coagulation function, rise in core body temperature, and bile output from the graft are indicators of a healthy graft.

Postoperative Complications
Early postoperative hemorrhage due to anastomotic leaks or laceration of the liver surface or coagulopathy results in reoperation in about 10% of transplanted patients. Vascular obstructive complications, particularly hepatic artery thrombosis, are a dreaded complication with the incidence ranging up to 10% in adults and 20% in children (due to the smaller vessel diameter). Other surgical and medical complications following OLT are shown in Table 7.

Postoperative management includes correction of coagulopathy, maintaining adequate volume status for vital organ perfusion, monitoring urine output, and prevention of infection. Immunosuppression is needed to prevent

Table 7 Postoperative Complications after Hepatic Transplantation

Surgical complications	Medical complications	Immunological complications
Anastomotic or implantation site bleed	Early postoperative infections causing pneumonia and sepsis	Acute rejection
Hepatic artery/portal vein thrombosis	Acute cholangitis	Subacute rejection and graft dysfunction
Supra/infra hepatic vena caval obstruction	Viral infections especially CMV	Recurrence of Hep B and C
Biliary leakage/strictures	Immunosuppression-related toxicity	Recurrence of autoimmune hepatitis, primary biliary cirrhosis, and primary sclerosing cholangitis
Wound infections, injury to bowel or other intra-abdominal organs	Acute renal failure	Chronic rejection

Abbreviations: CMV, cytomegalovirus; Hep, hepatitis.

Table 8 Immunuosuppressive Medications after Liver Transplantation

Drugs	Mechanism of action	Side effects
Corticosteroids	Suppress macrophage activation, powerful anti-inflammatory effect which suppresses immune response and acute graft rejection	Dose-related; fluid retention diabetes mellitus, osteoporosis, osteonecrosis, cataract, skin thinning Main concern: cardiovascular complications and promotion of virus replication in patients with viral hepatitis
Antimetabolites		
Azathioprine	Cytotoxic agents interfere with DNA and RNA synthesis of T and B lymphocytes	Bone marrow suppression, nausea, diarrhea
Mycophenolate	Interferes with synthesis of guanine nucleotides and DNA replication	
Calcineurin inhibitors		
Cyclosporine A	Inhibits calcineurin affecting T-cell activation	Renal dysfunction, diabetes, hypertension, headache and GI problems
Tacrolimus	Blocks T-cell proliferation and thereby interleukin synthesis	
Rapamycin	Blocks ligation of interleukin 2 to its receptor	Thrombocytopenia and hyperlipidemia
Monoclonal antibodies		
OKT3	Directed against CD3 complex of T cells	Diarrhea, nausea, myalgia, fever, tachycardia, dyspnea
Chimeric basiliximab	Selectively target the IL 2 receptor on activated T cells	Low toxicity and minor side effects
Humanized Daclizumab		

Abbreviations: DNA, deoxyribonucleic acid; RNA, ribonucleic acid.

allograft rejection. These include corticosteroids, antimetabolites, calcineurin inhibitors, and monoclonal antibodies (Table 8).

Success of liver transplantation for FHF patients depends upon the status of both, the recipient, and the graft. A review has shown that the severity of multiorgan failure at the time of transplantation was the single best predictor of patient survival. Another analysis of 116 patients showed markedly poor outcomes in patients receiving marginal, size reduced, or ABO incompatible grafts.

EYE TO THE FUTURE

Patient survival for deceased donor liver transplant recipients based on the annual report by the OPTN/SRTR registry was 86% by one year, 78% at three years, and 72% at five years after transplantation (94). The shortage of grafts, compared to the long list of waiting recipients, is causing many to expire prior to transplant.

Marginal and split grafts, living related donation, xenotransplantation, and stem-cell-derived organs are future options that need to be further explored due to the small pool of donor organs and the ever-increasing demand for organs. In reduced size liver transplantations, the left lateral segments and left lobe grafts are used for pediatric recipients. In split liver transplantation, the left graft is used for a pediatric patient and the right graft is placed into an adult recipient. The use of a single donor for two recipients has clear advantages, and some centers have shown improvement in outcomes with this technique. Long-term prevention of graft rejection is an important goal of liver transplantation and aside from refinement of pre-existing drugs there are several new drugs with specific

mechanisms of action under investigation. Basiliximab, a chimeric monoclonal antibody, has shown favorable outcomes, and may potentially reduce the need for maintenance immunosuppressants following transplantation (95). Gene therapy may soon open unexpected possibilities of immediate and long-term survival of the transplanted organ.

Continued evaluation and development of support technologies such as the biological and nonbiological liver support systems will allow more patients to survive long enough for spontaneous recovery of liver function or successful hepatic transplantation. Improving the supply and distribution of donor livers for patients with FHF is another area requiring ongoing emphasis.

SUMMARY

FHF is a life-threatening condition that requires prompt diagnosis and rapid initiation of therapy to avoid deterioration in liver function, particularly in cases of acetaminophen toxicity. FHF patients require complex, coordinated critical care which is best provided in specialized centers especially for those patients who require liver transplantation.

Aggressive treatment of hepatic encephalopathy with control of ICP and management of cerebral perfusion is crucial in severe cases. This is accomplished in concert with adequate hemodynamic resuscitation and respiratory support. Six areas in which treatment advances have led to improved outcomes over the last 10 years include: awareness of ICP considerations, airway protection, infection standards, metabolic control (aggressive pharmacologic treatment of hypoglycemia), maintenance of MAP (avoidance of hypo- and hypertension), and institution of moderate hypothermia. More recently, additional measures have been recognized as important for improving outcomes in all critically ill patients: use of high-intensity physician staffing, small tidal volume mechanical ventilation, use of low-dose corticosteroids, monitoring activated protein C, "tight" glucose control, and low-dose vasopressin. By using these measures in liver disease, improvements can be made to overall patient care (96).

Although early recognition and aggressive medical management may improve outcomes in subsets of FHF patients, liver transplantation has significantly improved the survival odds in these patients. Following investigation of etiology and careful consideration of prognostic indicators, all patients with FHF should be evaluated for transplant suitability although only 30% get transplanted.

KEY POINTS

- A rapid diagnosis and identification of the etiologic agent increases the likelihood that specific therapy will be beneficial in the treatment of FHF.
- Accurate assessment of severity and prognosis in FHF is particularly important for identifying those patients requiring liver transplantation.
- Hepatic encephalopathy is a defining feature of fulminant liver failure.
- Because of the potential for complications, ICP monitoring remains controversial in managing patients with stage III and IV encephalopathies.
- The most important aspect of treatment for encephalopathy in FHF is control or elimination of factors known to increase ICP and cerebral edema.
- Hypothermia has emerged as an integral supportive maneuver in the care of FHF patients.
- Circulatory abnormalities in liver failure include a decreased effective intravascular volume, vasodilation, and a hyperdynamic circulation.
- Hemodynamic management in ALF is aimed at providing adequate cerebral perfusion in the setting of intracranial hypertension, avoiding hemodynamically mediated deterioration in hepatic function, and preventing multiple organ failure.
- Maintaining intravascular volume and therefore cardiac preload is essential to preserve cardiac output and oxygen delivery.
- Hypotension not responding to fluid therapy should be treated with vasoactive drug infusion.
- Gas exchange abnormalities in FHF result from transpulmonary shunting, and in some cases aspiration pneumonia, atelectasis, acute lung injury, or hepatopulmonary syndrome.
- Correction of coagulation and platelet abnormalities is necessary in bleeding patients and those undergoing invasive procedures such as ICP monitor placement or surgery.
- Potentially reversible hepatorenal syndrome occurs in a significant proportion of FHF patients with renal dysfunction.
- Patients with ALF develop multiple metabolic and electrolyte abnormalities including hypoglycemia, hypokalemia, hypomagnesemia, hypophosphatemia, and metabolic acidosis.
- Sudden massive blood loss can occur intraoperatively and this in conjunction with baseline hyperfibrinolysis, coagulation factor deficiencies, and thrombocytopenia

results in the need for massive blood and blood product transfusions that have potentially severe consequences.
- Early postoperative hemorrhage due to anastomotic leaks or laceration of the liver surface or coagulopathy results in reoperation in about 10% of transplanted patients.

REFERENCES

1. Trey C, Lipworth L, Chalmers TC, et al. Fulminant hepatic failure: presumable contribution to halothane. N Engl J Med 1968; 279:798–801.
2. Trey C, Davison CS. The management of fulminant hepatic failure. In: Popper H, Shaffner F, eds. Progress in Liver Disease. New York: Grune and Stratton, 1970:282.
3. Belle SH, Beringer KC, Detre KM. An update on liver transplantation in the United States: recipient characteristics and outcome. In: Teraski PI, Cecka JM, eds. Clinical Transplants. Los Angeles: UCLA Tissue Typing Laboratory, 1995:19.
4. Ostapowicz G, Lee WM. Acute hepatic failure: a Western perspective. J Gastroenterol Hepatol 2000; 15(5):480–488.
5. Schiodt FV, Atillasoy E, Shakil AO, et al. Etiology and outcome for 295 patients with acute liver failure in the United States. Liver Transpl Surg 1999; 5(1):29–34.
6. Seef LB, Cuccherini BA, Zimmerman HJ, et al. Acetaminophen toxicity in alcoholics: a therapeutic misadventure. Ann Intern Med 1986; 104(3):399–404.
7. Murphy R, Swartz R, Watkins PB. Severe acetaminophen toxicity in a patient receiving isoniazid. Ann Intern Med 1991; 114(3):253.
8. Bernau J, Rueff B, Benhamou JP. Fulminant and subfulminant liver failure: definitions and causes. Semin Liver Dis 1986; 6(2):97–106.
9. O'Grady JG, Schalm SW, Williams R. Acute liver failure: redefining the syndromes. Lancet 1993; 342(8884): 1421–1422.
10. O'Grady JG, Alexander GJ, Hayllar KM, Williams R. Early indicators of prognosis in fulminant hepatic failure. Gastroenterology 1989; 97(2):439–445.
11. Adams RD, Foley JM. The neurological disorders associated with liver disease. Proc Assoc Res Nerv Ment Dis 1952; 32:198–237.
12. Lockwood AH, McDonald JM, Reiman RE, et al. The dynamics of ammonia metabolism in man: effects of liver disease and hyperammonemia. J Clin Invest 1979; 63(3):449–460.
13. Conn HO, Lieberthal MM. The Hepatic Coma Syndromes and Lactulose. Baltimore, MD: Williams and Wilkins, 1978.
14. Pappas SC, Ferenci P, Schafer DF, et al. Visual evoked potentials in a rabbit model of hepatic encephalopathy II. Comparison of hyperammonemic encephalopathy, postictal coma and coma induced by synergistic neurotoxins. Gastroenterology 1984; 86(3):546–551.
15. Ha JH, Basile AS. Modulation of ligand binding to components of the GABAA receptor complex by ammonia: implications for the pathogenesis of hyperammonemic syndromes. Brain Res 1996; 720(1–2):35–44.
16. Clemmesen JO, Larsen FS, Knondrup J, et al. Cerebral herniation in patients with acute liver failure is correlated with arterial ammonia concentration. Hepatology 1999; 29:646–648.
17. Jones EA. Pathophysiology of liver disease. Pathogenesis of hepatic encephalopathy. Clin Liver Dis 2000; 4(2):467–485.
18. Basile AS, Jones EA. Ammonia and GABA-ergic neurotransmission: interrelated factors in the pathogenesis of hepatic encephalopathy. Hepatology 1997; 25(6)1303–1305.
19. Basile AS, Hughes RD, Harrison PM, et al. Elevated brain concentrations of 1,4 benzodiazepines in fulminant hepatic failure. N Engl J Med 1991; 325(7):509–511.

20. Bansky G, Meier PJ, Riederer E, et al. Effects of the benzo-diazepine receptor antagonist flumazenil in hepatic encephalopathy in humans. Gastroenterology 1989; 97(3):744–750.

21. Cordoba J, Blei AT. Brain edema and hepatic encephalopathy. Semin Liver Dis 1996; 16(3):271–280.

22. Gazzard BG, Portmann B, Murray-Lyon IM, Williams R. Causes of death in fulminant hepatic failure and relationship to quantitative histological assessment of parenchymal damage. Q J Med 1975; 44(176):615–626.

23. Munoz SJ, Robinson M, Northrup B, et al. Elevated intracranial pressure and computed tomography of the brain in fulminant hepatocellular failure. Hepatology 1991; 13(2):209–212.

24. Blei AT, Olaffson S, Webster S, Levy R. Complications of intracranial pressure monitoring in fulminant hepatic failure. Lancet 1993; 341(8838):157–158.

25. Wendon JA, Harrison PM, Keays R, Williams R. Cerebral blood flow and metabolism in fulminant liver failure. Hepatology 1994; 19(6):1407–1413.

26. Larsen FS, Strauss G, Knudsen GM, et al. Cerebral perfusion, cardiac output and arterial pressure in patients with fulminant hepatic failure. Crit Care Med 2000; 28(4):996–1000.

27. Aggarwal S, Kramer D, Yonas H, et al. Cerebral hemodynamic and metabolic changes in fulminant hepatic failure: a retrospective study. Hepatology 1994; 19(1):80–87.

28. Sidi A, Mahla ME. Noninvasive monitoring of cerebral perfusion by transcranial Doppler during fulminant hepatic failure and liver transplantation. Anesth Analg 1995; 80(1):194–200.

29. Ellis AJ, Wendon JA, Williams R. Subclinical seizure activity and prophylactic phenytoin infusion in acute liver failure: a controlled clinical trial. Hepatology 2000; 32(3):536–541.

30. Lidofsky SD, Bass NM, Prager MC, et al. Intracranial pressure monitoring and liver transplantation for fulminant hepatic failure. Hepatology 1992; 16(1):1–7.

31. Shakil AO, Mazariegos GV, Kramer DL. Fulminant hepatic failure. Surg Clin North Am 1999; 79(1):77–108.

32. Munoz SJ. Difficult management problems in fulminant hepatic failure. Semin Liver Dis 1993; 13(4):395–413.

33. Canalese J, Gimson AE, Davis, et al. Controlled trial of dexamethasone and mannitol for the cerebral edema of fulminant hepatic failure. Gut 1982; 23(7):625–629.

34. Jalan R, Rose C. Hypothermia in acute liver failure. Metab Brain Dis 2004; 19(3–4):215–221.

35. Roberts DR, Manas D. Induced hypothermia in the management of cerebral oedema secondary to fulminant liver failure. Clin Transplant 1999; 13(6):545–547.

36. Larsen FS, Gottstein J, Blei AT. Cerebral hyperemia and nitric oxide synthase in rats with ammonia-induced brain edema. J Hepatol 2001; 34:548–554.

37. Ferenci P, Grimm G. Benzodiazepine antagonist in the treatment of human hepatic encephalopathy. Adv Exp Med Biol 1990; 272:255–265.

38. Walsh TS, Hopton P, Philips BJ, et al. The effect of N-acetylcysteine on oxygen transport and uptake in patients with fulminant hepatic failure. Hepatology 1998; 27(5):1332–1340.

39. Weston MJ, Talbot IC, Horoworth PJ, et al. Frequency of arrhythmias and other cardiac abnormalities in fulminant hepatic failure. Br Heart J 1976; 38(11):1179–1188.

40. Kowalski HJ, Abelmann WH. The cardiac output at rest in Laennec's cirrhosis. J Clin Invest 1953; 32:1025–1033.

41. Baudouin SV, Howdle P, O'Grady JG, Webster NR. Acute lung injury in fulminant hepatic failure following paracetamol poisoning. Thorax 1995; 50(4):399–402.

42. Weston MJ, Langley PG, Williams R. Proceedings: defective platelet function with deficiency of sticky platelets in fulminant hepatic failure. Gut 1975; 16(5):405–408.

43. Pernambuco JR, Langley PG, Hughes RD, et al. Activation of the fibrinolytic system in patients with fulminant liver failure. Hepatology 1993; 18(6):1350–1356.

44. O'Grady JG, Gimson AES, O'Brien CJ, et al. Controlled trials of charcoal hemoperfusion and prognostic factors in fulminant hepatic failure. Gastroenterology 1988; 94:1186–1192.

45. O'Grady JG, Gimson AES, O'Brien CJ, et al. Cirrhosis: a comparison between incidence, types and prognosis. Gut 1981; 22:585–591.

46. Ring-Larsen H, Palazzo U. Renal failure in fulminant hepatic failure and terminal cirrhosis: a comparison between incidence, types and prognosis. Gut 1981; 22:585–591.

47. Harrison PM, Keays R, Bray GP, et al. Improved outcome of paracetamol-induced fulminant hepatic failure by late administration of acetylcysteine. Lancet 1990; 335(8705): 1572–1573.

48. Davenport A, Will EJ, Davison AM, et al. Early changes in intracranial pressure during haemofiltration treatment in patients with grade 4 hepatic encephalopathy and acute oliguric renal failure. Nephron 1989; 53(2):142–146.

49. Murphy ND, Kodakat SK, Wendon JA, et al. Liver and intestinal lactate metabolism in patients with acute hepatic failure undergoing liver transplantation. Crit Care Med 2001; 29(11):2111–2118.

50. Bihari D, Gimson AE, Lindridge J, Williams R. Lactic acidosis in fulminant hepatic failure. Some aspects of pathogenesis and prognosis. J Hepatol 1985; 1(4):405–416.

51. Rolando N, Philpott-Howard J, Williams R. Bacterial and fungal infection in acute liver failure. Semin Liver Dis 1996; 16(4):389–402.

52. Rolando N, Harvey F, Brahm J, et al. Prospective study of bacterial infection in acute liver failure: an analysis of fifty patients. Hepatology 1990; 11(1):49–53.

53. Jollow DJ, Mitchell JR, Potter WZ, et al. Acetaminophen-induced hepatic necrosis. II. Role of covalent binding in vivo. J Pharmacol Exp Ther 1973; 187(1):195–202.

54. Smilkstein MJ, Knapp GL, Kulig KW, Rumack BH. Efficacy of oral N-acetylcysteine in the treatment of acetaminophen overdose: analysis of the national multicenter study. N Engl J Med 1988; 319(24):1557–1562.

55. Pinna AD, Rakela J, Demetris AJ, Fung JJ. Five cases of fulminant hepatitis due to herpes simplex virus in adults. Dig Dis Sci 2002; 47(4):750–754.

56. Keefee EB, Dieterich DT, Han S.HB, et al. A treatment algorithm for the management of chronic hepatitis B virus infection in the United States. Clin Gastroenterol Hepatol 2004; 2:87–106.

57. Lok AS, Lai CL, Leung N, et al. Long-term safety of lamivudine treatment in patients with chronic hepatitis B. Gastroenterology 2003; 125(6):1714–1722.

58. Yu ML, Hou NJ, Dai, CY, et al. Successful treatment of fulminant hepatitis C by therapy with alpha interferon and ribavirin. Antimicrob Agents Chemother 2005; 49:3986–3987.

59. Diaz JH. Syndromic diagnosis and management of confirmed mushroom poisonings. Crit Care Med 2005; 33(2):427–436.

60. Hruby K, Csomos G, Fuhrmann M, Thaler H. Chemotherapy of amanita phalloides poisoning with intravenous silibinin. Hum Toxicol 1983; 2(2):183–195.

61. Enjalbert F, Rapior S, Nouguier-Soule J, et al. Treatment of amatoxin poisoning: 20-year retrospective analysis. J Toxicol Clin Toxicol 2002; 40:715–757.

62. Rozga J, Umehara Y, Trofimenko A, et al. A novel plasma filtration therapy for hepatic failure: preclinical trials. Ther Apher Dial 2006; 10(2):138.

63. Covic A, Goldsmith DJA, Gusbeth-Tatomir P, et al. Successful use of molecular absorbent regenerating system (MARS) dialysis for the treatment of fulminant hepatic failure in children accidentally poisoned by toxic mushroom ingestion. Liver Int 2003; 23(s3):21–27.

64. Johnson PJ, McFarlane IG, Williams R. Azathioprine for long-term maintenance of remission in autoimmune hepatitis. N Engl J Med 1995; 333:958–963.

65. Krawitt EL. Autoimmune hepatitis. N Engl J Med 2006; 354(1):54–66.

66. Freeman JG, Matthewson K, Record CO. Plasmapheresis in acute liver failure. Int J Artif Organs 1986; 9(6):433–438.

67. Singer AL, Olthoff KM, Kim H, et al. Role of plasmapheresis in the management of acute hepatic failure in children. Ann Surg 2001; 234(3):418–424.

68. Stange J, Hassanein TI, Mehta R, et al. The molecular adsorbents recycling system as a liver support system based on albumin dialysis: a summary of preclinical investigations, prospective, randomized controlled clinical trial and clinical experience from 19 centers. Artif Organs 2002; 26(2):103–110.

69. Ellis AJ, Hughes RD, Wendon JA, et al. Pilot-controlled trial of the extracorporeal liver assisted device in acute liver failure. Hepatology 1996; 24(6):1446–1451.

70. Stockmann HB, Hiemstra CA, Marquet RL, et al. Extracorporeal perfusion for the treatment of acute liver failure. Ann Surg 2000; 231(4):460–470.

71. Strom SC, Fischer RA, Thompson MT, et al. Hepatocyte transplantation as a bridge to orthotopic liver transplantation in terminal liver failure. Transplantation 1997; 63(4):559–569.

72. Kanai N, Platt JL. Xenotransplantation of the liver. Clin Liver Dis 2000; 4(3):731–746.

73. Jain AJ, Reyes J, Kashyap R, et al. Long-term survival after liver transplantation in 4000 consecutive patients at a single center. Ann Surg 2000; 232(4):490–500.

74. Azoulay D, Samuel D, Ichai P, et al. Auxillary partial orthotopic versus standard orthotopic whole liver transplantation for acute liver failure: a reappraisal from a single center by case-control study. Ann Surg 2001; 234(6):723–731.

75. Belle SH, Detre KM. Report from the PITT-UNOS liver transplant registry. Transplant Proc 1993; 25(1):1137–1142.

76. Bernal W, Wendon J. Liver transplantation in adults with acute liver failure. J Hepatol 2004; 40:192–197.

77. CDC and the National Center for Injury Prevention and Control. Web based injury statistics query and reporting system. Available at http://www.cdc.gov/ncipc/wisqars/.

78. Lee W. Acute liver failure in the United States. Semin Liver Dis 2003; 23:217–226.

79. Fujiwara K, Mochida S. Indications and criteria for liver transplantation for fulminant hepatic failure. J Gastroenterol 2002; 37:74–77.

80. Anand AC, Nightingale P, Neuberger P. Early indicators of prognosis in fulminant hepatic failure: an assessment of King's criteria. J Hepatol 1997; 26:62–68.

81. Ostapowicz G, Fontana RJ, Schiodt FV, et al. Results of a prospective study of acute liver failure at 17 tertiary care centers in the United States. Ann Intern Med 2002; 137:947–954.

82. Bailey B, Amre DK, Gaudreault P. Fulminant hepatic failure secondary to acetaminophen poisoning: a systematic review and meta analysis of prognostic criteria determining the need for liver transplantation. Crit Care Med 2003; 31:299–305.

83. Kamath PS, Wiesner RH, Malinchoc M, et al. A model to predict survival in patients with end stage liver disease. Hepatology 2001; 33:464–470.

84. Wiesner RH. MECD/PECD and the allocation of decreased donor livers for status 1 recipients with acute fulminant hepatic failure, primary nonfunction, hepatic artery thrombosis, and acute Wilson's disease. Liver Transpl 2004; 10(suppl 2): 517–522.

85. Amin M, Wolf M, Tenbrook J, et al. Expanded criteria donor grafts for deceased donor liver transplantation under the MELD system: a decision analysis. Liver Transp 2004; 10(12): 1468–1475.

86. Lodge JP, Jonas S, Jones RM, et al. rFVIIa OLT Study Group. Efficacy and safety of repeated perioperative doses of recombinant factor VIIa in liver transplantation. Liver Transpl 2005; 11(8):973–979.

87. Lodge JP, Jonas S, Oussoultzoglou E. Recombinant coagulation factor VIIa in major liver resection: a randomized, placebo-controlled, double-blind clinical trial. Anesthesiology 2005; 102(2):269–275.

88. Kalicinski P, Markiewicz M, Kaminski A, et al. Single pretransplant bolus of recombinant activated factor VII ameliorates influence of risk factors for blood loss during orthotopic liver transplantation. Pediatr Transpl 2005; 9(3):299–304.

89. Gillies BS. Thromboelastography and liver transplantation. Rev Semin Thromb Hemost 1995; 21(4):45–49.

90. Harding SA, Mallett SV, Peachey TD, Cox DJ. Use of heparinase modified thromboelastography in liver transplantation. Br J Anaesth 1997; 78(2):175–179.

91. Xia VW, Steadman RH. Antifibrinolytics in orthotopic liver transplantation: current status and controversies. Liver Transpl 2005; 11(1):10–18.

92. Bulkley GB. Reactive oxygen metabolites and reperfusion injury: aberrant triggering of reticuloendothelial function. Lancet 1994; 344(8927):934–936.

93. Chui AK, Shi L, Tanaka K, et al. Post reperfusion syndrome in orthotopic liver transplantation. Transpl Proc 2000; 32(7):2116–2117.

94. OPTN. Liver only National Data 1989–2002: Organ procurement and Transplantation Network (Accessed June 2003).

95. Marino IR, Doria C, Scott VL, et al. Efficacy and safety of basiliximab with a tacrolimus-based regimen in liver transplant recipients. Transplantation 2004; 78(6):886–891.

96. Barshes NR, Lee TC, Balkrishnan R, et al. Risk stratification of adult patients undergoing orthotopic liver transplantation for fulminant hepatic failure. Transplantation 2006; 81(2):195–201.

37

The Cirrhotic Patient

Marie L. Borum, Christopher R. Entwisle, and Todd N. Witte

Division of Gastroenterology and Liver Diseases, Department of Medicine, George Washington University, Washington, D.C., U.S.A.

INTRODUCTION

Cirrhosis is the irreversible, final common pathway of many chronic progressive liver diseases. The incidence of cirrhosis in Western countries is approximately 15 to 25 per 100,000 people (1). It is the 10th leading cause of all mortality, and in individuals aged 45 to 64 years it is the fifth leading cause of death. Finally, cirrhosis is implicated in approximately 30,000 deaths each year in the United States alone (2,3).

Although patients with chronic liver diseases are often managed in the outpatient setting with occasional acute hospitalizations, it is not uncommon for the cirrhotic patient to be hospitalized in the surgical intensive care unit (SICU). Life-threatening conditions such as variceal hemorrhage, hepatic encephalopathy, or hepatorenal syndrome (HRS) frequently necessitate SICU management. If not involved earlier, critical care physicians may become involved with a cirrhotic patient postoperatively. Additionally, such physicians will manage a cirrhotic patient who has been involved in a trauma. In general, individuals with chronic liver disease and cirrhosis who require admission to an intensive care unit often have poor outcomes, as can be predicted by established scoring systems such as Child–Pugh or acute physiology, age, and chronic health evaluation (APACHE) (4,5).

In an era of rapidly expanding medical knowledge and rising healthcare costs, the critical care physician is expected to care effectively and efficiently for the cirrhotic patient. This chapter provides an overview of the pathophysiology, underlying conditions, presentation, complications, and management critical to caring for the critically ill cirrhotic patient.

PATHOPHYSIOLOGY
Basic Science

Cirrhosis is a fibrosis of the liver parenchyma that occurs as a response to liver injury from a variety of agents and results in a broad range of clinical manifestations. It is classified histologically as either macronodular (>3 mm nodules) or micronodular (<3 mm nodules) (6).

The normal liver has an extracellular matrix consisting of collagens, glycoproteins, and proteoglycans. This matrix is critical to the functions of the liver. The development of fibrosis in chronic liver injury causes this matrix to transform from a low-density matrix to a high-density matrix (Fig. 1). There are several factors involved in this process. During injury, there is a downregulation of matrix metalloproteinase-1 and upregulation of gelatinase A and gelatinase B, resulting in breakdown of basement membrane collagen and an amassing of interstitial collagens. As the hepatic environment changes, stellate cells become activated.

Stellate cells are found in the subendothelial space of Disse and are the principal storage site for retinoids. Stellate cells can also migrate to areas of injury through several potential chemoattractants including platelet-derived growth factor (PDGF) and monocyte chemotactic peptide-1 (7). Upon activation, the stellate cell transitions into a proliferative, fibrogenic, and contractile myofibroblast (8). This may be initiated by paracrine stimuli from surrounding cells. Endothelial cells may convert latent transforming growth factor-β1 (TGF-β1) to a profibrogenic form through the activation of plasmin (Table 1) (9). Hepatocytes produce lipid peroxides that may also promote activation. Kupffer cells can stimulate matrix synthesis, cell proliferation, and release of retinoids by stellate cells (10). Platelets produce and release several important mediators including PDGF, TGF-β1, and epidermal growth factor. In addition, during early activation there is an upregulation of the NF-kappa-gene expression, which can lead to the activation of a number of genes, including the transcription factor AP-1, c-Jun kinase, and matrix metalloproteinase-2 (11,12).

The hepatic stellate cells can progress into a perpetuation stage (13). This may result from an upregulation of many mitogenic factors and their receptors. In addition, PDGF, a potent mitogen, and its receptors are upregulated during injury. Other mitogens that may be involved include endothelin-1, thrombin, and fibroblast growth factor (11,12).

The contraction of hepatic stellate cells is likely the mechanism for the development of portal hypertension by impedance of portal blood flow. Endothelin-1 appears to be an important contractile stimulus to stellate cells (14). Nitric oxide (NO) is a physiologic antagonist to endothelin-1 and may be less active in portal hypertension (15,16). Alpha smooth muscle actin levels have also been found to be increased during stellate cell activation and may participate in their contractility.

⚲ **The fibrotic tissue in cirrhosis consists of extracellular matrix molecules, collagen types I and III, sulfated proteoglycans, and glycoproteins.** ⚲ TGF-β1 is the most potent fibrogenic factor in the liver and is upregulated during injury (17).

Etiologies

There are a large number of potential causes of cirrhosis (Table 2). Major categories include toxins (such as alcohol), viral hepatitis, metabolic disorders, autoimmune etiologies, nonalcoholic steatohepatitis (NASH), and miscellaneous

Normal   Fibrotic

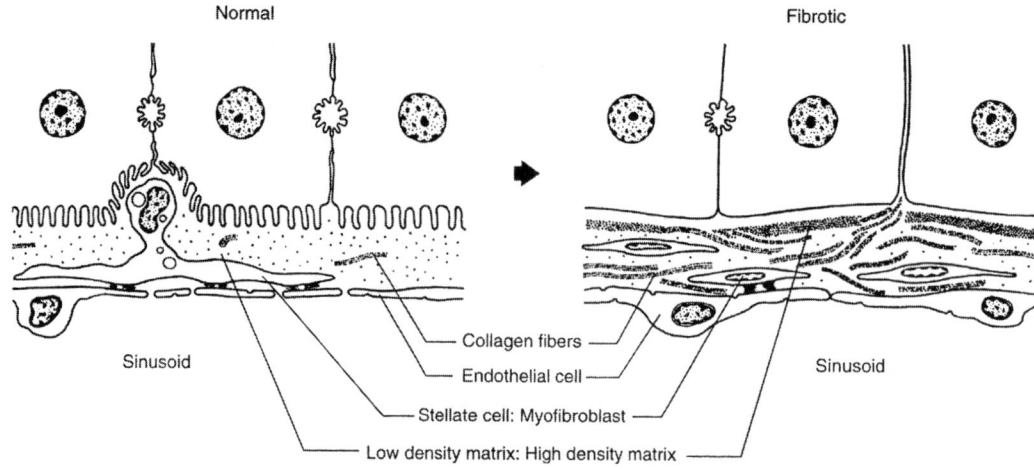

Sinusoid   Sinusoid

—— Collagen fibers ——
—— Endothelial cell ——
—— Stellate cell: Myofibroblast ——
—— Low density matrix: High density matrix ——

Figure 1 Fibrotic changes occurring in the space of Disse in cirrhosis. The figure shows the morphologic changes associated with stellate cell activation and collagenization of the space of Disse, namely loss of endothelial fenestrae and flattening of the microvillus border of the hepatocyte. *Source:* From Ref. 174.

causes, the common thread being injury to hepatocytes followed by scarring of residual tissue.

Fibrosis is a normal component of repair following injury. It provides a structural scaffold and temporary support during repair, and also interacts with other cells to signal remodeling and other events involved in the healing process. When injury is limited in duration, the fibrotic scaffolding is dismantled by matrix proteinases during final stages of healing at six to seven weeks (Fig. 2). However, in the setting of multiple recurrent injuries, or chronic inflammation, pathologic fibrosis is propagated, and residual fibrous remains when the next cycle of injury occurs. Ultimately fibrotic processes become dominant and too extensive for suitable remodeling, and cirrhosis results. A discussion of the major causes of cirrhosis is offered.

Alcohol-Induced Cirrhosis

Consumption of ethanolic [exposed to alcohol (ETOH)] alcohol can lead to a variety of hepatic changes, ranging from fatty liver to cirrhosis. Steatosis or fatty liver can develop after even a single ETOH binge and is likely to progress with continued alcohol use (18). Accumulation of membrane-bound fat droplets, proliferation of smooth endoplasmic reticulum, and gradual distortion of mitochondria can occur (19). Increased lipolysis and reduced oxidation

of hepatic fatty acids contribute to its development (20). Alcoholic hepatitis may develop with continued alcohol ingestion. Patients may present with fever, hepatomegaly, jaundice, and anorexia. The hallmarks of this disease include liver cell necrosis, the presence of Mallory bodies and neutrophils, and a perivenular distribution of inflammation (21). In alcoholic cirrhosis, perivenular inflammation becomes fibrosis and can progress to panlobular cirrhosis (6).

Table 2 Causes of Cirrhosis

Cause	Examples
Drugs	Alcohol
	Amiodarone
	Isoniazid
	Methyldopa methotrexate
	Vitamin A
Infection	Hepatitis B
	Hepatitis C
	Schistosomiasis
	Syphilis
Biliary obstruction	Cholangiocarcinoma
	Cystic fibrosis
	Pancreatitis (chronic)
	Pancreatic carcinoma
	Primary biliary cirrhosis
	Sclerosing cholangitis
	Strictures
Cardiovascular	Budd–Chiari syndrome
	Right heart failure (chronic)
	Veno-occlusive disease
Metabolic	Alpha-1-antitrypsin
	E. protoporphyria
	Hemochromatosis
	Wilson's disease
Miscellaneous	Sarcoidosis
	Hereditary hemorrhagic telangiectasia
	Cryptogenic
	Nonalcoholic steatohepatitis
	Autoimmune hepatitis

Table 1 Summary of Cirrhosis Pathophysiology

The stellate cell is the major cell involved in the process of liver fibrosis. It becomes a proliferative, fibrogenic, and contractile myofibroblast

TGF-β1 is the most potent fibrogenic factor in the liver

Example of alcohol induced cirrhosis

    Alcohol → fatty liver → alcoholic hepatitis → alcoholic cirrhosis

Hallmarks of alcoholic cirrhosis

    Liver cell necrosis

    Presence of Mallory bodies and neutrophils

    Perivenular distribution of inflammation

Abbreviation: TGF-β1, transforming growth factor-β1.

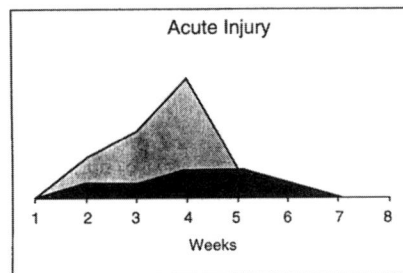
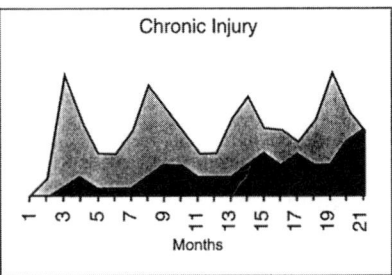

Figure 2 Schematic representation of inflammation (*lighter area*) and fibrosis (*darker area*) in acute or chronic liver injury. When inflammation is limited in time (acute injury), fibrosis resolves completely after approximately seven weeks. When inflammation is chronic with recurrent exacerbations, the level of fibrosis varies but rises over time. Examples of chronic exposure causing cirrhosis include heavy alcohol use with periods of heavy binges, or recurrent hepatitis from chronic active hepatitis B. *Source*: From Ref. 175.

There are several theories related to the pathogenesis of alcohol-mediated liver injury. The metabolism of ethanol acetaldehyde increases lobular oxygen consumption which may cause hypoxia and cell damage in the pericentral zones. The neutrophils present during alcohol-induced fibrosis may cause hepatocyte injury via cytokines and proteases. Additionally, acetaldehyde–protein adducts may serve as neoantigens causing an autoimmune reaction against hepatocytes. Alternative pathways for ethanol metabolism may also generate free radicals (6).

Infections

A number of infectious agents have been reported as potential etiologies for the development of cirrhosis. The most important infectious causes of cirrhosis in the United States include the hepatotropic viruses, hepatitis B and C. Less common, but important other viral etiologies of hepatitis include cytomegalovirus, Epstein-Barr, herpesvirus-6, and varicella zoster. Additionally, tertiary *Syphilis* and *Schistosoma japonicum* have been reported to cause hepatic fibrosis and cirrhosis; however, these infectious agents are infrequent causes of cirrhosis in the United States.

Chronic infections with both the hepatitis B and C viruses can lead to liver cirrhosis. Approximately 85% of patients infected with hepatitis C will develop a chronic infection, with up to 50% of these developing cirrhosis (22–24). ☞ **The development of cirrhosis is most often silent until complications of significant hepatic dysfunction occurs (22).** ☞ Several host factors are important determinants of disease progression in hepatitis C virus (HCV)-infected individuals. Coinfected HIV patients may progress more rapidly (25,26). Infection via blood transfusion has been reported to increase the risk of disease progression (27,28). Infection after the age of 40 years may be associated with a more rapid course (29,30). Coinfection of hepatitis C with hepatitis B is likely to accelerate the progression. Alcohol consumption has also been reported to promote the progression of chronic hepatitis C infection and should be avoided in all patients with this infection (29).

Chronic hepatitis B virus infection results in cirrhosis less commonly than hepatitis C in the United States. It is estimated to occur in approximately 15% to 40% of individuals infected with hepatitis B. The rate of progression to cirrhosis is determined by the replicative activity of the virus and whether there is a superinfection with another hepatotropic virus, such as hepatitis delta virus or hepatitis C (31).

Drug-Induced

Liver damage from pharmacologic agents accounts for about 2% to 5% of patients requiring hospitalization for jaundice and 10% of cases of hepatitis in all adults (32). Drug-induced injury can result in severe necrosis with the development of cirrhosis. Some agents are intrinsic hepatotoxins and may result in both aminotransferase elevations up to 500 times normal. Examples are carbon tetrachloride, chloroform, tannic acid, and troglitazone, which have been voluntarily removed from the market (33). Other drugs show a dose-related toxicity. These include acetaminophen, ethanol, methotrexate, intravenous tetracycline, and azathioprine (34). In addition, a hypersensitivity reaction may occur with many pharmacologic agents, resulting in eosinophilic or granulomatous inflammation with hepatocyte necrosis and cholestasis. These may include phenytoin, amoxicillin-clavulanate, sulfonamides, halothane, and dapsone (35). Liver injury may also be secondary to abnormal drug metabolism in which toxic metabolites may accumulate and lead to cellular necrosis. Agents such as ketoconazole, diclofenac, valproate, propylthiouracil, isoniazid, and amiodarone may cause hepatic toxicity through abnormal drug metabolism (33,36).

Hereditary (Inborn) Errors of Metabolism

There are multiple metabolic causes of liver disease. Hereditary enzymatic abnormalities can lead to accumulation of toxic substances resulting in liver damage, injury, and cirrhosis. Hemochromatosis, Wilson's disease, and alpha-1-antitrypsin (AAT) deficiency are the most often cited metabolic abnormalities that cause cirrhosis. *Erythropoietic protoporphyria* has also been reported as an etiology of cirrhosis. Other causes of cirrhosis in pediatric patients include galactosemia, hereditary fructose intolerance, glycogen storage disease type IV, and tyrosinosis.

Hereditary Hemochromatosis

Hereditary hemochromatosis (HHC) leads to an abnormal accumulation of iron in parenchymal organs, including the liver, heart, and pancreas. It is the most common genetic disorder among caucasians and is inherited as an autosomal-recessive trait on chromosome 6. Although the exact pathophysiology is unknown, the mutation may cause abnormal cell interaction with β2-microglobulin resulting in increased iron absorption with accumulation in the liver. Classically, patients present in the third and fourth decades with hepatomegaly, skin pigmentation, arthritis, and weakness. A fasting serum transferrin saturation greater than 60% in men or 50% in women is highly specific for HHC. Serum ferritin is often elevated. Liver biopsy with a measurement of hepatic iron concentration is the most sensitive diagnostic test. Individuals with HHC are at ~200-fold increased risk for developing hepatocellular carcinoma. Early diagnosis is essential to prevent progression to cirrhosis in the patient with hemochromatosis. Therapeutic phlebotomy remains the mainstay of therapy. Iron chelation, with agents such as deferoxamine, may be useful in anemic patients. Newer oral agents, such as deferasirox, are also being investigated (37). Liver transplantation is indicated for individuals who progress to end-stage liver disease (38).

Wilson's Disease

Wilson's disease is an autosomal-recessive disorder of reduced biliary excretion which results in copper accumulation. It is estimated to occur worldwide in 30 people per million population (39). Copper is normally incorporated into copper-containing enzymes, including ceruloplasmin, in the liver. Excess copper is normally excreted in the bile. The defective gene product is a P-type ATPase which is referred to as Wilson's disease. This is normally a copper transporter and is necessary for copper incorporation into ceruloplasmin and excretion into bile. In Wilson's disease, ceruloplasmin levels and copper bile concentrations are reduced. Copper eventually appears in dense granules in lysosomes and leads to chronic hepatitis and fibrosis. Over time the liver is progressively damaged and eventually becomes cirrhotic. Liver disease is often the presenting manifestation, but neuropsychiatric disease may also be the presenting feature in up to 10% of cases. The type of the liver disease can be highly variable, ranging from only biochemical abnormalities to fulminant hepatic failure.

Fulminant hepatic failure, sometimes referred to as a Wilsonian crisis, has characteristic features which include Coombs-negative hemolytic anemia with bilirubinemia, coagulopathy, renal failure, low alkaline phosphatase (Alk phos), and elevated aminotransferases. A useful clue to this disease may be the ratio of Alk phos (IU/L) to total bilirubin (T-bili) (mg/dL) of less than 2 (40).

Measurement of hepatic tissue copper concentration will provide the diagnosis in most patients, however, this requires a biopsy. A low ceruloplasmin is supportive, but not specific. An elevated serum copper and 24-hour urine copper level may be helpful as a screening test. Kayser–Fleischer rings may support the diagnosis, but such ophthalmologic findings may be absent in 50% of patients (40). Copper chelators, such as penicillamine and trientine, are the mainstays of therapy and are more effective when combined with a low copper diet (41). Patients with fulminant hepatitic failure require urgent liver transplantation to survive.

Alpha-1-Antitrypsin

AAT deficiency is a homozygous disorder affecting multiple organ systems. In adults, the most common manifestation is asymptomatic cirrhosis. Although there are many different alleles in AAT, the M and Z alleles have been shown to confer a risk for the development of liver disease. From 10% to 15% of at-risk newborns develop hepatic disease (42). Although the exact mechanism is unclear, the pathogenesis is thought to be related to the accumulation of AAT molecules in the rough endoplasmic reticulum of hepatocytes (43).

Autoimmune Hepatitis

Autoimmune hepatitis is a chronic inflammation of the liver of unknown etiology. There is continued hepatocellular injury that can progress to necrosis, with fibrosis that may ultimately lead to cirrhosis and liver failure. It may present with a variety of clinical features, histologic findings, immunogenetic phenotypes, and circulating autoantibodies. It most often occurs in female adolescents and women, although the disease can occur in males. The classic characteristic laboratory feature is an elevation in antinuclear or antismooth muscle antibodies with elevated serum globulins, particularly gamma globulins (44). Immunosuppressant therapy with steroids and/or azathioprine is the mainstay of therapy.

Biliary Obstruction

Diseases that cause chronic biliary destruction can result in hepatocellular injury with fibrosis that can progress to cirrhosis. Primary biliary cirrhosis (PBC) and primary sclerosing cholangitis (PSC) are presumed immunomediated diseases can that result in significant hepatocellular injury. Other acquired disorders that produce chronic biliary obstruction can also result in cirrhosis.

Primary Biliary Cirrhosis

Primary biliary cirrhosis is an immune-mediated disorder that is characterized by a T-lymphocyte-mediated injury affecting the intralobular bile ducts (6). The presence of antimitochondrial antibodies is the hallmark of this disorder. The cause of this injury remains unknown, but most likely involves both genetic and environmental factors. As the biliary ducts are destroyed, impairment of biliary flow develops. This can result in portal and parenchymal inflammation, liver cell necrosis, scarring, and eventually to cirrhosis and liver failure (45). The mainstay of therapy includes ursodeoxycholic acid and liver transplantation.

Primary Sclerosing Cholangitis

PSC is a chronic cholestatic disease affecting the liver and bile ducts. Patients will often present with pruritus, steatorrhea, and symptoms of vitamin deficiencies. Antinuclear and anticytoplasmic antibodies with a perinuclear staining pattern (P-ANCA) occur in up to 80% of patients with PSC. There is a strong association with inflammatory bowel disease, particularly ulcerative colitis. The diagnosis can often be made by cholangiography that shows diffuse, multifocal strictures, and focal dilation of the bile ducts (46). At present there are no pharmacologic agents that have been conclusively proven to decrease the progression of the disease; however, high-dose ursodeoxycholic acid (20–30 mg/kg/day) is being further studied based on encouraging preliminary results (47,48).

Nonalcoholic Steatohepatitis (NASH)

With rising obesity rates in the United States and other industrialized countries, about 20% to 30% of adults have excess fat in the liver, called nonalcoholic fatty liver disease (NAFLD). At least 10% of these individuals meet histologic criteria for NASH (49). The prevalence of this disease may be markedly higher in select patients with the risk factors of severe obesity, diabetes mellitus, hyperlipidemia, and metabolic syndrome (50). By definition, patients do not drink significant amounts of alcohol. There is great variability as to what is considered significant intake, however, a level of two drinks per day has been suggested (49).

Although progression to cirrhosis is rare in mild NAFLD, excess fat accumulation in the liver may sensitize the liver to injury from other causes. This is summarized by the multihit hypothesis, in which insulin resistance is believed to be central to the first hit of hepatic steatosis (51). There is no conclusive therapy for NASH, although modification of risk factors, such as obesity, hyperlipidemia, and poor diabetic control are generally used. Lifestyle modification being a challenge, sustained liver injury leads to progressive fibrosis and cirrhosis in up to one third of patients with NASH (49).

The evolution of NAFLD to NASH and subsequently cirrhosis may be accompanied by a loss of the typical histologic features, which include hepatic steatosis with mixed lobular inflammation and hepatocellular ballooning (49,52,53). Thus, as much as 80% of cases of cryptogenic cirrhosis likely represent burned-out NASH (52,54–56).

PHYSICAL EXAM AND STUDIES

An assessment of the cirrhotic patient begins with obtaining a thorough history. The patient will frequently be able to provide information that can offer insight into the etiology of the liver disease. Details regarding comorbid medical conditions, medications, previous blood transfusions, alcohol and intravenous drug use, and toxin exposure may also assist in the differential diagnosis of possible etiologies. Family history can be important to assess for potential familial disorders, such as Wilson's disease, hemochromatosis, or autoimmune liver diseases. Important key points in the history are summarized in Table 3. A review of systems should seek symptoms of malignancy such as weight loss or anorexia.

There are several physical stigmata on the examination of the cirrhotic patient that may indicate the presence of liver disease. (Fig. 3) The patient's mental status may be altered due to advanced liver disease and hepatic encephalopathy. A flapping tremor of asterixis can be seen. Jaundice, including icterus, typically occurs when the total serum bilirubin is above 3 mg/dL. Clubbing can also occur with advanced liver disease. Purpura and bruising can be present in the cirrhotic patient with coagulopathy.

In men, cirrhosis results in hypogonadism with a decrease in serum testosterone and a relative increase in circulating estrogens. The clinical features of this feminization can be demonstrated by decreased muscle mass, testicular atrophy, gynecomastia, and reduced secondary sexual hair. Telangectasias, known as spider angiomas, may be seen on the upper body while erythema is seen on the thumbs, proximal phalanges, and palms.

Table 3 Important Historical Clues to Cirrhosis

Patient's understanding of the etiology
Comorbid medical conditions
Medications
Transfusion history
Use of alcohol
Use of intravenous drugs
Family history of liver disorders
Recent weight loss or anorexia

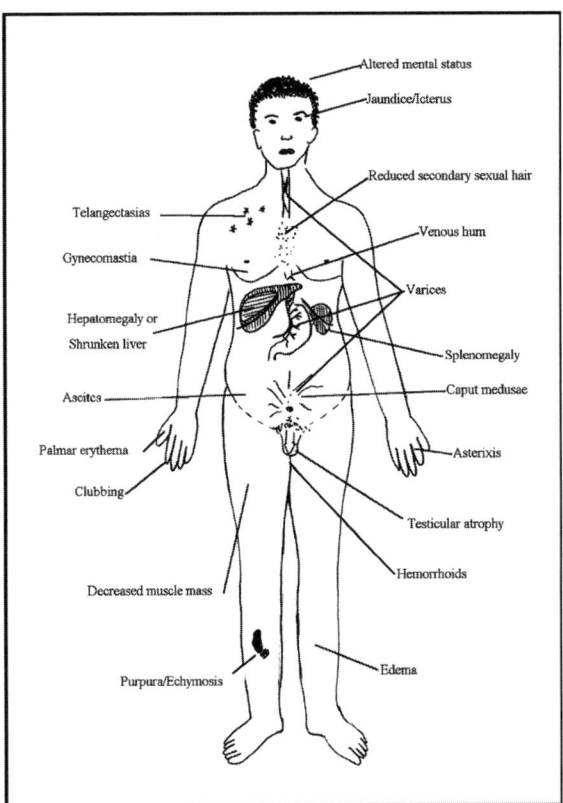

Figure 3 Physical stigmata found in cirrhosis. Every organ system is affected, and many of the stigmata are seen in the body habitus, and external surface of the patient. Others (e.g., varices) are seen within the gastrointestinal tract. *Source*: Drawing by Todd N. Witte.

Portal hypertension with resultant portosystemic shunting through umbilical and paraumbilical veins causes the classically distended abdominal wall veins, or "caput medusae," seen radiating outwards from the umbilicus. Less commonly, hemorrhoidal varices can be appreciated. Hypoalbuminemia will exacerbate any degree of peripheral edema, and when the serum albumin is low enough, edema develops de novo. The liver may be enlarged in early cirrhosis, but is more commonly shrunken in advanced disease. Auscultation over the liver, xiphoid process, or umbilicus may reveal a venous hum signifying portal hypertension. Splenomegaly may also occur in individuals with portal hypertension (57,58).

Laboratory abnormalities frequently seen in the routine investigation of the cirrhotic patient may include abnormal aspartate amino transferase (AST), alanine aminotransferase (ALT), Alk phos, and T-bili (Table 4). The ratio of AST to ALT can often be a clue to the underlying etiology of the disorder as an AST/ALT ratio greater than two is classically seen in acute alcoholic hepatitis. AST/ALT is usually less than one in patients with other etiologies of chronic hepatitis and cholestatic liver diseases, however the transaminases can return to near normal values in patients with cirrhosis. In this setting, the AST/ALT is often greater than 1 (59). Anemia, thrombocytopenia, elevated prothrombin time (PT), and an extended bleeding time are also not uncommon. The definitive diagnosis of cirrhosis is made by histologic exam of liver biopsy specimen.

Table 4 Laboratory Abnormalities Frequently Found in Cirrhosis

---

↑ AST
↑ ALT
AST/ALT > 2.0 = consistent with alcoholic hepatitis
↑ Alk phos
↑ T-bili
↓ hemoglobin
↓ platelets
↑ PT
↑ Bleeding time

Abbreviations: AST, aspartate amino transferase; ALT, alanine aminotransferase; Alk Phos, alkaline phosphatase; T-bili, total bilirubin; PT, prothrombin time.

ASCITES

Ascites, the accumulation of fluid in the peritoneal cavity, is the most common complication of cirrhosis (60). It can be complicated by spontaneous bacterial peritonitis (SBP), hyponatremia, HRS, and other fluid collections (e.g., pleural and pericardial effusions).

Pathophysiology

Portal hypertension is present in all patients with ascites. A portal pressure gradient greater than 12 mmHg is required for ascites to develop (61). There are three major theories regarding the pathogenesis of ascites formation. These theories are the underfill theory, the overflow theory, and the arterial vasodilation hypothesis. Although each theory may be relevant, the arterial vasodilation hypothesis has become the most accepted.

The underfill theory suggests that fluid is collected in the splanchnic vascular bed. The kidneys then act upon a perceived decrease in intravascular volume, resulting in sodium and water retention. The overflow theory proposes that the primary abnormality is in the kidneys. It is hypothesized that despite a normal intravascular volume, the kidneys retain sodium and water (62). The arterial vasodilation hypothesis is based upon hemodynamic findings in cirrhotic patients. Both the systemic vascular resistance (SVR) and mean arterial pressure (MAP) are decreased, whereas their cardiac output (Q̇) is increased (63). Vasodilation of the splanchnic circulation is likely responsible for these pressure changes (64). Several mechanisms of vasodilation have been proposed. Opening of portosystemic collaterals may contribute to decreases in SVR, as well as the presence of multiple circulating vasodilators (65). Agents such as glucagon, vasoactive intestinal peptide, substance P, platelet-activating factor, prostaglandins, prostacyclin, and NO have all been studied (61,66). The vasodilation results in an apparent hypovolemia, activating the renin-angiotensin system, the sympathetic nervous system, and the release of antidiuretic hormone (67). This results in sodium and water retention. Renal sodium excretion may fall to less than 10 meq/day and may result in an increased total body sodium with a dilutional hyponatremia (68).

Additional factors that may play a role in ascites development include increased central sympathetic outflow, increased hydrostatic pressures within the splanchnic capillary bed and hypoalbuminemia from decreased synthesis with reduced plasma oncotic pressure.

Treatment

ʘ **The mainstays of ascites management consist of dietary sodium restriction and diuretics.** ʘ When dietary sodium intake exceeds urinary sodium output, total body sodium, and water may further increase resulting in worsening ascites and peripheral edema. A diet with ~88 meq, or 2000 mg, of sodium each day is a practical initial goal. Reducing dietary intake to 44 to 66 meq/day may be necessary to manage ascites in up to 10% of patients (69).

When pharmacologic intervention is necessary, the most successful diuretic regimen consists of spironolactone and furosemide. Spironolactone 100 mg a day and furosemide 40 mg a day is a common initial dose (70). However, these doses may be doubled if there is no obvious response after several days. Spironolactone inhibits the sodium–potassium exchange in the distal tubule, thereby increasing sodium excretion. Furosemide will potentiate this effect by blocking the Na–K–2Cl cotransport in the loop of Henle. Furosemide alone will deliver more sodium to the distal tubule and typically should not be used as a sole agent to manage ascites (69). The maximum recommended doses are spironolactone 400 mg/day and furosemide 160 mg/day (71).

Ten to twenty percent of patients with ascites will be refractory to diet and diuretic therapy. One therapeutic option in these patients is large volume paracentesis. The removal of five or more liters as often as necessary is an effective means of ascites management. Controversy exists regarding the necessity to administer albumin with paracenteses that remove more than 5 L. Several studies have shown more stable renin and aldosterone levels after large volume paracentesis with the addition of albumin, with concomitant decreases in morbidity or mortality (69).

Distal surgical portosystemic shunts are an option for individuals with ascites who are refractory to diuretic therapy, and those with recurrent variceal hemorrhage. There is a high incidence of hepatic encephalopathy, and a high mortality following portosystemic shunts. Furthermore, central portosystemic shunts should be avoided if the possibility of liver transplantation exists. Another effective shunting procedure is the transjugular intrahepatic portosystemic shunt (TIPS). These procedures reduce sinusoidal pressure and increase the effective arterial blood volume by diverting blood from the liver, and reducing ascites formation. The major complications of the TIPS procedure include hepatic encephalopathy and liver failure (69).

Complications

Spontaneous Bacterial Peritonitis

ʘ **SBP is an infection of ascitic fluid without a recognizable secondary cause of bacterial peritonitis. About 10% to 25% of patients with cirrhosis and ascites admitted to the hospital will have SBP.** ʘ

Classically, SBP is a monobacterial infection, with aerobic Gram-negative organisms accounting for up to 80% of cases. *Escherichia coli* accounts for 50% of cases. Gram-positive cocci may also be involved, with *Streptococcus pneumoniae* being the most common.

Clinical features include fever, leukocytosis, abdominal pain, and mental status changes. Although these signs and symptoms may be helpful, an abdominal paracentesis must be performed to make the diagnosis. An ascitic fluid absolute neutrophil count greater than 250 cells/mm³ is sufficient for a presumptive diagnosis (72). Cultures and a gram stain should be performed. Inoculating blood culture bottles at the bedside can enhance the likelihood of obtaining a positive culture (73). Decreased ascitic fluid total protein, glucose, and lactate dehydrogenase may prove helpful in confirming the presence of SBP.

Empiric therapy with cefotaxime, or a similar third-generation cephalosporin, should be started as soon as possible as initial treatment (72). As the culture results become available, the antibiotic coverage should be tailored based upon the specific organism present. Based on a single study (74) in which patients who received intravenous albumin (1.5 g/kg initially followed by 1 g/kg on day 3) were significantly less likely to develop renal impairment, many authorities advocate its use as part of the treatment of SBP. Antibiotic prophylaxis should be considered in patients at high risk for SBP such as those with a prior episode of SBP, ascitic fluid total protein concentration of less than 1.0 g/dL, or cirrhotic patients with gastrointestinal bleeding (75,76). The two currently recommended prophylactic regimens are either ciprofloxacin, 750 mg once a week, or trimethoprim-sulfamethoxazole, one double-strength tablet (sulfamethoxazole 800 mg and trimethoprim 160 mg) five days a week (69).

Hepatorenal Syndrome

HRS, a potential complication of portal hypertension, is defined as renal failure associated with severe liver disease in the absence of an intrinsic kidney abnormality. ✒ **The severe splanchnic vasodilatation with a reduced effective arterial blood volume seen in end-stage cirrhosis can result in extreme renal artery vasoconstriction and renal failure.** ✒ The risk of HRS in patients with ascites is ~27% at one year and ~40% at five years. Renal failure of other etiologies must also be considered in patients with deteriorating renal function (Volume 2, Chapters 40 and 41). Patients with HRS have a very poor prognosis and liver transplantation remains a suitable therapy. The use of TIPS may be of some benefit, but further trials are needed (69). In critically ill patients, particularly those who are candidates for liver transplantation, early continuous renal replacement therapy is an important option (Volume 2, Chapter 43).

Hepatopulmonary Syndrome

✒ **Hepatopulmonary syndrome (HPS) is a condition that consists of a triad of (*i*) liver dysfunction, (*ii*) hypoxemia with an increased alveolar-arterial (A-a) gradient, and (*iii*) intrapulmonary vascular dilatation.** ✒ Although cirrhotic patients may be mildly hypoxic due to diaphragmatic excursion from ascites, severe hypoxemia (PaO$_2$ <50 mmHg) in the absence of cardiopulmonary disease in a cirrhotic patient suggests the presence of HPS. Individuals with HPS are frequently dyspneic, and may also display platypnea (increased dyspnea when upright and relieved with recumbency) or orthodeoxia (desaturation when upright and relieved with recumbency) (77). Key points of HPS are summarized in Table 5.

The precise mechanism of HPS is unclear, although it is believed that the intrapulmonary vascular dilatation is largely caused by failure of the cirrhotic liver to clear NO. Patients may benefit from supplemental oxygen. Other therapies have been tried unsuccessfully. Mortality has been estimated at 41% in patients who have been followed for over 2.5 years (2,77,78). At present, liver transplantation appears to be the most effective treatment for HPS in patients with severe hypoxemia.

Table 5 Summary Findings in Hepatopulmonary Syndrome

Hepatopulmonary syndrome triad
  Liver dysfunction
  Hypoxemia with wide A-a gradient
  Intrapulmonary vascular dilation
Severe hypoxemia in the absence of cardiopulmonary disease suggests HPS
Clinical signs consistent with the degree of HPS
  Platypnea = increased dyspnea when upright and relieved when supine
  Orthodeoxia = desaturation when upright and relieved when supine

Hyponatremia

Hyponatremia is a common problem in advanced cirrhosis. The reduction in SVR and MAP in cirrhosis leads to activation of the renin-angiotensin system and the sympathetic nervous system and increases levels of antidiuretic hormone. This results in renal sodium and water retention (38). This inability to excrete water results in dilutional hyponatremia (58,79). ✒ **The severity of the hyponatremia is proportional to the degree of cirrhosis and is of prognostic value (60).** ✒

The standard therapy in nontrauma or surgical patients is restriction of water intake to create a negative water balance. Providing oral or parenteral salt is only indicated if the hyponatremia is symptomatic. However, in trauma or critically ill postsurgical patients, salt-containing fluids often need to be administered to replete lost fluids and guard against further deletion of intravascular volume.

HEPATIC ENCEPHALOPATHY

Hepatic encephalopathy or portosystemic encephalopathy is a spectrum of neuropsychiatric abnormalities occurring in patients with advanced liver failure.

Pathogenesis

✒ **Although the precise mechanisms of hepatic encephalopathy are unknown, there are several theories regarding the pathogenesis. Ammonia, metabolic changes, cerebral edema, impaired perfusion, and changes in neurotransmitter systems may all be involved.** ✒

Ammonia acts as a neurotoxin in hepatic encephalopathy. It is produced by urease splitting colonic bacteria from nitrogenous sources such as protein, blood following upper GI hemorrhage, and by enterocytes from glutamine. Normally, the liver clears almost all the ammonia in the portal vein by converting it into glutamine. The arterial concentration of ammonia is increased in about 90% of patients with hepatic encephalopathy (80). Hyperammonemia can increase the cerebral concentration of neutral amino acids which may affect the synthesis of several neurotransmitters (81). Cerebral edema is also seen during hyperammonemia. This may be secondary to increased glutamine production from the metabolism of ammonia resulting in an increase in intracellular osmolarity (82). Ammonia may also directly affect neuronal electrical activity by inhibiting postsynaptic potentials (83–85).

Another metabolite that may be involved in the development of hepatic encephalopathy is oxindole. It is created by bacteria in the intestines and is a product of tryptophan with neurodepressant effects. It can cause sedation, weakness, hypotension, and coma. Greatly increased plasma concentrations of oxindole have been found in patients with hepatic encephalopathy (86).

Impaired neurotransmission may be a component in the pathogenesis of hepatic encephalopathy. Both the Gamma-aminobutyric acid-benzodiazepine and glutamatergic neurotransmission systems have been studied. Astrocytic benzodiazepine receptors may be increased in patients with hepatic encephalopathy resulting in accumulation of cholesterol and neurosteroids (87). Astrocytes appear to have a reduced ability to reuptake neuronally released glutamate during hepatic encephalopathy and may play a role in its pathogenesis (88,89).

Several catecholamines may also be implicated in hepatic encephalopathy. Reduced norepinephrine concentrations in the brain are routinely found in liver failure. Significantly increased levels of the serotonin metabolite, 5-hydroxyindoleacetic acid, are a consistent finding in hepatic encephalopathy (90). Additionally, alterations in the blood–brain barrier, as well as changes in cerebral energy metabolism may prove to be important in the pathogenesis, but require more study (91,92).

Signs and Symptoms

Patients with hepatic encephalopathy usually have advanced liver disease and will likely display many of the signs and symptoms associated with hepatic dysfunction.

The changes in mentation seen in hepatic encephalopathy are often preceded by sleep disturbances. This may be either insomnia or hypersomnia. Changes in cognition, personality, intellectual function, behavior, and eventually consciousness may then develop (45). A commonly used grading system for hepatic encephalopathy uses these changes to place patients into stages, from I to IV (Table 6) (93). This may be useful to follow the course of the illness and its response to therapy. Other clinical signs include the presence of asterixis, hyperactive deep tendon reflexes, and even focal neurologic deficits.

The diagnosis of hepatic encephalopathy is one of exclusion. Other causes of a change in mental status, such as electrolyte disturbances, drugs, infarction, uremia, and infection must first be excluded. There is no laboratory or radiologic test that is diagnostic of hepatic encephalopathy. Although ammonia may be involved in the pathogenesis, neither venous nor arterial serum levels are appropriate screening tests (94). Likewise, serum NH_3 levels have not been shown to correlate with the severity of clinical symptoms. The electroencephalogram may be used to evaluate the degree of encephalopathy. Although not specific, a bilaterally synchronous decrease in wave frequency and an increase in wave amplitude may be seen in hepatic encephalopathy (95).

Treatment

In managing the patient with hepatic encephalopathy, potential precipitating causes, such as gastrointestinal bleeding, high protein intake, infection, and benzodiazepine use, must first be identified and treated.

Many therapies target ammonia production or absorption. Reducing dietary protein to less than 70 g/day is an effective way to decrease ammoniagenic substrates (96). Oral and rectal lactulose are a mainstay of treatment. The bacterial flora in the gastrointestinal tract convert lactulose into a short-chain fatty acid which lowers the intestinal pH. This favors the conversion of ammonia to a nonabsorbable form, ammonium. The dose should be titrated to cause two to three stools each day (97). Lactitol, another synthetic disaccharide, appears to be as effective as lactulose and may have fewer side effects (98–100). The use of antibiotics has also been studied as a means to inhibit ammonia production. The poorly absorbed aminoglycoside neomycin has been shown to be effective, but ototoxicity and nephrotoxicity limit its use as a long-term treatment. Additionally, oral enterococcus faecium SF68, which may alter the gastrointestinal flora to a more urease-negative form, was shown to be as effective as lactulose in a small, randomized study (101). More recently, the minimally absorbed antibiotic rifaximin shows promise for its safety and efficacy in treating hepatic encephalopathy (102). Agents such as ornithine-aspartate, which may increase ammonia removal by stimulating glutamine synthesis, and sodium benzoate, which may increase urinary ammonia excretion, may prove useful, but need more study (103). Studies on branched-chain amino acid infusions, as well as agents that target the neurotransmitter systems (e.g., flumazenil),

Table 6   West Haven Staging for Hepatic Encephalopathy

Stage	Mental status	Intellectual function	Asterixis/reflexes	EEG
I	Euphoria or depression, mild confusion, slurred speech, disordered sleep	Short attention	+Tremor and incoordination +Mild astrexis	Usually normal
II	Lethargy, moderate confusion	Disoriented	+Hyperreflexia ++Astrexis	Abnormal Triphasic slowing (5 cps)
III	Marked confusion, incoherent speech, sleeping but arousable	Loss of meaningful communication	++Hyperreflexia +++Astrexis	Abnormal Triphasic slowing (5cps)
IV	Coma; initially responsive to noxious stimuli, later unresponsive	Absent	+++(Ankle clonus) +Decerebrate +Babinski	Abnormal Very slow (2–3 cps) (delta waves)

may be involved in hepatic encephalopathy and have yielded conflicting results (104,105).

ESOPHAGEAL VARICES AND UPPER GI BLEED

Esophageal variceal hemorrhage, a major complication of portal hypertension from cirrhosis, accounts for significant morbidity and mortality in the cirrhotic patient. This condition accounts for 10% to 30% of all upper gastrointestinal hemorrhages, but accounts for nearly 80% to 90% of bleeding episodes in patients with cirrhosis. ◢ **Variceal hemorrhage occurs in approximately one-third of patients with cirrhosis. Thirty to fifty percent of these bleeds are fatal.** ◢ Slightly more than two-thirds of those that do survive the first bleed are likely to have a recurrence, with an increased mortality as high as 50% (106,107).

In managing a cirrhotic patient with a variceal hemorrhage, it is important to consider four principal areas: prediction of the at-risk patient, prophylaxis, treatment of the acute bleed, and secondary prevention.

Predicting the Risk of Variceal Hemorrhage

Varices form in response to the increased obstruction of the portal vein outflow caused by the cirrhotic liver. ◢ **The formation of varices occurs when the portal vein to hepatic vein pressure gradient exceeds 12 mmHg (108).** ◢ Although this measurement may not be routinely performed, there are clinical and endoscopic factors that are useful for predicting which patients with cirrhosis are at highest risk for variceal hemorrhage (Table 7).

Clinical Factors

A greater degree of liver dysfunction, as measured by the Child–Pugh classification (Table 8), is associated with a greater risk of ruptured varices. In addition, a previous variceal bleed predicts a 70% likelihood of a second bleeding episode. The risk of rebleeding is greatest within the first six weeks of the initial bleeding episode. Approximately, 50% of rebleeds occur within the first 48 hours. Other clinical risk factors include presence of ascites and continued alcohol consumption (109).

Endoscopic Factors

Varices can develop anywhere along the gastrointestinal tract, but are most often identified in the esophagus. However, gastric and rectal varices can be found in cirrhotic patients. In the esophagus, varices which develop in the submucosa become more superficial and have less connective tissue in the distal aspect of the esophagus

Table 7 Risk Factors for Variceal Hemorrhage

Increased portal pressure (>12 mmHg)
Recent bleed (within 48 hr to 6 wk)
Severity of initial bleed
Size of varix
Erythema or "red wales"
Continued alcohol abuse
Active bleeding seen on endoscopy
Location of varices near the gastroesophageal
   junction
High Child–Pugh score (Table 8)

Table 8 Modified Child–Pugh Classification of the Severity of Cirrhosis

Variable	Score		
	1	2	3
Ascites	None	Mild	Moderate–severe
T-bili (mg/dL)	<2	2–3	>3
Albumin (g/dL)	>3.5	2.8–3.5	<2.8
INR	<1.7	1.8–2.3	>2.3
Encephalopathy[a]	None	Grade 1–2	Grade 3–4
Classification	Total score	1 yr survival	2 yr survival
A	5–6	100	85
B	7–9	80	60
C	10–15	45	35

[a]Encephalopathy grade refers to West Haven hepatic encephalopathy score (Table 6).
Abbreviations: INR, international normalization ratio; T-bili, total bilirubin.
Source: From Ref. 108.

(Fig. 4A). Therefore, varices near the gastroesophageal junction are more likely to rupture. Varices may also develop in the stomach. Gastric varices tend to bleed less frequently, but can bleed more severely (110). Rectal varices can also develop and may bleed. Laplace's Law suggests that a small increase in the vessel wall radius results in a significant increase in the wall tension and supports the finding that larger varices are at an increased risk of rupturing (106). Endoscopic identification of erythema, red spots, or red streaks (so called "red wales") can independently predict a higher likelihood of hemorrhage (110).

Prophylaxis

Portal hypertension results from increased portal venous inflow and/or increased resistance to portal outflow. Pharmacologic prophylaxis is aimed at reducing the inflow (Fig. 4B). Nonselective β-blockers (e.g., propranolol or nadolol) result in unopposed α-mediated vasoconstriction of the splanchnic arteries, thereby decreasing portal inflow. The β-blocker should be titrated to achieve a 25% decrease in resting heart rate or a pulse of 50 to 60 beats/min (Table 9) (106).

The potential side effects of blockers (especially the noncardioselective ones) include hypotension and bronchoconstriction which may limit the use of these agents in select patients. Although nitrates can decrease portal pressure, this class of drug is not recommended as single-agent prophylaxis because of concerns of an increased mortality in those over 50 years of age (111).

Combined therapy of β-blocker and a long-acting nitrate (e.g., isosorbide mononitrate) can be considered in patients who cannot achieve the desired pulse or response to β-blockers alone. In patients who can tolerate the combination of β-blockers and nitrates, the combination appears to offer greater benefit than β-blockers alone and without an increase in mortality (112). In patients who cannot tolerate pharmacologic prophylaxis, endoscopic sclerotherapy, or band ligation is a clinically effective means of prophylaxis

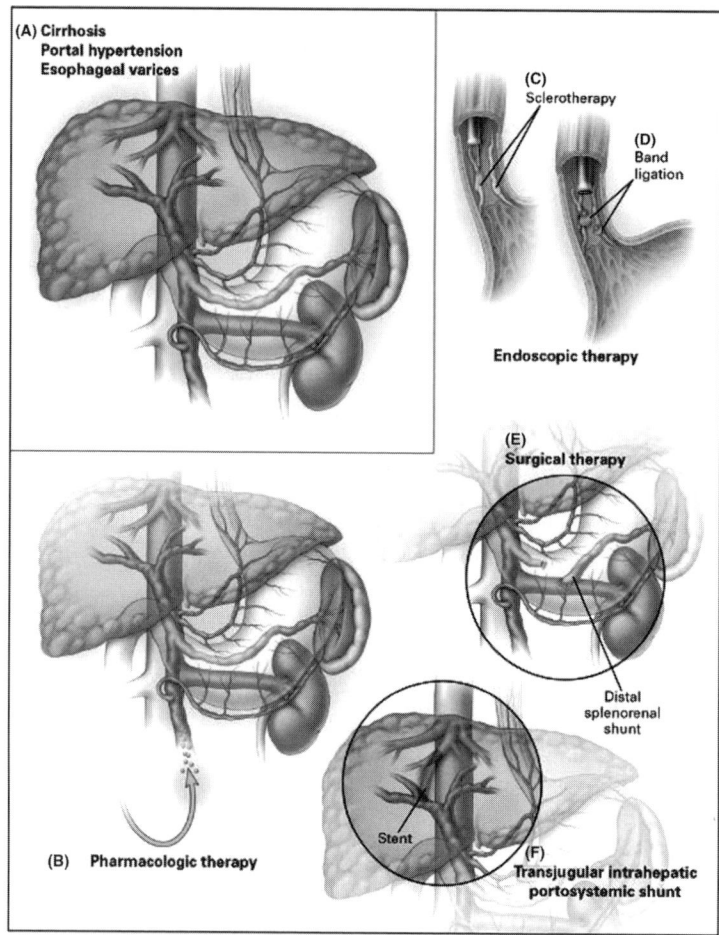

Figure 4 Pictorial representations. (**A**) Overview of cirrhosis, portal hypertension, and esophageal varices. (**B**) Pharmacologic therapy. (**C**) Sclerotherapy. (**D**) Band ligation. (**E**) Surgical therapy. (**F**) TIPS. *Abbreviation*: TIPS, transjugular intrahepatic portostemic shunt. *Source*: From Ref. 105.

(113). These procedures have typically been reserved for individuals who have already experienced an episode of bleeding. Although currently the standard practice, further studies are needed to determine whether endoscopic intervention should be advocated for use as a primary prevention.

Management of Variceal Hemorrhage

Variceal hemorrhage typically presents as severe acute hematemesis. Individuals typically require intensive care management. Pharmacologic therapy, endoscopic intervention, balloon tamponade, and TIPS are often used in the management of variceal bleeding (Table 10) (106).

Table 9 Variceal Hemorrhage Prophylaxis

Nonselective B-blocker titrated to pulse 50–60 or 25% decrease of
  resting heart rate
Nonselective B-blocker plus long-acting nitrate
Band ligation

Pharmacotherapy

Intravenous vasopressin constricts splanchnic arterioles and reduces portal pressure. Although this agent can achieve hemostasis, the benefit is limited by extrasplanchnic vasoconstriction that can result in myocardial and mesenteric ischemia. In addition, intracranial pressure can be increased in cirrhotics with cerebral edema and increased cerebral blood flow due to vasopressin-induced hypertension. The concurrent use of intravenous nitroglycerine results in improved hemostasis and a reduction in complications (114).

Somatostatin, or the synthetic longer acting octreotide, can reduce portal pressure via inhibition of vasoactive peptides. Somatostatin is approximately twice as effective in

Table 10 Management of Active Variceal Hemorrhage

Octreotide
Sclerotherapy
Band ligation
Balloon tamponade
Transjugular intrahepatic portosystemic shunt
Surgery

achieving initial hemostasis than vasopressin. Side effects can include mild hyperglycemia and abdominal cramping, but it is generally well tolerated (115).

Endoscopic Therapy

☞ **Endoscopic therapy is the preferred treatment for active variceal hemorrhage. Sclerotherapy or band ligation can result in a cessation of bleeding in 80% to 90% of patients. This is an important change to make because band ligation is actually preferred over sclerotherapy because of band ligations fever complications. Sclerotherapy is rarely done in this country any more. (Fig. 4C).** ☞ Its advantages include its wide availability, ease of use, and low cost. Its disadvantages include complications such as perforation, ulceration, and stricture formation (106).

Endoscopic variceal band ligation, involving the placement of an elastic band around the varices, is equally as effective as sclerotherapy with fewer reported complications, and is therefore in favor. Frequently individuals will require a combination of pharmacologic and endoscopic therapy (Fig. 4D) (116).

Balloon Tamponade

In situations where pharmacotherapy and endoscopic therapy have failed to control bleeding, balloon tamponade can be utilized to stabilize a patient during acute hemorrhage. An inflatable balloon attached to a nasogastric tube applies direct pressure to the bleeding site. The risk of rebleeding is high, once the balloon is deflated. However, this technique can be an effective method to achieve rapid, short-term hemostasis until more definitive treatment can be instituted. The patient should be intubated to protect the airway when this procedure is used for management of varices because of the increased risk of aspiration and tube migration. In addition, balloon tamponade has been associated with lethal complications including esophageal rupture (106). The benefits and disadvantages of the various nonoperative techniques for treatment of variceal hemorrhage are summarized in Table 11.

Transjugular Intrahepatic Portosystemic Shunt

☞ **TIPS creates a low-resistance pathway between the hepatic and portal veins by angiographic insertion of a metal stent in liver parenchyma (Fig. 4E).** ☞ This procedure can be performed when pharmacologic and endoscopic treatments are unsuccessful, which can occur in 10% to 20% of cases. TIPS has been shown to markedly improve short-term survival (117). Potential complications of TIPS include stent stenosis, encephalopathy, hemolytic anemia, and infection (118).

Surgical Therapy

The reported morbidity associated with surgical shunting and TIPS are comparable. However, the complications of surgery appear to be more immediate than the complications of TIPS placement. The decision to perform surgery or use TIPS is primarily based upon the experience and skills of available physicians (106,119).

Secondary Prevention

Approximately one-third of patients with esophageal varices will experience an episode of rebleeding within six weeks. One-third of individuals who have variceal bleeding will experience recurrent variceal bleeding with a 50% mortality at six weeks (119,120). Secondary prevention, using pharmacologic, endoscopic, or surgical intervention, is frequently employed to decrease the incidence of recurrent variceal bleeding with a potential reduction in morbidity and mortality in cirrhotic patients.

HEMOSTASIS

Numerous elements in the coagulation system are dysfunctional in the cirrhotic patient, including platelet number and function, increased fibrinolysis, and deficiencies in clotting factors (Table 12). The common causes and treatments for each of these abnormalities are discussed below.

Table 11 Benefits and Disadvantages of Various Nonoperative Techniques for the Control of Variceal Hemorrhage

Therapy	Advantages	Disadvantages
Sclerotherapy	Effective Widely available Inexpensive	Perforation Ulceration Stricture formation
Band ligation	Equally or more effective Fewer complications	More challenging procedure Better visibility required
Balloon tamponade	Effective Quick	Esophageal rupture possible Temporary Frequently rebleeds when removed Intubation required
TIPS	An option when all else fails Improves short term survival	In stent stenosis Encephalopathy Hemolytic anemia Infection

Abbreviation: TIPS, transjugular intrahepatic portosystemic shunt.

Table 12 Coagulation System Abnormalities and Cirrhosis

Abnormality	Laboratory finding	Treatment
Thrombocytopenia	Platelet count $<100,000\ \mu L^{-1}$	Platelet transfusion, splenic embolization
Platelet dysfunction	Bleeding time >10 min, impaired aggregation	Platelet transfusion, desmopressin
Increased fibrinolysis	Normal or low fibrinogen, increased fibrin split products, increased D-dimer	Supportive care, correct underlying abnormalities

Abnormal Platelet Number or Function

✍ **The severity of cirrhosis is directly related to the extent of thrombocytopenia and platelet dysfunction.** ✍ Approximately 40% of cirrhotic patients are thrombocytopenic with platelet counts of less than 100,000 mm^{-3} or have abnormal platelet function with a bleeding time of greater than 10 minutes (121,122). Thrombocytopenia can be explained by portal hypertension induced splenomegaly that causes sequestration of platelets from the circulation (121). Platelet-associated IgG in cirrhotic patients can play a role in immunologic platelet destruction (123). In addition, the cirrhotic liver may synthesize less thrombopoietin, a peptide that is responsible for platelet production (124). Cirrhosis is also independently associated with worsening of platelet function (122).

In the critical care setting, thrombocytopenia and thrombodysfunction are typically managed with platelet transfusion. Desmopressin may be helpful for management of prolonged bleeding times. Splenic embolization has been used to control the platelet sequestration and immunologic destruction. However, the use of splenic embolization to decrease morbidity associated with thrombocytopenia has declined with the increasing availability of transplantation (121).

Increased Fibrinolysis

Although the mechanisms are not clear, there appears to be an increase in fibrinolysis in cirrhotic patients. This is evidenced by increased levels of fibrin split products, D-dimers, and tissue plasminogen activator. Impaired clearance of tissue plasminogen activators and impaired synthesis of fibrinolytic inhibitors have been implicated. Severe dysfibrinogenemia can lead to disseminated intravascular coagulopathy (DIC). Treatment of this condition is challenging and largely aimed at supportive care and correcting other underlying abnormalities. At present, use of antifibrinolytic drugs is not recommended except in cases of intraoperative bleeding or liver transplantation (121).

Deficient Synthesis of Clotting Factors

The liver parenchyma cells produce most of the factors involved in the coagulation cascade. Individuals with cirrhosis can have progressive decrease in hepatocyte synthetic function. The production of vitamin K-dependent factors II, VII, IX, X, and proteins S and C can be significantly decreased. This results in impaired coagulation of the intrinsic and extrinsic coagulation pathways. The short four to seven hours half-life of factor VII results in early impairment of PT (120).

✍ **Urgent treatment of coagulopathy in the cirrhotic patient consists of administration of fresh frozen plasma (FFP).** ✍ This may need to be administered every 6 to 12 hours because of its short half-life. Additionally, vitamin K should be given to ensure optimization of carboxylation of the vitamin-K dependent clotting factors, although the effect will not be seen for at least six hours (121,125).

HEPATOCELLULAR CARCINOMA

Hepatocellular carcinoma (HCC) is a malignant tumor derived from hepatocytes. It is most frequently associated with chronic liver disease with cirrhosis (126). ✍ **The occurrence of hepatocellular carcinoma should be considered in patients with longstanding and recently decompensated chronic liver disease.** ✍ The association between hepatitis B and HCC is clearly established, with newer evidence suggesting that the relative risk of HCC is correlated with the serum level of hepatitis B virus DNA (HBV DNA) (127). This is in contrast to hepatitis C whereby HCC occurs almost exclusively in those with cirrhosis (27,128). The combination of HCV and HBV infections increases the relative risk of HCC. HCC is one reason for the interest in the continued improvement of the efficacy and tolerability of medical therapy for chronic viral hepatitis.

Epidemiology

Primary hepatocellular carcinoma results in between 250,000 and one million deaths globally per year. It is by far the most common primary malignancy of the liver, accounting for over 80% of these tumors. Its incidence varies widely according to geographic location, ethnicity, and sex. High incidence regions include sub-Saharan Africa, China, Hong Kong, and Taiwan. Low incidence areas include North and South America, most of Europe and Australia, but the incidence has been increasing in the United States (129). Men are more likely to develop hepatocellular carcinoma compared with females, with a ratio of 3:1 (126). The majority of cases occur in patients with chronic liver disease and cirrhosis. The mean age at presentation is between 50 and 60 years of age (129).

Etiology

A variety of risk factors have been identified for the development of hepatocellular carcinoma. Patients with chronic liver disease of any etiology have an increased incidence of hepatocellular carcinoma. Compensated cirrhotics have a 3% to 4% annual incidence of hepatocellular carcinoma (130,131). ✍ **Chronic hepatitis C infection, chronic hepatitis B and the carrier state, aflatoxins, and liver cirrhosis of any etiology are the most frequently reported etiologies of hepatocellular carcinoma.** ✍ Other less common associations that have been reported include AAT deficiency, hemochromatosis, oral contraceptives, and porphyria (126). Cigarette smoking appears to be an additional independent risk factor for hepatocellular carcinoma development. The role of alcohol may only be in the development of cirrhosis and not directly in the pathogenesis of hepatocellular carcinoma (130).

Clinical Features

✍ **Decompensation of a previously compensated cirrhotic patient is suspicious for malignancy.** ✍ The signs and symptoms of hepatocellular carcinoma are often similar to those caused by chronic liver disease and cirrhosis. General malaise, upper abdominal pain, anorexia, abdominal fullness, weight loss, ascites, nausea, vomiting, jaundice, and wasting may all be presenting symptoms (126). This may represent invasion of the hepatic or portal veins or arteriovenous shunting induced by the tumor (132). Severe abdominal pain with or without hypotension may be indicative of intraperitoneal bleeding secondary to tumor rupture (126). Watery diarrhea has been shown to be significantly more common among cirrhotics with hepatocellular carcinoma than those without (133).

Diagnosis

Several serum markers have been investigated for use in the diagnosis of hepatocellular carcinoma. Alpha-fetoprotein

(AFP) is a glycoprotein whose serum concentration is often elevated in patients with hepatocellular carcinoma. Levels do not correlate with tumor size, stage, or prognosis. AFP levels greater than 500 g/L (normal, 10–20 g/L) in a high-risk patient is essentially diagnostic of hepatocellular carcinoma (134). Des-gamma-carboxy prothrombin has also been evaluated as a potential marker in the diagnosis of hepatocellular carcinoma. Elevated levels are common in patients with hepatocellular carcinoma, but much less frequently with tumors less than 3 cm in size (135).

Ultrasound, computed tomography (CT), and magnetic resonance imaging (MRI) are all commonly used to help diagnose hepatocellular carcinoma. Ultrasound is noninvasive and can assess for vascular invasion, but cannot distinguish various types of solid tumors (136). Multiple studies have placed its sensitivity from 40% to 75% (137–139). Helical CT scan has greatly improved the sensitivity of this test. Hypervascular tumors as small as 3 mm may be detected with this method. Current sensitivity estimates are as high as 90% (140). MRI has a similar sensitivity as the helical CT scan in detection of hepatocellular carcinoma. Hepatocellular carcinoma has high density on T2-weighted images and low intensity on T1-weighted images (126). MRI is often used in patients with renal insufficiency, contrast allergies, and those with an inconclusive CT scan (141).

An ultrasound or CT-guided biopsy can be performed in patients with a lesion in whom the diagnosis is uncertain. The histology of the tumor can vary from well-differentiated to poorly differentiated lesions with large multinucleate anaplastic giant cells. The risks of biopsy should be considered before the procedure and include bleeding and seeding of the tumor along the needle track (142).

Treatment

Treatment of hepatocellular carcinoma can include hepatic resection, orthotopic liver transplantation, percutaneous ethanol injection, transarterial chemoembolization, radiofrequency thermal energy, and chemotherapy.

Partial hepatectomy is the mainstay treatment for those patients with preserved hepatic function, no evidence of portal hypertension, and a solitary lesion (143). Unfortunately, most patients do not meet these criteria. Tumors greater than 5 cm in diameter are not resected due to an increased likelihood of distant metastasis. Notably, patients who undergo surgical resection have recurrence rates ranging from 38% to 68% (44). Postoperative systemic chemotherapy evaluated with a meta-analysis has shown no improvement in survival and potentially an increase in mortality in patients with underlying cirrhosis (144).

Orthotopic liver transplantation may be appropriate and effective in certain patients (Volume 2, Chapter 36). Patients had a greater than 90% four-year survival after transplantation if there is a single lesion less than 5 cm in diameter or no more than three lesions that are less than 3 cm in diameter. Liver transplantation cannot be performed if there is evidence of vessel, node, or extrahepatic involvement (145). A primary concern with transplantation in patients with hepatocellular carcinoma is the prolonged waiting period that may result in the progression of the disease and disqualify the patient for transplantation. Percutaneous 95% ethanol injections into lesions are typically reserved for patients with small tumors who are not surgical candidates. This procedure can cause tumor shrinkage, necrosis, and may improve survival (146). The major side effects are intraperitoneal hemorrhage and hepatic or renal failure, which can occur in less than 5% of individuals (147). Transarterial chemoembolization involves the injection of chemotherapy into the hepatic artery and is often followed by occlusion of the artery. Lipiodol (iodized poppy seed oil) may be included to help tumor retention of the chemotherapy. In patients with large, unresectable lesions, using chemoembolization may reduce tumor size, but it has not been shown to improve survival (148). The use of radiofrequency thermal energy to induce tumor necrosis has received mixed reviews. While achieving similar success rates when compared with percutaneous ethanol injections, side effects are more common and may include death, hemorrhage, and tumor seeding (149). Most studies involving various combinations of systemic chemotherapy have yielded poor results. Agents such as doxorubicin, 5-fluorouracil, and gemcitabine have all been studied and shown minimal response with very short response durations (150–152).

THE CIRRHOTIC TRAUMA PATIENT

✍ **The cirrhotic patient with the same Injury Severity Score as a noncirrhotic patient has a fourfold increase in mortality and a higher mortality than predicted by scoring systems such as the APACHE II.** ✍ In the individual with cirrhosis who experiences trauma, there is little time for optimization of the hepatic function prior to the performance of potentially life-saving procedures or surgeries. Clinical outcome is correlated with the extent of the operation required to correct the sustained injury, with worse outcomes occurring in cirrhotic patients who have injuries that involve the abdomen. The pretrauma medical condition correlates with clinical outcome. The American College of Surgeons has recommended that prehospital providers transport a cirrhotic patient experiencing a traumatic emergency directly to a major trauma center (3,153).

It is specifically worth noting that hemoperitoneum is a commonly occurring complication of blunt traumatic injury in the cirrhotic patient. ✍ **Acute traumatic hemoperitoneum in a cirrhotic patient is a life-threatening condition and warrants the need for prompt surgical exploration (154).** ✍ Spontaneous hemoperitoneum can occur in 5% of cirrhotics. But hemoperitoneum is much more common after a trauma involving the liver or the often enlarged spleen. Occasionally, hemoperitoneum can develop insidiously without hemodynamic instability. When an adequate history may be unattainable, this insidious development of hemoperitoneum can go unrecognized without a high index of suspicion. Blood may only be a minor peritoneal irritant in this circumstance, resulting in the absence of peritoneal signs. The degree of abdominal pain in an individual with hemoperitoneum is related to the extent and rapidity of blood extravasation.

The diagnosis of hemoperitoneum is confirmed by an abdominal paracentesis revealing hemorrhagic (>50,000 RBC/mL or a hematocrit of ≥0.5%) ascitic fluid. It has been suggested that a second paracentesis be performed at another site to exclude the possibility of having punctured a dilated vessel during the first procedure. Hemorrhagic ascitic fluid should not be removed even in tense ascites as this may be acting to tamponade active bleeding. An abdominal CT scan is a sensitive and specific (≥95%) test to locate the site of bleeding (154). However, clinical evaluation rather than radiologic findings should determine the need for surgical exploration.

PREOPERATIVE EVALUATION AND RISK ASSESSMENT

Cirrhotic patients who require surgery are at an increased risk for complications depending on the severity of liver disease and type of surgery and anesthesia required.

A number of preoperative morbidities are associated with increased complications. Cirrhotic patients should be assessed for conditions that can complicate perioperative management. The coexisting diseases that may significantly impact upon clinical outcomes include chronic renal insufficiency, chronic obstructive pulmonary disease, pneumonia, congestive heart failure, ischemic heart disease, insulin-dependent diabetes mellitus, infection, and upper gastrointestinal tract bleeding. One study documented a perioperative complication rate of 30% in individuals with cirrhosis with significant comorbidities (155). However, cirrhosis by itself results in a higher perioperative morbidity.

Additional risk factors for perioperative complications are male gender, high Child–Pugh score, elevated PT, low serum albumin, elevated creatinine, presence of ascites, presence of varices, and an etiology of cirrhosis other than primary biliary cirrhosis. Postoperative complications in the cirrhotic patient, in order of frequency, include pneumonia, ventilatory dependence, infection, worsened ascites, and dysrhythmias.

The type of surgery required by a cirrhotic patient has an important role in determining the degree of postoperative hepatic dysfunction. 🗡 **Several studies have documented an approximately 5 to 20 times higher perioperative mortality risk associated with cirrhotic patients undergoing various surgical procedures (155–159).** 🗡 Procedures associated with more postoperative complications include: (*i*) emergent surgeries; (*ii*) laparotomy or other intraabdominal procedures requiring significant abdominal traction; (*iii*) procedures associated with significant blood loss, making the risk of hepatic ischemia more likely; (*iv*) surgery that encounters vascular adhesions from prior procedures which can bleed extensively; (*v*) extensive cardiac surgery for patients with a Child-Pugh class B or greater.

Risk factors for complications concerning anesthesia management include a high American Society of Anesthesiologists (ASA) physical status classification, emergency surgery, intraoperative hypotension, and general anesthesia (155).

INTRAOPERATIVE MANAGEMENT CONSIDERATIONS

Hepatic blood flow is altered during anesthesia and surgery. 🗡 **Compromise in hepatic blood flow can result in significant postoperative hepatic insufficiency and a potential increase in mortality in patients with cirrhosis.** 🗡 The liver receives approximately half of its oxygen supply from the hepatic artery and half from the portal vein. During periods of reduced portal inflow, the hepatic artery is able to provide additional oxygenation ("reciprocity of flow") by vasodilating. Intraoperative changes in blood pressure or cardiac output, as well as surgical manipulation can result in decreased portal inflow. However, the hepatic artery's ability to vasodilate can be blunted by certain anesthetics or high anesthetic concentrations (155). One study documented a 16% reduction in hepatic blood flow associated with anesthesia and mechanical ventilation (160). This can be identified by transient elevations of liver associated enzymes. 🗡 **In the cirrhotic patient, the reciprocity of flow between the hepatic artery and portal vein is disturbed, making the cirrhotic liver more prone to ischemia, with potential release of inflammatory mediators, and multiorgan system failure (155).** 🗡 There is no evidence that cirrhosis is a predisposing factor to anesthesia induced hepatotoxicity. However, cirrhotic livers are at greater risk of ischemic injury from low perfusion (hypotension, hypovolemia) states as frequently occur following trauma, some surgical procedures, and critical illness.

Mechanical Ventilation

🗡 **Cirrhotic patients may have respiratory failure for a number of reasons including atelectasis, pleural effusions, pulmonary hypertension, or HPS.** 🗡 Hypercarbia should be avoided as it decreases portal blood flow by sympathetically stimulating splanchnic circulation-resulting in vasoconstriction (161). One should also exercise caution with the use of positive end expiratory pressure (PEEP) in the patient with cirrhosis because it can potentially decrease hepatic blood flow as a result of impaired venous return. It is theorized that the decrease in hepatic blood flow related to PEEP may be further exacerbated by preportal venoconstriction (160).

Medications

Patients with liver dysfunction have an unpredictable response to medications. Altered response to medications can be the result of altered pharmacokinetics relating to alterations in drug plasma binding, volume of distribution, liver blood flow, drug metabolism, and degree of liver dysfunction. All medications should be administered with caution in patients with cirrhosis. The effects of specific classes of medications have been studied in patients with cirrhosis. Barbiturates, benzodiazepines, narcotics, propofol, neuromuscular blocking agents, ketamine, dopamine, dobutamine, and sodium nitroprusside will be discussed.

The safety of barbiturates in patients with hepatic dysfunction is well studied. Barbiturate-related rise in cytochrome P450 may result in increased toxic metabolites. Thiopental and methohexital have preserved clearance in cirrhotics, however, dosages should be decreased in cirrhotic patients with low albumin to account for a decrease in volume of distribution and protein binding.

Benzodiazepines can have prolonged effects in patients with liver dysfunction owing to their low hepatic clearance rate. Dosages of benzodiazepines need to be adjusted according to the degree of hepatic compromise. Narcotics may have potentiated effects in cirrhotic patients. Morphine has been reported to have both unaltered as well as reduced clearance in cirrhotics. Although its clearance is dependent on blood flow, extrahepatic conjugation may aid in its elimination. Hypoalbuminemia and hyperbilirubinemia, however, decrease protein binding of morphine, making more free drugs available for neurological side effects. Fentanyl, on the other hand, has the least effect on hepatic hemodynamics, and is thus the narcotic of choice in patients with liver dysfunction (160).

The metabolism of propofol is unchanged in uncomplicated cirrhotics. However, the effect of propofol upon systemic pressure may impact the hepatic blood flow. In general, propofol has been well tolerated when used on compensated cirrhotic patients (160,162). Neuromuscular blocking agents may have prolonged effects in cirrhotic patients based upon a decrease in excretion and an increase in the volume of distribution. Ketamine does not affect portal or hepatic flow, although it does decrease oxygen transport by increasing oxygen consumption of preportal organs. It is well-tolerated in cirrhotic patients (160).

Dobutamine causes increased total hepatic and portal venous blood flow. However, the improved hepatic oxygen delivery is counteracted by an increase in hepatic oxygen uptake. This results in no improvement in hepatic oxygen supply–uptake ratio. Dopamine and norepinephrine increase hepatic venous oxygen saturation. Sodium nitroprusside does not result in a change in hepatic portal flow despite a significant reduction in blood pressure, as long as the cardiac index is maintained (160). High antidiuretic hormone concentrations are usually seen in patients with decompensated cirrhosis, presumably reflecting vasodilatation and reduced effective intravascular volume. Vasopressin reduces portal blood flow via splanchnic vasoconstriction; however, this medication is not used to control variceal bleeding due to its side effect profile, which includes an increased risk of myocardial infarction and mesenteric ischemia (163).

Volatile Anesthetics

Volatile anesthetics reduce hepatic blood flow in a dose-dependent fashion via their effect on cardiac output and blood pressure.

Halothane significantly reduces cardiac function and thus results in impaired hepatic circulation. One animal study demonstrated that a 30% reduction in systolic blood pressure resulted in a 50% reduction in hepatic blood flow in addition to an increased oxygen extraction. Additionally fulminant hepatic failure can occur in patients receiving repeated doses of halothane. For equipotent doses, enflurane reduces hepatic blood flow to a lesser degree than halothane. ☞ **Isoflurane maintains the reciprocity of liver blood flow and can preserve hepatic perfusion, making it a preferred agent in patients with liver disease.** ☞ Nitrous oxide has also been used in patients with liver disease and has not been shown to have to contribute to worsening function (160).

POSTOPERATIVE MANAGEMENT

The postoperative management of a cirrhotic patient requires an understanding of the altered hepatic physiology, complications that can result from hepatic dysfunction, and the potential impact of coexisting disorders. In patients with cirrhosis, there can be postoperative worsening of ascites or the development of anasarca following the receipt of intraoperative intravenous fluid. The sodium content of all intravenous fluids should be closely monitored. Treatment of an infection or prophylaxis against SBP may be necessary in the postoperative cirrhotic patient. Careful consideration of the sodium content of intravenous fluids used for antibiotic administration is also necessary. Serum creatinine should be monitored to assess for worsening renal function and the potential development of HRS. Coagulopathy and bleeding tendency of the patient with cirrhosis should be considered throughout the perioperative period. It is important to consider the altered pharmacologic effects in the patient with compromised hepatic function.

Significant proportions of individuals with cirrhosis are malnourished. ☞ **Malnourishment in patients with chronic liver disease or cirrhosis can be the result of a combination of poor diet, malabsorption, maldigestion, increased catabolism, decreased protein synthesis, or a product of medication side effects (164).** ☞ It is no longer recommended that cirrhotic patients be protein restricted; rather an intake of 1 to 1.5 g/kg protein is advised in the nonencephalopathic patient. A minimum of 0.5 to 0.7 g/kg protein is suggested in the encephalopathic patient, with upward titration as tolerated (164,165). In addition, cirrhotic patients typically have an increased caloric need and perioperatively may require significant nutritional support (163). It is recommended that 25 to 40 kcal/kg body weight a day be administered to the critically ill patient, depending upon clinical status. A diet with 2 g of sodium/day is typically recommended in effort to balance a low-sodium diet with the need to offer a diet that is palatable. If adequate intake cannot be achieved orally, perioperative tube-feeding or parenteral feeding should be considered (164). Notably, percutaneous endoscopic gastrostomy tube is contraindicated in patients with ascites.

Nutritional support has been shown to be particularly beneficial in cirrhotic patients undergoing hepatectomy or liver transplantation, and is generally used both pre- and postoperatively. It aims to preserve protein synthesis, prevent hepatocellular dysfunction, and optimize hepatocyte repair and regeneration (164,166). The role of perioperative nutritional support targeted to liver dysfunction is an area of continued research.

EYE TO THE FUTURE

Liver biopsy is currently the gold standard for diagnosis of cirrhosis, but is inexact and invasive. Less invasive, more rapid, and reproducible diagnostic tools are in development to accurately evaluate the spectrum of hepatic fibrosis and cirrhosis. Transient elastography (FibroScan®, Echosens, France) is one example, in which ultrasound is used to measure the velocity of an induced low-amplitude, low-velocity vibratory elastic shear wave transmitted through the liver. The ultrasound follows the propagation of the wave and therein measures the liver's "stiffness." The greater the fibrosis, the stiffer the tissue, and the faster the wave propagates. Although further validation is needed, the device appears to perform well for advanced fibrosis, but is limited by a patient's obesity and ascites (167).

Understanding the fibrogenic process has led to the development of noninvasive tests (e.g., FibroTest–ActiTest®, Biopredictive, Paris, France) for the measurement of numerous matrix proteins, enzymes, and cytokines involved in the process. Although we may be nearing a time when serum biomarkers are integral to the assessment of patients with chronic liver disease, the current ability of these assays to differentiate the stages of fibrosis is less than that clinically required (168).

With the significant progress made in recent years in the understanding of fibrosis/cirrhosis, a field dedicated to therapeutic antifibrotics has emerged. The principal event in fibrogenesis appears to be activation of hepatic stellate cells; accordingly, recent efforts have focused on the hepatic stellate cell and its role in matrix deposition and the cascade of events with liver injury. A recent concept is that the fibrosis is dynamic and may be reversible. Although current therapy focuses on the removal of the underlying disease process (e.g., virus in hepatitis B, obesity in NASH), the future will likely include therapies targeted directly at the fibrotic lesion—likely directed at the stellate cell (169).

Owing to an inadequate supply of donors to meet the growing need, at least one-third of patients are dying while waiting for a liver transplant (170). Moreover, the critically ill patient often has a comorbid relative contraindication for transplantation. For this reason, there continues to be research into liver support systems. These can be categorized into: (*i*) noncell-based systems, which include plasmapheresis and charcoal-based hemoadsorption and (*ii*) systems with living hepatocytes, the so-called bioartificial support systems (171). Although these techniques are currently not indicated for routine clinical use, as we improve our understanding of the requirements of a liver support system, these may offer an alternative to acute liver transplantation in the future.

There is a need for improved stratification of surgical risk in patients with cirrhosis (especially in management of blunt abdominal trauma, as well as more routine surgical procedures) (172). In addition, as the frequency of hepatic infarction may be increasing because of more widespread use of laparoscopic surgery, hepatic artery chemoemboliza-tion, liver transplantation, and the hypoperfused cirrhotic patient, further research into augmenting hepatic perfusion is indicated. Finally, as we face the pandemic of obesity, we must be prepared for the growing challenges of caring for the morbidly obese cirrhotic patient (173).

SUMMARY

Cirrhosis represents the irreversible final common pathway of chronic progressive liver disease, and is a costly condition with a high morbidity and mortality. There are numerous etiologies for cirrhosis including infections, metabolic diseases, genetic conditions, drugs, and toxins. The therapy and outcomes vary according to the etiology and comorbidities.

A thorough history and physical examination can be helpful in patients suspected of being cirrhotic. Laboratory evaluation can also be suggestive of cirrhosis, although definitive diagnosis is currently made only by liver biopsy. Newer diagnostic modalities may allow earlier diagnosis.

As the end stage of progressive hepatic fibrosis, the complications of cirrhosis can include ascites, SBP, hepatic encephalopathy, HRS, HPS, varices, poor hemostasis, and hemorrhage. Individuals with cirrhosis are also at an increased risk for hepatocellular carcinoma.

The individual with cirrhosis who experiences trauma has a higher perioperative morbidity and mortality risk than noncirrhotic individuals. There is seldom time for optimiz-ation of the hepatic function prior to the performance of potentially life-saving procedures or surgeries in the cirrho-tic trauma patient. Yet these patients have additional con-siderations beyond the normal trauma patient. Particular focus is given to: (*i*) repletion of coagulation factors with FFP, and platelet transfusions to correct thrombocytopenia; (*ii*) close intraoperative monitoring of follow-up coagulation studies; (*iii*) alterations in hemodynamic response due to the baseline peripheral vasodilation and impaired ability to compensate for hemorrhage and third spacing; (*iv*) under-standing of splanchnic hypoperfusion and the particular vulnerability of the cirrhotic patient, emphasizing the need for vigorous fluid repletion and invasive monitoring; (*v*) and baseline metabolic alterations imposed by liver

dysfunction (e.g., hyponatremia, hypoalbuminemia, and impaired lactate clearance ability) all serve to exacerbate the severity of trauma shock in these patients.

The response to medications can be the result of altered pharmacokinetics relating to alterations in drug plasma binding, volume of distribution, liver blood flow, drug metab-olism, and degree of liver dysfunction. Various factors, includ-ing the Child–Pugh score, can be helpful in predicting clinical outcomes for the individual with cirrhosis. It is critical that the management of the cirrhotic patient be adjusted to encompass the altered hepatic physiology.

KEY POINTS

- The fibrotic tissue in cirrhosis consists of extracellular matrix molecules, collagen types I and III, sulfated proteoglycans, and glycoproteins.
- The development of cirrhosis is most often silent until complications of significant hepatic dysfunction occurs.
- The mainstays of ascites management consist of dietary sodium restriction and diuretics.
- SBP is an infection of ascitic fluid without a recogniz-able secondary cause of bacterial peritonitis. About 10% to 25% of patients with cirrhosis and ascites admitted to the hospital will have SBP.
- The severe splanchnic vasodilatation with a reduced effective arterial blood volume seen in end-stage cirrho-sis can result in extreme renal artery vasoconstriction and renal failure.
- Hepatopulmonary syndrome (HPS) is a condition that consists of a triad of (*i*) liver dysfunction, (*ii*) hypoxe-mia with an increased alveolar-arterial (A-a) gradient, and (*iii*) intrapulmonary vascular dilatation.
- The severity of the hyponatremia is proportional to the degree of cirrhosis and is of prognostic value.
- Although the precise mechanisms of hepatic encephalo-pathy are unknown, there are several theories regard-ing the pathogenesis. Ammonia, metabolic changes, cerebral edema, impaired perfusion, and changes in neurotransmitter systems may all be involved.
- Variceal hemorrhage occurs in approximately one-third of patients with cirrhosis. Thirty to fifty percent of these bleeds are fatal.
- The formation of varices occurs when the portal vein to hepatic vein pressure gradient exceeds 12 mmHg.
- Endoscopic therapy is the preferred treatment for active variceal hemorrhage. Sclerotherapy or band ligation can result in a cessation of bleeding in 80% to 90% of patients. This is an important change to make because band ligation is actually preferred over sclerotherapy because of band ligations fewer complications. Scler-otherapy is rarely done in this country any more. (Fig. 4C)
- TIPS creates a low-resistance pathway between the hepatic and portal veins by angiographic insertion of a metal stent in liver parenchyma (Fig. 4E).
- The severity of cirrhosis is directly related to the extent of thrombocytopenia and platelet dysfunction.
- Urgent treatment of coagulopathy in the cirrhotic patient consists of administration of fresh frozen plasma (FFP).
- The occurrence of hepatocellular carcinoma should be considered in patients with longstanding and recently decompensated chronic liver disease.

✒ Chronic hepatitis C infection, chronic hepatitis B and the hepatitis B carrier state, aflatoxins, and liver cirrhosis of any etiology are the most frequently reported etiologies of hepatocellular carcinoma.

✒ Decompensation of a previously compensated cirrhotic patient is suspicious for malignancy.

✒ The cirrhotic patient with the same Injury Severity Score as a noncirrhotic patient has a fourfold increase in mortality and a higher mortality than predicted by scoring systems such as the APACHE II.

✒ Acute traumatic hemoperitoneum in a cirrhotic patient is a life-threatening condition and warrants the need for prompt surgical exploration.

✒ Several studies have documented an approximately 5 to 20 times higher perioperative mortality risk associated with cirrhotic patients undergoing various surgical procedures.

✒ Compromise in hepatic blood flow can result in significant postoperative hepatic insufficiency and a potential increase in mortality in patients with cirrhosis.

✒ In the cirrhotic patient, the reciprocity of flow between the hepatic artery and portal vein is disturbed, making the cirrhotic liver more prone to ischemia, with potential release of inflammatory mediators, and multiorgan system failure.

✒ Cirrhotic patients may have respiratory failure for a number of reasons including atelactasis, pleural effusions, pulmonary hypertension, or HPS.

✒ Isoflurane maintains the reciprocity of liver blood flow and can preserve hepatic perfusion, making it a preferred agent in patients with liver disease.

✒ Malnourishment in patients with chronic liver disease or cirrhosis can be the result of a combination of poor diet, malabsorption, maldigestion, increased catabolism, decreased protein synthesis, or a product of medication side effects.

REFERENCES

1. Hayes PC. Cirrhosis. In: Shearman DJC, Finlayson N, Camilleri M, Carter D, eds. Diseases of the Gastrointestinal Tract and Liver. 3rd ed. Livingstone, NY: Churchill, 1997:915–928.
2. Saab S, Han SH, Martin P. Liver transplantation: selection, listing criteria, and preoperative management [review] [138 refs]. Clin Liver Dis 2000; 4(3):513–532.
3. Tinkoff G, Rhodes M, Diamond D, Lucke J. Cirrhosis in the trauma victim: effect on mortality rates. Ann Surg 1990; 211(2):172–177.
4. Shellman RG, Fulkerson WJ, DeLong E, Piantadosi CA. Prognosis of patients with cirrhosis and chronic liver disease admitted to the medical intensive care unit [see comment]. Crit Care Med 1988; 16(7):671–678.
5. Zimmerman JE, Wagner DP, Seneff MG, Becker RB, Sun X, Knaus WA. Intensive care unit admissions with cirrhosis: risk-stratifying patient groups and predicting individual survival. Hepatology 1996; 23(6):1393–1401.
6. Cecil RL. ed. Cecil Textbook of Medicine. 21st ed. Philadelphia: WB Saunders, 2000 (Chapter 153).
7. Marra F, Valente AJ, Pinzani M, Abboud HE. Cultured human liver fat-storing cells produce monocyte chemotactic protein-1: regulation by proinflammatory cytokines. J Clin Invest 1993; 92(4):1674–1680.
8. Friedman SL. Seminars in medicine of the Beth Israel hospital, Boston: the cellular basis of hepatic fibrosis: mechanisms and treatment strategies [review] [74 refs]. N Engl J Med 1993; 328(25):1828–1835.
9. Okuno M, Moriwaki H, Imai S, et al. Retinoids exacerbate rat liver fibrosis by inducing the activation of latent TGF-beta in liver stellate cells [see comment]. Hepatology 1997; 26(4):913–921.
10. Hines JE, Johnson SJ, Burt AD. In vivo responses of macrophages and perisinusoidal cells to cholestatic liver injury. Am J Pathol 1993; 142(2):511–518.
11. Friedman SL. Cytokines and fibrogenesis [review] [156 refs]. Semin Liver Dis 1999; 19(2):129–140.
12. Pinzani M, Marra F, Carloni V. Signal transduction in hepatic stellate cells [review] [86 refs]. Liver 1998; 18(1):2–13.
13. Friedman SL. Molecular regulation of hepatic fibrosis, an integrated cellular response to tissue injury [review] [57 refs]. J Biol Chem 2000; 275(4):2247–2250.
14. Rockey D. The cellular pathogenesis of portal hypertension: stellate cell contractility, endothelin, and nitric oxide [review] [43 refs]. Hepatology 1997; 25(1):2–5.
15. Yu Q, Shao R, Qian HS, George SE, Rockey DC. Gene transfer of the neuronal NO synthase isoform to cirrhotic rat liver ameliorates portal hypertension. J Clin Invest 2000; 105(6): 741–748.
16. Rockey DC, Chung JJ. Reduced nitric oxide production by endothelial cells in cirrhotic rat liver: endothelial dysfunction in portal hypertension. Gastroenterology 1998; 114(2):344–351.
17. Castilla A, Prieto J, Fausto N. Transforming growth factors beta 1 and alpha in chronic liver disease: effects of interferon alfa therapy [see comment]. N Engl J Med 1991; 324(14): 933–940.
18. Teli MR, Day CP, Burt AD, Bennett MK, James OF. Determinants of progression to cirrhosis or fibrosis in pure alcoholic fatty liver [see comment]. Lancet 1995; 346(8981): 987–990.
19. Rubin E, Lieber CS. Alcohol-induced hepatic injury in non-alcoholic volunteers. N Engl J Med 1968; 278(16):869–876.
20. Zakim D, Alexander D, Sleisenger MH. The effect of ethanol on hepatic secretion of triglycerides into plasma. J Clin Invest 1965; 44:1115.
21. Baptista A, Bianchi L, deGroote J, et al. Alcoholic liver disease: morphological manifestations: review by an international group. Lancet 1981; 1(8222):707–711.
22. Tong MJ, el-Farra NS, Reikes AR, Co RL. Clinical outcomes after transfusion-associated hepatitis C [see comment]. N Engl J Med 1995; 332(22):1463–1466.
23. Takahashi M, Yamada G, Miyamoto R, Doi T, Endo H, Tsuji T. Natural course of chronic hepatitis C. Am J Gastroenterol 1993; 88(2):240–243.
24. Yano M, Kumada H, Kage M, et al. The long-term pathological evolution of chronic hepatitis C. Hepatology 1996; 23(6):1334–1340.
25. Soto B, Sanchez-Quijano A, Rodrigo L, et al. Human immunodeficiency virus infection modifies the natural history of chronic parenterally-acquired hepatitis C with an unusually rapid progression to cirrhosis [see comment]. J Hepatol 1997; 26(1):1–5.
26. Garcia-Samaniego J, Soriano V, Castilla J, et al. Influence of hepatitis C virus genotypes and HIV infection on histological severity of chronic hepatitis C: the Hepatitis/HIV Spanish study group. Am J Gastroenterol 1997; 92(7):1130–1134.
27. Fattovich G, Giustina G, Degos F, et al. Morbidity and mortality in compensated cirrhosis type C: a retrospective follow-up study of 384 patients [see comment]. Gastroenterology 1997; 112(2):463–472.
28. Gordon SC, Bayati N, Silverman AL. Clinical outcome of hepatitis C as a function of mode of transmission [see comment]. Hepatology 1998; 28(2):562–567.
29. Poynard T, Bedossa P, Opolon P. Natural history of liver fibrosis progression in patients with chronic hepatitis C: the OBSVIRC, METAVIR, CLINIVIR, and DOSVIRC groups. Lancet 1997; 349(9055):825–832.
30. Seeff LB. Natural history of hepatitis C [review] [63 refs]. Hepatology 1997; 26(3, suppl 1):21S–28S.
31. Lok ASF. Perspective: chronic hepatitis B. N Engl J Med 2002; 346(22):1682–1683.
32. Ishak KG. Drug-induced liver injury pathology. In: Clinical and Pathological Correlations in Liver Disease: Approach to the

Next Millennium. Postgraduate Course ed. Am Assoc Study Liver Dis, 1998:236.

33. Lewis JH. Medication-related and other forms of toxic liver injury. In: Brandt LJ, ed. Clinical Practice of Gastroenterology Philadelphia: Churchill Livingstone, 1998:855.

34. Drug-induced liver injury. Proceedings of the Clinical and Pathological Correlations in Liver Disease: Approaching the Next Millennium, American Association for the Study of Liver Diseases Postgraduate course, 1998.

35. Castell JV. Allergic hepatitis: a drug-mediated organ-specific immune reaction [review] [47 refs]. Clin Exp Allergy 1998; 28(suppl 4):13–19.

36. Boelsterli UA. Diclofenac-induced liver injury: a paradigm of idiosyncratic drug toxicity. Toxicol Appl Pharmacol 2003; 192(3):307–322.

37. Cappellini MD, Cohen A, Piga A, et al. A phase 3 study of deferasirox (ICL670), a once-daily oral iron chelator, in patients with beta-thalassemia. Blood 2006; 107(9):3455–3462.

38. Tung BY, Kowdley KV. Clinical management of iron overload [review] [86 refs]. Gastroenterol Clin North Am 1998; 27(3):637–654.

39. Frydman M. Genetic aspects of Wilson's disease. J Gastroenterol Hepatol 1990; 5(6):697–699.

40. Roberts EA, Schilsky ML. A practice guideline on Wilson disease. Hepatology 2003; 37(6):1475–1492.

41. Cuthbert JA. Wilson's disease: update of a systemic disorder with protean manifestations [review] [121 refs]. Gastroenterol Clin North Am 1998; 27(3):655–681.

42. Birrer P, McElvaney NG, Chang-Stroman LM, Crystal RG. Alpha 1-antitrypsin deficiency and liver disease [review] [64 refs]. J Inherit Metab Dis 1991; 14(4):512–525.

43. Lomas DA, Finch JT, Seyama K, Nukiwa T, Carrell RW. Alpha 1-antitrypsin siiyama (Ser53→Phe): further evidence for intracellular loop-sheet polymerization. J Biol Chem 1993; 268(21):15333–15335.

44. Thiele DL. Autoimmune hepatitis. Clin Liver Dis 2005; 9(4):635–646.

45. Kaplan MM, Gershwin ME. Primary biliary cirrhosis [review] [98 refs]. N Engl J Med 2005; 353(12):1261–1273.

46. Lee YM, Kaplan MM. Primary sclerosing cholangitis [review] [141 refs]. N Engl J Med 1995; 332(14):924–933.

47. Mitchell SA, Bansi DS, Hunt N, Von Bergmann K, Fleming KA, Chapman RW. A preliminary trial of high-dose ursodeoxycholic acid in primary sclerosing cholangitis. Gastroenterology 2001; 121(4):900–907.

48. Harnois DM, Angulo P, Jorgensen RA, Larusso NF, Lindor KD. High-dose ursodeoxycholic acid as a therapy for patients with primary sclerosing cholangitis [see comment]. Am J Gastroenterol 2001; 96(5):1558–1562.

49. Neuschwander-Tetri BA, Caldwell SH. Nonalcoholic steatohepatitis: summary of an AASLD single topic conference [erratum appears in Hepatology 2003; 38(2):536] [review] [237 refs]. Hepatology 2003; 37(5):1202–1219.

50. Ong JP, Younossi ZM. Approach to the diagnosis and treatment of nonalcoholic fatty liver disease [review] [106 refs]. Clin Liver Dis 2005; 9(4):617–634.

51. Day CP, James OF. Steatohepatitis: a tale of two "hits?" Gastroenterology 1998; 114(4):842–845.

52. Powell EE, Cooksley WG, Hanson R, Searle J, Halliday JW, Powell LW. The natural history of nonalcoholic steatohepatitis: a follow-up study of forty-two patients for up to 21 years [see comment]. Hepatology 1990; 11(1):74–80.

53. Adams LA, Sanderson S, Lindor KD, Angulo P. The histological course of nonalcoholic fatty liver disease: a longitudinal study of 103 patients with sequential liver biopsies [see comment]. J Hepatol 2005; 42(1):132–138.

54. Caldwell SH, Oelsner DH, Iezzoni JC, Hespenheide EE, Battle EH, Driscoll CJ. Cryptogenic cirrhosis: clinical characterization and risk factors for underlying disease. Hepatology 1999; 29(3):664–669.

55. Poonawala A, Nair SP, Thuluvath PJ. Prevalence of obesity and diabetes in patients with cryptogenic cirrhosis: a case-control study. Hepatology 2000; 32(4, pt 1):689–692.

56. Ong J, Younossi ZM, Reddy V, et al. Cryptogenic cirrhosis and posttransplantation nonalcoholic fatty liver disease. Liver Transpl 2001; 7(9):797–801.

57. Summerfield JA. Diagnosis of cirrhosis and portal hypertension. In: Blumgart LH, Fong Y, eds. Surgery of the Liver and Biliary Tract. 3rd ed. London: W.B. Saunders Company, 2001:1815–1824.

58. Shankar A, Taylor I. Clinical examination and investigation. In: Blumgart LH, Fong Y. eds. Surgery of the Liver and Biliary Tract. 3rd ed. 2001:217–225.

59. Williams AL, Hoofnagle JH. Ratio of serum aspartate to alanine aminotransferase in chronic hepatitis: relationship to cirrhosis. Gastroenterology 1988; 95(3):734–739.

60. Runyon BA. Care of patients with ascites [see comment]. N Engl J Med 1994; 330(5):337–342.

61. Gines P, Fernandez-Esparrach G, Arroyo V, Rodes J. Pathogenesis of ascites in cirrhosis [review] [183 refs]. Semin Liver Dis 1997; 17(3):175–189.

62. Podolsky DK, Isselbacher KJ. Major complications of cirrhosis. In: Fauci AS, Braunwald E, Isselbacher KJ, et al. Harrison's Principles of Internal Medicine. 14th ed. 1998:1712–1713.

63. Abelmann WH. Hyperdynamic circulation in cirrhosis: a historical perspective [comment] [review] [48 refs]. Hepatology 1994; 20(5):1356–1358.

64. Schrier RW, Arroyo V, Bernardi M, Epstein M, Henriksen JH, Rodes J. Peripheral arterial vasodilation hypothesis: a proposal for the initiation of renal sodium and water retention in cirrhosis. [see comment] [review] [92 refs]. Hepatology 1988; 8(5):1151–1157.

65. Groszmann RJ. Hyperdynamic circulation of liver disease 40 years later: pathophysiology and clinical consequences [comment] [review] [64 refs]. Hepatology 1994; 20(5):1359–1363.

66. Guarner C, Colina I, Guarner F, Corzo J, Prieto J, Vilardell F. Renal prostaglandins in cirrhosis of the liver. Clin Sci (Colch) 1986; 70(5):477–484.

67. Henriksen JH, Bendtsen F, Gerbes AL, Christensen NJ, Ring-Larsen H, Sorensen TI. Estimated central blood volume in cirrhosis: relationship to sympathetic nervous activity, beta-adrenergic blockade and atrial natriuretic factor. Hepatology 1992; 16(5):1163–1170.

68. Asbert M, Gines A, Gines P, et al. Circulating levels of endothelin in cirrhosis [see comment]. Gastroenterology 1993; 104(5):1485–1491.

69. Wongcharatrawee S, Garcia-Tsao G. Clinical management of ascites and its complications [review] [87 refs]. Clin Liver Dis 2001; 5(3):833–850.

70. Fogel MR, Sawhney VK, Neal EA, Miller RG, Knauer CM, Gregory PB. Diuresis in the ascitic patient: a randomized controlled trial of three regimens. J Clin Gastroenterol 1981; 3(suppl 1):73–80.

71. Runyon BA. Management of adult patients with ascites caused by cirrhosis [review] [78 refs]. Hepatology 1998; 27(1):264–272.

72. Such J, Runyon BA. Spontaneous bacterial peritonitis [review] [12 refs]. Clin Infect Dis 1998; 27(4):669–674.

73. Runyon BA, Canawati HN, Akriviadis EA. Optimization of ascitic fluid culture technique. Gastroenterology 1988; 95(5):1351–1355.

74. Sort P, Navasa M, Arroyo V, et al. Effect of intravenous albumin on renal impairment and mortality in patients with cirrhosis and spontaneous bacterial peritonitis [see comment]. N Engl J Med 1999; 341(6):403–409.

75. Rolachon A, Cordier L, Bacq Y, et al. Ciprofloxacin and long-term prevention of spontaneous bacterial peritonitis: results of a prospective controlled trial. Hepatology 1995; 22(4, pt 1):1171–1174.

76. Bernard B, Grange JD, Khac EN, Amiot X, Opolon P, Poynard T. Antibiotic prophylaxis for the prevention of bacterial infections in cirrhotic patients with gastrointestinal bleeding: a meta-analysis. Hepatology 1999; 29(6):1655–1661.

77. Castro M, Krowka MJ. Hepatopulmonary syndrome: a pulmonary vascular complication of liver disease [review] [81 refs]. Clin Chest Med 1996; 17(1):35–48.

78. Battaglia SE, Pretto JJ, Irving LB, Jones RM, Angus PW. Resolution of gas exchange abnormalities and intrapulmonary shunting following liver transplantation [see comment]. Hepatology 1997; 25(5):1228–1232.

79. Porcel A, Diaz F, Rendon P, Macias M, Martin-Herrera L, Giron-Gonzalez JA. Dilutional hyponatremia in patients with cirrhosis and ascites. Arch Intern Med 2002; 162(3):323–328.

80. Zieve L, Doizaki WM, Zieve J. Synergism between mercaptans and ammonia or fatty acids in the production of coma: a possible role for mercaptans in the pathogenesis of hepatic coma. J Lab Clin Med 1974; 83(1):16–28.

81. James JH, Ziparo V, Jeppsson B, Fischer JE. Hyperammonaemia, plasma aminoacid imbalance, and blood–brain aminoacid transport: a unified theory of portal-systemic encephalopathy. Lancet 1979; 2(8146):772–775.

82. Blei AT, Olafsson S, Therrien G, Butterworth RF. Ammonia-induced brain edema and intracranial hypertension in rats after portacaval anastomosis. Hepatology 1994; 19(6):1437–1444.

83. Raabe W. Ammonium ions abolish excitatory synaptic transmission between cerebellar neurons in primary dissociated tissue culture. J Neurophysiol 1992; 68(1):93–99.

84. Raabe W. Effects of hyperammonemia on neuronal function: NH4+, IPSP and cl(−)-extrusion [review] [83 refs]. Adv Exp Med Biol 1993; 341:71–82.

85. Allert N, Koller H, Siebler M. Ammonia-induced depolarization of cultured rat cortical astrocytes. Brain Res 1998; 782(1–2):261–270.

86. Moroni F, Carpenedo R, Venturini I, Baraldi M, Zeneroli ML. Oxindole in pathogenesis of hepatic encephalopathy. Lancet 1998; 351(9119):1861.

87. Butterworth RF. The astrocytic ("peripheral-type") benzodiazepine receptor: role in the pathogenesis of portal-systemic encephalopathy [review] [37 refs]. Neurochem Int 2000; 36(4–5):411–416.

88. Michalak A, Rose C, Butterworth J, Butterworth RF. Neuroactive amino acids and glutamate (NMDA) receptors in frontal cortex of rats with experimental acute liver failure. Hepatology 1996; 24(4):908–913.

89. Oppong KN, Bartlett K, Record CO, al Mardini H. Synaptosomal glutamate transport in thioacetamide-induced hepatic encephalopathy in the rat. Hepatology 1995; 22(2):553–558.

90. Yurdaydin C, Hortnagl H, Steindl P, et al. Increased serotoninergic and noradrenergic activity in hepatic encephalopathy in rats with thioacetamide-induced acute liver failure. Hepatology 1990; 12(4, pt 1):695–700.

91. Horowitz ME, Schafer DF, Molnar P, et al. Increased blood–brain transfer in a rabbit model of acute liver failure. Gastroenterology 1983; 84(5, pt 1):1003–1011.

92. Mans AM, Biebuyck JF, Davis DW, Bryan RM, Hawkins RA. Regional cerebral glucose utilization in rats with portacaval anastomosis. J Neurochem 1983; 40(4):986–991.

93. Conn HO, Lieberthal MM. The Hepatic Coma Syndromes and Lactulose. Baltimore: Williams and Wilkins, 1979.

94. Stahl J. Studies of the blood ammonia in liver disease. Its diagnostic, prognostic, and therapeutic significance. Ann Intern Med 1963; 58:1–24.

95. Amodio P, Marchetti P, Del Piccolo F, et al. Spectral versus visual EEG analysis in mild hepatic encephalopathy. Clin Neurophysiol 1999; 110(8):1334–1344.

96. Plauth M, Cabre E, Riggio O, Assis-Camilo M, Pirlich M, Kondrup J. ESPEN guidelines on enteral nutrition: liver disease. Clin Nutr 2006; 25(2):285–294.

97. Ferenci P, Herneth A, Steindl P. Newer approaches to therapy of hepatic encephalopathy [review] [71 refs]. Semin Liver Dis 1996; 16(3):329–338.

98. Morgan MY, Hawley KE. Lactitol vs. lactulose in the treatment of acute hepatic encephalopathy in cirrhotic patients: a double-blind, randomized trial. Hepatology 1987; 7(6):1278–1284.

99. Blanc P, Daures JP, Rouillon JM, et al. Lactitol or lactulose in the treatment of chronic hepatic encephalopathy: results of a meta-analysis. Hepatology 1992; 15(2):222–228.

100. Camma C, Fiorello F, Tine F, Marchesini G, Fabbri A, Pagliaro L. Lactitol in treatment of chronic hepatic encephalopathy: a meta-analysis. Dig Dis Sci 1993; 38(5):916–922.

101. Loguercio C, Abbiati R, Rinaldi M, Romano A, Del Vecchio Blanco C, Coltorti M. Long-term effects of enterococcus faecium SF68 versus lactulose in the treatment of patients with cirrhosis and grade 1–2 hepatic encephalopathy. J Hepatol 1995; 23(1):39–46.

102. Mas A, Rodes J, Sunyer L, et al. Comparison of rifaximin and lactitol in the treatment of acute hepatic encephalopathy: results of a randomized, double-blind, double-dummy, controlled clinical trial [see comment]. J Hepatol 2003; 38(1): 51–58.

103. Stauch S, Kircheis G, Adler G, et al. Oral L-ornithine-L-aspartate therapy of chronic hepatic encephalopathy: results of a placebo-controlled double-blind study. J Hepatol. 1998; 28(5):856–864.

104. Ferenci P. Critical evaluation of the role of branched chain amino acids in liver disease. In: Thomas JC, Jones EA, eds. Recent Advances in Hepatology. New York: Churchill Livingstone, 1986:137.

105. Van der Rijt CC, Schalm SW, Meulstee J, Stijnen T. Flumazenil therapy for hepatic encephalopathy: a double-blind cross over study. Gastroenterol Clin Biol 1995; 19(6–7):572–580.

106. Sharara AI, Rockey DC. Gastroesophageal variceal hemorrhage [see comment]. [review] [111 refs]. N Engl J Med 2001; 345(9):669–681.

107. Navarro VJ, Garcia-Tsao G. Variceal hemorrhage [review] [171 refs]. Crit Care Clin 1995; 11(2):391–414.

108. Garcia-Tsao G, Groszmann RJ, Fisher RL, Conn HO, Atterbury CE, Glickman M. Portal pressure, presence of gastroesophageal varices and variceal bleeding. Hepatology 1985; 5(3):419–424.

109. de Franchis R, Primignani M. Why do varices bleed? [review] [89 refs]. Gastroenterol Clin North Am 1992; 21(1):85–101.

110. Sarin SK, Lahoti D, Saxena SP, Murthy NS, Makwana UK. Prevalence, classification and natural history of gastric varices: a long-term follow-up study in 568 portal hypertension patients. Hepatology 1992; 16(6):1343–1349.

111. Angelico M, Carli L, Piat C, Gentile S, Capocaccia L. Effects of isosorbide-5-mononitrate compared with propranolol on first bleeding and long-term survival in cirrhosis [see comment]. Gastroenterology 1997; 113(5):1632–1639.

112. Merkel C, Marin R, Sacerdoti D, et al. Long-term results of a clinical trial of nadolol with or without isosorbide mononitrate for primary prophylaxis of variceal bleeding in cirrhosis [see comment]. Hepatology 2000; 31(2):324–329.

113. Sarin SK, Lamba GS, Kumar M, Misra A, Murthy NS. Comparison of endoscopic ligation and propranolol for the primary prevention of variceal bleeding [see comment]. N Engl J Med 1999; 340(13):988–993.

114. Gimson AE, Westaby D, Hegarty J, Watson A, Williams R. A randomized trial of vasopressin and vasopressin plus nitroglycerin in the control of acute variceal hemorrhage. Hepatology 1986; 6(3):410–413.

115. Imperiale TF, Teran JC, McCullough AJ. A meta-analysis of somatostatin versus vasopressin in the management of acute esophageal variceal hemorrhage. Gastroenterology 1995; 109(4):1289–1294.

116. Laine L, Cook D. Endoscopic ligation compared with sclerotherapy for treatment of esophageal variceal bleeding: a meta-analysis [see comment]. Ann Intern Med 1995; 123(4):280–287.

117. Sanyal AJ, Freedman AM, Luketic VA, et al. Transjugular intrahepatic portosystemic shunts for patients with active variceal hemorrhage unresponsive to sclerotherapy. Gastroenterology 1996; 111(1):138–146.

118. Freedman AM, Sanyal AJ, Tisnado J, et al. Complications of transjugular intrahepatic portosystemic shunt: a comprehensive review [review] [55 refs]. Radiographics 1993; 13(6):1185–1210.

119. Graham DY, Smith JL. The course of patients after variceal hemorrhage. Gastroenterology 1981; 80(4):800–809.

120. Burroughs AK. The natural history of varices [review] [12 refs]. J Hepatol 1993; 17(suppl 2):S10–S13.
121. Fitz G. Systemic complications of liver disease. In: Sleisenger MH, Feldman M, Scharschmidt BF. eds. Sleisenger and Fordtran's Gastrointestinal and Liver Disease. 6th ed. Philadelphia: WB Saunders, 1998:1334–1353.
122. Violi F, Leo R, Vezza E, Basili S, Cordova C, Balsano F. Bleeding time in patients with cirrhosis: relation with degree of liver failure and clotting abnormalities: C.A.L.C. group: coagulation abnormalities in cirrhosis study group. J Hepatol 1994; 20(4):531–536.
123. Kajiwara E, Akagi K, Azuma K, Onoyama K, Fujishima M. Evidence for an immunological pathogenesis of thrombocytopenia in chronic liver disease. Am J Gastroenterol 1995; 90(6):962–966.
124. Peck-Radosavljevic M, Zacherl J, Meng YG, et al. Is inadequate thrombopoietin production a major cause of thrombocytopenia in cirrhosis of the liver? J Hepatol 1997; 27(1):127–131.
125. Chung RT, Jaffe DL, Friedman LS. Complications of chronic liver disease [review] [179 refs]. Crit Care Clin 1995; 11(2):431–463.
126. Molmenti EP, Marsh JW, Dvorchik I, Oliver JH III, Madariaga J, Iwatsuki S. Hepatobiliary malignancies: primary hepatic malignant neoplasms [review] [32 refs]. Surg Clin North Am 1999; 79(1):43–57.
127. Chen CJ, Yang HI, Su J, et al. Risk of hepatocellular carcinoma across a biological gradient of serum hepatitis B virus DNA level. J Am Med Assoc 2006; 295(1):65–73.
128. Tradati F, Colombo M, Mannucci PM, et al. A prospective multicenter study of hepatocellular carcinoma in Italian hemophiliacs with chronic hepatitis C: the study group of the association of Italian hemophilia centers. Blood 1998; 91(4):1173–1177.
129. Munoz N, Bosch X. Epidemiology of hepatocellular carcinoma. In: Okuda K, Ishak KG. eds. Neoplasms of the Liver. Tokyo: Springer, 1989:3.
130. Tsukuma H, Hiyama T, Tanaka S, et al. Risk factors for hepatocellular carcinoma among patients with chronic liver disease [see comment]. N Engl J Med 1993; 328(25):1797–1801.
131. Colombo M, de Franchis R, Del Ninno E, et al. Hepatocellular carcinoma in Italian patients with cirrhosis [see comment]. N Engl J Med 1991; 325(10):675–680.
132. Sugano S, Miyoshi K, Suzuki T, Kawafune T, Kubota M. Intrahepatic arteriovenous shunting due to hepatocellular carcinoma and cirrhosis, and its change by transcatheter arterial embolization. Am J Gastroenterol 1994; 89(2):184–188.
133. Bruix J, Castells A, Calvet X, et al. Diarrhea as a presenting symptom of hepatocellular carcinoma. Dig Dis Sci 1990; 35(6):681–685.
134. Wu JT. Serum alpha-fetoprotein and its lectin reactivity in liver diseases: a review [review] [34 refs]. Ann Clin Lab Sci 1990; 20(2):98–105.
135. Weitz IC, Liebman HA. Des-gamma-carboxy (abnormal) prothrombin and hepatocellular carcinoma: a critical review [review] [47 refs]. Hepatology 1993; 18(4):990–997.
136. Ishiguchi T, Shimamoto K, Fukatsu H, Yamakawa K, Ishigaki T. Radiologic diagnosis of hepatocellular carcinoma [review] [17 refs]. Semin Surg Oncol 1996; 12(3):164–169.
137. Sherman M, Peltekian KM, Lee C. Screening for hepatocellular carcinoma in chronic carriers of hepatitis B virus: incidence and prevalence of hepatocellular carcinoma in a north American urban population. Hepatology 1995; 22(2):432–438.
138. Dodd GD III, Miller WJ, Baron RL, Skolnick ML, Campbell WL. Detection of malignant tumors in end-stage cirrhotic livers: efficacy of sonography as a screening technique. AJR Am J Roentgenol 1992; 159(4):727–733.
139. Pateron D, Ganne N, Trinchet JC, et al. Prospective study of screening for hepatocellular carcinoma in Caucasian patients with cirrhosis [see comment]. J Hepatol 1994; 20(1):65–71.
140. Hollett MD, Jeffrey RB Jr, Nino-Murcia M, Jorgensen MJ, Harris DP. Dual-phase helical CT of the liver: value of arterial phase scans in the detection of small (<or = 1.5 cm)

141. malignant hepatic neoplasms. AJR Am J Roentgenol 1995; 164(4):879–884.
141. Lencioni R, Mascalchi M, Caramella D, Bartolozzi C. Small hepatocellular carcinoma: differentiation from adenomatous hyperplasia with color Doppler US and dynamic gd-DTPA-enhanced MR imaging. Abdom Imaging 1996; 21(1):41–48.
142. John TG, Garden OJ. Needle track seeding of primary and secondary liver carcinoma after percutaneous liver biopsy [review] [24 refs]. HPB Surg 1993; 6(3):199–203.
143. Bruix J. Treatment of hepatocellular carcinoma [review] [37 refs]. Hepatology 1997; 25(2):259–262.
144. Ono T, Yamanoi A, Nazmy El Assal O, Kohno H, Nagasue N. Adjuvant chemotherapy after resection of hepatocellular carcinoma causes deterioration of long-term prognosis in cirrhotic patients: metaanalysis of three randomized controlled trials. Cancer 2001; 91(12):2378–2385.
145. Mazzaferro V, Regalia E, Doci R, et al. Liver transplantation for the treatment of small hepatocellular carcinomas in patients with cirrhosis [see comment]. N Engl J Med 1996; 334(11):693–699.
146. Okuda K. Intratumor ethanol injection. J Surg Oncol Suppl 1993; 3:97–99.
147. Livraghi T, Benedini V, Lazzaroni S, Meloni F, Torzilli G, Vettori C. Long term results of single session percutaneous ethanol injection in patients with large hepatocellular carcinoma. Cancer 1998; 83(1):48–57.
148. Pelletier G, Ducreux M, Gay F, et al. Treatment of unresectable hepatocellular carcinoma with lipiodol chemoembolization: a multicenter randomized trial: groupe CHC. J Hepatol 1998; 29(1):129–134.
149. Curley SA, Izzo F, Ellis LM, Nicolas Vauthey J, Vallone P. Radiofrequency ablation of hepatocellular cancer in 110 patients with cirrhosis. Ann Surg 2000; 232(3):381–391.
150. Cheng AL, Yeh KH, Fine RL, et al. Biochemical modulation of doxorubicin by high-dose tamoxifen in the treatment of advanced hepatocellular carcinoma. Hepatogastroenterology 1998; 45(24):1955–1960.
151. Porta C, Moroni M, Nastasi G, Arcangeli G. 5-fluorouracil and *d,l*-leucovorin calcium are active to treat unresectable hepatocellular carcinoma patients: preliminary results of a phase II study. Oncology 1995; 52(6):487–491.
152. Yang TS, Lin YC, Chen JS, Wang HM, Wang CH. Phase II study of gemcitabine in patients with advanced hepatocellular carcinoma. Cancer 2000; 89(4):750–756.
153. Wahlstrom K, Ney AL, Jacobson S, et al. Trauma in cirrhotics: survival and hospital sequelae in patients requiring abdominal exploration. Am Surg 2000; 66(11):1071–1076.
154. Akriviadis EA. Hemoperitoneum in patients with ascites [review] [87 refs]. Am J Gastroenterol 1997; 92(4):567–575.
155. Ziser A, Plevak DJ, Wiesner RH, Rakela J, Offord KP, Brown DL. Morbidity and mortality in cirrhotic patients undergoing anesthesia and surgery. Anesthesiology 1999; 90(1):42–53.
156. Aranha GV, Sontag SJ, Greenlee HB. Cholecystectomy in cirrhotic patients: a formidable operation. Am J Surg 1982; 143(1):55–60.
157. Leonetti JP, Aranha GV, Wilkinson WA, Stanley M, Greenlee HB. Umbilical herniorrhaphy in cirrhotic patients. Arch Surg 1984; 119(4):442–445.
158. Rice HE, O'Keefe GE, Helton WS, Johansen K. Morbid prognostic features in patients with chronic liver failure undergoing nonhepatic surgery. Arch Surg 1997; 132(8):880–884.
159. Klemperer JD, Ko W, Krieger KH, et al. Cardiac operations in patients with cirrhosis. Ann Thorac Surg 1998; 65(1):85–87.
160. Melendez JA, Fischer M. Anesthesia and postoperative intensive care. In: Blumgart LH, Fong Y. eds. Surgery of the Liver and Biliary Tract. 3rd ed. 2001:545–555.
161. Maze M. Anesthesia and the liver. In: Miller RD, ed. Anesthesia. 4th ed. Edinburgh: Churchill Livingstone, 1994:1969.
162. Moysey J, Freeman JW. Liver transplantation: anesthesia, perioperative management and postoperative intensive care. In:

Blumgart LH, Fong Y, eds. Surgery of the Liver and Biliary Tract. 3rd ed. 2001:2035–2051.

163. Ferguson JW, Therapondos G, Newby DE, Hayes PC. Therapeutic role of vasopressin receptor antagonism in patients with liver cirrhosis [review] [60 refs]. Clin Sci (Colch) 2003; 105(1):1–8.

164. Brown ML, Fong Y, Helton WS. Pre- and postoperative nutrition in hepatobiliary surgery. In: Blumgart LH, Fong Y. eds. Surgery of the Liver and Biliary Tract. 3rd ed. 2001: 532–541.

165. Lochs H, Plauth M. Liver cirrhosis: rationale and modalities for nutritional support: the European society of parenteral and enteral nutrition consensus and beyond [review] [22 refs]. Curr Opin Clin Nutr Metab Care 1999; 2(4):345–349.

166. Fan ST. Review: nutritional support for patients with cirrhosis [review] [55 refs]. J Gastroenterol Hepatol 1997; 12(4):282–286.

167. Ziol M, Handra-Luca A, Kettaneh A, et al. Noninvasive assessment of liver fibrosis by measurement of stiffness in patients with chronic hepatitis C. Hepatology 2005; 41(1):48–54.

168. Thuluvath PJ, Krok KL. Noninvasive markers of fibrosis for longitudinal assessment of fibrosis in chronic liver disease:

are they ready for prime time? [comment]. Am J Gastroenterol 2005; 100(9):1981–1983.

169. Rockey DC. Antifibrotic therapy in chronic liver disease [review] [123 refs]. Clin Gastroenterol Hepatol 2005; 3(2):95–107.

170. Bauer M, Winning J, Kortgen A. Liver failure. Curr Opin Anaesthesiol 2005; 18(2):111–116.

171. Wigg AJ, Padbury RT. Liver support systems: promise and reality [review] [67 refs]. J Gastroenterol Hepatol 2005; 20(12):1807–1816.

172. Perkins L, Jeffries M, Patel T. Utility of preoperative scores for predicting morbidity after cholecystectomy in patients with cirrhosis. Clin Gastroenterol Hepatol 2004; 2(12):1123–1128.

173. Roth J, Qiang X, Marban SL, Redelt H, Lowell BC. The obesity pandemic: where have we been and where are we going? [review] [134 refs]. Obes Res 2004; 12(suppl 2):88S–101S.

174. Bissell DM. Cell–matrix interaction and hepatic fibrosis. Prog Liver Dis 1990; 9:143–155.

175. Bissell DM, Maher JJ. Hepatic fibrosis and cirrhosis; In: Zakim D, Boyer TD, eds. Hepatology: A Textbook of Liver Disease. 4th ed. Philadelphia PA: Saunders, 2003.

38

Artificial Liver and Blood Cleansing Techniques

Tarek Hassanein

Division of Hepatology and Liver Transplantation, Department of Medicine, UC San Diego Medical Center,
San Diego, California, U.S.A.

Jan Stange

Division of Gastroenterology, Department of Internal Medicine, University of Rostock School of Medicine, Rostock, Germany

Sangeeta N. Bhatia

Department of Electrical Engineering and Computer Science, Massachusetts Institute of Technology,
Cambridge, Massachusetts, U.S.A.

INTRODUCTION

Blood purification techniques have been used to supplement the treatment of hepatic failure for 50 years. However, a suitable complete liver replacement device remains elusive. This is mainly due to the complex anatomy, physiology, and biometabolic properties of the liver. The devices that have been employed are capable of providing certain functions but not all. Investigators and clinicians are still struggling to provide a system that supplies the full gamut of liver functions required to keep a patient with liver failure alive (1).

Liver Support Devices must not only remove toxic metabolites (e.g., ammonia, lactate, and toxins), but also provide metabolic functions (e.g., carbohydrate metabolism), immunologic support (e.g., production of complement, and serve as a filter system with its kupffer cells, etc.), a synthetic system for carrier proteins, albumin, and coagulation factors, finally the biliary functions of the liver need to be replicated as well (2).

Extracorporeal liver support systems usually process the blood of the patient using artificial filters and sieves, but to provide full replacement function will need to perform all activities of a hepatocyte. If the system does not contain active cells, it is classified as a nonbiological device; however, if the system contains active cells or tissue that provide some metabolic functions, they are classified as biological devices. In vivo hepatocyte transplantation can be considered as another method to support a failing liver, although they are not considered "classical" liver support systems (3).

This chapter reviews, briefly, the anatomy and physiology of the liver, the definition of liver failure, and the conventional support therapies as a refresher for the novice. Next, the early approaches to blood purification are reviewed, and a survey of current therapies is provided. The basic concepts of various techniques being studied to form a bioartificial liver are provided along with the current hurdles and successes. Finally, the reader is provided a glimpse into current research techniques in the "Eye to the Future" section.

REVIEW OF LIVER ANATOMY AND PHYSIOLOGY
Organ and Segmental Anatomy

The liver is the largest solid organ in the body. It weighs 1600 g in men and around 1400 g in women. The liver receives blood through the portal vein (75%) and the hepatic artery (25%). It drains bile through the biliary system into the duodenum. The liver has eight functional segments based on its vascular distribution (Fig. 1). Venous drainage is through the hepatic veins into the inferior vena cava. The caudate lobe of the liver has its own vascular supply and drainage. The liver has a complicated structure, which allows both hepatic and portal blood to reach the hepatocytes.

The functional unit of the liver is the hepatic lobule (Fig. 2) in which the central venule is in the center of the lobule and the portal tracts are in the corners. Accordingly, hepatocytes are described to be centrilobular around the central vein (zone 3), or perilobular around the portal tracts (zone 1) (4).

Hepatocytes

The liver cell (hepatocyte) occupies 80% to 90% of the total liver volume in humans. Cells are arranged in plates with their sinusoidal (basolateral) surface projecting into the presinusoidal Space of Disse in direct contact with plasma, and the lateral wall opens in an intercellular canalicular space formed with the adjacent cells. Other cells in the liver include nonparenchymal cells, which account for 20% to 30% of the total number of liver cells (5).

Hepatocytes residing in zone 1 of the liver have large mitochondria, as this is the dominant region for gluconeogenesis, beta-oxidation of fatty acids, amino acid catabolism, urea and cholesterol syntheses, and bile excretion. Whereas hepatocytes residing in zone 3 have more endoplasmic reticulum and large nuclei, it is the dominant region for glycolysis, lipogenesis, biotransformation of drugs, detoxification, and clearance of ammonia.

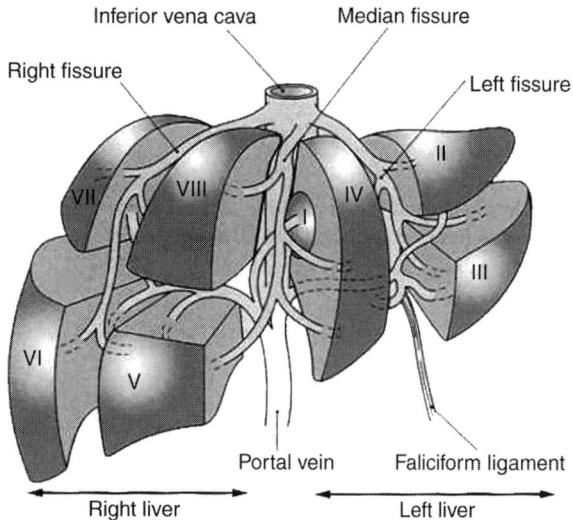

Figure 1 Functional segments of the liver. The eight hepatic functional segments are based on vascular distribution. *Source*: From Ref. 4.

☞ Certain hepatic injuries affect specific zones. ☞

Acetaminophen toxicity predominantly induces zone 3 necrosis. Iron deposition diseases such as hemochromatosis are predominately manifested in zone 1. Viral hepatitis tends to present with spotty necrosis in all zones. Hypotension and systemic hypoperfusion classically produce zone 3 necrosis, while in disseminated intravascular coagulation (DIC, Volume 2, Chapter 58), fibrin deposition occurs in the sinusoids of zone 1 hepatocytes, causing ischemic injury to these cells.

Nonparenchymal Cells

Other nonparenchymal cells residing within the liver include the endothelial cells, kupffer cells, stellate cells (fat-storing cells or Ito cells), and liver-associated lymphocytes (Pit cells). These cells are all directly in contact with blood in the

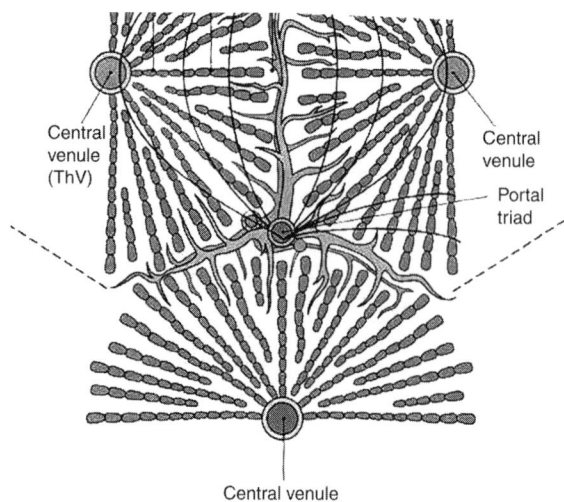

Figure 2 Hepatic lobule. The central vanule is the core of the hepatic lobule, portal tracts comprise the corners. *Source*: O'Grady JG, Lake JR, Howdle PD. Comprehensive Clinical Hepatology 2000; Chapter 1, p 1.7.

sinusoids. Endothelial cells line the sinusoids forming a barrier between the blood and the hepatocytes. Only plasma proteins leak through the fenestrae of the endothelial cells and get in contact with parenchymal cells in the Space of Disse. Endothelial cells have endocytolic activities and can secrete a wide variety of proteins, including interleukins, interferons, TNF-α, and others. Some of these cytokines play a role in the defense mechanism of the liver.

Kupffer cells are the macrophages of the liver. Kupffer cells are attached to the endothelial cells by long cytoplasmic processes. They spread along the sinusoids. They remove particles, toxins, foreign substances, immune complexes, and endotoxins from the blood. They produce vasoactive mediators, and are the main defensive cells of the liver.

Stellate cells (fat-storing cells), are located in the Space of Disse in contact with the parenchymal cells, contain vitamin A rich lipids, and are considered fibroblasts. In liver disease, the cells start proliferating actively, lose their lipid droplets and acquire the morphology of myofibroblast, synthesize and secrete extracellular matrix proteins, which play a major role in liver fibrosis (6).

Liver-associated lymphocytes (Pit cells) are recruited from the blood to the sinusoids to be activated into natural killer cells. These "Pit cells" reside within the sinusoids, and possess strong cytotoxic and antiviral activities, and support differentiation of liver cells (Fig. 3) (7).

Functions of the Liver

☞ The liver is a complex metabolic factory (biochemical reactor) and performs a number of other functions including protein synthesis, immuno protection, and bile formation– related tasks. ☞

The functions of the liver originate from the functions of its cells. It includes regulation of solutes in blood that affect the performance of other systems of the human body; neurological (brain, nerves), cardiovascular (heart, vessels), musculoskeletal (muscles, bones), and excretory systems (biliary, kidneys). The functions involve uptake, metabolism, biotransformation, storage, synthesis, and secretion, in addition to its role in support of the immune system.

Metabolic Functions

The liver is essential for the metabolism of lipids, carbohydrates, and proteins. It plays a major role in biotransformation of drugs, which subsequently are excreted in the urine or bile. Its role in ammonia metabolism is central. Ammonia

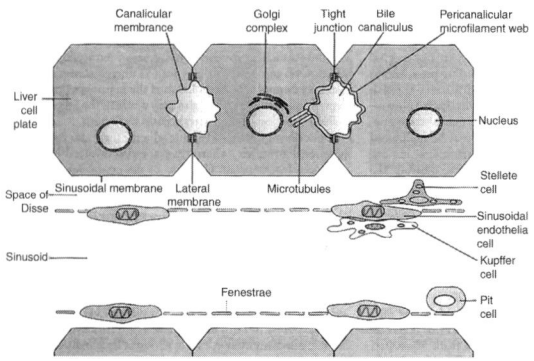

Figure 3 Pit cells. Liver-associated lymphocytes ("pit cells") reside within the hepatic sinusoids serving immunoprotective functions, and also serving to support hepatic cellular differentiation. *Source*: O'Grady JG, Lake JR, Howdle PD. Comprehensive Clinical Hepatology 2000; Chapter 3, p 3.1.

and nitrogenous compounds are removed from the circulation and metabolized into urea via the Krebs cycle in the periportal hepatocytes or glutamine in the perivenular hepatocytes.

Synthetic Functions

The liver synthesizes albumin (12 g/day), which is critical in the maintenance of plasma, oncotic pressure, and is a binder and transporter of many drugs and hormones. Other important synthetic products of the liver include the coagulation factors, antithrombin III, and protein C and S, which maintains the normal balance between blood coagulation and fibrinolysis without the deleterious occurrence of spontaneous thrombosis.

Immunologic Functions

The liver is exposed to influxes of nutrients, particulates, bacteria, viruses, parasites, endotoxins, and others. Both kupffer cells and pit cells constitute the main defense line of the liver against infection. In their role to defend the host, these cells become activated by different stimuli and induce their effects through the production of cytokines, eicosanoids, reactive oxygen intermediaries, extracellular matrix component, nitric oxide among others (8).

Role of Bile Formation

The liver forms bile (500 mL/day), which is composed of water, inorganic electrolytes, proteins, amino acids, lipids, steroids, vitamins, heavy metals, drugs, and toxins. Bile secretion is a complex metabolic process, which is essential for eliminating toxic lipophylic compounds, the excretion of cholesterol, and also facilitates the digestion and absorption of fats and fat-soluble vitamins in the intestine (9).

LIVER FAILURE: DEFINITION AND CONVENTIONAL THERAPIES

Liver failure is a process in which the different functions of the liver fall below the level required to maintain body homeostasis. It is termed acute if it occurs within days to weeks (<24 weeks) in a previously normal liver and is termed acute-on-chronic if it occurs in a patient with pre-existing chronic liver disease. Liver failure presents clinically as hepatic encephalopathy, hemodynamic instability, electrolyte and renal dysfunction (hepato-renal syndrome), severe coagulopathy, bleeding, and frequently results in sepsis and death from brain edema or multi-organ dysfunction syndrome (MODS).

Liver failure can result from numerous etiologies. ☞ **The most common cause of acute liver failure is drug-related hepatotoxicity, which comprises more than 50% of acute cases.** ☞ Acute liver failure occurs in approximately 2000 cases per year in the United States (10). However, death from chronic liver disease is estimated to occur in over 30,000 patients per year. The majority of these cases are due to acute events resulting in decompensation of the liver function in patients with pre-existing chronic liver disease and cirrhosis. In these situations, correcting the precipitating events responsible for the acute decompensation is the mainstay of therapy to give the liver an opportunity to regain its functions (11).

There are few toxin-specific treatment options for particular etiologies of liver failure. These options offer improvement in the liver's detoxification abilities, such as N-acetylcysteine in patients with acetaminophen toxicity and silymarin for patients with mushroom poison-

ing. Unfortunately, complications arising from the acute insult to liver functions compromise liver regeneration and recovery and result in patient death, unless the liver functions are replaced by performing a liver transplant.

Liver transplantation survival has improved, and remains the gold standard for treating patients with liver failure. However, liver grafts are not readily available. Waiting for a liver transplant can extend over a period of days to weeks. During that time, most patients die from complications of liver failure, or become inappropriate candidates for liver transplantation. Therefore, the goal of managing patients with liver failure is to keep them in a stable condition that could support liver regeneration and recovery, or maintain their transplant candidacy until a liver graft becomes available (12).

Coagulopathy and bleeding resulting from liver failure are controlled by plasma and platelet transfusions and replacement of deficient clotting factors, such as recombinant factor VII. Endoscopy and sclerotherapy or band ligation of varices and transjugular intrahepatic portosystemic shunt (TIPS) control variceal bleeding. Antibiotics and antifungals help in reducing the risk of systemic infection and sepsis. Renal therapies and ventilatory support help to regulate electrolyte and pH disturbances. However, accumulation of toxins resulting from the necrosis of hepatic cells and failure of the detoxification powers of the liver exacerbate and prolong the syndrome of liver failure. Approaches directed toward detoxification of the blood are the main goal of liver support systems.

☞ **Liver failure is associated with a significant compromise of metabolic regulation, protein synthesis, detoxification, and immunological defense mechanisms executed by the liver.** ☞ The clinically predominant consequences of lacking metabolic regulation are hypoglycemia and lactic acidosis. Predominant consequences of lacking protein synthesis are coagulopathy, hypoalbuminemia, and complement factor deficiencies. Insufficient detoxification results in the endogenous accumulation of toxic molecules, producing hepatic coma, hemodynamic instability, renal failure, blood cell and bone marrow toxicity, suppression of regeneration, and progression of hepatocyte apoptosis and necrosis. The immunological disturbances associated with liver failure include reduced clearance of microorganisms and their fragments and the subsequent increased exposure of the systemic circulation to infection and bacterial toxins emanating from the splanchnic bed and the portal venous drainage (11).

EARLY APPROACHES TO BLOOD PURIFICATION
Exchange Transfusions

In 1957, Lee and Tink treated a 13-year-old child with hepatic coma with a whole blood exchange transfusion. After two exchange transfusions with an exchange volume of 3 L each, the patient recovered from hepatic coma (13). Nine years later, in 1966, Trey et al. (14) reported 11 exchanges in patients with hepatic coma with seven survivors. Since then, this technique has been used widely. The advantages are toxin removal from the circulation and substitution by fresh blood and plasma components including coagulation factors. The best results were seen if direct transfusion from a donor to a recipient was performed. However, this is not a practical solution as several donors with the same blood group would be needed for every treatment. Thus citrated or heparinized blood has to be used which results in acidosis, hyperkalemia, high citrate levels, and hyperammonemia in patients with failing livers. The initial optimism concerning the effect on survival in liver failure was replaced by more realistic estimates as the results of larger patient data sets became available, indicating a survival rate below 25% (15,16). Thus no significant increase of survival could be demonstrated using exchange transfusion, and the main cause of death often reported was brain edema (17).

Therapeutic Plasma Exchange

In therapeutic plasma exchange (TPE), the blood of the patient is either centrifuged or filtered to separate the blood cells from the plasma. The patient's plasma is then replaced by fresh frozen plasma (FFP) of healthy donors and then both the blood cells and the plasma are transfused back to the patient. The goal is to remove toxic plasma compounds and supply plasma factors. An advantage over exchange transfusion is that FFP is easier to obtain and handle than whole blood. It can be performed daily and for a longer period of time. Moreover, larger plasma volumes can be exchanged (up to 2 L/hr) (18). Since the first report of successful use of TPE in hepatic coma by Cree and Berger in 1968, total survival rates differed extensively between the many groups that performed TPE studies (19). Buckner et al. reported in a study of TPE for acute liver failure, survival of 41 patients out of 138 patients (29.7%). Decisive for the poor outcome was the high complication rate of bacterial infections, lung edema and hemorrhage, and acute respiratory distress syndrome (ARDS) (18). One of the concerns of TPE is the removal of growth factors (HGF, IGF, EGF, TGF) produced by the injured liver and other tissues such as the pancreas, intestinal tract, and platelets during the process of plasma exchange (20,21). Yamazaki et al. reported survival rates of 34% in patients with FHF, who were treated with repeated 5 L plasma exchange compared with 14% survival in control patients (22). However, his study was not randomized and not controlled with respect to etiology and severity of FHF.

High-Volume Plasmapheresis

High-volume plasmapheresis involves exchange of large plasma volumes of (9.9 L per treatment) to remove toxins distributed throughout the body and not only in the plasma pool. Investigators have reported successfully bridging patients to transplantation using this approach (23).

Total Body Washout

The total body washout method was first attempted by Klebanoff et al. (24) in 1972 for a case with hepatic coma. The patient's blood was totally washed out of the body and continuously replaced by Ringer's lactate solution over 40 minutes while the core temperature was maintained around 21°C. The system was driven by a heart-lung machine with a flow rate of 2200 to 2300 mL/min. Then the circulation was filled with whole blood again. The patient regained consciousness and abnormal serum parameters returned to normal. Liver biopsy taken days after the treatment showed marked histological improvement. However, days later the patient died from respiratory failure and gram-negative sepsis.

In another trial the same group added albumin to the substitution fluid and reported better survival. Nine patients survived out of 13 treated for hepatic coma (25). Tobias and Isom (26) confirmed the success of total body washout in the treatment of hepatic coma secondary to fulminant viral hepatitis (2 long-term survivors out of 3 treated). However, this approach had not been pursued any further.

Hemoperfusion over Activated Charcoal and/or Resins

☞ **Hemoperfusion using activated charcoal was shown to have beneficial effects in patients with severe poisoning (8).** ☞ Chang (27) in 1972, reported the first clinical use of this technique in hepatic coma. In 1974, Gazzard et al. (28) treated 31 patients with grade III hepatic coma due to paracetamol-induced hepatic failure with coated charcoal columns. He achieved long-term survival in 11 patients. Using hemoperfusion over activated charcoal the outcome seems to be greatly influenced by the etiology of hepatic failure. The best survival was reported in patients with fulminant hepatic failure from acute hepatitis A infection (67%), followed by acetaminophen toxicity (53%), and was the lowest in acute hepatitis B infection (20%), and halothane and other drug induced acute liver failure (12%) (29).

Ion exchange resins can attract protein bound substances and, therefore, are of interest in the treatment of hepatic failure (30,31). Its clinical use was hampered by bioincompatability which could only be avoided by isolated plasma (plasmaperfusion) over the resins following plasma separation (32). However, the main disadvantages of hemoperfusion are the lack of selectivity with the adsorption of hormones, vitamins, immunoglobulins, drugs, and other important plasma components to the resins. It can also cause activation of the complement cascade, thrombocytopenia, and leukocyte margination. The approach of coating the charcoal particles could mitigate hemocompatability.

High-Flux Dialysis

Hemodialysis had been used in treatment of hepatic failure, but was abandoned because of failure to improve survival (33). The introduction of large-pore dialysis membrances improved the results of hemodialysis in hepatic failure patients. Opolon et al. treated 39 patients with FHF and coma with 164 hemodialysis sessions using the high-flux membrane AN69 (polyacrylonitrile) and a closed loop dialysate circuit containing sterile acetate buffered dialysafe. Recovery of consciousness was reported in 18% of the patients dialyzed versus 0% in the comparable group that was not dialyzed. Total survival was 23% in the dialysis group versus 18% in the undialyzed group. Silk and Williams (34) had long-term survival of 31% in 65 patients with hepatic failure treated with the same method. The initial rationale for the use of polyacrylonitrile membranes was the removal of middle molecular weight molecules up to 5000 Da. Indeed some of the "middle molecules" and substances known to accumulate in liver failure like ammonia and phenol-acids are partially removable by high-flux dialysis. Although this technique might improve hepatic encephalopathy, it does not promote liver regeneration or survival (35). High-flux dialysis cannot remove hydrophobic and/or protein-bound substances like short- and middle-chain fatty acids, mercaptans, or bilirubin.

Hemofiltration

Long-term hemofiltration was used in the treatment of fulminant hepatic failure. Opolon (36) reported hemofiltration in 10 patients with hepatic failure. The mean duration of treatment was 92 hours with a total hemofiltrate of 248 L. Five patients survived. In a further study, which included the following nine patients, he reported 10% survival in patients over 30 years of age, whereas with patients under 30 years of age, their survival was 25% with conventional intensive care, 35% with high-flux dialysis, and 57% with long-term hemofiltration.

CURRENT THERAPIES

Hemodiadsorption

✐ **Hemodiadsorption is "a process during which blood passes through dialysis membrane packages surrounded by a suspension of fine sorbent particle" (37).** ✐ Hemodiadsorption combines sieving (dialysis) and adsorption to remove toxins normally metabolized by the liver. Ash et al. (38) used a sorbent suspension dialysis system where a cellulosic flat membrane dialyzer is perfused by the patient's blood on one side and by a dialysate containing a mixture of charcoal and anion-exchange resin particles on the other. Employing a clamp mechanism, the entire system is driven by pumps on the dialysate side only, thus diminishing mechanical stress on the blood cells. The system has been available for several years in the United States and is FDA approved. Pilot trails showed its efficacy in improving hepatic encephalopathy in a subgroup of patients with liver failure. In a study of 15 patients with liver failure and hepatic encephalopathy grade III/IV, five patients survived; one of them had a liver transplant following treatment with the device. Improvement of neurological status occurred in 13 of the patients. In a randomized controlled trial of 10 patients with FHF and hepatic coma, only one patient survived in the device group versus three in the control group (39). Konstantin et al. (40) used hydrophobic polysulfone hollow-fiber membranes that were filled with paraffin oil. Blood was passed through the hollow fiber. An alkaline acceptor solution (NaO) was recirculated along the dialysate side of the membranes. Although removal of otherwise non-dialyzable toxins (e.g., mercaptans) could be demonstrated in vivo, no improvement in survival was shown (41).

Extracorporeal Albumin Dialysis

✐ **A number of extracorporeal albumin dialysis (ECAD) devices have been introduced in the last decade, and preliminary data demonstrate that these can be used as support systems for the failing liver or as a bridge to transplantation in selected patients.** ✐ The various ECAD devices do clean the blood from different toxins. These devices do not provide the metabolic functions of the liver, but do provide detoxification of the blood. The two commercially available devices with the greatest degree of research data are presented subsequently.

Molecular Adsorbent Recirculating System

Molecular adsorbent recirculating system (MARS) is another modification of hemodiadsorption which uses a new type of highly permeable hollow-fiber dialyzer. The MARS dialyzers are capable of loosening the albumin-toxin binding by physiochemical interaction. It also provides a closed-loop dialysate circuit containing standard dialysate with 15% to 20% human serum albumin, which acts as a molecular adsorbent. The on-line purified dialysate albumin accepts albumin-bound toxins (ABTs) from the blood side (e.g., free fatty acids, aromatic amino acids, bile acids, and bilirubin). It is then perfused over a charcoal and a resin column to remove albumin bound toxins from the albumin and dialyzed through a regular dialysis membrane to remove water-soluble toxins (urea, ammonia) (42). The MARS system is available in Europe and Asia, and was recently approved by the FDA for use in drug poisoning. The concept of extracorporeal albumin dialysis using the MARS device is currently in a multi-center trial in the United States for hepatic encephalopathy and its role on survival is being investigated in Europe in patients with fulminant hepatic failure and in patients with acute liver decompensation complicating end-stage liver disease (Fig. 4)

Fractional Plasma Separation and Adsorption

✐ **Fractional plasma separation and Adsorption (FPSA) is a form of albumin dialysis in which a filter with a cutoff of 250,000 Dalton (250KD) is used.** ✐ This technique was first introduced by Falkenhagen et al. in 1999 (43). Albumin and protein bound toxins pass through the membrane from the blood side into a secondary circuit. The filtered albumin-rich plasma flows through two adsorbers in a row where toxins are directly adsorbed. The purified plasma then returns to the blood side of the albumin filter, back to the patient via a conventional high-flux dialyzer to eliminate water-soluble toxins. A commercial version of this device is called "Prometheus®." A recent study by Rifai et al. (44) showed that Prometheus® is a safe supportive therapy for patients with liver failure. Randomized controlled trial using the Prometheus® device is underway.

Biological Liver Support Systems

In parallel to the developments of devices, biological liver support systems have been in development and testing. Biologicals combine synthetic components (an apparatus, a polymer membrane, etc.) with biologically active cells, tissue slices or liver lobules in a bioreactor aiming to provide most functions of the liver if possible. However, until today, the ideal biological liver replacement is a human liver transplant. But, as transplants are not readily available, extracorporeal liver support systems could provide enough liver function to keep the patients alive until recovery of their liver injury or until they get a liver transplant. This concept started as early as the 1960s when Burnell et al. performed the homologous blood cross circulation between a liver failure patient and a healthy "donor" with identical blood group, thus providing metabolic support for the patient given by a healthy individual with a healthy liver (45,46). Because that concept did not improve the survival rates but was accompanied with

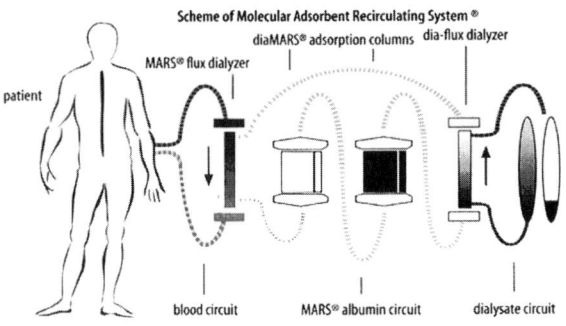

Figure 4 MARS device. The molecular adsorbent recirculating system (MARS) is a form of extracorporeal albumin dialysis, which can serve as a temporary bridge to transplantation. *Source*: From Ref. 139.

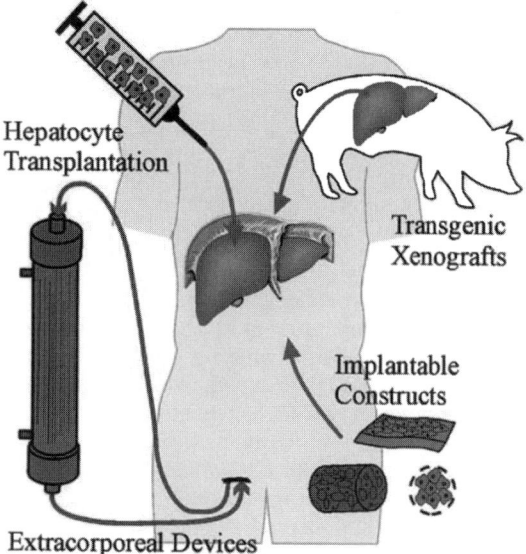

Figure 5 Bioartificial liver devices currently available. Cellular based extracorporeal devices perfuse the patient's blood through bioreacters containing hepatocytes, such as immortalized human dell lines that have been transplanted directly or implanted on scaffolds. Transgenic animals have also been raised to harvest humanized livers. *Source*: Allen JW, Hassanein T, Bhatia SN. Advances in bioartificial liver devices. Hepatology 2001; 34(3):447–455.

immunological complications and hazards for the healthy "donor," it was abandoned (47,48). To eliminate the disadvantage of risks for a healthy human donor several efforts were made to replace that donor by baboons (49–51). In that concept, a total blood exchange in the animals was performed against human blood in the hope to subsequently prevent immunological risks for the patient (48). However, because of the difficulty of the method and ethical aspects regarding the use of primates on the one hand and poor survival rates on the other, that concept was also abandoned.

The first generation of the bioartificial liver, as we know it today, is the extracorporeal isolated liver perfusion, which has been performed with pig and bovine livers with poor results (52,53). However, when primate livers were perfused, better survival rates were achieved (47,54,55). In the last decade, highly sophisticated bioreactors have been developed, which are populated by different cell lines. A discussion of these systems and its components will follow.

BIOARTIFICIAL LIVERS

Just as with dialytic therapies for renal failure, techniques for supporting liver failure and are continuing to undergo evolution with ongoing research and development. Renal failure patients can have their blood cleansed three times a week, and receive supplemental medications to help deal with some of the problems that are not directly addressed by dialysis (e.g., erythropoetin administration to assist with anemia). Similar efforts are likely to occur with liver failure (i.e., we may be able to supplement clotting factors, albumin, etc.—but this is expensive). This section reviews the currently available techniques.

Basic Concepts of Currently Available Techniques

⚡ The most common cell-based liver support designs incorporate hepatocytes in hollow fiber cartridges borrowed from hemodialysis (1). ⚡ Hollow fiber membranes provide a scaffold for cell attachment, immunoisolation, and are well characterized in a clinical setting but may not provide adequate nutrient transport or the proper environmental cues for long-term hepatocyte stabilization. In attempts to improve the hepatocyte microenvironment, investigators have used microcarriers (56), gel entrapment both intralumenally (57) and in the extracapillary space (58), multicompartment interwoven fibers (59), and multi-coaxial configurations (60).

Cellular Components

The full complement of cellular functions required in bioartificial liver devices to affect positive clinical outcomes has not been determined. To address this problem, "surrogate" markers of each class of liver-specific functions typically are characterized, including: synthetic, metabolic, detoxification (phase I and II pathways), and biliary excretion. The implicit assumption is that hepatocytes capable of a wide array of known functions will also express those unmeasured (or unknown) functions that are central to their metabolic role. Table 1 describes cell types that have been used and are currently being evaluated for use in cell-based systems. Each of these—primary hepatocytes, cell lines, and stem cells—should be evaluated on the basis of availability, potential adverse interactions, and efficacy in providing liver-specific function.

Primary porcine hepatocytes are most commonly used in devices undergoing preclinical and clinical evalution. Studies have also been conducted with cells isolated from rabbit (61), canine (62), and rodent species (63). In general, primary hepatocytes are well known to require specific microenvironmental cues to maintain the hepatic phenotype in vitro, and it is likely that a more detailed investigation of culture conditions will improve the stability of porcine hepatocytes in vitro as has been the case for rodent hepatocytes.

Primary human cells would be ideal, but like whole organs, they are in limited supply. They have been used for bioartificial liver application (Gerlach, personal communication), as well as for hepatocyte transplantation (64). A persistent paradox of human hepatocytes is their facile proliferation in vivo but static nature in culture, despite significant progress in stimulating DNA synthesis of rodent hepatocytes in culture (65–67). Recent reports regarding underlying differences in telomerase expression in humans and rodents may play a role in this phenomenon (68).

The growth limitations of primary cells has spurred attempts to develop cell lines that can proliferate in culture while maintaining liver-specific functions. Many cell lines have been established by retroviral transduction or lipofection of the simian virus 40 tumor antigen gene (SV40Tag) whose gene product binds to cell cycle regulator proteins Rb and p53. Spontaneous immortalization has been documented as a result of collagen gel sandwich cultures or co-cultures (69). Cell lines derived from hepatic tumors, such as C3A (a subclone of Hep G2), have already been used in clinical trials (70). The risk of transmitting oncogenic substances or cells into the patient's circulation remains a concern. Efforts to improve the control and safety of cell-based therapies with immortalized cells has resulted in the use of temperature-sensitive SV40Tag (71),

Table 1 Cell Sources for Liver Therapies

Cell source	Critical issues

Primary
  Human, xenogenic
	Sourcing, expansion,
	  safety (PERV), phenotypic
	  stability, immunogenicity

Immortalized
  SV40, telomerase,
  tumor-derived,
  spontaneously
  immortalized
	Safety (suicide genes,
	  tumorgenicity)
	  function, efficacy

Stem cells
  liver progenitor,
  embryonic,
  transdifferentiation
  (HSC, pancreas)
	Sourcing (cadaveric),
	  differentiation,
	  screening, phenotypic stability,
	  safety (tumorgenicity),
	  immunogenicity

Abbreviations: HSC, hematopoietic stem cells; PERV, porcine endogenous retrovirus; SV40, simian virus 40.

Cre-loxP-mediated oncogene excision (72), and integration of suicide genes such as HSV-tk. (73). In the case of tumor-derived cell lines, filters preventing transmission have been implemented in the bioartificial liver design as an extra precaution. Finally, stem cells are being considered for therapy of liver disease. Potential sources include embryonic stem cells, adult liver progenitors, and transdifferentiated nonhepatic cells (58,74–82).

Stabilization of Primary Hepatocytes

Although primary hepatocytes represent the most direct approach to replacing liver function in hepatic failure, they are anchorage-dependent cells and notoriously difficult to maintain in vitro.

When enzymatically isolated from the liver and cultured in monolayer or suspension cultures, they rapidly lose adult liver morphology and differentiated functions. Typical approaches to stabilizing liver-specific functions involve manipulation of the extracellular matrix environment, media composition, or promotion of cell–cell interaction (both homotypic and heterotypic). Extracellular matrix (ECM) modulation has included both variations in composition and topology (83–90). Sandwich culture (87) was designed to mimic the microenvironment of the adult hepatocyte where cells are sandwiched by extracellular matrix in the Space of Disse. Cells in the configuration stably express many liver-specific functions; however, attempts to scale-up this culture method have been met with limited success thus far.

Modifications such as hormonally defined media (80,91) and addition of low concentrations of dimethyl sulfoxide (92) or dexamethasone (93) are known to help stabilize hepatocyte morphology, survival, and liver-specific functions. However, these approaches are inapplicable to bioartificial liver designs because of systemic exposure of patients to these specialized and nonphysiological media components.

Finally, liver-specific functions are stabilized in hepatocytes that are cocultured with nonparenchymal cells ("heterotypic interaction"—see Bhatia et al., 1999 for review) (94). Although the precise molecular mechanisms that underlie the "coculture" effect are not known, it is likely that a highly conserved signaling pathway is involved.

While this concept has not been applied to a bioartificial liver device, it merits consideration.

Bioreactor Designs

Continued innovation in engineering and material science has contributed greatly to the development of an extracorporeal liver-assist device. Coupled with new discoveries in cell sourcing and hepatocyte stabilization, bioartificial liver devices tailored for use with hepatocytes are becoming a reality. Table 2 summarizes the bioreactor designs that have been proposed and studied. **There are four main types of hepatic bioreactors, each with inherent advantages and disadvantages: hollow fiber, flat plate and monolayer, perfused beds or scaffolds, and beds with encapsulated or suspended cells.** A successful and clinically effective bi-device should satisfy a few key criteria: adequate bidirectional mass transport, maintained cell viability and function, and potential for scale-up to therapeutic levels.

Bidirectional Mass Transfer

In bioartificial liver devices, bidirectional mass transfer is needed to provide nutrients to sustain cell viability and allow export of therapeutic cell products. Although most device designs address this, there are important limitations involving the use of membranes, diffusivity of key solutes, and spatial uniformity.

Semi-permeable membranes provide selectivity for the size of biological molecules that will be exchanged between the patient and the device. They are inherent in hollow-fiber devices but have been used also in flat-plate and perfusion systems (95,96). In many hollow-fiber devices, the membrane must simultaneously function as a perm-selective barrier and as a scaffold for cell attachment. As noted earlier, the interaction of the hepatocyte with its microenvironment dramatically affects stability and function. Therefore, this design may not allow for optimization of both function and transport. Conversely, hollow-fiber designs provide a larger surface area-to-volume ratio than flat designs thus improving metabolite transport and minimizing dead volume.

The membrane in a bioartificial liver device is typically characterized by its molecular weight cutoff (MWCO), which is selected both to prevent the exposure of bioreactor cells to components of the immune system and to block the transport of larger xenogenic substances into the circulation. The aim of allowing free transport of larger carrier proteins such as albumin ($\sim$60 kDa) while preventing transport of immunoglobulins ($\sim$150 kDa), complement ($>$200 kDa) or viruses has led most groups to choose a membrane MWCO of 100 to 150 kDa. Membranes also prevent the migration of cells into the patient's circulation, although case reports of cellular translocation exist. Although transport in bioartificial liver devices is a combination of convective and diffusional phenomena, mass transfer limitations of key nutrients to and from the cellular compartment often arise due to diffusion resistances. In contrast, transport in the liver is achieved primarily by convection along the sinusoid with short diffusion distances ($<$5 μm) across the Space of Disse. Barriers to diffusive transport include membranes, collagen gels, and nonviable cells. Some designs use encapsulated cells in perfusion systems, which provide immunoisolation, but also increases diffusion resistance (56,57,97). Packed bed reactors offer improved mass transfer by allowing direct contact of cells on microcarriers or packing material with the perfusing media (59,60,62,98).

Table 2 Bioreactor Designs

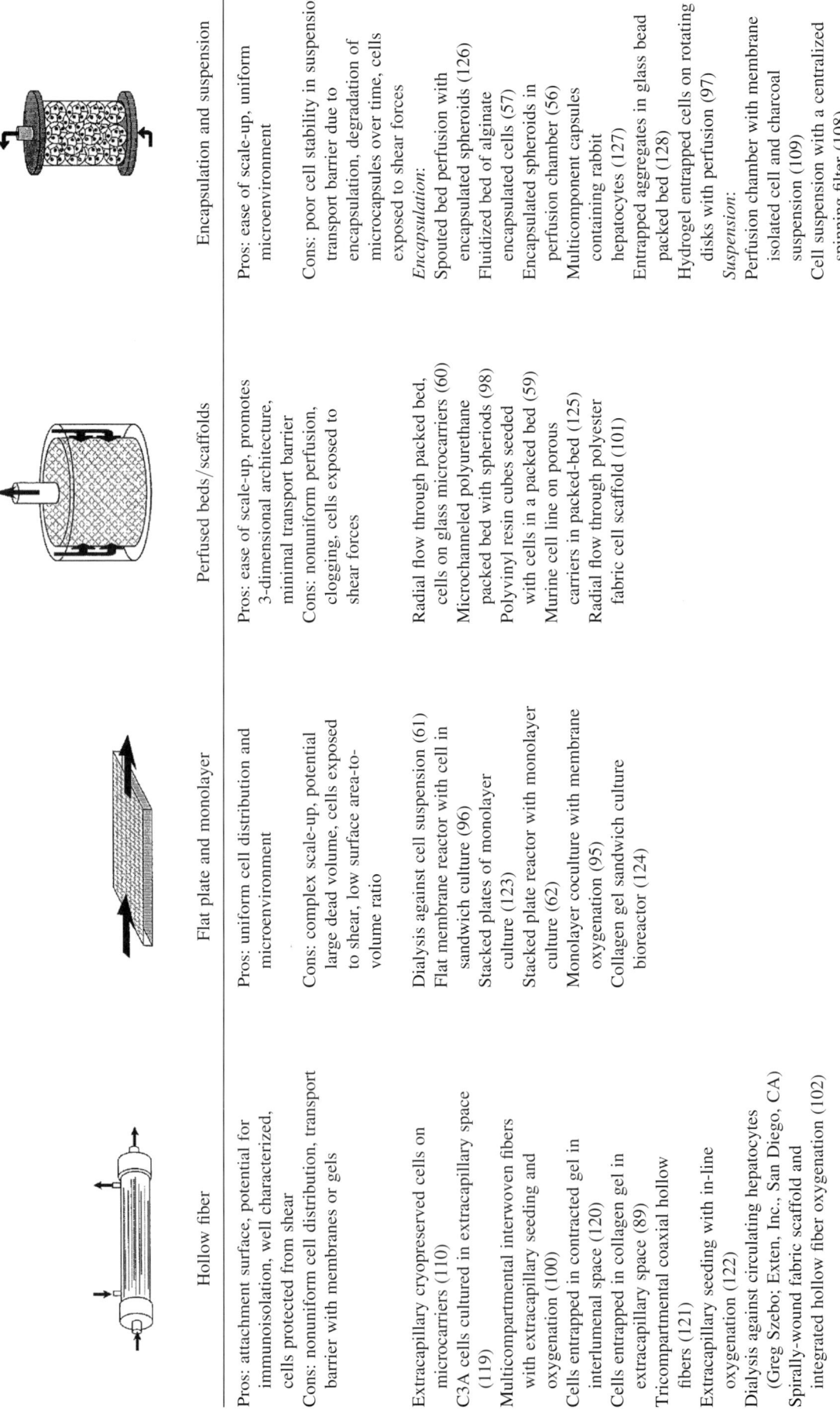

Hollow fiber	Flat plate and monolayer	Perfused beds/scaffolds	Encapsulation and suspension
Pros: attachment surface, potential for immunoisolation, well characterized, cells protected from shear	Pros: uniform cell distribution and microenvironment	Pros: ease of scale-up, promotes 3-dimensional architecture, minimal transport barrier	Pros: ease of scale-up, uniform microenvironment
Cons: nonuniform cell distribution, transport barrier with membranes or gels	Cons: complex scale-up, potential large dead volume, cells exposed to shear, low surface area-to-volume ratio	Cons: nonuniform perfusion, clogging, cells exposed to shear forces	Cons: poor cell stability in suspension, transport barrier due to encapsulation, degradation of microcapsules over time, cells exposed to shear forces
Extracapillary cryopreserved cells on microcarriers (110)	Dialysis against cell suspension (61)	Radial flow through packed bed, cells on glass microcarriers (60)	*Encapsulation:*
C3A cells cultured in extracapillary space (119)	Flat membrane reactor with cell in sandwich culture (96)	Microchanneled polyurethane packed bed with spheriods (98)	Spouted bed perfusion with encapsulated spheroids (126)
Multicompartmental interwoven fibers with extracapillary seeding and oxygenation (100)	Stacked plates of monolayer culture (123)	Polyvinyl resin cubes seeded with cells in a packed bed (59)	Fluidized bed of alginate encapsulated cells (57)
Cells entrapped in contracted gel in interlumenal space (120)	Stacked plate reactor with monolayer culture (62)	Murine cell line on porous carriers in packed-bed (125)	Encapsulated spheroids in perfusion chamber (56)
Cells entrapped in collagen gel in extracapillary space (89)	Monolayer coculture with membrane oxygenation (95)	Radial flow through polyester fabric cell scaffold (101)	Multicomponent capsules containing rabbit hepatocytes (127)
Tricompartmental coaxial hollow fibers (121)	Collagen gel sandwich culture bioreactor (124)		Entrapped aggregates in glass bead packed bed (128)
Extracapillary seeding with in-line oxygenation (122)			Hydrogel entrapped cells on rotating disks with perfusion (97)
Dialysis against circulating hepatocytes (Greg Szebo; Exten, Inc., San Diego, CA)			*Suspension:*
Spirally-wound fabric scaffold and integrated hollow fiber oxygenation (102)			Perfusion chamber with membrane isolated cell and charcoal suspension (109)
			Cell suspension with a centralized spinning filter (108)

Sourec: From Ref. 1.

Biliary Excretion Consideration

☞ **A continuing conundrum in current bioartificial liver designs is the universal absence of functional biliary excretion into an isolated compartment.** ☞ In current configurations, even primary hepatocytes that regain polarity in vitro (e.g., spheroids, coculture) excrete biliary constituents into the surrounding fluid, which then recirculate continuously. In this regard, addition of a nonbiological adjunct such as an albumin dialysis module may complement many existing bioartificial liver devices. In the long term, culture environments that promote a separate functional biliary compartment will greatly improve the design of these devices.

Oxygenation is key to hepatocyte function and may be suboptimal in current bioartificial liver devices (99–104). Hollow fiber compartments (100) or nonwoven fabric scaffolds (101) with fibers for gas delivery (102) may improve oxygen delivery. Geometric constraints also may affect mass transport in a bioartificial liver. Cell distribution and flow should be uniform. A single monolayer culture is easily perfused, but a series of stacked plates may introduce "shunting" through regions of low resistance. Hollow fiber devices present difficulty in achieving homogeneous cell distribution during inoculation through the tight matrix of capillaries. Uniform perfusion of packed-bed reactors is a classic engineering problem. Distribution of fluid flow is greatly dependent on the characteristic of the packing material. Larger, rigid particles will yield well-distributed flow but a decreased surface area for cells, while smaller, porous packing will result in clogging and fluid channeling (105). A packed bed reactor built around a microchanneled scaffold is an example of one designed explicitly to reduce heterogeneous perfusion and improve the transport characteristics of the devices (98).

Cell Viability and Function

☞ **One of the major obstacles to bioartificial liver offering long-term treatment is the inability to maintain highly functional hepatocytes in vitro.** ☞ Current device designs do very little to integrate an appropriate microenvironment for hepatocytes. Gel entrapment and use of spheroidal aggregates has been introduced into various membrane-based systems to provide chemical and topological ECM cues or cell–cell interaction; however, this introduces an additional diffusion barrier (56,89,106–108). Single cell suspensions, used in some devices because of their desirable transport properties, quickly lose metabolic capacity (109). Some packed bed designs (59,60) and one hollow-fiber device (110) seed cells on microcarriers before device assembly. While microcarriers provide a substrate for anchorage, data from hepatocyte cell culture suggests that these cells will likely detach in a few days and die as they do in monolayers. Along with providing adequate attachment, future devices should consider integrating engineering strategies for efficient transport with environments that optimize cell–ECM interactions, cell–cell interactions, and integrate relevant chemical stimuli.

Scale-Up

In order for a device to become a clinical reality, it must be scaled to a size that provides effective therapy. Studies indicate that between 10% and 30% of normal liver mass is needed to sustain life, which in adults, corresponds to 150 to 450 g of cells. Clinically tested devices incorporate between 1 g and 500 g of hepatocyte mass. The current solution for scaling up hollow fiber devices involves increasing cartridge size 101 and using multiple cartridges (112). Systems using spheroids or microcarriers are easily scaled to the needed cell mass but may entrain a considerable dead volume ("priming volume"). Flat or stacked plate designs raise similar concerns as well as the problem of heterogeneous flow distribution and channeling upon scale up.

Review of Recent Trials Evaluating Liver Support Systems

Experimental devices using suspended primary hepatocytes were some of the first to be used with human patients in the late 1980s, but have met with limited success (112,113). Presently, several hollow-fiber devices are under evaluation in clinical trials (Table 3). The most extensively tested device, the HepatAssist System from Circe Biomedical, recently completed phase II/III trials. The trial was the first prospective, randomized, controlled trial of a biological liver support system in patients with liver failure. It included 171 patients with either fulminant or subfulminant hepatic failure and primary graft nonfunction following liver transplantation. Eighty-five patients received bioartificial liver while 86 patients were controls. Their results showed 30-day survival of 71% for bioartificial liver versus 62% for control ($p = 0.26$). When survival was analyzed after accounting for the confounding factors (such as liver transplantation, time to transplant, disease etiology, disease severity, and treatment site), there was no difference between the two groups. However, survival in the fulminant/subfulminant liver failure patients was significantly higher in the bioartificial liver group compared with the control ($p = 0.048$). Though an examination of study subpopulations and secondary endpoints shows moderate benefit, a conclusive measure of efficacy is confounded by factors such as transplantation, disease etiology, and stage of encephalopathy. Critical evaluation of the complete results of the HepatAssist trial should provide valuable insight for future large-scale clinical studies (114). Careful consideration needs to be given to treatment indications, clinical end points, and device regulation in clinical trial design so that clear evidence of treatment efficacy may be established. Ongoing clinical experience with extracorporeal support will likely play a key role in the improvement of next generation devices.

EYE TO THE FUTURE

A difficulty that arises when examining the current clinical data is the inability to determine the role of live, functional hepatocytes as opposed to extracorporeal perfusion itself, given that some bioartificial liver designs incorporate charcoal filtration. Ideally, a protective comparison should be made between charcoal filtration alone, dead or nonhepatocyte cells, and live hepatocytes given that nonhepatocytes and dead hepatocytes provided survival benefit in some animal models of ALF (115).

Also inherent in the present data are a number of practical issues: Are the cells fresh or frozen? Should the device be perfused with plasma or whole blood? What is the role of heparin versus citrate anticoagulation? These issues are critical both for patient well-being and for survival of hepatocytes in the device. The limited function of cryopreserved hepatocytes has been well-documented, yet

Table 3 Current Clinical Trials of Extracorporeal Support Devices

Company	Indication—no. of patients	% Recovery[a]	Average bridge—hours[b]	Device	Phase	Comments
Biological devices						
Vaital Therapies (ELAD)	FHF (25)	Dbd			Chinese Trials 2006 US III 2006	C3A cell line, continuous treatment up to 10 days, ultrafiltrate perfusion, 150–300 mL/min, heparin, 4 replicable cartridges, cell mass: 4 × 200 g (70, 29, 130, 138)
Vitagen (ELAD) Hepatix (1991–1996) (ELAD)	FHF (25) FHF (23)	92% OLT/NR 54% OLT/NR	NA 56hrs	Sussman et al. (119)	I/II multicenter	
Circe Biomedical (HepatAssist®)	FHF (36) AoC (10) PNF (3)	80%OLT/NR 20% OLT 100% OLT	45hrs 89hrs 83hrs	Rozga et al. (110)	II/III multicenter	Cryopreserved porcine, treatment 3–6 for 1–5 days, 400 mL/min, citrate, charcoal column, centrifugal plasmapheresis, cell mass: 50 g (131,132)
Algenix (LIVERx 2000®)	FHF, Grade II	—	—	Nyberg et al. (120)	I 1 center	Primary porcine, whole blood perfusion, heparin anticoagulation, cell mass: 70 g
Excorp Medical (BLSS)	FHF (2) AoC (3)	50% OLT 33% OLT	NA	Patzer et al. (122)	I 1 center	Primary porcine, treatment 6–30, whole blood perfusion, heparin anticoagulation cell mass: 100 g
Charite Virchow Clinic–Berlin (MELS)	FHF (8) AoC	100% OLT	27hrs	Gerlach et al. (100)	I/II multicenter	Primary porcine, continuous treatment up to 3 days, filtration plasmapheresis, 100mL/min, heparin anticoagulation, cell mass: 500 g
Nonbiological devices						
Teraklin (MARS)	AoC (64) FHF (12) PNF (14) Other (13)	~70% OLT/NR	NA	Stange et al. (133)	I/II/II CE approved multicenter	Dialysis against recycle albumin, 6 treatments over 2–14 days, heparin anticoagulation (134, 135)
HemoTherapies (BioLogic-DT)	FHF (39) AoC (71)	56% OLT/NR 77% OLT/NR	NA	Ash et al. (136)	FDA-approved multicenter	Dialysis against charcoal suspension, treatment 2–6 hours for 2–5 consecutive days, 200–250mL/min, heparin anticoagulation (137)

[a]Percent survival with OLT or without.
[b]Time between initial treatment and OLT.
Abbreviations: FHF, fulminant hepatic failure; AoC, acute on chronic; FHF, fulminant hepatic failure; OLT, orthotopic liver transplantation; PNF, primary nonfunction; NA, not available; NR, native recovery.
Source: From Ref. 1.

ryopreservation offers flexibility in timing and scheduling of therapies (117).

The use of whole blood has the advantage of erythrocytes as oxygen-delivery vehicles for the bioartificial liver, although leukocyte activation and cell damage may occur. Conversely, plasmapheresis and plasma perfusion preserve the viability of hematopoietic cells, yet the solubility of oxygen in plasma is very low. Similarly, heparin anticoagulation has been shown in some studies to cause lipid accumulation and deleterious effect on otherwise phenotypically stable hepatocytes (117). Each group has grappled with these trade-offs, and the outcome remains to be seen. Even if these trials do not prove the efficacy of bioartificial liver devices, the knowledge gained along with future improvements in cell sourcing and stability will positively impact the next generation of devices.

In a recent review of all published data by the Cochrane Group, it was concluded that artificial support systems reduce mortality in acute-on-chronic liver failure compared with standard medical therapy; however, artificial and bioartificial support systems so far did not appear to affect mortality in acute liver failure. Hence, randomized trials on artificial or bioartificial support systems versus standard medical therapy for liver failure are still required (118).

Recently the ELAD® (Extracorporeal Liver Assist Device®)—Vital Therapies, Inc (San Diego, CA, USA) received US Federal Drug Administration (FDA) approval to ship units to China for clinical trials beginning in early 2006. The ELAD® system comprises four cartridges containing cloned human hepatocytes of the C3A cell line. Each of the four cartridges serves as a hollow fiber membrane bioreactor.

These cells function like normal human liver cells metabolizing toxins, removing waste products, and producing essential proteins that enter the plasma. The cartridges are incorporated into a blood pumping system and provide continuous treatment for up to 12 days.

Vital Therapies Inc. has completed phase I & II trails in the US and will start phase III trials in the US in 2007 after the clinical trails commencing in China (138).

SUMMARY

The liver is an essential organ that cannot currently be supported for long when failure occurs. The numerous roles of the liver including synthetic, metabolic, detoxification, and biliary excretion constitute one hurdle in developing a viable artificial liver. Other hurdles are technical in nature and relate to maintaining hepatocytes stabilized within artificial perfusion chambers ensuring viability of cells and the ongoing bidirectional mass transfer of nutrients and hepatocyte products, as well as the ability to handle bile production and excretion. Although numerous obstacles remain, solutions to these problems are being approached in numerous research laboratories around the globe.

Our prediction is that the next decade will see bioartificial liver therapies becoming more commonplace, though the solution to total compatibility and portability is still sometime off into the future.

ACKNOWLEDGMENTS

SNB thanks Jared Allen for his contribution to the review of cell-based systems and NIDDK for financial support.

KEY POINTS

- Certain hepatic injuries affect specific zones.
- The liver is a complex metabolic factory (biochemical reactor) and performs a number of other functions including protein synthesis, immuno protection and bile formation related tasks.
- The most common cause of acute liver failure is drug-related hepatotoxicity, which comprises more than 50% of acute cases.
- Liver failure is associated with a significant compromise of metabolic regulation, protein synthesis, detoxification and immunological defense mechanisms executed by the liver.
- Hemoperfusion using activated charcoal was shown to have beneficial effects in patients with severe poisoning.
- Hemodiadsorption is "a process during which blood passes through dialysis membrane packages surrounded by a suspension of fine sorbent particles."
- A number of Extra-Corporeal Albumin Dialysis (ECAD) devices have been introduced in the last decade, and preliminary data demonstrate that these can be used as support systems for the failing liver or as a bridge to transplantation in selected patients.
- Fractional plasma separation and adsorption (FPSA) is a form of albumin dialysis in which a filter with a cutoff of 250,000 Dalton (250KD) is used.
- The most common cell-based liver support design incorporates hepatocytes in hollow fiber cartridges borrowed from hemodialysis.
- Although primary hepatocytes represent the most direct approach to replacing liver function in hepatic failure, they are anchorage-dependent cells and notoriously difficult to maintain in vitro.
- There are four main types of hepatic bioreactors, each with inherent advantages and disadvantages: hollow fiber, flat plate and monolayer, perfused beds or scaffolds, and beds with encapsulated or suspended cells.
- A continuing conundrum in current bioartificial liver designs is the universal absence of functional biliary excretion into an isolated compartment.
- One of the major obstacles to bioartificial liver offering long-term treatment is the inability to maintain highly functional hepatocytes in vitro.

REFERENCES

1. Allen JW, Hassanein T, Bhatia SN. Advances in bioartificial liver devices. Hepatology 2001; 34(3):447–455.
2. Patzer RF. Advances in bioartifical liver assist devices. Ann N Y Acad Sci 2001; 944:320–333.
3. Bertani H, Gelmini R, Del Buono MG, et al. Literature overview on artificial liver support in fulminant hepatic failure: a methodological approach. Int J Artif Organs 2002; 903–910.
4. Portmann BC. Anatomy of the normal liver. In: OGrady, Lake, Howdle, ed. Comprehensive Clinical Hepatology. London: Mosby, 2000:1–1.14.
5. Desmet VJ. Organizational Principles in the Liver: Biology and Pathobiology. 3rd ed. New York: Raven Press Ltd, 1994:3–11.
6. Gressner AM. The cell biology of liver fibrogenesis an imbalance of proliferation, growth arrest and apoptosis of myofibroblasts. Cell Tissue Res 1998; 292:447–452.
7. Bouwens L, DeBless P, VenderKerken K, et al. Liver cell heterogenicity: functions of non-parenchymal cells. Enzyme 1992; 46:155–168.

8. Vale JA, Rees AJ, Widdop B, Goulding R. Use of charcoal haemoperfusion in the management of severely poisoned patients. BMJ 1975; I:5–9.

9. Mosely RH. Function of the normal liver. In: OGrady, Lake, Howdle, ed. Comprehensive Clinical Hepatology. London: Mosby, 2000:3.1–3.16.

10. Ostapowicz G, Fontana RF, Schindt EV, et al. Results of a prospective study of acute liver failure at 17 tertiary care centers in the United States. Ann Intern Med 2002; 137:947–954.

11. Jalan R, Williams R. Acute-on-chronic liver failure: pathophysiological basis of therapeutic options. Blood Purif 2002; 20:252–261.

12. Lee, WM, Schiodt FV. Fulminant hepatic failure. In: Schiff ER, Sorrell MF, Maddrey WC, eds. Schiffs Diseases of the Liver. Philadelphia: Lippincott-Raven, 1999:879–895.

13. Lee C, Tink A. Exchange transfusion in hepatic coma: report of a case. Med J Aust 1958; 45:40–42.

14. Trey C, Burns PG, Saunders SJ. Treatment of hepatic coma by exchange blood transfusion. N Engl J Med 1996; 274:473–481.

15. Bioartificail livertzer G, Dölle W, Bär, Becker K, Clodic PH. Austauschtransfusion bei akuten Leberversagen. Dtsch med Wschr 1971; 96:1329–1333.

16. Williams R. Treatment of fulminant hepatic failure. Clinical syndroma and basis of therapy. BMJ 1971; I:213–215.

17. Fiasse R, Collignon R, Bietlot A, et al. Le traitement des hépatites fulminates avec coma par exanguino- transfusions. Etude de neuf patients dont l'un a présenté des séqulles neruologiques au niveau des fonctions corticales. Acta gastro-ent Belg 1974; 37:12–39.

18. Buckner CD, Clift RA, Volwiler W, et al. Plasma exchange in patients with fulminant hepatic failure. Arch intern Med 1973; 132:487–492.

19. Cree JO, Berger SA. Plasmapheresis and positive-pressure ventilation in hepatic coma with respiratory arrest. Lancet 1968; II:976–977.

20. Strain AJ, Ismail T, Tsubouchi H, et al. Native and recombinant human hepatocyte growth factors are highly potent promoters of DNA synthesis in both human and rat hepatocytes. J Clin Invest 1991; 87:1853–1857.

21. Lindroos, PM, Zarnegar R, Michalopoulos GK. Hepatic growth factor (hepatopoietin A) rapidely increases in plasma before DNA synthesis and liver regeneration stimulated by partial hepatectomy and carbon tetrachloride administration. Hepatology 1991; 13:743–750.

22. Yamazaki Z, Kani F, Idezuki Y, Inoue N. Extracorporeal methods of liver failure treatment. Biomater Artif Cells Artif Organs 1987; 15:667–675.

23. Kaihara S, Vacanti JP. Tissue engineering—Toward new solutions for transplantation and reconstructive surgery. Arch Surg 1999; 134:1184–1188.

24. Klebanoff G, Hollander D, Cosimi B, et al. Asanguineous hypothermic total body perfusion (TBW) in the treatment of stage IV hepatic coma. J Surg Res 1972; 12:1–7.

25. Klebanoff G. Early experience with total body washout for hepatic coma. Gastroenterology 1973; 64:156.

26. Tobias H, Isom W. Total body perfusion in the treatment of hepatic coma secondary to fulminant hepatitis. Gastroenterol 1973; 64:157.

27. Chang TMS. Hemoperfusions over microencapsulated adsorbent in a patient with hepatic coma. Lancet 1972; II:1371–1372.

28. Gazzard BG, Portman B, Weston MJ, et al. Charcoal hemoperfusion in the treatment of fulminant hepatic failure. Lancet 1974; I:1301–1307.

29. OGrady JG, Gimson AES, OBrien CJ, et al. Controlled trials of charcoal hemoperfusion and prognostic factors in fulminant hepatic failure. Gastroenterol 1988; 94:1186–1192.

30. Weston MJ, Gazzard BG, Buxton BH, et al. Effects of haemoperfusion through charcoal or XAD-2 resin on an animal model of fulminant liver failure. Gut 1974; 15:482–486.

31. Willson RA, Hofman AF, Kuster GGR. Towards an artificial liver: II. Removal of cholephilic anions from dogs with biliary obstruction by haemoperfusion through charged and uncharged resins. Gastroenterol 1974; 66:93–107.

32. Weston MJ, Mellon PJ, Langley PG, et al. Biocompatibility of resins in relation to the use of the celltrifuge. In: Williams R, Murray-Lyon IM, eds. Artificial Liver Support. London: Pitman Medical Publishing Co., 1975:127–133.

33. Kiley JE, Welch H, Pender J. Removal of blood ammonia by hemodialysis. Proc Soc Exp Biol Med 1956; 91:489.

34. Silk DBA, William R. Experiences in the treatment of fulminant hepatic failure by conservative therapy, charcoal haemoperfusion and polyacrylonitrile haemodialysis. Internat J Artif Org 1978; 1:29–33.

35. Denis J, Opolon P, Nusinovici V, et al. Treatment of encephalopathy during fuminant hepatic failure by haemodialysis with high permeability membrane. Gut 1978; 78:87–793.

36. Opolon P. Large-pore hemodialysis in fulminant hepatic. In: Brunner G, Schmidt FW, eds. Artificial Liver Support. New York: Springer, Berlin, Heidelberg, 1981:41–146.

37. Ash SR. Hemodiabsorption in treatment of acute hepatic failure and chronic cirrhosis with ascites. Artif Organs 1994:355–362.

38. Ash SR, Blake DE, Carr DJ, et al. Clinical effects of a sorbent suspension dialysis system in the treatment of hepatic coma (the BioLogic-DT). Internat J Artif Organs 1992; 15:151–161.

39. Khanna HJ, Glenn JG, Klein MD, Matthew HWT. Polysaccharide scaffolds for hepatocyte transplantation: Design, seeding, and functional evaluation. Tissue Eng 2000; 6:670.

40. Konstantin P, Chang J, Otto V, Brunner G. Artificial liver. Artif Organs 1992; 16:235–242.

41. Konstantin P, Chang J, Otto V, Brunner G. Artificial liver support. Blood Purif 1992; 10:103.

42. Stange J, Mitzner S, Ramlow W, et al. A new procedure for the removal of protein bound drugs and toxins. ASAIO J 1993; 39:M621–M625.

43. Falkenhagen D, Strobl W, Vogt G, et al. Fractionated plasma separation and adsorption system: a novel system for blood purification to remove albumin bound substances. Artif Organs 1999; 231:81–86.

44. Rifai K, Ernst T, Kretschmer U, et al. Prometheus—a new extracorporeal system for the treatment of liver failure. J Hepatol 2003; 39:984–990.

45. Burnell GM, Thomas ED, Ansell JS, et al. Observations on cross-circulation in man. Am J Med 1965; 38:832–841.

46. Muller JM, Guignier M, Cordonnier D. Behandlung von komatösen Kranken mittels gekreuztem Kreislauf MMW 1969; 111:1827–1828.

47. Lie TS. Die extrakorporale Vitalleberperfusion zur Behandlung des akuten Leberversagens. Med Klin 1978; 73(4):124–129.

48. Zipprich B. Möglichkeiten und Grenzen des temporären Leberersatzes. Anaesth u Reanimation 1981; suppl 5:103–128.

49. Abouna GM. Cross-circulation between man and baboon in hepatic coma. Lancet 1968; II:729–730.

50. Hume DM, Gayle WE, Williams GM. Cross circulation of patients in hepatic coma with baboon partners having human blood. Surg Gynecol Obst 1969; 128:495–517.

51. Saunders SJ, Terblanche J, Bosman SCW, et al. Acute hepatic coma treated by cross-circulation with a baboon and by repeated exchange transfusions. Lancet 1968; II:585–588.

52. Tunk LC. Erfahrungen ber die Behandlung des akuten Leberversagens mit extrakorporaler Schweineleberperfusion. In: Eckert P, Liehr H, Hrsg. Intensivmed Notfallmed Anaesthesiol, Stuttgart-New York: Thieme, 1981; Bd25:25–28.

53. Zipprich B, Nilius R, Baust G, et al. Untersuchungen zur Funktionstchtigkeit mit Humanblut perfundierter Schweinelebern im maschinellen Rezirkulationsversuch. Zschr Inn Med 1976; 31(11):364–373.

54. Fischer M, Bottermann P. Extrakorporale Perfusion mit Pavianlebern zur Behandlung des Leberzerfallskomas. Dtsch med Wschr 1977; 102:1862.

55. Lie TS, Dengler HJ, Gutgemann A, et al. Die extrakorporale Perfusion mit Pavianlebern zur Behandlung des Leberzerfallskomas. Dtsch med Wschr 1977; 102:1506–1511.

56. Dixit V, Gitnick G. The bioartificial liver: state-of-the-art. Eur J Surg Suppl 1998; 36:71–76.

57. Doré, Legallais C. A new concept of bioartificial liver based on a fluidized bed bioreactor. Ther Apher 1999; 3:264–267.

58. Theise ND, Badve S, Saxena R, et al. Derivation of hepatocytes from bone marrow cells in mice after radiation-induced myeloablation. Hepatology 2000; 31:235–240.
59. Yanagi K, Miyoshi H, Ohshima N. Improvement of metabolic performance of hepatocytes cultured in vitro in a packed-bed reactor for use as a bioartificial liver. Asaio J 1998; 44:M436–M440.
60. Kawada M, Nagamori S, Aizaki H, et al. Massive culture of human liver cancer cells in a newly developed radial flow bioreactor system: ultrafine structure of functionally enhanced hepatocarcinoma cell lines. In vitro Cell Dev Biol Anim 1998; 34:109–115.
61. Matsumura KN, Guevara GR, Huston H, et al. Hybrid bioartificial liver in hepatic failure: preliminary clinical report. Surgery 1987; 101:99–103.
62. Uchino J, Tsuburaya T, Kumagai F, et al. A hybrid bioartificial liver composed of multiplated hepatocyte monolayers. ASAIO Trans 1988; 34:972–977.
63. Roger V, Ladur P, Honiger J, et al. Internal bioartificial liver with xenogeneic hepatocytes prevents death from acute liver failure: an experimental study. Ann Surg 1998; 228:1–7.
64. Strom SC, Fisher RA, Rubinstein WS, et al. Transplantation of human hepatocytes. Transplant Proc 1997; 29:2103–2106.
65. Tateno C, Takai-Kajihara K, Yamasaki C, et al. Heterogeneity of growth potential of adult rat hepatocytes in vitro. Hepatology 2000; 31:65–74.
66. Mitaka T. The current status of primary hepatocyte culture. Int J Exp Pathol 1998; 79:393–409.
67. Block GD, Locker J, Bowen WC, et al. Population expansion, clonal growth, and specific differentiation patterns in primary cultures of hepatocytes induced by hgf/sf, egf and tgf-alpha in a chemically defined (hgm) Medium. J Cell Biol 1996; 132:1133–1149.
68. Kodama S, Mori I, Roy K, et al. Culture condition-dependent senescence-like growth arrest and immortalization in rodent embryo cells. Radiat Res 2001; 55:254–262.
69. Kono Y, Yang SY, Letarte M, Roberts EA. Establishment of a human hepatocyte line derived from primary culture in a collagen sandwich culture system. Exp Cell Res 1995; 221:478–485.
70. Sussman NL, Gislason GT, Conlin CA, Kelly JH. The hepatix extracorporeal liver assist device—initial clinical experience. Artif Organs 1994; 18:390–396.
71. Yanai N, Suzuki M, Obinata M. Hepatocyte cell lines established from transgenic mice harboring temperature-sensitive simian Virus-40 large T-antigen gene. Exp Cell Res 1991; 197:50–56.
72. Kobayashi N, Noguchi H, Fujiwara T, Tanaka N. Establishment of a reversibly immortalized human hepatocyte cell line by using Cre/LoxP site-specific recombination. Transplant Proc 2000; 32:1121–1122.
73. Cai J, Ito M, Westerman KA, et al. Construction of a non-tumorigenic rat hepatocyte cell line for transplantation: reversal of hepatocyte immortalization by site-specific excision of the SV40 T antigen. J Hepatol 2000; 33:701–708.
74. Thomson JA, ItskovitzEldor J, Shapiro SS, et al. Embryonic stem cell lines derived from human blastocytes. Science 1998; 282:1145–1147.
75. Shamblott MJ, Axelman J, Wang SP, Bugg EM, Littlefield JW, et al. Derivation of pluripotent stem cells horn cultured human primordial germ cells. Proc Natl Acad Sci USA 1998; 95:13726–13731.
76. Petersen BE, Zajac VF, Michalopoulos GK. Hepatic oval cell activation in response to injury following chemically induced periportal or pericentral damage in rats. Hepatology 1998; 27:1030–1038.
77. Love W. Incara Pharmaceuticals. January 10, 2001.
78. Agelli M, DelloSbarba P, Halay ED, et al. Putative liver progenitor cells: conditions for long-term survival in culture. Histochem J 1997; 29:205–217.
79. Brill S, Zvibel I, Reid LM. Expansion conditions for early hepatic progenitor cells from embryonal and neonatal rat livers. Digest Dis Sci 1999; 44:364–371.
80. Kubota H, Reid LM. Clonogenic hepatoblasts, common precursors for hepatocytic and biliary lineages, are lacking classical major histocompatibility complex class I antigen. Proc Natl Acad Sci USA 2000; 97:12132–12137.
81. Thorgeirsson SS. Hepatic stem cells in liver regeneration. FASEB J 1996; 10:1249–1256.
82. Rudolph KL, Chang S, Millard M, et al. Inhibition of experimental liver cirrhosis in mice by telomerase gene delivery. Science 2000; 287:1253–1258.
83. Michalopoulos G, Pitot HC. Primary culture of parenchymal liver cells on collagen membranes. Morphological and biochemical observations. Exp Cell Res 1975; 94:70–78.
84. Bissel DM, Arenson DM, Maher JJ, Roll FJ. Support of cultured hepatocytes by a laminin-rich gel. Evidence for a functionally significant subendothelial matrix in normal rat liver. J Clin Invest 1987; 79:801–812.
85. Rojkind M, Gatmaitan Z, Mackensen S, et al. Connective tissue biomatrix: its isolation and utilization for long-term cultures of normal rat hepatocytes. J Cell Biol 1980; 87:255–263.
86. Landry J, Bernier D, Ouellet C, et al. Spheroidal aggregate culture of rat liver cells: histotypic reorganization, biomatrix deposition, and maintenance of functional activities. J Cell Biol 1985; 101:914–923.
87. Dunn JC, Tompkins RG, Yarmush ML. Long-term in vitro function of adult hepatocytes in a collagen sandwich configuration. Biotechnol Prog 1991; 7:237–245.
88. Akaike T, Tobe S, Kobayashi A, et al. Design of hepatocyte-specific extracelluler matrices for hybrid artificial liver. Gastroenterol Jpn 1993; 28(suppl):45–56.
89. Naka S, Takeshita K, Yamamoto T, et al. Bioartificial liver support system using porcine hepatocyte entrapped in a three-dimensional hollow fiber module with collagen gel: an evaluation in the swine acute liver failure model. Artif Organs 1999; 23:822–828.
90. Suzuki M, Takeshita K, Yamamoto T, et al. Hepatocyte entrapped in collagen gel following 14 days of storage at 4 degrees C: preservation of hybrid artificial liver. Artif Organs 1997; 21:99–106.
91. Dich J, Vind C, Grunnet N. Long-term culture of hepatocytes: effect of hormones on enzyme activities and metabolic capacity. Hepatology 1988; 8:39–45.
92. Isom HC, Secott T, Georgoff I, et al. Maintenance of differentiated rat hepatocyte in primary culture. Proc Natl Acad Sci USA 1985; 82:3252–3256.
93. Berry M, Edwards A, Barritt G. Monolayer culture of hepatocytes. Isolated hepatocytes. Preparation, properties, and application. Amsterdam:Elsevier, 1991; 265–354.
94. Bhatia SN, Yarmush ML, Toner M. Effect of cell–cell interactions in preservation of cellular phenotype: Cocultivation of hepatocytes and nonparenchymal cells. FASEB J 1999; 13:1883–1900.
95. Tilles AW, Balis UJ, Baskaran H, et al. Internal membrane oxygenation removes substrate oxygen limitations in a small-scale hepatocyte bioreactor. In: Proceedings of Tissue Engineering Therapeutic Uses. Tokyo, Japan: Elsevier, 2001:76–91.
96. De Bartolo L, Jarosch-Von Schweder G, Haverich A, Bader A. A novel full-scale flat membrane bioreactor utilizing porcine hepatocytes: cell viability and tissue-specific functions. Biotechnol Prog 2000; 16:102–108.
97. Yanagi K, Ookawa K, Mizuno S, Ohshima N. Performance of a new hybrid artificial liver support system using hepatocyte entrapped within a hydrogel. ASAIO Trans 1989; 35:570–572.
98. Gion T, Shimada M, Shirabe K, et al. Evaluation of a hybrid artificial liver using a polyurethane foam packed-Bed culture system in dogs. J Surg Res 1999; 82:131–136.
99. Hay PD, Veitch AR, Smith MD, et al. Oxygen transfer in a diffusion-limited hollow fiber bioartificial liver. Artif Organs 2000; 24:278–288.
100. Gerlach JC, Encke J, Hole O, et al. Bioreactor for a large scale hepatocyte in vitro perfusion. Transplantation 1994; 58:984–988.
101. Naruse K, Sakai Y, Nagashima I, et al. Development of a new bioartificial liver module filled with porcine hepatocytes

immobilized on non-woven fabric. Int J Artif Organ 1996; 19:347–352.

102. Flendrig LM, IaSoe JW, Jorning GGA, et al. In vitro evaluation of a novel bioreactor based on an integral oxygenator and a spirally wound nonwoven polyester matrix for hepatocyte culture as small aggregates. J Hepatol 1997; 26:1379–1392.

103. Jungermann K, Kietzmann T. Oxygen: modulator of metabolic zonation and disease of the liver. Hepatology 2000; 31:255–260.

104. Bhatia SN, Toner M, Foy BD, et al. Zonal liver cell heterogeneity: Effects of oxygen on metabolic functions of hepatocytes. Cell Eng 1996; 1:125–135.

105. Doran PM. Bioprocess Engineering Principles. London: Academic Press, 1995; 349.

106. Nyberg SL, Peshwa MV, Panye WD, et al. Evolution of the bioartificial liver: the need for randomized clinical trails. Am J Surg 1993; 166:512–521.

107. Bader A, Knop E, Boker K, et al. A novel bioreactor design for in vitro reconstruction of in vivo liver characteristics. Artif Organs 1995; 19(4):368–374.

108. Sakai Y, Naruse K, Nagashima I, et al. A new bioartificial liver using porcine hepatocyte spheroids in high-cell-density suspension perfusion culture: in vitro performance in synthesized culture medium and in 100% human plasma. Cell Transplant 1999; 8:531–541.

109. Margulis MS, Erukhimov EA, Andreiman LA, Viksna LM. Temporary organ substitution by hemoperfusion through suspension of active hepatocyte in a total complex of intensive therphy in patients with acute hepatic insufficiency. Resuscitation 1989; 18:85–94.

110. Rozga J, Podesta L, Lepage E, et al. A bioartificial liver to treat severe acute liver failure. Ann Surg 1994; 219:538–546.

111. Maguire PJ, Stevens C, Shander A, et al. Bioartificial organ support for hepatic, renal, and hematologic failure. Crit Care Clin 2000; 16:681–694.

112. Margulis MS, Erukhimov EA, Andreiman LA, Viksna LM. Temporary organ substitution by hemoperfusion through suspension of active donor hepatocytes in a total complex of intensive therapy in patients with acute hepatic insufficiency. Resuscitation 1989; 18:85–94.

113. Matsumura KN, Guevara GR, Hutson H, et al. Hybrid bioartificial liver in hepatic failure: preliminary clinical report. Surgery 1987; 101:99–103.

114. Demetrious AA, Brown RS Jr, Busuttil RW, et al. Prospective, randomized, multicenter, controlled trail of a bioartificial liver in treating acute liver failure. Ann Surg 2004; 239(5):660–670.

115. Makowka L, Rotstein LE, Falk RE, et al. Reversal of toxic and anoxic induced hepatic failure by syngeneic, allogeneic, and xenogeneic hepatocyte transplantation. Surgery 1980; 88:244–253.

116. Hengstler JG, Utesch D, Steinberg P, et al. Cryopreserved primary hepatocytes as a constantly available in vitro model for the evaluation of human and animal drug metabolism and enzyme induction. Drug Metab Rev 2000; 32:81–118.

117. Matthew HWT, Sternberg J, Stefanovich P, et al. Effects of plasma exposure on cultured hepatocytes—implications for bioartificial liver support. Biotechnol Bioeng 1996; 51:100–111.

118. Liu JP, Gluud LL, Als-Nielson B, Gluud C. Artificial and bioartificial support systems for liver failure. The Cochrane Database of Systematic Reviews 2004, Issue 1. Art. No.: CD003628.pub2. DOI: 10.1002/14651858.CD003628.pub2.

119. Sussman NL, Gislason GT, Kelly JH. Extracorporeal liver support. Application to fulminant hepatic failure. J Clin Gastroenterol 1994; 18:320–324.

120. Nyberg SL, Shirabe K, Peshwa MV, et al. Extracorporeal application of a gel-entrapment, bioartificial liver: demonstration of drug metabolism and other biochemical functions. Cell Transplant 1993; 2:441–452.

121. Macdonald JM, Grillo M, Schmidlin O, Tajiri DT, James TL. NMR spectroscopy and MRI investigation of a potential bioartificial liver. Nmr Biomed 1998; 11:55–66.

122. Patzer JF II, Mazariegos GV, Lopez R, et al. Novel bioartificial liver support system: preclinical evaluation. Ann NY Acad Sci 1999; 875:340–352.

123. Sheil AGR, Sun J, Wang L, et al. Biodialysis: a new liver support system. Transplant Proc 1999; 31:3258–3259.

124. Taguchi K, Matasushita M, Takahashi M, Uchino J. Development of a bioartificial liver with sandwiched-cultured hepatocytes between two collagen gel layers. Artif Organs 1996; 20:178–185.

125. Fassnacht D, Roessing S, Stange J, Poertner R. Long-term cultivation of immortalised mouse hepatocytes in a high cell density, fixed-bed reactor. Biotechnol Tech 1998; 12:25–30.

126. Takabatake H, Koide N, Tsuji T. Encapsulated multicellular spheroids of rat hepatocytes produce albumin and urea in a spouted bed circulating culture system. Artif Organs 1991; 15:474–480.

127. Matthew HWT, Basu S, Peterson WD, et al. Performance of plasma-perfused, microencapsulated hepatocytes—prospects for extracorporeal liver support. J Pediatr Surg 1993; 28:1423–1428.

128. Li AP, Barker G, Beck D, et al. Culturing of primary hepocytes as entrapped aggregates in a packed bed bioreactor: a potential bioartificial liver. In vitro Cell Dev Biol 1993; 29A:249–254.

129. Millis JM, Maguire PJ, Cronin HC, et al. Contiuous human liver support as a bridge to transplantation. Hepatology 1999; 30:168A.

130. Ellis AJ, Hughes RD, Wendon JA, et al. Pilot-controlled trial of the extracorporeal liver assist device in acute liver failure. Hepatology 1996; 24:1446–1451.

131. Demetriou AA. Clinical experience with a bioartificial liver in the treatment of severe liver failure: a phase I clinical trial—discussion. Ann Surg 1997; 225:493–494.

132. Mullon C, Pitkin Z. The hepat assist bioartificial liver support system: clinical study and pig hepatocyte process. Exp Opin Invest Drugs 1999; 8:229–235.

133. Stange J, Ramlow W, Mitzner S, et al. Dialysis against a recycled albumin solution enables the removal of albumin-bound toxins. Artif Organs 1993; 17:809–813.

134. Stange J, Mitzner SR, Risler T, et al. Molecular adsorbent recycling system (MARS): clinical results of a new membrane-based blood purification system for bioartificial liver support, Artif Organs 1999; 23:319–330.

135. Stange J, Hassanein T, Mehta R, et al. The molecular Adsorbents Recycling System (MARS) as a liver support system based on albumin dialysis—a summary of preclinical investigations, prospective, randomized, controlled clinical trial and clinical experience from 19 centers. Arif Organs 2002; 26:103–110.

136. Ash SR, Blake DE, Carr DJ, et al. Clinical effects of a sorbent suspension dialysis system in treatment of hepatic coma (the Biologic-Dt). Int J Artif Organs 1992; 15:151–161.

137. Ash S, Kuczek T, Foster D, et al. Liver dialysis in treatment of hepatic failure and hepatorenal failure: randomized clinical trails and recent improvements. Int J Artif Organs 2000; 23:534.

138. Vital Therapies Inc. web site. http://www.vitaltherapies.com/ Accessed March 16, 2006.

139. Wigg AJ, Padburg PT. Liver support systems: Promise and reality. J Gastroenterol Hiepatol 2000; 20:1807–1816.

39

Acute Pancreatitis and Pancreatic Injuries

Matthew H. Katz, A. R. Moossa, and Michael Bouvet

Department of Surgery, UC San Diego Medical Center, San Diego, California, U.S.A.

INTRODUCTION

Acute pancreatitis and trauma to the pancreas can result in varying degrees of secondary injuries due to pancreatic and peripancreatic inflammatory processes. Patients with acute pancreatitis may have a mild form of the disease, which is associated with minimal organ dysfunction, and they typically undergo a rapid, uneventful recovery. Others may acquire a severe, necrotizing pancreatitis characterized by glandular necrosis and infection in association with failure of multiple organ systems, requiring weeks of treatment in the intensive care unit (ICU). Similarly, patients with pancreatic trauma may have a simple pancreatic contusion, which can be treated nonoperatively, or a severe pancreatic ductal disruption with associated injury to the duodenum or other vital structures requiring immediate surgery and prolonged hospitalization. While mild pancreatic inflammation and injury are easily treated and carry a low rate of morbidity and mortality, fulminant pancreatic disease can be catastrophic and is associated with mortality rates up to 50% despite maximal medical and surgical therapy. It is an essential clinical challenge, therefore, not only to diagnose patients with these diseases, but also to rapidly identify that subset of patients with severe disease that will require management in the ICU and/or surgical treatment.

PANCREATIC ANATOMY AND BASIC PHYSIOLOGY
Anatomy
Surgical Anatomy and Related Structures
The pancreas is a soft, tan gland that weighs from 60 to 100 grams and measures approximately 12 to 15 centimeters long (1). It lies transversely in the retroperitoneum of the upper abdomen, at approximately the level of vertebrae L1 to L3, and has some of the most complex anatomical relationships in the human body. These relationships account for many of the symptoms and signs of pancreatic trauma and benign pancreatic disease, and are responsible for the technically demanding surgical operations which may be required for the treatment of patients with these problems.

Located directly behind the parietal peritoneum of the lesser sac, the pancreas is intimately related to several vital intra-abdominal organs. Lying to the right of the superior mesenteric vessels, the pancreatic head is cradled by the first three segments of the duodenum, and comes in contact with the right kidney, the vena cava, and the distal common bile duct. The posterior portion of the head may give rise to an uncinate process, which passes behind the superior mesenteric vessels along the third portion of the duodenum, directly anterior to the aorta and vena cava.

The neck of the pancreas overlies the superior mesenteric vessels and is intimately related to the portal confluence, wherein the portal vein is established from the superior mesenteric and splenic veins. The pancreatic body lies to the left of the superior mesenteric vessels, crossing transversely across the floor of the omental bursa. The root of the transverse mesocolon is attached at its inferior border. Posterior, it is associated with the renal vessels, left kidney and left adrenal gland. The body is arbitrarily divided from the tail, which is associated with the splenic flexure of the colon and the spleen.

Pancreaticobiliary Ductal Anatomy
The secretions of the exocrine pancreas are drained into the duodenum by two major ducts that are variable in their anatomy. The main pancreatic duct runs transversely through the length of the gland, turning inferiorly in the pancreatic head to open into the duodenum at the ampulla of Vater along with the distal common bile duct. The main pancreatic duct routinely drains the body, tail and uncinate body of the gland. The accessory pancreatic duct, which typically drains the pancreatic head, is more variable (2).

The ampulla of Vater (3) is a common pancreaticobiliary channel which lies on the posteromedial wall of the second portion of the duodenum and receives drainage from both the common bile duct and the main pancreatic duct. The ampulla surrounds a complex of sphincter muscles, the sphincter of Oddi (4), which regulates flow from these ducts into the small intestine, and prevents reflux of secretions from one system into another. In approximately one-third of patients, a true common channel is formed by the junction of the pancreatic and biliary ducts within the duodenal wall; other variations of distal ductal anatomy are common but rarely clinically relevant.

Arterial Supply and Venous Drainage
The pancreas receives its arterial supply from both the celiac and the superior mesenteric arteries. The head of the gland is supplied mainly from the pancreaticoduodenal arcades, the superior branches of which are derived from the celiac trunk via the gastroduodenal artery, and the inferior branches which receive flow from the superior mesenteric artery. The arcades course along the groove between the duodenal C-loop and the pancreatic head, and support a rich network of vessels, which are the predominant blood supply to both of these entities. The shared blood supply of the pancreatic head and the second and third portions of the duodenum imply that simultaneous surgical resection of both is compulsory.

The body and tail of the gland are mainly supported by branches of the splenic artery. This vessel travels transversely along the superior aspect of the pancreas, and gives rise to up to 10 branches which course inferiorly through the pancreatic parenchyma and anastomose with the transverse pancreatic artery running transversely over the inferoposterior surface of the gland.

The venous drainage of the pancreas is to the portal vein. This occurs via the splenic vein, the superior mesenteric vein and the inferior mesenteric vein. The portal confluence is located posterior to the neck of the pancreas and is created by the union of the superior mesenteric and splenic veins.

Surgical Access to the Pancreas

✍ **Three surgical maneuvers must be performed to completely evaluate the pancreas: (*i*) entry into the lesser sac via the gastrocolic ligament, (*ii*) division of the leinorenal ligament with full mobilization of the pancreatic tail, and (*iii*) mobilization of the duodenum and pancreatic head with a Kocher maneuver.** ✍ Because of the retroperitoneal location of the pancreas and its complex anatomical relationships with adjacent vital organs and blood vessels, surgical access to, and resection of the gland is technically demanding. Access to the pancreatic body may be achieved through the omental bursa by incising the gastrocolic omentum along the greater curvature of the stomach just distal to the gastroepiploic vessels, or along the avascular plane found between the posterior leaf of the gastrocolic omentum and its insertion on the transverse colon. The stomach is then retracted superiorly, while the transverse colon is retracted inferiorly, yielding an unobstructed view of the anterior surface of the gland. Inspection of the posterior aspect of the body and tail requires division of the leinorenal ligament and full mobilization of the spleen and pancreatic tail. To adequately visualize and palpate the anterior and posterior aspects of the head of the pancreas, a Kocher maneuver may be performed by mobilizing the right colon at its lateral border and then retracting the hepatic flexure inferomedially. The peritoneum overlying the second portion of the duodenum can then be incised. Blunt dissection is used to separate the head of the pancreas and duodenum from underlying structures.

Basic Pancreatic Physiology

Functionally and histologically, the pancreas is divided into endocrine and exocrine components. Of these, the exocrine component predominates, accounting for over 90% of the gland by weight. The functional unit of the exocrine pancreas is the acinus, composed of multiple acinar cells arranged around a central lumen, which empties into the pancreatic ductal system. The acinar cells are responsible for both production and secretion of pancreatic digestive enzymes, including amylases, lipases and proteases, which facilitate digestion of carbohydrates, fats, and proteins. Another component of the pancreatic acinus, the centroacinar cells, secrete bicarbonate and other electrolytes into a fluid that carries the digestive enzymes to their site of action in the duodenum.

Secretion of pancreatic digestive enzymes occurs primarily upon stimulation by cholecystokinin, which is released by the small intestine in response to an intraluminal meal. Acetylcholine release from vagal fibers also induces stimulation. With the exception of amylase, pancreatic digestive enzymes are secreted into the pancreatic ducts in an inactive form, and require subsequent activation by the protease trypsin to perform their digestive functions. This activation occurs in the duodenum and is accelerated by the presence of the duodenal enzyme enterokinase and a fall in the pH below 7.0. Within the substance of the pancreas, premature activation of digestive enzymes is prevented by a system of antiproteolytic enzymes also secreted by the acinar cells as well as by the presence of the bicarbonate-rich fluid secreted by the pancreatic centroacinar cells and ductal epithelium which maintains an alkaline pH in the pancreatic ducts.

The endocrine functions of the pancreas are performed by so-called islets of cells which are dispersed throughout the pancreatic parenchyma. These islets contain four types of cells, A, B, D, and F, which produce and secrete glucagon, insulin, somatostatin and pancreatic polypeptide, respectively. These hormones are responsible for maintaining intravascular and intracellular glucose levels and regulating gastric, pancreatic, and biliary secretions. Their functions are important to keep in mind, because major destruction of the pancreas, as may occur with severe pancreatitis or traumatic injury, may disrupt the homeostasis established by each of these endocrine mechanisms.

ACUTE PANCREATITIS IN THE CRITICALLY ILL PATIENT

Acute pancreatitis is defined as an acute inflammatory process of the pancreas, with variable involvement of other regional tissues or remote organ systems (5). The disease is characterized by the presence of varying degrees of pancreatic and peripancreatic inflammation, autodigestion and necrosis. Of the 185,000 patients newly diagnosed and hospitalized with acute pancreatitis in the United States each year (6), most will have a mild form of the disease which may be treated successfully with simple, conservative measures. In this subset of patients, pancreatic necrosis is minimal and the disease is typically self-limiting over two to five days, with a mortality rate less than one percent. In contrast, approximately 15% to 20% of patients develop severe acute pancreatitis, associated with widespread pancreatic necrosis, failure of multiple organ systems, and serious local and systemic complications. These patients will require a protracted course of therapy in the ICU and may need one or more surgical operations to eliminate necrotic and potentially infected pancreatic debris.

Etiology

✍ **The two leading causes for acute pancreatitis are biliary tract stones and alcohol abuse, which together account for over 90% of cases.** ✍ Hypotheses of the mechanisms by which gallstones induce pancreatitis center on the anatomic confluence of the common bile duct and the main pancreatic duct at the ampulla of Vater (7). Gallstones impacted at this site could induce pancreatic ductal obstruction and subsequent hypertension, leading to premature activation of digestive enzymes in the acinar cell. Ampullary inflammation and edema caused during the passage of a stone from the bile duct into the duodenum could cause similar effects; this is likely the more frequent mechanism (8).

Alcohol is the primary cause of acute pancreatitis in many parts of the world, including the United States. It has been suggested that alcohol exerts its toxic effects on the pancreas through the production of protein precipitates that block small pancreatic ducts and induce pancreatic

Table 1 Etiologies of Pancreatitis

Major causes	Subcategories
Biliary stone disease	
Alcohol	
Drugs	Salicylates
	Sulfa-containing agents
	Diuretics
	Didanosine (DDI)
Trauma	Blunt
	Penetrating
	Iatrogenic (ERCP)
Metabolic abnormalities	Hyperlipidemia
	Hypercalcemia
Infections	
Periampullary tumors	
Hereditary/congenital	Hereditary pancreatitis
	Cystic fibrosis
	Pancreas divisum
Idiopathic	Autoimmune

Many etiologies for acute pancreatitis exist. Alcohol and biliary tract disease account for approximately 90% of cases.
Abbreviations: DDI, diuretics didanosine; ERCP, endoscopic retrograde cholangiopancreatography.

ductal hypertension. This effect may be aggravated by the spasmogenic effects of alcohol on the sphincter of Oddi. Alcohol, its metabolites and metabolic by-products also appear to have a direct toxic effect on the enzyme-secreting acinar cells. Whatever the etiology, the incidence of pancreatitis caused by alcohol is proportional to the level of alcohol consumption, suggesting that the effects of alcohol on the pancreas are cumulative and dose related (9).

While gallstones and alcohol are responsible for the majority of cases of acute pancreatitis, several less frequent etiologies are well described (Table 1). Pancreatitis can be associated with congenital or hereditary conditions such as pancreas divisum or cystic fibrosis (10). Penetrating and blunt abdominal trauma are associated with acute pancreatitis in approximately 2% of cases, due to direct injury to the pancreatic parenchyma and ducts and to the premature release of activated digestive enzymes. Periampullary tumors may incite pancreatitis by obstructing the main pancreatic duct. Several drugs can induce pancreatitis, as can infection with certain parasites and the venom of rare varieties of scorpions and spiders. Often, a specific precipitating factor cannot be identified.

One final cause of pancreatitis deserves special mention. Iatrogenic injury to the pancreas may occur as a complication of several therapeutic interventions. It is well known that endoscopic retrograde cholangiopancreatography (ERCP) (11) carries a predictable risk of pancreatitis of approximately 5% overall (12). Pancreatitis in this setting is due to direct manipulation of the gland and pancreaticobiliary ducts; evidence suggests that this complication is more frequent when ERCP is performed by inexperienced operators (13). Severe pancreatic inflammation may also occur after other surgical procedures and interventions that do not involve the gland directly, such as cardiac (14) or aortic (15) operations, percutaneous liver biopsy (16), and gastric surgery. The mechanism by

which pancreatitis occurs in these settings is not always evident.

Pathophysiology and Natural History

Whatever its cause, the inflammatory process of pancreatitis is initiated by the final common pathway of premature and inappropriate activation of trypsin and other digestive enzymes, which subsequently induce autodigestion of the pancreas and peripancreatic tissues (17). Normally, the pancreas is protected from autodigestion by trypsin-inhibiting enzymes such as pancreatic secretory trypsin inhibitor, and trypsinogen-degrading enzymes such as mesotrypsin. Additionally, the bicarbonate-rich secretions of the exocrine pancreas typically prevent inappropriate enzyme activation by maintaining an alkaline pH. In pancreatitis, these protective mechanisms appear to be disrupted and overwhelmed, and activation of enzymatic proteases occurs. As pancreatic acinar cells are damaged by this initial insult, they discharge their enzymes, further exacerbating local injury.

For approximately 75% of patients, locoregional injury to the pancreas and peripancreatic tissues is the only manifestation of their disease. These patients may be described to have mild acute pancreatitis, as classified by the Atlanta Convention in 1992 (5). The predominant histological feature of this process is interstitial edema; microscopic areas of necrosis in the pancreatic parenchyma are occasionally found, but widespread pancreatic necrosis is conspicuously absent. Distant organ failure does not occur. ☛ **Treatment of patients with mild acute pancreatitis can be accomplished on a general medical or surgical ward, and the disease is typically self-limiting, resulting in an uneventful recovery.** ☚

Progressive injury to the pancreatic acini induces the overexpression of inflammatory mediators which may exacerbate both local and systemic injury. TNF-α is one of the most active of these mediators. Derived predominantly from activated macrophages, expression of this protein increases rapidly over the first several hours of pancreatitis (18) and induces an inflammatory syndrome clinically indistinguishable from that of shock. The inflammatory effects of TNF-α are exacerbated by IL-1 (19), which is also involved in the activation of leukocytes and in the upregulation of endothelial adhesion factors. Combined with mediators such as IL-6, the complement cascade and platelet activating factor (PAF), these agents are responsible for both the local and systemic manifestations of severe disease, which result from the effects of impaired microcirculatory perfusion of organs and capillary endothelial leak.

Severe acute pancreatitis is the clinical manifestation of local pancreatic and peripancreatic destruction, combined with distant organ failure and complications due to systemic cytokine release. Histologically, the pancreas shows evidence of parenchymal and peripancreatic necrosis, which may be widespread; a direct correlation exists between the amount of necrosis present and patient prognosis. Necrosis typically involves the acinar cells, islet cells and ductal system. Hemorrhage in these tissues is variable, but not uncommon. Systemic features of the disease include the cytokine-induced multiple organ dysfunction syndrome (MODS), with distant organ systems such as the kidneys, lungs and heart involved. Superinfection of the pancreatic necrosis is variable, but devastating.

As could be predicted, the course of patients with severe disease is protracted, and these are the patients who will require care in the ICU. The natural history of their disease can be described as having two stages (20). The first two weeks of hospitalization reflect the early local and systemic inflammatory response, and is characterized by cytokine release, systemic inflammation and injury, and failure of multiple organ systems. Patients who survive this initial insult often develop superinfection of their pancreatic necrosis in the second and third weeks, with associated sepsis and the potential for further decompensation.

Because the natural history of acute pancreatitis in the general population varies so widely, particular emphasis must be placed on the early identification of individual patients with severe disease, so that proper therapeutic interventions can be performed.

Diagnosis

While diagnosing this disease, the clinician should attempt to determine the following: (*i*) a clear diagnosis of pancreatitis, (*ii*) its etiology, and (*iii*) an individual assessment of disease severity. Accurate determination of all three of these may be difficult, even using all of the following diagnostic tools.

Clinical History and Physical Findings

The patient with acute pancreatitis may have several complaints, none of which is specific to this disease. Upper abdominal pain, which may radiate to the back, is the most common symptom. The pain is variable in severity, ranging from mild discomfort to severe pain that may be confused with peritonitis. Nausea and vomiting frequently occur. Fever is a part of the clinical presentation of over half of all the patients, but neither its presence nor magnitude correlate with severity of the disease (21). Other nonspecific complaints such as anorexia or lethargy may or may not be present.

The initial physical exam of patients with pancreatitis is also characteristically nonspecific. Patients may be febrile, tachycardic and in extremis, or may be hemodynamically stable. Abdominal findings are variable. Periumbilical and flank bruising (Cullen's and Grey Turner's signs) are often touted as evidence of severe pancreatitis, but these are very rare and can be seen in any hemorrhagic abdominal disorders. It is important to emphasize that the signs and symptoms of pancreatitis are variable, nonspecific, and may mimic other abdominal problems. Additional data must be accumulated to definitively diagnose the disease and to establish its severity.

Biochemical Studies
Amylase
Serum amylase is used universally in the diagnosis of acute pancreatitis (22). This pancreatic digestive enzyme is normally secreted by pancreatic acini; large amounts are released into the systemic circulation in states in which disruption or dysfunction of the pancreatic ductal system occurs. The serum amylase level typically rises steadily over the first 12 hours of an attack of pancreatitis, returning to normal over the next five days (23). Its peak may usually be measured within the first 48 hours. If a patient presents to the hospital late in the course of the disease, this peak may have passed and the amylase level may be normal (24). Normoamylasemia in the presence of pancreatitis may also occur in patients with an alcoholic etiology for their disease (25), and in states of chronic or severe necrotizing pancreatitis in which widespread acinar cell destruction has occurred.

While fairly sensitive, an elevated serum amylase is not specific to the diagnosis of acute pancreatitis. Serum amylase may rise in response to several other abdominal disorders, including trauma, appendicitis, perforated bowel and mesenteric ischemia. Similarly, salivary isoforms of the enzyme may lead to false positive elevations when patients present with inflammation of the salivary glands. Finally, because amylase is in large part cleared from the circulation by the kidneys, renal insufficiency may lead to an elevated amylase level.

Nonetheless, measurement of serum amylase is key to the diagnosis of acute pancreatitis. Differentiation from other extrapancreatic conditions can typically be made if the serum amylase is greater than five times normal, which rarely occurs when hyperamylasemia occurs from a nonpancreatic source. Though not routinely performed, salivary and pancreatic amylase isoforms may be measured in certain situations. Calculation of the fractional renal clearance of amylase, in which renal clearance of the enzyme is compared to that of creatinine, may be useful to confirm the diagnosis. A fractional clearance in excess of 4% is suggestive of acute pancreatitis.

It should be noted that no correlation has been found between the level of amylase elevation and magnitude of disease. ☞ **Serum amylase and lipase are used to diagnose pancreatitis, but their magnitudes are not predictive of disease severity.** ☞

Lipase
The serum lipase level may also be used to assist in the diagnosis of acute pancreatitis, and may be a more specific test than amylase (26,27), particularly if elevated greater than three times normal. Concentrations of the enzyme in serum increase within the first eight hours after the onset of symptoms, peak within the first 24 hours, and return to baseline over the following two weeks (28). Lipase concentrations may therefore be elevated long after serum amylase levels have returned to normal. Nonetheless, an increase in lipolytic activity is not specific to pancreatitis, and elevations can be seen in other conditions such as trauma, intestinal obstruction, cholecystitis, and esophagitis. As with amylase, the level of lipase elevation cannot be used to assess the severity of disease.

☞ **Whether amylase or lipase is more accurate in the diagnosis of pancreatitis is debatable; in clinical practice, serum levels of both are typically ordered. Concomitant elevation of both enzymes is good evidence for the diagnosis, especially in conjunction with a consistent history and physical examination.** ☞

Other Diagnostic Laboratory Tests
Other laboratory markers, such as trypsin, elastase, phospholipase A-2, trypsinogen-2, pancreas, associated peptide (PAP), and C-reactive protein (CRP) have been reported as possible adjuncts to the laboratory diagnosis of acute pancreatitis (29,30). None of these has been studied as thoroughly as CRP. CRP is an acute phase protein, produced in the liver upon inflammatory stimuli by cytokines (31), such as occurs in the early stages of acute pancreatitis. Unlike other markers of pancreatitis, CRP has been shown to reliably differentiate mild from severe acute pancreatitis with a high degree of specificity (32). Unfortunately, the clinical utility of CRP is undermined by the fact that its levels in serum do not spike until two to four days after the onset of the disease (33) and thus it cannot be used on admission, when its value would be most appreciated. The

marker is thus rarely used in the diagnosis and staging of acute pancreatitis in the United States.

Associated Biochemical Findings

Other laboratory findings consistent with a diagnosis of acute pancreatitis include hyperglycemia, hypocalcemia, hyperlipidemia, leukocytosis, an elevation in hepatic transaminases, elevated hematocrit, and derangements in the arterial blood gas. None of these markers can be used either to diagnose the disease or to assess its severity.

Imaging Studies

Ultrasound and Endoscopic Ultrasound

Transabdominal ultrasound (US) plays little role in the detection or grading of pancreatic necrosis. The gland is poorly visualized in up to 25% of cases, often due to the effects of intestinal ileus and superimposed bowel gas (34). Moreover, ultrasound cannot reliably distinguish between necrotic pancreatic parenchyma and surrounding tissues, and is unable to accurately identify pancreatic infection. Nonetheless, transabdominal ultrasound is generally recommended as an initial imaging study in patients suspected of having acute pancreatitis. Because of its excellent ability to assess the biliary tract and gallbladder, the primary role of US is identification or exclusion of biliary tract disease as a causal factor (35). It is also useful to demonstrate fluid collections and identify extrapancreatic spread of inflammation (36). ⚬⚬ **Ultrasound may also be used to assess complications of acute pancreatitis, such as pseudocyst and aneurysm formation.** ⚬⚬

The role of endoscopic US (EUS) is not yet well established (Fig. 1). This modality appears to be more sensitive than either transabdominal ultrasound or computed tomography (CT) scan, and as sensitive as ERCP, in the identification of both cholelithiasis and choledocholithiasis (37,38). Because it is less invasive than ERCP, it has been suggested that EUS be performed early for diagnosis of acute biliary pancreatitis, relegating ERCP to a purely therapeutic role (39). Nonetheless, no large studies have definitively established its role in the diagnosis or staging of acute pancreatitis. At present, its use must be viewed as experimental.

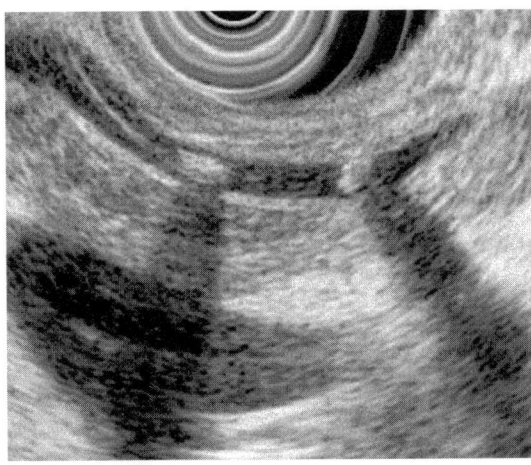

Figure 1 Endoscopic ultrasonography demonstrating choledocholithiasis. Two gallstones are visualized in the common bile duct using endoscopic ultrasonography. Information regarding the presence or amount of pancreatic necrosis is not provided, using this imaging modality.

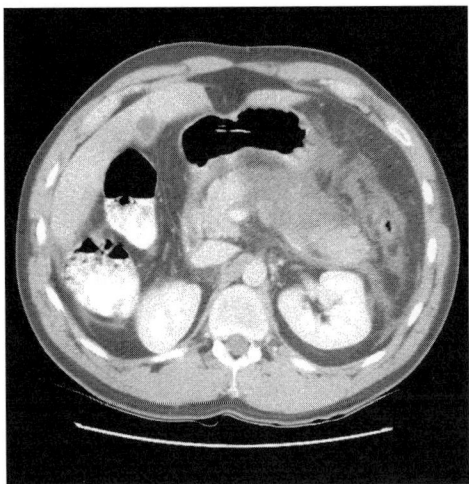

Figure 2 Computed tomography demonstrating pancreatic necrosis. Baseline contrast-enhanced computed tomography scan performed on admission of a 34-year-old male diagnosed with severe acute pancreatitis. Impaired perfusion reflects widespread pancreatic necrosis.

Computed Tomography

A contrast enhanced CT scan is the imaging modality of choice for both the diagnosis of severe acute pancreatitis and for the assessment of the severity of disease (40). Poorly perfused areas of pancreatic necrosis are easily identified on CT as areas of nonenhancement during the arterial phase of intravenous contrast administration (Fig. 2). The unperfused areas of pancreatic tissue seen on CT scan are detected with an overall accuracy of up to 90%, as confirmed by surgical exploration (41,42). Other possible CT findings in pancreatitis include diffuse or partial pancreatic enlargement, fluid collections, and obliteration of the peripancreatic fat planes.

Due to its ability to accurately identify and quantify pancreatic necrosis, and because pancreatic necrosis is one of the most important determinants of prognosis for patients with the disease, CT staging of disease severity has gained widespread acceptance. Several scoring systems, such as Balthazar's CT severity index (43) have been established; such systems have enabled accurate prediction of a patient's prognosis using CT findings alone. CT scanning is the diagnostic modality of choice, and a good baseline CT scan is therefore recommended upon admission to the ICU in all patients suspected of having severe disease. ⚬⚬ **Subsequent imaging may be performed later in the patient's hospital course to follow the course of treatment.** ⚬⚬

Endoscopic Retrograde Cholangiopancreatography

While ERCP may be used successfully to treat patients with choledocholithiasis and cholangitis, its role in the diagnosis and treatment of acute pancreatitis without biliary obstruction is, at best, controversial (44). ERCP is unable to assess or quantify pancreatic necrosis, and is therefore unsuitable for the diagnosis and staging of the disease. Several large studies have examined the outcomes of patients with pancreatitis treated with early ERCP and sphincterotomy compared with patients treated conservatively, with conflicting results (45,46). These results must be balanced with the known complications associated with ERCP, which include trauma to the ampulla of Vater, contamination of the main pancreatic duct and exacerbation of pancreatitis. The routine use of ERCP therefore cannot be justified in either the diagnosis or the treatment of acute pancreatitis. In cases where it is appropriate, such as in the presence of a gallstone clearly impacted at the ampulla of Vater, ERCP should be performed by an experienced endoscopist.

Magnetic Resonance Cholangiopancreatography
Accumulating evidence suggests that, like EUS, noninvasive MR imaging of the pancreas may eventually obviate the use of diagnostic ERCP. Magnetic resonance cholangiopancreatography (MRCP) (47) appears to be a safe imaging modality that gives reliable information about the patency of the pancreaticobiliary ductal system (48–50), and may therefore be useful in selecting out those few patients who truly require therapeutic ERCP. MRCP is able to differentiate pancreatic and peripancreatic necrosis from adjacent viable tissue, and may be as good as contrast-enhanced CT in this regard (51). It can also accurately identify peripancreatic fluid collections, and may be superior to CT in determining their contents and identifying their suitability for radiological drainage (52). At present, however, CT is more widely accessible, less expensive to perform, and should be regarded as the imaging modality of choice.

Fine Needle Aspiration for the Diagnosis of Infected Necrosis
☞ **Distinguishing between sterile and infected necrosis is imperative.** ☞ Typically, patients with severe but sterile necrotizing pancreatitis can be managed conservatively in the ICU, while patients with contaminated necrosis will ultimately require surgery (discussed subsequently). Many groups prefer to take a nonaggressive approach, and use clinical evidence of sepsis as an indicator of the presence of pancreatic contamination (53). Fine Needle Aspiration (FNA) may also be used to establish a definitive diagnosis, and has been generally accepted as safe and effective. Using ultrasound or CT guidance, a needle is inserted into the pancreatic parenchyma. Aspirated tissue may be sent for culture, yielding a sensitivity of detection of infected necrosis up to 90% (54). It must be remembered, however, that FNA is an invasive technique, and is associated with morbidity and mortality including bowel perforation, pancreatitis and hemorrhage. Clinical judgment must therefore be used in its application.

Assessment of Severity
Because the natural history of acute pancreatitis in those patients with mild disease is so different from that in patients with necrotizing pancreatitis, the early identification of patients who will develop severe disease is crucial. Unfortunately, staging of the severity of acute pancreatitis is notoriously difficult; using clinical data alone, even experienced examiners can predict patients' prognosis in only 39% of cases (55). Multifactorial scoring systems to predict the natural history of acute pancreatitis have therefore been established, the first of which was developed by Ranson in 1974 (Table 2) (56). In this system, five laboratory and clinical parameters are measured on admission, and six more are assessed over the course of the first 48 hours of hospitalization to estimate a likelihood of ultimate mortality. Validated by the Atlanta Convention, severe disease is frequently associated with three or more positive Ranson findings, and studies have confirmed an acceptable sensitivity for diagnosing severe disease (57). Unfortunately, the criteria require a full 48 hours to establish, and thus are not useful for diagnosis in the most crucial early hours.

Table 2   Ranson Criteria

On admission
  Age >55 years
  White blood cell count >16,000 mm³
  Serum glucose >200 mg/dL
  Lactate dehydrogenase (LDH) >350 IU/dL
  Aspartate aminotransferase (AST) >250 IU/L
Within 48 hours
  Hematocrit decrease >10%
  Blood urea nitrogen (BUN) increase >5 mg/dL
  Serum calcium <8 mg/dL
  Arterial pO_2 <60 mmHg
  Base deficit >4 mmol/L
  Fluid sequestration >6L

Ranson's criteria for the assessment of severity in acute pancreatitis. The presence of three of the above criteria is associated with severe disease according to the Atlanta Convention. If less than three criteria are present, the likelihood of mortality is approximately 1%. The original report focused on alcohol-induced pancreatitis; slight modifications have been adopted for patients with biliary etiology. *Source*: From Ref. 56

The acute physiology and chronic health evaluation (APACHE) II, (Table 3) (58), and more recently III (59) scores can be used to measure the severity of a variety of critical illnesses, and have the advantage that they may be used earlier in a patient's hospital course than the Ranson system (60) to predict prognosis in an attack of acute pancreatitis. While the system is able to predict severe disease with an overall accuracy approaching 90% within the first 24 hours, it is complicated to use in the clinical setting. No advantages to the use of APACHE III over APACHE II have yet been demonstrated.

Because of the cumbersome nature of these multifactorial systems, attempts have been made to estimate prognosis using a single clinical or laboratory indicator. The most successful of these attempts has been with CT scanning. By assessing the degree of pancreatic and peripancreatic inflammation, the presence of associated fluid collections and the presence and degree of pancreatic necrosis, scoring systems such as the Balthazar CT severity index (Table 4) can be used to reliably predict disease severity with an accuracy equal to, or even greater than, the previously described multifactorial systems (57,61).

Nonoperative Management Guidelines
Resuscitation
Initial therapy for patients diagnosed with severe acute pancreatitis has two aims: (*i*) to provide cardiocirculatory support and (*ii*) to prevent and to minimize the complications of multi-organ system failure (62). Patients identified as having severe disease should be admitted to the ICU and continuously monitored. ☞ **Fluid resuscitation with crystalloid solutions is the cornerstone of management, because immense volume shifts can lead to depletion of the intravascular volume.** ☞ Pulse, blood pressure, urine output and the base deficit determined by arterial blood gas can serve as markers of resuscitation in many patients; in the elderly or more tenuous patients a central venous catheter or pulmonary artery catheter should be inserted so that central venous pressure, pulmonary artery wedge pressure, cardiac output and systemic vascular resistance can be recorded. Electrolyte levels should be continuously monitored throughout the resuscitation.

Table 3 The Acute Physiology and Chronic Health Evaluation II Scoring System

Physiologic variables	Method of scoring	Reference range
	Score 0–4 points according to deviation of value from normal reference range unless otherwise stated	
Rectal temperature (°C)		36.0–38.4
Mean arterial pressure (mmHg)		70–109
Heart rate (beats/min)		70–109
Respiratory rate (breaths/min)		12–24
Oxygenation (mmHg)		$PaO_2 >70$ and FiO_2 <0.5 or $(A\text{-}a)O_2$ <200 and $FiO_2 >0.5$
Arterial pH		7.33–7.49
Serum sodium (mmol/L)		130–149
Serum potassium (mmol/L)		3.5–5.4
Serum creatinine (mg/dL)	Score doubled if patient in renal failure	0.6–1.4
Hematocrit		30–45.9
Leukocyte count ($\times 10^9$/L)		3–14.9
Glasgow Coma Scale (GCS)	Subtract GCS from total score	
Age	Score 0 if age <=44 Score 2 if age 45–54 Score 3 if age 55–64 Score 5 if age 65–74 Score 6 if age >=75	
Operative status and chronic health	Score 0–5 depending on operative status (nonoperative, emergency postoperative, felective postoperative) and presence of severe organ insufficiency	

Factors measured in the APACHE II Scoring System, which may be applied to many critical illnesses including pancreatitis. Up to four points are ascribed to each physiologic variable listed according to its most abnormal value within the first 24 hours of hospitalization. Additional points are given for older age, history of previously diagnosed medical conditions and surgical status. The magnitude of the APACHE index, from 0–71, correlates with an increased severity of disease and a greater risk of in-hospital death.
Abbreviation: APACHE, acute physiology and chronic health evaluation computed tomography.
Source: From Ref. 58.

The systemic cytokine release in the early stages of the disease, combined with the effects of massive fluid shifts, frequently lead to dysfunction of other organ systems. Renal failure is a frequent complication of severe disease (63) that carries a particularly poor prognosis (64). Continuous hemodialysis may be required. Acute lung injury and ARDS, found in up to one-third of patients with severe acute pancreatitis, account for 60% of deaths within the first week of diagnosis (65,66). Endotracheal intubation and respiratory support should be provided early in the face of impending respiratory failure. Routine strategies such as the use of low tidal volume mechanical ventilation, permissive hypercapnia, and proning may be used in patients with severe lung disease.

Despite maximal supportive therapy, the prognosis of patients with severe acute pancreatitis who develop multiple organ failure is poor (67). It is incumbent upon the clinician, therefore, to practice an aggressive policy of prevention and early detection.

Nutritional Support
Over the past two decades, the traditional tenets of restricting enteral nutrition and decompressing the stomachs of patients with severe acute pancreatitis have been challenged and largely discounted. Nasogastric decompression in

Table 4 The Balthazar Computed Tomography Severity Score

	Score	CT appearance
CT grade		
A	0	Normal
B	1	Pancreatic enlargement
C	2	Peripancreatic inflammation
D	3	Single fluid collection
E	4	Multiple fluid collections
Gland necrosis		
None	0	Normal pancreatic enhancement
<30%	2	Nonenhancement of <30% of pancreas
30%–50%	4	Nonenhancement of 30%–50% of pancreas
>50%	6	Nonenhancement of >50% of pancreas

Balthazar's index predicts severe pancreatitis based on an assessment of peripancreatic inflammation, associated fluid collections, and degree of pancreatic necrosis as seen on the admission computed tomography scan. Scores range from 0 to 10; patients with scores <3 have a 2% morbidity and essentially 0% mortality, while those with a score greater than 7 have a 17% mortality and a complication rate of 92%.
Source: From Ref. 43.

particular has been shown to have no positive effect on the clinical course of these patients (68,69), and may in fact have contradictory effects in terms of perceived pain, resumption of bowel function and length of hospital stay. ⚔ **Nasogastric suction should not be used routinely, and is limited to those patients who have a high risk of aspiration, or who suffer from a concomitant ileus or bowel obstruction.** ⚔

In contrast, the use of aggressive nutritional support is a fundamental part of treatment that should be provided to each patient with severe disease. The cytokine release initiated by pancreatic inflammation induces a metabolic state similar to that of sepsis, characterized by hypermetabolism, catabolism, and negative nitrogen balance. Patients' resting energy expenditures may reach 150% of normal as predicted by the Harris-Benedict equations (70,71), with catabolism contributing to nitrogen losses up to 40 g/day (72). Untreated, these metabolic derangements will lead to loss of lean body mass and malnutrition.

In the past, nutritional replacement has been accomplished using total parenteral nutrition (TPN) (73). The parenteral route was justified by the belief that enteral feeding would stimulate proteolytic pancreatic secretions and thus exacerbate pancreatic autodigestion and inflammation. Initial studies suggested that patients receiving TPN early in their hospital course for severe acute pancreatitis could enjoy a reduction in complications and a survival advantage compared to controls. Nonetheless, several disadvantages to its use were identified. First administration of concentrated dextrose solutions requires the introduction of a central venous catheter, which is itself associated with complications such as pneumothorax and catheter-related sepsis (74). Parenteral administration may lead to electrolyte imbalances and may exacerbate metabolic disturbances. Finally, neglect of the alimentary tract may lead to mucosal atrophy, increased intestinal permeability, and bacterial translocation (75). This may lead to contamination of pancreatic and peripancreatic necrosis or outright sepsis.

The use of enteral feeding for nutritional support for patients with severe pancreatitis has been justified by several recent studies, and has now replaced parenteral nutrition as the primary method of nutritional replacement for patients with this disease. Enteral feedings are typically performed through a nasojejunal feeding tube, the tip of which is endoscopically or radiographically placed beyond the ligament of Treitz, although recent studies suggest that intragastric feeding may also be acceptable (76). Use of the enteral route is safe and well tolerated by patients, and is not associated with an increase in pancreatic inflammation or necrosis, as previously supposed. In fact, enteral feeding appears to be associated with an improvement in disease severity, a decrease in the rate of complications, sepsis and organ failure, and a reduction in the length of ICU hospitalization compared to parenteral nutrition (77–79). Moreover, enteral feeding does not induce the atrophy and adverse functional changes in intestinal mucosa seen in patients treated with parenteral nutrition (80). This likely contributes to a reduction in the frequency of gut-derived systemic toxicity, a phenomenon seen both clinically and experimentally (81). Finally, enteral nutrition is also far less expensive to administer than TPN. For these reasons, current recommendations include the early use of enteral nutrition for patients with severe acute pancreatitis. ⚔ **The use of TPN should be relegated to the small subset of patients who do not tolerate enteral feedings.** ⚔

Prophylactic Antibiotics

Due to advances in critical care methods and care, the mortality rate from multiorgan system failure in the first stages of severe pancreatic illness has fallen. Septic complications, typically occurring later in the patients' hospital course, now account for approximately 80% of deaths from severe acute pancreatitis (20,82). Infection of pancreatic and peripancreatic necrosis, in particular, is recognized as the most important risk factor for death from the disease (83). Unfortunately, infections occur in up to 40% of patients who have over 30% necrosis of the pancreas. Prevention and diagnosis of infection are thus of utmost importance in the treatment of critically ill patients with acute pancreatitis.

Bacterial contamination of pancreatic necrosis can occur through several routes (84). The use of central venous catheters, endotracheal tubes, indwelling urinary catheters and nasogastric tubes can introduce bacteria into the bloodstream. Reflux of contaminated bile into the pancreatic duct may occur. Uncommonly, microorganisms can also ascend into the main pancreatic duct from the duodenum. The most important portal of entry, however, appears to be the colon, across which bacteria and endotoxins can translocate into the systemic circulation through an injured and hyperpermeable mucosal barrier (85). Injury to the mucosa may occur by several mechanisms, including hypoperfusion and ischemia, reperfusion injury, and bacterial overgrowth. Mucosal atrophy, as occurs during prolonged use of parenteral feeding, can contribute to the problem, as can mechanical injury to the bowel that may occur concomitantly with blunt or penetrating pancreatic trauma. Once the function of the mucosal barrier has failed, bacteria may translocate to intra-abdominal ascites, the systemic circulation, or to the pancreatic necrosis directly (84).

The theory of gut-derived sepsis in acute pancreatitis is supported by several lines of evidence. Experimental evidence has clearly demonstrated that splanchnic hypoperfusion during the early stages of pancreatitis can lead to gut barrier dysfunction (86). This dysfunction is associated with an increase in the permeability of enteric mucosa to bacteria and macromolecules such as bacterial endotoxin, which have been identified in high levels in the blood of patients during severe pancreatic attacks (87). Perhaps most compelling, prior to widespread use of antibiotics, gram-negative and other enteric bacteria such as *Escherichia coli*, *Enterobacter* spp, *Pseudomonas* spp, and *Bacteroides* spp were the most common organisms recovered from pancreatic necrosis; these organisms are still all too prevalent in patients with severe disease, particularly when due to biliary stones (88).

The use of prophylactic broad-spectrum antibiotics in patients with severe pancreatitis to reduce pancreatic contamination from the gut and other sources is now well established. The agents imipenem and ciprofloxacin have satisfactory efficacy against enteric organisms, and have been shown to achieve high levels in pancreatic secretions and peripancreatic tissues. These agents have been demonstrated to reduce both the frequency of complications and the rate of mortality in patients with severe disease (89,90).

⚔ **Current recommendations now support the early administration of prophylactic imipenem (or ciprofloxacin) in patients with severe pancreatitis and high levels of pancreatic necrosis. Because the rate of pancreatic infection in patients with minimal necrosis is very low, the use of prophylactic agents in patients with mild pancreatitis is not warranted.** ⚔

The prophylactic use of broad spectrum antibiotics has been shown to be associated with fungal infections, and therefore the administration of these agents must not be taken lightly. Several studies have demonstrated not only a strong association between the protracted use of prophylactic antibiotics and the occurrence of fungal contamination of pancreatic necrosis, but also an increased mortality rate in patients with this complication (91–94). No data yet support the routine use of prophylactic fluconazole in the treatment regimen for patients with severe disease, but this agent may be administered upon suspicion or diagnosis of fungal infection.

Somatostatin and Octreotide
For the last two decades, the role of somatostatin in the treatment of acute pancreatitis has been controversial. First described as a potential treatment for severe pancreatitis in 1980 (95), somatostatin is an endogenously produced antisecretory hormone secreted by D cells of the pancreatic islets. Octreotide, a somatostatin analog, was subsequently evaluated for use in these patients. While early studies demonstrated conflicting results in terms of the efficacy of these agents (96–98), recent studies suggest that no benefits exist (99). The use of somatostatin and octreotide therefore cannot be recommended for routine use in the treatment of patients with acute pancreatitis.

Several recent reports have also suggested that prophylactic somatostatin might play a role in reducing the incidence of pancreatitis after ERCP; results have been contradictory (100,101), and therefore their routine use is not recommended in this setting, either.

Surgical Treatment
Indications and Timing of Surgical Intervention
Three established indications for surgical intervention in severe pancreatitis exist: (*i*) the presence of infected pancreatic necrosis, (*ii*) failure to improve after a long period of conservative management, and (*iii*) acute abdominal catastrophe.

Infection of pancreatic necrosis occurs in up to 70% of patients with severe necrotizing pancreatitis (83), and its frequency correlates with the duration of the disease as well as the amount of necrotic tissue present. Left untreated, infected necrosis carries a high mortality rate approaching 100% (84,102) due to sepsis-induced organ failure initiated by the necrotic focus of infection. With appropriate surgical management, these patients fare better, with mortality rates in the order of 20% (103,104). The presence of infected pancreatic necrosis is therefore universally accepted as an absolute indication for surgical intervention.

Sterile necrosis, in contrast, is typically not an indication for surgery (105), and can be managed successfully using the nonoperative methods described in III.D.1. Several reports have validated the use of nonoperative therapy in these patients (104,106). In addition to conferring no benefit in the majority of these cases, operative manipulation of the sterile necrosis may actually contaminate it, leading to higher mortality rates.

In the case of infected necrosis, operation should be delayed as long as possible, with broad spectrum antibiotics used in the period of conservative management. Improved outcomes have been achieved with late compared to early surgical intervention (107,108). This phenomenon is attributed to the clear demarcation between viable and nonviable pancreatic tissues that occurs over time, enabling precise

necrosectomy when performed later in the disease course. Moreover, by waiting, patient stability can be maximized using nonoperative interventions. In cases of early operation, patients are frequently unstable, and the identification at laparotomy of truly necrotic tissues in the pancreatic bed is difficult, leading to unnecessary removal of potentially viable tissue. These drawbacks of early intervention appear to outweigh any advantages achieved by the early removal of the septic focus.

The second indication for surgical intervention in acute pancreatitis is failure of a patient to improve despite continued support for a prolonged period, typically three to four weeks. Often, these patients will demonstrate signs of increasing toxicity in the absence of proven infection; failure of multiple organ systems is a frequent complication. Evidence suggests that operating in these cases may be beneficial (109,110). Unfortunately, the timing of surgery in these patients is not clear; good surgical judgment remains the only way to select that subset of patients who will benefit from surgical management.

The final indication for operative management in patients with acute pancreatitis is in the presence of an acute abdominal catastrophe, such as rupture of a peripancreatic fluid collection or intra-abdominal bleeding from erosion of a major vessel (2). In these unusual cases, the surgeon may be forced to operate immediately.

Although these indications for operation serve as a guide, the following advice of the eminant pancreatic surgeon Dr. Kenneth Warren remains instructive: "the two most common mistakes made in the treatment of acute pancreatitis are to operate too early and do too much and to operate to late and do too little." The underlying wisdom of these remarks derive from the recognition that choosing the right operative path is based upon careful and repetitive examinations of the patient, and re-evaluation of all data (i.e., CT scans, amylase, etc.) in the setting of an optimally resuscitated patient.

Operative Techniques
Necrosectomy
The preferred surgical treatment for necrotizing pancreatitis involves necrosectomy, in which devitalized pancreatic parenchyma and peripancreatic tissues are debrided from the retroperitoneum (111). The abdomen is opened according to the preference of the surgeon, typically through a vertical upper abdominal or bilateral subcostal incision to facilitate exposure. Access to the pancreatic bed is achieved through the maneuvers described previously. Removal of necrotic tissue can then be accomplished using blunt finger dissection and irrigation with a balloon syringe. A sample of tissue should be sent for culture. All peripancreatic fluid collections are gently opened and drained. Perioperative oozing, which may be copious, is controlled by pressure with moist laparotomy pads.

Once the necrotic debris is entirely removed, the residual cavity must be drained in order to remove serum, blood, and pancreatic secretions. This may be accomplished using a closed technique in which saline is irrigated daily into the pancreatic bed through a series of catheters and then removed through another set of drains (103,112). Other authors perform a closed technique in which the residual cavity is packed with penrose drains stuffed with gauze, which are subsequently withdrawn over time (113). If the residual cavity is very large, or contains extensive necrosis, open drainage may be performed (114). In such methods, laparotomy pads are placed into the lesser sac and the abdominal wound is loosely approximated in a temporary closure. Daily packing changes can be performed using sterile technique in the operating room until the wound begins to granulate. With any of these methods, complete necrosectomy may require multiple explorations. These may be scheduled or may be performed on an as-needed basis dictated by the clinical condition of the patient.

The choice of technique depends in large part on the choice and comfort of the surgeon. Satisfactory results have been demonstrated using all of the above methods in which successful debridement and drainage of the lesser sac are effected.

Percutaneous Drainage

As experience with interventional radiology has grown, so too has interest in using percutaneous techniques in the treatment of acute pancreatitis. While percutaneous drainage clearly has a role in the treatment of peripancreatic fluid collections (115), abscesses (116), and pseudocysts (117), such techniques have not yet proven useful in the removal of pancreatic necrosis. ☞ **Open surgery remains the primary approach for pancreatic necrosis; interventional radiological techniques may subsequently be used successfully to drain residual fluid collections.** ☞

Late Complications and Sequelae

Although they are relatively common, the late complications and sequelae of acute pancreatitis and its treatment typically occur weeks after the acute event. They are therefore infrequently part of the course of treatment of patients with acute pancreatitis during their ICU hospitalization.

Pancreatic pseudocysts are cystic lesions that arise secondary to disruption of the pancreatic ductal system with subsequent leakage of pancreatic fluid and enzymes into surrounding tissues (Fig. 3). These lesions form over a protracted four to six weeks course after an initial attack, and can be diagnosed by their appearance on CT scan and their absence of an epithelial lining on histological analysis.

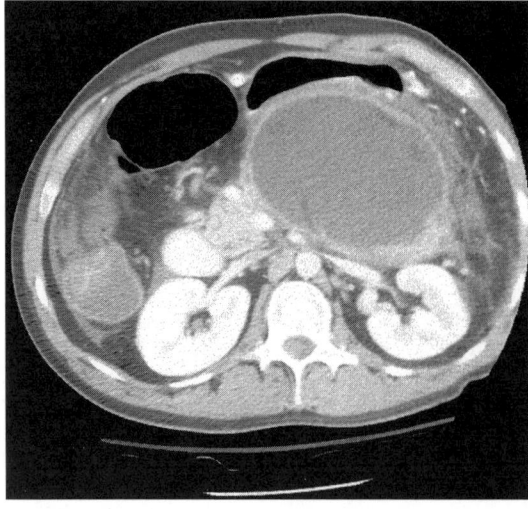

Figure 3 Computed tomography demonstrating a pancreatic pseudocyst. Computed tomography scan of the same patient as seen in Figure 2, performed seven weeks after the onset of symptoms. A large pancreatic pseudocyst was identified, which was subsequently treated by operative internal drainage into the stomach.

Pseudocysts occur in approximately 6% of cases of acute pancreatitis (20), and are more common in severe cases. Most cases resolve spontaneously, particularly when less than 6 cm in diameter. Drainage can be performed for large or symptomatic lesions, using surgical, endoscopic or percutaneous techniques.

Less common, yet more concerning, is the development of a pancreatic abscess (118). Like pseudocysts, these lesions occur late in the course of disease, but differ in that their contents are highly purulent. They are typically not associated with active pancreatic necrosis. Although drainage may be successfully accomplished percutaneously in a subset of patients, many patients will benefit from definitive surgical management (119).

Fistulas originating from the pancreas may occur despite therapy for acute pancreatitis, and typically communicate externally to the skin (120). Initial treatment for this complication is conservative, with endoscopic management or surgical treatment used only in cases that are unresponsive.

PANCREATIC INJURIES

Although relatively uncommon, the incidence of pancreatic trauma has risen over the past several decades due to an increase in the frequency of automobile accidents and major gunshot wounds. The considerable morbidity and mortality associated with pancreatic trauma is due in large part to the frequency with which it is associated with other severe intra-abdominal injuries. Nonetheless, pancreatic injuries run the gamut of severity from minor contusions and lacerations to major ductal disruptions. Left untreated, these injuries can lead to devastating sequelae and complications. This is further complicated by the fact that identification of pancreatic injury is often delayed, particularly when associated with a blunt abdominal trauma in the otherwise stable patient.

Etiology

Pancreatic injury may occur as a result of either blunt or penetrating mechanisms, and is a component of up to 12% of major abdominal injuries (121). Stab wounds and gunshot injuries are common penetrating etiologies of pancreatic injury, and occur as a result of direct mechanical disruption to the gland. In contrast, blunt injuries resulting in pancreatic injury are typically the result of high-energy transfer, in which the gland is compressed posteriorly against the spinal column. In adults, up to 60% of these injuries occur in automobile accidents, as a result of compression of the steering wheel against the anterior abdomen (122). In children, blunt pancreatic trauma is attributed to bicycle handlebar injuries in as many as 75% of cases (123).

Diagnosis

Isolated penetrating pancreatic injuries are uncommon (124) because of the gland's retroperitoneal location in close proximity to major blood vessels and other vital organs (Table 5). Penetrating pancreatic trauma is therefore typically identified intraoperatively upon laparotomy performed for other indications, such as evidence of hemorrhage or peritonitis, or identification of a stab wound which is found on digital examination to penetrate the anterior abdominal fascia. Gunshot wounds to the abdomen are themselves an indication for operation in most centers. Rarely, if ever, is emergent laparotomy performed because of isolated

Table 5 Intra-abdominal Injuries Associated with Pancreatic Trauma

Intra-abdominal organ	Percent of injuries (%)
Stomach	53
Liver	52
Diaphragm	44
Kidney	39
Major vascular	37
Minor vascular	31
Spleen	26
Small bowel	23
Large bowel	23
Duodenum	21
Extrahepatic biliary	8
Ureter	2

Additional intra-abdominal injuries found in association with pancreatic injury upon exploration for penetrating abdominal trauma in a series of 62 patients compiled over 11 years in a single, high-volume Level I trauma center.
Source: From Ref. 124.

concern for pancreatic injury (125). Patients requiring laparotomy for the treatment of penetrating abdominal trauma require no additional preoperative evaluation for the specific detection of pancreatic injury. ☞ **Pancreatic injuries secondary to penetrating abdominal trauma are best diagnosed within the critical first six hours of injury.** ☞

For the same reasons, identification of pancreatic injury in the unstable patient with blunt abdominal trauma is routinely made in the operating room. In contrast, the diagnosis of blunt pancreatic trauma in the relatively stable patient with no immediate indication for exploration is more difficult, frequently leading to significant delays in definitive diagnosis and treatment. Several factors contribute to this difficulty. First, clinical findings and laboratory values in cases of blunt pancreatic injury are nonspecific. Patients frequently present with abdominal pain, but this is common in trauma patients. Pain out of proportion to physical exam has been suggested as a clue to retroperitoneal injury; this finding is nonspecific and unreliable. Serum hyperamylasemia may be present, but amylase may be normal in as high as 34% of patients with blunt abdominal injury (125). In addition, random elevations in both serum amylase and lipase are frequently found in patients with blunt abdominal trauma but no pancreatic injury (126). Although additional sensitivity may be achieved by performing serial abdominal exams and measuring serial serum amylase levels, this implies a diagnostic and therapeutic delay.

Another factor contributing to a difficulty in diagnosing blunt pancreatic injury is the retroperitoneal location of the gland. Massive retroperitoneal injury may be present in the face of a normal diagnostic peritoneal lavage, which is most suitable for the diagnosis of intraperitoneal injury (127). Likewise, trauma ultrasound is typically used to identify free fluid in the intraperitoneal cavity; it is not as sensitive in the diagnosis of retroperitoneal injury (128).

For these reasons, blunt pancreatic trauma is frequently diagnosed using CT scan, which has a sensitivity of upwards of 80% in the diagnosis of these injuries. Findings suggestive of pancreatic injury on CT include the presence of a parenchymal laceration, peripancreatic fluid collections and hematoma, hemorrhage into the peripancreatic tissues, and focal or diffuse enlargement of the gland

(121). Nonetheless, the use of CT is associated with certain caveats.

☞ **Although CT scans are crucial to the early diagnosis of pancreatic injuries, the scans of patients with significant pancreatic injury may be entirely normal, particularly within the first 12 hours of injury.** ☞ As concerning, CT scan is notoriously inaccurate in its ability to diagnose major ductal injuries, and therefore often understages pancreatic injuries compared to findings made at laparotomy (121,129). CT scan should thus be viewed as a valuable tool in the diagnosis of pancreatic trauma, but should not be a substitute for clinical judgment and frequent physical examinations.

Classification and Assessment of Severity

Commonly used systems of classification of pancreatic injuries reflect the mechanism of an injury, its anatomic location, and its extent, and therefore both facilitate estimation of the severity of injury and help to guide its treatment. The classification system in most widespread use is that of the American Association for the Surgery of Trauma (AAST) (130), in which injuries are graded as follows (Table 6). Grade I injuries consist of minor pancreatic contusions or superficial lacerations without evidence of ductal injury. Grade II injuries represent major contusions or lacerations without ductal injury or substantial loss of tissue. Grade III injuries are those that involve distal transection or major parenchymal injuries that involve the pancreatic ducts. Transections of the gland that are more proximal are named Grade IV injuries, as are major parenchymal injuries that involve the ampulla of Vater. Massive disruptions of the pancreatic head are Grade V.

Treatment

Up to 75% of trauma victims who die with a pancreatic injury do so within the first 48 hours, often due to exsanguination from associated vascular injuries. Moreover, less than 10% of deaths in patients with pancreatic injury can be attributed directly to the pancreatic injury itself (122). Treatment of patients with abdominal trauma should therefore be initiated with proper resuscitation using standard Advanced Trauma Life Support® (ATLS®) protocols. Surgical procedures should likewise have, as their initial focus, the

Table 6 American Association for the Surgery of Trauma Classification of Pancreatic Injuries

Grade	Type	Description
I	Hematoma	Minor contusion without duct injury
	Laceration	Superficial laceration without duct injury
II	Hematoma	Major contusion without duct injury or significant tissue loss
	Laceration	Major laceration without duct injury or significant tissue loss
III	Laceration	Distal transection or parenchymal injury with duct involved
IV	Laceration	Proximal transection or parenchymal injury involving ampulla of Vater
V	Laceration	Massive disruption of the pancreatic head

Classification of pancreatic injuries based on mechanism, location of injury, and involvement of the pancreatic duct or ampulla of Vater. In general, a higher score is associated with a higher magnitude of severity.
Source: From Ref. 130.

identification and treatment of associated life-threatening injuries to the vasculature and other solid organs. Control of contamination from intestinal injuries is also of paramount importance. On occasion, this may require a damage control approach, wherein the patient's bleeding is controlled in a first operation and definitive treatment is accomplished in a second operation, performed after hypothermia, acidosis and coagulopathy are corrected in the ICU (131). ☞ **Only after the patient is stabilized should attention be turned to the pancreas.** ☞

Patients in whom pancreatic injury is suspected should undergo a complete surgical assessment of the gland, using the surgical maneuvers described above. Careful attention should be paid to the possibility of injury to the pancreatic duct, as its presence has an impact on both morbidity and surgical technique. In general, patients with class I and II injuries which do not disrupt the pancreatic duct require only external drainage, typically to closed suction Jackson Pratt-type drains. Injuries that involve the pancreatic duct, in contrast, may require additional procedures, which are dictated by the location of the injury. Injuries to the left of the superior mesenteric vessels, that is, those in the body or tail of the gland, may be treated successfully by distal pancreatectomy. Although splenic salvage can be attempted in these cases, undue effort should not be used to save the spleen in the unstable patient. If pancreatic duct injury is suspected but cannot be grossly identified, transduodenal pancreatography can be performed, but some authors prefer instead to assume a duct injury exists, because the morbidity of distal pancreatectomy is low and the morbidity of a duodenotomy can be substantial.

In cases in which injuries to the pancreatic head cause disruptions of the main pancreatic duct to the right of the superior mesenteric vessels, treatment may consist of pyloric exclusion or duodenal diverticulization, if the injury is associated with duodenal trauma. These procedures need not be performed for isolated injury to the pancreatic head, for which aggressive external drainage is the favored therapeutic technique. ERCP and stent placement may be used postoperatively to provide proximal drainage of pancreatic secretions. Only in rare circumstances must formal resection of the pancreatic head and duodenum, the "Trauma Whipple," be performed.

Overall, appropriate treatment of pancreatic trauma is associated with satisfactory results (124,132). ☞ **The most common complication following operative management of pancreatic trauma is the formation of a pancreatic fistula, which emphasizes the fundamental need for external drainage as part of any surgical operation on the gland.** ☞ Even despite such treatment, pancreatic fistula may occur in up to 25% of patients postoperatively. Treatment of this complication is typically conservative, although the use of ERCP for decompression has been successful in decreasing fistula output. Octreotide does not appear to play a role in management (133). Peripancreatic pseudocyst may also occur as a result of inadequate drainage. Abscess formation, pancreatitis, and pancreatic hemorrhage are other less common complications.

EYE TO THE FUTURE

Evolution in the care of patients with severe acute pancreatitis and pancreatic trauma is ongoing. Major advances in the fields can be grouped into those pertaining to the diagnosis of these diseases and those dealing with their medical and surgical treatment.

In both pancreatitis and pancreatic trauma, novel diagnostic modalities that could reliably diagnose and predict the severity of disease would be most welcome. To this end, current research is looking at early inflammatory mediators as potential markers for pancreatic inflammation, necrosis, and infection. Elevations in procalcitonin and IL-6 have been recently identified as having a predictive value for the ultimate occurrence of infected necrosis in severe acute pancreatitis (134). Measurement of urinary trypsin activation peptide (TAP), which is released upon activation of trypsinogen to trypsin, has also been shown to be an effective predictor of severe disease, and can be applied within the first 24 hours after its onset (135,136). Assays to measure these and other potential early indicators of severe disease are at present costly and require specialists to both perform and interpret. As experience grows, their acceptance and use should become more widespread.

Similar advances are also being made in the field of pancreatic imaging. MRCP appears to hold particular promise in the diagnosis of benign pancreatic disease. Currently, the use of MRCP is limited due to artifacts that compromise image quality, but improvements in technology should eliminate these problems. While the technique has questionable utility in the care of the acute trauma patient, similar advances in ultrasound and CT diagnostics will likely enable more rapid and definitive diagnosis of patients with pancreatic injury (137).

That these diagnostic advances may improve outcomes of patient's with severe acute pancreatitis, and pancreatic injury is unquestioned. It remains to be seen if advances in surgical technique will likewise have an effect on morbidity and survival. Laparoscopic necrosectomy (138,139), as performed using transgastrocolic or transgastric approaches, has been performed in small groups of patients, in an attempt to successfully debride the pancreas and create effective drainage without the morbidity of a laparotomy. Early results are enticing, but further studies are needed to perfect the procedures and to definitively identify a subgroup of patients for whom this minimally-invasive approach would be beneficial. Laparoscopic abdominal exploration in trauma is also gaining popularity in certain situations, with use of laparoscopy in the diagnosis and definitive treatment of injuries to the pancreas in its infancy (140).

Finally, elucidation of the pathogenic mechanisms behind acute pancreatitis and its effects on distant organ systems has driven investigation into the ability of immunomodulatory therapies, such as the platelet activating factor antagonist lexipafant (141), and drotrecogin alfa (recombinant human activated protein C) (142), to prevent catastrophic local and systemic complications. While no such therapies are currently in use, they represent potentially important novel strategies in the critical care management of pancreatitis.

SUMMARY

Acute pancreatitis ranges in severity from very mild to catastrophically severe. Patients with severe disease must be identified early. Although measurements such as the APACHE II score can be used for this purpose, the identification of widespread necrosis on an initial CT scan is just as reliable, and thus all patients suspected of having severe disease should receive a baseline CT scan on admission.

Those patients found to have a poor prognosis should be triaged to the ICU. Initial treatment is medical, and should focus on cardiopulmonary support and the prevention of injury to other organ systems. Patients that survive this first phase of treatment frequently develop superinfected pancreatic necrosis and must undergo an operation designed to remove the infected focus and drain the residual cavity. Although late sequelae are not uncommon, long-term morbidity and mortality have been reduced to acceptable levels using this course of therapy.

Morbidity from pancreatic injuries may likewise be substantial. While these injuries may be detected upon laparotomy performed for other indications, the diagnosis of pancreatic trauma is frequently difficult. A high level of suspicion should be maintained. If diagnosed, treatment depends on the severity and location of the injury, as well as on the presence or absence of involvement of the main pancreatic duct. In all cases, aggressive drainage is required to prevent complications such as fistula or pseudocyst formation.

KEY POINTS

- Three surgical maneuvers must be performed to completely evaluate the pancreas: (1) entry into the lesser sac via the gastrocolic ligament, (2) division of the leinorenal ligament with full mobilization of the pancreatic tail, (3) mobilization of the duodenum and pancreatic head with a Kocher maneuver.
- The two leading causes for acute pancreatitis are biliary tract stones and alcohol abuse, which together account for over 90% of cases.
- Treatment of patients with mild acute pancreatitis can be accomplished on a general medical or surgical ward, and the disease is typically self-limiting, resulting in an uneventful recovery.
- Serum amylase and lipase are used to diagnose pancreatitis, but their magnitudes are not predictive of disease severity.
- Whether amylase or lipase is more accurate in the diagnosis of pancreatitis is debatable; in clinical practice, serum levels of both are typically ordered. Concomitant elevation of both enzymes is good evidence for the diagnosis, especially in conjunction with a consistent history and physical examination.
- Ultrasound may be used to assess complications of acute pancreatitis, such as pseudocyst and aneurysm formation.
- CT scanning is the diagnostic modality of choice, and a good baseline CT scan is therefore recommended upon admission to the ICU in all patients suspected of having severe disease.
- Distinguishing between sterile and infected necrosis is imperative.
- Fluid resuscitation with crystalloid solutions is the cornerstone of management, because immense volume shifts may lead to a depletion of the intravascular volume.
- Nasogastric suction should not be used routinely, and is limited to those patients who have a high risk of aspiration, or who suffer from a concomitant ileus or bowel obstruction.
- The use of TPN should be relegated to the small subset of patients who do not tolerate enteral feedings.
- Current recommendations now support the early administration of prophylactic imipenem (or ciprofloxacin) in patients with severe pancreatitis and high levels of pancreatic necrosis. Because the rate of pancreatic infection in patients with minimal necrosis is very low, the use of prophylactic agents in patients with mild pancreatitis is not warranted.
- Three established indications for surgical intervention in severe pancreatitis exist: (1) the presence of infected pancreatic necrosis, (2) failure to improve after a long period of conservative management, (3) acute abdominal catastrophe.
- Open surgery remains the primary approach for pancreatic necrosis; interventional radiological techniques may subsequently be used successfully to drain residual fluid collections.
- Pancreatic injuries secondary to penetrating abdominal trauma are best diagnosed within the critical first six hours of injury.
- Although CT scans are pivotal in the early diagnosis of pancreatic injuries, the scans of patients with significant pancreatic injury may be entirely normal, particularly within the first 12 hours of injury.
- Only after the patient is stabilized should attention be turned to the pancreas.
- The most common complication following operative management of pancreatic trauma is the formation of a pancreatic fistula, which emphasizes the fundamental need for external drainage as part of any surgical operation on the gland.

REFERENCES

1. Gray H. Anatomy of the human body. Philadelphia: Lea & Febiger, 1918.
2. Moossa AR, Bouvet M, Gamagami R. Disorders of the pancreas. In: Cuschieri A, Steele R, Moossa A, eds. Essential Surgical Practice: Higher Surgical Training in General Surgery. London: Arnold, 2002:477–525.
3. Michels N. Blood supply and anatomy of the upper abdominal organs. Philadelphia: JB Lippincott, 1955.
4. Boyden E. The pars intestinalis of the common bile duct, as viewed by the older anatomists (Vesalius, Glisson, Bianchi, Vater, Haller, Santorini, etc). Anat Rec 1936; 66:217.
5. Bradley EL. 3rd. A clinically based classification system for acute pancreatitis. Ann Chir 1993; 47:537–541.
6. Imrie CW. Underdiagnosis of acute pancreatitis. Adv Acute Pancreatitis 1997; 1:3–5.
7. Forsmark CE. The clinical problem of biliary acute necrotizing pancreatitis: epidemiology, pathophysiology, and diagnosis of biliary necrotizing pancreatitis. J Gastrointest Surg 2001; 5:235–239.
8. Acosta JM, Pellegrini CA, Skinner DB. Etiology and pathogenesis of acute biliary pancreatitis. Surgery 1980; 88:118–125.
9. Apte M, Wilson J. Alcohol-induced pancreatic injury. Best Pract Res Clin Gastroenterol 2003; 17:593–612.
10. Jackson WD. Pancreatitis: etiology, diagnosis, and management. Curr Opin Pediatr 2001; 13:447–451.
11. Testoni PA. Preventing post-ERCP pancreatitis: where are we? JOP 2003; 4:22–32.
12. Gottlieb K, Sherman S. ERCP and biliary endoscopic sphincterotomy-induced pancreatitis. Gastrointest Endosc Clin N Am 1998; 8:87–114.
13. Loperfido S, Angelini G, Benedetti G, et al. Major early complications from diagnostic and therapeutic ERCP: a prospective multicenter study. Gastrointest Endosc 1998; 48:1–10.
14. Halm MA. Acute gastrointestinal complications after cardiac surgery. Am J Crit Care 1996; 5:109–118; quiz 119–120.
15. Hashimoto L, Walsh RM. Acute pancreatitis after aortic surgery. Am Surg 1999; 65:423–426.

16. Van Os EC, Petersen BT. Pancreatitis secondary to percutaneous liver biopsy-associated hemobilia. Am J Gastroenterol 1996; 91:577–580.

17. Bhatia M, Brady M, Shokuhi S, Christmas S, Neoptolemos JP, Slavin J. Inflammatory mediators in acute pancreatitis. J Pathol 2000; 190:117–125.

18. Norman JG, Fink GW, Franz MG. Acute pancreatitis induces intrapancreatic tumor necrosis factor gene expression. Arch Surg 1995; 130:966–970.

19. Okusawa S, Gelfand JA, Ikejima T, Connolly RJ, Dinarello CA. Interleukin 1 induces a shock-like state in rabbits. Synergism with tumor necrosis factor and the effect of cyclooxygenase inhibition. J Clin Invest 1988; 81:1162–1172.

20. Beger HG, Rau B, Mayer J, Pralle U. Natural course of acute pancreatitis. World J Surg 1997; 21:130–135.

21. Bohidar NP, Garg PK, Khanna S, Tandon RK. Incidence, etiology, and impact of fever in patients with acute pancreatitis. Pancreatology 2003; 3:9–13.

22. Smotkin J, Tenner S. Laboratory diagnostic tests in acute pancreatitis. J Clin Gastroenterol 2002; 34:459–462.

23. Zieve L. Clinical value of determinations of various pancreatic enzymes in serum. Gastroenterology 1964; 46:62–71.

24. Clavien PA, Robert J, Meyer P, et al. Acute pancreatitis and normoamylasemia. Not an uncommon combination. Ann Surg 1989; 210:614–620.

25. Spechler SJ, Dalton JW, Robbins AH, et al. Prevalence of normal serum amylase levels in patients with acute alcoholic pancreatitis. Dig Dis Sci 1983; 28:865–869.

26. Chase CW, Barker DE, Russell WL, Burns RP. Serum amylase and lipase in the evaluation of acute abdominal pain. Am Surg 1996; 62:1028–1033.

27. Gumaste VV, Roditis N, Mehta D, Dave PB. Serum lipase levels in nonpancreatic abdominal pain versus acute pancreatitis. Am J Gastroenterol 1993; 88:2051–2055.

28. Frank B, Gottlieb K. Amylase normal, lipase elevated: is it pancreatitis? A case series and review of the literature. Am J Gastroenterol 1999; 94:463–469.

29. Hedstrom J, Kemppainen E, Andersen J, Jokela H, Puolakkainen P, Stenman UH. A comparison of serum trypsinogen-2 and trypsin-2-alpha1-antitrypsin complex with lipase and amylase in the diagnosis and assessment of severity in the early phase of acute pancreatitis. Am J Gastroenterol 2001; 96:424–430.

30. Schroder T, Kivilaakso E, Kinnunen PK, Lempinen M. Serum phospholipase A2 in human acute pancreatitis. Scand J Gastroenterol 1980; 15:633–636.

31. Stahl WM. Acute phase protein response to tissue injury. Crit Care Med 1987; 15:545–550.

32. Wilson C, Heads A, Shenkin A, Imrie CW. C-reactive protein, antiproteases and complement factors as objective markers of severity in acute pancreatitis. Br J Surg 1989; 76: 177–181.

33. Sandberg AA, Borgstrom A. Early prediction of severity in acute pancreatitis. Is this possible? JOP 2002; 3:116–125.

34. McKay AJ, Imrie CW, O'Neill J, Duncan JG. Is an early ultrasound scan of value in acute pancreatitis? Br J Surg 1982; 69:369–372.

35. Gandolfi L, Torresan F, Solmi L, Puccetti A. The role of ultrasound in biliary and pancreatic diseases. Eur J Ultrasound 2003; 16:141–159.

36. Bennett GL, Hann LE. Pancreatic ultrasonography. Surg Clin North Am 2001; 81:259–281.

37. Chak A, Hawes RH, Cooper GS, et al. Prospective assessment of the utility of EUS in the evaluation of gallstone pancreatitis. Gastrointest Endosc 1999; 49:599–604.

38. Sugiyama M, Atomi Y. Acute biliary pancreatitis: the roles of endoscopic ultrasonography and endoscopic retrograde cholangiopancreatography. Surgery 1998; 124:14–21.

39. Romagnuolo J. "Noninvasive vs. selective invasive biliary imaging for acute biliary pancreatitis: an economic evaluation by using decision tree analysis" Gastrointest Endosc 2005; 61(1):86–97.

40. Balthazar EJ, Ranson JH, Naidich DP, et al. Acute pancreatitis: prognostic value of CT. Radiology 1985; 156:767–772.

41. Beger H, Maier W, Block S, Buchler M. How do imaging methods influence the surgical strategy in acute pancreatitis? In: Malfertheiner P, Ditschuneit H, eds. Diagnostic Procedures in Pancreatic Disease. Berlin: Springer, 1986.

42. Bradley EL, 3rd, Murphy F, Ferguson C. Prediction of pancreatic necrosis by dynamic pancreatography. Ann Surg 1989; 210:495–503; discussion 503–504.

43. Balthazar EJ, Robinson DL, Megibow AJ, Ranson JH. Acute pancreatitis: value of CT in establishing prognosis. Radiology 1990; 174:331–336.

44. NIH state-of-the-science statement on endoscopic retrograde cholangiopancreatography (ERCP) for diagnosis and therapy NIH Consens State Sci Statements. 2002; 19(1):1–26.

45. Neoptolemos JP, Carr-Locke DL, London NJ, et al. Controlled trial of urgent endoscopic retrograde cholangiopancreatography and endoscopic sphincterotomy versus conservative treatment for acute pancreatitis due to gallstones. Lancet 1988; 2:979–983.

46. Folsch UR, Nitsche R, Ludtke R, et al. Early ERCP and papillotomy compared with conservative treatment for acute biliary pancreatitis. The German Study Group on Acute Biliary Pancreatitis. N Engl J Med 1997; 336:237–242.

47. Semelka RC, Ascher SM. MR imaging of the pancreas. Radiology 1993; 188:593–602.

48. Hall-Craggs MA, Allen CM, Owens CM, et al. MR cholangiography: clinical evaluation in 40 cases. Radiology 1993; 189:423–427.

49. Sica GT, Braver J, Cooney MJ, et al. Comparison of endoscopic retrograde cholangiopancreatography with MR cholangiopancreatography in patients with pancreatitis. Radiology 1999; 210:605–610.

50. Makary MA. The role of magnetic resonance cholangiography in the management of patients with gallstone pancreatitis. Ann Surg 2005; 241(1):119–124.

51. Ward J, Chalmers AG, Guthrie AJ, et al. T2-weighted and dynamic enhanced MRI in acute pancreatitis: comparison with contrast enhanced CT. Clin Radiol 1997; 52:109–114.

52. Robinson PJ, Sheridan MB. Pancreatitis: computed tomography and magnetic resonance imaging. Eur Radiol 2000; 10: 401–408.

53. Bouvet M, Moossa AR. Pancreatic abscess. In: Cameron JL, ed. Current Surgical Therapy, 2004.

54. Rau B, Pralle U, Mayer JM, Beger HG. Role of ultrasonographically guided fine-needle aspiration cytology in the diagnosis of infected pancreatic necrosis. Br J Surg 1998; 85: 179–184.

55. McMahon MJ, Playforth MJ, Pickford IR. A comparative study of methods for the prediction of severity of attacks of acute pancreatitis. Br J Surg 1980; 67:22–25.

56. Ranson JH, Rifkind KM, Roses DF, et al. Prognostic signs and the role of operative management in acute pancreatitis. Surg Gynecol Obstet 1974; 139:69–81.

57. Chatzicostas C, Roussomoustakaki M, Vlachonikolis IG, et al. Comparison of Ranson, APACHE II and APACHE III scoring systems in acute pancreatitis. Pancreas 2002; 25: 331–335.

58. Knaus WA, Draper EA, Wagner DP, Zimmerman JE. APACHE II: a severity of disease classification system. Crit Care Med 1985; 13:818–829.

59. Knaus WA, Wagner DP, Draper EA, et al. The APACHE III prognostic system. Risk prediction of hospital mortality for critically ill hospitalized adults. Chest 1991; 100:1619–1636.

60. Larvin M, McMahon MJ. APACHE-II score for assessment and monitoring of acute pancreatitis. Lancet 1989; 2:201–205.

61. Simchuk EJ, Traverso LW, Nukui Y, Kozarek RA. Computed tomography severity index is a predictor of outcomes for severe pancreatitis. Am J Surg 2000; 179:352–355.

62. Bradley EL, 3rd. Complications of Pancreatitis: medical and surgical management. Philadelphia: WB Saunders, 1982.

63. Company L, Saez J, Martinez J, et al. Factors predicting mortality in severe acute pancreatitis. Pancreatology 2003; 3: 144–148.

64. Tran DD, Oe PL, de Fijter CW, van der Meulen J, Cuesta MA. Acute renal failure in patients with acute pancreatitis: prevalence, risk factors, and outcome. Nephrol Dial Transplant 1993; 8:1079–1084.

65. Shields CJ, Winter DC, Redmond HP. Lung injury in acute pancreatitis: mechanisms, prevention, and therapy. Curr Opin Crit Care 2002; 8:158–163.

66. Jacobs ML, Daggett WM, Civette JM, et al. Acute pancreatitis: analysis of factors influencing survival. Ann Surg 1977; 185:43–51.

67. Tran DD, Cuesta MA, Schneider AJ, Wesdorp RI. Prevalence and prediction of multiple organ system failure and mortality in acute pancreatitis. J Crit Care 1993; 8:145–153.

68. Sarr MG, Sanfey H, Cameron JL. Prospective, randomized trial of nasogastric suction in patients with acute pancreatitis. Surgery 1986; 100:500–504.

69. Navarro S, Ros E, Aused R, et al. Comparison of fasting, nasogastric suction and cimetidine in the treatment of acute pancreatitis. Digestion 1984; 30:224–230.

70. Bouffard YH, Delafosse BX, Annat GJ, et al. Energy expenditure during severe acute pancreatitis. JPEN J Parenter Enteral Nutr 1989; 13:26–29.

71. Dickerson RN, Vehe KL, Mullen JL, Feurer ID. Resting energy expenditure in patients with pancreatitis. Crit Care Med 1991; 19:484–490.

72. Abou-Assi S, O'Keefe SJ. Nutrition support during acute pancreatitis. Nutrition 2002; 18:938–943.

73. Kalfarentzos FE, Karavias DD, Karatzas TM, et al. Total parenteral nutrition in severe acute pancreatitis. J Am Coll Nutr 1991; 10:156–162.

74. Clark-Christoff N, Watters VA, Sparks W, et al. Use of triple-lumen subclavian catheters for administration of total parenteral nutrition. J Parenter Enteral Nutr 1992; 16: 403–407.

75. Kotani J, Usami M, Nomura H, et al. Enteral nutrition prevents bacterial translocation but does not improve survival during acute pancreatitis. Arch Surg 1999; 134:287–292.

76. Eatock FC. A randomized study of early nasogastric versus nasojejunal feeding in severe acute pancreatitis. Am J Gastroenterol 2005; 100(2), 432–439.

77. Kalfarentzos F, Kehagias J, Mead N, et al. Enteral nutrition is superior to parenteral nutrition in severe acute pancreatitis: results of a randomized prospective trial. Br J Surg 1997; 84:1665–1669.

78. McClave SA, Greene LM, Snider HL, et al. Comparison of the safety of early enteral vs. parenteral nutrition in mild acute pancreatitis. J Parenter Enteral Nutr 1997; 21:14–20.

79. Windsor AC, Kanwar S, Li AG, et al. Compared with parenteral nutrition, enteral feeding attenuates the acute phase response and improves disease severity in acute pancreatitis. Gut 1998; 42:431–435.

80. Buchman AL, Moukarzel AA, Bhuta S, et al. Parenteral nutrition is associated with intestinal morphologic and functional changes in humans. J Parenter Enteral Nutr 1995; 19: 453–460.

81. Qin HL, Su ZD, Hu LG, et al. Effect of early intrajejunal nutrition on pancreatic pathological features and gut barrier function in dogs with acute pancreatitis. Clin Nutr 2002; 21:469–473.

82. Yousaf M, McCallion K, Diamond T. Management of severe acute pancreatitis. Br J Surg 2003; 90:407–420.

83. Beger HG, Bittner R, Block S, Buchler M. Bacterial contamination of pancreatic necrosis. A prospective clinical study. Gastroenterology 1986; 91:433–438.

84. Hartwig W, Werner J, Uhl W, Buchler MW. Management of infection in acute pancreatitis. J Hepatobiliary Pancreat Surg 2002; 9:423–428.

85. Marotta F, Geng TC, Wu CC, Barbi G. Bacterial translocation in the course of acute pancreatitis: beneficial role of nonabsorbable antibiotics and lactitol enemas. Digestion 1996; 57: 446–452.

86. Rahman SH, Ammori BJ, Holmfield J, et al. Intestinal hypoperfusion contributes to gut barrier failure in severe acute pancreatitis. J Gastrointest Surg 2003; 7:26–35; discussion 35–36.

87. Ammori BJ, Leeder PC, King RF, et al. Early increase in intestinal permeability in patients with severe acute pancreatitis: correlation with endotoxemia, organ failure, and mortality. J Gastrointest Surg 1999; 3:252–262.

88. Raty S, Sand J, Nordback I. Difference in microbes contaminating pancreatic necrosis in biliary and alcoholic pancreatitis. Int J Pancreatol 1998; 24:187–191.

89. Sharma VK, Howden CW. Prophylactic antibiotic administration reduces sepsis and mortality in acute necrotizing pancreatitis: a meta-analysis. Pancreas 2001; 22:28–31.

90. Golub R, Siddiqi F, Pohl D. Role of antibiotics in acute pancreatitis: A meta-analysis. J Gastrointest Surg 1998; 2:496–503.

91. Gloor B, Muller CA, Worni M, et al. Pancreatic infection in severe pancreatitis: the role of fungus and multiresistant organisms. Arch Surg 2001; 136:592–596.

92. Robbins EG, Stollman NH, Bierman P, et al. Pancreatic fungal infections: a case report and review of the literature. Pancreas 1996; 12:308–312.

93. Isenmann R, Schwarz M, Rau B, Trautmann M, et al. Characteristics of infection with Candida species in patients with necrotizing pancreatitis. World J Surg 2002; 26:372–376.

94. Grewe M, Tsiotos GG, Luque de-Leon E, Sarr MG. Fungal infection in acute necrotizing pancreatitis. J Am Coll Surg 1999; 188:408–414.

95. Limberg B, Kommerell B. Treatment of acute pancreatitis with somatostatin. N Engl J Med 1980; 303:284.

96. Binder M, Uhl W, Friess H, et al. Octreotide in the treatment of acute pancreatitis: results of a unicenter prospective trial with three different octreotide dosages. Digestion 1994; 55:20–23.

97. Choi TK, Mok F, Zhan WH, et al. Somatostatin in the treatment of acute pancreatitis: a prospective randomised controlled trial. Gut 1989; 30:223–227.

98. D'Amico D, Favia G, Biasiato R, et al. The use of somatostatin in acute pancreatitis—results of a multicenter trial. Hepatogastroenterology 1990; 37:92–98.

99. Uhl W, Buchler MW, Malfertheiner P, et al. A randomised, double blind, multicentre trial of octreotide in moderate to severe acute pancreatitis. Gut 1999; 45:97–104.

100. Andriulli A, Leandro G, Niro G, et al. Pharmacologic treatment can prevent pancreatic injury after ERCP: a meta-analysis. Gastrointest Endosc 2000; 51:1–7.

101. Andriulli A, Caruso N, Quitadamo M, et al. Antisecretory vs. antiproteasic drugs in the prevention of post-ERCP pancreatitis: the evidence-based medicine derived from a meta-analysis study. JOP 2003; 4:41–48.

102. Bradley EL, 3rd. Operative vs. nonoperative therapy in necrotizing pancreatitis. Digestion 1999; 60:19–21.

103. Buchler MW, Gloor B, Muller CA, et al. Acute necrotizing pancreatitis: treatment strategy according to the status of infection. Ann Surg 2000; 232:619–626.

104. Bradley EL, 3rd, Allen K. A prospective longitudinal study of observation versus surgical intervention in the management of necrotizing pancreatitis. Am J Surg 1991; 161:19–24; discussion 24–25.

105. Banks PA. Practice guidelines in acute pancreatitis. Am J Gastroenterol 1997; 92:377–386.

106. Uomo G, Visconti M, Manes G, et al. Nonsurgical treatment of acute necrotizing pancreatitis. Pancreas 1996; 12:142–148.

107. Mier J, Leon EL, Castillo A, et al. Early versus late necrosectomy in severe necrotizing pancreatitis. Am J Surg 1997; 173:71–75.

108. Hartwig W, Maksan SM, Foitzik T, et al. Reduction in mortality with delayed surgical therapy of severe pancreatitis. J Gastrointest Surg 2002; 6:481–487.

109. Rattner DW, Legermate DA, Lee MJ, et al. Early surgical debridement of symptomatic pancreatic necrosis is beneficial irrespective of infection. Am J Surg 1992; 163:105–109; discussion 109–110.

110. Rau B, Pralle U, Uhl W, et al. Management of sterile necrosis in instances of severe acute pancreatitis. J Am Coll Surg 1995; 181:279–288.

111. Traverso LW. Pancreatic necrosectomy: definitions and technique. J Gastrointest Surg. 2005; 9(3):436–439.

112. Rau B. Surgical treatment of necrotizing pancreatitis by necrosectomy and closed lavage: changing patient characteristics and outcome in a 19-year, single-center series. Surgery. 2005; 138(1):28–39.

113. Fernandez-del Castillo C, Rattner DW, Makary MA, et al. Debridement and closed packing for the treatment of necrotizing pancreatitis. Ann Surg 1998; 228:676–684.

114. Bradley EL, 3rd. Management of infected pancreatic necrosis by open drainage. Ann Surg 1987; 206:542–550.

115. Szentkereszty Z, Kerekes L, Hallay J, et al. CT-guided percutaneous peripancreatic drainage: a possible therapy in acute necrotizing pancreatitis. Hepatogastroenterology 2002; 49: 1696–1698.

116. vanSonnenberg E, Wittich GR, Chon KS, et al. Percutaneous radiologic drainage of pancreatic abscesses. Am J Roentgenol 1997; 168:979–984.

117. Andersson R, Cwikiel W. Percutaneous cystogastrostomy in patients with pancreatic pseudocysts. Eur J Surg 2002; 168:345–348.

118. Srikanth G, Sikora SS, Baijal SS, et al. Pancreatic abscess: 10 years experience. ANZ J Surg 2002; 72:881–886.

119. Baril NB, Ralls PW, Wren SM, et al. Does an infected peripancreatic fluid collection or abscess mandate operation? Ann Surg 2000; 231:361–367.

120. Bassi C, Butturini G, Salvia R, et al. A single-institution experience with fistulojejunostomy for external pancreatic fistulas. Am J Surg 2000; 179:203–206.

121. Cirillo RL, Jr, Koniaris LG. Detecting blunt pancreatic injuries. J Gastrointest Surg 2002; 6:587-598.

122. Jurkovich GJ, Carrico CJ. Pancreatic trauma. Surg Clin North Am 1990; 70:575–593.

123. Takishima T, Sugimoto K, Asari Y, et al. Characteristics of pancreatic injury in children: a comparison with such injury in adults. J Pediatr Surg 1996; 31:896–900.

124. Vasquez JC, Coimbra R, Hoyt DB, Fortlage D. Management of penetrating pancreatic trauma: an 11-year experience of a level-1 trauma center. Injury 2001; 32:753–759.

125. Wisner DH, Wold RL, Frey CF. Diagnosis and treatment of pancreatic injuries. An analysis of management principles. Arch Surg 1990; 125:1109–1113.

126. Buechter KJ, Arnold M, Steele B, et al. The use of serum amylase and lipase in evaluating and managing blunt abdominal trauma. Am Surg 1990; 56:204–208.

127. Gomez GA, Alvarez R, Plasencia G, et al. Diagnostic peritoneal lavage in the management of blunt abdominal trauma: a reassessment. J Trauma 1987; 27:1–5.

128. Dolich MO, McKenney MG, Varela JE, et al. 2,576 ultrasounds for blunt abdominal trauma. J Trauma 2001; 50:108–112.

129. Jeffrey RB, Jr, Federle MP, Crass RA. Computed tomography of pancreatic trauma. Radiology 1983; 147:491–494.

130. Moore EE, Cogbill TH, Malangoni MA, et al. Organ injury scaling, II: Pancreas, duodenum, small bowel, colon, and rectum. J Trauma 1990; 30:1427–1429.

131. Johnson JW, Gracias VH, Schwab CW, et al. Evolution in damage control for exsanguinating penetrating abdominal injury. J Trauma 2001; 51:261–269; discussion 269–271.

132. Farrell RJ, Krige JE, Bornman PC, et al. Operative strategies in pancreatic trauma. Br J Surg 1996; 83:934–937.

133. Nwariaku FE, Terracina A, Mileski WJ, et al. Is octreotide beneficial following pancreatic injury? Am J Surg 1995; 170: 582–585.

134. Riche FC, Cholley BP, Laisne MJ, et al. Inflammatory cytokines, C reactive protein, and procalcitonin as early predictors of necrosis infection in acute necrotizing pancreatitis. Surgery 2003; 133:257–262.

135. Neoptolemos JP, Kemppainen EA, Mayer JM, et al. Early prediction of severity in acute pancreatitis by urinary trypsinogen activation peptide: a multicentre study. Lancet 2000; 355: 1955–1960.

136. Johnson CD. Urinary trypsinogen activation peptide as a marker of severe acute pancreatitis. Br J Surg 2004; 91(8): 1027–1033.

137. Gupta A. Blunt trauma of the pancreas and biliary tract: a multimodality imaging approach to diagnosis. Radiographics 2004; 24(5): 1381–1395.

138. Ammori BJ. Laparoscopic transgastric pancreatic necrosectomy for infected pancreatic necrosis. Surg Endosc 2002; 16:1362.

139. Pamoukian VN, Gagner M. Laparoscopic necrosectomy for acute necrotizing pancreatitis. J Hepatobiliary Pancreat Surg 2001; 8:221–223.

140. de Wilt JH, van Eijck CH, Hussain SM, Bonjer HJ. Laparoscopic spleen preserving distal pancreatectomy after blunt abdominal trauma. Injury 2003; 34:233–234.

141. Abu-Zidan FM. Lexipafant and acute pancreatitis: a critical appraisal of the clinical trials. Eur J Surg. 2002; 168(4): 215–219.

142. Jamdar S. Drotrecogin alfa (recombinant human activated protein C) in severe acute pancreatitis. Crit Care. 2005; 9(4): 321–322.

40

Oliguria: Renal Failure vs. Renal Success

Emilio B. Lobato

Department of Anesthesiology and Critical Care Medicine, University of Florida College of Medicine, Malcolm B. Randall VA
Medical Center, Gainesville, Florida, U.S.A.

Robert R. Kirby

University of Florida College of Medicine, and the Malcolm B. Randall VA Medical Center, Gainesville, Florida, U.S.A.

INTRODUCTION

"All we really know for certain about the kidney is that it produces urine" (1). This statement by the eminent twentieth century renal physiologist and philosopher, Homer Smith, epitomizes the complexity of urine formation. Clinicians often rely on adequate urine output as a sign of tissue perfusion and renal function. Normal urine production (about 1–2 L per day) is the result of a delicate balance between renal and extrarenal factors. This balance is frequently disrupted in patients following trauma and critical illness, which leads to decreased urinary output, or oliguria (oligio = few, small, or little).

Oliguria may be one of the first clinical clues heralding inadequate renal perfusion in trauma and critically ill patients. Understanding the definition, verification process, differential diagnosis and treatment priorities for oliguria constitutes essential fundamental knowledge required of all trauma intensivists. Because oliguria is a normal compensatory response to acute hypovolemia, it has been deemed by some as a sign of renal success rather than renal failure (2).

In the past, oliguria associated with a disease process was viewed by many as a primary renal event that heralded a dysfunctional kidney (renal failure); thus, therapy usually was directed towards restoration of normal urinary output. The concept that during illness or trauma, oliguria may also represent an adaptive mechanism by the kidney in its efforts to restore homeostasis (renal success) was introduced later (2,3).

However, there is a narrow window (approximately 30–60 minutes) between the onset of the protective compensation (renal conservation of sodium and water, resulting in oliguria), and the initiation of ischemic acute tubular necrosis (ATN) in the setting of severe renal hypoperfusion. Because of the short time span following hypoperfusion of the kidneys and progression to ATN, especially in the setting of pre-existing renal insufficiency, or concomitant toxic exposure, other (indirect) but earlier indicators of renal perfusion (or underperfusion) must be relied upon in order to protect patients and their kidneys from perioperative renal doom.

☞ **Oliguria is often an early sign of renal compromise, representing either a compensatory mechanism for hypoperfusion (hypovolemia and/or hypotension) or an acute renal insult.** ☞ Renal compensatory mechanisms are limited and progression to overt renal insufficiency can occur over a short period of time (minutes to hours), thus providing a small window for therapeutic intervention (4,5).

This chapter provides an overview of oliguria along with the background knowledge required to understand and promote renal viability following trauma and critical illness. Identifiable factors known to increase the risk for renal insufficiency, and the maneuvers that should be taken to limit renal injury in these susceptible patients are reviewed. The physiology of urine formation, and the pathogenesis of ARF are described.

The appropriate evaluation and treatment of the oliguric patient requires an understanding of the mechanisms involved in urine production, the risk factors, and the pathophysiological entities responsible for oliguria and ARF. An organized approach to the diagnosis and treatment of reversible causes of oliguria must be initiated expeditiously, in order to prevent the poor prognosis of acute renal failure (6,7).

DEFINITION AND CLASSIFICATION
Definition of Oliguria

The standard definition of oliguria in an adult is a urine output <400 mL/day (approximately 15 mL/hr) (8). This volume is based on the amount of maximally concentrated urine required to excrete the normal daily solute load including nitrogenous waste products. In certain clinical conditions (e.g., administration of osmotic diuretics, severe hyperglycemia), a patient may be considered oliguric despite a higher urinary output. Similarly, patients with pre-existing renal dysfunction may be unable to effectively concentrate the urine and thus require a higher urinary output to maintain homeostasis.

Definition of Acute Tubular Necrosis

Acute tubular necrosis (ATN) is the death of tubular cells as occurs following prolonged ischemia (hypotension and hypovolemia chiefly) or exposure to toxins (rhabdomyolysis, IV contrast, aminolycosides, etc.). The pathophysiology of ATN is not completely understood, but a recent review by Gill is recommended (8).

Classification of Acute Renal Failure

Traditionally acute renal failure (ARF) has been separated into three major categories: Prerenal, intrinsic renal, and

Table 1   Major Categories of Oliguria in Trauma and Critical Care

Class	Cause	Examples/comments
Prerenal	Hypovolemia	Blood loss, fluid loss, third space sequestration
	Hepatorenal syndrome	Liver failure and decreased effective intravascular volume
	Cardiac and cardiovascular failure	Infarction, tamponade, arrhythmia, sepsis, anaphylaxis
	Vascular obstruction	Thrombosis (arterial or venous), embolus, aneurysm, amyloidosis
Renal	Hemolysis	Transfusion and immune reactions, malaria
	Rhabdomyolysis	Trauma, muscle damage, heat stroke, malignant hyperthermia
	Nephrotoxins	Radiocontrast, aminoglycosides
	Vasculitis acute, diffuse	Periarteritis
	Pyelonephritis antibiotics	
Postrenal	Obstruction	Catheterized patients: kinked catheter, clot obstruction, false passage
		Non-catheterized patients: calculi, stricture, neoplasms
	Extravasation	Bladder rupture

postrenal (Table 1) (9,10). This is an incomplete classification system because prerenal oliguria initially is reversible, but when hypoperfusion is allowed to persist for too long, intrinsic renal injury in the form of ATN will occur. Post (or obstructive) renal failure is also initially reversible but when prolonged can cause intrinsic renal injury and failure. Nephrotoxic drugs and pre-existing renal disease can increase the risk of ATN with all these entities. A wide variety of medical conditions not unique to trauma or critical care can also cause renal failure.

PATHOPHYSIOLOGY

☞ **When the kidneys sense abnormalities in extracellular fluid volume or osmolality, they respond by increasing or decreasing the amount of urine excreted.** ☞ Marked reduction or cessation of urinary output in a trauma or critically ill patient can occur suddenly or over a period of several hours to days. Oliguria may be the harbinger of ATN. Correct diagnosis and treatment are paramount to prevent significant morbidity and mortality.

If oliguria is associated with a prerenal state, a measurable decrease in urine output is present and blood urea nitrogen (BUN) rises to a greater degree than does the serum creatinine, as the kidneys produce concentrated urine to conserve intravascular volume. As renal conservation mechanisms become exhausted, renal failure supervenes, function deteriorates and abnormal serum biochemical values develop. ☞ **Significant oliguria implies a state of renal dysfunction, since a urine output of ≤400 mL/day is inadequate for excretion of the daily solute load of 650 to 750 mOsm (normal diet) in a maximally concentrated urine (1.2 mOsm/mL).** ☞ Since renal failure also may be associated with a high urine output, both oliguric and polyuric states represent the extremes of a continuum. Thus, a diagnosis of renal failure must take into account the quality of urine excreted as well as the quantity produced.

Physiology of Urine Formation

160 to 180 L of water, each containing approximately 300 mOsm of solute, are filtered daily through the glomeruli of a healthy adult in a 24-hour period. As the filtrate passes through the proximal convoluted tubules, sodium is actively resorbed into the renal cortical interstitium, chloride follows passively, and water is reabsorbed by osmosis. Ions and water deposited in the interstitium are rapidly removed by blood perfusing the cortical capillaries, thereby reducing the fluid volume in the proximal tubules by approximately 75%. However, the osmolar concentration remains unchanged.

As fluid flows through the thin, descending limbs of Henle's loops, water diffuses out into the hypertonic interstitium of the medulla and papilla, and sodium and chloride diffuse in. The volume of tubular fluid decreases, and the osmotic pressure progressively increases. In the thick part of the ascending limb of Henle's loops, chloride is extruded into the interstitium. Since water cannot pass through the ascending limbs, the osmolar concentration of the tubular fluid is reduced.

Fluid entering the distal convoluted tubules is hypotonic compared to the surrounding cortical interstitial fluid, and its volume is reduced to 15% of the original glomerular filtrate. Tubular fluid is isotonic with cortical interstitial fluid when it reaches the middle of the distal segment. Active extrusion of sodium and passive osmotic diffusion of water are resumed in the distal tubule, and the volume of tubular fluid volume entering the collecting duct is reduced to approximately 1% of the original glomerular filtrate. Collecting duct fluid, which initially is iso-osmotic, becomes progressively concentrated as it descends through the hypertonic medullary and papillary interstitium.

As water diffuses out of the descending limbs of Henle's loops and the collecting ducts, it is removed by blood flow through the vasa recti of the medulla and papilla. These vessels reduce the loss of osmotically active solutes from the medulla and papilla. Once urine exits the kidney, it is transported to the bladder via ureteral peristalsis, initiated in pacemaker sites located at the junction of the ureter and the renal pelvis.

Renal Perfusion

The kidneys receive approximately one-fifth the total resting cardiac output ($\dot{Q}$). However, their oxygen consumption ($\dot{V}O_2$) is rather low (about 10% of total body $\dot{V}O_2$) (11). The three main determinants of renal blood flow are: (*i*) $\dot{Q}$, (*ii*) renal perfusion pressure, and (*iii*) local hemodynamic factors such as afferent versus efferent arteriolar tone.

Renal blood flow is preferentially directed to the cortex (90–95%), where most glomeruli are located, in order to optimize filtration and reabsorption. Unlike the cortex, the medulla receives only a fraction of flow (5–10%), to preserve the osmotic gradient required to concentrate the urine (12). Medullary cells (particularly those on the ascending limb) have a higher oxygen extraction than cortical cells (80% vs. 20%) (13). ♂ **The high metabolic rate in combination with a lower blood supply places the medullary tubular cells at a higher risk for hypoxic damage, despite what would be perceived as adequate renal blood flow. (Fig. 1).** ♂

Renal blood flow is constant over a wide range of mean arterial pressures (MAPs) (Fig. 2). The predominant mechanism involves changes in glomerular arteriolar tone with consequent variations in renal vascular resistance. Decreased renal perfusion may occur with low $\dot{Q}$ (e.g., hypovolemia), decreased perfusion pressure (MAP) despite adequate $\dot{Q}$ (e.g., sepsis), or due to local redistribution of blood flow (as occurs with hepatorenal syndrome). Hypotension due to hypovolemia causes a greater reduction in renal blood flow than hypotension (of a similar magnitude) due to impaired left ventricular (LV) function (14). This difference is caused by the release of atrial and brain natriuretic peptides from the left atrial and ventricular endocardium in response to increased filling pressures (15). These protective endogenous peptides are important renal vasodilators, which also increase GFR and sodium excretion.

The response to renal hypoperfusion is complex and multifactorial, as the kidneys "attempt" to preserve GFR.

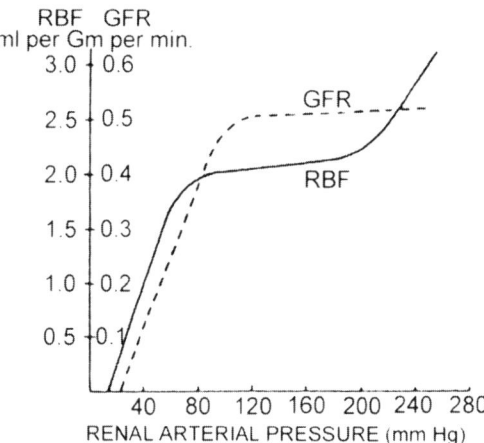

Figure 2 Autoregulation of glomerular filtration rate (GFR) and renal blood flow (RBF), based on the original data of Shipley and Study, GFR and RBF remain constant between a renal arterial pressures of 80 to 180 mmHg. *Source*: From Ref. 137.

Both neurohormonal and hemodynamic factors (local and systemic) are involved (16–18) and include: (*i*) afferent arteriolar dilatation that, when combined with efferent arteriolar constriction, increases filtration fraction; and (*ii*) activation of the renin-angiotensin aldosterone (RAA) axis, with increased sodium reabsorption and efferent arteriolar resistance. A low cardiac output will trigger the release of ADH with consequent reabsorption of water in the collecting duct (19). The accompanying sympathetic response produces a further increase in arteriolar resistance.

Intrarenal production of prostaglandins E_2, D_2, and I_2, each play an important role in local autoregulation of blood flow by acting as renal vasodilators. In the presence of decreased renal blood flow, the release of PGE_2 counteracts the renal vasoconstrictive effects of angiotensin and norepinephrine to preserve renal blood flow (20). Certain nonsteroidal anti-inflammatory agents (NSAIDs) decrease the synthesis of PGE_2 by inhibiting the activity of cyclooxygenase, thereby increasing the risk of renal ischemia in susceptible patients (21).

♂ **Oliguria in response to hypoperfusion is the result of the kidneys' self-preservation to circumvent renal failure.** ♂ Unless the primary insult is corrected, however, these mechanisms eventually become overwhelmed, and tubular necrosis occurs.

DIFFERENTIAL DIAGNOSIS
Prerenal Oliguria

Oliguria in trauma and postsurgical patients is most commonly associated with inadequate renal perfusion, stemming from hypotension and inadequate *circulating blood volume secondary to hemorrhage* and/or shift of third space fluids. Other contributors, including nephrotoxic drugs, cardiac failure or preexisting diseases can also be involved, especially during the critical illness. The abdominal compartment syndrome can also play an important role (Chapter 34). When renal blood flow is minimally or moderately depressed, a compensatory increase in filtration fraction occurs, and GFR and urine formulation remain relatively unaffected. However, when depression of renal

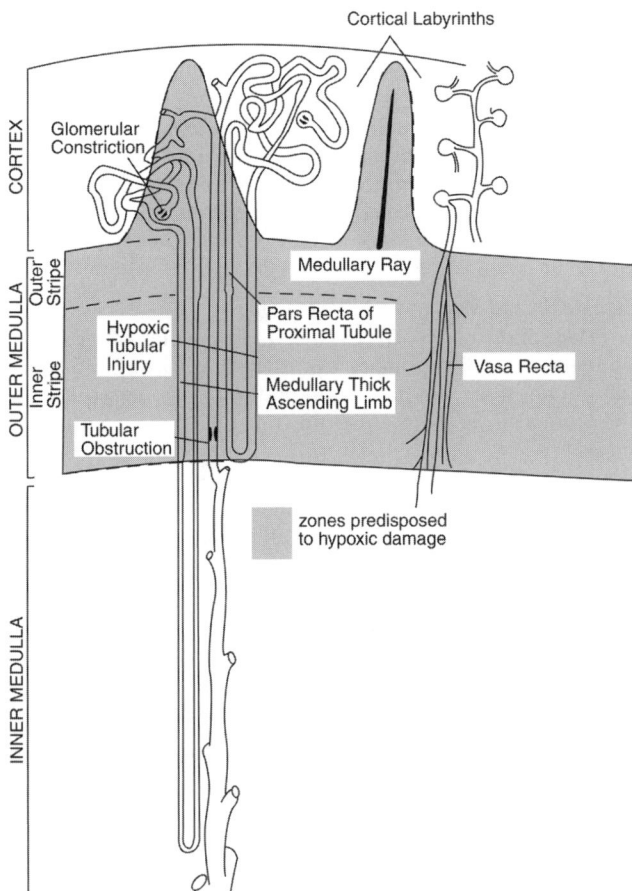

Figure 1 Anatomy of intrarenal zones predisposed to hypoxic injury in acute renal failure. *Source*: From Ref. 136.

blood flow is marked, GFR, urine formation, and electrolyte excretion also are significantly reduced.

Oliguria caused by blood loss, sequestration of fluid into a surgical third space, dehydration, or gastrointestinal loss is a complex problem. If hypovolemia is severe and persistent enough to cause renal ischemia, functional lesions acquire a renal morphological component. In extreme cases, simple prerenal oliguria is transformed into oliguric renal failure (22).

Extravasation of urine outside the bladder following pelvic trauma (Volume I, Chapter 28), may be associated with oliguria. Pelvic fractures are associated with 9% to 15% incidence of a ruptured bladder (23). The uterers are rarely injured, except from direct trauma during surgery.

Intrinsic Renal Disease (Acute Tubular Necrosis)

Renal causes of oliguria are also known as intrinsic renal failure, implying a nonprerenal etiology. This is not necessarily true in trauma patients. Indeed, renal oliguria in trauma and postsurgical patients usually results from uncorrected renal hypoperfusion, leading to ATN. Although primary renal oliguria is not usually associated with trauma and surgery, in certain clinical conditions, oliguria occurs as a result of a toxic insult to the kidney despite adequate renal perfusion.

Ischemia

Prolonged prerenal state, hypotension, hypovolemia, and hypoxia are all common conditions in the critically ill trauma patient and all can cause ATN. Many disparate etiologies, including various nephrotoxins, can lead to ATN via a mechanism involving reduced total or segmental renal blood flow with resultant ischemic injury.

The mortality associated with this syndrome has remained high despite 50 years of improvements in management. This is largely because modern resuscitation practices now prevent ATN in less severely ill patients, and saves the lives of those critically ill patients who formerly would have died. Thus ATN is seen in a progressively sicker subset of patients.

Ischemia causes changes in tubular cell polarity; loss of integrity of the tubular epithelial barrier; necrotic and apoptotic cell death; loss of both viable and nonviable cells, which lift off the basement membrane; and expression of genes characteristic of the embryonic kidney mesenchyme (24,25). The damaged kidney epithelium, however, in contrast to heart or brain, can be completely restored in structure and function.

The kidney possesses a remarkable regenerative capacity after acute ischemic and/or toxic injury. This regenerative capacity manifests itself by proliferation and migration of poorly differentiated cells along the denuded basement membrane of injured tubular segments within a few days after ischemic insult (26). In animal models of repair following ischemic injury, proliferation is observed to be maximal in the straight segment of the proximal tubule located in the outer medulla, where damage is most apparent. The damaged areas of the nephron are repopulated initially by poorly differentiated proliferating cells that have features of epithelial precursors, such as a less well-developed brush border, downregulation of the transcription factor kid-1 (27), and expression of the intermediate filament protein vimentin, which is normally undetectable in the adult proximal tubule epithelium but is expressed in the embryonic metanephric mesenchyme (26). There are several possibilities for the origin of these regenerating epithelial

cells: (*i*) epithelial cells may dedifferentiate, proliferate, then redifferentiate into mature tubular cells, as a survival response to injury; (*ii*) bone marrow stem cells (BMSCs) may home to the injured epithelium, where local cues trigger differentiation; or (*iii*) a population of renal mesenchymal stem cells exists that may replenish the epithelial cell population after injury.

In addition to tubular cell injury, the peritubular vasculature undergoes changes in response to ischemia associated with ATN. These changes range from activation of inflammatory genes, cell swelling, and disruption of endothelial junctions to detachment of live and dead cells from the basement membrane (28). These endothelial changes, together with persistent, inappropriate vasoconstriction, lead to reduction of peritubular blood flow, which contributes to extension of the initial ischemic insult (29). Although replacement of the lost tubular cells is essential for nephron regeneration, the return of blood flow, which is dependent upon endothelial cell integrity, is also essential for recovery. Recently, it has been suggested that cells repopulating the ischemically injured tubule derive from bone marrow stem cells. More recently Duffield et al. (30–34), showed that these bone marrow-derived cells do not make a significant contribution to the restoration of epithelial integrity after an ischemic insult (30). It is likely that intrinsic tubular cell proliferation accounts for functionally significant replenishment of the tubular epithelium after ischemia.

Nephrotoxic Drugs

Intravenous contrast agents (ionic worse than nonionic) are common causes of ATN. The agents are used in digital vascular imaging and selective renal angiography (31,32). Contrast induced nephropathy is classically oliguric and occurs within 24 hours of use. NSAIDs such as phenylbutazone, ibuprofen, and indomethacin (33,34), and aminoglycoside antibiotics may lead to oliguria and renal insufficiency. The latter agents account for 5% to 10% of all hospital-acquired acute renal failure (35), but ATN does not usually occur with these drugs until >5–7 days of use.

Myoglobin and Stroma-Free Hemoglobin

☞ Reduction of the GFR rather than tubular obstruction appears to be the primary event leading to oliguric renal failure when stroma-free hemoglobin or myoglobin enters the glomeruli (36,37). ☞ Also, the transfusion of incompatible blood leads to disseminated intravascular coagulation, with deposition of fibrin in renal tubules. Red cell membranes are thought to initiate the coagulation process, ultimately leading to a decrease in platelets, fibrinogen, and factors II, V, and VII (38). Rhabdomyolysis and Myoglobinuria following extensive, crushing-type muscle injuries also may lead to oliguric renal failure (38,39). The mechanism is probably similar as that for stroma-free hemoglobin.

Oliguria and azotemia have occurred after captopril therapy (40,41) or following treatment with amphotericin B. In the latter situation, renal vasoconstriction is thought to occur concomitantly with nephrotoxicity. Acute oliguria can also occur from thrombosis of the glomerular afferent arterioles following chemotherapy with vinblastine, bleomycin, or cisplatin (42).

Although degradation of sevoflurane to a compound (compound A) that is nephrotoxic in rats has been demonstrated (43), low-flow isoflurane and sevoflurane do not appear to alter renal function in patients with preexisting stable renal disease (44). With the exception of methoxyflurane (no longer used), anesthetic-induced changes of renal function are readily reversed when administration of the agent is discontinued (45–48).

Intratubular obstruction and backflow of filtrate into damaged tubules may be causative factors (36). Most common in the pathogenesis of ATN is the suppression of glomerular filtration (37). However, light and electron microscopic studies of glomeruli generally failed to reveal structural abnormalities; thus the likelihood is that reduced glomerular filtration is caused by vasomotor phenomena (49).

Postrenal Oliguria

Obstruction of normal urinary outflow is the most significant disorder in this category. It leads to an increase in hydrostatic pressure in the urinary tract proximal to the obstruction and, ultimately, a marked decrease in GFR. Morphologic damage to the renal parenchyma is related to the degree and duration of obstruction and related factors such as the virulence of associated pyelonephritis, which may develop as a result of urinary stasis.

Extrinsic obstruction can result from the abdominal compartment syndrome (50), retroperitoneal malignancies, rapidly growing cervical carcinomas, massive uterine fibromyomata, complete bilateral ureteral obstruction owing to lymphomatous or leukemic involvement of the lymph nodes (51), giant intra-abdominal cysts (52), and inadvertent ligation of or trauma to the ureters. The latter mishaps occur in 0.1% to 0.25% of patients undergoing gynecologic surgery (53,54). ☞ **Approximately 20% to 25% of ureteral injuries are bilateral, resulting in immediate anuria.** ☞ Fecal impaction in elderly patients can produce obstructive uropathy and oliguria.

Intrinsic obstruction results from blood clots, calculi, prostatic obstruction, neoplasms, fungus balls, bilharziasis, amyloidosis, and benign prostatic enlargement in older patients following operations around the groin or rectum (55–61). Intermittent anuria or oliguria may occur in patients with bladder stones if the calculus acts as a ball valve. Kidney transplant recipients also may develop obstructive uropathy with oliguria (60).

RISK FACTORS FOR ACUTE RENAL FAILURE

Appropriate management for high-risk patients depends on identifying and minimizing important risk factors for complications, and quickly treating problems when they occur. Accordingly, the first step is to identify the patient at high risk for ARF. Next, evaluate the intravascular volume status and optimize management of preexisting medical conditions (particularly cardiovascular disease). Finally, employ a review of medications and a strict avoidance of any nonessential medications associated with renal insufficiency.

In a recent meta-analysis of preoperative risk factors for postoperative renal failure (involving 28 studies and 10,865 patients), preexisting renal disease emerges as the most important preoperative risk factor for the development of postoperative ARF. Unfortunately, few studies use the same criteria for ARF, and there is a lack of consistent criteria for establishing risk factors. Furthermore, the literature provides little quantitative information concerning the degree of risk associated with most risk factors. However, certain systemic diseases, several known nephrotoxic

drugs, and certain surgical procedures or conditions are associated with an increased risk of renal failure (Table 2).

Clinical Assessment

In the majority of trauma and postsurgical patients, oliguria signifies renal hypoperfusion often due to either decreased effective circulating blood volume, renal perfusion pressure, or both. At present, no true monitor of renal perfusion exists for clinical use, although some authors have demonstrated that intrarenal blood flow can be evaluated with esophageal Doppler ultrasound (62) (Fig. 3). In practice, one must rely on evaluation of effective circulating blood volume as an indirect surrogate of renal perfusion by measuring arterial blood pressure, LV preload, and $\dot{Q}$.

Mean Arterial Pressure

☞ **The MAP provides an estimate of renal perfusion pressure, whereas the systolic blood pressure variation (SPV) during positive-pressure ventilation may provide information on effective circulating volume (63).** ☞

Left Ventricular Preload

Because a reliable method to determine intravascular volume is not currently available, clinicians must depend on measurements of cardiac filling pressures or LV size to estimate effective circulating volume. Central venous pressure (CVP) provides an estimate of right ventricular (RV) preload. In the presence of normal left heart function, one can expect a reasonable correlation between CVP and left atrial pressure. This relationship is lost when there is significant LV dysfunction, mitral valve disease, or pulmonary hypertension. Pulmonary artery catheterization can provide indirect estimates of LV filling by measuring pulmonary artery occlusion pressure (PAOP), while cardiac output can be measured intermittently or continuously to determine the response to treatment. Several investigators, however, have shown a poor correlation in critically ill patients between PAOP (as a surrogate of LV diastolic pressure) and direct measurement of LV diastolic volume (64–66). This observation results from changes in ventricular compliance that affects the LV end-diastolic pressure/volume relationship.

Echocardiography can provide visual estimates of ventricular preload and global and regional function. Transthoracic echocardiography (TTE) in the perioperative period is confined to the ICU environment, although the inability to obtain useful acoustic windows (e.g., chest tubes, dressings) significantly limits its usefulness (67,68). Transesophageal echocardiography (TEE), although more invasive, is the technique of choice, particularly in intubated patients. Once the transducer is inserted, evaluation of ventricular function can be performed rapidly and expeditiously (Chapter 21). Additionally, Doppler technology allows measurement of $\dot{Q}$ and estimates of filling pressures (69,70). While the role of TEE as a continuous monitor in the operating room is well established, the discomfort associated with the large size gastroscope limits its current use as a diagnostic tool in the ICU unless patients are heavily sedated.

Cardiac Output

☞ **Measurement of $\dot{Q}$ in combination with MAP determinations is, at present, the most reliable way to evaluate renal perfusion clinically.** ☞ Thermodilution $\dot{Q}$ obtained via a pulmonary artery catheter is considered the gold standard; however, it is an invasive technique, and its use is

Table 2 Risk Factors for Perioperative Acute Renal Failure

Category	Disorder/drug/procedure/comments
Pre-existing renal insufficiency	↓'d GFR, ↓'d renal reserve (likely more sensitive to all renal insults)
Prolonged hypovolemia or hypotension during resusc.	Prolonged hypotension or hypovolemia can cause ARF in normal patients, and exacerbates the renal effects of all the above conditions
Procedures associated with ARF	Biliary surgery
	Burns/trauma
	Cardiac surgery
	Genitourinary/obstetric
	Transplant
	Vascular surgery (especially suprarenal x-clamp)
Systemic diseases asociated with chronic renal failure	CAD, congestive heart failure
	Diabetes
	Hypertension (especially renovascular hypertension)
	Liver failure, jaundice
	Peripheral vascular disease,
	Polycystic kidney disease
	Scleroderma
	SLE
	Rheumatoid arthritis
	Wegner's granulomatosis
Nephrotoxic drug exposure	Acetaminophen (usually with hepatotoxicity)
	ACE II inhibitors (impairs renal autoregulation)
	Allopurinol
	Aminoglycosides (proximal tubule necrosis)
	Amphotericin B (GN and ATN)
	Asparaginase
	Cephalosporins (especially with aminoglycosides)
	Cisplatin (ATN)
	Cimetadine, ranitidine (interstitial nephritis)
	Cyclosporin-A, tacrolimis
	IV radiocontrast (oliguria within 24 hrs)
	Methotrexate
	Metoclopramide (inhibits renal D_2 receptors)
	Nitrosoureas
	NSAIDs (especially phenacetin, indomethacin, toradol) [less with selective cyclooxygenase$_2$ (cox$_2$) inhibitors]
	Penicillins, sulfonamides, (interstitial nephritis)

Abbreviations: ↓'d, decreased; GFR, glomerular filtration rate; ARF, acute renal failure; x-clamp, cross clamp; CAD, coronary artery disease; SLE, systemic lupus erethematosis; GN, glomerulonephritis; ATN, acute tubular necrosis; IV, intravenous; NSAIDs, nonsteroidal anti inflammatory drugs.

associated with complications. Recently, less invasive methods have been developed which utilize CO_2 rebreathing (71,72), esophageal Doppler (73), or arterial thermodilution (74). Early results have shown that these techniques compare favorably with pulmonary arterial thermodilution and may be considered a viable alternative in certain patient populations (75–77).

Laboratory Data
Blood Urea Nitrogen and Creatinine
Large amounts of protein, catabolic states, anabolic steroids, and blood in the gut increase urea nitrogen production. Urea nitrogen is freely filterable by the kidneys and is both secreted and reabsorbed by the tubules. In general, an inverse relationship between GFR and BUN exists. ☞ **Oliguria,**

hypercatabolism, and blood in the gut may increase the BUN independent of a decrease in GFR. ☞

Serum creatinine is also inversely proportional to GFR. Creatinine is produced by muscle, and its rates of production and release are related to muscle mass. Creatinine is freely filtered by the glomeruli, a small amount is also secreted by the tubules. Serum creatinine × GFR is a constant in steady state conditions; if GFR is halved, serum creatinine doubles (Table 3). If GFR ceases, the serum creatinine rises about 0.5 to 1.0 mg/dL/day. The increase is much greater following severe trauma with resultant muscle damage, or in rhabdomyolysis. Because creatinine production is related to muscle mass, loss of muscle tissue with renal failure may result in a deceptively low serum creatinine level. In this setting, BUN and serum creatinine values do not accurately reflect acute changes in GFR.

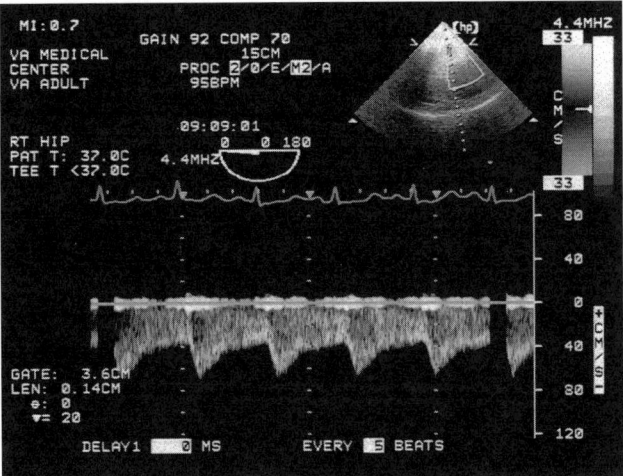

Figure 3 Pulsed-wave Doppler spectral array of the left renal artery. The negative orientation of the waveform velocities indicates flow away from the transducer. The area within the trace is used to calculate mean velocity. Peak systolic and diastolic values are obtained to calculate pulsatility index (peak systolic velocity – diastolic velocity/mean velocity) and resistive index (peak systolic velocity–diastolic velocity/peak systolic velocity).

Table 4 shows conditions associated with acute elevations in BUN and creatinine.

Urinalysis

Complete anuria is unusual (78). Causes include cortical necrosis, vascular accident, glomerulitides, vasculitides, and severe intra-abdominal hypertension. Urinary tract obstruction may result in anuria, but is usually incomplete as the obstructing body changes position. Urine composition may be helpful to distinguish prerenal oliguria from that due to established acute tubular necrosis.

Urinary Composition

Amber color urine with a high specific gravity (≥ 1.030) suggests preservation of the concentrating ability of the kidney and points towards a prerenal cause. Similarly, urinary indices, such as a low fraction excretion of sodium and high osmolar clearance, suggest a prerenal etiology (Table 5), with the exception of hepatorenal syndrome. This form of renal failure is due to local redistribution of blood flow and is invariably associated with a very low urinary sodium concentration.

The fractional excretion of sodium, the renal failure index, and other urinary indices for differentiating prerenal

Table 3 Relationship Between Serum Creatinine and Glomerular Filtration Rate

Creatinine (mg/dL)	Glomerular filtration rate (mL/min)
1	100
2	50
4	25
8	12.5
16	6.25

Table 4 Conditions Associated with an Elevated and a Low Serum BUN/Creatinine Ratio

>10	<10
Increased protein intake	Starvation/ketosis
Tissue necrosis	Liver disease
Sepsis	Rhabdomyolysis
Corticosteroids	Postdialysis
Trauma	Renal oliguria
Prerenal oliguria	Cimetidine, trimetoprim
Postrenal oliguria	

failure from acute tubular necrosis are of limited clinical value in the operating room. In the ICU, these indicies are often useful, particularly when a nephrology consultation is being obtained. Urine and plasma samples for analysis must be collected before any diuretic agents are administered. Similarly, the diagnostic utility of urinary indices is diminished in the presence of preexisting renal dysfunction or chronic diuretic use.

☞ **In the absence of lower urinary tract trauma, a positive heme result on a dipstick suggests the presence of free hemoglobin or myoglobin in the urine. The latter is characterized by the absence of red cells on urinalysis. ☞**

Urinary Sediment

Hyaline and finely granular casts are common in prerenal oliguria; coarse and cellular casts are rarely seen. Oliguria associated with acute tubular necrosis is characterized by dirty, brown cellular casts and numerous epithelial cells and casts. A paucity of formed elements suggests obstruction.

Imaging Studies

Supine abdominal radiographs help to determine kidney size and to visualize calcified stones. Further differentiation usually requires more specialized techniques. Urographic studies are used to exclude obstruction and, with modern techniques, are reasonably safe even in acute oliguric renal failure (31,79).

Intravenous pyelography will reveal an immediate, dense, and persistent nephrogram in patients with acute tubular necrosis and pyelonephritis, but not with other forms of oliguria. In prerenal oliguria, the pyelogram is normal; in established oliguric renal failure, the pyelogram is not seen, but the nephrogram may be dense enough to

Table 5 Urinary Indices and Oliguria

Parameter	Prerenal	Renal
U/P Osm	>1.5	≈1
U/P Cr	>30	<10
C H_2O	Negative values	Zero to positive values
U Na^+	<20	>40
$FENa^+$ (%)	<1	>2
RFI	<1	>2

Abbreviations: U/P Osm, ratio of urinary and plasma osmolarity; U/P Cr, ratio of urinary/plasma creatinine; C H_2O, (free water clearance; mL/min), U/P Osm, X urinary volume; U Na^+, urine Na^+ (mEq/L); $FENa^+$, fraction of excretion of sodium, $[(U_{Na^+} \cdot P_{Cr})/(P_{Na^+} \cdot U_{Cr})] \times 100$; RFI, renal failure index, U $Na^+/(U_{Cr}/P_{Cr})$.

demonstrate filling defects (retrograde urography may be necessary for precise localization).

Sonography and computed tomography are integral to the evaluation of oliguria (80). Radionuclide studies are useful in the diagnosis of renal artery stenosis, chronic pyelonephritis, and lymphomatous infiltration of the kidney. These studies also may provide functional information for each kidney without resorting to invasive measures (81).

TREATMENT
Repletion of Intravascular Volume

⚲ Maintenance or prompt restoration of adequate renal perfusion is paramount to minimize the risk of ATN. ⚲ In patients at risk for contrast nephropathy, appropriate hydration is necessary in order to minimize the renal effects of the contrast material. In addition, several other measures have been tested with varying success (Table 6). Recently, N-acetylcystine has been shown to prevent renal failure in high risk those with preexisting renal insufficiency (82,83).

Restoration of Circulating Blood Volume

Restoration of circulating blood volume to values as near normal as possible is a major goal in hypovolemic patients, regardless of the etiology of the deficit. During surgery, additional fluid losses may occur owing to hemorrhage, formation of a surgical third space, or evaporative loss from exposed intestinal surfaces. Postoperative hypovolemia should be avoided as carefully as during the preoperative or intraoperative periods.

As a general rule, replacement fluid should match the type of fluid that has been lost. The importance of intravascular volume replacement in surgery, shock, and trauma is obvious. Exsanguination necessitates blood volume replacement. When blood loss is less severe, or when hypovolemia has been present for a prolonged period, options other than blood replacement alone should be considered.

Hypertonic solutions are beneficial in resuscitation from shock and trauma. Compared to isotonic solutions, the lesser volumes required are associated with equivalent or improved systemic blood pressure, cardiac output, and survival in experimental animals. A positive cardiac inotropic effect results, as well as a decrease in systemic vascular resistance. Restoration of normal cellular transmembrane potential is enhanced, indicating a reversal of the cellular abnormalities induced by hemorrhagic shock. As long as 24 hours after the shock episode, blood pressure is maintained more efficiently than with Ringer's lactate alone or a combination of Ringer's lactate with added mannitol.

7.5% saline has been shown to be more beneficial with respect to survival than 0.9%, 5% or 10% saline solutions. Improved tissue perfusion occurs, as indicated by reduced lactate values. An early increase in urine output, decreased fluid retention, and improved late pulmonary function are also demonstrable. Currently, only 3% solutions are available "off-the-shelf" in the United States.

RescueFlow® (BioPhausia, Knivsta, Sweden) is a 250 mL solution containing 7.5% sodium chloride and 6% dextran 70. It represents a "new concept" drug for "Small Volume Resuscitation," is currently registered in 14 European countries, and is recommended as a volume substitution solution in trauma. However, this is not a new concept (as claimed by the manufacturer), having been promulgated in the early 1970s for burn therapy. Nevertheless, a prepackaged resuscitation solution combining the advantages of crystalloid and colloid is certainly convenient and probably useful. The increased intravascular volume provided by 250 mL of RescueFlow® is alleged to be two to three times the infused volume, equivalent to the increase in volume resulting from intravenous administration of 3 L of crystalloid solution. Treatment benefits have been observed in patients with severe injuries such as penetrating injury requiring surgery and for patients requiring intensive care (84). Application for FDA approval in the United States has been submitted.

More recently hypertonic saline (HS) along with the phosphodiesterase inhibitor HPX has shown less organ damage in gut and lung (Volume 1, Chapter 11) (85). However, the effect on renal function has not yet been studied.

Although the administration of hypertonic crystalloid solutions can produce hypernatremia, this condition will not have an adverse effect on renal function and oliguria as long

Table 6   Preventive Strategies During Administration of Contrast Dye

#	Strategy	Rationale
1	Vigorous hydration before, during, and after the procedure	Decrease osmotic stress; Nephrol Clin Pract 2003; 93: C29–C34
2	Prevention of hypotension	Prevent renal hypoperfusion; <counteracts #1 above>
3	Use of low contrast volume (<5 ml/kg ÷ [Cr])	Decrease toxic load; Am J Cardiol 2002; 90:1068–1073
4	Low osmolality contrast	Radiology 1993; 188:171–178
5	N-acetyl cystine 600 mg orally every 12–48 hrs	Antioxidant and vaso dilation effects; Nephrol 2004; 15:251–260
6	Consider alkalinization of urine	Decreasing pH dependent free radicals; JAMA 2004; 291:2328–2334
7	Avoidance of mannitol and loop diuretics in the presence of renal dysfunction	Can counteract (1–3)
8	Peri procedure hemofiltration	N Engl J Med 2003; 349:1333–1340
9	Administration of DA1 receptor agonists (e.g., fenoldopam)	Not proven to help but probably won't hurt

Abbreviations: Cr, creatinine, DAI, dopaminergic type 1.

Source: Data from multiple sources cited previously in this chapter, beyond the references provided in this table. *Additional resources*. From Ref. 138.

as the serum osmolality stays <330 mosm/dl. ☞ **Conversely, if hypotonic solutions are administered in large amounts (as frequently happens following resuscitation when 0.45% saline or dextrose solution is ordered), the resultant hyponatremia and water intoxication may essentially "shut down" the kidneys.** ☞ This situation was clearly described in 1951 (86). Earlier, in 1944, the surgical admonition was to avoid the use of any saline-containing solutions on the day of surgery and the first two postoperative days (87). It was felt that major surgery and anesthesia altered renal function so severely that the kidneys could not tolerate a salt and water load (Table 7). Indeed, the postoperative oliguria noted seemed, superficially, to support this concept. However, the changes, which at that time were thought to represent potential cardiac decompensation, actually reflected the water intoxication syndrome subsequently described by Bristol (Table 8) (86).

Finally, bear in mind that relative hypovolemia in conditions such as the abdominal compartment syndrome (Chapter 34) can play a role in the patient's problem. Emergency decompression may be necessary in order to restore renal blood flow (88).

Drugs that Increase Renal Perfusion

There are a series of clinically available drugs that increase renal perfusion. These do not necessarily increase renal function or systemic perfusion, and have not been shown to improve outcomes or decrease the rate of renal failure. None of these drugs should be contemplated in the hypovolemic patient. After restoration of intravascular volume and systemic perfusion, some of these drugs may ultimately be found to be beneficial (as of yet this has not been shown).

Dopaminergic Agents
Dopamine

It is generally accepted that Dopamine in doses between 1 and 5 μg/kg/min causes renal and splanchnic vasodilation from stimulation of dopaminergic type 1 (DA1) receptors (89–91). In animals and healthy humans, as well as those with severe LV dysfunction, infusion of dopamine at doses <5 μg/kg is associated with diuresis, increased renal blood flow and GFR. ☞ **Although it has been used for many years to improve renal perfusion and facilitate diuresis, no convincing evidence has yet shown "renal dose" dopamine to be renal protective.** ☞ Recent reviews of the published literature in oliguric critically ill patients suggest a lack of benefit and possibly harmful effects associated with dopamine administration (92,93). Possible reasons include the greater variability of dopamine levels (94), which may induce renal vasoconstriction from stimulation of vascular

Table 7 Decreasing Ability to Excrete an Administered Water Load Following Acute Water Intoxication and Progressive Hyponatremia

Serum sodium (mMol/L)	% of administered water load excreted
140	71
135–139	60
130–134	48
125–129	43
120–124	43
110–119	30

Table 8 Signs and Symptoms of Acute Water Intoxication

Weakness
Lethargy
Disorientation
Nausea, vomiting
Abdominal distention
Oliguria
Coma
Death

α receptors (94,95); the lack of efficacy with high renin levels (95); and the development of tolerance to the drug (96).

Dopexamine

Dopexamine is a dopamine analog with predominant affinity for DA1 and β-2 receptors (97,98). Its overall effects include systemic vasodilatation, mild inotropy, and increased cardiac output. In healthy volunteers, dopexamine was shown to increase renal blood flow, independent of systemic hemodynamic effects (99). Doses between 1 and 4 μg/kg are associated with a proportional reduction in renal vascular resistance up to 30% (100). In surgical patients, the evidence of a direct renal effect is mixed (101,102).

Fenoldopam

Fenoldopam is a synthetic catecholamine with selective affinity for the DA1 receptor (103,104). At low doses (0.03 μg/kg/min), fenoldopam acts as a renal vasodilator, whereas higher doses (0.1 to 0.3 μg/kg/min) decrease venous capacitance and modestly reduces systemic vascular resistance with a concomitant increase in cardiac output (105). Fenoldopam also increases GFR and diuresis. Increase in renal blood flow occurs in the absence of systemic hemodynamic effects, thus confirming fenoldopam's direct effects on the renal vasculature (106,107).

Natriuretic Peptides
Atrial Natriuretic Peptide

Atrial natriuretic peptide (ANP) is a polypeptide hormone found mainly in the left atrium. It is released in response to atrial stretching, and thus to elevated blood pressure (108). ANP reduces blood pressure by stimulating the rapid excretion of sodium and water in the kidneys (reducing blood volume), relaxing vascular smooth muscle (causing vasodilation), and through actions on the brain and adrenal glands. It appears to inhibit renin secretion, decrease aldosterone release, and may have a mutually antagonistic interaction with endothelin (109).

Administration of ANP increases GFR and may reverse renovascular hypertension. Animal studies suggest that it decreases azotemia and renal histologic damage in renal failure (110,111). A recent study in critically ill patients demonstrated improved renal function and increased dialysis-free periods in patients with oliguria who were treated with ANP; however, a followup study failed to demonstrate any difference (112). Blood pressure is less affected in oliguric renal failure than in nonoliguric states.

Brain Natriuretic Peptide

Peptide plasma brain natriuretic peptide (BNP) is a 32-amino acid polypeptide. The cardiac ventricles are the major source of plasma BNP. This circulating peptide has been used as a marker to assist in the diagnosis of congestive heart failure (113). In general, plasma BNP levels correlate positively with the degree of LV dysfunction, but they are sensitive to other biological factors such as age, sex, and diastolic dysfunction. Plasma BNP levels greater than 100 mg per mL are reported to support a diagnosis of abnormal or symptomatic heart failure. The pharmacological actions of BNP include vasodilation, increased GFR (due to afferent arteriolar vasodilation and efferent arteriolar vasoconstriction), decreased secretion of aldosterone, and inhibition of tubular reabsorption of sodium (114,115).

Synthetic BNP (Nesiritide) is available for clinical use in the treatment of decompensated congestive heart failure. Diuretic effects are seen at doses ranging from 0.015 $\mu g/kg/min$ to 0.3 $\mu g/kg/min$ (116).To date, no studies have been performed in oliguric critically ill patients.

Diuretics

As with drugs (discussed above) that increase renal perfusion, diuretics should never be administered to patients, who are prerenal (i.e., hypovolemic). The efficacy of diuretics in the treatment of critically ill patients with oliguria is variable. Because these agents are potentially harmful, their mechanisms of action must be understood if they are to be employed in the treatment of oliguria.These drugs should only be administered in patients who are intravascularly replete. A common error occurs when clinicians note that a patient is total body fluid overloaded but fail to recognize that the patient is also intravascularly depleted. When these patients are treated with diuretics, they can trigger conversion from prerenal oliguria to ATN and hence renal failure.

Loop Diuretics

Loop diuretics such as furosemide, bumetanide, and indapamide are commonly used in an effort to "convert" an oliguric patient to a nonoliguric state. Loop diuretics block sodium reabsorption in the loops of Henle and distal convoluted tubules. Furosemide is also a modest vasodilator of the renal vasculature (117), thus contributing to redistribution of intrarenal blood flow independent of the action of prostaglandin E_2 (118). It may modulate renin secretion by the macula densa, thereby preventing the harmful effects of vasoconstriction on the glomerular apparatus.

If diuretics are not completely effective, they still may improve the clinical situation by converting oliguric renal failure to high output renal failure.The latter condition seems to be more easily managed than the former, although data supporting this concept are questionable. In addition, there appears to be no difference in outcome (119).

Osmotic Diuretics

Drugs such as mannitol produce diuresis because they are filtered by the glomerulus but not reabsorbed in the renal tubule; thus, they obligate the excretion of water. Besides inducing an osmotic diuresis, other renal actions of mannitol include: (*i*) decreased renovascular resistance with consequent increase in blood flow, (*ii*) increased GFR, (*iii*) diuresis and natriuresis due to inhibition of tubular reabsorption of salt and water, (*iv*) decreased medullary hypertonicity with impairment of urinary concentration, (*v*) increased renal interstitial and intratubular pressure, (*vi*) release of ANP and renal prostaglandins, and (*vii*) scavenging of O_2 radicals (120,121). Because of the accompanying increase in blood volume, osmotic diuretics are contraindicated in patients with oliguria and congestive heart failure.

Distal Tubule Diuretics

The use of distal tubule diuretics such as thiazides and metolazone is reserved to provide synergism to loop diuretics. These agents can only be administered orally, and thus their absorption may be unpredictable in some patients. Features of various diuretics utilized in the treatment of oliguria are shown in Table 9.

Table 9 Classification of Diuretic Agents

Class	Examples	Site of action	Mechanisms	FENa	K	HCO$_3^-$
Loop diuretics	Furosemide, ethacrynic acid, bumetanide	MTAL	Inhibits Na-2K-2Cl symporter	20–25%	+	−
Thiazides	Chlorothiazide, hydrochlorthiazide, metolozone	Early distal tubule	Inhibit NaCl uptake	5–8%	++	+/−
Plasma-sparing	Triamterene, amiloride	Late distal tubule, collecting ducts	Inhibit Na uptake	<5%	−	−
	Spironolactone	Late distal tubule, collecting ducts	Aldosterone antagonism	<5%	−	−
Carbonic anhydrase inhibitors	Acetazolamide	Proximal tubule	Decreased intracellular H$^+$ formation (bicarbonate loss)	<5%	+	+++
Osmotic diuresis	Mannitol	Throughout tubule	Osmotic pressure: prevention of H$_2$O absorption by permeable segments of the nephron	<5%	+	+/−

Abbreviations: +, increased urinary loss; −, decreased or no urinary loss; Cl, chloride; FENa, fractional excretion of sodium (sodium clearance/creatinine clearance × 100%); H$^+$, hydrogen ion; HCO$_3^-$, bicarbonate; K, potassium; mTAL, medullary thick ascending loop of Henle; Na, sodium.
Source: From Ref. 139.

Spironolactone

In the hepatorenal syndrome, the effects of diuretic agents are variable, depending upon the degree of disease (110). In the earliest stages of cirrhosis, urinary sodium excretion is plentiful, and salt balance can be controlled by adjusting dietary intake. As the disease progresses, increased salt retention accompanies a progressive decline in renal function. Eventually, the filtered load of sodium becomes completely reabsorbed by the tubules, and the final urine becomes virtually devoid of salt.

When the filtered load is completely reabsorbed proximal to the thick ascending limb of Henle, the patient is resistant to the effects of diuretics and requires more invasive procedures such as repetitive large volume paracentesis or AV hemofiltration to remain in salt balance. However, mortality and hepatic regeneration do not appear to be affected by such interventions (111). In the terminal stages, the GFR falls to such a degree that oliguria, azotemia, and eventually uremia lead to the diagnosis of hepatorenal syndrome. Renal vasoconstriction at this point is severe and irreversible. Only after a successful liver transplant can restoration of near normal renal function be obtained.

Diuretic Resistant Oliguria

Lack of response following incremental doses of diuretics characterizes this abnormality (122,123). The most common condition in the acute setting is renal hypoperfusion due to decreased circulating volume, leading to increased sodium and water reabsorption from the renal tubules. This condition is not uncommon in critically ill patients.

Diuretic resistance can also be seen in patients receiving long term diuretics due to hypertrophy of the cells of the medullary ascending limb (124). In patients with chronic failure of the heart, liver or kidneys, a lack of response may be seen due to decreased renal perfusion (ACE inhibitors and diuretics), decreased delivery of either sodium or diuretic to the limb cells, or impaired cellular function (125).

The following therapeutic strategy is suggested: (*i*) Restore renal perfusion by optimizing hemodynamic function and intravascular volume, (*ii*) Administer a high dose of diuretic (furosemide, 100–200 mg or bumetanide, 4–5 mg) once and observe for response (126). The lack of response may indicate a severe renal insult, and further doses must be avoided to prevent toxic side effects. Alternatively, a continuous infusion (furosemide 5–20 mg/hr) may achieve better results by maintaining a steady concentration and delivery of the drug to the kidney (127,128), (*iii*) Concomitant administration of diuretics with different mechanisms of action. The purpose of this strategy is to block the various segments of the nephron engaged in tubular reabsorption. A popular combination is the administration of Metolazone (blocks the reabsorption of sodium in the distal tubule) with a loop diuretic. Acetazolamide (proximal tubular blocker) and spironolactone are not routinely used because they can exacerbate acidosis and hyperkalemia, (*iv*) Patients with liver disease may benefit from the concomitant administration of albumin and furosemide due to increased delivery of the drug to the kidney (129), (*v*) A trial of fenoldopam or nesiritide by infusion may be indicated. Increased diuresis is usually seen after a couple of hours. The infusion probably should be stopped if no measurable response is seen after six hours.

Miscellaneous Agents

Despite salutary effects associated with the use of some diuretics and renal vasodilators, their effects on outcome have been disappointing. Thus, the search for newer agents continues. ⚔ **Since the pathogenesis of acute oliguria is multifactorial, a targeted approach involving drugs with various mechanisms of action may be indicated.** ⚔ Adenosine receptor antagonists, calcium channel blockers, endothelin antagonists, and phosphodiesterase inhibitors conceivably can improve renal flow (130–133). Lazaroids and antioxidants (e.g., acetylcysteine) may prevent and decrease reperfusion injury (134). Small peptides such as arginine-aspartate-glycine decrease cell adhesion and may decrease tubular obstruction (135). Although animal models and small clinical trials have shown some promising results, their future clinical use must await the results of well-conducted clinical outcome studies.

Relief of Renal Obstruction

In the treatment of postobstructive uropathy, prompt intervention is essential, because prolonged ureteral obstruction may result in irreversible loss of renal function. The degree of renal damage is related to the degree of obstruction, its duration, and the presence or absence of infection (31).

Bladder Catheterization

If the patient is in severe pain, or if the bladder appears to be overdistended, a single in-and-out catheterization is appropriate. If too much time is permitted to elapse before the first postoperative voiding, the bladder becomes grossly overdistended and atonic. In this situation, an indwelling catheter should be inserted for five to seven days.

Surgical Considerations

Complicated cases of postrenal oliguria often require surgical intervention. Percutaneous nephrostomy may be necessary in high obstruction, while suprapubic cystostomy may be satisfactory for bladder obstruction. ⚔ **Massive diuresis occasionally follows relief of obstruction, and thus signs of hypovolemia and electrolyte imbalance must be monitored in these patients.** ⚔ Hypotension sometimes follows rapid decompression of an over-distended bladder.

EYE TO THE FUTURE

Our understanding of the mechanisms that lead to perioperative oliguria and renal failure has increased significantly. Although initial enthusiasm for new agents has been tempered by rather unimpressive results, new approaches continue to be examined. Similarly, the widespread use of time-honored techniques (e.g., dopamine, loop diuretics) may be limited to special circumstances due to a lack of overall efficacy and possible harm.

The importance of risk factors for acute oliguria and renal failure, such as renal medullary hypoperfusion and renal atheroembolism, is now increasingly recognized. The role of esophageal ultrasonography as a real-time monitor of renal blood flow is beginning to be evaluated. Since the etiology of perioperative oliguria is more often multifactorial, it is not surprising that a multifaceted approach will be necessary in order to show a benefit in outcome.

SUMMARY

Acute oliguria is a common finding in patients undergoing major surgery or after significant trauma. Identifying risk factors and understanding the mechanisms of urine formation are essential steps in the prevention and management of oliguric patients.

In the majority of surgical patients, renal hypoperfusion and nephrotoxins play a significant role. Thus, prompt restoration of adequate renal perfusion and limiting the effects of toxins on the nephron are essential components of therapy that should be carried out before irreversible damage occurs. Since a reliable monitor for renal perfusion is not widely available, the clinician must rely on frequent evaluation of hemodynamic status and indirect measures of renal function for the prevention and timely management of oliguria.

Similarly, knowledge of the mechanism of action of the various pharmacological agents is necessary in order to maximize renal protection while minimizing side effects. Strategies such as the indiscriminate use of diuretics to convert patients to a nonoliguric state or the use of low-dose dopamine, have failed to demonstrate a favorable outcome. Conversely, osmotic diuretics and DA1 receptor agonists may help to preserve renal function in some patients. At present, avoidance of hypovolemia and maintenance of adequate renal perfusion are the cornerstones of therapy to preserve renal function in high-risk patients.

KEY POINTS

- Oliguria is often an early sign of renal compromise, representing either a compensatory mechanism for hypoperfusion (hypovolemia and/or hypotension) or an acute renal insult.
- When the kidneys sense abnormalities in extracellular fluid volume or osmolality, they respond by increasing or decreasing the amount of urine excreted.
- Significant oliguria implies a state of renal dysfunction, since a urine output of ≤ 400 mL/day is inadequate for excretion of the daily solute load of 650 to 750 mOsm (normal diet) in a maximally concentrated urine (1.2 mOsm/mL).
- The high metabolic rate in combination with a lower blood supply, places the medullary tubular cells at a higher risk for hypoxic damage, despite what would be perceived as adequate renal blood flow.
- Oliguria in response to hypoperfusion is the result of the kidneys' self-preservation to circumvent renal failure.
- Reduction of the GFR rather than tubular obstruction appears to be the primary event leading to oliguric renal failure when stroma-free hemoglobin or myoglobin enters the glomeruli (32,33).
- Approximately 20% to 25% of ureteral injuries are bilateral, resulting in immediate anuria.
- The MAP provides an estimate of renal perfusion pressure, whereas the systolic blood pressure variation (SPV) during positive-pressure ventilation may provide information on effective circulating volume (63).
- Measurement of $\dot{Q}$ in combination with MAP determinations is, at present, the most reliable way to evaluate renal perfusion clinically.
- Oliguria, hypercatabolism, and blood in the gut may increase the BUN independent of a decrease in GFR.

- In the absence of lower urinary tract trauma, a positive heme result on a dipstick suggests the presence of free hemoglobin or myoglobin in the urine. The latter is characterized by the absence of red cells on urinalysis.
- Maintenance or prompt restoration of adequate renal perfusion is paramount to minimize the risk of ATN.
- Conversely, if hypotonic solutions are administered in large amounts (as frequently happens following resuscitation when 0.45% saline or dextrose solution is ordered), the resultant hyponatremia and water intoxication may essentially "shut down" the kidneys.
- Although it has been used for many years to improve renal perfusion and facilitate diuresis, no convincing evidence has yet shown "renal dose" dopamine to be renal protective.
- Loop diuretics such as furosemide, bumetanide, and indapamide are commonly used in an effort to "convert" an oliguric patient to a nonoliguric state.
- Drugs such as mannitol produce diuresis because they are filtered by the glomerulus but not reabsorbed in the renal tubule; thus, they obligate the excretion of water.
- Since the pathogenesis of acute oliguria is multifactorial, a targeted approach involving drugs with various mechanisms of action may be indicated.
- Massive diuresis occasionally follows relief of obstruction, and thus signs of hypovolemia and electrolyte imbalance must be monitored in these patients.

REFERENCES

1. Smith HW. Renal physiology between two wars. In: Lectures on the Kidney. Lawrence, KS: University of Kansas; 1943; 75.
2. Wilson WC, Aronson S. Oliguria: A sign of renal success or impending renal failure? Anesthesiol Clin North Am 2001; 19:841–882.
3. Thurau K, Boylan JW. Acute renal success: The unexpected logic of oliguria in acute renal failure. Am J Med 1976; 61:308–315.
4. Anderson RJ, Schrier RW. Acute renal failure. In: Schrier RW, Gottschalk CW eds. Diseases of the Kidney, Boston: Little Brown; 1997; 1069–1113.
5. Star RA. Treatment of acute renal failure. Kidney Int 1998; 54:1817–1831.
6. Thadhani R, Pascual M, Bonventre JV. Acute renal failure. N Engl J Med 1996; 334:1448–1460.
7. Wardle EN. Acute renal failure and multiorgan failure. Nephron 1994; 66:380–385.
8. Gill N, Nally JV, Falica RA. Renal failure secondary to acute tubular necrosis: epidemiology, diagnosis, and management. Chest 2005; 128:2847–2863.
9. Harrington JT, Cohen JC. Acute oliguria. Medicine 1984; 63:161–181.
10. Brezis M, Rosen S, Epstein FH. Acute renal failure. In: Brenner BM, Rector FC Jr, eds. The Kidney. 3rd ed. Philadelphia: WB Saunders, 1986:745–799.
11. Sladen RN. Effect of anesthesia and surgery on renal function. Crit Care Clin 1987; 3:373–393.
12. Aukland K. Methods for measuring renal blood flow: Total flow and regional distribution. Ann Rev Physiol 1980; 42:543–555.
13. Brezis M, Rosen S. Hypoxia of the renal medulla—its implications for disease. N Engl J Med 1995; 332:647–655.
14. Gorfinkel HS, Szidon JP, Hirsch LJ, Fishman AP. Renal performance in experimental cardiogenic shock. Am J Physiol 1972; 222:1260–1268.
15. Christensen G. Cardiovascular and renal effects of atrial natriuretic factor. Scand J Clin Lab Invest 1993:53:203–209.

16. Schrier RW. Effects of the adrenergic nervous system and catecholamines on systemic and renal hemodynamics, sodium and water excretion and renin secretion. Kidney Int 1974; 6:291–306.
17. Boventure JV. Mechanism of ischemic acute renal failure. Kidney Int 1993; 43:1160–1178.
18. Bersten AD, Holt AW. Vasoactive drugs and the importance of renal perfusion pressure. New Horiz 1995; 3:650–661.
19. Robertson GL. Thirst and vasopressin function in normal and disordered states of water balance. J Lab Clin Med 1983; 101:351–371.
20. Anggard E, Oliw E. Formation of prostaglandins in the kidney. Kidney Int 1981; 19:771–780.
21. Garella S, Matarese RA. Renal effects of prostaglandins and clinical adverse effects of nonsteroidal anti-inflammatory agents. Medicine 1984; 63:165–181.
22. Barry KG, Malloy JP. Oliguric renal failure. JAMA 1962; 179:510–513.
23. Derrick F, Kretkowski RC. Trauma to kidney, ureter, bladder and urethra. Diagnosis and management. Postgrad Med 1974; 55:183–192.
24. Thadhani R, Pascual M, Bonventre, JV. Acute renal failure. N Engl J Med 1996 334:1448–1460.
25. Zuk A, Bonventre JV, Brown D, Matlin KS. Polarity, integrin, and extracellular matrix dynamics in the postischemic rat kidney. Am J Physiol 1998; 275:C711–C731.
26. Witzgall R, Brown D, Schwarz C, Bonventre JV. 1994. Localization of proliferating cell nuclear antigen, vimentin, c-Fos, and clusterin in the postischemic kidney. Evidence for a heterogenous genetic response among nephron segments, and a large pool of mitotically active and dedifferentiated cells. J. Clin. Inves 1994; 93:2175–2188.
27. Witzgall R, Obernuller N, Balitz U, et al. 1998. Kid-1 expression is high in differentiated renal proximal tubule cells and suppressed in cyst epithelia. Am J Physiol 275:F928–F937.
28. Sutton TA, Fisher CJ, Molitoris BA. 2002. Microvascular endothelial injury and dysfunction during ischemic acute renal failure. Kidney Int. 62:1539–1549.
29. Conger J, Robinette, J, Villar A, Raij L, Shultz P. 1995. Increased nitric oxide synthase activity despite lack of response to endothelium-dependent vasodilators in postischemic acute renal failure in rats. J. Clin. Invest. 96:631–638.
30. Duffield JS, Park KM, Hsiao L-L, et al. Restoration of tubular epithelial cells during repair of the post ischemic kidney occurs independently of bone marrow-derived stem cells. J Clin Invest. 2005; 115:1743–1755.
31. Parfrey PS, Griffiths SM, Barrett BJ, et al. Contrast material-induced renal failure in patients with diabetes mellitus, renal insufficiency, or both: A prospective controlled study. N Engl J Med 1989; 320:143–149.
32. Walshe JJ, Venuto RC. Acute oliguric renal failure induced by indomethacin: possible mechanisms. Ann Intern Med 1979; 91: 47–49.
33. Brandstetter RD, Mar DD. Reversible oliguric renal failure associated with ibuprofen treatment. Br Med J 1978; 2(6146): 1194–1195.
34. Hou SH, Burshinsky DA, Wish JB, Cohen JJ, Harrington JT. Hospital-acquired renal insufficiency: a prospective study. Am J Med 1983; 74:243–248.
35. Birndor N. DIC and renal failure. J Lab Invest 1971; 24:314–318.
36. Ruiz-Guinazu A, Coelho JB, Paz RA. Methemoglobin-induced acute renal failure in the rat: in vivo observation, histology and micropuncture measurements of intratubular and postglomerular vascular pressures. Nephron 1967; 4:257–275.
37. Flanigan WJ, Oken DE. Renal micropuncture study of the development of anuria in the rat with mercury-induced renal failure. J Clin Invest 1965; 44:449–457.
38. Huang KC, Lee TS, Lin YM, Shu KH. Clinical features and outcome of crush syndrome caused by the Chi-Chi earthquake. J Formos Med Assoc 2002; 101:249–256.
39. Better OS. The crush syndrome revisited (1940–1990). Nephron 1990; 55:97–103.
40. Hricik DE, Browning PJ, Kopelman R, Goomo WE, Madias NE, Dzau VJ. Captopril-induced functional renal insufficiency in patients with bilateral renal artery stenosis or renal artery stenosis in a solitary kidney. N Engl J Med 1983; 308:373–376.
41. Farrow PR, Wilkinsin R. Reversible renal failure during treatment with captopril. Br Med J 1979; 1(6179):1680.
42. Harrel RM, Sibley R, Vogelzang NJ. Renal vascular lesions after chemotherapy with vinblastine, bleomycin, and cisplatin. Am. J Med 1982; 73:429–433.
43. Gonsowski CT, Laster MJ, Eger EI, Ferrell LD, Kerschman RL. Toxicity of compound A in rats: effect of a 3-hour administration. Anesthesiology 1994; 80:556–565.
44. Conzen PF, Kharasch ED, Czemer SF, et al. Low-flow sevoflurane compared with low-flow isoflurane anesthesia in patients with stable renal insufficiency. Anesthesiology 2002; 97: 578–584.
45. Habif DV, Papper EM, Fitzpatrick HF, Lawrence P, McSmythe C, Bradley SE. The renal and hepatic blood flow, glomerular filtration rate, and urinary output of electrolytes during cyclopropane, ether, and thiopental anesthesia, operation, and the immediate postoperative period. Surgery 1951; 30:241–255.
46. Deutsch S, Goldberg M, Stephen GW, Wu WH. Effects of halothane anesthesia on renal function in normal man. Anesthesiology 1966; 27:793–804.
47. Mazze RI, Cousins MJ, Barr GA. Renal effects and metabolism of isoflurane in man. Anesthesiology 1974; 40:536–542.
48. Cousins MJ, Greenstein LR, Hitt BA, Mazze RL. Metabolism and renal effects of enflurane in man. Anesthesiology 1976; 44:44–53.
49. Olsen ST, Skjoldborg H. The fine structure of the renal glomerulus in acute anuria. Acta Pathol Microbiol Scand 1967; 70:205–214.
50. Grubben AC, van Baardwijk AA, Broering DC, Hoofwijk AG. Pathophysiology and clinical significance of the abdominal compartment syndrome. Zentralbl Chir 2001; 126:605–609.
51. Swaminathan A, Tzamaloukas AH, Clark DA, McLemore JL, McKinney DR, Crooks LA. Oliguric acute renal failure in mycosis fungoides with lymphomatous infiltrates in the kidneys. Int Urol Nephrol 2002; 33:149–155.
52. Oray-Schrom P, St Martin D, Bartelloni P, Amoateng-Adjepong Y. Giantnonpancreatic pseudocyst causing acute anuria. J Clin Gastroent 2002; 34:160–163.
53. Charles AH. Some hazards of pelvic surgery. Proc R Soc Med 1967; 60:656–658.
54. Mate-Kole MO, Yeboah ED, Affram RK, Ghosh TS. Anuric acute renal failure due to bilateral accidental ureteric ligation during abdominal hysterectomy. Int J Gynaecol Obstet 1993; 41:67–73.
55. Chisholm GD, Shackman R. Malignant obstructive uraemia. Br J Urol 1968; 40:720–726.
56. Wanuck S. Carcinoma of pancreas causing ureteral obstruction. J Urol 1973; 110:395–396.
57. Fall M, Petterson S. Ureteral complications after intravenous formalin instillation.J Urol 1979; 122:160–163.
58. Elem B, Sinha SN. Ureterocele in bilharziasis of the urinary tract. Br J Urol 1981; 53:428–429.
59. Biggers R, Edwards J. Anuria secondary to bilateral ureteropelvic fungus balls. Urol 1980; 15:161–163.
60. Mundy AR, Podesta ML, Bewick M, Rudge CJ, Ellis FG. The urological complications of 1000 renal transplants. Br J Urol 1981; 53:397–402.
61. Mariani AJ, Barrett DM, Kurtz SB, Kyle RA. Bilateral localized amyloidosis of the ureter presenting with anuria. J Urol 1978; 120:757–759.
62. Garwood S, Davis E, Harris S. Intraoperative transesophageal ultrasonograpy can measure renal blood flow. J Cardiothorac Vasc Anesth 2001; 15:65–71.

63. Perel A, Pizov R, Cotev S. The systolic pressure variation is a sensitive indicator of hypovolemia in ventilated dogs subjected to gradual hemorrhage. Anesthesiology 1987; 67:498–501.

64. Fontes ML, Bellows W, Ngo L, Mangano DT. Assessment of ventricular function in critically ill patients: limitation of pulmonary artery catheterization. Institutions of the McSPI group. J Cardiothorac Vasc Anesth 1999; 13:521–527.

65. Benjamin E, Griffin K, LebowitzAB, et al. Goal-directed transeso-phageal echo-cardiography performed by intensivists to assess left ventricular function: comparison with pulmonary artery catheterization. J Cardiothorac Vasc Anesth 1998; 12:10–15.

66. Greim RC, Roewer N, Apfel G, Laux G, Schulte AM, Esch J. Relationship of echocardiographic preload indices to stroke volume in critically ill patients with normal and low cardiac index. Intensive Care Med 1997; 23:411–416.

67. San Fillipo AJ, Weyman AE. The role of echocardiography in managing critically ill patients. J Crit Illness 1988; 3:27–44.

68. Parker MM, Cunnion RE, Parillo JE. Echocardiography and nuclear imaging in the critical care unit. JAMA 1985; 254: 2935–2939.

69. Polaert JI, Trouerbach J, De Buyzere M, Everaert J, Colardyn FA. Evaluation of transesophageal echocardiography as a diagnostic and therapeutic aid in a critical care setting. Chest 1995; 107:774–779.

70. Tabata T, Thomas JD, Klein AL. Pulmonary venous flow by Doppler echocardiography: revisited 12 years later. J Am Coll Cardiol 2003; 41:1243–1250.

71. Jaffe MB. Partial CO_2 rebreathing cardiac output-operating principles of the NICO system. J Clin Monit Comp 1999; 15:387–401.

72. Haryadi D, Orr JA, Kuck K, McJames S, Westenskow DR. Partial CO_2 rebreathing indirect Fick technique for non-invasive measurement of cardiac output. J Clin Monit Comp 2000; 16:361–374.

73. Laupland KB, Bands CJ. Utility of esophageal Doppler as a minimally invasive hemodynamic monitor: a review. Can J Anaesth 2002; 49:393–401.

74. Zollner C, Haller M, Weis M, et al. Beat-to-beat measurement of cardiac output by intravascular pulse contour analysis: a pro-spective criterion standard study in patients after cardiac surgery. J Cardiothorac Vasc Anesth 2000; 14:125–129.

75. Odenstedt H, Stenqvist O, Lundin S. Clinical evaluation of a partial CO_2 rebreathing technique for cardiac output monitor-ing in critically ill patients. Acta Anaesthesiol Scand 2002; 46:152–159.

76. Marik PE. Pulmonary artery catheterization and esophageal doppler monitoring in the ICU. Chest 1999; 116:1085–1091.

77. Rauch H, Muller M, Fleischer F, Bauer H, Martin E, Bottiger BW. Pulse contour analysis versus thermodilution in cardiac surgery patients. Acta Anaesthesiol Scand 2002; 46:424–429.

78. Swann RC, Merrill JP. The clinical course of acute renal failure. Medicine 1953; 32:215–292.

79. Manske CL, Sprafka JM, Strony JT, Wang Y. Contrast nephropa-thy in azotemic diabetic patients undergoing coronary angio-graphy. Am J Med 1990; 89:615–620.

80. Balfe DM, McClennan BL. CT of the retroperitoneum in urosur-gical disorders. Surg Clin North Am 1982; 62:919–939.

81. Sherman RA, Byun KJ. Nuclear medicine in acute and chronic renal failure. Sem Nucl Med 1982; 12:265–279.

82. Tepel M, Van Der Giet M, Schwarzfeld C, Laufer U, Liermann D, Zidek W. Prevention of radiographic-contrast-agent-induced reductions in renal function by acetylcysteine. N Engl J Med. 2000; 343:180–184.

83. Diaz-Sandoval LJ, Kosowsky BD, Losordo DW. Acetylcysteine to prevent angiography-related renal tissue injury (The APART Trial). Am J Cardiol 2002; 89:356–358.

84. http://www.rescueflow.com/ (accessed 9/15/2002).

85. Coimbra R, Porcides R, Loomis W, et al. HSPTX protects against hemorrhagic shock resuscitation induced tissue injury: an attractive alternative to ringers lactate. J Trauma 2006; 60(1); 41–51.

86. Bristol WR. Relation of sodium chloride depletion to urine excretion and H2O intoxication.Am J Sci 1951; 221:412–416.

87. Coller FA, Campbell KN, Vaughan HH, et al. Postoperative salt intolerance. Ann Surg 1944; 119:533–542.

88. Chang MC, Miller PR, D'Agostino R, Meredith JW. Effects of abdominal decompression on cardiopulmonary function and visceral perfusion in patients with intra-abdominal hyperten-sion. J Trauma 1998; 44:440–445.

89. Carcoanna OV, Hines RL. Is renal dose dopamine protective or therapeutic? Yes, Crit Care Clin 1996; 12:677–685.

90. McDonald RH, Goldberg LI, McNay JL, et al. Effects of dopa-mine in man: augmentation of sodium excretion, glomerular filtration rate and renal plasma flow. J Clin Invest 1964; 43:1116–1124.

91. Lee MR. Dopamine and the kidney: ten years on. Clin Sci 1993; 84:357–375.

92. Philip W, Perdue MD, Blaser JR, Lipsett PA, Breslow MJ. "Renal dose" dopamine in surgical patients. Dogma or science? Ann Surg 1998; 227:470–473.

93. Holmes CL, Walley KR. Bad medicine: low-dose dopamine in the ICU. Chest 2003; 123:1266–1275.

94. Juste RN, Moran L, Hooper J, Soni N. Dopamine clear-ance in critically ill patients. Intensive Care Med 1998; 24: 1217–1220.

95. Marik PE. Low-dose dopamine in critically ill oliguric patients: the influence of the renin-angiotensin system. Heart Lung 1993; 22:171–175.

96. MacCannell KL, Giraud GD, Hamilton PL. Haemodynamic responses to dopamine and dobutamine infusions as a function of duration of infusion. Pharmacology 1983; 26:29–39.

97. Stephan H, Sonntag H, Henning H, Yoshimine K.Cardiovascu-lar and renal haemodynamic effects of dopexamine: compari-son with dopamine. Br J Anaesth 1990; 65:380–387.

98. Jamison M, Widerhorn J, Weber L, et al. Central and renal hemodynamic effects of a new agonist at peripheral dopamine-and beta-2 adrenoreceptors (dopexamine) in patients with heart failure. Am Heart J 1989; 117:607–614.

99. Foulds RA. Clinical development of dopexamine hydrocholor-ide (Dopacard) and an overview of its hemodynamic effects. Am J Cardiol 1988; 62:41C–45C

100. Olsen NV, Lund J, Jensen PF, et al. Dopamine, dobutamine and dopexamine: A comparison of renal effects in unanesthetized human volunteers. Anesthesiology 1993; 79:685–694.

101. MacGregor DA, Butterworth JF 4th, Zaloga CP, Prielipp RC, James R, Royster RL. Hemodynamic and renal effects of dopex-amine and dobutamine in paitents with reduced cardiac output following coronary artery bypass grafting. Chest 1994; 106:835–841.

102. Sherry E, Tooley MA, Bolsin SN, Monk CR, Willcox J. Effect of dopexamine hydrochloride on renal vascular resistance index and haemodynamic responses following coronary artery bypass graft surgery. Eur J Anaesthesiol 1997; 14:184–189.

103. Allison NL, Cubb JW, Ziemniak JA, Alexander F, Stote RM. The effects of fenoldopam, a dopaminergic agonist on renal hemodynamics. Clin Pharmacol Ther 1987; 41:282–287.

104. Aronson S, Goldberg LI, Glock D. Effects of fenoldopam on renal blood flow and systemic hemodynamics during isoflur-ane anesthesia. J Cardiothorac Vasc Anesth 1991; 5:29–32.

105. Murphy MB, McCoy CE, Weber RR, Frederickson EF, Douglas FL, Goldberg LI. Augmentation of renal blood flow and sodium excretion in hypertensive patients during blood pressure reduction by intravenous administration of the dopamine agonist fenoldopam. Circulation 1987; 76:1312–1318.

106. Garwood S, Hines R. Perioperative renal preservation. Dopexamine and fenoldopam- new agents to augment renal performance. Semin Anesth Periop Med Pain 1998; 17:308–318.

107. Singer I, Epstein M.Potential of dopamine A-1 agonists in the management of acute renal failure. Am J Kidney Dis 1998; 31:743–755.

108. Rankin AJ. Mechanisms for the release of atrial natriuretic peptide Can J Physiol Pharmacol 1987; 65:1673–1679.

109. Levin ER, Gardner DG, Samson WK. Natriuretic peptides. N Engl J Med 1998; 339:321–328.

110. Conger JD, Falk SA, Hammond WS. Atrial natriuretic peptide and dopamine in established acute renal failure in the rat. Kidney Int 1991; 40:21–28.

111. Seki G, Suzuki K, Nonaka T, et al. Effects of atrial natriuretic peptide on glycerol-induced acute renal failure in the rat. Jpn Heart J 1992; 33:383–393.

112. Allgren RL, Marbury TC, Rahman SN, et al. Anaritide in acute tubular necrosis. Auriculin Anaritide Acute Renal Failure Study Group. N Engl J Med 1997; 336:828–834.

113. Dhingra H, Roongsritong C, Kurtzman NA. Brain natriuretic peptide: role in cardiovascular and volume homeostasis. Semin Nephrol 2002; 22:423–437.

114. Abraham WT, Lowes BD, Ferguson DA, et al. Systemic hemodynamic, neurohormonal, and renal effects of a steady state infusion of human brain natriuretic peptide in patients with hemodynamically decompensated heat failure. J Card Fail 1998; 4:37–44.

115. Schrier RW. Hormones and hemodynamics in heart failure. N Engl J Med 1999; 341:577–585.

116. Rayburn BK, Bourge R. Nesiritide: a unique therapeutic cardiac peptide. Rev Cardiovasc Med 2001; 2(2):S25–S31.

117. Lindner A. Synergism of dopamine and furosemide in diuretic-resistant, oliguric acute renal failure. Nephron 1983; 33:121–126.

118. Kramer HJ, Schumann J, Wassermann C, Dusing R. Prostaglandin-independent protection by furosemide from oliguric ischemic renal failure in conscious rats. Kidney Int 1980; 17: 455–464.

119. Mehta RL, Pascual MT, Soroko S, Chertow GM; Picard Study Group. Diuretics, mortality, and nonrecovery of renal function in acute renal failure. JAMA 2002; 288:2547–2553.

120. Valdes ME, Landau SE, Shah DM, et al. Increased glomerular filtration rate following mannitol administration in man. J Surg Res 1979; 26:473–477.

121. Better OS, Rubinstein I, Winaver JM, Knochel JP. Mannitol therapy revisited (1940–1997). Kidney Int 1997; 51:886–894.

122. Sladen RN. Oliguria in the ICU. Anesthesiol Clin North Am 2000; 18:739–752.

123. Brater DC. Diuretic resistance: mechanisms and therapeutic strategies. Cardiology 1994; 84(2):57–67.

124. Sica DA, Gehr TW. Diuretic combinations in refractory oedema states: pharmacokinetic-pharmacodynamic relationships. Clin Pharmcokinet 1996:30:229–249.

125. Sjostrom PA, Odlind BG, Beermann BA, Hammarlund-Udenaes M. On the mechanism of acute tolerance to furosemide diuresis. Scand J Urol Nephrol 1988; 22:133–140.

126. Klahr S, Miller SB. Acute oliguria. New Engl J Med 1998; 388:671–675.

127. Pivac N, Rumboldt Z, Sardelic S, et al. Diuretic effects of furosemide infusion versus bolus injection in congestive heart failure. Int J Clin Pharmacol Res 1998; 18:121–128.

128. Keiseb J, Moodley J, Connolly CA. Comparison of the efficacy of continuous furosemide and low-dose dopamine infusion in preeclampsia/eclampsia-related oliguria in the immediate postpartum period. Hypertens Pregnancy 2002; 21:225–234.

129. Elwell RJ, Spencer AP, Eisele G. Combined furosemide and human albumin treatment for diuretic-resistant edema. Ann Pharmacother 2003; 37:695–700.

130. Tanahashi M, Hara S, Yoshida M, Suzuki-Kusaba M, Hisa H, Satoh S. Effects of rolipram and cilostamide on renal functions and cyclic AMP release in anesthetized dogs. J Pharmacol Exp Ther 1999; 289:1533–1538.

131. Parker MR, Willatts SM. A pilot study to investigate the effects of an infusion of aminophylline on renal function following major abdominal surgery. Anaesthesia 2001; 56:670–675.

132. Ruggenenti P, Perico N, Mosconi L, et al. Calcium channel blockers protect transplant patients from cyclosporine-induced daily renal hypoperfusion. Kidney Int 1993; 43:706–711.

133. Roux S, Qiu C, Sprecher U, Osterwalder R, Clozel JP. Protective effects of endothelin receptor antagonists in dogs with aortic cross-clamping. J Cardiovasc Pharmacol 1999; 34:199–205.

134. Brophy DF. Role of N-acetylcysteine in the prevention of radiocontrast-induced nephropathy. Ann Pharmacother 2002; 36: 1466–1470.

135. Venkataraman R, Kellum JA. Novel approaches to the treatment of acute renal failure. Expert Opin Investig Drugs 2000; 9:2579–2592.

136. Heyman SN, Fuchs S, Brezia M. The role of medullary ischemia in acute renal failure. New Horiz 1995; 3:597–607.

137. Pitts RF. Physiology of the Kidney and Body Fluids. 3rd ed. Chicago: Year Book Medical Publishers, Inc, 1974.

138. Barrett BJ, Parfrey PS. Preventing nephropathy induced by contrast medium. N Engl J Med 2006; 354:379–386.

139. Sladen RN. Diuretics. In: Bovill JG, Howie MB, eds. Clinical Pharmacology for Anaesthetists. London: WB Saunders, 1999:281.

41

Pathogenesis and Evaluation of Renal Failure

Lakhmir Chawla

Department of Anesthesiology and Critical Care Medicine, George Washington University Medical Center, Washington, D.C., U.S.A.

William C. Wilson

Department of Anesthesiology and Critical Care, UC San Diego Medical Center, San Diego, California, U.S.A.

INTRODUCTION

Acute renal failure (ARF) is a syndrome characterized by the rapid (hours to days) loss of glomerular filtration and the accumulation of nitrogenous waste products (1). Unlike the acute respiratory distress syndrome (ARDS), which has a clinical consensus definition (2), ARF continues to be defined differently by various investigators. For this reason, the precise incidence of ARF is unknown; however, amongst the published studies, using a variety of definitions, the estimated incidence of ARF in critically ill patients ranges between 15% and 30%, and portends an increased mortality in affected patients by as much as 40% to 60% (3–6). Recently, a group of international nephrology leaders have been meeting to develop a consensus definition of ARF amongst other issues, and it is likely that standards for the diagnosis of ARF will soon be in place (7), and the term acute kidney injury (AKI) may become used in place of ARF.

The etiology of ARF is often multi-factorial, and aside from renal replacement therapy and improved general supportive care there is yet to be an effective therapy introduced which significantly alters the morbidity or mortality of ARF. Numerous drug interventions, including dopamine, insulin-like growth factor, and anaritide (synthetic atrial naturetic peptide), have failed to show significant benefit (see Chapter 42) (8–10). Renal replacement therapies and transplantation are associated with a number of comorbidities, and are imperfect solutions. Thus, prevention of ARF and early recognition of renal insufficiency are the most important goals of renal management (11).

Over the past couple of decades, multiple organ dysfunction syndrome (MODS) has become a common pathway toward death for critically ill patients, including those who are septic (12,13). The kidney is nearly always one of the organs that fail in MODS. ☞ **Recent studies indicate that an increased relative risk of death is associated with kidney failure when adjusted for a wide range of covariates (14,15). Accordingly, early and accurate indicators of renal insufficiency or failure are essential to the management of critically ill patients.** ☞

This chapter briefly surveys the pathogenesis of acute tubular necrosis (ATN), which is the chief cause of ARF in trauma and critically ill patients, and emphasizes the role of the prerenal state. Next, the role of various renal toxins are reviewed, followed by a summary of the basic diagnostic approach. Both direct and indirect measures of renal function are clinically useful, and these are emphasized. Finally, specific renal failure scenarios of significance for trauma and critical care are reviewed in order to highlight the diagnostic clues, which assist in early recognition and treatment. The "Eye to the Future" section emphasizes newer diagnostic tests, which may become useful in the diagnosis of ARF and in the monitoring of renal well-being.

PATHOGENESIS: ROLE OF HYPOPERFUSION

Of the numerous mechanisms of renal compromise that can lead to ARF, the most prominent is hypoperfusion. Indeed, hypoperfusion is a frequent element in two of the three major classes of ARF.

Those three traditional categories of ARF are prerenal, intrarenal, and postrenal. When clearance is limited by factors that decrease renal perfusion, the syndrome is classified as "prerenal failure" or "prerenal azotemia." When dysfunction is due to damage within the kidney itself (e.g. ATN), it is termed "intrarenal" or "intrinsic" renal failure. If renal dysfunction occurs as a consequence of obstruction of the urinary outflow tract, then it is classified as "postrenal failure." Obstructive uropathy is rarely the etiology of ARF following trauma or critical injury, unless there has been disruption of the ureters.

☞ **Intrinsic or intrarenal ARF has many causes, but in trauma and critical care settings, the great majority of cases are due to acute tubular necrosis (ATN) following on from a prerenal hypoperfusion state.** ☞

Initially the underperfused kidney is still capable of physiologic adaptation, conserving salt and water to create a urine of high osmolality and low sodium content. This is the picture typical of the prerenal state. As hypoperfusion continues, however, the renal tubular cell mass, which has a high metabolic requirement, begins to fail in its tasks of urinary concentration and sodium reabsorption. Thus the urine osmolality begins to fall; initially during this phase, correction of prerenal deficits still has a good chance of restoring renal function. But with further progression, the urine osmolality falls further, approaching that of the plasma ("isosthenuria"), signifying serious tubular damage and the onset of ATN. Additional factors, such as tubular obstruction from sloughed renal tubular cells, and inhibition of glomerular filtration by the tubulo-glomerular feedback system, then come in to play, reducing the glomerular filtration rate (GFR) further. The kidney then cannot even reabsorb sodium effectively, leading to the established picture of ATN, with high fractional excretion of sodium, low urine osmolality, and usually oliguria (16). Established ATN begins to heal only when good renal perfusion is reestablished, and usually takes a period of many days to weeks to recover. Prerenal causes are responsible for more than 90% of perioperative ARF (17). This is why perioperative renal function monitoring, and early treatment of oliguria (Chapter 40) are paramount clinically.

In trauma and critically ill patients with inadequate blood flow (prerenal), injury is often triggered by an additional assault on the nephron from harmful drugs (altering intrarenal distribution of blood flow by abnormal hemodynamics) or by pre-existing disease (e.g., diabetes) (18). Patients with pre-existing renal insufficiency, for example, are especially prone to develop ARF during cardiovascular surgery. Patients with diabetes mellitus and renal insufficiency are especially vulnerable to radiocontrast agents (19). Intrinsic renal causes that result in ARF are described according to the primary lesion (i.e., tubules, interstitium, vessels, or glomerulus). Tubular injury is the most common type seen in trauma and post-surgical patients (20).

Normally, the RBF is about 20% to 25% of the total cardiac output. The amount of blood the kidneys receive in the resting state (1000–1250 mL/min) far exceeds that needed to provide their intrinsic oxygen requirement. Essentially, all blood passes through glomeruli, and about 10% of RBF is filtered (resulting in a GFR of approximately 125 mL/min in the normal adult). The basal normal blood flow is 3 to 5 mL/min/g of tissue. This average primarily reflects blood flow in the cortical glomeruli, because perfusion to the inner medulla and papilla is only about one tenth of the total flow (21).

Renal clearance is determined by the delivery of waste products to the kidney (i.e., RBF) and the kidney's ability to extract them (GFR). When RBF is decreased (hypotension, hypovolemia), a series of systemic and renal compensatory responses are activated initially to preserve ultrafiltration and renal clearance. ☞ **The hallmark that underscores experimental models of hemodynamically mediated ARF is a reduction of RBF (injury generally results when RBF is reduced by more than 50%) for at least 40 to 60 minutes.** ☞ Once a decrease in renal perfusion is established, then glomerular filtration is disproportionately depressed, compared with the decrease in blood flow. Indeed, it has been observed that when RBF is decreased sufficiently to cause depression of glomerular filtration to less than 5% of normal, blood flow may only be depressed 25% to 50% of normal (20). Hence, although deceased RBF is the initiating event, most of the time other factors (e.g., tubular pathology) can sustain abnormal filtration, besides decreased RBF.

The renal cortex contains most of the glomeruli and receives the majority of the RBF, optimizing glomerular filtration and solute reabsorption. In contrast, blood flow to the medulla is lower, and this relationship helps to preserve the osmotic gradient required to maximally concentrate the urine.

During ischemic hypoxia, the renal cortical structures can become injured, particularly the pars recta portion of the proximal tubules. However, it is the medullary thick ascending limb (mTAL) of the Loop of Henley that is at greatest risk of hypoxic injury. This is because the mTAL cells are the most rapidly metabolizing cells in the nephron, and because they exist in an environment, which teeters on the

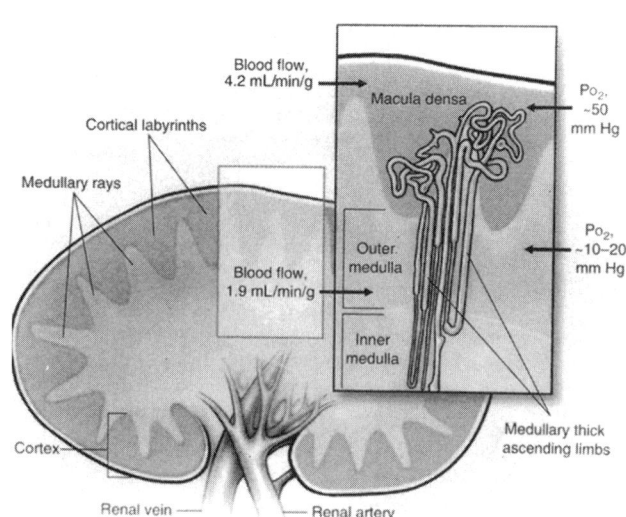

Figure 1   Anatomical and physiologic features of the renal cortex and medulla. The cortex receives ample blood supply, optimizing glomerular filtration. Accordingly, it is generally well oxygenated (except for the medullary-ray areas, which are devoid of glomeruli and are supplied by venous blood ascending from the medulla). The medulla possesses a meager blood supply and is poorly oxygenated. Medullary hypoxia results both from countercurrent exchange of oxygen within the recta and from the consumption of oxygen by the medullary thick ascending limbs. Renal medullary hypoxia is an obligatory consequence of the process of urinary concentration. *Abbreviation*: PO_2, partial pressure of oxygen. *Source*: From Ref. 26.

verge of hypoxia at baseline (Fig. 1). Thus, heterogeneity of intrarenal blood flow and cellular metabolic rate contribute to the pathophysiology of ischemic acute renal failure.

Furthermore, an imbalance between the intrarenal vasodilators [nitric oxide, prostaglandin-E_1 (PGE_1), prostaglandin-E_2 (PGE_2), and adenosine] (22) and the vasoconstrictors (endothelin, angiotensin II, vasopressin, etc.) can also impair medullary blood flow and contribute to tubular-cell damage (23). In the outer medulla, where the high oxygen consuming mTAL cells reside, ischemia causes swelling of tubular and endothelial cells as well as adherence of neutrophils to capillaries and venules (24,25). The resultant vascular congestion and reduced blood flow further impairs the balance between oxygen supply and demand. The role of renal medullary hypoxia in ATN has been recently reviewed by Brezis and Rosen (26).

In general, the response to renal hypoperfusion involves three major regulatory mechanisms that support renal function in the setting of decreased RBF: afferent arteriolar dilation increases the proportion of cardiac output that perfuses the kidney; efferent arteriolar resistance increases the filtration fraction; and hormonal and neural responses improve renal perfusion pressure by increasing intravascular volume, thereby indirectly increasing cardiac output (27). The afferent arterioles react to reductions in perfusion pressure by relaxing their smooth muscle elements to decrease renal vascular resistance. This property represents a relaxation response or myogenic reflex to reduced transmural pressure across the arteriolar wall.

The kidney also possesses a tubuloglomerular feedback system, which maintains the homeostasis of salt and water excretion. Decreased solute delivery to the macula densa in the cortical portion of the thick ascending loop of Henle results in relaxation of the juxtaposed afferent arteriolar smooth muscle cells, thus improving glomerular perfusion and filtration. The macula densa also increases renin release from the granular cells of juxtaglomerular apparatus in response to reduced sodium delivery.

A selective increase in efferent arteriole resistance decreases glomerular plasma flow, thereby preserving GFR. Glomerular filtration is augmented because capillary pressure upstream from the site of vasoconstriction tends to increase. This mechanism enables the kidney to offer high organ vascular resistance, thereby contributing to the maintenance of systemic blood pressure (BP) without compromising its function of filtration. Studies using specific inhibitors of angiotensin II have shown that efferent arteriolar resistance is largely caused by the action of angiotensin II. At low concentrations, norepinephrine has a vasoconstrictive effect on efferent arterioles, indicating that the adrenergic system may also be important for maintaining the renal compensatory response.

There is abundant evidence to support the notion that reductions in cardiac output are also accompanied by the release of vasopressin and by an increase in activity of the sympathetic nervous system and the renin–angiotensin–aldosterone (RAA) system (Fig. 2).

High concentrations of aldosterone stimulate reabsorption of sodium and water, primarily in the distal tubule and collecting ducts. Aldosterone is produced by the adrenal cortex in response to the feedback from the RAA system. Reduced delivery of sodium of the macula densa causes release of renin from the granular cells of the justaglomerular apparatus. Renin, in turn, catalyzes the release of angiotensin I from angiotensinogen. Angiotensin I then is transformed into angiotensin II in the lungs, catalyzed by angiotensin-converting enzyme (ACE). Angiotensin II stimulates the production of aldosterone (Fig. 2).

Antidiuretic hormone (ADH), or vasopressin, acts primarily on the collecting ducts to increase water reabsorption. An elevated level of ADH results in the excretion of small volumes of concentrated urine. The ADH is released from the posterior pituitary gland in response to increased blood osmolarity, which stimulates osmoreceptors in the hypothalamus (28). The ADH is inhibited by stimulation of the atrial baroreceptors or increased atrial volume. The ADH release is also increased by stress, pain, fear, and increased $PaCO_2$. However, plasma osmolality is the most potent regulator. The common denominator of these regulatory mechanisms to preserve RBF is salt and water conservation.

The control of blood delivery to the kidney, the fraction of plasma filtered, and the amount of volume returned to the systemic circulation are all determined by regulatory mechanisms within the kidney that attempt to preserve filtration function during compromised circulation. However, these compensatory mechanisms have limits. Excess vasoconstrictive forces may eventually induce a decrease in zfiltration function (29). If left unabated, the mechanisms that influence efferent vasoconstriction ultimately will overwhelm the system and cause afferent arteriolar vasoconstriction as well. The resulting decrease in filtration fraction is the hallmark of ischemic ARF.

Early cell changes following ischemia are reversible, such as the swelling of cell organelles, especially in the mitochondria. As ischemia progresses, lack of adenosine triphosphate interferes with the sodium pump mechanism, causing water and sodium to accumulate in the endoplasmic reticulum of tubular cells, and the cells themselves begin to swell (24).

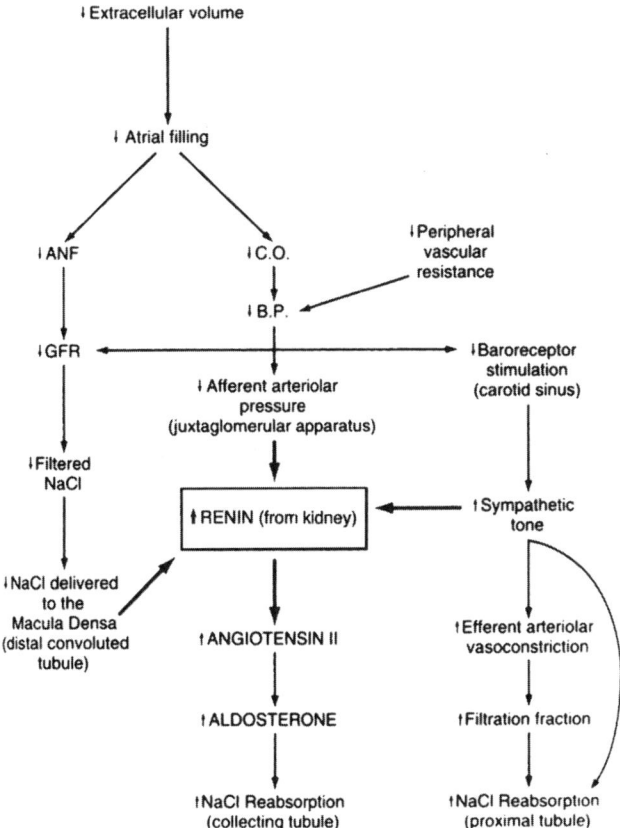

Figure 2 Mechanism of renal sodium and volume regulation. The regulation of intravascular volume and tonicity involves the complex interaction of atrial volume receptors, carotid and aortic body receptors, which stimulates the elaboration of renin. Renin promotes the conversion of angiotensinogen into angiotensin I (not shown). Angiotensin I is converted into angiotensin II in the liver, which increases blood pressure and aldosterone production. Aldosterone increases sodium reabsorption, potassium excretion, and hydrogen ion excretion. An additional mechanism regulating osmolality (not shown) involves the elaboration of antidiuretic hormone when osmoreceptors detect an eleveated osmolality, which leads to water retention until the target osmolality is reached. *Abbreviations*: ANF, atrial natriuretic factor; BP, blood pressure; CO, cardiac output; GFR, glomerular filtration rate; NaCl, sodium chloride. *Source*: From Ref. 166.

The time of onset for tubular damage in experimental models of ARF is usually within 25 minutes of ischemia, as the microvilli of the proximal tubular cell brush borders begin to change. Within an hour, they slough off into the tubular lumen, and membrane bullae protrude into the straight portion of the proximal tubule. After a few hours, intratubular pressure increases and tubular fluid passively flows backward. Within 24 hours, obstructing casts appear in the distal tubular lumen. Even when RBF is completely restored after 60 to 120 minutes of ischemia, GFR may not immediately improve. Ischemic tubular damage may eventually be exacerbated further by an imbalance between oxygen supply and demand. Most vulnerable to the imbalance are the mTAL cells (26). In ischemia-induced ARF, lesions are unevenly distributed among the nephrons, probably reflecting variability in blood flow (27). ☞ **Urine output is not always the best measure of renal wellbeing. Rather,** indirect measures are at times more reliable during resuscitation of a trauma patient (i.e., mean arterial pressure, preload, and cardiac output). ☞

In the clinical setting of hypotension, the kidney appears to have a distinct susceptibility to injury. The reason for this susceptibility is not apparent when reviewing RBF alone. Indeed, total RBF is normally high and oxygen supply far exceeds the requirements for oxygen utilization, even in moderate hypovolemia. The kidneys receive nearly one quarter of the cardiac output and extract relatively little oxygen (thus the discrepancy between cortical and medullary blood flow) and oxygen consumption is marked (30). The apparent overabundance of blood flow to the cortex maximizes flow-dependent functions, such as glomerular filtration and tubular reabsorption. In the medulla, blood flow and oxygen supply are restricted by a tubular vascular anatomy specifically designed for urinary concentration. Normally, approximately 90% to 95% of blood flow is delivered to the cortex compared with 5% to 10% delivered to the medulla. Average blood flow is 5.0 and 0.03 mL/g/min for the cortex and medulla, respectively, whereas the oxygen extraction ratio (i.e., O_2 consumption $[\dot{V}O_2] \div O_2$ delivery $[\dot{D}O_2]$) is 0.18 and 0.79 for the cortex and medulla, respectively. Normally, the PO_2 is approximately 55 mmHg in the cortex and 8 to 15 mmHg in the medulla, making the mTAL cells the most vulnerable to tissue hypoxia (26).

Therefore, severe hypoxia may easily develop in the medulla with what otherwise would seem to be adequate total RBF. The initial response to decrease RBF is increased sodium absorption in the ascending loop of Henle, which coincidentally increases oxygen demand in the region most vulnerable to decreased oxygen delivery. To compensate for this, sympathoadrenal mechanisms promote cortical vasoconstriction and oliguria, which tend to redistribute blood flow away from the outer cortex to the inner cortex and medulla.

At the same time, decreased sodium delivery to the macula densa causes afferent arterial constriction. With afferent arterial vasoconstriction, glomerular filtration decreases, and consequently, solute reabsorption in the loop of Henle and oxygen consumption are also reduced. The severity of cellular injury appears to be related to the degree of imbalance between cellular oxygen supply and demand. In the hypoperfused-kidney preparation, oxygen-enriched perfusion reduces cellular damage, hypoxic perfusion increases it, and complete cessation of perfusion (glomerular filtration zero, preventing ultrafiltration) is associated with less cellular injury than hypoxic perfusion. Afferent arterial vasoconstriction and consequent oliguria may be a normal protector response to acute tubular injury. By reducing ultrafiltration, energy-dependent ischemic injury to medullary tubular cells is prevented, even at the cost of retaining nitrogenous waste.

When RBF is compromised, blood flow and glomerular filtration in the outer cortical nephrons decline first because of the redistribution of blood toward the inner cortical and medullary regions. This cortical-to-medullary redistribution of RBF protects the vulnerable medullary oxygen balance (26). Decreased glomerular filtration during compromised flow thus appears to be protective, because decreased urine delivery to the tubules requires less reabsorptive work and prevents further oxygen supply–demand imbalance. Modulation by various drugs or compensatory mechanisms can reduce tubular workload and prevent medullary hypoxic cellular injury. Among the

compensatory mechanisms that reduce cellular injury is reduced tubular transport of glomerular filtration. Thus, temporarily, the oliguria may protect against ARF.

☞ Ischemic ATN is typically seen after a prolonged episode of hypotension, particularly when the blood flow to the kidney is interrupted (e.g., aortic crossclamp) (31–34). ☞ Experimental models of ATN indicate that ischemia damages the medullary tubular segments of the nephron, causing intratubular obstruction, consequent backleak, and increased intramedullary vascular resistance (35,36). The aggregate effect of this cascade is a profound reduction in GFR and a sustained maintenance phase of ARF after the ischemic injury (37). Despite the severe decrement in glomerular filtration, the kidney is quite resilient, and in the absence of further insults, usually recovers function within 7 to 21 days (27).

PATHOGENESIS: ROLE OF RENAL TOXINS

Nephrotoxic ARF is commonly encountered in trauma and critically ill postsurgical patients. The kidney is responsible for clearing a vast number of drugs and toxins. Many of these drugs have nephrotoxic properties themselves, while others become injurious when used in combination with other drugs. The mechanism by which nephrotoxins injure the renal parenchyma include intra-arterial vasoconstriction [e.g., contrast media, catecholamines, and nonsteroidal anti-inflammatory drugs (NSAIDs)], direct tubular injury (e.g., aminoglycosides and amphotericin), and intratubular obstruction (e.g., acyclovir and sulfonamides) (38–41). As in ischemic ATN, if the offending insult is removed and further insults are avoided in a previously healthy kidney, normalization of renal function is the rule after a maintenance phase (37).

The natural history of ATN is triphasic, and interpretation of urine output requires knowledge of these phases. It begins with an insult or initiation phase followed by a maintenance phase, which is typically oliguric (though not always), followed by a diuretic or recovery phase. The maintenance phase lasts between 7 to 21 days, but in rare circumstances, it can last as long as 11 to 12 months before recovery. The diuretic phase continues, until tubular function is restored and the kidney regains its concentrating ability. Ischemic ATN follows this paradigm more consistently, whereas nephrotoxic ATN is more variable depending on the duration and severity of nephrotoxic exposure (37,42,43).

In addition to a wide range of compounds that are nephrotoxic, there are also a large number of agents that can cause interstitial nephritis (44–46). Drugs or toxins generally induce acute interstitial nephritis (AIN), but various infectious agents can also cause AIN (47). The AIN can cause modest renal insufficiency, which is clinically silent, or can progress to ARF. Edema and interstitial infiltrate mark the resultant lesion seen in AIN. Clinically, fever, skin rash, rising creatinine, pyuria, and white cell casts are a typical presentation (47,48). Eosinophiluria, which are seen in most but not all patients, is a common finding, but the diagnostic value of this test in isolation is uncertain (49,50). An abbreviated list of medications commonly used in the ICU that can cause AIN is provided in Table 1. AIN ordinarily occurs within three to five days of initiation of the medication, and withdrawal of the offending agent is often adequate therapy (51). However, in some cases, AIN can lead to ARF of sustained duration (52).

Table 1 Drugs Commonly Used in the Intensive Care Unit that Have Been Reported to Cause Acute Interstitial Nephritis

Ciprofloxacin
Nitrofurantoin
Halothane
Sulfonamides
Penicillins
Cephalosporins
Tetracycline
Diazepam
Thiazides
Furosemide
NSAIDs

Abbreviation: NSAIDs, nonsteroidal anti-inflammatory drugs.
Source: From Refs. 45, 62, 160–165.

PATHOGENESIS: OTHER CAUSES

Occlusion of the renal arterial or venous vasculature is an uncommon cause of ARF, but any process that compromises the arterial supply (e.g., aortic dissection, vasculitis, ather-oemboli, thromboembolism, microangiopathic hemolytic anemia (MAHA), malignant hypertension, and hyper-viscosity syndromes) can rapidly cause ARF (53,54). Renal vein thrombosis is rare, primarily occurring in patients suffering from severe nephrotic syndrome, hypercoaguable state (e.g., cancer), or trauma where the kidney suffers direct trauma or a torsion injury (55–59). In order for there to be a significant clinical effect causing ARF from a vascular injury, there must be an underlying renal disease, both kidneys must be involved, or else one kidney must have been damaged previous to the new insult to the contralateral kidney (60).

Glomerular disease is an uncommon cause of ARF in the SICU, usually presenting over a more chronic course. Glomerular disease is invariably marked by significant proteinuria (>1 g/day) and hypertension. The major exception to this chronic course is rapidly progressive glomerular nephritis (RPGN), which can present with multi-system disease and can cause a brisk decline in GFR. Causes of RPGN that require ICU admission include but are not limited to Goodpasture's disease, Churg-Strauss disease, Wegner's granulomatosis, endocarditis, polyarteritis nodosa (PAN), and severe systemic lupus erythematosus (SLE). Identification of RPGN is explained in more detail subsequently.

Obstruction is an uncommon cause of ARF, but is seen more frequently in postoperative patients and trauma patients than medical patients in the ICU. In order for obstruction to cause ARF, the obstruction must be distal to the bladder neck (e.g., prostatic hypertrophy), involve some aspect of both ureters, or create unilateral obstruction with the contralateral kidney previously damaged or dysfunctional. If the obstruction is not chronic (<2 weeks), relieving the obstruction restores function promptly. As the duration of the obstruction lengthens, so does the delay in return of function and increases the amount of post obstructive tubular dysfunction.

GENERAL DIAGNOSTIC APPROACH

Although a consensus definition for ARF does not exist, ☞ most nephrologists would agree that doubling of the

Table 2 Definitions of Acute Renal Failure

Increase in serum creatinine of 1.0 mg/dL with clinical scenario consistent with ATN
Oliguria or elevated serum creatinine
Sudden rise in serum creatinine of greater than 2.0 mg/dL or greater than 50% in patients with baseline serum creatinine of 3.0 mg/dL

Abbreviation: ATN, acute tubular necrosis.
Source: From Refs. 8, 9, 124.

serum creatinine or the rising of serum creatinine of 1.0 mg/dL per day over two to three days would constitute a patient in ARF (Table 2). ☞ A recent categorization ("Rifle" system) has been proposed (Fig. 3). For purposes of this discussion, any rise of serum creatinine or indication of insufficient or unexpectedly poor clearance (e.g., elevated serum phosphorus and an elevated trough level of a renally excreted antibiotic that was dosed correctly) of a renally

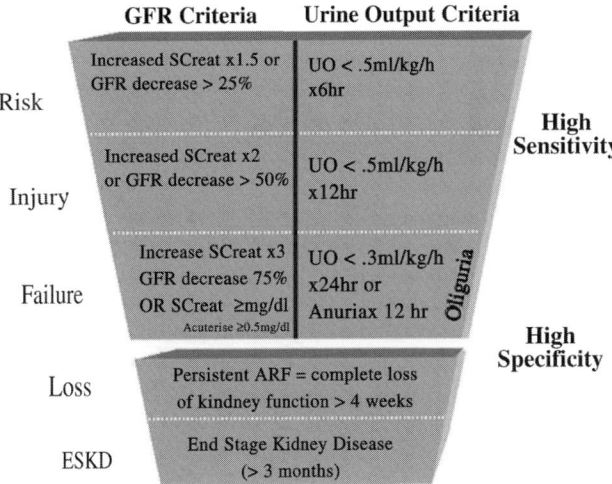

Figure 3 RIFLE (Risk, Injury, Failure, Loss, End-stage kidney Disease) criteria for acute renal failure. Proposed classification scheme for acute renal failure. The acronym RIFLE derives from the first letter of the following phrases: *R*isk of renal dysfunction; *I*njury to the kidney; *F*ailure of kidney function; *L*oss of kidney function; *E*nd-stage kidney disease. The classification system includes separate criteria for creatinine and urine output (UO). A patient can fulfil the criteria through changes in serum creatinine (SCreat) or changes in urine output, or both. The criteria that lead to the worst possible classification should be used. Note that the F component of RIFLE "Failure of kidney function" is present even if the increase in serum creatinine is under three-fold, as long as the new serum creatinine is greater than 4.0 mg/dL (350 μmol/L) in the setting of an acute increase of at least 0.5 mg/dL (44 μmol/L). The designation RIFLE-F should be used in this case to denote "acute-on-chronic" disease. Similarly, when the RIFLE-F classification is achieved by urine output criteria, a designation of RIFLE-F O should be used to denote oliguria. The shape of the figure denotes the fact that more patients (high sensitivity) will be included in the mild category, including some without actually having renal failure (less specificity). In contrast, at the bottom of the figure, the criteria are strict and therefore specific, but some patients will be missed. *Abbreviations*: ARF, acute renal failure; GFR, glomerular filtration rate.

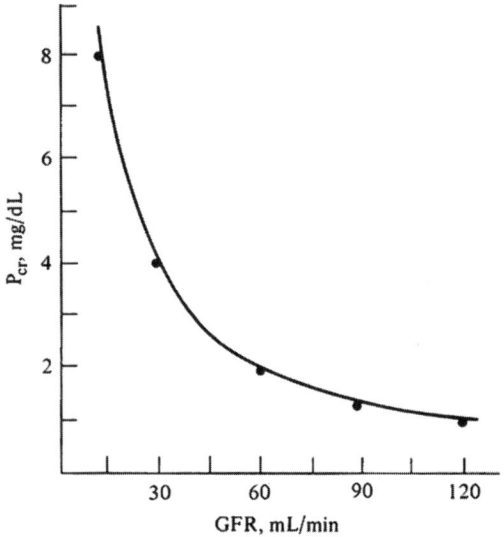

Figure 4 The glomerular filtration rate (GFR) creatinine graph. Steady-state relationship between the plasma creatinine concentration (P_{cr}), blood urea nitrogen, and the GFR. *Abbreviation*: GFR, glomerular filtration rate.

Table 3 Initial Survey

Complete blood count with differential
Urine electrolytes (sodium, potassium, and chloride)
Urine creatinine, urine protein, and urine eosinophils
Urinalysis with cell count, urine sediment assessment
Foley catheter placement, intra-abdominal pressure measurement
Renal U/S (assess kidney size and presence of obstruction)
Serum CPK, serum albumin
Correction of hypovolemia and hypotension
Discontinuation of any obvious nephrotoxic drugs (especially NSAIDs)

Abbreviations: CPK, creatine phosphokinase; NSAIDs, nonsteroidal anti-inflammatory drugs.

excreted substance should raise concern. If these abnormalities are not explained upon re-examination of the clinical picture, a formal diagnostic evaluation should begin.

Most clinicians use the blood urea nitrogen (BUN) and serum creatinine as their markers of renal function. However, these are both late markers of decreased GFR. Figure 4 shows the relationship between GFR decline and the rise of serum creatinine. As the figure illustrates, rise in serum creatinine is a late marker for the decrement in GFR. BUN is similarly unreliable due to its tendency to rise in conditions where the kidney is functioning adequately (e.g., hypermetabolic state, gastrointestinal bleeding, and high protein diet). Whenever the serum creatinine doubles within a 24-hour period, and the patient becomes oliguric, renal replacement therapy is often required, as the creatine cannot increase much faster and the value during this nonsteady state is no longer predictive of GFR.

Once ARF is suspected or in progress, the assessment of the cause of ARF should begin in a systematic fashion. Many clinicians rule out prerenal and postrenal (obstructive) etiologies and then begin to assess for renal causes of ARF. This approach does not work as well in the ICU; patient's disease processes evolve too fast to wait for investigative tests to be done. Like the shock/systemic inflammatory response syndrome (SIRS) mode or trauma model, treatment and diagnosis in critical illness must often occur simultaneously. Because prerenal and postrenal etiologies are the easiest to reverse, they should be assessed and immediately corrected if they are found (similar to the initial survey taken for a trauma patient) while other etiologies are evaluated.

Immediate interventions include correction of volume deficits, correction of hypotension or relative hypotension (for patients who have a normal mean arterial pressure (MAP), but are normally hypertensive), placement of Foley catheter, and cessation of known nephrotoxins (if clinically feasible) and basic urine and serum studies should be sent [i.e., urinalysis, urine electrolytes, urine protein, urine creatinine, urine eosinophils, urine osmolarity, and complete blood count with differential and serum creatine

phosphokinase (CPK) level]. Table 3 lists the initial steps that should be taken during the initial survey.

While these lab tests are drawn and sent, the next step is to play detective and "round up the usual suspects" of clinical disorders and agents that are often implicated in ARF. These agents are contrast media, NSAIDs, and angiotensin converting enzyme inhibitors (ACEi). The nephrotoxicity seen with all of these agents is potentiated by hypovolemia, and the typical course of events is that the patient is exposed to one or more of these agents while hypovolemic.

Other medications that often cause ARF via ATN or AIN include, antibiotics, antifungal, and antiviral agents. Penicillins, cephalosporins, aminoglycosides, vancomycin (alone or in combinations with other antibiotics), quinolones, rifampin, aztreonam, sulfonamides, tetracycline, amphotericin, foscarnet, and acyclovir have all been reported to cause ARF (61–70). In each individual case, the value of continuing an antimicrobial agent must be weighed versus the likelihood of that agent causing or contributing to ARF.

DIRECT AND INDIRECT ASSESSMENT OF RENAL STATUS

Monitoring urine output as a sign of the adequacy of renal perfusion is easy and assumes that patients with diminished renal perfusion excrete a low volume of concentrated urine. The level of nitrogenous wastes in the blood depends on both systemic production and renal clearance. Renal clearance is determined by the delivery of these waste products to the kidney (RBF) and the ability of the kidney to extract them (GFR). The kidney also concentrates the ultrafiltrate; when able to maximally concentrate, a total of 400 to 500 mL of urine is required in order to clear the daily obligatory nitrogenous wastes. Injured kidneys require more urine output to clear the daily obligate solute load. Traditionally, inadequate urinary volume, or oliguria, is defined as urinary output of less than 0.5 mL/kg/hr. Multiple studies, however, have shown no correlations between urine volume and histologic evidence of ATN, GFR, creatinine clearance, or changes from preoperative to postoperative levels of BUN and creatinine in patients with burn injury, trauma, cardiovascular surgery, and shock status. Moreover, measurement of mean and lowest hourly urinary output during aortic vascular surgery has not been predictive of postoperative renal insufficiency (71).

Oliguria may reflect a variety of factors independent of GFR, and a normal hourly urine output does not preclude the absence of renal failure. Among these factors is tubular excretion of solute and water, which is determined by local and systemic levels of renin, aldosterone, and ADH. In addition, patients in the OR are often not hemodynamically stable; decreased blood volume or cardiac output, fluctuating hormone levels (aldosterone, renin, and ADH), and increased catecholamine concentrations, with the effects of general anesthesia, can alter GFR. The data does not support oliguria as a reliable sign of pending renal dysfunction.

Monitoring Urine Output

A clinically robust intraoperative measure of renal function does not yet exist. The Foley catheter provides an acceptable reflection of intravascular volume in patients with normal renal function, normal serum osmolality (absence of hyperglycemia, alcohol intoxication, and mannitol therapy) and in the absence of other diuretics (e.g., caffeine, lasix).

☞ **Decreased urine output, and rising serum BUN and creatinine are the standard indicators for the development of worsening ARF.** ☞ Creatinine (which is neither secreted nor reabsorbed to any appreciable amount) is a good inverse measure of GFR. However, creatinine elevations occur after the renal insult has occurred, and only reflect the degree of renal insufficiency once a steady state is achieved. Indeed, a doubling of serum creatinine generally represents a 50% decrease in GFR at steady state. However, creatinine may double from 0.8 to 1.6 in a 24-hour period in a patient with essentially zero GFR, because this duration is required for creatinine to accumulate in the blood in essentially anephric patients. Serial determination of creatinine clearance is currently the most sensitive test for predicting the onset of perioperative renal dysfunction; however, the test is not practical for measuring renal function under OR conditions (72).

Urine output measurements recorded every 15 to 60 minutes, are most useful in determining renal perfusion. In the future, the ability to measure intrarenal blood flow distribution may ultimately improve our predictive and diagnostic abilities to assess perioperative ARF. However, methodological constraints limit its use at this time. During acute events, common during surgery (massive exanguination, clamping of major vascular structures), more direct and rapidly responsive measures of arterial perfusion and central venous pressure (CVP) are required. Although these pressures are directly measured, and are excellent indicators of intravascular pressure and volume, they are indirect measures of renal perfusion.

Indirect Measures of Renal Perfusion: Blood Pressure and Volume Status

Invasive Arterial Blood Pressure Monitoring

☞ **An arterial line serves the dual purpose of providing access for repetitive ABG samples, as well as continuous beat-to-beat measurement of arterial BP throughout resuscitation, operative management, and critical care.** ☞

Continuous BP monitoring is useful for surgical procedures where major intravascular volume shifts are likely to cause acute, profound changes in arterial BP. Not only does the absolute systolic, diastolic, and mean arterial pressure have important clinical relevance, but the information contained in the arterial pressure waveform has important hemodynamic information (including rate, rhythm, preload, afterload, and contractility) (73–75).

Any large peripheral artery can be used for catheterization. The risk of radial artery cannulation with a 20 g Teflon catheter is extremely low in adults (76). However, in certain situations (severe vasoconstriction or severe vasodilation), the femoral arterial catheter will more closely reflect the aortic pressure than the radial catheter (77). In addition, certain procedures (e.g., thoracic aortic aneurysm repair) are best managed with pressure measurements obtained above (right radial) and below (either femoral artery) the lesions (78). The complication rate from percutaneous cannulation of the femoral artery is no greater than that of radial artery (79,80).

☞ **Systolic pressure variation (SPV) is a technique for gauging intravascular volume status, which is very useful in renal failure patients.** ☞ Arterial BP has long been known to decrease with positive pressure ventilation. The SPV is a method of quantifying these changes. Perel has shown in both animal experiments and clinical studies that SPV directly correlates with intravascular depletion (81,82). Indeed, when the systolic pressure (delta down component) decreases by more than 10 mmHg in patients ventilated with 10 to 15 cc/kg, these patients are clinically volume under resuscitated (Fig. 5).

Systolic Pressure Variation Monitoring Indications

The CVP monitoring is considered a second-tier-monitoring device (recommended if the patient is sick or is undergoing a high risk procedure). The CVP reflects the relationship between the patient's blood volume, venous tone, and right ventricular performance. In patients without significant cardiac disease or pulmonary hypertension, the CVP also provides a useful reflection of right (and left) ventricular preload. Additionally, it provides a port for the administration of cardiovascular drugs, and the insertion of a pulmonary artery (PA) catheter or transvenous pacemaker. For the CRF patient receiving a renal transplant, one of the most important determinants of immediate post transplant renal viability and avoidance of ATN is the adequacy of perfusion to the newly transplanted kidney at the time the vascular clamps are released (83). The CVP (or pulmonary artery pressure (PAP) in patients with left ventricle (LV) dysfunction) should be used to guide therapy in these patients.

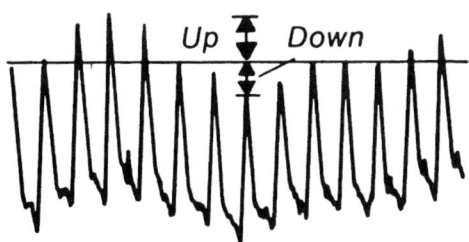

Figure 5 Systolic arterial blood pressure (BP) variation. The systolic arterial pressure variation (SPV) can be used as a measure of ventricular responsiveness to volume. The arterial BP wave form can be divided into a delta-up component and a delta-down component when observed during mechanical ventilation. When the SPV (delta-down component) varies more than 10 mmHg, with a positive pressure breath (tidal volumes 10–15 mL/kg), there is a relative paucity in left ventricular filling and reflects the need for additional intravascular volume administration. The SPV can be used in the operating room or in the surgical intensive care unit to assist in establishing the optimum intravascular volume. Also see Volume 2, Chapter 3. *Source*: From Ref. 81.

🖎 Trauma and critically ill patients with renal insufficiency should have their CVP maintained on the high side to protect against the prerenal state. 🖎

Indications for Pulmonary Arterial Catheterization

The PA catheterization is a second- or third-tier monitor reserved for patients in whom the CVP poorly reflects intravascular volume status (impaired LV function, severe coronary artery disease, known PA hypertension, and mitral or tricuspid valve pathology). In addition, PA catheters are indicated for high-risk procedures (thoracic aorta cross clamping), or when measurement of ventricular performance (SV) or systemic perfusion (cardiac output) is warranted.

Information available from PA catheters includes left-sided filling pressures, measurement of cardiac output, sampling mixed venous blood, calculation of systemic and pulmonary vascular resistances, and PA and wedge pressure waveform analysis. The PA catheter provides estimates of left ventricular (LV) preload [i.e., left ventricular end-diastolic volume (LVEDV)] by measuring left ventricular end-diastolic pressure (LVEDP). This LVEDP/LVEDV relationship is altered by changes in LV compliance (e.g., myocardial ischemia, tissue edema, etc.). Many investigators have demonstrated a poor correlation between pulmonary capillary wedge pressure (PCWP) and LVEDV in acutely ill patients (84). However, a recent study demonstrated reduced mortality in severely injured trauma patients who were monitored with a PA catheter (85). 🖎 **In situations where assessment of LVEDV is critical (e.g., hypotension, low cardiac output, and normal- or high-filling pressures by CVP and PACWP), using a transesophageal echocardiography (TEE) provides the more accurate and direct view of LV preload and contractility (86).** 🖎

Role of Transesophageal Echocardiography

TEE is an established monitoring and diagnostic tool for the cardiothoracic anesthesiologist. Techniques for insertion, interpretation, and complications have been comprehensively reviewed in Chapter 21. The main benefits in TEE lies in the fact that a picture can truly be worth a thousand words. Direct visualization of both ventricular and atrial chambers provide instantaneous information on preload. Contractility is also directly visualized using the short-axis view (87). Monitoring for ischemia and wall motion abnormalities is excellent with TEE, and automated real-time technologies are emerging (88). Valvular function can be assessed using color-labeled directional flow and Doppler techniques. Pericardial effusions and their effect on atrial and ventricular function are well visualized. Abnormal holes [(atrial septal defect (ASD) and ventricular septal defect (VSD)] can be detected via direct view or administration of agitated saline.

Renal Function Testing in ARF

Evaluating the urine takes time. Therefore, the traumatologist must measure and optimize indirect measures of renal wellbeing (arterial BP, CVPs, and cardiac output) before, or simultaneously with diagnostic studies. Direct visualization and dipstick testing are the first tests that should be done, as both are quick to perform. Next, specific gravity measurement, and then microscopy of the urinary sediment should be employed. Finally, a spot urine test and serum sample of sodium creatinine and BUN should be done. With these studies, most causes of oliguria will become elucidated.

Visual Inspection and Dipstick Evaluation of Urine

Urine color should be noted and a dip test performed (occult blood, bile, glucose, and protein) to determine if the urine is concentrated. If the urine is dark, it could be concentrated, have bile, or blood. A dipstick positive for occult blood, when there are no red blood cells (RBCs) seen on microscopy is consistent with rhabdomyolysis. This would occur in the setting of a crush injury, compartment syndrome, and severe flame or electrical burns. However, intravascular hemolysis will present in the same manner (rare in noncardiac surgery, common following cardiopulmonary bypass (CPB), especially if hemofiltration is used). When hemolysis occurs in association with blood transfusion, the transfusion must be stopped, and both the patient's blood sample and the partially transfused blood sample should be sent back to the blood bank to determine if there is a cross match, or clerical error. Other rare causes of hemolysis, such as cold aglutinans in a hypothermic patient, should also be considered. If the dipstick is positive for glucose, the patient may not have concentrated urine despite being severely volume-depleted (they would unlikely manifest oliguria in this setting as well).

Specific Gravity Evaluation of Urine

Next, the specific gravity of urine should be assessed. Dilute urine has a specific gravity <1.010, whereas concentrated urine in the setting of hypovolemic oliguria has a specific gravity >1.030.

Microscopic Evaluation of Urine Sediment

In many instances, renal sediment reveals evidence of intrinsic renal dysfunction. Microscopy of the spun urine pellet reveals an expansive array of information. The importance of the presence or absence of RBCs is mentioned earlier. The presence of tubuloepithelial cells with epithelial cell casts is pathognomonic for ATN.

Spot Urine and Serum Sodium, Creatinine, and Urea Nitrogen

A urine sample should be sent to the lab to determine urinary sodium and creatinine [a concomitant blood sample should also be sent to measure serum creatinine and sodium, and to evaluate the fractional excretion of sodium (FENa)—described subsequently]. The previously normal patient with oliguria from renal hypoperfusion should produce a small volume of concentrated urine with a low sodium concentration. Because sodium reabsorption increases and sodium excretion decreases in the setting of hypovolemia (and normal kidneys), the urinary sodium concentration should be less than 20 mEq/L (<10 mEq/L if the patient is seriously prerenal and the kidneys still can maximally concentrate urine).

However, if the patient has a prerenal condition superimposed on existing intrinsic renal dysfunction, or has received a high osmotic load (mannitol, ethanol intoxication), or has received another diuretic (furosomide, caffine, etc.), the urine may be paradoxically dilute in the setting of severe intravascular depletion.

Volume Challenge for Perfusion Pressure Augmentation

Immediately after documenting oliguria, but before completing the diagnostic work up described earlier, relative intravascular volume depletion should be presumed and treatment instituted. It is far easier to treat a modest episode of pulmonary edema than it is to treat ARF.

DIAGNOSTIC FEATURES OF COMMON SYNDROMES

After completing the initial survey, a full history and physical examination should be conducted, and an assessment of the laboratory data should be done. First, any aspect of the patient's history that could indicate a likely etiology of ARF should be evaluated. Examples include recent trauma, mechanism of trauma (clues to vascular, contusion, torsion injuries of the kidney, or crush injury predisposing a patient to rhabdomyolysis), recent procedures (a clue to cholesterol atheremboli from angiography, obstruction for cystoscopy, or intra-abdominal surgery), and constitutional symptoms that might suggest a systemic process or past history of renal disease (which could suggest previous unilateral kidney disease or underlying chronic renal insufficiency). If the patient's history and physical examination does not suggest an etiology, then the results of the initial survey should help determine possible etiologies.

Prerenal vs. ATN
A bland urinalysis (few cells and minimal or no proteinuria) is consistent with prerenal causes or ATN. However, the way to differentiate between the two etiologies is the assessment of renal concentrating function. Decreased renal perfusion pressure, which is the hallmark of prerenal azotemia, causes a volume retention effect in a normal kidney. The kidneys become sodium avid and the serum ADH rises in response to volume depletion. This results in urine, which has a low sodium concentration (U Sodium < 20 mEq/dL), a low fractional excretion of sodium (FeNa < 1%), an elevated urine osmolarity (Uosm > 450), and an elevated specific gravity (SG > 1.020) (89). In addition, in normal kidneys, the BUN to creatinine ratio will often rise to >20:1 (90). This ratio can be helpful when there are no other reasons for the increased ratio (see Table 4 for a complete list). Although these commonly used indicies are often useful in delineating between prerenal and other causes of ARF, they have three distinct limitations. First, if the patient has an underlying renal disease, these parameters may not be accurate. Second, other pathologic processes that cause intra-renal vasoconstriction (e.g., contrast media, vasopressors, and hepatorenal syndrome) will confound these values even if the patient is euvolemic, particularly the low FeNa and low urine sodium concentration. Third, when patients are given diuretics as a clinical challenge to increase urine output, it is difficult to reliably interpret the results of these tests. ☞ **The most clinically useful way to diagnose ATN is the evaluation of the urine sediment. The presence of brown granular casts and epithelial cells, singly or in casts, is seen in 80% of**

Table 4 Causes of Increased Blood Urea Nitrogen:Creatinine Ratio

High protein diet
Gastrointestinal bleeding
Steroid use
Hypercatabolic state
Decreased renal perfusion pressure

patients with ATN (91). However, the absence of casts does not preclude ATN. It is for this reason that patients with ARF should be assumed to have a prerenal state, and pre-emptive correction should be initiated if the patient's clinical condition can tolerate the restoration of renal perfusion pressure (91). ☞

Proteinuric Diseases
AIN or a glomerular process should be suspected if the urinalysis shows proteinuria. If the urine protein to urine creatinine ratio [(urine protein) mg/dL divided by (urine creatinine)] mg/dL is greater than 1, a glomerular disease is likely. In most such cases, proteinuria will be found to pre-date the ARF, and to be due to a chronic glomerular disease, such as diabetic nephropathy, a chronic form of glomerulonephritis, or lupus nephritis. This underscores the importance of knowing the baseline urinalysis findings, either the pre-operative result in a surgical patient, or the initial urine obtained from a trauma victim.

New-onset proteinuria with a urine protein-to-creatinine ratio of less than one is typical of AIN; there may also be microscopic hematuria, and pyuria in the absence of urinary infection. AIN is further suggested by the presence of urine eosinophils, white cell casts, and an offending agent known to cause AIN (92). Though AIN is usually associated with a modest amount of proteinuria, NSAID-induced AIN can occasionally cause proteinuria in the nephrotic range (>3 gms protein/d)(93). Unlike AIN from other agents, NSAID-induced AIN does not cause eosinophiluria. Treatment of AIN is supportive and requires withdrawal of the offending agent. Some studies suggest that steroids may be helpful, but this remains controversial (46).

A less common cause of new-onset proteinuria and microscopic hematuria is acute glomerulonephritis. RBC casts in the urine and persistent hypertension further suggest this diagnosis. Visible (macroscopic) hematuria, if it is not due to traumatic Foley catheterization or urinary infection, could suggest an acute glomerulonephritic or vasculitic illness. When these are a strong consideration, urgent consultation from the nephrology service would be warranted, particularly if the patient's serum creatinine is rising rapidly. Additional serologic tests are required for the work-up of glomerulonephritis and renal vasculitis.

Vascular Causes of Acute Renal Failure
Vascular insults uncommonly cause ARF, but in scenarios where one kidney is previously damaged or when bilateral vascular insults occur, modest proteinuria and significant hematuria are often present. Arterial insults (infarction) often result in flank or back pain. Though nonspecific, active urine sediment, flank or back pain, and an appropriate history (atrial fibrillation, recent aortic manipulation) might suggest a vascular insult (94–96). If the renal infarct is large enough, GFR may be completely compromised and no hematuria will be seen. However, if renal infarction has occurred, the serum lactate dehydrogenase (LDH) should be significantly elevated (97). In one small study, acute renal artery occlusion could be predicted when the urine concentrations of sodium, urea, and creatinine were the same as the serum concentration, along with the FeNa approaching 100% (98). Renal artery occlusion can usually be confirmed by Doppler ultrasound or radionucleotide scanning.

Medical therapy with anticoagulation is usually the preferred therapy if diagnosis is made within 24 to 48 hours. If the diagnosis is made promptly, there are many case reports of renal tissue salvage with thrombolytic, interventional, or surgical techniques as far as 35 hours after occlusion (94,96,99).

Atheremboli from cholesterol plaques can cause ARF, and usually has systemic findings. Eosinophilia, eosinophiluria, ARF, livedo reticularis, and evidence of peripheral cyanosis or infarction are all associated with atheroembolic disease (100–102). Risk factors for cholesterol embolization are aortic manipulation (surgical or angiographic) and recent anticoagulation. This process is seen more commonly in patients with large plaque burden, and in some cases can have a subacute course evolving over three to six weeks. Although proteinuria and hematuria are seen with severe cholesterol embolization, the urine can be bland as well, and a high index of suspicion is required to make the diagnosis. Treatment is largely supportive, and cessation of anticoagulation is recommended (103).

Renal vein thrombosis is rare. It is seen almost exclusively in patients with nephrotic syndrome or patients with underlying hypercoaguable state (55,57–59,104). Sporadic cases of bilateral RVT have been reported in patients with underlying nephrotic syndrome and hypercoaguable pathology (105–110). Rarely, RVT is seen as a consequence of trauma and has been reported in pediatric burn patients (56, 111,112). RVT presents usually without any specific symptoms; often, the presenting diagnosis is pulmonary embolization from inferior vena cava thrombosis that has extended from the renal vein (107). Rarely, elevated serum LDH and proteinuria are seen; this is often seen when RVT converts to renal infarction. Investigative studies include Doppler ultrasound, computed tomography (CT), magnetic resonance imaging (MRI), and caval venography. Many nephrologists treat RVT conservatively, because some trials have suggested no long-term benefit using thrombolytics and surgical embolectomy (113–115). However, thrombolytics and surgical thrombectomy have also been applied successfully (107,109,116,117).

Pigment Induced Causes of ARF

Another cause of ARF that can masquerade as hematuria is pigment-induced ARF. These two disorders are rhabdomyolysis and hemoglobinuria. Both disorders cause ATN via pigment-induced damage of the tubular cells. Both can cause the urine dipstick to be positive for blood; however, microscopic evaluation shows few to no RBCs. When assessing a urinalysis, the actual cell count should be noted. Rhabdomyolysis is caused by muscle necrosis that release myoglobin into the bloodstream, which is then filtered into the tubules, causing ATN. Rhabdomyolysis classically presents with brown-colored urine, pigmented casts in the urine, and an elevated CPK. Rhabdomyolysis can be seen in patients suffering from crush injury, compartment syndrome, operative cases with relative hypovolemia, and in alcoholics who have hypophosphatemia, or myositis (91,118). Many medications can cause high serum CPK levels, including but not limited to: HMG CoA reductase inhibitors (lovastatin), itraconazole, cyclosporine, zidovudine (AZT), amphetamines, and cocaine (119–121). Because rhabdomyolysis can be caused by such a wide variety of mechanisms, and because it is one the few treatable forms of ARF, serum CPK is included in the initial survey. Although no absolute level of CPK elevation correlates to ARF, most clinicians use the 10,000 u/L as a cut-off. One study showed the cut-off to be 16,000 u/L to predictive of patients who would develop ARF (122). If the serum CPK

is elevated in a patient, serial measurements should be performed to determine if a rising trend is developing. Initial muscle damage may not reveal an elevated CPK, until volume is restored and the CPK washes out of the muscle tissue. Patients with rhabdomyolysis can sequester enormous amounts of volume in their damaged tissue, and volume resuscitation is the cornerstone of therapy. Once the patient is volume replete, studies in crush patients have shown that maintaining urine flow with mannitol and alkalization of the urine is helpful. Alkalization of the urine is quite difficult and requires significant amounts of sodium bicarbonate. This creates a substantial volume load, and should not be continued if urine flow cannot be established because the patient may become volume overloaded (123). Hemoglobinuria is uncommon and occurs after massive hemolysis. Free hemoglobin is a large molecule and rapidly bound by haptoglobin. In order for hemoglobin to be freely filtered by the glomerulus, the amount of hemolysis must first overwhelm the haptoglobin buffering system. Treatment for hemoglobinuria is therapy targeted at stopping the hemolysis and maintaining urine flow.

Obstructive Causes of ARF

Obstruction is an uncommon cause of ARF (5–10% of cases), yet because it is reversible and treatable, it should be ruled out in the initial survey (124). In patients who have a clinical history that is highly suggestive of obstruction, an ultrasound that fails to show hydronephrosis should not lead to the abandonment of obstruction as an etiology. If the patient is volume depleted, if the collecting system is encased in fibrosis or malignancy, or if the obstruction is mild, the renal pelvis may not dilate (125). If obstruction is strongly suspected and the renal ultrasound is nondiagnostic, imaging with a repeat ultrasound after volume is given, CT, and/or renal radionucleotde scanning are appropriate steps for confirmation (126).

SPECIFIC RENAL SYNDROMES

There are clinical contexts when uncommon renal syndromes that cause ARF become more likely. Four pathologic processes that can cause ARF in the patients admitted to the ICU are abdominal compartment syndrome (ACS), microangiopathic hemolytic syndromes, hepatorenal syndrome, and the acute development of anuria.

Abdominal Compartment Syndrome

Postoperative ICU considerations relevant to renal monitoring and protection include close control of fluid, solute, and acid base status, monitoring for and prevention of bleeding and shock, coagulopathy, and special conditions that can further impair renal reserve (sepsis, MOSF, and additional toxin exposure, such as aminoglycosides, radiocontrast, etc). An additional postoperative complication, which can impair renal function known as "ACS," has been increasingly recognized in the last decade.

ACS results from increased intra-abdominal pressure (IAP), usually due to bowel and interstitial tissue edema, following laparotomy in patients with shock and massive fluid resuscitation (127). The increased IAP results in impairment of circulation, decreased tissue perfusion, and renal as well as other organ dysfunction (cardiovascular, gut, and pulmonary) (128). The tense abdomen leads to increased peak airway pressures, hypercarbia, and oliguria. Decreased thoracic venous return, with decreased cardiac output and decreased renal function due to hypoperfusion, are components of the syndrome. Additionally, increased IAP causes decreased tidal volume, increased ventilatory pressures, and increased atelectasis. Increased IAP can also cause venous hypertension and elevate ICP.

Abdominal compartment pressures may be measured by attaching an indwelling Foley catheter to a pressure transducer, leveled to the symphysis pubis (129). Pressures greater than 20 to 25 mmHg require abdominal decompression (130). Normal postoperative abdominal pressure is 0 to 5 mmHg. At pressures greater than 10 mmHg, hepatic arterial blood flow decreases; at 15 to 20 mmHg, oliguria and cardiovascular changes occur; and at pressures between 20 and 40 mmHg, anuria is typical (131).

Patients with abdominal pressures greater than 20 to 25 mmHg require emergency decompressive laparotomy to relieve the pressure and restore renal perfusion. However, extensive delay will lead to renal failure. Furthermore, opening the abdomen results in a rapid decrease in IAP with a resultant reperfusion syndrome that must be anticipated by the anesthesiologist. The reperfusion syndrome following abdominal decompression can lead to life-threatening hypotension, unless proper preparation occurs. Indeed, Morris (132) described asystole, following decompression in 4 of 16 patients who underwent rapid decompression.

Preparation for decompression of ACS involves maneuvers similar to those taken immediately prior to clamp removal during a thoracic aortic aneurysm repair: (*i*) intravascular volume is increased, (*ii*) dopamine (or other inotrope and vasopressors) are in line and running, and (*iii*) acidosis (if severe) is treated with sodium bicarbonate. An increase in minute ventilation is occasionally needed to eliminate CO_2 (neutralize lactate eminting from gut, and increased CO_2 from administered bicarbonate). Calcium chloride is administered to protect against increased potassium (washed out from gut). Calcium is also useful to bolster the transient hypocalcemia, following sodium bicarbonate administration. Morris et al. (132) recommends two liters of normal saline, with 50 g mannitol and 50 mEq sodium bicarbonate per liter prior to abdominal wall release.

Although ACS is thought of as a complication seen in surgical patients, it is becoming recognized as a process that affects many critically ill patients. It is classically described in postoperative trauma patients who have received a massive volume resuscitation, but it also has been reported in patients with decreased abdominal compliance (e.g., burn patients, tight surgical skin closures), pancreatitis, massive ascites, intractable constipation, peritonitis, and retroperitoneal bleeding (133–138). The IAP is usually quite low; however, as IAP increases the abdomen distends to accommodate the increased pressure. As the abdominal wall reaches the limits of its compliance, the IAP increases dramatically. This increased pressure is transmitted to the inferior vena cava and to the renal veins. As these veins are compressed, venous return to the heart diminishes and functional bilateral occlusion of the renal veins ensues. In addition to decreased mesenteric perfusion, renal function rapidly declines and ARF occurs. Various organ systems have different thresholds for dysfunction secondary to increased IAP; the kidneys show signs of oliguria at 15 mmHg and anuria at 30 mmHg (139). If ACS is suspected based on the patient's clinical context, direct IAP monitoring should be done. This can be easily and reliably achieved with intravesicular pressure transduction via a Foley catheter (129,140–143). A bladder pressure less than 10 mmHg rules out ACS, and a pressure of greater than 25 mmHg is highly suggestive of ACS (143). If ACS is confirmed by clinical and objective assessment, decompression of the abdomen should commence without delay (141,143).

Microangiopathic Hemolytic Anemia

MAHA is usually a result of hemolytic-uremic syndrome (HUS) or thrombotic thrombocytopenic purpura (TTP). The HUS presents with ARF and MAHA. In children, this disease is associated with an antecedent diarrheal infection, particularly *Escherichia coli* H7 : O157. The diagnosis is confirmed by the presence of anemia, elevated serum LDH, and schistocytes on peripheral smear (144). TTP classically presents as a pentad: fever, ARF, neurologic deficit (stroke, seizure, and delirium), thrombocytopenia, and MAHA. It is important to recognize the possibility of these syndromes because both (TTP in particular) can cause irreversible damage and/or rapid death. Frequently, patients present with a seizure or cerebrovascular accident (CVA) and they are admitted to the ICU for their neurologic presentation. The remainder of their disease becomes evident later in their hospital course. Although most patients will not present with the full pentad, the hallmark of this disease is MAHA as evidenced by evidence of anemia, elevated serum LDH, and schistocytes on peripheral smear (145). This finding in conjunction with thrombocytopenia, ARF, or neurologic findings should raise the suspicion for this diagnosis, and an urgent hematology consultation should be obtained. Treatment of TTP and HUS in adults consists of fresh frozen plasma administration and plasma exchange (144). Platelet infusions should be avoided because they have been associated with worsening of the disease process, resulting in death (146).

Hepato-renal Syndrome

Hepato-renal syndrome (HRS) is a syndrome in which the kidneys remain histologically normal and are within the spectrum of prerenal azotemia. Patients with severe liver impairment develop a low systemic vascular resistance state, where the incremental increase of renin and angiotensin from hypotension create intrarenal vasoconstriction and profound prerenal azotemia. This disorder is often misdiagnosed in patients with liver disease. Patients with liver disease are also susceptible to other forms of ARF as well, and other etiologies must be ruled out before a diagnosis of HRS is made. The diagnosis of HRS is made by documentation of serum creatinine >1.5 mg/dL, urine sodium <10 mEq/L, absence of other causes of ARF (ATN, nephrotoxic agents, absence of bacterial infection, proteinuria <500 mg/day, and no evidence of obstruction), and no improvement in renal function after withdrawal of diuretic and volume challenge of 1.5 L of normal saline (147). There are two type of HRS, Type I and Type II. Type I is defined by a drop in GFR <20 mL/min, a serum creatinine >2.5 occurring over less than two weeks. These patients are usually oliguric or anuric. Type II HRS is marked by less renal impairment, but those patients have ascites that are diuretic resistant. If the diagnosis of Type I HRS is made, the only definitive treatment is liver transplant. If Type II HRS is present, the role of long-term dialysis, colloid expansion, and porto-systemic shunts is under evaluation (148).

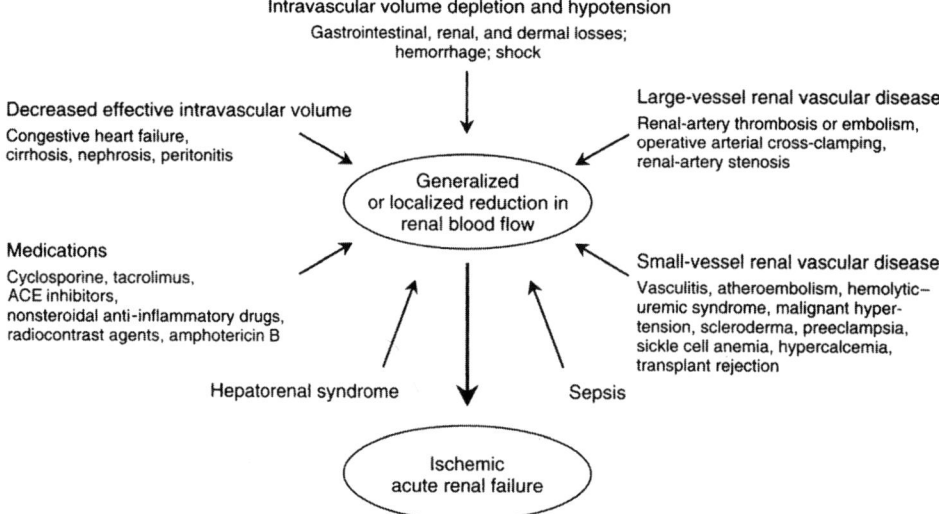

Figure 6 Summary of conditions that lead to ischemic acute renal failure. A variety of clinical conditions results in a reduction in renal blood flow; however, intravascular volume depletion and hypotension are the predominant culprits. When combined with the wide spectrum of additional toxic insults, renal blood flow can be so severely impaired that acute tubular necrosis results. *Abbreviation*: ACE, angiotensin-converting enzyme. *Source*: From Ref. 27.

Acute Development of Anuria

The acute development of anuria is rare in clinical practice and has few etiologic agents. If a patient who was previously nonoliguric becomes anuric, four etiologies should be investigated: (*i*) obstructive uropathy, (*ii*) massive ATN, (*iii*) acute cortical necrosis (ACN), and (*iv*) acute renal artery occlusion. All of these entities have been discussed earlier except ACN. The ACN is a rare result of profound renal ischemia and/or thrombosis. The most common cause worldwide is obstetrical complications, and is also seen as a consequence in patients who develop SIRS, suffer snakebites and HUS (149–153). Diagnosis is usually confirmed by CT or radionucleotide scanning. There is no treatment except hemodynamic support. The most common presenting symptom is anuria, and patients who suffer ACN are often dialysis-dependent for life (154).

EYE TO THE FUTURE

Investigations into the prediction of ARF have yielded early predictive markers that could assist in identifying kidney damage. In a study by McLaren et al. (155), it was found that the protein P53 was directly correlated with the cellular changes seen in ATN. Another study done by Parikh et al. (156) found that elevated levels of the biochemical marker, IL-18 correlated with ATN in mice. Other studies found that IL-18 was also a reliable marker in predicting acute kidney injury (157,158). The benefits of using these markers to test for kidney injury are that they are reliable, inexpensive, and easy to perform. Furthermore, the elevated levels in IL-18 are seen much earlier than elevations in creatinine.

SUMMARY

Limiting renal impairment begins with identifying patients at increased risk for renal dysfunction (monitoring of renal function is particularly important in these patients), and understanding the physiology of urine formation, the influence of

vasoactive drugs, and intraoperative events on the physiology and pathophysiology of renal function (Fig. 6).

The fundamental principles emphasized include (*i*) avoidance of hypovolemia or renal hypoperfusion (hypotension or decreased cardiac output) in patients at risk (either due to pre-existing disease or the nature of the operative procedure) and (*ii*) limitation of toxins that might jeopardize residual renal function (159).

Unfortunately, direct monitors of renal wellbeing are still in the rudimentary stage of development. Accordingly, indirect measures of renal function (CVP and MAP) are relied upon on a minute-to-minute basis, whereas the clinical measurement of urine output is still relied upon when evaluating renal function over longer time intervals.

To date, only one drug (*N*-acetylcystine) has proven to prophylactically improve renal outcome, following a high-risk procedure (radiocontrast administration). Manipulation of autorenal regulatory vasodilators (nitric oxide and PGE2) and vasoconstrictors (endothelin, vasopressin, and AII) may prove helpful in the future. However, at this time, maintenance of adequate intravascular volume, MAP, and cardiac output are the most important renal protective measures an anesthesiologist can provide for high-risk patients.

KEY POINTS

- ☞ Recent studies indicate that an increased relative risk of death is associated with kidney failure when adjusted for a wide range of covariates (14,15). Accordingly, early and accurate indicators of renal insufficiency or failure are essential to the management of critically ill patients.
- ☞ Intrinsic or intrarenal ARF has many causes, but in trauma and critical care settings, the great majority of cases are due to acute tubular necrosis (ATN) following on from a prerenal hypoperfusion state.
- ☞ The hallmark that underscores experimental models of hemodynamically mediated ARF is a reduction of RBF (injury generally results when RBF is reduced by more than 50%) for at least 40 to 60 minutes.

☞ Urine output is not always the best measure of renal wellbeing. Rather, indirect measures are at times more reliable during resuscitation of a trauma patient (i.e., mean arterial pressure, preload, and cardiac output).

☞ Ischemic ATN is typically seen after a prolonged episode of hypotension, particularly when the blood flow to the kidney is interrupted (e.g., aortic cross-clamp) (31–34).

☞ Most nephrologists would agree that doubling of the serum creatinine and the rising of serum creatinine of 1.0 mg/dL per day over two to three days would constitute a patient in ARF (Table 2).

☞ Decreased urine output, and rising serum BUN and creatinine are the standard indicators for the development of worsening ARF.

☞ An arterial line serves the dual purpose of providing access for repetitive ABG samples, as well as continuous beat-to-beat measurement of arterial BP throughout resuscitation, operative management, and critical care.

☞ SPV is a technique for gauging intravascular volume status, which is very useful in renal failure patients.

☞ Trauma and critically ill patients with renal insufficiency should have their CVP maintained on the high side to protect against the prerenal state.

☞ In situations where assessment of LVEDV is critical (e.g., hypotension, low cardiac output, and normal or high filling pressures by CVP and PACWP), using a TEE provides the more accurate and direct view of LV preload and contractility (86).

☞ The most clinically useful way to diagnose ATN is the evaluation of the urine sediment. The presence of brown granular casts and epithelial cells, singly or in casts, is seen in 80% of patients with ATN (94).

REFERENCES

1. Brady HR, Brenner BM, Clarkson MR, Lieberthal W. Acute renal failure. In: Brenner BM, ed. The Kidney. Philadelphia, PA: WB Saunders Company, 2000:1203.

2. Bernard GR, Artigas A, Brigham KL, et al. The American-European Consensus Conference on ARDS. Definitions, mechanisms, relevant outcomes, and clinical trial coordination. Am J Respir Crit Care Med 1994; 149(3 Pt 1):818–824.

3. Andersson LG, Ekroth R, Bratteby LE, Hallhagen S, Wesslen O. Acute renal failure after coronary surgery—a study of incidence and risk factors in 2009 consecutive patients. Thorac Cardiovasc Surg 1993; 41(4):237–241.

4. Firmat J, Zucchini A, Martin R, Aguirre C. A study of 500 cases of acute renal failure (1978–1991). Ren Fail 1994; 16(1):91–99.

5. Groeneveld AB, Tran DD, van der MJ, Nauta JJ, Thijs LG. Acute renal failure in the medical intensive care unit: predisposing, complicating factors and outcome. Nephron 1991; 59(4):602–610.

6. Guerin C, Girard R, Selli JM, Perdrix JP, Ayzac L. Initial versus delayed acute renal failure in the intensive care unit. A multi-center prospective epidemiological study. Rhone-Alpes Area Study Group on Acute Renal Failure. Am J Respir Crit Care Med 2000; 161(3 Pt 1):872–879.

7. Bellomo R, Ronco C, Kellum JA, Mehta RL, Palevsky P, and the ADQI Workgroup. Acute renal failure—definition, outcome measures, animal models, fluid therapy and information technology needs: the Second Internation Consensus Conference of the Acute Dialysis Quality Initiative (ADQI) Group. Crit Care 2004; 8(4):R204–R212.

8. Allgren RL, Marbury TC, Rahman SN, et al. Anaritide in acute tubular necrosis. Auriculin Anaritide Acute Renal Failure Study Group. N Engl J Med 1997; 336(12):828–834.

9. Bellomo R, Chapman M, Finfer S, Hickling K, Myburgh J. Low-dose dopamine in patients with early renal dysfunction: a placebo-controlled randomised trial. Australian and New Zealand Intensive Care Society (ANZICS) Clinical Trials Group. Lancet 2000; 356(9248):2139–2143.

10. Hirschberg R, Kopple J, Lipsett P, et al. Multicenter clinical trial of recombinant human insulin-like growth factor I in patients with acute renal failure. Kidney Int 1999; 55(6):2423–2432.

11. Pascual M, Theruvath T, Kawai T, et al. Strategies to improve long-term outcomes after renal transplantation. N Engl J Med 2002; 346(8):580–590.

12. Junger A, Engel J, Benson M, et al. Discriminative power on mortality of a modified Sequential Organ Failure Assessment score for complete automatic computation in an operative intensive care unit. Crit Care Med 2002; 30(2):338–342.

13. Cook R, Cook D, Tilley J, Lee K, Marshall J. Multiple organ dysfunction: baseline and serial component scores. Crit Care Med 2001; 29(11):2046–2050.

14. Levy EM, Viscoli CM, Horwitz RI. The effect of acute renal failure on mortality. A cohort analysis. J Am Med Assoc 1996; 275(19):1489–1494.

15. Chertow GM, Levy EM, Hammermeister KE, Grover F, Daley J. Independent association between acute renal failure and mortality following cardiac surgery. Am J Med 1998; 104(4):343–348.

16. Iken DR. Hemodynamic basis for human acute renal failure. Am J Med 1984; 76:702–710.

17. Novis BK, Roizen MF, Aronson S, et al. Association of preoperative risk factors with postoperative acute renal failure. Anesth Analg 1994; 78:143–149.

18. Davidman M, Olson P, Kohen J, et al. Iatrogenic renal disease. Arch Intern Med 1991; 151:1809–1812.

19. Shersterman N, Strom BL, Murray TG, et al. Risk factors and outcome of hospital acquired acute renal failure. Clinical epidemiologic study. Am J Med 1987; 83:65–71.

20. Badr KF, Ichikawa I. Prerenal failure. A deleterious shift from renal compensation to decompensation. N Engl J Med 1988; 319:623–629.

21. Boventure JV. Mechanism of ischemic acute renal failure. Kidney Int 1993; 43:1160–1178.

22. Morrissey JJ, McCracken R, Kaneto H, Vehaskari M, Montani D, Klahr S. Location of an inducible nitric oxide synthase mRNA in the normal kidney. Kidney Int 1994; 45:998–1005.

23. Chan L, Chittinandana A, Shapiro JI, Shanley PF, Schrier RW. Effect of an endothelin-receptor antagonist on acute renal failure. Am J Physiol 1994; 266:F135–F138.

24. Mason JC, Joeris B, Welsch J, Kriz W. Vascular congestion in ischemic renal failure: the role of cell swelling. Miner Electrolyte Metab 1989; 15:114–124.

25. Schmid-Schonbein GW. Capillary plugging by granulocytes and the no-reflow phenomenon in the microcirculation. Fed Proc 1987; 46:2397–2401.

26. Brezis M, Rosen S: Hypoxia of the renal medulla—its implications for disease. N Engl J Med 1995; 332:647–655.

27. Thadhani R, Pascual M, Bonventre JV: Acute renal failure. N Engl J Med 1996; 334:1448–1460.

28. Robertson GL. Thirst, and vasopressin function in normal and disordered states of water balance. J Lab Clin Med 1983; 101:351.

29. Myers BD, Moran SM. Hemodynamically mediated acute renal failure. N Engl J Med 1986; 314:97–105.

30. Shaw SG, Weidmann P, Hodler J, et al. Atrial Naturetic peptide protects against acute renal failure in the rat. J Clin Invest 1987; 80:1232–1237.

31. Gornick CC Jr, Kjellstrand CM. Acute renal failure complicating aortic aneurysm surgery. Nephron 1983; 35(3):145–157.

32. Hilberman M, Myers BD, Carrie BJ, Derby G, Jamison RL, Stinson EB. Acute renal failure following cardiac surgery. J Thorac Cardiovasc Surg 1979; 77(6):880–888.

33. Hou SH, Bushinsky DA, Wish JB, Cohen JJ, Harrington JT. Hospital-acquired renal insufficiency: a prospective study. Am J Med 1983; 74(2):243–248.

34. Luft FC, Hamburger RJ, Dyer JK, Szwed JJ, Kleit SA. Acute renal failure following operation for aortic aneurysm. Surg Gynecol Obstet 1975; 141(3):374–378.

35. Olsen S, Solez K. Acute renal failure in man: pathogenesis in light of new morphological data. Clin Nephrol 1987; 27(6): 271–277.

36. Racusen LC. Pathology of acute renal failure: structure/function correlations. Adv Ren Replace Ther 1997; 4(2 suppl. 1): 3–16.

37. Hall JW, Johnson WJ, Maher FT, Hunt JC. Immediate and long-term prognosis in acute renal failure. Ann Intern Med 1970; 73(4):515–521.

38. Abramowicz M, Edelmann CM Jr. Nephrotoxicity of anti-infective drugs. Clin Pediatr (Phila) 1968; 7(7):389–390.

39. Deray G, Baumelou B, Martinez F, Brillet G, Jacobs C. Renal vasoconstriction after low and high osmolar contrast agents in ischemic and nonischemic canine kidney. Clin Nephrol 1991; 36(2):93–96.

40. Solomon R. Radiocontrast-induced nephropathy. Semin Nephrol 1998; 18(5):551–557.

41. Aronoff GR. Nonsteroidal anti-inflammatory drug induced renal syndromes. J Ky Med Assoc 1992; 90(7):336–339.

42. Siegler RL, Bloomer A. Acute renal failure with prolonged oliguria. An account of five cases. J Am Med Assoc 1973; 225(2):133–136.

43. Chew SL, Lins RL, Daelemans R, De Broe ME. Outcome in acute renal failure. Nephrol Dial Transplant 1993; 8(2):101–107.

44. Andrews PA, Robinson GT. Intravascular haemolysis and interstitial nephritis in association with ciprofloxacin. Nephron 1999; 83(4):359–360.

45. Chandra M, Chandra P, McVicar M, Susin M, Teichberg S. Rapid onset of co-trimoxazole induced interstitial nephritis. Int J Pediatr Nephrol 1985; 6(4):289–292.

46. Kleinknecht D, Vanhille P, Morel-Maroger L, et al. Acute interstitial nephritis due to drug hypersensitivity. An up-to-date review with a report of 19 cases. Adv Nephrol Necker Hosp 1983; 12:277–308.

47. Cushner HM, Copley JB, Bauman J, Hill SC. Acute interstitial nephritis associated with mezlocillin, nafcillin, and gentamicin treatment for Pseudomonas infection. Arch Intern Med 1985; 145(7):1204–1207.

48. Drago JR, Rohner TJ Jr, Sanford EJ, Engle J, Schoolwerth A. Acute interstitial nephritis. J Urol 1976; 115(1):105–107.

49. Buysen JG, Houthoff HJ, Krediet RT, Arisz L. Acute interstitial nephritis: a clinical and morphological study in 27 patients. Nephrol Dial Transplant 1990; 5(2):94–99.

50. Corwin HL, Korbet SM, Schwartz MM. Clinical correlates of eosinophiluria. Arch Intern Med 1985; 145(6):1097–1099.

51. Linton AL, Clark WF, Driedger AA, Turnbull DI, Lindsay RM. Acute interstitial nephritis due to drugs: review of the literature with a report of nine cases. Ann Intern Med 1980; 93(5): 735–741.

52. Handa SP. Drug-induced acute interstitial nephritis: report of 10 cases. CMAJ 1986; 135(11):1278–1281.

53. Abdulkader RC, Avila MO, Saldanha LB, Ab'Saber AM, Burdmann EA. Acute bilateral renal artery occlusion due to granulomatous and necrotizing vasculitis. Ren Fail 1998; 20(1):157–162.

54. Jones RE, Tribble CG, Tegtmeyer CJ, Craddock GB Jr, Mentzer RM Jr. Bilateral renal artery embolism: a diagnostic and therapeutic problem. J Vasc Surg 1987; 5(3):479–482.

55. Asherson RA, Lanham JG, Hull RG, Boey ML, Gharavi AE, Hughes GR. Renal vein thrombosis in systemic lupus erythematosus: association with the "lupus anticoagulant". Clin Exp Rheumatol 1984; 2(1):75–79.

56. Berkovich GY, Ramchandani P, Preate DL Jr, Rovner ES, Shapiro MB, Banner MP. Renal vein thrombosis after martial arts trauma. J Trauma 2001; 50(1):144–145.

57. Chan HH, Douketis JD, Nowaczyk MJ. Acute renal vein thrombosis, oral contraceptive use, and hyperhomocysteinemia. Mayo Clin Proc 2001; 76(2):212–214.

58. Ellis D. Recurrent renal vein thrombosis and renal failure associated with antithrombin-III deficiency. Pediatr Nephrol 1992; 6(2):131–134.

59. Llach F, Koffler A, Massry SG. Renal vein thrombosis and the nephrotic syndrome. Nephron 1977; 19(2):65–68.

60. Cagnoli L, Viglietta G, Madia G, et al. Acute bilateral renal vein thrombosis superimposed on calcified thrombus of the inferior vena cava in a patient with membranous lupus nephritis. Nephrol Dial Transplant 1990; 5(suppl. 1):71–74.

61. Alexopoulos E. Drug-induced acute interstitial nephritis. Ren Fail 1998; 20(6):809–819.

62. Bihorac A, Ozener C, Akoglu E, Kullu S. Tetracycline-induced acute interstitial nephritis as a cause of acute renal failure. Nephron 1999; 81(1):72–75.

63. Feinfeld DA, Ansari N, Nuovo M, Hussain A, Mir R. Tubulointerstitial nephritis associated with minimal self reexposure to rifampin. Am J Kidney Dis 1999; 33(5):e3.

64. Frye RF, Job ML, Dretler RH, Rosenbaum BJ. Teicoplanin nephrotoxicity: first case report. Pharmacotherapy 1992; 12(3):240–242.

65. Helmink R, Benediktsson H. Ciprofloxacin-induced allergic interstitial nephritis. Nephron 1990; 55(4):432–433.

66. Hsu SI. Biopsy-proved acute tubulointerstitial nephritis and toxic epidermal necrolysis associated with vancomycin. Pharmacotherapy 2001; 21(10):1233–1239.

67. Pazmino P. Acute renal failure, skin rash, and eosinophilia associated with aztreonam. Am J Nephrol 1988; 8(1):68–70.

68. Fanos V, Cataldi L. Amphotericin B-induced nephrotoxicity: a review. J Chemother 2000; 12(6):463–470.

69. Cacoub P, Deray G, Baumelou A, et al. Acute renal failure induced by foscarnet: 4 cases. Clin Nephrol 1988; 29(6):315–318.

70. Becker BN, Fall P, Hall C, et al. Rapidly progressive acute renal failure due to acyclovir: case report and review of the literature. Am J Kidney Dis 1993; 22(4):611–615.

71. Aronson S. Monitoring renal function. In: Miller RD, ed. Anesthesia. 4th edn. New York: Churchill Livingstone, 1994: 1293–1317.

72. Kellen M, Aronson S, Roizen MF, Barnard J, Thisted RA. Predictive and diagnostic tests of renal failure: a review. Anesth Analg 1994; 78(1):134–142.

73. Coriat P, Vrillon M, Perel A, et al. A comparison of systolic blood pressure variations and echocardiographic estimates of end-systolic left ventricular size in patients after aortic surgery. Anesth Analg 1994; 78:46–53.

74. Weissman C, Ornstein E, Young W. Arterial pulse contour analysis trending of cardiac output: hemodynamic manipulations during cerebral arteriovenous malformation resection. J Clin Monit 1993; 9:347–353.

75. Young C, Mark J, White W, et al. Clinical evaluation of continuous noninvasive blood pressure monitoring: accuracy and tracking capabilities. J Clin Monit 1995; 11:245–252.

76. Bedford RF, Wollman H. Complications of percutaneous radial artery cannulation: an objective prospective evaluation in man. Anesthesiology 1973; 38:228.

77. Rulf ENR, Mitchell MM, Prakash O, et al. Measurement of arterial pressure after cardiopulmonary bypass with long radial artery catheters. J Cardiothoracic Anesth 1990; 4(1): 19–244.

78. Kopman E, Ferguson TB. Intraoperative monitoring of femoral artery pressure during replacement of aneurysm of descending thoracic aorta. Anesth Analg 1977; 56:603.

79. Russell JA, Joel M, Hudson RJ, et al. Prospective evaluation of radial and femoral artery catheterization sites in critically ill patients. Crit Care Med 1983; 11:936.

80. Gurman GM, Kriemerman S. Cannulation of big arteries in critically ill patients. Crit Care Med 1985, 13:217.

81. Perel A, Pizov R, Cotev S. The systolic pressure variation is a sensitive indicator of hypovolemia in ventilated dogs subjected to graded hemorrhage. Anesthesiology 1987; 67: 498–502.

82. Pizov R, Segal E, Kaplan L, et al. The use of systolic pressure variation in hemodynamic monitoring during deliberate hypotension in spine surgery. J Clin Anesth 1990; 2:96–100.

83. Carlier M, Souifflet JP, Pierson Y, et al. Maximal hydration during anesthesia increases pulmonary arterial pressures and improves early function of human transplants. Transplantation 1982; 34:201–204.

84. Raper R, Sibbald WJ. Misled by the wedge. Chest 1986; 89:427.

85. Friese RS, Shafi S, Gentilello LM. Pulmonary artery catheter use is associated with reduced mortality in severely injured patients: A National Trauma Data Bank Analysis of 53,312 patients. Crit Care Med 2006; 34(6):1597–1601.

86. Cheung AT, Savino JS, Weiss, et al. Echocardiographic and hemodynamic indexes of left ventricular preload in patients with normal and abnormal ventricular function. Anesthesiology 1994; 81:376.

87. Clements FM, Harpole DH, Quill T, et al. Estimation of left ventricular volume and ejection fraction by two-dimensional transesophageal echocardiography: comparison of short axis imaging and simultaneous radionucleotide angiography. Br J Anaesth 1990; 64:331.

88. Cahalan MK, Ionescu P, Melton HJ, et al. Automated real time analysis of intraoperative transesophageal echocardiograms. Anesthesiology 1993; 78:477.

89. Miller TR, Anderson RJ, Linas SL, et al. Urinary diagnostic indices in acute renal failure: a prospective study. Ann Intern Med 1978; 89(1):47–50.

90. Dossetor JB. Creatininemia versus uremia. The relative significance of blood urea nitrogen and serum creatinine concentrations in azotemia. Ann Intern Med 1966; 65(6):1287–1299.

91. Klahr S, Miller SB. Acute oliguria. N Engl J Med 1998; 338(10):671–675.

92. Shibasaki T, Ishimoto F, Sakai O, Joh K, Aizawa S. Clinical characterization of drug-induced allergic nephritis. Am J Nephrol 1991; 11(3):174–180.

93. Porile JL, Bakris GL, Garella S. Acute interstitial nephritis with glomerulopathy due to nonsteroidal anti-inflammatory agents: a review of its clinical spectrum and effects of steroid therapy. J Clin Pharmacol 1990; 30(5):468–475.

94. Fu GY, Candela RJ, Mishkind M, Obarski T, Yakubov SJ. Bilateral renal artery occlusion: an unusual presentation of atrial fibrillation and hypertrophic cardiomyopathy. Clin Cardiol 1994; 17(11):631–633.

95. Levin M, Nakhoul F, Keidar Z, Green J. Acute oliguric renal failure associated with unilateral renal embolism: a successful treatment with iloprost. Am J Nephrol 1998; 18(5):444–447.

96. Morris D, Kisly A, Stoyka CG, Provenzano R. Spontaneous bilateral renal artery occlusion associated with chronic atrial fibrillation. Clin Nephrol 1993; 39(5):257–259.

97. Lessman RK, Johnson SF, Coburn JW, Kaufman JJ. Renal artery embolism: clinical features and long-term follow-up of 17 cases. Ann Intern Med 1978; 89(4):477–482.

98. Liano F, Gamez C, Pascual J, et al. Use of urinary parameters in the diagnosis of total acute renal artery occlusion. Nephron 1994; 66(2):170–175.

99. Salam TA, Lumsden AB, Martin LG. Local infusion of fibrinolytic agents for acute renal artery thromboembolism: report of ten cases. Ann Vasc Surg 1993; 7(1):21–26.

100. Hauben M, Norwich J, Shapiro E, Reich L, Petchel KS, Goldsmith D. Multiple cholesterol emboli syndrome—six cases identified through the spontaneous reporting system. Angiology 1995; 46(9):779–784.

101. Scolari F, Bracchi M, Valzorio B, et al. Cholesterol atheromatous embolism: an increasingly recognized cause of acute renal failure. Nephrol Dial Transplant 1996; 11(8):1607–1612.

102. Kasinath BS, Corwin HL, Bidani AK, Korbet SM, Schwartz MM, Lewis EJ. Eosinophilia in the diagnosis of atheroembolic renal disease. Am J Nephrol 1987; 7(3):173–177.

103. Modi KS, Rao VK. Atheroembolic renal disease. J Am Soc Nephrol 2001; 12(8):1781–1787.

104. Ko WS, Lim PS, Sung YP. Renal vein thrombosis as first clinical manifestation of the primary antiphospholipid syndrome. Nephrol Dial Transplant 1995; 10(10):1929–1931.

105. Pohl M, Zimmerhackl LB, Hausser I, et al. Acute bilateral renal vein thrombosis complicating Netherton syndrome. Eur J Pediatr 1998; 157(2):157–160.

106. Pohl M, Zimmerhackl LB, Heinen F, Sutor AH, Schneppenheim R, Brandis M. Bilateral renal vein thrombosis and venous sinus thrombosis in a neonate with factor V mutation (FV Leiden). J Pediatr 1998; 132(1):159–161.

107. Markowitz GS, Brignol F, Burns ER, Koenigsberg M, Folkert VW. Renal vein thrombosis treated with thrombolytic therapy: case report and brief review. Am J Kidney Dis 1995; 25(5):801–806.

108. Sciacca V, Mingoli A, Cavallaro A. Renal vein thrombosis with involvement of the vena cava: report of a case. Ital J Surg Sci 1985; 15(1):79–83.

109. Crowley JP, Matarese RA, Quevedo SF, Garella S. Fibrinolytic therapy for bilateral renal vein thrombosis. Arch Intern Med 1984; 144(1):159–160.

110. Sutherland RD, Anthony WA, Martinez HE, Guynes WA. Bilateral renal vein and inferior vena cava thrombosis with nephrotic syndrome treated by thrombectomy: case report with 3-year follow-up. J Urol 1976; 116(4):510–511.

111. Waymack JP, Tweddell JS, Warden GD. Renal vein thrombosis in burned children. J Burn Care Rehabil 1988; 9(5):472–473.

112. Laakso M, Pentikainen PJ, Lampainen E, Romppanen T, Naukkarinen A, Collan Y. Trauma, renal vein thrombosis and subsequent nephrotic syndrome. Ann Clin Res 1982; 14(3): 140–144.

113. Kumar A, Chaudhary D, Bhargava V. Recovery from bilateral renal vein thrombosis on supportive management alone. Indian J Pediatr 1995; 62(2):251–252.

114. Laville M, Aguilera D, Maillet PJ, Labeeuw M, Madonna O, Zech P. The prognosis of renal vein thrombosis: a re-evaluation of 27 cases. Nephrol Dial Transplant 1988; 3(3):247–256.

115. Miller RA, Tremann JA, Ansell JS. The conservative management of renal vein thrombosis. J Urol 1974; 111(5): 568–571.

116. Burrow CR, Walker WG, Bell WR, Gatewood OB. Streptokinase salvage of renal function after renal vein thrombosis. Ann Intern Med 1984; 100(2):237–238.

117. Wu ZL, Zhou KR, Liao L. Renal vein thrombosis and selective arterial or venous thrombolytic therapy. J Thromb Thrombolysis 1996; 3(1):67–70.

118. Zager RA. Rhabdomyolysis and myohemoglobinuric acute renal failure. Kidney Int 1996; 49(2):314–326.

119. Richards JR. Rhabdomyolysis and drugs of abuse. J Emerg Med 2000; 19(1):51–56.

120. Sheikh RA, Yasmeen S, Munn R, Ruebner BH, Ellis WG. AIDS-related myopathy. Med Electron Microsc 1999; 32(2):79–86.

121. Segaert MF, De Soete C, Vandewiele I, Verbanck J. Drug-interaction-induced rhabdomyolysis. Nephrol Dial Transplant 1996; 11(9):1846–1847.

122. Ward MM. Factors predictive of acute renal failure in rhabdomyolysis. Arch Intern Med 1988; 148(7):1553–1557.

123. Vanholder R, Sever MS, Erek E, Lameire N. Rhabdomyolysis. J Am Soc Nephrol 2000; 11(8):1553–1561.

124. Liano F, Pascual J. Epidemiology of acute renal failure: a prospective, multicenter, community-based study. Madrid Acute Renal Failure Study Group. Kidney Int 1996; 50(3):811–818.

125. Rascoff JH, Golden RA, Spinowitz BS, Charytan C. Nondilated obstructive nephropathy. Arch Intern Med 1983; 143(4):696–698.

126. Webb JA. The role of ultrasonography in the diagnosis of intrinsic renal disease. Clin Radiol 1994; 49(9):589–591.

127. Reeves ST, Pinosky ML, Byrne TK, Norcross ED. Abdominal compartment syndrome. Can J Anaesth 1997; 44(3):308–312.

128. Wilson WC, Patel N, Hogt DB, Murphy MT. Anesthesia for abdominal trauma. In: Grande CM, Smith CE, eds. Trauma. Anesthesiol Clin North America 1999; 17(1):29–75; Philadelphia: WB Saunders & Co.

129. Iberti TJ, Kelly KM, Gentili DR, Hirsch S, Benjamin E. A simple technique to accurately determine intra-abdominal pressure. Crit Care Med 1987; 15(12):1140–1142.

130. Kron IL, Harman PK, Nolan SP. The measurement of intra-abdominal pressure as a criteria for abdominal re-exploration. Ann Surg 1984; 199:28.

131. Schein M, Wittmann DH, Aprahamian CC, Condon RE. The abdominal compartment syndrome: the physiological and clinical consequences of elevated intra-abdominal pressure. J Am Coll Surg 1995; 180:745–753.

132. Morris JA Jr, Eddy VA, Blinman TA, et al. The staged celiotomy for trauma. Issues in unpacking and reconstruction. Ann Surg 1993; 217:576–586.

133. Blevins DV, Khanduja KS. Abdominal compartment syndrome with massive lower-extremity edema caused by colonic obstruction and distention. Am Surg 2001; 67(5):451–453.

134. Carlo VM, Ramirez SG, Suarez IG, Villareal OD, Camps BJ, Medina TA. The abdominal compartment syndrome: a report of 3 cases including instance of endocrine induction. Bol Asoc Med P R 1998; 90(7–12):121–125.

135. Dabney A, Bastani B. Enoxaparin-associated severe retroperitoneal bleeding and abdominal compartment syndrome: a report of two cases. Intensive Care Med 2001; 27(12):1954–1957.

136. Gorecki PJ, Kessler E, Schein M. Abdominal compartment syndrome from intractable constipation. J Am Coll Surg 2000; 190(3):371.

137. Morken J, West MA. Abdominal compartment syndrome in the intensive care unit. Curr Opin Crit Care 2001; 7(4):268–274.

138. Saggi BH, Sugerman HJ, Ivatury RR, Bloomfield GL. Abdominal compartment syndrome. J Trauma 1998; 45(3):597–609.

139. Bloomfield GL, Blocher CR, Fakhry IF, Sica DA, Sugerman HJ. Elevated intra-abdominal pressure increases plasma renin activity and aldosterone levels. J Trauma 1997; 42(6):997–1004.

140. Iberti TJ, Lieber CE, Benjamin E. Determination of intra-abdominal pressure using a transurethral bladder catheter: clinical validation of the technique. Anesthesiology 1989; 70(1):47–50.

141. Burch JM, Moore EE, Moore FA, Franciose R. The abdominal compartment syndrome. Surg Clin North Am 1996; 76(4):833–842.

142. Gallagher JJ. Description of the procedure for monitoring intra-abdominal pressure via an indwelling urinary catheter. Crit Care Nurse 2000; 20(1):87–91.

143. Ivatury RR, Sugerman HJ, Peitzman AB. Abdominal compartment syndrome: recognition and management. Adv Surg 2001; 35:251–269.

144. Ruggenenti P, Noris M, Remuzzi G. Thrombotic microangiopathy, hemolytic uremic syndrome, and thrombotic thrombocytopenic purpura. Kidney Int 2001; 60(3):831–846.

145. George JN, Gilcher RO, Smith JW, Chandler L, Duvall D, Ellis C. Thrombotic thrombocytopenic purpura-hemolytic uremic syndrome: diagnosis and management. J Clin Apheresis 1998; 13(3):120–125.

146. Harkness DR, Byrnes JJ, Lian EC, Williams WD, Hensley GT. Hazard of platelet transfusion in thrombotic thrombocytopenic purpura. JAMA 1981; 246(17):1931–1933.

147. Gines P, Arroyo V. Hepatorenal syndrome. J Am Soc Nephrol 1999; 10(8):1833–1839.

148. Wong F, Blendis L. New challenge of hepatorenal syndrome: prevention and treatment. Hepatology 2001; 34(6):1242–1251.

149. Morel–Maroger L. Adult hemolytic-uremic syndrome. Kidney Int 1980; 18(1):125–134.

150. Amaral CF, Da Silva OA, Goody P, Miranda D. Renal cortical necrosis following Bothrops jararaca and B. jararacussu snake bite. Toxicon 1985; 23(6):877–885.

151. Chugh KS, Jha V, Sakhuja V, Joshi K. Acute renal cortical necrosis—a study of 113 patients. Ren Fail 1994; 16(1):37–47.

152. Fox JG, Sutcliffe NP, Boulton-Jones JM, Imrie CW. Acute pancreatitis and renal cortical necrosis. Nephrol Dial Transplant 1990; 5(7):542–544.

153. Grunfeld JP, Pertuiset N. Acute renal failure in pregnancy: 1987. Am J Kidney Dis 1987; 9(4):359–362.

154. Kleinknecht D, Grunfeld JP, Gomez PC, Moreau JF, Garcia-Torres R. Diagnostic procedures and long-term prognosis in bilateral renal cortical necrosis. Kidney Int 1973; 4(6):390–400.

155. McLaren BK, Zhang PL, Herrera GA. P53 protein is a reliable marker in identification of renal tubular injury. Appl Immunohistochem Mol Morphol. 2004; 12(3):225–229.

156. Parikh CR, Jani A, Melnikov VY, et al. Urinary interleukin-18 is a marker of human acute tubular necrosis. Am J Kidney Dis 2004; 43(3):405–414.

157. Parikh CR, Mishra J, Thiessen-Philbrook H, et al. Urinary IL-18 is an early predictive biomarker of acute kidney injury after cardiac surgery. Kidney International 2006; 70(1):199–203.

158. Mehta RL. Urine IL-18 levels as a predictor of acute kidney injury in intensive care patients. Nat Clin Practice Nephrol 2006; 2:252–253.

159. Cranshaw J, Holland D. Anaesthesia for patients with renal impairment. Br J Hosp Med 1996; 55(4):171–175.

160. Jennings M, Shortland JR, Maddocks JL. Interstitial nephritis associated with frusemide. J R Soc Med 1986; 79(4): 239–240.

161. Magil AB. Drug-induced acute interstitial nephritis with granulomas. Hum Pathol 1983; 14(1):36–41.

162. Revai T, Harmos G. Nephrotic syndrome and acute interstitial nephritis associated with the use of diclofenac. Wien Klin Wochenschr 1999; 111(13):523–524.

163. Hadimeri H, Almroth G, Cederbrant K, Enestrom S, Hultman P, Lindell A. Allergic nephropathy associated with norfloxacin and ciprofloxacin therapy. Report of two cases and review of the literature. Scand J Urol Nephrol 1997; 31(5):481–485.

164. Kahn SR. Acute interstitial nephritis associated with nitrofurantoin. Lancet 1996; 348(9035):1177–1178.

165. McNeil PE. Acute tubulo-interstitial nephritis in a dog after halothane anaesthesia and administration of flunixin meglumine and trimethoprim-sulphadiazine. Vet Rec 1992; 131(7): 148–151.

166. Aronson S. Renal function monitoring. In: Miller RD, ed. Anesthesia. 5th edn. Philadelphia, PA: Churchill Livingstone, 2000:1298.

42

Renal Protective Agents in Trauma and Critical Care

Ludwig H. Lin and A. Sue Carlisle

Department of Anesthesiology and Critical Care Medicine, UC San Francisco Medical Center, San Francisco, California, U.S.A.

INTRODUCTION

Acute renal failure (ARF) is a commonly seen complication of critical illness, and carries an additional grave prognosis for its sufferers. It occurs in about 5% of all general hospital patients. By various reports, the frequency of ARF among patients is 1% at the time of admission, 2% to 5% during hospitalization, and as high as 4% to 15% after cardiopulmonary bypass. It is associated with a greater than 50% mortality rate, and increases the relative risk of death by 6.2-fold (1). Even in patients who survive hospitalization and ARF to discharge, duration of stay is prolonged, adding additional costs to their medical care. Between 20% and 60% of patients with ARF would develop end-stage renal disease (ESRD), requiring long-term dialysis, which adds further to healthcare costs and significantly affects the quality of life (2).

In order to provide optimal care to the critically ill population, to decrease their mortality and morbidity, and to reduce the already overburdened healthcare budget, the prevention of ARF is of utmost importance to be able to prevent the development of ARF as a comorbidity, or barring that, to be able to treat it. ARF in trauma and critical illness is often reversible, if recognized early and appropriate treatment is promptly instituted. This chapter briefly summarizes the pathophysiology of the common causes of ARF in this population, and then reviews the various prophylactic and/or treatment measures for them.

PATHOPHYSIOLOGY OF ACUTE RENAL FAILURE IN TRAUMA/CRITICAL CARE

The definition of ARF is imprecise, and various standards exist in the literature. Commonly used definitions include a change in serum creatinine of >0.5 mg/dL (44 µmol/L), an increase of more than 50% over the baseline value, a reduction in the calculated creatinine clearance by 50%, or a need for dialysis (see Volume 2, Chapters 40 and 41).

♂ **ARF in the critically ill is often a multifactorial process, but usually involves a combination of hypoperfusion and local hypoxic injury, from inflammatory stress due to toxins or oxygen free radicals.** ♂ The causes of ARF in the surgical intensive care unit (SICU) and/or trauma setting are numerous. However, the list of etiologies is slightly narrower than the differential affecting patients with ARF at the time of admission to the hospital. In addition, as many as a third of patients who develop ARF have some degree of chronic kidney disease as a result of organ damage from pre-existing diabetes, hypertension, or renal vascular atheromatous disease. The renal injury

ranges from an easily treated prerenal azotemia to acute tubular necrosis (ATN) to cortical necrosis.

Many drugs used in the diagnosis or treatment of the critically ill population, such as anti-inflammatory agents, antimicrobials, immunosuppressants, and radiocontrast agents, can induce ARF, and do so by affecting renal blood flow (RBF) and by direct tissue toxicity (Table 1).

Hypoperfusion

Maintenance of the intravascular volume and preservation of renal perfusion is essential to the well-being of the kidneys. Adequate perfusion ensures two factors for the kidney: that the glomerular filtration rate (GFR) is maintained, which allows for proper homeostasis of electrolytes and fluid balance, and that oxygen delivery is adequate. The partial pressure of oxygen in the renal medulla is actually already quite low at baseline, ranging around 20 torr, compared with 50 torr in the cortex (3). Therefore, any further decrease in its perfusion pressure and oxygen delivery can be devastating. Once hypoxic injury occurs, the resulting necrosis and inflammatory responses are likely to prolong the deleterious effects.

♂ **Endocrine and autocrine functions act reflexively in the renal vasculature to adjust for hypoperfusion.** ♂ The kidney can adapt for brief periods to changing perfusion conditions. The macula densa in the juxtaglomerular apparatus provides a constant feedback to regulate the GFR; it does this by secreting paracrine signals, such as prostaglandins to vasodilate, and adenosine to vasoconstrict the afferent renal arteriole, in response to changing perfusion pressures. Afferent vasodilation increases the perfusion pressure, and thus the GFR; afferent vasoconstriction does the opposite (4). Further endocrine functions follow, such as the activation of the renin-angiotension II-aldosterone system for blood pressure regulation and increased water and sodium resorption.

Drugs and Toxic Exposure

Various conditions and therapeutic maneuvers occurring in trauma and critically ill patients can disrupt the baseline regulatory process (Table 2). Rhabdomyolysis, with free myoglobin acting as a scavenger of nitric oxide (NO), promotes afferent and intramedullary vasoconstriction (2,3,5). Rhabdomyolysis may account for nearly 5% of the causes of ARF in critically ill patients. Sepsis and septic shock, while having a direct effect of hypoperfusing the kidneys, probably also exert additional deleterious effects by increasing the amount of inflammatory and prothrombotic signals present, leading to renal microvascular injury, thromboemboli formation, and increased vasoconstriction.

Table 1 Common Mechanisms of Acute Renal Failure in Trauma and Critical Care

Hypoperfusion	Hypovolemic shock
	Hypotensive shock
	Sepsis
	Thromboemboli
	Afferent renal artery
	vasoconstriction
	(from toxins and drugs)
	Rhabdomyolysis
	NSAIDs
	Contrast dye
	ACE-inhibitor agents
	Amphotericin
	Cyclosporine
	FK-506
Direct renal tubular injury	Drugs
	Aminoglycosides
	Contrast dye
	Amphotericin
	Cyclosporine
	FK-506
	Hypoxia
	Inflammatory processes

Abbreviations: ACE, angiotensin-converting enzyme; NSAIDs, nonsteroidal anti-inflammatory drugs.

Sepsis syndromes are associated with more than 50% of all cases of ARF in critically ill patients.

Use of nonsteroidal anti-inflammatory drugs (NSAIDs) and cyclooxygenase-2 (COX-2) inhibitors decrease the amount of prostaglandins being produced in the macula densa (4). Prostaglandins are responsible for continued sodium resorption, potassium excretion, and afferent vasodilation. When prostaglandin-mediated afferent arterial vasodilation is disrupted, the decreased arteriolar caliber can lead to decreased tubular perfusion, especially in situations where the patient is also hypovolemic. Amphotericin and contrast dye agents have a similar effect in promoting afferent arteriolar vasoconstriction (6–8). Amphotericin also increases the release of thromboxane A2 to contribute to hypoperfusion.

Cyclosporine and FK-506 (tacrolimus), both exert a similar afferent renal arteriolar vasoconstrictive effect. The mechanisms are unclear, but part of the phenomenon

Table 2 Conditions and Agents Disrupting Afferent Arterial Vasodilation and Causing Direct Tubular Injury

Agents disrupting afferent renal artery vasodilation (i.e., cause vasoconstriction)	Agents causing direct renal tubular injury
Rhabdomyolysis	Aminoglycosides
NSAIDs	Contrast dye
Contrast dye	Amphotericin
ACE-inhibitor therapy	Cyclosporine
Amphotericin	FK-506
Cyclosporine	Diuretics
FK-506	

Abbreviations: ACE, angiotensin-converting enzyme; NSAIDs, nonsteroidal anti-inflammatory drugs.

involves the initiation and expression of the renin-angiotensin system. Endothelial activation also appears to be involved, and chronic administration of these agents leads to intimal proliferation of the renal arterioles.

In drug-induced renal toxicity, tubular cell damage occurs as a result of a multipronged injury cascade: direct injury to the tubular cells, disruption of their ion exchange function, as well as increased local concentration of oxygen free radicals (2,7,8). Compounds like peroxynitrite, and products of lipid peroxidation, are noted to be increased in the renal tissue, when aminoglycosides and radiocontrast agents are administered (7–9). They induce direct cellular damage, by damaging the cellular components, and by inactivating enzymes, including mitochondrial respiratory enzymes and membrane pumps, damaging DNA. These agents also deplete the stores of glutathione and endogenous NO to further impair renal perfusion. Amphotericin and aminoglycosides also directly increase the oxygen demand of tubular cells. Cyclosporine and FK-506 both seem to increase the expression of transforming growth factor-β (TGF-β), a signal for proliferation of fibroblast and endothelial cells. This results in arteriopathies, as mentioned earlier, and also in tubulointerstitial fibrosis and subsequent renal dysfunction.

The use of diuretics, particularly those affecting the loop of Henle have been promoted to preserve urine output in critically ill patients with ARF. Theoretically, loop diuretics may protect the loop of Henle by reducing its transport-related workload through inhibition of the Na+/K+/Cl− pump. However, clinical trials have not shown a renal protective benefit to loop diuretics. Other effects of diuretics include the reduction of volume overload and control of hyperkalemia and acidosis.

☞ **While diuretics have been used to convert oliguric ARF to nonoliguric ARF, the outcomes have not been improved with their use.** ☞ The Project to Improve Care in Acute Renal Disease (PICARD) study group performed a cohort study between October 1989 and September 1995, and analyzed 552 patients with ARF in intensive care units. Their observation was that diuretic use at the time of consultation (of the nephrology specialist) for the management of ARF was associated with a significant increase in the risk of death or nonrecoverable renal function. While the authors of the study stressed against any inference that diuretics themselves caused harm, they did note that such a lack of support for the use of diuretics to improve morbidity and mortality means that their use should be discouraged (10).

POTENTIAL PROPHYLACTIC REGIMENS

In order to actively pursue a principle of "renal protection" for trauma and SICU patients, the intensivist must maintain adequate renal perfusion, limit toxic exposure, and consider utilization of renal protective drugs. Furthermore, renal protective strategies should be instituted in high-risk patients, targeting each of the aforementioned mechanisms. Such a multifaceted plan consists of: preservation of perfusion via euvolemia, maintenance of renal arteriolar patency, and decreasing tissue damage from toxins and oxygen free radicals. Various agents have been employed as prophylactic treatment of ARF and are discussed as follows.

Preservation of Perfusion
Fluids
☞ **One of the best renal protective maneuvers is aggressive fluid resuscitation and maintenance of euvolemia.** ☞ In a

recent study of aggressive fluid resuscitation in septic patients, overall survival improved by 30% (30% vs. 46.5% mortality) (11). For the critically ill patient with multisystem organ dysfunction, the importance of preserving organ perfusion cannot be stressed enough (also see Volume 2, Chapters 40 and 41). For the kidney, especially, euvolemia is essential, and will effectively prophylax against many side effects of the toxins mentioned previously. For example, hydration has been demonstrated to prevent the decreased RBF in patients being given NSAIDs and COX-2 inhibitors (4), as well as amphotericin (12) and contrast dye agents (7,8). Goals of volume and fluid replacement for critically ill patients are shown in Table 3 (13).

Dopamine

Dopamine, mannitol, and diuretics are probably the classic examples of "renal protection." A combination of these agents is often used in the surgical setting, in patients undergoing high-risk procedures for renal damage, such as abdominal aortic aneurysm repair. In many critical care units a "low-dose" dopamine infusion (1–3 mcg/kg/min) is often used as a renal protective agent (2,5). There is some physiologic basis to support this empirical use, though more recently, its efficacy has been refuted. Dopaminergic receptors exit in the central nervous system as well as the renal circulation, and the DA-1 receptors on the renal vasculature effect vasodilation, and thus theoretically preserve renal perfusion (14). Dopamine has different effects on the various catecholamine receptors at varying concentrations. In the range of 1 to 3 mcg/kg/min, dopamine is primarily an agonist for dopamine$_1$ (D$_1$) receptors, and in higher doses (4–9 mcg/kg/min) can act as β-adrenergic agents to increase cardiac contractility and output, or in extremely high doses (10–20 mcg/kg/min) will exert α_1-adrenergic effects to increase the systemic vascular resistance via peripheral vasoconstriction. In fact, 25% of dopamine is converted to norepinephrine in the circulation, which probably also partially explains this dose-responsive differential effect (1).

To date, not a single large randomized controlled trial (RCT) has demonstrated a positive outcome (in terms of renal protection, morbidity, or mortality) with the use of renal dose (1–3 mcg/kg/min) dopamine infusion. It is not clear that dopamine infusion has long-term benefits. In both animal and human studies, RBF does increase with low dose dopamine. Urine output increases as well, and probably does so as a result of dopamine's stimulation of natriuresis, rather than the simple explanation of an increased RBF. There are numerous studies supporting this observation, and low-dose dopamine has been successfully used in conjunction with norepinephrine or epinephrine

Table 3   Goals of Volume and Fluid Replacement for Critically Ill Patients

Achieve and maintain normovolemia and hemodynamic stability
Optimize oxygen delivery and oxygen consumption
Restore fluid homeostasis in the different fluid compartments
Ensure adequate plasma COP
Improve microcirculatory perfusion
Ensure appropriate inflammatory response and endothelial
   cell–leukocyte interactions

Abbreviation: COP, colloid osmotic pressure.
Source: Adapted from Ref. 13.

infusions, for example, to provide for "renal vasodilation" during systemic hemodynamic support (15). In a direct comparison to dobutamine, dopamine was associated with better diuresis, kaliuresis, and natriuresis at the same hemodynamic parameters. In dog models, low-dose dopamine therapy seemed to lead to improved urine excretion of sodium, more so in the ischemic injury model of renal failure than the nephrotoxic injury models.

However, none of the small studies demonstrate a long-term benefit and improved survival of patients with ARF following renal dose dopamine administration. Although a few studies were indeed positive, their results could not be duplicated by other investigators (1). The best arguments for the continued use of low-dose dopamine may be that: (*i*) conversion from oliguric ARF to non-oliguric ARF does improve survival (50–80% vs. 15–20%) (16–18), and perhaps an increase in the GFR; and (*ii*) as long as low-dose dopamine does no harm to the patient, some clinicians advocate its continued use in selected patients (19).

Mannitol

While loop diuretics are not helpful, the osmotic diuretic agent mannitol may provide modest benefit by reducing oxidant activity. As discussed earlier, nephrotoxicity from oxygen-free radical damage follows from both ischemic and numerous toxic insults to the renal parenchyma. Mannitol, by forcing diuresis and scavenging oxygen-free radicals, is theoretically beneficial.

There is a small amount of data in the rhabdomyolysis literature to support these claims (20). Mannitol is often used along with fluid repletion, and sodium bicarbonate in the treatment of rhabdomyolysis. With free myoglobin accumulating in the renal tubules, sludging results, and oliguric ARF rapidly develops (21). Myoglobin catalyzes the metabolism of NO, and thus rhabdomyolysis produces a secondary injury through renal arteriolar vasoconstriction and decreased renal perfusion (3).

☞ **In rhabdomyolysis, aggressive intravenous fluid hydration, to maintain a urine output greater than 200 mL/ hr, is the recommended first priority (21).** ☞ Sodium bicarbonate and mannitol are often added to the regimen, with a small study showing some potential benefit (20). While the antioxidant and diuretic activity of mannitol and the alkalinization of urine by sodium bicarbonate to prevent urate and myoglobin crystal formation, may indeed be helpful, the conventional thinking is that the intravascular volume expansion, supplied by their administration, probably provides the greatest benefit.

Fenoldopam

☞ **Fenoldopam, a DA-1-specific dopaminergic agonist, actually has documented benefit, in that it improves renal hemodynamics, function, and histology (14).** ☞ Fenoldopam exerts renal vasodilation effects, improving both cortical and renal medullary blood flow and decreasing sodium reabsorption in the proximal tubule. Fenoldopam appears to lead to long-term improvement in patients who are receiving amphotericin B or cyclosporine. In a study comparing fenoldopam or placebo in treating patients recovering from thoracoabdominal aortic aneurysm, the survival of patients treated with prophylactic fenoldopam was 93%, compared with 80% for placebo (22). While the number of patients in this study was limited (*n* = 58), the data do suggest that there may be an advantage to fenoldopam that was not demonstrated with dopamine. Larger studies and trials that seek to duplicate the previous positive results with fenoldopam are needed before any conclusions can be drawn.

Atrial Natriuretic Peptide

Atrial natriuretic peptide (ANP) and its synthetic siblings, urodilatin and anaritide, are all potent renal artery renal vasodilators. ANP is a potent antagonist of renal vasoconstrictor signals (23). In animal models, it reduced the incidence of ARF in both ischemic (24) and toxic (25) models. In a small open label human study; involving 53 patients, it was demonstrated that a 24-hour infusion of ANP resulted in a statistically significant increase in creatinine clearance (26). In the subgroup of patients with nonoliguric ARF, ANP was associated with a significant increase in dialysis-free survival.

Urodilatin may be better than ANP, because it has more potent natriuretic and diuretic abilities, resists rapid breakdown, and does not exhibit tachyphylaxis (27). Some preliminary studies looking at prophylactic use of urodilatin as a renal protective agent, following transplant surgery (cardiac and liver), have been done (28,29), demonstrating favorable results in the small sample sizes used. In these investigations, fewer patients required dialysis, and nonoliguric patients had higher urine flow rates.

An early report found that anaritide treatment did not improve the dialysis-free survival rate in critically ill patients with ATN (30). In fact, it was associated with decreased survival. However, a more recent study showed that anaritide, administered to patients with ischemic ARF sustained as a complication of cardiac surgery, significantly increased renal function and decreased the need for dialysis (31).

Vasopressin

A recent study compared the outcome of fluid resuscitation with vasopressin following liver trauma. Treatment with vasopressin showed improved blood flow, and also prevented further blood loss. It also significantly improved short-term survival, when compared with fluid therapy (32,33). A unique feature of vasopressin, not shared by other vasopressors, is that it causes vasodilation in the renal vasculature. Vasopressin causes vasodilation in key vascular beds, including the pulmonary, cerebral, renal, and coronary circulations—unique features of vasopressin not shared by other vasoconstrictor agents. One mechanism of vasopressin-induced vasodilation is the activation of oxytocin endothelial receptors, which in turn trigger activation of endothelial isoforms of NO synthase (33). Thus vasopressin, at low doses, may have a sparing effect on key vascular beds.

Prevention/Reduction of Renal Injury Due to Drugs/Toxins
Avoidance of Hyperglycemia

The strict control of plasma glucose in patients with septic shock has yielded the stunning results of reduced mortality (from the septic shock), as well as decreased incidence of ARF (see Volume 2, Chapter 60) (34,35). Indeed, for the critically ill patient population, the use of aggressive insulin infusion regimens to maintain a glucose level between 80 and 110 mg/dL should now be regarded as a standard element in the prevention of ARF. These beneficial effects of normoglycemia were initially thought to be a secondary effect of the insulin administration, that perhaps the growth-factor-like properties of insulin were responsible.

Interestingly, in a follow-up multivariate analysis, the authors of the initial study demonstrated that the reduction in sepsis mortality was independently associated with the glucose level, whereas the beneficial differences in the incidence of ARF were due to the amount of insulin administered as an independent factor. Therefore, the benefits of insulin administration versus euglycemia need to be clarified in the prophylaxis of renal injury. ☞ **Tight control of glucose between 80 and 110 mg/dL, via the use of insulin infusions, is useful to prevent renal failure in the septic patient population.** ☞

Daily Dosing of Aminoglycosides

Altered administration regimens of nephrotoxic drugs have also been found to be helpful. With aminoglycosides, the literature supports utilizing a daily dose, rather than divided doses to deliver the daily total, in order to reduce nephrotoxicity (36). Recent studies have shown that aminoglycoside toxicity is higher when these drugs are administered in the setting of low urine pH, while it is the lowest when administered immediately after a meal, when the urine pH is the highest (6).

Radiocontrast Agent Dosing and N-Acetylcysteine Pretreatment Regimens

Antioxidant agents are being used to treat renal toxicity induced by specific drugs. *N*-acetylcysteine (NAC) is probably the most well known. In the literature, it has been effectively used prophylactically in patients receiving gentamicin or radiocontrast agents (7–9). Using it for contrast dye administration, NAC is given as an oral drug, 600-mg PO BID, for 24 hours, along with ample hydration with intravenous saline (7,8). The NAC dosing is continued for 24 hours after exposure to the radiocontrast agent. In one prospective study (8), the incidence of an increase in creatinine greater than 0.5 mg/dL was 2% in the NAC-treated group compared with 12% in the placebo (half-normal saline) treated group. The absolute creatinine levels achieved were also higher in the placebo group. Numerous studies have also demonstrated the efficacy of hydration protocols, and the use of nonionic isomolar contrast media.

The use of NAC in animal models of gentamicin treatment demonstrate a similar type of prophylactic effect in renal protection (9). On pathology slides, sections demonstrate that animals who received NAC had less tubular necrosis and cast formation. *N*-acetylcysteine treatment also decreases the levels of malondialdehyde and myeloperoxidase, which are involved in lipid peroxidation and oxygen free radicals (9).

The mechanism of action is complicated. *N*-acetylcysteine has direct vasodilatory properties by regenerating endogenous NO at the endothelium. Furthermore, as mentioned in the previous paragraph, it reduces the levels of enzymes responsible for lipid peroxidation and oxygen free radical generation. *N*-acetylcysteine reduces poly (ADP-ribose) synthase expression, meaning that the nuclear enzyme cannot deplete its substrate; nicotinamide adenine dinucleotide (NAD+) and nicotinamide adenine dinucleotide phosphate (NADP) are two important coenzymes found in cells. NADH is the reduced form of NAD+, and NAD+ is the oxidized form of NADH. Nicotinamide adenine dinucleotide is converted to NADP with the addition of a phosphate group to the 2' position of the adenosyl nucleotide through an ester linkage. In the setting of hypoperfusion or hypoxia, ATP levels are decreased and anaerobic metabolism is favored. In the presence of NADH, pyruvate is converted to lactate (anaerobic conditions), whereas in the presence of NAD+, pyruvate is converted to acetyl coA (aerobic conditions) to enter Krebs cycle and ATP is produced. Some investigators feel that in the setting of dangerously low ATP levels, increased glycolysis and decreased aerobic metabolism leads to apoptosis and renal tubular necrosis.

Finally, NAC upregulates antioxidant systems, such as superoxide dismutase and glutathione peroxidase, and may enhance oxygen consumption. In summary, NAC is active in all the various mechanisms responsible for renal toxicity: it counteracts vasoconstriction and decreased renal oxygen delivery; it counteracts the direct cellular toxicity of certain drugs; and it decreases the amount of secondary damage by oxygen free radicals (also see Volume 2, Chapter 40, Table 6).

 ☞ *N*-acetylcysteine should be used to prevent drug-induced nephrotoxicity caused by radiocontrast, aminoglycosides, and other susceptible agents. ☜

The methylxanthines, theophylline, and aminophylline, antagonists of adenosine, have also been considered in treating radiocontrast-induced nephropathy. Adenosine's role in RBF regulation is complex, because it is responsible not only for afferent arteriolar vasoconstriction, but also cortical arteriolar vasodilation (3). Because adenosine is expressed in the juxtaglomerular apparatus and the renal mesangial cells vasoconstrict (37), the thinking is that the methylxanthine compounds can counteract the vasoconstrictive phenomenon, caused by radiocontrast agents. That theory is clinically seen; some trials do suggest a slight benefit to aminophylline/theophylline administration (38–40). However, other studies have not demonstrated the same benefit. Comparing the methylxanthines to NAC, the latter compound demonstrates greater clinical efficacy.

Additional experimental drugs have been mentioned in the recent literature as possible prophylactic agents. These have yet to come into clinical practice. Prostaglandin analogs, such as prostacyclin and alprostadil (prostaglandin E1), have been studied in surgical patients undergoing orthotopic liver transplantation and cardiopulmonary bypass (41,42). Results do not consistently demonstrate benefit, although decreased postoperative creatinine levels and trends toward lesser incidence of dialysis-dependent renal failure were noted in some of the studies. It may be that prostaglandins, with their potent systemic vasodilator effects, have differing effects on renal perfusion, depending on the balance between selective renal arteriolar vasodilation versus systemic hypotension, and a resulting decrease in renal perfusion pressure, so that positive benefits from their administration depend on a detailed administration algorithm. Tirilazad mesylate, a 21-aminosteroid, has been tested for pharmacokinetics and safety in healthy human volunteers (43,44). In rat models, 21-aminosteroids are effective in attenuating the increase in postinjury serum creatinine and improving animal survival (45). They achieve these effects through their role in inhibiting lipid peroxidation, by scavenging lipid radicals and by inhibiting lipid–radical chain reaction, and by inducing NO synthase (46).

Amphotericin-B Formulations and Administration Regimens

In many immunosuppressed patients, severe fungal infections are an often lethal complication, and necessitate the utilization of the most efficacious antifungal agent, amphotericin. Amphotericin is a potent nephrotoxin, decreasing renal function in up to 80% of patients; the risk appears to be linked to the cumulative dose given (47). The more serious fungal infections requiring amphotericin treatment, such as fungemia, require a higher dose of amphotericin, and thus increase the risk of developing renal insufficiency, and the concomitant presence of other sequelae of critical illness (diuretic use, abnormal serum creatinine at baseline, use of other nephrotoxic drugs) in a patient requiring amphotericin increases the risk as well (48).

To reduce its toxicity, amphotericin can be given as a constant infusion rather than a bolus dose (12); this produces an increased serum creatinine in 33% versus 58% of the patients (49). Sodium infusion, with 1-L 0.9% saline load prior to amphotericin administration, has been used clinically, and a randomized, double-blinded placebo-control study demonstrated efficacy to prevent creatinine rise (50). In addition, various liposomal formulations, which are less nephrotoxic, are now being used. These liposomal amphotericin formulations reduce direct toxicity to the tubular cells, although the mechanism is unclear. The clinical data is scant regarding liposomal amphotericin, but seem to show equivalent efficacy with standard amphotericin, while reducing renal toxicity by 50% (51–56). ☞ **By utilizing different drug formulations and/or different dosing regimens for antimicrobials, like aminoglycosides, amphotericin, and radiocontrast agents, one can decrease their nephrotoxicity. ☜**

EYE TO THE FUTURE

The current research is focused on studying the molecular pathophysiology, to attempt to block the cascades responsible for renal injury. At the same time, the mechanism for inflammatory injury is being elucidated for possible therapeutic intervention. With advances in continuous renal replacement therapy (CRRT) and hemodialysis, further improvements, such as renal tubule assist devices, can help decrease the extent of renal injury. In addition, there is growing interest in blood purification systems to remove circulating mediators in sepsis, which may confer benefit in septic patients.

Molecular Pathophysiology

Lysophosphatidic acid (LPA) binds to a family of G protein-coupled receptors, and has effects on cell proliferation, cell differentiation, survival, and apoptosis suppression. It also functions as an inflammatory mediator. Reperfusion injury of the kidney is correlated with persistently increased levels of LPA (57–59). Three subtypes of LPA receptors exist, and LPA3 receptor antagonism has demonstrated, in the mouse experimental model, to lead to decreased renal ischemia-reperfusion injury (60). The same investigators applied a LPA3 receptor agonist to mouse kidneys, and found an enhanced level of renal injury. These data suggest that an LPA3 receptor antagonist compound could serve as treatment of ischemic ARF.

In addition, studies are examining the clinical utility of antagonists to the A_{2A} adenosine receptor. It is one of the four subtypes of adenosine receptors, and appears to function via the G protein-coupled effects on adenylyl cyclase to vasodilate the renal vasculature, and increase RBF and GFR (61). Activation of A_{2A} receptors on neutrophils also reduces neutrophil oxidative activity and decreases neutrophil adherence to endothelial cells. The combined effect is that of reduced tissue damage from neutrophil infiltration and the resulting oxidative damage (58,59).

Immunology

Investigators (62) recently demonstrated that T and B cells were important mediators of renal injury following whole body ischemia. When T-cell-deficient mice were exposed to whole body ischemia conditions, the rise in serum creatinine and tubular injury were significantly decreased. B-cell-deficient mice also had reduced rates of postischemic injury, via a pathway independent of T-cell function (63). Soluble mediators and changes in the expression of adhesion molecules like ICAM-1 are part of the mechanism. Once they are more clearly delineated, these systems may be the targets for future therapy.

Tissue Engineering

Tissue engineering may be used in the future, for either prophylaxis or treatment of renal injury. A group of investigators (64) treated pigs, inoculated with *Escherichia coli* with CRRT, including a filter with renal proximal tubule cells, forming a "renal tubule assist device" (RTAD), to prophylactically treat for ATN. The results demonstrated decreased plasma levels of IL-6 and gamma interferon, and the treated animals doubled their survival time compared with the sham control group. This result suggests that the idea of utilizing high-volume hemofiltration and other CRRT options may indeed lead to reduced levels of inflammatory cytokines and better survival.

Other Novel Drugs

One study found fructose-1,6-diphosphate (FDP) to be beneficial in preventing cell edema and protecting renal cells from ischemic damage. This study also suggests that treatment with FDP may, in some cases, be superior to treatment with mannitol (65). Early trials have indicated that recombinant human atrial natriuretic peptides (rhANP) and insulin-like growth factor 1 (IGF-1) may be beneficial in primary prevention of ARF (66,67). Further research is also needed to determine the effects of anti-inflammatory agents in the prophylaxis and treatment of ARF. Specific inducable nitric oxide synthose (iNOS) inhibitors, N-iminoethyl-L-lysine (L-NIL), and α-melanocyte-stimulating hormone (αMSH) have exhibited some protective properties against ARF (68,69).

Finally, a study aimed at evaluating the effectiveness of treating kidney trauma with a caffeic acid phenethyl ester (CAPE) found that this treatment provided significant protection against further injury (70).

SUMMARY

Many cases of ARF in critically ill patients are attributed to nonpreventable causes. Pathological processes, such as septic, hemorrhage, or cardiogenic shock are associated with ARF. In addition, the many diagnostic and therapeutic maneuvers instituted to stabilize and treat critically ill patients also introduce nephrotoxicity via a variety of mechanisms. In most situations of ARF, the etiology is multifactorial, but includes the common final pathways of renal hypoperfusion, oxygen-free radical injury and, in many cases, direct cellular toxicity from a specific nephrotoxic property of the compound administered. In these situations, certain prophylactic and treatment measures can be taken to increase chances of renal recovery. While some are only in preliminary clinical studies and others are pure theories, there are strategies and agents available now with documented clinical efficacy. Their use should definitely enter into the management plan of a critically ill patient, who has risk factors for developing ARF.

KEY POINTS

- ☞ ARF in the critically ill is often a multifactorial process, but usually involves a combination of hypoperfusion and local hypoxic injury, from inflammatory stress due to toxins or oxygen-free radicals.
- ☞ Endocrine and autocrine functions act reflexively in the renal vasculature to adjust for hypoperfusion.
- ☞ While diuretics have been used to convert oliguric ARF to nonoliguric ARF, the outcomes have not been improved with their use.
- ☞ One of the best renal protective maneuvers is aggressive fluid resuscitation and maintenance of euvolemia.
- ☞ In rhabdomyolysis, aggressive intravenous fluid hydration, to maintain a urine output greater than 200 mL/hr, is the recommended first priority (21).
- ☞ Fenoldopam, a DA-1-specific dopaminergic agonist, actually has documented benefit, in that it improves renal hemodynamics, function, and histology (14).
- ☞ Tight control of glucose between 80 and 110 mg/dL, via the use of insulin infusions, is useful to prevent renal failure in the septic patient population.
- ☞ *N*-acetylcysteine should be used to prevent drug-induced nephrotoxicity caused by radiocontrast, aminoglycosides, and other susceptible agents.
- ☞ By utilizing different drug formulations and/or different dosing regimens for antimicrobials, like aminoglycosides, amphotericin, and radiocontrast agents, one can decrease their nephrotoxicity.

REFERENCES

1. O'Hara JF, Jr. Low-dose "renal" dopamine. Anesthesiol Clin North America 2000; 18:835–851, ix.
2. Thadhani R, Pascual M, Bonventre JV. Acute renal failure. N Engl J Med 1996; 334:1448–1460.
3. Brezis M, Rosen S. Hypoxia of the renal medulla—its implications for disease. N Engl J Med 1995; 332:647–656.
4. Breyer MD, Hao C, Qi Z. Cyclooxygenase-2 selective inhibitors and the kidney. Curr Opin Crit Care 2001; 7:393–400.
5. Klahr S, Miller SB. Acute oliguria. N Engl J Med 1998; 338:671–675.
6. Beauchamp D, Labrecque G. Aminoglycoside nephrotoxicity: do time and frequency of administration matter? Curr Opin Crit Care 2001; 7:401–408.
7. Tepel M, van der Giet M, Schwarzfeld C, Laufer U, Liermann D, Zidek W. Prevention of radiographic-contrast-agent-induced reductions in renal function by acetylcysteine. N Engl J Med 2000; 343:180–184.
8. Tepel M, Zidek W. Acetylcysteine for radiocontrast nephropathy. Curr Opin Crit Care 2001; 7:390–392.
9. Mazzon E, Britti D, De Sarro A, Caputi AP, Cuzzocrea S. Effect of *N*-acetylcysteine on gentamicin-mediated nephropathy in rats. Eur J Pharmacol 2001; 424:75–83.
10. Mehta RL, Pascual MT, Soroko S, Chertow GM. Diuretics, mortality, and nonrecovery of renal function in acute renal failure. Jama 2002; 288:2547–2553.
11. Rivers E, Nguyen B, Havstad S, et al. Early goal-directed therapy in the treatment of severe sepsis and septic shock. N Engl J Med 2001; 345:1368–1377.
12. Costa S, Nucci M. Can we decrease amphotericin nephrotoxicity? Curr Opin Crit Care 2001; 7:379–383.

13. Ragaller MJR, Theilen H, Koch T. Volume replacement in critically ill patients with acute renal failure. J Am Soc Nephrol 2001; 12:S33–S39.

14. Murphy MB, Murray C, Shorten GD. Fenoldopam: a selective peripheral dopamine-receptor agonist for the treatment of severe hypertension. N Engl J Med 2001; 345:1548–1557.

15. Schaer L, Mitchell P, Parrillo J. Norepinephrine alone versus norepinephrine plus low-dose dopamine: enhanced blood flow with combination pressor therapy. Crit Care Med 1985; 13:492.

16. Rahman S, Conger JD. Glomerular and tubular factors in urine flow rate of acute renal failure patients. Am J Kidney Dis 1994; 23:788–793.

17. Anderson R, Schrier R. Acute tubular necrosis. In: Schrier R, Gottschalk C, eds. Diseases of the Kidney. Boston: Little, Brown, 1993:1287–1318.

18. Anderson R, Linas S, Berns A, et al. Nonoliguric acute renal failure. N Engl J Med 1977; 296:1134–1138.

19. Conger J. Interventions in clinical acute renal failure: what are the data? Am J Kidney Dis 1995; 26:565–576.

20. Eneas JF, Schoenfeld PY, Humphreys MH. The effect of infusion of mannitol-sodium bicarbonate on the clinical course of myoglobinuria. Arch Int Med 1979; 139:801–805.

21. Warren JD, Blumbergs PC, Thompson PD. Rhabdomyolysis: a review. Muscle Nerve 2002; 25:332–347.

22. Sheinbaum R, Safi H, Ignacio C, et al. Renal protection and improved outcome by utilization of a DA-1 agonist (fenoldopam) in TAAA repair. Anaesth Analg 2000; 90:SCA31.

23. Maack T, Camargo M, Kleinert H. Atrial natriuretic factor: structure and functional properties. Kidney Int 1985; 27:607–615.

24. Nakamoto M, Shapiro J, Shanley P. In vitro and in vivo protective effect of atriopeptin III on ischemic acute renal failure. J Clin Invest 1987; 80:698–705.

25. Capasso G, Rosati C, Cianii F. The beneficial effects of atrial natriuretic peptide on cyclosporin toxicity. Am J Hypertens 1990; 3:204.

26. Rahman S, Kim G, Mathew A, et al. Effects of atrial natriuretic peptide in clinical acute renal failure. Kidney Int 1994; 45:1731–1738.

27. Garwood S. New pharmacologic options for renal preservation. Anesthesiol Clin North Am 2000; 18:753–771.

28. Hummel M, Kuln M, Bub A. Urodilatin, a new peptide with beneficial effects in the postoperative therapy of cardiac transplant recipients. Clin Invest 1992; 70:674–682.

29. Cecedi C, Kuse E-R, Meyer M. Treatment of acute postoperative renal failure after liver and heart transplantation by Urodilatin. Clin Invest Med 1993; 71:435–436.

30. Allgren RL, Marbury TC, Rahman SN, et al. Anaritide in acute tubular necrosis. Auriculin Anaritide Acute Renal Failure Study Group. N Engl J Med 1997; 336:828–834.

31. Sward K, Valsson F, Odencrants P, et al. Recombinant human atrial natriuretic peptide in ischemic acute renal failure: a randomized placebo-controlled trial. Crit Care Med 2004; 32:1310–1315.

32. Raedler C, Voelckel WG, Wenzel V, et al. Treatment of uncontrolled hemorrhagic shock after liver trauma: fatal effects of fluid resuscitation versus improved outcome after vasopressin. Anesth Analg 2004; 98:1759–1766.

33. Holmes CL, Russell JA. Vasopressin. Semin Resp Crit Care Med 2004; 25(6):705–711.

34. van den Berghe G, Wouters PJ, Bouillon R, et al. Outcome benefit of intensive insulin therapy in the critically ill: insulin dose versus glycemic control. Crit Care Med 2003; 31:359–366.

35. van den Berghe G, Wouters P, Weekers F, et al. Intensive insulin therapy in the critically ill patients. N Engl J Med 2001; 345:1359–1367.

36. Bennett W, Plamp C, Gilbert D, et al. The influence of dosage regimen on experimental gentamicin nephrotoxicity: dissociation of peak serum levels from renal failure. J Infect Dis 1979; 140:576–580.

37. Gouyon JB, Guignard JP. Functional renal insufficiency: role of adenosine. Biol Neonate 1988; 53:237–242.

38. Shammas NW, Kapalis MJ, Harris M, McKinney D, Coyne EP. Aminophylline does not protect against radiocontrast nephropathy in patients undergoing percutaneous angiographic procedures. J Invasive Cardiol 2001; 13:738–740.

39. Erley CM, Duda SH, Rehfuss D, et al. Prevention of radiocontrast-media-induced nephropathy in patients with pre-existing renal insufficiency by hydration in combination with the adenosine antagonist theophylline. Nephrol Dial Transplant 1999; 14:1146–1149.

40. Kolonko A, Wiecek A, Kokot F. The nonselective adenosine antagonist theophylline does prevent renal dysfunction induced by radiographic contrast agents. J Nephrol 1998; 11:151–156.

41. Klein A, Cofer JB, Pruett T, et al. Pruett T. Prostaglandin E1 administration following orthotopic liver transplantation: a randomized, prospective multicenter trial. Gastroenterology 1996; 110(3):710–715.

42. Manasia A, Leibowitz A, Miller C. Postoperative intravenous infusion of alprostadil (PGE1) does not improve renal function in hepatic transplant patients. J Am Coll Surg 1996; 182:347–352.

43. Fleishaker J, Peters G, Cathcard K. Evaluation of the pharmacokinetics and tolerability of tirilizad mesylate, a 21-aminosteroid free radical scavenger: multiple-dose administration. J Clin Pharmacol 1993; 33:182–190.

44. Fleishaker J, Peters G, Cathcard K. Evaluation of the pharmacokinetics and tolerability of tirilizad mesylate, a 21-aminosteroid free radical scavenger: single-dose administration. J Clin Pharmacol 1993; 33:175–181.

45. Stanley J, Goldblum J, Frank T. Attenuation of renal reperfusion in rats by the 21-aminosteroid U74006F. J Vasc Surg 1993; 17:685–689.

46. Bruagher J, Pregenzer J, Chase R. Novel 21-aminosteroids as potent inhibitors of iron-dependent peroxidation. Biol Chem 1987; 262:10438–10440.

47. Anaissie D, Vartivarian S, Abi-Said D. Fluconazole vs. amphotericin B in the treatment of hematogenous candidiasis: a matched cohort study. Am J Med 1996; 101:170–176.

48. Luber AD, Maa L, Lam M, Guglielmo BJ. Risk factors for amphotericin B-induced nephrotoxicity. J Antimicrob Chemother 1999; 43:267–271.

49. Sabra R, Zeinoun N, Sharaf LH, Ghali R, Beshara G, Serhal H. Role of humoral mediators in, and influence of a liposomal formulation on, acute amphotericin B nephrotoxicity. Pharmacol Toxicol 2001; 88:168–175.

50. Llanos A, Cieza J, Bernardo J, et al. Effect of salt supplementation on amphotericin B nephrotoxicity. Kidney Int 1991; 40(2):302–308.

51. Leenders AC, Reiss P, Portegies P, et al. Liposomal amphotericin B (AmBisome) compared with amphotericin B both followed by oral fluconazole in the treatment of AIDS-associated cryptococcal meningitis. Aids 1997; 11:1463–1471.

52. Leenders AC, Daenen S, Jansen RL, et al. Liposomal amphotericin B compared with amphotericin B deoxycholate in the treatment of documented and suspected neutropenia-associated invasive fungal infections. Br J Haematol 1998; 103:205–212.

53. Walsh TJ, Finberg RW, Arndt C, et al. Liposomal amphotericin B for empirical therapy in patients with persistent fever and neutropenia. National Institute of Allergy and Infectious Diseases Mycoses Study Group. N Engl J Med 1999; 340:764–771.

54. White MH, Bowden RA, Sandler ES, et al. Randomized, double-blind clinical trial of amphotericin B colloidal dispersion vs. amphotericin B in the empirical treatment of fever and neutropenia. Clin Infect Dis 1998; 27:296–302.

55. Sharkey PK, Graybill JR, Johnson ES, et al. Amphotericin B lipid complex compared with amphotericin B in the treatment of cryptococcal meningitis in patients with AIDS. Clin Infect Dis 1996; 22:315–321.

56. Prentice HG, Hann IM, Herbrecht R, et al. A randomized comparison of liposomal versus conventional amphotericin B for the treatment of pyrexia of unknown origin in neutropenic patients. Br J Haematol 1997; 98:711–718.

57. Okusa MD. The inflammatory cascade in acute ischemic renal failure. Nephron 2002; 90:133–138.

58. Okusa MD. A(2A) adenosine receptor: a novel therapeutic target in renal disease. Am J Physiol Renal Physiol 2002; 282: F10–F18.

59. Okusa MD, Linden J, Huang L, Rieger JM, Macdonald TL, Huynh LP. A(2A) adenosine receptor-mediated inhibition of renal injury and neutrophil adhesion. Am J Physiol Renal Physiol 2000; 279:F809–F818.

60. Okusa MD, Linden J, Macdonald T, Huang L. Selective A2A adenosine receptor activation reduces ischemia-reperfusion injury in rat kidney. Am J Physiol 1999; 277:F404–F412.

61. Levens N, Beil M, Jarvis M. Renal actions of a new adenosine agonist, CGS 21680A selective for the A2 receptor. J Pharmacol Exp Ther 1991; 257:1005–1012.

62. Burne-Taney MJ, Kofler J, Yokota N, Weisfeldt M, Traystman RJ, Rabb H. Acute renal failure after whole body ischemia is characterized by inflammation and T cell-mediated injury. Am J Physiol Renal Physiol 2003; 285:F87–F94.

63. Burne-Taney MJ, Ascon DB, Daniels F, Racusen L, Baldwin W, Rabb H. B cell deficiency confers protection from renal ischemia reperfusion injury. J Immunol 2003; 171:3210–3215.

64. Humes HD, Buffington DA, Lou L, et al. Cell therapy with a tissue-engineered kidney reduces the multiple-organ consequences of septic shock. Crit Care Med 2003; 31:2421–2428.

65. Antunes N, Martinusso CA, Takiya CM, et al. Fructose-1,6 diphosphate as a protective agent for experimental ischemic acute renal failure. Kidney I 2006; 69:68–72.

66. Sward K, Valsson F, Odencrants P, et al. Recombinant human atrial natriuretic peptide in ischemic acute renal failure: a randomized placebo-controlled trial. Crit Care Med 2004; 32: 1310–1315.

67. Hirschberg R, Kopple J, Lipsett P et al. Multicenter clinical trial of recombinant human insulin-like growth factor I in patients with acute renal failure. Kidney Int 2003; 64:593–602.

68. Schwartz D, Mendonca M, Schwartz I, et al. Inhibition of constitutive nitric oxide synthase (NOW) by nitric oxide generated by inducible NOS after lipolysaccharide administration provokes renal dysfunction in rats. J Clin Invest 1997; 100:439–448.

69. Chio H, Kohda Y, McLeroy P, et al. Alpha-melanocyte-stimulating hormone protects against renal injury after ischemia in mice and rats. J Clin Invest 1997; 99:1165–1172.

70. Ozguner F, Armagan A, Koyu A, et al. A novel antioxidant agent caffeic acid phenethyl ester prevents shock wave-induced renal tubular oxidative stress. Urol Res 2005; 33: 239–243.

43

Dialysis Therapies

Omaran Abdeen

Division of Nephrology and Hypertension, Department of Medicine, UC San Diego Medical Center, and
VA Medical Center, San Diego, California, U.S.A.

Shamik Shah

Division of Nephrology and Hypertension, Department of Medicine, UC San Diego Medical Center, San Diego, California, U.S.A.

Ravindra Mehta

Division of Nephrology and Hemodialysis Services, Department of Medicine,
UC San Diego Medical Center, San Diego, California, U.S.A.

INTRODUCTION

During the past decades, a number of advances have been made in the field of renal replacement therapy (RRT). In addition, clinicians have gained a better appreciation of the need for early and aggressive management of patients with renal failure in the intensive care unit (ICU) (1). Although a number of treatment modalities exist, there seems to be continued controversy about selection of the most appropriate modality for an individual patient. This chapter briefly reviews the clinical spectrum of renal failure in the ICU, the indications for initiating dialysis, the general principles of dialysis therapy, and unique features, advantages, disadvantages, and utility of various renal replacement modalities.

DIVERSITY OF CLINICAL RENAL FAILURE IN THE ICU

Appropriate modality selection requires an understanding of the clinical spectrum of renal failure in the ICU. The incidence of acute renal failure (ARF) in the ICU is approximately 10–25% (2,3). Most (70%) of the critically ill patients who develop ARF require dialysis, and most do not survive (50–90% death rate) (2–4). Uncomplicated ARF refers to an acute and transient decline in glomerular filtration rate (GFR) without clinically apparent complications. Dialytic support is often unnecessary in such patients, or may be required for a single indication such as hyperkalemia. In contrast, complicated ARF is characterized by multiple metabolic and volume status perturbations. Often, the patient is oliguric, and the renal failure may be present in association with the multiple organ dysfunction syndrome (MODS). This is the type of renal failure most commonly seen in patients, who suffer from acute trauma or develop postoperative renal failure. The threshold for initiation of dialysis and the choice of dialytic modality will differ depending on associated complications and comorbid conditions.

INDICATIONS FOR INITIATION OF DIALYSIS

Although there has been an increased appreciation for the need for early and aggressive management of ARF in the ICU setting, there are no standards for initiation of dialysis and many nephrologists avoid dialysis initiation for as long as possible. Two major factors contribute to the tendency to delay dialysis. First, the dialysis procedure itself has associated risks. Hypotension, dysrrhythmias, and complications of vascular access placement are common (5,6). Second, there is a concern that dialysis can delay recovery of renal function (7,8). This contention is supported by animal data in which hypotension resulted in recurrent renal ischemia (9), and human studies that showed a decline in GFR during and after an intermittent hemodialysis session (10,11).

Several factors need to be considered when making the decision to provide RRT. First, it is important to recognize that in the ICU patient, ARF usually does not occur in isolation from other organ system dysfunction. Consequently, providing dialysis can be viewed as a form of renal support for multiorgan dysfunction rather than mere renal replacement (Table 1) (12). For example, in the presence of oliguric renal failure, administration of large volumes of fluid to patients with MODS may lead to impaired oxygenation. In such a setting, early intervention with extracorporeal therapies for management of fluid balance may significantly impact the function of other organs even in the absence of traditional indices of renal failure, such as marked azotemia.

ℴ **Indications for dialysis generally fall into one of three broad categories: solute indications such as marked azotemia, volume indications such as fluid overload, or both.** ℴ Often the patient who has suffered acute trauma receives large volumes of blood products, fluids, and nutrition. Such therapy is acutely life-saving, but may result in the manifestation of an indication for dialysis, such as fluid overload or hyperkalemia.

The indication for initiation of dialysis influences outcome. We showed in a randomized controlled trial comparing intermittent therapies with continuous therapies that patients dialyzed for solute control had a better outcome than those dialyzed for volume control (13). Moreover, patients dialyzed for both solute and volume control had the worst outcome. Therefore, it appears that volume overload tends to confer a poorer prognosis. This notion is supported by a number of observational studies. For

Table 1   Indications and Timing of Dialysis for Acute Renal Failure: Renal Replacement vs. Renal Support

Reason for dialysis	Renal replacement	Renal support
Therapeutic goal	Replace renal function	Support other organs
Timing of intervention	Based on level of biochemical markers	Based on organs involved (e.g., lungs, brain, and so on), and clinical needs
Indications for dialysis	Narrow	Broad
Dialysis dose	Extrapolated from ESRD	Targeted for overall support

Abbreviation: ESRD, end-stage renal disease.
Source: Adapted from Ref. 108.

example, recent studies have suggested that achieving a negative fluid balance in the first three days of admission for septic shock is a predictor of better survival (14). Moreover, hypervolemia is a common accompaniment to perioperative ARF. Mukau et al. (15) showed that 95% of their patients with postoperative acute renal failure had fluid excesses of more than 10 L at initiation of dialysis.

Consequently, fluid regulation ought to be an important consideration when deciding to initiate dialysis in the ICU patient with ARF. Such renal support provides volume "space," which permits for the administration of adequate nutritional support without limitations (16). In addition to volume overload, solute disturbances such as hyperkalemia may predispose to life-threatening dysrrhythmias, and uncontrolled uremia may lead to a variety of serious complications. Thus, maintaining electrolyte, acid–base, and solute homeostasis is another important factor when considering initiation of dialysis.

PRINCIPLES OF DIALYSIS
Overview
Dialysis is a process in which molecules in solution "A" (blood) diffuse across a semipermeable membrane into solution "B" (dialysate) (6). The transfer of solute across the membrane is determined by membrane characteristics and the solute concentration on the two sides of the membrane. Diffusive clearance denotes the movement of small molecular weight solutes from plasma to dialysate under the driving force of an electrochemical gradient. Convective clearance (ultrafiltration, UF) occurs when water is driven across the membrane by either a hydrostatic or an osmotic force. Those solutes that can pass through the membrane pores move along with the water (solute drag).

Determinants of Diffusive Clearance
Membrane characteristics play a major role in determining the efficacy of diffusive clearance. For example, membranes with larger pores, larger surface area, and a specific geometrical configuration have greater permeability to small and middle molecular weight solutes than membranes with smaller pores and smaller surface area. Most hemodialysis membranes in use today are of the synthetic type and are more permeable than older cellulose-based membranes. Flow rates of blood and dialysate and dialysis time are the principal determinants of diffusive solute clearance. Direction of blood and dialysate flow is also a major determinant of solute diffusion capacity. ☞ **Currently, all**

hemodialysis modalities employ a countercurrent mechanism in which the direction of dialysate flow is opposite that of the blood flow. ☞ Countercurrent flow serves to maximize the concentration gradient between the blood and dialysate throughout the length of the membrane (6).

Determinants of Convective Clearance
Because convective clearance is achieved mainly by solute drag during UF, the rate at which UF occurs is the major determinant of convective clearance. Ultrafiltration rate is, in turn, determined by transmembrane pressure, water permeability, pore size, surface area, membrane geometry, and thickness. Moreover, enhanced blood flow rates will increase UF rates because higher blood flow rates prevent the stagnant accumulation of proteins that cannot cross membranes at the surface of UF. As the transmembrane pressure difference increases, more fluid and accompanying solute will be removed. However, the maximum transmembrane pressure that can be applied is limited by the tensile strength of the membrane. The size of solutes that can be "dragged" during convection is determined in large part by the size selectivity of the membrane. In general, convection is more efficient than diffusion at removing middle and large molecular weight solutes (6).

Vascular Access
In order for blood to be removed from the patient, circulated through the dialyzer, and then returned to the patient, access to the vasculature is required. Although arteriovenous fistulas and grafts are used in chronic dialysis patients, it is more common to use a catheter for vascular access in the acute setting. When arteriovenous acute dialysis was still commonly used, patients would receive one catheter in a major artery and another in a major vein. This type of vascular access has fallen out of favor because of the multitude of complications that arise from the use of chronic indwelling arterial catheters.

Currently, most patients who require acute dialysis receive a dual-lumen venous catheter placed in either the femoral, internal jugular, or subclavian vein. The design of these catheters is such that blood is withdrawn from a proximal opening and returned to a more distal opening. Because of this design, some of the blood returned to the vein will "recirculate" into the withdrawing port and into the hemofilter again, reducing the efficiency of dialysis.

☞ **Recirculation associated with dual-lumen venous catheters have been shown to be worse in the femoral**

(16%) when compared with the subclavian catheter (4%, $p = 0.0001$) location (17). ♂

Anticoagulation

In order to avoid clotting of blood in the dialysis membrane, circuit tubing, or at the vascular access, patients who receive dialysis will generally require anticoagulation. Although a variety of anticoagulants have been used, including low molecular weight heparin, prostacyclin, and nafomostat, systemic unfractionated heparin anticoagulation, regional citrate anticoagulation, and frequent saline flushing of the system are the most commonly used methods (18).

Heparin anticoagulation is easy to use, but has the disadvantage of necessitating anticoagulation of the entire patient. At our institution we have favored the use of regional citrate anticoagulation (19,20). The use of protocol-driven monitoring and adjustment of anticoagulation has improved the efficiency of both the nursing staff and the physicians. In addition, we have been able to provide dialysis to patients at high risk of bleeding with minimal complications. Citrate anticoagulation works by binding ionized calcium, thereby decreasing its ability to act in the clotting system. Some specific considerations for citrate coagulation include the need for liver function to convert citrate to bicarbonate, and the risk of hypocalcemia (especially in the setting of liver failure).

DEFINITION OF TERMS
Intermittent Therapy

An intermittent therapy is defined as any extracorporeal dialysis therapy in which the patient is treated for less than 24 hours (Table 2). Included in this category are patients treated with intermittent hemodialysis (IHD), sorbent IHD, intermittent hemodiafiltration (IHDF), intermittent ultrafiltration (IUF), extended daily dialysis (EDD), and sustained low efficiency dialysis (SLED), also termed slow continuous dialysis (SCD) (21).

Continuous Therapy

A continuous therapy is defined as any extracorporeal dialysis therapy in which the patient is treated for 24 hours or

Table 2 Dialysis Modalities for Acute Renal Failure

Intermittent therapies (treatment duration < 24 hours)	Continuous therapies (treatment duration 24 hours per day)
Hemodialysis	Peritoneal dialysis
Single pass	Ultrafiltration (SCUF)
Sorbent based	Hemofiltration (CAVH, CVVH)
Hemodiafiltration	Hemodialysis (CAVHD, CVVHD)
Ultrafiltration	Hemodiafiltration (CAVHDF, CVVHDF)
Extended daily dialysis	
Slow continuous dialysis	

Abbreviations: SCUF, slow continuous ultrafiltration; CAVH, continuous arteriovenous hemofiltration; CVVH, continuous venovenous hemofiltration; CAVHD, continuous arteriovenous hemodialysis; CVVHD, continuous venovenous hemodialysis; CAVHDF, continuous arteriovenous hemodiafiltration; CVVHDF, continuous venovenous hemodiafiltration.
Source: Adapted from Ref. 108.

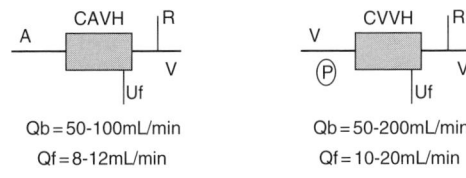
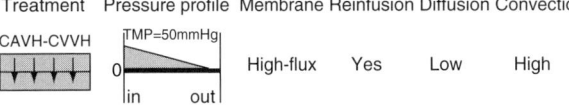

Figure 1 Continuous renal replacement techniques: continuous arteriovenous hemofiltration and continuous venovenous hemofiltration. *Abbreviations*: A, artery; V, vein; Uf, ultrafiltrate; R, replacement fluid; P, peristaltic pump; Q_b, blood flow; Q_f, ultrafiltration rate; TMP, transmembrane pressure. *Source*: Adapted from Ref. 23.

longer. Included in this category are a number of modalities that will be defined in the following (Table 2).

Continuous Arteriovenous Hemofiltration

Continuous arteriovenous hemofiltration (CAVH) is a form of continuous RRT (CRRT) whereby blood is driven by the patient's blood pressure through a filter containing a highly permeable membrane via an extracorporeal circuit originating from an artery and terminating in a vein (Fig. 1). The ultrafiltrate produced is replaced in part or completely with appropriate replacement solution to achieve blood purification and volume control (22,23).

Continuous Venovenous Hemofiltration

Continuous venovenous hemofiltration (CVVH) is a form of CRRT whereby blood is driven through a highly permeable membrane by a peristaltic pump via an extracorporeal circuit originating from a vein and terminating in a vein (Fig. 1). The ultrafiltrate produced is replaced in part or completely with appropriate replacement solution to achieve blood purification and volume control (22,23).

Slow Continuous Ultrafiltration

Slow continuous ultrafiltration (SCUF) is a form of CAVH or CVVH not associated with fluid replacement often used in the management of refractory edema with or without renal failure (Fig. 2). The primary aim of SCUF treatment is fluid removal (22,23).

Continuous Arteriovenous Hemodialysis

Continuous arteriovenous hemodialysis (CAVHD) is a form of CRRT in which the extracorporeal circuit includes slow countercurrent dialysate flow into the ultrafiltrate–dialysate compartment of the hemofilter (Fig. 3). Blood flow through the blood compartment of the membrane is driven by the patient's blood pressure through a circuit beginning in an artery and terminating in a vein. Fluid replacement is not routinely administered and solute clearance is mostly diffusive (22,23).

Continuous Venovenous Hemodialysis

Continuous venovenous vemodialysis (CVVHD) is a form of CRRT in which the extracorporeal circuit includes slow countercurrent dialysate flow into the ultrafiltrate–dialysate compartment of the hemofilter (Fig. 3). Blood flow through

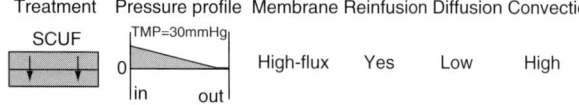

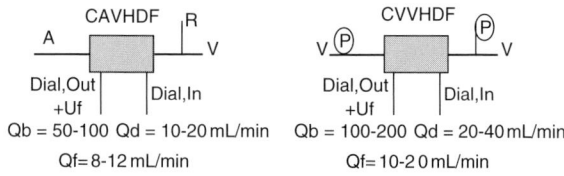

Figure 2 Continuous renal replacement techniques: slow continuous ultrafiltration. *Abbreviations*: A, artery; V, vein; Uf, ultrafiltrate; P, peristaltic pump; Q_b, blood flow; Q_f, ultrafiltration rate; TMP, transmembrane pressure; UFC, ultrafiltration control system. *Source*: Adapted from Ref. 23.

Figure 4 Continuous renal replacement techniques: continuous arteriovenous hemodiafiltration and continuous venovenous hemodiafiltration. *Abbreviations*: A, artery; V, vein; Uf, ultrafiltrate; P, peristaltic pump; Q_b, blood flow; Q_f, ultrafiltration rate; TMP, transmembrane pressure; in, dialyzer inlet; out, dialyzer outlet; Dial., dialysate; Q_d, dialysate flow rate. *Source*: Adapted from Ref. 23.

the blood compartment of the membrane is driven by a peristaltic pump through a circuit beginning and terminating in a vein. Fluid replacement is not routinely administered and solute clearance is mostly diffusive (22,23).

Continuous Arteriovenous Hemodiafiltration

Continuous arteriovenous hemodiafiltration (CAVHDF) is a form of CRRT whereby the CAVH circuit is modified by the addition of slow countercurrent dialysate flow into the ultrafiltrate–dialysate compartment of the hemofilter (Fig. 4). Ultrafiltration volumes are optimized to exceed the desired weight loss to take advantage of convection. Fluid replacement is routinely administered as clinically indicated to replace fluid losses either in part or completely. Solute removal is both diffusive and convective (22,23).

Continuous Venovenous Hemodiafiltration

Continuous venovenous hemodiafiltration (CVVHDF) is a form of CRRT whereby the CVVH circuit is modified by the addition of slow countercurrent dialysate flow into the ultrafiltrate–dialysate compartment of the hemofilter (Fig. 4). Ultrafiltration volumes are optimized to exceed the

desired weight loss to take advantage of convection. Fluid replacement is routinely administered as clinically indicated to replace fluid losses either in part or completely. Solute removal is both diffusive and convective (22,23).

DIALYSIS MODALITIES IN THE SICU
Intermittent Therapies
Intermittent Hemodialysis

Intermittent hemodialysis is the procedure that has been widely used over the past four decades in patients with end-stage renal disease (ESRD) and those with ARF (24). The vast majority of IHD is performed using a single pass of dialysate at flow rates greater than that of blood. Several important technological advances have made the procedure safer and more suited for the ARF patient. The availability of variable sodium concentrations in the dialysate, biocompatible membranes, bicarbonate-based dialysate, and volumetrically controlled UF offer certain advantages that are particularly well suited to the ARF patient (25,26). Nevertheless, most centers use a fairly standard regimen for administration of the therapy.

Because of limitations imposed by the use of dual-lumen catheters for vascular access, only moderate blood flow rates (200–300 mL/min) can be achieved. The standard dialysate flow rate used is 500 mL/min. IHD offers the advantage of providing for rapid correction of electrolyte and acid–base disturbances. A major disadvantage of IHD is the limited time (usually three to four hours) of total therapy per day. As a result, the patient will remain without renal support for the majority of the day during which fluid regulation, acid–base balance, and electrolyte homeostasis are not controlled.

☞ **The most significant disadvantages of IHD in the critically ill patient with ARF are related to hypotension and the possibility of worsening the severity of the renal injury.** ☞ Critically ill patients with hemodynamic instability may not tolerate the higher blood flow rates needed to achieve adequate levels of diffusive clearance in the limited duration (three to four months typically) of the treatment. More importantly, is the demonstration that intradialytic hypotension can contribute to delayed renal recovery

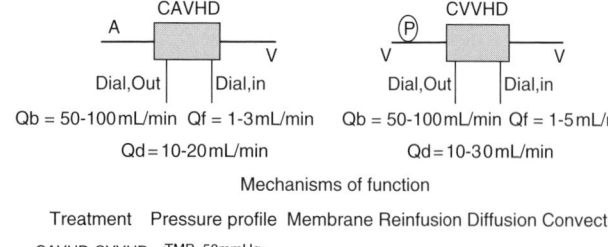

Figure 3 Continuous renal replacement techniques: continuous arteriovenous hemodialysis and continuous venovenous hemodialysis. *Abbreviations*: A, artery; V, vein; Uf, ultrafiltrate; P, peristaltic pump; Q_b, blood flow; Q_f, ultrafiltration rate; TMP, transmembrane pressure; in, dialyzer inlet; out, dialyzer outlet; Dial., dialysate; Q_d, dialysate flow rate. *Source*: Adapted from Ref. 23.

(7,8). Of interest is the demonstration by Schortgen et al. (27) that implementation of strict guidelines for the management and prevention of intradialytic hypotension helped reduce the incidence of such episodes, but did not affect overall mortality.

Sorbent System Intermittent Hemodialysis

Sorbent system IHD is a dialysis system in which dialysate is regenerated by passage through a sorbent cartridge that contains five distinct layers (28,29). The first layer contains activated carbon, the second contains urease, which converts urea to ammonium carbonate, and the third layer contains zirconium phosphate in which cations, such as potassium, calcium, and magnesium are adsorbed and exchanged for hydrogen and sodium ions. The fourth layer of the cartridge contains hydrated zirconium oxide to which phosphate and fluoride are adsorbed and exchanged for acetate. The fifth layer contains activated carbon, which removes creatinine and other waste products. Although this system is used infrequently, it provides the advantage of obviating the need for a source of pure water and providing a highly portable system. In addition, because of the unique characteristics of the regenerating system, sorbent IHD allows for greater flexibility in custom tailoring the dialysate. The biggest disadvantage of the sorbent system is that it is less efficient than single-pass IHD. The slower flow rate of dialysate and the overall adsorptive capacity of the sorbent cartridge impose the main limitations on efficiency of diffusive clearance.

Intermittent Hemodiafiltration

Intermittent hemodiafiltration (IHDF) uses convective clearance for solute removal. The main disadvantage of IHDF is the need for large volumes of sterile replacement fluid. Therefore, the expense associated with IHDF has limited its use in the United States. Proponents of the therapy claim that it offers greater hemodynamic stability and improved middle molecule clearance. Because of these advantages, IHDF has been used extensively in Europe (21,30).

Intermittent Ultrafiltration

Intermittent ultrafiltration utilizes the same device used for IHD, but differs in that the main utility of IUF is fluid removal. Typically, the procedure is used for treatment of pulmonary edema or severe cardiomyopathy with resistant fluid overload. Because the same machine used for IHDF is also used for IUF, some centers use a combination of IUF and IHD in series. Such an approach provides for greater hemodynamic stability and the ability to quickly treat volume overload. A major disadvantage is the loss of time available for diffusive solute clearance.

Extended Daily Dialysis

Extended daily dialysis (EDD) has recently been described by Kumar et al. (31). They treated 25 patients with daily IHD for a duration of six to eight hours during daylight at a blood flow rate of 200 mL/min and a dialysate flow rate of 100–300 mL/min. In comparison with a similar group of patients treated with CVVH, they demonstrated that less total daily heparin was needed and less intensive nursing commitments were required. However, no outcome measures such as survival or renal recovery were assessed. In a similar study using a single-batch dialysis system, Lonnemann et al. described treating 20 patients with ARF for 18 hours at blood flow rates of 70 mL/min and dialysate flow rates of 70 mL/min. Adequate urea clearance rates were achieved, but there was no control group and no clinical outcome data was reported (32).

Slow Continuous Dialysis/Sustained Low Efficiency Dialysis

The terms SCD and SLED have been used interchangeably within the medical literature; and, this dialytic modality was first reported by Schlaeper et al. in 1999 (33). With this technique, blood flow rates were 100–200 mL/min and dialysate flow rates were also 100–300 mL/min. Patients were treated for 12 hours during the day or evening (33). The procedure was felt to be safe, efficient, and relatively simple to use. More recently, Lornoy et al. (34) showed similar results. Marshal et al. (35) recently reported their experience with SLED in 37 critically ill patients who failed IHD. Adequate urea clearance and volume control were achieved. Mortality in the patients was not different than historical controls with a similar APACHE II score. A major disadvantage experienced in this study was the need for early termination of the procedure in one-third of the treatments because of hypotension or blood clotting. Hypokalemia and hypophosphatemia requiring replacement were also reported (35).

Continuous Therapies
Peritoneal Dialysis

Peritoneal dialysis was the first "continuous" form of dialysis therapy used in the acute setting. In peritoneal dialysis, the patient's peritoneum acts as the semipermeable dialysis membrane. Dialysate consists of a sterile, lactate-based solution inserted via a peritoneal catheter into the abdominal cavity. Diffusion occurs from the blood perfusing the peritoneum to the fluid in the abdominal cavity across the peritoneum. Once the dialysate becomes saturated (three to four hours), it is removed and fresh dialysate is instilled. Fluid removal is achieved by using an osmotic pressure mechanism in which varying dextrose concentrations in the dialysate provide an osmotic gradient for water flow from the patient's blood to the peritoneal cavity. The process of dialysate instillation and removal can be automated with a device known as a cycler. The main advantages of peritoneal dialysis are that it is less labor-intensive than hemodialysis, it does not require anticoagulation, and may be better tolerated hemodynamically than IHD. The major disadvantage is that dialysis is relatively inefficient because total solute removal is limited by total peritoneal effluent. In addition, transfer across the peritoneum is highly influenced by both the anatomy of the peritoneum and the underlying hemodynamic status of the patient. Another major disadvantage is that the procedure requires the placement of a peritoneal catheter into the abdominal cavity, which may add to the morbidity of the already compromised ICU patient (36). This later complication is often a major limiting factor in patients who have sustained trauma or have undergone abdominal surgery.

Continuous Renal Replacement Therapies
Overview

Over the last decade, a number of CRRTs have emerged. The definitions of the various therapies were given earlier. All forms of CRRT utilize membranes that are highly permeable to water and low molecular weight solutes. The various forms of CRRT differ in how the vasculature is accessed and the mechanism by which solute clearance is achieved.

The use of continuous arteriovenous modalities has fallen out of favor largely because of the complications associated with indwelling arterial catheters. The various venovenous modalities differ primarily by their mechanisms of solute removal. In SCUF, there is minimal solute removal, but adequate fluid removal. In CVVH, the removal is primarily by convection. In CVVHD, the removal is primarily by diffusion, and in CVVHDF, solute removal is by both diffusive and convective mechanisms.

Operational Characteristics
CRRT mechanisms have a number of operational characteristics that distinguish them from IHD. The blood flow rate is usually much lower (100–200 mL/min) as is the dialysate flow rate (1–2 L/hr or 17–34 mL/min). Because of the lower dialysate flow rate, the dialysate becomes saturated quickly and is a limiting factor in diffusive clearance capacity. As CUF will result in the loss of significant volumes of plasma water (often 1 L/hr), administration of replacement fluids is necessary. The composition of the replacement solution can be varied depending on the needs of the patient. ☞ **Continuous renal replacement therapy is unique in that solute removal is, in effect, dissociated from fluid removal.** ☞ Varying the composition of the dialysate or replacement fluid allows for accurate control of solute balance while fluid removal can be manipulated independently by varying the amount of replacement fluid administered. Net fluid removal during a given time period (e.g., each hour) is equal to the ultrafiltrate volume during that time period minus the amount of replacement fluid administered. Another unique feature of CRRT is the fact that the time available for either solute or fluid management is no longer a limiting factor (Table 3) (21,37). ☞ **CRRT provides improved hemodynamic stability, continuous electrolyte control, improved dialysis adequacy, and easier control of volume status.** ☞

*Potential Advantages of Continuous
Renal Replacement Therapies*
Hypotensive patients may not tolerate the rapid solute shifts associated with the higher blood flow rates required for IHD. Therefore, approximately 10% of all patients with ARF who require dialysis cannot be treated with IHD because of hemodynamic instability (5,10,38–41). Paganini et al. (42) were the first to show that 23 patients who were too unstable to tolerate IHD could be dialyzed with CRRT. Later,

Davenport et al. (39) showed that CRRT was superior to IHD in maintaining hemodynamic stability. Manns et al. (5) and Bellomo et al. (43) showed similar results. However, data from Misset et al. (41) showed no difference between CRRT and IHD with regard to hemodynamic stability. Because of the continuous nature of CRRT, lower blood and dialysate flow rates can be used to achieve blood purification without hemodynamic compromise.

☞ **Rapid alterations in sodium and fluid status have been shown to occur in IHD. Such alterations are implicated as a cause for the cerebral edema that can be observed in IHD.** ☞ Moreover, such fluctuations are avoided in CRRT as electrolyte and fluid changes are more gradual (39).

Dialysis dosing will be discussed next in greater detail, but a major advantage of CRRT is the more efficient removal of middle and large molecular weight solutes. Such solutes are removed inefficiently with IHD which utilizes primarily diffusive clearance, but can be cleared more effectively by CRRT modalities that incorporate convective clearance (21,44,45). The efficiency of diffusive small solute removal is less with CRRT, but because of the extended time of treatment and small solute removal with UF overall clearance is similar to IHD.

As fluid balance can be managed on an hour-by-hour basis, CRRT allows for the administration of large volumes of fluids. Of particular importance in this regard is the ability to administer adequate parenteral nutrition to the critically ill patient without concern for exacerbating fluid overload. It is well established that the increased catabolism seen in critically ill patients requires more aggressive nutrition management (46). Several studies have shown that CRRT allows patients with multi-organ failures (MOF) to benefit from adequate nutritional support (16,47,48). A recent study by Tremblay et al. in 12 burn patients showed that patients had gained an excess of 10 kg in weight prior to CRRT initiation, but that the fluid had been removed within a short period of time, allowing for improved nutritional support without compromising overall fluid status (48). In addition, several studies have shown that intermittent procedures often necessitate suboptimal nutrition because of fear of interdialytic volume overload (46) (Table 4).

*Potential Disadvantages of Continuous
Renal Replacement Therapies*
A number of disadvantages and potential complications also exist for CRRT. Cost, nursing support, anticoagulation, and

Table 3   Continuous Renal Replacement Therapy (Comparison of Techniques)

	SCUF	CAVH	CVVH	CAVHD	CAVHDF	CVVHD	CVVHDF	PD
Access	A-V	A-V	V-V	A-V	A-V	V-V	V-V	Peritoneal catheter
Pump	No	No	Yes	No	No	Yes	Yes	No[b]
Filtrate (mL/hr)	100	600	1000	300	600	300	800	500
Dialysate flow (L/hr)	0	0	0	1	1	1	1	2.0[c]
Replacement fluid (L/day)	0	12	21.6	4.8	12	4.8	16.8	0
Urea clearance (mL/min)	1.7	10	16.7	21.7	26.7	21.7	30	8.5
Simplicity[a]	1	2	3	2	2	3	3	2
Cost[a]	1	2	4	3	3	4	4	3

[a]1, most simple and least expensive; 4, most difficult and most expensive.
[b]Cycler can be used to automate exchanges, however it adds to the cost and complexity.
[c]2.0-L exchanges.
Abbreviations: SCUF, slow continuous ultrafiltration; CAVH, continuous arteriovenous hemofiltration; CVVH, continuous venovenous hemofiltration; CAVHD, continuous arteriovenous hemodialysis; CVVHD, continuous venovenous hemodialysis; CAVHDF, continuous arteriovenous hemodiafiltration; CVVHDF, continuous venovenous hemodiafiltration; PD, peritoneal dialysis.
Source: Adapted from Ref. 108.

Table 4 Relative Advantages of Continuous Renal Replacement Therapy (CRRT) and Intermittent Hemodialysis (IHD)

Parameter	CRRT	IHD
Continuous renal replacement	+	−
Hemodynamic stability	++	+
Fluid balance easily achieved	+	−
Unlimited nutritional supplementation	++	−
Superior metabolic control	+	−
Continuous removal of potential toxins	+	−
Relatively simple to perform	+	−
Rapid removal of poisons, electrolytes	−	+
Limited anticoagulation	−	+
Intensive care unit nursing support	++	−
Hemodialysis nursing support	+	++
Patient mobility	−	+

Source: Adapted from Ref. 108.

electrolyte disturbances are some of the main disadvantages or potential complications that may be encountered.

The required nursing support and cost of CRRT may be greater than that needed for intermittent techniques; however, this has not been clearly demonstrated. The requirement for specific nursing training and skills is important, but adequate training can be achieved (49,50). See the section on "Logistical Factors" that follows for a more in-depth discussion of this important topic.

Continuous renal replacement therapies require continuous anticoagulation to avoid clotting of the dialysis filter and tubing. Several choices exist for anticoagulation, but the most widely used anticoagulants are heparin, saline flushes, and citrate. Heparin is easy to use, but the patient is, by necessity, exposed to the anticoagulant for a prolonged period of time. As many patients who suffer from trauma or are in a postoperative state are at increased risk for bleeding, such patient exposure to heparin may be harmful. In our series, we showed that 26% of patients dialyzed with heparin anticoagulation experienced bleeding compared with 0% in citrate anticoagulated treatments (19,20).

Saline flushes were also associated with a low bleeding risk, but filter clotting occurred in 12% of cases and treatments were terminated because of clotting in 28% of cases (19,20). Consequently, we have found the use of regional citrate anticoagulation to be more advantageous in certain patients at high risk for bleeding complications.

Anticoagulation with citrate is achieved by the binding of citrate to ionized calcium, an essential cofactor for coagulation. The citrate is introduced into the circuit as the blood exits the patient and travels through the filter where some of it is removed; most of it enters the patient's systemic circulation. Postfilter-ionized calcium levels are lowered to 0.25 mmol/L in order to maintain system patency. ☞ **Systemic citrate is normally metabolized in the liver, liberating three bicarbonate ions for each citrate molecule.** ☞ Because of the mechanism of action and subsequent metabolism, citrate anticoagulation requires careful attention to acid–base balance and serum calcium levels. The use of citrate also requires the preparation of specialized solutions, which may not be available in all centers (18–20). Although frequent saline flushes have been used in CRRT, the filter life under such circumstances is markedly reduced. Filter life with heparin is also less than that achieved with citrate.

A number of electrolyte abnormalities are seen during CRRT. Although hyperkalemia and hyperphosphatemia are common complications of ARF, both IHD and CRRT are effective at adequately controlling both electrolytes. However, during CRRT hypokalemia and hypophosphatemia occur, commonly owing to the removal of both solutes during UF and diffusion, while replacing removed ultrafiltrate with solutions that do not contain either electrolyte. ☞ **Phosphate control is achieved faster with CRRT and phosphate reductions are often more profound than those seen with IHD (51).** ☞ The treatment for either hypokalemia or hyperphosphatemia is to replace the electrolytes with either potassium chloride, potassium phosphate, or sodium phosphate, depending on the need.

☞ **Hypocalcemia is a major concern in patients receiving CRRT with citrate anticoagulation (52,53).** ☞ Because citrate complexes ionized calcium, its administration often requires that the patients receive a calcium chloride infusion into a vein outside of the dialysis circuit in order to maintain appropriate systemic calcium levels. Normally, metabolism of citrate liberates the bound calcium, thus limiting overall ionized calcium declines. However, in patients with liver disease and reduced capacity to metabolize citrate, severe hypocalcemia may occur if inadequate calcium chloride replacement is not administered. Conversely, aggressive calcium chloride administration may result in hypercalcemia (52). This is particularly noted when patients with temporary liver dysfunction recover their ability to metabolize citrate liberating large amounts of ionized calcium. In most cases, stopping the calcium infusion and continuation of dialysis are sufficient to control hypercalcemia.

Acidosis is treated by a variety of mechanisms in CRRT. Most dialysate solutions contain either lactate or bicarbonate and thus limit bicarbonate diffusion in acidemic patients. The use of bicarbonate-based replacement solutions allow for delivery of large amounts of bicarbonate without causing volume overload or sodium overload. The exact effect of using bicarbonate replacement on outcomes has not been systematically studied. The use of citrate anticoagulation also delivers bicarbonate to the patient once the citrate is metabolized. Overall, CRRT seems to result in more rapid and normalized correction of electrolyte abnormalities when compared with IHD (52).

Intraoperative Dialysis
Overview
The use of dialysis in the operating room has emerged recently as a potentially important therapy for intraoperative management of both solute and volume control. The use of SCUF in cardiothoracic surgery has been in place for many years and has been successful at controlling fluid overload. Recently, the use of intraoperative CRRT in patients with combined liver and renal failure undergoing orthotopic liver transplantation (OLT) has gained acceptance.

Potential Advantages
☞ **Tight control of both intravascular volume and plasma solute concentration constitute the major advantages of intraoperative CRRT.** ☞ Often, patients require infusion of large volumes of blood products, colloids, and crystalloids during lengthy operative procedures in which hemodynamic instability is common, such as in OLT. The use of intraoperative CRRT may prove beneficial in such patients. Previously, we published our experience with the use of intraoperative CRRT in OLT and showed that the typical

patient required approximately 35 units of packed red blood cells and 4–5 L of crystalloid (54). In the setting of renal failure, administration of such large volumes may cause respiratory compromise.

Hyperkalemia secondary to administration of large volume of blood products is better controlled with intra-operative CRRT in oliguric patients. Moreover, recent studies have shown that during OLT there is a predictable pattern of cytokine release that may correlate with hemo-dynamic instability. Specifically, Miki et al. (55) showed that during the anhepatic phase and up to four hours after reperfusion of the allograft serum levels of interleukin (IL)-1 and IL-6 are increased two to three times the baseline values. Potentially, CRRT may be advantageous if limitation of such rises in cytokine levels can be achieved.

Potential Disadvantages

☞ **The important disadvantages of intraoperative CRRT include the need for anticoagulation of the circuit, and logistics.** ☞ The use of heparin would be contraindicated during surgery, but regional citrate anticoagulation described here may be safer. We reported our experience with the use of regional citrate anticoagulation in 13 patients undergoing OLT (54). The main disadvantage was transient changes in ionized calcium concentrations that were related to either excessive exogenous calcium administration or excessive citrate administration with blood products (54). Protocol-driven adjustments in citrate and calcium administration may be safer for maintaining adequate circuit anticoagulation while avoiding significant serum calcium changes.

The use of CRRT in operations requires the presence of a dialysis machine in what is already a fairly limited space. More important is the need for a well-coordinated multi-disciplinary team composed of nephrologists, anesthesiologists, dialysis nurses, operating room nurses, and ICU nurses to ensure that all facets of dialysis, including UF, anticoagulation, vascular access function, and machine troubleshooting are addressed.

SELECTION OF DIALYSIS MODALITY
Overview

In general, the goal of dialysis is to provide adequate renal replacement and/or support while minimizing complications of therapy. Unfortunately, there is no consensus regarding the timing, duration, frequency, and amount of dialysis to be administered for patients with ARF in the ICU. Thus, in current practice, modality choice is dictated by the experience of the provider and the availability of various modalities (56). In a recent survey of nephrologists in the United States, IHD was used most commonly for ARF in the ICU followed by CRRT and peritoneal dialysis (PD) (57). Of those who used IHD most commonly, familiarity with the procedure, efficacy, and ease of use were cited as the main reasons for choosing IHD. Continuous renal replacement therapy techniques were reserved, in large part, for patients with hemodynamic instability or those in need of aggressive nutritional support. The few who preferred PD felt that it offered several unique advantages. Most notably, it provides dialysis with remarkable hemodynamic stability. In addition, PD does not require the use of anticoagulation.

It is clear that the choice of modality must be tailored to the needs of each patient. The factors that influence the selection of dialysis modality can be divided into three main categories: those specific to the patient, those specific to the

modality, and those specific to the practice environment. ☞ **The recognition that CRRT provides the greatest advantages in critically ill patients has fostered an increased trend toward the use of this technique, especially in those with hemodynamic instability, those with traumatic brain injury (TBI), and/or sepsis/systemic inflammatory response syndrome (SIRS).** ☞

Patient Factors
Indications for Renal Replacement Therapy

The indications for dialysis in the ICU are both diverse and prone to modification over the course of the disease. Consequently, the indication for initiating dialysis will influence the type of modality selected. Certain modalities are more efficient at solute control while others are more efficient at controlling fluid balance. For example, if the main indication for initiation of dialysis is hyperkalemia in a hemodynamically stable patient, then IHD is the modality of choice. Conversely, if volume overload is the main indication for dialysis, particularly in the setting of hemodynamic instability, CRRT may be the preferred modality (10,38,39,41). In many cases, however, the indications are multiple and often include solute and fluid components. In such cases, the time course of the desired response will influence the choice of modality. It is important to recognize that indications and modality selection do influence outcome. In our randomized controlled trial comparing CRRT with IHD, patients dialyzed for solute control had a better outcome than those dialyzed predominantly for volume control (13). Patients dialyzed for both solute and volume control had the worst outcome. The use of protocol-driven hour-by-hour fluid balance management in CRRT affords more sustained and predictable control of volume status. In addition, Bellomo et al. (58) showed that CVVHDF was superior to IHD at controlling azotemia 24 hours after initiation of RRT in ICU patients with ARF (58).

In a recent study of ARF resulting from rhabdomyolysis in victims of the 1999 Marmara earthquake in Turkey, only 15% of patients with ARF died. Dialysis was a predictor of worse outcome with a mortality rate of 17% of those who required dialysis compared with only 9% of those who did not require dialysis. Interestingly, most of the deaths occurred in patients with coexisting thoracic or abdominal trauma and in patients who required an amputation. The level of creatine phosphokinase (CPK) rise did not correlate with mortality (59). A recent report from the experience of the 1999 Taiwan earthquake showed that ARF occurred in 55% of the 90 rhabdomyolysis cases requiring dialysis that were identified. Acute renal failure was associated with a higher mortality (17% vs. 0%), but CPK values were unrelated to mortality. Of the 52 patients with ARF, 32 required dialysis with either IHD or CRRT, but further details are not provided in the report (60).

Presence of Other Organ Failure

The presence of nonrenal organ failure concomitantly with ARF has a major impact on outcome. Data from the European Dialysis and Transplant Association (EDTA) has shown that patients with isolated ARF experienced a mortality of only 8% (61). Moreover, several investigators have shown that the greater the number of failing organ systems in MODS, the greater the mortality. Lohr et al. (62) described a clinical index to predict survival in patients with ARF undergoing dialysis. These investigators found that the presence of associated organ system failure worsened mortality.

Moreover, the presence of other organ failures in the setting of ARF can influence the choice of modality selection. For example, patients with an abdominal surgery, such as an abdominal aortic aneurysm repair or perforated duodenal ulcer will not be candidates for peritoneal dialysis. Patients with severe hypotension will not be likely to tolerate IHD. Additionally, the impact of anticoagulation is an important consideration. PD and IHD can both be performed without anticoagulation; however, CRRT usually requires some form of anticoagulation (18). The influence of the therapy itself on the function of other compromised organs is another important consideration. For example, IHD, but not CRRT, is often associated with changes in intracranial pressure (ICP) (63,64).

Continuous therapies generally do not compromise hemodynamic stability; however, if not monitored closely volume depletion can ensue from lack of adequate replacement fluid administration. A recent report by Stoves et al. (65) showed that bradykinin release at the start of CRRT was correlated with initiation of hypotension. Interestingly, hypotension was uncommon in patients with sepsis receiving pressor support. Peritoneal dialysis may contribute to worsening hypoalbuminemia in patients with liver disease and may not be the modality of choice in that patient population (36). Moreover, PD is often associated with the enhanced removal of albumin-bound drugs, a problem (or benefit) not associated with hemodialysis (36).

Vascular Access

The ability to obtain appropriate vascular access is one of the most important factors affecting the ability to provide adequate dialysis therapy. The use of arterial vascular access catheters has fallen out of favor because of the many complications encountered with these catheters. A number of complications can limit the ability to use a venous catheter adequately. Clotting or malpositioning of the catheter in the vein can lead to unforeseen reductions in blood flow rate. Currently used peristaltic blood pumps are usually set to withdraw blood from the access at a certain rate. However, in the presence of partial clotting, actual blood flow may be lower than the dialed rate. Such a complication may go unnoticed for many hours. Another important complication is the presence of recirculation in which a portion of "clean" blood returned to the patient from the dialyzer is redrawn by the peristaltic pump before it enters the patients' overall blood pool (17). Such recirculation will limit the efficacy of dialysis, as the same portion of blood is dialyzed repeatedly.

Infectious and thrombotic complications of dialysis catheters are an additional important consideration. A recent report showed that femoral catheters were associated with increased infectious and thrombotic complications when compared with subclavian catheters (66). In general, subclavian catheters are discouraged in patients with ARF, because stenosis of the subclavian vein may limit the ability to place arm vascular access in the future if the patient survives, but does not recover renal function.

Mobility

In cases where a patient will need to be moved from the bedside for imaging studies, surgery, and so on, it may be difficult to perform CRRT. It is usually not possible to transfer CRRT equipment with the patient because most current CRRT machines are not equipped with a battery-operated module. Disconnecting the patient from CRRT will deprive the patient of important dialysis and UF time, lowering the efficacy of the treatment. Moreover, because of the need for more intensive nursing monitoring with CRRT, patients who are not in an ICU setting where there is no one-to-one nursing are not candidates for CRRT.

Dialysis Modality Factors
Membrane Choice

There are two factors to consider when choosing the type of membrane used for dialysis: biocompatibility and cytokine removal efficiency. The first issue (membrane biocompatibility) has several ramifications (67–70). Complement activation and neutrophil sequestration are known to occur in IHD with the use of certain membranes. However, because in CRRT the patient's blood is exposed to the membrane for a prolonged time, the issue of membrane interactions is of paramount importance. Polysulfone and polyacrylnitrile membranes do not seem to activate complement and are often used in CRRT (71). In addition, biocompatible membranes seem to be associated with improved renal recovery (68,69,71–73). However, a recent study comparing cellulose acetate membranes with polysulfone membranes for acute IHD showed no difference in survival or renal recovery (72). A meta-analysis by Subramanian et al. (74) showed that synthetic membranes confer a significant survival advantage over cellulose-based membranes.

The second issue concerning membrane selection is the finding that membranes differ in their capacity to clear certain cytokines, such as TNFα, IL-1β, and IL-6. Conceivably, removal of these cytokines at a critical stage of disease progression may influence outcome. An in vitro model of CAVHD showed that a polyacrylnitrile membrane was two- to threefold more efficient at removing TNFα when compared with a polysulfone or polyamide membrane (75,76). Nevertheless, human studies have shown the ability to remove cytokines in CRRT, but blood levels of cytokines remain unchanged in adults (77–79). This is likely related to the membrane surface area compared with the volume of total body water and solute (which is larger in adults than in children). Although this remains an active area of research, it is not yet a factor that can be consistently used in modality selection at the current time.

Dose of Dialysis

Unfortunately, there are no standard methods for the assessment of dialysis dose in ARF. In ESRD patients, dialysis dose is assessed by using urea kinetic modeling. In such a model, the basic elements measured are the urea levels prior to and after dialysis. Many formulae exist that incorporate weight, UF volume, time, and change in blood urea nitrogen (BUN) for assessment of dialysis dose. A main assumption of these models is that ESRD patients have a relatively constant urea generation rate and are at steady state. Because of this assumption, the method of dialysis dose determination used in ESRD is not directly applicable to patients with ARF. ARF patients tend to have fluctuating body fluid composition and varying urea generation rates. Nevertheless, a number of factors are related to the dialysis dose delivered. For example, in intermittent therapies, higher blood flow rates and longer durations of therapy are associated with an increased dose of dialysis delivered. In some studies, changes in BUN have been used as a surrogate for dose intensity. Clark et al. (44) compared IHD with CRRT using a computer model to determine the number of IHD sessions that would be required to achieve equivalent control of uremia. They found that for a 50-kg male, an average of

4.4 sessions of IHD per week was required to achieve the same uremic control obtained with CRRT. However, in patients with a weight of greater than 90 kg, equivalent uremic control could not be achieved with even daily IHD. Bellomo et al. (58) showed that in similar critically ill patients CRRT was more effective at control of azotemia than IHD.

Although it is difficult to measure dose per se, many have studied the factors that influence dose and their effects on outcomes. In hemofiltration techniques, the amount of ultrafiltrate generated per kilogram of body weight per unit time is associated with dose. Ronco et al. (80) have shown that in patients treated with hemofiltration techniques, a filtration rate of 35 ml/hr/kg was associated with improved 15-day survival. Honore et al. (81) showed that short-term high-volume hemofiltration (35 L in the first four hours) improved survival in patients with septic shock. Schiffl et al. (82) compared, prospectively, daily hemodialysis with every other day treatments. They showed an improvement in survival among patients on daily hemodialysis (15% vs. 22%, $p < 0.05$). Paganini et al. (83,84) showed that approximately 65% of IHD patients received a dialysis dose as measured by urea kinetic modeling that was lower than prescribed. The nonsurvivors in that group of patients had significantly lower actual dose delivered compared with survivors. However, another study by Bouman et al. (85) showed no improvement in 28-day mortality and recovery from renal failure when early initiation of hemofiltration and high ultrafiltrate volumes were used. While the results are provocative, they need to be confirmed in a well-designed large multicenter trial. Such a trial is in progress [The VA/NIH Acute Renal Failure Trian Network Study (ATN)]. The ATN study is a multicenter, randomized controlled trial comparing two dosing strategies for RRT in ARF. In both treatment arms patients move freely between IHD and CRRT and SLED, as determined by their hemodynamic status. In the intensive therapy arm, IHD and SLED are provided on a basis of six times per week with a target K_t/V of 1.2–1.4 per treatment. Continuous renal replacement therapy is provided with an effluent flow rate of 35 ml/kg/hr. In the less intensive therapy arm, the same modalities of treatment are used; however, IHD and SLED are provided on a basis of three times per week, and CRRT is provided with an effluent flow rate of 20 ml/kg/hr. The primary study endpoint is 60-day all-cause mortality. Target enrollment is 1164 patients.

Intermittent vs. Continuous Therapies

Because of the heterogeneity of ARF patients with respect to illness severity and comorbidities, it is difficult to adequately assess the effect of a particular renal replacement modality on survival. Nevertheless, a number of studies have compared IHD with CRRT in an effort to delineate whether one modality is superior to another with regard to survival. Several retrospective analyses in the early 1990s showed that it was likely that CRRT offered a survival advantage when compared with IHD (43,47,86,87).

In 1986, Mauritz et al. (88) compared IHD with either CAVH or CVVH and found no difference in survival between the groups. In 1992, Bellomo et al. (38,47) compared survival in 84 critically ill patients treated with conventional dialysis with 83 age-matched, APACHE II score-matched, and number of organs failing-matched patients treated with either CAVHDF or CVVHDF. Overall survival was 30% and 41% in the conventional dialysis and CRRT groups, respectively ($p = $ NS).

The same group then compared a prospectively treated group with the same conventional dialysis control group in their initial study. In this second study, patients treated with CVVHDF had better survival if they had two, three, or four organs failing or an APACHE II score of 24–29 (87). However, at the extremes of illness severity survival was not different. This study is difficult to interpret in view of the use of a retrospective control group. In 1993, Kruczynski et al. (89) reported a retrospective analysis of 12 patients treated with CAVH versus 23 patients treated with conventional hemodialysis. Survival was better in the CAVH compared with the conventional dialysis group (25% vs. 82%, $p < 0.001$). However, patients in the conventional dialysis group were significantly older.

In 1991, Kierdorf (90) retrospectively compared 73 patients treated with CVVH with 73 age-matched controls treated with IHD and found a significant survival advantage in the CVVH group. In 1995, van Bommel et al. (91,92) retrospectively compared 34 patients treated with IHD to 60 patients treated with CAVHDF. The CAVHDF had a higher APACHE II score, but survival was not different between the two groups. A recent retrospective analysis by Jacka et al. (93) showed better renal recovery in patients initially treated with CRRT. However, mortality was not affected significantly by RRT mode (93). Thus, the data from retrospective analyses is conflicting, with some studies showing a survival advantage and others showing no advantage for CRRT. A comprehensive review of multiple studies showed that no survival advantage was conferred with the use of continuous therapies (94).

To date there are about six prospective, randomized trials comparing IHD with CRRT. The first study by Kierdorf and Sieberth had a target enrollment of 400 patients (95). An interim analysis of 100 patients showed a survival of 39.6% in the CVVH group and 34.1% in the IHD group. However, five patients in the IHD group were excluded from the analysis as they failed to complete the therapy because of "hemodynamic instability." The final results of this study were not published. In our study, 166 patients with ARF requiring dialysis were randomized to either CRRT ($n = 84$) or IHD ($n = 82$) (13). Patients with a mean arterial pressure (MAP) of less than 70 were excluded. Patients in the two groups were similar except that there were more males in the CRRT group and the APACHE II and III scores were higher in the CRRT group. Intensive care unit (59% vs. 41%, $p < 0.02$) and hospital (65% vs. 47%, $p < 0.02$) mortality was worse in the CRRT group. However, group analysis showed a preponderance of nonrenal conditions associated with a higher mortality in the CRRT group. When logistic regression was applied to adjust for this bias, the odds ratio for death with CRRT was 1.3 (95% CI, 0.6–2.7, $p = $ NS). Subgroup analysis showed that renal recovery was improved in survivors of CRRT when compared with survivors of IHD (92% vs. 59%, $p = 0.01$). One of the main limitations of the study was the exclusion of patients with a MAP of less than 70 mmHg, a group that is likely to benefit the most from CRRT.

One multicenter prospective survey of 28 ICUs in France demonstrated that CRRT was used in 60% of patients dialyzed for ARF. Patients on CRRT had a greater number of organ dysfunction and higher mortality than IHD (79% vs. 59%) (96). More recently, Uehlinger et al. (97) randomized 125 patients over a 30-month period to treatment with either CVVHDF or IHD from a total of 191 patients with ARF in a tertiary-care university hospital ICU and analyzed the impact on in-hospital mortality, recovery from renal failure, and length of hospitalization. The two groups were comparable at the start of RRT with respect to age (62 ± 15 vs. 62 ± 15 years, CVVHDF vs. IHD), gender (66% vs. 73% male sex), number of failed organ systems (2.4 ± 1.5 vs. 2.5 ± 1.6), Simplified Acute Physiology Scores (57 ± 17 vs. 58 ± 23), septicaemia (43% vs. 51%), shock (59% vs. 58%), or previous surgery (53% vs. 45%). Mortality rates in the hospital (47% vs. 51%, CVVHDF vs. IHD, $p = 0.72$) or in the ICU (34% vs. 38%, $p = 0.71$) were independent of the technique of RRT applied. Hospital length of stay in the survivors was comparable in patients on CVVHDF [median (range) 20 (6–71) days, $n = 36$] and in those on IHD [30 (2–89) days, $n = 27$, $p = 0.25$]. The duration of RRT required was the same in both groups. The authors concluded that there was no evidence for a survival benefit of continuous versus intermittent RRT in ICU patients with ARF (97).

A meta-analysis of continuous versus intermittent therapies looking at all randomized and observational studies and applying strict selection criteria showed several interesting results (98). Overall, CRRT was associated with a lower risk of hospital death (RR 0.48, CI 0.34–0.69, $p < 0.0005$) than IHD when studies in which patients with a similar baseline severity of illness was present. Overall mortality was similar when the two modalities were compared and even after adjustment for a number of factors including quality of the study, underlying condition of the patient, and type of membrane used. The main conclusion of the authors was that "current evidence is insufficient to draw strong conclusions regarding the mode of replacement therapy for ARF." The authors did note that their analysis did not show that CRRT was worse than IHD even after numerous adjustments (98). Another meta-analysis by Tonelli et al. (99) showed that in comparison with IHD therapy, CRRT does not improve survival or renal recovery in unselected critically ill patients with ARF.

Although there is no definitive evidence that CRRT is superior to IHD, it may be inherently invalid to make such a broad comparison. It might be more appropriate to categorize patients into subgroups. For example, patients with heart failure may have a different outcome with CRRT than patients with sepsis or trauma. Similarly, patients with end-stage liver disease who do not receive a transplant will have a grave outcome irrespective of the modality used (64). Selection of modality based on the anticipated duration of therapy is better judged by the needs of the patients at the time of initiation. In hemodynamically unstable patients in whom fluid control is the main indication, it may be more appropriate to initiate CRRT, whereas in the trauma patient with isolated extremity injuries and rhabdomyolysis-mediated ARF and hyperkalemia and normal blood pressure, an intermittent modality may be preferable.

Logistic Factors
Cost
It remains unclear whether CRRT is more expensive than IHD. Some studies have suggested that CRRT may be slightly more expensive (100,101). The higher cost of CRRT can be accounted for in large part by the higher price of the hemofilters that are generally different than those used for IHD. The filters used for IHD are cheaper because they are purchased in bulk for use in the ESRD population. This disparity in cost may be reduced if CRRT is used more frequently and if filter life is extended by adequate anticoagulation. Physician time spent per patient is increased for CRRT;

however, this can be reduced as the physician gains familiarity with the procedure. At our institution, standardized protocols for fluid, electrolyte, and anticoagulation management have markedly reduced the time spent on monitoring and adjusting the CRRT prescription.

Nursing Expertise and Other Support
Unlike IHD and PD, CRRT requires active participation of the critical care nurse caring for the patient. Consequently, nurses who are unfamiliar with CRRT may have difficulty managing the accurate fluid and electrolyte monitoring that is required to minimize complications (49,50). The availability of simple, easy to understand flow sheets, instructional booklets, and backup support serves to minimize errors related to nursing involvement (49). One of the main advantages of CRRT is the ability to provide the patient with improved nutrition. As a result, involvement of clinical nutrition personnel in the care of the patient becomes essential. Preparation of custom dialysate and replacement fluid, as well as drug dosing adjustment will require the involvement of skilled pharmacists who are familiar with the pharmacokinetics associated with the different dialysis modalities.

     ☛ **Selection of dialysis modality depends on patient, modality, and logistic factors.** ☛

Summary of Modality Selection
A number of factors play a role in the process of deciding which dialysis modality is most appropriate for a particular clinical situation. Consequently, it is important for the intensivist to become familiar with the various modalities available and to gain some understanding of the differences between the modalities and their relative advantages and disadvantages. Table 5 summarizes recommendations regarding the choice of dialysis modality in common clinical circumstances.

DIALYTIC REMOVAL OF CYTOKINES FOR SEPSIS

☛ **The sepsis syndrome is associated with the presence of high levels of circulating and tissue cytokines that result in impairment of vascular permeability, hypotension, and renal failure.** ☛ Removal of such cytokines is a potentially attractive therapy for the sepsis syndrome. TNF-α and IL-1 are important mediators of the sepsis response. Early in vitro studies showed that TNF-α was mainly adsorbed to the dialysis membrane and very little was actually filtered (102–104). Hoffman et al. (78) showed that TNF-α levels did not change after hemofiltration in patients with sepsis.

In contrast, Millar et al. (105) and Journois et al. (106) showed that hemofiltration reduced TNF-α levels in pediatric patients undergoing cardiopulmonary bypass surgery. Silvester (103) showed that reductions in TNF-α can be achieved after four hours of hemofiltration if a polyacrylnitrate (PAN) filter was used as opposed to a polysulfone filter. The reports for IL-1 are similarly inconclusive. Lonnemann et al. (102) showed that IL-1 is adsorbed onto PAN filters, but not filtered. Human studies failed to show a reduction in IL-1 levels, irrespective of the dialyzer type.

More recent studies compared CVVH with CVVHD with a polysulfone dialyzer and blood and dialysate flow rates of 70 mL/min in the treatment of patients with sepsis.

Table 5   Recommendation for Initial Choice of Dialysis Modality for Acute Renal Failure (ARF)

Indication	Clinical condition	Preferred therapy
Uncomplicated ARF	Antibiotic nephrotoxicity	IHD, PD
Fluid removal	Cardiogenic shock, CP bypass	SCUF, CAVH
Uremia	Complicated ARF in intensive care unit	CVVHDF, CAVHDF, IHD
Increased intracranial pressure	Subarachnoid hemorrhage, hepatorenal syndrome	CVVHD, CAVHD
Shock	Sepsis, ARDS	CVVH, CVVHDF, CAVHDF
Nutrition	Burns	CVVHDF, CAVHDF, CVVH
Poisons	Theophylline, barbiturates	IHD, CVVHDF
Electrolyte abnormalities	Marked hyperkalemia	IHD, CVVHDF
ARF in pregnancy	Uremia in second, third trimester	PD

Abbreviations: ARDS, acute respiratory distress syndrome; CAVH, continuous arteriovenous hemofiltration; CAVHDF, continuous arteriovenous hemodiafiltration; CVVH, continuous venovenous hemofiltration; CVVHD, continuous venovenous hemodialysis; CVVHDF, continuous venovenous hemodiafiltration; CAVHD, continuous arteriovenous hemodialysis; PD, peritoneal dialysis; SCUF, slow continuous ultrafiltration.
Source: From Ref. 108.

These studies showed that blood from patients treated with CVVH or CVVHD had a reduced capacity to generate TNF-α in a cell culture model. The implication of these studies was that blood treated with CVVH or CVVHD had a reduced capacity to generate proinflammatory cytokines. Interestingly, the effect was more profound in the CVVHD group. Spent dialysate from the CVVHD-treated patients was able to suppress TNF-α production in donor blood by 33%, whereas no suppression was seen from ultrafiltrate obtained from the CVVH patients (107). The use of high-volume CVVH with ultrafiltrate volumes of 8 L/hr was shown to be beneficial in patients with sepsis and renal failure.

When high-volume CVVH was applied to 20 patients with severe septic shock, responders were noted to have received the therapy earlier and had higher UF volumes when compared with nonresponders. In this study, response was defined as an improvement in cardiac index, mixed venous O_2 saturation, pH, and a reduction in pressor dose. Overall, data regarding the utility of conventional CRRT techniques in the treatment of sepsis are lacking and its use for the sole purpose of treatment of sepsis cannot be recommended at this time.

Emerging dialysis techniques, such as high-flux CVVHD and high-volume CVVH may have some application to the treatment of sepsis in the future. Randomized clinical trials to evaluate the efficacy of extracorporeal treatments for sepsis are needed.

EYE TO THE FUTURE

The determination of the optimal dialysis modality for various clinical presentations of ARF is an area of active investigation. Continuous therapies will likely take the lead role as the dialysis modality of choice for patients with hemodynamic instability, bleeding risk, and possibly the sepsis syndrome. Intermittent therapies will continue to play an important role in patients with isolated ARF, hemodynamic stability, and severe electrolyte abnormalities that require immediate correction. The expansion of dialysis to include treatment of nonrenal conditions is an expanding field. It is conceivable that dialysis may be used more extensively for treatment of the sepsis syndrome, certain intoxications, and heart failure.

SUMMARY

Acute renal failure in the ICU is a clinically diverse entity. Consequently, the indications for initiation of dialysis therapy are varied. In general, the indications are either solute control, volume control, or both. A variety of dialysis modalities are available to the intensivist and nephrologist; however, there is no consensus as to the optimal modality for any particular group of patients. Nevertheless, a careful understanding of the particular benefits, limitations, and potential complications of each modality coupled with a thorough assessment of individual patient needs formulate the basis for dialysis modality selection. In certain circumstances, the more conventional intermittent therapies are sufficient, whereas in other settings, CRRT techniques are advantageous. The impact of modality selection on outcome remains an area of significant controversy. Future studies in which more uniformity within specific subgroups of patients with ARF is sought may shed light on the optimal modality for a particular patient group. Newer therapies aimed at more optimal and more specific blood purification may prove promising in the management of complex critically ill patients with ARF and other comorbid conditions.

KEY POINTS

- Indications for dialysis generally fall into one of three broad categories: solute indications such as marked azotemia, volume indications such as fluid overload, or both.
- CRRT provides improved hemodynamic stability, continuous electrolyte control, improved dialysis adequacy and easier control of volume status.
- Recirculation associated with dual-lumen venous catheters have been shown to be worse in femoral (16%) when compared with the subclavian catheters (4%, $p = 0.0001$) location (17).
- The most significant disadvantages of IHD in the critically ill patient with ARF are related to hypotension and the possibility of worsening the severity of the renal injury.

- Continuous renal replacement therapy is unique in that solute removal is, in effect, dissociated from fluid removal.
- CRRT provides improved hemodynamic stability, continuous electrolyte control, improved dialysis adequacy and easier control of volume status.
- Rapid alterations in sodium and fluid status have been shown to occur in IHD. Such alterations are implicated as a cause for the cerebral edema that can be observed in IHD.
- Systemic citrate is normally metabolized in the liver liberating three bicarbonate ions for each citrate molecule.
- Phosphate control is achieved faster with CRRT and phosphate reductions are often more profound than those seen with IHD (51).
- Hypocalcemia is a major concern in patients receiving CRRT with citrate anticoagulation (52,53).
- Tight control of both intravascular volume and plasma solute concentration constitute the major advantages of intraoperative CRRT.
- The important disadvantages of intraoperative CRRT include the need for anticoagulation of the circuit, and logistics.
- The recognition that CRRT provides the greatest advantages in critically ill patients has fostered an increased trend toward the use of this technique, especially in those with hemodynamic instability, those with TBI, and or sepsis/SIRS.
- Selection of dialysis modality depends on patient, modality, and logistic factors.
- The sepsis syndrome is associated with the presence of high levels of circulating and tissue cytokines that result in impairment of vascular permeability, hypotension, and renal failure.

REFERENCES

1. Biesenbach G, Zazgornik J, Kaiser W et al. Improvement in prognosis of patients with acute renal failure over a period of 15 years: an analysis of 710 cases in a dialysis center. Am J Nephrol 1992; 12:319–325.
2. Brivet F, Kleinknecht D, Loirat P et al. Acute renal failure in intensive care units—causes, outcome and prognostic factors of hospital mortality. Critical Care Med 1996; 24:192–198.
3. Liano F, Junco E, Pascual J et al. The spectrum of acute renal failure in the intensive care unit compared with that seen in other settings. Kidney Int 1998; 66:S16–S24.
4. Hou S, Bushinsky D, Wish J et al. Hospital-acquired renal insufficiency: a prospective study. Am J Med 1983; 74: 243–248.
5. Manns M, Sigler M, Teehan B. Intradialytic renal haemodynamics—potential consequences for the management of the patient with acute renal failure [editorial]. Nephrol, Dial, Transplant 1997; 12(5):870–2.
6. Yeun J, Depner T. Principles of dialysis. In: Owen WF, Pereira BJ, Sayegh MH, eds. Dialysis and Transplantation: A companion to Brenner & Rector's The Kidney, 1st edn. Philadelphia: WB Sanders, 2000:1–32.
7. Conger JD. Does hemodialysis delay recovery from acute renal failure. Semin Dial 1990; 3:146–150.
8. Solez L, Morel-Maroger L, Sraer J. The morphology of acute tubular necrosis in man: analysis of 57 renal biopsies and comparison with the glycerol model. Medicine 1979; 58:362–367.
9. Kelleher S, Robinette J, Conger JD. Effect of hemorrhagic reduction in blood pressure on recovery from acute renal failure. Kidney Int 1987; 31:725–730.
10. Manns M, Sigler MH, Teehan BP. Advantages of continuous venovenous hemodialysis (CVVHD) in acute renal failure. (Abstract 905) J Am Soc Nephrol 1995; 6(3):470.
11. Manns M, Sigler M, Teehan B. Factors influencing the residual kidney function during intermittent hemodialysis (IHD) in acute renal failure (ARF). (Abstract) Nephrol, Dial, Transplant 1995; 10 (6):1018.
12. Mehta RL. Indications for dialysis in the ICU: renal replacement vs. renal support. Blood Purification 2001; 19(2):277–232.
13. Mehta R, McDonald B, Gabbai F et al. A randomized clinical trial of continuous versus intermittent dialysis for acute renal failure. Kidney Int 2001; 60:1154–1163.
14. Alsous F, Khamiees M, DeGirolamo A. Negative fluid balance predicts survival in patients with septic shock. Chest 2000; 117(6):1749–1754.
15. Mukau L, Latimer RG. Acute hemodialysis in the surgical intensive care unit. Am Surg 1988; 54(9):548–552.
16. Weiss L, Danielson B, Wikstrom B, et al. Continuous arteriovenous hemofiltration in the treatment of 100 critically ill patients with acute renal failure: report on clinical outcome and nutritional aspects. Clin Nephrol 1989; 31(4):184–189.
17. Leblanc M, Fedak S, Mokris G et al. Blood recirculation in temporary central catheters for acute hemodialysis. Clin Nephrol 1996; 45(5):315–319.
18. Mehta RL. Anticoagulation strategies for continuous renal replacement therapies: what works? Am J Kid Dis 1996; 28(5) (Suppl 3):S8–S14.
19. Ward D. The approach to anticoagulation in patients treated with extracorporeal therapy in the intensive care unit. Adv Renal Replace Ther 1997; 4(2):160–173.
20. Ward D, Mehta RL. Extracorporeal management of acute renal failure patients at high risk of bleeding. Kidney Int 1993; 43 (Suppl 41):S237–S244.
21. Mehta RL, Chertow GM. Selection of dialysis modality. In: Owen WF, Pereira BJ, Sayegh MH, eds. Dialysis and Transplantation: A Companion to Brenner & Rector's The Kidney, 1st edn. Philadelphia: WB Sanders, 2000:403–417.
22. Bellomo R, Ronco C. Continuous renal replacement therapy in the intensive care unit. Intensive Care Med 1999; 25:781–789.
23. Bellomo R, Ronco C, Mehta RL. Nomenclature for continuous renal replacement therapies. Am J Kid Dis 1996; 28(5) (Suppl 3): S2–S7.
24. Lameire N, Van Biesen W, Vanholder R et al. The place of intermittent hemodialysis in the treatment of acute renal failure in the ICU patient. Kidney Int 1998; 53 (Suppl 66): S110–S119.
25. De Vries P, Olthof CG, Solf A et al. Fluid balance during hemodialysis and hemofiltration: the effect of dialysate sodium and a variable ultrafiltration rate. Nephrol, Dial, Transplant 1991; 6:257–263.
26. Karsou S, Jaber B, Pereira B. Impact of intermittent hemodialysis variables on clinical outcomes in acute renal failure. Am J Kidney Dis 2000; 35:980–991.
27. Schortgen F, Soubrier N, Delclaux C et al. Hemodynamic tolerance of intermittent hemodialysis in critically ill patients. Am J Respir Crit Care Med 2000; 162:197–202.
28. Roberts M, Daugirdas J. REDY sorbent hemodialysis. In: Daugirdas JT, Ing TS, eds. Handbook of Dialysis, 2nd edn. Boston: Little, Brown and Company, 1994:198–217.
29. Shapiro W. The current status of sorbent hemodialysis. Semin Dial 1990; 3:40–45.
30. Botella J, Ghezzi P, Sanz-Moreno C et al. Multicentric study on paired filtration dialysis as a short, highly efficient dialysis technique. Nephrol Dial Transplant 1991; 6:715–721.
31. Kumar V, Craig M, Depner T et al. Extended daily dialysis: a new approach to renal replacement for acute renal failure in the intensive care unit. Am J Kidney Dis 2000; 36(2):294–300.
32. Lonnemann G, Floege J, Kliem V. Extended daily veno-venous high-flux haemodialysis in patients with acute renal failure and multiple organ dysfunction syndrome using a single batch dialysis system. Nephrol Dial Transplant 2000; 15:1189–1193.

33. Schlaeper C, Amerling R, Manns M et al. High clearance continuous renal replacement therapy with a modified dialysis machine. Kidney Int 1999; 56 (Suppl 72):S20–S23.

34. Lornoy W, De Meester J, Demeyer I et al. Outcome of critically ill patients with acute renal failure treated with slow, extended daily, on-line hemodiafiltration (Abstract 21). In Abstracts of the Sixth International Conference on Continuous Renal Replacement Therapies (CRRT), Blood Purification 2001; 19:338.

35. Marshall M, Golper T, Shaver M et al. Sustained low-efficiency dialysis for critically ill patients requiring renal replacement therapy. Kidney International, 2001; 60:777–785.

36. Kronfol N. Acute peritoneal dialysis prescription. In: Daugirdas JT, Ing TS, eds. Handbook of Dialysis, 2nd edn. Boston: Little, Brown and Company, 1994:301–309.

37. Mehta RL. Continuous dialysis therapeutic techniques. In: Henrich WL, ed. Principles and Practice of Dialysis, 2nd edn. Baltimore: Williams & Wilkins, 1999:141–159.

38. Bellomo R, Parkin G, Love J. Use of continuous haemodiafiltration: an approach to the management of acute renal failure in the critically ill. Am J Nephrol 1992; 12:240–245.

39. Davenport A, Will E, Davidson A. Improved cardiovascular stability during continuous modes of renal replacement therapy in critically ill patients with acute hepatic and renal failure. Crit Car Med 1993; 21:328–338.

40. John S, Griesbach D, Baumgärtel M et al. Effects of continuous haemofiltration vs. intermittent haemodialysis on systemic haemodynamics and splanchnic regional perfusion in septic shock patients: a prospective, randomized clinical trial. Nephrol, Dial, Transplant 2001; 16:320–327.

41. Misset B, Timsit J, Chevret S et al. A randomized cross-over comparison of the hemodynamic response to intermittent hemodialysis and continuous Hemofiltration in ICU patients with acute renal failure. Intensive Care Med 1996; 22:742–746.

42. Paganini E, O'Hara P, Nakamoto S. Slow continuous ultrafiltration in hemodialysis resistant oliguric acute renal failure patients. Trans Am Soc Artif Intern Organs 1984; 30:173–178.

43. Bellomo R, Farmer M, Parkin G et al. Severe acute renal failure: a comparison of acute hemodiafiltration and conventional dialytic therapy. Nephron 1995; 71:59–64.

44. Clark WR, Mueller B, Kraus A et al. Extracorporeal therapy requirements for patients with acute renal failure. J Am Soc Nephrol 1997; 8:804–812.

45. Clark WR, Ronco C. CRRT efficiency and efficacy in relation to solute size. Kidney Int 1999; 56 (Suppl 72):S3–S7.

46. Monson P, Mehta RL. Nutrition in acute renal failure: a reappraisal for the 1990s. J Ren Nutr 1994; 4:58–77.

47. Bellomo R, Mansfield D, Rumble S et al. Acute renal failure in critical illness: Conventional dialysis versus acute continuous hemodiafiltration. ASAIO J 1992; 38:M654–M657.

48. Tremblay R, Ethier J, Querin S et al. Veno-venous continuous renal replacement therapy for burned patients with acute renal failure. Burns 2000; 26:638–643.

49. Baldwin I. Training, management, and credentialing for CRRT in the ICU. Am J Kidney Dis 1997; 30(5) (Suppl 4):S112–S116.

50. Baldwin I, Bellomo R. Blood flow reduction associated with nursing care activities during continuous renal replacement therapy (Abstract 33). In Abstracts of the Sixth International Conference on Continuous Renal Replacement Therapies (CRRT), Blood Purification 2002; 19:343.

51. Tan K, Bellomo R, M'Pis D et al. Phosphatemic control during acute renal failure: intermittent hemodialysis versus continuous Hemodiafiltration. Int J Artif Organs 2001; 24(4):186–91.

52. Uchino S, Bellomo R, Ronco C. Intermittent versus continuous renal replacement therapy in the ICU: impact on electrolyte and acid-base balance. Intensive Care Med 2001; 27:1037–1043.

53. Meier-Kriesche H, Finkel K, Gitomer J et al. Unexpected severe hypocalcemia during continuous Venovenous hemodialysis with regional citrate anticoagulation. Am J Kidney Dis 1999; 33(4):1–4.

54. Abdeen O, Kohler G, Mehta R et al. Intraoperative continuous renal replacement therapy (IO-CRRT) during liver transplantation. J Am Soc Nephrol 2001; 161A–162A.

55. Miki C, Iriyama K, Mayer AD et al. Energy storage and cytokine response in patients undergoing liver transplantation. Cytokine 1999; 11(3):244–248.

56. Ronco C, Brendolan A, Bellomo R. Continuous renal replacement techniques. Contrib Nephrol 2001; (132):236–51.

57. Mehta RL, Letteri JM. Current status of renal replacement therapy for acute renal failure. A survey of US nephrologists. The National Kidney Foundation Council on Dialysis. Am J Nephrol 1999; 19(3):377–382.

58. Bellomo R, Farmer M, Bhonagiri S et al. Changing acute renal failure treatment from intermittent hemodialysis to continuous hemofiltration: impact on azotemic control. Int J Artif Organs 1999; 22:145–150.

59. Erek E, Sever M, Serdengecti K et al. An overview of morbidity and mortality in patients with acute renal failure due to crush syndrome: the Marmara earthquake experience. Nephrol, Dial, Transplant 2002; 17:33–40.

60. Hwang S, Shu K, Lain J et al. Renal replacement therapy at the time of the Taiwan Chi-Chi earthquake. Nephrol Dial Transplant 2001; 16 (Suppl 5):78–82.

61. Wheeler DC, Feehally J, Walls J. High risk acute renal failure. Q J Med 1986; 234:977–984.

62. Lohr J, McFarlane M, Grantham JJ. A clinical index to predict survival in acute renal failure requiring dialysis. Am J Kidney Dis 1988; 11:254–259.

63. Davenport A, Will E, Davison A. Effect of renal replacement therapy on patients with combined acute renal and fulminant hepatic failure. Kidney Int 1993; 43 (Suppl 41):S245–S251.

64. Fraley D, Burr R, Bernardini J et al. Impact of acute renal failure on mortality in end-stage liver disease with or without transplantation. Kidney Int 1998; 54:518–524.

65. Stoves J, Goode N, Visvanathan R et al. The bradykinin response and early hypotension at the introduction of continuous renal replacement therapy in the intensive care unit. Artif Organs 2001; 25(12):1009–1021.

66. Merrer J, De Jonghe B, Golliot F et al. Complications of femoral and subclavian venous catheterization in critically ill patients. JAMA 2001; 286(6):700–707.

67. Cheung A. Biocompatibility of hemodialysis membranes. J Am Soc Nephrol 1990; 1:150–161.

68. Himmelfarb J, Tolkoff R, Chandran P et al. A multicenter comparison of dialysis membranes in the treatment of acute renal failure requiring dialysis. J Am Soc Nephrol 1998; 9:257–266.

69. Schiffl H. The role of dialyzer biocompatibility in acute renal failure. Blood Purification 2001; 19(1):70–72.

70. Schiffl H, Sitter T, Lang S et al. Bioincompatible membranes place patients with acute renal failure at increased risk of infection. ASAIO J 1995; 41:M709–M712.

71. Schiffl H, Lang SM, Haider M. Biocompatibility of dialyzer membranes may have a negative impact on outcome of acute renal failure, independent of the dose of dialysis delivered: a retrospective multicenter analysis. ASAIO J 1998; 44(5):M418–M422.

72. Albright R, Smelser J, McCarthy J et al. Patient survival and renal recovery in acute renal failure: randomized comparison of cellulose acetate and polysulphone membrane dialyzers. Mayo Clin Proc 2000; 75:1141–1147.

73. Hartman J, Fricke H, Schiffl H. Biocompatible membranes preserve residual renal function in patients undergoing regular hemodialysis. Am J Kidney Dis 1997; 30(3):366–373.

74. Subramanian S, Venkataraman R, Kellum JA. Influence of dialysis membranes on outcomes in acute renal failure: a meta-analysis. Kidney Int 2002; 62(5):1819–1823.

75. Brown A, Mehta RL. Effect of CAVH membranes on transmembrane flux of TNF alpha. J Am Soc Nephrol 1991; 2:316.

76. Barrera P, Janssen E, Demacker P. Removal of interleukin-1 beta and tumor necrosis factor from human plasma by in vitro dialysis with polyacrylnitrate membranes. Lymphokine Cytokine Res 1992; 11:99–104.

77. Hoffman J, Hartl W, Deppisch R et al. Hemofiltration in human sepsis: evidence for elimination of immunomodulatory substances. Kidney Int 1995; 48:1563–1570.

78. Hoffman J, Hartl W, Deppisch R et al. Effect of hemofiltration on hemodynamics and systemic concentrations of anaphylatoxins and cytokines in human sepsis. Intensive Care Med 1996; 22:1360–1367.

79. Ronco C, Ricci Z, Bellomo R. Importance of increased ultrafiltration volume and impact on mortality: sepsis and cytokine story and the role of continuous veno-venous haemofiltration. Curr Opin Nephrol Hypertens 2001; 10:755–761.

80. Ronco C, Bellomo R, Homel P et al. Effects of different doses in continuous veno-venous haemofiltration on outcomes of acute renal failure: a prospective randomised trial. Lancet 2000; 356:26–30.

81. Honore P, Jamek J, Wauthier M et al. Prospective evaluation of short-term, high-volume isovolemic hemofiltration on the hemodynamic course and outcome in patients with intractable circulatory failure resulting from septic shock. Crit Care Med 2000; 28(11):3581–3587.

82. Schiffl H, Lang SM, Konig A et al. Dose of intermittent hemodialysis and outcome of acute renal failure: A prospective randomized study. J Am Soc Nephrol 1997; 8:290A–291A.

83. Paganini E, Pudelski B, Bednarz D. Dialysis delivery in the ICU: Are patients receiving the prescribed dose? (Abstract). J Am Soc Nephrol 1992; 3:384.

84. Leblanc M, Tapolyai M, Paganini E. What dialysis dose should be provided in acute renal failure? A review. Adv Ren Replace Ther 1995; 2(3):255–264.

85. Bouman CS, Oudemans-Van Straaten HM, Tijssen JG, Zandstra DF, Kesecioglu J. Effects of early high-volume continuous venovenous hemofiltration on survival and recovery of renal function in intensive care patients with acute renal failure: a prospective, randomized trial. Crit Care Med 2002; 30(10):2205–2211.

86. Bellomo R, Boyce N. Continuous venovenous hemodiafiltration compared with conventional dialysis in critically ill patients with acute renal failure. ASAIO J 1993; 39:M794–M797.

87. Bellomo R, Ronco C. Continuous versus intermittent renal replacement therapy in the intensive care unit. Kidney Int 1998; 53 (Suppl 66): S125–S128.

88. Mauritz W, Sporn P, Schindler I et al. Acute renal failure in abdominal infection: comparison of hemodialysis and continuous arteriovenous hemofiltration. Anesthes Intensive notfallmed 1986; 21:212–217.

89. Kruczynski K, Irvine-Bird K, Toffelmire E et al. A comparison of continuous arteriovenous hemofiltration and intermittent hemodialysis in acute renal failure patients in the intensive care unit. ASAIO J 1993; 39(21):M778–M781.

90. Kierdorf H. Continuous versus intermittent treatment: clinical results in acute renal failure. Contrib Nephrol 1991; 93:1–12.

91. Van Bommel E, Bouvy N, So K et al. Acute dialytic support for the critically ill: intermittent versus continuous arteriovenous hemodiafiltration. Am J Nephrol 1995; 15:192–200.

92. Van Bommel E, Ponssen HH. Intermittent versus continuous treatment for acute renal failure: where do we stand? Am J Kidney Dis 1997; 30(5) (Suppl 4): S72–S79.

93. Jacka MJ, Ivancinova X, Gibney RT. Continuous renal replacement therapy improves renal recovery from acute renal failure. Can J Anaesth 2005; 52(3):327–332.

94. Jakob S, Frey F, Uehlinger D. Does continuous renal replacement therapy favourably influence the outcome of the patients? Nephrol, Dial, Transplant 1996; 11:1250–1255.

95. Kierdorf H, Sieberth H. Continuous renal replacement therapies versus intermittent hemodialysis in acute renal failure: what do we know? Am J Kidney Dis 1996; 28(5) (Suppl 3):S90–S96.

96. Guerin C, Girard R, Selli JM, Ayzac L. Intermittent versus continuous renal replacement therapy for acute renal failure in intensive care units: results from a multicenter prospective epidemiological survey. Intensive Care Med 2002; 28(10): 1411–1418.

97. Uehlinger DE, Jakob SM, Ferrari P, Eichelberger M, Huynh-Do U, Marti HP et al. Comparison of continuous and intermittent renal replacement therapy for acute renal failure. Nephrol Dial Transplant. 2005; 20(8):1630–7.

98. Kellum J, Angus D, Johnson J et al. Continuous versus intermittent renal replacement therapy: a meta-analysis. Intensive Care Med 2002; 28:29–37.

99. Tonelli M, Manns B, Feller-Kopman D. Acute renal failure in the intensive care unit: a systematic review of the impact of dialytic modality on mortality and renal recovery. Am J Kidney Dis 2002; 40(5):875–885.

100. Hoyt D. CRRT in the area of cost containment: is it justified? Am J Kidney Dis 1997; 30(5) (Suppl 4):S102–S108.

101. Mehta RL, Turner D, Black E. Cost effectiveness of intermittent versus continuous renal replacement therapy in the treatment of acute renal failure: a preliminary report. Abstracts of the Xth Intensivists Congress on Nephrology, 1989:325.

102. Lonnemann G, Schindler R, Dinarello C et al. Removal of circulating cytokines by hemodialysis membranes in vitro. In: Faist K, Meakins D, Schildberg D, eds. Host Defense Dysfunction in Trauma, Shock and Sepsis. Germany: Springer-Verlag, 1993.

103. Silvester W. Mediator removal with CRRT: complement and cytokines. Am J Kidney Dis 1997; 30(5) (Suppl 4):S38–S43.

104. Lonnemann G, Bechstein M, Linnenweber S et al. Tumor necrosis factor-α during continuous high-flux hemodialysis in sepsis with acute renal failure. Kidney International 1999; 56 (Suppl 72):S84–S87.

105. Millar A, Armstrong L, van der Linden J et al. Cytokine production and hemofiltration in children undergoing cardiopulmonary bypass. Ann Thorac Surg 1993; 56:1499–1502.

106. Journois D, Pouard P, Greeley W et al. Hemofiltration during cardiopulmonary bypass in pediatric cardiac surgery. Effect on hemostasis and complement components. Anesthesiology 1994; 81:1181–1189.

107. Heering P, Morgera S, Schmitz F et al. Cytokine removal and cardiovascular hemodynamics in septic patients with continuous venovenous hemofiltration. Intensive Care Med 1997; 23:288–296.

108. Mehta RL. Supportive therapies: intermittent hemodialysis, continuous renal replacement therapies, and peritoneal dialysis. In: Schrier RW, ed. Atlas of Diseases of the Kidney. Philadelphia: Current Medicine, 1998.

44

Fluid and Electrolyte Disorders

Amy A. McDonald and Charles J. Yowler

Department of Surgery, MetroHealth Medical Center, Case Western Reserve University, Cleveland, Ohio, U.S.A.

INTRODUCTION

Cellular function is dependent on the proper electrolyte content of the intracellular fluid (ICF) and the extracellular environment. The body has an elaborate mechanism to sustain homeostasis, which includes feedback mechanisms involving the pituitary and renal systems. Significant electrolyte imbalance is rare in a patient with normal renal function and free access to water and nutrients.

However, fluid and electrolyte balance is often disrupted following trauma and during critical illness. The most common initial change is the loss of voluntary intake of food and water, as the patient becomes entirely dependent on the doctor to supply these needs. If the treating physician is unaware of or miscalculates the fluid and electrolyte losses, the resultant imbalance of the internal milieu can further exacerbate the degree of cellular dysfunction. Fluid and electrolyte therapy is, therefore, an essential component of the management of these critically ill patients.

Although significant improvements in the understandings of the clinical effects of various fluid and electrolyte disorders has occurred in the last decade (1,2), the basic physiology and biochemistry have been known for much longer, and the approach to myriad factors, causing fluid and electrolyte disorders, still follows the classification scheme developed by Narins et al. (3) in the late 1970s and early 1980s. The specific injuries resulting from trauma and critical care continue to be elucidated (4).

This chapter begins with a review of the normal distribution of fluid and electrolytes among the different compartments of the body, and then details diagnosis and management of fluid and electrolyte disorders commonly encountered in trauma and critical care. Rather than providing an encyclopedic list of disease states, this review stresses the application of pathophysiologic principles in the classification and diagnosis of fluid and electrolyte disorders, and emphasizes those most commonly encountered in trauma and critical care.

FLUIDS
Distribution of Body Fluids

Total body water (TBW) varies according to lean body mass and age (Fig. 1). Adipose tissue and bone have relatively low water content compared with muscle and solid organ mass. Using indicator dilution methods, TBW approximates 60% of body weight in men, or 42 L in a 70-kg

adult male, and 50% in women (i.e., 35 L). Thin patients may have a 5% to 10% increase in TBW, whereas obese patients have a 10% to 20% decrease on a per-kilogram basis. Age also plays a role with the decrease in lean body mass in the elderly, decreasing TBW by 10–15% of body weight.

The TBW is distributed between the intracellular and extracellular compartments (Fig. 2). Approximately two-thirds of the TBW exists in the intracellular compartment (approximately 28 L in a 70-kg man), and one-third is contained in the extracellular compartment (14 L in 70-kg man). The extracellular fluid (ECF) is further subdivided into the intravascular, interstitial, and transcellular fluid. The intravascular compartment contains the plasma volume, which is approximately 5% of the TBW and 25% of the ECF (i.e., approximately 3.5 L in a 70-kg male). The interstitial compartment is comprised mainly of the acellular tissue matrix surrounding the cells, and equilibrates rapidly with the remainder of the extracellular water. The free phase, which contains water, is freely exchangeable. The free phase, which contains water, is freely exchangeable. The gel phase represents water that is bound as a matrix with hydrophilic components, such as glycosaminoglycans and mucopolysaccharides. The transcellular fluid compartment includes pleural, pericardial, peritoneal, cerebrospinal, synovial, intraocular, and glandular fluids, all of which are poorly exchangeable. It is important to note that TBW, contained in the intracellular, interstitial, and transcellular compartments, is in dynamic equilibrium; hence, a change in one compartment causes compensatory alterations in the others (1–4).

Composition of Body Fluids

The chemical compositions of the ECF and the ICF differ in regard to cations, anions, organic acids, and proteins (Table 1). Sodium and potassium are the principle cations within the body. Sodium is mainly relegated to the ECF space, whereas potassium is predominantly contained within the ICF compartment. The sodium content in the average adult is approximately 60 meq/kg; however, about 25% to 30% of this is confined to bone and is not freely exchangeable. Of the exchangeable portion, about 85% is found in the ECF. Potassium, magnesium, and calcium make up the remainder of the cations in the ECF.

⚓ **Only a fraction of the total body potassium (about 4 meq/L, or approximately 14 meq in a 70-kg patient) is normally present in the plasma.** ⚓ Most of the total body potassium, approximately 150 meq/L, is contained within the 28 L of ICF (approximately 4200 meq in total) and is

Total Body Water as a Percentage of Total Body Weight

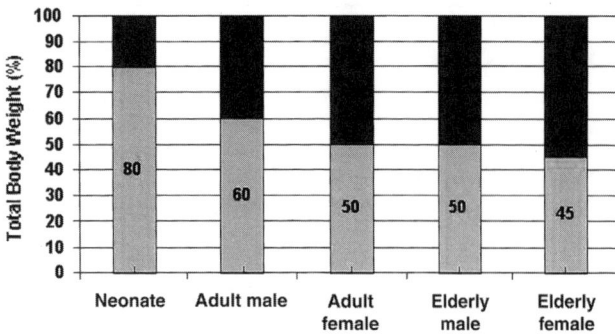

Figure 1   Total body water as a percentage of body weight. The number on the bar lists the average percentage of body weight that is accounted for by total body water for various genders and ages of individuals.

freely exchangeable. Smaller amounts of magnesium and sodium are also found in the ICF. The concentration gradient between the ECF and ICF is maintained by an adenosine triphosphate (ATP)-dependent sodium/potassium pump in the cellular membrane.

Chloride is the principal anion in the ECF, with a normal plasma chloride of 103 meq/L (Table 1). The remainder of the anionic content of the ECF consists of bicarbonate, phosphates, anionic proteins, and sulfates.

The primary intracellular anion is phosphate, with a concentration of 116 meq/L. The remainder of the intracellular anionic load is controlled by anionic proteins, with chloride and bicarbonate contributing negligible amounts.

Concentration of Body Fluids

Although the ECF and ICF differ in relation to ions and proteins, water is evenly distributed throughout in all compartments, and diffuses freely across the semipermeable

Distribution of Total Body Water as a Percentage of Total Body Weight

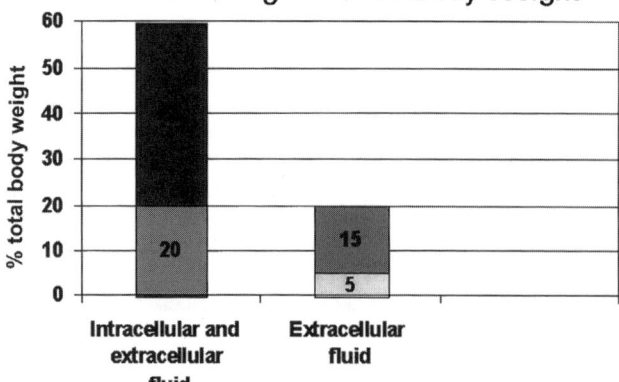

Figure 2   Distribution of total body water (TBW) as a percentage of body weight. Two-thirds of the TBW resides in the intracellular space, and one-third is in the extracellular space. Of the extracellular water, 25% is located within the blood vessels as plasma (approximately 3.5 L in a 70-kg patient).

Table 1   Composition of Body Fluids

Component	Plasma	Interstitial	Intracellular
Na^+	140	140	12
K^+	4	4	150
Cl^-	103	114	3
HCO_3^-	24	27	10
Ca^{2+}	5	3	0
Mg^{2+}	2	1	7
SO_4^{2-}	1	1	0
HPO_4^{2-}	2	2	116
Protein	16	5	40
Organic anions	5	5	0

All values are given in meq/L.

cellular membranes, balancing the osmotic forces. Accordingly, a given bolus of water does little to expand the intravascular compartment. In contrast, sodium-containing fluids expand the ECF, typically expanding the interstitial fluid compartment three times as much as the intravascular compartment, due to the relative volumes of the two compartments.

Osmolality is defined as the number of osmotically active solute particles per kilogram of water, whereas osmolarity is expressed as the number of osmotically active solutes per liter, and the usual units are milliosmoles per liter (mOsm/L). Particles that freely dissociate in water in 1:1 ratio, such as sodium chloride (NaCl), produce 2 Osm. This is in contrast to glucose, which does not freely dissociate, and produces only 1 Osm per molecule. Because water moves freely between the compartments, the tonicity or the relative osmolarity between the ECF and the ICF is maintained between 280 and 290 mOsm/L in normal healthy patients. Isotonic solutions, such as 0.9% NaCl, do not cause the movement of water between ECF and ICF. Urea and alcohol also have little effect of water movement, because they are freely permeable across the cellular membrane; that is, they increase osmolarity without increasing tonicity. However, glucose and mannitol are not freely permeable across the cell membrane, and increase both osmolarity and tonicity.

☞ **Plasma osmolarity (Posm) is generally a good estimate of total body osmolarity, because isosmotic conditions are maintained through fluid shifts.** ☞ Plasma osmolarity can be roughly calculated by the following:

$$Posm(mOsm/L) = 2 \times serum[Na^+] + glucose/18 + BUN/2.8$$

The [Na^+] is usually expressed in meq/L, whereas the glucose and BUN concentrations are provided in mg/dL. Accordingly, these concentrations must be divided by one-tenth of their molecular weights to convert into units mOsm/L.

☞ **When the calculated Posm differs by >15 mOsm from the laboratory-measured value, an osmolar gap exists.** ☞ In this case, other uncalculated, osmotically active molecules are present. Osmotically active particles that are not normally calculated, but commonly measured in the serum of trauma victims, include ethanol, methanol, mannitol, or polyethylene glycol. Certain disease states may also lead to an increase in osmolar gap. For example, multiple myeloma proteins or hypertriglyceridemia can both cause this phenomenon. These substances cause an artifical osmolar gap by reducing the plasma water fraction.

Osmolarity is regulated by arginine vasopressin (AVP), also known as antidiuretic hormone (ADH). After being synthesized in the hypothalamus, ADH is stored in the posterior pituitary. The secretion of ADH is stimulated by osmoreceptors, located in the brainstem, and also by baroreceptors, situated in the heart and vasculature. Antidiuretic hormone enhances the water permeability of the collecting ducts in the kidney, resulting in more concentrated urine. When serum osmolarity is <280 mOsm/L, the secretion of ADH is entirely suppressed. When serum osmolarity is ≥280 mOsm/L, osmoreceptors stimulate the posterior pituitary to release ADH into the bloodstream. The rate of ADH release is normally directly proportional to the serum osmolarity, once it is ≥280 mOsm/L.

The baroreceptors also stimulate ADH release, in response to reduced intravascular volume or decreased mean arterial pressure (MAP). Although the chief stimulus for ADH synthesis and release is serum osmolarity. The baroreceptor response can stimulate ADH release in the absence of any osmoreceptor-mediated response. Therefore, ADH-regulated renal water reabsorption will continue to occur, despite a serum osmolarity <280 mOsm/L in the presence of hypovolemia and/or hypotension. Other nonosmotic mechanisms that also stimulate ADH release include pain and emotional stress.

Disturbances in plasma tonicity and electrolytes are dependent on the volume and electrolyte composition of the fluid gained or lost. By far the most common disturbance in surgical patients is the loss of isotonic fluids. This may result from blood loss, interstitial fluid loss, or sequestration of fluid due to infection or injury. Restoration of these deficits requires isotonic fluids, such as lactated Ringer's (LR) or 0.9% saline (NS). The loss of hypotonic fluids requires replacement based on the expected concentration of cations and anions in these fluids. "Third space" losses develop when cellular and capillary permeability increase, resulting in loss of fluid from the intravascular compartment. Common clinical conditions associated with "third-space" fluid losse, include burns, poly trauma, and sepsis.

Fluid and solutes are exchanged between the intravascular and interstitial fluid compartments. There is a net unidirectional flow of these substances, including albumin and plasma proteins, from the intravascular space to the interstitium, and then back to the intravascular space via lymphatics, helping to maintain physiologic fluid and solute balance. The flux of water through the interstitium is largely determined by capillary hydrostatic pressure. Hydostatic pressure is a function of intravascular volume and vascular tone. Opposing the force of hydrostatic pressure is colloid oncotic pressure, the major determinant of which is albumin.

Molecules, such as water, glucose, urea, and electrolytes pass freely through the capillary membrane. Their concentrations in the intravascular and interstitial compartments are essentially equal. The passage of other molecules is dependent upon the relative permeability (or porosity) of the capillary membrane to those substances. Large molecules, such as albumin, fibrinogen, immunoglobulins, and other proteins do not pass readily through the capillary membrane. Accordingly, the concentration of these osmotically active substances is generally higher in plasma than in interstitial fluid and lymph.

The baseline porosity of capillary membranes varies between tissues. For instance, the liver is very porous, whereas, the muscle capillary membranes are generally nonporous. Capillary permeability can also change, in response to the hormonal and autocrine influences of bradykinin and histamine.

The complex movement of fluid across the capillary membrane is described by Starling's equation.

$$Q = K_f[(P_c - P_i) - \sigma (COP_p - COP_i)]$$

where Q is the net rate of transcapillary fluid movement (mL/min/100 g), K_f is the capillary filtration coefficient, $P_c - P_i$ is the hydrostatic pressure gradient, σ is the reflection coefficient, and $COP_p - COP_i$ is the colloid oncotic pressure gradient.

K_f, or the capillary filtration coefficient, depends on the tissue and surface area. It can also be influenced by atrial natriuretic factor and platelet activating factor. The reflection coefficient, σ, varies from zero to one and represents the ability of capillary membranes to prevent plasma proteins from crossing the membrane. Values closer to zero are highly permeable, whereas values approaching one are highly impermeable. The hydrostatic pressure gradient ($P_c - P_i$) is largely dependent on arteriolar and venous vasomotor tone.

This complex interaction is autoregulated. If there is an increase in hydrostatic pressure with net fluid movement into the interstitium, the protein concentration in the interstitium will decrease. This would cause a higher oncotic pressure in the plasma, further retarding fluid movement into the interstitium. If there is a decrease in plasma colloid oncotic pressure, leading to increased water in the interstitium, more fluid dilutes the interstitial oncotic pressure, reducing oncotic forces.

In the setting of edema, or abnormal accumulation of excess fluid in the interstitium, there is increased permeability of the capillary membrane to plasma proteins. The movement of fluid into the interstitium, however, dilutes the interstitial protein concentration such that further fluid movement is counteracted. Diuresis removes excess interstitial fluid and eventually restores protein distribution to normal.

Maintenance Therapy

Maintenance therapy provides for the loss of water and electrolytes expended during normal physiologic activities. This consists of sensible and insensible losses. Sensible losses, such as urine and stool can be measured. Insensible losses consist of water vapor lost through the lungs and skin. The rate of insensible loss depends on the water vapor tension of the environment, air movement, rate and volume of respiration, and metabolic rate. Insensible losses increase by 10% for each 1°C above 37.2°C. The repletion of water losses, both sensible and insensible, is based on weight (kg).

The electrolyte composition of maintenance fluids is based on weight, and estimated quantity of electrolytes present in fluids lost during normal physiologic conditions. The concentration of electrolytes depends on the source of the fluid. Urine can have varying amounts of sodium, chloride, and potassium. Urinary excretion depends on the overall electrolyte and volume status of the patient, and the balance of hydrogen ion, phosphates, sulfates, and organic acids. Approximately 800 to 1500 mL of water is required to excrete the normal daily solute load. The kidney excretes all sodium in excess of the body's need, but is less efficient with potassium. Urine sodium concentration can decrease to as low as 1 meq/day. Stool contains a larger amount of potassium, with only small amounts of sodium and chloride. In general, daily sodium requirements are 1–2 meq/kg/day and daily potassium requirements are 0.5–1.0 meq/kg/day. Repletion of calcium, magnesium, and phosphorus is unnecessary in patients with adequate stores of these electrolytes. However, critically ill patients, often require repletion of these on a daily basis. Glucose is typically added to maintenance fluids in order to help maintain tonicity and prevent proteolysis. An appropriate daily maintenance fluid in the 70-kg adult without abnormal sensible or insensible losses is approximately 2 L of D5 $\frac{1}{2}$ NS + 20-meq KCl/L (1–3).

Replacement Therapy

Acute volume deficits, resulting in hemodynamic instability, are generally replaced via bolus infusion with isotonic fluids (Table 2). Crystalloid and colloid solutions can both be used, but there has been considerable debate regarding which is optimal during resuscitation and maintenance in trauma patients. ☞ **Crystalloids should be the initial resuscitation fluid administered in most situations.** ☞ Both LR and 0.9% NS are suitable crystalloid resuscitation solutions. Aggressive resuscitation with NS can result in hyperchloremic metabolic acidosis (4). Lactated Ringer's contains a more physiologic array of electrolytes than NS, and is a commonly employed crystalloid solution for blunt and penetrating noncerebral trauma. However, LR may lead to increased inflammatory activity of leukocytes (see Volume 1, Chapter 11). In addition, NS is preferred by many neurosurgeons for resuscitation from cerebral trauma, because it is slightly more hypertonic than LR and normal plasma.

Hypertonic saline solutions (HTS) are currently being studied for their utility in head-injured (5) and nonhead-injured trauma patients (6), as well as burn patients. The major advantage appears to be the attainment of hemodynamic stability with less volume. Animal models have demonstrated the advantages and disadvantages of HTS in hemorrhagic shock. It seems most useful in controlled hemorrhagic shock (CHS) rather than uncontrolled hemorrhagic shock (UCHS). HTS may increase blood loss in UCHS, due to the effects on blood pressure, vasodilatation, coagulation, and blood rheology. Human studies with HTS, thus far, have shown no statistically significant increase in survival. However, there may be a subpopulation that could benefit, such as those with severe traumatic brain injuries Glasgow Coma Scale (GCS < 8). Hypertonic saline

solutions, in both in-vitro and animal studies of hemorrhagic shock, have an immunomodulatory effect that can attenuate the adverse effects of the systemic inflammatory response and ischemia/reperfusion on the host (7–9). However, it also has been shown, in vitro and in animal studies, to alter platelet and plasma coagulation (10). Its exact role in the resuscitation of the trauma patient has yet to be defined.

There are several colloid solutions available for fluid resuscitation. The most commonly used solutions are albumin and hydroxyethlyl starch (HES). The benefit of colloids is theoretically based on their ability to expand the intravascular volume more efficiently. Microvascular permeability of colloids is dependent on the molecular size, shape, and ionic charge of the particles, as well as the porosity of the microvascular membrane. In the presence of injury and shock, microvascular porosity is often increased. Colloid can therefore more easily enter the interstitial space, bringing with it increased oncotic pressure and attendant water. This appears to be more of a problem with albumin (low molecular weight) and polymers of hydroxyethyl starch, with low and medium molecular weights. High-molecular-weight hydroxyethyl starch has, however, been shown to cause a coagulopathy by reducing factor VIII and von Willebrand's factor. The medium- and low-molecular-weight hydroxyethyl starches have less of an effect on coagulation. A newer formulation of hydroxyethyl starch, Hextend® (Abbott Laboratories, Chicago, IL, USA) contains a lactate-buffered balanced salt and glucose solution. Clinical studies on this solution have shown less of an effect on coagulation than the NS-based solutions (11). Anaphylactic reactions have also occurred with albumin and HES. According to a study in France of 19,593 patients, the incidence of allergic reactions was 0.099% for albumin and 0.058% for HES (12).

The crystalloid–colloid debate continues (see Volume 1, Chapter 11). Several studies, including meta-analyses, have tried to address this issue (13). A Cochran meta-analysis addressed the crystalloid–colloid question by addressing three categories of patients: (*i*) surgery or trauma, (*ii*) burns, and (*iii*) hypoalbuminemia (14). They demonstrated no survival difference in the surgery/trauma group, but showed an increased mortality following albumin administration for burns and in hypoalbuminemic patients (14). This report changed practice, until a more complete meta-analysis was conducted by Wilkes and Navickis (15). The Wilkes and Navickis evaluation included all of the trials surveyed by the Cochran group, along with several others. They also divided the subgroup analysis into six categories (the original three groups from Cochran, plus a three others: high-risk neonates, ascites, and other indications) (15). The Wilkes and Navickis

Table 2 Parenteral Fluids

Fluid	Na (meq/L)	K (meq/L)	Ca (meq/L)	Cl (meq/L)	Lactate (meq/L)	Dextrose (g/L)	Osm (mEq/L)	pH
Lactated Ringer's	130	4	2.7	109	28	0	273	6.5
0.9% NaCl	154	0	0	154	0	0	308	6.0
D5 0.45% NaCl	77	0	0	77	0	50	406	4.0
3% NaCl	513	0	0	513	0	0	1027	5.0
25% mannitol	0	0	0	0	0	0	1372	4.5–7.0
5% albumin	145	<2.5	0	0	0	0	330	7.4
25% albumin	130–160	<1	0	0	0	0	269	6.4–7.4
6% hetastarch (Hespan®)	154	0	0	154	0	0	310	5.9
Hextend (buffered Hespan)	143	3	5	124	28	0.99	307	5.9

meta-analysis revealed no overall effect of albumin on mortality, but some of the better-conducted studies showed a possible survival benefit from albumin therapy (15).

These disparate results promulgated the American Thoracic Society-Critical Care Group (ATS-CCG) to develop a working group to study the problem, and a consensus statement was published in December 2004 (16). The ATS-CCG working group reviewed the published literature (including all publications between 1996 and 2002) by performing a systematic search of MEDLINE and the Cochran Databases. Their particular focus was on patients in medical, surgical, and cardiovascular intensive care units, and excluded burn injuries and pediatric patients (16). Evidence was graded for a clinically important outcome, according to a standard hierarchical schema (Table 3) (17).

The ATS-CCG Consensus Statement main points are provided in Table 4, and their therapeutic recommendations are summarized in Table 5. In summary, they found no clear advantage of commercially available colloids over crystalloids in the resuscitation of the trauma patient. Crystalloid solutions, due to low cost and absence of significant adverse effects, remain the mainstay of fluid resuscitation in the trauma patient. The role of HTS in trauma and critical care resuscitation is still evolving, as numerous clinical studies are ongoing.

SODIUM DISORDERS

Sodium is the primary determinant of serum osmolarity, and thus pivotal in body fluid homeostasis (18). If changes in TBW occur without a corresponding alteration in total body sodium content, the serum osmolarity changes. Therefore, the manifestations of hyper- or hyponatremia reflect disturbances in water homeostasis. ☞ **Hypernatremia almost always represents a hyperosmolar or hypertonic state, whereas hyponatremia can be present in a hypertonic, isotonic, or hypotonic state.** ☞

Hypernatremia
Causes

Hypernatremia is defined as a serum $[Na^+] > 145$ meq/L. The most common cause for hypernatremia is inadequate replacement of free water losses. The physiologic response to this loss is the activation of thirst sensation and concentration of urine at the renal tubule (through ADH secretion). Thus, the hospitalized patient who has decreased alertness, and may not be on an oral diet, is vulnerable to the increased free water losses of fever, diarrhea, burns, and/or diuretic therapy. Both the thirst mechanism and renal concentrating capacity are diminished in elderly patients (see Volume 1, Chapter 37), making them more vulnerable to hypernatremia (19).

The release of ADH is the normal response to the increased osmolarity of hypernatremia. However, brain injury or hypothalamic-pituitary dysfunction, secondary to infection, inflammation, ischemia, or mass lesions, may impair ADH release, resulting in central diabetes insipidus (DI). Drugs, such as ethanol and phenytoin may also inhibit ADH release. Conversely, the ADH receptor at the renal tubule may be impaired, resulting in nephrogenic DI. Acquired nephrogenic DI may be due to obstructive uropathy, a chronic tubulointerstitial disorder, hypovolemia or hypercalcemia. Drugs, such as lithium, demeclocycline, amphotericin B, and foscarnet may also cause nephrogenic DI.

Symptoms

Clinical manifestations of hypernatremia generally relate to the effect of decreased water content in brain cells. This includes symptoms of restlessness, irritability, confusion, seizures, lethargy, coma, muscle twitching, spasticity, and hyper-reflexia. Intracerebral hemorrhage can result from cell shrinkage and subsequent traction on cerebral vasculature. These symptoms generally do not appear unless the Na^+ is greater than 160 meq/L or serum osmolarity exceeds 320 mOsm/L (20).

☞ **The work-up for hypernatremia starts with the determination of intravascular volume status, based on history, physical examination, and laboratory data.** ☞ The initial laboratory tests include urine and Posm and urine sodium. High urine osmolarity in the setting of low urine sodium usually means extrarenal losses of free water. Low urine osmolarity with hypernatremia usually means inappropriate renal losses of free water (Table 6).

Treatment

Treatment of hypernatremia varies according to the etiology. Hypovolemic hypernatremia requires expeditious replacement of intravascular volume with isotonic fluids (e.g., NS). In this condition, a total body sodium deficiency is present in addition to the free water deficit. Hypotonic fluids, such as 0.45% NS should never be used to rapidly correct significant intravascular volume deficits. Free water deficits need to be replaced slowly to prevent deleterious cellular edema, especially in the brain. Furthermore, chronic hypernatremia should be treated more slowly than acute hypernatremia. In general, after significant intravascular volume deficits have been replaced, the free water deficiency is corrected.

Table 3 Grades of Evidence for the Quality of Clinical Study Design

Grade	Criteria/description
I	Evidence obtained from at least one properly randomized, controlled trial
II-A	Evidence obtained from well-designed controlled trials without randomization or randomized trials, without blinding
II-B	Evidence obtained from well-designed cohort or case-control analytic studies, preferably from more than one center or research group
II-C	Evidence obtained from multiple time series with or without intervention, uncontrolled cohort studies, and case series
III	Opinions of respected authorities, based on clinical experience; descriptive studies, and case reports; or reports of expert committees
NR	Evidence not rated for clinically nonrelevant outcome

Source: Adapted from Ref. 17.

Table 4   American Thoracic Society 2004 Consensus Statement on Colloid Use in Critical Care: Summary Points

#	Summary point comments and (level of evidence)
1	Colloids have various nononcotic properties that may influence vascular integrity, inflammation, and pharmacokinetics, although the clinical relevance of these properties has not been elucidated (NR)
2	All colloids affect the coagulation system, with dextran and starch solutions having the most potent antithrombotic effects (II-A)
3	HES may be deposited in the reticuloendothelial tissues for prolonged periods; the clinical significance of this is unknown (II-C)
4	Colloids restore intravascular volume and tissue perfusion more rapidly than crystalloids in all shock states, regardless of vascular permeability (II-A)
5	There is conflicting evidence that HES increases the risk of bleeding after cardiopulmonary bypass surgery (I)
6	Although hydrostatic pressure is more important than COP for accumulation of pulmonary edema, colloid administration reduces tissue edema and may ameliorate pulmonary edema as a consequence of shock resuscitation (II-A)
7	There is no evidence of a benefit of colloids in treating ischemic brain injury (I) or subarachnoid hemorrhage (II-A). Colloids may adversely impact survival in traumatic brain injury (I).
8	Hydroxyethlyl starch administration may increase the risk of acute renal failure in patients with sepsis (II-A)
9	Treatment of dialysis-related hypotension with colloids is superior to crystalloids for chronic dialysis patients; presumably, colloids are similarly superior for acutely ill patients (II-A)
10	Colloids are superior to crystalloids in intravascular volume replacement with large-volume paracentesis (II-A) and as adjunctive therapy to antibiotics in treating spontaneous bacterial peritonitis (II-A)
11	Meta-analyses of critical care colloid use are conflicting because of entry trial heterogeneity and varied analytic techniques, and a large prospective trial suggests a neutral influence of colloids on clinical outcomes

Abbreviations: COP, colloid oncotic pressure; HES, hydroxyethlyl starch.
Source: Adapted from Ref. 16.

The free water deficit is calculated as follows:

$$\text{Free water deficit} = \frac{(\text{plasma}[Na^+] - 140)}{140} \times TBW$$

$$\text{Total body water (TBW)} = \text{body weight (kg)} \times 0.60$$

One-half of the deficit should be replaced over the first 24 hours. The next half should be replaced over the next 48–72 hours. Hypervolemic hypernatremia is rare, but occurs when excess hypertonic or NS is used to replace free water loss. This may occur in the setting of burn injury, and following 3% NS administration for traumatic brain injury (TBI). In the absence of TBI, treatment involves diureses with partial replacement of urine losses using D_5W, or additional free water via tube feeding. In the setting of TBI, acute treatment should be deferred until brain swelling has decreased, intracranial pressure (ICP) has normalized, and the patient is hemodynamically stable.

Diabetes insipidus classically causes euvolemic or (if allowed to persist untreated) hypovolemic hypernatremia. ☞ **In complete central DI, the urinary osmolality is** **<150 mOsm/L, but may be higher in partial DI.** ☞ In the setting of hypernatremia ($[Na^+] > 150$ meq/L) and polyuria, a urinary osmolality <290 mOsm/L is virtually diagnostic of DI, as this constellation of factors is unusual for any other disease process (Table 7). Central DI can be treated with exogenous vasopressin and free water replacement. The usual dose for aqueous vasopressin is 5–10 units every four to six hours. D-des-argenine-vasopressin [desmopressin (ddAVP)] has a longer half-life, and can be used in chronic cases of central DI. The usual dose of ddAVP is $20\mu g$ intranasal every 12–24 hours. Other drugs used in the treatment of central DI are carbamazepine, clofibrate, and chlorpropamide.

Nephrogenic DI is much less common in trauma and surgical critical care. Although most cases of nephrogenic DI are acquired (secondary to various drug use), there is a congenital form. Treatment of nephrogenic DI requires correction of calcium and potassium deficits, discontinuation of offending drugs, low-sodium diet, and thiazide diuretics. Amiloride can be used for lithium-induced DI. The risk of DI resulting from amphotericin B can be

Table 5   American Thoracic Society 2004 Consensus Statement on Colloid Use in Critical Care: Therapeutic Implications

#	Therapeutic implication(s) and (level of evidence)
1	Crystalloids should be administered first in nonhemorrhagic shock resuscitation (III)
2	Hydroxyethyl starch solutions should be used with caution in cardiopulmonary bypass (meta-analysis) and in patients with sepsis (II-A)
3	Colloids should be avoided or used with caution in patients with traumatic brain injury (I)
4	Fluid restriction is appropriate for patients with hemodynamically stable ALI/ARDS (II-A); the combination of colloids and diuretics may be considered in patients with hypo-oncotic ALI/ARDS (III)
5	Colloids are preferred for treating dialysis-associated hypotension, and in maintaining hemodynamics to achieve dialysis goals (II-A)
6	Hyperoncotic albumin should be administered in conjunction with large-volume paracentesis for diuretic-refractory ascites (II-A)
7	Albumin may be administered in conjunction with antimicrobial therapy to patients with spontaneous bacterial peritonitis (II-A)

Abbreviations: ALI = acute lung injury; ARDS = acute respiratory distress syndrome.
Source: Adapted from Ref. 16.

Table 6 Causes and Characteristics of Hypotonic (<280 mOsm/L) Hyponatremia

Variable	Extracellular fluid volume status		
	Hypovolemic	Euvolemic	Hypervolemic
Causes	GI losses, excess sweating/poor H$_2$O intake (e.g., desert exposure) excess diuretic use, CSW syndrome[a]	SIADH, hypothyroidism, adrenal insufficiency	CHF, cirrhosis, nephrotic syndrome
Urine volume	Decreased	Varies with intake	Usually decreased
Urine osmolarity[b]	>500 mOsm/L	>100 mOsm/L	>100 mOsm/L
Urine [Na$^+$]	<20 meq/L[a]	>40 meq/L	<20 meq/L[c]
Response to 0.9% saline infusion	Clinical and biochemical improvement	No change or worsening hyponatremia	Minimal change in hyponatremia, worsening edema

[a]The urine [Na$^+$] would be >40 meq/L in CSW; thus the most important differentiating factor between CSW syndrome and SIADH is that the intravascular volume is decreased with CSW syndrome and normal with SIADH. The urine [Na$^+$] would be >20 meq/L with ongoing diuretic use as well.
[b]Urine osmolarity <100 mOsm/L would indicate appropriate antidiuretic hormone and renal response to hyponatremia, and would be expected in the setting of iatrogenic hyponatremia or psychogenic polydipsia (rare in critical care).
[c]The urine [Na$^+$] would be >20 meq/L when the hypervolemic condition was renal failure, but in this condition, the serum sodium is less often low.
Abbreviations: CHF, congestive heart failure; CSW, cerebral salt wasting syndrome; SIADH, syndrome of inappropriate antidiuretic hormone secretion.

minimized by using the liposomal formulation. (see Volume 2, Chapter 53).

Hyponatremia
Causes

The normal serum sodium concentration is 140 meq/L. Hyponatremia is defined as a serum [Na$^+$] of less than 135 meq/L.

Hyponatremia is usually associated with a state of hypotonicity. However, it can also occur in the setting of normal tonicity and hypertonicity (when other osmotically active solutes are present in elevated concentrations). Additionally, a clinical entity, known as pseudohyponatremia, can exist in the setting of normal tonicity. Pseudohyponatremia (measured hyponatremia in association with normal tonicity) is usually due to a laboratory measurement error. The most common causes of pseudohyponatremia are hyperproteinemia or hyperlipidemia, and as such, symptoms of hyponatremia do not occur.

Hypertonic hyponatremia occurs whenever there is an increase in nonsodium serum osmoles, most commonly hyperglycemia, but can also exist in the setting of alcohol intoxication or concurrent mannitol use. In this state, excess intravascular solute particles cause a shift of water from the intracellular to extracellular space. This can also result from methanol or ethylene glycol intoxication. In these hypertonic states, total body sodium often remains normal.

Hypotonic hyponatremia, the most common form, can be associated with hypovolemia, euvolemia, or hypervolemia (21,22). In all states, there is excess free water relative to sodium in the extracellular space. Clinical assessment of volume status, urine osmolarity, and urine sodium concentration can aid in assessing the etiology of hyponatremia (Table 7). Renal losses of sodium are suggested by a urine sodium level >20 to 40 meq/L, whereas extrarenal losses are suggested by a urine sodium level <20 meq/L. In the setting of euvolemia, iatrogenic or psychogenic polydipsia is suggested by a

urine osmolarity <100 mOsm/L (this is an unusual etiology in critically ill trauma patients).

The syndrome of inappropriate antidiuretic hormone (SIADH) can occur as a result of cerebral or pulmonary pathology (i.e., trauma, tumor, or infection), as well as various tumors of the pancreas, duodenum, bladder, and prostate. The postoperative and postinjury states often result in transient inappropriate (for serum osmolarity) ADH secretion. It can be further exacerbated by the infusion of hypotonic fluids (23). **☞ The diagnosis of SIADH is suggested by the finding of urine osmolarity >100 mOsm/L and urine sodium >40 meq/L in the setting of hyponatremia (23). ☞**

Hypervolemic hyponatremia occurs in patients with edema and ascites, due to congestive heart failure, nephrotic syndrome, or cirrhosis. A state of total body sodium excess exists; however, TBW is present in excess to an even greater degree. In these states, total effective circulating volume is decreased, thus creating a nonosmotic stimulus for ADH production. Renal hypoperfusion exacerbates the problem with resultant antidiuresis and water retention.

Hypovolemic hyponatremia results from pathologic losses of sodium-rich body fluids (gastrointestinal or biliary losses from tubes, drains, fistulas, vomiting, or diarrhea), which are replaced with inadequate volumes of sodium-deficient fluids. The pediatric patient with severe vomiting from pyloric stenosis or duodenal obstruction may present with hypovolemic hypernatremia, if losses are inadequately replaced with NS, or with hypovolemic hyponatremia, if his losses are replaced with inadequate amounts of dextrose in one-fourth or one-half NS. This emphasizes the fact that Na$^+$ concentration is generally independent of volume status. Similar conditions can exist in the adult patient with high-volume gastrointestinal or biliary fistulas, depending on the adequacy of fluid and Na$^+$ replacement.

A unique entity, referred to as cerebral salt wasting (CSW) syndrome, can occur in neurosurgical patients, and presents as a hypovolemic hyponatremia (24). The mechanism for the decreased absorption of sodium in the kidney is thought to be due to the release of a brain natriuretic peptide

Table 7 Evaluation of Hypernatremia (Plasma [Na$^+$] >145 to 150 meq/L)

Variable	Extracellular fluid volume status		
	Hypovolemic	Euvolemic	Hypervolemic

Mechanism	Loss of H$_2$O and Na$^+$
	  H$_2$O Loss > Na$^+$ Loss
		Loss of water	Gain of H$_2$O and Na$^+$
			  Na$^+$ gain > H$_2$O gain

Clinical causes	Chronic diuretic use, vomiting, or diarrhea	DI, diuresis, or excessive evaporative loss	Aggressive administration of NaCl or NaHCO$_3$
Pretreatment urine volume	Low	High	Usually high
Urine osmolarity[a]	Nonrenal H$_2$O losses >400 mOsm/L Renal H$_2$O losses < 300 mOsm/L	Nonrenal H$_2$O losses >400 mOsm/L DI[b] and other renal H$_2$O losses <290 mOsm/L	Iatrogenic causes variable mineralocorticoid excess >300 mOsm/L
Urine [Na$^+$][a]	Nonrenal H$_2$O losses <10–15 meq/L Renal H$_2$O losses >20 meq/L	Nonrenal H$_2$O losses variable DI[b] and other renal H$_2$O losses <10–15 meq/L	Iatrogenic causes variable Mineralocorticoid excess >20 meq/L
Treatment	Replete intravascular volume with normal saline Then, more slowly, replace free H$_2$O deficit	Replace urinary losses with one-half normal saline If DI, treat with vasopressin or ddAVP Slow free H$_2$O replacement later if needed	Loop diuretics Replace urinary losses with one-half normal saline, or add free H$_2$O to tube eedings If renal failure, Rx with dialysis

[a]The values for urine osmolarity and urine [Na$^+$] are taken from Ref. 41.
[b]In the case of DI, urine osmolality is usually <150 mOsm/L and urine [Na$^+$] <10 meq/L.
Abbreviations: ddAVP, desmopressin; DI, diabetes insipidus; Rx, treatment.

(BNP), which acts on the nephron to decrease sodium reabsorption (probably at the proximal tubule) (25). Atrial natriuretic peptide (ANP) and BNP are capable of decreasing autonomic outflow at the level of the brain stem, and thus may have a dual affect, causing hyponatremia (i.e., decreasing neural input to the kidney, and directly inhibiting sodium reabsorption) (26).

In contrast to ANP (secreted mainly by human atria), BNP is secreted by the brain, and also by human ventricles, during times of increased pressure or stretch (27). The increased BNP release, seen in patients with congestive heart failure (CHF), has been used as a measure of left ventricular failure. Recently, a rapid BNP immunoassay (Triage Assay, Biosite Diagnostics, Inc, San Diego, CA, USA) was approved by the Food and Drug Administration for point-of-care testing, returning results within 15 minutes (27). This assay is being used in CHF patients, but has not yet been studied in head injured patients, who may be at risk of CSW syndrome. ☞ **CSW syndrome must be differentiated from SIADH, because their treatments are divergent, and directly effect outcome.** ☞ Heretofore, the distinction was made by noting that euvolemia favored SIADH, and hypovolemia was consistent with CSW syndrome; additionally, the urine osmolarity would be >500 mOsm/L in CSW syndrome (Table 7). The measurement of BNPs may soon be useful in differentiating these entities (but this must be prospectively studied first). In the case of CSW syndrome,

both Na$^+$ and intravascular volume must be repleted. This can be accomplished by the administration of 3% NS. In CSW syndrome, fluid restriction (the normal treatment for SIADH) would likely be detrimental to neurological recovery.

Symptoms

☞ **Symptoms secondary to acute hyponatremia typically do not arise until the serum [Na$^+$] is less than 125 meq/L in acute hyponatremic states, or less than 120 meq/L in more chronic conditions.** ☞ The symptoms of hyponatremia are primarily due to the associated hypotonicity, with resultant cellular swelling. The most pronounced effect of cellular swelling is cerebral edema. The resultant symptoms include headache, nausea, vomiting, lethargy, and confusion. If the fall in serum Na$^+$ continues, seizures, coma, and respiratory arrest may occur.

Rapid development of hyponatremia may result in irritability and seizures. This most commonly occurs in the setting of unrecognized SIADH with hypotonic fluid replacement.

Treatment

The hyponatremia treatment plan must address multiple issues, including an estimate of the sodium deficit, and a calculation of the sodium repletion rate that prevents the occurrence of osmotic demyelination, often referred to as central pontine myelinolysis (CPM) (28). Osmotic demyelination results from rapid transfer of water out of central nervous tissue cells. The injury and symptoms are often delayed for two to six days after the abrupt elevation of serum sodium has occurred. The structural damage and symptoms resulting from CPM are usually irreversible, and can consist of dysarthria, dysphagia, para- or quadraparesis, lethargy, coma, respiratory arrest, and seizures.

The term CPM refers to the earliest descriptions demonstrating demyelination, chiefly in the pons (29,30). However, more recently, it has become recognized that the demyelination occurs along most of the myelinated nerve tracts (31). Because of the rich concentration of myelinated fibers in the pons, lesions do predominate there (65% of cases), but other commonly involved sites include the cerebral periventricular and subcortical white matter, thalami, basal ganglia, internal capsule, and the cerebellar peduncles and white matter (31). All of these commonly demyelinated sites contain interdigitated gray and white matter. This interdigitation may interfere with the diffusion of hypertonic edema fluid into adjacent white matter, making these areas particularly vulnerable to rapid fluid and electrolyte changes.

Conventional computed tomography and magnetic resonance imaging findings lag behind the clinical manifestations of CPM. However, using MR diffusion-weighted imaging, lesions within the central pons have been identified within 24 hours of the onset of patient tetraplegia and before findings are conspicuous with conventional MR imaging sequences (32).

↗ **Experimental studies in animals and observations in humans suggest that the rate of hyponatremia correction in the first 24 hours is the major determinant for the development of osmotic demyelination (28–33).** ↗ It is more common when the plasma sodium concentration is raised by more than 20 meq/L in the first 24 hours, and rare when raised less than 10 to 12 meq/L over the first day (33). The rate of correction must reflect the presence or absence of symptoms, and the duration of hyponatremia (Table 8). Longstanding hyponatremia should be corrected over a long period (i.e., five to seven days), and should not be corrected faster than 0.25 meq/L per hour, whereas acute hyponatremia can be corrected more aggressively (but should not be corrected faster than 0.5 meq/L per hour, unless symptomatic). Symptomatic patients require more rapid correction, and may require correction rates of 0.5 to 1 meq/L per hour for the first two to three hours or until symptoms resolve. However, the total 24-hour raise in serum sodium should still not be greater than 12 meq/L.

The treatment of hyponatremia further depends upon the volume status and the presence or absence of symptoms (21,22). As described earlier, the treatment of CSW syndrome requires increased intravascular volume and Na^+ (either as 3% NS, or supplemental dietary salt, if tolerating enteral nutrition), whereas water restriction is the primary therapy for asymptomatic SIADH. Symptomatic SIADH requires more aggressive initial therapy, which may include diuresis with the addition of 3% NS. Serum sodium levels need to be obtained every two to four hours to prevent too rapid a rise in serum sodium as detailed earlier. Demeclocycline 600 to 1200 mg/day can also be utilized in SIADH resulting from chronic conditions.

Fluid restriction plus diuresis is necessary in hypervolemic edematous states, such as CHF, renal failure, and cirrhosis. Loop diuretics are the preferred agents, whereas thiazide diuretics should be avoided, as they may exacerbate the hyponatremia. Overly aggressive fluid restriction and diuresis must be avoided, because the resultant decrease in effective circulating volume can exacerbate the stimulus for ADH release and renal conservation of water. The correction of excess free water may take days to weeks, depending upon the rate of mobilization from the extracellular compartment.

Table 8 Rules for Sodium Correction for Hyponatremia

Rule priority	Sodium correction guidelines	Rationale/comments
1	Correct no more than 12 meq/L in the first 24 hrs of treatment	No patients receiving corrections this slow or slower developed CPM in a recent study
2	Correct no faster than 0.25 meq/L per hour in asymptomatic chronically hyponatremic patients, and complete normalization of sodium in these patients over five to seven days	Chronic hyponatremia results in brain intracellular volume adaption, and redistribution of osmotically active particles from the brain. It takes at least five days to rebuild the stores of the brain's idiogenic osmoles
3	Correct no faster than 0.5 meq/L per hour in asymptomatic acutely hyponatremic patients, and complete normalization of sodium in these patients over 2–3 days	Acute hyponatremia (occurring over 12–24 hr) does not allow time for loss of brain idiogenic osmoles, and patients are theoretically at less risk of demyelination
4	If symptoms are severe (i.e., seizures have occurred), more rapid correction is appropriate (i.e., 0.5–1 meq/L per hour) for the first 2–3 hr or until symptoms abate	Severe symptoms (especially seizures), require prompt treatment to avoid brain injury. These patients should also receive an antiseizure drug (e.g., ativan)
5	Isotonic (0.9%) saline should be utilized for asymptomatic and mildly symptomatic patients. Hypertonic (3%) saline should be reserved for severe symptoms and CSW syndrome	Isotonic (0.9%) saline should raise the serum sodium concentration 1–2 meq/L for each liter infused into a 70-kg patient. Hypertonic (3%) saline, run at a rate of 25–30 mL/hr, will increase the serum sodium 8–10 mEq/L in a 70-kg patient
6	In ECF volume contraction, isotonic (0.9%) saline should be used to expand the ECF volume. Three percent saline is reserved for CSW syndrome, and to supplement other low ECF hyponatremic states	Expanding the ECF volume leads to decreased antidiuretic hormone release, which serves to help correct the serum $[Na^+]$

Abbreviations: CPM, central pontine myelinolysis; CSW, cerebral salt wasting; ECF, extracellular fluid.

Hypovolemic hyponatremia requires volume repletion with isotonic saline. The degree to which a liter of any given solution would increase serum sodium can be estimated by the following equation (which can be used in hypernatremic conditions as well):

$$\Delta \text{in serum}[Na^+] = \frac{\text{infusate}[Na^+] - \text{initial serum}[Na^+]}{\text{Total body water} + 1}$$

This formula demonstrates how little the serum $[Na^+]$ changes with only 1 L of fluid. To calculate the total number of liters needed to change a hyponatremic condition $([Na^+] = 130 \text{ meq/L})$ to a normal serum sodium state $([Na+] = 140 \text{ meq/L})$ by administering NS $([Na^+] = 154 \text{ meq/L})$, simply add up the aggregate changes predicted by the earlier equation, in repetitive fashion, until the normal value is being approached.

For a 70-kg patient with TBW = 42 L, the first-liter NS changes the serum sodium from 130 to 130.56 meq/L, the second liter of NS brings the serum sodium from 130.56 to 131.11 meq/L, and so on. The aggregate number of liters of NS, calculated to bring the serum sodium to normal, divided by 24 provides the hourly infusion rate, if the intention is to make the change in a single day.

Serial measurements of sodium are essential, because the formula has several limitations. The equation does not account for shifts of body water, urinary losses, insensible losses, increases in sodium excretion in the setting of SIADH, or the effects of potassium and other osmotically active solutes.

POTASSIUM DISORDERS

The average 70-kg adult male contains approximately 60 meq/kg of potassium $[K^+]$. Most of the potassium is intracellular $(28 \text{ L} \times 150 \text{ meq/L} = 4200 \text{ meq})$, with less than 2% extracellular $(14 \text{ L} \times 4.5 \text{ meq/L} = 63 \text{ mEq})$. The intracellular predominance of potassium limits the value of serum potassium in estimating total body potassium stores, except during steady states. ☞ **Because the extracellular concentration of potassium changes most quickly, it has the greatest effect on cell membrane function, and is particularly important for cardiac and nerve tissues.** ☞ A sodium–potassium membrane pump $(Na^+/K^+ \text{ ATPase})$ maintains a gradient of 30:1 to 40:1 of intracellular to extracellular potassium, causing a transmembrane potential of approximately -90 mV, as per the Nernst Equation.

On the whole, potassium balance is dependent on intake and both renal and extrarenal losses. The kidney secretes approximately 90% of ingested potassium, whereas the remainder is excreted in sweat and feces. The net secretion of potassium by the kidney is determined by many factors, including the amount of urine flow, amount of sodium delivery to the distal nephron, plasma potassium concentration, and acid–base status. An increase in urine flow, sodium content, or plasma potassium increases the amount of potassium excreted.

☞ **The acid–base status of the patient affects potassium through the reciprocal relationship between the hydrogen [H$^+$] and potassium [K$^+$] ions.** ☞ Acidosis increases intracellular H^+ and K^+ flows into the plasma to maintain ionic balance, resulting in serum hyperkalemia. Alkalosis decreases intracellular H^+ and plasma K^+ moves

into the cell to maintain ionic balance, resulting in serum hypokalemia. The Na^+/K^+ ATPase pump is stimulated by insulin, thyroid hormone, and β-adrenergic catecholamines, resulting in cellular uptake of potassium.

Hyperkalemia
Causes

Hyperkalemia is usually defined by a serum $K^+ > 5.5 \text{ meq/L}$. In the critically ill patient, the most common cause of hyperkalemia is renal insufficiency, though an acute rise in extracellular potassium levels can also occur following crush injuries (rhabdomyolysis), or other forms of cellular destruction, and reperfusion injury can also result in hyperkalemia. Other causes include acidemia, hormone abnormalities, and drugs. Drugs can cause hyperkalemia through various mechanisms (Table 9), including transcellular shifts, involving hormonal, renal, or cellular membrane pump effects (34).

The use of succinylcholine, the depolarizing neuromuscular blockade drug, will transiently increase the serum K^+ concentration by 0.5–1 meq/L in most patients, including those with renal failure. However, patients who have sustained major burns or upper motor neuron trauma (head injuries and spinal cord injuries), as well as those who have been at chronic bed rest, often have an exaggerated release of K^+, due to the development of extrajunctional neuromuscular junction (NMJ) receptors (Volume 2, Chapter 6). The degree of K^+ elaboration may be enough to cause ventricular dysrhythmias, including asystole, which can only be treated by cardiopulmonary resuscitation, the administration of calcium chloride (to stabilize cellular membranes), alkalinization (to decrease the plasma $[K^+]$), by dialysis, if necessary.

Symptoms

☞ **The clinical manifestations of hyperkalemia are related to cellular membrane depolarization, the most serious of which involves cardiac muscle.** ☞ Hyperkalemia shortens

Table 9   Drug-Induced Hyperkalemia

Increased potassium intake
    Potassium supplements
    Herbal and nutritional supplements
    Packed red blood cells
    Penicillin G potassium

Transcellular shift
    Beta blockers
    IV amino
    Succinylcholine
    Digoxin intoxication

Impaired renal excretion
    Potassium-sparing diuretics (i.e., spironolactone)
    Nonsteroidal anti-inflammatory drugs
    Angiotensin converting enzyme inhibitors
    Angiotensin-II receptor blockers
    Trimethoprim
    Pentamidine acids
    Tacrolimus
    Heparin
    Cyclosporine

the duration of the cardiac action potential, decreases resting membrane potential (which depolarizes the membrane), and suppresses automaticity of cardiac pacemakers. The earliest electrocardiographic (ECG) manifestations are high-peaked T waves, usually first evident in the precordial leads. As the potassium level rises, this progresses to the prolongation of the P-R interval, flattening of the P wave, widening of the QRS complex with the merging of the T wave into a sine-wave configuration, with eventual ventricular fibrillation and cardiac standstill. Peripheral muscle can also be affected by moderate to severe hyperkalemia. Ascending muscular paresis can progress to flaccid quadriplegia and respiratory paralysis.

Treatment

Treatment depends on the degree of hyperkalemia. Mild hyperkalemia can usually be treated by hydration and the use of loop diuretics, which will increase potassium excretion, or treatment of volume, acid–base, or hormonal disturbances.

The presence of symptoms or ECG abnormalities demands more immediate, aggressive therapy. Immediate treatment with calcium salts will stabilize the cardiac membrane. Using 10 ml of 10% calcium gluconate, given intravenously over 3–5 minutes, provides 4.7 meq of calcium; whereas, 10 ml of 10% calcium chloride given intravenously over 10 minutes, provides 13.6 meq of calcium, but is best administered through a central line because of it's damaging effects on small vessels. The effect of calcium salts is temporary, lasting for about 30 minutes. Sodium bicarbonate can also be given to temporarily shift potassium into cells. Insulin and glucose therapy begins immediately, but may require an hour or more to demonstrate a significant effect; likewise, the serum [K$^+$] only decreases temporarily via this treatment modality.

Longer lasting therapies that actually decrease total potassium levels from the body include hemodialysis, potassium-exchange resins, and loop diuretics. Onset of action of these therapies on hyperkalemia is slower, and the aforementioned methods should be instituted for immediate relief when necessary. The usual dose of a potassium-exchange resin, such as sodium polystyrene, is 0.5 to 1 g/kg, which is usually dissolved in a sorbitol solution, and can be given orally or rectally.

Hypokalemia
Causes
✍ **Hypokalemia, usually defined as a serum K$^+$ <3.5 meq/L, is the most common electrolyte disorder in hospitalized patients (35), and is associated with hypomagnesemia, and can result from decreased potassium intake or increased renal or extrarenal potassium losses.** ✍

The most common source for extrarenal losses is the gastrointestinal tract. Drugs can cause hypokalemia through increased renal losses (e.g., diuretics) or transcellular shift (e.g., β-agonists and methylxanthines). Metabolic alkalosis, associated with excessive abnormal hydrochloric acid losses from vomiting or nasogastric suctioning can also exacerbate hypokalemia. As renal chloride levels decrease, the chloride-linked reabsorption of sodium in the proximal nephron decreases. Increased delivery of sodium to the distal convoluted tubule, in addition to the alkalemia, results in aldosterone-driven sodium reabsorption and potassium (and H$^+$) excretion. This situation drives both the hypokalemia and the alkalosis. The hypokalemic alkalosis

due to excessive gastric HCL losses is termed chloride sensitive, and can be treated with the administration of potassium chloride (no more than 40 meq/hr via a central vein). Non-chloride-sensitive metabolic alkalosis, such as hyperaldosteronism, usually results from increased distal nephron absorption of sodium. Any mineralocorticoid excess can potentially cause hypokalemia through this mechanism. In either case, magnesium is also usually very low, and must be replaced as well.

Symptoms
The symptoms of hypokalemia can be found in skeletal, smooth, and cardiac muscle, and include muscle weakness and paralysis, absent deep tendon reflexes, paralytic ileus, and cardiac conduction abnormalities. In the average individual with a normal heart, clinical manifestations usually do not occur unless the potassium level is less than 3.0 meq/L.

In patients with underlying heart disease, and especially those on digitalis, even mild hypokalemia can cause cardiac dysrhythmias. The toxic effects of digitalis are potentiated by hypokalemia, secondary to the inhibitory action of digitalis on the Na$^+$/K$^+$ ATPase pump. Electrocardiographic manifestations include progressive depression of the S-T segment and a decrease in T-wave amplitude. The U-wave amplitude and Q-T interval increase. A-V conduction prolongation and both ventricular and supraventricular dysrhythmias can result.

Treatment
✍ **Treatment of hypokalemia requires an understanding that a steady-state serum deficiency of 1 meq/L can translate to a total body deficit of >1000 meq.** ✍ However, no more than 40 meq should be administered per hour to a 70-kg patient (always administer via a central line to avoid peripheral vein sclerosis). Intravenous replacement is required if the patient is unable to take oral supplementation or if ECG changes are present. In general, potassium is replaced as a chloride, which is especially useful in the presence of alkalemia. Replacement via a peripheral vein should occur at a rate no faster than 10 meq per hour, and should rarely ever exceed 20 meq per hour. Cardiac monitoring is required for rates faster than 20 meq per hour.

CALCIUM DISORDERS

Calcium is a divalent cation. A normal adult contains 1 to 2 kg of calcium, of which the vast majority is deposited in bone (~99%) as hydroxyapatite crystals. Calcium homeostasis depends on bone exchange, renal excretion, and intestinal absorption (36). Calcium influx into the cell occurs through specific voltage-dependent calcium channels, or through receptor-mediated G-protein-linked channels. These G-protein-linked channels are activated through various membrane receptors that respond to endocrine and paracrine substances. Very small amounts of calcium leak passively through the cell membrane. Calcium in the cells functions as a second messenger, and is found in the cytosol and various organelles. Normally, energy is expended to pump calcium out of the cytosol and into the organelles and ECF. However, in the setting of shock with depletion of intracellular energy, calcium accumulates in the cells and has adverse effects, which can lead to widespread organ dysfunction and death.

Calcium exists in three forms in the ECF: ionized calcium, protein-bound calcium, and nonprotein anion calcium complexes. The ionized form functions as the most physiologically active, and comprises about 45% of total serum calcium. About 40% of serum calcium is protein bound. The majority of this calcium is bound to albumin, whereas the remainder is bound to the globulins. The remaining 15% of serum calcium is complexed to nonprotein anions, such as phosphate, citrate, sulfate, bicarbonate, and lactate. Extracellular calcium is tightly regulated, and is determined by a calcium receptor (first described in 1993), several hormones, and calcium itself. The most important hormones in calcium regulation are parathyroid hormone (PTH) and 1,25-dihydroxy vitamin D. Parathyroid hormone secretion is inversely related to serum calcium levels, and regulates calcium through several mechanisms. Within minutes, PTH decreases renal tubular reabsorption of phosphate, and causes an increase in distal tubular Ca reabsorption through a cyclic adenine monophosphate (cAMP)-mediated process. Within hours, PTH causes release of Ca^{+2} from the bone through osteoclast activation, serving as the main reservoir for calcium exchange in the body. As hypocalcemia persists, PTH stimulates renal transformation of circulating prohormone 25-hydroxy vitamin D into 1,25-dihydroxy vitamin D, the active form. This hormone facilitates the reabsorption of calcium by the proximal small bowel. 1,25-dihydroxy vitamin D also stimulates bone reabsorption. The hormone calcitonin, secreted by C cells of the thyroid, only moderately affects calcium metabolism.

Normal values of total serum calcium usually range between 8.5 and 10.5 mg/dL. Following trauma and critical care, patients have decreased albumin levels, making the total serum calcium measurement less useful. ☞ **In the setting of trauma and critical illness, the free ionized (physiologically active) form of calcium is the relevant value that should be measured.** ☞ The ratio of free calcium to protein-bound calcium is dependent on several factors. For instance, in the setting of low albumin levels, the total serum calcium level will also be low, whereas the ionized or free amount of calcium may remain near normal. There are formulas that exist to correct serum calcium to albumin level; however, in critically ill patients, they are inaccurate. As a general rule in the critically ill patient, therapeutic decisions should be based on the level of ionized calcium alone (rather than total serum calcium).

Hypercalcemia

Primary hyperparathyroidism is the most common chronic cause of hypercalcemia. Malignancy, caused by bony metastases and/or by a parathyroid hormone-related protein (PTHrP), is the second most common cause. This protein binds to PTH receptors in bone and kidney. Breast, lung, and renal cell carcinoma are the most common solid tumors that can cause hypercalcemia. Multiple myeloma causes hypercalcemia through bony destruction, as a result of inflammatory mediators (IL-1, IL-6, and TNF- σ). In both Hodgkin's and non-Hodgkin's lymphoma, hypercalcemia results from increased conversion of 25-hydroxy-cholecalciferol to calcitriol by tumor cells. Other common causes include granulomatous diseases (i.e., sarcoidosis), drugs (i.e., thiazide diuretics, vitamin A or vitamin D intoxication).

Symptoms

Symptomatology is often related to the degree and acute nature of the hypercalcemia. Most cases of mild hypercalcemia (levels ≤ 12 mg/dL) are asymptomatic, but once calcium levels are above 12 mg/dL, neurologic, gastrointestinal, and renal symptoms usually appear. Neurologic symptoms can begin with mild drowsiness, progressing to weakness, depression, and coma. Gastrointestinal symptoms can involve constipation, nausea, vomiting, anorexia, and peptic ulcer disease. Renal manifestations include nephrocalcinosis, nephrolithiasis, and nephrogenic DI. Serum calcium levels above 13.5 mg/dL generally constitute a medical emergency.

Treatment

Treatment of hypercalcemia initially involves volume loading with NS and diuresis (usually furosemide). The resulting natriuresis is accompanied by calciuresis. Depending on the degree of hypercalcemia, urine volumes should range from 2 to 3 L/day, up to 6 L/day. The patient must remain euvolemic, as hypovolemia will exacerbate the problem.

The etiology of the hypercalcemia must then be determined. Most cases of severe hypercalcemia are caused by malignancy. Bisphosphonates, which have made mithramycin relatively obsolete, are utilized in the setting of increased osteoclastic activity, such as malignancy. If primary hyperparathyroidism is the underlying etiology, serious consideration should be given to urgent parathyroid surgery after initial patient stabilization. Parathyroidectomy may also be useful in cases of secondary or tertiary hyperparathyroidism. Glucocorticoids have been shown to be helpful in cases of hypercalcemia, secondary to sarcoidosis, hematologic malignancies, and vitamin D intoxication. Hemodialysis, with a low- or no-calcium bath, is also an available treatment modality. Thiazide diuretics and digitalis are contraindicated in the setting of hypercalcemia, as thiazides can decrease calciuria, and digitalis can cause cardiac arrest.

Hypocalcemia
Causes

Hypocalcemia is defined as a decrease in the ionized fraction of total serum calcium. ☞ **Hypocalcemia is a common entity in critically ill patients (37). It is estimated that about 70% to 90% of critically ill patients have decreased total serum calcium levels, and ionized calcium levels are deficient in 15% to 50%.** ☞ The etiology is often multifactorial.

There appears to be a relationship between sepsis and critical illness, and altered PTH secretion and peripheral action. Inflammatory mediators, such as TNF- σ, IL-1, and IL-6 have also been implicated. Chelating substances, such as phosphate, bicarbonate, citrate, and even radiocontrast dye can decrease ionized calcium levels. Hypocalcemia is a particular problem during the anhepatic stage of liver transplant (following massive blood and factor transfusion), and during continuous veno-veno hemodialysis (CVVHD) in patients with severe liver failure in the intensive care unit (ICU). In all these cases the citrate used for chelating calcium (to keep blood products from clotting, and to keep blood on the CVVHD machine from clotting) is not being metabolized by a normal liver, and thus very large quantities of calcium gluconate, and/or calcium chloride are needed to restore the ionized calcium concentration.

Postoperative hypocalcemia can occur following parathyroid, thyroid, or radical neck surgery. This decrease is exacerbated following surgery for hyperparathyroidism, due to the "hungry bone syndrome," which causes a rapid accretion of calcium into bone as PTH levels fall to normal or subnormal levels, which may result in profound hypocalcemia.

Conditions of rapid cell destruction, such as rhabdomyolysis or tumor lysis syndrome, which result in hyperphosphatemia, can cause hypocalcemia. This is due to phosphate binding to calcium. Other conditions that are associated with increased organic anions (i.e., citrate toxicity) or free fatty acids (acute pancreatitis) can also decrease serum calcium levels. Renal and hepatic insufficiency can result in hypocalcemia owing to their effects on vitamin D metabolism. Hypomagnesemia interferes with PTH secretion and possibly its peripheral action. Therefore, correction of magnesium deficits is essential in the treatment of hypocalcemia.

Symptoms

Symptoms of neuromuscular irritability predominate in the setting of hypocalcemia. These symptoms include numbness, paresthesias (typically circumoral and digital), muscle cramps, Chvostek's and Trousseau's signs, laryngospasm, tetany, and seizures. Chvostek's sign is a facial twitch, elicited by tapping the facial nerve just below the zygomatic arch with the mouth open. Trousseau's sign is induction of wrist and metacarpophalangeal joint flexion, hyperextension of fingers, and flexion of thumb and palm with brachial artery occlusion for three minutes. Hypocalcemia also may cause Q-T prolongation on the ECG, and this can progress to heart block or ventricular fibrillation.

Treatment

Treatment of hypocalcemia depends upon the acuteness, severity, and etiology. The normal serum ionized calcium concentration is 1.13 to 1.32 mmol/L (4.52–5.28 mg/dL). In severe hypocalcemia (<0.6–0.8 mmol/L), as seen with citrate toxicity from massive blood product administration, and/or hepatic dysfunction in the setting of citrate-anticoagulated CVVHD, aggressive calcium administration is warranted. For this condition, 500 to 1000 mg (elemental calcium equivalent) IV push via a central line, followed by infusion at rates as high as 50 to 100 mg per minute, may be required. In this setting, continuous infusions and frequent (every 15–30 minutes) arterial blood gasses with concomitant ionized calcium values should be obtained to titrate therapy.

Note that in the presence of excess unmetabolized citrate, a safe level of ionized calcium (>1.0 mmol/L or >4mg/dL) will require the total blood calcium to be supranormal. Indeed, in this setting, >17 mg/dL has been recorded with massive transfusion during liver transplantation (36). This concurrence of a low ionized calcium and a high total calcium ("calcium gap") allows recognition of the citrate accumulation syndrome. If severe, it may prompt a decision to minimize administration of additional citrate-containing products. Otherwise, when the calcium citrate complexes are subsequently metabolized, ionized calcium levels may rise to high levels.

In the less acute setting, symptomatic hypocalcemia and ionized calcium levels of less than 1.0 μmol/L should be treated, but less aggressively. The amount of parenteral calcium given initially in this less acute setting is 100 mg (elemental calcium equivalent) over 5 to 10 minutes. This is followed by an infusion of 0.5 to 2.0 mg/kg/hr.

Magnesium and phosphorus levels, and if clinically indicated, PTH and vitamin D levels, should be determined. Magnesium should be supplemented and phosphorus lowered if indicated. Calcium administration in the setting of hyperphosphatemia can result in metastatic calcium phosphate precipitation. In general, phosphorus levels should be below 6 mg/dL prior to calcium administration. Parenteral calcium is given for acute symptomatic hypocalcemia. Oral supplementation and vitamin D are given for chronic hypocalcemia.

There are different preparations for infusion of elemental calcium. The most commonly used preparations are calcium gluconate and calcium chloride. Calcium gluconate 10% solution contains 93 mg of elemental calcium, whereas calcium chloride 10% solution contains 272 mg. The higher the amount of elemental calcium, the more irritating it is to the veins. Calcium should be infused through a central vein, if possible. There are various oral calcium preparations available. Acute oral therapy generally involves 0.5 to 1.0 g every six hours. Vitamin D_3 or calcitriol can also be given to increase calcium reabsorption from the gut. Of note, there is an increasing body of evidence that cellular calcium overload is detrimental. Therefore, a mild ionized hypocalcemia may be desirable in acute inflammatory states (37).

MAGNESIUM DISORDERS

Magnesium is the second most abundant intracellular ion. It is an essential cofactor in many enzymatic reactions, including the transfer of phosphate groups (energy metabolism), replication and transcription of DNA and translation of mRNA, membrane stabilization, nerve conduction, ion transport, and calcium channel activity. Total body magnesium content is about 21 to 28 g, most of which is in the skeletal bone mass (>50%). Less than 1% is located in the extracellular space. Normal serum levels range from 1.5 to 2.5 mg/dL. The total body magnesium balance is mainly dependent on gastrointestinal absorption and renal excretion. Bone is an extremely slow exchangeable source of magnesium. Approximately 55% of extracellular magnesium exists in the free ionized form, with the remainder complexed to anions and proteins (38,39).

Hypermagnesemia
Causes

The most common cause of elevated serum magnesium levels is acute or chronic renal insufficiency. This may be exacerbated by the use of magnesium-containing antacids and laxatives in the setting of impaired renal function. Hypermagnesemia may also occur secondary to rhabdomyolysis following burn or crush injuries.

Symptoms

Clinical manifestations relate to neuromuscular depression. Synaptic acetylcholine release is inhibited by hypermagnesemia. Loss of deep tendon reflexes occurs at levels of about 8 mg/dL. As levels increase above this, paralysis and coma can occur. Cardiovascular effects consist of hypotension and cardiac conduction disturbances. The P-R interval, in addition to widening of the QRS complex and elevated T waves, can eventually lead to cardiac arrest.

Treatment

Treatment involves repleting extracellular volume deficits, correcting acidosis, withholding exogenous magnesium intake, and occasionally hemodialysis. Loop diuretics can also increase magnesium renal excretion. Because hypermagnesemia is generally a rather benign condition (especially in intubated patients), the need for specific therapy is exceedingly rare. However, acute symptomatology in nonintubated patients or hypotensive patients can be temporarily controlled by slow intravenous administration of 5 to 10 meq/L of calcium, which antagonizes the neuromuscular effects of magnesium.

Hypomagnesemia
Causes

Poor intake alone is rarely a cause of hypomagnesemia, because of the ability of the kidneys to conserve magnesium. Most states of deficiency result from decreased intake, in addition to increased gastrointestinal losses. Other causes include prolonged intravenous fluid replacement without magnesium replacement, chronic loop diuretic use, and certain drugs, such as cisplatin, aminoglycosides, cyclosporine, amphotericin B, insulin, and mannitol. ☛ **It is estimated that about >25% of patients on a medical-surgical ward and >75% on the postoperative ICU setting are hypomagnesemic.** ☛ Serum levels of magnesium correlate poorly with total body stores, which may be reduced despite normal serum levels.

Symptoms

Most states of magnesium deficiency are asymptomatic. When symptoms do occur, a severe deficiency usually exists. Neuromuscular symptoms mirror hypocalcemia, with hyperreflexia, tremors, tetany, and positive Chvostek's and Trousseau's sign. Seizures can ensue, as can life-threatening cardiac dysrhythmias. Early ECG changes include prolonged P-R and Q-T intervals and atrial tachydysrhythmias. More life threatening dysrhythmias may result with ventricular tachycardia, including polymorphic ventricular tachycardia (torsades de pointes) and ventricular fibrillation (Volume 2, Chapter 20).

Treatment

Acute therapy involves 1 to 2 g of intravenous magnesium sulfate (8–16 meq) over 5 to 10 minutes, followed by an infusion of 0.5 to 1.0 g/hr. Sulfate can bind both calcium and potassium, and therefore, levels of these ions should be measured during therapy. During treatment, clinically significant hypermagnesemia can result. However, the therapeutic window for magnesium is quite large, and the treatment of hypermagnesemia is seldom required (and when needed consists mainly of supportive care). Nonetheless, it is helpful to have calcium gluconate or calcium chloride available for nonintubated patients, who become symptomatic. Magnesium oxide is the preferred agent for oral supplementation.

PHOSPHORUS DISORDERS

Phosphorus is primarily contained in the ICF, but is involved in both cellular and extracelluar processes. Cellular energy is generated through phosphate bonds (i.e., ATP, creatine phosphate). In addition, phosphate functions as an oxygen carrier in hemoglobin [as a component of 2,3-diphosphoglycerate (2,3-DPG)], and serves as an integral component of cAMP, cGMP, and inositol polyphosphates. Phosphorus is also involved in the processing and synthesis of DNA, mRNA, and proteins. It is likewise important in acid–base balance, glycolysis, vitamin D metabolism, and in the structure of bone and cell membranes (phospholipids).

Normal total serum phosphorus levels range between about 2.5 and 4.5 mg/dL, though serum levels are not necessarily reflective of total body stores. Fifty-five percent of total serum phosphorus exists in the ionized form. Phosphorus homeostasis is dependent upon intestinal absorption, renal excretion, and bone mineralization/resorption. The kidneys are the primary regulators, and renal phosphorus excretion is increased by PTH, calcitonin, vasopressin, ANP, dopamine, metabolic acidosis, volume expansion, glucose, amino acids, NS, and ketones. Renal phosphorus excretion is decreased by vitamin D, growth hormone, IGF-1, glucocorticoids, thyroid hormone, and metabolic alkalosis. In addition, PTH decreases, and vitamin D increases the intestinal absorption of phosphate.

Hyperphosphatemia
Causes

Hyperphosphatemia can result from diminished renal excretory capacity, increased exogenous phosphate or vitamin D load, and transcellular shift. Renal failure is the most common cause of hyperphosphatemia. Initially, in mild-to-moderate renal failure, hyperphosphatemia leads to increased PTH secretion. The increase in PTH leads to decreased renal tubular reabsorption and increased urinary excretion. In severe renal failure (usually glomerular filtration rate <25 mL/min), this mechanism often fails and hyperphosphatemia is almost a universal finding. Cell lysis of any etiology can cause intracellular release of phosphorus to the extracellular space. Acidosis of either a metabolic or respiratory etiology causes the transcellular shift of phosphate with resultant extracellular hyperphosphatemia. Hypoparathyroidism, hyperthyroidism, and acromegaly cause hyperphosphatemia through decreased phosphaturia. Treatment with bisphosphonates can also cause hyperphosphatemia, but this is believed to be secondary to both transcellular shift and decreased renal excretion. Exogenous etiologies of hyperphosphatemia include laxative phosphate salts and phosphate-containing enemas. Patients most susceptible to exogenous hyperphosphatemia are those with intravascular depletion, renal insufficiency, bowel mucosal abnormalities, bowel obstruction, or ileus.

Symptoms

The clinical manifestations of hyperphosphatemia are a result of the consequent hypocalcemia and precipitation of calcium phosphate in soft tissues. Hyperphosphatemia causes hypocalcemia by decreasing the renal conversion of vitamin D, decreasing the production of calcitriol, and precipitation. When the calcium–phosphorus product exceeds 70, precipitation in the soft tissues is likely to occur.

Treatment

Treatment involves correcting the underlying disorder, elimination of exogenous phosphate sources, increased phosphorus excretion, and treatment of associated hypocalcemia (39). Renal phosphorus excretion is facilitated by NS loading and loop diuretics. Gut absorption is decreased by the use of phosphate binders. Aluminum phosphate binders should only be used for short periods in patients with renal failure, as aluminum accumulation can be detrimental with long term therapy. Calcium levels need to be monitored closely when calcium carbonate is used, because hypercalcemia can result, and if calcium is given when the phosphorus level is greater than 7 mg/dL, calcium phosphate is likely to precipitate. Hemodialysis is very effective in patients with renal failure. As a temporizing measure, insulin and glucose can cause transcellular shift of phosphorus from the extracellular to the intracellular compartment, but potassium monitoring in this setting is mandatory.

Hypophosphatemia
Causes
☞ **Transcellular shift is the most common mechanism of acute hypophosphatemia, though chronic total body hypophosphatemia results from decreased intake and/or increased renal or gastrointestinal losses.** ☞ Clinical situations associated with transcellular shift generally involve conditions that stimulate glycolysis. During glycolysis, phosphorylated glucose compounds are generated and utilized. Refeeding syndromes (in malnourished and chronic alcoholic patients), insulin administration during diabetic ketoacidosis, corticosteroid or catecholamine administration, and CVVHD (with the massive quantities of glucose containing fluids administered) can all cause hypophosphatemia.

Hungry bone syndrome following parathyroidectomy results in massive deposition of phosphorus into bone. Increased urinary losses of phosphorus accompany renal tubular defects, increased PTH, vitamin D deficiency, acidosis, and diuretic use. Up to 30% of patients with malignancy have increased urinary losses of phosphorus. Increased intestinal losses accompany chronic diarrhea, steatorrhea, fistulas, and dietary intake of phosphate binders (i.e., magnesium or aluminum hydroxide). Decreased intestinal vitamin D absorption often accompanies these conditions and exacerbates the problem.

Chronic alcoholic patients are especially susceptible to hypophosphatemia for a multitude of reasons, including dietary deficiency, decreased intestinal absorption (secondary to increase antacid use), vomiting, magnesium deficiency, refeeding syndrome, and renal phosphorus wasting. Diabetic patients are prone to increased renal phosphorus wasting, secondary to accompanying insulin deficiency, glycosuria, ketonuria, and acidosis.

Symptoms
Clinical manifestations generally do not occur unless the serum phosphorus level is less than 1 mg/dL. As phosphorus is involved in many cellular and extracellular processes, the clinical manifestations can be profound and quite diverse, and can include muscle weakness, respiratory insufficiency, tremors, paresthesias, encephalopathy, ataxia, coma, seizures, anorexia, rhabdomyolysis, hemolysis, thrombocytopenia, immune cell dysfunction, insulin resistance, impaired gluconeogenesis, impaired vasopressor response, and cardiac, renal, and hepatic insufficiency.

Treatment
Phosphorus repletion is always indicated when the level is less than 1 mg/dL and generally indicated when it is less than 1.5 mg/dL (39). A level of 1.5 mg/dL or above usually does not require supplementation in the absence of other clinical evidence of phosphate depletion. The safest mode

for phosphate repletion is oral, and usual doses are 1 to 3 g/day. Intravenous phosphorus replacement is recommended for levels less than 1 mg/dL. Great care must be taken with intravenous supplementation, as it can precipitate a hypocalcemic crisis, and as such, calcium levels should be followed with appropriate supplementation. Usually the phosphorus is administered as a sodium or potassium salt in NS at 2.5 mg/kg over six hours. Parenteral administration should discontinue when levels are greater than 2 mg/dL.

EYE TO THE FUTURE

Currently, research appears concentrated in the early detection of electrolyte disorders. Point of care laboratory testing is currently available with resultant reductions in the turn-around time for electrolyte determinations. However, the cost effectiveness of such testing for widespread ICU use remains to be determined.

Indwelling electrodes have been tested that give continuous read-outs of selected serum electrolytes. However, determination of electrolyte replacement requires knowledge of factors other than the serum electrolyte concentration (i.e., volume status, albumin concentration, etc.). The electrodes are also invasive and a potential source of infection.

Additionally, clinical trials are needed to determine the clinical significance of basic science properties specific to the various crystalloid solutions, colloids, and blood products, including their modulation of vascular permeability and systemic inflammation. Outcome-focused clinical trials powered to discern a mortality benefit for various resuscitation fluids in septic shock and/or hemorrhagic shock are needed, along with integrated acid base and systemic electrolyte analyses. Furthermore, well-designed clinical trials are required to evaluate the physiologic effects of colloids and crystalloids, electrolyte and acid–base disturbances with respect to individual organ function (including lung-fluid balance in patients at risk for or with established ALI/ARDS, renal function in patients at risk for renal insufficiency/failure, gut and liver function in patients with pre-existing liver injury or ileus and those at high risk for shock liver, the immune and reticuloendothelial system in patients suffering from sepsis or at risk for sepsis) and the effect on the immune system, and the central nervous system in terms of both short- and long-term outcomes.

Another area of interest is the important problem of CSW syndrome, and the differentiation from SIADH. We believe the rapid determination of BNP (via newly released bedside immunoassay, currently used for CHF) holds promise in more quickly diagnosing CSW syndrome, and beginning important NS and volume repletion therapy (27).

In addition, the problem of CPM, resulting from too rapid a correction of hyponatremia, continues to be a clinically important problem, which may be limited by better understanding of the pathophysiology, and more frequent and earlier measures of serum sodium, so as to protect from the development of the entity in the first place.

SUMMARY

Fluid and electrolyte disorders are common in the ICU. Their management requires more than the determination of serum chemistries. Proper management of Na$^+$ disorders requires the knowledge of volume status and sources of continued fluid and/or Na$^+$ losses. Similarly, management of K$^+$ disorders requires a determination of the sources of K$^+$ loss (diuretics, diarrhea, etc.) or accumulation (renal failure, crush injury). The interpretation of Ca^{2+} and Mg^{2+} serum concentrations must include the etiology of the disorder and serum albumin concentrations. Phosphorus concentrations are dependent on renal function and calcium homeostasis.

Thus, an approach to fluid and electrolyte disorders that is narrowly based solely on the determinations of serum chemistries will often inadequately correct the abnormality and may, in fact, exacerbate the disorder. Instead, proper treatment requires an in-depth determination of volume status, renal function, serum albumin, and a review of current drug therapy that may be contributing to the disorder. Only then can a plan for the correction of the given disorder be properly formulated.

The initial choice of fluid administration is guided by the goal of optimizing perfusion of tissues; however, there is still limited data that can predict which fluids (colloids or crystalloids) are best in any particular scenario (Volume 1, Chapter 11). There is an increasing amount of information available regarding the physiochemical and biological properties of various colloid and crystalloid fluids available (40). Yet, the goals of providing adequate tissue perfusion (with appropriate levels of intravascular volume), and optimum cellular function (by maintaining normal values of serum chemistries), has not substantially changed in the last decade. The best way to achieve these goals is by frequent measurements of the intravascular volume and plasma solute concentrations, and by both anticipating and monitoring expected perturbations. Frequent monitoring in concert with frequent alterations in the fluid and electrolytes being administered represents the optimum strategy for care. It is more likely that new monitoring modalities will provide a greater impact on trauma and critical care management than the development of new fluid and electrolyte formulations.

KEY POINTS

↪ Only a fraction of the total body potassium, about 4 mEq/dL (approx 67 meq in a 70 kg patient), is in the blood.

↪ Plasma osmolarity (Posm) is generally a good estimate of total body osmolarity, because isosmotic conditions are maintained through fluid shifts.

↪ When the calculated Posm differs by >15 mOsm from the laboratory-measured value, an osmolar gap exists.

↪ Crystalloids should be the initial resuscitation fluid administered in most situations.

↪ Hypernatremia almost always represents a hyperosmolar or hypertonic state, whereas hyponatremia can be present in a hypertonic, isotonic, or hypotonic state.

↪ The work-up for hypernatremia starts with determination of intravascular volume status, based on history, physical examination, and laboratory data.

↪ In complete central DI, the urinary osmolality is <150 mOsm/L, but may be higher in partial DI.

↪ The diagnosis of SIADH is suggested by the finding of urine osmolarity >100 mOsm/L and urine sodium >40 meq/L in the setting of hyponatremia.

↪ Cerebral salt wasting syndrome must be differentiated from SIADH, because their treatments are divergent, and directly effect outcome.

↪ Symptoms secondary to acute hyponatremia typically do not arise until the serum [Na$^+$] is less than 125 mEq/L in acute hyponatremic states, or less than 120 meq/L in more chronic conditions.

↪ Experimental studies in animals and observations in humans suggest that the rate of hyponatremia correction in the first 24 hours is the major determinant for the development of osmotic demyelination.

↪ Because the extracellular concentration of potassium changes most quickly, it has the greatest effect on cell membrane function, and is particularly important for cardiac and nerve tissues.

↪ The acid–base status of the patient affects potassium through the reciprocal relationship between the hydrogen [H$^+$] and potassium [K$^+$] ions.

↪ The clinical manifestations of hyperkalemia are related to cellular membrane depolarization, the most serious of which involves cardiac muscle.

↪ Hypokalemia, usually defined as a serum K$^+$ < 3.5 meq/L, is the most common electrolyte disorder in hospitalized patients (35), and is associated with hypomagnesemia, and can result from decreased potassium intake or increased renal or extrarenal potassium losses.

↪ Treatment of hypokalemia requires an understanding that a steady-state serum deficiency of 1 meq/L can translate to a total body deficit of >1000 meq.

↪ In the setting of trauma and critical illness, the free ionized (physiologically active) form of calcium is the relevant value that should be measured.

↪ Hypocalcemia is a common entity in critically ill patients (37). It is estimated that about 70 to 90% of critically ill patients have decreased total serum calcium levels, and ionized calcium levels are deficient in 15–50%.

↪ It is estimated that about >25% of patients on a medical-surgical ward and >75% on the postoperative ICU setting are hypomagnesemic.

↪ Transcellular shift is the most common mechanism of acute hypophosphatemia, though chronic total body hypophosphatemia results from decreased intake and/or increased renal or gastrointestinal losses.

REFERENCES

1. Malangoni MA, Yowler CJ. Electrolytes and electrolyte dysfunction. In: Argenta ed. Basic Science for Surgeons: A Review. Philadelphia: Elsevier, 2004.
2. McHenry CR, Weinstein LS. Fluid and electrolyte therapy. In: Cameron JL, ed. Current Surgical Therapy. 7th ed. St. Louis: Mosby, 2001.
3. Narins RG, Jones ER, Stom MC, et al. Diagnostic strategies in disorders of fluid, electrolyte and acid-base homeostasis. Am J Med 1982; 72:496–520.
4. Ho AM, Karmaker MB, Contardi LH, Ng SS, Hewson JR. Excessive use of normal saline in managing traumatized patients in shock: a preventable contributor to acidosis. J Trauma 2001; 51:173–177.
5. Shackford SR, Bourguignon PR, Wald SL, et al. Hypertonic saline resuscitation of patients with head injury: a prospective, randomized clinical trial. J Trauma 1998; 44:50–58.
6. Krausz MM. Controversies in shock research: hypertonic resuscitation—pros and cons. Shock 1995; 3:69–72.

7. Rizoli SB, Kapus JF, Li YH, Marshall JC, Rotstein OD. Immunomodulatory effects of hypertonic resuscitation on the development of lung inflammation following hemorrhagic shock. J Immunol 1998; 161:6288–6296.

8. Corso CO, Okamoto S, Leiderer R, Messmer K. Resuscitation with hypertonic saline dextran reduces endothelial cell swelling and improves hepatic microvascular perfusion and function after hemorrhagic shock. J Surg Res 1998; 80:210–220.

9. Cushcieri J, Gourlay D, Garcia I, et al. Hypertonic preconditioning inhibits macrophage responsiveness to endotoxin. J Immunol 2002; 168:1389–1396.

10. Wilder DM, Reid TJ, Bakaltcheva IB. Hypertonic resuscitation and blood coagulation. In vitro comparison of several hypertonic solutions for their action on platelets and plasma coagulation. Thromb Res 2002; 107:255–261.

11. Roche AM, James MFM, Grocott MPW, Mythen MG. Coagulation effects of in vitro serial haemodilution with balanced electrolyte hetastarch solution compared with a saline-based hetastarch solution and lactated Ringer's solution. Anaesthesia 2002; 57:950–955.

12. Treib J, Baron JF, Grauer MT, Strauss RG. An international view of hydroxyethyl starches. Intensive Care Med 1999; 25:258–268.

13. Schierhout G, Roberts I. Fluid resuscitation with colloid or crystalloid solution in critically ill patients: a systematic review of randomized trials. Br Med J 1998; 316:961–964.

14. Cochrane Injuries Group Albumin Reviewers. Human albumin administration in critically ill patients: systematic review of randomised controlled trials. BMJ 1998; 317:235–240.

15. Wilkes MM, Navickis RJ. Patient survival after human albumin administration: a meta-analysis of randomized, controlled trials. Ann Intern Med 2001; 135:149–164.

16. Martin GS, Matthay MA (for the working group of the Critical Care Assembly of the American Thoracic Society): Evidence-based colloid use in the critically ill: American Thoracic Society Consensus Statement. Am J Respir Crit Care Med 2004; 170(11):1247–1259.

17. U.S. Preventive Services Task Force. Guide to clinical preventive services: report of the U.S. Preventive Services Task Force. 2d ed. Baltimore, MD: Williams & Wilkins, 1996.

18. Kumar S, Berl T. Sodium. Lancet 1998; 352:220–228.

19. Kugler JP, Hustead T. Hyponatremia and hypernatremia in the elderly. Am Family Physician 2000; 61:3623–3630.

20. Riggs JE. Neurologic manifestations of electrolyte disturbances. Neurol Clin 2002; 20:227–239.

21. Adrogué HJ, Madias NE. Hyponatremia. N Engl J Med 2000; 342:1581–1589.

22. Yeates KE, Singer M, Morton AR. Salt and water: a simple approach to hyponatremia. Can Med Assoc J 2004; 170:365–369.

23. Abboud CF, Laws ER. Clinical endocrinological approach to hypothalamic-pituitary disease. J Neurosurg 1979; 51:271–291.

24. Palmer BF. Hyponatremia in neurosurgical patients: syndrome of inappropriate antidiuretic hormone versus cerebral salt wasting. Nephrol Dial Transplant 2000; 15:262–268.

25. Berendes E, Walter M, Cullen P, et al. Secretion of brain natriuretic peptide in patients with aneurysmal subarachnoid haemorrhage. Lancet 1997; 349:245–249.

26. Levin ER, Gardner DG, Samson WK. Natriuretic peptides. N Engl J Med 1998; 339: 321–328.

27. Prahash A, Lynch T. B-type natriuretic peptide: a diagnostic, prognostic, and therapeutic tool in heart failure. Am J Crit Care 2004; 13:46–53.

28. Laureno R, Karp BI. Myelinolysis after correction of hyponatremia. Ann Intern Med 1997; 126:57–62.

29. Adams RA, Victor M, Mancall EL. Central pontine myelinolysis: a hitherto undescribed disease occurring in alcoholics and malnourished patients. Arch Neurol Psychiatry 1959; 81:154–172.

30. Endo Y, Oda M, Hara M. Central pontine myelinolysis: a study of 37 cases in 1000 consecutive autopsies. Acta Neuropathol 1981; 53:145–153.

31. Tarhan NC, Agildere AM, Benli US, et al. Osmotic demyelination syndrome in end-stage renal disease after recent hemodialysis: MRI of the brain. Am J Roentgenol 2004; 182(3): 809–816.

32. Ruzek KA, Campeau NG, Miller GM. Early diagnosis of central pontine myelinolysis with diffusion-weighted imaging AJNR. Am J Neuroradiol 2004; 25(2):210–213.

33. Sterns RH, Cappuccio JD, Silver SM, Cohen EP. Neurologic sequelae after treatment of severe hyponatremia: a multicenter perspective. J Am Soc Nephrol 1994; 4:1522–1530.

34. Perazella MA. Drug-induced hyperkalemia: old culprits and new offenders. Am J Med 2000; 109:307–314.

35. Gennari JF. Hypokalemia. N Engl J Med1998; 339:451–458.

36. Abdeen O, Kohler G, Mehta R, et al. Intraoperative continuous renal replacement therapy (IO-CRRT) during liver transplantation. J Am Soc Nephrol 2001; 12(9):161A-162A.

37. Carlstedt F, Lind L. Hypocalcemic syndromes. Crit Care Clin 2001; 17:139–153.

38. Fox C, Ramsoomair D, Carter C. Magnesium: its proven and potential clinical significance. Southern Med J 2001; 94:1195–1201.

39. Weisinger JR, Bellorin-Font E. Magnesium and phosphorus. Lancet 1998; 352:391–396.

40. Grocott MPW, Mythen MG, Gan TJ: Perioperative fluid management and clinical outcomes in adults. Anesth Analg 2005; 100:1093–106.

41. Prough DS, Mathru M. Acid-base, fluids and electrolytes. In: Barash PG, Cullen BF, Stoelting RK, eds. Clinical Anesthesia, 4th ed. Philadelphia: JB Lippincott, 2001:165–200.

45

Acid–Base Disorders

Lewis J. Kaplan

Section of Trauma, Critical Care, and Surgical Emergencies, Yale University School of Medicine, New Haven, Connecticut, U.S.A.

John A. Kellum

Departments of Critical Care Medicine and Medicine, University of Pittsburgh, Pittsburgh, Pennsylvania, U.S.A.

INTRODUCTION

The invention of the pH probe ushered in a new era of critical care medicine where a definable physiologic endpoint became possible. A series of somewhat contradictory theories regarding acid–base interpretation were developed culminating in the great "Trans-Atlantic Debate" which occurred in the wake of the pH probe's creation (1). Most of the controversy revolves around the explanation of the metabolic component (i.e., what causes hydrogen ions [H^+] to increase, decrease, or be buffered). The period during the late 1960s and early 1970s witnessed the evolution of the "classic model" based on the Henderson–Hasselbach relationship and the "standard base excess" (SBE) concept whose roots trace back to standard bicarbonate and buffer base (BB). Both of these models evolved into the establishment of nomograms and formulas for guiding acid–base management.

During the 1980s, Stewart (Canadian born, American physiologist) (2) proposed a new theory of acid–base physiology that challenged the existing paradigm. Stewart's theory is based on physicochemical principles and direct observation of charge dynamics in various solutions, including plasma. Stewart's term strong ion difference (SID) utilizes concepts similar to the BB principle developed earlier by Singer and Hastings (3), though they used different nomenclature.

Despite acceptance of the underlying principles involving Stewart's method, some traditionalists of acid–base balance (ABB) prefer to use the more familiar HCO_3^- or SBE approach or derived nomograms to evaluate acid–base disorders. All of these approaches, when applied correctly will result in correct ABB determinations for simple disorders. However, the HCO_3^- and SBE are not dependent variables but rather associated variables that correlate with changes in ABB.

This chapter will explore the Stewart SID paradigm that is increasingly used, along with the more traditional methods of acid–base evaluation. These techniques will be explained so the reader will be able to investigate the common acid–base disturbances that arise de novo or iatrogenically during the care of trauma and critically ill patients.

In a recent review, Schlichtig et al. (4) provide in-depth derivations, explanations, and comparisons of the various techniques for evaluating the metabolic component of ABB reviewed in this chapter, and they also appropriately emphasize that all of these methodologies are internally consistent. Readers interested in reviewing a more traditional (i.e., HCO_3^-) approach to acid–base disturbances and their analysis are referred to the classic landmark article by Narins and Emmett (5). A shorter, more practical, and clinically based approach utilizing the Narins principles is offered in the review by Haber (6). Other excellent reviews are also recommended for those seeking greater understanding of the traditional acid–base models (7–13).

In addition to the formal derivation of the SID, which some find complicated, the practical graphical approach of ABB presented by Schlichtig et al. (4,14) is also reviewed in this chapter, because its simplicity appeals to graphically minded clinicians. The rules-based approach suggested by Haber (6) is also provided here because it represents the simplest application of the classic approach using the standard concepts put forward by Narins and Emmet (5).

Each phase of trauma care from resuscitation through convalescence can be accompanied by prototypical acid–base derangements. This chapter will help the reader to recognize, characterize, and remedy the common acid–base disorders identified in trauma patients, as well as tertiary acid–base derangements. This chapter will also provide ample examples of clinical conditions where ABB may be perturbed and where application of the SID concept will best explain the acid–base disorder and its treatment.

ACID–BASE OVERVIEW AND NOMENCLATURE
Overview of Acid–Base Balance

By convention, ABB is measured and analyzed from arterial blood samples. However, the data are clinically interpreted to apply to the entire volume of extracellular fluid (ECF). ABB reflects the hydrogen ion concentration in blood and depends upon three independent factors: (i) *respiratory component*, where pulmonary ventilation results in CO_2 elimination and controls the arterial P_{CO_2} (Pa_{CO_2}); (ii) *metabolic component*, primarily affected by tissue metabolism and gastrointestinal output and renal regulatation; and (iii) *nonvolatile weak acid buffers*: phosphate and proteins (predominantly albumin and in the case of whole blood, hemoglobin). For the student of ABB, most confusion stems from explanations and interpretations of the metabolic component. ☞ **The three major presentations of the metabolic component are (i) bicarbonate ion [HCO_3^-], (ii) SBE, and (iii) the SID between plasma strong cations and anions.** ☞

The final result of ABB is the regulation of H^+ ion concentration in blood (normal [H^+] = 40 nM/L). The [H^+] is normally presented as pH, where pH equals the negative logarithm (base 10) of [H$^+$]. Accordingly, the normal [H$^+$] of 40 nM/L corresponds to a pH of 7.40 (Fig. 1). During acidemia, [H$^+$] increases and pH decreases <7.35. During alkalemia, [H$^+$] decreases and pH increases >7.45. The use of logarithmic notation to characterize blood acid–base state is conceptually attractive because the effective range of a buffer generates a characteristic "S" shape when acid or base concentration is plotted against pH, but not when plotted against [H$^+$]. The logarithmic scale for [H$^+$] is analogous to the Richter scale for earthquake intensity, an integer increase in pH (e.g., 7 to 8) means a 10-fold reduction in [H$^+$]. A doubling of [H$^+$] (e.g., 40 nM/L to 80 nM/L) decreases the pH by 0.3 (e.g., 7.40 to 7.10).

☞ **ABB is regulated by the respiratory center of the medulla (respiratory component) and by the liver and kidneys (metabolic and weak acid components).** ☞ First, we will examine the effects of changing dissolved CO_2 in blood (changing P_{CO_2} by changing alveolar ventilation). Second, we will examine metabolic effects on ABB. Third, we will examine the buffer capacity of blood and ECF.

Respiratory Component (P_aCO_2)

Dissolved CO_2 is measured as the partial pressure of CO_2 in arterial blood (Pa_{CO_2}). Alveolar ventilation determines the level of Pa_{CO_2}. Hyperventilation leads to CO_2 elimination, and hypoventilation leads to CO_2 retention. ☞ **The Pa_{CO_2} level is regulated by the medulla, which governs the alveolar ventilation.** ☞

The concentration of dissolved CO_2 is linearly related to P_{CO_2} by its solubility ([dissolved CO_2] = $P_{CO_2} \cdot Sol_{CO_2}$, where Sol_{CO_2} = 0.0306 mM/mmHg). CO_2 reacts reversibly with water to generate carbonic acid (H_2CO_3), which immediately dissociates into hydrogen and bicarbonate ions:

$$CO_2 + H_2O \leftrightharpoons H_2CO_3 \leftrightharpoons H^+ + HCO_3^-. \qquad (1)$$

The hydration of CO_2 is rapid in red blood cells (RBCs) because they contain the enzyme carbonic anhydrase.

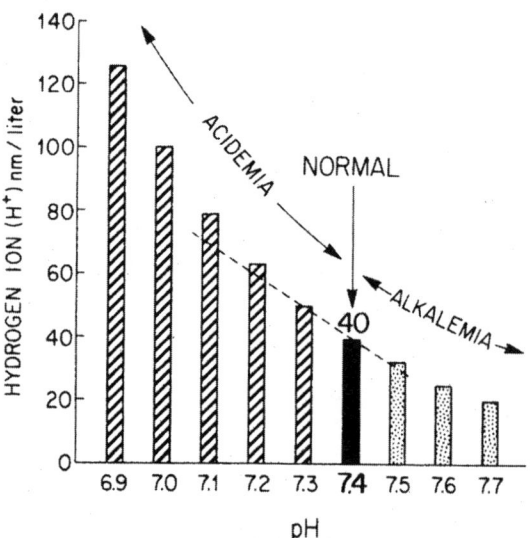

Figure 1   Relationship of pH to hydrogen concentration. Broken line is drawn to emphasize the (approximately) linear relationship between hydrogen ion concentration and pH over the pH range of 7.1 to 7.5.

According to the law of mass action, the dissociation of carbonic acid may be written as

$$K[H_2CO_3] = [H^+][HCO_3^-], \qquad (2)$$

where K is the dissociation constant.

It is almost impossible to measure the concentration of undissociated carbonic acid (H_2CO_3) in solution because it rapidly dissociates into dissolved CO_2 and H_2O as well as $H^+ + HCO_3^-$. However, the amount of dissolved CO_2 is easily measured, and the amount of undissociated H_2CO_3 is proportional to the amount of dissolved CO_2. The rate and depth of breathing is dependent upon the medulla's set pH point and upon its ability to measure pH levels in the blood.

Also, by substituting $P_{CO_2} \cdot Sol_{CO_2}$ for H_2CO_3 in Equation 2, and by taking the negative logarithm of both sides of Equation 2, and solving for pH, the familiar Henderson–Hasselbalch equation can be derived:

$$pH = pK' + \log\left(\frac{[HCO_3^-]}{(Sol_{CO_2} \cdot P_{CO_2})}\right)$$
$$= 6.1 + \log\left(\frac{[HCO_3^-]}{(0.0306 \cdot P_{CO_2})}\right) \qquad (3)$$

The Henderson–Hasselbalch equation assumes that all dissolved CO_2 exists as H_2CO_3, although only 0.33% is actually hydrated, and the pK' is 6.1. The true pK of H_2CO_3 is actually about 3.1.

High P_{CO_2} [e.g., alveolar hypoventilation during chronic obstructive pulmonary disease (COPD)] will cause respiratory acidosis by driving Equation 1 to the right. In the Henderson–Hasselbalch equation (Equation 3), increased P_{CO_2} will decrease the log expression and decrease pH. P_{CO_2} is directly measured in blood gas and pH analyzer machines with a CO_2 electrode.

Metabolic Component

Changes to the metabolic component result from the addition of strong acids or bases to the acid-base system, where strong acid or base means always ionized, that is, always dissociated from H^+ or OH^-. ☞ **As opposed to ventilation for elimination of CO_2, strong acids or bases require either elimination by the kidney (inorganic acids such as HCl or bases such as NaOH, KOH) or gastrointestinal tract, or through metabolism, often in the liver (organic acids such as lactate$^-$, acetoacetate$^-$, and β-hydroxybutyrate$^-$).** ☞

Hepatic ammoniagenesis (and glutaminogenesis) is important for systemic ABB. Nitrogen metabolism by the liver can result in the formation of urea, glutamine, or NH_4^+. Normally, the liver releases only a small amount of free NH_4^+, as most of this nitrogen is incorporated into urea or glutamine. The produced urea or glutamine is subsequently used by the kidney to generate NH_4^+ and to facilitate the excretion of Cl$^-$. Thus, the production of glutamine can be seen as having an alkalinizing effect on plasma pH (15).

Examination of Equation 1 reveals that [HCO$_3^-$] by itself would be a poor discriminator of the metabolic component. However, Equation 1 does not act in isolation, nor does any acid base system in the body. Furthermore, the ratio of P_{CO_2} to HCO$_3^-$ does indeed describe the [H$^+$] both in theory (e.g., Equation 3) and in clinical practice.

☞ **The parameter, SBE, has been introduced to measure the purely metabolic component of ABB in the**

ECF. A negative SBE occurs during metabolic acidosis and a positive SBE is obtained during metabolic alkalosis. ↗ The SBE (mM) estimates the amount of strong acid or base that would be needed to correct a metabolic disturbance. Mathematical calculation of the SBE by hand is complicated, but it is automatically computed by most blood gas and pH analyzers from directly measured P_{CO_2} and pH.

Once the SBE is determined, the millimoles of $NaHCO_3$ required to normalize the pH can be estimated as $0.3 \cdot Weight$ (kg) $\cdot SBE$, where $0.3 \cdot Weight$ (kg) estimates the ECF space in liters. For example, a 70 kg man with a SBE $= -8$ would require $(70 \cdot 0.3 \cdot 8) = 168$ mM of sodium bicarbonate ($NaHCO_3$) to correct the acidosis. However, in practice the "bicarbonate space" is not as easily defined. The apparent volume of distribution of $NaHCO_3$ varies depending on the nature of the acid–base disorder and, as detailed below, is a rather dubious concept to begin with. ↗ **Clinicians should be aware that the administration of $NaHCO_3$ is almost always a temporizing maneuver while simultaneously working to correct the primary disorder causing the metabolic acidosis.** ↗ Furthermore, full correction is seldom advisable.

The Weak Acid Buffers

A buffer is a molecule that takes up H^+ ions when they are in excess and releases H^+ ions in times of acid deficit, thus preventing marked changes in $[H^+]$ and hence pH. Three major buffer systems maintain the pH balance in mammals (the bicarbonate, phosphate, and protein buffer systems). The most powerful buffers are those that have the pK at or near the pH of interest (7.40 for humans) and are present in large concentration.

By this standard, the bicarbonate system is not powerful (the pK is 6.1, and the $[HCO_3^-]$ and $[CO_2]$ are not present in high concentrations). However, the bicarbonate system is the most important buffer system in the body, because $[CO_2]$ and hence $[HCO_3^-]$ can be rapidly altered by the respiratory system. Although $[HCO_3^-]$ can also be altered directly by the kidneys, the relative impact compared to ventilation renders the renal effect meaningless in buffering against an acute H^+ ion excess. Instead, the kidneys influence ABB predominately by regulating the plasma concentration of strong acids and bases and phosphate.

The other buffers in the plasma are weak acids and since their pKs are all close to 6.8, they can be lumped together under the term total weak acids or A_{TOT}. A_{TOT} includes phosphate, albumin, hemoglobin, etc., but not HCO_3^- (this is discussed below). The phosphate buffer system is one such weak acid, but its concentration in the ECF is low, only 1/12 that of the bicarbonate system, and hence its power is relatively limited. The most plentiful buffer system of the body is that provided by the proteins located in the cells and plasma.

Hemoglobin is the principle protein buffer system in whole blood. Proteins are made up of various amino acids, some of which have the ability to dissociate their H^+ ion. Histadine is the predominant amino acid possessing this property, and the most important amino acid in the blood with regard to pH buffering. The pKa for histadine is around 6.8. Because the proteins are so ubiquitous in the blood, they play the greatest role in buffering, especially ex vivo (without the ability of the lungs to ventilate off excess CO_2). For example, when a strong acid is added to blood, the hemoglobin buffer system can reduce the change in pH by 90%, compared to the condition when blood (and

hemoglobin) is absent. In the plasma, albumin is the principal buffer and, like hemoglobin, the histidine moieties on its surface supply most of its buffer capacity.

The fact that hemoglobin is contained within circulating RBCs provides another important element impacting the interaction between the bicarbonate system and the protein buffer systems in the transport of CO_2 from its tissue sites of cellular production to the lungs for excretion. Briefly, CO_2 diffuses out of metabolizing tissues into the capillary venous flow where it penetrates the RBC membrane. Inside the RBC, the enzyme carbonic anhydrase catalyzes the hydration of CO_2 into H_2CO_3, which immediately ionizes into H^+ and HCO_3^- (as per Equation 1). The histidine moiety of hemoglobin absorbs the H^+, whereas the HCO_3^- exits the RBC in exchange for entering chloride (so called "chloride shift"). The reverse occurs in the capillary bed of the lungs where the lower P_{CO_2} in alveolar air enables the diffusion of CO_2 from the hypercapnic mixed venous blood, of the pulmonary artery capillaries, into the alveolus.

The SBE represents the metabolic component by assuming that the mean buffer strength of the human ECF equals that of blood with 5 g/dL hemoglobin. Despite individual variation of hemoglobin, the effective buffer system changes little.

Four Primary Acid–Base Conditions

Four primary acid–base derangements are classically described: metabolic acidosis, metabolic alkalosis, respiratory acidosis, and respiratory alkalosis. The preceding overview helps one understand these four basic conditions prior to identifying and repairing complex disorders such as tertiary acid–base disorders. The clinical history is exceedingly helpful in determining the cause and each of the four primary acid–base conditions can be acute or chronic (Table 1).

Metabolic Acidosis

↗ **Metabolic acidosis exists when there is more metabolic acid present than can be balanced by the available BB.** ↗ This is analogous to having inadequate positive charge in the serum or a reduced SID (as with Cl^- loading). When metabolic acidosis is the only process, the HCO_3^- is lower than normal. The respiratory compensation for metabolic acidosis is CO_2 elimination. The observed pH is lower than expected for the observed P_{CO_2} (for every 10 torr change in P_{CO_2} there is a reciprocal and inverse change of 0.08 pH units).

Metabolic Alkalosis

This state stems from having an excess of base relative to the available acid. It is analogous to having too much serum positive charge (increased SID) leading to proton consumption (as in Cl^- loss or Na^+ loading). This concept is critical to understanding how sodium bicarbonate ($NaHCO_3$) raises pH. According to Stewart (2), HCO_3^- is a dependent variable and does not set pH. Rather, the pH is set by the three independent variables of P_{CO_2}, A_{TOT}, and the SID. Thus, $NaHCO_3$ raises pH by increasing the serum sodium concentration since it delivers Na^+ without another negatively charged strong ion; since HCO_3^- is not a strong ion, it does not influence the SID or the pH. Therefore, with $NaHCO_3$ administration, the serum becomes more positive and proton consumption is the expected mechanism to restore electrical homeostasis. At the same time, each liberated HCO_3^- ion combines with an H^+ ion and as per Equation 1 is converted

Table 1 Medical Conditions, Historical and Physical Findings Suggesting Particular Acid–Base Disturbances

Acute	Chronic
Respiratory acidosis $(PaCO_2 \geq 45)$	**Compensation:** $\uparrow$ HCO_3^-
Respiratory arrest	COPD (increased baseline $[HCO_3^-]$)
Opioid or sedative drug overdose	Increased V_D/V_T (can be acute also)
Under ventilation	
Exacerbation of asthma	
Respiratory alkalosis $(PaCO_2 \leq 35)$	**Compensation:** $\downarrow$ HCO_3^-
Pain, fear, anxiety, hypoxia	Cerebrovasclar accident
Fever, pneumonia	Recovery from head injury
Congestive heart failure	Jaundice, cirrhosis
Salicylate overdose (and metacidosis)	Pregnancy (until post partum)
Sepsis	Hyperthyroidism
Metabolic acidosis $(SBE \leq -4)$	**Compensation:** $\downarrow$ $PaCO_2$
Shock (hemorrhagic, septic, cardiogenic)	Chronic renal failure
Seizures (lactate)	Renal tubular acidosis
Ketosis, toxins	
Diarrhea, acetazolamide	
Sulfamylon (burn patient)	
Acute renal failure	
Malignant hyperthermia	
Iatrogenic (e.g., NSS resuscitation)	
Metabolic alkalosis $(SBE \geq 4)$	**Compensation:** $\uparrow$ $PaCO_2$
Chloride responsive: $\downarrow$'d $[K^+]$, $\downarrow$'d $[Cl^-]$	Chloride unresponsive (usually increased intravascular volume)
Contraction alkalosis (may need Mg^{2+} also)	
Vomiting	Chronic diuretic use (lasix)
NG aspirate	Hyper aldosteroneism
Past excessive diuretic use	Cushing's syndrome
Posthypercapnea	Exogenous steroid use
	Licorice (inhibits cortisol degradation)
	Barters syndrome (hyper rennin)
	Citrate (postmassive blood products)

to H_2CO_3 and then to CO_2 (eliminated in the lungs) and water. The clinical outcome is the development of metabolic alkalosis.

Respiratory Acidosis

Respiratory acidosis is identified as a $Pa_{CO_2} > 42$ torr. This state generally emerges during clinical decompensation of a trauma patient from respiratory failure due to increased work of breathing [e.g., due to pulmonary contusion, bronchospasm, acute respiratory distress syndrome (ARDS)] or due to decreased ability to do the work (e.g., flail chest), decreased drive to breath (e.g., opioid intoxication), or decreased neuromuscular function (e.g. spinal cord injury). Respiratory acidosis also occurs as an expected condition when using permissive hypercapnia to manage acute lung injury (ALI)/ARDS (16).

In patients with an intact CO_2 response mechanism, CO_2 retention triggers an increase in the respiratory rate, which serves to normalize the Pa_{CO_2}. In cases where excessive CO_2 is being produced (e.g., fever or other causes of hypermetabolism), respiratory rate must increase significantly to normalize the Pa_{CO_2}. This is also the case in situations where the alveolar dead space is increased (e.g., pulmonary embolus). Thus, fever, hypermetabolism, and increased alveolar deadspace situations are counterproductive when attempting to liberate a patient from mechanical ventilation.

The renal compensation for respiratory acidosis is slower as it requires altering the SID (i.e., HCO_3^- reabsorption). One should note that the deliberate induction of a metabolic alkalosis (increasing the SID) during weaning of a COPD patient (who retains CO_2) can occasionally facilitate liberation from mechanical ventilation because the metabolic alkalosis helps normalize the pH change caused by respiratory acidosis and decreases the V_E required to normalize CO_2, thereby reducing the work of breathing.

Respiratory Alkalosis

Respiratory alkalosis is present when a primary process causes the Pa_{CO_2} to be <38 mmHg. It is commonly associated with hypercatecholamine states (e.g., pain, fear, and anxiety). In the case of metabolic acidosis, compensatory hyperventilation will decrease the Pa_{CO_2} and decrease water dissociation via the law of mass action on Equation 1. A secondary respiratory alkalosis is also associated with sepsis for the same reason (compensation for metabolic acidosis). The clinician identifies this compensation as hyperventilation in the nonintubated patient or as increased minute ventilation ($\dot{V}_E$) in the spontaneously breathing mechanically ventilated patient.

☞ **Tachypnea and respiratory alkalosis commonly occur in compensation for a primary metabolic acidosis in the early post-trauma time frame, typically due to hypoperfusion or iatrogenic hyperchloremia.** ☞ This finding may be one of the first signs to herald metabolic acidosis of numerous etiologies [e.g., diabetic ketoacidosis (DKA), alcoholic ketoacidosis, lactic acidosis, hyperchloremic acidosis, and various poisons]. Tachypnea is prominent in severe shock; however, when there is insufficient energy and/or cerebral blood flow to fuel the respiratory compensation or when there is a superimposed primary respiratory acidosis (e.g. opioid intoxication, spinal cord injury lung injury), respiratory compensation can fail and acidosis will worsen.

☞ **Metabolic alkalosis is more commonly seen in the postresuscitation phase of trauma patients, commonly during induced diuresis with a loop diuretic (induced by the net effect of Cl^- loss in the urine).** ☞ One should note that in elderly patients on daily doses of loop diuretics, metabolic alkalosis may be a pre-existing state prior to the traumatic injury. In this scenario, development of an acute metabolic acidosis will often initially be occult due to the elevated baseline SID and $[HCO_3^-]$. Accordingly, the initial compensatory respiratory alkalosis will be blunted compared to what would normally be expected based, for example, on the patient's lactate concentration.

CLINICAL MODELS OF ACID–BASE BALANCE

The Classical or Henderson–Hasselbalch Model

The classical model of ABB based on the Henderson–Hasselbalch equation has been the most widely accepted (especially in North America) and is well incorporated into medical education and practice. It holds that the pH and thus the proton concentration (H^+) is related to a balance between protons and the bicarbonate ion in relation to the BB that is in plasma and the red cell mass (17). Directly related to the Henderson–Hasselbalch equation are the "Six Bostonian Rules" of acute versus chronic primary acid–base disorders (Table 2), as well as the well-known acid–base nomogram (Fig. 2). The so-called Bostonian Rules characterize the expected human metabolic or respiratory compensation for primary acid–base disorders. In the case of metabolic acidosis or alkalosis, the respiratory compensation occurs quickly, thus there is only one compensation formula needed for each entity. In the case of respiratory disorders, the renal compensation takes longer, thus there is an expected acute response, and a chronic response, associated with each primary disorder.

The Standard Base Excess and Graphical Approaches to Acid–Base Analysis

ABB can be depicted using a graphical relationship (Fig. 2) charting two of three interdependent variables: (*i*)

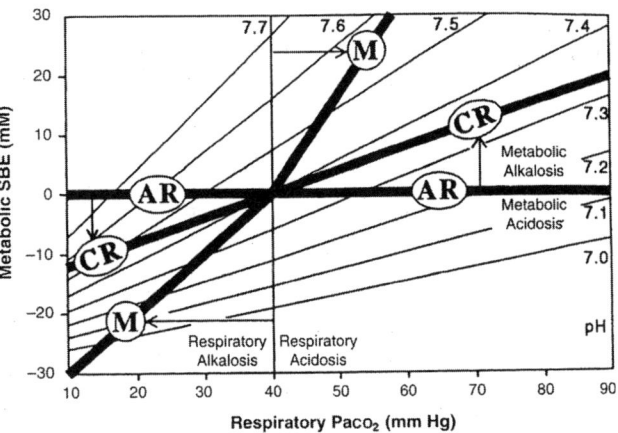

Figure 2 Detailed clinical map of the average or typical human compensations for acid–base imbalances. Arrows show direction of compensatory changes from uncompensated acid base imbalances. Linear pH isopleths permit location of a patient data set on the diagram when only a pH and PaCO$_2$ are known. Solid lines have these slopes. Primary respiratory: PaCO$_2$ affects SBE: Acute = AR (SBE = 0) and chronic = CR (ΔSBE = 0.4 ΔPCO$_2$). Primary metabolic: SBE affects PaCO$_2$: acidosis (*lower line*) = M (ΔPCO$_2$ = 1.0 ΔSBE) and alkalosis (*upper line*) = M (ΔPCO$_2$ = 0.6 ΔSBE). *Abbreviations*: M, metabolic acidosis or alkalosis; AR, acute respiratory acidosis or alkalosis; CR, chronic respiratory acidosis or alkalosis; SBE, standard base excess; PaCO$_2$, arterial PCO$_2$. *Source*: From Ref. 60.

Table 2 Expected Human Metabolic or Respiratory Compensation to Acid–Base Disorders

Expected metabolic compensation for a change in PaCO$_2$

(assume starting $[HCO_3^-]$ = 24 mEq/dL)

Acute respiratory acidosis or alkalosis 0.1 · ΔPaCO$_2$ (e.g., PaCO$_2$ = 60 mmHg $\Rightarrow$ HCO$_3^-$ = 26)

Chronic respiratory acidosis or alkalosis 0.4 · ΔPaCO$_2$ (e.g., PaCO$_2$ = 60 mmHg $\Rightarrow$ HCO$_3^-$ = 32)

For every 10 mmHg increase in PaCO$_2$, the pH will decrease 0.08 pH units (e.g., when PaCO$_2$ increases from 40 to 70 mmHg, the pH will decrease from 7.40 to 7.16) (Providing no other concomitant disorders are occurring, i.e., this is a primary disorder)

Expected respiratory compensation for a change in SBE

(assume starting PaCO$_2$ = 40 mmHg)

Metabolic alkalosis ΔPaCO$_2$ = 0.6 · ΔSBE (e.g., +5 SBE $\Rightarrow$ PaCO$_2$ = 43 mmHg)

Metabolic acidosis ΔPaCO$_2$ = 1.0 · SBE (e.g., −5 SBE $\Rightarrow$ PaCO$_2$ = 35 mmHg)

For a pure metabolic acidosis, Winter's formula predicts the respiratory compensation:

PCO$_2$ = 1.5 * HCO$_3^-$ + 8 (±2) (e.g., HCO$_3^-$ = 19 $\Rightarrow$ PaCO$_2$ = 35–37 mmHg)

Alternatively

PCO$_2$ = 40 + SBE (±2)

Note: Also note that some references will list greater metabolic compensation for a respiratory acidosis than for a respiratory alkalosis. The table provides just one number to simplify memorization, and the ranges provided are adequate for clinical decision-making. Also note that this table provides some metabolic compensation for an acute respiratory process. This is because whenever CO$_2$ is added to the system both HCO$_3^-$ and H$^+$ are increased (Equation 1). However, the pH decreases because the proportion of PaCO$_2$ to HCO$_3^-$ is increased (Equation 3). Although this is a departure from other standard reference tables, it is more accurate.

Abbreviations: "Δ" denotes change in variable; SBE, standard base excess; Pa$_{CO_2}$, arterial blood PaCO$_2$.

Source: From Ref. 14.

respiratory Pa$_{CO_2}$ (mmHg, *x*-axis) and (*ii*) metabolic SBE (mM, *y*-axis). When using the graphical method, P$_{CO_2}$ is plotted against calculated SBE, and pH isopleths are plotted on the same graph. A change in ventilation (respiratory component) moves the intersection of P$_{CO_2}$ and SBE horizontally rightward (respiratory acidosis) or leftward (respiratory alkalosis). A metabolic change moves the point upward (alkalosis) or downward (acidosis).

During acute respiratory acid–base disturbances, SBE equals zero because there has not been time for metabolic compensation to occur; this is reflected graphically by acute respiratory changes occurring along the SBE = 0 line of Figure 2. Chronic respiratory aberrations lie vertically between no metabolic compensation (SBE = 0) and complete compensation (pH = 7.40). The kidney eventually increases or decreases SBE (by altering SID) but rarely to the point of complete compensation. Metabolic disturbance lie horizontally between zero to complete respiratory compensation. Respiratory compensation for simple, primary metabolic disorders is generally immediate. Table 2 summarizes the mathematical relationships governing the amount of respiratory or metabolic compensation in response to a disturbance to the other variable.

One of the pitfalls of the graphical approach occurs when chronic (compensated) respiratory acidosis is superimposed with an acute metabolic acidosis. Chronic hypoventilation results in decreased pH due to increased P$_{CO_2}$. The metabolic compensation increases SBE to partially correct pH. Then, a superimposition of a metabolic acidosis could normalize SBE. However, the continued increase in P$_{CO_2}$ and decrease in pH would suggest only acute respiratory acidosis, masking the serious presence of the acute, and clinically relevant, metabolic (e.g., lactic) acidosis. In this situation, clinical presentation may help make the diagnosis. Also, examination of the anion gap (AG) or strong ion gap (SIG) (both defined below) would detect the presence of unmeasured anion (in this example, lactate$^-$).

Another pitfall of the SBE approach to patient management involves the following common clinical example: A 70 kg patient, with normal kidneys and tissue perfusion, undergoes a 12-hour bladder resection and urinary diversion procedure, involving a 3000 mL estimated blood loss. The losses are replaced with six units of packed RBCs, and 12 L of 0.9% saline. Blood pressure and heart rate are stable throughout the case, urine output is 150 cc per hour. The arterial blood gas and electrolytes at the end of the case are: pH = 7.36, Pa_{CO_2} = 31 mmHg, [HCO_3^-] = 15 mmol/L, [Na^+] = 140 mmol/L, and [Cl^-] = 115 mmol/L. Using the SBE, a significant base deficit (of −8 to −10) would be obtained and could trigger additional needless fluid resuscitation or bicarbonate administration. Review of the electrolytes reveals a normal AG = 10 mmol/L, thus eliminating lactate and underperfusion as the etiology of the acidosis. This scenario represents a case of iatrogenic hyperchloremic metabolic acidosis, which will resolve by itself (if the kidneys are provided time to excrete the elevated Cl^- and reabsorb HCO_3^-).

Another limitation to the SBE approach is that SBE is slightly unstable as P_{CO_2} changes (Fig. 3). Furthermore, the SBE equation assumes a normal A_{TOT}. When albumin or phosphate is decreased, a common scenario in the critically ill and injured, SBE will result in even more instability (Fig. 3). Although recent attempts to correct the SBE for changes in A_{TOT} have resulted in a formula that agrees much more closely with experimental data in humans, this formula has not yet been widely applied.

$$\text{Corrected SBE}$$
$$= (HCO_3^- - 24.4) + ([8.3 \times \text{albumin} \times 0.15] \quad (4)$$
$$+ [0.29 \times \text{phosphate} \times 0.32]) \times (pH - 7.4)$$

Albumin is expressed in g/dL and phosphate in mg/dL.

Importance of the Anion Gap in Acid–Base Analysis

The AG concept is based upon electroneutrality of total anions and cations in solution (5). The importance of the AG in clinical medicine is underscored by the two examples

provided above and will be developed further in this section. The addition of 1 mmol of acid to blood results in approximately 1 mmol of bicarbonate consumption and replacement of the lost bicarbonate with approximately 1 mmol of anion. The character of the substituted anion influences the pattern of normally measured serum electrolytes and has important diagnostic and therapeutic value. The AG is the difference between the concentration of cation (sodium and potassium) and anion (chloride and bicarbonate) concentrations in plasma:

$$[AG] = ([Na^+] + [K^+] - ([Cl^-] + [HCO_3^-])$$
$$= 14 \pm 2 \text{ mEq/L} \quad (5)$$

Because the changes in serum potassium concentration compatible with life are relatively small, some authors omit the potassium from AG calculation, resulting in an expected AG of 10 ± 2 mEq/L. The "normal" AG occurs because of the normally unmeasured anions [mostly due to albumin, PO_4^{2-}, SO_4^{2-}, and some normal organic acids (Fig. 4)].

☞ **The normal AG is up to 14 ± 2 (if [K^+] is included) and 10 ± 2 (when [K^+] omitted), and assumes a normal albumin concentration and a P_{CO_2} of 40 torr (15,18).** ☞ Recall that the AG represents the negative charge that is contributed by anions that are not measured in the usual chemistry panel, but are necessarily present to balance the existing positive charge in the plasma. The remainder of this discussion assumes the [K^+] is included in the calculation of the AG.

The expected or normal range for AG must be corrected when A_{TOT} is abnormal. There are several ways to calculate this correction (15). A reasonable approximation is to assume that the expected AG should equal [alb] × 2.5 (where [alb] is expressed in g/dL). A more precise method

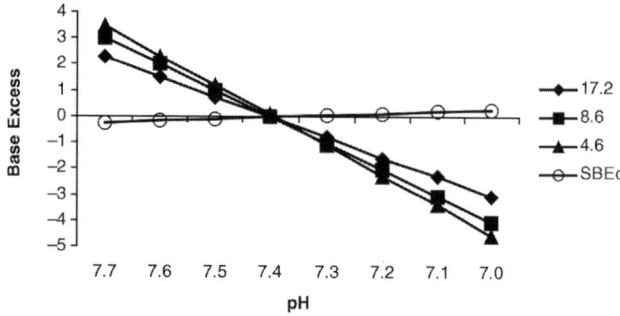

Figure 3 Carbon dioxide titration curves. Computer simulation of in vivo CO_2 titration curves for human plasma using the traditional Van Slyke equation and various levels of A_{TOT} (total weak acids) from normal (17.2) to 25% of normal. Also shown is the titration curve using the A_{TOT} corrected standard base excess.

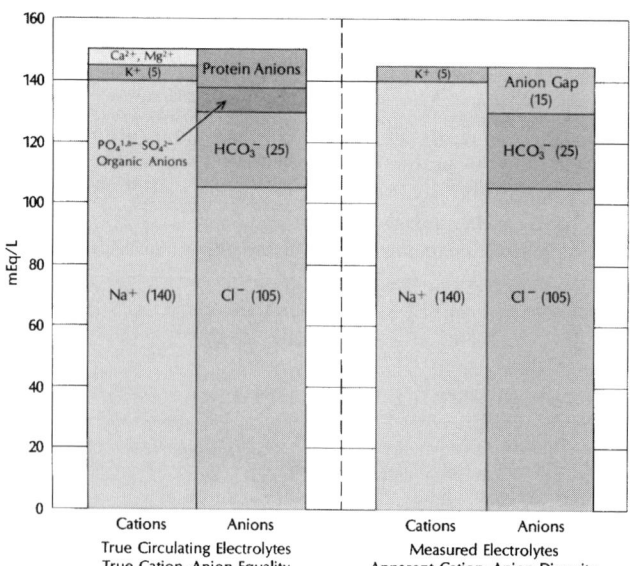

Figure 4 Circulating cations always counterbalance circulating anions, thereby maintaining electroneutrality (*left*). In routine electrolyte assays, however, only a portion of circulating anions is measured, and an apparent cation–anion disparity exists (*right*). This difference, in mEq/L, is termed the anion gap.

incorporates the affect of phosphate levels, as shown in Equation 6.

$$\text{Expected AG} = 2[\text{alb}(\text{g/dL})] + 0.5[\text{PO}_4^{2-} (\text{mg/dL})] \pm 2 \tag{6}$$

Failure to use the correct expected AG when A_{TOT} is reduced will result in the failure to identify an AG acidemia when it is present (unless it is very large). For example, an AG of 12 mEq/L in a patient with a serum albumin concentration of 2 g/dL and PO_4^{2-} of 2 mg/dL and metabolic acidosis by arterial blood gas (ABG) analysis might be initially attributed to a nongap cause. However, the expected normal range for the AG in this patient with low levels of albumin and PO_4^{2-} is $2(2) + 0.5(2) = 5 \pm 2$ and thus a measured AG of 12 indicates that 5 to 9 mEq of unmeasured anion exists. Accordingly, the clinician needs to employ the AG differential diagnosis (Table 3).

Not only will the baseline AG will be lower than normal in hypoalbuminemia states, it will also be low in the setting of excess positively charged "para-proteins" (e.g., Waldenstrom's macroglobinemia). An increase in a patient's AG from baseline reflects anions contributed by an acid other than HCl (since Cl^- ion is measured and will thus not raise the AG). An increase in the AG helps detect the presence of significant unmeasured anions, such as lactate$^-$, α-ketogluterate, β-hydroxybutyrate$^-$, and those associated with other organic acidosis syndromes listed in Table 3. ☞ **The use of the AG in acid–base analysis is critical in order to detect most of the acute disturbances requiring immediate therapy (Table 3).** ☞

Metabolic acidosis is generally separated into two categories: (*i*) non-AG (hyperchloremic), meaning that the AG is normal, and (*ii*) AG metabolic acidosis, where the AG is greater than normal. Following a rigorous rules-based approach to acid–base analysis (including determination of the AG) will diminish the chance of misdiagnosing a metabolic acidosis. Some have dismissed the utility of the AG in acid–base analysis because it is often insensitive in the critically ill and injured (19). Adjusting the expected or "normal" range of the AG for the patient's albumin and phosphate concentrations as described above (Equation 6) will avoid this insensitivity.

Hyperchloremic metabolic acidosis most commonly results from the excess administration of Cl^- ions (e.g., NaCl). However, hyperchloremia may be due to renal tubular acidosis (RTA) in which ion handling by the kidney is impaired or as result of ion loss (as can occur with profound diarrhea). Table 4 lists the common causes of hyperchloremic metabolic acidosis.

The Stewart Model

The Stewart model of ABB is compatible with other models which all hold that electrical balance is related to ionic balance and therefore, proton concentration. However, the Stewart approach emphasizes the importance of independent versus dependent variables and that only three independent variables control pH (P_{CO_2}, A_{TOT}, and SID). All three of these factors affect the mechanism for proton generation via water dissociation. Understanding how water dissociation is controlled is essential to comprehending pH control in the Stewart model.

There are three independent control mechanisms for water dissociation. The first is the reaction that occurs when CO_2 combines with H_2O to generate carbonic acid which then dissociates into bicarbonate and a proton (Equation 1).

The second is the sum of the weak acid buffers (A_{TOT}) which may exist in a form associated with a proton (AH) or in the dissociated state (A^-). In healthy humans, the charge of A_{TOT} is approximately 16–20 mEq/L and is principally derived from the histidine residues on albumin ($\sim$78%), phosphate ($\sim$20%), and other proteins ($\sim$2%). The negatively charged portion of A_{TOT} (A^-) together with the negative change of bicarbonate is counterbalanced by a positive charge from excess of strong cations in plasma, the SID.

Strong ions are those that are completely (or nearly completely) dissociated from their partners at physiologic pH. The principal strong ions are Na^+, K^+, Ca^{2+}, Mg^{2+}, Cl^-, and lactate. Unlike the others, lactate is only partially dissociated, although at pH 7.4 only 1 in 3000 ions is not dissociated; thus, for all intents and purposes, lactate can be considered a strong ion. ☞ **The SID is the difference between the strong cations and strong anions (Equation 7) and in health has an approximate value of 40 to 42 mEq/L.** ☞

$$\text{SID} = (Na^+ + K^+ + Ca^{2+} + Mg^{2+}) - (Cl^- + \text{lactate}) \tag{7}$$

There is a parallel similarity between SID and the AG, which are offset by approximately 25 mEq/L, which is the sum of the $[HCO_3^-]$ plus the difference between the normally circulating strong ions and cations that are not included in the normal AG calculation (i.e., Ca^{2+}, Mg^{2+}, lactate, urate).

Only three variables, P_{CO_2}, A_{TOT}, and SID set the proton concentration in plasma, as these three are the only independent control mechanisms; all other entities that have been traditionally thought important in pH regulation are actually dependent variables (e.g., $[HCO_3^-]$). The SID's positive charge is counterbalanced by the charge carried by the BB (HCO_3^- plus A^-). It is the relative balance of the total plasma charge that determines water dissociation.

For example, in patients with hypoalbuminemia, the decreased quantity of negative charges results in a net excess of plasma positive charge compared to the SID. A chemical response to this imbalance is proton consumption, which decreases the plasma positive charge and generates a metabolic alkalosis. Similarly, a patient with a normal albumin, but acute Cl^- loss (e.g., gastric outlet obstruction, excessive vomiting, or NG suction without proton generation blockade) would have a net excess of plasma positive charge due to the loss of an anion that cannot be regenerated (Cl^-). Once again, the acute chemical response is to reduce the plasma positive charge by proton consumption.

More germane to trauma patients is the addition of excess Cl^- in the form of large amounts of 0.9% NS, and to a lesser extent, even large amounts of LR during resuscitation (20). Each of these intravenous fluids (IVFs) are hyperchloremic with regard to plasma normal saline solution (NS): 154 mEq Cl^-/L; lactated Ringer's solution (LR): 110 mEq Cl^-/L; plasma: 100 mEq Cl^-/L. Large volume resuscitation (i.e., 5–10 L or more) will raise the Cl^- out of proportion to plasma Na^+ creating an excess of negative charge (Example 1). The effect is to generate protons to counterbalance the excess negative charge, leading to the well-identified hyperchloremic metabolic acidosis (21).

Of course, one must recognize that acidosis is not an invariable response to hyperchloremia secondary to crystalloid resuscitation. There are accompanying reductions in the weak acids (albumin, phosphate) and in many cases strong acids such as lactate are reduced, first through

Table 3 Elevated Anion Gap Metabolic Acidosis

Acidosis type	Offending acid	Clinical setting	Associated findings	Treatment
Lactic	Lactic	Shock, sepsis, hypoxia, seizure, drugs, liver failure, etc.	↓ Cardiac function ↓ BP ↑ LFTs (if liver failure)	O_2, ↑ volume, ↑ $\dot{D}O_2$ to tissues, remove toxins, liver transplant (if liver failure does not recover)
DKA	Acetoacetate, b-hydroxybuterate	Diabetes, stress (including sepsis)	↑ Glucose, falsely elevated creatinine	↑ volume repletion, insulin titrated [glucose], electrolyte repletion (especially, Mg^{2+}, K^+)
AKA	Acetoacetate, b-hydroxybuterate	Chronic excessive alcohol intake	Glucose may be normal or low, PO_4^{2-}, K^+	↑ volume repletion, PO_4^{2-}, K^+, Mg^{2+} repletion
Uremic	Phosphoric, sulfuric, mixed organic	End stage renal failure, worse with: catabolism, SO_4^{2-} diet, infrequent dialysis	↑ BUN and creatinine ↑ Osm., 'd SO_4^{2-} ↑ PO_4^{2-} (mixed gap, non-gap)	Dialysis, improve nutrition (catabolism increases acid load), minimize sulfur containing amino acids in diet, oral supplementation of HCO_3^-
Methanol	Formic	Toxic ingestion of methyl alcohol	↑ Osmolality, ↑ Amylase, retinal (papillary) edema	Ethanol (ETOH competes with alcohol dehydrogenase—the enzyme that converts methanol to the toxic formic acid). Hemodialysis if severe
Ethylene glycol	Glycolic	Toxic ingestion of ethylene glycol (active ingredient in antifreeze)	↑ Osmolality, calcium oxalate crystalluria, cerebral edema, direct injury to kidneys, lungs, liver, heart, muscles, retinas	Ethanol or Fomepizole (ETOH competes with alcohol dehydrogenase—the enzyme that converts ethylene glycol to glycoaldehyde (precursor to the toxic glycolic acid). Fomepizole directly inhibits the enzyme.
Propylene glycol	Lactic, pyruvate	Prolonged etomidate infusion. Propylene glycol is an alcohol vehicle used for some hydrophobic drugs	↑ Osmolality, protamine like effects, intravascular hemolysis, perception deafness, skin irritation, renal insufficiency	Stop etomidate infusion. ↑ volume, supportive care Renal function improves with etomidate cessation. Other drugs (phenytoin, diazepam, pentobarbital) using propylene glycol as a vehicle, can cause propylene glycol toxicity (unusual when normal doses used)
Aspirin	Salicylate	Toxic ingestion of aspirin (children most prone)	Rapid deep respiration, confusion, coma, vomiting, sweating, dehydration	O_2, ↑ volume, K^+, Cl^-, Mg^{2+} repletion alkalinization of the urine, hemodialysis if severe
Iron	Lactic, mixed organic and inorganic (hydration of Fe^{3+})	Toxic ingestion of $FeSO_4$ (children most prone)	Vomiting (blood from gastric erosions), shock, coma, liver failure, renal failure	O_2, ↑ volume, desferroxamine (chelation therapy), whole bowel irrigation (GoLytely®), supportive care
Paraldehyde	Mixed organic	Sedative hypnotic—no longer used in USA	Coma, paraldehyde odor	O_2, ↑ volume, supportive care

Abbreviations: AKA, alcoholic (starvation) ketoacidosis; DKA, diabetic ketoacidosis; LFT, liver function test; ↑, increased; ↓, decreased.

simple dilution and second by restoring tissue perfusion. These reductions lead to the commonly identified hypoalbuminemia and hypophosphatemia that characterize the significantly resuscitated trauma patient. However, these compensatory reductions in negative charge are generally insufficient to offset the increased negative charge from the added Cl^- (particularly in the case of NS), thus resulting in a clinically relevant increase in proton concentration which creates a state of hyperchloremic metabolic acidemia.

Table 4 Common Causes of Normal (i.e., Non-) Anion Gap Metabolic Acidosis

Fistulae (pancreatic)
Uretero-enteric fistulae
Saline (0.9 or 3% NaCl administration or saline-based TPN)
Endocrine (hyperparathyroidism)
Diarrhea
Carbonic anhydrase inhibitors (e.g., Diamox®, Sulfamylon®)
Argenine, lysine, chloride (total parenteral nutrition with excess)
Renal tubular acidosis
Spirinolactone

Note: The mnemonic F-Used Cars are sometimes used to remember this list.
Abbreviation: TPN, total parenteral nutrition.

The transparency and simplicity of the Stewart model is appealing to many students and researchers of ABB. For clinicians, understanding how an acid–base derangement is created allows one to select a repair strategy, as well as to understand how that repair strategy works. More importantly, understanding these principles allows one to select appropriate plasma volume expanders to minimize the impact on ABB as a consequence of resuscitation (i.e., avoid hyperchloremic metabolic acidosis).

Another application of the Stewart model is the SIG. The SIG is the difference or "gap" between the SID calculated from Equation 7 and BB calculated from HCO_3^- and A_{TOT}. The SIG is similar to, but distinct from the AG (22). The BB is a term used by Singer and Hastings, and is equal to the sum of the weak acids (chiefly albumin, PO_4^{2-}, SO_4^{2-}) or A_{TOT}, and $[HCO_3^-]$

$$[SIG] = [SID] - [BB] \qquad (8)$$

The SIG identifies unmeasured ions that are not accounted for by any other method (Fig. 5) (22). The SIG is normally near zero (<4 mEq/L in healthy humans). When abnormal, it is usually positive (indicating excess unmeasured anions) but may be negative (indicating excess unmeasured cations). Several clinical conditions have been associated with the genesis of unmeasured ions including liver failure, trauma, resuscitation, and shock (15,23).

The entire source of these unmeasured ions is incompletely understood. Strong ions (e.g., D-lactate, ketones, sulphate) appear to be responsible for at least half. The residual portion may be related to intracellular or transmembrane proteins that are released during apoptosis-triggered cell death or other types of cell destruction. What is increasingly clear is that unmeasured ions are useful markers of deranged physiology. Accordingly, the utility of the SIG as a predictive tool with regard to mortality in trauma patients has been explored for those with major vascular injury, and a high correlation with the risk of death has been shown (24). Indeed, SIG is a more powerful predictor of outcome in this population than lactate or injury severity score.

Reconciling Different Acid–Base Models

Given the wide range of seemingly contradictory inferences that can be drawn from the three models of ABB presented in this chapter, it is easy to see why "opposing camps" have been formed, each advocating one approach over the others, often with a zeal that could only be described as religious. To the casual observer, this may seem inevitable but in fact all three models are fully compatible and no model is

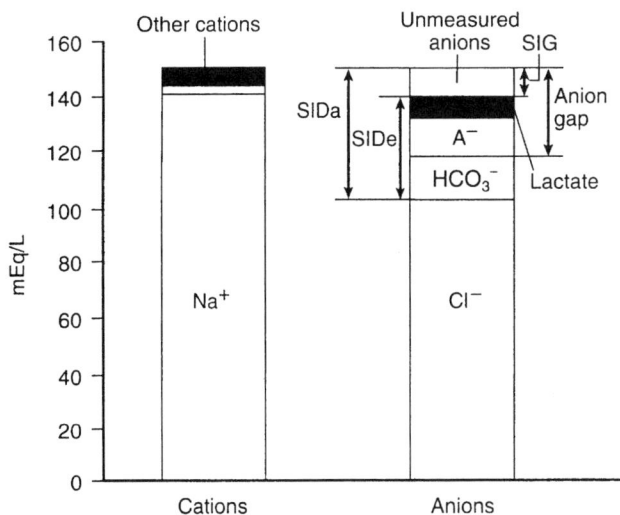

Figure 5 Charge balance in blood plasma. "Other cations" include Ca^{2+} and Mg^{2+}. The strong ion difference (SID) is always positive (in plasma) and SID–SIDe (effective) must equal zero. Any difference between SID apparent (SIDa) and SIDe is the strong ion gap and must represent unmeasured anions.

perfect. Although we believe that Stewart's quantitative physical chemical model yields predictions that are more consistent with experimental data, we do not deny that the more traditional approaches are valid and may have value in certain situations. Moreover, all three models have important common elements and apparent differences are fairly easy to resolve. The classical model uses the Henderson–Hasselbalch equation as a guide and then uses a set of "rules" to analyze ABB. The SBE model builds on the classical model by conceptualizing nonvolatile ABB as changes in BB. Finally, the Stewart model takes this one step forward by using the term SID in place of BB and by no longer assuming that weak acids are either normal or constant as the other models do. Thus, a change in SID is equal to a change in BB which is equal to SBE. A^- (the charged portion of A_{TOT}) is equal to the AG. In this way, the Stewart model is merely a more complete model of ABB.

A PARADIGM FOR EVALUATING AN ACID–BASE DISORDER
Clinical Setting

☞ An initial step in the evaluation of an acid–base disorder is to assess the clinical circumstance of the patient and to develop an initial differential diagnosis based upon the likely acid–base disorders associated with the clinical picture. ☞ The injury history is essential in making this determination (i.e., large volume blood loss, hypothermia, toxic ingestion, etc.). The assessment is then tempered by physical examination evidence.

Physical Exam

☞ Cool extremity temperature has been validated as an indicator of hypoperfusion (excluding exposure to hypothermic environments and peripheral vascular disease with arterial insufficiency). ☞

The physical examination usually provides important indicators of a patient's underlying condition and acid–base status. A patient with hemorrhagic shock is expected to demonstrate signs and symptoms of impaired perfusion, including cool extremities, confusion, tachycardia, narrowed pulse pressure, and ultimately hypotension. Low or unreadable pulse oximetry is a common finding as well (25). These patients evidence lactic acidosis and an elevated AG.

The acid–base analysis becomes more complex when the trauma patient also suffers from chronic renal failure, as a pre-existing elevated AG acidosis (elevated $[SO_4^{2-}]$) and a non-AG acidosis (renal tubular defects) will be present. Conversely, pre-existing chloride loss from excessive vomiting will create a metabolic alkalosis, where normalization will hinge on Cl^- replacement. Chloride replacement may be best achieved using KCl, but 0.9% NS may be more appropriate, especially when fluid resuscitation is also required.

Also, as discussed above, the AG may appear normal with conditions that create albumin loss (nephrotic syndrome, cirrhosis with hypoproteinemia, massive crystalloid resuscitation, chronic disease) necessitating that a corrected range for expected or normal AG be used.

In the intensive care unit (ICU), physical examination has long been used, and recently validated as a sensitive and specific means to detect hypoperfusion (26). The value of combining the presence of a cool peripheral extremity examination with a decreased $[HCO_3^-]$ level was that this combination strongly predicted an increased arterial lactate concentration and a low cardiac index. In contrast, warm extremity examination and a normal or increased $[HCO_3^-]$ was strongly predictive of a normal lactate level and a normal or elevated cardiac index. Two confounders were also identified: (*i*) hyperlactatemia from hypermetabolism in a patient with warm extremities and a normal or elevated cardiac index and (*ii*) distributive or "warm" shock where the extremities are warm and accompanied by an increased cardiac index but low bicarbonate and high arterial lactate concentrations. This method has not been validated in patients with peripheral vascular occlusive disease, an important consideration in geriatric trauma patients.

Biochemical Evaluation

The next step in the evaluation is to assess the serum chemistries and the arterial blood gases. The first step is to determine whether the P_{CO_2} is normal or abnormal. There is a reciprocal relationship between P_{CO_2} and pH such that for each 10 torr ΔP_{CO_2} there is an inverse $\Delta 0.08$ pH. Thus, one can determine whether the ΔpH is entirely attributable to the ΔP_{CO_2}. When the pH is not explained by the P_{CO_2}, one must explore further.

Next, the SBE must be determined. The SBE is an excellent indicator of the presence or absence of nonvolatile acidosis prior to resuscitation. Assuming a constant A_{TOT}, the SBE defines the amount that the SID must be changed in order to restore the pH to 7.40 assuming a P_{CO_2} of 40 (15). ☞ **The value of the SBE (in isolation) as an indicator of lactic acidosis is corrupted following resuscitation because the electrolyte composition of the IVF will significantly impact pH and therefore, the SBE.** ☞ Using an initial SBE, one then assesses whether there is an acidosis (a base deficit more negative than −4). Alternatively, one can examine the serum $[HCO_3^-]$; if less than 22 in a patient with a low pH, then a metabolic acidosis is present (though other processes can also be occurring). However, unlike SBE or SID, the change in $[HCO_3^-]$ does not quantify the amount of acidosis only that it is present.

If a metabolic acidosis is present, the next step is to calculate the AG to determine whether there is an "AG" or "non-AG" metabolic acidosis. ☞ **The differential diagnosis**

for an AG acidosis can be remembered using the mnemonic "MUD PILES" and include methanol, uremia, dehydration, paraldehyde, INH, lactate, ethylene glycol, and salicylates. However, the differential diagnosis also includes other conditions including ketoacidosis, sepsis, and liver failure, making the mnemonic somewhat incomplete (Table 3). ☞ The differential diagnosis of non-AG acidosis is even more broad (Table 4). Metabolic alkaloses may be grouped into two classifications based upon their chloride responsiveness (Table 1).

Recall that the normal range for the AG should be corrected (Equation 6) when the protein concentration is less than normal. If the measured gap exceeds this value, then a positive AG acidosis is present.

Next, one must assess for the presence of any of the known causes of an increased AG. Most clinical laboratories can also provide an arterial lactate value using the ABG machine. If this is elevated, then one must ask whether the increase in the AG is due to the lactate (a 1:1 relationship exists). If it is not, then other unmeasured ions are also present. Rarely, even the corrected AG can miss small quantities (usually less than 5 mEq/L) of unmeasured anions. The SIG, though more cumbersome to calculate, can provide a more accurate quantification of missing anions.

The standard biochemical means of detecting acid–base disorders regardless of time frame requires a serum chemistry panel and an arterial blood gas sample. New monitoring systems will allow the clinician to obtain serum chemistries and ABG analysis every two to five minutes using an indwelling catheter attached to an automated sampling system and point-of-care testing device. New instrumentation allows this kind of device to be similar in size to an alphanumeric pager. These two tests will cover the basic disorders of metabolic acidemia or alkalemia and respiratory acidemia or alkalemia. A brief discussion of the basic derangements was provided above.

There remains significant controversy regarding the pH that is deemed dangerous. Previous data suggested that at a pH < 7.25, catecholamine efficiency was reduced and that a return to normal pH range was indicated (27). This notion has been challenged by more recent data (28). Nonetheless, the recent data fail to supplant the observation that mean arterial pressure commonly increases with NaHCO₃ administration to the hypotensive and pressor dependent patient. The reader should recognize that this observed manipulation of mean arterial pressure has not been demonstrated to confer a survival advantage. Yet, in the authors' experiences, failure to respond to the administered NaHCO₃ often portends impending death.

Differential Diagnosis
Graphical Evaluation

The graphical methodology of Grogono et al. (Fig. 2) has been explained above. This method works well for visual thinkers, especially when the acid–base disorder is simple. However, for complex acid–base disorders, the rules-based approach using HCO_3^-, or SBE along with a calculation of AG, and/or employing the SID method of Stewart are recommended.

Rules-Based Approach Using HCO_3^- vs. SBE Along with AG

☞ **Although algorithms and nomograms are useful (if present at the bedside), the most important factor in evaluating acid–base perturbations is to understand how they occur in the human body and to take a systematic approach in diagnosis.** ☞ The technique of Haber (6) involves a simple, easy to remember, rules-based approach incorporating the concepts developed by Narins and Emmit and represents a practical clinical approach.

Step 1 Look at the pH, determine if acidemia (pH < 7.38) or alkalemia (pH > 7.42) is present. This step is based upon the principle that the human body does not fully compensate, and never overcompensates, for any primary acid–base disturbance.

Step 2 Determine the AG (Equations 5 and 6)

If the AG is increased, refer to Table 3 for sources.

If the AG normal, but the patient has a metabolic acidosis (negative SBE), the patient has a non-gap metabolic acidosis (refer to Table 4 for sources).

If the AG is significantly increased (>5 mEq/L above expected), a primary metabolic acidosis is present regardless of the pH, base excess, or HCO_3^-. This is because the body does not generate a large AG to compensate for a primary disorder (6).

Step 3 Calculate the excess AG (the calculated AG from Step 2 minus the normal expected AG (from Equation 6) is added to the value of the measured [HCO_3^-]).

If the excess AG is significantly greater than the normal serum [HCO_3^-] of 24 mmol/L (i.e., >30 mmol/L), there is an additional underlying metabolic alkalosis.

If the excess AG is significantly lower than the normal serum [HCO_3^-] (i.e., <20 mmol/L), there is an additional underlying nongap metabolic acidosis.

This third step is based upon the physical chemical principle that 1 mmol of unmeasured acid will titrate 1 mmol of HCO_3^- (6). Using this technique, mixed acid–base disorders can be identified. However, it must be emphasized that neither nomograms, nor graphs, nor a series of rules can be used in isolation. The history and physical exam should suggest a differential diagnosis, and the acid–base analysis (as provided above) should corroborate the clinical suspicion. Table 1 provides a list of historical and physical findings, which suggests a classic acid–base disturbance. In addition, Tables 3 and 4 provides clinical information that is useful in diagnosing AG and non-AG metabolic acidosis conditions.

Stewart Approach

Although some clinicians, using programmable calculators, calculate SID and A_{TOT} at the bedside, a simpler approach is as follows. First, one can evaluate PCO_2 as described above. Next, one can assess the approximate change in SID, if any, by examining the SBE. This method is superior to calculating the apparent SID (Equation 6) because the SIG may be increased or A_{TOT} may be decreased, both of which will alter the interpretation of SID. If SBE is increased either the SID has increased or A_{TOT} has decreased or both have occurred. If the SBE is decreased, the answer is usually that the SID has decreased since an increase in A_{TOT} is unusual.

Next, one can estimate the SIG by comparing the measured AG to the normal expected value from Equation 6. In health, SIG is near zero and the measured AG will equal the normal value. The differential diagnosis for an increased SIG is shown in Table 3, whereas a metabolic acidosis (decreased SID) without an increased SIG is shown in Table 4. The primary value of the Stewart model

is that it is completely quantitative; thus, even a triple acid–base disorder can easily be broken down.

Clinical Example Using Stewart Approach

A 75-year-old female was struck by a bus and was run over. She was hypotensive in the field and her trachea was intubated. She underwent evaluation in the Trauma Resuscitation Suite, where a positive focused assessment by sonography in trauma (FAST) examination revealed free abdominal fluid and she was taken to the operating room (OR). A ruptured right hemidiaphragm, multiple rib fractures, as well as a devascularized right lobe of the liver were identified. She underwent large volume resuscitation after controlling hemorrhage with a Pringle maneuver and a partial hepatic resection, diaphragm repair, and the placement of a tube thoracostomy. She received 8 L of LR, 8 U packed red blood cells (PRBC), 6 U fresh frozen plasma (FFP), 750 cc Cell saver, and 2 L of 0.9% NS; her abdomen was packed and a temporary abdominal wall closure was placed. She returned to the surgical intensive case unit (SICU) about 1.5 hours after arrival in the hospital.

Her extremities were cool and slightly clammy. An active convective external warming device was placed to manage hypothermia (core temperature = 94.6 F), and additional warmed fluid resuscitation was undertaken. Her ABG was as follows: 7.18/34/518 (FIO_2 = 1.0). The SBE = −15 and thus the SID is markedly decreased and there is a metabolic acidosis.

The electrolytes and derived values are as follows:

Na^+ 138	Cl^- 115	BUN 9	iCa^{2+} 1.0	Mg^{2+} 1.3	PO_4^{2-} 1.0	Alb 2.3
K^+ 3.8	HCO_3^- 12	Cr 0.5	Gluc 88	Lactate 2.9		

According to Equation 5, the above electrolyte values show a calculated AG = 14, whereas Equation 6 predicts that the adjusted normal range for this patient (with low albumin and PO_4^{2-}) is 5.1 ± 2. The lactate is 2.9 and thus, the SIG is approximately 6 mEq/L (14—5.1—2.9) and there is an increased SIG acidosis. Therefore, another mechanism besides lactic acid (LA) is responsible for the acidosis. However, this patient appears to have a hyperchloremic metabolic acidosis as well, since the SBE is −15, the SIG is only 6, and lactate is only 2.9 (i.e., 6.1 mEq are from a non-SIG, non-LA source).

Finally, there is a respiratory disorder as well. Expected PCO_2 should equal 40 + SBE (−15) = 25, yet the P_{CO_2} is 34 indicating a respiratory acidosis as well. In summary, this patient has at least three sources for the metabolic acidosis and a concomitant respiratory acidosis. The Stewart SID methodology facilitated identification of these various disturbances.

A calculator capable of performing this sort of analysis is downloadable from the internet at the Acid–Base Phorum (30). Inputting the data from above allows one to derive the following values: SID SIG, AG, expected PCO_2, and SBE. One can readily determine that there are unmeasured anions and that the patient has a tertiary acid–base disorder: a respiratory acidosis, a metabolic acidosis (LA and SIG), and a hyperchloremic metabolic acidosis. This knowledge is imperative insofar as it prompts a change in therapy. Failure to discern and understand this information would lead to a standard response to the presence of a metabolic acidosis, such as providing additional IVF and Cl^-. This hypothetical patient does need additional resuscitation, but not additional Cl^- as it would accelerate the metabolic acidosis by further reducing the SID. It is not possible to change the presence of unmeasured anions, thus compensation for them must be initiated by using a low Cl^- resuscitation fluid. Therefore, a colloid for resuscitation could be used to limit Cl^- loading—a departure from the standard high Cl^- crystalloid resuscitation paradigm.

Trauma patients frequently have pre-existing or concurrent illness. The patient in the preceding example may have hyperchloremia secondary to NS resuscitation or she may have had an underlying RTA. The respiratory acidosis may be due to chest wall and/or lung injury or sedation, or it may be due to respiratory muscle failure in the setting of profound hypophosphatemia. The increased SIG is an ominous prognostic finding. In one series, trauma patients had nearly 100% mortality when their initial SIG was greater than 7 mEq/L. This may be due to acute phase stress response protein release by injured cells. However, poisoning including methanol and ethylene glycol (alcoholics) and toluene (glue sniffing) is also occasionally seen in this population.

ACID–BASE STATUS AS A MEASURE OF RESUSCITATION
Effect of Acidosis on Urine Output
☞ **Urine output can be quite deceptive as a measure of resuscitation success and as a guide to ABB.** ☞ However, acid–base disorders may influence urine output. It has been demonstrated that infusion of large volumes of highly hyperchloremic solutions (0.9% NS) will decrease glomerular filtration rate, renal blood flow, and the rate of urine flow compared to a less hyperchloremic solution (lactated Ringer's solution) (31). Moreover, acidotic disorders such as DKA may artificially elevate the urine output due to osmotic diuresis. The K_m for renal glucose transport is breached at about 180 mg% in the healthy adult. Therefore, glucose containing solutions should not be used for resuscitation so as to not overwhelm renal transport mechanisms and initiate an osmotic diuresis.

End-Tidal CO_2 Measurements
The use of monitoring devices to track the success of resuscitation is common. Recent data have validated the ability to detect a pulse oximetry signal as a valid tracking measure of progress in resuscitation (25). The pulse oximeter signal amplitude has also been studied as an indicator of the adequacy of resuscitation. In addition, routine application of end-tidal CO_2 ($P_{ET}CO_2$) analysis may aid in evaluating cardiac performance. Abnormalities of $P_{ET}CO_2$ tracings, not recorded values, have correlated well with the failure or success of cardiopulmonary cerebral resuscitation (CPR) and trauma resuscitation (32), although this device seems best suited to identifying instances of abnormal perfusion (i.e., low cardiac output), rather than when it is inadequately high (i.e., high cardiac index, but persistent lactic acidemia).

Sublingual CO_2
A relatively new device, the sublingual CO_2 oximeter (SLCO$_2$) shows promise in the early detection of poor perfusion (SLCO$_2$ > 70) (33). However, the value may return to normal more rapidly than the establishment of a truly adequate cardiac profile. The near infrared spectrometer (NIS) has also been successfully utilized to track the adequacy of resuscitation using a thigh muscle monitoring site as an indicator of limb perfusion (34). In this study, the NIS method was more sensitive than SvO$_2$ and the gastric-mucosal CO_2 gap obtained via gastric tonometry

(Chapter 10). This device shows promise, but needs additional investigation prior to recommending it as a first-line source of information. The role of the pulmonary artery (PA) catheter in the acute setting remains controversial. At least one study in trauma patients observed reductions in morbidity with routine use, but failed to demonstrate a survival advantage (35).

Invasive Monitoring Tools
However, central venous pressure (CVP) monitoring in combination with ABG and vital sign-derived indices have shown strong correlations with determining fluid requirements for critically ill patients with sepsis in the Emergency Department; unsurprisingly, morbidity and mortality reductions were observed for the better and earlier resuscitated group (36). This observation underscores the need for timely identification of hypoperfusion and rapid reversal of inadequate oxygen delivery and consumption. A host of sophisticated monitoring devices using the combination of a CVP line and an arterial catheter are available (i.e., PICCO, Metracor, etc.). Despite the attractiveness of an easily inserted monitoring system, its efficacy in reducing mortality in the trauma setting remains undetermined.

ACID–BASE DISORDERS IN TRAUMA PATIENTS
Lactic Acidosis and Hypoperfusion
Acid–base disorders in trauma patients may be conveniently divided into several phases including prehospital, resuscitation suite, OR, ICU, and then general ward/convalescence (37). Generally, the first three time frames are quite similar and may be considered together. Recall that, based on changes in cytokine levels, trauma resuscitation may be divided into a flow and ebb phase or an early and late phase. When one evaluates the phase of care with regard to mortality, there is an early phase (<72 hours posttrauma) and a late phase (more than seven days posttrauma) that correspond to defined mortality time-points on the continuum of trauma care. One must recognize that the majority of late-phase deaths are related to multisystem organ failure (MSOF) and occur in the ICU. The impact of iatrogenic acid–base disturbances is important during both phases, but may not be as appreciated during the early resuscitative phase as during the late time frame.

☞ **The early phases of the postinjury period are often dominated by lactic acidosis.** ☞ Lactate has been identified as an important marker for mortality since the early work of Abramson at Kings County Hospital where he identified reduced survivorship in patients admitted to a trauma center who failed to clear their lactate in less than 24 hours (38). These findings helped establish a paradigm of initial hypoperfusion reflected by lactic acidosis that could be corrected by volume resuscitation and hemorrhage control. The correlation is that by so doing, survivorship would improve. This paradigm was recently buttressed by Claridge et al. (39) and Blow et al. (40) as they noted that survivorship and morbidity were related to failed lactate clearance whether overt or occult. Consequently, the rather surgical notion of massive volume resuscitation as a salubrious maneuver was born and then deeply entrenched in surgical dogma. The side effects of massive volume resuscitation outside of pulmonary edema, abdominal hypertension, and subcutaneous edema have only been examined at cursory levels. Furthermore, although lactic acidosis may indicate hypoperfusion, it is neither sensitive nor specific. Integrating the information from clinical examination and hemodymanic monitoring with ABB will greatly enhance both sensitivity and specificity.

Hyperchloremic Acidosis Following Saline Resuscitation

✍ **A negative side effect of massive volume resuscitation is hyperchloremic metabolic acidosis, which principally occurs during the perioperative and ICU phase of trauma therapy (21).** ✍ This finding has long been recognized in the anesthesia literature as an expected consequence of massive volume resuscitation. However, only in the past decade have surgical manuscripts addressed this problem. In Example 1 (discussed earlier), we demonstrated that the addition of 10 L of 0.9% NSS could significantly increase $[Cl^-]$ and induce acidosis in a healthy individual. If this acidosis was initiated in a patient with pre-existing lactic acidemia from hypoperfusion related to hypovolemic shock, then the resultant pH may be dangerously low particularly if lactic acidosis does not resolve quickly with resuscitation.

Relationship Between Acidosis and Acute Lung Injury

✍ **Recent work has demonstrated a strong relationship between large volume resuscitation and the development of ALI (41).** ✍ Patients who developed ALI received larger volumes and evidenced a lower pH than their counterparts who did not develop ALI. One must question whether the low pH was due to the addition of greater amounts of Cl^- in the group who received larger volumes of crystalloid resuscitation and whether the ALI was related to the increased minute ventilation ($\dot{V}_E$) needed to blow off the excess CO_2 and buffer the acidosis. Unfortunately, the study by Eberhard et al. was not reported in sufficient detail to answer these questions. Instead, the study assessed the ability of different kinds of fluids to trigger a white cell immune activation response and found crystalloids to be potent triggers indeed (41). Data from isolated cells in culture suggest that acidosis itself may result in inflammatory effects.

Acidosis and Coagulopathy

The clotting cascade is comprised of serine proteases whose activity is pH dependent. It has been widely established that acidosis is a common consequence of acute injury (locally and systemically). It is also known that severe acidosis impairs the efficiency of the clotting cascade. Thromboelastography (TEG) is a sensitive means of assessing the interaction of all parts of the clotting cascade as they work in concert (42). In a large trial of general surgery patients undergoing large volume blood loss surgery (>500 cc), the presence of hyperchloremic acidosis correlated with the development of coagulopathy. Ex vivo data evaluating the impact of high chloride solutions on the TEG profile also indicates clotting dysfunction when the serine proteases are in a Cl^- rich and acidemic environment (43). Gross measures such as prothrombin time (PT) and aPTT are also deranged by raising the Cl^- concentrations in ex vivo specimens by 16 to 20 mEq/L above baseline with 0.9% NSS or 3% NSS (44).

The Lethal Triad and Damage Control Surgery

The triad of acidosis, hypothermia, and coagulopathy (the so-called "lethal triad") has been well reviewed by Spahn and Rossaint (45). Acidosis-related coagulopathy is further exacerbated by the presence of hypothermia (Volume 1, Chapter 40). Much like enzyme activity is related to pH, it is also intimately related to temperature. In fact, a core temperature of 33°C is equivalent to a clinically relevant,

functional factor deficiency despite normal factor levels (46). ✍ **The presence of hypothermia (in combination with metabolic markers of acidemia) has been identified as a trigger to pursue damage control (DC) surgery instead of a definitive procedure (47).** ✍

Ideally, a DC procedure (Volume 1, Chapter 21) should be decided upon at the initiation of surgery, rather than identified as an appropriate strategy at the end. The goals of DC surgery are to arrest hemorrhage, control gastrointestinal (GI) contamination, and deliver a viable patient to the ICU for ongoing resuscitation and metabolic restoration. The DC surgery time frame limits the time in the OR with an open major body cavity and reduces heat loss. DC surgery also potentially reduces the extent of coagulopathy by limiting the blood loss that could accrue from ongoing blood loss while attempting to achieve complete surgical repair in partly resuscitated patients.

Acidosis in the Elderly

The geriatric patient population presents unique challenges that can compound the impact of lactic acidemia on outcome (Volume 1, Chapter 37). This patient population is likely to present with multiple comorbidities including coronary artery disease, hypertension, chronic renal impairment, hepatic failure, and peripheral vascular disease (48). Each of these entities may impair the patient's ability to tolerate hypoperfusion and repair trauma or resuscitation-related acidosis. These sequelae are identified as persistent acidosis and a failure of lactate clearance. Recent data have shown survivorship of elderly patients is directly related to their injury complex as well as the number of comorbidities at the time of injury (48).

The term elderly as utilized by the American College of Surgeons Committee on Trauma (ACS-COT) is in part derived from the data of Rutherford et al. (49) where an lethal dose (LD_{50}) for base deficit was influenced by the presence of absence of TBI. Patients younger than 55 years old developed the same mortality curve as those older than 55 years if the younger patients also had brain trauma. The reason for this observation is unclear, but may be related to the elaboration of apoptotic triggers following the induction of secondary brain damage. Furthermore, in a large database analysis of US trauma centers, the ACS-COT identified that the mortality rate for men acutely rose at the age of 55 (50). Thus, despite a general trend in the literature to define elderly as ≥60 to 65 (Volume 1, Chapter 37), there may be a re-evaluation and reduction in the elderly age designation to 55.

Lactate Clearance and Mortality

Interestingly, not all patients who fail to clear their lactate levels in 24 hours die. It remains unclear from the current literature whether this represents persistent lactic acidemia, or the more subtle entity, hyperlactatemia. It has been well documented that plasma epinephrine levels may remain elevated (up to 4000 pcg/mL; normal <200 pcg/mL) for several weeks after injury (51). This is especially true in chronically stressed patients who are under-resuscitated and/or inadequate analgesia. The effect of the elevated epinephrine levels is to increase metabolic rate and induce a catabolic state. The increased flux through the Krebs cycle increases the total lactate production, but does so in proportion to pyruvate. Thus, the lactate/pyruvate ratio remains constant. Arterial lactate, when measured in this circumstance, will be greater than normal.

An additional confounder to lactate interpretation is that lactate may be released from the lungs of patients with ALI or ARDS (52). This lactate release does not represent systemic hypoperfusion and does not need to be treated as such. In fact, treating such a patient with additional volume loading may worsen the lung injury and aggravate the lactate output. This diagnosis is suggested by identifying an elevated lactate level in a patient who appears to be well resuscitated, but who has a lung injury. Drawing an arterial lactate and comparing it to a lactate level from mixed venous blood obtained from a pulmonary artery catheter (PAC) will establish the diagnosis. The lactate from the PAC will be higher than that from the peripheral artery. In a patient with an increasing arterial lactate level, a positive gradient across the lung indicates pulmonary lactate release.

Multiple Organ Dysfunction Syndrome and Acidosis

The late phase of trauma care is dominated by acid–base derangements related to organ failure as well as to iatrogenic acid–base disturbances. The ultimate pH is determined by the proportion of acidosis or alkalosis that is generated by the individual organ failure in relation to the prevailing electrolyte content and protein content of the patient's blood plasma. Acidemia from renal or hepatic failure is commonly mixed with alkalemia from the use of loop diuretics. Dilutional hyponatremia coupled with hyperchloremia leads to a narrow SID and a metabolic acidemia. It is not uncommon to identify complex acid–base disorders during the late phase of trauma care for these reasons. Identifying these disorders has important implications for IVF administration, total parenteral nutrition (TPN) composition, as well as enteral formulation selection, as the electrolyte composition of a patient's plasma is variable while the protein composition is not (acutely). Thus, the patient's ABB is directly related to both intrinsic disease and clinician intervention.

FLUID ADMINISTRATION AND ACID–BASE BALANCE

Volume 1, Chapter 11 reviews the relative merits of crystalloids versus colloids and their meta-analyses, whereas this chapter focuses only on the relative effect of different plasma volume expanders on lactate clearance, Cl^- loading, and induced acidemia.

Earlier, we reviewed the effect of loading a patient with 10 L of 0.9% NSS with regard to the SID and pH. ☞ **The degree to which hyperchloremic metabolic acidosis occurs following significant resuscitation is related to the total fluid volume and the SID of the fluid in relation to the patient's SID and any electrolyte losses.** ☞ Solutions that are rich in Cl^- (relative to plasma) will predictably produce hyperchloremia. However, metabolic acidosis occurs as function of the SID of the solution and volume infused. Since no crystalloid contains albumin, A_{TOT} will always decrease as a result of crystalloid resuscitation and will always have a mildly alkalinizing effect. A stronger effect on ABB comes from the change in SID. A solution with a SID of 0 (e.g., NS) will reduce the plasma SID and this has a stronger acidifying effect relative to the alkalinizing effect of reducing A_{TOT}. Compared to 0.9% NS (Cl^- 154, SID 0), LR has a more physiologic Cl^- concentration 110 and a higher SID (20). Of note, the SID of LR is equal to its lactate concentration (28 mEq/L) provided that the lactate is metabolized. Lactate will be metabolized quickly

in most situations, but if lactate is not metabolized the SID of LR is 0, just like NS.

Since one may utilize colloids suspended in low Cl^- vehicles, and colloids achieve a 3:1 superiority over crystalloids with regard to retained intravascular volume, resuscitation with colloid in a low Cl^-, higher SID solution would markedly reduce the total Cl^- load. This strategy would be expected to improve ABB relative to a high Cl^-, low SID strategy.

Evidence Supporting Lactated Ringer's Solution

The above hypotheses are validated by data derived from large volume blood loss surgery. In two studies, one conducted in the United States and one in the U.K., patients resuscitated with Cl^- rich, low SID fluids were found to have metabolic acidosis when they were resuscitated with NS-based IVF or NS-based colloid solution relative to LR or an LR-like vehicle for colloid delivery (53,54). Moreover, gastric tonometry derived gut perfusion was improved in the low Cl^- group, as was lactate clearance. Importantly, one of the studies identified the tripartite association of hyperchloremic acidemia, NS-based resuscitation, and impaired clotting identified by TEG.

☞ **Hyperchloremia is known to independently diminish measures of renal function, including glomerular filtration rate (GFR), urine flow, and creatinine clearance (30,55). It has been identified to be the factor most important for induced acidosis not associated with lactate in the OR.** ☞ Moreover, volume loading of healthy volunteers with either 0.9% NS or LR (50 cc/kg bw) at equivalent rates leads to a longer time to urine generation and abdominal pain in the NS group, as well as central nervous system (CNS) changes (55). It is suggestive that the abdominal pain may be related to intestinal perfusion since the above studies in the elderly identified markedly improved gastric tonometry values in the group resuscitated with a lower Cl^- regimen.

An Empiric Approach to Minimize Cl^-

Alterations of daily practice paradigms would appear to be in order. On the basis of the above data, it is appropriate to avoid large volume Cl^- loading of trauma patients to avoid compounding an existing lactic acidosis with one stemming from hyperchloremia. For those patients who have already undergone significant fluid resuscitation and have an extant hyperchloremic metabolic acidosis, reducing Cl^- and increasing the SID in their maintenance fluid is a reasonable approach. The authors employ solutions containing 25 to 150 mEq/L $NaHCO_3$, even as maintenance fluid in select patients. Since HCO_3^- is converted to CO_2 and removed almost instantly by ventilation, it has no real role in determining pH; thus this solution is a Na^+ delivery vehicle with the intent being to increase the plasma SID. This induces proton consumption and reverses the hyperchloremic metabolic acidosis. Ongoing restoration of the effective circulating (a.k.a. "stressed") volume can be accomplished by colloid in a balanced salt solution (BSS) solution to minimize the total amount of Cl^- that is delivered during resuscitation. However, no prospective studies have yet shown benefit to this practice.

Effect of Fluids and Acid–Base Balance on Coagulation

The clotting cascade is dependent on a series of serine proteases (Chapters 58 and 59). Recall that enzymes demonstrate a pH-dependent activity profile and, as such, evidence diminished activity when their microenvironment shifts outside of the pH optimum. This concerns many topics of this chapters regarding independent control mechanisms of pH to bear upon the problem of trauma-related coagulopathy. It is reasonable to hypothesize that the induction of hyperchloremia and the accompanying acidosis may induce coagulopathy. Coagulopathy is most commonly assessed by gross measures such as PT and aPTT, associated elements such as platelets and fibrinogen, but most sensitively by TEG. The TEG assesses all of the elements involved in coagulation and displays these data by means of a strain gauge coupled to a computer deflection trace. Delayed clotting is most clearly obvious as an increased time to clot formation, as well as decreased maximal amplitude of the trace.

Recent data address these hypotheses. In an ex vivo whole blood model, the deliberate induction of hyperchloremia with either 0.9% saline or 3% saline predictably decreased pH (30). Using 3% saline allowed the Cl^- to be changed without altering the concentration of the clotting cascade proteins. As a control, Hetastarch (HES) in 0.9% NS or HES in a balanced salt solution were added to separate tubes; no significant pH abnormalities were identified. This observation stems from the much smaller Cl^- load that was delivered to the system in the HES groups. Importantly, the crystalloid groups consistently demonstrated a prolonged PT and aPTT at Cl^- increases >20 mEq/L. Since neither HES group demonstrated coagulopathy, this observation cannot be related to the presence of Ca^{2+} in the HES in BSS group since there is no Ca^{2+} in the HES in 0.9% NS arm. A limitation of this study is the lack of TEG analysis.

TEG data have been provided for serial dilutions of blood with LR, HES in 0.9% NS, and HES in a balanced salt solution. It is clearly demonstrated that progressive dilution of blood with a chloride-rich solution results in multiple TEG abnormalities (43). Further data stem from an FDA phase III trial in which HES in BSS was found free of coagulation abnormalities up to 5000 cc in a 24-hour period, whereas HES in NS was clearly associated with TEG abnormalities (54). This further implicates Cl^- as an important arbiter of coagulopathy, as the main difference between the two regimens was the Cl^- content. Nonetheless, the potential role of Ca^{2+} must be evaluated. Since none of the patients in either group was receiving a massive transfusion, the role of induced hypocalcemia is unlikely in explaining the abnormal TEG profile.

TOXIN-INDUCED ACID–BASE DERANGEMENTS

Acute intoxications with agents other than alcohol derive their acid–base imbalance from their effect in their native state, or more commonly, as they are degraded by hepatic metabolism and exert deleterious effects upon the liver or the kidney (Volume 1, Chapters 30 and 31). The most common finding is metabolic acidosis, stemming from one of a variety of causes including (but not limited to) direct acid loading, tissue destruction, induction of lactate, induction of hypoperfusion from cardiovascular failure, poisoning of mitochondrial metabolism, decreased level of consciousness with hypoventilation and subsequent hypoxemia (respiratory and metabolic acidosis), and the induction of hepatic and renal failure.

Therapy consists of supportive measures including the standard care directed by Advanced Trauma Life Support (ATLS). However, certain intoxicants are removed by dialysis or charcoal hemoperfusion, whereas others are remedied by antitoxins (i.e., marine toxin envenomation) or antivennins (i.e., snake or spider bites) (Volume 1, Chapter 32).

EYE TO THE FUTURE

There is surprisingly much to discover about acid–base physiology, despite this topic having been the subject of intense scrutiny over the past several decades since the development of the practical hospital-based blood gas analyzing machine. The exact identity of the unmeasured ions remains obscure. Intense investigative efforts have explored whether the unmeasured ions are lectins, serum proteins, lysed cells, or denatured circulating proteins.

The most likely answer appears to be that the etiology of increases in SIG is multifactorial, and different acids are present in different patients. Similarly, the unmeasured ions have demonstrated remarkable correlation with poor outcome in some sepsis studies, while not in others. However, in trauma patients, the presence of an SIG ≥ 7 prior to fluid therapy strongly correlated with 72-hour mortality regardless of mechanism of injury (24,56). In an animal model of endotoxemia, where it was predicted that the gut and liver would be primary sources of unmeasured ions, the liver was either neutral or took up ions (baseline) and then released anions during early endotoxemia. In contrast, at baseline, the gut was neutral to anions, but then consumed anions as endotoxemia progressed. The lung and kidney were neutral to anions, neither generating nor consuming in this model (57). The author has embarked upon a search into the natural history of unmeasured ions, as well as the development of a prognostic model for those admitted to the critical care area.

Alterations of plasma volume expansion with agents that are constructed to minimize acid–base derangements may represent a major advance in altering the course of trauma patients during the acute resuscitation phase, especially in the areas of ALI, coagulation abnormalities, and immune activation. Moreover, programs using colloid resuscitation that are aimed at reducing the need for blood product administration are being jointly developed with the U.S. military. One such program, STORM ACT (Strategies to Reduce Military and Civilian Transfusion), is supported in part by the International Trauma Anesthesia and Critical Care Society (ITACCS), as well as a variety of other academic organizations and trauma societies. A number of forward thinking articles have been published speculating how trauma resuscitation will progress over the next decade (58). However, only multi-institutional trials that are sufficiently powered to enable outcome analysis will serve to accurately guide advances in resuscitation and ABB.

SUMMARY

Three widely used approaches to acid–base physiology have been reviewed in this chapter. Each utilizes specific variables to assess changes in ABB. Complete parity can be brought to all three acid–base approaches. Conversion between the descriptive approaches using HCO_3^- or SBE and AG and the quantitative approach using SID and SIG are fairly straightforward and have been recently reviewed elsewhere (59).

The authors favor the use of the Stewart model because it explains the mechanisms that underpin each acid–base abnormality, in terms of independent and dependent control mechanisms, and thus best guides therapeutic intervention. Understanding the concepts of SID and SIG allows one to rationally select appropriate resuscitation fluids to achieve effective resuscitation while minimally impacting pH. These concepts have also been applied to common acid–base problems that occur during trauma resuscitation and subsequent care to illustrate the improved control of metabolic derangements possible for insults resulting as a consequence of injury, as well as those that stem from the therapy for those conditions.

KEY POINTS

- The three major presentations of the metabolic component are (*i*) bicarbonate ion (HCO$_3^-$), (*ii*) SBE, and (*iii*) the SID between plasma strong cations and anions.
- ABB is regulated by the respiratory center of the medulla (respiratory component) and by the liver and kidneys (metabolic and weak acid components).
- The PaCO$_2$ level is regulated by the medulla, which governs the alveolar ventilation.
- As opposed to ventilation for elimination of CO$_2$, strong acids or bases require either elimination by the kidney (inorganic acids such as HCl or bases such as NaOH, KOH) or gastrointestinal tract or through metabolism, often in the liver (organic acids such as lactate$^-$, acetoacetate$^-$, and β-hydroxybutyrate$^-$).
- The parameter, SBE, has been introduced to measure the purely metabolic component of ABB in the ECF. A negative SBE occurs during metabolic acidosis and a positive SBE is obtained during metabolic alkalosis.
- Clinicians should be aware that the administration of NaHCO$_3$ is almost always a temporizing maneuver, while simultaneously working to correct the primary disorder causing the metabolic acidosis.
- Metabolic acidosis exists when there is more metabolic acid present than can be balanced by the available BB.
- Tachypnea and respiratory alkalosis commonly occur in compensation for a primary metabolic acidosis in the early post-trauma time frame due to hypoperfusion or iatrogenic hyperchloremia.
- Metabolic alkalosis is more commonly seen in the post-resuscitation phase of trauma patients, commonly during induced diuresis with a loop diuretic (induced by the net effect of Cl$^-$ loss in the urine).
- The normal AG is up to 14 $\pm$ 2 (if [K$^+$] is included) and 10 $\pm$ 2 (when [K$^+$] omitted), and assumes a normal albumin concentration and a PCO$_2$ of 40 torr (15,18).
- The use of the AG in acid–base analysis is critical in order to detect most of the acute disturbances requiring immediate therapy.
- The SID is the difference between the strong cations and strong anions (Equation 7) and in health has an approximate value of 40 to 42 mEq/L.
- An initial step in the evaluation of an acid–base disorder is to assess the clinical circumstance of the patient and to develop an initial differential diagnosis based upon the likely acid–base disorders associated with the clinical picture.
- Cool extremity temperature has been validated as an indicator of hypoperfusion (excluding exposure to hypothermic environments and peripheral vascular disease with arterial insufficiency).
- The value of the SBE (in isolation) as an indicator of lactic acidosis is corrupted following resuscitation because the electrolyte composition of the IVF will significantly impact pH and therefore, the SBE.

- The differential diagnosis for an AG acidosis can be remembered using the mnemonic "MUD PILES" and include methanol, uremia, dehydration, paraldehyde, INH, lactate, ethylene glycol, and salicylates. However, the differential diagnosis also includes other conditions including ketoacidosis, sepsis, and liver failure, making the mnemonic somewhat incomplete (Table 3).
- Although algorithms and nomograms are useful (if present at the bedside), the most important factor in evaluating acid–base perturbations is to understand how they occur in the human body and to take a systematic approach in diagnosis.
- Urine output can be quite deceptive as a measure of resuscitation success and as a guide to ABB.
- The early phases of the postinjury period are often dominated by lactic acidosis.
- A negative side effect of massive volume resuscitation is hyperchloremic metabolic acidosis, which principally occurs during the perioperative and ICU phase of trauma therapy (21).
- Recent work has demonstrated a strong relationship between large volume resuscitation and the development of ALI (40).
- The presence of hypothermia (in combination with metabolic markers of acidemia) has been identified as a trigger to pursue DC surgery instead of a definitive procedure (46).
- The degree to which hyperchloremic metabolic acidosis occurs following significant resuscitation is related to the total fluid volume and the SID of the fluid in relation to the patient's SID and any electrolyte losses.
- Hyperchloremia is known to independently diminish measures of renal function including GFR, urine flow, and creatinine clearance (30,54). It has been identified to be the factor most important for induced acidosis not associated with lactate in the OR.

REFERENCES

1. Van Slyke DD. Some points of acid–base history in physiology and medicine. Ann NY Acad Sci 1966; 133(1):5–14.
2. Stewart PA. Modern quantitative acid–base chemistry. Can J Physiol Pharmacol 1983; 61(12):1444–1461.
3. Singer RB, Hastings AB. Improved clinical method for estimation of disturbances of acid–base balance of human blood. Medicine. 1948; 27:232–242.
4. Schlichtig R, Grogono AW, Severinghaus JW. Current status of acid–base quantitation in physiology and medicine. In: Breen PH, ed. Respiration in Anesthesia: Pathophysiology and Clinical Update. WB Saunders: Philadelphia, 1998. Anesthesiol Clin N Am 1998; 16:259–293.
5. Narins RG, Emmett M. Simple and mixed acid–base disorders: A practical approach. Medicine 1980; 59:161–187.
6. Haber RJ. A practical approach to acid–base disorders. West J Med 1991; 155:146–151.
7. Brewer ED. Disorders of acid–base balance. Ped Clin NA 1990; 37:429–447.
8. Fencl V, Leith DE. Stewart's quantitative acid–base chemistry: applications in biology and medicine. Respir Physiol 1993; 91:1–16.
9. Fencl V, Rossing TH. Acid–base disorders in critical care medicine. Ann Rev Med 1989; 40:17–29.
10. Gluck SL. Acid–Base. Lancet 1998; 352:474–479.
11. Hood VL, Tannen RL. Protection of acid–base balance by pH regulation of acid production. N Eng J Med 1998; 339:819–826.
12. Kassirer JP: Serious acid–base disorders. N Eng J Med 1974; 291:773–776.

13. Preuss HG. Fundamentals of clinical acid–base evaluation. Clin Lab Med 1993; 13:103–116.

14. Schlichtig R, Grogono AW, Severinghaus JW. Human Pa_{CO_2} and standard base excess compensation for acid–base imbalance. Crit Care Med 1998; 26:1173–1179.

15. Kellum JA. Determinants of plasma acid–base balance. Criti Care Clin 2005; 21(2):329–346.

16. Ni Chonghaile M, Higgins B, Laffey JG. Permissive hypercapnia: role in protective lung ventilatory strategies. Curr Opin Crit Care 2005; 11(1):56–62.

17. Harrison RA. Acid–base balance. Respir Care Clin N Am 1995; 1(1):7–21.

18. Hatherill M, Waggie Z, Purves L, et al. Correction of the anion gap for albumin in order to detect occult tissue anions in shock. Arch Dis Child 2002; 87(6):526–529.

19. Salem MM, Mujais SK. Gaps in the anion gap. Arch Intern Med 1993; 152:1625–1629.

20. Scheingraber S, Rehm M, Sehmisch C, Finsterer U. Rapid saline infusion produces hyperchloremic acidosis in patients undergoing gynecologic surgery. Anesthesiology 1999; 90(5):1265–1270.

21. Koch SM, Taylor RW. Chloride ion in intensive care medicine. Crit Care Med 1992; 20(2):227–240.

22. Kellum JA, Kramer DJ, Pinsky MR. Strong ion gap: a methodology for exploring unexplained anions. J Crit Care 1995; 10(2):51–55.

23. Kellum JA, Bellomo R, Kramer DJ, Pinsky MR. Hepatic anion flux during acute endotoxemia. J Appl Physiol 1995; 78(6):2212–2217.

24. Kaplan LJ, Kellum JA. Initial pH, base deficit, lactate, anion gap, strong ion difference, and strong ion gap predict outcome from major vascular injury. Crit Care Med 2004; 32(5):1120–1124.

25. Kober A, Scheck T, Lieba F, et al. The influence of active warming on signal quality of pulse oximetry in prehospital trauma care. Anesth Analg 2002; 95(4):961–966.

26. Kaplan LJ, McPartland K, Santora TA, Trooskin SZ. Start with a subjective assessment of skin temperature to identify hypoperfusion in intensive care unit patients. J Trauma 2001; 50(4):620–627.

27. Shepherd JT, Vanhoutte PM. Local modulation of adrenergic neurotransmission in blood vessels. J Cardiovasc Pharmacol 1985; 7(suppl 3):S167-S178.

28. Schomig A, Richardt G, Kurz T. Sympatho-adrenergic activation of the ischemic myocardium and its arrhythmogenic impact. Herz 1995; 20(3):169–186.

29. Slutsky AS. Lung injury caused by mechanical ventilation. Chest 1999; 116(1 suppl):9S–15S.

30. www.ccm.upmc.edu/education/resources/phorum.html.

31. Wilcox CS. Regulation of renal blood flow by plasma chloride. J Clin Invest 1983; 71(3):726–735.

32. Kober A, Schubert B, Bertalanffy P, et al. Capnography in nontracheally intubated emergency patients as an additional tool in pulse oximetry for prehospital monitoring of respiration. Anesth Analg 2004; 98(1):206–210.

33. Marik PE. Regional carbon dioxide monitoring to assess the adequacy of tissue perfusion. Curr Opin Crit Care 2005; 11(3):245–251.

34. McKinley BA, Marvin RG, Cocanour CS, Moore FA. Tissue hemoglobin O_2 saturation during resuscitation of traumatic shock monitored using near infrared spectrometry. J Trauma 2000; 48(4):637–642.

35. Ivanov R, Allen J, Calvin JE. The incidence of major morbidity in critically ill patients managed with pulmonary artery catheters: a meta-analysis. Crit Care Med 2000; 28(3):615–619.

36. Magder S. How to use central venous pressure measurements. Curr Opin Crit Care 2005; 11(3):264–270.

37. Kaplan LJ, Bailey H, Kellum J. The etiology and significance of metabolic acidosis in trauma patients. Curr Opin Crit Care 1999; 5(6):458–463.

38. Abramson D, Scalea TM, Hitchcock R, et al. Lactate clearance and survival following injury. J Trauma 1993; 35(4):584–588; discussion 588–589.

39. Claridge JA, Crabtree TD, Pelletier SJ, et al. Persistent occult hypoperfusion is associated with a significant increase in infection rate and mortality in major trauma patients. J Trauma 2000; 48(1):8–14.

40. Blow O, Magliore L, Claridge JA, et al. The golden hour and the silver day: detection and correction of occult hypoperfusion within 24 hours improves outcome from major trauma. J Trauma 1999; 47(5):964–969.

41. Eberhard LW, Morabito DJ, Matthay MA, et al. Initial severity of metabolic acidosis predicts the development of acute lung injury in severely traumatized patients. Crit Care Med 2000; 28(1):125–131.

42. Luddington RJ. Thromblelastography/thromboelastometry. Clini Lab Haematol 2005; 27(2):81–90.

43. Roche AM, James MF, Grocott MP, Mythen MG. Coagulation effects of in vitro serial haemodilution with a balanced electrolyte hetastarch solution compared with a saline-based hetastarch solution and lactated Ringer's solution. Anaesthesia 2002; 57(10):950–955.

44. Patterson T, Bailey H, Kaplan LJ. Hyperchloremia induces acidosis, increases the strong ion gap, and impairs coagulation. Crit Care Med 2000; 28(12):A118.

45. Spahn DR, Rossaint R. Coagulopathy and blood component transfusion in trauma. Br J Anaesth 2005; 95(2):130–139.

46. DeLoughery TG. Coagulation defects in trauma patients: etiology, recognition, and therapy. Crit Care Clin 2004; 20(1):13–24.

47. Krishna G, Sleigh JW, Rahman H. Physiological predictors of death in exsanguinating trauma patients undergoing conventional trauma surgery. Aust NZ J Surg 1998; 68(12): 826–829.

48. Grossman MD, Miller D, Scaff DW, Arcona S. When is an elder old? Effect of preexisting conditions on mortality in geriatric trauma. J Trauma 2002; 52(2):242–246.

49. Rutherford EJ, Morris JA Jr, Reed GW, Hall KS. Base deficit stratifies mortality and determines therapy. J Trauma 1992; 33(3):417–423.

50. The American college of Surgeons Committee on Trauma National Trauma Databank. www.facs.org/trauma/ntdb.html.

51. James JH, Luchette FA, McCarter FD, Fischer JE. Lactate is an unreliable indicator of tissue hypoxia in injury or sepsis. Lancet 1999; 354(9177):505–508.

52. Kellum JA, Kramer DJ, Mankad S, et al. Release of lactate by the lung in acute lung injury. Adv Exp Med Biol 1997; 411: 281–285.

53. Wilkes NJ, Woolf R, Mutch M, et al. The effects of balanced versus saline-based hetastarch and crystalloid solutions on acid-base and electrolyte status and gastric mucosal perfusion in elderly surgical patients. Anesth Analg 2001; 93(4): 811–816.

54. Gan TJ, Bennett-Guerrero E, Phillips-Bute B, et al. a physiologically balanced plasma expander for large volume use in major surgery: a randomized phase III clinical trial. Hextend Study Group. Anesth Analg 1999; 88(5):992–998.

55. Williams EL, Hildebrand KL, McCormick SA, Bedel MJ. The effect of intravenous lactated Ringer's solution versus 0.9% sodium chloride solution on serum osmolality in human volunteers. Anesth Analg 1999; 88(5):999–1003.

56. Kaplan LJ, Bailey H, Klein A, et al. Strong ion gap: a predictor of early mortality following blunt or penetrating trauma. Crit Care Med 1999; 27(12):A42.

57. Bellomo R, Kellum JA, Pinsky MR. Transvisceral lactate fluxes during early endotoxemia. Chest 1996; 110(1):198–204.

58. Tisherman SA. Trauma fluid resuscitation in 2010. J Trauma 2003; 54(5 suppl):S231–S234.

59. Kellum JA. Clinical review: Reunification of acid–base physiology. Crit Care 2005; 9:500–507.

60. Schlichtig R, Grogon AW, Severinghaus JW. Human PaCO2 and standard base excess compensation for acid–base imbalance. Crit Care Med. In press.

46

Fever in Trauma and Critical Illness

John B. Cone
Department of Surgery, University of Arkansas, Little Rock, Arkansas, U.S.A.

William C. Wilson
Department of Anesthesiology and Critical Care, UC San Diego Medical Center, San Diego, California, U.S.A.

Charles L. James
Division of Infectious Diseases, Departments of Medicine and Pharmacy, UC San Diego Medical Center, San Diego, California, U.S.A.

INTRODUCTION

Humanity has but three great enemies; fever, famine and war; of these, by far the greatest, by far the most terrible, is fever.

—Sir William Osler

The ability to elevate body temperature in a controlled manner in response to injury or infection is highly conserved throughout both vertebrate and invertebrate species. Even the single-celled paramecium is capable of a regulated increase in its core temperature (a febrile response) (1). It seems unlikely that such an energy-expensive response would be so near universally present in the animal kingdom if it were not beneficial. Fever has been both deliberately induced and aggressively suppressed, and considered both a good and a bad prognostic sign. Accordingly, core temperature is one of the vital signs routinely monitored in trauma and critically ill patients.

Numerous causes of fever exist; these are generally classified into noninfectious and infectious etiologies. The two can also coexist in trauma and critically ill postsurgical patients. Differentiating the causes of fever and determining the proper treatments can be quite vexing in this patient population. Elevations in temperature often provoke elaborate and expensive diagnostic evaluations, fever control therapies, and empiric antibiotic administration.

Although the importance of treating fever varies with the clinical situation, the main virtue in quickly evaluating a new fever is that it frequently reflects an inflammatory state owing to an infectious or noninfectious etiology, which may or may not be life threatening.

This chapter reviews the clinical significance, diagnosis, and treatment of fever in trauma and critically ill surgical patients. The historical accounts of fever and its interpretation over time is initially surveyed and the basic physiology of thermoregulation is reviewed. Because fever occurs so commonly in the first couple of days following noninfectious tissue injury and inflammatory conditions associated with trauma, these are discussed first. The infectious causes of fever rarely occur less than three to five days following trauma or surgery. However, after five to seven days infections are the most common causes of fever. These are discussed roughly in the order of their frequency and/or urgency for treatment. Some disease processes are more fully discussed in other dedicated chapters, and the reader is referred there as appropriate.

BRIEF HISTORY OF FEVER

Elevations in body temperature were probably one of the first symptoms of disease recognized by early man (2). The Edwin Smith papyrus (circa 2500 BC) records symptoms complicating a wound to the shoulder that likely represented infectious-related fever. References to a "hot disease" were described in Assyria (circa 670 BC) and first century BC China. Pictographs representing this term were typically based on fire or a brazier (3). The same term was often used for wound infections, inflammation, or fever from systemic illness, depending on whether the condition was localized or generalized.

The scientific understanding of fever began with the development of the thermometer, which provided physicians with the ability to quantify body temperature (4). Philo of Byzantium and Hero of Alexandria in the second or first century BC are credited with the first written descriptions of devices that reflected the expansion or contraction of air that occurs with changes in temperature using devices called thermoscopes (5). Sanctorius (1561–1636), a colleague of Galileo, was the first to apply quantitative determinations to the thermoscope and actually make a crude thermometer (6). The term thermometer first appeared in the literature in Leurechon's "Récréation Mathématique" (1624) (6), as a device to test the intensity of fever.

But it was Sanctorius, a man with a passion to quantify all aspects of human physiology, who recognized that the human body has a normal temperature and that variations in temperature could be an aid in diagnosis. Two centuries later, Carl Rheinhold August Wunderlich (1815–1877) quantified temperature in a large patient population. His 1868 *opus magnus, Das Verhalten der Eigenwärme in Krankenheiten* (The Course of Temperature in Diseases), evaluated the results of over a million temperature measurements in 25,000 patients in a Leipzig clinic (7). He described the diurnal variation in body temperature and that "normal temperature" varied among individuals with 98.6°F (37°C) being the average "normal body temperature." He also established 100.4°F (38°C) as the upper limit of this normal range and by doing so offered the first quantitative definition of fever.

Efforts to suppress fever were also employed by antiquarian physicians; indeed, cooling measures utilized to treat the fever of Alexander the Great in 323 BC, using water baths, are well documented (8). Cooling cloths or cool baths were also used to provide symptomatic relief from the headache, myalgias, and arthralgias associated with fever. Pharmacologic treatment of fever was also known to the ancients. Hippocrates wrote of a bitter powder derived from the bark of the willow tree, as did texts from Egypt, Samaria, and Assyria. This substance was first made available commercially in 1899, with the introduction of the minimally toxic agent "aspirin."

Conversely, fever has also been induced in an effort to treat disease, a practice which can also be traced back to the era of Hippocrates. Fever was popularly applied to the treatment of syphilis as early as 1659. Following the extensive studies of Julius Wagner-Jauregg in the 1880s, fever therapy for syphilis (alone or in combination with drugs) became widely accepted. Indeed, this approach was so well received that Wagner-Jauregg received the Nobel Prize for this work in 1927 (9). Fever therapy has also been employed to treat multiple sclerosis, tuberculosis, and rheumatic fever, among other conditions. Interestingly, induced malaria was the standard means of creating a fever, but hot baths, hot air, heat cabinets, and heat lamps were also employed. The development of effective drug therapy along with the complications of fever therapy led to the abandonment of this form of treatment.

DEFINITION OF FEVER

☞ **Fever is perhaps best defined as: "an elevation in core body temperature >1°C above the patient's thermoregulatory set point (TRSP)."** ☞ However, clinicians seldom know what a patient's TRSP is prior to trauma or critical illness. Therefore, most traumatologists will define fever according to a set temperature criterion (e.g., 38.5°C). ☞ **In a joint statement of the Society of Critical Care Medicine (SCCM) (10) and the Infectious Disease Society of America (IDSA) (11), fever is defined as a temperature greater than or equal to 38.3°C (≥101°F).** ☞

Wunderlich was the first to emphasize that fever was a sign of illness, and not a disease in itself. His definition of fever is still in use today, both by the medical profession and the general public. In the 1870s, Liebermeister suggested that fever was not a result of the host's inability to regulate temperature, but rather that a higher TRSP was set (12). Today, most investigators working in the field of temperature regulation agree with the Liebermeister concept (13,14).

THERMODYNAMICS AND THERMOREGULATION
Thermodynamics

Biological organisms are energy converters and as such are subject to the same fundamental laws of thermodynamics as are inanimate objects. Energy derived from foodstuffs is converted to high-energy bonds such as ATP for storage. These high-energy storage molecules then supply energy for cellular transport, movement, synthesis, and so on. These intracellular chemical reactions are not perfectly

efficient. Most such reactions dissipate 50–75% of the available energy as heat. For temperature to be maintained at a constant level, heat loss must equal heat production. Humans are capable of manipulating both variables in this relationship to maintain a stable core temperature.

When heat production needs to be increased quickly and significantly, as required following exposure to a cold environment, shivering is the primary method for rapid increases in heat production. Under hypothalamic control, skeletal muscle rhythmically and rapidly contracts, generating large amounts of heat. Heat production can be supported or even stimulated by catecholamines, thyroxine, glucocorticoids, or insulin. A second chemical mechanism of generating additional heat, so-called nonshivering thermogenesis, exists but is most significant in the first year of life (13–15). Nonshivering thermogenesis occurs primarily in brown fat, a specialized tissue that largely disappears in humans after infancy.

The body loses heat to its environment via one of four mechanisms: conduction, convection, radiation, and evaporation as described in Volume 1, Chapter 40 and Chapter 11 in this Volume (15). The rate of heat loss is subject to manipulation by both physiologic and behavioral means. For example, in a cold environment, cutaneous vessels constrict, skin temperature is reduced, and less heat is lost via radiation, conduction, and convection (Volume 1, Chapter 40).

Clinicians frequently speak of body temperature as though it was a single number but there is no unique temperature that represents the body as a whole. The core or central compartment consists of the brain, heart, and the other viscera. The temperature of this core is best measured by a thermistor on a pulmonary artery catheter, nasopharyngeal, or esophageal probes. The tympanic membrane also reflects core temperature. Oral, rectal, bladder, axillary, and skin temperatures correlate with the core, but may be offset, and often lag behind core temperature changes (also see Volume 2, Chapter 11).

Body temperature is a reflection of the thermal energy stored in the body. The heat content of any object is determined by its mass, temperature, and specific heat. The specific heat of biologic tissues varies depending on the tissue in question, but the average specific heat for mammalian tissue is 0.83 kcal/kg (15). The higher the specific heat of a material, the more energy must be added to raise its temperature.

Thermoregulation

Body temperature, like many physiologic systems, is regulated by a negative feedback control system. Hammel et al. (16) first proposed a model involving the hypothalamus to explain this feedback to the control system. Essential to this model is the concept of a reference TRSP. Feedback signals from several core and peripheral receptors are continuously compared with the TRSP. However, the TRSP can be altered by physiologic conditions such as sleep, the administration of sedatives or analgesics, as well as pathologic conditions such as inflammation from both infectious, and noninfectious causes.

If this thermostat in the anterior hypothalamus is heated, heat loss mechanisms (e.g., peripheral vasolidation) are invoked. Conversely, if this area of the hypothalamus is cooled, heat production is stimulated (13,14). Temperature control involves a hierarchy of regional inputs from various central and peripheral thermoreceptors (refer Volume 1, Chapter 40) (13–15). Although certain neural lesions lead to varying degrees of dysfunction in thermoregulation, they seldom completely abolish thermoregulation in the absence of total brain and brainstem death. Skin temperature primarily influences the gain of the system. For example, when the skin is relatively cold, a small decrement in hypothalamic temperature produces a larger response than if the skin were warm.

The effectiveness of this system is demonstrated by the observation that man's core body temperature rarely varies more than $\pm 1°C$, despite large changes in environmental temperatures. This tight control is expensive in terms of energy demands (17). The high-energy expenditure is beneficial to the mammalian internal milieu by helping to maintain enzyme reaction rates and substrate needs relatively constant, providing a degree of biochemical stability.

The mechanism by which localized or even generalized infection or inflammation leads to an elevation in body temperature has been the source of much investigation. The current understanding of this process involves a release of soluble mediators, referred to as pyrogens, from cells involved in the inflammatory process (18,19). These pyrogens travel to the central nervous system (CNS), either crossing or interacting with the blood–brain barrier (BBB) and altering the hypothalamic thermostat so that the TRSP is raised. When the TRSP is raised, both autonomic and volitional heat conservation mechanisms are invoked. These responses include shivering, vasoconstriction of the skin, and behavioral changes such as seeking a warmer environment or more cover. This reset thermostat explains why patients may feel subjectively cold despite having elevated core temperatures.

Pyrogens can be classified into two groups: exogenous and endogenous. The exogenous pyrogens arise from bacteria, viruses, or foreign bodies causing fever (and inflammation), while the endogenous pyrogens arise from the host's own cells. The most extensively studied exogenous pyrogens are endotoxins derived from the cell wall of Gram-negative bacteria. However, Gram-positive bacteria, viruses, and even antigen–antibody complexes also have the capability to induce fever.

Most if not all exogenous sources of fever also act via the production of endogenous pyrogens by the host's immune cells (14,15). Such endogenous pyrogens include interleukin-1 (IL-1), tumor necrosis factor-alpha (TNF-α), and IL-6. It has been widely believed that these pyrogens cause the synthesis or release of other mediators (prostaglandin E) at a circumventricular area such as the *organum vasculosum laminae terminalis* (OVLT) (15), which is located near the preoptic region of the hypothalamus and has a more permeable BBB than other regions. Endogenous pyrogens differ in several significant ways from endotoxin and other exogenous pyrogens. The endogenous pyrogens are small proteins produced by various leukocyte populations, predominantly polymorphonuclear leukocytes (PMNs) and macrophages as components of the inflammatory response.

It has long been known that neuronal changes combine to raise the hypothalamic TRSP, inducing a febrile response (16). Prostaglandin E_2 (PGE$_2$) and the cyclooxygenase$_2$ (COX$_2$) pathways are known to be centrally involved in fever. Prostaglandin E_2 binds to thermoregulatory neurons in the hypothalamus; mice lacking the COX$_2$ enzyme do not mount fever following exposure to exogenous pyrogens (20). However, additional influences beyond prostaglandins are involved in the febrile response. Neuronal responses to PGE$_2$ may be activated by pyrogens, and some pyrogens may directly inhibit warm-sensitive and stimulate cold-sensitive neurons in the preoptic area of the hypothalamus (21).

BENEFITS AND ADVERSE CONSEQUENCES OF FEVER
Beneficial Role of Fever in Host Defense

No convincing study in humans has yet established that fever is either beneficial or detrimental to patients. Such studies are difficult to perform as temperature is essentially never the only variable involved in illness, or its treatment. For example, administration of an anti-inflammatory, antipyretic drug such as ibuprofen reduces fever but also reduces inflammatory and other components of the acute phase response (APR). The use of external cooling reduces fever but imposes additional stresses on the host, including increased muscular activity such as shivering, which can confound experimental observations.

Investigators of elevated temperature on host defense have examined individual components of the immune response in vitro and have utilized animal models with a standardized infection. However, neither approach provides perfect experimental conditions; accordingly, contradictory results have occurred.

PMNs have been shown to accelerate chemotaxis at 42°C compared with 37°C (22). Phagocytosis and killing of pathogens by PMNs from human blood is enhanced at 40°C compared with that found at 37°C (22). Yet, at higher temperatures PMN chemotaxis is reduced (23). However, others have not confirmed these results (24). Although less well studied, mononuclear phagocytes (25) and complement (26) probably behave in a similar manner.

T-cell proliferation in response to mitogens is known to increase when cultured at 39°C compared with 37°C (27). In other studies, this enhancement occurred at 38.5°C, but not at 40°C. There appears to be an augmentation of the lymphocyte response with moderate temperature increases above normal, but these are blunted or eliminated when the temperature is increased still further. Antibody production is also enhanced, and the timing of the temperature increase relative to antigen exposure appears to be critical (28).

The release and activity of most cytokines and pyrogens is also temperature sensitive. In some cell lines, TNF-α protein synthesis is stimulated at increased temperature, but the associated m-RNA is less stable leading to an augmented, but less persistent TNF-α effect (26).

In summary, the body's immunoinflammatory responses become more robust with a modest increase in core temperature (1.5–2.0°C), indicating that modest fever during infection is likely beneficial, but that higher fevers are less helpful to the host. Because higher fevers are associated with more severe infection and inflammatory states, uncertainty is added to the question of whether fever benefits the host or not.

Fever is just one component of the APR (29). The most familiar components of this response include: increased metabolic rate, protein catabolism, leuko- and thrombocytosis, alterations in protein and hormone synthesis, and release as well as changes in various minerals such as zinc and copper. These changes appear to result from resets of other "homeostats" by cytokines such as IL-1, IL-6, and TNF-α in a manner similar to resetting of the hypothalamic thermostat to produce fever (29,30).

Adverse Consequences of Fever

Despite the apparent benefits of fever, it is often accompanied with malaise, lethargy, anorexia, somnolence, and subjective discomfort including headache, arthralgia, and myalgia. Changes in the TRSP often lead to severe chills, shivering, and profuse sweating (13). The subjective findings, while not life threatening, can produce significant discomfort for the conscious patient. Furthermore, when fever becomes very high seizures can occur, and/or somnolence can progress to stupor and coma, both conditions requiring airway management.

The febrile response is associated with an increase in metabolic rate (oxygen consumption, nutritional need, or heat production) of 7–8% per degree centigrade increase in core temperature. In addition, fever is usually associated with an increase in the pulse of eight beats per minute for each degree centigrade of temperature increase (Liebermeister's rule). Such increased oxygen needs (and myocardial work) may be difficult for a patient with limited cardiopulmonary reserve to meet. The associated increase in CO_2 production requires an increase in minute ventilation. Fever is also directly associated with increases in intracranial pressure (ICP) at the same time that CNS oxygen demands are increased. Temperatures greater than 41°C have the ability to produce direct damage to sensitive tissues, particularly in the CNS.

INITIAL FEVER EVALUATION

The differential diagnosis of fever should take into account the many conditions that can alter a critically ill patient's body temperature and include environmental factors (large volumes of fluids, dialysis, hot lights, heating, or cooling devices) as well as clinical factors that may point to the etiology. Fever is generally divided into infectious and noninfectious causes (31).

☞ **Fever is frequently seen in the initial 48 hours after trauma, burns or surgery; however, such fevers are usually noninfectious in origin.** ☞ Blood cultures, chest X-rays, and urine studies are usually not necessary in this circumstance unless the physician has a particular reason for concern. A careful examination of the patient is warranted with particular attention to traumatic and surgical wounds, the chest examination, as well as any indwelling devices such as central lines. Particular attention should be devoted to the patient's history including events prior to admission as well as anything that might suggest increased bacterial numbers or virulence (e.g., barnyard injuries, open fractures, witnessed aspiration, or immunosuppression).

Routine cultures are not necessary but removal of the dressing and frequent careful inspection of all wounds is mandatory. ☞ **Although infection is unlikely in the first 48 hours following injury, Group A streptococcal infections and Clostridial myonecrosis represent uncommon, but important, exceptions which can present within this time period.** ☞

The longer the patient has been in the intensive care unit (ICU), the greater the probability that the fever is secondary to infection, and the more aggressively the diagnosis of infection should be pursued. Evaluation of the source of fever following trauma and critical care includes ruling out of the etiologies shown in Tables 1 and 2. In addition, the greatest focus needs to be on eliminating particularly virulent infections and the noninfectious etiologies with greatest mortality.

Examination of the patient includes scrutiny of the entire body surface, along with every orifice, every tube (or other foreign body passing through the skin), and

Table 1   Noninfectious Causes of Fevers

Cause	Example and comments
Tissue injury	Trauma, burns, postsurgical
Cerebral hemorrhage	Tissue trauma, inflammatory mediators
Reabsorption of hematoma	DVT, PE[a], procedure-related (e.g., groin), spontaneous (e.g., retroperitoneal, rectus)
ARDS	Fibroproliferative phase of disease
Alcohol or other drug withdrawal	Increased adrenergic state, leads to hypermetabolism
Fat embolus PE[a]	Release of pyrogens in the pulmonary circulation beyond normal hematoma reabsorption-related factors
Drug related (nonallergic)	MH, NMS, nonallergic drug toxicity serotonin syndrome, atropine, cocaine, methamphetamines
Allergic	Antiseizure drugs (DPH)
Pancreatitis	Inflammatory SIRS
Adrenal insufficiency	Hemorrhage, chronic use of corticosteroids, metastatic malignancy
Thyroid storm	Excessive metabolic heat thyrotoxicosis
Transfusion-related	WBC membrane-related, and release of cellular constituents
Other causes	Post MI, autoimmune, malignancy

[a]PE can cause fever through a number of mechanisms. Some are similar to those occurring with the reabsorption of any hematoma. Other mechanisms include the elaboration of inflammatory mediators into the pulmonary circulation.
Abbreviations: DVT, deep venous thrombosis; PE, pulmonary embolus; ARDS, acute respiratory distress syndrome; MH, malignant hyperthermia; NMS, neuroleptic malignant syndrome; DPH, Diphenylhydantion (phenytoin); SIRS, systemic inflammatory response syndrome; MI, myocardial infarction.

Table 2 Most Frequent Sites of Infection in Trauma Patients Admitted to the Surgical Intensive Care Unit (SICU)

Site of infection	Comments
Lower respiratory	Ventilator-associated pneumonia is most common cause of fever in SICU
Urinary tract	Although a common site of infection, urinary tract infections rarely cause SICU fever
Surgical wound	Rarely a cause of early (<72 hours postoperation) fever. However, these are responsible for approximately 25% of the nosocomial infections occurring in trauma and postsurgical patients[a]
Line sepsis	Approximately 70% of bloodstream infections are associated with invasive lines
Blood stream	All sources of invasive infection can cause bacteremia. Endocarditis is rarely the initial cause of infection or fever in trauma and surgical critical care
Intra-abdominal	3–15% of surgical injuries to the gastrointestinal tract can become infected (Volume 2, Chapter 50)

[a]Adapted from Ref. 119.

every wound on the body. The extremities can be quickly eliminated as a source of fever, if they are free of cellulitis, lymphagitis, lymphadenitis, or swelling (associated with DVT). Next the head can be evaluated for sinusitis (as described in the following), parotiditis (ruled out if parotid glands are normal), intracranial causes [ruled out if neurological status, head computed tomography (CT), and cerebrospinal fluid (CSF) studies are all normal]. The neck should be evaluated for swelling, including lymph nodes, and any internal or external jugular lines examined for signs of infection.

If all of these are negative, attention can then be directed solely on the torso. A complete examination of lungs, heart, abdomen, and pelvis is essential. The skin should be surveyed for rash, lesions, or decubitus ulcers. A rectal exam can rule out perirectal abscess, and the genitalia should be examined for various forms of infection. The chest should also be evaluated with chest radiography, chest CT, or bronchoscopy, as appropriate (32,33). A chest CT may be useful to evaluate pneumonia, emypema (34), and noninfectious causes of fever, and infiltrates such as pulmonary contusion, hemothorax, pulmonary embolus, and so on. The abdomen, pelvis, and retro-peritoneum can be evaluated by CT scan as well (see Volume 2, Chapter 50). Generally, at least one week should have elapsed since operation or the last abdominal CT scan for useful information to be provided using this imaging modality (35).

With these physical and imaging studies, most localized causes of infection will be suggested (36–38). Gram stain supplements this and helps suggest empiric antibiotic therapy (if indicated); culture data later confirms diagnosis and allows for narrowing of antibiotic coverage. When these evaluations are negative, and/or the patient has any other features (e.g., rash, muscle rigidity, and the like), then noninfectious etiologies may be identified. The most common of these will be reviewed in the next section.

NONINFECTIOUS CAUSES OF FEVER

Noninfectious fever is common following trauma, burns, and surgical procedures. The list shown in Table 1 is far from complete, but includes some of the more frequently encountered possibilities as well as those that require specific and urgent treatment. Noninfectious causes of fever rarely lead to temperatures greater than 38.9°C (102°F). ☛ **If the temperature exceeds 38.9°C, the patient**

should be considered to have an infectious etiology until negative cultures demonstrate otherwise. ☛ Exceptions to this generalization include drug fevers, transfusion reactions, malignant hyperthermia (MH), neuroleptic malignant syndrome (NMS), and heatstroke (36).

Tissue Injury

Trauma, burns, and surgery all cause tissue destruction; the more severe, the greater the associated injury. Along with the tissue trauma, inflammatory mediators are released into the circulation, some of which are pyrogens. In addition, macrophages and other cells that clear cellular debris also release cytokines.

Cerebral Hemorrhage—Hematoma

Cerebral hematomas release brain tissue thromboplastin and other toxins into the circulation, lending to an increased risk of disseminated intravascular coagulation (DIC), inflammation, and fever. When blood is released into the subarachnoid space, fever occurs, probably because of the release of pyrogens that enter the hypothalamus.

Noncerebral Hematoma

Hematomas located anywhere in the body, including deep venous thrombosis (DVT), pulmonary embolus (PE), and those occurring in tissue (because of trauma, procedure-related, or spontaneous), all release inflammatory mediators, cytokines, and pyrogens.

Drug-Related (Nonallergic)
Malignant Hyperthermia

The syndrome of MH typically occurs soon following induction of anesthesia with volatile anesthetics or succinylcholine (39,40). Extremely rapid temperature increases are the hallmark of MH; it can also have an insidious and delayed onset (41). Malignant hyperthermia is characterized by elevated core temperature, muscle rigidity, tachycardia, and excess CO_2 production. Hyperthermia, hyperkalemia, and lactic acidosis are common. Hypoglycemia is often present as well. Malignant hyperthermia is a genetic disease of skeletal muscle with variable patterns of inheritance (42–44). The pathophysiology involves the uncontrolled increase in intracellular calcium in skeletal muscle resulting in intense and sustained muscle contraction, with resulting increase in heat production and temperature. The molecular basis of MH is more fully discussed in Volume 1, Chapter 40.

Treatment consists of discontinuation of the causative agent if still in use, immediate administration of 100% O_2, and dantrolene sodium. In addition, aggressive volume replacement and control of acidosis and hyperkalemia are key elements of care, along with the institution of core temperature cooling measures. External cooling should be instituted immediately with ice packs, cooling blankets, iced saline lavage, and so on, and continuous core temperature monitoring is critical.

Neuroleptic Malignant Syndrome

The NMS is a relatively rare but potentially lethal drug-related complication that includes fever and muscle rigidity, and frequently is associated with the use of neuroleptic drugs (e.g., haloperidol) (45–47). In addition, creatine phosphokinase (CPK) values may be elevated secondary to rhabdomyolysis. The muscle rigidity is of the "lead pipe" variety. The resulting chest wall involvement may result in tachypnea and hypoventilation, even requiring mechanical ventilatory support. Extrapyramidal symptoms such as dyskinesia and dysarthria may also be seen. Leukocytosis is a common finding.

A wide variety of drugs are associated with NMS including phenothiazines and butyrophenones (48). Alcoholic patients, sicker patients, and those with underlying infection or organic neuromuscular diseases appear to be at increased risk of developing NMS. The pathophysiology of NMS is not clearly established, but it is related to a functional dopamine$_2$ (D_2) deficiency resulting from either the use of a drug with anti-D_2 side effects (e.g., haloperidol), or from the abrupt discontinuation of a D_2 agonist (e.g., Sinemet) in patients with Parkinson's disease (45–49).

Successful management of NMS requires prompt recognition, immediate withdrawal of D_2 antagonists, and if appropriate the reintroduction of D_2 agonist. Supportive care also requires hydration, support of respiration, treatment of acidosis, and reduction of fever. Although not proven to enhance survival, specific therapy appears to significantly shorten the course of NMS in comparison with supportive care alone (47). The D_2 agonist bromocriptine mesylate (Parlodel®) has also been shown to reduce rigidity and temperature. Hypotension is the usual limiting side effect of this therapy. Dantrolene sodium, the drug of choice for malignant hyperthermia (discussed earlier), decreases the calcium available for muscle contraction and leads to improvement in the rigidity, which in turn leads to less heat production and a decrease in the temperature. Clinical improvement in patients treated with either of these two agents begins within hours in contrast to days required with supportive care alone. Other D_2 agonists such as amantadine and carbidopa have also been used successfully (45–49). Rechallenge with neuroleptic drugs after NMS may or may not result in recurrence of the syndrome (45). If the use of such drugs is necessary, re-exposure can usually be accomplished safely with either less potent drugs or lower initial doses in the closely monitored patient.

Nonallergic Drug Toxicity

Nonallergic drug toxicity is common when patients are administered high levels of drugs with CNS effects, or side effects. Common drugs in this category are the anticholinergics (atropine, scopolamine), drugs of abuse (e.g., cocaine, methamphetamines, and the like), as well as elevated doses of drugs prescribed for depression particularly selective serotonin reuptake inhibitors (SSRIs) with monoamine oxidase inhibitors (MAOIs) or MAOIs along with tricyclic antidepressants (TCAs).

Serotonin syndrome (SS) is a recently recognized source of temperature elevation that occurs most frequently as a result of combination therapy with psychotropic medications that increase brain serotonin activity (50,51). ☞ **The SS is usually associated with combinations of SSRIs with MAOIs, or MAOIs with TCAs (50,51).** ☞ Illicit drugs such as MDMA (ecstasy) have also been associated with the syndrome. Patients with SS usually respond to discontinuation of the offending agent and general supportive care. However, antiserotonin therapy with cyproheptadine or methysergide and/or propranolol may be indicated in severe cases (50–52).

Allergy-Related Fevers

Numerous drugs used in trauma and critically ill patients can cause fever. There is no absolute physical finding or laboratory test to confirm the diagnosis of drug fever. Drug fevers are often high, spiking fevers with associated chills (53). Leukocytosis and eosinophilia may be present but are not consistent; maculopapular rash may be present as well. Drug fevers can only be diagnosed after excluding likely infectious causes and stopping the drug in question, hence drug fever is often referred to as a "diagnosis of exclusion." ☞ **After stopping a drug responsible for fever, 48–72 hours are usually required for the temperature to fully normalize.** ☞ The β-lactam antibiotics and diphenylhydantoin are probably the two most frequent causes of drug-induced fevers in the surgical intensive care unit (SICU), but other common causes include other antibiotics, dobutamine (54), and antidysrhythmics (53). Many other medications have been implicated in drug fevers and include those that may be easily overlooked, such as pain medications, sedatives, and sulfa-containing stool softeners (Table 3).

Alcohol and drug use and abuse are common in the trauma patient population. Patients and families should be questioned carefully for any history of alcohol or drug use but often this use is minimized or denied. Patients who develop disorientation, tremor, hyperarousal, or hallucinations one to three days or more after admission should be evaluated for withdrawal and managed appropriately. Findings that may suggest withdrawal include fever, tachycardia, hypertension, agitation, and delirium.

Pancreatitis

☞ **Pancreatitis is one of the classic inflammatory conditions that can cause significant noninfectious fever, with signs similar to sepsis.** ☞ Fortunately, the majority of patients with pancreatitis have minimal organ dysfunction and recovery is uneventful. However, approximately 20% of patients may go on to develop systemic inflammatory response syndrome (SIRS), leading to a fulminant course with pancreatic necrosis and multiorgan failure. The SIRS state is partly caused by activation of the inflammatory cascade mediated by cytokines, immunocytes, and the complement system (Volume 2, Chapters 47 and 63) (55). Many of the cytokines associated with disease progression are also known to be major causes of SIRS, evoking a febrile response (e.g., IL-1, IL-6, and TNF) (14,15).

Because the development of infected pancreatic necrosis significantly increases the mortality in patients with acute pancreatitis, much attention has been given to the prevention and early identification of patients at risk

Table 3 Drugs Commonly Implicated in the Development of Fever

Common	Less common	Rare
Antidysrhythmics	Allopurinol	Antacids
Amphotericin B	Azothioprine	Antihistamines
Barbiturates	H$_2$ blockers	Insulin
Methyldopa	Hydralazine	Corticosteroids
Penicillins	Iodides	Aminoglycosides
Cephalosporins	Isoniazid	Macrolides
Phenytoin	Rifampin	Tetracyclines
Diuretics	Carbapenems	Clindamycin
Sleep medications	Vancomycin	Vitamin preparations
Sulfonamides	Nifedipine	
(including sulfa-containing laxatives)	Nonsteroidal anti-inflammatory drugs	

Source: Adapted from Refs. 120 and 121.

of developing Gram-negative pancreatitis sepsis. The major source of Gram-negative bacteria is the gut, hence empiric antibiotic therapy targeted at these organisms is often employed (56).

Adrenal Insufficiency

☞ **Patients who have a vasodilated picture suggestive of sepsis but in whom sepsis is unlikely may have adrenal insufficiency. Serum cortisol determination, a cosyntropin stimulation test or even empiric corticosteroid administration may be indicated.** ☞ Fever associated

with adrenal insufficiency in the trauma ICU patient is most often secondary to chronic use of corticosteroids with resulting adrenal suppression. Primary adrenal failure can occur as a result of adrenal hemorrhage associated with sepsis, coagulopathy, or other conditions (57). This diagnosis should be considered in any patient with sudden hemodynamic collapse. A history of previous corticosteroid use, anticoagulants, metastatic malignancy, or other medical conditions may help to suggest the diagnosis but cannot exclude it.

Suggestive laboratory abnormalities include hyponatremia, hyperkalemia, hypoglycemia, and prerenal azotemia. Eosinophilia can be present. Patients with adrenal insufficiency can develop hyperdynamic shock (58), manifested by elevated cardiac index ($\geq$4 L/min/m^2), tachycardia, hypotension and low systemic vascular resistance, and a high pulmonary capillary wedge pressure. A random serum cortisol <10 μg/dL is sufficient to confirm the diagnosis while a level of 10–15 μg/dL is suggestive (59).

These standard diagnostic criteria are not sufficient to exclude adrenal insufficiency in the ICU population. The "normal" cortisol level in critically ill patients has not been well established. Furthermore, relative adrenal insufficiency may play a role in the critically ill. In this condition, cortisol levels are elevated above the normal range, but metabolic needs may require an even higher cortisol level. The cosyntropin (ACTH) stimulation test can help with the recognition of these patients (60). Because untreated adrenal insufficiency is almost 100% fatal in critically ill patients in shock, it is appropriate to initiate therapeutic steroid replacement without waiting for the results of the cortisol assay or the cosyntropin stimulation test.

Thyrotoxicosis

Thyroid storm results from excessive metabolic heat production (61,62). It is most often characterized by fever, and tachycardia in the presence of an enlarged thyroid gland. Tachydysrhythmias, particularly atrial fibrillation, are common. Treatment includes large doses of glucocorticoids combined with propylthiouracil and iodine (62). Propranolol antagonizes the peripheral effects of thyrotoxicosis. The combined β1- and β2-blockade is preferable to the more selective β1 antagonism seen with esmolol or metoprolol. The metabolic effects of thyroid hormone are in part mediated by the β2 receptors. Supportive measures should include surface cooling, acetaminophen, and volume replacement.

Transfusion-Related Fevers

Transfusion-related fever is caused by cellular constituents contained in blood products, and can occur with packed red blood cells, fresh frozen plasma, platelets, or cryoprecipitate (63). ☞ **Most febrile reactions following transfusions are related to white blood cells (WBC), as leukocyte-depleted blood products have a low rate of this complication (64).** ☞ However, WBC cell wall components and various antigen–antibody complexes can also have an immunological involvement, possibly involving circulating immune cells.

Other Noninfectious Causes

Numerous other noninfectious causes of fever exist, including postmyocardial infarction syndromes (65), autoimmune disorders (66), and various forms of malignancy (67).

IMPORTANT INFECTIONS IN TRAUMA AND CRITICAL CARE

Although a host of noninfectious conditions can cause fever in the ICU (Table 1), infections represent the most common cause, particularly after the first 48–72 hours. More than 50% of trauma patients admitted to the ICU develop an infection. In general, fevers caused by infection will have clinical findings indicating the source (if a thorough exam is employed). To an extent, higher temperatures are most often because of infection. Miller et al. (31) found that temperatures greater than or equal to 102°F predicted infection with a sensitivity of 72% and a specificity of 83%. However, when the temperature is >41°C, MH, NMS, heat stroke, and other drug-related causes should also be considered (Volume 1, Chapter 40).

The infections reviewed in this chapter constitute the most troublesome, either in terms of their prevalence (e.g., nosocomial pneumonia, line sepsis, and abdominal abscesses), rapidity of progression (e.g., necrotizing fasciitis, meningococcemia), or uniqueness to the trauma population (e.g., orthopedic fracture prophylaxis and postsplenectomy prophylaxis). These infections are reviewed in terms of the organisms involved, their virulence factors, and the appropriate antibiotics for each condition (Volume 2, Chapter 53).

Blood cultures should be performed on patients with new fever unless there is strong reason to doubt an infectious cause, such as is an early post-trauma or postoperative patient without evidence of wound infection. The SCCM/IDSA guidelines suggest no more than three blood samples (in most cases two are sufficient) for culture during the initial 24 hours of fever (10,11). A second pair of cultures should be obtained in the second 24 hours if the fever persists. Additional cultures are usually needed only if the suspicion of bacteremia or fungemia is strong. A common source of bacteremia is central venous lines. The highest risk is with noncuffed temporary hemodialysis catheters and the lowest risk is for small peripheral catheters. However, catheters placed in field are at high risk for infection, and should be replaced within 24 hours of admission. Femoral lines are also associated with increased risk of DVT, and should be considered for replacement on a daily basis. Multiple other sites of possible infection exist (Table 4). Rational diagnostic approaches have been described (10,11,36–38), and will not be reviewed further here.

Atelectasis has been widely credited as a cause of fever but proof for this remains elusive (68). Experimental atelectasis usually does not produce fever although levels of some pyogenic cytokines are elevated (69). ☞ **Most investigators now recognize that atelectasis does not cause fever in the absence of infection.** ☞ However, patients with alveolar collapse are more prone to developing subsequent infections, owing to the interruption of normal cleansing of secretions, as microinfections (which would normally be cleared) become established as a result of stagnant clearance. Therefore, while the pathophysiologic connection between atelectasis and fever is not fully understood, patients with atelectasis demonstrated by diminished breath sounds or typical chest X-ray findings should receive aggressive pulmonary toilet and re-expansion of alveolar volume to decrease the risk of subsequent infection.

Nosocomial and Ventilator-Associated Pneumonia

☞ **The most common infectious cause of fever in critically ill patients is ventilator-associated pneumonia (VAP).** ☞ Members from the American Thoracic Society (ATS) and the IDSA have recently published a consensus document containing recommendations for the management of hospital-acquired pneumonia (HAP) and VAP in adults (70). Nosocomial HAP is divided into two categories, early-onset HAP, which occurs within the first five days of hospitalization, and late-onset HAP, which occurs after the fifth hospital day. As a generality, the organisms that cause pneumonia that develops within the first few days of hospitalization are essentially the same organisms that are associated with community-acquired pneumonia (CAP): pneumococci, *Hemophilus influenzae*, so-called atypical pathogens such as *Chlamydia pneumoniae*, *Mycoplasma* spp., and *Legionella* spp., along with viral pathogens. When patients develop late-onset nosocomial pneumonia, multiresistant bacterial pathogens are much more likely to be the microbiologic cause of pneumonia. Common pathogens include methicillin-resistant *Staphylococcus aureus* (MRSA), *Pseudomonas aeruginosa*, *Acinetobacter* spp., Gram-negative enteric flora such as *Klebsiella* spp. or *Enterobacter* spp., which may contain the genetic capability to express extended spectrum beta-lactamases (ESBLs).

Oral anaerobes are only rarely involved as pathogens in late-onset HAP. The change in species distribution results from changes in bacterial colonization of the buccal mucosa that occurs in all patients within 48–72 hours, after hospitalization for an acute illness. The appearance of novel binding sites on mucosal cells, specific for enteric Gram-negative organisms and pseudomonal species, allows these organisms to completely replace the normal flora, resulting in the virtual disappearance of viridans streptococci and obligate anaerobes from the mouth. Aerobic Gram-negative rods are the most common class of organisms causing nosocomial aspiration pneumonia. Ventilator-associated pneumonia is a subset of nosocomial pneumonia but is extremely important because of the associated high morbidity and mortality.

Proper treatment for early-onset HAP comprises use of the same antibiotics recommended in modern guidelines for CAP, including a third-generation cephalosporin in combination with either a macrolide, a quinolone, or doxycycline (71). Methicillin-sensitive *Staphylococcus aureus* (MSSA), especially secondary to a viral respiratory illness like influenza can also present as an early-onset pneumonia and can be treated with semisynthetic antistaphylococcal penicillin or cephalosporin (71).

As late-onset HAP and especially VAP are more likely to result from multidrug-resistant organisms, the antibiotic recommendations for empiric treatment differ from those of early-onset HAP (70). Treatment for Gram-negative rods should always include the possibility of pseudomonal infections. Initially, treatment with two drugs in different drug classes is indicated because of the possibility of resistance to at least one of the agents. In general, the recommended strategy is to combine a beta-lactam agent with either an antipseudomonal fluoroquinolone (e.g., ciprofloxacin or levofloxacin), or with an aminoglycoside.

Third-generation cephalosporins such as ceftazidime or cefepime are good beta-lactam choices; aztreonam should be selected in patients with severe penicillin allergies. Alternative treatment strategies include the use of carbapenems or beta-lactam/beta-lactamase inhibitors (e.g., piperacillin/tazobactam). Among the carbapenems, imipenem and meropenem are first choices, as ertapenem lacks significant effective antipseudomonal activity. Of the available beta-lactam/beta-lactamase inhibitors, piperacillin/tazobactam is the most effective antipseudomonal drug combination. As anaerobic organisms are of only minor significance in late-onset HAP and VAP (unless associated with postextubation

Table 4 Less Frequent Sites of Infection in Intensive Care Unit Trauma Patients

Sinusitis
Colitis (i.e., *Clostridium difficile*)
Acute cholecystitis
Decubitus
Hepatitis
Central nervous system (i.e., meningitis or encephalitis)

aspiration), empiric anaerobic treatment is only required if aspiration is the source of pneumonia.

Alternatively, a beta-lactam drug can be used with either a fluoroquinolone or an aminoglycoside for the first several days. Owing to the increased prevalence of multiply-resistant Gram-negative organisms, the rationale for dual therapy is to use at least one drug that is active against the infecting bacteria. Ciprofloxacin and levofloxacin have been widely preferred over aminoglycosides for this purpose because they are easier to dose (drug level monitoring not required), and because they have almost no nephrotoxicity. However, as the level of fluoroquinolone resistance among *P. aeruginosa* has risen, in some places to over 30% of isolates, they are becoming less effective as first-line therapy. Aminoglycosides are an alternative despite toxicity and a relatively poor distribution into lung tissues compared with other tissues.

The need for dual antibiotic coverage in nosocomial pneumonia is much debated. Available studies suggest that outcomes are similar with either dual antibiotic therapy or monotherapy as long as the causative microorganism is sensitive to the single drug used. Therefore, in those situations where two drugs are used initially, one can be discontinued when the final culture with sensitivities are known. When these drugs are used for pneumonia, the doses are generally higher than when used for other diseases.

As pneumonia caused by *S. aureus* and especially by MRSA is an important concern in an ICU, initial empiric coverage should include linezolid or vancomycin. Although recent data suggest that survival is improved with the use of linezolid instead of vancomycin in MRSA pneumonia, inadequately low doses of vancomycin were used as the comparator drug in some of the studies. Vancomycin is a large molecule, and its distribution into the lung parenchyma is low. As a result, the current guidelines recommend that trough levels of vancomycin should be between 15 and 20 mg/L rather than the usual 5–10 mg/L. The increase in dosage will require monitoring and carries the risk of increased nephrotoxicity.

Of important note, daptomycin probably results in the greatest killing of MRSA in all cavities of the body except for the lungs, where the surfactant has been found to inactivate it. Accordingly, daptomycin is contraindicated in pneumonia.

Patients who receive early and appropriate therapy have better survival than those who receive inappropriate antibiotics. This emphasizes the need to obtain cultures early, preferably before starting therapy, and with a technique such as bronchoalveolar lavage or protected brush specimen. Duration of therapy should be for a period of seven to ten days (also refer Volume 2, Chapters 48 and 53) (72).

Aspiration Pneumonia

Aspiration and subsequent aspiration pneumonia are common in patients who have experienced multiple trauma (73). Aspiration can occur in the field, especially during a period of decreased level of consciousness, or during emergent intubation, either in the field or on arrival to the trauma unit, or following extubation in debilitated patients. In some cases, the aspirated material contains stomach contents, including previously eaten food remnants. In addition, it may contain hydrochloric acid and digestive proteolytic enzymes which can both cause an inflammatory chemical pneumonitis. In addition to gastric contents, the patient can aspirate the bacterial flora residing in the buccal cavity. The organisms that cause disease are predominately microaerophilic streptococci and oral anaerobes; most of these bacteria live in the gingival crevice. As a result, therapy should be directed against this set of organisms. Antianaerobic therapy may not be necessary in edentulous patients. As they lack a gingival crevice, they have a much diminished anaerobic microbial burden in the mouth.

Penicillin had been the mainstay of treatment for aspiration pneumonia, and can be effective as a single therapy, but clindamycin has resulted in slightly better outcomes and fewer relapses (73). Ceftriaxone also has antianaerobic activity and provides a more than adequate coverage as a single agent. Combination therapy with ceftriaxone and clindamycin, though common, has not been demonstrated to be more effective than either drug alone. Quinolones with antianaerobic activity, such as moxifloxacin, are also effective. Metronidazole is also effective against oral anaerobes; as it has no activity against aerobic Gram-negative or Gram-positive bacteria, it must be combined with another agent (e.g., cefazolin or ceftriaxone) that is active against those organisms.

Invasive Line Sepsis

Infections associated with peripheral intravenous catheters can cause cellulitis, thromboplebitis and, if untreated, severe infections. When extremity infections are becoming severe, lymphangitis and lymphadenitis are typically present, and should be specifically assessed for. If these signs of advancing local infections are present, systemic manifestations (fever and leukocytosis) are common, and generally represent strong corroborative evidence for the source of infection. As discussed earlier, the extremities should be closely examined in the fever work-up. If a source is found, the offending catheter should be removed and antibiotics started.

Central venous catheters are a considerable source of morbidity and mortality in ICU patients (Volume 2, Chapter 49). ☞ **Seventy percent of nosocomial blood stream infections occur in patients with central venous catheters.** ☞ As these catheters pierce the skin to enter the vasculature, the skin break itself is the usual portal of entry for microorganisms. However, there is not always a good correlation between cultures of the skin site and cultures from the catheter tip. Studies have demonstrated that the catheter hub lumen is also a common source of contamination (74,75).

The predominant organisms associated with vascular catheter infections are skin flora. Indeed, coagulase-negative staphylococci and *S. aureus* comprise 90% of all isolates from both peripheral and central line infections. The coagulase-negative staphylococci secrete biofilms that allow the bacteria to survive in sites that are protected from host defenses and antibiotics; biofilms containing other species have also been described. Gram-negative rods such as *Escherichia coli* and other Enterobacteriaceae are the third most common group of infecting microbes. *Candida* spp., which was uncommon in previous decades, has become the fourth most common organism in line-related infections, and is becoming an increasing problem in critically ill patients.

Infections can also be caused by contamination of the infusate and any intravenous fluid can potentially become contaminated. The most notable of these are infections with lipid-dependent yeasts like *Malassezia furfur* and *Candida parapsilosis*, which are associated with contaminated lipid emulsions in total parenteral nutrition (TPN).

Determining whether a central venous catheter is infected is not always straightforward. Data exists to support the use of semiquantitative cultures of the catheter tips (76), the differential time to culture positivity in blood samples drawn from the central lines and from peripheral sites (77), and the use of quantitative blood cultures (78). A recent meta-analysis suggests that quantitative cultures, comparing colony forming units per milliliter of blood in central line and peripheral blood samples, have the best sensitivity and specificity (78).

As Gram-positive cocci are the largest group of infecting microbes, empiric treatment should target staphylococci. The vast majority of coagulase-negative staphylococci are methicillin-resistant (MRSAE), and because of the increasing prevalence of MRSA, vancomycin should be used as initial empiric therapy. Daptomycin, linezolid, and quinupristin/dalfopristin and, perhaps, tigecycline are alternative initial empiric choices. If the organisms are methicillin-sensitive, first-generation cephalosporins or antistaphylococcal penicillins are therapy of choice.

When Gram-negative line-associated bacteremia is a possibility, or is associated with greatly increased mortality (e.g., a neutropenic patient), therapy should include an antipseudomonal beta-lactam/beta-lactamase inhibitor, carbapenem, or cephalosporin, possibly in combination with an aminoglycoside. If a patient remains febrile for several days after initiating broad antibacterial treatment, the practitioner should consider the possibility of line-associated candidemia.

Removal of infected central venous catheters is generally mandatory, especially with *S. aureus*, Gram-negative bacilli, and *Candida* spp. Successful short-term salvage of lines is possible with coagulase-negative staphylococci, but recurrences of bacteremia are nearly universal, making this an unattractive option.

Wound Infection

✒ Surgical wound infections should be considered in all critically ill trauma patients, and postoperative surgical patients with fever, especially when beginning >48–72 hours following surgery or trauma. ✒ Although wound infections rarely develop prior to this period, dressing should be taken down and wounds examined to rule out necrotizing soft tissue infections (discussed next). Infected surgical wounds manifest all the cardinal signs of inflammation, *rubor, color, dolor, tumor,* and *functio laesa* (redness, heat, pain, swelling, and loss of function), as were known since the times of Hippocrates and Galen. In addition, infected wounds will usually be associated with a discharge of infected fluid or pus. Occasionally, no discharge is present when the infection is deep, and the skin site still closed. Whenever wound infection is diagnosed, the wound should be opened to express the purulent material and the patient should go to the OR for complete incision and drainage. Appropriate antibiotics are also administered.

Necrotizing Soft Tissue Infections

In contrast to a simple cellulitis which only involves the cutaneous layers of the skin, necrotizing soft tissue infections rapidly spread, often along the deep fascia with secondary necrosis of the fascia, subcutaneous tissues, and occasionally muscles (79). The presence of gas-forming organisms classically results in subcutaneous air in the tissues that may be palpated on physical examination or seen radiographically, on plain films or by CT scan (though these signs are often absent). Because the infection spreads along the deep fascial

planes and the overlying skin is less involved, the extent of the infection is often underappreciated with regards to its severity and lethality. Thus, a high index of suspicion is necessary to make the diagnosis and promptly initiate therapy.

The bacteria associated with necrotizing fasciitis produce toxins including cytolysins and sphingomyelinases, which destroy tissue and allow rapid progression along tissue planes. The fascial necrosis is followed by thrombosis of the arterioles that bridge the space between the skin and the fascial layer, causing loss of blood flow and oxygen to the skin, resulting in death of the overlying skin. Necrotizing soft tissue infections are fully discussed in Volume 1, Chapter 29 (extremity trauma) only the salient points are provided here. Soft tissue infections are often associated with a paucity of inflammatory cells, which presumably are killed by the bacterial hemolysins. The inability to deliver antibiotics to the involved areas of muscle fascia and the overlying skin make cure with antimicrobials alone futile, and surgical resection (usually wide and extensive) is the only effective therapy.

Necrotizing soft tissue infections can occur following trauma (especially involving puncture wounds, and following IV drug abuse), but can also occur following surgery contaminated with organisms that flourish in the relatively anaerobic environment of the surgical wound, or deep fascial planes. It is more common in situations involving unrecognized foreign bodies, delayed presentation to medical care, and in patients with immunosuppressive conditions (e.g., diabetes, alcoholism, peripheral vascular disease, HIV, neutropenia, renal failure, and so on).

Classically, necrotizing soft tissue infections are associated with anaerobic organisms, specifically *Clostridia* spp. and particularly *Clostridium perfringens*, the organism most commonly associated with gas gangrene, especially from battlefield wounds. *Streptococcus* spp. are the second most common group of organisms isolated from wounds (79). *Staphylococcus aureus* or facultative aerobic Gram-negative rods like *E. coli* are rarely isolated as the single etiologies of necrotizing fasciitis, but are often found in combination with other organisms and may be facultative in some mixed infections (79,80).

Mixed synergistic necrotizing fasciitis can involve a combination of bacteria, including anaerobic pathogens such as *Bacteroides, Clostridium, Peptostreptococcus* as well as enteric Gram-negative rods like *E. coli, Proteus, Serratia, Enterobacter,* and *Klebsiella. Pseudomonas* is also occasionally seen. Mixed infections usually arise from the traumatic implantation of foreign material (e.g., oral flora in a drug addict's needle) or in proximity to the bowel.

Swabbing of deep wounds, as apposed to superficial wounds, followed by immediate Gram stain can provide a presumptive microbiologic diagnosis, which can be used to guide empiric therapy, but operative debridement is the most important factor.

The selection of empiric antimicrobials will also depend on anatomic location, mechanism of infection, and Gram stain results. High-dose penicillin in combination with clindamycin is appropriate (unless *Bacteroides fragilis* is presumed or documented). Aggressive fluid repletion and immediate wide surgical debridement is mandatory to save the life of an individual with established necrotizing fasciitis caused by clostridial spp. and by beta-hemolytic streptococci.

Infections with *S. aureus* alone are an unusual cause of necrotizing fasciitis although there are a few case reports describing this (80,81). When *S. aureus* is the etiologic organism, treatment with vancomycin or an antistaphylococcal penicillin or cephalosporin is indicated. Because of the high prevalence of MRSA (in many hospitals it is above 50%), vancomycin should be part of the initial antibiotic treatment. In cases of mixed synergistic infection, appropriate coverage for facultative aerobic Gram-negative rods and obligate anaerobes will include a carbapenem, a beta-lactam/beta-lactamase inhibitor, or a third- or fourth-generation cephalosporin in combination with metronidazole.

As many of the manifestations of necrotizing soft tissue infection are toxin-mediated, clindamycin should be used in conjunction with other antibiotics because, as a protein synthesis inhibitor, it shuts down further production of toxins; it is also active in situations of high bacterial density (i.e., in wounds) where beta-lactams and vancomycin may not be—a phenomenon known as the "Eagle Effect" (82). As an adjunctive measure, hyperbaric oxygen (Volume 2, Chapter 73) has been shown to be effective in delaying or stopping progression of the affected areas in necrotizing fasciitis (83), but operative debridement should occur first.

Interestingly, a high proportion of community-acquired MRSA (CA-MRSA) strains (nearly 100%) express a unique hemolysin, the Panton-Valentine leukocidin (PVL), which contributes to virulence by causing lysis of WBCs, specifically PMNs, thereby crippling the immune response. Typically, only about 2% of *S. aureus* express this toxin. In addition, PVL also affects cells other than WBCs and causes separation of tissue layers, contributing to the spread of the infection in the host. Vancomycin is the antimicrobial of choice against these infections, but newer antibiotics such as daptomycin, linezolid, and tigecycline are also effective. Rifampin, in combination with vancomycin, can provide synergistic antibacterial action.

Orthopedic Fracture Infections and Prophylaxis

Open orthopedic fractures constitute a surgical emergency, and are prone to infections. Accordingly, these patients should receive antibiotic prophylaxis. The most common system used to classify orthopedic fractures and the associated risk of infection are those that have been modified from that of Gustilo and Anderson (83).

This system divides fractures into three grades and further subdivides grade 3 fractures, the most severe fracture, into three subtypes. All grades can become infected, but the prevalence of infection is higher with more severe injury.

Grade 1 fractures are usually simple transverse or oblique fractures that result from low-energy injuries with skin wounds less than 1 cm in length. Grade 2 fractures result from an injury with more energy absorption and cause some degree of comminution and moderate crushing component along with a skin wound that is larger than 1 cm. Grade 3 injuries are usually the result of significant mechanical injury, such as gunshot wound, motor vehicle injuries, especially motorcycle injuries, and other traumatic injuries. These injuries usually have extensive soft tissue damage, severe comminution, and large areas of denuded skin. These wounds are likely to be contaminated with external debris, like soil, from the site of the accident. Grade 3A injuries generally do not require extensive reconstructive surgery to provide skin coverage to the injured site. Grade 3B injuries, on the other hand, have more extensive soft tissue and periosteal injury and require major reconstructive plastic surgery to provide a flap for cutaneous coverage.

Grade 3C fractures are associated with vascular compromise and may necessitate vascular reconstruction.

The key therapeutic principles in treating actual or potentially infected fractures are extensive and include: adequate debridement of all infected and necrotic tissue, removal of foreign bodies, copious irrigation of the wound, management of dead space and coverage of exposed bone with appropriate flaps, and minimizing the time to operation (84). Prophylactic antibiotics are adjunctive in the sense that they decrease the incidence of wound infection and osteomyelitis, but do not entirely prevent all infections.

A large meta-analysis and Cochrane review demonstrated that single-dose antibiotic prophylaxis significantly decreased superficial and deep wound infections by about 60% (85). Prolonged treatment did not yield a better outcome than single-dose prophylaxis. In a similar meta-analysis, the data also supports the efficacy of prophylactic antibiotics in preventing infections in patients with open fractures (86). Most infections are caused by skin flora, primarily by coagulase-negative staphylococci and *S. aureus*, but aerobic Gram-negative rods and soil anaerobes are increasingly frequent with more traumatic, open fractures.

In general, first-generation cephalosporins, antistaphylococcal penicillins, and vancomycin are effective prophylactic antibiotics for closed fractures and grades 1 and 2 fractures. For grade 3 fractures, aminoglycosides and clindamycin are useful additions (Volume 2, Chapter 53). ✄ **Despite antibiotic prophylaxis, patients with open fractures and fever should have their wounds examined for infections, and if present, incision and drainage should be performed.** ✄

Abdominal Infections: Following Trauma/Surgery with Colonic Contamination

Abscesses following abdominal trauma result from injuries to the bowel and spillage of intestinal contents into the peritoneal cavity. In blunt trauma, the organisms that cause disease derive from the normal commensal flora. In penetrating trauma (e.g., gunshot wounds or shrapnel), additional organisms can be directly implanted at the time of injury. In addition, when a projectile travels through soiled clothing before it penetrates the victim, it carries the environmental flora living on the clothing that enters the wound.

The most common classes of organisms causing abdominal infections in previously healthy trauma victims are enterococci, Gram-negative enteric organisms, and intestinal anaerobes. The types of organisms that predominate in a particular patient also depend on which portion of the intestine is injured. A stomach injury can cause gross contamination following a large meal, or may release essentially sterile contents if injured between meals after prior contents have been bathed in hydrochloric acid and proteolytic enzymes. *Candida albicans* is usually a component of the mouth; it is present normally in the esophagus and often survives in the stomach because it is moderately acid-tolerant. If the patient is taking medications that decrease the gastric pH, that is, antacids, H_2-blockers, or proton pump inhibitors, oral flora, particularly oral anaerobes, and streptococci may colonize the stomach.

The small intestine is normally colonized with facultative anaerobic Enterobacteriaceae, like *E. coli*, and enterococcal spp. In biliary trauma, the same organisms will most likely be involved; the presence of anaerobes is unusual. As one progresses distally along the bowel, one finds an increasing proportion of anaerobic bacteria, such as *Bacteroides*, *Prevotella*, and *Peptostreptococci*. In the colon, greater than 99.99% of the bacteria are anaerobic.

The Surgical Infection Society and the IDSA have recently published guidelines for treating intra-abdominal infections (87,88). In general, regimens that treat enterococcal spp. have no better outcomes than those that do not. This is because of the relative avirulence of the enterococci, especially in nonimmunocompromised individuals. Similarly, although *Pseudomonas* can be an intestinal colonizer, especially in children, it is not necessary to use antibiotics effective against *Pseudomonas* in an empiric fashion for intra-abdominal infections. In the past, studies showed that second-generation anaerobic cephalosporins, like cefoxitin, were as effective as monotherapy. However, there has been a steady increase in the number of *B. fragilis* group organisms that are resistant to these agents. Accordingly, cefoxitin should no longer be used alone for empiric treatment of intra-abdominal infections. Adding metronidazole to both second- and third-generation cephalosporins is now necessary to provide adequate treatment for *B. fragilis*. The newer fluoroquinolones (e.g., moxifloxacin and gatifloxacin) possess intrinsic activity against intestinal anaerobes; however, the prevalence of fluoroquinolone-resistant *Bacteroides* has increased to >50% in some countries. Accordingly, abdominal infection treatment with fluoroquinolones should occur only in combination with metronidazole (88). Metronidazole remains the backbone of treatment regimens for intra-abdominal sepsis. Additionally, monotherapy with either carbapenems or beta-lactams/beta-lactamase inhibitors is an attractive alternative strategy because of simplicity. Of note, none of these therapies adequately treats MRSA, but MRSA is not generally a cause of intra-abdominal infection in previously healthy individuals. If the patient is at high risk for MRSA, for example, in an SICU after a surgical procedure, then vancomycin or other drugs effective against MRSA should be used. If the presence of vancomycins resistant enterococcus, vancomycin intermediate sensitivity. *Staphyloccus aureus*, or vancomycin resistant *Staphylococcus aureus* complicates an abdominal infection, then linezolid, daptomycin, tigecycline, or dalfopristin/quinupristin should be used.

Isolation of fungi from intraoperative peritoneal cultures is increasingly common (89), especially in patients with renal failure who are being treated with chronic ambulatory peritoneal dialysis (CAPD). *Candida* spp. cause the vast majority of fungal peritoneal infections as it is a normal constituent of the gastrointestinal (GI) flora, but other fungi such as *Aspergillus* spp. and zygomycetes (e.g., mucor) have also been reported in association with CAPD catheter infections. Most of the candidal isolates are fluconazole-susceptible *C. albicans*, but the use of fluconazole as prophylaxis is changing the epidemiology of candidal infections so that fluconazole-resistant *Candida* spp. are causing a greater proportion of invasive candidiasis. For patients who have not received prophylactic azoles, fluconazole is an effective empiric treatment in most cases. If the patient has received prophylaxis, then voriconazole, an echinocandin (caspofungin, micafungin, anidulafungin) or amphotericin should be used. Antibiotic treatment is an adjunct to and not a replacement for proper surgical drainage of abscess collections.

Sinusitis

Sinusitis can occur in critically ill trauma patients with tubes or packing in their noses, or those who have sustained nasal trauma prior to admission (90). The paranasal sinuses are four paired structures with drainage ostea in the nose. The sinuses are lined with ciliated pseudostratified columnar epithelium. The cilia of the sinus mucosa propel secretions, bacteria, and foreign material toward their ostea in the nose. When the ostea becomes obstructed because of foreign bodies (tubes/packing) or swelling (direct trauma), the bacteria are not cleared and begin to proliferate, causing a clinical sinusitis infection (90).

Common bacteria involved in nosocomial sinusitis are quite different from those of community-acquired (91). In most reports, the etiology is usually polymicrobial with about one-third being Gram-positive and two-thirds Gram-negative organisms. *Staphylococcus aureus* is by far the predominant Gram-positive organism and *Pseudomonas* spp. are the leading Gram-negative organisms. While highly resistant organisms, such as MRSA, VRE, and *Acinetobacter* spp. have not been reported in this disease; with their increasingly important roles in nosocomial infections these organisms must be considered when selecting antibiotics for treatment.

Diagnosis includes, fever, purulent nasal discharge, tenderness to percussion over the sinus (often notable in sedated or obtunded critically ill patients). Further clinical features, diagnostic work-up (including use of nasal endoscopy and imaging studies), and treatment recommendations are provided in Volume 2, Chapter 51 (90,91).

Urosepsis

Urinary tract infections (UTI) are the most common nosocomial infection in the United States (causing about a third of the infections in hospitals and nursing homes) (92). However, UTI is an infrequent cause of fever or sepsis following trauma and critical care. Almost all UTIs occurring in critical care are associated with instrumentation of the bladder.

In the normal, uncatheterized bladder, several mechanisms allow for clearing uropathogens from the urinary tract. These include: Tamm-Horsfall protein, glycosaminoglycans, and an intact bladder mucosa. Micturition alone will remove 99.9% of all microbes that enter the bladder. A catheter overcomes these protective mechanisms by providing a direct conduit to the bladder from outside; the presence of a foreign object can also irritate and disrupt the uroepithelial mucosa. Once a catheter is in place, microbes can enter the bladder either extra- or intraluminally. Estimates are that about one-quarter of urinary tract colonization is intraluminal with the remaining occurring extraluminally (i.e., between the urethral epithelium and the catheter). Some uropathogens, such as *E. coli* K1, have specialized fimbriae that allow attachment to uroepithelial cells. Additionally, the presence of a glycocalyx or biofilm along the catheter surface can allow colonization and persistence of bacteria in the presence of both host immune effectors and antibiotics (93).

Risk factors for catheter-associated bacteriuria or funguria include: (*i*) the length of catheterization, (*ii*) absence of a urinometer or drip chamber, (*iii*) colonization of the drainage bag, (*iv*) diabetes, (*v*) abnormal renal function, and (*vi*) breaks in proper catheter care (92). If bacteria or yeast are in the urine cultures of an afebrile patient, the first step in management is to change the catheter and repeat the urinalysis and culture.

Dysuria, suprapubic pain and tenderness, back pain and costovertebral angle tenderness may be clinical clues to a diagnosis in a cognitively aware patient. However, assessment of these signs and symptoms in an SICU setting is difficult in sedated patients and in those with altered mental status. Fever is the most common sign. On occasion, physical exam is useful when one finds an enlarged epididymis on the testis or a soft, mushy prostate, but diagnosis usually is dependent on the results of urinalysis and urine culture.

The majority of microbes that colonize the urinary tract are the host's resident flora, usually deriving from the GI tract. These are predominantly facultative anaerobic enteric Gram-negative rods, Pseudomonads, *Enterococci*, and *Candida* spp. Truly anaerobic colonic bacteria rarely cause UTIs in the absence of a direct connection from the urinary tract to the GI tract, as in the case of an enterovesicular fistula. The most common organisms are Gram-negative rods (94–96).

Aminoglycosides are an attractive first choice because they are excreted renally and are concentrated in the urine; bactericidal levels of drug can be present for days after even a single dose. Third-generation cephalosporins and quinolones are second-line options. Carbapenems can be used for multidrug-resistant organisms. Enterococcal spp. are generally sensitive to ampicillin and vancomycin and should be used first. Approximately 30% of a linezolid dose is excreted into the urine unchanged and can be used to treat vancomycin-resistant organisms. Daptomycin, active against VRE is 80% renally excreted and is an alternative choice. *Candida* spp. also can cause UTIs and are an increasingly common problem. Fluconazole is the only antifungal drug that achieves significant levels in the urine and is, therefore, the drug of choice to treat candiduria. The echinocandins and voriconazole do achieve measurable amounts in the kidney parenchyma, but only about 3% of either drug is excreted into the urine itself. Changing the catheter is the first step in managing candiduria and may, by itself, be therapeutic. Alternatively, amphotericin B bladder washes can also be effective (97).

Postsplenectomy Sepsis and Prophylaxis

Asplenic patients are at higher risk for bacteremia and fulminant septic shock, known as overwhelming postsplenectomy sepsis (OPSS) (98). Asplenic patients include not only post-splenectomy patients but also those individuals who are functionally asplenic, such as those with sickle-cell anemia (owing to repetitive infarct-mediated autosplenectomy), infiltrative disorders with splenomegaly (e.g., myelodysplastias), or deficiencies in the terminal components of the complement (99). The microorganisms that cause these syndromes are usually those with polysaccharide capsules that resist phagocytosis by PMNs and macrophages unless they are bound by anticapsular antibody or compliment (i.e., opsonized). The most common organisms include *Streptococcus pneumoniae*, *Haemophilus influenzae*, and *Neisseria meningitides*. Of these, the pneumococcus is the most common organism causing OPSS, having a case-fatality rate as high as 60%. Vaccines exist against all of these species, and their use is recommended (as described in Volume 2, Chapter 52 (100).

Many hyposplenic individuals will also have received prophylactic antibiotics, usually penicillin, either orally or sometimes in monthly injections. In many cases, they will have prescriptions for another class of antibiotics, like fluoroquinolones. ☞ **Postsplenectomy patients should be instructed to keep antiencapsulated bacteria antibiotics readily available, to take them at the onset of an acute, febrile illness, and to also seek medical evaluation at that time.** ☞ When these patients are sick enough to be admitted to the SICU, therapy should be directed against the most likely organisms; third-generation cephalosporins or quinolones are drugs of choice. Postsplenectomized trauma patients should also be given a card and med-alert bracelet declaring their condition.

Meningococcemia

The term meningococcemia is used here to describe the fulminant septic disease complicated by hemorrhage, purpura, and thrombosis-associated tissue infarcts (often involving distal extremity) (101).

The typical patient presents with fever, generalized weakness and malaise, headache, skin rashes, and the abrupt onset of hypotension and sepsis requiring admission in the SICU or burn unit. A number of authors have described a prominent rubella-like maculopapular rash, which is initially painless, nonpruritic, and temporary. Most commonly, the initial rash consists of 1–2-mm petechial lesions that are usually seen on the trunk and lower extremities, but may occur in places like the palpebral conjunctiva or the buccal mucosa. Often the rash is prominent under belts or on areas that are subject to pressure. Gradually, the petechiae enlarge and coalesce to form larger ecchymotic lesions. The petechial bleeding is a result of thrombocytopenia. The rapid evolution from petechiae to large ecchymotic lesions is known as purpura fulminans. ☞ **The pathophysiology of fulminant meningococcemia results from sepsis, vascular collapse, shock, disseminated intravascular coagulation (DIC), and tissue infarcts (101).** ☞

Some manifestations of purpura fulminans result from damage to the vascular endothelium and protein C levels are decreased, participating in the debilitating microvascular infarcts of digits and extremities. Accordingly, some have hypothesized that the use of activated protein C (APC) might improve the outcome (102). Although, the number of patients studied in prospective randomized controlled trials (RCTs) with APC is low, the available series suggest that APC does provide benefit. If APC is employed, it should be administered early and judiciously because of the increased risk of bleeding associated with it's use (103; refer to Volume 2, Chapters 47 and 63).

Meningitis

There are a myriad of causes of infective meningitis. Organisms of all classes, including viruses, typical bacteria, mycobacteria, spirochetes, Rickettsial spp., fungi and sometimes parasites, including protozoa and helminths, have all been described as causes of meningitis (104). Meningitis can also follow trauma by direct implantation of foreign matter and can occur as a complication of therapeutic and diagnostic intracranial devices (e.g., ventriculostomy).

Correct management of meningitis requires establishing an etiologic diagnosis. The use of CT scan or magnetic resonance imaging may show diffuse meningeal enhancement, but this is not specific for any particular organism (104).

The key procedure for establishing a diagnosis of meningitis is sampling of the CSF. Examination of the CSF should include assays for glucose, total protein, differential cell counts, and Gram stain and routine culture (104). If appropriate, there are stains for fungi (e.g., India ink for *Cryptococcus neoformans*) and mycobacteria. Latex agglutination assays are routinely available to detect the capsular polysaccharides of *Cryptococcus*, *Hemophilus* type B., the *Meningococcus*, and the pneumococcus in CSF. Advances in molecular biology-based techniques, such as polymerase chain reaction are now available for the diagnosis of enterovirus, cytomegalovirus (CMV), Epstein-Barr virus (EBV), herpes simplex viruses (HSV), and others.

The *Pneumococcus*, the *Meningococcus*, enteroviruses, and herpes simplex virus are the most common causes of meningitis in immunologically normal hosts (104). Selected hosts have an increased predisposition to infections with other organisms, such as *Cryptococcus neoformans* in AIDS patients, and other immunocompromised patients and *Listeria monocytogenes* in pregnancy (104). In trauma patients with CNS shunts or ICP monitoring devices, the most common organisms are *Staphylococci* (implicated in ~80% of shunt infections). Gram-negative aerobic bacilli comprise the great bulk of the remainder of the causes. True anaerobes comprise only a small percentage of the remainder of organisms; if they are present, especially in patients with ventriculoperitoneal shunts, it is strongly suggestive of intestinal perforation at the abdominal end of the shunt with ascending infection.

Empiric therapy should be directed against the most likely causative organism. Identification of a specific pathogen allows de-escalation to a specifically targeted regimen. The ability of an individual antibiotic to cross the BBB is a primary determinant for the outcome (104).

Most antibiotics do not cross the BBB in the absence of inflammation. With inflammation, the levels of drugs like penicillin and ceftriaxone increase markedly, but higher doses are still a requirement to exceed the minimum inhibitory concentrations of most pathogens. For acute bacterial meningitis, ceftriaxone at a dose of 2 g IV every 12 hours provides adequate therapy for the *H. influenzae*, the *Meningococcus*, and penicillin-sensitive pneumococci. In hospitals with a high prevalence of penicillin-resistant *S. pneumoniae*, most authorities recommend the addition of vancomycin to the regimen. Corticosteroids are useful therapeutic adjuncts in cases of meningitis caused by *S. pneumoniae*, *H. influenzae*, and *Mycobacterium tuberculosis* (105–107).

For patients with infected intracranial devices, targeted therapy based on initial Gram stain is the best. As most organisms are nosocomially acquired and drug-resistant, vancomycin is the initial drug of choice. However, vancomycin does not penetrate BBB well. As drug levels may be subtherapeutic even in the presence of inflammation, intrathecal administration of vancomycin may be the preferred route.

If the organisms are methicillin-sensitive, it is wise to switch to antistaphylococcal penicillin; rifampin may be a useful synergistic agent in the presence of prosthetic material. Aminoglycosides, colistin, and amphotericin can also be administered intrathecally.

For Gram-negative bacteria, ceftazidime and meropenem achieve therapeutic levels of drug in the CSF. Shunt removal is usually necessary for cure of the infection. The most efficacious strategy seems to be externalization of the shunt, treatment with antibiotics, and replacement of the shunt after an adequate duration of therapy. Duration of antibiotic administration depends on the infecting organisms; *S. aureus* may need 10 days of therapy before replacement of the shunt. Gram-negative organisms may require 14–21 days of therapy (104).

TREATMENT OF FEVER

✍ **In the absence of traumatic brain injury (TBI) or other CNS injury, temperature elevation between 37°C and 39.5°C may be beneficial.** ✍ Side effects of fever including tachycardia and increased ICP will benefit from lowering

body temperature. In the conscious patient, fever is usually associated with malaise, headache, myalgias, and/or arthralgias. In such patients, symptomatic relief may be obtained by reducing the fever.

The most extensively studied and utilized method of reducing temperature is to reset the thermostat downward and let the body correct the temperature. This approach employs drugs classified as antipyretics, such as aspirin and ibuprofen. Other options to lower temperature require either reducing heat production or increasing the rate of heat loss. Heat production can be lowered somewhat by reducing or eliminating skeletal muscle activity, reducing pain, and anxiety, and so on. Increasing heat loss can be accomplished by sponging with cool liquid, cold baths, cooling blankets, fans, or ice packs. Each of these techniques has pros and cons.

Antipyretic Drug Therapy

Antipyretic agents can be classified into three types: the largest class includes aspirin, ibuprofen, and other nonsteroidal anti-inflammatory drugs (NSAIDs); while corticosteroids and acetaminophen are each in a class by themselves (108). The NSAIDs are inhibitors of both central and peripheral COX. Acetaminophen decreases the production of prostaglandins in the brain but does not inhibit COX at peripheral sites. Corticosteroids are thought to interfere with fever by blocking transcription of IL-1 and by inhibiting phospholipase A_2 (108). Without a doubt, the high fevers seen in heat stroke, MH, and NMS ($\geq 42°C$.) are inherently damaging to tissues, but these temperatures are unresponsive to antipyretics. Regulated fevers such as seen with inflammatory processes rarely exceed 41°C (109). However, specific subgroups benefit from antipyretic therapy, including those with CNS pathology and critically ill patients with cardiopulmonary dysfunction (limiting oxygen delivery).

Both animal and human studies of brain injury indicate that fever is common and associated with a worse prognosis (110). However, the use of antipyretic drugs to lower temperature has not been shown to reduce brain injury and is not always effective (111,112). Regarding the safety of NSAIDs in TBI patients, hypotension with reduced CPP, along with nephrotoxicity and oliguria, have been reported (113). Acetaminophen is comparable with NSAIDs in its ability to reduce temperature in TBI patients. Although corticosteroids have been studied in TBI (and found to be efficacious), there are little or no data on their use specifically as an antipyretic. Clinical studies demonstrate a positive correlation between ICP and brain temperature (114). Simultaneous measurement of core and brain temperature demonstrated that in some patients core temperature significantly underestimated brain temperature, suggesting that if antipyretic therapy is to be utilized in patients with brain injury it may be more effective if based on brain temperature (114). ✍ **The administration of antipyretics to ICU patients in an effort to reduce fever is common practice, but data proving a benefit to this practice is lacking.** ✍ Very few studies have addressed the use of antipyretics such as acetaminophen in the ICU patients. The data available suggests only a limited efficacy for antipyretics in critically ill patients (115). The risks of GI bleeding, acute renal failure, platelet dysfunction, and the like should be considered when reducing fever to decrease metabolic demand, or ICP.

External Cooling Techniques

External cooling reduces body temperature by increasing heat loss but does not change the TRSP. Therefore, the hypothalamus sends out feedback stimulation to return core temperature to the TRSP via means such as shivering and vasoconstriction. The net effect can more than offset the gains made by lowering temperature. Accordingly, when external cooling techniques are employed, sedatives and analgesics (which decrease the TRSP) should be used.

Although several single institution trials of hypothermia have shown it to be advantageous in brain-injured patients (116), a larger, prospective, randomized multicenter trial failed to demonstrate such a benefit to hypothermia (117). This negative trial has not eliminated the use of hypothermia to treat brain injury. ☞ **Antipyretics are usually the initial treatment for a febrile ICU patient because they are convenient and well tolerated by patients, but external cooling has generally been more successful at lowering core temperature (115).** ☞

External cooling is widely employed for all patient types in critical care units, sometimes by nursing personnel without physician participation in the decision. External cooling in the absence of sedation and/or neuromuscular blockade often results in shivering and increased peripheral vasoconstriction, making it ineffective at lowering temperature. But, if adequate sedation analgesia and/or muscle relaxants are employed, metabolic demands, cardiac output, and heart rate can all be reduced (118). Frequent monitoring of core temperature is required during external cooling to achieve appropriate temperature goals.

EYE TO THE FUTURE

A number of fundamental questions regarding fever remain unanswered. Of greatest importance to the clinician is whether fever should be treated or not. A major difficulty in answering this question is the difficulty in maintaining close control of the temperature. Failure to eliminate the fever or overly aggressive efforts and hypothermia complicate the interpretation of the results. This is exemplified by studies in TBI patients in whom fever is known to be detrimental, and hypothermia is associated with its own set of complications. Future studies will need to ensure that cooling is initiated early enough, and continues long enough with greater CNS effect (i.e., case of cooling helmet) and use of sedatives and analgesics to drop temperature.

SUMMARY

Elevation in body temperature has been recognized as a significant diagnostic and therapeutic finding since the beginning of recorded medical history. The obvious diagnostic value of fever in the ICU patient is often complicated by the numerous confounding problems leading to expensive and sometimes excessive testing and the risks of inappropriate antibiotic therapy.

Both fever and infections are common complications in critically ill trauma patients. In this group, temperatures greater than 102°F have a high probability of being the result of an infection, and should be assumed infectious until proven otherwise. A short list of noninfectious causes of fever must also be ruled out in the setting of high fevers (MH, NMS, SS, and the like).

Despite a long history of experimental study, we still cannot say with certainty how we should respond therapeutically to the febrile patient. Only in cases of extreme temperature elevation, such as MH, NMS, or heat stroke, or in patients with acute TBI, or other brain injury, or limited cardiopulmonary reserve should temperature elevations be routinely treated. The optimal method of treating such temperature elevations remains uncertain.

KEY POINTS

☞ Fever is perhaps best defined as: "an elevation in core body temperature >1°C above the patient's thermoregulatory set point (TRSP)."

☞ In a joint statement of the Society of Critical Care Medicine (SCCM) (10) and the Infectious Disease Society of America (IDSA) (11), fever is defined as a temperature greater than or equal to 38.3°C (≥101°F).

☞ Fever is frequently seen in the initial 48 hours after trauma, burns or surgery; however, such fevers are usually noninfectious in origin.

☞ Although infection is unlikely in the first 48 hours following injury, Group A streptococcal infections and Clostridial myonecrosis represent uncommon but important exceptions which can present within this time period.

☞ If the temperature exceeds 38.9°C, the patient should be considered to have an infectious etiology until negative cultures demonstrate otherwise.

☞ The SS is usually associated with combinations of SSRIs with MAOIs, or MAOIs with TCAs (50,51).

☞ After stopping a drug responsible for fever, 48–72 hours are usually required for the temperature to fully normalize.

☞ Pancreatitis is one of the classic inflammatory conditions that can cause significant noninfectious fever, with signs similar to sepsis.

☞ Patients who have a vasodilated picture, suggestive of sepsis, but in whom sepsis is unlikely, may have adrenal insufficiency. Serum cortisol determination, a cosyntropin stimulation test or even empiric corticosteroid administration may be indicated.

☞ Most febrile reactions following transfusions are related to white blood cells (WBC), as leukocyte-depleted blood products have a low rate of this complication (64).

☞ Most investigators now recognize that atelectasis does not cause fever in the absence of infection.

☞ The most common infectious cause of fever in critically ill patients is ventilator-associated pneumonia (VAP).

☞ Seventy percent of nosocomial blood stream infections occur in patients with central venous catheters.

☞ Surgical wound infections should be considered in all critically ill trauma patients, and postoperative surgical patients with fever, especially when beginning >48–72 hours following surgery or trauma.

☞ Despite antibiotic prophylaxis, patients with open fractures and fever should have their wounds examined for infections, and if present, incision and drainage should be performed.

☞ Postsplenectomy patients should be instructed to keep antiencapsulated bacteria antibiotics readily available, to take them at the onset of an acute, febrile illness, and to also seek medical evaluation at that time.

☞ The pathophysiology of fulminant meningococcemia results from sepsis, vascular collapse, shock, disseminated intravascular coagulation (DIC), and tissue infarcts (101).

✒ In the absence of TBI or other CNS injury, temperature elevation between 37°C and 39.5°C may be beneficial.

✒ The administration of antipyretics to ICU patients in an effort to reduce fever is common practice but data proving a benefit to this practice is lacking.

✒ Antipyretics are usually the initial treatment for a febrile ICU patient because they are convenient and well tolerated by patients, but external cooling has generally been more successful at lowering core temperature (115).

REFERENCES

1. Kluger MJ. Protozoan thermoregulation. In: Kluger MJ, ed. Fever: Its Biology, Evolution and Function. Princeton, NJ: Princeton University Press, 1979:17–18.
2. Majno G. The Healing Hand. Cambridge, MA: Harvard University Press, 1975.
3. Majno G. Inflammation and infection: historic highlights. In: Majno G, Cofran R, Kaufman N, eds. Current Topics in Inflammation and Infection. Baltimore, MD: Williams and Wilkins, 1982.
4. Mackowiak PA. History of clinical thermometry. In: Mackowiak PA, ed. Fever: Basic Mechanisms and Management. 2nd ed. Philadelphia, PA: Lippincott-Raven Publishers, 1997:1–10.
5. Berger RL, Clem TR, Harden VA, Mangum BW. Historical development and newer means of temperature measurements in biochemistry. Methods Biochem Anal 1984; 30:269–331.
6. Bolton HC. Evolution of the thermometer 1592–1743. Easton, PA: Chemical Publishing, 1900.
7. Wunderlich CA. Das Verhalten der Eigenwarme in Krankenheiten. Leipzig: Otto Wigard, 1868.
8. Oldach DW, Borza EN, Benitez RM. A mysterious death. NEJM 1998; 338:1764–1769.
9. Whitrow M. Wagner-Jauregg and fever therapy. Med History 1990; 34:294–310.
10. O'Grady NP, Barie PS, Bartlett JG et al. Practice guidelines for evaluating new fever in critically ill adult patients. Crit Care Med 1998; 26(2):392–407.
11. O'Grady NP, Barie PS, Bartlett JG et al. Practice guidelines for evaluating new fever in critically ill adult patients. Clin Inf Dis 1998; 26:1042–1059.
12. Liebermeister C. Vorlesungen uber specielle pathologie und therapie. Leipzig: Verlag von F.C.W. Vogel, 1887.
13. Sessler DI. Temperature monitoring. In: Miller RD, ed. Anesthesia. 6th ed. New York: Churchill Livingstone, 2005:1571–1597.
14. Bernheim HA, Block LH, Atkins E. Fever: pathogenesis, pathophysiology and purpose. Ann Int Med 1979; 91:261–270.
15. Boulant JA. Thermoregulation. In: Mackowiak PA, ed. Fever: Basic Mechanisms and Management. 2nd ed. Philadelphia, PA: Lippincott-Raven Publishers, 1997:35–58.
16. Hammel HT, Jackson DC, Stolwijk JAJ, Hardy JD et al. Temperature regulation by hypothalamic proportional control with an adjustable set point. J Appl Physiol 1963; 18:1146–1154.
17. Kluger MJ. Regulation of body temperature in the vertebrates. In: Kluger MJ, ed. Fever: Its Biology, Evolution and Function. Princeton, NJ: Princeton University Press, 1979:3–50.
18. Dinarello CA, Wolff SM. Pathogenesis of fever in man. NEJM 1978; 298:607–612.
19. Mackowiak PA. Concepts of fever. Arch Intern Med 1998; 158:1870–1881.
20. Steiner AA, Rudaya AY, Robbins JR et al. Expanding the febrigenic role of cyclo oxygenase-2 to the previously overlooked responses. Am J Physiol Regul Integr Comp Physiol 2005; 289:R1253–R1257.
21. Székely M, Balaskó M, Kulchitsky VA et al. Multiple neural mechanisms of fever. Auton Neurosci 2000; 85:78–82.
22. Bryant RE, DesPrez RM, VanWay MH, Rogers DE. Studies on human leukocyte motility. I. Effects of alterations in pH, electrolyte concentration and phagocytosis on leukocytosis migration, adhesiveness, and aggregation. J Exp Med 1966; 124:483–499.
23. van Oss CJ, Absolom DR, Moore LL, Park BH et al. Effect of temperature on the chemotaxis, phagocytic engulfment, digestion and O_2 consumption of human polymorphonuclear leukocytes. J Reticuloendothel Soc 1980; 27:561–565.
24. Sebag J, Reed WP, Williams RC. Effect of temperature on bacterial killing by serum and by polymorphonuclear leukocytes. Infect Immun 1977; 16:947–954.
25. Bruggen IV, Robertson TA, Papadimitriou JM. The effect of mild hyperthermia on the morphology and function of murine resident peritoneal macrophages. Exp Mol Pathol 1991; 55:119–134.
26. Hasday JD. The influence of temperature on host defenses. In: Mackowiak PA, ed. Fever: Basic Mechanisms and Management. 2nd ed. Philadelphia, PA: Lippincott-Raven Publishers, 1997:177–196.
27. Duff GW, Durum SK. Fever and immunoregulation: hyperthermia, interleukins 1 and 2, and T-cell proliferation. Yale J Biol Med 1982; 55:437–442.
28. Saririan K, Nickerson DA. Enhancement of murine in vitro antibody formation by hyperthermia. Cell Immunol 1982; 74:306–312.
29. Pannen BHJ, Robotham JL. The acute phase response. New Horizons 1995; 3:183–197.
30. Kushner I. The phenomenon of the acute phase response. Ann NY Acad Sci 1982; 389:39–48.
31. Miller PR, Munn DD, Meredith JW, Chang MC. Systemic inflammatory response syndrome in the trauma intensive care unit: who is infected? J Trauma 1999; 47:1004–1008.
32. Fagon JY, Chastre J, Hance AJ. Detection of nosocomial lung infection in ventilated patients. Use of a protected specimen brush and quantitative culture techniques in 147 patients. Am Rev Respir Dis 1988; 138:110–116.
33. Pugin J, Auckenthaler R, Mili N et al. Diagnosis of ventilator-associated pneumonia by bacteriologic analysis of bronchoscopic and nonbronchoscopic "blind" bronchoalveolar lavage fluid. Am Rev Respir Dis 1991; 143:1121–1129.
34. Gross BH, Spizarny DL. Computed tomography of the chest in the intensive care unit. Crit Care Clin 1994; 10:267–275.
35. Norwood SH, Civetta JM. Abdominal CT scanning in critically ill surgical patients. Ann Surg 1985; 202(2):166–175.
36. Marik PE. Fever in the ICU. Chest 2000; 117:855–869.
37. Green RJ, Clarke DE, Fishman RS, Raffin TA. Techniques for evaluating fever in the ICU. J Crit Illness 1995; 10:67–71.
38. Cunha BA, Shea KW. Fever in the intensive care unit. Inf Dis Clin North Am 1996; 10:185–209.
39. Gronert GA. Malignant hyperthermia. Anesthesiology 1980; 53:395–423.
40. Gronert GA, Pessah IN, Muldoon SM, Tautz TJ. Miller Ronal D, ed. Malignant Hyperthermia in Miller's Anesthesia. 6th ed. New York: Churchill Livingstone, 2005:1169–1190.
41. Hoenemann CW, Halene-Holtgrave TB, Booke M et al. Delayed onset of malignant hyperthermia in desflurane anesthesia. Anasthes Analg 2003; 96:165–167.
42. Jurkat-Rott K, McCarthy T, Lehmann-Horn F. Genetics and pathogenesis of malignant hyperthermia. Muscle Nerve 2000; 23:4–17.
43. Loke JC, Kraev N, Sharma P et al. Detection of a novel ryanodine receptor subtype 1 mutation (R328W) in a malignant hyperthermia family by sequencing of a leukocyte transcript. Anesthesiology 2003; 99:297–302.
44. Sambuughin N, Holley H, Muldoon S et al. Screening of the entire ryanodine receptor type 1 coding region for sequence variants associated with malignant hyperthermia susceptibility in the North American population. Anesthesiology 2005; 102(3):515–521.
45. Adnet P, Lestavel P, Krivosic-Horber R. Neuroleptic malignant syndrome. Br J Anaesthes 2000; 85:129–135.
46. Levenson JL. Neuroleptic malignant syndrome. Am J Psychiatry 1985; 142:1137–1145.

47. Rosenberg MR, Green M. Neuroleptic malignant syndrome: review of response to therapy. Arch Intern Med 1989; 149: 1927–1931.

48. Guze BH, Baxter LR Jr. Neuroleptic malignant syndrome. N Engl J Med 1985; 313:163–166.

49. Caroff SN, Mann SC. Neuroleptic malignant syndrome. Med Clin North Am 1993; 77:185–202.

50. Sporer KA. The serotonin syndrome: implicated drugs, pathophysiology and management. Drug Saf 1995; 13:94–104.

51. Boyer EW, Shannon M. The serotonin syndrome. N Engl J Med 2005; 352:1112–1120.

52. Simon HB. Current concepts: hyperthermia. N Engl J Med 1993; 329:483–487.

53. Mackowiak PA, LaMaistre CF. Drug fever: a critical appraisal of conventional concepts; and analysis of 51 episodes in two Dallas hospitals and 97 episodes reported in the English literature. Ann Intern Med 1987; 106:728–733.

54. Chapman SA, Stephan T, Lake KD, Sonnesyn SW, Emery RW. Fever induced by dobutamine infusion. Am J Cardiol 1994; 74:517.

55. Mitchell RMS, Byrne MF, Baillie J. Pancreatitis. Lancet 2003; 361:1447–1455.

56. Lankisch PG, Lerch MM. The role of antibiotic prophylaxis in the treatment of acute pancreatitis. J Clin Gastroenterol 2006; 40(2):149–155.

57. Rao RH, Vagnucci AH, Amico JA. Bilateral massive adrenal hemorrhage: early recognition and treatment. Ann Intern Med 1989; 110:227–235.

58. Dorin RI, Kearns PJ. High output circulatory failure in acute adrenal insufficiency. Crit Care Med 1988; 16:296–297.

59. Oelkers W. Adrenal insufficiency. NEJM 1996; 355:1206–1211.

60. Baldwin WA, Allo M. Occult hypoadrenalism in critically ill patients. Arch Surg 1993; 128:673–676.

61. Tietgens ST, Leinung MC. Thyroid storm. Med Clin North Am 1995; 79:169–184.

62. Sarlis NJ, Gourgiotis L. Thyroid emergencies. Rev Endocr Metab Disord 2003; 4(2):129–136.

63. Snyder EL, Stack G. Febrile and nonimmune transfusions reactions. In: Rossi EC, Simon TL, Moss GS, eds. Principles of Transfusion Medicine. Baltimore, MD: Williams and Wilkins, 1991.

64. Barton JC. Nonhemolytic, noninfectious transfusion reactions. Semin Hematol 1981; 18:95–121.

65. Spodick DH. Decresed recognition of the postmyocardial infarction (Dressler) syndrome in the postinfarct setting: does it masquerade as "idiopathic pericarditis" following silent infarcts? Chest 2004; 126(5):1410–1411.

66. Carsons SE. Fever in rheumatic and autoimmune disease. Infect Dis Clin North Am 1996; 10(1):67–84.

67. Mendelson M. Fever in the immunocompromised host. Emerg Med Clin North Am 1998; 16(4):761–779.

68. Engoren M. Lack of association between atelectasis and fever. Chest 1995; 107:81–84.

69. Kisala JM, Ayala A, Stephan RN. A model of pulmonary atelectasis in rats: activation of alveolar macrophage and cytokine release. Am J Physiol 1993; 264:R610–614.

70. American Thoracic Society; Infectious Diseases Society of America. Guidelines for the management of adults with hospital-acquired, ventilator-associated, and healthcare-associated pneumonia. Am J Respir Crit Care Med 2005; 171: 388–416.

71. Menedez R, Torres A et al. Guidelines for the treatment of community-acquired pneumonia: predictors of adherence and outcome. Am J Respir Crit Care Med 2005; 3, E-pub.

72. Mandell, LA, Bartlett JG et al. Update of practice guidelines for the management of community-acquired pneumonia in immunocompetent adults. Clin Infect Dis 2003; 37:1405–1433.

73. Marik PE. Aspiration pneumonitis and aspiration pneumonia. N Engl J Med 2001; 344:655–671.

74. O'Grady, NP, Alexander M et al. Guidelines for the prevention of intravascular catheter-related infections. Clin Infect Dis 2002; 35:1281–1307.

75. Mermel LA, Farr BM et al. Guidelines for the management of intravascular catheter-related infections. Clin Infect Dis 2001; 32:1249–1272.

76. Maki D, Weise C, Sarafin H. A semiquantitative method for identifying intravenous catheter related-infection. N Engl J Med 1977; 296:1305.

77. Safdar N, Fine JP, Maki DG. Meta-analysis: methods for diagnosing intravascular device-related bloodstream infection. Ann Intern Med 2005; 142:451–466.

78. Seifert H, Cornely O, Seggewiss K et al. Bloodstream infection in neutropenic cancer patients related to short-term nontunnelled catheters determined by quantitative blood cultures, differential time to positivity, and molecular epidemiological typing with pulsed-field gel electrophoresis. J Clin Microbiol 2003; 41:118.

79. Hasham S, Matteucci P et al. Necrotizing fasciitis. BMJ 2005; 330:830–833.

80. Bluman EM, Mechrefe AP, Fadale PD. Idiopathic *Staphylococcus aureus* necrotizing fasciitis of the upper extremity. J shoulder Elbow Surg 2005; 14:227–230.

81. Miller LG, Perdreau-Remington F et al. Necrotizing fasciitis caused by community-associated methicillin-resistant *Staphylococcus aureus* in Los Angeles. N Engl J Med 2005; 352: 1445–1453.

82. Stevens DL, Gibbons AE, Bergstrom R et al. The Eagle Effect revisitied: efficacy of clindamycin, erythromycin, penicillin in the treatment of streptococcal myositis. J Infect Dis 1988; 158(1):23–28.

83. Gustilo RB, Anderson JT. Prevention of infection in the treatment of one thousand and twenty-five open fractures of long bones; restrospective and prospective analysis. J Bone Joint Surg A, 1976; 58:453–458.

84. Skaggs DL, Friend L et al. The effect of surgical delay on acute infection following 554 open fractures in children. J Bone Joint Surg Am 2005; 87:8–12.

85. Gillespie WJ, Walenkamp G. Antibiotic prophylaxis for surgery for proximal femoral and other closed long bone fractures. Cochrane Database Syst Rev 2001; 1:CD000244.

86. Gosselin RA, Roberts I, Gillespie WJ. Antibiotics for preventing infection in open limb fractures. Cochrane Database Syst Rev 2004; 1:CD003764.

87. Mazuski JE, Sawyer RG, Nathens AB et al. The surgical infection society guidelines on antimicrobial therapy for intra-abdominal infections: evidence for the recommendations. Surg Infect 2002; 3(3):175–233.

88. Solomkin JS, Mazuski JE, Baron EJ et al. Guidelines for the selection of anti-infective agents for complicated intra-abdominal infections. Clin Infect Dis 2003; 37:997–1005.

89. Salvaggio MR, Pappas PG. Current concepts in the management of fungal periotonitis. Curr Infect Dis Rep 2003; 5: 120–124.

90. Talmor M, Li P, Barie PS. Acute paranasal sinusitis in critically ill patients: guidelines for prevention, diagnosis, and treatment. Clin Infect Dis 1997; 25(6):1441–1446.

91. Stein M, Caplan ES. Nosocomial sinusitis: a unique subset of sinutitis. Curr Opin Infect Dis 2005; 18:147–150.

92. Platt R, Polk BF, Murdock B et al. Risk factors for nosocomial urinary tract infection. Am J Epidemiol 1986; 124:977–985.

93. Trautner BW, Darouiche RO. Role of biofilms in catheter-associated urinary tract infection. Am J Infect Control 2003; 32:177–183.

94. Nicolle LE, Bradley S et al. Infectious Diseases Society of America guidelines for the diagnosis and treatment of asymptomatic bacteriuria in adults. Clin Infect Dis 2005; 40: 643–654.

95. Tambyah PA. Catheter-associated urinary tract infections: diagnosis and prophylaxis. Int J Antimicrob Agents 2004; 24S:S44–S48.

96. Trautner BW, Huff RA, Darouiche RO. Prevention of catheter-associated urinary tract infection. Curr Opin Infect Dis 2005; 18:37–41.

97. Jacobs LG, Skidmore EA, Freeman K et al. Oral fluconazole compared with bladder irrigation with amphotericin B for treatment of fungal urinary tract infections in elderly patients. Clin Infect Dis 1996; 22:30–35.

98. Melles DC, de Marie S. Prevention of infections in hyposplenic and asplenic patients: an update. Neth J Med 2004; 62:45–52.

99. Castagnola E, Fioredda F. Prevention of life-threatening infections due to encapsulated bacteria in children with hyposplenia or asplenia: a brief review of current recommendations for practical purposes. Eur J Haematol 2003; 71:319–326.

100. Sherpa TY, Leaf HL. Pneumococcal vaccination in adults. Curr Infect Dis Rep 2005; 7:211–217.

101. Singh J, Arrieta AC. Management of meningococcemia. Indian J Pediatr 2004; 71:909–913.

102. Weisel G, Joyce D et al. Human recombinant activated protein C in meningococcal sepsis. Chest 2002; 121:292–295.

103. Alberio L, Laemmle B, Esmon CT: Protein C replacement in severe meningococcemia: rationale and clinical experience. Clin Infect Dis 2001; 32:1338–1346.

104. Tunkel AR, Hartman BJ et al. Practice guidelines for the management of bacterial meningitis. Clin Infect Dis 2004; 39:1267–1284.

105. van de Beek D, de Gans J. Adjunctive corticosteroids in adults with bacterial meningitis. Curr Infect Dis Rep 2005; 7:285–291.

106. Thwaites GE, Nguyen DB et al. Dexamethasone for the treatment of tuberculous meningitis in adolescents and adults. N Engl J Med 2004; 351:1741–1751.

107. de Gans J, van de Beek D. European dexamethasone in Adulthood Bacterial Meningitis Study Investigators. Dexamethasone in adults with bacterial meningitis. N Engl J Med 2002; 347:1549–1556.

108. Mackowiak PA, Plaisance KI. Benefits and risks of antipyretic therapy. Ann NY Acad Sci 1998; 856:214–223.

109. Mackowiak PA, Boulant JA. Fever's upper limit. In: Mackowiak PA, ed. Fever: Basic Mechanisms and Management. 2nd ed. Philadelphia, PA; Lippincott-Raven Publishers, 1997:147–163.

110. Kilpatrick MM, Lowry DW, Firlik AD et al. Hyperthermia in the neurosurgical intensive care unit. Neurosurgery 2000; 47:850–856.

111. Henker R, Rogers S, Kramer DJ et al.: Comparison of fever treatments in the critically ill: a pilot study. Am J Crit Care 2001; 10:276–280.

112. Stocchetti N, Rossi S, Zanier ER et al. Pyrexia in head-injured patients admitted to intensive care. Int Care Med 2002; 28:1555–1562.

113. Boyle M, Hundy S, Torda TA. Paracetamon administration is associated with hypotension in the critically ill. Aust Crit Care 1997; 10:120–122.

114. Rossi S, Zanier ER, Mauril, Columbo et al. Brain temperature, body core temperature, and intracranial pressure in acute cerebral damage. J Neurol Neurosurg Psychiatry 2001; 71:448–454.

115. Poblete B, Romand JA, Pichard C et al. Metabolic effects of IV propacetamol, metamizol or external cooling in critically ill febrile sedated patients. Br J Anaesthes 1997; 78:123–127.

116. Marion DW, Penrod LE, Kelsey SF et al. Treatment of traumatic brain injury with moderate hypothermia. NEJM 1997; 336:540–546.

117. Clifton GL, Miller ER, Choi SC et al. Lack of effect of induction of hypothermia after acute brain injury. NEJM 2001; 344:556–563.

118. Manthous CA, Hall JB, Olson D et al. Effect of cooling on oxygen consumption in febrile critically ill patients. Am J Respir Crit Care Med 1995; 151:10–14.

119. Haley RW, Culver DH, White JW, Morgan WM, Emori TG. The nationwide nosocomial infection rate: a new need for vital statistics. Am J Epidemiol 1985; 121:159–167.

120. Johnson D, Cunha B. Drug fever. Infect Dis Clin North Am 1996; 10(1):85–91.

121. Cunha B. Drug fever. Postgraduate Med 1986; 80(5):123–129.

47

Sepsis

Theo N. Kirkland

Division of Infectious Diseases, Departments of Pathology and Medicine, UC San Diego School of Medicine,
San Diego, California, U.S.A.

Jeanne Lee

Division of Trauma, Burns, and Critical Care, Department of Surgery, UC San Diego Medical Center, San Diego, California, U.S.A.

INTRODUCTION

The development of antibiotics in the second half of the twentieth century led to dramatic reductions in the mortality rates of many infectious diseases. However, the mortality rate of a subset of acute infections associated with shock and organ dysfunction remains high at about 30% to 60% despite modern antibiotics and critical care (1). Septic shock is a relatively common problem; there are about 750,000 cases of severe sepsis due to bacterial or fungal infections each year in the United States (1). The incidence of septic shock is increasing. From 1979 to 1987 the percentage of infectious disease diagnoses that included sepsis increased from approximately 10% to 25% (1). This increase may be due to the increased use of cytotoxic and immunosuppressive drugs, aging of the patient population, the increased use of invasive medical devices, and an increase in antibiotic resistant organisms.

This chapter will review the definition and pathophysiology of sepsis and its molecular mechanisms, as well as the clinical signs and symptoms, laboratory characteristics, inciting infections and therapeutic options. This summary will also include a discussion on the recent successful activated protein C trial for sepsis, as well as a review of several of the trials that failed to improve outcome. Finally, we will present a brief glimpse at promising therapies still on the clinical horizon in the "Eye to the Future" section.

DEFINITION OF SEPSIS AND RELATED SYNDROMES

In the past, the diagnosis of sepsis required the presence of a positive blood culture in the setting of fever, leukocytosis, and a hemodynamic profile consistent with hypotension or shock. However, disagreements over the essential diagnostic features, variations in sepsis research entry criteria, and the recognition that the systemic response to infection is what differentiates sepsis from mere bacteremia, led to much confusion and debate about diagnostic criteria. In an effort to bring order to this subject, Roger Bone and others organized a consensus conference in 1991 involving the American College of Chest Physicians (ACCP) and the Society of Critical Care Medicine (SCCM) to propose new definitions for sepsis and the related syndromes (Table 1).

The attendees concluded that sepsis is the systemic inflammatory response to documented infection, but also acknowledged, and emphasized, that this response may be observed in a number of other clinical conditions not involving infection (see also Volume 2, Chapter 63). According to the 1991 ACCP/SCCM criteria, sepsis is a subset of the systemic inflammatory response syndrome (SIRS). Similarly, severe sepsis is a subset of sepsis, and septic shock a subset of severe sepsis (Table 1). An individual patient may meet all of these definitions as time progresses. The 1991 ACCP/SCCM criteria have also been widely used to describe SIRS resulting from trauma, surgery, burns, pancreatitis, etc., in the absence of infectious diseases. Because the definition of SIRS is very broad, its clinical utility has been challenged (2,3). In 2001, another consensus conference was convened to review the 1991 ACCP/SCCM definitions and address methods to improve their diagnostic accuracy (4). The group of experts from the SCCM, European Society of Intensive Care Medicine (ESICM), ACCP, American Thoracic Society (ATS) and the Surgical Infection Society (SIS) concluded that there was insufficient data to change the 1991 ACCP/SCCM definitions (4). However, they did recommend expanding the list of signs and symptoms used as diagnostic criteria for sepsis because (i) the clinical presentation is variable and (ii) they resolved that accurate bedside diagnosis was of a higher priority than clear and simple entry criteria for clinical trials (4). The newly expanded diagnostic criteria for sepsis are shown in Table 2.

The 2001 SCCM/ESICM/ACCP/ATS/SIS consensus conference also concluded that the use of biomarkers for diagnosing sepsis may soon be available, but their use is currently premature. Despite this proclamation, they specifically included the biomarkers procalcitonin (PCT) and C-reactive protein (CRP) in their discussions, in their expanded diagnostic criteria for sepsis (Table 2), and in their first iteration of the new staging system for sepsis called PIRO (Table 3) (4). The PIRO system stratifies patients by their "P" predisposing conditions, the nature and extent of the insult (in the case of sepsis "I" infection), the nature and magnitude of the "R" host response and the degree of "O" organ dysfunction.

The PIRO staging system aims to stratify patients by both their baseline risk of an adverse outcome, and their potential to respond to therapy (4). The PIRO system is a work in progress. The inaugural version ranks the patient's predisposition, insult infection, response, and degree of organ dysfunction in terms of currently available factors,

Table 1 1991 ACCP/SCCM Definitions and Criteria for SIRS/Sepsis and Related Syndromes

SIRS/sepsis category	Criteria/comments
SIRS	A widespread inflammatory response to a variety of severe clinical insults (infectious or noninfectious)
	Recognized by the presence of two or more of the following:
	Temperature >38°C or <36°C
	Heart rate >90 beats/min
	Respiratory rate >20 breaths/min or $PaCO_2$ <32 mmHg
	WBC >12,000 cells/μL, <4000 cells/μL, or with >10% immature (band) forms
Sepsis[a]	The systemic response to infection
	If patient has sepsis, they will then have the clinical signs of SIRS with concrete evidence of infection
Severe sepsis	Associated with organ dysfunction hypoperfusion, or hypotension
	Clinical manifestations of hypoperfusion may include lactic acidosis, oliguria, or an acute alteration in mental status
Septic shock	Sepsis with hypotension, despite adequate fluid resuscitation, combined with perfusion abnormalities that may include, but are not limited to, lactic acidosis, oliguria, or an acute alteration in mental status
	Patients who require inotropic or vasopressor support, despite adequate fluid resuscitation, are in septic shock
Hypotension	Defined as a systolic BP of <90 mmHg or a reduction of >40 mmHg from baseline in the absence of other causes for the fall in blood pressure
Multiple organ failure	The presence of an altered organ function in acutely ill patient such that homeostasis cannot be maintained without intervention

[a]Note the criteria for sepsis was expanded in 2001 (Table 2).
Abbreviations: BP, blood pressure; SIRS, systematic inflammatory response syndrome; WBC, white blood cell.
Source: From Ref. 2.

Table 2 2001 SCCM/ESICM/ACCP/ATS/SIS **Diagnostic Criteria for Sepsis[c]**

Diagnostic criteria	Clinically acceptable definitions, and diagnostic ranges
Infection[a]	Documented or suspected, and some of the following[b]
General variables	Fever (core temperature >38.3°C)
	Hypothermia (core temperature <36°C)
	Heart rate >90/min or >2 SD above the normal value for age
	Tachypnea
	Altered mental status
	Significant edema or positive fluid balance (>20 mL/kg over 24 hr)
	Hyperglycemia (plasma glucose >120 mg/dL or 7.7 mmol/L) in the absence of diabetes
Inflammatory variables	Leukocytosis (WBC count >12,000/μL)
	Leukopenia (WBC count <4000/μL)
	Normal WBC count with >10% immature forms
	Plasma C-reactive protein >2 SD above the normal value
	Plasma procalcitonin >2 SD above the normal value
Hemodynamic variables	Arterial hypotension[b] (SBP <90 mmHg, MAP <70 mmHg, or an SBP decrease >40 mmHg in adults or <2 SD above normal for age)
	Svo_2 >70%[b]
	Cardiac index > 3.5 L/min/M² [b,c]
Organ dysfunction variables	Arterial hypoxemia (PaO_2/F_{IO_2} <300)
	Acute oliguria (urine output <0.5 mL/kg/hr)
	Creatinine increase >0.5 mg/dL
	Coagulation abnormalities (INR >1.5 or aPTT >60 sec)
	Ileus (absent bowel sounds)
	Thrombocytopenia (plasma count <100,000/μL)
	Hyperbilirubinemia (plasma total bilirubin >4 mg/dL or 70 mmol/L)
Tissue perfusion variables	Hyperlactatemia (>3 mmol/L)
	Decreased capillary refill or mottling

[a]Infection defined as a pathologic process induced by a microorganism.
[b]Svo_2sat >70% is normal in children (normally, 75–80%).
[c]CI 3.5–5.5 is normal in children; therefore, NEITHER should be used as signs of sepsis in newborns or children.
Note: Diagnostic criteria for sepsis in the pediatric population are signs and symptoms of inflammation plus infection with hyper- or hypothermia (rectal temperature >38.5°C or <35°C), tachycardia (may be absent in hypothermic patients), and at least one of the following indications of altered organ function: altered mental status, hypoxemia, increased serum lactate level, or bounding pulses.
Abbreviations: aPTT, activated partial thromboplastin time; INR, international normalized ratio; MAP, mean arterial blood pressure; SBP, systolic blood pressure; S_{VO_2}, mixed venous oxygen saturation; WBC, white blood cell; SD, standard deviation.
Source: From Ref. 4.

as well as considerations and criteria that are not yet available, but are on the horizon (Table 3).

SIRS and sepsis are usually thought of as an overexuberant inflammatory response, which is then followed by an anti-inflammatory response. Therefore, many of the attempts to treat sepsis have been directed at blunting the inflammatory response. More recently, some authors have stressed the anti-inflammatory and apoptotic elements of SIRS and sepsis, and suggested that these aspects of sepsis may be suitable targets for therapy (2,3). ☞ **SIRS and sepsis are such global responses that focusing on one or a few aspects of the response necessarily oversimplifies the true pathophysiology of the disease.** ☞ Nevertheless, targeted therapy can influence the outcome of SIRS and sepsis (see below). SIRS and sepsis affect many organs.

Table 3 The PIRO System for Staging Sepsis

Domain	Present	Future	Rationale
Predisposition	Premorbid illness with reduced probability of short term survival. Cultural or religious beliefs, age, sex.	Genetic polymorphisms in components of inflammatory response (e.g., TLR, TNF, IL-1, CD14); enhanced understanding of specific interactions between pathogens and host diseases.	In the present, premorbid factors impact on the potential attributable morbidity and mortality of an acute insult; deleterious consequences of insult heavily dependent on genetic predisposition (future).
Insult infection	Culture and sensitivity of infecting pathogens; detection of disease amenable to source control.	Assay of microbial products (LPS, mannan, bacterial DNA); gene transcript profiles.	Specific therapies directed against inciting insult require demonstration and characterization of that insult.
Response	SIRS, other signs of sepsis, shock, CRP.	Nonspecific markers of activated inflammation (e.g., PCT or IL-6) or impaired host responsiveness (e.g., HLA-DR); specific detection of target of therapy (e.g., protein C, TNF, PAF).	Both mortality risk and potential to respond to therapy vary with nonspecific measures of disease severity (e.g., shock); specific mediator-targeted therapy is predicated on presence and activity of mediator.
Organ dysfunction	Organ dysfunction as number of failing organs or composite score (e.g., MODS, SOFA, LODS, PEMOD, PELOD).	Dynamic measures of cellular response to insult—apoptosis, cytopathic hypoxia, cell stress.	Response to pre-emptive therapy (e.g., targeting microorganism or early mediator) not possible if damage already present; therapies targeting the injurious cellular process require that it be present.

Abbreviations: CRP, C-reactive protein; HLA-DR, human leukocyte antigen-DR; IL, interleukin; LODS, logistic organ dysfunction system; LPS, lipopolysaccharide; MODS, multiple organ dysfunction syndrome; PAF, platelet-activating factor; PCT, procalcitonin; PELOD, pediatric logistic organ dysfunction; PEMOD, pediatric multiple organ dysfunction; SIRS, systemic inflammatory response syndrome; SOFA, sepsis-related organ failure assessment; TLR, toll-like receptor; TNF, tumor necrosis factor.
Source: From Ref. 4.

Table 4 lists some of the more prominent organs involved in sepsis and their role in mediating SIRS. The inflammatory nature of SIRS (without regard to etiology) is the subject matter of Volume 2, Chapter 63, whereas this chapter focuses mainly on the infectious disease etiology of sepsis.

PATHOGENESIS OF SEPSIS

A major early insight into the molecular mechanisms of sepsis occurred following the recognition that the bacterial cell wall constituents reproduced many of the signs and symptoms of sepsis. Abraham Braude demonstrated that infusion of blood contaminated with cold-growing bacteria, (i.e., unable to grow in vivo) caused sepsis just as effectively as spontaneous bacteremia with organisms that grow at body temperature. He reasoned that bacterial products had to be responsible for sepsis. He focused on bacterial lipopolysaccharide (LPS) because of the epidemiologic association between septic shock and Gram-negative bacteremia that was seen in the 1960s. We now realize that Gram-positive, Gram-negative bacteria and fungi are all associated with septic shock.

☞ **The constituents of microbial organisms that elicit inflammatory responses are collectively known as Pathogen Associated Molecular Patterns (PAMPs) (5).** ☜ Pathogens have molecular structures that are not shared by mammals, but are shared by related pathogens, and are relatively invariant (i.e., do not evolve rapidly). These structures are known as PAMPs. Examples of PAMPs include flagellin of bacterial flagella, LPS of Gram-negative bacteria, and peptidoglycan of Gram-positive bacteria.

We have recently come to appreciate that the PAMPs are recognized by mammalian Pattern Recognition Receptors (PRRs) that signal the responding cells that PAMPs are present in the environment (6–8). PRRs are found on many cell types, including monocytes, macrophages, dendritic cells, polymorphonuclear phagocytes (PMNs), endothelial cells and some types of epithelial cells. One increasingly understood family of PRRs are the Toll-Like Receptors (TLRs). These evolutionary conserved receptors are homologues of the Drosophila Toll gene, and thus named after them. TLRs identify the nature of the pathogen and turn on an effector response appropriate for dealing with it. Mammals have 11 known TLRs, each of which specializes in a subset of PAMPs (often with the aid of accessory molecules). Binding of the pathogen molecule (PAMP) to the TLR initiates a signaling pathway leading to the activation of nuclear factor-κB (NF-κB). NF-κB turns on genes needed for cell proliferation, adhesion, and angiogenesis. NF-κB also turns on various cytokine genes. A new TLR (TLR-11) is expressed in liver, bladder, and kidney and may have a role in protecting against uropathogenic bacteria. Table 5 lists the currently known TLRs and associated PAMPs.

Lipopolysaccharide, also known as endotoxin, is a major constituent of the cell wall of Gram-negative bacteria. It is a glycolipid that usually has a large sugar component on the extracellular face of the cell membrane linked to a glycolipid region that provides osmotic stability to the

Table 4 Organ Systems Involved in Sepsis and Their Role in Mediating the Inflammatory Response

Organ system	Mediations involved in SIRS and sepsis	
Hypothalamic-pituitary adrenal corticoid axis	ACTH → Cortisol	
CNS	Fever, obtundation	
Peripheral sympathetic and parasympathetic nervous system	Epinephrine Norepinephrine Acetylcholine	
Endothelial cells	Early	Tissue factor ICAM, VCAM TNF, IL-1, IL-6, NO
	Late	Apoptosis, IL-10, TNF receptors
Monocytes/ macrophages	Early	TNF, IL-1, IL-6 Tissue factor MHC class II
	Late	IL-4, IL-10 IL-13 Apoptosis
Liver	Acute phase proteins C-reactive protein IL-6, LPS-binding protein many others	
Lung	Acute lung injury ARDS	
Kidney	Acute tubular necrosis	

Abbreviations: ACTH, adrenocorticotropic hormone; ARDS, acute respiratory distress syndrome; CNS, central nervous system; ICAM, intracellular adhesion molecule; IL, interlukin; LPS, lipopolysaccharide; MHC, major histocompatability complex; NO, nitric oxide; SIRS, systematic inflammatory response syndrome; TNF, tumor necrosis factor; VCAM, vascular cellular adhesion molecule.

organism. The glycolipid region, known as lipid A, is responsible for the toxicity of LPS. Infusion of LPS into human volunteers elicits many of the signs and symptoms of septic shock (9). Peptidoglycan is a complex sugar consisting of N-acetylglucosamine and N-acetylmuramic acid units cross linked by pentapeptides. Peptidoglycan is found both in gram-negative and gram-positive bacteria. Lipoteichoic acid is limited to gram-positive bacteria, whereas lipoproteins and flagella are found in both gram-positive and Gram-negative bacteria.

Some of the interactions between PAMPs and PRRs are complex. Optimal recognition of LPS requires a plasma protein that binds LPS (known as LPS binding protein or LBP) (10). LBP catalytically transfers the LPS to a second protein known as CD14 (11). This protein exists both on the surface of macrophages and PMN and circulates in the plasma. Membrane CD14 is part of the macrophage receptor LPS receptor; soluble CD14 is part of the endothelial cell LPS receptor. CD14 binds LPS very well and is needed for a robust LPS response, but it cannot signal the cell that LPS is present, because it lacks a transmembrane region. CD14 associates with PRRs known as Toll-Like Receptor 4 (TLR-4) and an associated protein MD-2 (12,13). TLR-4 is responsible for signaling the interior of the cell that LPS is present by forming clusters of protein that activate intracellular kinases. Some of the other PAMPs react with more than one type of TLR, so that combinations of PRRs can signal the presence of a specific PAMP (14). Once the TLR has signaled that PAMPs are present within the environment, a complex series of intracellular signaling events is triggered (15). The end result of these signals is the transcriptional activation of many genes. Studies in human dendritic cells demonstrated that roughly 10% of the genes measured had significant changes in transcription levels after exposure to whole *E. coli* bacteria (16). Some of the specific genes that are affected by PAMP interaction with PRR will be discussed.

Table 5 Pathogen-Associated Microbial Patterns and Their Specialized Toll-Like Receptor

TLR #	PAMP	Comments
TLR-1	Lipoproteins	Also bound by TLR-1 and TLR-6
TLR-2	Peptidoglycan, lipoproteins, lipoteichoic acid glucan (fungal)	Peptidoglycan is a cell wall constituent of gram-positive bacteria (e.g., Staph and Strep). Lipoteichoic acid is a constituent of the cell wall. Glucan is a fungal constituent. Another receptor binding glucan is dectin
TLR-3	Double-stranded RNA (dsRNA)	dsRNA genomes belong to such viruses as the Colorado tick fever virus
TLR-4	LPS also known as endotoxin	LPS is located in the outer membrane of gram-negative bacteria (e.g., *E. coli*, *Salmonella*) Other receptors also binding to LPS include MD-2, CD-14, LPS-binding protein
TLR-5	Flagellin	Flagellin is a constituent of the flagella found on many motile bacteria (e.g., Listeria)
TLR-6	Lipoproteins	Also bound by TLR-1 and TLR-2
TLR-7	Single-stranded RNA (ssRNA)	ssRNA genomes belong to such viruses as influenza, measles, and mumps
TLR-8	Single-stranded RNA (ssRNA)	(see above)
TLR-9	Unmethylated CpG of the DNA	CpG islands in mammals are located around "promoters" of genes, and tend to have methyl groups attached.
TLR-10	Unknown	Similar in structure to TLR-1 and TLR-6
TLR-11	Unknown	Found in liver, bladder, and kidney, may have a role against uropathogenic bacteria (i.e., *E. coli*)

Abbreviations: CpG, cytosine phosphodiester guanine (a specific dinucleotide motif of DNA); LPS, lipopolysaccharide; PAMP, pathogen associated microbial patterns; TLR, toll-like receptor.

The Mammalian Response to Pathogen-Associated Microbial Patterns: The Cells

☞ **A wide variety of mammalian cells respond to PAMPs. These include PMNs, blood monocytes, tissue macrophages and dendritic cells.** ☞ All these cells express CD14 and TLRs and are major participants in the inflammatory response to PAMPs and microbial infection. The endothelial cell is also responsive to PAMPs. Though it lacks CD14, it responds to LPS via soluble CD14 and TLR-4; the endothelial cell also expresses the other TLRs important for responses to PAMPs (15,17). Epithelial cells, such as respiratory epithelial cells, bladder epithelial cells and many other types of epithelial cells susceptible to infectious organisms, are also responsive to various microbial derived products. Vascular smooth muscle cells, cardiac myocytes and a wide of other cell types also respond to PAMPs.

Mammalian Response to Pathogen-Associated Microbial Patterns: Genes and Protein Induction

As mentioned above, the transcriptional response to PAMPs is very dramatic. To briefly summarize the response of macrophages, there is a decrease in the transcription of genes associated with phagocytosis and genes coding for PRR (16). Conversely, there is a transient, but dramatic, increase in cytokines (e.g., TNF-α, IL-1α and β, IL-6, IFN-γ), chemokines (e.g., IL-8) and receptors for these proteins. Tissue factor expression is also up-regulated. In addition, there is an up-regulation of genes coding for antigen presentation molecules, and genes for enzymes that make reactive oxygen intermediates and reactive nitrogen intermediates. As time progresses, expression of the anti-inflammatory cytokine IL-10 develops, as does expression of genes involved in programmed cell death or apoptosis (16).

The response of endothelial cells is similar with early increases in expression of cytokines and chemokines and increased expression of the surface adhesion molecules. Two of the most well described adhesion molecules are the intercellular adhesion molecule (ICAM) and the vascular cell adhesion molecule (VCAM). In the case of ICAM and VCAM, these adhesion molecules bind to integrins located upon the cell surface of circulating leukocyte (Fig. 1). The binding of these receptors allows the leukocyte to undergo other modifications involved in the immune response to infection.

Other adhesion molecules include tissue factor, and inducible nitric oxide synthase (iNOS) (18–20). Many of the activated genes express proteins that act to stimulate cells further. For example, TNF-α stimulates macrophages and endothelial cells to produce more TNF-α, IL-1α, IL-6, and to activate expression of genes leading to apoptosis, or programmed cell death. The response to microbial infection changes with time: early on, there is a prominent inflammatory response, but as time progresses the response changes to an anti-inflammatory one, with IL-10 production and apoptosis of many cell types becoming predominant (discussed further in Volume 2, Chapter 63).

The induction of inducible iNOS probably plays a major role in the early "warm shock" state sometimes seen. This is low systemic vascular resistance (SVR) in the face of hypotension; often good perfusion of the skin is seen when the central organs are not being adequately perfused. Nitric Oxide (NO) made by iNOS diffuses from the endothelial cell into the adjacent vascular smooth muscle cell and triggers muscle relaxation.

Induction of tissue factor on the surface of endothelial cells and macrophages triggers the coagulation pathway. The expression of tissue factor activates Factor VII to VIIa, which stimulates the coagulation cascade leading to the formation of fibrin clots. This is the major mechanism by which sepsis triggers disseminated intravascular coagulation (DIC).

Bacterial surfaces, LPS, peptidoglycan and immune complexes activate the complement cascade. This leads to activation of C5 to C5a, which is an anaphylotoxin. This protein elicits PMN chemotaxis, release of granular enzymes from phagocytic cells, vasodilatation, and increased vascular permeability (21).

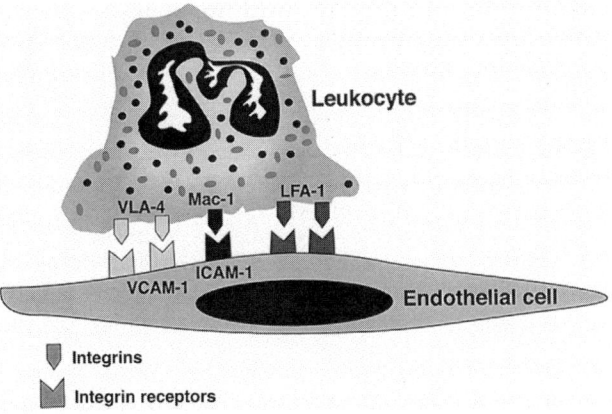

Figure 1 Binding of leukocyte and its integrins to the endothelial cell by way of immunoglobulin adhesion molecules during the process of neutrophil migration. During inflammation adhesion molecules promote leukocyte emigration from capillaries through a series of steps involving various adhesion molecules. Rolling of the leukocyte upon the endothelial occurs after binding L-, P-, and E-selectins (not shown). The leukocyte is stopped by binding to ICAM-1 and VCAM-1 (as shown). Shape change and aggregation occurs after binding with LFA-1 receptors (shown in figure). Migration through the endothelial cell wall occurs after binding of ICAM-1, and VCAM-1, as well as others not shown. *Abbreviations*: ICAM-1, intercellular adhesion molecule; LFA, lymphocyte functional antigen; Mac-1, macrophage antigen-1, CD11b/CD18; VCAM-1, vascular cell adhesion molecule; VLA-4, very late antigen 4 or CD49d/CD29. *Source*: From Ref. 46.

DIAGNOSIS OF SEPSIS
The Clinical Presentation

All physicians have been trained to recognize sepsis. It is a problem that does not respect medical or surgical boundaries. However, definitions tend to be fairly broad. The current and most widely used definitions are shown in Table 1. SIRS has a very broad definition that includes most people with significant infections. In addition, people with pancreatitis, severe trauma or thermal burns can present with SIRS (see Volume 2, Chapter 63). Only a subset of patients with SIRS has sepsis. Conversely, not all patients who are septic have SIRS. Patients who are elderly, those who are chronically ill, and those on corticosteroids or other immunosuppressive drugs tend not to generate as robust of an inflammatory response as young, healthy individuals.

There are a few clinical clues to sepsis that deserve mention. Patients frequently present with an intense feeling of anxiety. Altered mental status is also a condition that should trigger suspicions of sepsis as well as central nervous system disease. Tachypnea is another very early sign of sepsis; tachypnea with a low PaCO$_2$ and a normal pH suggests that lactic acidosis is occurring. All patients with SIRS should have a complete and careful physical examination in search of signs of infection and possible sources. The "classic" presentation of septic shock is as "warm shock," where the patient is hypotensive with warm and well perfused skin and extremities. This state is due to a high cardiac output and low SVR. Later in the course of sepsis, or in patients who can't increase their cardiac output, the hypotension may become associated with peripheral vasoconstriction, and petechial lesions suggest DIC (e.g., meningococcemia). A complete physical may suggest a source of infection that will help focus efforts to collect appropriate cultures and or drain an abscess. Frequent sources of infection in critically ill trauma patients include the lungs (pneumonia), invasive lines, the abdomen (if injured or operated upon—especially if known fecal contamination occurred), and the urinary tract, among others (Table 6). Areas that are often forgotten include the paranasal sinuses (Volume 2, Chapter 51), the throat, the joints, the sacrum (decubitus ulcers), and rectum (peri-rectal abscess).

The Laboratory Examination
Standard Laboratory Tests
Patients with SIRS typically have an elevated WBC count with a shift toward immature band forms. However, in some cases the WBC count falls rather than rises (Table 2). The platelet count is variable; low counts suggest DIC (Volume 2, Chapter 58) while high platelet counts are associated with the inflammatory response (Volume 2, Chapter 63). The erythrocyte sedimentation rate (ESR) has long been used as a nonspecific indication of infection or inflammation. Both the ESR and CRP are acute phase proteins, and tend to be elevated, just like those that play a role in the pathogenesis of

sepsis, such as LPS binding protein. Recent studies have tested the ability of other markers to predict the development of septic shock in patients with SIRS. The proteins IL-6, IL-8, and procalcitonin have been investigated as markers of sepsis. One group has shown that an elevated procalcitonin level is a good predictor of sepsis and septic shock (22). These tests are not widely available, and others have suggested that clinical parameters are perfectly adequate predictors (23). The current understanding of CRP and procalcitonin in sepsis and SIRS is more fully developed in Volume 2, Chapter 63.

Currently, there is no clinically useful test for LPS in the blood. Potential reasons for this include the high degree that LPS is bound to serum lipoproteins and a short circulating half-life. Furthermore, since Gram-positive bacteria can cause septic shock, a useful test for LPS could miss as many as 50% of the cases, making LPS a less useful universal test for sepsis, even if available.

In severe sepsis there is a tendency for lactic acid to accumulate so the patient presents with an anion gap metabolic acidosis. Often the patient will have a compensatory tachypnea, lowering the $PaCO_2$ and almost normalizing the pH. If organ damage develops the laboratory signs of that damaged organ are seen.

☛ **The timely and appropriate collection of cultures is a mainstay of diagnostic management of sepsis.** ☛ The results of cultures are not available immediately, but if cultures are not collected before antibiotics are administered, it is impossible to clinically distinguish patients with bacteremia from those with SIRS due to noninfectious causes. All patients with a diagnosis of SIRS should have blood and urine cultured. If there is a pulmonary infiltrate, sputum Gram stain and cultures should also be obtained.

Table 6   Sources of Infection in Trauma and Critical Care

Source	Diagnostic criteria[a]	Comments/clinical examples
Lungs (pneumonia) (see Volume 2, Chapter 48)	Pulmonary infiltrate, sputum gram stain and culture identifying specific organism	Aspiration may occur at scene or during resuscitation ALI, ARDS from TRALI, fat emboli, pulmonary contusion, Later >3–5 days, nosocomial. organisms (e.g., Pseudomonas, Enterobacter)
Invasive lines (Line sepsis) (see Volume 2, Chapter 49)	Differential blood cultures (catheter and peripheral site), pus and erythema around skin entry site (unless immunosuppressed)	Catheters should be removed whenever infection suspected (do not change over wire).
Abdomen (peritonitis) (see Volume 2, Chapter 50)	Obvious acute abdominal source. Not tolerating tube feeding	Rare unless prior ABD trauma, or prior ABD operation (risk ↑ with spilled visceral contents.) or in cirrhotic patients.
Urinary tract infection (UTI) (see Volume 2, Chapter 46)	Dysuria, frequency, urgency, bacteriuria	Bacterial colonization is common in catheterized patients. Significant UTI more common in immunosuppressed, or those with stone, tumor, clots, or obstruction.
Soft tissue (Abscess → necrotizing fasciitis Volume 1, Chapter 29)	Tenderness, swelling eryethema over site, becomes fluctuant with abscess, subcutaneous emphysema and disruption of fascial plane with necrotizing fasciitis	Many sources of skin disruption following trauma and critical care; ↑ risk in diabetes, and immunosuppressed.
Sinus tract (sinusitis) (see Volume 2, Chapter 51)	Headache, purulent nasal discharge, pain over involved sinus(s)	Presence of tubes in nares prolonged supine position all ↑ risk.
Acalculous cholecystitis (see Volume 2, Chapters 35 and 50)	Tenderness over G.B. bed ("Murphy's Sign"), G.B. wall thickening and sludge on ultrasound	Prolonged GI tract disuse. ↑ risk (i.e., npo +/− TPN).

[a]Fever and leukocytosis are common diagnostic finds for each of these sources.

Abbreviations: ALI, acute lung injury; ARDS, acute respiratory distress syndrome; TRALI, transfusion associated lung injury; ABD, abdomen; GB, gall bladder; npo, non per os (nothing per oral route); TPN, total parenteral nutrition; ↑, increased.

Microbiology

✍ **In the setting of trauma, most patients with SIRS do not have an infectious source.** ✍ Overall, only about 30% to 40% of trauma patients with SIRS turn out to have an infection (24). In these patients, there is roughly a 50% incidence of infections due to Gram positive bacteria and 50% incidence of infections due to Gram negative bacteria (1,24–26). A breakdown of the most common organisms found in bacteremic sepsis in one typical study is shown in Table 7 (24). The most prevalent organisms are *E. coli* and *Staphylococcus* (aureus or coagulase negative, depending on the study). In some ICU settings, yeasts account for 10% of the cases of septicemia, with the majority of these being *Candida albicans* (26). Meningococcemia and streptococcemia, classic causes of sepsis, are rare compared to these organisms. The primary sources of bloodstream infections are typically the pulmonary tree (40%), the abdomen (32%), urinary system (8%), soft tissue (5%), and intravenous catheters (4%) (24). Patients do not have to be bacteremic to develop sepsis.

Fungemia is a growing cause of sepsis in the ICU setting. This is almost always due to Candida species, usually *C. albicans*. Candidemia is most often a nosocomial infection in a patient receiving broad spectrum antibiotics, which affects the normal gastrointestinal flora and allows overgrowth of the yeast. As colonization spreads from the GI tract to the airway, the skin, and the urinary tract, the probability of candidemia increases. Blood cultures for yeast often take several days to be recognized as positive.

The most common parasitic cause of septic shock is malaria. *Plasmodium falciparum* is a very common cause of sepsis in the endemic area and should be considered in travelers to the tropics. The other species of Plasmodium are usually not associated with shock.

Viruses are uncommon causes of sepsis except in young children.

TREATMENT
Antibiotic Therapy for Sepsis

One of the first tasks in managing patients with trauma and SIRS is to assess the patient and decide whether they have SIRS or sepsis. Most patients with trauma and SIRS on

Table 7 Blood Culture Isolates from Patients with Bacteremic Sepsis

	No.	Percentage
Gram positive (n = 473)		
Staphylococcus aureus	180	20
Coagulase-negative Staph.	90	10
Pneumococcus	74	8
Enterococci	46	5
β-hemolytic streptococci	34	4
Gram negative (n = 406)		
E. coli	246	28
Klebsiella sp.	36	4
Enterobacter, Citrobacter, Serratia spp.	28	3
Pseudomonas	32	4
Other organisms (n = 44)		
Candida	14	2
Anaerobes	27	3

Source: From Ref. 24.

admission to the hospital do not have sepsis (24). Those with a fever, an elevated WBC count with a left shift or signs and symptoms of a localized infection are more likely to have sepsis. Elevated plasma levels of procalcitonin have also been found by one group to be associated with sepsis in patients with trauma (22). The development of SIRS in the hospital raises the level of suspicion that an infection has developed, either as a result of the trauma or a nosocomial infection.

✍ **There is no evidence that antibiotic therapy improves the outcome of SIRS in the absence of sepsis.** ✍ A great deal of money is spent on prophylactic antibiotics in patients with SIRS and these antibiotics have an adverse effect on the antibiotic resistance profile of organisms found in the ICU.

✍ **The distinction between SIRS and sepsis is critical because it triggers the decision tree for the administration of antibiotic therapy.** ✍ Patients with presumed sepsis should all receive antibiotics, while those with SIRS alone should not. The choice of antibiotics depends upon the presumed or known microbiologic source of sepsis (Table 6), the antibiotic sensitivity profile of bacteria in the hospital, allergies affecting that patient, and the antibiotic choices offered by the hospital formulary. For example, in patients with sepsis and evidence of a urinary tract infection, coverage should be focused on Gram-negative rods and/or Enterococci. If there is no clear source of infection, antibiotic coverage should include both Gram-positive and Gram-negative bacteria. The incidence of Methicillin-resistant *Staphylococcus aureus* (MRSA) varies greatly from area to area. In most urban centers, however, the incidence of MRSA is high enough (>15%) to warrant the initial use of vancomycin (until isolates demonstrate sensitivities). Similarly, the antibiotic sensitivity pattern of Gram-negative bacteria is highly variable. In general, a third-generation cephalosporin or an anti-pseudomonal penicillin with a beta-lactamase inhibitor (with or without a quinolone) are reasonable choices for Gram-negative organisms. The low incidence of obligate anaerobes in the bloodstream (Table 7) is probably due to the source of the cultures; in patients with an abdominal source of sepsis obligate anaerobes should be covered as well.

Regarding fungal sepsis, fluconazole is adequate therapy for candida colonization and prophylaxis. However, candida species other than albicans are not reliably sensitive to fluconazole. Sepsis due to filamentous fungi is very uncommon, and only occurs in the immunocompromised. Invasive fungal infections require treatment with amphotericin-B, an echinocandin (e.g., caspofungin), or voriconazole (see Volume 2, Chapter 53).

Clinicians should develop reasonable antibiotic treatment strategies to achieve microbial coverage for commonly encountered pathogens and use those antibiotics in the majority of situations. That allows the physician to become familiar with the antibiotic dosages and side effects. One should avoid using unfamiliar or novel antibiotics unless there is a clear rationale for their use. Just as importantly, the results of cultures should be used to modify decisions. If the patient has bacteremic sepsis without a clear source, the antibiotic use can be tailored to treat the organism causing the bacteremia. Volume 2, Chapter 53 provides a review of antibiotic selection for various causes of sepsis. If the patient has no positive cultures and the SIRS are improving, antibiotics can be stopped.

✍ **A major source of sepsis in the ICU is IV catheters.** ✍ Care should be taken to insert all catheters aseptically, and catheter care should be a part of the daily routine. If the patient develops sepsis in the hospital, blood cultures should be drawn through the central venous and arterial catheters as well as from a peripheral vein. If a decision is made to change an IV catheter a new puncture site should be used to insert the new catheter; changing a catheter over a wire does not decrease the chance of catheter-related bacteremia. Prevention of ventilator-associated pneumonia and urinary tract infections associated with Foley catheters is also important.

Early Goal-Directed Therapy of Fluids and Vasopressors

A recent study has emphasized the usefulness of early, aggressive and structured therapy with crystalloid and vasopressive agents (27). The study randomized patients to "early goal-directed" therapy versus standard therapy. In those who were treated with the goal-directed therapy, a central venous catheter capable of sensing mixed venous O_2 (ScvO$_2$) and an intra-arterial catheter were inserted in the Emergency Ward. The patients were given fluids, vasopressors, or vasodilators to maintain the central venous pressure between 8 and 12 mmHg, the mean arterial pressure between 65 and 90 mmHg, and urine output >0.5 ml/kg/hr and the ScvO$_2$ >70%. Once these parameters were achieved, SaO$_2$ >93%, hematocrit >30%, and the cardiac index was maximized by blood transfusion and use of dobutamine in increments of 2.5 μg/kg/min (adjusted every 30 min) to maintain the central venous oxygen saturation at 70% or higher with a maximal dose of 20 μg/kg/min. If these parameters could not be achieved, the patients were sedated and mechanical ventilation was started to decrease oxygen consumption. This therapy was done in the Emergency Ward. After six hours of therapy, the two groups of patients were treated identically. The mortality rate was monitored for 60 days. The group treated with early goal-directed therapy had a dramatically lower in-hospital mortality (30.5%) compared to the standard therapy group (46.5%). The 28- and 60-day mortality rates were also better in the early goal-directed therapy group. This was a relatively small study (263 patients total), but this approach makes a great deal of common sense, should be easy to implement, and is inexpensive.

Glucose Management

✍ An important recent discovery impacting outcome in sepsis is the importance of tight glucose control in the surgical ICU population (28). ✍ Patients who were treated with an insulin drip to maintain their blood sugar between 80 and 110 mg/dl had a significantly better survival than patients whose blood sugar was allowed to rise to 180 mg/dl before insulin therapy was stated. The incidence of sepsis was also lower in the tight glucose control group (see Volume 2, Chapter 60).

Corticosteroids

The role of corticosteroids has been studied intermittently for 40 years. It is clear that high dose steroids are not helpful in sepsis. More recently, the finding that some patients had "relative" adrenal insufficiency revived the notion that low dose corticosteroids might be helpful in sepsis. The concept of "relative" adrenal insufficiency is somewhat fuzzy. Patients with SIRS or sepsis tend to have elevated baseline cortisols, which may explain their poor

response to adrenocorticotropic hormone (ACTH). One small clinical trial has suggested that patients with a blunted response to ACTH (75% of the total) had a lower mortality rate than controls if they were treated with 50 mg hydrocortisone IV every six hour and 50 mg of fludrocortisone orally every day for seven days (29). All patients were enrolled within eight hours of admission to the ICU. There was no difference in the mortality rates in those patients without relative adrenal insufficiency but there was a difference in mortality rate in the whole patient population. This paper supports the use of low dose corticoid therapy. However, it is a single, relatively small study. There is no clear consensus definition of a blunted response to ACTH. The incidence of blunted responses in this study seems extraordinarily high. For all these reasons, the routine use of steroids cannot be recommended. In patients who are on chronic steroids, or those who have adrenal insufficiency, stress dose steroids should be administered.

Adjunctive Therapies for Sepsis
Activated Protein C- PROWESS Trial

✍ Activated protein C is the first useful adjunctive therapy for sepsis documented in a large, international randomized clinical trial (PROWESS: Protein C Worldwide Efficacy Trial in Severe Sepsis) (30). ✍ The rationale for this therapy was that activated protein C (APC) inhibits the clotting cascade at several points and has anti-inflammatory properties (31). The levels of APC are depressed in patients with meningococcal sepsis, and those patients are not able to activate exogenous protein C (32). In the PROWESS trial, patients had to be enrolled within 24 hour of onset of SIRS. Patients with <30,000 platelets, or on therapeutic doses of anticoagulant, those with recent surgery, head trauma, GI bleeding, chronic renal failure, cirrhosis, bone marrow transplants, or HIV infection were excluded. APC was given as a 96 hour continuous infusion. The study showed that 25% of the patients treated with APC died by 28 days after treatment compared to 31% in the control group (P = 0.005). The levels of D-dimer and IL-6 were significantly lower in the APC group than in the control patients. APC therapy improved the outcome in patients with both Gram-positive and Gram-negative sepsis. Those patients older than 50 and with more than one dysfunctional organ had maximum benefit. The incidence of serious bleeding was higher in the APC group than in the control group (3.5% vs. 2%), but did not quite reach statistical significance (P = 0.06).

The PROWESS trial indicates that APC is a useful adjunctive therapy for the treatment of septic shock. There is disagreement among experts about how widely APC should be used. The Food and Drug Administration (FDA) has approved APC for the therapy of septic shock in patients with an Acute Physiological and Chronic Health Evaluation (APACHE II) score >25. There are many issues left unresolved. The drug is expensive, costing $6000/patient, so it should not be given to patients with SIRS without strong evidence of an infection. Furthermore, many of the exclusion criteria are common clinical situations. If a patient has DIC and platelets of <30,000, should they be excluded? What about patients with chronic renal failure on dialysis, or those who have been treated with a bone marrow transplant? These questions remain unanswered.

It is interesting that another inhibitor of the coagulation pathway, anti-thrombin III, is not an effective therapy for sepsis (33). There is no clear reason why APC is effective and anti-thrombin III is not.

Failed Attempts of Adjunctive Therapy

There have been many other randomized trials of adjunctive therapies for sepsis over the past 30 years and almost all of them have failed to demonstrate any benefit. There are several excellent reviews of these trials (21,34–39). Problems that all of these trials face include heterogeneity of the patient population, uncertainty of the optimal timing of the administration of the potential therapy, uncertainty of the optimal dose of the potential therapy and the use of "all cause mortality" as an endpoint. These trials are also now facing the reduction in mortality rate of sepsis to 30%. Given the severity of some cases of sepsis, it is not clear how much lower the mortality rate can be expected to fall, even with effective adjunctive therapy. The decreasing mortality rate for sepsis increases the number of patients that must be enrolled in a given clinical trial, and therefore, increases the expense and time involved. It is no wonder that the "nearly 40-year history of clinical trials of anti-inflammatory strategies for the treatment of sepsis has been referred to as a 'graveyard' for pharmaceutical companies . . ." (21).

Marshall has suggested a rational approach to deciding what compounds should be tested in clinical sepsis trials and how those trials should be done (34). These include testing in a panel of animal models of sepsis, including endotoxinemia and sepsis, to ensure that the intervention actually has some promise in preclinical studies. He also suggests that physiologic testing be done for patients with sepsis before an efficacy trial is considered. He also proposes that morbidity, as well as mortality, be considered as an endpoint. We will not extensively review the unsuccessful treatments here, but will briefly touch on a few of the most prominent trials.

Anti-endotoxin Therapy with Antibody

The first trial of anti-endotoxin strategy was done using polyclonal antiserum to a whole bacterial vaccine, using an *E. coli* strain that lacked most of its polysaccharide (40). Patients with Gram-negative sepsis were the population treated, and there was a statistically significant decrease in the mortality rate in those given immune serum compared to those given preimmune serum. This led to the creation of a monoclonal antibody to the lipid A region of LPS, known as HA-1A. HA-1A was tested in two trials. In the first, patients with Gram-negative sepsis were thought to benefit from antibody therapy (41). In a second clinical trial there was no benefit seen (42). Since only 50% of the patients with septic shock have Gram-negative infections, it is perhaps not surprising that this therapy was not effective in the total population. However, subsequent in vitro experiments suggested that the monoclonal antibody bound to LPS poorly and did not neutralize its biological activity (43). There are naturally occurring LPS binding proteins. One of these is called bactericidal/permeability-increasing protein (BPI). This is a protein naturally found in the granules of neutrophils. A recombinant fragment of BPI was found to have some activity in meningococcal sepsis, using morbidity as an endpoint (44). The study was underpowered to detect differences in mortality, primarily because so many patients died or became moribund before the study drug could be administered. This study does validate the concept that anti-LPS therapy might work in a disease where endotoxin is the primary PAMP, such as meningococcal disease.

Anti-tumor Necrosis Factor Therapy

The most extensively studied adjunctive treatment for sepsis has been anti-TNF therapy, with either monoclonal antibodies or soluble TNF receptors. The 10 studies investigating anti-TNF therapies have been recently reviewed by Marshall (34). Though some small studies show a trend toward benefit, larger studies show no effect. In one study using a tumor necrosis factor:Fc receptor fusion protein, higher doses of the protein appeared to be associated with increased mortality (45).

Nitric Oxide Synthase Inhibitors

Since Nitric Oxide is a potent vasodilator, there was initially a great hope that inhibition of its formation would be an effective therapy for septic shock. Unfortunately, several different types of NO synthase inhibitors have been tested and found to improve blood pressure and decrease the need for vasopressors but not improve the mortality in sepsis (34).

EYE TO THE FUTURE

Bacterial resistance to antibiotics is an increasing problem in medicine. Improved understanding of the receptors allowing bacterial adherence and virulence are yielding multiple promising areas to focus treatment of sepsis. Indeed, we may soon have techniques for manipulating surface adhesion molecules to either promote leukocyte migration or inhibit bacterial adherence in the first place (46). In addition, the recent success of the PROWESS trial and progress made in understanding the molecular basis of septic and inflammatory mediators has fostered a renewed enthusiasm in the pharmaceutical industry to investigate therapies for sepsis. The interest of physicians in this problem remains high because of the large number of patients who die every year. We will briefly discuss a few promising ideas that are on the clinical horizon, but have not yet been tested in clinical trials.

Extracorporeal Blood Purification

The idea of purifying blood of inflammatory mediators and/or PAMPs by hemofiltration or hemadsorption is an intuitively appealing one. There are a variety of techniques that could be used. Some of these are used in septic patients with renal failure, and they seem to be safe. However, there are no clinical trials to formally assess safety or efficacy (47).

High Mobility Group B1 Protein

High mobility group B1 (HMGB1) protein was initially identified as a nuclear binding protein. It also binds to the macrophage and endothelial cell receptor for advanced glycation end products and activates those cells to produce inflammatory cytokines (36,48). In mouse models of endotoxinemia and peritonitis, antibody to HMGB1 protein improved survival (48,49). HMGB1 protein levels are high in patients with sepsis, and in one very small sample, appeared to be correlated with mortality. There are no intervention studies (or clinical trials) in nonhuman primates.

Complement C5a and C5a Receptor

The mannose on bacterial surfaces activates complement through the classical pathway via the mannose binding protein, and LPS activates the alternative complement pathway. Both pathways generate the C5 peptide fragment C5a, which is a chemoattractant and a pro-inflammatory peptide. Antibody to C5a improved survival in a rat model of peritonitis (50). There are no studies in humans or non-human primates. An obvious hurdle is that C5a at the site of infection is beneficial only for a brief window of time (when sepsis syndrome is overwhelming but bacterial burden is low).

Apoptosis

The idea that apoptosis of immune cells, antigen presenting cells, and epithelial cells is a critical part of sepsis has become recognized over the past several years (3,51,52). One intriguing finding is that activated protein C activates anti-apoptotic genes in endothelial cells, which may partially explain its activity in sepsis (31). Specific caspase inhibitors have been shown to improve survival in a mouse model of peritonitis (53). This protection appeared to be dependent upon lymphocytes, though lymphocyte-deficient mice were much more susceptible to peritonitis compared to controls.

Two recent studies in septic rodents demonstrated significant survival benefit by inhibiting apoptosis (54,55). The first utilized the knowledge that the protease inhibitor (PI) class of antiretroviral agents is known to prevent apoptosis in vitro, and was evaluated in a mouse cecal perforation and ligation (CPL) sepsis model in regards to lymphocyte apoptosis and consequent cytokine production (54). The investigators used a PI mixture consisting of 125 mg/kg nelfinavir (Agouron Pharmaceuticals, La Jolla, CA, U.S.A.) and 13 mg/kg ritonavir (Abbott Pharmaceuticals, Abbott Park, IL, U.S.A.) in 2% ethanol in distilled water or vehicle control (2% ethanol). Mice pretreated with PIs demonstrated improved survival (67%; P < 0.0005) compared with controls (17%) and a significant (P < 0.05) reduction in lymphocyte apoptosis. Even mice receiving therapy beginning four hours after perforation demonstrated improved survival (50%; P < 0.05) compared with controls.

PI therapy is also associated with an increase in the Th1 cytokine TNF-α (P < 0.05) early in sepsis and a reduction in the Th2 cytokines IL-6 and IL-10 (P < 0.05) late in sepsis; despite no intrinsic antibacterial effects, PI also reduced quantitative bacterial blood cultures. The beneficial effects of PI appear to be specific to lymphocyte apoptosis, as lymphocyte-deficient Rag1-/- mice did not experience benefit from treatment with PI. Thus, inhibition of lymphocyte apoptosis by PI is a candidate approach for the clinical treatment of sepsis (54).

The second study demonstrated that the serine threonine kinase Akt over expressed in lymphocytes prevents sepsis-induced apoptosis, causes a Th1 cytokine propensity, and improves survival (55). Findings from this study strengthen the concept that a major defect in sepsis is impairment of the adaptive immune system, and further bolsters the concept that strategies to prevent lymphocyte apoptosis represent an important new avenue of sepsis therapy. Once again, there are no studies of this promising approach in nonhuman primates or human beings.

SUMMARY

Sepsis continues to be an important problem responsible for the majority of deaths in the ICU. As we enter a new millennium, the mortality rate is at 30% in the most aggressively and carefully managed patients. It is likely that further progress in this syndrome will be incremental, rather than dramatic. The most important keys to the management of patients with sepsis are careful attention to their fluid and pressor management and judicious use of appropriate antibiotics. Adjunctive therapy with activated protein C should be strongly considered in patients who meet the admission criteria and should be thoughtfully contemplated in some patients who would have been excluded. As in all phases of medicine, prevention is superior to therapy, so preventing nosocomial infections should also be a focus of the ICU practice.

KEY POINTS

- SIRS and sepsis are such global responses that focusing on one or a few aspects of the response necessarily oversimplifies the true pathophysiology of the disease.
- The constituents of microbial organisms that elicit inflammatory responses are collectively known as PAMPs.
- A wide variety of mammalian cells respond to PAMPs. These include PMNs, blood monocytes, tissue macrophages and dendritic cells.
- The timely and appropriate collection of cultures is a mainstay of diagnostic management of sepsis.
- In the setting of trauma, most patients with SIRS do not have an infectious source.
- There is no evidence that antibiotic therapy improves the outcome of SIRS in the absence of sepsis.
- The distinction between SIRS and sepsis is critical because it triggers the decision tree for the administration of antibiotic therapy.
- A major source of sepsis in the ICU is I.V. catheters.
- An important recent discovery impacting outcome in sepsis is the importance of tight glucose control in the surgical ICU population.
- Activated protein C is the first useful adjunctive therapy for sepsis documented in a large, international randomized clinical trial (PROWESS: Protein C Worldwide Efficacy Trial in Severe Sepsis).

REFERENCES

1. Annane D, Aegerter P, Jars-Guincestre MC, Guidet B, Network C.-R. Current epidemiology of septic shock: the CUB-Rea network. Am J Respir Crit Care Med 2003; 168(2):165–172.
2. Bone RC, Balk RA, Cerra FB, et al. American College of Chest Physicians/Society of Crit Care Med Consensus Conference: Definitions for sepsis and organ failure and guidelines for the use of innovative therapies in sepsis. Chest 1992; 101:1644–1655.
3. Hotchkiss RS, Karl IE. The pathophysiology and treatment of sepsis. N Eng J Med 2003; 348(2):138–150.
4. Levy MM, Fink MP, Marshall JC, et al. 2001 SCCM/ESICM/ACCP/ATS/SIS international sepsis definitions conference. Crit Care Med 2003; 31(4):1250–1256.
5. Janeway CA. The immune system evolved to discriminate infectious non-self from noninfectious self. Immunol Today 1992; 13:11–16.
6. Medzhitov R, Preston-Hurlburt P, Janeway CA. A human homologue of the *drosophila* toll protein signals activation of adaptative immunity. Nature 1997; 388:394–397.
7. Aderem A, Ulevitch RJ. Toll-like receptors in the induction of the innate immune response. Nature 2000; 406:782–787.

8. Akira S, Takeda K, Kaisho T. Toll-like receptors: critical proteins linking innate and acquired immunity. Nature Immunol 2001; 2(8):675–680.

9. Taveira da Silva AM, Kaulbach HC, Chuidian FS, DLambert DR, Suffredini AF, Danner Rl. Brief Report: Shock and multiple-organ dysfunction after self-administration of salmonella endotoxin. N Eng J Med 1993; 328(20): 1457–1460.

10. Tapping RI, Tobias PS. Cellular binding of soluble CD14 requires lipopolysaccharide (LPS) and LPS-binding protein. J Biol Chem 1997; 272:23157–23164.

11. Wright SD, Ramos RA, Tobias PS, Ulevitch RJ, Mathison JC. CD14, a receptor for complexes of lipopolysaccharide (LPS) and LPS binding protein. Science 1990; 249: 1431–1433.

12. Poltorak A, He S, Smirnova I, et al. Defective LPS signaling in C3H/HeJ and C57BL/10ScCr mice: Mutations in Tlr4 gene. Science 1998; 282:2085–2088.

13. Shimazu R, Akashi S, Ogata H, et al. MD-2, a molecule that confers lipopolysaccharide responsiveness on toll-like receptor 4. J Exp Med 1999; 189(11):1777–1782.

14. Ozinsky A, Underhill DM, Fontenot JD, et al. The repertoire for pattern recognition of pathogens by the innate immune system is defined by cooperation between toll-like receptors. PNAS 2000; 97(25):13766–13771.

15. Takeda K, Kaisho T, Akira S. Toll-like receptors. Ann Rev Immunol 2003; 21:335–376.

16. Huang Q, Liu D, Majewski P, et al. The plasticity of dendritic cell responses to pathogens and their components. Science 2001; 294:870–875.

17. Pugin J, Schurer-Maly CC, Leturcq D, Moriarty A, Ulevitch RJ, Tobias PS. Lipopolysaccharide activation of human endothelial and epithelial cells is mediated by lipopolysaccharide-binding protein and soluble CD14. PNAS 1993; 90:2744–2748.

18. Gerritsen ME, Bloor CM. Endothelial cell gene expression in response to injury. FASEB J 1993; 7:523–532.

19. Pober JS, Cotran RS. Cytokines and endothelial cell biology. Physiol Rev 1990; 70:427–451.

20. Aird WC. The role of the endothelium in severe sepsis and multiple organ dysfunction syndrome. Blood 2003; 101(10):3765–3777.

21. Riedemann NC, Guo R, Ward PA. The enigma of sepsis. J Clin Invest 2003; 112(4):460–467.

22. Harbarth S, Holeckova K, Froidevaux C, Pittet D, Ricou B, Grau GE, Vadas L, Pugin J. Geneva Sepsis Network. Diagnostic value of procalcitonin, interleukin-6, and interleukin-8 in critically ill patients admitted with suspected sepsis. Am J Respir Crit Care Med 2001; 164(3):396–402.

23. Bossink AW, Groeneveld AB, Koffeman GI, Becker A. Prediction of shock in febrile medical patients with a clinical infection. Crit Care Med 2001; 29(1):25–31.

24. Brun-Buisson C. The epidemiology of the systemic inflammatory response. Inten Care Med 2000; 26(Suppl 1): S64–S74.

25. Kieft H, Hoepelman AIM, Zhou W, Rozenberg-Arska M, Struyvenberg A, Verhoef J. The sepsis syndrome in a Dutch University Hospital. Clinical observation. Arch Intern Med 1993; 153(19):2241–2247.

26. Aledo A, Heller G, Ren L, Gardner S, Dunkel I, McKay SW, Flombaum C, Brown AE. Septicemia and septic shock in pediatric patients: 140 consecutive cases on a pediatric hematology-on oncology service. J Pediatr Hematol Oncol 1998; 20(3):215–221.

27. Rivers E, Nguyen B, Havstad S, Ressler J, Muzzin A, Knoblich B, Peterson E, Tomlanovich M. Goal-Directed Therapy Collaborative Group. Early goal-directed therapy in the treatment of severe sepsis and septic shock. N Eng J Med 2002; 345(19):1368–1377.

28. Van Den Berghe G, Wouters P, Weekers F, et al. Intensive insulin therapy in critically ill patients. N Eng J Med 2001; 345(19):1359–1367.

29. Annane D, Sebille V, Charpentier C, et al. Effect of treatment with low doses of hydrocortisone and fludrocortisone on mortality in patients with septic shock. JAMA 2002; 288(7):862–871.

30. Bernard GR, Vincent J, Laterre P, et al. Efficacy and safety of recombinant human activated protein C for severe sepsis. N Eng J Med 2001; 344(10):699–709.

31. Joyce DE, Gelbert L, Ciaccia A, DeHoff B, Grinnell BW. Gene expression profile of antithrombotic protein C defines new mechanisms modulating inflammation and apoptosis. J Biol Chem 2001; 276(14):11199–11203.

32. Faust SN, Levin M, Harrison OB, et al. Dysfunction of endothelial protein C activation in severe meningococcal sepsis. N Eng J Med 2001; 345(6):408–416.

33. Warren RL, Eid A, Singer P, et al. Caring for the critically ill patient. High-dose antithrombin III in severe sepsis: a randomized controlled trial. JAMA 2001; 286(15):1869–1878.

34. Marshall JC. Such stuff as dreams are made of: mediator-directed therapy in sepsis. Nat Rev 2003; 2:391–405.

35. Vincent JL, Sun Q, Dubois MJ. Clinical trials of immunomodulatory therapies in severe sepsis and septic shock. Clin Infect Dis 2002; 34(8):1084–1893.

36. Riedmann NC, Guo RF, Ward PA. Novel strategies for the treatment of sepsis. Nat Med 2003; 9(5):517–524.

37. Sessler CN, Shepherd W. New concepts in sepsis. Curr Opin Crit Care 2002; 8(5):465–472.

38. Patel GP, Gurka DP, Balk RA. New treatment strategies for severe sepsis and septic shock. Curr Opin Crit Care 2003; 9(5):390–396.

39. Cross AS, Opal SM. A new paradigm for the treatment of sepsis: Is it time to consider combination therapy? Ann Intern Med 2003; 138:502–505.

40. Ziegler EJ, McCutchan JA, Fierer J, et al. Treatment of gram-negative bacteremia and shock with human antiserum to a mutant *Escherichia coli*. N Eng J Med 1982; 307(20):1225–1230.

41. Ziegler EJ, Fisher CJ, Sprung CL, et al. Treatment of gram-negative bacteremia and septic shock with HA-1A human monoclonal antibody against endotoxin. A randomized, double-blind, placebo-controlled trial. The HA-1A Sepsis Study Group. N Eng J Med 1991; 324(7):429–436.

42. McCloskey RV, Straube RC, Saunders C, Smith SM, Smith CR, Group MCTS. Treatment of septic shock with human monoclonal antibody HA-1A: A randomized, double-blind, placebo-controlled trial. Ann Intern Med 1994; 121(1):1–5.

43. Warren HS, Amato SF, Fitting C, et al. Assessment of ability of murine and human anti-lipid A monoclonal antibodies to bind and neutralize lipopolysaccharide. J Exp Med 1993; 177(1):89–97.

44. Levin M, Quint PA, Goldstein B, et al. Recombinant bactericidal/permeability-increasing protein (rBPI$_{21}$) as adunctive treatment for children with severe meningococcal sepsis: a randomised trial. Lancet 2000; 356(9234):961–967.

45. Fisher CJ, Agosti JM, Opal SM, et al. Treatment of septic shock with the tumor necrosis factor receptor:Fc fusion protein. N Eng J Med 1996; 334(26):1697–1702.

46. Martinez-Mier G, Toledo-Pereyra LW, Ward PA: Adhesion molecules and hemorrhagic shock. J Trauma 2001; 51(2): 408–415.

47. Venkataraman R, Subramanian S, Kellum JA. Clinical review: extracorporeal blood purification in severe sepsis. Crit Care 2003; 7(2):139–145.

48. Wang H, Bloom O, Zhang M, et al. HMG-1 as a late mediator of endotoxin lethality in mice. Science 1999; 285:248–251.

49. Yang H, Ochani M, Li J, et al. Reversing established sepsis with antagonists of endogenous high-mobility group box 1. Proc Natl Acad Sci 2004; 101(1):296–301.

50. Czermak BJ, Sarma V, Pierson CL, et al. Protective effects of C5a blockade in sepsis. Nat Med 1999; 5(7):788–792.

51. Oberholzer C, Oberholzer A, Clare-Salzler M, Moldawer LL. Apoptosis in sepsis: a new target for therapeutic exploration. FASEB J 2001; 15(6):879–892.

52. Munshi N, Fernandis AZ, Cherla RP, Park I-W, Ganju RK. Lipopolysaccharide-induced apoptosis of endothelial cells and its inhibition by vascular endothelial growth factor. J Immunol 2002; 168(168):5860–5866.

53. Hotchkiss RS, Chang KC, Swanson PE, et al. Caspase inhibitors improve survival in sepsis: a critical role of the lymphocyte. Nat Immunol 2000; 1(6):496–501.

54. Weaver JGR, Rouse MS, Steckelberg JM, et al. Improved survival in experimental sepsis with an orally administered inhibitor of apoptosis. FASEB J 2004; 18: 1185–1191.

55. Bommhardt U, Chang KC, Swanson PE, Wagner TH. Akt decreases lymphocyte apoptosis and improves survival in sepsis. J Immunol 2004; 172:7583–7591.

48

Ventilator-Associated Pneumonia

Thomas Genuit

Department of Surgery, R Adams Cowley Shock-Trauma Center, Baltimore, Maryland, U.S.A.

Lena M. Napolitano

Department of Surgery, University of Michigan School of Medicine, Ann Arbor, Michigan, U.S.A.

INTRODUCTION

Hospital-acquired or nosocomial pneumonia is the second most common nosocomial infection in the United States and is associated with substantial morbidity and mortality (1). Conservative analyses estimate the cost related to increased length of hospital stay and resource utilization to over $1.5 billion annually (2).

Most hospitalized patients who develop pneumonia have one or more risk factors, including the age of 65 years or more, immuno-suppression, altered-sensorium, significant pre-existing cardiac or pulmonary disease, or have undergone major thoraco-abdominal surgical procedures (3).

Ventilator-associated pneumonia (VAP) is defined as nosocomial pneumonia (NP) in patients who have received mechanical ventilation for a time period of more than 48 hr and did not demonstrate any prior signs or symptoms of pneumonia (4). Although individuals receiving mechanical ventilation do not comprise the largest subgroup among all patients that develop NP, they are at the highest individual risk for this infection. Mechanical ventilation increases the risk for NP in a time dependent fashion by a factor of 6–21 (5).

Recent data from the Centers for Disease Control (CDC) National Nosocomial Infection Surveillance (NNIS) group documents that trauma patients have one of the highest VAP rates (16.2/1000 ventilator days, Table 1) amongst critically ill patients (6).

Therapy of VAP can be difficult due to the involvement of resistant organisms and overall reduced state of health of the host. This contributes to the significant morbidity and high mortality rates. Prevention of VAP through an organized multimodality approach is one of the most important goals in patients receiving mechanical ventilation.

PATHOPHYSIOLOGY OF VENTILATOR-ASSOCIATED PNEUMONIA

The pathophysiology of VAP is complex and includes host-related, equipment-related, and microbial factors that promote colonization of the tracheobronchial tree, impaired clearance of micro-organisms, and alteration of the local immune response, ultimately leading to pulmonary infection (Fig. 1).

Ventilator Equipment and Health Care Worker Cross Contamination

Ventilzator equipment and health care worker cross contamination have long been implicated in the pathogenesis of VAP via means of aerosolization and inhalation of micro-organisms. The relative risk of contamination contributed by each component in the chain of infection is reviewed in Table 2. Although there are numerous possible equipment related sources of infection, healthcare worker cross contamination is generally a far more important contributor.

Because of the use of filters, the internal machinery of mechanical ventilators is not considered an important source of bacterial contamination of the inhaled gas. Routine sterilization or high-grade disinfection is currently not recommended (7–9). The current generation of filters is capable of protecting the internal pathways from colonization. However, these filters require periodic replacement. Furthermore, if patients are ventilated without the filters in place, high-grade disinfection of the internal machinery is required.

Studies have shown, however, that the external breathing circuit may become colonized with bacteria within 8 to 24 hours of use (9). In an attempt to decrease the rate of VAP the impact of scheduled circuit changes at frequencies ranging from daily to weekly have been studied. No consistent benefit could be demonstrated with these changes and there is some evidence that changes more often than every 48 hours may actually increase the incidence of VAP (10–12). At the same time no data exists that delineates the maximum safe duration of use for the circuit tubing. Given the significant materials and labor costs, routine circuit changes are currently not recommended and when used should not be done more frequently than every 48 hours (13–17).

One of the mechanisms believed important in contaminating the patient's tracheo-bronchial tree is related to accidental spillage of contaminated condensate in the tubing by improper handling. Spillage of condensate should be avoided. No studies have shown consistent benefits of condensate traps versus periodic drainage of the condensate (18,19).

Most hospitals in the US currently use bubble-through or wick humidifiers, which does not produce significant amounts of aerosols. Although inspiratory-phase tubing condensate formation may be increased, there is no data to convincingly show an increase in the rate of VAP. The water in these devices is usually heated to temperatures that reduce bacterial growth; however, it is currently

Table 1 Ventilator-Associated Pneumonia in the Intensive Care Setting[a]

Type of ICU	Number of ICU's	Ventilator days[b]	Mean VAP rate[c]	Median VAP rate[d]
Respiratory	7	24,519	4.3	—
Pediatric	75	285,607	4.9	3.9
Medical	134	636,355	7.3	6.0
Coronary	100	173,668	8.4	7.1
Medical-surgical[e]	179	674,536	8.7	7.6
Medical-surgical[f]	121	494,941	10.5	9.4
Cardio-thoracic	64	251,034	10.5	9.5
Surgical	152	638,321	13.2	11.6
Neurosurgical	46	107,820	14.9	11.9
Burn	18	28,935	15.9	—
Trauma	25	106,884	16.2	15.3

[a]Pooled data from the Centers for Disease Control National Nosocomial Infection Surveillance report, issued August 2001.
[b]Pooled total number of ventilator days.
[c]VAP rate per 1000 ventilator days (mean).
[d]50% percentile (median) of all units reported.
[e]Nonteaching hospitals.
[f]Major teaching hospitals.
Source: From Ref. 233.

recommended to use sterile or distilled water when operating these devices to avoid contamination with more temperature resistant species that may be found in tap water (20–24). High-grade disinfection between uses in different patients is recommended (21–25). Condensate formation may be reduced by using heat-moisture exchangers (HME) or hygroscopic condenser humidifiers (HCH, "artificial nose"). Some of these devices are equipped with bacterial filters. The advantage of using such filters is not known, and all of these devices can increase the anatomic dead space and resistance of breathing. Respiratory secretions may lead to partial or complete obstruction and frequent device surveillance is required (26–32). Another relatively new attempt of decreasing inspiratory-phase condensate formation is made through use of heated circuit tubing. To date no studies adequately assess its effect on VAP.

Small volume in-line and hand-held nebulizers for the application of medications can produce bacterial aerosols if they or their circuit access site becomes contaminated through improper handling. It is currently recommended to use sterile fluids for nebulization, disinfect and air dry

the devices between uses, maintain strict aseptic technique when accessing the circuit, and avoid multi-dose vials whenever possible. Under these circumstances these devices are not considered a significant source of aerosol contamination (33–34). It is currently recommended to avoid large volume nebulizers (greater than 500 cc in volume) whenever possible. When used, all equipment should be sterilized or high-grade disinfected between uses or at least every 24 hours (35–38).

☞ **Health care worker (HCW) cross contamination has been shown to play an important role in the pathogenesis of VAP.** ☞ The pathogens that cause NP are ubiquitous in the hospital environment, especially in critical care areas. Transmission occurs via the hands of HCW, improper access to the circuit or patient's tracheo-bronchial tree, as well as improper care of respiratory equipment (3). It is of utmost importance to maintain an aseptic technique when accessing the circuit for the administration of medications, tracheal suctioning, or other manipulations. Washing hands before and after contact and wearing of gloves must be strictly enforced, and spillage of circuit condensate into the patient's tracheobronchial tree should be avoided (39–41).

With regard to tracheobronchial suctioning, no studies clearly support the preferential use of multi-use closed system catheters over open systems [single-use catheters, as long as sterile technique (catheter, gloves)] is maintained when using open systems (42–45).

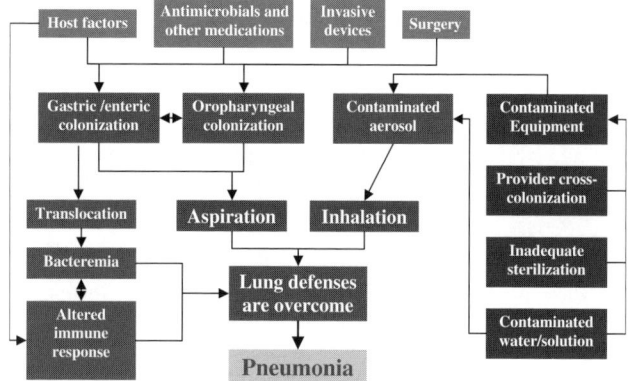

Figure 1 Pathophysiology of ventilator-associated pneumonia.

Endotracheal Tube and Tracheal Colonization

☞ **Endotracheal tube (ETT) bio-film formation and tracheal colonization have been acknowledged as potentially significant factors leading to (chronic) tracheo-bronchitis and subsequent lower airspace infection.** ☞ Certain organisms, particularly *Haemophilus influenzae* and Streptococci (group I pathogens, early VAP) as well as *Staphylococcus* spp., *Pseudomonas* spp. and other enteric gram negative bacteria (group II pathogens, delayed VAP) seem to have a greater propensity to colonize the ETT bio-film.

Table 2 Ventilator Equipment and Health Care Worker Cross-Contamination as a Source of Ventilator-Associated Pneumonia

Cross-contamination mechanism	Relative importance as a contamination-source—comments
Internal machinery of mechanical ventilation	Not a significant source as long as filters are in place.
External breathing circuit	Source of bacterial colonization after 24 hr of use. But not a significant source as long as condensate is frequently emptied (see below) and only one patient is assigned to be ventilated on each breathing circuit.
Spillage of condensate	Large quantities of condensate and exhaled secretions can mix in external tubing. If spilled into patient's trachea, this can represent a large inoculum. Condensate must be emptied frequently.
Humidifiers	Humidifiers can become contaminated. However, with proper disinfection between patients, the use of sterile or distilled water, and frequent emptying of condensate (see above), contamination is minimized.
In-line hand-held nebulizers	In-line nebulizers have been a source of contamination. However, when sterile fluids and strict aseptic techniques are used, these are not a significant source of contamination.
	If MDIs are used one MDI is issued per patient.
Tracheal–bronchial suctioning	As long as sterile technique is maintained, not a source of contamination.
Healthcare worker cross-contamination	This is the dominant source of patient cross contamination!
	Infectious secretions can be accessed by the health care worker from all of the above sources, and carried secretions from one patient to the next.
	Strict hand washing and the use of gloves are mandatory when touching these items, and any others that may be contaminated.

Abbreviation: MDI, metered dose inhalers.

Colonization of the tracheo-bronchial tree was found to precede the development of VAP in the majority of patients (46). In one study, over 70% of patients that developed VAP had identical bacterial isolates recovered from cultures of the ETT bio-film and tracheo-bronchial suctioning. This correlation was not found in patients that did not develop VAP (47). Similar to the ventilator circuit, colonization of the ETT polyvinyl chloride (PVC) material begins within hours after intubation. In this process the bacteria change from a suspension-type to a sessile-type growth mode with formation of a protective glycocalyx layer. Layering of bacteria and polymorphnuclear neutrophils suggests a progressive accretion of respiratory secretions. The sessile bacteria demonstrate greater resistance [higher minimal inhibitory concentration (MIC)] against commonly used antibiotics (48). Local disinfectants (chlorhexidine, hexetidine) demonstrate greater bactericidal activity than standard antibiotic agents against these sessile bacterial concreations (49). Infection of the lower airspaces is believed to result from a progressive descending spread rather than aerosolization of bio-film material. Distal spread is aided by trans-ETT airway manipulations (suctioning) and impaired muco-ciliary clearance of the proximal airways (50). Early colonization (<24 hours) was found to be a significant risk factor (odds ratio 4.1) for VAP in trauma patients (51). Head trauma patients were found to have more than 60% colonization within 24 hours, which may partially explain the higher VAP rates in these patients (52). Late colonization with group II pathogens in some studies has been linked to the prior use of systemic antibiotics; the use of these agents predicted the development of late-onset VAP with an odds ratio of 9.2 (53). Currently, only preliminary data on the use of alternative ETT materials (i.e., silver-coating) is available; although these materials seem to reduce bacterial growth in vitro, their in vivo effect on the incidence of VAP is not clear (54). All of these devices are associated with significant cost and have not yet found widespread utilization in routine clinical practice (54).

Tracheostomies

The early use of tracheostomies has been proposed as an alternative to ETT to reduce the incidence of VAP. In certain patient populations (neurosurgical patients with Glasgow Coma Scale (GCS) less than nine, multiple-trauma patients, burn patients with inhalations injury) a 20–40% reduction of the mean duration of mechanical ventilation was shown by some authors through the use of early (day 3–10 of mechanical ventilation) tracheostomy (55–58). However, no consistent differences in the incidence of VAP or mortality rates have been demonstrated. Furthermore, in a large prospective study on a mixed ICU cohort, the presence of a tracheostomy carried a significantly increased risk for the development of VAP (odds ratio 6.7) (59).

With a tracheostomy in place the air stream bypasses the physiologic filter and immune surveillance organs of the upper airways. Similar rates of airway colonization and impairment of muco-ciliary clearance as those found with ETTs have been demonstrated (60). In addition, tracheostomies, like ETTs, have low-pressure cuffs and do not prevent (micro-) aspiration of pooled oropharyngeal secretions (61–63). These findings may in part explain the offset of results that could be expected from a reduction in duration of mechanical ventilation. The technique of placement (open surgical vs. percutaneous) does not alter outcomes and both can be associated with significant complications (64). To date no universal recommendations can be made as to when and in what patient population to consider for early tracheostomy (65).

Oropharyngeal/Gastrointestinal Colonization and (Micro-) Aspiration

Oropharyngeal and gastrointestinal colonization and (micro-) aspiration have long been implicated in the pathogenesis of VAP. The most commonly found organisms in patients with

VAP are believed to be endogenously acquired, and are part of the enteric flora. In radioisotope tracer studies, healthy non-intubated adults were found to aspirate gastric contents 45% of the time (66). The aspiration rate is believed higher in intubated patients, particularly in the presence of oral or nasogastric tubes, with evidence of gastrointestinal dysmotility (i.e., after abdominal procedures), and in those patients with swallowing abnormalities (i.e., prolonged intubation, and depressed consciousness) (67–73).

☞ **Increased colonization of the esophagus and stomach with a bacterial shift towards pathogenic enteric gram-negative species and candida has been demonstrated in critically ill patients.** ☜

Gastric pH Elevation vs. Sucralfate for Ulcer Prophylaxis

Gastric pH elevation (above four) facilitated by antacid, H_2-blockade, or proton pump-inhibition has been used as ulcer prophylaxis or therapy. However, pH elevation regiments and continuous gastric tube feeding with duodenal-gastric reflux has been shown to lead to gastric bacterial overgrowth (74–76).

A few small clinical trials assessing VAP risk, using sucralfate as an alternative regimen for peptic ulcer prophylaxis, demonstrated lower gastric bacterial counts and a trend towards lower VAP rates with sucralfate use (77–79). Meta-analyses did not show a strong correlation and one study suggested that there might not be a difference in early onset (<4 days) VAP but a significant reduction in late-onset VAP (5% w. sucralfate vs. 16% w. antacids and 21% w. H_2-blockers) (80–82).

☞ **It is currently recommended to use agents that do not raise the gastric pH in patients with low to moderate risk of upper GI bleeding. Drugs that lower pH are recommended for patients at high risk of upper gastrointestinal bleeding.** ☜

Indeed, it has been well-documented that patients with respiratory failure requiring mechanical ventilation for more than 48 hours have a 15.6-fold increased risk of developing a gastrointestinal bleed, compared with other ICU patients (total study cohort = 2252), and therefore appropriate stress ulcer prophylaxis is of paramount importance (79). In the largest prospective randomized (sucralfate vs. ranitidine) study done to date (n = 1200 patients requiring mechanical ventilation), sucralfate was associated with a higher risk of stress-ulcer-related bleeding (3.8 vs. 1.7%, p = 0.02) and no difference in pneumonia rates was identified (p = 0.19) (83).

Selective Decontamination of the Digestive Tract

Selective decontamination of the digestive tract (SDD) has been suggested for two decades as alternative strategy to address gastro-enteric bacterial colonization and risk reduction for VAP (84–86). Optimal SDD regimens are aimed at reducing colonization with aerobic gram-negative bacilli and *Candida* spp. without altering the (protective) anaerobic flora. Various regimens have used combinations of nonabsorbable antibiotics (i.e., aminoglycosides, polymyxin) or quinolones with Amphotericin B or nystatin, applied (as paste or solution) to the oropharynx or enterally via oral or nasogastric tube, as well as combinations with prophylactic systemic agents (i.e., 2nd or 3rd generation cephalosporins, trimethoprim) (87–92). Two early, prospective, randomized, double-blind trials using broncho-alveolar lavage (BAL) or protected specimen brushing (PSB) for the diagnosis of VAP failed to demonstrate any

significant benefit from SDD in terms of duration of mechanical ventilation, incidence of VAP, or mortality (93,84). However, most studies, including several recent meta-analyses, have shown an overall decrease in nosocomial infections (particularly after abdominal procedures) using SDD. The overall impact of SDD on VAP has been difficult to fully assess because of differences in study designs and populations, as well as non-stringent criteria for the diagnosis of VAP and, for the most part, short follow-up periods (95–97). Formal cost-benefit analyses have not yet been performed, and the development of antibiotic resistance continues to be a theoretical concern. Because of the unknown cost-benefit equation, and the concern for resistant organisms, the recent evidence based guidelines on VAP developed by the Canadian Critical Society did not recommend SDD (98).

Enteral Feeding

Enteral feeding (Volume 2, Chapter 32) has been demonstrated to be beneficial in terms of overall infection rates, organ dysfunction, nutritional status, and outcome in critically ill patients (99–103). However, the presence of oral or nasoenteric tubes and increases of gastric pH caused by continuous gastric feeding have been implemented in the development of VAP. It is currently recommended to routinely verify the position of these tubes in all patients prior to starting feeds; the patient's enteric motility should be assessed routinely by clinical examination and documentation of gastric residuals. Although gastric feeds should be withheld upon evidence of significant gastric pooling (despite motility agents), no data demonstrates a universal benefit of post-pyloric tubes. Similarly, no clear benefit has been demonstrated through use of small-bore tubes. Further distal tubes (i.e., jejunal) and tubes with the combined ability to feed distally and decompress the gastric reservoir (i.e., gastro-jejunostomy) that bypass the oropharyngeal-esophageal route may be beneficial but have not been studied adequately. All transesophageal feeding tubes should be removed as soon as clinically feasible (69,100). Acidification of gastric feeds has been demonstrated to reduce bacterial colonization of the stomach (104), but no significant difference in the incidence of VAP was demonstrated in a prospective randomized multicenter trial (105). Likewise, no data to date convincingly demonstrates a difference in VAP with the use of bolus versus continuous enteral feeds (106,107). Randomized trials show that the semi-recumbent position (elevating the head of bed ≥30°) compared with the supine position is associated with less gastroesophageal aspiration and pneumonia in patients receiving mechanical ventilation (102,107,108).

Oropharyngeal Colonization, Pooling of Secretions, and Micro-Aspiration

More recently the concept of oropharyngeal colonization, pooling of secretions, and micro-aspiration in the pathogenesis of VAP has drawn some attention. Studies have shown that the currently used high-volume low-pressure ETT cuffs do not prevent leakage of secretions into the trachea. Although the pathogens most commonly responsible for VAP are found only infrequently and in low numbers in the pharynx of healthy individuals, a bacterial shift and colonization similar to that of the stomach occurs in the critically ill (109,110). The likelihood of (early) colonization substantially increases with depressed consciousness, immunosupression, shock, renal failure, malnutrition, and placement of oral or nasogastric tubes (111). Bacterial (adherence) factors and alteration of the patient's mucosal defense (surface proteins and polysaccharides, IgA, pH, etc.) improve bacterial adherence and growth (112–115).

♂ **Recent studies have demonstrated significant reductions in VAP (37–69%) and mortality (40–45%) in critically ill surgical and cardiac surgery patients by improving oral hygiene through frequent suctioning of pooled secretions and the use of the topical disinfectant chlorhexidine (116–118). ♂**

Specialized Hi-Lo Evac Endotracheal Tubes Assist with Continuous Aspiration of Sub-glottic Secretions

In mechanically ventilated patients, subglottic secretions pool above the ETT cuff, where they can contaminate the lower respiratory tract and cause pneumonia (119). Recently, a specialized ETT with an additional lumen that terminates in the sub-glottic space above the ETT cuff has been developed to allow for continuous aspiration of sub-glottic secretions (CASS) (120). The Malencrodt Hi-Lo Evac ETT utilizes the CASS principle, and compared to a standard ETT has been shown to reduce the incidence of VAP by up to 75% (120).

However, these tubes are associated with increased material costs, some problems still exist with occlusion of the suction port by respiratory secretions, and benefits for patients that are intubated for less than 72 hours may be questionable (121,122).

Pulmonary De-recruitment

♂ **Pulmonary de-recruitment (atelectasis, alveolar collapse) begins early and is progressive in supine patients receiving mechanical ventilation.** ♂ The weight of the abdominal contents is transmitted preferentially though elevation and dysfunction of the posterior diaphragm to the posterior inferior lung aspects. At the same time the weight of the mediastinum is transmitted posteriorly. This leads to a shift in the ventilation-perfusion (VQ) zones and relative under-ventilation and vascular congestion of the posterior lung aspects. Thoracic and abdominal procedures significantly interfere with chest and abdominal wall compliance and function and aggravate this problem. The use of higher FiO_2 with associated nitrogen washout as well as loss of surfactant associated with more severe respiratory failure augments the alveolar collapse. Atelectatic areas of the lung are at higher risk for bacterial infection due to increased build up of stagnant secretions. Conventional mode ventilation (low inspiratory to expiratory [I:E] time ratio) and use of positive end-expiratory pressure (PEEP) do not reliably prevent progression of this process. Several strategies have been employed to address this problem but none have been studied rigorously.

Inverse I:E ventilation, higher levels of PEEP, and alternative modes like Airway Pressure Release Ventilation (APRV) may offer strategies for the prevention of progressive de-recruitment in individual patients with adult respiratory distress syndrome (ARDS).

Kinetic Beds [continuous lateral rotational therapy (CLRT)] has been shown to be beneficial (123–128). Turn continuously and slowly between 40–60° off the neutral position to either side along the long axis. Some beds incorporate vibration elements to simulate the effects of chest physiotherapy. The few studies on this subject have yielded variable results and suffered from small patient numbers and flawed design (no randomization, no clear definitions of pneumonia, no adjustment for confounding factors); these beds carry a significant cost, impose added difficulties in routine patient care, and currently cannot be recommended for routine use (123–128).

Prone positioning therapy has recently evolved as an alternative means to counteract posterior lung de-recruitment and attempt to reverse V/Q mismatching. Patients are positioned on special bed frames that can rotate 180° along the longitudinal axis and are designed to allow access to the face in the prone position (i.e., Stryker frame) or turned and positioned in conventional hospital beds. Several studies have shown improved PaO_2/FiO_2 ratios, decreased barotrauma and reversal of diffuse posterior atelectasis, faster weaning from mechanical ventilation, and improved outcomes in patients with severe respiratory failure (129,130). However, no studies to date have specifically looked at the impact of this mode of therapy on the incidence of VAP.

Duration of Mechanical Ventilation

♂ **Duration of mechanical ventilation itself may be the single most important risk factor for the development of pneumonia.** ♂ The risk for VAP increases in a time dependent fashion (5). Daily cumulative hazard rates are quoted between 1.3% and 3.3% and the overall risk approached 100% after 30 days of ventilation (131). The time dependent risk increase of VAP does not follow a linear pattern. There is an early steep rise in the incidence of VAP during the first 5–10 days (early VAP) and a second phase of more gradual risk increase at two to three weeks of mechanical ventilation (late VAP). Several studies have now shown clear benefits in terms of VAP reduction (40–60%) and outcome improvement (reduced mortality by more than 40%), employing strategies designed to decrease the duration of mechanical ventilation (132).

The best results may be achieved by combining several preventative strategies that address different aspects of the pathophysiology of VAP. Standardized weaning protocols based on physiologic parameters (Volume 2, Chapter 28) help decrease the duration of ventilation particularly in patients with mild to moderate reversible respiratory failure (133). Intensive chest physiotherapy, patient positioning, and ventilator recruitment maneuvers decrease the progression of atelectasis. Improved oropharyngeal hygiene through suctioning, topical chlorhexidine, semirecumbency, and possibly CASS decrease the impact of upper gastrointestinal (GI) colonization and micro-aspiration. Appropriate nutritional support (avoidance of large gastric volumes, enteral feeding access, motility agents) helps to avoid the complications associated with malnutrition and aspiration. Strict compliance with contamination precautions and aseptic techniques when handling airway-related equipment will decrease tracheo-bronchial inoculation. Prevention of VAP is the foremost goal in any patient receiving mechanical ventilation and requires implementation of institutional multi-specialty programs (118,119,131–134).

DIAGNOSIS OF VENTILATOR-ASSOCIATED PNEUMONIA
Clinical Diagnosis

Consensus regarding the diagnosis of ventilator-associated pneumonia has been difficult to reach in the past. ♂ **The clinical diagnosis of VAP is based on the appearance of new infiltrates on plain chest radiographs, new or altered** appearance of respiratory secretions, and general signs of infection (i.e., leukocytosis and fever). ☞

Radiographic Evaluation of Lung Parenchyma

Critics of this purely clinical diagnosis concept point out several problems: Plain film chest radiographs are not sensitive and are often inaccurate for the assessment of pulmonary infiltrates (Volume 1, Chapter 16). In the ICU setting the chest radiographs are most often done as portable anterior-posterior films with the patient in a supine position [Figs. 2(top) and 3(top)]. The anterior and posterior costodiaphragmatic as well as the retro-cardiac and lingular lung areas are difficult to assess. Critically ill patients receiving mechanical ventilation may develop significant regional lung collapse (atelectasis) that can mimic infiltrates on plain chest films. This de-recruitment may be so extensive that patients require increased ventilatory support, develop (low grade) elevated temperatures, and in the past have been labeled with the diagnosis ARDS (Volume 2, Chapter 24) (135–140). Computed Tomography (CT) of the chest better delineates the distribution of parenchymal changes but cannot reliably differentiate between collapse and infiltration (Fig. 3) (141,142).

Changed Respiratory Secretions

As outlined before, essentially all mechanically ventilated patients develop bacterial tracheo-bronchial colonization and altered muco-ciliary clearance with subsequent changes in respiratory secretions (increased amount, purulent appearance, numerous PMNs). Although not well studied in ventilated patients, changes in the character and color of sputum correlates with the degree of bacterial proliferation in the airways. In a recent study in bronchitic patients, "purulent" sputum was much more likely to have pathogenic bacterial growth than "mucoid." Additionally, a darkening of the sputum color (from yellowish to brownish) was associated with an increased yield of gram-negative organisms (143). Although tracheo-bronchitis does not necessarily represent pneumonia, the majority of critically ill patients with purulent sputum and tracheo-bronchitis should receive appropriate antibiotic therapy (see Volume 2, Chapter 53).

Fever and Leukocytosis

Fever and leukocytosis are common in critically ill patients and may represent a systemic inflammatory response syndrome (SIRS) due to the underlying illness or trauma (Volume 2, Chapter 46). Other potential sources of infection, particularly of the blood stream (i.e., intravenous catheter related), urinary tract, wounds, and intra-abdominal infections are common in this patient population and must be sought diligently.

Transtracheal Aspiration of Sputum and Blood Cultures

In the past, transtracheal aspiration specimen of sputum and blood cultures have been the gold standard to solidify the diagnosis of NP and VAP (Table 3). The use of blood cultures is problematic for several reasons: The majority of patients who develop VAP (at least initially) do not have a concomitant bacteremia; and at the same time the false negative rate of "routine" blood cultures (most often obtained after a temperature spike to ≥38.5°C) is significant (144). The use of qualitative

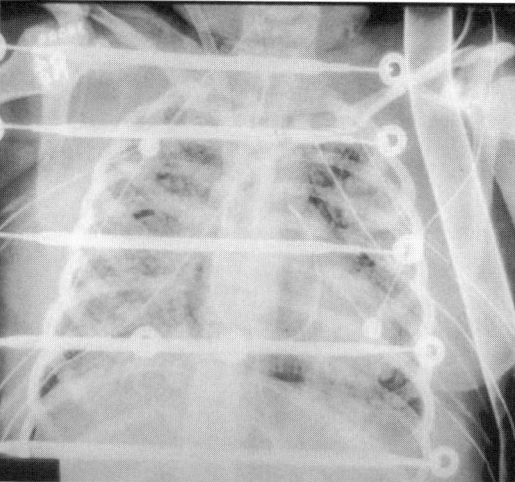
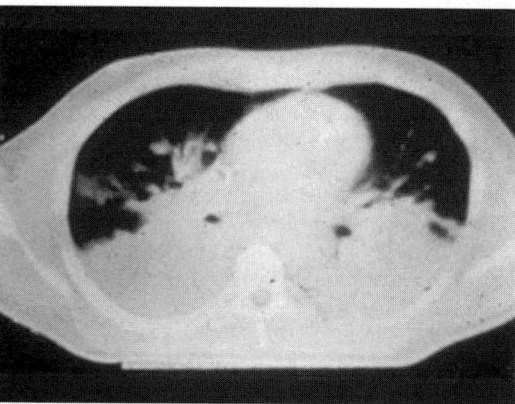
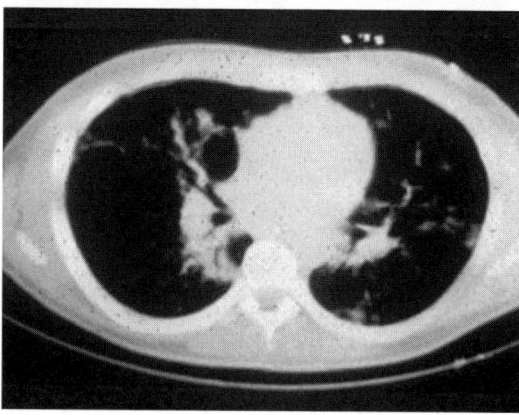

Figure 2 Pulmonary infiltrates representing retained secretions and atelectasis. This series of images depicts a patient a few days after significant blunt torso and extremity trauma. The patient required increasing ventilator support and was (low grade) febrile. The supine anterior-posterior projection plain film chest radiograph (*top*) shows bilateral opacifications in both upper and lower lung fields, consistent with pneumonia or ARDS. The computed tomography (CT) image of the patient's chest (*middle*) shows predominant posterior consolidation consistent with pneumonia of dependent atelectasis. A repeat CT of the same patient after 48 hours (*bottom*) of intermittent prone position therapy and intensive chest physiotherapy demonstrates near complete resolution of the above changes. The patient did not require antibiotic therapy. *Abbreviation*: ARDS, adult respiratory distress syndrome.

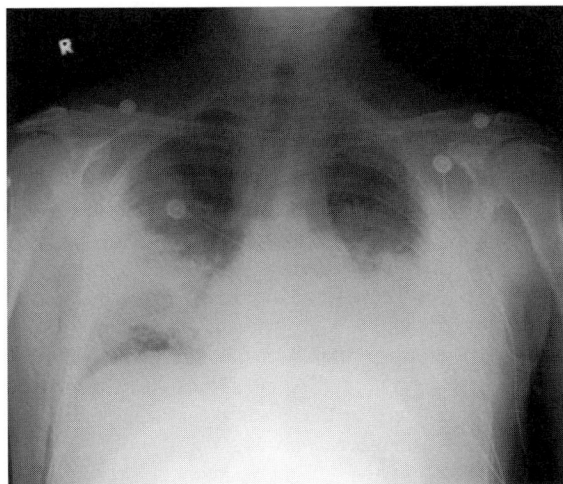
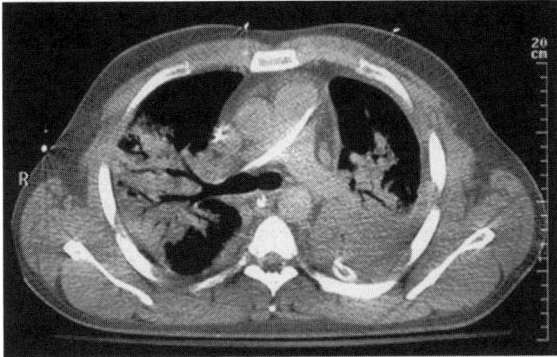

Figure 3 Pulmonary infiltrates representing pneumonia. This series of images depicts a patient after motor vehicle crash with significant blunt injury to the head and extremities. The supine anterior-posterior projection plain film chest radiograph (*top*) shows right middle and left lower lobe consolidation. The patient was febrile, and demonstrated leukocytosis and increased sputum production. Aggressive chest physiotherapy did not significantly change the patient's clinical picture. A computer tomographic image of the patient's chest (*bottom*) demonstrates the consolidation and air-bronchograms consistent with pneumonia.

sputum cultures obtained via standard trans-endotracheal tube suctioning techniques is likewise flawed. It is impossible to reliably guide the suction catheter (blindly) to the area in question [segment with infiltrate on chest x-ray (CXR)]; the so-obtained specimen may become contaminated with colonized tracheobronchial secretions. Although, in the presence of late VAP, there may be a $\geq 70\%$ correlation between the pathogens recovered in tracheo-bronchial secretions and those responsible for pneumonia (145), this correlation is less reliable in early VAP and the true presence of VAP is difficult to establish. Several studies have noted variable sensitivities (44–86%) and specificities (95–52%) with accuracies between 61% and 82% for quantitative endotracheal aspirate cultures (cut-off levels between 10^3 and 10^7 cells/ml) when compared to histopathologic findings at autopsy (146–150).

In a study of 255 patients, the statistical agreement of classical CDC NNIS diagnosis, Johanson Criteria and MD Probable diagnostic criteria was analyzed (151). Agreement was poor (kappa < 0.3) for any comparison of diagnostic tools and VAP diagnosis rates varied from 4% to 48% on the same patient set (151).

Bronchoscopic Guided Protected Specimen Brushing and Bronchoalveolar Lavage

Bronchoscopic guided PSB and BAL both employ the use of bronchoscopy to reach the pulmonary segment(s) of interest. With these techniques, the amount and quality of secretions can be assessed visually at the (sub-) segmental level.

For BAL a known quantity of sterile physiologic saline solution (between 50 and 150 cc) is injected into the (sub-) segmental bronchus and retrieved after three to four respiratory cycles via suction aspiration into a sterile container attached to the bronchoscope (152). In order to obtain a representative specimen, one-fourth to one-third of irrigate must be recovered (152). The lavage fluid is sent for a cell count and differential as well as gram stain and quantitative culture. In prospective studies comparing bronchoscopically guided BAL results, with postmortem histopathologic evaluation sensitivities of $>80\%$ and specificities of 75% to 100% with positive predictive values of up to $\sim$95% and negative predictive values of up to $\sim$89%, were found using quantitative culture cut-off levels between 10^3 and 10^4 CFU/mL (150). Gram staining of the BAL effluent was negative in $\sim$94% of patients without VAP and similar results were achieved using cell count and differential with cut-off points of 400,000 cells/mL ($\geq 50\%$ neutrophils) (153). Other studies found similar sensitivities and specificities for BAL quantitative cultures when comparing it to various methods of clinical diagnosis but less sensitivity ($\sim$75%) for initial Gram stain and differential cell count for the diagnosis of early VAP (positive predictive value 100%, negative predictive value $\sim$75%) (152,154).

In PSB a special catheter containing a telescoping brush (covered by a coated tip) is advanced into the segment of interest. Pushing off the protective tip deploys the brush and a sample of the distal airway secretions is obtained. The brush is retracted back into the catheter and removed. Quantitative cultures from the brush specimen, using similar cut-off levels as those for BAL, have yielded 75–100% sensitivity and 90–100% specificity for the correct diagnosis of VAP when compared with histopatholic findings (150–165). Critics have argued that guided PSB and BAL are invasive, require a skilled operator, and are associated with significant cost.

Nonbronchoscopic Protected Catheter Aspirate and Bronchoalveolar Lavage

Recently, non-bronchoscopic protected catheter aspirate and broncho-alveolar lavage have evolved as alternative diagnostic methods (166). Sensitivities for these blind sampling methods have been reported as being somewhat lower (61–72%) than those of the bronchoscopic PSB and BAL, but specificities ranged at a comparable 84–99% in the initial studies (167). Qualitative concordance of the predominant pathogen was demonstrated in 83–93% (kappa > 0.8) when comparing invasive with noninvasive PSB and BAL. Problems with these non-guided techniques are related to the inability to reliably direct the sampling tool to the area of interest and, in the case of BAL, to a higher rate of

Table 3   Centers for Disease Control Definition of Nosocomial Pneumonia 2002

	Main Criterion[a,b]	Sub Criterion
Criterion 1	Patient has rales or dullness to percussion on physical examination of the chest and at least one sub criterion	New onset of purulent sputum or Change in character of sputum Organisms cultured from blood Isolation of an etiologic agent from a specimen obtained by transtracheal aspirate, bronchial brushing, or biopsy
Criterion 2	Patient has a chest radiographic examination that shows new or progressive infiltrate, consolidation, cavitation, or pleural effusion and at least one sub criterion	New onset of purulent sputum or change in character of sputum Organisms cultured from blood Isolation of an etiologic agent from a specimen obtained by transtracheal aspirate, bronchial brushing, or biopsy Isolation of a virus or detection of viral antigen in respiratory secretions Diagnostic single antibody titer (IgM) or fourfold increase in paired sera (IgG) for pathogen Histopathologic evidence of pneumonia

[a]Pneumonia must meet at least one of the main criteria
[b]*Comments*: Expectorated sputum cultured are *not* useful in the diagnosis of pneumonia but may help identify the etiologic agent and provide useful antimicrobial susceptibility data. Findings from serial chest x-rays may be more helpful than a single x-ray.
Source Notes: Nosocomial infection is defined as a localized or systemic condition (*i*) that results from adverse reaction to the presence of an infectious agent(s) or its toxin(s) and (*ii*) that was not present or incubating at the time of admission to the hospital (see reference below). The information used to determine the presence and classification of an infection should be a combination of clinical findings and results of laboratory data and other tests.
Source: From Ref. 234.

inadequate sampling (return of inadequate fluid amount, differential cell count demonstrates >5% bronchial epithelial cells) (147,155,168–170).

☞ **To avoid therapy delay, several studies suggest the use of an initial Gram stain obtained via guided or non-guided BAL or PSB as guide to initiate therapy. Sensitivity and specificity are slightly lower than those of quantitative cultures, but positive and negative predictive values are between 70% and 90% (152,160,171).** ☞

In today's clinical practice a uniform consensus as to which criteria to use for the diagnosis of NP and VAP has not been reached. It is recognized that the early correct diagnosis and initiation of appropriate antibiotic therapy improves outcome (171,172). Similarly, over-diagnosis and indiscriminate use of antibiotics are associated with increased cost and complications. An evidence-based assessment of diagnostic tests for VAP in 2000 concluded that insufficient high-level evidence was available to indicate that quantitative testing produced better clinical outcomes than empiric treatment, and recommended formal outcome research with randomized, controlled trials to assess various diagnostic and management strategies for VAP (171). However, a recent prospective randomized multi-center study from France compared "invasive" (broncho-scope guided) BAL to standard clinical criteria (including suction catheter aspirate) for diagnosis of pneumonia in 413 patients (164). The use of an invasive diagnostic strategy was associated with a decreased mortality at day 14 (16.2% vs. 25.8%, p = 0.022); decreased mean Sepsis-related Organ Failure (SOFA) occurs at day 3 and 7, and decreased antibiotic use at day 14 with more antibiotic-free days at day 28 (11.5 ± 9.0 vs. 7.5 ± 7.6, p < 0.001) (164). The Canadian Critical Care Trials Group documented similar reductions

of antibiotic usage in a prospective multi-center study on 92 patients receiving mechanical ventilation (173). In that study no difference in ICU length of stay but a decrease in mortality (18.5% vs. 34.7%, p = 0.03) were noted. These studies also demonstrated that the clinical diagnosis of VAP could not be confirmed by microbiological data from invasive diagnostic techniques in 22% to 60% and that the initial antibiotic therapy was inadequate in 24–39% of those patients with confirmed VAP (most often due to resistance of Gram negative pathogens to 3rd generation cephalosporins) (173). A Spanish study demonstrated no difference in outcome regardless of the method of microbiological diagnosis (174).

CDC NNIS Pneumonia Flow Diagram

In an effort to resolve some of the above issues and to create a common language that can be used to compare the results of future studies, the CDC, through the NNIS, has developed a new pneumonia flow diagram that incorporates classic (clinical) diagnostic elements, PSB and BAL as well as the immune status of the host to define four types of pneumonia (175,176) (Fig. 4).

☞ **Invasive diagnosis with BAL or PSB may not be necessary in the normal host that has clear clinical evidence of VAP, an absence of other potential sources of infection, and who responds appropriately to a course of antibiotic therapy. Invasive diagnosis should be considered early in patients that have equivocal clinical signs, in the immuno-compromised host, in patients with evidence of severe infection, in patients with ARDS and suspected VAP, in patients who develop late VAP and those who do not respond to therapy.** ☞

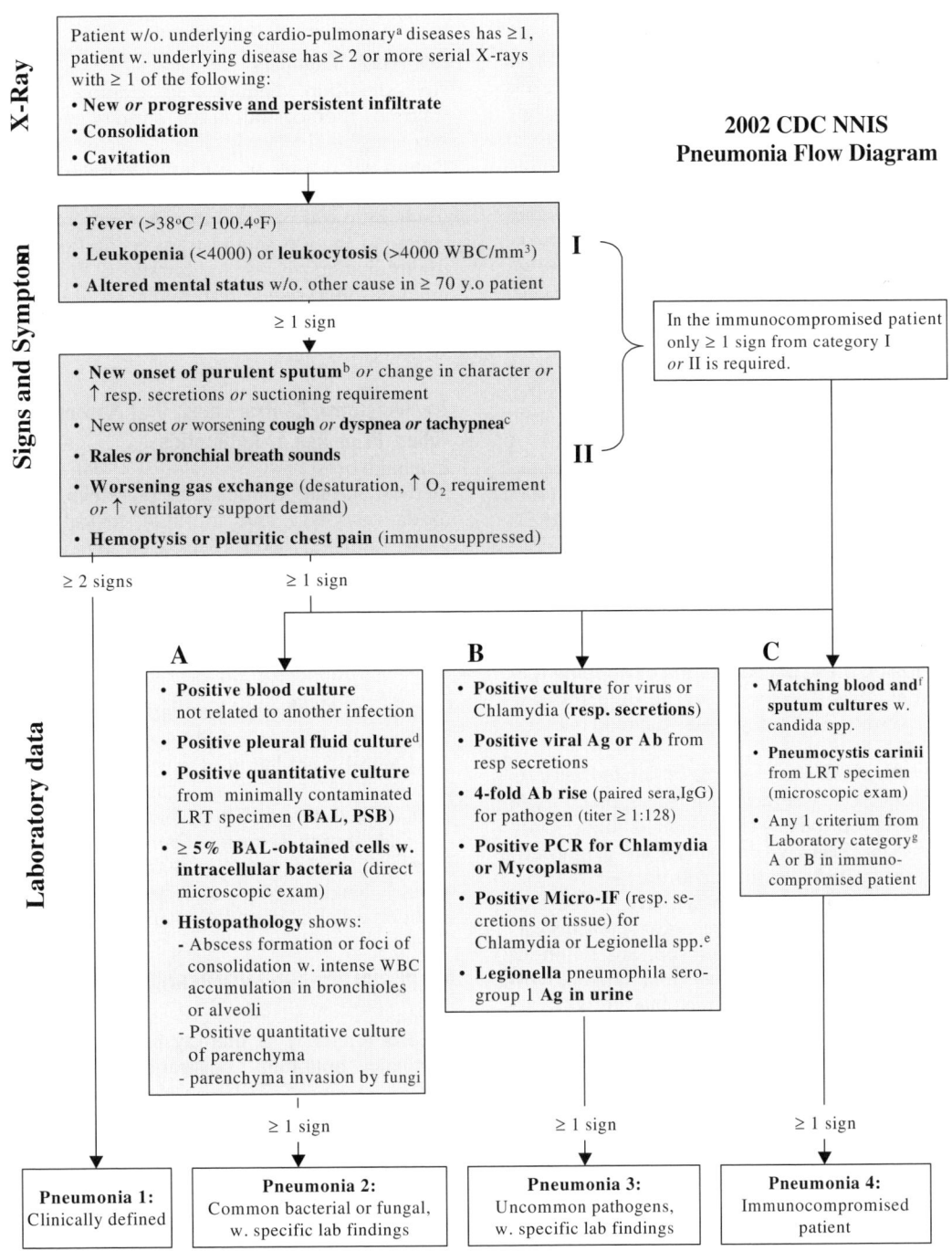

X-Ray

Patient w/o. underlying cardio-pulmonary[a] diseases has ≥1, patient w. underlying disease has ≥ 2 or more serial X-rays with ≥ 1 of the following:
- **New *or* progressive <u>and</u> persistent infiltrate**
- **Consolidation**
- **Cavitation**

2002 CDC NNIS Pneumonia Flow Diagram

Signs and Symptom

- **Fever** (>38°C / 100.4°F)
- **Leukopenia** (<4000) or **leukocytosis** (>4000 WBC/mm³)
- **Altered mental status** w/o. other cause in ≥ 70 y.o patient

I

≥ 1 sign

In the immunocompromised patient only ≥ 1 sign from category I *or* II is required.

- **New onset of purulent sputum**[b] *or* change in character *or* ↑ resp. secretions *or* suctioning requirement
- New onset *or* worsening **cough** *or* **dyspnea** *or* **tachypnea**[c]
- **Rales** *or* **bronchial breath sounds**
- **Worsening gas exchange** (desaturation, ↑ O₂ requirement *or* ↑ ventilatory support demand)
- **Hemoptysis or pleuritic chest pain** (immunosuppressed)

II

≥ 2 signs   ≥ 1 sign

Laboratory data

A
- **Positive blood culture** not related to another infection
- **Positive pleural fluid culture**[d]
- **Positive quantitative culture** from minimally contaminated LRT specimen (**BAL, PSB**)
- **≥ 5% BAL-obtained cells w. intracellular bacteria** (direct microscopic exam)
- **Histopathology** shows:
  - Abscess formation or foci of consolidation w. intense WBC accumulation in bronchioles or alveoli
  - Positive quantitative culture of parenchyma
  - parenchyma invasion by fungi

B
- **Positive culture** for virus or Chlamydia (**resp. secretions**)
- **Positive viral Ag or Ab** from resp secretions
- **4-fold Ab rise** (paired sera,IgG) for pathogen (titer ≥ 1:128)
- **Positive PCR for Chlamydia or Mycoplasma**
- **Positive Micro-IF** (resp. secretions or tissue) for Chlamydia or Legionella spp.[e]
- **Legionella** pneumophila serogroup 1 **Ag in urine**

C
- **Matching blood and**[f] **sputum cultures** w. candida spp.
- **Pneumocystis carinii** from LRT specimen (microscopic exam)
- Any 1 criterium from Laboratory category[g] A or B in immunocompromised patient

≥ 1 sign   ≥ 1 sign   ≥ 1 sign

Pneumonia 1: Clinically defined

Pneumonia 2: Common bacterial or fungal, w. specific lab findings

Pneumonia 3: Uncommon pathogens, w. specific lab findings

Pneumonia 4: Immunocompromised patient

Figure 4 2002 CDC NNIS Pneumonia Flow Diagram.

[a]Cardio-pulmonary diseases to be considered: congestive heart failure, interstitial lung disease, bronchio-pulmonary dysplasia, respiratory distress syndrome, chronic obstructive pulmonary disease, smoke inhalation, pulmonary injury, etc.

[b]Purulent sputum contains ≥25 PMNs and ≤10 epithelial cells per low power field; pure qualitative clinical description is insufficient. A single notation of change in character is not meaningful, repeated notations in a 24 hours period are more indicative of an infectious process

[c]In adults, tachypnea is >25 breaths/min.

[d]Scant or watery sputum is often seen with pneumonia due to viruses and mycoplasma; influenza and RSV may produce copious sputum.

[e]Few bacteria may be seen on stains from resp. secretions from patients with pneumonia due to *Legionella* spp., mycoplasma or viruses.

[f]Semiquantitative or nonquantitative cultures of sputum obtained by aspiration or lavage are acceptable; when sputum and blood cultures are matched, specimen needs to be obtained within 48 hours of each other.

[g]Imunnocompromised patients are those with neutropenia (<500WBC/mm³), leukemia, lymphoma, HIV infection w. CD₄-counts <200, post splenectomy, post organ transplantation, on cytotoxic chemotherapy, on high dose steroids (>40 mg Prednisone/day or its equivalent) (See Volume 2, Chapter 52).

Abbreviations: Ab, antibody; Ag, antigen; BAL, bronchoalveoar lavage; CDC, centers for disease control; IF, immunofluorescence; LRT, lower respiratory tract; PSB, protected brush specimen; PCR, polymerase chain reaction.

ACUTE RESPIRATORY DISTRESS SYNDROME AND VENTILATOR-ASSOCIATED PNEUMONIA

The diagnosis and therapy of VAP in patients with ARDS is particularly difficult. These patients often require high levels of ventilatory support for prolonged periods of time. They demonstrate diffuse patchy bilateral pulmonary infiltrates on plain chest films. CT scanning is only moderately accurate in differentiating ARDS-related infiltrates from pneumonia with 70% true negative and 60% true positive ratings when evaluated by skilled radiologists (141,142). Fever and leukocytosis from SIRS or an underlying infectious process (often the inciting event for the development of ARDS) are exceedingly common, and a significant proportion of these patients have received prior/concomitant antibiotic therapy. Similarly, patients with ARDS often develop inflammatory-type respiratory secretions and bacterial tracheo-bronchitis, making the interpretation of standard endotracheal aspirate Gram stains and cultures difficult (139).

In a multi-center study by the ARDS Study Group, the incidence of VAP (diagnosed by invasive techniques) among ARDS patients was about 60% higher than that of non-ARDS patients (36.5–55% vs. 23–28%) receiving mechanical ventilation (135). ☞ **In ARDS, the combination of an altered local immune response, loss of alveolar wall integrity, and collapse or consolidation of parenchyma with subsequent under-ventilation of these areas are thought to act synergistically in predisposing these patients to the development of VAP.** ☞ Pneumonia may develop in several different lung areas at the same time and 40% of patients develop bilateral bacterial growth (137).

Patients with ARDS often require prolonged periods of mechanical ventilation. The incidence of late pneumonia as well as recurrent episodes of infection is high. Only ~10% of the first episodes of VAP occur (or are diagnosed) before day 7 of mechanical ventilation (mean 9.8 +/−5.7 days) (138). Non-fermenting Gram-negative rods and problem pathogens like (multi-drug resistant) *Pseudomonas* spp., *Ancinetobacter*, and *Staphylococcus* spp. are found in over 50% of these patients (144). Patients with bilateral involvement are more likely to have polymicrobial growth and >10^5 CFU/mL in the BAL fluid (140).

It is unclear as to what extent the development of VAP influences the overall outcome of ARDS. Some authors suggest no significant differences in overall mortality whereas others found ARDS mortality increases by a factor of 1.5–2 in patients with VAP (138). We believe it important to maintain a high level of suspicion for VAP in patients with ARDS that develop clinical signs of infection or fail to improve gradually with intensive medical support. Invasive diagnostic methods should be employed early to ensure diagnosis. Empiric antibiotic therapy should cover the common drug resistant pathogens and should be tailored according to culture results as soon as possible (4).

RISK ASSESSMENT
Host-Related Factors
Independent risk factors for the development of VAP include host related factors, like age greater than 65, a higher degree of severity of the acute illness (i.e., APACHE II >20, odds ratio 4.8), evidence of immunosuppresion (i.e., diabetes, steroid use, moderate to severe malnutrition, HIV, bone marrow diseases and organ transplantation), and

significant pre-existing cardiac, renal, vascular, or pulmonary co-morbidity (3).

Admission Diagnosis
An admission diagnosis of trauma (particularly head trauma), thoraco-abdominal surgery, or significant burns increase the risk for VAP by a factor of 3–5 (177). Other factors, soon after or during admission, that increase the risk of VAP include the need for emergent intubation (odds ratio 6.4) or re-intubation (odds ratio 2.9) during the course of the illness and frank aspiration before or during the intubation process (odds ratio 12.7) (178). The development of initial severe respiratory failure ($PaO_2/FiO_2 < 200$, odds ratio 3.5), severe acute lung injury (ALI), and ARDS raises the risk of VAP in a similar fashion (179).

Tracheostomy, Central Lines, Oral Nasoenteric Tubes, Prior Use of Antibiotics
In a large prospective study on 3171 patients admitted to the medical and surgical ICU, the placement of a tracheostomy (odds ratio 6.7) and multiple central venous catheters (odds ratio 4.2) also increased the risk for development of VAP (180). Likewise the presence of oral or nasoenteric feeding tubes and prior use of systemic antibiotic therapy has been linked to the development of VAP (see previous paragraphs) (181–184).

Duration of Mechanical Ventilation
VAP risk is not static but increases with the duration of mechanical ventilation. Daily hazard rates are quoted between 1.3% and 3.3% and overall risk approaches 100% after 30 days of ventilation (Fig. 5) (179).

Most of these factors cannot be altered acutely in any given patient, but knowledge of the patient's potential risk should heighten the clinician's vigilance to minimize additional risk and employ available preventive strategies.

MICROBIOLOGY AND ANTIMICROBIAL THERAPY

☞ **The mainstay of therapy in NP and VAP is adequate systemic antibiotic coverage. The antibiotics used**

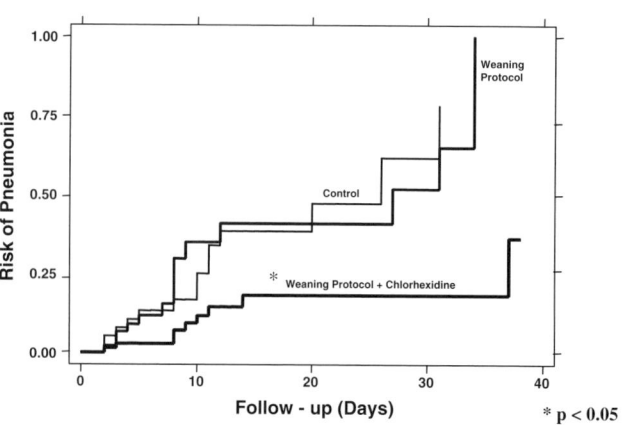

Figure 5 Ventilator-associated pneumonia and duration of mechanical ventilation. Cox regression analysis of the risk for development of ventilator-associated pneumonia in relation to the duration of mechanical ventilation. *Source*: From Ref. 116.

should be bactericidal to the suspected pathogen(s), and reach adequate tissue levels in the lung. ☞ In general it is believed that a large portion of the pathogens responsible for VAP is acquired endogenously, mostly from the patient's enteric Gram negative flora (185).

In 1995 the American Thoracic Society published a set of guidelines for the (initial empiric) treatment of NP, based on the severity of infection, presence of risk factors for specific organisms, and timing of NP occurrence (186). Although the concept may be valid and is still used throughout the country, there are several problems with these guidelines: the original recommendations do not include data derived from the multiple studies on invasive diagnostic techniques, the original selection of antibiotics is outdated since many new agents have been Food Drug Administration (FDA) approved, microbial resistance patterns have shifted, and no specific recommendations regarding duration of therapy were made.

A decade later the updated 2005 Guidelines for the Management of Adults with Hospital-acquired Pneumonia, Ventilator-associated Pneumonia, and Healthcare-associated Pneumonia was published (4). These guidelines are evidence-based and were prepared by an expert committee sponsored by the American Thoracic Society (ATS) and the Infectious Diseases Society of America (IDSA) (4).

☞ **There is a striking difference in the prevalence of individual pathogens between countries, hospitals, and even individual patient care units within each hospital.** ☞ Moreover, studies and aggregate data from the NNIS (Table 4) demonstrate an alarming increase in drug resistant pathogens in the United States (4,6,185).

Patient-related factors, including preexisting pulmonary disease, immune status, type of surgery, prior antibiotic exposure, the timing of the VAP (early vs. late), as well as the severity of the infection, all further influence the spectrum of most likely pathogens (4,186–190).

Inadequate initial therapy (even when begun early) is associated with worse outcomes (191). Therefore, it is of utmost importance to know the patient's clinical history,

severity, and timing of VAP, and locale-specific data prior to making the choice for empiric therapy. Other factors that must be considered include the patient's allergies and cross-allergenicity of certain antibiotic classes, the patient's hepatic and renal function (for dose adjustments), potential interactions of certain antibiotics with other medications, and specific contraindications (i.e., pregnancy, neuromuscular disease, cardiac disease) for certain agents (see Volume 2, Chapter 53 for specific antibiotic guidelines).

In general, antimicrobial therapy is begun empirically when clinical suspicion of pneumonia arises in the ventilated patient. Several studies have demonstrated that early therapy improved outcome (192). Although there is no clear cut-off point, the data suggests that the maximum benefit is achieved when therapy is begun within 8–12 hours of the initial diagnosis (suspicion). Delays of >48 hr have been associated with increased mortality (4,191,182). The current antibiotic guidelines for VAP are summarized in Table 5.

Early Ventilator-Associated Pneumonia

☞ **Early VAP (occurrence in less than 5–7 days), particularly in trauma patients, is associated most commonly with *Streptococcus pneumoniae* (SP), *Haemophilus influenzae* (HI), Enteric gram-negative bacilli (GNB) and Methicillin Sensitive Staphylococci (MSSA). A prolonged hospital stay prior to intubation and exposure to (broad-spectrum) antibiotics are linked to a higher incidence of *Pseudomonas aeruginosa* (PA), *Acinetobacter* spp., other resistant staphylococci (MRSA) and, possibly, vancomycin resistant *Enterococcus* spp. (VRE).** ☞ In absence of these factors, monotherapy with a ß-lactum/ß-lactamase inhibitor (with or without antipseudomonal activity), 2nd or 3rd-generation cephalosporin (with or without antipseudomonal activity), newer generation quinolone, or carbapenem all demonstrate equal success rates (4,6,185–189,193).

Table 4 Ventilator-Associated Pneumonia: Microbial Isolates and Resistance

Organism isolates	NNIS aggregate data			
	1984	1986–89	1990–96	1999
Pseudomonas aeruginosa	17	17	17	18
Staphylococcus aureus	13	16	19	18
Klebsiella pneumoniae	12	7	8	7
Enterobacter	9	11	11	12
Echerichia coli	6	6	4	4
Haemophilus influenzae	–	–	5	5
Candida albicans	–	–	–	4
Others	43	43	36	32
Resistance patterns	**Antibiotic**	**% Resistance**	**No. cases**	**% Change**
Staphyloccocus aureus	Methicillin	55.3	5070	+29
Pseudomonas aeruginosa	Imipenem	17.7	1848	+23
	Quinolone	27.3	2530	+53
	3rd Cephalosporin	26.4	2945	+24
Enterobacter spp.	3rd Cephalosporin	34.9	1811	−1
Klebsiella pneumoniae	3rd Cephalosporin	11.2	1659	+5

Source: From Ref. 235.

Table 5 Therapy of Ventilator-Associated Pneumonia According to Severity, Risk Factor, Onset, and Most Likely Pathogens

Severity of illness[a]	Risk factors[b]	Onset	Most likely organisms	Core antibiotics
Mild/ moderate	Yes	Any time	*Pseudomonas aeruginosa* (and related species) w. prolonged ICU stay, steroids, prior antibiotics, structural lung disease)	Antipseudomonal cephalosporin (ceftazidime, cefepime) or Antipseudomonal carbapenem (imipenem, meropenem) or B-lactam/B-lactamase inhibitor (piperacillin/tazobactam) PLUS Antipseudomonal fluoroquinolone (ciprofloxacin, levofloxacin) or Aminoglycoside (gentamicin, tobramycin, amikacin)
			Anaerobes- w. recent abdominal surgery or witnessed aspiration	Metronidazole clindamycin is only useful for anaerobic infections above the diaphragm (see Volume 2, Chapter 53)
			Staphylococcus aureus w. coma, head trauma	+/− Vancomycin or linezolid until MRSA excluded; +/− Rifampin
			Legionella on high-dose steroids	Azithromycin or levofloxacin
	No	Any time	Enteric gram-negative bacilli (Non-Pseudomonal) *Enterobacter spp.* *Escherichia coli* *Klebsiella spp.* *Proteus spp.* *Serratia marcescens* *Haemophilus influenzae*	Ceftriaxone or ampicillin/sulbactam or ertapenem
			Gram-positive organisms *Staphylococcus aureus* (MSSA)- *Streptococcus pneumoniae*	Vancomycin plus antipneumococcal fluroquinolone (levofloxacin, moxifloxacin)
	Yes	Any time	*Pseudomonas aeruginosa* (and related species.) *Acinetobacter* spp.	See mild/moderate; Positive risk factors
Severe	No	Late onset	*Staphylococcus aureus* (MRSA)	
		Early onset	See: mild/moderate; no risk factors	

[a]Definition of severe hospital-acquired pneumonia:
Admission to the intensive care unit with:
  Respiratory failure (need for FiO$_2$ >35% to maintain SaO$_2$ >90% or need for mechanical ventilation
    Severe sepsis w. hypotension (SBP <90 mmHg or DBP <60 mm Hg, requirement of pressors >4 hr) and/or endorgan dysfunction (i.e., acute renal failure w. urine output <20 ml/hr for >4 hr)
Rapid radiographic progression, multilobar pneumonia, or cavitation of a lung infiltrate
[b]Patient-related risk factor include severe acute/chron. illness, coma, malnutrition, prolonged hospitalization, hypotension, smoking, COPD, diabetes mellitus, alcoholism, renal failure, advanced age.
[b]Infection control-related risk factor include poor infection control measures, lack of hand washing/universal precautions.
[b]Intervention-related risk factor include medications (sedatives, steroids, antibiotics, antacids, H$_2$-blockers), thoraco-abdominal procedures, intubation, nasogastric tubes, and others.
Source: Modified from Guidelines for the management of adults with hospital-acquired, ventilator-associated, and healthcare-associated pneumonia. Am J Resp Crit Care Med 2005; 171:388–415.

Late Ventilator-Associated Pneumonia Due to Problem Pathogens

In presence of the above factors and with late VAP (occurrence more than 10–14 days), the initial antibiotic coverage should include activity against pseudomonas and take local resistance patterns into strong consideration.

According to a recent international consensus conference, the high prevalence of resistant PA, *Klebsiella pneumoniae* (KP), *Acinetobacter* spp. and *Enterobacter* spp. in these patients may be better treated initially with a combination regimen (aminoglycoside or quinolone plus an anti-pseudomonal extended spectrum ß-lactam or carbapenem) (194).

This recommendation has been made despite the lack of large prospective trials comparing mono- to combination therapy with regard to efficacy and outcomes, using clinical and invasive microbiological data (194).

Pseudomonas

VAP due to *Pseudomonas aeruginosa* is associated with a high mortality (195–197). The organism produces several exotoxins and causes invasive infections (195–197,198). The most recent NNIS data demonstrate an alarming 30–50% increase in resistance to the most commonly used antibiotics (Table 4) (6). Monotherapy may lead to a higher incidence of resistance and higher mortality rates in pseudomonal VAP. To date there is still considerable debate as to which combination regimen is best. Aminoglycosides have good bactericidal activity and a prolonged post-antibiotic effect but a narrow therapeutic range, poor penetration into lung parenchyma, and decreased activity with lower pH (abscess) (193). These factors may be responsible for the synergistic advantage found in vitro which is not as obvious in vivo. On the other hand, the combination of ß-lactam and quinolone does not demonstrate similar synergistic effects in vitro, but has similar efficacy in vivo (199). Fluoroquinolones reach high levels in most tissues, including lung, pulmonary immune cells and respiratory secretions (200). Antipseudomonal cephalosporins (e.g., ceftazidime or cefepime) and carbapenems have been reserved by most clinicians as second line agents for specific indications. With multi-drug resistant strains of *Pseudomonas aeruginosa*, the use of polymyxin B and/or colistimethate (colistin) may be the only alternative (201). Bacterial eradication may take a long time and overall outcome in resistant pseudomonas cases is worse (197–203).

Acinetobacter

Similar to PA, VAP due to *Acinetobacter baumanii* (AB) is challenging due to extensive resistance (up to >70% to any of the mainstream antibiotic agents) and high mortality rates (198,204–208). The prevalence of this pathogen is highly different between individual units; AB VAP occurs predominantly in patients with significant pre-existing lung disease and after prior antibiotic exposure; it should be suspected mainly in late VAP, with failure to respond to standard treatment regimen and patients with severe infections. Septic shock in these patients is thought to be associated with production of a cell wall endotoxin (204). Like pseudomonas, acinetobacter has the ability to survive in a wide variety of contaminated materials and easily spreads among patients. Treatment must be individualized according to microbiologic data, as soon as possible; most authors agree on the use of combination regimen. Isolation of these patients is important to prevent spread.

Extended Spectrum Beta-Lactamase Producing Klebsiella pneumoniae

Extended Spectrum Beta-Lactamase (ESBL) producing KP is a problem directly related to the extensive use of 3rd-generation cephalosporins (particularly ceftazidime) in the ICU (209,210). Whereas resistance was prevalent in 2% of strains in 1989, to date it has risen five fold. ESBL confers resistance to essentially all 3rd generation cephalosporins, extended-spectrum penicillins and the monobactam, aztreonam. Recent data demonstrates emerging resistance to the quinolones as well (208). In these cases carbapenems become the drug of choice; however, the first

reports on resistance to these drugs are already emerging (209). Interestingly, efforts to reduce the use of ceftazidime (and other 3rd generation cephalosporins) have led to dramatic reductions (from 20–40% to 0–14%) in KP multi-drug resistance over a relatively short time period (207–210).

Anaerobes

Anaerobes may be found in up to 35% of NP but the incidence of VAP is significantly lower (1.1–3.5%). Although it is important to pay attention to adequate sampling (PSB sampling has been recommended) and proper transport (<30 min) and processing of the specimen to avoid false negative results, routine therapy for VAP does not need to include specific anaerobic coverage (211–213).

Methicillin-Resistant Staphylococcus

MRSA is encountered mainly in patients with prior colonization, prolonged hospital stay or duration of mechanical ventilation (>7 days), prior exposure to antibiotics or steroid therapy and significant pre-existing lung disease (COPD) (214). Prior antibiotic exposure and significant COPD were the factors most often associated with MRSA infection (215). The overall incidence of MRSA in VAP is 15–18% (NNIS) and primary empiric therapy with vancomycin or linezolid is probably warranted in patients with the above-mentioned risk factors (6,186,188,195,207, 214–217). A recent prospective study in 340 patients with gram-positive VAP documented that *S. aureus* was the most frequent pathogen isolated, and 68% were MRSA (218). In a double blind study of MRSA VAP with patients randomized to linezolid versus vancomycin, with aztreonam for Gram-negative coverage (219). The cure rates in clinically evaluable patients were 57% for linezolid-treated patients and 60% for vancomycin-treated patients. Although this study demonstrated the relative equivalence of the two drugs, lack of clinical response after five to seven days of treatment using therapeutic levels of vancomycin warrants a switch to linezolid.

Interestingly, patients with altered mental state (i.e., head trauma) are at increased risk of developing (early) infections with MSSA, which is better treated with the semi-synthetic penicillins oxacillin or nafcillin (6,220).

Candida spp.

Candida spp. is often recovered in the respiratory specimen of critically ill ventilated patients who have received prior antibiotic therapy. In non-immunosuppressed patients candida seldom causes VAP even when recovered in high colony numbers. One of the important modes of therapy in candidal colonization/suspected infection is to remove foreign bodies (central venous lines, urinary catheters, ETT) and reduce or stop systemic broad-spectrum antibiotics as soon as feasible. Routine antifungal coverage is not warranted, unless the patient is neutropenic or otherwise significantly immunosuppressed (uncontrolled diabetes, high-dose corticosteroid therapy, HIV) or candida is found in multiple sites (i.e., urine, abdominal, blood). Fluconazole (at appropriate doses) will treat all candida species except *C. krusei* and *C. lusitaniei* (194,221).

Duration of Antibiotic Therapy

One of the most important questions regarding VAP treatment relates to the optimal duration of antibiotic therapy. Most studies report treatment courses between 7 and 14 days (4). Longer courses are usually related to selective (resistant) pathogens or lack of overall patient improval. Prolonged courses of antibiotic therapy and indiscriminate broad-spectrum coverage are linked to increased adverse effects from the drugs, increased cost, opportunistic infections with resistant bacteria and fungi, *Clostridium difficile* entero-colitis, and overall worse outcomes (4). However, short courses of therapy may be related to treatment failure or relapse, particularly with pathogens that are difficult to eradicate (PA, MRSA, AB, VRE).

In a randomized trial of patients with ventilator-associated pneumonia, Chastre et al. reported patients who received eight days of antibiotic therapy had fever recurrences and less resistance overall than did patients who received 15 days of therapy (222).

In this context, the importance of obtaining unequivocal microbiological data (BAL or PSB) and adjustment of empiric therapy to local/individual resistance patterns and clinical response to therapy cannot be overemphasized. The adjustment (de-escalation of therapy) should be made as soon as culture results are available (within <72 hours of initiation of therapy).

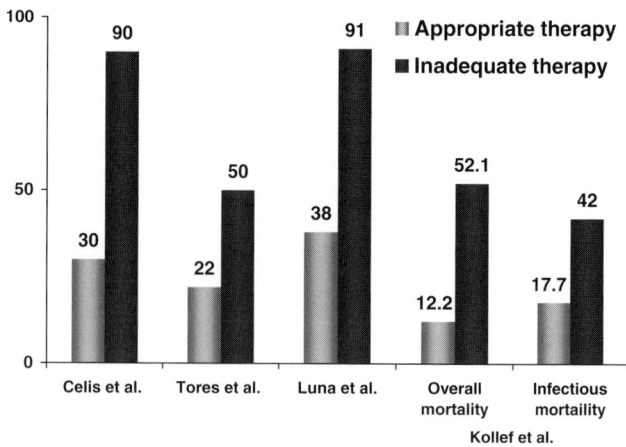

Figure 6   Therapy-dependent ventilator-associated pneumonia mortality. VAP-associated mortality (in %, *y*-axis) depending on inadequate or adequate systemic anti-microbial therapy. *Source*: From Ref. 236, 69, 71, 237.

OUTCOMES

The development of NP and VAP is associated with significant morbidity and mortality. Crude mortality rates of 20–50% have been documented (4). Attributable mortality rates are reported to be ~30%, and patients that develop VAP demonstrate a 30–50% higher mortality (relative risk increase) than those who require mechanical ventilation but do not develop VAP (223). VAP significantly increases the duration of mechanical ventilation and ICU length of stay (mean two to seven days), and thereby the amount of resource utilization and cost (224). Studies investigating various strategies of VAP prevention (i.e., weaning protocols, chlorhexidine oral decontamination) have demonstrated a reduction in overall mortality by 35% to 60% related to similar decreases in the incidence of VAP in their respective patient populations (118,119,177).

The reported impact on outcome in studies investigating the use of early aggressive invasive diagnosis has been variable. Fagon et al. demonstrated in a large prospective multicenter trial that invasive diagnosis and management reduced death from any cause at day 14 (16 vs. 26%) as well as organ failure scores at days 3 and 7 (225). In that study the group managed by invasive diagnostic strategy had significantly more antibiotic-free days (11.5 vs. 7.5, p < 0.001) compared to the clinical group. Several other studies have clearly demonstrated that delays in initiation of appropriate antibiotic therapy (for as little as 48 hr) increased crude morality rates 20–30% (odds ratio 1.72) (164,172,174). In addition to the early initiation of antibiotic therapy, concentrations of drugs must be adequate, and the choice of antimicrobial agent must be appropriate for the organism(s) present. Indeed, most studies have shown a 50% or more reduction in mortality when appropriate antibiotics are used compared to inadequate therapy (Fig. 6).

To improve outcomes it is important to combine several strategies in the diagnosis and therapy of VAP: in the normal host and in absence of significant confounding factors (i.e., ARDS, significant chronic lung disease, prolonged intubation, prior antimicrobial therapy, or potential other sources of infection) the clinical diagnosis of VAP

and confirmation with qualitative endotracheal aspirate cultures may be adequate to guide therapy. In all other patients, particularly those with late or recurrent episodes of VAP, consideration should be given to early invasive diagnosis. The decision-making process for initial empiric antibiotic regimen should include microbial data for the specific unit location of the patient, the time point of occurrence (early vs. late), as well as prior patient-specific culture data and antibiotic usage when available. Antibiotic therapy should be combined with intensive chest physiotherapy and strategies designed to wean the patient off mechanical ventilation (4,223–225).

EYE TO THE FUTURE

Future research in VAP is focused in three main areas: early accurate diagnosis of VAP with microbiology, reduction of duration of antimicrobial therapy for VAP treatment, and, most importantly, prevention of VAP.

Early Accurate Diagnosis of Ventilator-Associated Pneumonia

Multiple studies have defined that both bronchoscopic and non-bronchoscopic BAL are significantly more sensitive and specific than non-quantitative endotracheal aspirate cultures in the microbiological diagnosis of pneumonia in mechanically ventilated patients. Non-bronchoscopic BAL is a simple, safe, inexpensive bedside procedure, and should be examined in a large multi-center trial to determine if it has equal sensitivity and specificity compared with bronchoscopic BAL. This would greatly simplify the optimal procedure for diagnosis of VAP, and would potentially become a standard for use in all future clinical trials in VAP. At present, VAP studies are a mix of those that use the CDC clinical definition for VAP versus bronchoscopic BAL, making these studies difficult to compare.

Significant advances have been made in the rapid detection of resistant organisms, such as MRSA. A rapid procedure, providing results in less than six hours, was recently reported using mutiplex quantitative PCR for the identification of MRSA directly from sterile sites or mixed flora samples, such as nasal swabs (226). A 96-well format assay allowed analysis of 30 swab samples per run and detection of MRSA with exquisite sensitivity compared to optimal culture-based techniques that require two to three days. New rapid diagnostic technology such as this will allow us to minimize overuse of antibiotics, and employ targeted antibiotic therapy, in attempts to prevent widespread antimicrobial resistance.

Reduced Duration of Antibiotic Therapy for Ventilator-Associated Pneumonia Treatment

It is clearly evident from the research to date that it is imperative to prescribe initial appropriate antibiotic therapy in VAP treatment, but duration of therapy for VAP treatment remains controversial. Clinicians have commonly used arbitrary durations of antimicrobial treatment ranging from 10 to 21 days. Recent data suggest that other endpoints for defining duration of VAP treatment can be considered, such as the clinical pulmonary infection score (CPIS) (227). Serial measurements of CPIS in VAP patients may help define strategies to shorten duration of therapy for VAP.

Prevention of Ventilator-Associated Pneumonia

Traditional strategies aimed at prevention of VAP include the use of ventilator weaning protocols to reduce duration of mechanical ventilation and the semi-recumbent position to decrease aspiration incidence. All ICUs should aim to achieve full compliance with these standards that have been documented to reduce VAP.

Recent studies have focused on other innovative strategies to reduce bacterial colonization (228). Modified endotracheal tubes with a port for continuous suctioning of accumulated secretions in the subglottic space (CASS, continuous aspiration of subglottic secretions) have demonstrated potential benefit in small studies, but a large multi-center randomized study has not yet been accomplished. The efficacy of silver-coated endotracheal tubes is being investigated, using silver and hydrogel technology that is commonplace in the use of urinary catheters, and has been associated with reduced incidence of urinary tract infections (229). This has been hypothesized to occur due to the antibacterial properties of silver and its ability to prevent bio-film formation (229). It is well known that bio-films harbor large concentrations of bacteria that display an inherent resistance to therapy with systemically administered antibiotics.

Similarly, other strategies to reduce bacterial colonization in the posterior pharynx have been investigated, including the use of chlorhexidine gluconate oral rinse and protegrins (230). Protegrins are extremely broad-spectrum antimicrobial peptides, active against many bacterial and fungal species, including those resistant to conventional antimicrobial drugs, by attaching to and destroying the integrity of the lipid cell membrane (230). The first protegrin to undergo clinical trial is iseganan hydrochloride oral solution, and is in phase II/III clinical trials for the prevention of VAP (230). Inhaled protegrins are also being investigated for the active treatment respiratory tract infections in cystic fibrosis patients (230).

Noninvasive positive pressure ventilation (NPPV) has been documented to reduce VAP in patients with acute respiratory failure caused by exacerbations of chronic pulmonary disease. Cost reduction associated with NPPV in this group is attributed to the prevention of VAP by avoidance

of endotracheal intubation (230). The benefit of NPPV for patients with acute nonhypercarbic hypoxemic respiratory failure is less clear, and more clinical studies are necessary in this area. The CDC and the Healthcare Infection Control Practices Advisory Committee have developed a comprehensive Guideline for the Prevention of Healthcare-associated Pneumonia 2003, which reviews all potential therapies for prevention of VAP and the available evidence supporting their use (232).

SUMMARY

Hospital-acquired or nosocomial pneumonia is the second most common nosocomial infection in the United States and is associated with substantial morbidity and mortality. VAP significantly increases the duration of mechanical ventilation and ICU length of stay, and thereby the amount of resource utilization and cost. Most hospitalized patients who develop pneumonia have one or more risk factors, including ages above 65 yr, immunosuppression, altered sensorium, and significant pre-existing cardiac or pulmonary disease, or have undergone major thoraco-abdominal surgical procedures. The pathophysiology of VAP is complex and includes host-related, equipment-related, and microbial factors that promote colonization of the tracheo-bronchial tree, impaired clearance of microorganisms, and alteration of the local immune response, ultimately leading to pulmonary infection. The most important factors contributing to the development of VAP include oro-pharyngeal colonization and micro-aspiration, pulmonary de-recruitment and decreased clearance, prolonged mechanical ventilation, and development of ARDS.

Consensus regarding the diagnosis of ventilator-associated pneumonia has been difficult to reach in the past. The clinical diagnosis is based on the appearance of new infiltrates on plain chest radiographs, new or altered appearance of respiratory secretions, and general signs of infection (i.e., leukocytosis and fever). While this approach may be sufficient for the normal host and in absence of significant confounding factors (i.e., ARDS, significant chronic lung disease, prolonged intubation, prior antimicrobial therapy, or potential other sources of infection), pneumonia is often over diagnosed in critically ill patients, using clinical criteria alone. Protected specimen brushing, and bronchoscopic and nonbronchoscopic bronchoalveolar lavage (BAL) are significantly more sensitive and specific than nonquantitative endotracheal aspirate cultures in the microbiological diagnosis of pneumonia in mechanically ventilated patients and are becoming the standard of care for critically ill patients.

Organized strategies for the prevention of pneumonia in mechanically ventilated patients are of paramount importance, should address various aspects of the pathophysiology of VAP simultaneously, and include most importantly the use of ventilator weaning protocols to reduce duration of mechanical ventilation, the semi-recumbent position to decrease aspiration incidence, the use of improved oro-pharyngeal hygiene (chlorhexidine), and prevention of progressive pulmonary de-recruitment (chest physiotherapy, positioning therapy). Studies have demonstrated reduction in overall mortality by 35% to 60% using these strategies. All ICUs should aim to achieve full compliance with these standards that have been documented to reduce VAP.

The mainstay of therapy in NP and VAP is adequate systemic antibiotic coverage. The antibiotics used should be bactericidal to the suspected pathogen(s) and reach adequate tissue levels in the lung. There is a striking difference in the prevalence of individual pathogens between individual patient care units within each hospital, and studies and aggregate data from the NNIS demonstrate an alarming increase in drug resistance and prevalence of the problem pathogens in the United States. Patient factors (i.e., pulmonary disease, type of surgery, immune status, and prior antibiotic exposure) and the timing of the occurrence (early vs. late) of VAP, as well as the severity of the infection, further influence the spectrum of most likely pathogens. Inadequate initial therapy, even when begun early, is associated with worse outcomes. Therefore, it is of utmost importance to know the patient's clinical history, severity and timing of VAP, and locale-specific data prior to making the choice for empiric therapy. Empiric therapy should be tailored to the patient-specific pathogens as soon as culture data are available. Duration of therapy for VAP treatment remains controversial; currently arbitrary durations of antimicrobial treatment range from 7 to 21 days. Recent data suggest that shorter duration of therapy may be feasible in uncomplicated VAP and that end-points such as serial measurements of the clinical pulmonary infection score (CPIS) may help define strategies to shorten duration of therapy for VAP (222).

KEY POINTS

✎ Health care worker (HCW) cross contamination has been shown to play an important role in the pathogenesis of VAP.

✎ Endotracheal tube (ETT) bio-film formation and tracheal colonization have been acknowledged as potentially significant factors leading to (chronic) tracheo-bronchitis and subsequent lower airspace infection.

✎ Increased colonization of the esophagus and stomach with a bacterial shift towards pathogenic enteric gram negative species and candida has been demonstrated in critically ill patients.

✎ It is currently recommended to use agents that do not raise the gastric pH in patients with low to moderate risk of upper GI bleeding. Drugs that lower pH are recommended for patients at high risk of upper gastrointestinal bleeding.

✎ Recent studies have demonstrated significant reductions in VAP (37–69%) and mortality (40–45%) in critically ill surgical and cardiac surgery patients by improving oral hygiene through frequent suctioning of pooled secretions and the use of the topical disinfectant chlorhexidine.

✎ Pulmonary de-recruitment (atelectasis, alveolar collapse) begins early and is progressive in supine patients receiving mechanical ventilation.

✎ Duration of mechanical ventilation itself may be the single most important risk factor for the development of pneumonia.

✎ The clinical diagnosis of VAP is based on the appearance of new infiltrates on plain chest radiographs, new or altered appearance of respiratory secretions, and general signs of infection (i.e., leukocytosis and fever).

✎ To avoid therapy delay, several studies suggest the use of an initial Gram stain obtained via guided or non-guided BAL or PSB as a guide to initiate therapy. Sensitivity and specificity are slightly lower than those of quantitative cultures, but positive and negative predictive values are between 70% and 90%.

✎ Invasive diagnosis with BAL or PSB may not be necessary in the normal host that has clear clinical evidence of VAP, has an absence of other potential sources of infection, and responds appropriately to a course of antibiotic therapy. Invasive diagnosis should be considered early in patients that have equivocal clinical signs, in the immunocompromised host, in patients with evidence of severe infection, in patients with ARDS and suspected VAP, in patients who develop late VAP, and in those who do not respond to therapy.

✎ In ARDS, the combination of an altered local immune response, loss of alveolar wall integrity, and collapse or consolidation of parenchyma with subsequent under-ventilation of these areas is thought to act synergistically in predisposing these patients to the development of VAP.

✎ The mainstay of therapy in NP and VAP is adequate systemic antibiotic coverage. The antibiotics used should be bactericidal to the suspected pathogen(s), and reach adequate tissue levels in the lung.

✎ There is a striking difference in the prevalence of individual pathogens between countries, hospitals, and even individual patient care units within each hospital.

✎ Early VAP (occurrence <5–7 days), particularly in trauma patients, is associated most commonly with Streptococcus pneumoniae (SP), Haemophilus influenzae (HI), enteric Gram negative bacilli (GNB) and methicillin sensitive Staphylococci (MSSA). A prolonged hospital stay prior to intubation and exposure to (broad-spectrum) antibiotics are linked to a higher incidence of *Pseudomonas aeruginosa* (PA), *Acinetobacter* spp., and other resistant Staphylococci (MRSA) and, possibly, vancomycin resistant *Enterococcus spp.* (VRE).

REFERENCES

1. Richards MJ, Edwards JR, Culver DH, et al. Nosocomial infections in medical intensive care units in the United States. Crit Care Med 1999; 27(5):887–892.
2. Wilbin R. Nosocomial pneumonia. In: Wenzel R., ed. Prevention and control of nosocomial infections. Baltimore: Williams and Wilkins, 1997:807–819.
3. Kollef MH. Prevention of hospital-associated pneumonia and ventilator-associated pneumonia. Crit Care Med 2004; 32(6):1396–1405.
4. Hospital-acquired Pneumonia Guideline Committee of the American Thoracic Society & Infectious Diseases Society of America. Guidelines for the management of adults with hospital-acquired pneumonia, ventilator-associated pneumonia, and healthcare-associated pneumonia – 2005. Am J Resp Crit Care Med 2005; 171:388–416.
5. Centers for Disease Control and Prevention. Guidelines for prevention of nosocomial pneumonia. MMWR Recomm Rep 1997; 46:1–79.
6. Centers for Disease Control and Prevention NNIS System. National Nosocomial Infections Surveillance (NNIS) system report, data summary from January 1992–June 2001, Issues August 2001. Am J Infect Control 2001; 29:404–421.
7. Reinarz JA, Pierce AK, Mays BB, Sanford JP. The potential role of inhalation therapy equipment in nosocomial pulmonary infection. J Clin Invest 1965; 44:831–839.
8. Pierce AK, Sanford JP, Thomas GD, Leonard JS. Long-term evaluation of decontamination of inhalation-therapy equipment and the occurrence of necrotizing pneumonia. N Engl J Med 1970; 292:528–531.
9. Comhaire A, Lamy RM. Contamination rate of sterilized ventilators in an ICU. Crit Care Med 1981; 9:546–548.

10. Craven DE, Connolly MG, Lichtenberg DA, et al. Contamination of mechanical ventilators with tubing changes every 24 or 48 hr. N Engl J Med 1982; 306:1505–1509.

11. Lareau SC, Ryan KJ, Diener CF. The relationship between frequency of ventilator circuit changes and infectious hazard. Am Rev Resp Dis 1978; 118:493–496.

12. Han JN, Liu YP, Ma S, et al. Effects of decreasing the frequency of ventilator circuit changes to every 7 days on the rate of ventilator-associated pneumonia in a Bejing hospital. Resp Care 2001; 46:888–890.

13. Cook D, Ricard JD, Reeve B, et al. Ventilator circuit and secretion management strategies: a Franco–Canadian survey. Crit Care Med 2000; 28:3547–3554.

14. Salemi C, Padilla S, Canola T, Reynolds D. Heat-and-moisture exchangers used with biweekly circuit tubing changes: effect on costs and pneumonia rates. Infect Control Hosp Epidemiol 2000; 21:737–739.

15. Long MN, Wickstrom G, Grimes A, et al. Prospective, randomized study of ventilator-associated pneumonia in patients with one *versus* three ventilator circuit tubing changes per week. Infect Control Hosp Epidemiol 1996; 17:14–19.

16. Kollef MH, Shapiro SD, Fraser VJ, et al. Mechanical ventilation with or without 7-day circuit changes. A randomized controlled trial. Ann Intern Med 1995; 124:168–174.

17. Stamm AM. Ventilator-associated pneumonia and frequency of circuit changes. Am J Infect Control 1998; 26:71–73.

18. Gorman LJ, Sanai L, Notman AW, Grant IS, Masterton RG. Cross infection in an intensive care unit by Klebsiella pneumoniae from ventilator condensate. J Hosp Infect 1993; 23:27–34.

19. Craven DE, Goularte TA, Make BA. Contaminated condensate in mechanical ventilator circuits—risk factor for nosocomial pneumonia? Am Rev Resp Dis 1984; 129:625–628.

20. Arnow PM, Chou T, Weil D, Shapiro EN, Kretzschmar C. Nosocomial Legionnaires' disease caused by aerosolized tap water from respiratory devices. J Infect Dis 1982; 146:460–467.

21. Goularte TA, Manning M, Craven DE. Bacterial colonization in humidifying cascade reservoirs after 24 and 48 hr of continuous mechanical ventilation. Infect Control 1987; 8:200–203.

22. Vesley D, Anderson J, Halbert MM, Wyman L. Bacterial output from three respiratory therapy humidifying devices. Resp Care 1979; 24:228–234.

23. Rhame FS, Streifel A, McComb C, Boyle M. Bubbling humidifiers produce microaerosols which can carry bacteria. Infect Control 1986; 7:403–407.

24. Pierce AK, Sanford JP. Bacterial contamination of aerosols. Arch Intern Med 1973; 131:156–159.

25. Favero MS, Bond WW. Clinical disinfection of medical and surgical materials. In: Block S, ed. Disinfection, Sterilization, and Preservation. 4th ed. Philadelphia: Lea and Febiger, 1991:617–641.

26. Tomachot L, Vialet R, Arnaud S, et al. Do the components of heat and moisture exchanger filters affect their humidifying efficacy and the incidence of nosocomial pneumonia? Crit Care Med 1999; 27:923–928.

27. Kollef MH, Shapiro SD, Boyd V, et al. A randomized trial comparing an extended-use hygroscopic condenser humidifier with heated water humidification in mechanically ventilated patients. Chest 1998; 113:759–767.

28. Das I, Fraise AP. How useful are microbial filters in respiratory apparatus? J Hosp Infect 1997; 37:263–272. Comment in J Hosp Infect 1998; 39:331–332.

29. Make BJ, Craven DE, O'Donnell C. Clinical and bacteriologic comparison of hygroscopic and cascade humidifiers in ventilated patients [Abstract]. Am Rev Resp Dis 1987; 135:A212.

30. Roustan JP, Kienlen J, Aubas P, et al. Comparison of hydrophobic heat and moisture exchanger with heated humidifier during prolonged mechanical ventilation. Inten Care Med 1992; 18:97–100.

31. Misset B, Escudier B, Rivara D, et al. Heat and moisture exchanger vs. heated humidifier during long-term mechanical ventilation: a prospective randomized study. Chest 1991; 100:160–163.

32. Martin C, Perrin G, Gevaudan MJ, et al. Heat and moisture exchangers and vaporizing humidifiers in the intensive care unit. Chest 1990; 97:144–149.

33. Craven DE, Lichtenberg DA, Goularte TA, et al. Contaminated medication nebulizers in mechanical ventilator circuits. Am J Med 1984; 77:834–838.

34. Moffet HL, Williams T. Bacteria recovered from distilled water and inhalation therapy equipment. Am J Dis Child 1967; 114:7–12.

35. Ringrose RE, McKown B, Felton FG, et al. A hospital outbreak of Serratia marcescens associated with ultrasonic nebulizers. Ann Intern Med 1968; 69:719–729.

36. Rhoades ER, Ringrose R, Mohr JA, et al. Contamination of ultrasonic nebulization equipment with gram negative bacteria. Arch Intern Med 1971; 127:228–232.

37. Moffet HL, Allan D. Survival and dissemination of bacteria in nebulizers and incubators. Am J Dis Child 1967; 114:13–20.

38. Seto WH, Ching TY, Yuen KY, Lam WK. Evaluating the sterility of disposable wall oxygen humidifiers, during and between use on patients. Infect Control 1990; 11:604–605.

39. Larson E. Persistent carriage of gram-negative bacteria on hands. Am J Infect Control 1981; 9:112–119.

40. Doebbeling BN, Stanley GL, Sheetz CT, et al. Comparative efficacy of alternative hand-washing agents in reducing nosocomial infections in intensive care units. N Engl J Med 1992; 327:88–93.

41. Simmons B, Bryant J, Neiman K, et al. The Role of hand washing in prevention of endemic intensive care unit infections. Infect Control Hosp Epidemiol 1990; 11:589–594.

42. Kollef MH, Prentice D, Shapiro SD, et al. Mechanical ventilation with or without daily changes of in-line suction catheters. AM J Resp Crit Care Med 1997; 156:466–472.

43. Combes P, Fauvage B, Oleyer C. Nosocomial pneumonia in mechanically ventilated patients, a prospective randomized evaluation of the Stericath closed suctioning system. Inten Care Med 2000; 26:878–882.

44. Decker MD, Lancaster AD, Latham RH, et al. Influence of closed suctioning system on ventilator-associated pneumonias. Third Annual Meeting of the Society for Hospital Epidemiology of America, 1993:A6 (Abstract).

45. Johnson KL, Kearney PA, Johnson SB, et al. Closed *versus* open endotracheal suctioning: costs and physiologic consequences. Crit Care Med 1994; 22:658–666.

46. Gorman SP, McGovern JG, Woolfson AD, et al. The concomitant development of poly(vinyl-chloride)-related biofilm and antimicrobial resistance to ventilator-associated pneumonia. Biomaterials 2001; 22:2741–2747.

47. Inglis TJ, Lim TM, Ng MI, et al. Structural features of tracheal tube biofilm formed during prolonged mechanical ventilation. Chest 1995; 108:1049–1052.

48. Wallace WC, Cinat M, Gornick WB, et al. Nosocomial infections in the intensive care unit: a difference between trauma and surgical patients. Am Surg 1999; 65:987–990.

49. Adair CG, Gorman SP, Feron BM, et al. Implications of endotracheal biofilm for ventilator-associated pneumonia. Inten Care Med 1999; 25:1072–1076.

50. Ahmed QA, Niederman MS. Respiratory infection in the critically ill patient. Ventilator-associated pneumonia and tracheobronchitis. Clin Chest Med 2001; 22:71–85.

51. Berthelot P, Grattard F, Mahul P, et al. Prospective study of nosocomial colonization and infection due to Pseudomonas aeruginosa in mechanically ventilated patients. Inten Care Med 2001; 27:503–512.

52. Sirvent JM, Torres A, Vidaur L, et al. Tracheal colonization within 24 hr of intubation in patients with head trauma: risk factor for developing early-onset ventilator-associated pneumonia. Inten Care Med 2000; 26:1369–1372.

53. Ewig S, Torres A, El-Ebiary M, et al. Bacterial colonization patterns in mechanically ventilated patients with traumatic and medical head injury. Incidence, risk factors, and association

with ventilator-associated pneumonia. Am J Resp Crit Care Med 1999; 159:188–198.

54. Hartmann M, Guttmann J, Muller B, et al. Reduction of bacterial load by the silver-coated endotracheal tube (SCET), a laboratory investigation. Technol Healthcare 1999; 7:359–370.

55. Teoh WH, Goh KY, Chan C. The role of early tracheostomy in critically ill neurosurgical patients. Ann Acad Med Singapore 2001; 30:324–328.

56. Brook AD, Sherman G, Malen J, Kollef MH. Early versus late tracheostomy in patients who require prolonged mechanical ventilation. Am J Crit Care 2000; 9:352–359.

57. Barret JP, Desai MH, Herndon DN. Effects of tracheostomies on infection and airway complications in pediatric burn patients. Burns 2000; 26:190–193.

58. Kollef MH, Ahrens TS, Shannon W. Clinical predictors and outcomes for patients requiring tracheostomy in the intensive care unit. Crit Care Med 1999; 27:1714–1720.

59. Sugerman HJ, Wolfe I, Pasquale MD, et al. Multicenter, randomized, prospective trial of early tracheostomy. J Trauma 1997; 43:741–747.

60. Kane TD, Rodriguez JL, Luchette FA. Early versus late tracheostomy in the trauma patient. Resp Care Clin N Am 1997; 3:1–20.

61. Kluger Y, Paul DB, Lucke J, et al. Early tracheostomy in trauma patients. Eur J Emerg Med 1996; 3:95–101.

62. Zeitouni AG, Kost KM. Tracheostomy: a retrospective review of 281 cases. J Otolaryngol 1994; 23:61–66.

63. Johanson WG. Tracheostomy risks outweigh benefits in preventing pneumonia. J Crit Illn 1993; 8:656–657.

64. Lesnik I, Rappaport W, Fulginiti J, Witzke D. The role of early tracheostomy in blunt, multiple organ trauma. Am Surg 1992; 58:346–349.

65. Bonten MJ, Gaillard CA, de Leeuw PW, Stobberingh EE. Role of colonization of the upper intestinal tract in the pathogenesis of ventilator-associated pneumonia. Clin Infect Dis 1997; 24:309–319.

66. Huxley EJ, Viroslav J, Gray WR, Pierce AK. Pharyngeal aspiration in normal adults and patients with depressed consciousness. Am J Med 1973; 64:564–568.

67. Torres A, El-Ebiary M, Soler N, et al. Stomach as source of colonization of the respiratory tract during mechanical ventilation: association with ventilator-associated pneumonia. Eur Resp J 1996; 9:1729–1735.

68. de Latorre FJ, Pont T, Ferrer A, et al. Pattern of tracheal colonization during mechanical ventilation. Am J Resp Crit Care Med 1995; 152:1028–1033.

69. Torres A, Aznar R, Gatell JM, et al. Incidence, risk, and prognosis factors of nosocomial pneumonia in mechanically ventilated patients. Am Rev Resp Dis 1990; 142:523–528.

70. Craven DE, Kunches LM, Kilinsky V, Lichtenberg DA, Make BJ, McCabe WR. Risk factors for pneumonia and fatality in patients receiving continuous mechanical ventilation. Am Rev Resp Dis 1986; 133:792–796.

71. Celis R, Torres A, Gatell JM, et al. Nosocomial pneumonia—a multivariate analysis of risk and prognosis. Chest 1988; 93:318–324.

72. Spray SB, Zuidema GD, Cameron HL. Aspiration pneumonia: incidence of aspiration with endotracheal tubes. Am J Surg 1976; 131:701–703.

73. Cameron JL, Reynolds J, Zuidema GD. Aspiration in patients with tracheostomies. Surg Gynecol Obstet 1973; 136:68–70.

74. Cook D, Guyatt G, Marshall J, et al. A comparison of sucralfate and ranitidine for the prevention of upper gastrointestinal bleeding in patients requiring mechanical ventilation. Canadian Critical Care Trials Group. N Engl J Med 1998; 19:338.

75. Bonten MJ, Gaillard CA, van der Geest S, et al. The role of intragastric acidity and stress ulcer prophylaxis on colonization and infection in mechanically ventilated ICU patients. A stratified, randomized, double-blind study of sucralfate versus antacids. Am J Resp Crit Care 1995; 152:1825–1834.

76. Pingleton SK, Hinthron DR, Liu C. Eternal nutrition in patients receiving mechanical ventilation: Multiple sources of tracheal colonization include the stomach. Am J Med 1986; 80:827–832.

77. Kappstein I, Friedrich T, Hellinger P. Incidence of pneumonia in mechanically ventilated patients treated with sucralfate or cimetidine as prophylaxis for stress bleeding: bacterial colonization of the stomach. Am J Med 1991; 91(Suppl 2A):125S–131S.

78. Driks MR, Craven DE, Celli BR, et al. Nosocomial pneumonia in intubated patients given sucralfate as compared with antacids or histamine type 2 blockers. N Engl J Med 1987; 317:1376–1382.

79. Cook DJ, Fuller HD, Guyatt GH, et al. Risk factors for gastrointestinal bleeding in critically ill patients. Canadian Critical Care Trials Group. N Engl J Med 1994; 330:377–381.

80. Daschner F, Kappstein I, Reuschenbach K, et al. Stress ulcer prophylaxis and ventilation pneumonia: prevention by antibacterial cytoprotective agents? Infect Control 1988; 9:59–65.

81. Prod'hom G, Leuenberger PH, Koerfer J, et al. Nosocomial pneumonia in mechanically ventilated patients receiving antacid, ranitidine, or sucralfate as prophylaxis for stress ulcer. Ann Intern Med 1994; 120:653–662.

82. Cook DJ, Laine LA, Guyatt GH, Raffin TA. Nosocomial pneumonia and the role of gastric pH. A meta-analysis. Chest 1991; 100:7–13.

83. Pickworth KK, Falcone RE, Hoogeboom JE, Santanello SA. Occurrence of nosocomial pneumonia in mechanically ventilated trauma patients: a comparison of sucralfate and ranitidine. Crit Care Med 1993; 21:1856–1862.

84. Stoutenbeek CP, Van Saene HKF, Miranda DR, Zandstra DF. The effect of selective decontamination of the digestive tract on colonisation and infection rate in multiple trauma patients. Inten Care Med 1984; 10:185–192.

85. Ledingham IM, Alcock SR, Eastaway AT, et al. Triple regimen of selective decontamination of the digestive tract, systemic cefotaxime, and microbiological surveillance for prevention of acquired infection in intensive care. Lancet 1988; i:785–790.

86. Ulrich C, Harinck-de Weerd JE, Bakker NC, et al. Selective decontamination of the digestive tract with norfloxacin in the prevention of ICU-acquired infections: a prospective randomized study. Inten Care Med 1989; 15:424–431.

87. Flaherty J, Nathan C, Kabins SA, Weinstein RA. Pilot trial of selective decontamination for prevention of bacterial infection in an intensive care unit. J Infect Dis 1990; 162:1393–1397.

88. McClelland P, Murray AE, Williams PS, et al. Reducing sepsis in severe combined acute renal and respiratory failure by selective decontamination of the digestive tract. Crit Care Med 1990; 18:935–939.

89. Rodriguez-Roldan JM, Altuna-Cuesta A, Lopez A, et al. Prevention of nosocomial lung infection in ventilated patients: use of an antimicrobial pharyngeal nonabsorbable paste. Crit Care Med 1990; 180:1239–1242.

90. Aerdts SJA, van Daelen R, Clasener HAL, et al. Antibiotic prophylaxis of respiratory tract infection in mechanically ventilated patients: A prospective, blinded, randomized trial of the effect of a novel regimen. Chest 1991; 100:783–791.

91. Blair P, Rowlands BJ, Lowry K, et al. Selective decontamination of the digestive tract: A stratified, randomized, prospective study in a mixed intensive care unit. Surgery 1991; 110:303–310.

92. Hartenauer U, Thulig B, Diemer W, et al. Effect of selective flora suppression on colonization, infection, and mortality in critically ill patients: A one-year, prospective consecutive study. Crit Care Med 1991; 19:463–473.

93. Vandenbroucke-Grauls CMJE, Vandenbroucke JP. Effect of selective decontamination of the digestive tract on respiratory tract infections and mortality in the intensive care unit. Lancet 1991; 338:859–862.

94. Cockerill FR, Muller SM, Anhalt JP, et al. Prevention of infection on critically ill patients by selective decontamination of the digestive tract. Ann Intern Med 1992; 117:545–553.

95. Gastinne H, Wolff M, Destour F, et al. A controlled trial in intensive care units of selective decontamination of the digestive tract with nonabsorbable antibiotics. N Engl J Med 1992; 326:594–599.

96. van Nieuwenhoven CA, Buskens E, van Tiel FH, et al. Relationship between methodological trial quality and the effects of selective digestive decontamination on pneumonia and mortality in critically ill patients. JAMA 2001; 286:335–340.

97. Liberati A, D'Amico R, Pifferi, Torri V. Antibiotic prophylaxis to reduce respiratory tract infections and mortality in adults receiving intensive care. Cochrane Database Syst Rev 2004; 000022 [PMID: 14973945].

98. Dodek P, Keenan S, Cook D, et al. Evidence-based clinical practice guideline for the prevention of ventilator-associated pneumonia. Ann Intern Med 2004; 141:305–313.

99. Kearns PJ, Chin D, Mueller L, et al. The incidence of ventilator-associated pneumonia and success in nutrient delivery with gastric versus small intestinal feeding: a randomized clinical trial. Crit Care Med 2000; 28:1742–1746.

100. Ibanez J, Penafiel A, Marse P, et al. Incidence of gastroesophageal reflux and aspiration in mechanically ventilated patients using small-bore nasogastric tubes. JPEN 2000; 24:103–106.

101. Olivares L, Segovia A, Revuelta R. Tube feeding and lethal aspiration in neurologic patients: A review of 720 autopsy cases. Stroke 1974; 5:654–657.

102. Drakulovic MB, Torres A, Bauer TT, et al. Supine body position as risk factor for nosocomial pneumonia in mechanically ventilated patients: a randomized trial. Lancet 1999; 354:1851–1858.

103. Treolar DM, Stechmiller J. Pulmonary aspiration of tube-fed patients with artificial airways. Heart Lung 1984; 13:667–671.

104. Heyland D, Bradley C, Mandell LA. Effect of acidified enteral feedings on gastric colonization in the critically ill patient. Crit Care Med 1992; 20:1388–1394.

105. Heyland DK, Cook DJ, Schoenfeld PS, et al. The effect of acidified enteral feeds on gastric colonization in critically ill patients: results of a multicenter randomized trial. Canadian Critical Care Trials Group. Crit Care Med 1999; 27:2399–2406.

106. Bonten MJM, Gaillard CA, Van der Juist R, et al. Intermittent enteral feeding: The influence on respiratory and digestive tract colonization in mechanically ventilated Intensive care unit patients. Am J Resp Crit Care Med 1996; 154:394–399.

107. Lee B, Chang RWS, Jacobs S. Intermittent nasogastric feeding: A simple and effective method to reduce pneumonia among ventilated ICU patients. Clin Inten Care 1990; 1:100–102.

108. Cook DJ, Meade MO, Hand LE, et al. Toward understanding evidence uptake: semirecumbency for pneumonia prevention. Crit Care Med 2002; 30:1472–1477.

109. Reynolds HY. Bacterial adherence to respiratory tract mucosa: A dynamic interaction leading to colonization. Seminars Resp Infect 1987; 2:8–19.

110. Rosenthal S, Tager IB. Prevalence of gram-negative rods in the normal pharyngeal flora. Ann Intern Med 1975; 83:355–357.

111. Valenti WM, Trudell RG, Bentley DW. Factors predisposing to oropharyngeal colonization with gram-negative bacilli in the aged. N Engl J Med 1978; 298:1108–1111.

112. Niederman MS. Bacterial adherence as a mechanism of airway colonization. Eur J Clin Microbiol Infect Dis 1989; 8:15–20.

113. Johanson WG Jr, Higuchi JH, Chaudhuri TR. Bacterial adherence to epithelial cells in bacillary colonization of the respiratory tract. Am Rev Resp Dis 1980; 121:55–63.

114. Niederman MS, Merrill WW, Polomski LM, Reynolds HY, Gee JBL. Influence of sputum IgA and elastase on tracheal cell bacterial adherence. Am Rev Resp Dis 1986; 133:255–260.

115. Palmer LB, Merrill WW, Niederman MS, et al. Bacterial adherence to respiratory tract cells: Relationships between in vivo and in vitro pH and bacterial attachments. Am Rev Resp Dis 1986; 133:784–788.

116. Genuit T, Bochicchio G, Napolitano LM, et al. Prophylactic Chlorhexidine oral rinse decreases ventilator-associated pneumonia in surgical ICU patients. Surg Infections 2001; 2:5–18.

117. DeRiso AJ, Ladowski JS, Dillon TA, et al. Chlorhexidine gluconate 0.12% oral rinse reduces the incidence of total nosocomial respiratory infection and nonprophylactic antibiotic use in patients undergoing heart surgery. Chest 1996; 109:1556–1561.

118. Pugin J, Auckenthaler R, Lew DP, Suter PM. Oropharyngeal decontamination decreases incidence of ventilator-associated pneumonia: A randomized, placebo-controlled, double-blind clinical trial. JAMA 1991; 265:2704–2710.

119. American Thoracic Society. Consensus statement: Hospital-acquired pneumonia in adults: diagnosis, assessment of severity, initial antimicrobial therapy, and prevention strategies. Am Resp Crit Care Med 1996; 151:1711–1725.

120. Vallas J, Artigas A, Rello J, et al. Continuous aspiration of subglottis secretions in preventing ventilator-associated pneumonia. Ann Intern Med 1995; 122:179–186.

121. Shorr AF, O'Malley PG. Continuous subglottic suctioning for the prevention of ventilator-associated pneumonia: potential economic implications. Chest 2001; 119:228–235.

122. Kollef MH, Skubas NJ, Sundt TM. A randomized clinical trial of continuous aspiration of subglottic secretions in cardiac surgery patients. Chest 1999; 116:1339–1346.

123. Kelley RE, Vibulsresth S, Bell L, Duncan RC. Evaluation of kinetic therapy in the prevention of complications of prolonged bed rest secondary to stroke. Stroke 1987; 18:638–642.

124. Gentilello L, Thompson DA, Tonnesen AS, et al. Effect of a rotating bed on the incidence of pulmonary complications in critically ill patients. Crit Care Med 1988; 16:783–786.

125. Summer WR, Curry P, Haponik EF, et al. Continuous mechanical turning of intensive care unit patients shortens length of stay in some diagnostic-related groups. J Crit Care 1989; 4:45–53.

126. Fink MP, Helsmoortel CM, Stein KL, et al. The efficacy of an oscillating bed in the prevention of lower respiratory tract infection in critically ill victims of blunt trauma: a prospective study. Chest 1990; 97:132–137.

127. Nelson LD, Choi SC. Kinetic therapy in critically ill trauma patients. Clin Inten Care 1992; 37:248–252.

128. deBoisblanc BP, Castro M, Everret B, et al. Effect of air-supported, continuous, postural oscillation on the risk of early ICU pneumonia in nontraumatic critical illness. Chest 1993; 103:1543–1547.

129. Tobin A, Kelly W. Prone positioning—it's time. Anaesth Inten Care 1999; 27:194–201.

130. Webster NR. Ventilation in the prone position. Lancet 1997; 349:1638–1639. Comments: Gattinoni et al. Ventilation in the prone position. The prone position Study Collaborative Group. Lancet 1997; 350:815; Lavender et al. Regional ventilation in the prone position. Lancet 1997; 350:1117.

131. Marelich GP, Murin S, Battistella F, et al. Protocol weaning of mechanical ventilation in medical and surgical patients by respiratory care practitioners and nurses: effect on weaning and the incidence of ventilator-associated pneumonia. Chest 2000; 118:459–467.

132. deBoisblanc MW, Goldman RK, Mayberry JC, et al. Weaning injured patients with prolonged pulmonary failure from mechanical ventilation in a non-intensive care unit setting. J Trauma 2000; 49:224–230.

133. Kollef MH, Horst HM, Prang L, Brock WA. Reducing the duration of mechanical ventilation: three examples of change in the intensive care unit. New Horiz 1998; 6:52–60.

134. Kollef MH. Current concepts: the prevention of ventilator-associated pneumonia. N Engl J Med 1999; 340(8):627–634.

135. Markowicz P, Wolff M, Dejedaini K, et al. Multicenter prospective study of ventilator-associated pneumonia during acute respiratory distress syndrome. Incidence, prognosis, and risk

factors. ARDS Study Group. Am J Resp Crit Care Med 2000; 161:1942–1948.

136. Croce MA. Diagnosis of acute respiratory distress syndrome and differentiation from ventilator-associated pneumonia. Am J Surg 2000; 179(Suppl 2A):26S–30S.

137. Meduri GU, Reddy RC, Stanley T, El-Zeky F. Pneumonia in acute respiratory distress syndrome. A prospective evaluation of bilateral bronchoscopic sampling. Am J Resp Crit Care Med 1998; 158:870–875.

138. Chastre J, Trouillet JL, Vuagnat A, et al. Nosocomial pneumonia in patients with respiratory distress syndrome. Am J Resp Crit Care Med 1998; 157:1165–1172.

139. Delcaux C, Roupie E, Blot F, et al. Lower respiratory tract colonization and infection during severe acute respiratory distress syndrome: incidence and diagnosis. Am J Resp Crit Care Med 1997; 156:1092–1098.

140. Headley AS, Tolley E, Meduri GU. Infections and the inflammatory response in the acute respiratory distress syndrome. Chest 1997; 111:1306–1321.

141. Hahn U, Pereida P, Heininger A, et al. Value of CT diagnosis of respirator-associated pneumonia. Rofo fortschr Geb Rontgenstr Neuen Nildgeb Verfahr 1999; 170:150–155.

142. Winer-Muram HT, Steiner RM, Gurney JW, et al. Ventilator-associated pneumonia in patients with adult respiratory distress syndrome: CT evaluation. Radiology 1998; 208:193–199.

143. Allegra L, Blasi F, Diano PL, et al. Sputum color as a marker of acute bacterial exacerbations in chronic obstructive pulmonary disease. Resp Med 2005; 99:742–747.

144. Luna CM, Videla A, Mattera J, et al. Blood cultures have limited value in predicting the severity of illness and as a diagnostic tool in ventilator-associated pneumonia. Chest 1999; 116:1075–1084.

145. El-Ebiary M, Torres A, Gonzales J, de la Bellacasa JP, et al. Quantitative cultures of endotracheal aspirates for the diagnosis of ventilator-associated pneumonia. Am Rev Resp Dis 1993; 148:1552–1557.

146. Torres A, de la Bellacasa J, Rodruigez-Roisin R, et al. Diagnostic value of telescoping plugged catheters in mechanically ventilated patients with bacterial pneumonia using the Metras catheter. Am Rev Resp Dis 1988; 138:117–120.

147. Jorda R, Parras F, Ibanez J, et al. Diagnosis of pneumonia in mechanically ventilated patients by the blind protected telescoping catheter. Inten Care Med 1993; 19:377–382.

148. Salata RA, Lederman MM, Shlaes DM, et al. Diagnosis of nosocomial pneumonia in intubated, intensive care unit patients. Am Rev Resp Dis 1987; 135:426–432.

149. Jourdain B, Novara A, Joly-Guillou ML, et al. Role of quantitative cultures of endotracheal aspirates in the diagnosis of nosocomial pneumonia. Am J Resp Crit Care 1995;15:241–246.

150. Balthazar AB, Von Nowakonski A, De Capitani EM, et al. Diagnostic investigation of ventilator-associated pneumonia using bronchalveolar lavage: comparative study with postmortem lung biopsy. Braz J Med Biol Res 2001; 34:993–1001.

151. Minei JP, Hawkins K, Moody B, Bottini PV, et al. Alternative case definitions of ventilator-associated pneumonia identify different patients in a surgical intensive care unit. Shock 2000; 14:331–336; discussion: 336–337.

152. Duflo F, Allaouchiche B, Debon R, et al. An evaluation of the Gram stain in protected bronchoalveolar lavage fluid for the early diagnosis of ventilator-associated pneumonia. Anaesth Analg 2001; 92:442–447.

153. Woske HJ, Roding T, Schulz I, Lode H. Ventilator-associated pneumonia in a surgical intensive care unit: epidemiology, etiology and comparison of three bronchoscopic methods for microbiological specimen sampling. Crit Care 2001; 5:167–173.

154. Mayhall CG. Ventilator-associated pneumonia or not? Contemporary diagnosis. Emerg Infect Dis 2001; 7:200–204.

155. Bregeon F, Papazian L, Thomas P, et al. Diagnostic accuracy of protected catheter sampling in ventilator-associated bacterial pneumonia. Eur Resp J 2000; 16:969–975.

156. Pittet D, Bonten MJ. Towards invasive diagnostic techniques as the standard of management of ventilator-associate pneumonia. Lancet 2000; 356:874; comment in Lancet 2000; 356:2011.

157. Torres A, Fabregas N, Ewig S, et al. Sampling methods for ventilator-associated pneumonia: validation using different histologic and microbiological references. Crit Care Med 2000; 28:2799–2804.

158. Souweine B, Veber B, Bedos JP, et al. Diagnostic accuracy of protected specimen brush and bronchoalveolar lavage in nosocomial pneumonia: impact of previous antimicrobial treatments. Crit Care Med 1998; 26:236–244.

159. Rodriguez de Castro F, Sole-Violan J, Aranda Leon A, et al. Do quantitative cultures of protected brush specimens modify the initial empirical therapy in ventilated patients with suspected pneumonia? Eur Resp J 1996; 9:37–41.

160. Sole-Violan J, Rodriguez de Castro F, Rey A, Martin-Gonzalez JC, Cabrera-Navarro P. Usefulness of microscopic examination of intracellular organisms in lavage fluid in ventilator-associated pneumonia. Chest 1994; 106:889–894.

161. Sole Violan J, Rodriguez de Castro F, Caminero Luna J, et al. Comparative efficacy of bronchoalveolar lavage and telescoping plugged catheter in the diagnosis of pneumonia in mechanically ventilated patients. Chest 1993; 103:386–390.

162. Waterer GW, Wunderink RG. Controversies in the diagnosis of ventilator-acquired pneumonia. Med Clin North Am 2001; 85:1565–1581.

163. Fagon JY, Chastre J. Management of suspected ventilator-associated pneumonia. Ann Intern Med 2000; 133:1009.

164. Fagon JY, Chastre J, Wolff M, et al. Invasive and noninvasive strategies for management of suspected ventilator-associated pneumonia. A randomized trial. Ann Intern Med 2000; 132:621–630.

165. Chastre J, Fagon JY, Bornet-Lecso M, et al. Evaluation of bronchoscopic techniques for the diagnosis of nosocomial pneumonia. Am J Resp Crit Care Med 1995; 152:231–240.

166. Baughman RP, Spencer RE, Kleykamp BO, et al. Ventilator-associated pneumonia: quality of nonbronchoscopic bronchoalveolar lavage sample affects diagnostic yield. Eur Resp J 2000; 16:1152–1157.

167. Flanagan PG, Findlay GP, Magee JT, et al. The diagnosis of ventilator-associated pneumonia using nobronchoscopic, non-directed lung lavages. Inten Care Med 2000; 26:20–30.

168. Casetta M, Blot F, Antoun S, et al. Diagnosis of nosocomial pneumonia in cancer patients undergoing mechanical ventilation: a prospective comparison of the plugged telescoping catheter with the protected specimen brush. Chest 1999; 115:1641–1645.

169. Kollef MH, Ward S. The influence of mini-BAL cultures on patient outcomes: implications for the antibiotic management of ventilator-associated pneumonia. Chest 1998; 113:412–420.

170. Wearden PD, Chendrasekhar A, Timberlake GA. Comparison of nonbronchoscopical with bronchoscopic brushing in the diagnosis of ventilator-associated pneumonia. J Trauma 1996; 41:703–707.

171. Grossman RF, Fein A. Evidence-based assessment of diagnostic tests for ventilator-associated pneumonia; Executive summary. Chest 2000(April Supplement); 117(4): 117S–181S. http://www.chestnet.org/guidelines/pneumonia/

172. Sole Violan J, Fernandez JA, Benitez AB, et al. Impact of quantitative invasive diagnostic techniques in the management and outcome of mechanically ventilated patients with suspected pneumonia. Crit Care Med 2000; 28:2737–2741.

173. Heyland DK, Cook DJ, Marshall J, et al. The clinical utility of invasive diagnostic techniques in the setting of ventilator-associated pneumonia: Canadian Critical Care Trials Group. Chest 1999; 115:1076–1084.

174. Ruiz M, Torres A, Ewig S, et al. Noninvasive versus invasive microbial investigation in ventilator-associated pneumonia: evaluation of outcome. Am J Resp Crit Care Med 2000; 162:119.

175. http://www.cdc.gov/ncidod/hip/nnis/members/pneumonia/adult-instructions.pdf

176. http://www.cdc.gov/ncidod/hip/nnis/members/pneumonia/adult-flow-diagram.pdf

177. Ibrahim EH, Tracy L, Hill C, et al. The occurrence of ventilator-associated pneumonia in a community hospital: risk factors and clinical outcome. Chest 2001; 120:555–561.

178. Torres A, Gatell JM, Aznar E, et al. Re-intubation increases the risk of nosocomial pneumonia in patients needing mechanical ventilation. Am J Resp Crit Care Med 1995; 152:137–141.

179. Richardson CJ, Rodriguez JL. Identification of patients at highest risk for ventilator-associated pneumonia in the surgical intensive care unit. Am J Surg 2000; 179:8–11.

180. Akca O, Koltka K, Uzel S, et al. Risk factors for early-onset, ventilator-associated pneumonia in critical care patients: selected multiresistant versus nonresistant bacteria. Anaesthesiology 2000; 93:638–645.

181. Sofianou DC, Constandinidis TC, Yannacou M, et al. Analysis of risk factors for ventilator-associated pneumonia in a multi-disciplinary intensive care unit. Eur J Clin Microbiol Infect Dis 2000; 19:460–463.

182. Cook DJ, Walter SD, Cook RJ, et al. Incidence of and risk factors for ventilator-associated pneumonia in critically ill patients. Ann Intern Med 1998; 129:433–440.

183. Cook D, De Jonghe B, Brochard L, Brun-Buisson C. Influence of airway management on ventilator-associated pneumonia: evidence from randomized trials. JAMA 1998; 279:781–787; erratum in JAMA 1999; 281:2089.

184. Kollef MH, Silver P, Murphy DM, Trovillion E. The effect of late-onset ventilator-associated pneumonia in determining patient mortality. Chest 1995; 108:1655–1662.

185. Waterer GW, Wunderink RG. Increasing threat of Gram-negative bacteria. Crit Care Med 2001; 29:75–81.

186. American Thoracic Society. Hospital acquired pneumonia in ventilated patients: diagnosis, assessment of severity, initial antimicrobial therapy and preventive strategies. Am J Resp Crit Med 1995; 153:1711–1725.

187. Rello J, Ausina V, Ricart M, et al. Impact of previous antimicrobial therapy on the etiology and outcome of ventilator-associated pneumonia. Chest 1993; 104:1230–1235.

188. Trouillet JL, Castre J, Vuagnat A, et al. Ventilator-associated pneumonia caused by potentially drug-resistant bacteria. Am J Resp Crit Med 1998; 157:531–539.

189. Rello J, Quintana E, Ausina V, et al. Incidence, etiology and outcome of nosocomial pneumonia in mechanically ventilated patients. Chest 1991; 100:439–444.

190. Bartlett JG, O'Keefe P, Tally FP, et al. Bacteriology of hospital-acquired pneumonia. Arch Int Med 1986; 146:868–871.

191. Ibrahim EH, Sherman G, Ward S, et al. The influence of inadequate antimicrobial treatment of bloodstream infections on patient outcomes in the ICU setting. Chest 2000; 118:146–155.

192. Koontz CS, Chang MC, Meredith JW. Effects of empiric antibiotic administration for suspected pneumonia on subsequent opportunistic infections. Am Surg 2000; 66:1110–1114.

193. Malangoni MA. Single versus combination antimicrobial therapy for ventilator-associated pneumonia. Am J Surg 2000; 179(Suppl):58–62.

194. Rello J, Paiva JA, Baraibar J, et al. International conference for the development of consensus on the diagnosis and treatment of ventilator-associated pneumonia. Chest 2001; 120:955–970.

195. Brewer SC, Wunderink RG, Jones CB, et al. Ventilator associated pneumonia due to Pseudomonas aeruginosa. Chest 1996; 109:1019–1029.

196. Rello J, Rue M, Jubert P, et al. Survival in patients with nosocomial pneumonia: impact of severity of illness and etiologic agent. Crit Care Med 1997; 25:1862–1867.

197. Rello J, Jubert P, Valles J, et al. Evaluation of outcome for intubated patients with pneumonia due to pseudomonas aeruginosa. Clin Infect Dis 1996; 23:973–978.

198. Fagon JY, Chastre J, Domart Y, et al. Mortality due to ventilator-associated pneumonia or colonization with Pseudomonas or Acinetobacter species: assessment by quantitative culture of samples obtained by a protected specimen brush. Clin Infect Dis 1996; 23:538–542.

199. Fink MP, Snyderman DR, Niederman MS, et al. Treatment of severe pneumonia in hospitalized patients: results of a multi-center, randomized, double-blind trail comparing intravenous ciprofloxacin with imipenem-cilastin. Antimicrob Agents Chemother 1994; 38:1309–1313.

200. Forrest A, Nix DE, Ballow CH, et al. Pharmacodynamics if intravenous ciprofloxacin in seriously ill patients. Antimicrob Agents Chemother 1993; 37:1073–1081.

201. Evans ME, Feola DJ, Rapp RP. Polymyxin B sulfate and colistin: old antibiotics for emerging multiresistant gram-negative bactria. Ann Pharmacother 1999; 33:960–967.

202. Chan EL, Zabrinsky RJ. Determination of synergy by two methods with eight antimicrobial combinations against tobramycin-susceptible and tobramycin-resistant strains of Pseudomonas aeruginosa. Diagn Microbiol Infect Dis 1987; 6:157–164.

203. Brun-Buisson C, Sollet JP, Schweich H, et al. Treatment of ventilator-associated pneumonia with piperacillin-tazobactam/amicacin versus ceftazidime/amicacin: a multicenter, randomized controlled trial. VAP Study Group. Clin Infect Dis 1998; 26:346–354.

204. Garcia-Garmendia JL, Ortiz-Leyba C, Garnacho-Montero J, et al. Mortality and increased length of stay attributable to the acquisition of Acinetobacter in critically ill patients. Crit Care Med 1999; 27:1794–1799.

205. Bergogne-Berezin E. The Increasing role of acinetobacter species as nosocomial pathogens. Curr Infect Dis Rep 2001; 3:440–444.

206. Bergogne-Berezin E, Towner KJ. *Acinetobacter* spp. as nosocomial pathogens: microbiological, clinical, and epidemiological features. Clin Microbiol Rev 1996; 9:148–165.

207. Lesch CA, Itokazu GS, Danzinger LH, Weinstein RA. Multi-hospital analysis of antimicrobial usage and resistance trends. Diagn Microbiol Infect Dis 2001; 71:149–154.

208. Itokazu GS, Quinn JP, Bell-Dixon C, et al. Antimicrobial resistance rates among aerobic Gram-negative bacilli recovered from patients in intensive care units: evaluation of a national post-marketing surveillance program. Clin Infect Dis 1996; 23:779–784.

209. Koh TH, Sng LH, Babini GS, et al. Carbapenem-resistant Klebsiella pneumoniae in Singapore producing IMP-1 beta-lactamase and lacking an outer membrane protein. Antimicrob Agents Chemother 2001; 45:1939–1940.

210. Babini GS, Livermore DM. Antimicrobial resistance amongst Klebsiella *spp.* collected from intensive care units in Southern and Western Europe in 1997–1998. J Antimicrob Chemother 2000; 45:183–189.

211. Marik PE, Careau P. The role of anaerobes in patients with ventilator-associated pneumonia and aspiration pneumonia: a prospective study. Chest 1999; 115:178–183.

212. Dore P, Robert R, Grollier G, et al. Incidence of anaerobes in ventilator-associated pneumonia with use of a protected specimen brush. Am J Resp Crit Care Med 1996; 153:1292–1298.

213. Robert R, Grollier G, Dore P, et al. Nosocomial pneumonia with isolation of anaerobe bacteria in ICU patients: therapeutic considerations and outcome. J Crit Care 1999; 14:114–119.

214. Gonzales C, Rubio M, Romero-Vivas J, et al. Bacteremic pneumonia due to Staphylococcus aureus: a comparison of disease caused by methicillin-resistant and methicillin-susceptible organisms. Clin Infect Dis 1999; 29:1171–1177.

215. Pujol M, Corbella X, Pena C, et al. Clinical and epidemiological findings in mechanically ventilated patients with methicillin-resistant Staphylococcus aureus pneumonia. Eur J Microbiol Infect Dis 1998; 17:622–628.

216. Rello J, Torres A, Ricard M, et al. Ventilator-associated pneumonia by Staphylococcus aureus: comparison of methicillin-resistant and methicillin-sensitive episodes. Am J Resp Crit Care Med 1994; 150:1545–1549.

217. Rello J, Quintana E, Ausina V, et al. Risk factors for Staphylococcus aureus nosocomial pneumonia in critically ill patients. Am Rev Resp Dis 1990; 142:1320–1324.

218. Heyland DK, Cook DJ, Griffith L, et al. The attributable mortality of ventilator-associated pneumonia in the critically ill patient. The Canadian Critical Care Trials Group. Am J Resp Crit Care Med 1999; 159:1249–1256.

219. Wunderink RG, Rello J, Cammarata SK, et al. Linezolid vs. Vancomycin analysis of two double-blinded studies of patients with methicillin—resistant staphylococcus aureus noscomial pneumonia. Chest 2003; 124:1789–1797.

220. Relo J, Ausina V, Castella J, et al. Nosocomial respiratory tract infections in multiple trauma patients: influence of level of consciousness with implications for therapy. Chest 1992; 102:525–529.

221. El-Ebiary M, Torres A, Fabergas N, et al. Significance of the isolation of Candida species from respiratory samples in critically ill non-neutropenic patients. Am J Resp Crit Care Med 1997; 156:583–590.

222. Chastre J, Wolff M, Fagon JY, et al. Companion of 8 vs. 15 days of antibiotic therapy for ventilator-associated pneumonia in adults: a randomized trial. JAMA 2003; 290(19):2588–2598.

223. Fagon JY, Chastre J, Vuagnat A, et al. Nosocomial pneumonia and mortality among patients in intensive care units. JAMA 1996; 275:866–869.

224. Dupont H, Mentec H, Sollet JP, Bleichner G. Impact of appropriateness of initial antibiotic therapy on the outcome of ventilator-associated pneumonia. Inten Care Med 2001; 27:355–362.

225. Fagon JY, Chastre J, Hance AJ, et al. Nosocomial pneumonia in ventilated patients: a cohort study evaluating attributable mortality and hospital stay. Am J Med 1993; 94:281–288.

226. Francois P, Pittet D, Bento M, Pepey B, Vaudaux P, Lew D, Schrenzel J. Rapid detection of methicillin-resistant Staphylococcus aureus directly from sterile or nonsterile clinical samples by a new molecular assay. J Clin Microbiol 2003; 41:254–260.

227. Luna CM, Blanzaco D, Miederman MS, et al. Resolution of ventilator-associated pneumonia: Prospective evaluation of the clinical pulmonary infection score as an early clinical predictor of outcome. Crit Care Med 2003; 31:676–682.

228. Smulders K, van der Hoeven H, Weers-Pothoff I, Vandenbroucke-Grauls C. A randomized clinical trial of intermittent subglottic secretion drainage in patients receiving mechanical ventilation. Chest 2002; 12:858–862.

229. Olson ME, Harmon BG, Kollef MH. Silver-coated endotracheal tubes associated with reduced bacterial burden in the lungs of mechanically ventilated dogs. Chest 2002; 121:863–870.

230. Bellm L, Lehrer RI, Ganz T. Protegrins: new antibiotics of mammalian origin. Expert Opin Investig Drugs 2000; 9:1731–1742.

231. Sinuff T, Cook DJ. Health technology assessment in the ICU: Noninvasive positive pressure ventilation for acute respiratory failure. J Crit Care 2003; 18:59–67.

232. Tablan OC, Anderson LJ, Besser R, et al. Centers for disease control and prevention. Recommendations of CDC and the Healthcare Infection Control Practices Advisory Committee: Guidelines for preventing healthcare-associated pneumonia, 2003. MMWR 2004; 53(RR-3):1–36.

233. Centers for Disease Control and Prevention NNIS System. Am J Infect Control 2001;29:404–421. www.cdc.gov/ncidod/hip/NNIS/2001nnis_report.pdf

234. Horan TC, Gaynes R. Surveillance of nosocomial infections. In: Mayhall CG, ed. CDC Definitions of Nosocomial Infections. Hospital epidemiology and infections control. Philadelphia: Lippincott Williams & Wilkins, 2004:1659–1702; Updated PDF file available at Centers for Diseases Control and Prevention (CDC) web site: http://www.cdc.gov/ncidod/hip/NNIS/NosInfDefinitions.pdf

235. National Nosocomial Infections Surveillance (NNIS) System Report, Issued August 2001; AM J Infect Control 2001; 29: 404–421; On the Web at http://www.cdc.gov/ncidod/hip/surveill/NNIS.htm Table 3A denotes the incidence of certain pathogens (in %) in VAP, during various analysis intervals; Table 3B denotes the overall pathogen resistance in 2000 and change (in %) to 1995–99 Report.

236. Kollef MH, et al. Inadequate antimicrobial therapy of infections: a risk factor for hospital mortality among critically ill patients. Chest 1999; 115(2):462–474.

237. Luna CM, et al. Impact of BAL on the therapy and outcome of ventilator-associated pneumonia. Chest 1997; 111:676–685.

49

Indwelling Vascular Catheter–Related Infection and Sepsis

Michael G. Seneff and Ahmet Can Senel

Department of Anesthesiology and Critical Care Medicine, George Washington University Medical Center,
Washington, D.C., U.S.A.

INTRODUCTION

Vascular catheterization is the most common procedure performed in critically ill patients (1). Sites of catheterization include the peripheral veins, central veins, large systemic arteries, and pulmonary arteries. Insertion of peripheral venous catheters is usually performed by nonphysician support staff and managed by protocol that includes removal within 72 hours. Limiting peripheral venous catheters to 72 hours or less has virtually eliminated these catheters as a significant source of infectious complications (2,3).

Indwelling central venous catheters are indispensable in caring for the critically ill and are inserted in the majority of patients admitted to the ICU. However, their use comes with the cost of several important complications including catheter-related infection (CRI) and sepsis (4). A developing evidence base supports the use of catheter management protocols. However, many ICUs still do not have modern protocols governing insertion technique, maintenance of catheters, duration of catheterization, or indications for removal. Surveys of catheter management demonstrate a continued wide diversity of practice between institutions, and among ICUs within the same institution, and even among practitioners in the same ICU (5). For example, practices such as routine guidewire exchanges and change of catheter site after 72–96 hours still occur, even though these practices have been shown not to decrease, and in some cases increase, infectious and mechanical complications (6). We believe this diversity in clinical management, frequently involving techniques and practice patterns at odds with a large evidence base, is a result of a concentration on the art (and not the science) of insertion, unstructured methods of teaching, under-appreciation of risks, and habitual physician behavior. This approach can lead to less than optimal ICU management.

Vascular catheterization is an art and a science, but any individual with a reasonable amount of dexterity can learn to insert catheters. Management of catheters in a given patient is a more difficult, decision-making task and requires a physician well versed with recent methodological and technological advances. CRI prolongs hospital stay and increases cost; in the worst case the patient may suffer significant morbidity and even mortality. In this chapter, we focus primarily on percutaneously inserted central venous catheters because they are associated with the highest infectious complication rate. Appropriate, arterial catheters and pulmonary artery catheters (PACs) are also discussed. Surgically implanted central venous catheters and peripherally inserted central catheters are also placed in ICU patients, but usually for special situations in the chronically critically ill and the interested reader is referred elsewhere for a review of these catheters (7,8). We first define and review the epidemiology of CRI, followed by a discussion of the pathophysiology of and ways to prevent CRI. We then discuss the treatment of established CRI, provide a look at future developments, and conclude with a plea that every ICU director study the literature, establish strict catheter protocols, and monitor adherence in their own units.

DEFINITIONS, INCIDENCE, AND IMPACT OF CATHETER-RELATED INFECTION

Part of the problem in communication regarding CRI is the disparity in definitions and methods of diagnosis. When does catheter colonization become catheter infection? What's the best method of diagnosing catheter infection? Are blood cultures drawn through central catheters valid? Although controversies still exist, some uniformity and agreement has emerged regarding important concepts. ☙ **Semi-quantitative catheter segment cultures are easier to perform, but less specific than quantitative culture techniques for diagnosis of CRI.** ❧

Of several methods exist for catheter segments and hubs, including direct gram staining (9), acridine-orange staining (10–12), qualitative broth culture (13), semi-quantitative catheter segment culture (14), and quantitative catheter cultures (15); the latter two are the most commonly utilized and documented in published studies. Rolling a catheter segment on an agar plate performs semi-quantitative cultures, while submerging the catheter segment in broth performs quantitative cultures. Semi-quantitative cultures are generally easier to perform, but are less sensitive and less specific for diagnosing true CRI and bacteremia (16), due in part to the fact that quantitative cultures sample both the external and intra-luminal parts of the catheter. Both of these techniques involve removal of the catheter. However, the "paired" quantitative blood culturing technique has been developed for diagnosis of CRI without removing the catheter, as might be indicated in a patient with limited access. This technique involves paired blood samples, one obtained through the central catheter and the other from a peripheral venipuncture site. Approximately 1.0 ml of the drawn blood is then added to a molten agar pour plate. The number of colonies of bacteria growing on the pour plate from each sample is compared. In some studies, time elapsed before the culture becomes positive is also evaluated (17,18).

Definitions

The spectrum of CRI includes catheter colonization, catheter infection, and catheter-related bacteremia (CRB), as described in Table 1. The term catheter-related sepsis is typically reserved for patients with sepsis [i.e., systemic inflammatory response syndrome (SIRS) due to infection] caused by CRI.

Catheter colonization is defined as ≥ 15 colony forming units (CFU) on semi-quantitative or $\geq 10^3$ on quantitative culture of the intradermal or distal catheter segment, in the absence of accompanying signs of inflammation at the catheter site. Catheter infection (also referred to as local CRI) is defined as ≥ 15 CFU with accompanying signs of inflammation, such as erythema, warmth, swelling, and tenderness. Local CRI can be limited to the exit site and involve the pocket of a totally implantable device or the subcutaneous tunnel of a surgically implanted catheter. Catheter-related bacteremia is present when a peripheral blood sample and a catheter segment culture are positive for the same organism, in a patient with clinical symptoms of bloodstream infection and no other apparent source of infection. If paired quantitative blood cultures are being utilized, catheter infection is considered present if the central catheter sample is positive and the peripheral sample negative, while CRB is diagnosed if the colony count from the central catheter is five to tenfold greater than the peripheral blood colony count (19).

Incidence of Catheter-Related Infection

It is difficult to define the true overall incidence of CRI because it is impacted by so many different variables, including type of ICU, type and composition of catheter, duration of catheterization, method of insertion, and site of insertion. That is part of the reason CRI rates vary greatly between reports and institutions, but some estimates are possible, and all of the figures are staggering. Utilizing the above definitions, CRI occurs in 3% to 9% of all percutaneously inserted catheters in the ICU, and 90% of these are related to central venous catheters. This translates into between two and eight episodes of infections per 1000 central catheter days, the most relevant benchmark (20,21). Arterial catheters have a much lower incidence of infection, whereas specialty catheters, such as hemodialysis catheters, are associated with an increased incidence of infection. Pulmonary artery catheter infection rates are similar, assuming they are removed within 72–120 hour (21).

Magnitude of Morbidity from Catheter-Related Infection

Approximately 5 million central venous catheters are inserted annually, accounting for 15 million central venous catheter days, which means there are between 150,000 and 450,000 episodes of CRI each year. On average, CRI, and especially CRB, are associated with considerable morbidity, including an attributable mortality of zero to 30%, prolonged hospitalization (up to 7 days), and thousands of dollars (one estimate as much as $ 50,000 per episode) in increased costs (22–26).

☞ **Seventy per cent of nosocomial bloodstream infections occur in patients with central venous catheters.** ☜

An analysis of the data by Wenzel and Edmond is particularly eye opening (27). They report that of the 200,000 nosocomial bloodstream infections (NBSI) that occur annually, 70% occur in patients with central venous catheters. Assuming an attributable mortality of 10% to 30%, NBSI represent the fourth to thirteenth leading cause of death in the U.S., a large percentage of these directly a result of central venous catheters. They also put into perspective the importance of measures proven to reduce CRI and NBSI, estimating that the use of new catheter technologies (antiseptic or antibiotic-coated and impregnated) could result in 4,000–9,000 lives saved annually (Table 2) (27,28). By their estimates, simple measures such as increased hand-washing could save between 1000–2000 lives annually (27,29). Even using the most conservatives figures, it is obvious that every ICU, and especially surgical and trauma units where CRI rates usually trend higher (30), should have strict catheter protocols and strategies in place to minimize the incidence of CRI.

PATHOPHYSIOLOGY OF CATHETER-RELATED INFECTION/SEPSIS

☞ **Most CRI is initiated by skin (site) colonization, followed by migration down the catheter tract, involving the bio-film**

Table 1 Definitions of Catheter-Related Infection

Infection Type	Definition
Catheter colonization	>15 colony forming units (cfu) (semiquantitative culture) or $>10^3$ (quantitative culture) of a catheter segment (or hub) without associated clinical symptoms of infection
Catheter infection	
Exit-site infection	Erythema, tenderness, warmth, induration, or purulence involving only the catheter skin exit site
Pocket infection	Erythema, tenderness, and/or necrosis of the skin over the reservoir of a totally implanted device and/or purulent exudate in the subcutaneous pocket
Tunnel infection	Erythema, tenderness, warmth, and induration involving the subcutaneous tract of a tunneled catheter
Bloodstream infection	
Infusate-related	Growth of the same organism from infusate and from separate percutaneous blood cultures, with no other identifiable source of infection. Often an unusual gram negative organism in an epidemic setting
Catheter(device)-related	Growth of the identical organism on a catheter segment and from a separate percutaneous blood culture in a patient with clinical symptoms of infection and no other identifiable source

Table 2 Estimate of Potential Number of Lives Saved Using New Catheter Technologies

Attributable mortality rate (%)	Expected central venous catheter-related deaths from blood stream infection	No. of deaths assuming new catheters prevent 45% of deaths	No. of lives saved
15	10,500	5755	4745
20	14,000	7700	6300
25	17,500	9625	7875
30	21,000	11,550	9450

Note: See text for details.
Source: From Ref. 27.

surrounding the catheter and ultimately infection of the catheter tip, bacteremia, and metastatic infection. ☞

The pathogenesis of CRI has been better elucidated in recent years. Most CRI (60–75%) is initiated by skin colonization, followed by migration of the infecting organism around the catheter through the intra-dermal tract (30–34). The organism(s) then become part of a bio-film coating the catheter, and once the catheter and tract are involved, quickly migrate to the catheter tip. Once infected, the catheter acts as an intra-vascular source of infection with potentially continuous bacteremia and risk for metastatic infection. Colonization of the hub and intra-luminal migration of bacteria may be more important in long term catheters, but represents the etiology of CRI in only about one fourth of infected percutaneous catheters (35–37). Secondary infection of catheters from bacteremia of another source, or contaminated infusate, occurs much less frequently.

An understanding of the pathophysiology explains many clinical features of CRI and why certain preventive strategies are effective. Catheters associated with thrombosis are more likely to be infected because the clot is part of the biofilm, supports growth, and impedes defense mechanisms (38–40). Triple lumen catheters have a higher rate of CRI than single lumen catheters, but it is not three times higher and may be more related to disease severity (41,42). Catheters inserted through or adjacent to a highly contaminated or abnormal skin site, such as burns or tracheostomies, have a higher incidence of infection. Finally, any intervention that more thoroughly sterilizes the skin site (chlorhexidine) (43), impedes migration of bacteria (silver-impregnated cuffs) (32,44), prevents formation of a bio-film (catheter composition, heparin), or inhibits bacterial growth on the catheter (antiseptic and antibiotic coated and impregnated catheters) (45) logically should reduce the overall incidence of CRI. Most of the recent advances in catheter maintenance discussed below were developed with the primary pathogenesis of CRI in mind.

PREVENTION OF CATHETER-RELATED INFECTION

☞ **Simple measures of prevention such as handwashing with an alcohol-based solution or gel could save 1000–2000 lives annually.** ☞

Strict adherence to hand-washing and aseptic technique remains the cornerstone to prevention of CRI (46,47). Catheters inserted under suboptimal conditions (such as in

an emergency) should be removed as soon as feasible (within 24 hours at the latest). Additional strategies shown to minimize CRI are summarized in Table 3, and discussed in greater detail below.

Operator Education and Standardization

Numerous studies have demonstrated the effectiveness of educational and quality improvement programs for physicians and nurses in reducing CRI (5,48–50). These programs educate caregivers about recent improvements in infection control and lead to standardization in technique and catheter maintenance. Whether hospitals- or specifically ICU-based, these programs should be mandatory for any physician inserting catheters, and updated on an annual basis. At our hospital, we incorporate a catheter education program during hospital house-staff orientation, reinforce concepts during ICU rotation with specific lectures and supervision, and monitor continuously for compliance. Likewise, an active surveillance program for CRI and overall infection control is instrumental in early recognition of CRI. Each institution should have their CRI rates expressed in per 1000 catheter days to measure the impact of institutional

Table 3 Steps to Minimize Catheter-Related Infection

Strict adherence to catheter insertion and maintenance protocols
Site preparation with chlorhexidine-based preparation
Appropriate site selection, avoiding heavily colonized or anatomically abnormal areas; use subclavian veins for anticipated catheterization of >5 days
Maximal barrier precautions during catheter insertion
Use of antiseptic or antibiotic impregnated/coated catheter for anticipated duration of >4 days
Remove pulmonary artery catheters/introducers after 5 days
Use multilumen catheters only when indicated, remove when no longer needed
Avoid routine guidewire exchanges
Use surgically implantable catheters or peripherally inserted central catheters for anticipated long term (>2–3 weeks) catheterization
Hospital-wide CRI reduction education programs
Active infection control and quality improvement programs

Note: Strategies demonstrated to decrease the incidence of CRI. See text for details.

protocols, new catheter technologies, and for comparison to national benchmarks (21).

Strict Indications for Central Access Limits Catheter-Related Infection

The best way to prevent CRI is not to insert a central venous catheter. Central and arterial catheters are over-utilized and often placed for convenience or as an auto-matic/habitual behavior. Indications for gaining central venous access are shown in Table 4, and should be fol-lowed closely. The table is important as much for what is not listed as what is. Fluid resuscitation alone is a less robust indication for central venous catheters because it can be accomplished quicker in emergencies using peripheral catheters. Determination of CVP as a sole indication for central venous catheters is controver-sial, given the limitations of CVP as a reflection of intra-vascular blood volume. Pulmonary artery catheters are probably also overutilized, and should be reserved for established indications (51). Most importantly, patients should be monitored daily as to continued need for central venous catheters, arterial cathers, or PAC, and these catheters should be withdrawn immediately when no longer indicated.

Site Selection

✄ **The sub-clavian approach is preferred for limiting CRI, because it can be performed (or supervised) safely by experi-enced operators and is associated with a lower incidence of CRI than jugular or femoral catheters.** ✄

Although there are many technical variations, most central venous catheters and PACs are inserted with a sub-clavian, jugular, femoral, or antecubital (peripherally inserted central catheters) approach, and arterial catheters with a radial, ulnar, femoral, dorsalis pedis, or brachial approach. Which site is chosen in any given patient depends on many variables, including operator experi-ence, indication for catheterization, presence or absence of pulmonary disease, and local skin conditions (Table 4). Whenever possible the sub-clavian approach is preferred for moderate to long duration cathererization, because it can be performed (or supervised) safely by experienced operators and is associated with a lower inci-dence of CRI than jugular or femoral catheters (52–56). We reserve the jugular approach for shorter duration use and typically remove after 5–7 days. We utilize the femoral vein mainly for emergency resuscitation and tem-porary hemodialysis. The lower incidence of CRI with sub-clavian catheters is likely due to the lower baseline skin colony counts, and because the area is easier to main-tain, and farther away from potentially highly contami-nated sites, such as a body orifice or airway appliance. Whether peripherally inserted central catheters have a lower rate of CRI in the critically ill is controversial (57) but they are generally much less useful in the acute setting and usually reserved for rehabilitation and chronic care (58).

Infectious considerations have no bearing on the choice of arterial catheterization site. Arterial catheters have a low overall incidence of significant infection, and there is not a substantial difference between sites (59–61). We reserve the use of brachial catheters to specialized situations or in patients with limited arterial access (62).

Barrier Protection During Catheter Insertion

Maximal barrier protection, including gloves, gown, and mask for the operator and a large sterile body drape for the field, regardless of the site of catheterization and area in the hospital (i.e., operating room *vs.* ICU), reduces the overall rate of CRI for central venous catheters (63,64). This rule needs to be strictly enforced, especially in academic centers where house officers frequently have their own ideas about the need for gowns and drapes. Peripheral arter-ial catheters can be inserted using gloves (after excellent hand-washing) and local aseptic technique during insertion, but we recommend maximal barrier protection for insertion of femoral arterial catheters (63). The emergency department or resuscitation suite should change catheters placed in the field within 24 hour.

Table 4   Indications, Site Selection, and Recommended Duration of Central Venous Catheter

Indication for central venous catheter	Preferred site	Recommended duration
Central venous access for vasoactive agents, caustic medications, concentrated agents, inability to perform peripheral catheterization	SV	Indefinite, change for specific indication
Total parenteral nutrition–long term	SV SV (surgically implanted)	Indefinite
Preoperative preparation	IJV or SV	Indefinite
Acute renal replacement therapy	IJV or FV	Change to new site after 7 days
Emergency airway management	FV or SV	Change FV catheters ASAp
Transvenous pacemaker	R IJV	Change to new site after 7 days
Inability to lie supine	FV	Change to new site after 7 days
Cardiopulmonary arrest	FV or SV	Change FV catheter ASAP
Pulmonary artery catheterization	RIJV L SV	Change to new site after 5 days
Coagulopathy	IJV, EJV. FV SV[a]	Change to new site after 7 days

[a]SV catheters can often be placed safely in patients with coagulopathy, but the clinical situation should dictate choice. Recommendations are based on the literature and authors' experience. See text for details.
Abbreviations: FV, femoral vein; IJV, internal jugular vein; R, right; L, left; SV, subclavian vein.

Skin Site Preparation and Care

Proper skin cleansing/antisepsis of the insertion site are one of the most important measures for preventing CRI. Commonly used antiseptics are 10% povidone–iodine, 70% alcohol, tincture of iodine, and 2% aqueous chlorhexadine. Although comparative data is not extensive, it appears that 2% aqueous chlorhexidine is the superior agent in preventing central venous and arterial CRI (43,65). We use a Chloraprep® One-Step applicator that is a combination of 2% chlorhexidine and 70% isopropyl alcohol. Proper application involves repeated back and forth strokes for 30–60 sec, and then drying for 30 sec.

During catheter maintenance, there are many potential measures to reduce CRI, but most have not been definitively shown to be effective. Application of antimicrobial ointments to the catheter site at the time of insertion or dressing change is a common practice, but has not convincingly decreased CRI and may increase fungal contamination (66,67). A recently developed chlorhexidine patch that can be applied to the catheter site was effective in reducing epidural catheter colonization and may be effective for vascular catheters (68). The type of dressing used probably has little bearing on the incidence of CRI (69). Transparent dressings that allow moisture to evaporate are not associated with a lower CRI rate than gauze and tape, but they are more versatile, secure the site better, permit visual inspection, and do not have to be changed as frequently. Other maintenance issues, such as routine tubing and administration set changes, stopcocks versus needle-less systems, type of infusate or flush, and in-line filters, probably have no significant bearing on CRI (as long as sterile technique is maintained for entering system) and their use should be dictated by institutional protocols (21).

Catheter Types and Technology

Catheter type is correlated with incidence of CRI (70). In general, specialty catheters such as temporary dialysis and PAC introducers have higher CRI rates due to host and treatment related factors. These catheters generally must be removed sooner than central venous catheters (Table 4). Triple lumen catheters have higher rates than single lumen, although not three times higher, and should only be placed when actually needed for optimal patient care (41). However, it is a frequently quoted fallacy that the use of single lumen catheters is needed for total parenteral nutrition or the infusion of a special drug. Single lumen catheters are rarely indicated in the SICU because most patients require several lines and to insert several single lumen central lines actually would increase the complication rate (mechanical and infectious) as compared to using multiport central venous catheters.

✍ **New catheter technologies that incorporate antibiotic-bonding or impregnation, or infection resistant materials, reduce CRI and allow for longer duration of catheterization.** ✍

New catheter technologies that reduce the rate of CRI include antiseptic-bonded and impregnated catheters, antibiotic-impregnated catheters, and most recently, catheters designed with a trimetal (silver, carbon and platinum) compound inherently resistant to infection (46,71–75). Most of the discussion regarding these new catheters is whether they are cost-effective and which technology reduces CRI the most, but it cannot be denied that they do effectively reduce CRI rates and can safely remain in place longer (53,76,77). Concerns regarding the risks of allergic reactions or induction

of resistance have so far not nearly outweighed the benefits of reduced CRI (78,79). Impregnated catheters protect both the inner and outer surface, and logically will be most effective, but available evidence does not definitively justify one catheter type or manufacturer over another. However, in our opinion, available data strongly support the routine use of one of these catheters for prolonged catheterization (more than 3 days). Indeed, in other institutions and ours, the use of catheters has been strongly cost-effective with a significant drop in CRI rates (77) (data on file).

Duration of Catheterization

Obviously, individual factors and situations impact on the CRI risk for any given catheter, and risk/benefit decisions to withdraw or leave catheters in place must be individualized. A single lumen catheter placed in the SV utilized expressly for TPN and no other purpose can remain for weeks, while a triple lumen catheter placed in the IJV in a shocked patient with multiple infusions is at risk for significant CRI within a week. Any ICU can decrease its episodes of infection per 1000 catheter days by using all preventive strategies and routinely changing the catheter site every three days, but this is neither practical nor cost-effective, and will increase noninfectious complications. Still, for infection control, it is important that each ICU have guidelines governing, *in general*, the duration of catheterization and other decisions, such as when it is appropriate to change over a guide-wire.

✍ **Colonization of the skin site initiates most CRI, and in the presence of adequate site care, colonization is not necessarily going to necessarily be time-dependent, prevented by guide-wire exchanges, or change to another site.** ✍ The presence of guidelines standardizes care, sets a baseline on which recommendations for changes can be made, and acts as a benchmark for continuous quality improvement. Luckily, recently completed clinical trials provide an adequate evidence base to make recommendations. These trials have demonstrated that (*i*) SV catheters have a lower incidence of CRI than FV or IJV catheters (33,52,55,56,80); (*ii*) routine guidewire exchanges do not prevent, and may increase, CRI (6); (*iii*) scheduled changes of catheter site (e.g., at 3 or 7 days) does not lower overall complications (81,82); (*iv*) the use of preventive strategies safely prolongs the duration of catheterization at any given site (53,83); and (*v*) there is not a linear association between duration of catheterization and risk for CRI (84). When one remembers the pathophysiology of CRI, these results are logical.

Critical care physicians and surgeons are strong willed, and habits die hard, thus, not all ICUs have adapted guidelines incorporating all the above evidence. However, it is important that every ICU have well delineated and publicized guidelines for catheter duration that are enforced and monitored (Table 4). Guidelines should be dynamic and reassessed frequently, and changes implemented in a quality improvement program that is based on valid infection control data (48–50,83).

DIAGNOSIS AND TREATMENT OF CATHETER-RELATED INFECTION

Inevitably, even with best practices, CRI occurs and will require evaluation and treatment. CRI can be uncomplicated and resolve with removal of the catheter, or associated with catastrophic complications such as shock, septic thrombophlebitis, or endocarditis, requiring weeks of antibiotics. Management and decision making is complex because there are invariably potential non-catheter sources of fever and infection, and patients may be at high risk for catheter change or replacement. In this section, we review the diagnosis and treatment of CRI, again concentrating on percutaneously inserted central venous catheters, since they constitute 90% of all relevant CRI (43). Arterial catheters, perhaps because of the high flow, are much less likely to be the source of CRB, but the principles discussed here also apply to their management (85). Cuffed, tunneled, and peripherally inserted central catheters are specialized catheters intended to remain in place longer, and although the diagnosis of CRI is made in a similar fashion, decisions to remove these catheters are a bit more complex. In general, long term catheters may not require removal for uncomplicated CRI, but should be removed if associated with shock, septic thrombosis, endocarditis, recurrent bacteremia, or with candida and gram negative infection (19,21).

Pathogens
Gram-Positive Cocci
Coagulase-Negative Staphylococci
Coagulase negative staphylococci, especially *S. epidermidis*, are the quintessential microbial pathogens associated with device-related infections (Table 5). Staphylococci constitute the most frequent cause of CRI because these organisms are ubiquitous in the ICU, exist in the normal skin flora, and elaborate a slime factor that enables them to thrive on the surface of catheters (34,86). CRIs due to coagulase-negative staphylococci often present with fever alone, are sometimes associated with inflammation at the insertion site, and rarely are complicated by severe sepsis (87,88). Treatment approaches vary among institutions, and there are no randomized clinical trials that offer strong guidance (89). Clearly, some of these infections will resolve with removal of the catheter only, but many experts recommend treatment with an appropriate antibiotic such as vancomycin or alternatively, linezolid (these organisms are almost always methicillin-resistant) for 5–7 days (19). Patients who develop recurrent bacteremia, have prosthetic heart valves, infection induced organ failure, or other complications require a longer duration of therapy.

Staphylococcus aureus
✍ Recently completed studies suggest that low risk patients with CRI caused by *Staphylococcus aureus* can be safely treated with 10–14 days of antibiotic therapy. ✍ *S. aureus*

constitutes the second most common cause of CRI in critical care units, and is far more consequential than coagulase-negative Staphylococcal infections. *S. aureus* infections of percutaneously inserted central venous catheters mandate removal of the catheter and appropriate antibiotic therapy (90,91). Many of these infections are caused by methicillin resistant *S. aureus* (MRSA) (92,93), and longer durations of antibiotic therapy are frequently indicated. The primary decision is whether to treat with 7 to 14 days (short course) or 28 to 42 days (long course) of therapy. Recently completed studies suggest that low risk patients, identified by a physiologic response to therapy within 48 to 72 hours (fever defervescence and white blood cell count decreased organ function stable or improving, and no valvular abnormalities by echocardiogram) can be safely treated with 10 to 14 days of appropriate therapy (19,94–97). For MSSA, nafcillin alone is usually adequate, whereas vancomycin or linezolid is required for MRSA. For vancomycin intermediate sensitive (VISA) or resistant (VRSA) *S. aureus*, linezolid or daptomycin should be used. The addition of rifampin is usually not necessary for uncomplicated, low-risk patients.

High risk patients are individuals who do not respond quickly to therapy, have persistent bacteremia, evidence of metastatic infection, septic thrombosis, indwelling prosthetic material, or are immuno-compromised. High-risk CRI should be treated with an extended duration of antibiotics, usually 28 days. Infective endocarditis, best diagnosed using transesophageal echocardiogram (TEE) (96), usually requires 6 weeks of therapy, frequently with the addition of rifampin for at least part of the time (19).

Enterococci
✍ VRE is usually identified in patients with prolonged, complicated ICU stays who have received multiple courses of antibiotics. ✍ Enterococci are as frequent a cause of CRI as *S. aureus* and perhaps more important because of the emergence of vancomycin-resistant enterococci (VRE) (98). Vascular catheters are the most frequent source of VRE bacteremia in the ICU, and although these infections are usually not highly virulent, they are problematic because of infection control issues. VRE is usually identified in patients with prolonged, complicated ICU stays and multiple courses of antibiotics (99). Treatment is not standardized, and there are no randomized controlled studies to guide therapy. We usually treat low risk patients by removing the catheter, treating with 14 days of linezolid, and documenting sterile blood and stool cultures. High-risk patients warrant longer durations of therapy, and

Table 5 Common Pathogens Causing CRI and Associated Mortality Rates

Pathogen	1986–1989 (%)	1992–1999 (%)	Crude mortality (%)
Coagulase-negative Staphylococci	27	37	21
S. aureus	16	13	25
Enterococcus spp.	8	13	32
Candida spp.	8	8	40
Gram-negative rods	19	14	37

Note: Most frequent organisms causing CRI.
Source: Adapted from Ref. 29.

consultation with an infectious disease expert is frequently indicated (100–102).

Gram-Negative Organisms

Catheter-related infection due to gram-negative organisms is not common but is increasing in frequency, especially in immunocompromised patients with tunneled catheters. Gram-negative infections of percutaneous catheters mandate removal of the device and antibiotic therapy for 10 to 14 days (low risk patients) or 4 to 6 weeks (high risk). Gram negative infections of surgically implanted and other tunneled catheters do not necessarily mandate removal of the catheter, and management should be individualized, based on the physiologic status of the patient and early response to therapy (19). However, we almost always remove catheters infected with gram-negatives, because of their virulence, difficulty in clearing these organisms, and the high rate of recurrence.

Fungal Species

☞ **Some of the patient factors that increase the likelihood of fungal-related CRI are abdominal surgery, total parenteral nutrition, hyperglycemia, extended length of stay, and exposure to multiple antibiotics.** ☞ Candida is the most common fungal source of CRI (103). Anti-fungal therapy is mandatory for all instances of CRI caused by candida species. On occasion, when the catheter tip but not peripheral blood is positive for *Candida albicans*, antifungal therapy may not be necessary—but we treat all of these patients to avoid the late recurrences which may have devastating consequences (104–109). Patient factors that increase the likelihood of fungal-related CRI are abdominal surgery, total parenteral nutrition, hyperglycemia, extended length of stay, and exposure to multiple antibiotics.

Treatment of fungal CRI involves removal of the catheter and treatment with antifungal therapy for 14 days beyond the date of the last positive blood culture. The biggest decision regarding therapy is whether to use amphotericin with all of its attendant complications, or fluconazole, which is better tolerated but carries a greater risk of resistance. *Candida tropicalis* and *C. krusei* are inherently resistant to fluconazole, and in some hospitals, as much as 20–40% of albicans are resistant.

High risk, hemodynamically unstable, and previously fluconazole-treated patients should initially be started on amphotericin or an echinocandin until cultures and sensitivities are available to guide therapy. In patients with renal insufficiency, lipid preparations of amphotericin are appropriate. When fluconazole is used, we favor doses at least as high as 400 mg daily, the dose found to be as effective as amphotericin dosed at 0.5 mg/kg/day (106). Newer antifungal agents, such as caspofungin, are significant advances with high potency and low side effects, and will likely be increasingly utilized for CRI caused by candida species, especially as an alternative to lipid preparations of amphotericin.

Unusual Pathogens

☞ **Some unusual organisms, such as *Corynebacterium* JK-1, *Malassezia furfur*, *Candida parapsilosis*, and *mycobacteria species*, are uniquely associated with CRI, usually in the setting of long-term catheterization in immunocompromised patients.** ☞ When an unusual pathogen is isolated from a catheter tip, it often represents a contaminant unless it is an organism known to be associated with CRI. Obviously, if catheter-related bacteremia is identified, any organism should be regarded as a pathogen and treated appropriately, including removal of the catheter and initiation of appropriate antibiotic therapy (110–116).

Management of the Febrile Catheterized Patient

Because it is such a frequent occurrence, management of the febrile patient with one or more indwelling vascular catheters deserves special comment (Fig. 1). The majority of fevers in catheterized patients are not secondary to CRI but rather the myriad of other potential causative factors in ICU patients (117). In general, management decisions should be individualized and the decision to discontinue a catheter is impacted by the duration of catheterization (CRI is very unusual in catheters less than 96 hour old inserted under sterile conditions), type of catheter (non-tunneled catheters are easier to remove than tunneled/surgically implanted catheters), and physiological status of the patient (fever alone versus organ dysfunction/shock) (117). Figure 1 summarizes our approach to the febrile patient with non-tunneled catheters, and we discuss below what changes to this approach are necessary when surgically implanted catheters are involved. ☞ **The decision to discontinue a catheter is impacted by the duration of catheterization (CRI is very unusual in catheters less than 96 hour old inserted under sterile conditions), type of catheter (non-tunneled catheters are easier to remove than tunneled/surgically implanted catheters), and physiological status of the patient** *(When in doubt-pull it out!).* ☞

For catheters inserted by surgery or interventional radiology (Permacath, Quinton, Mediport, etc.) the approach is similar, but a more concentrated effort at catheter salvage is warranted. Evidence of complicated device infection, such as tunnel infection, port abscess, or extensive cellulitis, mandate catheter removal and 7 to 14 days of antibiotic therapy; likewise, evidence for systemic or metastatic infection also require removal of the catheter and a longer course of antibiotics, as much as 4 to 6 weeks for septic thrombosis and infective endocarditis (118). In our experience, CRI due to non-staphylococcal organisms almost always requires catheter removal, although in rare instances and only when the patient is stable, the organism can be cleared with the catheter in place utilizing antibiotic lock therapy (19). Uncomplicated CRI caused by *S. aureus* can sometimes be cleared without catheter removal, but relapses are common and the clinician must be vigilant for recurrent bacteremia and systemic complications (97). In the presence of uncomplicated infection due to coagulase-negative staphylococcus, the catheter can be retained if there is no evidence of persisting or relapsing bacteremia.

Catheter colonization occurs when the catheter tip or segment is positive for more than 15 cfu. but blood cultures remain negative. Again, it is difficult to make general recommendations and each episode should be evaluated individually. Coagulase negative staphyloocous generally does not need to be treated, but other pathogens should be respected and, if necessary, treated with a relatively short course (5–7 days) of appropriate antibiotics. Repeat blood cultures should be drawn to ensure clearance of the pathogen. If the catheter was exchanged over a guide-wire and the old catheter segment is positive, the new catheter should be removed.

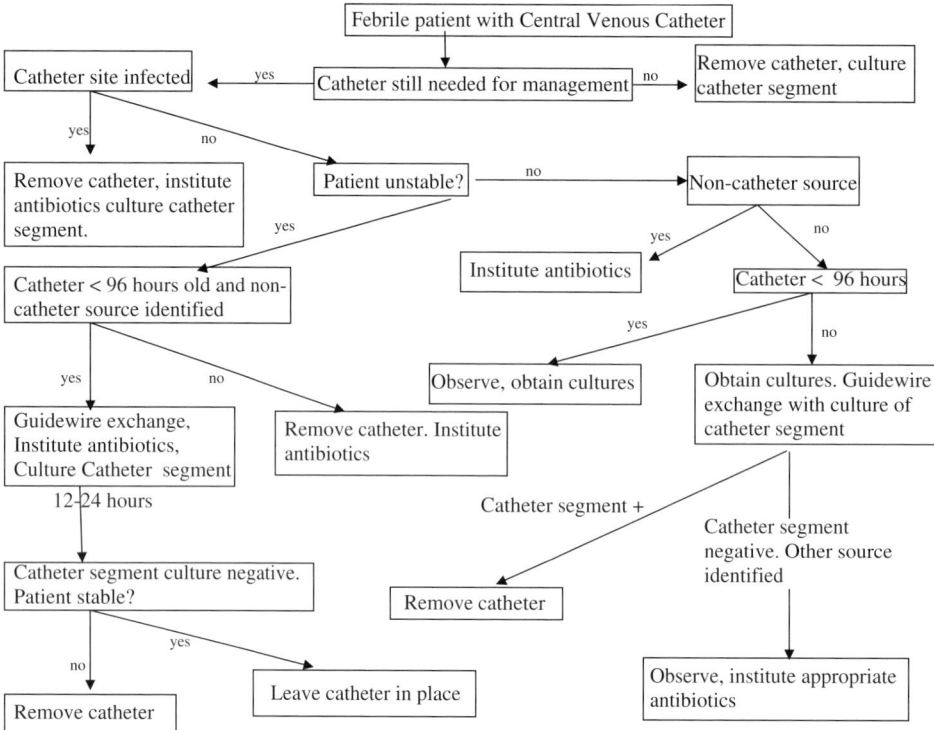

Figure 1   General approach to the patient with fever and central venous catheter(s). Many exceptions apply. Catheter segment can be tip or indradermal. See text for details.

EYE TO THE FUTURE

A zero incidence of CRI is a holy grail that will be difficult to obtain. However, improvements to catheter technology, site preparation, insertion technique, and catheter management protocols have resulted in trends of longer catheterization durations with fewer infectious complications. In addition, advancements in non-invasive technologies have decreased the frequency of central catheterization requirements, thereby exposing fewer patients to its risks (119–121). Future improvements in catheter technology will likely center on novel infection and thrombosis-resistant materials, and development of new anti-microbial strategies (122–125). Barrier devices, such as the collagen cuff and chlorhexidine patch, will see improvements in design, and concomitant increases in utilization (32,68,126). Site decontamination will be improved by greater availability of user friendly, existing antiseptics, and undoubtedly, development of new, broader spectrum and longer-acting preparations (65). Insertion techniques that may further reduce CRI include emphasis on the sub-clavian route, subcutaneous tunneling for internal jugular and femoral catheters, and changes to standardized kits, such as sutureless securement devices, needle-less systems, and bloodless syringes (21,127–130).

Perhaps the greatest challenge in the future, and an area for which there may be the biggest impact, is preventing the emergence of resistant organisms. Vascular catheters are one of the most important sources of VRE, MRSA, VISA, VRSA and fluconazole-resistant candida (especially non-albicans species) (46), and it is likely that other resistant pathogens will appear in the future.

Prevention of resistant organisms in the modern day ICU is a complex exercise that involves all aspects of catheter insertion and management, including institutional antibiotic policies. Rapid and accurate diagnosis of CRI will lead to more timely, earlier, appropriate use of antibiotics, measures which are proven to reduce infectious morbidity and mortality (131–132). Equally as important, an ability to rapidly exclude CRI will also reduce the amount of antibiotic empiricism, and decrease the overall exposure to antimicrobials. The accurate diagnosis of CRI may be improved by better culture techniques and, potentially, by the use of specific serum markers (133–138). Better institutional-wide infection control programs incorporating new technologies will improve physician compliance with existing protocols, and allow for more rapid adoption of emerging technologies. As advances occur, it will ultimately remain the responsibility of the treating physician to incorporate these changes into daily practice, with an overall goal of lessening the aggregate burden of infectious diseases, while likewise limiting other complications and cost.

SUMMARY

Infections caused by invasive devices continue to be an important nosocomial complication in critically ill patients. It is the mandate of all physicians practicing in ICUs to minimize this expensive and sometimes fatal event. Technological improvements have dramatically reduced the incidence of CRI, and it is likely that there will be additional developments in catheter composition, site preparation, and barrier devices that will further reduce the incidence of CRI. However, physician practices continue to be the greatest source of CRI, which is inexcusable and must be a result of under-appreciation of factors leading to the development of CRI. Every critical care unit should have strict catheter insertion and maintenance policies in effect, based upon the most recent evidence-based literature (Table 4). An active infection control program monitors CRI and benchmarks to regional/national standards, and measures the impact of changes or quality improvements. When CRI does occur, rapid diagnosis and appropriate therapy limits the impact of infection and reduces the likelihood of emergence of resistance. Treatment should be individualized based on virulence of the organism, patient physiology, catheter type, and presence of complications. It is only through the implementation of a comprehensive catheter insertion and management protocol, as reviewed in this chapter, that ICU managers can begin to approach the ideal of a zero incidence in device related infection.

KEY POINTS

- ✍ Semi-quantitative catheter segment cultures are easier to perform, but less sensitive than quantitative culture techniques for diagnosis of CRI.
- ✍ 70% of nosocomial bloodstream infections occur in patients with central venous catheters.
- ✍ Most CRI is initiated by skin (site) colonization, followed by migration down the catheter tract, involving the biofilm surrounding the catheter, and ultimately infection of the catheter tip, bacteremia, and metastatic infection.
- ✍ Simple measures of prevention, such as hand-washing with an alcohol-based solution or gel, could save 1000–2000 lives annually.
- ✍ The subclavian approach is preferred for limiting CRI, because it can be performed (or supervised) safely by experienced operators and is associated with a lower incidence of CRI than jugular or femoral catheters.
- ✍ New catheter technologies that incorporate antibiotic-bonding or impregnation, or infection resistant materials, reduce CRI and allow for longer durations of catheterization.
- ✍ Colonization of the skin site initiates most CRI, and in the presence of adequate site care, colonization is not necessarily going to be time-dependent, prevented by guidewire exchanges, or change to another site.
- ✍ Recently completed studies suggest that low risk patients with CRI caused by *Staphylococcus aureus* can be safely treated with 10–14 days of antibiotic therapy.
- ✍ VRE is usually identified in patients with prolonged, complicated ICU stays who have received multiple courses of antibiotics.
- ✍ Some of the patient factors that increase the likelihood of fungal-related CRI are abdominal surgery, total parenteral nutrition, hyperglycemia, extended length of stay, and exposure to multiple antibiotics.
- ✍ Some unusual organisms, such as *Corynebacterium* JK-1, *Malassezia furfur, Candida parapsilosis,* and *mycobacteria species,* are uniquely associated with CRI, usually in the setting of long-term catheterization in immunocompromised patients.
- ✍ The decision to discontinue a catheter is impacted by the duration of catheterization (CRI is very unusual in catheters <96 hour old inserted under sterile

conditions), type of catheter (non-tunneled catheters are easier to remove than tunneled/surgically implanted catheters) and physiological status of the patient *(When in doubt-pull it out!)*.

REFERENCES

1. Shapiro CL. Central venous access catheters. Surg Oncol Clin North Am 1995; 4:443–451.
2. Maki DG, Ringer M. Risk factors for infusion-related phlebitis with small peripheral venous catheters. A randomized controlled trial. Ann Intern Med 1991; 114(10):845–854.
3. Lai KK. Safety of prolonging peripheral cannula and i.v. tubing use from 72 hr to 96 hr. Am J Infect Control 1998; 26(1):66–70.
4. McGee DC, Gould MK. Preventing complications of central venous catheterization. NEMJ 2003; 348: 1113–1123.
5. Sherertz RJ, Ely EW, Westbrook DM, et al. Education of physicians-in-training can decrease the risk for vascular catheter infection. Ann Intern Med 2000; 132(8):641–648.
6. Cook D, Randolph A, Kernerman P, et al. Central venous catheter replacement strategies: a systematic review of the literature. Crit Care Med 1997; 25(8):1417–1424.
7. Clarke DE, Raffin TA. Infectious complications of indwelling long-term central venous catheters. Chest 1990; 97(4):966–972.
8. Groeger JS, Lucas AB, Thaler HT, et al. Infectious morbidity associated with long-term use of venous access devices in patients with cancer. Ann Intern Med 1993; 119(12):1168–1174.
9. Cooper GL, Hopkins CC. Rapid diagnosis of intravascular catheter-associated infection by direct Gram staining of catheter segments. N Engl J Med 1985; 312(18):1142–1147.
10. Kite P, Dobbins BM, Wilcox MH, McMahon MJ. Rapid diagnosis of central-venous-catheter-related bloodstream infection without catheter removal. Lancet 1999; 354(9189): 1504–1507.
11. Dobbins BM, Kite P, Wilcox MH. Diagnosis of central venous catheter related sepsis—a critical look inside. J Clin Pathol 1999; 52(3):165–172.
12. Dobbins BM, Kite P. Endoluminal brushing in catheter-related sepsis: a "sweeping" statement. Nutrition 1999; 15(1):66–67.
13. Haslett TM, Isenberg HD, Hilton E, et al. Microbiology of indwelling central intravascular catheters. J Clin Microbiol 1988; 26(4):696–701.
14. Maki DG, Weise CE, Sarafin HW. A semiquantitative culture method for identifying intravenous-catheter-related infection. N Engl J Med 1977; 296(23):1305–1309.
15. Cleri DJ, Corrado ML, Seligman SJ. Quantitative culture of intravenous catheters and other intravascular inserts. J Infect Dis 1980; 141(6):781–786.
16. Raad II, Sabbagh MF, Rand KH, Sherertz RJ. Quantitative tip culture methods and the diagnosis of central venous catheter-related infections. Diagn Microbiol Infect Dis 1992; 15(1):13–20.
17. Blot F, Schmidt E, Nitenberg G, et al. Earlier positivity of central-venous- versus peripheral-blood cultures is highly predictive of catheter-related sepsis. J Clin Microbiol 1998; 36(1):105–109.
18. Fan ST, Teoh-Chan CH, Lau KF. Evaluation of central venous catheter sepsis by differential quantitative blood culture. Eur J Clin Microbiol Infect Dis 1989; 8(2):142–144.
19. Mermel LA, Farr BM, Sherertz RJ, et al. Guidelines for the management of intravascular catheter-related infections. Infect Control Hosp Epidemiol 2001; 22(4):222–242.
20. Mermel LA. Prevention of intravascular catheter-related infections. Ann Intern Med 2000; 132(5):391–402.
21. O'Grady NP, Alexander M, Dellinger EP, et al. Guidelines for the prevention of intravascular catheter-related infections. Centers for Disease Control and Prevention. MMWR Recomm Rep 2002; 51(RR–10):1–29.
22. Pittet D, Tarara D, Wenzel RP. Nosocomial bloodstream infection in critically ill patients. Excess length of stay, extra costs, and attributable mortality. JAMA 1994; 271(20):1598–1601.

23. Dimick JB, Pelz RK, Consunji R, et al. Increased resource use associated with catheter-related bloodstream infection in the surgical intensive care unit. Arch Surg 2001; 136(2):229–234.

24. Rello J, Ochagavia A, Sabanes E, et al. Evaluation of outcome of intravenous catheter-related infections in critically ill patients. Am J Resp Crit Care Med 2000; 162(3 Pt 1):1027–1030.

25. Collignon PJ. Intravascular catheter associated sepsis: a common problem. The Australian Study on Intravascular Catheter Associated Sepsis. Med J Aust 1994; 161(6):374–378.

26. Soufir L, Timsit JF, Mahe C, et al. Attributable morbidity and mortality of catheter-related septicemia in critically ill patients: a matched, risk-adjusted, cohort study. Infect Control Hosp Epidemiol 1999; 20(6):396–401.

27. Wenzel RP, Edmond MB. The impact of hospital-acquired bloodstream infections. Emerg Infect Dis 2001; 7(2):174–177.

28. Darouiche RO, Raad II, Heard SO, et al. A comparison of two antimicrobial-impregnated central venous catheters. Catheter Study Group. N Engl J Med 1999; 340(1):1–8.

29. Doebbeling BN, Stanley GL, Sheetz CT, et al. Comparative efficacy of alternative hand-washing agents in reducing nosocomial infections in intensive care units. N Engl J Med 1992; 327(2):88–93.

30. CDC. National Nosocomial infections surveillance (NNIS) system report, data summary from January 1992–June 2001, issued August 2001. Am J Infect Control 2001; 6:404–421.

31. Cooper GL, Schiller AL, Hopkins CC. Possible role of capillary action in pathogenesis of experimental catheter-associated dermal tunnel infections. J Clin Microbiol 1988; 26(1):8–12.

32. Maki DG, Cobb L, Garman JK, et al. An attachable silver-impregnated cuff for prevention of infection with central venous catheters: a prospective randomized multicenter trial. Am J Med 1988; 85(3):307–314.

33. Mermel LA, McCormick RD, Springman SR, Maki DG. The pathogenesis and epidemiology of catheter-related infection with pulmonary artery Swan-Ganz catheters: a prospective study utilizing molecular subtyping. Am J Med 1991; 91(3B):197S–205S.

34. Passerini L, Lam K, Costerton JW, King EG. Biofilms on indwelling vascular catheters. Crit Care Med 1992; 20(5):665–673.

35. Raad I, Costerton W, Sabharwal U, et al. Ultrastructural analysis of indwelling vascular catheters: a quantitative relationship between luminal colonization and duration of placement. J Infect Dis 1993; 168(2):400–407.

36. Linares J, Sitges-Serra A, Garau J, et al. Pathogenesis of catheter sepsis: a prospective study with quantitative and semiquantitative cultures of catheter hub and segments. J Clin Microbiol 1985; 21(3):357–360.

37. Sitges-Serra A, Linares J, Garau J. Catheter sepsis: the clue is the hub. Surgery 1985; 97(3):355–357.

38. Stillman RM, Soliman F, Garcia L, Sawyer PN. Etiology of catheter-associated sepsis. Correlation with thrombogenicity. Arch Surg 1977; 112(12):1497–1499.

39. Raad II, Luna M, Khalil SA, et al. The relationship between the thrombotic and infectious complications of central venous catheters. JAMA 1994; 271(13):1014–1016.

40. Randolph AG, Cook DJ, Gonzales CA, Andrew M. Benefit of heparin in central venous and pulmonary artery catheters: a meta-analysis of randomized controlled trials. Chest 1998; 113(1):165–171.

41. Farkas JC, Liu N, Bleriot JP, et al. Single- *versus* triple-lumen central catheter-related sepsis: a prospective randomized study in a critically ill population. Am J Med 1992; 93(3):277–282.

42. Miller JJ, Venus B, Mathru M. Comparison of the sterility of long-term central venous catheterization using single lumen, triple lumen, and pulmonary artery catheters. Crit Care Med 1984; 12(8):634–637.

43. Chaiyakunapruk N, Veenstra DL, Lipsky BA, Saint S. Chlorhexidine compared with povidone-iodine solution for vascular catheter-site care: a meta-analysis. Ann Intern Med 2002; 136(11):792–801.

44. Flowers RH, III, Schwenzer KJ, Kopel RF, et al. Efficacy of an attachable subcutaneous cuff for the prevention of intravascular catheter-related infection. A randomized, controlled trial. JAMA 1989; 261(6):878–883.

45. Veenstra DL, Saint S, Saha S, et al. Efficacy of antiseptic-impregnated central venous catheters in preventing catheter-related bloodstream infection: a meta-analysis. JAMA 1999; 281(3):261–267.

46. Eggimann P, Pittet D. Infection control in the ICU. Chest 2001; 120(6):2059–2093.

47. Eggimann P, Pittet D. Nonantibiotic measures for the prevention of Gram-positive infections. Clin Microbiol Infect 2001; 7(Suppl 4):91–99.

48. Civetta JM, Hudson-Civetta J, Ball S. Decreasing catheter-related infection and hospital costs by continuous quality improvement. Crit Care Med 1996; 24(10):1660–1665.

49. Coopersmith CM, Rebmann TL, Zack JE, et al. Effect of an education program on decreasing catheter-related bloodstream infections in the surgical intensive care unit. Crit Care Med 2002; 30(1):59–64.

50. Parras F, Ena J, Bouza E, et al. Impact of an educational program for the prevention of colonization of intravascular catheters. Infect Control Hosp Epidemiol 1994; 15(4 Pt 1):239–242.

51. Bernard GR, Sopko G, Cerra F, et al. Pulmonary artery catheterization and clinical outcomes: National Heart, Lung, and Blood Institute and Food and Drug Administration Workshop Report. Consensus Statement. JAMA 2000; 283(19):2568–2572.

52. Goetz AM, Wagener MM, Miller JM, Muder RR. Risk of infection due to central venous catheters: effect of site of placement and catheter type. Infect Control Hosp Epidemiol 1998; 19(11):842–845.

53. Norwood S, Wilkins HE III, Vallina VL, et al. The safety of prolonging the use of central venous catheters: a prospective analysis of the effects of using antiseptic-bonded catheters with daily site care. Crit Care Med 2000; 28(5):1376–1382.

54. Pearson ML. Guideline for prevention of intravascular device-related infections. Hospital Infection Control Practices Advisory Committee. Infect Control Hosp Epidemiol 1996; 17(7):438–473.

55. Ruesch S, Walder B, Tramer MR. Complications of central venous catheters: internal jugular *versus* subclavian access—a systematic review. Crit Care Med 2002; 30(2):454–460.

56. Merrer J, De Jonghe B, Golliot F, et al. Complications of femoral and subclavian venous catheterization in critically ill patients: a randomized controlled trial. JAMA 2001; 286(6):700–707.

57. Ng PK, Ault MJ, Maldonado LS. Peripherally inserted central catheters in the intensive care unit. J Inten Care Med 1996; 11(1):49–54.

58. Heffner JH. A guide to the management of peripherally inserted central catheters. J Crit Illness 2000; 15(3):165–169.

59. Norwood SH, Cormier B, McMahon NG, et al. Prospective study of catheter-related infection during prolonged arterial catheterization. Crit Care Med 1988; 16(9):836–839.

60. Russell JA, Joel M, Hudson RJ, et al. Prospective evaluation of radial and femoral artery catheterization sites in critically ill adults. Crit Care Med 1983; 11(12):936–939.

61. Soderstrom CA, Wasserman DH, Dunham CM, et al. Superiority of the femoral artery of monitoring. A prospective study. Am J Surg 1982; 144(3):309–312.

62. Macon WL, Futrell JW. Median nerve neuropathy after percutaneous puncture of the brachial artery in patients receiving anticoagulants. New Engl J Med 1973; 288:1396–1398.

63. Maki DG. Yes, Virginia, aseptic technique is very important: maximal barrier precautions during insertion reduce the risk of central venous catheter-related bacteremia. Infect Control Hosp Epidemiol 1994; 15(4 Pt 1):227–230.

64. Raad II, Hohn DC, Gilbreath BJ, et al. Prevention of central venous catheter-related infections by using maximal sterile

barrier precautions during insertion. Infect Control Hosp Epidemiol 1994; 15(4 Pt 1):231–238.

65. Maki DG, Ringer M, Alvarado CJ. Prospective randomised trial of povidone-iodine, alcohol, and chlorhexidine for prevention of infection associated with central venous and arterial catheters. Lancet 1991; 338(8763):339–343.

66. Maki DG, Band JD. A comparative study of polyantibiotic and iodophor ointments in prevention of vascular catheter-related infection. Am J Med 1981; 70(3):739–744.

67. Zinner SH, Denny-Brown BC, Braun P, et al. Risk of infection with intravenous indwelling catheters: effect of application of antibiotic ointment. J Infect Dis 1969; 120(5):616–619.

68. Shapiro JM, Bond EL, Garman JK. Use of a chlorhexidine dressing to reduce microbial colonization of epidural catheters. Anesthesiology 1990; 73(4):625–631.

69. Hoffmann KK, Weber DJ, Samsa GP, Rutala WA. Transparent polyurethane film as an intravenous catheter dressing. A meta-analysis of the infection risks. JAMA 1992; 267(15): 2072–2076.

70. McKinley S, Mackenzie A, Finter S. Incidence and predictors of central venous catheter-related infection in intensive care patients. Anaesth Inten Care 1999; 27:164–169.

71. Hanley EM, Veeder A, Smith T, et al. Evaluation of an antiseptic triple-lumen catheter in an intensive care unit. Crit Care Med 2000; 28(2):366–370.

72. Maki DG, Stolz SM, Wheeler S, Mermel LA. Prevention of central venous catheter-related bloodstream infection by use of an antiseptic-impregnated catheter. A randomized, controlled trial. Ann Intern Med 1997; 127(4):257–266.

73. Raad I, Darouiche R, Dupuis J, et al. Central venous catheters coated with minocycline and rifampin for the prevention of catheter-related colonization and bloodstream infections. A randomized, double-blind trial. The Texas Medical Center Catheter Study Group. Ann Intern Med 1997; 127(4):267–274.

74. Marin MG, Lee JC, Skurnick JH. Prevention of nosocomial bloodstream infections: effectiveness of antimicrobial-impregnated and heparin-bonded central venous catheters. Crit Care Med 2000; 28(9):3332–3338.

75. Ranucci M, Isgro G, Giomarelli PP, Pavesi M, Luzzani A, Cattabriga I, Carli M, Giomi P, Campostella A, Digito A, Mangari V, Silvestri V, Mondelli E. Impact of oligon central venous catheters in catheter colonization and catheter-related bloodstream infection. Crit Care Med 2003; 31:52–59.

76. Marik PE, Abraham G, Careau P, Varon J, Fromm RE, Jr. The ex vivo antimicrobial activity and colonization rate of two antimicrobial-bonded central venous catheters. Crit Care Med 1999; 27(6):1128–1131.

77. Veenstra DL, Saint S, Sullivan SD. Cost-effectiveness of antiseptic-impregnated central venous catheters for the prevention of catheter-related bloodstream infection. JAMA 1999; 282(6):554–560.

78. Oda T, Hamasaki J, Kanda N, Mikami K. Anaphylactic shock induced by an antiseptic-coated central venous [correction of nervous] catheter. Anesthesiology 1997; 87(5):1242–1244.

79. Pearson ML, Abrutyn E. Reducing the risk for catheter-related infections: a new strategy. Ann Intern Med 1997; 127(4): 304–306.

80. Trottier SJ, Veremakis C, O'Brien J, Auer AI. Femoral deep vein thrombosis associated with central venous catheterization: results from a prospective, randomized trial. Crit Care Med 1995; 23(1):52–59.

81. Cobb DK, High KP, Sawyer RG, et al. A controlled trial of scheduled replacement of central venous and pulmonary-artery catheters. N Engl J Med 1992; 327(15):1062–1068.

82. Eyer S, Brummitt C, Crossley K, et al. Catheter-related sepsis: prospective, randomized study of three methods of long-term catheter maintenance. Crit Care Med 1990; 18(10): 1073–1079.

83. Eggimann P, Harbarth S, Constantin MN, et al. Impact of a prevention strategy targeted at vascular-access care on incidence of infections acquired in intensive care. Lancet 2000; 355(9218):1864–1868.

84. Moro ML, Vigano EF, Cozzi LA. Risk factors for central venous catheter-related infections in surgical and intensive care units. The Central Venous Catheter-Related Infections Study Group. Infect Control Hosp Epidemiol 1994; 15(4 Pt 1):253–264.

85. Maki DG. Nosocomial bacteremia. An epidemiologic overview. Am J Med 1981; 70(3):719–732.

86. Christensen GD, Simpson WA, Bisno AL, Beachey EH. Adherence of slime-producing strains of Staphylococcus epidermidis to smooth surfaces. Infect Immun 1982; 37(1):318–326.

87. Christensen GD, Bisno AL, Parisi JT, et al. Nosocomial septicemia due to multiply antibiotic-resistant Staphylococcus epidermidis. Ann Intern Med 1982; 96(1):1–10.

88. Sattler FR, Foderaro JB, Aber RC. Staphylococcus epidermidis bacteremia associated with vascular catheters: an important cause of febrile morbidity in hospitalized patients. Infect Control 1984; 5(6):279–283.

89. Thylefors JD, Harbarth S, Pittet D. Increasing bacteremia due to coagulase-negative staphylococci: fiction or reality? Infect Control Hosp Epidemiol 1998; 19(8):581–589.

90. Knudsen AM, Rosdahl VT, Espersen F, et al. Catheter-related *Staphylococcal aureus* infections. J Hosp Inf 1993; 23:123–131.

91. Marr KA, Sexton DJ, Conlon PJ, et al. Catheter-related bacteremia and outcome of attempted catheter salvage in patients undergoing hemodialysis. Ann Intern Med 1997; 127(4): 275–280.

92. Harbarth S, Rutschmann O, Sudre P, Pittet D. Impact of methicillin resistance on the outcome of patients with bacteremia caused by Staphylococcus aureus. Arch Intern Med 1998; 158(2):182–189.

93. Mulligan ME, Murray-Leisure KA, Ribner BS, et al. Methicillin-resistant Staphylococcus aureus: a consensus review of the microbiology, pathogenesis, and epidemiology with implications for prevention and management. Am J Med 1993; 94(3):313–328.

94. Ehni WF, Reller LB. Short-course therapy for catheter-associated Staphylococcus aureus bacteremia. Arch Intern Med 1989; 149(3):533–536.

95. Raad II, Sabbagh MF. Optimal duration of therapy for catheter-related Staphylococcus aureus bacteremia: a study of 55 cases and review. Clin Infect Dis 1992; 14(1):75–82.

96. Rosen AB, Fowler VG Jr, Corey GR, et al. Cost-effectiveness of transesophageal echocardiography to determine the duration of therapy for intravascular catheter-associated Staphylococcus aureus bacteremia. Ann Intern Med 1999; 130(10):810–820.

97. Jernigan JA, Farr BM. Short-course therapy of catheter-related Staphylococcus aureus bacteremia: a meta-analysis. Ann Intern Med 1993; 119(4):304–311.

98. Murray BE. Vancomycin-resistant enterococci. Am J Med 1997; 102(3):284–293.

99. Edmond MB, Ober JF, Weinbaum DL, et al. Vancomycin-resistant Enterococcus faecium bacteremia: risk factors for infection. Clin Infect Dis 1995; 20(5):1126–1133.

100. Hoge CW, Adams J, Buchanan B, Sears SD. Enterococcal bacteremia: to treat or not to treat, a reappraisal. Rev Infect Dis 1991; 13(4):600–605.

101. Lai KK. Treatment of vancomycin-resistant Enterococcus faecium infections. Arch Intern Med 1996; 156(22):2579–2584.

102. Vergis EN, Hayden MK, Chow JW, et al. Determinants of vancomycin resistance and mortality rates in enterococcal bacteremia. a prospective multicenter study. Ann Intern Med 2001; 135(7):484–492.

103. Franson TR, Zak O, van den Broek P. Evaluation of new anti-infective drugs for the treatment of vascular access device-associated bacteremia and fungemia. Clin Infect Dis 1993; 17:789–793.

104. Lazzarini L, Luzzati R. Removal of central venous catheters from patients with candidemia. Clin Infect Dis 2002; 35(8):1021.

105. Nucci M, Anaissie E. Should vascular catheters be removed from all patients with candidemia? An evidence-based review. Clin Infect Dis 2002; 34(5):591–599.

106. Rex JH, Bennett JE, Sugar AM, et al. A randomized trial comparing fluconazole with amphotericin B for the treatment of

candidemia in patients without neutropenia. Candidemia Study Group and the National Institute. N Engl J Med 1994; 331(20):1325–1330.

107. Rose HD. Venous catheter-associated candidemia. Am J Med Sci 1978; 275(3):265–269.

108. Walsh TJ, Rex JH. All catheter-related candidemia is not the same: assessment of the balance between the risks and benefits of removal of vascular catheters. Clin Infect Dis 2002; 34(5):600–602.

109. Wenzel RP. Nosocomial candidemia: risk factors and attributable mortality. Clin Infect Dis 1995; 20(6):1531–1534.

110. Friedland G, von Reyn CF, Levy B, Arbeit R, Dasse P, Crumpacker C. Nosocomial endocarditis. Infect Control 1984; 5(6):284–288.

111. Lau SK, Woo PC, Woo GK, Yuen KY. Catheter-related Microbacterium bacteremia identified by 16S rRNA gene sequencing. J Clin Microbiol 2002; 40(7):2681–2685.

112. Rozdzinski E, Kern W, Schmeiser T, Kurrle E. Corynebacterium jeikeium bacteremia at a tertiary care center. Infection 1991; 19(4):201–204.

113. Rupp ME, Stiles KG, Tarantolo S, Goering RV. Central venous catheter-related Corynebacterium minutissimum bacteremia. Infect Control Hosp Epidemiol 1998; 19(10):786–789.

114. Schoch PE, Cunha BA. The JK diphtheroids. Infect Control 1986; 7(9):466–469.

115. Schwartz MA, Tabet SR, Collier AC, et al. Central venous catheter-related bacteremia due to Tsukamurella species in the immunocompromised host: a case series and review of the literature. Clin Infect Dis 2002; 35(7):e72–e77.

116. Wang CC, Mattson D, Wald A. Corynebacterium jeikeium bacteremia in bone marrow transplant patients with Hickman catheters. Bone Marrow Transplant 2001; 27(4):445–449.

117. O'Grady NP, Barie PS, Bartlett J, et al. Practice parameters for evaluating new fever in critically ill adult patients. Task Force of the American College of Critical Care Medicine of the Society of Critical Care Medicine in collaboration with the Infectious Disease Society of America. Crit Care Med 1998; 26(2):392–408.

118. Mayhall CG. Diagnosis and management of infections of implantable devices used for prolonged venous access. Curr Clin Top Infect Dis 1992; 12:83–110.

119. Shoemaker WC, Wo CC, Chan L, et al. Outcome prediction of emergency patients by noninvasive hemodynamic monitoring. Chest 2001; 120:528–539.

120. Velmahos GC, Wo CC, Demetriades D, Shoemaker WC. Early continuous noninvasive haemodynamic monitoring after severe blunt trauma. Injury 1999; 30:209–214.

121. Valtier B, Cholley BP, Belot JP, de la Coussage JE, et al. Noninvasive monitoring of cardiac output in critically ill patients using transesophageal doppler. Am J Respir Crit Care Med 1998; 158:77–83.

122. Theaker C, Juste R, Lucas N, et al. Comparison of bacterial colonization rates of antiseptic impregnated and pure polymer central venous catheters in the critically ill. J Hosp Infect 2002; 52:310–312.

123. Crnich CJ, Maki DG. The promise of novel technology for the prevention of intravascular device-related bloodstream infection. I. Pathogenesis and short term devices. Clin Infect Dis 2002; 34:1232–1242.

124. Crnich CJ, Maki DG. The promise of novel technology for the prevention of intravascular device-related bloodstream infection. II. Long-term devices. Clin Infect Dis 2002; 34:1362–1368.

125. Raad II, Hanna HA. Intravascular catheter-related infections: new horizons and recent advances. Arch Intern Med 2002; 182:871–878.

126. Groeger JS, Lucas AB, Coit D, et al. A prospective, randomized evaluation of the effect of the silver impregnated cuffs for preventing tunneled chronic venous access catheter infections in cancer patients. Ann Surg 1993; 218:206–210.

127. Timsit JF, Bruneel F, Cheval C, et al. Use of tunneled femoral catheters to prevent catheter-related infection. Ann Int Med 1999; 130:729–735.

128. Randolph AG, Cook DJ, Gonzales CA, Brun-Buisson C. Tunneling short-term central venous catheters to prevent catheter-related infections: a meta-analysis of randomized, controlled, trials. Crit Care Med 1998; 26:1452–1457.

129. Yamamoto AJ, Solomon JA, Soulen MC, Tang J, Parkinson K, Lin R, Shears GJ. Sutureless securement device reduces complications of peripherally inserted central venous catheters. J Vasc Intervent Radiol 2002; 13:77–81.

130. Seymour VM, Dhallu TS, Moss HA, et al. A prospective clinical study to investigate the microbial contamination of a needleless connector. J Hosp Infect 2000; 45:165–168.

131. Ibrahim EH, Sherman G, Ward S, et al. The influence of inadequate antimicrobial treatment of bloodstream infections on patient outcomes in the ICU setting. Chest 2000; 118: 146–155.

132. Valles J, Rello J, Ochagavia A, et al. Community-acquired bloodstream infection in critically ill adult patients. Impact of shock and inappropriate antibiotic therapy on survival. Chest 2002; 123:1615–1624.

133. Lannergard A, Hersio K, Larsson A, et al. Evaluation of laboratory markers for the detection of infections in open-heart surgery patients. Scand J Infect Dis 2003; 35:121–126.

134. Shafazand S, Weinacker AB. Blood cultures in the critical care unit: Improving utilization and yield. Chest 2002; 122: 1727–1736.

135. Mermel LA, Maki DG. Detection of bacteremia in adults: Consequences of culturing an inadequate volume of blood. Ann Intern Med 1993; 119:270–272.

136. Beutz M, Sherman G, Mayfield J, et al. Clinical utility of blood cultures drawn from central vein catheters and peripheral venipuncture in critically ill medical patients. Chest 2003; 123:854–861.

137. Safdar N, Fine JP, Maki DG. Meta-analysis: Methods for diagnosing intravascular device-related blood stream infections. Ann Intern Med 2005; 142:451–466.

138. von Eiff C, Jansen B, Kohnen W, et al. Infections associated with medical devices: Pathogenesis, management and prophylaxis. Drugs 2005; 65(2):179–214.

50

Abdominal Infections in Trauma and Critical Care

Bruce Potenza

Division of Trauma, Burns, and Critical Care, Department of Surgery, UC San Diego Medical Center, San Diego, California, U.S.A.

Jason Marengo and Sara Minasyan

Department of Surgery, UC San Diego Medical Center, San Diego, California, U.S.A.

INTRODUCTION

In a busy surgical intensive care unit (SICU), 25% to 40% of the patients present with or develop intra-abdominal disease (including infections) requiring medical or surgical attention. Patients with suspected intra-abdominal pathology may have signs and symptoms referable to a primary intra-abdominal process or referred pain secondary to medical disease (1).

Some patients admitted to the SICU with a primary diagnosis of an intra-abdominal infection can be managed with medical therapy alone. Common examples include: (i) the cirrhotic with spontaneous bacterial peritonitis; (ii) fulminant pancreatitis; and (iii) nonperforated diverticulitis. However, most will need antibiotics and decompressive or operative therapy. Some can be treated by interventional radiologic procedures for decompression or drainage of localized suppurative disease process, such as those seen with a pelvic abscess or complicated cholecystitis and ascending cholangitis. Some patients will need operative therapy. Deciding which patient requires operative intervention, determining the timing, and selecting which operation is to be performed are challenging decisions.

The development of sepsis or low cardiac output states can result in splanchnic hypoperfusion. Resuscitation and treatment of the underlying circulatory dysfunction often resolves the end-organ ischemia. Conversely, if the patient does not demonstrate signs of clinical improvement, concern over continued intestinal ischemia may prompt surgical intervention.

Other patients admitted to the surgical critical care unit are recent postoperative cases. These patients may develop complications as a direct consequence of their operative procedures, resulting in an intra-abdominal infection (2). Examples include failure of the primary surgical procedure, an anastomotic leak or breakdown, a complication of surgery such as a small bowel obstruction, unanticipated complication of the surgical procedure such as an enterotomy, or colotomy with leak or devascularization of a mesenteric segment of the bowel. Patients may also develop medical complications while recovering from their surgery. These include acalculous cholecystitis, pancreatitis, ileus, bowel obstruction, and gastrointestinal bleeding (Table 1).

Not all intra-abdominal infections are created equal. Intra-abdominal infections that are community-acquired have lower morbidity and mortality associated with them than hospital-acquired infections (3). Factors contributing to increased mortality include the nature of the abdominal complication, physiologic status of the host, comorbid disease, and microbiology of the infectious process (4). Christou et al. reported a 32% mortality rate in patients who developed a postoperative intra-abdominal complication. If the patient required a reoperation, the mortality increased to 42% (5). If patients developed secondary peritonitis due to a prior surgical procedure, the mortality rate was 50% (6). The development of tertiary peritonitis in a postoperative patient increases the mortality rate to 60% (7). Other factors adding to the morbidity include advancing age, male gender, shock, poor nutritional status, multisystem organ failure, emergency surgical procedures, and multiple surgical procedures (8).

The traditional presentation of abdominal infections and other diseases is often altered in critically ill patients due to changes in a patient's neurologic status from traumatic brain injury (TBI), drug intoxication, or the development of metabolic disorders (liver or renal failure), or due to the administration of sedatives, analgesics, or neuromuscular blockade (NMB) drugs. The altered mental status from trauma or critical illness makes obtaining the chief complaint and historical information difficult as well.

Distracting postoperative pain and pain associated with trauma can also mask or delay the recognition of abdominal distress. The use of NMB drugs, and/or presence of spinal cord injury (SCI) also hinder the practitioner's ability to accurately examine the patient's abdomen for signs of peritonitis. ☞ **The first clues to the development of an intra-abdominal infection may be the new onset of fever, leukocytosis, intolerance to oral feedings, abdominal distension, or deterioration in the patient's hemodynamic status (7).** ☞

Intra-abdominal infection remains an important clinical entity. ☞ **Familiarity with the normal postoperative course as well as the timing and presentation of postoperative complications assist in the management of critically ill patients.** ☞ Prompt recognition and correction of these problems may mitigate untoward effects and lead to a better outcome. This chapter will discuss the pathophysiology, diagnosis, and methods of treatment of intra-abdominal infections. The concept of source control will be discussed, as it pertains to intra-abdominal infections and disease.

PERITONEAL PHYSIOLOGY AND BACTERIAL CLEARANCE

The peritoneal membrane is the natural barrier between the abdominal cavity and the blood-soft tissue interface of the

Table 1 Etiologies of Abdominal Infection

Primary peritonitis
  Spontaneous bacterial peritonitis
  Peritoneal dialysis catheter infection
  Childhood spontaneous peritonitis
Perforated abdominal viscous
  Appendicitis
  Diverticulitis
  Strangulated bowel
    Strangulated hernias
    Volvulus
  Trauma
  Ischemia based on a vascular etiology
  Gastrointestinal tumor erosion into adjacent abdominal organs
Tertiary peritonitis
  Nosocomial infection
  Opportunistic infection
Retroperitoneal abscess
  Psoas abscess
  Osteomyelitis of the spine
Solid organ infection
  Liver or splenic abscess
  Bacterial or protozoan
  Pancreatitis
  Pyelonephritis
Post operative complications: anastomotic breakdown or leak
GI or GU infection
  Pyelonephritis
  Tubo-ovarian abscess
  Pelvic inflammatory disease
  Septic abortion

Abbreviation: GU, genitourinary.

surrounding abdominal support structures. In the healthy adult, the peritoneal surface closely approximates the total body surface area of skin, measuring approximately 1.7 cm (2). The peritoneum is divided into the visceral (covering the internal structures of the abdomen) and the parietal peritoneum, which covers the outer lining of the abdomen. This peritoneal membrane is composed of mesenchymal cells (9). The peritoneal lining is semipermeable, consisting of multiple small fenestrations that permit the passage of fluid and small solutes into and out of the peritoneal cavity. These fenestrations, located within the basement membrane, permit the bidirectional passage of fluid and small solutes (10). The bidirectional flow is influenced by the solute concentration, temperature, vasoactive compounds, local perfusion, tonicity, and volume of the peritoneal fluid.

A small amount of intra-abdominal fluid (50–100 mL) is normally found within the abdominal cavity. This fluid acts as a lubricant between visceral and parietal structures and assists with the intraperitoneal immunologic function. The predominant cells found within the fluid consist of macrophages (50%) and lymphocytes (40%). The constant motion of the diaphragm exerts a gentle counterclockwise movement of this fluid within the abdomen. Fluid initially found in the infrahepatic area will migrate in this pattern until it has moved inferiorly through the pelvis and then superiorly into the left upper quadrant.

☞ **The peritoneum acts as a semipermeable membrane allowing for the passage of both fluid and solutes.** ☞ Intra-abdominal and intravascular hydrostatic

pressure and oncotic pressure gradients effect movement of intra-abdominal fluid. The movement of fluid into and out of the peritoneal cavity is a dynamic process.

Lymphatic drainage occurs via the peritoneal-lymphatic complex at the undersurface of the diaphragm. This complex is composed of peritoneal mesothelial cells with intervening stomata, which cover a fenestrated basement membrane and the inner layer of the lymphatic endothelium. The degree of opening at the stomata varies with diaphragmatic movement, and changes with intrathoracic and intraperitoneal pressure. The presence of valves in the draining lymphatics prevents reversal of flow back into the abdominal cavity. The constant motion of the diaphragm facilitates the passage of these substances into the thoracic duct (11). Thus, there is a constant movement of fluids and solutes throughout the abdomen at any time (3).

Histologically, these mesenchymal cells are filled with extensive rough endoplasmic reticulum and multiple cytoplasmic lipid inclusions, which support the active metabolic function of the peritoneum (12). The peritoneum is very biochemically active, secreting interleukin-1 (IL-1), and interleukin-6 (IL-6), monocyte attractant proteins, transforming growth factors, granulocyte, monocyte, and macrophage colony stimulating factor.

Contamination from a viscous perforation results in a bacterial challenge to the abdomen. The key goals in the management of these patients is to prohibit further intra-abdominal contamination, obtain source control, administer antibiotic therapy to prevent secondary infection, and perform definitive therapy for the underlying intra-abdominal disease process.

The initiation of the inflammatory response of the abdominal cavity generates an intense cascade of cellular events, which effectively attempt to contain the site of infection (13). The immune response to infection includes both humeral and cellular activation. The increased permeability of the peritoneal membrane facilitates an influx of polymorphonuclear cells, cytokines, and fluid. Macrophages secrete proinflammatory products. Within 24 to 48 hours, levels of IL-1, IL-6, and tumor necrosis factor alpha (TNF-α) can be measured in the peritoneal fluid.

The coagulation cascade is also amplified. Fibrinogen and prothrombin are released into the peritoneal cavity. In addition, the release of tissue thromboplastin, by stimulated mesenchymal cells, promotes the conversion of fibrinogen to fibrin. As the fibrin polymerizes, the viscous fluid promotes the development of adhesions and thick fibrinous peel. Bacteria become trapped within the reticulum. The development of an ileus places the bowel wall in close proximity to the site of infection, permitting the adherence of omentum or loops of small and large bowel, which may wall off an infection. If successful, the infectious process will be sequestered, permitting phagocytosis of bacteria by macrophages and polymorphonuclear cells (14–16). If the area of infection can be sequestered, then an abdominal abscess will form; however, if the host is unable to contain the area of infection then a diffuse peritonitis may occur.

Systemic manifestations, such as fever (Volume 2, Chapter 46) and leukocytosis (Volume 2, Chapter 57) develop. Inflammation of the somatic nerves within the peritoneal membrane due to abdominal distension or peritoneal irritation will lead to subjective complaints of abdominal tenderness. The physiologic alterations of diffuse peritonitis are similar to those that are seen with a 50% total body surface area burn. Rapid exudation of fluid and solutes into the peritoneal cavity result in the decrease of circulating intravascular volume. An initial rise in the systemic vascular resistance and secondary tachycardia develop in order to augment cardiac output. The picture of uncontrolled abdominal infection is likely to follow a predictable course.

After the initial infectious insult and the inability of the host to control the infection, a hyperdynamic phase develops. Oxygen delivery is increased. Cutaneous vasodilatation and erythema is noticed, signifying the typical "warm phase of shock." As the systemic inflammatory response worsens, sepsis and systemic inflammatory response syndrome (SIRS) can progress to septic shock. If the infection is not controlled by antibiotics, surgery, or drainage, then a hypodynamic phase develops. Worsening systemic vascular resistance, poor tissue perfusion, and the uncoupling of the ATP cytochrome system renders the cells incapable of handling the oxygen. Microcapillary and intracellular shunting occurs, resulting in systemic acidosis and septic shock (17). If this is not reversed, multisystem organ dysfunction (MODS) or death can occur.

ABDOMINAL INFECTIONS FOLLOWING TRAUMA AND SURGERY
Scope and Pathophysiology

Intra-abdominal infections are an important complication in critically ill, postsurgical, and trauma patients (18,19). These infections range from an isolated intra-abdominal abscess to diffuse infectious peritonitis. These conditions may have a primary focus emanating from the abdomen or may be due to a local, regional, or hematogenous spread. The host may respond with traditional signs of infection, progress to SIRS, or develop frank sepsis (20–22).

ⅇ **In a study of 2457 consecutive surgical infections at the University of Virginia, 10% (252/2457) were due to intra-abdominal infections (23).** ⅇ The leading sources of abdominal infection were the colon (29%), the stomach (21%), the hepatobiliary tract (16%), and the small bowel (15%). Mortality was directly related to or was complication of the infectious process in 25% (614 patients) with surgical infections. Twenty-four percent of the cultured organisms demonstrated resistance to typical antibiotic regimens. Organisms with a high resistance rate included *Staphylococcus epidermidis* (67%), *Staphylococcus aureus* (49%), and *Pseudomonas aeruginosa* (51%) (24). Treatment failures and mortality were higher in the patients infected with resistant bacteria.

Bochud et al. (25), reported an abdomen source of sepsis in 27% (2430/9000) of the patients in intensive care. In another study of 465 patients with an intra-abdominal infection, 72% presented with primary abdominal pathology, whereas a nosocomial intra-abdominal infection occurred in 28%. Barie et al. (27), described the colon as the etiologic agent in 50% of all abdominal infections in the ICU. A localized process resulting in an intra-abdominal abscess was seen in 22% of the patients. Those patients who developed a diffuse peritonitis were sicker, older, and had a higher rate of MODS (1).

Factors Promoting Abscess Formation

Although bacteria resistance is one factor that contributes to treatment failure, the status of the host plays an important role in treatment success or failure. If the host is not capable of controlling or sequestering an infection, spread may occur by direct extension into contiguous tissues. This may result in a larger abscess or erosion into a contiguous

organ. In the latter instance, a fistula may develop (entercutaneous, colocutaneous, colovaginal, or colovesical) fistula. A disseminated infection may occur if an abdominal source of infection is not controlled, resulting in a systemic inflammatory response or sepsis (28).

Certain physiologic environments hinder the host's ability to fight infection. Local and regional perfusion abnormalities, due to hypotension, impair the delivery of cell mediators of inflammation as well as the clearance of bacterial-laden leukocytes. The presence of an intra-abdominal hematoma acts as a good culture medium. Antibiotic penetration into an abscess cavity is impaired and efficacy is reduced due to the acidic environment of an abscess cavity. Necrotic tissue may be a nidus for bacterial growth while hindering phagocytosis.

Role of Antibiotics and Source Control

Once the diagnosis of an intra-abdominal infection has been made, the selection of an appropriate therapeutic regimen is essential. Antibiotics, percutaneous drainage, or surgery of an infected intra-abdominal infection are the mainstay of therapy (Fig. 1). The application of these modalities remains challenging. Appropriate antibiotic selection, length of therapy, microbial resistance patterns, and combination versus mono drug regimens remain as the key issues to this therapeutic arm. Does the patient have an identifiable abscess collection? Does the abscess require drainage? How should the abscess cavity be drained, percutaneously or surgically? (29).

In most patients with a contained small intra-abdominal abscess, a combination of antibiotics with either percutaneous drainage or surgery is the preferred modality of treatment. A favorable response to the outlined treatment plan may yield a resolution of the intra-abdominal infection; however, continued fever, leukocytosis, and abdominal pain may herald an incompletely treated intra-abdominal infection, which may need more intervention. Due to the high likelihood that many intra-abdominal infections derive their source from a perforation or discontinuity of the gastrointestinal tract, therapy must be directed to the primary etiologic anatomic area. One of the key concepts of intra-abdominal infection management is source control. If there

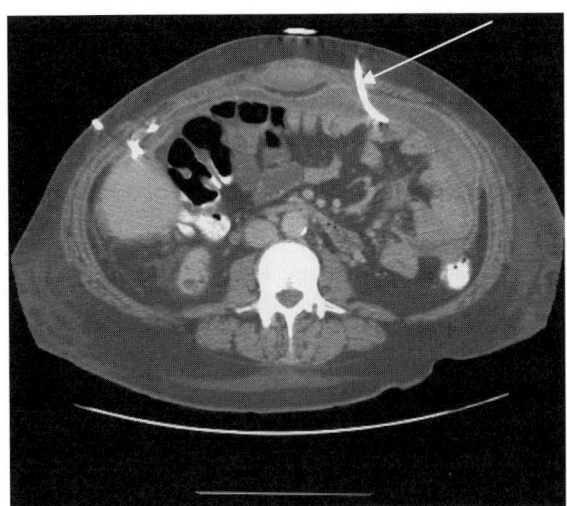

Figure 1 Percutaneous drainage of anterior abdominal fluid collection (*arrow*).

is an ongoing intra-abdominal contamination from a perforated viscous, there can be neither control of the infection nor eradication of the disease.

Imaging for Intra-abdominal Processes

✒ **Adjunct imaging studies are critical to the diagnosis of intra-abdominal infections, postoperative complications, or missed traumatic injuries.** ✒ These studies may include the acute abdominal radiograph series, ultrasound (US), computerized tomography (CT), magnetic resonance imaging (MRI), and nuclear scanning. Which of these modalities is best for a specific patient is predicated on many considerations. Familiarization and knowledge of relative perioperative complications and time of presentation facilitate appropriate use of these diagnostic modalities.

The acute abdominal series (flat plate, upright, or lateral decubitus films) may demonstrate free air, ascites, renal or hepatobiliary stone disease, or bowel obstruction. However, it has limited utility in critically ill patients. US, on the other hand, is portable, noninvasive, reproducible, and carries no radiation risk to the patient. Specific pathology, such as hepatobiliary disease (acute cholecystitis, cholangitis, and pancreatitis) are imaged well by US. Extra or intrahepatic ductal dilatation can be identified suggesting biliary outflow obstruction. Biliary stones greater than 2 mm in diameter can be visualized in the common bile duct. Cholelithiasis, abnormal gall bladder wall thickening (≥ 3.5 mm), gall bladder wall enhancement, and pericholecystic fluid are suggestive of gall bladder pathology. Repeat US examination can delineate structure-specific changes, such as organ size, dilatation, luminal diameter, and wall thickness. US is also useful in the diagnosis of free fluid and acute appendicitis (30). Renal evaluation for obstruction or intraparenchymal abscess is also accomplished with US. Doppler US can be utilized to evaluate vascular flow or obstruction.

✒ **The abdominal CT scan has greatly advanced our ability to diagnose intra-abdominal pathology (31).** ✒ The delineation of anatomic structures continues to improve with each advancing generation of scanners. Multidetector scanning with 16, 32, or 64 slides per revolution yields improved definition and resolution of intra-abdominal pathology. Adjacent structure review and analysis aids the clinician in the planning of interventional procedures.

In addition to soft tissue and intra-abdominal pathology, abdominal CT scanning is useful to study vital retroperitoneal structures, such as the major vessels, the kidney, and the pancreas. In patients with acute pancreatitis who are not progressing as expected in the SICU, an abdominal CT scanning may demonstrate the complications of the disease. CT findings may demonstrate the presence of pancreatic inflammation, peripancreatic abscess, pseudocyst, or evidence of pancreatic necrosis. Retroperitoneal abscess or vascular abnormalities are also best visualized by CT scanning. Finally, bowel obstruction or compromise is also well-imaged by CT.

A pelvic CT is useful when intra-abdominal pathology is suspected within the pelvis and mandatory when peritonitis or abscess location is being evaluated. In this area, transabdominal US is limited due to the distance between the abdominal wall and deeper pelvic pathology. Often gas within the superiorly resting bowel will obscure deeper abdominal pathology. Transrectal and transvaginal US are methods to circumvent these problems, and are used in the diagnosis and management of deep pelvic pathology. CT of the area of concern will provide a detailed picture of the underlying disease process and surrounding anatomy (32).

Arterial and venous phase CT angiography is now available at most institutions. Determination of vascular integrity, perfusion characteristics, or occlusion of vessels is now possible with faster scanning techniques. Both arterial and venous flow protocols exist to image during the appropriate vascular phase. In addition to vascular integrity, organ perfusion can be determined. Areas of focal perfusion defects suggest local thrombosis or embolism. Multiple areas of poor perfusion suggest low cardiac output that may be due to a cardiac etiology, hypovolemia, or shock.

A clinical example of the utility of abdominal CT scanning in ICU patients was performed by Velmahos et al. This was a prospective study to determine if an intra-abdominal infection was responsible for the clinical deterioration in 86 critically ill trauma patients (33). The patients had unexplained fever (>38.0), leukocytosis ($>12,000$), and abnormal Swan-Ganz readings, suggestive of sepsis or a clinical suspicion of an ongoing intra-abdominal process. Eighty-two percent of these patients were postoperative patients from abdominal exploration. Major surgical findings included gastric trauma, small intestine perforation (46%), or colonic perforation (19%), with intraperitoneal fecal contamination. Forty-five of these patients had abnormal (initial) CT scans with 41 patients having their management changed based on the CT scan. Thirty-five had CT-guided drainage of fluid collections. Thirty had positive bacterial cultures representative of an intra-abdominal abscess. Three patients underwent a second abdominal operation and three patients had their antibiotic regimen changed. The mean time for a CT scan was nine days. Overall the abdominal CT demonstrated a sensitivity of 97.5% and a specificity of 87.5%. Forty patients underwent a second abdominal CT scan. Eight patients had their management altered or avoided a second abdominal exploration. Fifteen patients underwent a third abdominal CT. Two patients underwent CT-guided aspiration with one requiring abdominal exploration. Most of the patients who developed an intra-abdominal infectious complication did so by the ninth postoperative day.

Nuclear medicine techniques have a limited role in the diagnosis and management of patients with intra-abdominal pathology (34). Nuclear medicine uses radionuclide agents, such as Technetium-99 (Tc-99) sulfur colloid scintigraphy, to demonstrate the function of an organ in question. Evaluation of hepatobiliary integrity and function can be performed in this fashion.

Radionucleotide scanning can also be utilized on recently transplanted organs to evaluate tissue blood flow through the demonstration of normal versus pathologic perfusion patters. However, solid organ transplants are currently most commonly evaluated with ultrsound. Abnormalities may suggest arterial or venous anastomotic problems due to thrombosis inflow or outflow obstruction.

✒ **The use of radionuclide scanning with Gallium-67 citrate or Indium-111 to detect areas of active inflammation or infection are less commonly used today, due to the advancements in multisliced CT scanning.** ✒ However, in selected patients these scans may be used to either identify an area of increased uptake, suggestive of a pathologic process, or monitor the treatment plan to eradicate an infectious process.

MRI offers improved visualization of soft tissue and vascular structures (35). When gadopentetate dimeglumine is used for contrast, the risk of contrast administration nephrotoxicity or allergic reaction can be avoided. A magnetic resonance cholangiogram may be performed to evaluate the hepatobiliary system in lieu of the more invasive endoscopic retrograde cholangiogram. Expense, unavailability of 24-hour accesses, difficult radiographic interpretation for the average physician, and the need for long scanning times in areas that offer little ability to administer ICU care make this a second-line diagnostic tool.

DEFINITIONS
Source Control

↗ **Local source control is paramount in order to manage intra-abdominal infections; without it, fluid resuscitation, antibiotic therapy, and critical care are unlikely to succeed (36).** ↗ Although source control may be specific for each abdominal infection, the principles remain constant (37). Perforations of hollow organs must be repaired or diverted. Ongoing ischemia must be reversed with the reestablishment of adequate perfusion. Discrete collections of infected material (abscesses) must be drained percutaneously or surgically. Devitalized or necrotic tissue must be considered for resection.

Abscess Cavity

An abscess is a collection of infected material, cellular debris, and components of leukocytes that are contained within a fibrinous capsule. The abscess may be located within the proper abdominal cavity, soft tissue or bone. Its characteristics are determined by the material within the abscess cavity, viscosity, and complexity, as determined by loculations. The location of the abscess contributes to the ability to percutaneously or surgically drain the cavity. The abscess cavity may remain as a singular entity, enlarge, or fistulize into a surrounding organ if not treated appropriately. Abscess cavities tend to be relatively protected by the fibrinous capsule that had formed to sequester the infection. Within the cavity are bacteria, necrotic tissue, and pus. The fibrinous capsule also hinders antibiotic penetration, and the antibiotic entry into the deeper areas of large abscess cavity is the poorest of all. As abscess cavities enlarge or become multiloculated, alternative methods of management become necessary (38).

Phlegmon

Phlegmon is the term used to describe a collection of tissues that have been inflamed and now has the characteristics of an amorphous tissue collection. The tissue is not infected by definition, but may become infected by hematogenous seeding or seeding from an adjacent organ. An example of this is the retroperitoneal pancreatic phlegmon that occurs with necrotizing pancreatitis. It is often difficult to determine if a phlegmon is infected. Fine needle aspiration may assist in this decision.

Devitalized Tissue

Necrotic or traumatized tissue that is unlikely to repair itself represents the tissue that should be removed in the face of an infection. This tissue has the potential to be a "safe harbor" for bacteria due to poor perfusion. Antibiotic penetration and activity is impaired as well as native, immune, and phagocytic activities. This tissue most often needs to be débrided or excised.

Unencapsulated Free Purulent Fluid

Free infected fluid within the abdomen is seen when the host is unable to sequester or encapsulate a collection of suppurative fluid due to ongoing purulent drainage or host immunoincompetence. The result may be a freely flowing collection of pus located within a dependent portion of the abdomen or pelvis.

Soft Tissue Infections

The infection of soft tissue may involve the superficial layers of the epidermis and dermis, as in cellulites, or involve deeper structures such as a superficial abscess within the layers deeper, than the dermis. Once the infection has spread deeper it may extend to the fascial layer and track the infection along this layer causing necrotizing fasciitis. If the infection goes deeper it may enter into the muscle compartment and result in a localized abscess cavity or an infectious myonecrosis.

Fistula

This represents a tract usually lined with pseudoepithelium, which connects a perforation in a hollow viscous with another structure. The fistula may track to a second structure and result in a colovesical or rectovaginal fistula. It may also track to the soft tissue through the epidermis to form an enterocutaneous or colocutaneous fistula.

Foreign Body Infection

Foreign body infections can occur following implantation of materials or shrapnel from external penetration during trauma or from infection secondary to an implantable biocompatible device. Examples of the latter include heart valves, peritoneal dialysis catheters, stents, and orthopedic implants. Two modes of therapy exist for these devices. One can attempt to eradicate the infection with antibiotic therapy or one can remove the device. The latter can be done if the antibiotic therapy does not succeed. Some devices can be removed easily and replaced at a later date when the infection has subsided. Other devices such as heart valves are difficult to replace and must be immediately replaced. These considerations as well as the species of the infecting organism must be taken into account when managing patients with infected implantable devices.

SOURCE CONTROL STRATEGIES

↗ **Source control is the process by which a site of infection (intra-abdominal or otherwise) is controlled so that further contamination of the surrounding tissues ceases.** ↗ Options of drainage, diversion, and definitive management of the infection vary with the organ injured or infected, the degree of infection, and the physiologic condition of the host (Table 2). The initial therapy may only serve the temporary goal of controlling the infection. After additional resuscitation, antibiotics and intensive care therapy, definitive treatment can be more safely accomplished in the physiologicall stronger host (28). Systemic antibiotics and drainage may control the infection and permit a definitive procedure to be performed at a later time when the situation has been optimized. In this case, a one-stage colonic resection with primary anastomosis may be performed in patients successfully managed with percutaneous drainage. On the other hand, diffuse abdominal soilage with peritonitis due to uncontrolled infection may require source control of the

Table 2 Source Control Strategies

Strategy	Examples
Drainage	
Percutaneous	Cholecystostomy, liver abscess drainage
	Perforated diverticulitis with localized abscess
Surgical	Diffuse peritonitis or suppuration
	Abscess inaccessible to percutaneous drainage
Diversion	Ileostomy or colostomy
Debridement/ peritoneal toilette infection	Pancreatitis with necrosis, soft tissue
Deciding on the extent of surgery	Can the patient tolerate a definitive procedure
	Do they need a temporizing procedure to
	Control of gastrointestinal spillage
	Peritoneal toilette vs. a definitive procedure
Device removal	Removal of peritoneal dialysis catheter
Definitive care	Diverticulitis with perforation (peritoneal toilette, bowel resection, and colostomy vs. primary repair)

initial problem and an abdominal washout at one or more settings. This is seen when the host is not capable of sequestering the infectious process. In this situation a definitive procedure may need to be delayed due to the degree of tissue inflammation and adhesions that one may encounter during a definitive procedure. Postponing may permit a resolution of the intense inflammation and permit safer operative dissection at a later date. "Time and Mother Nature are the surgeon's two greatest allies, and many a seemingly impossible situation can be converted to one that is merely a challenge by careful patience" (39).

Drainage

Drainage can be accomplished surgically or percutaneously. Recent advances in interventional radiologic techniques now make percutaneous drainage of deep-seated intra-abdominal or solid organ abscesses a viable option. Criteria for the use of percutaneous drainage include accessibility to the abscess via the percutaneous route. Relative contraindications to percutaneous drainage include the sites generally inaccessible to catheter drainage (i.e., include interloop abscesses), the presence of continued leakage into the abscess cavity from an uncontrolled gastrointestinal perforation, or the presence of multiloculated abscess or one that has a highly viscous fluid or cellular debris (40).

Diversion

The need to divert a source of infection is dependent upon the organ injured, the location of the injury, the physiologic condition of the patient, and knowledge of the natural history of the problem. Most diversion procedures are done on the gastrointestinal tract; however, diversion of the genitourinary tract is also performed. The gastrointestinal tract may be obstructed, perforated, infarcted or involved with an inflammatory process, making definitive therapy, including excision, difficult if not dangerous.

Diversion with a loop ileostomy will prevent distal movement of gastrointestinal succus into an area of perforation. Similarly proximal large bowel diversion will prevent a distal perforation from continued leakage. In certain situations, the distal pathology may remain if the involved area is so inflamed as to make operative resection dangerous. More often, the distal lesion is resected and a diverting small bowel or large bowel stoma is created. At a later date, when the inflammation and infection have resolved, a primary anastomosis is performed similar to what is done in a two-set procedure for perforated diverticulitis.

Debridement and Peritoneal Toilette

Indications to surgically debride the source of abdominal infection include the presence of diffuse peritonitis with free fluid that is suspected to be purulent, an abscess that is inaccessible to percutaneous drainage, and a complex abscess defined as one with multiple loculations, highly viscous material, or full of cellular debris. In these situations surgical debridement and peritoneal toilette is carried out. ☞ **The intent of peritoneal toilette is to drain the abscess, debride devitalized tissue, and remove gross fecal material and foreign bodies.** ☞ The goal is to reduce the burden of infected and devitalized tissue so the host's defense mechanisms will be able to eradicate the remaining infection. Free-flowing infected peritoneal ascites or pus is suctioned and irrigated.

There appears to be no benefit to attempt to remove fibrinous material from the partial or visceral surfaces of the abdomen and its contents. Clearly necrotic or devitalized tissue should be removed. At the end of the case, the abdomen should be suctioned so that large amounts of fluid do not remain. Although one can anticipate postoperative ascites to develop, leaving lavage fluid has the theoretical disadvantage of inhibiting macrophage function as well as other important advantageous inflammatory processes.

In staged procedures, the patient's initial physiology may be so deranged and tenuous that a prolonged procedure would adversely affect the outcome. Similar to damage control in the trauma setting, an initial debridement lavage and diversion (if necessary) is performed. Re-exploration within the next 24 to 48 hours is undertaken for a second look, lavage, and debridement. Staged abdominal repair is performed in situations where source control has not been possible at the initial operative settings. The abdomen is left open, that is, without closure of the fascia or skin. A temporary closure is placed, thus saving the fascia for the final operative procedure and closure (41).

No irrigation technique seems to be superior to another. A key point to remember is that in order for the abdominal immunologic defense mechanisms to work, there should be no residual irrigation fluid. Leaving irrigant fluid would simulate an ascites situation where it is known that the host's defense mechanisms are diminished. The macrophage in particular does not function well in an ascitic fluid medium. The addition of antibiotics to the irrigant has not been shown to be superior to simple saline solution. If one is going to lavage or irrigate the abdomen then the best method is to use multiple small aliquots of irrigate and then suction the fluid rather than the usual "pour and agitate" technique seen in most operating rooms.

Removal of Implanted Devices

The rationale to remove these sources of infection is dependent upon a number of factors. These include the etiology of the infecting organism and the likelihood of a therapeutic response and resolution with antibiotic therapy, the morbidity of removing the devices, and the ability of the host to survive without the device. ☞ **The presence of a foreign body significantly lowers the quantity of micro-organisms needed to produce infection (42).** ☞ Depending upon the timing of the infection, certain organisms predominate. Early graft infections are typically *S. epidermidis*. This organism is known for its propensity to produce a biofilm layer on a prosthetic device, which becomes adherent to the organism. Eradication of this infection becomes more difficult in this situation as the organism is "protected" within this layer from phagocytosis (43).

Determining the Extent of Surgery

The extent of the surgical procedure is determined by the underlying pathophysiology, the patient's condition, and knowledge of the natural history of the surgical disease. Early in the course of a surgical disease it may be possible to operate and achieve source control, as well as correct the primary problem. In the later stages of a disease time course, tissue inflammation, adhesions, or complex abscess formations may make it difficult if not unwise to attempt a curative and definitive procedure on the patient. The operative time spent with tedious lysis of adhesions, in order to separate component anatomic structures, may be prohibitive in a critically ill patient. The added operative time may tax the patients' underlying physiologic reserve, add to the perioperative fluid requirements, and may result in excess blood loss due to the highly inflamed nature of the hostile abdomen. In other patients, comorbid disease and poor physiology may render a definitive procedure unsafe. In these instances, temporizing measures of repair, diversion, or exclusion of an injured segment without definitive reconstruction may be warranted.

Definitive Care

Definitive care simply encompasses all of those therapeutic modalities, medical and surgical, which will be utilized in the overall treatment of the patient. Although many patients will have a stepwise approach to the eradication of their intra-abdominal infection, the sum total of these will leave the patient free of infectious disease with restored intra-abdominal continuity or semi, or permanent diversion (Table 3).

ANTIBIOTIC THERAPY FOR INTRA-ABDOMINAL INFECTIONS

In most cases of intra-abdominal infections of surgical patients the use of antibiotics is an adjunct of therapy. Control of the source of infection by drainage, debridement, diversion, or resection is the essential component of the treatment plan. ☞ **The choice of antibiotics is predicated upon thoughtful consideration of the patient's surgical infection in conjunction with the patient's underlying physiologic state as well as comorbid disease.** ☞ The benefits of appropriate antibiotic usage include eliminating causative bacterial pathogens, prevention of the spread of disease to distant sites, prevention of recurrent infection, and shortening the time for the patient to resolve the signs and symptoms of disease. The main questions to be answered, which aid in the determination of antibiotic treatment, include the following: (*i*) What is the etiology of the surgical infection? (*ii*) What are the likely bacterial pathogens associated with the disease process? (*iii*) How long has the infection been active? (*iv*) What is the degree of contamination or spread of the disease? (*v*) Is the infection community or hospital acquired? (*vi*) What are the antibiotic susceptibility and resistance patterns at your hospital? (*vii*) What is the duration of antibiotic therapy? and (*viii*) What are the potential side effects and medication interactions that might affect antibiotic selection? In an era where there is increasing bacterial resistance to antibiotic therapy, judicious and appropriate use of these agents, in addition to sound surgical practice, afford the best outcomes for these patients. It cannot be stressed that the successful treatment of an intra-abdominal infection is predicated upon adequate source control.

☞ **Significant factors that have been shown to increase patient morbidity and mortality include a higher severity of illness age greater than 50, an [acute physiology and chronic health evaluation (2nd edition) APACHE II] score of >8, poor nutritional status, significant cardiovascular disease, inadequate source control, and the presence of multidrug-resistant organisms (44).** ☞ When there is an intra-abdominal perforation, how the patient's defense mechanisms are able to cope with the infection fundamentally defines the outcome. Patient outcome is better if the contamination is small and the patient is able to localize the infection into an abscess rather than if the spillage is large and diffuse. Patients with generalized peritonitis have a two-fold increase in death than if the patient has a confined intra-abdominal abscess (21). In a study by Merlino et al. (45), 70% of those patients with localized

Table 3 Source Control Options in Common Intra-abdominal Infections

Disease	Temporizing	Definitive care
Perforated peptic ulcer	Omental patch Omental patch with HSV	Vagotomy/ pyloroplasty
Perforated gallbladder	Cholecystostomy	Cholecystectomy
Perforated stomach	Oversewing	Wedge resection
Perforated intestine	Resection and exclusion	Resection, ostomy, or primary repair
Perforated diverticulitis		
Free fluid	Abdominal washout	Abdominal washout, resection with ostomy or primary repair
With abscess	Percutaneous drainage	Surgical drainage, resection with ostomy, or primary repair

Abbreviation: HSV, highly selective vagotomy.
Source: From Ref. 150.

intra-abdominal abscess were treatment successes, whereas those patients who presented with diffuse peritonitis had a treatment failure rate of 70%. Treatment failures may result in a worsening of the patient's clinical condition. This in turn may lead to a prolonged hospitalization due to an additional antibiotic course, reoperation, multisystem organ failure, and (rarely) death (46). Those factors known to increase the likelihood of developing sepsis include age greater than 40 years, perforation of a hollow viscus (nonappendiceal), the presence of diffuse peritonitis, and pre-existing organ dysfunction (47). In a study by Mulier et al., all patients died in whom source control of a gastrointestinal perforation failed. Likewise, all patients died if source control was achieved, but clinical signs of peritonitis did not resolve (48).

☞ **The microbiology of intra-abdominal infections has remained remarkably stable over the last 30 years.** ☞ The choice of antibiotics is directed by the type and expected microbiology of the infection. Gram-positive, gram-negative anaerobic, and aerobic organisms abound in the gastrointestinal and gynecologic tract; however, the anatomic location determines the specific makeup and concentration of the microbe flora. The normal upper gastrointestinal tract has only 10^3 organisms proximal to the ligament of Treitz. In patients on antacid therapy, the microflora is colonized with up to 10^6 organisms including *Enterobacteriaceae* and *Candida albicans.*

Distal to the ligament of Treitz, the bacterial counts increase, and the predominant microflora changes from gram-positive organisms to enteric gram-negative rods and anaerobic bacteria. Once the terminal ileum and cecum are reached, logarithmic increases in the concentrations of gram-negative and anaerobic organisms occur. Movement into the colon alters the microflora to predominantly gram-negative organisms. Within the colon, over 400 discrete bacterial species can be isolated. Concentrations of microbes within the large bowel reach 10^{12} to 10^{13} mL bacteria per gram of feces. In the large bowel the concentration of facultative anaerobes reach 10^{12}, whereas the concentration of anaerobic organisms concentrations are 10^8. *Escherichia coli* constitute less than 0.1% of the intracolonic flora; however, with a colonic perforation, the concentration of *E. coli* rapidly increases in the peritoneum to levels of 33 times than that found in the intracolon. This is due in part to the endotoxin, adherence characteristics, and virulence of *E. coli* within the peritoneum. Fifty percent of abdominal cultures after colonic perforation will demonstrate the presence of *E. coli.* It is important to note that of all the bacterial species found within the colon only a small number are actually found in the culture. This may be in part due the virulence of the organism as well as the local intra-abdominal conditions, such as local tissue oxygen tension and the inability of the less virulent organism to coexist with rapid proliferation of *E. coli* and other gram-negative organisms (49).

As seen with obstruction, gastrointestinal stasis will promote overgrowth of bacteria irrespective of the location of the obstruction. Bacterial colony concentration and representative species are altered, setting the stage for a more virulent inoculum, if there is a perforation. Familiarity with the most likely microbes involved in the infectious process is important in the choice of antibiotic therapy. The distinction between a community-acquired versus a hospital-acquired intra-abdominal infection is also important. Hospital-acquired infections, due to postoperative surgical complications or due to complications of other medical disease processes, have a different bacteria profile than community-acquired intra-abdominal infections. The microbiology of hospital (nosocomial) infections demonstrate a more resistant microflora including *P. aeruginosa, Enterobacter,* Enterococci, and *Proteus* species, as well as methicillin resistant *S. aureus* and candida (50). The choice of empiric antibiotic therapy in this group should be broader than in the community-acquired group. Consideration of antifungal therapy should be given in the setting of chronic illness, surgical relapse, or in the face of an immunosuppressed patient.

☞ **The use of antibiotics directed against anaerobic bacteria (*Bacteroides fragilis*) in colonic perforation is an established principle.** ☞ These anaerobic antibiotics do not change the short-term morbidity of the patient, but rather decrease the change in the development of a late abdominal abscess formation (51).

The predominant antibacterial agents for treatment of intra-abdominal infections include the semisynthetic penicillins, cephalosporins, carbapenems, quinolones, and anaerobic agents such as clindamycin and metronidazole. Vancomycin and newer agents for use with methicillin-resistant staphylococci include linezolid, tigecycline, and daptomycin (see Volume 2, Chapter 53). Therapy with aminoglycosides has been declining due to the use of other less toxic antimicrobial agents.

Single-agent coverage is reserved for shorter duration of therapy as well as less serious infections. These agents tend to be either semisynthetic penicillin with beta-lactamase inhibitors, such as piperacillin/tazobactam, or a cephalosporin, such as cefoxitin. They afford broad aerobic and limited anaerobic antimicrobial coverage. Broader spectrum agents such as the carbapenems are reserved for serious intra-abdominal infections. These include meropenem and imipenem. Combination therapy provides additional coverage for anaerobes with the addition of clindamycin or metronidazole to any of the other antibiotics. Synergistic antipseudomonal coverage includes semisynthetic penicillin or a third-generation cephalosporin plus a quinolone or an aminoglycoside. The Society for Surgical Infections has recommended single- and double-coverage antimicrobial regimens for intra-abdominal infections, which are listed in Table 4. They have also developed broad guidelines for who should receive antibiotics, as well as the duration of

Table 4 Antibiotic Regimens for Intra-abdominal Infections

Single agents
Extended spectrum penicillins
    Ampicillin/sulbactam
    Piperacillin/tazobactam
Cephalosporins
    Cefoxitin
    Cefotetan
Carbapenems
    Imipenem/cilastatin
    Meropenem

Combination agents (all include anaerobic coverage)
Aztreonam plus clindamycin
Ciprofloxacin plus metronidazole
Cefuroxime plus metronidazole
Third generation cephalosporin plus metronidazole
Aminoglycide plus metronidazole

Source: Adapted from Ref. 55.

antibiotic therapy for intra-abdominal infections. Those patients for whom antibiotic therapy is recommended for ≤24 hours include the following: (*i*) patients with iatrogenic or traumatic enteric perforations with peritoneal contamination, who are able to be operated upon within 12 hours, (*ii*) patients with gastroduodenal perforation operated on within 24 hours, (*iii*) patients with acute or gangrenous appendicitis or cholecystitis without perforation, and (*iv*) patients with transmural bowel necrosis without bowel perforation, peritonitis, or abscess formation. In these patients a single dose of preoperative antibiotics are indicated. A second group of patients for whom antibiotic therapy would be indicated for ≥24 hours include those patients with established surgical intra-abdominal infections or more extensive intraoperative findings than the former described group of patients (52–55).

The efficacy of the overall treatment plan should yield an improvement in the patient's overall condition. Although there is no definitive duration of antibiotic therapy, the improvement of the clinical course, resolution of leukocytosis, a normalization of temperature, and return of their gastrointestinal function are good markers of infection control. Those patients may have their antibiotics ceased 24 to 48 hours after these markers have been achieved. In the patient with a favorable clinical response a total time of antibiotic therapy should be no longer than five to seven days.

In those patients with compromised immune systems, a longer time frame should be established. In some patients (i.e., a periappendiceal abscess), a shorter course may be sufficient. Use of antibiotics in trauma where there has been abdominal contamination is dependent upon the amount and duration of spillage. Typically the duration of time is short unless the injury has been missed and the patient's infection is well established. Trauma patients with a perforation of a hollow viscus and surgical repair within 12 hours, show no benefit from antibiotic therapy for longer than 24 hours of antibiotic therapy (52). A course of 24 hours of antibiotics appears to be as good when compared to a three- to five-day course of antibiotics. In trauma patients with established infections such as those with missed intra-abdominal injuries, therapy should be carried out for five to seven days as in other established gastrointestinal perforations (52,54,56). Lack of clinical response, suggested by persistent fever, leukocytosis, prolonged fluid requirements, and gastrointestinal dysfunction suggest ongoing infection and the need to be reevaluated after five to seven days of appropriate treatment. Complicated intra-abdominal infections with ongoing contamination, organ infection (pancreatitis), or an open abdomen may need prolonged antibiotic therapy. The duration in this group of patients is dictated more on the clinicians' impression as to patient progression or deterioration.

Whether or not there is a need to culture all peritoneal fluid or aspirate remains a debated topic (57,58). Reasons for the routine use of intra-abdominal cultures would be to identify bacteria that are not suspected in the infectious process or to identify resistant bacteria to the treatment regimen (58,59). Those who oppose the use of routine cultures claim that the bacteria profile of the intra-abdominal infection can be predicted with a great degree of certainty, and routine cultures are neither sensitive nor specific enough to guide therapy.

There may be subsets of patients where routine intra-abdominal cultures may be efficacious. These include immunocompromised patients, hospitalized patients, patients already on antibiotics who then present with an intra-abdominal infection, patients who develop postoperative abdominal complications, or patients who fail to clear their initial intra-abdominal infections. Intraoperative cultures can assist in appropriate antibiotic selection. There is a 15% to 20% incidence of resistant bacteria found in an intra-abdominal infection, and knowledge of this fact along with sensitivities of the organism may alter antibiotic therapy. Routine cultures of intra-abdominal fluid remain an unresolved issue; perhaps a middle-of-the-road approach to selective culturing of infected abdominal fluid in higher risk patients may be of benefit.

Certain bacteria and fungi are sometimes present in the intra-abdominal cultures. The significance of these organisms remains a pertinent question for the practitioner. Organisms such as Enterococci, Candida, and methicillin-resistant *S. aureus* are common isolated bacteria. Enterococcus has been found in 5% to 20% of patients with peritonitis; yet, large-scale studies have described successful treatment for intra-abdominal infections without specific antibiotic coverage for Enterococci (60,61). In most instances, it functions as a copathogen rather than the active infectious agent. In community-acquired abdominal infections, there appears to be no role for antimicrobial coverage for Enterococci (60,62). Hospital-acquired (nosocomial) infections, such as those seen in postoperative patients, are circumstances where Enterococci may play an active role and are not simply co-pathogens (63–65). Recent studies have demonstrated an increased risk of postoperative complications and a higher mortality rate in subgroups of patients with Enterococci cultured (66). These include patients with peritonitis who are immunocompromised, a prosthetic heart valve, severe sepsis, prior cephalosporin therapy, or persistent intra-abdominal collection without clinical improvement (63,67). These patients may benefit from enterococcal antibiotic coverage. The choice of antibiotic should be driven by culture sensitivities and institutional protocols, but would include monotherapy with vancomycin, ampicillin, an aminoglycoside, or linezolid. Linezolid and daptomycin are newer agents for soft tissue infections with Enterococci (68).

The isolation of candida has been associated with an increase in morbidity as well as mortality in intra-abdominal infections (69). Yet in a large series of patients with *C. albicans* and intra-abdominal infection, there appeared to be no difference in clinical outcome if antifungal treatment of candida was undertaken (70). One explanation for this finding may be that what most cultures represented was colonization with candida, rather than a true infection with candida. Again, in subgroups of patients with intra-abdominal candida, the outcome seems to have been dependent upon early administration of antifungal therapy (71). Patients likely to be included in the latter group include those with recurrent gastrointestinal perforation, patients with postoperative complications of acute pancreatitis surgery, or patients with repeated positive intra-abdominal cultures (72). Present therapeutic strategies include fluconazole, amphotericin, or liposomal amphotericin for those patients with renal insufficiency.

In summary, the Surgical Infection Society guidelines aid in the choice and duration of antibiotic therapy (68). These include: (*i*) Those patients undergoing an elective gastrointestinal surgery should receive a bowel preparation. (*ii*) Patients in whom source control is achieved at the first operation can be treated for 24 hours and then discontinued (53). (*iii*) Trauma patients with a perforated abdominal viscus can be treated for 24 hours. (*iv*) Patients with an established abdominal infection should undergo antibiotic therapy for five to seven days. If the patient develops signs or symptoms suggestive of an ongoing abdominal infection then prompt diagnostic workup should be initiated. (v) The use of antifungal therapy should be withheld unless the patient is at risk of development of a fungal infection.

SPECIFIC ABDOMINAL INFECTIONS
Peritonitis

There are three forms of peritonitis: primary, secondary, and tertiary. Primary peritonitis, also called spontaneous bacterial peritonitis (SBP), may be due to an inflammatory or infectious process. Secondary peritonitis is due to breakdown, perforation, or leak of an intra-abdominal hollow organ or viscus that permits contamination of the abdomen. Tertiary peritonitis is a latent infection seen in chronically ill or immunosuppressed critically ill patients. It tends to be due to atypical nonpathogenic organisms and is not due to a disruption of the gastrointestinal tract or other solid organs.

Primary Peritonitis

☞ **SBP is infectious in origin and is usually seen in patients with cirrhosis and ascites (73).** ☞ The ascites become infected without evidence of an intra-abdominal source. The bacterial flora typically has only one bacterial species, which is often due to gram-positive organisms, such as *Staphylococcus sp.* and *Streptococcus sp.*, or gram-negative organisms, such as *E. coli* or *Klebsiella*.

Speculation as to the source of the infection includes translocation through the gastrointestinal wall or hematogenous spread from distant foci, such as the genitourinary track or skin infection. Patients with indwelling peritoneal dialysis catheters may develop peritonitis due to a break in the sterile technique. The dialysis fluid may become infected during changing of the peritoneal dialysate or due to a dialysis catheter. A sterile form of primary peritonitis may be due to the presence of blood, bile, or urine within the peritoneum. Many episodes of blood or bile in the peritoneum do not lead to peritonitis. Release of pancreatic enzymes into the peritoneum during acute pancreatitis will most certainly result in peritoneal inflammation and abdominal pain. Granulomatous peritonitis is less common, but may result from an infectious source, such as tuberculosis, or from a chemical source, such as talc from surgical gloves.

The diagnosis of primary peritonitis is usually made by documentation of ascites, by physical examination or US. Paracentesis is performed and the fluid sent for cell count and culture. Leukocytes (WBC) of 500 or polymorphoneutrophils (PMNs) of 250 or greater are diagnostic. Gram stain and culture will help direct appropriate antibiotic coverage. In the case of a peritoneal dialysis infection both systemic administration and intraperitoneal administration of antibiotics are the mainstays of treatment. If there is a true dialysis catheter infection, the treatment remains the same. Clinical response to antibiotic therapy is reflected by an improvement in the patients' condition and a clearing of purulent exudate from the peritoneal fluid within 48 to 72 hours. A negative peritoneal culture is obtained at the end of the treatment. In patients failing to improve, the peritoneal dialysis catheter must be removed.

The outcome of primary peritonitis in cirrhotic patients is variable and dependent upon whether this occurred in the outpatient setting or as an inpatient. In outpatient cirrhotic patients there is a 3.5% incidence of SBP

with a corresponding one-year survival of 67% (74). In a group of hospitalized patients the prevalence of SBP was 10% to 20% with an in-hospital mortality of 20% to 30% (75). The presence of acute renal failure increases the mortality rate to 58% if the renal failure is at steady state, versus nearly 100% for those patients with permanent renal failure (76–78).

Secondary Peritonitis

☞ **Secondary peritonitis is a result of a break in the intra-abdominal viscera integrity (13).** ☞ Perforation or transmural necrosis of a hollow viscus may lead to spillage of gastrointestinal contents into the abdomen. These leaks may occur from perforated, gastric or duodenal ulcers, perforated small bowel, appendicitis, inflammatory bowel disease, ischemia, or diverticulitis. Spillage of gastrointestinal contents may occur due to abdominal trauma, operative procedures (enterotomies), or anastomotic leaks. Although gastric perforations may have low bacteria concentrations, progression from proximal to distal in the gastrointestinal tract demonstrates increasing bacterial counts and the presence of anaerobic microbes.

The diagnosis of secondary peritonitis is suspected in a patient with fever, leukocytosis, abdominal peritoneal findings, unexplained hypotension, or intolerance to oral nutrition. An abdominal radiograph may demonstrate pneumo-peritoneum, intestinal wall thickening, pneumocystis intestinalis, or thumb printing. In other patients, abdominal and pelvis CT scans may detect free fluid in the presence of free abdominal air, focal area of intestinal edema, pneumatosis intestinalis, or an abscess. Patients with a localized abscess may develop localized findings without systemic signs or symptoms of illness. They may be treated with percutaneous catheter drainage (66,79).

The initial therapy of the patients is fluid resuscitation. Secondly, control of the intra-abdominal source of infection is obtained. This may include a definitive procedure such as resection of the affected segment of sigmoid diverticulitis with primary anastomosis. Conversely, it may involve a temporizing measure with a diverting colostomy. The abdomen is then cleaned of any purulent material via controlled lavage. If there is no evidence of elevated intra-abdominal pressures, the fascia is approximated. The wound is left open to heal with a delayed primary closure, wet-to-dry bandages, or a vacuum-assisted closure. Lastly, the prevention of further intra-abdominal infection and faster resolution of active disease symptoms are facilitated by antibiotic administration (36,80). In patients with severe diffuse peritonitis, a single operation to control the source of infection was successful in 88% of the patients. In other patients reoperation at 24 to 48 hours or open abdominal management with repeated staged operative procedures is indicated.

In some patients, a single definitive operation is not possible. Declining physiologic reserve, hypothermia, coagulopathy, and acidosis are conditions where damage control surgical principles should be employed (81). In severely compromised patients, a shorter operative procedure, both in time and in scope, may be beneficial. The correction of hypotension, coagulopathy, and hypothermia could be accomplished in the SICU (82). In certain patients, abdominal edema due to fluid resuscitation and the systemic inflammatory response may limit the surgeon's ability to close the abdomen safely (Table 5).

In some patients, the degree of abdominal soilage and contamination is so great that a second-look operation with

Table 5 Indications for Open Abdomen Management

Excessive bowel, peritoneal and soft tissue edema
Massive soft tissue loss to the abdominal wall
Inability to obtain source control
Need for a second look procedure (to assess bowel perfusion)
Damage control surgery (hypothermia, coagulopathy, or acidosis)
Abdominal compartment syndrome

further debridement and lavage may be indicated. Source control can usually be controlled with two to three operative procedures (80). At some point if the abdomen cannot be surgically closed, temporary mesh and skin grafting or a component closure may be necessary.

There is a cost to abdominal reexploration that can be measured in increased patient morbidity and mortality (83). Mortality rates for reoperation range between 30% and 52% (82). Each trip back to the operating room extolls a physiologic price on the patient. It has the potential to incite the second hit, which may trigger a broader inflammatory response such as SIRS. Patients who require additional operative interventions seem to do better with reoperation, based on demand rather than simply planned at some time interval. Those patients with a planned reoperation developed SIRS (21%) versus reoperation on demand patients (13%). Similarly, multisystem organ failure developed in 68% of patients with planned reoperation versus 39% if the reoperation was performed on demand (32,84,85). If a second-look operation is necessary, mortality is reduced if the procedure is undertaken within 48 hours of the first procedure.

Frequent abdominal reoperations are associated with the development of intense inflammation of the bowel and subject it to ongoing tissue trauma. The rate of intestinal fistulae formation, perforation, and anastomotic leaks increase with each subsequent operative procedure (86). This observation can be readily seen by the operating surgeon. The bowel becomes more edematous and adhesions grow denser with each operation. An intense serositis develops on the bowel wall. Dissection of free tissue plains within the abdomen becomes difficult. At this point, it is probably better to attempt to secure some type of abdominal closure rather than continue to reoperate, if possible (85,87).

The decision for temporizing surgery rather than definitive surgery is determined by intra-operative evaluation of the three key areas: (*i*) evaluation of the overall physiologic status of the patient, (*ii*) evaluation of the condition of the surgical anatomy, and (*iii*) knowledge of the natural history and course of the disease encountered.

Tertiary Peritonitis

Tertiary peritonitis occurs in critically ill patients. These patients tend to be immuno-compromised or have been hospitalized for a long period of time. In the latter group of patients, they are often not clinically improving and have gone from one medical or surgical problem to the next, never seeming to fully recover (88). These patients have poor physiologic reserve and nutritional status. Tertiary peritonitis is not a common disease, but is often seen in patients who were originally seen with secondary peritonitis. In the medical ICU, patients may develop tertiary peritonitis without any antecedent operative therapy. The recovery in these patients is hindered by recurrent infections, which are dominated by nosocomial bacteria and opportunistic

infections. Mortality for this disease ranges from 30% to 60% (89).

The diagnosis of tertiary peritonitis is difficult to make (90). There are a paucity of clinical signs, symptoms, and findings to direct the clinician. Suspicion of tertiary peritonitis may be initiated by a gradual downward course of a patient without an obvious etiology, heralded by fever and leukocytosis. Fluid collections are aspirated and therapy directed by gram stain and culture. In these patients, *S. epidermidis*, *Pseudomonas* spp., and *Candida* spp. are frequent pathogens. These patients are succumbing to pathogens that are typically nonpathogenic to the immunocompetent host. Their ultimate demise is not due to the organisms, but to multisystem organ failure.

Perforated Abdominal Viscous

The management of a perforated abdominal viscus follows the same basic treatment principle of source control. Perforations must be contained either through normal host defense mechanisms, drainage, or surgery. If there is to be spontaneous healing or sequestration of a perforation, the surrounding tissue must be of good quality so that an inflammatory reaction may develop and sequester the infection. All but small (3–5 mm) intra-abdominal abscesses should be considered for drainage. Diffuse peritonitis with accompanying free suppurative abdominal fluid most often requires operative intervention.

The most common etiologies of upper gastrointestinal sources of abdominal perforations are gastric and duodenal ulcers. Unfortunately, currently, many patients are on antacids that effectively bypass the stomach's natural defense mechanism. In these patients, the upper gastrointestinal contents are of higher bacterial concentrations and often contain atypical bacteria and fungi.

The diagnosis of an upper gastrointestinal perforation may be heralded by epigastric pain, fever, and leukocytosis. The pain is constant and may radiate into the posterior epigastrium or right upper and lower quadrants. Nausea and vomiting may accompany these symptoms. Physical examination may reveal abdominal pain or guarding in the epigastrium and right upper quadrant. Plain films of the abdomen, including upright and lateral decubitus films may reveal free intra-abdominal air. If a CT of the abdomen is performed, both free air and free fluid may be seen. Additionally, local tissue edema may be seen near the area of perforation. If oral contrast was administered it may be seen outside the confines of the stomach or duodenum.

☞ **Primary repair of gastroduodenal ulcer perforation is dependent upon the etiology of the perforation.** ☞ Simple perforated ulcers may be repaired by oversewing and Graham patch. More complex ulcers, such as giant ulcers or ulcers due to gastric cancer, may require resection and anastomosis. Definitive surgical anti-ulcer therapy needs to be weighed against this benchmark. More and more younger people are using nonsteroidal anti-inflammatory agents. The incidence of *Helicobacter pylori*-associated gastrointestinal perforation is rising. A study by Tokunaga et al. (91), and another by Ng et al. (92), discovered that 80% to 90% of patients with a perforated ulcer were found to test positive for *H. pylori*. In these patients simple oversewing with a patch and treatment with antibiotics effective against *H. pylori* was sufficient to control the disease process (92). Hydrogen pump inhibitors are very effective acid-reducing agents. In selected patients (the elderly or critically ill) these pump inhibitors may be more beneficial than the morbidity of a larger resection.

Small bowel perforation is unusual and is often times a result of inflammatory bowel disease, obstruction, or trauma. Large bowel perforation is more common and includes the additional differential diagnosis of diverticulitis, volvulus, and malignancy. Within the colon the concentrations of anaerobic organisms increase so that one gram of stool contains 10^{12} anaerobes and 10^8 aerobes (93).

Management is specific to the disease process. Ischemic or infarcted bowel is resected and usually reconstructed with a primary repair at the first operation if the patient's physiology permits it. Revascularization of mesentery vessels may be indicated in the presence of a proximal obstruction due to embolic or occlusive disease. Intestinal obstruction is relieved as adhesions are lysed or hernias reduced. If the bowel is viable then no gastrointestinal surgery is performed. Inflammatory bowel problems may present with bleeding, obstruction, or perforation.

Surgical repair is directed toward the correction of the underlying problem, with the understanding that most of the inflammatory diseases are chronic and recurring. Surgical repair of traumatic small bowel injuries are the mainstay after debriding any nonviable tissue from the site of injury. Primary repair of large bowel perforations has become the first line of therapy in patients who can tolerate the added time to the initial operation (94). In those patients who physiologically cannot tolerate a longer operation can be surgically temporized by leaving a segment of bowel in discontinuity to be repaired at a second-stage operation or by diversion ostomy (95).

Intra-abdominal Infections Due to Trauma

The management of seriously injured patients is complex. Operative versus nonoperative strategies, use of adjunct angiographic procedures, and supportive critical care are commonplace in the management of these patients. Overall, 25% of postoperative trauma patients develop an intra-abdominal infection (Table 6). Surgical wound complications occur in 12% and intra-abdominal abscess formation develops in 9% of patients. The remaining patients develop

Table 6   Traumatic Etiologies of Abdominal Infections

Incomplete peritoneal toilette with residual peritoneal
   contamination
Continued lack of source control
Gastrointestinal anastomosis leak
Gastrointestinal repair leak
Gastrointestinal fistula
Gastrointestinal ischemia with perforation
Hepatic abscess due to trauma
Infected biloma
Missed injury with continued peritoneal contamination
Soft tissue infection
Postoperative intra-abdominal abscess
Postoperative pancreatitis or leak with infection
Infected vascular prosthesis
Infectious complications due to open abdomen management
Tertiary peritonitis
Retained foreign body infection (bullet, explosive fragments)
Incomplete tissue debridement
Delayed gastrointestinal perforation after blunt trauma

diffuse peritonitis, solid organ, or retroperitoneal abscesses. In the multicenter trial of the American Association for the Surgery of Trauma (AAST), 297 patients underwent laparotomy for bowel perforation, 19% (55) patients developed an intra-abdominal abscess, 9% (27) patients developed fascial dehiscence, and 4.3% (13) patients developed a colonic leak. Primary infectious sources include gross fecal contamination, hepatic, gastric, enteric, and colonic perforation. Intra-abdominal complications may also occur as a result of treatment, delay in diagnosis, or due to missed injuries. Sometimes, the gastrointestinal injury may not result in immediate perforation. Rather, ongoing tissue injury from ischemia, intramural hematoma or acute distension of a partial thickness bowel injury may result in a late complication. Medical complications, secondary to critical illness, such as pancreatitis or cholecystitis are seen in 14% of the cases (96). The nonoperative management of selected abdominal trauma is associated with the development of intra-abdominal complications.

Over the last 20 years, there has been a paradigm shift to the nonoperative management of liver injuries. Mortality from higher-grade injuries, the AAST Grade 4 and 5, has decreased. Yet, this has not come without a cost. Morbidity from the nonoperative management of liver injuries includes intra-abdominal complications (97,98). Bile leaks may progress to form a biloma, become infected, or develop diffuse peritonitis. Devitalized hepatic tissue may become infected and develop an intrahepatic or intra-abdominal abscess.

In a study by Wahl et al. (99), 33% (94/281) of patients with hepatic injuries developed an intra-abdominal complication. These complications were bile leak, liver abscess, or an intra-abdominal abscess. Patients who developed a complication had higher liver Abbreviated Injury Scores (AIS ≥ 4). Almost half of the patients who underwent operative therapy developed a liver-related complication. Fifty-three percent of the patients who underwent simple angiography and 60% of those with angioembolization developed a complication. In the nonoperative and nonprocedure group only 1.5% of the patients developed a complication. Presenting symptoms included unexplained fever, leukocytosis, or peritonitis. The diagnosis was confirmed with a hepato-iminodiacetic acid (HIDA) scan using Tc-99. The sensitivity and specificity of this test were both 100%. Treatment consisted of laparoscopic drainage or abdominal washout and placement of a closed suction drain.

Complications increase with increasing severity of hepatic injury. Patients with AAST Grade 3 liver injuries experience a 4.7% chance of developing an intra-abdominal infection. This increases to 21% with Grade 4 injuries and 63% of Grade 5 injuries (100,101). Options of treatment include percutaneous drainage, endoscopic retrograde cholangiography (ERCP) with stent placement, laparoscopic drainage, and washout or open exploration.

Splenic injuries do not have the same complication profile. Here, recurrent hemorrhage rather than infection appears to be the main complication with nonoperative management. Those patients managed nonoperatively, and who undergo angiography, seem to have a slight increase in the risk of developing an infectious complication. Recently, there have been case reports and small series of splenic abscess formation (6%) after angioembolization of ongoing splenic hemorrhage (102).

From a surgical standpoint, one of the most dreaded complications has been the breakdown or leak of a gastrointestinal primary repair or anastomosis. The stomach, due to the rich vascular supply, tolerates repair well. Caveats to obtaining a good repair are adequate debridement of the injured tissue, standard repair techniques, and postoperative gastric decompression. Leak rates are less than 6%.

The evolution from diversion colostomy to primary repair of colon injuries has been a slow process. During World War II, both British and American surgeons performed these procedures as a standard of care for battlefield colonic injuries. With improved technique, antibiotics, rapid evacuation, and perioperative care, surgeons gradually tested primary repair of the colon. From 1949 to 1990, there were 26 studies examining this premise. Leak rates from the primary closure of traumatic colonic injuries were 1.3% (20/1507). Leaks from resection and anastomosis were 5.7% (19/335). Some of these studies were retrospective and many not randomized. In four prospective studies, where patients received primary colonic repair without exclusionary criteria, there were no leaks in the simple suture repair group and there was a leak rate of 3.7% in the resection and anastomosis group (103). In a large multicenter trail of 297 patients with colonic injury, an abdominal complication occurred in 24% of the cases (104). There was no statistical difference between the primary anastomosis (22%) and the diversion group (27%). Independent risk factors for the development of an abdominal complication included severe fecal contamination, transfusion of RBCs of ≥4 units in the first 24 hours or single-agent antibiotic prophylaxis. Current recommendation is to consider primary gastrointestinal repair or resection and anastomosis in most trauma patients. In a study by Sasaki et al. (105,106), there was no difference in septic complications in the primary repair group versus the diversion colostomy group.

With these statistics in mind it is important to put this knowledge in a conceptual postoperative timeframe. Behrman et al. (107), examined the temporal frame of development of the intra-abdominal infection after a leak. In 222, intestinal repairs were done in 171 patients. There were 11 complications (5%) that occurred in 11 patients. There were four duodenal, four small bowel, and three colon-failed repairs that were diagnosed on an average on postoperative day 15. The four duodenal leaks (4 of 12) were in primary enterorrhaphies with associated pancreatic injury. The small and large bowel leaks all occurred in patients with resection and primary anastomosis. In three of the four small bowel leaks the patients had developed abdominal compartment syndrome. Overall complications were associated with more seriously ill patients, with higher blood transfusion and fluid requirements during the initial resuscitation and operation.

Missed abdominal injuries are seen at variable rates in the literature (0.3–31.4%) (108,109). The higher missed injury rates were reported by institutions with relatively low volume; less than 200 patients per year (110). Other institutions reported a much lower incidence. Buduhan et al. (111), reported an abdominal missed injury rate of 1.6% which was a splenic laceration. Data from our own institution examining over 13,000 patients over a 12-year period, revealed an overall missed injury rate of 3% (all anatomic areas). Missed abdominal injuries were diagnosed in 0.5% (65 patients). Most of these missed abdominal injuries were due to a false initial read on the CT of a solid organ (liver and spleen). This did not impact on immediate care as these were managed nonoperatively. Other abdominal injuries resulted in 38% of (22/65) of patients requiring operative intervention. These included small bowel perforations (11), diaphragm (9), splenic injury (1), stomach (1), and perforated duodenal ulcer (2). Thus 0.3% of all the trauma patients admitted to our center had missed abdominal injury (stomach, bowel, or duodenal) that had the potential to cause an intra-abdominal infectious process (112).

Acute Appendicitis

Complicated cases of appendicitis may send a patient to the SICU with a diagnosis of abdominal sepsis. Acute appendicitis begins with obstruction of the lumen of the appendiceal orifice. Secondary bacterial overgrowth occurs with distension of the appendix.

Simple appendicitis can become a suppurative appendicitis. In addition, a perforated appendicitis can develop into a periappendiceal abscess. Diffuse peritonitis may occur in a patient who is unable to sequester the suppurative process. This may be seen in the immunoincompetent or elderly patient. These patients are at risk of developing sepsis due to an uncontrolled intra-abdominal source. Complicating the diagnosis sometimes is a redundant sigmoid colon with diverticula. This situation may resemble acute diverticulitis; however, the management of these two conditions in the early stages is very similar. Although US imaging may demonstrate a distended appendix, CT scans better delineate the anatomy of the disease process. The sensitivity of the abdominal CT was 94% with a sensitivity of 95%. US had a sensitivity of 86% with a sensitivity of 81% (113). Radiographic findings on CT for acute appendicitis include appendiceal wall thickening >5 mm, periappendiceal inflammation or fat streaking, nonfilling of the appendix, the presence of a fecalith, or a periappendiceal mass or abscess.

Simple appendicitis and suppurative appendicitis are treated surgically by appendectomy. An appendiceal abscess is typically drained percutaneously or treated operatively. Perforated appendicitis is managed operatively unless there is a periappendiceal abscess. Localized abscesses may be drained percutaneously. If the abscess cavity is small and adjacent to the appendix, both may be operatively resected. On the other hand, if there is a complex picture of inflamed bowel and a large abscess then percutaneous drainage may be more beneficial. Early operation on stable patients with this ileocecal inflammation has been shown to increase the likelihood of complications and more extensive operative intervention. Appropriate antibiotics include second-generation cephalosporins or quinolones or semisynthetic penicillin. Improvement in the patient's condition at 48 hours should be demonstrated. If not, rescanning for an undrained abscess or operation is necessary. Complex abscesses or regional peritonitis is best managed by operation. A patient with an appendiceal phlegmon is probably best treated conservatively with antibiotics and an interval appendectomy at six weeks (114). However, if patients do not undergo interval appendectomy, only 20% go on to develop signs and symptoms of a second episode of appendicitis. The majority of these cases will present within one year of the first episode and tend to be uncomplicated (115). Therefore, there are advocates of watching and waiting rather than performing an interval appendectomy. If this management strategy is utilized in patients over the age of 40, then screening colonoscopy is recommended at a later date to exclude other significant colonic pathology such as colon cancer or inflammatory bowel disease.

Appendectomy can be performed via the open technique or laparoscopically. In patients whom the diagnosis is not known for certain, the laparoscopic approach affords the opportunity to visually explore the abdomen (116).

Acute Cholecystitis

Over 90% of the patients with acute cholecystitis have associated cholelithiasis. The remaining patients have acalculous cholecystitis, a disease primarily of critically ill patients. Calculous cholecystitis is secondary to cystic duct obstruction with secondary gall bladder dilatation.

Signs and symptoms of acute cholecystitis include right upper quadrant pain and referred pain to the right scapula and back. There may be associated nausea and vomiting. The pain tends to be unremitting in contradistinction to biliary colic that waxes and wanes, but subsides typically in six hours.

US is the primary diagnostic procedure as it is noninvasive, quick, and offers no risk to the patient. Typical findings include cholelithiasis, a distended gall bladder (>5 mm) with wall thickening (>3.5 mm), and pericholecystic fluid (32). In some cases, there may be mucosal wall separation or intramural air. A HIDA scan will demonstrate nonvisualization of the gall bladder. Care must be used in the interpretation of a nonvisualized gall bladder in a fasting critically ill patient. The gall bladder may be contracted due to disuse and not pick up the technetium contrast material and give a false positive result (117).

☞ **Acalculous cholecystitis is rarely seen outside of the SICU. It typically occurs in very ill patients who have been receiving parenteral nutrition.** ☞ The pathophysiologic mechanism of acalculous cholecystitis appears to be an alteration to the microcirculation of the mucosa of the gall bladder wall. This in turn leads to gall bladder wall ischemia, inflammation, bacterial invasion, necrosis, and possibly perforation (118). Risk factors for this process include recent hypotension, as seen with septic and burn patients, or prolonged biliary stasis (total parenteral nutrition). The diagnosis of this condition is more difficult to make and is often inferred. A critically ill patient who suddenly decompensates without an obvious cause, a newly developed intolerance to feedings, development of an ileus and unexplained fever or leukocytosis should prompt consideration of acalculous cholecystitis. Serum chemistries may be misleading with relatively normal liver function tests. Only a mild-to-moderate leukocytosis may be present.

A right upper quadrant US may demonstrate all the findings seen with calculous cholecystitis, except for the stones (Fig. 2). More often, the only ultrasonic finding will be a distended gall bladder. The additional finding of a thickened gall bladder wall (>3.5 mm) is supportive evidence for acalculous cholecystitis. Serial USs may demonstrate an enlarging gall bladder with some pericholecystic fluid or some slough in the gall bladder.

Surgical treatment is the mainstay for both acalculous and calculous cholecystitis. Both open surgical as well as laparoscopic surgical approaches have been utilized (119). Due to the intense inflammatory nature of this process one needs to exercise caution and sound surgical judgment when utilizing the laparoscopic approach. Conversion to an open surgical procedure may be indicated in patients in whom the anatomy is distorted or the inflammation prohibitive for a safe dissection (120).

Antibiotics are administered in the perioperative period and consist of a second-generation cephalosporin. If the patient is stable, laparoscopic cholecystectomy with cholangiography as indicated should be carried out. Patients whose symptoms have been present for longer than three to four days may have a very inflamed gall bladder that would make operative resection difficult. In these patients, a delayed surgical procedure after antibiotics and a cooling

down period may make a laparoscopic procedure feasible. Conversion rates of <2% are seen in acute cholecystitis of less than two days duration. More advanced cholecystitis is associated with an 11% to 32% conversion rate to open cholecystectomy (121).

In those patients with an intense inflammatory reaction of the gall bladder, partial cholecystectomy is an alternative. Here the posterior wall of the gall bladder can be left on the liver and it is safer to dissect the gall bladder in a retrograde fashion from the fundus toward the neck. Transection of the gall bladder is performed when it is deemed too treacherous to dissect further. Attempts to perform a cholangiogram through the proximal gall bladder may be of benefit in these circumstances. Otherwise, the remaining gall bladder wall is oversewn and a closed suction drain is placed in the Morison's pouch. If the gall bladder cannot be sutured, the placement of a drain should suffice in the absence of common bile duct obstruction. In the case of an obstructed common bile duct, an ERCP can be employed postoperatively to clear the duct.

(A)
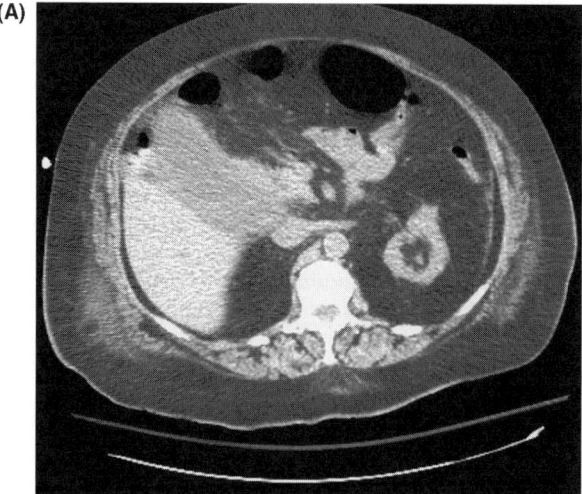

(B)
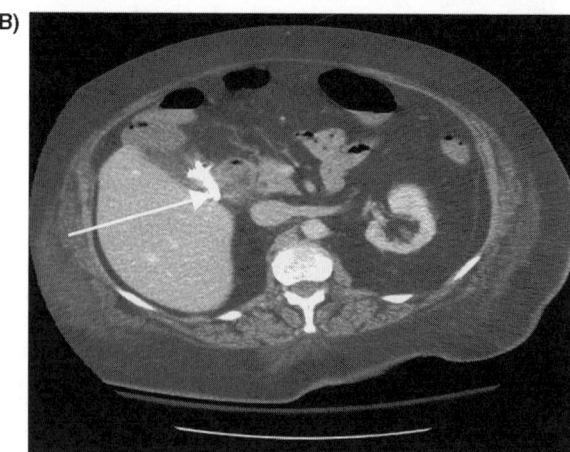

Figure 2   Acalculous cholecystitis. (**A**) Acalculous cholecystitis-distended gallbladder with pericholecystic fluid and edema. (**B**) Percutaneous drain placed demonstrating collapsed gallbladder (*arrow*).

If a patient is critically ill, and has acalculous cholecystitis, consideration of a percutaneous drainage of the gall bladder is possible. A note of caution is that the ischemia to the gall bladder walls may lead to necrosis and eventual perforation. ☞ **The presence of gall bladder wall necrosis may be missed on both CT and US; therefore, if a percutaneous drain is placed, the patient needs to be observed closely over the next two to three days to ensure clinical improvement.** ☞ Antibiotics are generally continued for a 7 to 14-day course in these patients. If the patient improves an interval cholecystectomy can be performed (122).

Acute Cholangitis

Acute cholangitis is an ascending infection of the hepatobiliary tree caused by obstruction of the common bile duct. The resulting stasis of bile behind an obstruction is fertile material for bacteria to colonize. Biliary obstruction may be acute or more indolent. The most common cause of obstruction in North America is due to choledocholithiasis (30–60%) (123). Hemobilia may be seen in trauma and transplant patients, leading to occlusion of the bile duct due to the RBC. Biliary strictures due to malignancy, ischemia, sclerosing cholangitis, or recurrent episodes of pancreatitis may cause obstruction. Malignant strictures are associated with infected bile in 25% to 33% of the cases. Infection of the biliary tree may also follow manipulation from ERCP. Common bile duct stents as well as biliary decompressive tubes may become infected. Extrinsic compression of the common bile duct may be seen with pancreatic cancer, gastric cancer, duodenal hematomas, and lymphomas. Patients who have undergone a biliary decompressive surgery with a choly-enteric anastomosis are at an increased risk for biliary infection.

Signs and symptoms are manifested by Charcot's triangle of right upper quadrant pain, jaundice, and fever. In 15% of the patients a more severe ascending cholangitis is seen with accompanying hypotension and mental status changes. The addition of the mental status changes and septic picture along with Charcot's triad, form the Reynold's pentad (124).

Laboratory tests demonstrate an elevated WBC (12,000–22,000), total and direct bilirubin, alkaline phosphatase, [alanine aminotransferase (ALT) also known as serum glutamic pysuvic transaminase (SGPT)] and [aspartate aminotransferase (AST) also known as serum glutamic oxaloacetic transaminase (SGOT)]. The degree of hyperbilirubinemia is proportional to the length of time and completeness of the obstruction. Diagnostic tests include US, HIDA scan, and CT scan. US is usually the first test of choice. The US typically demonstrates a dilated common bile duct with associated intrahepatic ductal dilatation. There is usually evidence of cholelithiasis, and choledocholithiasis may be demonstrated. Stones >2 mm can be visualized by the US, if imaged in the appropriate plan.

A HIDA scan will demonstrate filling of the liver and gall bladder without emptying of the Tc-99 into the duodenum. CT scans are beneficial when malignancy is suspected. Magnetic resonance cholangiopancreatography (MRCP) also visualizes the hepatobiliary tree, but a secondary test is usually reserved for patients who cannot tolerate an ERCP. An ERCP is both diagnostic and therapeutic in most cases.

Biliary stones can be retrieved with a basket or crushed. A sphincterotomy may be done to accommodate the passage of larger stones or a stent may be placed if a stricture is present to relieve the infected obstruction. Biopsies may be taken if there is suspicion of cholangiocarcinoma or ampullary carcinoma. The most common bacteria found in these infections are *E. coli*, *Klebsiella pneumoniae*, and *Enterococcus faecalis*. In two-thirds of the cases there is a mixed flora. Anaerobes are uncommonly found in this type of infection.

☞ **Treatment of ascending cholangitis is a medical emergency and requires prompt decompression.** ☞ Antibiotic therapy should be started with a broad-spectrum antibiotic, such as second- or third-generation cephalosporin or semi-synthetic penicillin. Septic patients may benefit from dual antibiotic coverage. A quinolone may be started in the penicillin-allergic patient. Fluid resuscitation should be instituted immediately. Seventy percent to 85% of the patients will respond favorably to this initial treatment. After 24 to 48 hours of clinical improvement, ERCP is attempted to relieve the obstruction. This management scheme is successful in 85% to 90% of the cases. Cannulation of the common bile duct and identification of the obstruction are diagnostic.

In patients in whom there is no clinical improvement in 24 hours, surgical decompression with cholecystectomy and common bile duct exploration should be considered (125). Morbidity and mortality are greatly increased in this patient population and correspond to the patient's underlying physiologic state [and approach 30% to 40% (126)]. Those patients who present in shock with comorbid disease are at higher risk. These patients are quite ill and typically require an open procedure rather than a laparoscopy. If surgical decompression is unsuccessful, placement of a T-tube for drainage also affords the interventional radiologist a chance to retrieve a stone in six weeks, when the T-tube track may be sequentially cannulated and dilated. Outcomes of mild-to-moderate ascending cholangitis are excellent. Severe cholangitis or a poor host has significant morbidity and mortality associated with this disease. Patients in septic shock have a 20% to 25% mortality rate associated with this disease (127).

Acute Diverticulitis

The presence of fever, leukocytosis and CT evidence of free fluid, abscess, hemoperitoneum or micro deposits of free air around the inflamed colon signify a more serious case of diverticulitis (128). Advanced diverticulitis may present with a localized abscess, peritonitis, or fistula formation. The latter may present as colocutaneous, colovaginal, colovesical, or coloenteric fistula. ☞ **Patients with diverticulitis who are unable to sequester the infection can develop peritonitis.** ☞ Indications for operative care of diverticulitis include: (*i*) diffuse peritonitis, (*ii*) unresolving obstruction, (*iii*) fistula, (*iv*) symptomatic stricture, (*v*) failure to improve on medical therapy, (*vi*) recurrent attacks, (*vii*) inability to exclude carcinoma, (*viii*) bleeding, and (*ix*) immunosuppression (129). Patients may be admitted to the SICU with newly diagnosed diverticulitis after percutaneous drainage of an abscess or in the perioperative period. These patients are typically elderly and have a more advanced disease. Their needs include ongoing fluid resuscitation, control of heart rate, ventilation, or general supportive critical care measures. Patients returning from the operating room will have undergone resection of the affected segment of colon, drainage, and debridement of the surrounding abscess cavity and a diverting colostomy with a Hartman's procedure. In selected patients, primary colonic anastomosis in the setting of an unprepped bowel may be considered (130). Choosing the proper patients for a primary repair is dependent upon the patient's physiologic state, nutritional state, and added operating time (36,95). The abdomen may be left open with only a fascial closure.

OTHER INTRA-ABDOMINAL INFECTIOUS PROCESSES
Clostridium difficile Colitis

Clostridium difficile is a gram-positive, spore forming, anaerobic bacillus. The primary source of infection is nosocomial. It is estimated that 20% to 30% of patients will test positive for *C. difficile* after admission to the hospital, compared to 2% of healthy individuals in the community. The spores from *C. difficile* are resistant to oxygen, desiccation, and many disinfectants facilitating the nosocomial transmission of *C. difficile* via the fecal–oral route.

In order for clinical *C. difficile* colitis to develop, alterations in the normal colonic microenvironment must be changed to favor this proliferation of *C. difficile*. Antibiotics are the most common cause for this alteration. Although all medications have been associated with *C. difficile* colitis, including vancomycin and metronidazole, those most commonly linked are clindamycin, cephalosporins, quinolones, amoxicillin, and ampicillin. Antibiotic factors associated with clinical disease include the dose and frequency of antibiotic use, route of administration (oral most associated), and the bactericidal effect of the antibiotic to anaerobes.

☞ **Only one-third of the hospitalized patients who become colonized with *C. difficile* will go on to have clinical manifestations of colitis (131).** ☞ Fifty percent of all colonized patients will harbor the toxigenic strains. The host immune system is thought to play a significant role in who becomes symptomatic. Significant correlation has been found between high levels of IgG Anti-Toxin A and asymptomatic carriers. Higher levels of anti toxin IgG may play a role in lessening risk of onset and/or clinical severity of the patient's disease (132). The pathogenicity of the *C. difficile* strain is also an important factor. *C. difficile* becomes pathogenic when it acquires the ability to produce Toxin A or Toxin B. These toxins incite an inflammatory reaction in the lamina propria, and recruit proinflammatory cells (133).

Risk factors of clinical disease are: duration of hospital stay, an ICU admission, use of multiple antibiotics, and duration of antibiotic exposure. Increased age and severity of underlying illness were also found to be important and correlated with an eight-time increase in the likelihood of clinical infection. *C. difficile* colitis occurring in the absence of antibiotics has also been reported in the chemotherapy and Hirschsprung disease population.

Given that antibiotics are one of the leading risk factors for developing *C. difficile* colitis, prolonged surgical antibiotic prophylaxis should be avoided. Antibiotics continued postoperatively versus a single or three-dose prophylaxis regimen have been found to significantly increase the incidence of *C. difficile* infections. Prophylaxis preop with metronidazole has not been found to be effective in protection against *C. difficile*.

The spectrum of clinical disease varies widely. As previously discussed there is a significant hospitalized population who becomes colonized with pathogenic strains of *C. difficile*, but remain asymptomatic. These patients are without clinical symptoms, and will require no further diagnostic testing or treatment.

Antibiotic-associated diarrhea is the most common clinical manifestation of intestinal *C. difficile* disease. This is usually manifested by watery nonbloody diarrhea without true systemic signs of infection, such as fever or leukocytosis. Endoscopic findings vary from a normal to a mildly edematous-appearing colonic mucosa. These cases typically resolve after the offending antibiotic has been stopped. In more advanced clinical *C. difficile* colitis cases, the colon will demonstrate luminal inflammation, edema, and in severe cases, the classical pseudomembrane. These changes may endoscopically appear to be continuous or present as patchy areas of colonic involvement (134). These patients usually have watery mucoid diarrhea, and possibly hemoccult positive stool. Frank blood is rare. Often patients complain of abdominal pain with distension and systemic signs (nausea, low grade fevers, leukocytosis, and fatigue). The preferential areas of colonic disease are usually limited to the sigmoid and rectum. In some patients, the colitis is limited to the cecum and right colon. These patients may present with abdominal distension, ileus, and minimal diarrhea.

Fulminant pseudomembranous colitis is a rare consequence of *C. difficile* intestinal infection. These patients may present with any combination of signs and symptoms from abdominal pain and watery diarrhea to abdominal distension and a paralytic ileus. In the most severe cases, patients may present with a toxic megacolon, signs of a systemic inflammatory response, tachycardia, and hypotension. *C. difficile* colitis should be considered in any patient who has recently received antibiotics and presents with toxic megacolon of unknown etiology. Cytomegalovirus (CMV) colitis must also be in the differential, especially if the patient is immunocompromised and presents with symptoms of pseudomembranous colitis with negative *C. difficile* toxin assays (135).

A suspicion of *C. difficile* colitis should be raised if antibiotics have been used in the last three months or if the patient has been hospitalized for greater than 72 hours. The gold standard diagnostic test is a stool sample cytotoxicity assay for Toxin B. This test is costly and requires several days for results. An ELISA for Toxin A or B is more rapid, with sensitivities and specificities similar to the gold standard. Endoscopic evaluation is indicated if significant disease is present and stool labs are repeatedly negative, or if a rapid diagnosis is required. ☞ **On endoscopy, the presence of pseudomembranes correlates with a >95% chance of *C. difficile* infection.** ☞ Flexible sigmoidoscopy or colonoscopy is indicated as 20% of pseudomembranes are beyond 25 cm from the anal verge. A CT scan of the abdomen will demonstrate a thickened colonic wall in involved regions, and may show pneumatosis or perforation in advanced cases.

No benefit has been found in the treatment of asymptomatic carriers with antimicrobials. Treatment of mild-to-moderate disease should focus on fluid and electrolyte replacement, discontinuation of antibiotic regimen, and avoidance of medications that impair gastrointestinal peristalsis (narcotics/antidiarrheal agents). Drugs that impair gastrointestinal motility impair the clearance of *C. difficile* toxin and allow more time for the toxin to incite an inflammatory reaction in the gastrointestinal tract. High-risk antibiotics should be discontinued if possible or substituted with those that are less likely to contribute to *C. difficile* colitis. Clinical improvement is seen in 15% to 25% of patients after discontinuing the inciting antibiotics.

If symptoms continue despite discontinuing or changing antibiotics, and *C. difficile* infection has been confirmed, then either metronidazole or vancomycin is indicated. Oral metronidazole is the first drug of choice with a dose of 500 mg TID for 10 to 14 days. In patients unable to take oral metronidazole, intravenous therapy should be attempted for a longer course of 14 days. Attempts to coadminister oral metronidazole via a nasogastric tube can be undertaken. With this regimen, greater than 90% of cases of *C. difficile* will resolve. Metronidazole has been found to be therapeutically equivalent to vancomycin in the treatment of *C. diffucile*, is less expensive, and carries a theoretically decreased risk of creating vancomycin resistant strains of Enterococcus. Oral vancomycin (125 mg TID) is indicated as a first line medication in pregnant females, children under ten, and those who fail a course of metronidazole.

The treatment of severe/fulminant pseudomembranous colitis is not standardized. Although this represents 3% to 5% of *C. difficile* associated disease, the mortality rate is 65%. Oral vancomycin is recommended as the initial pharmacologic intervention, along with fluid and electrolyte replacement, and discontinuing high-risk antibiotics as discussed above. Although vancomycin and metronidazole have been shown to be therapeutically equivalent, some feel that patients respond more rapidly to oral vancomycin. Because decreased gastrointestinal motility may interfere with drug delivery, many increase the dose of vancomycin to 500 mg every 6 hr and deliver it via a nasogastric or nasointestinal tube. A few small studies have also reported infusing vancomycin via colonic catheters during colonoscopy. Passive immunization with anti *C. difficile* toxin immunoglobulin has also been reported as effective, but needs further investigation via controlled studies.

Surgery is required in approximately 5% of *C. difficile* cases. Generally, these fall into the severe/fulminant category, which is initially unresponsive to medical treatment and in those patients who present with perforation. There is no consensus as to how long medical treatment should be continued before declaring failure and pursuing surgical options. If possible, a therapeutic course of 48 to 72 hours of medical treatment should be attempted if the patient's condition permits before proceeding onto a surgery. Some of these patients may present as an "acute surgical abdomen" and undergo a laparotomy prior to establishment of the *C. difficile* diagnosis. The most common complications in these patients who ultimately require surgery for fulminant colitis include toxic megacolon with perforation, volvulus, and complicated acute diverticulitis. Plain films often demonstrate dilated small or large bowel, mucosal edema with thumb printing, and intramural gas, which may be indistinguishable from obstruction or ischemic bowel. A CT scan is also usually unhelpful in establishing the diagnosis of *C. difficile* fulminant colitis. Bowel thickening with pericolic streaking and possible ascites may be present with a classic cloverleaf or accordion sign in 20% of the cases. Severity of clinical disease has not been found to correlate with CT appearance. Colonoscopy may be helpful in decompressing a dilated colon, but increases the risk of perforation.

At laparotomy, the external wall of the involved bowel may appear normal. Because of this deceptive appearance of "healthy bowel," some have been tempted to perform segmental resection with reanastomosis (136). Several studies, although with smaller number of patients, have found a decreased mortality rate with subtotal colectomy versus segmental resection or colostomy (137). The failure rate of subtotal colectomy has been reported to be 24% versus that of segmental resection and diverting stomas, which are 40% and 75%, respectively (138).

✐ *C. difficile* will recur in 16% to 20% of patients who initially responded to treatment. ✐ No difference in recurrence exists between patients initially treated with vancomycin versus metronidazole. Risk factors for recurrence include treatment with additional antibiotics and history of a previous recurrence. Although recurrence may be due to reactivation of persistent *C. difficile* spores in the colon, approximately 50% of recurrences are a consequence of reinfection with a different *C. difficile* strain. These patients may simply be retreated with the same agent (metronidazole or vancomycin). Patients with a second relapse should be on vancomycin 125 mg QID for six weeks of therapy. Multiple recurrences are seen in 8% of the treated patients.

Anion-binding resins have also been used in the treatment of *C. difficile* colitis. Cholestyramine binds *C. difficile* toxin and helps with elimination of the toxin. Anion-binding resins also bind vancomycin, and should not be given within three hours of one another. Probiotics have also been investigated in an attempt to establish a colonic microenvironment, which limits *C. difficile* overgrowth. *Saccharomyces boulardii* has been found, in a recent European study of 124 patients, to significantly decrease recurrences of *C. difficile* in patients with a history of multiple recurrences when used in conjunction with vancomycin or metronidazole. No difference in recurrence rates was discovered when used in the patients' first episodes of *C. difficile*.

Cytomegalovirus Colitis

CMV is a DNA virus belonging to the herpes family that is clinically active in critically ill patients with acquired immuno deficiency syndrome (AIDS) and organ transplantation. CMV is ubiquitous, and seropositivity for CMV ranges from 30% to 100% depending on the population studied (139). CMV is present in most bodily secretions including urine, feces, semen, saliva, breast milk, blood, cervical, and vaginal secretions. The initially asymptomatic inoculation and infection is followed by a period of latency that can last for the life of the patient if they remain immunocompetent. Immunosuppression or immunodeficiency allows for reactivation of the disease.

Patient populations found to be particularly at risk include AIDS and transplant patients, as well as patients on immunosuppression for inflammatory bowel disease (140). Ninety percent of patients with AIDS, at autopsy, have been found to have disseminated CMV. The most common infectious complication of solid organ transplant remains CMV, occurring in 60% to 70% of patients. Ten percent of these patients manifest clinical CMV colitis. ✐ **Symptomatic CMV infection rates for solid organ transplantation have been as follows; kidney (8%), liver (29%), heart (25%), and heart–lung transplant recipients (39%) (141).** ✐ The two major factors that seem to correlate with symptomatic CMV colitis in transplant patients include exposure to CMV prior to transplantation and the degree of immunosuppression after transplantation. Many transplant patients are placed on prophylactic antiviral regimens, such as ganciclovir 3 gm/day or acyclovir 3.2 gm/day for disease prevention (142).

✐ **Although CMV colitis typically presents with watery diarrhea, 30% of patients may have fever and weight loss without diarrhea and some may present simply with bloody stools and no diarrhea.** ✐ Associated symptoms are nausea, vomiting, fever, weight loss, and gastrointestinal bleeding. CMV infection of the colon causes vasculitis, and may result in bowel ischemia and a clinical presentation, which mimics surgical acute abdomen. Toxic megacolon, perforation, and hemorrhage have been reported as complications of intestinal CMV infection. The Wilson group reported that the most common reason for AIDS patients receiving abdominal surgery was CMV colitis. Antiviral therapy has been effective in reducing the incidence of the most severe complications associated with CMV colitis and have made surgery for this disease uncommon.

CMV colitis may be difficult to distinguish from other causes of colitis. On endoscopy, friable mucosa, erythema, and isolated shallow or deep coalescing ulcers are present. Submucosal hemorrhage may also be present, and is a result of CMV-induced vasculitis. These lesions are usually patchy and limited to one region of the colon. Isolated right colonic lesions are reported in the literature from 13% to 40%, underscoring the importance of full colonoscopic evaluation versus sigmoidoscopy. Endoscopic biopsy with demonstration of CMV inclusion bodies is the gold standard of diagnosis (143). In addition, 25% of patients may have mucosa that appears grossly normal. Random biopsies of inflamed and noninflamed regions from the cecum, ascending, transverse, descending, and sigmoid are important. Although uncommon, CMV has been isolated from grossly normal bowel.

Biopsies typically demonstrate an inflammatory infiltrate consisting of leukocytes, lymphs, and plasma cells. Enlarged mucosal cells with basophilic intranuclear inclusions are pathognomonic for CMV. CMV cultures of stool have not consistently been found to be predictive of active infection and are not advised. Polymerase chain reaction of patient serum is the best method of diagnosis and monitoring therapy. CT scan generally shows nonspecific colonic thickening consistent with colitis, and is often a nonspecific diagnostic tool.

Most patients with CMV colitis are managed medically. Typically an initial treatment regimen includes ganciclovir (5 mg/kg IV q 12 hours). Improvements in histological samples have been seen within three weeks. Complete response to therapy is seen in about 90% of patients. If complete response is not achieved, Foscarnet (60–90 mg/kg IV TID) is initiated. The lowest recurrence rates in patients with AIDS-associated CMV colitis have been those on protease inhibitors. The "outcome of AIDS-associated CMV colitis in the era of potent antiretroviral therapy" was examined by Bini et al. (144). The patient population consisted of severely immunocompromised AIDS patients. Although rectosigmoid colon was most commonly affected, 29% on endoscopy had disease limited to the right side of the colon. Bini felt strongly that full colonoscopy was important in AIDS patients with chronic unexplained diarrhea or gastrointestinal bleeding. Recurrent CMV infection has been found in up to 75% of patients.

➤ **Indications for the surgical management of CMV colitis include perforation, massive gastrointestinal bleeding, and toxic megacolon.** ➤ Patients with mild signs of peritoneal irritation with no free air and strong likelihood of CMV colitis should initially be treated medically. Patients who require surgery should have segmental resection of the colon without reanastomosis at the initial surgery. Surgical mortality of AIDS patients undergoing emergency bowel resection was 28% on the first postoperative day. One-month mortality rose to 71%. Six-month mortality was 86%. Death was usually due to sepsis and *Pneumocystis carinii* pneumonia.

Genitourinary Infections

Genitourinary infections that may present in the critically ill patient include simple urinary tract infections, perinephric abscess, acute focal bacterial nephritis, and renal abscess

(145). Urinary tract infections (UTI) present no differently than in noncritically ill patients and are suspected with a change in the color of the urine, cloudy sediment, or hematuria. Under normal conditions, the genitourinary tract is sterile. In the face of obstruction, secondary infection may develop. Urinalysis may demonstrate the presence of leukocytes, bacteria, or test positive for leukocyte esterase or nitrate, which are supportive evidence of an infection. Urine cultures confirm that the diagnosis may be classified as a solitary carbuncle or multifocal medullary abscess.

➤ **Ascending infections, pyelonephritis, and medullary abscess are usually accompanied by history of reflux, calculi, or obstruction due to previous surgery.** ➤ Urinalysis usually demonstrates pyuria and bacteria. Medullary abscess may present as acute pyelonephritis. Classically with this presentation, fever and leukocytosis continue after initiation of antibiotics (146).

Hematogenous spread of bacteria to the kidneys is also possible. Primary sources of infection include infected skin wounds, osteomyelitis, and use of contaminated intravenous devices via intravenous drug use or hemodialysis. Currently, the most common etiology of renal abscesses is ascending urinary tract infection usually associated with "renal tubular obstruction from previous infection or calculi" (147).

Clinical presentation usually includes fever, chills, flank pain, and occasionally weight loss and malaise. Important historical points are recent Staph infection (within last 1–8 weeks), recent history of urinary stasis, calculi, pregnant neurogenic bladder, and diabetes. Typically, renal abscess due to hematogenous spread presents with acute onset of fever, chills, flank pain without history of UTI, and usually demonstrates no growth on urine culture. The cutaneous Staph infection that leads to hematogenous seeding may occur up to eight weeks prior to the renal symptoms.

Urinary cultures correlate well with the etiologic agent of the renal abscess. Although pyuria and proteinuria are common, one-third of the urinalysis will be normal and 40% of urine cultures will have no growth. One-third of patients will have positive blood cultures, whereas anemia and azotemia are present in 40% and 25%, respectively.

Radiographic data may be helpful in establishing the diagnosis. Plain film is a nonspecific tool, but may demonstrate obliteration of the psoas shadow or enlargement of the kidney. A CT scan is the diagnostic procedure of choice and will best define the relationship of the abscess with the surrounding structures. The appearance of the infectious process will depend on its stage of development. In the early stages of infection, a "focal region of decreased attenuation" will be present. In the next few days, the focus of infection becomes walled off. When the chronic abscess is established, surrounding tissue planes are obliterated, Gerota's fascia appears thickened, and the abscess is a "low attenuating mass with a ring of higher attenuation which represents the inflamed wall." This is known as the ring sign. Generally, renal carbuncles appear as solitary space-occupying lesions, whereas medullary abscesses appear as small multifocal lesions or simply as a poorly functioning kidney.

Treatment of the infection depends on its size. Abscesses less than 3 cm that are discovered early may be treated with intravenous antibiotics and close observation. Percutaneous drainage becomes necessary when abscesses are 3 to 5 cm or if the patient is either immunocompromised or unresponsive to antibiotics and close observation. Surgical drainage is required when abscesses are greater then 5 cm.

Tubo-ovarian Abscess

Tubo-ovarian abscess (TOA) is a major complication of pelvic inflammatory disease. The history of prior pelvic inflammatory disease is elicited from 30% to 50% of the patients with a tubo-ovarian abscess. Tubo-ovarian abscess occurs most frequently in the third and fourth decades of life. Abdominal and pelvic pain present in greater than 90% of tubo-ovarian abscesses in the literature. This is usually accompanied by fever, chills, and occasional vaginal discharge and/or bleeding, and nausea. Twenty to thirty-five percent of these patients may present afebrile with a normal white count. The clinical picture of the tubo-ovarian abscess may be further complicated by some presenting as uncomplicated pelvic inflammatory disease. ☞ **The key to diagnosis of tubo-ovarian abscess is "inflammatory adnexal mass." Because physical exam alone may be inadequate, when suspicion arises, imaging test should be used.** ☞

US or CT is the most appropriate investigation for imaging a potential pelvic/intra-abdominal abscess. US will not only localize the mass, but also provide information as to its complexity. Transabdominal US has 90% sensitivity for diagnosing pelvic abscess. Endovaginal US has improved on both sensitivity and specificity. An additional use for US is its ability to determine efficacy of therapy once antibiotics or drainage has been employed.

In most patients, the tubo-ovarian abscess is composed of mixed aerobic and anaerobic bacterial flora. The predominant organisms discovered, in a recent study, by the Landers group included *E. coli* (37%), *B. fragilis* (22%), Prevotella (26%), aerobic streptococci, Peptococcus (11%), and Peptostreptococcus (18%). Although pelvic inflammatory disease is a key risk factor for tubo-ovarian abscess, *Neisseria gonorrhoeae* and *Chlamydia trachomatis* are rarely isolated from the tubo-ovarian abscess. Most infections are polymicrobial and contain anaerobes. Similar to intra-abdominal infections, it is the anaerobic bacteria that are responsible for abscess formation within the oviducts and ovaries.

With an unruptured tubo-ovarian abscess and concerns regarding future reproductive ability and maintenance of the hormonal axis, a conservative medical approach is initially pursued. If there is no clinical response to antibiotics (persistent fever, persistent leukocytosis), if the patient's condition worsens (increased size of tubo-ovarian abscess, increased sedimentation rate), or a suspicion of rupture exists in the first 48 to 72 hours, then surgery is indicated. In young nulliparous women, some allow for an additional 24 to 48 hours before declaring a failure of antibiotic therapy. The presence of an adnexal mass >8 cm and/or bilateral adnexal involvement were predictive of medical failure. Degree of leukocytosis, fever, and past history of pelvic inflammatory disease (PID) were not predictive of medical failure. Response to medical therapy ranges from 16% to 95% in the literature with a mean of 69.4% (148). Broad-spectrum antimicrobial agents with anaerobic coverage are indicated for these infections (149).

☞ **Indications for surgical management of TOAs include rupture and suspicion of rupture. Delay in treatment of TOA significantly increases mortality.** ☞ The surgical approach to unruptured tubo-ovarian abscess includes extraperitoneal drainage, drainage via posterior colpotomy or vaginal colpotomy, total hysterectomy with bilateral adnexectomy, unilateral adnexectomy, percutaneous drainage, and laparoscopic drainage. Extraperitoneal drainage requires the "adherence of parietal and visceral peritoneum" to be effective. This modality is infrequently used because better results have been achieved with laparoscopic and percutaneous techniques. Posterior colpotomy is used primarily for "fluctuant abscess in the midline, which dissects the rectovaginal septum and is firmly attached to the parietal peritoneum." This specific indication has limited the number of tubo-ovarian abscesses, which would benefit from this procedure. A danger of peritoneal sepsis also exists as a potential complication from this approach. Vaginal colpotomy is rarely used and carries a high complication rate. Aggressive debridement with total hysterectomy and bilateral adnexectomy has been advocated by some. Unilateral adnexectomy is recommended to maintain fertility and a normal hormonal axis. Seventeen percent of patients after this procedure required additional surgery at a later date and 14% had subsequent intrauterine pregnancies. Studies that support this approach are retrospective and lack significant long-term follow-up.

CT-guided drainage is usually carried out via the transgluteal approach that often causes significant patient discomfort. Endovaginal and transrectal US guided drainage have demonstrated good results in the limited number of cases that have been reported. The additional benefit of CT and US are that they can later be used to evaluate the effectiveness of the therapeutic drainage. Reported cases of laparoscopic drainage are also encouraging, but are limited in number.

EYE TO THE FUTURE

Better understanding of the perioperative course of a critically ill surgical patient affords the clinician the best opportunity to provide high quality care. Improved diagnostic equipment, such as abdominal CT scans with 32 and 64 arrays, produce a more comprehensive scan. Multiplanar scanning and computerized reconstruction will produce body images of a quality not yet achieved.

Antibiotic resistance is an ever-increasing problem. Clinicians will need to embrace evidence-based recommendations for surgical antibiotic therapy. These recommendations describe which patients would benefit from antibiotic therapy and specify the duration of therapy. The recommendations must become widespread, rather than each clinician basing antibiotic therapy on personal experience.

Source control will remain the cornerstone of abdominal infection control. Basic principles of drainage, diversion, debridement, and definitive care are essential to eradicate any infection. Patient physiology will continue to drive the intraoperative surgical decision-making. Whether the patient has the reserve to continue on the operating table or if the patient should undergo a temporizing procedure will remain a difficult and crucial question. Ultimately, patient care will depend upon thoughtful consideration of these choices often made under very difficult circumstances.

SUMMARY

Intra-abdominal infections remain a significant problem. Knowledge of the normal and abnormal postoperative period is essential for the clinician taking care of critically ill patients. ICU patients are often unable to demonstrate the typical signs and symptoms of intra-abdominal disease. Attention to the patient's progression in the perioperative period is essential, to notice subtle changes in the gastrointestinal function, which may be the only harbinger of abdominal disease.

The abdominal and pelvic CT have done more to aid in the diagnosis of an intra-abdominal infection than any other diagnostic modality. Often times, not only is the abdominal pathology visualized but important information concerning the adjacent structures is obtained. This facilitates better operative planning and patient management. In trauma patients, the delineation of bowel wall characteristics suggestive of injury are now becoming commonplace. Thin cuts through the hepatobiliary system aids in the diagnosis of injury. The use of the CT angiography to identify vascular flow within intra-abdominal organs and vessels greatly assists in our diagnostic abilities. Perfusion of organs, such as the pancreas in disease, is much better delineated so as to determine the viability of this organ.

Antibiotic selection and duration of antibiotic therapy is an important issue particularly in light of the increasing pattern of microbial resistance. Those patients for whom antibiotic therapy is recommended for ≤24 hours include the following: (i) patients with iatrogenic or traumatic enteric perforations, with peritoneal contamination, who are able to be operated upon within 12 hours; (ii) patients with gastroduodenal perforation operated on within 24 hours; (iii) patients with acute or gangrenous appendicitis or cholecystitis without perforation; and (iv) patients with transmural bowel necrosis, without bowel perforation, peritonitis, or abscess formation. In these patients single dose of preoperative antibiotics are indicated. A second group of patients for whom antibiotic therapy would be indicated for ≥24 hours include those patients with established surgical intra-abdominal infections or more extensive intraoperative findings than the former described group of patients.

The ultimate resolution of an intra-abdominal infection is predicated upon adequate source control. Methods include drainage, diversion, debridement, and definitive care. The choice of which modality to use is determined by the underlying disease process, likelihood of establishing source control, and patient physiology.

Paradigm shifts to the nonoperative management of solid organ injury has generated a new set of complications. High grade liver injuries (4–5) are associated with the formation of a bile leak, biloma, hepatic, or intra-abdominal abscess. Suspicion of these problems by day 4 postinjury should prompt the clinician for a workup, which may include an US or CT. Drainage and possible washout of bile collections is usually performed in these patients.

Missed injuries in trauma patients represent only a small area for which intra-abdominal infections occur. Constant vigilance to potential injuries that may present in a delayed fashion should be suspected in selected patients. Yet, it is clear that missed abdominal injuries that result in gastrointestinal perforation result in increased morbidity and mortality if there is a delay in diagnosis. If a patient unexpectedly deteriorates, appropriate diagnostic testing should be performed and resuscitative measures taken.

Other disease entities may cause intra-abdominal infection. These include colitis, genitor-urinary infection, and gynecologic infections. C. difficile colitis, in particular, is a great masquerader. Patients should be suspected with this disease in situations where they have been on long-term antibiotics or have long-term hospitalizations. The disease is readily treatable, however, when a toxic

colitis has developed, treatment options are limited and the end result may be a subtotal colectomy with diverting ileostomy.

Overall, a fundamental understanding of the perioperative course of a surgical patient and recognition of deviations from this is essential to provide critical care. Armed with this knowledge a physician can act upon subtle clinical signs and disease presentation to rapidly diagnose and treat an underlying intra-abdominal infection.

KEY POINTS

- The first clues to the development of an intra-abdominal infection may be the new onset of fever, leukocytosis, intolerance to oral feedings, abdominal distension, or deterioration in the patient's hemodynamic status (7).
- Familiarity with the normal postoperative course as well as the timing and presentation of postoperative complications assist in the management of critically ill patients.
- The peritoneum acts as a semipermeable membrane allowing for the passage of both fluid and solutes.
- In a study of 2457 consecutive surgical infections at the University of Virginia, 10% (252/2457) were due to intra-abdominal infections (23).
- Adjunct imaging studies are critical to the diagnosis of intra-abdominal infections, Postoperative complications, or missed traumatic injuries.
- The abdominal CT scan has greatly advanced our ability to diagnose intra-abdominal pathology (31).
- The use of radionuclide scanning with Gallium-67 citrate or Indium-111 to detect areas of active inflammation or infection is less commonly used today, due to the advancements in multisliced CT scanning.
- Local source control is paramount in order to manage intra-abdominal infections; without it, fluid resuscitation, antibiotic therapy, and critical care are unlikely to succeed (36).
- Source control is the process by which a site of infection (intra-abdominal or otherwise) is controlled so that further contamination of the surrounding tissues ceases.
- The intent of peritoneal toilette is to drain the abscess, debride devitalized tissue, and remove gross fecal material and foreign bodies.
- The presence of a foreign body significantly lowers the quantity of micro-organisms needed to produce infection (42).
- The choice of antibiotics is predicated upon thoughtful consideration of the patient's surgical infection in conjunction with the patient's underlying physiologic state as well as comorbid disease.
- Significant factors that have been shown to increase patient morbidity and mortality include a higher severity of illness, age greater than 50, an APACHE II score of >8, poor nutritional status, significant cardiovascular disease, inadequate source control, and the presence of multidrug-resistant organisms (44).
- The microbiology of intra-abdominal infections has remained remarkably stable over the last 30 years.
- The use of antibiotics directed against anaerobic bacteria (B. fragilis) in colonic perforation is an established principle.
- SBP is infectious in origin and is usually seen in patients with cirrhosis and ascites (73).
- Secondary peritonitis is a result of a break in the intra-abdominal viscera integrity (13).
- Primary repair of gastroduodenal ulcer perforation is dependent upon the etiology of the perforation.

- Acalculous cholecystitis is rarely seen outside of the SICU. It typically occurs in very ill patients who have been receiving parenteral nutrition.

- The presence of gall bladder wall necrosis may be missed on both CT and US; therefore, if a percutaneous drain is placed the patient needs to be observed closely over the next two to three days to ensure clinical improvement.

- Treatment of ascending cholangitis is a medical emergency and requires prompt decompression.

- Patients with diverticulitis who are unable to sequester the infection can develop peritonitis.

- Only one-third of the hospitalized patients who become colonized with *C. difficile* will go on to have clinical manifestations of colitis (152).

- On endoscopy, the presence of pseudomembranes correlates with a >95% chance of *C. difficile* infection.

- Treatment of ascending cholangitis is a medical emergency and requires prompt decompression.

- Symptomatic CMV infection rates for solid organ transplantation have been as follows: kidney (8%), liver (29%), heart (25%), and heart–lung transplant recipients (39%) (162).

- Although CMV colitis typically presents with watery diarrhea, 30% of patients may have fever and weight loss without diarrhea and some may present simply with bloody stools and no diarrhea.

- Indications for the surgical management of CMV colitis include perforation, massive gastrointestinal bleeding, and toxic megacolon.

- Ascending infections, pyelonephritis and medullary abscess are usually accompanied by history of reflux, calculi, or obstruction, due to previous surgery.

- The key to diagnosis of tubo-ovarian abscess is "inflammatory adnexal mass." Because physical exam alone may be inadequate, when suspicion arises, imaging test should be used.

- Indications for surgical management of TOAs include rupture and suspicion of rupture. Delay in treatment of TOA significantly increases mortality.

REFERENCES

1. Martin RF, Flynn R. The acute abdomen in the critically ill patient. Surg Clin N Am 1997; 77(6):1455–1464.
2. Sleeman D, Norwood S. The complicated postoperative abdomen. In: Civetta JM, Taylor RW, Kirby RR, eds. Critical Care, 3rd ed. Philadelphia, PA: Lippincott-Raven Publishers, 1997:1109–1414.
3. Marshall JC. Intra-abdominal infections. Microbes Infect 2004; 6:1015–1025.
4. Marshall JC, Innes M. Intensive care unit management of intra-abdominal infection. Crit Care Med 2003; 31(8):2228–2237.
5. Christou NV, Barie PS, Dellinger EP, Waymack JP, Stone HH. Surgical infection society intra-abdominal infection study-prospective evaluation of management techniques and outcome. Arch Surg 128(2):193–199.
6. Nathans AB, Rotstein OD, Marshall JC. Tertiary peritonitis: clinical features of a complex nosocomial infection. World J Surg 1998; 22:158–163.
7. Evans HL, Raymond DP, Pelletier SJ, Crabtree TD, Pruett T, Sawyer RG. Diagnosis of intra-abdominal infection in the critically ill patient. Curr Opin Crit Care 2001; 7:117–121.
8. Stafford RE, Weigelt JA. Surgical infections in the critically ill. Curr Opin Crit Care 2002; 8:449–452.
9. Nance FC. Diseases of the peritoneum, mesentery, and omentum. In: Bockus J, ed. Gastroenterology. 4th ed. Vol. 7. Philadelphia: W.B. Saunders, 1985:4177–4179.
10. Levinson ME, Bush LM. Peritonitis and other intra-abdominal infection. In: Mandell GL, Bennet JE, Dolin R, eds. Principles and Practice of Infectious Disease. 5th ed. New York: Churchill Livingston, 2000:821–848.
11. Glasgow RE, Mulviihill SJ. Abdominal pain including the acute abdomen. In: Feldman M, Sleisenger MH, Scharschmidit BF, eds. Gastrointestinal and Liver Disease. Philiadelphia: W.B. Saunders, 1998:80–84.
12. Broche F, Tellado JM. Defense mechanisms of the peritoneal cavity. Curr Opin Crit Care 2001; 7:105–116.
13. Marshall JC, Netto FS. Secondary bacterial peritonitis problems. Gen Surg 2002; 19(1):54–64.
14. Rotstein OD, Nathens AB. Peritonitis and intra-abdominal abscesses. In: Willmore DW, Cheung LY, Harken AH, et al., eds. ACS Surgery Principles and Practice. New York: Webb MD, 2002:1250–1251.
15. Heemken R, Gandawidjaja L, Hau T. Peritonitis: pathophysiology and local defense mechanisms. Hepato-gatroenterology 1997; 44(16):927–936.
16. Dunn DL. The biological rational. In: Schein M, Marshall JC, eds. Source Control—A Guide to the Management of Surgical Infections. New York: Springer Publishers, 2002:9–16.
17. Wang P, Chaudry IH. Experimental models of source control. In: Schein M, Marshall JC, eds. Source Control—A Guide to the Management of Surgical Infections. New York: Springer Publishers, 2002:17–24.
18. Liolios A, Oropello JM, Benjamin E. Gastrointestinal complications in the intensive care unit. Clin Chest Med 1999; 20(2):329–345.
19. Merrell RC. The Abdomen as source of sepsis in critically ill patients. Crit Care Clin 1995; 11(2):255–272.
20. Calandra T, Cohen J. The international sepsis consensus conference on definitions of infection in the intensive care unit. Crit Care Med 2005; 33(7):1538–1548.
21. Cheadle WG, Spain DA. The continuing challenge of intra-abdominal infection. Am J Surg 2003; 186(5A):S15–S22.
22. Bartlett JG. Intra-abdominal sepsis. Med Clin North Am 1995; 79(3):599–617.
23. Sawyer RG, Raymond DP, Pelletier SJ, Crabtree TG, Pruett TL. Implications of 2,457 consecutive surgical infections entering year 2000. Ann Surg 2001; 232(6):867–874.
24. Stephan F, Cheffi A, Bonnet F. Nosocomial infections and outcome of critically ill elderly patients after surgery. Anesthesiology 2001; 94(3):407–414.
25. Bochud PY, Glauser MP, Calandra T. Antibiotics in sepsis. Intensive Care Med 2001; 27:S33–S48.
26. Danielson D, West MA. Recent developments in clinical management of surgical sepsis. Curr Opin Crit Care 2001; 7:367–370.
27. Barie PS, Hydo LJ, Eachempath SR. Longitudinal outcomes of intra-abdominal infection complicated by critical illness. Surg Infect 2004; 5(4):365–373.
28. Reed RL. Contemporary issues with bacterial infection in the intensive care unit. Surg Clin N Am 2000; 80(3):895–909.
29. Duszak RL, Levy JM, Akin EW, et al. Percutaneous catheter drainage of infected intra-abdominal fluid collections. American College of Radiology: Appropriateness Criteria. Radiology 2000; 215(suppl):1067–1075.
30. Puylaert JB. Ultrasonography of the acute abdomen: gastrointestinal conditions. Radiol Clin North Am 2003; 31:1227–1242.
31. Kundra V, Silverman PM. Impact of multislice CT imaging of acute abdominal disease. Radiol Clin North Am 2003; 41:1083–1093.
32. McDowell RK, Dawson SL. Evaluation of the abdomen in sepsis of unknown orgin. Radiol Clin North Am 1996; 34(1):177–190.
33. Velmahos GC, Akamel E, Berne T, et al. Abdominal computerized scan of the abdomen in critically injured patients—fishing the murky waters. Arch Surg 1999; 134:831–838.
34. Zudkier LS, Freeman LM. Selective role of nuclear medicine in evaluating the acute abdomen. Radiol Clin North Am 2003; 41:1275–1288.
35. Pedrosa I, Rofsky NM. MR imaging in abdominal emergencies. Radiol Clin North Am 2003; 41:1243–1273.

36. Jimenez MF, Marshall JC. Source control in the management of sepsis. Intens Care Med 2001; 27:S49–S62.

37. Bohnen JM, Marshall JC, Fry DE, Johnson SB, Solomkin JS. Clinical and scientific importance of source control in abdominal infections: summary of a symposium. Can J Surg 1999; 42:122–126.

38. Sirinek KR. Diagnosis and treatment of intra-abdominal abscesses. Surg Infect 2000; 1(1):31–38.

39. Marshall JC, Schein M. In: Schein M, Marshall JC, eds. Source Control—A Guide to the Management of Surgical Infections. New York: Springer Publishers, 2002:5–12.

40. Gang GI, Moulton JF, Solomkin JS. Drainage. In: Schein M, Marshall JC, eds. Source Control: A Guide to the Management of Infections. New York: Springer 2003.

41. Moore EE, Burch JM, Franciose RJ, Offner PJ, Biffl WL. Staged physiologic restoration and damage control surgery. World J Surg 1998; 22:1184–1191.

42. Doughery SH. Pathobiology of infection in prosthetic devices. Rev Infect Dis 1988; 10:1102–1117.

43. Patrick CC, Plaunt MR, Hetherington SV, May SM. Pole of the Staphylococcus epidermidis slime layer in experimental tunnel tract infections. Infect Immun 1992; 60:1363–1367.

44. Mazuski JE. Clinical challenges and unmet needs in the management of complicated intra-abdominal infections. Surg Infections 2005; 6(S2):Supp 49–66.

45. Merlino JI. Malangoni MA. Smith CM, Lang RL. Prospective randomized trials affect the outcomes of intra-abdominal infection. Ann Surg 2001; 233(6):839–866.

46. Falagas ME, Barefoot L, Griffith J, Ruthazar R, Snydman DR. Risk factors leading to clinical failure in the treatment of intra-abdominal or skin/soft tissue infections. Eur J Clin Microbiol Infect Dis 1996; 15(12):913–921.

47. Anaya DA, Nathens AB. Risk factors for severe sepsis in peritonitis. Surg Infect 2003; 4(4):355–362.

48. Mulier S, Penninckx F, Verwaest C, et al. Factors affecting mortality in generalized postoperative peritonitis: multivariate analysis in 96 patients. World J Surg 2003; 27:379–384.

49. Malangoni MA. Contributions to the management of intra-abdominal infections. Am J Surg 2005; 190:255–259.

50. Tellado JM, Wilson SE. Empiric treatment of nosocomial intra-abdominal infections: a focus on carbapenems. Surg Infect 2005; 6(3):329–343.

51. Fry DE. Basic aspects of and general problems in surgical infections. Surg Infect 2001; 2(suppl 1):S3–S11.

52. Fabian T, Croce MA, Payne LW, Minard G, Pritchard FE, Kudsk KA. Duration of antibiotic therapy for penetrating abdominal trauma: a prospective trial. Surgery 1992; 112:788–794.

53. Kirton OC, O'Neill PA, Kestner M, Tortella BJ. Perioperative antibiotic use in high-risk penetrating hollow viscus injury: a prospective randomized, double-blind, placebo-control trial of 24 hours versus 5 days. J Trauma 2000; 49(5):822–832.

54. Luchette FA, Borzotta AP, Croce MA, et al. Practice management guidelines for prophylactic antibiotic use in penetrating abdominal trauma the EAST practice management guidelines work group. J Trauma 2000; 48(3):508–518.

55. Solomkin JS, Mazuski JE, Baron EJ, et al. Guidelines for the selection of anti-infective agents for complicated intra-abdominal infections. Clin Infect Dis 2003; 37(15):97–1005.

56. Cornwell EE 3rd, Dougherty WR, Berne TV, et al. Duration of antibiotic prophylaxis in high-risk patients with penetrating abdominal trauma: a prospective randomized trial. J Gastrointest Surg 1999; 3(6):648–653.

57. Bilik R, Burnweit C, Shanding B. Is abdominal cavity culture of any value in appendicitis? Am J Surg 1988; 175:267–270.

58. Nathens AB. Relevance and utility of peritoneal cultures in patients with peritonitis. Surg Infect 2001; 2(2):153–162.

59. Christou NV, Turgeon P, Wassef R, et al. Management of intra-abdominal infections. The case for intraoperative cultures and comprehensive broad spectrum antibiotic coverage. Arch Surg 1996; 131:1193–1201.

60. Barie PS, Christou NV, Dellinger EP, et al. Pathogenicity of the Enterococcus in surgical infections. Ann Surg 2000; 212:155–159.

61. Nichols RL, Muzik AC. Enterococcal infections in surgical patients: the mystery continues. Clin Infect Dis 1992; 15:72–76.

62. Rohrborn A, Wacha H, Schoffel U, et al. Coverage of enterococci in community acquired secondary peritonitis: results of a randomized trial. Surg Infect 2000; 1:95–107.

63. Harbarth SC, Uckay I. Are there patients with peritonitis who require empiric therapy for Enterococcus? Eur J Clin Microbiol Infect Dis 2004; 23:73–77.

64. Burnett RJ, Kenney PR, Slotman GJ, et al. Enterococcal bacteremia in surgical patients. Arch Surg 1985; 120:57–63.

65. Burnett RJ, Haverstock DC, Dellinger EP, et al. Definition of the role of enterococcus in intra-abdominal infection: analysis of a prospective randomized trail. Surgery 1995; 118:716–721.

66. Sotto A, Lefrant JY, Fabbro-Peray P, et al. Evaluation of antimicrobial therapy management of 120 consecutive patients with secondary peritonitis. J Antimicrob Chemother 2000; 50: 569–576.

67. Sitges-Serra A, Lopez MJ, Girvent M, et al. Postoperative enterococcal infection after treatment of complicated intra-abdominal sepsis. Br J Surg 2002; 89:361–367.

68. Mazuski JE, Sawyer RG, Nathans AB, et al. The surgical infection society guidelines on antimicrobial therapy for intra-abdominal infections: evidence for the recommendations. Surg infect 2002; 3(3):124.

69. Hoerarf A, Hammer S, Muller-Myshok B, et al. Intra-abdominal Candida infection during acute necrotizing pancreatitis has a high prevalence and is associated with increased mortality. Crit Care Med 1998; 26:2010–2015.

70. Sandven P, Qvist H, Skovland P, et al. Significance of Candida recovered from intra-abdominal specimens in patients with intra-abdominal perforations. Crit Care Med 2002; 30: 541–547.

71. Solomkin JS, Flohr AB, Quie PG, et al. The role of Candida in intraperitoneal infections. Surgery 1980; 88:524–530.

72. Calandra T, Bille J, Schneider R, et al. Clinical significance of Candida isolated from peritoneum in surgical patients. Lancet 1989; 2:1437–1440.

73. Johnson DH, Cunha BA. Infections in cirrhosis. Infect Dis Clin North Am 2001; 15(2):363–371.

74. Ramachandran A, Balasubramanian KA. Intestinal dysfunction in liver cirrhosis: its role in spontaneous bacterial peritonitis. J Gastroenterol Hepatol 2001; 16:607–612.

75. Kramer L, Drumi W. Ascites and intraabdominal infection. Curr Opin Crit Care 2004; 10:146–151.

76. Perdomo CG, Alves de Mattos A. Renal impairment after spontaneous bacterial peritonitis: incidence and prognosis. Can J Gastroenterol 2003; 17:187–190.

77. Cheung AHS, Wong LMF. Surgical infections in patients with chronic renal failure. Infect Dis Clin North Am 2001; 15(3):775–796.

78. Levi D, Goodman ER, Patel M, Savransky Y. Critical care of the obese and bariatric surgical patient. Crit Care Clin 2003; 19:11–32.

79. Abrams JH. Bacterial secondary peritonitis. Surg Clin N Am 1997; 77(6):1395–1417.

80. Wittmann DH, Schein M, Condon RE. Management of secondary peritonitis. Ann Surg 1996; 224(1):10–18.

81. Bunt TJ. Non-directed relaparotomy for intra-abdominal sepsis. Am Surg 1986; 52:294–298.

82. Bosscha K, Hulstaert PF, Visser MR, et al. Open Management of the abdomen and planned reoperations in severe bacterial peritonitis. Eur J Surg 2000; 166:44–49.

83. Anderson ID, Fearson JCH, Grant IS. Laparotomy for abdominal sepsis in the critically ill. Br J Surg 1996; 83:535–539.

84. Koperna T, Schultz F. Relaparotomy in peritonitis: prognosis and treatment of patients with persisting intraabdominal infection. World J Surg 2002; 24:32–37.

85. Hau T, Wolmershauser A, Wacha H, Yang Q. Planned relaparotomy vs relaparotomy on demand in the treatment of intraabdominal infections. The peritonitis study group of the surgical infection society-Europ. Arch Surg 1995; 130:1193–1197.

86. Klausner JM, Rozin RR. Late abdominal complications in war wounded. J Trauma 1995; 38(2):313–317.

87. Pusajo JF, Bumaschny E, Doglio GR, et al. Postoperative intra-abdominal sepsis requiring reoperation. Arch Surg 1993; 128:218–223.

88. Malangoni MA. Evaluation and management of tertiary peritonitis. Am Surg 2000; 66:157–161.

89. Johnson CC, Baldessarre J, Levison ME. Peritonitis: update on pathophysiology, clinical manifestations, and management. Clin Infect Dis 1997; 24:1035–1045

90. Rosengart MR, Nathens AB. Tertiary peritonitis problem. Gen Surg 2002; 19(1):65–71.

91. Tokunaga Y, Hata K, Ryo J, et al. Density of Helicobacter pylori infection in patients with peptic ulcer perforation. J Am Coll Surg 1998; 186:659–663.

92. Ng EK, Lam YH, Sung JJ, et al. Eradication of Helicobacter pylori prevents recurrence of ulcer after simple closure of duodenal ulcer perforation: randomized controlled trail. Ann Surg 2000; 231:153.

93. Bosscha K, van Vroonhoven MV, van der Weren Ch. Surgical management of severe secondary peritonitis. Br J Surg 1999; 86:1371–1377.

94. Espinoza R, Rodriguez A. Traumatic and nontraumatic perforation of hollow viscera. Surg Clin N Am 1997; 77(6):1291–1304.

95. Schilling MK, Maurer CA, Kollmar O, et al. Primary vs. secondary anastomosis after sigmoid colon resection for perforated diverticulitis (Hinchey Stage III and IV): a prospective outcome and cost analysis. Dis Colon Rectum 2001; 44:699–703.

96. Choi KC, Peek-Asa C, Lovell M, et al. Complications after therapeutic trauma laparotomy. J Am Coll Surg 2005; 201(4):546–553.

97. Fingerhut A, Trunkey D. Surgical management of liver injuries in adults-current indications and pitfalls of operative and non-operative policies: a review. Eur J Surg 2000; 166:676–686.

98. Mohr AM, Lavery RF, Barone A, et al. Angiographic embolization for liver injuries; low mortality, high morbidity. J Trauma 2003; 55:1077–1082.

99. Wahl WL, Brandt MM, Hemmila MR, Arbabbi S. Diagnosis and management of bile leaks after blunt liver trauma. Surgery 2005; 138:742–748.

100. Hsieh CH. Liver abscess after non-operative management of blunt liver injury. Langenbecks Arch Surg 2003; 387:343–347.

101. Kozar RA. Complications of non-operative management of high grade blunt hepatic injuries. J Trauma 2005; 59(5):1066–1071.

102. Akpofure PE, Mc Carthy MC, Woods RJ, Haley E. Complications arising from splenic embolizations after blunt splenic trauma. Am J Surg 2005; 189:335–339.

103. Curran TJ, Borzotta AP. Complications of primary repair of colon injury: literature review of 2,964 cases. Am J Surg 1999; 177:42–47.

104. Demeriades D, Murray JA, Ordonez CK, et al. Penetrating colon injuries requiring resection: diversion or primary anastomosis? An AAST prospective multicenter study. J Trauma 2001; 50(5):765–775.

105. Sasaki LS, Mittal V, Allaben RD. Primary repair of colon injuries: a retrospective analysis. Am Surg 1994; 60:522–527.

106. Sasaki LS, Allaben RD, Golwala R, et al. Primary repair of colon injuries: a prospective randomized study. J Trauma 1119; 39:895–901.

107. Behrman SW, Bertken KA, Stefanacci HA, Parks SN. Breakdown of intestinal repair after laparotomy for trauma: incidence, risk factors and strategies for prevention. J Trauma 1998; 45(2):227–233.

108. Hoyt DB, Hollingsworth-Fridlund P, Forlage D, et al. An evaluation of provider–related and disease-related morbidity in a level 1 university trauma service: directions for quality improvement. J Trauma 1992; 33:586–601.

109. Vles WJ, Veen EJ, Roukema JA, et al. Consequences of delayed diagnoses in trauma patients: a prospective study. J Am Coll Surg 2003; 197:596–602.

110. Houshian S, Larsen MS, Holm C. Missed Injuries in a level 1 trauma center. J Trauma 2002; 52:715–719.

111. Buduhan G, McRitchie DI. Missed injuries in patients with multiple trauma. J Trauma 2000; 49:600–605.

112. Hoyt DB, Coimbra RC, Potenza BM, et al. A twelve year analysis of disease and provider complications on an organized level 1 trauma service: as good as it gets? J Trauma 2003; 54: 26–37.

113. Teruhiko T, Blackmore C, Bent S, Kohlwes J. Systematic Review: Computed tomography and ultrasonography to detect acute appendicitis in adults and adolescents Ann Inter Med 2004; 141:537–546.

114. Oliak D, Yamini D, Udani VM, et al. Initial nonoperative management for periappendiceal abscess. Dis Colon Rectum 2001; 44:936.

115. Mazziotti MV, Marley EF, Winthrop AL, et al. Histopathologic analysis of interval appendectomy specimens: support for the role of interval appendectomy. J Pediatr Surg 1197; 32:806.

116. Piskun G, Kozik D, Rajpal S, Shaftan G, Fogler R. Comparison of laparoscopic, open, and converted appendectomy for perforated appendicitis. Surg Endosc 2001; 15:660–662.

117. Dawes LG. Biliary tract infections problems. Gen Surg 2002; 19(1):81–91.

118. Barie PS, Fischer E. Acute acalculous cholecystitis. J Am Coll Surg 1995; 180:232–244.

119. Chandler CF, Lan JS, Ferguson P, Thompson JE, Ashley SW. Prospective evaluation of early versus delayed laparoscopic cholecystectomy for treatment of acute cholecystitis. Am Surg 2000; 66:896–900.

120. Willsher PC, Sanabria JR, Gallinger S, et al. Early laparoscopic cholecystectomy for acute cholecystitis: a safe procedure. J Gastrointest Surg 1999; 3:50–53.

121. Lo CM, Lai EC, Fan ST, Liu CL, Wong J. Laparoscopic cholecystectomy for acute cholecystitis in the elderly. World J Surg 1996; 20:983–986.

122. Berer E, Eingle KL, String A, et al. Selective use of cholecystostomy with interval laparoscopic cholecystectomy in acute cholecystitis. Arch Surg 2000; 135:346.

123. Barkun JS, Lewis RT. Infections in the upper abdomen: biliary tract, pancreas, liver, and spleen. ACS Surg Princ Pract 2002; 83:1263–1278.

124. Hanau LH, Steigbigel NH. Infections of the liver. Acute (ascending) Cholangitis. Infect Dis Clin North Am 2000; 14(3):521–546.

125. Lillemoe KD. Surgical treatment of biliary tract infections. Am Surg 2000; 66:138–144.

126. Lai EC, Tam PC, Paterson IA, et al. Emergency surgery for severe cholangitis: the high risk patients. Ann Surg 1990; 117:437.

127. Yusoff IF, Barkun JS, Barkun AN. Diagnosis and management of cholecystitis and cholangitis. Gastroenterol Clin North Am 2003; 32:1145–1168.

128. Arnell TD, Stabile BE. Acute colonic diverticulitis problems. Gen Surg 2002; 19(1):109–120.

129. Wong RJ, Wexner SD, Lowry A, et al. Practice parameters for the treatment of sigmoid diverticulitis-supporting documentation. The standards task force. The American society of Colon and Rectal Surgeons. Dis Colon Rectum 2000; 43:290–297.

130. Gooszen AW, Tollenaar RA, Geelkerken RH, et al. Prospective study of primary anastomosis following sigmoid resection for suspected acute complicated diverticular disease. Br J Surg 2001; 88:693–697.

131. Mazuski JE, Longo WE. Clostridium difficile colitis problems. Gen Surg 2002;19(1):121–132.

132. Kyne L, Farrell RJ, Kelly CP. Clostridum difficile. Review in: Gastroenterol Clin North Am (W.B. Saunders) 2001; 30(3):753–777.

133. Dallal RM, Harbrecht BG, Boujoukas AJ, et al. Fulminant Clostridium difficile: an under appreciated and increasing cause of death and complications. Ann Surg 2002; 235(3):363–372.

134. Kent KC, Rubin MS, Wroblewski L, et al. The impact of Clostridium difficile on a surgical service: a prospective study of 374 patients. Ann Surg 1998; 227(2):296–301.

135. Johnson S, Gerding DN. Clostridium difficile-associated diarrhea. Clin Infect Dis 1998; 26:1027–1034.

136. Bradbury AW, Barrett S. Surgical aspects of Clostridium difficile colitis. Review in: Br J Surg 1997; 84:150–159.

137. Medich DS, Lee KKW, Simmons RL. Laparotomy for fulminate Pseudo membranous colitis. Arch Surg 1992; 127:847–853.

138. Longo WE, Mazurski JE, Virgo KS, et al. Outcome after colectomy for Clostridium difficile colitis. Dis Colon Rectum 2004; 47:1620–1626.

139. Page MJ, Dreese JC, Poritz LS, et al. Cytomegalovirus enteritis: A highly lethal condition requiring early detection and intervention. Dis Colon Rectum 1998; 41(5):619–623.

140. Helderman JH, Goral S. Gastrointestinal complications of transplant immunosuppression. J Am Soc Nephrol 2002; 13(1):277–287.

141. Kaufman HS, Kahn AC, Iacobuzio-Donahue C, et al. Cytomegaloviral enterocolitis. Dis Colon Rectum 1999; 42(1):24–30.

142. Kalil AC, Levitsky J, Lyden E, Stoner J, Freifeld AG. Meta-analysis: the efficacy of strategies to prevent organ disease by cytomegalovirus in solid organ transplant recipients. Ann Intern Med 2005; 143:870–880.

143. Al-Kawas FH, Baillie J, Kalloo AN, et al. An endoscopic approach. In: DiMarino AJ, Benjamin SB, eds. 2nd ed. Gastrointestinal Disease. Thorofare, NJ: Slack Corporation, 2002.

144. Bini EJ, Gorelick SM, Weinshel EH. Outcome of AIDS-associated cytomegalovirus colitis in the era of potent antiretroviral therapy. J Clin Gastroenterol 2000; 30(4):414–419.

145. Siroky MB, Edelstein RA, Krane RJ. Manual of Urology: Diagnosis and Therapy. 2nd ed. Philadelphia, PA: Lippincott Williams & Wilkins, 1999.

146. Gillenwater JY, Grayhack JT, Howards SS, et al. Adult and Pediatric Urology. 4th ed. Vol. 1. Philadelphia, PA: Lippincott Williams & Wilkins, 2002.

147. Walsh PC, Retik AB, Vaughan Jr ED, et al. Campbell's Urology, 8th ed. Philadelphia, PA: Elsevier Inc., 2002.

148. Sweet RL, Gibbs RS. Infectious Disease of the Female Genital Tract. 4th ed. Philadelphia, PA: Lippincott Williams & Wilkins, 2002.

149. Duff P. Antibiotic selection in obstetric patients. Infect Dis Clin North Am 1997; 11:1–12.

150. Fry DE. Definitive versus temporizing therapy. in: Schein M, Marshall JC, eds. Source Control: A Guide to Management of Surgical Infections. New York: Springer-Verlag, 2002.

51

Sinusitis

Quyen T. Nguyen and Terence M. Davidson

Department of Otolaryngology–Head and Neck Surgery, UC San Diego Medical Center, and San Diego VA Healthcare System, San Diego, California, U.S.A.

INTRODUCTION

Paranasal sinusitis is an important potential cause of fever in the intensive care unit (ICU) (1). The pathophysiology of sinusitis in the ICU setting is similar to that of outpatient sinusitis and is related to obstruction of the osteomeatal complex (OMC), or to disruption of normal mucociliary transport. This is true for the critically ill trauma patient who often has additional risk factors beyond simple inflammatory sinus obstruction, for example, structural injury and disruption of the sinus drainage system. Patients in the ICU often have complicating debilitating medical issues such as nosocomial colonization and immune suppression. Paranasal sinusitis in this setting may lead to severe complications including pneumonia, meningitis, and sepsis (2–5). Thus, when there is clinical concern of sinusitis in the ICU setting, it is evaluated and treated aggressively. This chapter will review the anatomy, pathophysiology, microbiology, diagnosis, and treatment of sinusitis in the critically ill patient. A typical case will be presented to illustrate the key points of diagnosis and treatment.

ANATOMY

The paranasal sinuses consist of four paired pneumatized cavities of the skull and facial bones with ostia that drain into the nose (Fig. 1). These are named from top-medial to bottom-lateral as the frontal, ethmoid, sphenoid, and maxillary sinuses. The ethmoid sinuses are unique in that they are composed of 18 to 20 small air cells (like a honeycomb) rather than a single large cavity. The ethmoids are divided into anterior cells, which drain into the middle meatus, and the posterior cells, which drain into the superior meatus. The sphenoid sinus drains via the superior meatus. The frontal, maxillary, and anterior ethmoids all drain via the middle meatus. All of the paranasal sinuses are lined with ciliated pseudostratified columnar epithelial cells (6). The cilia of the sinus mucosa propel a mucus blanket of secretions, bacteria, and purulence toward the ostia. In normal adults, approximately 1500 cc of fluid is produced each day from the epithelium of the nose and paranasal sinuses. Mucociliary transport is estimated to be at a speed of 0.5 cm/min in normal conditions (7). The combination of a large fluid production and a healthy active mucous transport system keeps the bacterial colony count low in normal healthy patients.

The most frequently diseased paranasal sinuses are those that drain into a small region in the middle meatus called the ethmoid infundibulum, a part of the OMC. This small space has a maximal volume of 2.88 cc (7) and contains multiple small narrow clefts that can be easily occluded and obstructed. Obstruction and consequent inhibition of the mucociliary transport system causes decreased ventilation, leading to stagnation of the secretions, resulting in an infection commonly called sinusitis.

PATHOPHYSIOLOGY

The area of the middle meatus where the sinus ostia drain from the frontal, maxillary, and anterior ethmoid sinus is called the OMC. Nasogastric (NG) tubes can physically obstruct the ostia or paralyze the mucocilliary transport system. The anterior ethmoid and maxillary sinuses are the most commonly involved paranasal sinuses in patients with nosocomial sinusitis. However, many patients with radiologic maxillary sinusitis also have abnormalities of the posterior ethmoid, frontal, and sphenoid sinuses.

Mechanical Obstruction

↗ **The single most important factor in the development of sinusitis is the disruption of the mucociliary transport system, typically from obstruction of the normal drainage pathways, the OMC of the paranasal sinuses.** ↗ In the intensive care setting, mucociliary transport from the paranasal sinuses is commonly obstructed in the nasal cavity by NG tubes or nasotracheal intubation. These tubes may directly obstruct the sinus osteum, or cause swelling of the nasal osteum via inadvertent trauma occurring during insertion (8). However, impaired mucociliary clearance or changes in the mucous composition in states of dehydration, chronic disease, and mechanical ventilation also lead to mucociliary stasis, obstruction of sinus ventilation, and impaired mucous outflow. Trauma to the nasal mucosa leads to mucosal edema and inflammation that can impair mucociliary clearance. Interestingly, no difference in sinusitis rates was seen in critically ill patients who were intubated via the nasal route compared to orally intubated patients (9). This is partly explained by the fact that most

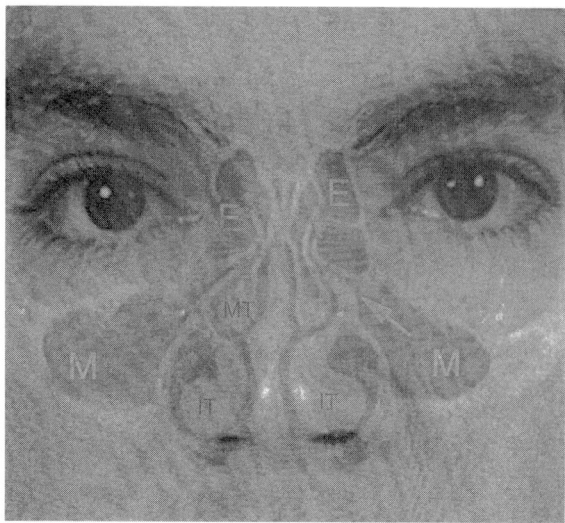

Figure 1 Superimposition of coronal computed tomographic image through paranasal sinuses on photograph of male patient. The paranasal sinuses occupy a large volume within the human head and produce a large amount of mucus each day. However, the drainage outflow from these sinuses must pass through narrow clefts that are easily obstructed. *Note:* The outflow tract (*arrow*) is in the superior medial aspect of the maxillary sinus; thus gravity has a limited role in the drainage of mucosal secretions. *Arrow,* maxillary sinus ostia through which mucus secreted by maxillary sinus mucosa must pass. *Abbreviations:* E, ethmoid sinus; IT, inferior turbinate; M, maxillary sinus; MT, medial turbinate.

of the orally intubated patients also had nasal tubes for GI decompression or enteral feeding.

Non-mechanical Factors

The composition of the sinonasal mucus is sensitive to multiple factors. Changes in the mucous viscosity can affect mucociliary clearance (10). In acutely ill patients, dehydration, chronic disease, or mechanical ventilation may lead to thickened mucus, mucociliary stasis, and consequent sinusitis (11). Even in patients without nasal tubes, the supine position and limitation of head movements in the ICU setting impedes the natural sinus drainage facilitated by gravity (12). Furthermore, the supine position is associated with decreased venous drainage from the head and neck regions, leading to increased nasal congestion and mucosal edema, further obstructing mucociliary transportation. In the intubated patient, positive pressure ventilation may compound this problem by raising central venous pressure (5).

Trauma-Related Risk Factors

Patients in the trauma ICU often have additional risk factors that predispose them to developing paranasal sinusitis. For example, craniofacial trauma can lead to the presence of blood and bony debris in the nose and paranasal sinuses, which predispose the patient to bacterial sinusitis. Furthermore, fractures of the facial bones may lead to mechanical obstruction of the OMC, with resultant development of ostial obstruction, mucous stasis, and sinusitis (13).

Pre-existing Conditions

There are a number of additional pre-existing conditions completely unrelated to trauma or critical illness that increases the risk of sinusitis. These include anatomic abnormalities such as congenital choanal atresia, septal deviation, foreign bodies, and tumors. In addition, allergic rhinitis causes nasal mucosal swelling and predisposes the patient to sinusitis. Similarly, patients with prolonged and repeated infections, chronic or recurrent sinusitis may undergo changes in the mucosal lining of the sinuses. These patients may undergo replacement of the normal ciliated epithelium with stratified squamous epithelium that does not maintain normal sinus sterility and these patients are prone to congestion stagnation and exacerbation of the underlying sinus disease (14). Immuno compromised and out of control diabetics are not only prone to sinusitis but also fungal diseases such as mucormycosis.

MICROBIOLOGY
Bacterial Sinusitis

Community-acquired acute sinusitis is usually of viral origin. Additionally, less than 2% of all upper respiratory tract infections in adults are complicated by bacterial sinusitis (15,16). Thus, antibiotic treatment for community-acquired sinusitis is only recommended if symptoms persist for more than seven days, and in patients with clinical symptoms of purulent nasal secretions, maxillary facial or tooth pain, or tenderness (15).

When cultures are taken in patients with community-acquired sinusitis, only 15% demonstrate a viral origin, the remainder being caused by bacterial organisms. The most common bacteria cultured from community-acquired sinusitis are pneumococcus and *Haemophilus influenzae*, with almost no isolates from *Pseudomonas* spp, *Acinetobacter* spp, or *Escherichia coli* (15,16). This contrasts sharply with the findings in nosocomial sinusitis.

Sinus infection isolates from ICU patients have a distinctly different profile. ☛ **Nosocomial sinusitis may be caused by both gram-negative bacilli and gram-positive cocci, with 20% being polymicrobial (14).** ☛ Thus antibiotics with broad coverage directed at gram-positive as well as gram-negative bacteria with efficacy against *Pseudomonas* should be initiated when treating nosocomial sinusitis. More virulent, gram-negative bacilli (*Pseudomonas* spp., *Acinetobacter* spp., etc.,) were found in 47% of cases of bacterial sinusitis documented with transnasal puncture, with *P. aeruginosa* being the most common. *Staphylococcus aureus* was found in 35% of the cases, and fungus in 8% (Table 1). Fungal sinusitis should be considered when the patient does not improve clinically despite removal of inciting agents and broad-spectrum antibiotic coverage.

Fungal Sinusitis

In rare situations, usually involving immunosuppression, fungi may be the causative organisms. In the outpatient setting, fungal sinusitis is rare and usually caused by Aspergillus found in soil and decaying plant matter. Fungal sinusitis with Aspergillus is rarely invasive and is usually treated with immunotherapy and/or corticosteroids (17). However, in immune-compromised patients (e.g., patients in the ICU setting) and in patients with poorly controlled diabetes, fungal infection of the paranasal sinuses caused by Mucor and Rhizopus fungal species is extremely serious

Table 1 Microbial Flora of Sinusitis

	Community-acquired (%)	Nosocomial (%)
Streptococcus pneumoniae	31	
Haemophilus influenzae	21	
Moraxella catarrhalis	2	
Group A streptococcus	2	
Anaerobes	6	
Viruses	15	
Staphylococcus aureus	4	35
Gram-negative bacilli		47
(*Pseudomonas* spp., *Acinetobacter* spp., *Escherichia coli*)		
Fungus		8

Source: Adapted from Refs. 15, 16.

and often fatal (18). Granulocytopenic patients are most vulnerable to these invasive fungi. Thus, there should be a high index of suspicion for fungal sinusitis in patients in the ICU that do not respond to medical control, especially in the setting of granulocytopnea or periorbital inflammation (19).

DIAGNOSIS
Clinical Presentation
☞ **The usual clinical symptoms and signs of sinusitis seen in otherwise healthy outpatients may be missed in critically ill patients.** ☞ Acute sinusitis in the normal population usually presents with headache, facial pain, nasal obstruction, mucopurulent nasal discharge, malaise, and lethargy. Many ICU patients are sedated and analgesed to such a degree that fever, purulent nasal discharge, or air-fluid levels on sinus imaging may provide the first clinical indication of sinusitis. Interestingly, fever is present in less than 50% of patients with acute (community-acquired) sinusitis. Thus, the presence of fever and radiographic evidence of sinusitis does not necessarily indicate that sinusitis is the cause of fever in the ICU patient.

Nosocomial sinusitis is fairly common in the ICU setting, ranging from 5% to 35% of patients (20–25). Indeed, nosocomial pneumonia, sinusitis, and bloodstream infections are the most common infectious sources of fever in ICU patients (1). However, given the multitude of additional potential sources of fever, the presence of sinusitis alone does not mean that sinusitis is the cause of fever in the ICU patient (26).

☞ **An important risk factor for the development of sinusitis in the ICU setting is the presence of nasal tubes.** ☞ Unfortunately, in this patient population, localized symptoms of infection (headache, facial pain, malaise, and lethargy) are difficult to elicit and the presence of purulent discharge may only be present in a minority (∼25%) of patients (5). When sinusitis is in the differential for fever, computed tomography (CT) scans are the most useful tool for imaging the paranasal sinuses, and is better than magnetic resonance imaging (MRI), which has false positives. Plain films have no value in the assessment of sinusitis.

Diagnostic Significance of Fever
The Society of Critical Care Medicine defines fever in the ICU as a temperature of $>38.3°C$ ($>101.0°F$) (27,28). Any disease process that results in the release of proinflammatory cytokines IL-1, IL-6, and TNF-α may result in the development of fever (29). Thus infectious as well as a large list of noninfectious inflammatory conditions [including trauma, burns, and systemic inflammatory response syndrome (SIRS)] may result in a febrile response (see Volume 2, Chapter 46 for evaluation of febrile ICU patient).

Historically, especially in the preantibiotic era, increased body temperature has been shown to be associated with improved outcome (including survival) from infectious diseases (30–33). ☞ **The acute development of fever in a previously stable and afebrile ICU patient must immediately trigger a search for a treatable infection.** ☞ Indeed, infection is the most common cause of delayed morbidity in trauma patients. Furthermore, elevated body temperature is associated with a number of additional deleterious effects such as increased cardiac output, oxygen consumption, carbon dioxide production, and energy expenditure (34). Additionally, fever is associated with a worse neurologic outcome following traumatic brain injury (TBI) (35,36). Accordingly, these deleterious side effects far outweigh any potential benefit of fever in the ICU setting.

☞ **Sinusitis is only one of a host of infectious etiologies of fever in critically ill patients (see Volume 2, Chapter 46).** ☞ Unfortunately, many of the normal diagnostic clues to sinusitis will be absent in critically ill patients, due to sedation or neurologic injury. In the ICU setting, fever may be the only indication that sinusitis is present.

Imaging Studies
One-third of patients with radiologic evidence of sinusitis (e.g., air-fluid levels or mucosal thickening in head CT) have clinically significant infectious sinusitis documented by bacterial cultures (22). Thus, the clinical importance of radiologic data in isolation is unknown, and should never be assumed to be the sole source of a fever in a critically ill patient until cultures are obtained and other sources of fever are excluded.

Plain Film Radiography
Plain film radiography was historically used in the outpatient setting for the diagnosis of acute sinusitis. Although the specificity of plain films is adequate, the sensitivity has been shown to be unacceptably low as compared to that of CT (37) and thus is not used as a tool in the diagnosis of sinusitis either in the clinic or in the ICU. Furthermore, as plain film radiography cannot clearly delineate the relationship between soft tissue and the bony sinus framework, it is not very helpful for diagnosis in the setting of bony trauma or anatomic abnormalities. However, some critically ill patients are too unstable to transport to the CT scanner; for these patients plain film radiography may be considered.

The four standard radiographic projections are as follows: occipitofrontal ("Caldwell's view"), occipitomental ("Water's view"), lateral, and submental vertex (axial view). Because the maxillary sinuses are most commonly involved, and are best seen on the Water's view, some advocate this simple projection, rather than all four.

Computed Tomography
☞ **CT is the most useful radiographic method to evaluate the presence of sinusitis in the paranasal sinuses.** ☞ CT

is the preferred imaging study for paranasal sinuses because it clearly delineates the relationship between the soft tissue density of paranasal sinus mucosa, the integrity of the bony framework, and the presence or absence of air/fluid within the sinuses (38). Mucosal thickening, opacification, or air-fluid levels suggest infection (Fig. 2) (22). CT scans should be obtained, 5 × 5 mm with coronal views without contrast. Air-fluid levels on CT are not pathognomonic for acute sinusitis, because blood in the sinuses (resulting from head trauma) can also appear as an air-fluid level. Using sterile technique and a diagnostic threshold of 10,000 colony-forming units/milliliter (cfu/mL), sinus cultures should be obtained, when both clinical and radiologic evidence of sinusitis exists. ☞ **Significant infection as diagnosed by positive sinus culture is only found in 38% of patients with radiologic (CT) evidence of sinusitis.** ☞ Bacteremia with the same microbial flora was found in 17% to 25% of patients with nosocomial sinusitis (22).

Sinus Ultrasound

Sinus ultrasound is another emerging technique that has been shown to be useful in the evaluation of acute sinusitis. A prospective trial comparing the accuracy of sinus ultrasound to that of standard sinus radiography revealed more than 92% sensitivity and specificity for the diagnosis of maxillary sinusitis in the outpatient setting (39) as well as in the ICU setting with mechanically ventilated patients (40). However, the use of sinus ultrasound in the diagnosis of sinusitis requires training and has not gained popularity in the United States, despite its common usage in other countries (39,40).

Diagnostic Procedures
Nasal Endoscopy

Nasal endoscopy is emerging as an important new tool in the evaluation of paranasal sinusitis. This technique has been shown to be both sensitive and specific in predicting a positive bacterial culture from paranasal sinusitis. In a prospective study involving 141 patients in the ICU, Skoulas et al. found that plain film radiography and CT scans were only 41% and 47% accurate, respectively, in predicting the presence of maxillary sinus purulence. However, the presence of purulent exudates emanating from the middle meatus seen by nasal endoscopy was 78% accurate in predicting a positive culture (41). Given the need to have a significant

clinical suspicion for sinusitis prior to confirming the diagnosis with an invasive procedure such as antral puncture and culture, nasal endoscopy is increasingly utilized.

Antral Puncture

☞ **The gold standard for the diagnosis of sinusitis is maxillary sinus puncture (antral puncture), aspiration, Gram stain, and culture (Fig. 3) (42).** ☞ This technique involves accessing the maxillary sinus through the bony maxillary (canine) fossa, is invasive, time-consuming, and carries the risk of orbital hemorrhage, infection, and blindness (43,44). However, it has been shown that a change in antibiotic therapy guided by culture of maxillary sinus aspirate results in improved patient outcome (45). Thus, the question of when to perform maxillary sinus tap remains controversial. Recent studies suggest that nasal endoscopy should be performed first and antral punctures should only be performed if purulence is seen in the middle meatus (41).

TREATMENT
Removal of Intranasal Tubes and Promotion of Nasal Drainage

☞ **The most important factor in treating nosocomial sinusitis in the ICU setting is the removal of inciting factors causing impairment of mucociliary transportation and paranasal sinus ventilation.** ☞ Thus, if the patient has any foreign bodies within the nasal passages such as nasotracheal or NG tubes, these should be removed completely or switched over to the other nasal passage. This is a difficult decision for it may mean that if a patient is nasally intubated, one must transfer these tubes to the oral cavity or neck, that is, consider tracheostomy. If a patient requires enteral feeding, consider an orogastric tube, a cervicogastric tube, or a gastric feeding tube. To further facilitate mucociliary transport, mucosal congestion can be reduced with topical decongestants, elevating the head of the bed 30°, and improving hydration of the patient (both intravascular and with humidified oxygen if extubated).

Antibiotics

Acute bacterial sinusitis is routinely treated in the outpatient setting with amoxicillin, doxycycline, or erythromycin (15).

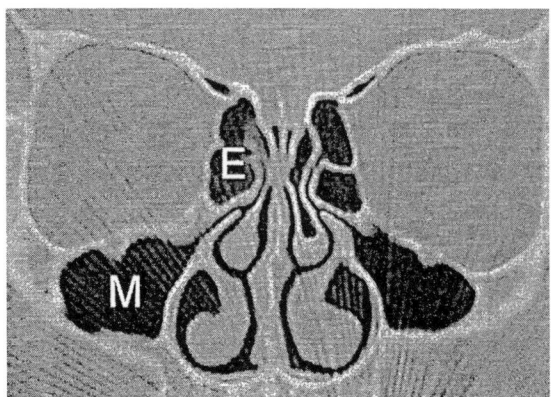 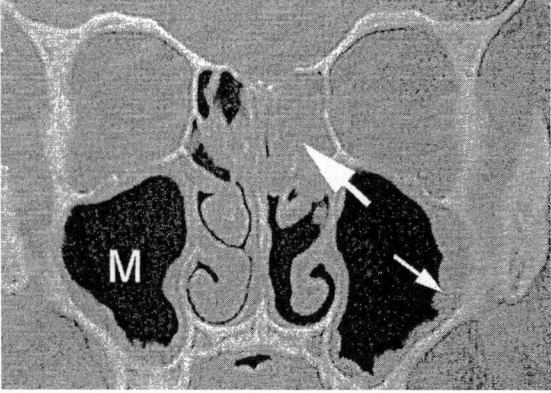

Figure 2   Coronal computed tomographic (CT) images of paranasal sinuses. On the *left* is a coronal CT image showing the maxillary (M) and ethmoid (E) sinuses in a healthy patient. Note that the sinuses are air-filled cavities (*black*) enclosed by bony walls (*white*). On the *right* is a coronal CT image showing paranasal sinuses in a patient with maxillary sinus mucosal thickening (*small arrow*) and ethmoid sinus opacification (*large arrow*).

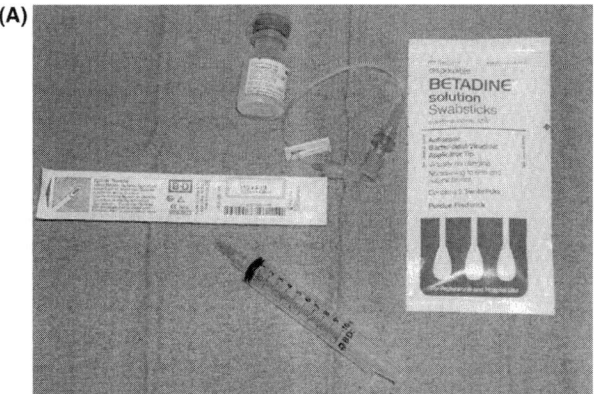

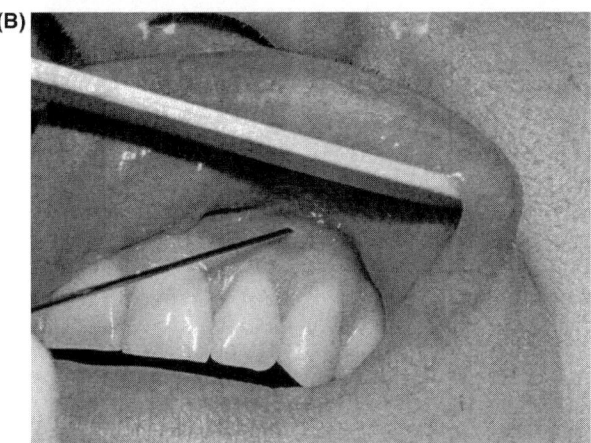

Figure 3 Sinus cavity aspiration equipment and technique.
(**A**) The equipment necessary to perform a sinus aspiration:
betadine swab, 18-gauge spinal needle, 10-cc syringe, intravenous
tubing, and injectable sterile saline without preservatives.
(**B**) Following infiltration with a local anesthetic/vasoconstrictor
(lidocaine 1% with epinephrine 1:100,000), the superior
gingivolabial groove at the level of the canine fossa is prepared
with betadine. The 18-gauge spinal needle is advanced through
the mucosa and bone superior to the root of the canine tooth,
medial to the zygomatic buttress, and lateral to the piriform
aperture. Advance the needle until the sinus mucosa is penetrated,
and then remove the introducer. Aspirate a sterile sample for
gram stain, culture, and sensitivities. Irrigate the sinus with
sterile saline solution, which allows flow of purulent secretions
through the natural ostium. Irrigation should commence only
once the position of the spinal needle is confirmed to be in the
antrum by aspiration of air or purulent fluid.

However, sinusitis occurring in the ICU requires broad-
spectrum antibiotics due to the increased incidence of
gram-negative and polymicrobial organisms. ☞ **Initial
empiric antimicrobial therapy requires coverage of both
gram-positive and gram-negative bacteria (with adequate
pseudomonas coverage) (Table 2).** ☞ If clinical assessment
reveals inadequate improvement following antibiotic
therapy along with the removal of the inciting agents (naso-
tracheal/NG tubes), the antibiotic regimen can be changed
either empirically or with guidance by nasal endoscopy,
with culture or direct aspirate via antral puncture (46). As
mentioned above, although direct aspirate via antral puncture has traditionally been the gold standard for establishing
a diagnosis of bacterial sinusitis (15,45), multiple recent
studies indicate that cultures obtained with swab via nasal

endoscopy are equally specific and sensitive as are cultures
derived from antral punctures with direct aspiration (47,48).

Surgery

As the majority of patients develop nosocomial sinusitis in
the ICU setting as a consequence of foreign bodies blocking
normal drainage of the paranasal sinuses, the removal of
these foreign bodies is usually adequate treatment. Thus,
all foreign bodies should be removed from the nasal cavities, topical decongestants used to minimize mucosal congestion, and adequate hydration insured. Surgery in the
absence of invasive fungal sinusitis or central nervous
system/orbital complication has a limited indication in the
setting of ICU sinusitis. Antibiotics are used when
deemed clinically indicated. Surgical drainage is rarely
indicated in the setting of nosocomial sinusitis in the
absence of anatomic abnormalities, sepsis, or secondary
complications (49).

CLINICAL PERSPECTIVE: CASE ANALYSIS

The clinical lessons described herein are further emphasized
with the following case presentation. This is a typical critical
care trauma patient with fever, upon whom an ear, nose, and
throat (ENT) consult was obtained to rule out sinusitis. The
patient is a 35-year-old male with closed head injury and
fever of 39.2°C.

One week prior to consult, the patient was involved in
a motor vehicle accident and suffered a closed head injury
with subdural hematoma. The patient was intubated orally
in the field because of loss of consciousness and brought to
the hospital by the emergency medical services. Following
surgical evacuation of the subdural hematoma, the patient
remained intubated and was brought to the surgical ICU.
Despite withdrawal of all sedatives, the patient remained
unresponsive and ventilator-dependent. A soft, small-diam-
eter NG tube was placed on the left side on hospital day 2 to
initiate enteral nutrition. On hospital day 6, the patient
developed fever of 39.2°C.

This patient is otherwise healthy without any significant prior medical or surgical conditions, has no history
of prior sinusitis, is not taking any medication other
than phenytoin for seizure prophylaxis, and is not allergic
to medicines.

The physical examination reveals that the patient has a
Glasgow Coma Scale (GCS) equivalent to 9-T. He can open
his eyes spontaneously, can localize pain with all extremities,
but does not follow commands, and cannot vocalize (endotracheal tube in place). His head, eyes, ears, nose, and
throat examination reveals the craniotomy incision for evacuation of subdural hematoma; the wound is clean and
dry, no obvious nasal discharge is noted, but left serous
otitis media is noted with otoscope. An NG tube is seen
passing through the left nare, the nasal mucosa is edematous, and no evidence of purulent discharge is detected.
His extraoccular muscles and pupillary examination are
normal. The chest examination reveals diffuse rhonchi bilaterally. The heart examination is normal, the abdomen is soft
and nondistended, there is no organomegaly, and he is tolerating his enteral nutrition. His extremity examination reveals
a left antecubital IV without erythema or induration, a right
radial arterial line, and there is no lymphadonopathy in
either axilla. A Foley catheter is in place.

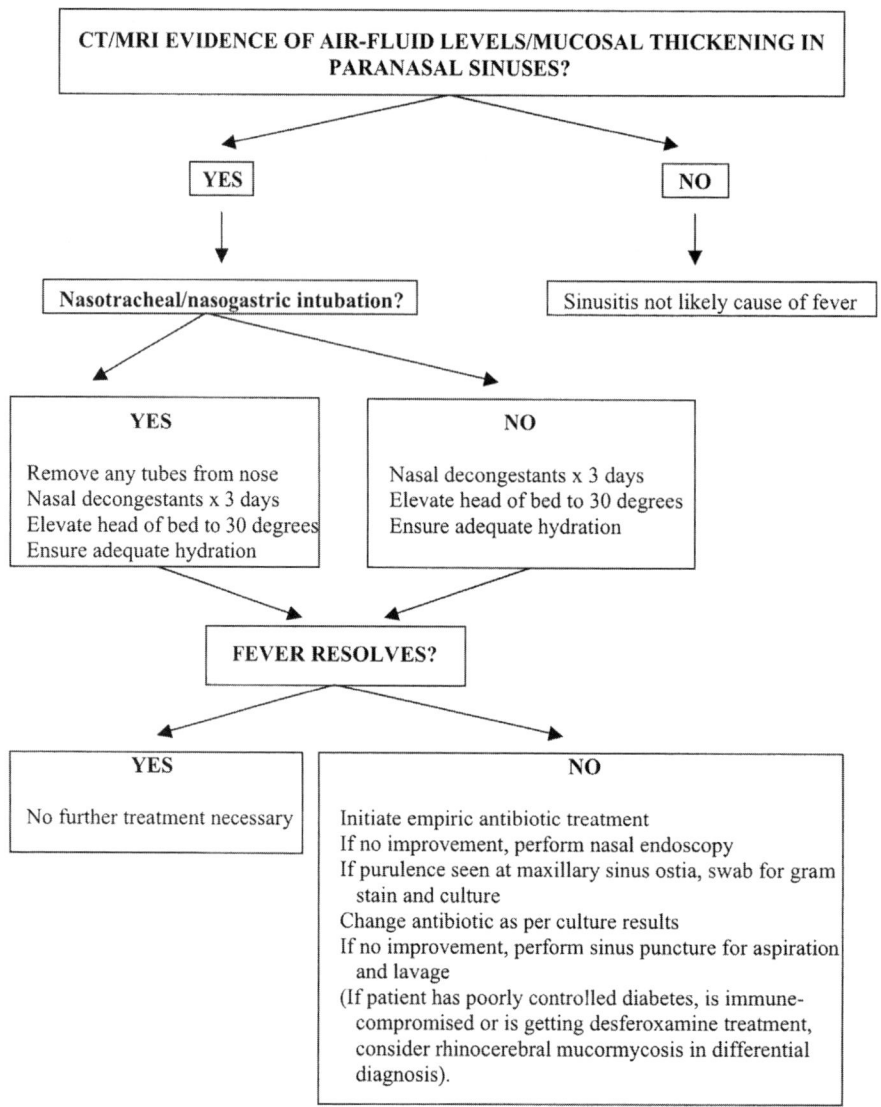

Figure 4   Diagnostic and treatment algorithm for the febrile intensive care unit patient.

Table 2   Antimicrobial Therapy for Sinusitis

	Community-acquired	Nosocomial
Primary treatment	Amoxicillin (500 mg PO tid × 10 d)	Piperacillin and Tazobactam
	Amoxicillin/clavulanic acid	3.375 gm IV q6 hr
	(875 mg/125 mg PO bid or	Imipenem (0.5 mg IV q6 hr)
	500 mg/125 mg PO tid × 10 d)	Meropenem (0.5 mg IV q6 hr)
	Cefdinir	
	(300 mg PO bid or 600 mg PO qd × 10 d)	
	Cefpodoxime (200 mg PO bid)	
Alternate treatment		Amphotericin B (for
(resistant disease/		mucormycosis)
penicillin allergy)	Levofloxacin (500 mg PO qd × 10 d)	(0.8–1.5 mg/kg/d IV)
	Moxifloxacin (400 mg PO qd × 10 d)	

Abbreviations: IV, intravenously; PO, per OS (orally).
Source: Adapted from Refs. 15, 16.

His white blood cell count is 14.7% with 87% segmented neutrophils. His chest radiograph is clear except for a left lower lobe atelectasis, which comes and goes periodically. The abdominal CT from admission (one week ago) is negative. A sinus CT is ordered by the head and neck surgery consultant revealing both left maxillary and ethmoid sinuses' mucosal thickening and opacity, with an air-fluid level in the left maxillary sinus. Initial assessment by the ENT consultant (based upon above data, without culture data) was as follows: "Radiologic evidence of left maxillary and ethmoid sinusitis in febrile patient with NG tube in place." Suggestions to the critical care team included: (*i*) change NG tube to orogastric tube, (*ii*) start oxymetazoline topical decongestant for three days, and (*iii*) elevate head of bed to 30°.

Twenty-four hours following removal of NG tube and initiation of the oxymetazoline topical decongestant, the patient defervesced to 38.2°C. However, over the ensuing 48 hours, the patient became febrile again with Tmax of 39.4°C. Nasal endoscopy was performed revealing purulent material at the maxillary sinus ostia bilaterally. Following disinfection with betadine, maxillary sinus puncture was performed and aspirate sent for Gram stain and culture. Gram stain revealed Gram-negative bacilli and multiple polymorphonucleocytes. Intravenous ciprofloxacin was initiated. Cultures subsequently became positive for *P. aeruginosa*. Twenty-four hours following the initiation of antibiotics, the patient defervesced to 37.4°C and remained afebrile.

Lessons from the case report include: (*i*) Most patients with a nasal tube >72° will have air-fluid levels and (*ii*) nasal endoscopy is simple and noninvasive and should have been performed on the initial consultation. When purulent discharge is seen in the sinus ostia, cultures should be obtained and antibiotics started.

EYE TO THE FUTURE

Although the gold standard in the diagnosis of paranasal sinusitis has been maxillary sinus puncture, aspiration, and culture, this technique is fairly invasive, time-consuming, and painful in the nonsedated patient. Recent advances in nasal endoscopy have shown that it is a useful tool for the diagnosis of paranasal sinusitis. The advantage of this noninvasive technique is that it can be performed quickly and is not operator-dependent. Further studies will be needed to confirm the correlation between nasal endoscopy and antral puncture. Continued development of endoscope technology has notably improved the image quality and ability to visualize the sinus ostia. Additional developments in ENT will improve the ability to diagnose and manage nasal sinusitis including continued development of imaging capabilities with both spiral CT scans and MRI. Increasing recognition of the morbidity of large nasal tubes in critically ill patients should also have a beneficial effect on lowering the incidence of disease. Ultrasonography may play a future role in the evaluation of paranasal sinusitis.

SUMMARY

Paranasal sinusitis is a known cause of fever in the ICU. The pathophysiology of acute paranasal sinusitis is usually due to decreased muciliary clearance leading to OMC obstruction, mucous stasis, and consequent infection. The treatment of paranasal sinusitis is fairly straightforward—eliminate the source of OMC obstruction (i.e., intranasal intubation) and improve intranasal mucous drainage (head elevation and topical decongestants).

Acute bacterial sinusitis in the community is chiefly due to *Streptococcus pneumoniae* and *H. influenzae* (50), whereas sinusitis in critically ill patients generally results from *S. aureus*, *Acinetobacter* spp., *Pseudomonas* spp., and, up to 8% of the time, fungi (Table 1). The majority of ICU patients with bacterial paranasal sinusitis respond appropriately to antibiotics.

The most common clinical dilemma involving sinusitis in the ICU revolves around determining in which patient sinusitis is a significant contributing factor to fever, when so many other conditions following trauma and critical care also elevate the temperature (Volume 2, Chapter 46). Increased use of nasal endoscopy and study of the correlation between CT scan images, surgical culture data, and antral culture may clarify the future therapy of this vexing condition.

KEY POINTS

- ☞ The single most important factor in the development of sinusitis is the disruption of the mucociliary transport system, typically from obstruction of the normal drainage pathways, the OMC of the paranasal sinuses.
- ☞ Nosocomial sinusitis may be caused by both gram-negative bacilli and gram-positive cocci, with 20% being polymicrobial (14).
- ☞ The usual clinical clues of sinusitis seen in otherwise healthy outpatients may be missed in critically ill patients.
- ☞ An important risk factor for the development of sinusitis in the ICU setting is the presence of nasal tubes.
- ☞ The acute development of fever, in a previously stable and afebrile ICU patient must immediately trigger a search for a treatable infection.
- ☞ Sinusitis is only one of a host of infectious etiologies of fever in critically ill patients (see Volume 2, Chapter 46).
- ☞ CT is the most useful radiographic method to evaluate the presence of sinusitis in the paranasal sinuses.
- ☞ Significant infection as diagnosed by positive sinus culture is only found in 38% of patients with radiologic (CT) evidence of sinusitis.
- ☞ The gold standard for the diagnosis of sinusitis is maxillary sinus puncture (antral puncture), aspiration, Gram stain, and culture (Fig. 3) (42).
- ☞ The most important factor in treating nosocomial sinusitis in the ICU setting is the removal of inciting factors causing impairment of mucociliary transportation and paranasal sinus ventilation.
- ☞ Initial emperic antimicrobial therapy requires coverage of both gram-positive and gram-negative bacteria (with adequate pseudomonas coverage) (Table 2).

REFERENCES

1. Marik PE. Fever in the ICU. Chest 2000; 117:855–869.
2. Arens FJ, LeJeune FE, Webre DR. Maxillary sinusitis, a complication of nasotracheal intubation. Anesthesiology 1974; 4: 415–416.

3. O'Reilly MJ, Reddick EJ, Black W, et al. Sepsis from sinusitis in nasotracheally intubated patients. Am J Surg 1984; 147: 601–604.

4. Mevio E, Benazzo M, Quaglieri S, Mencherini S. Sinus infection in intensive care patients. Rhinology 1996; 34(4):232–236.

5. Torres A, el-Ebiary M, Rano A. Respiratory infectious complications in the intensive care unit. Clin Chest Med 1999; 20(2):287–301, viii.

6. Wake M, Takeno S, Hawke M. The early development of sinonasal mucosa. Laryngoscope 1994; 104:850–855.

7. Stamberger H, Hasler G. Functional Endoscopic Sinus Surgery: The Messerklinger Technique. Philadelphia, PA: Mosby, 1991.

8. Elwany S, Mekhamer A. Effect of nasotracheal intubation on nasal mucociliary clearance. Br J Anaesth 1987; 59(6): 755–759.

9. Holzapfel L, Chevret S, Madinier G, et al. Influence of long-term oral or nasotracheal intubation on nosocomial maxillary sinusitis and pneumonia: results of a prospective randomized clinical trial. Crit Care Med 1993; 21:1132–1138.

10. Rubin BK, MacLeod PM, Sturgess J, King M. Recurrent respiratory infections in a child with fucosidosis: is the mucus too thin for effective transport? Pediatr Pulmonol 1991; 10(4): 304–309.

11. Antonelli M, Conti G, Rocco M, et al. A comparison of noninvasive positive-pressure ventilation and conventional mechanical ventilation in patients with acute respiratory failure. N Engl J Med 1998; 13:339(7):429–435.

12. Lew HL, Han J, Robinson LR, et al. Occult maxillary sinusitis as a cause of fever in tetraplegia: 2 case reports. Arch Phys Med Rehabil 2002; 83(3):430–432.

13. Bell RM, Page GV, Bynoe RP, et al. Post-traumatic sinusitis. J Trauma 1988; 28(7):923–930.

14. Caplan ES, Hoyt NH. Nosocomial sinusitis. JAMA 1982; 24:639–641.

15. Snow V, Mottur-Pilson C, Hickner J. Principles of appropriate antibiotic use for acute sinusitis in adults. Annals of Internal medicine 2001; 134:495–497.

16. Talmor M, Lichtman P, Barie PS. Acute paranasal sinusitis in critically ill patients: guidelines for prevention, diagnosis and treatment. Clin Infect Dis 1997; 25:1441–1446.

17. Marple B. Allergic fungal rhinosinusitis: current theories and management strategies. Laryngoscope 2001; 111:1006–1019.

18. deShazo RD, O'Brien M, Chapin K, et al. A new classification and diagnostic criteria for invasive fungal sinusitis. Arch Otolaryngol Head Neck Surg 1997; 123(11):1181–1188.

19. deShazo RD, Chapin K, Swain RE. Fungal sinusitis. N Engl J Med 1997; 337:254–259.

20. Le Moal G, Lemerre D, Grollier G, et al. Nosocomial sinusitis with isolation of anaerobic bacteria in ICU patients. Intensive Care Med 1999; 25:1066–1071.

21. Holzapfel L, Chastang C, Demingeon G, et al. A randomized study assessing the systematic search for maxillary sinusitis in nasotracheally mechanically ventilated patients: influence of nosocomial maxillary sinusitis on the occurrence of ventilator-associated pneumonia. Am J Respir Crit Care Med 1999; 159:695–701.

22. Rouby JJ, Laurent P, Gosnach M, et al. Risk factors and clinical relevance of nosocomial maxillary sinusitis in the critically ill. Am J Respir Crit Care Med 1994; 150:776–783.

23. George DL, Falk PS, Meduri GU, et al. Nosocomial sinusitis in patients in the medical intensive care unit: a prospective epidemiological study. Clin Infec Dis 1998; 27:463–470.

24. Geiss HK. Nosocomial sinusitis. Intensive Care Med 1999; 25:1037–1039.

25. Westergren V, Lundblad L, Hellquist HB, et al. Ventilator-associated sinusitis: a review. Clin Infec Dis 1998; 27:851–864.

26. Borman KR, Brown PM, Mezera KK, Jhaveri H. Occult fever in surgical intensive care unit patients is seldom caused by sinusitis. Am J Surg 1992; 164:412–415; discussion 415–416.

27. Dinarello CA, Cannon JG, Mancilla J. Interleukin-6 as an endogenous pyrogen: induction of prostaglandin E2 in brain but not peripheral blood mononuclear cells. Brain Res 1991; 562:199–206.

28. Dinarello CA, Olff SM. The role of interleukin-1 in disease. N Engl J Med 1993; 328:106–113.

29. Leon LR, White AA, Kluger MJ. Role of IL-6 and TNF in thermoregulation and survival during sepsis in mice. Am J Physiol 1998; 275:R269–R277.

30. Bernheim HA, Kluger MJ. Fever: effect of drug-induced antipyresis on survival. Science 1976; 193:237–239.

31. Kluger MJ, Ringler DH, Anver MR. Fever and survival. Science 1975; 188:166–168.

32. Carmichael LE, Barnes FD, Percy DH. Temperature as a factor in resistance of young puppies to canine herpesvirus. J Infect Dis 1969; 120:669–678.

33. Bryant RE, Hood AF, Hood CE, et al. Factors affecting mortality of gram-negative rod bacteremia. Arch Intern Med 1971; 127:120–128.

34. Manthous CA, Hall JB, Olson D, et al. Effect of cooling on oxygen consumption in febrile critically ill patients. Am J Respir Crit Care Med 1995; 151:10–14.

35. Wass CT, Lanier WL, Hofer RE, et al. Temperature Changes of greater or equal to 1°C alter functional neurologic outcome and histopathology in a canine model of complete cerebral ischemia. Anesthesiology 1995; 83:325–335.

36. Warner DS, McFarlane C, Todd MM, et al. Sevoflurane and halothane reduce focal ischemic brain damage in the rat. Possible influence on thermoregulation. Anesthesiology 1993; 79(5):985–992.

37. Aalokken TM, Hagtvedt T, Dalen I, Kolbenstvedt A. Conventional sinus radiography compared with CT in the diagnosis of acute sinusitis. Dentomaxillofac Radiol 2003; 32(1):60–62.

38. Josephson J, Rosenberg S. Sinusitis. Clin Symp 1994; 46(2):1–32.

39. Varonen H, Savolainen S, Kunnamo I, et al. Acute rhinosinusitis in primary care: a comparison of symptoms, signs, ultrasound, and radiography. Rhinology 2003; 41(1):37–43.

40. Hilbert G, Vargas F, Valentino R, et al. Comparison of B-mode ultrasound and computed tomography in the diagnosis of maxillary sinusitis in mechanically ventilated patients. Crit Care Med 2001; 29(7):1337–1342.

41. Skoulas IG, Helidonis E, Kountakis SE. Evaluation of sinusitis in the intensive care unit patient. Otolaryngol Head Neck Surg 2003; 128(4):503–509.

42. Benninger MS, Holzer SE, Lau J. Diagnosis and treatment of uncomplicated acute bacterial rhinosinusitis: summary of the Agency on Health Care Policy and Research Evidence Based Report. Otolaryngol Head Neck Surg 2000; 122:1–7.

43. Tolstov IuP, Ryzhanov EA. Cerebral hemorrhage as a complication of puncture of the maxillary sinus. Vestn Otorinolaringol 1966; 28(5):108–109.

44. Burakova ZN, Zagainova NS. Infection as a complication of puncture of the maxillary sinus. Vestn Otorinolaringol 1976; (6):69–70.

45. Ramadan HH, Owens RM, Tiu C, Wax MK. Role of antral puncture in the treatment of sinusitis in the intensive care unit. Otolaryngol Head Neck Surg 1998; 119(4):381–384.

46. Kountakis SE, Burke L, Rafie J-J, et al. Sinusitis in the intensive care unit patient. Otolaryngol Head Neck Surg 1997; 117: 362–366.

47. Casiano RR, Cohn S, Villasuso E 3rd, et al. Comparison of antral tap with endoscopically directed nasal culture. Laryngoscope 2001; 111(8):1333–1337.

48. Tantilipikorn P, Fritz M, Tanabodee J, et al. A comparison of endoscopic culture techniques for chronic rhinosinusitis. Am J Rhinol 2002; 16(5):255–260.

49. Kronberg FG, Goodwin WJ Jr. Sinusitis in intensive care unit patients. Laryngoscope 1985; 95(8):936–938.

50. Picarrelo JF. Acute Bacterial Sinusitis. N Engl J Med 2004; 351:902–910.

52

Immunity and Immunodeficiency in Trauma and Critical Care

Elizabeth H. Sinz

Departments of Anesthesiology and Neurosurgery, Penn State College of Medicine, Penn State University Hospital, Hershey, Pennsylvania, U.S.A.

William C. Wilson

Department of Anesthesiology and Critical Care, UC San Diego Medical Center, San Diego, California, U.S.A.

Vishal Bansal

Division of Trauma, Burns, and Critical Care, Department of Surgery, UC San Diego Medical Center, San Diego, California, U.S.A.

INTRODUCTION

By their very nature, traumatic injuries commonly break down our most important barriers to infection: the external skin and endothelium of the gut, lung, and genito-urinary systems. Even in "closed" injuries such as bony fractures or head injuries, many of our supportive and resuscitative therapies violate these barriers, for example, placement of central venous catheters, endotracheal intubation, and surgical repairs. The experienced physician is mindful of the potential harm that may result from invasive interventions, as well as the anticipated benefits.

As we learn more about the immune system, we are discovering that major immunological changes are triggered by traumatic injury, some of which enhance the immune response, and others that seem to suppress it. Old ideas become new again as we marvel at the complexity of regulatory mechanisms involved in immunity, and strive to understand the variations of the immunological response to similar antigens under varying conditions. Other elements of treatment including antibiotics, nutrition, and ventilation strategies are also known to affect immunity.

This chapter reviews the human immune system and the effects of trauma, burns, and critical illness. The chapter also reviews the effect of some common systemic diseases on the immune system, including an illuminating section on autoimmunity, presently an area of intense research. Autoimmunity has been discovered to play an important role in otherwise idiopathic disorders such as inflammatory bowl disease, myasthenia gravis, rheumatoid arthritis, and other ailments previously known as "collagen vascular diseases." A specific section is dedicated to human immunodeficiency virus (HIV) infection in trauma and critical care. Next, the most common infectious agents that afflict immunocompromised patients are surveyed, followed by a brief review of the considerations for immunosuppressed solid organ transplantation. Section "Eye to the Future" provides a glimpse at the considerable research ongoing in the area of immune modulation in trauma and critical care.

REVIEW OF THE HUMAN IMMUNE SYSTEM
Anatomic Barriers

The first line of defense against infection includes the normal anatomic barriers of the skin, airway, and gut. These defenses are often disrupted by traumatic injuries or by invasive therapies intended to treat critically ill patients. Because of the physical barriers provided by keratinized epithelium, bacteria seldom survive in large numbers on the skin surface. In addition, the direct antibacterial effects of lactate and fatty acids in sweat and sebaceous secretions decrease the pH and generate an external surface that is hostile to most bacteria. An exception is *Staphylococcus aureus*, which often invades the hair follicles and sweat glands.

Protection is also provided by the antimicrobial mucous lining the inner surfaces of the body, including the gut and airway epithelium. Special antimicrobial protection factors such as immunoglobulin A (IgA) and complement also help kill invading microbes. Bactericidal factors are also provided by gastric acid, spermine and zinc in semen, lactoperoxidase in breast milk, and lysozyme in tears, nasal secretions, and saliva. Lactic acid produced by commensal organisms in the vagina also helps protect against pathogenic bacteria. Microbial invaders are often trapped in the mucus and removed mechanically by cilia, coughing, and sneezing. Other mechanical factors include washing by tears, saliva, and urine. Langerhans cells in skin, and dendritic cells in the interstitium of various tissues, are also constantly on the prowl for foreign invaders.

☞ **Once a pathogen has overcome the primary barrier of the skin, respiratory, gastrointestinal (GI), or genito-urinary epithelium, the immune system must then combat the invader.** ☞

The natural or innate immunity process refers to the older, nonspecific immune system that involves recruitment and release of macrophages, neutrophils, natural killer (NK) cells, cytokines, some cellular receptors, and the complement system (1–3). Adaptive or acquired immunity involves recognition of specific antigen and confers both specificity and a "memory effect" by T- and B-lymphocytes. The acquired immune system can be further divided into the humoral and cellular immune systems, both of which communicate through the influence of cytokines. The complement system is also active in both cellular and

Table 1 Leukocytes Involved in the Immune System

Cell type	Function	Surface marker	Special traits
T helper (Th)	Stimulate B-cells: provides specific and nonspecific cytokine signals for activation and differentiation	CD3+, CD4+, CD8−	MHC class II markers restrict activation Th2 activates B-cells, makes IL-4
	Activate macrophages: cytokines provide message for activation	CD3+, CD4+, CD8−	MHC class II markers restrict activation Th1 activates macrophages, makes interferon-γ
T cytotoxic (T_C)	Lyse antigen expressing cells: such as those infected by virus, or allografts	CD3+, CD4−, CD8+	MHC class I markers restrict activity
T supressor (T_S)	Downregulates cellular and humoral immunity	Can be CD3+ or CD3− Usually CD4−, CD8+	
T regulator (T_{REG})	Suppresses T-cell-mediated inflammation	CD4+, CD25+	Diminishes autoimmunity
NK	Spontaneous lysis of tumor cells, Ab-dependent cellular cytotoxicity	Fc receptor for IgG	MHC class I markers restrict activity
NK T-cells	Amplify both cell-mediated and humoral immunity	CD4+	Express a restricted subset of surface markers ($V\alpha$)
B cells	Ab Production, and presents antigen to T-cells	Fc and C3d receptors MHC class II	Differentiate into plasma cells (which produce Ab)
Macrophages (monocytes)	Phagocytosis, secretion of cytokines to activate T-cells (e.g., IL-1), neutrophils	Macrophage surface antigens, and "armed" with Ab binding to Fc receptors	Express surface receptors for C3a, kill ingested bacteria by oxidative bursts
PMN (neutrophils)	Phagocytosis killing	Can be "armed" with Ab	Protective in parasitic infections, but adverse effects (e.g., granuloma) can occur

Abbreviations: Ab, antibody; C3a, activated third component of complement; IL, interleukin; MHC, major histocompatibility complex; PMN, polymorphonuclear; NK, natural killer.

Cellular Immunity

humoral immunity, and serves as an interface between the innate and adaptive immune systems.

A large array of white blood cells (WBCs), or leukocytes, are involved in the immune system (Table 1). Cellular immunity is mediated by thymus derived (T) lymphocytes. The T-cells constitute approximately 65% of the circulating lymphocytes. Each T-cell is genetically programmed to recognize and bind to specific cell-bound antigens by way of an antigen-specific T-cell receptor (TCR). Each antigen-specific TCR is linked to a cluster of nonvariable polypeptides referred to as the CD3 molecular complex. The CD3 proteins are involved in signal transduction into the T-cell after the antigen-specific TCR binds antigen. In addition to CD3 proteins, T-cells express a variety of nonpolymorphic-function-associated proteins, of which CD4 and CD8 are particularly important.

☞ **The CD4 and CD8 proteins are expressed on two mutually exclusive sets of T-cells, and are co-receptors of T-cell activation.** ☞ During antigen expression, CD4 molecules bind to the nonpolymorphic portions of major histocompatibility complex (MHC) class II molecules on the antigen-presenting cells. In contrast, CD8 molecules bind to the nonpolymorphic portions of MHC class I molecules. The CD4+ T-cells are referred to as helper T-cells, and the CD8+ T-cells are known as cytotoxic/suppressor T-cells. The CD4+ T-cells are the major regulators of cellular immunity. The CD4+ T-cells secrete cytokines influencing virtually every cell type in the immune system including other T-cells, B-cells, macrophages, and NK cells. ☞ **The important regulatory role of CD4+ T-cells is evident when HIV infects the host and selectively kills CD4+ T-cells**

(described subsequently). ☞ The CD8+ T-cells secrete cytokines as well, but are mainly cytotoxic cells.

The bone marrow derived (B) lymphocytes constitute approximately 15% of the peripheral circulating lymphocytes. In mature patients, they are found in the bone marrow, lymphocytes, spleen, tonsils, and extralymphatic organs (including Peyer's patches in the ileum). After antigen stimulation, B-cells transform into plasma cells and secrete immunoglobulins, which are the main mediators of humoral immunity.

☞ **Immunoglobulin M (IgM) is present on the surface of all B-cells, comprising the antigen-binding component of the B-cell receptor.** ☞ Like the T-cells, the B-cell receptor has antigen specificity, partly due to the IgM molecular structure. In addition to the IgM molecule, the B-cell has a nonpolymorphic transmembrane protein similar to the CD3 proteins of the TCR. B-cells have other nonpolymorphic receptors required for function including complement receptors, Fc receptors and CD40. Interestingly, the B-cell complement receptor (CD21) binds Epstein-Barr virus (EBV), explaining why EBV often infects B-cells. Additionally, the CD40 molecule is a member of the tumor necrosis factor-α (TNF-α) family of receptors, and is instrumental in interactions between the CD4+ T-helper cells and B-cells. Activated T-helper cells express the CD40 ligand that binds CD40 expressed on B-cells, and are required for mature plasmacytes to secrete IgG, IgE, and IgA. Patients with a mutation in the CD40 ligand do not secrete sufficient immunoglobulins and have a defined immunodeficiency called X-linked hyper-IgM syndrome.

Macrophages are part of the mononuclear phagocyte system involved in both inflammation and immunity. ☞ **The first cells to migrate to areas of injury following trauma are**

the polymorphonuclear neutrophils (PMNs) with quantities peaking in the first 24 hours, followed by the macrophages, which reach their zenith at 72 hours. ☞ Macrophages play a key role in the immune response and, initially, the macrophages process and present antigens to T-cells. Additionally, in the presence of certain cytokines from the CD4+ T-cells, macrophages will kill tumor cells and other benign cells. Macrophages are also important in humoral immunity as they phagocytose bacteria and other microbes that have been opsonized (coated) by IgG or C3b (a factor in complement). Dendritic cells have antigen-presenting roles and are so-named because of the cytoplasmic extensions, extending from the main cell body. Langerhans cells are dendritic cells located in the epidermis that may be killed during severe burns. Dendritic cells are widely distributed within lymphoid tissues and within non-lymph interstitial space of tissues such as lung and heart. In the spleen and lymph nodes, dendritic cells are referred to as follicular dendritic cells and express IgG Fc receptors serving to trap antigen opsonized by these antibodies.

NK cells comprise approximately 10% of the peripheral lymphocytes. These NK cells are larger than most lymphocytes, they possess Fc receptors that bind to IgG and kill opsonized cells. However, NK cells have another method of seeking out and killing foreign cells. The NK cells have a receptor mechanism that recognizes MHC class I molecules (which are on the surface of all normal mammalian cells) and do not attack these. However, cells lacking the MHC class I molecule (e.g., bacteria, tumors) are attacked by perforating the cell membrane with a molecular punch called "perforin," and injecting cell destructive proteins called "granzymes." NK cells are part of the innate immune system. Additionally, NK cells may attack some host cells with MHC class I molecules associated with other surface molecules that indicate to the NK cells that the host cell has been infected by a virus. MHC class II molecules are restricted to lymphocytes, macrophages, and (antigen-presenting) dendritic cells.

Erythrocytes and platelets also have a role in the immune system, which is not often acknowledged. Both red blood cells and platelets have receptors for complement, and platelets in addition have IgG Fc receptors. Thus, they could play a role in clearing immune complexes and antigens that have been opsonized by complement.

Humoral Immunity

Passive humoral immunity is conferred when preformed antibodies are obtained from an external source. This occurs naturally during human gestation by the transfer of maternal IgG. Maternal IgG is gradually lost over the first year of life. Breast-fed babies also obtain maternal IgA affording local protection particularly to the gut. Beyond infancy, passive humoral immunity can be conferred by parenterally administered human immunoglobulin.

In contrast, active humoral immunity develops when the immune system encounters an antigen either due to natural infection or by vaccination. The relative serum concentrations and characteristics of separate classes of immunoglobulins are summarized in Table 2. Antigen may be categorized as thymus-independent (TI) type 1 or type 2 and thymus dependent (TD) based on its predominant mechanism of B-cell activation. TI-type 1 antigens are microbial or vegetable molecules that bind to B-cells and stimulate proliferation and differentiation of specific or nonspecific antibody responses. TI-type 2 antigens elicit predominantly antigen-specific antibody responses. Most protein and glycoprotein antigens encountered by the immune system are TD antigens. Two types of cellular interactions are required for antibody responses to TD antigens. T-cells must recognize antigen associated with MHC class II molecules on the surface of the antigen-presenting cell. Next, the B-cell and T-helper cell interact, and the B-cell internalizes antigen. Once the antigen is processed and associated with the MHC class II molecules, the T-helper cell is able to recognize appropriate cells to deliver its stimulating signal.

☞ **When the host has pre-existing circulating antibodies due to vaccination or prior infection, microbial replication can be halted at the onset of infection.** ☞ This secondary antibody response results from activation of a memory B-cell. Memory cells typically circulate widely and survive for long periods of time. Upon interaction with antigen, antibodies (predominately IgG, IgA, and IgE) are rapidly produced. In contrast, the primary humoral immune response (predominately IgM) may be too slow to protect against many pathogens (1).

The Complement System

The complement system consists of a group of plasma proteins, which are essential for antibodies to achieve destruction of foreign cells, bacteria, and apoptotic cells. The complement proteins lack immunologic specificity, but comprise a highly complex cascade system consisting of 35 discrete proteins (12 of which are directly involved in the complement pathways, while the rest have regulatory functions) (4).

Table 2 Structural and Biological Properties of Human Immunoglobulins

Property	IgG	IgA	IgM	IgD	IgE
Approximate mass (Da)	150,000	160,000 460,000	900,000 memb. 180,000	180,000	190,000
Serum concentration (mg/mL)	15	3.5	2.0	0.003	0.0005
Serum half-life (days)	23	6	5	2–8	1–5
Exist as polymer	0	+	++	0	0
Agglutinating	0	0	++	?	?
Complement fixation	+	0	+++	0	0
Reagenic activity	?	0	0	0	+++
Lysis of bacteria	+	+	+++	?	
Antiviral activity	+	+++	+	?	?
Present in secretions	0	+++	0	0	0
B-cell receptor for antigen	+ (memory)	+ (memory)	+ (primary)	+ (primary)	+ (memory)
Placental transfer	+	0	0	0	0

Abbreviations: Ig, immunoglobulin; ?, unknown.

The protein components of complement are numbered in the order of their discovery rather than the sequence in which they are activated. ☞ **Although there is no immunologic specificity in complement activation, or in its effects, there are several immunological methods by which the complement system can be activated.** ☞ Some complement components enhance the effects of antigen–antibody interactions (as occurs with opsonization), whereas others increase the inflammatory response by stimulating the release of vasoactive substances, and by stimulating chemotaxis of leukocytes (Table 3) (4).

Three biochemical pathways can activate the complement system (all converging at C3): (1) the classic pathway, (2) the alternative complement pathway, and (3) the mannan-binding lectin (MBL) pathway (4). All three pathways generate homologous variants of C3-convertase. The enzyme, C3-convertase initiates the membrane-attack pathway culminating with the assembly of the membrane-attack complex (MAC), the cytolytic endproduct of the complement cascade consisting of C5b, C6, C7, C8, and polymeric C9. The MAC pentamer inserts into the cell membrane and forms a transmembrane channel which causes osmotic lysis of the target cell.

Classic Pathway

The classic complement pathway is initiated by antigen–antibody complexes involving IgM or IgG, either by binding to C1 at their Fc portions or by direct binding of C1 to the pathogen surface. The C1 complex is inhibited by C1-inhibitor. The C1 complex now binds to and splits C2 and C4 into C2a and C4b. C4b and C2a bind to form C3-convertase (C4b2a complex). Production of C3-convertase signals the start of the membrane-attack pathway (the final common pathway of all three activation routes).

Alternative Pathway

The alternative pathway is more primitive than the classical pathway, and does not require the presence of antibody. Instead, C3 can be hydrolyzed directly by endotoxin, or following contact with bacterial cell wall constituents, aggregated IgA, or as a form of amplification feedback following activation of C3 by any of the three major complement pathways. In the alternative pathway, C3 is split into C3a and C3b. Some of the C3b is bound to the pathogen where it will bind to factor B; this complex will then be cleaved by factor D into Ba and the alternative pathway C3-convertase,

Bb. In other words, after hydrolysis of C3, C3b complexes to form C4b2a3b, which cleaves C5 into C5a and C5b. C5a and C3a are known to trigger mast cell degranulation and release histamine among other products (see Volume 1, Chapter 33). C5b, together with C6, C7, C8, and C9, form the MAC (C5b6789).

Lectin Pathway

The lectin pathway is homologous to the classical pathway, but with the opsonin, MBL, instead of C1. This pathway is activated by binding MBL to mannose residues on the microbial cell walls, which activates the MBL-associated serine proteases, MASP-1 and MASP-2, which can then split C4 and C2 into C4b and C2a, which then binds together to form C3-convertase, as in the classical pathway.

Complement Involvement in Immunologic Diseases

The complement system plays a role in numerous immunologic diseases including anaphylaxis, asthma, systemic lupus erythematosus (SLE), and various forms of arthritis, autoimmune heart disease, and multiple sclerosis. Additionally, deficiencies of the constituents in the terminal portion of the complement pathway predispose to infections, particularly meningitis, and infections due to encapsulated bacteria requiring opsonization for death (e.g., Pneumococcus, *Neisseria*, and *Haemophilus influenzae*) (4,5).

Immunologic Regulation and Tolerance

Immune effector mechanisms are powerful processes that can lead to cell and tissue destruction; therefore, close control of immune system activation is essential. T-cells regulate both humoral and cellular effector mechanisms. The division of CD4+ helper T (Th) cells into two functional subsets, Th1 and Th2, is a paradigm for understanding how autoimmune inflammation is orchestrated by cytokines and chemokines. The cytokines interleukin (IL)-12 and interferon-α, secreted by antigen-presenting cells, promote proinflammatory and cytodestructive Th1 responses via secretion of interferon-α and TNF-α, whereas IL-4 promotes Th2 responses with activation of B-cells. Chemokines are chemotactic proteins secreted by various cell types and, through their interaction with specific receptors, direct the selective traffic of leukocytes throughout the lymphoid system and into inflammatory sites. Once activated, large numbers of

Table 3 The Three Main Physiologic Functions of the Complement System

Function	Mechanism of action	Complement protein responsible for activity
Host defense against infection	Opsonization	Covalently bound C3 and C4 fragments
	Chemotaxis and leukocyte activation	Anaphylatoxins (C5a, C3a, and C4a); leukocyte anaphylatoxin receptors
	Lysis of bacteria and cells	MAC (C5b–C9)
Interface between innate and adaptive immunity	Augmentation of antibody response	C3b and C4b bound to immune complexes and to antigen; C3 receptors on B-cells and antigen-presenting cells
	Enhancement of immunologic memory	C3b and C4b bound to immune complexes and to antigen; C3 receptors on follicular dendritic cells
Disposal of waste	Clearance of immune complexes from tissues	C1q; covalently bound fragments of C3 and C4
	Clearance of apoptotic cells	C1q; covalently bound fragments of C3 and C4

Abbreviation: MAC, membrane-attack complex.
Source: From Ref. 4.

Table 4 Gell and Coombs Classification of Immune-Mediated Hypersensitivity Reactions

Hypersensitivity class	Prototype disorder	Immune mechanism
I—Anaphylactic	Anaphylaxis, some forms of bronchial asthma	Formation of IgE (cytotropic) antibody → immediate release of vasoactive amines and other mediators from basophils and mast cells followed by recruitment of other inflammatory cells
II—Cytotoxic	Autoimmune hemolytic anemia, erythroblastosis fetalis, Goodpasture syndrome	Formation of IgG, IgM → binds to antigen on target cell surface → phagocytosis or lysis of target cell by C8,9 fraction of complement or antibody-dependent cellular cytotoxicity
III—Immune complex	Arthus reaction, serum sickness, SLE, certain forms of acute glomerulonephritis	Antigen–antibody complexes → activated complement → attracted neutrophils → release of lysosomal enzymes and other toxic moieties. Failure of complement to clear
IV—Cell-mediated (delayed)	Tuberculosis, contact dermatitis, transplant rejection	Sensitized T lymphocytes → release of lymphokines and T-cell-mediated cytotoxicity

Abbreviations: Ig, Immunoglobulin; SLE, systemic lupus erythematosus.

cytokine-producing cells are produced; therefore, it is essential that the process be self-limited to avoid excessive injury.

The immune system is closely regulated by a process termed "tolerance." In vertebrates, tolerance occurs at multiple levels. One of the most fundamental is the presence of "self"-markers on the native cell membranes, for example, the MHC class I binding structures described above. Cells without the MHC class I "self"-protein are attacked as foreign.

Another mechanism of negative regulation is activation-induced cell death, a form of apoptosis that eventually kills the cells (2). The complement system plays an integral role in the clearance of apoptotic cells and the immune complexes from plasmas and tissues. Some other negative feedback signals include prostaglandins produced by macrophages, transforming growth factor-β, and IL-10, which deactivates macrophages, in turn decreasing cytokine production by T-cells. Disruption of any or all of these tolerance systems or other immune system control mechanisms leads to autoimmune disease (described further below).

☞ **Hypersensitivity reactions are exuberant, improperly regulated immunological responses to various antigenic molecules resulting in tissue injury to the host.** ☞ These have been classified into four major types by Gell and Coombs based upon the mechanism of tissue injury (Table 4). In Type I disease, the antigen triggers an IgE-mediated anaphylactic response (Volume 1, Chapter 33). Type II disorders involve the formation of antibodies against native tissues, so-called cytotoxic response, as seen in Goodpasture Syndrome. Type III hypersensitivity disease is caused by immune complexes that fail to clear properly, thereby causing tissue injury as seen with SLE. Type IV disorders involve delayed tissue injury that is mediated by sensitized T-lymphocytes.

EFFECT OF TRAUMA, BURNS, AND CRITICAL ILLNESS ON IMMUNITY
Overview of Immune Modulation Following Injury
The effects of severe trauma and burns are often manifest as an overwhelming "systemic inflammatory response syndrome" (SIRS) followed by a relatively immunodepressed state during which life-threatening infections may occur (6).

This period of recovery from systemic inflammation is called the "counter-regulatory anti-inflammatory response" (CARS). A traumatic insult typically initiates an inflammatory state that will establish a balance between the beneficial effects of controlled inflammation and potential injurious effects such as "adult respiratory distress syndrome" (ARDS) and "multi-organ dysfunction syndrome" (MODS) due to uncontrolled inflammation. The normal initial result of massive injury and shock can be an excessive inflammatory response; this is commonly called the "one-hit" model. In other cases, this response may result from a "two-hit" model where the patient receives a relatively mild initial inflammatory stimulus that would normally resolve, followed by a second hit such as a surgical procedure or an infection that leads to hyperstimulation of the immune system. In either case, the innate immune system including macrophages, leukocytes, NK cells, IL-8, and complement components are excessively activated leading to SIRS and MODS.

The opposite may also occur in which the initial inflammatory response is relatively mild yet the recovery response is marked by excessive immunosuppression. Patients may have inadequate neutrophil chemotaxis, phagocytosis, lysosomal enzyme content, and respiratory burst. This relatively immunosuppressed state following trauma likely contributes to an increased risk of infection following traumatic injury. The production of immunoglobulins and interferon falls and many patients become anergic. In the context of excessive CARS, infection and sepsis become more likely and mortality increases. The cytokine profile and interplay ultimately determines whether SIRS or CARS will manifest.

Several studies support the notion that the immune response is suppressed following severe trauma. There is evidence that levels of some naturally occurring anti-inflammatory mediators, such as soluble TNF-α receptor and IL-1 receptor antagonist are increased during the 14 days following severe traumatic injury. There were higher levels in patients with more severe injury, and patients with higher levels had higher mortality (7). Likewise, the ability of peripheral blood mononuclear cells to respond to endotoxin is reduced in severely injured patients. In these patients with an average injury severity score (ISS) of 39, release of proinflammatory cytokines (TNF-α, IL-1β, IL-6, IL-8, IL-12, and IFN-α) in response to stimulation with lipopolysaccharide was inhibited compared with healthy controls (8). It has been demonstrated previously that following burn injury, PMN function is impaired (9). Significant traumatic injury can influence leukocyte function and cytokine expression leading to both immunoactivation and immunosuppression. In fact, the optimal goal of therapy may be best understood in terms of the goal of restoring the balance between immunostimulation and immunosuppression (10).

As our ability to measure inflammatory mediators has improved, there have been many studies attempting to determine serum markers of patients at highest risk. For example, C-reactive protein is typically elevated within the first two days following traumatic injury. However, it is nonspecific and has not been shown to predict complications (11). Another marker, procalcitonin, is produced in the thyroid and not detected in normal individuals. Although it is elevated after trauma or infection, there is no consensus on its usefulness as a marker (12). TNF-α is one of the central regulators in the acute phase response involved in leukocyte chemotaxis, fever, hypotension, and endothelial cell adhesion. Persistently elevated levels are associated with poor outcome. Its usefulness as a marker has been inconsistent and treatment with anti-TNF-α has not proven successful (13–15). IL-1 and IL-8 have also been unreliable as markers. IL-6 and IL-10 may be more reliable (16,17), and in one study the ratio of IL-6 to IL-10 was recommended as a useful marker to predict the degree of injury following trauma (18).

Measures of Immunocompetence

Cell-mediated immunity is most commonly evaluated clinically by placing an anergy panel in which small quantities of common antigens are injected intradermally, to see if induration occurs within 48 to 72 hours. Common antigens used to assess cell-mediated immunity include proteins from tetanus toxoid, diphtheria toxoid, *Candida*, *Tricophyton*, *Streptococcus*, and *Proteus*. If no response occurs within 72 hours, the patient is said to be anergic, and is probably unable to mount an adequate immune response to foreign invaders. Many institutions have stopped performing these in conjunction with ppd testing, but anergy panels remain a clinically sound method to determine a patient's cell-mediated immune status.

Of the markers of cellular activity, monocyte human leukocyte antigen (HLA)-DR class II molecules seem to most consistently serve as an index of antigen-presenting capacity(19–21). HLA-DR class II molecules mediate antigen processing which allows cellular immunity to proceed. As an index of antigen-presenting capacity, it stands to reason that their decline and recovery rates are closely linked to clinical outcome. In fact, multiple measures of PMN function are altered in ways that would seem to increase the likelihood of infection (22). The infectious agents commonly found in these patients include opportunistic organisms such as *Pseudomonas aeruginosa*, *Staphylococcus epidermidis*, *S. aureus*, and *Candida albicans*. In many cases, the source of infection may be distant from the initial wound, further indicating that there is systemic dysfunction of the immune system.

One study of chest trauma demonstrated an aggressive inflammatory response locally at the source of the injury, followed by systemic immunosuppression (23). Therefore, the innate systemic phagocytic cells, particularly PMNs and monocytes, appear to become suppressed following traumatic injury (24).

Other cellular markers such as endothelial adhesion molecules (ICAM-1, L-selectin) and the CD11b leukocyte receptor have received some attention but results have been mixed (25,26). As other markers are characterized, the ability to predict and intervene before specific complications arise for a particular patient will likely be enhanced.

Treatment-Related Immunomodulation

In addition to the disruption of barriers and tissues from the initial trauma and the response of the immune system to the inflammatory cascade, the treatments applied to traumatically injured patients can also influence infection risk. Something as simple as intravenous (IV) access can have a profound impact on the patient's infection risk due to type of access, location of placement, and line care both during and after placement (Volume 2, Chapter 49).

The timing of surgical intervention may have a profound effect on the immune response to trauma. In patients with limited orthopedic injuries, early total care allows rapid mobilization and restoration of function. However, in patients who are more severely injured, limiting primary surgery to only essential, life-saving interventions gives the patient the best chance of recovery. Early surgical repair of bony fractures in these patients may be associated with a massively increased inflammatory response leading to SIRS, ARDS, and MODS (27–29). ☞ **Damage control surgery in severely injured patients was first applied to abdominal surgery (Volume 1, Chapter 21), and is now known to improve outcome for orthopedic trauma surgery as well (29).** ☞

Severe traumatic injury is related to an increase in gut permeability (30–32), allowing translocation of gut flora into the systemic circulation (33,34). The gut has emerged as a target for immunomodulation; glutamine, arginine, Ω-3 fatty acids, and nucleotides have been added to enteral feeding as a means to enhance the patient's immune response (35–37). Early enteral nutrition is an important element of prophylaxis against nosocomial infections (see Volume 2, Chapter 32).

Patients in the hospital, particularly in the intensive care unit (ICU), are sleep-deprived both in quantity and quality of sleep. Sedatives and narcotics are known to interfere with the quality of sleep as well. There appears to be a relationship, possibly involving the autonomic nervous and neuroendocrine systems, between sleep deprivation and the immune system that might lead to increased risk of infection (38).

Patients who are intubated are at increased risk for ventilator-associated pneumonia (Volume 2, Chapter 48). Treatment decisions, such as the timing of a tracheostomy, can influence the rate of infection and mortality (39). Ventilator settings with lower tidal volumes can reduce the inflammatory response in acute lung injury and has been shown to reduce mortality in the setting of ARDS (40,41).

Other commonly employed treatments have also been shown to have adverse effects on the immune system. Blood transfusions have been shown to correlate with an increase in infection rate in a dose-dependent manner (42,43), although there remains controversy if this is causal or a marker of injury severity (44). Hypertonic saline may even have an immunosuppressive effect, possibly beneficial in blunting the immune hyperstimulation typical of the acute phase of resuscitation (45). Many, if not all of the vasoactive agents that are used in critically ill patients, also have immunologic activity. The interactions of this therapy

Table 5 Postsplenectomy Vaccination Guidelines

Vaccine name (bacterial species covered)	Adult dose	Pediatric dose	Optimum timing/comments
Pneumovax 23 (pneumococcal vaccine with antigens for 23 most common pneumococcal strains)	0.5 mL IM/SC	0.5 mL IM/SC (contraindicated for age <2 years)	For traumatic splenectomy: administer immediately upon arrival (prior to splenectomy). For elective splenectomy at least 2 weeks prior to scheduled surgery
MCV4-conjugate MPSV4-old formulation [tetravalent meningococcal vaccine, including capsular polysaccharide antigens (groups A, C, Y, and W-135) of *Neisseria meningitidis*]	0.5 mL SC	0.5 mL SC (contraindicated for age <2 years)	Same as above MCV4—licensed in 2005 confers longer lasting immunity. MPSV4—available since 1970s provides only short (<1 year) immunity
ActHIB, HibTITER, PedvaxHIB (Haemophilus B conjugate vaccine)	Not indicated	Age and Hib titer dependent (see package insert)	Initial Rx is same as above, but requires repeated doses per schedule

Abbreviations: HIB, *Haemophilus influenzae*-type B; IM, intramuscular; MCV4, meningococcal tetravalent conjugate vaccine; MPSV4, meningococcal tetravalent polysaccharide antigen vaccine; SC, subcutaneous.
Source: Data for pneumococcal, meningococcal, and hemophilus from Refs. 145–147.

with the patient's immune system is only beginning to be understood (46).

Agranulocytosis, a syndrome characterized by severe neutropenia, was first reported to be associated with medication exposure in 1934 (47). A host of pharmacologic agents, for example, antibiotics, antidysrhythmics, and anti-seizure medications, can cause marrow suppression and agranulocytosis (see Table 6 in Volume 2, Chapter 57) (48,49). Severe neutropenia ($<0.5 \times 10^9$ neutrophils/L) is a life-threatening disorder, rendering the patient unable to battle infection. The agents most frequently implicated are antibiotics, antithyroid drugs, antiplatelet agents, and neuroleptic and antiepileptic agents, although drug-induced agranulocytosis is a rare event with an incidence around 3 to 12 cases per million population (for a more complete list and explanation, see Volume 2, Chapter 57) (49). Risk increases with increasing age and drug exposure and appears to be more common in women than men (50). Treatment with hematopoietic growth factors such as granulocyte colony-stimulating factor has been shown to shorten the duration of neutropenia (51).

Splenectomy—Special Case of Immune Component Removal

The spleen is the most commonly injured intra-abdominal organ (see Volume 1, Chapter 27), and a missed splenic injury is the most common cause of preventable death in trauma patients (see Volume 1, Chapter 42). The optimal management of splenic trauma has shifted during the last two decades from nearly uniform splenectomy to an emphasis on spleen salvage (52). Part of the reason for this trend is the decreased post-trauma morbidity observed with properly staged nonoperative treatment. Another major factor driving nonoperative management of spleen injuries is the increasingly recognized immunological importance of the organ (especially in children <5 years of age) (52–54).

The most worrisome infectious complication following splenectomy is overwhelming postsplenectomy sepsis (OPSS). Chronic thrombocytosis (see Volume 2, Chapter 55) is the most common long-term effect of splenectomy, but it is clinically benign. Though relatively rare, OPSS has a high mortality (50%) (52). ✇ **The risk of OPSS is particularly high following splenectomy in children under five years of age (especially infants splenectomized for trauma, with reported infection rates of >10%) (53).** ✇ Infection most commonly occurs with encapsulated organisms (*Streptococcus pneumoniae*, *Neisseria meningitidis*, *Haemophilus influenzae*-type B). Encapsulated organisms are problematic because the spleen is integral in the removal of opsonized microbes such as these bacteria (54). Early antibiotic therapy is essential to avoid death from a rapidly progressive infection.

Protection against OPSS involves vaccination and less commonly antibiotic prophylaxis (Volume 2, Chapter 53). The optimal timing of vaccination has long been a subject of debate. Shatz et al. demonstrated that a 14-day delay in vaccination after emergent splenectomy resulted in improved antibody response, but that total postvaccination IgG levels were not significantly different from normal control subjects regardless of the time of vaccination (1, 7, or 14 days following splenectomy). The better functional antibody responses occurred against the serogroup and serotypes studied with delayed (14-day) vaccination, but not all serotypes were studied (55). In a follow-up study, antibody response was not improved any further by delaying vaccination to 28 days (56).

Although the antibody response may be better two weeks after splenectomy, if a delayed vaccination strategy is used, many patients would be discharged home from the hospital prior to receiving vaccination, and either miss immunization completely due to loss to follow-up, or develop infection prior to immunization. Many trauma surgeons in North America (44.1%) vaccinate their patients within the first week after emergent splenectomy, chiefly for this reason (57).

Table 6 Autoimmune Diseases with Immunomodulating Treatments in Use or Being Developed

Disease	Autoimmunological mechanism of disease	Treatment(s)
Myasthenia gravis	Antibodies nicotinic Ach receptors in muscle disrupt transmission at the NMJ	Anticholinesterase drugs (e.g., pyridostigmine, neostigmine), thymectomy (improves 80%), plasmapharesis
Multiple sclerosis	Anti-myelin antibodies	Interferon β-1a (inhibits IL-12)
SLE	Auto-antibodies to numerous structures including DNA, nuclei, immune complex nephritis, etc (due to IL-2 inhibition)	Steroids, and other immunosuppressive therapies. Soon, may have IL-s2 boosting therapy for defective cells. Administration of complement may be therapeutic (SLE is more common and severe in complement deficiencies)
Rheumatoid arthritis	Auto-antibodies to numerous structures including synovium. TNF-α activated macrophages contribute to synovial inflammation	Methotrexate and blockade of TNF-α receptor (etanercept) or a monoclonal antibody against TNF-α (infliximab)
Inflammatory bowel disease	CD4 + CD45RO+ T-cell migration into inflamed mucosa elevated IL-2, IL-7, IL-10 production	Corticosteroids; aminosalicylates; anti-TNF-α agent (infliximab); inhibition of leukocyte migration into inflamed intestine by blocking integrins (cellular adhesion molecules)
Psoriasis	T-lymphocyte-based immunopathogenesis with Munro microabscesses below the stratum corneum	Alefacept, efalizumab, and etanercept, monoclonal antibodies, cytokines, and fusion proteins (see text for explanation)
Pemphigus	IgG anti-BM auto-antibodies, anti-BPAG$_1$, and anti-BPAG$_2$ produced, and T-cells are	Immunosuppressive agents (e.g., azathioprine, mycophenolate mofetil, or cyclophosphamide), plasmapharesis to remove anti-BPAG$_1$ and anti-BPAG$_2$
Addison's disease	21-Hydroxylase auto-antibodies impair adrenocortical function (takes years)	Corticosteroid replacement (targeted immunosuppressive regimens being developed)
Type 1A diabetes	Anti-insulin antibodies as well as transglutaminase auto-antibodies	Immunosuppressive regimens

Abbreviations: Ach, acetylcholine; BPAG$_1$, bullous pemphigoid antigen$_1$; BPAG$_2$, bullous pemphigoid antigen$_2$; CD45RO, markers on cell surface; CD4 + CD45RO+ T-cell, T helper cell with CD4 marker; IL, interleukin; NMJ, neuromuscular junction; SLE, systemic lupus erythematosus; TNF-α tumor necrosis factor alpha.

☞ **The current vaccination recommendations for traumatic splenectomy patients call for administration of indicated vaccines as soon as possible, preferably prior to splenectomy (58).** ☞ Pneumococcal vaccine should be administered at least two weeks before an elective splenectomy. If the above time frames are not practical for various reasons, the patient should be immunized as soon as possible after recovery and before discharge from the hospital to minimize the possibility that the patient will be lost to follow-up prior to vaccination (58).

The three commonly administered vaccines used in the post-traumatic splenectomy patient are summarized in Table 5. Pneumococcal vaccine (Pneumovax 23) contains capsular polysaccharide antigens of 23 pneumococcal types, comprising 98% of pneumococcal disease isolates (59). As one might predict, the most virulent pneumococcal serotypes tend to be the least immunogenic. Unfortunately, vaccine efficacy is poorest in younger patients, who are at higher risk. However, under ideal conditions in a healthy immunocompetent host, the vaccine offers a 70% protection rate.

Amoxicillin is recommended for antibiotic prophylaxis against encapsulated bacteria in asplenic children, especially for the first two years after splenectomy (60). Patients who are allergic to penicillin should be offered erythromycin. Some investigators advocate continuing antibiotic prophylaxis in children for at least 5 years after splenectomy or until aged 16 (61), however, long term antibiotics are less frequently utilized.

PRE-EXISTING IMMUNOSUPPRESSIVE MEDICAL DISEASES

It is intuitive that known immunosuppression should adversely affect outcome in traumatic injury, and this is often the case. Disorders of the immune system can result from hypersensitivity reactions, such as anaphylaxis (Volume 1, Chapter 33), or from numerous triggers for SIRS (Volume 2, Chapter 63). Autoimmune diseases and immunodeficiency syndromes are also debilitating. Additionally, several important systemic diseases (including diabetes, renal failure, and liver failure) impair the native immune system, and will be briefly reviewed here.

Diabetes

It has long been known that hyperglycemia and diabetes predispose patients to infection (see Volume 2, Chapter 60). However, the role of diabetes and hyperglycemia in trauma-associated infections is just now becoming elucidated. In a large retrospective review of the Pennsylvania trauma registry over a two-year period, the group of patients with a history of diabetes had an increased risk of sepsis (odds ratio, 1.61) (62).

Several immunological mechanisms are distorted by hyperglycemia and diabetes. The release of IL-1 and oxygen radicals by macrophages and neutrophils is inhibited, and phagocytosis by macrophages is impaired (63). Conversely, tight glycemic control improves the leukocyte oxidative burst and phagocytic activity (64). Therefore, it is not surprising that tight glucose control with IV insulin in diabetic critically ill postoperative open-heart cardiac surgery patients demonstrated a reduced incidence of deep sternal wound infections (0.8% vs. 2% for subcutaneous insulin injections) (65) and decreased mortality overall (66,67). ☞ **The incidence of bacteremia is reduced by almost 50%, and sepsis-associated mortality is similarly reduced when critically ill patients are intensively treated with exogenous insulin to maintain normoglycemia.** ☞

The link between hyperglycemia and increased risk of serious infections, regardless of a previous history of diabetes, was provided only recently (see Volume 2, Chapter 60). Improved capacity to clear bacterial invaders with euglycemia was observed in a novel rabbit model of prolonged critical illness (68). In this study, Weekers et al. (68) demonstrated that aggravation of insulin resistance and hyperglycemia likely plays a role in the reduced phagocytosis capacity and impaired bacterial killing of monocytes, and that this can be ameliorated with insulin administration and tight blood sugar control. Diabetic patients have additional stigmata that may increase their risk of infection such as arteriolar sclerosis which decreases tissue perfusion to various vascular beds. However, titrating insulin to maintain tight blood glucose control at normal levels appears to markedly enhance the immune system of critically ill patients.

Renal Failure

Chronic renal failure (CRF), particularly in patients who are hemodialysis-dependent, results in considerable immunosuppression (69,70). Additionally, these patients have decreased perfusion to numerous tissue beds, and increased blood sugar, both of which favor microbial growth rather than host defense. Furthermore, these patients require specialized vascular access that can readily become seeded with infection with bacteremia (71).

☞ **Immune dysfunction in patients with renal failure involves both cellular (PMNs, T-cells, B-cells, dendritic cells), and humoral systems (alterations in complement, immunoglobulin levels, and cytokines) (72).** ☞ The accumulation of both low- and high-molecular-weight uremic toxins (e.g., *p*-cresol, guanidine compounds, oxidation products, and granulocyte inhibitory proteins) are believed to be causal. Additionally, the secondary hyperparathyroidism associated with CRF is also thought to play an immuno-inhibitory role. With the frequent co-morbidity of malnutrition, the immune system is even more profoundly impaired.

Of the known uremic retention solutes, *p*-cresol dose dependently decreases PMN function by depressing the respiratory burst activity at concentrations commonly found in CRF patients (73,74). The toxicity of *p*-cresol is greater in the setting of hypoalbuminemia, a common problem following trauma and critical illness (75). Additionally, a factor removed by continuous ambulatory peritoneal dialysis but not by conventional hemodialysis was found to inhibit the function of PMNs in CRF patients (76). Whether these "toxic factors" are cleared by continuous renal replacement therapies has not yet been fully established.

Intracellular calcium plays an important role in many cellular functions, and increased cytosolic calcium is associated with secondary hyperparathyroidism of CRF, and with alterations in PMN function (77). Interestingly, normalization of cytosolic calcium by treatment with a calcium channel blocker (verapamil) resulted in improved PMN function without influencing the elevated parathyroid levels (78).

Liver Failure

☞ **The immune system is altered in liver failure due to chronic inflammation, decreased production of proteins including complement with increased circulating TNF-α, and increased production of cytokines by the Kupffer cells.** ☞ Accordingly, bacterial infection is a frequent complication of cirrhosis, particularly in those patients with GI bleeding or ascites (79). Additionally, these patients often have other co-existing disease such as malnutrition and diabetes that further impair their immunologic response. Infection in patients with fulminant hepatic failure is a major source of morbidity as 44% to 80% of patients with fulminant hepatic failure develop bacterial infections. Empiric broad-spectrum antibiotics should be initiated on clinical suspicion of infection (80).

Bacterial and fungal infections are common in acute liver failure for a number of reasons. Patients with acute liver failure have diminished serum opsonic activity (81), faulty PMN leukocyte function (82), and impaired cell-mediated and humoral immunity (especially alcoholic cirrhosis) (83). Bacteremia is common because patients are comatose, have numerous indwelling catheters, and may be receiving H2-receptor blockers, steroid therapy, or broad-spectrum antibiotics. In one prospective study of 50 patients, 80% had culture-proven infection, and in half of the remaining patients, infection was suspected (though cultures were negative) (84). Gram-positive organisms, mainly streptococci and *S. aureus*, predominate in acute liver failure, suggesting that the entry through the skin is more important than GI entry (the pathway of Gram-negative organisms) (85). Regular microbial surveillance and aggressive treatment of presumed infection are essential, since prophylactic antibiotic regimens have shown little benefit (86). A finding of disseminated fungemia is particularly ominous (87).

Autoimmune Diseases

☞ **Autoimmune diseases result from a failure of immune tolerance; the immune system fails to recognize native cells and tissues as "self," instead treating these structures as though they are foreign invaders.** ☞ Damage occurs to native cells and organs due to activation of T-cells and/or B-cells, in the absence of an ongoing infection or other discernible cause (88). There are a number of known ways in which tolerance of self-tissues is bypassed and autoimmune disease occurs. Genetics is involved, and there is an increased incidence in females (approximately 75% of autoimmune diseases) (89). However, environmental triggers are also exceedingly important (and almost universally required). A typical environmental trigger is infection. For example, following Group A Streptococci infection, patients may develop rheumatic fever due to cross-reaction between the bacterial antigens and myocardial tissue. Additionally, viral infections can lead to gene insertions or immunogenic circulating proteins that can trigger immune cross reactivity. Some autoimmune diseases such as pemphigoid may result as a paraneoplastic syndrome (90). Finally, several putative autoimmune diseases may have an immunological component that is not antiself. For example, women with scleroderma who have had children have significantly higher levels of fetal WBCs circulating in their blood decades after pregnancy than do mothers without the disease (89). Perhaps, scleroderma will eventually become re-categorized as graft-versus-host disease.

Because autoimmune diseases can cause significant organ failure, it is not uncommon for these patients to become critically ill. When such patients are injured, their course is complicated by their unique organ system dysfunction and immunological dysregulation. Moreover, the heavy use of glucocorticoids potentiates overall immunosuppression. A complete review of these processes is beyond the scope of this text, and the reader is referred to a recent review by Davidson and Diamond for a more comprehensive discussion (88). Table 6 summarizes briefly the selected autoimmune diseases.

While the best remedy is treating the root cause of autoimmune disease (i.e., blocking the specific cytokines or chemokines produced by improperly regulated T- or B-cells), symptomatic relief is particularly important when the structure attacked by the immune system involves the central nervous system (CNS), or neuromuscular junction (e.g., myasthenia gravis). Plasma exchange and administration of IV immunoglobulin (IVIG) are both effective in many autoimmune neurologic diseases (91). However, the specificity of IVIG can vary, and the proper patient selection in terms of initiation and duration of long-term maintenance requires additional randomized clinical trials. Clinical symptom relief for myasthenia gravis is provided by administration of anticholinesterase drugs, such as pyridostigmine and neostigmine. Psoriasis is an example of an autoimmune disease where immunomodulation has been employed at several levels of the disease including: (*i*) inhibition of T-cell activation; (*ii*) depletion of pathogenic T-cells (high-affinity IL-2 receptor or CD4); (*iii*) inhibition of key adhesion molecules, for example, selectins or integrins [Integrins are adhesion molecules that confer mechanical stability between the cells and their environment (92). They also act as cellular sensors and signaling molecules. Adhesion molecules can be inhibited by drugs such as efalizumab, a monoclonal antibody that interferes with adhesion mediated by leukocyte-function-associated antigen 1]; (*iv*) inhibition of key inflammatory cytokines (the monoclonal antibodies infliximab and adalimumab, as well as the fusion proteins etanercept and onercept all focus upon TNF-α); and (*v*) shifting the cytokine milieu dominated by Th1 cells to a milieu weighted with Th2 cells, thus alleviating psoriasis by minimizing the IL-10 and IL-4 levels (93). There are no current studies reviewing the morbidity and mortality of pre-existing autoimmune diseases in trauma patients, but those with pre-existing organ dysfunction will have a more complicated course.

Elderly

Elderly patients who sustain traumatic injuries and burns have a higher mortality. One reason commonly cited is their compromised immune response (94–97). The elderly are also at increased risk for diabetes, renal insufficiency, liver insufficiency, and malnutrition, all associated with immune impairment. In addition, there is considerable evidence that both chronic and acute ingestion of ethanol causes suppression of the immune response as well as impaired intestinal immunity and barrier function (98,99). **With regard to malnutrition, a recent mouse perforated bowel study showed that malnutrition was an independent risk factor for infection and mortality (100).**

HIV/AIDS AND TRAUMA OR CRITICAL ILLNESS
Brief Review of HIV/AIDS

The acquired immunodeficiency syndrome (AIDS) is a profound immunosuppression state resulting from infection with HIV, causing opportunistic infections, secondary neoplasms, and neurological manifestations. The virus is transmitted inside infected CD4+ T-cells and macrophages. Clinically, the disease is spread sexually or through blood or blood products as encountered by IV drug abusers.

Two genetically distinct but related forms of HIV (HIV-1 and HIV-2) have been isolated from patients with AIDS. HIV-1 is the predominant source of AIDS in the United States, Europe, and Central Africa (where it likely originated from the chimpanzee) (101). HIV-2 is more prevalent in West Africa, where it likely emerged from the sooty mangabey monkeys indigenous there (102).

HIV infection targets the immune system along with the CNS. **The CD4 molecule is a high affinity receptor for HIV, explaining the tropism of the virus for CD4+ T-cells and other CD4+ cells (i.e., monocytes/macrophages, and Langerhans cells/dendritic cells). The loss of these cells leads to profound immunosuppression, primarily cell-mediated immunity.**

Early in the disease, HIV colonizes the lymphoid organs (spleen, lymph nodes, tonsils) producing over 100 billion viral particles per day, and killing one to two billion CD4+ T-cells daily. Initially, the immune system can regenerate the dying T-cells, and the CD4+ T-cell loss appears deceptively low. The Center for Disease Control classification of HIV stratifies patients into three categories on the basis of CD4+ T-cell counts: CD4+ ≥500, 200 to 499, and <200 cells/μL. Patients in the first group are usually asymptomatic, those with levels from 200 to 499 are associated with early symptoms, and levels below 200 are associated with severe immunosuppression; the last group is conventionally considered to have AIDS.

The HIV epidemic continues to expand globally, especially in third world countries (103). The U.S. statistics demonstrate that AIDS- and HIV-related deaths peaked in 1993, but that the prevalence of HIV continues to increase (104). Indeed, in December 2004, the estimated prevalence of HIV infected individuals was near one million persons (including 180,000–280,000 who do not know they are infected) (105).

Trauma and Critical Illness Involving HIV+ Patients

As the prevalence of HIV increases, traumatologists will become increasingly involved in the care of HIV-positive (HIV+) patients. A recent study of HIV infection in trauma patients demonstrated a prevalence of 0.3% (106). Most other North American trauma centers have reported a higher prevalence of HIV infection ranging between 0.96% and 4.3% (107,108). In one study, male patients from an urban area who were victims of interpersonal violence had an HIV prevalence of 3.5% (107).

HIV and AIDS can undoubtedly affect outcome in trauma patients. Much has been written about the prevalence of HIV infection in trauma patients, however, little is known about how the infection affects morbidity and mortality in these patients. Similarly, the stresses of trauma may affect the progression of HIV disease, yet little is actually known about these relationships either. Indeed, no randomized prospective trials have been conducted in trauma patients to evaluate the effects of HIV disease.

Patients who were identified as being immunosuppressed (AIDS, HIV+, routine steroid use, transplants, or active chemotherapy) have a markedly increased risk of sepsis (odds ratio, 4.43) (62). In other studies, HIV+ patients have been more likely to develop infection after bony fracture (109), and HIV+ burned patients were more likely to develop systemic infections with higher associated mortality (110). In contrast, those patients who did not develop infection had similar length of stay and recovery characteristics as non-HIV+ patients, also the case in a study of nonburn traumatic injury (106). Another study showed no increased mortality in burned patients with HIV infection compared with previously healthy controls (111).

A recent Pennsylvania trauma outcome study (PTOS), retrospectively evaluated the status of HIV disease in trauma (106). PTOS reported some anticipated results, for example, that the majority of HIV+ patients were male, with a mean age of 39 years. The study also showed higher rates of penetrating trauma among HIV+ patients than in control patients, a pattern previously reported by others (112,113).

However, PTOS has made a first estimation at quantifying the various risk factors and co-morbidities. Compared with age-matched controls, HIV+ trauma patients were significantly more likely to suffer from chronic drug and alcohol use; neurologic disorders; renal, pulmonary, GI, and liver disease; non-HIV hematologic disease; and a history of psychiatric diagnosis (all $P < 0.01$) (106).

The HIV+ status was also associated with significantly longer hospital length of stay (10.2 days vs. 6.8 days for controls, $P = 0.001$). Additionally, HIV+ patients spent more days in the ICU ($P < 0.02$), and were more likely to remain in the ICU for >7 days (106). These observations are partly explained by the greater overall number of complications in the HIV+ group.

Although there was no overall statistical difference in mortality between the two groups (3.6% vs. 3.1%, $P = 0.6447$), infection/sepsis and pulmonary complications were associated with significant mortality in HIV+ patients. HIV+ patients also underwent more thoracostomies (7.5% vs. 4.4%, $P < 0.03$) and exploratory laparotomies (7.0% vs. 2.4%, $P < 0.001$) (106).

The greater proportion of pulmonary complications in HIV+ patients occurred despite lack of significant difference in abbreviated injury scale score for the chest between the two groups. In a separate study by Rosen et al. (114) involving 63 HIV+ patients admitted to an ICU, 44% of those patients required mechanical ventilation, with a 57% associated mortality.

The PTOS study authors speculated that the incidence of post-traumatic complications may be related to the greater frequency of pre-existing conditions in the HIV+ trauma population. Although exact diagnoses are not reported in the PTOS database, HIV+ patients had nearly double the rate of pre-existing pulmonary disease compared with control patients. In the Rosen study of HIV+ ICU patients, 16 of 25 patients who died had primary pulmonary diagnosis and 3 of 25 died as a result of sepsis (114). In another study, mortality with a pleural effusion was two times higher for HIV+ patients with pleural effusion than for those without effusion (115). Others showed that the incidence of bacterial infectious complications in trauma patients was tied to increasing ISS and not the CD4 count (116).

HIV+ patients in the PTOS study underwent more operative procedures than the control group, and had nearly twice the frequency of exploratory laparotomy and chest tubes, and more frequent laparoscopy and thoracotomy (106). Hebra et al. (117) examined the types of procedures performed on 150 HIV+ patients admitted to the hospital for various surgical procedures (including trauma, general surgical, orthopedic, cardiac, thoracic, and vascular procedures). They found that nearly half of 30 operations performed on their patients were performed to treat AIDS-related complications or to facilitate the workup of AIDS patients (117). In contrast, a study in burn patients showed similar number of procedures in HIV+ and control groups (118). The disparity of these results (especially without reporting absolute CD4+ T-cell numbers) emphasize the current inability to predict the relative detrimental outcome weight that HIV+ status connotes for various injuries.

Although the overall HIV+ patient mortality was not statistically different from the control group in the PTOS study, the operative mortality for HIV+ patient was 5.6%. Other studies agree with this finding, with mortality rates ranging from 3.8% to 5% (116,119). Additionally, having the stigmata of AIDS increases mortality (118,119). In a small study involving 10 general surgical patients with AIDS who underwent emergency laparotomy, Burack et al. (120) reported a 70% mortality in the postoperative period.

Although it has been suggested that major surgery or trauma can advance a patient's HIV stage as measured using the World Health Organization HIV clinical staging system (120–122), PTOS did not investigate this phenomenon. Other significant limitations of this study include its retrospective nature, inability to distinguish asymptomatic HIV from symptomatic AIDS, and lack of information on CD4+ count and retroviral or antimicrobial therapies used.

HIV Drugs During Trauma and Critical Care

Complex treatment regimens are frequently required to manage unique infectious diseases and medical problems in HIV+ patients (123). However, there have not been any recent reviews in medical management for the HIV+ trauma patient in a decade (124).

The most common current therapy for HIV+ patients include the protease inhibitors that block the protease enzyme used by HIV to infect new cells. Protease inhibitors can reduce the amount of virus in the blood and increase CD4+ T-cell counts. In some cases, these drugs have improved CD4+ T-cell counts, even when they were very low or zero.

With the advent of protease inhibitors in combination with other drugs, the number of HIV+ patients who became ill from opportunistic infections, or died from AIDS, dropped by about 70%. However, some HIV strains have become resistant to protease inhibitors. Thus, it is recommended that protease inhibitors be taken in combination with at least two other anti-HIV drugs. This is called highly active anti-retroviral therapy or HAART, which increases the anti-HIV effect, and helps prevent resistance.

Nine Food and Drug Administration (FDA) approved protease inhibitors are available: darunavir (Prezista®), indinavir (Crixivan®), lopinavir/ritonavir (Kaletra®), ritonavir (Norvir®), saquinavir (Fortovase® and Invirase®), nelfinavir (Viracept®), and atazanavir (Rayataz®), tipranavir (Aptivus®), and fosamprenavir (Lexiva®).

Because of the rapidly expanding array of anti-HIV drugs, and the rapidity with which research results are changing in this area, any recommendations regarding the general treatment of HIV+ patients is likely to become quickly obsolete. Accordingly, readers are referred to the latest recommendations from the International AIDS Society—USA Panel (123). In addition, when HIV+ patients are admitted to the trauma unit or surgical ICU, it is

Table 7 Categories of Micro-organisms Responsible for Sepsis in Immunocompromised Patients According to Various Etiologies of Impaired Immunity

Cause of impaired immune status	Gram-positive bacteria	Gram-negative bacteria	*Listeria, Legionella, Mycobacteria*	CMV and other HSV	Respiratory viruses	*Candida* species	Aspergillus and other molds
Sepsis	++	+	−	+/−	+/−	++	+
Glucocorticoids	+	+	++	+/−	+/−	+++	++
Neutropenia	++	+++	−	−	+	+++	++
HIV/AIDS	++	++	++	+	+/−	++	++
Solid organ transplant	+	+	+	+++	+	+++	+++
HSCT	+	+	+	+++	+++	++	+++

Abbreviations: CMV, cytomegalovirus; AIDS, autoimmune deficiency syndrome; HIV, human immunodeficiency virus; HSCT, hematopoietic stem cell transplant; HSV, herpes simplex virus; −, not a significant problem; +, occasional problem; +/−, may become a problem; ++, significant problem; +++, major problem.
Source: From Ref. 125.

recommended that an HIV specialist be immediately consulted to assist with the decisions regarding antiretroviral, and other immunological therapy.

INFECTIOUS DISEASES IN THE IMMUNOCOMPROMISED

A consensus document was published in 2004 by an international group of critical care and infectious disease experts containing management guidelines for sepsis associated with immunosuppressive medications (125). The most commonly described infectious complications of immunosuppressive therapy are summarized in Table 7. The most common immunosuppressant medications are corticosteroids, cytoreductive agents such as methotrexate, immunophilin-binding agents such as tacrolimus, mycophenolate, anti-TNF agents, and other monoclonal antibodies and fusion proteins. Agents are commonly used in combination making the exact risk of infection for any one agent or patient difficult to discern. Nevertheless, patterns of infection have been noted and Table 7 shows the likely categories of micro-organisms for different types of patients.

It is very important to make the correct diagnosis to appropriately direct therapy at the causative organism. The preferred methods for diagnosis of the common pathogens infecting immunocompromised patients are summarized in Table 8. Interestingly, various categories of immunosuppressive drugs are associated with a specific set of infectious organisms that are normally suppressed by pathways they disrupt (Table 9). Finally, treatment recommendations based upon the status of the patient are given in Table 10.

It is useful to recognize that no unique combination of antibiotics is universally appropriate in this setting. The prevalent pathogens in a given ICU and antibiotics currently being administered must be put into the context of the patient's immunocompromised status and infectious symptoms. Prompt initiation of adequate antimicrobial coverage is of utmost importance; any delay results in worse outcome for the patient (126–129). Therefore, most experts in the management of immunocompromised patients tend to use very broad-spectrum coverage initially when dealing with severe sepsis of unknown origin in this patient population. Once the pathogens have been accurately identified, the coverage can be tailored more specifically. The reader is referred to Volume 2, Chapter 53 for a more complete review of the antimicrobial options.

TRANSPLANTATION AND TRAUMA

Although the number of trauma patients presenting with a history of organ transplantation is small, these patients have a more complicated interaction between immunosuppression and inflammation than others. The risk of infection is related to the patient's overall immune state, including patient factors and medication effects, and the intensity of exposure to potential pathogens (130). In the hospital, these patients may become infected more easily from exposure to pathogens from other patients as well as contamination of air, water, or equipment in the building. Given the fact that steroids are the mainstay of most immunosuppressive regimens following transplant, these patients are at increased risk for osteoporosis and bony fractures (131–134). It is reasonable to assume that transplant recipients will be a small, but regular clientele on the trauma service. The typical timing of certain types of infection after transplant is reviewed below.

1. *First month following transplantation* ✔ **During the first month after solid organ transplantation, the infections usually encountered in transplant recipients are the same as those found in a typical surgical population (135).** ✔ Like other cases, the most important factors determining the incidence of infections are the type of operation, the technical skill applied to the operation, and the postoperative care of the patient. Duration of vascular access, use of drainage catheters, duration of intubation, and presence of indwelling stents, devitalized tissue, or fluids will all increase infection risk. Although uncommon, primary infection may be transmitted from the donor with the allograft. Opportunistic infections are also uncommon during the first month after transplant. If opportunistic infections occur during the first post-transplant month, it likely indicates significant environmental exposure, immunosuppressive state prior to transplant, or pre-existing infection in the donor or recipient (130).

2. *Second through sixth month following transplantation* ✔ **After the first month, the immunomodulating viruses can become clinically significant, in addition to residual agents from prior infections and events.** ✔ The combination of sustained immunosuppression and viral infection with cytomegalovirus (CMV), EBV, hepatitis B virus (HBV), hepatitis C virus (HCV), or HIV makes infection with opportunistic infections *Pneumocystis carinii*, Aspergillus, Candida, and *Listeria monocytogenes* more likely. This time period is when immunosuppression is typically at the highest.

Table 8 Diagnostic Methodology for Selected Pathogens in Immunocompromised Patients

Suspected pathogen	Method of diagnosis	Alternate diagnosis	Comments
Bacteria			
Fastidious or unusual bacteria	Two to three BCs using aerobic and anaerobic bottles containing resin or charcoal neutralization particles	Standard aerobic, anaerobic BC bottles	Prolonged (i.e., 7–14 days incubation required
Legionella species	BAL or sputum Cx. *Legionella* may not be seen in Gram stain or DFA of respiratory secretions	Urinary antigens PCR promising, but no standardized assay available	Urinary antigen detects only *Legionella pneumophila* serotype 1
Nocardia	Modified acid-fast stain or GMS of respiratory secretions or tissue Bx	Blood culture (note these may frequently be negative)	Beaded branching gram-positive bacilli should raise suspicion
Mycobacterium tuberculosis	Fluorochrome stain of BAL or sputum; amplification of rRNA or DNA using TB rapid broth Cx (Bactec, BactAlert, ESP systems)	Transbronchial Bx in case of negative BAL; bone marrow Bx if disseminated "miliary" TB	Disseminated TB may have skin lesions amenable to Bx. QuantiFERON-TB®Gold (QFT) can measure TB proteins in blood
Nontuberculous mycobacteria	Sputum/BAL in case of lung lesions	BC (isolator or rapid mycobacterial bottle); Bx of skin lesions	Bone marrow Cx is not more sensitive than BC, but may allow for earlier Dx
Fungi			
Pneumocystis jiroveci (formerly *Pneumocystis carinii*)	Direct fluorescence antibody from induced sputum or BAL	Silver stain from induced sputum or BAL	PCR may be more sensitive, particularly in non-HIV patients
Candida species	Bx of suspicious lesions; 2–3 aerobic BCs plus Cx of catheters	Funduscopic exam may be suggestive; CT scan helpful in chronic disseminated candidiasis	BCs may be negative in acute, and are typically negative in chronic disseminated candidiasis
Cryptococcus neoformans	EIA detection of cryptococcal antigen in serum or CSF	Two to three BCs; CSF India ink and Cx	
Histoplasma capsulatum	Stain of tissue Bx, two lysis-centrifugation (isolator) BCs	EIA detection of histoplasma antigen in urine; two aerobic BCs	Urine antigen positive only in disseminated disease
Mold infections (*Aspergillus* species, *Fusarium* species, etc)	BAL; biopsy of any suspicious lesion; sputum, tracheal aspirate, bronchial brush	Plasma galactomannan antigenemia (but this cross reacts with some other molds such as *Penicillium*)	Isolation of molds from sputum indicates high risk of invasive disease—not to be ignored
Viruses			
CMV	CMV antigen detection, CMV PCR, shell vial from BAL	Viral Cx; cytopathic effect seen in cells from BAL suggests pneumonia	CMV antigen in the blood, and CMV PCR in the BAL does not mean CMV is causing disease
EBV	Quantitative PCR in blood (also useful for monitoring viral load)	Bx with immunohistochemistry is required for Dx of EBV lymphoproliferative disease	EBV causes lymphoproliferative disease in some transplant patients
Human herpes virus 6	PCR (preferably quantitative) detection of DNA in CSF	Serology (usually EIA) for IgM antibody; IgG only confirms previous infection	Detection of human herpes virus 6 by PCR in serum does not mean there is active disease
Adenovirus	Direct immunofluorescence staining and cell Cx (or shell vial) of secretions; BAL or blood PCR	Electron microscopy of respiratory secretions	Disseminated infection is Dx'd when adenovirus is found in the blood by PCR or if isolated from three different body sites

(Continued)

Table 8   Diagnostic Methodology for Selected Pathogens in Immunocompromised Patients (*Continued*)

Suspected pathogen	Method of diagnosis	Alternate diagnosis	Comments
Parasites			
Toxoplasma gondii	PCR detection of DNA in blood, BAL, or lung tissue; cysts may occasionally be seen on Giemsa staining of lung or other tissues	Serology—IgM often negative, presence of IgG only confirms previous infection	Ninety percent of toxoplasmosis disease in critical illness is reactivation; septic shock can occur in AIDS and transplant patients
Strongyloides hyperinfection	First-stage "filariform" larvae in BAL, sputum, and feces; detection of adult larvae and eggs in intestine Bx (obtained by EGD)	Serology; migration test of larvae by plating stool on blood agar plate	The clinical syndrome of *Strongyloides* hyperinfection includes recurrent polymicrobial bacteremia with enteric bacteria

Abbreviations: AIDS, acquired immunodeficiency syndrome; BAL, bronchoalveolar lavage; BC, blood culture; Bx, biopsy; CMV, cytomegalovirus; CSF, cerebral spinal fluid; CSF, colony-stimulating factor; CT, computed tomography; Cx, culture; DFA, direct fluorescent assay; Dx, diagnosis; EGD, esophagogastroduodenoscopy; EIA, enzyme-linked immunoassay; GMS, Gomori methenamine silver; IgM, immunoglobulin M; PCR, polymerase chain reaction; rRNA, recombinant RNA; TB, *Mycobacterium tuberculosis*.
Source: From Ref. 125.

3. *Beyond 6 Months* Most transplant patients are maintained on minimal long-term immunosuppressive therapy with good allograft function after 6 months. The most common infection in these patients is respiratory and is generally similar to what is seen in the general community. Opportunistic infections are rare unless there has been an unusually intense exposure (130). A small group of patients will have ongoing viral infection with human papillovavirus, HBV, HCV, CMV, or EBV. The most challenging patients are those who develop recurrent or chronic rejection requiring an escalation in the use of immunosuppressive agents and a corresponding increased risk of chronic viral infections. These patients are very prone to opportunistic infections and must be guarded carefully.

A few other considerations in transplant recipients are worth mention. Transplant patients who are seronegative for varicella-zoster virus should receive varicella immune globulin and antiviral prophylaxis if exposed to varicella-zoster virus. These people are at risk for developing chronic active infection if exposed. The use of prophylactic therapy such as trimethoprim-sulfamethoxazole during the first 4 to 12 months after transplantation has markedly reduced the incidence of *P. carinii*, other respiratory infections, and urinary tract infections. When antibiotics are needed for transplant patients, the interactions with the immunosuppressive regimen must be carefully considered. Some combinations are particularly problematic and can cause excessive toxicity. Aggressive modes of diagnosing infection in immunocompromised patients are warranted, such as bronchoalveolar lavage for pulmonary infiltrates (136), because the patient's presentation may be altered due to their immunocompromised status. Consultation with experts in transplantation and infectious disease may be very helpful.

EYE TO THE FUTURE

An area of great promise is that of human genomics and the possibility of identifying patients at high risk for either excessive immunoactivation or immunosuppression at the time of presentation after traumatic injury occurs (137,138).

This may permit patient-specific interventions to modify the natural response to the patient's benefit (139). In fact, it is already known that gender can play a role in outcome after traumatic injury. It seems that females are immunologically in a better position to recover from a septic insult than males (62,140).

Some of the potentially promising new treatment options are interference with MIF, HMGB1, C5a, or TREM-1 signal transduction pathways and an inhibition of apoptosis (141). These interventions, or others, may improve the prognosis of septic patients in the future. Simple measures including thorough irrigation and debridement of contaminated wounds will likely continue to be a mainstay of therapy, just as proper immunizational prophylaxis against tetanus continues to be important (142).

The relationships between the neuroendocrine and immune systems is another area of future interest as we learn how these systems interact (143). Indeed, some are attempting to develop a unifying theory of post-traumatic inflammation with the hope that this might better guide our research efforts and make sense of the many components. One such theory is based on the nutritional needs of cells following traumatic injury (144). Early immunonutrition may after the cytokine balance preventing SIRS and/or CARS. It is hoped that this type of immunity-based thinking will improve the treatment of our patients, by giving rise to new ideas and therapies.

SUMMARY

Traumatic injuries disrupt natural barriers to infection. Immunocompetent patients who sustain these injuries are likely to experience an acute inflammatory response that is proportional to the degree of tissue destruction, followed by a more prolonged immunosuppressed state. Patients suffering trauma with a pre-existing immunosuppressed state may not have as exuberant of an initial inflammatory response, but are at increased risk of infection and involvement of atypical organisms.

Table 9 Association Between Immunosuppressive Drugs and Specific Infections

Agent	Mechanism of action	Infection	Comments
Corticosteroids	Prevents release of IL-1 and IL-2 from macrophages; inhibits phagocytosis by macrophages and PMNs; prevents T-cell proliferation and Ig production	Bacterial infection most common; HSV, fungi (*Candida, Aspergillus, Cryptococcus, Pneumocystis*), and *Strongyloides* superinfection	No increased risk with <10 mg of prednisone equivalent per day or <700 mg cumulative; aspergillosis risk after allogeneic BMT increases with ≥1 mg/kg prednisone equivalent for ≥1 week
Calcineurin inhibitors [Cyclosporine A (CsA), Tacrolimus]	CsA binds to cyclophilin-A; tacrolimus binds to FKBP12; inhibiting calcineurin and decreasing IL-2 gene transcription and T-cell proliferation	No specific association with severe infection	Role of CsA and tacrolimus alone is difficult to quantitate, but appear to be associated with the smallest risk of infection compared with other agents
Sirolimus (rapamycin)	Inhibits lymphocyte proliferation	Decreased risk of CMV infection compared with CsA and tacrolimus	One study reported increased risk of invasive aspergillosis
Cyclophosphamide	Inhibits lymphocyte proliferation	Bacterial complications of neutropenia, herpes zoster	
Azathioprine	Inhibits lymphocyte proliferation	Bacterial complications of neutropenia	No difference in infection rate between methotrexate with azathioprine in rheumatoid arthritis
Mycophenolate (MMF)	Antilymphoproliferative agent (purine synthesis inhibition)	Increased incidence of CMV disease, VZV	No increase in bacterial or fungal infections; less frequency of *Pneumocystis*
Methotrexate	Inhibits lymphocyte proliferation	*Histoplasmosis, Listeria, Pneumocystis*	*Pneumocystis* is the most common opportunistic infection associated with methotrexate
Anti-TNF-α agents (etanercept, infliximab)	Infliximab is a chimeric Ab against human TNF-α, and can fix complement and lyse target cells; etanercept is a modified soluble TNF-α receptor	Bacteremia, *Listeria*, tuberculosis, cryptococcosis, aspergillosis, CMV	Severe infection most common with infliximab; also, diminished signs and symptoms of infection until they are very advanced
Anti-CD25 antibodies (daclizumab, basiliximab)	Blocks high-affinity IL-2 receptors	No increase in bacterial, fungal, or viral infections	Delayed wound healing described by manufacturer
Purine analogues (2-chlorodeoxyadenosine, fludarabine)	Inhibits DNA synthesis	*Cryptococcus, Listeria*, herpes virus	Used in hematologic malignancies (themselves immunosuppressive)
Alemtuzumab (campath)	Anti-CD52, targets T- and B-lymphocytes, monocytes	Respiratory virus, adenovirus, CMV	Reactivation of CMV is common; CMV disease is rare except with HSCT

Abbreviations: BMT, allogeneic bone marrow transplantation; CMV, cytomegalovirus; CNV, choroidal neovascularization; FKBP, FK-site binding protein; HSCT, hemopoietic stem cell transplantation; HSV, herpex simplex virus; IL, interleulcin; PMN, polymorphonuclear neutrophil; TNF, tumor necrosis factor; VZV, varicella-zoster virus.

The balance between the inflammatory and immunosuppressive responses can also be affected by the type and timing of therapeutic interventions employed, including surgery, transfusion, and IV access choices. Indeed, each of these interventions primarily intended to treat the patient with traumatic injuries can increase the likelihood of associated infectious complications.

A significant number of patients are at increased risk of infectious complications due to immunocompromise-related illness such as renal failure, liver failure, diabetes, HIV, malignancy, autoimmune disease, malnutrition, or therapies including use of steroids, chemotherapy, or splenectomy. These patients deserve special attention in regards to infectious complications. Broad-spectrum antibiotic coverage should be started without delay in immunocompromised patients who demonstrate evidence of sepsis.

Understanding the balance between inflammation and immunosuppression following trauma will likely lead to improved treatment modalities. The current goals of therapy may be best approached in terms of restoring appropriate balance between immunostimulation and immunosuppression.

Table 10 Immunocompromised States and Empirical Antibiotic Recommendations

Cause of immunosuppression	Pathogens causing severe sepsis	Recommended empirical antimicrobials[a]	Comments
Neutropenia	Enteric gram-negative bacilli, *Pseudomonas aeruginosa*, viridans group streptococci, *Candida* species	Carbapenem or cefepime or piperacillin/tazobactam + a quinolone or aminoglycoside ± vancomycin	Antifungal coverage should be added if shock develops late in the course of neutropenia or if there is evidence of Candida colonization
Splenectomy	*Streptococcus pneumoniae*, *Haemophilus influenzae*, meningococcus, others	Third generation cephalosporin + vancomycin	Patients should be vaccinated against encapsulated organisms (Table 6)
HIV/AIDS	*P. aeruginosa*, *Staphylococcus aureus*, *S. pneumoniae*, *Salmonella enteritidis*, *Cryptococcus neoformans*; rarely: *Toxoplasma gondii*, Helicobacter, *Mycobacterium tuberculosis*	Ceftazidime or fluoroquinolone + vancomycin ± amphotericin B lipid formulation	Stage of disease and associated risk factors also to be considered: IVDA is risk factor for *S. aureus*; Neutropenia for *Pseudomonas*; only advanced AIDS increases risk for septic shock due to *Cryptococcus* and *Toxoplasma*
Solid organ transplant— early	Surgical site source: gram-negative bacilli (including *Pseudomonas*), *S. aureus*, and VRE	Antipseudomonal beta-lactam + linezolid	
Solid organ transplant— late	Pathogens related to defect in cell-mediated immunity (e.g., *Legionella*, *Listeria*, etc.)	Flouroquinolone ± vancomycin	
HSCT—pre-engraftment	See "neutropenia" above	See "neutropenia" above	See "neutropenia" above
HSCT—early (<day 100)	Without GVHD: catheter-related *Staphylococcus epidermidis*, *S. aureus*, nonfermentative gram-negative bacilli; with acute GVHD: enteric gram-negative bacilli, fungi	Too diverse for sole recommendation; combination therapy appropriate in septic shock	When considering antifungal coverage, septic shock is more commonly caused by *Candida* sp., than with mold infections; consider azole-resistant Candida
HSCT—late (≥100 days)	Chronic GVHD: combination of splenectomized and steroid-recipients	Third generation cephalosporin + vancomycin	Consider specific immunosuppressive agents being used

[a]These recommendations are based upon expert opinion and present a logical empirical approach. Local microbial resistance patterns, or known colonization with resistant pathogens should also be considered.
Abbreviations: AIDS, acquired immunodeficiency syndrome; GVHD, graft-versus-host disease; HIV, human immunodeficiency virus; HSCT, hematopoietic stem cell transplant; IVDA, intravenous drug abuse; VRE, vancomycin-resistant enterococcus.
Source: From Ref. 125.

KEY POINTS

- Once a pathogen has overcome the primary barrier of the skin, respiratory, GI, or genito-urinary epithelium, the immune system must then combat the invader.
- The CD4 and CD8 proteins are expressed on two mutually exclusive sets of T-cells, and are co-receptors of T-cell activation.
- The important regulatory role of CD4+ T-cells is evident when HIV infects the host and selectively kills CD4+ T-cells.
- Immunoglobulin M (IgM) is present on the surface of all B-cells, comprising the antigen-binding component of the B-cell receptor.
- The first cells to migrate to areas of injury following trauma are the polymorphonuclear neutrophils (PMNs) with quantities peaking in the first 24 hours, followed by the macrophages, which reach their zenith at 72 hours.

- When the host has pre-existing circulating antibodies due to vaccination or prior infection, microbial replication can be halted at the onset of infection.
- Although there is no immunologic specificity in complement activation, or in its effects, there are several immunological methods by which the complement system can be activated.
- Hypersensitivity reactions are exuberant, improperly regulated immunological responses to various antigenic molecules resulting in tissue injury to the host.
- Damage control surgery in severely injured patients was first applied to abdominal surgery (Volume 1, Chapter 21), and is now known to improve outcome for orthopedic trauma surgery as well (29).
- The risk of OPSS is particularly high following splenectomy in children under five years of age (especially infants splenectomized for trauma, with reported infection rates of >10%) (53).

✎ The current vaccination recommendations for traumatic splenectomy patients call for administration of indicated vaccines as soon as possible, preferably prior to splenectomy (58).

✎ The incidence of bacteremia is reduced by almost 50%, and sepsis-associated mortality is similarly reduced when critically ill patients are intensively treated with exogenous insulin to maintain normoglycemia.

✎ Immune dysfunction in patients with renal failure involves both cellular (PMNs, T-cells, B-cells, dendritic cells), and humoral systems (alterations in complement, immunoglobulin levels, and cytokines) (72).

✎ The immune system is altered in liver failure due to chronic inflammation, decreased production of proteins including complement with increased circulating TNF-α, and increased production of cytokines by the Kuppfer cells.

✎ Autoimmune diseases result from a failure of immune tolerance: the immune system fails to recognize native cells and tissues as "self," instead treating these structures as though they are foreign invaders.

✎ With regard to malnutrition, a recent mouse perforated bowel study showed that malnutrition was an independent risk factor for infection and mortality (100).

✎ The CD4 molecule is a high affinity receptor for HIV, explaining the tropism of the virus for CD4+ T-cells and other CD4+ cells (i.e., monocytes/macrophages, and Langerhans cells/dendritic cells). The loss of these cells leads to profound immunosuppression, primarily cell-mediated immunity.

✎ During the first month after solid organ transplantation, the infections usually encountered in transplant recipients are the same as those found in a typical surgical population (135).

✎ After the first month, the immunomodulating viruses can become clinically significant, in addition to residual agents from prior infections and events.

REFERENCES

1. Delves PJ, Roitt IM. The immune system. First of two parts. N Engl J Med 2000; 343:37–49.
2. Delves PJ, Roitt IM. The immune system. Second of two parts. N Engl J Med 2000; 343:108–117.
3. Luster AD. Chemokines–chemotactic cytokines that mediate inflammation. N Engl J Med 1998; 338:436–445.
4. Walport MJ. Advances in immunology: complement. First of two parts. N Engl J Med 2001; 344:1058–1066.
5. Walport MJ. Advances in immunology: complement. Second of two parts. N Engl J Med 2001; 344:1140–1144.
6. Giannoudis PV. Current concepts of the inflammatory response after major trauma: an update. Injury 2003; 34:397–404.
7. Ertel W, Keel M, Bonaccio M, et al. Release of anti-inflammatory mediators after mechanical trauma correlates with severity of injury and clinical outcome. J Trauma 1995; 39:879–885; discussion 885–887.
8. Keel M, Schregenberger N, Steckholzer U, et al. Endotoxin tolerance after severe injury and its regulatory mechanisms. J Trauma 1996; 41:430–437; discussion 437–438.
9. Rodeberg DA, Meyer JG, Babcock GF. Heat shock response: presence and effects in burn patient neutrophils. J Leukoc Biol 1999; 66:773–780.
10. Menger MD, Vollmar B. Surgical trauma: hyperinflammation versus immunosuppression? Langenbecks Arch Surg 2004; 389:475–484.
11. Giannoudis PV, Smith MR, Evans RT, Bellamy MC, Guillou PJ. Serum CRP and IL-6 levels after trauma. Not predictive of septic complications in 31 patients. Acta Orthop Scand 1998; 69:184–188.
12. Wanner GA, Keel M, Steckholzer U, Beier W, Stocker R, Ertel W. Relationship between procalcitonin plasma levels and severity of injury, sepsis, organ failure, and mortality in injured patients. Crit Care Med 2000; 28:950–957.
13. Oberhoffer M, Karzai W, Meier-Hellmann A, Bogel D, Fassbinder J, Reinhart K. Sensitivity and specificity of various markers of inflammation for the prediction of tumor necrosis factor-alpha and interleukin-6 in patients with sepsis. Crit Care Med 1999; 27:1814–1818.
14. Reinhart K, Menges T, Gardlund B, et al. Randomized, placebo-controlled trial of the anti-tumor necrosis factor antibody fragment afelimomab in hyperinflammatory response during severe sepsis: the RAMSES study. Crit Care Med 2001; 29:765–769.
15. Abraham E. Why immunomodulatory therapies have not worked in sepsis. Intensive Care Med 1999; 25:556–566.
16. Giannoudis PV, Smith RM, Perry SL, Windsor AJ, Dickson RA, Bellamy MC. Immediate IL-10 expression following major orthopaedic trauma: relationship to anti-inflammatory response and subsequent development of sepsis. Intensive Care Med 2000; 26:1076–1081.
17. Pape HC, van Griensven M, Rice J, et al. Major secondary surgery in blunt trauma patients and perioperative cytokine liberation: determination of the clinical relevance of biochemical markers. J Trauma 2001; 50:989–1000.
18. Taniguchi T, Koido Y, Aiboshi J, Yamashita T, Suzaki S, Kurokawa A. The ratio of interleukin-6 to interleukin-10 correlates with severity in patients with chest and abdominal trauma. Am J Emerg Med 1999; 17:548–551.
19. Cheadle WG, Hershman MJ, Wellhausen SR, Polk HC Jr. HLA-DR antigen expression on peripheral blood monocytes correlates with surgical infection. Am J Surg 1991; 161:639–645.
20. Hershman MJ, Cheadle WG, Wellhausen SR, Davidson PF, Polk HC Jr. Monocyte HLA-DR antigen expression characterizes clinical outcome in the trauma patient. Br J Surg 1990; 77:204–207.
21. Giannoudis PV, Smith RM, Windsor AC, Bellamy MC, Guillou PJ. Monocyte human leukocyte antigen-DR expression correlates with intrapulmonary shunting after major trauma. Am J Surg 1999; 177:454–459.
22. Babcock GF. Predictive medicine: severe trauma and burns. Cytometry B Clin Cytom 2003; 53:48–53.
23. Keel M, Ecknauer E, Stocker R, et al. Different pattern of local and systemic release of proinflammatory and anti-inflammatory mediators in severely injured patients with chest trauma. J Trauma 1996; 40:907–912; discussion 912–914.
24. Ayala A, Ertel W, Chaudry IH. Trauma-induced suppression of antigen presentation and expression of major histocompatibility class II antigen complex in leukocytes. Shock 1996; 5:79–90.
25. Maekawa K, Futami S, Nishida M, et al. Effects of trauma and sepsis on soluble L-selectin and cell surface expression of L-selectin and CD11b. J Trauma 1998; 44:460–468.
26. Weigand MA, Schmidt H, Pourmahmoud M, Zhao Q, Martin E, Bardenheuer HJ. Circulating intercellular adhesion molecule-1 as an early predictor of hepatic failure in patients with septic shock. Crit Care Med 1999; 27:2656–2661.
27. Giannoudis PV, Abbott C, Stone M, Bellamy MC, Smith RM. Fatal systemic inflammatory response syndrome following early bilateral femoral nailing. Intensive Care Med 1998; 24:641–642.
28. Pape HC, Schmidt RE, Rice J, et al. Biochemical changes after trauma and skeletal surgery of the lower extremity: quantification of the operative burden. J Orthop Trauma 2004; 18:S24–S31.
29. Harwood PJ, Giannoudis PV, van Griensven M, Krettek C, Pape HC. Alterations in the systemic inflammatory response after early total care and damage control procedures for femoral shaft fracture in severely injured patients. J Trauma 2005; 58:446–452; discussion 452–454.

30. Pape HC, Dwenger A, Regel G, et al. Increased gut permeability after multiple trauma. Br J Surg 1994; 81:850–852.

31. Samonte VA, Goto M, Ravindranath TM, et al. Exacerbation of intestinal permeability in rats after a two-hit injury: burn and *Enterococcus faecalis* infection. Crit Care Med 2004; 32:2267–2273.

32. Alexander JW, Boyce ST, Babcock GF, et al. The process of microbial translocation. Ann Surg 1990; 212:496–510; discussion 511–512.

33. Gianotti L, Alexander JW, Pyles T, Gennari R, Babcock GF. Translocation and survival of *Bacteroides fragilis* after thermal injury. J Burn Care Rehabil 1995; 16:127–131.

34. Gianotti L, Alexander JW, Pyles T, James L, Babcock GF. Relationship between extent of burn injury and magnitude of microbial translocation from the intestine. J Burn Care Rehabil 1993; 14:336–342.

35. Gianotti L, Alexander JW, Gennari R, Pyles T, Babcock GF. Oral glutamine decreases bacterial translocation and improves survival in experimental gut-origin sepsis. JPEN J Parenter Enteral Nutr 1995; 19:69–74.

36. McCowen KC, Bistrian BR. Immunonutrition: problematic or problem solving? Am J Clin Nutr 2003; 77:764–770.

37. Bistrian BR. Practical recommendations for immune-enhancing diets. J Nutr 2004; 134:2868S–2872S; discussion 2895S.

38. Bryant PA, Trinder J, Curtis N. Sick and tired: does sleep have a vital role in the immune system? Nat Rev Immunol 2004; 4:457–467.

39. Moller MG, Slaikeu JD, Bonelli P, Davis AT, Hoogeboom JE, Bonnell BW. Early tracheostomy versus late tracheostomy in the surgical intensive care unit. Am J Surg 2005; 189:293–296.

40. Parsons PE, Eisner MD, Thompson BT, et al. Lower tidal volume ventilation and plasma cytokine markers of inflammation in patients with acute lung injury. Crit Care Med 2005; 33:1–6; discussion 230–232.

41. Amato MB, Barbas CS, Medeiros DM, et al. Effect of a protective-ventilation strategy on mortality in the acute respiratory distress syndrome. N Engl J Med 1998; 338:347–354.

42. Claridge JA, Sawyer RG, Schulman AM, McLemore EC, Young JS. Blood transfusions correlate with infections in trauma patients in a dose-dependent manner. Am Surg 2002; 68:566–572.

43. Gianotti L, Pyles T, Alexander JW, Babcock GF, Carey MA. Impact of blood transfusion and burn injury on microbial translocation and bacterial survival. Transfusion 1992; 32:312–317.

44. Hughes MG, Evans HL, Lightfoot L, et al. Does prior transfusion worsen outcomes from infection in surgical patients? Surg Infect (Larchmt) 2003; 4:335–343.

45. Kolsen-Petersen JA. Immune effect of hypertonic saline: fact or fiction? Acta Anaesthesiol Scand 2004; 48:667–678.

46. Oberbeck R. Therapeutic implications of immune–endocrine interactions in the critically ill patients. Curr Drug Targets Immune Endocr Metabol Disord 2004; 4:129–139.

47. van der Klauw MM, Wilson JH, Stricker BH. Drug-associated agranulocytosis: 20 years of reporting in The Netherlands (1974–1994). Am J Hematol 1998; 57:206–211.

48. Andres E, Kurtz JE, Maloisel F. Nonchemotherapy drug-induced agranulocytosis: experience of the Strasbourg teaching hospital (1985–2000) and review of the literature. Clin Lab Haematol 2002; 24:99–106.

49. Andres E, Noel E, Kurtz JE, Henoun Loukili N, Kaltenbach G, Maloisel F. Life-threatening idiosyncratic drug-induced agranulocytosis in elderly patients. Drugs Aging 2004; 21:427–435.

50. van Staa TP, Boulton F, Cooper C, Hagenbeek A, Inskip H, Leufkens HG. Neutropenia and agranulocytosis in England and Wales: incidence and risk factors. Am J Hematol 2003; 72:248–254.

51. Andres E, Kurtz JE, Martin-Hunyadi C, et al. Nonchemotherapy drug-induced agranulocytosis in elderly patients: the effects of granulocyte colony-stimulating factor. Am J Med 2002; 112:460–464.

52. Knudson MM, Maull KI. Nonoperative management of solid organ injuries. Past, present, and future. Surg Clin North Am 1999; 79:1357–1371.

53. Peitzman AB, Ford HR, Harbrecht BG, Potoka DA, Townsend RN. Injury to the spleen. Curr Probl Surg 2001; 38:932–1008.

54. Pachter HL, Guth AA, Hofstetter SR, Spencer FC. Changing patterns in the management of splenic trauma: the impact of nonoperative management. Ann Surg 1998; 227(5):708–719.

55. Shatz DV, Schinsky MF, Pais LB, et al. Immune responses of splenectomized trauma patients to the 23-valent pneumococcal polysaccharide vaccine at 1 versus 7 versus 14 days after splenectomy. J Trauma 1998; 44:760–766.

56. Shatz DV, Romero-Steiner S, Elie CM, et al. Antibody responses in postsplenectomy trauma patients receiving the 23-valent pneumococcal polysaccharide vaccine at 14 versus 28 days postoperatively. J Trauma 2002; 53(6):1037–1042.

57. Shatz DV. Vaccination practices among North American trauma surgeons in splenectomy for trauma. J Trauma 2002; 53(5):950–956.

58. Waghorn DJ. Overwhelming infection in asplenic patients: current best practice preventive measures are not being followed. J Clin Pathol 2001; 54:214–218.

59. Kaplan LJ, Coffman D. Splenomegally, Oct 5, 2004, e-Medicine (http://www.emedicine.com/med/topic2156.htm) accessed November 21, 2005.

60. Cavill I. Guidelines for the prevention and treatment of infection in patients with an absent of dysfunctional spleen. BMJ 1996; 312:430–434.

61. Cavill I. (for the Working Party of the British Committee for Standards in Haematology). Guidelines for the prevention and treatment of infection in patients with an absent or dysfunctional spleen. BMJ 1996; 312(7028):430–434.

62. Osborn TM, Tracy K, Dunne JR, Pasquale M, Napolitano LM. Epidemiology of sepsis in patients with traumatic injury. Crit Care Med 2004; 32:2234–2240.

63. Rassias AJ, Marrin CA, Arruda J, Whalen PK, Beach M, Yeager MP. Insulin infusion improves neutrophil function in diabetic cardiac surgery patients. Anesth Analg 1999; 88:1011–1016.

64. Rassias AJ, Givan AL, Marrin CA, Whalen K, Pahl J, Yeager MP. Insulin increases neutrophil count and phagocytic capacity after cardiac surgery. Anesth Analg 2002; 94:1113–1119.

65. Furnary AP, Zerr KJ, Grunkemeier GL, Starr A. Continuous intravenous insulin infusion reduces the incidence of deep sternal wound infection in diabetic patients after cardiac surgical procedures. Ann Thorac Surg 1999; 67:352–360; discussion 360–362.

66. Furnary AP, Gao G, Grunkemeier GL, et al. Continuous insulin infusion reduces mortality in patients with diabetes undergoing coronary artery bypass grafting. J Thorac Cardiovasc Surg 2003; 125:1007–1021.

67. Furnary AP, Wu Y, Bookin SO. Effect of hyperglycemia and continuous intravenous insulin infusions on outcomes of cardiac surgical procedures: the Portland Diabetic Project. Endocr Pract 2004; 10 (suppl 2):21–33.

68. Weekers F, Giulietti AP, Michalaki M, et al. Metabolic, endocrine, and immune effects of stress hyperglycemia in a rabbit model of prolonged critical illness. Endocrinology 2003; 144:5329–5338.

69. Carracedo J, Ramirez R, Madueno JA, et al. Cell apoptosis and hemodialysis-induced inflammation. Kidney Int 2002; 61:589–593.

70. Carracedo J, Ramirez R, Soriano S, et al. Monocytes from dialysis patients exhibit characteristics of senescent cells: does it really mean inflammation? Contrib Nephrol 2005; 149:208–218.

71. Cheung AH, Wong LM. Surgical infections in patients with chronic renal failure. Infect Dis Clin North Am 2001; 15:775–796.

72. Horl WH. Immune dysfunction in hemodialysis and peritoneal dialysis patients. In: Lameire N, Mehta RL, eds. Complications of Dialysis. New York: Marcel Dekker Inc., 2000:389–404.

73. Vanholder R, De Smet R, Lameire N. Protein-bound uremic solutes: the forgotten toxins. Kidney Int Suppl 2001; 78:S266–S270.

74. Vanholder R, De Smet R, Waterloos MA, et al. Mechanisms of uremic inhibition of phagocyte reactive species production: characterization of the role of p-cresol. Kidney Int 1995; 47:510–517.

75. De Smet R, Van Kaer J, Van Vlem B, et al. Toxicity of free p-cresol: a prospective and cross-sectional analysis. Clin Chem 2003; 49:470–478.

76. Porter CJ, Burden RP, Morgan AG, Daniels I, Fletcher J. Impaired polymorphonuclear neutrophil function in end-stage renal failure and its correction by continuous ambulatory peritoneal dialysis. Nephron 1995; 71:133–137.

77. Shurtz-Swirski R, Shkolnik T, Shasha SM. Parathyroid hormone and the cellular immune system. Nephron 1995; 70:21–24.

78. Haag-Weber M, Mai B, Horl WH. Normalization of enhanced neutrophil cytosolic free calcium of hemodialysis patients by 1,25-dihydroxyvitamin D3 or calcium channel blocker. Am J Nephrol 1993; 13:467–472.

79. Deschenes M, Villeneuve JP. Risk factors for the development of bacterial infections in hospitalized patients with cirrhosis. Am J Gastroenterol 1999; 94:2193–2197.

80. Marrero J, Martinez FJ, Hyzy R. Advances in critical care hepatology. Am J Respir Crit Care Med 2003; 168:1421–1426.

81. Almasio PL, Hughes RD, Williams R. Characterization of the molecular forms of fibronectin in fulminant hepatic failure. Hepatology 1986; 6:1340–1345.

82. Bailey RJ, Woolf IL, Cullens H, Williams R. Metabolic inhibition of polymorphonuclear leucocytes in fulminant hepatic failure. Lancet 1976; 1:1162–1163.

83. Tilg H, Diehl AM. Cytokines in alcoholic and nonalcoholic steatohepatitis. N Engl J Med 2000; 343:1467–1476.

84. Rolando N, Harvey F, Brahm J, et al. Prospective study of bacterial infection in acute liver failure: an analysis of fifty patients. Hepatology 1990; 11:49–53.

85. Wyke RJ, Canalese JC, Gimson AE, Williams R. Bacteraemia in patients with fulminant hepatic failure. Liver 1982; 2:45–52.

86. Rolando N, Gimson A, Wade J, Philpott-Howard J, Casewell M, Williams R. Prospective controlled trial of selective parenteral and enteral antimicrobial regimen in fulminant liver failure. Hepatology 1993; 17:196–201.

87. Walsh TJ, Hamilton SR. Disseminated aspergillosis complicating hepatic failure. Arch Intern Med 1983; 143:1189–1191.

88. Davidson A, Diamond B. Autoimmune diseases. N Engl J Med 2001; 345:340–350.

89. Goldsmith MF. Are autoimmunologists in many women's future? JAMA 2001; 285:1433–1434.

90. Yancey KB, Egan CA. Pemphigoid: clinical, histologic, immunopathologic, and therapeutic considerations. JAMA 2000; 284:350–356.

91. Dalakas MC. Intravenous immunoglobulin in autoimmune neuromuscular diseases. JAMA 2004; 291:2367–2375.

92. von Andrian UH, Engelhardt B. Alpha4 integrins as therapeutic targets in autoimmune disease. N Engl J Med 2003; 348:68–72.

93. Schon MP, Boehncke WH. Psoriasis. N Engl J Med 2005; 352:18.

94. Butcher SK, Lord JM. Stress responses and innate immunity: aging as a contributory factor. Aging Cell 2004; 3:151–160.

95. Butcher S, Chahel H, Lord JM. Review article: ageing and the neutrophil: no appetite for killing? Immunology 2000; 100:411–416.

96. Butcher SK, Chahal H, Nayak L, et al. Senescence in innate immune responses: reduced neutrophil phagocytic capacity and CD16 expression in elderly humans. J Leukoc Biol 2001; 70:881–886.

97. Butcher SK, Killampalli V, Chahal H, Kaya Alpar E, Lord JM. Effect of age on susceptibility to post-traumatic infection in the elderly. Biochem Soc Trans 2003; 31:449–451.

98. Choudhry MA, Ba ZF, Rana SN, Bland KI, Chaudry IH. Alcohol ingestion before burn injury decreases splanchnic blood flow and oxygen delivery. Am J Physiol Heart Circ Physiol 2005; 288:H716–H721.

99. Choudhry MA, Rana SN, Kavanaugh MJ, Kovacs EJ, Gamelli RL, Sayeed MM. Impaired intestinal immunity and barrier function: a cause for enhanced bacterial translocation in alcohol intoxication and burn injury. Alcohol 2004; 33:199–208.

100. Nimmanwudipong T, Cheadle WG, Appel SH, Polk HC Jr. Effect of protein malnutrition and immunomodulation on immune cell populations. J Surg Res 1992; 52:233–238.

101. Gao F, Bailes E, Robertson DL, et al. Origin of HIV-1 in the chimpanzee Pan troglodytes troglodytes. Nature 1999; 397:436–441.

102. Hahn BH, Shaw GM, De Cock KM, Sharp PM. AIDS as a zoonosis: scientific and public health implications. Science 2000; 287:607–614.

103. Gayle HD, Hill GL. Global impact of human immunodeficiency virus and AIDS. Clin Microbiol Rev 2001; 14:327–335.

104. Twenty-five years or HIV/AIDS-United States, 1981–2006, vol. 55, No MM21; 555, June 2, 2006. Acquired immunodeficiency deficiency syndrome—United States, 2001, Morb Mortal Wkly Rep, Centers for Disease Control, 2001: 430–434.

105. Epidomiology of HIV/AIDS-United States, 1981–2005, Vol 55, No MM21:559, June 2, 2006. Diagnoses of HIV/AIDS in 32 States, 2000–2003, Morb Mortal Wkly Rep, Centers for Disease Control, 2004: 1106–1110.

106. Stawicki SP, Hoff WS, Hoey BA, Grossman MD, Scoll B, Reed JF III. Human immunodeficiency virus infection in trauma patients: where do we stand? J Trauma 2005; 58:88–93.

107. Rudolph R, Bowen DG, Boyd CR, Jurgensen P. Seroprevalence of human immunodeficiency virus in admitted trauma patients at a southeastern metropolitan/rural trauma center. Am Surg 1993; 59:384–387.

108. Sloan EP, McGill BA, Zalenski R, et al. Human immunodeficiency virus and hepatitis B virus seroprevalence in an urban trauma population. J Trauma 1995; 38:736–741.

109. Harrison WJ, Lewis CP, Lavy CB. Open fractures of the tibia in HIV positive patients: a prospective controlled single-blind study. Injury 2004; 35:852–856.

110. James J, Hofland HW, Borgstein ES, Kumiponjera D, Komolafe OO, Zijlstra EE. The prevalence of HIV infection among burn patients in a burns unit in Malawi and its influence on outcome. Burns 2003; 29:55–60.

111. Sjoberg T, Mzezewa S, Jonsson K, Salemark L. Immune response in burn patients in relation to HIV infection and sepsis. Burns 2004; 30:670–674.

112. Kelen GD, Fritz S, Qaqish B, et al. Unrecognized human immunodeficiency virus infection in emergency department patients. N Engl J Med 1988; 318:1645–1650.

113. Kelen GD, Fritz S, Qaquish B, et al. Substantial increase in human immunodeficiency virus (HIV-1) infection in critically ill emergency patients: 1986 and 1987 compared. Ann Emerg Med 1989; 18:378–382.

114. Rosen MJ, Clayton K, Schneider RF, et al. Intensive care of patients with HIV infection: utilization, critical illnesses, and outcomes. Pulmonary Complications of HIV Infection Study Group. Am J Respir Crit Care Med 1997; 155:67–71.

115. Afessa B. Pleural effusion and pneumothorax in hospitalized patients with HIV infection: the pulmonary complications, ICU support, and prognostic factors of hospitalized patients with HIV (PIP) study. Chest 2000; 117:1031–1037.

116. Guth AA, Hofstetter SR, Pachter HL. Human immunodeficiency virus and the trauma patient: factors influencing postoperative infectious complications. J Trauma 1996; 41:251–255; discussion 255–256.

117. Hebra A, Adams DB, Holley HP Jr. Human immunodeficiency virus and the surgeon. JSC Med Assoc 1990; 86:479–483.

118. Edge JM, Van der Merwe AE, Pieper CH, Bouic P. Clinical outcome of HIV positive patients with moderate to severe burns. Burns 2001; 27:111–114.

119. Carrillo EH, Carrillo LE, Byers PM, Ginzburg E, Martin L. Penetrating trauma and emergency surgery in patients with AIDS. Am J Surg 1995; 170:341–344.

120. Burack JH, Mandel MS, Bizer LS. Emergency abdominal operations in the patient with acquired immunodeficiency syndrome. Arch Surg 1989; 124:285–286.

121. Whitney TM, Brunel W, Russell TR, Bossart KJ, Schecter WP. Emergent abdominal surgery in AIDS: experience in San Francisco. Am J Surg 1994; 168:239–243.

122. Okong P. Response of HIV positive patients to surgery. Proc Assoc Surg East Afr 1988; 11:41.

123. Hammer SM, Saag MS, Schechter, et al. Treatment of adult HIV infection: 2006 recommendations of the International AIDS Society—USA panel. JAMA 2006; 296(7):827–843.

124. Quebbeman EJ. Care of the trauma patient in the age of the human immunodeficiency virus. Surg Clin North Am 1995; 75:327–334.

125. Gea-Banacloche JC, Opal SM, Jorgensen J, Carcillo JA, Sepkowitz KA, Cordonnier C. Sepsis associated with immunosuppressive medications: an evidence-based review. Crit Care Med 2004; 32:S578–S590.

126. Ibrahim EH, Sherman G, Ward S, Fraser VJ, Kollef MH. The influence of inadequate antimicrobial treatment of bloodstream infections on patient outcomes in the ICU setting. Chest 2000; 118:146–155.

127. Iregui M, Ward S, Sherman G, Fraser VJ, Kollef MH. Clinical importance of delays in the initiation of appropriate antibiotic treatment for ventilator-associated pneumonia. Chest 2002; 122:262–268.

128. Kollef MH, Sherman G, Ward S, Fraser VJ. Inadequate antimicrobial treatment of infections: a risk factor for hospital mortality among critically ill patients. Chest 1999; 115: 462–474.

129. Kolleff MH. Appropriate antibiotic therapy for ventilator-associated pneumonia and sepsis: a necessity, not an issue for debate. Intensive Care Med 2003; 29:147–149.

130. Fishman JA, Rubin RH. Infection in organ-transplant recipients. N Engl J Med 1998; 338:1741–1751.

131. Cohen A, Sambrook P, Shane E. Management of bone loss after organ transplantation. J Bone Miner Res 2004; 19:1919–1932.

132. Compston JE. Osteoporosis after liver transplantation. Liver Transpl 2003; 9:321–330.

133. de Nijs RN, Jacobs JW, Algra A, Lems WF, Bijlsma JW. Prevention and treatment of glucocorticoid-induced osteoporosis with active vitamin D3 analogues: a review with meta-analysis of randomized controlled trials including organ transplantation studies. Osteoporos Int 2004; 15:589–602.

134. Zimakas PJ, Sharma AK, Rodd CJ. Osteopenia and fractures in cystinotic children post renal transplantation. Pediatr Nephrol 2003; 18:384–390.

135. Toivonen HJ. Anaesthesia for patients with a transplanted organ. Acta Anaesthesiol Scand 2000; 44:812–833.

136. Jain P, Sandur S, Meli Y, Arroliga AC, Stoller JK, Mehta AC. Role of flexible bronchoscopy in immunocompromised patients with lung infiltrates. Chest 2004; 125:712–722.

137. O'Keefe GE, Hybki DL, Munford RS. The G → A single nucleotide polymorphism at the −308 position in the tumor necrosis factor-alpha promoter increases the risk for severe sepsis after trauma. J Trauma 2002; 52:817–825.

138. Scott MJ, Hoth JJ, Gardner SA, Peyton JC, Cheadle WG. Genetic background influences natural killer cell activation during bacterial peritonitis in mice, and is interleukin 12 and interleukin 18 independent. Cytokine 2004; 28:124–136.

139. Cobb JP, O'Keefe GE. Injury research in the genomic era. Lancet 2004; 363:2076–2083.

140. Oberholzer A, Keel M, Zellweger R, Steckholzer U, Trentz O, Ertel W. Incidence of septic complications and multiple organ failure in severely injured patients is sex specific. J Trauma 2000; 48:932–937.

141. Weigand MA, Horner C, Bardenheuer HJ, Bouchon A. The systemic inflammatory response syndrome. Best Pract Res Clin Anaesthesiol 2004; 18:455–475.

142. Rhee P, Nunley MK, Demetriades D, et al. Tetanus and trauma: a review and recommendations. J Trauma 2005; 58(5):1082–1088.

143. Maddali S, Stapleton PP, Freeman TA, et al. Neuroendocrine responses mediate macrophage function after trauma. Surgery 2004; 136:1038–1046.

144. Aller MA, Arias JL, Arias J. Post-traumatic inflammatory response: perhaps a succession of phases with a nutritional purpose. Med Hypotheses 2004; 63:42–46.

145. Prevention of pneumococcal disease: recommendations of the Advisory Committee on Immunization Practices (ACIP). MMWR April 4, 1997; 46(RR-8):1–24.

146. Bilukha OO, Rosenstein N. Prevention and Control of Meningococcal Disease: Recommendations of the Advisory Committee on Immunization Practices (ACIP). MMWR May 27, 2005; 54(RR-7):1–21.

147. Weniger BG. Combination vaccines for childhood immunization: recommendations of the Advisory Committee on Immunization Practices (ACIP), the American Academy of Pediatrics (AAP), and the American Academy of Family Physicians (AAFP) MMWR May 14, 1999; 48(RR05):1–15.

53

Antimicrobial Therapy

Charles L. James and Leland S. Rickman

Division of Infectious Diseases, Departments of Medicine and Pharmacy, UC San Diego Medical Center, San Diego, California, U.S.A.

Mark A. Swancutt

Departments of Microbiology and Medicine, Southwestern Medical Center, Dallas, Texas, U.S.A.

INTRODUCTION

Infections occurring in the intensive care unit (ICU) almost always involve nosocomial organisms, which are more resistant and more virulent than those typically acquired in the community. Nosocomial infections develop in approximately 24% of medical ICU patients, and 31% of surgical ICU patients (1), increasing morbidity (2), and prolonging hospital stay (3).

Trauma related injuries are the second largest source of health care costs in the United States (US) (3), and account for a significant portion of morbidity and mortality in all regions of the world (4,5). Infections in trauma patients can increase mortality up to three-fold (6).

The principles of antimicrobial use and the mechanisms of antibacterial resistance are reviewed in the first two sections of this chapter. Next, the factors increasing the risk of infectious disease following trauma and critical care are reviewed. The remainder of the chapter reviews the important clinical considerations for the various antimicrobial drugs currently in use.

All antibiotics must be evaluated in terms of their antimicrobial spectra, toxicities, and pharmacokinetic and pharmacodynamic attributes. Susceptibility results of antimicrobials reflect in vitro properties and do not always correlate with clinical results. Hence the reader is advised to consider many factors during antimicrobial selection (7). Several antibiotic choices are usually effective in the treatment of most infections. The recommendations listed here reflect the perspectives of two infectious diseases physicians and an infectious diseases pharmacist specialist.

PRINCIPLES OF ANTIMICROBIAL USE

☞ Antimicrobial selection for trauma and critical care is based on the following seven considerations: (*i*) whether the antibiotics are planned for prophylaxis or treatment of an established infection; (*ii*) the anatomic site of infection; (*iii*) whether the infection is community-acquired or nosocomial; (*iv*) best guess of the most probable causative microorganism (based upon geographical and institutional isolate profiles); (*v*) the patient's innate immunological status; (*vi*) the severity of the infection and general condition of the patient; and (*vii*) financial cost. ☞

General Rules for Selecting Single vs. Multiple Antibiotics

On some occasions, a single antibiotic is appropriate, for example, the treatment of cellulitis with cefazolin. However, there are several circumstances where combination antimicrobial treatment should be employed. The first is the prevention of the emergence of resistant organisms while on therapy; an example is the absolute necessity to use an antistaphylococcal agent, like nafcillin, in combination with rifampin to prevent the emergence of rifampin-resistant mutations, which are single-step mutations to full resistance in the gene that encodes the bacterial RNA polymerase, the rifampin site of action. A second example is with polymicrobial infections (e.g., intraperitoneal and pelvic infections). The flora causing these infections includes gram-negative enteric rods, a multiplicity of different obligately anaerobic species, as well as enterococci and, occasionally, yeast. A third circumstance where antimicrobial combinations is in empiric therapy where early aggressive treatment improves survival and mixed microbial infection is probable, for example, necrotizing fasciitis.

Antibiotic Synergy vs. Antagonism

In order to use combinations of antimicrobial drugs properly, the prescriber should be familiar with the concepts of antibiotic synergy and antagonism. Synergy occurs when the use of one antibiotic enhances the antimicrobial activity of another. In general, synergy occurs when the agents of any particular combination act on different biochemical pathways of the microorganism or act sequentially along the same metabolic pathway; an example of the first is the use of ampicillin (or vancomycin) and gentamicin against enterococci. Aminoglycosides are ineffective as single drugs in treating gram-positive organisms because they cannot penetrate the thick peptidoglycan cell wall to reach their site of action at the ribosome within the bacterial cytoplasm. The combination of ampicillin (or vancomycin) and gentamicin is synergistic for enterococci because ampicillin (and vancomycin) damage the bacterial cell wall (as their antimicrobial mechanism of action) thereby allowing the aminoglycoside to penetrate into the cell. Clinical studies have shown that the addition of gentamicin to ampicillin significantly improves outcome in patients with enterococcal endocarditis, even though enterococci are relatively resistant to ampicillin (8). Similar effects are noted with the combination of antistaphylococcal penicillins (or vancomycin) combined with an aminoglycoside against *Staphylococcus aureus*, but the magnitude of the effect is less. Another clinical example of synergism involves the use of anti-pseudomonal beta-lactams such as piperacillin or ticarcillin in combination with aminoglycosides to treat serious infections with *Pseudomonas aeruginosa* (9).

The combination drug trimethoprim-sulfamethoxazole (Bactrim or Septra) is an example of synergism resulting from using two antibiotics that act sequentially in the same pathway. Sulfamethoxazole acts first and trimethoprim (TMP) second in the microbial pathway for de novo synthesis of folic acid, which is necessary for synthesizing precursors for DNA and other molecules involved in bacterial intermediary metabolism. For treating fungi, 5-FC is not used alone because of the development of rapid resistance. However, the combination of 5-FC and amphotericin is synergistic in vitro, and this combination is commonly used clinically to treat cryptococcal meningitis (10).

Antagonism occurs when the combination of antibiotics is less effective than either agent alone. For example, the use of bacteriostatic drugs such as tetracycline or chloramphenicol that inhibit protein synthesis generally decrease the effectiveness of beta-lactam drugs that act on the cell wall (11). Another example of antagonism in vitro involves the use of azoles like fluconazole in combination with amphotericin. Ergosterol, a sterol in the fungal plasma membrane, is the target site of amphotericin; azole drugs inhibit the enzyme necessary for ergosterol synthesis and decreases the amount of ergosterol present in the plasma membrane, thereby decreasing the target of action for amphotericin and making it potentially less effective.

MECHANISMS OF ANTIBIOTIC RESISTANCE

Factors influencing the emergence of resistance in microorganisms include: (*i*) the indiscriminant use of broad-spectrum antibiotics in medicine, (*ii*) the widespread use of antibiotics in animal husbandry and fisheries, (*iii*) prolonged hospitalizations, (*iv*) the increasing numbers of immunocompromised patients, (*v*) international travel, and (*vi*) medical progress resulting in increased use of invasive procedures and devices.

Bacteria evade antimicrobial action by diverse mechanisms. These mechanisms include changes in permeability of the bacterial cell wall and plasma membrane to the antibiotic, antibiotic efflux from bacterial cells, inactivation of the antibiotic (usually enzymatically), modification or elimination of the target site(s) for the antibiotic, and the development of auxotrophs (bacterial strains with growth requirements different from those of the wild-type strains) which can bypass steps inhibited by antibiotics. Understanding the general mechanism of resistance has clinical relevance when choosing a specific antibiotic for a specific organism. For example, methicillin-resistant *S. aureus* (MRSA) is resistant to beta-lactam agents by virtue of possessing an altered penicillin-binding protein (PBP), the target of all beta-lactams. Therefore, combination products increasing the duration of beta-lactam activity with a beta-lactamase inhibitor, (e.g., piperacillin/tazobactam or ampicillin/sulbactam) will not demonstrate any activity against MRSA (12–17).

☞ **A primary tenet of antimicrobial therapy is to use the narrowest spectrum antibiotic possible, rather than a broad-spectrum agent.** ☞ Empiric treatment (prior to the final identification of specific microorganisms) is by necessity broad-spectrum, and the antibiotic selection is based upon several features. These include the location where the suspected infection developed (e.g., community vs. hospital-acquired), the anatomic site involved (e.g., oropharynx vs. colon), suspected organisms (based on prior literature and local experiences), the local antibiotic sensitivity and resistance patterns, the current gram stain and prior culture results, patient allergies, renal/hepatic function, and other clinical factors. Emergent, empiric antimicrobial treatment is indicated in only a few situations, including, for example, suspected sepsis, bacterial meningitis, some fulminant pneumonias (i.e., *Bacillus anthracis*) and some severe soft-tissue infections (i.e., necrotizing fasciitis). There is usually adequate time for a thorough clinical evaluation of a patient in other circumstances, including the collection of adequate specimens (for gram stain and culture) prior to the institution of antibiotics. Fever alone in a clinically stable patient can result from either an infection or a myriad of other causes (e.g., major trauma, burns, surgery, hematoma in soft tissue or subarachnoid blood, etc.), and frequently does not require antimicrobial therapy. (Volume 2, Chapter 46) Hence the dictum "antibiotics are not the antipyretic of choice."

Prophylactic antibiotic use in surgery should be limited to proven indications and duration. A good example of this principle are the recently published guidelines for the appropriate use of vancomycin to reduce the emergence of vancomycin-resistant enterococci (VRE) and possible vancomycin-resistant *S. aureus* (VRSA) (16). These guidelines discourage the use of vancomycin except for limited situations, which include: (*i*) severe beta-lactam allergy, (*ii*) infections caused by gram-positive cocci that are resistant to beta-lactams, (*iii*) empiric use in circumstances where there is a high institutional prevalence of MRSA, (*iv*) life threatening infections until definitive culture results return, and (*v*) the oral treatment of *Clostridium difficile* colitis (only when there is a failure of metronidazole) (16).

RISK FACTORS FOR INFECTIONS IN TRAUMA AND CRITICAL CARE

Many factors increase the infection risk in trauma and critical illness. Defects in the mucosal and skin surfaces after trauma allow microbes to bypass initial defenses. Chest tubes, endotracheal tubes, catheters, and drains facilitate pathogen entry. Devitalized tissues and obstruction of drainage ports (e.g., sinusitis) increase the bacterial count, impair the normal self-cleansing of bacteria, and decrease the ability of white blood cells (WBC) to have access to bacteria—all serving to increase the risk of infection. Within a few days, patients lose the normal protective skin and gut flora and become colonized with nosocomial organisms, which subsequently cause hospital-acquired infections with microbes that are often resistant to many antibiotics.

The most basic question to be answered by the physician contemplating antibiotics in a critically ill patient is whether the patient is in fact infected. The cardinal signs and symptoms of infection (elevated WBC count, fever, hyperdynamic state), and inflammation (rubor et tumor cum calore et dolore [from Celsus]—redness and swelling with heat and pain) are also common accompaniments of acute trauma, and therefore, do not necessarily indicate an infection (18). These signs can persist for days after admission, especially with multiple fractures, burns, or diffuse soft tissue injury. Further complicating infection evaluations in this patient population are patient care devices, limited mobility, and ventilators. Another clinical conundrum is deciding whether a patient is colonized or actually infected, once organisms have been isolated. This can be especially problematic when the culture isolate was derived from suctioned sputa or previously placed drains.

Infection control measures are vitally important to mitigate the spread of resistant organisms. ☞ **As Ignaz Phillip Semmelweis discovered 150 years ago, the most important means of preventing the transmission of microorganisms from one patient (via the doctor or nurse) to another patient is strict hand washing (and now, the use of clean disposable gloves).** ☞

Bacterial organisms commonly responsible for infections in trauma and critically ill patients are divided into three main classes: aerobic gram positive, aerobic gram negative, and anaerobic. The common gram-positive pathogens and the currently recommended antibiotics for these organisms are listed in Table 1. The recommendations provided in this and other tables in this chapter reflect general sensitivity and resistance patterns as of the publication of this textbook, and local conditions may be different.

Organisms causing infections in trauma patients have changed over time. ☞ **At present, the majority of infections occurring in hospitalized trauma patients are due to gram-positive organisms (19), for example, MRSA and VRE, and to a lesser extent, multi-resistant gram-negative rods (20).** ☞ This is in sharp contrast to a few decades ago where gram-negative organisms prevailed.

Gram-negative organisms include many of the enteric bacteria and some of these are developing extended spectrum beta lactamases (ESBLs), especially the so called

"SPACE" organisms (*Serratia* spp., *Pseudomonas* spp., *Acinetobacter* spp., *Citrobacter* spp., *Enterobacter* spp). The common gram negative aerobic bacteria, along with the antimicrobial drugs of choice, are summarized in Table 2.

With appropriate antibiotic use, fungal infections are still rare in trauma injured patients, excluding catheter-related urinary tract infections. Judicious prophylactic antibiotic use in the trauma setting is generally accepted practice in specific situations (21–24).

☞ **Penetrating intra-abdominal injury, perforated abdominal viscera, and open fractures all warrant antibiotic prophylaxis (22–25).** ☞

Infections involving the mouth and gastrointestinal tract (including most intraabdominal abscesses) involve anaerobic bacteria, in addition to aerobic gram-positive and gram-negative organisms. The common anaerobic pathogens involved in trauma and critical care are summarized in Table 3. In general, infections involving anaerobic organisms that occur above the diaphragm, or in the vagina, can be treated with clindamycin or metronidazole. However, those occurring from organisms native to the colon (e.g., *Bacteroides fragilis*) are best treated by metronidazole.

A complete survey of infectious and non-infectious sources of fever is provided in Volume 2, Chapter 46. Sepsis and SIRS are reviewed in great detail in Volume 2, Chapters 47 and 63, respectively. The most common

Table 1 Antimicrobial Drugs of Choice Against Aerobic Gram-Positive Bacteria

Microorganisms	Drug of choice	Alternative agents
Staphylococcus aureus		
Non-penicillinase-producing	Penicillin	Vancomycin, cephalosporin
Penicillinase producing	Nafcillin, oxacillin	Vancomycin, cephalosporin, erythromycin, clindamycin
MRSA	Vancomycin[a]	Linezolid, quinupristin/dalfopristin, tigecycline
VISA	Daptomycin[b]	Quinupristin/dalfopristin, linezolid
VRSA	Daptomycin[b]	Quinupristin/dalfopristin, linezolid
Alpha-streptococci (*Streptococcus viridans*)	Penicillin	Cephalosporin
Beta-streptococci (A, B, C, G)	Penicillin	Cephalosporin, erythromycin
Streptococcus bovis	Penicillin	Vancomycin, cephalosporin
Streptococcus pneumoniae (pneumococcus)		
PCN-susceptible (MIC <0.1 mcg/mL)	Penicillin or amoxicillin	Cephalosporin, erythromycin, azithromycin, clarithromycin, levofloxacin, moxifloxacin, carbapenems, clindamycin, tetracycline
PCN-intermediate resistance (MIC = 0.1–2 mcg/mL)	Penicillin or ceftriaxone, cefotaxime	Levofloxacin, gatifloxacin, moxifloxacin, clindamycin, vancomycin
PCN-high-level resistance (MIC >2 mcg/mL)	Meningitis: vancomycin + ceftriaxone or cefotaxime other indications: vancomycin + ceftriaxone or cefotaxime, linezolid, levofloxacin, gatifloxacin, moxifloxacin	Carbapenems, quinupristin/dalfopristin
Enterococcus spp.		
Serious infection	Ampicillin + gentamicin or streptomycin	Vancomycin + gentamicin or streptomycin; linezolid; quinupristin/dalfopristin
Uncomplicated UTI	Ampicillin	Nitrofurantoin; ciprofloxacin, levofloxacin; fosfomycin
VRE	Linezolid	Daptomycin; quinupristin/dalfopristin

[a]Some studies show that linezolid was superior to vancomycin for ventilator associated pneumonia due to MRSA. However, the doses of vancomycin in these studies were subtherapeutic.
[b]Daptomycin contraindicated in pneumonia (surfactant inhibits daptomycin). For pneumonia, due to VISA, or VRSA use quinupristin/dalfopristin, or linezolid.
Abbreviations: MIC, minimum inhibitory concentration; MRSA, methicillin-resistant *S. aureus*; PCN, penicillin; UTI, urinary tract infection; VISA, vancomycin intermediate sensitive *S. aureus*; VRE, vancomycin-resistant enterococcus; VRSA, vancomycin-resistant *S. aureus*.

Table 2 Antimicrobial Drugs of Choice Against Aerobic Gram-Negative Bacteria

Microorganisms	Drug of choice	Alternative agents
Acinetobacter spp.	Imipenem, meropenem	Aminoglycoside, ciprofloxacin, cotrimoxazole, ceftazidime
Aeromonas	Cotrimoxazole	Aminoglycoside, imipenem, fluoroquinolone
Enterobacter spp.	Imipenem, meropenem	Aminoglycoside, ciprofloxacin, cotrimoxazole, cefepime
Escherichia coli	Ceftriaxone, cefotaxime	Aminoglycoside, imipenem, meropenem, ceftazidime, cefepime, cotrimoxazole, fluoroquinolone, aztreonam, piperacillin/tazobactam
Haemophilus influenzae	Second- or third-generation cephalosporin	Fluoroquinolone, cotrimoxazole
Klebsiella pneumoniae	Ceftriaxone, cefotaxime	Aminoglycoside, carbapenems, ceftazidime, aztreonam, cefepime, cotrimoxazole, fluoroquinolone, piperacillin/tazobactam
Legionella spp.	Azithromycin or a fluoroquinolone ± rifampin	Doxycycline ± rifampin, cotrimoxazole, erythromycin
Proteus mirabilis	Ampicillin	Cephalosporin, cotrimoxazole, aminoglycosides, carbapenem, fluoroquinolone, aztreonam
Other *Proteus* spp.	Ceftriaxone, cefotaxime, ceftazidime, cefepime	Imipenem, meropenem, fluoroquinolones, piperacillin/tazobactam, cotrimoxazole, aminoglycoside
P. aeruginosa	Ceftazidime + an aminoglycoside or cipro	Carbapenems, cefepime, aztreonam, levoflox, piperacillin
Salmonella spp.	Fluoroquinolone or ceftriaxone	Cotrimoxazole
Stenotrophomonas maltophilia	Cotrimoxazole	Fluoroquinolone
Serratia spp.	Carbapenem	Aminoglycoside, aztreonam, third- or fourth-generation cephalosporin, cotrimoxazole, piperacillin/tazobactam, fluoroquinolone

sources of infection in trauma and critical care also have specific chapters dedicated to them, including ventilator associated pneumonia (Volume 2, Chapter 48), indwelling catheter related infections (Volume 2, Chapter 49), abdominal sources of infection (Volume 2, Chapter 50), and sinusitis (Volume 2, Chapter 51). The remainder of this chapter reviews the antimicrobials most frequently used for trauma and critical care.

PENICILLINS
History/Description
Dr. Alexander Fleming discovered penicillin in 1929, while working on unrelated influenza research. Fleming happened upon his discovery when he observed that one of his staphylococcal culture plates became contaminated with

Table 3 Antimicrobial Drugs of Choice Against Anaerobic Bacteria

Microorganisms	Drug of choice	Alternative agents
Prevotella melanogenica	Penicillin G; or clindamycin	Metronidazole
Bacteroides fragilis	Metronidazole	Carbapenems, cefoxitin, ampicillin/sulbactam, piperacillin/tazobactam
Clostridium perfringens	Penicillin or clindamycin	Metronidazole, carbapenems, chloramphenicol
Clostridium tetani	Metronidazole	Penicillin, a tetracycline
Clostridium difficile	Metronidazole	Vancomycin (oral)

a mould, and that surrounding the fungi was a ring-like bacteria-free zone. Fleming subsequently diluted the mould more than 800 times, and still it retained the antibacterial effect. With the assistance of a mycologist colleague, the mould was identified as a *Penicillium*, and Fleming subsequently named the antibacterial active substance penicillin. His publication in 1929 describing this research received little attention until World War II, when penicillin use became widespread. In 1945, Fleming received the Nobel Prize for his discovery. Since that time, penicillin and its derivatives have remained the drug of choice for many bacterial infections, and modifications of its chemical structure has led to the development of numerous other beta-lactam derived antimicrobials (26–28).

Mechanism of Action, Pharmacology, Administration, and Dosage
Penicillin and other beta-lactam related antibiotics (e.g., cephalosporins, monobactams, and carbapenems) all have similar mechanisms of action, primarily targeting the peptidoglycan cell wall; these actions are characterized by enzymatic inhibition of cell wall synthesis and turnover with the resultant destruction of bacteria through autolytic enzymes. For the available penicillin agents, modifications of the side-chain results in a wide variety of pharmacokinetic properties and antimicrobial activities (Table 4).

Most penicillin antibiotics are widely distributed however, penetration across the blood-brain barrier and into the cerebrospinal fluid (CSF) and into the vitreous humor is poor, and levels are significantly lower than serum concentrations, except in the presence of inflammation. Therefore, relatively high doses of penicillins are required to treat infections in these "protected" sites.

Table 4 The Penicillins: Selected Dosing and Need for Adjustment Based Upon Renal or Hepatic Dysfunction

Penicillin sub-type	Typical adult IV dose range and intervals	Requires dose adjustment for renal insufficiency (CrCl <30 mL/min)	Requires dose adjustment for hepatic failure
Aqueous crystalline penicillin G	1–4 million units every 4–6 hr	Yes	No
Ampicillin	1–2 g every 4–6 hr	Yes	No
Ampicillin/sulbactam	1.5–3 g every 6–8 hr	Yes	No
Piperacillin	3–5 g every 4–8 hr	Yes	No
Piperacillin/tazobactam	3.375–4.5 g every 4–6 hr	Yes	No
Oxacillin	1–2 g every 4–6 hr	Yes	No
Nafcillin	1–2 g every 4–6 hr	Yes	No

Abbreviation: IV, intravenously.

Antimicrobial Activity/Spectrum/Resistance

Differential bacterial cell wall permeability, binding site affinity and susceptibility to bacterial enzymes (e.g., beta-lactamases) account for the various susceptibility patterns among different penicillins, and other beta-lactams (Tables 1–3). Bacterial production of beta-lactamases, which enzymatically destroy beta-lactam antibiotics, represent the most common mechanism of antimicrobial resistance. Gram-positive organisms usually secrete beta-lactamases extracellularly, whereas gram-negative organisms secrete small quantities of beta-lactamases within the periplasmic space. There are several types of beta-lactamases, each with various binding affinities to enzymes required for the reproduction of specific microorganisms. With this in mind, the development of beta-lactamase inhibitors, in combination with specific penicillins, provides the rationale for the clinical use of combinations (i.e., ticarcillin-clavulanate, piperacillin-tazobactam, and ampicillin-sulbactam).

Narrow–spectrum penicillins, such as penicillin G or ampicillin, remain the drug of choice for most streptococci, enterococci, and oral anaerobic bacteria. The semi-synthetic penicillins, such as nafcillin or oxacillin, were designed specifically for *S. aureus* and have neither anaerobic nor enterococcal activity, and have reduced streptococcal activity. They also lack activity against gram-negative rods. Extended spectrum penicillins, (e.g., piperacillin, mezlocillin, and ticarcillin) have improved activity against not only *P. aeruginosa* but also against additional community and hospital-acquired gram-negative rods. ☞ **The addition of a beta-lactamase inhibitor to beta-lactam antibiotics produces efficacy against beta-lactamase-producing organisms such as *S. aureus*, *Escherichia coli*, and most anaerobic bacteria. However, these combination products add no additional activity against *P. aeruginosa* and have no activity against MRSA.** ☞ MRSA specifically lack the binding proteins for these beta lactams, and are intrinsically resistant regardless of the concentration or duration of high drug levels of beta lactams.

Adverse Effects and Drug Interactions

Hypersensitivity reactions are the most common adverse effects encountered with the use of penicillins. These reactions range from minor, such as rash, to potentially life-threatening such as anaphylaxis (Volume 1, Chapter 33). A few unique adverse effects are seen with specific penicillins, such as platelet dysfunction with piperacillin and a high incidence of rash with ampicillin and amoxicillin. The management of adverse effects and allergy testing is discussed below (Beta-Lactam Allergy). No clinically important drug interactions occur with the penicillins.

Therapeutic/Clinical Uses

Because of their long history of clinical safety, efficacy, and availability, the penicillins are frequently used in the critically ill patient. As seen in Table 1–3, the penicillins are the drugs of choice for many infections commonly encountered in these patients.

CEPHALOSPORINS
History/Description

Cephalosporins are a group of natural and semi-synthetic compounds that are structurally similar to penicillins and have been in clinical use since the 1960s. The cephalosporins are categorized into first-to-fourth "generation," based upon antimicrobial spectrum. Table 5 lists the four generations of cephalosporins (29–32).

Mechanism of Action, Pharmacology Administration, and Dosage

Cephalosporins, like penicillins, enzymatically inhibit bacterial cell wall synthesis. Therapeutic cephalosporin concentrations are reached in many body sites; however, cefazolin and cephalothin do not provide adequate enough concentrations in the CSF to treat bacterial meningitis. However, several of the third and fourth generation cephalosporins reach sufficient concentrations in the CSF for therapeutic utility. These include ceftriaxone, cefotaxime, ceftizoxime, ceftazidime, and cefepime. Table 5 delineates the dosing considerations for the most commonly used cephalosporins. Uniquely, among the cephalosporins, ceftriaxone has the longest half-life and may be dosed on a once-daily basis in most clinical circumstances.

Antimicrobial Activity/Spectrum/Resistance

☞ **In general, as one selects a second, third, or fourth generation cephalosporin, there is increased activity against aerobic gram-negative bacteria and less activity against gram-positive organisms.** ☞ Although ceftriaxone, ceftizoxime, and cefotaxime retain excellent gram-positive activity, the cephalosporins, as a class, do not have activity against

Table 5 The Cephalosporins: Selected Dosing and Need for Adjustment Based Upon Renal or Hepatic Dysfunction

Cephalosporin generation and sub-type	Typical adult IV dose range and intervals	Requires dose adjustment for renal insufficiency (CrCl <30 mL/min)	Requires dose adjustment for hepatic failure
First generation			
Cephalothin	1–2 g every 4–6 hr	Yes	No
Cefazolin	1–2 g every 8 hr	Yes	No
Second generation			
Cefoxitin	1–2 g every 6 hr	Yes	No
Cefuroxime	0.75–1.5 g every 8–12 hr	Yes	No
Third generation			
Cefoperazone	1–2 g every 12 hr	Yes	No
Cefotaxime	1–2 g every 4–8 hr	Yes	No
Ceftriaxone	1–2 g every 12–24 hr	Yes	No
Ceftazidime	1–2 g every 8 hr	Yes	No
Fourth generation			
Cefepime	1–2 g every 12 hr	Yes	No

Abbreviation: IV, intravenously.

enterococci, MRSA, or *Listeria monocytogenes*. For activity against *P. aeruginosa*, the use of ceftazidime or cefepime is usually required. Because of their broad activity against most aerobic gram-positive cocci (except enterococci), and gram-negative bacilli (except *P. aeruginosa*), the third generation cephalosporins (ceftriaxone, cefotaxime and ceftizoxime) are commonly used in the critically ill patient.

The first generation cephalosporins, such as cefazolin, have a wide-range of activity against almost all aerobic cocci, including MSSA (but not enterococci or MRSA) and some gram-negative bacilli (with the exception of *P. aeruginosa* and some other gram-negative rods).

☞ The cephamycins, specifically cefoxitin and cefotetan, have unique broad-spectrum activity against most anaerobic organisms. However, there are increasing resistant forms of *B. fragilis.* ☞ *B. fragilis* resistance has risen to such a degree that both the Infectious Disease Society of America and the Surgical Infection Society now recommend against these drugs as single agents for intra-abdominal infections (23,24,33).

Adverse Effects and Drug Interactions

The adverse effects of the cephalosporins are similar to those of the penicillins. Additionally, certain drug–drug interactions occur with cephalosporins and cephamycins, which have a methyl-thio-tetrazole side chain (cefotetan, cefoperazone, cefamandole, and moxalactam). This class of cephalosporins can produce a disulfiram-like reaction when administered with alcohol. In addition, these antibiotics can prolong the INR via inhibition of vitamin K metabolism.

Therapeutic/Clinical Uses

The third generation cephalosporins (ceftriaxone, cefotaxime, and ceftizoxime) have broad activity against most aerobic gram-positive cocci and gram-negative bacilli, (except *P. aeruginosa*), and are very commonly used for empiric therapy for Ventilator-associated pneumonia (VAP) in critical care units. Ceftazidime also has excellent activity against *P. aeruginosa* but only marginal activity against gram-positive cocci.

Advantages of the cephalosporins include their relatively low toxicity, especially compared to the aminoglycosides, their activity against certain hospital-acquired, multi-drug resistant bacteria, and the opportunity to administer a single agent rather than multiple antibiotics. Cephalosporins are not superior to the older, narrow-spectrum, and less-expensive antimicrobials. Thus, extended-spectrum cephalosporins are rarely the drug of choice for any infection. In addition, the emergence of resistance during therapy with these newer cephalosporins has been shown, including VRE, MRSA, and *C. difficile* through selection pressures.

OTHER BETA-LACTAM ANTIBIOTICS AND ADVERSE REACTIONS

Monobactams

Aztreonam is a synthetic monocyclic B-lactam (monobactam) antibiotic, and was the first approved for clinical use in the US (34,35). Monobactams differ structurally from penicillins and cephalosporins because of their monocyclic rather than a bicyclic nucleus; this novel structure explains why aztreonam has little cross-allergenicity with the bicyclic B-lactams. Although skin rashes have occurred occasionally with the use of aztreonam, the drug has been given safely to patients with immediate-type hypersensitivity reactions (e.g., anaphylaxis and urticaria) to both penicillins and cephalosporins (36). Other adverse effects are similar to those of other B-lactam drugs.

☞ Aztreonam is devoid of antibacterial activity against gram-positive and anaerobic bacteria. ☞ Aztreonam is clinically effective against most facultative aerobic Gram-negative bacilli. The spectrum and potency of aztreonam is similar to the third generation cephalosporin ceftazidime (37) as both contain the same 2-aminothiazolyl with a propyl-carboxy addition to its side-chain (38). Aztreonam adequately crosses the blood brain barrier and is highly active against *Haemophilus influenza* and *N. gonorrhoeae* (including beta-lactamase-producing strains), and against most of the Enterobacteriaceae (including *E. coli*, *Klebsiella*,

Table 6 Monobactams and Carbapenems (Beta Lactam-like Drugs): Selected Dosing and Need for Adjustment Based Upon Renal or Hepatic Dysfunction

Beta lactam-like drug classification and name	Typical adult IV dose range and intervals	Requires dose adjustment for renal insufficiency (CrCl <30 mL/min)	Requires dose adjustment for hepatic failure
Monobactams			
Aztreonam	1–2 g every 8 hr	Yes	No
Carbapenems			
Imipenem/cilastatin	0.5–1.0 g every 6–8 hr	Yes	No
Meropenem	0.5–1.0 g every 6–8 hr	Yes	No
Etrapenem	1 g every 24 hr	Yes	No

Abbreviation: IV, intravenously.

Proteus, Serratia, Shigella, and *Salmonella* species). Aztreonam is slightly less potent than imipenem or ceftazidime against *P. aeruginosa*. The usual dosage of aztreonam is 1 to 2 g intravenously given every eight hours. Refer to Table 6 for selected dosing and route of administration.

Carbapenems

Carbapenems are a class of antimicrobials created by a simple substitution of a sulfur atom for a carbon atom of the beta-lactam nucleus, and the addition of a double bond to the 5-member ring comprising the penicillin nucleus (7). The first clinically available carbapenem for use in the United States was imipenem, released in 1985 followed a decade later by meropenem (released in 1996) and shortly thereafter ertapenem. Imipenem is marketed as a combination drug with cilastatin (which inhibits the renal hydrolysis of imipenem). Meropenem and ertapenem, the other currently available carbapenems, are not combined with cilastatin.

    Carbapenems are the class of antibiotics with the greatest activity spectrum of any class of antibiotics for systemic use in humans. They are active against gram-positive (except MRSA), gram-negative, and anaerobic bacteria. These agents (except ertapenem) are particularly useful for hospital-acquired infections where bacterial resistance (other than MRSA and VRE) may be a concern.

Similar to the beta-lactam agents (especially the cephalosporins) the carbapenems have no activity against MRSA, *Enterococcus faecium*, and *Legionella* spp. In addition, the carbapenems have no activity against *Stenotrophomonas* (formerly *Pseudomonas) maltophilia*. The activity of ertapenem does not include *P. aeruginosa* or *Acinetobacter* spp., two organisms commonly involved in hospital-acquired infections. The carbapenems, imipenem and meropenem, are considered the drugs of choice for extended-spectrum beta-lactamase (ESBL) producing organisms.

The mechanism of action is similar to that of other beta-lactam antibiotics and the toxicities are similar. In addition, imipenem is associated with an increased risk of seizures when administered in large doses to patients with renal insufficiency, a side effect caused by the cilistatin component (which decreases the seizure threshold). Refer to Table 6 for selected dosing, route of administration, and need for dose adjustment for the carbapenems. The pharmacology of meropenem has recently been reviewed (7,39).

Beta-Lactam Allergy

Beta-lactam antibiotics are the most common class of antibiotics associated with adverse reactions partly because they are the most frequently used class of antibiotics. It was previously estimated that 1% to 10% of patients receiving penicillins will develop an adverse effect (40). However, that estimate was probably high, and the incidence of potentially life-threatening anaphylactic reactions is far lower (41).

Beta-lactam allergies are classified as immediate, accelerated, or delayed. Immediate reactions are of rapid onset occurring usually <30 minutes after administration, with the clinical manifestations of laryngeal edema, bronchospasm, hypotension, urticaria (hives), pruritus, and occasionally, anaphylactic shock. These reactions are IgE-mediated (Volume 1, Chapter 33).

Accelerated reactions occur from 1 to 72 hours after antibiotic administration, with the clinical manifestations of urticaria and angioedema. Delayed reactions are those occurring 3 days to several weeks after exposure, with rash being the most common, but they may also include serum sickness, hemolytic anemia, interstitial nephritis, arthralgias, and urticaria. Only the immediate and accelerated reactions have major clinical significance in terms of antibiotic selection.

Patients with a history of an immediate or accelerated reaction to penicillins manifesting as laryngeal edema, hypotension, urticaria, and/or angioedema, should not receive penicillins or any other beta-lactam antibiotics. In the event that a patient must be given penicillin, a penicillin skin test should be performed for patients with accelerated reactions, and if positive, then desensitization is required. If negative, these agents may be given cautiously. **Patients with a history of penicillin allergy due to rash or pruritus only occurring more than 3 days after administration are no more likely to have any allergic reaction to a cephalosporin than patients without a history of penicillin allergy and can safely receive cephalosporins.**

Recent studies indicate that the incidence of cross-reactivity to cephalosporins in penicillin-allergic patients is probably not more than two percent (42). Cross-reactions between penicillins and carbapenems occur much more frequently. **There is up to a 50% chance of developing a rash to carbapenems in patients with a history of rash to penicillins.** Aztreonam, a monobactam, does not appear to have any cross-reactivity in patients with immediate reactions to beta-lactams and is a useful therapeutic option when an antibiotic possessing excellent gram-negative rod activity is indicated in a beta-lactam allergic patient. **Aztreonam is** considered a safe alternative in patients allergic to penicillins or cephalosporins requiring gram-negative coverage, and vancomycin is the recommended choice when these patients require gram-positive coverage. ♂

AMINOGLYCOSIDES
History/Description

Aminoglycosides are naturally occurring antibacterial compounds produced by members of the Actinomycetes family that are filamentous bacteria that resemble fungi. Streptomycin (derived from *Streptomyces griseus*) was discovered in 1943, followed in 1963 by gentamicin (derived from *Actinomycetes* spp.), and tobramycin (derived from *Streptomyces tenebrarius*). The use of aminoglycosides has declined in recent years due to nephrotoxicity and the development of less toxic alternatives. However, the ability to dose these medications once daily and the relatively low level of resistance keeps the aminoglycosides in the clinical arena as a useful class of antibiotics (43,44).

Mechanism of Action, Pharmacology, Administration, and Dosage

Aminoglycosides bind to the 30S ribosomal subunit of bacteria, thereby inhibiting protein synthesis. The ability of aminoglycosides to reach ribosomes, which are intracellular, is facilitated by the concurrent use of antibiotics that inhibit the synthesis of the bacterial cell wall, such as the beta-lactam antibiotics and vancomycin. This synergistic activity accounts for the clinical use of combination of an aminoglycoside with a penicillin beta-lactam or vancomycin for serious enterococcal infections.

The aminoglycosides exert concentration-dependent killing. They also have a prolonged post-antibiotic effect that allows for once-daily dosing in many patients. Aminoglycosides have poor oral absorption and therefore are administered parenterally. Changes in the extracellular fluid compartment, as in congestive heart failure, ascites, or dehydration, will alter the volume of distribution and necessitate dosage modifications. Aminoglycosides have negligible protein binding. The average half-life for aminoglycosides in patients with normal renal function is approximately two hours. Aminoglycosides are significantly removed by hemodialysis but to a much lesser extent via peritoneal dialysis. Aminoglycosides do not cross the blood brain barrier, even in the presence of inflamed meninges.

A loading dose is often administered in the critically ill; 1.5 to 2 mg/kg for gentamicin or tobramycin and 7.5 to 15 mg/kg for amikacin (Table 7). Interpatient variability in volume of distribution and renal function in the critically ill population necessitates monitoring of aminoglycoside concentrations in the serum. Ideally, peak concentrations should be obtained 30 minutes after a 30-minute infusion. Trough concentrations should be drawn as close as possible prior to the start of the next dose. Recent studies suggest that single daily dosing is at least as effective as traditional dosing (due to the prolonged post-antibiotic effect) and may be less toxic (because the kidneys are allowed some recovery time between doses, when the blood concentration is low) (45).

Antimicrobial Activity/Spectrum/Resistance

Aminoglycosides are active against aerobic gram-negative bacilli and certain mycobacteria (including *Mycobacterium tuberculosis*) and have in vitro activity against many Staphylococcus species. Despite in vitro activity, aminoglycosides are not useful as single agents in treating gram-positive infections. However, aminoglycosides can be used synergistically with either beta-lactams or glycopeptides in patients with either *S. aureus* or enterococcal infections. *Burkholderia* (formerly *Pseudomonas cepacia*) and *Stenotrophomonas* (formerly *Pseudomonas* or *Xanthomonas*) *maltophilia* are typically resistant to all aminoglycosides. This rather narrow spectrum of activity is reflected in Tables 1 and 2 showing aminoglycosides as mainly alternative agents to first-line therapy.

The most common mechanism of aminoglycoside resistance is the production of plasmid-mediated aminoglycoside-modifying enzymes. Resistance of enterococci to gentamicin was first reported in the United States 15+ years ago. A survey of eight United States tertiary-care hospitals demonstrated that 25% of enterococci had high-level resistance to gentamicin. These organisms are generally resistant to all other aminoglycosides, but occasionally are susceptible to streptomycin.

Adverse Effects and Drug Interactions

♂ All aminoglycosides are nephrotoxic and ototoxic and can prolong the duration of neuromuscular blockade drugs. ♂ Aminoglycosides are reabsorbed by the proximal tubule accumulating in the renal cortex. This accounts for the nephrotoxicity, which is reportedly most common for gentamicin and least common for streptomycin, with amikacin and tobramycin being intermediate. Clinical nephrotoxicity does not usually occur until after at least 1 week of therapy, and is nonoliguric. Nephrotoxicity is typically reversible; however, ototoxicity (either vestibular or auditory) is generally permanent. Potentiation of neuromuscular blockade may also occur with the aminoglycosides, even after copious peritoneal irrigation with an aminoglycoside

---

Table 7 Aminoglycosides: Selected Dosing and Need for Adjustment Based Upon Renal or Hepatic Dysfunction

Aminoglycoside drug name	Typical adult IV dose range and intervals	Requires dose adjustment for renal insufficiency (CrCl <30 mL/min)	Requires dose adjustment for hepatic failure
Gentamicin	1.5–2.5 mg/kg q12 hr or 5 mg/kg q24 hr	Yes	No
Tobramycin	1.5–2.5 mg/kg q12 hr or 5 mg/kg q24 hr	Yes	No
Amikacin	7.5 mg/kg q12 hr or 15 mg/kg q24 hr	Yes	No
Streptomycin	10–15 mg/kg q24 hr	Yes	No

Abbreviation: IV, intravenously.

(Volume 2, Chapter 6). It is treated primarily by supportive means (airway protection or ventilation).

The ototoxicity seen with furosemide is additive when administered concomitantly with aminoglycosides. Bumetanide is less ototoxic and should be considered when concomitant use of aminoglycosides and diuretics are needed.

Age greater than 60 and co-administration of other nephrotoxic drugs can exacerbate the nephrotoxicity due to aminoglycosides. Examples of these drugs include: amphotericin B, vancomycin, parenteral bacitracin, capreomycin, cidofovir, cisplatin, cyclosporine, foscarnet, ganciclovir, IV pentamidine, polymyxin B, streptozocin, or tacrolimus.

Therapeutic/Clinical Uses
Gentamicin
Gentamicin is used alone primarily for urinary tract infections. It is also typically used in conjunction with extended-spectrum penicillins for nosocomial infections caused by *Enterobacter* spp. and *P. aeruginosa*. Combination therapy including an aminoglycoside with agents that provide gram-positive or anaerobic activity is frequently used in potentially polymicrobial infections when gram-negative rods may be playing a role. An aminoglycoside is used in combination therapy with either ampicillin or vancomycin for several different types of endocarditis, most commonly those that are due to enterococci.

Tobramycin
Tobramycin has essentially the same parenteral uses as gentamicin. It has greater activity against *Acinetobacter* spp. and *P. aeruginosa* but less activity against *Serratia marcescens* than gentamicin does. If organisms are resistant to gentamicin, they will likely be resistant to tobramycin. Inhaled tobramycin has been associated with improved pulmonary function and decreased hospitalization in patients with cystic fibrosis.

Amikacin
Amikacin is useful primarily for organisms that are resistant gentamicin and tobramycin. It is also used in combination with other antibiotics, for example, for infections due to *Nocardia asteroides* and occasionally for infections due to *M. tuberculosis* or *M. avium* complex.

Streptomycin
Streptomycin is sometimes used (as part of combination therapy) in the treatment of multidrug-resistant tuberculosis and may be useful in the treatment of some gentamicin-resistant enterococcal infections. It is also the drug of choice for several potential bacterial agents in bioterrorism, such as tularemia and plague, although gentamicin can be used alternatively.

TETRACYCLINES AND GLYCYLCYCLINES
History/Description
The tetracyclines were isolated from *Streptomyces* spp., first used clinically over 50 years ago. ✍ **Tetracycline has a broad spectrum of activity against gram-positive, gram-negative, and anaerobic bacteria as well as rickettsiae, mycoplasma, chlamydiae, protozoa, actinomycetes, and even certain viruses.** ✍ Tetracyclines are infrequently used in the ICU setting. However, when they are employed, it is usually to combat pneumonia due to presumed or known "atypical" agents (Table 8). Doxycycline and, to a lesser extent, minocycline are the most commonly used drugs of this class. The tetracyclines are still commonly used for community acquired pathogens, and have recently been reviewed in depth (46,47).

Mechanism of Action, Pharmacology, Administration, and Dosage
The tetracyclines are similar in mechanism of action to aminoglycosides, as both antimicrobials inhibit bacterial protein synthesis at the ribosomal level. However, in regard to spectrum of activity, the tetracyclines more closely resemble the macrolides. The tetracyclines are typically bacteriostatic rather than bactericidal. Tetracycline is excreted in the urine and should be avoided in renal insufficiency, because high concentrations of the accumulated drug are hepatotoxic. In contrast to tetracycline, doxycycline, and minocycline are eliminated through hepatobiliary processes and can be used in patients with renal insufficiency.

Doxycycline and other tetracyclines can be administered either parenterally or orally, and because of the long half-life, can be administered once or twice daily. Refer to Table 9 for tetracycline dosing and need for dose adjustment.

Antimicrobial Activity/Spectrum/Resistance
The tetracyclines are currently utilized for the empiric treatment of community-acquired pneumonia because of their activity against both many pyogenic bacteria and "atypical" organisms, such as *Mycoplasma spp.*, *Chlamydia* spp., or *Legionella* spp. They also have utility in the treatment of infections

Table 8 Antimicrobial Drugs of Choice Against Atypical Organisms

Microorganisms	Drug of choice	Alternative agents
Mycoplasma pneumoniae	Azithromycin or a tetracycline	Fluoroquinolone, erythromycin, clarithromycin
Chlamydia psittaci	Flourquinolone or doxycycline	Chloramphenicol
Chlamydia pneumoniae	Azithromycin or tetracycline	Fluoroquinolone, erythromycin, clarithromycin
Ehrlichia spp.	Doxycycline	
Rickettsia spp.	Doxycycline	Chloramphenicol, rifampin, fluoroquinolone
Borrelia burgdorferi (Lyme disease)	Amoxicillin or doxycycline	Ceftriaxone, cefotaxime, azithromycin, clarithromycin
Leptospira	Penicillin	A tetracycline, ceftriaxone
Treponema pallidum (syphilis)	Penicillin	Ceftriaxone, a tetracycline, erythromycin
Actinomyces spp.	Penicillin	A tetracycline, erythromycin, clindamycin
Nocardia spp.	Co-trimoxazole	A tetracycline, carbapenem, linezolid

Table 9 Antibacterial Agents: Requiring Selected Dosing and Need for Adjustment Based Upon Renal or Hepatic Dysfunction

Misc. drug name	Typical adult IV dose range and intervals	Requires dose adjustment for renal insufficiency (CrCl <30 mL/min)	Requires dose adjustment for hepatic failure
Mimocycline	100 mg every 12 hr	No	±
Doxycycline	100 mg every12 hr	No	±
Erythromycin	0.5–1 g every 6 hr	No	±
Azithromycin	0.25–0.5 g every 24 hr	No	No
Clarithromycin	500 mg orally every 12 hr	Yes	No
Clindamycin	600 mg every 8 hr	No	No
Metronidazole	500 mg every 8–12 hr	No	Yes
Quinupristin/dalfopristin	7.5 mg/kg every 8 hr	No	±
Linezolid	600 mg every12 hr	No	±
Vancomycin	15 mg/kg every 12 hr	Yes	No
Daptomycin	4–6 mg/kg every 24 hr	Yes	No
Rifampin	600 mg every 24 hr	No	Yes
Tmp/sulfamethoxazole	5 mg/kg of tmp every 8–12 hr	Yes	±
Aminoglycosides	Table 7	Yes	No
Tigecycline	100 mg once followed by 50 mg every 12 hr	No	Yes

Note: ± indicates although specific dosage guidelines are not available, a reduced dosage may be necessary.
Abbreviations: Tmp, trimethoprim; IV, intravenously.

due to *Brucella* spp., rickettsiae, chlamydiae, syphilis, *Borrelia burgdorferi* (the agent of Lyme infection), *Vibrio* spp., *Yersinia* spp., *Francisella tularensis*, *Leptospira* spp., and genital infections. The tetracycline group is also useful in the treatment of some nontuberculous mycobacterial infections (such as *Mycobacteria marinum*). Tetracyclines were originally the only drugs available to treat VRE, however, linezolid, daptomycin, and quinopristiry/dalfopristin have been recently used as well.

Adverse Effects and Drug Interactions
The tetracyclines are generally well tolerated with two important exceptions: photosensitivity and discoloration of developing teeth and bones in children. Minocycline is also associated with vestibular toxicity and a blue-tinged hyperpigmentation of the skin and mucous membranes.

Milk, antacids, iron supplements, and probably other agents with divalent cations decrease the gastrointestinal absorption of orally administered tetracyclines and should be ingested several hours before or after the administration of tetracycline (which is best taken on an empty stomach). These oral divalent cations have less effect on the oral absorption of doxycycline and minocycline.

Therapeutic/Clinical Uses
As a result of the broad spectrum of the tetracyclines as noted above, these agents are useful in a wide variety of infections; however, they are rarely indicated as the drug of choice in the critically ill patient except for the treatment of rickettsial infections and pulmonary infections due to "atypical" agents (Table 8).

Tigecycline, a glycine derivative of minocycline, received FDA approval for skin and skin structure infections and complicated intra abdominal infections in 2005. Like the tetracyclines, tigecycline has a broad spectrum of activity (48,49). It is active against gram-positive organisms,

gram-negative aerobes, anaerobes, and "atypical" organisms like Chlamydiae and Mycoplasma. It also has activity against organisms that are tetracycline resistant and is also active against MRSA, MRSE, VRE, and penicillin-resistant pneumococci. A notable gap in its spectrum is a lack of activity against *P. aeruginosa*, which could limit the use of tigecycline in the treatment of nosocomial infections, especially HAP. However, since it is much more potent than other tetracyclines, which are bacteriostatic, tigecycline will likely find use in non-pseudomonal HAP. The major side effect noted in early phase trials is nausea and vomiting in patients (20–35%). Tigecycline is only available as an intravenous preparation due to poor oral bioavailability. Its potential place in the therapeutic armentarium is yet undefined.

MACROLIDES
History/Description
Erythromycin was the first clinically available macrolide antibiotic, and was introduced clinically in the 1950s. Erythromycin is derived from the soil fungus, *Streptomyces erythreus*. Modifications of the erythromycin chemical structure have led to two new macrolides (azithromycin and clarithromycin). Both azithromycin and clarithromycin possess better gastrointestinal tolerability and a somewhat broader spectrum of activity than erythromycin, although at a greatly increased cost. The macrolides are reviewed in several recent articles (50–52).

Mechanism of Action, Pharmacology, Administration, and Dosage
The macrolides all act at the ribosome by inhibiting RNA-dependent protein synthesis. Azithromycin and clarithromycin are acid-stable and well absorbed from the gastrointestinal tract, irrespective of the presence of food.

Erythromycin, which is inactivated by stomach acids, requires enteric coating to increase its efficacy. All macrolides are rapidly absorbed and concentrate well within tissues, including phagocytes. The high concentration of macrolides within phagocytes serves as a delivery system of the drug to the site of infection. ☞ **Azithromycin has an extremely long intracellular dwell time, permitting once daily (or less often) dosing.** ☞ Indeed, azithromycin is often used once weekly for the prophylaxis of mycobacterial infections in patients with AIDS.

Various erythromycin products are available for both oral and parenteral administration. Intravenous administration of erythromycin is associated with thrombophlebitis, and intramuscular injections should be avoided due to pain. Oral and intravenous azithromycin are also available. A parenteral form of clarithromycin is currently not available. Dosing guidelines are shown in Table 9.

Antimicrobial Activity/Spectrum/Resistance

Erythromycin, clarithromycin, and azithromycin all have bacteriostatic activity against gram-positive organisms, such as *Streptococcus pneumoniae* and some *S. aureus*. These agents also have good in vitro and clinical activity against Mycoplasma, Legionella, syphilis, and chlamydiae. Of note, both clarithromycin and azithromycin have activity against some mycobacteria (including *M. avium* complex) and *Helicobacter* spp. Erythromycin lacks activity against *H. influenzae*, whereas both azithromycin and clarithromycin are efficacious against this agent. The macrolides are frequently used in patients with allergies to beta-lactams, especially for infections due to gram-positive bacteria. However, they have very limited activity against MRSA and enterococcus, and a significant proportion of *S. pneumoniae* are resistant to the macrolides in some locales.

Adverse Effects and Drug Interactions

Gastrointestinal intolerance is a frequent complication of oral erythromycin products, whereas the other macrolides tend to be much better tolerated. One advantage of azithromycin over the other macrolides is the absence of clinically significant drug–drug interactions involving the cytochrome P-450 system (CP450) (Volume 2, Chapter 4).

Therapeutic/Clinical Uses

Macrolides are commonly used for community-acquired pneumonias and in patients who are allergic to penicillins. The promotility side effect of low-dose erythromycin is increasingly utilized as a promotility agent in critically ill patients with gastroparesis.

LINCOSAMIDES (CLINDAMYCIN)
History/Description

Clindamycin, a lincosamide derivative, has been in clinical use since the mid-1960s. Although clindamycin is associated with *C. difficile* colitis, it remains one of the mainstays in the treatment of serious anaerobic infections, and as an alternative agent for some *S. aureus* infections (51,53,54).

Mechanism of Action, Pharmacology, Administration, and Dosage

Clindamycin inhibits RNA-dependent protein synthesis acting at the ribosomal level (infusion similar to macrolides). Although oral and intravenous preparations of clindamycin

penetrate most body tissues (including lung, liver, bone, and extra-cranial abscesses), it does not easily cross the blood-brain barrier or enter the CSF, even when the meninges are inflamed. Thus, metronidazole, which fully penetrates the CSF, should be used for any CNS infections involving anaerobic organisms (other than CNS toxoplasmosis—which can be treated with clindamycin). Dosing guidelines are shown in Table 9.

Antimicrobial Activity/Spectrum/Resistance

Clindamycin has a spectrum of activity that includes many anaerobes, especially oral flora; some aerobic gram-positive cocci, including most strains of pneumococci; other streptococci; *S. aureus*; *Pneumocystis carinii*; and *Toxoplamsa gondii*. Clindamycin has no activity against enterococci and has limited activity against most MRSA. The majority of aerobic gram-negative bacilli are intrinsically resistant to clindamycin. Most intestinal *Bacteroides* spp., especially of *B. fragililis* are resistant to clindamycin (55). Clindamycin, therefore, should not be a first-line antianaerobic agent to treat infections below the diaphragm.

Adverse Effects and Drug Interactions

Clindamycin exerts a direct muscular depressant effect, and may prolong the duration of neuromuscular blockage (56). Diarrhea is a common side effect of clindamycin, even in the absence of colitis, and the potential for the development of *C. difficile* colitis makes the use of this antibiotic complicated, limiting its use to severe infections with clear indications for use.

Clindamycin has no clinically significant drug–drug interactions.

Therapeutic/Clinical Uses

Clindamycin is used most commonly for infections outside of the CNS (except cerebral toxoplasmosis) that are thought to include anaerobes, especially *B. fragilis* and other penicillin-resistant anaerobes. Clindamycin is utilized in some pulmonary infections, especially aspiration pneumonia that is community-acquired and also as a useful alternative to penicillin.

Clindamycin has been successfully used in the treatment of pelvic inflammatory disease (PID) for years. This success probably relates to the fact that vaginal anaerobic flora are more similar to oral anerobes than to colonic anerobes in general. However, if the PID infection involves *B. fragilis*, metronidazole is a better choice. Although sexually transmitted pathogens can cause PID, these infections tend to become polymicrobial, involving aerobes and anaerobes. Clindamycin is frequently used with other antibiotics that have gram-negative bacillary activity. Since clindamycin is a protein synthesis inhibitor and can act even when cells are in stationary phase, it has utility in the treatment of bacterial toxidromes and in situations such as necrotizing fasciitis. ☞ **Because of its gram-positive and anaerobic coverage, clindamycin is useful (with combination gram-negative therapy) for necrotizing fasciitis, most oral and vaginal anaerobic infections, and diabetic foot infections, which tend to be polymicrobial and virulent.** ☞

METRONIDAZOLE
History/Description

Metronidazole is a nitroimidazole drug first synthesized in the 1950s and was originally recognized as being effective against certain protozoa. In the 1960s metronidazole was recognized to also possess excellent anaerobic antimicrobial activity (53,57). ☞ **Metronidazole is indicated for the treatment of serious polymicrobial infections involving anaerobes (e.g., necrotizing fasciitis and infections involving contamination from the GI tract). Importantly, other agents with aerobic gram-positive and gram-negative coverage must be co-administered.** ☞

Mechanism of Action, Pharmacology, Administration, and Dosage

Metronidazole enters the cell by passive diffusion where its nitro group is reduced by electron transport proteins with low redox potential. This process produces metabolites that alter the helical structure of DNA and subsequently causes cell death (58).

Metronidazole is rapidly absorbed in the gut. Indeed, serum levels are similar following oral and intravenous administration. Although metronidazole is almost completely absorbed after oral administration, critically ill patients should receive therapy via the intravenous route until stable (59). When the patient is stable, and the gut is functional, administration should be converted to the enteral route for cost saving since it is nearly 100% bioavailable. The liver metabolizes metronidazole into a water-soluble metabolite, and both this metabolite and the un-metabolized metronidazole are excreted in the urine. No dosage adjustment is required in those with renal insufficiency, but dosage should be reduced in patients with hepatic insufficiency. Therapeutic drug levels are attained in most tissues; excellent levels are found in the CSF.

In severe anaerobic infections, metronidazole is administered as a loading dose of 15 mg/kg intravenously followed by 7.5 mg/kg every six to eight hours. This typically equates to 1 g followed by 500 mg every six to eight hours.

Antimicrobial Activity/Spectrum/Resistance

Metronidazole is active against certain protozoa, including *Trichomonas*, *Giardia*, and *Entamoeba* however; its primary role in the critically ill patient is as an extremely active agent against obligate anaerobic bacteria and is the antimicrobial agent most reliably active against *B. fragilis* (60). Resistance has been reported in Europe and Africa but is very uncommon (53). When metronidazole resistance does occur, it is most commonly attributable to the presence of one of the five known *nim* nitroreductase genes (61). Metronidazole resistance had not previously been reported in *B. fragilis* isolates from the Western Hemisphere, recently a serious infection involving a metronidazole-resistant *B. fragilis* isolate was recovered from a patient in Seattle, Washington in 2004 with the *nim*A nitroreductase gene (61).

Adverse Effects and Drug Interactions

The most severe adverse effect seen with metronidazole, although rare, involves the central nervous system and may include seizures, encephalopathy, cerebellar dysfunction, and peripheral neuropathy (57). More commonly, metronidazole causes minor gastrointestinal side effects such as nausea, diarrhea, a metallic taste, stomatitis, and dry mouth (57). Alcohol should be avoided while receiving metronidazole because it can induce a disulfiram-like reaction (57,62). Metronidazole inhibits the metabolism of warfarin and will prolong the prothrombin time and INR in patients taking coumarin-type anticoagulants (63).

Therapeutics/Clinical Use

In general, as a result of its spectrum of activity, metronidazole is extremely useful in most anaerobic infections with the important exceptions of those due to *Actinomyces* spp. and *Propionobacterium acnes* (57). The excellent penetration of metronidazole into all tissues combined with its bactericidal activity makes it effective for the treatment of most serious anaerobic infections (57). Many serious anaerobic infections are polymicrobial, therefore, additional agents with better coverage against gram-positive aerobes and gram-negative organisms are also necessary. ☞ ***B. fragilis* is probably the most frequently encountered clinically significant anaerobe where metronidazole should be considered the drug of choice, especially in intra-abdominal infections (57).** ☞ Metronidazole is also the drug of choice for the treatment of pseudomembranous colitis due to *C. difficile* (54). Oral vancomycin is an alternative in seriously ill patients with pseudomembranous colitis.

QUINUPRISTIN/DALFOPRISTIN (SYNERCID®)
History/Description

The evolution of multi-drug resistant bacteria, including MRSA and VRE faecium, has created a pressing need for effective alternative antibiotics, hence the utility of the streptogramins (i.e., quinupristin/dalfopristin), linezolid, and daptomycin.

The streptogramins are a family of compounds isolated from *Streptomyces pristinaespiralis*. The family is divided into group A and group B based on molecular structure. Dalfopristin is a derivative of a group A streptogramin, and quinupristin is a group B streptogramin. These two streptogramins have been combined in a commercially available injectable form at a 30:70 weight-to-weight ratio. Individually, these compounds demonstrate only modest in vitro activity. However, the combination is synergistic. Unfortunately, in vitro studies also demonstrate that the combination of quinupristin and dalfopristin is not bactericidal against all species and strains of common gram-positive organisms.

Quinupristin/dalfopristin, a combination product known as "Synercid," has demonstrated activity against most strains of aerobic gram-positive microorganisms, both in vitro and in clinical infections, including; *E. faecium* (vancomycin-resistant and multi-drug resistant strains only), *S. aureus* (both MSSA and MRSA), and *Streptococcus pyogenes* (group A beta-hemolytic streptococci) (64,65). This compound is bacteriostatic against *E. faecium* and bactericidal against strains of methicillin-susceptible and methicillin-resistant *Staphylococci* spp. Importantly, dalfopristin/quinupristin has no activity against *Enterococcus faecalis*. A post-antibiotic effect has been demonstrated for *S. aureus*: seven hours for methicillin-susceptible strains; five hours for methicillin-resistant strains. Since the mode of action of streptogramins differs from other classes of antibacterial agents, there is no cross-resistance.

Mechanism of Action, Pharmacology, Administration, and Dosage

Quinupristin and dalfopristin bind to sequential sites located on the 50S subunit of the bacterial ribosome. Dalfopristin binding causes a conformational change in the ribosome that subsequently increases the binding of quinupristin. The binding of both agents to the ribosome constricts the exit channel on the ribosome through which nascent polypeptides are extruded; proper functioning of the ribosome is blocked and transfer RNA (tRNA) synthetase activity is inhibited leading to a decrease in free tRNA within the cell. Without these tRNAs, the bacterial cell cannot properly incorporate amino acids into peptide chains leading to bacterial cell death.

Quinupristin/dalfopristin undergoes hepatic metabolism, and both compounds have active metabolites. However, no increase in adverse events has been reported in patients with hepatic impairment, and no dosage reduction is required in these patients. The parent drugs and major metabolites are eliminated primarily by fecal excretion (75%) with a small portion of unchanged quinupristin and dalfopristin (15–19%) eliminated renally. In patients with a creatinine clearance <29 mL/min, a 30% increase in the combined AUC of quinupristin/dalfopristin and their metabolites has been observed, but the manufacturer has not established guidelines for dosage reduction. The manufacturer's recommended intravenous dose of quinupristin/dalfopristin in adults is 7.5 mg/kg given over 60 minutes every eight hours preferably through a central line.

Antimicrobial Activity/Spectrum/Resistance

Resistance to the streptogramins has been reported (66,67). The most common expression of bacterial resistance to streptogramins is through conformational alterations in ribosomal target binding sites. However, it appears that multiple point mutations are required for drug resistance to this combination product to develop.

Adverse Effects and Drug Interactions

The most common adverse effects with quinupristin/dalfopristin are infusion-site reactions. Non-infusion related reactions including nausea, diarrhea, vomiting, rash, headache, pain, and pruritus were reported with similar frequency as comparator antibiotics in one trial. Elevations in liver enzymes (2–7%), increases in total and direct bilirubin (1–5%), thrombocytopenia (2%), and decreases in hemoglobin of <8–mg/dl (2.6%) have also been reported.

Quinupristin/dalfopristin is an inhibitor of Cytochrome P450 (CP450) 3A4 enzyme. One study demonstrated a two-fold increase in cyclosporine levels within two to five days of concomitant use. Caution is recommended when concomitantly administering other agents that are eliminated via the CP450-3A4 isoenzyme pathway with quinupristin/dalfopristin (Volume 2, Chapter 4).

Therapeutic/Clinical Uses

Quinupristin/dalfopristin is the most expensive parenteral antibacterial currently on the market. ☞ **The greatest utility of quinupristin/dalfopristin, daptomycin, and linezolid is in the management of patients with multi-resistant enterococci (VRE) or MRSA infections for which limited alternatives exist.** ☞ The treatment of VRE infections has been recently reviewed (68,69).

LINEZOLID (ZYVOX®)
History/Description

Linezolid is one of a new class of synthetic antibiotics known as fluorinated oxazolidinones (70,71). This drug is designed to target MRSA; it also provides good activity against other gram-positive organisms, including penicillin-resistant pneumococci and VRE (72). This drug now provides an alternative to vancomycin therapy in an oral formulation.

Mechanism of Action, Pharmacology, Administration, and Dosage

Linezolid inhibits bacterial protein synthesis by interfering with translation. Linezolid binds to a site on the bacterial 23S ribosomal RNA of the 50S subunit; this action prevents the formation of a functional 70S initiation complex, an essential step in the bacterial translation process. The action of linezolid is considered to be bacteriostatic against Staphylococci and Enterococci, but is bacteriocidal against the majority of Streptococcal strains tested.

Following oral administration, absorption of linezolid appears to be rapid with a peak plasma concentration (t_{max}) of one to two hours (73). The oral bioavailability is approximately 100% and as such linezolid may be administered orally or intravenously without dosage adjustment (73). Linezolid is distributed extensively to various tissues. Linezolid appears to partition into the central nervous system at a CSF: serum ratio of 0.65:1; it has been used to successfully treat ventriculoperitoneal shunt infections caused by VRE or coagulase-negative Staphylococci. Of major importance in critical care, linezolid penetrates into bronchoalveolar lavage fluid and lung tissue more effectively than vancomycin (74).

The recommended adult dosage is 600 mg intravenous or orally every 12 hours for all indications except uncomplicated skin and soft-tissue infections, for which the recommended dosage is 400 mg orally every 12 hours. Elimination of linezolid is primarily (65%) nonrenal. Clearance is mediated by non-enzymatic chemical oxidation, which results in the formation of two major inactive metabolites, which are excreted renally (75).

Dosage adjustments are not necessary in renal insufficiency or mild to moderate hepatic dysfunction. Approximately 30% of a dosage of linezolid is removed by hemodialysis. For this reason, patients should receive their linezolid doses post-dialysis.

Antimicrobial Activity/Spectrum/Resistance

Soon after linezolid became FDA-approved in the US, reports of linezolid-resistant VRE organisms were identified at several institutions. Resistance with linezolid has been observed in 15 patients with enterococcal infections, and a vancomycin-resistant strain of *E. faecium* with reduced susceptibility to linezolid (MIC = 8 mg/mL) has been isolated. Preliminary reports suggest that most cases of resistance to linezolid occur when the drug is used for prolonged periods of time in patients with prosthetic devices. Resistance to linezolid is usually associated with single-point mutations in 23S rRNA. Studies suggest the frequency of spontaneous resistance to linezolid is $<10^{-9}$.

Adverse Effects and Drug Interactions

The most frequently reported adverse events with linezolid in one study were diarrhea (8.3%), nausea (6.6%), headache (6.4%), and vomiting (4.3%). In another study, tongue discoloration (2.5%), oral candidiasis (2.3%), and injection-site pain (1.4%) were also reported. Thrombocytopenia (platelet count <75% of the lower limit of normal and/or baseline) was reported in 2.4% of patients who received linezolid in clinical trials. Linezolid-related thrombocytopenia appears to be associated with prolonged duration of therapy (>2 weeks) and is generally reversible on discontinuation.

Linezolid is metabolized via oxidation of its morpholine ring, independent of CP450 activities. It is 31% protein bound; therefore, interactions via displacement from protein binding sites are unlikely. Linezolid is a weak, reversible inhibitor of human monoamine oxidase A. Consequently, it has the potential to interact with adrenergic and serotonergic agents, leading to hypertensive crises (Volume 2, Chapter 17) and serotonin syndrome (Volume 1, Chapter 40 and Volume 2, Chapter 46). Mean increases in systolic blood pressure of 32 and 38 mmHg have been observed in normotensive subjects taking linezolid concomitantly with pseudoephedrine and phenylpropanolamine, respectively.

Therapeutic/Clinical Uses

Linezolid is an expensive drug; one day of linezolid costs roughly the same amount as 500 days of either doxycycline or co-trimoxazole. Although this antibiotic represents the first in a unique class of antibiotics (the oxazolidinones), more clinical experience and formal pharmacoeconomics data should be obtained prior to its widespread clinical use. Linezolid should be reserved for the treatment of documented serious VRE or MRSA infections, or when oral therapy is an option. Since it appears to achieve high levels in the lungs, it may soon become the drug of choice to treat MRSA pneumonia (74).

VANCOMYCIN
History/Description

Vancomycin is a bactericidal glycopeptide derived from the soil fungus *Streptomyces orientalis* and was first introduced in 1956. Within two years, vancomycin use was superseded by methicillin and cephalothin, which had fewer side effects. In the late 1970s, MRSA began to emerge, and vancomycin returned to the clinical arena to treat these threats. Recent improvements in manufacturing have increased its purity and reduced the nephrotoxicity of vancomycin (75–78). However, the histaminereleasing effect responsible for "red man" syndrome and hypotension during administration still persist. Teicoplanin, a related compound, is at least as efficacious and less toxic. Teicoplanin has been used for years in Europe, but it is not currently available in the US.
☞ **Vancomycin is most often used parenterally to treat MRSA, empirically in life-threatening infections, and orally for *C. difficile* colitis.** ☞

Mechanism of Action, Pharmacology, Administration, and Dosage

Vancomycin exerts its effect by binding to the precursor units of bacterial cell walls, known as peptidoglycans, inhibiting their synthesis. This binding occurs at a different site of action from that of penicillin. The net result is an alteration of bacterial cell wall permeability. In addition, RNA synthesis is inhibited. Gram-negative organisms are not sensitive to vancomycin, because porin channels in their cell wall do not accommodate the large, bulky vancomycin molecule.

Vancomycin is about 55% protein bound. Vancomycin penetrates most body tissues including the brain when the meninges are inflamed. Vancomycin also distributes well into pericardial, pleural, ascitic, and synovial fluids. Intravenous vancomycin is primarily excreted unchanged by the kidneys. Vancomycin has poor oral bioavailability with oral doses remaining intraluminal in the intestine until eliminated in the feces; this also explains its oral use in *C. difficile* colitis. Vancomycin has a half-life of approximately six hours in a patient with normal renal function. However, in anuric patients, the half-life can be prolonged to approximately 7.5 days. Vancomycin is not removed by hemodialysis or peritoneal dialysis, unless F60 or F80 polysulfone filters are used (Volume 2, Chapter 43). In patients with normal renal function, vancomycin is dosed at 1 g IV every 12 hours, and levels are tested. Teicoplanin is dosed on an every 24-hour basis. In those patients with known or suspected renal impairment, an initial vancomycin dose of 15 mg/kg should be given, and the dosage interval increased. The appropriate dosage interval should be further determined using therapeutic drug level monitoring. When vancomycin is given with an aminoglycoside, increased incidence of nephrotoxicity is possible. For pseudomembranous colitis, a dosage of 125–500 mg orally every six hours for 7–10 days is appropriate.

Antimicrobial Activity/Spectrum/Resistance

Vancomycin is bactericidal against essentially all staphylococci (both *S. aureus* and coagulase-negative Staphylococci), all *S. pneumoniae*, *S. pyogenes*, and *S. viridans*. It is bacteriostatic against most Enterococcus and most *Corynebacterium* spp. A few anaerobes are susceptible, but virtually no gram-negative organisms are susceptible to vancomycin. Vancomycin has achieved a prominent role in therapy of critically ill patients due to the large prevalence of MRSA in hospitals. To an increasing extent, critically ill patients have temporary or permanent foreign bodies implanted as pacemakers, vascular access, valves, or shunts. These devices are particularly predisposed to infection by Staphylococci, including *S. aureus* and coagulase-negative Staphylococci, an increasing fraction of which is methicillin-resistant.

Vancomycin intermediate-susceptible *S. aureus* (VISA) is used to describe decreased susceptibility of *S. aureus* to vancomycin (79,80). In 1997, the first strain of *S. aureus* with reduced susceptibility to vancomycin was reported from Japan (81). The Clinical and Laboratory Standards Institute (CLSI) defines Staphylococci requiring concentrations of vancomycin of ≤4 mcg/mL for growth inhibition as susceptible, those requiring 8 to 16 mcg/mL as intermediate (VISA) (79,80), and those requiring concentrations of >32 mcg/mL as resistant (VRSA) (82). Implications of multi-drug resistant organisms make therapeutic choices much more difficult and reinforce the need to control the use of vancomycin and other antibiotics (16). Infections with these vancomycin resistant microorganisms are usually sensitive to linezolid, daptomycin, or dalfopristin/quinupristin.

The proportion of Enterococci isolated from ICUs that were resistant to vancomycin increased from 0.3% in 1989 to almost 24% in 1998. Enterococci are able to build cell walls in the presence of glycopeptide antibiotics because they can bypass an intermediate molecule to which the glycopeptide binds (83). Risk factors for the emergence of VRE include exposure to broad spectrum cephalosporins, vancomycin, or antibiotics with significant anaerobic activity; and prolonged hospital and/or ICU stay. The empiric use of vancomycin should be limited to life threatening infections in order to reduce the emergence of VRE.

Adverse Effects and Drug Interactions

Vancomycin is now considered approximately 95% free of impurities; therefore the incidence of adverse effects has declined (84). However, phlebitis still occurs with peripherally administered vancomycin in approximately 13% of patients. Hypotension, flushing, tingling, and erythema affecting upper trunk, face, and arms (red person syndrome) are associated with rapid infusion in 3% to 11% of patients, especially if 1-g doses are used. Treatments with fluid administration, antihistamines, and corticosteroids have been suggested, as well as slowing the infusion. Rash unrelated to "red person syndrome" is also seen in about 2% to 5% of patients. The rash is often described as maculopapular, but rare cases of Stevens-Johnson have been reported, Neutropenia occurs in approximately 2% of patients (84), the onset typically being delayed up to 30 days after commencing the drug. Nephrotoxicity and ototoxicity are uncommon if peak serum levels are maintained <50 mcg/mL, but more likely to occur if vancomycin is administered with other nephro- or ototoxic compounds, and more common in critically ill patients.

Drugs that increase the risk of nephrotoxicity when co-administered with vancomycin include: amphotericin B, aminoglycosides, parenteral bacitracin, capreomycin, cidofovir, cisplatin, cyclosporine, foscarnet, ganciclovir, IV pentamidine, polymyxin B, streptozocin, and tacrolimus. The combined use of vancomycin and cidofovir is contraindicated. Vancomycin should be discontinued seven days prior to beginning cidofovir.

Orally administered vancomycin should not be used with cholestyramine or colestipol. These anion-exchange resins can bind vancomycin and reduce its effectiveness. Since these drugs are sometimes used to treat *C. difficile* colitis by binding the toxin in the intestinal lumen, patients may be taking vancomycin and one of the resins simultaneously. If patients must take both drugs, doses should be administered several hours apart.

Vancomycin should be used cautiously with other ototoxic drugs such as aminoglycosides, aspirin or other salicylates, capreomycin, ethacrynic acid, furosemide, or paromomycin. Vancomycin may potentiate the neuromuscular effects of nondepolarizing neuromuscular blockers (Volume 2, Chapter 6). Vancomycin, when used concomitantly with metformin, may increase the risk of lactic acidosis. Vancomycin can decrease metformin elimination by competing for common renal tubular transport systems, necessitating careful monitoring while on concurrent therapy.

Therapeutic Drug Level Monitoring

The ideal vancomycin-dosing regimen is one that results in peak vancomycin concentrations that are less than 30 to 50 mg/L and trough concentrations that are in the range of 5 to 15 mg/L. Therapeutic drug monitoring of vancomycin remains controversial (85). Vancomycin exhibits concentration-dependent killing, requiring a serum concentration >1 mg/L. Therefore, higher concentrations are not necessarily associated with improved bactericidal effects (especially in the lung)! For MRSA pneumonia vancomycin troughs should be >15 to 20 mg/L. Most clinicians believe patients at high risk for therapeutic failure or potential toxicity should have both peak and trough values monitored. These patients include the elderly, those with poor renal function, or patients with suspected alteration in their volume of distribution; this includes the critically ill.

Therapeutic/Clinical Uses

The primary indication for vancomycin is for MRSA infections, and empiric administration in critically ill patients with significant infections or sepsis until culture results return. Other indications for vancomycin include Staphylococcal and Streptococcal infections in patients allergic to penicillins, and as an alternative to penicillin for the prophylaxis of bacterial endocarditis. Vancomycin is being used in conjunction with ceftriaxone in locales with high prevalence rates of highly penicillin-resistant pneumococcal meningitis. For organisms susceptible to beta-lactams, clinical experience has demonstrated improved patient outcome with the use of beta-lactams rather than with vancomycin. Vancomycin is also useful in oral therapy against *C. difficile* colitis.

DAPTOMYCIN
History/Description

Daptomycin is the first antibacterial agent from a novel class of drugs, the cyclic lipopeptides (derived from *Streptomyces roseosporus*). Discovered more than 20 years ago, its clinical research was halted due to concerns of skeletal muscle toxicity. However, development resumed in response to the increasing demand for bactericidal antibiotics effective against VRE and VRSA (86). Daptomycin is now approved for the treatment of complicated skin and skin structure infections caused by gram-positive bacteria. It recently received FDA approval for use in the treatment of bacteria and endocarditis (87). Because of inactivation by alveolar surfactant, daptomycin is not effective in the treatment of pneumonia. However, it has excellent concentrations in all other tissues (88–90).

Mechanism of Action, Pharmacology, Administration, and Dosage

Daptomycin works by binding to and interfering with the integrity of cell wall structure in gram-positive bacteria but does not penetrate the bacterial cytoplasm. Upon binding, transmembrane channels are formed, causing rapid depolarization of membrane potential and inhibition of protein, DNA, and RNA synthesis, resulting in bacterial cell death. It has a concentration-dependent bactericidal activity.

Daptomycin is poorly absorbed orally and should be administered intravenously only. Direct toxicity to muscles prohibits intramuscular injection. Daptomycin is highly bound to human plasma protein (92%), primarily to serum albumin. The serum half-life is eight to nine hours in normal subjects, allowing once daily administration. Approximately 80% of the administered drug is excreted unchanged by the kidney with a smaller portion (6%) excreted in the feces. Dosage adjustment is required for creatinine clearance below 30 mL/min. Daptomycin is removed by hemodialysis and the dose should be administered immediately following dialysis.

Antimicrobial Activity/Spectrum/Resistance

Daptomycin is unable to permeate the outer membrane of gram-negative bacteria, thus its spectrum of activity is limited to gram-positive organisms only. Daptomycin is active in vitro against both antibiotic-susceptible and resistant gram-positive bacteria, including Staphylocci (MSSA, MRSA, VISA, and VRSA), *S. pyogenes, Streptococcus agalactiae, Streptococcus dysgalactiae* subspecies *equismilis*, and Enterococci (both *E. faecalis*, and *E. faecium* including (VRE), and *S. pneumoniae* (including penicillin-resistant).

In an in vitro comparative study with vancomycin, linezolid, and quinupristin/dalfopristin, daptomycin was found to have the most rapid bactericidal activity and approximately 8- to 30-fold greater activity against MSSA and MRSA than the other products (90,91). Against VISA, quinupristin/dalfopristin was the most active agent, followed by daptomycin, linezolid, and vancomycin (92). The activity of daptomycin against both VRE vancomycin-sensitive *E. faecalis* was greater than all the other agents tested (92,93).

Bacteria in the stationary growth phase (as occurs in endocarditis and foreign body infections) are killed faster with daptomycin than with vancomycin or nafcillin. To date, no mechanism of resistance to daptomycin or cross-resistance with other antimicrobials has been reported.

Adverse Effects and Drug Interactions

The most frequently reported side effects with daptomycin use are headache, constipation, and rash. Initial development of daptomycin was suspended in the early 1980s due to concerns of skeletal muscle toxicity. With less frequent administration (98 hour vs. daily), clinical toxicity has not been seen. Elevations in serum creatine phosphokinase (CPK) have been reported in patients receiving daptomycin. Accordingly, weekly CPK levels should be monitored, and patients should be examined for muscle pain or weakness throughout therapy. Daptomycin should be used cautiously in patients with a history of myopathy or peripheral neuropathy. Although no drug–drug interactions have been identified, patients receiving medications that have the potential to cause rhabdomyolysis, such as HMG-CoA reductase inhibitors, should be closely monitored during daptomycin use. Daptomycin does not inhibit or induce the C-P450 enzymes.

Therapeutic/Clinical Uses

Daptomycin is indicated for treatment of complicated skin and skin structure infections caused by MSSA and MRSA, VISA, and VRSA strains, hemolytic streptococci, and vancomycin-susceptible enterococci and VRE. A recent clinical trial demonstrated that daptomycin is noninferior to comparator agents (vancomycin and semi-synthetic penicllins) for the treatment of bacteremia and right-sided endocarditis due to *Staphylococcus aureus*; The drug recently received FDA approval for these indications. Daptomycin is uniquely ineffective for the treatment of pneumonia due to its inactivation by surfactant, and is not appropriate for this infection.

SULFONAMIDES AND TRIMETHOPRIM
History/Description

Sulfonamides are derived from sulfonic acid, and were discovered in 1932. Sulfamethoxazole (SMX) and Sulfadiazine remain the most useful members of this class of antibiotics. Trimethoprim (TMP) was first used for the treatment of infections in humans in 1962, and it was registered for clinical use in combination with SMX in 1968 (94,95).

Mechanism of Action, Pharmacology, Administration, and Dosage

TMP and SMX in combination have synergistic effects. The optimal ratio of serum concentrations of TMP to SMX against most bacteria is 1:20. Both drugs inhibit bacterial folic acid synthesis at different steps in the pathway. SMX inhibits dihydropteroate synthetase, which catalyzes the formation of dihydrofolate from para-aminobenzoic acid. In the subsequent step of the pathway, TMP inhibits

dihydrofolate reductase, which catalyzes the formation of tetrahydrofolate from dihydrofolate.

TMP is 45% and SMX is 66% bound to plasma proteins. In patients with normal renal function, the half-lives of TMP and SMX are approximately 11 and 9 hours, respectively. When the creatinine clearance decreases to less than 30 mL/min, the dosage of TMP/SMX should be adjusted.

TMP/SMX (trade names Bactrim® or Septra®) is available in a single strength tablet, containing 80 mg TMP and 400 mg of sulfamethoxazole; a double strength tablet, containing 160 mg TMP and 800 mg of sulfamethoxazole; as an oral suspension; and intravenous solution. Dosing equivalents for TMP/SMX are one DS tablet equivalent to 10 mL intravenous solution, equivalent to 20 mL oral suspension. For most indications, one double-strength tablet is administered twice daily for 7 to 14 days depending on the type and severity of the infection. For the treatment of *Pneumocystis carinii* pneumonia (PCP) the administration of dosages of 15 mg/kg of TMP daily, is recommended typically divided into three doses for 21 days. PCP prophylaxis may be achieved with 1 double-strength tablet daily or every other day.

Antimicrobial Activity/Spectrum/Resistance

Many aerobic gram-positive and gram-negative bacteria, *Pneumocystis carinii*, and several protozoa are inhibited or killed by clinically achievable concentrations of TMP/SMX. Certain nosocomial pathogens, such as *Burkholderia cepacia*, *Stenotrophomonas maltophilia*, and *Serratia* spp. are frequently susceptible to SMZ-TMP. In immunosuppressed individuals, some microorganisms of particular concern such as *Nocardia asteroides* and *Listeria monocytogenes* are also usually inhibited by TMP/SMX.

Important pathogens that are usually resistant to TMP/SMX are *P. aeruginosa*, *B. fragilis*, and most other obligatory anaerobic bacteria. Additionally, *M. tuberculosis*, *Campylobacter* spp., *Treponema pallidum*, and *Rickettsiae* are resistant to SMZ-TMP. MRSA is variably susceptible, and most penicillin-resistant pneumococci are resistant. The clinical use of TMP/SMX has gradually declined during recent decades as a result of growing resistance to this agent among most major bacterial pathogens (96).

Adverse Effects and Drug Interactions

SMX can cause blood dyscrasias. Hypersensitivity reactions may also occur with this medication, most commonly manifested as rashes, but may include erythema multiforme major (Stevens-Johnson syndrome). TMP has fewer life-threatening side effects than do the sulfonamides. However, TMP has been shown to cause drug-induced aseptic meningitis. TMP/SMX is contraindicated in pregnancy. TMP/SMX may potentiate the effects of warfarin, phenytoin, tolbutamide, and chlorpropamide.

Therapeutic/Clinical Uses

Growing resistance and potential toxicity has led to the decreased use of TMP/SMX. However, this agent is still used in the treatment and prophylaxis of urinary tract infections, treatment and prevention of PCP, shigellosis, and otitis media. Of note, TMP/SMX is being used more frequently in the treatment of severe Staphylococcal infections (97). ☞ **TMP/SMX may be extremely useful in severe infections caused by susceptible organisms in the critically ill patient, especially those infections caused by *Enterobacter*** *sp.*, and other gram-negative rods that may be multi-resistant to beta-lactam drugs. ☞

QUINOLONES
History/Description
Nalidixic acid, the first quinolone, was developed in 1962 as a byproduct of chloroquine synthesis, and was only useful in urinary tract infections. Its poor pharmacokinetic profile and its toxicity led to the development of the 6-fluorine-substituted quinolones in the 1980s. The fluoroquinolones are reviewed in references (98–100).

Mechanism of Action, Pharmacology, Administration, and Dosage
The quinolones have a novel mechanism of action. These compounds target bacterial topoisomerases II and IV. Topoisomerase II (also known as DNA gyrase) is responsible for nicking and sealing DNA, as well as regulating supercoiling. Topoisomerase IV separates the DNA daughter molecules after DNA replication.

The quinolones have excellent oral bioavailability (approximately 90–99%), which allows for early conversion from intravenous to oral formulations. All are available as tablets or capsules. Parenteral formulations of ciprofloxacin, gatifloxacin, ofloxacin, levofloxacin, moxifloxacin, and trovafloxacin (as the pro-drug alatrofloxacin) are also available. Administering the fluoroquinolones with food delays the absorption, but does not alter its extent . However, concomitant administration of divalent ions such as aluminum, magnesium, zinc, iron, and/or calcium may block absorption.

The quinolones have a post-antibiotic effect of approximately one to two hours, similar to the aminoglycosides, but greater than that with the beta-lactam antibiotics (101). Gemifloxacin and trovafloxacin have a greater tendency to bind to proteins than the other quinolones (approximately 70% vs. less than 50% for the other quinolones), but are not likely to displace other protein-bound drugs.

Routes of metabolism vary greatly between the different quinolones. Moxifloxacin and trovafloxacin undergo extensive hepatic metabolism; however, the metabolites are less active than the parent compounds. Ciprofloxacin, gatifloxacin, gemifloxacin, levofloxacin, lomefloxacin, and ofloxacin are renally eliminated. The fluoroquinolones have elimination half-lives of approximately 3 to 20 hours. Please refer to Table 10 for dosing of the commercially available quinolones.

Antimicrobial Activity/Spectrum/Resistance
☞ **Quinolone antibiotics, similar to the cephalosporins, are traditionally categorized into first to fourth generations based upon spectrum of activity. In general, the second, third, and fourth generations have enhanced gram-positive cocci activity (except ciprofloxacin) and gram-negative rod activity. Excellent anaerobic activity is seen with trovafloxacin and moxifloxacin.** ☞

In 1995, an alarming trend toward increased resistance to ciprofloxacin was noted in *S. aureus*, *E. coli*, *Citrobacter freundii*, *S. marcescens*, and *P. aeruginosa*. The activity of the fluoroquinolones against gram-positive bacteria has been reviewed (102). Approximately 28% of the fluoroquinolone-resistant enteric bacilli also demonstrated aminoglycoside and B-lactam resistance. Multiple mechanisms, many of which are bacteria-specific have been identified in fluoroquinolone resistance, and different bacteria may acquire more than one mutation to confer resistance. Because mutations in the genes that code for the subunits of topoisomerase II and IV vary between bacteria, patterns of quinolone resistance will vary.

Adverse Effects, Drug Interactions
About 5% of patients experience GI side effects with the fluoroquinolones (100). CNS effects (headache, dizziness, insomnia, and nervousness) are also noted with some of

Table 10 Quinolones: Dosing

Quinolone	Dosage form	Dose (mg)	Dosing interval (hours)	Adjust dose (for renal impairment)	Dosage adjustment
First generation					
Nalidixic acid	PO	250, 500, 1000	6	None	None
Second generation					
Ciprofloxacin	PO	250, 500, 750	8, 12	CrCl <30 mL/min, HD[a]	250–500 mg q18 hr 250–500 mg q24 hr, after HD[a]
	IV	200, 400	8, 12	CrCl <30 mL/min	200–400 mg q18–24 hr
Third generation					
Levofloxacin	PO	500, 750	24	CrCl 20–50 mL/min	500–750 mg LD, then 250–500 mg q24 hr
	IV	500, 750	24	CrCl <20 mL/min	500–750 mg LD, then 250–500 mg q48 hr
Fourth generation					
Trovafloxacin[a]	PO	200	24	Hepatic	Avoid if possible, if not, half-dose
	IV	300	24	Impairment	
Moxifloxacin	PO	400	24	Hepatic	Not studied
	IV	400	24	Impairment	
Gemifloxacin	PO	320	24	CrCl <40 mL/min	320 mg LD, then 160 mg qd

[a]Trovafloxacin should only be used in hospitalized patients when the potential benefits are greater than the risks. See text.
Abbreviations: HD, hemodialysis; IV, intravenously; LD, loading dose; PO, per OS.

the quinolones, primarily at higher dosages. Allergic reactions occur in 1% to 2% of patients. Phototoxicity is a possible side effect with fluoroquinolone therapy. Although taking the medication at bedtime can reduce this effect, patients should remain indoors and away from ambient light while on this drug.

Maintaining adequate hydration and urine acidity will prevent crystalluria, an infrequent effect of the fluoroquinolones. Laboratory test abnormalities, including hematologic, hepatic, and renal function markers, occur at a rate of approximately 11.6%. Both hypoglycemia and hyperglycemia have been reported with all the quinolones.

Animal studies have shown that the fluoroquinolones have a propensity to cause toxicity to chondrocytes (103). Tendon rupture has also been described with many of the fluoroquinolones (104–116). Recent research indicates that oxidative stress is involved (103). There is an increased risk in the elderly, those on steroids, and those with renal failure (105). For this reason, fluoroquinolones should be avoided in the elderly when other options exist; and those who must take a flouroquinolone should be advised to avoid heavy exercise. If a patient complains of tendon pain, fluoroquinolones should be discontinued unless there are very compelling indications for their use. Additionally, flouroquinolones should not be prescribed for pregnant and breast-feeding women, and only used for specific indications for children. Trovafloxacin has also been found to cause rare but fatal cases of liver toxicity. Therefore the FDA has asked that it be reserved for short-term intravenous use for life-threatening infections in hospitalized patients.

In contrast to ciprofloxacin, the third- and fourth-generation quinolones do not seem to inhibit theophylline or caffeine metabolism. Although a modest increase in digoxin concentrations was noted in studies with gatifloxacin, no change in the renal elimination of digoxin was noted, therefore no dosage adjustments appear necessary for either drug (117).

QT_c prolongation has been reported at a rate of less than 1% for nearly all the quinolones, but the manufacturer reports an incidence 1.3% for sparfloxacin. Torsades de pointes have been reported with all quinolones but seem to occur more frequently with levofloxacin, gatifloxacin, sparfloxacin, and moxifloxacin. The potential for QT_c prolongation with sparfloxacin and moxifloxacin suggests concomitant Class IA and Class III anti-dysrhythmic drugs should be avoided (Volume 2, Chapter 20). Case reports with ciprofloxacin had noted increased levels of cyclosporine and decreased levels of phenytoin. Levels of these medications should be carefully monitored with ciprofloxacin administration.

Therapeutic/Clinical Uses

All of the newer quinolones offer lower MICs against various streptococcal species, particularly *S. pneumoniae* although there are reports of *S. pneumococcus* resistance to levofloxacin (118). Compared with the newer entities, ciprofloxacin retains equal or better activity against enteric gram-negative rods (especially *P. aeruginosa*). As a result of their anaerobic activity, several of the fluoroquinolones may be useful in the treatment of both community-acquired and hospital-acquired aspiration pneumonia (119), although older agents of different classes still remain useful with more clinical experience. Trovafloxacin, gatifloxacin, and moxifloxacin have enhanced in vitro activity against anaerobes, a property not demonstrated by previous fluoroquinolones. Resistance

in anaerobic bacteria, most importantly of the *B. fragilis* group, is increasingly common. The newer agents appear to also have activity against atypical bacteria, such as *Legionella* spp. and *Mycoplasma pneumoniae*. The fluoroquinolones, especially moxifloxacin, gatifloxacin, and levofloxacin (in this order) are sometimes useful in the treatment of mycobacterial infections (120).

TOPICAL ANTIMICROBIALS FOR BURN WOUNDS
General Considerations

Burns impair the skin integrity, allowing infectious organisms to invade deeper tissues. Within hours of sustaining a burn, gram-positive organisms populate the wound. After several days, more virulent gram-negative organisms replace the gram-positive ones. The most commonly isolated gram-negative organisms include *P. aeruginosa*, *Proteus* spp., and *Klebsiella* spp (121). The gram-negative organisms have greater morbidity, possess many antibiotic resistance mechanisms, and have the ability to secrete collagenases, proteases, lipases, and elastases, enabling them to proliferate and penetrate into the subeschar space (122). If host defenses are inadequate, invasion of viable tissue occurs. Please refer to Volume 1, Chapter 34 and the following references for additional information about topical antimicrobials and burns (123–127).

Topical antimicrobials are applied after injury to limit bacterial colonization. Established infection requires use of topical agents that can penetrate the eschar to reduce microbial counts and to prevent systemic dissemination. Systemic agents are instituted for cellulitic wound infections, gram-positive suppurative infections, extensive fungal invasion, or systemic spread.

Mafenide (Sulfamylon)

Mafenide was discovered by German scientists just before World War II but was not used clinically until the early 1960s after Robert Lindberg demonstrated its ability to control *P. aeruginosa* infections in a rat-burn model.

Mafenide is a topical sulfonamide formulated as an 11.1% suspension in a water-soluble cream base. It diffuses rapidly and freely into the eschar, and is detected in the systemic circulation. Mafenide is renally metabolized to an inactive salt. The salt itself constitutes a large osmotic load, promoting an osmotic diuresis. Mafenide is also metabolized to a carbonic anhydrase inhibitor that may result in a clinically significant metabolic acidosis.

Mafenide should be avoided in patients with renal impairment. Occlusive dressings should not be used, as the drug is usually applied every 12 hours, but it dissipates from the wound surface after approximately three hours (due to its excellent absorption), leaving up to nine hours of bacterial proliferation time on the wound surface. However, tissue levels remain adequate for 9 to 10 hours after application.

Mafenide has excellent bacteriostatic activity against most gram-positive species, including clostridia, but has limited activity against some *S. aureus*, particularly methicillin resistant strains. Mafenide is highly effective against gram-negative organisms, including *Pseudomonas* spp., but has minimal antifungal activity.

Pain or burning frequently occurs upon application to partial thickness burns. The pain is hypothesized to result from the hyperosmotic properties of the preparation, as well as some irritating quality of the drug itself. Hypersensitivity reactions may also occur in up to 50% of patients treated with this agent (124), and rashes may mimic cellulitis (127).

Mafenide may still be the most useful agent for the treatment of invasive burns because of its superior eschar penetration, but careful monitoring of pulmonary function and acid-base status is critical.

Silver Nitrate

Silver nitrate solutions had been used for centuries as an incompletely understood antiseptic. In 1965, Moyer (128) reintroduced topical use of silver nitrate to burn wound management where it is typically employed as a 0.5% solution. The precise mechanism of action is unknown, but ionic silver is known to exert bacteriostatic activity via several potential mechanisms.

Silver nitrate does not penetrate the burn eschar because silver chloride and other silver salts are highly insoluble and precipitate on the wound surface. Application with silver nitrate is relatively painless, but requires frequent nursing attention, as the dressing cannot be allowed to dry. The dressing must be rewetted every two to three hours with fresh 0.5% silver nitrate solution, otherwise the concentration of silver nitrate rises to caustic levels.

Silver nitrate is effective against most strains of *S. aureus* and coagulase-negative Staphylococci, and it also has activity against *P. aeruginosa*. It has less activity against other gram-negative species such as *Enterobacter* spp. and *Klebsiella* spp. An advantage of this compound is the infrequent emergence of silver-resistant bacteria.

Silver nitrate's insolubility requires it be prepared with distilled water. This results in a hypotonic compound. This hypotonicity causes electrolyte abnormalities as the silver removes electrolytes from the wound. Hyponatremia is the most common electrolyte disturbance. Hyponatremia can become significant, even fatal, when children with large burns are treated for long periods with silver nitrate and do not have their serum sodium monitored or replaced. Silver nitrate also stains everything it comes into contact with brown-black. Methemoglobinemia can occur with silver nitrate but is a rare complication, related to bacterial oxidation of nitrate to nitrite. The organism most often involved when patients have developed methemoglobinemia is, *Enterobacter cloacae*, as this organism efficiently metabolizes nitrate (NO_3^-) to nitrite (NO_2^-) and in so doing oxidizes the iron heme moiety hemoglobin from ferrous (Fe^{++}) to ferric (Fe^{+++}).

The vigilant nursing attention required with this compound, coupled with the fact that silver nitrate does not penetrate the eschar, means this compound should be avoided in very deep burns or in wounds where topical care has been delayed and the wounds are already heavily colonized. However, silver nitrate is attended with rapid debridement of the eschar, and less hypertrophic scar is seen than with other compounds.

Silver Sulfadiazine (Silvadene)

Silver sulfadiazine (SSD) was formulated in 1967 by mixing the weakly acidic sulfadiazine with silver nitrate. It was initially thought that both the silver ion and sulfadiazine had antimicrobial properties; however more recent work suggests sulfadiazine is simply an effective means of delivering silver to the wound. Penetration of SSD into the wound is intermediate between the readily absorbed mafenide and minimally absorbed silver nitrate. Unlike mafenide, the application of SSD is painless. Its antibacterial activity

lasts up to 24 hours, but like most burn agents, it is often applied every 12 hours coupled with daily wound debridement.

SSD has bactericidal activity against many gram-positive and gram-negative bacteria, as well as yeast. SSD has excellent activity against *P. aeruginosa* and *S. aureus*. Generally, more organisms are resistant to SSD than mafenide. And although SSD-resistant strains of *P. aeruginosa* and enteric gram-negative rods have been reported, the incidence of infection with these resistant organisms is not increasing.

SSD is contraindicated for pregnant or breast feeding women because of the possibility of kernicterus in the infant. SSD should also be used with caution in patients with G6PD deficiency and renal insufficiency. This compound may induce leukopenia as a result of direct bone marrow suppression, but this generally resolves over 72 to 96 hours without discontinuing the medication with no concomitant increase in morbidity or mortality in studies. Hypersensitivity reactions are relatively uncommon with cutaneous reactions occurring in fewer than 5% of patients (124). SSD may cause sulfa crystal formation in the urine, but this is less of a problem when patients are adequately hydrated. Absorption of propylene glycol (the vehicle) has also been reported to cause problems in evaluating the patient's serum osmolality, as this causes an osmolar load. The effect of proteolytic enzymes (collagenase, papain, sutilains) is reduced when used concomitantly with SSD. ✍ **SSD represents a compromise between the high efficacy of mafenide and the high maintenance of silver nitrate. It is therefore the most commonly employed topical antimicrobial agent in the burn patient, and frequently used as combination treatment (often alternating every 12 hours) with mafenide.** ✍

ANTI-MYCOBACTERIAL AGENTS
General

✍ **Although many anti-TB agents are available, the most important drugs for therapy of critically ill patients are commonly known as "RIPE" which stands for: rifampin, isoniazid, pyrazinamide, and ethambutol (49,50).** ✍ Certain other antituberculosis agents also have an important role and include streptomycin and certain fluoroquinolone antibiotics (129,130). Linezolid also has antimycobacterial activity, but its expense precludes its frequent use. The first two agents of RIPE, namely, rifampin and isoniazid, a few of the fluoroquinolone antibiotics, and numerous aminoglycoside agents are available for parenteral administration. With the recent epidemic spread of TB in the United States and worldwide (131) and the fear of multi-drug resistant TB, critical care clinicians are likely to use these drugs with increasing frequency. The "gold standard" recommendations for the treatment of TB infections emanate from the American Thoracic Society and the Centers for Disease Control and Prevention (132–134).

Treatment Recommendations

Treatment recommendations typically include isoniazid (INH), rifampin, pyrazinamide, and ethambutol (Table 11).

INH is the hydrazine of isonicotinic acid, and is bactericidal against replicating mycobacteria (including *M. tuberculosis*, and some atypical mycobacteria). It appears to work by inhibiting mycolic acid formation in the cell wall.

Table 11 First-Line Anti-TB Medications, Dosage, and Adjustment for Renal and Hepatic Insufficiency

Anti-TB drug name	Dosage form	Standard dose	Dosing interval	Requires dose adjustment for renal insufficiency (CrCl <30 mL/min)	Requires dose adjustment for hepatic failure
INH	PO or IM	300 mg (5 mg/kg)	Every 24 hr	No	Yes
RIF	PO or IV	600 mg (10 mg/kg)	Every 24 hr	No	Yes
RFB	PO	300 mg (5 mg/kg)	Every 24 hr	No	Yes
PZA	PO	2000 mg (25 mg/kg)	Every 24 hr	Yes	Yes
EMB	PO	1000 mg (15–25 mg/kg)	Every 24 hr	Yes	No
SM	IM or IV	1000 mg (12–15 mg/kg)	Every 24 hr	Yes	No

Abbreviations: EMB, ethambutol; IM, intramuscular; INH, isoniazid; IV, intravenously; PO, per OS; PZA, pyrazinamide; RIF, rifampin; RFB, rifabutin; SM, streptomycin.

Approximately one in 10^5 TB organisms is genetically resistant (intrinsic resistance) to INH.

INH is well absorbed enterally, and therapeutic levels are obtained in all body tissues, including the CSF. The drug is acetylated and hydrolyzed and then excreted in the urine. Acetylation is genetically determined, and INH serum concentration is 50% to 80% lower in rapid acetylators than in slow acetylators.

INH-induced side effects develop in approximately 5% of patients and may include rash, peripheral neuritis, fever, hypersensitivity reactions (including an SLE-type reaction), and jaundice arthritis. Peripheral neuritis can be prevented with concurrent administration of pyridoxine (vitamin B$_6$). Hepatic injury due to INH is the most common concern with its use. A mild increase in hepatic transaminases (ALT and AST two to three times the upper limit of normal) is common and does not predict more serious hepatic injury. The drug need not be stopped in these patients as long as they are monitored. In contrast, the drug should be discontinued immediately in patients with symptoms of hepatitis (nausea, malaise, anorexia, and jaundice) including those whose transaminases are above five times normal. The risk of hepatitis is increased in people who drink large quantities of alcohol and in patients with chronic hepatitis from other causes. Older patients are also at higher risk for both neuritis and hepatic damage, but isoniazid should not be withheld in the elderly if they have recent skin test conversion or active TB despite the hepatitis risk.

Rifampin is just as potent as isoniazid for TB. Rifampin is also active against many gram-positive and gram-negative organisms in addition to *M. tuberculosis* by inhibiting the bacterial DNA-dependent RNA polymerase, which suppresses the initiation of RNA chain synthesis. A single point mutation in the target enzyme is sufficient to confer resistance, and resistance occurs quickly when it is used as a single agent, therefore, the drug must be combined with other antibiotics.

Rifampin is well absorbed orally and distributes widely in body tissues, including the CSF. Rifampin is metabolized in the liver by active deacetylation and is ultimately excreted via the bile in the gastrointestinal tract. Adverse effects due to rifampin occur in about 4% of patients and include fever, rash, jaundice, GI upset, and hypersensitivity reactions.

Rifampin increases the metabolism of numerous drugs, including some B-blockers, corticosteroids, oral contraceptives, warfarin, some oral hypoglycemics, some antiarrhythmics, various immunosuppressants (cyclosporine, tacrolimus, sirolimus), clarithromycin, triazole antifungals, protease inhibitors, methadone, theophylline, and phenytoin (135). Reduced drug levels may cause serious problems unless the affected drug dose is appropriately adjusted. Conversely, caution must be exercised when discontinuing rifampin therapy to avoid supratherapeutic and/or toxic effects. Rifabutin can be used as an alternative to rifampin. It can be given less frequently and has fewer drug interactions than rifampin.

Rifaximin, an analog of rifampin, was recently approved by the FDA for traveler's diarrhea. Of note, it is devoid of *M. tuberculosis* activity. In the ICU, rifaximin (400 mg orally three times daily) has been used enterally in place of neomycin for hepatic encephalopathy (134). Both neomycin and rifaximin are minimally absorbed enterally, and both inhibit the urease-producing bacteria responsible for intestinal ammonia production. Neomycin can cause ototoxic and nephrotoxic effects, especially if used over several months. Rifaximin is not approved in the US for this indication; however, it is increasingly employed to protect against hepatic encephalopathy because it is not associated with either renal toxicity or ototoxicity (136).

Pyrazinamide is an analog of nicotinamide and is well absorbed orally, and penetrates tissues throughout the body (129). Pyrazinamide is a pro-drug and is metabolized to pyranizoic acid, which is bactericidal against intracellular replicating organisms. The exact mechanism of action is unknown; pyrazinamide is hydrolyzed by the liver and is excreted primarily by renal glomerular filtration. Hepatotoxicity is the most common side effect and has been reported in approximately 15% of patients who received 40 to 50 mg/kg/day, a regimen used previously. With current dosages of 15 to 30 mg/kg/day, pyrazinamide toxicity is substantially lessened. The drug can also cause hepatitis, arthralgias, and nausea.

Ethambutol is an orally active compound with excellent tuberculostatic activity. The drug widely distributes throughout the body, including the CSF. Approximately 50% of the dose is excreted unchanged in the urine. Optic neuritis occurs rarely with the standard dose of 15 mg/kg/day. Patients should be tested for visual acuity and green color perception before and periodically during ethambutol therapy. If a dosage of more than 15 mg/kg/day adjusted for renal function is used, tests should be conducted monthly. Other adverse effects are rare.

Streptomycin is an aminoglycoside antibiotic long used to treat tuberculosis, and is tuberculocidal. Vestibular toxicity, auditory toxicity, and to a lesser degree than the

Table 12 Clinically Significant Fungi and Their Antimicrobial Drugs of Choice

Microorganism	Drug of choice[a]	Alternative agents
Aspergillus sp.	Voriconazole	Itraconazole, amphotericin B, an echinocandin[b]
Candida sp.	An echinocandin[b]	Fluconazole, voriconazole, amphotericin B
Coccidioides immitis	Amphotericin B	Fluconazole, itraconazole, voriconazole, posaconazole?
Cryptococcus neoformans	Amphotericin B plus flucytosine	Fluconazole plus flucytosine
Histoplasma capsulatum	Amphotericin B	Itraconazole, voriconazole
Mucor-Absidia-Rhizopus (Zygomycetes)	Amphotericin B	Posaconazole?

[a]Amphotericin lipid formulations are less toxic.
[b]An echinocandin = anidulafungin, caspofungin, micafungin.

other aminoglycosides, nephrotoxicity has been reported with streptomycin use. Amikacin is sometimes used in place of streptomycin to treat tuberculosis.

Various fluoroquinolones, namely, moxifloxacin, gatifloxacin, and levofloxacin, have been used as second line therapy in the treatment of tuberculosis in combination with other antituberculosis agents, but their efficacy for the treatment of tuberculosis is not entirely clear (101).

ANTIFUNGALS
History/Description
Introduced in 1960. Amphotericin B was the first clinically useful anti-fungal agent for the treatment of systemic fungal infections. Subsequently, lipid-based preparations of amphotericin B (with diminished toxicities) has made therapy safer. Additionally, the introduction of agents with different mechanisms of action (i.e., 5-flucytosine, miconagole, voriconazole, and the echinocandins), have increased the ability to treat serious fungal infections (137–140). The major fungi responsible for human disease and their antifungal drugs are summarized in Table 12.

Mechanism of Action, Pharmacology, Administration, and Dosage
Amphotericin B and all of the lipid-based preparations bind to ergosterol, an essential component of the fungal cell wall, with the resultant membrane permeability leading to cell death. Nystatin is in the same class of antifungal drugs as amphotericin but is not given systemically and is used primarily topically (e.g., swish and swallow) and for oral and esophageal candidiasis. Table 13 shows the characteristics of various amphotericin B formulations. Liposomal amphotericin B is better tolerated than other formulations of amphotericin B (141). The azoles, including the triazoles, inhibit the fungal cytochrome P450 enzymes responsible for the conversion of lanosterol to ergosterol, an essential compound for fungal replication and the target upon which amphotericin acts. Table 14 compares the various azole agents. Refer to Tables 13 and 14 for dosing guidelines of the various preparations of amphotericin and the azoles, respectively.

Caspofungin, the first licensed drug in the class of echinocandins, inhibits cell wall synthesis by acting upon the beta-1,3 glucan synthase (142). Some fungi have cell wall glucans, which are glucose polymers akin to cellulose in plant cell walls; other fungi have chitin, which is a polymer of glucosamine. Echinocandins are not active against fungi that have chitin in the cell wall; this property restricts the range of fungi that can be targets for this class of drug.

Caspofungin, only available in a parenteral formulation, is given as a loading dose of 70 mg/kg, followed by 50 mg per day with dose adjustment for hepatic insufficiency. Caspofungin can cause some hepatic toxicity with elevation of liver enzymes and bilirubin. There is no dosage adjustment for renal insufficiency; safety data shows that it can be used in patients with mild to moderate hepatic disease (Child-Pugh class B), but its safety in patients with severe liver disease is untested (143). The FDA approved a second echinocandin drug, micafungin, for the

Table 13 Characteristics of Various Amphotericin Formulation Preparations

Characteristic	Amphotericin B deoxycholate	Amphotericin B cholesteryl sulfate	Amphotericin B lipid complex	Liposomal Amphotericin B
Brand name	Fungizone®	Amphotec®	Abelcet®	AmBisome®
Chemical composition	Micelle	Lipid disks	Ribbons and sheets	Liposomes
Relative infusion-related toxicity	++++	++	++	+
Relative nephrotoxicity	++++	+	+	+
Dosage (mg/kg/day)	0.5–1	3–4	5	3–5

Note: Relative infusion-related toxicity and relative nephrotoxicity are in comparison with amphotericin B deoxycholate, and range from + (mild) to ++++ (severe).

Table 14 Major Pharmacologic Properties of Azole Antifungals

Factor	Ketoconazole	Fluconazole	Itraconazole	Voriconazole
Brand name	Nizoral®	Diflucan®	Sporanox®	Vfend®
Oral absorption decreased by H2-blocking agent or antacid	Yes	No	Capsule—yes; suspension—no	No
Half-life (hours)	9	25	15–42	6
Clearance	Hepatic	Renal	Hepatic	Hepatic
Urinary levels of active drug	Low	High	Low	Low
Penetration of CSF[a]	Poor	Excellent	Poor	Unknown
Typical dose	200 mg PO q12 hr	400 mg PO/IV q24 hr	200 mg PO/IV q12 hr	200 mg PO/IV q12 hr

[a]Penetration into CSF does not always correlate with clinical efficacy in meningitis.
Abbreviations: CSF, cerebrospinal fluid; IV, intravenously; PO, per OS.

use in treating esophageal candidiasis and febrile neutropenia in recipients of hematologic stem cell transplants. It has not received approval yet for invasive candidiasis or invasive aspergillosis. However, its mechanism of action and its in vitro spectrum of activity are identical to those of caspofungin, so it will probably be used for these purposes (144). Another echinocandin, anidulafungin, anidulafungin, the third FDA approved echinocandin; it has the same spectrum of activity and mechanism of action as caspofungin (145). Neither micafungin or anidulafungin requires dose adjustments for end stage renal disease or end stage liver disease, including Child-Pugh "Class C" disease.

Flucytosine inhibits the formation of fungal RNA and DNA. Inside fungal cells, 5-FC is converted to 5-fluorouracil, which interferes with pyrimidine metabolism and decreases the pool of precursors for incorporation into DNA and RNA, thereby inhibiting DNA replication and fungal cell multiplication. 5-FC is readily bioavailable when given orally. It distributes widely to body tissues, including the central nervous system. It is not metabolized by humans and is excreted unchanged in the urine, so it must be used cautiously in patients with renal insufficiency. Levels must be monitored so that steady state levels are from 25 to 100 mcg/mL to avoid toxicity.

Antimicrobial Activity/Spectrum/Resistance

Amphotericin B remains the reference standard by which all anti-fungal agents are measured because it has the broadest spectrum, and has been available for the longest period of time. Amphotericin B has activity against most fungi and yeasts; however, several organisms that are not usually pathogens in the ICU display intrinsic resistance, including *Cladosporium* spp. and *Fonsecaea* spp., and it has variable activity against *Fusarium* spp., *Scedosporium* spp. and *Sporothrix schenckii*. Alternative anti-fungals for these organisms include voriconazole in most cases, or sometimes flucytosine (which should not be used as a single agent). Because of these resistance patterns in these relatively unusual molds, it is increasingly important that complete identification of clinically important fungi and yeasts be performed. Some *Candida albicans* have developed resistance to fluconazole, some have unpredictable resistance patterns (*C. glabrata*), and certain non-albicans Candida are intrinsically resistant to the fluconazole (such as *C. krusei*).

Itraconazole is effective against *Candida* spp. Additionally, it has activity against *Aspergillus* spp. and some of the organisms that cause endemic mycoses, such as *Coccidioides immitis* and *Histoplasma capsulatum*. Its major drawback is poor bioavailability; the capsules do not dissolve in the

absence of gastric acid, and the drug is poorly absorbed. The suspension is well-absorbed, but it is unpalatable.

Voriconazole is effective against most strains of fluconazole-resistant *C. albicans* and *C. glabrata*. In contrast to the other azoles, it is fungicidal for Aspergillus, Scedosporium, and Fusarium, although it has poor activity against Zygomycetes (which includes mucor), where amphotericin B remains the drug of choice (146). The efficacy and safety of voriconazole in the treatment of acute invasive aspergillosis was recently reviewed by Denning et al. (147) Voriconazole was recently shown to have better responses and improved survival against invasive aspergillosis, and have fewer severe side effects than the standard therapy of amphotericin B (148). In addition, an oral formulation of voriconazole is available with excellent oral bioavailability, making itraconazole and voriconazole the only oral agents with activity against *Aspergillus* sp.

Posaconazole is a new triazole drug that has received FDA approval for treatment of candida infections and for prophylaxis of invasive fungal infections, specifically in the setting of cancer chemotherapy and transplantation (149). Posaconazole is promising because it has activity against the zygomycetes, which are the cause of invasive mucormycosis (150). One potential disadvantage to the use of posaconazole is that there is no intravenous formulation. It does come as a suspension and may be given orally or down a nasogastric tube. Ravuconazole is another triazole in phase III testing (151). It also has activity against Candida and Aspergillus; it is not as active against zygomycetes as posaconazole. They both may be useful for treating fungi that are resistant to some of the older azole drugs.

Caspofungin is only clinically effective for infections due to *Aspergillus* spp. and *Candida* spp. Caspofungin has been shown to be at least as effective as amphotericin B for the treatment of invasive candidiasis, and candidemia (152). It is also as effective as liposomal amphotericin in the treatment of aspergillosis and has fewer side effects. Caspofungin is not active against *Cryptococcus* spp. (142,143), despite the fact that this organism has a polyglucan cell wall; the large capsule that surrounds the Cryptococcus sterically prevents the drug from reaching its site of action.

Adverse Effects and Drug Interactions
Amphotericin

Amphotericin B has immediate (infusion-related toxicities) and delayed nephrotoxic effects. Infusion-related toxicities include fever, chills, rigors, myalgia, malaise, nausea, and vomiting. Pre-medication with acetaminophen, diphenhydramine, and low-dose meperidine (for rigors) may mitigate these responses. Hypotension, bradycardia, and ventricular dysrhythmias may also occur and are related to the infusion rate of amphotericin. All of the amphotericin preparations can cause these infusion-related adverse effects; however, they tend to be less frequent and less severe with the lipid preparations than with the deoxycholate formulation (140). The major delayed adverse effects of amphotericin B involve the kidney, and these can become permanent. These effects include nephrotoxicity, electrolyte abnormalities (especially hypokalemia and hypomagnesemia), and renal tubular acidosis. Amphotericin B deoxycholate is more nephrotoxic than the other lipid-based preparations of amphotericin B; however, these other agents still exhibit dose and time-dependent nephrotoxicity. Co-administration of corticosteroids or ACTH can exacerbate hypokalemia. Anemia is sometimes seen, and bone marrow toxicity of ganciclovir is exacerbated by amphotericin B. Finally, probenecid may increase the plasma levels of amphotericin B.

Azoles

The most common side effects for all of the azoles include anorexia, nausea, and vomiting. Other side effects include rash, headache, and potential hepatotoxicity (especially with ketoconazole). The azoles should be used with caution, in patients on medications metabolized via the CP450 system, due to their numerous clinically significant interactions (153). Unique adverse effects from specific azoles include: diminished testosterone and cortisol levels with ketoconazole; mineralocorticoid excess with itraconazole (less so with ketoconazole); cardiac dysrhythmias with itraconazole; and transient, reversible visual changes (seen only with voriconazole).

Echinocandins

Caspofungin is generally well tolerated with minimal side effects. Caspofungin interacts with cyclosporine (increasing the risk of liver toxicity), and tacrolimus (increasing clearance, thereby decreasing available tacrolimus). Minor dosage adjustments are necessary with these drugs and are outlined in the package insert. Micafungin and anidulafungin have none of the above listed drug interactions. Anidulafungin must be reconstituted in alcohol for infusion and, therefore, risks inducing a disulfiram-like reaction if given to a patient also receiving metronidazole; administration of anidulafungin also required a larger volume (up to 500 mL) for infusion, which may present a problem for fluid management in an ICU patient.

Therapeutic/Clinical Uses

The choice of anti-fungal therapy may be complex due to the numerous anti-fungal agents with different mechanisms of action, spectrum of activity, various adverse effects, and the paucity of comparative studies. ☞ **Amphotericin B remains the reference standard by which all anti-fungals are measured. For fungi known to be resistant, other agents including the azoles and echinocandins may be considered in the treatment of systemic infections (154).** ☞ The option of treating with enteral antifungals has also been recently recognized with agents that have excellent oral bioavailability (fluconazole, itraconazole suspension, and voriconazole).

The newer liposomal preparations of amphotericin B are significantly more expensive than amphotericin B deoxycholate but are also less toxic. Caspofungin and micafungin are similar in expense to liposomal amphotericin B. The

Table 15 Antimicrobial Drugs of Choice Against Selected Viruses (Tables 16–18)

Microorganisms	Drug of Choice	Alternative agents
Cytomegalovirus	Ganciclovir	Foscarnet, cidofovir, valganciclovir
Herpes simplex	Acyclovir	Ganciclovir, foscarnet, valacyclovir, famciclovir
Herpes zoster	Acyclovir	Foscarnet, penciclovir, famciclovir, valacyclovir
Influenza	Oseltamavir, rimantidine	Zanamavir, amantadine

enterally effective azoles are much less expensive alternatives via that route. Therefore, the choice of antifungal agent(s) must take into account the specific mold or yeast suspected or proven, local epidemiologic patterns (especially non-albicans *Candida* spp. infection), severity of illness, ability to take oral medication, toxicities, allergies, drug–drug interactions, and cost.

Guidelines for the treatment of Aspergillus infections have recently been reviewed (155,156), and practice guidelines for the treatment of Candida infections have also been published (157,158).

There are no prospective RCTs available that describe the use of putatively synergistic combinations of antifungals although these treatment strategies appear reasonable based upon the respective mechanisms of action. For instance, the combination of an azole, like voriconazole, with caspofungin make intuitive sense since the azoles inhibit ergosterol synthesis and caspofungin works on the cell wall, which are separate biochemical pathways. In a similar vein, the combination of caspofungin and amphotericin formulations would appear to be a useful combination. The use of multiple anti-fungal agents has been used anecdotally in case reports and case series (159,160). However, azoles should not be used together with amphotericin B because they are antagonistic.

ANTIVIRALS

Antiviral agents will be discussed in terms of viral infections that are commonly seen in the critical care unit (Table 15). Antiretroviral agents, used for patients infected with the human immunodeficiency virus (HIV), will not be discussed, but the interested reader may refer to recently published treatment guidelines (161–163). Antimicrobials useful for the prophylaxis of opportunistic infections in patients with HIV infection were recently reviewed (164).

☞ **Currently there are more than a dozen antiviral drugs commercially available in the US for the treatment and/or prophylaxis of viral infections. Most of these drugs function as nucleoside analogs and can be conveniently divided into drugs useful for herpes virus infections, influenza infection (165), hepatitis viruses (166), and miscellaneous viral infections.** ☞ Several recent reviews of antiviral drugs are noted (167–169).

Herpes Virus Antivirals

The most common viral infections seen in the ICU are due to one or more of the herpes viruses that include herpes simplex virus (HSV) (Table 16), Varicella-zoster virus

Table 16 Antiviral Agents for Herpes Simplex Virus Infections

Viral infection	Drug	Route	Usual dosage
Genital herpes[a]	Acyclovir	PO or IV	400 mg tid for 5–10 days
	Famciclovir	PO	250 mg tid for 7–10 days
	Valacyclovir	PO	1 g bid for 10 days
Herpes encephalitis	Acyclovir	IV	10 mg/kg every 8 hr in 1-h infusion for 14–21 days
Mucocutaneous disease in immunocompromised hosts	Acyclovir	IV	5 mg/kg every 8 hr for 7–14 days
		PO	400 mg five times daily for 7–14 days
	Ganciclovir	IV	5 mg/kg every 8–12 hr for 7 days
	Famciclovir	PO	500 mg bid for 7 days
Orolabial herpes	Penciclovir 1%	Topical	q2 hr while awake for 4 days
Keratoconjunctivitis[b]	Trifluridine 1%	Topical—solution	One drop, every 2 hr up to 9 drops/day
	Vidarabine 3%	Topical—ointment	1/2 inch ribbon five times daily

[a]In acyclovir-resistant in HSV or VZV infections, IV foscarnet 40 mg/kg every 8 hr appears beneficial.
[b]Treatment of HSV ocular infections should be supervised by an ophthalmologist.
Abbreviations: HSV, herpes simplex virus; IV, intravenously; PO, per OS; VZV, varicella–zoster virus.

Table 17 Antiviral Agents for Varicella–Zoster Virus Infections[a]

Viral infection	Drug	Route	Usual dosage
Varicella in normal adults	Acyclovir	PO	20 mg/kg up to 800 mg qid for 5 days
Varicella in immunocompromised hosts	Acyclovir	IV	500 mg every 8 hr for 7–10 days
Zoster in normal hosts	Acyclovir	PO	800 mg five times daily for 7–10 days
	Valacyclovir	PO	1 g tid for 7 days
	Famciclovir	PO	500 mg tid for 7 days
Zoster in immunocompromised hosts	Acyclovir	IV	10 mg/kg every 8 hr in 1-hr infusion for 7 days

[a]In acyclovir-resistant in HSV or VZV infections, IV foscarnet 40 mg/kg every 8 hr appears beneficial.
Abbreviations: HSV, herpes simplex virus; IV, intravenously; PO, per OS; VZV, varicella–zoster virus.

(VZV) (Table 17), (reviewed in Gnann) (170) and cytomegalovirus (CMV) (Table 18). There are a variety of antivirals available for the treatment and/or prophylaxis of the various herpes virus infections.

Acyclovir, the first orally available anti-herpes drug, is a nucleoside analog and is available in both enteral and parenteral forms. Because of its poor oral bioavailability, a unique pro-drug, a covalent conjugate of valine and acyclovir, has been developed into the pro-drug valacyclovir (the pro-drug). Valacyclovir is converted to acyclovir by a host enzyme in the intestinal mucosa, leading to improved bioavailability of acyclovir. Similarly, famciclovir, which is available only in an oral preparation, is a pro-drug of penciclovir.

Famciclovir has essentially the same spectrum of activity as acyclovir but with improved oral bioavailability.

Ganciclovir differs only slightly from acyclovir structurally and, in addition to the herpes virus spectrum of acyclovir, also is active against CMV. An oral preparation of ganciclovir is available; however, its poor oral bioavailability recently led to the development of valganciclovir, an orally available pro-drug of ganciclovir, which is metabolized in the same manner as valacyclovir.

Foscarnet is an analog of inorganic pyrophosphate and complexes with DNA polymerase, thereby inhibiting viral DNA synthesis. This agent is useful against all of the herpes viruses, including CMV. Its clinical use is not

Table 18 Antiviral Agents for CMV Infections

Viral infection	Drug	Route	Usual starting dosage
CMV retinitis	Ganciclovir	IV	5 mg/kg every 12 hr in 1-hr infusion for 14–21 days
	Ganciclovir	Oral	1000 mg every 8 hr for 21 days
	Valganciclovir	Oral	900 mg every 12 hr for 21 days
	Cidofovir	IV	5 mg/kg weekly for two doses
	Formivirsen	Intravitreal	330 μg every 2 weeks
	Foscarnet	IV	60 mg/kg every 8 hr in 1–2 hr infusion for 14–21 days
CMV pneumonia	Ganciclovir	IV	5 mg/kg every 12 hr in 1-hr infusion + IV immunoglobulin for 14–21 days (in BMT patients)

Abbreviations: BMT, bone marrow transplant; CMV, cytomegalovirus; IV, intravenously.

Table 19 Antiviral Agents for Hepatitis B and C Infections

Viral infection	Drug	Route	Usual dosage
Chronic hepatitis B	Interferon-α	SC	10 MU three times weekly or 5 MU daily
	Lamivudine	PO	100 mg/day
	Adefovir	PO	10 mg/day
	Entecavir	PO	0.5–1 mg/day
Chronic hepatitis C	Peginterferon alfa-2a	SC	180 mcg weekly
	$\pm$ Ribavirin	PO	800–1200 mg/day depending on weight and genotype
	Pegylated interferon alfa-2b $\pm$	SC	1.0–1.5 mcg/kg weekly
	Ribavirin	PO	800–1200 mg/day depending on weight and genotype
	Interferon alfa-2a	SC/IM	3 MU three times weekly
	Interferon alfa-2b	SC/IM	3 MU three times weekly
	Interferon alfacon-1	SC	9 mcg three times weekly

Abbreviations: IM, intramuscular; PO, per OS; SC, subcutaneously.

popular, however, because of its toxicities (nephrotoxicity and electrolyte abnormalities), and it is generally reserved for mainly for acyclovir-resistant HSV and CMV infections.

Cidofovir is a phosphonate nucleotide analog that is available intravenously for the treatment of cytomegalovirus infection. It is only useful intravenously. Its use is complicated by nephrotoxicity and renal tubular acidosis, and it is generally reserved for patients who have failed or have a contraindication to ganciclovir. Dosing guidelines for drugs used to treat HSV and CMV infections are shown in Tables 16 to 18.

Hepatitis B and C Antivirals

Hepatitis B and C are notable causes of chronic hepatitis and cirrhosis. Treatment for acute hepatitis is generally supportive in nature. Many patients in an ICU setting having liver disease and antiviral treatment for hepatitis B and C are discussed in this context. Ribavirin is a guanosine analog that inhibits ribonucleoprotein synthesis, is active against many RNA viruses, including infections caused by hepatitis C virus (especially in combination with interferon), and hemorrhagic fever viruses. Its major toxicity is anemia that can be clinically quite significant. Lamivudine (3TC) is a nucleoside that is useful for both HIV infection and hepatitis B virus infection. Adefovir, which was originally used for HIV but taken off the market due to nephrotoxicity at higher doses, can be used in much lower doses to treat hepatitis B. Tenofovir, a congener of adefovir, can also be used for

both hepatitis B and HIV. Interferon-alpha and polyethylene glycol-conjugated forms of interferon are also used as antivirals for infections caused by hepatitis B and hepatitis C infections. They are generally poorly tolerated, must be given parenterally (subcutaneously), must be taken over a long period of time, and frequently cause a flu-like syndrome. Treatment of hepatitis B and C are reviewed elsewhere (171–174). Refer to Table 19 for antiviral drug useful in the treatment of Hepatitis B and Hepatitis C infections.

Influenza Antivirals

Influenza, (and its sequelae) is the major cause of respiratory failure in and outside of the US. Influenza vaccines, which are manufactured annually, according to which subtypes are judged to be the most likely epidemic strains, can prevent a large majority of the cases of severe illness. There are also several drugs that are available for the prophylaxis and treatment of influenza virus infections. Two of the older drugs, amantadine and rimantadine are oral agents that inhibit the replication of only influenza A virus but not influenza B virus. Two newer agents inhibit the replication of both influenza A and B viruses: oral oseltamivir (Tamiflu®) and inhaled zanamivir (Relenza®). Please refer to Table 20 for dosing guidelines recommendations.

IMMUNOMODULATORS: ACTIVATED PROTEIN C
History/Description

Despite advances in critical care, the rate of death from severe sepsis still ranges from 30% to 50%. Though all the mechanisms of sepsis have yet to be elucidated, our understanding of this complex condition has greatly increased in the past decade (Volume 2, Chapter 47). This has led to the development of compounds that interrupt the detrimental inflammatory and coagulation process involved in sepsis. One such development is drotrecogin alfa (Xigris®), a recombinant version of natural human plasma-derived activated protein C (APC). Several studies have reviewed this agent (175–177). Kox (178) recently reviewed other immunomodulator agents for sepsis and two reviews of the treatment of sepsis were recently published by Wheeler (179) and Healy (180) and will not be discussed further. Refer also to Volume 2, Chapter 47 for a discussion on sepsis and Volume 2, Chapter 63 for a review of SIRS.

Table 20 Antiviral Agents for Treatment of Influenza Virus Infections[a]

Viral infection	Drug	Route	Usual dosage
Influenza A or B virus	Oseltamivir	PO	75 mg bid for 5 days
	Zanamivir	Aerosol	10 mg bid by inhaler for 5 days
Influenza A virus	Amantadine	PO	100 mg bid for 5 days for treatment
	Rimantadine	PO	200 mg/day for 5 days for treatment

[a]Different doses used for prophylaxis.
Abbreviation: PO, per OS.

Mechanism of Action, Pharmacology, Administration, and Dosage

The antithrombotic effects of APC are mediated by inactivation of clotting factors Va and VIIIa. APC also increases fibrinolytic activity by inhibiting plasminogen-activator inhibitor 1 (PAI-1), which increases endogenous tissue-plasminogen activator (t-PA). In vitro data suggests that APC exerts anti-inflammatory effects by inhibiting the production of the inflammatory cytokines TNF-α, interleukin-1 (IL-1), and interleukin-6 (IL-6) by monocytes and by limiting the rolling of monocytes and neutrophils along injured endothelium.

The average half-life after a 24 mcg/kg/hour infusion of APC is 1.2 hours. This is five times longer than the average half-life of native APC. APC is metabolized and inactivated by endogenous plasma protease inhibitors. There is a linear relationship between APC concentrations and activated partial thromboplastin time (aPPT) response in healthy patients. To date, no patients with sepsis have been re-administered APC. Antibodies to the recombinant APC (drotrecogin alfa) have been detected in two patients during phase II and III trials. One of the patients with neutralizing antibodies developed superficial and deep vein thrombi and died of multi-organ failure.

The dosage of APC is 24 mcg/kg/hour infused intravenously for 96 hours. The drug must be infused within 24 hours from the time of reconstitution or preparation. Patients with end-stage renal disease were excluded from phase III studies. However, in six non-septic ESRD patients, APC was not cleared by dialysis, and patients had clearance rate similar to patients without ESRD.

Adverse Effects and Drug Interactions

The most common adverse event associated with APC is bleeding, which is consistent with the drug's antithrombotic activity. Bleeding occurred in 25% of treated patients and 18% of placebo-treated patients in the Efficacy and Safety of Recombinant Human Activated Protein C for Severe Sepsis (PROWESS) trial. However, the frequency of serious bleeding with APC was only 3.5%, compared to 2.0% in the placebo-treated patients, but this difference was not clinically or statistically ($P = 0.06$) significant (177). Serious bleeding tended to occur mostly during the infusion period and in patients with predisposing conditions such as gastrointestinal ulceration, traumatic injury to a blood vessel, highly vascular organ injury, or markedly abnormal coagulation values. Relatively uncommon side effects found in phase I trials included headache, ecchymoses, diarrhea, and pain at the site of injection.

Because the major adverse effect of APC is bleeding, concomitant administrations of medications that also increase the risk of bleeding are relatively contraindicated. These medications include the use of unfractionated heparin at >15,000 units/day within eight hours of drug infusion; LMWH at any dose higher or more frequent than recommended by their package inserts within 12 hours of drug administration; warfarin if used within seven days of APC infusion or warfarin-type medications within <5 half-lives at the time of drug administration and the PT >13.3 seconds, and/or INR > 3.0; antiplatelet drugs (ticlopidine or clopidogrel) or ASA >650 mg/day or compounds that contain ASA >650 mg/day within seven days prior to drug administration; thrombolytic therapy (unless used to treat an intra-catheter thrombosis) within three days of drug administration (e.g., streptokinase, tPA, rPA, and urokinase); glycoprotein IIb/IIIa antagonists (abciximab, eptifibatide, tirofiban) within seven days of drug administration; antithrombin infusion of >10,000 units received within 12 hours of drug administration; and protein C concentrate infusion within 24 hours of drug administration.

Therapeutic/Clinical Uses

♂ The PROWESS study demonstrated a statistically significant decrease in 30-day mortality in septic patients treated with APC. ♂ However, safety and economic concerns have led to the development of strict usage criteria for APC at most institutions. There are absolute and relative contraindications to the use of APC. Absolute contraindications are active bleeding, epidural anesthesia, intracranial hemorrhage, retroperitoneal bleeding, and recent major surgery. Relative contraindications include those patient populations excluded from the PROWESS trial and for which no data exist. These relative contraindications include pregnant or breastfeeding mothers, platelet count <30,000/mm^3, and age <18 years. The cost of a complete course of APC therapy is approximately $7,000 to $10,000.

EYE TO THE FUTURE

Microbes are developing resistance to a number of previously efficacious antimicrobials. Accordingly, new modalities are being explored and developed to combat microbial pathogens. New vaccines targeted at nosocomial pathogens are being assessed that may lead to infection prevention in this patient population (181,182). Antibiotics specifically designed with activity against emerging resistant organisms are currently under investigation (183). Antibacterial agents in development showing clinical promise include fluoroquinolones (184–186), ketolides (187,188), oxazolidinones (189–193), everninomycins (194), carbapenems (195–198), glycopeptides (199–201), and glycylcyclines (202–203). Likewise, many new and novel antifungal (204–208) and antiviral (209–213) agents are in clinical development.

A potentially helpful addition to preventing staphylococcal infections has emerged recently with the use of a vaccine (StaphVAX®) for the prevention of S. aureus infections in chronic dialysis patients, a group of patients who are susceptible to repeated line associated infections (214). The vaccine consists of a mixture of type 5 and type 8 capsular polysaccharides conjugated to a carrier protein, and immunization of dialysis patients decreased S. aureus infections by 64% at 32 weeks post immunization as compared to controls. Unfortunately, immunity wanes within a year, so annual vaccinations are necessary. Future vaccines might contain more serotypes. Further, it remains an open question as to whether the protection seen in patients with chronic renal failure can be extended to other sets of patients.

Better insight into the understanding of septic shock will bring us additional agents targeted to alter the natural history of this most feared complication of infection (215–219). In addition, many immunomodulatory therapies are being investigated for severe sepsis and septic shock (220,221). To date, more than 70 phase II and phase III RCTs have been performed evaluating the potential role of adjuvant mediator-targeted therapy in patients with sepsis. A great deal has been learned from these investigations and the future of sepsis research holds not only the prospect of fundamental new insights into the interaction of the host, the environment, and medical intervention in disease pathogenesis, but also the possibility that a major cause of global morbidity and mortality can be successfully confronted (222).

Adjunctive immune therapy using immunomodulatory therapies and combination antifungal therapy are being explored to help combat the ever-increasing spectra of encountered fungal infections (223–229). Resolution of invasive fungal infections is dependant on host defenses. Clinical trials utilizing granulocyte colony-stimulating factor and interferon products are currently underway that will hopefully establish whether immunotherapy is of clinical value in the treatment of invasive fungal infections (229).

Newly discovered antimicrobial peptides (AMPs) are being studied to help overcome bacterial resistance that currently hampers our ability to treat many hospital-acquired infections (230–232). AMPs have a broad antimicrobial spectrum and lyse microbial cells by interaction with biomembranes. They also have multiple roles as mediators of inflammation that can influence diverse processes such as cell proliferation, immune induction, wound healing, cytokine release, chemotaxis, and protease-antiprotease relationship. Studies are currently ongoing investigating the biology of AMPs that will hopefully determine their place in therapeutics for infectious and inflammatory diseases (231).

In addition, exciting research is currently underway investigating the newly discovered Type III secretion systems common to several important bacteria and may prove to be a beneficial new target for combating these

Table 21 Antibiotic Guidelines for Trauma Patients

Site/diagnosis	Potential organisms	Primary therapy	Alternative therapy
Aspiration pneumonia during traumatic event	Oral flora	Clindamycin or third-generation cephalosporin[a]	Fluoroquinolone + clindamycin or metronidazole
Closed head injury with ventriculostomy	*Staphylococcus aureus*, coagulase-negative staphylococci	Need for prophylaxis controversial	Oxacillin[b] or cefazolin or vancomycin
Open head injury	*S. aureus*, GNR	Ceftriaxone + oxacillin[b]	Vancomycin
Post-brain injury abscess	*S. aureus*, GNR (including *Pseudomonas*), anaerobes	Ceftazidime + metronidazole + oxacillin[b]	Meropenem + vancomycin
Blunt chest trauma	n/a	Antibiotics not recommended	n/a
Chest tube prophylaxis	n/a	Antibiotics not recommended	n/a
Blunt abdominal trauma			
Without visceral penetration	n/a	Antibiotics not recommended	n/a
With visceral penetration	Enteric GNR, enterococcus	Ampicillin + third-generation cephaolspoin[a] + metronidazole	Vancomycin + fluorquinolone or aminoglycoside[c] + metronidazole or carbapenem or piperacillin/tazobactam
If gastric rupture involvement	*Candida albicans*	Fluconazole	Voriconazole or caspofungin or amphotericin B
Gunshot wound abdomen	GNR, anaerobes, anaerobes, enterococcus	Ampicillin + third-generation cephalosporin or fluoroquinolone + metronidazole	Vancomycin or piperacillin/ tazobactam or carbapenem ± aminoglycoside[c] + metronidazole
Biliary trauma	GNR, enterococci, anaerobes (less often)	Ampicillin or piperacillin + an aminoglycoside[c]	Add metronidazole if initial therapy is unsuccessful
Renal trauma			
Nicked ureter	n/a	Antibiotics not recommended	n/a
Nicked kidney	Follow urine cultures and treat accordingly	n/a	n/a
Orthopedic			
Grade I	*S. aureus*	Cephalosporin[b,d]	Oxacillin or vancomycin
Grade II	*S. aureus*	Cephalosporin[b,d] + aminoglycoside[c]	Oxacillin or vancomycin + an aminoglycoside[c]
Grade III	*S. aureus*; GNR; possible anaerobes	Cephalosporin[b,d] + an aminoglycoside[c] ± metronidazole or clindamycin	Vancomycin + an aminoglycoside[c] ± metronidazole or clindamycin
Acute burns			
Topical	*S. aureus*	Topical sulfadiazine or sulfamylon	Nitrofurazone
Inhalational	n/a	Antibiotics not recommended	n/a

[a]Cefotaxime, ceftriaxone, ceftazidime.
[b]Vancomycin if methicillin-resistant *S. aureus* is common.
[c]Gentamicin, tobramycin, amikacin.
[d]First-generation cephalosporin (cefazolin, cephalothin).
Abbreviation: GNR, gram-negative rods.

pathogenic bacteria. In the 1980s and 1990s researchers studying Yersinia (the causative agent of bubonic plague) discovered that these organisms utilized a syringe-like injection system to deliver virulence factors inside the mammalian host cell (233). These have since been called Type III secretion systems, and significant homology exists across several species of pathogenic gram-negative organisms (including *Yersinia, E. coli, P. aeruginosa, B. pertussis, Salmonella, Shigella,* as well as *Chlamydia* spp, and various plant and fish pathogens) (234). Further study of these flagella-like structures likely be a source of anti-infective therapy in the not so distant future (235).

Finally, the field of pharmacogenomics is a rapidly emerging discipline of interest in medicine and pharmaceutical research and development. Pharmacogenomics may have considerable and significant impact on infectious disease therapy, including antibiotic therapy. The last few years have witnessed an enormous increase in genomic-related technologies as they apply to antibacterial therapies (237). Pharmacogenomics has the potential to revolutionize the prevention, diagnosis, and treatment of infectious diseases (238–245).

SUMMARY

Many patients with severe illness or conditions like multiple trauma and severe burns are susceptible to infection due to their depressed immune function. The goal of antimicrobial therapy is to prevent an infection from developing or to treat an existing infection. In this chapter we have reviewed a multitude of antimicrobials, including antibacterials, antifungals, and antivirals, that are currently available to the clinician for utilization in preventing or treating infections

Table 22 Empiric Antibiotic Therapy for the Critically Ill Intensive Care Unit Patient

Anatomic site/diagnosis	Potential organism	Primary therapy	Alternative therapy
Blood/bacteremia — line associated— endocarditis	*Staphylococcus aureus* coagulase-negative-staphylococci GNR	Oxacillin[a] or nafcillin[a] + an aminoglycoside[b] (if enterococcus is suspected, add ampicillin)	Vancomycin or cephalosporin[d] + an aminoglycoside[b]
		A third-generation cephalosporin[c] + aminoglycoside[b]	Imipenem or meropenem or piperacillin/tazobactam or azteonam or fluorquinolone + aminoglycoside[b]
CNS/meningitis	*Streptococcus pneumoniae*	Ceftriaxone + vancomycin[e]	Imipenem or meropenem
	Neisseria meningitides	Penicillin	Ceftriaxone or imipenem
	GNR, *S. aureus*	Oxacillin[a] or nafcillin[a] + ceftriaxone + an aminoglycoside[b] or use ceftazidime in place of ceftriaxone if Pseudomonas suspected	Vancomycin + ceftriaxone + an aminoglycoside[b]
Intracranial/acute abscess	*S. aureus*	Oxacillin[a] or nafcillin[a] + an aminoglycoside[b]	Vancomycin
	Anaerobes (commonly subacute)	Add metronidazole	Chloramphenicol
Lungs/pneumonia	*S. aureus*	Oxacillin[a] or nafcillin[a]	Cephalosporin[d] or vancomycin or linezolid
	GNR, oral anaerobes	Third-generation cephalosporin[c] + metronidazole	Fluoroquinolone or imipenem or piperacillin (+clindamycin) or piperacillin/tazobactam + an aminoglycoside[b]
Abdomen/peritonitis, abscess	GNR, anaerobes, enterococci	Ampicillin or piperacillin + metronidazole + an aminoglycoside[b] (if Pseudomonas)	Vancomycin in place of penicillin + metronidazole + an aminoglycoside[b] or third-generation cephalosporin[c]; imipenem or piperacillin/tazobactam
Abdomen/biliary tract	GNR, enterococci, anaerobes (occur late and in the elderly)	Ampicillin or piperacillin + an aminoglycoside[b]	Add metronidazole if initial therapy is unsuccessful
Pelvis/PID	GNR/anaerobes	Gentamicin and clindamycin	Cefoxitin and doxycycline
Urinary tract/pyelonephritis	GNR, enterococci	Ampicillin or vancomycin + an aminoglycoside[b]	Third-generation cephalosporin (with ampicillin or vancomycin if enterococcus suspected)

[a]Vancomycin if methicillin-resistant *S. aureus* common.
[b]Gentamicin, tobramycin, amikacin.
[c]Cefotaxime, ceftriaxone, ceftazidime.
[d]First-generation cephalosporin (cefazolin, cephalothin).
[e]In areas with high incidence of penicillin-resistant *S. pneumoniae*, vancomycin should be added.
Abbreviations: GNR, gram-negative rods; PID, pelvic inflammatory disease.

in critically ill patients. In addition, we have highlighted many areas currently being investigated with the quest of identifying additional agents to assist in the control of antibiotic-resistant bacteria and opportunistic infections.

Antibiotic use should be planned deliberately from the time of admission in hospitalized patients. Prophylactic antibiotic use should be restricted to a specific diagnosis and exceptional conditions. The antibiotic choice should be determined based on prevailing, institution-specific bacterial resistance patterns. Only through judicious antimicrobial use can prevention of the development of multi-resistant pathogens be realized. The choice of antimicrobial agent must be influenced by a clinician's familiarity with the available drugs. Empiric guidelines for Trauma patients are provided in Table 21, and those for critically ill patients of trauma, surgical, or medical origin are shown in Table 22.

ACKNOWLEDGMENTS

The authors wish to dedicate this chapter to their colleague, Lee Rickman, who tragically died during the preparation of this manuscript. We also wish to recognize his immense contributions to patient care in San Diego, infectious disease education around the world, and to his insightful and enthusiastic assistance with this chapter prior to his passing.

KEY POINTS

- Antimicrobial selection for trauma and critical care is based on the following seven considerations: (*i*) whether the antibiotics are planned for prophylaxis or treatment of an established infection; (*ii*) the anatomic site of infection; (*iii*) whether the infection is community-acquired or nosocomial; (*iv*) best guess of the most probable causative microorganism (based upon geographical and institutional isolate profiles); (*v*) the patient's innate immunological status; (*vi*) the severity of the infection and general condition of the patient; and (*vii*) financial cost.
- A primary tenet of antimicrobial therapy is to use the narrowest spectrum antibiotic possible, rather than a broad-spectrum agent.
- As Ignaz Phillip Semmelweis discovered 150 years ago, the most important means of preventing the transmission of micro-organisms from one patient (via the doctor or nurse) to another patient is strict hand washing (and now, the use of clean disposable gloves).
- At present, the majority of infections in hospitalized trauma patients are due to gram-positive organisms (19) for example, MRSA and VRE and to a lesser extent, multi-resistant gram-negative rods (20).
- Penetrating intra-abdominal injury, perforated abdominal viscera, and open fractures, all warrant antibiotic prophylaxis(22–25).
- The addition of a beta-lactamase inhibitor to beta-lactam antibiotics produces efficacy against beta-lactamase producing organisms, such as *S. aureus*, *E. coli* and most anaerobic bacteria. However, these combo products add no additional activity against *Pseudomonas aeruginosa* and have no activity against MRSA.
- In general, as one selects a second, third or fourth generation cephalosporin, there is increased activity

against aerobic gram-negative bacteria and less activity against gram-positive orgamisms.
- The cephamycins, specifically cefoxitin and cefotetan, have unique broad-spectrum activity against most anaerobic organisms (except there are increasing resistant forms of *B. fragilis*).
- Aztreonam is devoid of antibacterial activity against gram-positive and anaerobic bacteria.
- Carbapenems are the class of antibiotics with the greatest spectrum activity of any class of antibiotics for systemic use in humans. They are active against gram-positive (except MRSA), gram-negative, and anaerobic bacteria. These agents (except ertapenem) are particularly useful for hospital-acquired infections where bacterial resistance (other than MRSA and VRE) may be a concern.
- Patients with a history of penicillin allergy due to rash or pruritus only occurring more than three days after administration are no more likely to have any allergic reaction to a cephalosporin than patients without a history of penicillin allergy, and can safely receive cephalosporins.
- There is up to a 50% chance of developing a rash to carbapenems in patients with a history of rash to penicillins.
- Aztreonam is considered a safe alternative in patients allergic to penicillins or cephalosporins requiring gram-negative coverage, and vancomycin is the recommended choice for those patients requiring gram-positive coverage.
- All aminoglycosides are nephrotoxic and ototoxic and can prolong the duration of neuromuscular blockade drugs.
- Tetracycline has a broad spectrum of antimicrobial activity including gram-positive, gram-negative, and anaerobic bacteria, as well as rickettsias, mycoplasma, chlamydias, protozoa, actinomycetes, and certain viruses.
- Azithromycin has an extremely long intracellular dwell time, permitting once daily (or less often) dosing.
- Because of its gram-positive and anaerobic coverage, clindamycin is useful (with combination gram-negative therapy) for necrotizing fasciitis, most oral and vaginal anaerobic infections, and diabetic foot infections, which tend to be polymicrobial and virulent.
- Metronidazole is indicated for the treatment of serious polymicrobial infections involving anaerobes (e.g., necrotizing fasciitis and infections involving contamination from the GI tract). Importantly, other agents with aerobic gram-positive and gram-negative coverage must be coadministered.
- *Bacteroides fragilis* is probably the most frequently encountered clinically significant anaerobe and metronidazole should be considered the drug of choice, especially in intra-abdominal infections (57).
- The greatest utility of quinupristin/dalfopristin, daptomycin, and linezolid is in the management of patients with VRE or MRSA infections for which limited alternatives exist.
- Vancomycin is most often used parenterally to treat MRSA, empirically in life-threatening infections, and orally for *C. difficile* colitis.
- TMP/SMX may be extremely useful in severe infections caused by susceptible organisms in the critically ill patient, especially those infections caused by *Enterobacter* sp., and other gram-negative rods that may be multi-resistant to beta-lactam drugs.
- Quinolone antibiotics, similar to the cephalosporins, are traditionally categorized into first to fourth generations based upon spectrum of activity. In general, the second, third, and fourth generations have enhanced

gram-positive cocci activity (except ciprofloxacin) and gram-negative rod activity. Excellent anaerobic activity is seen with trovafloxacin and moxifloxacin.

✍ SSD represents a compromise between the high efficacy of mafenide and the high maintenance of silver nitrate. It is therefore the most commonly employed topical antimicrobial agent in the burn patient, and frequently used as combination treatment (often alternating every 12 hours) with mafenide.

✍ Although many anti-TB agents are available, the most important drugs for therapy of critically ill patients are commonly known as "RIPE" which stands for: rifampin, isoniazid, pyrazinamide, and ethambutol (49,50).

✍ Amphotericin B remains the reference standard by which all anti-fungals are measured. For fungi known to be resistant, other agents including the azoles and echinocandins may be considered in the treatment of systemic infections (151).

✍ Currently there are more than a dozen antiviral drugs commercially available in the United States for the treatment and/or prophylaxis of viral infections. Most of these drugs function as nucleoside analogs and can be conveniently divided into drugs useful for herpes-virus infections, influenza infection (162) hepatitis viruses (163), and miscellaneous viral infections.

✍ The PROWESS study demonstrated a statistically significant decrease in 30-day mortality in septic patients treated with APC.

REFERENCES

1. Crawford GE. Empiric selection of antibiotics. Probl Crit Care 1992; 6(1):1–20.
2. Craven DE, Kunches LM, Lichtenberg DA, et al. Nosocomial infection and fatality in medical and surgical intensive care unit patients. Arch Intern Med 1998; 148:1161–1168.
3. Harlan LC, Harlan WR, Parsons PE. The economic impact of injuries: a major source of medical costs. Am J Public Health 1990; 80:453–459.
4. Murray CJ, Lopez AD. Alternative projections of mortality and disability by cause: 1990–2020: global burden of disease study. Lancet 1997; 349:1498–1504.
5. Murray CJ, Lopez AD. Mortality by cause for eight regions of the world: global burden of disease study. Lancet 1997; 349:1269–1276.
6. Dinkel RH, Lebok U. A survey of nosocomial infections and their influence on hospital mortality rates. J Hosp Infect 1994; 28:297–304.
7. Hessen MT. Principles of selection and use of antibacterial agents. In vitro activity and pharmacology. Infect Dis Clin North Am 2000; 14(2):265–279.
8. Le T, Bayer AS. Combination antibiotic therapy for infective endocarditis. Clin Infect Dis 2003; 36:615–621.
9. Hilf M, Yu VL, Shart JA, et al. Antibiotic therapy for *Pseudomonas aerginosa* bacteremia: outcome correlations in a prospective study of 200 patients. Am J Med 1989; 87: 540–546.
10. Brouwer AE, Rajanuwong A, Chierakul W, et al. Combination antifungal therapies for HIV = associated cryptococcal meningitis: a randomized trial. Lancet 2004; 363:1764–1767.
11. Asmar BI, Prainito M, Dajani AS. Antagonostic effects of chloramphenicol in combination with cefotaxime or ceftriaxone. Antimicrob Agents Chemother 1988; 32(9):1375–1378.
12. Kaye KS. Pathogens resistant to antimicrobial agents. Epidemiology, molecular mechanisms, and clinical management. Infect Dis Clin North Am 2000; 14(2):293–319.
13. Virk A, Steckelberg JM. Clinical aspects of antimicrobial resistance. Mayo Clin Proc 2000; 75:200–214.
14. Dever LA, Dermody TS. Mechanisms of bacterial resistance to antibiotics. Arch Intern Med 1991; 151:886–895.
15. Gold HS, Moellering RC. Drug therapy: antimicrobial-drug resistance. N Engl J Med 1996; 335:1445–1453.
16. Centers for Disease Control and Prevention. Recommendations for preventing the spread of vancomycin resistance: recommendations of the Hospital Infection Control Practices Advisory Committee (HICPAC). MMWR 1995; 44(RR12):1–13.
17. Cunha BA. Antibiotic resistance. Med Clin North Am 2000; 84:1407–1429.
18. Schwenzer KJ, Gist A, Durbin CG. Can bacteremia be predicted in surgical intensive care unit patients? Intensive Care Med 1994; 20:425–430.
19. Sands KE, Bates DW, Lanken PN, et al. Epidemiology of sepsis syndrome in eight academic medical centers. JAMA 1997; 278(3):234–240.
20. Rapp RP. Overview of resistant gram-positive pathogens in the surgical patient. Surg Infect 2000; 1(1):39–46.
21. Malangoni MA, Jacobs DG. Antibiotic prophylaxis for injured patients. Infect Dis Clin North Am 1992; 6(3):627–642.
22. Dellinger EP. Antibiotic prophylaxis in trauma: penetrating abdominal injuries and open fractures. Rev Infect Dis 1991; 13(suppl 10):847–857.
23. Mazuski JE, Sawyer RG, Nathens AB, et al. The surgical infection society guidelines on antimicrobial therapy for intra-abdominal infections: evidence for the recommendations. Surg Infect 2002; 3(3):175–233.
24. Solomkin JS, Mazuski JE, Baron EJ, et al. Guidelines for the selection of anti-infective agents for complicated intra-abdominal infections. Clin Infect Dis 2003; 37:997–1005.
25. Luchette FA, Bone LB, Born CT, et al. Practice management guidelines for prophylactic antibiotic use in open fractures. Available online at http://www.east.org. Accessed on October 5, 2003.
26. Bush LM. Ureidopenicillins and beta-lactam/beta-lactamase inhibitor combinations. Infect Dis Clin North Am 2000; 14(2):409–433.
27. Wright AJ. The penicillins. Mayo Clin Proc 1999; 74:290–307.
28. Chambers HF. Penicillins. In: Mandell, Douglas, and Bennett's Principles and Practice of Infectious Diseases, 6th ed. Mandell GL, Bennett JE, and Dolin R, eds. Philadelphia: Churchill Livingstone, 2005:281–293.
29. Asbel LE. Cephalosporins, carbapenems, and monobactams. Infect Dis Clin North Am 2000; 14(2):435–447.
30. Andes DR, Craig WA. Cephalosporins. In: Mandell, Douglas, and Bennett's Principles and Practice of Infectious Diseases, 6th ed. Mandell GL, Bennett JE, and Dolin R, eds. Philadelphia: Churchill Livingstone, 2005:294–310.
31. Marshall WF, Blair JE. The cephalosporins. Mayo Clin Proc 1999; 74:187–195.
32. Cunha BA, Gill MV. Cefepime. Med Clin North Am 1995; 79:721–732.
33. Nguyen MH, Yu VL, Morris AJ, et al. Antimicrobial resistance and clinical outcome of *Bacteroides bacteremia*: findings of a multicenter prospective observational trial. Clin Infect Dis 2000; 30:870–876.
34. Sykes RB, Bonner DP. Discovery and development of the monobactams. Rev Infect Dis 1985; 7(suppl 4):s579–s593.
35. Chambers HF. Other β-lactam antibiotics. In: Mandell GL, Bennett JE, Doling R, eds. Mandell, Douglas, and Bennett's Principles and Practice of Infectious Diseases, 6th ed. Philadelphia: Churchill Livingstone, 2005:311–317.
36. Saxon A, Hassner A, Swabb EA, et al. Lack of cross-reactivity between aztreonam, a monobactam antibiotic, and penicillin in penicillin-allergic subjects. J Infect Dis 1984; 149:16–22.
37. Brogen RN, Heel RC. Aztreonam, a review of its antibacterial activity, pharmacokinetic properties and therapeutic use. Drugs 1986; 31:96–130.
38. Bonner DP, Sykes RB. Structure–activity relationships among the monobactams. J Antimicrob Chemother 184; 14:313–327.
39. Craig WA. The pharmacology of meropenem: a new carbapenem antibiotic. Clin Infect Dis 1997; 24(suppl 2):s266–s275.

40. Saxon A, Gliden EN, Rohr AS, et al. Immediate hypersensitivity reactions to beta-lactam antibiotics. Ann Intern Med 1987; 107:204–215.
41. Salkind AR, Cuddy PG, Foxworth JW. Is this patient allergic to penicillin? An evidence-based analysis of the likelihood of penicillin allergy. JAMA 2001; 285:2498–2505.
42. Kelkar PS, Li JT-C. Current concepts: cephalosporin allergy. N Engl J Med 2001; 345:804–809.
43. Edson RS, Terrell CL. The aminoglycosides. Mayo Clin Proc 1999; 74:519–528.
44. Gilbert DN. Aminoglycosides. In: Mandell GL, Bennett JE, Doling R, eds. Mandell Douglas and Bennett's Principles and Practice of Infectious Diseases, 6th ed. Philadelphia: Churchill Livingstone, 2005:328–355.
45. Fisman DN. Once-daily dosing of aminoglycoside antibiotics. Infect Dis Clin North Am 2000; 14:475–487.
46. Meyers B, Salvatore M. Tetracyclines and chloramphenicol. In: Mandell GL, Bennett JE, Doling R, eds. Mandell Douglas and Bennett's Principles and Practice of Infectious Diseases, 6th ed. Philadelphia: Churchill Livingstone, 2005:356–373.
47. Smilack JD. The tetracyclines. Mayo Clin Proc 1999; 74: 727–729.
48. Zhanel GG, Homenuik K. The glycylcyclines: a comparative review with the tetracyclines. Drugs 2004; 64:63–88.
49. Rubinstein E, Vaughan D. Tigecycline: a novel glycylcycline. Drugs 2005; 65(10):1317–1336.
50. Zuckerman JM. The newer macrolides: azithromycin and clarithromycin. Infect Dis Clin North Am 2000; 14:449–462.
51. Alvarez-Elcoro S, Enzler MJ. The macrolides: erythromycin, clarithromycin and azithromycin. Mayo Clin Proc 1999; 74:613–634.
52. Sivapalasingam S, Steigbigel NH. Macrolides, Clindamycin, and Ketolides. In: Mandell, Douglas, and Bennett's Principles and Practice of Infectious Diseases, 6th ed. Mandell GL, Bennett JE, and Dolin R, eds. Philadelphia: Churchill Livingstone, 2005:396–416.
53. Kasten MJ. Clindamycin, metronidazole, and chloramphenicol. Mayo Clin Proc 1999; 74:825–833.
54. Bartlett JG. Antibiotic-associated diarrhea. N Engl J Med 2002; 346:334–339.
55. Aldridge KE, Ashcraft D, Cambre K, et al. Multicenter survey of the changing in vitro antimicrobial susceptibilities of clinical isolates of Bacteroides fragilis group, Prevotella, Fusobacterium, Porphyromonas, and Peptostreptococcus species. Antimicrob Agents Chemother 2001; 45:1238–1243.
56. Fogdall RP, Miller RD. Prolongation of a pancuronium-induced neuromuscular blockade by clindamycin. Anesthesiology 1974; 41:407–408.
57. Salvatore M, Meyers B. Metronidazole. In: Mandell, Douglas, and Bennett's Principles and Practice of Infectious Diseases, 6th ed. Mandell GL, Bennett JE, and Dolin R, eds. Philadelphia: Churchill Livingstone, 2005:388–395.
58. Eggleston M. Metronidazole. Infect Control 1986; 7:514–518.
59. Tally FP, Sullivan CE. Metronidazole: in vitro activity, pharmacology and efficacy in anaerobic bacterial infections. Pharmacotherapy 1981; 1:28–38.
60. Finegold SM. Metronidazole. Ann Intern Med 1980; 93: 585–587.
61. Schapiro JM, Gupta R, Stefansson E, et al. Isolation of metronidazole-resistant Bacteroides fragilis carrying the nimA nitroreductase gene from a patient in Washington State. J Clin Microbiol 2004; 42:4127–4129.
62. Cina SJ, Russell RA, Conradi SE. Sudden death due to metronidazole/ethanol interaction. Am J Forensic Med Pathol 1996; 17:343–346.
63. Kazmier FJ. A significant interaction between metronidazole and warfarin. Mayo Clin Proc 1976; 51:782–784.
64. Allington DR, River MP. Quinupristin/dalfopristin: a therapeutic review. Clin Therapeut 2001; 23(1):24–44.
65. Lamb HM, Figgitt DP, Faulds D. Quinupristin/dalfopristin. A review of its use in the management of serious gram-positive infections. Drugs 1999; 58:1061–1097.
66. McDonald LC, Rossiter S, MacKinson C, et al. Quinupristin/dalfopristin resistant Enterococcus faecium on chicken and in human stool specimens. N Engl J Med 2001; 345(18):1155–1160.
67. Thal LA, Zervos MJ. Occurrence and epidemiology of resistance to Virginiamycin and Streptogramin. J Antimicrob Chemother 1997; 43:171–176.
68. Murray BE. Drug therapy: vancomycin-resistant enterococcal infections. N Engl J Med 2000; 342:710–721.
69. Kerr K, Reeves D. Vancomycin resistance in enterococci: a clinical challenge. J Antimicrob Chemother 2003; 51(suppl 2): 1–35.
70. Fung HB, Kirschenbaum HL, Ojofeitimi BO. Linezolid: an oxazolidinone antimicrobial agent. Clin Therapeut 2001; 23(3):356–389.
71. Clemett D, Markham A. Linezolid. Drugs 2000; 69:815–827.
72. Bain KT, Wittbrodt ET. Linezolid for the treatment of resistant gram-positive cocci. Ann Pharmacother 2001; 35:566–575.
73. Dresser LD, Rybak MJ. The pharmacologic and bacteriologic properties of oxazolidinones: a new class of synthetic antimicrobials. Pharmacotherapy 1998; 18:456–462.
74. Kollef MH, Rello J, Cammarata SK, et al. Clinical cure and survival in gram-positive ventilator-associated pneumonia retrospective analysis of two double-blind studies comparing linezolid with vancomycin. Intensive Care Med 2004; 30(3):388–394.
75. Slatter JC, Staker DJ, Feenstra KL, et al. Pharmacokinetics, metabolism, and excretion of linezolid following an oral dose of [(14)C] linezolid to healthy human subjects. Drug Metab Dispos 2001; 29(8):1136–1145.
76. Lundstrom TS. Antibiotics for gram-positive bacterial infections. Vancomycin, teicoplanin, quinupristin/dalfopristin, and linezolid. Infect Dis Clin North Am 2000; 14(2):463–474.
77. Cunha BA. Vancomycin. Med Clin North Am 1995; 79(4): 817–831.
78. Wilhelm MP, Estes L. Vancomycin. Mayo Clin Proc 1999; 74:928–935.
79. Sieradzki K, Roberts RB, Haber SW, Tomasz A. Brief report: the development of vancomycin resistance in a patient with methicillin-resistant Staphylococcus aureus infection. N Engl J Med 1999; 340:517–523.
80. Smith TL, Pearson ML, Wilcox K, et al. Emergence of vancomycin resistance in Staphylococcus aureus. The glycopeptide-intermediate Staphylococcus aureus working group. N Engl J Med 1999; 340:493–501.
81. Tenover FC, Biddle JW, Lancaster MV. Increasing resistance to vancomycin and other glycopeptides in Staphylococcus aureus. Emerg Infect Dis 2001; 7(2):327–332.
82. Centers for Disease Control and Prevention. Public health dispatch: vancomycin-resistant Staphylococcus aureus—Pennsylvania, 2002. MMWR 2002; 51(40):902.
83. Murray BE, Weinstock GM. Enterococci: new aspects of an old organism. Proc Assoc Am Physician 1999; 111(4):328–334.
84. Duffull SB, Begg EJ. Vancomycin toxicity. What is the evidence for dose dependency? Adverse Drug React Toxicol Rev 1994; 13(2):103–114.
85. Andres I, Lopez R, Pou L, Pinol F, Pascual C. Vancomycin monitoring: one or two serum levels? Therapeut Drug Monit 1997; 19(6):614–619.
86. Stephenson J. Researchers describe latest strategies to combat antibiotic-resistant microbes. JAMA 2000; 285:2317–2318 [Editorial].
87. Fowler VG, Boucher HW, Corey GR, et al. Daptomycin versus standard therapy for bacteremia and endocarditis caused by Staphylococcus aureus. N Engl J Med. 2006; 355:653–665.
88. Carpenter CF, Chambers HF. Daptomycin: another novel agent for treating infections due to drug-resistant Gram-positive pathogens. Clin Infect Dis 2004; 38:994–1000.
89. Fenton C, Keating GM, Curran MP. Daptomycin. Drugs 2004; 64(4):445–455.
90. Tedesco KL, Rybak MJ. Daptomycin. Pharmacotherapy 2004; 24(1):41–57.

91. Cubicin® (daptomycin) package insert. Lexington, MA: September 2006. Cubist Pharmaceuticals Inc.

92. Rybak MJ, Hershberger E, Moldovan T, et al. In vitro activities of daptomycin, vancomycin, linezolid, and quinupristin/dalfopristin against staphylococcus and enterococci, including vancomycin-intermediate and –resistant strains. Antimicrob Agents Chemother 2000; 44:1062–1066.

93. Barry AL, Fuchs PC, Brown SD. In vitro activities of daptomycin against 2,789 clinical isolates from 11 North American medical centers. Antimicrob Agents Chemother 2001; 45: 1919–1922.

94. Zinner SH, Mayer KH. Sulfonamides and Trimethoprim. In: Mandell, Douglas, and Bennett's Principles and Practice of Infectious Diseases, 6th ed. Mandell GL, Bennett JE, and Dolin R, eds. Philadelphia: Churchill Livingstone, 2005: 440–450.

95. Smilack JD. Trimethoprim-sulfamethoxazole. Mayo Clin Proc 1999; 74:730–734.

96. Huovinen P. Resistance to trimethoprim-sulfamethoxazole. CID 2001; 32:1608–1614.

97. Adra M, Lawrence KR. Trimethoprim/sulfamethozaxole for treatment of severe *Staphylococcus aureus* infections. Ann Pharmacotherapy 2004; 387:338–341.

98. Hooper DC. Quinolones. In: Mandell GL, Bennett JE, Doling R, eds. Mandell, Douglas, and Bennett's Principles and Practice of Infectious Diseases, 6th ed. Philadelphia: Churchill Livingstone, 2005:451–472.

99. O'Donnell JA. Fluoroquinolones. Infect Dis Clin North Am 2000; 14(2):489–513.

100. Walker RC. The fluoroquinolones. Mayo Clin Proc 1999; 74:1030–1037.

101. Ginsburg AS, Grossett JH, Bishai WR. Fluoroquinolones, tuberculosis, and resistance. Lancet Infect Dis 2003; 3(7): 432–442.

102. Eliopoulos GM. Activity of newer fluoroquinolones in vitro against gram-positive bacteria. Drugs 1999; 58:23–28.

103. Pouzaud F, Bernard-Beaubois K, Thevenin M, et al. In vitro discrimination of fluoroquinolones toxicity on tendon cells: involvement of oxidative stress. J Pharmacol Exp Ther 2004; 308:394–402.

104. van der Linden PD, van Puijenbroek EP, Feenstra J, et al. Tendon disorders attributed to fluoroquinolones: a study on 42 spontaneous reports in the period 1988 to 1998. Arth Care Res 2001; 45:235–239.

105. van der Linden PD, Sturkenboom MCJM, Herings RMC, et al. Increased risk of Achilles tendon rupture with quinolone antibacterial use, especially in elderly patients taking oral corticosteroids. Arch Intern Med 2003; 163:1801–1807.

106. Haddow LJ, Chandra Sekhar M, Hajela V, et al. Spontaneous Achilles tendon rupture in patients treated with levofloxacin. J Antimicrob Chemother 2003; 51:747–748.

107. Chhajed PN, Plit ML, Hopkins PM, et al. Achilles tendon disease in lung transplant recipients: association with ciprofloxacin. Eur Respir J 2002; 19:469–471.

108. van der Linden PD, Sturkenboom MCJM, Herings RMC, et al. Fluoroquinolones and risk of Achilles tendon disorders: case–control study. BMJ 2002; 324:1306–1307.

109. Williams RJ, Attia E, Wickiewicz TL, Hannafin JA. The effect of ciprofloxacin on tendon, paratenon, and capsular fibroblast metabolism. Am J Sports Med 2000; 28:364–369.

110. Maffulli N. Current concepts review—rupture of the Achilles tendon. J Bone Joint Surg 1999; 81:1019–1036.

111. Simonin MA, Gegout-Pottie P, Minn A, et al. Pefloxacin-induced Achilles tendon toxicity in rodents: biochemical changes in proteoglycan synthesis and oxidative damage to collagen. Antimicrob Agents Chemother 2000; 44:867–872.

112. Szarfman A, Chen M, Blum MD. More on fluoroquinolone antibiotics and tendon rupture [letter]. N Engl J Med 1995; 332:193.

113. Pierfitte C, Royer RJ. Tendon disorders with fluoroquinolones. Therapie 1996; 51:419–420.

114. Ribard P, Audisio F, Kahn MF, et al. Seven Achilles tendinitis including 3 complicated by rupture during fluoroquinolone therapy. J Rheumatol 1992; 19:1479–1481.

115. Zabraniecki L, Negrier I, Vergne P, et al. Fluoroquinolone induced tendinopathy: report of 6 cases. J Rheumatol 1996; 23:516–520.

116. Mathis AS, Chan V, Gryszkiewicz M, et al. Levofloxacin-associated Achilles tendon rupture. Ann Pharmacother 2003; 37(7):1014–1017.

117. Fish DN, North DS. Gatifloxacin, an advanced 8-methoxy fluoroquinolone. Pharmacotherapy 2001; 21(1):35–59.

118. Davidson R, Cavalcanti R, Brunton JL, et al. Brief report: resistance to levofloxacin and failure of treatment of pneumococcal pneumonia. N Engl J Med 2002; 346:747–750.

119. Marik PE. Primary care: aspiration pneumonitis and aspiration pneumonia. N Engl J Med 2001; 344:665–671.

120. Jacobs MR. Activity of quinolones against mycobacteria. Drugs 1999; 58:19–22.

121. Monafo WM, West MA. Current treatment recommendations for topical burn therapy. Drugs 1990; 40(3):364–373.

122. Schwartz K, Dulchavsky S. Burn wound infections. eMed J 2001; 2(6):1–9.

123. Mayhall CG. The epidemiology of burn wound infections: then and now. Clin Infect Dis 2003; 37:543–550.

124. Kaye ET. Topical antibacterial agents. Infect Dis Clin North Am 2000; 14(2):321–339.

125. O'Donnell JA, Tunkel AR. Topical antibacterials. In: Mandell GL, Bennett JE, Dolin R. Mandell, Douglas, and Bennett's Principles and Practice of Infectious Diseases, 6th ed. Philadelphia: Churchill Livingstone, 2005:478–488.

126. Boswick JA. The art and science of burn care (chapter 23). In: Peterson HD, ed. Topical Antibacterials. Rockville, MD: Aspen Publishers, 1987:181–187.

127. Shusterman EM, Rickman LS, Tenenhaus M. Pseudochondritis of the burned ear. Infect Dis Clin Pract 1999; 8(3):166–170.

128. Moyer CA, Brentano L, Grovens DL, et al. Treatment of large human burns with 0.5% silver nitrate solution. Arch Surg 1965; 90:812–867.

129. Van Scoy RE, Wilkowske CJ. Antimycobacterial therapy. Mayo Clin Proc 1999; 74:1038–1048.

130. Wallace RJ, Griffith DE. Antimycobacterial agents. In: Mandell GL, Bennett JE, Dolin R. Mandell, Douglas, and Bennett's Principles and Practice of Infectious Diseases, 6th ed. Philadelphia: Churchill Livingstone, 2005:489–501.

131. Espinal MA, Laszlo A, Simonsen L, et al. Global trends in resistance to antituberculosis drugs. The World Health Organization–International Union against Tuberculosis and Lung Disease Working Group on Anti-Tuberculosis Drug Resistance Surveillance. N Engl J Med 2001; 344:1294–1303.

132. Centers for Disease Control and Prevention (CDC). Core curriculum on tuberculosis. What the clinician should know, 4th ed. Atlanta, GA: US Department of Health and Human Services, CDC, 2000.

133. American Thoracic Society and Centers for Disease Control and Prevention. Treatment of tuberculosis and tuberculosis infections in adults and children. Am J Respir Crit Care Med 2003; 167:603–662.

134. Small PM, Fujiwara PI. Medical progress: management of tuberculosis in the United States. N Engl J Med 2001; 345:189–200.

135. Strayhorn VA, Baclewicz AM, Self TH. Update on rifampin drug interactions. III. Arch Intern Med 1997; 157: 2453–2458.

136. Bucci L, Palmieri GC. Double-blind, double-dummy comparison between treatment with rifaximin and lactulose in patients with medium to severe degree hepatic encephalopathy. Curr Med Res Opin 1993; 13:109–118.

137. Rex JH, Stevens DA. Systemic Antifungal Agents. In: Mandell, Douglas, and Bennett's Principles and Practice of Infectious Diseases, 6th ed. Mandell GL, Bennett JE, and Dolin R, eds. Philadelphia: Churchill Livingstone, 2005:502–513.

138. Patel R. Antifungal agents. Part I. Amphotericin preparations and flucytosine. Mayo Clin Proc 1999; 74:1205–1225.

139. Terrell CL. Antifungal agents. Part II. The azoles. Mayo Clin Proc 1999; 74:1205–1225.

140. Arathoon EG. Clinical efficacy of echinocandin antifungals. Curr Opin Infect Dis 2001; 14:685–691.

141. Walsh TJ, Finberg RW, Arndt C, et al. Liposomal amphotericin B for empirical therapy in patients with persistent fever and neutropenia. The National Institute of Allergy and Infectious Diseases Mycoses Study Group. N Engl J Med 1999; 340: 764–771.

142. Letscher-Bru V, Herbrecht R. Caspofungin: the first representative of a new antifungal class. J Antimicrob Chemother 2003; 51:513–521.

143. Denning DW. Echinocandin antifungal drugs. Lancet 2003; 362:1142–1151.

144. Zaas AK, Steinbach WJ. Micafungin: the US perspective. Expert Rev Anti Infect Ther 2005; 3:183–190.

145. Raasch RH. Anidulafungin: review of a new echinocandin antifungal agent. Expert Rev Anti Infect Ther 2004; 2:499–508.

146. Espinel-Ingroff A, Boyle K, Sheehan DJ. In vitro antifungal activities of voriconazole and reference agents as determined by NCCLS methods: review of the literature. Mycopathologia 2001; 150(3):101–115.

147. Denning DW, Ribaud P, Milpied N, et al. Efficacy and safety of voriconazole in the treatment of acute invasive aspergillosis. Clin Inf Dis 2002; 34:563–571.

148. Herbrecht R, Denning DW, Patterson TF, et al. Voriconazole versus amphotericin B for primary therapy of invasive aspergillosis. The invasive fungal infections group of the European organization for research and treatment of cancer and the global aspergillus study group. N Engl J Med 2002; 347: 408–415.

149. Schering-Plough Corporation. Noxafil (Posaconazole) package insert. Kenilworth, NJ, September 2006.

150. van Burik JA, Hare RS, Solomon HF, et al. Posaconazole is effective as salvage therapy in zygomycosis: a retrospective summary of 91 cases. Clin Infect Dis 2006; 42(7):61–65.

151. Chen A, Sobel JD. Emerging azole antifungals. Expert Opin Emerg Drugs 2005; 10:21–33.

152. Mora-Duarte J, Betts R, Rotstein C, et al. Comparison of caspofungin and amphotericin B for invasive candidiasis. N Engl J Med 2002; 347:2020–2029.

153. Lomaestro BM, Piatek MA. Update on drug interactions with azole antifungal agents. Ann Pharmacother 1998; 32(9):915–928.

154. Denning DW, Kibbler CC, Barnes RA. British society for medical mycology proposed standards of care for patients with invasive fungal infections. Lancet Infect Dis 2003; 3: 230–240.

155. Stevens DA, Kan VL, Judson VL, et al. Practice guidelines for diseases caused by *Aspergillus*. Clin Infect Dis 2000; 30: 696–709.

156. Patterson TF, Kirkpatrick WR, White M, et al. Invasive aspergillosis: disease spectrum, treatment practices, and outcomes. Medicine 2000; 79:250–260.

157. Rex JH, Walsh TJ, Sobel JD, et al. Practice guidelines for the treatment guidelines of candidiasis. Clin Infect Dis 2000; 30:662–678.

158. Pappas PG, Rex J, Sobel J, et al. Guidelines for treatment of candidiasis. Clin Infect Dis 2004; 38:161–189.

159. Johnson MD, MacDonald C, Ostrosky-Zeichner L, et al. Combination antifungal therapy. Antimicrob Agents Chemother 2004; 48(3):693–715.

160. Cuenca-Estrella M. Combinations of antifungal agents in therapy—what value are they? J Antimicrob Chemother 2004; 54:854–869.

161. Centers for Disease Control and Prevention. Guidelines for using antiretroviral agents among HIV-infected adults and adolescents. Recommendations of the Panel on Clinical Practices for Treatment of HIV. MMWR 2002; 51(RR-7):1–55.

162. Yeni PG, Hammer SM, Carpenter CCJ, et al. Antiretroviral treatment for adult HIV infection in 2002. Updated recommendations of the International AIDS Society—USA panel. JAMA 2002; 288:222–235.

163. Kress KD. HIV update: emerging clinical evidence and a review of recommendations for the use of highly active antiretroviral therapy. Am J Health Syst Pharm 2004; 61:s3–s16.

164. Kovacs JA, Masur H. Drug therapy: prophylaxis against opportunistic infections in patients with human immunodeficiency virus infection. N Engl J Med 2000; 342:1416–1429.

165. Couch RB. Drug therapy: prevention and treatment of influenza. N Engl J Med 2000; 343:1778–1787.

166. Forton D, Karayiannis P. Established and emerging therapies for the treatment of viral hepatitis. Dig Dis 2006; 24(1–2): 160–173.

167. Hayden FG. Antiviral drugs (other than antiretrovirals). In: Mandell GL, Bennett JE, Dolin R. Mandell, Douglas, and Bennett's Principles and Practice of Infectious Disease, 6th ed. Philadelphia: Churchill Livingstone, 2005:514–550.

168. Balfour HH. Antiviral drugs. N Engl J Med 1999; 340: 1255–1268.

169. Keating MR. Antiviral agents for non-immunodeficiency virus infections. Mayo Clin Proc 1999; 74:1266–1283.

170. Gnann JW, Whitley RJ. Herpes Zoster. N Engl J Med 2002; 347:340–346.

171. Lok AS, McMahon BJ. Practice guidelines committee, American Association for the Study of Liver Diseases (AASLD). Chronic hepatitis B: update of recommendations. Hepatology 2004; 39(3):857–861.

172. Straley SD, Terrault NA. Chronic hepatitis B. Curr Treat Option Gastroent 2004; 7:477–489.

173. Strader DB, Wright T, Thomas DL, et al. American Association for the Study of Liver Diseases (AASLD). Diagnosis, management, and treatment of hepatitis C. Hepatology 2004; 39(4):1147–1171.

174. Pearlman BL. Hepatitis C treatment update. Am J Med 2004; 117(5):344–352.

175. Grinnell BW, Joyce D. Recombinant human activated protein C: a system modulator of vascular function for treatment of severe sepsis. Crit Care Med 2001; 29(suppl 7):s53–s61.

176. Kanji S, Devlin JW, Piekos KA, Racine E. Recombinant human activated protein C, drotecogin alfa (activated): a novel therapy for severe sepsis. Pharmacotherapy 2001; 21(11): 1389–1402.

177. Bernard GR, Vincent JL, Laterre PF. Efficacy and safety of recombinant human activated protein C for severe sepsis (PROWESS). N Engl J Med 2001; 344(10):699–709.

178. Kox WJ, Volk T, Cox SN, et al. Immunomodulator therapy in sepsis. Intensive Care Med 2000; 26(suppl 1):s124–s128.

179. Wheeler AP, Bernard GR. Current concepts: treating patients with severe sepsis. N Engl J Med 1999; 340:207–214.

180. Healy DP. New and emerging therapies for sepsis. Ann Pharmacother 2002; 36:648–654.

181. Sela M, Arnon R, Schechter B. Therapeutic vaccines: realities of today and hopes for the future. Drug Discovery Today 2002; 7(12):664–673.

182. Plotkin SA. Vaccines in the 21st century. Inf Dis Clin North Am 2001; 15(1):307–328.

183. Bronson JJ, Barrett JF. Quinolone, everninomycin, glycylcycline, carbapenem, lipopeptide and cephem antibacterials in clinical development. Curr Med Chem 2001; 8(14): 1775–1793.

184. Emmerson AM, Jones AM. The quinolones: decades of development and use. J Antimicrob Chemother 2003; 51(suppl S1):S13–S20.

185. Reeves D, Spencer RC. Antimicrobial development; quinolones past, present and future. J Antimicrob Chemother 2003; 51(suppl 1):1–47.

186. Van Bambeke F, Michot JM, Van Eldere J, et al. Quinolones in 2005; an update. Clin Microbiol Infect 2005; 11(4): 256–280.

187. Leclercq R. Overcoming antimicrobial resistance: profile of a new ketolide antibacterial, telithromycin. J Antimicrob Chemother 2001; 48(suppl T1):9–23.

188. Ackermann G, Rodloff AC. Drugs of the 21st century: telithromycin (HMR 3647)—the first ketolide. J Antimicrob Chemother 2003; 51:497–511.

189. Reeves D, Wilson P. Linezolid: a novel oxazolidinone antimicrobial for the treatment of serious Gram-positive infections. J Antimicrob Chemother 2003; 51(suppl 2):1–53.

190. Wilcox MH. Update on linezolid: the first oxazolidinone antibiotic. Expert Opin Pharmacother 2005; 6(13):2315–2326.

191. Moellering RC. Linezolid: the first oxazolidinone antimicrobial. Ann Intern Med 2003; 138(2):135–142.

192. Johnson AP. The future prospects of oxazolidinones. Idrugs 2003; 6(3):240–245.

193. Abbanat D, Macielag M, Bus K. Novel antibacterial agents for the treatment of serious gram-positive infections. Expert Opin Investig Drugs 2003; 12(3):379–399.

194. Ganguly AK. Ziracin, a novel oligosaccharide antibiotic. J Antibiot 2000; 53(10):1038–1044.

195. Goa KL, Noble S. Panipenem/betamipron. Drugs 2003; 63(9):913–925.

196. Odenholt I. Ertapenem: a new carbapenem. Expert Opin Investig Drugs 2001; 10(6):1157–1166.

197. Sader HS, Gales AC. Emerging strategies in infectious diseases: new carbapenem and trinem antibacterial agents. Drugs 2001; 61(15):553–564.

198. Perry CM, Ibbotson T. Biapenem. Drugs 2002; 62(15): 2221–2234.

199. Van Bambeke F, Van Laethem Y, Courvalin P, et al. Glycopeptide antibiotics from conventional molecules to new derivatives. Drugs 2004; 64(9):913–936.

200. Malabarba A, Ciabatti R. Glycopeptide derivatives. Curr Med Chem 2001; 8:1759–1773.

201. Pace JL, Yang G. Glycopeptides: Update on an old successful antibiotic class. Biochem Pharmacol 2006; 71(7):968–980.

202. Chopra I. Glycylcyclines: third-generation tetracycline antibiotics. Curr Opin Pharmacol 2001; 1(5):464–469.

203. Zhanel GG, Homenuik K, Nichol K, et al. The glycylcyclines: a comparative review with the tetracyclines. Drugs 2004; 64(1):63–88.

204. Selitrennikoff CP, Nakata M. New cell wall targets for antifungal drugs. Curr Opin Investig Drugs 2003; 4(2):200–205.

205. Spanakis EK, Aperis G, Mylonakis E. New agents for the treatment of fungal infections: clinical efficacy and gaps in coverage. Clin Infect Dis 2006; 43(8):1060–1068.

206. Gupte M, Kulkarni P, Ganguli BN. Antifungal antibiotics. Appl Microbiol Biotechnol 2002; 58(1):46–57.

207. Wiederhold NP, Lewis RE. The echinocandin antifungals: an overview of the pharmacology, spectrum and clinical efficacy. Expert Opin Investig Drugs 2003; 12(8):1313–1333.

208. Sundriyal S, Sharma RK, Jain R. Current advances in antifungal targets and drug development. Curr Med Chem 2006; 13(11):1321–1335.

209. Wilson JC, von Itzstein M. Recent strategies in the search for new anti-influenza therapies. Curr Drug Targets 2003; 4(5): 389–408.

210. Villarreal EC. Current and potential therapies for the treatment of herpesvirus infections. Prog Drug Res 2003; 60:263–307.

211. De Clercq E. Antivirals and antiviral strategies. Nat Rev Microbiol 2004; 2(9):704–720.

212. Coen DM, Schaffer PA. Antiherpesvirus drugs: a promising spectrum of new drugs and drug targets. Nat Rev Drug Discov 2003; 2(4):278–288.

213. Emery VC, Hassan-Walker AF. Focus on new drugs in development against human cytomegalovirus. Drugs 2002; 62(13): 1853–1858.

214. Fattom AL, Horwith G, Fuller S, Propst M, Naso R. Development of StaphVAX, a polysaccharide conjugate vaccine against S. aureus infection; from the lab bench to phase III clinical trials. Vaccine 2004; 22(7):880–887.

215. Sharma VK, Dellinger RP. Treatment options for severe sepsis and septic shock. Expert Rev Anti Infect Ther 2006; 4(3):395–403.

216. Rice TW, Bernard GR. Therapeutic intervention and targets for sepsis. Annu Rev Med 2005; 56:225–248.

217. Nasraway SA. The problems and challenges of immunotherapy in sepsis. Chest 2003; 123(suppl 5):451s–459s.

218. Vincent JL, Abraham E, Annane D, et al. Reducing mortality in sepsis: new directions. Crit Care 2002; 6(suppl 3):s1–s18.

219. Cross AS, Opal SM. A new paradigm for the treatment of sepsis: is it time to consider combination therapy? Ann Intern Med 2003; 138(6):502–505.

220. Vincent JL, Sun Q, Dubois MJ. Clinical trials of immunomodulatory therapies in severe sepsis and septic shock. Clin Infect Dis 2002; 34:1084–1093.

221. Marshall JC. Sepsis: current status, future prospects. Curr Opin Crit Care 2004; 10:250–264.

222. Russell JA. Management of sepsis. N Engl J Med 2006; 355(16): 1699–1713.

223. Casadevall A, Pirofski L. Adjunctive immune therapies for fungal infections. Clin Infect Dis 2001; 33:1048–1056.

224. Steinbach WJ, Stevens DA. Review of newer antifungal and immunomodulatory strategies for invasive aspergillosis. Clin Infect Dis 2003; 37(suppl 3):s157–s187.

225. Steinbach WJ, Stevens DA, Denning DW. Combination and sequential antifungal therapy for invasive aspergillosis: review of published in vitro and in vivo interactions and 6281 clinical cases from 1966 to 2001. Clin Infect Dis. 2003; 37(suppl 3):s188–s224.

226. Fohrer C, Fornecker L, Nivoix Y, et al. Antifungal combination treatment: a future perspective. Int J Antimicrob Agents 2006; 27 Suppl 1:25–30.

227. Baddley JW, Pappas PG. Antifungal combination therapy: clinical potential. Drugs 2005; 65(11):1461–1480.

228. Mukherjee PK, Sheehan DJ, Hitchcock CA, et al. Combination treatment of invasive fungal infections. Clin Microbiol Rev 2005; 18(1):163–194.

229. Jenssen H, Hamill P, Hancock RE. Peptide antimicrobial agents. Clin Microbiol Rev 2006; 19(3):491–511.

230. Bradshaw J. Cationic antimicrobial peptides: issue for potential clinical use. BioDrugs 2003; 17(4):233–240.

231. Koczulla AR, Bals R. Antimicrobial peptides: current status and therapeutic potential. Drugs 2003; 63(4):389–406.

232. Tincu JA, Taylor SW. Antimicrobial peptides from marine invertebrates. Antimicrob Agents Chemother 2004; 48(10): 3645–3654.

233. Michiels T, Vanooteghem JC, Lambert de Rouvroit C, et al. Analysis of virC, an operon involved in the secretion of Yop proteins by Yersinia enterocolitica. J Bacteriol 1991; 73(16): 4994–5009.

234. Galan JE, Collmer A. Type III secretion machines: bacterial devices for protein delivery into host cells. Science 1999; 284:1322–1333.

235. Stevens MP, Haque A, Atkins T, et al. Attenuated virulence and protective efficacy of a Burkholderia pseudomallei bsa type III secretion mutant in murine models of melioidosis. Microbiology 2004; 150:2669–2676.

236. Cornelis GR. The type III secretion injectisome. Nat Rev Microbiol 2006; 4(11):811–825.

237. Mills SD. The role of genomics in antimicrobial discovery. J Antimicrob Chemother 2003; 51:749–752.

238. Davison DB, Barrett JF. Antibiotics and pharmacogenomics. Pharmacogenomics 2003; 4(5):657–665.

239. Hayney MS. Pharmacogenomics and infectious diseases: impact on drug response and applications to disease management. Am J Health Syst Pharm 2002; 59:1626–1631.

240. Kirchheiner J, Fuhr U, Brockmoller J. Pharmacogenetics-based therapeutic recommendations—ready for clinical practice? Nat Rev 2005; 4:639–647.

241. Pang T. Impact of pharmacogenomics on neglected diseases of the developing world. Am J Pharmacogenomics 2003; 3(6):393–398.

242. Ziebuhr W, Xiao K, Coulibaly B, et al. Pharmacogenomic strategies against resistance development in microbial infections. Pharmacogenomincs 2004; 5(4):361–379.

243. Zhang R, Zhang CT. The impact of comparative genomics on infectious disease research. Microbes Infect 2006; 8(6):1613–1622.

244. Boshoff HI, Manjunatha UH. The impact of genomics on discovering drugs against infectious diseases. Microbes Infect 2006; 8(6):1654–1661.

245. Bissonnette L, Bergeron MG. Next revolution in the molecular theranostics of infectious diseases: microfabricated systems for personalized medicine. Expert Rev Mol Diagn 2006; 6(3): 433–450.

54

Anemia: Diagnosis and Treatment

Debra L. Malone

Department of Surgery, University of Maryland School of Medicine, R Adams Cowley Shock-Trauma Center,
Baltimore, Maryland, U.S.A.

Lena M. Napolitano

Department of Surgery, University of Michigan School of Medicine, Ann Arbor,
Michigan, U.S.A.

INTRODUCTION

✴ **Anemia is common in the intensive care unit (ICU), and blood transfusions are often used to treat anemia in critical care.** ✴ Anemia in the critically ill can result from trauma, surgical intervention, occult gastrointestinal (GI) bleeding, repeated phlebotomy for diagnostic testing, and chronic diseases. Critically ill patients often have impaired erythropoiesis due to blunted endogenous erythropoietin (EPO) production, direct inhibition from inflammatory cytokines and certain drugs, or nutritional deficiencies (iron, folate, vitamin B_{12}). Shortened red cell life span can result from consumptive problems, such as disseminated intravascular coagulation (DIC).

This chapter reviews the definition and diagnosis as well as the classification of anemia in specific patient populations (including trauma and critical illness). In addition, the normal physiologic adaptation to anemia and its impact on patient outcome is reviewed. Finally, strategies for preventing and treating anemia are discussed.

DEFINITION OF ANEMIA

Anemia can be defined technically as a hemoglobin (Hb) concentration below the normal laboratory range. The World Health Organization (WHO) defines anemia as a Hb concentration <12 g/dL (women) and <13 g/dL (men). Hemoglobin concentration is determined by hemoglobin mass and plasma volume (1). ✴ **Low Hb concentration typically accompanies a decreased red blood cell (RBC) count and a decrease in packed cell volume, although these indices may be normal in an anemic patient with low Hb levels alone.** ✴

Age influences "normal" Hb concentrations. An evaluation of 420,000 healthy Swedes found significant age-related decline in Hb from age 70 to 88, particularly among men (2). In addition, Hb levels considered "optimal" in a stable condition are not necessarily adequate or "normal" in pathologic conditions (e.g., heart failure), or in certain environments (i.e., high altitude).

DIAGNOSIS OF ANEMIA
Clinical Signs and Symptoms
✴ **Symptoms are dictated by the etiology, severity, and chronicity of the anemia.** ✴ Weakness, fatigue, and lethargy are common. Cardiac symptoms include palpitations, angina pectoris, or dyspnea. Patients may complain of headaches and visual disturbances.

Signs of anemia include pallor, tachypnea, dyspnea, tachycardia, a "thready" pulse, and confusion, perhaps indicating cardiac failure. Alternatively, bounding pulse and systolic flow murmur can signify chronic anemia. Signs of specific causes of anemia may be evidence, for example, koilonychia with iron (Fe) deficiency.

Laboratory Diagnosis
✴ **Evaluation of red cell indices is the most clinically relevant measurement tool.** ✴ Mean corpuscular volume (MCV) is a measure of the average size of the RBC. Mean corpuscular hemoglobin (MCH) is a measure of the amount of Hb per RBC. Both the MCV and the MHC are used to classify anemia as microcytic/hypochromic, normocytic/normochromic, or macrocytic. Concomitant leukopenia and thrombocytopenia indicates pancytopenia, suggesting bone marrow disease or cell sequestration (hypersplenism) or hemodilution. Granulocytosis and thrombocytosis often occur after significant hemorrhage (as occurs with trauma), and with hemolysis.

The reticulocyte count can assist in the diagnosis of anemia. The normal reticulocyte count is 0.5 to 2.5% with an absolute count of 25 to 125×10^9/L. The reticulocyte count should rise in anemia due to EPO increase; the more severe the anemia, the greater the usual increase in a reticulocyte count. Thus, a relatively low reticulocyte count suggests bone marrow dysfunction and/or impaired EPO response.

The reticulocyte count directly reflects effective bone marrow erythrocyte production, while the proportion of circulating macroreticulocytes (red cells with high RNA content) reflects the intensity of EPO stimulation (3). This tool may differentiate between bone marrow erythrocyte production and intensity of EPO stimulation. In states of chronic hemolysis, the bone marrow demonstrates erythroid hyperplasia accounting for increased EPO and rapid increases in reticulocyte count. This is in contrast to the slower response that occurs after trauma and major hemorrhage. After significant hemorrhage, in a patient with no previous hematological disease, the marrow demonstrates an EPO response in approximately six hours. The reticulocyte count begins to increase in two to three days, maximizes in 6 to 10 days and remains elevated until the Hb level returns to normal.

Blood smear examination is helpful for the diagnosis of anemia. Besides assessing red cell morphology and presence of inclusions, white cell and platelet abnormalities also provide useful information.

Examination of the bone marrow aspirate can assess normoblastic versus megaloblastic erythropoiesis, and quantitate proportions of different cell lines (myeloid:erythroid ratio) and iron stores. Bone marrow biopsy reveals architecture, cellularity, and presence of fibrosis or malignant cells.

In ICU settings, measurement of Hb (g/dL) or hematocrit (Hct, %) are the red cell indices most utilized, with typical causes of anemia being acute hemorrhage (after trauma or surgery) or anemia of chronic illness (prolonged ICU stay). A reduction in plasma volume, as seen in dehydration or acute hemorrhage, can mask anemia until normal plasma volume is restored. Dehydration can even cause hemoconcentration (pseudo-polycythemia), with normal total red cell volume. This is particularly common following major burns, and differs from acute hemorrhage wherein proportional losses of blood volume and Hb occur.

☞ Laboratory evaluation of nutritional deficiencies that cause anemia should also be considered. ☞ A recent study of 184 ICU patients found 13% to have potential deficiencies, including iron (9%), vitamin B_{12} (2%), and folate (2%) (4). However, as serum iron and total iron binding capacity (TIBC) levels were low, and serum ferritin levels high, iron deficiency was not necessarily present.

The laboratory diagnosis of iron deficiency can be made by multiple criteria: saturation of transferrin (TrfS) ≤15%, hypochromic erythrocytes ≥ 10%, and a serum ferritin concentration ≤ 50 μg/L. A high plasma transferrin receptor (sTfR) concentration is useful in distinguishing iron deficiency anemia from anemia of chronic disease (ACD) (5).

The ratio of sTfR to serum ferritin (R/F ratio) is used to estimate body Fe stores, and can be used to evaluate the degree to which Fe deficiency complicates the anemia of critical illness. High levels of sTfR, and R/F ratios above 500 are generally correlated with deficiency of tissue iron storage (6). The R/F ratio is not influenced by the use of recombinant human EPO (rHuEPO). However, inflammatory conditions and the use of parenteral Fe supplementation may interfere with this metabolic relationship (7). Recent studies have suggested that erythrocyte zinc protoporphyrin may be a superior test for assessment of iron deficiency in critically ill and injured patients (8). In iron deficiency, zinc protoporphyrin (ZPP) is produced instead of heme, and the ZPP concentration in erythrocytes is increased (normal ≤ 40 μmol/mol heme) (9).

☞ The endogenous hormone erythropoietin is critical for the normal bone marrow response to anemia. ☞ EPO synthesis is increased in states of anemia, when Hb is unable to release oxygen appropriately, when oxygen levels are low, or when there is low cardiac output. Increased severity of anemia typically results in higher plasma EPO concentrations (inverse correlation between plasma EPO and Hb concentrations). Plasma concentrations of EPO assess the individual response to anemia. Endogenous EPO deficiency is a fundamental factor in the pathophysiology of the anemia of critical illness (10).

ANEMIA CLASSIFICATIONS
Microcytic/Hypochromic
Microcytic/hypochromic anemia is characterized by a decrease in MCV, MCH, and mean corpuscular hemoglobin

concentration (MCHC). Red cells are small (microcytic) and pale (hypochromic) due to reduced Hb synthesis. The most common etiology world-wide is Fe deficiency, with chronic inflammation or malignancy ("chronic disease") and thalassemia also important causes.

Iron deficiency is caused by chronic blood loss, increased demand, malabsorption or poor diet. In developed countries, the most common cause is chronic blood loss, usually from the uterus or GI tract, whereas in developing countries, dietary deficiency predominates. Fe deficiency due to increased Fe demand usually occurs during times of growth (childhood and adolescence), pregnancy, lactation, or menses.

Critically ill patients can have microcytic/hypochromic anemia, but the platelet count is often increased, especially following hemorrhage (see Volume 2, Chapter 55). The blood film may demonstrate target cells and poikilocytes alongside the small, poorly-hemoglobinized red cells. In a patient with recent iron therapy or blood transfusion, macrocytic cells can coexist together with microcytic cells.

Serum ferritin levels reflect tissue Fe stores. Ferritin is low in Fe deficiency anemia, whereas elevated levels are seen in Fe overload, following excessive tissue damage, during the acute phase response, and in ACD. Low serum Fe and elevated TIBC are characteristic of Fe deficiency anemia, whereas both are low in ACD.

Normocytic/Normochromic
Normocytic/normochromic anemia is characterized by an MCV 80 to 95 fl, and MCH >26 pg/cell. Causes include acute hemorrhage, renal disease, hemolysis, and bone marrow failure (e.g., hypoplasia, post-chemotherapy, infiltration by carcinoma).

Macrocytic
Macrocytic anemias are so named because of the large RBC size, that is, an MCV >95 fl. These anemias are further classified as megaloblastic or non-megaloblastic.

Megaloblastic anemias are characterized by abnormal erythroblasts ("megaloblasts") in the bone marrow. Nuclear chromatin appears open and "lace-like." Normal Hb formation progresses in the cytoplasm, whereas nuclear maturation is delayed due to abnormal DNA synthesis. The macrocytes are oval and the bone marrow is hypercellular. Giant megamyelocytes ("giant bands") are also characteristic. Increased unconjugated bilirubin and lactate dehydrogenase reflect increased turnover of RBCs and Hb within the marrow. Megaloblastic anemia is most often caused by vitamin B_{12} or folate deficiency, with rare explanations including congenital abnormalities of vitamin B_{12} or folate metabolism.

Vitamin B_{12} deficiency can occur in adults due to pernicious anemia (most common), GI bacterial overgrowth, or loss of ileal function. Pernicious anemia is impaired vitamin B_{12} absorption due to loss of intrinsic factor activity. Intrinsic factor is a glycoprotein secreted by the gastric parietal cells. It then binds dietary vitamin B_{12}, facilitating its uptake by cells located in the terminal ileum. Common causes of pernicious anemia in surgical or critically ill patients include partial or total gastrectomy, intestinal blind loop syndrome, ileal resection, and Crohn's disease. Dietary deficiency of vitamin B_{12} is rare; it typically takes two years to deplete body stores in the absence of dietary intake.

Elevated homocysteine levels (potential vascular risk factor) are associated with low folate, vitamin B_{12}, and vitamin B$_6$ levels. Prophylactic vitamin administration should be considered in hyperhomocysteinemic patients, although benefits remain to be established.

Non-megaloblastic macrocytic anemias can be caused by liver disease, excess alcohol ingestion (even in the absence of liver disease), myxoedema, primary marrow disorders (aplasia, myelodysplasia, myeloproliferative disorders), pregnancy, and ingestion of certain drugs, notably phenytoin and azathioprine.

EPIDEMIOLOGY OF ANEMIA IN TRAUMA AND CRITICAL CARE

Anemia is a common diagnosis following trauma and during critical illness and results in a large burden of patients requiring blood transfusion. ☞ **It is important to understand the epidemiology of anemia in trauma and critical care in order to appreciate the large number of patients that require treatment for anemia.** ☞

Two recent large multicenter prospective observational studies have examined the prevalence of anemia in the ICU: the Anemia and Blood Transfusion in Critical Care (ABC) trial (11) (Europe) and the CRIT study (12) (U.S.A.). The ABC trial included 3534 patients from 146 ICUs. The mean Hb concentration at ICU admission was 11.3 ± 2.3 g/dL (29% of patients had level <10 g/dL). Overall, 37.0% were transfused, with differences among specific subgroups, for example, emergency surgery (57.5%), trauma (48%), elective surgery (42.1%), and medical (32%). Older patients and those with longer length of stay (LOS) were more often transfused. Of patients with ICU stays beyond seven days, 73% were transfused. The overall mean pretransfusion Hb was 8.4 ± 1.3 g/dL.

The CRIT study enrolled 4892 patients from 284 ICUs (12). Its goal was to quantify the incidence of anemia and RBC transfusion in critically ill patients and to examine the relationship of anemia and RBC transfusion to clinical outcomes. Mean baseline Hb concentration on admission to the ICU was 11.0 ± 2.4 g/dL, and mean Hb decreased to 9.8 ± 1.4 g/dL by the end of the study ($P < 0.0045$). Of patients evaluated, 44% were transfused (mean 4.6 ± 4.9 units) during their ICU stay. Patients with an ICU LOS stay

of seven days or longer were more commonly transfused (63.0%) than patients with shorter stays (33.4%; $P < 0.0001$). Mean pretransfusion Hb was 8.6 ± 1.7 g/dL.

A Canadian multicenter cohort study examined RBC transfusion in 5298 consecutive patients admitted to six tertiary level ICUs (13). One-quarter of the patients received red cell transfusions, with the number of transfusions per patient-day averaging 0.95 ± 1.39 (range 0.82 ± 1.69 to 1.08 ± 1.27 between institutions; $P < 0.001$). Independent predictors of pre-transfusion Hb thresholds included patient age, admission Acute Physiology and Chronic Health Evaluation (APACHE) II score, and the institution ($P < 0.0001$). The most frequent reasons for administering red cells were acute bleeding (35%) and to augment oxygen delivery (25%). This study documented significant institutional variation in ICU transfusion practice, with many intensivists adhering to a 10 g/dL threshold despite contrary published guidelines.

Another prospective observational study assessing transfusion practice in critically ill patients in the UK found that 53% of 1247 consecutive patients received RBC transfusions (14). Transfused patients had higher mortality but they also had higher APACHE II scores and longer durations of stay. The average pre-transfusion Hb concentration was below 9 g/dL in 75% of transfusion episodes. The common indications for transfusion were low Hb (72%) and hemorrhage (25%).

Table 1 reveals common features of these studies examining anemia and transfusion practice in the ICU among different countries. First, the most critically ill patients have anemia at ICU admission. Second, the transfusion trigger is a Hb of approximately 8.5 g/dL. Third, RBC transfusion rates increase with greater LOS stay and increased patient age. Finally, the most common indication for RBC transfusion was the treatment of anemia.

ANEMIA IN SPECIFIC TRAUMA AND CRITICALLY ILL POPULATIONS
Anemia Due to Acute Hemorrhage

Anemia is common in critically injured trauma patients. A post hoc analysis of a subset of trauma patients ($n = 576$) from the CRIT study documented a high incidence of

Table 1 Results of Epidemiologic Studies on Anemia and Blood Transfusions in Critical Care

	ABC Trial [2] (western Europe)	CRIT Study [3] (U.S.A.)	TRICC Investigators [9] (Canada)	North Thames Blood Interest Group [5] (U.K.)
n	3534	4892	5298	1247
Mean admission hemoglobin (g/dL)	11.3 ± 2.3	11.0 ± 2.4	9.9 ± 2.2	–
Percentage of patients transfused in ICU	37%	44.1%	25%	53.4%
Mean transfusions per patient (units)	4.8 ± 5.2	4.6 ± 4.9	4.6 ± 6.7	5.7 ± 5.2
Mean pretransfusion hemoglobin (g/dL)	8.4 ± 1.3	8.6 ± 1.7	8.6 ± 1.3	8.5 ± 1.4
Mean ICU length of stay (days)	4.5	7.4 ± 7.3	4.8 ± 12.6	–
ICU mortality	13.5%	13%	22%	21.5%
Hospital mortality	20.2%	17.6%	–	–
Admission APACHE II (mean)	14.8 ± 7.9	19.7 ± 8.2	18 ± 11	18.1 ± 9.1

Data is expressed as mean $\pm$ standard deviation.
Abbreviations: ABC, Anemia and Blood Transfusion in Critical Care; APACHE, Acute Physiology and Chronic Health Evaluation; ICU, intensive care unit; TRICC, Transfusion Requirements in Critical Care.
Source: From Refs. 11–14, 188.

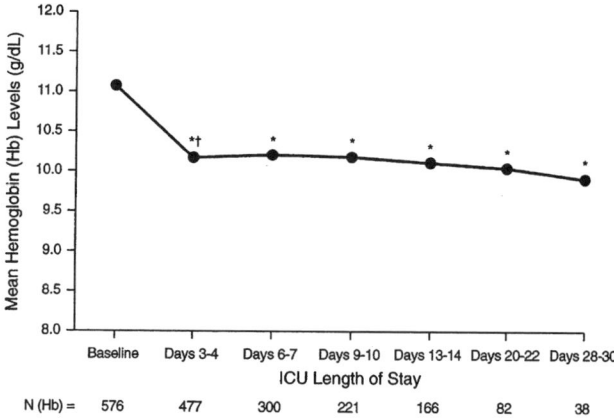

Figure 1 Hemoglobin levels in the intensive care unit (ICU) in trauma patients (*n* = 576). Note that the largest drop in hemoglobin occurred within the first four days of ICU stay. *The difference is significant at *P* < 0.0045 (using analysis of variance and Bonferroni adjustment) compared with baseline. †The difference is significant at *P* < 0.0045 (Bonferroni adjustment) compared with previous ICU stay group. *Source*: From Ref. 15.

anemia (15). Mean baseline Hb was 11.1 ± 2.4 g/dL and patients remained anemic throughout the study, with or without transfusion (Fig. 1). Transfusions (mean, 5.8 ± 5.5 units) were given to 55.4% of patients (43.8% had an ICU LOS ≥7 days). Mean pre-transfusion Hb was 8.9 ± 1.8 g/dL. However, blood transfusion was also common in patients with a Hb greater than 10 g/dL (Fig. 2). Compared with the full study population, trauma patients were more likely to be transfused (55.4% vs. 44%) and received an average of one additional unit of blood.

Severe trauma is associated with major blood loss leading to progressive anemia during fluid resuscitation.

☞ An acute normocytic, normochromic anemia is associated with systemic blood loss. ☞ The degree of anemia correlates directly with the volume of blood lost. Besides their anemia resulting from early blood loss, trauma victims regularly exhibit persisting low red cell counts and low Hb levels during their ICU stay, without necessarily having ongoing bleeding.

☞ In trauma, hemorrhagic shock and tissue injury also result in an acute inflammatory response, and the anemia associated with inflammation (or critical illness) rapidly ensues. ☞ This was shown in a study of 23 patients with severe trauma (injury severity score ≥ 30) (16). Hb levels were low on admission (mean, 10.0 g/dL; range, 6.8–12.9 g/dL) and did not increase to day 9. Serum EPO levels were low (mean 49.8 U/L) on post-injury day 1 and did not show significant increase thereafter. In contrast, acute blood loss in healthy individuals and in animal models leads within minutes to an increase in serum EPO; these increased levels persist for at least one to two days, stimulating erythropoiesis.

The normal inverse correlation between EPO and Hb concentrations was missing in these trauma patients (Fig. 3). Possible explanations for the inadequate EPO response in trauma includes inflammatory mediators that inhibit EPO (17), such as the cytokines IL-1α, IL-1β, and TNF-α, which suppress EPO gene expression and production. Table 2 shows the time course of proinflammatory cytokines following severe trauma. IL-6 levels are high at admission, and do not decrease thereafter. Neopterin, a marker for the activation of the cellular immune system known to suppress EPO production, increased 4.3-fold. Furthermore, neopterin stimulates the release of nitric oxide (suppressor of EPO production) by the activation of inducible nitric oxide synthase. Thus, the inadequate EPO response to anemia in severe trauma may result from the systemic inflammatory response resulting from trauma and its effects on inhibiting EPO production.

Anemia in trauma patients is also characterized by disturbed iron homeostasis (Table 3). During the

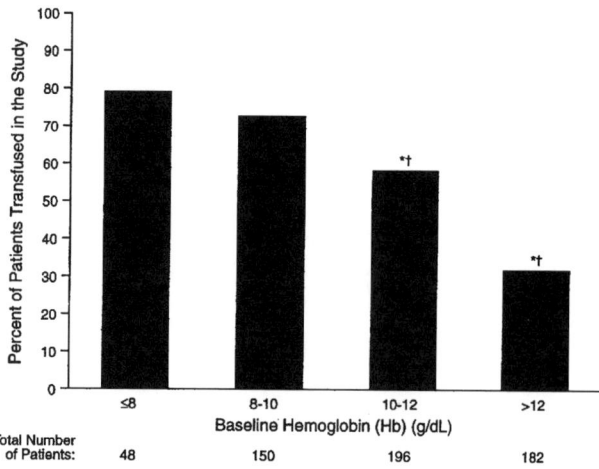

Figure 2 Intensive care unit transfusion rates by baseline hemoglobin levels in trauma patients (*n* = 576). Note that a large number of transfusions (in over 50% of trauma patients) were administered when the hemoglobin concentration was >10 g/dL. *The difference is significant at *P* < 0.01 (Bonferroni adjustment) compared with the first baseline hemoglobin group. †The difference is significant at *P* < 0.01 (Bonferroni adjustment) compared with the previous baseline hemoglobin group. *Source*: From Ref. 15.

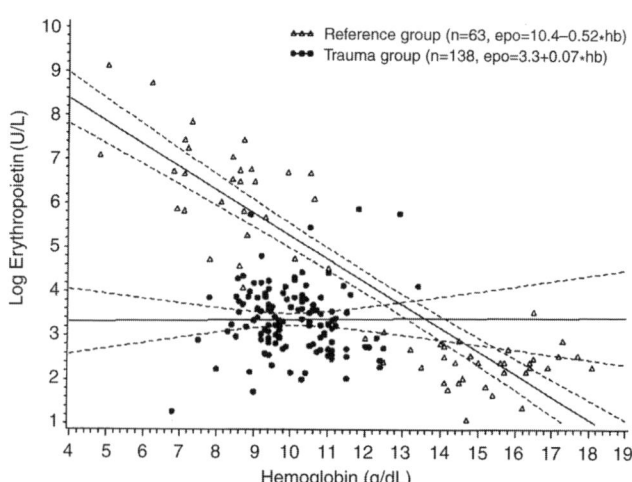

Figure 3 Semilogarithmic presentation of the exponential increase in serum erythropoietin with the degree of anemia as shown by the hemoglobin concentration in 63 subjects (normal persons and patients with primary hemopoietic disorders; *triangles*) and the missing correlation in the 23 multiple traumatized patients (*black dots*; pooled data for all collection times). *Abbreviations*: EPO, erythropoietin; hb, hemoglobin. *Source*: From Ref. 17.

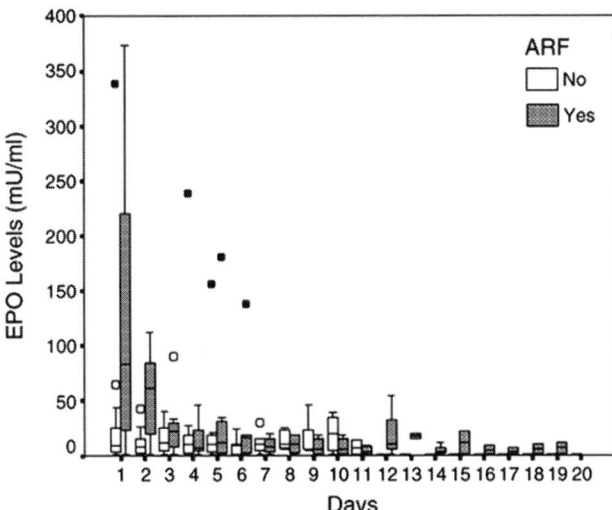

Figure 4 Reduced erythropoietin concentrations in critically ill patients. Box and whisker plot of erythropoietin (EPO) concentrations against time for all patients. Hollow circles indicate outliers (cases with values of the variable between 1.5 and 3 times the length of the corresponding box for that day and group); filled circles indicate extreme values (cases with values greater than three times the corresponding box for that day and group). *Abbreviation*: ARF, acute renal failure. *Source*: From Ref. 10.

inflammatory response, iron is incorporated into the storage protein, ferritin, resulting in low serum Fe concentrations. Serum Fe decreases on day two post-trauma, and remains low, as do transferrin levels (17). Serum ferritin is already elevated on admission and remains so until at least day nine. Proinflammatory cytokines enhance iron uptake by the reticuloendothelial system via enhanced transferrin-receptor expression and stimulate the transcription of ferritin, causing hypoferremia. Thus, this study shows that anemia in severe trauma results from the interplay of bleeding, blunted EPO response to low Hb levels, proinflammatory mediators, and a resulting hypoferremic state. Anemia in trauma patients thus shares a common pathophysiology with anemia of chronic inflammatory disease.

A recent study examined bone marrow and hematopoietic function in trauma patients (18). The mean Hb concentration and reticulocyte counts of the trauma patients were $8.6 \pm 1.0 \, \text{g/dL}$ and $2.75 \pm 0.7\%$, respectively. Bone marrow aspirates and peripheral blood were obtained between day 1 and 7 following injury from 45 multiple trauma patients. Normal volunteers served as controls. Peripheral blood and bone marrow were cultured for various types of hematopoietic progenitor cells. Bone marrow progenitor cells were reduced, whereas peripheral blood progenitor cells were increased in the trauma patients, compared with controls. Bone marrow stroma failed to grow to confluence by day 14 in >90% of trauma patients (confluent growth was always observed in controls). This study thus identified profound changes in bone marrow function after traumatic injury.

Anemia of Critical Illness

Several factors contribute to anemia in the ICU, including pre-existing anemia, blood loss (e.g., GI bleeding), repeated phlebotomy for diagnostic tests, reduced RBC life span, impaired Fe/vitamin B_{12}/folate availability, organ dysfunction (renal,

Table 2 Time Course of Proinflammatory Cytokines, Cytokine Receptor Antagonists, and Neopterin After Severe Trauma

	Day 1	Day 2	Day 4	Day 6	Day 9	P Value
TNF-α, pg/mL [<10]	18 (2–59)	17 (0–40)	18 (0–64)	29 (3–172)	25 (6–86)	NS
sTNF-rI, pg/mL [750–2000]	2979 (260–6000)	3201 (710–6700)	4518 (247–29,000)	6564 (589–51,000)	6882 (1496–5100)	0.003
ILl-ra, pg/mL [106–1550]	3825 (355–10000)	3023 (233–9500)	2534 (329–9400)	3275 (633–9100)	3250 (267–9100)	NS
IL-6, pg/mL [<6]	913 (34–3500)	969 (22–3200)	390 (10–2400)	452 (65–2300)	344 (67–2310)	NS
Neopterin, nmol/L [<10]	6.0 (2.2–20.9)	10.1 (3.8–24.5)	12.7 (4.7–33)	22.2 (5–119)	25.5 (5.7–120)	<0.001

Data are given as mean values and range, respectively. Normal values are shown in square brackets. The P value indicates the time dependence of the measured parameters as analyzed by means of an analysis of variance for repeated measures. A P value < 0.05 was considered statistically significant. Blood was collected within 12 hours after trauma and in the morning on days 2, 4, 6, and 9 after admission to the intensive care unit. Changes in TNF-α, sTNF-rI, IL1-ra, and IL-6 are presented in *Table 2*. TNF α was detectable in all trauma patients at admission, but it did not show significant alterations. In contrast to TNF α, its soluble receptor sTNF-rI increased significantly 2.3-fold until day 9. On day 1, IL1-ra was above normal and remained high thereafter. IL-6 was very high at admission and did not change further. Serum neopterin was low after admission and increased significantly until day 9.

Abbreviations: TNF-α, tumor necrosis factor-α; sTNF-R1, soluble tumor necrosis factor receptor I; IL1-ra, interleukin 1-receptor antagonist; IL-6, interleukin 6.
Source: From Ref. 17.

Table 3 Variables of Iron Status During the First Nine Days After Severe Trauma

	Day 1	Day 2	Day 4	Day 6	Day 9	P Value
s-Fe, μmol/L [9.5–30]	9.5 (1.6–22.9)	3.9 (0.5–18.1)	3.4 (1.1–16.9)	4.0 (1.4–16.8)	5.0 (2.3–16)	0.0043
Transferrin, mg/dL [200–360]	166 (87–268)	166 (114–242)	155 (102–245)	162 (110–243)	161 (96–219)	NS
Ferritin, μg/L [20–300]	832 (76–3137)	547 (143–2035)	466 (251–1054)	530 (368–1261)	842 (406–2931)	NS

Data are given as mean values and range, respectively. Normal values are shown in square brackets. The *P* value indicates the time dependence of the measured parameters as analyzed by means of an analysis of variance for repeated measures. A *P* value <0.05 was considered statistically significant. Blood was collected within 12 hours after trauma and in the morning on days 2, 4, 6, and 9 after admission to the intensive care unit.

Serum iron was significantly decreased on day 2 post-trauma and remained low during the study. In contrast, no change in serum transferrin was observed. Ferritin values were already elevated at admission and remained above the normal range for healthy subjects.

Abbreviation: s-Fe, serum iron.

Source: From Ref. 17.

hepatic), and direct inhibition of erythropoiesis by inflammatory cytokines (19,20). Biochemical and clinical markers of systemic inflammation include proinflammatory cytokines and multiple organ dysfunction syndrome (MODS), respectively. The pathogenesis of anemia in nontraumatized critically ill patients is complex, and generally is a mix of ACD and continued blood loss from GI sources and phlebotomy.

⟁ **Phlebotomy is a significant contributor to ICU-acquired anemia.** ⟁ A recent prospective observational study of 1136 patients from 145 European ICUs demonstrated that the average total volume of blood drawn per patient was 41.1 mL during a 24-hour period (mean volume per blood draw, 10.3 mL) (21). A positive correlation between organ dysfunction and the number of blood draws (and total volume drawn) was shown. An earlier study (22) documenting an even greater daily blood draw (61–70 mL) found that phlebotomy accounted for half the variation in amount of RBCs transfused.

A blunted EPO response was observed in 36 critically ill, non-hypoxic patients who stayed more than seven days in an ICU (though not in the non-septic subgroup with preserved renal function) (23). Thus, EPO deficiency can contribute to ICU-acquired anemia.

⟁ **A blunted EPO response is commonly seen in critically ill or injured patients.** ⟁ This blunted EPO response is not age-dependent, as it is also seen in pediatric ICU patients (24). Serum EPO concentrations in the acutely anemic group were significantly lower than in the chronically anemic group, and were similar to levels in the critically ill control and acutely hypoxemic groups.

Similar to the findings in trauma patients, the blunted endogenous EPO response in critically ill patients is due to the inflammatory response. Abnormal cytokine elaboration has been associated with diseases associated with hematopoietic insufficiency and anemia (25,26). ACD, commonly observed in patients with chronic infections, malignancy, trauma, and inflammatory disorders, is a well-known clinical entity. Recent evidence shows that the inflammatory cytokine IL-6 induces production of hepcidin, an iron-regulatory hormone that may account for some features of this disorder (27).

Recent evidence suggests an association between the activation of the immune system and the development of anemia in critically ill patients. Similar to events that occur in trauma, immune activation induces oxidative stress and leads to a shift of Fe from the circulation into storage sites, thus decreasing bioavailability of free Fe for erythropoiesis. Moreover, released proinflammatory cytokines inhibit erythroid precursor cells and reduce the formation of EPO. The combination of low EPO values (for the degree of anemia), increased production of proinflammatory cytokines, and low serum Fe despite adequate stores that is characteristic of ACD has been identified in patients with the anemia of critical illness.

Anemia of Chronic Disease

⟁ **ACD is encountered frequently in surgery and critical care, and may exacerbate acute anemia associated with trauma and hemorrhage.** ⟁ This condition is common, and is most often associated with inflammatory processes (infectious and non-infectious), renal failure, and malignancy. Laboratory and histological features include normocytic and normochromic (or slightly hypochromic) indices and RBC morphology; reduced serum Hb, Fe and TIBC; and normal or increased serum ferritin (reflecting normal or increased Fe stores).

Repletion of serum Fe does not improve ACD, whereas rHuEPO may benefit. The best treatment is to cure or control the underlying disease.

The pathogenesis of ACD involves decreased RBC life span, inadequate erythropoiesis due to inflammatory mediator release, and decreased release of Fe from macrophages. Hepcidin is an acute-phase reactant that could be a key mediator of ACD. It is an antibacterial protein produced in the liver that can be found in blood or urine, and that participates in host defense. Recent studies demonstrate that hepcidin is a key regulator of Fe balance in the intestinal mucosa, and that abnormalities in hepcidin gene expression are associated with clinical abnormalities in Fe parameters and, in some cases, with anemia (28).

Anemia Associated with Renal Disease

Most patients with renal failure have associated normochromic anemia (approximate 2 g/dL Hb decrease for a 10 mmol/L increase in blood urea). Reduced EPO production by the kidneys is the major explanation for decreased RBC production. Uremia also shortens RBC life span, perhaps related to abnormal RBC morphology (spur and burr cells). RBC levels of 2,3-diphosphoglycerate (2,3-DPG) and uremic acidosis shift the Hb dissociation curve to the right, accounting for only mild symptoms in relation to the degree of anemia. Exacerbation of anemia due to Fe deficiency (e.g., blood losses during hemodialysis or bleeding secondary to platelet dysfunction), folate deficiency, and/or aluminum excess (inhibitor of erythropoiesis) are all contributory. Treatment with rHuEPO after repletion of Fe and folate can correct the anemia.

Increased cardiac output induced by anemia is associated with left ventricular hypertrophy and cardiac disease in renal patients (29). Impaired endothelium-induced vasodilation, impaired angiogenesis, and atherosclerosis can result.

Anemia Associated with Cardiac Disease

Anemia occurs in 10% to 20% of patients with chronic heart failure (30), compromising oxygen-carrying capacity and contributing independently to increased mortality. Causes of anemia include ACD, decreased EPO production (renal insufficiency), and perhaps other poorly defined mechanisms. Treatment with rHuEPO and Fe improves symptoms and exercise capacity (31). rHuEPO supplementation also improves the functional capacity of the failing myocardium, and potentially reverses detrimental myocardial remodeling, thereby reducing mortality and morbidity among patients receiving maximal pharmacologic therapy for heart failure.

Anemia Associated with Liver Disease

Mild macrocytic anemia is associated with chronic liver disease. Contributing factors include blood loss (increased bleeding tendency) and deficiency of vitamin K, Fe, and/or folate. Hemolytic anemia can be seen in end-stage liver disease, Wilson's disease, or due to (autoimmune hemolysis) in some patients with chronic hepatitis. Aplastic anemia rarely complicates acute viral hepatitis.

Anemia Associated with Thyroid Disease

Thyroxine augments EPO and thus thyroid disease associated with decreased thyroxine can result in a macrocytic anemia. Thyroxine therapy benefits the anemia and often reduces the MCV. In addition autoimmune thyroiditis is associated with anemia (see Volume 2, Chapter 52).

ADAPTATION AND RESPONSE TO ANEMIA

✍ **The physiological response to anemia is dictated by the etiology and rapidity of onset of the anemia and the age and general state of health of the patient.** ✍ The cardiovascular compensation for anemia involves tachycardia and increased stroke volume, coordinated with vascular changes serving to boost preload. Peripheral resistance may be decreased and oxygen extraction from Hb increased to augment tissue oxygen delivery (29). Immunological compensation includes cytokine and neuroendocrine changes. Hypoxia inducible factors are associated with the transcriptional activation of genes involved in these adaptive mechanisms (29). At the red cell level, anemia is associated with an increase in 2,3-DPG and a shift of the O_2 dissociation curve to the right so that oxygen is delivered to tissues expeditiously.

Inducing acute severe isovolemic anemia (Hb about 5 g/dL) in 95 healthy, unmedicated volunteers (32) reveals an inverse linear relationship between heart rate and Hb concentration that exhibits greater slope among females. The relationship between anemia and heart rate resembles that found in conscious dogs, but differs from the pattern reported in anesthetized humans, in which either no change or a decreased heart rate is seen.

A study (33) compared 41 elderly patients (mean age 70 years) with chronic severe anemia (mean Hb 6.3 g/dL) and no history of cardiac disease with 63 healthy age- and sex-matched controls. Although heart rates were similar between patients and controls, mean arterial blood pressures were significantly lower in the anemic patients (92.7 vs. 102.1 mmHg, $P < 0.001$). No patient had congestive heart failure (CHF). Thus, in the absence of cardiac disease, chronic severe anemia is well tolerated by the aging heart.

In general, more rapid onset of anemia causes more symptoms, as the compensatory physiological processes have less time to adapt. Although symptoms are uncommon until the Hb falls below 9 to 10 g/dL, older patients may be quite symptomatic at these levels. In contrast, gradual onset of anemia in a young, otherwise healthy patient may not produce symptoms and signs even with a Hb of 6.0 g/dL.

Anesthesia reduces the typical cardiac output response to anemia (34). Anesthetized patients have significantly smaller increases in cardiac index (resulting from increased stroke volume), whereas awake patients have increases both in heart rate and in stroke volume (34).

The normal physiologic response to anemia is to increase erythropoiesis, a complex process regulated by EPO, an erythropoietic hormone primarily produced (90%) in the peritubular interstitial cells of the kidney in response to low tissue oxygen tension. EPO stimulates erythropoiesis by shifting hematologic progenitor cells towards greater production of erythrocytes, resulting in expansion of marrow eythroid cells, which in extreme states of chronic anemia can lead to erythropoiesis even within extramedullary sites.

✍ **Adaptation to anemia and hypoxia results in the induction and regulation of a number of physiologically relevant genes in response to changes in intracellular oxygen tension.** ✍ These include genes encoding EPO, vascular endothelial growth factor, and tyrosine hydroxylase. Studies on the regulation of the EPO gene have provided insights into the common mechanism of oxygen sensing and signal transduction, leading to activation of the hypoxia-inducible transcription factor 1 (HIF-1) (35).

ANEMIA AND PATIENT OUTCOME

☞ **Anemia adversely affects patient mortality and morbidity.** ☞ However, in many critically ill populations, transfusions are associated with worse outcomes than occurs in anemic patients who are not transfused (see later). Patient outcomes will be reviewed by specific patient group.

TRAUMA

A study of over 15,000 trauma patients found that anemia (Hct < 36%) was an independent risk factor for blood transfusion, mortality, ICU admission and LOS, hospital LOS after controlling for indices of shock and blood product transfusion (36).

A prospective observational cohort study of 550 hip fracture surgery patients found anemia (Hb <12.0 g/dL) in 40.4% of patients on admission, in 45.6% at the presurgery nadir, rising to 93.0% at the postsurgery nadir, and in 84.6% near discharge (37). In multivariate analyses, higher Hb levels on admission were associated with shorter LOS and lower odds of death and readmission. Previous studies in hip fracture patients revealed similar findings (38).

Critical Care
Anemia is associated with adverse outcome in critically ill patients, but it remains uncertain whether adverse outcomes are related to anemia alone, or to the resulting use of blood transfusions.

The CRIT study evaluated the association of anemia to outcome in critically ill patients (12). Baseline Hb in ICU patients was related to the number of RBC transfusions but was not an independent predictor of LOS or mortality. However, a nadir Hb concentration of <9 g/dL was a predictor of increased LOS and mortality.

In the ABC trial, anemia was associated with adverse outcome. The 28-day survival curves differed significantly by admitting Hb category in transfused patients (Kaplan–Meier log rank = 30.3, $P < 0.001$), but not in nontransfused patients (11). Moreover, mortality rates were higher in transfused than in nontransfused patients at every Hb category.

Surgery
In the largest study of surgical patients, prospective data from the National Veterans Administration Surgical Quality Improvement Program identified a high rate of perioperative anemia in 6301 noncardiac surgical patients over a five-year period (39). Preoperative anemia (Hct < 36%) was found in 33.9% and postoperative anemia was found in 84.1% of the study cohort. Multiple logistic regression analysis documented that low preoperative Hct, low postoperative Hct, and increased blood transfusion rates were associated with increased mortality ($P < 0.01$), increased postoperative pneumonia ($P < 0.05$), and increased LOS ($P < 0.05$).

Prior studies in surgical patients documented similar findings. A retrospective cohort study in surgical patients ($n = 1958$) who declined blood transfusion for religious reasons documented a higher mortality associated with preoperative anemia (40). The overall 30-day mortality was 3.2% (95% CI 2.4–4.0); however, the mortality was only 1.3% (0.8–2.0) in patients with preoperative Hb 12 g/dL or greater, but 33.3% (18.6–51.0) in patients with preoperative

Hb less than 6 g/dL. The increase in risk of death with anemia was more pronounced in patients with cardiovascular disease. The effect of blood loss on mortality was greater in patients with low preoperative Hb. Thus, decisions about blood transfusion in the perioperative period should consider cardiovascular status in addition to Hb levels and operative blood loss.

Geriatrics
The appropriateness of using WHO criteria for anemia (Hb <12 g/dL for women; <13 g/dL for men) in older populations is debatable, as the incidence of anemia rises with age (41). Additionally, anemia is more often symptomatic in the elderly, and is associated with increased mortality in people more than 85 years of age (42). A retrospective review of 900 long-term residents in skilled-nursing facilities (median age 82 years) that applied the WHO criteria for anemia found a prevalence of 48%, with a higher hospitalization rate among those with more severe anemia (43).

Chronic Heart Failure
Anemia is also common in chronic forms of CHF, and is more frequent in patients with more severe CHF (44). Patients with both CHF and anemia have a poorer quality of life, reduced exercise tolerance, higher hospital admission rates, and other adverse outcomes. Although treatment of anemia can result in improved symptoms, it may also provoke hypertension or thrombosis in this patient population.

A recent prospective study of 912 patients, the Randomized Etanercept North American Strategy to Study Antagonism of Cytokines (RENAISSANCE) trial, investigated the relationship between anemia, CHF severity, and clinical outcomes (45). Anemia (Hb ≤12.0 g/dL) was present in 12% of subjects. Regression analysis indicated that for every 1 g/dL-higher baseline Hb, the risk of mortality was 15.8% lower ($P = 0.0009$) and the risk of mortality or hospitalization for CHF was 14.2% lower ($P < 0.0001$). Greater CHF severity was associated with lower Hb concentrations. Investigations of a 69 patient subgroup who underwent cardiac MRI (at randomization and 24 weeks later) showed an increase in Hb over time associated with a decrease in left ventricular mass and lower mortality, whereas a decrease in Hb over time associated with an increase in left ventricular mass and higher mortality. In multivariate analysis, anemia remained a significant, independent predictor of death or hospitalization for CHF.

Acute Ischemic Cardiac Disease
The impact of anemia in patients with acute myocardial infarction (MI) undergoing percutaneous coronary intervention (PCI) was recently evaluated (46). In the Controlled Abciximab and Device Investigation to Lower Late Angioplasty Complications (CADILLAC) trial, 2082 patients with MI undergoing primary PCI were randomized to balloon angioplasty versus stenting, each with or without abciximab. Outcomes were stratified by presence of anemia at baseline (WHO criteria). Anemia was present in 12.8% of randomized patients. Patients with baseline anemia more frequently developed in-hospital hemorrhagic complications (6.2% vs. 2.4%, $P = 0.002$), had higher rates of blood transfusions (13.1% vs. 3.1%, $P < 0.0001$), and had prolonged (median 4.1 vs. 3.5 days, $P < 0.0001$) index hospitalization. Anemic patients also had higher mortality during hospitalization

(4.6% vs. 1.1%, $P = 0.0003$), at 30 days (5.8% vs. 1.5%, $P < 0.0001$), and at one year (9.4% vs. 3.5%, $P < 0.0001$), as well as higher rates of disabling stroke at 30 days (0.8% vs. 0.1%, $P = 0.005$) and at one year (2.1% vs. 0.4%, $P = 0.0007$). Anemia independently predicted in-hospital (hazard ratio, 3.26; $P = 0.048$) and one-year mortality (hazard ratio, 2.38; $P = 0.016$).

Anemia is also an independent risk factor for mortality in patients requiring PCI, based on a study (47) examining outcomes of 6116 patients in relation to the pre-procedural Hb value. Anemia was associated with higher 30-day major adverse cardiac events, greater post-PCI peak troponin and creatine kinase-MB fraction, and longer LOS. The adverse impact of anemia on survival was observed irrespective of whether patients presented with stable or unstable angina, or with MI.

A recent study (48) examining the relation between blood transfusion and mortality among patients with acute coronary syndrome (ACS) raises concerns about possible adverse consequences of transfusion. The post hoc analysis included 24,112 enrollees in three large international clinical trials of ACS patients, of whom 2401 (10.0%) received at least one blood transfusion. Patients who underwent transfusion were older and had more comorbid illness at presentation. They also had a significantly higher unadjusted 30-day mortality rate (8.0% vs. 3.1%; $P < 0.001$) and MI rate (25.2% vs. 8.2%; $P < 0.001$), compared with patients who did not undergo transfusion. The relationship between blood transfusion and increased mortality persisted after adjustment for other predictive factors. Given the limitations of post hoc analysis, a randomized controlled trial (RCT) of transfusion strategies is warranted. However, routine use of blood to maintain an arbitrary Hct level in a stable patient with ischemic heart disease probably should be avoided.

Chronic Renal Disease

Anemia is strongly associated with morbidity and mortality in hemodialysis patients, as documented in the Dialysis Outcomes and Practice Patterns Study (DOPPS) (49). The DOPPS study also documented inconsistencies in anemia management practices, despite availability of consensus guidelines. Greater efforts to attain the recommended Hb concentrations may improve patient outcomes, as with rHuEPO therapy. For example, a RCT of early versus deferred initiation of rHuEPO in non-diabetic patients with chronic renal insufficiency and anemia (50) found that early treatment (50 U/kg/wk of rHuEPO alpha aiming for Hb ≥ 13 g/dL) significantly slowed the progression of renal disease compared with later therapy (initiated only when the Hb fell to <9 g/dL).

Malignancy

Anemia is highly prevalent in patients with cancer, in part because of anti-cancer therapy. The resulting decrease in oxygen carrying capacity of blood manifests as fatigue, dyspnea, palpitations, anorexia, cold hypersensitivity, and general weakness (51).

☞ **Anemia in cancer patients correlates with poor clinical outcome, including reduced tumor response to anti-cancer therapy and mortality.** ☞ Since anemia compromises both quality of life and survival, effective and well-tolerated treatment strategies are needed (52). A Cochrane meta-analysis of 19 RCTs of rHuEPO involving 2865 cancer patients showed improved survival with rHuEPO. A more recent meta-analysis of nine RCTs of epoetin beta

($n = 1413$) suggested that this therapy may reduce tumor progression, but had no favorable survival effect (52). Unlike the potential survival benefit of rHuEPO, blood transfusion has not been shown to improve patient survival.

PREVENTION OF ANEMIA
Control of Hemorrhage

☞ **Cessation of active bleeding is a key component in the prevention of anemia due to acute hemorrhage.** ☞ Maneuvers associated with control of active hemorrhage can be life-saving. Most often, hemorrhage is controlled by direct digital or hand compression of bleeding soft tissue and/or control of a distinct bleeding vessel. Definitive control often requires more advanced procedural or surgical intervention. Recently there has been increased interest in other methods of hemorrhage control, including pharmacological approaches.

Tourniquets

The most widely used mechanical systems incorporate use of a tourniquet. The use of tourniquets in the prehospital setting is primarily associated with the military, rather than the civilian, emergency medical system, primarily due to the longer medical evacuation times in the military (particularly during battle), and the increased frequency of life-threatening extremity wounds in recent armed conflicts.

A four-year retrospective analysis of tourniquet applications by Israeli Defense Force soldiers demonstrated that a total of 78% of applications were effective, with higher success rates for medical staff compared with soldiers (53). These researchers concluded that tourniquet application is an effective method for preventing exsanguination in the military prehospital setting. One-handed tourniquets have recently been developed.

Recent experience with elastic adhesive dressings for the treatment of bleeding wounds in trauma patients has demonstrated efficacy in emergency situations (54). A similar elastic bandage was used to avoid fasciotomy in treating upper extremity compartment syndrome (55). Tourniquets are also used for elective surgery when limited blood flow to an extremity is needed.

Damage Control and Packing

Damage control surgery, such as packing liver injuries, limits bleeding and permits resuscitation "catch-up," and helps to protect against anemia (56). ☞ **Damage control concepts, including early control of hemorrhage and delay of definitive treatment or reconstruction, have now been applied to areas of trauma care beyond abdominal injuries, including treatment of thoracic injuries where hemorrhage control is quickly established (57,58)** ☞ (Volume 1, Chapter 21 reviews the concepts and application of damage control).

Angiographic Embolization

Angiographic embolization is an adjunctive strategy to treat hemorrhage from injured organs (e.g., liver, spleen) and pelvic fractures (59–61). It is safe and effective for controlling bleeding after blunt and penetrating intra- and retroperitoneal injuries.

Pharmacological Interventions

Pharmacologic agents that inhibit fibrinolysis (aprotinin, ϵ-aminocaproic acid, tranexamic acid) or increase von Willebrand factor release (desmopressin) are used to decrease bleeding and blood product use in selected clinical settings. For example, aprotinin is well-established in reducing bleeding with cardiac surgery (62). Tranexamic acid was shown to reduce blood loss by 30% and drainage volume by 50%, with reduced transfusion requirements, in a study of knee arthroplasty (63). However, particularly in settings of acute trauma, interest in recent years has focused on recombinant factor VIIa (rFVIIa).

rFVIIa is approved for treatment of bleeding in hemophilia patients with inhibitors to factors VIII and IX. It is also used during surgery in these patients to control hemorrhage (64–66). Hemostasis is initiated by formation of a complex between tissue factor (TF), exposed by blood vessel wall injury, and activated FVII (FVIIa), normally present in circulating blood (66). TF-FVIIa complexes then convert FX to FXa on TF-bearing cells; FXa then activates prothrombin to thrombin, with thrombin clotting fibrinogen, activating several coagulation factors (VIII, V, XI), and activating platelets. The activated platelets undergo a conformational change, and form a template for coagulation factor assembly and full thrombin generation, which is needed to produce the fibrin component of the hemostatic plug. If thrombin generation is impaired, the fibrin plugs are loose and permeable, and readily dissolved by normal fibrinolytic activity. The addition of rFVIIa normalizes fibrin clot permeability in vitro and tightens the fibrin structure (66,67).

Recently, rFVIIa was found to be efficacious in both surgical and trauma patients with profuse bleeding (68–73). It has also been used to correct warfarin-related coagulopathy in preparation for emergency surgery (74,75). Based upon its mechanism of action, it is expected that its hemostatic effects are mainly limited to the site of injury, without systemic activation of coagulation (76). rFVIIa also appears to be efficacious in moderate hypothermia, but not in severe acidosis (72,77).

rFVIIa demonstrated a significant reduction of perioperative blood loss in patients undergoing radical retropubic prostatectomy (78). Median perioperative blood loss was 1235 mL and 1089 mL in groups given rFVIIa 20 and 40 μg/kg, respectively, compared with 2688 mL in placebo controls ($P = 0.001$). Seven of twelve placebo-treated patients were transfused, whereas none who received 40 mg/kg rFVIIa needed blood.

Trauma-associated bleeding can be reduced by rFVIIa (68,69). Seven massively bleeding, coagulopathic, multi-transfused trauma patients treated with rFVIIa (median, 120 μg/kg) achieved cessation of diffuse bleeding, reduction in blood requirements, and shortening of prothrombin and activated partial thromboplastin times (68). Similar results were seen in 19 critically-ill, multi-transfused trauma patients (70), as well as in a series of 21 Australian patients with life-threatening hemorrhage due to trauma or surgery (79). Few thrombotic events directly attributable to rFVIIa have occurred. rFVIIa also has been shown to correct the coagulopathy associated with traumatic brain injury more effectively than plasma infusion, allowing for earlier placement of invasive monitors (80). Animal models of hemorrhagic shock indicate that early rFVIIa administration decreases bleeding and improves survival without producing thrombosis in vital organs (65,81,82).

Recently, results of an international multicenter, double-blind, placebo-controlled RCT of rFVIIa in trauma ($n = 301$) were reported (83). Patients with blunt or penetrating trauma requiring transfusion of eight units RBC were randomized to three infusions of rFVIIa (200, 100, and 100 μg/kg) or placebo at entry, one hour and three hours.

In blunt trauma, after excluding early deaths, rFVIIa resulted in a significant decrease in the number of RBC transfusions within 48 hours, and a trend to reduced MOF and ARDS.

Topical Fibrin Sealant

Fibrin sealant (FS) is a prohemostatic agent initially created by combining human fibrinogen concentrate with thrombin solutions containing calcium (84). More recent products also contain factor XIII and aprotinin. The components are combined and applied to tissue with instantaneous formation of a coagulum. The fibrinogen is obtained from single donor plasma. FS can be applied topically or injected into organ parenchyma.

FS has been used to control bleeding in trauma and surgery patients for many years (85). Animal studies demonstrate effective hemostasis of superficial and deep hepatic injuries (86–90), control of arterial injuries without compromising blood flow (91), and control of renal bleeding (92). Dry FS dressings provide rapid hemorrhage control and improved survival in swine with grade V liver injuries (93). Clinical studies suggest efficacy in trauma as well (84,94,95). FS use in thermally-injured patients led to reduced need for blood transfusion (96). A multicenter trial of FS for topical hemostasis in skin grafting demonstrated its safety and suggested it may have contributed to accelerated scar maturation (97).

FS has demonstrated efficacy in a multitude of surgical procedures. It has been used to seal esophageal, gastric, colonic, or rectal anastomoses, and provided a 41% reduction in incidence of air leakage when added to suture lines in patients undergoing pulmonary resection (98). It has been utilized to seal cerebrospinal fluid leaks in neurosurgery, and has attenuated bleeding after dental extraction (98). Endoscopic injection of FS was superior to sclerotherapy in a RCT of 805 patients with bleeding peptic ulcer (98). FS was found to be a safe, simple and efficacious endoscopic treatment option in patients with gastric variceal bleeding (99). FS also has been shown to decrease blood loss and transfusion requirements in major joint replacement surgery (100–102). FS was more effective than bipolar or needle point coagulation for hemostasis in tonsillectomy and adenoidectomy (103).

Reduction of Blood Loss Due to Phlebotomy

Multiple studies have documented that ICU patients are phlebotomized about 40 to 70 mL/day (11,104). ☞ **Repeated phlebotomy for diagnostic laboratory testing contributes significantly to blood loss in critically ill patients.** ☞ Simple strategies to reduce such blood loss include the use of blood conservation devices, low-volume adult (or pediatric) sampling tubes, and minimizing diagnostic testing.

A RCT in 100 medical ICU patients found that a blood conservation device incorporated into the arterial pressure monitoring system reduced the total volume of discarded blood from 103.5 ± 99.9 mL to 19.4 ± 47.4 mL ($P < 0.0001$) (105). Discarded blood volume proved to be an independent predictor of Hb concentration decline.

A survey of 280 ICUs throughout England and Wales found that few measures were taken to reduce diagnostic blood loss from arterial blood sampling (106). The average volume of blood withdrawn to clear the arterial line before sampling was 3.2 mL, which was subsequently returned to the patient in only 18.4% of ICUs. Specific measures to reduce the blood sample size by the routine use of pediatric sample tubes occurred in only 9.3% of adult ICUs. In pediatric ICUs, the average volume withdrawn was 1.9 mL, which was routinely returned in 67% of units.

Strategies to reduce blood loss related to diagnostic phlebotomy, including use of pediatric tubes, low-volume adult tubes, and blood conservation devices, should be implemented in all ICUs, thereby reducing the incidence of anemia and need for blood transfusion (107).

Prophylaxis for Stress-Related Mucosal Damage

GI bleeding in ICU patients, both occult and overt, is commonly related to stress-related mucosal disease (SRMD), representing a continuum ranging from stress-related injury (superficial mucosal damage) to stress ulcers (focal deep mucosal damage) (108,109). Pharmacologic prophylaxis to prevent SRMD includes histamine-2-receptor antagonists, proton pump inhibitors, sucrulate, misoprostol, enteral nutrition, and antacids, though few modern ICUs still use anatacid titration approaches.

Patients with coagulopathy and respiratory failure are at highest risk for SRMD. Other risk factors include head and spinal cord injury, multiple trauma, sepsis, and steroid therapy. All high-risk patients should be started on enteral nutrition as soon as possible and receive concomitant pharmacologic prophylaxis (see Volume 2, Chapter 30).

TREATMENT OF ANEMIA
Correction of Nutritional Deficiencies

When present, correction of nutritional deficiency (Fe, folate, or B_{12}) is imperative to correct the anemia.

Erythropoietin

⚔ **Recombinant human erythropoietin (rHuEPO) rapidly produces erythropoiesis, and is used for treatment of anemia and to reduce the need for RBC transfusions.** ⚔ The use of rHuEPO is approved by the FDA for treatment of anemia in many patients, including those with renal disease, cancer, HIV, and before surgery. Treatment with rHuEPO should be supplemented with Fe and vitamin C for optimal efficacy. The first prospective study evaluating rHuEPO in critically ill patients was conducted in trauma patients with MODS (110). Patients received either 600 IU/kg intravenous rHuEPO three times weekly ($n = 9$) or saline control ($n = 10$). Whereas serum EPO concentrations in controls remained low, the active treatment group achieved pharmacologic EPO blood levels, and showed significantly increased reticulocyte counts compared with controls and baseline. Subsequently, several RCTs have evaluated rHuEPO for treating anemia in critically ill patients. The studies vary with respect to rHuEPO (and concurrent Fe) dosing, patient characteristics, and transfusion thresholds.

In 1999, the first large-scale RCT ($n = 160$) of rHuEPO for preventing anemia in critically ill patients was published (111). Study drug (300 units/kg of rHuEPO or placebo) was given by subcutaneous injection beginning ICU day three and continuing daily for five days; subsequently, dosing was every-other-day (target Hct >38%), with study drug given a minimum of two weeks (or until ICU discharge) up to six weeks post-randomization. This study demonstrated that rHuEPO decreased by 50% the number of packed red blood cells (PRBCs) transfused (166 vs. 305 units) and increased the HCT compared to placebo, without increase in adverse events.

The response to rHuEPO was carefully evaluated in a study of 36 anemic ICU patients in a single-center, open-label trial (112). The patients were divided into three groups: one group received rHuEPO (epoetin alfa, 300 IU/kg subcutaneously) plus intravenous Fe on days 1, 3, 5, 7, and 9, another group received intravenous Fe alone, and the third group (controls) received no additional therapy (all patients received folate). Serum EPO concentrations were inappropriately low for the degree of anemia at baseline irrespective of renal status. EPO concentrations increased among rHuEPO-treated patients from 23 ± 13 to a maximum of 166 ± 98 IU/L on day 10 ($P < 0.05$). The reticulocyte count increased exclusively in the rHuEPO group from $56 \pm 33 \times 10^9$/L to a maximum of 189 ± 97 on day 13 ($P < 0.05$). Serum transferrin receptor levels rose only in the rHuEPO group, indicating increased erythropoiesis. Interestingly, this study identified an increased zinc protoporphyrin concentration in the rHuEPO group, suggesting iron deficiency, despite the concurrent Fe supplementation.

The efficacy of weekly rHuEPO administration to decrease RBC transfusion was examined in a large multicenter RCT (113). ICU patients ($n = 1303$) expected to be in the ICU for at least two days were randomized to receive either 40,000 IU of rHuEPO or placebo. rHuEPO was started on day 3 and doses continued weekly for a total of three doses (patients remaining in the ICU on day 21 received a fourth dose). Patients treated with rHuEPO were less likely to undergo transfusion compared with placebo (50.5% vs. 60.4%; $P < 0.001$), with an overall 19% reduction in total units of RBCs transfused (1590 vs. 1963 units) and reduction in RBC units transfused per day alive (ratio of transfusion rates, 0.81). Increase in Hb from baseline to study end was greater in the rHuEPO group (1.32 vs. 0.94 g/dL; $P < 0.001$). Mortality (14% for rHuEPO and 15% for placebo) and adverse clinical event rates did not differ, however. The lower efficacy of rHuEPO in reducing blood transfusion in this study (113) [19% vs. 50% reduction (111)] could be due to the shorter study duration (28 vs. 42 days), lower rHuEPO dose (40,000 IU weekly), and inclusion of a transfusion protocol.

rHuEPO treatment can cause hypertension, particularly in uremic patients (29). Potential explanations include increased blood viscosity, reversal of hypoxic vasodilation, increased blood volume, and impaired nitric oxide synthesis. Antibody-associated pure red-cell aplasia (PRCA) has also been reported as a rare but serious adverse event (114). Between January 1998 and April 2004, 175 cases of rHuEPO-associated PRCA were reported for Eprex, 11 cases for Neorecormon (a formulation of epoetin beta), and five cases for Epogen. Over half occurred in France, Canada, the United Kingdom, and Spain. After adoption of procedures to ensure appropriate storage, handling, and administration of Eprex, the exposure-adjusted incidence decreased by 83% worldwide.

Blood Transfusion

The transfusion of ABO/Rhesus-matched PRBCs is the mainstay of therapy for many anemic patients.

Transfusion Triggers

In the late 1990s, research trials were undertaken to determine the optimal Hb/Hct level at which transfusion of blood products should occur. Too often, ICU patients received blood transfusions based on an arbitrary transfusion trigger or simply a "below normal" Hb level rather than a physiological need for blood (104).

One of the earliest studies evaluating physician response to various Hb levels divided the patient population into three groups based on the following Hb levels: 7.5 to 7.9, 7.0 to 7.4, and <7.0 g/dL (115). Approximately the same number of patients was transfused in each group. Patients in the progressively more anemic groups received slightly more transfused units and the post-transfusion IIb increase was higher in more anemic patients. The physicians surveyed indicated that the Hb critical limit could be lowered without adverse consequence. These investigators concluded that the transfusion trigger and low critical limit for Hb are distinct entities (115).

In 1999, the Canadian Critical Care Trials Group published the results of the only RCT, named the Transfusion Requirements in Critical Care (TRICC) trial (117), which compared two transfusion "triggers" with the primary outcomes of mortality and severity of organ dysfunction. Critically ill patients ($n = 838$) with euvolemia after initial treatment for Hb concentrations less than 9 g/dL within 72 hours following ICU admission were enrolled. Patients were randomized to a *restrictive strategy* of transfusion, in which PRBCs were transfused if the Hb concentration dropped below 7 g/dL, with Hb maintained at 7 to 9 g/dL, or to a *liberal strategy*, in which transfusions were given when the Hb fell below 10 g/dL, and Hb concentrations maintained at 10 to 12 g/dL. Overall, there was a trend to lower 30-day mortality in the restrictive transfusion strategy group (18.7% vs. 23.3%, $P = 0.11$). Moreover, mortality was significantly lower with the restrictive strategy among less acutely ill patients (APACHE II score of ≤ 20; 8.7% vs. 16.1%, $P = 0.03$) and in patients less than 55 years of age (5.7% vs. 13.0%; $P = 0.02$), but not among patients with clinically significant cardiac disease (20.5% vs. 22.9%; $P = 0.69$). The in-hospital mortality rate was significantly lower in the restrictive strategy group (22.3% vs. 28.1%, $P = 0.05$). In a post hoc analysis of 257 patients with severe ischemic heart disease, there were no statistically significant differences in any survival measures; the restrictive group had a lower, but nonsignificant, absolute survival rate compared with patients in the liberal group (117). **A restrictive strategy of red cell transfusion is at least as effective as and probably superior to a liberal transfusion strategy in critically ill patients, with the possible exception of patients with acute MI or unstable angina.**

Subsequent analysis of the TRICC trial patient cohort requiring mechanical ventilation ($n = 713$) found no evidence that a liberal PRBC transfusion strategy for treating anemia decreased the duration of mechanical ventilation (118). Similarly, analysis of the cohort of trauma patients in the TRICC trial showed no significant differences in mortality, MODS severity or change, or in ICU or hospital LOS (119). Nevertheless, the number of PRBCs transfused per patient was significantly less in the restrictive transfusion group (2.3 ± 4.4 vs. 5.4 ± 4.3; $P < 0.0001$), indicating that a restrictive PRBC transfusion strategy appears safe for critically ill trauma patients.

A meta-analysis (120) of 10 trials with 1780 patients demonstrated that restrictive transfusion strategies reduced PRBC transfusion by 42% (mean, 0.93 units per patient). Mortality, cardiac events, and hospital LOS were unaffected. The authors conclude that the use of restrictive transfusion triggers is appropriate in patients free of serious cardiac disease, although they cautioned that most of the data were generated by one trial.

Most stable critically ill patients can probably be managed using a restrictive transfusion strategy (121).

Indeed, abnormally high Hb levels may be detrimental in the critically ill patient. High Hb levels upon entry into the ICU were associated with increased mortality, increased incidence of MI, and with more severe left ventricular dysfunction in 2202 cardiac patients who underwent coronary artery bypass graft surgery (CABG) (122). In contrast, low intraoperative HCT (<0.22) was associated with stroke, MI, sepsis, and MODS in another study (123), indicating the need for further studies of optimal transfusion thresholds (124). Despite studies supporting a transfusion threshold between 7 and 8 g/dL for most patients, actual clinical practice continues to vary widely (125).

Correcting decreased oxygen delivery by transfusing an anemic patient has been hypothesized to help in weaning from mechanical ventilation. However, Hebert et al. (118) found that a liberal transfusion strategy did not decrease the duration of mechanical ventilation.

Nontraditional Transfusion Triggers

The concept of a viscosity trigger has been evaluated. Theoretically, hemodilution to a Hb level of 7 to 8 g/dL might not compromise oxygen delivery and consumption; however, the corresponding reduced blood viscosity might not transmit adequate pressure to the capillaries, causing functional capillary density (FCD) to decrease and jeopardizing organ function through the inadequate extraction of products of metabolism from the tissue by the capillaries (126). Previous studies in hemorrhagic shock have demonstrated that survival is primarily determined by maintenance of FCD and secondarily by tissue oxygenation; thus, increasing plasma viscosity may extend the transfusion trigger and reduce the use of blood transfusions.

The use of an oxygen extraction ratio of 50% as a transfusion trigger has been shown to lead to a reduction in allogeneic blood transfusion in postoperative CABG patients (127). Oxygen saturation may also be used as a transfusion trigger. A recent study using near-infrared spectroscopy measured regional Hb oxygen concentration from the cerebral cortex and gastrocnemius muscle, as well as arterial oxygen saturation, end-tidal carbon dioxide tension, mean arterial pressure, and Hb concentration, in patients undergoing acute normovolemic hemodilution (128). Hb concentration and blood loss volume correlated with both cerebral cortex and gastrocnemius oxygen saturation.

Complications Associated with Utilization of Blood Products

The transfusion of blood products has been associated with worse clinical outcome in numerous studies (36,129,130). One explanation could be transfusion-induced immunomodulation (131), such as decreased T-cell-mediated immunity (132) observed with both autologous and allogeneic blood (133). Blood transfusion is associated with an increase in serum and soft tissue tumor necrosis factor α (TNF-α), interleukin (IL)-1β, IL-6, IL-8, and other cytokines and their soluble receptors (134–138). Blood transfusion enhances inflammatory mediator release from normal neutrophils incubated with plasma from stored blood (139). Cardiac surgery patients demonstrated increased levels of IL-6 and bactericidal permeability increasing protein in relation to the number of PRBCs transfused (135). Release of IL-8, IL-1β, and TNF-α and secretory phopholipase is amplified by older (>14 days) blood (140).

Transfusion of blood products in the perioperative period has also been associated with cancer recurrence, as demonstrated in patients undergoing hepatic resection for hepatocellular carcinoma (141), and those undergoing colon cancer resection. In this latter group, perioperative blood transfusion was associated with a significant decrease in overall survival (3 years vs. 4.6 years for non-transfused patients) (142).

☞ **Blood transfusion is associated with increased risk for death, perioperative infection, MODS, and ICU admission in the trauma patient population (129,143–146).** ☞ Blood transfusion within the first 24 hours of admission was a significant independent risk factor for SIRS, mortality, and ICU admission and LOS in 9569 acute trauma patients (147). Age (>15 days storage) of blood was also an independent predictor of increased ICU admission and LOS and hospital LOS in a study evaluating >15,000 acute trauma patients (148).

☞ **Blood product age correlates with mortality in patients admitted to the ICU with severe sepsis.** ☞ In one study (149), the median age of blood was 17 days for survivors versus 25 days for non-survivors. Age of blood was also associated with worse outcome in a study of 416 patients (269 transfused) who underwent CABG (150). The risk of postoperative pneumonia increased 1% per day of increase in mean storage time of PRBCs and increased 5% per unit of PRBCs or platelets transfused.

Blood transfusion is associated with increased risk for infection. In a study of trauma patients, transfusion of PRBCs within the first 48 hours of admission was associated with an increase in infection rate (33.0% for patients receiving at least one blood transfusion vs. 7.6% in patients not transfused) (146). Transfusion was associated with a 1.35-fold increased risk for bacterial infection and a 1.52-fold increased risk for pneumonia in a retrospective cohort study of 9598 consecutive hip fracture patients who underwent surgical repair (144). A dose–response relationship between blood transfusion, bacterial infection, and pneumonia was also observed. Allogeneic blood transfusion was a dose-dependent, independent predictor of postoperative bacterial infection and mortality in a prospective analysis of 1349 patients (282 transfused) who underwent colorectal surgery (151). Transfused medical-surgical ICU patients had a significantly higher rate of nosocomial infections when 1717 patients were stratified for severity of illness, age, and gender (145). A dose–response relationship was established between number of units of PRBCs transfused and risk for nosocomial infection. The odds of infection were increased by a factor of 1.5 for each unit of blood transfused. In another cohort study of 738 surgical patients, transfusion of four or more units led to an increased risk for severe postoperative infection and nosocomial pneumonia (152). Preoperative anemia and intraoperative blood transfusion were independent predictors of postoperative pneumonia in 6301 non-cardiac surgical patients in a prospective observational trial (153).

Leukodepletion

Leukocytes present in RBC and platelet concentrates have been implicated in several immunological and infective complications of blood transfusion (154). Transfusion can result in persistent survival of donor leukocyte subpopulations in the recipient (microchimerism), a phenomenon that likely reflects engraftment within the recipient of donor hematopoietic stem cells. Microchimerism is very uncommon following transfusion for elective surgery,

sickle cell anemia, thalassemia, and HIV, but occurs significantly more often in trauma patients. A recent prospective study of 45 transfused trauma patients found that 53% had evidence of microchimerism by polymerase chain reaction (155). The long-term sequelae of microchimerism in trauma patients are unknown.

Leukodepletion is a process whereby filtration is used to remove the vast majority of white blood cells from blood products, typically resulting in less than 5×10^6 residual leukocytes per transfused unit. This is typically accomplished soon after collection (prestorage leukodepletion), although it can be done at the bedside. However, bedside leukofiltration can be associated with bradykinin-induced hypotension (156) that results when platelets are exposed to negatively charged leukocyte filters.

In a recent study evaluating leukodepletion filters, IL-8 levels were lower on storage days 1 and 35 in filtered concentrates compared with control (unfiltered) counterparts (157). In another study, leukodepletion during CABG led to reduced need for blood transfusion and crystalloid infusion in the postoperative period compared to controls (158).

Whether or not *universal* leukoreduction of blood products should be performed is controversial. The largest RCT of universal leukodepletion failed to establish efficacy (159). Patients ($n = 2780$) received either unmodified blood components or stored leukocyte-reduced RBCs and platelets. Three prespecified primary outcome measures did not differ between the leukodepletion and control groups (respectively), namely in-hospital mortality (9.0 vs. 8.5% control; $P = 0.64$), hospital LOS post-transfusion (median days, 6.3 vs. 6.4; $P = 0.21$), and total hospital costs (median, \$19,200 vs. \$19,500; $P = 0.24$). Secondary outcomes (ICU LOS, postoperative LOS, antibiotic usage, and readmission rate) also did not differ. Subgroup analysis based on patient age, gender, amount of blood transfused, or type of surgery showed no effect. However, patients receiving leukodepleted blood had a lower incidence of febrile reactions ($P = 0.06$).

Saline Washing

Saline washing refers to rinsing of donor RBCs in isotonic sodium chloride, thereby depleting the PRBCs of leukocytes, microaggregates and nearly all of the plasma (160). The optimal number of washings needed is controversial. One study that measured total protein, immunoglobulin levels, and complement factor C3 content, along with RBC osmotic fragility in whole blood washed anywhere from one to six times (161) found that protein, immunoglobulin, and C3 levels decreased precipitously after the first two washing procedures, without significant effect from subsequent washes. Interestingly, more washes were needed when storage time was greater. RBC osmotic fragility increased with each wash and with greater storage time. These researchers concluded that optimal results were obtained when a one to two week old unit of whole blood was washed two to three times. As the immunomodulatory effects of RBC transfusion include neutrophil priming for cytotoxicity (an effect exacerbated by longer storage times), post-storage saline washing abrogates neutrophil priming (162).

Hemoglobin-Based Oxygen Carriers

☞ **Increasing demand for blood products and safety concerns have stimulated the search for alternative erythrocyte transfusion strategies such as the development of hemoglobin-based oxygen carriers (HBOCs) (163,164).** ☞

Several unforeseen adverse effects have kept blood substitutes "out of reach" (165). Agents under investigation are pathogen-free, have acceptable side effect profiles, and long shelf lives. Two HBOCs include polymerized bovine Hb (HBOC-201, Hemopure, Biopure Corporation, Cambridge, MA) and human polymerized Hb (PolyHeme, Northfield Laboratories, Evanston, IL).

Hemopure—Polymerized Bovine Hemoglobin (Hemoglobin-Based Oxygen Carriers-201)

Phase III trials with polymerized bovine Hb demonstrate that allogeneic blood transfusions can be reduced in certain perioperative settings (166,167). This product has also been used to enhance oxygen delivery in a severely anemic Jehovah's Witness pending response to high-dose rHuEPO (168). HBOC can reach post-stenotic or other poorly perfused tissues where erythrocytes cannot pass, thus enhancing tissue oxygenation (163). Compared with PRBC transfusion, low doses of HBOC-201 maintained enhanced oxygen extraction after extended hemodilution, and provided a faster and higher increase in muscular tissue PO$_2$ in animal studies (169).

PolyHeme—Polymerized Human Hemoglobin

PolyHeme is a chemically-modified Hb solution derived from outdated human blood developed as an alternative to transfused blood (170). As single Hb molecules are toxic to the kidneys and cause vasoconstriction, the Hb molecules are polymerized to create small chains of linked tetramers.

Initial studies of PolyHeme demonstrated that it was safe when used in patients with acute blood loss, reducing the use of allogeneic blood (171). In a recent RCT, PolyHeme given in lieu of PRBCs to trauma patients requiring urgent transfusion avoided the neutrophil priming seen in other patients who had received PRBCs (172). Utilization of PolyHeme could therefore decrease risk for MODS in this patient population.

Another recent study comparing survival in 171 trauma or urgent surgical patients with life-threatening anemia given PolyHeme to historical controls (300 similarly anemic patients refusing transfusion) found increased survival with Polyheme (173). Johnson et al. (174) measured serial pro- and anti-inflammatory cytokine levels in critically injured patients resuscitated either with PRBCs or with PolyHeme, and found higher cytokine levels among patients who received PRBCs, with exaggerated levels of these cytokines associated with adverse outcomes.

EYE TO THE FUTURE

Continued advances are being made in the pathogenesis, diagnosis, and treatment of anemia associated with trauma and critical illness, including the development of nontransfusional therapies.

Hepcidin

Hepcidin is a recently discovered hepatic peptide that regulates intestinal absorption and placental transport of Fe. It probably also affects release of Fe from hepatic stores and from macrophages involved in the recycling of Fe from Hb. Hepcidin is a key mediator of hypoferremia of inflammation, contributing to pathogenesis of ACD (175). The inflammatory cytokine IL-6 induces production of hepcidin

(Fig. 5). Studies of human liver cell cultures, mice, and human volunteers indicate that IL-6 is the necessary and sufficient cytokine for the induction of hepcidin during inflammation, indicating that the IL-6-hepcidin axis is responsible for the hypoferremia of inflammation (176).

Decreased hepcidin leads to tissue Fe overload, while hepcidin overproduction causes hypoferremia and ACD. Ferroportin is an Fe exporter present on the surface of absorptive enterocytes, macrophages, hepatocytes, and placental cells. A recent study determined that hepcidin is bound to ferroportin in tissue culture cells (177). Following binding, ferroportin was internalized and degraded, leading to decreased export of cellular Fe. The post-translational regulation of ferroportin by hepcidin may thus complete a homeostatic loop whereby Fe regulates secretion of hepcidin, which in turn controls the concentration of ferroportin on the cell surface.

If inflammatory induction of hepcidin causes hypoferremia, it is logical to predict that inhibition of hepcidin expression or activity would ameliorate the anemia of inflammation. Would that be advantageous? We know that patients and mice lacking hepcidin have increased intestinal Fe absorption and increased serum Fe, and this is unlikely to be harmful in the short term. However, there may be cause for concern in patients with infections or malignancy, as decreased serum Fe contributes to host defense against invading pathogens and tumor cells, while hepcidin itself has antimicrobial properties (178).

"Old" Blood and Free Hemoglobin

Increased blood storage time leads to increased hemolysis, producing free Hb within the unit of PRBC. Stroma-free plasma Hb rapidly destroys nitric oxide by oxidation to met-Hb and nitrate ions (Fig. 6). Cell-free Hb, due to its low molecular weight, may also diffuse into extravascular spaces where it can bind nitric oxide as well. Limited nitric oxide bioavailability under these conditions promotes systemic vasoconstriction and organ dysfunction.

Similarly, first-generation HBOCs were associated with adverse events, including severe hypertension and renal failure as a result of severe vasoconstriction due to nitric oxide binding by cell-free Hb monomers and dimers.

Under normal circumstances, confinement of Hb within RBCs reduces the rate of reaction of Hb with nitric oxide by a factor of 1000 or greater, because the RBC membrane creates a barrier to the diffusion of nitric oxide. Furthermore, in rapidly flowing arterial blood, the streaming of plasma along the endothelium separates nitric oxide from

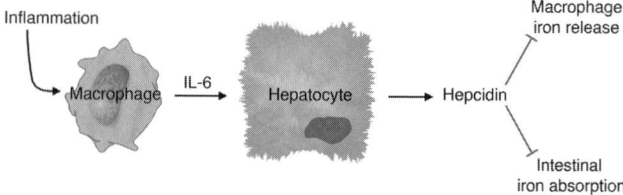

Figure 5 Hepcidin and the anemia of critical illness. Regulation of hepcidin production in inflammation. Inflammation leads to macrophage elaboration of IL-6, which acts on hepatocytes to induce hepcidin production. Hepcidin inhibits macrophage iron release and intestinal iron absorption, leading to hypoferremia. *Source*: From Ref. 178.

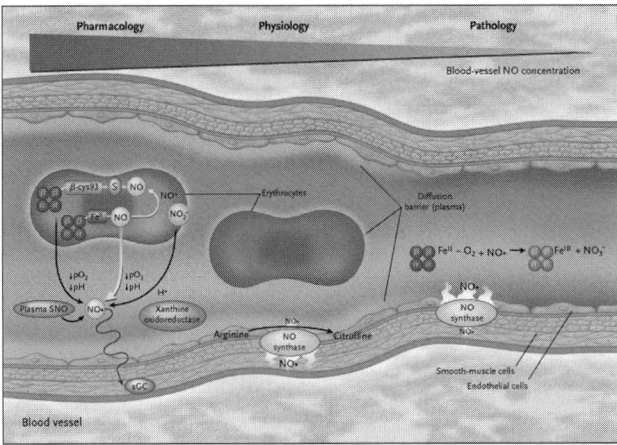

Figure 6 A model of the interactions of nitric oxide with erythrocytes (RBCs) and cell-free hemoglobin in an arterial blood vessel. The diagram illustrates the major processes regulating nitric oxide (NO) levels in blood vessels during pharmacologic NO delivery (left), under normal conditions (center), and under pathologic conditions, such as acute or chronic hemolysis (right). The overall blood-vessel NO concentration is depicted by the width of the blue band above the vessel. Within the vessel, smooth-muscle cells and a layer of endothelial cells are shown. Under normal conditions (*center*), NO produced by endothelial NO synthase with arginine as a substrate (and also producing citrulline) diffuses into smooth muscle to activate soluble guanylyl cyclase (sGC) to form cyclic guanosine monophosphate and thus maintain basal vascular tone. Intravascular destruction of NO by intraerythrocytic hemoglobin is limited by diffusional barriers in the red-cell–free layer adjacent to the endothelium and factors in and around the erythrocyte membrane that slow nitric oxide transit. Note shading around the RBCs and endothelium. However, sufficient NO is consumed to limit its activity to the local environment. When NO is administered by inhalation or infusion (left), high intravascular nitric oxide concentrations promote nitric oxide reactions, with erythrocyte hemoglobin and plasma proteins that can either protect it, thereby promoting systemic vasodilatation, or destroy it. Possible mechanisms of protection and delivery of nitric oxide from iron-nitrosyl hemoglobin (Fe^{II}-NO) and S-nitrosohemoglobin (β-cys93-SNO) within erythrocytes and from plasma nitric oxide species (including nitric oxide gas [NO^-], plasma SNO, and nitrite ions [NO_2^-]) are shown, as are conditions that may promote these reactions, including low oxygen tension ($\downarrow PO_2$) and low pH ($\downarrow$ pH). Of considerable recent interest is the possible bioactivity of nitrite ions, since they can be converted to nitric oxide by enzymatic reactions (including by xanthine oxidoreductase or heme proteins) or nonenzymatic reactions. The extent to which these processes occur in normal physiology is not yet clear. During hemolysis (right) or the infusion of hemoglobin-based blood substitutes, cell-free ferrous hemoglobin (shown as a protein tetramer with one Fe^{II}-O_2 molecule) in the plasma rapidly destroys nitric oxide by being oxidized to methemoglobin (Fe^{III}) and nitrate ions. Owing to its low molecular weight, cell-free hemoglobin (especially as a dimer subunit) may diffuse into extravascular spaces. Limited nitric oxide bioavailability under these conditions promotes systemic vasoconstriction and organ dysfunction.
Source: From Ref. 189.

much of the red cell mass, thereby reducing its contact with oxy-Hb. Further study is needed to optimize methods to reduce storage-associated hemolysis, or to remove free Hb.

Prehospital Trials of Hemoglobin-Based Oxygen Carriers

The management of uncontrolled bleeding in trauma patients is difficult in the prehospital setting. Current prehospital therapies (low volume resuscitation, compression of external bleeding sites, mobilization of fractures to reduce bleeding) do not include blood transfusion due to logistics and storage. HBOCs exhibit many desirable characteristics that make them potential therapeutic agents in this setting. These compounds do not need cross-matching, have favorable oxygen dissociation characteristics, long half-lives, do not transmit infectious disease, appear less immunoreactive than blood, and do not require refrigeration. An RCT in the prehospital setting has been initiated, entitled "A Phase III, Randomized, Controlled, Open-Label Multicenter, Parallel Group Study Using Provisions for Exception from Informed Consent Requirements Designed to Evaluate the Safety and Efficacy of Poly SFH-P Injection [Polymerized Human Hemoglobin (Pyridoxylated) PolyHeme®] When Used to Treat Patients in Hemorrhagic Shock Following Traumatic Injuries Beginning in the Prehospital Setting."

In this study, patients in hemorrhagic shock will begin to receive either the standard of care with crystalloid fluid resuscitation (control) or PolyHeme. Treatment would begin before arrival at the hospital, and continue during a 12-hour post-injury period. In the hospital, patients in the control group will receive crystalloid for resuscitation and blood transfusion if necessary, as required. Patients in the treatment group will receive crystalloid for resuscitation and PolyHeme® instead of blood transfusion. The maximum dose of PolyHeme will be six units during the first 12 hours. Blood will be used thereafter, if oxygen delivery levels need to be increased. Information regarding this trial is available at http://www.northfieldlabs.com/amb_trial.html.

Similarly, plans are underway to conduct an RCT of Hemopure for out-of-hospital resuscitation of patients with severe hemorrhagic shock. Entitled "Restore Effective Survival in Shock" (RESUS), the trial is intended to support an indication for out-of-hospital military and civilian trauma applications. The scientific advisory committee for this protocol includes Navy, Army, and Air Force medical researchers and academic experts in trauma, emergency medicine, critical care, and statistics. Because the proposed RESUS protocol involves waiver of patient informed consent (WIC), regulations require the submission of a separate investigational new drug application (IND). Once a new IND is assigned and the final protocol is agreed upon with the FDA, the participating hospitals' internal review boards must approve the protocol. This process may require obtaining separate approvals at each trial site for the WIC community notification program, which begins prior to patient enrollment, and for the actual initiation of patient enrollment. Further information regarding this study is at http://www.biopure.com/shared/home.cfm?CDID=2&CPgID=19.

Recombinant Human Hemoglobin

A considerable problem with human or bovine HBOCs is procuring an adequate supply, since human HBOC derives from outdated human blood, and bovine HBOC is made from a U.S. cattle source. The recent development of a recombinant human Hb (rHb 2.0) that has reduced reactivity with nitric oxide is exciting, since it would potentially provide limitless HBOC supply.

A recent study evaluated the efficacy of this second-generation HBOC for resuscitation in a swine model of uncontrolled perioperative hemorrhage (179). After instrumentation, animals underwent splenectomy and rapid hemorrhage to a systolic blood pressure of 35 mmHg and isoelectric electroencephalography; 15 minutes of shock was followed by resuscitation over 30 minutes. rHb2.0 for injection performed as well as heterologous blood, did not cause sustained pulmonary hypertension, maintained adequate cardiac output and oxygen delivery, and was superior to either LR or the first-generation HBOC, diaspirin-cross-linked Hb. No human studies of rHb2.0 have yet been undertaken.

Perfluorocarbons

Significant efforts have been made over the past 70 years to find an oxygen-carrying solution that could substitute for blood (180). During this time, the focus has shifted to developing a solution capable of delivering oxygen to the tissues. Perfluorocarbons (PFCs) are highly inert solutions with a high solubility for all gases, making them a prime candidate to become such an oxygen delivery agent. Although research efforts with these agents continue, the rapid disappearance of emulsified PFCs from the vascular space, and their accumulation in the liver and spleen, limit their usefulness as transfusion substitutes.

Because of their ability to dissolve significant quantities of oxygen and carbon dioxide, these agents may be more attractive as oxygen delivery agents during periods of local or global organ ischemia, including preservation of organs for transplantation. PFCs have also been tested in animal models of cardiopulmonary bypass, and may be efficacious in adsorbing the gases present in air emboli.

Recently a second class of oxygen therapeutics (allosteric modifiers) has been developed, and these agents enhance oxygen delivery by shifting the oxygen dissociation curve to the right, thus increasing tissue PO_2. Allosteric modifiers have been shown to shift the p50 of Hb 10 mmHg at clinically relevant dosages, reduce (in animal models) cerebral infarct size following carotid ligation, and improve myocardial performance following myocardial ischemia. Despite significant research efforts, however, none of the solutions under development are currently approved for clinical use, with the exception of myocardial contrast imaging agents.

The oxygen transport capacity of PFCs was recently investigated in the hamster chamber window model microcirculation to determine the rate at which oxygen is delivered to the tissue in conditions of extreme hemodilution (Hct = 11%) (181). It was found that systemic and microvascular oxygen delivery was 25% and 400% higher in the PFC animals compared with Hydroxyethylstarch (HES) control animals, respectively, showing that PFCs deliver oxygen to the tissue when combined with hyperoxic ventilation in the present experiments, with no evidence of vasoconstriction or impaired microvascular function. Oxygen ventilation (100%) led to a positive base excess for the PFC group (5.5 $\pm$ 2.5 mmol/L) versus a negative balance (-0.8 ± 1.4 mmol/L) for the HES group, suggesting that microvascular findings corresponded to systemic events.

Liposome-Encapsulated Hemoglobin and Hemoglobin Vesicles

Besides HBOCs and PFCs, liposome-encapsulated Hb, Hb with low oxygen affinity (P50 = 40–50 mmHg), and Hb vesicles (phospholipid vesicles encapsulating concentrated human Hb) are candidate blood substitutes (182).

Animal studies have documented that hemodilution with liposome-encapsulated low-oxygen-affinity Hb facilitates rapid recovery from incomplete forebrain ischemia in the rat (183). On the basis of circulation kinetics, the half-life of 99mTc-LEH in blood was determined to be 30 and 39.8 hours in rats and rabbits, respectively (184). Most recently, the effect of hemodilution with NeoRedCell (NRC, liposome-encapsulated Hb) on myocardial perfusion was evaluated in rat hearts under 300 bpm pacing and 100 mmHg perfusion pressure (185). The results suggested that NRC is superior to erythrocytes in terms of the homogenization of oxygen delivery, indicating its potential therapeutic value in myocardial microcirculatory failure.

Hb vesicles are produced from outdated human blood, and are stable in long-term storage, with a Hb concentration of 8.6 g/dL. Hb vesicles are similar to RBCs, since both have lipid bilayer membranes that prevent direct contact of Hb with endothelium and scavenging of nitric oxide. The oxygen transport capacity of phospholipid vesicles encapsulating purified Hb produced with a P50 of 8 mmHg and 29 mmHg were investigated in the hamster chamber window model using microvascular measurements to determine oxygen delivery during extreme hemodilution (186). This study documented that improved tissue PO_2 was obtained when red blood cells deliver oxygen in combination with an oxygen carrier with high rather than low oxygen affinity.

In a recent study using a rat hemorrhagic shock model, resuscitation with Hb-vesicle suspended in recombinant human serum albumin (HbV/rHSA) at an Hb concentration of 8.6 g/dL was compared with shed autologous blood (187). HbV suspended in rHSA provided restoration from hemorrhagic shock comparable with that using shed autologous blood.

SUMMARY

Anemia is a common problem in trauma and critical care, and has significant consequences, including the high prevalence of blood transfusion and associated adverse outcomes. In trauma and critical care, multiple strategies for preventing anemia, including reduction in diagnostic phlebotomy, pharmacologic prophylaxis for stress-related mucosal damage and GI bleeding, and efforts to reduce blood loss in renal replacement therapy should be initiated. Furthermore, the use of blood transfusion for treatment of anemia should be considered only for manifestations of physiologic intolerance of anemia. Alternatives to blood transfusion are undergoing active investigation, including rHuEPO and HBOCs.

KEY POINTS

- Anemia is common in the intensive care unit (ICU), and blood transfusions are often used to treat anemia in critical care.
- Low Hb concentration typically accompanies a decreased red blood cell (RBC) count and a decrease

in packed cell volume, although these indices may be normal in an anemic patient with low Hb levels alone.

✔ Symptoms are dictated by the etiology, severity, and chronicity of the anemia.

✔ Evaluation of red cell indices is the most clinically relevant measurement tool.

✔ Laboratory evaluation of nutritional deficiencies that cause anemia should also be considered.

✔ The endogenous hormone erythropoietin is critical for the normal blood marrow response to anemia.

✔ It is important to understand the epidemiology of anemia in trauma and critical care in order to appreciate the large numbers of patients that require treatment for anemia.

✔ An acute normocytic, normochromic anemia is associated with systemic blood loss.

✔ In trauma, hemorrhagic shock and tissue injury also result in an acute inflammatory response, and the anemia associated with inflammation (or critical illness) rapidly ensues.

✔ Phlebotomy is a significant contributor to ICU-acquired anemia.

✔ A blunted erythropoietin response is commonly seen in critically ill or injured patients.

✔ Anemia from chronic disease is encountered frequently in surgery and critical care, and may exacerbate acute anemia associated with trauma and hemorrhage.

✔ The physiological response to anemia is dictated by the etiology and rapidity of onset of the anemia and the age and general state of health of the patient.

✔ Adaptation to anemia and hypoxia results in the induction and regulation of a number of physiologically relevant genes in response to changes in intracellular oxygen tension.

✔ Anemia adversely affects patient mortality and morbidity.

✔ Anemia in cancer patients correlates with poor clinical outcome, including reduced tumor response to anticancer therapy and mortality.

✔ Cessation of active bleeding is a key component in the prevention of anemia due to acute hemorrhage.

✔ Damage control concepts, including early control of hemorrhage and delay of definitive treatment or reconstruction, have now been applied to many areas of trauma care other than laparotomy and solid organ injuries, including treatment of thoracic injuries where hemorrhage control is quickly established.

✔ Repeated phlebotomy for diagnostic laboratory testing contributes significantly to blood loss in critically ill patients.

✔ Recombinant human erythropoietin (rHuEPO) rapidly produces erythropoiesis, and is used for treatment of anemia and to reduce the need for red blood cell transfusions.

✔ A restrictive strategy of red cell transfusion is at least as effective as and probably superior to a liberal transfusion strategy in critically ill patients, with the possible exception of patients with acute MI or unstable angina.

✔ The transfusion of blood products has been associated with worse clinical outcome in numerous studies.

✔ Blood transfusion is associated with increased risk for death, perioperative infection, MODS, and ICU admission in the trauma patient population.

✔ Blood product age correlates with mortality in patients admitted to the ICU with severe sepsis.

✔ Increasing demand for blood products and safety concerns have stimulated the search for alternative

erythrocyte transfusion strategies such as the development of hemoglobin-based oxygen carriers (HBOCs).

REFERENCES

1. Hoffbrand AV, Pettit JE, Moss PAH. Essential Haematology. Malden, MA: Blackwell Science Ltd, 2001.
2. Nilsson-Ehle H, Jagenburg R, Landahl S, Svanborg A. Blood haemoglobin declines in the elderly: implications for reference intervals from age 70 to 88. Eur J Haematol 2000; 65(5):297–305.
3. d'Onofrio G, Kuse R, Foures C, et al. Reticulocytes in haematological disorders. Clin Lab Haematol 1996; 18 (suppl 1):29–34.
4. Rodriguez RM, Corwin HL, Gettinger A, et al. Nutritional deficiencies and blunted erythropoietin response as causes of the anemia of critical illness. J Crit Care 2001; 16(1):36–41.
5. Das Gupta A, Abbi A. High serum transferrin receptor level in anemia of chronic disorders indicates coexistent iron deficiency. Am J Hematol 2003; 72(3):158–161.
6. Cook JD, Flowers CH, Skikne BS. The quantitative assessment of body iron. Blood 2003; 101(9):3359–3363.
7. Kaltwasser JP, Gottschalk R. Erythropoietin and iron. Kidney Int Suppl 1999; 69:S49–S56.
8. Labbe RF, Dewanji A. Iron assessment tests: transferring receptor vis-a-vis zinc protoporphyrin. Clin biochem 2004; 37(3):165–174.
9. Hastka J, Lasserre JJ, Schwarzbeck A, Hehlmann R. Central role of zinc protoporphyrin in staging iron deficiency. Clin Chem 1994; 40(5):768–773.
10. Elliot JM, Virankabutra T, Jones S, et al. Erythropoietin mimics the acute phase response in critical illness. Crit Care 2003; 7(3):R35–R40.
11. Vincent JL, Baron J-F, Reinhart K, et al. Anemia and blood transfusion in critically ill patients. JAMA 2002; 288:1499–1507.
12. Corwin HL, Gettinger A, Pearl RG, et al. The CRIT study: Anemia and blood transfusion in the critically ill: current clinical practice in the United States. Crit Care Med 2004; 32:39–52.
13. Hebert PC, Wells G, Martin C, et al. Variation in red cell transfusion practice in the intensive care unit: a multicentre cohort study. Crit Care 1999; 3(2):57–63.
14. Rao MP, Boralessa H, Morgan C, et al. Blood component use in critically ill patients. Anaesthesia 2002; 57:530–534.
15. Shapiro MJ, Gettinger A, Corwin HL, et al. Anemia and blood transfusion in trauma patients admitted to the intensive care unit. J Trauma 2003; 55(2):269–273.
16. Jelkmann W. Erythropoietin: structure, control of production, and function. Physiol Rev 1992; 72:449–489.
17. Hobisch-Hagen P, Wiedermann F, Mayr A, et al. Blunted erythropoietic response to anemia in multiply traumatized patients. Crit Care Med 2001; 29(4):743–747.
18. Livingston DH, Anjaria D, Wu J, et al. Bone marrow failure following severe injury in humans. Ann Surg 2003; 238(5):748–753.
19. Tan IK, Lim JM. Anaemia in the critically ill—the optimal haematocrit. Ann Acad Med Singapore 2001; 30(3):293–299.
20. Baginski S, Korner R, Frei U, Eckardt KU. Anemia and erythropoietin in critically ill patients. Zentralbl Chir 2003; 128(6):487–492.
21. Vincent JL, Baron JF, Reinhart K, et al. Anemia and blood transfusion in critically ill patients. JAMA 2002; 25; 288(12):1499–1507.
22. Corwin HL, Parsonnet KC, Gettinger A. RBC transfusion in the ICU. Is there a reason? Chest 1995; 108(3):767–771.
23. Rogiers P, Zhang H, Leeman M, et al. Erythropoietin response is blunted in critically ill patients. Intensive Care Med 1997; 23(2):159–162.
24. Krafte-Jacobs B, Levetown ML, Bray GL, et al. Erythropoietin response to critical illness. Crit Care Med 1994; 22(5):821–826.
25. Brugnara C. Iron deficiency and erythropoiesis: new diagnostic approaches. Clin Chem 2003; 49(10):1573–1578.

26. Schwarzmeier JD. The role of cytokines in haematopoiesis. Eur J Haematol Suppl 1996; 60:69–74.

27. Weinstein DA, Roy CN, Fleming MD, et al. Inappropriate expression of hepcidin is associated with iron refractory anemia: implications for the anemia of chronic disease. Blood 2002; 100(10):3776–3781. Epub 2002 Jun 28.

28. Means RT Jr. Hepcidin and anaemia. Blood Rev 2004; 18(4):219–225.

29. Eckardt KU. Anaemia in end-stage renal disease: pathophysiological considerations. Nephrol Dial Transplant 2001; 16 (suppl. 7):2–8.

30. Crosato M, Steinborn W, Anker SD. Anemia in chronic congestive heart failure: frequency, prognosis, and treatment. Heart Fail Monit 2003; 4(1):2–6.

31. McBride BF, White CM. Anemia management in heart failure: a thick review of thin data. Pharmacotherapy 2004; 24(6): 757–767.

32. Weiskopf RB, Feiner J, Hopf H, et al. Heart rate increases linearly in response to acute isovolemic anemia. Transfusion 2003; 43(2):235–240.

33. Aessopos A, Deftereos S, Farmakis D, et al. Cardiovascular adaptation to chronic anemia in the elderly: an echocardiographic study. Clin Invest Med 2004; 27(5):265–273.

34. Ickx BE, Rigolet M, Van Der Linden PJ. Cardiovascular and metabolic response to acute normovolemic anemia. Effects of anesthesia. Anesthesiology 2000; 93(4):1011–1016.

35. Zhu H, Jackson T, Bunn HF. Detecting and responding to hypoxia. Nephrol Dial Transplant 2002; 17(suppl 1):3–7.

36. Malone DL, Dunne J, Tracy JK, Putnam AT, Scalea TM, Napolitano LM. Blood Transfusion, independent of shock severity, is associated with worse outcome in trauma. J Trauma 2003; 54(5):898–907.

37. Halm EA, Wang JJ, Boockvar K, et al. The effect of perioperative anemia on clinical and functional outcomes in patients with hip fracture. J Orthop Trauma 2004; 18(6):369–374.

38. Gruson KI, Aharonoff GB, Egol KA, et al. The relationship between admission hemoglobin level and outcome after hip fracture. J Orthop Trauma 2002; 16(1):39–44.

39. Dunne JR, Malone D, Tracy JK, et al. Perioperative anemia: an independent risk factor for infection, mortality, and resource utilization in surgery. J Surg Res 2002; 102(2):237–244.

40. Carson JL, Duff A, Poses RM, et al. Effect of anaemia and cardiovascular disease on surgical mortality and morbidity. Lancet 1996; 348(9034):1055–1060.

41. Beghe C, Wilson A, Ershler WB. Prevalence and outcomes of anemia in geriatrics: a systematic review of the literature. Am J Med 2004 5; 116 (suppl 7A):3S–10S.

42. Izaks GGJ, Westendorp RG, Knook DL. The definition of anemia in older persons. JAMA 1999; 281(18):1714–1717.

43. Artz AS, Fergusson D, Drinka PJ, et al. Prevalence of anemia in skilled-nursing home residents. Arch Gerontol Geriatr 2004; 39(3):201–206.

44. Felker GM, Adams KF Jr, Gattis WA, O'Connor CM. Anemia as a risk factor and therapeutic target in heart failure. J Am Coll Cardiol 2004; 44(5):959–966.

45. Anand I, McMurray JJ, Whitmore J, et al. Anemia and its relationship to clinical outcome in heart failure. Circulation 2004; 110(2):149–154.

46. Nikolsky E, Aymong ED, Halkin A, et al. Impact of anemia in patients with acute myocardial infarction undergoing primary percutaneous coronary intervention: analysis from the Controlled Abciximab and Device Investigation to Lower Late Angioplasty Complications (CADILLAC) Trial. J Am Coll Cardiol 2004; 44(3):547–553.

47. Lee PC, Kini AS, Ahsan C, et al. Anemia is an independent predictor of mortality after percutaneous coronary intervention. J Am Coll Cardiol 2004; 44(3):541–546.

48. Rao SV, Jollis JG, Harrington RA, et al. Relationship of blood transfusion and clinical outcomes in patients with acute coronary syndromes. JAMA 2004; 292(13):1555–1562.

49. Locatelli F, Pisoni RL, Akizawa T, et al. Anemia management for hemodialysis patients: Kidney Disease Outcomes Quality Initiative (K/DOQI) guidelines and Dialysis Outcomes and Practice Patterns Study (DOPPS) findings. Am J Kidney Dis 2004; 44(5 suppl 3):27–33.

50. Gouva C, Nikolopoulos P, Ioannidis JP, Siamopoulos KC. Treating anemia early in renal failure patients slows the decline of renal function: a randomized controlled trial. Kidney Int 2004; 66(2):753–760.

51. Pujade-Lauraine E, Gascon P. The burden of anaemia in patients with cancer. Oncology 2004; 67(suppl 1):1–4.

52. Glaspy J, Dunst J. Can erythropoietin therapy improve survival? Oncology 2004; 67(suppl 1):5–11.

53. Lakstein D, Blumenfeld A, Sodolov T, et al. Tourniquets for hemorrhage control on the battlefield: a 4–year accumulated experience. J Trauma 2003; 54(suppl 5):S221–S225.

54. Naimer SA, Chemla F. Elastic adhesive dressing treatment of bleeding wounds in trauma victims. Am J Emerg Med 2000; 18(7):816–819.

55. Shah JS, Anagnos D, Norfleet EA. Elastic tourniquet technique for decompression of extremity compartment syndrome. J Clin Anesth 2002; 14(7):524–528.

56. Brasel KJ, Weigelt JA. Damage control in trauma surgery. Curr Opin Crit Care 2000; 6(4):276–280.

57. Rotondo MF, Bard MR. Damage control surgery for thoracic injuries. Injury 2004; 35(7):649–654.

58. Loveland JA, Boffard KD. Damage control in the abdomen and beyond. Br J Surg 2004; 91(9):1095–1101.

59. Wahl WL, Ahrns KS, Chen S, et al. Blunt splenic injury: operation versus angiographic embolization. Surgery 2004; 136(4):891–899.

60. Haan JM, Biffl W, Knudson MM, et al. Western Trauma Association Multi-Institutional Trials Committee. Splenic embolization revisited: a multicenter review. J Trauma 2004; 56(3):542–547.

61. Velmahos GC, Chahwan S, Falabella A, et al. Angiographic embolization for intraperitoneal and retroperitoneal injuries. World J Surg 2000; 24(5):539–545.

62. Kovesi T, Royston D. Pharmacological approaches to reducing allogeneic blood exposure. Vox Sang 2003; 84(1):2–10.

63. Good L, Peterson E, Lisander B. Tranexamic acid decreases external blood loss but not hidden blood loss in total knee replacement. Br J Anaesth 2003; 90(5):596–599.

64. Carr ME Jr, Loughran TP, Cardea JA, et al. Successful use of recombinant factor VIIa for hemostasis during total knee replacement in a severe hemophiliac with high-titer factor VIII inhibitor. Int J Hematol 2002; 75(1):95–99.

65. Schreiber MA, Holcomb JB, Hedner U, et al. The effect of recombinant factor VIIa on coagulopathic pigs with grade V liver injuries. J Trauma 2002; 53(2):252–257.

66. Hedner U: General Haemostatic agents—fact or fiction? Pathophysiol Haemost Thromb 2002; 32(suppl 1):33–36

67. Allen GA, Hoffman M, Roberts HR, Monroe DM III. Recombinant activated factor VII: its mechanism of action and role in the control of hemorrhage. Can J Anaesth 2002; 49(10):S7–S14.

68. Martinowitz U, Kenet G, Segal E, et al. Recombinant activated factor VII for adjunctive hemorrhage control in trauma. J Trauma 2001; 51(3):431–439.

69. Aldouri M. The use of recombinant factor VIIa in controlling surgical bleeding in non-haemophiliac patients. Pathophysiol Haemost Thromb 2002; 32 (suppl 1):41–46.

70. Matinowitz U, Kenet G, Lubetski A, et al. Possible role of recombinant activated factor VII (rFVIIa) in the control of hemorrhage associated with massive trauma. Can J Anaesth 2002; 49(10):S15–S20.

71. Murkin JM. A novel hemostatic agent: the potential role of recombinant activated factor VII (rFVIIA) in anesthetic practice. Can J Anaesth 2002; 49(10):SS21–SS26.

72. Dutton RP, Hess JR, Scalea TM. Recombinant factor VIIa for control of hemorrhage: early experience in critically ill trauma patients. J Clin Anesth 2003; 15(3):184–188.

73. Bouwmeester FW, Junkhoff AR, Verheijen RH, van Geijn HP. Successful treatment of life-threatening postpartum hemorrhage with recombinant activated factor VII. Obstet Gynecol 2003; 101(6):1174–1176.

74. Veshchev I, Elran H, Salame K. Recombinant coagulation factor VIIa for rapid preoperative correction of warfarin-related coagulopathy in patients with acute subdural hematoma. Med Sci Monit 2002; 8(12):CS98–CS100.

75. Lin J, Hanigan WC, Tarantino M, Wang J. The use of recombinant activated factor VII to reverse warfarin-induced anticoagulation in patients with hemorrhages in the central nervous system: preliminary findings. J Neurosurg 2003; 98(4):737–740.

76. Erhardtsen E. Ongoing NovoSeven trials. Intensive Care Med 2002; 28(suppl 2):S248–S255.

77. Meng ZH, Wolberg AS, Monroe DM III, Hoffman M. The effect of temperature and pH on the activity of factor VIIa: implications for the efficacy of high-dose factor VIIa in hypothermic and acidotic patients. J Trauma 2003; 55(5):886–891.

78. Friederich PW, Henny CP, Messelink EJ, et al. Effect of recombinant activated factor VII on perioperative blood loss in patients undergoing retropubic prostatectomy: a double-blind placebo-controlled randomised trial. Lancet 2003 18; 361(9353):201–205.

79. Eikelboom JW, Bird R, Blythe D, et al. Recombinant activated factor VII for the treatment of life-threatening haemorrhage. Blood Coagul Fibrinolysis 2003; 14(8):713–717.

80. Morenski JD, Tobias JD, Jimenez DF. Recombinant activated factor VII for cerebral injury-induced coagulopathy in pediatric patients. RrHuEPOrts of three cases and review of the literature. J Neurosurg 2003; 98(3):611–616.

81. Lynn M, Jerokhimov I, Jewelewicz D, et al. Early use of recombinant factor VIIa improves mean arterial pressure and may potentially decrease mortality in experimental hemorrhagic shock: a pilot study. J Trauma 2002; 52(4):703–707.

82. Jeroukhimov I, Jewelewicz D, Zaias J, et al. Early injection of high-dose recombinant factor VIIa decreases blood loss and prolongs time from injury to death in experimental liver injury. J Trauma 2002; 53(6):1053–1057.

83. Boffard kD, Riou B, Warren B, et al. For the Novoseven Trauma study Group. Recombinant factor VIIa as adjunctive therapy for bleeding control in severely injured trauma patients: two paralled randomized, placebo-controlled, double–blind clinical trials. J Trauma 2005; 54(1):8–18.

84. Ochsner MG, Maniscalco-Theberge ME, Champion HR. Fibrin glue as a hemostatic agent in hepatic and splenic trauma. J Trauma 1990; 30(7):884–887.

85. Goudarzi YM. Segmental resection of the spleen as function-preserving therapy in pediatric rupture of the spleen. Sealing of the resected surface with fibrin glue, collagen fleece and dexon net. Aktuelle Traumatol 1986; 16(5):186–189.

86. Kram HB, Hino ST, Harley DP, et al. Use of concentrated fibrinogen in experimental splenic trauma. J Biomed Mater Res 1986; 20(5):547–553.

87. Kram HB, Reuben BI, Fleming AW, Shoemaker WC. Use of fibrin glue in hepatic trauma. J Trauma 1988; 28(8):1195–1201.

88. Cohn SM, Cross JH, Ivy ME, et al. Fibrin glue terminates massive bleeding after complex hepatic injury. J Trauma 1998; 45(4):666–672.

89. Holcomb JB, Pusateri AE, Harris RA, et al. Effect of dry fibrin sealant dressings versus gauze packing on blood loss in grade V liver injuries in resuscitated swine. J Trauma 1999; 46(1): 49–57.

90. Feinstein AJ, Varela JE, Cohn SM, et al. Fibrin glue eliminates the need for packing after complex liver injuries. Yale J Biol Med 2001; 74(5):315–321.

91. Jackson MR, Friedman SA, Carter AJ, et al. Hemostatic efficacy of a fibrin sealant-based topical agent in a femoral artery injury model: a randomized, blinded, placebo-controlled study. J Vasc Surg 1997; 26(2):274–280.

92. Griffith BC, Morey AF, Rozanski TA, et al. Central renal stab wounds: treatment with augmented fibrin sealant in a porcine model. J Urol 2004; 171(1):445–447.

93. Holcomb JB, Pusateri AE, Harris RA, et al. Dry fibrin sealant dressings reduce blood loss, resuscitation volume, and improve survival in hypothermic coagulopathic swine with grade V liver injuries. J Trauma 1999; 47(2):233–240.

94. de la Garza JL, Rumsey E Jr. Fibrin glue and hemostasis in liver trauma: a case rrHuEPOrt. J Trauma 1990; 30(4):512–513.

95. Okada S, Ishimori S, Yamagata S, et al. A thoracosopic technique with fibrin glue and polyglycolic acid mesh for the injured lung during thoracoscopic operation. Kyobu Geka 2003; 56(11):913–917.

96. McGill V, Kowal-Vern A, Lee M, et al. Use of fibrin sealant in thermal injury. J Burn Care Rehabil 1997; 18(5):429–434.

97. Greenhalgh DG, Gamelli RL, Lee M, et al. Mulicenter trial to evaluate the safety and potential efficacy of pooled human fibrin sealant for the treatment of burn wounds. J Trauma 1999; 46(3):433–440.

98. Dunn CJ, Goa KL. Fibrin sealant: a review of its use in surgery and endoscopy. Drugs 1999; 58(5):863–886.

99. Datta D, Vlavianos P, Alisa A, Westaby D. Use of fibrin glue (beriplast) in the management of bleeding gastric varices. Endoscopy 2003; 35(8):675–678.

100. Levy O, Martinowitz U, Oran A, et al. The use of fibrin tissue adhesive to reduce blood loss and the need for blood transfusion after total knee arthroplasty. A prospective, randomized, multicenter study. J Bone Joint Surg Am 1999; 81(11): 1580–1588.

101. Wang GJ, Hungerford DS, Savory CG, et al. Use of fibrin sealant to reduce bloody drainage and hemoglobin loss after total knee arthroplasty: a brief note on a randomized prospective trial. J Bone Joint Surg Am 2001; 83–A(10):1503–1505.

102. Wang GJ, Goldthwaite CA Jr, Burks S, et al. Fibrin sealant reduces perioperative blood loss in total hip replacement. J Long Term Eff Med Implants 2003; 13(5):399–411.

103. Vaiman M, Eviatar E, Shlamkovich N, Segal S. Effect of modern fibrin glue on bleeding after tonsillectomy and adenoidectomy. Ann Otol Rhinol Laryngol 2003; 112(5):410–414.

104. Corwin HL, Parsonnet KC, Gettinger A. RBC transfusion in the ICU. Is there a reason? Chest 1995; 108(3):767–771.

105. Peruzzi WT, Parker MA, Lichtenthal PR, et al. A clinical evaluation of a blood conservation device in medical intensive care unit patients. Crit Care Med 1993; 21:501–506.

106. O'Hare D, Chilvers RJ. Arterial blood sampling practices in intensive care units in England and Wales. Anaesthesia 2001, 56:568–571. Critl Care June 2004 Vol. 8 Suppl 2 Napolitano.

107. Fowler RA, Berenson M. Blood conservation in the intensive care unit. Crit Care Med 2003; 31(Suppl 12):S715–S720.

108. Spirt MJ. Stress-related mucosal disease: risk factors and prophylactic therapy. Clin Ther 2004; 26(2):197–213.

109. Steinberg KP. Stress-related mucosal disease in the critically ill patient: risk factors and strategies to prevent stress-related bleeding in the intensive care unit. Crit Care Med 2002; 30(suppl 6):S362–S364.

110. Gabriel A, Kozek S, Chiari A, et al. High-dose recombinant human erythropoietin stimulates reticulocyte production in patients with multiple organ dysfunction syndrome. J Trauma 1998; 44(2):361–367.

111. Corwin HL, Gettinger A, Rodriguez RM, et al. Efficacy of recombinant human erythropoietin in the critically ill patient: a randomized, double-blind, placebo-controlled trial. Crit Care Med 1999; 27(11):2346–2350.

112. van Iperen CE, Gaillard CA, Kraaijenhagen RJ, et al. Response of erythropoiesis and iron metabolism to recombinant human erythropoietin in intensive care unit patients. Crit Care Med 2002; 28(8):2773–2778.

113. Corwin HL, Gettinger A, Pearl RG, et al. Efficacy of recombinant human erythropoietin in critically ill patients: a randomized controlled trial. JAMA 2002 11; 288(22):2827–2835.

114. Bennett CL, Luminari S, Nissenson AR, et al. Pure red-cell aplasia and rHuEPOetin therapy. N Engl J Med 2004 30; 351(14):1403–1408.

115. Lum G. Should the transfusion trigger and hemoglobin low critical limit be identical? Ann Clin Lab Sci 1997; 27(2): 130–134.

116. Hebert PC, Wells G, Blajchman MA, et al. A multicenter, randomized, controlled clinical trial of transfusion requirements in critical care. Transfusion Requirements in Critical Care Investigators, Canadian Critical Care Trials Group. N Engl J Med 1999 11; 340(6):409–417.

117. Hebert PC, Yetisir E, Martin C, et al. Is a low transfusion threshold safe in Critically ill patients with cardiovascular diseases? Crit Care Med 2001; 29(2):227–234.

118. Hebert PC, Blajchman MA, Cook DJ, Yetisir E, Wells G, Marshall J, et al. Transfusion requirements in critical care investigators for the Canadian critical care trials group. Do blood

transfusions improve outcomes related to mechanical ventilation? Chest 2001; 119(6):1850–1857.

119. McIntyre L, Hebert PC, Wells G, et al. Is a restrictive transfusion strategy safe for resuscitated and critically ill trauma patients? J Trauma 2004; 57(3):563–568.

120. Hill SR, Carless PA, Henry DA, et al. Transfusion thresholds and other strategies for guiding allogeneic red blood cell transfusion. Cochrane Database Syst Rev 2002; (2):CD002042.

121. McLellan SA, McClelland DB, Walsh TS. Anaemia and red blood cell transfusion in the critically ill patient. Blood Rev 2003; 17(4):195–208.

122. Spiess BD, Ley C, Body SC, et al. Hematocrit value on intensive care unit entry influences the frequency of Q-wave myocardial infarction after coronary artery bypass grafting. The Institutions of the Multicenter Study of Perioperative Ischemia (McSPI) Research Group. J Thorac Cardiovasc Surg 1998; 116(3):460–467.

123. Habib RH, Zacharias A, Schwann TA, et al. Adverse effects of low hematocrit during cardiopulmonary bypass in the adult: should current practice be changed? J Thorac Cardiovasc Surg 2003; 125(6):1438–1450.

124. Freudenberger RS, Carson JL. Is there an optimal hemoglobin value in the cardiac intensive care unit? Curr Opin Crit Care 2003; 9(5):356–361.

125. Petrides M. Red cell transfusion "trigger": a review. South Med J 2003; 96(7):664–667.

126. Tsai AG, Intaglietta M. High viscosity plasma expanders: volume restitution fluids for lowering the transfusion trigger. Biorheology 2001; 38(2–3):229–237.

127. Sehgal LR, Zebala LP, Takagi I, et al. Evaluation of oxygen extraction ratio as a physiologic transfusion trigger in coronary artery bypass graft surgery patients. Transfusion 2001; 41(5):591–595.

128. Torella F, Haynes SL, McCollum CN. Cerebral and peripheral near-infrared spectroscopy: an alternative transfusion trigger? Vox Sang 2002; 83(3):254–257.

129. Moore FA, Moore EE, Sauaia A. Blood transfusion. An independent risk factor for postinjury multiple organ failure. Arch Surg 1997; 132(6):620–624.

130. Napolitano LM, Corwin HL. Efficacy of red blood cell transfusion in the critically ill. Crit Care Clin 2004; 20:255–268.

131. Dzik S, Blajchman MA, Blumberg N, Kirkley SA, Heal JM, Wood K. Current research on the immunomodulatory effect of allogeneic blood transfusion. Vox Sang 1996; 70:187–194.

132. Innerhofer P, Luz G, Spotl, et al. Immunologic changes after transfusion of buffy coat-poor versus white cell-reduced blood to patients undergoing arthroplasty. Transfusion 1999; 39:1089–1096.

133. Heiss MM, Fraunberger P, Delanoff C, et al. Modulation of immune response by blood transfusion: evidence for a differential effect of allogeneic and autologous blood in colorectal cancer surgery. Shock 1997; 8(6):402–408.

134. Bengtsson A, Avall A, Hyllner M, Bengston JP. Formation of compliment split products and proinflammatory cytokines by reinfusion of shed autologous blood. Toxicol Lett 1998; 100–101:129–133.

135. Fransen E, Maessen J, Dentener M, et al. Impact of blood transfusions on inflammatory mediator release in patients undergoing cardiac surgery. Chest 1999; 116:1233–1239.

136. Avall A, Hyllner M, Bengston JP, et al. A. postoperative inflammatory response after autologous and allogeneic blood transfusion. Anesthesiology 1997; 87:511–516.

137. Schmidt H, Bendtzen K, Mortensen PE. The inflammatory cytokine response after autotransfusion of shed mediastinal blood. Acta Anaesthesiol Scand 1998; 42:558–564.

138. Haynes SL, Wong JC, Torella F, et al. The influence of homologous blood transfusion on immunity and clinical outcome in aortic surgery. Eur J Vasc Endovasc Surg 2001; 22:244–250.

139. Zallen G, Moore EE, Ciesla DJ, et al. Stored red blood cells selectively activate human neutrophils to release IL-8 and secretory PLA-2. Shock 2000; 13:29–33.

140. Biffl WL, Moore EE, Zallen G, et al. Neutrophils are primed for cytotoxicity and resist apoptosis in injured patients at risk for multiple organ failure. Surgery 1999; 126:198–202.

141. Makino Y, Yamanoi A, Kimoto T, et al. The influence of perioperative blood transfusion on intrahepatic recurrence after curative resection of hepatocellular carcinoma. Am J Gastroenterol 2000; 95:1294–1300.

142. Mynster T, Nielson HJ. Storage time of transfused blood and disease recurrence after colorectal cancer surgery. Dis Colon Rectum 2001; 44:955–964.

143. Dresner SM, Lamb PJ, Shenfine J, et al. Prognostic significance of perioperative blood transfusion following radical resection for oesophageal carcinoma. Eur J Surg Oncol 2000; 26:492–497.

144. Carson JL, Altman DG, Duff A, et al. Risk of bacterial infection associated with allogeneic blood transfusion among patients undergoing hip fracture repair. Transfusion 1999; 39:694–700.

145. Taylor RW, Manganaro LA, O'Brien J, et al. Impact of allogeneic packed red blood cell transfusion on nosocomial infection rates in the critically ill patient. Crit Care Med 2002; 30:2249–2254.

146. Claridge JA, Sawyer RG, Schulman AM, et al. Blood transfusion correlates with infections in trauma patients in a dose-dependent manner. Am Surg 2002; 68:566–572.

147. Malone D, Kuhls D, Napolitano L, et al. Blood transfusion in the first 24 hours is associated with systemic inflammatory response syndrome (SIRS) and worse outcome in trauma. Crit Care Med 2000; 28(suppl):A138.

148. Malone D, Edelman B, Hess J, et al. Age of blood transfusion in trauma: Does it alter outcome? Crit Care Med 30(12) (suppl)72, A21, Society of Critical Care Medicine 2003.

149. Purdy FR, Tweeddale MG, Merrick PM. Association of mortality with age of blood transfused in septic ICU patients. Can J Anaesth 1997; 44:1256–1261.

150. Vamvakas EC, Carven JH. Transfusion and postoperative pneumonia in coronary artery bypass graft surgery: effect of the length of storage of transfused red cells. Transfusion 1999; 39(7):701–710.

151. Chang H, Hall GA, Geerts WH, et al. Allogeneic red blood cell transfusion is an independent risk factor for the development of postoperative bacterial infection. Vox Sang 2000; 78:13–18.

152. Leal-Noval SR, Rincon-Ferrari MD, Garcia-Curiel A, et al. Transfusion of blood components and postoperative infection in patients undergoing cardiac surgery. Chest 2001; 119(5):1461–1468.

153. Malone D, Gannon C, Dunne J, et al. Risk factors for postoperative pneumonia: the role of anemia and blood transfusion [abstr. 349/S140]. Crit Care Med 2001; 29(12, suppl.):A107.

154. Norfolk DR, Williamson LM. Leukodepletion of blood products by filtration. Blood Rev 1995; 9(1):7–14.

155. Utter GH, Owings JT, Lee TH, et al. Blood transfusion is associated with donor leukocyte microchimerism in trauma patients. J Trauma 2004; 57(4):702–708.

156. Cross MH. Cell salvage and leukodepletion. Perfusion 200; 16 Suppl:61–66.

157. Seghatchian J, Krailadsiri P, Dilger P, et al. Cytokines as quality indicators of leukoreduced red cell concentrates. Transfus Apheresis Sci 2002; 26(1):43–46.

158. Stefanou DC, Gourlay T, Asimakopoulos G, Taylor KM. Leucodepletion during cardiopulmonary bypass reduces blood transfusion and crystalloid requirements. Perfusion 2001; 16(1):51–58.

159. Dzik WH, Anderson JK, O'Neill EM, et al. A prospective, randomized clinical trial of universal WBC reduction. Transfusion 2002; 42(9):1114–1122.

160. Toth CB, Kramer J, Pinter J, et al. IgA content of washed red blood cell concentrates. Vox Sang 1998; 74(1):13–14.

161. Sachs V, Dorner R, Rehder V. Washed erythrocyte concentrates. A contribution to the problem of the effect of wash procedures and storage time on erythrocytes in the preparation of blood. Infusionstherapie 1988; 15(6):240–243.

162. Biffl WI, Moore EE, Offner PJ, et al. Plasma from aged stored red blood cells delays neutrophil apoptosis and primes for cytotoxicity: abrogation by postorage washing but not prestorage leukoreduction. J Trauma 2001; 50(3):426–431.

163. Standl T. Haemoglobin-based erythrocyte transfusion substitutes. Expert Opin Biol Ther 2001; 1(5):831–843.

164. Vaslef SN, Kaminski BJ, Talarico TL. Oxygen transport dynamics of cellular hemoglobin solutions in an isovolemic hemodilution model in swine. J Trauma 2001; 51(6):1153–1160.

165. Wahr JA. Clinical potential of blood substitutes or oxygen therapeutics during cardiac surgery. Anesthesiol Clin North America 2003; 21(3):553–568.

166. Sprung J, Kindscher JD, Wahr JA, et al. The use of bovine hemoglobin glutamer-250 (Hemopure) in surgical patients: results of a multicenter, randomized single-blinded trial. Anesth Analg 2002; 94:799–808.

167. Levy JH, Goodnough LT, Greilich PE, et al. Polymerized bovine hemoglobin solution as a replacement for allogeneic red blood cell transfusion after cardiac surgery: results of a randomized, double-blind trial. J Thorac Cardiovasc Surg 2002; 124:35–42.

168. Gannon CJ, Napolitano LM. Severe anemia after gastrointestinal hemorrhage in a Jehovah's witness: new treatment strategies. Crit Care Med 2002; 30(8):1893–1895.

169. Standl T, Freitag M, Burmeister MA, et al. Hemoglobin-based oxygen carrier HBOC-201 provides higher and faster increase in oxygen tension in skeletal muscle of anemic dogs than do stored red blood cells. J Vasc Surg 2003; 37(4):859–865.

170. Human haemoglobin—northfield. BioDrugs 2003; 17(4): 296–298.

171. Gould SA, Moore EE, Hoyt DB, et al. The first randomized trial of human polymerized hemoglobin as a blood substitute in acute trauma and emergent surgery. J Am Coll Surg 1998; 187(2):113–120.

172. Johnson JL, Moore EE, Offner PJ, et al. Resuscitation with a blood substitute abrogates pathologic postinjury neutrophil cytotoxic function. J Trauma 2001; 50(3): 449–455.

173. Gould SA, Moore EE, Hoyt DB, et al. The life-sustaining capacity of human polymerized hemoglobin when red cells might be unavailable. J Am Coll Surg 2002; 195(4):445–452.

174. Johnson JL, Moore EE, Gonzalez RJ, et al. Alteration of the postinjury hyperinflammatory response by means of resuscitation with a red cell substitute. J Trauma 2003; 54(1):133–139.

175. Ganz T. Hepcidin in iron metabolism. Curr Opin Hematol 2004; 11(4):251–254.

176. Nemeth E, Rivera S, Gabayan V, et al. IL-6 mediates hypoferremia of inflammation by inducing the synthesis of the iron regulatory hormone hepcidin. J Clin Invest 2004; 113(9):1271–1276.

177. Nemeth E, Tuttle MS, Powelson J, et al. Hepcidin Regulates Iron Efflux by Binding to Ferroportin and Inducing Its Internalization. Science 2004; 306(5704):2090–2093.

178. Andrews NC. Anemia of inflammation: the cytokine-hepcidin link. J Clin Invest 2004; 113(9):1251–1253.

179. Malhotra AK, Kelly ME, Miller PR, et al. Resuscitation with a novel hemoglobin-based oxygen carrier in a Swine model of uncontrolled perioperative hemorrhage. J Trauma 2003; 54(5):915–924.

180. Wahr JA. Clinical potential of nonhemoglobin oxygen therapeutics in cardiac and general surgery. Am J Cardiovasc Drugs 2002; 2(2):69–75.

181. Cabrales P, Tsai AG, Frangos JA, et al. Oxygen delivery and consumption in the microcirculation after extreme hemodilution with perfluorocarbons. Am J Physiol Heart Circ Physiol 2004; 287(1):H320–H330.

182. Stowell CP. Hemoglobin-based oxygen carriers. Curr Opin Hematol 2002; 9(6):537–543.

183. Oda T, Nakajima Y, Kimura T, et al. Hemodilution with liposome-encapsulated low-oxygen-affinity hemoglobin facilitates rapid recovery from ischemic acidosis after cerebral ischemia in rats. J Artif Organs 2004;7(2):101–106.

184. Awasthi VD, Garcia D, Klipper R, et al. Kinetics of liposome-encapsulated hemoglobin after 25% hypovolemic exchange transfusion. Int J Pharm 2004 28; 283(1–2):53–62.

185. Asano T, Matsumoto T, Tachibana H, et al. Myocardial microvascular perfusion after transfusion of liposome-encapsulated hemoglobin evaluated in cross-circulated rat hearts using tracer digital radiography. J Artif Organs 2004; 7(3):145–148

186. Cabrales P, Sakai H, Tsai AG, et al. Oxygen transport by low and normal P50 hemoglobin-vesicles in extreme hemodilution. Am J Physiol Heart Circ Physiol 2004; 24.

187. Sakai H, Masada Y, Horinouchi H, et al. Hemoglobin-vesicles suspended in recombinant human serum albumin for resuscitation from hemorrhagic shock in anesthetized rats. Crit Care Med 2004; 32(2):539–545.

188. Napolitano LM. Scope of the problem: Epidemiology of anemia and use of blood transfusions in critical care. Crit Care 2004; 8(suppl2):S1–S8.

189. Schechter AN, Gladwin MT. Hemoglobin and the paracrine and endocrine functions of Nitric oxide. N Engl J Med 2003; 348(15):1483–1485.

55

Thrombocytopenia and Thrombocytosis

Donald M. Arnold
Section of Transfusion Medicine, Department of Medicine, McMaster University, Hamilton, Ontario, Canada

Theodore E. Warkentin
Departments of Pathology and Molecular Medicine, McMaster University School of Medicine, and the Transfusion Medicine Service, Hamilton Health Sciences, Hamilton, Ontario, Canada

PLATELET PHYSIOLOGY
Platelet Production
Normal Platelet Count Range

♂ **The normal platelet count is generally between 150 and 400 $\times$ 10⁹/L. Although this is a wide normal range, the platelet count tends to remain fairly constant during the lifetime of an individual (1).** ♂ However, as will be discussed later, the normal platelet count range is much higher (about $250–1000 \times 10^9$/L) during the second week following an acute, reversible thrombocytopenia (2), because of transient platelet overproduction ("post-thrombocytopenia thrombocytosis"; discussed below).

The Megakaryocyte

Platelets originate from megakaryocytes, the largest cells resident within the bone marrow. Although platelets constitute about 5% of circulating blood cells, megakaryocytes are relatively infrequent, making up only 0.05% of nucleated marrow cells (3). However, each of the 40 million megakaryocytes can make 2000 to 3000 platelets (4). As the average human has about one trillion circulating platelets, and another one-half trillion platelets exchangeably sequestered within the spleen, the normal 10-day platelet survival indicates that about 150 billion platelets are manufactured daily. ♂ **Normal platelet survival is approximately 10 days.** ♂

Megakaryocytes develop in stages (5): the earliest committed megakaryocyte precursor in adult marrow is the burst-forming unit-megakaryocyte, followed by the colony-forming unit-megakaryocyte. These progenitor cells, which cannot be recognized morphologically, represent intermediate stages between the multipotential stem cell and megakaryocytes. Subsequent intermediate stages (megakaryoblast, basophilic megakaryocyte) can be identified morphologically.

Megakaryocytes are large multilobed cells that average 35 μm in diameter (6). They exhibit a unique biologic process known as *endomitosis*, that is, repeated nuclear replication in the absence of cytoplasmic division, leading to polyploidy. Although present in largest numbers within the marrow, megakaryocytes are also found in extravascular sites, such as the spleen and lungs.

Complex cytoplasmic changes occur during megakaryocyte development. The most unique and dramatic is the formation of extensive tubular, membrane-like organelles (the demarcating membrane system), which are involved in platelet formation (7). Microtubule bundles form within the megakaryocyte to create organelle-containing extensions called proplatelets. The demarcation membranes act as a reservoir, continuously providing membrane for the growing cytoplasmic proplatelet projections, which ultimately form both the internal (open canalicular system) and external platelet membranes (8). Specific platelet granules that contain adhesive and other platelet proteins are also formed.

Megakaryocytes are located in the extravascular marrow space. To what extent platelets are released from megakaryocytes directly into the marrow sinuses, versus release of intact proplatelets that subsequently fragment into platelets, and to what extent such fragmentation might occur in the circulation outside the marrow—or even within the pulmonary capillary bed (9)—remain uncertain.

Platelet Heterogeneity

Platelets exhibit remarkable size heterogeneity (10). The normal platelet size histogram is right-skewed, that is, there is a prominent "tail" of large-sized platelets. This size distribution can be normalized statistically by converting the platelet volume determinations to log values ("lognormal distribution") (10). Platelet size can change somewhat under different situations: for example, animal models of acute thrombocytopenia demonstrate rapid increase in mean platelet volume (MPV) that indicates the capacity to modify platelet production rapidly (11). Platelets are also heterogeneous with respect to activation response to chemical agonists (12,13).

Platelet Distribution

Although the spleen normally receives only 5% of the cardiac output, at any one time about one-third of the circulating platelets are present within the spleen (splenic "sequestration" or "pooling") (14,15). This relationship is explained by the relatively long splenic transit time (about 10 minutes) (16) compared with the average time a platelet takes to traverse other organs during the average circulatory pass (only about 1 minute) (Fig. 1).

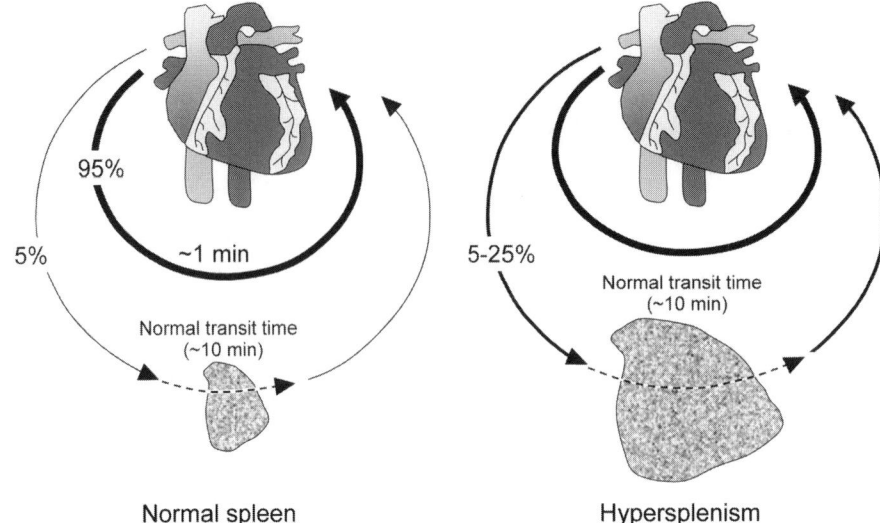

Normal spleen   Hypersplenism

Figure 1 Physiologic and pathologic platelet splenic sequestration. Normally, about 5% of cardiac output is to the spleen; however, a platelet that enters the spleen spends about 10 minutes there (splenic transit time ∼10 minutes). In contrast, it usually takes only about one minute for a platelet to make a circulatory pass elsewhere. Thus, about one-third of the platelets at any one time are located within the spleen: (5% × 10 minutes):(95%×1 minutes), or a ∼1:2 ratio. In hypersplenism, the splenic blood flow can increase by a factor of 5, that is, from 5% to 25% of total blood flow per minute. Thus, even without increase in splenic transit time, up to 70% or more of the platelets can be exchangeably sequestered within the spleen.

☞ **Normally, about one-third of the circulating platelets are exchangeably sequestered within the spleen; increased spleen size leads to greater splenic pooling and thus thrombocytopenia ("hypersplenism").** ☞

In pathologic states associated with splenomegaly, the splenic pool contains up to 70% or more of the platelet mass (hypersplenism). Two factors determine the extent of splenic pooling (17): splenic blood flow and splenic transit time. The most important determinant of splenic blood flow is the spleen size, and the most important determinant of splenic transit time is splenic perfusion (spleen blood flow/spleen volume) (16–18). However, as disorders that alter splenic transit time (e.g., congestive heart failure, rheumatologic disorders) usually have counterbalancing effects on splenic blood flow (17), in practical terms, spleen size correlates well with splenic platelet pooling. Thus, radiologic imaging of spleen size is indicated when assessing whether thrombocytopenia is caused by hypersplenism. A more recent concept is that reduced hepatic production of thrombopoietin (TPO) also contributes to the thrombocytopenia of hypersplenism secondary to liver disease (19).

Thrombopoietin
Thrombopoietin Structure, Regulation, and Function
Cytokines such as granulocyte-macrophage colony-stimulating factor and interleukin-3 (IL-3), and hormones, notably TPO (20), maintain the platelet count under tight regulatory control. TPO, which was cloned in 1994, consists of a 353-amino acid polypeptide, including a 21-amino acid secretory leader sequence, a 155-amino acid amino (N)-terminal domain, and a 177-amino acid carboxyl (C)-terminal domain. The N-terminal region has extensive homology with erythropoietin, and is responsible for binding of TPO to its cellular receptor. The C-terminal region, which has no homology with any known protein, is responsible for the long elimination half-life (30 hours), which exceeds that of any other hematopoietic factor.

TPO exhibits relative specificity for the megakaryocyte lineage of hematopoietic stem cells. TPO binds a specific receptor (c-Mpl) on megakaryocytes and platelets (20). TPO binding to megakaryocyte receptors leads to megakaryocyte differentiation and proliferation. In contrast, binding of TPO to platelet receptors results in the degradation of TPO and its removal from circulation. Basal levels of TPO are produced constitutively by the liver (major source) and kidneys, which results in a constant level of TPO under steady-state conditions (Fig. 2) (21,22). During thrombocytopenia, the decreased platelet mass results in higher levels of free TPO, stimulating megakaryocytes to proliferate, differentiate, and shed new platelets. In thrombocytosis, the increased platelet mass acts as a "sink" for TPO and blood levels of the hormone decline. Thus, TPO concentrations are inversely related to platelet and megakaryocyte mass, forming a primitive feedback loop.

During thrombocytopenic "stress," TPO can also be produced to a minor extent by the bone marrow and spleen (23). Thus, both constitutive and inducible TPO production elements contribute to platelet count regulation. TPO also "primes" platelets, making them more sensitive to platelet agonists (24).

Perhaps surprisingly, TPO levels are decreased in chronic platelet destructive disorders, such as chronic immune thrombocytopenic purpura (ITP), even when the platelet count is very low (25). It appears that the high platelet turnover in these disorders, which are characterized by increased megakaryocyte mass and increased platelet production, leads to considerable removal of TPO from the circulation, despite the chronic thrombocytopenia. In contrast, TPO levels are high in thrombocytopenic patients with megakaryocyte hypoplasia, for example, aplastic anemia, postchemotherapy, or postradiation therapy.

Post-thrombocytopenia Thrombocytosis
The primitive TPO feedback loop (Fig. 2) ensures that acute thrombocytopenia associated with trauma, whether caused

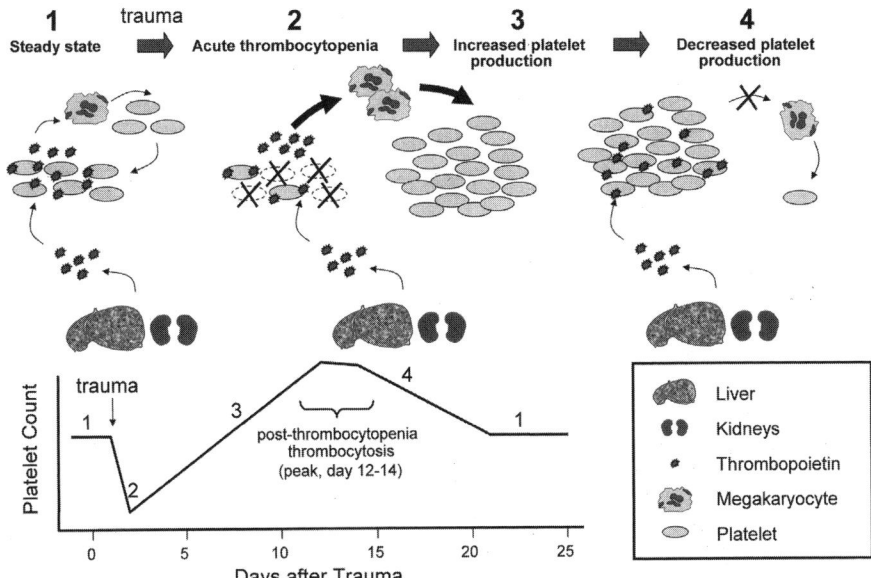

Figure 2 Thrombopoietin (TPO) physiology and post-thrombocytopenia thrombocytosis. TPO binds to platelets and megakaryocytes via a specific receptor (c-Mpl, not shown). The receptor-bound TPO is removed from circulation and degraded. The level of circulating TPO is thus inversely related to the mass of platelets and megakaryocytes. In thrombocytopenia, fewer binding sites are available, and free TPO levels are high, stimulating megakaryocyte proliferation and differentiation and leading to increased platelet production. In thrombocytosis, the high platelet mass acts as a "sink" for removing TPO, with decreased stimulus for platelet production. Thus, following acute thrombocytopenia, TPO levels rise about two-fold, leading to increased platelet production that begins on days 2 to 4, with resulting thrombocytosis that generally peaks about days 12–14 (post-thrombocytopenia thrombocytosis), and returns to baseline by about day 21.

by fluid resuscitation (hemodilution) and/or effects of the of the injury itself (DIC), leads to transient increase in blood TPO levels (about two-fold) (26). Because of the prolonged biological effects of TPO—due to its long elimination half-life (~30 hours) and its stimulation of both primitive and mature thrombopoietic cells—this acute thrombocytopenia will generally be followed by increased platelet count production that is first evident three to four days post-trauma, when the platelet count is first observed to begin to increase from the post-trauma nadir usually seen on day 2 or 3. Subsequently, thrombocytosis results, with the peak platelet count observed about 12 to 14 days post-trauma. At this point, the elevated platelet numbers lead to decreased TPO levels, reduced platelet production, and the platelet count returns to the normal baseline by about 3 weeks post-trauma (Fig. 2). If the platelet count fails to follow this normal recovery pattern, it often indicates complications of trauma, e.g., septicemia or SIRS.

ơ⁺ **Acute decrease in the platelet count in trauma leads to increase in TPO levels. The long half-life of TPO (30 hours) and its effects on early megakaryocyte progenitors mean that this trauma-associated thrombocytopenia is invariably followed by thrombocytosis from day 7 to 21 (peak, days 12–14), unless clinical complications lead to ongoing platelet consumption.** ơ⁺

Therapy with Thrombopoietin

Two forms of TPO have undergone clinical investigation: (a) TPO (full-length polypeptide) and (b) a truncated form consisting only of the receptor-binding moiety chemically modified by addition of polyethylene glycol (PEG). Unfortunately, commercial development of the latter preparation (PEG-conjugated recombinant human megakaryocyte

growth and development factor) was abandoned because of the occurrence of cross-reactive anti-TPO antibodies that caused long-term thrombocytopenia in some human volunteers (27). Unlike the experience with erythropoietin, clinical benefit of TPO even in patients with severe cancer-associated thrombocytopenia remains to be established. Ironically, platelet transfusions given to severely thrombocytopenic patients binds the TPO administered, thus negating its therapeutic effects.

Platelet Function
Platelet Adhesion (Primary Hemostasis)

Platelets provide the initial hemostatic response to vessel injury by adhering to subendothelial molecules (*primary hemostasis*). Adhesion is mediated by a platelet surface glycoprotein (GP) complex (GP Ib–IX–V) and the multimeric adhesion protein, von Willebrand factor (vWF) (28). Once tethered to the subvessel tissues, irreversible adhesion contacts form between platelet integrins and specific subendothelial matrix proteins, leading to platelet activation and aggregation. Besides normal quantities of platelets and vWF, a normal hematocrit is also important for maintaining primary hemostasis (Fig. 3).

ơ⁺ **Three components are required for normal primary hemostasis: (*i*) platelets, (*ii*) vWF, and (*iii*) normal hematocrit. In trauma, acquired thrombocytopenia and anemia lead to impaired primary hemostasis.** ơ⁺

In trauma patients, acquired anemia and thrombocytopenia lead to impaired primary hemostasis. The common congenital bleeding disorder—type 1 von Willebrand disease (vWD-1), which occurs to a mild extent in 1% to 2% of the population, is not a common cause of bleeding

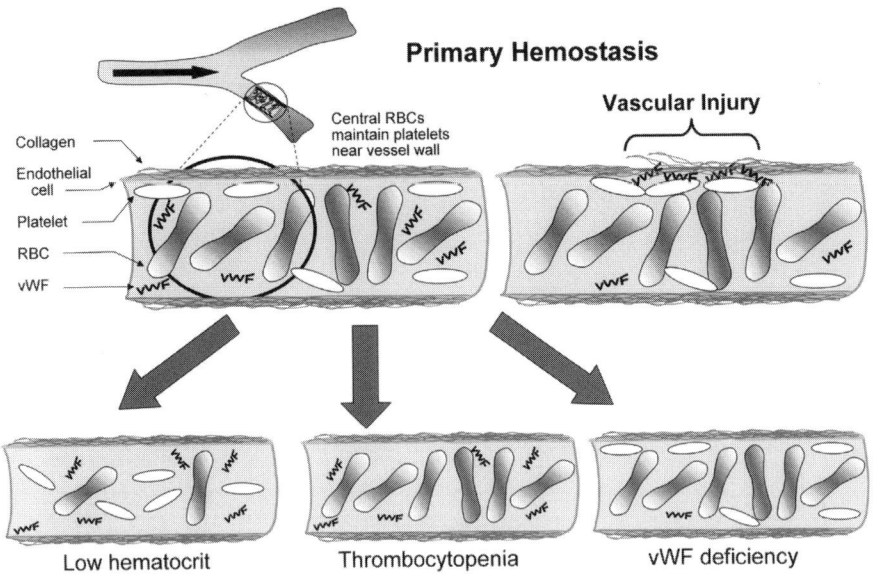

Figure 3 Three determinants of primary hemostasis. In the microcirculation, the central location of the red blood cell column maintains platelets near the vessel wall, contributing to increased platelet–subendothelial interaction during vessel injury. Thus, a low hematocrit is one factor that leads to impaired primary hemostasis, for example, prolonged bleeding time, increased microvascular bleeding. Other factors include thrombocytopenia and deficiency in von Willebrand factor (VWF). Very rarely, congenital absence of the platelet surface glycoprotein complex (GP Ib–IX–V)—a disorder known as Bernard–Soulier syndrome (not shown)—explains inability of the platelets to bind to vWF, and thus impaired primary hemostasis. *Abbreviations*: RBC, red blood cell; vWF, von Willebrand factor.

post-trauma, because the physiologic response to injury includes release of endothelial stores of vWF (29).

Platelet Aggregations and Platelet Procoagulant Activity (Secondary Hemostasis)

Following adhesion, platelets undergo aggregation and various "procoagulant" membrane changes (secondary hemostasis). A recent cell-based hemostasis model views three overlapping phases of coagulation, beginning when injury results in blood coming into contact with cells such as fibroblasts that are rich in tissue factor (TF) (Fig. 4) (30,31). The initiation phase of coagulation occurs when zymogen (proenzyme) factor VII binds to TF, leading to formation of activated factor VII (VIIa). The amplification phase results when small amounts of thrombin first generated on TF-bearing cells now activate cofactors (V to Va and VIII to VIIIa) and XI (to XIa) on the platelet surface. In the final propagation phase, the active serine proteases (Xa and IXa) combine with their cofactors (Va and VIIIa, respectively) to generate the "tenase" and "prothrombinase" complexes on platelet surfaces, producing the "thrombin burst" that leads to fibrin polymerization.

The Fixed Platelet Requirement

The ongoing physiologic role of platelets in maintenance of hemostasis is illustrated by the concept of the "fixed platelet requirement," that is, the constant homeostatic platelet losses needed to maintain vascular integrity. For example, radiolabeled platelet lifespan studies demonstrate an apparent reduction in platelet survival in all severely thrombocytopenic patients, including patients with impaired platelet production. To explain this, it has been proposed that a minimal, fixed number of platelets (7×10^9/L, or about 20% of normal platelet turnover) is removed from the circulation each day independent of the platelet count (32). Although such platelet losses,

which are believed to contribute to maintaining vascular integrity via platelet–endothelial interactions, represent only a small part of normal platelet turnover, they constitute a relatively large component of platelet loss in patients with severely impaired platelet production.

This physiologic role of platelets in maintaining vascular integrity means that profound thrombocytopenia is incompatible with life. For example, a >99% decline to "only" 10 billion circulating platelets (i.e., a platelet count of $1–2 \times 10^9$/L or less) presents a major risk of fatal hemorrhage. Usually, such severe thrombocytopenia occurs only in patients with primary hematologic disorders, for example, severe ITP. However, in the context of a trauma patient, thrombocytopenia of even a moderate degree can contribute to bleeding because of the impairment in hemostasis that additionally results from injury to vessels, coagulopathy, and reduced hematocrit.

THROMBOCYTOPENIA

Thrombocytopenia indicates reduced numbers of blood platelets. The term is derived from three Greek roots: *thrombo* = clot, *cyto* = hollow vessel (i.e., cell), and *penia* = poverty or need. Thus, the rough literal meaning—"need for a clotting cell"—is apropos to the context of thrombocytopenia complicating trauma, where platelet transfusions may be needed to prevent or treat bleeding.

Trauma often occurs to young and otherwise healthy individuals. Thus, pre-existing, chronic thrombocytopenia is uncommon in this patient population. Rather, thrombocytopenia in trauma is generally acute, either from direct effects of tissue injury leading to accelerated platelet consumption [e.g., disseminated intravascular coagulation (DIC)] or indirect effects of resuscitation (i.e., hemodilution). Besides initial thrombocytopenia, trauma patients are also at

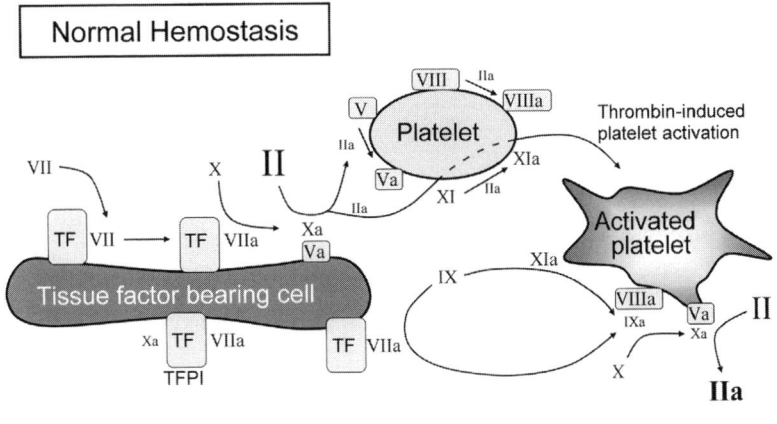

Figure 4 Cell-based model of hemostasis. Hemostasis is usually initiated when zymogen VII in blood contacts a TF-bearing cell, such as a fibroblast. Ultimately, small amounts of thrombin (IIa) are formed from prothrombin (II), leading to thrombin-induced platelet activation. The surface of activated platelets binds several active coagulation factors (Va, VIIIa, XIa), leading to propagation of coagulation, culminating in the "thrombin burst" that clots fibrinogen. During therapy with rVIIa, direct binding of VIIa to activated platelet surfaces may lead directly to thrombin generation on platelet surfaces (not shown). *Abbreviation*: TFPI, tissue factor pathway inhibitor.

risk for delayed onset of thrombocytopenia, in which later platelet count declines can indicate common complications such as septicemia or systemic inflammatory response syndrome (SIRS), or rare events such as drug-induced immune thrombocytopenia.

⚓ **Four general mechanisms for thrombocytopenia exist: (*i*) decreased platelet production, (*ii*) increased platelet consumption (or destruction), (*iii*) hemodilution, and (*iv*) hypersplenism. Only two mechanisms—increased platelet consumption and hemodilution—are common in acute trauma. However, decreased production can develop following critical illness, or (along with hypersplenism) can be present as a pre-existing condition.** ⚓

APPROACH TO THROMBOCYTOPENIA
Platelet Count Measurements (via Automated Particle Counters)
Blood count determinations are generally made using electronic particle counters, which provide the hemoglobin count, white blood count, and platelet count. In addition, various cell indices are provided, such as red cell volume (mean corpuscular volume) and platelet size (MPV). There is no single normal range for the MPV because this parameter varies with the platelet count: The normal MPV for a platelet count of 150×10^9/L is 9 to 12 femtoliters (fL), whereas for a platelet count of 400×10^9/L, it is 7.5–10 fL (33).

The MPV may assist the clinician in classifying the thrombocytopenic disorder (33). For example, thrombocytopenia caused by increased platelet destruction with a normal megakaryocyte response is characterized by a higher MPV (and more hemostatically effective platelets) than disorders of impaired platelet production or hypersplenism. However, the practical significance of these observations remains uncertain, and we believe that the MPV is only modestly helpful in classifying thrombocytopenia.

Occasionally, electronic particle counters will falsely under- or overestimate the true platelet count. Whenever this is suspected, a hematologist should review the peripheral blood smear, to evaluate platelet morphology and perform a manual platelet count. This is discussed further below in the section on "Pseudothrombocytopenia and Pseudothrombocytosis."

History and Physical Examination
Platelet Count History
As platelet counts are generally stable over an individual's lifetime, one can usually obtain a patient's "baseline" platelet count from their family physician's office, or from records of prior hospitalizations. This can help in determining whether the patient has pre-existing chronic thrombocytopenia (see the section on "Pre-existing Thrombocytopenia") or a prior episode of acute thrombocytopenia. Information about any previous bleeding, transfusion, or thrombotic events should be sought.

Physical Examination
The clinical impact of thrombocytopenia usually is apparent from the physical examination. ⚓ **The hallmark of severe thrombocytopenia is *mucocutaneous bleeding*, particularly pin-point intradermal hemorrhages known as *petechiae*.** ⚓ These are non-raised, non-blanching, and represent capillary hemorrhages. Petechiae are most common in dependent areas, for example, the legs and feet in outpatients, and the back and posterior thighs in bedridden patients, because hydrostatic pressure contributes to the microvascular bleeding.

Oozing at intravascular catheter sites, or hemorrhage from the nose, genito-urinary tract, or other mucosal sites, can indicate severe thrombocytopenia. For example, "blood blisters" (hemorrhagic vesicles of the oral mucosa or tongue) are sometimes seen when the platelet count is 10×10^9/L or less, particularly if caused by autoimmune or drug-induced immune thrombocytopenia.

Ecchymosis denotes intradermal hemorrhage greater than 2 mm (larger than petechiae). However, ecchymoses are less specific for thrombocytopenic bleeding than are petechiae.

Examining the Blood Film
Pseudothrombocytopenia and Pseudothrombocytosis
Review of the blood film occasionally reveals spurious thrombocytopenia or thrombocytosis. For example, "pseudothrombocytopenia," which occurs in about 0.1%

of complete blood counts, is caused by naturally occurring antibodies that lead to platelet clumping or (more rarely) to platelet "rosetting" around white blood cells. This phenomenon occurs under the low-calcium conditions of anticoagulated blood, for example, ethylene-diaminetetraacetic acid (EDTA)-induced pseudothrombocytopenia (34,35). Thus, the electronic particle counter underestimates the true platelet count. The major clinical significance is the risk for falsely diagnosing thrombocytopenia that is not present, or in causing difficulty in determining the true platelet count in a patient who also has true thrombocytopenia. Usually, collecting the blood into one of several alternative anticoagulants (heparin, sodium citrate, acid-citrate dextrose) and maintaining the temperature of the blood at 37°C until testing yield an accurate count. Additionally, the platelet count can be estimated by review of the blood film.

☞ "Pseudothrombocytosis" occurs in patients with severe burns (36): Thermal injury to red cells produces microspherocytes that can be falsely identified as platelets by the electronic particle counter, and thus suggest apparent thrombocytosis when the patient may actually suffer acute burn-induced thrombocytopenia and DIC. ☞

Morphologic Clues to Diagnosis

Examining the peripheral blood film can provide important diagnostic clues in evaluating thrombocytopenia. Paradoxically, inspection of the red and white cells is usually more helpful than looking at the platelets. In a trauma patient, the presence of red blood cell (RBC) fragments suggests DIC, as the red cells are "scissored" by intravascular fibrin strands (37,38). Nucleated RBCs (normoblasts) and "left-shift" of leukocytes ("bands," myelocytes, etc.) indicate a "leukoerythoblastic" picture that can be seen in severe shock or hemolysis. Granulocytes that contain "toxic" granules, cytoplasmic vacuolation, and pale blue cytoplasmic inclusions (Döhle bodies) strongly suggest septicemia. Pre-morbid hematologic disorders might also be suggested by the blood film, for example, macrocytic red cells suggestive of alcohol consumption or megaloblastic anemia, "tear drop" cells consistent with marrow fibrosis, red cell spherocytes indicating hereditary spherocytosis or immune hemolysis, dysplastic white cells suggesting myelodysplasia, etc.

Hemostasis Testing
Screening Assays

In a trauma patient, acute thrombocytopenia can indicate DIC, hemodilution secondary to fluid resuscitation, or both. Table 1 lists coagulation assays helpful for evaluating the presence of DIC, such as the prothrombin time (PT)—usually expressed as the international normalized ratio (INR)—the activated partial thromboplastin time (aPTT), fibrinogen, thrombin clotting time (TCT), and cross-linked fibrin degradation products (fibrin D-dimer). Generally, an increase in fibrin D-dimers or a positive "paracoagulation" assay (e.g., protamine sulfate test) suggests DIC (although both hemodilution and DIC cause abnormalities in routine coagulation assays, such as the INR, aPTT, TCT, and fibrinogen levels, hemodilution does not result in increased fibrin D-dimer or a positive protamine sulfate test). Nowadays, however, few hospital laboratories perform paracoagulation tests (38,39). DIC is more fully discussed in Volume 2, Chapter 58.

☞ Coagulation testing is needed to distinguish whether thrombocytopenia is caused by hemodilution or acute DIC in a patient with trauma. Generally, increase in

fibrin D-dimers or a positive paracoagulation assay (e.g., protamine sulfate test) is confirmatory of DIC. Both hemodilution and DIC can cause abnormalities in routine coagulation assays, such as the INR, aPTT, TCT, and fibrinogen levels. ☞

Specialized Assays

The bleeding time is sometimes used to estimate the clinical significance of thrombocytopenia, although it is doubtful whether this provides information beyond that gleaned from the magnitude of the patient's thrombocytopenia and

Table 1 Hemostasis Testing Appropriate in a Trauma Patient

Test	Comments
CBC	Hemoglobin/hematocrit and platelet counts are important for assessing primary hemostasis
PT (often expressed as the INR[a])	Assesses function of the "extrinsic" pathway factor (VII) and subsequent common pathway factors (X, V, II)
aPTT	Assesses function of the "intrinsic" pathway factors, including the contact factors[b], VIII, and IX, as well as the subsequent common pathway factors (X, V, II)
Fibrinogen	Direct measurement of fibrinogen is useful because the INR and aPTT do not increase in hypofibrinogenemia unless the fibrinogen is severely reduced
TCT	Assesses fibrinogen levels and/or presence of heparin (which has antithrombin activity)
Fibrin D-dimer	Detects cross-linked fibrin degradation products which are formed when thrombin and plasmin have acted sequentially upon fibrinogen
Protamine sulfate or ethanol gel "paracoagulation" test	Semi-quantitative assay in which incubation of plasma with protamine sulfate (positively charged protein) leads to gelling of plasma in presence of clinically significant concentrations of fibrin monomer and fibrin degradation products (thus, the assay is fairly specific assay for DIC)
Bleeding time	Assesses "primary hemostasis" (Fig. 3); infrequently performed in a trauma patient

[a]The INR is determined by the patient's prothrombin time (PT), the control PT, and a constant International Sensitivity Index (ISI) that is determined for the thromboplastin reagent and the coagulation analyzer used, as follows: $INR = (PT_{patient}/PT_{control})^{ISI}$.
[b]There are four contact factors: XI, XII, prekallikrein, and high-molecular-weight kininogen; only deficiency of factor XI is associated with bleeding.
Abbreviations: CBC, complete blood count; DIC, disseminated intravascular coagulation; PT, prothrombin time; INR, international normalized ratio; aPTT, activated partial thromboplastin time; TCT, thrombin clotting time.

signs of hemostatic impairment on physical examination. Occasionally, other specialized coagulation tests provide useful information. For example, severe depletion in natural anticoagulants such as antithrombin or protein C can explain microvascular thrombosis and acral limb ischemia in a patient with DIC (38).

Pre-existing Thrombocytopenia
Immune Thrombocytopenic Purpura
Acute and chronic thrombocytopenia is often caused by autoantibodies that bind to platelet membrane GPs, leading to premature platelet destruction by the macrophages of the reticuloendothelial system (40–42). Treatment is generally avoided unless the patient has symptomatic thrombocytopenia, which usually occurs only when the platelet count is $30 \times 10^9/L$ or less. Thus, there is the potential for marked thrombocytopenia in a trauma patient who has pre-existing chronic ITP. Although platelet transfusions are rarely indicated in chronic ITP (because antiplatelet antibodies limit their survival and clinical efficacy), their use is appropriate in emergency situations such as trauma. Adjunctive medical therapies that raise the platelet count within 24 to 48 hours include high-dose corticosteroids and high-dose intravenous gammaglobulin (IVIgG; 1 g/kg given over 6 to 8 hours intravenously on two consecutive days). Although Rh immune globulin administered to an Rh(D)-positive individual also raises the platelet count, this effect is generally slower than with IVIgG, and so anti-D is usually not given in emergency situations such as post-trauma. Also, anti-D is ineffective in patients who have previously undergone splenectomy for chronic ITP. Splenectomy is a relatively common therapy for chronic ITP, as it has a 75% probability of effecting long-term "cure" or amelioration of chronic thrombocytopenia.

Hereditary Thrombocytopenia
These are relatively rare disorders that sometimes exhibit characteristic syndromes, e.g., thrombocytopenia-absent radii syndrome (marked reduction in megakaryocytes, deformed forearms and hands secondary to absent radii) and Wiskott-Aldrich syndrome (very small platelets, eczema, immunodeficiency, X-linked inheritance). Most often, patients with hereditary thrombocytopenia have very large platelets ("macrothrombocytopenia"), normal numbers of marrow megakaryocytes, and autosomal-dominant inheritance (43). In some families with macrothrombocytopenia, white cell inclusions are evident on microscopy, either without other somatic abnormalities (Sebastian syndrome) or with clinical features such as glomerulonephritis and deafness (Fechtner's syndrome). No specific therapy is available for these disorders, and platelet transfusions should be reserved for life-threatening bleeding.

Hypersplenism
Any cause of splenomegaly can cause chronic pancytopenia secondary to splenic sequestration of blood cells (see the section on "Platelet Distribution" and Fig. 1). Usually, mild-to-moderate thrombocytopenia and leukopenia are observed that parallel each other in severity; the reduction in hemoglobin is usually less marked. In western societies, the most common cause of hypersplenism is alcohol-induced cirrhosis, and so coagulopathy secondary to hepatic cellular dysfunction can coexist. Platelet transfusion response is often suboptimal in hypersplenism, because the transfused platelets become sequestered in the spleen to the same extent as the patient's own platelets. Patients with splenomegaly and particularly severe thrombocytopenia $(20–50 \times 10^9/L)$ probably also have impaired platelet production secondary to decreased hepatic TPO production (19).

Alcohol-Induced Thrombocytopenia
Very heavy alcohol consumption has the potential to cause severe, isolated thrombocytopenia due to a direct toxic effect on megakaryocytes (44). Upon ceasing alcohol, the platelet count begins to increase after two to three days, typically leading to thrombocytosis by 10 to 17 days.

Clonal Marrow Disorders
Demographics trends—particularly the "graying" of the population—suggest that increasing numbers of elderly patients will become victims of trauma. The elderly are at particular risk for one or more chronic cytopenias—often including thrombocytopenia—caused by clonal marrow disorders, for example, myelodysplasia ("preleukemia") (45) or chronic lymphoid leukemia. In contrast, clonal myeloproliferative disorders often produce thrombocytosis (see the section on "Physiologic vs. Pathologic"). Platelet dysfunction in some patients with myelodysplasia may cause greater bleeding than expected for the degree of thrombocytopenia. Even in the absence of later transformation to acute leukemia, patients with myelodysplasia are at increased risk for death from infection, bleeding, or transfusional iron overload.

Platelet Dysfunction
✍ Platelet dysfunction in trauma patients is often the result of renal failure (uremia) or drug effects (e.g., aspirin, clopidogrel). ✍ Less often, marrow disorders, gammopathy, cirrhosis, and post-cardiopulmonary bypass (CPB) status are possible explanations.

Uremia
Acute or chronic renal failure causes bleeding diathesis characterized by prolonged bleeding time and various platelet function abnormalities (46). Defective primary hemostasis is partly explained by a low hematocrit, particularly in chronic renal failure (low erythopoietin levels), which explains why transfusing red cells can dramatically lower the bleeding time (47–49). Table 2 lists various strategies to reduce the uremic bleeding defect (46–62).

Drugs
Antiplatelet agents, such as aspirin [acetyl-salicylic acid (ASA)] and clopidogrel, are increasingly used to prevent vascular thrombosis. Both can prolong the bleeding time and increase surgical bleeding (63,64). Although ASA and clopidogrel inhibit different aspects of platelet physiology [cyclooxygenase-1 (COX-1) and the adenosine diphosphate receptor, respectively], their effects are irreversible for the duration of the platelet lifespan; accordingly, platelet dysfunction lasts for up to 10 days even after stopping either drug (65). This contrasts with reversible COX inhibitors (e.g., nonsteroidal antiinflammatory agents, such as indomethacin, ibuprofen, and naproxen), in which platelet function recovers within hours after stopping the drug. Selective COX-2 inhibitors (e.g., celecoxib, rofecoxib) do not affect platelet function (66).

Platelet transfusions are indicated for life-threatening bleeding if clinical suspicion for significant drug-induced

Table 2   Treatment of Abnormal Hemostasis Complicating Acute or Chronic Renal Failure

Treatment	Comment
Red cell transfusions (47–49) and/or erythropoietin (50) (target hematocrit >0.30)	Raised hematocrit improves hemostasis via enhanced platelet–subendothelial interaction (Fig. 3)
Increased intensity of hemodialysis	Removal of uremic "toxins" that impair platelet function
Desmopressin (L-deamino-8-D-arginine vasopressin), 0.3 μg/kg (maximum, 20 μg) in 50 mL normal saline over 30 min IV (51); may repeat once 8–12 hr later	Induces release of vWF[a] from endothelial stores; thus, less effective with repeated doses (tachyphylaxis) (52); hemostatic effect begins 30–60 min post-infusion and lasts for 8–12 hr
Conjugated estrogens, for example, Emopremarin, 0.6 mg/kg OD IV for 5 days (53–55); or Premarin, 50 mg po OD until bleeding time corrects (up to 9 days) (56)	Mechanism unknown, but possibly by reducing endothelial nitric oxide (physiologic platelet inhibitor) [57]; effect of 5-day course begins 6 hr after first dose, peaks at 5–7 days, and lasts for 14 days
Cryoprecipitate, 10 units (52,58)	Provides vWF[a] and fibrinogen; variable benefit (59); usually used only if patient does not respond to desmopressin and estrogens (60)
Platelet transfusions (for bleeding or shortly before invasive procedure)	Usually used only if patient does not respond to desmopressin and conjugated estrogens
rVIIa, 90 μg/kg IV once (30,61)	May enhance coagulation reactions on platelet surfaces in the absence of TF; anecdotal experience only; very expensive

[a]Abnormal vWF multimer distribution in uremic platelets and plasma has been reported (62).
Abbreviations: rVIIa, recombinant factor VIIa; TF, tissue factor; vWF, von Willebrand factor.

platelet dysfunction exists. Indeed, transfusing 5 to 10 units of platelets largely corrects ASA-induced platelet dysfunction, because the transfused platelets can provide thromboxane A_2 to the patient's aspirin-treated platelets via transcellular metabolic pathways.

Miscellaneous Disorders

Platelet dysfunction is a common feature of certain acquired bone marrow disorders, such as myelodysplasia and myeloproliferative disorders. Marked elevations in monoclonal or polyclonal immunoglobulin levels (gammopathy) also can lead to impaired platelet function. Cirrhosis is another explanation for platelet dysfunction that can be transiently benefitted by desmopressin (67); however, most patients with advanced liver disease also have thrombocytopenia, deficient coagulation factors, and hyperfibrinolysis. Heart surgery utilizing CPB leads to impaired hemostasis via transient platelet dysfunction, hyperfibrinolysis, and thrombocytopenia. Antifibrinolytic agents, especially when given during CPB, ameliorate bleeding.

Rare congenital disorders with abnormal platelet structure [e.g., Bernard–Soulier syndrome (absent platelet GP Ib–IX–V receptor complexes), Glanzmann's thrombasthenia (absent platelet GP IIb/IIIa receptors)] can be associated with severe abnormalities in platelet function. More common are poorly characterized platelet function disorders that may prompt consideration for platelet transfusions and/or desmopressin following trauma, particularly if one obtains a history of chronic mucocutaneous bleeding in the patient or family members.

ABRUPT ONSET OF THROMBOCYTOPENIA AFTER TRAUMA

Hemodilution

General Principles

A platelet count decline that is roughly proportional to the amount of crystalloid, colloid, or red cell concentrates administered is known as dilutional thrombocytopenia. Even in the absence of ongoing platelet losses, thrombocytopenia persists for two to four days, prior to platelet count increase and subsequent thrombocytosis resulting from increased platelet production (Fig. 2). Dilutional coagulopathy generally accompanies thrombocytopenia. However, acute DIC frequently coexists, and thus frequent CBC and coagulation testing is important for assessment of hemostatic compromise (Table 3).

Table 3   Interpretation of Platelet Count and Coagulation Test Results

Test	Approximate normal range	Patient #1	Patient #2
Platelet count	$150–400 \times 10^9$/L	50	50
INR	0.9–1.2	1.6	1.6
aPTT	26–38 sec	50	50
TCT[a]			
10 unit	7–11 sec	15	15
2 unit	20–30 sec	40	40
Fibrinogen (clottable)	1.6–4.2 g/L	0.8	0.8
Fibrin D-dimer[b]	<500 μg/L	500	>2000
Protamine sulfate test[b]			
15 min	Negative	Negative	2 +
30 min	Negative	Negative	3 +
Interpretation		*Hemodilution*	*DIC (±hemodilution)*

[a]Different concentrations of thrombin can be used to perform the thrombin clotting time (TCT). The lower the thrombin concentration, the more sensitive the assay is to the presence of heparin in the blood sample.
[b]Generally, an increase in fibrin D-dimers or a positive paracoagulation assay (e.g., protamine sulfate test) is needed to diagnose DIC, as hemodilution can lead to abnormalities in routine coagulation assays, such as the INR, aPTT, TCT, and fibrinogen levels.
Abbreviations: aPTT, activated partial thromboplastin time; DIC, disseminated intravascular coagulation; INR, international normalized ratio; TCT, thrombin clotting time.

☞ **Dilutional thrombocytopenia related to fluid resuscitation is the most common cause of thrombocytopenia in a trauma patient. Repeated CBC and coagulation testing is important to assess the presence and severity of coexisting DIC.** ☜

Massive Transfusion

Massive transfusion is generally defined as replacement of a patient's blood volume within 24 hours, that is, about 3000 mL or 10 units of red cell concentrates in an average-size individual (68,69). Trauma accounts for at least one-third of massive transfusion situations (68,69). At one time, "formulaic" approaches to massive transfusion were advocated, that is, the automatic transfusion of platelets and fresh frozen plasma (FFP) after every 'nth' unit of red cells or whole blood. However, a randomized trial of prophylactic platelet transfusion and FFP during massive transfusion did not show improved outcomes using this approach (70). Further, diffuse microvascular bleeding is relatively uncommon even when serious derangements in platelet count and coagulation tests result (70,71), and the correlation between units of red cells transfused and laboratory abnormalities observed is poor (68). Thus, "automatic" platelet transfusions are not generally advised. However, aggressive correction of platelet and coagulation abnormalities was associated with improved survival in one retrospective study (72). ☞ **When diffuse bleeding is evident or relatively severe thrombocytopenia is documented (generally, less than $50 \times 10^9/L$), platelet transfusion support is appropriate (73–75). A higher platelet count threshold (i.e., $100 \times 10^9/L$) is a more appropriate transfusion trigger for certain conditions (e.g., traumatic brain injury).** ☜

Acute Disseminated Intravascular Coagulation

DIC is a clinicopathologic disorder in which systemic generation of intravascular thrombin leads to a generalized derangement of the hemostatic mechanism via consumption of coagulation factors and platelets, and generation of intravascular fibrin and fibrinogen/fibrin degradation products (76–79). Bleeding can result from depletion of procoagulant factors and platelets, and from parallel generation of plasmin (the enzyme that degrades the fibrin clot). Formation of intravascular fibrin is one mechanism to account for multiple-organ dysfunction syndrome (MODS). Occasionally, depletion of natural anticoagulant factors (e.g., antithrombin, protein C) leads to dramatic syndromes of micro- or macrovascular thrombosis. The clinical spectrum of DIC is wide, ranging from laboratory abnormalities without clinical sequelae, to severe bleeding caused by depletion of coagulation factors and platelets and/or hyperfibrinolysis, to organ dysfunction and skin necrosis resulting from microvascular thrombosis.

Thrombocytopenia in DIC probably results at least in part from platelet activation and consumption caused by thrombin, the major physiologic platelet agonist. Indeed, thrombin concentrations as low as 0.15 nmol/L can activate platelets without any effect on fibrin generation (80). Thrombin-induced platelet activation also leads to formation of procoagulant platelet-derived microparticles, suggesting that platelet activation directly promotes the consumption of the coagulation factors in acute DIC.

DIC in trauma is usually multifactorial. For example, an early event in many trauma patients is vascular disruption, which causes blood to become exposed to extravascular TF (81). This leads directly to activation of coagulation via the "extrinsic" system: TF:VII(a) complexes directly activate factor X to Xa on TF-bearing cells (Fig. 4). In some patients, procoagulant substances are liberated through massive red cell membrane disruption, for example, burn-associated hemolysis. Subsequent events such as shock and acidosis lead to further procoagulant changes on endothelium. Finally, generation of cytokines and other proinflammatory mediators characteristic of SIRS occurs, often with concomitant MODS and adult respiratory distress syndrome (ARDS) (82,83).

Figure 5 lists various coagulation assays that can be used for rapid laboratory assessment of DIC. An important tenet of viewing DIC as a clinicopathologic disorder is that no single laboratory profile is diagnostic of DIC. For example, a routine postcardiac surgery patient will have laboratory abnormalities that resemble that for DIC, so interpretation of test results in the clinical context is paramount. Similarly, fluid resuscitation will cause a trauma patient to have prolonged INR and aPTT assays, reduced fibrinogen, thrombocytopenia, and so on. However, greatly increased fibrin D-dimer levels and a strongly positive ethanol gel or protamine sulfate paracoagulation assay (38,39) suggest intravascular fibrin formation and hence have greater specificity for indicating the presence of DIC (Table 3).

Management of DIC includes treating the cause (where possible) and any potentiating factors. Thus, treating hypovolemia, acidosis, hypoxemia, infection, and so on are mandatory. In addition, red cell, plasma, and platelet transfusions for patients with coagulopathic bleeding or severe derangement in laboratory parameters may also improve outcomes. Diagnosis and management of DIC are discussed further in Volume 2, Chapter 58.

Systemic Inflammatory Response Syndrome

Severe trauma complicated by DIC often leads to early death from MODS. In less serious trauma, systemic inflammation

Tests for DIC

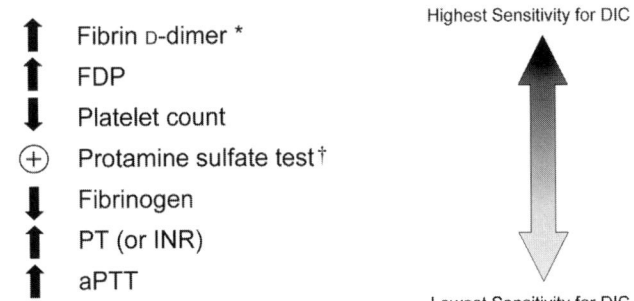

*most specific for DIC
†usually positive in clinically-significant DIC (see text)

Figure 5 Sensitivity and specificity of routine coagulation assays for DIC. In the authors' opinion, the protamine sulfate paracoagulation assay for fibrin monomer has a relatively high sensitivity and specificity for clinically significant DIC, that is, DIC complicated by thrombosis or bleeding. However, this assay is no longer widely performed. *Abbreviations*: DIC, disseminated intravascular coagulation; FDP, fibrin(ogen) degradation products; INR, international normalized ratio; PT, prothrombin time; aPTT, activated partial thromboplastin time; ↑, increased, ↓, decreased; +, positive.

associated with activation of coagulation and fibrinolysis is self-limited, and initially abnormal hemostasis parameters, including the platelet count, normalize. However, there remain a sizeable group of trauma patients who develop SIRS (83). In these patients, laboratory abnormalities consistent with DIC persist. Microvascular thrombosis secondary to DIC is associated with MODS and ARDS. Associated hemostasis abnormalities include persisting thrombocytopenia, elevated fibrin D-dimers, elevated plasminogen activator inhibitor-1 (PAI-1) levels, and decrease in natural coagulation inhibitors (antithrombin, protein C). These abnormalities appear to be related to proinflammatory cytokines such as tumor necrosis factor-α, interleukin-6, and interleukin-8, that promote TF-mediated DIC and increased PAI-1 levels. The strong association between thrombocytopenia and SIRS is one reason why persisting thrombocytopenia is a simple, but strong, risk factor associated with increased mortality following trauma (82,83).

Mechanical Assist Devices

Platelet consumption from intravascular devices such as the intra-aortic balloon pump or left (or right) ventricular assist devices may contribute to thrombocytopenia (84,85). However, the extent to which the mechanical device directly contributes to platelet consumption vis-a-vis platelet activation related to shock, ARDS, and so on, is difficult to ascertain. Heparin is generally given with these devices, and so an important issue is whether the thrombocytopenia may be caused by immune heparin-induced thrombocytopenia (HIT) (see the section on "Immune Heparin-induced").

Hypothermia

Thrombocytopenia of mild-to-moderate severity that corrects with rewarming has been observed in humans undergoing planned or accidental hypothermia. Platelet kinetic studies in cooled dogs demonstrate reversible hepatic and splenic platelet sequestration (86,87). Indirect evidence suggests that decreased platelet production may contribute to this phenomenon as well (88).

DELAYED ONSET OF THROMBOCYTOPENIA AFTER TRAUMA
Septicemia

Infection is a relatively common cause of unexpected thrombocytopenia that occurs during the hospitalization of a trauma patient. Usually, thrombocytopenia in this setting indicates microbial invasion of the blood, that is, bacteremia, fungemia, and so on. Thus, blood cultures should be drawn in any patient with unexpected thrombocytopenia. Examination of the blood film often reveals other evidence for infection, that is, left-shift in the white blood cells, "toxic" changes such as vacuolation, and dark granules in neutrophils. These findings may be evident even when the total leukocyte count is not increased. Coagulation assays for DIC should also be ordered, although in many patients with septicemia-associated thrombocytopenia, evidence for DIC is limited to elevated fibrin D-dimer levels, with normal INR, aPTT, fibrinogen, and protamine sulfate paracoagulation test results.

↙ Late onset of thrombocytopenia in a trauma patient can indicate acute bacteremia, so blood cultures should always be drawn in this situation. ↗

The pathogenesis of thrombocytopenia is multifactorial, and includes platelet activation by thrombin (89),

increased platelet clearance by reticuloendothelial cells (90), decreased marrow platelet production, and direct and indirect effects of microbial toxins (91,92). Elevation in PAI-1 may contribute to hypofibrinolysis, with increased risk for MODS.

Aggressive treatment of the infection is crucial. Prophylactic platelet transfusions are usually given for severe thrombocytopenia (e.g., platelet count less than 20×10^9/L), although a higher platelet count threshold (e.g., 50×10^9/L) is appropriate if the patient is bleeding or an invasive procedure is planned.

Drug-Induced Thrombocytopenia

Table 4 lists various drug-induced thrombocytopenic syndromes. In general, drug-induced thrombocytopenia is rare, and is most unlikely to be the cause of thrombocytopenia in a trauma patient. The major exception to this rule is immune HIT, which can explain thrombocytopenia in about 1% to 3% of patients treated with unfractionated heparin (UFH) for more than one week (2,93).

Immune Heparin-Induced Thrombocytopenia

↙ HIT is by far the most common drug-induced, immune-mediated thrombocytopenia. Paradoxically, HIT is associated with thrombosis rather than bleeding (2). ↗ Typical sequelae of HIT include: venous thromboembolism (deep-vein thrombosis, pulmonary embolism), thrombosis of large arteries (lower limb > cerebrovascular > coronary > other), and other complications such as skin lesions and acute inflammatory or cardiorespiratory reactions post-heparin bolus (Table 5) (94). Hypotension and/or abdominal pain suggests adrenal hemorrhagic infarction, which typically is bilateral and therefore results in acute and chronic adrenal insufficiency (Fig. 6) (94). By recognizing this syndrome, the clinician can prevent death from adrenal failure by administering corticosteroid replacement.

↙ Hypotension and/or abdominal pain in a thrombocytopenic patient treated with heparin suggests bilateral adrenal hemorrhagic infarction with acute adrenal failure: Corticosteroid replacement therapy can be life-saving. ↗

HIT can be difficult to diagnose in trauma patients, for several reasons. First, trauma patients often have multiple alternative explanations for thrombocytopenia (DIC, ARDS, septicemia, etc.). Second, thrombocytopenia is usually not very severe in HIT: The platelet count nadir falls between 30 and 100×10^9/L in about 60% of HIT patients, which is similar to that observed in DIC, ARDS, septicemia, and so on (Fig. 7) (94). Third, even when HIT antibodies are detected in the laboratory, these are not specific for HIT, as many patients who receive heparin develop subclinical seroconversion (generation of non-pathogenic antibodies) (2,93). Particularly in a trauma patient—where multiple alternative explanations for thrombocytopenia may exist—the lack of diagnostic specificity is problematic. An important clinical clue indicates that HIT is the onset of an unexpected fall in the platelet count beginning 5 to 10 days after beginning a course of heparin (94).

Pathogenesis (Fig. 8): The pathogenic HIT antibodies recognize a "self" protein, platelet factor 4 (PF4) (95,96). PF4 is a tetrameric, positively charged protein found within platelet α granules. Neoepitopes are formed when PF4 binds to heparin (negatively charged mucopolysaccharide) (97). When multimolecular complexes of heparin, PF4, and the pathogenic IgG antibodies form on platelet surfaces, the Fc "tails" of the HIT-IgG interact with a low-affinity class

Table 4 Syndromes of Drug-Induced Thrombocytopenia

Syndrome	Implicated drugs	Comments
Immune HIT	UFH; LMWH; certain polyanion but non-heparin drugs (e.g., pentosan polysulfate)	Most common immune drug reaction; prothrombotic; typically causes mild-to-moderate thrombocytopenia
D-ITP	Quinine, quinidine, gold salts, vancomycin, rifampicin, sulfa drugs (e.g., sulfamethoxazole-trimethoprim), naproxen, pentamidine, acetaminophen, aspirin, carbamazepine, carbimazole, cefotetan, etc.	Very rare; severe thrombocytopenia with mucocutaneous bleeding (platelet count nadir typically less than $20 \times 10^9/L$); treatment may include platelet transfusions and high-dose IVIgG
Abrupt D-ITP caused by platelet GP IIb/IIIa inhibitors	Abciximab (Reopro®), eptifibatide (Integrelin) tirofiban (Aggrastat®)	Moderate-to-severe thrombocytopenia that occurs abruptly in ~1–2% of patients
Drug-induced platelet agglutination	Protamine sulfate, porcine vWF, hematin, others	Mild platelet fall that is not clinically significant
Drug-induced microangiopathy (TTP or HUS)	Mitomycin C, cyclosporine, quinine, ticlopidine, clopidogrel	Antibodies against vWF-cleaving metalloproteinase have been reported in ticlopidine-associated TTP
Drug metabolite-dependent decrease in platelet production (?)	Valproic acid	Mild thrombocytopenia without clinical relevance; thrombocytopenia correlates with levels of valproate metabolite

Abbreviations: D-ITP, drug-induced immune thrombocytopenic purpura; HIT, heparin-induced thrombocytopenia; HUS, hemolytic uremic syndrome; LMWH, low-molecular-weight heparin; TTP, thrombotic thrombocytopenic purpura; UFH, unfractionated heparin; vWF, von Willebrand factor.

of platelet Fc receptors, causing the platelets to activate. Heparin chains that are at least 10 monosaccharide units in length bind to PF4 (98), perhaps explaining why UFH causes HIT antibody formation, and clinical HIT, more often than does low-molecular-weight heparin (2,93).

HIT is a hypercoagulability disorder, that is, there is increased thrombin generation in vivo (99). Activation of coagulation occurs by formation of procoagulant platelet-derived microparticles during platelet activation, as well as activation of endothelium and monocytes. Nevertheless,

"overt" DIC—manifesting either hypofibrinogenemia or elevated INRs—occurs in only 5% to 10% of HIT patients. Once triggered, the prothrombotic nature of HIT persists for a few weeks, even despite stopping heparin (100).

The systemic activation of coagulation explains the association between HIT and venous thrombosis, as well as the risk for progressive microvascular thrombosis during acute protein C depletion (warfarin-associated venous limb gangrene complicating HIT) (99). Thus, warfarin should be avoided during acute HIT, among other "treatment

Table 5 Clinical Sequelae of Immune HIT

Venous thrombosis	Arterial thrombosis	Miscellaneous

DVT
  Lower-limb
    (often bilateral)
  Upper-limb DVT (usually at
    intravascular catheter site)
  Phlegmasia cerulea dolens[a]
  Coumarin (warfarin)-associated
    venous limb gangrene[b]
Pulmonary
  embolism
Cerebral dural sinus thrombosis
Adrenal hemorrhagic infarction
  acute and/or chronic adrenal
  insufficiency
	Aorto-iliofemoral thrombosis
	Limb ischemia/
	  necrosis
	Paralysis
	Thrombotic stroke
	Myocardial
	  infarction
	Intracardiac thrombosis (atrial,
	  ventricular)
	Miscellaneous thrombosis involving:
	  mesenteric arteries, renal arteries,
	  spinal arteries, brachial arteries and
	  so on
		Heparin-induced skin lesions[c]
		Coumarin (warfarin)-induced skin
		  necrosis[b]
		Acute systemic reaction post-intravenous
		  heparin bolus
		    Inflammatory reaction: fever, chills,
		      flushing
		    Cardiorespiratory reaction, for example,
		      cardiac or respiratory arrest
		    Gastrointestinal: vomiting, diarrhea
		    Neurologic: transient global amnesia
		DIC (risk for microvascular
		  thrombosis)

[a]Inflamed, blue, painful limb, that is, venous ischemia (prodrome to venous limb gangrene); in heparin-induced thrombocytopenia (HIT)-associated deep vein thrombosis, progression to venous limb gangrene has been linked to warfarin therapy causing depletion of the vitamin K-dependent natural anticoagulant, protein C (99).
[b]Warfarin-induced necrosis is more likely to manifest as venous limb gangrene (acral necrosis) than as "classic" skin necrosis (central sites, e.g., breast, abdomen, thigh) when it complicates a platelet activation disorder such as immune HIT.
[c]Occurs at heparin injection sites, and ranges from erythematous plaques to frank necrosis.
Abbreviations: DVT, deep-vein thrombosis; HIT, heparin-induced thrombocytopenia; DIC, disseminated intravascular coagulation.

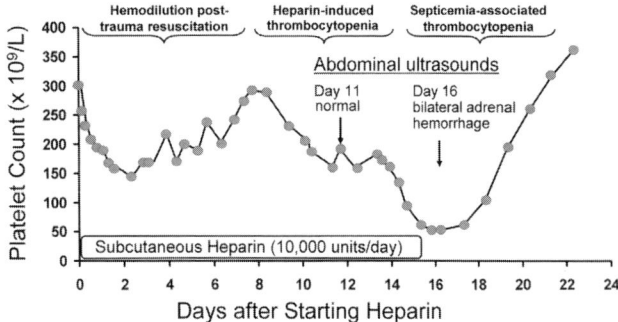

Figure 6 Bilateral adrenal hemorrhagic infarction complicating HIT and septicemia. Abdominal ultrasonography on day 16 showed massive bilateral adrenal hemorrhages that were not evident on imaging performed five days earlier. In such a patient, corticosteroid therapy can be life-saving. *Abbreviation*: HIT, heparin-induced thrombocytopenia.

paradoxes" (Table 6). Currently, treatment of HIT involves substitution of heparin with another anticoagulant that inhibits thrombin directly (lepirudin, argatroban) or that reduces thrombin generation by inhibition of factor Xa (danaparoid) (Fig. 9) (95,101). Lepirudin is renally excreted, and thus is relatively contraindicated in renal failure, which occurs commonly in ill post-trauma patients.

Drug-Induced Immune Thrombocytopenic Purpura

There are several drugs for which severe immune-mediated thrombocytopenia can occur, albeit rarely (Table 4). Typically, platelet count nadirs are less than 20×10^9/L. For example, sulfamethoxazole-trimethoprim causes D-ITP in about 1/15,000 to 1/25,000 patients, and quinidine in about 1/1,000 patients (102). For patients with life-threatening thrombocytopenia, platelet transfusions along with reticuloendothelial blockade with high-dose IVIgG is appropriate. The rarity of these reactions means that they will almost

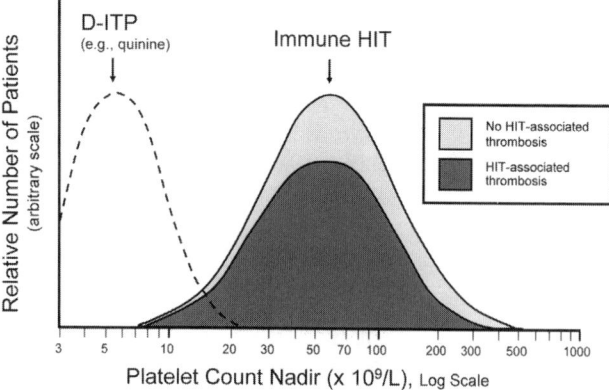

Figure 7 Severity of thrombocytopenia in drug-induced immune thrombocytopenia: comparison of D-ITP and immune HIT. Note that the relative risk of HIT-associated thrombosis increases as the platelet count nadir decreases. Note also that the median platelet count nadir in HIT (about 60×10^9/L) resembles that seen in many other causes for thrombocytopenia in a patient with trauma, for example, DIC, ARDS, SIRS, and so on. *Abbreviations*: D-ITP, drug-induced immune thrombocytopenic purpura; HIT, heparin-induced thrombocytopernia.

never explain thrombocytopenia in a critically ill trauma patient.

Miscellaneous Drug-Induced Thrombocytopenia

Table 4 also lists other distinct drug-induced thrombocytopenic syndromes (102,103). In general, these syndromes are unlikely to cause significant thrombocytopenia in a trauma population.

Nutritional Thrombocytopenia

Acute folic acid deficiency is a possible explanation for acquired thrombocytopenia in a trauma patient who has increased metabolic demands following tissue injury and blood losses, and who may not be receiving adequate nutrition following the injury (104,105).

Thrombocytopenia Following Blood Transfusion

Paradoxically, blood transfusion therapy itself can result in severe thrombocytopenia. Three examples that are discussed later in this chapter (see the section on Contradictions to platelet transfusion") include (in decreasing order of frequency): transfusion-associated bacteremia, post-transfusion purpura (PTP), and passive alloimmune thrombocytopenia (PAT). A more common situation is that the clearance of transfused platelets over 24 to 48 hours after platelet transfusion mimics new-onset thrombocytopenia (Fig. 9).

PLATELET TRANSFUSION THERAPY
Overview

In general, life-threatening bleeding caused by thrombocytopenia is rare. Indeed, mortality usually results from the underlying cause of the thrombocytopenia, rather than from thrombocytopenic bleeding itself. This is evident in trauma patients, where severe injury that results in thrombocytopenia can cause death via any of a large number of mechanisms other than bleeding, particularly given the wide availability of platelet transfusions for preventing and treating thrombocytopenic bleeding of numerous etiologies. Indeed, some 8 million units of platelets are transfused each year in the United States (106).

The following section will outline aspects of the preparation of platelet products and safety issues. The expected therapeutic response to transfusion, important contraindications to platelet transfusions, and complications will also be reviewed.

Platelet Preparation
Pooled Platelets vs. Single-Donor Plateletpheresis

Platelets are usually prepared by separating the platelet component from random-donor whole blood donations. Each "unit" of platelet concentrate is stored for up to five days, and then (usually) five units of platelets, each from a different donor, are pooled shortly before use. After pooling, a standard 5-unit "dose" of platelets contains about 300×10^9 platelets, that is, about one-fifth the normal number of circulating platelets in an average-size adult. This product also contains about 250 to 300 mL plasma (each platelet donor contributes about 50–60 mL plasma) and (if unfiltered) also contains about 0.5×10^9 leukocytes.

Alternatively, platelets can be collected from a single donor using apheresis ("plateletpheresis"), whereby an efferent venous catheter channels whole blood from the donor into a blood separator where the platelet component is collected; the remaining (platelet-poor) blood flows back

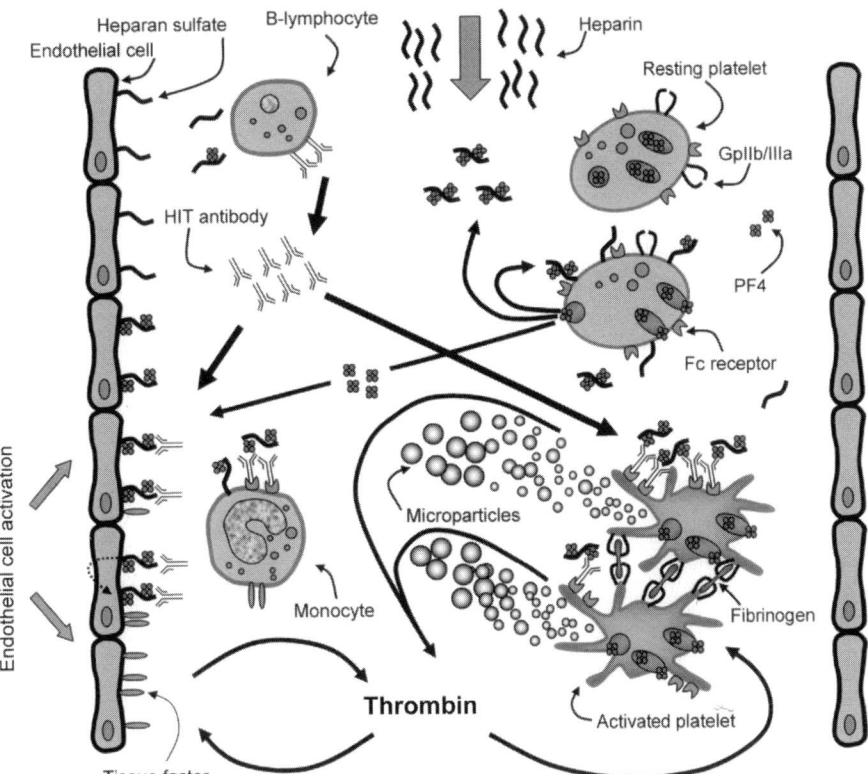

Figure 8 Pathogenesis of HIT: a central role for thrombin generation. The target antigen of HIT is a "self" protein, platelet factor 4, that expresses one or more neoepitopes when bound to heparin. HIT-IgG antibodies lead to increased thrombin generation, by activating platelets via their Fc receptors (which results in formation of procoagulant, platelet-derived microparticles), as well as activating endothelium and monocytes. *Abbreviation*: HIT, heparin-induced thombocytopenia.

Table 6 Paradoxes in the Treatment of HIT

Treatment	Paradox	Comments
Stop heparin	Risk for thrombosis persists for days to weeks	Use alternative anticoagulant[a] even for "isolated HIT"
Warfarin	Warfarin-induced venous limb gangrene or skin necrosis	Avoid warfarin unless satisfactorily anticoagulated with alternative anticoagulant[a] and thrombocytopenia has substantially recovered (platelet count $>150 \times 10^9$/L)
LMWH	Although less likely to cause HIT than UFH, LMWH is contraindicated to treat HIT	Approximately 50% risk of thrombocytopenia and/or thrombosis if LMWH is used to treat HIT caused by UFH
Platelet transfusions	May increase risk for thrombosis	Spontaneous bleeding rare and platelet transfusions theoretically confer risk
Dosing of alternative anticoagulant	"Therapeutic" dosing of anticoagulation is appropriate even when preventing thrombosis in acute HIT	Prophylactic-dose for danaparoid (750 Units bid s.c.) is suboptimal for preventing thrombosis in HIT; therapeutic doses are recommended (initial 2250 unit bolus for average-size adult, then 3600–4800 Unit 24 hr); argatroban and lepirudin are also generally prescribed in therapeutic doses
Repeat use of heparin	Re-exposure to heparin is appropriate under exceptional circumstances	Negligible risk of acute HIT once antibodies are no longer detectable

[a]Alternative anticoagulants include: lepirudin, bivalirudin, argatroban, and danaparoid (danaparoid has been withdrawn from the U.S. market, but is available in Canada, Europe, Japan, Australia, and New Zealand.
Abbreviations: HIT, heparin-induced thrombocytopenia; LMWH, low-molecular-weight heparin; UFH, unfractionated heparin.

Typical-Onset HIT

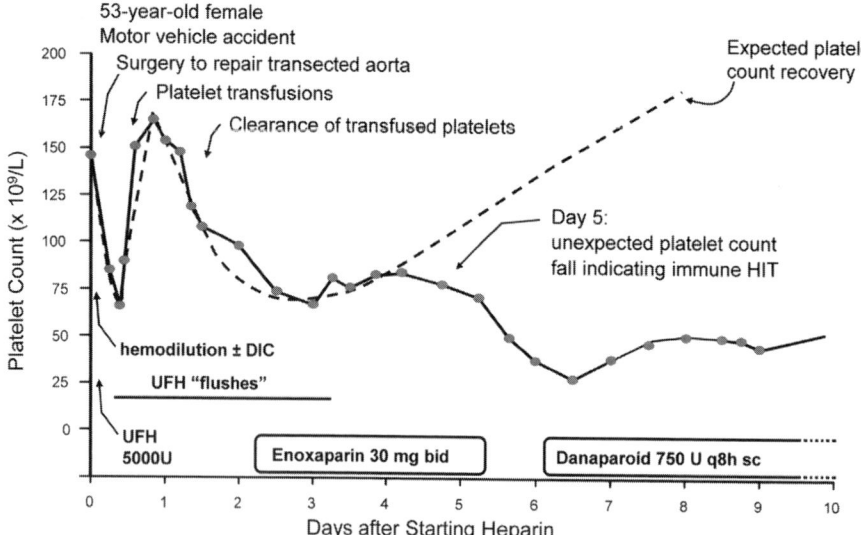

Figure 9 Typical-onset HIT in a trauma patient. The initial platelet count fluctuations are explained, in sequence, by: hemodilution ± DIC, platelet transfusions, and clearance of the transfused platelets. The dotted line indicates the expected platelet count sequence in this patient. Thus, the unexpected platelet count fall on day 5 indicates immune HIT, which was confirmed by strong positive testing for HIT antibodies. The patient received prophylactic-dose danaparoid sodium, although therapeutic-dose anticoagulation would have been preferred in this situation (102). (*Note*: Danaparoid is no longer available in the United States, as it was withdrawn by the manufacturer in April 2002.) *Abbreviation*: HIT, heparin-induced thrombocytopenia.

to the donor via an afferent venous catheter. The volume of platelet concentrate can be predetermined prior to platelet-pheresis, but in general, the equivalent of five units of random-donor platelets are collected from a single apheresis donor. Following collection, the platelets are also stored for up to five days prior to use.

Both types of platelet concentrate are equally effective in raising the platelet count (107,108), with an equivalent incidence of nonimmune refractoriness (109). However, febrile non-hemolytic transfusion reactions (FNHTR, "febrile reactions") occur less often with apheresis platelets (110), an effect that may have been due to differences in storage times in comparative studies (111). Obviously, the risk of infectious disease transmission with pooled platelets from multiple donors is greater (about five-fold). However, the current rates of viral disease transmission are so low that the absolute risk-reduction using single-donor apheresis platelets is negligible (112). The incidence of bacterial contamination appears to be lower with apheresis platelets as well (113), although fatal septicemia has occurred with both preparations.

Limiting exposure to multiple donors also has the advantage of decreasing the likelihood of HLA alloantibody formation by the blood recipient, thus potentially reducing subsequent immune-mediated platelet transfusion refractoriness. However, removing the white blood cells (which cause alloimmunization) by filters is also effective at preventing HLA alloimmunization, and much more cost-effective. Leukoreduction of platelet and red cell products is even standard in Canada, with filtration performed soon after blood collection ("universal pre-storage leukodepletion"). However, avoiding HLA alloimmunization is not a major issue in the trauma patient, in contrast to patients who require long-term platelet transfusion support (e.g., cancer patients).

Platelets collected by apheresis also have a place in specialized transfusion situations, for example, when a patient must receive HPA-1b homozygous platelets (only 2% of Caucasians) because of PTP.

Platelet Storage

Platelets can be stored at room temperature for up to five days; if not transfused by that time, they are discarded. Prior to 1985, platelet storage up to seven days was permitted by the FDA. However, the risk of bacterial contamination in platelets rises with increasing storage time, especially since platelets—unlike other blood products—are stored at room temperature (114). Platelet viability is lost if they are cooled, and they are stored with constant agitation to inhibit clumping. Also, with prolonged storage, function and viability of platelets are adversely affected (115,116).

The plasma component within a platelet product is responsible for producing most febrile reactions, due to the presence of proinflammatory cytokines such as interleukin-1β and interleukin-6 produced during platelet storage by residual white cells (117). This explains why prestorage leukodepletion reduces the frequency of these reactions (118), whereas bed-side filtration does not (the cytokines pass through the filter). In special transfusion situations, platelets can be washed to remove the plasma.

Leukocytes are the vector for certain transmissible viruses, including cytomegalovirus, human T-cell leukemia/lymphoma virus I and II, and Epstein–Barr virus (119), and so leukofiltration theoretically reduces the risk of transmitting these diseases. White cells can also be killed by ultraviolet-B irradiation, which should be administered to blood products prior to their administration to severely immunocompromised patients, so as to avoid transfusion-related graft versus host disease. Blood irradiation also reduces HLA alloimmunization, and associated alloimmune platelet transfusion refractoriness, to an equivalent extent as does leukodepletion by filtration (120).

Therapeutic Effects
Expected Platelet Count Increments Post-transfusion

Although a normal platelet has a lifespan of about 8 to 10 days (16), routine collection and storage result in transfused platelets having a lower survival (about 2–3 days) compared with the expected survival (4–5 days). The rise in platelet count after a platelet transfusion can be expressed as the "percent platelet recovery" (PPR), defined as (120a):

$$\text{PPR} = \frac{\text{platelet increment} \times 10^9 \times \text{blood volume (as 75 mL/kg)} \times 100\%}{\text{number of platelets transfused} (\times 10^{11}) \times 0.67 \times 10^{-3}}$$

The expected PPR is about $66 \pm 8\%$ (121). (The PPR is not 100%, reflecting exchangeable splenic sequestration of about one-third of the transfused platelets.)

Another measure of the platelet count increment is the "corrected count increment" (CCI), which normalizes the platelet count response for the patient blood volume and platelet dose, as follows (120b):

$$\text{CCI} = \frac{\text{platelet count increment (per } \mu\text{L)} \times \text{body surface area (m}^2) \times 10^{11}}{\text{number of platelets transfused} (\times 10^{11})}$$

Thus, a 6-foot male trauma patient weighing 78 kg (body surface area = 2.0 m^2) whose platelet count rose from 50,000 to 80,000 per μL (50 to 80 $\times$ 10^9/L) after receiving five random donor units (containing a total of about 3.0 $\times$ 10^{11} platelets) would have a PPR of 87% and a CCI of 20,000.

The expected CCI between 10 minutes and one hour post-tranfusion is >7500. The CCI measured at 18 to 24 hours after transfusion should be >4500 (122). However, both the PPR and CCI require measuring the platelet count in the platelet product itself (not routinely performed), and are seldom used outside of research purposes.

☞ **For an average-size adult, the usual platelet dose (300–400 × 10^9) within 5 units of pooled random-donor platelets, or one single-donor (plateletpheresis) product, is expected to raise the platelet count approximately 50 × 10^9/L immediately after transfusion. However, in an observational study (122a) of platelet transfusions in critically ill patients, the median post-transfusion platelet count rise was much lower at 14 × 10^9/L.** ☞ In a trauma setting, a suboptimal platelet count rise probably reflects ongoing platelet consumption or hemodilution, although in other patient settings (e.g., cancer patients) alloimmune refractoriness may be operative.

Platelet Transfusion Refractoriness

If the post-transfusion platelet count is less than expected (e.g., CCI < 7500 at 1 hour) on two consecutive transfusions, the patient is considered "refractory" to platelet transfusion. This is generally caused by shortened survival of transfused platelets (123). Reasons for refractoriness are often multifactorial, and can be classified by non-immune and immune causes (Table 7) (124–126). In the trauma patient, the most common explanation probably is accelerated platelet

Table 7 Nonimmune and Immune Causes of Platelet Transfusion Refractoriness

Nonimmune	Immune
Platelet quality (storage lesion)	HLA alloimmunization
DIC[a]	ABO incompatibility[a]
Sepsis[a]	Allo- or isoantibodies against platelet-specific allo(iso)antigens[b]
Fever[a]	
Splenomegaly	
Amphotericin B	
Post-bone marrow transplantation	

[a]DIC, sepsis, and fever are common in trauma patients; however, it should be noted that these factors were identified in studies (124–126) of cancer patients, rather than trauma patients.
[b]allo-or isoantibodies are a rare from of immune-mediated platelet dysfunction.
Abbreviation: DIC, disseminated intravascular coagulation.

destruction associated with DIC, SIRS, and so on. In contrast, immune causes of refractoriness predominate in multiply transfused patients (e.g., cancer patients). However, a multiparous female trauma victim with multiple HLA alloantibodies (resulting from previous pregnancies) could have immune refractoriness. The standard practice of administering "incompatible" platelets (e.g., from a blood group A donor to a group O recipient) can also lead to a blunted platelet count response, particularly if the recipient has high-titer (>1:64) anti-A antibodies (127).

Platelet Transfusion Triggers

Therapeutic platelet transfusion indicates when platelets are given to treat clinically important bleeding in the context of thrombocytopenia. Prophylactic platelet transfusion denotes their use in preventing bleeding in thrombocytopenic patients. Platelet count thresholds below which the potential risk of hemorrhage is judged to outweigh the risks associated with platelet transfusions (discussed later in the section on "Complications of Platelet Transfusions") are known as "platelet triggers." However, appropriate triggers vary broadly among various clinical situations (Table 8), and further require individualized assessment of patient risk (73–75,128–133).

Platelet transfusion triggers have been evaluated most extensively in cancer patients receiving myeloablative chemotherapy, particularly adults with acute leukemia. In this patient population, a platelet threshold of 10 × 10^9/L is believed to be safe, unless there is concomitant bleeding or fever, in which case a threshold of 20 × 10^9/L is used (128). In 2001, the American Society of Clinical Oncology (ASCO) published guidelines for platelet transfusion that included recommended platelet count thresholds for thrombocytopenic patients undergoing invasive procedures (129). These guidelines are largely based on retrospective reviews, as few (if any) randomized trials have been done. The ASCO guidelines state that, in the absence of other coagulopathies, a platelet count of at least 40 to 50 × 10^9/L is sufficient to perform major invasive procedures, including placement of central venous catheters, lumbar punctures, endoscopic transbronchial and esophageal biopsies, fiberoptic bronchoscopy and broncholaveolar lavage, and even major surgery. Certain procedures are safe at even lower platelet counts, e.g., most hematologists do not transfuse

Table 8   Platelet Transfusion Triggers

Clinical scenario	Platelet transfusion trigger ($\times 10^9$/L)
Neurosurgery/head trauma	$\leq$100
Major surgery	$\leq$50
Massive transfusion	$\leq$50
Central venous catheter insertion	$\leq$50
Transbronchial and gastrointestinal endoscopy with biopsy[a]	$\leq$50
Liver biopsy	$\leq$50
Lumbar puncture	$\leq$20
Acute leukemia (with fever or bleeding)	$\leq$10 ($\leq$20)

Triggers are based on the authors' interpretation of various published studies and reviews (73–75,128–133).

[a]Prophylactic platelet transfusions may not be necessary for endoscopy even if the platelet count is $<20 \times 10^9$/L, provided that biopsy is not performed (133).

Table 9   Risk of Infection per Unit of Blood

Transmissible infectious disease	Approximate risk
HIV[a]	1/1,930,000 (134)
Human T-cell leukemia/ lymphoma virus	Negligible (with leukodepletion)
Hepatitis A	Very rare
Hepatitis B	1/138,700 (134)
Hepatitis C[a]	<1/543,000 (134)
Syphilis	Extremely rare
Septicemia	1/10,000 septic episodes per unit of platelets transfused (114)

[a]Blood screening includes NAT for viral genetic material and thus gives greater sensitivity for detecting HIV and hepatitis C than serology alone. *Abbreviations*: HIV, human immunodeficiency virus; NAT, nucleic acid testing.

platelets before performing a bone marrow aspirate and biopsy even when the platelet count is less than 20×10^9/L (129). Liver biopsy was judged to be relatively safe at a platelet count of at least 50×10^9/L (129), based upon a retrospective study in which patients with moderate thrombocytopenia (50 to 99×10^9/L) had a bleeding incidence similar to controls without thrombocytopenia (130).

Prophylactic platelet transfusion after massive transfusion did not show improved outcomes in a randomized control trial (70). However, aggressive correction of thrombocytopenia and coagulopathies was associated with improved survival in one retrospective study (72). In general, when bleeding is evident or severe thrombocytopenia is present (generally, less than 50×10^9/L), platelet transfusion support is considered appropriate (73–75). An even higher platelet count threshold (100×10^9/L) is suggested prior to neurosurgical procedures (74,132), suggesting a similar trigger may be appropriate in trauma patients with serious head injury or evidence for intracranial bleed. Table 8 lists the platelet transfusion triggers for various clinical scenarios.

Contraindications to Platelet Transfusions

For some thrombocytopenic patients, platelet transfusions are contraindicated (73,95). For example, immune HIT and thrombotic thrombocytopenic purpura (TTP) are characterized by in vivo platelet activation and vWF-dependent platelet agglutination, respectively. Theoretically, platelet transfusions could increase the risk for vessel occlusion in these patients. Platelet transfusions are also contraindicated when the patient has pseudothrombocytopenia, as the actual circulating platelet count is normal.

Complications of Platelet Transfusion
Infection
Viral Infection
Continuing improvements in screening for transmissible infectious disease in the developed world have greatly reduced the risk for blood-borne infection (Table 9) (134). As most platelet transfusions are pooled from five or more different donors, they carry a greater relative risk of

viral contamination than individual red cells or plasma transfusions, but the difference in absolute risk remains negligible. Transfusion-transmitted Creutzfeld–Jacob disease (prion disease) has also been reported.

Bacterial Contamination
Currently, the most common cause of mortality directly attributable to a platelet transfusion is bacterial contamination leading to septicemia (114,135). This is because platelets—unlike red cells and plasma—are stored at room temperature, making a fertile culture medium for bacteria. The reported incidence of bacterial contamination of platelets is about 1/3000, but usually without clinical consequence as few organisms are actually transfused (114). Overt sepsis is estimated at about 1/50,000 per platelet unit transfused (114), with significant risk for morbidity and mortality. Besides fever and chills, clinical features that suggest bacterial contamination of a blood product include hypotension/shock, vomiting, and respiratory distress beginning within two hours of transfusion (114).

Non-infectious
Febrile Non-hemolytic Transfusion Reactions (FNHTR)
This is the most common complication of platelet transfusion, with an overall frequency of about 25% to 30% (117,136,137): The reaction is about five times more common following platelet than red cell transfusions. Typically, symptoms occur toward the end of the transfusion, and include a rise in temperature by at least 1°C, often accompanied by chills, rigors, feelings of discomfort, nausea and vomiting. Sometimes, these symptoms are present without a rise in temperature. The reaction is self-limiting, and responds to antipyretics. If the reaction is very severe or accompanied by hypotension or respiratory distress, bacterial contamination must be suspected, the transfusion immediately stopped, and the unit(s) returned for culture. FNHTR appears to be caused by leukocyte-derived proinflammatory cytokines (e.g., interleukin-6) (137), and thus occurs more often with older platelet units (136), and much less often when the blood product has undergone prestorage leukodepletion (118).

Allergic and Anaphylactic Reactions

Allergic reactions after platelet (or other blood component) transfusions are due to plasma proteins within the blood product reacting with pre-existing IgE antibodies in the recipient. This results in a type I hypersensitivity reaction and the release of histamine and prostaglandins from mast cells. Symptoms and signs include cutaneous reactions (urticaria, pruritus, erythema, flushing), cardiorespiratory complications (laryngeal edema with the potential for upper airway obstruction, wheezing, chest tightness, chest pain), gastrointestinal complaints (nausea, vomiting, abdominal cramps), and hypotension. Urticaria (hives) occur in about 3% of blood transfusions (138), and usually respond to antihistamines. Other preventative measures for recipients that have experienced less severe anaphylactic reactions include washed blood products that are deplete of plasma proteins and premedication with antihistamines and/or steroids (138). For mild reactions, the transfusion can be resumed as the symptoms abate.

Anaphylactic reactions are characterized by intractable hypotension and shock, often with a component of airway obstruction; fever is usually not seen. This syndrome is caused by IgG anti-IgA antibodies that can occur in IgA-deficient patients (139), as small quantities of IgA are present in the blood product. The frequency is about 1/20,000 to 1/50,000 units of blood products transfused (140). Anaphylactic transfusion reactions usually begin very soon after initiating transfusion. Treatment involves immediate discontinuation of the transfusion, subcutaneous epinephrine, intravenous fluids, and other measures appropriate for shock. The patient's pretransfusion serum must be tested for the presence of anti-IgA antibody and if present, blood products from IgA-deficient blood donors, or washed blood products, can be given.

Alloimmune Thrombocytopenia

There are two rare situations in which blood products—including platelets—can paradoxically cause thrombocytopenia: PTP and PAT (141). PTP typically begins about 1 week after blood transfusion, and is characterized by generally severe thrombocytopenia and mucocutaneous hemorrhage. Typically, affected patients are elderly parous women who are homozygous for the HPA-1b alloantigen on platelets, and they form strong anti-HPA-1a alloantibodies (also known as anti-Zw^a and anti-Pl^{A1} alloantibodies), although other alloantigen systems have also been implicated. For uncertain reasons, these alloantibodies lead to transient destruction of the patient's own platelets. IVIgG with or without platelet transfusions (ideally, giving HPA-1a negative platelets) is used for treatment. The timeframe of PTP closely resembles immune HIT, with which it can be confused (142).

In contrast, PAT is characterized by abrupt onset of severe thrombocytopenia following a blood transfusion (141,143). It is caused by the passive administration of antiplatelet alloantibodies that were present in the plasma of the blood donor, for example, if the donor was sensitized to a platelet alloantigen such as HPA-1a during previous pregnancy, and the blood product recipient is HPA-1a positive. In contrast to PTP, this syndrome resolves within a few days.

Transfusion-Related Acute Lung Injury

Transfusion-related Acute Lung Injury (TRALI) is a very rare but life-threatening acute lung injury caused by plasma-containing blood components. Clinically and radiologically, TRALI resembles ARDS, with typical onset between one and six hours after transfusion. The mortality rate is about 5% to 10% (cf. ARDS: 40–50% mortality), with the survivors usually recovering within 48 to 96 hours (144–146). Passive transfer of complement-fixing alloantibodies against granulocyte-specific or HLA antigens present within donor plasma is believed to cause this syndrome. Other possible mechanisms of pulmonary injury include neutrophil-priming lipids which may develop during routine storage of blood components (147,148) and cytokine-mediated injury, e.g., tumor necrosis factor. Although very rare, TRALI is the third most common cause of transfusion-related death (after ABO hemolytic reaction and bacteremia). Aggressive supportive treatment, including mechanical ventilation, is often needed for this transient but life-threatening syndrome.

THROMBOCYTOSIS

Physiologic vs. Pathologic

☞ **Thrombocytosis in the trauma patient typically represents an appropriate physiologic response to initial acute thrombocytopenia, and thus is normal and expected in the second or third week post-trauma (Fig. 2) (149–151).** ☞ Indeed, lack of thrombocytosis during this time period may indicate ongoing complications (septicemia, SIRS, ARDS, etc). This is consistent with a retrospective study (152) that found thrombocytosis in critical care patients to be associated with lower mortality despite longer intensive care unit (ICU) stays, that is, the longer ICU stay provided sufficient time to observe the expected increase in platelet count in a recovering patient. Table 10 lists the differential diagnosis of thrombocytosis.

Two studies of platelet counts following orthopedic surgery indicate the magnitude of post-thrombocytopenia thrombocytosis that can be expected following trauma (2,151). The median peak platelet count in a post-orthopedic

Table 10 Causes of Thrombocytosis

Physiologic

Post-thrombocytopenia thrombocytosis (common during second and third week post-trauma)

Post-splenectomy or congenital/acquired asplenia (the peak postoperative platelet count in a trauma patient who undergoes splenectomy typically reaches 500 to 1500 × 10^9/L; subsequently, the platelet count declines to a normal range that is about one-third higher than in normal, non-splenectomized patients, reflecting absence of splenic pooling

Hereditary or familial thrombocytosis

Pathologic

Inflammatory/infectious (polymyalgia rheumatica, rheumatoid arthritis, polyarteritis nodosa, inflammatory bowel disease, tuberculosis, chronic infection)

Neoplastic (myeloproliferative disorders, e.g., polycythemia rubra vera, chronic myeloid leukemia; essential thrombocythemia, myeloid metaplasia; myelodysplasia, e.g., 5q- syndrome, refractory anemia with ringed sideroblasts; solid tumors, especially metastatic)

Iron deficiency

Hemolytic anemia

Pseudothrombocytosis (e.g., burns)

patient population is about 400 to 500×10^9/L, with the upper 2 SD value approximately 1000×10^9/L.

Post-splenectomy

Dramatic thrombocytosis is common following splenectomy performed following trauma, for example, for splenic rupture. This is because physiologic thrombocytosis that follows acute trauma-associated thrombocytopenia is exacerbated by the lack of splenic sequestration of platelets, which normally represents about one-third of the platelet distribution. Thus, platelet counts as high as 1500×10^9/L can occur, usually peaking about 12 to 14 days following trauma, occasionally later. It is unknown whether physiologic thrombocytosis imparts a greater risk for postoperative thrombosis compared with a similar patient who has a less marked platelet count rise. ☞ **Long-term, the loss of platelet sequestration means that the platelet count of the post-splenectomy patient is about 30% higher than the preoperative platelet count, baseline (153).** ☞

EYE TO THE FUTURE

Platelets are extraordinarily complex "cells" that provide effective hemostasis in response to day-to-day tissue injury and in response to major trauma. Platelets serve as the major effectors of primary hemostasis by forming the platelet plug at the site of injury, and they are crucial for proper secondary hemostasis by providing the proper phospholipid membrane surface for coagulation reactions. At present, the only routine source of exogenous platelets are pooled concentrates from allogeneic donors or apheresis platelets, stored at room temperature for a maximum of five days. Despite advances in safety processing and storage of conventional platelet concentrates, there are still important shortcomings, including short supply. There is much interest in developing novel platelet products and platelet substitutes, and some of these products are entering phase III clinical trials.

Novel platelet products include frozen platelets, cold-liquid stored platelets, photochemically treated platelets (a strategy for pathogen inactivation), platelet-derived microparticles, lyophilized platelets, and platelets cultured from megakaryocytes in vitro (154). Frozen platelets are currently the only viable alternative to fresh platelets, but cryopreservation is cumbersome and expensive, and offers little advantage over standard platelet products.

Various platelet substitutes are under current investigation (154). "Thromboerythrocytes" are red cells with surface-bound fibrinogen or surface-bound arginine-glycine-aspartic acid (fibrinogen-mimicking) peptides. Fibrinogen-coated albumin microcapsules/microspheres are albumin-based microspheres coated with fibrinogen. These platelet substitutes promote hemostasis by enhancing platelet activation and aggregation at sites of vessel injury. Liposome-based hemostatic agents include plateletsomes, which are extracts of platelet membranes contained within a lipid vesicle, and vesicles that contain phospholipid with or without Factor Xa. These products have only undergone preclinical testing (animal models).

Finally, one possible alternative approach for otherwise uncontrollable bleeding in a trauma patient may become available: recombinant factor VIIa (rVIIa, NovoSeven, Novo Nordisk, Denmark). This agent is believed to promote hemostasis either by facilitating tissue factor-mediated initiation of coagulation, or by binding directly to the surface of activated platelets, where it directly activates factor X in the absence of TF (30,31). The latter mechanism does not require coagulation factors VIII or IX, and may explain why rVIIa in high doses is effective for bleeding patients with hemophilia A or B (lacking factor VIII or IX, respectively) who have developed inhibitory antibodies against the factor they lack. Although rVIIa is currently approved only for hemophiliacs with inhibitors, its investigational and "off-label" use as a general procoagulant agent in a variety of challenging hemostatic crises—including patients with severe coagulopathy and bleeding secondary to trauma—is increasing (155–159).

Unfortunately, this agent is extremely expensive: the approximate per-patient cost for one regimen under study for bleeding following trauma (200 μg/kg first dose, with two subsequent 100 μg/kg doses one and three hr later) is about US \$20,000 (assumes an 80-kg recipient, and an approximate cost of CDN \$1/μg rVIIa) (160).

Recently, Dutton et al. showed that rFVIIa therapy led to an immediate clinical reduction of coagulopathic hemorrhages in a retrospectively reviewed series of trauma cases conducted at the Maryland Shock-Trauma Center (161). More recently, two prospective placebo-controlled, double-blind RCTs, one in blunt trauma ($n = 143$) and the other in penetrating trauma ($n = 134$) were completed (162). The studies suggest that rFVIIa may decrease transfusion requirements, particularly in patients with blunt trauma.

In another retrospective study, Dutton's group showed that profound acidosis and severe shock may predict failure of rFVIIa therapy for trauma-related coagulopathy, and suggest that these variables should be considered as potential contraindications to the use of rFVIIa (163). Although earlier administration of rFVIIa, before the development of massive blood loss and severe shock, may increase the rate of clinical response, few would administer this very expensive drug unless some of these poor prognosticating signs were present.

Accordingly, further research is required to identify those bleeding trauma patients in whom this therapy is safe and effective; in addition, the optimum dose and duration of rFVIIa therapy requires further clarification.

SUMMARY

Platelets are produced in the bone marrow by the megakaryocyte, and normally survive for about 10 days. In normal individuals, the platelet count is usually fairly constant within a broad normal range (about $150–400 \times 10^9$/L). The megakaryocyte-stimulating hormone, TPO, contributes to platelet count regulation via a primitive feedback loop. Normally, about 30% of circulating platelets are exchangeably sequestered within the spleen (splenic pooling).

In trauma patients, initial thrombocytopenia is usually caused by increased platelet consumption (DIC) or hemodilution (fluid resuscitation). Thrombocytopenia that persists or that begins later during the hospitalization often indicates complications, such as septicemia, SIRS, ARDS, or drug reactions, particularly immune HIT. Blood levels of TPO increase after trauma-induced thrombocytopenia, which leads to transient thrombocytosis that peaks about 14 days post-trauma, before returning to baseline during the third week. If a trauma patient undergoes splenectomy, the platelet counts are about 30% greater than expected because of the absence of physiologic splenic platelet pooling.

Investigating thrombocytopenia in a trauma patient includes: assessing the temporal features of the thrombocytopenia (early thrombocytopenia: DIC and/or hemodilution; late thrombocytopenia: bacteremia, SIRS, ARDS, drug reaction, etc.); clinical evidence for impaired hemostasis (petechiae, ecchymoses, line-site oozing, etc); severity of the thrombocytopenia (e.g., prophylactic platelet transfusions often are appropriate for platelet count thresholds between 50 and 100×10^9/L, depending on the perceived bleeding risk); and coagulation assays, including testing for DIC (e.g., fibrin D-dimers). Impaired primary hemostasis results from thrombocytopenia and anemia, as adequate red cell numbers are required in the microcirculation to optimize platelet–subendothelial interactions. Even though mild von Willebrand disease is a common congenital bleeding disorder, it only rarely contributes to bleeding in these patients, as vWF levels can increase dramatically during the acute "stress" associated with trauma.

Blood cultures are appropriate in patients with unexpected "late" thrombocytopenia. Immune HIT is a prothrombotic adverse reaction of heparin that mandates cessation of heparin, and usually also requires substitution with an alternative anticoagulant. However, warfarin is contraindicated during acute HIT because it paradoxically increases the risk for thrombosis, particularly microvascular thrombosis associated with limb loss (syndrome of warfarin-associated venous limb gangrene complicating immune HIT).

KEY POINTS

- The normal platelet count range is between 150 and 400×10^9/L. Although this is a wide normal range, the platelet count tends to remain fairly constant during the lifetime of an individual (1).
- Normal platelet survival is approximately 10 days.
- Normally, about one-third of the circulating platelets are exchangeably sequestered within the spleen; increased spleen size leads to greater splenic pooling and thus thrombocytopenia ("hypersplenism").
- Acute decrease in the platelet count in trauma leads to increase in TPO levels. The long half-life of TPO (30 hours) and its effects on early megakaryocyte progenitors mean that this trauma-associated thrombocytopenia is invariably followed by thrombocytosis from day 7 to 21 (peak, days 12–14), unless clinical complications lead to ongoing platelet consumption.
- Three components are required for normal primary hemostasis: (*i*) platelets, (*ii*) vWF, and (*iii*) normal hematocrit. In trauma, acquired thrombocytopenia and anemia lead to impaired primary hemostasis.
- Four general mechanisms for thrombocytopenia exist: (*i*) decreased platelet production, (*ii*) increased platelet consumption (or destruction), (*iii*) hemodilution, and (iv) hypersplenism. Only two mechanisms—increased platelet consumption and hemodilution—are common in acute trauma. However, decreased production can develop following critical illness, or (along with hypersplenism) can be present as a pre-existing condition.
- The hallmark of severe thrombocytopenia is mucocutaneous bleeding, particularly pin-point intradermal hemorrhages known as *petechiae*.
- "Pseudothrombocytosis" occurs in patients with severe burns (36): Thermal injury to red cells produces microspherocytes that can be falsely identified as platelets by the electronic particle counter, and thus suggest apparent thrombocytosis when the patient may actually suffer acute burn-induced thrombocytopenia and DIC.
- Coagulation testing is needed to distinguish whether thrombocytopenia is caused by hemodilution or acute DIC in a patient with trauma. Generally, increase in fibrin D-dimers or a positive paracoagulation assay (e.g., protamine sulfate test) is confirmatory of DIC. Both hemodilution and DIC can cause abnormalities in routine coagulation assays, such as the INR, aPTT, TCT, and fibrinogen levels.
- Platelet dysfunction in trauma patients is often the result of renal failure (uremia) or drug effects (e.g., aspirin, clopidogrel).
- Dilutional thrombocytopenia related to fluid resuscitation is the most common cause of thrombocytopenia in a trauma patient. Repeated CBC and coagulation testing is important to assess the presence and severity of coexisting DIC.
- When diffuse bleeding is evident or relatively severe thrombocytopenia is documented (generally, less than 50×10^9/L), platelet transfusion support is appropriate (73–75). A higher platelet count threshold (i.e., 100×10^9/L) is a more appropriate transfusion trigger for certain conditions (e.g., traumatic brain injury).
- Late onset of thrombocytopenia in a trauma patient can indicate acute bacteremia, so blood cultures should always be drawn in this situation.
- HIT is by far the most common drug-induced, immune-mediated thrombocytopenia. Paradoxically, HIT is associated with thrombosis rather than bleeding.
- Hypotension and/or abdominal pain in a thrombocytopenic patient treated with heparin suggests bilateral adrenal hemorrhagic infarction with acute adrenal failure: Corticosteroid replacement therapy can be life-saving.
- For an average-size adult, the usual platelet dose ($300–400 \times 10^9$) within five units of pooled random-donor platelets, or one single-donor (plateletpheresis) product, is expected to raise the platelet count approximately 50×10^9/L immediately after transfusion.
- However, in an observational study (122a) of platelet transfusions in critically ill patients, the median post-transfusion platelet count rise was much lower at 14×10^9/L.
- Thrombocytosis in the trauma patient typically represents an appropriate physiologic response to initial acute thrombocytopenia, and thus is normal and expected in the second or third week post-trauma (Fig. 2) (149–151).
- Long-term, the loss of platelet sequestration means that the platelet count of the post-splenectomy patient is about 30% higher than the preoperative platelet count baseline.

REFERENCES

1. Brecher G, Schneiderman M, Cronkite EP. The reproducibility and constancy of the platelet count. Am J Clin Pathol 1953; 23:15–26.
2. Warkentin TE, Levine MN, Hirsh J, et al. Heparin-induced thrombocytopenia in patients treated with low-molecular-weight heparin or unfractionated heparin. N Engl J Med 1995; 332:1330–1335.
3. Harker L. Megakaryocyte quantitation. J Clin Invest 1968; 47:452–457.

4. Long MW. Megakaryocyte differentiation events. Semin Hematol 1998; 35:192–199.

5. Bruno E, Hoffman R. Human megakaryocyte progenitor cells. Semin Hematol 1998; 35:183–191.

6. Berkow RL, Straneva JE, Bruno E, Beyer GS, Burgess JS, Hoffman R. Isolation of human megakaryocytes by density centrifugation and counterflow centrifugal elutriation. J Lab Clin Med 1984; 103:811 818.

7. Nurden P, Poujol C, Nurden AT. The evolution of megakaryocytes to platelets. Baillieres Clin Haematol 1997; 10:1–27.

8. Italiano JE Jr, Lecine P, Shivdasani RA, Hartwig JH. Blood platelets are assembled principally at the ends of proplatelet processes produced by differentiated megakaryocytes. J Cell Biol 1999; 147:1299–1312.

9. Zucker-Franklin D, Philipp CS. Platelet production in the pulmonary capillary bed. New ultrastructural evidence for an old concept. Am J Pathol 2000; 157:69–74.

10. Paulus JM. Platelet size in man. Blood 1975; 46:321–326.

11. Corash L, Chen HY, Levin J, Baker G, Lu H, Mok Y. Regulation of thrombopoiesis: effects of the degree of thrombocytopenia on megakaryocyte ploidy and platelet volume. Blood 1987; 70:177–185.

12. Warkentin TE, Powling MJ, Hardisty RM. Measurement of fibrinogen binding to platelets by flow cytometry in whole blood: a micromethod for the detection of platelet activation. Br J Haematol 1990; 76:387–394.

13. Opper C, Schuessler G, Kuschel M, et al. Analysis of GTP-binding proteins, phosphoproteins, and cytosolic calcium in functional heterogeneous human blood platelet subpopulations. Biochem Pharmacol 1997; 54:1027–1035.

14. Aster RH. Pooling of platelets in the spleen: role in the pathogenesis of "hypersplenic" thrombocytopenia. J Clin Invest 1966; 45:645–657.

15. Harker LA, Finch CA. Thrombokinetics in man. J Clin Invest 1969; 48:963–974.

16. Wadenvik H, Jacobsson S, Kutti J, Syrjala M. In vitro and in vivo behavior of ^{111}In-labelled platelets: an experimental study of healthy male volunteers. Eur J Haematol 1987; 38:415–425.

17. Peters AM, Saverymuttu SH, Wonke B, Lewis SM, Lavender JP. The interpretation of platelet kinetic studies for the identification of sites of abnormal platelet destruction. Br J Haematol 1984; 57:637–649.

18. Wadenvik H, Denfors I, Kutti J. Splenic blood flow and intrasplenic platelet kinetics in relation to spleen volume. Br J Haematol 1987; 67:181–185.

19. Peck-Radosavljevic M. Hypersplenism. Eur J Gastroenterol Hepatol 2001; 13:317–323.

20. Kaushansky K. Thrombopoietin. N Engl J Med 1998; 339:746–754.

21. de Sauvage FJ, Hass PE, Spencer SD, et al. Stimulation of megakaryocytopoiesis and thrombopoiesis by the c-Mpl ligand. Nature 1994; 369:533–538.

22. Lok S, Kaushansky K, Holly RD, et al. Cloning and expression of murine thrombopoietin cDNA and stimulation of platelet production in vivo. Nature 1994; 369:565–568.

23. McCarty JM, Sprugel KH, Fox NE, Sabath DE, Kaushansky K. Murine thrombopoietin mRNA levels are modulated by platelet count. Blood 1995; 86:3668–3675.

24. Chen J, Herceg-Harjacek L, Groopman JE, Grabarek J. Regulation of platelet activation in vitro by the c-Mpl ligand, thrombopoietin. Blood 1995; 86:4054–4062.

25. Emmons RV, Reid DM, Cohen RL, et al. Human thrombopoietin levels are high when thrombocytopenia is due to megakaryocyte deficiency and low when due to increased platelet destruction. Blood 1996; 87:4068–4071.

26. Hobisch-Hagen P, Jelkmann W, Mayr A, et al. Low platelet count and elevated serum thrombopoietin after severe trauma. Eur J Haematol 2000; 64:157–163.

27. Li J, Yang C, Xia Y, et al. Thrombocytopenia caused by the development of antibodies to thrombopoietin. Blood 2001; 98:3241–3248.

28. Dopheide SM, Yap CL, Jackson SP. Dynamic aspects of platelet adhesion under flow. Clin Exp Pharmacol Physiol 2001; 28:355–363.

29. Siemiatkowski A, Kloczko J, Galar M, Czaban S. von Willebrand factor antigen as a prognostic marker in posttraumatic acute lung injury. Haemostasis 2000; 30:189–195.

30. Monroe DM, Hoffman M, Allen GA, Roberts GA. The factor VII-platelet interplay: effectiveness of recombinant factor VIIa in the treatment of bleeding in severe thrombocytopathia. Semin Thromb Hemost 2000; 26:373–377.

31. Hoffman M, Monroe DM. A cell-based model of hemostasis. Thromb Haemost 2001; 85:958–965.

32. Hanson SR, Slichter SJ. Platelet kinetics in patients with bone marrow hypoplasia: evidence for a fixed platelet requirement. Blood 1985; 66:1105–1109.

33. Bessman JD, Gilmer PR, Gardner FH. Use of mean platelet volume improves detection of platelet disorders. Blood Cells 1985; 11:127–135.

34. Bizzaro N. EDTA-dependent pseudothrombocytopenia: a clinical and epidemiological study of 112 cases, with 10-year follow-up. Am J Hematol 1995; 50:103–109.

35. Fiorin F, Steffan A, Pradella P, Bizzaro N, Potenza R, De Angelis V. IgG platelet antibodies in EDTA-dependent pseudothrombocytopenia bind to platelet membrane glycoprotein IIb. Am J Clin Pathol 1998; 110:178–183.

36. Lawrence C, Atac B. Hematologic changes in massive burn injury. Crit Care Med 1992; 20:1284–1288.

37. Rosner F, Rubenberg ML. Erythrocyte fragmentation in consumption coagulopathy [letter]. N Engl J Med 1969; 280:219–220.

38. Spero JA, Lewis JH, Hasiba U. Disseminated intravascular coagulation. Findings in 346 patients. Thromb Haemost 1980; 43:28–33.

39. Niewiarowski S, Gurewich V. Laboratory identification of intravascular coagulation: the serial dilution protamine sulfate test for the detection of fibrin monomer and fibrin degradation products. J Lab Clin Med 1971; 77:665–676.

40. George JN, Woolf SH, Raskob GE, et al. Idiopathic thrombocytopenic purpura: a practice guideline developed by explicit methods for the American Society of Hematology. Blood 1996; 88:3–40.

41. Cines DB, Blanchette VS. Immune thrombocytopenic purpura. N Engl J Med 2002; 346:995–1008.

42. Warkentin TE. Management of immune thrombocytopenia. In: Simon TL, Dzik WH, Snyder EL, Stowell CP, Strauss RG, eds. Rossi's Principles of Transfusion Medicine, 3rd ed. Philadelphia: Williams & Wilkins, 2002:367–395.

43. Mhawech P, Saleem A. Inherited giant platelet disorders. Classification and literature review. Am J Clin Pathol 2000; 113:176–190.

44. Lindenbaum J, Lieber CS. Hematologic effects of alcohol in man in the absence of nutritional deficiency. N Engl J Med 1969; 281:333–338.

45. Menke DM, Colon-Otero G, Cockerill KJ, Jenkins RB, Noel P, Pierre RV. Refractory thrombocytopenia. A myelodysplastic syndrome that may mimic immune thrombocytopenic purpura. Am J Clin Pathol 1992; 98:502–510.

46. Weigert AL, Schafer AI. Uremic bleeding: pathogenesis and therapy. Am J Med Sci 1998; 316:94–104.

47. Livio M, Gotti E, Marchesi D, Mecca G, Remuzzi G, de Gaetano G. Uraemic bleeding: role of anaemia and beneficial effect of red blood cell transfusions. Lancet 1982; 2:1013–1015.

48. Fernandez F, Goudable C, Sie P, et al. Low hematocrit and prolonged bleeding time in uraemic patients: effect of red cell transfusions. Br J Haematol 1985; 59:139–148.

49. Boneu B, Fernandez F. The role of the hematocrit in bleeding. Transfus Med Rev 1987; 1:182–185.

50. Moia M, Mannucci PM, Vizzotto L, Casati S, Cattaneo M, Ponticelli C. Improvement in the haemostatic defect of uraemia after treatment with recombinant human erythropoietin. Lancet 1987; 2:1227–1229.

51. Mannucci PM, Remuzzi G, Pusineri F, et al. Deamino-8-D-arginine vasopressin shortens the bleeding time in uremia. N Engl J Med 1983; 308:8–12.

52. Canavese C, Salomone M, Pacitti A, Mangiarotti G, Calitri V. Reduced response of uraemic bleeding time to repeated doses of desmopressin [letter]. Lancet 1985:1:867–868.

53. Lin YK, Kosfeld RE, Marcum SG. Treatment of uraemic bleeding with conjugated oestrogens. Lancet 1984; 2:887–890.

54. Livio M, Mannucci PM, Viganò G, et al. Conjugated estrogens for the management of bleeding associated with renal failure. N Engl J Med 1986; 315:731–735.

55. Vigano G, Gaspari F, Locatelli M, Pusineri F, Bonati M, Remuzzi G. Dose–effect and pharmacokinetics of estrogens given to correct bleeding time in uremia. Kidney Int 1988; 34:853–858.

56. Shemin D, Elnour M, Amarantes B, Abuelo JG, Chazan JA. Oral estrogens decrease bleeding time and improve clinical bleeding in patients with renal failure. Am J Med 1990; 89:436–440.

57. Zoja C, Noris M, Corna D, et al. L-Arginine, the precursor of nitric oxide, abolishes the effect of estrogens on bleeding time in experimental uremia. Lab Invest 1991; 65:479–483.

58. Janson PA, Jubelirer SJ, Weinstein MJ, Deykin D. Treatment of the bleeding tendency in uremia with cryoprecipitate. N Engl J Med 1980; 303:1318–1322.

59. Triulzi DJ, Blumberg N. Variability in response to cryoprecipitate treatment for hemostatic defects in uremia. Yale J Biol Med 1990; 63:1–7.

60. Humphries JE. Transfusion therapy in acquired coagulopathies. Hematol/Oncol Clin North Am 1994; 8:1181–1201.

61. Révész T, Arets B, Bierings M, van den Bos C, Duval E. Recombinant factor VIIa in severe uremic bleeding [letter]. Thromb Haemost 1998; 80:353.

62. Casonato A, Pontara E, Vertolli UP, et al. Plasma and platelet von Willebrand factor abnormalities in patients with uremia: lack of correlation with uremic bleeding. Clin Appl Thromb Hemost 2001; 7:81–86.

63. Bashein G, Nessly ML, Rice AL, Counts RB, Misbach GA. Preoperative aspirin therapy and reoperation for bleeding after coronary artery bypass surgery. Arch Intern Med 1991; 151:89–93.

64. Yende S, Wunderink RG. Effect of clopidogrel on bleeding after coronary artery bypass surgery. Crit Care Med 2001; 29: 2271–2275.

65. Bennett JS. Novel platelet inhibitors. Annu Rev Med 2001; 52:161–184.

66. Geis GD. Update on clinical developments with celecoxib, a new specific COX-2 inhibitor: what can we expect? Scand J Rheumatol 1999; 28(suppl):31–37.

67. Mannucci PM, Vicente V, Vianello L, et al. Controlled trial of desmopressin in liver cirrhosis and other conditions associated with a prolonged bleeding time. Blood 1986; 67:1148–1153.

68. Harvey MP, Greenfield TP, Sugrue ME, Rosenfeld D. Massive blood transfusion in a tertiary referral hospital. Clinical outcomes and haemostatic complications. Med J Aust 1995; 163:356–359.

69. Sawyer PR, Harrison CR. Massive transfusion in adults. Diagnoses, survival and blood bank support. Vox Sang 1990; 58:199–203.

70. Reed LR, Ciavarella D, Heimbach DM, et al. Prophylactic platelet administration during massive transfusion: a prospective randomized double-blind clinical study. Ann Surg 1986; 203:40–48.

71. Harrigan C, Lucas CE, Ledgerwood AM, Walz DA, Mammen EF. Serial changes in primary hemostasis after massive transfusion. Surgery 1985; 98:836–844.

72. Cinat ME, Wallace WC, Nastanski F, et al. Improved survival following massive transfusion in patients who have undergone trauma. Arch Surg 1999; 134:964–970.

73. British Committee for Standards in Haematology, Blood Transfusion Task Force. Guidelines for the use of platelet transfusions. Br J Haematol 2003; 122:10–23.

74. Rebulla P. Platelet transfusion trigger in difficult patients. Transfus Clin Biol 2001; 8:249–254.

75. Rao MP, Boralessa H, Morgan C, et al. Blood component use in critically ill patients. Anaesthesia 2002; 57:530–534.

76. Kitchens CS. Disseminated intravascular coagulation. Curr Opin Hematol 1995; 2:402–406.

77. Levi M, ten Cate H. Disseminated intravascular coagulation. N Engl J Med 1999; 341:586–592.

78. Levi M, de Jonge E, van der Poll T, ten Cate H. Advances in the understanding of the pathogenetic pathways of disseminated intravascular coagulation result in more insight in the clinical picture and better management strategies. Semin Thromb Hemost 2001; 27:569–575.

79. Bakhtiari K, Meijers JC, de Jonge E, Levi M. Prospective validation of the International Society of Thrombosis and Haemostasis scoring system for disseminated intravascular coagulation. Crit Care Med 2004; 32:2416–2421.

80. Jamieson GA. The activation of platelets by thrombin: a model for activation by high and moderate affinity receptor pathways. In: Jamieson GA, ed. Platelet Membrane Receptors: Molecular Biology, Immunology, Biochemistry, and Pathology. Prog Clin Biol Res 1988; 283:137–158.

81. Gando S, Nanzaki S, Morimoto Y, Ishitani T, Kemmotsu O. Tissue factor pathway inhibitor response does not correlate with tissue-factor induced disseminated intravascular coagulation and multiple organ dysfunction syndrome in trauma patients. Crit Care Med 2001; 29:262–266.

82. Gando S, Nanzaki S, Kemmotsu O. Disseminated intravascular coagulation and sustained systemic inflammatory response syndrome predict organ dysfunctions after trauma. Ann Surg 1999; 229:121–127.

83. Gando S. Disseminated intravascular coagulation in trauma patients. Semin Thromb Hemost 2001; 27:585–592.

84. Addonizio VP, Colman RW. Platelets and extracorporeal circulation. Biomaterials 1982; 3:9–15.

85. Vonderheide RH, Thadhani R, Kuter DJ. Association of thrombocytopenia with the use of intra-aortic balloon pumps. Am J Med 1998; 105:27–32.

86. Pina-Cabral JM, Amaral I, Pinto MM, Gerra LH. Hepatic and splenic platelet sequestration during deep hypothermia in the dog. Haemostasis 1974; 2:235–244.

87. Hessel EA II, Schmer G, Dillard DH. Platelet kinetics during deep hypothermia. J Surg Res 1980; 28:23–34.

88. Holm IA, McLaughlin JF, Feldman K, Stone EF. Recurrent hypothermia and thrombocytopenia after severe neonatal brain infection. Clin Pediatr 1988; 27:326–329.

89. Neame PB, Kelton JG, Walker IR, et al. Thrombocytopenia in septicemia: the role of disseminated intravascular coagulation. Blood 1980; 56:88.

90. François B, Trimoreau F, Vignon P, Fixe P, Praloran V, Gastinne H. Thrombocytopenia in the sepsis syndrome: role of hemophagocytosis and macrophage colony-stimulating factor. Am J Med 1997; 103:114–120.

91. Arvand M, Bhakdi S, Dahlbäck B, Preissner KT. Staphylococcus aureus α-toxin attack on human platelets promotes assembly of the prothrombinase complex. J Biol Chem 1990; 265:14377–14381.

92. Lopez Diez F, Nieto ML, Fernandez-Gallardo S, Gijon MA, Sanchez Crespo M. Occupancy of platelet receptors for platelet-activating factor in patients with septicemia. J Clin Invest 1989; 83:1733–1740.

93. Lee DH, Warkentin TE. Frequency of heparin-induced thrombocytopenia. In: Warkentin TE, Greinacher A, eds. Heparin-Induced Thrombocytopenia, 3rd ed. New York: Marcel Dekker, 2004:107–148.

94. Warkentin TE. Clinical picture of heparin-induced thrombocytopenia. In: Warkentin TE, Greinacher A, eds. Heparin-Induced Thrombocytopenia, 3rd ed. New York: Marcel Dekker, 2004:53–106.

95. Greinacher A, Warkentin TE. Treatment of heparin-induced thrombocytopenia: an overview. In: Warkentin TE, Greinacher A, eds. Heparin-induced Thrombocytopenia, 3rd ed. New York: Marcel Dekker, 2004:335–370.

96. Amiral J, Bridey F, Dreyfus M, et al. Platelet factor 4 complexed to heparin is the target for antibodies generated in heparin-induced thrombocytopenia [letter]. Thromb Haemost 1992; 68:95–96.

97. Li ZQ, Liu W, Park KS, et al. Defining a second epitope for heparin-induced thrombocytopenia/thrombosis antibodies

using KKO, a murine HIT-like monoclonal antibody. Blood 2002; 99:1230–1236.

98. Visentin GP, Moghaddam M, Beery SE, McFarland JG, Aster RH. Heparin is not required for detection of antibodies associated with heparin-induced thrombocytopenia/thrombosis. J Lab Clin Med 2001; 138:22–31.

99. Warkentin TE, Elavathil LJ, Hayward CPM, Johnston MA, Russett JI, Kelton JG. The pathogenesis of venous limb gangrene associated with heparin-induced thrombocytopenia. Ann Intern Med 1997; 127:804–812.

100. Warkentin TE, Kelton JG. A 14-year study of heparin-induced thrombocytopenia. Am J Med 1996; 101:502–507.

101. Warkentin TE. Heparin-induced thrombocytopenia: yet another treatment paradox? Thromb Haemost 2001; 85:947–949.

102. Warkentin TE, Kelton JG. Platelet life cycle: quantitative disorders. In: Handin RI, Lux SE, Stossel TP, eds. Blood: Principles and Practice of Hematology, 2nd ed. Philadelphia: Lippincott, Williams & Wilkins, 2003:983–1047.

103. Medina PJ, Sipols JM, George JN. Drug-associated thrombotic thrombocytopenic purpura–hemolytic uremic syndrome. Curr Opin Hematol 2001; 8:286–293.

104. Mant MJ, Connolly T, Gordon PA, King EG. Severe thrombocytopenia probably due to acute folic acid deficiency. Crit Care Med 1979; 7:297–300.

105. Ibbotson RM, Colvin BT, Colvin MP. Folic acid deficiency during intensive therapy. Br Med J 1975; 4:145.

106. Wallace EL, Chruchill WH, Surgenor DM, et al. Collection and transfusion of blood and blood components in the United States, 1992. Transfusion 1995; 35: 802–812.

107. Anderson NA, Gray S, Copplestone JA, et al. A prospective randomized study of three types of platelet concentrates in patients with haematological malignancy: corrected platelet count increments and frequency of nonhaemolytic febrile transfusion reactions. Transfus Med 1997; 7:33–39.

108. Kelley DL, Fegan RL, Ng AT, et al. High-yield platelet concentrates attainable by continuous quality improvement reduce platelet transfusion cost and donor exposure. Transfusion 1997; 37:482–486.

109. Legler TJ, Fischer I, Dittmann J, et al. Frequency and causes of refractoriness in multiply transfused patients. Ann Hematol 1997; 74:185–189.

110. Chambers LA, Kruskall MS, Pacini DG, Donovan LM. Febrile reactions after platelet transfusions: the effect of single versus multiple donors. Transfusion 1990; 30:219–221.

111. Sarkodee-Adoo CB, Kendall JM, Sridhara R, Lee EJ, Schiffer CA. The relationship between the duration of platelet storage and the development of transfusion reactions. Transfusion 1998; 38:229–235.

112. Sweeney JD, Petrucci J, Yankee R. Pooled platelet concentrates: maybe not fancy, but fiscally sound and effective. Transfus Sci 1997; 18:575–583.

113. Chambers LA, Herman JH. Considerations in the selection of a platelet component: apheresis versus whole blood-derived. Transfus Med Rev 1999; 13:311–322.

114. Blajchman MA, Goldman M. Bacterial contamination of platelet concentrates: incidence, significance, and prevention. Semin Hematol 2001; 38 (suppl 11):20–26.

115. Seghatchian J, Krailadsiri P. The platelet storage lesion. Transfus Med Rev 1997; 11:130–144.

116. Rinder HM, Murphy M, Mitchell JG, Stocks J, Ault KA, Hillman RS. Progressive platelet activation with storage: evidence for shortened survival of activated platelets after transfusion. Transfusion 1991; 31:409–414.

117. Heddle NM, Klama L, Singer J, et al. The role of the plasma from platelet concentrates in transfusion reactions. N Engl J Med 1994; 331:625–628.

118. Patterson BJ, Freedman J, Blanchette V, et al. Effect of premedication guidelines and leukoreduction on the rate of febrile nonhaemolytic platelet transfusion reactions. Transfus Med 2000; 10:199–206.

119. Bordin JO, Heddle NM, Blajchman MA. Biologic effects of leukocytes present in transfused cellular blood products. Blood 1994; 84:1703–1721.

120. Pamphilon DH. The treatment of blood components with ultraviolet-B irradiation. Vox Sang 1998; 74 (suppl 2):15–19.

120a. Petz LD, Garratty G, Calhoun L, et al. Selecting donors of platelets for refractory patients on the basis of HLA antibody specificity. Transfusion 2000; 40(12):1446–1456.

120b. Davis KB, Slichter SJ, Corash L. Corrected count increment and percent platelet recovery as measures of posttransfusion platelet response: problems and a solution. Transfusion 1999; 39(6):586–592.

121. Harker LA. The role of the spleen in thrombokinetics. J Lab Clin Med 1971; 77:247–253.

122. Bishop JF, Matthews JP, Yuen K, McGrath K, Wolf MM, Szer J. The definition of refractoriness to platelet transfusions. Transfus Med 1992; 2:35–41.

122a. Arnold DM, Crowther MA, Cook RJ, et al. Utilization of platelet transfusions in the intensive care unit: indications, transfusion triggers, and platelet count responses. Transfusion 2006; 46(8):1286–1291.

123. Delaflor-Weiss E, Mintz PD. The evaluation and management of platelet refractoriness and alloimmunization. Transfus Med Rev 2000; 14:180–196.

124. Bishop J, McGrath K, Wolf MM, et al. Clinical factors influencing the efficacy of pooled platelet transfusions. Blood 1988; 71:383–387.

125. McFarland JG, Anderson AF, Slichter SJ. Factors influencing the transfusion response to HLA-selected apheresis donor platelets in patients refractory to random platelet concentrates. Br J Haematol 1989; 73:380–386.

126. Bishop JF, Matthews JP, McGrath K, Yuen K, Wolf MM, Szer J. Factors influencing 20-hour increments after platelet transfusion. Transfusion 1991; 31:392–396.

127. Heal J, Rowe J, McMican A, Masel D, Finke K, Blumberg N. The role of ABO matching in platelet transfusion. Eur J Haematol 1993; 40:110–117.

128. Rebulla P, Finazzi G, Marangoni F, et al. The threshold for prophylactic platelet transfusions in adults with acute myeloid leukemia. N Engl J Med 1997; 337:1870–1875.

129. Schiffer CA, Anderson KC, Bennett CL, et al. Platelet transfusion for patients with cancer: clinical practice guidelines of the American Society of Clinical Oncology. J Clin Oncol 2001; 19:1519–1538.

130. McVay PA, Toy PT. Lack of increased bleeding after liver biopsy in patients with mild hemostatic abnormalities. Am J Clin Pathol 1990; 94:747–753.

131. National Institutes of Health Consensus Conference. Platelet transfusion therapy. Transfus Med Rev 1987; 1:195–200.

132. Chan KH, Mann KS, Chan TK. The significance of thrombocytopenia in the development of postoperative intracranial hematoma. J Neurosurg 1989; 71:38–41.

133. Chu DZJ, Shivshanker K, Stroehlein JR, Nelson RS. Thrombocytopenia and gastrointestinal hemorrhage in the cancer patient: prevalence of unmasked lesions. Gastrointest Endosc 1983; 29:269–272.

134. Dodd RY. Germs, gels, and genomes: a personal recollection of 30 years in blood safety testing. In: Stramer SL, ed. Blood Safety in the New Millenium. Bethesda, MD: American Association of Blood Banks, 97–122.

135. Williamson LM, Lowe S, Love EM, et al. Serious hazards of transfusion (SHOT) initiative: analysis of the first two annual reports. BMJ 1999; 319:16–19.

136. Heddle NM, Klama LN, Griffith L, Roberts R, Shukla G, Kelton JG. A prospective study to identify the risk factors associated with acute reactions to platelet and red cell transfusions. Transfusion 1993; 33:794–797.

137. Heddle NM, Klama L, Meyer R, et al. A randomized controlled trial comparing plasma removal with white cells reduction to prevent reactions to platelets. Transfusion 1999; 39:231–238.

138. Vamvakas E, Pineda A. Allergic and anaphylactic reactions. In: Popovsky MA, ed. Transfusion Reactions, 2nd ed. Bethesda, MD: AABB Press, 2001: 83–127.

139. Sandler SG, Mallory D, Malamut D, Eckrich R. IgA anaphylactic transfusion reactions. Transfus Med Rev 1995; 9:1–8.

140. Pineda AA, Taswell HF. Transfusion reactions associated with anti-IgA antibodies: report of four cases and review of the literature. Transfusion 1975; 15:10–15.

141. Warkentin TE, Smith JW. The alloimmune thrombocytopenic syndromes. Transfus Med Rev 1997; 11: 296–307.

142. Lubenow N, Eichler P, Albrecht D, et al. Very low platelet counts in post-transfusion purpura falsely diagnosed as heparin-induced thrombocytopenia. Report of four cases and review of literature. Thromb Res 2000; 100:115–125.

143. Warkentin TE, Smith JW, Hayward CPM, Ali AM, Kelton JG. Thrombocytopenia caused by passive transfusion of anti-glycoprotein Ia/IIa alloantibody (anti-HPA-5b). Blood 1992; 79:2480–2484.

144. Popovsky MA, Chaplin HC Jr, Moore SB. Transfusion-related acute lung injury: a neglected, serious complication of chemotherapy. Transfusion 1992; 32:589–592.

145. Popovsky MA. Transfusion-related acute lung injury. Curr Opin Hematol 2000; 7:402–407.

146. Silliman CC. Transfusion-related acute lung injury. Transfus Med Rev 1999; 13:177–186.

147. Lenahan SE, Domen RE, Silliman CC, Kingsley CP, Romano PJ. Transfusion-related acute lung injury secondary to biologically active mediators. Arch Pathol Lab Med 2001; 125: 523–526.

148. Silliman CC, Voelkel NF, Allard JD, et al. Plasma and lipids from stored packed red blood cells cause acute lung injury in an animal model. J Clin Invest 1998; 101:1458–1467.

149. Schafer AI. Thrombocytosis and thrombocythemia. Blood Rev 2001; 15:159–166.

150. Folman CC, Ooms M, Kuenen B, et al. The role of thrombopoietin in post-operative thrombocytosis. Br J Haematol 2001; 114:126–133.

151. Bunting RW, Doppelt SH, Lavine LS. Extreme thrombocytosis after orthopaedic surgery. J Bone Joint Surg Br 1991; 73:687–688.

152. Gurung AM, Carr B, Smith I. Thrombocytosis in intensive care. Br J Anaesth 2001; 87:926–928.

153. Lipson RL, Bayrd ED, Watkins CH. The postsplenectomy blood picture. Am J Clin Pathol 1959; 32:526–532.

154. Lee DH, Blajchman MA. Novel treatment modalities: new platelet preparations and substitutes. Br J Haematol 2001; 114:496–505.

155. Kenet G, Walden R, Eldad A, Martinowitz U. Treatment of traumatic bleeding with recombinant factor VIIa. Lancet 1999; 354:1879.

156. Martinowitz U, Michaelson M, and the Israeli Multidisciplinary rFVIIa Task Force. Guidelines for the use of recombinant activated factor VII (rFVIIa) in uncontrolled bleeding: a report by the Israeli Multidisciplinary rFVIIa Task Force. J Thromb Haemost 2005; 3:640–648.

157. Levi M, Peters M, Buller HR. Efficacy and safety of recombinant factor VIIa for treatment of severe bleeding: a systematic review. Crit Care Med 2005; 33:883–890.

158. Wilson SJ, Bellamy MC, Giannoudis PV. The safety and efficacy of the administration of recombinant activated factor VII in major surgery and trauma patients. Expert Opin Drug Saf 2005; 4:557–570.

159. Holcomb JB. Use of recombinant activated factor VII to treat the acquired coagulopathy of trauma. J Trauma 2005; 58:1298–1303.

160. Hardy JF. Managing uncontrolled hemorrhage in trauma and surgery: a novel and promising approach. Can J Anesth 2002; 49:S4-S6.

161. Dutton RP, McCunn M, Hyder M, et al. Factor VIIa for correction of traumatic coagulopathy. J Trauma 2004; 57(4): 709–719.

162. Boffard KD, Riou B, Warren B, et al. Recombinant factor VIIa as adjunctive therapy for bleeding control in severely injured trauma patients: two parallel randomized, placebo-controlled, double-blind clinical trials. J Trauma 2005; 59(1):8–18.

163. Stein DM, Dutton RP, O'Connor J, et al. Determinants of futility of administration of recombinant factor VIIa in trauma. J Trauma 2005; 59(3):609–615.

56

Venous Thromboembolism

Niten Singh

Division of Vascular Surgery, Department of Surgery, USUHS Medical Center, Bethesda, Maryland, and the Madigan Army Medical Center, Tacoma, Washington, D.C., U.S.A.

Jon C. White

Department of Surgery, VA Medical Center, George Washington University, Washington, D.C., U.S.A.

INTRODUCTION

Venous thromboembolism (VTE) is a term used to describe thromboses that may occur in any vein as well as the emboli that result when one of these thrombi breaks off and migrates to other areas in the systemic venous network, most notably the pulmonary circulation. When the veins involved are superficial, the resultant superficial phlebitis may be painful, but is of minor consequence. When the affected veins are located in the deep system, the phenomenon is termed deep venous thrombosis (DVT), which has more serious implications than its superficial counterpart.

The occurrence of VTE is of particular significance in patients following trauma or in those with critical illness for several reasons. First, these patients are at high risk for VTE, often due to hypercoagulability, intimal injury, or stasis, all of which predispose to formation of venous thrombosis and propagation of pre-existing thrombi. Secondly, the compromise of hemodynamics and organ perfusion caused by venous and/or pulmonary arterial obstruction is more deleterious in a patient whose cardiopulmonary function is already compromised. These facts help to explain why pulmonary embolus (PE) is the third major cause of death following trauma in those who survive longer than 24 hours after injury (1,2).

Since the lower extremities are the usual areas affected with thrombosis, the term DVT is often used in reference to lower extremity thromboses alone. However, following trauma and critical care, upper extremity DVTs may also have clinical significance. Accordingly, we will consider the pathophysiology of all DVTs in this chapter and also review the prophylaxis, diagnosis, and treatment of PE. Finally, recent guidelines from the Seventh America College of Chest Physicians (ACCP) Conference on Antithrombotic and Thrombolytic Therapy will be provided (3). These will be evaluated within the context of the previously published trauma VTE recommendations by the EAST Workgroup, (4) and more recent data summarized by Knudson et al. from the American College of Surgeons National Trauma Data Bank (ACS-NTDB) (5).

PATHOGENESIS

☞ The components of Virchow's triad (hypercoagulation, endothelial injury, and venous stasis) have long been recognized as the etiological factors for VTE. When one or more of these factors are present, initiation of the coagulation cascade is increased, as is the risk of clot formation. ☞

Normal Clot Formation

When the integrity of the endothelial lining of the blood vessels is disrupted, platelets in the blood become exposed to the collagen of the vessel wall. Contact with the collagen causes the usually smooth-surfaced (resting) platelet (Fig. 1A) to become irregular and "sticky" (activated) (Fig. 1B) as it adheres to the area of the injury. The activated platelet secretes a number of factors including von Willebrand factor (vWF), which recruits more platelets to the area of injury and stimulates them to adhere. Other factors released by the platelets initiate the coagulation cascade.

Coagulation occurs via two main pathways, the intrinsic and extrinsic pathway (Fig. 2). The intrinsic pathway is primarily triggered by the disruption of vascular endothelial integrity exposing blood vessel collagen to circulating blood. The extrinsic pathway is more often activated in conditions such as sepsis, infection, and trauma, where tissue factor and factor VII initiate coagulation without necessarily exposing endothelial collagen. Regardless of which pathway initiates coagulation, the final common event is the conversion of prothrombin to thrombin (factor II), which catalyzes the conversion of soluble fibrinogen (factor I) to insoluble fibrin filaments. These filaments form a net, trapping additional blood cells and platelets and causing the clot to form, grow, and mature.

Like many other physiologic responses in the body, clotting has its own negative feedback controls. ☞ As soon as clot formation begins, processes are initiated to turn off (or down-regulate) clotting [antithrombin III (AT III) and proteins C and S] or dissolve the already formed clots (plasmin and tissue plasminogen activator). Proper regulation of clotting and clot dissolution will minimize the risk of VTE. ☞

These two interactive systems may be grouped together as the coagulofibrinolytic system (Fig. 3). The balance of the coagulation and fibrinolytic arms of this system is especially important for critically ill trauma patients because its homeostasis may be disturbed by injury, surgery, sepsis, the systemic inflammatory response syndrome, and multiple organ dysfunction syndrome. The recent PROWESS study demonstrated that treatment with activated protein C reduced

(A)

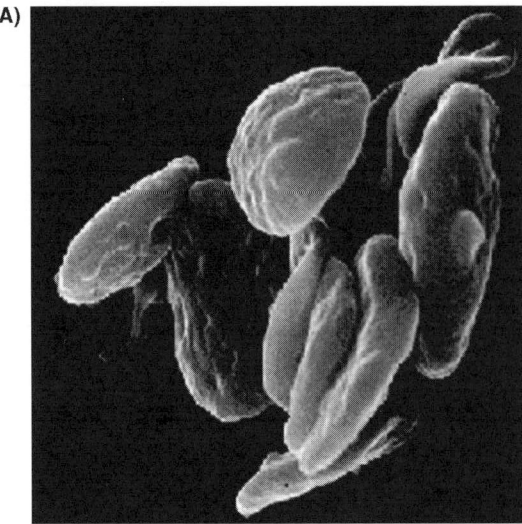

(B)

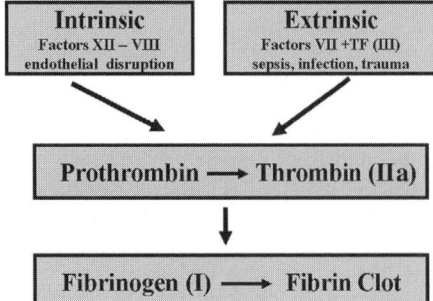

Figure 1 Resting platelets (**A**) are smooth and travel through the blood vessels unimpeded. When platelets adhere to areas of endothelial injury, they become activated (**B**), undergo shape change, and form platelet aggregates.

thrombosis and conferred a survival advantage in septic patients (see Volume 2, Chapters 56 and 63) (6).

Hypercoagulation

The body forms a clot in response to an injury that causes loss of blood from the vascular system. The system is also programmed to dissolve that clot after it has served its purpose. It should not form unnecessary clots, such as

Coagulation Cascade

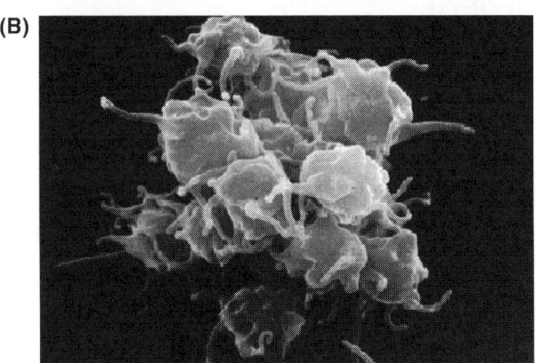

Figure 2 The coagulation cascade is activated through the intrinsic or extrinsic pathways. Both pathways convert prothrombin to thrombin, which stimulates the polymerization of soluble fibrinogen to an insoluble fibrin clot.

Coagulofibrinolytic System

Clotting Coagulation Fibrin formation	Clot Prevention Anti-coagulation Fibrinolysis
Factors I-XIII Thrombin vWF Platelets	Plasmin Anti-thrombin tPA Proteins C + S

Figure 3 The coagulofibrinolytic system includes factors that stimulate clotting and fibrin formation and opposing factors that antagonize coagulation and stimulate fibrinolysis. *Abbreviation*: vWF, von Willebrand factor.

those that cause DVTs, and should be able to dissolve unwanted clots when they do occur. ♂ **Overactivity of the procoagulant system or underactivity of the anticlotting or fibrinolytic systems results in a hypercoagulable state, also termed thrombophilia (Table 1).** ♂

Examples of procoagulant overactivity include the presence of factor V Leiden, or very high levels of homocysteine; factors VIII, IX, or XI, thrombin activatable fibrinolysis inhibitor (TAFI); or fibrinogen (7). There are certain acquired conditions such as pregnancy, malignancy, trauma, surgery, heparin-induced thrombocytopenia (HIT), and ingestion of oral contraceptives that also result in overactivity of the coagulation cascade. Of note, many of these conditions are found in the critically ill patient.

Examples of underactivity of the anticlotting system are deficiencies of protein C, protein S, plasminogen, factor XII, AT III, or heparin cofactor II (8). In the trauma patient, VTE has a 13-fold increased incidence compared to normal patients (9). The increased risk results from systemic hypercoagulation that manifests itself locally in areas of stasis induced by immobilization (10). The hypercoagulability is due to both activation of coagulation and reduced levels of coagulation inhibitors and increased levels of fibrinolytic inhibition (11).

Endothelial Damage

Endothelial damage is a key element of Virchow's triad, yet is difficult to separate out as an independent risk factor in patients following trauma or surgery who may have other predisposing factors, such as immobility, that lead to clot formation. It is clear, however, from the discussion below of indwelling catheters that intimal damage done by

Table 1 Hereditary Causes of Hypercoagulation

Increased levels or activity	Decreased levels or activity
Factor V Leiden	Protein S
Factor IX	Protein C
Factor XI	Antithrombin III
Thrombin activatable fibrinolysis inhibitor	Heparin cofactor II Plasminogen
Fibrinogen	Factor XII
Homocysteine	
Prothrombin gene variant	

penetration of the vein wall or its continuous irritation with an indwelling foreign body predisposes to clot formation. Of all the major operations performed, the ones that involve the major blood vessels of the pelvis and lower extremities, such as hip arthroplasty, cystectomy, major vascular procedures, and total knee arthroplasty (12), carry the highest risk of VTE that develops in this area. This suggests that injury to these vessels confers an independent risk factor. Intravenous drug abuse, which is not associated with the major morbidity of surgery or trauma, has also been shown to be associated with DVT, indicating that intimal damage alone can lead to clot formation (13).

Venous Stasis

ợ**⁴ Venous stasis is probably the most important risk factor for VTE in patients who are critically ill or recovering from trauma or surgery. Since these patients are often bedridden, sedated, or paralyzed, they have sluggish blood flow and poor venous return. Blood flow may also be compromised by low cardiac output, abdominal compartment syndrome, and elevated intravenous pressure from right heart failure (14). ợ⁴**

Indeed, all of the conditions that contribute to patient immobility, such as mechanical ventilation, complex drains, paralytic drugs, sedatives, indwelling catheters, or traction, have been associated with an increased risk for VTE (15). Knudson et al. recently completed a retrospective analysis of the risk factors associated with VTE in 1602 trauma patients (Table 2) of the >450,000 patients in the ACS-NTDB (5). Days on mechanical ventilation and venous injury emerged as the most significant risk factors. Other risk factors that have traditionally been considered important [e.g., spinal cord injury (SCI), pelvic fractures, etc.] were also found to be important, but not to the same degree of significance (5).

The diagnosis of VTE is difficult to make in critically ill patients because their comorbidity often leads to edema, respiratory compromise, decreased sensorium, pain, decreased perfusion, and other signs that are important clinical indicators of DVT or the resultant emboli. Estimates of VTE range from 5% to 35% in ICU patients (14). However, these percentages likely underestimate the true incidence of VTE due to the reasons enumerated earlier. It is clear, however, that one or more elements of Virchow's triad are present in the majority of critically ill patients, making diagnosis, prevention, and treatment of this disorder a top priority for these patients.

Nontrauma-specific medical conditions that affect critically ill patients also come into play. A rare prothrombotic risk factor is the presence of a congenital or acquired venous malformation, which decreases venous return. Examples of this phenomenon are IVC webs seen in Budd–Chiari syndrome (BCS) and left common iliac occlusions seen with May–Thurner sydrome, both of which are discussed later.

UPPER EXTREMITY

DVT of an upper extremity may result from an indwelling foreign body, such as an intravenous catheter, or may occur spontaneously (i.e., Paget–Schroetter syndrome). Of the two entities, the former is of far greater significance for critically ill trauma patients. Indeed, these patients often have catheters placed in their central veins for intravenous resuscitation, administration of medications, parenteral nutrition, hemodynamic monitoring, cardiac pacing, or hemodialysis. The two veins most commonly involved are the axillary and subclavian, therefore, the term axillosubclavian vein thrombosis (ASVT) is generic for this condition.

The incidence of upper extremity venous thrombosis has been reported to occur in 0.06% of unselected hospitalized patients (16). This incidence is higher in selected populations such as those with indwelling central venous catheters or malignancy (17).

Catheter-Induced Vein Thrombosis

Because of its relative ease of performance, central access is usually obtained via percutaneous puncture of veins in the groin, antecubital fossa, subclavian region, or base of the neck. This leads to direct damage to and the presence of a foreign body adjacent to the intima of the femoral, brachial, axillary, subclavian, or superior vena caval veins. When thromboses result, the consequences range from minor swelling of an extremity to life-threatening superior vena cava (SVC) syndrome.

The incidence of ASVT is highest in patients with indwelling intravenous catheters. The incidence in this subset of patients is related to the material used for the catheter as well as the position of the catheter. ợ**⁴ Polyethylene and polyvinyl chloride catheters are more prone to pulmonary emboli than polyurethane or siliconized catheters (18), whereas the heparin-bonded catheters seem to be better than those without heparin bonding (19). Additionally, catheters placed so that the tips are in the SVC or the right atrium have a lower incidence of thrombi than those placed in the innominate or subclavian veins. ợ⁴**

Spontaneous Thrombosis

Spontaneous thrombosis of the upper extremity (Paget–Schroetter syndrome) is most often seen in young, active people who use their upper arms and shoulders in repetitive sports or professional activities. The thrombogenic state is believed to result principally from overuse of an upper extremity; hence, it is also called "effort thrombosis." Alternatively, when clotting occurs in the axillary vein due to anatomic compression as the vein passes through the thoracic outlet, it may be called "thoracic outlet" syndrome (though this term is usually used to describe subclavian arterial obstruction). In any case, "spontaneous thrombosis" may be a misnomer insofar as a predisposing condition is

Table 2 Risk Factors Associated with Venous Thromboembolism (Univariate Analysis)

Risk factor (number with risk)	Odds ratio (95% confidence interval)[a]
Age ≥ 40 yrs (*n* = 178,851)	2.29 (2.07–2.55)
Pelvic fracture (*n* = 2707)	2.93 (2.01–4.27)
Lower extremity fracture (*n* = 63,508)	3.16 (2.85–3.51)
Spinal cord injury with paralysis (*n* = 2852)	3.39 (2.41–4.77)
Head injury (AIS ≥ 3) (*n* = 52,197)	2.59 (2.31–2.90)
Ventilator days >3 (*n* = 13,037)	10.62 (9.32–12.11)
Venous injury (*n* = 1450)	7.93 (5.83–10.78)
Shock on admission (BP <90 mm Hg) (*n* = 18,510)	1.95 (1.62–2.34)
Major surgical procedure (*n* = 73,974)	4.32 (3.91–4.77)

[a]*P* <0.0001 for all factors.
Abbreviation: AIS, abbreviated injury scale.
Source: From Ref. 5.

often identified. Often, more than one thrombogenic condition will be present, for example, a tennis player with a vein compressed by a small thoracic outlet.

Spontaneous thrombosis has no particular significance for the critically ill patient, but must be differentiated from catheter-related thromboses described earlier. It is important to search for hypercoagulable states in all patients who develop DVT and treat promptly because it may otherwise progress to long-term disability (20).

Clinical Signs

The clinical signs and symptoms of upper extremity DVT are chiefly pain and swelling. In critically ill or sedated patients, swelling may be the only clue. Fever is also associated, but is nonspecific, because it is often present for other reasons following trauma and critical care. Occasionally, thrombi, even when they totally occlude the vein, may be asymptomatic. This is more likely to occur in a critically ill patient with other comorbidities and unable to recognize that an arm is swollen or painful (i.e., the head-injured patient). In these patients, signs such as asymmetric arm edema or distended upper arm and chest wall veins may be seen. Less commonly, venous thrombus of the upper extremity may present as PE, which occurs in 20% of catheter-related thrombi (21). Similar to DVT in the lower extremities, emboli that break off of upper extremity thrombi can also travel through a right to left shunt in the left heart to embolize to the brain or coronary arteries (22). ☞ **When emboli originate from the vessel wall they are termed mural thrombi. When emboli originate from an indwelling catheter they are termed sleeve emboli. Sleeve emboli have a greater chance of embolizing. ☞**

Diagnosis

Diagnosis of an intravenous thrombosis is most easily made in patients who have the thrombosis related to the presence of an indwelling catheter. In these patients, it is not possible to withdraw blood from the catheter. Although this phenomenon may be caused by catheter kinking, it is more often caused by an intravenous thrombus. Regardless of etiology, the first diagnostic test of upper extremity vein thrombosis should be venous Doppler ultrasound (VDU) which has high specificity (94–100%) but only moderate sensitivity (56–100%) (23). This test is noninvasive, portable, and relatively inexpensive. It can be used for initial diagnosis and may be used sequentially to follow the progress of the disease or monitor the efficacy of treatment.

The gold standard for diagnosing upper (and lower) extremity thrombi is venography. ☞ **Although a properly performed venogram has close to 100% sensitivity and 100% specificity, it is done only infrequently because VDU is safer, less expensive, and usually sufficient. ☞**

Venography is an invasive procedure, which carries risks such as renal toxicity and allergic reactions. It may also be difficult to access small veins in the hand or distal extremity to inject contrast material. Digital subtraction venography allows studies to be done with less contrast material and is associated with fewer side effects than plain venography (24). Venography is more comprehensively reviewed in the section devoted to diagnostic tests of the lower extremity, but the upper extremity is particularly suited to this modality because of the inaccessibility of the axillary, subclavian, and innominate veins to physical examination and other noninvasive tests.

Treatment

☞ **When the thrombi occur as a result of an indwelling catheter, the cornerstone of treatment is removal of the catheter and anticoagulation (when not contraindicated). ☞**

Of course, this removes access to the central circulation, which may cause problems in itself. For these patients, there must also be a strategy for obtaining alternative access to the circulation if it is still needed. Another strategy is to leave the catheter in place and keep the patient anticoagulated (25). Patients who do not respond to anticoagulation alone may have a fibrinolytic agent infused through the catheter (26). However, fibrinolytics are associated with more bleeding complications than heparin alone, and are relatively contraindicated following acute trauma to the central nervous system. Prior to surgical treatment of an anatomic obstruction, fibrinolysis must be initiated acutely to prevent a chronic disability. Surgical procedures for the upper extremity are usually reserved for conditions caused by extrinsic compression such as effort vein thrombosis (27) or thoracic outlet syndrome. If the injury is recognized and treated promptly with fibrinolysis, surgical opening of the thoracic outlet is usually successful (28). If the injury is recognized late, vein patch angioplasty or replacement of permanently damaged subclavian or axillary vein with saphenous grafts may be necessary. Although thrombosis caused by intimal damage, such as occurs with ASVT, may go on to produce permanent problems, surgical intervention is not usually necessary unless there are predisposing anatomic problems that must be addressed (29).

Otherwise, treatment for upper extremity thrombi is similar to treatment of lower extremity thrombi discussed later. Medical treatment consists of acute anticoagulation with unfractionated heparin (UFH) or low molecular weight heparin (LMWH) followed by chronic anticoagulation by warfarin. Intravascular filters may be placed to prevent embolization (30), but the possibility of creating a swollen extremity is more debilitating when it occurs in an upper extremity. Dissolution of the clot with a fibrinolytic agent such as tissue-type plasminogen activator or recombinant urokinase may be done in the upper extremity as well as the lower extremity. However, these drugs are generally contraindicated within a few days after acute trauma.

SUPERIOR VENA CAVA

Although thrombosis can occur anywhere in the vena cava, it is more likely to occur in areas of low flow and/or partial obstruction. A variety of medical etiologies besides trauma and/or catheter-related conditions are known to increase the risk of VTE, each requiring a different treatment depending on their location (Table 3). SVC syndrome may be caused by thrombi originating within the SVC or may be initiated by external compression of the SVC. It is a relatively common complication of thoracic or mediastinal malignancies, but there are other benign causes of this syndrome as well (31). More recently, the increased use of intravenous catheters has made intrinsic causes of thrombi more common so that a careful workup must be done before definitive treatment can be initiated.

Malignancies

Malignancy is still the most common cause of SVC syndrome. The malignant conditions most often associated with SVC syndrome are bronchogenic carcinoma and

Table 3 Medical Etiologies and Treatment of Vena Cava Thromboses

Location	Etiology	Treatment
Superior vena cava	Malignancy	Treat malignancy
	Bronchogenic CA	Endoluminal stenting
	Lymphoma	Thrombolysis
Inferior vena cava	BCS	Anticoagulation
		Thrombolysis
		TIPPS (BCS)
		Surgery
	Nephrotic syndrome	Anticoagulation
		Thrombolysis
		Surgical thrombectomy
	Behcet's disease	Variable

Abbreviations: BCS, Budd–Chiari syndrome; CA, cancer; TIPPS, transjugular intrahepatic portosystemic shunting.

lymphoma. The etiology of the SVC obstruction in patients with these diseases is almost always external compression by a tumor or direct growth of the tumor into the SVC. Thus, DVT does not play a major etiologic role in the development of this syndrome for these malignancies. Recent advances in endoluminal stenting, however, have made thrombolysis and stent placement an alternative treatment for this condition (32). Stenting may be particularly appropriate for critically ill patients who are too ill to wait for resolution of symptoms of SVC syndrome by radiation or chemotherapy and cannot undergo surgical procedures.

Catheter-Related Superior Vena Cava Syndrome

⚡ **Although catheter-related thrombosis represents a relatively small percentage of patients who develop SVC syndrome, it is commonly seen in critically ill trauma patients who have multiple indwelling catheters for fluids, monitoring, pacemakers, and cardiac defibrillators.** ⚡ Although the phenomenon of catheter-related thrombus was described in the section on upper extremity DVT, SVC thrombosis is more serious than upper extremity thrombosis because of the hemodynamic consequences of an obstructed SVC.

Catheter-related obstructions are true thrombi and are important to recognize early because they can be treated effectively by catheter removal or thrombolytics. If the clot is diagnosed within five days of symptoms, then it can usually be lysed successfully (33). It is also important to diagnose catheter-related SVC syndrome because it usually develops acutely. When SVC syndrome develops slowly, as occurs with many malignant conditions, collateral circulation, especially through the azygous system, may develop to return blood to the right atrium. When the clot forms acutely around an indwelling line collaterals do not have time to develop and the hemodynamic consequences of the obstruction are more severe.

Other Benign Conditions

Historically, infectious conditions such as syphlitic aortic aneurysms and untreated fungal conditions caused most SVC obstructions. Although improved antimicrobial treatment has decreased the number of patients who present with these causes of SVC syndrome, there are still patients who develop the syndrome from fibrosing mediastinitis,

usually related to untreated or under-treated granulomatous and fungal conditions (34,35).

INFERIOR VENA CAVA

⚡ **Thrombosis may occur anywhere in the inferior vena cava (IVC), such as with Behcet's disease (36). However, most IVC clotting occurs near the hepatic veins as a consequence of BCS or adjacent to the renal veins as a consequence of nephrotic syndrome.** ⚡

Budd–Chiari Syndrome

Although BCS may be loosely defined as any process that causes obstruction of hepatic blood outflow, it is more typically reserved for thrombosis of the hepatic veins and adjacent IVC (37). Numerous inciting events can lead to veno-occlusive disease of the hepatic veins, including myeloproliferative disorders, malignancies, infections, oral contraceptives, and other conditions causing hypercoagulable states (38). Mechanical obstruction may play a role in some of these conditions; however, hypercoagulability is the primary etiologic factor leading to BCS.

BCS may present as an acute or chronic condition. When it is acute there is often hepatomegaly and severe right upper quadrant pain. The chronic form presents more gradually and patients may complain only of vague abdominal pain. These patients usually have a better prognosis (39). Ascites and variceal bleeding may occur with either presentation; however, the pattern of biochemical test abnormalities differs. Patients with acute BCS have elevations of their aminotransferases and alkaline phosphatases, whereas those with chronic disease experience hypoalbuminemia and elevated prothrombin times.

As with deep vein thrombosis in other anatomic locations, diagnosis is most easily made with noninvasive studies such as Doppler ultrasonography, magnetic resonance imaging, and computed tomography (CT). The gold standard for diagnosis remains venography that may be needed when the noninvasive tests are inconclusive. Liver biopsy is also helpful and may be needed to determine the extent of cirrhosis and to guide treatment.

Treatment options for thromboses in other anatomic locations are similar and include medical management, anticoagulation, radiographic interventions, and surgical procedures. Due to the unique involvement of the liver in this condition, the medical management includes controlling symptoms of liver failure. Radiographic treatment of BCS includes transjugular intrahepatic portosystemic shunting (TIPSS) as well as all of methods described later such as thrombolysis, stenting, and angioplasty. Surgical approaches to BCS are particularly challenging because of the inaccessible location of the hepatic veins and the retrohepatic IVC. Portosystemic shunting and liver transplantation, however, do offer some hope for these patients (40).

Nephrotic Syndrome

Nephrotic syndrome is characterized by proteinuria greater than $3.5 \, g/m^2/day$. Hypoalbuminemia, edema, hyperlipidemia, and lipiduria may also be seen but are variable in expression. ⚡ **There is a high incidence of renal vein thrombosis with nephrotic syndrome for reasons that are not clear. Patients with nephrotic syndrome are hypercoagulable and have an increased occurrence of generalized arterial and venous thromboemboli; however,**

the incidence of clotting is highest in the renal veins. ☞
This may be due to the decreased perfusion of the kidneys
seen in NS and resultant low flow and hemoconcentration
in the postglomerular circulation.

Diagnosis of renal vein thrombosis is similar to that of
BCS insofar as noninvasive ultrasonography is the preferred
screening technique (41), whereas invasive venography has
the highest sensitivity and specificity.

Treatment of thromboembolism for nephrotic
syndrome is similar to that of BCS when the IVC is involved.
Treatment for renal vein thrombosis, however, is limited to
anticoagulation and, in unusual circumstances, surgical
thrombectomy (42).

LOWER EXTREMITY AND PELVIC VEINS

The lower extremity has two systems of venous drainage,
the deep and superficial systems. The superficial system is
comprised of the lesser and greater saphenous veins
(GSVs), and the deep system is comprised of paired
common femoral veins (CFVs), superficial femoral
veins, profunda femoral veins, popliteal veins, and tibial
veins (43). The superficial veins communicate with the
deep system via venous perforators and directly at the
saphenofemoral junction. Thrombosis of the deep veins of
the lower extremity can propagate into the iliac system
and further into the IVC. DVTs are also classified by
the location in the lower extremity with proximal (thigh)
veins being considered more clinically important
than distal (calf) veins in terms of potential for subsequent
PE (44).

Thrombosis of the iliac veins has the greatest risk of
massive PE. ☞ **DVTs occur more commonly in the left
common iliac vein. This is explained anatomically because
the right common iliac artery compresses the left common
iliac vein as it crosses over it. Repetitive pulsations may
cause a "web" or "spur" to form and make this vein more
prone to thrombosis. This condition has been termed
May–Thurner syndrome (45).** ☞

Diagnostic Tests

The diagnostic workup of suspected VTE must be initiated
based on clinical suspicion and must proceed systematically
from bedside examination to noninvasive [i.e., impedance
plethysmography (IPG) or VDU] and, in some circumstances, invasive testing (Table 4).

Physical Exam

Classic findings of DVT are the following: pain, swelling,
and variable discoloration of the involved extremity. In the
ICU setting, symptoms may be difficult to illicit from a
sedated, paralyzed, or endotracheally intubated patient.
Therefore, a high index of suspicion must be maintained
and physical examination revealing unilateral swelling, a
palpable cord, or superficial venous dilation must be
followed by further testing (46,47). Clinical examination
and grouping patients into low, moderate, and high-risk
groups prior to testing (Table 5) has been shown to increase
diagnostic accuracy (48,49).

Ultrasound/Duplex

VDU examination of the lower extremity is useful in that it is
noninvasive and can be done at the bedside, thus eliminating

Table 4   Diagnostic Tests of Lower Extremity
Deep Venous Thrombosis

Test	Findings
Physical exam	Pain
	Swelling
	Discoloration
	Unilateral swelling
	Palpable cord
VDU	Visualization of clot
	Response to compression
	Echodensity
	Duplex flow
IPG	Resistance related to obstruction
Venography	Normal anatomy
	Intraluminal filling defect

Abbreviations: IPG, impedance plethysmography; VDU,
venous Doppler ultrasound.

the need to transport critically ill patients. Venous interrogation is most accurate when compression ultrasonography
(50,51) is used. The vein is identified and followed along
its course until the thrombus is found. The chronicity of
the thrombus can be inferred from its appearance on
ultrasonography as older clots have a more echodense
appearance (52). Finally, the vein is compressed during
duplex scanning to determine if there is an appropriate
flow response. The obvious limitation of compression ultrasonography is in imaging veins that cannot be compressed
by the probe, such as those above the inguinal ligament.

Table 5   Pretest Probability of Deep Vein Thrombosis

Clinical feature	Score[a]
Active cancer (treatment ongoing or within the previous 6 mo or palliative)	1
Paralysis, paresis, or recent plaster immobilization of the lower extremities	1
Recently bed-ridden for more than 3 days or major surgery, within 4 wks	1
Localized tenderness along the distribution of the deep venous system	1
Entire leg swollen	1
Calf swelling by more than 3 cm when compared to the asymptomatic leg (measured below tibial tuberosity)	1
Pitting edema (greater in the symptomatic leg)	1
Collateral superficial veins (nonvaricose)	1
Alternative diagnosis as likely or more likely than that of deep venous thrombosis	−2

Note: This clinical model has been modified to take one other clinical
feature into account: a previously documented deep vein thrombosis
(DVT) is given the score of 1. Using this modified scoring system, DVT
is either likely or unlikely as: DVT likely = 2 or greater; DVT unlikely = 1
or less.
[a]A score of 3 or higher indicates that the probability of deep vein thrombosis is likely; a score of 1 or 2 indicates that the probability is moderate; and a
score of 0 or less indicates that the probability is very unlikely.
Source: Adapted from Ref. 115.

✍ Serial VDU studies should be performed if the initial exam is negative because 2% of patients with an initially negative study will have a positive result when studied seven days later (3,53). ✍ A carefully done ultrasound examination has been found in one series to have a 100% sensitivity and 99% specificity (54).

Impedence Plethysmography

IPG is another noninvasive test, which is useful to define venous obstruction. A pneumatic cuff is placed around a patient's thigh and two electrodes are placed on the calf. The cuff is inflated and then rapidly deflated while the resistance between the electrodes is measured. The outflow fraction, which is related to the degree of obstruction, may be calculated (55).

The sensitivity and specificity of this technique is 91% and 96% in some series (56); however, significant variabilities have been demonstrated in the same patient (57). In addition, patients must be correctly positioned and immobile for two minutes, which might be difficult in an agitated ICU patient. Finally, as the success of ultrasound increases, the use of plethysmography decreases and fewer people are familiar with the technique.

Venography

Contrast venography is still the "gold standard" for the diagnosis of DVT. Adequate imaging requires visualization of the deep venous structures from the calf veins to the IVC. ✍ **The most reliable venographic finding indicating a DVT is an intraluminal filling defect seen on two or more views of the same area (58).** ✍ In one study, only 1.3% of patients developed a DVT following an initially negative venogram over a six-month follow-up (59). However, due to the invasive nature of the study and the need to transport ICU patients to an interventional suite, venography is not the first choice of studies for critically ill patients. If the ultrasound is read as inconclusive (such as "suspicious for but not diagnostic" of iliac or pelvic vein thrombosis) or is unavailable, then contrast venography can be used. It is also not recommended for patients with renal insufficiency unless other studies are inconclusive and the risk of empiric anticoagulation is great.

Prevention and Treatment

The prevention and treatment of DVT should be considered for every hospitalized patient. The approaches used vary from simple preventative measures such as anticoagulation and early ambulation to more invasive treatments such as mechanical devices, interventional radiology, and surgery (Table 6). In the absence of a major contraindication, LMWH is indicated for the prophylaxis of trauma patients with at least one risk factor for VTE (3). Those with a contraindication to LMWH because of active bleeding or high risk of hemorrhage should receive mechanical prophylaxis (described later).

DVT is the most common complication of HIT, and, therefore, symptoms or signs of DVT in a patient receiving antithrombotic prophylaxis with UFH or LMWH should prompt consideration of this diagnosis, including determination of the platelet count and comparison with previous values.

Anticoagulants

Primary therapy for DVT centers on anticoagulation and there is a wide variety of anticoagulants available that

Table 6 Prevention/Treatment of Lower Extremity Deep Vein Thrombosis

Anticoagulation	UFH
	LMWH
	Heparinoids
	Thrombin inhibitors
	Enzyme inhibitors
	Factor inhibitors
	Warfarin
Mechanical devices	Elastic stockings
	Sequential compression
	Intravascular filters
Interventional radiology	Fibrinolysis
	Balloon angioplasty
	Stenting
	Clot extraction
Surgery	Direct thrombectomy
	Cross-over saphenous bypass
Early ambulation	Postoperative protocols
	Travel ambulation

Abbreviations: DVT, deep vein thrombosis; UFH, unfractionated heparin; LMWH, low molecular weight heparin.

vary in dosing, monitoring, and limitations (Table 7). The main anticoagulant used is UFH, which is an indirect thrombin inhibitor, as it combines with AT III to accelerate the inactivation of thrombin and factor Xa. This inactivation involves the formation of a ternary complex in which heparin binds to both AT III and to thrombin. This requires an adequate saccharide length, which occurs commonly in UFH preparations, but less so with LMWH (60).

✍ **UFH is the first choice in treatment for DVT but has limitations, which include a narrow therapeutic window and variable dose–response that requires frequent monitoring.** ✍ The half-life of UFH is approximately 30 to 60 minutes (61). The dosing of UFH usually involves a weight-adjusted nomogram (Table 8) with an initial bolus of 80 units/kg followed by 18 units/kg/hour (62). The rate is then adjusted to maintain an activated partial thromboplastin time (APTT) that is about 1.5 to 2.3 times higher than normal. However, in patients in whom there is a concern for bleeding (e.g., a recent postoperative patient), a smaller bolus or no bolus may be used. Complications of UFH include bleeding, immune HIT, and, with chronic use, osteoporosis. Bleeding can occur without a supratherapeutic APTT, especially in patients who have undergone trauma or surgery (63). If a patient is bleeding while receiving UFH, protamine sulfate can reverse the anticoagulant effects using a dose of 1 mg of protamine sulfate for every 100 units of heparin administered within the past few hours.

Two types of HIT are known. Type I is not immune-mediated and is manifested by a fall in the platelet count within 48 hours with a return to normal with or without discontinuation of heparin. Type II is immune-mediated and is caused by antibodies that recognize a platelet granule protein (platelet factor 4) complexed to heparin. Usually, platelets do not recover unless heparin is discontinued. Thrombotic events rather than bleeding are typical for type II HIT. Two to five percent of patients receiving UFH and 0–1% of patients receiving LMWH for one to two weeks develop immune HIT. ✍ **All forms of heparin (including LMWH) should be discontinued when HIT is diagnosed**

Table 7 Anticoagulants

Agent	Dosage[a]	Monitoring	Limitations
UFH	80 units/kg/hr, IV bolus 18 units/kg continuous IV	APTT	IV infusion HIT

LMWH
  Enoxaparin
  Daltiparin
  Tinzaparin
	1.5–2 mg/kg/day, SQ	None needed	HIT (less than with UFH)

Heparinoids Danaparoid	2250 units SQ, BID	Antifactor Xa assay	Expensive (but less than thrombin inhibitors) No antidote

Thrombin inhibitors
  Lepirudin (hirudin)
  Bivalirudin
  Argatroban
	Variable	APTT	Expensive
			No antidote

Warfarin	2–10 mg, QD or QOD[b]	PT	Variable dose–response slow to reverse

[a]Therapeutic, rather than prophylactic, dosing is shown.
[b]The first dose of warfarin should not exceed 5 mg.
Abbreviations: APTT, activated partial thromboplastin time; BID, 2 times per day; HIT heparin-induced thrombocytopenia; IV, intravenous; LMWH, low molecular weight heparin; PT, prothrombin time; QD, once daily; QOD, 4 times per day; SQ, subcutaneous; UFH, unfractionated heparin.

and nonheparin based anticoagulation should be instituted (64). ☞

The other commonly employed forms of heparin are LMWHs. These smaller molecules are made by treating UFH with a variety of depolymerization reactions. The ones that are currently approved for use by the FDA include enoxaparin, dalteparin, and tinzaparin. Like UFH, they are all indirect factor Xa inhibitors, but in contrast to UFH, LMWHs inhibit thrombin to a lesser extent (binding poorly to AT III) and, as a result, do not usually prolong the APTT. LMWHs are given subcutaneously and their anti-Xa activities correlate well with body weight, allowing a fixed dosing regimen to be used. Laboratory monitoring is not necessary unless the patient is pregnant or has renal insufficiency. Additionally, LMWHs cause less immune

Table 8 Weight-Based Nomogram for Intravenous Heparin Infusion

Initial dose	80 U/kg bolus, then 18 U/kg/hr

APTT < 35 sec
  (< 1.2 × control)
	80 U/kg bolus, then increase infusion
	  rate by 4 U/kg/hr

APTT 35–45 sec
  (1.2–1.5 × control)
	40 U/kg bolus, then increase infusion
	  rate by 2 U/kg/hr

APTT 46–70 sec (1.5–2.3 × control)	No change
APTT 71–90 sec (2.3–3.0 × control)	Decrease infusion rate by 2 U/kg/hr

APTT > 90 sec
  (>3.0 × control)
	Hold infusion 1 hr, then decrease
	  infusion rate by 3 U/kg/hr

Note: Each laboratory should establish the appropriate APTT range that corresponds to a therapeutic level of heparin (which may or may not correspond to the APTT ranges used in the nomogram shown above).
Abbreviation: APTT, activated partial thromboplastin time.
Source: From Ref. 116.

thrombocytopenia. Normal dosing for full anticoagulation is 1 mg/kg twice per day or 1.5 mg/kg once a day (65). Although LMWHs can be given subcutaneously, UFH is usually given by a constant IV infusion, making conversion to an oral anticoagulant necessary for outpatient treatment.

Nonheparin agents may be used for anticoagulation and are particularly helpful when HIT develops. Two large classifications of agents are the heparinoids and the direct thrombin inhibitors (DTIs). Danaparoid is a low molecular weight heparinoid that is a more selective factor Xa inhibitor than LMWH. Its activity can be measured by a chromogenic antifactor Xa assay. Unlike heparin, danaparoid is not effectively neutralized by protamine. Danaparoid is not available in the United States. Currently, the two FDA-approved anticoagulants for treatment of HIT are DTIs, lepirudin and argatroban. Lepirudin is a recombinant form of hirudin, the natural polypeptide anticoagulant from the saliva of the medicinal leech. Argatroban is a synthetic small-molecule thrombin inhibitor derived from arginine. A third DTI available in the United States, bivalirudin (analogue of hirudin), is not approved for treatment of HIT, but has, except during angioplasty, seen limited use for this indication. Unlike other anticoagulants, these drugs are sometimes difficult to monitor with standard laboratory tests, as the APTT does not always reliably estimate drug levels. No antidotes exist for these DTIs (66).

The standard oral anticoagulation drug is the vitamin K antagonist, warfarin. Its mechanism of action is to reduce the synthesis of functional levels of the vitamin K-dependent procoagulant factors, II (prothrombin), VII, IX, and X. There is the potential for a hypercoagulable effect occurring within the first few days after initiating treatment due to the reduction in synthesis of two vitamin K-dependent anticoagulant factors, protein C and protein S; this results particularly from the relatively short half-life of protein C compared with the other vitamin K-dependent factors. The peak effect of anticoagulation does not occur with warfarin until 36 to 72 hours after the first dose, but the effect on the individual factors varies (Fig. 4). Dosing is monitored using the prothrombin time, expressed as the International Normalized Ratio (INR), which is usually maintained at 2.0 to 3.0 for DVT therapy. Complications include bleeding (especially with excessive INR prolongation) or necrosis (either skin necrosis or venous limb gangrene, which are secondary to microvascular thrombosis related to warfarin-associated decreases in protein C and/or protein S). To avoid complications of warfarin-induced hypercoagulation, UFH and LMWH are usually overlapped for at least five days with warfarin. If a patient requires immediate reversal of anticoagulation while receiving warfarin, fresh frozen plasma or prothrombin complex concentrates should be administered. Rapid (within a few hours) reversal of anticoagulation can be achieved by slow (over 30–60 minutes) intravenous infusion of vitamin K (67).

Mechanical Devices

Intermittant Pneumatic Compression

☞ **Intermittent pneumatic leg compression has both local and systemic effects. Locally, it acts by simulating the calf muscle pump and, thus, preventing venous stasis. Systemically, it acts by inhibiting plasminogen activator inhibitor-1 (68) and increasing the body's fibrinolytic activity.** ☞ For this reason, compression devices placed on an arm may convey some benefit in preventing clot formation in the lower extremities.

Although there is little risk in using pneumatic leg compression devices, they should be used with caution in patients with severe peripheral vascular occlusive disease. In addition, some clinicians believe they should not be started on patients who have been at bed rest for greater than 72 hours prior to obtaining a noninvasive evaluation of pre-existing DVT, due to the possible dislodging of a previously formed clot. The literature has clearly demonstrated benefits of intermittent pneumatic leg compression

in moderate risk patients following trauma, and those undergoing general surgical, cardiac, and neurosurgical procedures (69,70). Compression should be initiated preoperatively in elective cases and be used throughout the postoperative period until the patient is ambulatory.

Intravascular Filters

Interruption of the IVC was first described by Trousseau in 1868 (71). Since that time IVC filters have evolved and are routinely placed in high risk trauma patients, and those with DVT but a contraindication to anticoagulation. There are many different types of IVC filters which are all designed to trap clots but allow blood flow (Fig. 5). As the technology has advanced, the delivery system has become smaller, making deployment of the filters easier. The use of IVC filters in addition to anticoagulation has been investigated and found to cause a decrease in incidence of short-term PE but no difference in incidence of long-term PE or survival (72). IVC filters are not routinely used for patients without evidence of thromboembolism. ☞; **The indications for placement of filters are the following: (*i*) acute VTE in a patient who has a contraindication for anticoagulation, (*ii*) VTE in a patient who is already anticoagulated, (*iii*) patients who have a compromised pulmonary vascular bed in whom a VTE would not be tolerated, (*iv*) patients with a high fall risk in whom anticoagulation could cause bleeding, and (*v*) trauma patients with a prolonged high risk for VTE due to prolonged immobility (e.g., quadriplegia) and severe traumatic brain injury (TBI) (73).** ☞

Retrievable vena cava filters are now clinically available for use in patients with a short anticipated duration of need for protection against PE. One such device is the Günther Tulip™ Vena Cava Filter (Cook, Inc., Bloomington, IN, US) (Fig. 6). Because these devices are still under study, and complications have been reported, retrievable venacaval filters are discussed later in the "Eye to the Future."

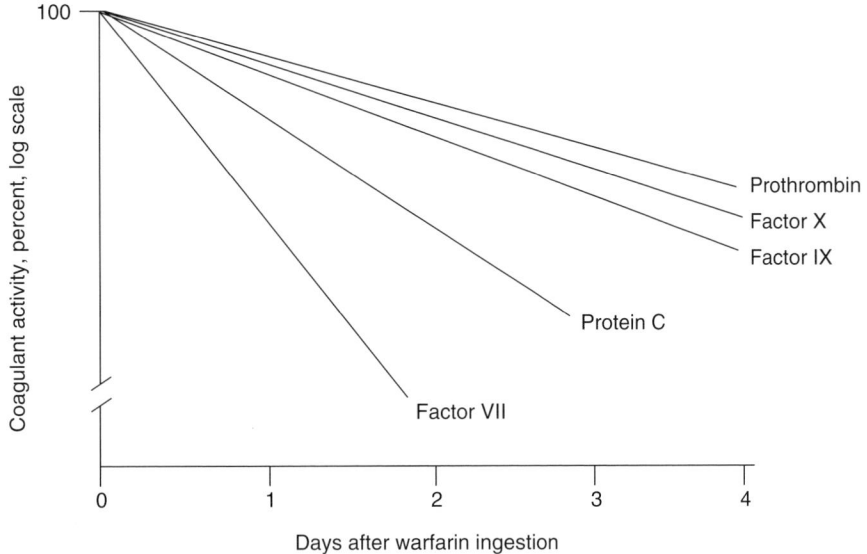

Figure 4 Effect of warfarin on blood-clotting proteins. The activity of various clotting proteins (logarithmic scale) is shown here as a function of time after ingestion of warfarin (10 mg/day PO for four consecutive days) by a normal subject. Factor VII activity, to which the prothrombin time is most sensitive, is the first to decrease. Full anticoagulation, however, does not occur until factors IX, X, and prothrombin are sufficiently reduced (at least four days). Protein C activity falls quickly, and, in some patients, a transient hypercoagulable state may ensue resulting in microvascular thrombosis (e.g., coumarin necrosis). The half-life of protein S (not shown) resembles that of prothrombin (60 hours).

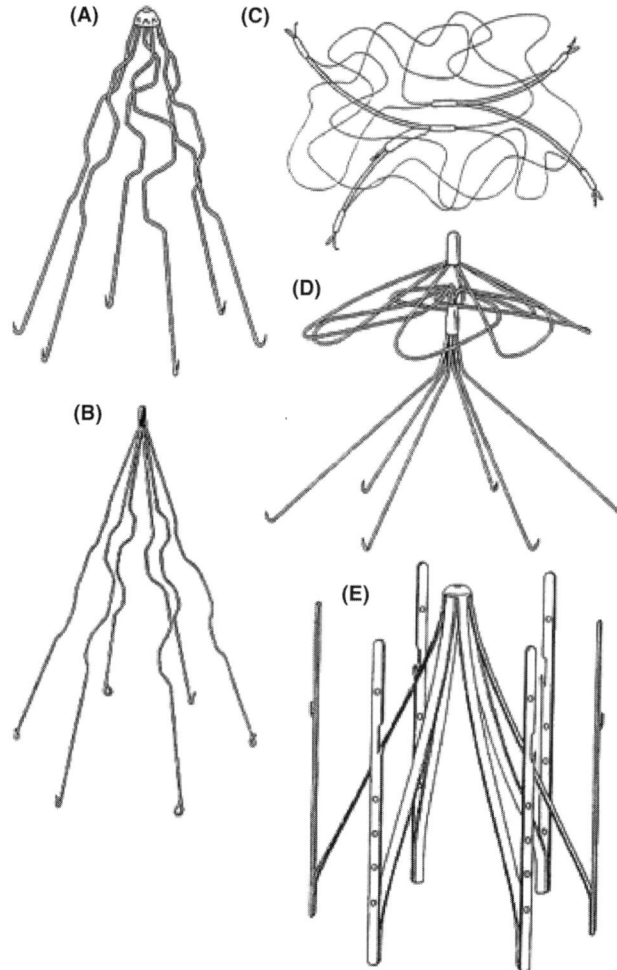

Figure 5   Inferior vena cava filter models. (**A**) Stainless steel Greenfield filter, (**B**) modified-hook titanium Greenfield filter, (**C**) bird's nest filter, (**D**) Simon nitinol filter, (**E**) Vena Tech® filter. *Source*: From Ref. 117.

systemic dosing and several series have reported excellent success rates (78,79).

DVTs are more frequently located in the left lower extremity due to the anatomic compression resulting in the May–Thurner syndrome (80) as described earlier. Treatment of a thrombus at this location usually involves catheter-directed thrombolysis, balloon angioplasty, and placement of a stent due to the recurrent nature of thrombosis. May–Thurner syndrome and acute DVTs causing a threatened limb (phlegmasia cerulea dolens) are the two most common indications for peripheral thrombolytics (81). Thrombolytic therapy also increased thrombin generation, and thus conco-mitant anticoagulation, at least in low doses, is usually given.

☞ **In addition to May–Thurner syndrome, endolum-inal stenting and balloon angioplasty have been described in other types of iliofemoral venous occlusive disease. Although these procedures are uncommonly performed, they offer nonsurgical options for trauma and critically ill patients with VTE disease.** ☞

Surgery
In the situation of a threatened limb such as phlegmasia cerulea dolens, in which the patient cannot wait for cath-eter-directed thrombolysis, surgical thrombectomy should be considered. The GSV is identified and followed to the saphenofemoral vein junction. The CFV is then opened and a Fogarty catheter is used to extract the thrombus while the patient is under general endotracheal anesthesia. Some recommend a pulmonary end expiratory pressure of 10 cm water to decrease the risk of PE (though this mechan-ism is entirely speculative). After the thrombus is removed, the GSV is attached to the femoral artery to create an AV fistula to help keep the vein open. A completion venogram is performed to ensure the patency of the thrombectomized vein. The procedure should include fasciotomies to relieve a potential compartment syndrome and anticoagulation is continued throughout the postoperative period (82).

If the thrombus is chronic and the vessel cannot be surgically recanalized, other surgical procedures such as the crossover saphenous vein bypass (Palma procedure) can be performed. This procedure involves dissecting the contralateral GSV but keeping it attached to its saphenofe-moral junction. It is then tunneled to the affected groin where an anastamosis is made to the CFV proximal to the occlusion. In addition, an end-to-side anastomosis between the ipsilateral saphenous vein and adjacent femoral artery is performed to create an arteriovenous fistula to keep the outflow tract open (83).

In this era of interventional radiology and other non-surgical alternatives, however, surgical thrombectomy should be reserved for dire circumstances and the unusual cases noted earlier.

Early Mobilization
Of the triad of risk factors Virchow identified as causative for VTE, the one that is most easily addressed is venous stasis. It is also the risk factor that is most often seen in criti-cally ill, traumatized, anesthetized, or postoperative patients. It is clear that prevention is the most important strategy to use against the development of VTE and the prevention of venous stasis should be the primary focus of this strategy.

☞ **Although elastic compression and pneumatic compression devices restore some of the lost blood flow, mobilization and, specifically, ambulation provides**

Interventional Radiology
Although there have been controlled trials for the use of thrombolytics in patients who have suffered a VTE, the data on its use in DVT alone are minimal. The potential benefits of complete clot lysis, the lower incidence of post-phlebitic syndrome, and reduced chances for potential PE must be weighed against the potential bleeding compli-cations that may occur with thrombolytics. In addition, many patients may not be candidates for thrombolysis, such as those who have undergone recent surgery or trauma (74). The main thrombolytic agents that have been studied are streptokinase, urokinase, and tissue plasmino-gen activator. Most of studies are small and conclusions about optimal dosing and expected results cannot be drawn (75–77).

In the setting of acute DVT, the use of catheter-directed thrombolysis is becoming more popular. This technique is commonly employed for iliofemoral DVT by passing a wire across the thrombus, placing an infusion catheter with side-holes, and infusing a thrombolytic substance directly into the thrombus. By employing this method, the amount of thrombolytic agent given is less than with

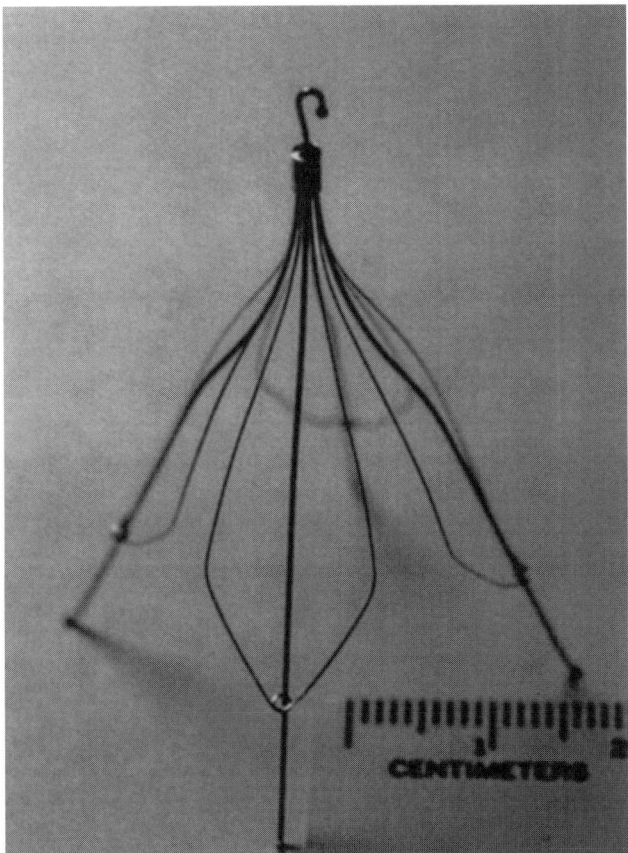

Figure 6 Günther Tulip™ retrievable vena cava filter (Cook, Inc., Bloomington, Indiana, U.S.A.). The Günther Tulip filter is conical in shape and consists of four legs that contain additional wire loops attached to each leg. A hook is present at the apex of the filter, which is used in the retrieval process. It can be placed via a femoral or jugular vein approach. However, inferior vena cava filters must be retrieved from the jugular approach. *Source*: From Ref. 106.

complete restoration of flow and the greatest protection against VTE. ☞ Although there are numerous studies demonstrating the protective effects of prophylactic anticoagulation and mechanical compression, there is very little documentation of the benefits of early ambulation. This effect of ambulation must be inferred from studies that show that lack of ambulation in patients with no other comorbid conditions, such as those who have prolonged periods of sitting, traveling, or lying in a bed, results in stasis and VTE (84,85). This information is the basis for many surgical protocols which call for early ambulation. Despite many protocols calling for early operative intervention and early restoration of ambulation in bedridden patients, there has been no convincing evidence that this approach decreases VTE (86). The recent interest in minimally invasive surgical procedures is partially inspired by the benefits of reduced postoperative morbidity leading to early ambulation.

There is another aspect of ambulation that has been studied in a more systematic way. Early ambulation versus bed rest after a DVT has developed has been subjected to several recent studies. These studies challenge the previously held notion that patients should be sedentary until a clot becomes adherent to the vein to prevent it from dislodging and embolizing. ☞ **There have been several recent** studies that have demonstrated that bed rest does not decrease the incidence of PE following DVT (87). Future prospective studies will have to be conducted to determine whether a period of bed rest or early ambulation should be recommended for patients with documented DVT. ☞

PULMONARY EMBOLISM

Of all the complications caused by DVT, PE is the most serious, with 500,000 cases diagnosed per year in the United States alone (88). Untreated PE is associated with a 30% mortality. When timely diagnosis and treatment occurs, mortality is reduced to approximately 5% (89). Much of the diagnosis, prevention, and treatment of DVT is, therefore, aimed at decreasing the incidence and lethal consequences of PE.

Diagnosis

The most common clinical findings in PE are related to obstructed blood flow through the heart and lungs and the resultant compromise of oxygen delivery. The signs and symptoms of this disorder include tachypnea, rales, tachycardia, fourth heart sound, pleuritic chest pain, dyspnea, cough, hemoptysis, and mild fever. Unfortunately, these findings are relatively nonspecific (and may be completely absent) so that confirmatory testing is almost always warranted when PE is clinically suspected. When one or more of these signs is present in a patient at risk for VTE, an arterial blood gas (ABG), chest X ray (CXR), and electrocardiogram (EKG) are commonly obtained. Although the ABG typically shows hypoxemia, hypocapnia, and a respiratory alkalosis, a major PE may lead to hypercapnia and respiratory acidosis. Other patients with PE have close to normal oxygenation. Other lab values such as WBC, ESR, LDH, SGOT, troponin, and brain natriuretic protein may be elevated, but the utility of these nonspecific findings is questionable. The most frequently observed CXR pattern with PE is atelectasis or a pulmonary parenchymal injury, which has been observed almost as frequently in patients who were determined not to have a PE (90). Findings on electrocardiography such as nonspecific ST segment and T wave changes are frequently found but are also insensitive and nonspecific. The greatest utility of EKG in diagnosing PE may be to rule out other cause of chest pain such as myocardial ischemia.

Because of the nonspecificity of the clinical findings, and of these routinely ordered lab tests, further diagnostic testing is usually warranted. In patients with essentially normal chest radiographs, a ventilation perfusion ($\dot{V}/\dot{Q}$) scan is a useful screening test. This test may be read as high probability (80–90% probable), moderate probability (40% probable), or low probability (15% probable). In the setting of patients with initially abnormal chest radiographs (i.e., most critically ill trauma patients), $\dot{V}/\dot{Q}$ scans are rarely helpful. Furthermore, $\dot{V}/\dot{Q}$ results may not be sensitive or specific enough to direct treatment such as anticoagulation, which can be associated with significant morbidity.

Helical CT, especially when complemented with intravenous contrast administration (CT angiography), is currently the most commonly employed study to diagnose PE. The technique, however, is operator-dependent and only experienced centers show sensitivities and specificities approaching pulmonary angiography (91). Emboli that occlude segmental and larger vessels are more likely to be detected by helical CT scanning, whereas emboli in subsegmental vessels may easily be missed.

Pulmonary angiography, similar to venography for DVT, remains the "gold standard" for diagnostic tests of PE but is decreasingly used. It is the most invasive and expensive test and should only be used when other tests (including helical CT) are nondiagnostic, and making the diagnosis is important enough to justify the potential complications of the procedure. Complications of pulmonary angiography include injuries related to catheter placement, contrast reactions, cardiac dysrhythmias, or respiratory compromise (73).

The risks and benefits of all diagnostic tests should be weighed carefully for critically ill patients with suspected PE. A combination of clinical signs, lab tests, EKG findings, and a documented DVT by methods outlined in the previous sections may be enough to start treatment for PE. V̇/Q̇ scanning and helical CT may be used in situations where there is uncertainty about the initial diagnosis, the patient is stable enough to be transported to the radiology suite, and the risk of treatment (e.g., anticoagulation) outweighs the risk of the added diagnostic techniques. In a minority of patients with suspected PE (about 20%), pulmonary angiography will be needed to make a definitive diagnosis.

The occurrence of PE in a patient receiving UFH or LMWH antithrombotic prophylaxis should prompt consideration of HIT, and warrants measurement of the platelet count, as HIT confers a 40-fold increased risk of PE (by odds ratio) and requires use of a nonheparin anticoagulant such as lepirudin or argatroban.

Treatment

Treatment for documented PE embolus is similar to treatment for documented DVT and includes anticoagulation, thrombolytic therapy, invasive radiology, and, rarely, surgical intervention. Anticoagulation following PE is no different from that described earlier for DVT except that the duration of anticoagulation after a documented PE is somewhat longer. Those patients with a known risk factor for PE (e.g., postoperative patients) should be anticoagulated for three to six months if the risk factor is reversed. If there are no known risk factors, then anticoagulation should be continued for the entire six months. If there is a risk factor that cannot be reversed, then anticoagulation should be permanent (92).

Thrombolysis, similar to its employment for DVT, is used only when there is a severe compromise of blood flow in the pulmonary arteries that cannot wait for the body's natural fibrinolytic system to clear the obstruction. It requires catheterization of the pulmonary arteries and direct infusion of a thrombolytic agent, such as streptokinase, urokinase, or tissue plasminogen activator, adjacent to or into the blood clot. As well as the acute resolution of hemodynamic and radiographic abnormalities, there is some evidence that patients who receive thrombolytic therapy have lower pulmonary artery pressures and lower pulmonary artery resistances years after treatment when compared to those who receive anticoagulation alone (93). IVC filters, which are described earlier, are usually placed for the prevention of initial or recurrent PE.

When the patient has significant hemodynamic compromise from a large embolus and thrombolysis is contraindicated, interventional radiologists may use a variety of catheters to both fragment and aspirate the clot (94). Similar to treatment of DVT, surgical intervention is usually the last option. Surgical removal of a clot from the pulmonary artery is a heroic maneuver with very high morbidity and mortality. Although it is easiest to do on cardiac bypass, it has been done without extracorporeal circulation (95).

There is a risk of mortality and morbidity associated with every treatment used for PE. For this reason, some investigators have suggested that treatment for PE may be withheld in patients who have a small embolus, adequate cardiopulmonary reserve, and a contraindication to anticoagulation (96). These patients should be followed with serial noninvasive leg studies to demonstrate the absence of recurrent DVT. This strategy should be considered experimental and must be evaluated further before it is used outside of a clinical trial.

AMERICAN COLLEGE OF CHEST PHYSICIANS RECOMMENDATIONS FOR VENOUS THROMBOEMBOLISM PROPHYLAXIS FOLLOWING TRAUMA

Decision-making regarding VTE prophylaxis in trauma patients has been recently reviewed by "the Seventh ACCP Conference on Antithrombotic and Thrombolytic Therapy: Evidence-Based Guidelines" published their evidence-based recommendations (Table 9) (3).

The strength of their recommendations was assigned a numerical grade (1 or 2) based upon the trade-off between the benefits of a therapy and the risks and burdens (and costs) of that treatment. If the benefits outweigh the risks, burdens, and costs, treatment is recommended.

The uncertainty associated with the risk/benefit (R/B) equation determined the strength of the recommendations. If the R/B equation was clearly demonstrated in the literature, a strong recommendation (Grade 1) was assigned. When they were less certain of the R/B equation, a weaker (Grade 2) recommendation was assigned.

The methodological quality of their recommendations was also assigned an alphabetical grade as follows: Randomized clinical trials (RCTs) with consistent results and a low likelihood of bias are classified as Grade A, whereas, RCTs with inconsistent results, or with major methodological weaknesses, were assigned Grade B recommendations. Grade C recommendations come from observational studies or from a generalization from one group of patients in an RCT to a different (similar) group of patients who did not participate in the trials. When the generalization from RCTs was considered secure, or the data from observational studies overwhelmingly compelling, the Grade of C+ was assigned. Otherwise, a simple grade of C was assigned.

Most of the recommendations in the ACCP Guidelines are supported by this review and are in concert with the EAST guidelines released two years prior (4). Both our review of the literature and the EAST guidelines suggest a slightly more aggressive rule for IVC filters (Table 8). Accordingly, we have supplemented recommendation 5a with 5b, which we believe reflects the current thinking. Additionally, the role of retrievable IVC filters is evolving (see Eye to the Future).

In the most extensive review of the ACS-NTDB to date, Knudson et al. reviewed the risk factors associated with VTE in 1602 trauma patients (5). The list of risk factors evaluated was developed by prospective studies conducted at San Francisco General Hospital and also identified by a consensus panel of VTE experts led by Dr. Lazar Greenfield. Of

Table 9 Recommendations for Prevention of Venous Thromboembolism Following Trauma

Topic	Recommendation[a]	Grade
≥1 Risk factor	Trauma patients with at least one risk factor for VTE should receive thromboprophylaxis, if possible.	1A
LMWH indications	In the absence of a major contraindication, LMWH prophylaxis is indicated starting as soon as it is considered safe to do so.	1A
Mechanical prophylaxis	Mechanical prophylaxis with IPC devices, or possibly with GCS alone should be used if LMWH prophylaxis is delayed or if it is currently contraindicated due to active bleeding or a high risk for hemorrhage.	1B
VDU screening	VDU screening in patients who are at high risk for VTE (e.g., in the presence of a SCI, lower extremity or pelvic fracture, major TBI, or an indwelling femoral venous line) and who have received suboptimal prophylaxis or no prophylaxis.	1C
IVCF Indications	Per the ACCP recommendations, IVCFs should not be used as primary prophylaxis in trauma patients.	1C
EAST[b] rec's and Our view	The EAST recommendations, and the view of the authors of this review, are that high-risk patients (see VDU) with contraindication to LMWH should receive an IVCF. When the high risk for VTE is anticipated to be of short duration (e.g., severe polytrauma including pelvic fracture and thoracic injuries, but without SCI or TBI), a retrievable IVCF may be best.	1C See ETTF
Prophylaxis duration (normal mobility)	Thromboprophylaxis should continue until hospital discharge, including the period of inpatient rehabilitation.	1C +
Prophylaxis duration (impaired mobility)	Thromboprophylaxis should continue after hospital discharge with LMWH or a VKA (target INR, 2.5; INR range, 2.0–3.0) in patients with major impaired mobility.	2C

[a]Recommendations mainly distilled from Ref. 3.
[b]EAST recommendations from Ref. 4.
Abbreviations: ACCP, American College of Chest Physicians; EAST, Eastern Association for the Surgery of Trauma; rec, recommendations; GPC, graduated compression stockings; INR, international ratio; IPC, intermittent pneumatic compression; IVCF, inferior vena cava filter; LMWH, low molecular weight heparin; SCI, spinal cord injury; TBI, traumatic brain injury; VDU, venous doppler ultrasound; VKA, vitamin K antagonists; VTE, venous thromboembolism.

the total 450,375 patients studied, 1602 had VTE (998 had a DVT, 522 had a PE, 82 had both). Nine risk factors were significantly associated with VTE using univariate analysis ($P < 0.0001$), summarized in Table 2 (5). However, only six risk factors were identified as independently significant using multivariate logistic regression (Table 10). Days requiring mechanical ventilation >3 and venous injury carried the highest individual risk (by odds ratio). Knudson et al. utilized the data garnered in this comprehensive analysis, along with a complete review of the literature including most of the references cited by the ACCP recommendations (3) and the EAST Guidelines (4) to develop an algorithm for VTE prophylaxis (Fig. 7) (5). This algorithm is supported by the reviewed literature in this chapter and represents the current state of practice at most Level I trauma centers. The only caveat being the emphasis on temporary (retrievable) IVC filters.

Our expectation is that the "very high risk factor" arm of the algorithm will be further modified based upon prospective data now being gathered regarding these removable IVC filters. One of the key questions beyond safety is the expected duration that very high risk factors persist. For example, patients age ≥ 40 years with SCI might benefit more from a permanent IVC filter, whereas, a 20 year old with, SCI might be best served with a retrievable IVC filter until other risk factors have abated. The ultimate answers to these questions await RCTs. Another important question is the maximum time these "retrievable" filters may remain in place before they can no longer be removed (discussed further in Eye to the Future).

EYE TO THE FUTURE
Medical Treatment

LMWH is increasingly viewed as the anticoagulant of choice for DVT prophylaxis (97). Many are commercially available now and undoubtedly many more will be developed and marketed in the future.

As the coagulation cascade has become better understood, the problems that lead to thrombophilia have been addressed more directly. The newest generation of antithrombotic agents target single elements of the procoagulant cascade such as thrombin (e.g., hirudin, lepirudin, argatroban, bivalrudin) and factor Xa (e.g., fondaparinux). Although some are in use now, many more are in development. These anticoagulants, due to their specificity,

Table 10 Independent Risk Factors for Venous Thromboembolism (Multivariate Logistic Regression)

Risk factor	Odds ratio (95% CI)	P value
Age ≥40 yr	2.01 (1.74–2.32)	<0.0001
Lower extremity fracture (AIS ≥3)	1.92 (1.64–2.26)	<0.0001
Head injury (AIS ≥3)	1.24 (1.05–1.46)	0.0125
Ventilator days >3	8.08 (6.86–9.52)	<0.0001
Venous injury	3.56 (2.22–5.72)	<0.0001
Major operative procedure	1.53 (1.30–1.80)	<0.0001

Note: Presents independent risk factors for venous thromboembolism (multivariate analysis).
Abbreviations: AIS, abbreviated injury scale; CI, confidence interval.

have efficacy and safety profiles that are better than conventional anticoagulants (98).

Other factors involved in the coagulation scheme such as tissue factor, factor VII, factor V, and factor VIII will be targets for future anticoagulation strategies. Agents that inhibit these molecules are in development or in active trials now and will certainly be part of the VTE prevention and treatment armamentarium of the future.

Hyperhomocysteinemia is known to be associated with thrombophilia. Trials are under way now to determine if treatment with folate, which decreases homocysteine levels in the blood, will reverse the thrombophilia (99).

Diagnostic Studies

Ultrasonography is the best screening test for DVT whereas venography has the highest sensitivity and specificity. Other noninvasive imaging studies such as magnetic resonance imaging and CT have not proven to be very useful due to their low sensitivity, especially in the case of nonocclusive mural thrombi (100). In the situation where a patient is being scanned for other reasons, one

of these imaging studies may occasionally prove useful for making the diagnosis of DVT, but they should not be considered screening studies or primary diagnostic modalities. As the sensitivities of these procedures increase, however, they may find uses in diagnosing DVT in patients who have absolute or relative contraindications for venography.

Computerized tomography pulmonary angiography (CTPA) is a test that is often used in patients with suspected PE. Many of the current protocols for CTPA now involve scanning through the pelvis and upper thigh as well as the chest. DVTs in the pelvic and lower extremity vessels have been identified using this technique (101); however, it is not used in most cases of suspected DVT because it requires a significant contrast load. It is a useful adjunct, however, and should be reserved for situations when all other tests are inconclusive and the suspicion of DVT is high.

Another promising imaging test is magnetic resonance venography. Studies comparing it to contrast venography have been small, but indicate that the test is very accurate (102). The main limitations to this study are transport issues in critically ill patients and the cost of the study.

Retrievable Inferior Vena Cava Filters

Interventional radiologists routinely place IVC filters, but because these filters are associated with complications such as iliofemoral and IVC thrombosis (103), there has been interest in removable IVC filters, especially in trauma patients. Critically ill trauma patients at high risk for VTE of short anticipated duration (e.g., severe polytrauma including pelvic fracture and thoracic injuries, but without SCI or TBI) are candidates for a retrievable IVC filters (Fig. 6). The Günther Tulip™ Vena Cava Filter (Cook, Inc., Bloomington, IN, U.S.) has been used in Europe since 1992 as a retrievable filter (104), and has begun to be used in the United States over the last couple years in selected cases. However, several aspects of its use are not yet known.

Recently, Yamagami studied the deployment and retrieval of the Günther Tulip™ in 10 patients being

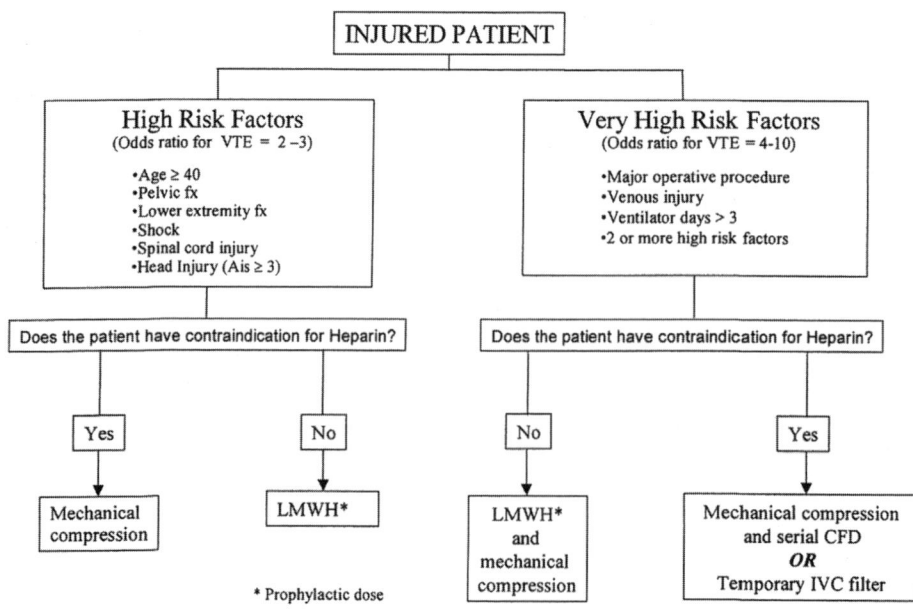

Figure 7 Algorithm for VTE prophylaxis proposed by Eastman AB (based upon data generated in Ref. 4). *Abbreviations*: VTE, venous thromboembolism; LMWH, low molecular weight heparin; IVC, inferior vena cava.

treated for DVT (105). All were successfully retrieved and there were no complications. In a larger study involving 55 trauma patients among 130 studied, Morris et al. showed the Günther Tulip™ to be relatively safe with only one major complication in 130 patients and 136 filter placements (106). The average duration between placement and removal was 19 days (range, 11–41 days). The mean age of patients selected prospectively for filter removal (29 years; range, 18–71 years) was significantly lower than the mean age (49 years; range, 19–82 years) of trauma, surgical, and intracranial hemorrhage patients selected for placement of prophylactic permanent filters (*P* < 0.002; 95% confidence interval, 18.0–22.4) (106).

The maximum duration that these "removable" filters can remain in place, and still be retrievable, is not yet known. The manufacturer suggests that the Günther Tulip filter can be safely removed within 14 days of implantation or it can remain in place as a permanent filter. However, numerous investigators have now reported removal of the filter far beyond the 14 days recommended by the manufacturer. In an effort to address this question, Terhaar et al. evaluated the Gunther Tulip vena cava filter with regard to ease of retrieval over relatively long time periods (107). Nineteen patients underwent attempted retrieval of their filter. Sixteen attempts were successful (84%). In three patients, the filter could not be removed due to extensive filter thrombus in two patients and firm attachment to the wall in one patient. Median implantation time for retrievable filters was 34 days (range, 7–126 days) (107). In the study by Morris et al., the longest duration of deployment prior to removal was 41 days (106). However, Binkert et al. recently reported retrieval of an IVC filter 317 days after deployment. Clearly, the maximum duration is unknown, and the time before removal generally becomes technically difficult requires additional study (108).

Another important question under study is the period of time a patient remains at risk for VTE and PE following trauma. Greene et al. recently recommended that the IVC filter should not be removed until the patient has fully recovered from the trauma and critical illness, or that there is objective data to show that the VTE risk is low (generally at least 30 days after the trauma) (109). Accordingly, there is much still to be learned about these retrievable filters, including the migration rate to the right ventricle and pulmonary artery in large populations of mobile patients. Furthermore, there is a trend toward placing these filters at the bedside in critically ill ICU patients (i.e., too unstable for transport to radiology) (110).

Percutaneous Mechanical Thrombectomy

More recently, the use of mechanical thrombectomy devices has been employed to remove thrombus from the vein. The advantage of these devices is that their use avoids the use of thrombolytics with their attendant bleeding complications and, if successful early in the course of the disease, will prevent development of postphlebitic syndrome (111).

Percutaneous mechanical retrieval of venous thrombi is usually not necessary due to dissolution that occurs following anticoagulation therapy. However, systemic anticoagulation is often contraindicated in severely injured trauma patients. When a large, potentially lethal DVT is diagnosed in a trauma patient with contraindications to anticoagulation, an IVC filter is generally placed (as discussed earlier). However, occasionally, the thrombus extension may be so severe that venous drainage from

vital organs (e.g., liver, kidneys), becomes obstructed, or lower extremity swelling becomes so significant that healing and clearance of infection is impaired. In these conditions, clot retrieval via percutaneous devices may become useful (112). Percutaneous mechanical thrombectomy devices fall into two categories: rotational and hydrodynamic.

Rotational thrombectomy devices use a high-speed rotating basket or impeller to fragment the thrombus. The ground thrombus particles then travel to the pulmonary circulation (suboptimal for critically ill patients with impaired pulmonary function) (113). Examples of rotational thrombectomy instruments are the Amplatz thrombectomy device (Microvena), the Arrow-Trerotola percutaneous thrombolytic device (Arrow), and the Cragg-Castaneda thrombolytic brush (Microtherapeutics) (112).

Hydrodynamic, or "jet," devices are based on the Venturi effect created by high-speed saline jets directed retrograde. The jets fragment the thrombus and the material is then aspirated into the device. Devices based on this mechanism are presumed to produce less endothelial damage than rotational thrombectomy instruments, but this has not been studied. Examples of hydrodynamic recirculation devices include the AngioJet (Possis), the Hydrolyzer (Cordis), and the Oasis Thrombectomy System (Boston Scientific Corporation). In a study of 37 patients, Kasirajan et al. reported >50% thrombus extraction in 59% of patients treated with these devices and symptomatic improvement in 82% (111).

The Bacchus Trellis (Bacchus Vascular) is a relatively recent device, consisting of a catheter with proximal and distal occlusion balloons and a sheath designed to aspirate contents between the balloons (114). A sinusoidal nitinol wire placed within the catheter is rotated to mix the blood between the balloons. The Trellis device combines a high concentration of thrombolytic drug with mechanical disruption of the clot and has been shown to rapidly remove thrombus in patients with DVT (114). The occlusive balloons limit leakage of thrombolytic drug into the systemic circulation, reducing the risk of bleeding complications, whereas the central balloon is engineered to reduce embolization of particulate debris into the pulmonary circulation. A combination of these technologies may be useful in the management of high-risk critically ill trauma patients in the future.

SUMMARY

VTE refers to thrombi forming in the venous system and the emboli that may become dislodged from these thrombi and travel to other areas of the venous network. The pelvis and lower extremities are the most common places for DVTs to develop, although DVTs may occur in the upper extremities, SVC, and IVC. Embolization of a DVT to the pulmonary circulation and the PE syndromes are the most dreaded complications of VTE.

Venous thrombus forms in veins when one or more of three causative factors (Virchow's triad) are present. These factors (hypercoagulation, intimal injury, and venous stasis), occur commonly in post-trauma, postoperative, systemically inflamed, infected, or anesthetized patients. Clotting is stimulated by a series of procoagulant events that are counteracted by coordinated anticlotting and fibrinolytic activities. The balance between these events will determine whether clots will form and enlarge or will be lysed. Hypercoagulation occurs when the procoagulant system is hyperactive or when the anticlotting or lytic systems are underactive. Examples of the former are the presence of factor V Leiden or high levels of homocysteine, Factors VIII, IX, and XI, TAFI, and fibrinogen. Examples of the latter are deficiencies of protein C, protein S, plasminogen, factor XII, or heparin cofactor II.

The endothelial damage that occurs with operations or penetrating trauma predispose to VTE. Patients who have trauma to the pelvis and lower extremities, in particular, have a greater risk for developing clots in these areas. Intimal damage alone has been reported to result in DVT. Hypercoagulation is another important cause of DVT, which is seen quite often in critically ill patients. Strategies aimed at restoring blood flow with vein compression or early ambulation have been successful in decreasing the incidence of DVT. This clinical triad of findings for DVT may be masked by the presence of edema, pain, discoloration, dyspnea, hypotension, tachycardia, and other clinical signs often seen in critically ill patients. Because the consequences of a missed diagnosis may be devastating, critical-care practitioners must have a high index of suspicion and employ prophylactic measures to prevent or minimize VTE.

In the upper extremities, the axillary and subclavian veins are most often involved with DVT and the clots are usually caused by indwelling catheters. Spontaneous clots caused by anatomic variations such as a narrowed thoracic outlet have no particular significance for the ICU patient other than that they must be differentiated from the thrombi caused by indwelling catheters. Similar to lower extremity thrombi, upper extremity thrombi may embolize to the lungs. Diagnosis of an upper extremity thrombus is usually made by ultrasonography, but venography is occasionally required. The area of the shoulder and neck is less accessible and the full range of diagnostic maneuvers such as compression ultrasound and plethysmography that are used in the lower extremities is not possible. Catheter-related thrombi can usually be treated by removing the catheter. Clot lysis using the catheter to deliver the thrombolytic agents is another strategy that is particularly helpful when the catheter cannot be removed for therapeutic reasons.

The SVC is another anatomic location for clot formation. Many of these are formed around catheter tips and the diagnosis and treatment of these clots are similar to those that form in the more peripheral veins. Of note, catheters that end in the subclavian or innominate veins are more likely to form clots than those positioned with their tips in the SVC close to the right atrial junction. SVC obstruction can also be caused by malignancies of the mediastinum that either compress or invade the SVC. Although DVT is not the primary etiology of these obstructions, clotting may be secondarily involved, making stenting and thrombolysis therapeutic alternatives for critically ill patients.

IVC thrombus is typically seen with BCS or nephrotic syndrome. The prognosis in both cases is more dependent on the effect of the diseases on hepatic and renal function, respectively. Clots in the IVC are not easily accessible and treatment usually involves anticoagulation, thrombolysis, and only rarely, surgical intervention.

Most DVTs occur in the veins of the pelvis and lower extremities. The iliac veins have the greatest risk of massive embolism to the lungs. Clots form more often in the left iliac vein due to compression on this side by the right iliac artery. The diagnosis of a lower extremity DVT may be accomplished by careful physical exam, but in the case of critically ill patients with significant comorbidity, other methods may be required. Ultrasonography, combined with Doppler technology and physical maneuvers such as compression, is the best screening exam. It has the advantages of being relatively inexpensive and portable. IPG is also useful, but has been largely supplanted by ultrasound. Contrast venography is the most sensitive and specific exam; however, it is invasive and is associated with a number of complications, such as renal failure.

Prevention and treatment of lower extremity VTE generally starts with anticoagulation. UFH is used most often for acute situations, but it requires lab tests for monitoring and an intravenous drip for full therapeutic anticoagulation. LMWH preparations are now available that may be given by subcutaneous injection without lab monitoring, making them useful for outpatient management. Both forms of heparin can cause immune thrombocytopenia (less so with LMWH) so alternative medications such as DTIs are sometimes required. VTE is the most common sequela of HIT, and thus signs or symptoms of DVT or PE in a patient receiving antithrombotic prophylaxis with UFH or LMWH should prompt diagnostic consideration of HIT.

Mechanical devices that prevent or treat VTE include elastic or pneumatic compression stockings and a variety of intravenous filters. Interventional radiologists have developed a number of strategies for dealing with venous obstruction related to DVTs. Catheter-directed thrombolysis using urokinase, tissue plasminogen activator, or streptokinase is the mainstay of radiographic intervention. Thrombolytics may be delivered directly adjacent to the clots or sometimes within the clot, with a side-holed catheter. Balloon angioplasty and stenting may be added to thrombolysis in circumstances when a stricture or narrowing may compromise flow. Surgery is not done very commonly due to the success of the less invasive procedures noted earlier. When surgery is necessary (e.g., an acutely threatened limb), thrombectomy of the ipsilateral side or venous bypass to the contralateral side is possible. Despite the large number of therapeutic options available, the major thrust of treatment should be preventative. For this reason, prevention of venous stasis by early ambulation should be encouraged in all bed-bound or minimally ambulatory patients.

KEY POINTS

- The components of Virchow's triad (hypercoagulation, endothelial injury, and venous stasis) have long been recognized as the etiological factors for VTE. When one or more of these factors are present, there is an initiation of the coagulation cascade and increased risk of clot formation.
- As soon as clot formation begins, processes are initiated to turn off (or downregulate) clotting [AT III and proteins C and S] or dissolve the already formed clots (plasmin and tissue plasminogen activator). Proper regulation of clotting and clot dissolution will minimize the risk of VTE.
- Overactivity of the procoagulant system or underactivity of the anticlotting or fibrinolytic systems results in a hypercoagulable state, also termed thrombophilia (Table 1).
- Venous stasis is probably the most important risk factor for VTE in patients who are critically ill or recovering from trauma or surgery. Since these patients are often bed-ridden, sedated, or paralyzed, they have sluggish blood flow and poor venous return. Blood flow may also be compromised by low cardiac output, abdominal

compartment syndrome, and elevated intravenous pressure from right heart failure (14).

- Polyethylene and polyvinyl chloride catheters are more prone to pulmonary emboli than polyurethane or siliconized catheters, whereas the heparin-bonded catheters seem to be better than those without heparin bonding. Catheters placed so that the tips are in the SVC or the right atrium have a lower incidence of thrombi than those placed in the innominate or subclavian veins.

- When emboli originate from the vessel wall they are termed mural thrombi. When emboli originate from an indwelling catheter they are termed sleeve emboli. Sleeve emboli have a greater chance of embolizing.

- Although a properly performed venogram has close to 100% sensitivity and 100% specificity, it is done only infrequently because VDU is safer, less expensive, and usually sufficient.

- When the thrombi occur as a result of an indwelling catheter, the cornerstone of treatment is removal of the catheter and anticoagulation (when not contraindicated).

- Stenting may be particularly appropriate for critically ill patients who are too ill to wait for resolution of symptoms of SVC syndrome by radiation or chemotherapy and cannot undergo surgical procedures.

- Although catheter-related thrombosis represents a relatively small percentage of patients who develop SVC syndrome, it is commonly seen in critically ill trauma patients who have multiple indwelling catheters for fluids, monitoring, pacemakers, and cardiac defibrillators.

- Thrombosis may occur anywhere in the IVC, such as with Behcet's disease. However, most IVC clotting occurs near the hepatic veins as a consequence of BCS or adjacent to the renal veins as a consequence of nephrotic syndrome.

- There is a high incidence of renal vein thrombosis with nephrotic syndrome for reasons that are not clear. Patients with nephrotic syndrome are hypercoagulable and have an increased occurrence of generalized arterial and venous thomboemboli; however, the incidence of clotting is highest in the renal veins.

- DVTs occur more commonly in the left common iliac vein. This is explained anatomically because the right common iliac artery compresses the left common iliac vein as it crosses over it. Repetitive pulsations may cause a "web" or "spur" to form and make this vein more prone to thrombosis. This condition has been termed May–Thurner syndrome (45).

- Serial VDU studies should be performed if the initial exam is negative because 2% of patients with an initially negative exam will have a positive study when studied seven days later (3,51).

- The most reliable venographic finding indicating a DVT is an intraluminal filling defect seen on two or more views of the same area (58).

- UFH is the first choice in treatment for DVT but has limitations, which include a narrow therapeutic window and variable dose–response that requires frequent monitoring.

- All forms of heparin (including LMWH) should be discontinued when HIT is diagnosed and nonheparin based anticoagulation should be instituted (64).

- Intermittent pneumatic leg compression has both local and systemic effects. Locally, it acts by simulating the calf muscle pump and, thus, preventing venous stasis. Systemically, it acts by inhibiting plasminogen activator inhibitor-1 and increasing the body's fibrinolytic activity.

- The indications for placement of filters are the following: (*i*) acute VTE in a patient who has a contraindication for anticoagulation, (*ii*) VTE in a patient who is already anticoagulated, (*iii*) patients who have a compromised pulmonary vascular bed in whom a VTE would not be tolerated, (*iv*) patients with a high fall risk in whom anticoagulation could cause bleeding, and (*v*) trauma patients with a prolonged high risk for VTE due to prolonged immobility (e.g., quadriplegia) and severe traumatic brain injury (TBI) (73).

- In addition to May–Thurner syndrome, endoluminal stenting and balloon angioplasty have been described in other types of iliofemoral venous occlusive disease. Although these procedures are uncommonly performed, they offer nonsurgical options for trauma and critically ill patients with VTE disease.

- Although elastic compression and pneumatic compression devices restore some of the lost blood flow, mobilization and, specifically, ambulation provides complete restoration of flow and the greatest protection against VTE.

- There have been several recent studies that have demonstrated that bed rest does not decrease the incidence of PE following DVT.

REFERENCES

1. Knudson MM, Ikossi DG. Venous thromboembolism after trauma. Curr Opin Crit Care 2004; 10:539–548.
2. Eastman AB. Venous thromboembolism prophylaxis in trauma patients. Tech Orthop 2004; 19(4):293–299.
3. Geerts WH, Pineo GF, Heit JA, et al. Prevention of venous thromboembolism: the seventh ACCP conference on antithrombotic and thrombolytic therapy. Chest 2004; 126: 338S–400S.
4. Rogers FB, Cipolle MD, Velmahos G, et al. Practice management guidelines for the prevention of venous thromboembolism in trauma patients: the EAST practice management work group. J Trauma 2002; 53:142–164.
5. Knudson MM, Ikossi DG, Khaw L, et al. Thromboembolism after trauma: an analysis of 1602 episodes from the American College of Surgeons National Trauma Data Bank. Ann Surg 2004; 240:490–498.
6. Bernard GR, Vincent JL, Laterre PF, et al. Efficacy and safety of recombinant human activated protein C for severe sepsis. N Engl J Med 2001; 344:699–709.
7. deLange M, Snieder H, Ariens RA, et al. The genetics of haemostasis: a twin study. Lancet 2001; 357:101–105.
8. Mateo J, Oliver A, Borrell M, et al. Laboratory evaluation and clinical characteristics of 2,132 consecutive unselected patients with venous thromboembolism—results of the Spanish Multicentric Study on Thrombophilia (EMET-Study). Thromb Haemost 1997; 77:444–451.
9. Heit JA, Silverstein MD, Mohr DN, et al. Risk factors for deep vein thrombosis and pulmonary embolism: a population based case-control study. Arch Intern Med 2000; 160:809–815.
10. Meissner MH, Chandler WL, Elliott JS. Venous thromboembolism in trauma: a local manifestation of systemic hypercoagulability. J Trauma 2003; 54:224–231.
11. Boldt J, Papsdorf M, Rothe A, et al. Changes of the hemostatic network in critically ill patients: is there a difference between sepsis, trauma, and neurosurgery patients? Crit Care Med 2000; 28:445–450.
12. White RH, Zhou H, Romano PS. Incidence of symptomatic venous thromboembolism after different elective or urgent surgical procedures. Thromb Haemost 2003; 90:446–455.
13. McColl MD, Tait RC, Greer IA, Walker ID. Injecting drug use is a risk factor for deep vein thrombosis in women in Glasgow. Br J Haematol 2001;112:641–643.

14. Williams MT, Aravindan N, Wallace MJ, et al. Venous thromboembolism in the intensive care unit. Crit Care Clin 2003; 19:185–207.

15. Cook D, Attia J, Weaver B, et al. Venous thromboembolic disease: an observational study in medical-surgical intensive care unit patients. J Crit Care 2000; 15:127–132.

16. Otten TR, Stein PD, Patel KC, et al. Thromboembolic disease involving the superior vena cava and brachiocephalic veins. Chest 2003; 123:809–812.

17. Lokich JJ, Becker B. Subclavian vein thrombosis in patients treated with infusion chemotherapy for advanced malignancy. Cancer 1983; 52:1586–1589.

18. Monreal M, Raventos A, Lerma R, et al. Pulmonary embolism in patients with upper extremity DVT associated to venous central lines—a prospective study. Thromb Haemost 1994; 72:548–550.

19. Pierce CM, Wade A, Mok Q. Heparin-bonded central venous lines reduce thrombotic and infective complications in critically ill children. Intensive Care Med 2000; 29:967–972.

20. Haire WD. Arm vein thrombosis. Clin Chest Med 1995; 16:341–351.

21. Sivaram CA, Craven P, Chandrasekaran K. Transesophageal echocardiography during removal of central venous catheter associated with thrombus in superior vena cava. Am J Card Imaging 1996; 10:266–269.

22. Harvey JR, Teague SM, Anderson JL, et al. Clinically silent atrial septal defects with evidence for cerebral embolization. Ann Int Med 198; 105:695–697.

23. Mustafa BO, Rathbun SW, Whitsett TL, Raskob GE. Sensitivity and specificity of ultrasonography in the diagnosis of upper extremity deep vein thrombosis: a systematic review. Arch Int Med 2002; 162:401–404.

24. Andrews JC, Williams DM, Cho KJ. Digital subtraction venography of the upper extremity. Clin Radiol 1987; 38:423–424.

25. Moss JF, Wagman LD, Rijhmaki DU, Terz JJ. Central venous thrombosis related to the silastic Hickman/Broviac catheter in an oncologic population. JPEN 1989; 13:397–400.

26. Haire WD, Lieberman RP, Lund GB, et al. Obstructed central venous catheters. Restoring function with a 12 hour infusion of low-dose urokinase. Cancer 1990; 66:2279–2285.

27. Molina JE. Surgery for effort thrombosis of the subclavian vein. J Thorac Cardiovasc Surg 1992; 103:341–346.

28. Urschel HC, Razzuk MA. Paget–Schroetter syndrome: what is the best management? Ann Thorasc Surg 2000; 69:1663–1668.

29. Donayre CE, White GH, Mehringer SM, Wilson SE. Pathogenesis determines late morbidity of axillosubclavian vein thrombosis. Am J Surg 1986; 152:179–184.

30. Spence LD, Gironta MG, Malde HM, et al. Acute upper extremity deep venous thrombosis: safety and effectiveness of superior vena caval filters. Radiology 1999; 210:53–58.

31. Markham M. Diagnosis and management of superior vena cava syndrome. Clev Clin J Med 1999; 66:59–61.

32. Chatzioannou A, Alexopoloulos T, Mourikis D, et al. Stent therapy for malignant superior vena cava syndrome: should be first line therapy or simple adjunct to radiotherapy. Eur J Radiol 2003; 47:247.

33. Gray BH, Olin JW, Graor RA, et al. Safety and efficacy or thrombolytic therapy for superior vena cava syndrome. Chest 1991; 99:54–59.

34. Lagerstrom CF, Mitchell HG, Graham BS, Hammon JW. Chronic fibrosing mediastinitis and superior vena caval obstruction from blastomycosis. Ann Thorac Surg 1992; 54:764–765.

35. Ramakantan R, Shah P. Dysphagia due to mediastinal fibrosis in advanced pulmonary tuberculosis. Am J Roentgenol 1990; 154:61–63.

36. Bayraktar Y, Balkanci F, Bayraktar M, Calguneri M. The Budd–Chiari syndrome: a common complication of Behcet's Disease. Am J Gastroenterol 1997; 92:858–862.

37. Menon KV, Shah V, Kamath PS. The Budd–Chiari syndrome. N Engl J Med 2004; 350:578–585.

38. Dilawari JB, Bambery P, Chawla Y, et al. Hepatic outflow obstruction (Budd–Chiari syndrome): experience with 177 patients and a review of the literature. Medicine 1994; 73:21–36.

39. Hadengue A, Poliquin M, Vilgrain V, et al. The changing scene of hepatic vein thrombosis: recognition of asymptomatic cases. Gastroenterology 1994; 106:1042–1047.

40. Klein AS, Molmenti EP. Surgical treatment of Budd–Chiari syndrome. Liver Transpl 2003; 9:891–896.

41. Platt JF, Ellis JH, Rubin JM. Intrarenal arterial Doppler sonography in the detection of renal vein thrombosis of the native kidney. Am J Roentgenol 1994; 162:1367–1370.

42. Duffy JL, Letteri J, Clinque T, et al. Renal vein thrombosis and the nephrotic syndrome. Report of two cases with successful treatment of one. Am J Med 1973; 54:663–672.

43. Mozes P and Gloviczki P. New discoveries in anatomy and new terminology of leg veins: clinical implications. Vasc Endovasc Surg 2004; 38:367–374.

44. Moser KM, Lemoine JR. Is embolic risk conditioned by localization of deep venous thrombosis? Ann Intern Med 1981; 94:439.

45. Kibbe MR, Ujiki M, Goodwin L, et al. Iliac vein compression in an asymptomatic patient population. J Vasc Surg 2004; 39:937–943.

46. Cranley JJ, Canos AJ, Sull WJ. The diagnosis of deep venous thrombosis: fallibility of clinical symptoms and signs. Arch Surg 1976; 111:34–36.

47. Hirsh J, Hull RD, Raskob GE. Clinical features and diagnosis of venous thrombosis. J Am Col Card 1986; 8:114B–127B.

48. Geerts WH, Heit JA, Claggett GP, et al. Prevention of venous thromboembolism. Chest 2001; 119:132S–175S.

49. Wells PS, Anderson DR, Rodger M, et al. Evaluation of D-Dimer in the diagnosis of suspected deep-vein thrombosis. N Engl J Med 2003; 349:1227–1235.

50. Comerota AJ, Katz ML. The diagnosis of acute deep venous thrombosis by duplex venous imaging. Semin Vasc Surg 1988; 1:32–39.

51. Mattos MA, Londrey GL, Leutz DW, et al. Color-flow duplex scanning for the surveillance and diagnosis of acute deep venous thrombosis. J Vasc Surg 1992; 15:366–375.

52. Peter DJ, Flanagan LD, Cranley JJ. Analysis of blood clot echogenicity. J Clin Ultra 1986; 14:111–116.

53. Kearon C, Ginsberg JS, Hirsh J. The role of venous ultrasonography in the diagnosis of suspected deep venous thrombosis and pulmonary embolism. Ann Int Med 1998; 129:1044–1049.

54. Lensing AW, Prandoni P, Brandjes D, et al. Detection of deep-vein thrombosis by real time B-mode ultrasonography. N Engl J Med 1989; 320:342–345.

55. Hull R, Hirsh J, Sackett DL, et al. Replacement of venography in suspected venous thrombosis by impedance plethysmography and 125 I-fibrinogen leg scanning. Ann Int Med 198; 94:12–15.

56. Hull RD, Hirsh J, Carter CJ. Diagnostic efficacy of impedance plethysmography for clinically suspected deep vein thrombosis. A randomized trial. Ann Int Med 1985; 102:21–28.

57. Comerota AJ, Katz ML, Grossi RJ, et al. The comparative value of noninvasive testing for diagnosis and surveillance of deep venous thrombosis. J Vasc Surg 1988; 7:40–49.

58. Rubinov K, Paulin S. Roentgen diagnosis of venous thrombosis of the leg. Arch Surg 1972; 104:134–144.

59. Hull RD, Hirsh J, Sackett DL, et al. Clinical validity of a negative venogram in patients with clinically suspected venous thrombosis. Circ 1981; 64:622–626.

60. Hirsh J, Warkentin TE, Shaughnessy SG, et al. Heparin and low-molecular-weight heparin: mechanisms of action, pharmacokinetics, dosing, monitoring, efficacy, and safety. Chest 2001; 119:64S–94S.

61. Hirsh J, Anand SS, Halperin JL, Fuster V. Guide to anticoagulant therapy: Heparin: a statement for healthcare professionals

from the American Heart Association. Circulation 2001; 103:2994–3018.

62. Cruickshank MK, Levine MN, Hirsh J, et al. A standard nomogram for the management of heparin therapy. Arch Intern Med 1991; 151:333–337.

63. Juergens CP, Semsarian C, Keech AC, et al. Hemorrhagic complications of intravenous heparin use. Am J Cardiol 1997; 80:150–154.

64. Warkentin TE, Greinacher A. Heparin-induced thrombocytopenia: recognition, treatment, and prevention. The seventh ACCP conference on antithrombotic and thrombolytic therapy. Chest 2004; 126:311S–337S.

65. Weitz JI. Low molecular weight heparins. N Engl J Med 1997; 337:688–698.

66. Weitz JI, Hirsh J, Samama MM. New anticoagulant drugs: the Seventh ACCP conference on antithrombotic and thrombolytic therapy. Chest 2004: 126:265S–286S.

67. Hirsh J, Dalen J, Anderson DR, et al. Managing oral anticoagulant therapy. Chest 2001; 119:22S–38S.

68. Comerota AJ, Chouhan V, Harada RN, et al. The fibrinolytic effects of intermittent pneumatic compression: mechanism of enhanced fibrinolysis. Ann Surg 1997; 226:306–313.

69. Turpie AG, Delmore T, Hirsh J, et al. Prevention of venous thrombosis by intermittent sequential calf compression in patients with intracranial disease. Thromb Res 1979; 15:611–616.

70. Ramos RS, Salem BI, De Pawlikowski MP. The efficacy of pneumatic compression stockings in the prevention of pulmonary embolism after cardiac surgery. Chest 1996; 109:82–87.

71. Streiff MD. Vena caval filters: a review for the intensive care specialist. J Intensive Care Med 2003; 18:59–79.

72. Decousus H, Leizorovicz A, Parent F, et al. A clinical trial of vena caval filters in the prevention of pulmonary embolism in patients with proximal deep-vein thrombosis. N Engl J Med 1998; 338:409–415.

73. Hyers TM, Agnelli G, Hull RD, et al. Antithrombotic therapy for venous thromboembolic disease. Chest 2001; 119: 176S–193S.

74. Markel A. Manzo RA, Strandness DE. The potential role of thrombolytics therapy in venous thrombosis. Arch Intern Med 1992; 152:1265–1267.

75. Rogers LQ, Lutcher CL. Streptokinase therapy for deep venous thrombosis: a comprehensive review of the literature. Am J Med 1990; 88:389–395.

76. O'Meara JJ, Mcnutt RA, Evans AT. A decision analysis of streptokinase plus heparin as compared with heparin alone for deep-vein thrombosis. N Engl J Med 1994; 330:1864–1869.

77. Turpie AG, Levine MN, Hirsh J, et al. Tissue-plasminogen activator versus heparin in deep venous thrombosis. Results of a randomized trial. Chest 1990; 97:172S–175S.

78. Mewissen MW, Seabrook GR, Meissner MH. Catheter directed thrombolysis for lower extremity deep venous thrombosis: report of a national multicenter registry. Radiology 1999; 211:39–49.

79. Hood DB, Alexander JQ. Endovascular management of iliofemoral venous occlusive disease. Surg Clin North Am 2004; 84:1381–1396.

80. Ouriel K, Green R, Greenberg RK, Clair DG. The anatomy of deep venous thrombosis of the lower extremity. J Vasc Surg 2000; 31:895–900.

81. Comerota AJ, Aldridge SC, Cohen G, et al. A strategy of aggressive regional therapy for acute iliofemoral venous thrombosis with contemporary venous thrombectomy or catheter-directed thrombolysis. J Vasc Surg 1994; 20:244–254.

82. Rutherford RB, Eklof B, Mewissen M. Interventional treatments for iliofemoral venous thrombosis. In: Rutherford RD, ed. Vascular Surgery, 5th ed. Philadelphia, PA: W.B. Saunders; 2000:1959–1968.

83. Reber PU, Patel, AG, Genyk, I, Kniemeyer. Crosover saphenous vein bypass (Palma) in phlegmasia cerulea dolens caused by total iliac outflow obstruction. J Am Coll Surg 1999; 189:527–529.

84. Beasley R, Raymond N, Hill S, et al. Thrombosis: the 21st century variant of venous thromboembolism associated with immobility Eur Respir J 2003; 21:374–376.

85. Kiekegaard A, Norgren L, Olsson CG, et al. Incidence of deep vein thrombosis in bed-ridden non-surgical patients. Acta Med Scand 1987; 222:409–414.

86. Orosz GM, Magaziner J, Hannan EL, et al. Association of timing of surgery for hip fracture and patient outcomes. JAMA 2004; 291:1738–1743.

87. Partsch H. Bed rest versus ambulation in the initial treatment of patients with proximal deep vein thrombosis, Curr Opin Pulm Med 2002; 8:389–393.

88. Horlander KT, Mannino DM, Leeper KV. Pulmonary embolism mortality in the United States, 1979-1998: an analysis using multi-cause mortality data. Arch Intern Med 2003; 163:1711–1717.

89. Goldhaber SZ, Visani L, DeRosa M. Acute pulmonary embolism: clinical outcomes in the International Cooperative Pulmonary Embolism Registry (ICOPER). Lancet 1999; 353: 1386–1389.

90. Stein PD, Terrin ML, Hales CA, et al. Clinical, laboratory, roentgenographic, and electrocardiographic findings in patients with acute pulmonary embolism and no pre-existing cardiac or pulmonary disease. Chest 1991; 100: 598–603.

91. Perrier A, Howarth N, Didier D, et al. Performance of helical computed tomography in unselected outpatients with suspected pulmonary embolism. Ann Intern Med 2001; 135:88–97.

92. Hudson ER, Smith TP, McDermott VG, et al. Pulmonary angiography performed with iopamidol: complications in 1,434 patients. Radiology 1996; 198:61–65.

93. Sharma GV, Folland ED, McIntyre KM, Sasahara AA. Long-term benefit of thrombolytic therapy in patients with pulmonary embolism. Vasc Med 2000; 5:91–95.

94. Tajima H, Murata S, Kumazaki T, et al. Hybrid treatment of massive pulmonary thromboembolism by mechanical fragmentation with a modified rotating pigtail catheter, local fibrinolytic therapy, and clot aspiration followed by systemic fibrinolytic therapy. AJR Am J Roentgenol 2004; 183:589–595.

95. Hirnle T, Hirnle G. A case of surgical treatment of acute pulmonary embolism without the use of extracorporeal circulation. Surgery 2004; 135:461–462.

96. Stein PD, Hull RD, Raskob GE. Withholding treatment in patients with acute pulmonary embolism who have a high risk of bleeding and a negative serial noninvasive leg tests. Am J Med 200; 109:301–306.

97. Fareed J, Ma Q, Florian M, et al. Differentiation of low-molecular weight heparins: impact on the future of the management of thrombosis. Semin Thromb Hemostat 2004; 30:89–104.

98. Andersen JC. Advances in anticoagulation therapy: the role of selective inhibitors of factor Xa and thrombin in thromboprophylaxis after major orthopedic surgery. Semin Thromb Hemostat 2004; 30:609–618.

99. Willems HP, Heijer M, Bos GM. Homocysteine and venous thrombosis: outline of a vitamin intervention trial. Semin Thromb Hemostat 2000; 26:297–304.

100. HaireWD, Lynch TG, Lund GB, Edney JA. Limitations of magnetic resonance imaging and ultrasound-directed (duplex) scanning in the diagnosis of subclavian vein thrombosis. J Vasc Surg 1991; 13:391.

101. Yankelevitz DF, Gamsu G, Shah A, et al. Optimization of combined CT pulmonary angiography with lower extremity CT venography. Am J Roentgen 2000; 174:67–69.

102. Carpenter JP, Holland GA, Baum RA, et al. Magnetic resonance venography for the detection of deep venous thrombosis: comparison with contrast venography and duplex Doppler ultrasonography. J Vasc Surg 1993; 18:734–741.

103. Blebea J, Wilson R, Waybill P, et al. Deep venous thrombosis after percutaneous insertion of vena caval filters. J Vasc Surg 1999; 30:831–838.

104. Kinney TB. Update on inferior vena cava filters. J Vasc Interv Radiol. 2003; 14:425–440.

105. Yamagami T, Kato T, Iida S, et al. Retrievable vena cava filter placement during treatment for deep venous thrombosis. Br J Radiol 2003; 76(910):712–718.

106. Morris CS, Rogers FB, Najarian KE, et al. Current trends in vena caval filtration with the introduction of a retrievable filter at a level I trauma center. J Trauma 2004; 57(1):32–36.

107. Terhaar OA, Lyon SM, Given MF, et al. Extended interval for retrieval of Gunther Tulip filters. J Vasc Interv Radiol 2004; 11:1257–1262.

108. Binkert CA, Bansal A, Gates JD. Inferior vena cava filter removal after 317-day implantation. J Vasc Interv Radiol 2005; 16(3):395–398.

109. Greene FL, Sing RF, Mostafa G, et al. Letter to the editor. J Trauma 2005; 58(5):1091.

110. Rosenthal DR, Wellons ED, Levitt AB, et al. Role of prophylactic temporary inferior vena cava filters placed at the ICU bedside under intravascular ultrasound guidance in patients with multiple trauma. J Vasc Surg 2004; 4440:958–964.

111. Kasirajan K, Gray B, Ouriel K. Percutaneous AngioJet thrombectomy in the management of extensive deep venous thrombosis. J Vasc Intervent Rad 2001; 12:179–185.

112. Augustinos P, Ouriel K. Invasive approaches to treatment of venous thromboembolism. Circulation 2004; 110(9 suppl 1): I27–I34.

113. Delomez M, Beregi JP, Willoteaux S, et al. Mechanical thrombectomy in patients with deep venous thrombosis. Cardiovasc Intervent Radiol 2001; 24:42–48.

114. Ramaiah V, Del Santo PB, Rodriguez-Lopez JA, et al. Trellis thrombectomy system for the treatment of iliofemoral deep venous thrombosis. J Endovasc Ther 2003; 10:585–589.

115. Wells PS, Anderson DR, Bormanis J, et al. Lancet 1997; 350:1795 and Wells PS, Anderson DR, Rodger M, et al. N Engl J Med 2003; 349:1227.

116. Raschke RA, Reilly BM, Guidry JR, et al, Ann Intern Med 1993; 199:874.

117. Streiff MB: Vena cava filters: a comprehensive review. Blood 2000; 95(12):2669–2677.

57

Leukocytosis and Leukopenia

Theodore E. Warkentin

Departments of Pathology and Molecular Medicine, McMaster University School of Medicine,
and the Transfusion Medicine Service, Hamilton Health Sciences,
Hamilton, Ontario, Canada

INTRODUCTION

☞ **Leukocytosis or leukopenia is often the first clue that a post-trauma or critically ill patient has an infection or a severe inflammatory process.** ☞ Leukocytosis is an abnormally high white blood count (WBC), whereas leukopenia denotes a reduced WBC (1–3); either laboratory finding constitutes a potentially consequential event in a critically ill patient. For example, abrupt onset of leukopenia could signify acute bacterial invasion of the blood, or perforation of a viscus; the decrease in leukocyte count reflects margination of neutrophils and their egress into tissues, a process that is sufficiently rapid so as to precede the (eventual) leukocytosis expected from increased production and release of granulocytes from the marrow storage pool. In other situations, however, abrupt and transient leukopenia is not unusual or unexpected, such as during the initial phase of cardiopulmonary bypass (CPB) (4).

The ubiquity of automated cell counters, with their computerized digital and graphical displays summarizing patient laboratory data, facilitates clinician awareness and interpretation of such important *quantitative* leukocyte changes. However, evaluation of *qualitative* leukocyte abnormalities requires nonautomated human action; indeed, the review of a peripheral blood film by an experienced "morphologist" is the single most useful laboratory evaluation performed in hematology (1). It is crucial that important information regarding leukocyte abnormalities evident within the blood film be communicated from the laboratory to the critical care practitioner.

This chapter reviews quantitative leukocyte disorders of particular relevance to the post-trauma and critically ill postsurgical patient. The reader should consult other sources for detailed information on pre-existing leukocyte disorders, particularly of neoplastic origin (leukemia, lymphoma, myeloma, etc.).

DEFINITION OF LEUKOCYTOSIS AND LEUKOPENIA

☞ **Leukocytosis is defined as a WBC count above the upper limit of the normal laboratory range (about 11×10^9/L), whereas leukopenia is defined as a WBC count below the lower limit of the normal laboratory range (about 4.0×10^9/L).** ☞ Higher leukocyte counts are normal in children, especially neonates; moreover, the relative proportion of lymphocytes is greater in children (2). Proper evaluation of leukocytosis and leukopenia requires consideration of the relative distribution of the various types of leukocytes (i.e., evaluation of the differential leukocyte count) and any abnormal morphological features.

LEUKOCYTE CLASSIFICATION

Leukocytes are classified by their morphologic appearance into granulocytes, monocytes, and lymphocytes (Fig. 1) (1–3). Table 1 lists terms used to describe specific quantitative abnormalities of the various leukocyte types. Table 2 lists an overview of trauma-associated and other diagnostic considerations based upon the type of leukocyte involved in the quantitative abnormality.

Granulocytes

Granulocytes (polymorphonuclear leukocytes) consist of neutrophils, eosinophils, basophils, and their respective morphologically distinguishable precursors within the bone marrow. Mature neutrophils are about 13 μm in diameter, and circulate in the peripheral blood in the largest relative numbers [40% to 80%; percentages relate to the fraction of the total WBC count (absolute: $1.5–8.0 \times 10^9$/L)]. They are also known as "polys" or "segmented" leukocytes, based upon the characteristic appearance of the nucleus, which consists of 2 to 5 lobes separated by thin chromatin strands (1,3). A somewhat earlier stage, known as band cells (or "bands"), possesses the horseshoe-shaped nucleus that precedes nuclear segmentation seen in the polys. These cells are normally absent or found in low levels (<5%) in the peripheral blood, but their increase is a characteristic early finding in infections or inflammatory states. Normal polys and bands have light pink cytoplasm and fine azurophilic granules. Progressively more immature granulocytes (metamyelocytes, myelocytes, promyelocytes, myeloblasts) are only found in the bone marrow in normal situations. The production of neutrophils involves several growth factors, primarily granulocyte colony-stimulating factor (G-CSF), and to a lesser extent, granulocyte-macrophage colony-stimulating factor (GM-CSF), and macrophage colony-stimulating factor (M-CSF).

Other granulocytes that circulate normally in the peripheral blood in small numbers are eosinophils [1% to 5% (absolute: <0.4%)], characterized by their numerous orange/red-staining granules, and basophils [<1%; (absolute: <0.2%)], which have darkly-staining purple-black granules (2,3). Eosinophils contain three different types of granules, but their characteristic appearance results from

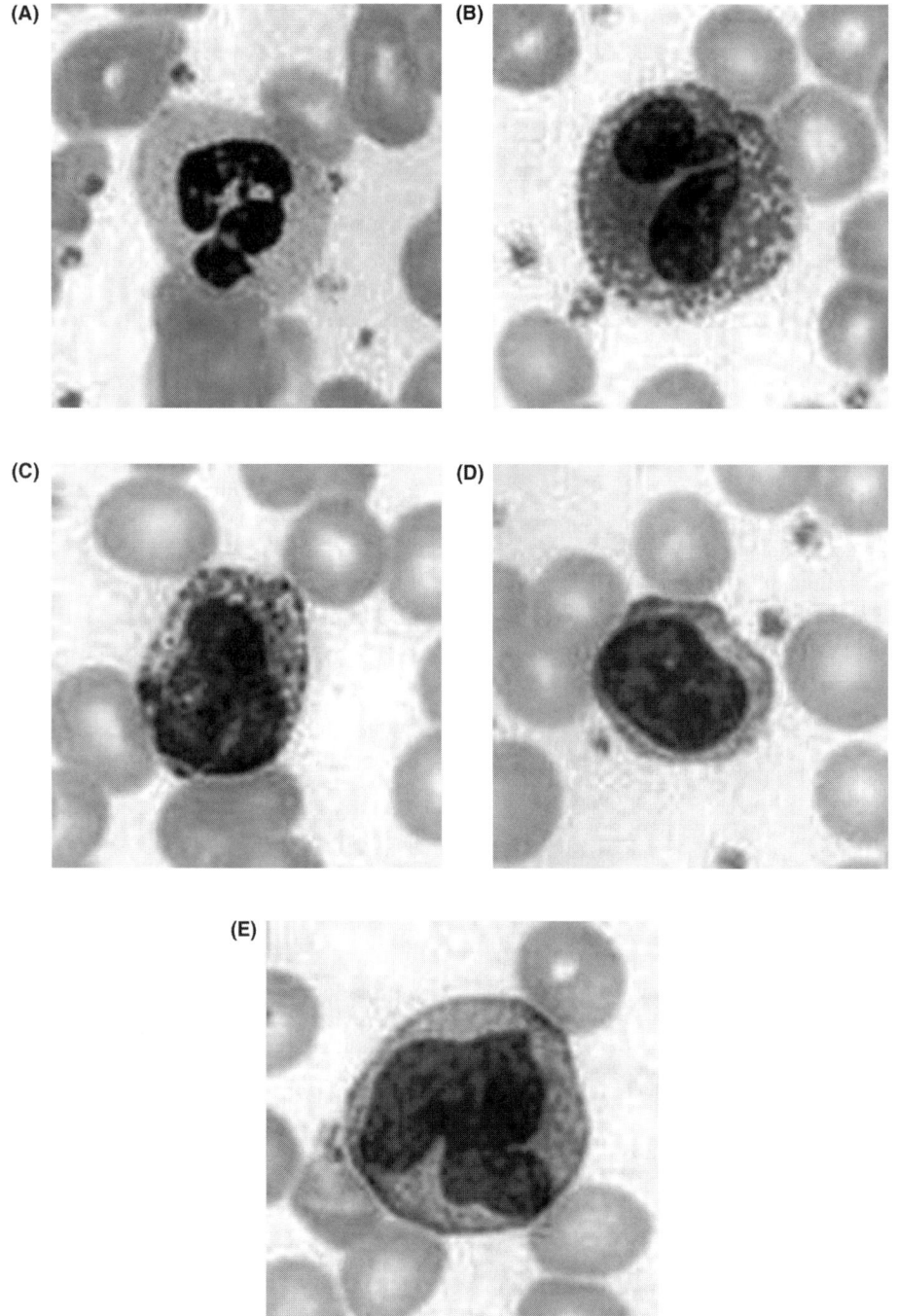

Figure 1   (**A**) Neutrophil granulocyte, (**B**) eosinophil granulocyte, (**C**) basophil granulocyte, (**D**) lymphocyte, (**E**) monocyte.

so-called "specific" (secondary) granules bearing proteins, toxic to metazoan parasites [major basic protein (MBP), eosinophil cationic protein (ECP), eosinophil derived neurotoxin (EDN)]. Eosinophils (and their precursors) resemble morphologically their neutrophil counterparts, except for their distinct granules and bilobed nuclei. They play a major role in the pathogenesis of several allergic, parasitic, and malignant disease processes.

Previously, basophils were regarded simply as circulating tissue mast cells. However, basophils mature in the bone marrow and then circulate in the peripheral blood, whereas mast cells mature in the tissues. Like eosinophils, basophils (and mast cells) have roles in mediating certain types of allergic and inflammatory diseases, and in defense against parasites. Basophils are the only peripheral blood mononuclear cells with the ability to release preformed IL-4 rapidly in response to appropriate stimuli, such as cell surface IgE cross-linking, which may play a role in amplifying ongoing immune response to helminth infections in the presence of antigen-specific IgE (5).

Monocytes

Monocytes [2% to 10% (absolute: $0.2–1.0 \times 10^9/L$)] are of similar size as granulocytes, but have oval, lobulated nuclei with a slate-grey, convoluted cytoplasm containing a

Table 1 Hematologic Terms Used to Describe Various Profiles of Leukocyte Increase and Decrease

Type of leukocyte	Increased number	Decreased number
Leukocyte	Leukocytosis	Leukopenia
Granulocyte[a]	Granulocytosis	Granulocytopenia
		Agranulocytosis[b]
Neutrophil[a]	Neutrophilia	Neutropenia
Eosinophil[a]	Eosinophilia	Eosinopenia
Basophil[a]	Basophilia	Basopenia
Monocyte[a]	Monocytosis	Monocytopenia
Lymphocyte	Lymphocytosis	Lymphocytopenia

[a]Myeloid cells consists of granulocytes and monocytes, as well as red cells and platelets, and their precursors, all arising from a common committed progenitor cell, the colony-forming unit, granulocyte/erythroid/monocyte/megakaryocyte (CFU-GEMM).
[b]Agranulocytosis indicates complete or near-complete absence of granulocytes, especially neutrophils and their immediate precursors.

few, very fine granules (1,3). Monocytes can be identified also by their staining positive for nonspecific esterase. Cytoplasmic vacuolation, which can occur ex vivo as monocytes, adhere to the glass slide and undergoes activation occurs normally with monocytes, whereas its presence is abnormal in granulocytes. Following their release into the circulation, some monocytes will migrate into tissues, where they attain a larger size, transforming into long-lived tissue macrophages.

Lymphocytes

Lymphocytes (20% to 40% [absolute: $1.5-4.0 \times 10^9$/L]) comprise two morphologically-distinct forms (1). Most lymphocytes are small, with a diameter similar to that of red cells (about 8 μm), and with a central round nucleus surrounded by a thin light blue cytoplasmic rim. About 10% of lymphocytes are larger (diameter 8–16 μm), with the nucleus occupying only about half the cell, and usually containing 5–10 large azurophilic granules. This latter type of lymphocyte

is also called a "large granular lymphocyte" and corresponds to the "natural killer" (NK) cell.

LEUKOCYTE PRODUCTION AND FUNCTION
Hematopoietic Stem Cells

☞ All blood cells ultimately are derived from self-renewing pluripotential stem cells that are able to differentiate into lineage-committed stem cells that themselves differentiate into mature blood cells (6). ☞ Normal human marrow contains only about one million of the earliest such cells. Previously, their existence was inferred by patterns of growth of cellular "colonies," e.g., burst-forming unit-erythroid (BFU-E), but now cell surface markers (particularly, high expression of CD34 antigen) can identify cells that are likely to represent true stem cells.

Myeloid cells (red cells, neutrophils, eosinophils, basophils, monocytes-macrophages, platelets, and their precursors) are derived from a pluripotent stem cell known as colony-forming unit, granulocyte/erythrocyte/monocyte/megakaryocyte (CFU-GEMM). The more committed stem cell, colony-forming unit, granulocyte/monocyte (CFU-GM), can give rise to either the neutrophil or monocytic pathways, depending on cytokines and growth factors.

Lymphocytes are also cells of the hematopoietic system, but the lymphoid lineage diverges at an early time point from the myeloid lineage (7). There are three classes of lymphocytes: T (thymus-derived) cells, which confer cellular immunity; B (bone marrow-derived) cells, which provide humoral immunity; and NK cells, which are able to kill cells infected by microbes that try to evade immune recognition by downregulating the cell's major histocompatibility complex class I molecules. Historically, the "B" in B cells refers to the bursa of Fabricius in which the corresponding avian cells develop.

Granulocyte Production and Function

A normal bone marrow has about a 3:1 ratio of myeloid to erythroid cells. However, about 95% and 5% of peripheral blood cells are erythrocytes and platelets, respectively, and

Table 2 Differential Diagnosis Based upon Type of Increased Leukocyte

Type of leukocyte	Clinical interpretation
Neutrophilia	Trauma-associated: bacterial infection (most common cause; viral infections generally do not cause neutrophilia); fungemia (can cause marked neutrophilia); inflammation; surgery/postoperative state; physiologic stress; postsplenectomy; corticosteroids; epinephrine; hemolysis (see Table 4 for less common causes, as well as nontrauma-associated causes)
Eosinophilia	Trauma-associated: drug-induced allergic (or hypersensitivity) reaction; corticosteroid-induced reactivation of latent parasitic infection
	Other: parasitic infections; atopic/allergic disorders (e.g., asthma); vasculitis; pulmonary and cutaneous eosinophilic disorders; hypereosinophilic syndrome; myeloid leukemia; lymphoma (especially Hodgkin's disease)
Basophilia	Trauma-associated: post-splenectomy
	Other: myeloproliferative disorders; urticaria; hypothyroidism; ulcerative colitis; drug reactions
Monocytosis:	Trauma-associated: bacterial infection, including chronic infections (abscess); post-splenectomy
	Other: infection (e.g., rickettsia, brucellosis, tuberculosis, syphilis, subacute bacterial endocarditis, malaria); autoimmune disorders (e.g., systemic lupus erythematosus, rheumatoid arthritis); vasculitis; ulcerative colitis; sarcoidosis; malignancy; chronic severe neutropenia
Lymphocytosis	Trauma-associated: marker of severe trauma; transfusion-associated cytomegalovirus infection; post-splenectomy
	Other: viral and nonviral infections (e.g., pertussis, tuberculosis, brucellosis); allergic drug reactions; dermatitis herpetiformis; hyperthyroidism

only about 0.5% are leukocytes. The high relative numbers of mature granulocytes and their precursors within the bone marrow, and their relative paucity within the peripheral blood, attests to their short physiologic lifespan within the circulation and, consequently, very rapid cell turnover (more than 100 billion granulocytes are synthesized daily). ☞ **The brief neutrophil lifespan within the circulation (about 6–8 hours) is one major reason why granulocyte transfusions are impracticable.** ☞

Granulocytes are an important component of the innate host defense, providing a "first line of defense" against invading microbial pathogens through their primary function of phagocytosis (2,3). Unlike macrophages, which are resident phagocytic cells within certain organ and tissue sites including alveoli, liver, spleen, or bone marrow, granulocytes are circulating marauders that travel through the bloodstream, thus focusing their antimicrobial activities to sites of infection (2).

Most (75%) of the 90 billion granulocytes within an average-sized adult are mature and maturing neutrophils within the marrow storage pool, with most of the remainder (about 20%) in the myeloid precursor pool also within the marrow. About 3% comprise the marginated (endothelium-adherent) pool (3%), leaving only 2% to circulate within the blood. Awareness of this distribution helps in understanding various explanations for neutrophilia and neutropenia, such as increased demargination and mobilization of marrow storage pool neutrophils (e.g., corticosteroid therapy) or increased margination and neutrophil egress into tissue sites (e.g., burns, systemic complement activation). Increased granulocyte production (e.g., infection, inflammation, myeloproliferative disorders) or decreased granulocyte production (e.g., drug-induced agranulocytosis) are other causes of granulocytosis and granulocytopenia, respectively.

Neutrophils ultimately effect their primary role of phagocytosis through multiple complex processes (3). These include cell-cell and cell-matrix adhesion (e.g., allowing margination to endothelium and subsequent entry into tissues); chemotaxis (chemically-directed cell movement, as in migration of neutrophils toward microbes or sites of inflammation); recognition by neutrophils of immunoglobulin and/or complement-tagged (opsonized) microbes through specialized neutrophil immunoglobulin and complement surface receptors; associated triggering of complex downstream cell signaling events (e.g., immunoglobulin receptor cross-linking induced tyrosine phosphorylation); degranulation and secretion (release of storage granules into phagocytic vacuoles and into the extracellular space, respectively); and phagocytic killing.

Neutrophil mediated phagocytic killing is accomplished by (*i*) synthesis of highly toxic, microbicidal derivatives of molecular O_2 species [superoxide anion (O_2^-), hydrogen peroxide (H_2O_2) and, especially, hydroxyl radical (OH^-)], through activation of the normally latent NADPH oxidase system ("the respiratory burst"), (*ii*) generation of highly-reactive nitric oxide (NO) through nitric oxide synthase (NOS), and (*iii*) the delivery of stored neutrophil microbicidal proteins (both nonenzymic, e.g., bacterial permeability-increasing protein [BPI], defensins, lactoferrin, and enzymic, e.g., proteinase 3, cathepsin, azurocidin, lysozyme, elastase) into the vacuoles containing engulfed microbes (3). Some of these mechanisms are also responsible for clearing senescent and apoptotic cells, and in mediating effects of inflammation even in the absence of infection (3).

Eosinophils are derived from myeloid precursors in response to several T-cell derived cytokines and growth factors, most notably IL-5, whereas for basophils, the major growth and differentiation factor is IL-3 (3).

Monocyte Production and Function

Monocytes are the circulating version of the tissue macrophage; together with their bone marrow progenitors, they comprise the mononuclear phagocyte system (MPS; formerly known as the reticuloendothelial system). Monocytes and tissue monocyte-macrophages play an important role in host defense, although it is worth noting that monocytopenia does not connote the high risk of infection that neutropenia does. Production of monocytes is regulated by IL-3 and GM-CSF produced by T-lymphocytes, and M-CSF produced by endothelium and monocytes themselves. This may help explain the association of monocytes with certain chronic infections in which T-lymphocyte activity has been increased (8).

Macrophages reside predominantly within certain organ and tissue sites including alveoli, liver, spleen, or bone marrow. Exposure of macrophages to cytokines, growth factors, and environmental stimuli from microorganisms will lead to their activation, which stimulates their proliferation, phagocytic, and microbicidal activities.

Lymphocyte Production and Function

Lymphocytes are usually long-lived cells which confer certain special properties, e.g., long-lived immunologic "memory." They are produced mostly in lymphoid organs, such as lymph glands, splenic "white" pulp, and certain regions of the small bowel. Immune specificity is conferred through T-cell receptor and immunoglobulin gene rearrangements, which create molecules with reactivity against foreign antigens (and, sometimes, autoantigens). Volume 2, Chapter 52 provides more information regarding immune system function and dysfunction in normal states and in the critically ill trauma patient.

LABORATORY EVALUATION
Leukocyte Differential

☞ **The first step in evaluating any abnormal increase or decrease in WBC is to determine the leukocyte differential, and thereby classify the process as a neutrophilia, eosinophilia, monocytosis, or lymphocytosis (marked basophilia is rare) or, conversely, a neutropenia or lymphopenia (monocytopenia, eosinopenia, and basopenia are rare).** ☞ Previously, the differential was determined by a morphologist who counted 200 to 300 leukocytes, but now automated assessment is routine. However, for reliable detection of abnormal circulating cells, such as nucleated red cells (normoblasts) or leukemic cells, manual assessment of the blood film is required.

Morphologic Abnormalities

Manual assessment of a peripheral blood film by a technologist and/or hematologist (hematopathologist) is the only way that important leukocyte morphologic abnormalities can be recognized. These features often provide important diagnostic clues regarding infection or severe inflammation in post-trauma or critically-ill patients (Table 3). ☞ **Morphologic granulocyte abnormalities, such as shift-to-the-left, toxic granulation, pale blue cytoplasmic inclusions**

Table 3 Morphologic Features Seen in Peripherical White Blood Cells Indicating Infection or Inflammatory Processes

Morphologic feature[a]	Description
Shift-to-the-left	Relative increase in young polymorphonuclear leukocytes, most often band cells, occasionally also metamyelocytes and myelocytes, and in extreme situations, promyelocytes and myeloblasts
Toxic granulation	Increase in number and size of cytoplasmic granules within granulocytes
Döhle bodies	Small, pale blue $1-2$ μm cytoplasmic inclusions
Vacuolation	Open spaces in cytoplasm of polymorphonuclear leukocytes
Leukemoid reaction	Leukocytosis $>50 \times 10^9/L$
Leukoerythroblastosis	Circulating nucleated red cells (normoblasts) and granulocytic shift-to-the-left (additional presence of "tear drop" red cells suggests infiltrative marrow process)
Pelger-Huët anomaly	Benign variant of autosomal dominant inheritance and 1/6000 frequency in which the neutrophils have a "pince nez" (spectacles clipped to the bridge of the nose) appearance that can resemble bands and thus mimic a left-shift

[a]These features are generally seen in non-neoplastic inflammatory conditions.

(Döhle bodies), or vacuoles can indicate serious infectious/ inflammatory problems. ☞ The shift-to-the-left most commonly presents as an increase in bands, but can also involve the appearance of the earlier granulocytes, metamyelocytes and myelocytes, and in extreme infectious/inflammatory situations (or with certain hematologic neoplasia), promyelocytes and myeloblasts. Sometimes, these abnormal cells are seen even when the WBC is normal. The more "toxic" the overall leukocyte picture, the more likely the patient has a bacteremia/fungemia or noninfective but severe proinflammatory picture (e.g., systemic inflammatory response syndrome (SIRS).

☞ **Severe proinflammatory states can produce a "leukemoid reaction," defined as a leukocyte count above $50 \times 10^9/L$. ☞** Leukoerythroblastosis indicates the presence of granulocytic shift-to-the-left and circulating nucleated red cells (normoblasts), and can be seen in overwhelming pathophy- siologic "stress" (e.g., severe lactic acidosis or hypoxemia, severe hemolysis); the additional presence of "tear drop" red cells suggests an infiltrative marrow process (e.g., metastatic carcinoma).

A major increase in eosinophils or basophils typically indicates allergic reaction/parasitic infestation/neoplastic hypereosinophilia or myeloproliferative/systemic mast cell disorder, respectively. Abnormal monocytes can indicate certain monocytic leukemias, whereas increased numbers of normal-appearing monocytes are seen in certain infections or inflammatory disorders. In some acute viral infections, or certain autoimmune disorders, lymphocytes transform towards plasma cells ("plasmacytoid lymphocytes"), and show evidence of immunoglobulin synthesis (eccentric nucleus implying presence of Golgi apparatus; dark blue cytoplasm inferring the presence of ribosomes producing immunoglobulin).

Ancillary Investigations

Besides WBC quantitation by automated or manual determination of the leukocyte differential, and manual assessment of leukocyte morphologic abnormalities, there are relatively few routine studies to evaluate leukocyte abnormalities. The bone marrow aspirate is often performed to diagnose drug-induced agranulocytosis (in which normal or increased marrow cellularity, with "maturation arrest" at the metamyelocyte or band stage is characteristic), or to investigate any other unexplained persistent neutropenia. Both marrow aspiration and biopsy are usually performed when hematologic neoplasm is suspected. Cell marker studies,

performed with leukocyte-containing fluid (blood, marrow, pleural, peritoneal, cerebrospinal), can detect neoplastic clones [e.g., clonally-restricted (κ or λ light chain-bearing) lymphocytes or plasma cells indicating a neoplastic lymphoproliferative disorder or plasma cell dyscrasia, respectively; absence of CD59 antigen on a clonal population of red cells and granulocytes indicates paroxysmal nocturnal hemoglobulinuria (PNH)]. Measuring leukocyte alkaline phosphatase ("LAP score") can help distinguish a neoplastic myeloproliferative disorder from a "reactive" process, with the former situation having an abnormally low score; unfortunately, a patient with an underlying myeloproliferative syndrome who is post-trauma or critically ill can develop a normal (or even elevated) LAP score, limiting its diagnostic usefulness in this setting. In unusual situations, specialized investigations may be required [detection of antineutrophil antibodies in severe neutropenia; measurement of neutrophil capacity to reduce nitroblue tetrazolium (NBT slide test), which is impaired in chronic granulomatous disease]. Although elevated serum lysozyme or lactoferrin levels corroborate increased neutrophil destruction in many acquired neutropenias, these tests are not of practical help.

DIAGNOSTIC CONSIDERATIONS

Leukocytosis and Leukopenia

As highlighted earlier, the first step in evaluating any abnormal increase or decrease in WBC count is to determine the leukocyte differential. Both neutrophilia and lymphocytosis can occur abruptly in a patient with severe trauma, although the former suggests acute infection, most often with bacteria. A moderate leukopenia may be the first clue that the patient has virtually no circulating neutrophils (but normal lymphocyte numbers), thus suggesting the diagnosis of acute drug-induced agranulocytosis. ☞ **Leukopenia must prompt evaluation of the leukocyte differential to determine the absolute neutrophil level, since acquired severe neutropenia in a hospitalized patient usually signifies drug-induced agranulocytosis, a life-threatening adverse drug reaction. ☞**

The magnitude and rate of leukocyte increase or decrease should be considered. Sometimes, obtaining previous complete blood counts (CBCs) from hospital or family physician records reveals that an abnormal leukocyte count preceded hospitalization.

☞ **Pre-existing causes of leukocytosis in a trauma patient could include a chronic myeloproliferative or**

lymphoproliferative disorder; splenomegaly is often present in this situation. Pre-existing causes of leukopenia in a trauma patient can include hypersplenism (usually due to chronic liver disease), HIV-associated, Felty's syndrome (autoimmune neutropenia complicating rheumatoid arthritis), or benign chronic neutropenia (normal variant). ⚓

Evaluation for infection (fever? chills? tachycardia? hypotension? organ dysfunction? mottling? obvious source?) should be sought, and blood along with other appropriate fluids (e.g., CSF, ascites, pleural fluid, respiratory secretions, nasal sinus secretions, synovial fluid, etc.) cultured. Hematologist or pathologist review of a peripheral blood film can help in quickly pointing to whether leukocytosis is likely to be "reactive" or neoplastic. Splenomegaly and leukocytosis often indicate a neoplastic myeloproliferative or lymphoproliferative syndrome, although in a post-trauma setting various non-neoplastic explanations are plausible (e.g., hypersplenism and superimposed infection, nosocomial bacterial endocarditis). Leukopenia is a common feature of acquired immunodeficiency syndrome, and often reflects multiple causative factors (virus-induced lymphopenia, drug-induced cytopenia, antineutrophil antibodies, hypersplenism, etc.) (9,10).

Neutrophilia

In general, the more rapid and marked the leukocyte increase, the more severe the proinflammatory stimulus. The more marked the leukocyte morphologic abnormalities (leukocyte shift-to-the-left < toxic granulation < Döhle bodies < cytoplasmic vacuolation < leukoerythroblastosis), the more severe the infectious or proinflammatory process.

Common causes of neutrophilia are listed in Table 4. Acute infection, particularly with bacteria, leads to increased production and release of the marrow storage pool of maturing granulocytes, and is a common cause of neutrophilia, especially when there is concomitant shift-to-the-left and other morphological evidence of granulocytic response. Some scenarios representative of post-trauma patients include: sinusitis complicating nasotracheal or nasogastric tube use (11), esophageal rupture (12), intra-abdominal abscesses posthepatic trauma (13), post-traumatic acalculous cholecystitis (14), among many others. To some extent, viral and fungal infections also can produce granulocytosis.

Numerous inflammatory disorders, both acute and chronic, can result in increased numbers of neutrophils. Blunt trauma, such as might lead to rupture of an internal organ (15) or viscus, can lead to rapid changes in neutrophil count that precede establishment of infection. Chronic inflammatory processes, such as abscesses, can produce neutrophilia and/or monocytosis. Numerous acute and chronic noninfectious inflammatory disorders, ranging from acute gout (16) or acute pancreatitis to chronic non-neoplastic [e.g., giant cell arteritis (17)] to neoplastic [e.g., lung carcinoma (18)] can also produce significant neutrophilia.

"Stress" situations commonly lead to neutrophilia, at least in part as a result of neutrophil demargination, ranging from mild [e.g., exercise (19), catecholamine injection (20)] to moderate [e.g., postoperative state (21)] to marked [e.g., status epilepticus (22), heat stroke, neuroleptic malignant syndrome (23) see Volume 1, Chapter 40].

Certain drugs cause neutrophilia, most notably corticosteroids (24) (via demargination and increased mobilization of marrow storage pool neutrophils) and lithium (25). Tetracyclines have also been implicated in a drug-induced leukemoid reaction (26).

Granulocytosis is a feature of marrow stimulation, e.g., in marked hemolysis (27,28) and recovery from myelosuppression, including from antineoplastic chemotherapy or drug-induced agranulocytosis (29).

Neutrophilia and thrombocytosis are characteristically seen in a patient with hyposplenia or asplenia (because of decreased splenic pooling) (30,31). However, marked granulocytosis and left-shift could indicate the rare, but highly lethal complication of overwhelming post-splenectomy sepsis (OPSS) (32). The vaccination principles aimed at decreasing the risk of OPSS in postspleenectomy trauma patients are discussed in Volume 2, Chapter 52.

Table 4 Causes of Neutrophilia

Category	Description and comments
Secondary (thus, more likely to occur in trauma patients)	Acute or chronic infection
	Acute or chronic inflammatory disorders (including nonhematologic malignancy such as lung carcinoma)
	"Stress" (e.g., exercise, catecholamines, surgery/postoperative period, postictal state, heatstroke, neuroleptic malignant syndrome)
	Drugs (e.g., corticosteroids, lithium, tetracycline)
	Asplenia (e.g., s/p splenectomy/hyposplenia)
	Increased general marrow response (e.g., hemolysis, recovery from myelosuppression)
Primary (unlikely to be present in a trauma patient)	Chronic myeloproliferative disorders
	Chronic myeloid leukemia
	Polycythemia vera
	Essential thrombocythemia
	Agnogenic myeloid metaplasia
	Hereditary neutrophilia
	Congenital anomalies (with leukemoid reaction)
	Idiopathic
	Leukocyte adhesion deficiency
	Familial cold urticaria and leukocytosis

Table 5 Causes of Neutropenia in Trauma Patients

Frequency	Cause and comments
Common	Hemodilution from resuscitation or surgery
	Acute infection (usually transient)
	Acute, severe inflammatory process (e.g., perforation of a viscus, aspiration pneumonitis)
	Complement-mediated (e.g., acute burns, hemodialysis, membrane oxygenator, cardiopulmonary bypass, transfusion reactions)
Occasional	Drug-induced agranulocytosis
	Drug-induced aplastic anemia
	Megaloblastic anemia (e.g., folate deficiency, nitrous oxide anesthesia)
	Aplastic anemia (e.g., from radiation injury, or drug-induced aplastic anemia)
Pre-existing causes of neutropenia (selected list)	Common: Hypersplenism (usually secondary to cirrhosis)
	Myelodysplasia
	HIV-associated
	Rare: Autoimmune neutropenia (e.g., Felty's syndrome, systemic lupus erythematosus, other collagen vascular diseases), pure white cell aplasia
	Large granular lymphocytosis (T-lymphoproliferative syndrome; some have rheumatoid arthritis, splenomegaly)
	Neoplastic marrow disorders (e.g., paroxysmal nocturnal hemoglobulinuria)
	Congenital and familial neutropenias [multiple, rare syndromes, e.g., Kostmann syndrome (congenital agranulocytosis), cyclic neutropenia]

Neutropenia

⚡ **Neutropenia is classified based on the absolute neutrophil count as mild ($1.0-1.5 \times 10^9$/L), moderate ($0.5-1.0 \times 10^9$/L), or severe ($<0.5 \times 10^9$/L). Infection risk increases exponentially with decreasing neutrophil numbers.** ⚡ However, this relationship is seen most clearly when neutropenia results from impaired marrow production, rather than immune-mediated destruction or margination (2).

A classification system for neutropenia occurring in post-trauma patients is provided in Table 5. Categories are separated according to the estimated frequency of occurrence, and whether the neutropenia predates admission to hospital. A common cause of neutropenia in a post-trauma patient is an abrupt-onset infectious or severe inflammatory process, such as acute bacteremia, aspiration pneumonitis, or rupture of a viscus. Such events lead to neutrophil margination and their rapid egress into tissues. The resulting leukopenia and neutropenia are usually mild-to-moderate and transient, with recovery usually seen within 24 to 48 hours, as increased granulocyte production and mobilization from the marrow storage pool leads to subsequent leukocytosis and neutrophilia. Hemodilution during trauma resuscitation from rapid large-volume replacement by crystalloids, colloids, and blood products also can contribute to transient neutropenia.

Complement activation with generation of C5a leads to neutrophil activation, margination, adherence, and aggregation (including within the pulmonary circulation), resulting in usually transient neutropenia (33,34). This can result from acute burns, hemodialysis, membrane oxygenators, CPB, and transfusion reactions.

An occasional cause of acquired neutropenia in a critically ill post-trauma patient includes acute folate deficiency (35). In folate deficient patients, neutropenia can potentially be exacerbated by megaloblastosis induced by prolonged exposure to nitrous oxide during anesthesia (36).

Prominent neutropenia as a component of pancytopenia is a feature of aplastic anemia from radiation injury (37), or as a very rare adverse immune-mediated drug reaction (discussed subsequently) (38–42). One of the most common causes of neutropenia, antineoplastic chemotherapy or radiation, is an uncommon factor in the trauma or normal post surgical patient.

Agranulocytosis

⚡ **Severe neutropenia (neutrophil $<0.5 \times 10^9$/L) that begins during hospitalization is a life-threatening emergency usually resulting from an immune-mediated adverse drug effect (drug-induced agranulocytosis) (38–42).** ⚡ A thorough drug history, particularly focused on agents newly started in the past two weeks and known to cause agranulocytosis (Table 6) is important when reviewing a patient with leukopenia, especially if the neutropenia is severe (43,44). The most commonly implicated drugs are antithyroid agents (e.g., carbamizole, methimazole) and sulfonamides, but other reported triggers that could be used in a trauma patient include other antibiotics (e.g., penicillins, cephalosporins, chloramphenicol), antiseizure medications (e.g., carbamazepine, valproate, phenytoin) and, possibly H_2 antagonists (e.g., ranitidine, cimetidine) (2,38–44). The antipsychotic, clozapine, has an exceptionally high incidence of agranulocytosis estimated at 1%, and has a genetic, rather than immune, basis (42). The mortality rate is about 10%, but is higher if the occurrence of septicemia precedes recognition and discontinuation of the causative agent. ⚡ **Hematopoietic growth factors such as granulocyte colony-stimulating factor (G-CSF) appear to hasten recovery from agranulocytosis (45).** ⚡

Eosinophilia and Basophilia

⚡ **Eosinophilia that develops in a post-trauma or critically ill patient usually signifies an allergic drug reaction.** ⚡ In some instances, the eosinophilic response is sufficiently dramatic to be termed an eosinophilic leukemoid reaction, as has been reported for carbamazepine (46) and minocycline (47). Nonhematologic effects, such as exfoliative

Table 6 Drugs Known to Cause Agranulocytosis

Drug class	Drugs
Analgesics and NSAIDs	Aminopyrine, benoxaprofen, diclofenac, diflunisal, dipyrone, fenoprofen, indomethacin, ibuprofen, noramidopyrine, phenylbutazone, piroxicam, sulindac, tenoxicam, tolmetin
Antibiotics	Cephalosporins, chloramphenicol, ciprofloxacin, clindamycin, tetracyclines, ethambutol, gentamicin, imipenem, isoniazid, lincomycin, metronidazole, nitrofurantoin, novobiocin, penicillins, rifampicin, sulfamethoxazole, streptomycin, thiacetazone, tinidazole, vancomycin
	Chloroquine, flucytosine, dapsone, hydroxychloroquine, levamizole, mebendazole, pyrimethamine, quinine, quinacrine
	Acyclovir, zidovudine, terbinafine
Anticonvulsants	Carbamazepine, ethosuximide, phenytoins, trimethadione, valproic acid
Antihistamines	Brompheniramine, chlorpheniramine, cimetidine, famotidine, methaphenilene, ranitidine, tripelenamine, thenalidine
Antipsychotics, sedatives, antidepressants	Amoxapine, chlordiazepoxide, clozapine, diazepam, haloperidol, imipramine, meprobamate, phenothiazines, risperidone, tiapridal, upstene
Antiplatelet agents	Ticlodipine, aspirin
Antithyroid drugs	Carbimazole, methimazole, potassium perchlorate, thiocynate, thiouracils
Cardiovascular drugs	Aprindine, captopril, flubiprofen, furosemide, hydralazine, methyldopa, nifedipine, phenindione, procainamides, propafenone, propanolol, quinidine, spironolactone, thiazide diuretics, ticlopidine, lisinopril
Heavy metals	Arsenic compounds, gold, mercurial diuretics
Others	Acetazolamide, allopurinol, aminoglutethimide, benzafibrate, colchicine, flutamide, methazolamide, levodopa, oral hypoglycemic agents, penicillamine, retinoic acid, most sulfamides, tamoxifen, deferiprone Chinese herbal medicines, DDT, dinitrophenol, hair dye, insecticides, mustard

Abbreviations: NSAIDs, nonsteroidal anti-inflammatory drugs; DDT, dichloro-diphenyl-trichloroethane.
Source: From Refs. 43 and 44.

dermatitis or hepatitis, can be present (47). Another potential explanation for eosinophilia in a patient who has resided in certain third-world environments is reactivation of a dormant parasitic infection following the administration of corticosteroids or some other immunosuppressive agents in a trauma patient. For example, disseminated strongyloidiasis can present as colonic infiltration and bleeding can present as eosinophilia or even as gram-negative meningitis due to polymicrobial colonic invasion (48).

Uncommon causes of eosinophilia in a trauma patient, but which could represent a pre-existing disorder, include various parasitic infections, allergic disorders (including atopic asthma), various pulmonary or cutaneous eosinophilic disorders, vasculitis, hypereosinophilic syndrome, myeloid leukemia, lymphoma, and so forth (3).

Basophilia is most commonly seen in patients with myeloproliferative disorders, such as chronic myeloid leukemia. Rare forms of acute leukemia have high basophil levels. Other non-neoplastic causes include ulcerative colitis and myxedema. Transient basophilia can accompany recovery from acute illness or with drug reactions (3).

Monocytosis

Some degree of monocytosis is observed in about 30% of patients with acute bacterial infection (49). The frequency and degree of monocytosis may even be higher in certain chronic infections mediated by T-lymphocytes, such as tuberculosis and syphilis (50), as well as subacute bacterial endocarditis. ☞ **Monocytosis that develops in a post-trauma or critically ill patient can signify the development of a "chronic" inflammatory process, such as abscess. ☞**

Monocytosis is a feature of certain autoimmune disorders (e.g., systemic lupus erythematosus, rheumatoid arthritis), vasculitis (e.g., temporal arteritis, polyarteritis),

miscellaneous inflammatory disorders (e.g., ulcerative colitis, sarcoidosis, myositis), neoplasia (e.g., monocytic leukemia/myelodysplasia, lymphoma, histiocytosis, carcinoma), and postsplenectomy (3). Monocytosis can occur as a secondary response in a large proportion of patients with congenital or chronic autoimmune neutropenia (51). Interestingly, even though intense hematophagocytosis, as shown by bone marrow macrophages engulfing normoblasts, neutrophils, and platelets is a feature of severe infection-associated cytopenias, patients do not necessarily evince peripheral monocytosis, despite the suspected pathogenesis of infection-associated increase in M-CSF (52).

Lymphocytosis and Lymphopenia

☞ **Trauma can cause a rapid increase in lymphocyte number, which reflects an increase in T-lymphocytes and NK cells (53–55). ☞** The presence of trauma-associated lymphocytosis appears to confer an adverse prognosis (55). Acute viral infections, such as transfusion-associated cytomegalovirus infection, can produce very high lymphocyte counts in a post-trauma patient (56). Nonmalignant causes of lymphocytosis include certain nonviral infections that are rare in trauma patients (e.g., pertussis, tuberculosis, brucellosis, syphilis, cat scratch fever, toxoplasmosis), as well as allergic drug reactions, post-splenectomy, dermatitis herpetiformis, and hyperthyroidism (7).

Lymphopenia is found in many diverse clinical settings, ranging from many types of infection, nutritional deficiency, uremia, neoplasia, autoimmune disorders, myasthenia gravis, aplastic anemia, sarcoidosis, severe right heart failure, and numerous other acute and chronic illnesses (7). Lymphopenia can also occur transiently through lymphocyte redistribution as a result of corticosteroid therapy, or chronically in various rare primary immunodeficiency disorders.

THERAPEUTIC CONSIDERATIONS
Leukocytosis
There are few specific therapeutic implications of leukocytosis besides the goal of treating the underlying cause, such as treatment of infection. Leukopheresis is a rarely applied therapy that may be indicated in extreme leukocytosis associated with neoplasia, and is essentially never appropriate in non-neoplastic situations. Consultation with a hematologist is indicated when the cause of leukocytosis is inapparent, or if neoplasia is suspected.

Leukopenia
Treatment of the underlying cause of acute leukopenia is the major therapeutic intervention. Administration of folate or vitamin B_{12} is indicated when either deficiency is suspected to be the cause of leukopenia.

In suspected drug-induced agranulocytosis, it is important to discontinue promptly all plausible causal agents. Empiric use of broad-spectrum antibiotics is indicated pending neutrophil recovery. The use of hematopoietic growth factors [e.g., G-CSF (Filgrastim)] may reduce the mortality associated with this disorder (45). G-CSF may also be helpful in selected patients with other severe neutropenic disorders (e.g., autoimmune neutropenia, HIV-associated, congenital neutropenia).

Granulocytes are very labile, difficult to separate from other blood cells, and have short circulating lifespans (57). "Buffy coats" from at least ten blood donors are required to produce a single therapeutic dose of granulocytes for an adult recipient, which will be "contaminated" by the two units of red cells and 2.5 pools of platelets. Thus, for practical reasons, granulocytes concentrates obtained from single donors using apheresis is the only satisfactory way to obtain a therapeutic dose for a neutropenic patient, and this is rarely performed. Administration of G-CSF and corticosteroids to leukocyte donors increases yield about 10-fold.

EYE TO THE FUTURE

Relatively few developments appear imminent in relation to diagnosis or management of leukocytosis or leukopenia. Automated detection of important leukocyte morphologic abnormalities could hasten communication to the clinician that a patient has a severe developing infection or inflammatory process. Rapid nucleotide-based blood or tissue analyses may help determine whether an infection is present, and which type of microbe in particular could be responsible for neutrophilia. The "holy grail" of achieving satisfactory granulocyte transfusions on a large scale for severely-infected, neutropenic patients could represent a major therapeutic advance. Perhaps, leukocytes harvested from the peripheral blood stem cells of the patient or (related or unrelated) donors could be transfused. Newer and more effective preparations of hematopoietic growth factors could be developed.

SUMMARY

Leukocytosis and leukopenia are common and important clues suggesting that a trauma patient may have a serious infection or inflammatory state. Evaluation of quantitative leukocyte abnormalities requires determination of the leukocyte differential, whereas examination of the blood film by an experienced physician or technician morphologist is necessary to recognize important qualitative granulocyte abnormalities such as shift-to-the-left, toxic granulation, Döhle bodies, cytoplasmic vacuolation, and leukoerythroblastosis. Neutrophilia, especially when accompanied by some of these qualitative abnormalities, most commonly indicates the presence of infection (usually bacterial) or a severe inflammatory process. Leukopenia requires determination of the leukocyte differential, as it could indicate severe neutropenia indicating the life-threatening syndrome of drug-induced agranulocytosis. Sometimes, increased number of a less common type of leukocyte has diagnostic significance, e.g., eosinophilia indicating allergic drug reaction or corticosteroid-induced reactivation of a latent parasitic infection.

KEY POINTS

- Leukocytosis or leukopenia is often the first clue that a post-trauma or critically ill patient has infection or a severe inflammatory process.
- Leukocytosis is defined as a WBC count above the upper limit of the normal laboratory range (about $11 \times 10^9/L$), whereas leukopenia is defined as a WBC count below the lower limit of the normal laboratory range (about $4.0 \times 10^9/L$).
- All blood cells ultimately are derived from self-renewing pluripotential stem cells that are able to differentiate into lineage-committed stem cells that themselves differentiate into mature blood cells (6).
- The brief neutrophil lifespan within the circulation (about 6–8 hours) is one major reason why granulocyte transfusions are impracticable.
- The first step in evaluating any abnormal increase or decrease in WBC is to determine the leukocyte differential, and thereby classify the process as neutrophilia, eosinophilia, monocytosis, or lymphocytosis (marked basophilia is rare) or, conversely, neutropenia or lymphopenia (monocytopenia, eosinopenia, and basopenia are rare).
- Morphologic granulocyte abnormalities, such as shift-to-the-left, toxic granulation, pale blue cytoplasmic inclusions (Döhle bodies), or vacuoles, can indicate serious infectious/inflammatory problems.
- Severe proinflammatory states can produce a "leukemoid reaction," defined as a leukocyte count above $50 \times 10^9/L$.
- Leukopenia must prompt evaluation of the leukocyte differential to determine the absolute neutrophil level, since acquired severe neutropenia in a hospitalized patient usually signifies drug-induced agranulocytosis, a life-threatening adverse drug reaction.
- Pre-existing causes of leukocytosis in a trauma patient could include a chronic myeloproliferative or lymphoproliferative disorder; splenomegaly is often present in this situation. Pre-existing causes of leukopenia in a trauma patient can include hypersplenism (usually

due to chronic liver disease), Felty's syndrome (auto-immune neutropenia complicating rheumatoid arthritis), or benign chronic neutropenia (normal variant).

☞ Neutropenia is classified based on the absolute neutrophil count as mild ($1.0-1.5 \times 10^9/L$), moderate ($0.5-1.0 \times 10^9/L$), or severe ($<0.5 \times 10^9/L$). Infection risk increases exponentially with decreasing neutrophil numbers.

☞ Severe neutropenia (neutrophil $<0.5 \times 10^9/L$) that begins during hospitalization is a life-threatening emergency, usually resulting from an immune-mediated adverse drug effect (drug-induced agranulocytosis) (38–42).

☞ Hematopoietic growth factors such as granulocyte colony-stimulating factor (G-CSF) appear to hasten recovery from agranulocytosis (45).

☞ Eosinophilia that develops in a post-trauma or critically ill patient usually signifies an allergic drug reaction.

☞ Monocytosis that develops in a post-trauma or critically ill patient can signify the development of a "chronic" inflammatory process, such as abscess.

☞ Trauma can cause a rapid increase in lymphocyte number, which reflects an increase in T-lymphocytes and NK cells (53–55).

REFERENCES

1. Weatherall DJ. In: Warrell DA, et al. eds. Oxford Textbook of Medicine, 4th ed. Oxford, UK: Oxford University Press, 2003:501–507.
2. Curnutte JT, Coates TD. Disorders of phagocyte function and number. In: Hoffman R, et al. eds. Hematology: Basic Principles and Practice, 3rd ed. New York: Churchill Livingstone, 2000:720–762.
3. Ravandi F, Hoffman R. Phagocytes. Hoffbrand AV, et al. eds. Postgraduate Haematology, 5th ed. Malden MA: Blackwell Publishing, 2005:277–302.
4. Hammerschmidt DE, Stroncek DF, Bowers TK, et al. Complement activation and neutropenia occurring during cardiopulmonary bypass. J Thorac Cardiovasc Surg 1981; 81(3):370–377.
5. Mitre E, Nutman TB. Basophils, basophilia and helminth infections. Chem Immunol Allergy 2006; 90:141–156.
6. Byrne JL, Russell NH. Haemopoietic growth factors. In: Hoffbrand AV, Catovsky D, Tuddenham EGD, eds. Postgraduate Haematology, 5th ed. Malden MA: Blackwell Publishing, 2005:303–317.
7. Drayson MT, Moss PAH. Normal lymphocytes and non-neoplastic lymphocyte disorders. In: Hoffbrand AV, Catovsky D, Tuddenham EGD, eds. Postgraduate Haematology, 5th ed. Malden MA: Blackwell Publishing, 2005:330–357.
8. Cannistra S, Griffin J. Regulation of the production and function of granulocytes and monocytes. Semin Hematol 1988; 25(3):173–188.
9. Frontiera M, Myers AM. Peripheral blood and bone marrow abnormalities in the acquired immunodeficiency syndrome. West J Med 1987; 147(2):157–160.
10. McCance-Katz E, Hoecker J, Vitale N. Severe neutropenia associated with anti-neutrophil antibody in a patient with acquired immunodeficiency syndrome-related complex. Pediatr Infect Dis J 1987; 6(4):417–418.
11. Caplan ES, Hoyt NJ. Nosocomial sinusitis. JAMA 1982; 247(5):639–641.
12. Popovsky J. Perforations of the esophagus from gun shot wounds. J Trauma 1984; 24(4):337–339.
13. Scott CM, Grasberger RC, Heeran TF, et al. Intra-abdominal sepsis after hepatic trauma. Am J Surg 1988; 155(2):284–288.
14. Branch Jr CL, Albertson DA, Kelly DL. Post-traumatic acalculous cholecystitis on a neurosurgical service. Neurosurgery 1983; 12(1):98–101.
15. Dodds WJ, Taylor AJ, Erickson SJ, Lawson TL. Traumatic fracture of the pancreas: CT characteristics. J Comput Assist Tomogr 1990; 14(3):375–378.
16. Craig MH, Poole GV, Hauser CJ. Postsurgical gout. Am Surg 1995; 61(1):56–59.
17. Gonzalez-Gay MA, Lopez-Diaz MJ, Barros S, et al. Giant cell arteritis: laboratory tests at the time of diagnosis in a series of 240 patients. Medicine 2005; 84(5):277–290.
18. Ascensao JL, Oken MM, Ewing SL, et al. Leukocytosis and lung cell cancer. A frequent association. Cancer 1987; 60(4):903–905.
19. Brenner I, Shek PN, Zamecnik J, Shephard RJ. Stress hormones and the immunological responses to heat and exercise. Int J Sport Med 1998; 19(2):130–143.
20. Berkow RL, Dodson RW. Functional analysis of the marginating pool of human polymorphonuclear leukocytes. Am J Hematol 1987; 24(1):47–54.
21. Jakobsen B, Pedersen J, Egeberg B. Postoperative lymphocytopenia and leucocytosis after epidural and general anaesthesia. Acta Anaesthesiol Scand 1986; 30(8):668–671.
22. Aminoff MJ, Simon RP. Status epilepticus. Causes, clinical features and consequences in 98 patients. Am J Med 1980; 69(5):657–666.
23. Vincent FM, Zimmerman JE, Van Haren. Neuroleptic malignant syndrome complicating closed head injury. Neurosurgery 1986; 18(2):190–193.
24. Hetherington SV, Quie PG. Human polymorphonuclear leukocytes of the bone marrow, circulation, and marginated pool: function and granule protein content. Am J Hematol 1985; 20(3):235–246.
25. Boggs DR, Joyce RA. The hematopoietic effects of lithium. Semin Hematol 1983; 20(2):129–138.
26. Chatham WW, Ross DW. Leukemoid blood reaction to tetracycline. South Med J 1983; 76(9):1195–1196.
27. Porter WG, Lyle CB Jr. Leukemoid reaction: an unusual manifestation of autoimmune hemolytic anemia. South Med J 1974; 67(1):79–80.
28. Stroncek D, Procter JL, Johnson J. Drug-induced hemolysis: cefotetan-dependent hemolytic anemia mimicking an acute intravascular immune transfusion reaction. Am J Hematol 2000; 64(1):67–70.
29. Levine PH, Weintraub LW. Pseudoleukemia following recovery from dapsone-induced agranulocytosis. Ann Intern Med 1968; 68(5):1060–1065.
30. McBride JA, Dacie JV, Shapley R. The effect of splenectomy on the leucocyte count. Br J Haematol 1968; 14(2):225–231.
31. Spencer RP, McPhedran P, Finch SC, Morgan WS. Persistent neutrophilic leukocytosis associated with idiopathic functional asplenia. J Nucl Med 1972; 13(3):224–226.
32. Neilan BA. Late sequelae of splenectomy for trauma. Postgrad Med 1980; 68(3):207–210.
33. Jacob HS. Granulocyte-complement interaction. A beneficial antimicrobial mechanism that can cause disease. Arch Intern Med 1978; 138(3):461–463.
34. Craddock PR, Hammerschmidt DE, Moldow CF, et al. Granulocyte aggregation as a manifestation of membrane interactions with complement: possible role in leukocyte margination, microvascular occlusion, and endothelial damage. Semin Hematol 1979; 16(2):140–147.
35. Geerlings SE, Rommes JH, van Toorn DW, Bakker J. Acute foliate deficiency in a critically ill patient. Neth J Med 1997; 51(1):36–38.
36. Amos RJ, Amess JA, Hinds CJ, Mollin DL. Incidence and pathogenesis of acute megaloblastic bone-marrow change in patients receiving intensive care. Lancet 1982; 2(8303): 835–838.
37. Champlin R. Bone marrow aplasia due to radiation accidents: pathophysiology, assessment and treatment. Baillieres Clin Haematol 1989; 2(1):69–82.
38. Asconape JJ. Some common issues in the use of antiepileptic drugs. Semin Neurol 2002; 22(1):27–39.
39. Patton WN, Duffull SB. Idiosyncratic drug-induced haematological abnormalities. Incidence, pathogenesis, management and avoidance. Drug Saf 1994; 11(6):445–462.

40. Van der Klauw MM, Wilson JH, Stricker BH. Drug-induced agranulocytosis: 20 years of reporting in The Netherlands (1974–1994). Am J Hematol 1998; 57(3):206–211.

41. Van der Klauw MM, Goudsmit R, Halie MR, et al. A population-based case-cohort study of drug-associated agranulocytosis. Arch Intern Med 1999; 159(4):369–374.

42. Berliner N, Horwitz M, Loughran TP Jr. Congenital and acquired neutropenia. Hematology (Am Soc Hematol Educ Program) 2004; 63–79.

43. Andres E, Kurtz JE, Maloisel F. Nonchemotherapy drug-induced agranulocytosis: experience of the Strasbourg teaching hospital (1985–2000) and review of the literature. Clin Lab Haematol 2002; 24:99–106.

44. Andres E, Noel E, Kurtz JE, Henoun Loukili N, Kaltenbach G, Maloisel F. Life-threatening idiosyncratic drug-induced agranulocytosis in elderly patients. Drugs Aging 2004; 21: 427–435.

45. Sprikkelman A, de Wolf JT, Vellenga E. The application of hematopoietic growth factors in drug-induced agranulocytosis: a review of 70 cases. Leukemia 1994; 8(12):2031–2036.

46. Laad G, Miranda MF. Eosinophilic leukemoid reaction associated with carbamazepine hypersensitivity. Indian J Dermatol Venereol Leprol 2005; 71(1):35–37.

47. MacNeil M, Haase DA, Tremaine R, Marrie TJ. Fever, lymphadenopathy, eosinophilia, lymphocytosis, hepatitis, and dermatitis: a severe adverse reaction to minocycline. J Am Acad Dermatol 1997; 36(2):347–350.

48. Kimmelstiel F, Lange M. Fatal systemic strongyloidiasis following corticosteroid therapy. N Y State J Med 1984; 84(8):399–401.

49. Myhre EB, Braconier JH, Sjogren U. Automated cytochemical differential leucocyte count in patients hospitalized with acute bacterial infections. Scand J Infect Dis 1985; 17(2): 201–208.

50. Maldonado J, Hanlon D. Monocytosis: a current appraisal. Mayo Clin Proc 1965; 40:248–259.

51. Bux J, Kissel K, Nowak K, Spengel U, Mueller-Eckhardt C. Autoimmune neutropenia: clinical and laboratory studies in 143 patients. Ann Hematol 1991; 63(5):249–252.

52. Francois B, Trimoreau F, Vignon P, et al. Thrombocytopenia in the sepsis syndrome: role of hemophagocytosis and macrophage colony-stimulating factor. Am J Med 1997; 103(2): 114–120.

53. Thommasen HV, Boyko WJ, Montaner JS, et al. Absolute lymphocytosis associated with nonsurgical trauma. Am J Clin Pathol 1986; 86(4):480–483.

54. Teggatz JR, Parkin J, Peterson L. Transient atypical lymphocytosis in patients with emergency medical conditions. Arch Pathol Lab Med 1987; 111(8):712–714.

55. Pinkerton PH, McLellan BA, Quantz MC, Robinson JB. Acute lymphocytosis after trauma—early recognition of the high-risk patient? J Trauma 1989; 29(6):749–751.

56. Baumgartner JD, Glauser MP, Burgo-Black AL, et al. Severe cytomegalovirus infection in multiply transfused, splenectomized trauma patients. Lancet 1982; 2(8289):63–66.

57. Contreras M, Tahlor CPF, Barbara JA. Clinical blood transfusion. In: Hoffbrand AV, Catovsky D, Tuddenham EGD, eds. Postgraduate Haematology, 5th ed. Malden MA: Blackwell Publishing, 2005:249–276.

58

Disseminated Intravascular Coagulation

Joanne Ondrush and Christopher Junker

Department of Anesthesiology and Critical Care Medicine, George Washington University Hospital,
Washington, D.C., U.S.A.

INTRODUCTION

Disseminated intravascular coagulation (DIC) is a condition whereby the coagulation cascade is activated in an accelerated and uncontrolled manner. The resulting intravascular fibrin deposition and microvascular thrombosis leads to tissue ischemia and multiple organ dysfunction syndrome (MODS). Clot production is magnified through the generation of serine proteases whose interactions with proinflammatory mediators are a key component of the organ dysfunction seen with DIC (1).

While the precise definition of DIC varies among different investigators, with some focusing more upon the bleeding sequale, the majority have emphasized the clotting aspects of the syndrome. The Subcommittee on DIC of the International Society on Thrombosis and Hemostasis (ISTH) has suggested the following definition for DIC: "An acquired syndrome characterized by the intravascular activation of coagulation with loss of localization arising from different causes. It can originate from and cause damage to the microvasculature, which if sufficiently severe, can produce organ dysfunction (2)."

The loss of regulatory mechanisms that normally control coagulation further exacerbates the thrombotic process. The consumption of platelets and coagulation factors ultimately results in bleeding from multiple sites, a common clinical finding with severe DIC. However, it is the clotting of microvascular beds that underlies most of the long-term damages associated with DIC. Indeed, it is the failure to perfuse tissues of critical organ systems that leads to ischemia and ultimately to MODS.

This chapter reviews the normal physiology of hemostasis, as well as the major pathologic conditions that alter coagulation, including the common etiologies of the DIC. The clinical presentation, laboratory diagnosis, and management of DIC are surveyed. Finally, new drugs and diagnostic techniques are reviewed in the "Eye to the Future" section.

NORMAL PHYSIOLOGY OF HEMOSTASIS

Normal coagulation can be conceptualized as occurring in overlapping phases. Vascular injury prompts platelets to become "sticky" and coalesce into a plug at the site of injury. Formation of this "platelet plug" is propagated by a series of enzyme amplifications as part of the coagulation cascade. The clot is normally prevented from occupying the entire vascular bed by antithrombotic control mechanisms, and removal of excess clot debris through fibrinolysis.

The Coagulation System

The coagulation cascade is traditionally divided into "intrinsic" and "extrinsic" pathways (Fig. 1). This division actually reflects the laboratory measurements of the coagulation system components to a greater degree than it describes the specific physiology of clotting. The two limbs of the coagulation cascade can be activated by various triggers. The "intrinsic pathway" is activated by endothelial damage or contact with a foreign surface, as with the use of glass in the measurement of activated partial thromboplastin time (aPTT). The "extrinsic pathway" is activated by "tissue factor" exposed at the site of injury.

The intrinsic and extrinsic pathways join in a common activation of factor X. In Figure 1, note the multiple feedback loops that accelerate the process, amplifying the original stimulus many times over accelerating the process of hemostasis. Factor Xa binds with factor Va, calcium, and phospholipid to form a complex that converts prothrombin into thrombin. Thrombin (factor IIa) then acts to cleave fibrinogen into fibrin. In Figure 2, note the central role of thrombin in upregulating the coagulation cascade as well as activating protein C in the anticoagulation response.

The Anticoagulation System
Protein C, Protein S, Antithrombin

The anticoagulant pathways regulate the production of thrombin. The plasma protein, antithrombin (AT; formerly antithrombin III) normally circulates as a weak inhibitor of thrombin. The reactive portion of AT is an arginine residue that is normally in a "low-activity" conformation. However, in the presence of heparin (which binds to a lysine site on AT), a conformational change occurs and AT becomes very active, with its arginine reactive center binding to the serine moiety of thrombin, inhibiting it as well as other serine proteases involved in the coagulation cascade (including IXa, Xa, XIa, XIIa, and plasmin). When AT binds to free thrombin, thrombin-AT complexes are formed, permanently disabling thrombin's proteolytic activity (3).

In addition, thrombomodulin forms a complex with thrombin, which activates protein C. When "activated protein C" (APC) is bound with its cofactor, protein S, it degrades activated factors Va and VIIIa (3). Lastly, tissue factor pathway inhibitor (TFPI), expressed on the microvascular endothelium, also plays a role in the inhibition of the coagulation pathway (4). The pathogenic pathways involved in DIC are illustrated in Figure 3, including exuberant formation of fibrin and (in some patients) inhibition of the fibrinolytic system, thereby resulting in decreased removal of fibrin.

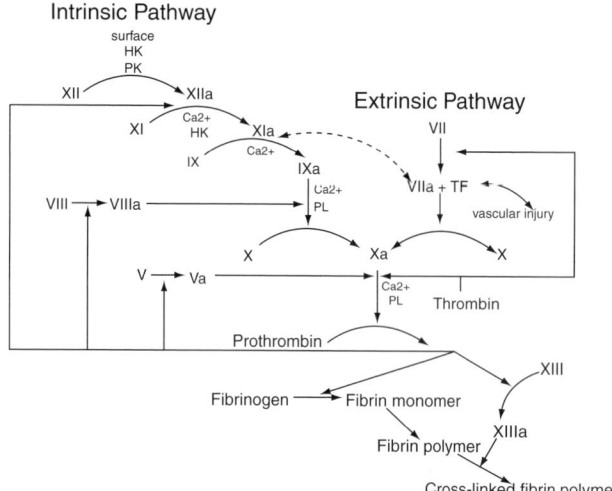

Intrinsic Pathway

Extrinsic Pathway

Figure 1   The coagulation cascade. The coagulation cascade has multiple interacting components and two major routes of activation: the intrinsic (i.e., contact activation) pathway and the extrinsic (i.e., tissue factor) pathway, both leading to fibrin formation. It was previously believed that two arms of the coagulation cascade were of equal importance. It is now recognized that the primary pathway responsible for the imitation of blood coagulation is the tissue factor (extrinsic) pathway. Note the major role played by thrombin as the enzyme responsible for converting fibrinogen to fibrin monomer, as well as its involvement at numerous other areas of factor conversion to the activated form. *Abbreviations*: HK, high molecular weight kininogen (aka HMWK); PK, prekallikrein; TF, tissue factor.

The Fibrinolytic System and Its Inhibitors

The fibrinolytic system normally prevents excessive clot formation, and helps eliminate old clot during tissue repair through the degradation of fibrin. Plasmin, the activated form of plasminogen, is synthesized in the liver and is the key protein in fibrinolysis. Circulating fibrin, produced in clot formation, binds plasminogen. The resulting fibrin-plasminogen complex accelerates endothelial cell release of tissue plasminogen activator (tPA), and fibrin plasminogen

tPA complexes form. Within these ternary complexes, the conversion of plasminogen to its active form, plasmin, proceeds.

In the absence of fibrin, tPA does not activate plasminogen, limiting fibrinolysis to the sites of fibrin deposition (3). Plasmin is a proteolytic enzyme that degrades fibrin into small fragments known as D-dimers (5). Plasmin also cleaves fibrinogen and other plasma proteins and clotting factors (5). In addition, fibrinolysis is triggered by the intrinsic coagulation pathway as kallikrein converts plasminogen to plasmin.

The inhibitors of the fibrinolytic pathway, which include plasminogen activator inhibitor and alpha 2-anti-plasmin, serve to further regulate fibrinolysis. Plasminogen activator inhibitor, which is released from platelets and endothelium, binds to tPA, thus preventing its binding to, and activation of, plasminogen to plasmin. Alpha 2-antiplasmin binds and neutralizes plasmin (6). Exogenous agents such as streptokinase, which causes an alteration of the plasminogen active site, and urokinase, which has direct proteolytic activity on plasminogen, can also alter fibrinolysis. This complex system of amplification feedback loops and inhibition is extraordinarily stable in the healthy subject. However, in catastrophic illness or trauma the clotting system can go wildly out of control, and become very difficult to restore to order, without first resolving the primary underlying insult.

Just as inflammatory mediators can serve as triggers for DIC, it is not uncommon in coagulopathic states for inflammatory mediators to be markedly elevated, as there is extensive "cross-talk" between these two systems, as illustrated in Figure 4. Indeed, patients with severe coagulophatic states and DIC can proceed to the systemic inflammatory response syndrome (SIRS) (7). The critical initiator of inflammation-induced thrombin generation is tissue factor, and its inhibition abrogates inflammation-induced coagulation activation (7). Proinflammatory cytokines (TNF-α, IL-1β, and IL-6) increase coagulation and will be described in greater detail below (also see Volume 2, Chapters 47 and 63) (7).

PATHOPHYSIOLOGY OF DISSEMINATED INTRAVASCULAR COAGULATION
Tissue Factor

☞ Tissue factor is expressed on the surface of activated monocytes and endothelial cells activating the extrinsic pathway by complexing with factor VII. The uncontrolled release of tissue factor appears to be one of the principal initiating steps in DIC (3,4). ☞ Primate studies suggest that only small amounts of tissue factor circulate in healthy animals (8). In trauma conditions, tissue factor is an important trigger, especially the release of brain tissue thromboplastin in severe traumatic brain injury (TBI) (9), or massive tissue destruction (e.g., crush injury). In patients with endotoxemia, trauma, neoplasm, and other severe disorders, this prothrombotic protein complexes with factor VII and begins the coagulation cascade. In baboons, infusion with *Escherichia coli* or endotoxin results in activation of the coagulation cascade, as indicated by elevated levels of fibrin degradation products (FDPs), protein C, and thrombin-antithrombin complexes (10). Infusion of monoclonal antibody to tissue factor inhibits the augmentation of thrombin generation (7,11–14). Many diseases associated with DIC also demonstrate increased tissue factor activity. For example, production or release of tissue factor from wounds sustained during trauma, or from leukemic cells

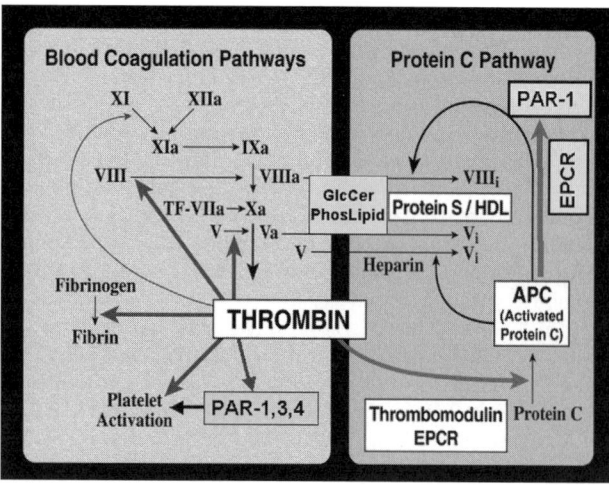

Figure 2   The central role of thrombin in upregulating the coagulation cascade and protein C. *Abbreviations:* EPCR, endothelial protein C receptor; GlcCer, glucosylceramide I, inactivated; PAR, protease-activated receptor.

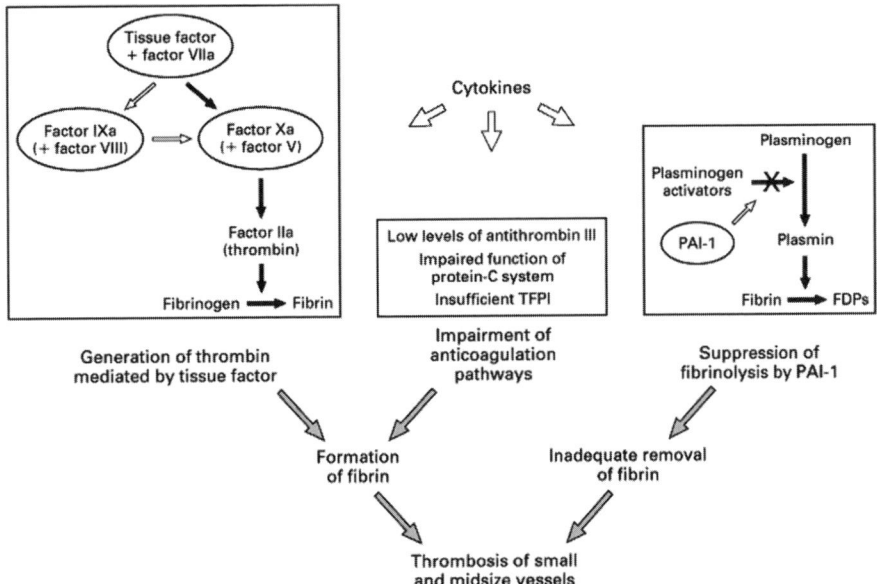

Figure 3 Pathogenetic pathways involved in DIC. Tissue factor, expressed on the surface of activated mononuclear cells and endothelial cells, binds and activates factor VII. The complex of tissue factor and factor VIIa can activate factor X directly (*black arrows*) or indirectly (*white arrows*) by means of activated factor IX and factor VIII. Activated factor X, in combination with factor V, can convert prothrombin (factor II) to thrombin (factor IIa). Simultaneously, all three physiologic means of anticoagulation, antithrombin (shown as the old term antithrombin III in this figure), protein C, and TFPI are impaired. The resulting intravascular formation of fibrin is not balanced by adequate removal of fibrin because endogenous fibrinolysis is suppressed by high plasma levels of plasminogen-activator inhibitor type 1 (PAI-1). The high levels of PAI-1 inhibit plasminogen-activator activity and consequently reduce the rate of formation of plasmin. The combination of increased formation of fibrin and inadequate removal of fibrin results in disseminated intravascular thrombosis. FDPs denote fibrin-degradation products. *Source*: From Ref. 36.

in acute leukemia, is associated with an increased incidence of DIC. Other triggers include thromboplastic substances released from the dead fetus in intrauterine fetal death, and endotoxin-mediated inflammation in sepsis (15).

Abnormalities in Coagulation Inhibitory Pathways

Abnormalities in coagulation inhibitory pathways also play a role in DIC. ☞ **Levels of coagulation pathway inhibitors including TFPI, AT, and Protein C are all decreased in patients with DIC, hence perpetuating thrombosis.** ☞

Tissue Factor Pathway Inhibitor

The primary site of TFPI elaboration is at the microvascular endothelium where it is released into the plasma and circulates in low concentrations, thereby serving to inhibit tissue factor/factor VIIa complexes at the initiation stage of the tissue factor pathway cascade (16). In patients with DIC, higher levels of TFPI are associated with a better outcome (17). It is unclear whether these observations represent a protective effect of TFPI, a different severity of disease, or different pools of circulating TFPI. Plasma levels of TFPI are an incomplete and thus inaccurate reflection of the true functional concentration. Trauma-associated coagulopathy (discussed below) is an entity with a few distinct differences from common DIC; measurement of factor VIIa levels may ultimately prove to be more predictive and useful in this condition (once they become available clinically).

Antithrombin

Most of the inhibitory effects of AT are exhibited during the propagation phase of coagulation, whereby it binds with thrombin (and other activated coagulation factors, e.g., factor Xa) during its rapid phase of production (16). Patients with DIC have increased concentrations of thrombin-AT complexes (18) and lower levels of AT are associated with poorer outcomes (8,19). Accordingly, patients with congenitally low AT are at increased risk for thrombotic complications [e.g., deep venous thrombosis (DVT)], and have a worse outcome with DIC and sepsis.

Protein C Anticoagulant Pathway

The protein C anticoagulant pathway plays a critical role in the regulation of coagulation, fibrinolysis, and inflammatory pathways. The complex formed by thrombin and the endothelial surface cofactor, thrombomodulin, increases the rate of protein C activation more than 1000-fold, while simultaneously blocking the ability of thrombin to catalyze fibrin formation, platelet activation, and feedback activation of coagulation cofactors (20). The APC binds with cofactor protein S, and this complex then inactivates factors Va and VIIIa, thus limiting the generation of thrombin (21).

☞ **Protein C levels are decreased in both sepsis and DIC (19,22,23). The decrease in sepsis-related mortality by using APC, as demonstrated in the PROWESS study (23), suggests the possibility of using it to treat DIC.** ☞

Activated Protein C—Profibrinolytic Effect

APC also has profibrinolytic activity by neutralizing plasminogen activator inhibitor 1 (PAI-1) and by preventing the thrombin activatable fibrinolysis inhibitor. PAI-1 is responsible for neutralizing tPA and plasmin (24) and increased levels of PAI-1 decrease in fibrinolysis and the ability to clear fibrin clots from circulation (20). In a

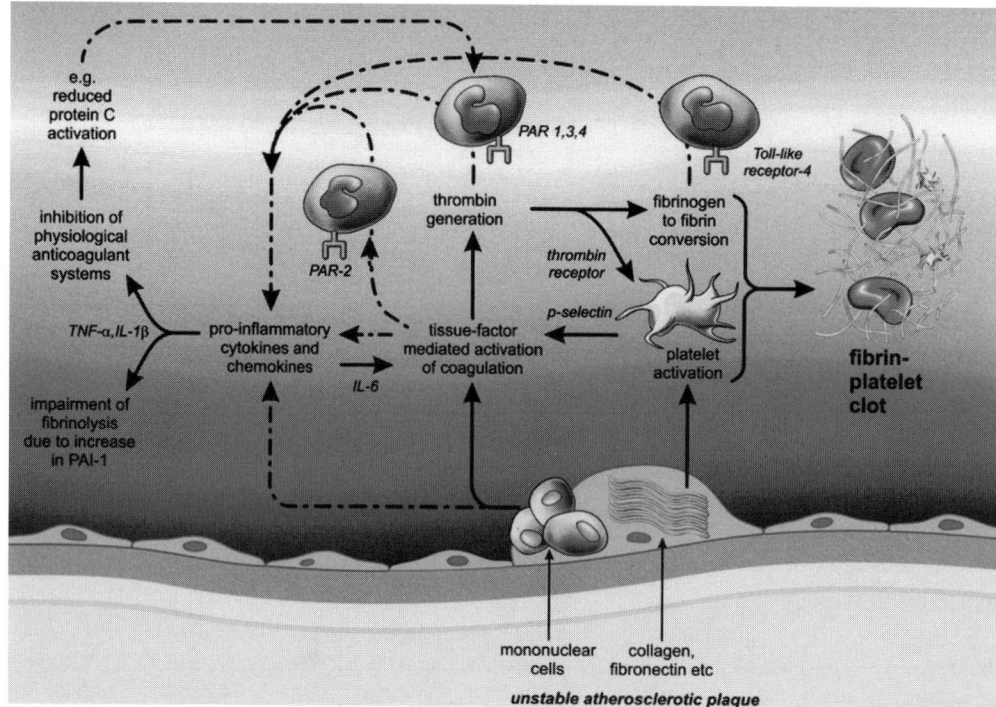

Figure 4 Schematic representation of activation of coagulation and inflammation. Exposure of tissue factor-bearing inflammatory cells to blood results in thrombin generation and subsequent fibrinogen to fibrin conversion. This example uses rupture of an atherosclerotic plaque, but the same mechanism would result from other causes of tissue injury. Simultaneously, activation of platelets occurs, both by thrombin and by exposure of collagen (and other subendothelial platelet-activating factors) to blood. Binding of tissue factor, thrombin, and other activated coagulation proteases to specific PARs on inflammatory cells may affect inflammation by inducing release of proinflammatory cytokines, which will subsequently further modulate coagulation and fibrinolysis. Coagulation pathways are indicated by straight arrows; inflammatory mechanisms by dashed arrows. *Source*: From Ref. 7.

chimpanzee sepsis model, PAI-1 levels remained elevated after injection of endotoxins, suppressing fibrinolytic activity (25). Elevated levels of PAI-1 have been associated with a poor prognosis in patients with DIC (8). In addition, depressed levels of plasmin–alpha 2 antiplasmin complexes, which inhibit the ability of plasmin to cleave fibrin, were found more often in DIC patients with multiple organ failure (26).

Consumption of Coagulation Factors

As these various cascades begin accelerating out of control, the consumption of coagulation factors and platelets depletes endogenous stores exceeding the body's regenerative ability to replace them. Quantitative studies have shown accelerated turnover rates for fibrinogen, platelets and prothrombin. ☞ **Plasma levels of factor V, factor VIII, prothrombin, and fibrinogen are universally reduced in severe DIC, though fibrinogen levels can be maintained until late in the process.** ☞

Thrombocytopenia, which can often be severe in DIC, is probably multifactorial. Platelets are consumed by the thrombotic lesions and adhere to damaged endothelial surfaces; megakaryocyte production is decreased (15). In the setting of trauma or other conditions involving hemorrhage, further platelet and coagulation factor loss occurs with shed blood. This depletion of coagulation factors and platelets magnifies the bleeding complications clinically manifested in DIC.

Impairment of Procoagulant Clearance

The impairment of clearance mechanisms of procoagulant material may also play a role in DIC. Products of intravascular coagulation (i.e., fibrin degradation products, tissue factor, endotoxin, activated coagulation factors, etc.) are removed from the circulation by the reticuloendothelial system, particularly, the Kupffer cells of the liver and splenic macrophages. It is hypothesized that some forms of DIC may saturate the system's ability to clear these products, due to its overwhelming production (27).

Proinflammatory Mediators and Coagulation

Our understanding of the interactions between proinflammatory mediators and coagulation is improving (13,28–30). Proinflammatory cytokines (IL-6 and IL-8) increase expression of tissue factor (28,29), and inhibit expression of thrombomodulin and endothelial cell protein C receptor; both are important regulators of the coagulation cascade (31). Elastase, released by activated neutrophils, destroys AT and C1 esterase inhibitor (32). C1 esterase inhibitor is responsible for regulation of the contact factors of the intrinsic clotting system. C-reactive protein, an acute phase reactant, promotes tissue factor expression and increases levels of α-1 antitrypsin, which decreases APC levels (33,34). The acute phase complement C4b binds to, and inactivates, protein S (33,35). Release of tumor necrosis factor (TNF-α) results in increased expression of PAI-1 and hence inhibition of fibrinolysis (36). All of these actions combine to form a hypercoagulable state.

Coagulation Mediated Proinflammatory Effects

Concurrently, coagulation can have many proinflammatory effects. The decreased levels of AT and protein C increase cytokine synthesis as well as increase neutrophil aggregation and adherence (31,37). APC inhibits both TNF-α and macrophage migration inhibitory factor in vitro (38). More importantly, APC has been shown to suppress nuclear factor κB (NF-κB), which is the principal nuclear regulatory mechanism that modulates expression of proinflammatory factors (24,39). Thrombin generation promotes upregulation of P-selectin and E-selectin, which result in increased neutrophil-platelet aggregation and neutrophil-endothelial interactions (30,40). Thrombin activatable fibrinolysis inhibitor inactivates C5a (which promotes neutrophil chemotaxis) (41,42). The relationship between the two complex systems of coagulation and inflammation remains under intense investigation.

Chronic or Compensated Disseminated Intravascular Coagulation

Chronic or compensated DIC is similar to acute DIC, except there tends to be a weak or intermittent stimulus (15). Chronic DIC has been associated with many conditions, including intrauterine fetal death, vasculitis, large abdominal aortic aneurysms, giant hemangiomas, amyloidosis, some malignancies, and hydatidiform moles. There is a wide spectrum of clinical and laboratory findings, and a high index of suspicion is required to make the diagnosis.

COMMON TRIGGERS OF DISSEMINATED INTRAVASCULAR COAGULATION

DIC is associated with many conditions found in trauma and critical illness. Table 1 lists many of them and the degree of DIC they are often associated with. ☞ **The persistence of SIRS, rather than the number of SIRS criteria met, appears to be a more important prognostic factor in determining which trauma patients develop DIC, emphasizing the importance of early appropriate treatment of these patients.** ☞

Tissue Injury

Major tissue injuries, such as severe head trauma (9,43–45), extensive burns, or soft tissue damage, and fat embolism from multiple fractures (46), are all associated with inflammatory activation of tissue factor and DIC. This can result from direct endothelial damage or release of fat and phospholipids from the tissue into the circulation (36). The persistence of SIRS rather than the number of SIRS criteria that are met appears to be a more important prognostic factor in determining which trauma patients develop DIC and, the development of DIC correlates well with the onset of MODS (42).

Severe Sepsis/Systemic Inflammatory Response Syndrome

☞ **DIC occurs in a variety of clinical settings associated with trauma, infection being one of the most common.** ☞ Recently, we have developed a better understanding of the complex physiology that occurs during severe sepsis and its activation of the coagulation and inflammatory cascades (see Volume 2, Chapters 47 and 63 for further discussion in the interaction between sepsis and SIRS) (7).

Table 1 Table of Diseases Associated with Disseminated Intravascular Coagulation

Fulminant DIC	Low-grade DIC
Burns	Cardiovascular diseases
Crush injuries and tissue necrosis	Autoimmune diseases
Trauma	Renal vascular disorders
Intravascular hemolysis	Hematologic disorders
Hemolytic transfusion	(e.g., HIT)
reactions	Inflammatory disorders
Major hemolysis	
(e.g., TTP)	
Massive transfusions	
Septicemia	
Gram-negative (endotoxin)	
Gram-positive	
(mucopolysaccharides)	
Acute liver disease	
Obstructive jaundice	
Acute hepatic failure	
Prosthetic devices	
Leveen or denver shunts	
Aortic balloon assist devices	
Obstetric accidents	
Amniotic fluid	
embolism abortion	
Retained fetus	
syndrome eclampsia	
Placental abruption	
Viremias	
HIV CMV hepatitis	
Varicella	
Metastatic malignancy	
Vascular disorders	

Abbreviations: CMV, cytomegalovirus; HIT, heparin-induced thrombocytopenia; TTP, thrombotic thrombocytopenic purpura.
Source: Adapted from Ref. 64a.

All microorganisms have the potential to cause DIC, however the release of endotoxin (the membrane constituent of gram-negative bacteria) is best recognized (46). Other bacterial triggers of activation are the mucopolysaccharide coats and exotoxin in gram-positive organisms (36). Viremias, including varicella, hepatitis, cytomegalovirus and HIV, have all been associated with DIC (47,48). The presence of DIC with severe sepsis confers a graver prognosis.

Obstetrical Complications Associated with Disseminated Intravascular Coagulation

There are numerous obstetrical complications associated with DIC. Amniotic fluid embolism (AFE) is one of the most catastrophic, accounting for 10% of maternal deaths in the United States (46). The syndrome presents an acute onset of respiratory distress and circulatory collapse. In 80% of patients, the syndrome presents during labor (49). AFE is caused by entry of amniotic fluid, (which includes tissue factor), entering the maternal circulation after rupture of the placental membranes. If meconium is present in the fluid, it can precipitate a more intense form of DIC (50). For those who survive the initial event, DIC typically follows within four hours (46). The mortality rate for the mother ranges between 60% and 80%, and approximately 50% of the survivors develop permanent neurologic sequelae (51). Abruptio placentae may also induce DIC through a similar mechanism, releasing tissue factor into the maternal circulation. Fortunately, rapid delivery of the fetus and removal of all placental material often halts the progression of DIC in this scenario (52,53).

Pre-eclampsia, eclampsia, and the "hemolysis, elevated liver enzymes, low platelets" (HELLP) syndrome, which can be considered as a continuum of one disease process, are also associated with DIC. Pre-eclampsia is characterized by hypertension and proteinuria; in the presence of seizures, the term is eclampsia. The pathophysiology is unclear, but endothelial dysfunction, as well as neutrophil and platelet activation may play a role (2). DIC is present in 11% of patients with eclampsia and often remains low-grade; however, in 10% to 15% of women, the process becomes fulminant (54–56). In addition, placental abruption will occur in approximately 16% of women with pre-eclampsia and eclampsia, further increasing the likelihood of DIC (56). Therapy usually involves immediate delivery, removal of the placenta, and supportive care.

Retained fetus syndrome usually presents as low-grade, compensated DIC. Fetal tissue slowly leaks into the maternal circulation, causing a smoldering procoagulant state that is somewhat compensated by the fibrinolytic system (46). If a dead fetus is retained in utero for longer than 5 weeks, the incidence of DIC approaches 50% (52,53,57). Women with a septic abortion are at risk for DIC, again because of entry of products of conception into the maternal circulation, as well as associated infection.

Malignancy

Patients with both solid tumors and hematologic malignancies have a high incidence of DIC. The type of tumor can determine the underlying pathophysiology and sometimes the clinical presentation (i.e., hemorrhage vs. thrombosis). Approximately 50% of acute leukemias will be complicated by DIC, most commonly promyelocytic leukemia. Leukemic (promyelocytes, myeloblasts) cells themselves release procoagulant material (58), contrasting with prostate cancer, which directly or indirectly stimulates the fibrinolytic system leading to a primary fibrinolytic syndrome. This explains why patients with prostate cancer and DIC present with hemorrhage instead of thrombosis (58). DIC has been described in carcinomas of the lung, breast, colon, ovary, stomach, and gallbladder, and malignant melanoma. In patients with adenocarcinoma-associated DIC complicated by thrombosis, heparin but not warfarin is often effective in managing thrombocytopenia and thrombosis. Initiation of chemotherapy is associated with acceleration of DIC, presumably related to accelerated thrombin generation from necrosis of the tumor (46).

Chronic Liver Disease and Other Inflammatory Conditions

Bleeding complications, and a low level of chronic DIC, are common findings in patients with chronic liver disease; however, this may not be solely attributable to diminished factor production. The inability to synthesize AT and loss of activated factor clearance from the liver are likely contributors to the increased susceptibility to DIC in this population (46). Other conditions known to cause DIC include large volume transfusions of blood products (59), giant hemangiomas, and large aortic aneurysms (36).

CLINICAL PRESENTATION

In the trauma patient, the development of DIC is multifactorial, likely resulting from a combination of direct tissue injuries and massive hemorrhage [with dilution and loss of endogenous factors, along with transfusions of exogenous clotting factors, platelets and packed red blood cells (PRBCs)]. All these factors lead to a rise in microvascular coagulation as DIC becomes established (the special case of trauma coagulopathy is further reviewed below).

Due to the multiple contributing factors, the trauma patient's course and presentation can be variable. Since acute DIC can present as bleeding or thrombosis, the key to making the diagnosis is having a high index of suspicion. Most patients with fulminant DIC will bleed from at least three unrelated sites simultaneously (58), frequently presenting with hemoptysis, hematuria, gastrointestinal bleeding, epistaxis, gingival bleeding, and/or oozing from indwelling needle or catheter sites. There may be petechiae, purpura, or generalized ecchymosis. Thrombosis often occurs in small distal vessels and can present as generalized mottling or as acral cyanosis, with discoloration of the fingers, toes, and ears (15).

End-organ damage can also be a manifestation of vessel occlusion, most commonly, renal, pulmonary, and neurologic dysfunction (58). In chronic or low-grade DIC, there is often minor bleeding from the skin or mucous membranes. Recurrent thrombophlebitis is an especially common presentation in patients with underlying adenocarcinoma (15).

LABORATORY DIAGNOSIS

✍ **The complex pathophysiology of DIC, and high prevalence of coagulopathy in trauma and critical care, makes it difficult for a single laboratory test to confirm the diagnosis.** ✍ The tests commonly used to diagnose DIC are listed in Table 2 in the order of reliability. However, not all tests listed are available with the rapid turnaround required in all locations. The combination of tests, the

Table 2   Reliability of Laboratory Tests in Disseminated Intravascular Coagulation (in Descending Order of Reliability)

Profragment 1 + 2
D-dimer
AT
Thrombin precursor protein[a]
Fibrinopeptide A
Platelet factor 4
FDP
Platelet count
Protamine test
Thrombin time
Fibrinogen
Prothrombin time
Activated PTT
Reptilase time

[a]ELISA for soluble fibrin monomer.

Table 3 Utility of Commonly Used Tests in the Diagnosis of Disseminated Intravascular Coagulation

Tests	Sensitivity (%)	Specificity (%)	Efficiency (%)
PT ($n = 82$)	91	27	57
PTT ($n = 82$)	91	42	57
TT ($n = 43$)	83	60	70
Fibrinogen ($n = 71$)	22	100	65
Platelet count ($n = 82$)	97	48	67
Schistocytes ($n = 80$)	23	73	51
FDP ($n = 71$)	100	67	87
D-dimer ($n = 44$)	91	68	80
AT ($n = 21$)	91	40	70
PT + PTT + TT ($n = 43$)	83	11	51
PT + PTT + fibrinogen ($n = 71$)	22	100	65
PT + PTT + FDP ($n = 71$)	91	71	86
FDP + D-dimer ($n = 39$)	91	94	95

Abbreviations: AT, antithrombin; FDP, fibrinogin/fibrin degradation products; PT, prothombin time; PTT, partial thromboplastin time; TT, thrombin time.
Source: From Ref. 61.

clinical presentation, and knowledge of the underlying disease increases the sensitivity and specificity of diagnosis. Table 3 lists the most common tests and their relative usefulness in diagnosing DIC, both individually and in combination. A proposed scoring system to integrate clinical events with laboratory findings is provided in Table 4.

Fibrin Degradation Products
The FDPs are elevated in virtually all patients with DIC (53,54). The FDPs represent the breakdown of fibrin(ogen) by plasmin, but are not specific for DIC as increased FDPs are also seen in DVT, pulmonary embolus, myocardial infarction, and oral contraceptive use (53,54). A somewhat

Table 4 Scoring System for Diagnosing Disseminated Intravascular Coagulation

Appropriate clinical settings	1 point
Thrombohemorrhagic events	1 point
Elevated PT or PTT or TT	1 point
Thrombocytopenia[a]	1 point
Decreased fibrinogen[b]	1 point
Elevated FDP[c]	1 point
Elevated D-dimer[d,e]	1 point
Low AT level[e,f]	1 point
Total score	8 points
Needed for the diagnosis of DIC	5 points

[a]Thrombocytopenia $<130,000/\text{mL}$
[b]Fibrinogen $<150 \text{ mg/dL}$
[c]Elevated FDP $>10 \text{ mg/mL}$
[d]Patients should be free of thrombolytic agents
[e]Elevated D-dimer $>0.25 \text{ mg/mL}$
[f]Low AT level $<75\%$
Abbreviations: AT, antithrombin; FDP, fibrinogen/fibrin degradation products; PT, prothombin time; PTT, partial thromboplastin time; TT, thrombin time.
Source: From Ref. 61.

more specific test is the D-dimer assay, which measures the product of plasmin digestion of cross-linked fibrin. ✄ **The D-dimer appears to be the most reliable of the commonly available tests for the diagnosis of DIC, and when combined with FDP has a sensitivity of 91% and specificity to 94% (60,61).** ✄

Low fibrinogen levels are relatively specific for DIC, but because it is an acute phase reactant, plasma levels may be in a normal range despite significant ongoing DIC, making it relatively insensitive (36). The protamine plasma paracoagulation (PPP) test is rapid, inexpensive, and may be the most specific assay for DIC, as it detects fibrin monomers in plasma. However, the PPP test is not widely used due to its semi-quantitative nature and significant operator-dependence.

Reliability of Prothrombin Time, Activated Partial Thromboplastin Time, and Thrombin Time
The use of PT and aPTT is unreliable in the setting of DIC. The PT may be prolonged in only 50% to 75% of patients with DIC, and the aPTT is prolonged in only 50% to 60% of patients (49). These low sensitivities may be related to the presence of circulating activated clotting factors that cause the test to register as normal (53,54). Prolonged PT and aPTT are more a reflection of the late consumptive stage of coagulation factors than the activation of the procoagulant system (61). Thrombin time has similar sensitivity as PT and PTT and can be normal, especially if the fibrinogen level is not decreased.

Thrombocytopenia, Antithrombin Assay, Schistocytes
Thrombocytopenia is a common finding in DIC. However, a progressive drop in platelet count is sensitive, but not specific, for DIC. The decline in numbers may represent ongoing thrombin-induced activation and platelet use or a reflection of the underlying disease process, such as sepsis or malignancy (36). AT is a low-specificity test for the diagnosis of DIC because levels decline in many systemic illnesses (61). However, there is some correlation between the severity of DIC and low levels of AT, as well as increased levels of thrombin-AT complexes (18,61). Schistocytes are seen in 50% of individuals with DIC (62). Table 5 displays a summary of laboratory tests by groups.

Molecular Markers
The protean laboratory and clinical findings in DIC has led to increasing interest in the use of molecular markers. Prothrombin fragment 1+2 is an intermediate product of the conversion of prothrombin to thrombin, now measurable by ELISA. Fibrinogen peptide A is a proteolytic compound of fibrinogen and may be used as a reliable marker for presence of thrombin acting on fibrinogen (63,64). Decreased levels of alpha-2-antiplasmin and increased levels of plasmin–alpha-2-antiplasmin complexes provide direct evidence of both fibrinolytic activation and inhibitor consumption (49).

DIFFERENTIAL DIAGNOSIS

The differential diagnosis for DIC includes hemodilution, primary fibrinolysis, chronic liver disease, and microangiopathic hemolytic anemias (MHA). Most of these diseases do not present with such an abrupt onset of bleeding, or with the wide array of coagulation abnormalities. Patients with fibrinogenolysis or primary fibrinolysis, which is an acquired condition, will have abnormal PT and PTT, decreased fibrinogen, and increased FDP. However, the

Table 5 Laboratory Diagnostic Criteria[a]

Procoagulant activation (group I tests)	Fibrinolytic activation (group II tests)
⇔ Prothrombin fragment 1 + 2	⇔ D-dimer
⇔ Fibrinopeptide A	⇔ FDP
⇔ Thrombin-antithrombin complex (TAT)	⇔ Plasmin
⇔ D-dimer[b]	⇔ Plasmin-antiplasmin complex (PAP)
⇔ Soluble fibrin monomer (TPP) ELISA	⇔ Soluble fibrin monomer (TPP) ELISA

Inhibitor consumption (group III tests)	End-organ damage (group IV tests)
⇔ AT	⇔ LDH
⇔ a-2-antiplasmin	⇔ Creatinine
⇔ Heparin cofactor II	⇔ pH
⇔ Protein C or protein S	⇐ paO$_2$
⇔ TAT complex	
⇔ PAP complex	

[a]Only one abnormality each is needed in groups I, II, and III and at least two abnormalities are needed in group IV tests to satisfy criteria for a laboratory diagnosis of DIC.

[b]The D-dimer is reliable only for this purpose if using the correct assay and monoclonal antibody.

Source: Adapted from Ref. 64a.

platelet count and D-dimer levels are often only mildly abnormal, helping to distinguish it from DIC (15).

Chronic Liver Disease

The laboratory findings in patients with chronic liver disease may be difficult to differentiate from DIC (36). Thrombocytopenia and coagulation abnormalities are common in this population and high levels of FDP are seen in patients with cirrhosis. However, unlike most causes of DIC, the D-dimers should be normal (or only mildly increased) in liver disease.

Microangiopathic Hemolytic Anemias

MHA, including thrombocytopenic thrombotic purpura (TTP) and hemolytic-uremic syndrome (HUS), may also mimic DIC. Clinically, the microthrombotic events may resemble DIC with the presence of thrombocytopenia and schistocytes. However, none of these conditions exhibits marked abnormalities in coagulation or fibrinolysis. Marked elevation in lactate dehydrogenase (LDH) indicating hemolysis is a useful differentiating laboratory parameter.

Heparin-Induced Thrombocytopenia

↻ Heparin-induced thrombocytopenia (HIT) can mimic the clinical appearance of DIC with thrombosis and thrombocytopenia. ↻ In its most severe form, HIT can result in overt (decompensated) DIC, with severe thrombocytopenia, elevated PT, hypofibrinogenemia, and schistocytes (65). Tests for HIT antibodies include antiplatelet factor 4/ heparin ELISA and washed platelet activation assays. HIT should be considered in any patient with falling platelet counts or thrombosis that begins 5–14 days after initiation

of heparin therapy (66). As DIC and HIT are not mutually exclusive, HIT should be considered in the appropriate clinical scenario even when DIC from another cause is a likely cause of thrombocytopenia (also see Volume 2, Chapter 55).

Inherited Disorders of Coagulation

Inherited disorders of coagulation can cause excessive bleeding in trauma and critically ill patients. Although patients with these life-long coagulation disorders are generally capable of alerting their doctors of their condition, this is not necessarily true in the acute trauma or emergency setting. Patients who present with obtunded mental status are unable to provide a history, and important underlying diagnosis (e.g., hemophilia) may not become known to the ED physician, anesthesiologist, or trauma surgeon, unless the patient is bearing a medication alert (med-alert) bracelet or card or other information.

The common inherited disorders of coagulation are summarized in Table 6. These coagulation disorders have specific trauma and perioperative management considerations, which are beyond the scope of this chapter, and which usually require hematologist consultation. However, the presence of some of these disorders can exacerbate the severity of DIC, and therefore the most common will be briefly summarized.

The hemophilias are inherited disorders resulting from the deficiency of specific coagulation factors. Increased bleeding is experienced following trauma, during surgery, or with conditions increasing the risk of developing a bleeding condition that can mimic DIC. Hemophilia A results from factor VIII deficiency, while hemophilia B is due to reduced levels of factor IX. Hemophilia C (factor XI deficiency) is an autosomal recessive condition occurring in approximately 5% of Ashkenazi Jews, whereas both hemophilias A and B are X-linked recessive disorders, and thus affect almost exclusively males.

von Willebrand disease results from abnormal production of von Willebrand factor (vWF), a protein produced in endothelial cells (and found in α granules of platelets). vWF serves as an adhesion molecule between platelets and the subendothelium, and as a carrier molecule for factor VIII.

von Willebrand disease is generally mild, and associated with bleeding only, following surgery or trauma. When severe, it can be associated with spontaneous hemarthroses and mucocutaneous bleeding. vWF is an acute phase reactant and is increased during pregnancy, thus women generally require no specific therapy for normal spontaneous vaginal delivery, or for Cesarian sections performed at term pregnancy. Additionally, desmopressin (DDAVP) 0.3 μg/kg can be administered 60 minutes preoperatively, increasing vWF and factor VIII to near normal values, although avoidance of free water administration is important to minimize risk of desmopressin-induced hyponatremia.

Trauma-Associated Coagulopathy vs. Disseminated Intravascular Coagulation

The development of coagulation abnormalities early after trauma is common, and is an independent predictor of mortality (67). Indeed, an initial elevated PT increases the adjusted odds of dying by 35% and an initial elevated PTT increases the adjusted odds of dying by 326% (67).

Table 6 Inherited Disorders of Hemostasis

Disorder	Factor(s) deficient	Inheritance pattern	Incidence per: million	Treatment
Hemophilia A	Factor VIII	X-linked recessive	100	For minor surgery DDAVP 0.3 μg/kg. For major surgery factor VIII concentrate or recombinant Factor VIII
Hemophilia B (Christmas disease)	Factor IX	X-linked recessive	20	Factor IX concentrate
Hemophilia C	Factor XI	Autosomal recessive	5% Ashkenazi Jews	FFP has adequate factor XI levels alternatively, factor XI concentrate (only target 70% normal factor IX levels)[a]
von Willebrand disease	vWF	Autosomal recessive or dominant	>100	DDAVP 0.3 μg/kg purified vWF if severe
Afibrinogenemia	Factor I		1	Per hematologist recommendations
Dysfibrinogenemia	Factor I	Autosomal dominant	1	
Prothrombin deficiency	Factor II	Autosomal recessive	1	
Factor V deficiency	Factor V	Autosomal recessive	1	
Factor V plus VIII deficiency	Factors V and VIII		1	
Factor VII deficiency	Factor VII	Autosomal recessive	1	
Factor X deficiency	Factor X	Autosomal recessive	1	
Factor XIII deficiency	Factor XIII		1	

[a]>70% factor XI repletion levels can cause a hypercoagulable state in hemophilia C patients.
Abbreviations: DDAVP, des-amino, D-arginine vasopressin (synthetic vasopressin analogue); vWF, von Willebrand's factor.

Coagulation abnormalities associated with acute trauma have several injury-specific factors (not typically seen with common DIC) that uniquely contribute to the acute trauma-associated coagulopathy, including: (*i*) hemorrhage—resulting in loss of factors to the external environment, without necessarily having an opportunity to be consumed in clot; (*ii*) hemodilution—due to resuscitation with noncoagulation factor containing fluids; (*iii*) acidosis—from under-perfusion of tissues (including liver), and (*iv*) hypothermia—due to environmental exposure and the administration of nonheated fluids.

At the same time, there are conditions occurring with trauma that are common to other forms of DIC. These include consumption of clotting factors and platelets at sites of vascular injury, the release of tissue thromboplastin (containing tissue factor), and other inflammatory and/or procoagulant factors. The release of these DIC triggers is particularly prominent in those who suffer massive crush injuries, fat embolus syndrome, or TBI (68).

Patients with severe TBI are at particular risk for the development of DIC, and the incidence increases with the severity of the cerebral insult. Thrombocytopenia and coagulopathy often occur upon admission in patients with particularly severe TBI. However, DIC can emerge on subsequent laboratory examinations in a number of patients with TBI who had documented normal coagulation studies on the initial blood draw in the resuscitation bay (69).

Trauma-associated coagulopathy can be further exacerbated by resuscitation with non-coagulation containing fluids (e.g., isotonic crystalloids, colloids, red cells) that dilute the supply of clotting factors, elevate blood pressure, and reduce viscosity, washing out previously formed clots and exacerbating hemorrhage. Some of these solutions (e.g., hetastarch) can directly impair coagulation (see Volume 1, Chapter 11) (69).

That a DIC state can occur in trauma patients prior to resuscitation with fluids was demonstrated in a recent retrospective evaluation of trauma patients admitted on a helicopter service. This study design incorporated appropriate physician review during the pre-hospital period, and demonstrated that acute traumatic coagulopathy [PT >18 seconds, APTT >60 seconds, or TT >15 seconds (1.5 times normal)] not related to fluid administration did occur early following severe trauma. Furthermore, coagulopathy was shown to be a marker of injury severity and mortality (70).

In an effort to determine the relative contributions of acidosis and hypothermia to coagulopathy, Martini et al. recently demonstrated that acidosis, hypothermia, or both caused the development of coagulopathy in pigs, as indicated by 47%, 57%, and 72% increases in splenic bleeding time ($P < 0.05$, pre- vs. post). Plasma fibrinogen concentration was decreased by 18% and 17% in the acidotic and combined groups, respectively, but not in the hypothermic pigs. Hypothermia caused a delay in the onset of thrombin generation, whereas acidosis primarily caused a decrease in thrombin generation rates (71). Additional research is required to further delineate the relative contributions of each of these many insults on trauma-associated coagulopathy.

MANAGEMENT

☞ **The cornerstone of treatment for DIC is an aggressive attempt to remove the underlying disorder or precipitating factor.** ☞

Removal of Underlying Disorder

Therapy for DIC begins with identification of the triggering etiology and treating or eliminating it. Common examples include debridement of necrotic and or infected tissues (e.g., abscess, necrotizing fasciitis, infected hematoma). Additional categories of DIC that can resolve within a few hours of removing the trigger factor include severe TBI and several obstetric causes (e.g., placental abruption). For many other conditions, such as sepsis, DIC can take days to fully resolve despite appropriate treatment of the underlying infection (72). Specific therapy varies based upon the severity and location of the primary process (TBI vs. pancreatitis vs. ischemic extremity with necrotic and infected tissues), as well as the general health of the patient.

A more complete understanding of the pathophysiology of DIC is beginning to emerge. In knowing that the key event in DIC is disregulated thrombin production, with resulting microvascular thrombosis, rational approaches at interrupting the intravascular clotting process have emerged. Pharmacologic treatment options for acute DIC are mostly supplementary to treatment of the primary disorder and include: (*i*) administering anticoagulants, (*ii*) supplementing missing inhibitors of coagulation (e.g., AT, APC), (*iii*) administering general inhibitors of coagulation (e.g., heparin), (*iv*) administering consumed blood components (e.g., fibrinogen, etc.), and (*v*) administering antifibrinolytics (which should be used rarely and with extreme caution, as discussed below).

♂ **Currently, heparin is the most common agent directed at DIC, typically administered as a low dose infusion with no loading dose.** ♂

Heparin

Heparin in its various forms has been the agent most commonly utilized, though seldom in controlled clinical trials. By binding to AT, heparin inhibits thrombin and its production. The use of low dose subcutaneous heparin has been effective in DIC, and is the first line agent for some because of the minimal chance of hemorrhage when administered in this fashion (49,54,73). Some clinicians advocate low molecular weight heparin (LMWH), with its lower risk of HIT, as it has been found to be efficacious in limited studies (52–54). The use of moderate dose heparin infusions have been successful in chronic DIC and in some animal studies (74), but results in acute DIC have been less conclusive (15,75). Although the theoretical risk of administering an anticoagulant to a bleeding patient in DIC exists, clinical studies have not shown an increased incidence of bleeding complications (15,36).

Activated Protein C

The role of APC and the possible benefits of supplementation in patients with DIC are currently being evaluated. APC has had some initial success in the treatment of sepsis through control of microvascular thrombosis and inflammation, and may hold promise for patients with DIC from other causes (20,24). The use of recombinant TFPI (rTFPI) to control coagulation associated with severe sepsis and subsequent DIC has been studied extensively (4,76–79). A recently completed phase II study showed a relative reduction in day 28 all-cause mortality in rTFPI treated patients when compared with placebo (80). Further studies are currently underway.

Thrombin Inhibitors (Antithrombin, Hirudin)

The use of AT concentrates in patients with DIC and sepsis has shown overall improvement in the DIC and organ dysfunction, with a modest reduction in mortality, often not

Table 7 Properties of Heparins and Hirudiens

Property	Heparins	Hirudins
Thrombin inhibition	Indirect (requires AT)	Direct
Clot-bound thrombin	Not inhibited	Inhibited
Immune thrombocytopnea	Associated	Not associated
Effect on PT	Weak	Moderate
Effect on aPTT	Yes (weak with LMWH)	Yes
Metabolism and/or excretion	Liver, kidney	Kidney
Antidote	Protamine (60% reversal of LMWH)	None

Abbreviations: AT, antithrombin; LMWH, low molecular weight heparin; PT, prothrombin time; aPTT, activated partial thromboplastin time.

reaching statistical significance (72,81–84). More recent trials have used supernormal levels of AT (36). Larger randomized control trials are necessary before this can be advocated as a standard therapy.

Hirudin, a thrombin inhibitor extracted from the salivary glands of the medicinal leech, *Hirudo medicinalis*, is currently under investigation as an AT agent to be used in the treatment of DIC (85–87). Hirudin is currently available in three different recombinant DNA forms: (*i*) recombinant hirudin (lepirudin, desirudin); (*ii*) hirugen; and (*iii*) bivalirudin.

Natural and recombinant hirudin binds to both the catalytic site and the fibrinogen binding exosite of thrombin, as is true for bivalirudin, whereas hirugen binds to only the exosite. These molecules inhibit thrombin conversion of fibrinogen to fibrin as well as thrombin-induced platelet aggregation (the advantages and disadvantages of various hirudins compared to heparin are shown in Table 7).

Replacement of Missing and Consumed Components

♂ **Repletion of coagulation factors should be limited to the treatment of clinically significant bleeding in conjunction with laboratory abnormalities. However, abnormal lab values alone should rarely be treated.** ♂

The replacement of missing and consumed components is controversial. The common belief that the infusion of products may actually exacerbate DIC has never been proven in clinical studies. While it is recognized that low levels of platelets and coagulation factors can contribute to bleeding in DIC, early or overzealous factor replacement can itself produce complications.

It is only when active bleeding is present, and not solely laboratory abnormalities, that platelets and fresh frozen plasma should be administered (72). Patients with DIC may have an acquired storage pool defect of platelets, as well as FDP inhibition of platelets, and may require a higher platelet count for adequate hemostasis (15). Repletion of fibrinogen with cryoprecipitate again should be reserved for patients with hypofibrinogenemia and significant bleeding. Transfusion of PRBC should, as always, be based on the severity of hemorrhage; target hematocrits should be dictated by symptoms and co-existing disease.

Antifibrinolytics—for Selected Cases Only

ᕰ Only in rare circumstances should inhibition of the fibrinolytic system with antifibrinolytic agents be considered for the treatment of DIC. ᕰ

In approximately 3% of patients with DIC, there is resolution of the intravascular coagulation and fibrin deposition but the patient continues to bleed due to secondary fibrinolysis (49). The agents currently available to inhibit inappropriate fibrinolysis include ε-aminocaproic acid (EACA) (49), tranexamic acid, and the protease inhibitor aprotinin (46). The therapeutic effects of these agents must clearly outweigh the risk of thromboembolic effects, prior to initiating therapy.

Aprotinin inhibits fibrinolysis by directly binding to plasmin, and also by inhibiting a series of other serine proteases, including kallikrein (88). Aprotinin is thought to reduce bleeding through inhibiting the contact phase activation of hemostasis, preventing fibrinolysis (89), and reducing thrombin generation (90). Aprotonin has been shown to decrease blood loss following cardiac surgery, including those at highest risk (re-do open heart surgeries) (91), and those on aspirin and with renal failure (92). EACA is a lysine analog that inhibits plasmin activity by preventing plasminogen from binding to fibrin, thereby suppressing fibrinolysis (93).

Tranexamic acid, or 4-(aminomethyl) cyclohexane carboxylic acid (AMCA), is another lysine analog with a similar mechanism of action, except AMCA has a seven-fold to 10-fold greater potency than EACA (94). These agents reduce blood loss in cardiothoracic surgery (95,96), following liver transplantation (97), and following orthopedic surgery.

In addition, recent attention has focused on its potential anti-inflammatory properties of the antifibrinolytic drugs in patients undergoing CPB because both plasmin and kallikrein amplify the inflammatory response by activating key components of the complement cascade (98–100). However, minimal work has been done to establish the safety and efficacy of any of these antifibrinolytic agents in the trauma setting (101).

The use of antifibrinolytic agents should be used with extreme caution, as they may lead to fatal disseminated thrombosis. This select trauma patient population should have been previously treated with heparin and have clear documentation that ongoing inappropriate fibrinolysis has continued (15).

Recombinant Activated Factor VII for Treatment of Trauma-Associated Coagulopathy

Recombinant activated factor VII (rFVIIa) is approved for the use in hemophilia (with inhibitors) in North America, and in Europe a few additional medical indications are also approved (102). The initial results of rFVIIa use in trauma have been very promising, although most studies have been limited to case series and anecdotal reports (102). Consequently, as of this printing, the use of rFVIIa for trauma patients remains investigational, or "off-label."

Recently, Dutton et al. showed that rFVIIa therapy lead to an immediate clinical reduction of coagulopathic hemorrhages in a retrospectively reviewed series of trauma cases conducted at the Maryland Shock-Trauma Center (103). Friederich et al. reported their successful experience in the first prospective double blinded, randomized controlled trial (RCT), describing use of rFVIIa in radical prostate surgery documenting reduced blood loss and decreased transfusion after a single preoperative dose (104).

Table 8 Causes of Disseminated Intravascular Coagulation

Category	Example
Trauma	Brain tissue destruction
	Extensive crush injury
	Severe burns
Infections	Meningococcemia
	Other gram negative or gram positive bacteria
	Rocky mountain spotted fever
	Viral
Environmental causes	Heat stroke
	Snake bites
Hemolytic transfusion reactions	ABO blood group incompatibility
Liver disease	Cirrhosis, acute hepatic necrosis
Obstetric complications	Amniotic fluid embolus
	Placental abruption
	Uterine rupture (Possibly 2° trauma)
	Retained dead fetus or septic abortion
Malignancy	Metastatic carcinoma (esp. adenocarcinoma)
	Hematological (especially PML)
Activation	Mechanical heart valves
Mechanical destruction	Aortic aneurysms
	CPB
Platelet activation disorders	Heparin-induced thrombocytopenia[a]
	Thrombotic thrombocytopenic purpura[a]

[a] Overt (decompensated) DIC is seen only in a minority of severely-affected patients.
Abbreviations: CPB, cardiopulmonary bypass; PML, promyelocytic leukemia.
Source: Adapted from Ref. 64a.

More recently, two prospective placebo-controlled, double-blind RCTs, one in blunt trauma ($n = 143$) and the other in penetrating trauma ($n = 134$) were completed by Boffard et al. in South Africa (105). In blunt trauma, PRBC transfusion was significantly reduced with rFVIIa relative to placebo (estimated reduction of 2.6 PRBC units, $P = 0.02$), and the need for massive transfusion (>20 units of PRBCs) was reduced (14% vs. 33% of patients; $P = 0.03$). In penetrating trauma, rFVIIa use resulted in similar trends toward reducing PRBC transfusion (estimated reduction of 1.0 PRBC units, $P = 0.10$) and massive transfusion (7% vs. 19%; $P = 0.08$). Trends toward a reduction in mortality and critical complications were observed. Adverse events including thromboembolic complications were evenly distributed between treatment groups (105). Additional studies are required to further clarify the dose, duration, and specific patient populations that will benefit the most from rFVIIa.

ᕰ While not recommended for all causes of DIC, rFVIIa appears to be useful in severe trauma-associated coagulopathy and diffuse hemorrhage. ᕰ

Treatment of Chronic Disseminated Intravascular Coagulation

As with acute DIC, first-line management of chronic DIC is to treat the underlying disorder. Processes such as aortic aneurysms may require operative management to cure. Malignancy and other chronic disorders may require ongoing therapy. Both unfractionated and LMWH have been used successfully in patient groups requiring long-term anticoagulation therapy. In circumstances where heparin or warfarin are contraindicated (e.g., brain metastases), antiplatelet agents such as clopidogrel and acetyl-salicylic acid have also been used (49).

EYE TO THE FUTURE

Through better understanding of the pathophysiology of DIC, advances continue to be made to identify this syndrome at its early stages via more sensitive laboratory tests and molecular markers. This may allow intervention before the procoagulant and inflammatory cascades advance beyond therapeutic benefit.

New assays are currently under investigation, including the thrombin precursor protein, performed by ELISA, which detects circulating soluble fibrin polymer, and a new radioimmunoassay of B-beta 15–42, which is a cleavage product of fibrinogen in the presence of plasmin. These tests, in addition to prothrombin fragment 1+2 and fibrinogen peptide A (previously mentioned) may become part of the standard work-up for DIC in the near future.

Hirudin and argatroban, direct thrombin inhibitors used in treatment of HIT, have shown promise in early studies of use in DIC (106,107). Defibrotide, a polydeoxyribonucleotide is an adenosine receptor agonist that increases endogenous prostaglandins (PGI_2 and E_2), stimulates expression of thrombomodulin in endothelial cells, modulates platelet activity, and increases the function of endogenous tPA while diminishing the activity of PAI-1. This compound has a relatively low risk of bleeding as a side effect of the drug and is in early studies for efficacy in DIC.

Finally, simplification of the scoring systems for DIC has been evolving over the last decade with the ISTH endorsing simpler systems, with the most recent iteration utilizing just platelet count and PT. While this system may work for most medical causes of DIC, it is not necessarily reliable in the trauma setting. Additional studies are underway.

SUMMARY

DIC is a complex syndrome, and only recently has a greater understanding of its pathophysiology emerged. Tissue factor, which is expressed on the surface of activated monocytes and endothelial cells, activates the extrinsic pathway, and its uncontrolled release appears to be one of the principal initiating steps in DIC. Inhibitors of the coagulation pathways, including TFPI, AT, and APC are present in lower levels in patients with DIC, hence perpetuating thrombosis. As protein C levels are decreased in both DIC and sepsis, and given the recent successful PROWESS trial of APC in severe sepsis (23), there is the potential for a similar benefit with APC for treating DIC of other causes. The persistence of SIRS, rather than the number of SIRS criteria met, appears to be a more important prognostic factor in determining which trauma patients develop DIC (emphasizing the importance of success in early treatment of these patients).

The complex pathophysiology of DIC and the high prevalence of coagulopathy in the ICU population make it difficult to rely on any single laboratory test to make the diagnosis of DIC. The D-dimer levels appear to be the most reliable of the commonly available tests for DIC, and the combination with FDP has a sensitivity of 91% and specificity to 94%. HIT can mimic DIC and should be considered in the setting of thrombosis and thrombocytopenia that bears a temporal relationship beginning 5 to 14 days after starting heparin.

The cornerstone of treatment for DIC is aggressive treatment of the underlying disorder. For some disorders, removing the precipitating factor can have dramatic effects. AT, APC, and other agents are being studied for use in DIC. Currently, heparin is the most common agent directed at DIC, most commonly as a low dose infusion with no loading dose. Some clinicians advocate LMWH, with its lower risk of HIT, for anticoagulation in DIC. Antifibrinolytic agents should be used rarely and with extreme caution. Replacement of coagulation factors should be limited to the treatment of clinically significant bleeding, not to correct laboratory abnormalities.

Despite improvements in understanding DIC and pharmacological developments in manipulating the coagulation and fibrinolytic systems, the mortality associated with this process has not changed substantially in the last decade. However, with new treatment modalities on the horizon, improved patient outcomes may also occur in the near future. Until more effective specific therapy becomes available, aggressive treatment of the underlying disease and early recognition of DIC remain the mainstay of therapy.

KEY POINTS

- Tissue factor is expressed on the surface of activated monocytes and endothelial cells activating the extrinsic pathway by complexing with factor VII. The uncontrolled release of tissue factor appears to be one of the principal initiating steps in DIC (7).
- Levels of coagulation pathway inhibitors including TFPI, AT, and protein C are all decreased in patients with DIC, hence perpetuating thrombosis.
- Protein C levels are decreased in both sepsis and DIC (19,22,23). The decrease in sepsis-related mortality by using APC, as demonstrated in the PROWESS study (23), suggests the possibility of using it to treat DIC.
- Plasma levels of factor V, factor VIII, prothrombin, and fibrinogen are universally reduced in severe DIC, though fibrinogen levels can be maintained until late in the process.
- The persistence of SIRS, rather than the number of SIRS criteria met, appears to be a more important prognostic factor in determining which trauma patients develop DIC, emphasizing the importance of early appropriate treatment of these patients.
- DIC occurs in a variety of clinical settings associated with trauma, infection being one of the most common.
- The complex pathophysiology of DIC, and high prevalence of coagulopathy in trauma and critical care, makes it difficult for a single laboratory test to confirm the diagnosis.
- The D-dimer appears to be the most reliable of the commonly available tests for the diagnosis of DIC, and

when combined with FDP has a sensitivity of 91% and specificity to 94% (60,61).

☞ Heparin induced thrombocytopenia (HIT) can mimic the clinical appearance of DIC with thrombosis and thrombocytopenia.

☞ The cornerstone of treatment for DIC is an aggressive attempt to remove the underlying disorder or precipitating factor.

☞ Currently, heparin is the most common agent directed at DIC, typically administered as a low dose infusion with no loading dose.

☞ Repletion of coagulation factors should be limited to the treatment of clinically significant bleeding in conjunction with laboratory abnormalities. However, abnormal lab values alone should rarely be treated.

☞ Only in rare circumstances should inhibition of the fibrinolytic system with antifibrinolytic agents be considered for the treatment of DIC.

☞ While not recommended for all causes of DIC, rFVIIa appears to be useful in severe trauma-associated coagulopathy and diffuse hemorrhage.

REFERENCES

1. ten Cate H, Schoenmakers SH, Franco R, et al. Microvascular coagulopathy and disseminated intravascular coagulation. Crit Care Med 2001; 29:S95–S97.
2. Taylor FB, Toh CH, Hoots WK, et al. (On behalf of the Scientific Subcommittee on Disseminated Intravascular Coagulation [DIC] of the International Society on Thrombosis and Haemostasis [ISTH]): Towards Definition, Clinical and Laboratory Criteria, and a Scoring System for Disseminated Intravascular Coagulation. Thromb Haemost 2001; 86:1327–1330.
3. Cummins D. Disseminated intravascular coagulation. In: Webb AR, Shapiro MJ, eds. Oxford Textbook of Critical Care. Oxford: Oxford University Press, 1999:668–670.
4. Bajaj MS, Bajaj SP. Tissue factor pathway inhibitor: potential therapeutic applications. Thromb Haemost 1997; 78(1):471–477.
5. Rosing J, van Rijn JL, Bevers EM, et al. The role of activated human platelets in prothrombin and factor X activation. Blood 1985; 65(2):319–332.
6. Arky RA. MKSAP: Hematology. American College of Physicians-American Society of Intern Med 2001:45–47.
7. Levi M, van der Poll T, Buller HR. Bidirectional relation between inflammation and coagulation. Circulation. 2004; 109(22):2698–2704.
8. ten Cate H. Pathophysiology of disseminated intravascular coagulation in sepsis. Crit Care Med 2000; 28(9):S9–S11.
9. Hulka F, Mullins RJ, Frank EH. Blunt brain injury activates the coagulation process. Arch Surg 1996; 131(9):923–927.
10. Taylor FB Jr, Wada H, Kinasewitz G. Description of compensated and uncompensated disseminated intravascular coagulation (DIC) responses (non-overt and overt DIC) in baboon models of intravenous and intraperitoneal *Escherichia coli* sepsis and in the human model of endotoxemia: toward a better definition of DIC. Crit Care Med 2000; 28:S12–S19.
11. Edgington TS, Mackman N, Fan ST, et al. Cellular immune and cytokine pathways resulting in tissue factor expression and relevance to septic shock. Nouv Rev Fr Hematol 1992; 34:S15–S27.
12. Levi M, ten Cate H, Bauer KA, et al. Inhibition of endotoxin-induced activation of coagulation and fibrinolysis by pentoxifylline or by a monoclonal anti-tissue factor antibody in chimpanzees. J Clin Invest 1994; 93(1):114–120.
13. Levi M, van Der PT, ten Cate H, et al. The cytokine-mediated imbalance between coagulant and anticoagulant mechanisms in sepsis and endotoxaemia. Eur J Clin Invest 1997; 27(1):3–9.
14. ten Cate H, Bauer KA, Levi M, et al. The activation of factor X and prothrombin by recombinant factor VIIa in vivo is mediated by tissue factor. J Clin Invest 1993; 92(3):1207–1212.
15. Wintrobe MM, Lee GR. Wintrobe's clinical hematology. 10th ed. Baltimore: Williams & Wilkins, 1999:1675–1687.
16. Mann KG, van't Veer C, Cawthern K, et al. The role of the tissue factor pathway in initiation of coagulation. Blood Coagul Fibrinolysis 1998; 9(11):S3–S7.
17. Shimura M, Wada H, Wakita Y, et al. Plasma tissue factor and tissue factor pathway inhibitor levels in patients with disseminated intravascular coagulation. Am J Hematol 1996; 52(3):165–170.
18. Hoek JA, Sturk A, ten Cate JW, et al. Laboratory and clinical evaluation of an assay of thrombin-antithrombin III complexes in plasma. Clin Chem 1988; 34(10):2058–2062.
19. Fourrier F, Chopin C, Goudemand J, et al. Septic shock, multiple organ failure, and disseminated intravascular coagulation. Compared patterns of antithrombin III, protein C, and protein S deficiencies. Chest 1992; 101(3):816–823.
20. Esmon CT. Protein C anticoagulant pathway and its role in controlling microvascular thrombosis and inflammation. Crit Care Med 2001; 29(7):S48–S51.
21. Esmon C. The protein C pathway. Crit Care Med 2000; 28(9):S44–S48.
22. Faust SN, Heyderman RS, Levin M. Coagulation in severe sepsis: a central role for thrombomodulin and activated protein C. Crit Care Med 2001; 29(7):S62–S67.
23. Bernard GR, Vincent J, Laterre P, et al. Efficacy and safety of recombinant human activated protein C for severe sepsis. N Engl J Med 2001; 344(10):699–709.
24. Grinnell BW, Joyce D. Recombinant human activated protein C: a system modulator of vascular function for treatment of severe sepsis. Crit Care Med 2001; 29(7):S53–S60.
25. Biemond BJ, Levi M, ten Cate H, et al. Plasminogen activator and plasminogen activator inhibitor I release during experimental endotoxaemia in chimpanzees: effect of interventions in the cytokine and coagulation cascades. Clin Sci (Lond) 1995; 88(5):587–594.
26. Asakura H, Ontachi Y, Mizutani T, et al. An enhanced fibrinolysis prevents the development of multiple organ failure in disseminated intravascular coagulation in spite of much activation of blood coagulation. Crit Care Med 2001; 29(6):1164–1168.
27. Oka K, Shimamura K, Nakazawa M, et al. The role of Kupffer's cells in disseminated intravascular coagulation. A morphologic study in thrombin-infused rabbits. Arch Pathol Lab Med 1983; 107(11):570–576.
28. Johnson K, Choi Y, DeGroot E, et al. Potential mechanisms for a proinflammatory vascular cytokine response to coagulation activation. J Immunol 1998; 160(10):5130–5135.
29. Neumann FJ, Ott I, Marx N, et al. Effect of human recombinant interleukin-6 and interleukin-8 on monocyte procoagulant activity. Arterioscler Thromb Vasc Biol 1997; 17(12):3399–3405.
30. Opal SM. Phylogenetic and functional relationships between coagulation and the innate immune response. Crit Care Med 2000; 28(9):S77–S80.
31. Conway EM, Rosenberg RD. Tumor necrosis factor suppresses transcription of the thrombomodulin gene in endothelial cells. Mol Cell Biol 1988; 8(12):5588–5592.
32. Giebler R, Schmidt U, Koch S, et al. Combined antithrombin III and C1-esterase inhibitor treatment decreases intravascular fibrin deposition and attenuates cardiorespiratory impairment in rabbits exposed to *Escherichia coli* endotoxin. Crit Care Med 1999; 27(3):597–604.
33. Vervloet MG, Thijs LG, Hack CE. Derangements of coagulation and fibrinolysis in critically ill patients with sepsis and septic shock. Semin Thromb Hemost 1998; 24(1):33–44.
34. Lorente JA, Garcia-Frade LJ, Landin L, et al. Time course of hemostatic abnormalities in sepsis and its relation to outcome. Chest 1993; 103(5):1536–1542.
35. Xu J, Esmon NL, Esmon CT. Reconstitution of the human endothelial cell protein C receptor with thrombomodulin in

phosphatidylcholine vesicles enhances protein C activation. J Biol Chem 1999; 274(10):6704–6710.

36. Levi M, ten Cate H. Disseminated intravascular coagulation. N Engl J Med 1999; 341(8):586–592.

37. Grinnell BW, Hermann RB, Yan SB. Human protein C inhibits selectin-mediated cell adhesion: role of unique fucosylated oligosaccharide. Glycobiology 1994; 4(2):221–225.

38. Schmidt-Supprian M, Murphy C, While B, et al. Activated protein C inhibits tumor necrosis factor and macrophage migration inhibitory factor production in monocytes. Eur Cytokine New 2000; 11(3):407–413.

39. Abraham E. NF-kappaB activation. Crit Care Med 2000; 28(4):N100–N104.

40. Bajzar L, Morser J, Nesheim M. TAFI, or plasma procarboxy-peptidase B, couples the coagulation and fibrinolytic cascades through the thrombin-thrombomodulin complex. J Biol Chem 1996; 271(28):16603–16608.

41. Wolbink GJ, Bossink AW, Groeneveld AB, et al. Complement activation in patients with sepsis is in part mediated by C-reactive protein. J Infect Dis 1998; 177(1):81–87.

42. Dries DJ. Activation of the clotting system and complement after trauma. New Horiz 1996; 4(2):276–288.

43. Churliaev I, Lychev VG, Epifantseva NN, et al. [Clinico-pathogenetic variants of DIC syndrome in patients with severe craniocerebral trauma]. Anesteziol Reanimatol 1999; (3):35–37.

44. Kaufman HH, Timberlake G, Voelker J, et al. Medical complications of head injury. Med Clin North Am 1993; 77(1):43–60.

45. Zolotokrylina ES. [Stages of disseminated intravascular coagulation after resuscitation in patients with massive hemorrhage and severe multiple trauma]. Anesteziol Reanimatol 1999; (1):13–18.

46. McKenna R. Abnormal coagulation in the postoperative period contributing to excessive bleeding. Med Clin North Am 2001; 85(5):1277–1310, viii.

47. Linder M, Muller-Berghaus G, Lasch HG, et al. Virus infection and blood coagulation. Thromb Diath Haemorrh 1970; 23(1): 1–11.

48. McKay DG, Margaretten W. Disseminated intravascular coagulation in virus diseases. Arch Intern Med 1967; 120(2):129–152.

49. Bick RL. Syndromes of disseminated intravascular coagulation in obstetrics, pregnancy, and gynecology. Objective criteria for diagnosis and management. Hematol Oncol Clin North Am 2000; 14(5):999–1044.

50. Petroianu GA, Altmannsberger SH, Maleck WH, et al. Meconium and amniotic fluid embolism: effects on coagulation in pregnant mini-pigs. Crit Care Med 1999; 27(2):348–355.

51. Locksmith GJ. Amniotic fluid embolism. Obstet Gynecol Clin North Am 1999; 26(3):435–444.

52. Bick RL, Arun B, Frenkel EP. Disseminated intravascular coagulation. Clinical and pathophysiological mechanisms and manifestations. Haemostasis 1999; 29(2-3):111–134.

53. Bick RL. Disseminated intravascular coagulation. Objective laboratory diagnostic criteria and guidelines for management. Clin Lab Med 1994; 14(4):729–768.

54. Bick RL. Disseminated intravascular coagulation. Objective criteria for diagnosis and management. Med Clin North Am 1994; 78(3):511–543.

55. Mjahed K, Hammamouchi B, Hammoudi D, et al. [Critical analysis of hemostasis disorders in the course of eclampsia. Report of 106 cases]. J Gynecol Obstet Biol Reprod (Paris) 1998; 27(6):607–610.

56. Orozhanova V, Bozhinova S, Khristova V. [The perinatal outcome in adolescents with eclampsia and the HELLP syndrome]. Akush Ginekol (Sofiia) 1996; 35(1-2):14–16.

57. Baker WF Jr. Clinical aspects of disseminated intravascular coagulation: a clinician's point of view. Semin Thromb Hemost 1989; 15(1):1–57.

58. Bick RL, Strauss JF, Frenkel EP. Thrombosis and hemorrhage in oncology patients. Hematol Oncol Clin North Am 1996; 10(4):875–907.

59. Drummond JC, Petrovitch CT. The massively bleeding patient. Anesthesiol Clin North America 2001; 19(4):633–649.

60. Bick RL, Kunkel LA. Disseminated intravascular coagulation syndromes. Int J Hematol 1992; 55(1):1–26.

61. Yu M, Nardella A, Pechet L. Screening tests of disseminated intravascular coagulation: guidelines for rapid and specific laboratory diagnosis. Crit Care Med 2000; 28(6): 1777–1780.

62. Heyes H, Kohle W, Slijepcevic B. The appearance of schistocytes in the peripheral blood in correlation to the degree of disseminated intravascular coagulation. An experimental study in rats. Haemostasis 1976; 5(2):66–73.

63. Cronlund M, Hardin J, Burton J, et al. Fibrinopeptide A in plasma of normal subjects and patients with disseminated intravascular coagulation and systemic lupus erythematosus. J Clin Invest 1976; 58(1):142–151.

64. Bick RL. The clinical significance of fibrinogen degradation products. Semin Thromb Hemost 1982; 8(4):302–330.

64a. Bick RL. Disseminated intravascular coagulation: a review of etiology, pathophysiology, diagnosis, and management: guidelines for care. Clin Appl Thromb Hemost 2002; 8(1):1–31.

65. Warkentin TE, Bernstein RA. Delayed-onset heparin-induced thrombocytopenia and cerebral thrombosis after a single administration of unfractionated heparin. N Engl J Med 2003; 348:1067–1068.

66. Warkentin TE. Heparin-induced thrombocytopenia: pathogenesis and management. Br J Haematol 2003; 121(4):535–555.

67. MacLeod J, Lynn M, McKenney MG. MD Early Coagulopathy Predicts Mortality in Trauma. J Trauma 2003; 55(1):39–44.

68. Armand R, Hess JR. Treating coagulopathy in trauma patients. Transfusion Med Rev. 2003; 17:223–231.

69. Carrick MM, Tyroch AH, Youens C A, Handley T. Subsequent development of thrombocytopenia and coagulopathy in moderate and severe head injury: support for serial laboratory examination. J Trauma 2005; 58(4):725–730.

70. Brohi K, Singh J, Heron M, Coats T. Acute Traumatic Coagulopathy. J Trauma 2003; 54(6):1127–1130.

71. Martini WZ, Pusateri AE, Uscilowicz JM, et al. Independent contributions of hypothermia and acidosis to coagulopathy in swine. J Trauma 2005; 58(5):1002–1010.

72. Levi M, de Jonge E, van Der PT, et al. Novel approaches to the management of disseminated intravascular coagulation. Crit Care Med 2000; 28(9 suppl):S20–S24.

73. Bick RL. Disseminated intravascular coagulation. Hematol Oncol Clin North Am 1992; 6(6):1259–1285.

74. du Toit HJ, Coetzee AR, Chalton DO. Heparin treatment in thrombin-induced disseminated intravascular coagulation in the baboon. Crit Care Med 1991; 19(9):1195–1200.

75. Feinstein DI. Diagnosis and management of disseminated intravascular coagulation: the role of heparin therapy. Blood 1982; 60(2):284–287.

76. Abraham E. Tissue factor inhibition and clinical trial results of tissue factor pathway inhibitor in sepsis. Crit Care Med 2000; 28(9):S31–S33.

77. Creasey AA, Chang AC, Feigen L, et al. Tissue factor pathway inhibitor reduces mortality from *Escherichia coli* septic shock. J Clin Invest 1993; 91(6):2850–2856.

78. de Jonge E, Dekkers PE, Creasey AA, et al. Tissue factor pathway inhibitor dose-dependently inhibits coagulation activation without influencing the fibrinolytic and cytokine response during human endotoxemia. Blood 2000; 95(4):1124–1129.

79. Paramo JA, Montes R, Hermida MJ, et al. [Inhibitor of the extrinsic pathway of coagulation and cytokines in patients with sepsis]. Sangre (Barc) 1995; 40(1):59–62.

80. Abraham E, Reinhart K, Svoboda P, et al. Assessment of the safety of recombinant tissue factor pathway inhibitor in patients with severe sepsis: a multicenter, randomized, placebo- controlled, single-blind, dose escalation study. Crit Care Med 2001; 29(11):2081–2089.

81. Baudo F, Caimi TM, de Cataldo F, et al. Antithrombin III (ATIII) replacement therapy in patients with sepsis and/or postsurgical complications: a controlled double-blind, randomized, multicenter study. Intensive Care Med 1998; 24(4):336–342.

82. Blauhut B, Kramar H, Vinazzer H, et al. Substitution of antithrombin III in shock and DIC: a randomized study. Thromb Res 1985; 39(1):81–89.

83. Eisele B, Lamy M, Thijs LG, et al. Antithrombin III in patients with severe sepsis. A randomized, placebo-controlled, double-blind multicenter trial plus a meta-analysis on all randomized, placebo-controlled, double-blind trials with antithrombin III in severe sepsis. Intensive Care Med 1998; 24(7):663–672.

84. Fourrier F, Chopin C, Huart JJ, et al. Double-blind, placebo-controlled trial of antithrombin III concentrates in septic shock with disseminated intravascular coagulation. Chest 1993; 104(3):882–888.

85. Markwardt F. Development of hirudin as an antithrombotic agent. Semin Thromb Hemost 1989; 15(3):269–282.

86. Munoz MC, Montes R, Hermida J, et al. Effect of the administration of recombinant hirudin and/or tissue-plasminogen activator (t-PA) on endotoxin-induced disseminated intravascular coagulation model in rabbits. Br J Haematol 1999; 105(1):117–121.

87. Talbot M. Biology of recombinant hirudin (CGP 39393): a new prospect in the treatment of thrombosis. Semin Thromb Hemost 1989; 15(3):293–301.

88. de Haan J, van Oeveren W. Platelets and soluble fibrin promote plasminogen activation causing downregulation of platelet glycoprotein Ib/IX complexes: Protection by aprotinin. Thromb Res 1998; 92:171–179.

89. Blauhut B, Gross C, Necek S, et al. Effects of high-dose aprotinin on blood loss, platelet function, fibrinolysis, complement, and renal function after cardiopulmonary bypass. J Thorac Cardiovasc Surg 1991; 101:958–967.

90. Dietrich W, Dilthey G, Spannagl M, et al. Influence of high-dose aprotinin on anticoagulation, heparin requirement, and celite- and kaolin-activated clotting time in heparin-pretreated patients undergoing open-heart surgery: A double-blind, placebo-controlled study. Anesthesiology 1995; 83:679–689.

91. Royston D, Bidstrup BP, Taylor KM, et al.: Effect of aprotinin on need for blood transfusion after repeat open-heart surgery. Lancet 1987, 2:1289–1291.

92. Royston D, Taylor KM, Sapsford RN: Aprotinin (Trasylol) reduces bleeding after open-heart surgery in patients taking aspirin and those with renal failure. Anesthesiology 1989, 71(A6).

93. Verstraete M. Clinical application of inhibitors of fibrinolysis. Drugs 1985; 29:236–261.

94. Okamoto S, Sato S, Takada Y, et al. An active stereoisomer (transform) of AMCHA and its antifibrinolytic (antiplasmic) action in vitro and in vivo. Keio J Med 1964, 13:177.

95. Katsaros D, Petricevic M, Snow NJ, et al. Tranexamic acid reduces postbypass blood use: a double-blinded, prospective, randomized study of 210 patients. Ann Thorac Surg 1996, 61:1131–1135.

96. Vander Salm TJ, Kaur S, Lancey RA, et al. Reduction of bleeding after heart operations through the prophylactic use of epsilon-aminocaproic acid. J Thorac Cardiovasc Surg 1996, 112:1098–1107.

97. Boylan JF, Klinck JR, Sandler AN, et al. Tranexamic acid reduces blood loss, transfusion requirements, and coagulation factor use in primary orthotopic liver transplantation. Anesthesiology 1996; 85:1043–1048.

98. Mojcik CF, Levy JH. Aprotinin and the systemic inflammatory response after cardiopulmonary bypass. Ann Thorac Surg 2001; 71:745–754.

99. Laffey JG, Boylan JF, Cheng DC. The systemic inflammatory response to cardiac surgery: Implications for the anesthesiologist. Anesthesiology 2002; 97:215–252.

100. Greilich DE, Brouse CF, Rinder CS, et al. Effects of epsilon-aminocaproic acid and aprotinin in leukocyte-platelet adhesion in patients undergoing cardiac surgery. Anesthesiology 2004; 100:225–233.

101. Chiu J, Ketchum LH, Reid TJ. Transfusion-sparing hemostatic agents. Current Opinion in Hematology 2002; 9(6):544–550.

102. Holcomb JB. Use of Recombinant Activated Factor VII to Treat the Acquired Coagulopathy of Trauma. J Trauma 2005; 58(6):1298–1303.

103. Dutton RP, McCunn M, Hyder M, et al. Factor VIIa for Correction of Traumatic Coagulopathy. J Trauma 2004; 57(4):709–719.

104. Friederich PW, Henny CP, Messelink EJ, et al. Effect of rFVIIa on perioperative blood loss in patients undergoing retropubic prostectomy. Lancet 2003; 361:201–205.

105. Boffard KD, Riou B, Warren B, et al. Recombinant factor VIIa as adjunctive therapy for bleeding control in severely injured trauma patients: two parallel randomized, placebo-controlled, double-blind clinical trials. J Trauma 2005; 59(1):8–18.

106. Pernerstorfer T, Hollenstein U, Hansen JB, et al. Lepirudin blunts endotoxin-induced coagulation activation. Blood 2000; 95(5):1729–1734.

107. Mukundan S, Zeigler ZR. Direct antithrombin agents ameliorate disseminated intravascular coagulation in suspected heparin-induced thrombocytopenia thrombosis syndrome. Clin Appl Thromb Hemost 2002; 8(3):287–289.

59

Rational Use of Blood Products for Trauma and Critical Care

Colin F. Mackenzie
Department of Anesthesiology, University of Maryland School of Medicine, Baltimore, Maryland, U.S.A.

Daniel Scheidegger
Department of Anesthesiology, University of Basel School of Medicine, Basel, Switzerland

INTRODUCTION

Blood transfusion is the most important medical advance of World War I (1). The quantity of blood shipped (2000 units a day) to U.S. troops during World War II in March 1945 is the highest rate of blood transported in U.S. military history, and was required to support the 12 million military personnel who sustained 30,000 casualties in that month alone (2,3). The benefits of blood in saving lives of those injured were fully recognized by British and American medical units, yet the United States entered the Korean War without a formal military blood program. In Vietnam, the most frequent mode of transfusion was two to five units of red blood cells (RBCs), usually given as packed RBCs (PRBCs), but small amounts of fresh whole blood were drawn on site for production of platelets or direct administration to coagulopathic casualties. More than 100,000 universal donor group O uncross-matched RBCs were transfused in Vietnam without a single fatal hemolytic transfusion reaction. The nine reported fatal transfusion reactions all followed misidentified cross-matched blood (4). Although small stores of PRBCs are available, large quantities of blood are also collected and administered as whole blood to military trauma victims.

☞ **The requirement for blood in military and disaster situations is largely determined by the number of injured that survive long enough to present for care.** ☜

In Vietnam, only 16% of casualties required transfusion. In Iraq and Afghanistan, the transfusion rates are likely to be in a similar range, though current numbers are not available. In modern civilian trauma centers the transfusion rates are lower. Only 9% of trauma patients admitted to the University of Maryland Shock Trauma Center in 2000 required transfusion. One to two units of blood transfusions are the most frequent mode of military and civilian trauma center blood transfusions (2).

This chapter reviews the current transfusion triggers for blood transfusion in trauma and critical care, as well as the monitoring considerations for tissue oxygenation and perfusion. The various blood components that are available for transfusion are surveyed, and distinctions are made regarding the special situations of emergency and massive transfusion conditions. The complications of blood transfusion, along with newer data on the tolerance for acute anemia, are also included. The "Eye to the Future" section previews newer artificial blood now under development.

TRANSFUSION TRIGGERS

The traditional indication for administration of blood to trauma patients occurs when hemoglobin (Hb) values fall below 10 g/dL (5). This became known as the *transfusion trigger* and was used by clinicians to guide their decision about whether or not to administer blood. More recently, the benefits of blood transfusion have been questioned. The concept of a single laboratory value as a rigid transfusion guide has been reassessed due to the belief that the decision to transfuse is influenced by many factors including co-morbidities (especially cardiac and diabetes), age, the acuteness of blood loss, expectations for continued future blood loss, and the physiological changes that the current amount of blood loss has produced (6).

Recent transfusion practices among U.S. anesthesiologists indicate that more than half of them measure Hb or hematocrit (Hct) values before red cell transfusion (7): Among the 862 survey respondents, 6% indicated that they transfuse when Hb falls below 10 g/dL (or Hct <30%), 39% indicated they would transfuse when Hb <8 g/dL (or Hct <24%), and 6% indicated that they would transfuse when Hb <6 g/dL (or Hct <18%). The remaining 46% indicated "other" with conditional responses due to the factors identified above as influencing their transfusion decision (7).

Liberal vs. Restrictive Transfusion Practices in Critical Care

The Canadian Critical Care Trials group compared the outcome of a liberal strategy to a restrictive strategy of blood transfusion (8,9). In the first study of euvolemic critically ill patients, they compared mortality in just over 400 patients randomized to each of two groups, one to be transfused if Hb was less than 7 g/dL within 72 hours after their admission, the other if their Hb fell below 10 g/dL. They found that overall 30-day mortality was similar (18.7% vs. 23.3%) (8). However, mortality rates were significantly lower with the restrictive transfusion strategy among patients who were less acutely ill [with Acute Physiology and Chronic Health Evaluation (APACHE) score ≤20] and among patients less than 55 years of age. The in-hospital mortality rate during hospitalization was also significantly lower in those randomized to the restrictive strategy. Although the restrictive strategy appears superior to the liberal transfusion protocol, patients with acute myocardial infarction and unstable angina can be exceptions to this rule.

In their follow-up study of critically ill patients with cardiovascular disease, they again compared restrictive and liberal transfusion strategies (9). Mortality rates were similar in the two groups. However, changes from baseline in the multiple organ dysfunction scores were significantly less in the restrictive group (transfusion trigger of 7 g/dL). In 257 patients with severe ischemic heart disease, the restrictive group had a lower but nonsignificant absolute survival rate compared to patients in the liberal group. Further, the restrictive policy in these patients significantly reduced the average number of red cells transfused from 5.2 ± 5.0 units to 2.4 ± 4.1—a 53% reduction.

General Transfusion Guidelines

The transfusion guideline produced by the National Institutes of Health (NIH) Consensus Panel, published in 1988, was that red cell transfusion should occur at a Hb value of 7 g/dL in patients free of cardiac and cerebral disease (10). The American College of Physicians, with many of the same participants, also identified 7 g/dL, as an appropriate level for red cell transfusion (11). The American Society of Anesthesiology (ASA) proposed a range of 6 g/dL, when blood must be transfused, to 10 g/dL, when it should not be transfused (12). The recently published survey of U.S. Anesthesiologists suggests that current transfusion practices are, in general, consistent with ASA guidelines (7). The Canadian Medical Association identified 8 g/dL as the guideline for transfusion (13). Thus, the consensus panels are inconsistent, further discrediting the concept of a single laboratory value to guide the need for transfusion. The College of American Pathologists Practice Guidelines recommends that in acute anemia, a fall in Hb below 6 g/dL or a rapid blood volume loss of more than 30% to 40% requires RBC transfusion in most patients (14).

Transfusion Trends in Trauma Patients

Another way to examine guidelines for transfusion in trauma patients is to review actual clinical practice. Compared to other populations, trauma patients are more likely to be transfused (15). In an article from the Trauma Program at the University of Toronto, Farion et al. (16) described trends in the use of blood among adults admitted during 1991, 1993, and 1995 (Fig. 1). On admission in each year, there were between 500 and 560 patients with similar Hb levels and injury severity scores. A significant reduction was found in the average 24-hour Hb levels, the lowest Hb levels, and the discharge Hb concentrations during the years 1993–1995. Discharge Hb levels fell significantly from 11.5 to 11.0 g/dL, lowest Hb levels from 9.6 to 9.2 g/dL (Fig. 2) (16). These trends indicated significant reductions in both the number of trauma patients receiving blood products and the total number of units transfused. More than 300 fewer blood units were transfused when 60 more patients were treated in 1995 with similar injury severity scores compared to 1991 (Fig. 1). There was also more cross-matched blood and less type-specific and uncross-matched blood used in 1995, indicating that clinicians had become more tolerant of acute anemia.

Recent studies continue to indicate that blood transfusion is a confirmed independent predictor of mortality in trauma patients (17). Indeed, a recent retrospective evaluation of 316 patients with blunt hepatic and/or splenic injuries, after being controlled for shock and injury severity, found both mortality and hospital length of stay to be sig nificantly increased with each unit of blood transfused

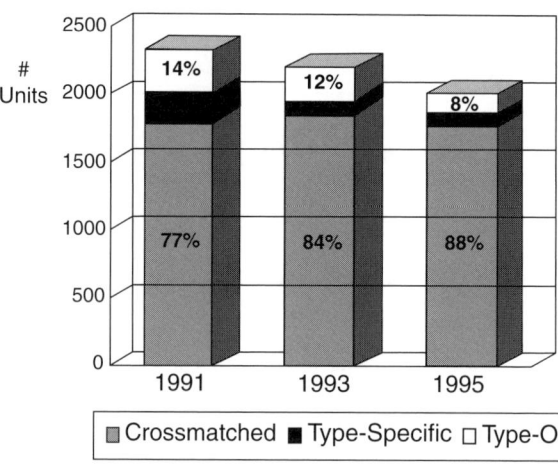

Figure 1 Trends in the type of blood transfused at the University of Toronto Trauma Program in 1991–1995 as a proportion of total blood. A reduction is seen in the use of type-specific and type O blood as well as a reduction in overall cross-matched blood administration between the three years. *Source*: From Ref. 16.

($p < 0.001$ and $p = 0.005$, respectively) (18). Yet, once the threshold of massive transfusion was reached (discussed below) other factors such as base deficit became stronger predictors of mortality (19). Indeed, Vaslef et al. (19) found that among trauma patients who had received >50 units of blood products, mortality rates were not different between those who received 51 to 75 units and those who received >75 units on the first day of admission.

☞ **The concept of a single transfusion trigger is flawed. Comorbidities, especially cardiac, age, injury severity, and magnitude of hemorrhage should all be considered.** ☞

Strategy for the Bleeding Trauma Patient

The low limits of Hb used in restrictive transfusion strategies, whereas generally being acceptable in elective surgical

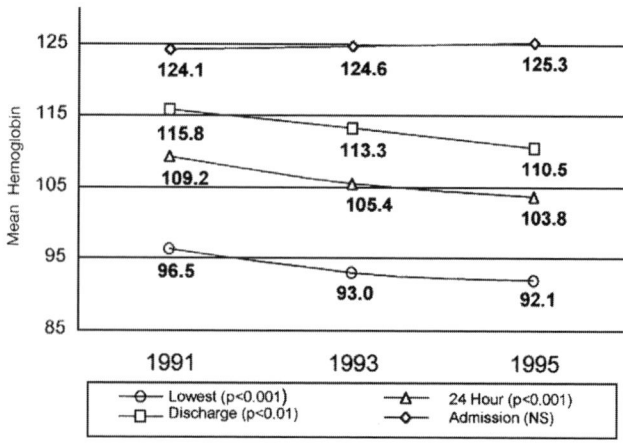

Figure 2 The mean hemoglobin concentration of trauma patients on admission, after 24 hours, on hospital discharge as well as their hemoglobin nadirs among the University of Toronto Trauma Program 1991–1995. Patient discharge hemoglobin levels fell significantly over these years. *Source*: From Ref. 16.

cases or in a nonischemic critical care patient, may not be appropriate in the management of a bleeding trauma patient for the following reasons. First, cardiac output may be inadequate in the bleeding trauma patient because of a low circulating blood volume as occurs with hemorrhagic shock. Second, in low cardiac output states with low circulating blood volume, the maldistribution of blood flow potentially places vital organs at risk for ischemia (20). Third, ongoing blood loss will continue to stress the patient. Some of this blood loss may be hidden when in association with fracture sites or may result from coagulopathies—especially likely when associated with hypothermia and/or prolonged high blood loss surgery. Fourth, multiple trauma patients exhibit inadequate erythropoiesis in response to low hemoglobin, and have a hypoferric state secondary to a complex network of bleeding and inflammatory mediators appearing within 12 hours of injury and lasting for more than nine days (Fig. 3) (21). Finally, there is always an element of uncertainty in estimating future blood loss.

MONITORING OXYGENATION AND PERFUSION
Organ-Specific Monitors of Oxygenation and Perfusion Are Lacking

The two major organs at risk for impaired oxygenation are the brain and the heart. The brain is not usually monitored in any quantitative way during anesthesia; although transcranial cerebral oximetry and jugular venous oximetry may have some merit, these are not often monitored in the acute setting (22). And although cardiac ischemia can be followed by ST segment analysis transesophageal echocardiography and troponin measurements, very few clinicians actually do this in the midst of a busy resuscitation or anesthetic for a patient with significant bleeding.

Monitoring of urine output is an imprecise indicator of renal resuscitation. Indeed urine production can be high despite intravascular depletion in the setting of hyperglycemia, alcohol intoxication, and mannitol or other diuretic usage. Further, in more chronic settings, high output renal failure (the frequent precursor to oliguric renal failure) is accompanied by increased urine flow in combination with decreased creatinine clearance (23).

The gut has less autoregulation capability than other organs. Accordingly, when blood pressure falls in a bleeding trauma patient, the bowel becomes ischemic with the resulting changes likely to contribute to multi-organ dysfunction syndrome and peritonitis. The gut can be monitored by tonometers, but these require initial and sometimes repeated calibration, and more stable conditions than are usually present during trauma resuscitation. Thus, clinicians tend to err on the cautious side of 8 to 10 g/dL Hb levels during management of the acutely bleeding trauma patient.

Global Indicators of Oxygenation and Perfusion

In an NIH sponsored study, the accuracy of common physiological parameters was evaluated, in relation to their predictability of actual blood loss during progressive blood removal in awake, chronically instrumented dogs. In the perfect model, the measure shown on the horizontal axis of these graphs (Fig. 4) would be related to the volume of blood loss (shown on the vertical axis of the graph) by a line of identity. The correlation between hemorrhage volume and base deficit was best during progressive increments of blood loss. Even though there is a wide variance, the trend in each individual animal relates base-deficit to blood loss.

In another study in which animals were bled to different levels of O_2 debt, base deficit was an excellent predictor of different levels of O_2 debt (with -17 base deficit and 9.40

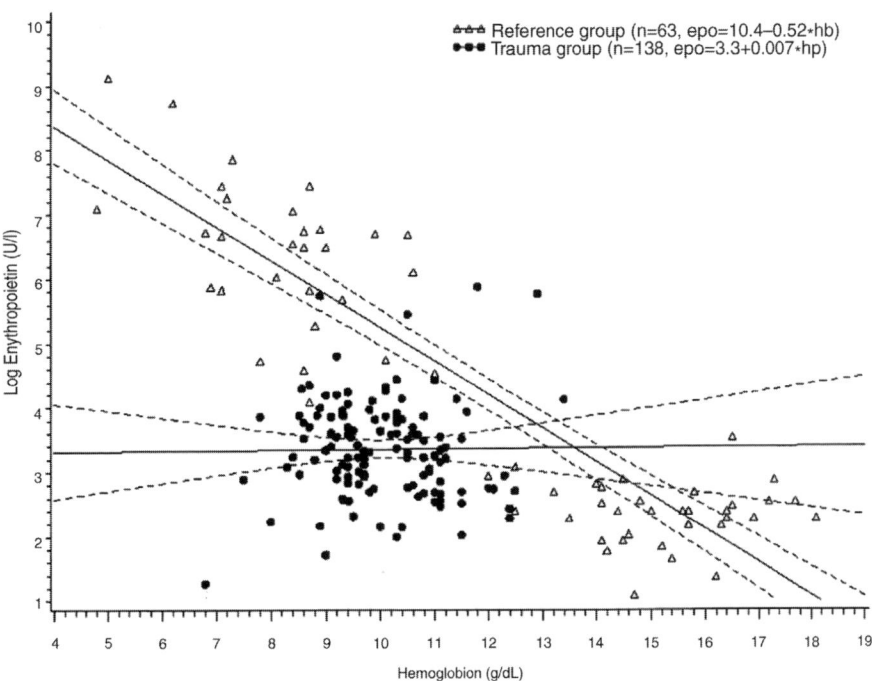

Figure 3 The *y*-axis shows a log plot of erythropoietin (μ/L) and the *x*-axis is hemoglobin in g/dL. Sixty-three patients with primary hemopoietic disorders (triangles) are compared to 138 multiple trauma patients (black dots). As hemoglobin decreases in patients with primary hemopoietic disorders, so erythropoietin levels rise (line of identity shown) exponentially. For trauma patients, there is no increase of erythropoietin as hemoglobin levels decrease. *Source*: From Ref. 21.

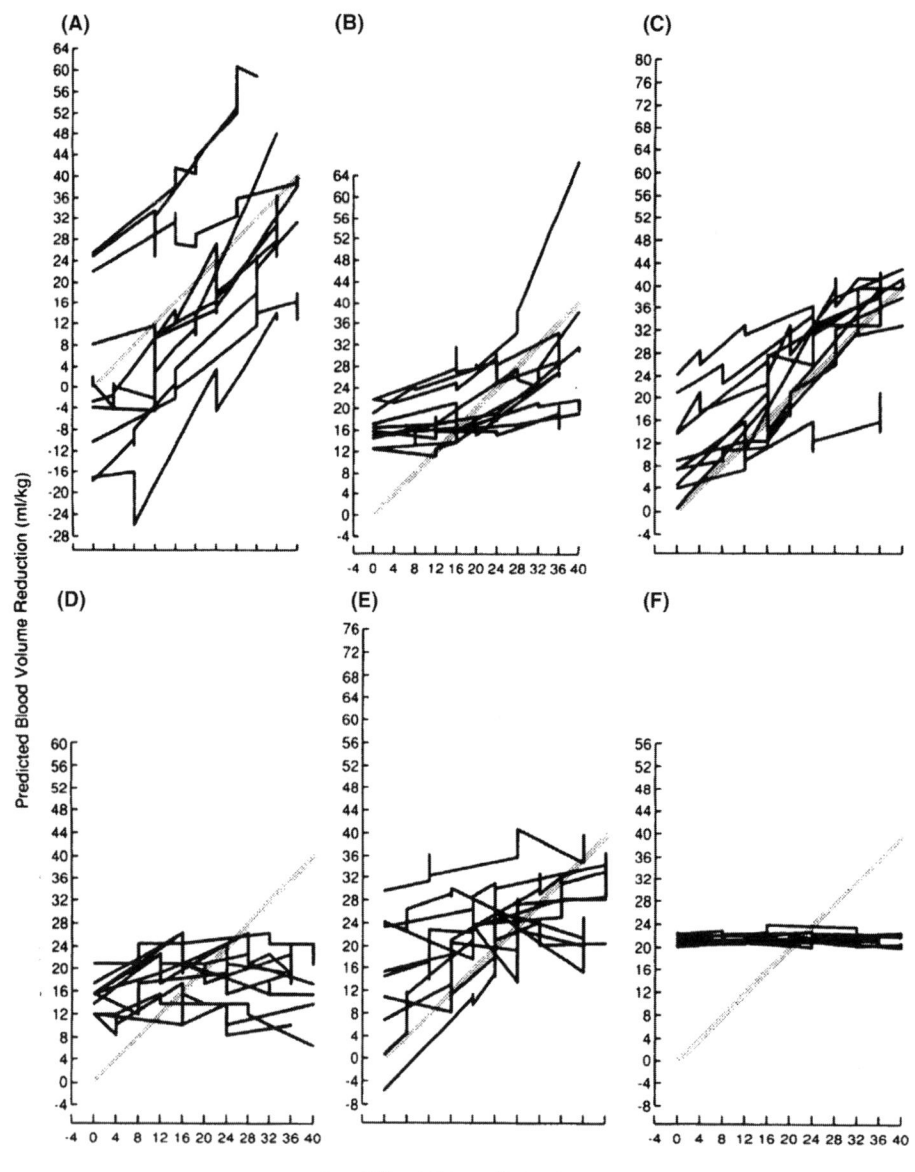

Figure 4   Comparison of model predictions versus actual blood volume reductions for six representative parameters [arterial base deficit (**A**), arterial lactate (**B**), mean arterial pressure (**C**), heart rate (**D**), hemoglobin (**E**), and mixed venous PCO_2 (**F**)]. Solid black lines represent individual animal ($n = 10$). Gray bar represents an ideal model slope in which model predictions equal actual blood volume reductions. For mean arterial pressure, predictions at large volume hemorrhage were more accurate than predictions with small volume bleeds. Models such as heart rate and lactate both showed significant variability before hemorrhage among animals and flat slopes (e.g., mixed venous PCO_2) indicated fixed-volume predictions regardless of actual degree of hemorrhage. *Source*: From Ref. 24.

lactate levels being associated with 25% mortality) (25). The correlation coefficient with hemorrhage volume was higher with base deficit than with lactate in both studies. Arteriovenous pH and PCO_2 differences, as a measure of adequacy of resuscitation, was also useful as a simple evaluation of the onset of tissue ischemia (26). In animal data both arteriovenous pH and arterio-venous CO_2 differences have a high correlation with critical O_2 delivery ($\dot{D}O_2$) and lactate (Fig. 5) (26). The practical measurement of these values is easy with venous samples for pH and P_vCO_2 being obtained from a central vein, not the pulmonary artery. The use of a colorimetric hemoglobin meter in the operating room for serial monitoring of Hb concentration is also a sensible monitor of the anemia status. In addition to the above

measures, a fiberoptic intramucosal PCO_2 monitor sublingual PCO_2, transcranial cerebral oximetry, and ST segment analysis capability on the electrocardiogram (ECG) monitor, provide optimum current state-of-the-art monitoring for management of the hemorrhaging patient following trauma.

BLOOD AND COMPONENTS FOR TRANSFUSION
Red Blood Cells

RBCs can be stored in several different ways, including whole blood, PRBCs, frozen, and lyophilized cells. Whole blood is rarely needed or available in civilian practice but

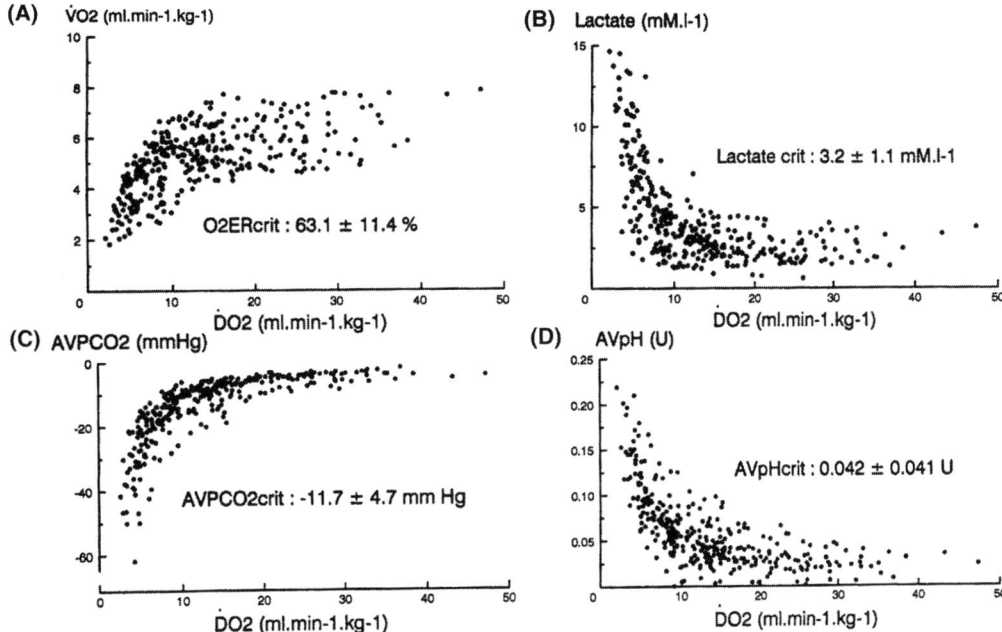

Figure 5 (**A**) and (**B**): Pooled response of $\dot{V}O_2$ and AV PCO_2 to the progressive reduction in $\dot{D}O_2$. O_2Ercrit and AV PCO_2crit were determined in each animal. (**C**) and (**D**): Pooled response of blood lactate and AV pH to the progressive reduction in $\dot{D}O_2$. Lactate crit and AV pHcrit were determined in each animal. *Abbreviations*: AV PCO_2, arteriovenous gradient for PCO_2; AV PCO_2crit, arteriovenous gradient for PCO_2 at critical point; AV pH, arteriovenous gradient for pH; AV pHcrit, arteriovenous gradient for pH at critical point; $\dot{D}O_2$, oxygen delivery; Lactate crit, blood lactate level at critical point; O_2Ercrit, O_2 extraction ratio at critical point; $\dot{V}O_2$, oxygen uptake. *Source*: From Ref. 26.

is used in military situations when it is drawn on site from military personnel (2). In austere situations, whole blood transfusion may be the only effective way to obtain platelets and clotting factors. Frozen RBC storage at $-80°C$, with the high-glycerol method to prevent red cell lysis, allows storage for several years. However, deglycerolization is very resource intensive, needing several hours of preparation before these red cells can be transfused (27). Rapid freeze-drying of red cells (lyophilization) also results in the need to process the product before it can be transfused. Recent advances in storage of PRBC by use of additive solution EAS-76 with 45 mEq/L NaCl allows RBC storage for 12 weeks with acceptable recovery, and 0.6% hemolysis and normal 2,3-diphosphoglycerate (2,3-DPG) concentrations for two weeks (28). Specialized blood units, such as cytomegalovirus negative, irradiated, and leukoreduced preparations have not been shown to be generally required in adult trauma. However, leukoreduction is beneficial for limiting febrile reactions, and irradiation can decrease graft versus host disease (GVHD). Irradiation decreases blood storage time and increases the potassium concentration of each unit, so it is best done immediately prior to transfusion (a process that could slow availability of the blood by approximately 15 minutes).

Platelets

The normal adult platelet count is in the range of 150 to 400×10^9/L. During trauma, platelets are lost with shed blood, consumed in wounds, and diluted by resuscitation fluids (see Volume 1, Chapters 11 and 12). The anticipated platelet count decline is difficult to predict during massive hemorrage due to the multifactorial nature of the losses. Once the patient's blood losses are controlled, and in the absence of ongoing platelet losses, thrombocytopenia

persists for two to four days. Subsequently, the platelet count should begin to increase, resulting in a thrombocytosis from increased marrow production (see Volume 2, Chapter 55).

Activity, Administration, and Half-Life

One platelet concentrate unit will generally increase the platelet count by approximately 5 to 10×10^9/L in the average adult. Because the usual therapeutic dose is one platelet concentrate per 10 kg body weight, typically, 10 concentrate units are pooled and administered at a time.

Apheresis (single-donor) platelet units also have wide variation in platelet yield. The content of each random-donor unit may vary from 5.5 to 8.5×10^{10}/L platelets (29). The American Association of Blood Banks' standards require a minimum of 3.0×10^{11}/L platelets in each plateletpheresis collection (30). When yields are greater than 6×10^{10}/L, the collections are often split into two "doses" (31). The in vivo activity of stored platelets in a recipient is estimated to be reduced by 75% to 80% of their activity on collection. Platelets should be given through an unused infusion set with a 170 micron filter. The transfused platelets have a half-life of only about two days (32).

↪ **One platelet concentrate increases the platelet count by 5 to 10×10^9/L. In vivo platelet activity is decreased 75% from collected activity. Transfused platelets have a half-life of about two days.** ↩

Single vs. Pooled Platelet Donors

The advantages of single-donor platelets over pooled random-donor platelets include reduction in the rate of alloimmunization and transfusion transmitted infection, fewer transfusion reactions, and easier logistics (33). The risk of bacterial contamination is lower in single-donor platelets than in pooled random-donor platelets, but nevertheless was 0.42% in one study (34). White blood cell reduction appears to be related causally to a reduction in alloimmunization, regardless of whether single or pooled concentrates of platelets are used (35). The NIH consensus document on platelet transfusion therapy is under revision (36).

   ✔ **Single-donor platelets have a lower rate of alloimmunization, transmitted infections, and transfusion reactions.** ✔

Platelet Transfusion Trigger

The consensus is that a platelet count of 10×10^9/L (10,000/mm^3) provides a safe lower limit for the prescription of prophylactic platelet transfusion in a routine (nontrauma, noncritical illness) setting (31,33). A threshold of 20×10^9/L should be used for those with fever, infection, and related conditions, with a therapeutic threshold of 50×10^9/L for surgery or invasive procedures (31). Although the ASA believes that this level should be taken into consideration, counts between 50 and 100×10^9/L should merit platelet transfusion on the basis of individual patient risk for bleeding (13). If thrombocytopenia occurs due to massive transfusion or persists in the intensive care unit, platelet infusion will be required. Thrombocytopenia due to consumption or dilution of dysfunctional platelets may increase morbidity and mortality from surgical and traumatic hemorrhage.

   In nonsurgical and some nontrauma patients, spontaneous microvascular bleeding from gums, submucosa, and percutaneous catheter sites rarely occur with platelet counts above 20×10^9/L (37). In massively transfused patients receiving more than 20 units of blood, 75% had platelet counts less than 50×10^9/L, whereas no patients receiving less than 20 units had counts less than 50×10^9/L (38).

   Since six units of platelets contain the equivalent of 1.5 to 2 units of fresh frozen plasma (FFP), clotting and coagulation improvement following platelet transfusion may not be solely due to platelets (39). Forty-one patients randomized to receive platelets ($n = 22$) or FFP ($n = 19$), 32 of whom were trauma patients, were prospectively studied after an average of more than 20 units of modified whole blood units (range 12–39 for platelet group and 14–41 units for FFP group). One patient randomized to FFP had microvascular bleeding after 20 units of modified whole blood (from which platelets and/or cryoprecipitate are salvaged before storage), which was thought to be due to dilutional thrombocytopenia (40). Two patients receiving platelets and one other patient receiving FFP required multiple doses of platelet concentrates and the authors concluded that prophylactic platelet administration was not warranted in massive transfusion (40). However, patients with massive transfusion beyond that studied would likely need platelet transfusion.

   The ASA task force concluded that the need for platelet transfusion is dependent on multiple risk factors, and not a single laboratory value such as platelet count. The risk for surgical patients is defined by the type and extent of surgery, the ability to control bleeding, the consequences of uncontrolled bleeding, the actual and anticipated rate of bleeding, and the presence of other factors adversely affecting platelet function (12). Although the ASA task force did not single out trauma patients separately from surgical patients, these conclusions seem applicable to nonsurgical bleeding trauma patients. Their final conclusion is that platelet transfusion is justified in bleeding patients, despite an apparently adequate platelet count, if there is known platelet dysfunction, microvascular bleeding, or otherwise increased risk of bleeding.

   ✔ **Transfusion of greater than 20 units of blood will reduce platelets to less than 50×10^9/L in 75% of patients. The decision to transfuse platelets is usually based on evidence of microvascular bleeding or in a patient judged to be at high risk of bleeding, rather than on the level of the platelet count per se.** ✔

   In certain groups of trauma patients, including those with intracranial bleeding or those who require intracranial or intraocular surgery, it is recommended by the British Committee for Standards in Haematology that efforts should be made to maintain platelet counts above 100×10^9/L (41). Clinicians appear to support this recommendation, if intracranial bleeding is deemed a possibility (31,42). Clinicians also identified difficulty obtaining platelets in emergencies for trauma patients in Britain (32). In the United States, an audit of underutilization of platelets at one hospital was defined as failure to administer platelets when the platelet count was less than 10×10^9/L, but this was found in only one patient among 89 during the 14-month period when 3967 units of apheresis platelets were transfused (43).

   ✔ **In the setting of acute intracranial bleeding, platelet counts greater than 100×10^9/L should be maintained.** ✔

Drug-Induced Thrombocytopenia and Platelet Dysfunction

Immune-mediated thrombocytopenia can be induced by heparin and other drugs (44,45). However, the clinical picture and therapeutic implications of heparin-induced thrombocytopenia (HIT) differ considerably from other drug-induced immune thrombocytopenic purpura (D-ITP). Whereas HIT tends to give a moderate thrombocytopenia (median platelet count nadir, 60×10^9/L, with a range between 15 and 150×10^9/L in 90% of affected patients), the majority of patients with D-ITP have a platelet count nadir below 15×10^9/L (46). Moreover, patients with HIT do not have petechiae or mucocutaneous bleeding, whether or not such clinical evidence of thrombocytopenic bleeding is typical of D-ITP. Further, HIT is a hypercoagulability state with greatly increased risk of venous and arterial thrombosis (47). Platelet transfusions are considered to be *contraindicated* in HIT, as they may confer greater risk of thrombosis or other complications (48). In contrast, platelet transfusions (with or without high-dose intravenous gammaglobulin) would be an appropriate treatment option in a symptomatic patient with severe D-ITP. Although HIT induced by unfractionated heparin is a relatively common adverse drug reaction (46), D-ITP is very rare (frequency <1000–10,000), but has been implicated with several drugs (e.g., quinine, quinidine, sulfa antibiotics, vancomycin, carbamazepine, certain penicillins and cephalosporins, rifampin, ibuprofen, ranitidine, among others).

   Ketamine inhibits agonist-induced aggregation by suppression of platelet inositol 1,4,5-triphosphate formation, guanosine 5-triphophatase activity, and calcium currents (49). The in vitro concentrations to produce the inhibition were in excess of the in vivo clinical concentrations; accordingly clinical relevance is indeterminate (50). Other intravenous induction agents, volatile anesthetics, and local anesthetics may also modestly inhibit platelet function. However, these effects are not thought to be clinically relevant under normal conditions. Aspirin clearly has antiplatelet action and may worsen bleeding in trauma patients.

However, in elective coronary artery by-pass graft (CABG) patients, it remains unclear to what extent aspirin increases bleeding complications (51).

Thrombocytopenia Associated with Massive Transfusion

Thrombocytopenia associated with trauma and massive transfusion is almost always due to platelet consumption, blood loss, and hemodilution. The relative rate of bleeding and mechanism of injury determine which of these etiologies is most predominant (see Volume 2, Chapter 55).

Prostaglandin E_1 (PGE$_1$) is a vasodilator with antiplatelet and anti-inflammatory properties. PGE$_1$ was tested to see if such an infusion would prevent thrombocytopenia in association with massive transfusion for major orthopedic surgery (52). PGE$_1$ infusion resulted in decreased platelet aggregation and prevented decline in platelet count. The 22 patients who received PGE$_1$ in doses up to 30 ng/kg/min for 72 hours after surgery had no reduction in platelet counts after more than 10 units of red cell infusion, whereas the control groups of 23 patients had a significant drop in platelet counts three and five days after surgery, necessitating platelet transfusion. The PGE$_1$ treated group was more stable and required fewer postoperative blood transfusions, suggesting that PGE$_1$ might inhibit transfusion-induced coagulation disturbances (53). Although this orthopedic surgery patient study is intriguing, its application to less controlled trauma situations is unknown, and potentially dangerous.

Fresh Frozen Plasma

FFP contains all of the major plasma proteins, including the labile factors (V, VIII). In 1997, 3,320,000 units of FFP/single-donor plasma were transfused in the United States. A recent audit, using the Canadian Medical Association's published recommendations, found that FFP transfusions were appropriate for 167 patients (47%), probably appropriate for 31 (9%), and inappropriate for 160 (45%) (54,55). The Canadian Medical Association guidelines recommended transfusion of FFP in three specific situations: (*i*) for patients with significant coagulopathy because of acquired deficiencies of multiple coagulation factors in whom serious bleeding has occurred or for whom emergency surgery or other procedures are planned, (*ii*) for treatment of thrombotic thrombocytopenic purpura (TTP), and (*iii*) for treatment of acquired single factor deficiencies where a product containing the single factor is unavailable or ineffective (55).

An NIH consensus conference concluded that FFP was indicated for documented coagulation protein deficiencies, for selected patients with massive transfusion as well as patients with multiple coagulation defects (e.g., liver disease) in conjunction with therapeutic plasma exchange for TTP, for infants with protein losing enteropathy, and for selected patients with other immunodeficiencies. FFP use in other situations was discouraged (56). They noted that there was little scientific evidence to support the increasing clinical use of FFP.

The Canadian Committee stated that use of FFP as a volume expander or for wound healing was contraindicated (55). The British Committee for Standards in Haematology noted that four units of FFP will usually promote coagulation in adults (41). The ASA task force recommended FFP for correction of microvascular bleeding secondary to coagulation factor deficiency in patients transfused with more than one blood volume or for correction of bleeding in the presence of elevated (>1.5 times normal)

prothrombintime (PT) or partial thromboplastin time (PTT) (12). The dose should be that to achieve a minimum of 30% of plasma factor concentration (usually achieved with administration of 10 to 15 mL/kg FFP). The ASA Task Force notes that four to five platelet concentrates, one unit of single-donor apheresis platelets, or one unit of whole blood provide a quantity of coagulation factors similar to that found in one unit FFP (12).

In contrast, during elective surgical conditions where normovolemia and normal core temperature are maintained, FFP transfusions are seldom required. However, during rapid or massive blood loss conditions associated with trauma, more liberal use of FFP is warranted. Indeed, once one blood volume has been replaced, consideration should be given to administering PRBCs and FFP together in a 1:1 ratio (57).

> ⚡ **An FFP dose of 10 to 15 mL/kg will usually increase plasma coagulation factor concentration by 30% (the minimum level required for hemostasis for most of the coagulation factors).** ⚡

Cryoprecipitate

In 1997, 816,000 units of cryoprecipitate were transfused (58). Cryoprecipitate contains factor VIII, fibrinogen, fibronectin, Von Willebrand factor, and factor XIII, and is used for correction of inherited and acquired coagulopathies. One unit of cryoprecipitate per 10 kg body weight raises the fibrinogen concentration by approximately 50 mg/dL. The Canadian Committee recommended cryoprecipitate transfusion in bleeding patients with hypofibrinogenemia, Von Willebrand disease, and patients with hemophilia A (when factors VIII concentrate is not available) (55). The British Committee recommends that cryoprecipitate should also be given to massively transfused patients when fibrinogen is less than 80 mg/dL.

The ASA Task Force had three recommendations about cryoprecipitate: (*i*) prophylaxis in nonbleeding perioperative or peripartum patients with congenital fibrinogen deficiencies, or Von Willenbrand disease unresponsive to desmopressin—in consultation with a hematologist; (*ii*) bleeding patients with Von Willebrand disease; and (*iii*) correction of microvascular bleeding in massively transfused patients with fibrinogen concentrations less than 80 to 100 mg/dL or when fibrinogen concentrations cannot be measured in a timely fashion (12). After the loss of 1.5 blood volumes, in massively bleeding patients, cryoprecipitate (10–12 cryoprecipitate packs) should be administered after every 10 to 15 units of PRBCs and FFP to maintain fibrinogen levels.

> ⚡ **One unit cryoprecipitate per 10 kg body weight increases fibrinogen 50 mg/dL in stable patients, and is indicated for massively bleeding or transfused patients with fibrinogen below 80 to 100 mg/dL.** ⚡

Recombinant Factor VIIa

Recombinant factor VIIa (rFVIIa) induces coagulation at the sites of vascular injury where it reacts with exposed tissue factor to induce platelet activation and allow the platelet plug to form and reduce bleeding (59). Initially it was used to treat hemophiliac patients with inhibitors to factor VIII. A potential adverse effect is promotion of thrombosis (60). In a prospective, randomized trial in prostatectomy patients, rFVIIa was shown to decrease blood loss (61).

The use of rFVIIa in trauma patients is usually restricted to situations in which conventional means of hemorrhage control, including surgery and angiographic embolization, have failed. The appropriate dose and time of administration remains uncertain. Early experience was reported by Dutton et al. (62), where its use was generally found to be beneficial. A subsequent report by this group wherein 81 patients were treated with rFVIIa showed that 61 (75%) had sustained improvements in their coagulation status and 20 had persistent coagulaopathy ("nonresponders") (63). The nonresponders were significantly more acidotic and had lower platelet counts than the responders (63).

In a recent multicenter randomized trial, rFVIIa was found to significantly decrease RBC transfusion in both blunt ($p = 0.03$) and penetrating trauma ($p = 0.08$) (64). The incidence of adverse events did not significantly increase in the study population, but then mortality did not significantly improve either (64). In summary, rFVIIa is effective in achieving hemostasis in a large number of trauma patients, but additional studies are required to clarify target population, dosing, efficacy, and safety (65).

EMERGENCY AND MASSIVE TRANSFUSION
Emergency Transfusion
In a trauma setting, several administrative decisions should be made jointly by the clinicians and the blood bank regarding policy and procedures for emergency compatibility testing (ABO and Rh typing, antibody screening, and cross-matching). In decreasing order of preference, options include: type-specific, partially cross-matched blood; type-specific uncross-matched blood; and, lastly, type O Rh-negative ("universal donor"), uncross-matched blood (66,67).

Partially cross-matched blood includes ABO–Rh typing and an "immediate-spin" cross-match that takes one to five minutes and eliminates serious hemolytic reactions due to errors in ABO typing. Type-specific uncross-matched blood requires a blood sample from the patient to determine ABO and Rh type. This blood will be released by the blood bank if the physician indicates the emergency need for blood. Meanwhile, compatibility testing is completed while the blood is being transfused. An advantage of type-specific blood is that it saves type O/Rh-negative blood. As many as 1 in 1000 patients have antibodies detected on cross-match that may make transfusion of ABO–Rh type specific uncross-matched blood hazardous; previous exposure to RBC antigens increases this risk tenfold (66,67).

Universal donor (type O) blood, which lacks both A and B antigens, avoids risk of ABO-mediated hemolysis in a blood group A, B, or AB recipient who has the antithetical anti-B or anti-A (or both) alloantibodies. In many trauma centers, O-negative blood is available in the trauma patient resuscitation area, which can be transfused emergently once a sample of patient blood is withdrawn for transfusion investigations. This patient blood sample is essential for subsequent units to be type-specific, and to determine if significant red cell alloantibodies are present (68). After administration of uncross-matched universal donor blood, the decision to transfuse the patient's corresponding ABO/Rh blood type is made when the blood bank determines that passively transfused anti-A and/or anti-B antibodies have fallen to levels low enough to permit the safe transfusion of type-specific blood. At the Shock Trauma Center in Baltimore in 2000, 161 of 501 patients who received blood products were given at least one unit of uncross-matched group O, including 52 of the 80 blood transfused patients

who died within the first 24 hours after admission. The maximum number of uncross-matched units administered to any one patient was 14, and a total of 581 units were given to the 161 patients. These 581 units represented 11% of all PRBCs administered at the Shock Trauma Center and 18% of those given in the first 24 hours to those patients who had a mortality of 45% (69).

Massive Transfusion
Massive transfusion is defined as replacement of a patient's blood volume within 24 hours, for example, about 5000 mL blood or 3000 mL (10 units) of PRBCs in an average-size adult (70,71). Trauma accounts for at least one-third of massive transfusion situations (70,71). In the United States, 10% to 15% of all PRBCs transfused are used to treat injured patients. Massive transfusion protocols in trauma centers support the transfusion service and their activation identifies a need for better hemorrhage control modalities. These massive transfusion protocols include use of additional personnel and provide rapid infusion system technicians to enable administration of large quantities of warmed blood. Massive transfusion protocols ensure that cross-matching policies are streamlined, automated thawing of FFP is initiated, and platelets become readily available (66,67).

Massive Transfusion Protocols
Massive transfusion protocols should be invoked judiciously, as it may limit blood transfusion services to other patients in need. A massive transfusion protocol used by the UCSD trauma center mobilizes 45 units of blood (66). The initial four units may be O Rh negative. Following this, type-specific blood will be used to the extent possible, with the decision to use compatible but nontype-specific blood (e.g., O for type B recipient; A or O for type AB recipient) made by the blood bank. Due to limited supplies of Rh-negative blood, it may be necessary to use Rh-positive blood in an Rh-negative individual, especially in males or post-menopausal females, for whom implications of Rh-sensitization is less of a concern. To prevent confusion, a single individual on the trauma team should be designated to communicate with the blood bank. Following the immediate resuscitation period, standard procedures for blood ordering should be followed (66).

Hemostasis and Component Therapy During Massive Transfusion
Hemostatic defects are often related to dilution and consumption of platelets and coagulation factors. In the absence of trauma, disseminated intravascular coagulation (DIC), or pre-existing coagulopathy, patients who bleed up to 1.5 blood volumes (in a 70 kg male approximately 15 units of PRBC and 3–5 L crystalloid) generally do not have clinically relevant hemostatic defects. Consequently, prophylactic transfusion of platelets, FFP, or cryoprecipitate should not be given to patients simply because they have received 10 to 15 units of PRBC (67).

However, the presence of a pre-existing coagulopathy, acute trauma with extensive tissue damage, or DIC increases the likelihood that hemostatic support will be required (72). Trauma patients whose blood loss is >1.5 blood volume should be carefully monitored for clinical signs of microvascular bleeding (i.e., oozing from IV sites or wounds), as well as by laboratory monitoring. When the coagulation assays are abnormal (PT >17 seconds, PTT >55 seconds; fibrinogen <150 mg/dL, platelets <75 × 10^9/L), empirical use of FFP in a 1:1 ratio of FFP to PRBCs in the setting of ongoing massive bleeding (57). Platelets contain associated plasma factors equivalent to one to two units of FFP for each plateletpheresis bag.

Following initial therapy, it is important to evaluate clinical and laboratory parameters for response. There is no universal formula to guide hemostatic replacement therapy. However, in patients who bleed in excess of two blood volumes (>20 units of PRBC), it is prudent to transfuse sufficient platelets to keep the platelet count $>75 \times 10^9$/L, and sufficient FFP to maintain fibrinogen >150 mg/dL, and/or the PT <18 seconds; PTT <55 seconds.

It is usually not necessary to give cryoprecipitate unless there is a disproportionate decrease in fibrinogen or factor VIII, for example, in the setting of DIC, because a unit of FFP supplies about twice as much fibrinogen and factor VIII as a unit of cryoprecipitate. The most common error in the management of massively bleeding patients is to apply outdated, rote formulae without monitoring Hct, platelet, and coagulation factor levels. This results in inadequate replacement therapy in some, whereas others are treated unnecessarily (66).

COMPLICATIONS OF BLOOD TRANSFUSION

☞ **Inadvertent transfusion of ABO incompatible blood and transfusion-associated acute lung injury (TRALI) are life-threatening, noninfectious hazards of blood transfusion.** ☜

Infections
More than 12 million units of blood are transfused annually in the United States (73,74). In 1999, the risks for acquiring viral infection from a unit of blood were: <1/1,000,000 for HIV, 1:103,000 for hepatitis C, and 1:63,000 for hepatitis B (Fig. 6) (73). The incidence of viral transmission from blood transfusion is decreasing, with current infection rates even lower (73). Indeed, the risk of viral infection from blood is much lower than the risk of a patient being given the wrong unit of blood due to clerical error within the blood bank or in the ward, which occurs at a rate of about 1:37,000, resulting in one fatality per 1.8 million units transfused (75,76).

Noninfectious Hazards of Transfusion
Besides inadvertent transfusion of ABO-incompatible blood, hemovigilance programs in the United Kingdom, France, and the United States demonstrate that patients suffer other significant noninfectious transfusion-related morbidity and mortality (77), an issue that has gained increasing attention, given the dramatic reduction in viral transmission from blood (e.g., 10,000-fold reduced risk of HIV and hepatitis over the past few decades) (76).

Current data probably underestimate noninfectious transfusion risk. Febrile nonhemolytic transfusion reactions are common, occurring in up to 10% to 30% of transfusions, especially with nonleukoreduced platelet transfusions (78).

A prospective study of transfusions identified substantial underreporting of bedside transfusion errors in Belgium with a rate of unintended recipients of RBCs being one in 400 units (79). This Belgian study concluded that current passive reporting systems underestimate the true frequency of hazard from blood transfusion by 30-fold. Even fatal transfusion mishaps are significantly underreported. In a study of 355 transfusion-associated deaths from 1976–1985, no fatalities were reported to the

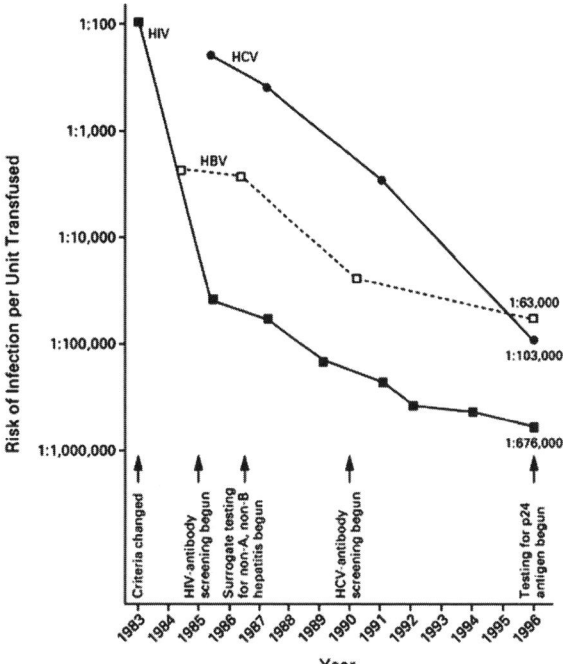

Figure 6 The risks of transfusion-related transmission of human immunodeficiency virus (HIV), hepatitis B virus (HBV), and hepatitis C virus (HCV) in the United States. Each unit represents exposure to one donor. The risk of each of these infections has declined dramatically since 1983, the year the criteria for donor screening were changed; at that time the prevalence of HIV infection among donors was approximately 1%. Further declines have resulted from the implementation of testing of donor blood for antibodies to HIV beginning in 1985; surrogate testing for non-A, non-B hepatitis beginning in 1986–1987; testing for antibodies to HCV beginning in 1990; and testing for HIV p24 antigen beginning in late 1995. *Source*: From Ref. 74.

FDA (80). Yet, the FDA-reported transfusion-related death rate due to hemolytic reactions alone was two times that due to all infectious hazards combined (81).

Circulatory overload is a significant problem in trauma, and may be associated with red cell transfusion. A seven-year retrospective study at a single institution found the incidence to be 1:3168 patients (82). In another study, 1% of orthopedic surgery patients developed circulatory overload, sometimes necessitating transfer to an intensive care unit (83). Extrapolating these data nationally, it has been estimated that 30,000 to 40,000 patients annually might have circulatory overload as an avoidable complication of transfusion (82,83). When two groups of critical care unit patients were randomized to a liberal or restrictive use of blood, the patients randomly assigned to a more liberal strategy had a significantly higher incidence of cardiac and pulmonary morbidity (8).

☞ **Noninfectious transfusion risk exceeds infectious hazard by 100- to 1000-fold.** ☜

Transfusion-Related Acute Lung Injury
TRALI is defined as acute post-transfusion noncardiogenic pulmonary edema, and is characterized by severe bilateral patchy pulmonary alveolar infiltrates, hypoxia, tachycardia, and fever. It clinically resembles adult respiratory distress syndrome (ARDS). TRALI occurs one to six hours after transfusion of blood products, especially FFP. TRALI often

requires mechanical ventilation, and may be fatal. It was the third most common cause reported of transfusion-related mortality (84,85). In the FDA reports, 31 cases (9%) were attributed to acute pulmonary dynfunction (85). In another study, 46 of 2430 platelet transfusions (2%) were associated with severe respiratory reaction over a two-year period (86). The FFP donated by women with a history of ≥ 3 pregnancies resulted in a significantly lower oxygen extraction ratio, and in four out of 100 patients an acute pulmonary transfusion reaction was noted, suggesting an immunological etiology (antigranulocyte alloantibodies) (also see Volume 2, Chapter 52) (87).

The development of ARDS following transfusion in trauma patients has recently been prospectively reviewed (88). The amount of transfused blood in these patients was independently associated with both the development of ARDS and hospital mortality. ARDS developed in 21% of severe trauma patients who received zero to five units of PRBCs, in 31% of those who received 6 to 10 units, and in 57% of those who received >10 units ($p = 0.007$) (88). The association between the amount of transfused blood and the development of ARDS remained significant even after accounting for differences in the severity of illness, type of trauma, race, gender, and base deficit ($p = 0.002$; odds ratio, 14.4; 95% confidence interval, 3.2–78.7). Patients who received more units of PRBCs during the first 24 hours also had a higher hospital mortality rate ($p = 0.03$) (88).

Graft vs. Host Disease

Over 200 cases of transfusion-associated GVHD have been reported, with a fatality rate of about 90% (89). In contrast to TRALI, where the etiology appears to involve passively-acquired antigranulocyte alloantibodies and possibly other toxins, GVHD is related to transfusion of live white blood cells that become engrafted within the recipient. In a recent prospective study by Utter et al. (90), 53% (24 of 45) trauma patients who received >2 units of PRBCs developed evidence of microchimerism when studied using polymerase chain reaction technology. However, clinically-evident GVHD is one of the rarest of transfusion reactions. Irradiating cellular blood components will prevent this problem, but irradiation has detrimental effects on erythrocytes and there is no current standard for irradiation dosing.

    ✄ **Transfusion-associated GVHD has high mortality (>90%), but is extremely rare; irradiating blood components can prevent this complication, but is not practical in the acute trauma setting.** ✄

Exchange Transfusion

In neonates, exchange transfusion increases existing metabolic derangements and causes hypoglycemia (91). Among pediatric recipients of massive transfusion, hyperkalemia and hypocalcemia are more common, and when untreated may cause cardiac arrest. Among 140 exchange transfusions that included 106 neonates, more than 34% of the infants had documented hypoglycemia, 1/20 had ECG changes related to hypocalcemia, and one had a cardiac arrest. In 25 ill neonates, 12% had severe complications (including two deaths) attributed to transfusion (92).

Undertransfusion

Undertransfusion indicates risk for morbidity and mortality associated with a lack of transfusion when Hb concentration was less than 6 g/dL. This issue is complex, because, in one

study, mortality was even lower in patients transfused when Hb was <7.0 g/dL compared to <10 g/dL (93).

However, evidence for risk of undertransfusion was seen in one study of 190 patients undergoing radical prostatectomy in which myocardial ischemic episodes occurred in 61 (34%) of 181 evaluable patients (94). After adjustments for other risk factors, the authors concluded that a Hct <28% was independently associated with a risk for myocardial ischemia during and after noncardiac surgery.

In cardiac bypass patients randomly assigned to receive either blood and colloid or crystalloid fluids, the patients given crystalloids had delayed myocardial lactate extraction compared to the patients receiving blood, indicating that anemia had a potentially deleterious effect on the heart (95).

In peripheral vascular surgery, among 13 of 27 patients with a Hct <28%, 10 patients had myocardial ischemia and six sustained a morbid cardiac event, and there was an overall incidence of 37% cardiac ischemia (96). A Hct of <28% was significantly associated with myocardial ischemia and morbid cardiac events.

    ✄ **Blood transfusion does not reduce mortality in stable critically ill patients with Hb 8 to 10 g/dL, except for a subset with coronary artery disease.** ✄

Inappropriate Transfusion

Transfusion of blood products has come under increased scrutiny because of concerns over safety, product shortages, rising costs of specialized blood components, and questions about transfusion efficacy. The usefulness of behavioral interventions to reduce inappropriate transfusion was reviewed by Wilson et al. (97). They identified nine studies describing different types of interventions: prospective audit ($n = 2$), education ($n = 4$), transfusion algorithm ($n = 1$), retrospective audit ($n = 1$), and patient-specific decision support ($n = 1$). Using Hct levels >36% as an indicator for overtransfusion, all studies showed an impact of the intervention on reducing inappropriate transfusion.

Compared to 1994, the gross domestic blood supply in the United States, in 1997 (12,602,000 units) decreased by 5.5% (97). The 1997 collection included 11,741,000 units allogeneic community blood, 643,000 units autologous blood (5.5% of total), and 205,000 units of allogeneic-directed donation. The rate of whole blood collections in 1997 per 1000 members of the population aged 18 to 65 years was 12.6% lower than 1994. However, the red-cell transfusion rate per 1000 members of the population in 1997 remained nearly unchanged, raising concerns about progressive supply shortfalls (97).

    ✄ **Blood collection in 1997 fell 12.6%, but the rate of transfusion remained the same as in 1994.** ✄

Blood Storage Abnormalities

Progressive deterioration in blood quality occurs upon storage and may impair flow through the microcirculation and decrease cellular $\dot{D}O_2$. Increased splanchnic ischemia occurs following transfusion with old blood in patients with ischemia (98). In septic rats, old blood failed to increase $\dot{V}O_2$, whereas fresh blood caused $\dot{V}O_2$ to increase (99). Storing blood decreases 2,3-DPG concentration, reducing the deformability of the red cell and increasing aggregation, thereby decreasing flow through the microcirculation and impairing cellular $\dot{D}O_2$ (100).

Immunosuppression

Transfusion-induced immunosuppression is increasingly being recognized as an important adverse effect of blood. Decreased cell-mediated immunity occurs by reducing nonkiller cell activity, suppressing macrophage antigen presentation, altering T-cell ratios, and decreasing the concentrations of cytokines (TNF, IFN-8, and GM-CSF) vital to the immune response (101). There is evidence linking this immunosuppression to white cells within the transfused blood. Transfusion of leukodepleted blood to patients undergoing colorectal surgery resulted in a lower incidence of postoperative infection (102). There is a significant association between the number of blood transfusions and the risk of subsequent infection in burn patients and a variety of elective and significant emergency procedures. This increased morbidity is associated with longer hospital stays and higher costs. In addition, patients with malignancy may have sooner recurrences and lower survival rates when they receive blood transfusion (105).

TOLERANCE FOR ACUTE ANEMIA

Compensatory Mechanisms

There are three main mechanisms by which global $\dot{D}O_2$ is maintained during acute, progressive anemia: (*i*) increased O_2 extraction, (*ii*) reduction in O_2 affinity with shift of the oxy-hemoglobin disassociation curve to the right due to increased 2,3-DPG (Fig. 7), and (*iii*) increased cardiac output. A fourth mechanism is the use of 100% O_2 to increase the amount of oxygen carried in the plasma. In hemodiluted children undergoing orthopedic surgery, 37% of the oxygen delivered came from the plasma (106). In fact, at a Hb of 3 dg/dL and normal cardiac output, 62% of the actual $\dot{V}O_2$ can be provided by O_2 dissolved in the plasma. In addition, extraction of O_2 from plasma is much more efficient than from Hb exceeding 85% removal (Table 1). As with the acellular hemoglobin-based O_2 carrying solutions, the presence of larger quantities of O_2 in solution facilitates the diffusion of O_2 into the mitochondria by minimizing the O_2 gradient between Hb in the red cell and tissues (106,107). So, high

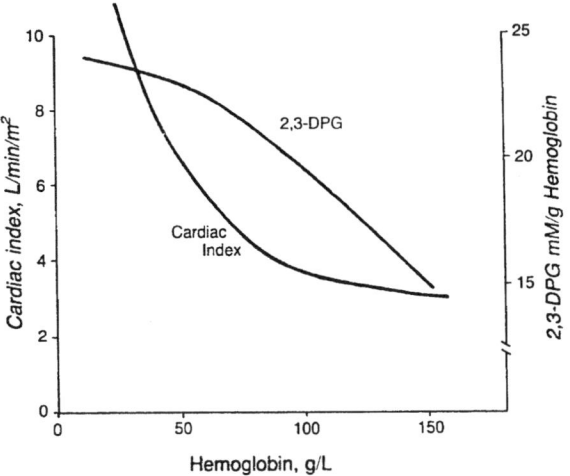

Figure 7 Shows the relationship between cardiac index, hemoglobin levels, and 2,3-dipophoglycerate (2,3-DPG). At a hemoglobin level of 8 to 9 g/dL cardiac index remains low, while 2,3-DPG levels are greater than 18 mM/g hemoglobin. *Source*: From Ref. 121.

FiO_2 in excess of 80% should be used when Hb is low. There is value in small quantities of added nitrogen, such as are found in air, to minimize the microatelectasis that occurs with 100% inspired O_2 caused by the resulting alveolar nitrogen washout with 100% O_2. Thus, 100% O_2 should not be used unless the Hb concentration is below about 5 g/dL (108).

Human Data on Anemia Tolerance (Jehovah's Witnesses)

Jehovah's Witness patients comprise a group of patients in whom effects of extremely low Hb levels can be observed. Since blood transfusions are not permitted, treatment approaches include deep sedation, mechanical ventilation, and avoiding unnecessary blood sampling. Although erythropoietin is often given, reticulocyte counts begin to improve only after two to three weeks. There is a reported 20% mortality rate associated with a Hb concentration of 5 g/dL. However, there are a few reports of Jehovah's Witnesses surviving with a Hb concentration near 3 g/dL, but most patients with a Hb concentration of 3 g/dL die (109).

In some settings, very low Hb levels occur because of a lack of available blood or refusal to receive blood. In one report, pregnant women in West Africa with Hb values greater than 4.5 g/dL had no mortality or cardiac failure (110). In another study in Romania, there was no postoperative mortality in 72 patients with Hb levels above 5 g/dL (111). In one of two studies in the Unites States, 48 pediatric patients undergoing cardiac surgery had no mortality despite blood being withheld, provided Hb was greater than 7 g/dL (Table 2). In the other U.S. study, 59 patients successfully underwent surgery after refusing transfusion, with no postoperative mortality when the blood loss was less than 500 mL and Hb greater than 8 g/dL (112,113).

Critical Oxygen Delivery in Hemodiluted Animals

In animals that were hemodiluted and monitored at intervals, as Hb decreased from 14 to 10, 8, 5, and then 2.4 g/dL, it was only at a Hb of 2.4 g/dL that a significant difference in brain pH and pCO2 was detected compared with baseline. At the 2.4 g/dL Hb level, there was also a significant decrease in mean arterial pressure and increase in central venous pressure (Table 3). Brain O_2 consumption (cerebral oxygen metabolism) was also significantly lower and cerebral blood flow significantly higher than baseline. Both were restored to normal baseline ranges by transfusion.

Critical Hct values for intestinal O_2 consumption were measured by Van Bommel et al. and compared with the critical values for intestinal microvascular O_2 (uPO2). The critical values were almost identical at 15.8 ± 4.6 and 16.0 ± 3.5 uPO2 respectively. These Hcts represent a Hb value just above 5 g/dL (Fig. 8) (106).

Critical Oxygen Delivery in Anesthetized Humans

At the Children's National Medical Center, eight ASA I children undergoing scoliosis correction surgery were hemodiluted by exchanging whole blood for 5% albumin in 0.7% saline. On 100% O_2 ventilation, Hb fell from 10 to 3 g/dL, while mixed venous O_2 saturation decreased from 90% to 72%, and O_2 extraction increased from 17% to 44%, and $\dot{D}O_2$ decreased from 532 mL/min/M² (Fig. 9). When hemodiluted, one child had Hb fall to 2.1 g/dL and this was associated with ST segment depression, which resolved on re-infusion of autologous blood. The authors concluded

Table 1 Hemoglobin, Hematocrit, and Acid–Base Status During Hemodilution and Reinfusion

Variable (range)	T_0	T_1	T_2
Hct (%)	29.5 ± 4.8 $(20.3–36.1)$	9.0 ± 2.2^a $(6.3–13.3)$	16.7 ± 3.1^a $(12.2–21.6)$
Hgb (g/dL)	10.0 ± 1.6 $(7.0–12.4)$	3.0 ± 0.8^a $(2.1–4.5)$	5.6 ± 1.0^a $(4.1–7.1)$
Lactate (mmol/L)	1.3 ± 0.2 $(1.0–1.5)$	1.4 ± 0.5 $(0.9–1.95)$	1.5 ± 0.5 $(1.0–2.2)$
Arterial pH	7.42 ± 0.05 $(7.33–7.50)$	7.33 ± 0.08^a $(7.25–7.49)$	7.37 ± 0.06 $(7.26–7.45)$
Venous pH	7.39 ± 0.05 $(7.34–7.46)$	7.28 ± 0.07^a $(7.22–7.42)$	7.33 ± 0.06 $(7.22–7.42)$
P_aCO_2	34.1 ± 6.5 $(25.1–46.1)$	37.9 ± 3.4 $(32.1–42.7)$	39.2 ± 4.1 $(33.6–45.0)$
P_vCO_2	38.3 ± 4.0 $(32.5–43.3)$	43.4 ± 2.5^a $(39.3–45.9)$	44.8 ± 4.3 $(39.2–50.8)$
ABE (mmol/L)	-1.1 ± 2.3 $(-6.1–0.6)$	-50 ± 3.6^a $(-8.4–2.4)$	-1.8 ± 2.5 $(-5.4–2.1)$
VBE (mmol/L)	-0.6 ± 1.1 $(-2.5–1.0)$	-6.0 ± 3.5^a $(-8.9–1.4)$	-2.3 ± 2.5^a $(-5.5–2.1)$

Note: [a]Significant difference ($p < 0.05$) from the mean value at the previous stage.
Abbreviations: ABE, arterial base excess; Hb, hemoglobin; Hct, hematocrit; P_aCO_2, arterial partial pressure of carbon dioxide; P_vCO_2, mixed venous partial pressure of carbon dioxide; T_0, immediately prior to hemodilution; T_1, the lowest hemoglobin level reached; T_2, end of surgery; VBE, mixed venous base excess.
Source: From Ref. 106.

that Hb of 3 g/dL was safe in anesthetized and monitored children, and that one should not hemodilute below a mixed venous saturation of 60% as levels above this have never been shown to produce lactic acidosis or compromise cardiac function (114). The "critical point" of global $\dot{D}O_2$ below which $\dot{V}O_2$ becomes linearly dependent on $\dot{D}O_2$ in anesthetized humans is estimated at 330 mL/min/m^2 by Shibutani (115), as 300 mL/min/m^2 by Komatsu et al. (116), while Van Woerkens (117) found that critical $\dot{D}O_2$ was lower in hemodilution when cardiac output was maintained. Rheological changes in blood were impaired with hemodilution and increased capillary O_2 delivery and a critical value of 184 mL/min/m^2 was obtained in a patient with a Hb of 4 g/dL (Table 4). However, these studies were carried out either in anesthetized humans or when cardiac output was maintained. Such states are not representative of recently injured patients who may be hypovolemic and have significant catecholamine and other stress responses activated. Whether the existence of critical $\dot{D}O_2$ states can be identified in such trauma patients also remains controversial. Recently, a study in animals showed that multivariable analysis of critical delivery may help determine the physiological oxygenation boundary at the whole body level (118). This may assist in finding therapeutic triggers on an individual basis using systemic markers of the transition from aerobic to anaerobic metabolism (118).

Relationship Between Oxygen Delivery and Consumption

Some patients may benefit from the increased $\dot{D}O_2$ that is expected to occur after blood transfusion. The anticipated, concomitant increase in O_2 consumption has only been shown in a limited number of studies, possibly in part due to the frequency of such studies being carried out in septic patients rather than in impaired $\dot{D}O_2$ settings such as hemorrhagic shock. Surrogate markers to quantitate benefit from blood transfusion have been suggested, including lactate washout and decrease in O_2 debt, but confounding variables occur because when blood is infused reperfusion occurs and lactate rises (119,120). States with impaired O_2 extraction (e.g., sepsis) limit the usefulness of such surrogate measures. The relationship of transfusion for anemia or ischemia with oxygen metabolism is shown in Figure 10. Factors alleviating ischemia include increased O_2 supply (and by inference, but not always true, reduced O_2 debt) and decreased O_2 demand, such as can occur with sedation, anesthesia, and decreased cardiac afterload (11). Increased afterload, increased blood viscosity, and decreased 2,3-DPG levels in stored blood will aggravate ischemia. Hemoglobin levels per se are nonlinearly related to cardiac index and 2,3-DPG with lowest cardiac index associated with greatest 2,3-DPG levels occurring about 8 g/dL (Fig. 7) (121). Because data on O_2 extraction are difficult to obtain in humans in emergency circumstances, much of this work has been done on animals. There are

Table 2 Natural History of Untreated Anemia

Study (reference)	Year	Patients, n	Site	Setting	Finding
Fullerton and Turner (59)	1969	Unknown	West Africa	Pregnant woman; no available transfusions	No mortality or cardiac failure in patients with hemoglobin >4.5 g/L
Gollub and Bailey (61)	1966	5	New York City	Jehovah's Witness patients undergoing cardiac surgery	No postoperative mortality in patients with hemoglobin >7.0 g/L
Alexiu et al. (62)	1975	72	Romania	Patients with bleeding ulcers undergoing surgery without transfusion	No postoperative mortality in patients with hemoglobin >5.0 g/L
Kawaguchi et al. (64)	1984	44	Buffalo	Pediatric patients undergoing cardiac surgery	No mortality in patients for whom blood was withheld for hemoglobin >7.0 g/L
Carson et al. (60)	1988	59	New Jersey	Patients undergoing surgery who refused transfusion	No postoperative mortality in patients with blood loss <500 mL and hemoglobin >8.0 gL

Table 3 Physiological Variables at Baseline and During Anemia

	Baseline	D1	D2	D3	D4	I1
Hemoglobin (g/dL)	14.2 ± 0.7	10.4 ± 0.6[a]	7.7 ± 0.6[a]	5.0 ± 0.5[a]	2.4 ± 0.3[a]	5.7 ± 0.3[a]
pH	7.34 ± 0.02	7.31 ± 0.01	7.28 ± 0.01	7.27 ± 0.01	7.25 ± 0.02[a]	7.26 ± 0.02
P_aCO_2 (mm Hg)	36.0 ± 0.3	36.1 ± 0.4	36.5 ± 0.4	38.3 ± 0.3	37.8 ± 0.6[a]	36.7 ± 0.5
P_aO_2 (mm Hg)	89 ± 2	88 ± 2	88 ± 3	86 ± 4	94 ± 6	88 ± 3
Temp (Brain) (°C)	37.6 ± 0.4	37.6 ± 0.4	37.6 ± 0.5	37.7 ± 0.4	37.6 ± 0.05	37.8 ± 0.5
MAP (mm Hg)	81 ± 3	77 ± 3	74 ± 3	70 ± 2	63 ± 1[a]	68 ± 2
CVP (mm Hg)	6 ± 0	6 ± 1	6 ± 0	7 ± 1	9 ± 1[a]	9 ± 1

Note: Values are mean ± SEM; D1–D4, hemodilution; I1–I3, red blood cell infusion. Physiological variables measured in anesthetized rabbits during progressive hemodilution from baseline of Hb 14.2 g/dL to the nadir of 2.4 g/dL at time point D_4 before infusion of red cells at I1. Brain tissue pO_2 fell from 27 to 12 mmHg and brain pH decreased from 7.22 to 7.12 (Fig. 11 for cerebral blood flow changes).
[a]Significant difference versus baseline ($p < 0.025$); $n = 12$.
Abbreviations: CVP, central venous pressure; MAP, mean arterial pressure; P_aCO_2, arterial carbon dioxide tension; P_aO_2, arterial oxygen tension.
Source: From Ref. 131.

extraordinary compensatory abilities in the hemorrhagic shock model. O_2 extraction increased to more than 70% in anesthetized dogs exsanguinated of more than 60% of their estimated blood volume during a two hour period when systolic blood pressure was maintained at 50 mmHg (122). Resuscitation with volumes of shed blood or Hb-based O_2 carrying solutions produced supranormal cardiac index with all these fluids, but only blood normalized O_2 extraction and cardiac index six hours later. Total Hb concentration fell with the O_2 carrying solutions due to endothelial and other interactions causing red cell sequestration.

Anemia and the Brain

The other major organ besides the heart, at risk during anemia, is the brain. In a study in rabbits, Morimoto et al. (123) continuously monitored brain tissue pH PCO_2 and PO_2 during production of anemia (Table 3). They found that as Hb progressively fell from 10 to 7, to 5, and then to a mean low of 2.4 g/dL, brain tissue PO_2 fell from 27 to 12 mmHg, pH decreased from 7.22 to 7.12, cerebral blood flow almost doubled to 66 mL/100 g/min, and cerebral metabolic rate more than halved to under 2 mL/100 g/min. At this level of anemia (2.4 g/dL), the authors concluded that increases in cerebral blood flow and cerebral O_2 extraction were only partially able to compensate for the decreased O_2 carrying capacity (Fig. 11). Postoperative visual loss has been associated with many factors including anemia, blood loss, and hypotension (124,125).

Anemia in Trauma and Critically Ill Patients

In bleeding but otherwise healthy trauma patients, cardiovascular compensation should be adequate for Hb levels as low as 5 g/dL. As blood loss continues and Hb falls further, compensatory responses begin to fail (126,127). Mortality rates range from 50% to 95% when the Hb falls below 3.5 g/dL (126,128). Anemia is a common problem in critically ill patients. In part, anemia can be explained by an average of 41 ± 39.7 mL blood samples drawn per 24 hours. In a major European study involving 3534 patients, there was a positive correlation between organ dysfunction and the number of blood draws and volume drawn. The mean Hb on critical care unit admission was 11.3 ± 2.3 g/dL with 29% (963/3295) having a Hb <10 g/dL. The transfusion rate was 37% (1307/3534). Older patients and those with longer critical care unit stay were more commonly transfused. Both critical care unit and overall mortality rates were significantly higher in patients who received a transfusion (critical care unit rates 18.5% vs. 10.1%; overall mortality 29% vs. 14.9%). For similar degrees of organ dysfunction, patients who had a transfusion also had a higher mortality rate. For matched patients, the 28-day mortality was 22.7% among patients receiving blood transfusions and 17.1% among those without ($p = 0.02$) (129).

☞ **In bleeding, otherwise healthy trauma patients, cardiovascular compensation may be adequate to a Hb as low as 5 g/dL. However, any further compensation is inadequate with mortality 50% to 95% at Hb <3.5 g/dL.** ☜

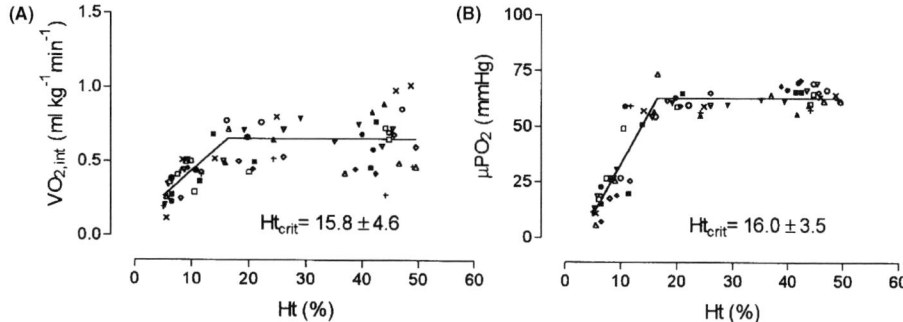

Figure 8 (**A**) Critical hematocrit value for the intestinal oxygen consumption. (**B**) Critical hematocrit value for the intestinal microvascular oxygen partial pressure. Critical values were determined in each animal separately and are represented here as mean ± SD. Data originating from the same animal are represented by a similar symbol. *Abbreviations*: μPO$_2$, intestinal microvascular oxygen partial pressure; Ht$_{crit}$, critical hematocrit value; VO$_{2,int}$, intestinal oxygen consumption. *Source*: From Ref. 106.

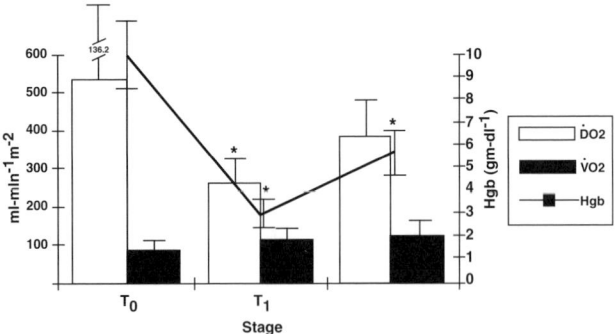

Figure 9 Relationship between oxygen delivery, oxygen consumption, and hemoglobin concentration (Hgb) during the stages prior to hemodilution (T_o), the lowest Hgb reached (T_1), and at the end of surgery (T_2). Values are mean $\pm$ SD. * represents significant difference ($P < 0.05$) from the mean value at the previous stage. *Abbreviations*: $\dot{D}O_2$, oxygen delivery; Hgb, hemoglobin concentration; $\dot{V}O_2$, oxygen consumption. *Source*: From Ref. 114.

Risk of Mortality with Anemia

In a study of 2738 sequential isolated coronary artery bypass surgery patients, there was a significantly increased risk of mortality for Hct <14%. For high risk patients, Hct <17% had increased mortality after adjusting for other risk factors (130). A meta-analysis of several studies of Jehovah's Witnesses found that of 50 reported deaths, 23 were primarily due to anemia. Except for three patients who died after cardiac surgery, all other patients died with Hb concentrations <5 g/dL (109).

EYE TO THE FUTURE

Progress is needed not only in the avoidance of complications of blood transfusion, but also in strategies to reduce the need for blood and component therapy. The potential methods of achieving this include: improved

Table 4 Critical Limit Global O_2 Delivery by Various Authors

Study	$\dot{D}O_2$ limit	Comments
Shinbutani et al. (115)	330 mL/min/M^2	In anesthetized man
Komatsu et al. (116)	300 mL/min/M^2	After CPB
Von Woerkens et al. (117)	184 mL/min/M^2	In hemodiluted man

Abbreviation: CPB, cardiopulmonary bypass; $\dot{D}O_2$, oxygen delivery.

methods of hemostasis at the sites of injury; pharmacological and physical means for restricting blood flow to hemorrhage sites; increased tolerance of organs and tissues for hypoxia; and improved fluid and blood flow distribution to conserve function of vital organs, such as the brain and heart. The future of blood and component transfusion includes prolongation of storage of red cells, improved uptake and release of oxygen, and avoidance of allogeneic and other transfusion reactions. On the horizon, ongoing work will reduce ABO incompatibility issues by changing all blood to universal donor group O. Major advances are being made in blood safety and these will continue in the future with special emphasis on problems related to human error and the improved culture of patient safety for blood transfusion. Screening tests for West Nile Virus will be developed and earlier detection of HIV will occur. Hepatitis and other blood borne infections will continue to decline in frequency because of better detection tools and viral inactivation methods.

O_2 carrying solutions will eventually receive FDA approval and may be used as substitutes for the O_2 carrying capacity of blood. Because they are acellular, these solutions may be used like a drug to facilitate O_2 diffusion into the mitochondria for many purposes including ischemia, and trauma resuscitation, and to enhance the effectiveness of radiation therapy. Control of O_2 affinity for these O_2 carrying solutions may enable better tissue oxygenation with hemoglobinopathies such as sickle cell anemia. Endothelial interactions and binding of nitric oxide by free hemoglobin O_2 carrying solutions will be mitigated.

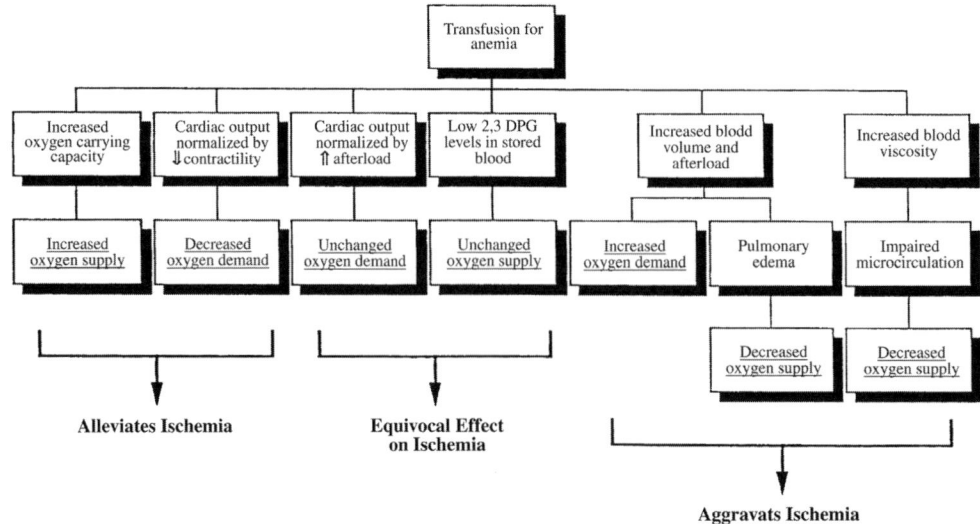

Figure 10 The effects of red cell transfusion for anemia, or the many variables that can impact myocardial oxygen metabolism and the ultimate impact on myocardial ischemia. *Abbreviation*: 2,3-DPG, 2,3-disphosphoglycerate. *Source*: From Ref. 11.

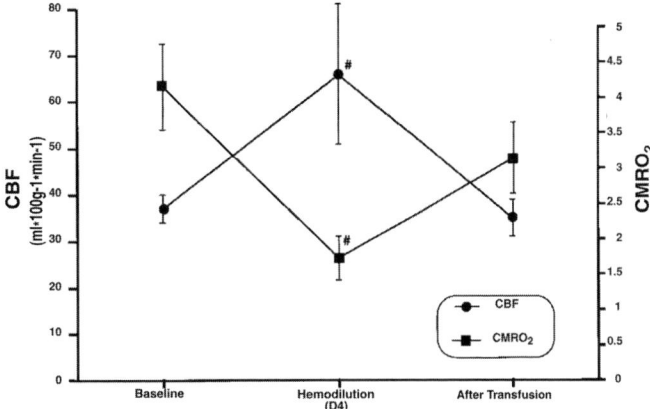

Figure 11 The time course of cerebral blood flow (CBF), cerebral oxygen metabolism (CMRO$_2$), and cerebral oxygen transport (CTO$_2$). Data are expressed as mean $\pm$ SEM. # represents significant difference ($P < 0.05$) versus baseline. Hemodilution = fourth blood draw; after transfusion = third red blood infusion. D$_4$ corresponds to the physiological variables listed under D$_4$ in Table 3. *Source*: From Ref. 123.

The indications for RBCs, platelets, FFP, and cryopreci-pitate transfusions will become more individualized than the current numerical transfusion triggers. Evidence-based practices will minimize overtransfusion and identify a constellation of indications for red cell and component therapy. Monitoring of ischemia and quantification of the results of increased O$_2$ carriage will better indicate the cir-cumstances in which red cell transfusion may be beneficial. The brain and heart, as organs at risk from acute lack of oxygen, will be targets for improved monitoring during trauma patient resuscitation.

SUMMARY

The concept of a single transfusion "trigger" is flawed. Rather, comorbidities should be taken into consideration in erring on the side of Hct >28%. These comorbidities include cardiac risk (unstable angina, myocardial infarction), age >55, and the acuteness of ongoing hemorrhage and expectations for future blood loss. Blood loss in excess of one blood volume in six hours indicates a need to monitor Hb levels frequently. Clinicians should be aware that in 75% of patients receiving 20 units of blood, thrombocytope-nia will occur; FFP may be needed should microvascular bleeding occur, or PT and PTT may need to be prolonged 1.5 times or more. Cryoprecipitate is indicated in trauma patients whose fibrinogen is decreased below 80 to 100 mg/dL with massive transfusion. Transfusion trends in many trauma centers have changed with much less O uni-versal donor uncross-matched blood being administered, as well as less type-specific blood, indicating that clinicians have increased anemia tolerance in this patient population.

Noninfectious hazards of blood transfusion—includ-ing ABO/Rh incompatibility due to human error and TRALI that have become relatively more important compli-cations of blood transfusion than infectious complications—have diminished in frequency (75–78). Errors occur in one out of 37,000 transfusions and cause 1 fatality/1.8 million transfusions (79–81). Generally, these noninfectious compli-cations of transfusion are thought to be under-reported by 30%. It is estimated that circulatory overload may occur in 30,000 to 40,000 patients/yr (77). Base deficit, serum lactate, arterio-venous pH, and pCO$_2$ differences appear to be the

simplest and most practical measures for quantifying the shock state and blood loss in hemorrhaging trauma patients (26). Sublingual pCO$_2$ monitoring may be a useful real-time monitor to assess the progress of resuscitation from shock. Real-time identification of lack of $\dot{D}O_2$ to the brain and heart needs more sophisticated monitors than are currently routinely in use (22). Blood collection of about 12.5 million units in 1997 was 12.6% lower/1000 population than in 1994, yet blood transfusion rates remain the same, raising concerns about progressive supply shortfalls (58). Tolerance for acute anemia is considerable in otherwise healthy indi-viduals. Data from Jehovah's Witness patients indicate that mortality rates are 20% when Hb is around 5 g/dL, increas-ing to 90% to 95% when the Hb falls below 3.5 g/dL. Brain oxygenation becomes critical in normo-volemic animals at 2.4 g/dL (109,126). Hemodiluted anesthetized human chil-dren at Hb of 2.1 g/dL showed evidence of myocardial ische-mia (114). Critical $\dot{D}O_2$ in anesthetized humans and animals varies between 330 mL/min/m^2 and 184 mL/min/m^2 (115–117).

Compensatory mechanisms to anemia include increased O$_2$ extraction (up to 70%), reduced O$_2$ affinity, increased cardiac output, and more O$_2$ dissolved in plasma with supplementary oxygen. Blood transfusion, although increasing O$_2$ carriage, does not necessarily increase tissue $\dot{V}O_2$. Particularly in sepsis, and maybe even in other shock states, O$_2$ extraction does not increase with increased hemo-globin (119–123,127). Red cell transfusion in critically ill patients with no cardiac or cerebrovascular disease, when hemogoblin is 7 g/dL or above, increases mortality and pro-longs hospital stay (128–130). The therapeutic threshold for platelets is 50×10^9/L for most elective surgical settings. For emergency surgery or for acutely traumatized patients with many potential bleeding sites, platelet counts of 100×10^9/L or even higher may indicate the need for platelets when associ-ated with clinically apparent microvascular bleeding. Dilu-tional thrombocytopenia is less common than may be suspected. In 75% of patients receiving more than 20 units of blood, platelet transfusion will be required. The usual platelet dose is one platelet concentrate/10 kg body weight. Thrombo-cytopenia may be prevented in massive transfusion by prosta-glandin E$_1$ infusion. FFP is administered in a dose of 10 to 15 mL/kg for PT and PTT values more than 1.5 times the normal. One single-donor apheresis platelet, four to five platelet concentrates, or one unit of whole blood provides one unit of FFP. Cryoprecipitate is indicated in massively transfused patients with fibrinogen concentrations of below 80 to 100 mg/dL or to correct microvascular bleeding. Factor VIIa appears to have a potential benefit for emergency use, in patients bleeding uncontrollably.

KEY POINTS

- The requirement for blood in military and disaster situations is largely determined by the number of injured that survive long enough to present for care.
- The concept of a single transfusion trigger is flawed. Comorbidities, especially cardiac, age, injury severity, and magnitude of hemorrhage should all be considered.
- One platelet concentrate increases the platelet count by 5 to $10 \times 10^9/L$. In vivo platelet activity is decreased 75% from collected activity. Transfused platelets have a half-life of about two days.
- Single-donor platelets have a lower rate of alloimmunization, transmitted infections, and transfusion reactions.
- Transfusion of greater than 20 units of blood will reduce platelets to less than $50 \times 10^9/L$ in 75% of patients. The decision to transfuse platelets is usually based on evidence of microvascular bleeding or in a patient judged to be at high risk of bleeding, rather than on the level of the platelet count per se.
- In the setting of acute intracranial bleeding, platelet counts greater than $100 \times 10^9/L$ should be maintained.
- An FFP dose of 10 to 15 mL/kg will usually increase plasma coagulation factor concentration by 30% (the minimum level required for hemostasis for most coagulation factors).
- One unit cryoprecipitate per 10 kg body weight increases fibrinogen 50 mg/dL in stable patients, and is indicated for massively bleeding or transfused patients with fibrinogen 80 to 100 mg/dL.
- Inadvertent transfusion of ABO incompatible blood and transfusion-associated acute lung injury (TRALI) are life-threatening, noninfectious hazards of blood transfusion.
- Noninfectious transfusion risk exceeds infectious hazard by 100- to 1000-fold.
- Transfusion-associated GVHD has high mortality (>90%), but is extremely rare; irradiating blood components can prevent this complication, but is not practical in the acute trauma setting.
- Blood transfusion does not reduce mortality in stable critically ill patients with Hb 8 to 10 g/dL (except for a subset with coronary artery disease).
- Blood collection in 1997 fell 12.6%, but the rate of transfusion remained the same as in 1994.
- In bleeding, otherwise healthy trauma patients, cardiovascular compensation may be adequate to a Hb as low as 5 g/dL. However, any further compensation is inadequate with mortality 50% to 95% at Hb <3.5 g/dL.

REFERENCES

1. Blood Transfusion. In: History of the Great War, Medical Services and Surgery in the War. London: HMSO; 1922: 108–128.

2. Hess JR, Thomas MJG. Blood use in war and disaster: Lessons from the past century. Transfusion 2003; 43:1622–1633.
3. Kendrick, DB. Blood program in World War II. Washington Medical Department. US Army, 1964.
4. Camp FR, Conte NR, Braver JR. Military blood banking 1941–1973. Fort Knox (KY): US Army Medical Research Lab, 1973:20.
5. Allen JB. The minimum acceptable level of hemoglobin. Int Anesthesiol Clin 1982; 20:1–22.
6. McCrossan L, Masterson G. Editorial III: Blood transfusions in critical illness. Brit J Anaesth 2002; 88:6–10.
7. Nuttall GA, Stehling LC, Beighley CM, et al. Current transfusion practices of members of the American Society of Anesthesiologists. Anesthesiology 2003; 99:1433–1443.
8. Herbert PC, Wells G, Blajchman MA, et al. A multicenter, randomized controlled clinical trial of transfusion requirements in critical care. N Engl J Med 1999; 340:409–417.
9. Herbert PC, Yetisir E, Martin C, et al. Schweitzer I and the transfusion requirements in critical care investigations for the Canadian Critical Care Trials Group. Crit Care Med 2000; 29:227–234.
10. Perioperative Red Blood Cell Transfusion Consensus Conference. Office of Medical Application of Research. National Institutes of Health. Perioperative red cell blood transfusion. JAMA 1988; 260:2700.
11. Welch HG, Mehan VR, Goodnough LT. Prudent strategies for elective and red cell transfusion. Ann Intern Med 1992; 116:393–402.
12. Practice Guidelines for Blood Component Therapy. A report by the American Society of Anesthesiologists Task Force on blood component therapy. Anesthesiology 1996; 84:732–744.
13. Guidelines for Red Cell and Plasma Transfusion for Adults and Children. Suppl J Can Med Assoc J 1997; 156(111):S1–S40.
14. Simon TL, Alverson DC, AuBullion J, et al. Practice parameter for the use of red cell transfusions. Arch Pathol Lab Med 1998; 122:130–138.
15. Shapiro MJ, Gettinger A, Corwin HL, et al. Anemia and blood transfusion in trauma patients admitted to the intensive care unit. J Trauma 2003; 55(2):269–274.
16. Farion KJ, McLellan BA, Boulanger BR, Szalai JP. Changes in red cell transfusion practice among adult trauma victims. J Trauma 1998; 44:583–587.
17. Malone DL, Dunne J, Tracy JK, et al. Blood transfusion, independent of shock severity, is associated with worse outcome in trauma. J Trauma 2003; 54(5):898–907.
18. Robinson, WP, Ahn J, Stiffler A, et al. Blood transfusion is an independent predictor of increased mortality in nonoperatively managed blunt hepatic and splenic injuries. J Trauma 2005; 58(3):437–445.
19. Vaslef SN, Knudsen NW, Neligan PJ, et al. Massive transfusion exceeding 50 units of blood products in trauma patients. J Trauma 2002; 53(2):291–296.
20. Mirhashemi S, Brect GA, Chavez Chavez RH, Inteliglietta M. Effects of hemodilution on skin microcirculation. Am J Physiol 1988; 25:4411–4416.
21. Hobisch-Hagen PP, Widermann F, Mayr A, et al. Blunted erythropoetic response to anemia in multiply traumatized patients. Crit Care Med 2001; 29:743–747.
22. Kaminogo M, Ochi M, Ouizuka M, et al. All additional monitoring of regional cerebral oxygen saturation with HMPAOS-PECT Study during balloon test occlusion. Stroke 1993; 30:407–413.
23. Shin B, Mackenzie CF, Helrich M. Creatinine clearance for early detection of post-traumatic renal dysfunction. Anesthesiology 1096; 64:605–609.
24. Waisman Y, Eichacker PQ, Bansk SM, et al. Acute hemorrhage in dogs: Construction and validation of models to quantify blood loss. J Appl Physiol 1993; 74:510–519.
25. Dunham CM, Siegel JH, Weireter L, et al. Oxygen debt and metabolic academia as quantitative predictors of mortality and the severity of the ischemic insult in hemorrhagic shock. Crit Care Med 1991; 19:231–243.
26. Van der Linden P, Rausin I, Deltell A, et al. Detection of Tissue hypoxia by arteriovenous gradient for pCO2 and pH in

anesthetized dogs during progressive hemorrhage. Anesth Analg 1995; 80:269–275.

27. Moss GS, Valeri CR, Brodine CE. Clinical experiences in the use of frozen blood in combat casualties. N Engl J Med 1968; 278:747–732.

28. Hess, Jr, Hill HR, Oliver CK, et al. Twelve-week RBC storage. Transfusion 2003; 43:867–872.

29. Kellen DL, Fegan AT, Kennedy MK, et al. High-yield platelet concentrates attainable by continuous quality improvement reduce platelet transfusion cost and donor exposure. Transfusion 1997; 37:482–486.

30. Menitove JE. Standards for blood banks and transfusion services. 18th ed. Bethesda: American Association of Blood Banks, 1997.

31. Menitove JE, Snyder EL. Platelet transfusion practice: time for renewed consensus. Transfusion 1998; 38:707–709.

32. Horsey PJ. Editorial: Multiple trauma and massive transfusion. Anaesthesia 1997; 52:1027–1029.

33. Royal College of Physicians of Edinburgh. Final statement from the consensus conference on platelet transfusion 1997. Transfusion 1998; 38:796–797.

34. Illert WE, Sanger W, Weise W. Bacterial contaminations of single-donor blood components. Transfus Med 1995; 5:57–61.

35. VandeWatering LM, Hermans J, Houbierg JA. Beneficial effects of leukocyte depletion of transfused blood on postoperative complications in patients undergoing cardiac surgery: a randomized clinical trial. Circulation 1998; 97:562–568.

36. Aster RH. Platelet transfusion therapy: consensus conference. JAMA 1987; 257:1777–1780.

37. Bishop JF, Schiffer CA, Aisner J, Matthews JP, Wiernik PH. Surgery in acute leukemia; A review of 167 operations in thromboctopenic patients. Am J Hematol 1987; 26:147–155.

38. Leslie SD, Toy PTCY. Laboratory hemostatic abnormalities in massively transfused patients given red blood cells and crystalloid. Am J Clin Pathol 1991; 96:770–773.

39. Reed RL, Heimbach DM, Counts RB, et al. Prophylactic platelet administration during massive transfusion. Ann Surg 1986; 203:40–48.

40. Slichter SJ, Counts RB, Henderson R, Haker LA. Preparation of cryoprecipitate factor VIII concentrates. Transfusion 1976; 16:616–626.

41. British Committee for Standards in Hematology: Guidelines for platelet transfusion. Transfus Med 1992; 2:311–318.

42. Murphy WG, Davies MJ, Eduardo A. The hemostatic response to surgery and trauma. Br J Anaesth 1993; 70:205–213.

43. Saxena S, Wehrli G, Makarewicz K, et al. Monitoring for under-utilization of RBC components and platelets. Transfusion 2001; 41:587–590.

44. Warkentin TE, Kelton JG. Temporal aspects of heparin-induced thrombocytopenia. N Engl J Med 2001; 344(17):1286–1292.

45. Warkentin TE. Clinical presentation of heparin-induced thrombocytopenia. Semin Hematol 1998; 35(suppl 5):9–16.

46. Warkentin TE. Heparin-induced thrombocytopenia: pathogenesis and management. Br J Haematol 2003; 121:535–555.

47. Warkentin TE. Management of heparin-induced thrombocytopenia: a critical comparison of lepirudin and argatroban. Thromb Res 2003; 110:73–82.

48. Warkentin TE, Greinacher A. Heparin-induced thrombocytopenia: Recognition, treatment, and prevention. The Seventh ACCP Conference on Antithrombotic and Thrombolytic Therapy. Chest 2004; 126(suppl 3):311S–337S.

49. Aoki M, Mizobe T, Nozuchi S, Huramatsu N. In vivo and in vitro studies of the intubation effect of propofol on human platelet aggregation. Anesthesiology 1998; 88:362–370.

50. Faraday N. Platelets, perioperative hemostasis and anesthesia. Anesthesiology 2002; 96:1042–1043.

51. Sun JCJ, Crowther MA, Warkentin TE, Lamy A, Teoh KHT. Should aspirin by discontinued before coronary artery bypass surgery? Circulation 2005; 112:e85–e90.

52. Himmelreich G, Hundt K, Neuhans P, Bechstein WO, Rossant R, Riess H. Evidence that intraoperative prostaglandin E1, infusion reduces impaired platelet aggregation after reperfusion in orthoptic liver transplantation. Transplantation 1993; 55:819–826.

53. Locker GJ, Standinger J, Knapp S, et al. Prostaglandin E1, inhibits platelet decrease after massive blood transfusion during major surgery: influence on coagulation cascade. J Trauma 1997; 42:525–531.

54. Luk C, Eckert KM, Barr RM, Chin-Ye JH. Prospective audit of the use of fresh frozen plasma based on Canadian Medical Association Transfusion Guidelines. Can Med Assoc J 2002; 166:1539–1540.

55. Expert Working Group. Guidelines for red blood cell and plasma transfusion for adults and children. Can Med Assoc J 1997; 156 (suppl 11):S1–S24.

56. Tullies JL. Fresh frozen plasma. Indication and risk. JAMA 1985; 253:551–553.

57. Ho AMH, Karmakar MK, Dion PW. Are we giving enough coagulation factors during major trauma resuscitation. Am J Surg 2005; 190:479–484.

58. Sullivan MJ, McCullough J, Schreiber GB, Wallace EL. Blood collection and transfusion in the United States in 1997. Transfusion 2002; 42:1253–1260.

59. Monroe DM, Hoffman M, Oliver JD, Robert HR. Platelet activity of high dose factor VIIa is independent of tissue factor. Br J Haematol 1997; 99:544–547.

60. O'Connell KA, Wood JJ, Wise RP, Lozier JN, Braun MM. Thromboembolic adverse events after use of recombinant human coagulation factor VIIa. JAMA 2006; 295:293–298.

61. Friederich PW, Henny CP, Messelink EJ, et al. Effect of recombinant activated factor VII on perioperative blood loss in patients undergoing retropubic prostatectomy: a double-blind placebo-controlled randomized trial. Lancet 2003; 361:201–205.

62. Dutton RP, Hess JR, Scalea TM. Recombinant factor VIIa for control of hemorrhage: Early experience in critically ill trauma patients. J Clin Anesth 2003; 19:184–188.

63. Stein M, Dutton, RP, O'Connor J, et al. Determinants of Futility of Administration of Recombinant Factor VIIa in Trauma. J Trauma 2005; 59(3):609–615.

64. Boffand KD, Riou B, Warren B, et al. Recombinant factor VIIa as adjunctive therapy for bleeding control in severely injured trauma patient: two parallel randomized, placebo-controlled, double-blind clinical trials. J Trauma 2005; 59:8–18.

65. Batletta JF, Ahrens CL, Tyburski JG, et al. A review of recombinant factor VII for refractory bleeding in nonhemophilic trauma patients. J Trauma 2005; 58(3):646–651.

66. Lane TA. Blood Bank Handbook. UCSD Medical Center Hospitals available at http://medicine.ucsd.edu/blood bank.

67. Stainsky D, MaLennar S, Hamilton PJ. Management of massive blood loss: A template guideline. Brit J Anaesth 2000; 85:487–491.

68. Regan F, Taylor C. Recent developments: Blood transfusion medicine. Br Med J 2002; 325:143–147.

69. Coma JJ, Dutton RP, Scalea TM, Edelman BE, Hess R. Blood transfusion rates in the care of acute trauma. Tranfusion 2004; 44:809–813.

70. Harvey MP, Greenfield TP, Sugrue ME, Rosenfeld D. Massive blood transfusion in a tertiary referral hospital. Clinical outcomes and haemostatic complications. Med J Aust 1995; 163:356–359.

71. Codner P, Cinat M. Massive transfusion for trauma is appropriate. ITACCS TraumaCare 2005; 15(3):148–152.

72. Brohi K, Singh J, Heron M, Coats T. Acute traumatic coagulopathy. J Trauma 2003; 54(6):1127–1130.

73. Goodnough LT, Brecher ME, Kanter MH, AuBuchon JP. Transfusion medicine—blood transfusion-first of two parts. N Engl J Med 1999; 340(6):438–447.

74. Goodnough LT, Brecher ME, Kanter MH, AuBuchon JP. Transfusion medicine—blood conservation-second of two parts. N Engl J Med 1999; 340(7):525–533.

75. America's Blood Centers. Hemolytic transfusion reactions, Part 1: biological product deviations (errors and accidents). ABC Blood Bull 3, No. 3, Nov. 2000.

76. Williamson L, Cohen H, Love E, Jones H. Todd A, Soldan K. The serious hazard of transfusion (SHOT) initiative. The UK approach to hemovigilance. Vox Sang 2000; 78(suppl 2):291–295.

77. Klein HG, Lipton KS. Noninfectious serious hazard of transfusion (NISHOT). Amer Assoc Blood Bank Bull 2001; (June 01–04):1–10.

78. Heddle NM, Kellon JG. Febrile nonhemolytic transfusion reactions. In: Popvosky MA, ed. Transfusion Reactions. 2nd ed. Bethesda, Maryland: AABB Press, 2001:47–85.

79. Baele PL, de Bruyeire M, Deneys V, Dupont E, Flament J, Lamberamont M. Bedside transfusion errors. A prospective study by the Belgium SANGUIS Group. Vox Sang 1994; 66:117–121.

80. Sazama K. Reports of 355 transfusion-associated deaths: 1976 through 1985. Transfusion 1990; 30:583–590.

81. Linden JV, Wagner K, Voytovich AE, Sheenan J. Transfusion errors in New York State: An analysis of 10 years' experience. Transfusion 2000; 40:1207–1213.

82. Popovsky MA, Taswell H. Circulatory overload: An under-diagnosed consequence of transfusion (abstract). Transfusion 1985; 25:469.

83. Audet AM, Popovsky MA, Andrzejewski C. Current transfusion practice in orthopedic surgery patients (abstract). Blood 1995; 86(suppl):853a.

84. Whitsett CF, Robichaux MB. Assessment of blood administration incident report. Transfusion 2001; 41:581–586.

85. Clarke G, Podlosky L, Petrie L. Boshov L. Severe respiratory reactions to random donor platelets: an incidence and nested case control study (abstract). Blood 1994; 84(suppl):465a.

86. Palfi M, Berg S, Ernerudh J, Berlin G. A controlled randomized study on tranfusion-related acute lung injury (abstract). Vox Sang 2000; 78:51.

87. Audet A-M, Goodnough LT. Practice Strategies for elective Red Blood Cell Transfusion. Ann Intern Med 1992; 116:403–406.

88. Silverboard H, Aisiku I, Martin GS, Adams S. The role of acute blood transfusion in the development of acute respiratory distress syndrome in patients with severe trauma. J Trauma 2005; 59(3):717–723.

89. Ohto H, Anderson KC. Survey of transfusion-associated graft vs. host disease in immuno-competent recipients. Transfus Med Rev 1996; 10:31–43.

90. Utter GH, Owings JT, Lee T-H, et al. Blood transfusion is associated with donor leukocyte microchimerism in trauma patients. J Trauma 2004; 57(4):702–708.

91. Mahon PM, Jones ST, Kovar IZ. Hypoglycemia and blood transfusion in the newborn (correspondence). Lancet 1985; 2:388.

92. Jackson JC. Adverse events associated with exchange transfusion in healthy and ill newborns. Pediatrics 1977; 99:7.

93. Carson JL, Duff A, Berlin JA, et al. Perioperative blood transfusion and postoperative mortality. JAMA 1988; 279:199–205.

94. Hogue CW Jr, Goodnough LT, Monk TG. Perioperative myocardial ischemic episodes are related to hematocrit levels in patients undergoing radical prostatectomy. Transfusion 1998; 38:924–931.

95. Weisel RD, Charlesworth DC, Mickleborough LL, et al. Limitations of blood conservation. J Thorac Cardiovasc Surg 1984; 84:26–38.

96. Nelson DH, Fleisher LA, Rosenbaum SH. Relationship between postoperative anemia and cardiac morbidity in high-risk vascular patients in the critical care unit. Crit Care Med 1993; 21:860–866.

97. Wilson K, MacDougall H, Ferguson P, Graham I, Tinmouth A, Herbert PC. The effectiveness of interventions to reduce physician's levels of inappropriate transfusion: What can be learned from a systematic review of the literature. Transfusion 202; 42:1224–1229.

98. Mark PE, Sibbald WJ. Effects of stored blood transfusion on oxygen delivery in patients with sepsis. JAMA 1993, 269:3024–3029.

99. Fitzgerald RDS, Martin CM, Dietz GE, Doig GS, Potter RF, Sibbald WJ. Transfusion of red blood cells stored in citrate phosphate dextrose adenine-1 for 28 days fails to improve tissue oxygenation in rats. Crit Care Med 1997; 20:726–732.

100. Hovav T, Yedgar S, Manny N, Barshtein G. Alteration of red cell aggregability and shape during blood storage. Transfusion 1999; 39(3):277–281.

101. Kaplan J, Sarnack S. Gitlin J. Diminished helper/suppressor lymphocyte ratios and natural killer activity in recipients of repeated blood transfusions. Blood 1986; 64:308–310.

102. Jenson LS, Kissmyeer-Nielsen P, Wolff B, Qvist N. Randomized comparison of leucocyte-depleted versus buffy-coat-poor blood transfusion and complications after colorectal surgery. Lancet 1996; 348:841–845.

103. Tom-Harold F, Tormod B. Association between blood transfusion and infection in injured patients. J Trauma 1992;33:659–661.

104. Triulzi DJ, Vanek K, Ryan DH, Blumberg N. A clinical and immunological study of blood transfusion and post-operative bacterial infection in spinal surgery. Transfusion 1992; 32:517–524.

105. Kirkley SA. Proposed mechanisms of transfusion-induced immunomodulation. Clin Diag Lab Immun 1999; 6(5):652–657.

106. Van Bommel J, Siegemund M, Henry CP, Trouwborst A, Ince C. Critical hematocrit in intestinal tissue oxygenation during severe normovolemic hemodilution. Anesthesiology 2001; 94:152–160.

107. Hughes GSJ, Yancey EP, Albrecht R, et al. Hemoglobin-based oxygen carrier preserves submaximal exercise capacity in humans. Clin Pharmacol Ther 1995; 58:434–443.

108. Browne DR, Rockford J, O'Connell V, Jones JG. The incidence of post-operative atelectasis in the dependant lung following thoractomy: the value of added nitrogen. Br J Anesth 1970; 42:340–346.

109. Viele MK, Weiskopf RB. What can we learn about the need for transfusion from patients who refuse blood? The experience with Jehovah's Witnesses. Transfusion 1994; 34:396–401.

110. Fullerton WT, Turner AG. Exchange transfusion in treatment of severe anemia in pregnancy. Lancet 1962; 75–78.

111. Alexiu O, Mircea N, Balaban M, Furtunescua B. Gastrointestinal hemorrhage from peptic ulcer. An evaluation of bloodless transfusion and early surgery. Anaesthesia 1975; 30:609–615.

112. Kawaguchi A, Bergland J, Subramanian S. Total bloodless open heart surgery in the pediatric age group. Circulation 1984; 70(suppl I):30–34.

113. Carson JL, Poses RM, Spence RK, Bonavita G. Severity of anemia and operative mortality and morbidity. Lancet 1988; 727–729.

114. Fontana JL, Welborn L, Morgan PD, Sturin P, Martin G, Bunger R. Oxygen consumption and cardiovascular function in children during profound intraoperative normovolemic hemodilution. Anesth Analg 1995; 80:219–225.

115. Shibutani K, Komatzu T, Kubal K, Sanchala V, Kumar V, Bizzarri DV. Critical level of oxygen delivery in anesthetized man. Crit Care Med 1983; 11:640–643.

116. Komatsu T, Shibutani K, Okamoto K, et al. Critical level of oxygen delivery after cardiopulmonary bypass. Crit Care Med 1987; 15:194–197.

117. Von Woerkens EC, Trouwborst A, van Lanschoff JJ. Profound hemodilution: What is the critical level of hemodilution at which oxygen delivery-dependent oxygen consumption starts in an anesthetized human? Anesth Analg 1992; 75:818–821.

118. Filho IPT, Spiess BD, Pittman R, et al. Experimental analysis of critical oxygen delivery. Am J Physiol Heart Circ Physiol 2005; 288:1071–1079.

119. Lorente JA, Landin LO, De Pablo R, Renes E, Rodriguez-Diaz R, Liste D. Effects of blood transfusion on oxygen transport variables in severe sepsis. Crit Care Med 1993; 21:1312–1318.

120. Conrad SA, Dietrich KA, Herbert CA, Romero MD. Effect of red cell transfusion on oxygen consumption following fluid resuscitation in septic shock. Circ Shock 1990; 31:419–429.

121. Finch CA, Lenfant C. Oxygen transport in man. N Engl J Med, 1972; 286:407–415.

122. Sprung J, Mackenzie CF, Barnas GM, Williams JE, Parr M. Oxygen transport and cardiovascular effects of resuscitation from severe hemorrhagic shock using hemoglobin solutions. Crit Care Med 1995; 23:1540–1553.

123. Morimoto Y, Mathru M, Martinez-Tica JC, Zornow MH. Effects of profound anemia on brain tissue oxygen tension, carbon dioxide tension and pH in rabbits. J Neurosurg Anesthesiol 2001; 13:33–39.

124. Petrozza PH. Major spine surgery. Anesthesiol Clin North America, 2002; 20:405–415.

125. Remigio D, Westenbaker C. Post-operative bilateral visual loss. Surv Opthalmol 2000; 44:426–432.

126. Gould SA, Moore EE, Hoyt DB, et al. The life-sustaining capacity of human polymerized hemoglobin when red cells might be unavailable. J Am Coll Surg 2002; 195:445–455.

127. Weiskopf RB, Viele MK, Feiner J, et al. Human cardiovascular and metabolic response to acute severe isovolemic anemia. JAMA 1998; 279:217–221.

128. Wilkerson DK, Rosen AL, Sehgal LR, Gould SA, Sehgal HL, Moss GS. Limits of cardiac compensation in anemic baboons. Surgery 1988; 103:665–670.

129. Vicent JL, Baron J-F, Reinhart K, et al. Anemia and blood transfusion in critically ill patients. JAMA 2002; 288: 1499–1507.

130. Fang WC, Helm RE, Kreiger KH, et al. Impact of minimum hematocrit during cardiopulmonary bypass on mortality in patients underging coronary artery surgery. Circulation 1997; 96(suppl 9):194–199.

60

Glucose and Insulin Management in Critical Care

Dieter Mesotten, Ilse Vanhorebeek, and Greet Van den Berghe

Department of Intensive Care Medicine, University Hospital Gasthuisberg, Catholic University of Leuven, Leuven, Belgium

INTRODUCTION

The discovery of insulin by Banting and Best in 1922 was a revolutionary breakthrough in the treatment and outcome of patients with Type 1 diabetes mellitus, a previously lethal disorder due to the development of ketoacidosis. In the late 19th century, Claude Bernard described the association of acute trauma with the occurrence of hyperglycemia, which was considered to be an adaptive stress response proceeding irrespective of underlying diabetes. In addition to trauma, hyperglycemia also commonly develops during other types of critical illness. Whereas hyperglycemia in critical illness was treated conventionally only when blood glucose levels became excessively elevated, the beneficial effects of treating even moderate hyperglycemia in critically ill patients have recently been established (1).

ALTERED GLUCOSE REGULATION IN TRAUMA AND CRITICAL ILLNESS

The concept "stress diabetes" or "diabetes of injury" has been in the literature for almost 150 years. **The stress-induced hyperglycemia, seen following severe trauma, burns and critical illness results from the combined action of hormonal, cytokine, and nervous "counter-regulatory" signals on glucose metabolic pathways.** In the acute stage of the disease, both hepatic gluconeogenesis and glycogenolysis are enhanced in the critically ill patient. Hepatic gluconeogenesis is assumed to be upregulated by increased levels of glucagon (2), cortisol (3), and growth hormone. Hepatic glycogenolysis is stimulated by the catecholamines epinephrine and norepinephrine, which are released in response to acute injury (4). In addition, both these hyperglycemic responses may be enhanced directly or indirectly by the cytokines interleukin-1, interleukin-6, and tumor necrosis factor (5–7). The evolution of intensive care medicine during the last three to four decades has fostered a dramatic increase in the survival of patients under conditions of multiple trauma, extensive burns, and severe sepsis, among others. Hence, patients now frequently enter a chronic phase of critical illness (8). How maintenance of hyperglycemia is regulated during protracted critical illness remains less clear. In comparison to the acute phase, growth

hormone, cortisol, catecholamine, and cytokine levels are usually decreased in the more chronic phase of critical illness, but the changes in glucagon levels are not well documented (9,10). In addition to the increased synthesis of glucose, its uptake mechanisms are also affected during critical illness. In the first place, the immobilization of the patient leads to complete loss of the important exercise-stimulated glucose uptake in skeletal muscle. In addition, the insulin-stimulated glucose uptake by glucose transporter-4 (GLUT-4) as well as glycogen synthase activity are inhibited, together compromising the insulin-stimulated glucose uptake (11,12). Conflicting data have been reported on glucose oxidation through pyruvate produced in the glycolytic pathway, with some studies showing decreased oxidation rates (13), whereas the opposite effect was found by others (14). However, the decrease in insulin-stimulated glucose uptake in skeletal muscle and adipose tissue is completely offset by a massive increase in total body glucose uptake, of which the mononuclear phagocyte system in liver, spleen, and ileum is the main receiver (15). The overall increased peripheral glucose uptake (16) in light of hyperglycemia only underscores the pivotal role of increased hepatic glucose production during critical illness, which cannot be suppressed by exogenous glucose (17). Under normal circumstances, hepatic synthesis of glucose by gluconeogenesis and glycogenolysis is inhibited by insulin. **The combined picture of increased serum insulin levels, impaired peripheral glucose uptake, and elevated hepatic glucose production indicates the development of insulin resistance during critical illness (18).**

HISTORICAL RATIONALE FOR HYPERGLYCEMIC INTENSIVE CARE UNIT MANAGEMENT

In normal individuals, blood glucose levels are tightly regulated within the narrow range of 60–140 mg/dL (3.3–7.7 mmol/L) both in fed and fasted states. According to the definition given by the World Health Organization, fasting and fed blood glucose levels rise to, respectively, 110 mg/dL (6.1 mmol/L) or higher and 147 mg/dL (8.1 mmol/L) or higher in patients with diabetic hyperglycemia. The reported prevalence of hyperglycemia in critically ill patients ranges from 3% to 71% (19). This large variation results from the divergent diagnostic criteria to define hyperglycemia in critically ill patients, in contrast to the clear guidelines set for diabetes mellitus. Until recently, it was considered state of the art to tolerate blood glucose levels up to 220 mg/dL (12 mmol/L) in fed critically ill patients (20), and treatment of hyperglycemia was only initiated when glucose levels exceeded this value. The primary motivation for this treatment was the occurrence of hyperglycemia-induced osmotic diuresis and fluid shifts, once glycemia exceeds that threshold. Secondly, it was known that uncontrolled and pronounced hyperglycemia predisposes to infectious complications, as shown by data regarding diabetic hyperglycemia (21,22). A third argument for tolerating glucose levels up to 220 mg/dL (12 mmol/L) was found in the commonly accepted view that moderate hyperglycemia in critically ill patients is "beneficial" for organs such as the brain and the blood cells that largely rely on glucose for their energy supply but do not require insulin for glucose uptake. Finally, many clinicians feared that tight glucose management might occasionally cause hypoglycemia and brain injury; moderate hyperglycemia was viewed as a buffer against this occurrence.

STRICT MAINTENANCE OF NORMOGLYCEMIA DEMONSTRATED TO IMPROVE OUTCOME IN CRITICALLY ILL PATIENTS

Recently, the classical dogma that stress-induced hyperglycemia is beneficial to the critically ill patient has been challenged by an extended prospective, randomized, controlled clinical trial, studying the effects of strict glycemic control on mortality and morbidity of these patients (1). A total of 1548 mechanically ventilated patients who were admitted to the ICU, predominantly after extensive or complicated surgery or trauma, were enrolled in the study and randomly subdivided into two groups. In the intensive insulin therapy, group blood glucose levels were kept tightly between 80–110 mg/dL (4.4–6.1 mmol/L) by exogenous insulin infusion, while in the conventional treatment group insulin was only administered if blood glucose levels exceeded 220 mg/dL (12 mmol/L). ☞ **Strict maintenance of normoglycemia by intensive insulin therapy markedly reduced intensive care mortality of critically ill patients (Fig. 1), particularly in the patient population with prolonged critical illness where mortality was reduced from 20.2% to 10.6% (P = 0.005).** ☞ The superiority of intensive insulin therapy was also demonstrated by the higher mortality even of patients with only moderate hyperglycemia of 110–150 mg/dL (6.1–8.3 mmol/L) in the conventional treatment group, compared to the patients receiving the intensive insulin therapy and having blood glucose levels below 110 mg/dL (6.1 mmol/L) (23). The extreme importance of this observation is illustrated by the lack of any intervention with such a pronounced beneficial effect on intensive care mortality since the introduction of mechanical ventilation. Intensive insulin therapy also improved several morbidity-related factors, including a reduction in the need for prolonged ventilatory support, the duration of intensive care stay, and the number of blood transfusions. In addition, a lower incidence of blood stream infections, extreme inflammation and, even more strikingly, of acute renal failure and critical illness polyneuropathy was observed. Insulin therapy also protected the central and peripheral nervous

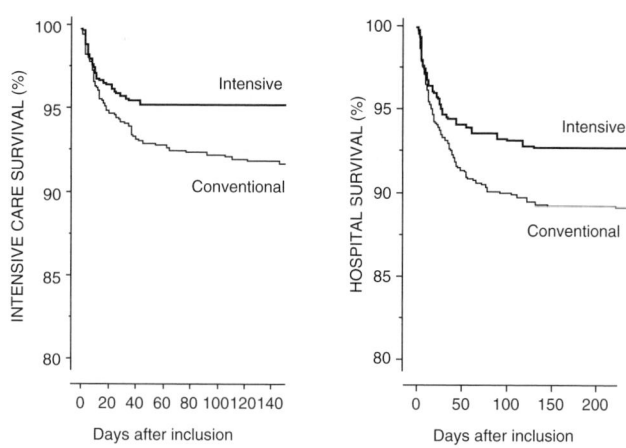

Figure 1   Kaplan–Meier cumulative survival plots for intensive care and in-hospital survival, showing the effect of intensive insulin treatment in a study of 1548 critically ill patients. Patients discharged alive from intensive care (*left panel*) and hospital (*right panel*), respectively, were considered survivors. *P*-values were obtained by log rank (Mantel-Cox) significance testing. The difference between the intensive insulin group and the conventional group was significant for intensive care survival (unadjusted *P* = 0.005; adjusted *P* < 0.04) and for hospital survival (unadjusted *P* = 0.01). *Source*: Reproduced, From Ref. 1.

system from secondary insults and improved long-term rehabilitation of patients with isolated brain injury (24). Importantly, in a large randomized controlled trial, the Leuven protocol of glycemic control in a predominantly surgical patient population (1) was recently proven to be similarly effective in a strictly medical ICU patient population (25).

In the intention-to-treat population of 1200 patients, in-hospital mortality was reduced from 40.0% to 37.3%. The difference did not reach statistical significance, but this was not surprising as the study was not powered for this mortality endpoint. However, in the target group of long-stay patients needing at least a third day of intensive care, for which the study had been powered based on the results of the surgical study, tight glycemic control with insulin significantly reduced in-hospital mortality from 52.5% to 43.0%. Morbidity was significantly reduced in the intention-to-treat group of patients receiving intensive insulin therapy. New development of kidney injury occurred less frequently, the therapy allowed earlier weaning from mechanical ventilation and earlier discharge from the ICU and from the hospital, and the patients less frequently developed hyperbilirubinemia. The reduction in morbidity was even more striking in the target group of patients remaining in ICU for at least a third day. These patients were discharged from the hospital alive on average 10 days earlier than on conventional insulin therapy. In contrast to the surgical patients, there was no difference in bacteremia or prolonged antibiotic therapy requirement, but the number of long-stay patients with hyperinflammation was also reduced.

An earlier observational study also largely confirmed the clinical benefits of the surgical ICU trial (1) in "real life" intensive care of a heterogeneous medical/surgical population with glucose levels targeted below 7.8 mmol/L with insulin (26). A small prospective, randomized, controlled trial that aimed to control glucose levels below 120 mg/dL (6.7 mmol/L) showed a decreased incidence of nosocomial infections in a predominantly general surgical ICU patient population (27).

SPECIFIC MORBIDITIES ASSOCIATED WITH HYPERGLYCEMIA
Diabetic Patients Have Improved Outcomes with Tight Glycemic Control

The question whether tight glycemic control is beneficial for subjects with Type 1 diabetes was the subject of vigorous debate until this issue was resolved in 1993 by the results of the diabetes control and complications trial (DCCT). The study demonstrated a highly significant decrease not only of the progression rates of diabetic retinopathy, the most prevalent complication in Type 1 diabetes, but also of the development of nephropathy and peripheral and autonomic neuropathy (28). Like for Type 1 diabetes, evidence for the importance of tight glycemic control in patients with Type 2 diabetes was provided by a large clinical trial. In the late 1990s, the United Kingdom Prospective Diabetes Study (UKPDS) showed that a 0.7% decrease in glycated hemoglobin (HbA1c) lowered the incidence of retinopathy by 21%, microalbuminuria by 33%, cataracts by 24%, myocardial infarction by 16%, and resulted in a nonsignificant 5% decrease in the incidence of cerebrovascular accident (29). In addition, a tendency toward a lower death-rate was observed when blood glucose levels were tightly controlled. However, neither the UKPDS nor the DCCT was appropriately powered to detect a significant decrease in diabetes-related mortality.

A history of diabetes strongly increases the risk for fatal outcome following acute myocardial infarction (AMI). More specifically, the risk of mortality is 1.5 to two times higher in this patient group than in nondiabetic patients (30). Moreover, in AMI patients without previously diagnosed diabetes, hyperglycemia on admission has been associated with larger infarct size, a higher incidence of cardiac failure, and decreased one-year survival (31). These findings suggested that strict glycemic control might improve the prognosis for diabetic patients with myocardial infarction. This has been investigated by a number of studies, of which the Diabetes and Insulin-Glucose infusion in Acute Myocardial Infarction (DIGAMI) Study was the largest and also covered the longest follow-up period (32). In that study, diabetic patients admitted to the hospital with an AMI were randomly assigned to standard treatment (at the physician's discretion), or to "intensive insulin therapy." The latter comprised an infusion of glucose and insulin, started as soon as possible and continued for 48 hours. Thereafter, the intensive insulin therapy patients were submitted to a "stricter" blood glucose control regimen (below 215 mg/dL [12 mmol/L]) with subcutaneous insulin continued for at least three months after discharge. Thirty day and long-term survival significantly improved under the intensive insulin treatment (29% relative risk reduction at one year) (33,34) and also, the risk for re-infarction and new cardiac failure was remarkably reduced (35). An observational study of patients with diabetes undergoing cardiac surgery showed that elimination of hyperglycemia with intravenous insulin infusion lowered in-hospital mortality compared to the historical control group and reduced the occurrence of deep sternal wound infections and length of hospital stay (36).

A significant correlation between on-admission hyperglycemia and adverse outcome has also been demonstrated for other clinical conditions. Thus, high blood glucose levels were associated with increased mortality and poorer neurological recovery after cerebrovascular ischemic insults (37,38). Similarly, hyperglycemia predicted increased morbidity and mortality after severe brain injury (39,40), trauma (41,42), and severe burn injury (43), as well as in critically ill children with widely varying pathology (44). Retrospective analysis of a heterogeneous population of critically ill patients revealed that even a modest degree of hyperglycemia was associated with substantially increased hospital mortality (45).

Although data from different studies appear controversial, administration of insulin in a glucose-insulin-potassium (GIK) regimen has shown to improve myocardial function and to protect the myocardium during AMI, open heart surgery, endotoxic shock, and other critical conditions (46,47). Lack of glucose control might explain the controversy surrounding GIK using different protocols (48–50). Indeed, direct anti-apoptotic properties of insulin, independent of glucose uptake and involving insulin signalling, have been shown to play a role in the cardio-protective action of insulin (46,51,52), but such effects may be counteracted by elevated levels of blood glucose (46). This is in line with the lack of tight glucose control and the disappointing results of the recent DIGAMI-2 trial in patients with diabetes and AMI (48), and the large randomized CREATE-ECLA trial on GIK infusion in patients with AMI (49). These studies failed to show an effect of this intervention on survival, cardiac arrest, and cardiogenic shock. Likewise, GIK infusion for 24 hours after acute stroke failed to realize a significant reduction in glycemia or mortality, as examined in the glucose-insulin in stroke trial (GIST) (53).

Critical Illness–Associated Renal Failure: Role of Hyperglycemia

The pathophysiology of diabetic and critical illness-associated nephropathy is presumably different. While in diabetic nephropathy the glomerulus is mainly affected, in the critically ill renal failure mostly results from acute tubular necrosis. Taking measures to prevent deterioration of renal function in critically ill patients is of crucial importance. This is illustrated by the lack of any therapeutic option besides bridging time to spontaneous recovery by extracorporeal hemofiltration or dialysis, with the continuous veno-venous mode being the preferred method for unstable critically ill patients (54). These preventive strategies include maintaining or optimizing renal perfusion, diligence with monitoring of nephrotoxic therapies such as aminoglycosides, and limiting the use of nonionic radiocontrast materials. Intensive insulin therapy has emerged as a specific preventive measure for acute renal failure in critical illness, with the demonstration of a 42% reduction in the number of patients that required extracorporeal replacement therapy to compensate for loss of renal function (1).

Critical Illness–Associated Neuropathy: Role of Hyperglycemia

In the diabetic patient, distal sensory neuropathy with the classic stocking distribution is the most frequent presentation of neuropathies (55). Protracted critically ill patients often suffer from a diffuse axonal polyneuropathy (56), which presents as a tetraparesis with muscle atrophy, but requires confirmation by electromyography (EMG). Although the course of critical illness neuropathy usually is self-limited and a good recovery should be expected once the underlying critical illness is overcome, it severely delays weaning from the ventilator and mobilization of the patient (57). Several factors, including sepsis, the use of high dose corticosteroids, and the use of neuromuscular blocking agents, have been implicated in the etiology of critical illness polyneuropathy (see Volume 2, Chapter 6). However, the exact pathogenesis of critical illness polyneuropathy is still not understood (58). This lack of knowledge for a long time hampered specific prevention of, or treatment for, this complication.

However, ☞ **strong indications recently became available that underscore the importance of blood glucose levels in relation to the development of critical illness polyneuropathy.** ☞ In that regard, Bolton described a strong link between, on one hand, the risk of critical illness polyneuropathy and, on the other hand, increased blood glucose and decreased serum albumin levels, which are both metabolic manifestations of multiple organ failure and sepsis. Sepsis, and the accompanying release of cytokines, was considered to be the causal factor (59). Cytokines may indeed induce microangiopathy, which may play a role, as in diabetic polyneuropathy. In addition, the Leuven study on intensive insulin therapy in the ICU convincingly demonstrated that strict glycemic control with insulin infusion has an important preventive effect on the occurrence of critical illness polyneuropathy, which was associated with a decrease in duration of mechanical ventilation of protracted critically ill patients (1).

Infectious Disease/Immune System Impairment by Hyperglycemia

It has long been known that hyperglycemia of diabetes predisposes to infection (21). Several mechanisms could account for this phenomenon. ☞ **Hyperglycemia inhibits the release of interleukin-1 by macrophages and oxygen radicals by neutrophils (60). In addition, phagocytosis by macrophages is impaired under hyperglycemic conditions (61,62).** ☞ Importantly, tight glycemic control was able to ameliorate the leukocyte oxidative burst and phagocytotic activity (63,64). In diabetic critically ill patients, such as those after open-heart surgery, an association between higher risk of infectious complications (65), and blood glucose levels higher than 200 mg/dL (11 mmol/L) has been documented. A follow-up study demonstrated that continuous intravenous insulin infusion reduced the incidence of postcardiac surgery deep sternal wounds (0.8% vs. 2% for subcutaneous insulin injections) (66). Also in patients with severe burn injuries, failure of skin graft take and outcome seemed to be related to uncontrolled hyperglycemia (43). Again, the causal link between hyperglycemia and higher risk of serious infections, regardless of a previous history of diabetes, was provided only recently by the Leuven insulin in ICU study (1). Indeed, the incidence of bacteremia was reduced by almost 50% and sepsis-associated mortality was largely prevented when critically ill patients were intensively treated with exogenous insulin to maintain normoglycemia. Hence, these observations suggest that insulin-titrated blood glucose control enhances the immune system. Improved capacity to clear bacterial invaders was recently shown to mediate this benefit in a novel rabbit model of prolonged critical illness (67,68).

Lipid Metabolism—Impairment by Critical Illness and Hyperglycemia

Parallel to what is observed in diabetic patients (69), lipid metabolism is severely disturbed during critical illness, in addition to the presence of abnormally high glucose levels (70–72). The most characteristic abnormalities are elevated triglyceride levels, due to an increase in very-low-density lipoprotein (VLDL) and low circulating high-density lipoprotein (HDL) cholesterol (73). The levels of low-density lipoprotein (LDL) cholesterol are also decreased (73), but this is offset by an increase in circulating small dense LDL particles (74) that presumably are more proatherogenic than the medium and large LDL particles (75). ☞ **The derangement in serum lipid profiles seen during critical illness is partially counteracted by intensive insulin therapy; specifically, the hypertriglyceridemia is completely eliminated, and serum levels of HDL and LDL are substantially increased, though not fully normalized (76).** ☞ The role of triglycerides in energy provision and the coordinating position of the lipoproteins in transportation of lipid components (cholesterol, triglycerides, phospholipids, lipid-soluble vitamins) are well established (77). In addition, lipoproteins have recently been shown to possess endotoxin-scavenging potential, and in that way are able to prevent death in animal models (78,79). For that reason, intensive insulin therapy may improve the overall endotoxin scavenging function. Considering these data, intensive insulin therapy would be a more integrated approach to correct the abnormal serum lipid profile when compared to the proposed infusions of lipoproteins (73,80). This was indeed demonstrated by the multivariate logistic regression analysis in which the improvement of the deranged lipidemia explained a significant part of its beneficial effect on mortality and organ failure and, surprisingly, surpassed the effect of glycemic control and insulin dose. Likewise, the effect of intensive insulin therapy on inflammation, reflected by a lowering of the serum C-reactive protein (CRP) concentrations (81), was no longer independently related to the outcome benefit when the changes in lipid metabolism were taken into account. In that way, a link may be put forward between the anti-inflammatory effect of intensive insulin therapy and its amelioration of the lipid profile. However, a mechanistic explanation for the dominant effect of serum lipid correction still needs to be delineated.

Inflammation, Endothelium, and Coagulation Effects of Critical Illness and Insulin

Critical illness also resembles diabetes mellitus in the activation of the inflammatory cascade. Here too, intensive insulin therapy has been proved beneficial, as it prevented excessive inflammation in critically ill patients subjected to this treatment (1,81), a finding that was confirmed in an experimental rabbit model of prolonged critical illness (68). ☞ **Although the anti-inflammatory effect of insulin has clearly been established, the exact underlying mechanisms have not yet elucidated been (82).** ☞ However, several factors can be considered, such as suppression of the secretion and antagonism of the harmful actions of tumor necrosis factor-α (83,84), macrophage migration-inhibitory factor (85), and superoxide (86).

As in patients with diabetes mellitus, endothelial dysfunction is present in critically ill patients (87–91). Importantly, maintaining normoglycemia with intensive insulin therapy protected the endothelium, likely in part via inhibition of excessive inducible nitric oxide synthase (iNOS)-induced nitric oxide release and hereby contributed to prevention of organ failure and death with this intervention (92).

Furthermore, diabetes mellitus and critical illness both are hyper-coagulable states (93,94). Putative causes in diabetes include vascular endothelium dysfunction (95), increased blood levels of several clotting factors (96,97), elevated platelet activation (98,99), and inhibition of the fibrinolytic system (97). Levels of the anticoagulant protein C are also decreased (100). Considering the similarities with critical illness (101,102) and the powerful preventive effect of intensive insulin therapy on septicemia, multiple organ failure, and mortality (1), investigating the influence of this simple and cheap metabolic intervention on the balance between coagulation and fibrinolysis in the critically ill is strongly recommended.

HYPER-, NORMO-, OR HYPOCALORIC NUTRITION?

When hypercaloric nutrition (35–40 kcal/kg) is administered to critically ill patients, this "hyperalimentation" leads to a higher incidence of infections and severe metabolic complications, ranging from hyperglycemia, hypertriglyceridemia, and azotemia to hepatic steatosis, fat-overload syndrome, and hypertonic dehydration (103,104). Nowadays, serious complications of feeding have been drastically reduced thanks to the introduction of more accurate means to estimate energy expenditure and a cautious approach toward obese or highly oedematous patients.

McCowen et al. (105) compared the efficacy of hypocaloric total parenteral nutrition (TPN) feeding (14 kcal/kg) with a standard weight-based regimen (18 kcal/kg) in relation to the occurrence of hyperglycemia or infections. Surprisingly, hypocaloric nutrition did not lower these parameters. In fact, caloric restriction only seems to be effective in conjunction with a hyperproteinic approach (about 1.8 g protein per kg ideal body weight (IBW), compared to 1.2 g/kg IBW) (106). Similar results were obtained with a hypocaloric parenteral regimen with 2 g protein/kg IBW in patients with morbid obesity (107). However, a clear-cut benefit of hypocaloric over normocaloric nutrition was not consistently present. This might be attributed to the ineffectiveness of hypocaloric nutrition to lower blood glucose levels.

In view of the described morbidities associated with hyperglycemia, the importance of glycemic control is becoming increasingly clear. As indicated, hypercaloric feeding in combination with insulin infusion (GIK) should simultaneously target normoglycemia, in order to result in clinical benefits for the patients (see section "Specific Morbidities associated with Hyperglycemia").

Recently, interest in preoperative carbohydrate loading has been rekindled through the studies of Ljungqvist et al. which revealed that carbohydrate treatment instead of overnight fasting before surgery reduces postoperative insulin resistance and length of hospital stay (108).

INTENSIVE INSULIN THERAPY METHOD: TARGET GLUCOSE <110 MG/DL FOR ALL CRITICALLY ILL PATIENTS

Since the effect of intensive insulin therapy on morbidity and mortality of critically ill patients was equally present among those with and without previously diagnosed diabetes (1), the authors believe that strict normoglycemia below 110 mg/dL (6.1 mmol/L) should be the therapeutic goal, irrespective of diabetic condition. ☞ **The best way to achieve blood glucose control during intensive care is by continuous insulin infusion for both diabetic and nondiabetic**

critically ill patients. In addition, oral antidiabetic agents should be discontinued during critical illness. ☞

Nutrition of critically ill patients, either with enteral nutrition, TPN or with a combination of parenteral and enteral feeding, is typically administered as a continuous process. Consequently, it is intuitive that insulin should be administered in a continuous way as well. In addition, intravenous administration is more reliable and consistent than subcutaneous injections. Titrating of a continuous insulin infusion is preferred to sliding scales as the former not only provides a baseline insulin level but also can be more easily and precisely titrated in response to the actual blood glucose levels. Because of its short intravenous half-life, insulin administration via infusion also allows rapid cessation of insulin action in case the patient develops hypoglycemia.

This risk of hypoglycemia is a major concern on intensive insulin therapy during critical illness. Clinical symptoms of the autonomic response (sweating, tachycardia, tremor) and central nervous symptoms like dizziness, blurred vision, altered mental acuity, confusion, and eventually convulsions may be masked by concomitant diseases and by inherent intensive care treatments such as sedation, analgesia, and mechanical ventilation. Severe (<30 mg/dL) (<1.67 mmol/L) or prolonged hypoglycemia can lead to irreversible brain damage. Another insidious complication of hypoglycemia is the induction of cardiac dysrhythmias ranging from abnormal QT-intervals (109) and sinus bradycardias (110) to ventricular tachycardias (111).

Measures taken to prevent hypoglycemia in the critically ill are the administration of insulin together with carbohydrates, either intravenous dextrose or tube feeds, and close monitoring of blood glucose levels. Specifically in the Leuven insulin in ICU study (1), blood glucose levels were measured every one or two hours during the first 12–24 hours after the patient's admission to the ICU. Once the targeted blood glucose level was reached on a stable insulin dose, measurements were scaled down to every four hours. In case hypoglycemia did develop, this usually took place after the first week of ICU stay, at a time when blood glucose levels were stable. The precipitating factor of this complication was often found in inadequate insulin dose reduction during interruption of enteral feeding. Clearly, the hazard of hypoglycemia warrants a strict and detailed insulin titration protocol, combined with sufficient training of the nursing and medical staff.

EYE TO THE FUTURE

Future studies will help elucidate whether the beneficial effects of intensive insulin therapy during critical illness (1) derive from the maintenance of normoglycemia or rather result directly from the insulin infusion itself. There are data supporting the notion that both effects provide benefit (23,112,113).

Insulin may have played a direct role in the functional improvement of the insulin-sensitive organs. In a normal individual, the heart and skeletal muscles are responsible for the majority of the insulin-stimulated glucose uptake. In addition, muscle catabolism is aggravated in hyperglycemic conditions. This could partially explain the beneficial effects of intensive insulin therapy on duration of mechanical ventilation of the critically ill patients in the intensive insulin therapy trial. At the molecular level, the higher steady-state mRNA levels of GLUT-4 and hexokinase II (HXK-II) found in skeletal muscle after intensive insulin therapy suggests that peripheral glucose uptake is stimulated in these patients, in comparison to the conventional treatment group (76).

The liver, the major site for gluconeogenesis, is another important insulin-sensitive organ that could be involved in the improved outcome of the patients intensively treated with insulin. However, a recent study showed that serum and gene expression levels of insulin-like growth factor binding protein-1 (IGFBP-1) and gene expression levels of phosphoenolpyruvate carboxykinase (PEPCK), the rate-limiting enzyme in the gluconeogenesis, are not regulated by insulin in critically ill patients. This may indicate that controlling gluconeogenesis was not the major factor in the normalization of blood glucose levels with exogenous insulin in the critically ill (114), although true glucose kinetics can only be estimated by glucose turn-over studies.

Nevertheless, such a study, using a well-designed canine model of critical illness, recently endorsed our findings to a great extent (115). After induction of a sublethal hypermetabolic infection in the dogs, hepatic glucose uptake was decreased and unresponsive to insulin administration. In contrast, peripheral glucose uptake did respond to insulin infusion. Contrary to our findings, insulin therapy suppressed hepatic glucose production. This occurred apparently by inhibition of glycogenolysis rather than diminished hepatic uptake of gluconeogenic amino acids and gluconeogenesis. The lack of insulin responsiveness in liver suggests that beneficial effects of insulin therapy in the this organ are mediated by avoiding hyperglycemia. In this regard, we recently demonstrated a protective effect of intensive insulin therapy on hepatocytic mitochondria of critically ill patients, where no effect was seen on the mitochondrial compartment in skeletal muscle (116). The tissue-specific effect combined with different glucose uptake mechanisms in these tissues is consistent with the direct effect of avoiding glucose toxicity on the hepatocytic mitochondria rather than of insulin.

Another major insulin-responsive organ is the adipose tissue. The increased serum free fatty acid and triglyceride levels present during critical illness and the relative accretion of adipose tissue as compared with lean body mass (muscle and bone tissue) with feeding in the protracted critically ill patient both point to a deranged lipid metabolism. This imbalance in serum lipids was partially restored by intensive insulin therapy, which significantly contributed to the reduced ICU mortality. However, its direct effects on the adipocytes remain to be investigated (76).

On the other hand, Finney et al. (117) recently published results showing that increased insulin administration is positively associated with death in the ICU regardless of the prevailing blood glucose level. Although this was an observational study mainly confirming the association of insulin resistance and risk of death, the data are in line with the previous interpretation (23) that metabolic control, rather than the absolute amount of exogenous insulin, explains the mortality benefit associated with intensive insulin therapy demonstrated by others in a randomized study (1).

Intensive insulin therapy is beneficial to kidney function and also decreases the incidence of critical illness polyneuropathy. This may in part be explained by maintenance of normoglycemia, as both organs are supposedly, at least in part, insulin-insensitive. Here, although on a totally different time scale, a parallel with Type 2 diabetes emerges. Long-term studies have indeed demonstrated that meticulous blood glucose control reduces the incidence and the severity of diabetic nephropathy—and the onset of diabetic neuropathy, and that "glucose-toxicity" may be the underlying mechanism. However, the rapid onset of critical illness polyneuropathy and of acute renal failure suggest that other factors, which predispose the critically ill to the toxic effects of hyperglycemia on neurons and kidneys, must play a role.

In a similar fashion, avoiding hyperglycemia may be important for prevention of bloodstream infections. The suppression of the immune system conceivably results in increased risk of postoperative infections, as discussed precedingly. However, the exact underlying mechanisms of the clinical benefits of intensive insulin therapy in critically ill patients remain incompletely understood at this stage (112,113).

Other areas of intensive insulin therapy that have been studied with direct relevance to the critically ill trauma patient are those who undergo cardiopulmonary bypass (CPB) for myocardial revascularization, as numerous stresses in trauma critical illness can lead to myocardial ischemia. It is already known that hyperglycemia is an independent risk factor for perioperative morbidity and mortality in both diabetic and nondiabetic patients undergoing CPB (118).

In a recent prospective trial, 280 nondiabetic adult patients undergoing first-time coronary artery bypass grafting at a single university hospital were randomized to receive GIK infusion or placebo (dextrose 5%) before, during, and for six hours after surgical intervention (119). The GIK group experienced higher cardiac indices ($P < 0.001$) throughout infusion, but also a decreased systemic vascular resistance (thus, the effect on contractility is unclear). However, of particular note is that the incidence of low cardiac output episodes was 16% (22/138) in the GIK group and 28% (39/142) in the placebo group ($P = 0.021$). Furthermore, inotropes were required in only 18.8% (26/138) of the GIK and 40.8% (58/142) of the placebo group ($P < 0.001$). Of greatest interest to the general trauma critical care population, patients in the GIK group had approximately half the rate of significant perioperative myocardial injury (16/133) versus the placebo group (32/137) ($P = 0.017$) (119).

Additional clinical and laboratory studies are required to explain the underlying molecular basis for these improved outcomes associated with aggressive insulin administration and tight blood glucose control. In addition, the benefit of aggressive insulin and tight glucose during the initial prehospital and resuscitation stages is yet to be determined.

Finally, finding the best method for maintaining tight glucose control while avoiding episodes of hypoglycema remains an important goal. Ultimately, computerized algorithms will likely perform better than insulin sliding scales administered by the bedside nurse, who can be occupied with other important patient care duties (120).

SUMMARY

In summary, hyperglycemia is a well-known accompaniment of trauma, burns, and critical illness resulting from the combined action of "counter-regulatory" hormones, cytokines, and nervous signals on glucose metabolic pathways. In addition, insulin resistance develops during critical illness, and is manifested by increased serum insulin levels, impaired peripheral glucose uptake, and elevated hepatic glucose production (18).

Recently, Van den Berghe, et al. (1) demonstrated that strict maintenance of normoglycemia by intensive insulin therapy markedly reduces mortality of ICU patients, particularly those with prolonged critical illness (mortality was reduced by half). Furthermore, the intensive insulin therapy was protective against acute renal failure, with a 42% reduction in dialytic therapy for loss of renal function (1). They also documented a decrease in the development of critical illness polyneuropathy.

Hyperglycemia has also been shown to impair immunity, and is known to inhibit the release of interleukin-1 by macrophages and oxygen radicals by neutrophils (60), and to impair phagocytosis by the macrophages (61,62). Hyperglycemia is also associated with a deranged serum lipid profile of critically ill patients. This can be partially counteracted by intensive insulin therapy, totally eliminating hypertriglyceridemia and substantially increasing the serum levels of HDL and LDL (76). Insulin is also known to have an anti-inflammatory effect; however, the exact mechanism has yet to be elucidated (82).

The authors believe blood glucose should be tightly controlled between 80 and 110 mg/dL, by continuous insulin infusion for both diabetic and nondiabetic critically ill patients. Blood sugars should be measured every one hour until stable, then weaned to sampling every four hours. Although most agree that continuous insulin infusion is superior to intermittent subcutaneous dosing, the perfect method for titrating of the insulin therapy may involve computerized protocols (120). Ultimately, bedside testing coupled with servo-controlled insulin administration devices coordinated by computer derived protocols will likely be utilized in the near future.

Caution must be observed when infusing intravenous insulin to eliminate the possibility of hypoglycemic complications. In particular, insulin must be weaned down or off whenever discontinuing enteral nutrition or peripheral glucose-containing solutions. In addition, oral anti-diabetic agents should be discontinued during critical illness.

KEY POINTS

- ☞ The stress-induced hyperglycemia, seen following severe trauma, burns, and critical illness results from the combined action of hormonal, cytokine, and nervous "counter-regulatory" signals on glucose metabolic pathways.
- ☞ The combined picture of increased serum insulin levels, impaired peripheral glucose uptake, and elevated hepatic glucose production indicates the development of insulin resistance during critical illness (18).
- ☞ Strict maintenance of normoglycemia by intensive insulin therapy markedly reduced intensive care mortality of critically ill patients (Fig. 1), particularly in the patient population with prolonged critical illness where mortality was reduced from 20.2% to 10.6% (*P* = 0.005).
- ☞ Intensive insulin therapy has emerged as a specific preventive measure for acute renal failure in critical illness, with the demonstration of a 42% reduction in the number of patients that required extracorporeal

replacement therapy to compensate for loss of renal function (1).
- ☞ Strong indications recently became available that underscore the importance of blood glucose levels in relation to the development of critical illness polyneuropathy.
- ☞ Hyperglycemia inhibits the release of interleukin-1 by macrophages and oxygen radicals by neutrophils (60). In addition, phagocytosis by macrophages is impaired under hyperglycaemic conditions (61,62).
- ☞ The derangement in serum lipid profiles seen during critical illness is partially counteracted by intensive insulin therapy; specifically, hypertriglyceridemia is completely eliminated, and serum levels of HDL and LDL are substantially increased, though not fully normalized (76).
- ☞ Although the anti-inflammatory effect of insulin has clearly been established, the exact underlying mechanisms have not yet been elucidated (82).
- ☞ The best way to achieve blood glucose control for both diabetic and nondiabetic critically ill patients. during intensive care is by continuous insulin infusion. In addition, oral anti-diabetic agents should be discontinued during critical illness.

REFERENCES

1. Van den Berghe G, Wouters P, Weekers F, et al. Intensive insulin therapy in critically ill patients. N Engl J Med 2001; 345(19):1359–1367.
2. Hill M, McCallum R. Altered transcriptional regulation of phosphoenolpyruvate carboxykinase in rats following endotoxin treatment. J Clin Invest 1991; 88(3):811–816.
3. Khani S, Tayek JA. Cortisol increases gluconeogenesis in humans: its role in the metabolic syndrome. Clin Sci (Lond) 2001; 101(6):739–747.
4. Watt MJ, Howlett KF, Febbraio MA, et al. Adrenaline increases skeletal muscle glycogenolysis, pyruvate dehydrogenase activation and carbohydrate oxidation during moderate exercise in humans. J Physiol 2001; 534(Pt 1):269–278.
5. Flores EA, Istfan N, Pomposelli JJ, et al. Effect of interleukin-1 and tumor necrosis factor/cachectin on glucose turnover in the rat. Metabolism 1990; 39(7):738–743.
6. Sakurai Y, Zhang XJ, Wolfe RR, et al. TNF directly stimulates glucose uptake and leucine oxidation and inhibits FFA flux in conscious dogs. Am J Physiol 1996; 270(5 Pt 1):E864–E872.
7. Lang CH, Dobrescu C, Bagby GJ, et al. Tumour necrosis factor impairs insulin action on peripheral glucose disposal and hepatic glucose output. Endocrinology 1992; 130(1):43–52.
8. Van den Berghe G, de Zegher F, Bouillon R, et al. Clinical review 95: acute and prolonged critical illness as different neuroendocrine paradigms. J Clin Endocrinol Metab 1998; 83(6):1827–1834.
9. Damas P, Reuter A, Gysen P, et al. Tumor necrosis factor and interleukin-1 serum levels during severe sepsis in humans. Crit Care Med 1989; 17(10):975–958.
10. Van den Berghe G, Weekers F, Baxter RC, et al. Five-day pulsatile gonadotropin-releasing hormone administration unveils combined hypothalamic-pituitary-gonadal defects underlying profound hypoandrogenism in men with prolonged critical illness. J Clin Endocrinol Metab 2001; 86(7):3217–3226.
11. Stephens JM, Bagby GJ, Pekala PH, et al. Differential regulation of glucose transporter gene expression in adipose tissue or septic rats. Biochem Biophys Res Commun 1992; 183(2): 417–422.
12. Virkamaki A, Yki-Jarvinen H. Mechanisms of insulin resistance during acute endotoxemia. Endocrinology 1994; 134(5): 2072–2078.
13. Stoner HB, Little RA, Frayn KN, et al. The effect of sepsis on the oxidation of carbohydrate and fat. Br J Surg 1983; 70(1):32–35.

14. Gore DC, Jahoor F, Hibbert JM, et al. Lactic acidosis during sepsis is related to increased pyruvate production, not deficits in tissue oxygen availability. Ann Surg 1996; 224(1):97–102.

15. Meszaros K, Lang CH, Bagby GJ, et al. In vivo glucose utilization by individual tissues during nonlethal hypermetabolic sepsis. FASEB J 1988; 2(15):3083–3086.

16. Meszaros K, Lang CH, Bagby GJ, et al. Contribution of different organs to increased glucose consumption after endotoxin administration. J Biol Chem 1987; 262(23):10965–10970.

17. Long CL, Schiller WR, Geiger JW, et al. Gluconeogenic response during glucose infusions in patients following skeletal trauma or during sepsis. J Parenter Enteral Nutr 1978; 2(5):619–626.

18. Mizock BA, Sugawara J, Tazuke SI, et al. Alterations in fuel metabolism in critical illness: hyperglycemia. Best Pract Res Clin Endocrinol Metab 2001; 15(4):533–551.

19. Capes SE, Hunt D, Malmberg K, et al. Stress hyperglycemia and increased risk of death after myocardial infarction in patients with and without diabetes: a systematic overview. Lancet 2000; 355(9206):773–778.

20. Boord JB, Graber AL, Christman JW, et al. Practical management of diabetes in critically ill patients. Am J Respir Crit Care Med 2001; 164(10 Pt 1):1763–1767.

21. Pozzilli P, Leslie RD. Infections and diabetes: mechanisms and prospects for prevention. Diabet Med 1994; 11(10):935–941.

22. McCowen KC, Malhotra A, Bistrian BR et al. Stress-induced hyperglycemia. Crit Care Clin 2001; 17(1):107–124.

23. Van den Berghe G, Wouters PJ, Bouillon R, et al. Outcome benefit of intensive insulin therapy in the critically ill: insulin dose versus glycemic control. Crit Care Med 2003; 31(2): 359–366.

24. Van den Berghe G, Schoonheydt K, Becx P, et al. Insulin therapy protects the central and peripheral nervous system of intensive care patients. Neurology 2005; 64(8):1348–1353.

25. Van den Berghe G, Wilmer A, Hermans G, et al. Intensive insulin therapy in the medical ICU. N Engl J Med 2006; 354(5):449-461.

26. Krinsley JS. Effect of an intensive glucose management protocol on the mortality of critically ill adult patients. Mayo Clin Proc 2004; 79(8):992–1000.

27. Grey NJ, Perdrizet GA. Reduction of nosocomial infections in the surgical intensive-care unit by strict glycemic control. Endoc Pract 2004; 10(2):46–52.

28. The effect of intensive treatment of diabetes on the development and progression of long-term complications in insulin-dependent diabetes mellitus. The Diabetes Control and Complications Trial Research Group. N Engl J Med 1993; 329(14):977–986.

29. Intensive blood-glucose control with sulphonylureas or insulin compared with conventional treatment and risk of complications in patients with type 2 diabetes (UKPDS 33). UK Prospective Diabetes Study (UKPDS) Group. Lancet 1998; 352(9131):837–853.

30. Mukamal KJ, Nesto RW, Cohen MC, et al. Impact of diabetes on long-term survival after acute myocardial infarction: comparability of risk with prior myocardial infarction. Diabetes Care 2001; 24(8):1422–1427.

31. Bolk J, van der Ploeg T, Cornel JH, et al. Impaired glucose metabolism predicts mortality after a myocardial infarction. Int J Cardiol 2001; 79(2–3):207–214.

32. Malmberg K, McGuire DK. Diabetes and acute myocardial infarction: the role of insulin therapy. Am Heart J 1999; 138(5 Pt 1):S381–S386.

33. Malmberg K, Ryden L, Efendic S, et al. Randomized trial of insulin-glucose infusion followed by subcutaneous insulin treatment in diabetic patients with acute myocardial infarction (DIGAMI study): effects on mortality at 1 year. J Am Coll Cardiol 1995; 26(1):57–65.

34. Malmberg K. Prospective randomised study of intensive insulin treatment on long term survival after acute myocardial infarction in patients with diabetes mellitus. DIGAMI (Diabetes Mellitus, Insulin Glucose Infusion in Acute Myocardial Infarction) Study Group. BMJ 1997; 314(7093): 1512–1515.

35. Malmberg K, Ryden L, Hamsten A, et al. Effects of insulin treatment on cause-specific one-year mortality and morbidity in diabetic patients with acute myocardial infarction. DIGAMI Study Group. Diabetes Insulin-Glucose in Acute Myocardial Infarction. Eur Heart J 1996; 17(9):1337–1344.

36. Furnary AP, Wu Y, Bookin SO, et al. Effect of hyperglycemia and continuous intravenous insulin infusions on outcomes of cardiac surgical procedures: the Portland Diabetic Project. Endocr Pract 2004; 10(suppl 2):21–33.

37. Williams LS, Rotich J, Qi R, et al. Effects of admission hyperglycemia on mortality and costs in acute ischemic stroke. Neurology 2002; 59(1):67–71.

38. Capes SE, Hunt D, Malmberg K, et al. Stress hyperglycemia and prognosis of stroke in nondiabetic and diabetic patients: a systematic overview. Stroke 2001; 32(10):2426–2432.

39. Rovlias A, Kotsou S. The influence of hyperglycemia on neurological outcome in patients with severe head injury. Neurosurgery 2000; 46(2):335–342; discussion 42–43.

40. Jeremitsky E, Omert LA, Dunham M, et al. The impact of hyperglycemia on patients with severe brain injury. J Trauma 2005; 58(1):47–50.

41. Yendamuri S, Fulda GJ, Tinkoff GH, et al. Admission hyperglycemia as a prognostic indicator in trauma. J Trauma 2003; 55(1):33–38.

42. Laird AM, Miller PR, Kilgo PD, et al. Relationship of early hyperglycemia to mortality in trauma patients. J Trauma 2004; 56(5):1058–1062.

43. Gore DC, Chinkes D, Heggers J, et al. Association of hyperglycemia with increased mortality after severe burn injury. J Trauma 2001; 51(3):540.

44. Faustino EV, Apkon M. Persistent hyperglycemia in critically ill children. J Pediatr 2005; 146(1):30–34.

45. Krinsley JS. Association between hyperglycemia and increased hospital mortality in a heterogeneous population of critically ill patients. Mayo Clin Proc 2003; 78(12):1471–1478.

46. Das UN. Insulin: an endogenous cardio-protector. Curr Opin Crit Care 2003; 9(5):375–383.

47. Jonassen A, Aasum E, Riemersma R, et al. Glucose-insulin-potassium reduces infarct size when administered during reperfusion. Cardiovasc Drugs Ther 2000; 14(6):615–623.

48. Malmberg K, Ryden L, Wedel H, et al. Intense metabolic control by means of insulin in patients with diabetes mellitus and acute myocardial infarction (DIGAMI-2): effects on mortality and morbidity. Eur Heart J 2005; 26(7):650–661.

49. Mehta SR, Yusuf S, Diaz R, et al. The CREATE-ECLA Trial Group Investigators. Effect of glucose-insulin-potassium infusion on mortality in patients with acute ST-segment elevation myocardial infarction. The CREATE-ECLA randomized controlled trial. JAMA 2005; 293(4):437–446.

50. Bothe W, Olschewski M, Beyersdorf F, et al. Glucose-insulin-potassium in cardiac surgery: a meta-analysis. Ann Thorac Surg 2004; 78(5):1650–1657.

51. Gao F, Gao E, Yue T, et al. Nitric oxide mediates the anti-apoptotic effect of insulin in myocardial ischemia-reperfusion: the role of PI3-kinase, Akt and eNOS phosphorylation. Circulation 2002; 105(12):1497–1502.

52. Jonassen A, Sack M, Mjos O, et al. Myocardial protection by insulin at reperfusion requires early administration and is mediated via Akt and p70s6 kinase cell-survival signalling. Circ Res 2001; 89(12):1191–1198.

53. Scott JF, Robinson GM, French JM, et al. Glucose potassium insulin infusions in the treatment of acute stroke patients with mild to moderate hyperglycemia: the Glucose Insulin in Stroke Trial (GIST). Stroke 1999; 30(4):793–799.

54. Murray P, Hall J. Renal replacement therapy for acute renal failure. Am J Respir Crit Care Med 2000; 162(3 Pt 1): 777–781.

55. Boulton AJ. Clinical presentation and management of diabetic neuropathy and foot ulceration. Diabet Med 1991; 8(Spec No):S52–S57.

56. Hund E. Neurological complications of sepsis: critical illness polyneuropathy and myopathy. J Neurol 2001; 248(11): 929–934.

57. Leijten FS, De Weerd AW, Poortvliet DC, et al. Critical illness polyneuropathy in multiple organ dysfunction syndrome and weaning from the ventilator. Intensive Care Med 1996; 22(9):856–861.

58. Bolton CF, Young GB. Critical Illness Polyneuropathy. Curr Treat Options Neurol 2000; 2(6):489–498.

59. Bolton CF. Sepsis and the systemic inflammatory response syndrome: neuromuscular manifestations. Crit Care Med 1996; 24(8):1408–1416.

60. Nielson CP, Hindson DA. Inhibition of polymorphonuclear leukocyte respiratory burst by elevated glucose concentrations in vitro. Diabetes 1989; 38(8):1031–1035.

61. Kwoun MO, Ling PR, Lydon E, et al. Immunologic effects of acute hyperglycemia in nondiabetic rats. J Parenter Enteral Nutr 1997; 21(2):91–95.

62. Rassias AJ, Marrin CA, Arruda J, et al. Insulin infusion improves neutrophil function in diabetic cardiac surgery patients. Anesth Analg 1999; 88(5).1011–1016.

63. Rayfield EJ, Ault MJ, Keusch GT, et al. Infection and diabetes: the case for glucose control. Am J Med 1982; 72(3):439–450.

64. Rassias AJ, Givan AL, Marrin CA, et al. Insulin increases neutrophil count and phagocytic capacity after cardiac surgery. Anesth Analg 2002; 94(5):1113–1119.

65. Zerr KJ, Furnary AP, Grunkemeier GL, et al. Glucose control lowers the risk of wound infection in diabetics after open heart operations. Ann Thorac Surg 1997; 63(2):356–361.

66. Furnary AP, Zerr KJ, Grunkemeier GL, et al. Continuous intravenous insulin infusion reduces the incidence of deep sternal wound infection in diabetic patients after cardiac surgical procedures. Ann Thorac Surg 1999; 67(2):352–360; discussion 360–362.

67. Weekers F, Van Herck E, Coopmans W, et al. A novel in vivo rabbit model of hypercatabolic critical illness reveals a biphasic neuroendocrine stress response. Endocrinology 2002; 143(3):764–774.

68. Weekers F, Giulietti A, Michalaki M, et al. Metabolic, endocrine and immune effects of stress hyperglycemia in a rabbit model of prolonged critical illness. Endocrinology 2003; 144(12): 5329–5338.

69. Taskinen MR. Pathogenesis of dyslipidemia in type 2 diabetes. Exp Clin Endocrinol Diabetes 2001; 109(suppl 2):S180–S188.

70. Lanza-Jacoby S, Wong SH, Tabares A, et al. Disturbances in the composition of plasma lipoproteins during gram-negative sepsis in the rat. Biochim Biophys Acta 1992; 1124(3):233–240.

71. Khovidhunkit W, Memon RA, Feingold KR, et al. Infection and inflammation-induced proatherogenic changes of lipoproteins. J Infect Dis 2000; 181(suppl 3):S462–S472.

72. Carpentier YA, Scruel O. Changes in the concentration and composition of plasma lipoproteins during the acute phase response. Curr Opin Clin Nutr Metab Care 2002; 5(2):153–158.

73. Gordon BR, Parker TS, Levine DM, et al. Low lipid concentrations in critical illness: implications for preventing and treating endotoxemia. Crit Care Med 1996; 24(4):584–589.

74. Feingold KR, Krauss RM, Pang M, et al. The hypertriglyceridemia of acquired immunodeficiency syndrome is associated with an increased prevalence of low density lipoprotein subclass pattern B. J Clin Endocrinol Metab 1993; 76(6):1423–1427.

75. Kwiterovich PO Jr. Lipoprotein heterogeneity: diagnostic and therapeutic implications. Am J Cardiol 2002; 90(8A):1i–10i.

76. Mesotten D, Swinnen JV, Vanderhoydonc F, et al. The relative contribution of lipid and glucose control to the improved outcome of critical illness obtained by intensive insulin therapy. J Clin Endocrinol Metab 2004; 89(1):219–226.

77. Tulenko TN, Sumner AE. The physiology of lipoproteins. J Nucl Cardiol 2002; 9(6):638–649.

78. Harris HW, Grunfeld C, Feingold KR, et al. Human very low density lipoproteins and chylomicrons can protect against endotoxin-induced death in mice. J Clin Invest 1990; 86(3):696–702.

79. Harris HW, Grunfeld C, Feingold KR, et al. Chylomicrons alter the fate of endotoxin, decreasing tumor necrosis factor release and preventing death. J Clin Invest 1993; 91(3):1028–1034.

80. Harris HW, Johnson JA,Wigmore SJ, et al. Endogenous lipoproteins impact the response to endotoxin in humans. Crit Care Med 2002; 30(1):23–31.

81. Hansen TK, Thiel S, Wouters PJ, et al. Intensive insulin therapy exerts anti-inflammatory effects in critically ill patients and counteracts the adverse effect of low mannose-binding lectin levels. J Clin Endocrinol Metab 2003; 88(3):1082–1088.

82. Das UN. Is insulin an anti-inflammatory molecule? Nutrition 2001; 17(5):409–413.

83. Satomi N, Sakurai A, Haranaka K, et al. Relationship of hypoglycemia to tumor necrosis factor production and antitumor activity: role of glucose, insulin, and macrophages. J Natl Cancer Inst 1985; 74(6):1255–1260.

84. Fraker DL, Merino MJ, Norton JA, et al. Reversal of the toxic effects of cachectin by concurrent insulin administration. Am J Physiol 1989; 256(6 Pt 1):E725–E731.

85. Sakaue S, Nishihira J, Hirokawa J, et al. Regulation of macrophage migration inhibitory factor (MIF) expression by glucose and insulin in adipocytes in vitro. Mol Med 1999; 5(6):361–371.

86. Chen HC, Guh JY, Shin SJ, et al. Insulin and heparin suppress superoxide production in diabetic rat glomeruli stimulated with low-density lipoprotein. Kidney Int Suppl 2001; 78:S124–S127.

87. Cowley HC, Heney D, Gearing AJ, et al. Increased circulating adhesion molecule concentrations in patients with the systemic inflammatory response syndrome: a prospective cohort study. Crit Care Med 1994; 22(4):651–657.

88. Sessler, CN, Windsor AC, Schwartz M, et al. Circulating ICAM-1 is increased in septic shock. Am J Respir Crit Care Med 1995; 151(5):1420–1427.

89. Boldt J, Wollbruck M, Kuhn D, et al. Do plasma levels of circulating soluble adhesion molecules differ between surviving and nonsurviving critically ill patients? Chest 1995; 107(3):787–792.

90. Kayal S, Jais JP, Aguini N. Elevated circulating E-selectin, intercellular adhesion molecule 1, and von Willebrand factor in patients with severe infection. Am J Respir Crit Care Med 1998; 157(3 Pt 1):776–784.

91. Whalen MJ, Doughty LA, Carlos TM. Intercellular adhesion molecule-1 and vascular cell adhesion molecule-1 are increased in the plasma of children with sepsis-induced multiple organ failure. Crit Care Med 2000; 28(7):2600–2607.

92. Langouche L, Vanhorebeek I, Vlasselaers D, et al. Intensive insulin therapy protects the endothelium of critically ill patients. J Clin Invest 2005; 115(8):2277–2286.

93. Carr ME. Diabetes mellitus: a hyper-coagulable state. J Diabetes Complications 2001; 15(1):44–54.

94. Calles-Escandon J, Garcia-Rubi E, Mirza S, et al. Type 2 diabetes: one disease, multiple cardiovascular risk factors. Coron Artery Dis 1999; 10(1):23–30.

95. Williams E, Timperley WR, Ward JD, et al. Electron microscopical studies of vessels in diabetic peripheral neuropathy. J Clin Pathol 1980; 33(5):462–470.

96. Patrassi GM, Vettor R, Padovan D, et al. Contact phase of blood coagulation in diabetes mellitus. Eur J Clin Invest 1982; 12(4):307–311.

97. Carmassi F, Morale M, Puccetti R, et al. Coagulation and fibrinolytic system impairment in insulin dependent diabetes mellitus. Thromb Res 1992; 67(6):643–654.

98. Hughes A, McVerry BA, Wilkinson L, et al. Diabetes, a hyper-coagulable state? Hemostatic variables in newly diagnosed type 2 diabetic patients. Acta Haematol 1983; 69(4):254–259.

99. Garcia Frade LJ, de la Calle H, Alava I, et al. Diabetes mellitus as a hyper-coagulable state: its relationship with fibrin fragments and vascular damage. Thromb Res 1987; 47(5):533–540.

100. Vukovich TC, Schernthaner G. Decreased protein C levels in patients with insulin-dependent type I diabetes mellitus. Diabetes 1986; 35(5):617–619.

101. Garcia Frade LJ, Landin L, Avello AG, et al. Changes in fibrinolysis in the intensive care patient. Thromb Res 1987; 47(5): 593–599.

102. Mavrommatis AC, Theodoridis T, Economou M, et al. Activation of the fibrinolytic system and utilization of the coagulation inhibitors in sepsis: comparison with severe sepsis and septic shock. Intensive Care Med 2001; 27(12): 1853–1859.

103. Schloerb PR, Henning JF. Patterns and problems of adult total parenteral nutrition use in US academic medical centers. Arch Surg 1998; 133(1):7–12.

104. Klein CJ, Stanek GS, Wiles CE 3rd, et al. Overfeeding macronutrients to critically ill adults: metabolic complications. J Am Diet Assoc 1998; 98(7):795–806.

105. McCowen KC, Friel C, Sternberg J, et al. Hypocaloric total parenteral nutrition: effectiveness in prevention of hyperglycemia and infectious complications—a randomized clinical trial. Crit Care Med 2000; 28(11):3606–3611.

106. Patino JF, de Pimiento SE, Vergara A, et al. Hypocaloric support in the critically ill. World J Surg 1999; 23(6):553–559.

107. Choban PS, Burge JC, Scales D, et al. Hypo-energetic nutrition support in hospitalized obese patients: a simplified method for clinical application. Am J Clin Nutr 1997; 66(3):546–550.

108. Soop M, Nygren J, Myrenfors P, et al. Pre-operative oral carbohydrate treatment attenuates immediate postoperative insulin resistance. Am J Physiol Endocrinol Metab 2001; 280(4): E576–E583.

109. Landstedt-Hallin L, Englund A, Adamson U, et al. Increased QT dispersion during hypoglycemia in patients with type 2 diabetes mellitus. J Intern Med 1999; 246(3):299–307.

110. Pollock G, Brady WJ Jr, Hargarten S, et al. Hypoglycemia manifested by sinus bradycardia: a report of three cases. Acad Emerg Med 1996; 3(7):700–707.

111. Chelliah YR. Ventricular arrhythmias associated with hypoglycemia. Anaesth Intensive Care 2000; 28(6):698–700.

112. Van den Berghe G. How does blood glucose control with insulin save lives in intensive care? J Clin Invest 2004; 114(9):1187–1195.

113. Vanhorebeek I, Langouche L, Van den Berghe G, et al. Glycemic and nonglycemic effects of insulin: how do they contribute to a better outcome of critical illness? Curr Opin Crit Care 2005; 11(4):304–311.

114. Mesotten D, Delhanty PJD, Vanderhoydonc F, et al. Regulation of insulin-like growth factor binding protein-1 during protracted critical illness. J Clin Endocrinol Metab 2002; 87(12):5516–5523.

115. Donmoyer CM, Chen SS, Lacy DB, et al. Infection impairs insulin-dependent hepatic glucose uptake during total parenteral nutrition. Am J Physiol Endocrinol Metab 2003; 284(3):E574–E582.

116. Vanhorebeek I, De Vos R, Mesotten D, et al. Strict blood glucose control with insulin in critically ill patients protects hepatocytic mitochondrial ultrastructure and function. Lancet 2005; 365(9453):53–59.

117. Finney SJ, Zekveld C, Elia A, Evans TW, et al. Glucose control and mortality in critically ill patients. JAMA 2003; 290:2041–2047.

118. Doenst T, Wijeysundera D, Karkouti K, et al. Hyperglycemia during cardiopulmonary bypass is an independent risk factor for mortality in patients undergoing cardiac surgery. J Thorac Cardiovasc Surg 2005; 130(4):1144a–1144e.

119. Quinn DW, Pagano D, Bonser RS, et al. Improved myocardial protection during coronary artery surgery with glucose-insulin-potassium: a randomized controlled trial. J Thorac Cardiovasc Surg 2006; 131:34–42.

120. Plank J, Blaha J, Cordingley ME, et al. Multicentric, randomized, controlled trial to evaluate blood glucose control by the model predictive control algorithm versus routine glucose management protocols in intensive care unit patients. Diabetes Care 2006; 29(2):271–276.

61

Thyroid and Parathyroid Disorders in Critical Care

Jon C. White

Department of Surgery, VA Medical Center, George Washington University, Washington, D.C., U.S.A.

Eric S. Nylen

Department of Endocrinology, George Washington University, VA Medical Center, Washington, D.C., U.S.A.

INTRODUCTION

Most patients in intensive care units (ICU) with thyroid or parathyroid disorders do not have an endocrine abnormality as their primary problem. Indeed, most endocrine hormonal derangements observed in the ICU may be attributed to primary, nonendocrine illness(es) that promote a secondary adaptation in hormonal levels. The converse is also true; primary endocrine problems modulate a patient's response to nonendocrine illness. Trauma, in particular, is a global disorder, and the clinical course of individuals recovering from trauma is directly related to their pretraumatic state. Because the endocrine system plays such an important role in a patient's premorbid homeostasis, endocrine dysfunction places the trauma victim at greater risk for morbidity and mortality.

Usually the status of the endocrine system is assessed by measurement of hormone levels. In critical illness, however, these levels are frequently deranged as the endocrine system undergoes an adaptive response to reestablish homeostasis. Thus, a primary objective of this chapter is to provide guidance for determining whether abnormal thyroid or parathyroid hormone levels occur as a result of primary endocrine disorders or due to adaptive responses of the endocrine system to nonendocrine illness.

The endocrine system is made up of glands that produce and secrete hormones, which are transported by the bloodstream to act on specific target organs. These hormones are usually measured while in transit in the systemic circulation, where their levels are influenced, and are indicative of disordered physiological states. Serum levels of these hormones can be used for diagnosing both endocrine and nonendocrine illness. Either administration or blockade of these hormones may be used for therapeutic purposes. The thyroid and the parathyroid glands are representative of the endocrine system insofar as their hormone products have been used for both diagnosis and therapy. This chapter will first address problems related to thyroid dysfunction in the ICU (Section II) and then review the clinical manifestations of parathyroid dysfunction in critically ill patients (Section III). Future directions in the diagnosis and treatment of thyroid and parathyroid disorders are discussed in Section IV. Key points and important concepts presented in this chapter are summarized in Section V.

THYROID DYSFUNCTION IN THE ICU

Thyroid disorders in critically ill patients may present as "euthyroid sick syndrome," as myxedema in patients with pre-existing hypothyroidism, or as thyrotoxicosis in patients with pre-existing hyperthyroid states. The signs and symptoms of all three conditions are easy to confuse with the signs of other systemic illnesses. Thus, it is important to ascertain each patient's premorbid thyroid state and to understand the perturbations that the thyroid axis causes to patients with severe illness, if these thyroid disorders are going to be properly diagnosed and managed.

Anatomy and Physiology of the Thyroid Gland
Anatomy
The thyroid gland is a 15 to 20 gm, bilobed gland that lies directly anterior to the tracheal rings and cephalad to the thyroid cartilage. This position has clinical relevance insofar as thyroid enlargement may cause embarrassment to the aerodigestive tract and block emergent access to the trachea. The blood supply to the thyroid is abundant with paired inferior thyroid arteries, paired upper thyroid arteries, and occasionally a central thyroidea in an artery. The vascularity of the gland, plus its location adjacent to the parathyroid glands and next to the paired recurrent laryngeal nerves and paired superior laryngeal nerves (nerves of Galli-Curci), make surgical approaches to the gland challenging. The thyroid parenchyma is comprised mainly of follicular cells, which are arranged in acini and are responsible for the secretion of thyroid hormone. The less abundant parafollicular cells (C cells) are neuroendocrine cells, which are part of the APUD system (amine containing, precursor uptake, and decarboxylase). These cells secrete calcitonin (1), whose precursor molecule, procalcitonin, has recently been recognized as an important marker for a number of inflammatory states, often seen in critically ill patients (e.g., sepsis (1), pancreatitis (2), pneumonitis (3), smoke inhalation (4), and heat stroke (5).

The production, storage, and secretion of thyroid hormone (Fig. 1) are the most important functions of the thyroid gland (the designation of thyroid hormone in this section will refer to thyroxine and triiodothyronine rather than calcitonin). This is accomplished by concentrating

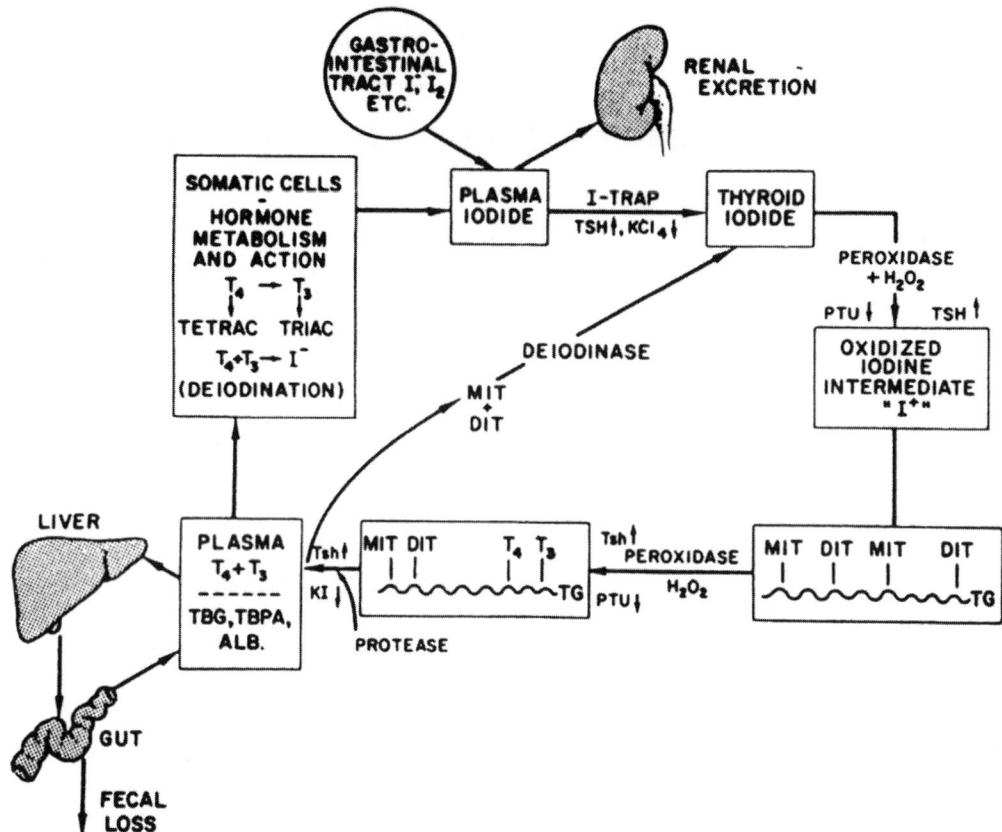

Figure 1 A diagram detailing the iodine cycle. Iodine from the gastrointestinal tract is trapped in the thyroid where it is bound to tyrosine to form either monoiodothyrosine (MIT) or diiodothyrosine (DIT). MIT and DIT are then coupled to form triiodothyronine (T3) or thyroxine (T4). Some T4 is deiodinated outside of the gland to form T3, the more active hormone. After T3 and T4 are utilized, they are deiodinated and the iodine is returned to the plasma where it is recycled.

plasma iodide in the gland via a specific and rate-limiting, ATP-dependent, sodium-iodide symporter protein, which can also transport monovalent anions and chemicals such as lithium. Following transport, the iodine is stored in thyroglobulin. Organification, performed by the enzyme thyroid peroxidase, occurs by iodinating tyrosine molecules to make monoiodotyrosine (MIT) and diiodotyrosine (DIT), and then combining these molecules to make the physiologically active hormones, triiodothyronine (T3), and thyroxine (T4). This entire process is stimulated by the pituitary peptide, thyrotropin, or thyroid-stimulating hormone (TSH). The hormonally active T3 and T4 are stored in the thyroid gland, bound to thyroglobulin and, in this state, form intrafollicular colloid. ☞ **Thyroxine, the prohormone, is the predominately released species upon TSH stimulation; most of the triiodothyronine, the bioactive hormone, is produced by extrathyroidal conversion.** ☞ The thyroid stores an enormous amount of thyroid hormone in colloid and can maintain a euthyroid state for several months without synthesis.

The mechanisms and regulations of thyroid secretion are complex, with the cerebral cortex stimulating thyrotropin-releasing hormone (TRH) from the hypothalamus, which in turn stimulates TSH release from the anterior pituitary. The feedback loops are both positive and negative, resulting in a very carefully regulated secretion of thyroid hormone from the thyroid gland (Fig. 2). The levels of iodide in the blood also influence the production of thyroid hormone; an important fact to keep in mind in

critically ill patients who may be administered medications high in iodine (e.g., amiodarone).

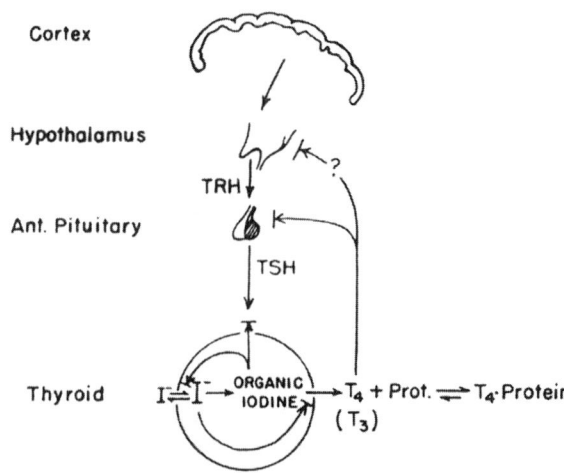

Figure 2 The mechanism of thyroid hormone regulation. The unbound fraction of thyroxine (T4) in the blood influences the secretion of thyroid stimulating hormone from the pituitary using a negative feedback mechanism. Although the control of thyroid releasing hormone secretion from the hypothalamus is unknown, it may also be subject to the same negative feedback mechanism by unbound T4 levels.

Metabolic Effects

The metabolic effects of thyroid hormone are considerable and affect most tissues in the body. In general, thyroid hormone promotes growth and maturation by increasing protein turnover, oxygen consumption, heat production, and oxidative phosphorylation. These anabolic functions, however, are of secondary importance during stress when most bodily functions are focused on responding to injury-related problems such as inflammation, hypotension, or shock. For this reason, the decreased level of thyroid hormone during stress may be a teleologically programmed adaptive response. ☞ **Levels of thyroid hormone should not necessarily be normalized during critical illness.** ☞

Pharmacology

Medications commonly used to treat hyperthyroidism block the synthesis of thyroid hormone, its release from the thyroid, or its peripheral conversion. Other medications used for hyperthyroidism treat the symptoms (Table 1).

As noted above, iodide (and its oxidized form iodine) influence the production of thyroid hormone. Small amounts increase the production of hormone while larger, pharmacological doses (e.g., potassium iodide or Lugol's solution) decrease the release of active hormone from the thyroid gland and can be used to treat thyrotoxicosis. ☞ **This biphasic response to iodide is important insofar as iodide administration can precipitate either hyperthyroidism or hypothyroidism.** ☞

There are multiple antithyroid medications. Potassium perchlorate interferes with the uptake of iodine by the thyroid, although it is used less often than the thionamides due to its unacceptable side effects. The thionamide derivatives propylthiouracil (PTU) and methyl-mercapto-imidazole (MMI) prevent oxidation of iodide to iodine and block the synthesis of the hormone. PTU also interferes with the peripheral conversion of T4 to T3, an important distinction between the two drugs. Lithium carbonate is a second-line antithyroid drug that decreases thyroidal secretion. Although lithium is not often used therapeutically for hyperthyroidism, its effect on thyroid hormone should be kept in mind when it is being used for nonthyroidal illnesses (discussed below). Beta-adrenergic blockers (e.g.,

propranolol) and, less commonly, alpha-adrenergic blockers (e.g., reserpine) are used to control the symptoms of thyrotoxicosis while waiting for other drugs to decrease hormone levels or for rapid control of symptoms prior to surgery.

Studies of Thyroid Function

Thyroid Function Tests

Thyroid function tests measure serum levels of T4, T3, and TSH (Table 2). As previously mentioned, T4 is considered a prohormone of T3. Although it is less potent, there is usually more T4 than T3 present. There are important circulating thyroid binding proteins, which can alter the measured total T4 or T3 levels. ☞ **Many problems seen in the ICU cause either increased or decreased binding of thyroid hormone to its binding proteins, which may make the total hormone levels abnormal while the free, active hormone levels are normal or vice versa.** ☞ Most laboratories now use two-step analog methods to establish the free (unbound) and hormonally active fraction of T4, thereby avoiding but not eliminating prior methods of protein binding. The more accurate equilibrium dialysis method of measuring the free T4 is cumbersome but more precise (6).

Due to the negative feedback by T4 on TSH, measurements of TSH have become the most useful tests in diagnosing hyper- and hypo-thyroid states as well as determining whether T4 administration is sufficient for suppression. Two-site noncompetitive immunometric monoclonal assays for TSH have now reached third-generation capability; i.e., the functional sensitivity is 0.01–0.02 µU/mL which can reliably separate euthyroid conditions from hyperthyroidism and subclinical hyperthyroidism, as well as nonthyroidal illness (NTI). This refinement in TSH measurement has resulted in this test becoming the initial and often the sole test to evaluate all thyroid abnormalities. Note, however, that the TSH test is not accurate in patients with pituitary insufficiency, due to either the pituitary pathology or the concurrent use of dopamine, dobutamine, or glucocorticoids.

Table 1 Drugs Used to Treat Hyperthyroidism and the Steps Blocked

Step blocked	TH synthesis	Thyroid secretion	Peripheral conversion of T4 to T3	Symptoms
Drugs used (dose, route, interval)	PTU[a] (100–150 mg, po, tid, acutely) MMI[b] (10–15 mg/day, po, tid, acutely) Potassium perchlorate (0.6–1 g, po, qd)	Iodides[c] (5 drops Lugols, po, qd) Ipodate sodium (0.5 g, po, qd) Lithium (300 mg, po, tid) Corticosteroids (see next column)	PTU[a] (100–300 mg, po, tid) Beta blockers (see next column) Ipodate sodium (0.5 g, po, qd) Lithium (300 mg, po, tid) Corticosteroids (see next column)	Beta-blockers (e.g., propanalol, 10–80 mg, po qid or 1–2 mg, q15 min, iv) Alpha-blockers (e.g., reserpine or guanethidine for gradual control) Corticosteroids (e.g., hydrocortisone, 100–500 mg, iv, bid)

[a]100–200 mg/day for maintenance.
[b]5–15 mg/day for maintenance.
[c]In thyroid storm a loading dose of PTU or MMI should be given before iodides are started.
Abbreviations: PTU, polythiouracil; MMI, mercapto-imidazole; po, by mouth; qd, once a day; tid, three times a day; qid, four times a day.

Table 2 Thyroid Assays

Peptide measured	Range of normal values conventional (SI units)	Assay, limitations
Total T4 (bound and free T4)	4.5–12.5 µg/dL (58–161 nmol/L)	RIA, hemolysis may cause a false decrease
Total T3	80–220 ng/dL (1.23–3.39 nmol/L)	RIA, no interference
Free T4	0.7–1.5 ng/dL (9.0–19.4 pmol/L)	Labeled antibody immunoassays (TS and AM). TS is comparable to ED, while AM often disagrees with ED in acute illness and other conditions, including NTI
Free T3	230–420 pg/dL (3.5–6.5 pmol/L)	RIA, heparin causes false low values
Reverse T3	80–350 ng/L (123–539 pmol/L)	RIA, no interference
TSH	0.3–5.0 µIU/mL (0.3–5.0 mIU/L)	The second-generation assay detects levels as low as 0.1–0.5 µIU/mL, so the range of subnormal values is limited. The third-generation assay measures levels as low as 0.01-0.05 µIU/mL which is more reliable for hyperthyroid states

Abbreviations: RIA, radioimmunoassay; TS, two-step; AM, analog method; ED, equilibrium dialysis; NTI, nonthyroidal illness.

Radioiodine

Radioactive isotopes (I^{131}, I^{123}, technetium^{99}) given orally or intravenously are concentrated in the thyroid and read by a gamma camera. Small amounts of these radioisotopes are used as tests to assess the function of the gland or localize ectopic thyroid tissue (e.g., thyroid cancer metastases), while administration of higher amounts of radioactivity can be used to ablate thyroid tissue. Although this is not a modality commonly used in the ICUs, patients who have been treated with radioactive iodine should be evaluated carefully for hypothyroidism.

Drugs that Interfere with Thyroid Studies

Patients in intensive care units often receive multiple medications. These medications may interfere with thyroid function itself, measurement of thyroid hormone, peripheral conversion of T4 to T3, or measurement of TSH. Drugs commonly used in the ICU that affect thyroid hormone status are shown on Table 3. In addition, phenytoin and carbamezapine both increase T4 metabolism and decrease T4 binding. Certain nonsteroidal anti-inflammatory drugs (and aspirin) displace T4 from binding proteins. Furosemide, at high doses used in renal insufficiency, lowers T4 levels. Several medications, such as dobutamine, dopamine, and glucocorticoids, decrease TSH levels, whereas propanolol and other b-blockers decrease the peripheral conversion of T4 to T3 (and are therapeutically useful in managing thyroid storm). These many drug interactions must be kept in mind when interpreting thyroid function tests in critically ill patients. Other commonly used medications, which affect thyroid function, are listed on Table 3.

Hypothyroid Disorders in Critically Ill Patients

Hypothyroidism is clinically expressed as lack of energy, intolerance to cold, weight gain, lethargy, dry skin, and prolongation of the relaxation phase of deep tendon reflexes (Table 4). When these symptoms are present and TSH levels are elevated (i.e., >20 µU/mL), the diagnosis is easy to make. When subclinical hypothyroidism exists, there are scant signs and symptoms, the free T4 level is normal, and the TSH is mildly elevated but usually less than 20 µU/mL. When overt hypothyroidism is recognized, it is easily treated with thyroid hormone replacement (approximately 1.2–1.6 µg/kg/d of levothyroxine). Subclinical hypothyroidism may also necessitate treatment. There are a number of conditions that cause hypothyroidism (Table 5). Importantly, some of these conditions may also cause hyperthyroidism.

Euthyroid Sick Syndrome

The euthyroid sick syndrome (ESS) is the most frequently encountered thyroid condition in the ICU. In this condition, abnormal thyroid function indices develop in otherwise euthyroid patients who have a variety of illnesses such as infections, renal failure, liver disease, stress, starvation, surgery, acute myocardial infarction, stroke, poorly-controlled diabetes, cancer, and burns (7,8). Although the etiology of ESS is unclear, other neuroendocrine systems, such as the hypothalamic-pituitary-gonadal and somatotropic axes, undergo parallel changes, which are thought to minimize the catabolic impact of severe illness and malnutrition. ☞ **In ESS, there are perturbations in the entire hypothalamic-pituitary-thyroid hormone system and it is unclear if these patients are truly euthyroid or**

Table 3 Effects of Drugs on Thyroid Function

Inhibit thyroid function	Increase binding protein	Decrease binding protein	Inhibit T4 to T3 conversion	Decrease TSH	Increase TSH
Iodine Lithium Sulfonylureas Interleukin-2	Estrogens Clofibrate Opiates 5-fluorouracil	Androgens Glucocorticoids Danazol L-asparaginase Salicylates	Glucocorticoids Ipodate Propranolol Amiodarone Propylthiouracil	Glucocorticoids Dopamine agonists Dobutamine Somatostatin	Iodine Lithium Dopamine agonists Cimetidine

Abbreviation: TSH, thyroid-stimulating hormone.

Table 4 Common Manifestations of Hyperthyroidism and Hypothyroidism

Organ system affected	Hyperthyroidism	Hypothyroidism
Central nervous system	Poor concentration, headache, confusion (with thyroid storm: agitated, delirious, tremulous)	Lethargy, may progress to myxedema coma
Cardiac rhythm	Palpitations, atrial fibrillation	Bradycardia
Cardiac musculature	Myopathy, heart failure	Nonpitting edema (myxedema)
Cardiopulmonary symptoms	Shortness of breath, (as GI fluid losses progresses, may develop hypotension and vascular collapse)	Hypotension, hypoventilation
Thyroid size	Goiter	Sometimes thyroid not palpable
Integumentary	Warm, moist, flushed skin (due to vasodilation)	Dry skin, brittle nails, puffy skin, palor, periorbital edema, patchy hair loss
Metabolism	Hyperactivity, weight loss, fever	Decreased activity, obesity, hypothermia
Musculo-skeletal system	Tetany, spasms, seizure	Malaise, fatigue, weakness, tremor, slow relaxation of deep tendon reflexes
Eyes	Lid retraction, exophthalmos	Cataracts
Gastrointestinal	Diarrhea	Mild constipation to severe obstipation
Menstruation	Decreased menstrual bleeding	Increased menstrual bleeding

perhaps have central hypothyroidism (9). For this reason, the term NTI may be more appropriate than ESS. The clinical expression in NTI follows a certain pattern, which is shown in Figure 3. In the early (or mild) phase, the T3 level is low with a parallel increase in reverse T3, the inert metabolite of T4 (low T3 syndrome). This is thought to be due to both inhibition of the enzyme 5'-iodinase and alternate metabolism of T4. These changes occur in the majority of hospitalized patients. With increased gravity of illness or disease progression, total T4 levels decrease (low T4 syndrome), despite normal or slightly elevated free T4 (measured by equilibrium dialysis). These changes occur due to increased T4 clearance, which is the result of abnormal production and binding of thyroid-binding protein. Low measured levels of both T3 and T4 portend a poor prognosis and parallel (inversely) APACHE II scores. In one study 84% of patients who had T4 levels <3 µg/dL died, although it is not clear whether these decreased levels of T4 contributed to morbidity or were only indicators of the severity of illness (10). Low T4 levels that persist for greater than one week also correlate with higher mortality. In NTI, the TSH is usually normal or slightly low which is detectable with the third-generation TSH assay. TSH may surge with recovery from the illness and reach levels seen in mild hypothyroidism, but usually stays <20 µg/dL (11).

Thus, there are several issues that must be kept in when caring for these challenging patients: (*i*) Serum thyroid hormone levels are fraught with interpretive problems making it difficult to determine which patients with hypothyroidism need urgent treatment. (*ii*) The NTI

Table 5 Conditions Causing Hypothyroidism

Drugs
 Thionamides
 Iodide[a]
 Amiodarone[a]
 Lithium[a]
Thyroiditis
 Hashimoto[a]
 Subacute (viral)
 Silent
Ablation of thyroid tissue
 Radioactive
 Surgical
Infiltrative diseases
 Sarcoidosis
 Lymphoma
 Metastatic malignancy[a]
Endocrine
 End stage Graves[a]
 TRH deficiency
 TSH deficiency
 TH resistance

[a]Also causes hyperthyroidism.

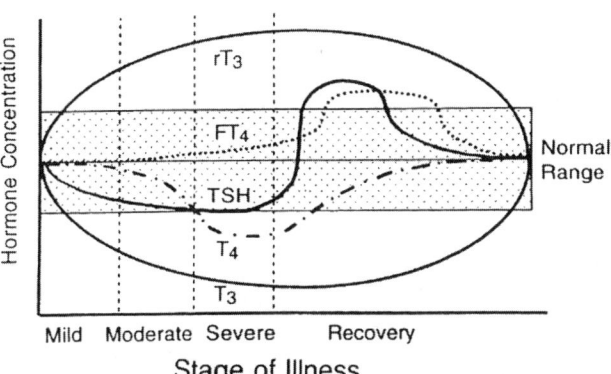

Stage of Illness

Figure 3 Serum levels of T3, T4, rT3, FT4, and TSH during euthyroid sick syndrome, also known as nonthyroidal illness (NTI). Early in the illness, levels of the active hormone (T3) are depressed while levels of the inactive metabolite (rT3) are high. This trend reverses as NTI resolves. TSH decreases as the illness worsens, but is transiently elevated during the recovery phase. T4 levels stay within the normal range unless NTI gets very severe, when they drop below the lower level of normal. Free T4 (FT4) also stays within the normal range except for a transient elevation during recovery.

response by the thyroidal axis may be an adaptive mechanism. (*iii*) Most importantly, attempts to treat routine NTI have not been successful and, in some circumstances, have been harmful (12). Considering the difficulty making this diagnosis, the clinician should not rely too heavily on laboratory measurements. Instead the focus of the evaluation should be on the physical examination and historical information relevant to thyroid disease. ☞ **The presence of a surgical scar, a goiter, unexplained atrial fibrillation, hyponatremia, or constipation may be important clues to NTI.** ☞ Although hormone levels appear to be predictive when NTI in the ICU is diagnosed, routine measurement of thyroid function tests in patients upon admission to the ICU does not predict outcome (13). Indeed, there is a great deal of controversy regarding whether thyroid hormones should be routinely measured or treated in the ICU. It also seems most prudent to withhold thyroid supplementation in the critical care setting in the absence of strong clinical or laboratory evidence for hypothyroidism (14).

Amiodarone

Amiodarone is an iodine-rich medication used frequently in the intensive care setting for controlling cardiac tachyarrythmias. ☞ **Approximately 15% to 20% of patients on long-term treatment with amiodarone develop thyroid abnormalities, especially if there is underlying thyroid pathology (15).** ☞ Because of its iodine content, amiodarone may prevent the oxidation of organic iodide, the first step in producing thyroid hormone (the Wolff-Chaikoff effect). This decrease in thyroid hormone production produces clinical hypothyroidism. On the other hand, the increased iodine may escape the Wolff-Chaikoff effect and cause increased synthesis of thyroid hormone and hyperthyroidism. Patients being treated with amiodarone may also develop an increase in T4 and a decrease in T3 due to the inhibition of 5'-iodinase. Less frequently, amiodarone induces thyroiditis which is associated with hyperthyroidism.

The treatment for amiodarone-induced hypothyroidism is thyroid hormone replacement. Treatment of amiodarone-induced thyrotoxicosis is more difficult, however, and often requires the use of antithyroid medications and potassium perchlorate (1 g/day) (16). Amiodarone may be continued in thyrotoxicosis or myxedema if the symptoms are mild and medically controlled. Amiodarone-induced thyrotoxicosis, however, can be life-threatening and may require aggressive treatment including ablative surgery (17).

Lithium

Lithium carbonate is a second-line medication when used to treat thyrotoxicosis and, when used for this purpose, it works by decreasing the release of iodothyronines. It is more commonly used in clinical practice to treat bipolar affective disorder. In either case, when high levels of lithium are being used, myxedema and goiter usually result. Less often, lithium therapy can cause hyperthyroidism, which may cause decreased renal clearance of lithium and increased lithium toxicity (18). Other symptoms of lithium toxicity include blurred vision, slurred speech, hand tremor and hypercalcemia. These symptoms are easy to miss in the ICU setting so thyroid function tests must be followed carefully in all ICU patients undergoing treatment with lithium for thyroidal or nonthyroidal illnesses.

Hashimoto Thyroiditis

Hashimoto thyroiditis is an autoimmune disease of the thyroid gland that is the most common cause of hypothyroidism, although rare patients with this disease have hyperthyroidism (i.e., Hashitoxicosis). Although its occurrence is not related to critical illness and its appearance in the ICU is not common, it should be identified as a premorbid condition. Critical illness, as noted above, may precipitate severe myxedema in patients who have pre-existing, poorly controlled hypothyroidism.

Patients with Hashimoto thyroiditis typically have firm goiters, although the glands can be almost normal in size. The diagnosis may be made immunologically with demonstration of TPO (thyroid peroxidase) antibodies in the serum. As with other causes of hypothyroidism in the ICU, establishing the diagnosis of Hashimoto thyroiditis is less important than recognition of the hypothyroidism (or hyperthyroidism) and instituting treatment for either condition before severe myxedema (or thyroid storm) develops.

Ablation

Two common causes of hypothyroidism include the administration of ablative radioactive iodine to control Grave's disease and total thyroidectomy. These are both circumstances where the ablation of all functional thyroid tissue was planned. In these cases, hypothyroidism should be anticipated and adequately treated before patients develop critical illness.

Myxedema Coma

The term "myxedema coma" does not connote a unique condition, but is simply the clinical expression of severe, uncompensated hypothyroidism. ☞ **When hypothyroidism is severe, it will result in hypothermia, hypo-ventilation, severe metabolic derangements, cardiovascular collapse, and eventually, coma.** ☞ It occurs most often in the elderly who have long-term, untreated hypothyroidism, but it may be seen in younger patients as well who have untreated hypothyroidism and are then subjected to severe physiological stresses, such as infection and invasive surgical procedures.

Historically, myxedema coma was associated with as high as 50% mortality. More recently, survival has increased with improved critical care and more successful treatment of the underlying disorders, although myxedema coma is still an ominous clinical entity. Treatment, as with other hypothyroid states, is mainly thyroid hormone supplementation. The hormone should probably be given intravenously to obviate the problems of uncertain enteric absorption. In severe uncomplicated hypothyroidism, the most common initial treatment is to give T4 (200–500 µg), to allow tissue conversion to the more active hormone, T3. (Some clinicians advocate an initial combination of T4 and T3, although high doses of T3 should be avoided.) It is also prudent to preadminister stress doses of glucocorticoids to patients who have other endocrine abnormalities (i.e., hormone deficiencies) and are at high risk for developing multiple hormone failure. After the initial dose, T4 is administered at about 50 µg daily.

Hyperthyroid Disorders in Critically Ill Patients

Hyperthyroidism is easier to identify than hypothyroidism. The signs and symptoms of hypothyroidism are usually subtle whereas those of hyperthyroidism are often more flagrant (Table 4). However, either condition may be difficult to identify in critically ill patients.

Table 6 Conditions Causing Hyperthyroidism

Drugs
  Amiodarone
  Lithium
  Iodide containing drugs
  Thyroxine (factitious)
Thyroid Neoplasia
  Single toxic adenoma (Plummer disease)
  Multi-toxic adenoma
  Metastatic thyroid carcinoma
Autoimmunity
  Toxic goiter (Graves disease)
  Hashimoto disease (Hashitoxicosis)
Thyroiditis
  Silent
  Postpartum
  Granulomatous
Endocrine
  Familial nonautoimmune hyperthyroidism
  Over-production of TRH
  Over production of TSH (pituitary and other sources)
  Pituitary resistance to thyroid hormone
  TSH resistance
Ectopic
  Trophoblastic tumors (high hCG)
  Struma ovarii

Abbreviations: TRH, thyrotropin-releasing hormone; TSH, thyroid-stimulating hormone.

There are multiple causes of thyrotoxicosis, which may be broken down into those caused primarily by thyroid tissue and those caused by nonthyroidal problems (19). In the first group are toxic goiter (Graves Disease), toxic adenoma (Plummer Disease), metastatic thyroid carcinoma, and thyroiditis. In the second group are factitious ingestion of thyroid hormone, administration of iodine-containing drugs, overproduction of TRH, and trophoblastic tumors that stimulate the thyroid and struma ovarii (Table 6).

Graves Disease

Graves disease is the most common cause of thyrotoxicosis. It is an autoimmune disorder that presents with symptoms of thyrotoxicosis and others not related to hyperthyroidism. The diagnosis is usually made by noting these nonthyroidal signs and symptoms (e.g., orbitopathy) in a patient with thyrotoxicosis and a symmetrically enlarged thyroid gland. In the critical care setting, establishing the diagnosis of Graves may not be as important as controlling the acute symptoms of thyrotoxicosis. Acutely controlling symptoms, such as tachycardia, atrial fibrillation, and heart failure, with adrenergic blockade is important (see thyroid storm, below). Controlling the production and release of more thyroid hormone may be achieved in the acute or chronic setting with the use of iodine (preceded by one to two doses of PTU) and prednisone (to decrease T4 to T3 conversion). In the chronic setting, antithyroid medications, such as PTU, play a more important role. After the initial stabilization of a patient with thyrotoxicosis, more permanent remission with radioactive iodine or surgery may be considered. ☞ **Although subtotal or total thyroidectomy immediately**

controls symptoms of Graves Disease, surgery should not be attempted unless chemical control of symptoms, and optimally, thyroid hormone levels have been achieved with antithyroid drugs. ☞

Iodinated Contrast Dyes and Other Agents

Critically ill patients are often given radiographic contrast material containing iodine. Although these radiographic contrast dyes have been reported to cause hyperthyroidism (i.e., jodbasedow phenomenon), the actual incidence is low. The practice of treating these patients with perchlorate or thionamide prophylactically is no longer recommended (20). It should be recognized that other iodine-containing drugs (amiodarone, betadine, iodo-niacin), which can cause hypothyroidism through mechanisms elucidated above, can also produce hyperthyroidism. This usually happens in iodine-deficient patients who may have pre-existing goiters, although this phenomenon has been reported in euthyroid patients as well (21).

Toxic Nodular Goiter and Thyroiditis

These conditions present with findings similar to those seen in Graves disease without the autoimmune features. When they affect the elderly, these patients may present with masked (i.e., apathetic) hyperthyroidism, in which the signs and symptoms are not obvious and the clinical picture is often dominated by cardiovascular compromise such as new onset atrial fibrillation.

In thyroiditis, hyperthyroidism may be due to a spontaneously resolving inflammation with a variable clinical course. Characteristically, there is associated thyroid tenderness, jaw pain, myalgias, and an enlarged, firm, tender thyroid. The thyroid uptake of radioactive iodine is decreased and these patients need supportive care with prednisone and aspirin.

Treatment of Hyperthyroidism

The other hyperthyroid states noted above may require different diagnostic tests to make the diagnosis (e.g., thyroid scans, sonography, CT scans, MRI); however, the treatment of these states is similar to that for Graves Disease. Treatment of life-threatening physiological derangements should be accomplished first. After the symptoms are controlled, efforts should be focused on controlling thyroid hormone production, release, and peripheral conversion. Finally, an attempt to control the source (e.g., thyroid lobectomy, excision of a diseased ovary, treatment of thyroid cancer metastases) may be appropriate if the patient is physiologically stable.

Thyroid Storm

Similar to what was stated above about myxedema coma, the term "thyroid storm" does not connote a unique disease process different from the other conditions causing thyrotoxicosis. Rather it suggests that the disease process causing thyrotoxicosis is severe. Severe thyrotoxicosis may be seen in patients who are undergoing thyroid surgery for hyperthyroidism or patients who are undergoing nonthyroid surgery and have coexisting hyperthyroidism that is either unrecognized or poorly controlled. It is also seen frequently in hyperthyroid patients with systemic illnesses, especially infections (22). Relatively minor trauma may trigger thyroid storm in a hyperthyroid patient (23). The syndrome is therefore part of the differential diagnosis of hyperpyrexia and tachycardia in the emergency department, where it must be distinguished from heat stroke, neuroleptic malignant syndrome, malignant hyperthermia, and serotonin syndrome (24). Thyroid storm is difficult to diagnose in patients who present to the hospital following trauma and have other reasons for hyperthermia, tachycardia, and mental obtundation.

The symptoms of thyroid storm, i.e., tachycardia, hyperthermia, sweating, and irritability, are not different from those of Graves Disease, but are much more pronounced. The tachycardia may become as severe as to precipitate congestive heart failure and pulmonary edema. These symptoms may be attributed to other systemic illnesses seen in the ICU, and if not recognized, may lead to hypotension, coma and, ultimately, death. Thus, an index of suspicion must always be maintained when these common symptoms occur if this important entity is to be recognized in critically ill ICU patients.

🖝 **The symptoms of thyroid storm are believed to be the result of the precipitous release or enhanced action of catecholamines by thyroid hormone. Thus, the immediate treatment is adrenergic blockade with agents such as propanolol, reserpine, and guanethidine.** 🖝 Supportive measures such as antipyretics, sedation, oxygen, glucose, sodium, and steroids should also be started early. Treatment of the thyroid hormone excess with antithyroid medications and iodine [iodine preferably after the antithyroid medications (19)] is secondary, but is also important. The best treatment however is prophylactic. Patients who are known to be hyperthyroid should be well-controlled on antithyroid medications before elective surgery or pregnancy.

Thyroid Axis in Critical Illness
Assessment
Disordered thyroid function can cause or contribute to critical illness, and critical illness can affect thyroid function. Although most critical illness, including burns (25), are associated with a low T3, hypothyroid state, there is evidence that there may be a biphasic response to acute traumatic injury with an immediate but short-lived "fight-or-flight" hyperthyroid response and a later adaptive, hypothyroid phase (26). Often, the cause and effect relationship between thyroid and nonthyroid disease is difficult to sort out. Nonetheless, the approach to both the problems is the same. Thyroid parameters must be evaluated to determine if treatment of the thyroid axis is appropriate. It must be kept in mind that the only hormonally active fragments are free T3 and, to a lesser extent, free T4. Determining if the levels of these hormones are appropriate requires an understanding of the measurement of these fractions, their protein binding, and the peripheral conversion of T4 to T3.

Treatment
It should also be recognized that the endocrine response to critical illness is different for acute and chronic diseases. 🖝 **When there is an acute metabolic or physiologic insult associated with trauma, sepsis, surgery, etc., the endocrine response can be characterized as actively secreting pituitary hormones with peripheral inactivation of the target organ hormones.** 🖝 For the thyroid, this is seen as normal or slightly high TSH levels but decreased conversion of T4 to T3 with a low T3 state. This is most likely a protective mechanism and should not be treated with supplemental hormone. On the other hand, chronic illness is associated

with a different endocrine picture characterized by a depression of anterior pituitary secretion with a resultant depression of target organ secretion. In this scenario, there may be a role for intervention. Use of the hypothalamic peptides is optimal, allowing the normal feedback inhibition to regulate hormone levels. Studies with infusion of TRH have been able to restore T3 levels, but its ultimate effect on survival is unknown (27). Administration of the active hormone itself should be considered dangerous, based on the adverse outcomes reported when patients were treated with other active hormones (e.g., growth hormone) in the ICU (28).

Neuroendocrine Function
Parafollicular Cells
The parafollicular cells (C cells) of the thyroid produce calcitonin, a 33 amino acid hormone that functions to maintain calcium homeostasis (discussed in greater detail below) and to protect the skeleton in times of increased need such as growth and pregnancy. As noted above, these cells are neuroendocrine cells and are a part of the APUD system. Calcitonin acts by inhibiting bone osteoclastic activity and decreasing serum levels of calcium. Salmon calcitonin is given to patients therapeutically to treat the hypercalcemia of malignancy and conditions such as Paget's disease. Most of the body's calcitonin is made by the C cells of the thyroid, but small amounts are made by other neuroendocrine cells located in the lungs, adrenal gland, hypothalamus, pituitary, etc.

Calcitonin and Procalcitonin
Calcitonin is made as a 116 amino acid prohormone, procalcitonin, which has recently been recognized as an important marker for inflammatory states (2–5). Furthermore, it is believed to be a mediator of inflammation (29). During inflammatory states, levels of procalcitonin increase as much as a 1000-fold and have prognostic significance (1,30). It has been determined, however, that most of this procalcitonin comes from nonthyroidal, nonneuroendocrine cells (31). Thus, although procalcitonin has become a marker (and perhaps mediator) that is measured often in ICU patients, the thyroid does not play a prominent role in the massive outpouring of procalcitonin seen during inflammation.

Postoperative Complications in the ICU
For many years, surgeons have been reporting almost no operative mortality in large series of patients undergoing thyroid surgery (32). Postoperative complications following thyroid surgery, however, are still a significant problem and include neck swelling, bleeding, thyroid storm, nerve injury, and hypocalcemia. The thyroid gland is vascular and, in many pathological states, becomes enlarged, engorged, and extremely friable. Good operative technique dictates a careful dissection with meticulous hemostasis. Nonetheless, bleeding and airway compromise in the postoperative period does occur, mandating careful monitoring of the airway in the post anesthesia care unit. 🖝 **Post thyroid surgery stridor is an airway emergency, most frequently due to bleeding into the wound or injury to the recurrent laryngeal nerves.** 🖝 In the case of post surgical bleeding, opening the neck wound and decompressing the expanding hematoma may be life saving.

Thyroid lobectomy or total thyroidectomy may result in damage to one or both of the recurrent laryngeal nerves

(RLN) or the superior laryngeal nerves (nerves of Galli-Curci). Superior laryngeal nerve injuries may impair the patient's ability to phonate or sing at high pitch, but is not an emergency. In contrast, bilateral RLN injuries can be life threatening as the patient's airway may become obstructed, requiring intubation or an emergent surgical airway, if unable to inubate. Obviously, a bilateral operation puts both nerves at risk. Recently, there has been a trend toward performing unilateral or minimally invasive operations to minimize injury to surrounding structures, including the RLNs. The risk for permanent unilateral injury to the RLN is often reported as less than 1% in first operations and as much as 5% in reoperations. Therefore, reoperative surgery and aggressive operations for undifferentiated thyroid malignancy are more often associated with nerve injuries.

Thyroid surgery can also precipitate thyroid storm in a patient with untreated or uncontrolled hyperthyroidism. This condition is usually recognized in the operating room and should be managed postoperatively in a critical care setting according to guidelines outlined in the section on thyroid storm.

Unlike hypocalcemia resulting from parathyroid surgery (see below), hypocalcemia related to thyroid surgery is usually transient and is more often an outpatient problem.

PARATHYROID DYSFUNCTION IN THE ICU
Anatomy and Physiology of the Parathyroid Glands
Anatomy

The parathyroid glands are 35 mg, flat, ovoid glands that lie posterior to the thyroid. The most important features of their anatomy are the variability in numbers of glands and the variability in their locations. In a large autopsy series, 80% of patients had four glands, 13% had three and 6% had five (33). The upper glands are more consistent in location with 75% occurring immediately above the inferior thyroid artery. The locations of the inferior glands are more variable and only 50% are found immediately below the inferior thyroid artery with some extending as low as the mediastinum (33).

The blood supply to the lower glands is usually from the inferior thyroid artery. The blood supply to the upper glands may be from the inferior or the superior thyroid artery. Since the glands are small, hypertrophy rarely causes obstruction and the only significance of their anatomic position relates to finding them during surgical exploration.

Calcium and Phosphate Homeostasis

The primary physiological role of the parathyroid glands is to maintain calcium levels. Calcium homeostasis is a complicated process which requires the participation of parathyroid hormone (PTH) and the metabolically active form of vitamin D [1,25 $(OH)_2D$], as noted in Figure 4. Calcium is an important constituent of all cells and serves as a major intracellular messenger. It is critically important for such vital functions as muscle contraction, membrane repolarization, bone mineralization, and clotting. Calcium homeostasis is characterized by: (*i*) multi-hormonal regulation, including PTH and vitamin D, (*ii*) a rapid response to changes in ambient calcium (e.g., a 1% to 2% reduction in ionized calcium leads to an increase in PTH within a few seconds), (*iii*) tight control of the extracellular calcium concentration, and (*iv*) an intracellular calcium concentration which is 10,000-fold lower than the extracellular calcium concentration. It should be noted that, while the intracellular calcium levels may be the most important for cell health, it is the extracellular levels that are tightly regulated. Intracellular calcium, on the other hand, varies widely.

Extracellular, circulating calcium levels are controlled by the interaction with a calcium sensing receptor on parathyroid cells. This cell surface protein binds extracellular calcium and is coupled to a G protein signaling system. The response of the calciumsensing receptor is coupled to PTH secretion so that a lowering of ambient calcium increases the synthesis and release of PTH. Both gain-of-function mutations (e.g., autosomal dominant hypocalcemia), which result in lower extracellular calcium, and loss-of-function mutations (e.g., familial hypocalciuric hypercalcemia), which result in increased extracellular calcium, have been identified. In addition, there are several

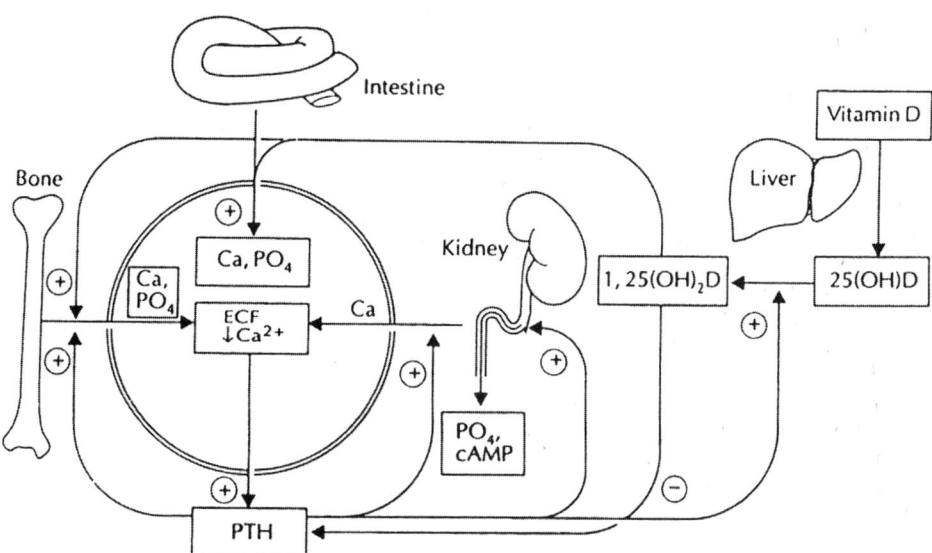

Figure 4 Calcium homeostasis. Calcium enters the extracellular fluid (ECF) compartment from the bone, kidney, and GI tract. Calcium levels are increased by the stimulatory effects of vitamin D, which is converted to its active form [1,25$(OH)_2D$] by the liver and kidney. Parathormone (PTH) stimulates bone to release calcium and the liver to produce 1,25$(OH)_2D$. When ECF calcium levels are low, PTH is stimulated, and calcium levels increase.

acquired conditions in which the calciumsensing receptor activity is altered (e.g., parathyroid adenomas, autoimmune hypoparathyroidism). PTH bioactivity involves mobilization of calcium from the skeleton via direct effects on osteoblasts and indirect effects on osteoclasts. PTH also acts on the kidney to reabsorb calcium and enhance excretion of phosphate. PTH also stimulates 1,25-$(OH)_2D$ hydroxylase, which converts 25-OHD to 1,25-$(OH)_2D$, the active form of vitamin D. Interestingly, 1,25-$(OH)_2D$ imparts negative feedback control on the secretion of PTH itself.

Another peptide, PTHrp (PTH-related protein), is a nonparathyroid peptide made by certain tumor cells and, via the PTH/PTHrp receptor, increases calcium levels in malignancy. It is also involved in calcium homeostasis in multiple tissues such as placenta, mammary gland, smooth muscle, skin, uterus, and cartilage, especially during neonatal life.

Measurement of Parathyroid Function and Calcium Homeostasis
Free and Total Calcium Levels
Ionized free bioactive calcium constitutes 45% of the total extracellular calcium pool, whereas albumin-bound calcium contributes 45%, and calcium complexed to anions accounts for another 10%. Therefore in patients with hypoalbuminemia, the total calcium levels will decrease without changing the ionized or active fraction. Thus, in hypoalbuminemia, a corrected total calcium level can be estimated by adding 0.8 mg/dL to the measured total calcium for every 1 g/dL decrease in the albumin below the normal 4 g/dL. However, changes in protein binding, pH, fatty acids, or other ions may also affect the levels of total, estimated, and ionized calcium. These changes often occur in the ICU, making measurement of ionized calcium necessary in circumstances where accurate calcium levels are important. ☞ **Acidosis increases the ionized calcium levels, and alkalosis reduces these levels (i.e., an increase of pH change by 0.1 decreases ionized calcium by 0.1 mg/dL and vice versa).** ☞ Also important in the ICU are sudden increases in phosphates, citrate, and bicarbonate, which significantly reduce the bioactive ionized calcium levels. For example, an acidotic hypotensive patient may receive several amps of sodium bicarbonate in an effort to improve pH and myocardial contractility. Unfortunately, the acute alkalosis may initially impair contractility (due to the decreased ionized calcium) to a greater extent than it restores contractility, and the patient can arrest in some situations. Accordingly, the clinician must be keenly aware of these effects, and consider supplementing the sodium bicarbonate with small (e.g., 250 mg) doses of calcium chloride or calcium glucinate (use separate syringes and I.V. lines to prevent calcium carbonate precipitation).

The most accurate ionized calcium levels are obtained in the fasting state and at a time when the patient is not hemoconcentrated. The use of a tourniquet should be avoided if possible. Drugs used often in the ICU which decrease total and ionized calcium measurements include carbamazepine, phenytoin, foscarnet, furosemide, glucocorticoids, and tetracycline.

Magnesium
Magnesium has important effects on calcium homeostasis. Modest magnesium deficiency increases levels of PTH, while severe magnesium deficiency causes a decrease in PTH. The resulting hypocalcemia may be severe (34). Similar to calcium, magnesium circulates in free, bound, and chelated forms. It is now possible to measure ionized magnesium and, although not universally available, ionized magnesium levels are available and being utilized in many critical care units. Unfortunately, serum magnesium does not adequately reflect tissue magnesium levels and the assays commonly employed can detect only severe hypermagnesemia. ☞ **Digitalis, cyclosporin, *cis*-platinum, diuretics, aminoglycosides, amphoterecin B, and citrate (in blood transfusions) will lower measured magnesium levels.** ☞

Intact Circulating Parathyroid Hormone
The majority of PTH circulates as fragments of the parent molecule. However the two-site, immunometric measurement of the intact (bioactive) PTH (1–84) molecule is now the standard by which parathyroid activity is assessed. The level of intact PTH typically increases up to two-fold in primary hyperparathyroidism and as much as 10-fold in acute hyperparathyroidism (also called parathyroid poisoning) and secondary hyperparathyroidism. PTHrp (parathyroid hormone-related protein) is a protein that is structurally related to PTH and is found in patients with certain malignancies. It has PTH-like properties, which are responsible for malignancy-related hypercalcemia. Similar to PTH, it is measured by a two-site, immunometric assay, but there is no cross-reactivity between the two peptides. PTHrp is very labile at room temperature.

Vitamin D
The measurement of vitamin D is important in assessing calcium homeostasis. Liver produces 25-OHD (25-hydroxyvitamin D), which is the precursor molecule for mature vitamin D. Phenytoin, carbamazepine, rifampin, and glucocorticoids decrease liver production of 25-OHD. 25-OHD is further hydroxylated in the kidney to form 1,25 $(OH)_2D$ (1,25-dihydroxy Vitamin D), the bioactive hormone, which rises sharply with pregnancy, lactation, and obesity. Isoretinonin and ketoconazole decrease renal production of the mature hormone.

Imaging
Ultrasound and techneitium Tc 99 m sestamibi scanning both image the parathyroid glands. Although they are both used to assess parathyroid function, they have limited utility other than localizing parathyroid glands for surgical treatment.

Hypocalcemic Disorders
There are many causes for hypocalcemia, which may be divided into those related to hypoparathyroidism and those caused by other conditions (Table 7). Hypocalcemia in the ICU is more often caused by conditions not related to parathyroid deficiency. ☞ **Both the absolute level and the rate of fall of calcium influence the clinical manifestations of hypocalcemia.** ☞

As many as 70% to 80% in the ICU experience hypocalcemia at some time during their hospital course, whether calcium levels are measured by a total calcium assay or are estimated using various formulae to calculate total calcium. Hypocalcemia appears to be particularly prevalent in patients with sepsis, but its etiology in this group is often multifactorial. Hypocalcemic signs and symptoms, which are related to disturbances of the neuromuscular, gastrointestinal (GI), central nervous system (CNS), and cardiovascular systems, may be present yet masked by the severity of the concurrent illness. The diagnosis may rely

Table 7 Conditions Causing Hypocalcemia

Parathyroid-related	Nonparathyroid
Postoperative	SIRS
Parathyroid	Pancreatitis
Thyroid	Malignancy
Other head and neck	Hypoproteinemia
Magnesium Deficiency	Hyperphosphatemia
PTH Failure	Necrotizing fasciitis
Genetic-DiGeorge,	Enteric fistulas
APECED	Vitamin D deficiency
Sporadic	Malabsortion
Hungry Bone Syndrome	Liver failure
PTH Resistance	Renal failure
Infiltrative	Vitamin D resistance
Hemachromatosis	Chelation
Wilson Disease	Hyperphosphatemia
Metastatic tumor	Hypoproteinemia
	(pseudohypocalcemia)
	Renal failure
	(acute and chronic)
	Rhabdomyolysis

Abbreviations: APECED, autoimmune polyendocrinopathy-cadidiasis-ectodermal dystrophy; SIRS, systemic inflammatory response syndrome.

on a careful physical exam and performance of confirmatory tests (Table 8).

Systemic Inflammatory Response Syndrome

Hypocalcemia is commonly associated with critical illness and the systemic inflammatory response syndrome (SIRS). Indeed, hypocalcemia is a prognostic factor in ICU patients with or without SIRS. Their hypocalcemia is thought to be due to multiple abnormalities such as hypomagnesemia, impaired vitamin D synthesis, impaired vitamin D action, calcium chelation, or calcium precipitation. Prior evidence implicating parathyroid insufficiency as the main causative factor for hypocalcemia in SIRS patients appears not to be correct. Indeed, PTH is frequently elevated during hypocalcemia and its levels often correlate to both the APACHE II scores and mortality.

Table 8 Signs and Symptoms of Hypocalcemia

Symptoms	Physical Finding	Tests
Circumoral numbness	Carpopedal spasm	Serum
Tingling in	Laryngospasm	hypocalcemia
extremities	Hyperactive	Increased ICP
Abdominal cramps	tendon reflexes	Somatosensory
Muscle cramping	Chvostek sign	EP changes
Fatigue	Trousseau sign	EKG changes
Anxiety	Papilledema	QT prolongation
Irritability	Dry skin	EEG
Depression	Coarse hair	
Seizures	Brittle nails	
(grand mal	(transverse	
and petit mal)	grooves)	
Dementia	Hypotension	
Steatorrhea	CHF	

Abbreviations: ICP, intracranial pressure; EKG, electrocardiogram; CHF, congestive heart failure; EEG, electroencephalogram.

Endotoxin causes ionized hypocalcemia, suggesting that proximal cytokines, stimulated by gram negative sepsis, may be involved. Another group of peptides, which are involved in the inflammatory response and may also influence calcium levels, are the so-called calcitonin precursors (CTpr). These are the peptide fragments derived from the procalcitonin molecule, including procalcitonin itself, which are released by both endotoxin and TNF. Levels of CTpr, but not PTH, correlate inversely to ionized hypocalcemia (35). As noted above, CTpr levels are valuable markers of the severity of stress and correlate with the severity of SIRS, sepsis, and septic shock state (1). The studies demonstrating that CTpr levels correlate with the degree of hypocalcemia provide further evidence that CTpr are mediators as well as markers of the inflammatory response (see calcitonin and procalcitonin above).

☞ **Administration of calcium in systemic inflammation has not been useful. In this regard, the hypocalcemia seen with SIRS may be part of the inflammatory response process and may be protective.** ☞ Extracellular hypocalcemia might even be a response to intracellular hypercalcemia, which is toxic to the cells.

Postsurgical

Hypocalcemia may result from surgery of the thyroid gland, parathyroid glands, or other head and neck structures (e.g., lymph nodes being dissected for oropharyngeal malignancy). When a parathyroid adenoma is removed, the resulting hypocalcemia is usually transient (about one week) and related to the preoperative atrophy of the remaining parathyroid glands. Occasionally, in cases of severe, preoperative osteoblastic overactivity, the hypocalcemia may be more profound due to the "hungry bone syndrome" (described below). Permanent hypocalcemia, which is rare, is usually due to the deliberate removal of all parathyroid tissues for hyperplasia or the inadvertent removal of all parathyroid tissues in very extensive head and neck operations.

☞ **Hypocalcemia from the hungry bone syndrome occurs following surgical resection of large adenomas, which had caused severe primary hyperparathyroidism.** ☞ Removal of the exuberant PTH elaboration (from the resected adenoma) results in disappearance of the osteoclasts in the bone and thus promotes rapid calcium deposition into the skeleton (along with phosphate and magnesium). The subsequent hypocalcemia can be severe, causing symptoms in the first 24 hours and reaching a nadir two to three days postoperatively. This effect may persist for as long as three months. Tetany, seizures, and CHF may accompany the hypocalcemia from hungry bone syndrome. Hypophosphatemia and hypomagnesemia may also manifest as concomitant electrolyte disturbances in the hungry bone syndrome. Risk factors for this form of hypocalcemia include the volume of the resected adenoma, the blood urea nitrogen level, the alkaline phosphatase level, and the patient's age. Interestingly, preoperative PTH level is not a risk factor.

Patients undergoing subtotal thyroid resection due to thyrotoxicosis may also experience transient hypocalcemia. The etiology of this phenomenon is unclear, although the hyperthyroid state is associated with increased bone turnover as well as elevated serum calcium.

Malignancy

Although malignancy is more often associated with hypercalcemia, osteoblastic metastases from prostate and breast cancer may also cause hypocalcemia. In addition, about

10% of cancer patients experience hypocalcemia due to hypoproteinemia. For others with malignancy, chemotherapy-induced rhabdomyolysis and tumor lysis precipitate a sudden influx of phosphate into the intravascular space, which lowers calcium. Oliguria may contribute to this occurrence, exacerbating the hypocalcemia. Although this cause for hypocalcemia is not specific for ICU patients, a similar drop in calcium is seen more often in the ICU with phosphate infusion.

Magnesium

Magnesium deficiency occurs in a variety of conditions and can cause reversible hypocalcemia. Severe hypomagnesemia decreases PTH secretion. Hypomagnesemia is also associated with abnormal PTH receptor action. Finally, hypomagnesemia can lower the production of 1,25-$(OH)_2$D. Alternatively, hypermagnesemia, as seen in the obstetric use of high-dose magnesium infusions, can also cause hypocalcemia. For these reasons, magnesium levels, which may be high or low in the intensive care unit, must be considered in the differential diagnosis of hypocalcemia in critically ill patients.

Vitamin D

Hypovitaminosis is common in hospitalized patients and especially those in the ICU who may have compromised nutrition. This is especially true for vitamin D, because of the restricted exposure to sunlight for patients residing in the ICU. In one study, 57% of 164 hospitalized patients had a 25-OHD level <15 ng/mL while 22% had levels <8 ng/mL (nl. Level >25 ng/mL) (36). These numbers are probably larger for ICU patients.

Deficiencies or impaired activity of vitamin D result in poor intestinal absorption of calcium and subnormal mobilization of calcium from bone. The resulting hypocalcemia may cause an adaptive elevation of PTH and low phosphate, which may be helpful in making the diagnosis. Malabsorption syndromes are associated with the lack of the parent vitamin D compound. In addition, liver disease is associated with the inability to form 25-OHD, while renal abnormalities are associated with inability to form 1,25-$(OH)_2$D. Renal disease is also associated with decreased calcium due to the elevated concentration of phosphate, resulting from decreased glomeruler filtration rate. Elevated phosphate decreases renal-associated hydroxylation of 25-OHD, resulting in decreased GI absorption of calcium. Similarly, hepatobiliary disease is associated with a specific deficiency in 25-OHD.

Pancreatitis

In acute pancreatitis, the destruction of pancreatic exocrine tissue leads to release of fatty acids with the precipitation and deposition of calcium salts in the damaged pancreatic tissue and surrounding fat. The resulting hypocalcemia correlates with the severity of pancreatitis and is a clinically useful indicator [Ranson criterion (37)] for predicting morbidity and mortality in patients with acute pancreatitis.

Idiopathic (Autoimmune, Genetic, Sporadic)

There are several other causes of hypocalcemia that may not be associated with the ICU illness per se but may be contributing factors. Idiopathic hypoparathyroidism may be sporadic or occur in a familial syndrome, which may involve multiple glands and be associated with other developmental abnormalities. For example, type 1 polyglandular syndrome, which has been given the acronym APECED for autoimmune polyendocrinopathy-candidiasis-ectodermal dystrophy typically occurs in early childhood followed by hypoparathyroidism and subsequent adrenal failure (38). Mutations in the AIRE (autoimmune regulator) gene, located on chromosome 21, have been reported in patients with APECED.

Idiopathic hypoparathyroidism may also occur as an isolated deficiency, not related to other endocrine disorders. These disorders, like APECED, usually involve antibodies that inhibit parathyroid secretion or destroy parathyroid tissue. They may occur at any time in life, but are most often seen before the age of 10 years.

Hypoparathyroidism may also occur due to agenesis or dysgenesis of the parathyroid glands. In the DiGeorge syndrome, under-developed third and fourth branchial pouches are associated with congenital absence of the parathyroid glands and thymus and characteristic facial anomalies (e.g., hypertelorism, antimongoloid slant of the eyes, asymmetric malformed ears). Children with the DiGeorge syndrome are susceptible to infections and cardiac failure and do not often survive into adulthood. This is not often a problem seen in adult ICUs, however it may be seen on pediatric wards or in pediatric ICUs.

Other

Rarely, infiltrative parathyroid conditions, including hemochromatosis, Wilson's disease, and metastatic tumors, may cause hypoparathyroidism. Even more rarely, exposure to I^{131} can cause postirradiation hypoparathyroidism. These conditions result in PTH-related hypocalcemia.

Hypocalcemia has also been associated with massive blood transfusions as well as volume expansion with associated hypoalbuminemia. These last two causes for hypocalcemia are seen frequently in ICU patients. Indeed, hypoalbuminemia for any reason is the most common cause for hypocalcemia in hospitalized patients. For these patients an ionized calcium determination or a calculated total calcium level is more clinically relevant than measured serum calcium levels. In addition, many of the drugs associated with hypocalcemia are used in the ICU.

There are several disorders that cause PTH receptor resistance and result in hypocalcemia with high PTH (39). These include the pseudohypoparathyroidism syndromes (1a, 1b, 1c, 2) as well as several hypomagnesemic conditions.

Treatment

Correction of hypocalcemia in sepsis and during the acute phase response is not always recommended. Although normalizing calcium levels may increase blood pressure regardless of the level of ionized calcium, it does not change cardiac index or oxygen delivery and may be associated with catecholamine resistance (40). Thus, treatment of mild to moderate ionized hypocalcemia (0.7–1.05 mmol/L) is generally not recommended. Instead, reducing aggravating conditions, such as loop diuretic administration, should be the clinical focus in caring for patients with moderately depressed levels of calcium. ☞ **Aggressive therapy should be reserved for severe ionized hypocalcemia, (<0.7 mmol/L), severe symptoms (Table 8), or antagonism of specific conditions such as hyperkalemia, hypermagnesemia, and calcium channel blocker toxicity.** ☞ If a patient with hypocalcemia is symptomatic, treatment may require intravenous calcium gluconate [initially 1–2 amps (90 mg Ca/amp) in

50 mL of D5 infused over 10–20 min until symptoms stabilize, followed by a maintenance infusion of five to six amps in 1L D5 infused at 100–125 mL/hr]. When the hungry bone syndrome is expected, such as in surgery for hyperparathyroidism and renal dysfunction, the patients need preoperative calcitriol (2 μg for about five days) along with oral calcium (2–3 g/day for about five days) to prevent the expected decline in calcium. Calcium levels can also be raised in renal failure patients by dialysis using a high calcium bath. Preoperative use of bisphosphonates appears to inhibit calcium mobilization from bone and thus decreases the impact of the acute PTH withdrawal that precipitates the hungry bone syndrome.

Routine administration of calcium with massive blood transfusions is controversial, however calcium is frequently useful if blood is administered rapidly and when ten or more units are administered (41). Measuring ionized calcium levels and electrocardiogram monitoring of QT intervals may be done and calcium administered only when hypocalcemia has been documented.

Because of the various effects of magnesium on calcium homeostasis, magnesium levels should be monitored and corrected in all hypocalcemic patients.

Osteoporosis

Although osteoporosis is not invariably associated with hypocalcemia, it is often seen in critically ill patients. ☞ **Severe illness, prolonged immobilization, low vitamin D levels, and aging all conspire to increase bone resorption.** ☞ These conditions usually respond to combined calcitriol and pamidronate treatment (42). Other factors that adversely impact the health of the skeleton include the use of glucocorticoids and anticonvulsants. In both the conditions, the prompt use of vitamin D and calcium may ameliorate the effects on the bone. In the case of glucocorticoids, the use of bisphosphonates or calcitonin should also be considered.

Table 9 Conditions Causing Hypercalcemia

Common	Rare
Hyperparathyroidism	Immobilization[a]
Primary	Familial hypocaliuric hypercalcemia
Secondary	Thyrotoxicosis
Ttertiary	Hypophosphatemia[a]
Ectopic	Addison disease
Drug-induced	Vipoma
Vitamins A and D	Parathyroid cysts
Thiazides	Milk-alkali syndrome
Lithium	Paget disease
Malignancy	Pheochromocytoma
Osteolytic lesions	
PTHrp	
Lymphoma	
Multiple myeloma	
Granulomatous disease	
Sarcoid	
Tuberculosis	

[a]Although immobilization and hypophosphatemia are often seen in critically ill patients and may contribute to the hypercalcemia caused primarily by other conditions, they are not often the sole cause of hypercalcemia.
Abbreviation: PTHrp, PTH-related protein.

Table 10 Signs and Symptoms of Hypercalcemia

Early	Late
Apathy	Obtundation
Lassitude	Severe weakness
Drowsiness	Coma
Headache	Stupor
Confusion	Depression
QT shortening	Death
Bowel hypomotility	Constipation
Nephrogenic diabetes	Dehydration
Polyuria	Obstructive uropathy
Polydipsia	Band keratopathy
Nephrocalcinosis	Pancreatitis, PUD
Calcium phosphate precipitation	Weight loss
Nausea, vomiting	Chondrocalcinosis
Anorexia	
Gout, pseudogout	

Abbreviation: PUD, peptic ulcer disease.

Other drugs used in the ICU which effect bones include long-term, high dose heparin (>15,000 IU/day) and possibly catecholamines. Acidosis and vitamin D deficiency predispose to osteomalacia characterized by bone pain, elevated alkaline phosphatase, and radiological abnormalities.

Hypercalcemic Disorders

Hypercalcemia may be caused by a multitude of conditions often seen in the ICU (Table 9). Hypercalcemia from any cause can be severe when renal elimination of calcium is impaired. In ICU patients, renal function is often compromised for a multitude of reasons, including dehydration, vomiting, drug toxicity, and multiple organ dysfunction syndrome. Immobilization, which is another problem for critically ill patients, also contributes to hypercalcemia.

The signs and symptoms of hypercalcemia start in ICU patients with nonspecific findings such as apathy, drowsiness, confusion, bowel hypomotility, and anorexia. As the hypercalcemia becomes more severe, these signs develop into more ominous conditions such as obtundation, coma, dehydration and death (Table 10).

Primary Hyperparathyroidism

Primary hyperparathyroidism, with elevated PTH levels, is most commonly due to a single adenoma or, less commonly, multiple adenomas. Primary hyperparathyroidism related to either single or multiple adenomas is more common than primary hyperparathyroidism caused by multiple gland hyperplasia. Hyperparathyroidism associated with a genetic syndrome (e.g., a MEN syndrome) is less common than sporadic cases. On the other hand, when hyperparathyroidism is part of a genetic syndrome, hyperplasia is the usual pathology. Secondary hyperparathyroidism is invariably caused by hyperplasia. Very rarely, hypercalcemia is due to parathyroid carcinoma.

Most patients with hyperparathyroidism are asymptomatic with modest elevations of serum calcium. The PTH levels in these patients are usually less than twice normal. Any patient, however, may decompensate to a life-threatening hypercalcemic crisis with PTH levels reaching 10–20 times normal. Almost 25% of these patients in crisis have chronic stable hypercalcemia characteristic of primary hyperthyroidism, prior to their decompensation. On the other hand, only 1% of patients with mild hyperparathyroidism develop crisis.

In patients with pre-existing hyperparathyroidism, the crisis may be precipitated by spontaneous hemorrhage and rupture of an adenoma (43). Another consequence of rupture of an adenoma is mediastinal hemorrhage with superior vena cava obstruction, mimicking a dissecting aortic aneurysm. Partial necrosis of parathyroid cysts accounts for another small percentage of patients experiencing hyperparathyroid crisis.

Malignancy

Malignant tumors, including lung cancer, breast cancer, lymphomas, and multiple myeloma, are associated with malignancy-related hypercalcemia. Some of these tumors produce PTHrp (see above), while others stimulate local osteolytic humoral factors. Approximately 80% of patients with solid tumors and hypercalcemia produce PTHrp (44), making this the most common cause for hypercalcemia in these patients. Those patients with concurrently elevated PTHrp have PTH levels which are suppressed, a finding which helps with the diagnosis. In addition, patients with malignancy-associated hypercalcemic crisis are often more debilitated and immobile, exacerbating their hypercalcemia. Although almost any cancer can be associated with life-threatening hypercalcemia, lung cancer, breast cancer, lymphoma (especially HTLV-1), and multiple myeloma are most commonly involved.

Disorders of Vitamin D

There are several conditions associated with endogenously-generated, excessive levels of vitamin D [1,25(OH)$_2$D]. In general, these are granulomatous disorders, such as sarcoidosis, tuberculosis, histoplasmosis, and coccidiomycosis, which have amplified macrophage-derived 1,25 (OH)$_2$D activity. In lymphoma, the lymphomatous tissue generates enhanced 1,25 (OH)$_2$D hydroxylase activity. HTLV-1 is associated with severe hypercalcemia, related to elevated levels of vitamin D. These conditions respond to glucocorticoid or hydroxychloroquin treatment, which impairs the hydroxylase enzyme activity.

Endocrine

Other endocrine conditions result in hypercalcemia. In thyrotoxicosis, hypercalciuria is commonly present and 20% also have transient hypercalcemia due to excessive bone remodeling by thyroxine. Pheochromocytoma and VIPomas can generate PTHrp and cause hypercalcemia through mechanisms outlined above. Severe Addison disease has been associated with hypercalcemia, perhaps mainly due to hemoconcentration. Familial hypocalciuric hypercalcemia is a loss-of-function mutation in the calcium-sensing receptor with resultant hypercalcemia, mildly elevated PTH, and hypermagnesemia. These patients typically are asymptomatic and, although the PTH levels may be high, the hypercalcemia does not respond to parathyroid surgery.

Drugs and Ingestion

As was the case with hypocalcemia, many drugs used in the ICU can lead to hypercalcemia. The thiazide diuretics reduce distal tubule reabsorption of calcium and may cause hypercalcemia. This condition may be exacerbated by diuretic-induced dehydration. Hypercalcemia develops in 10% to 15% of patients treated with lithium, which appears to reset the set point for PTH release, shifting the response curve to the right (45). These patients may also have hypocalciuria and hypermagnesemia. Recently, the milk-alkali syndrome is being seen more often, due to public health efforts to get people to increase dietary calcium or use antiosteoporotic calcium supplementation. Excessive vitamin A may also cause calcium toxicity related to increased osteclastic activity. This is a problem of intoxication and is not a problem when recommended daily allowances are observed.

Immobilization

Immobilization caused by a medical condition or a sedentary lifestyle is well known to exacerbate underlying positive calcium balance by increasing bone resorption. This is an under-appreciated yet important cause of hypercalcemia in the ICU that is usually masked by the hypocalcemia more often associated with critical illness. The resulting osteoporosis, however, is a significant clinical problem, which is often manifested by pathologic fractures following falls.

Treatment

The cornerstone for treatment in mild to moderate hypercalcemia involves rehydration, preferably using normal saline, sometimes supplemented with diuretics. For more rapid control, albeit with modest reductions, subcutaneous calcitonin injection may be administered twice per day at a dose range of 100–200 IU. Pamindronate inhibits bone resorption without inhibiting bone formation. It is useful for treatment for hypercalcemia due to malignancy, Paget disease, and osteoporosis. Bisphosphonates can also be very effective for osteoporosis and Paget disease, but take two to three days to act. Bisphosphonates must be used carefully in patients with renal failure and high phosphate levels.

☞ **The patient with "hypercalcemic crisis" often presents with signs and symptoms of severe hypercalcemia including severe fatigue, oliguria, anuria, somnolence, and coma.** ☞ In extreme cases, either emergency surgery or hemodialysis may be needed for a successful outcome. In cases with parathyroid carcinoma, there are often associated bone and kidney diseases and a palpable neck mass. Some of these patients need urgent surgery.

Postoperative Complications in the ICU

The postoperative complications in the ICU following parathyroid surgery are similar to those noted above for thyroid surgery and include neck swelling, bleeding, nerve injury, and hypocalcemia. Because the parathyroid glands are smaller than the thyroid, neck swelling and bleeding are not common problems following surgical exploration and excision. The parathyroid glands are more variable in location and an extensive exploration is sometimes necessary in the retro-thyroid space, making injury to the one or both of the recurrent laryngeal nerves more likely. Damage to a superior laryngeal nerve (nerve of Galli-Curci) is less common in parathyroid surgery because these nerves lie in close apposition to the superior thyroid artery, which does not have to be routinely divided as it does in thyroid surgery. Because the inferior parathyroid glands may be found in the mediastinum, parathyroid surgery may involve retrosternal or mediastinal exploration. These extended operations are certainly more complicated and carry increased risks of bleeding and aerodigestive tract compromise.

Hypocalcemia following thyroid surgery may occur, if all of the parathyroid glands are removed, injured, or devascularized. The hypocalcemia in these cases may take weeks to develop and is often transient. When a patient is being operated on for hyperparathyroidism, the responsible adenoma is removed or the hyperplastic tissue is reduced in volume. In these circumstances, the bones, which were previously decalcified by hyperparathyroidism, avidly take up calcium (hungry bone syndrome, discussed above). The serum calcium levels may plummet rapidly in these patients and require extremely aggressive intravenous calcium replacement with cardiac and hemodynamic monitoring in an ICU.

The trend toward minimally invasive procedures is revolutionizing parathyroid surgery. Adenomas can be localized with preoperative sestamibi scintigraphy, allowing a unilateral exploration through a minimal incision. Occasionally, a hand-held gamma camera is also used to further localize the adenoma. A rapid PTH assay is then used to document intraoperatively that the PTH levels normalize after removal of the adenoma. Minimally invasive parathyroid surgery is too recent to have long-term follow-up data, but initial results suggest that this approach has a 93% success rate in the 64% of patients who have hyperparathyroidism caused by sporadic adenomas (46).

EYE TO THE FUTURE
Thyroid

New, highly sensitive TSH assays have become the cornerstone of diagnostic testing used to evaluate the thyroid axis. Tests with the highest sensitivity can differentiate normal from hyperthyroid levels in virtually all cases, including acutely ill patients. Improved TSH sensitivity has also contracted the upper range of normal values. The majority (>95%) of euthyroid individuals have a serum TSH between 0.4 and 2.5 mU/L. Individuals with a TSH value above 2.5 mU/L may have the early stages of thyroid failure (47).

The isolation and genetic cloning of the sodium iodide symporter protein (NIS), which is important in iodide transport, has opened a new field in thyroid research. These ongoing studies involving the molecular mechanism of iodide transport have important implications for nuclear medicine evaluation and treatment of both benign and malignant thyroid diseases. Reduced NIS expression accounts for reduced iodide uptake in thyroid cancer cells. These cancer cells can be targeted to increase NIS expression and thereby enhance the effectiveness and scope of radioiodine therapy. Interestingly, it also appears that radioiodine could have a similar diagnostic and therapeutic role in breast cancer, as these cells also express NIS.

Another important advance in thyroid disease management has been the development and use of recombinant human thyrogen (i.e., TSH). The indications for thyrogen should increase depending on the results of several ongoing trials. Already, it has a role in assessing metastatic disease in lieu of the standard practice of body scanning following induced hypothyroidism. Combined with ultrasonography of the neck, it has the highest sensitivity for monitoring differentiated thyroid carcinoma (48). Future uses will most likely include therapeutic preparation of patients for radioiodine treatment.

Interventional radiology is being used more for the evaluation and treatment of endocrine disorders.

Minimally-invasive techniques for treating Graves disease are being developed using selective arteriography and arterial embolization of thyroid arteries using the Seldinger technique. These techniques are especially valuable in patients who have significant comorbidity, making their risk for surgery prohibitively high.

Following thyroidectomy for Graves disease, some investigators have advocated the combined administration of T4 and T3. To demonstrate the efficacy of thyroid hormone replacement in this situation, however, will require additional trials. Although surgery is no longer considered primary treatment for hyperthyroid Graves disease, thyroidectomy is still indicated in circumstances when patients cannot tolerate medical treatment or when rapid control of hyperthyroidism is deemed necessary. In these situations, rapid control of hyperthyroidism can be achieved with a combination of iopanoic acid and dexamethasone (49). Another area of controversy involves the use of thyroid hormone replacement in the so-called euthyroid sick syndrome. Thus, the data does not support such an approach. It appears, however, that better powered trials might be able to discern a potential role of thyroid hormones and/or thyroid hormone-like agents in this hypothyroid state.

Parathyroid

Hyperparathyroidism with normal calcium but elevated parathyroid hormone levels (without secondary hyperparathyroidism) is now more commonly recognized, due to more routine PTH screening. This probably represents detection of hyperparathyroidism at an early stage, before hypercalcemia develops. Because it may be associated with clinical problems such as osteoporosis, treatment of this early stage of hyperparathyroidism may be appropriate.

Parathyroid scintigraphy for the diagnosis and surgical location of hyperparathyroidism is evolving rapidly. Dual-tracer (subtraction) techniques using technetium-99 m sestamibi has become the standard mode of localizing parathyroid adenomas. Refinements, including the use of 99 m-tetrofosmin, single-photon emission tomography, and PET scanning are currently being evaluated. The availability of improved precision in the localization of a single adenoma has already changed the scope of surgery to include minimally invasive techniques utilizing a radio-guided surgical approach.

Another area of development involves the use of allosteric activators of the calcium sensing receptor, that is, calcimimetic agents. These small organic molecules lower the threshold for receptor activation by extracellular calcium and thereby diminish parathyroid hormone secretion. Their effectiveness in controlling parathyroid hormone levels has been shown in both primary and secondary hyperparathyroidism. These agents are alternatives to vitamin D and calcium therapy to treat the secondary hyperparathyroidism of renal failure. Notably they have also been reported to decrease the calcium-phosphorus product (50).

Other agents that control parathyroid hormone secretion are the modified vitamin D compounds. Although these agents are already important in secondary hyperparathyroidism due to end-stage renal disease, newer compounds with more potent effects on the secretion of parathyroid hormone are being developed.

Finally, the availability of parathyroid hormone itself, administered as a once-daily injection, will potentially revolutionize the anabolic approach to osteoporosis. Completed phase III trials demonstrate an impressive increase in bone mineral density as well as a decrease in bone fractures using PTH supplementation.

SUMMARY
Thyroid Dysfunction

The signs and symptoms of thyroid dysfunction may be confused with those caused by critical illness, and an understanding of thyroid hormone secretion and action is important in order to recognize thyroidal illness in ICU patients. The most important aspect of thyroid hormone physiology is the recognition that most of the biologically active hormone T3 is not secreted directly from the thyroid, but is produced by extrathyroidal conversion of T4. TSH, in general, relates inversely to the levels of T4, the inactive species, due to the negative feedback mechanism. When T4 is not converted to active T3, it may be converted to the inactive hormone, reverse T3 (rT3), therefore levels of T4 only bear an indirect relationship to levels of T3, the active hormone. Although the measurement of TSH is usually sufficient to determine whether thyroid hormone levels are adequate, because of the confusing metabolism and feedback of T3 and T4, it may be necessary to measure the levels of other hormones to assess the thyroidal axis in these challenging patients. When thyroid hormone levels are determined to be high or low, it is not necessarily beneficial to normalize these levels.

The most common thyroid problem seen in the ICU is "euthyroid sick syndrome," which represents abnormal laboratory tests that don't reflect primary thyroidal problems. Although some clinicians consider that patients with ESS may have clinical hypothyroidism, there is no role for therapeutic thyroid hormone supplementation in these patients. Several medications used in the ICU are commonly associated with hypothyroidism, including amiodarone and lithium. Other conditions encountered in ICU patients that may lead to hypothyroidism include Hashimoto thyroiditis and conditions requiring thyroid ablation by radioactive iodine or surgery. When hypothyroidism is severe it may lead to "myxedema coma" with cardiovascular collapse, severe metabolic derangements, and eventually, coma.

The signs and symptoms of hypothyroidism are usually subtle whereas those of hyperthyroidism are more flagrant and easy to recognize. The main cause of hyperthyroidism in the ICU as well as in the general population is Graves Disease. Although symptoms in Graves Disease may be severe, surgery, which controls the disease immediately, should not be attempted unless chemical control of the symptoms has been achieved with antithyroid drugs. Other less common but important causes of hyperthyroidism are use of iodinated contrast dyes, toxic nodular goiter, and thyroiditis. When hyperthyroidism is extreme, thyroid storm may be precipitated, which, if not recognized in critically ill patients, may lead to death. The symptoms of thyroid storm are believed to be related to the precipitous release of catecholamines. Thus the immediate treatment of this life-threatening condition is adrenergic blockade.

In general, there is an endocrine response to acute physiologic derangements seen in the ICU. This response is characterized by actively secreting pituitary hormones (e.g., TSH) with peripheral inactivation of the target organ hormones (e.g., T3). It is unclear whether this mechanism is harmful or protective. Treatment of these low hormone states with hormone supplementation has not been successful to date.

The parafollicular cells of the thyroid produce calcitonin and its prohormone, procalcitonin. Procalcitonin has become increasingly recognized as an important marker for inflammatory states such as sepsis. Most of the procalcitonin produced in these states are not produced in the thyroid, but originates in extrathyroidal, nonneuroendocrine cells.

Parathyroid Dysfunction

The parathyroid glands vary in number and in position for all patients, thus, an understanding of these variations is important before one embarks upon surgical exploration and removal of parathyroid tissue. The principal action of these glands is the regulation of calcium levels. It should be noted that although the intracellular levels of calcium may be most important for cell health, it is the extracellular levels that are tightly regulated by the parathyroid glands. Extracellular calcium exists as free active calcium, calcium bound to albumin and calcium complexed to anions. Because of changes in albumin and electrolytes in the ICU, measurement of ionized calcium is important to understand how much free bioactive calcium is present. Measurements of other serum levels such as magnesium, PTH, and Vitamin D are important to get a complete picture of calcium homeostasis and the role that the parathyroid glands play.

The rate at which calcium levels fall as well as the levels of hypocalcemia influence the clinical manifestations of hypocalcemia. There are many clinically-encountered conditions which lead to low serum levels of calcium, among which are postsurgery (parthyroidectomy), malignancy, hypomagnesemia, hypovitaminosis (Vitamin D), pancreatitis, autoimmune diseases (e.g., APECED), genetic diseases (e.g., diGeorge syndrome), infiltrative diseases (e.g., hemochromatosis), massive blood loss, and hypoalbuminemia. Some of these conditions, such as malignancy, can also be associated with hypercalcemia. Some, such as massive blood transfusion and hypoalbuminemia, are seen often in the ICU.

Calcium administration should be reserved for ionized levels less than 0.7 mmol/L, whereas mild hypocalcemia should be treated by measures such as withholding loop diuretics. Although massive blood transfusion may lead to hypocalcemia, calcium supplementation is usually not necessary unless ten or more units of banked blood have been transfused.

Hypercalcemia initially presents with nonspecific findings such as drowsiness, confusion, and anorexia, which are difficult to identify in ICU patients. Unrecognized hypercalcemia may become severe leading to more serious conditions such as obtundation, coma, and death. There are multiple etiologies for hypercalcemia including primary hyperparathyroidism, malignancy, hypervitaminosis (D and A), granulomatous disease, thyrotoxicosis, pheochromocytoma, thiazide diuretics, milk-alkali syndrome, and immobilization. Treatment of hypercalcemia usually requires only hydration and diuresis (saline diuresis). For severe hypercalcemia and hypercalcemia caused by specific disease processes, pamindronate, calcitonin, biphosphonates, and, in rare circumstances, surgery (parathyroidectomy) may be required. Surgery for both parathyroid and thyroidal illnesses relies on careful, meticulous technique and, when done correctly, is not associated with much morbidity or mortality. Nonetheless, recent advances in minimally invasive surgery have given surgeons more options for performing these delicate operations. The most commonly recognized problem for parathyroid (and less commonly, thyroid) surgery is hypocalcemia secondary to hypoparathyroidism. Significant acute hypocalcemia that might require ICU monitoring occurs only following removal of hyperactive parathyroid tissue causing "hungry bone syndrome."

KEY POINTS

✍ Thyroxine, the prohormone, is the predominately released species upon TSH stimulation; most of the triiodothyronine, the bioactive hormone, is produced by extrathyroidal conversion.

✍ Levels of thyroid hormone should not necessarily be normalized during critical illness.

✍ This biphasic response to iodide is important insofar as iodide administration can precipitate either hyperthyroidism or hypothyroidism.

✍ Many problems seen in the ICU cause either increased or decreased binding of thyroid hormone to its binding proteins, which may make the total hormone levels abnormal while the free, active hormone levels are normal or vice versa.

✍ In ESS, there are perturbations in the entire hypothalamic-pituitary-thyroid hormone system and it is unclear if these patients are truly euthyroid or perhaps have central hypothyroidism (9). For this reason, the term nonthyroidal illness (NTI) may be more appropriate than ESS.

✍ The presence of a surgical scar, a goiter, unexplained atrial fibrillation, hyponatremia, or constipation may be important clues to NTI.

✍ Approximately 15% to 20% of patients on long-term treatment with amiodarone develop thyroid abnormalities, especially if there is underlying thyroid pathology (15).

✍ When hypothyroidism is severe, it will result in hypothermia, hypo-ventilation, severe metabolic derangements, cardiovascular collapse, and eventually, coma.

✍ Although subtotal or total thyroidectomy immediately controls symptoms of Graves Disease, surgery should not be attempted unless chemical control of symptoms and, optimally, thyroid hormone levels have been achieved with antithyroid drugs.

✍ The symptoms of thyroid storm are believed to be the result of the precipitous release or enhanced action of catecholamines by thyroid hormone. Thus, the immediate treatment is adrenergic blockade with agents such as propanolol, reserpine, and guanethidine.

✍ When there is an acute metabolic or physiologic insult associated with trauma, sepsis, surgery, etc., the endocrine response can be characterized as actively secreting pituitary hormones with peripheral inactivation of the target organ hormones.

✍ Post thyroid surgery stridor is an airway emergency, most frequently due to bleeding into the wound or injury to the recurrent laryngeal nerves.

✍ Acidosis increases the ionized calcium levels, and alkalosis reduces these levels (i.e., an increase of pH change by 0.1 decreases ionized calcium 0.1 mg/dL and vice versa).

✍ Digitalis, cyclosporin, *cis*-platinum, diuretics, aminoglycosides, amphotericin B, and citrate (in blood transfusions) will lower measured magnesium levels.

✍ Both the absolute level and the rate of fall of calcium influence the clinical manifestations of hypocalcemia.

✍ Administration of calcium in systemic inflammation has not been useful. In this regard, the hypocalcemia seen with SIRS may be part of the inflammatory response process and may be protective.

✍ Hypocalcemia from the "hungry bone syndrome" occurs following surgical resection of large adenomas, which had caused severe primary hyperparathyroidism.

✍ More aggressive therapy should be reserved for severe ionized hypocalcemia (<0.7 mmol/L), severe symptoms (Table 8), or antagonism of specific conditions such as hyperkalemia, hypermagnesemia, and calcium channel blocker toxicity.

✍ Routine administration of calcium with massive blood transfusions is controversial; however, calcium is frequently useful if blood is administered rapidly and when ten or more units are administered (41).

✍ Severe illness, prolonged immobilization, low vitamin D levels, and aging all conspire to increase bone resorption.

✍ The patient with "hypercalcemic crisis" often presents with signs and symptoms of severe hypercalcemia including severe fatigue, oliguria, anuria, somnolence, and coma.

REFERENCES

1. Whang KT, Steinwald PM, White JC, et al. Serum calcitonin precursors in sepsis and systemic inflammation. J Clin Endocrinol Metab 1998; 83:3296–3301.
2. Neoptolemos JP. Procalcitonin strip test in the early detection of severe acute pancreatitis. Br J Surg 2001; 88:222–227.
3. Nylen ES, Snider RH, Rohatgi P, Becker KL. Pneumonitis-associated hyperprocalcitonemia. Am J Med Sci 1996; 312:12–18.
4. Nylen ES, O'Neill WJ, Jordan MH, Snider RH, Moore CF, Lewis MS. Serum calcitonin as an index of inhalational injury in burns. Horm Metab Res 1992; 24:439–443.
5. Nylen ES, Alafiri A, Snider RH, Becker K. The effect of classic heat stroke on serum procalcitonin. Crit Care Med 1997; 25:1362–1365.
6. Witherspoon LR, Schuler SE. RE: Clinical assessment of a radioimmunoassay for free thyroxine using a modified tracer. J Nucl Med 1984; 25:1150.
7. Wartofsky L, Burman KD. Alterations in thyroid functions in patients with systemic illness: "The euthyroid sick syndrome." Endocr Rev 1982; 3:164–168.
8. McIver B, Gorman CA. Euthyroid sick syndrome: an overview. Thyroid 1997; 7:125–132.
9. Chopra IJ. Clinical review: Euthyroid sick syndrome: is it a misnomer? J Clin Endocrinol Metab 1997; 82:329–334.
10. Slag MF, Morley JE, Elsson MK, Crowson TW, Nuttal FQ, Shafer RB. Hypothyroxemia in critically ill patients as a predictor of high mortality. JAMA 1981; 245:43–45.
11. Hamblin PS, Dyer SA, Mohr VS, LeGrand BA, Lim CF, Tuxen DV. Relationship between thyrotropin and thyroxine changes during recovery from severe hypothyroxinemia of critical illness. J Clin Endocrinol Metab 1986; 62:717–722.
12. Nylen ES, Zaloga G, Becker KL, Burman KD, Wartofsky L, Muller B. Endocrine therapeutics in critical illness. In: Becker KL, ed. Principles and Practice of Endocrinology and Metabolism. 3rd ed. Philadelphia: Lippincott, Williams & Wilkins, 2001:2108–2121.
13. Ray DC, Drummond GB, Wilkinson E, Beckett GJ. Relationship of admission thyroid function tests to outcome in critical illness. Anesthesia 1995; 50:1022–1025.
14. Stathatos N, Levetan C, Burman KD, Wartofsky L. The controversy of the treatment of critically ill patients with thyroid hormone. Best Pract Res Clin Endocrinol Metab 2001; 15:465–478.
15. Bogazzi F, Bartalena L, Gasperi M, Braverman LE, Martino E. The various effects of amiodarone on thyroid function. Thyroid 2001; 11:511–519.

16. Bartalena L, Brogioni S, Grasso L, Bogazzi F, Burelli A, Martino E. Treatment of amiodarone-induced thyrotoxicosis, a difficult challenge: results of a prospective study. J Clin Endocrinol Metab 1996; 81:2930–2933.

17. Meurisse M, Gollogly L, Degauque C, Fumal I, Defechereux T, Hamoir E. Iatrogenic thyrotoxicosis: causal circumstances, pathophysiology, and principles of treatment—review of the literature. Word J Surg 2000; 24:1377–1385.

18. Oakley PW, Dawson AH, Whyte IM. Lithium: thyroid effects and altered renal handling. J toxicol Clin Toxicol 2000; 38:333–337.

19. Burman KD. Hyperthyroidism. In: Becker KL, ed. Principles and Practice of Endocrinology and Metabolism, 3rd ed. Philadelphia: Lippincott, Williams & Wilkins, 2001:409–428.

20. Hintze G, Blombach O, Fink H, Burkhardt U, Kobberling J. Risk of iodine-induced thyrotoxicosis after coronary angiography: an investigation in 788 unselected subjects. Eur J Endocrinol 1999; 140:264–267.

21. Rajatanavin R, Safran M, Stoller WA, Mordes JP, Braverman LE. Five patients with iodine-induced hyperthyroidism. Am J Med 1984; 77:378–384.

22. Tietgens ST, Leinung MC. Thyroid storm. Med Clin No Am 1995; 79:169–184.

23. Van den Berghe G, de Zegher F, Baxter RC, Veldhuis JD, Wouters P, Schetz M. On the neuroendocrinology of prolonged critical illness: effect of continuous thyrotropin- releasing hormone infusion and its combination with growth hormone-secretagogues. J Clin Endocrinol Metab 1998; 83:309–319.

24. Yoshida D. Thyroid storm precipitated by trauma. J Emerg Med 1996; 14:697–701.

25. McGugan EA. Hyperpyrexia in the emergency department. Emerg Med 2001; 13:116–120.

26. Becker RA, Wilmore DW, Goodwin CW, Zitzka CA, Wartofsky L, Burman KD. Free T4, free T3, and reverse T3 in critically ill, thermally injured patients. J Trauma 1980; 20:713–721.

27. Vitek V, Shatney CH. Thyroid hormone alterations in patients with shock and injury. Injury 1987; 18:336–341.

28. Ruokonen E, Takala J. Dangers of growth hormone therapy in critically ill patients. Curr Opin Clin Nutr Metab Care 2002; 5:199–209.

29. Nylen ES, Whang KT, Snider RH, Steinwald PM, White JC, Becker KL. Mortality is increased by procalcitonin and decreased by an antiserum reactive to procalcitonin in experimental sepsis. Crit Care Med 1998; 26:1001–1006.

30. Steinwald PM, Whang KT, Becker KL, Snider RH, Nylen ES, White JC. Elevated calcitonin precursor levels are related to mortality in an animal model of sepsis. Crit Care 1999; 3:11–16.

31. Muller B, White JC, Nylen ES, Snider RH, Becker KL, Habener JF. Ubiquitous expression of the calcitonin-1 gene in multiple tissues in response to sepsis. J Clin Endocrinol Metab 2001; 86:396–404.

32. Colcock BP, King ML. The mortality and morbidity of thyroid surgery. SGO 1962; 114:131–143.

33. Gilmour, JR. The embryology of the parathyroid glands, the thymus, and certain associated rudiments. J Pathol 1937; 45:507–513.

34. Duran MJ, Borst GC, Osburne RC, Eil C. Concurrent renal hypomagnesemia and hypoparathyroidism with normal parathormone responsiveness. Am J Med 1984; 76:151–154.

35. Muller B, Becker KL, Kranzlin M, Schachinger H, Huber PR, Nylen ES. Disordered calcium homeostasis of sepsis: association with calcitonin precursors. Eur. J. Clin. Invest. 2000; 30:823–831.

36. Thomas MK, Lloyd-Jones DM, Thadani RI, et al. Hypovitaminosis D in medical inpatients. N Engl J Med 998; 338:777–783.

37. Ranson JHC, Pasternack BS. Statistical methods for quantifying the severity of clinical acute pancreatitis. J Surg Res 1977; 22:79–91.

38. Ahonen P, Myllarniemi S, Sipila I, Perheentupa J. Clinical variation of autoimmune polyendocrinopathy-candidiasis-ectodermal dystrophy (APECED) in a series of 68 patients. N Engl J Med 1990; 322:1829–1836.

39. Kerr D, Hosking DJ. Pseudohypoparathyroidism: clinical expression of PTH resistance. QJM 1987; 247:889–894; N Engl J Med 1990; 322:1829–1836.

40. Zaloga GP, Willey S, Malcolm D, Chernow B, Holaday JW. Hypercalcemia attenuates blood pressure response to epinephrine. J Pharmacol Exp Ther 1988; 247:949–952.

41. Valeri CR. Physiology of blood transfusion. In: Barie PS, Shires GT, eds. Surgical Intensive Care. Boston: Little Brown, 1993.

42. Nierman DM, Mechanick JI. Biochemical response to treatment of bone hyperresorption in chronically critically ill patients. Chest 2000; 118:761–766.

43. Nylen ES, Shah A, Hall J. Spontaneous remission of primary hyperparathyroidism from parathyroid apoplexy. J Clin Endocrinol Metab 1996; 81:1326–1328.

44. Stewart AF. Nonparathyroid hypercalcemia. In: Becker KL, ed. Principles and Practice of Endocrinology and Metabolism, 3rd ed. Philadelphia: Lippincott, Williams & Wilkins, 2001: 574–586.

45. Brown E. Lithium induces abnormal calcium-regulated PTH release in dispersed bovine cells. J Clin Endocrinol Metab 1981; 52:1046–1049.

46. Perrier ND, Ituarte PHG, Morita E, Hamill T, Gielow R, Duh QY. Parathyroid surgery: Separating promise from reality. J Clin Endocrinol Metab 2002; 87:1024–1029.

47. Baloch Z, Carayon P, Conte-Devolx B, Demers LM, Feldt-Rasmussen U, Henry JF. Laboratory medicine practice guidelines. Laboratory support for the diagnosis and monitoring of thyroid disease. Thyroid 2003; 13:3–126.

48. Pacini F, Molinaro E, Castana MG, Agate L, Elisei R, Ceccarelli C. Recombinant human thyroglobulin combined with neck ultrasonography has the highest sensitivity in monitoring differentiated thyroid carcinoma. J Clin Endocrinol Metab 2003; 88:3668–3673.

49. Panzer C, Beasley R, Braverman L. Rapid preoperative preparation for severe hyperthyroid Graves disease. J Clin Endocrinol Metab 2004; 89:2142–2144.

50. Block GA, Martin KJ, deFrancisco AL, et al. Cinacalcet for secondary hyperparathyroidism in patients receiving hemodialysis. New Engl J Med 2004; 350:1516–1525.

62

Adrenal Suppression and Crisis

Tareg Bey

Department of Emergency Medicine, UC Irvine Medical Center, Irvine, California, U.S.A.

Eleni Pentheroudakis

Department of Emergency Medicine, Drexel University College of Medicine, Philadelphia, Pennsylvania, U.S.A.

INTRODUCTION

The adrenal cortex produces steroids of three different types: glucocorticoids, mineralocorticoids, and steroidal sex hormones. The adrenal medulla produces the catecholamines adrenaline (aka epinephrine) and noradrenaline (aka norepinephrine). In the case of adrenal injury, failure of production or secretion of the glucocorticosteroid cortisol bears the most serious consequences (1–3). Hypocorticism is a rather rare disease and is, therefore, more difficult to diagnose. The absence of hydrocortisone in the critically ill patient can have catastrophic consequences (4).

σ⁺ **Adrenal crisis, also known as Addisonian crisis, in a critically ill patient is a medical emergency.** σ⁺ Fatalities have been described following inadequate hydrocortisone administration in patients severely stressed by acute illness and in those undergoing major surgery (1–4). The intensivist should be familiar with the classic presentation of adrenal crisis and be prepared to supplement the ill patient with adequate amounts of glucocorticoids. σ⁺ **Because adrenal crisis is a rare event, the diagnosis may be missed, unless the traumatologist/intensivist has a high index of suspicion.** σ⁺ Often empiric therapy is warranted due to the lack of history and time constraints, especially in the unconscious patient.

This chapter reviews the physiology of normal adrenal function and the associated hormones, the classic clinical presentation, and diagnostic and treatment options of adrenal crisis in the setting of the operating room and the intensive care unit (ICU). In addition, the effects of various exogenous steroids are provided, along with perioperative guidelines for exogenous steroid use in patients with presumed adrenal suppression.

ADRENAL GLAND ANATOMY

The adrenal glands are located in the retroperitoneal space above the superior pole of the kidneys. The adrenal glands are extremely well vascularized and consist of two distinct but interconnected endocrine organs of embriologically distinct origins: the adrenal cortex (derived from mesoderm), which produces three major categories of steroid hormones; and the adrenal medulla, derived from ectoderm (neural crest cells), which produces the catecholamines epinephrine and norepinephrine.

The medulla is perfused by a portal venous system that drains the cortex, providing a rich flow of glucocorticoids that induce enzymes responsible for catecholamine synthesis. The chromaffin cell is the principle cell type that synthesizes catecholamines from cholesterol. The medulla is richly innervated by preganglionic sympathetic nerve fibers, serving in essence as an extension of the sympathetic nervous system.

The adrenal cortex is divided into three layers: the outer zona glomerulosa, which produces and secretes the mineralocorticoid aldosterone; the middle zona fasciculata, which produces the glucocorticoid cortisol; and the inner zona reticularis, which produces androgens.

HYPOTHALAMIC-PITUITARY-ADRENAL AXIS PHYSIOLOGY

The production and release of glucocorticoids and androgens is regulated by the hypothalamic-pituitary-adrenal (HPA) axis (5). The hypothalamus is responsible for the production of corticotropin-releasing hormone (CRH). CRH, in turn, acts upon the anterior pituitary gland by signaling the release of adrenocorticotropic hormone (ACTH). ACTH regulates the synthesis and release of glucocorticoids and androgens in the adrenal cortex (6). The glucocorticoid cortisol is life maintaining, and its deficiency plays a central role in hypoadrenal crisis. In contrast, the androgens do not play a significant role. Both CRH and ACTH receive negative feedback regulation from cortisol (Fig. 1) (7).

ACTH and cortisol secretion have a diurnal pattern of variation, with maximum secretion between 2 a.m. and 8 a.m., and minimum availability around midnight. Normally, in the absence of any physical or psychological stressors, the body produces 15 to 20 mg of cortisol per day (8).

An abnormally flattened circadian cortisol cycle has been linked with chronic fatigue syndrome (9), insomnia (10), and "burnout" (11). Critically ill patients often manifest a slightly elevated but flattened curve as well (particularly when chronically stressed) (3–8).

Cortisol Production and Actions

Cortisol, like many other steroidal hormones, is an end product of cholesterol. Cholesterol is first metabolized in the adrenal gland to pregnenolone, which serves as a precursor for both cortisol and aldosterone, in two separate biochemical pathways. The last step of the synthesis of cortisol is the

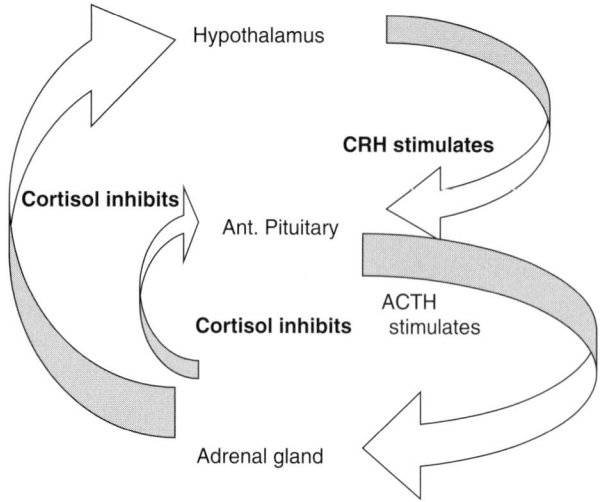

Figure 1   Hypothalamic-pituitary-adrenal axis. Hypothalamus releases corticotropin-releasing factor, stimulating the pituitary gland. The pituitary gland releases adrenocorticotropic hormone which stimulates the adrenal gland to produce cortisol. Cortisol exerts a negative feed back to the pituitary gland and the hypothalamus, and thus inhibits both their activity. *Abbreviations*: ACTH, adrenocorticotropic hormone; CRH, corticotropin-releasing hormone. *Source*: From Ref. 5.

conversion of 11-desoxycortisol to cortisol, under the influence of the enzyme 11β-hydroxylase (Fig. 2) (12). If one of the rate-limiting steps in the cortisol production is

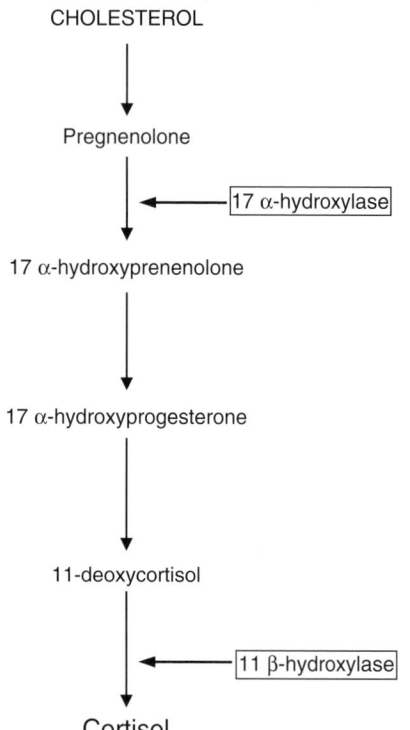

Figure 2   Etomidate inhibits in a dose-dependent fashion the enzyme 11β-hydroxylase, and to a lesser extent the enzyme 17α-hydroxylase. This leads to an excess of 11-deoxycortisol and a lack of cortisol. *Source*: From Ref. 12.

inhibited (as can occur with the drug etomidate), then the production and homeostasis of glucocorticoids is severely disturbed (13).

Cardiovascular Effects of Cortisol

☞ **Cortisol is essential in maintaining vascular tone and thus sustaining blood pressure; indeed, in the absence of cortisol, smooth muscle cells become unresponsive to catecholamines.** ☞ Cortisol both facilitates the vasoconstrictor actions of catecholamines, and has a permissive role on catecholamine synthesis (14,15). Classic mediators of septic shock, like interleukin-1 (IL-1) and interleukin-6 (IL-6), have been shown to stimulate the HPA axis and raise plasma cortisol levels by inducing the release of CRH (16).

Stress Hormone Role of Cortisol

Cortisol is considered a stress hormone and has a positive effect on mood, providing a sense of well being. Stress-mediated neuronal stimulation of the hypothalamus causes CRH release, which induces ACTH release and a subsequent raise in cortisol; this mechanism overrides the body's usual circadian rhythm of ACTH and cortisol secretion (17). Patients with an intact HPA axis are found to have elevated cortisol levels during periods of stress and illness (16). Serum cortisol increases by two to 10 times that of normal, depending on the nature of the stressor (1,8–19). For example, with the stress of surgery, cortisol requirements usually increase from 75 to 150 mg/day (6). The maximum release of cortisol does not exceed 300 mg. Even major surgery does not lead to more than 200 to 300 mg of cortisol secretion in the first 24 hours (6,18). Patients with adrenal insufficiency, by definition, fail to reach the normal increased physiologic levels in a stressed state (1,8).

Anatomical connections between the amygdala, hippocampus, and hypothalamus facilitate activation of the HPA axis (20). Sensory information arriving at the lateral aspect of the amygdala is processed and conveyed to the central nucleus, which hosts projections to several parts of the brain involved in the fear responses. At the hypothalamus, fear-signaling impulses activate both the sympathetic nervous system and the HPA axis (20–22). These neuroendocrinological connections involving the HPA axis are now thought to be integrally related to the development of post-traumatic stress disorder (PTSD), which is fully reviewed in Volume 2, Chapter 65 (20–22).

Glucocorticoids serve important functions, including modulation of stress reactions, but they can be damaging with chronic stimulation. ☞ **Atrophy of the hippocampus is seen in humans and animals exposed to severe stress, and believed to result from excessive stress-induced glucocorticoid levels.** ☞ Deficiencies of the hippocampus are believed to reduce the memory resources available to help a body formulate appropriate reactions to stress (23).

Metabolic Properties of Cortisol

Cortisol has metabolic and catabolic properties as well. It promotes glucose production through gluconeogenesis and antagonism of insulin action (1,8). It also promotes the breakdown of lipids and proteins, mobilizing these energy stores as substrate for gluconeogenesis.

Cortisol and other glucocorticoids affect bone and calcium homeostasis. Cortisol increases calcium reabsorption from bone and in excess can cause osteoporosis (1,2). Cortisol also inhibits intestinal calcium absorption and drives extracellular calcium into intracellular space. Cortisol and other glucocorticoids also inhibit ADH, and when in high concentrations, bind to mineralocorticoid receptors, providing an aldosterone-like effect (sodium reabsorption and potassium secretion).

ALDOSTERONE PRODUCTION REGULATION AND ACTION

The secretion of aldosterone is mainly under the control of the rennin-angiotensin-aldosterone system (RAAS). Aldosterone is the principle mineralocorticoid, although cortisol is said to have weak mineralocorticoid effects in nonrodent mammals. Aldosterone causes sodium reabsorption in conjunction with potassium and hydrogen ion excretion at the renal tubules, and serves as the primary controller of extracellular fluid and plasma volume (24,25). Also see Volume 2, Chapter 44.

A decrease in intravascular volume leads to increased secretion of renin by the juxtaglomerular apparatus (JGA), leading to increased conversion of angiotensinogen to angiotensin I, and then to angiotensin II. Angiotensin II acts on the adrenal zona glomerulosa to increase the activity of aldosterone synthase, and therefore, the secretion of aldosterone. Hyperkalemia also increases the activity of aldosterone synthase.

☞ **Aldosterone deficiency leads to hyponatremia, decreased plasma volume, hyperkalemia, and metabolic acidosis. In primary adrenal crisis, these effects exacerbate those due to cortisol deficiency and lead to profound cardiovascular collapse (24,25).** ☞

ADRENAL INSUFFICIENCY DEFINITIONS AND ETIOLOGIES

"Primary" adrenal insufficiency is defined as a deficiency of aldosterone, cortisol, and other adrenal hormones due to disease of, or direct trauma to, the adrenal glands themselves, or due to drugs that block the adrenal synthesis of cortisol. "Secondary" adrenal insufficiency is defined as a decrease in secretion of ACTH by the pituitary gland either due to direct pituitary pathology, or because of hypothalamic pathology resulting in decreased elaboration of CRH (though some term the hypothalamic causes as "Tertiary" adrenal insufficiency) (3). "Tertiary" adrenal insufficiency is generally referred to as that resulting from peripheral resistance to cortisol, and is by far the least common variety of adrenal insufficiency. The pathological entities that can result in primary and secondary adrenal insufficiency are extensive. Only the most common causes will be reviewed here.

Primary

Primary adrenal insufficiency, dysfunction of the adrenal glands themselves, is commonly referred to as Addison's disease. Though this term is probably best reserved for the autoimmune variety (the most common type), Addison's disease is reported to occur in 39 to 177 individuals per million population (26,27). The mean age at which it is diagnosed in adult patients is 40 years (range, 17–72 years old) (28). The estimates of occult adrenal insufficiency in critically ill patients and in the general population depend partly upon the criteria chosen and the tools used to diagnose the disease. Therefore, it is difficult to compare older with newer literature (29).

In one survey, over 80% of patients with adrenal insufficiency and who belonged to the National Adrenal Disease Foundation (NADF) had seen two or more physicians before the correct diagnosis was considered (30). The NADF estimates that approximately 10,000 individuals in the United States suffer with Addison's disease (30). The NADF points out that this figure most likely underestimates the prevalence of Addison's disease in the United States. The number of people who have subclinical secondary adrenal insufficiency that can be uncovered by stressful events is not included.

Autoimmune

Primary adrenal insufficiency, also known as Addison's disease, most commonly results from an autoimmune adrenalitis, accounting for about 70% to 90% of all cases of adrenal insufficiency in the United States (1–3,31,32). Autoimmune adrenalitis may present alone or along with other autoimmune endocrine diseases, and may be found as a component of type I or II polyglandular syndrome (1–3,31,32). The primary autoimmune etiology is the formation of autoantibodies against the 21-hydroxylase enzyme producing cells. Also, see Volume 2, Chapter 52 for a discussion of autoimmune disease in trauma and critical care.

Granulomatous Disease

Tuberculosis (TB) was once the most common cause of primary adrenal insufficiency (1). Granulomatous diseases (including TB), along with some fungal diseases (i.e., histoplasmosis, blastomycosis), can cause complete adrenal destruction (1). Other causes of primary adrenal insufficiency include acquired immunodeficiency syndrome (AIDS), metastatic carcinoma, and sepsis-related adrenal hemorrhage.

Trauma-Related Adrenal Hemorrhage

Adrenal hemorrhage can also result from abdominal trauma (33), and the risk is likely elevated in patients taking anticoagulants (33,34). Porter et al. (33) describe in a case series of blunt trauma deaths (mainly caused by motor vehicle accidents) with an adrenal hemorrhage incidence of 8% (21 of 269 patients). The authors suggest in this study that adrenal hemorrhage can result from direct injury itself, rather than as a terminal event involving the HPA axis, and that some patients with severe abdominal trauma may benefit from exogenous steroid administration (33).

In a case series of 14 patients with adrenal gland trauma by Gomez et al. (35), 12 patients required surgical exploration of the adrenal gland. In seven of the 12 patients, repair, rather than removal of the gland, was possible and no patient required adrenal corticosteroid replacement therapy (35). Webster and Bell (36) describe a young patient who developed primary adrenal insufficiency in a rehabilitation center one month after an isolated serious head injury and a complex ICU course. The patient's symptoms improved markedly under corticosteroid therapy (36).

Both blunt and penetrating abdominal trauma, as well as prolonged critical illness and stressful operations, have led to bleeding or dysfunction of the adrenal gland resulting in relative hypoadrenalism or adrenal insufficiency (so-called "Addisonian crisis") (1–3). However, primary injury to the adrenal glands is a far less common cause of adrenal insufficiency in critically ill trauma patients.

Human Immunodeficiency Virus and Miscellaneous Causes

Adrenal insufficiency is also the most serious endocrine complication that occurs in persons with human immunodeficiency virus (HIV) infection (37). In AIDS, the adrenal gland may be destroyed by opportunistic infections. Adrenal insufficiency develops in 30% of patients with advanced AIDS (1,31). Metastases to the adrenal gland most often originate from the lung, but also from other primary sites including the breast, kidney, stomach, pancreas, and colon.

Secondary Adrenal Insufficiency

Secondary adrenal insufficiency can result from any lesion to the pituitary (decreasing ACTH production) or the hypothalamus (impairing CRH). The most common cause is the abrupt discontinuation of exogenous glucocorticoid administration following long-term glucocorticoid therapy (38). Chronic glucocorticoid use results in prolonged suppression of CRH production and release. In the long-term glucocorticoid user, adrenal insufficiency clinically manifests itself in two circumstances: (*i*) when maintenance steroids are not increased in response to stress, or (*ii*) when chronic steroids are tapered too abruptly (1–3).

ADRENAL SUPPRESSION AND CRISIS IN CRITICAL ILLNESS

☞ **Secondary adrenal insufficiency is most commonly seen with long-term use of glucocorticoid usage. However, in critically ill patients, prolonged periods of elevated stress are also associated.** ☞

The patient postcessation of steroid therapy may be asymptomatic unless there is an acute stress. If the patient undergoes surgery or sustains an infection, it is critical to provide replacement steroids, otherwise circulatory collapse may result (5,16–19).

It may only take a few weeks of glucocorticoid administration to develop suppression of the HPA axis and relative adrenal insufficiency to occur (2). However, it can take six to 12 months postsuppression by exogenous steroids for the HPA axis to fully recover its function (39). Lamberts et al. (19) emphasize that the duration of recovery of the HPA can range from days to one year. Less common causes of secondary adrenal insufficiency include pituitary or metastatic tumors, hypothalamic tumors, craniopharyngioma, sarcoidosis, pituitary surgery or radiation, traumatic brain injury (TBI), and postpartum pituitary necrosis (Table 1) (1).

Glucocorticoids administered in equivalent doses of up to 5 mg of prednisone, for any given period of time, generally do not cause secondary adrenal insufficiency once the steroid is withdrawn (19,40). However, doses greater than 10 mg prednisone for extended periods may cause HPA suppression.

Trauma patients are prone to adrenal hemorrhage. Porter (33) describes a 7% incidence of adrenal hemorrhage in ultimately fatal motor vehicle accident victims. Adrenal injuries should also be considered in blunt and penetrating trauma (35). The incidence and response to treatment of adrenal insufficiency in high-risk postoperative patients was studied in a prospective observational case series by Rivers et al. (17). They found that 33% of patients, amongst 104 critically ill surgical patients over the age of 55, have abnormally low adrenal function. Although the study design did not test prospectively against a noncortisol treatment group, it appears that there was a trend toward earlier

Table 1   Factors Contributing to the Development of Relative Hypoadrenalism in Critically Ill Patients

Pre-existing or previously undiagnosed asymptomatic diseases of the adrenal gland
   Partial destruction of the adrenal cortex
   Autoimmune adrenalitis
   Tuberculosis
   Metastasis
Acute partial destruction of the adrenal glands
   Hemorrhage
      Massive retroperitoneal bleeding
      Thrombocytopenia
      Anticoagulant therapy
   Bacterial infection (meningococcemia), viral, or fungal infections
Previously unknown hypothalamic-pituitary disease resulting in undiagnosed secondary hypothalamic-pituitary-adrenal insufficiency
Cytokine-mediated inhibition of ACTH release during septic shock? (16)

Abbreviation: ACTH, adrenocorticotropic hormone.
Source: From Ref. 19. Courtesy of NEJM.

recovery from vasopressor therapy within 24 hours among the patients who received a hydrocortisone stress dose.

Critically ill patients with adrenal dysfunction and those with functional hypoadrenalism have a different response to fluid resuscitation and pressors than those with normal cortisol function (41). This is partly due to the low systemic vascular resistance (SVR) present with this condition. Seriously ill patients have a higher prevalence of adrenal insufficiency than the general population (4,41,42). Merry et al. (43) found that postoperative patients older than 55 also have a higher incidence of adrenal failure.

In critically ill patients with hemodynamic instability, a cortisol level and an ACTH test should be considered to test for the diagnosis of adrenal insufficiency (17). There is a wide variance of postoperative incidents of adrenal insufficiency and failure. One of the reasons for this wide discrepancy could be different patient populations, and different types and states of disease in various studies.

Routine screening for adrenal failure in the critically ill is therefore expensive, because with an incidence as low as 1%, it would take 99 patients without disease to find one ill patient with adrenal insufficiency. Patients with a high pretest probability such as old age, massive stress, laboratory abnormalities, and poor response to pressors and fluids should be considered as candidates for presumptive cortisol replacement and ACTH response testing.

DIAGNOSIS OF ADRENAL SUPPRESSION IN CRITICAL ILLNESS
Clinical Picture

In primary adrenal insufficiency, patients demonstrate depressed mentation, weakness, nausea, vomiting, diarrhea, pigmented skin, and eosinophilia. With secondary adrenal insufficiency, fluid and electrolyte disturbances are minimized, but hypoglycemia can be severe because both cortisol and (occasionally) growth hormone can be missing. These patients often lack the marked weight loss that is present in primary adrenal insufficiency and are not pigmented.

Table 2 Laboratory Finding with Primary Adrenal Insufficiency

Hyponatremia (frequent)
Hyperkalemia
Acidosis
Slightly elevated plasma creatinine
Hypoglycemia
Hypercalcemia (rare)
Normocytic anemia
Lymphocytosis
Mild eosinophilia

Source: From Ref. 25.

Fever, tachycardia, low SVR, and orthostatic hypotension are seen with both varieties.

Biochemical profiles usually show a prerenal azotemia, an abnormal hyponatremia, increased potassium levels initially, and hypoglycemia (Table 2). ✍ **The cardiovascular exam in adrenal-suppressed patients usually reveals tachycardia, a weak thready pulse, a small cardiac silhouette on chest X-ray (CXR), and an empty heart by transesophageal echocardiography (TEE); Swan-Ganz would show a low cardiac output (due to low stroke volume) despite a low SVR.** ✍

Baseline Laboratory Abnormalities

Adrenal insufficiency typically causes classic electrolyte abnormalities, which include hyponatremia, hyperkalemia, and hypercalcemia. Hypoglycemia is also common and a mild metabolic acidosis and azotemia may also occur (Table 1) (1). However, serum electrolyte levels may all be initially normal in the adrenal insufficient patient, particularly if the onset of adrenal insufficiency is abrupt.

The hyponatremia that may occur with Addison's disease is rarely less than 120 mEq/L. Hyperkalemia is rarely greater than 7 mEq/L. Hyponatremia results from both aldosterone and cortisol deficiency in primary adrenal insufficiency. Cortisol deficiency results in increased levels of antidiuretic hormone (ADH, also known as vasopressin), which prevents the excretion of free water. ✍ **Hyponatremia is less profound in secondary adrenal insufficiency because both RAASs are still typically intact.** ✍ Aldosterone deficiency, seen in primary adrenal insufficiency, results in sodium depletion with retention of potassium and hydrogen ions. In secondary adrenal insufficiency, the reasons for hyponatremia are due to cortisol deficiency, increased vasopressin secretion, and water retention (25).

Recognition of the above described laboratory/electrolyte abnormalities may be very helpful in establishing the diagnosis of adrenal insufficiency. However, it is important that the diagnosis of adrenal insufficiency not be excluded on the basis of normal electrolytes, because they may be relatively normal initially. In addition, electrolyte abnormalities alone do not constitute a basis for diagnosis.

Measurement of Cortisol Levels

A first step to evaluate a patient for adrenal insufficiency is to obtain a basal plasma cortisol level at 8 AM to 9 AM. If the basal cortisol level is less than 3 mcg/dL (83 nmol/L), the patient has primary adrenal insufficiency and no further testing is needed. A basal morning cortisol level of more than 19 mcg/dL (525 nmol/L) rules out a primary adrenal insufficiency (1–3,18,44). All other patients need dynamic testing with cosyntropin (synthetic ACTH) induced cortisol stimulation. For the critically ill patient, it is very important to recognize adrenal insufficiency. Acute adrenal insufficiency is now more commonly recognized in patients with sepsis and septic shock (17,42).

In the standard cosyntropin stimulation test, the plasma cortisol levels are measured before and after cosyntropin is administered. In this test, a high dose of 250 mcg is given intravenously before 10 AM, and plasma cortisol levels are measured prior to injection, as well as 30 and 60 minutes after injection (1). A response of more than 18 mcg/dL of cortisol is considered to be a normal test and should exclude primary adrenal insufficiency (Table 3) (44).

Because of erratic absorption via intramuscular injections in critically ill patients, this test should only be performed with intravenous administration of cosyntropin. Zaloga and Shenker believe that a high-dose cosyntropin ACTH stimulation test (250 mcg), normally used for noncritically ill patients, may not be appropriate for critically ill patients in an ICU (5,18).

Current data suggests that the cortisol response to critical illness should exceed 25 to 30 mcg/dL, which is higher than the 18 mcg/dL proposed by Grinspoon (5,44). Additionally, in critically ill patients with an acute onset of stress and illness, a normal response to exogenous ACTH can occur due to acute adrenal insufficiency, partial secondary adrenal insufficiency, and ACTH resistance. Furthermore, the standard ACTH stimulation test uses nonphysiologic high doses of cosyntropin, and should be replaced by lower doses of 1 to 2 mcg of cosyntropin since critically ill patients can develop ACTH resistance, which can be overcome with nonphysiologic high doses of cosyntropin (5,18).

Table 3 Considerations During Cortisol and Cosyntropin[a] Laboratory Testing in Critically Ill Patients

Basal cortisol level between 8 and 9 AM	Lower than 3 mcg/dL = primary adrenal insufficiency
	Higher than 18 mcg/dL = no primary adrenal insufficiency
Standard cosyntropin stimulation testing with 250 mcg i.v	Response of more than 18 mcg/dL cortisol is considered to be a normal test and should exclude primary adrenal insufficiency
	Problems
	250 mcg cosyntropin is unphysiologically high and it can miss ACTH resistance and partial secondary adrenal insufficiency
	Current data suggest that the cortisol response to the ACTH stimulation test in critical illness should exceed 25–30 mcg/dL
The standard dose of 250 mcg cosyntropin for the ACTH stimulation test should be replaced by 1–2 mcg by IV	1–2 mcg of cosyntropin is more physiologic and sensitive in critically ill patients

[a]Cosyntropin is synthetic adrenocorticotropic hormone (ACTH).
Abbreviation: ACTH, adrenocorticotropic hormone.

The insulin hypoglycemia or the metapyron test are better for testing for secondary adrenal insufficiency, but they are cumbersome and difficult to perform with an ICU patient (18). The considerations and potential pitfalls with the cortisol and cosyntropin laboratory testing in critically ill patients is reviewed in Table 3.

DRUG INTERACTIONS CAUSING ADRENAL SUPPRESSION

☞ **Certain drugs like etomidate or rifampin can cause adrenal insufficiency and potentially trigger or exacerbate an Addisonian crisis in a critically ill patient with pre-existing adrenal insufficiency.** ☞

Numerous drugs can interfere with the release, biosynthesis, metabolism, and receptor effects of glucocorticoids, which precipitate drug-induced adrenal insufficiency or adrenal crisis. Another factor can be an unrecognized use of steroids. The patient and the physician might not always be aware of previous steroid use. Intra-articular injections of corticosteroids have seldom caused HAA suppression and been associated with subsequent adrenal crisis, which rapidly improved with hydrocortisone therapy (45). Systemic glucocorticoid therapy is more likely to suppress the HPA axis than intra-articular, inhalation, or topical steroid use (46).

The most common cause of secondary adrenal insufficiency in the ICU is the withdrawal of exogenous glucocorticoids (47). Many surgical and medical patients enter the ICU because of an emergency without a detailed medical history and with the immediate need for critical and life-saving interventions like endotracheal intubation. In these cases, the health care personnel (physicians and nurses) have to investigate the patient's prior medication history. Adrenal insufficiency should always be a differential diagnosis in critically ill patients with a recent use of steroids and therapy-refractory hypotension. Classic examples for steroid use are asthma bronchiale, rheumatologic disease, and chronic inflammatory conditions.

There are many drugs which can lead to relative hypoadrenalism. Several drugs and medications interfere with corticosteroid homeostasis and therapy. Adrenal insufficiency under stress may simply be due to previously unknown glucocorticosteroid therapy. Patients with obvious Cushing syndrome should be considered at risk for relative adrenal insufficiency under medical or surgical stress. Relative deficiency of endogenous glucocorticosteroids or current steroid therapy can be a result of a drug–drug interaction, change in cortisol synthesis, glucocorticoid-receptor blockade or interference with ACTH action at the adrenal gland (1–4,19). Patients who are treated with phenytoin, rifampin, barbiturates, mitotane, and aminoglutethimide have increased steroid metabolism (Table 4) (19).

Rifampin is a good example for such a drug–drug interaction. Rifampin is a potent inducer of both gut and hepatic cytochrome P450 (CYP3A4) (31,47). The induction of this enzyme leads to a significant increase in the clearance of steroids and other drugs (47). Ketoconazole is an effective inhibitor of endogenous steroid production. Ketoconazole inhibits the synthesis of glucocorticoids by blocking the 17α-hydoxylase cytochrome P450 (CYP-17α), which is an important enzyme in steroidogenesis (48).

Mefipristone (RU 486), or the abortion pill as it is known, acts by blocking glucocorticoid receptors and was approved by the Food and Drug Administration (FDA) in

Table 4   Drug-Related Factors Contributing to the Development of Relative Hypoadrenalism in Critically Ill Patients

Previously unknown corticosteroid therapy

Medroxyprogesteron, megestrol acetate

Increased metabolism of cortisol: phenytoin, phenobarbital, rifampin

Changes in cortisol synthesis: ketoconazol, etomidate, aminogluthemite, metapyron, mitotane, trilostane

Interference with ACTH action: suramin

Peripheral glucocorticoid-receptor blockade

Abbreviation: ACTH, adrenocorticotropic hormone.
Source: From Ref. 19. Courtesy of NEJM.

2000 as an option for first-trimester abortions (49). Replacement therapy with glucocorticoids in patients with adrenal insufficiency receiving RU 486 may be insufficient, due to the steroid receptor blockade of this drug. Also, megestrol acetate, a synthetic pro-gestational agent used to increase appetite in cachexia-inducing illnesses, can suppress ACTH secretion at doses of >160 mg/day, leading to secondary adrenal insufficiency.

Etomidate is another example where a therapeutic drug interferes with steroidogenesis, and can lead to problems with the stress response of critically ill or injured patients in the perioperative period, or the ICU setting. Etomidate is a carboxylated imidazole-containing compound that is chemically unrelated to any other drug used for the induction of anesthesia. Following an induction dose of 0.3 mg/kg intravenously, the onset of unconsciousness occurs within one arm-to-brain circulation time. It is used in trauma because of its hemodynamic stability. Etomidate inhibits the 11β-hydroxylase and (to a lesser extent) the 17α-hydroxylase enzymes (Fig. 1) (12). After a single dose, adrenal suppression lasts only six to eight hours (13). However, with a prolonged infusion in critically ill trauma patients, Ledingham et al. (50) found an increased mortality compared to patients sedated with morphine and benzodiazepines. Fellows et al. (13) confirmed this observation in a small prospective study with six multiply injured patients in an ICU. All had in common a low adrenocortical function, and all received etomidate infusions for sedation. Another ICU study with similar patients, also receiving steroid replacement, did not experience increased mortality. Vitamin C restores the plasma cortisol level after etomidate (51,52).

DIFFERENTIAL DIAGNOSIS

The differential diagnosis for adrenal insufficiency, especially under medical or surgical stress, is broad. Often the patients are unconscious and cannot give a history of previous steroid use. This is true in patients with head injuries or other intracranial pathology such as subarachnoid bleed. Mental status changes should be investigated for other structural-anatomic or toxic metabolic causes. Patients with an unknown change of mentation should undergo advanced head imaging studies, such as computed tomography, as well as a full laboratory work-up including cultures of all body fluids in the febrile patient. A lumbar puncture should be performed in the absence of a classic contraindication.

New psychiatric changes, especially after the third life decade, should receive a full medical work-up, including an endocrine evaluation, since adrenal insufficiency can present as depression or apathy. Anytime a patient shows mental status or psychiatric changes accompanied with fluid and electrolyte imbalance and cardiovascular instability, adrenal insufficiency should be included in the differential diagnosis.

High fever without apparent cause and negative cultures that do not respond to antibiotics should generate a differential diagnosis of adrenal insufficiency (19). Unexplained circulatory instability (including low SVR) should raise suspicion for sepsis, unrecognized hypovolemia, unknown drug ingestion or medications, adrenal insufficiency, and other endocrinopathies. Hypoglycemia, hyponatremia, hyperkalemia, neutropenia, and eosinophilia can all be caused by adrenal insufficiency (Table 2). However, these symptoms can also be seen with diabetes mellitus, hypotonic dehydration, renal failure, chemo- and radiotherapy, and parasitic disease.

Skin changes like vitiligo, altered pigmentation, or cushingoid appearance with striae can be helpful in establishing a diagnosis of adrenal insufficiency, especially in the patient who cannot communicate. Physicians caring for seriously injured and unconscious patients should perform a careful inspection to look for a Medical-Alert ("Med-Alert") bracelet or necklace, which could warn of pre-existing medical conditions such as adrenal insufficiency.

TREATMENT
Adrenal Insufficiency/Crisis

Empiric steroid administration should be considered in the patient who is hemodynamically unstable despite adequate fluid resuscitation and the use of high dose vasopressors. Administration of glucocorticoids should not be delayed for testing in a crisis situation. However, moderately stable or "metastable" patients can generally tolerate a brief time delay (for testing) between corticosteroid administration. If the patient is dwindling, then dexamethasone (a corticosteroid that does not interfere with the cosyntropin test) can be immediately administered.

⚬ **The diagnosis and treatment of adrenal insufficiency in the "metastable" patient involves administration of dexamethasone sodium phosphate as the glucocorticoid of choice so as not to interfere with the cosyntropin stimulation test.** ⚬

A lack of cortisol response following the administration of cosyntropin (synthetic ACTH) confirms hypoadrenocorticism. The intravenous administration 0.9% sodium chloride will help repair the hyponatremia and hypovolemia.

Although there is no strict biochemical criteria for relative adrenal insufficiency (19), Lamberts et al. (19) emphasize that the diagnosis of adrenal insufficiency should be entertained if administration of hydrocortisone to severely ill patients is followed by a period of diminished or absent requirement for exogenous vasopressor administration. In addition, as Zaloga and Marik (7) point out, a therapeutic trail with hydrocortisone should not be withheld in patients with suspected adrenal insufficiency who have pending results of a diagnostic stress cortisol level or cosyntropin stimulation test.

⚬ **Emergency treatment for Addisonian crisis involves prompt intravenous administration of hydrocortisone, glucose, and 0.9% sodium chloride for shock and maintenance fluid volumes. Glucose and steroids will help to correct hypoglycemia.** ⚬ Fever etiologies should be

thoroughly evaluated with appropriate cultures. However, fever is an important element in the constellation of Addisonian crisis and will resolve with glucocorticoid replacement and rehydration.

Baldwin and Allo (41) report that the administration of 100 to 300 mg hydrocortisone in a 24-hour period decreased or eliminated the need for vasopressors in critically ill patients. This suggests the occurrence of previously unrecognized occult hypoadrenalism, which under conditions of stress manifests as adrenal crisis.

Perioperative Glucocorticoids for Suspected Hypothalamic-Pituitary-Adrenal Axis Suppression

Classically, a bolus of 100 mg hydrocortisone is administered intravenously immediately prior to a major operation, and again after eight and 16 hours (approximately 300 mg hydrocortisone) on the first perioperative day in patients with suspected HPA axis depression, with continued high dose therapy for an additional one to two days, and a taper over the subsequent five days. However, this aggressive approach may not be required in patients who are undergoing minimally invasive procedures.

A consensus paper by Salem et al. (6) provides less aggressive recommendations for the substitution and supplementation of hydrocortisone depending upon both the previous dose and the magnitude of the operation. For minor stress, 25 mg is considered sufficient, and for moderate stress, 50 to 75 mg is recommended. If the patient is subjected to major operative and perioperative stress, a dose of 100 to 150 mg hydrocortisone per day over a period of one to three days should be administered. Since the more seriously ill patients remain intubated postoperatively and cannot eat, the hydrocortisone should be administered intravenously (Table 5).

Jabbour (8) recommends tapering the corticosteroid pulse over a five-day period. It is emphasized that the patient has to be stable and stressors such as fever or vomiting have been resolved, otherwise the taper is extended over a longer duration (Table 6).

For children undergoing major surgery, Tan (53) recommends the administration of hydrocortisone 100 mg/m^2/day for 24 hours peri- and postoperatively before tapering over several days to a maintenance dose. After tapering, the patient needs to receive the regular maintenance dose. The authors point out that it is unnecessary to give mineralocorticoids over such periods if the patient starts

Table 5 Dosage Recommendations for Hydrocortisone Supplementation Based upon the Magnitude of the Surgical Stress

Magnitude of stress	Amount of hydrocortisone per day
Minor stress	25 mg
Moderate stress	50–75 mg
Major stress	100–150 mg

The recommended glucocorticoid dose should be given for one to three days depending on the clinical course. The glucocorticoids are administered in three divided doses over each 24-hour span. See Table 6 for recommendations on tapering. Topical steroid users: In patients who use topical steroids (like inhaled beclomethasone), hypothalamic-pituitary-adrenal axis suppression is very rare. They usually do not need glucocorticoid supplementation with minor or moderate stress if they are clinically asymptomatic.
Source: From Refs. 6, 31.

Table 6 Tapering Recommendations for Hydrocortisone Dosage Following Major Surgical Stress[a] in the Preoperative Phase for Patients with Hypothalamic-Pituitary-Adrenal Axis Suppression

Day of surgery	Dose of IV hydrocortisone per injection	Frequency of IV application
1	100 mg	Every 8 hr or tid
2	50 mg	Every 8 hr or tid
3	25 mg	Every 8 hr or tid
4	25 mg	Every 12 hr or bid
5	15–20 mg (AM) and 5–10 mg (PM)	Morning and evening dose

[a]Major surgical stress includes large scale tissue manipulation, cardiopulmonary bypass, major burns, massive trauma. Once fever and hemodynamic instability have resolved, the taper can be started.
Abbreviation: bid, twice a day; IV, intravenous; tid, three times a day.
Source: From Ref. 8.

the operation with adequate salt balance (43). This is in support of common practice in most hospitals, in that all patients with fluid and electrolyte imbalance, including those with adrenal insufficiency, should have their physiological status optimized before major surgery takes place.

Some controversy appears in the animal experimental literature: whether supraphysiologic doses of glucocorticoids, which are ten times the normal cortisol production rate, are really necessary to treat adrenal insufficiency during operative procedures to prevent hemodynamic instability (54).

EYE TO THE FUTURE

Newer methods of diagnosis and treatment of glucocorticoid deficiency are on the horizon. Diagnosis requires measurement of the serum cortisol levels and the response of cortisol to ACTH. Currently, these tests to measure mcg levels of hormones at specific times are time-consuming and expensive. Often, patients require a series of hormonal testing panels performed in different settings before a definitive diagnosis can be established. In the future, easier and less expensive testing will help to establish adrenal insufficiency in the perioperative trauma patient. Treatment depends upon the degree of adrenocortical dysfunction, response to stimulating hormones, and clinical presentation.

Testing of therapeutic drugs on their propensity to disrupt cortisol synthesis should be intensified in the future, prior to release by the FDA. Etomidate is a commonly used anesthetic drug that can significantly impair adrenal function, especially in compromised patients in stressful situations. Vitamin C has been shown to attenuate this response in laboratory animals, and should be administered to trauma patients requiring etomidate for induction.

Ongoing studies are currently evaluating the role of high dose glucocorticoids in the context of hemorrhagic shock and septic shock. No conclusive data currently justify the routine prophylactic use of high dose corticosteroids in adrenally noncompromised patients to improve outcome. However, this role of steroids and other

inflammation inhibitors will continue to be the subject of future clinical investigation.

One of the most common errors in diagnosing adrenal insufficiency, especially in the unconscious or mentally impaired patient, is failure to consider the pre-existing condition, or failure to recognize the disease stigmata amongst other life-threatening injuries. Beyond the obvious benefit of reviewing a Med-Alert bracelet or necklace, future selected patients might have a microchip implanted under their skin on a voluntary basis (55). Implanted microchips could store vital information including: allergies, medical history, and current therapy for pre-existing conditions. In the case of important allergic predispositions or pre-existing adrenal insufficiency, this information could be life saving.

SUMMARY

Glucocorticoids are life-sustaining steroids. Lack or relative lack of glucocorticoids can lead to therapy-refractory hypotension, imbalance of glucose, fluids, and electrolyte homeostasis in critically ill patients.

Life-threatening hypotension due to adrenal insufficiency constitutes adrenal ("Addisonian") crisis (1–3). In many cases patients with chronic steroid use cannot produce enough endogenous glucocorticoids to combat the stress of severe illness, surgery, or massive trauma.

A common reason for adrenal suppression is the chronic use of steroids (secondary adrenal insufficiency) (38). Other causes of adrenal insufficiency are destruction of the adrenal glands by infection (e.g., tuberculosis), metastasis, or hemorrhage (e.g., trauma) (31). It is crucial to identify patients with true adrenal insufficiency. A medical history and clinical awareness are important to make the correct diagnosis.

Often, the diagnosis of adrenal insufficiency or adrenal crisis in the ICU or in the operating room can only be made empirically by treating therapy-refractory hypotension with glucocorticoids. A full work-up in search of the precipitating illness has to be performed. Supportive care, fluid administration, and hydrocortisone of up to 300 mg intravenously are the mainstay of therapy to treat adrenal crisis.

KEY POINTS

- Adrenal crisis, also known as Addisonian crisis, in a critically ill patient is a medical emergency.
- Because adrenal crisis is a rare event, the diagnosis may be missed unless the traumatologist/intensivist has a high index of suspicion.
- Cortisol is essential in maintaining vascular tone and thus sustaining blood pressure; indeed in the absence of cortisol, smooth muscle cells become unresponsive to catecholamines.
- Atrophy of the hippocampus is seen in humans and animals exposed to severe stress and believed to result from excessive stress-induced glucocorticoid levels.
- Aldosterone deficiency leads to hyponatremia, decreased plasma volume, hyperkalemia, and metabolic acidosis. In primary adrenal crisis, these effects exacerbate those due to cortisol deficiency and lead to profound cardiovascular collapse.
- Secondary adrenal insufficiency is most commonly seen with long-term glucocorticoid usage. However, in

critically ill patients, prolonged periods of elevated stress is also associated.

✍ The cardiovascular exam in adrenal-suppressed patients usually reveals tachycardia, a weak thready pulse, a small cardiac silhouette on CXR, and an empty heart by TEE Swan-Ganz would show a low cardiac output (due to low stroke volume) despite a low SVR.

✍ Hyponatremia is less profound in secondary adrenal insufficiency because both RAASs are still typically intact.

✍ Certain drugs like etomidate or rifampin can cause adrenal insufficiency and potentially trigger or exacerbate an Addisonian crisis in a critically ill patient with pre-existing adrenal insufficiency.

✍ The diagnosis and treatment of adrenal insufficiency in the "metastable" patient involves administration of dexamethasone sodium phosphate as the glucocorticoid of choice, so as not to interfere with the cosyntropin stimulation test.

✍ Emergency treatment for Addisonian crisis involves prompt intravenous administration of hydrocortisone, glucose, and 0.9% sodium chloride for shock and maintenance fluid volumes. Glucose and steroids will help to correct hypoglycemia.

REFERENCES

1. Oelkers W. Adrenal insufficiency. N Engl J Med 1996; 335: 1206–1212.
2. Krasner AS. Glucocorticoid-induced adrenal insufficiency. JAMA 1999; 282:671–676.
3. Salvatori R. Adrenal insufficiency. JAMA 2005; 294(19): 2481–2488.
4. Nylen ES, Muller B. Endocrine changes in critical illness. J Intensive Care Med 2004; 19:67–82.
5. Zaloga GP. Sepsis-induced adrenal deficiency syndrome. Crit Care Med 2001; 29:688–690.
6. Salem M, Tainsh RE Jr, Bromberg J, Loriaux DL, Chernow B. Perioperative glucocorticoid coverage. A reassessment 42 years after emergence of a problem. Ann Surg 1994; 219: 416–425.
7. Zaloga GP, Marik P. Hypothalamic-pituitary-adrenal insufficiency. Crit Care Clin 2001; 17:25–41.
8. Jabbour SA. Steroids and the surgical patient. Med Clin North Am 2001; 85:1311–1317.
9. MacHale SM, Cavanagh JTO, Bennie J, et al. Diurnal variation of adrenocortical activity in chronic fatigue syndrome. Neuropsychobiology 1998; 38(4):213–217.
10. Backhaus J, Junghanns K, Hohagen F, et al. Sleep disturbances are correlated with decreased morning awakening salivary cortisol. Psychoneuroendocrinology 2004; 29(9):1184–1191.
11. Pruessner JC, Hellhammer OH, Kirschbaum C, et al. Burnout, perceived stress, and cortisol responses to awakening. Psychosom Med 1999; 61(2):197–204.
12. Reves JG, Glass PSA, Lubarsky DA. Nonbarbiturates intravenous anesthetics. In: Miller RD, ed. Anesthesia, 5th ed. Vol. 1. Philadelphia, PA: Churchill Livingstone, 2000:228–272.
13. Fellows IW, Byrne AJ, Allison SP. Adrenocortical suppression with etomidate. Lancet 1983; 2:54–55.
14. Kvetnansky R, Pacak K, Fukuhara K, et al. Sympathoadrenal system in stress. Interaction with the hypothalamic-pituitary-adrenocortical system. Ann NY Acad Sci 1995; 771:131–158.
15. Bollaert PE. Stress doses of glucocorticoids in catecholamine dependency: a new therapy for a new syndrome? Intensive Care Med 2000; 26:3–5.
16. Soni A, Pepper GM, Wyrwinski PM, et al. Adrenal insufficiency occurring during septic shock: incidence, outcome, and relationship to peripheral cytokine levels. Am J Med 1995; 98:266–271.
17. Rivers EP, Gaspari M, Saad GA, et al. Adrenal insufficiency in high-risk surgical ICU patients. Chest 2001; 119:889–896.
18. Shenker Y, Skatrud JB. Adrenal insufficiency in critically ill patients. Am J Respir Crit Care Med 2001; 163:1520–1523.
19. Lamberts SWJ, Bruining HA, De Jong FH. Corticosteroid therapy in severe illness. N Engl J Med 1997; 337:1285–1292.
20. Ehlert U, Gaab J, Heinrichs M. Psychoneuroendocrinological contributions to the etiology of depression, posttraumatic stress disorder, and stress-related bodily disorders: the role of the hypothalamus-pituitary-adrenal axis. Biol Psychol 2001; 57(1–3):141–152.
21. Bremner JD, Vythilingam M, Anderson G, et al. Assessment of the hypothalamic-pituitary-adrenal axis over a 24-hour diurnal period and in response to neuroendocrine challenges in women with and without childhood sexual abuse and posttraumatic stress disorder. Biol Psychiatry 2003; 54(7):710–718.
22. Duval F, Crocq MA, Guillon MS, et al. Increased adrenocorticotropin suppression following dexamethasone administration in sexually abused adolescents with posttraumatic stress disorder. Psychoneuroendocrinology 2004; 29(10):1281–1289.
23. Vasterling JJ, Duke LM, Brailey K, et al. Attention, learning, and memory performances and intellectual resources in Vietnam veterans: PTSD and no disorder comparisons. Neuropsychology 2002; 16(1):5–14.
24. Freel EM, Connell JMC. Mechanisms of hypertension: the expanding role of aldosterone. J Am Soc Nephrol 2004; 15:1993–2001.
25. Oelkers W. Hyponatremia and inappropriate secretion of vasopressin (antidiuretic hormone) in patients with hypopituitarism. N Engl J Med 1989; 321:492–496.
26. Lovas K, Husebye ES. High prevalence and increasing incidence of Addison's disease in western Norway. Clin Endocrinol (Oxf) 2002; 56:787–791.
27. Willis AC, Vince FP. The prevalence of Addison's disease in Coventry, UK. Postgrad Med J 1997; 73:286–288.
28. May ME, Vaughn ED. Adrenocortical insufficiency—clinical aspects. In: Vaughn ED, Carey RM, eds. Adrenal Disorders. New York: Thiema Medical, 1989:171–189.
29. Liddle GW. Pathogenesis of glucocorticoid disorders. Am J Med 1972; 53:638–648.
30. Margulies PL, Mullen J. National Adrenal Diseases Foundation North American Survey. http://www.medhelp.org/nadf/frameset.html.
31. Coursin DB, Wood KE. Corticosteroid supplementation for adrenal insufficiency. JAMA 2002; 287:236–240.
32. Peterson P, Uibo R, Krohn KJ. Adrenal autoimmunity: results and developments. Trends Endocrinol Metab 2000; 11: 285–290.
33. Porter JM, Muscato K, Patrick JR. Adrenal hemorrhage: a comparison of traumatic and nontraumatic deaths. J Natl Med Assoc 1995; 87:569–571.
34. Kovacs KA, Lam YM, Pater JL. Bilateral massive adrenal hemorrhage. Assessment of putative risk factors by the case-control method. Medicine (Baltimore) 2001; 80:45–53.
35. Gomez RG, McAninch JW, Carroll PR. Adrenal gland trauma: diagnosis and management. J Trauma 1993; 35:870–874.
36. Webster JB, Bell KR. Primary adrenal insufficiency following traumatic brain injury: a case report and review of the literature. Arch Phys Med Rehabil 1997; 78:314–318.
37. Eledrisi MS, Verghese AC. Adrenal insufficiency in HIV infection: a review and recommendations. Am J Med Sci 2001; 321:137–144.
38. Glowniak JV, Loriaux DL. A double-blind study of perioperative steroid requirements in secondary adrenal insufficiency. Surgery 1997; 121:123–129.
39. Rusnak RA. Adrenal and pituitary emergencies. Emerg Med Clin North Am 1989; 7:903–925.
40. LaRochelle GE Jr, LaRochelle AG, Ratner RE, Borenstein DG. Recovery of the hypothalamic-pituitary-adrenal (HPA) axis in patients with rheumatic diseases receiving low-dose prednisone. Am J Med 1993; 95:258–264.
41. Baldwin WA, Allo M. Occult hypoadrenalism in critically ill patients. Arch Surg 1993; 128:673–676.

42. Sibbald WJ, Short A, Cohen MP, Wilson RF. Variations in adrenocortical responsiveness during severe bacterial infections. Unrecognized adrenocortical insufficiency in severe bacterial infections. Ann Surg 1977; 186:29–33.

43. Merry WH, Caplan RH, Wickus GG, et al. Postoperative acute adrenal failure caused by transient corticotropin deficiency. Surgery 1994; 116:1095–1100.

44. Grinspoon SK, Biller BM. Clinical review 62: laboratory assessment of adrenal insufficiency. J Clin Endocrinol Metab 1994; 79:923–931.

45. Wicki J, Droz M, Cirafici L, Vallotton MB. Acute adrenal crisis in a patient treated with intraarticular steroid therapy. J Rheumatol 2000; 27:510–511.

46. Axelrod L. Glucocorticoid therapy. Medicine (Baltimore) 1976; 55:39–65.

47. Bryyny RL. Preventing adrenal insufficiency during surgery. Postgrad Med 1980; 67:219–225.

48. Schimmer BP, Parker KL. Adrenocorticotropic hormone; adrenocortical steroids and their synthetic analogs; inhibitors of the synthesis and actions of adrenocortical hormones. In: Hardman JG, Limbird LE, eds. Goodman & Gilman's. The Pharmacological Basis of Therapeutics. New York: McGraw-Hill, 1996:1459–1485.

49. Bamberger CM, Chrousos GP. The glucocorticoid receptor and RU 486 in man. Ann NY Acad Sci 1995; 761:296–310.

50. Ledingham IM, Finlay WEI, Watt I, McKee JI. Etomidate and adrenocortical function. Lancet 1983; 1:1434.

51. Boidin MP, Erdmann WE, Faithfull NS. The role of ascorbic acid in etomidate toxicity. Eur J Anaesthesiol 1986; 3:417–422.

52. Boidin MP. Steroid response to ACTH and to ascorbic acid during infusion of etomidate for general surgery. Acta Anaesthesiol Belg 1985; 36:15–22.

53. Tan S, New M, Maclaren N. Clinical review 130: Addison's disease 2001. J Clin Endocrinol Metab 2001; 86:2909–2922.

54. Udelsman R, Ramp J, Gallucci WT, et al. Adaptation during surgical stress. A reevaluation of the role of glucocorticoids. J Clin Invest 1986; 77:1377–1381.

55. Morton L, Murad S, Omar RZ, et al. Importance of emergency identification schemes. Emerg Med J 2002; 19:584–586.

Systemic Inflammatory Response Syndrome (SIRS): Cellular and Humoral Mediators

Debra L. Malone

Department of Surgery, University of Maryland School of Medicine, R Adams Cowley Shock-Trauma Center, Baltimore, Maryland, U.S.A.

Lena M. Napolitano

Department of Surgery, University of Michigan School of Medicine, Ann Arbor, Michigan, U.S.A.

INTRODUCTION

Systemic inflammation characterizes the nonspecific constitutional disturbance resulting from numerous insults including trauma, burns, major surgery, sepsis, and a variety of disease processes including pancreatitis. The cause of this postinjury systemic inflammatory response remains incompletely understood. The currently known inflammatory mediators involved in the systemic derangement involve multiple normally protective systems (including the immune and coagulation systems). The name given to this systemic maladaptive disturbance is the systemic inflammatory response syndrome (SIRS).

Whereas Volume 2, Chapter 47 (Sepsis) focuses mainly upon the infectious disease-related triggers and considerations for SIRS, this chapter highlights the fact that a variety of noninfective triggers can cause SIRS and reviews the many interrelated, cellular, and humoral (paracrine, autocrine, and endocrine) processes known to be involved. The chapter begins by reviewing the definition of SIRS, followed by a survey of the known contributors to SIRS, including in the immune system, cytokines, various markers of inflammation, the neuroendocrine system, and hormones. The increasingly appreciated interaction between inflammation and the coagulation system is reviewed subsequently. A theoretical construction is provided to incorporate the factors involved in the progression of SIRS to compensatory anti-inflammatory response syndrome (CARS) and multiple organ dysfunction syndrome (MODS). The presentation and progression of SIRS within specific populations (including trauma and critical care) is next examined, following which the effects of resuscitation, the gut, immunomodulation, and immunonutrition on SIRS are reviewed. Finally, the eye to the future section provides new definitions, improved diagnostic techniques, and emerging therapies still on the clinical horizon.

THE 1992 DEFINITION OF SYSTEMIC INFLAMMATORY RESPONSE SYNDROME AND ITS REVISION IN 2001

SIRS is a systemic response to nonspecific insults, which may include infections (Volume 2, Chapter 47), pancreatitis

(Volume 2, Chapter 39), trauma, and burns (Volume 1, Chapter 34). SIRS, as a constitutional disturbance frequently associated with sepsis and trauma, has been recognized clinically for over a century. However, operational definitions and descriptions were extremely variable. A consensus conference of the American College of Chest Physicians (ACCP) and the Society of Critical Care Medicine (SCCM) was convened in 1991 and developed a uniform definition in an effort to provide standardization of definitions for both SIRS and sepsis for use in clinical research (1,2). According to the 1991 ACCP/SCCM Consensus Conference Committee, SIRS is defined as a widespread inflammatory response to a variety of clinical insults (infectious and noninfectious). The 1991 ACCP/SCCM scoring system for SIRS has a range from 0 to 4, with 1 point for each variable present (Table 1). SIRS is diagnosed if two or more of the following criteria are present: fever or hypothermia (T > 38°C or T < 36°C), tachycardia (HR > 90), tachypnea respiratory rate (RR) > 20/min or $PaCO_2$ < 32], and abnormal white blood cell count (WBC >12,000/mm^3 or <4000/mm^3, or 10% bands).

☞ **SIRS has been classified as an early component of the sepsis syndrome. SIRS and sepsis commonly present as a continuum of disease states, with progression of SIRS to sepsis, severe sepsis, and septic shock.** ☞ "Sepsis" is defined as SIRS with a presumed or confirmed infectious process (see Volume 2, Chapter 47) (1). Sepsis can progress to "Severe Sepsis" that is defined as sepsis with evidence of organ dysfunction, hypoperfusion, or hypotension. "Septic shock" is defined as sepsis-induced hypotension persisting despite adequate fluid resuscitation, along with the presence of hypoperfusion abnormalities or organ dysfunction. The presence of altered organ function in an acutely ill patient with SIRS, often progresses to MODS (3).

In 2001, an international consensus was convened to review the 1991 definitions (4). The 2001 conference consensus included delegates from the SCCM, European Society of Intensive Care Medicine (ESICM), ACCP, American Thoracic Society (ATS), and the Surgical Infection Society (SIS) (4). They concluded that the current concepts of sepsis, severe sepsis, and septic shock seem robust and should remain as described 10 years prior. However, they also concluded that the diagnostic criteria for SIRS were overly sensitive

Table 1 American College of Chest Physicians/Society of Critical Care Medicine Scoring System for Systemic Inflammatory Response Syndrome (SIRS). SIRS Is Diagnosed if Two or More of the Following Criteria Are Present (SIRS Score ≥2)

SIRS score variables	Points
Fever or hypothermia (T ≥ 38°C or ≤36°C)	1
Tachycardia (HR >90)	1
Tachypnea (RR >20/min, $PaCO_2$ <32)	1
Abnormal WBC (WBC >12,000/mm³, or <4000/mm³, or 10% bands)	1
Maximum total SIRS score	4

Abbreviations: RR, respiratory rate; SIRS, systemic inflammatory response syndrome; WBC, white blood cell count, HR, heart rate.
Source: From Ref. 1.

and not specific (4). They proposed an expanded list of signs and symptoms of sepsis (provided in Volume 2, Chapter 47) and a staging system called PIRO (Predisposition, Infection, Response, and Organ dysfunction) (also provided in Volume 2, Chapter 47) (4). However, they do not provide any new guidance regarding noninfectious etiologies of SIRS. The 2001, SCCM/ESICM/ACCP/ATS/SIS summary recommendations are provided in Table 2 (4).

IMMUNE SYSTEM REVIEW AND ROLE IN THE SYSTEMIC INFLAMMATORY RESPONSE SYNDROME

The immune system is a complex network of diverse cells and proteins that continuously evolves in response to both innate and environmental stimuli. The individual cells communicate and collaborate with each other to modulate their own proliferation, and to coordinate the complex elaboration of compounds, which aid in the identification and destruction of foreign invaders and other compounds associated with survival, repair, and recovery after critical illness, surgery or trauma.

Initial Immune Response

The immune response is triggered when an antigen encounters antigen-presenting cells (APCs). APCs process a protein component of the antigen and present it to antigen-specific helper T lymphocytes. These helper T lymphocytes become activated and initiate an immune cascade (Fig. 1). This process involves the self-proliferation of helper T cells that then carry out their specific effector functions. These helper T cells subsequently activate other immune effector cells (B cells, cytotoxic T cells) as well as other systemic cascades (complement, kinin, fibrinolysis), which are described below. These interactions lead to phagocytosis, thrombosis, and ultimately structural repair under normal conditions. However, in certain individuals, and following certain major insults, these processes lead to an increased inflammatory state (which may be dysfunctional).

Lymphocytes, immunoglobulins, and APCs are considered the key components of the immune system in regards to finding and destroying "foreign" cells. However, the elaboration of certain humoral factors (e.g., cytokines) represents the most important immune system mediators of SIRS. Some cytokines are proinflammatory, whereas others are anti-inflammatory. Typically the proinflammatory mediators predominate during the acute phase, whereas the anti-inflammatory cytokines predominate in the later "chronic" phase of SIRS.

Inflammatory Response

The inflammatory response involves a complex network of interactions that proceeds along specific pathways delineated by distinct physiological and biochemical events. These events are controlled by cytokines and other regulatory molecules, known collectively as inflammatory

Table 2 2001 International Systemic Inflammatory Response Syndrome/Sepsis Conference Conclusions[a]

Consensus point	Conclusion/comments/examples
Current concepts of sepsis, severe sepsis, and septic shock are robust.	Should remain as described 10 years ago (1991 ACCP/SCCM definitions), until further evidence arises justifying alteration.
Current definitions do not allow precise staging of the host response to infection.	Staging system called PIRO proposed (see below), involves host response.
Signs and symptoms of sepsis are more varied than the initial criteria established in 1991.	In contrast to SIRS (which may be triggered by a variety of noninfectious processes), sepsis must be diagnosed promptly, because there are specific treatments (antibiotics, activated protein C, etc).
An expanded list of the signs and symptoms for the diagnosis of sepsis is presented.	See Volume 2, Chapter 47, Table 2
The future lies in developing a staging system that characterizes the progression of sepsis.	Staging system called PIRO proposed definition involves progression and the extent of the resultant organ dysfunction
SIRS remains a useful concept, but the diagnostic criteria published in 1992 are overly sensitive and nonspecific.	Biomarkers (e.g., IL-6, procalcitonins, and C-reactive protein) among others, should be used to document the degree of SIRS.

[a]The conference included delegates from the following organizations: SCCM, ESICM, ACCP, ATS, and SIS.
Abbreviations: ACCP, American College of Chest Physicians; ATS, American Thoracic Society; ESICM, European Society of Intensive Care Medicine; PIRO, stratifies patients on the basis of their Predisposing conditions, the nature and extent of the Insult (in the case of sepsis, infection), the nature and magnitude of the host Response, and the degree of concomitant Organ dysfunction; SCCM, Society of Critical Care Medicine; SIRS, systemic inflammatory response syndrome; SIS, Surgical Infection Society.
Source: From Ref. 4.

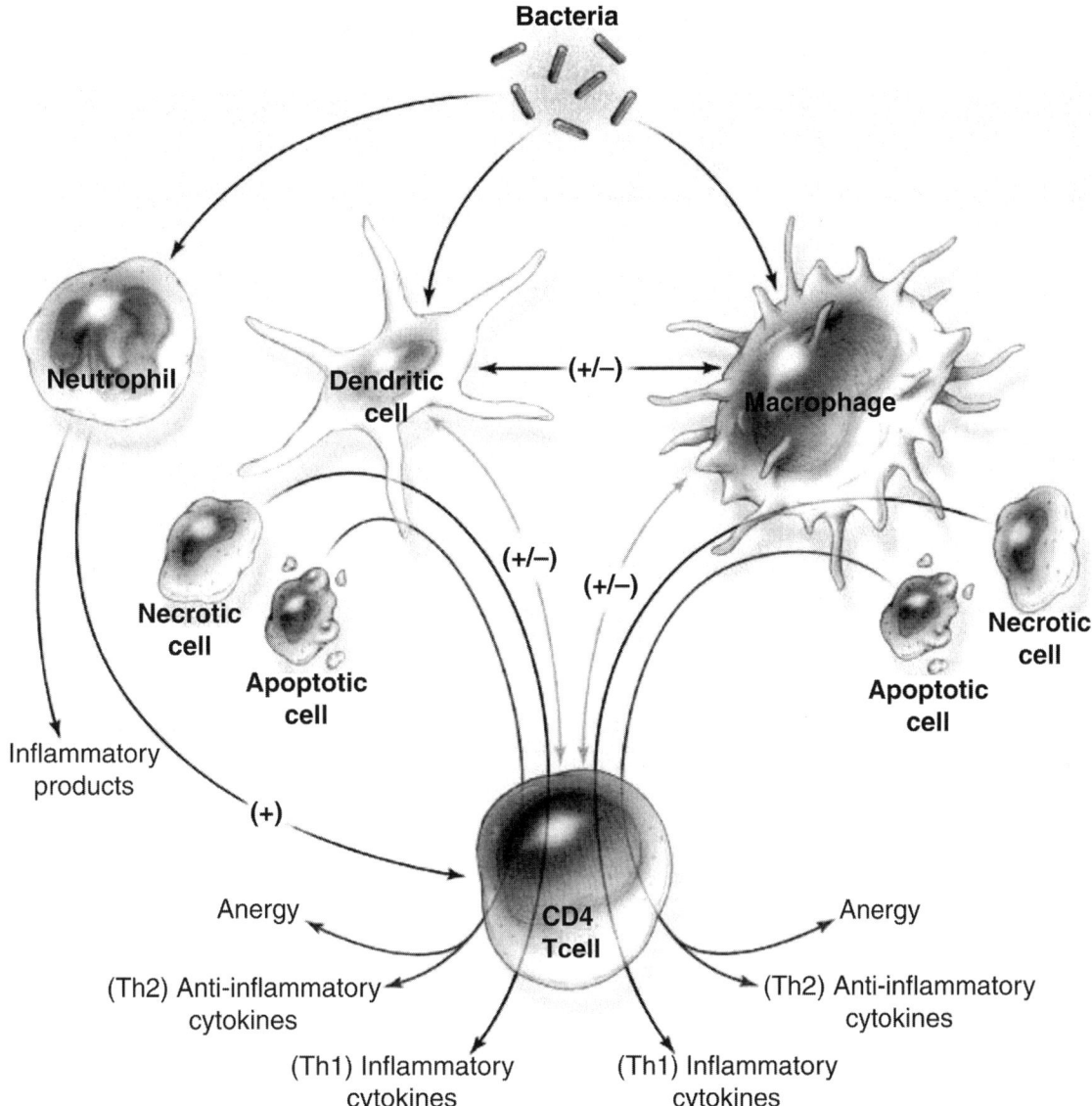

Figure 1 The response to pathogens in sepsis, involving "cross-talk" among many immune cells, including macrophages, dendritic cells, and CD4 T cells. Macrophages and dendritic cells are activated by the ingestion of bacteria, and by stimulation through cytokines (e.g., interferon) secreted by CD4 T cells. Alternatively, CD4 T cells that have an anti-inflammatory profile (type 2 helper T cells [Th2]) secrete interleukin-10, which suppresses macrophage activation. Macrophages and dendritic cells secrete interleukin-12, which activates CD4 T cells to secrete inflammatory (type 1 helper T-cell [Th1]) cytokines. Depending on numerous factors (e.g., the type of organism and the site of infection), macrophages and dendritic cells will respond by inducing either inflammatory or anti-inflammatory cytokines, or causing a global reduction in cytokine production (anergy). Other processes that release inflammatory cytokines (e.g., trauma/burns) may trigger some of these systems causing SIRS in the absence of infection. Macrophages or dendritic cells that have previously ingested necrotic cells will induce an inflammatory cytokine profile (Th1). Ingestion of apoptotic cells can induce either an anti-inflammatory cytokine profile, or anergy. A plus sign indicates upregulation, and a minus sign indicates downregulation; in cases where both a plus sign and a minus sign appear, either upregulation or downregulation may occur, depending on a variety of factors. *Abbreviations*: Th1, type 1 helper T cells; Th2, type 2 helper T cells. *Source*: From Ref. 187.

mediators. The inflammatory mediators include molecules operating as paracrine, autocrine, and endocrine effectors. ☛ **The outcome of inflammation may be beneficial (inactivation of injurious substances, initiation of repair) or deleterious (injury to tissue, interference with normal functions) to the host.** ☛

Inflammation may proceed along different pathways based upon the specific inciting event and, therefore, may present clinically with different signs and symptoms. When activation of the innate immune system is severe enough, the host response may propel the patient into SIRS, shock, and/or MODS (5). The mortality of patients with MODS increases linearly with the SIRS score (Table 3). SIRS and multiple organ failure (MOF) are observed in as many as 30% of all trauma patients and can result in a mortality rate as high as 80% (6). Most patients do survive the initial SIRS insult, but remain at risk for developing secondary or opportunistic infections because of a CARS, typically occurring later in the "chronic" phase.

Table 3 Mortality and Multiple Organ Dysfunction Syndrome are Significantly Correlated with Day 2 Systemic Inflammatory Response Syndrome Score in Surgical Intensive Care Unit Patients

SIRS score	APACHE III score	ICU stay (days)	MOD score	Mortality (%)
0	47.6	4.0	3.6	3.8
1	51.8	7.0	4.5	8.2
2	60.3	11.3	7.0	18.4
3	58.0	12.6	7.5	24.2
4	78.5	9.8	8.5	40.0

Abbreviations: APACHE III, Acute Physiologic and Chronic Health Evaluation; ICU, intensive care unit; MOD, multiple organ dysfunction; SIRS, systemic inflammatory response syndrome.
Source: From Ref. 83.

Acute Phase Response

☞ **Most soluble mediators of inflammation are present in minute concentrations under normal conditions. Elaboration of these mediators may dramatically increase when the body is exposed to infecting organisms, trauma, surgery, and/or critical illness.** ☞ With these insults, the liver responds by immediately increasing synthesis of key proteins, referred to as acute phase proteins. This process is designed to augment immune defense against invading organisms in the case of infection, and initiate the processes of stabilization and repair after surgery and trauma. Exposure to cytokines [primarily interleukin (IL)-1, IL-6, and tumor necrosis factor (TNF)-α], released via both paracrine and endocrine mechanisms, incites hepatocytes to initiate the acute phase response.

Lipopolysaccharide (LPS) is a potent stimulant for release of the above mentioned cytokines. The acute phase proteins as well as complement factors (particularly C3), mannan-binding lectin, LPS-binding protein, and C-reactive protein (CRP) are directly involved in antimicrobial activity and are also released. Other proteins involved in antimicrobial defense include coagulation factors (primarily fibrinogen), granulocyte colony-stimulating factor (GCSF), antioxidants, and metal-binding proteins. The cytokines involved in this process react systemically in concert with hormonal and neural factors to cause systemic symptoms including fever (mediated by the hypothalamus via induction of endogenous pyrogens), lethargy, malaise, and anorexia. Increased glucocorticoid release by the adrenals results from cytokine stimulation of the hypothalamus, which in turn increases the secretion of corticotropin-releasing factor, and adrenocorticotropic hormone from the pituitary. Prolongation of this response can lead to cachexia and anemia. The presence of the acute phase response can be determined by measurement of serum fibrinogen, CRP, procalcitonin (PCT), or the time-honored erythrocyte sedimentation rate.

Endothelial Activation

The endothelium contained within the human body covers approximately 4000 to 7000 m^2 of surface area (7). Endothelial cell properties vary widely depending upon the specific organ or blood vessel type and size. For example, hypoxia and/or acidosis in the systemic arterioles causes vasodilation, whereas the presence of these factors in the pulmonary vasculature leads to vasoconstriction. When surrounding tissue is stressed, endothelial cells (in particular, cells lining postcapillary venules) express high levels of specific adhesion molecules. This stress results from exposure to inflammatory mediators including cytokines, complement, histamines, LPS, or components of the coagulation system (7).

A recent study demonstrated that activated protein C (APC) signals through protease-activated receptor-1 (PAR-1), an endothelial cell protein required for the cytoprotective antiapoptotic effect (8). Two of the most commonly studied adhesion molecules include intercellular adhesion molecule 1 (ICAM-1, CD54) and vascular cell adhesion molecule 1 (VCAM-1) (see Volume 2, Chapter 47, Fig. 1). E-selectin and P-selectin (in the selectin family of carbohydrate-binding proteins) are also widely expressed on activated endothelium (discussed later in the section on adhesion molecules). These adhesion molecules have an affinity for surface molecules expressed by different leukocytes.

☞ **The selectin-phase is the first component of endothelial activation promoting neutrophil migration. In this phase, passing neutrophils or other leukocytes attach to P-selectin and E-Selectin molecules on the activated endothelium.** ☞ Leukocytes come into contact with inflammatory mediators (referred to as leukocyte chemotactic factors) elicited both locally and systemically. When these mediators bind to the leukocytes, the surface adhesion properties of the leukocytes change. One example is that L-selectin (typically present on neutrophils and all other leukocytes) is shed. At the same time, integrins located on the surface of leukocytes transform their molecular shape, enabling them to bind to specific endothelial glycoproteins. This endothelial surface interaction with integrin creates a stable bond that effectively stops neutrophil rolling, allowing the neutrophils to migrate out of vessels into adjacent tissue. Then, through the process of chemotaxis, neutrophils travel to the site of infection or injury.

The integrins are heterodimeric proteins, composed of α and β chain polypeptides, that can associate in different combinations to produce dimers with distinct binding properties that are expressed on different cell types. The integrins bind extracellular matrix proteins as well as nonintegrin adhesion molecules such as VCAM-1.

CYTOKINES
Cytokine Structure and Physiology

Cytokines are the soluble mediators involved in coordinating the immune inflammatory response. They are potent glycoproteins (MW 6000–60,000), involved in intercellular signaling. Acting in concentrations of 10^{-9} to 10^{-15} M, they bind to specific cell membrane receptors and influence intracellular processes ultimately leading to gene transcription and translation, creating the mediators (including other cytokines) that produce the biochemical/molecular cascade of events known as the inflammatory response.

It was initially believed that, unlike hormones which are preformed and secreted into the circulation to act systemically, cytokines were produced locally, and had their effect primarily in an autocrine or paracrine manner. However, recently, new cytokine assays have detected large concentrations of cytokines in serum under certain inflammatory conditions, suggesting that cytokines may play a key endocrine role as well (9).

Some cytokines cause cellular chemoattraction (these are known as chemokines). Others cause cellular proliferation or apoptosis. Others cause the release of bioactive substances (e.g., histamine from mast cells or basophils). The

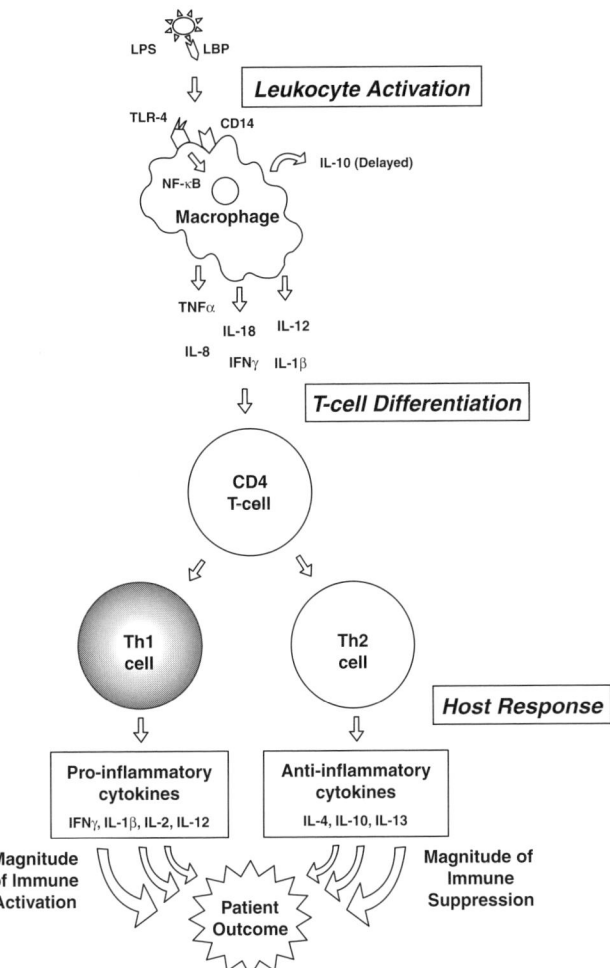

Figure 2 Balance of pro-inflammatory and anti-inflammatory cytokines. Simplified schematic, depicting initiation of host response to lipopolysaccharide (LPS) challenge by macrophages. Beyond this stage, the interaction and redundancy of host inflammatory and anti-inflammatory response is dependent on factors such as infectious cause, coexisting conditions, and genetics. *Abbreviations*: IFN, interferon; IL, interleukin; LBP, lipopolysaccharide-binding protein; Th1, type 1 helper T cells; Th2, type 2 helper T cells; TLR, Toll-like receptors; TNF, tumor necrosis factor. *Source*: From Ref. 73.

cytokines involved in systemic inflammation are considered either pro- or anti-inflammatory (Fig. 2). "Cross-talk" among many immune cells, including macrophages, lymphocytes, and endothelial and dendritic cells, is vitally important for a functional inflammatory response. ☞ **Pro-inflammatory cytokines are responsible for initiation and augmentation of inflammation and its sequelae, whereas anti-inflammatory cytokines are associated with moderation of the inflammatory response.** ☞ Recent studies have demonstrated that an imbalance between pro- and anti-inflammatory cytokines leads to worse outcome in these patients (10). An exuberant inflammatory response may cause SIRS, acute respiratory distress syndrome (ARDS), or MODS. Whereas an exaggerated anti-inflammatory response may lead to immune suppression and infection. TNF-α, IL-1α, IL-1-β, IL-2, IL-4, IL-6, IL-8, IL-10, IL-18, and transforming growth factor (TGF)β are the most frequently studied cytokines associated with trauma, surgery, and critical illness (Table 4). These and

other cytokines mediate the biological cascades associated with the inflammatory response.

Cytokine Receptors

Cytokine receptors and receptor antagonists have been studied extensively in recent years. Both membrane-bound and soluble receptors play key roles. It is apparent that acute utilization of membrane receptors and the release of soluble receptors and their receptor antagonists occur in specific sequences based on time-specific physiological cascades. It is therefore theorized that the receptors regulate the inflammatory response and that the balance between receptors for the pro- and anti-inflammatory cytokines more so than the serum level of these cytokines defines the immune response. Measurement of soluble receptors may be utilized to characterize the immune response and may serve as markers for SIRS and MODS (11).

Cytokine Measurements in Systemic Inflammatory Response Syndrome Patients

Cytokines signal the normal processes of inflammation and repair in all organs. Therefore, adequate measurement of cytokines is critical to adequately assess their role in this process. Plasma cytokine concentrations are at times difficult to detect, perhaps due to the methods of measurement. Enzyme-linked immunosorbent assay (ELISA) is the method utilized most often in research studies. It requires binding at two sites in order to detect the cytokines and, therefore, measures only free cytokines.

Most cytokines are bound to carrier proteins, frequently present in 10 to 1000 times the cytokine concentration, that block detection by two-site ELISAs. Therefore, a bound cytokine is 1000 times more apt to exist on the cellular receptor than the soluble species. Although bound cytokines are not measurable by ELISA, they are present in the circulation and have the potential to be active at the cellular level.

Recent evidence suggests that the total cytokine assay (a competitive immunoassay) has the highest detectability for cytokines in biological samples such as serum and plasma, since only one antibody site is required for capture and detection, thereby detecting essentially all the cytokine in the sample. Malone et al. (9) compared this new assay to ELISA in a study evaluating serum cytokine concentrations in trauma patients, and determined that no significant differences in mean serum cytokine concentrations were noted between trauma patients and normal controls for IL-1, IL-6, and IL-10 using ELISA. In contrast, trauma patients had significantly higher serum concentration of these cytokines on admission compared to normals using the "Total" cytokine immunoassay. Competitive immunoassays may be the method of choice when measuring cytokines in biological fluids, and new normal ranges for cytokines need to be established for future accurate research in systemic inflammation.

OTHER MARKERS OF INFLAMMATION
Procalcitonin (PCT) and C-Reactive Protein (CRP)

PCT and CRP can be utilized to determine the presence and severity of inflammation. These mediators differ in sensitivity and specificity, as related to the ability to differentiate between infectious versus noninfectious causes of SIRS, sepsis, and MODS. Both PCT and CRP are included in the

Table 4 Inflammatory and Anti-inflammatory Cytokines

	Principal source	Target cells	Function
IL-1α and β	Monocytes, macrophages, APCs, endothelial cells	T and B cells, hematopoietic cells	APCs and T cell stimulation B-cell proliferation Immunoglobulin production Phagocyte activation Inflammation
IL-2	Activated T cells, NK cells	T and B cells, NK cells	Activated T cell proliferation T cell growth factor T cell apoptosis (after repeated activation) NK cell activation B cell proliferation
IL-4	T cells (Th2), mast cells	T and B cells, mast cells	B cell activation and growth factor Class II MHC expression Th2 and CTL proliferation Mast cell and eosinophil proliferation Inhibition of monocyte proliferation
IL-6	Monocytes, macrophages, T cells (Th2), APCs, endothelial cells	T and B cells, fibroblasts, hematopoietic cells	B cell stimulation, proliferation and differentiation Synergism with IL-1 and TNF-α Acute phase response
IL-8	Monocytes, macrophages, endothelial cells	Neutrophils, basophils	Neutrophil activation and chemoattraction T cell chemoattraction Angiogenesis
IL-10	T (Th2, CD8) and B cells, macrophages	Monocytes, mast cells, T cells	Inhibition of cytokine production B cell proliferation Suppression of cell-mediated immunity
IL-18	Macrophages, keratinocytes, intestinal epithelial cells	T cells, NK cells	T cell (Th1) activation NK cell activation and proliferation IFNγ production Pro-inflammatory cytokine production
TNF-α	Macrophages, endothelial cells	T and B cells, monocytes, macrophages, neutrophils, endothelial cells, hematopoietic cells	T cell activation B cell proliferation Monocyte and macrophage chemoattraction Neutrophil activation and cytokine production Angiogenesis
TGF-β	Macrophages, T lymphocytes, platelets	Macrophages, T and B cells, endothelial cells, hematopoietic cells	Suppression of cytokine production Antiproliferation of T and B cells Neutrophil and monocyte chemoattraction

Abbreviations: APC, antigen presenting cell; IFN, interferon; MHC, major histocompatibility complex; NK, natural killer cell; TGF, transforming growth factor; TNF, tumor necrosis factor.

PIRO system of response assessment for sepsis (see Volume 2, Chapter 47, Table 3).

Elevated levels of PCT are associated with both systemic inflammation and sepsis. Experiments have demonstrated that serum levels are predictive of injury severity and mortality in clinical studies; however, no studies to date have elucidated the source of PCT and its mechanism of action in these inflammatory states. Indeed, some studies have actually suggested an anti-inflammatory role for this molecule. Some investigators have demonstrated that PCT may be a modulator that augments the inflammatory response, initiated by other mediators, to include LPS and cytokines (12).

Serum concentrations of PCT, compliment C3a, CRP, and elastase were evaluated for their ability to predict SIRS versus sepsis in medical intensive care unit (ICU) patients (13). In this study, serum PCT and C3a levels were shown to discriminate between sepsis and SIRS, whereas CRP and elastase (measured in some ICUs to evaluate systemic inflammation) did not.

Serum levels of PCT, cytokines, and acute phase proteins were measured in patients with postoperative SIRS, sepsis, limited wound infections, or pneumonia in another clinical study to determine if any of these inflammatory indices were more predictive of infection (14). PCT, when compared to these other markers, was more sensitive to systemic stimuli accompanying bacterial infection, most notably endotoxin. It was found to have much less sensitivity to nonbacterial stimuli after surgery or localized bacterial inflammation. Molter et al. (15) cautioned, however, that postoperative PCT plasma concentrations in patients without signs of infection are largely influenced by the type of surgical procedure. These investigators report that on postoperative days 1 and 2, PCT concentrations are more frequently elevated in patients after major abdominal, vascular, or thoracic surgery compared to patients undergoing minor procedures. Therefore, the "infection monitoring" capacity of PCT may be impeded during the first two postoperative days.

Furthermore, PCT may only be a useful marker in patients without leukopenia. Indeed, a recent study showed that PCT was not a sensitive marker for sepsis in leukopenic patients with WBC $<1.0 \times 10^9$ leukocytes/L (16). These authors determined that PCT had both high positive and negative predictive values in patients with WBC $>1.0 \times 10^9$/L.

PCT and CRP were assessed as markers for noninfectious SIRS versus sepsis, and as predictors of the severity of organ failure in critically ill patients (17). CRP levels were not found to be significantly different between the three groups. PCT levels differed significantly between the three groups and were determined to be a good indicator of severity of sepsis and organ failure in patients with severe SIRS. PCT was also found to be more predictive than CRP and WBCs in emergency department patients suspected of sepsis (18).

CRP, SIRS, temperature, and WBC were prospectively evaluated as predictors for infection in 74 medical ICU patients at admission and every four days thereafter (19). Multivariate analysis determined that CRP and SIRS were the only variables independently associated with the presence of infection. The combination of CRP and SIRS was significantly more predictive than any of the other indices. A decrease in CRP between admission and day 4 was the best predictor of recovery.

Preoperative elevations of serum CRP, without other indications of infection, were associated with worse outcome after cardiac surgery with CPB (20). Fifty patients with isolated preoperative CRP elevation were compared with matched (age, gender, and disease) patients who did not have preoperative elevations of CRP. Septic complications, prolonged catecholamine support, increased duration of respiratory support, and increased ICU length of stay were more frequently demonstrated in patients with preoperative elevations in CRP. ⚡ **It appears that patients without apparent infection who have increased CRP values preoperatively are at increased risk for infectious complications postoperatively.** ⚡

Nitric Oxide

Although nitric oxide (NO) does not itself cause inflammation, NO is increased in many SIRS and shock states, and has been shown to be the primary effector of vasolidation in endotoxin LPS-induced hypotension during sepsis (21). NO is an inhibitor of mitochondrial electron transport, an inducer of vascular leak, and a mediator of LPS-induced cytokine release. NO has also been shown to directly increase ileal mucosal membrane and enterocyte monolayer permeability, and bacterial translocation (22). These investigators demonstrated that increased NO production and inducible nitric oxide synthase (iNOS) mRNA expression is associated with endotoxin and/or cytokine-induced loss of enterocyte monolayer barrier function. Although a recent study indicates that iNOS activity may be compartmentalized at the site of infection in patients in septic shock (23), most studies demonstrate systemic release. Circulating peripheral neutrophils in postsurgical septic patients were compared to those from healthy controls after stimulation with LPS and/or TNFα, to determine if there were differences in iNOS expression and constitutive NO production (24). These authors demonstrated that neutrophils from septic patients expressed higher levels of iNOS mRNA than those patients with SIRS alone. Neutrophils from healthy controls did not express iNOS mRNA and did not produce NO. After in vitro stimulation with LPS and TNF-α, these neutrophils did produce iNOS mRNA and NO, indicating that activated neutrophils might be a source of NO in sepsis.

NO is also elevated in hemorrhagic shock with concurrent induction of iNOS along with cyclo-oxygenase (COX)-2 and CD14. This promotes inflammation by the immediate production of NO and prostaglandins. However, hemorrhagic shock patients do not manifest vasodilation during hemorrhagic shock, because more powerful vasoconstrictive forces are at play (centrally-mediated catecholamine elaboration from volume depletion). Another transcription factor, hypoxia-inducible factor-1 is thought to regulate the induction of iNOS during the ischemic phase of shock (25). NO acts as a signaling molecule involved in redox reactions to include activation of nuclear factor-κB (NF-κB) (25). This activation of NF-κB can also promote inflammatory cytokine expression during reperfusion, further contributing to organ injury after hemorrhagic shock.

Sepsis-induced hypotension is also related to impaired angiotensin II (AII)-mediated adrenal catecholamine release, despite the strong systemic activation of the renin-angiotensin system. This may be due to the down-regulation of the adrenal AII receptors (26).

Lipopolysaccharide-Binding Protein

Lipopolysaccharide-binding protein (LBP) is a humoral protein that recognizes and forms complexes with LPS, the macromolecule on the outer lipid layer of gram-negative bacteria. LBP activity has been historically associated with gram-negative bacterial sepsis. Specialized CD14 cell surface receptors on numerous cells (including human monocytes, neutrophils, and endothelial cells) bind with the LBP-LPS complex. This bond initiates the immunological steps that destroy these bacteria. CD14 is a 55 kD glycoprotein originally thought to promote differentiation of monocytes. CD14 is now known to have a glycosylphosphatidylinositol-anchor in the cell membrane, and requires interaction with transmembrane receptors (necessary for cell membrane signal transduction), including Toll-like receptors (TLRs) and certain integrins (e.g., CD18, CD55) to transmit signals into the cell. Recently, Trianafilou et al. (27) proposed a new model of LPS recognition upon discovery of a signaling complex of receptors involving heat shock proteins.

LBP, PCT, CRP, and IL-6 were studied as markers of inflammation in the first four postoperative days, in 12 adult male patients with SIRS, and at least two dysfunctional organs (MODS) following coronary artery bypass graft (CABG) surgery (28). Plasma PCT and IL-6 concentrations were significantly elevated in all MODS patients. PCT and LBP were markedly elevated in MODS patients with positive microbial findings. The authors concluded that LBP may be a marker for differentiation between noninfectious SIRS and ongoing bacterial sepsis in the early postoperative course following CABG while microbiological results are still pending.

In another study of 24 patients with severe sepsis, LBP serum levels from patients with gram-positive or fungal infections did not differ from those with gram-negative infections (29). When compared to LBP levels in healthy volunteers, levels were significantly increased in patients with sepsis regardless of bacterial etiology. In patients with multiple bouts of sepsis, the LBP response was of lesser magnitude with each subsequent episode. These data suggest that LBP may be a nonspecific marker of sepsis. An ongoing clinical study at our institution is examining the time-dependent changes LBP following trauma (29a).

Intestinal Fatty Acid Binding Protein

The intestinal fatty acid binding protein (IFABP) is a small protein uniquely located in the small intestine enterocyte, and is believed to be important for fatty acid transport and storage (6). IFABP is not typically detectable in serum and/ or urine of healthy individuals. It is, however, detectable after episodes of acute intestinal ischemia and inflammation, occurring most often at a time when the insult was still reversible. Urinary levels of IFABP were significantly elevated in critically ill patients with SIRS, and peaked 1.4 days before SIRS was diagnosed, suggesting that urinary levels of IFABP could be used to predict patients at risk for SIRS (30).

Adhesion Molecules

Adhesion molecules play a critical role in SIRS, sepsis, and MODS as described above in the section on endothelial activation. Figure 3 shows the sequential activation and engagement of various families of adhesion molecules (including L, P, and E-selectins). These adhesion molecules have been utilized as markers for ongoing systemic inflammation following injury. L-selectin (CD62L) surface expression on neutrophils, monocytes, and lymphocytes and soluble CD62L (sCD62L) plasma concentrations were measured in trauma patients at different time points after injury (31). Severe organ dysfunction in these patients was associated with altered CD62L expression on leukocytes and circulating sCD62L plasma concentrations. Nonsurvivors had decreased sCD62L on admission and T-cell CD62L expression after four hours. E-selectin (principle ligands are surface proteins on cutaneous lymphocytes)

and P-selectin (principle ligand is P-selectin glycoprotein ligand 1) activity was measured in ICU patients who had experienced cardiopulmonary resuscitation (CPR) to determine if there was an association between CPR, SIRS, and elaboration of these molecules (32). SIRS was a common occurrence after CPR (66% of all patients). Soluble P-selectin (sP-selectin) levels were higher in patients with SIRS compared to those without SIRS or with noncritically ill control patients. Soluble E-selectin (sE-selectin) levels were higher in patients with and without SIRS compared to noncritically ill patients, and were higher in nonsurvivors than in survivors. P-selectin was higher in patients who developed sepsis within one week after CPR. These authors concluded that SIRS was a nonspecific finding after CPR, and the determination of sP- and sE-selectin early after CPR might be utilized to identify patients at a high risk for sepsis or adverse outcome. E-selectin is so strongly expressed in sepsis states that its identification on intravascular, interstitial, or intra-alveolar leukocytes in postmortem exams is diagnostic of sepsis-induced fatalities (33). These authors determined that ICAM-1 is strongly expressed on endothelial cells of pulmonary vasculature, macrophages, and lymphocytes, and may be considered a marker for death due to sepsis. Most recently, a prospective, double-blind, randomized, placebo-controlled clinical trial evaluated the safety and efficacy of the humanized monoclonal anti-L-selectin antibody aselizumab in severely injured patients. Aselizumab was associated with a higher rate of infections and leukopenia, however, this difference was not significantly different compared with placebo (34).

NEUROENDOCRINE RESPONSE

☞ **Neurological and endocrine functions interact intimately with inflammatory mediators after injury or onset of illness.** ☞ Together, these systems modulate the immune system via release of neurotransmitters, neuropeptides, and endocrine hormones (6). The immunological response to the release of hormones associated with the hypothalamic-pituitary-adrenal axis after trauma-hemorrhage has been

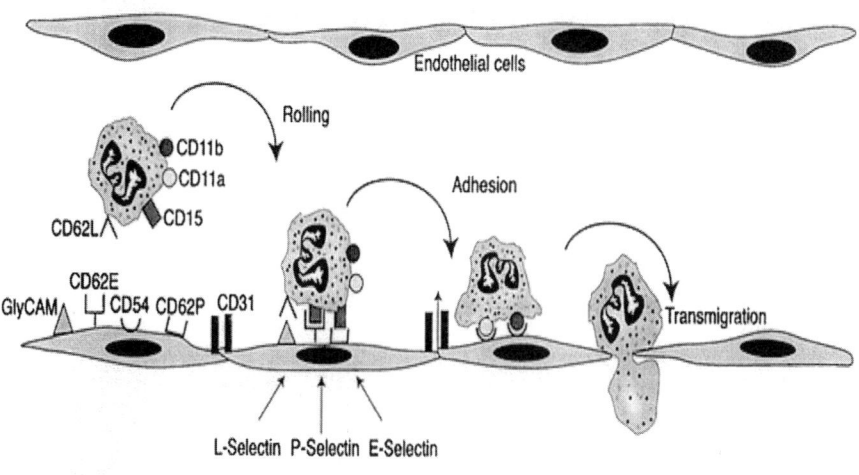

ADHESION MOLECULES CASCADE

Figure 3 Adhesion molecules-sequential engagement. Sequential activation and engagement of all the families of adhesion molecules, resulting in neutrophil migration onto tissue. *Source*: From Ref. 188.

studied. The administration of prolactin augmented spleno-cyte proliferation and splenocyte elaboration of IL-2 and IL-3 in mice, after trauma-hemorrhage (35). Prolactin also signifi-cantly improved macrophage IL-1 and IL-6 release after trauma hemorrhage, and demonstrated better survival after sepsis [cecal ligation and puncture (CLP) model] (36). These same investigators demonstrated that administration of metoclopramide, to augment circulating prolactin levels, exerted a beneficial cell-mediated immune response follow-ing hemorrhagic shock (37). Melatonin, the major hormone released by the pineal gland, maintains immune function in mice subjected to severe hemorrhage and soft tissue injury (6). Glucocorticoids, released by the adrenal glands, have demonstrated anti-inflammatory effects by interfering with leukocyte proliferation, and release of cytokines and other inflammatory mediators. These steroids have also been shown to limit TNFα production and enhance IL-10 synthesis in septic states (38).

Cells of both the central and peripheral nervous systems, as well as endocrine organs, are capable of produ-cing cytokines. Cytokines released under conditions of stress by these cells act in an autocrine or paracrine manner to stimulate organ-specific responses within the involved organ. This is evidenced by the adrenal expression of mRNA for IL-6 in cells of the cortex and the medulla in juxtaposition to cells responsible for catecholamine secretion (39). Furthermore, IL-6 and its receptors are expressed in adrenal cell cultures in the presence or absence of macro-phages (40). Under conditions of stress, these cytokines are also released systemically, eliciting an endocrine response.

Cells of the central nervous system (CNS) respond in similar fashion, demonstrating both the ability to release cytokines and express cytokine receptors, as well as react to systemically released cytokines. Cytokines play an important role in normal development of the brain (neuro-trophic) and the response to traumatic brain injury (TBI) (41). Levels of IL-6 in the CNS compared to measurement in other organs or plasma, after either local (into CSF) or sys-temic injection of cytokines to include IL-1α, IL-1β, and IL-6, indicate that the brain may be a significant source of this cytokine elaboration (42,43). Whether released locally or sys-temically, the cytokines act in an afferent manner, eliciting an efferent response to the stimulus. This efferent response is the brain-directed physiological sequelae to injury or illness.

Peripheral nerves are affected by the inflammatory response as well. Inflammatory mediators have been shown to alter neuronal phenotypes affecting growth and functional and electrical properties (44). Il-6 and IL-6 recep-tor expression, after neuronal injury has been associated with initiation of neural tissue repair (45).

Neurogenic inflammation is thought to originate from the release of substance P and other neurokinins encoded by the preprotachykinin A gene, from unmyelinated nerve fibers following noxious stimuli (46). This mechanism may account for respiratory distress in response to CNS injury. The airways have a complex network of sensory nerve fibers just below the epithelial surface. Conceivably, any change in the bronchial environment could stimulate the release of substance P (47). Piedimonte demonstrated this phenomenon in an animal study wherein the respiratory syncytial virus (RSV) caused a marked increase in airway vascular permeability, resulting in an increase in overall inflammation (47). He demonstrated that these changes were mediated by the high affinity receptor for substance P (neurokinin [NK-1]). T lymphocyte subpopulations within bronchial-associated lymphoid tissue in the lungs of RSV-infected rats also expressed high levels of the NK-1 receptor. This upregulation presumably occurs at the gene expression level, as NK-1 receptor mRNA levels were noted to increase significantly during RSV infection.

The neurological and endocrine systems work in col-laboration after either systemic or end-organ release of inflammatory mediators. Cytokines released by neurological cells act on those cells and others in the nervous system, but also on the endocrine organs. These endocrine organs secrete cytokines as well as hormones that act within the endocrine system, but also act as afferent stimuli for the nervous system. Recent evidence suggests that there is a specific afferent system directly connecting endocrine and CNS cells (48). This creates an intricate immunological cycle incorporating the CNS and the hypothalamic-pituitary-adrenal hormonal axis, wherein the systemic functional physiological outcome after trauma or illness may be orchestrated.

HORMONAL INVOLVEMENT

Animal studies utilizing trauma-hemorrhagic shock models have demonstrated gender differences in outcome. Females demonstrated enhanced immune function and better outcome compared with males following hemorrhagic shock and sepsis, whereas males demonstrated better out-comes following major burn injury. Clinical studies have been inconsistent in regard to outcome associated with gender. However, basic science studies have demonstrated sex hormonal differences that may explain the observed gender based survival variation.

IL-10 therapy has been shown to have a potential role in treatment of the early inflammatory state after hemorrha-gic shock in some animal studies. To determine whether gender impacted these results, male and female mice were subjected to hemorrhage or sham operation, and then received either recombinant murine IL-10 (rmIL-10) or placebo during the resuscitation phase (49). At 48 hours after resuscitation, peritoneal macrophages and splenocytes were harvested. IL-1β and IL-12 released by the macro-phages, and splenocyte proliferation, interferon (IFN)γ, and IL-2 release capacity was measured. IL-10 plasma levels were not increased after treatment. In males, the treat-ment with IL-10 restored the depressed immune response as evidenced by depressed splenocyte proliferation, IFNγ, and IL-1β. Only depression of splenocyte proliferation was demonstrated in female mice. Furthermore, sham-operated male mice treated with rmIL-10 demonstrated depressed immune responses compared with the placebo group.

Another recent study demonstrated female gender protection from sepsis following hemorrhage (50). In this study, both male and female mice were subjected to hemor-rhage or sham operation. All mice were then subjected to sepsis by CLP, and survival was assessed over 10 days. Male mice subjected to hemorrhage prior to CLP had higher mortality than shams. In contrast, mortality in female mice after CLP was comparable in both the hemor-rhage and sham groups. Plasma levels of the inflammatory mediators, IL-6 and TNF-α after CLP were increased in males subjected to hemorrhage, whereas these mediators were not increased in hemorrhaged females.

In contrast, Wichmann et al. (51) did not demonstrate gender differences regarding death from severe sepsis in almost 4000 human patients in a surgical ICU. In a smaller critical care population, female gender was associated with a lower mortality rate after severe sepsis (52). When patients were stratified by age and injury severity score (ISS), there were no gender differences in mortality in 18,892 blunt trauma patients (53). In this study, male gender was associated with an increased incidence of pneumonia after injury; however, females with pneumonia had higher mortality. Gannon et al. (54) studied 22,332 patients from 26 trauma centers. These researchers demonstrated that age, ISS, non-Caucasian race, blunt injury, revised trauma score, and pre-existing diseases were associated with increased risk for mortality. Gender was not associated with increased risk for mortality. Female patients represented 27% of the 17,589 trauma patients stratified by age, ISS, mechanism of injury, and gender in another study that evaluated outcome to include mortality (55). Females ≤40 years old had a survival advantage in the ISS 16 to 24 group; however, these patients had significantly less severe injury. Males had more infectious complications, and females with pneumonia had higher mortality. Interestingly, burn trauma shows an opposite gender dimorphic outcome response. With burn trauma, premenopausal women demonstrate worse outcome compared with age-matched males (see Volume 1, Chapter 34).

Estradiol

ơ⁺ **The hormone 17-beta-estradiol has been associated with female gender-specific protective effects from SIRS following trauma and hemorrhage in animal studies.** ơ⁺ The Kupffer cell is a major source of inflammatory cytokine release following trauma. Estradiol appears to directly attenuate Kupffer cell release of inflammatory mediators. To study this effect in an injury model, male mice were subjected to laparotomy and hemorrhage or sham operation (56). Two hours later, Kupffer cells were harvested and cultured with 17beta-estradiol, in the presence or absence of LPS stimulation. Kupffer cell production of IL-6 and TNF-α were increased following trauma and hemorrhage. Production of IL-6 was attenuated in all animals after incubation with 17-beta-estradiol in a dose-dependent manner. In contrast, the down-regulation of TNF-α was minimal. Continued synthesis of 17-beta-estradiol, in proestrus female mice, appears to be responsible for maintenance of T lymphocyte cytokine release associated with protection after trauma and hemorrhage (57). Specifically, it may be that estradiol in females may maintain type 1 helper T cells (Th1) cytokine release (e.g., IL-2, IFN-γ) after trauma and hemorrhage, whereas androgens are responsible for depressed Th1 cytokine release (58).

Testosterone

ơ⁺ **In contrast to the female sex hormone estradiol, increased levels of the male sex hormone testosterone are associated with decreased cell mediated immune response following trauma in animal studies. However, testosterone decreases muscle catabolism following burns.** ơ⁺ In multiple animal studies male mice exhibited significantly decreased levels of cytokine release from inflammatory cells after trauma and during severe sepsis (CLP) (6). Castration, leading to undetectable serum testosterone levels, was associated with conservation of cell-mediated immunity in these studies. To determine whether castration and testosterone inhibition was the causative factor in this immune response, flutamide, a testosterone receptor antagonist, was administered to male mice after trauma-hemorrhage (59). At 72 hours

postinjury and hemorrhagic shock, protection of cell-mediated immunity was observed in the flutamide treated males.

Studies have also demonstrated that flutamide was protective against the lethal effects of CLP after hemorrhagic shock (60). Yokoyama et al. (56) also demonstrated that castration or androgen receptor blockade with flutamide after trauma-hemorrhage in male mice presented beneficial effect. This group also demonstrated that administration of 17-beta estradiol or prolactin to male animals significantly improved immune function.

Some clinical studies have demonstrated abnormally low testosterone levels in males after trauma. Severely burned male mice were found to have abnormally low testosterone levels after injury (61). These mice were then treated with testosterone enanthate (1 dose/wk) for two weeks. Serum testosterone levels increased from baseline to low normal in one week, and to high normal range after two weeks. These investigators also measured protein synthesis over this time period, and found that protein synthetic efficiency increased two-fold, demonstrating that restoration of serum testosterone can ameliorate the muscle catabolism of severe burn injury. Abnormally low levels of testosterone were elaborated in male patients after traumatic injury, in a study that evaluated time-dependent changes in serum hormones (62). In this study, serum estradiol, progesterone, and testosterone were measured at admission and at 24 hours in male and female trauma patients. Estradiol levels were not significantly different at admission, but females had significantly higher levels at 24 hours. Progesterone levels were not different between the genders at admission or at 24 hours; however, male levels were noted to be abnormally high at admission. Males had significantly higher testosterone levels than females at admission, but not at 24 hours. Interestingly, testosterone levels were at a low normal value for males at admission and were below normal at 24 hours. There were no differences in outcome based on gender. Future studies must examine time-dependent changes in sex hormone concentrations at later time points, to further elucidate their role in gender-related outcome differences in human SIRS and sepsis following trauma.

Progesterone

To date, progesterone has not been studied as extensively as estradiol or testosterone. The main focus of some of the studies is modulation of the immune system. In one study, progesterone administration in a trauma-hemorrhage animal model was found to ameliorate the pro-inflammatory response (decreased IL-6 and TNF-α), and subsequently hepatocellular injury (decreased transaminases and reduced myeloperoxidase activity), compared to controls that received resuscitation fluid alone (63). Shear et al. (64) studied progesterone as a treatment for cerebral edema after TBI. These investigators determined that a single dose of progesterone can attenuate cerebral edema after TBI in rats, but didn't always lead to functional improvement. Regimens continued for three to five days reduced the size of injury-induced necrosis and cell loss, and a five-day regimen improved behavioral outcome.

Leptin

Leptin is an adipocyte-derived hormone whose serum levels are influenced by cytokines. It is thought to regulate immune function, food intake, and energy expenditure. Recent studies have demonstrated that hypercatabolism and immune dysfunction are closely associated with SIRS and

MODS. Papathanassoglou et al. studied leptin levels, nutritional indices, and outcome in critically ill patients (65). Critically ill patients exhibited higher serum levels of leptin, as well as IL-6, TNF-α, and cortisol than controls. The authors concluded that cytokines and cortisol up-regulate leptin levels that in turn may predispose the patients to hypercatabolism, wasting, and immune dysfunction. Serum leptin levels alone were not independently associated with severity of SIRS or MODS, or with mortality. Gender specific changes in leptin levels also require further elucidation.

SYSTEMIC INFLAMMATORY RESPIRATORY SYNDROME—COAGULATION SYSTEM INTERACTION

The increasingly appreciated molecular linkage between the procoagulant and inflammatory systems is one of the critical discoveries of the last 25 years (66). The coagulation system evolved as a mechanism to limit the loss of vital elements from the internal milieu following mechanical injury to the circulatory system. Whereas the innate immune system was developed as a rapid response mechanism for detection and clearance of microbial invaders that breach the integument, the coagulation and innate immunity systems co-evolved from a common ancestral substrate early in eukaryotic development, and these two systems retain a highly integrated and co-regulated circuitry of signals and control elements that defend the host following tissue injury and microbial invasion. Indeed, the ancestry may predate eukaryotic development, as primitive micro-organisms, lacking a circulatory system and thus without need for coagulation to stop bleeding, possess a coagulation system that is used to protect against microbial invasion (66).

Coagulopathy and systemic inflammation are almost universal findings in patients with sepsis. Septic patients are also known to have diminished concentrations of circulating antithrombin III (AT III), tissue plasminogen activator, and activated protein C (APC) (67).

In the landmark Protein C Worldwide Evaluation in Sepsis (PROWESS) trial, Bernard et al. (68) showed a significant decrease in mortality for septic patients treated with recombinant human APC compared to placebo. The PROWESS trial was very well conducted with a large sample number (1690 patients), demographic factors were similar in the treatment and placebo groups, and protein C deficiency was detected in 90% of the patients in which it was measured (68). The relative risk of death in the treated group was reduced by 20%. Furthermore, APC reduced mortality in almost every subgroup examined in the phase III trial. The only significant side effect of the drug is bleeding, and the treatment patients had a higher rate of bleeding episodes compared to placebo (3.5% vs. 2.0%), but this difference was not clinically or statistically significant ($p = 0.06$).

The administration of APC was associated with a reduction in plasma D-dimer levels, demonstrating that the procoagulant effects of sepsis were diminished by this therapy. A concomitant reduction in the serum levels of IL-6 and TNF-α indicated that treatment also attenuated the inflammatory cascade. The reduced TNF-α results are in concert with the evidence that APC reduces the production of TNF-α monocytes by inhibiting the coupling of endotoxin and CD14, without affecting the antimicrobial properties of monocytes (69).

Additionally, APC inhibits factors Va and VIIIa resulting in decreased thrombin generation, and increases the fibrinolytic response by reducing the levels of plasminogen activator inhibitor-1 and by preventing activation of thrombin–activatable fibrinolysis inhibitor (TAFI) (70). APC is also known to reduce interactions between neutrophils and endothelial cells, and to decrease tissue ischemia (71), in part by reducing the endothelial expression of E-selectin (72).

At present, no clinical studies have evaluated the use of agents that alter both coagulation and inflammation (such as APC) in patients with noninfectious causes of SIRS. Additionally, studies involving patients who are at increased risk of bleeding (omitted from the PROWESS trial) must be studied to better define the potential morbidity of APC therapy. Real-time protein detection technologies, which monitor a panel of sepsis-related bio-markers (including APC levels) will likely improve the targeting of this promising therapy (73). Optimal use of APC and other anti-coagulant agents in sepsis and SIRS requires additional basic research into the critical linkage between coagulation and innate immunity (73).

PROGRESSION OF SYSTEMIC INFLAMMATORY RESPONSE SYNDROME TO COMPENSATORY ANTI-INFLAMMATORY RESPONSE SYNDROME AND MULTIPLE ORGAN DYSFUNCTION SYNDROME

It is unclear whether SIRS serves a purposeful function, or merely represents an epiphenomenon resulting from severe tissue injury, induced by trauma, shock, and infection. However, we do know that the severity and intensity of the inflammatory response affects outcome, and appears to be determined by the balance between inflammatory and CARS. Bone was the first to propose the five-stage progression from SIRS to MODS (Fig. 4), in 1996 (74). At that time, considerable new evidence indicated that, in addition to a massive pro-inflammatory reaction, a compensatory anti-inflammatory response contributes to the onset of these disorders. The five stages summarized in Figure 4 are as follows: (i) local inflammatory response, (ii) systemic inflammatory response, (iii) massive systemic inflammatory response, (iv) immunologic paralysis, and (v) immune dissonance. If the last three phases do not quickly resolve, cell damage can be amplified thus perpetuating the inflammatory process and promoting infectious complications, resulting in MODS.

At a local site of injury or infection, and during the initial appearance of pro- and anti-inflammatory mediators in the circulation, the beneficial effects of these mediators typically outweigh their harmful effects. However, when the balance between these two forces is lost, widespread inflammation occurs and these mediators become harmful. Sequelae of an unbalanced systemic pro-inflammatory reaction include shock, organ dysfunction, and coagulation defects. An unbalanced systemic compensatory anti-inflammatory response can result in anergy and immunosuppression. This late immunosuppressive phase was termed the "CARS"—by Bone (Fig. 4). The pro- and anti-inflammatory forces may ultimately reinforce each other, creating a state of increasingly destructive immunologic dissonance. SIRS continues to be recognized as an ubiquitous early harbinger of MODS. Although these acronyms are clever and provide simplified understanding of the pathophysiology, they do not fully explain the complexity of the human response to injury.

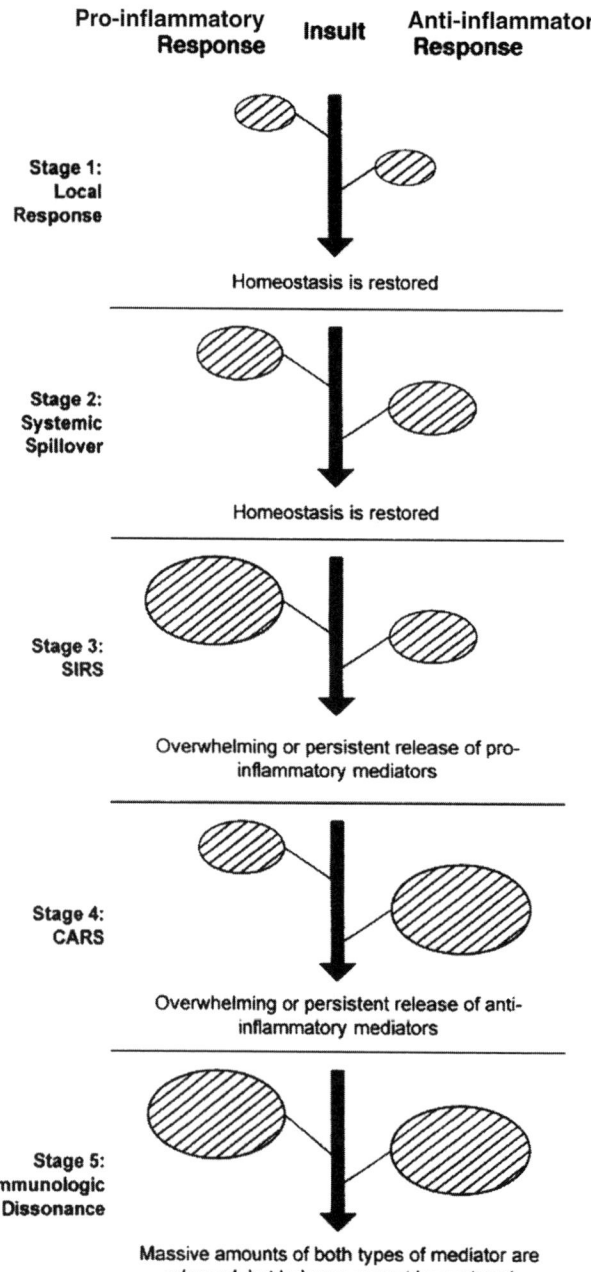

Figure 4   Progression from systemic inflammatory response syndrome (SIRS) to compensatory anti-inflammatory response syndrome (CARS) to multiple organ dysfunction syndrome (MODS). The five stages in the development of multiple organ dysfunction as postulated by Roger Bone. Stage 1 begins at a site of local injury or infection. Pro-inflammatory mediators are released locally to promote wound healing and to combat foreign organisms or antigens. Anti-inflammatory mediators are then released to downregulate this process. If the original insult is small and the patient is healthy, homeostasis will be quickly restored. Stage 2 occurs if local defense mechanisms are insufficient to correct the local injury, or eliminate the local infection. Through various mechanisms, pro-inflammatory mediators are released into the systemic circulation; these recruit additional cells to the local area of injury. Systemic release of anti-inflammatory mediators follows soon thereafter; under normal circumstances, these mediators ameliorate the pro-inflammatory reaction and restore homeostasis. Stage 3 occurs if the systemic release of pro-inflammatory mediators is too massive, or if the anti-inflammatory reaction is insufficient to permit downregulation. It is at this stage that most patients have symptoms of the SIRS, as well as incipient evidence of the MODS. Stage 4 can be represented by excessive systemic levels of anti-inflammatory mediators that develop as a response to a massive pro-inflammatory response; however, these levels can also develop de novo. Patients with a stage 4 CARS have marked immunosuppression and, thus, are at increased risk for infection. The body can re-establish homeostasis after stage 3 or 4 and improve. Others will advance to stage 5—the final phase of MODS. At this stage of immunologic dissonance, the balance between pro- and anti-inflammatory mediators has been lost, and many of these patients currently go on to die. Some patients may have persistent, massive inflammation; others may have ongoing immunosuppression and secondary infections. Still others may oscillate between periods of inflammation and immunosuppression. *Source*: From Ref. 74.

The human immune response is regulated by a highly complex and intricate network of control elements (many still unknown). Prominent among the known regulatory components are the anti-inflammatory cytokines and specific cytokine inhibitors (75). Under physiologic conditions, these cytokine inhibitors serve as immunomodulators limiting the potentially injurious effects of sustained or excess inflammatory reactions. Under pathologic conditions, these anti-inflammatory mediators may either: (*i*) provide insufficient control over pro-inflammatory activities in immune-mediated diseases; or (*ii*) overcompensate and inhibit the immune response, rendering the host at risk from systemic infection. A dynamic and ever-shifting balance exists between pro-inflammatory cytokines and anti-inflammatory components of the human immune system. The regulation of inflammation by these cytokines and cytokine inhibitors is further complicated by the fact that the immune system has redundant pathways with multiple elements having similar physiological effects.

SYSTEMIC INFLAMMATORY RESPONSE SYNDROME AND SPECIFIC PATIENT POPULATIONS
Trauma and Critical Illness
Traumatic injury immediately stimulates inflammation in order to save the individual and initiate repair. This inflammatory response is a cascading process involving a delicate balance between pro- and anti-inflammatory mediators, and components of all bodily systems. If the injured person does not die immediately, his morbidity and/or mortality may depend in large part on the degree to which systemic inflammation influences his clinical course. Basic and clinical science studies have demonstrated an intricate relationship between trauma, shock, SIRS, and sepsis (6). ☞ **Trauma, especially when complicated by hemorrhagic shock, may induce SIRS, potentially resulting in immunodepression, MODS, severe sepsis, or septic shock.** ☜ If severe enough, this inflammatory response may adversely affect organ systems not involved in the original traumatic injury. In this scenario, MODS typically follows a specific pattern affecting the lungs first, followed by the liver, gut, and kidneys (6). The presence of SIRS may provide insight into patients at risk, for progression to MODS.

A SIRS score of ≥2 at the time of admission has been shown to be an independent predictor of increased mortality and length of stay in trauma patients, suggesting that admission SIRS score may be used as a predictor of outcome and resource utilization (76). These findings were confirmed in 9539 trauma patients admitted to a level-one trauma center over a 30-month period (77). This study demonstrated that the SIRS score was an independent predictor of mortality and ICU length of stay, hypothermia (temperature <36°C) was the most significant predictor of mortality, and leukocytosis (neutrophil count >12,000/mm^3) was the most significant predictor of total hospital length of stay (LOS). Another study of 4887 blunt trauma patients admitted to a level one trauma center determined that admission SIRS score, independent of age and ISS, was an independent predictor of infection (78). Infected patients had statistically longer hospital lengths of stay and increased risk for mortality.

The predictive capability of daily SIRS scores and outcome in trauma patients admitted to an ICU has been evaluated (79). SIRS on hospital days 3 to 7 was a significant predictor of nosocomial infection and hospital length of stay. Persistent SIRS to hospital day 7 was associated with a significant risk for increased mortality. In another study, SIRS for ≥3 days in trauma patients was associated with an increased incidence of disseminated intravascular coagulation (DIC), the adult respiratory distress syndrome (ARDS), and MODS (80).

A review of published cohort studies, examining the septic syndromes with an emphasis on ICU patients revealed that the prevalence of SIRS is very high, affecting one-third of all in-hospital patients and >50% of all ICU patients (81). SIRS occurs in 80% of all surgical ICU patients. In this patient population, the prevalence of infection and bacteremia increases with the number of SIRS criteria met, as well as with increasing severity of the septic syndromes. Approximately one-third of patients with SIRS has, or evolves to, sepsis. Sepsis may occur in 25% of ICU patients, progressing to severe sepsis in >50% of the cases. Mortality rates increase with progression from SIRS to septic shock, and are similar within each stage whether infection is documented or not. Most deaths (3/4) occur during the first few months after sepsis, but there is also a 50% reduction of life expectancy over the following five years. When SIRS progresses to MODS and MOF, mortality rates increase substantially (30–80%), depending on the number of failed organs (82).

A prospective study evaluating daily SIRS scores and outcomes in 2300 surgical ICU admissions demonstrated that SIRS on postoperative day 2 (compared to the score on day 1) was a more accurate predictor of mortality and correlated better with Acute Physiologic and Chronic Health Evaluation III (APACHE III) and MODS scores (Table 3) (83). It was hypothesized that the effects of surgery, surgical stress, anesthesia, and ICU resuscitation in the first 24 hours may overestimate the pro-inflammatory response itself, making quantitation of the SIRS within that time period too sensitive.

The degree of metabolic stress among critically ill patients may be variable, and dependent upon whether or not SIRS is related to infection and/or sepsis (84). Moriyama et al. (84) demonstrated that oxygen consumption and resting energy expenditure were higher in SIRS patients with sepsis, compared to SIRS patients without sepsis.

Surgery
☞ **Surgical procedures are known to elicit systemic inflammation. The magnitude and duration of the procedure, comorbid diseases, and reperfusion injury are just a few of the variables that affect the inflammatory response.** ☜ Some operations are associated with specific procedures that directly affect the immune response. Knowledge of these potential inflammatory insults may lead to modification of certain surgical procedures and/or re-evaluation of their indications.

Cardiopulmonary bypass (CPB) and extracorporeal circulation have been associated with SIRS and MODS due to inflammatory mediator release. Survival in patients with MODS after CPB may be affected by the degree of inflammatory mediator release. A recent study determined that levels of IL-8, IL-18, and PCT could be used as parameters for the prognosis of patients with organ dysfunctions after cardiac surgery (85).

The inflammatory response associated with hepatic ischemia/reperfusion during liver resection and transplantation has been studied, though the clinical implications remain to be clarified. These findings may also be applicable to hepatic surgery associated with traumatic injury. The inflammatory cytokines TNF-α, IL-1β, IL-6, and IL-8 were measured in serial samples of portal and systemic blood before hepatic inflow clamping, at the end of clamping, one hour, and one day after continuous inflow occlusion in 25 patients undergoing elective hepatectomy (86). These investigators demonstrated that portal IL-6 levels during resection and at one hour after cessation of clamping significantly correlated with duration of hepatic inflow occlusion, portal venous pressure, and increase in postoperative serum transaminases and bilirubin. Increased levels of systemic IL-8 demonstrated increases in these same parameters, whereas portal IL-8 levels showed no such correlation. The one patient who died had elevated cytokine levels in the presence of elevated portal venous pressure. The authors proposed that hepatectomy that would require prolonged inflow occlusion be reconsidered when an enhanced acute generation of cytokines is anticipated, especially in the presence of markedly increased portal pressure.

Instrumentation is frequently utilized in orthopedic trauma surgery. The effects of instrumentation on postoperative inflammation in patients undergoing spinal injury were investigated by Takahashi et al. (87). The pro-inflammatory cytokines IL-6 and IL-8, the anti-inflammatory cytokines IL-10 and IL-1RA, and the soluble TNF-a receptors I and II were assayed in seven patients who underwent lumbar spinal posterior decompression, six patients with spinal decompression and posterolateral fusion without instrumentation, and seven patients with spinal decompression and posterolateral fusion with instrumentation. All cytokines increased significantly after spinal instrumentation on postoperative days 0 and 1. Seven days later, the inflammatory cytokines had normalized, but the anti-inflammatory cytokines remained elevated in this group. These findings suggest that patients undergoing instrumentation may be at higher risk for infection and/or SIRS and MODS, due to an exaggeration of the inflammatory response.

Extremity ischemia/reperfusion injury is frequently encountered in trauma and vascular surgery. Free radical release following ischemia/reperfusion leads to inflammation, and the patient's innate antioxidant system [total antioxidant capacity (TAC)] is the mode of defense. TAC was evaluated in patients with chronic leg ischemia who underwent femoral-distal bypass (88). Patients who developed SIRS following revascularization had a significantly reduced TAC, and increased lipid peroxidation and vascular permeability (measured by changes in the urinary albumin to creatinine ratio). TAC may represent a marker for patients at risk for SIRS, and the authors thought that augmentation with antioxidants may be utilized to augment their defense.

Levels of postoperative inflammatory cytokine levels have been shown to reflect the magnitude of surgical stress. Laparoscopically performed intra-abdominal surgery has been demonstrated to elicit lower postoperative levels of inflammatory cytokines (specifically IL-6 and IL-8) compared with open procedures, lending support to the use of this modality when technically and/or surgically feasible (89). Indications for the use of laparoscopic surgery in trauma are presently under investigation.

Anesthesia

☞ With the exception of anaphylaxis and allergy (see Volume 1, Chapter 33), anesthetics and analgesics by themselves are not initiators of SIRS. However, several anesthetics and analgesics have shown immunomodulatory effects, and may therefore have some effects on SIRS. ☞

Different anesthetic agents have different effects on the inflammatory response. The inflammatory response associated with Total Intravenous Anesthesia (TIVA) and Balanced Inhalation Anesthesia (BIA) was compared in patients undergoing elective lumbar discectomies (90). In the BIA group, the IL-6 plasma concentration was significantly elevated, but IL-2Rα and IL-1RA were reduced compared with the TIVA group. There was also a relatively greater increase in postoperative cortisol, epinephrine, and norepinephrine concentrations under BIA, perhaps representing an enhanced activation of the hypothalamic-pituitary-adrenal axis and the sympathetic nervous system. Ketamine reduced the CPB-induced IL-6 and IL-8 response in patients undergoing cardiac valve replacement (91). Anesthesia with ketamine/acepromazine/zylazine significantly blunted the LPS-induced plasma TNF-α release in an animal study (92). Preoperative administration of clonidine decreased both plasma and CSF concentrations of TNF-α (93). A large dose of clonidine resulted in no detectable TNF-α in the CSF. Clonidine also led to decreased catecholamine release in the periphery and CNS. Furthermore, patients who received clonidine preoperatively had lower pain scale scores and required less postoperative pain medications. Propofol inhibited IL-6 and IL-10 production by LPS-stimulated peripheral blood mononuclear cells and thiopental induced IL-10 production, when different IV anesthetics were compared (94). General anesthesia with propofol and fentanyl led to a decrease in circulating lymphocytes, characterized by a significant increase in the percentage of T lymphocytes in favor of CD4+ cells, increased B lymphocytes and a significant decrease in NK cells, suggesting promotion of a pro-inflammatory immune response in patients undergoing elective orthopedic surgery (95). These investigators also studied the immune response to whole blood stimulated with LPS in these patients. There was a significant enhancement of TNF-α and IL-1β release in these samples after induction of anesthesia. Synthesis of IL-10 decreased significantly in these LPS-stimulated cultures.

Inhalational (volatile) anesthetics utilized during GA have been studied for their effect on systemic inflammation and for effects on pulmonary tissue. Alveolar epithelial type II (AT II) cells are known to elicit cytokines when stressed and are exposed to volatile anesthetics when patients are under GA. Giraud et al. (96) studied the effects of halothane, enflurane, and isoflurane on rat AT II cells after stimulation with recombinant murine IL-1β (rmIL-1β). The volatile anesthetics decreased AT II secretions of inflammatory cytokines, but did not modify total protein secretion. Halothane exposure decreased the inflammatory response in a dose- and time-dependent manner. This inhibition was reversed between 4 and 24 hours postoperatively.

Thoracic epidural anesthesia utilized during cardiac surgery has been associated with a reduction in ischemia/reperfusion injury, which may in turn decrease the elaboration of pro-inflammatory cytokines (97). Epidural anesthesia with bupivacaine administered during CPB surgery led to an attenuated inflammatory response compared to patients who had GA alone (98).

Inflammatory mediators, when present in patients preoperatively, may adversely affect anesthesia. An animal study demonstrated that both central (via intracerebro-ventricular placement) and peripheral (via intraperitoneal placement) administration of TNF-α decreased anesthesia time induced by ketamine or propofol (99).

Cardiopulmonary Bypass

CPB has been the traditional methodology for providing oxygenated blood for tissue perfusion during cardiac surgery. CPB is associated with augmentation of the systemic inflammatory response. Okubo et al. (100) studied the immunological effect of CABG, with and without CPB. In this study, 10 patients who had CABG on pump, and 10 patients who underwent CABG without CPB, had peripheral blood sampled before and 6 hours after surgery. This blood was then evaluated for gene expression of cytokines, adhesion molecules, and vasoactive substances in the leukocytes. Postoperative expression of mRNA for IL-1, IL-8, IL-10, TNF-α, heme oxygenase-1, platelet endothelial cellular adhesion molecule, and Mac-1 increased significantly in the on-pump group, but not in the off-pump group. ☞ **Direct contact between patient blood and the synthetic surfaces of the CPB system, along with released intracellular elements of destroyed cells, are the most likely reasons for the increased inflammatory mediators seen with CPB.** ☜ In a review of alternatives to CPB, Ganapathy et al. (97) reported that beating heart surgery (without CPB) significantly attenuates the pro-inflammatory cytokine stress response. They reported that there is reduced renal dysfunction associated with beating heart surgery as well.

Dexamethasone given to patients prior to CABG surgery led to a relative decrease in inflammatory mediator release and an increase in anti-inflammatory mediators (101). Patients who had dexamethasone also had better outcome immediately postop, and shorter ICU lengths of stay. Dopexamine administered intravenously during cardiac surgery, and up to 18 hours postoperatively, led to a decrease in the pro-inflammatory immune response when compared to controls [normal saline (NS) infusion instead of dopexamine] (98).

EFFECTS OF RESUSCITATION ON INFLAMMATION

☞ **Resuscitation for trauma and surgery may affect an individual's innate immune response, as a result of the type, quantity, and timing of fluid resuscitation.** ☜ Controversy presently exists regarding the timing and titration of fluid resuscitation, as related to goal mean arterial pressure (MAP) and end-points of resuscitation (e.g., measurement of base deficit and/or lactate vs. other). There is also concern that certain IV fluids may be more efficacious and less immunogenic than others (see Volume 1, Chapter 11). As with all decisions in medicine, one must balance risks of fluid resuscitation with the benefits (102).

One of the concerns regarding fluid resuscitation in hemorrhagic shock is the potential to disrupt efficacious vascular clot. Animal studies have demonstrated that increasing IV rates/blood pressure in the presence of uncontrolled bleeding is accompanied by increased bleeding (102). Using a rat model of uncontrolled hemorrhage, Burris et al. (103) demonstrated that the group that had no fluids had the lowest survival rate. Groups resuscitated with lactated ringers (LR) to a MAP of 100 mmHg also had low survival rates. The highest survival rates were seen in rats resuscitated to a MAP of 80 mm Hg with LR or 40 mm Hg with 7.5% hypertonic saline (HS) and 6% hetastarch. Timing and volume of fluid resuscitation, cytokine elaboration, and mortality were evaluated in an animal model of hemorrhagic shock (104). Sprague-Dawley rats were hemorrhaged 35% of their total blood volume and then resuscitated with varying volumes of crystalloid either early (15 minutes), delayed (60 minutes), or not at all. These investigators determined that rats resuscitated early had decreased cytokine elaboration and decreased mortality. Interestingly, the delayed resuscitation group had increased mortality compared to both the early resuscitation and no resuscitation groups. Excessive fluid resuscitation in both early and late resuscitation groups resulted in increased inflammatory cytokine elaboration and increased mortality. The authors concluded that perhaps volume of fluid, rather than timing of initiation, is a more important determinant of outcome after hemorrhagic trauma.

The first study to evaluate low MAP resuscitation in humans was published in 1994 (105). These investigators randomized hypotensive penetrating trauma victims to routine fluid resuscitation or no fluid resuscitation, until surgical control of bleeding had been achieved. The results demonstrated a survival advantage in the group that had resuscitation withheld initially. However, when the data included those patients who "died in the field" on an intent-to-treat basis, no survival advantage was demonstrated when fluid was withheld. No survival advantage was demonstrated in a more recent study when 110 trauma patients presenting with hemorrhagic shock were randomized to receive resuscitation to either systolic blood pressure (SBP) > 100 mmHg (conventional) or SBP of 70 mmHg (low) (106). These investigators determined that the imprecision of SBP as a marker for tissue oxygen delivery might have accounted for these results. Clearly, large, multicenter prospective randomized studies need to be done to evaluate this more closely.

Resuscitation studies have also focused recently on the type of fluid used. Presently, isotonic fluids are given preferentially in resuscitation protocols. Normal saline (NS) or LR are the crystalloids most frequently utilized. Isotonic fluids are quickly distributed throughout the entire extracellular space, as unfortunately there is no predilection for the intravascular space. This results in fluid retention with an increased ratio of extracellular to plasma space; only 10% to 20% or less of infused isotonic fluids remain in circulation (107). Colloid solutions elicit an oncotic pressure similar to plasma (20–30 mmHg). Commonly used colloids include: albumin (20–25 mmHg), hetastarch (30–35 mmHg), and dextran 70 (60–75 mmHg) (107). Albumin expands plasma volume by 80% of infused volume, hetastarch expands plasma volume equal to the infused volume, and dextran expands plasma volume 20% to 50% more than the infused volume.

HS has been investigated extensively as both a fluid medium for resuscitation and as an anti-inflammatory agent in trauma and critical illness. It has demonstrated efficacy in the restoration of hemodynamic stability and microcirculatory support, in patients who are hypovolemic due to hemorrhagic shock (6). HS has been associated with decreased blood viscosity and improved microcirculation, when utilized as a resuscitation fluid. HS mobilizes an amount of cellular water proportional to osmotic load, and tends to reduce overall volume needs in perioperative patients (107). Cells become edematous during shock and surgical stress, and HS has been shown to normalize cell volume rather than reduce it below normal (107). HS resuscitation was associated with improvement in microcirculatory perfusion to the kidney and small bowel (108). Coimbra et al. (109) demonstrated decreased bacterial translocation and decreased incidence of lung injury associated with HS resuscitation. Resuscitation with HS was also associated with restoration of intestinal nutrient blood flow, prevention of gut barrier breakdown and bacterial translocation, and prevention of organ failure (110). Gurfinkel et al. (111) demonstrated improved tissue oxygenation and perfusion, and reduced SIRS when HS [compared with isotonic saline (IS)] was utilized for resuscitation in an animal model of hemorrhage/shock. These authors demonstrated that animals that received HS had higher oxygenation and perfusion indices, and lower arterial lactate, TNF-α, and IL-6 levels. These animals also demonstrated less pulmonary edema, polymorphonuclear cell (PMN) sequestration, and lower mortality compared with animals that received IS. HS (7.5%) was added to dextran 70 (HSD), by Kramer et al. (107), with the theory that HS would expand the vascular space by mobilizing cellular water and that a hyperoncotic colloid might selectively retain more of this water in the vascular space. Their work demonstrated significantly higher and more sustained cardiac output and MAP, and a lower total peripheral resistance compared with either compound alone. These results were repeated in multiple animal studies, some of which also demonstrated decreased mortality.

HS has demonstrated immune-enhancing properties when utilized for fluid resuscitation. Increasing sodium-chloride concentrations in resuscitation fluid was associated with increased T-cell proliferation and decreased levels of immunosuppressive mediators [e.g., prostaglandin E_2 (PGE_2)] (6). Neutrophil activation and associated release of oxygen radicals and proteases is associated with worse outcome after trauma-hemorrhage. Resuscitation with LR was associated with neutrophil activation and release of these harmful reactants, whereas resuscitation with HS was not in an awake-swine model of hemorrhagic shock (112). Junger et al. (113) demonstrated that increasing the tonicity of the saline resuscitation fluid led to a dose-dependent (saline concentration) decrease in N-formyl-methionyl-leucyl-phenylalanine activated human neutrophil release of proteases and oxygen radicals. When compared with LR in an animal model of trauma-hemorrhage, then sepsis (CLP), HS resuscitation was associated with decreased mortality (14.3%) compared to LR (76.9%) (108). These investigators also demonstrated less severe lung injury in animals resuscitated with HS. In another study, these same investigators demonstrated that pentoxifylline added to HS reduced bacterial translocation and lung injury in an animal model of hemorrhagic shock, compared to resuscitation with LR (114).

HS can reverse the immunosuppressive effects of trauma, and the mechanism may in part be due to altered neutrophil adhesion properties in the microcirculation (102). Preliminary human studies have demonstrated many of the same immunological benefits, but not all studies demonstrate clear-cut differences in the immune response to different fluids. Isotonic and hypertonic fluids were evaluated, to determine whether or not the differential effects elicited by these compounds were due to different cytokine gene elaboration profiles (115). All of the resuscitation fluids analyzed led to increased pro-inflammatory mediator gene expression (to include TNF-α, IL-1α, IL-6, and IL-10). There was no difference in the cytokine expression profile between isotonic and hypertonic fluids in this study. Likewise, multicenter trials that have studied the efficacy of HSD, compared to other crystalloids (e.g., LR), have not demonstrated an overall survival benefit, although a subgroup of patients who received HSD

and required surgery had a survival advantage (102). Clearly, human studies need to be undertaken to study this more in depth.

A recent clinical study, designed to determine if HSD was detrimental when administered to hypotensive patients after penetrating trauma to the torso, demonstrated that HSD resuscitation improved survival in the patients who required surgery (116). The study evaluated 230 patients. Overall survival in the 120 patients who received HSD was 82.5%, whereas survival was 75.5% in those who received an equivalent amount of NS ($p = 0.19$). Surgery was required in 157 patients (68%). Of these patients, 84 were resuscitated with HSD and 73 with NS. Survival was 84.5% in those patients who received HSD, compared with 67.1% in those resuscitated with NS ($p = 0.01$).

HS has become a mainstay of therapy for intracranial hypertension associated with TBI. HS decreases intracranial pressure, due to changes that primarily occur in areas of the brain that maintain intact blood-brain barriers (102). Different saline tonicities are also being investigated regarding efficacy in this scenario. A 7.5% saline solution in doses of 2 mL/kg per treatment was as (or more) efficacious than mannitol, for intracranial hypertension refractory to other standard methods of treatment (117). Other strategies most recently utilized along with HS for intracranial hypertension include mild hypothermia, and decompressive craniotomy (118).

THE ROLE OF THE GUT IN SYSTEMIC INFLAMMATORY RESPONSE SYNDROME AND SEPSIS

Under nonstressed conditions, gut integrity is well protected. Intraluminal contents (containing large quantities of bacteria) are kept within the confines of the bowel in multiple ways. An intact gastrointestinal (GI) mucosa via maintenance of tight intracellular junctions is one important method. Additionally, the GI tract has immunological tissue referred to as gut-associated lymphoid tissue (GALT). GALT includes Peyer's patches, mesenteric lymph nodes, and intraepithelial and lamina propria lymphocytes. These immunological cells represent the first line of defense against foreign proteins. Furthermore, surface immunoglobulin A is found in high concentrations amongst these cells. If foreign antigens transfer across the bowel wall, clearance through the portal system (including the mesenteric veins and lymphatics, liver, and spleen) should eliminate the toxic threat (Fig. 5). **A breakdown in any component of this GI defense system may contribute to bacteremia and sepsis, following injury or illness.** The transfer of bacteria across the bowel wall and into surrounding tissue and/or circulation is known as "bacterial translocation." When normal mesenteric processes tasked with controlling this bacterial load fail, overwhelming levels of local, and then circulating, endotoxin levels lead to SIRS, sepsis, and MODS. The pathophysiology of intestinal bacterial translocation is not entirely understood, but it is probably due in part to a breakdown at the local intestinal mucosal barrier from an imbalanced local inflammatory response, ischemia, malnutrition, or a combination of these. Gut associated immune cells release both pro- and anti-inflammatory cytokines when stressed (119). Animal studies have demonstrated significant changes in GALT after hemorrhagic shock and soft tissue trauma. Buzdon et al. (120) utilized a murine femur fracture model to demonstrate a significant

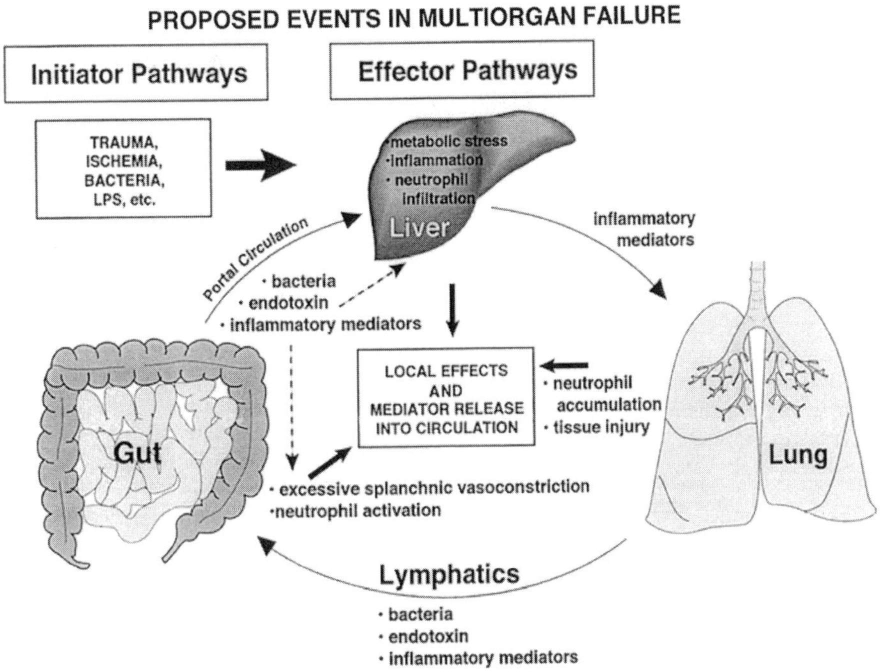

PROPOSED EVENTS IN MULTIORGAN FAILURE

Figure 5 Gut–liver–lung axis in response to shock and hemorrhage. The gut–liver–lung axis in response to hemorrhagic shock injury. These organs (gut, liver, and lung) seem to be the major target organs of systemic inflammatory response syndrome. Initiation of the inflammatory state can occur in any of these organs following trauma or shock. The gut can leak inflammatory mediators into the portal circulation, which will cause a response in the liver. Inflammatory mediators then travel in the hepatic vein to the inferior vena cava and to the lungs. The lungs may become injured, may inactivate some substances (not shown), or can release inflammatory substances themselves, which travel systemically to distant organs (including the gut). *Abbreviation*: LPS, lipopolysaccharide. *Source*: From Ref. 188.

increase in Peyer's patch lymphocyte CD3, CD4, and TCRαβ expression, as well as a significant decrease in Peyer's patch IL-10 protein expression. Secretion of the inflammatory cytokines TNF-α, IL-6, and IFNγ occurs in the small bowel and levels of IL-6 are increased in states of bacterial overgrowth (38). Ischemia/reperfusion may contribute to this insult. In exvivo human intestine, ischemia/reperfusion was associated with increased pro-inflammatory cytokine levels in venous effluent (38).

Basic science and clinical research have demonstrated that the GI tract plays a pivotal pathogenic role in the development of postinjury SIRS and MODS (121). These and other investigators have demonstrated the following findings: (*i*) shock with resulting gut hypoperfusion is an important inciting event; (*ii*) upon reperfusion, the gut is a source of pro-inflammatory mediators capable of amplifying SIRS and contributing to early MODS; (*iii*) early gut hypoperfusion causes an ileus in the stomach and small bowel that sets the stage for progressive gut dysfunction, so that the proximal gut becomes a reservoir for pathogens and toxins that contribute to late sepsis-associated MODS; and (*iv*) Late infections then cause worsening of the gut dysfunction. These findings elucidate the gut's role as both an initiator of inflammation and as a "victim" of SIRS/MODS.

The exact role of malnutrition in this scenario is unknown. Malnutrition has not been directly associated with bacterial translocation; however, there is evidence to suggest that it may make the gut more sensitive to inflammatory mediator release. Maintenance of bowel mucosal integrity in the setting of SIRS is a target of ongoing scientific investigation.

Selective decontamination of the digestive tract (SDD) is a process through which the intraluminal bacterial load is

decreased. A decreased bacterial load is theorized to modulate the inflammatory response to gut hypoperfusion after trauma or critical illness.

Male Wistar rats were divided into four groups in a study to determine the influence of SDD on the pro-inflammatory immune response of the gut (122). The rats were given either SDD or conventional rat chow, and underwent hemorrhage with withdrawal/reinfusion of shed blood or not. TNF-α and IL-6 were measured in portal and caval blood, splenic macrophages, and gut mononuclear cells. Mesenteric lymph nodes were harvested to determine bacterial translocation and a histological specimen was taken from the distal ileum. Feces were also examined to evaluate the effect of SDD. SDD eliminated gram-negative enteric bacteria, but had no influence on mucosal damage or on bacterial translocation in control animals and animals after hemorrhage. There was a significantly elevated LPS-induced pro-inflammatory cytokine release in portal blood, splenic macrophages, and gut mononuclear cells in animals subjected to hemorrhagic shock that were fed rat chow. Hemorrhagic shock after SDD led to suppressed or unchanged cytokine release in these organs, compared to unmanipulated animals receiving SDD. In unmanipulated animals, SDD itself induced a significant inflammatory response. Plasma concentrations of cytokines were significantly elevated in animals after hemorrhage and SDD, compared with animals after hemorrhage alone. The authors warn that SDD may induce an increased inflammatory response in some patients that can be augmented after an insult such as hemorrhagic shock.

Clinical trials have not demonstrated improved outcome after SDD. In a study of 78 consecutive cardiac surgery patients, Bouter et al. (123) demonstrated that SDD effectively reduced the percentage of gram-negative flora, but did not affect the incidence of postoperative endotoxemia and cytokine activation. SDD did not decrease bacterial colonization, nor did it decrease subsequent infectious episodes when severely burned pediatric patients were studied (124).

IMMUNOMODULATION: MODERATING THE INFLAMMATORY RESPONSE

✐ **Manipulation of immune pathway mediators may become a tool for modulating the balance between the pro-inflammatory and anti-inflammatory conditions.** ✐ The key is to balance the exuberant pro-inflammatory response (which may lead to SIRS) with selected anti-inflammatory modulators that decrease systemic inflammation, but do not decrease the necessary local antibacterial or inflammatory processes needed to control infection and promote healing. The ideal modulator would be effective when given after injury or onset of illness to regulate SIRS, and it would be readily available and economical.

Tumor Necrosis Factor α and Interleukin-1

TNF-α is a target of immunological research, as it initiates the pro-inflammatory response and is a key mediator in the development of sepsis. Despite continued investigation into the role of TNF-α in injury and sepsis and therapies designed to control its role in adverse physiological outcome, little progress has been achieved over the last decade.

Antibodies to TNF-α and IL-1 have been investigated as potential therapeutic agents, with encouraging results in preliminary studies but disappointing results in clinical trials, due to lack of efficacy and the occurrence of unwanted side-effects (125). Large clinical trials of anti-TNF-α monoclonal antibodies and soluble TNF-α receptors produced only small, insignificant beneficial trends in patients with sepsis (6). Furthermore, when investigated for its effects on cytokine release and physiological responses in patients with severe sepsis, there was no difference in overall pattern of cytokine activation or the physiological derangements associated with sepsis.

Pentoxifylline, a methyl-zanthine derivative, best known for successful treatment of atherosclerotic disease, inhibits the formation of TNF-α and has demonstrated efficacy in attenuating the inflammatory response in clinical trials (6). In a multitude of studies, it has been demonstrated to decrease the release of inflammatory cytokines that lead to neutrophil activation and superoxide radical release (6). It has been shown to improve erythrocyte flow and increase tissue oxygenation when added to resuscitation fluids (126–128). It has also been shown to restore effective hepatic blood flow after shock and resuscitation, perhaps by reducing neutrophil-endothelial cell interaction and activation (129).

TGFβ and corticosteroids as antagonists to these two agents have also been investigated. TGFβ does reduce IL-1 production, but it also induces production of IL–1RA (competitively binds to IL-1 receptors), making the immunosuppression overly toxic. Likewise, corticosteroids amplify immunosuppression by reducing production of IL-1 and TNF-α, but they also increase IL-1RII. This receptor preferably binds IL-1β and inhibits it.

GCSF, a growth factor, has been shown to modulate these two cytokines. GCSF supplementation suppresses the LPS-induced release of TNF-α and IL1β, and increases sTNF-R p75 and IL-1ra, thus enhancing anti-inflammatory activity (6). Growth factor was evaluated by Zhang et al. (130), who used rat acute necrotizing pancreatitis (ANP) models and measured serum levels of IL-6, IL-8, IL-10, and TNF-α. They also observed TNF-α mRNA in the liver, lung, kidney, and heart after ANP. Serum levels of these inflammatory cytokines were elevated in response to ANP, and this elevation led to the development of MODS. The administration of Somatostatin and growth hormone inhibited these inflammatory mediators and TNF-α mRNA over-expressions, reduced the risk of the MODS, and markedly increased survival.

Exciting work by Wang et al. (131) has demonstrated a key link between inflammation and the involuntary nervous system that may lead to new therapeutic options. These researchers discovered that the vagus nerve has receptors for inflammatory cytokines and, once stimulated, can suppress ongoing inflammation. In an animal study, this group electrically stimulated the vagus nerve after injecting LPS into rats (132). This stimulation prevented the release of TNF-α from macrophages and death. They characterized the macrophage nicotinic receptor that binds to the acetylcholine released by the vagus nerve, leading to suppression of TNF-α release. This receptor is comprised of five copies of the monomer α7. When this receptor was blocked, acetylcholine and nicotine were no longer able to prevent the release of TNF-α. This was confirmed by studying α7 deficient mice. These mice actually exhibited an exaggerated inflammatory response to LPS. Therapies involving vagus nerve and/or α7 stimulation should undergo further investigation.

Interleukin-2

Preoperative pretreatment with IL-2 has been shown to abrogate the immunosuppression associated with surgery. The cytokine mechanisms responsible for this effect were studied in colorectal cancer patients (133). Operable colorectal cancer patients ($n = 12$) pretreated with IL-2 were compared to 21 age- and disease-matched patients (controls) who underwent surgery without IL-2 pretreatment. Serum levels of IL-6 were measured before surgery, and then at days 3 and 7 in the postoperative period. A significant increase in mean serum levels of IL-6 occurred in the postoperative period in the control patients, whereas no significant difference was seen between presurgical and postsurgical IL-6 mean concentrations in the IL-2 pretreated groups, suggesting that the neutralization of surgery induced immunosuppression by IL-2 may, in part, be due to inhibition of IL-6.

Preoperative administration of IL-2 was also associated with attenuation of immunodysfunction after nephrectomy for renal cell carcinoma (134). In this study, postoperative levels of IL-6 and IL-10 were lower in the pretreated patients. T cell and activation markers were also decreased.

Cyclo-oxygenase Inhibitors

PGE$_2$ is known to disrupt cell-mediated immunity after severe trauma or hemorrhage (6). PGE$_2$ acts on the phosphokinase-A-phosphokinase-C pathway by cAMP. Prostaglandin inhibitors would therefore block this pathway or enhance cyclic guanosine monophosphate, which is protective.

Diclofenac, a COX inhibitor (and thus prostaglandin inhibitor), has been studied as a modulator of inflammatory cytokine release. In a double blind, placebo-controlled study, the administration of diclofenac in the perioperative period (of patients undergoing major urological surgery) was associated with lower IL-6 and IL-10 concentrations, lower leukocyte count, and CRP (135). It was concluded that Diclofenac might play an anti-inflammatory role in surgery.

Prostacyclin has been theorized as an anti-inflammatory option for patients undergoing CABG (136). In a randomized prospective double-blind study, 40 patients undergoing CABG were divided into four groups. One group served as a control, another group received prostacyclin, another group was given high-dose aprotinin, and the last group was treated with prostacyclin and aprotinin. Plasma elastase, PCT, C1-esterase inhibitor (CEI), and coagulation and fibrinolysis parameters were measured in the perioperative period. Levels of elastase increased significantly in the peri- and postoperative period in all patients, and were most pronounced in the control and aprotinin groups. The duration of myocardial ischemia could be directly correlated to elastase levels at the end of CPB. Elastase levels were significantly higher in patients who developed SIRS. These patients developed a hypercoagulatory state. PCT and CEI levels did not change significantly during and after CPB. These authors speculated that prostacyclin controlled the inflammatory effects of increased elastase release associated with CPB and myocardial ischemia.

Thymopentin stimulates cyclic guanosine monophosphate, and has been shown to result in improved in vitro lymphocyte proliferation compared to placebo-treated cardiac surgery patients (137). When combined with indomethacin, cardiac surgery patients who received this therapy demonstrated improved cell-mediated immunity (i.e., IL-1, IL-2, and IFNγ production and IL-2 receptor expression) and lymphocyte proliferation (138).

Nitric Oxide Inhibitors

Due to the extensive involvement of NO in the augmentation of inflammation following hemorrhagic shock and sepsis, it is a target for therapeutic intervention. Animal studies have demonstrated that NO scavengers may suppress proinflammatory signaling. Hierholzer et al. (139) studied NOX, an inhibitor of induced NO (iNO), in rats subjected to hemorrhagic shock. These rats were resuscitated and then examined 24 hours later for histological evidence of inflammatory lung injury. Nontreated animals demonstrated IL-6 localized to luminal sides of bronchial cells, and increased activation of NF-κB and Stat3 (IL-6 signaling intermediary). Administration of NOX beginning at 60 minutes of shock reduced all measured inflammatory parameters within lung tissue, and the authors concluded that NOX might prevent lung injury in this hemorrhagic shock model.

In contrast to short-term animal studies, long-term human studies have shown nonselective NO inhibition to increase mortality (140). A recent multicenter, randomized, two-stage, double-blind, placebo-controlled safety and efficacy study was performed to assess the safety and efficacy of the nonselective NO synthase inhibitor 546C88, in patients with septic shock in a total of 124 ICUs in Europe, North America, South America, South Africa, and Australia. A total of 797 patients with septic shock diagnosed for <24 hours were enrolled. Patients with septic shock were allocated to receive 546C88 or placebo (5% dextrose) for up to seven days (stage 1) or 14 days (stage 2) in addition to

conventional therapy. Study drug (546C88) was initiated at 2.5 mg/kg/hr and titrated up to a maximum rate of 20 mg/kg/hr to maintain MAP between 70 mmHg and 90 mmHg, while attempting to withdraw concurrent vasopressors.

The trial was stopped early, after review by the independent data safety monitoring board detected an increased mortality in the NO synthase inhibitor group (140). The day-28 mortality was 59% (259/439) in the 546C88 group, compared to 49% (174/358) in the placebo group ($p < 0.001$). The overall incidence of adverse events was similar in both groups, although a higher proportion of the adverse events were attributed to the study drug in the 546C88 group (140). Most of the events accounting for the disparity between the groups were associated with the cardiovascular system (e.g., decreased cardiac output, increased pulmonary and systemic hypertension, and increased heart failure). The causes of death in the study were consistent with those expected in patients with septic shock, although there was a higher proportion of cardiovascular deaths and a lower incidence of deaths caused by MOF in the 546C88 group (140).

Interestingly, sub-group analysis of the 312 patients with vasopressor-dependent septic shock treated with the NO synthase inhibitor 546C88 showed slightly improved resolution of shock, and an acceptable overall safety profile. Indeed, administration of 546C88 was associated with resolution of shock at 72 hours in 40% and 24% of the patients in the 546C88 and placebo cohorts, respectively ($p = 0.004$). There was no evidence that treatment with 546C88 had any major adverse effect on pulmonary, hepatic, or renal function. A decrease in cardiac index occurred, but stroke index was maintained. Day 28 survival was similar for both groups (141).

Antithrombin III

Experimental data and clinical observations suggest a therapeutic role for Antithrombin III (AT III) in sepsis, as its plasma concentration is commonly decreased in patients with sepsis or septic shock, and the degree of decrease of AT III is correlated with the severity of the clinical status (142).

AT III, a serine protease inhibitor, has been demonstrated to prevent the development of DIC, decrease the incidence of organ dysfunction during sepsis, and lower the mortality rate in septic animals (143). AT III may incur this effect by inhibiting the induction of iNOS, by inhibiting production of TNF-α (144). This effect may be mediated by the endothelial release of prostacyclin. In another animal study, Mizutani et al. (145) observed that AT III reduced ischemia/reperfusion renal injury by inhibiting leukocyte activation, and concluded that these therapeutic effects may be mediated by prostacyclin as well. AT III limited renal cellular injury by inhibiting LPS-induced iNOS expression in an obstructive jaundice model in rats (146). When recombinant human AT III was administered to baboons, the baboons demonstrated less severe coagulopathic pathology, and a significantly attenuated inflammatory response, compared to baboons that did not receive rhAT III after challenge with *Escherichia coli* (147). However, the rhAT III was given one hour before *E. coli* challenge.

AT III dosage may be the key determinant to its efficacy. AT III inhibited LPS-induced production of inflammatory cytokines when given at high concentrations (5 or 10 U/mL), and actually enhanced production of these cytokines at lower doses in a study utilizing vascular smooth muscle as a monoculture model (148). This effect of high dosage was demonstrated in CBA mice given different doses of AT III just prior to heart transplantation (149). A 50 U/kg dose induced a moderate increase in graft survival, whereas with a 500 U/kg dose, all grafts survived indefinitely and regulatory cells were generated. Invitro, the AT III suppressed the proliferation of mixed leukocyte responses and generation of IL-2.

The same results could not be duplicated in human studies. In the human studies, however, the dosages were much lower proportionally than those in the animals, and were started several hours after the onset of sepsis. In these patients, AT III was shown to improve laboratory values associated with DIC, but did not decrease mortality. A recent study of high-dose AT III (30,000 intravenously over 7 days in 2,314 patients with severe sepsis documented increased 90-day survival in the AT III group ($p = 0.04$) (150). Presently, AT III is indicated to treat AT III hereditary disorders, DIC, and lack of heparin effect due to low AT III levels. The potential therapeutic effects of AT III in patients with SIRS have yet to be demonstrated.

Protease Inhibitors

Because intestinal ischemia and mucosal injury are thought to be contributors to shock induced MODS, researchers hypothesized that pancreatic proteases may cause mucosal stress, or incite inflammatory mediators within ischemic intestine leading to SIRS, and that inhibition of pancreatic proteases may attenuate that response. In an animal study utilizing male Wistar rats, Fitzal et al. (151) demonstrated that intestinal ischemia and reperfusion-induced hypotension was accompanied by a significant increase in leukocyte–endothelium interactions, suggesting neutrophil cell activation. Lavage with the protease inhibitor gabexate mesilate resulted in a stable blood pressure throughout the experiment and essentially abolished cell activation, leukocyte-endothelial interactions, and cell death. The researchers concluded that pancreatic protease inhibition significantly attenuates intestinal ischemia-induced shock by reducing SIRS and gut injury. Much additional work needs to be done in this area prior to initiating human studies.

Platelet-Activating Factor

Platelet-activating factor (PAF) is a potent phospholipid autocoid with a major role in priming, amplification, and regulation of inflammatory mediator release in septic patients. PAF is thought to amplify the inflammatory response associated with SIRS, sepsis, and MODS. This may in part be due to acetylhydrolase, a lipoprotein-associated enzyme, that hydrolyzes PAF to an inactive form. Depressed activity of this enzyme has been correlated with death due to sepsis, suggesting that prolongation of the half-life of PAF contributes to the pathophysiology of fatal sepsis (6). Early studies of the PAF receptor antagonists failed to demonstrate a therapeutic benefit. Recently the PAF antagonist, TCV-309 was studied in a double-blind, randomized, placebo controlled multicenter trial to determine if this antagonist could reduce morbidity and mortality associated with septic shock (152). Though the overall survival was similar in treated versus placebo groups, the mean percentage of failed organs per patient and mean APACHE II scores were significantly lower in the treatment group. The number of patients who recovered from shock after 14 days was significantly higher in the TCV-309 treated group. The number of adverse events was not different between the groups. These findings led the investigators to conclude that TCV-309 can substantially reduce the organ dysfunction and morbidity associated with septic shock, without an increase in adverse events.

Opal et al. (153) recently reported the results of their phase III clinical trial of a recombinant human platelet-activating factor acetylhydrolase, in sepsis. No significant difference in 28-day mortality was identified. Of note, however, is that the anti-PAF agent used by Opal was not studied in a population with a mortality risk as high as in the APC trial. This is the seventh clinical sepsis trial studying the inhibition of the PAF inflammatory pathway. Analysis of the combined treatment effect from these seven trials of anti-PAF agents reveals a small, but nonsignificant improvement in survival rate (odds ratio of survival 1.10; 95% confidence interval, 0.93–1.30, $p = 0.28$) (154). These data stress the importance of the need for adequately powered clinical trials in high-risk patient populations to definitively determine efficacy.

Leukodepletion

As described previously, the interaction between PMNs and vascular endothelial cells is considered the stimulus for the development of SIRS and MODS. This concept is supported by the increased elaboration of PMN cell surface receptors and adhesion to endothelium in patients with SIRS. Leukodepletion filters have been evaluated as a means of removing activated PMNs from the blood of patients with SIRS. In a laboratory–designed extracorporeal circuit, passage of SIRS blood through leukodepletion filters resulted in a marked depletion of PMNs (155). Of the cells that remained in the blood, far fewer cells were adherent to cultured endothelial cells, compared with PMNs prior to leukofiltration (LF). LF was evaluated in a clinical study by Treacher et al. (156), who examined patients who developed SIRS after CPB. Patients randomized to receive LF underwent LF for 60 minutes every 12 hours while SIRS criteria were met. LF patients demonstrated improvement in respiratory and renal function, while demonstrating no improvement in mortality rate or ICU length of stay compared with controls.

Hypertonic Preconditioning

As a potential therapeutic agent, hypertonic preconditioning was hypothesized to impair subsequent inflammatory mediator signaling through a reduction in stress fiber polymerization and mitogen-activated protein kinase activity after LPS stimulation, in a study utilizing rabbit alveolar macrophages (157). Rabbit alveolar cells were stimulated with LPS. Selected cells were preconditioned with NaCl, mannitol, or urea and then returned to isotonic medium prior to LPS stimulation. Preconditioning of macrophages with NaCl or mannitol resulted in a dose dependent decrease in extracellular signal-related kinase, a dose-dependent attenuation of TNF-α production, and a failure of LPS-induced stress fiber polymerization. Urea (intracellular hypertonic condition) had no significant effect. These investigators concluded that HS or mannitol resuscitation might protect against MODS due to reduced pro-inflammatory responsiveness.

Anti-lipopolysaccharide Compounds

Different classes of compounds that bind directly to LPS, thereby neutralizing its effects, have been examined (158). These consist primarily of antiLPS monoclonal antibodies, naturally occurring proteins and their derivatives, including Limulus antiLPS factor (LALF), and antibiotics including polymyxin B and taurolidine. The LPS monoclonal antibodies failed to demonstrate clinical efficacy, but investigation of these compounds led to a better understanding of the biochemical interactions associated with LPS-induced inflammation and endotoxin antagonism.

Pituitary Adenylate Cyclase-Activating Polypeptide and Vasoactive Intestinal Peptide

Pituitary adenylate cyclase-activating polypeptide (PACAP) is a neuropeptide in the vasoactive intestinal peptide (VIP)/secretin/glucagon family of peptides. Recent research has demonstrated that this molecule is a potent anti-inflammatory mediator, functioning by regulating the production of both pro- and anti-inflammatory mediators. Delgado et al. (159) demonstrated that PACAP prevented the deleterious effects of arthritis by downregulating both the inflammatory and autoimmune components of the disease. These authors suggest that PACAP may be used as treatment for acute and chronic inflammatory and autoimmune diseases, including septic shock.

VIP and PACAP have been shown to have inhibitory effects on the production of pro-inflammatory mediators associated with microglia (160). Microglia have a central role in the regulation of immune processes, inflammation, and tissue remodeling in the CNS. Pathological activation of microglia is thought to contribute to progressive damage in neurodegenerative diseases, via the release of pro-inflammatory and cytotoxic factors. VIP and PACAP may, therefore, have therapeutic potential in the treatment of inflammatory or degenerative brain disorders.

IMMUNONUTRITION IN TRAUMA AND CRITICAL ILLNESS

Immunological dysregulation due to trauma and critical illness may complicate a patient's clinical course and result in sepsis and MOF. Immunomodulatory interventions aim to ameliorate the pro-inflammatory component of systemic inflammation. ✐ **Immunonutrition is a modulatory intervention intensively investigated over the past two decades (also see Volume 2, Chapters 31–33).** ✐ It is theorized that changes in the GALT may contribute to gut-derived sepsis, and enteral feeding supplemented with key nutrients may prevent that change. Bastian et al. (161) utilized a prospective, randomized, double-blind, controlled study to demonstrate that immunonutrition to include arginine, n-3 fatty acids, and nucleotides significantly reduced the number of SIRS days per patient and lowered MOF scores. Other studies have demonstrated reduction in septic complications, decreased antibiotic usage, decreases in hospital length of stay, and reduction in hospital costs when patients were randomized to receive immuno-enhancing diets (IED). The mechanism for the gut-protective effect of IED may be augmentation of blood flow to the GALT in the terminal ileum (162). This protection is in contrast to TPN, which has been associated with increased release of pro-inflammatory cytokines when compared to an enteral diet (163).

The amino acid L-glycine has demonstrated anti-inflammatory, immunomodulatory, and cytoprotective effects in recent immunonutrition research (164). Glycine protects against shock due to hemorrhage, endotoxin, and sepsis, and prevents multi-organ ischemia/reperfusion injury. It suppresses inflammatory cytokine release from inflammatory cells to include macrophages. In the plasma

membrane, it activates a chloride channel that stabilizes membrane potential. This suppresses the agonist-induced opening of calcium channels, thus preventing cellular calcium influx (believed to be an important component of the onset of inflammation).

Glutathione (GSH), an endogenous antioxidant believed to be an important defense against oxygen metabolites, was measured along with TNF-α and IL-6 in 28 trauma patients and 14 normal controls who were treated with recombinant human growth factor (rhGH) (165). All patients received total parenteral nutrition (TPN) starting after 48 hours. Plasma levels of GSH were not altered in the early catabolic phase, but TNF-α and IL-6 were elevated compared to controls. After seven days, GSH levels were enhanced with TPN alone, but these levels were two times higher in patients who also received rhGH. These patients also had higher levels of TNF-α, but no change in IL-6. These authors concluded that modification of plasma GSH and TNF-α, by adequate nutritional support with adjuvant rhGH, has a beneficial role in enhancing antioxidant defenses.

Zinc is essential for the proper functioning of all cells in the human immune system. These cells demonstrate decreased function in states of zinc depletion. Zinc depletion impairs all monocyte functions, decreases cytotoxicity in NK cells, reduces phagocytosis in neutrophils, and impairs T cell function (166). Autoreactivity and alloreactivity of T cells is increased, and B cells undergo apoptosis. These impaired immune functions can be reversed by adequate supplementation. However, overtreatment can induce negative effects on immune cells similar to those seen in zinc deficiency.

Animal studies have demonstrated the benefit of zinc therapy in inflammation. Zinc depletion sensitized mice to the deleterious effects of TNF-α, whereas pretreatment with zinc conferred protection against these deleterious effects in a study evaluating the role of metallothionein as a mediator in TNF-induced SIRS (167). Furthermore, co-treatment with zinc led to complete regression of inoculated tumors with TNF-α and INFγ, leading to significantly increased survival.

Selenium is an essential micronutrient associated with improvement in T cell function and reduced apoptosis in animal studies (166). It may enhance resistance to infections through modulation of IL-1, and the Th1/Th2 response. It upregulates IL-2 and increases the activation, proliferation, differentiation, and programmed cell death of T helper cells. Baum et al. (168) report that selenium supplementation may down-regulate the abnormally high levels of IL-8 and TNF-α in human immunodeficiency virus type 1 disease that has been associated with disease progression and increased viral replication.

Selenium has been shown to modulate cytokine-induced expression of the adhesion molecules ICAM-1, VCAM-1, and E-selectin, thus hindering the endothelial pro-inflammatory state (169). Selenium at physiological levels mediates the inhibition of the activation of NF-κB (the transcription factor that regulates the genes that encode for inflammatory cytokines), and the reduction of selenium induces the synthesis of CRP by hepatocytes during the acute phase response (170).

Selenium was investigated as an adjunct to treatment in children suffering from inflammatory surgical diseases and extended scalded skin, in an age and diagnosis-matched cohort study (169). All of the patients in the study had SIRS. Inflammatory mediators and acute phase reactants were measured on the first, second, third, sixth, and last treatment day. Levels of IL-6 and the acute phase reactants CRP and fibrinogen were similar in both groups. Plasma glutathione peroxidase activity increased significantly (representing cell membrane protection) in patients who received selenium, in comparison to those who did not. Malondialdehyde was initially elevated in all patients (representing raised lipid peroxidation), and then decreased to normal levels in the selenium treated group, thus supporting selenium as supportive therapy in children with SIRS.

EYE TO THE FUTURE

The concept of SIRS has been evolving for decades. The operational definition has recently come under great scrutiny (172–175). Bossink et al. (174) documented that SIRS is present in 95% of patients with fever, despite the fact that only 44% of patients had sepsis with a microbiologically confirmed infection. Earlier sections in this chapter described some of the recent research which has begun to elucidate the pathophysiology of SIRS. In this section, we would like to focus the interested reader on a few additional topics, which will play an increasing role in management of patients with SIRS in the near future, and also describe some promising areas of investigation, which may allow manipulation of SIRS in future patients. We will review the new PIRO staging system proposed for SIRS, the role of accurate ICD-9 coding, important advances in the pathophysiology of SIRS, and an area of potential treatment not discussed above, based upon vitamin supplementation.

New Predisposition, Infection, Response, and Organ Dysfunction Staging System for Systemic Inflammatory Response Syndrome and Sepsis

In 2001, an International Sepsis Definitions Conference was convened to review the strengths and weaknesses of the current definitions of sepsis and related conditions, identify ways to improve the current definitions, and identify methodologies for increasing the accuracy, reliability, and/or clinical utility of the diagnosis of sepsis (4). The primary consensus points of this conference are reviewed in Volume 2, Chapter 47. A new system, PIRO (Volume 2, Chapter 47, Table 3), has recently been proposed for characterizing and staging the host response to infection.

This newly developed conceptual framework for understanding sepsis, called the PIRO concept, is a classification scheme that could stratify patients on the basis of their predisposing conditions, the nature and extent of the insult (in the case of sepsis, infection), the nature and magnitude of the host response, and the degree of concomitant organ dysfunction (Volume 2, Chapter 47, Table 3). The PIRO system has been conceptually modeled from the TNM classification (tumor size, nodal spread, metastases) that has been successfully used in defining treatment and prognostic indicators in clinical oncology. PIRO was introduced as a hypothesis-generating model for future research and extensive testing will be necessary before it can be considered ready for routine application in clinical practice. It should be noted, however, that SIRS remains a prominent feature in the new PIRO paradigm as one of the earliest "Response" markers of sepsis. Furthermore, SIRS continues to be utilized as an excellent screening tool to enroll patients in clinical studies on SIRS and sepsis.

New ICD-9 Codes for Systemic Inflammatory Response Syndrome and Sepsis

In October 2002, the Centers for Medicare and Medicaid Services established new ICD-9 codes for SIRS and sepsis (Table 5). Prior to this, there were no ICD-9 codes for SIRS, and the only code for sepsis was "septicemia." As medical practitioners caring for critically ill trauma patients with SIRS and sepsis, it is important to utilize these codes. By so doing, additional information will be captured regarding the accurate incidence and outcome of patients with SIRS, sepsis, and severe sepsis that have sustained traumatic injury. Although these ICD-9 codes do not themselves shed light on the pathophysiology of SIRS, their correct application is mandatory for accurate epidemiological data and outcome studies in humans.

Advances in Pathophysiology of Systemic Inflammatory Response Syndrome

Additional advances continue to be made in understanding the pathophysiology of SIRS (176). The resemblance between SIRS and sepsis has long been recognized. In the case of sepsis, exogenous macromolecules such as LPS acting on TLRs trigger the SIRS response. What triggers SIRS in the absence of infection, however, has not been fully elucidated. A recent study reported that a SIRS-like response could be induced in mice by the administration of a soluble heparan sulfate and by elastase, both of which were dependent on functional TLR 4, because mutant mice lacking that receptor or its function do not develop SIRS (177). These important results provide an additional molecular explanation for the initiation of noninfectious SIRS.

Resolution of inflammation and infection involves removal of neutrophils and other inflammatory cells by the induction of apoptosis. Fas/Apo-1 is a widely occurring apoptotic signal receptor molecule expressed by almost any type of cell, which is also released in a soluble circulating form. A recent study investigated the role of circulating Fas/Apo-1 in patients with systemic SIRS. They evaluated 57 critically ill patients, 34 with infectious SIRS (sepsis and septic shock), and 23 patients with noninfectious SIRS (178). Levels of Fas/Apo-1 were significantly elevated in patients with infectious and noninfectious SIRS (10.4 +/− 8.1 pg/mL, controls: 5.0 +/− 0.7 pg/mL; $p < 0.0001$). In this small study, Fas/Apo-1 levels were not predictive of poor outcome of patients with SIRS. Importantly, these results show that increased levels of Fas/Apo-1 from patients with SIRS is a mechanism that contributes to

Table 5 New ICD-9 Codes for Systemic Inflammatory Response Syndrome and Sepsis

ICD-9 code	Diagnosis
995.90	SIRS, unspecified
995.91	SIRS due to infectious process without organ dysfunction
995.92	SIRS due to infectious process with organ dysfunction (severe sepsis)
995.93	SIRS due to noninfectious process without organ dysfunction
995.94	SIRS due to noninfectious process with organ dysfunction

Abbreviation: SIRS, systemic inflammatory response syndrome.

inflammatory response, through accumulation of neutrophils at sites of inflammation/infection.

Interestingly, two recent studies in septic rodents demonstrated significant survival benefit by inhibiting apoptosis (179,180). The first utilized the antiretroviral protease inhibitor nelfinavir® (Agouron Pharmaceuticals, La Jolla, California, U.S.A.), in a mouse cecal perforation and ligation sepsis model (179). Mice pretreated with nelfinavir® demonstrated improved survival (67%; $p < 0.0005$) compared with controls (17%), and a significant ($p < 0.05$) reduction in lymphocyte apoptosis.

The second study demonstrated that Akt (a serine/threonine kinase, and a key regulator of cell proliferation and death) overexpression in lymphocytes prevents sepsis-induced apoptosis, causes a Th1 cytokine propensity, and improves survival (180). Findings from this study strengthen the concept that a major defect in sepsis is impairment of the adaptive immune system, and further bolsters the concept that strategies to prevent lymphocyte apoptosis represents an important new strategy of sepsis therapy. Furthermore, it may turn out that in late SIRS (from sepsis or other sources), triggering apoptosis to occur may be actually beneficial. Much additional animal work needs to be done before aptotic control is studied in humans with SIRS.

Antioxidant Strategies: Vitamin Supplementation

We currently have few efficacious strategies to prevent the progression from SIRS to MODS. Early enteral nutrition and the use of immunonutrition have been discussed as an early preventive strategy in trauma. Two recent studies examined the use of antioxidant vitamin E and C supplementation as an additional preventive strategy to consider.

A recent prospective, randomized study compared outcomes in patients receiving early antioxidant supplementation versus those receiving standard care, with a cohort of 595 patients, 91% of whom were trauma victims (181). The treatment regimen included α-tocopherol (Aquasol-E 1000 IU q8 h via NGT) and ascorbate (1000 mg IV in 100 ml D5W q8 h) for the shorter duration of ICU stay or 28 days. Patients randomized to antioxidant supplementation had significantly decreased risk for pulmonary morbidity, including ARDS and pneumonia (RR 0.81, CI 0.60–1.1), and MOF (RR 0.43, CI 0.19–0.96). Patients randomized to antioxidant supplementation also had a shorter duration of mechanical ventilation and length of ICU stay. This important study documented that the early administration of antioxidant supplementation reduced the incidence of organ failure and shortened ICU length of stay in a cohort of critically ill surgical patients. Significant limitations of this study included lack of a placebo and lack of investigator blinding.

Oxidant stress has been implicated in SIRS both as a mechanism for direct cellular injury, as well as activation of intracellular signaling cascades within inflammatory cells, resulting in progression of the inflammatory response. Vitamin E is an inexpensive, nontoxic, chain-breaking antioxidant that has therapeutic potential in regulating this process. A recent review evaluated the current literature regarding the use of Vitamin E in controlling the excessive inflammation seen in SIRS and argued for further study of its therapeutic potential for critically ill and injured patients (182). Additional studies in this important area of investigation are clearly warranted.

Genetic Influences

Genetic epidemiologic studies suggest a strong genetic influence on the outcome from sepsis, and genetics may explain the wide variation in the individual response to infection that has long puzzled clinicians (176). Several candidate genes have been identified as important in the inflammatory response and investigated in case-controlled studies, including the TNF-α and TNF-β genes, positioned next to each other within the cluster of human leukocyte antigen class III genes on chromosome 6. Other candidate genes for sepsis and septic shock include the IL-1 receptor antagonist gene, the heat shock protein gene, the IL-6 gene, the IL-10 gene, the CD-14 gene, the TLR-4 gene, and the TLR-2 gene, to name a few. A number of recent comprehensive reviews have summarized the evidence for a genetic susceptibility to development of sepsis and death from sepsis (183–185). These reviews discuss candidate genes likely to be involved in the pathogenesis of sepsis, and review the potential for gene targeted therapy and prophylaxis against sepsis and septic shock (183–185). Few studies have examined genetic polymorphisms and genetic susceptibility for SIRS, and additional research in this area is also warranted (186).

SUMMARY

The systemic response to trauma, surgery, and critical illness is extremely complex and is a major factor affecting morbidity and mortality in trauma. The pathogenesis of SIRS and sepsis is becoming increasingly understood. When tissue injury is severe, a maladaptive dysregulation of the immune response occurs, which may lead to SIRS, and later to CARS and MODS.

Early in the course of severe injury, patients demonstrate an increase in inflammatory mediators, which may lead to complications (e.g., SIRS or ARDS). However, later in the course of severe illness following trauma, the immune system may become impaired (i.e., CARS), leading to other complications such as infections from organisms not normally encountered by immuno-competent individuals (Fig. 6). Research focusing upon manipulating the

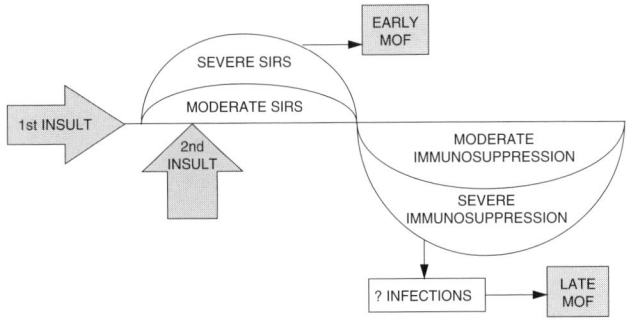

Figure 6 Progression from systemic inflammatory response syndrome (SIRS) to multiple organ dysfunction syndrome (MODS). Following major trauma, patients develop an early physiologic state of hyperinflammation (i.e., SIRS) due to a dysfunctional inflammatory response. This can lead to early multiple organ dysfunction or failure (MODS, MOF). Subsequently, the compensatory anti-inflammatory response is associated with significant immunosuppression and risk for infectious complications that is the most common cause of late MODS and MOF. *Source*: From Ref. 189.

immune system is ongoing. Decreasing the initial exuberant inflammatory state (SIRS), and/or increasing immuno-competence during the (later) immuno-impaired state (CARS) may result in significant improvement in morbidity and mortality.

Researchers and clinicians have made great strides in determining many of the key facets of the immunological system related to SIRS over the past few decades. Perhaps the most astounding finding is that systems previously believed to be entirely separate are now known to be intricately related (e.g., inflammation and coagulation). Furthermore, SIRS is not merely the result of a single dysfunctional cytokine, autocrine, paracrine, or endocrine response. Rather, it is now recognized as a complex phenomenon, involving all of the above mediators and perhaps many others (some still unrecognized).

Although numerous prior attempts to foil specific steps in the inflammatory response failed to improve patient outcomes, the PROWESS study has recently shown that mortality can be affected by inhibition of coagulation with APC therapy in severe sepsis. The benefit in SIRS patients without a septic etiology has not yet been studied. Additionally, the benefit of APC treatment in patients with various coagulation disorders is unclear. Answers to these questions, and review of numerous other novel treatments, are now being contemplated. Some of the newer potential remedies have been reviewed earlier in the Eye to the Future section (e.g., apoptosis manipulation, antioxidant administration, and genetic manipulations). As the frontiers of research push our knowledge forward, SIRS, sepsis, and organ failure are becoming increasingly understood.

KEY POINTS

- SIRS has been classified as an early component of the sepsis syndrome. SIRS and sepsis commonly present as a continuum of disease states, with progression of SIRS to sepsis, severe sepsis and septic shock.
- The outcome of inflammation may be beneficial (inactivation of injurious substances, initiation of repair) or deleterious (injury to tissue, interference with normal functions) to the host.
- Most soluble mediators of inflammation are present in minute concentrations under normal conditions. Elaboration of these mediators may dramatically increase when the body is exposed to infecting organisms, trauma, surgery, and/or critical illness.
- The selectin-phase is the first component of endothelial activation, promoting neutrophil migration. In this phase, passing neutrophils or other leukocytes attach to P-selectin and E-Selectin molecules on the activated endothelium.
- Pro-inflammatory cytokines are responsible for initiation and augmentation of inflammation and its sequelae, whereas anti-inflammatory cytokines are associated with moderation of the inflammatory response.
- It appears that patients without apparent infection who have increased CRP values preoperatively are at increased risk for infectious complications postoperatively.
- Neurological and endocrine functions interact intimately with inflammatory mediators after injury or onset of illness.

- The hormone 17-beta estradiol has been associated with female gender-specific protective effects from SIRS, following trauma and hemorrhage in animal studies.
- In contrast to the female sex hormone estradiol, increased levels of the male sex hormone testosterone are associated with decreased cell mediated immune response following trauma in animal studies. Testosterone also decreases muscle catabolism following burns.
- Trauma, especially when complicated by hemorrhagic shock, may induce SIRS, potentially resulting in immunodepression, MODS, severe sepsis, or septic shock.
- Surgical procedures are known to elicit systemic inflammation. The magnitude and duration of the procedure, comorbid diseases, and reperfusion injury are just a few of the variables that affect the inflammatory response.
- With the exception of anaphylaxis and allergy (see Volume 1, Chapter 33), anesthetics and analgesics by themselves are not initiators of SIRS. However, several anesthetics and analgesics have shown immunomodulatory effects, and may therefore have some effects on SIRS.
- Direct contact between patient blood and the synthetic surfaces of the CPB system, along with released intracellular elements of destroyed cells, are the most likely reasons for the increased inflammatory mediators seen with CPB.
- Resuscitation for trauma and surgery may affect an individual's innate immune response, as a result of the type, quantity, and timing of fluid resuscitation.
- A breakdown in any component of this GI defense system may contribute to gut-derived bacteremia and sepsis, after injury or illness.
- Key mediators in the immune pathways continue to be studied extensively in an effort to control or modulate the pro-inflammatory/anti-inflammatory response.
- Immunonutrition is a modulatory intervention intensively investigated over the past two decades (also see Volume 2, Chapters 31–33).

REFERENCES

1. Bone R, Balk R, Cerra F, et al. American College of Chest Physicians/Society of Critical Care Medicine Consensus Conference Committee: Definitions for sepsis and organ failure and guidelines for the use of innovative therapies in sepsis. Chest 1992; 101:1644–1655.
2. Bone R, Balk R, Cerra F, et al. The ACCP/SCCM Consensus Conference Committee: Definitions for sepsis and organ failure and guidelines for the use of innovative therapies in sepsis. Crit Care Med 1992; 20:864–974.
3. Kim P, Deutschman C. Inflammatory responses and mediators. Surg Clin North Am 2000; 80(3):885–894.
4. Levy MM, Fink MP, Marshall JC, et al. 2001 SCCM/ESICM/ ACCP/ATS/SIS international sepsis definitions conference. Crit Care Med 2003; 31(4):1250–1256.
5. Oberholzer A, Oberholzer C, Moldawer LL. Sepsis syndromes: understanding the role of innate and acquired immunity. Shock 2001; 16(2):83–96.
6. Napolitano L, Faist E, Wichmann M, Coimbra R. Immune Dysfunction in Trauma. Surg Clin North Am 1999; 79(6):1385–1416.
7. Arid WC. The role of the endothelium in severe sepsis and multiple organ dysfunction syndrome. Blood 2003; 101(10):3765–3777.
8. Cheng T, Liu D, Griffin JH, et al. Activated protein C blocks p53-mediated aptosis in ischemic human brain endothelium and is neuroprotective. Nat Med 2003; 9:338–342.

9. Malone D, Napolitano L, Genuit T, Bochicchio G, Kole K, Scalea T. "Total" Cytokine Immunoassay: A more accurate method of cytokine measurement. J Trauma 2001; 50(5):821–825.

10. Rodriguez-Gaspar M, Santolaria F, Jarque-Lopez A, et al. Prognostic value of cytokines in SIRS general medical patients. Cytokine 2001; 15(4):232–236.

11. el-Barbary M, Khabar KS. Soluble tumor necrosis factor receptor p55 predicts cytokinemia and systemic inflammatory response after cardiopulmonary bypass. Crit Care Med 2002; 30(8):1712–1716.

12. Hoffmann G, Czechowski M, Schloesser M, Schobersberger W. Procalcitonin amplifies inducible nitric oxide synthase gene expression and nitric oxide production in vascular smooth muscle cells. Crit Care Med 2002; 30(9):2091–2095.

13. Selberg O, Hecker H, Martin M, Klos A, Bautsch W, Kohl J. Discrimination of sepsis and systemic inflammatory response syndrome by determination of circulating plasma concentrations of procalcitonin, protein complement 3a, and interleukin–6.

14. Maruna P, Gurlich R, Frasko R, et al. Procalcitonin in the diagnosis of postoperative complications. Sb Lek 2002; 103(2): 283–295.

15. Molter GP, Soltesz S, Kottke R, Wilhelm W, Biedler A, Silomom M. Procalcitonin plasma concentrations and systemic inflammatory response following different types of surgery. Anaesthesist 2003; 52(3):210–217.

16. Svaldi M, Hirber J, Lanthaler AI, et al. Procalcitonin-reduced sensitivity and specificity in heavily leucopenic and immunosuppressed patients. Br J Haematol 2001; 115(1):53–57.

17. Yukioka H, Yoshida G, Kurita S, Kato N. Plasma procalcitonin in sepsis and organ failure. Ann Acad Med Singapore 2001; 30(5):528–531.

18. Guven H, Altintop L, Baydin A, et al. Diagnostic value of procalcitonin levels as an early indicator of sepsis. Am J Emerg Med 2002; 20(3):202–206.

19. Reny JL, Vuagnat A, Ract C, Benoit MO, Safar M, Fagon JY. Diagnosis and follow-up of infections in intensive care patients: value of C-reactive protein compared with other clinical and biological variables. Crit Care Med 2002; 30(3):529–535.

20. Boeken U, Feindt P, Zimmermann N, Kalweit G, Petzold T, Gams E. Increased preoperative C-reactive protein (CRP)-values without signs of an infection and complicated course after cardiopulmonary bypass (CPB)-operations. Eur J Cardiothorac Surg 1998; 13(5):541–545.

21. De Angelo J. Nitric oxide scavengers in the treatment of shock associated with systemic inflammatory response syndrome. Expert Opin Pharmacother 1999; 1(1):19–29.

22. Xu D, Lu Q, Deitch E. Nitric oxide directly impairs intestinal barrier function. Shock 2002; 17(2):139–145.

23. Annane D, Sanquer S, Sebill V, et al. Compartmentalized inducible nitric-oxide synthase activity in septic shock. Lancet 2000; 355(9210):1143–1148.

24. Tsukahara Y, Morisaki T, Kojima M, Uchiyama A, Tanaka M. iNOS expression by activated neutrophils from patients with sepsis. Aust N Z J Surg 2001; 71(1):15–20.

25. Hierholzer C, Billiar TR. Molecular mechanisms in the early phase of hemorrhagic shock. Langenbecks Arch Surg 2001; 386(4):302–308.

26. Bucher M, Hobbhahn J, Kurtz A. Nitric oxide-dependent down-regulation of angiotensin II type 2 receptors during experimental sepsis. Crit Care Med 2001; 29(9):1750–1755.

27. Triantafilou M, Triantafilou K. Lipopolysaccharide recognition: CD14, TLRs and the LPS-activation cluster. Trends Immunol 2002; 23(6):301–304.

28. Sablotzki A, Borgermann J, Baulig W, et al. Lipopolysaccharide-binding protein (LBP) and markers of acute-phase response in patients with multiple organ dysfunction syndrome (MODS) following open heart surgery. Thorac Cardiovasc Surg 2001; 49(5):273–278.

29. Blairon L, Wittebole X, Laterre PF. Lipopolysaccharide-binding protein serum levels in patients with severe sepsis due to gram-positive and fungal infections. J Infect Dis 2003; 187(2):287–291.

29a. Cunningham SK, Malone DL, Bochicchio GV, et al. Serum lipopolysaccharide binding protein concentrations in trauma victims. Surg Infect 2006; 7(3):251–261.

30. Lieberman J, Marks W, Cohn S, et al. Organ failure, infection, and the systemic inflammatory response syndrome are associated with elevated levels of urinary intestinal fatty acid binding protein: study of 100 consecutive patients in a surgical intensive care unit. J Trauma 1998; 45:900–906.

31. Kerner T, Ahlers O, Spielmann S, et al. L-selectin in trauma patients: a marker for organ dysfunction and outcome? Eur J Clin Invest 1999; 29(12):1077–1086.

32. Geppert A, Zorn G, Karth GD, et al. Soluble selectins and the systemic inflammatory response syndrome after successful cardiopulmonary resuscitation. Crit Care Med 2000; 28(7):2360–2365.

33. Tsokos M. Immunohistochemical detection of sepsis-induced lung injury in human autopsy material. Leg Med (Tokyo) 2003; 5(2):73–86.

34. Seekamp A, vanGriensven M, Dhondt E, et al. The effect of anti-L-selectin (aselizumab) in multiple traumatized patients—results of a phase II clinical trial. Crit Care Med 2004; 32(10):2021–2028.

35. Zellweger R, Wichmann M, Ayala A, DeMaso C, Chaudry I. Prolactin: A novel and safe immunomodulating hormone for the treatment of immunodepression following severe hemorrhage. J Surg Res 1996; 63:53–58.

36. Zellweger R, Zhu X, Wichmann M, Ayala A, DeMaso C, Chaudry I. Prolactin administration following hemorrhage shock improves macrophage cytokine release capacity and decreases mortality form subsequent sepsis. J Immunol 1996; 157:5748–5754.

37. Zellweger R, Wichmann M, Ayala A, Chaudry I. Metoclopramide: A novel and safe immunomodulating agent for restoring the depressed macrophage immune function following hemorrhage. J Trauma 1998; 44:70–77.

38. Corson J, Williamson R, eds. Surgery. USA: Mosby, 2001.

39. Gonzalez-Hernandez J, Bornstein S, Ehrhart-Bornstein M, Spath-Schwalbe E, Jirikowski G, Scherbaum W. Interleukin-6 messenger ribonucleic acid expression in human adrenal gland in vivo: new clue to a paracrine or autocrine regulation of adrenal function, J Clin Endocrinol Metab 1994; 79:1492.

40. Path G, Bornstein S, Ehrhart-Bornstein M, Scherbaum W. Interleukin-6 and the interleukin-6 receptor in the human adrenal gland: expression and effects on steroidogenesis. J Clin Endocrinol Metab 1997; 82:2343.

41. Sredni-Kenigsbuch D. TH1/TH2 cytokines in the central nervous system. Int J Neurosci. 2002; 112(6):665–703.

42. Reyes T, Coe C. The proinflammatory cytokine network: interactions in the CNS and blood of rhesus monkeys. Am J Physiol 1998; 274:R139.

43. Romero L, Kakucska I, Lechan R, Reichlin S. Interleukin-6 (IL-6) is secreted from the brain after intercerebroventricular injection of IL-1α in rats. Am J Physiol 1996; 270:R518.

44. Senba E, Kasiba K. Sensory afferent processing in multi-responsive DRG neurons. Prog Brain Res 1996; 113:387.

45. Hirota H, Kiyama H, Kishimoto T, Taga T. Accelerated nerve regeneration in mice by upregulated expression of interleukin (IL) 6 and IL-6 receptor after trauma. J Exp Med 1996; 183:2627.

46. Chavolla-Calderon M, Bayer M, Fontan J. Bone marrow transplantation reveals an essential synergy between neuronal and hemopoietic cell neurokinin production in pulmonary inflammation. J Clin Invest 2003; 111(7):973–980.

47. Piedimonte G. Contribution of neuroimmune mechanisms to airway inflammation and remodeling during and after respiratory syncytial virus infection. Pediatr Infect Dis J 2003; 22(suppl 2):S66–S74; discussion S74–S75.

48. Parslow T, Stites D, Terr A, Imboden J. Medical Immunology. 10th ed. USA: McGraw-Hill, 2001.

49. Kahlke V, Dohm C, Mees T, Brotzmann K, Schreiber S, Schroder J. Early interleukin-10 treatment improves survival and enhances immune function only in males after hemorrhage and subsequent sepsis. Shock 2002; 18(1):24–28.

50. Diodato MD, Knoferl MW, Schwacha MG, Bland KI, Chaudry IH. Gender differences in the inflammatory response and survival following haemorrhage and subsequent sepsis. Cytokine 2001; 14(3):162–169.

51. Wichmann M, Inthorn D, Schildberg F. Incidence and mortality of severe sepsis in surgical intensive care: influence of gender on disease process and outcome. Shock 1998; 10:3.

52. Schroder J, Kahlke V, Staubach K, Zabel P, Stuber F. Gender differences in human sepsis. Arch Surg 1998; 133:1200–1205.

53. Napolitano L, Greco M, Rodriguez A, Kufera J, West R, Scalea T. Gender differences in adverse outcomes after blunt trauma. J Trauma 2001; 50(2):274–280.

54. Gannon C, Napolitano L, Pasquale M, Tracy J, McCarter R. A state-wide population-based study of gender differences in trauma: validation of a prior single-institution study. J Am Coll Surg 2002; 195(1):11–18.

55. Croce M, Fabian T, Malhotra A, Bee T, Miller P. Does gender difference influence outcome? J Trauma 2002; 531(5):889–894.

56. Yokoyama Y, Kuebler J, Matsutani T, Schwacha M, Bland K, Chaudry I. Mechanism of the salutary effects of 17beta-estradiol following trauma-hemorrhage: direct downregulation of Kupffer cell proinflammatory cytokine production. Cytokine 2003; 21(2):91–97.

57. Samy TS, Zheng R, Matsutani T, Rue LW 3rd, Bland KI, Chaudry IH. Mechanism for normal splenic T lymphocyte functions in proestrus females after trauma: enhanced local synthesis of 17beta-estradiol. Am J Physiol Cell Physiol 2003; 285(1):C139–C149.

58. Angele MK, Knoferl MW, Ayala A, Bland KI, Chaudry IH. Testosterone and estrogen differently affect Th1 and Th2 cytokine release following trauma-haemorrhage. Cytokine 2001; 16(1):22–30.

59. Wichmann M, Angele M, Ayala A, Cioffi W, Chaudry I. Flutamide: A novel agent for restoring the depressed cell-mediated immunity following soft tissue trauma and hemorrhagic shock. Shock 1997; 8:242–248.

60. Angele M, Wichmann M, Ayala A, Cioffi W, Chaudry I. Testosterone receptor blockade after hemorrhage in males: Restoration of the depressed immune functions and improved survival following subsequent sepsis. Arch Surg 1997; 132:1207–1214.

61. Ferrando A, Sheffield-Moore M, Wolf S, Herndon D, Wolfe R. Testosterone administration in severe burns ameliorates muscle catabolism. Crit Care Med 2001; 29(10):1936–1942.

62. Malone D, Keledjian K, Tracy J, Scalea T, Napolitano L. Gender-related human sex hormone alterations after trauma. Crit Care Med 2003; 31(2):284/A59.

63. Kuebler JF, Yokoyama Y, Jarrar D, et al. Administration of progesterone after trauma and hemorrhagic shock prevents hepatocellular injury. Arch Surg 2003; 138(7):727–734.

64. Shear DA, Galani R, Hoffman SW, Stein DG. Progesterone protects against necrotic damage and behavioral abnormalities caused by traumatic brain injury. Exp Neurol 2002; 178(1):59–67.

65. Papathanassoglou ED, Moynihan JA, Ackerman MH, Matzoros CS. Serum leptin levels are higher but are not independently associated with severity or mortality in the multiple organ dysfunction/systemic inflammatory response syndrome: a matched case control and a longitudinal study. Clin Endocrinol (Oxf) 2001; 54(2): 225–233.

66. Opal SM. Interactions between coagulation and inflammation. Scand J Infect Dis 2003; 35(9):545–554.

67. Matthay MA. Severe sepsis—a new treatment with both anti-coagulant and anti-inflammatory properties. N Engl J Med 2001; 344:759–762.

68. Bernard GR, Vincent J-L, Laterre P-F, et al. Efficacy and safety of recombinant human activated protein C for severe sepsis. N Engl J Med 2001; 344:699–709.

69. Grey ST, Tsuchida A, Hau H, Orthner CL, Salem HH, Hancock WW. Selective inhibitory effects of the anticoagulant activated protein C on the responses of human mononuclear phagocytes to LPS, IFN-gamma, or phorbol ester. J Immunol 1994; 153:3664–3672.

70. Bernard GR. Drotrecogin alfa (activated) (recombinant human activated protein C) for the treatment of severe sepsis. Crit Care Med 2003; 31(suppl):S85–S93.

71. Hirose K, Okajima K, Taoka Y, et al. Activated protein C reduces the ischemia/reperfusion-induced spinal cord injury in rats by inhibiting neutrophil activation. Ann Surg 2000; 232:272–280.

72. Esmon CT. Introduction: are natural anticoagulants candidates for modulating the inflammatory response to endotoxin? Blood 2000; 95:1113–1116.

73. Carrigan SD, Scott G, Tabrizian M. Toward Resolving the Challenges of Sepsis Diagnosis. Clin Chem 2004; 50:1301–1314.

74. Bone RC. Immunologic dissonance: a continuing evolution in our understanding of the systemic inflammatory response syndrome (SIRS) and the multiple organ dysfunction syndrome (MODS). Ann Intern Med 1996; 125(8):680–687.

75. Opal SM, Depalo VA. Anti-inflammatory cytokines. Chest 2000; 117:1162–1172.

76. Napolitano L, Ferrer T, McCarter R, Scalea T. Systemic inflammatory response syndrome score at admission independently predicts mortality and length of stay in trauma patients. J Trauma 2000; 49(4):647–652.

77. Malone D, Kuhls D, Napolitano L, McCarter R, Scalea T. Back to basics: Validation of the admission systemic inflammatory response syndrome score in predicting outcome in trauma. J Trauma 2001; 51(3):458–463.

78. Bochicchio G, Napolitano L, Joshi M, McCarter R, Scalea T. Systemic inflammatory response syndrome score at admission independently predicts infection in blunt trauma patients. J Trauma 2001; 50(5):817–820.

79. Bochicchio G, Napolitano L, Joshi M, et al. Persistent systemic inflammatory response syndrome is predictive of nosocomial infection in trauma. J Trauma 2002; 53(2):245–250.

80. Gando S, Nanzaki S, Kemmotsu O. Disseminated intravascular coagulation and sustained systemic inflammatory response syndrome predict organ dysfunction after trauma: application of clinical decision analysis. Ann Surg 1999; 229(1):121–127.

81. Brun-Buisson C. The epidemiology of the systemic inflammatory response. Intensive Care Med 2000; 26(12):1870.

82. Baue AE, Durham R, Faist E. Systemic inflammatory response syndrome (SIRS), multiple organ dysfunction syndrome (MODS), multiple organ failure (MOF): Are we winning the battle? Shock 1998; 10(2):79–89.

83. Talmor M, Hydo L, Barie PS. Relationship of systemic inflammatory response syndrome to organ dysfunction, length of stay, and mortality in critical surgical illness: effect of intensive care unit resuscitation. Arch Surg 1999; 134(1):81–87.

84. Moriyama S, Okamoto K, Tabira Y, et al. Evaluation of oxygen consumption and resting energy expenditure in critically ill patients with systemic inflammatory response syndrome. Crit Care Med 1999; 27(10):2133–2136.

85. Sablotzki A, Dehne MG, Friedrich I, et al. Different expression of cytokines in survivors and nonsurvivors from MODS following cardiovascular surgery. Eur J Med Res 2003; 8(2): 71–76.

86. Kim YI, Song KE, Ryeon HK, et al. Enhanced inflammatory cytokine production at ischemia/reperfusion in human liver resection. Hepatogastroenterology 2002; 49(46): 1077–1082.

87. Takahashi J, Ebara S, Kamimura M, et al. Pro-inflammatory and anti-inflammatory cytokine increases after spinal instrumentation surgery. J Spinal Disord Tech 2002; 15(4):294–300.

88. Spark JI, Chetter IC, Gallavin L, Kester RC, Guillou PJ, Scott DJ. Reduced total antioxidant capacity predicts ischaemia-reperfusion injury after femorodistal bypass. Br J Surg 1998; 85(2):221–225.

89. Yahara N, Abe T, Morita K, Tangoku A, Oka M. Comparison of interleukin-6, interleukin-8, and granulocyte colony-stimulating factor production by the peritoneum in laparoscopic and open surgery. Surg Endosc 2002; 16(11): 1615–1619; Epub 2002 Jun 27.

90. Schneemilch CE, Bank U. Release of pro- and anti-inflammatory cytokines during different anesthesia procedures. Anaesthesiol Reanim 2001; 26(1):4–10.

91. Cao DQ, Chen YP, Zou DQ. Effects of katamine on cardiopulmonary bypass-induced interleukin-6 and interleukin-8 response and its significance. Hunan Yi Ke Da Xue Xue Bao 2001; 26(4):350–352.

92. Mastronardi CA, Yu WH, McCann S. Lipopolysaccharide-induced tumor necrosis factor-alpha release is controlled by the central nervous system. Neuroimmunomodulation 2001; 9(3):148–156.

93. Nader ND, Ignatowski TA, Kurek CJ, Knight PR, Spengler RN. Clonidine suppresses plasma and cerebrospinal fluid concentrations of TNF-alpha during the perioperative period. Anesth Analg 2001; 93(2):363–369.

94. Takaono M, Yogosawa T, Okawa-Takatsuji M, Aotsuka S. Effects of intravenous anesthetics on interleukin (IL)-6 and IL-10 production by lipopolysaccharide-stimulated mononuclear cells from healthy volunteers. Acta Anaesthesiol Scand 2002; 46(2):176–179.

95. Brand JM, Frohn C, Luhm J, Kirchner H, Schmucker P. Early alterations in the number of circulating lymphocyte subpopulations and enhanced pro-inflammatory immune response during opioid-based general anesthesia. Shock 2003; 20(3):213–217.

96. Giraud O, Molliex S, Rolland C, et al. Halogenated anesthetics reduce interleukin-1beta-induced cytokine secretion by rat alveolar type II cells in primary culture. Anesthesiology 2003; 98(1):74–81.

97. Ganapathy S, Murkin JM, Dobkowski W, Boyd D. Stress and inflammatory response after beating heart surgery versus conventional bypass surgery: the role of thoracic epidural. anesthesia. Heart Surg Forum 2001; 4(4):323–327.

98. Bach F, Grundmann U, Bauer M, et al. Modulation of the inflammatory response to cardiopulmonary bypass by dopexamine and epidural anesthesia. Acta Anaesthesiol Scand 2002; 46(10):1227–1235.

99. Yasuda T, Takahashi S, Matsuki A. Tumor necrosis factor-alpha reduces ketamine- and propofol-induced anesthesia time in rats. Anesth Analg 2002; 95(4):952–955.

100. Okubo N, Hatori N, Ochi M, Tanaka S. Comparison of m-RNA expression for inflammatory mediators in leukocytes between on-pump and off-pump coronary artery bypass grafting. Ann Thorac Cardiovasc Surg 2003; 9(1):43–49.

101. El Azab SR, Rosseel PM, de Lange JJ, et al. Dexamethasone decreases the pro- to anti-inflammatory cytokine ratio during cardiac surgery. Br J Anaesth 2002; 88(4):496–501.

102. Hoyt DB. Fluid resuscitation: the target from an analysis of trauma systems and patient survival. J Trauma 2003; 54:S31–S35.

103. Burris D, Rhee P, Kaufmann C, et al. Controlled resuscitation for uncontrolled hemorrhagic shock. J Trauma 1998; 46: 216–223.

104. Santibanez-Gallerani AS, Barber AE, Williams SJ, ZhaoB SY, Shires GT. Improved survival with early fluid resuscitation following hemorrhagic shock. World J Surg 2001; 25(5): 592–597.

105. Bickell W, Wall M, Pepe P, et al. Immediate versus delayed fluid resuscitation for hypotensive patients with penetrating torso injuries. N Engl J Med 1994; 331:1105–1109.

106. Dutton RP, Mackenzie CF, Scalea TM. Hypotensive resuscitation during active hemorrhage: impact on in-hospital mortality. J Trauma 2002; 52(6):1141–1146.

107. Kramer GC. Hypertonic resuscitation: physiologic mechanisms and recommendations for trauma care. J Trauma 2003; 54:S89–S99.

108. Behrman S, Fabian T, Kudsk K, Proctor K. Microcirculatory flow changes after initial resuscitation of hemorrhagic shock with 7.5% hypertonic saline/6% dextran 70. J Trauma 1991; 31:589–600.

109. Coimbra R, Hoyt D, Junger W, et al. Hypertonic saline resuscitation decreases susceptibility to sepsis after hemorrhagic shock. J Trauma 1997; 42:602–607.

110. Diebel L, Robinson S, Wilson R, Dulchavsky S. Splanchnic mucosal perfusion effects of hypertonic versus isotonic resuscitation of hemorrhagic shock. Am Surg 1993; 59:495–499.

111. Gurfinkel V, Poggetti RS, Fontes B, da Costa Ferreira Novo F, Birolini D. Hypertonic saline improves tissue oxygenation and reduces systemic and pulmonary inflammatory response caused by hemorrhagic shock. J Trauma 2003; 54(6):1137–1145.

112. Rhee P, Buris D, Kaufmann C. Lactated ringers solution resuscitation causes neutrophil activation after hemorrhagic shock. J Trauma 1998; 44:313–319.

113. Junger W, Hoyt D, Davis R, et al. Hypertonicity regulates the function of human neutrophils by modulating chemoattractant receptor signaling and activating mitogen-activated protein kinase p38. J Clin Invest 1998; 101:2768–2779.

114. Coimbra R, Yada M, Rocha-e-Silva M, et al. Hypertonic saline and pentoxifylline resuscitation reduce bacterial translocation and lung injury following hemorrhagic shock: Lactated Ringer's does not. Proceedings of the 75th Annual Meeting of the American Association for the Surgery of Trauma 1997; 285.

115. Gushchin V, Stegalkina S, Alam HB, Kirkpatrick JR, Rhee PM, Koustova E. Cytokine expression profiling in human leukocytes after exposure to hypertonic and isotonic fluids. J Trauma 2002; 52(5):867–871.

116. Wade CE, Grady JJ, Kramer GC. Efficacy of hypertonic saline dextran fluid resuscitation for patients with hypotension from penetrating trauma. J Trauma. 2003; 54(suppl 5):S144–S148.

117. Vialet R, Albanese J, Thomachot L, et al. Isovolume hypertonic solutes (sodium chloride or mannitol) in the treatment of refractory posttraumatic intracranial hypertension: 2 mL/kg 7.5% saline is more effective than 2 mL/kg 20% mannitol. Crit Care Med 2003; 31(6):1683–1687.

118. Bayir H, Clark RS, Kochanek PM. Promising strategies to minimize secondary brain injury after head trauma. Crit Care Med 2003; 31(suppl 1):S112–S117.

119. O'Farrelly C. Just how inflamed is the normal gut? Gut 1998; 42:603.

120. Buzdon M, Napolitano L, Shi H, Ceresoli D, Rauniya R, Bass B. Femur fracture induces site-specific changes in T-cell immunity. J Surg Res 1999; 82:201–208.

121. Hassoun HT, Kone BC, Mercer DW, Moody FG, Weisbrodt NW, Moore FA. Postinjury multiple organ failure: the role of the gut. Shock 2001; 15(1):1–10.

122. Kahlke V, Fandrich F, Brotzmann K, Zabel P, Schroder J. Selective decontamination of the digestive tract: impact on cytokine release and mucosal damage after hemorrhagic shock. Crit Care Med 2002; 30(6):1327–1333.

123. Bouter H, Schippers E, Luelmo S, et al. No effect of preoperative selective gut decontamination on endotoxemia and cytokine activation during cardiopulmonary bypass: a randomized, placebo-controlled study. Crit Care Med 2002; 30(1):38–43.

124. Barret JP, Jeschke MG, Herndon DN. Selective decontamination of the digestive tract in severely burned pediatric patients. Burns 2001; 27(5):439–435.

125. Vincent J. New therapies in sepsis. Chest 1997; 112:330S.

126. Ehrly A. The effect of pentoxifylline on the deformability of erythrocytes and on the muscular oxygen pressure in patients with chronic arterial disease. J Med 1979; 10:331–338.

127. Porter J, Cutler B, Lee B, et al. Pentoxifylline efficacy in the treatment of intermittent claudication: Multicenter controlled double-blind trial with objective assessment of chronic occlusive arterial disease patients. Am Heart J 1982; 104:66–72.

128. Waxman K, Clark L, Soliman M, Parazin S. Pentoxifylline in resuscitation of experimental hemorrhagic shock. Crit Care Med 1991; 19:728–731.

129. Flynn W, Cryer H, Garrison R. Pentoxifylline but not saralasin, restores hepatic blood flow after resuscitation from hemorrhagic shock. J Surg Res 1991; 50:616–621.

130. Zhang Q, Ni Q, Cai D, Zhang Y, Zhang N, Hou L. Mechanisms of multiple organ damages in acute necrotizing pancreatitis. Chin Med J (Engl) 2001; 114(7):738–742.

131. Wang H, Yu M, Ochani M, et al. Nicotinic acetylcholine receptor alpha 7 subunit is an essential regulator of inflammation. Nature 2003; 421(6921):384–388.

132. Borovikova L, Ivanova S, Zhang M, et al. Vagus nerve stimulation attenuates the systemic inflammatory response to endotoxin. Nature 2000; 405(6785):458–462.

133. Brivio F, Lissoni P, Perego MS, Lissoni A, Fumagalli L. Abrogation of surgery-induced IL-6 hypersecretion by presurgical immunotherapy with IL-2 and its importance in the preventiion of postoperative complications. J Biol Regul Homeost Agents 2001; 15(4):370–374.

134. Bohm M, Ittenson A, Schierbaum KF, Rohl FW, Ansorge S, Allhoff EP. Pretreatment with interleukin-2 modulates perioperative immuno-dysfunction in patients with renal cell carcinoma. Eur Urol 2002; 41(4):458–467; discussion 467–468.

135. Mahdy AM, Galley HF, Abdel-Wahed MA, el-Korny KF, Sheta SA, Webster NR. Differential modulation of interleukin-6 and interleukin-10 by diclofenac in patients undergoing major surgery. Br J Anaesth 2002; 88(6):797–802.

136. Boeken U, Feindt P, Schulte HD, Gams E. Elastase release following myocardial ischemia during extracorporeal circulation (ECC)—marker of ongoing systemic inflammation? Thorac Cardiovasc Surg 2002; 50(3):136–140.

137. Faist E, Ertel W, Salmen B, et al. The immune-enhancing effect of perioperative thymopentin administration in elderly patients undergoing major surgery. Arch Surg 1988; 123:1449–1453.

138. Faist E, Markewitz A, Fuchs D, et al. Immunomodulatory therapy with thymo-opentin and indomethacin: Successful restoration of interleikin-2 synthesis in patients with major surgery. Ann Surg 1991; 214(3):264–273.

139. Hierholzer C, Menezes JM, Ungeheuer A, Billiar TR, Tweardy DJ, Harbrecht BG. A nitric oxide scavenger protects against pulmonary inflammation following hemorrhagic shock. Shock 2002; 17(2):98–103.

140. Lopez A, Lorente JA, Steingrub J, et al. Multiple-center, randomized, placebo-controlled, double-blind study of nitric oxide synthase inhibitor 546C88: effect on survival in patients with septic shock. Crit Care Med 2004; 32(1):21–30.

141. Bakker J, Grover R, McLuckie A, et al. Glaxo Wellcome International Septic Shock Study Group. Administration of the nitric oxide synthase inhibitor NG-methyl-L-arginine hydrochloride (546C88) by intravenous infusion for up to 72 hours can promote the resolution of shock in patients with severe sepsis: results of a randomized, double-blind, placebo-controlled, multicenter study (study no. 144-002). Crit Care Med 2004; 32(1):1–12.

142. Baudo F, de Cataldo F. Antithrombin III concentrates in the treatment of sepsis and septic shock: indications, limits and future prospects. Minerva Anestesiol 2000; 66(11 suppl 1):3–23.

143. Kulka PJ, Tryba M, Lange S. Are there certified indications for the use of antithrombin III in intensive care? Anasthesiol Intensivmed Notfallmed Schmerzther 2001; 36(3):143–153.

144. Isobe H, Okajima K, Uchiba M, Harada N, Okabe H. Antithrombin prevents endotoxin-induced hypotension by inhibiting the induction of nitric oxide synthase in rats. Blood 2002; 99(5):1638–1648.

145. Mizutani A, Okajima K, Uchiba M, et al. Antithrombin reduces ischemia/reperfusion-induced renal injury in rats by inhibiting leukocyte activation through promotion of prostacyclin production. Blood 2003; 101(8):3029–3036; Epub 2002 Dec 12.

146. Pata C, Caglikulekci M, Cinel L, Dirlik M, Colak T, Aydin S. The effects of antithrombin-III on inducible nitric oxide synthesis in experimental obstructive jaundice. An immunohistochemical study. Pharmacol Res 2002; 46(4):325–331.

147. Minnema MC, Chang AC, Jansen PM, et al. Recombinant human antithrombin III improves survival, and attenuates inflammatory responses in baboons lethally challenged with *Escherichia coli*. Blood 2000; 95(4):1117–1123.

148. Totzke G, Schobersberger W, Schloesser M, Czechowski M, Hoffmann G. Effects of antithrombin III on tumor necrosis factor-alpha and interleukin-1beta synthesis in vascular smooth muscle cells. J Interferon Cytokine Res 2001; 21(12):1063–1069.

149. Aramaki O, Takayama T, Yokoyama T, et al. High dose of antithrombin III induces indefinite survival of fully allogeneic cardiac grafts and generates regulatory cells. Transplantation 2003; 75(2):217–220.

150. Wiedermann CJ, Hoffmann JN, Juers M, et al. High-doss antithrombin III in the treatment of severe sepsis in patients with a high risk of death: efficacy and safety. Crit Care Med 2006, 34(2):285–292.

151. Fitzal F, DeLano FA, Young C, Rosario HS, Schmid-Schonbein GW. Pancreatic protease inhibition during shock attenuates cell activation and peripheral inflammation. J Vasc Res 2002; 39(4):320–329.

152. Poeze M, Froon AH, Ramsay G, Buurman WA, Greve JW. Decreased organ failure in patients with severe SIRS and septic shock treated with the platelet-activating factor antagonist TCV-309: a prospective, multicenter, double-blind, randomized phase II trial. TCV-309 Septic Shock Study Group. Shock 2000; 14(4):421–428.

153. Opal SM, Laterre PF, Abraham E, et al. Recombinant human platelet-activating factor acetylhydrolase for the treatment of severe sepsis: Results of a phase III, multicenter, randomized, double-blind, placebo-controlled clinical trial. Crit Care Med 2004; 32:332–341.

154. Minneci PC, Deans KJ, Banks SM, Eichacker PQ, Natanson C. Should we continue to target the platelet-activating factor pathway in septic patients? Crit Care Med 2004; 32(3):585–588.

155. Brown KA, Lewis SM, Hill TA, et al. Leucodepletion and the interaction of polymorphonuclear cells with endothelium in systemic inflammatory response syndrome. Perfusion 2001; 16(suppl):75–83.

156. Treacher DF, Sabbato M, Brown KA, Gant V. The effects of leucodepletion in patients who develop the systemic inflammatory response syndrome following cardiopulmonary bypass. Perfusion 16 (suppl):67–73.

157. Cuschieri J, Gourlay D, Garcia I, Jelacic S, Maier RV. Hypertonic preconditioning inhibits macrophage responsiveness to endotoxin. J Immunol 2002; 168(3):1389–1396.

158. Dunn DL. Prevention and treatment of multiple organ dysfunction syndrome: lessons learned and future prospects. Surg Infect (Larchmt). 2002; 1(3):227–237.

159. Delgado M, Abad C, Martinez C, et al. PACAP in immunity and inflammation. Ann N Y Acad Sci 2003; 992:141–157.

160. Delgado M, Leceta J, Ganea D. Vasoactive intestinal peptide and pituitary adenylate cyclase-activating polypeptide inhibit the production of inflammatory mediators by activated microglia. J Leukoc Biol 2003; 73(1):155–164.

161. Bastian L, Weimann A. Immunonutrition in patients after multiple trauma. Br J Nutr 2002; 87(suppl 1):S133–S134.

162. Matheson PJ, Hurt RT, Mittel OF, Wilson MA, Spain DAG, Harrison RN. Immune-enhancing enteral diet increases blood flow and pro-inflammatory cytokines in the rat ileum. J Surg Res 2003; 110(2):360–370.

163. Lin MT, Saito H, Fukushima R, et al. Preoperative total parenteral nutrition influences postoperative systemic cytokine responses after colorectal surgery. Nutrition 1997; 13(1):8–12.

164. Zhong Z, Wheeler MD, Li X, et al. L-Glycine: a novel anti-inflammatory, immunomodulatory, and cytoprotective agent. Curr Opin Clin Nutr Metab Care 2003; 6(2):229–240.

165. Jeevanandam M, Begay CK, Shahbazian LM, Petersen SR. Altered plasma cytokines and total glutathione levels in parenterally fed critically ill trauma patients with adjuvant recombinant human growth hormone (rhGH) therapy. Crit Care Med 2000; 28(2):324–329.

166. Ibs KH, Rink L. Zinc-altered immune function. J Nutr 2003 May; 133(5 suppl 1):1452S–1456S.

167. Waelput W, Broekaert D, Vandekerckhove J, Brouckaert P, Tavernier J, Libert C. A mediator role for metallothionein in tumor necrosis factor-induced lethal shock. J Exp Med 2001; 194(11):1617–1624.

168. Baum MK, Miguez-Burbano MJ, Campa A, Shor-Posner G. Selenium and interleukins in persons infected with human immunodeficiency virus type 1. J Infect Dis 2000; 182(suppl 1):S69–S73.

169. Zhang F, Yu W, Hargrove JL, et al. Inhibition of TNF-alpha induced ICAM-1, VCAM-1, and E-selectin expression by selenium. Atherosclerosis 2002; 161(2):381–386.

170. Maehira F, Miyagi I, Eguchi Y. Selenium regulates transcription factor NF-kappaB activation during the acute phase reaction. Clin Chim Acta 2003; 334(1-2):163–171.

171. Borner J, Zimmermann T, Albrecht S, Roesner D. Selenium administration in children with SIRS. Med Klin 1999; 94(suppl 3):93–96.

172. Vincent JL. Dear SIRS, I'm sorry to say that I don't like you ... . Crit Care Med 1997; 25(2):372–374.

173. Opal S. The uncertain value of the definition for SIRS. Systemic inflammatory response syndrome. Chest 1998; 113(6):1442–1443.

174. Bossink AW, Groeneveld J, Hack CE, Thijs LG. Prediction of mortality in febrile medical patients: How useful are systemic inflammatory response syndrome and sepsis criteria? Chest 1998; 113(6):1533–1541.

175. Dellinger RP, Bone RC. To SIRS with love. Crit Care Med 1998; 26(1):178–179.

176. Watanabe E, Hirasawa H, Abe R, et al. Cytokine-related genotypic differences in the peak interleukin-6 blood levels of the patients with SIRS and septic complications. J Trauma 2004; 57:438.

177. Johnson GB, Brunn GJ, Platt JL. Cutting Edge: An endogenous pathway to systemic inflammatory response syndrome (SIRS)-like reactions through Toll-like receptor 4. J Immunol 2004; 172(1):20–24.

178. Torre D, Tambini R, Manfredi M, et al. Circulating levels of FAS/APO-1 in patients with the systemic inflammatory response syndrome. Diagn Microbiol Infect Dis 2003; 45(4):233–236.

179. Weaver JGR, Rouse MS, Steckelberg JM, et al. Improved survival in experimental sepsis with an orally administered inhibitor of apoptosis. FASEB J 2004; 18:1185–1191.

180. Bommhardt U, Chang KC, Swanson PE, Wagner TH. Akt decreases lymphocyte apoptosis and improves survival in sepsis. J Immunol 2004; 172:7583–7591.

181. Nathens AB, Neff MJ, Jurkovich GJ, et al. Randomized, prospective trial of antioxidant supplementation in critically ill surgical patients. Ann Surg 2002; 236(6):814–822.

182. Bulger EM, Maier RV. An argument for Vitamin E supplementation in the management of systemic inflammatory response syndrome. Shock 2003; 19(2):99–103.

183. Tabrizi AR, Zehnbauer BA, Freeman BD, Buchman TG. Genetic markers in sepsis. J Am Coll Surg 2001;192(1):106–117.

184. Kellum JA, Angus DC. Genetic variation and risk of sepsis. Minerva Anestesiol. 2003; 69(4):245–253.

185. Holmes CL, Russell JA, Walley KR. Genetic polymorphisms in sepsis and septic shock: role in prognosis and potential for therapy. Chest 2003; 124(3):1103–1115.

186. Child NJ, Yang IA, Pulletz MC, et al. Polymorphisms in Toll-like receptor 4 and the systemic inflammatory response syndrome. Biochem Soc Trans 2003; 31(Pt 3):652–653.

187. Hotchkiss RS, Karl IE. The pathophysiology, and treatment of sepsis. N Engl J Med 2003; 348(2):138–150.

188. Martinez-Mier G, Toledo-Pereyra LH, Ward PA. Adhesion molecules and hemorrhagic shock. J Trauma 2001; 51:408–415.

189. Partrick DA, Moore FA, Moore EE, Barnett CC, Silliman CC. Neutrophil priming and activation in the pathogenesis of postinjury multiple organ failure. New Horizons 1996; 4(2):194–210.

64

Providing Family-Centered Care

Catherine McCoy-Hill
School of Nursing, Azusa Pacific University, Azusa, California, U.S.A.

William C. Wilson
Department of Anesthesiology and Critical Care, UC San Diego Medical Center, San Diego, California, U.S.A.

INTRODUCTION

A family-centered approach to critical care is characterized by collaboration between the patient, family (or loved ones), and the health care providers. The important elements of family-centered care include: (*i*) respect for patient's values, beliefs, including their cultural and spiritual backgrounds; (*ii*) frequent communication and information sharing; and (*iii*) physician encouraged collaboration in the decision-making process (Table 1) (1). Caring for the needs of families is an important component of comprehensive trauma care and likely facilitates improved outcomes (1–3).

The American College of Surgeons Committee on Trauma (ACS-COT) has identified the provision of family services as an important measure for trauma programs process improvement (4). Providing family-centered care in trauma settings requires multidisciplinary support, including education of providers, and is facilitated when a dedicated case manager can oversee the process. Institutional guidelines that address family support, information sharing, and utilization of supportive resources can be developed and implemented from evidence-based models (1).

IMPACT OF TRAUMA AND CRITICAL ILLNESS ON FAMILY MEMBERS

☞ **Because the nature of trauma is sudden and unexpected and includes the potential for loss of life or significant disability, family systems are often stressed to their emotional limits.** ☞ Typical responses evoked by observing one's family member in a life-threatening situation include: shock, disbelief, helplessness, fear, and anxiety, as loved ones seek understanding of what has happened. Fears about death often predominate. Anxiety centers on concerns about the seriousness of the patient's condition as well as the quality of medical care being received.

Additional burdens impacting family members include financial hardships, loss of work, and concerns about the future. Often the family's entire lifestyle is disrupted, with resultant changes in roles, relationships, and usual routines. Lifelong goals and dreams may be shattered (5–7).

The circumstances surrounding the trauma as well as the nature and severity of the injury impact the family's ability to cope with the crisis. The nature of the trauma [e.g., unanticipated, violent, or stigmatizing (suicide attempts)] can provoke high degrees of stress on families.

Tragic insults such as spinal cord injury (SCI) and traumatic brain injury (TBI) are emotionally overwhelming, as they represent lifelong debility to the patient. Severe disfigurements from major burns, craniofacial injuries, amputations, etc., are similarly devastating and result in high levels of emotional distress to patients and their loved ones (7–9).

Acute grief responses can occur as members of the family are confronted with actual or potential loss of the patient's physical status, level of function, and future capabilities. Individual family member characteristics also influence their response to the crisis. These include: age and developmental stage, relationships and family demands, past experiences with illness or trauma, social support networks, cultural and spiritual values, as well as pre-existing states of mental health and coping abilities (7,9,10). Specific family members will also react differently based upon their relationship with the patient and their own emotional condition. When extreme emotional stresses are perceived by a family member, initial anxiety and grief can develop into an Acute Stress Disorder (ASD), or, if prolonged, to Post Traumatic Stress Disorder (PTSD), as described briefly later, and extensively in Volume 2, Chapter 65 (7–9).

FAMILY NEEDS FOLLOWING TRAUMA AND CRITICAL CARE

☞ **Evidence indicates that families exhibit a universally predictable set of needs when a loved one becomes critically ill** (7–10). ☞ Common family needs following injury or critical illness of a loved one include: (*i*) information, (*ii*) proximity (i.e., to "be with" the patient), (*iii*) emotional support (including reassurance that the patient is receiving optimal care), (*iv*) cultural sensitivity, and (*v*) spiritual support (Table 1) (10–16).

Communication and Information Sharing

The desire to obtain timely and accurate information about the patient's condition is the concern of family members most widely recognized. Informational needs are particularly important to families of trauma patients, as the unexpected injury evokes high levels of emotional distress (8,9). Sparse communication from physicians and the unfamiliar environment of the surgical intensive care unit (SICU) can intensify feelings of anxiety, uncertainty, worry, and fear. ☞ **Well-informed families report a greater sense of control, are more often able to accept the tragedy affecting their loved one, and participate more effectively in patient**

Table 1   Universal Family Needs During the Management of Trauma and Critical Care

Family needs	Elements of care emphasized, comments, and examples
Communication and information sharing	Information should be honest and sensitively communicated; Brief daily meetings should be scheduled for information exchange; The family should always be notified promptly following a change in the patient's condition; Regular (e.g., weekly) multidisciplinary family conferences are encouraged, especially regarding major changes in patient status or treatment direction; The family should be provided access to clinicians (phone number, pager etc.); Informational booklets should be utilized (e.g., SCCM brochure: *When your loved one is in the ICU*).
Proximity (need to be with the patient)	Liberalized, flexible visiting hours should be maintained; The family should be prepared for what to expect in terms of patient's condition and the ICU environment; Family members should be informed regarding what they can do for the patient at the bedside.
Emotional support	Reassure family optimal care is occurring; Provide anticipatory guidance re: treatment plan and expected outcomes; Assist in mobilizing family resources; Refer to social worker, clergy, mental health clinicians, etc. when indicated; Identify family members at risk for psychologic sequelae (i.e., depression, PTSD).
Cultural sensitivity	Accept and respect cultural differences; Adapt care to be congruent with cultural preferences when appropriate; Utilize translators when language barriers exist.
Spiritual support	Assessment of spiritual needs should be ongoing; Spiritual rituals should be allowed to occur whenever possible; Referrals should be made for spiritual support services whenever needs are identified (e.g., grave news, ethical dilemmas, at or near the end of life).

Abbreviations: SCCM, Society of Critical Care Medicine; PTSD, posttraumatic stress disorder.

care decision making (2,5,8). ☞ Understanding the patient's diagnosis, treatment plan, and likely outcome constitute essential information elements for families to develop realistic expectations regarding the patient's condition and prospects for recovery. Clinicians have an obligation not only to provide honest and timely information, but also to convey it in a sensitive and thoughtful manner. When patients are not capable of making their own decisions (e.g., coma, severe TBI), family members must be prepared to act as surrogate decision makers, regarding invasive procedures, life support, and end-of-life care (refer to Volume 2, Chapters 68 and 69).

Several studies have addressed how health care providers can best meet the informational needs of families (2,5). Findings indicate that most family members want and expect direct, specific information about the patient's condition and overall management goals to be delivered by the attending physician at least once a day. From nurses, families expect to be informed about the daily care of the patient, reasons for particular treatments, and general information regarding the critical care environment (staff roles, procedures, equipment, policies, etc.). Family members also place great importance on being promptly informed of any significant changes in the patient's condition (5–7). Many of the studies investigating family needs have used the Critical Care Family Needs Inventory (Table 2), originally developed by Molter in 1979 (12). This tool has been validated across multiple critical care and trauma settings (5,11–14).

Useful strategies to maintain communication include scheduling a specific time for daily updates, holding multidisciplinary family conferences (especially with changes in treatment direction), and providing family members with written information that outlines the communication process and lists the responsible physician and means of access (i.e., names, phone/pager numbers, etc.).

A number of hospitals have made loaner pager systems available to family members of unstable critical patients so that they can feel more comfortable in leaving the ICU, knowing they will be easily reached if the need arises. The Society of Critical Care Medicine (SCCM) and The American Association of Critical Care Nurses (AACN) have published brochures that provide useful information for families of critically ill patients, advising them of their rights and responsibilities along with a list of questions they should consider asking the doctors and nurses (15,16).

More recently, critical care family/visitor centers have been developed. These spaces often equipped with web-enabled computers providing access to informations (e.g., medical conditions, treatments, tests, drugs, etc.) (17). This concept has been implemented in a number of ICUs and is

Table 2   The Critical Care Family Needs Inventory[a]

Do you feel that the best possible care is being given to the patient?

Do you feel that the hospital personnel are courteous and care about the patient?

Have explanations about the patient's condition been in terms you can understand?

Do you feel that you have been given honest information about the patient's condition?

Do you believe that someone will notify you following a significant change in the patient's condition?

Have the staff members shown interest in how you are coping?

Have the hospital personnel explained the equipment being used?

Do you feel comfortable visiting with the patient in the intensive care unit?

Is the waiting room welcoming and comfortable?

[a]The listed questions are asked of the family members by the staff.
Source: Adapted from Refs. 12, 13.

expanding as individuals want access to knowledge sources and desire to be well informed. The reader is referred to Ref. 17 for an excellent resource sponsored by the SCCM, detailing implementation of a consumer medical information system in ICU settings (17). Ideally, the environment of waiting rooms should also be welcoming and comforting (furnishings, noise, lighting, refreshments, etc.) to visitors.

Communication is an ongoing process among the critical care team, the patient, and the patient's family members. Open exchange of information and regular access to the physician are vital to this process. ☞ **Although the physician's time is limited due to the complex demands of the trauma and critical care environment, consistent communication with the family and open access to informational resources are essential in meeting family needs.** ☞

When communicating with families, information should be presented at a level the family members can easily understand. The family's emotional status must also be considered, since denial or severe anxiety limits the amount of information that can be assimilated. ☞ **During serious discussions, family members may be intimidated or ashamed to admit that they do not fully understand what has been said. To avoid confusion, medical information should be clearly explained, and repeated as necessary. Technical language and euphemisms should be avoided, whereas clarifying questions should be encouraged.** ☞ Initial attention should be focused on listening to and addressing the most pressing concerns of the family. These discussions ideally occur in a comfortable, private place protected from the noise and chaos of the Trauma Resuscitation Suite (TRS), emergency department (ED), or SICU. Conflicts may arise when information given to families is inadequate, inconsistent, or is not clearly understood. Examples of inadequate communication include using phrases such as the patient is "stable" without further explanation of clinical status, or stating that certain physical findings have improved when, in fact, the patient's overall condition may be worsening. Inconsistencies occur when physicians from different specialties give contradictory information, or when there is a lack of consensus in the clinical management plan.

Proximity: Open Visitation Policy

The need for proximity (to be with the patient) reflects the desire of the family to be physically near the patient to maintain family relationships and provide emotional support to their loved one (10). Not long ago, critical care units maintained rigid visiting hours that limited family access to the patient and restricted visits by children or those beyond the immediate family. In most critical care units these traditions have given way to more liberalized visitation policies. ☞ **A flexible visitation policy has psychological benefits for both the patient and the family members, with a resultant positive influence on their overall satisfaction with care.** ☞

For family members, being physically present enables them to provide support to the patient and maintain family connections. Being at the bedside also provides assurance that their loved one is receiving the best possible care. Visitation policies should consider patient preferences, remain flexible to accommodate family needs, and convey the message that families are valued. Family presence is especially important in the acute phase, and whenever the family perceives the patient as being critically ill.

Prior to visiting, and especially at the initial visit, family members should be given explanations of the patient's medical status, appearance, and behavior, as well as a description of the bedside environment. Whenever possible, a nurse should remain with the family members to assess their level of distress and to provide information and emotional support. Families often require guidance regarding what they can do at the bedside, and should be encouraged to communicate with the patient even when the patient cannot respond.

Emotional Support

Family requirements for emotional support typically center on the tragedy of the trauma, and the universal wish to be assured that their loved one is receiving the best possible care. Family members also commonly perceive strong needs to maintain personal coping strength in order to "be there" for their ill-loved one. ☞ **Although family members give priority to the welfare of their relative, their own emotional needs become increasingly significant over time, while the quest for hope remains universal (11–14).** ☞

Other support needs emerge as family members of severely traumatized patients begin to redefine their hopes about the future, and as they begin to recognize the emotional toll that the injury experience has imposed upon them. The burden of having a traumatized family member impacts multiple domains within the family structure, including practical day-to-day concerns, financial worries, and material comfort needs. High levels of anxiety, depression, anticipatory grief, ASD, and later PTSD are frequently reported in patients with life threatening injuries (Volume 2, Chapter 65), and in their family members as well (7–9,18).

Interventions to assist family members include strengthening family-coping abilities and mobilizing resources to provide needed emotional support. Because of their 24-hour presence and close relationship with the patient, the bedside SICU nurse plays a critical role in the emotional well-being of family members by providing information, support, and encouragement. Often family members need someone to listen to them, acknowledge their feelings, and be sensitive to their concerns. Recognition by clinicians that this is an overwhelming and stressful time helps to "normalize" feelings of fear, anger, or helplessness.

Anticipatory guidance regarding the treatment plan and expected outcomes also helps relatives to better understand the nature and severity of the illness, and serves to foster more realistic expectations for recovery. When recovery is unlikely, families require the most intensive support and guidance during the difficult transition from curative to palliative care (3). Family members who are highly distressed or struggling to grasp the gravity of irrecoverable medical conditions benefit most from clear, direct explanations by the attending physician. ☞ **Occasionally, reviewing diagnostic images (e.g., brain computerized tomography scans, etc.) with family members helps to convey situations that are difficult to grasp by words alone.** ☞

Those family members who are highly distressed or unable to cope may need the support of social workers, mental health clinicians, or visitation by their spiritual leaders. Utilizing the expertise and resources of interdisciplinary specialized support services early in the process can help identify "at-risk family members," and allow for earlier implementation of supportive interventions.

In many centers, the trauma nurse coordinator or case manager acts as a liaison between the patient/family and the trauma team to monitor patient progress, coordinate implementation of care needs, and facilitate access to needed services throughout the continuum from admission, through discharge and follow-up.

Cultural Sensitivity

Changing demographics and the increasingly diverse cultural profiles of major city populations' worldwide (>300 languages are spoken in the US alone) mandates the provision of culturally sensitive and competent care by health providers. Culture refers to integrated patterns of behavior that include the language, beliefs, values, and customs of racial, ethnic, or social groups. ✍ **Cultural factors are recognized to have a strong influence on health practices, and to affect patient/family satisfaction with medical care, trust of healthcare providers, and adherence to treatment regimens (19,20).** ✍

In 2001, the Department of Health and Human Services published national standards for culturally and linguistically appropriate services (CLAS) in health care. These standards address the need for patients to receive effective, understandable, and respectful care compatible with their cultural health beliefs, practices, and preferred language. Cultural and linguistic competence refers to the ability of health care providers and their organizations to understand and respond effectively to these patient and family needs (21).

When language barriers are encountered, bilingual translators/interpreters should be utilized to obtain important clinical information and ensure accurate two-way communication. Family members or children should not be used as translators (unless requested by the patient), to avoid problems with confidentiality and impartiality.

In situations where patients or families have unique needs, it is appropriate to involve a social worker or patient advocate/ombudsperson with special expertise regarding unusual concerns. When important to the family, the patient's cultural traditions (e.g., healing rituals, ethnic customs, etc.) can often be integrated into the medical plan of care. Clinicians should also be sensitive to individual family dynamics (e.g., divorce, estrangement), as well as differences in educational and socioeconomic backgrounds amongst members within the family group. When families and their doctors have trouble agreeing, an ethics consult is often helpful in resolving conflict (Volume 2, Chapter 67).

Although difficult on a busy trauma service or critical care unit, knowledge and awareness of cultural factors not only improves diagnostic accuracy and decreases errors, but also improves therapeutic relationships by demonstrating understanding and acceptance of the unique concerns of patients and their families.

Spiritual Support

Assessment, recognition, and support of the spiritual concerns of patients and their families are important aspects of modern critical care. Indeed, assessing and acknowledging the patient's spirituality can provide vital information and guidance throughout their critical illness, from initial resuscitation management (e.g., Jehovah's Witness), to end of life decision making, including the withholding or withdrawal of life-sustaining therapy when further treatment is futile (also refer to Volume 2, Chapters 67–69) (22).

Spiritual support services have become an integral aspect of care provided in most western hospitals, and spiritually related issues can influence medical care and ethical decision-making (23). Spirituality is recognized as a universal human phenomenon that transcends biological and psychosocial realms. For many individuals, spirituality provides a sense of inner strength, meaning, and purpose in their lives (24). ✍ **Spiritual belief systems can influence a patient or family's explanation of injury causation, perceptions of severity, and acceptance of changes imposed by illness.** ✍ When faced with the crisis of critical illness, including patient suffering, fear of death or uncertain prognosis, spiritual concerns often arise. Ethical conflicts ensue when patient/family values or beliefs conflict with treatment plans, and/or with the healthcare professional's perceptions regarding quality of life (23,24).

While not endorsing any particular belief system, the Joint Commission on Accreditation of Healthcare Organizations (JCAHO) has identified the provision of spiritual support services as a requisite for quality, holistic patient care (25). Hospitals are expected to anticipate, plan for, and address patient/family spiritual needs. Ideally, requests or needs for spiritual care are assessed as part of the admission assessment, and on an ongoing basis as concerns arise. Upon request or when needs are expressed or identified, clinicians have a responsibility to make appropriate referrals (with patient/family permission) for spiritual support services (22,23).

As part of the healthcare team, pastoral care professionals (priests, rabbis, mullahs, pastors, etc.) can offer valuable support and assistance in addressing the diverse spiritual needs of patients and families. Considerations for referral include situations where grave news has been received, when ethical dilemmas present, and at or near the end of life (Volume 2, Chapter 68). Changes in a patient's emotional state (e.g., hopelessness, grief, or despair) may also warrant referrals.

COLLABORATING WITH FAMILIES

✍ **Collaboration between clinicians and family members is fundamental in meeting the emotional needs of patients and families.** ✍ Collaboration in care transcends the ICU stay, and continues into the recovery period when family members often assume the role of care provider for the patient.

The establishment of rapport begins at the initial contact with patients and families. Distress in family members can be reduced when clinicians are perceived as knowledgeable and professional, yet approachable, understanding, and empathetic (26). The ability to convey a sense of experienced professionalism at the same time as humility, openness, and unhurried compassion, results from years of experience in counseling families in crisis situations. This is why senior members of the trauma team should speak with the family about these important considerations.

Early and effective communication provides the foundation for developing a relationship of mutual trust, and influences the efficacy of future deliberations. Conversely, inadequate attention to the interpersonal relations between the trauma team and family can generate negative emotions, and can impair the family's ability to cope and participate effectively in decision-making. Poor communication also promotes family dissatisfaction with care (26,27).

Due to their condition, patients are often unable to participate in care; family members must be educated and empowered to act as advocates, and at times, as surrogate decision makers (5). As patients recover, family members often are the patient's most important source of support. Effective communication between family members and the healthcare team is strongly associated with empowerment and improved decision-making, yet suboptimal communication in trauma and ICU settings continues to be reported (2,26,27).

Ideally, collaborative discussions should take place with the trauma/critical care team (including house staff and nursing staff) prior to meeting with the family about major changes in patient condition or treatment plans, to ensure information consistency. The challenge for the attending physician is to synthesize all of the patient data and present it in a clear and understandable way that provides a full perspective of the patient's condition, while showing empathy and compassion to the family (6,28). In most cases it is best to have a designated family member serve as spokesperson, and as a primary point of contact to receive and relay information to other family members.

ACUTE GRIEF MANAGEMENT AND BEREAVEMENT SUPPORT
Acute Grief Management

Family members often require considerable levels of guidance and support to facilitate coping with the psychological stress associated with injury or impending death of a loved one. Patients themselves may manifest serious feelings of grief and/or guilt, especially those who were involved in motor vehicle collisions (or other traumas) where they may have been only minimally injured, whereas another family member was severely harmed or killed. The survivor guilt can become particularly profound when the minimally injured patient was directly responsible for the accident or injury (e.g., driving while intoxicated), or otherwise derelict in his or her duty (e.g., failure to use a car seat resulting in infant death). In all of these situations professional grief management should be employed. ☞ **Specialists trained in grief and bereavement management may not be available when most needed (e.g., in the middle of the night or on weekends). Accordingly, the physicians, and especially the nursing staff, often provide this essential supportive role.** ☞

The most important element in grief intervention is demonstrating compassion and genuine concern for the grieving patient as well as for their family and loved ones (29,30). When patients and family members perceive that the physicians and nurses are genuinely concerned about them, an unnecessary barrier to care is removed. Providing early and open emotional support positively impacts the patient and family's experience, and may decrease the development of ASD, and later PTSD, as discussed in Volume 2, Chapter 65 (31,32).

Notifying the Family About Bad News

Notifying families of trauma victims that a death has occurred is perhaps one of the most difficult challenges faced by the trauma team and minimal formal attention is typically given to this aspect of trauma management. Notification is best carried out by a senior physician on the trauma team who is experienced in handling this delicate task (3). The manner in which survivors are informed of a death in the family and the support provided at this time has an enduring impact on their grief response, and emotional healing process (29). Grief reactions of emotionally distraught family members can be mediated by receiving skilled, sensitive, and caring support from the trauma team. Strategies for conveying unpleasant news to families are summarized in Table 3.

Jurkovich et al. (2000) published the results of one of the first studies in the trauma literature that addressed the needs of bereaved family members of trauma victims (29). The study investigated "giving bad news," and identified characteristics valued by families whose loved one had died after a short stay in the ED or Trauma ICU. ☞ **Family perceptions regarding the most important elements of "giving bad news" include: (*i*) the attitude of the news-giver; (*ii*) the clarity of the information conveyed; and (*iii*) the ability to have questions answered.** ☞ Clinician behaviors found to be most comforting were: (*i*) the display of an empathetic and caring attitude, (*ii*) the deli-

Table 3 Strategies for Conveying "Bad News" (e.g., Poor Prognosis or Poor Outcomes) to Family Members and Loved Ones

Strategies	Comments and explanations
General approach	Display a compassionate and caring demeanor; a sensitive and thoughtful approach can positively impact the survivor's grief process.
Information-giving	Attending physician responsibility (delegation is discouraged); provide clear, direct, honest information in understandable terms, avoiding euphemisms; utilize translators as needed.
Anticipate grief reactions	Reactions can include: shock and disbelief, anger, extreme sadness, and occasionally violent behavior; assess coping abilities, mobilize resources as needed; identify those at risk for ASD (later PTSD) for early intervention.
Allow sufficient time	Maintain a non-hurried attitude allowing time for emotional responses and questions; allow loved ones to be with the patient before death if possible, and following death; ongoing clinician presence can provide comfort and guidance to distraught family members.
Provide emotional support	Reassure the family that the patient received the best possible care; acknowledge the sorrow of losing a loved one; respect spiritual and cultural traditions; provide privacy and physical comfort.
Follow-up and referral	Refer to interdisciplinary support services as indicated (trauma case manager, social service, pastoral care, bereavement specialist, etc); provide written informational resources; consider follow-up condolences with phone calls or correspondence.

Abbreviations: ASD, acute stress disorder; PTSD, post traumatic stress disorder.

very of a well-informed clear message, (*iii*) privacy of the conversation, and (*iv*) the allowance of sufficient time to answer questions and allow families to adjust to the emotional distress (29).

When a patient dies following trauma, the goals and efforts of the trauma team are directed toward comforting and supporting the family through the initial bereavement experience. Documented needs of families facing sudden bereavement include: (*i*) prompt and compassionate attention from professional staff immediately upon arrival to the hospital; (*ii*) notification of imminent or actual death in a sensitive and compassionate manner; (*iii*) opportunity to be with the patient before death, if possible, and in most cases, following death; (*iv*) to know the patient received the best possible care; (*v*) to have questions answered; (*vi*) to be advised on what to do next; and (*vii*) to be given support and follow-up resources (29,30).

Kenneth Iserson, MD in *Grave Words: Notifying Survivors About Sudden Unexpected Deaths,* outlines strategies to effectively communicate with and support survivors, emphasizing that delivering bad news with sensitivity and in the right context, including support and direction for continued assistance can attenuate the grief process (30). In most, cases, it is the responsibility of the trauma surgeon to notify the family of a death. The presence of a nurse, social worker, or clergy provides additional resources for emotional and spiritual support of the family.

When initial contact is made by phone, it is generally agreed that the relative should not be told over the phone that the patient has died. It is usually best to briefly describe the event, notify the family that the patient is "seriously injured" and ask them to come to the hospital as soon as possible, ideally with someone to drive and accompany them. In circumstances where informing of death by phone is unavoidable, the clinician should attempt to ensure that the individual receiving the news does so in the company of family or loved ones, and is not left alone. Follow-up communication should also be specifically arranged at that time. Extreme care must always be taken to accurately identify the deceased person and notify the appropriate family members (30,33).

Upon arrival to the resuscitation suite or SICU, a nurse or social worker should meet the family member(s), bring them to a private room, and remain with them. In communicating with the family, the attending physician can assess what is already known, and give a brief chronology of prehospital, resuscitation, and subsequent events. The deceased should always be referred to by name, and by use of clear words stating that the person has "died" rather than using terms such as "expired" or "succumbed" and so on (30,33,34).

Bereaved relatives have the right to thoughtful explanations of the circumstances surrounding their loved one's death, the efforts taken to save the person's life, and that everything possible was done by providers in both the prehospital and hospital settings (34,35). ☞ **Careful listening to the family's style of communication and vocabulary can help healthcare professionals develop a message that is clearly understandable.** ☞ Nonverbal communication gestures such as sitting together and speaking on the same physical level, maintaining eye contact, and a non-hurried attitude also enhance communication.

Bereavement Support

Clinicians must be prepared for the resultant, sometimes intense, expressions of grief and sadness following notification of a patient's death. Grief-stricken survivors are known

to experience a period of severe psychic pain, which usually lasts for 10 to 20 minutes (36). During this highly stressful time, the family's emotional reactions should be acknowledged, allowing time for responses and questions. Insensitive remarks such as "we all must deal with death" do little to console, and must be avoided. The clinician's remaining presence, expression of sorrow for the family's loss, and conveyance of empathy through physical touch when appropriate, and even tears, can provide immeasurable support and comfort to suffering and distraught family members.

Following the initial grief responses, the family should be given the option of spending time with the deceased. The physical appearance of the body should be made to look as attractive as possible prior to viewing, and relatives should be informed of what to expect ahead of time. This is especially important with disfiguring injuries, and when medical equipment (e.g., endotracheal tubes, etc.) is required to remain in place for postmortem exam. When viewing the deceased, staff should allow for privacy but remain nearby to answer questions and provide emotional support. Families can be encouraged to touch the body, and in the case of young children, to hold the child. It is essential to allow unrushed time for expression of mourning, and demonstrate respect for cultural and spiritual traditions, which may help survivors accept the loss of a loved one. A concluding process in which families are given "permission" to leave and guidance regarding what to do next is often helpful (33,35,36).

Requests for organ/tissue donation and autopsy requirements are best handled after the family has acknowledged the patient's death, in order to emotionally separate the issues. Personnel (usually from the regional organ procurement agency), skilled in approaching families and knowledgeable regarding procurement protocols should be utilized. Survivor grief may be facilitated by the sense of comfort associated with the decision to donate. When handled timely and sensitively, negative reactions are minimized and donation rates are improved (refer Volume 2, Chapter 16 for a discussion of the donor procurement process) (30,33).

When autopsy is indicated, requests for permission should involve an explanation of the reasons for postmortem exam, along with a brief description of procedures to dispel any misconceptions. When the cause of death is unclear, a specific determination of cause may help the family's grief process by reassuring them that nothing else could have been done to save the patient's life (33).

In medical examiner cases where authority to perform autopsy does not require consent, clinicians must clearly communicate mandates for medico-legal examination. In cases involving criminal investigation, notification of death may be under the jurisdiction of law enforcement, and viewing the body may be temporarily prohibited. Although complex situations can arise, the clinician's role is to provide necessary information in a compassionate and consoling manner.

The nature and circumstances of the death may also place survivors at greater risk for adverse psychological sequelae. Unexpected mortality (e.g., following acute trauma) is generally more difficult to assimilate than is a death resulting from chronic illness, and traumatic deaths are associated with higher rates of psychological morbidity in loved ones, including prolonged or pathologic grief, depression, and PTSD (35). Recognized risk factors for psychological morbidity include: death of a child; death or disability of more than one family member; traumatic, mutilating, or violent death; death by homicide or suicide; and death perceived as preventable. The bereaved may suffer from survivor guilt, believing that they could or should have done more to prevent the death; this is especially serious when the survivor was unintentionally responsible for the death. Individual characteristics such as prior mental health problems, multiple life stressors, conflicted or overly dependent relationships with the deceased, and limited social support networks increase vulnerability for psychological morbidity (31,32,37,38). Survivors who seem to be especially disturbed or those recognized to be at high-risk for pathologic grief should be identified and offered referral for early psychiatric intervention.

Bereaved survivors should be informed about the psychological impact of traumatic loss, the process of grieving, and available supportive resources. Written material for follow-up contacts, available hospital and community-based grief support systems, mental health services, and pastoral care (if indicated) should be provided in the hospital, and mailed out in the following weeks. Follow-up phone calls can also be made to express condolences (35,37). This provides families with a sense that clinicians "really care" and also affords an opportunity to assess the family's grief status, identify needs for ongoing support, and to make referrals if warranted.

☞ **A structured approach to bereavement care that is integrated into the spectrum of trauma services has great potential to reduce the stressors of the grief-stricken family members faced with the sudden, unexpected death of a loved one.** ☞ Resources have begun to appear in the trauma literature, and much can be learned from existing models in pediatrics and palliative care where family needs in bereavement have been more thoroughly investigated (3,35,38). Multidisciplinary teams comprised of trauma surgeons, intensivists, nurses, social workers, clergy, and psychiatric clinicians committed in providing family-centered care can have a positive impact on the grief experience of those loved ones who are the "secondary victims" of trauma.

FAMILY PRESENCE DURING RESUSCITATION

The presence of patients' families in the trauma resuscitation suite is a topic of recent and considerable debate. Controversy on this topic centers on medico-legal issues, fear of causing psychological trauma to witnessing family members, and practitioner concerns that family needs may compete with urgent patient care demands or scarce resources (39,40). Although mostly limited to small, noncontrolled studies, a growing body of research indicates that many families would elect to be present during resuscitative and invasive procedures, and when given the option, often choose to remain. ☞ **Almost universally, studies questioning family members who have experienced resuscitations have strongly supported family-witnessed resuscitation (FWR), and most would elect to do so again (41,42).** ☞ Although "media miracles" and glorified misinformation may be influential, lay surveys indicate that the majority of the general population also favors FWR (43,44).

Several investigators have reported that witnessing resuscitation has few adverse psychological effects, and that family members may benefit from the practice. Reported benefits include seeing that everything possible was being done, feeling they were able to support the patient, and in facilitating the grief process when death was imminent

(41,42,45). In the only study to date addressing patient preferences, Benjamin et al. in 2004 studied resuscitation survivors and reported that 72% (n of 200) of patients surveyed favored the presence of their families (46).

Several professional organizations (Emergency Nurses Association; American Association of Critical Nurses) have recommended that health care providers offer families the option to be present during both adult and pediatric resuscitations (47). In 2000, the *American Heart Association Guidelines for Emergency Cardiovascular Care and CPR* advocated family-witnessed resuscitation and recommended that family members be given the option to be present during CPR attempts (48). The American College of Emergency Physicians (ACEP) has made the following statement: "When no hospital policy exists, the decision should be based on the family's wish to remain with their loved one, the views of medical personnel, the reactions of family members and patients to the situation, and the nature of the emergency"(49). A few emergency departments and trauma centers (including Parkland Hospital in Dallas, Texas, U.S.A.) have adopted family presence protocols for FWR. The protocols generally involve pre-screening for suitability of family members (e.g., emotional stability, no hostile intent, no evidence of intoxication or drug use, etc.) and the agreement to follow all instructions and leave the resuscitation room if instructed to do so. A family facilitator is designated (usually a social worker or nurse) to prepare family members beforehand and remain present for guidance, information, and support (41)

Provider views on this issue are divergent, with nurses generally holding more favorable views of FWR than physicians, and less experienced clinicians more often preferring to avoid the practice (39). Geographic differences also exist, with Midwest professionals more likely to allow family presence, and northeastern states least likely to implement FWR (39). Pediatric providers have a longer history with FWR and are generally more supportive of family presence (40).

While opposing views are likely to remain, continued research exploring family presence is needed to evaluate outcomes of family witnessed resuscitation from patient, family, and provider perspectives (50). Not all resuscitations are amenable to family presence (e.g., resuscitative thoracotomy, open head injury, violent crime circumstances, etc.). Also, not all family members will choose this option.

Most importantly, staff resources and physical space must be available to screen, monitor, and provide support to the family. Protocols may be helpful, although their usefulness has not been well studied. Currently, research on FWR is still in early stages since the concept is relatively new. Many clinical, ethical, and legal/risk management issues surrounding FWR deserve further exploration, and research must specifically address outcomes in trauma settings. Both proponents and critics of FWR agree that an individualized rather than a prescribed approach is essential, and that multiple variables (patient needs, family characteristics, resource availability, clinician education, etc.) must be considered in decision-making and establishment of best practices.

ROLE OF THE CASE MANAGER

Successful achievement of family-centered care not only requires a dedicated staff trained in the various elements reviewed in this chapter but also is best facilitated by the establishment of a trauma case manager (often a clinical nurse specialist) who begins working with the family, patient, bedside nurse, and trauma/critical care team from, the initiation of admission to the unit through the hospital course of stay (51).

The trauma case manager helps both to standardize and optimize care by facilitating the communication and collaboration between patients and health professionals and between the health professionals themselves. Collaboration among health care disciplines is well supported as an effective solution to many problems, particularly fragmentation among complex patient groups (52).

Indeed, a recent study showed that the introduction of a trauma case manager system resulted in several benefits including: (*i*) a trend toward reduced length of stay (especially in older patients and those with higher injury severity scores), (*ii*) improved missed injury detection rates ($p < 0.0015$), (*iii*) more efficient coordination of allied health workers ($p < 0.0001$), and (*iv*) staff surveys exhibiting dramatic improvement in perceived effectiveness of patient care ($p < 0.0001$) (51). One criticism of the study is the absence of a survey comparing the family's perceptions before and after the program.

Despite these minor reservations, the introduction of the Trauma Case Management system provided greater continuity and familiarity for the patient and family. The unexpected benefit of improved missed injuries may have directly led to the overall trend toward decreased length of stay. Similar results have been achieved by others, particularly in terms of improving the ability to follow critical pathways in the management of critically ill patients (53). Additional randomized controlled studies are required to further validate this model.

EYE TO THE FUTURE

As trauma systems have matured, it is now recognized that the delivery of comprehensive trauma care extends across the continuum, from the acute phase of injury through critical care and rehabilitation and beyond, to the time when patients have returned to their families and communities. Advances in the long-term management of injury are occurring with increasing recognition of the importance of optimizing psychosocial and functional outcomes following trauma from both patient and family perspectives (54–56).

Over the past several decades, trauma outcomes research by Michaels (57), Holbrook (58), Zatrick (59), Richmond (54), and others has made significant contributions to understanding the long-term physical and psychological effects of trauma. These studies have examined pre-post, and injury-related factors influencing functional recovery (e.g., return to work, school, homemaking, etc.), psychological outcomes (e.g., emotional well-being, depression, PTSD, substance abuse, etc.), and health-related quality of life in trauma survivors. Evidence indicates that functional limitations and trauma-related emotional problems, especially PTSD and post injury depressions, are common across trauma populations, and are still under-recognized and poorly treated (57–60). Pre-existing and untreated psychiatric disorders as well as problems of substance abuse/dependence are also prevalent, and contribute to the recidivistic nature of certain types of trauma (57–60).

Trauma outcomes data suggest that psychological and functional recovery from trauma is not just related to injury severity and degree of physical disability, but that psychoso-

cial factors are additional important recovery predictors (54,56,61). Evidence suggests that positive family coping and adaptation may be associated with improved patient functioning, long-term outcomes, and directly influences treatment adherence (62,63). Further research is needed to specifically examine the mediating effects of family support in trauma recovery, and greater attention should be focused on investigating the social and psychologic factors surrounding injury.

With shortened hospital stays, a greater percentage of trauma recovery takes place at home; accordingly, family members frequently assume much of the responsibility for care, necessitating earlier intervention with families (56,61–63). Studies have begun to address the need to educate and adequately prepare patients and families to cope after discharge from hospitalization. These issues have been best studied in major burn victims and brain injured populations, where it has been demonstrated that patients and families benefit from education and guidance regarding the emotional, financial, and life disruptions they will likely experience. Findings indicate that patients and family caregivers frequently require more knowledge and assistance in accessing resources (e.g., counseling, financial, legal, etc.) and obtaining follow-up care than they usually receive (62,64–66). These studies suggest that educational and counseling interventions can positively impact patient and family functioning, and are most effective when begun early in rehabilitation and extended through recovery via formalized programs and services.

Research on the impact of sudden bereavement in trauma settings is also increasing. Previous literature on delivering grave news and providing bereavement support has been primarily anecdotal, with recommendations based on the experiences and opinions of experts. More recently, interventional studies in the emergency and trauma literature are contributing to a more evidence-based approach to the communication of bad news and the establishment of bereavement protocols following trauma-related deaths. Models of bereavement care, which are well established in palliative care settings, are becoming increasingly studied and implemented in trauma settings (3,29,37,67).

SUMMARY

Trauma services continue to be challenged to deliver holistic care including complex physiological and psychosocial support for their patients. Likewise, clinicians have a responsibility to address the needs of distressed and vulnerable family members who are the "secondary victims" of trauma. There is a compelling need to humanize the critical care unit, and create a more caring and supportive environment conducive to recovery and quality end-of-life care. Equally important is the obligation to assist patients and families to adapt and cope with the many potential long-term physical, psychological, and life-quality sequelae following trauma.

Future research will focus on evidence-based approaches to caring for relatives who are suddenly bereaved by the unexpected death of a loved one. These studies will include longitudinal studies to identify psychological and socioeconomic issues affecting the health and well-being of patients and families that often emerge after hospitalization and rehabilitation. In addition, the inclusion of greater numbers of well-designed trauma outcomes studies may provide a deeper understanding of the life experiences and perspectives of patients and their families following serious injury or death (68,69).

There are perhaps few situations in health care where the family suffers more than in trauma and critical care. As technological advances improve the ability to sustain life after critical injury, simultaneously the need to support patients and families faced with the acute and chronic burdens imposed by trauma increases (70). Recognition of the family's importance to a patient's recovery, and an understanding of the impact of critical injury on the family are essential prerequisites to establishing the systems and resources for providing comprehensive family-centered trauma care.

KEY POINTS

- Because the nature of trauma is sudden and unexpected with the potential for loss of life or significant disability, family systems are often stressed to their emotional limits.
- Evidence indicates that families exhibit a universally predictable set of needs when a loved one becomes critically ill.
- Well informed families report a greater sense of control, are more often able to accept the tragedy affecting their loved one, and participate more effectively in patient care decision making.
- Although the physician's time is limited, due to the complex demands of the trauma and critical care environment, consistent communication with the family and open access to informational resources are essential in meeting family needs.
- During serious discussions, family members may be intimidated or ashamed to admit that they do not fully understand what has been said. To avoid confusion, medical information should be clearly explained, and repeated as necessary. Technical language and euphemisms should be avoided, whereas clarifying questions should be encouraged.
- A flexible visitation policy has psychological benefits for both the patient and the family members, with a resultant positive influence on their overall satisfaction with care.
- Although family members give priority to the welfare of their relative, their own emotional needs become increasingly significant over time while the quest for hope remains universal.
- Occasionally reviewing diagnostic images (e.g., brain computed tomography scans, etc.) with family members helps to convey situations that are difficult to grasp by words alone.
- Cultural factors are recognized to have a strong influence on health practices, and to affect patient/family satisfaction of medical care, trust of healthcare providers, and adherence to treatment regimens.
- As with culture, spiritual beliefs systems can influence a patient or family's explanation of injury causation, perceptions of severity, and acceptance of changes imposed by illness.
- Collaboration between clinicians and family members is fundamental in meeting the emotional needs of patients and families.
- Specialists trained in grief and bereavement management may not be available when most needed (e.g., in the middle of the night or on weekends). Accordingly,

the physicians, and especially the nursing staff, often provide this essential supportive role.

- Family perceptions regarding the most important elements of "giving bad news" include: (*i*) the attitude of the news-giver, (*ii*) the clarity of the information conveyed, and (*iii*) the ability to have questions answered.
- Careful listening to the family's style of communication and vocabulary can help healthcare professionals develop a message that is clearly understandable.
- A structured approach to bereavement care that is integrated into the spectrum of trauma services has great potential to reduce the stressors of the grief-stricken family members faced with the sudden, unexpected death of a loved one.
- Almost universally, studies questioning family members who have experienced resuscitations have strongly supported FWR, and most would elect to do so again (41,42).

REFERENCES

1. Family-Centered Care: Changing Practice, Changing Attitudes. Bethesda, MD: Institute for family-centered care; 2004. Available at: The Institute for Family-Centered Care website (Accessed Feb. 9, 2006, at http://www.familycenteredcare.org/resources-frame.html).
2. Azoulay E, Pochard F, Chevret S, et al. Meeting the needs of intensive care unit patient families: A multicenter study. Am J Resp Crit Care Med 2001; 163(1):135–139.
3. Mosenthal AC, Murphy PA. J Trauma care and palliative care: Time to integrate the two? Am Coll Surg 2003; 197(3):509–516.
4. American College of Surgeons Committee on Trauma Performance Improvement Subcommittee. Trauma performance improvement reference manual. Chicago: ACS COT; Jan 2002. Available from the ACS-COT website. (Accessed Feb. 9, 2006, at: www.facs.org/trauma/publications/manual.pdf.).
5. Auerbach SM, Kiesler, DJ, Wartella J, et al. Optimism, satisfaction with needs met, interpersonal perceptions of the healthcare team, and emotional distress in patients' family members during critical care hospitalization. Am J Crit Care 2005; 14:202–210.
6. Kirchhoff KT, Song MK, Kehl K. Caring for the family of the critically ill patient. Crit Care Clinics 2004; 20(3):453–466.
7. Leske JS, Jiricka MK. The impact of family demands and family strengths and capabilities on family well-being and adaptation after critical injury. Am J Crit Care 1998; 7(5):383–392.
8. Van Horn E, Tesh A. The effect of critical care hospitalization on family members: stress and responses. Dimens Crit Care Nurs 2000; 19(4):40–49.
9. Perez-San Gregorio MA, Blanco-Picabia A, Murillo-Cabezas F, et al. Psychological problems in the family members of gravely traumatized patients admitted to an intensive care unit. Intensive Care Med 1992; 18:278–281.
10. Leske JS. Interventions to decrease family anxiety. Crit Care Nurse 2002; 22:61–65.
11. Leske JS. Needs of relatives of critically ill patients: a follow-up. Heart Lung 1986; 15(2):189–193.
12. Molter NC. Needs of relatives of critically ill patients: a descriptive study. Heart Lung 1979; 8(2):332–339.
13. Johnson D, Wilson M, Cavanaugh B, et al. Measuring the ability to meet family needs in an intensive care unit. Crit Care Med 1998; 26(2):266–271.
14. Price DM, Forrester DA, Murphy PA, Monaghan JF. Critical care family needs in an urban teaching medical center. Heart Lung 1991; 20:183–188.
15. Patient Family Support Committee of the Society of Critical Care Medicine. Participating in care: What questions should I ask? When a loved one is in the ICU what can you do to help? Des Plaines, IL: SCCM: 2002. Available at the SCCM

website (Accessed Feb. 9, 2006, at: http://www.sccm.org/patient_family_resources/index.asp).

16. American Association of Critical Care Nurses. When a loved one needs critical care. Aliso Viejo, CA: AACN: 2005. Available at the AACN website. (Accessed Feb. 9, 2006, at: http://www.aacn.org/AACN/mrkt.nsf/Files/IcuTip/$file/IcuTip.pdf.).

17. ICU-USA. The official patient and family website of the Society of Critical Care Medicine. Knowledge is the best medicine. St. Louis, MO: SCCM: 2005. Available at the ICU-USA website. (Accessed Feb. 9, 2006, at http://www.icu-usa.com/).

18. Jones C, Skirrow P, Griffiths RD, et al. Post-traumatic stress disorder related symptoms in relatives of patients following intensive care. Intens Care Med 2004; 30(3):456–460.

19. Anderson A, Scrimshaw SC, Fullilove MT, et al; and the Task Force on Community Preventive Services. Culturally competent healthcare systems: a systematic review. Am J Prevent Med 2003: 24(3S):68–77.

20. Betancourt JR, Green AR, Carrillo JE, Ananeh-Firempong O 2nd: Defining cultural competence: a practical framework for addressing racial/ethnic disparities in health and health care. Public Health Report 2003; 118(4):293–302.

21. US Department of Health and Human Services, Office of Minority Health. National standards on culturally and linguistically appropriate services (CLAS) in health care. Federal Register 2000; 65(247):80865–80879.

22. Killough WB. Acknowledging spiritual dynamics during trauma care. Topics in Emerg Med 2005; 27(3):183–185.

23. Koenig HG. Religion, spirituality, and medicine: research findings and implications for clinical practice. Southern Med J 2004; 97(12):1194–1200.

24. Anandarajah G, Hight E. Spirituality and medical practice: using the HOPE questions as a practical tool for spiritual assessment. Am Family Physician 2001; 63(1):81–89.

25. Clark PA, Drain M, Malone MP. Addressing patients emotional and spiritual needs. Joint Commission J on Quality and Safety 2003; 29(12):659–670.

26. Travaline JM. Communicating in the ICU: an essential component of patient care; strategies for communicating with patients and their families. J Crit Illness 2002; 17(11):451–456.

27. Heyland DK, Rocker GM, Dodek PM, et al. Family satisfaction with care in the intensive care unit: results of a multiple center study. Crit Care Med 2002; 30(7):1413–1418.

28. Azoulay E, Pouchard F, Chevret S, et al. Meeting the needs of intensive care unit patient families: a multicenter study. Am J Resp Crit Care Med 2001; 163(1):135–139.

29. Jurkovich GJ, Pierce B, Pananen L, Rivara FP. Giving bad news: the family perspective. J Trauma 2000; 48(5):865–873.

30. Iserson K. Grave words: Notifying survivors about sudden unexpected deaths. Tucson, Arizona, U.S.A.: Galen Press, 1999.

31. McLauchlan CAJ. Handling distressed relatives and breaking bad new. In: Skinner D. ed. ABC of Major Trauma. London: BMJ Publishing, 1991:102–106.

32. Kaltman S, Bonnano GA. Trauma and bereavement: examining the impact of sudden and violent death. J Anxiety Disord 2003; 17(2):131–147.

33. Olsen JC, Buenefe ML, Falco WD. Death in the emergency department. Ann of Emerg Med 1998; 31(6):758–765.

34. Rutkowski A. Death notification in the emergency department. Ann of Emerg Med 2002; 40: 521–523.

35. Williams AG, O'Brien DL, Laughton KJ, Jelinek GA. Improving services to bereaved relatives in the emergency department: making healthcare more human. Med J Aust 2000; 173:480–483.

36. Knazik SR, Gausche-Hill M, Dietrich AM, et al. The death of a child in the emergency department. Ann Emerg Med 2003; 42(4):519–529.

37. Bereavement practice guidelines for health care professionals in the emergency department. National Association of Social Workers and Health Resources and Services Administration. Washington, DC: HRSA, 1998.

38. Kaul RE. Coordinating the death notification process: the roles of the emergency room social worker and physician following a sudden death. Brief Treatment and Crisis Intervention, 2001 1(2):101–114.

39. McClenathan BM, Torrington KG, Uyehara CFT. Family Member presence during cardiopulmonary resuscitation: a survey of US and international critical care professionals. Chest 2002; 122(6):2204–2211.

40. Helmer SD, Smith RS, Dort JM, et al. Family presence during trauma resuscitation: a survey of AAST and ENA members. American Association for the Surgery of Trauma.and Emergency Nurses Association. J Trauma. 2000; 48:1015–1024.

41. Meyers TA, Eichorn DJ, Guzetta CE. Do families want to be present during CPR? A retrospective survey. J Emerg Nurs 1998; 24:400–405.

42. Robinson SM, Mackenzie-Ross S, Campbell-Hewson GL, et al. Psychological effect of witnessed resuscitation on bereaved relatives. Lancet 1998; 352(9128):614–617.

43. NBC Dateline Poll. Should family members of patients be allowed in the emergency department during emergency procedures? Available at the NBC website. www.nbc.com.

44. USA Today Poll. Would you want to be in the emergency department while doctors worked on a family member? Available at: www.USATODAY.com.

45. Mason DJ. Family presence: Evidence vs. tradition. Am J Crit Care 2003; 12(3):190–192.

46. Benjamin M, Holger J, Carr M. Personal preferences regarding family member presence during resuscitation. Acad Emerg Med 2004; 11(7):750–753.

47. Emergency Nurses Association. Presenting the option for family presence. 2nd ed. Des Plaines, Ill: Emergency Nurses Association, 2001. Available at: www.ena.org.

48. American Heart Association. Guidelines 2000 for Cardiopulmonary Resuscitation: Part 2. Ethical aspects of CPR and ECC. Circulation 2000; 102(suppl):112–121.

49. American College of Emergency Physicians. Critical issues in emergency medicine: family presence. ACEP; 2005.Available at: www.acep.org.

50. Boudreaux ED, Francis JL, Loyacano T. Family presence during invasive procedures and resuscitations in the emergency department: a critical review and suggestions for future research. Ann Emerg Med 2002; 40(2):193–205.

51. Curtis K, Lien D, Chan A, et al. The impact of trauma case management on patient outcomes. J Trauma 2002; 53(3):477–482.

52. Lindeke L, Block DE. Maintaining professional integrity in the midst of interdisciplinary collaboration. Nurs Outlook. 1998; 46:213–218.

53. Sesperez J, Wilson S, Jalaludin B, et al. Trauma case management and clinical pathways: prospective evaluation of their effect on selected patient outcomes in five key trauma conditions. J Trauma 2001; 50(4):643–649.

54. Richmond TS, Kauder D, Hinkle J, Shults J. Early predictors of long-term disability after injury. Am J Crit Care 2003; 12(3):197–205.

55. O' Donnell ML, Creamer M, Pattison P, Atkin C. Psychiatric morbidity following trauma. Am J Psychiatry 2004; 161(3):507–514.

56. Dimopoulou I, Anthi A, Mastora Z, et al. Health-related quality of life and disability in survivors of multiple trauma one year after intensive care unit discharge. Am J Phys Med Rehabil 2004: 83:171–176.

57. Michaels AJ, Michaels CE, Moon CH, et al. Posttraumatic stress disorder after injury: impact on general health outcome and early risk assessment. J Trauma 1999; 47:460–467.

58. Holbrook TL, Anderson JP, Sieber WJ, et al. Outcome after major trauma: 12-month and 18-month follow-up results from the Trauma Recovery Project. J Trauma 1999; 46:765–771; discussion, 771–773.

59. Zatrick DF, Kang SM, Muller HG, et al. Predicting posttraumatic distress in hospitalized trauma survivors with acute injuries. Am J Psychiatry 2002; 159(6):941–946.

60. Zatrick D, Jurkovich G, Russo J, et al. Posttraumatic distress, alcohol disorders, and recurrent trauma across level-1 trauma centers. J Trauma 2004; 57:360–366.

61. Michaels AJ, Michaels CE, Moon CH, et al. Psychosocial factors limit outcomes after trauma. J Trauma1998; 44(4): 644–648.

62. DePalma J, Fedorka P, Simko LC. Quality of life experienced by severely injured trauma survivors. AACN Clin Issues 2003; 14(1): 54–63.

63. Leske JS. Comparison of family stresses, strengths, and outcomes after trauma and surgery. AACN Clin Issues 2003; 14(1): 33–41.

64. Montgomery V, Oliver R, Reisner A, Fallat ME. The effect of severe traumatic brain injury on the family. J Trauma 2002; 52 (6):1121–1124.

65. Kalpakjian CZ, Lam CS, Toussaint LL, Hansen Merbitz NK. Describing quality of life and psychosocial outcomes after traumatic brain injury. Am J Phys Med Rehabil 2004; 83(4):255–265.

66. Wiechman SA, Patterson DR. ABC of burns: psychosocial aspects of burn injuries. BMJ 2004; 329(7642):391–393.

67. Oliver RC, Sturtevant J, Scheetz J, Fallat ME. Beneficial effects of a hospital bereavement intervention program after traumatic childhood death. J Trauma 2001; 50(3): 440–446.

68. Buchman TG, Ray SE, Wax MI, et al. Families' perceptions of surgical intensive care. J Am Coll Surg 2003; 196(6): 977–983.

69. Verhaeghe S, Defloor T, Van Zuuren F, et al. The needs and experiences of family members of adult patients in the intensive care unit: A review of the literature. J Clin Nurs 2005; 14(4):501–509.

70. Harvey MA. Evolving toward-but not to-meeting family needs. (Commentary). Crit Care Med 1998; 26(2):206–207.

Post-traumatic Stress Disorder in Trauma and Critical Care

Robert Stone

Department of Psychiatry, Post Traumatic Stress Disorder Unit, Oregon State Hospital, Salem, Oregon, U.S.A.

Catherine McCoy-Hill

School of Nursing, Azusa Pacific University, Azusa, California, U.S.A.

Troy L. Holbrook

Department of Family and Preventative Medicine, UC San Diego Medical Center, San Diego, California, U.S.A.

William C. Wilson

Department of Anesthesiology and Critical Care, UC San Diego Medical Center, San Diego, California, U.S.A.

David B. Hoyt

Department of Surgery, UC Irvine Medical Center, Irvine, California, U.S.A.

INTRODUCTION

Post-traumatic stress disorder ☞ **(PTSD) is a psychiatric ailment resulting from an individual experiencing or witnessing an actual or potential life-threatening event.** ☞ Symptoms include recurrent, intrusive recollections of the event (e.g., nightmares or flashbacks), avoidant behavior (e.g., emotional numbing), increased arousal (e.g., irritability, insomnia), and significant impairment in social and occupational functioning (1–8).

Both acute stress disorder (ASD) and PTSD are increasingly recognized to occur in trauma survivors, and each entity has specific Diagnostic and Statistical Manual of Mental Disorders, 4th edition (DSM-IV) criteria. To achieve the diagnosis of PTSD, the aforementioned symptoms must be present for more than one month. When these manifestations combine with dissociative symptoms and persist between two days and four weeks following the traumatic event, this entity is referred to as ASD. Being affected by ASD or PTSD significantly impacts the quality of life (QoL), emotional well being, and functional recovery outcomes of these patients (1,5).

The symptoms attributable to ASD and PTSD have been most closely associated with military combatants, and have been recognized in various forms for centuries. Myers ABR (1838–1921) (9) was the first to publish a clinical description of symptoms describing ASD and PTSD in his treatise "on the etiology and prevalence of diseases of the heart among soldiers" in 1870. Da Costa JM (1833–1921), (10) an American internist working at a Philadelphia military hospital, chronicled cases of PTSD that occurred during the American Civil War in 1871; consequently, for a time this entity was known as "Da Costa's Syndrome." Since then, symptoms of ASD and PTSD have been called by various terms including: (*i*) "Soldier's Heart" (Spanish American War), (*ii*) "Shell Shock" (World War I), and (*iii*) "Combat Fatigue" (World War II). During and after the Vietnam conflict, the recurrent nature of the reliving experiences became popularized by the symptom terminology known as "flashbacks." However, not until 1980 and the compilation of DSM-III was PTSD even listed as an official psychiatric disorder; it was at this time that the diagnostic criteria were initially specified. The formal diagnosis of ASD was not specified until 1994 and the publication of DSM-IV.

Post-traumatic stress symptomatology is not rare. ☞ **Research on trauma survivors cared for in U.S. Trauma Centers reveals that 10% to 40% develop symptoms of ASD and PTSD (1–8).** ☞ In addition, it is now recognized that ASD and PTSD can develop in loved ones or family members through "vicarious traumatization" mechanisms, when they are confronted with death or serious injury to significant others.

Fifty percent of American adults will experience a traumatic stressor significant enough to cause PTSD (11). Fifteen percent of those exposed will develop chronic symptoms of PTSD (12). Childhood trauma is also not uncommon (Volume 1, Chapter 36). Sixteen percent of women were sexually abused before the age of 18, (13) and probably half as many men. PTSD is about twice as common in women as men even after controlling for trauma rates for all causes of trauma except perhaps rape (Fig. 1A and B) (14). One million Americans were exposed to traumatic stress in Vietnam, and several hundred thousand more were exposed during the Gulf War and the antiterrorist campaigns in Afghanistan and Iraq.

☞ **Structural changes occur in the brains of patients whose PTSD symptoms have been allowed to persist untreated for too long.** ☞ The connection between exposure to traumatic stressors and the development of ASD/PTSD is becoming increasingly well characterized in psychological, neuroanatomical, and evolutionary terms. The mind/brain initially reacts to trauma by increasing the elaboration of stress hormones (e.g., cortisol, epinephrine, and norepinephrine) to marshal resources, direct attention, and increase awareness. However, if the stress hormones,

(A)

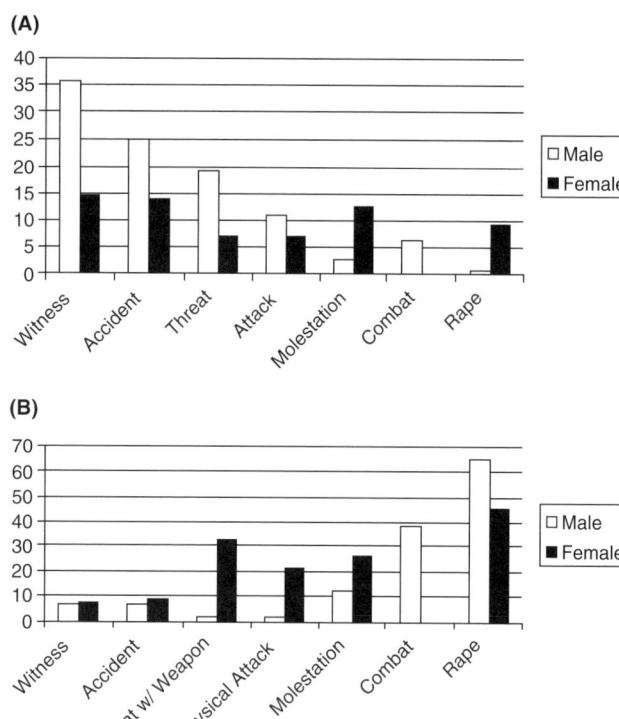

(B)

Figure 1 (A) Prevalence of trauma category according to gender. (B) Probability of developing post-traumatic stress disorder by type of trauma. *Source*: From Ref. 14.

which are beneficial during the acute trauma response, remain elevated for too long a time period, detrimental changes can occur including brain damage to memory centers and thought association loci. Chronic stress can also exacerbate the development of heart disease, gastric stress ulcers (Volume 2, Chapter 30), and immunosuppression (Volume 2, Chapter 52) (15,16).

This chapter provides a multidisciplinary approach to the pathophysiology, diagnosis, and treatment of ASD and PTSD in acutely injured trauma and critically ill patients. Post-trauma depression (PTD) is also briefly summarized. The neurobiological mechanisms underpinning ASD and PTSD are emphasized. Treatment modalities are reviewed, including the optimum timing for each type. Emphasis is placed on early recognition of risk factors and symptoms during initial hospitalization, with specific focus on interventions occurring in the Trauma Resuscitation Suite (TRS) and the surgical intensive care unit (SICU), when possible.

NEUROBIOLOGY OF POST-TRAUMATIC STRESS DISORDER
Anatomic Brain Regions Involved in Post-traumatic Stress Disorders

Several anatomic areas of the brain have been implicated in the pathophysiology of ASD and PTSD. ☞ **Four integral components of the limbic system are specifically involved in the pathophysiology of ASD/PTSD.** ☞ These include the hippocampus, the amygdala, the medial prefrontal cortex (MpFC) (cingulate gyrus), and the hypothalamus. The limbic system is an evolutionarily primitive portion of the brain involving memory, emotions and motivations, especially those involved in survival. Certain structures in the limbic system are critical for memory formation

(especially the hippocampus, the amygdala, and the hypothalamus), and likely play an important role in the pathophysiology of PTSD. The MpFC, rectifies thoughts that pass through the aforementioned structures, and also regulates the hypothalamic-pituitary-adrenal (HPA) axis under basal and stressful conditions.

The hypothalamus, like the MpFC, is involved in both the limbic system, and the neurohormonal regulation between the anterior pituitary gland and the adrenal glands (Volume 2, Chapter 62). Apart from cardiorespiratory and thermoregulation, the hypothalamus is an important attenuator of emotional output by adjusting the elaboration of hormones that cause joy, sadness, anger, and depression. Numerous studies implicate dysregulation of the HPA axis in PTSD, (17–22) along with impairments in cognitive function, (23) hippocampal tissue volume reduction, (24) and alterations in the neuronal circuitry of the limbic system (25). Recently Wang et al. (26) demonstrated axonal shrinkage, myelin deformation, and neuronal degeneration in both the hippocampal and hypothalamic structures of dogs following high-energy missile wounds to extremities, suggesting central nervous system (CNS) damage to limbic structures following distant injury.

The hippocampus is integral to learning, data acquisition, and memory of content, (27,28) and also records the emotions associated with memorized events (29–31). Structures within the hippocampal complex have access to virtually the entire brain, and create integrated records of various aspects of memory including visual, auditory, smell, and the somatosensory context. Permanent memory of any event typically takes at least 45 minutes, but final memory consolidation may take weeks or months. Hippocampal dysfunction or damage during consolidation can cause impaired memory of events surrounding and subsequent to a trauma. Furthermore, damage to the hippocampus can result in increased risk of subsequent ASD/PTSD, chronic memory loss, and a propensity to dissociate memory from experiences that occur later.

The amygdala is important in the acquisition of emotional memory experiences, but not for neutral memory. The amygdala is involved in producing an anger or fear response when a threat is detected. Its size is positively correlated with aggressiveness in humans, and shrinks by 30% following castration in men. The amygdala connects with many areas of the brain and causes the stress response by stimulating cortisol and epinephrine release (32). The amygdala also has critical functions affecting the conditioned fear response and emotional memory. Recently, Eric R Kandel's group identified the gene that codes for "stathmin," a protein highly expressed in the amygdala, which inhibits microtubule formation, and appears to be critical to the formation of the innate and acquired fear response. When knocked out in laboratory animals, fear was abolished (33).

The MpFC is important in regulating emotion and suppressing primitive brain reactions such as those emitted by the amygdala (35). Although the acute stress response following fearful situations is universal, PTSD patients fail to show remission of this response. The failure of higher brain centers to suppress amygdala activity is likely responsible for the exaggerated "startle response" that is often seen in PTSD (36–38). The suppressive function of the MpFC inhibits fear responses from the amygdala when no actual threat exists. In patients with PTSD, this suppressive response is altered, creating a tendency to respond to all threats as if they were real.

Neuroendocrine Changes

The neurobiological mechanisms mediating the response to stress include: (*i*) stimulation of the sympathetic nervous system, (*ii*) parasympathetic nervous system suppression, and (*iii*) activation of the HPA axis.

Adrenergic stimulation causes adrenal medullary release of epinephrine and norepinephrine with consequent increased heart rate (HR), contractility, blood pressure (BP), respiratory rate, and tidal volume coupled with a sharpening of mental focus and memory formation. HPA axis activation results in release of corticotropin releasing hormone (CRH) from the hypothalamus and subsequent secretion of adrenocorticotropic hormone (ACTH) from the anterior pituitary gland, which signals cortisol release from the adrenal cortex (Volume 2, Chapter 62).

Elevated hippocampal cortisol is thought to impair the formation of new memories, while epinephrine causes stronger memory formation and increased emotional intensity associated with specific memories. Increased norepinephrine levels also stimulate brain activity; however, excessive release of these endogenous catecholamines can lead to neurotransmitter overload, inhibiting the brain's ability to process information. These factors may partially account for the chaotic memory formation commonly surrounding trauma events, as well as the intrusive memories characteristic of PTSD.

☞ **Individuals with PTSD have dysregulation of the HPA axis (resulting in lower than normal cortisol levels), as well as an elevated basal adrenergic tone.** ☞ These initially beneficial survival mechanisms are likely deleterious in the chronic state. Long-term alterations of these neurotransmitters may be partly responsible for the structural changes detected in the brains of ASD and PTSD patients.

Several neuroendocrine studies have shown lower than normal cortisol levels in individuals with PTSD as well as an increased cortisol response (receptor sensitivity) to subsequent trauma events (Fig. 2) (20,39). Norepinephrine under extreme stress conditions may act longer or more intensely on the hippocampus, leading to abnormally strong memory formations. Since cortisol normally limits norepinephrine activation, low cortisol levels may increase adrenergic hyperarousal mechanisms (19–22). Long-term effects of elevated adrenergic levels have adverse cardiovascular effects whereas diminished baseline cortisol may have an impact on stamina, mood, and immune-mediated disorders (see Volume 2, Chapter 52) (15–16).

Other neurotransmitter functions are altered in PTSD. Benzodiazepine receptors are reduced in the frontal cortex of humans with PTSD (40). Opioid receptors appear to be stimulated during traumatic reminders in PTSD, creating decreased pain sensitivity during re-experiencing periods (41). Frontal cortex serotonin function is also dysregulated in PTSD. Animal studies indicate that serotonin may block frontal cortex stress responses (42). Selective serotonin reuptake inhibitor (SSRI) drugs are currently first line pharmacotherapy for PTSD (discussed later).

Structural Changes

It is now well established that structural and biochemical changes occur within the brain of trauma survivors supporting the mind/brain-integrated concept (43). Although experiencing the symptoms can be seen as psychological in origin, the neural circuitry underlying this is biological as are the consequent structural changes associated with ASD/PTSD.

The most significant structural damage that occurs after the stress of trauma is found in the hippocampus. The hippocampus is involved in recording the emotions associated with a traumatic event. Several well-controlled studies have demonstrated hippocampal volume shrinkage in PTSD populations (44,45,50–51). Hippocampal volume decrease is nearly always imageable by two years post-trauma, but has been seen as early as five to six months after trauma (46,48,52). Structural hippocampal changes including atrophy have been correlated with decreased capacity for hippocampal mediated memory tasks, indicating that the physiological damage is directly relevant to the clinical deterioration of memory functioning in PTSD patients (47,49).

Stress may also affect the expression of brain derived neurotrophic factor (BDNF), a protein necessary for neuronal survival, normal hippocampal activity, and long-term memory function. Decreased BDNF is probably associated with the cell atrophy and death seen in PTSD (53).

PET scans have identified an entire network of dysfunctional memory areas of the brain in PTSD patients including the hippocampus, amygdala, and the MpFC (38). The amygdala also exerts supernormal influence on the visual cortex, subcallosal gyrus, and anterior cingulate gyrus in PTSD compared to normal controls (54). In PTSD, the amygdala appears to be hyperreactive to trauma-related stimuli (55,56).

IMPACT OF TRAUMA INTERVENTIONS
Effect of Resuscitation, Anesthesia, and Critical Care on Acute Stress Disorder/Post-traumatic Stress Disorder

☞ **The initial resuscitation, anesthesia, and critical care experiences may contribute (negatively or positively) to the development of ASD/PTSD.** ☞ Because of the changing awareness of these patients (due to hypotension, anxiety, pain), their memories can become distorted. In addition, some of the drugs administered to alleviate stress and pain may contribute to memory impairment (and possibly ASD/PTSD).

Awareness under anesthesia, prolonged ICU treatment (ARDS, septic shock), and successful resuscitation after cardiac arrest are also linked to the development of PTSD. The prevalence of PTSD in these medical conditions lies around 10% to 20%; they are therefore considered important comorbidities (57,58).

Studies of former ICU patients utilizing a 10 item, the Post-traumatic Symptom Scale (PTSS), indicate 17% screen positive for probable PTSD, and just under 10% confirm positive for PTSD following rigorous clinical evaluation (58). Large level I trauma center studies have revealed higher rates of PTSD development ranging between 30% to 40% after severe injury (excluding those with moderate or severe brain injury) (1–8,59).

Treatment occurring in the critical care setting appears to further increase the risk of developing PTSD. In studies of patients undergoing treatment for myocardial infarction (MI), cardiac surgery, hemorrhage, stroke, burns, cancer, and awareness under anesthesia, the highest rates of PTSD were found in those whose course included treatment in ICUs (60). Postcardiac surgery patients show an 18% PTSD rate, which is highly correlated with the number of traumatic memories from their ICU/CCU treatment (61). Spinal cord injury (SCI) patients show a 10% to 20% PTSD rate (62), and rates of up to 51% have been seen in orthopedic trauma patients (63). ICU stays have also been shown to be

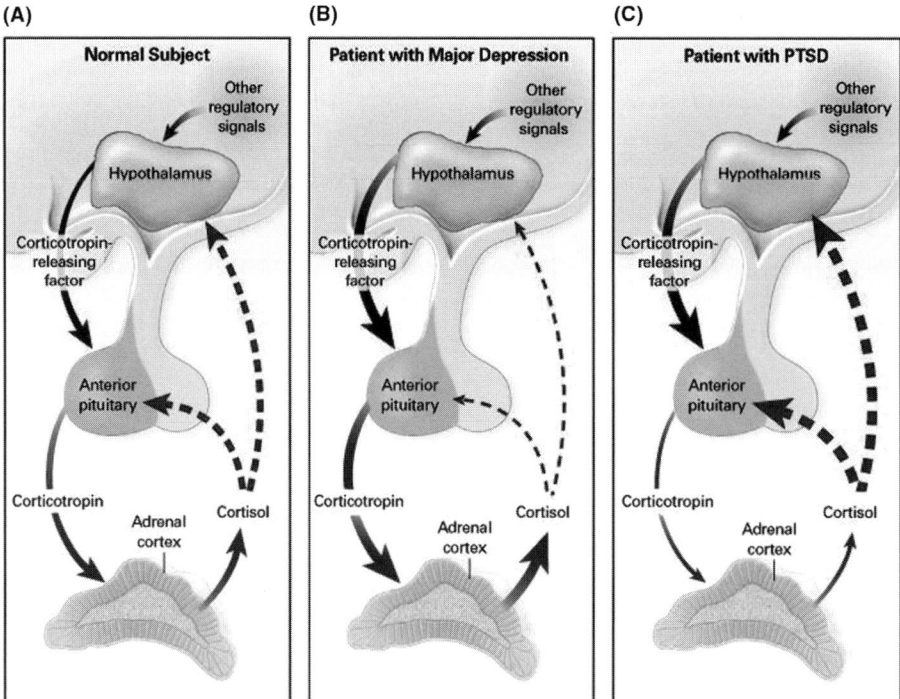

Figure 2   Response to stress in a normal subject (**A**), a patient with major depressive disorder (**B**), and a patient with post-traumatic stress disorder (PTSD) (**C**). In normal subjects (**A**) and in patients with major depression (**B**), brief or sustained periods of stress are typically associated with increased levels of both cortisol and corticotropin-releasing factor. In each panel the thickness of the interconnecting arrows denotes the magnitude of the biologic response. Corticotropin-releasing factor stimulates the production of corticotropin, which in turn stimulates the production of cortisol. Cortisol inhibits the release of corticotropin from the pituitary and the release of corticotropin-releasing factor from the hypothalamus. It is also responsible for the containment of many stress-activated, biologic reactions. In patients with PTSD (**C**), levels of cortisol are low and levels of corticotropin-releasing factor are high. In addition, the sensitivity of the negative-feedback system of the hypothalamic–pituitary–adrenal axis is increased in patients with PTSD rather than decreased, as often occurs in patients with major depression. *Source*: from Ref. 208; Photos courtesy of Ref. 20.

extremely stressful to relatives of trauma patients, and to relatives of patients undergoing elective cardiac surgery (64).

Duration of Mechanical Ventilation and Other Interventions

PTSD, which can develop as a result of traumatic experiences during ICU treatment, causes significant impairment, decreased QoL, and increased risk for comorbid mental health conditions (65). In a large review of long-term survivors of ICU-based ARDS treatment, 44% were found to meet criteria for PTSD upon hospital discharge. At eight year follow-up, 24% continued to suffer full-blown PTSD and an additional 20% had continuing post-traumatic symptoms (66). ☞ **In one large study of critically ill patients the risk of PTSD was directly correlated with the duration of mechanical ventilation and inversely related to patient age (67).** ☞ Questionnaires after discharge from ICU treatment indicated almost 40% had significant PTSD symptoms, and 14% met full diagnostic criteria for PTSD three months following discharge from the ICU (67).

Although trauma-inducing interventions during critical care treatment can increase PTSD rates, sedating patients throughout the critical care experience (using standard drugs) does not abolish it. In fact, daily sedation interruption for patients on mechanical ventilation was correlated with a lower incidence of PTSD (68).

☞ **Trauma outcomes researchers have consistently identified PTSD as a significant factor in functional limitations and diminished QoL above and beyond the medical** comorbities associated with their physical wounds **(7,62–67,69,70).** ☞

During and just after critical care treatment, patients can make incorrect subjective decisions about the need for psychiatric care (71). Trauma patients are often less able to communicate due to the need for mechanical ventilation soon following trauma, and are generally not interviewed about the need for psychiatric involvement unless the patient has a pre-existing psychiatric history or was injured during a suicide attempt. Following discharge, few patients seek mental health treatment; some fail to recognize they have a problem, others believe the symptoms will resolve on their own. Patients who seek care late more often present with somatic symptoms, sleep disorders, and increased rates of comorbid depression and substance abuse (59,60,71).

In a study of almost 100 people with civilian PTSD, more than half had some form of suicidal ideation, and almost 10% had made at least one suicide attempt. While PTSD is considered a significant risk factor for suicide (72), substantial disability and suicidal risk is also associated with those experiencing subdiagnostic post-traumatic symptoms (73).

ACUTE STRESS DISORDER (ASD)
Overview

Prior to 1994 (DSM-IV), severe psychological and emotional distress immediately following trauma was not a diagnostic entity. This led to delay in diagnosis and appropriate treatment. Currently, the diagnosis of ASD is made in individuals experiencing significantly distressing symptoms of re-experiencing, avoidance, and increased arousal within two days to four weeks of the traumatic event. ☛ **The diagnosis of ASD symptoms helps identify patients at risk for PTSD, in quantifying the severity of distress suffered by the trauma survivor during the first month following the event.** ☛

The diagnostic criteria for ASD include the presence of dissociative symptoms (not included in the criteria for PTSD). Dissociative symptoms by themselves are strong predictors of post-traumatic symptom severity. Several studies have documented that having ASD markedly increases the risk of subsequently developing PTSD. Approximately 50% of those with ASD will go on to develop PTSD (74). However, ASD does not necessarily need to be present prior to developing PTSD. One study of severely injured hospitalized trauma survivors found only 1% with ASD at day eight, while at months 3 and 12, the PTSD rates were 9% and 10% respectively (75). However, ASD appears to be a more accurate predictor of PTSD in females than males. (76).

In one study of motor vehicle crash (MVC) survivors, 78% of those who met criteria for ASD at one month were diagnostic for PTSD at six months. Sixty percent of those who met all but the dissociative criteria for ASD were also positive for PTSD at six months (77). This study has been supported by similar studies of MVC survivors who sustained mild traumatic brain injuries, (78,79) and in studies of sexual and physical assault victims (80).

Diagnostic and Statistical Manual of Mental Disorders, 4th Edition (DSM-IV) Diagnostic Criteria

Since patients without ASD symptoms may later develop PTSD, it is imperative to maintain a high index of suspicion, and utilize early and follow-up symptom screening. Those who meet criteria for ASD, with or without dissociative symptoms, need definitive treatment because of their higher risk of long-term pathology. The complete DSM-IV criteria for ASD are summarized in Table 1. Each of the specific symptom criteria is discussed subsequently.

Exposure (A₁) and Response (A₂) to Traumatic Stressor (Criterion A)

The DSM-IV Criterion A for the diagnosis of ASD requires the person to have been exposed to a traumatic event in which both of the following has occurred: (*i*) The person experienced, witnessed, or was confronted with an event or events that involved actual or threatened death or serious injury to self or others; and (*ii*) the person's response involved intense fear, helplessness, or horror. This trauma exposure criterion for ASD is the same as that required for PTSD.

Dissociative Symptoms (Criterion B)

Criterion B symptoms for ASD are dissociative in nature. Dissociation refers to an unconnectedness of things that should normally be linked. When experiences are not encoded correctly into memory, they do not contribute to the normal sense of self.

☛ **Dissociative symptoms contribute to discontinuities in memory, identity, and perception; these are required for the diagnosis of ASD but not PTSD. Re-experiencing, avoidant, and hyperarousal symptoms are characteristic of both entities.** ☛

A common manifestation of dissociative symptomatology is "emotional numbing" where the person may fully recall a trauma, but feels no emotions associated with it (81). Dissociative experiences are also commonly expressed in the opposite way, with strong and overwhelming emotions displayed without any obvious cognate memory. Some patients experience acting, feeling, or thinking as if "someone else" was actually carrying out their actions. Five main categories of dissociation are listed in DSM-IV Criterion B (Table 1): (*i*) subjective numbing, (*ii*) awareness reduction, (*iii*) derealization, (*iv*) depersonalization, and (*v*) dissociative amnesia. To meet the DSM-IV criteria for ASD, the victim must exhibit at least three of the five dissociative symptoms listed in Table 1.

The dissociative symptom load manifested by ASD patients is significant since three of the five listed symptom categories must be present for diagnosis. Subjective numbing can take several forms, including a lack of emotional response to the trauma, anhedonia (the inability to feel pleasure), or the experience of intense guilt. Reduced awareness can manifest as difficulty concentrating, missed social cues, and difficulty remembering post-trauma details. Derealization is the subjective experience that the world is not real; these patients often describe seeing things through a fog or a veil (82). Depersonalization is the subjective sense of being detached from one's own body. In extreme cases, patients may not even recognize themselves in the mirror (83). Dissociative amnesia is the inability to remember substantial details of the trauma and subsequent period. Episodes of amnesia can also occur well after the trauma, usually with a significant attempt on the part of the survivor to conceal their memory impairment from others.

Re-experiencing Symptoms (Criterion C)

Psychological re-experiencing of the traumatic event can be extremely debilitating. For the diagnosis of ASD, re-experiencing must occur in at least one of the following ways: recurrent images, thoughts, dreams, illusions, flashback episodes, a sense of reliving the experience, or distress with exposure to reminders of the traumatic event (Table 1). Images, thoughts, or flashbacks about the trauma can intrude forcefully on the person's awareness or they may experience dreams and nightmares with content related to the trauma. The re-experiencing criterion is considered positive whenever the person has significant emotional distress when confronted with a trigger stimulus or reminder of the traumatic event.

Avoidant Symptoms (Criterion D)

Avoidant symptoms describe the marked abstention from stimuli that arouse recollections of the trauma (including thoughts, feelings, conversations, activities, places, or people). The trauma survivor with ASD or PTSD goes to significant lengths to avoid anything that might cause the event(s) to be remembered. Often, the nature of protracted legal or medical procedures place the survivors into situations where they are unintentionally forced to remember the event. Avoidant symptoms can drive ASD/PTSD patients away from using beneficial services in an attempt to avoid retraumatization.

Hyperarousal/Anxiety Symptoms (Criterion E)

Symptoms of anxiety or increased arousal may include difficulty sleeping, irritability, poor concentration, hypervigilance,

Table 1   Acute Stress Disorder: Diagnostic Criteria

Criterion	Short title	Description
Criterion A	Exposure to traumatic stressor	The person has been exposed to a traumatic event where both of the following were present: The person experienced, witnessed, or was confronted with an event that involved actual or threatened death or serious injury, or a threat to the physical integrity of self or others The person's response involved intense fear, helplessness, or horror
Criterion B	Dissociative symptoms	Either while experiencing or after experiencing the distressing event, the individual has three (or more) of the following dissociative symptoms: A subjective sense of numbing, detachment, or absence of emotional responsiveness A reduction in awareness of his or her surroundings (e.g., "being in a daze") Derealization Depersonalization Dissociative amnesia
Criterion C	Re-experiencing symptoms	The traumatic event is persistently re-experienced in at least one of the following six ways: recurrent images, thoughts, dreams, illusions, flashback episodes, or a sense of reliving the experience, or distress on exposure to reminders of the traumatic event
Criterion D	Avoidant symptoms	Marked avoidance of stimuli that arouse recollections of the trauma (e.g., thoughts, feelings, conversations, activities, places, or people)
Criterion E	Anxiety/arousal symptoms	Marked symptoms of anxiety or increased arousal (e.g., difficulty sleeping, irritability, poor concentration, hypervigilance, exaggerated startle response, motor restlessness)
Criterion F	Distress level	The disturbance causes clinically significant distress or impairment in social, occupational, or other important areas of functioning or impairs the individual's ability to pursue some necessary task, such as obtaining necessary assistance or mobilizing personal resources by telling family members about the traumatic experience
Criterion G	Duration of symptoms	The disturbance lasts for a minimum of 2 days and a maximum of 4 wk and occurs within 4 wk of the traumatic event
Criterion H	Other etiologies	The disturbance is not due to the direct physiological effects of a substance (e.g., drug of abuse or medication) or a general medical condition, is not better accounted for by brief psychotic disorder or other Axis I or II, DSM-IV disorder

Abbreviation: DSM-IV, Diagnostic and Statistical Manual of Mental Disorders, 4th edition.
Source: Courtesy of DSM-IV.

exaggerated startle response, or motor restlessness. The criterion is specifically vague, as there are numerous ways hyperarousal can manifest in ASD.

Distress Level (Criterion F)
For diagnosis, the symptomatology disturbance must: (*i*) cause clinically significant distress or impairment in social, occupational, or other important areas of functioning, or (*ii*) impair the individual's ability to pursue some necessary task, such as obtaining assistance or mobilizing personal resources by telling family members about the traumatic experience.

Duration of Symptoms (Criterion G)
The disturbance must last for a minimum of two days to a maximum of four weeks and must occur within four weeks of the traumatic event to meet the criteria for ASD. Disturbances lasting beyond the four-week period become categorized as PTSD, providing the other criteria (see subsequently) are also present.

Absence of Other Etiologies (Criterion H)
The disturbance must not be due to the direct physiological effects of a substance (e.g., a drug of abuse or medication) or a general medical condition, and must not be better accounted for as a brief psychotic break, or an exacerbation of a pre-existing Axis I or Axis II DSM-IV disorder. Differential diagnosis can be difficult due to the high

prevalence of psychiatric comorbidities (i.e., major depressive and anxiety disorders) that may pre-exist or co-occur with PTSD.

POST-TRAUMATIC STRESS DISORDER (PTSD)
Overview
The factors underlying PTSD development are multiple, complex, and not entirely understood. These include pre-trauma individual differences (i.e. psychological, neurobiological, and genetic), peritrauma variables (e.g., characteristics of the trauma, responses to the event), and post-trauma factors (i.e. biological and environmental).

The DSM-IV criteria for the trauma exposure necessary for PTSD (Table 2) is identical to that required for ASD, and can usually be made based on clinical interview alone. However, if an evaluation of treatment efficacy is being conducted or prolonged therapy is contemplated, the diagnosis should be confirmed by a trained mental health professional.

DSM-IV Diagnostic Criteria
Exposure (A₁) and Response (A₂) to Traumatic Stressor (Criterion A)
To fulfill the DSM-IV (Criterion A_1) for PTSD, the person had to be exposed to a catastrophically traumatic event involving actual or threatened death or physical harm to him/herself or others (Table 2). The general injury types can be divided

Table 2 Post-traumatic Stress Disorder: Diagnostic Criteria

Criterion	Name	Description
Criterion A1	Involvement proximity and type of trauma	The person had to see or learn about a trauma that involved: Actual or threatened: death, serious injury, or violation of the body of self or others

Criterion A2	Reaction to trauma	The person had to react to the trauma with:
		    Intense fear,
		    Hopelessness, or
		    Horror

Criterion B	Re-experiencing symptoms	Five ways trauma can be relived. Only one is required for diagnosis:
		    Recurrent, intrusive recollections of the event
		    Recurrent, distressing dreams of the event
		    Acting or feeling as if the trauma were recurring [i.e., dissociative hallucinations, illusions, flashbacks, (including those occurring upon awakening or when intoxicated)].
		    Intense psychological distress upon exposure to internal or external cues that symbolize or resemble an aspect of the traumatic event
		    Physiological reactivity upon exposure to such internal or external cues

Criterion C	Avoidant symptoms	At least, three of these seven avoidance symptoms must have developed since the trauma, for diagnosis:
		    Efforts to avoid thoughts, feelings, or conversations associated with the trauma
		    Efforts to avoid activities, places, or people that arouse recollection of the trauma
		    Inability to recall important aspects of the trauma
		    Markedly diminished interest or participation in significant activities
		    Feeling of detachment or estrangement from others
		    Restricted range of effect (e.g., unable to have loving feelings)
		    Sense of foreshortened future (does not expect to have a career, marriage, children, or a normal life span)

Criterion D	Persistent increased arousal symptoms	At least, two of five types of persistent increased arousal must be experienced for diagnosis, with onset since the trauma:
		    Difficulty falling or staying asleep
		    Irritability or outbursts of anger
		    Difficulty concentrating
		    Hypervigilance
		    Exaggerated startle response

Criterion E	Duration of symptoms in B, C, and D	The symptoms of PTSD from criteria B, C, and D must be experienced for one month for diagnosis. Given this, the diagnosis of PTSD cannot be made prior to 1 mo after the trauma
Criterion F	Distress level	If all the criteria above are met, for the diagnosis of PTSD to be made, the symptoms must cause clinically significant distress or impairment in social, occupational, or other important areas of functioning

Abbreviations: DSM-IV, Diagnostic and Statistical Manual of Mental Disorder 4th edition; PTSD, post-traumatic stress disorder.
Source: Courtesy of DSM-IV.

into three groups: (*i*) intentional (including combat, abuse, criminal acts, and torture), (*ii*) unintentional human acts (e.g., industrial accidents, MVC), and (*iii*) surgery (the secondary harm is unintentional, though the surgery is intentional); and acts of nature, (e.g., hurricanes, tornados, floods, earthquakes, etc.). Traumas in the intentional category (especially involving interpersonal violence) are known to cause higher rates of PTSD than traumas in the other two categories.

Having been exposed to the trauma is not sufficient to meet DSM-IV criteria; the person must also have reacted to the trauma with intense fear, hopelessness, and/or horror (Criterion A$_2$).

Re-experiencing Symptoms (Criterion B)

The re-experiencing (Criterion B) symptoms associated with PTSD describes a condition where "to remember is to relive." That is, when survivors are remembering the trauma they are actually reliving it in their mind, complete with the full emotional impact. Indeed, PTSD is very much a derangement of memory, where recollections of the trauma intrude on the person against their will. Common re-experiencing symptoms include recurrent and intrusive recollections that involve images, thoughts, or perceptions of the trauma, as well as illusions, flashbacks, or distressing dreams of the event (as described above for ASD)(Table 2). Only one re-experiencing/reactivating symptom cluster is required to fulfill Criterion B.

  ↗ **Intrusive recollections are unwanted and unintentional memories of the trauma event that force themselves into awareness, and in so doing evoke panic, terror, dread, or grief.** ↗ Vivid nightmares in these patients are particularly troublesome because sleep difficulties are also specifically associated with PTSD (Criteria D), due to increased arousal symptoms. Although the subject matter is trauma-specific, these nightmares are otherwise subject to the same distortions and characteristics associated with normal dreams. Flashbacks can be particularly devastating because the individual feels as though the traumatic event is actually occurring again.

☞ **Triggers (e.g., experiences, sounds, smells) can generalize to such an extent that what is initiating a flash-back years after the event may not appear on the surface to be connected in any way to the original trauma.** ☞

In PTSD, the term "trigger" refers to anything that might initiate the recurrence of a memory or a re-experiencing symptom. These include any sensory experience, (i.e., the smell of gunpowder or fire, the sound of helicopters or gunshots). Anniversaries of previous traumas new stressful events associated with strong emotions can also trigger intrusive recollections. Initially, the triggers are obviously related to the trauma. Eventually, conditions that trigger a response become blurred and generalized (e.g., a woman may develop a fear of flying after going on a trip where she ran into someone who resembled her rapist) through a process of trigger generalization.

Avoidant Symptoms (Criterion C)

The Criterion C symptoms are "avoidant" in nature. Indeed, trauma survivors with PTSD will go out of their way to avoid anyone or any thing that reminds them of the trauma. Amnestic symptoms, with inability to recall important parts of the trauma, are experienced by many. The structural alteration of biological memory centers (i.e., hippocampus, amygdala), along with HPA axis dysregulation provides the anatomic neurohumoral explanation of why memory gaps of the event occur.

In addition, individuals can lose their ability to feel strong emotions or participate in meaningful interpersonal relationships. In order to fulfill Criterion C, the trauma survivor must experience at least three of seven specific avoidant symptoms (Table 2). Since a wide range of avoidant symptoms can occur, trauma survivors can present with a variety of cognitive, affective, and behavioral symptoms as part of avoidance mechanisms.

As with ASD, depressive symptoms (including restricted affect, anhedonia, detachment from others) can be experienced. Trauma survivors with PTSD often relate a sense of foreshortened future and beliefs that the positive aspects in life are unattainable. From an interpersonal perspective, these symptoms are particularly troubling, as they contribute to a decreased social support system when it is most needed.

Hyperarousal Symptoms (Criterion D)

While the individual's effect may be flattened, arousal levels are characteristically elevated. At least two of the five types of persistent hyperarousal symptoms listed in Table 2 must be present to fulfill Criterion D. Symptoms resemble those seen in panic and generalized anxiety disorders, including emotional irritability, concentration difficulties, and sleep disturbances. An exaggerated startle response to innocuous stimuli is common and may be one of the most pathognomic symptoms of PTSD. Hypervigilance is characteristic, with a sense that once something so horrible has been experienced, "constant guard" must be maintained during surveillance for anything even remotely similar.

These increased arousal symptoms are psychobiologically mediated. The amygdala and other structures frequently send out "beware of trauma" signals, which in PTSD are not appropriately suppressed by the higher-level

brain functions of the MpFC, resulting in high levels of arousal, emotionality, and hypervigilance. This is exemplified by combat veterans who talk about "walking the perimeter" at night and rape survivors who refer to keeping watch when "things just aren't safe."

Hyperarousal behaviors can include anger, hostility, and self-destructive behavior (e.g., acting out, dangerous behavior, substance abuse, etc.). Emotional reactivity can escalate to the level of rage and can be misdiagnosed as bipolar disorder, antisocial behavior, or erroneously attributed to agitated depression.

Duration of B, C, and D Symptoms (Criterion E)

The PTSD criteria B, C, and D symptoms must be experienced for at least one month to fulfill Criterion E of DSM-IV diagnostic requirements for PTSD. This does not mean that trauma survivors manifesting these symptoms cannot be identified or receive treatment prior to one month. Indeed, many patients can be identified early as having ASD, and with proper treatment, may not progress to full PTSD.

Distress (Criterion F)

In addition to the above criteria (A–E), for the diagnosis of PTSD to be made, the symptoms must cause clinically significant distress or impairment in social, occupational, or other important areas of functioning.

Additional DSM-IV Specifiers

PTSD is labeled "acute," if the symptoms are of less than three months in duration and modified as "chronic," if persisting beyond three months. Delayed onset PTSD can occur if the symptoms do not appear until six months or more after the trauma. Finally, the symptoms of PTSD must have developed since the trauma. Pre-existing symptoms are excluded from the diagnostic criteria.

"Complex" PTSD refers to PTSD symptoms that develop after extreme traumas, including childhood sexual abuse, torture, captivity, and other prolonged horrific experiences. In addition to the typical PTSD symptoms, complex PTSD is associated with substantial risk for other psychiatric comorbidities and can cause severe emotional dysregulation, dissociative symptoms, and increased risk for suicide.

Instruments to Assist in Diagnosis

In clinical studies, rigorous evaluations are time intensive and require specially trained staff. The gold standard for comprehensive evaluation is the Clinician Administered PTSD Scale (CAPS). Due to its statistical validity, intervention literature typically reports CAPS scores for diagnosis, severity, and improvement measurements (84,85).

The Post-traumatic Stress Disorder Checklist—Civilian

The PTSD Checklist-Civilian (PCL-C) is the clinical assessment instrument that can be used in the process of any mental health evaluation. It has shown correlations with the CAPS of over 0.9 in diagnostic and overall severity ratings (86). The PCL-C is an instrument developed by the National Center for PTSD Behavioral Science Division (87). Patients are asked to rate the severity of impact in the last month (on a scale of 1–5) for 17 PTSD symptoms (Table 3). Questions 1 to 5 refer to re-experiencing symptoms, 6 to 12 are avoidant in nature, and 13 to 17 focuses on hyperarousal symptoms. For critically ill trauma patients, these questions can be asked as soon as the "high-risk" patient becomes capable of answering questions. Although the PCL-C is

Table 3 The Post-traumatic Stress Disorder Checklist—Civilian

Question/symptom	1	2	3	4	5
1. Repeated, disturbing memories, thoughts, or images of a stressful experience from the past?					
2. Repeated, disturbing dreams of a stressful experience from the past?					
3. Suddenly acting or feeling as if a stressful experience were happening again (as if you were reliving it)?					
4. Feeling very upset when something reminded you of a stressful experience from the past?					
5. Having physical reactions (heart pounding, trouble breathing, sweating) when something reminded you of a stressful event of the past?					
6. Avoiding thinking about or talking about a stressful experience from the past or avoiding having feelings related to it?					
7. Avoiding activities or situations because they remind you of a stressful experience?					
8. Trouble remembering important parts of a stressful experience from the past?					
9. Loss of interest in activities that you used to enjoy?					
10. Feeling distant or cut off from other people?					
11. Feeling emotionally numb or being unable to have loving feelings for those close to you?					
12. Feeling as if your future will somehow be cut short?					
13. Trouble falling or staying asleep?					
14. Feeling irritable or having angry outbursts?					
15. Having difficulty concentrating?					
16. Being "super-alert" or watchful or on guard?					
17. Feeling jumpy or easily startled?					

Note: Rating, scale of 1 to 5.
Abbreviations: 1, not at all; 2, a little bit; 3, moderately; 4, quite a bit; 5, extremely.

specifically designed to evaluate the overall symptom burden, it has also been used as a general guide to monitor therapy in PTSD patients (88).

Trauma History Screen

A trauma patient's prior history of ASD/PTSD is generally unknown to SICU staff. The Trauma History Screen (Table 4) was developed for patients who are not critically ill; however, the 12 questions (or selected items as appropriate) can be asked by the critical care nursing staff to determine the emotional impact of prior events on the trauma survivor. The information gathered from this screen helps to determine if a subsequent full mental health evaluation for ASD or PTSD should be conducted.

EARLY RECOGNITION OF POST-TRAUMATIC STRESS DISORDER

Most critically ill trauma patients will by default meet ASD/PTSD Criterion A₁. If the patient's response to this event included significant horror or helplessness (Criterion A₂), the patient has both of the necessary prerequisites to diagnose ASD (symptoms <1 month) or PTSD (symptoms >1 month). Initially, trauma patients may not be able to convey their feelings about the event due to intubation and/or sedation. However, once the patient recovers and begins to follow commands, inquiries about the patient's emotional status should be sought.

In addition to the PCL-C and trauma history screen (mentioned above), the Impact of Events Scale (IES) can be used to measure early ASD/PTSD symptoms. Ideally this should be done at least, once prior to hospital discharge

(8,77). The IES is a well-validated 15-item symptom scale that measures subjective distress (related to intrusion and avoidance) surrounding traumatic events. The IES appears to be a very useful early screening tool in the acute care setting.

Trauma-Associated Risk Factors for Developing Acute Stress Disorder/Post-traumatic Stress Disorder
Prior Traumatic Exposure

Pretrauma factors have a significant influence on which patients develop PTSD following physical trauma. A major risk factor for developing PTSD is the experience of a previous traumatic stressor. In one study of Vietnam combat veterans, 37% of those with PTSD had a history of severe childhood abuse, while only 7% of those without PTSD had such a history (89). ⚘ **When previous trauma includes interpersonal violence, either as a child or adult, the risk of developing PTSD is particularly high following exposure to subsequent trauma.** ⚘ Domestic violence is another situation where numerous prior victimization factors increase the likelihood of developing PTSD. In one urban county medical facility for survivors of domestic violence, a two-year sample revealed that nearly 70% of the population met diagnostic criteria for PTSD (91).

Peritrauma Factors

⚘ **Peritrauma factors increasing the risk of PTSD development fall into three categories: characteristics of the trauma, survivor reactions, and psychosocial support.** ⚘ Although the degree of trauma is difficult to quantify, in general PTSD frequency and intensity increase with greater severity, duration, and repetitions of trauma events. Factors of the trauma

Table 4 Trauma History Screen

Instructions: These events may or may not have happened to you. Answer "Yes" if that kind of thing has happened to you and "No" if it has not

Event	Yes	No	If you answer YES, indicate the number of times something like that happened to you
1. A really bad car, boat, train, or airplane accident			
2. A really bad accident at work or home			
3. A hurricane, flood, earthquake, tornado, or fire			
4. Getting beat up or attacked—as a child			
5. Getting beat up or attacked—as an adult			
6. Forced sex—as a child			
7. Forced sex—as an adult			
8. Attack with a gun, knife, or weapon			
9. During military service, seeing something horrible or being badly scared			
10. Sudden death of close family or friend			
11. Seeing someone badly hurt or killed			
12. Some other event that scared you badly			

Answer the following questions for each event that happened to you, if it bothered you emotionally

Question	Answer	
1. When this happened, did anyone get hurt or killed?	Y	N
2. When this happened, were you afraid that you or someone else might get hurt or killed?	Y	N
3. When this happened, did you feel very afraid, helpless, or horrified?	Y	N
4. When this happened, did you feel unreal, spaced out, disoriented, or strange?	Y	N
5. After this happened, how long were you bothered by it?	a. Not at all,	
	b. 1 wk,	
	c. 2–3 wk, days $\geq$ 1 mo	
6. At the time, how much did it bother you emotionally?	a. Not at all	
	b. A little	
	c. Somewhat	
	d. Much	
	e. Very much	

associated with higher PTSD risk include: (*i*) intentional trauma, (*ii*) being wounded, (*iii*) seeing others killed (especially loved ones, particularly when the survivor is responsible for the death of another), and (*iv*) repetition or feared repetition of the trauma ☛ **Perceived threat to life (92) and injury due to penetrating trauma (93) are consistently identified as major predictors for the development of PTSD.** ☛

The presence of three or more ASD symptoms from the re-experiencing and hyperarousal categories has been found to be an accurate and strong predictor of future PTSD development (80).

Survivor reactions which include physiological hyperarousal and/or dissociation in the peritrauma period comprise the highest risk group for long-term symptoms, and are more likely to dissociate during traumatic reminders in the future (94,95).

Decreased or limited psychological and social support after a trauma is a major (underappreciated) risk factor for PTSD. This issue is further complicated in the critical care setting. The support systems and coping mechanisms that the patient relied on during the pretrauma phase can be disrupted. Characteristics of the SICU environment (e.g.,

constant noise, lights, unfamiliar people, frequent treatments, etc.) must be considered when evaluating the impact of critical care on the psychobiology of the survivor.

Other factors associated with greater risk of developing PTSD include: pre-existing mental health conditions, genetic predisposition, high levels of chronic stress, poor coping skills, lack of education, emotional immaturity, female gender, and family history of mental illness.

Predicting Likelihood of Acute Stress Disorder/ Post-traumatic Stress Disorder

Despite a large body of literature, predicting which patients will develop ASD and PTSD remains an illusive task. Several studies have shed important light, however, on this process and certain factors are known to increase the likelihood of developing ASD in accident victims. These include: prior trauma, stay in an ICU/CCU, pre-existing psychiatric disorders, perceived threat to life, appraisal of accident severity, preventability of accident, pain, and prognosis for physical recovery (96,97).

In women who were assaulted as adults, two factors predicted greater PTSD severity even after treatment: previous childhood trauma and sustaining physical injury during adult trauma (98). Younger age is also frequently cited as a risk factor for developing PTSD; a study of 400 adolescent trauma victims showed a long-term PTSD rate of 27% (99). Gender itself is a predictor; women develop significantly more PTSD than men, given the same trauma exposure. In a study of MVC survivors, 23% of females developed ASD compared to 8% of males, and PTSD was diagnosed in 38% of females and 15% of males. Females also had higher rates of dissociative symptoms; and, ASD like PTSD has a higher predictive value for females across all age groups (100–104).

Several studies have shown the presence of delusions in acutely traumatized patients as a significant predictor of developing ASD and PTSD. Factual memories of difficult trauma are less associated with PTSD than are delusions. In one study, well more than half of ICU patients had delusional memories of their ICU treatment and up to 10% had no factual memories of their time in the ICU/CCU (105).

In a study of burn patients, acute levels of anxiety, depression, and avoidant symptoms strongly predicted symptom levels at three months postburn. Perceived threat to life during the burn also predicted severity, but objective burn severity did not (106). In another study more than a quarter of burn patients were symptomatic in the first month, and 15% remained positive for PTSD at one year (107). Similarly, in MI survivors, perceived severity of MI predicted PTSD, while the actual severity did not (108).

In a large SCI study, perceived threat to life was a significant predictor of PTSD levels. Death awareness, pain level, and spiritual/religious coping were also significant predictors (109). In an orthopedic trauma sample, patients who answered yes to the question, "Do the emotional problems caused by the injury cause more difficulty than the physical problems?" had a very high correlation with the presence of PTSD (63). In accident victims, some evidence suggests that extended periods of trauma-induced unconsciousness actually decreases rates of PTSD (110).

Providing written information about psychological recovery from ICU stay was not shown, in one study, to be effective as a stand-alone intervention in decreasing patient or relative stress, anxiety, or PTSD rates (111). Further, studies are warranted regarding the efficacy of written educational interventions in the early post-trauma period in preventing PTSD.

Diagnosis and Evaluation in the Trauma/Surgical Intensive Care Unit Setting

Referral for mental health evaluation in the emergency department (ED) is rare, but more common when physicians are satisfied their institution provides qualified mental health services (112). Requests for formal psychiatric evaluation is similarly rare in the critical care setting, partly because psychiatrists are perceived as not being particularly receptive to interviewing patients in the SICU. This impression should be changed, as screening and awareness of ASD, PTSD, and post-traumatic depression is very important for the patient's ultimate recovery. ⚐ **Trauma surgeons and intensivists should develop a level of expertise in counseling patients with these disorders, in addition to requesting early psychiatric consultation when appropriate.** ⚐

The successful SICU/trauma center will require education of all staff as well as advanced collaboration with mental health professionals. SICU studies show that rates

of detection for mental health conditions are far less than the actual occurrence, and when diagnoses are made by critical care clinicians, there is low correlation with objective psychiatric assessment, (113) although diagnostic accuracy improves when the case specificities are more typical (114).

For the purpose of evaluating those at risk for PTSD, evaluations within the first week are sometimes futile. However, at one-week post-trauma, most studies show that a reasonable assessment can be made, providing the patient is awake and cooperative. In one relatively large-scale study it was found that surgical ward PTSD symptoms (though too early to meet DSM-IV criteria) were strong predictors of PTSD symptoms over the course of the year after injury (7). The one-week post-trauma time frame provides some guidance for trauma providers to determine when more formal evaluation and intervention might be warranted.

POSTINJURY DEPRESSION

Depression and PTSD are highly correlated. Depression has been found in numerous studies of trauma victims to be the most prevalent psychiatric condition occurring with PTSD (59). The associative mechanisms between PTSD and depression are not well understood. Current evidence suggests that pre-existing depression may render an individual more vulnerable to PTSD; conversely the presence of PTSD may increase the risk of depression. Studies also suggest that the PTSD/depression combination that occurs after a trauma is different from generalized depression postinjury that occurs without PTSD (115).

Some of the most in-depth studies of depression in critical care settings have been conducted on coronary artery bypass graft (CABG) patients. Typically, 20% of these patients are depressed. Depressed patients also have a higher late mortality (116–118) and a higher subsequent cardiac event rate (27% vs. 10% for nondepressed patients) (119,120). Depression one-month postsurgery was found to be a major indicator of cardiac morbidity five years later (121).

The subject of depression is of considerable clinical importance in traumatized populations, given the significance of depressive comorbidity in determining treatment options. Relationships between PTSD and postinjury depression (and other mental health sequelae) are becoming increasingly understood, but additional research is required to identify predictive patterns.

ACUTE STRESS DISORDER/POST-TRAUMATIC STRESS DISORDER TREATMENT

⚐ **Treatment goals in PTSD are aimed at: reducing core symptoms, improving stress resilience, improving QoL, and reducing disability and comorbidity.** ⚐

Early on, patients and families should be educated about why PTSD develops, the expected responses to trauma (psychological and physical), and that treatment is available to assist in the healing process. Education should be given in a way that is practical and easily understandable. Follow-up resources should be provided, as well as how and when to access needed support services.

For the SICU patient, recognition of risk factors, early symptom identification, management of distressing symptoms [pharmacological and nonpharmacological, and minimizing potential triggers (e.g., reducing loud noises, approaching the patients calmly)] are important initial interventions.

Early Interventions

Though many people show early signs of distress following a trauma most will resolve their symptoms and adapt within three months. This text deals with patients mainly in their first days and weeks following trauma. Those who have not resolved their symptoms by three months are at greatest risk for developing severe, chronic PTSD; their treatment should be coordinated by a mental health professional trained in managing PTSD (122,123).

Single Session Psychological Debriefing Is Worse Than No Debriefing

Psychological debriefing (PD) refers to the process of engaging in a single session with trauma survivors or witnesses, either individually or in groups. PD was previously advocated for stimulating emotional processing and normalizing reactions. After reviewing its implementation over many years, there is no evidence for PD effectiveness in preventing future psychopathology (124,125), and in several replicated studies, PD has been shown to actually exacerbate subsequent PTSD symptoms (126). Most experts have called for ceasing single session psychological debriefing interventions (64).

Critical Incident Stress Debriefing (CISD) is a common form of PD for families and loved ones of trauma victims. Originally intended for use with emergency medical services (EMS) personnel, its use has widened to other areas of trauma treatment. Cessation of CISD as a secondary PTSD prevention measure is supported by scientific review of the available data (128,129). Techniques for dealing with families and loved ones of trauma survivors are provided in Volume 2, Chapter 64.

Cognitive Behavioral Therapy ≥ 4 sessions

Controlled trials of brief Cognitive Behavioral Therapy (CBT) for recently traumatized individuals has shown great promise in functioning as a secondary prevention for PTSD. The initial trial compared assault victims who completed a four-session course of CBT with evaluation only controls. The treatment patients showed significantly less PTSD and depression symptoms two months postassault and a strong signal for a similar difference at 5.5 months (130). In another trial of five session CBT versus supportive counseling for MVC and industrial accident survivors with ASD, those who completed the brief CBT showed significant benefit with lower rates of subsequent PTSD and depression (131).

Psychological First Aid

Prior to September 11th, the American Red Cross and most other multinational relief agencies were not routinely providing psychological first aid (132). PTSD support researchers BA Hong, CS North (both from the Washington University, St. Louis, Montana, U.S.A.), were at that time developing an organized plan for the mental health needs of disaster survivors called "Project CREST"(132). Findings from studies of survivors of the September 11th 2001 terrorist attacks were coupled with those from survivors of the Oklahoma City bombing and experience of B. Pfefferbaum (University of Oklahoma) to develop a "Practical Front Line Assistance and Support for Healing®" (P-FLASH®). This is an empirically based rapid mental health intervention program suitable for use in disaster settings.

The focus of this front-line counseling (also known as "Psychological First Aid") is current symptom reduction and/or issue resolution. There are six major elements of front-line counseling (Table 5). These symptom reduction techniques are most relevant to acute trauma treatment and are likely to be helpful in both the prehospital setting as well as the TRS.

↙ **The patient and family (when appropriate) should be made aware that there is a normal biological basis for their symptoms and be reassured that treatment options are available to help them.** ↙

Symptom Management

Symptom management tools can have an immediate impact and can be taught by health care providers. The tools described below can often be implemented in the SICU as symptoms arise. The tools and skills are divided into two sets, based on the symptoms they address. The Criterion B (Re-experiencing), and D (Hyperarousal) symptoms have a specific set of treatment tools. The Criterion C (Avoidant symptoms) has a different set of management tools.

Post-traumatic Stress Disorder Criterion B (Re-experiencing) and D (Hyperarousal) Management

Symptom management tools for Criterion B (Re-experiencing) symptoms are provided in Table 6. In general, relaxation techniques and other nonpharmacologic treatments are preferred. Muscle relaxation skills first became a tool for stress reduction in the 1920s when it was shown that stress could be maintained in muscles, and that it was nearly impossible to remain stressed or anxious and be relaxed at the same time. Relaxation skills are typically

Table 5 Psychological First Aid: For Survivors of Trauma[a]

Element	Key points of psychological first aid
Supportive listening	Being present and demonstrating interest in listening to the patient is paramount.
Education and reassurance	Provide the patient with knowledge that ASD and PTSD symptoms are natural, understandable, and treatable.
Coping and stress management	Suggest nonpharmacological therapy first (e.g., sleep meditation, exercise, and relaxation training).
Problem solving	Refrain from pejorative counseling. Rather, use objective problem solving capabilities. Help them untangle their web of problems.
Finding meaning and perspective	Without imposing one's own belief-system on the patient, help them describe and find their own perspective.
Observation and reassessment	Continued observation and reassessment is required—patients may have a delayed onset of symptoms as well as intermittent set backs and exacerbations.

[a]Tools such as this may be most suitable for dealing with large casualty situations (e.g., Hurricane Katrina, 2005; Indian Ocean Tsunami, 2004).
Abbreviations: ASD, acute stress disorder; PTSD, post-traumatic stress disorder.

Table 6 Post-traumatic Stress Disorder Criterion B (Re-experiencing) and D (Hyperarousal) Symptom Management Tools

Management tools	Examples and comments
Skeletal muscle relaxation	Series of muscle group relaxation techniques: The process: Muscle groups are tensed, then relaxed in sequence as shown in Table 7.
Abdominal breathing	Instructions: Lay, supine, and calm, right hand on abdomen and left hand on chest. Both hands raise and fall with each breath. Diverts focus from PTSD trigger to abdominal breathing. Can be used during ventilator weaning (see text).
Guided imagery	Helps patient create a "safe place" (for mental refuge from the PTSD trigger). Use of a guided script helps change mental focus to a calming, relaxing one.
Systematic desensitization	A process of gradually exposing patients to stressful images and thoughts while they utilize a relaxing skill. Potentially dangerous (professional oversight recommended).
Thought stopping	A distraction technique used to overcome distressing thoughts by inwardly or outwardly shouting, "stop" as these thoughts are called to mind.
Cognitive reframing	A process of restructuring cognitions or conclusions, which have been drawn as a result of the trauma. Reframing assists the patient to develop a different, reality based cognition of the event.
Sleep hygiene	This refers to the optimal conditions in which to sleep and induce good (i.e., restful) sleep without nightmares.

Abbreviation: PTSD, post-traumatic stress disorder.

Table 7 The Short Muscle Group Relaxation Process

Tense the muscles as listed below. Hold the tension for 5 sec then relax for 15 sec, before proceeding to the next set of muscles. Do them in the order listed here.

Tighten both fists. Flex your arms all the way in, tightly.

With head back, scrunch up the muscles of your face. With neck muscles tightened, roll your head clockwise then counterclockwise.

Shoulders up, jaw clenched.

Arch your back gently, tense your back muscles and breath in deeply and hold.

Toes up with tight shin and calf muscles.

Toes down with tight calf, thigh and buttock muscles.

Note: Muscle tensing relaxation training must take into account the patient's physical condition and the other effects the muscle tension may have on body systems.

taught in two forms, skeletal muscle relaxation and breathing techniques.

Skeletal muscle relaxation is a process that involves intentional skeletal muscle tensing, followed by relaxation in a sequential and repetitive fashion. The skill can be quickly taught and begins helping immediately. The entire process is described in Table 7, can be completed within several minutes. Muscle relaxation training must take into account the patient's physical condition and associated fractures or dislocations, etc.

Considerable stress, tension, and anxiety can be maintained in the muscles of respiration and in the abdominal muscles. Abdominal breathing instructions are provided in Table 6. The abdominal breathing relaxation exercise can even be practiced by most mechanical ventilation dependent SICU patients when they have improved to the weaning phase guided imagery, systematic desensitization, thought stopping, cognitive reframing, and sleep hygiene are additional Criterion B and D management tools (Table 6).

Sleep hygiene is particularly important and relevant to the SICU, and refers to attempts at ensuring post-trauma

patients have normal restful sleep. Sedatives/hypnotics should be considered when the patient experiences difficulty in falling or remaining asleep.

Post-traumatic Stress Disorder Criterion C (Avoidant Symptom) Management

For the Criterion C (Avoidant) symptoms, treatment can be very complex. Because the manifestation of avoidant symptoms often involves major volitional components (i.e., deciding to stay home), avoidant symptoms are some of the most difficult PTSD symptoms to treat, and some of the worst in terms of long-term prognosis. Many of these symptoms may not emerge until the patient has left the SICU. Avoidant symptoms cause people to shun treatment, withdraw, and become unemotional. Trauma systems should have outreach programs to follow-up on those patients that fail to return to clinic (these may be the patients in greatest need). Selected tools for managing Avoidant (Criterion C) symptoms are provided in Table 8; many of these patients will also require antidepressant medications.

Acute Stress Disorder Criterion B (Dissociation) Interventions

Grounding techniques (Table 9) help to keep patients "in the present" when they are experiencing dissociative symptoms. The dissociation can take the form of flashbacks or alteration of one's sense of self, but distortions of awareness of space, time, and location are particularly in acute need of grounding. Grounding tools used in the acute trauma setting help to return the patients' awareness to the present from a dissociated state. These techniques can be performed by the bedside nurse and include sensory and cognitive grounding skills, which are described in Table 9.

Psychotherapy

Psychotherapy for PTSD can take many forms, including typical insight oriented therapy, CBT, and desensitization therapies (Table 10). Meta-analysis of studies from 1980–2003 of psychotherapy for PTSD showed that, as a whole, most patients treated with psychotherapy either recover or improve with treatment; however, a majority of patients continue to have substantial residual symptoms (133).

Table 8 Post-traumatic Stress Disorder (PTSD) Criterion C (Avoidant) Symptom Management Tools

Management tools	Examples and comments
Positive memory anchoring	Allows the patient to focus on a positive memory in their life that they can recall at any time.
	Helps switch out of an intrusive traumatic memory.
	Facilitates reconnection to positive events.
Resuming past positive activity	Helps overcome the psychobiological pressure to avoid all emotions.
	Involves engaging in previously pleasurable activities (chosen by the patient) without any association with the trauma.
Reconnecting with important relationships	Helps the patient heal the disruption in social interaction that develops with PTSD.
	Reconnection should occur in a safe setting.
	The safe setting (not associated with the trauma) helps avoid creating associations between significant relationships and the trauma.
Emotional literacy	Helping the patient to experience emotions not related to the event helps them acknowledge the existence of emotions outside the trauma.
	This skill encourages patients to recognize and identify sad and happy events in their life prior to the trauma.
	Eventually the patient should acknowledge these emotions in their current experience.

Table 9 Acute Stress Disorder Criterion B (Dissociative Symptoms) Interventions: Sensory and Cognitive Grounding Skills

Type of intervention	Examples and comments
Sensory grounding skills	Provides physical sensations, which will help the patient return their awareness to the present. These tools are facilitated by the bedside nurse
	Examples
	Open eyes, look at something; identify details of object
	Hold something; concentrate on physical sensation of touch
	Place a cool cloth on face; be aware of the cold sensation
	Listen to music that maintains awareness
	Place feet firmly on the ground; become aware of the sensation in feet and legs
	Focus on someone else's voice or concentrate on details in conversation
Cognitive grounding skills	The SICU nurse asks the patient a series of orientation questions. Later the patient is encouraged to ask themselves
	Where am I?
	What is today?
	What is the date?
	How old am I?
	What was the most recent holiday?

Abbreviation: SICU, surgical intensive care unit.

Cognitive Behavioral Therapy

CBT is a common and effective technique utilized in PTSD patients, and is probably the most researched intervention for treating post-traumatic symptoms. In one example study, MVC survivors were evaluated in a controlled trial of CBT versus supportive therapy. At one year follow-up, the CBT group met diagnostic criteria for PTSD significantly less than the control group (134). Another study of nearly 100 MVC survivors with PTSD found that 11% of those treated with CBT remained positive for PTSD at nine months, whereas 61% of those given a self-help booklet covering the same CBT information remained diagnostic for PTSD, demonstrating the importance of ongoing psychiatric intervention in this population (135).

Exposure based CBT techniques include: (*i*) gradual exposure, (*ii*) flooding, and (*iii*) systematic desensitization, which are used to help the patient confront the avoided fears directly. By exposing a person to traumatic memories in the safe setting of therapy, and usually combined with stress reduction techniques, the overwhelming fear is reduced or eliminated. Compared to other psychotherapies for PTSD, patients tend to follow-up with exposure-based CBT to about the same degree as with others (136).

Eye Movement Desensitization and Reprocessing

Eye movement desensitization and reprocessing (EMDR) is an evolving therapy for PTSD (Table 10). EMDR are thought (by some) to be analogous to rapid eye movement (REM), sleep related eye movements, and thereby could serve as a stress reducing function similar to sleep. Elements of exposure therapy are combined with physical actions (e.g., saccadic eye movements) in EMDR. Review of the randomized clinical trials of EMDR indicates symptom improvement duration of between three and nine months, but comparison study findings are equivocal with numerous methodological variations and small sample sizes (137,138).

Group Therapy and Brief Psychodynamic Psychotherapy

Survivors without major avoidant symptoms may feel more comfortable sharing their experiences and feelings with others who have been through similar events. Group therapy can help resolve issues of trust and improve interpersonal relations.

Brief psychodynamic psychotherapy focuses on the emotional aspects of the trauma, including their relation to early life experiences. Telling "one's story" and exploring the trauma in an empathic, nonjudgmental setting has been shown to have psychologic benefit in the aftermath of trauma.

Drug Therapy

Medication usage (Table 11) is best implemented when PTSD has been evaluated and a formal diagnosis has been made. Symptom severity should be initially assessed and serial measurements made to help to monitor the treatment process. The PCL-C is included in this chapter (Table 3), and allows for initial and repeated evaluation of PTSD severity from both a specific and global perspective by

Table 10 Post-traumatic Stress Disorder Psychotherapy Methodology

Type of therapy	Examples and comments
CBT	The cognitive part of CBT addresses cognitions (mental conclusions drawn about the self, the world, and other people). With PTSD some cognitions become distorted.
	CBT works when the therapist helps reorder cognitions for the patient.
	The behavioral parts of CBT consist of skills training to cope with anxiety, anger, stress reactions, and to relate effectively with others.
EMDR	Elements of exposure therapy are combined with physical actions (e.g., eye movements).
Group therapy	Some survivors may feel more comfortable sharing their experiences and feelings with others who have been through similar events.
	Can help heal issues of trust and interpersonal relations.
	Focuses on how members are successfully coping, which helps bring positive attention to the here and now.
Brief psychodynamic psychotherapy	Explores the trauma in an empathetic, nonjudgmental setting.
	Focuses on the emotional aspects of the trauma, including their relation to early life experiences.

Abbreviations: CBT, cognitive behavioral therapy; EMDR, eye movement desensitization and reprocessing; PTSD, post-traumatic stress disorder.

interrogating 17 areas, which address the triad of avoidant, arousal, and re-experiencing symptoms.

Initial Pharmacotherapy (First Month)

Medication is typically used within the first month for patients who have already had some other kind of intervention such as psychological first aid, CBT, or other individual or group therapy following trauma. No medications have yet been Food and Drug Administration (FDA) approved for ASD treatment, and treatment guidance is mainly extrapolated from PTSD studies.

Prior to receiving medication for ASD/PTSD the patient should receive thorough psychiatric and medical evaluations. In the critical care settings, collaborative assessment is required to determine which symptoms and findings are due to current medications, delirium, brain injury, or other nonpsychiatric etiology, and which are likely attributable to the ASD/PTSD spectrum of symptoms.

In general, two populations of acutely traumatized patients should receive medication: (*i*) those who have received a therapy oriented intervention but remain symptomatic; and (*ii*) those who have symptoms that in themselves warrant immediate pharmacological intervention, such as patients who are dangerous (suicidal or homicidal), extremely agitated, or exhibiting psychotic symptoms.

Symptoms of extreme arousal, including severe anxiety, panic, hyper-vigilance, and insomnia, typically require acute

medication. In the past, high potency neuroleptics such as haloperidol were used for early symptom reduction. In current practice some of the atypical antipsychotics (i.e., olanzapine, risperidone, and quetiapine) are legitimate considerations since they have shown robust effects on PTSD symptoms, and are highly effective in reducing agitative symptoms.

Benzodiazepines, which decrease acute anxiety, have been shown to decrease anxiety in ASD/PTSD (139). Benzodiazepines are frequently and effectively used for initial symptom management in the acute trauma/critical care setting. Benzodiazepines, however, are of limited value in treating core symptoms, and with prolonged use, have actually been associated with an increase in the rate of PTSD development (140). Benzodiazepines must be used cautiously, due to their abuse potential and withdrawal symptoms with discontinuation.

Alpha-2 agonists (e.g., clonidine), and both alpha-1 and beta-adrenergic blocking agents (e.g., prazosin and propanolol respectively) have been used successfully to decrease symptoms of hyperarousal in ASD/PTSD. One trial has shown a secondary PTSD prevention effect in patients who received a 10-day course of propranolol beginning within six hours of the event (141,142). Each of these agents must be used with caution in the critical care patient due to effects on cardiovascular functioning. Clonidine, and the newer α_2 agonist, dexmedetomidine may be particularly useful (research pending).

Selective Serotonin reuptake inhibitors (SSRIs) are the pharmacologic agents of choice in treating PTSD. SSRI antidepressants have shown efficacy in reducing symptoms in all three-symptom clusters, (Criteria B, C, and D) in multiple double-blind and open-label studies. ☞ **Although no medications are approved for ASD, sertraline, and paroxetine do have FDA indication for PTSD.** ☞ These agents are usually well tolerated with a low incidence of side effects. SSRIs are a first line treatment for PTSD after acute crisis management, and in conjunction with continued psychological therapy. Dosage of these medications should start low and be increased slowly with close monitoring of symptom response. Similar to their effect in anxiety disorders, SSRIs can cause CNS activation and anxiety in PTSD when first started or when doses are increased. Full effect of SSRI treatment takes from weeks to a few months and the magnitude of improvement may be insufficient to achieve full PTSD symptom resolution.

Maintenance Pharmacotherapy (After First Month)

After the first month, if PTSD symptoms either remain or develop, full psychiatric assessment is warranted. If PTSD or significant subsyndromal PTSD is present, a comprehensive treatment plan must be implemented. Acute trial literature indicates that either psychotherapy or psychopharmacology alone may leave significant residual symptoms even when effective (143). The most powerful combination is probably medication and psychotherapy, in conjunction with education and family support.

Only two medications (sertraline and paroxetine) have FDA approval for treatment of PTSD, but studies with other SSRIs and serotonin norepinephrine reuptake inhibitors (SNRIs) have also shown improvement. In addition to being first line pharmacotherapy for PTSD (144,145), the SSRIs are also useful in treating conditions, which frequently arise or coexist with PTSD (e.g., depression and panic disorder), and are effective in decreasing aggression and impulsivity. Beyond these medications, there is no definitive

Table 11 Drug Therapy for Post-traumatic Stress Disorder Symptomatology

Type	Drug	Examples and comments
Initial (first month)	Benzodiazepines	Used to decrease anxiety in ASD/PTSD.
		Should only be used briefly, if at all; other drugs may have a lower incidence of subsequent PTSD development.
	Antiadrenergics Clonidine	Have been used successfully to decrease symptoms of hyperarousal in chronic PTSD.
	Propranolol Prazosin	Must be used with caution in the critical care patient due to effects on cardiovascular functioning.
	SSRIs Setraline (Zoloft®)	Have shown effectiveness in improving PTSD symptoms in all three-symptom clusters, (Criteria B, C, and D).
	Paroxetine (Paxil®)	Full effect from SSRI treatment takes from weeks to a few months.
Maintenance (after first month)	SSRIs Setraline (Zoloft) Paroxetine (Paxil)	First line pharmacotherapy in PTSD. U.S. FDA approved—effective in all three clusters of PTSD symptoms, in civilian and combat populations, in men and women, and in short-term and long-term studies.
	Tricyclic antidepressants	Second line treatment after SSRI failure.
	Benzodiazepines	Do not specifically treat PTSD symptoms, but assists in anxiety and sleep improvement in the short-term.
	Antiadrenergic agents	Decrease hyperarousal symptoms.
	Prazosin Clonidine	Prazosin showed beneficial effect on nightmares in combat related PTSD.
	Anticonvulsants/mood stabilizers	Useful in patients who are labile, impulsive, or aggressive.
	Atypical antipsychotics Risperidone Olanzapine Quetiapine	Effective in acute psychiatric crisis. Atypical antipsychotics may be appropriate for patients with significant fear, hyper vigilant, paranoid, or psychotic PTSD symptoms.
Chronic	SSRIs Setraline (Zoloft) Paroxetine (Paxil)	Success shown using SSRIs for more than one year for the treatment of PTSD and prevention of relapse. Patients with a quick and robust response to treatment may need a shorter duration of therapy.

Abbreviations: ASD, acute stress disorder; PTSD, post-traumatic stress disorder; SSRIs, selective serotonin reuptake inhibitors; U.S. FDA, United States Food and Drug Administration

empirical evidence to guide second-line choices. Suggestions in the literature are made based on data available (146).

Twelve-week sertraline studies have shown 23% to 26% PTSD remission rates (147). Evaluating nearly 400 patients in sertraline trials, the average dose for response in PTSD was 125 mg and in PTSD with comorbid depression 147 mg daily. Average time to response was 4.5 weeks in PTSD and 5.5 in PTSD with comorbid depression (148). In depression, sertraline can be started as high as 100 mg daily. In PTSD, a starting dose of 50 mg is prudent; this may be decreased to 25 mg if necessary in order to reduce adverse effects, which are typically dose related.

Paroxetine has been well studied and shown to be effective in all three clusters of PTSD symptoms, in civilian and combat populations, in men and women, and in short-and long-term studies (149). In a landmark study, PTSD patients treated for one year with the SSRI paroxetine were shown to have an increase in hippocampal volume of 5% and an associated 35% increase in verbal declarative memory functioning (150). Effective doses of paroxetine are usually between 20 to 60 mg daily, often with a 10 mg starting dose.

Tricyclic antidepressants (TCAs) were used extensively prior to the introduction of SSRIs. They are still used in PTSD with SSRI failure, but remain second line due to their negative side effect profile, and their significantly increased lethality in overdose (151). There is also renewed interest in reversible monoamine oxidase inhibitors (MAOIs) with several studies showing promise in reducing PTSD symptomatology.

Benzodiazepines do not specifically treat PTSD symptoms, but may assist in anxiety and sleep improvement in the short-term (2–4 days). With prolonged use (greater than one week), there is a possibility of increasing the rate of PTSD development, possibly through blurring of reality with sedation-related dreams. Buspirone, has been studied (open label) as an alternative to benzodiazepines, and holds promise as an effective antianxiety agent in PTSD.

Antiadrenergic agents have shown to benefit treating hyperarousal symptoms and may be appropriate for patients with significant arousal or dissociation. Prazosin has been studied in combat PTSD, showing a beneficial effect on PTSD nightmares (152,153). Propranolol has shown some potential for use in the emergency department with acutely traumatized patients to reduce the acute stress response. Early administration may decrease future physiological reactivity to trauma stimuli and PTSD development.

Anticonvulsant/mood stabilizer medications have been used for some time in PTSD. These agents may be particularly useful in patients who are significantly labile, impulsive, or aggressive (154). Open label studies have shown positive results with carbamazepine, (155) valproic acid, (156,157) topiramate, (158) phenytoin, (159) and gabapentin (160,161). A small double-blind placebo-controlled study also supported the efficacy of lamotrigine (162). Valproic acid has been widely used in Veterans Administration (VA) treatment of combat-related PTSD. Dosing typically targets serum levels similar to those used for seizure control.

Atypical antipsychotics are effective for treating patients in acute psychiatric crisis. Atypical antipsychotics may be also be appropriate for patients with significant fear, hypervigilant, paranoid, or psychotic PTSD symptoms. Olanzapine has been studied in oral (PO) and intra-muscular (IM) formulations for stabilizing severely agitated patients (163–165). Olanzapine has shown efficacy in all three symptom clusters (166), and in treatment-resistant, combat-related PTSD (167,168). Doses up to 20 mg daily were studied in these chronic populations, while short-term use of doses as low as 2.5 mg daily were found effective in torture victims with acute PTSD (169). Risperidone has been studied in doses from 0.5 to 8 mg daily as monotherapy or more typically as an augmentation to an already stable regimen (170). The most typical dosing is between 2 and 6 mg daily in divided doses (171,172). Quetiapine has also shown symptom improvement in doses ranging from 75 to 300 mg (173,174). Psychotic symptoms in PTSD are not rare, and are particularly debilitating, given the overall symptom burden. Often, these symptoms go undetected due to the patient's reluctance to admit psychotic experiences (175).

Postsymptom Medication Continuation

✒ **Medication continuation beyond the symptom period may be prudent in PTSD, in order to reduce or prevent relapse.** ✒ Recent SSRI studies suggest that longer continuation therapy (at least one year) should be considered in treating PTSD. In a study of patients stabilized on sertraline within 36 weeks, those who continued on medication for an additional 28 weeks showed a 5% relapse rate compared to a 26% rate for patients who had been switched to placebo (176,177). Other studies have also supported the extended use of SSRIs for improved response rates and PTSD relapse prevention. Patients who have a very quick and robust response to treatment may need a shorter duration of therapy. As with other SSRI use, gradually tapering is suggested.

Multimodal Treatment

Multimodal treatment therapies may prevent or lessen PTSD symptoms. Combined therapeutic modalities may include, among others: CBT, pharmacotherapy, and collaborative care. In one study that compared patients who received standard therapy to those who received collaborative care, the latter showed decreased PTSD symptoms after one year as well as a 24% decrease in alcohol abuse. Usual care patients showed an increase in PTSD symptoms and a 13% increase in alcohol abuse (178).

Non-traditional Therapies

Based on research conducted in trauma survivors, several nontraditional therapies have shown promise (Table 12). Writing about one's emotional aspects of trauma has been shown to produce measurable changes in physical and mental health (179). Prospective diaries have resulted in greater understanding of events and responses in the SICU, and have helped patients and families set more realistic goals for recovery (180).

Table 12 Novel and Emerging Therapies

Type of therapy	Examples and comments
Writing exercises	Writing about the emotional aspects of trauma organizes thoughts, forces analysis.
	As little as 15–20 min/day for 3–4 days has produced measurable improvements in physical and mental health.
Meditation	Can help develop an accepting attitude of thoughts or emotions that arise during treatment.
	Effective in reducing chronic pain, stress, and anxiety in patients undergoing medical treatment.
VRET	VRET helps recreate trauma conditions such as combat and offers new potential in re-exposure therapy.
	VRET has been shown in small trials to decrease symptoms in all three clusters.
Hypnotherapy	Used in patients trying to access memories they cannot consciously recall or are too emotional to recall.
	No formal RCTs have shown hypnotherapy to be a beneficial treatment.
Peritrauma cortisol dosing	Recently, supplemental cortisol administration has been known to be protective of PTSD in certain populations.
	In a study of 91 patients undergoing cardiac surgery, half received a stress dose of hydrocortisone during the perioperative period and showed significant reduction of chronic stress and PTSD symptoms at 6 mo postsurgery.

Abbreviations: PTSD, post-traumatic stress disorder; RCTs, randomized clinical trials; VRET, virtual reality exposure therapy.

Meditation has been studied in numerous medical populations. Meditation has been shown to be effective in reducing chronic pain, stress, and anxiety in patients undergoing medical treatment (181). In postsurgical breast and prostate cancer patients, meditation-based stress reduction increased QoL, decreased stress, and had a potentially beneficial impact on the HPA axis functioning (182).

Virtual reality exposure therapy (VRET) helps recreate trauma conditions (e.g., combat) and offers new potential in re-exposure therapy. VRET has been shown in small trials to decrease PTSD symptoms in all three clusters (183,184). It has been used to treat survivors of the September 11 World Trade Center attack (183) and Vietnam veterans (184). The U.S. Navy is currently funding further research on VRET in veterans. VRET has not been tested in the SICU.

Hypnosis has been used for over a century in the attempt to treat post-traumatic symptoms. To date, no formal, randomized clinical trials have been completed to support its use as a definitive treatment in PTSD (185).

Another recent form of treatment is "Acceptance and Commitment Therapy." This is a therapeutic method designed to reduce experiential avoidance. It has been validated in randomized clinical trials to decrease self-harm among women with Borderline Personality Disorder (186), and in treating polysubstance abuse (187). It may be well suited for the use in PTSD populations (188).

Recently, supplemental cortisol administration has been shown to be protective of PTSD in certain populations of patients. In a study of 91 patients undergoing cardiac surgery, half received a stress dose of hydrocortisone during the perioperative period and showed significant reduction of chronic stress and PTSD symptoms at six months postsurgery (189). The same researchers completed similar studies on long-term survivors of ICU treatment, again showing a protective effect from a stress dose of cortisol (57,190). Another study of septic shock treatment showed promising results for hydrocortisone in reducing PTSD symptoms in these patients (191). Currently however, there is insufficient evidence to support the use of cortisol in PTSD prophylaxis.

LONG-TERM FOLLOW-UP
Observation and Reassessment During the First Month Following Trauma

Formal diagnostic assessment typically requires a week to have passed since the trauma. The suitability of the patient for psychiatric evaluation depends on many factors, including the level of critical care being received, the potential for further traumatic interventions, prognosis for recovery, psychological state, and willingness to participate in therapy. Serial formal assessments in high-risk patients provide data for longitudinal evaluation of the patient's condition and effectiveness of treatment. Collaborative efforts between in hospital and outpatient providers are essential to reduce the number of patients who drop out of treatment or are lost to follow-up.

Formal Post-traumatic Stress Disorder Screening and Diagnosis After the First Month

Screening for PTSD requires at least a month to have passed since the initial trauma. The setting a patient is in at the time of screening will have a significant impact on how formal screening is implemented. The National Center for PTSD promotes the Primary Care Screen (PC-PTSD) (192). The screening is designed for maximal sensitivity and is easily administered by appropriately trained healthcare providers at all levels. The screen consists of four questions (Table 13) that address the symptoms of hyperarousal, avoidance, and intrusive recollections. This screening is considered positive when the response to question three or any other two answers are positive.

Table 13 Post-traumatic Stress Disorder: Primary Care Screen

In your life, have you ever had any experience that was so frightening, horrible, or upsetting that in the past month, you:	Yes	No
1. Have had nightmares about it or thought about it when you did not want to?		
2. Tried hard not to think about it or went out of your way to avoid situations that remind you of it?		
3. Were constantly on guard, watchful, or easily startled?		
4. Felt numb or detached from others, activities, or your surroundings?		

Note: This screening is considered positive in two cases. First, if any two or more questions are answered yes, it is considered positive. Second, if question three is positive, even by itself, the screening is considered positive.
Source: From Ref. 1.

Prolonged Critical Illness and Post-traumatic Stress Disorder

✍ **Factors associated with prolonged critical illness may play a causative role in PTSD, and critical illness may, of itself, be considered a traumatic event.** ✍ The severity and number of traumas experienced in the hospital setting can be the nidus for PTSD or increase the likelihood of its development. For example, compared to all patients who experience myocardial infarction, those who suffer cardiac arrest are almost three times as likely to develop PTSD (193).

Critical care interventions need to be implemented with the utmost consideration for the psychobiological impact. This is especially important in situations, which may be perceived as a threat to life (e.g., invasive procedures). Clinician interventions, such as calming presence, simple and clear explanations, and remaining with the patient following treatment may help to mitigate anxiety and reduce the perceived level of threat. Pharmacotherapy with sedatives and antianxiety agents should be used as appropriate.

Permanent Disability and Post-traumatic Stress Disorder

Permanent disability adds another significant level of impact to the patient. In the case of someone who recovers from a severe MVC, the person can feel as though they are disabled and permanently broken. This can be due to the severity of the PTSD symptoms, which causes disability in itself, or it can be a cognitive distortion. Those who experience both a life threat and a traumatic loss are at highest risk for PTSD and for symptom severity (194,195).

Perceived threat to life has been noted in many traumatized populations to be strongly associated with PTSD development (92). Some large studies of war survivors have shown that PTSD rates of disabled trauma survivors are similar to nondisabled survivors (196). A study of disabled foreign war veterans who were treated in substandard rehabilitation facilities found that the PTSD rate more than doubled in five years and was related to inadequate social support at home and deficient psychological care (197).

Even though depression is common with PTSD, the depression rate for disabled patients with PTSD is even higher, and the associated suicide risk is increased as well (198). In physically disabled patients, there will be a significant period of grieving the loss of functionality during which recovery from ASD/PTSD symptoms may not be possible.

In studies of SCI patients PTSD symptoms can impact methods of adaptation to disability e.g., shock, anxiety, denial, depression, internalized anger, externalized hostility, acknowledgment, or adjustment (199). In this population, death anxiety is highly correlated with total post-traumatic stress levels experienced (199).

Importance of Long-Term Follow-Up Care

Long-term follow-up is essential to identify patients who are initially asymptomatic, or with latent PTSD onset (200). A study of 231 men who required trauma services due to interpersonal violence found that while the need for mental health services to treat their PTSD was high, the use of these services outside the acute care setting was low (200). Psychoeducation is required to increase the number of people who take advantage of the services they need. Critical care providers are in a unique position to provide brief, but powerful screenings, education, and referrals for specialized care and follow-up. Web-based education programs can help facilitate education and outreach for patients and families (201).

In relation to physical symptoms, trauma survivors with PTSD have significantly higher than normal rates of somatization, including conversion symptoms and chronic pain, even when compared to traumatized patients without PTSD (202–204). They are also at higher risk for developing physiological illnesses. Combat veterans with PTSD were found in a large study to have biological markers associated with cardiovascular and autoimmune inflammatory disorders (205).

Follow-up care providers must keep this in mind as they reassess for both physical and psychological effects of the trauma. Somatic complaints can lead to a seemingly endless series of medical evaluations and procedures. If the potential for a post-traumatic somatization etiology is not considered among the differential, the true cause of the symptoms may never be identified.

EYE TO THE FUTURE

Although many risk factors for ASD and PTSD have been identified, much still needs to be learned. Very little is currently known about the interaction of specific injury event-related phenomena and treatment in the prehospital, resuscitation, SICU, and rehabilitation phases of trauma care. For example, although PTSD onset is common after MVCs that result in serious injury, it is not yet known what specific collision or prehospital conditions, such as crash severity or extrication time, are significant risk factors. Also unknown is whether the contribution of resuscitation and trauma treatment, such as the role of specific drug treatments and environmental conditions during the treatment and institution of invasive procedures, are harmful or beneficial to the early development of ASD and subsequent PTSD. In conjunction with the elucidation of risk factors for ASD and PTSD, further research efforts must also be directed toward evaluating the efficacy of treatment protocols in trauma patients. Hypocortisolemia may become one of the diagnostic markers for PTSD (206). Furthermore, cortisol or hydrocortisone therapy may be used in patients with high risk for PTSD. Indeed, the use of stress doses of hydrocortisone in high-risk cardiac surgical patients reduces perioperative stress exposure, decreases chronic stress symptoms, and improves health-related QoL at six months after cardiac surgery (190, 207).

In the resuscitation and critical care settings, relatively little is known about the efficacy of combined pharmacological and psychological therapeutic approaches to treatment. The elucidation of effective early intervention therapies to control early ASD symptoms during hospitalization will be a crucial focus of future research in order to decrease or eliminate ASD and PTSD onset.

The strong association of PTSD with significant long-term deficits in QoL and functional status after serious injury further underscores the importance of early secondary prevention and effective treatment addressing the physical, psychological, and emotional responses to traumatic injury. Patients treated in the advanced trauma care setting may receive optimal clinical care, but may not be able to return to preinjury QoL without advances in awareness of psychiatric pathology, long-range trauma care, and rehabilitation and support services.

SUMMARY

Recent research has begun to elucidate the pathophysiology of ASD/PTSD and has increased our understanding of trauma on the brain's emotional and memory centers. An evolving understanding of the neurobiology of PTSD recognizes that structural changes in limbic system structures (chiefly hippocampus and the amygdala) along with neuro-hormonal changes in the HPA system are involved in the pathophysiology. The complex psychological and emotional factors that contribute to an individual's resiliency and adjustment following trauma are just now becoming elucidated. When making the formal diagnosis of ASD, PTSD is important for formulating proper treatment decisions, educating patients, and for research purposes. However, subdiagnostic acute stress symptoms constitute another important area of concern due to the physical and emotional distress to the patient, and the increased likelihood of progression to ASD or PTSD, if unchecked.

✒ **Although patient wishes regarding mental health intervention should be honored, formal diagnostic evaluation is indicated whenever ASD or PTSD symptoms are present and causing significant distress.** ✒ Practitioners caring for these patients should inform the patient and family about the common nature of the symptomatology in highly traumatized individuals. The symptoms and diagnoses should be destigmatized, given the high frequency with which these symptoms arise in trauma survivors who have experienced or perceived a major threat to their life or that of a loved one.

When patients are experiencing symptoms that are distressing, or causing functional impairment, specific treatment is warranted. ✒ **Optimum interventions for ASD and PTSD are symptom-targeted and should be individualized to the patient's phase of illness and overall clinical condition.** ✒

From the trauma survivor's perspective, PTSD symptomatology is often viewed as being far more significant than the nonpsychiatric medical and physical conditions resulting from injury. Accordingly, trauma care systems must adopt a more comprehensive conceptualization of trauma that extends beyond their fundamental *raison d'etre* (saving lives), and addresses the associated life-altering consequences of traumatic injury. Comprehensive trauma systems must be responsive, not only to the immediate physical outcomes, but also to the long-term emotional, psychological, and social outcomes of severely injured individuals.

KEY POINTS

✒ PTSD is a psychiatric ailment resulting from an individuals experiencing or witnessing of an actual or potential life-threatening event.

✒ Research on trauma survivors cared for in U.S. Trauma Centers reveals that 10% to 40% develop symptoms of ASD and PTSD (1–8).

✒ Structural changes occur in the brains of patients whose PTSD symptoms have been allowed to persist untreated for too long.

✒ Four integral components of the limbic system are specifically involved in the pathophysiology of ASD/PTSD.

✎ Individuals with PTSD have dysregulation of the HPA axis (resulting in lower than normal cortisol levels), as well as an elevated basal adrenergic tone.

✎ The initial resuscitation, anesthesia, and critical care experiences may contribute (negatively or positively) to the development of ASD/PTSD.

✎ In one large study of critically ill patients the risk of PTSD was directly correlated with the duration of mechanical ventilation and inversely related to patient age (67).

✎ Trauma outcomes researchers have consistently identified PTSD as a significant factor in functional limitations and diminished QoL above and beyond the medical comorbidities associated with their physical wounds (7,62–67,69,70).

✎ The diagnosis of ASD symptoms helps to identify patients at risk for PTSD, in quantifying the severity of distress suffered by the trauma survivor during the first month following the event.

✎ Dissociative symptoms contribute to discontinuities in memory, identity, and perception; these are required for the diagnosis of ASD but not PTSD. Re-experiencing, avoidant, and hyperarousal symptoms are characteristic of both entities.

✎ Intrusive recollections are unwanted and unintentional memories of the trauma event that force themselves into awareness and, in so doing, evoke panic, terror, dread, or grief.

✎ Triggers (e.g., experiences, sounds, smells) can generalize to such an extent that what is initiating a flashback years after the event may not appear on the surface to be connected in any way to the original trauma.

✎ When previous trauma includes interpersonal violence, either as a child or adult, the risk of developing PTSD is particularly high following exposure to subsequent trauma.

✎ Peritrauma factors increasing the risk of PTSD development fall into three categories: characteristics of the trauma, survivor reactions, and psychosocial support.

✎ Perceived threat to life (92) and injury due to penetrating trauma (93) are consistently identified as major predicators for the development of PTSD.

✎ Trauma surgeons and intensivists should develop a level of expertise in counseling patients with these disorders, in addition to requesting early psychiatric consultation when appropriate.

✎ Treatment goals in PTSD are aimed at: reducing core symptoms, improving stress resilience, improving QoL, and reducing disability and comorbidity.

✎ The patient and family (when appropriate) should be made aware that there is a normal biological basis for their symptoms, and be reassured that treatment options are available to help them.

✎ Although no medications are approved for ASD, sertraline and paroxetine do have FDA indication for PTSD.

✎ Medication continuation beyond the symptom period may be prudent in PTSD, in order to reduce or prevent relapse.

✎ Factors associated with prolonged critical illness may play a causative role in PTSD, and critical illness may, of itself, be considered a traumatic event.

✎ Although patient wishes regarding mental health intervention should be honored, formal diagnostic evaluation is indicated whenever ASD or PTSD symptoms are present and causing significant distress.

✎ Optimum interventions for ASD and PTSD are symptom targeted and should be individualized to the patient's phase of illness and overall clinical condition.

REFERENCES

1. Michaels AJ, Michaels CE, Moon CH, et al. Posttraumatic stress disorder after injury: impact on general health outcome and early risk assessment. J Trauma 1999; 47:460–466.
2. Michaels AJ, Michaels CE, Zimmerman MA, Smith JS, Moon CH, Petersen C. Posttraumatic stress disorder in injured adults: etiology by path analysis. J Trauma 1999; 47:867–873.
3. Michaels AJ, Michaels CE, Smith JS, Moon CH, Petersen C, Long WB. Outcome from injury: general health, work status, and satisfaction 12 months after trauma. J Trauma 2000; 48:841–850.
4. Holbrook TL, Anderson JP, Sieber WJ, Browner D, Hoyt DB. Outcome after major trauma: 12-month and 18-month follow-up results from the Trauma Recovery Project. J Trauma 1999; 46:765–773.
5. Holbrook TL, Hoyt DB, Anderson JP. The impact of major in-hospital complications on functional outcome and quality of life after trauma. J Trauma 2001; 50:91–95.
6. Zatzick D, Jurkovich G, Russo J, et al. Posttraumatic Distress, Alcohol Disorders, and Recurrent Trauma Across Level 1 Trauma Centers. J Trauma 2004; 57(2):360–366.
7. Zatzick DF, Kang SM, Muller HG, et al. Predicting posttraumatic distress in hospitalized trauma survivors with acute injuries. Am J Psychiatry 2002; 159:941–946.
8. Michaels AJ, Michaels CE, Moon CH, Zimmerman MA, et al. Psychosocial factors limit outcomes after trauma. J Trauma 1998; 44:644–648.
9. Myers ABR. On the etiology and prevalence of diseases of the heart among soldiers: the "Alexander" prize essay. London: John Churchill and Sons, 1870:92,39,1.
10. DaCosta JM. On irritable heart: A clinical study of a form of functional cardiac disorder and its consequences. American Journal of Medical Science 1871; 161:17–52.
11. Acierno R, Resnick H, Kilpatrick DG, et al. Risk factors for rape, physical assault, and posttraumatic stress disorder in women: examination of differential multivariate relationships. J Anxiety Disord 1999; 13(6):541–563.
12. Kulka RA, Schlenger WE, et al. Trauma and the Vietnam War Generation: Report of Findings from the National Vietnam Veterans Readjustment Study. New York: Brunner/Mazel, 1990.
13. McCauley J, Kern DE, Kolodner K, et al. Clinical characteristics of women with a history of childhood abuse: unhealed wounds. JAMA 1997; 277(17):1362–1368.
14. Kessler RC, Sonnega A, Bromet E, et al. Posttraumatic stress disorder in the National Comorbidity Survey. Arch Gen Psychiatry 1995; 52(12):1048–1060.
15. McEwen BS, Stellar E. Stress and the individual. Mechanisms leading to disease. Arch Intern Med 1993; 153(18):2093–2101.
16. Brass LM, Hartigan PM, Page WF, et al. Importance of cerebrovascular disease in studies of myocardial infarction. Stroke 1996; 27(7):1173–1176.
17. Bremner JD, Vythilingam M, Anderson G, et al. Assessment of the hypothalamic-pituitary-adrenal axis over a 24-hour diurnal period and in response to neuroendocrine challenges in women with and without childhood sexual abuse and posttraumatic stress disorder. Biol Psychiatry 2003; 54(7):710–718.
18. Duval F, Crocq MA, Guillon MS, et al. Increased adrenocorticotropin suppression following dexamethasone administration in sexually abused adolescents with posttraumatic stress disorder. Psychoneuroendocrinology 2004; 29(10):1281–1289.
19. Ehlert U, Gaab J, Heinrichs M. Psychoneuroendocrinological contributions to the etiology of depression, posttraumatic stress disorder, and stress-related bodily disorders: the role of the hypothalamus-pituitary-adrenal axis. Biol Psychol 2001; 57(1–3):141–152.

20. Yehuda R. Post-Traumatic Stress Disorder. N Engl J Med 2002; 346(2):108–114.

21. Yehuda R, Golier JA, Halligan SL, et al. The ACTH response to dexamethasone in PTSD. Am J Psychiatry 2004; 161(8): 1397–1403.

22. Marshall RD, Blanco C, Printz D, et al. A pilot study of noradrenergic and HPA axis functioning in PTSD vs. panic disorder. Psychiatry Res 2002; 110(3):219–230.

23. Vasterling JJ, Duke LM, Brailey K, et al. Attention, learning, and memory performances and intellectual resources in Vietnam veterans: PTSD and no disorder comparisons. Neuropsychology 2002; 16(1):5–14.

24. Hull AM. Neuroimaging findings in post-traumatic stress disorder. Systematic review. Br J Psychiatry 2002; 181:102–110.

25. Lanius RA, Williamson PC, Boksman K, et al. Brain activation during script-driven imagery induced dissociative responses in PTSD: a functional magnetic resonance imaging investigation. Biol Psychiatry 2002; 52(4):305–311.

26. Wang Q, Wang Z, Zhu P, et al. Alterations of myelin basic protein and ultrastructure in the limbic system at the early stage of trauma-related stress disorder in dogs. J Trauma 2004; 56(3):604–610.

27. Zola-Morgan SM, Squire LR. The prinate hippocampal formation: Evidence for a time-limited role in memory storage. Science 1990; 250:288–290.

28. McClelland JL, McNaughton BL, O'Reilly RC. Why there are complementary learning systems in the hippocampus and neocortex: insights from the successes and failures of connectionist models of learning and memory. Psychol Rev 1995; 102(3):419–457.

29. Phillips RG, LeDoux JE. Differential contribution of amygdala and hippocampus to cued and contextual fear conditioning. Behav Neurosci 1992; 106(2):274–285.

30. Bohbot VD, Jech R, Ruzicka E, et al. Rat spatial memory tasks adapted for humans: characterization in subjects with intact brain and subjects with selective medial temporal lobe thermal lesions. Physiol Res 2002; 51(suppl 1):S49–S65.

31. Nadel L, Bohbot V. Consolidation of memory. Hippocampus 2001; 11(1):56–60.

32. Gunne LM, Reis DJ. Changes in brain catecholamines associated with electrical stimulation of amygdaloid nucleus. Life Sci 1963; 11:804–809.

33. Shumyatsky GP, Malleret G, Shin RM, et al. *Stathmin*, a gene enriched in the amygdala, controls both learned and innate fear. Cell 2005; 123:697–709.

34. Cahill L. The neurobiology of emotionally influenced memory. Implications for understanding traumatic memory. Ann NY Acad Sci 1997; 821:238–246.

35. Hamner MB, Lorberbaum JP, George MS. Potential role of the anterior cingulate cortex in PTSD: review and hypothesis. Depress Anxiety 1999; 9(1):1–14.

36. Nutt DJ, Malizia AL. Structural and functional brain changes in posttraumatic stress disorder. J Clin Psychiatry 2004; 65 (suppl 1):11–17.

37. Bremner JD, Staib LH, Kaloupek D, et al. Neural correlates of exposure to traumatic pictures and sound in Vietnam combat veterans with and without posttraumatic stress disorder: a positron emission tomography study. Biol Psychiatry 1999; 45(7):806–816.

38. Bremner JD, Vythilingam M, Vermetten E, et al. Neural correlates of declarative memory for emotionally valenced words in women with posttraumatic stress disorder related to early childhood sexual abuse. Biol Psychiatry 2003; 53(10): 879–889.

39. Bremner JD, Licinio J, Darnell A, et al. Elevated CSF corticotropin-releasing factor concentrations in posttraumatic stress disorder. Am J Psychiatry 1997; 154(5):624–629.

40. Bremner JD, Innis RB, Southwick SM, et al. Decreased benzodiazepine receptor binding in prefrontal cortex in combat-related posttraumatic stress disorder. Am J Psychiatry 2000; 157(7):1120–1126.

41. van der Kolk BA, Greenberg MS, Orr SP, et al. Endogenous opioids, stress induced analgesia, and posttraumatic stress disorder. Psychopharmacol Bull 1989; 25(3):417–421.

42. Petty F, Kramer G, Wilson L. Prevention of learned helplessness: in vivo correlation with cortical serotonin. Pharmacol Biochem Behav 1992; 43(2):361–367.

43. Bremner JD. Does Stress Damage the Brain? Understanding Trauma-Related Disorders from a Mind-Body Perspective. Vol. xii. New York: W.W. Norton, 2002:311.

44. Lindauer RJ, Vlieger EJ, Jalink M, et al. Smaller hippocampal volume in Dutch police officers with posttraumatic stress disorder. Biol Psychiatry 2004; 56(5):356–363.

45. Villarreal G, Hamilton DA, Petropoulos H, et al. Reduced hippocampal volume and total white matter volume in posttraumatic stress disorder. Biol Psychiatry 2002; 52(2): 119–125.

46. Bremner JD. Neuroimaging studies in post-traumatic stress disorder. Curr Psychiatry Rep 2002; 4(4):254–263.

47. Bremner JD, Krystal JH, Southwick SM, et al. Functional neuroanatomical correlates of the effects of stress on memory. J Trauma Stress 1995; 8(4):527–553.

48. Bremner JD, Randall P, Vermetten E, et al. Magnetic resonance imaging-based measurement of hippocampal volume in posttraumatic stress disorder related to childhood physical and sexual abuse–a preliminary report. Biol Psychiatry 1997; 41(1):23–32.

49. Stein MB, Hanna C, Koverola C, et al. Structural brain changes in PTSD. Does trauma alter neuroanatomy? Ann N Y Acad Sci 1997; 821:76–82.

50. Bremner JD, Vythilingam M, Vermetten E, et al. MRI and PET study of deficits in hippocampal structure and function in women with childhood sexual abuse and posttraumatic stress disorder. Am J Psychiatry 2003; 160(5):924–932.

51. Gurvits TV, Shenton ME, Hokama H, et al. Magnetic resonance imaging study of hippocampal volume in chronic, combat-related posttraumatic stress disorder. Biol Psychiatry 1996; 40(11):1091–1099.

52. Wignall EL, Dickson JM, Vaughan P, et al. Smaller hippocampal volume in patients with recent-onset posttraumatic stress disorder. Biol Psychiatry 2004; 56(11):832–836.

53. Smith MA, Makino S, Kvetnansky R, et al. Stress and glucocorticoids affect the expression of brain-derived neurotrophic factor and neurotrophin-3 mRNAs in the hippocampus. J Neurosci 1995; 15(3 Pt 1):1768–1777.

54. Gilboa A, Shalev AY, Laor L, et al. Functional connectivity of the prefrontal cortex and the amygdala in posttraumatic stress disorder. Biol Psychiatry 2004; 55(3):263–72.

55. Shin LM, Wright CI, Cannistraro PA, et al. A functional magnetic resonance imaging study of amygdala and medial prefrontal cortex responses to overtly presented fearful faces in posttraumatic stress disorder. Arch Gen Psychiatry 2005; 62(3):273–281.

56. Protopopescu X, Pan H, Tuescher O, et al. Differential time courses and specificity of amygdala activity in posttraumatic stress disorder subjects and normal control subjects. Biol Psychiatry 2005; 57(5):464–473.

57. Krauseneck T, Rothenhausler HB, Schelling G, et al. PTSD in somatic disease. Fortschr Neurol Psychiatr 2005; 73(4):206–217.

58. Nickel M, Leiberich P, Nickel C, et al. The occurrence of posttraumatic stress disorder in patients following intensive care treatment: a cross-sectional study in a random sample. J Intensive Care Med 2004; 19(5):285–290.

59. O'Donnell ML, Creamer M, Pattison P, et al. Psychiatric morbidity following injury. Am J Psychiatry 2004; 161(3): 507–514.

60. Tedstone JE, Tarrier N. Posttraumatic stress disorder following medical illness and treatment. Clin Psychol Rev 2003; 23(3):409–448.

61. Schelling G, Richter M, Roozendaal B, et al. Exposure to high stress in the intensive care unit may have negative effects on health-related quality-of-life outcomes after cardiac surgery. Crit Care Med 2003; 31(7):1971–1980.

62. Lude P, Kennedy P, Evans M, et al. Post traumatic distress symptoms following spinal cord injury: a comparative review of European samples. Spinal Cord 2005; 43(2):102–108.

63. Starr AJ, Smith WR, Frawley WH, et al. Symptoms of posttraumatic stress disorder after orthopaedic trauma. J Bone Joint Surg Am 2004; 86(6):1115–1121.

64. Young E, Eddleston J, Ingleby S, et al. Returning home after intensive care: a comparison of symptoms of anxiety and depression in ICU and elective cardiac surgery patients and their relatives. Intensive Care Med 2005; 31(1):86–91.

65. Schelling G, Stoll C, Haller M, et al. Health-related quality of life and posttraumatic stress disorder in survivors of the acute respiratory distress syndrome. Crit Care Med 1998; 26(4):651–659.

66. Kapfhammer HP, Rothenhausler HB, Krauseneck T, et al. Post-traumatic stress disorder and health-related quality of life in long-term survivors of acute respiratory distress syndrome. Am J Psychiatry 2004; 161(1):45–52.

67. Cuthbertson BH, Hull A, Strachan M, et al. Post-traumatic stress disorder after critical illness requiring general intensive care. Intensive Care Med 2004; 30(3):450–455.

68. Kress JP, Gehlbach B, Lacy M, et al. The long-term psychological effects of daily sedative interruption on critically ill patients. Am J Respir Crit Care Med 2003; 168(12): 1457–1461.

69. Rothenhausler HB, Ehrentraut S, Kapfhammer HP, et al. Psychiatric and psychosocial outcome of orthotopic liver transplantation. Psychother Psychosom 2002; 71(5):285–297.

70. Stoll C, Schelling G, Goetz AE, et al. Health-related quality of life and post-traumatic stress disorder in patients after cardiac surgery and intensive care treatment. J Thorac Cardiovasc Surg 2000; 120(3):505–512.

71. Lennmarken C, Bildfors K, Enlund G, et al. Victims of awareness. Acta Anaesthesiol Scand 2002; 46(3):229–231.

72. Tarrier N, Gregg L. Suicide risk in civilian PTSD patients–predictors of suicidal ideation, planning and attempts. Soc Psychiatry Psychiatr Epidemiol 2004; 39(8):655–661.

73. Marshall RD, Olfson M, Hellman F, et al. Comorbidity, impairment, and suicidality in subthreshold PTSD. Am J Psychiatry 2001; 158(9):1467–1473.

74. Fuglsang AK, Moergeli H, Schnyder U. Does acute stress disorder predict post-traumatic stress disorder in traffic accident victims? Analysis of a self-report inventory. Nord J Psychiatry 2004; 58(3):223–229.

75. Creamer M, O'Donnell ML, Pattison P. The relationship between acute stress disorder and posttraumatic stress disorder in severely injured trauma survivors. Behav Res Ther 2004; 42(3):315–328.

76. Bryant RA, Harvey AG: Gender differences in the relationship between acute stress disorder and posttraumatic stress disorder following motor vehicle accidents. Aust N Z J Psychiatry 2003; 37(2):226–229.

77. Harvey AG, Bryant RA. The relationship between acute stress disorder and posttraumatic stress disorder: a prospective evaluation of motor vehicle accident survivors. J Consult Clin Psychol 1998; 66(3):507–512.

78. Harvey AG, Bryant RA. Acute stress disorder after mild traumatic brain injury. J Nerv Ment Dis 1998; 186(6): 333–337.

79. Harvey AG, Bryant RA. Two-year prospective evaluation of the relationship between acute stress disorder and posttraumatic stress disorder following mild traumatic brain injury. Am J Psychiatry 2000; 157(4):626–628.

80. Brewin CR, Andrews B, Rose S, et al. Acute stress disorder and posttraumatic stress disorder in victims of violent crime. Am J Psychiatry 1999; 156(3):360–366.

81. Anderson CL, Alexander PC. The relationship between attachment and dissociation in adult survivors of incest. Psychiatry 1996; 59(3):240–254.

82. Steinberg M, Steinberg A. Using the SCID-D to assess dissociative identity disorder in adolescents: three case studies. Bull Menninger Clin 1995; 59(2):221–231.

83. Guralnik O, Schmeidler J, Simeon D. Feeling unreal: cognitive processes in depersonalization. Am J Psychiatry 2000; 157(1):103–109.

84. Betemps EJ, Smith RM, Baker DG, et al. Measurement precision of the clinician administered PTSD scale (CAPS): a RASCH model analysis. J Appl Meas 2003; 4(1):59–69.

85. Blake DD, Weathers FW, Nagy LM, et al. The development of a clinician-administered PTSD scale. J Trauma Stress 1995; 8(1):75–90.

86. Blanchard EB, Jones-Alexander J, Buckley TC, et al. Psychometric properties of the PTSD Checklist (PCL). Behav Res Ther 1996; 34(8):669–673.

87. Weathers FW, Keane TM, Davidson JR. Clinician-administered PTSD scale: a review of the first ten years of research. Depress Anxiety 2001; 13(3):132–156.

88. Yao SN, Cottraux J, Note I, et al. Evaluation of Post-traumatic Stress Disorder: validation of a measure, the PCLS. Encephale 2003; 29(3 Pt 1):232–238.

89. Bremner JD, Southwick SM, Johnson DR, et al. Childhood physical abuse and combat-related posttraumatic stress disorder in Vietnam veterans. Am J Psychiatry 1993; 150(2): 235–239.

90. Stone RC. Psychiatric Diagnoses in Patients of an Urban County Domestic Violence Center. In Annual Meeting of the American Psychiatric Association, New Research. Philadelphia, PA, 2001.

91. True WR, Rice J, Eisen SA, et al. A twin study of genetic and environmental contributions to liability for posttraumatic stress symptoms. Arch Gen Psychiatry 1993; 50(4):257–264.

92. Holbrook TL, Hoyt DB, Stein MB, Sieber WJ. Perceived threat to life predicts posttraumatic stress disorder after major trauma: risk factors and functional outcome. J Trauma 2001; 51:287–293.

93. Greenspan AI, Kellermann AL. Physical and psychological outcomes 8 months after serious gunshot injury. J Trauma 2002; 53:709–716.

94. Bremner JD, Krystal JH, Putnam FW, et al. Measurement of dissociative states with the Clinician-Administered Dissociative States Scale (CADSS). J Trauma Stress 1998; 11(1):125–136.

95. Yehuda R, McFarlane AC, Shalev AY. Predicting the development of posttraumatic stress disorder from the acute response to a traumatic event. Biol Psychiatry 1998; 44(12):1305–1313.

96. Fuglsang AK, Moergeli H, Hepp-Beg S, et al. Who develops acute stress disorder after accidental injuries? Psychother Psychosom 2002; 71(4):214–222.

97. Schnyder U, Morgeli H, Nigg C, et al. Early psychological reactions to life-threatening injuries. Crit Care Med 2000; 28(1):86–92.

98. Hembree EA, Street GP, Riggs DS, et al. Do assault-related variables predict response to cognitive behavioral treatment for PTSD? J Consult Clin Psychol 2004; 72(3):531–534.

99. Holbrook TL, Hoyt DB, Coimbra R, et al. Long-term posttraumatic stress disorder persists after major trauma in adolescents: new data on risk factors and functional outcome. J Trauma 2005; 58(4):764–769; discussion 9–71.

100. Bryant RA, Harvey AG. Gender differences in the relationship between acute stress disorder and posttraumatic stress disorder following motor vehicle accidents. Aust N Z J Psychiatry 2003; 37(2):226–229.

101. Holbrook TL, Hoyt DB, Anderson JP. The importance of gender on outcome after major trauma: functional and psychologic outcomes in women versus men. J Trauma 2001; 50: 270–273.

102. Holbrook TL, Hoyt DB, Stein MB, Sieber WJ. Gender differences in long-term posttraumatic stress disorder after major trauma: women are at higher risk of adverse outcomes than men. J Trauma 2002; 53:882–888.

103. Holbrook TL, Hoyt DB. The impact of major trauma: quality-of-life outcomes are worse in women than in men, independent of mechanism and injury severity. J Trauma 2004; 56:284–290.

104. Holbrook TL, Hoyt DB, Coimbra R, et al. High rates of acute stress disorder impact quality-of-life outcomes in injured

adolescents: mechanism and gender predict acute stress disorder risk. J Trauma 2005; 59:1126–1130.

105. Jones C, Griffiths RD, Humphris G, et al. Memory, delusions, and the development of acute posttraumatic stress disorder-related symptoms after intensive care. Crit Care Med 2001; 29(3):573–580.

106. Willebrand M, Andersson G, Ekselius L. Prediction of psychological health after an accidental burn. J Trauma 2004; 57(2):367–374.

107. Van Loey NE, Maas CJ, Faber AW, et al. Predictors of chronic posttraumatic stress symptoms following burn injury: results of a longitudinal study. J Trauma Stress 2003; 16(4):361–369.

108. Ginzburg K, Solomon Z, Koifman B, et al. Trajectories of posttraumatic stress disorder following myocardial infarction: a prospective study. J Clin Psychiatry 2003; 64(10):1217–1223.

109. Martz E. Death anxiety as a predictor of posttraumatic stress levels among individuals with spinal cord injuries. Death Stud 2004; 28(1):1–17.

110. Glaesser J, Neuner F, Lutgehetmann R, et al. Posttraumatic stress disorder in patients with traumatic brain injury. BMC Psychiatry 2004; 4(1):5.

111. Jones C, Skirrow P, Griffiths RD, et al. Post-traumatic stress disorder-related symptoms in relatives of patients following intensive care. Intensive Care Med 2004; 30(3):456–460.

112. Lee S, Brasel K, Lee B. Emergency care practitioners' barriers to mental health assessment, treatment, and referral of post-injury patients. Western Med J 2004; 103(6):78–82.

113. Rincon HG, Granados M, Unutzer J, et al. Prevalence, detection and treatment of anxiety, depression, and delirium in the adult critical care unit. Psychosomatics 2001; 42(5):391–396.

114. Papa FJ, Stone RC, Aldrich DG. Further evidence of the relationship between case typicality and diagnostic performance: implications for medical education. Acad Med 1996; 71(suppl 1):S10–S12.

115. O'Donnell ML, Creamer M, Pattison P. Posttraumatic stress disorder and depression following trauma: understanding comorbidity. Am J Psychiatry 2004; 161(8):1390–1396.

116. Fraguas Junior R, Ramadan ZB, Pereira AN, et al. Depression with irritability in patients undergoing coronary artery bypass graft surgery: the cardiologist's role. Gen Hosp Psychiatry 2000; 22(5):365–374.

117. Baker RA, Andrew MJ, Schrader G, et al. Preoperative depression and mortality in coronary artery bypass surgery: preliminary findings. ANZ J Surg 2001; 71(3):139–142.

118. Blumenthal JA, Lett HS, Babyak MA, et al. Depression as a risk factor for mortality after coronary artery bypass surgery. Lancet 2003; 362(9384):604–609.

119. Connerney I, Shapiro PA, McLaughlin JS, et al. Relation between depression after coronary artery bypass surgery and 12-month outcome: a prospective study. Lancet 2001; 358(9295):1766–1771.

120. Ho PM, Masoudi FA, Spertus JA, et al. Depression predicts mortality following cardiac valve surgery. Ann Thorac Surg 2005; 79(4):1255–1259.

121. Borowicz L Jr, Royall R, Grega M, et al. Depression and cardiac morbidity 5 years after coronary artery bypass surgery. Psychosomatics 2002; 43(6):464–471.

122. Blanchard EB, Hickling EJ, Taylor AE, et al. Who develops PTSD from motor vehicle accidents? Behav Res Ther 1996; 34(1):1–10.

123. Koren D, Arnon I, Klein E. Acute stress response and posttraumatic stress disorder in traffic accident victims: a one-year prospective, follow-up study. Am J Psychiatry 1999; 156(3):367–373.

124. Bisson JI. Single-session early psychological interventions following traumatic events. Clin Psychol Rev 2003; 23(3):481–499.

125. Gist R, Devilly GJ. Post-trauma debriefing: the road too frequently traveled. Lancet 2002; 360(9335):741–742.

126. Bisson JI. Post-traumatic stress counseling. Br J Hosp Med 1997; 57(3):112.

127. Rose S, Bisson J, Churchill R, et al. Psychological debriefing for preventing post traumatic stress disorder (PTSD). Cochrane Database Syst Rev 2002;ISS2Art No:CD000560.

128. van Emmerik AA, Kamphuis JH, Hulsbosch AM, et al. Single session debriefing after psychological trauma: a meta-analysis. Lancet 2002; 360(9335):766–771.

129. Bledsoe BE. EMS mythology, Part 3. EMS myth #3: Critical incident stress management (CISM) is effective in managing EMS-related stress. Emerg Med Serv 2003; 32(5):77–80.

130. Foa EB, Hearst-Ikeda D, Perry KJ. Evaluation of a brief cognitive-behavioral program for the prevention of chronic PTSD in recent assault victims. J Consult Clin Psychol 1995; 63(6):948–955.

131. Bryant RA, Harvey AG, Dang ST, et al. Treatment of acute stress disorder: a comparison of cognitive-behavioral therapy and supportive counseling. J Consult Clin Psychol 1998; 66(5):862–866.

132. North CS, Hong BA. Project CREST: A new model for mental health intervention after a community disaster. Am J Publ Health 2000; 90:1057–1058.

133. Bradley R, Greene J, Russ E, et al. A multidimensional meta-analysis of psychotherapy for PTSD. Am J Psychiatry 2005; 162(2):214–227.

134. Blanchard EB, Hickling EJ, Malta LS, et al. One- and two-year prospective follow-up of cognitive behavior therapy or supportive psychotherapy. Behav Res Ther 2004; 42(7):745–759.

135. Ehlers A, Clark DM, Hackmann A, et al. A randomized controlled trial of cognitive therapy, a self-help booklet, and repeated assessments as early interventions for posttraumatic stress disorder. Arch Gen Psychiatry 2003; 60(10):1024–1032.

136. Hembree EA, Foa EB, Dorfan NM, et al. Do patients drop out prematurely from exposure therapy for PTSD? J Trauma Stress 2003; 16(6):555–562.

137. Shepherd J, Stein K, Milne R. Eye movement desensitization and reprocessing in the treatment of post-traumatic stress disorder: a review of an emerging therapy. Psychol Med 2000; 30(4):863–871.

138. Taylor S, Thordarson DS, Maxfield L, et al. Comparative efficacy, speed, and adverse effects of three PTSD treatments: exposure therapy, EMDR, and relaxation training. J Consult Clin Psychol 2003; 71(2):330–338.

139. Mellman TA, Byers PM, Augenstein JS. Pilot evaluation of hypnotic medication during acute traumatic stress response. J Trauma Stress 1998; 11(3):563–569.

140. Gelpin E, Bonne O, Peri T, et al. Treatment of recent trauma survivors with benzodiazepines: a prospective study. J Clin Psychiatry 1996; 57(9):390–394.

141. Vaiva G, Ducrocq F, Jezequel K, et al. Immediate treatment with propranolol decreases posttraumatic stress disorder two months after trauma. Biol Psychiatry 2003; 54(9):947–949.

142. Pitman RK, Sanders KM, Zusman RM, et al. Pilot study of secondary prevention of posttraumatic stress disorder with propranolol. Biol Psychiatry 2002; 51(2):189–192.

143. Marshall RD, Cloitre M. Maximizing treatment outcome in post-traumatic stress disorder by combining psychotherapy with pharmacotherapy. Curr Psychiatry Rep 2000; 2(4):335–340.

144. Foa EB, Keane TM, Friedman MJ, et al. Effective treatments for PTSD: practice guidelines from the International Society for Traumatic Stress Studies. Vol. xii. New York: Guilford Press, 2000:388.

145. Yehuda R. Treating trauma survivors with PTSD. Vol. Xvi. 1st ed. Washington, DC: American Psychiatric Pub, 2002:199.

146. Friedman MJ. Future pharmacotherapy for post-traumatic stress disorder: prevention and treatment. Psychiatr Clin North Am 2002; 25(2):427–441.

147. Davidson JR. Remission in post-traumatic stress disorder (PTSD): effects of sertraline as assessed by the Davidson Trauma Scale, Clinical Global Impressions and the Clinician-Administered PTSD scale. Int Clin Psychopharmacol 2004; 19(2):85–87.

148. Brady KT, Clary CM. Affective and anxiety comorbidity in post-traumatic stress disorder treatment trials of sertraline. Compr Psychiatry 2003; 44(5):360–369.

149. Davidson JR. Treatment of posttraumatic stress disorder: the impact of paroxetine. Psychopharmacol Bull 2003; 37(suppl 1):76–88.

150. Bremner JD, Vermetten E. Neuroanatomical changes associated with pharmacotherapy in posttraumatic stress disorder. Ann N Y Acad Sci 2004; 1032:154–157.

151. Stone RC. Tricyclics Versus SSRIs in Overdose: A Retrospective Study. In Annual Meeting of the American Psychiatric Association, New Research. Washington, D.C, 1999.

152. Brkanac Z, Pastor JF, Storck M. Prazosin in PTSD. J Am Acad Child Adolesc Psychiatry 2003; 42(4):384–385.

153. Raskind MA, Peskind ER, Kanter ED et al. Reduction of nightmares and other PTSD symptoms in combat veterans by prazosin: a placebo-controlled study. Am J Psychiatry 2003; 160(2):371–3.

154. Asnis GM, Kohn SR, Henderson M, et al. SSRIs versus non-SSRIs in post-traumatic stress disorder: an update with recommendations. Drugs 2004; 64(4):383–404.

155. Looff D, Grimley P, Kuller F, et al. Carbamazepine for PTSD. J Am Acad Child Adolesc Psychiatry 1995; 34(6):703–704.

156. Petty F, Davis LL, Nugent AL, et al. Valproate therapy for chronic, combat-induced posttraumatic stress disorder. J Clin Psychopharmacol 2002; 22(1):100–101.

157. Clark RD, Canive JM, Calais LA, et al. Divalproex in posttraumatic stress disorder: an open-label clinical trial. J Trauma Stress 1999; 12(2):395–401.

158. Berlant JL. Prospective open-label study of add-on and monotherapy topiramate in civilians with chronic nonhallucinatory posttraumatic stress disorder. BMC Psychiatry 2004; 4(1):24.

159. Bremner JD, Mletzko T, Welter S, et al. Treatment of posttraumatic stress disorder with phenytoin: an open-label pilot study. J Clin Psychiatry 2004; 65(11):1559–1564.

160. Malek-Ahmadi P. Gabapentin and posttraumatic stress disorder. Ann Pharmacother 2003; 37(5):664–666.

161. Hamner MB, Brodrick PS, Labbate LA. Gabapentin in PTSD: a retrospective, clinical series of adjunctive therapy. Ann Clin Psychiatry 2001; 13(3):141–146.

162. Hertzberg MA, Butterfield MI, Feldman ME, et al. A preliminary study of lamotrigine for the treatment of posttraumatic stress disorder. Biol Psychiatry 1999; 45(9):1226–1229.

163. Wagstaff AJ, Easton J, Scott LJ. Intramuscular olanzapine: a review of its use in the management of acute agitation. CNS Drugs 2005; 19(2):147–164.

164. Turczynski J, Bidzan L, Staszewska-Malys E. Olanzapine in the treatment of agitation in hospitalized patients with schizophrenia and schizoaffective and schizofreniform disorders. Med Sci Monit 2004; 10(5):I74–180.

165. Baker RW, Kinon BJ, Maguire GA, et al. Effectiveness of rapid initial dose escalation of up to forty milligrams per day of oral olanzapine in acute agitation. J Clin Psychopharmacol 2003; 23(4):342–348.

166. Petty F, Brannan S, Casada J, et al. Olanzapine treatment for post-traumatic stress disorder: an open-label study. Int Clin Psychopharmacol 2001; 16(6):331–337.

167. Jakovljevic M, Sagud M, Mihaljevic-Peles A. Olanzapine in the treatment-resistant, combat-related PTSD–a series of case reports. Acta Psychiatr Scand 2003; 107(5):394–396; discussion 6.

168. Pivac N, Kozaric-Kovacic D, Muck-Seler D. Olanzapine versus fluphenazine in an open trial in patients with psychotic combat-related post-traumatic stress disorder. Psychopharmacology (Berl) 2004; 175(4):451–456.

169. Stone RC. Olanzapine Treatment of Severe PTSD: A Case Series Report. In Annual Meeting of the American Psychiatric Association, New Research. 2000.

170. Hamner MB, Faldowski RA, Ulmer HG, et al. Adjunctive risperidone treatment in post-traumatic stress disorder: a preliminary controlled trial of effects on comorbid psychotic symptoms. Int Clin Psychopharmacol 2003; 18(1):1–8.

171. Bartzokis G, Lu PH, Turner J, et al. Adjunctive risperidone in the treatment of chronic combat-related posttraumatic stress disorder. Biol Psychiatry 2005; 57(5):474–479.

172. Reich DB, Winternitz S, Hennen J, et al. A preliminary study of risperidone in the treatment of posttraumatic stress disorder related to childhood abuse in women. J Clin Psychiatry 2004; 65(12):1601–1606.

173. Sokolski KN, Denson TF, Lee RT, et al. Quetiapine for treatment of refractory symptoms of combat-related post-traumatic stress disorder. Mil Med 2003; 168(6):486–489.

174. Hamner MB, Deitsch SE, Brodrick PS, et al. Quetiapine treatment in patients with posttraumatic stress disorder: an open trial of adjunctive therapy. J Clin Psychopharmacol 2003; 23(1):15–20.

175. Hamner MB, Frueh BC, Ulmer HG, et al. Psychotic features in chronic posttraumatic stress disorder and schizophrenia: comparative severity. J Nerv Ment Dis 2000; 188(4):217–221.

176. Davidson JR, Landerman LR, Farfel GM, et al. Characterizing the effects of sertraline in post-traumatic stress disorder. Psychol Med 2002; 32(4):661–670.

177. Rapaport MH, Endicott J, Clary CM. Posttraumatic stress disorder and quality of life: results across 64 weeks of sertraline treatment. J Clin Psychiatry 2002; 63(1):59–65.

178. Zatzick D, Roy-Byrne P, Russo J, et al. A randomized effectiveness trial of stepped collaborative care for acutely injured trauma survivors. Arch Gen Psychiatry 2004; 61(5):498–506.

179. Pennebaker JW. Writing to Heal: A Guided Journal for Recovering from Trauma & Emotional Upheaval. Vol. vi. Oakland, CA, [S.l.]: New Harbinger Publications, Distributed in Canada by Raincoast Books, 2004: 164.

180. Combe D. The use of patient diaries in an intensive care unit. Nurs Crit Care 2005; 10(1):31–34.

181. Grossman P, Niemann L, Schmidt S, et al. Mindfulness-based stress reduction and health benefits. A meta-analysis. J Psychosom Res 2004; 57(1):35–43.

182. Carlson LE, Speca M, Patel KD, et al. Mindfulness-based stress reduction in relation to quality of life, mood, symptoms of stress and levels of cortisol, dehydroepiandrosterone sulfate (DHEAS) and melatonin in breast and prostate cancer outpatients. Psychoneuroendocrinology 2004; 29(4):448–474.

183. Difede J, Hoffman HG. Virtual reality exposure therapy for world trade center post-traumatic stress disorder: a case report. Cyberpsychol Behav 2002; 5(6):529–535.

184. Rothbaum BO, Hodges LF, Ready D, et al. Virtual reality exposure therapy for Vietnam veterans with posttraumatic stress disorder. J Clin Psychiatry 2001; 62(8):617–622.

185. Cardena E. Hypnosis in the treatment of trauma: a promising, but not fully supported, efficacious intervention. Int J Clin Exp Hypn 2000; 48(2):225–238.

186. Gratz KL, Gunderson JG. Preliminary data on an acceptance-based emotion regulation group intervention for deliberate self-harm among women with Borderline Personality Disorder. Behavior Therapy 2006; 37:25–35.

187. Hayes SC, Wilson K. G, Gifford E, et al. The use of acceptance and commitment therapy and 12-step facilitation in the treatment of polysubstance abusing heroin addicts on methadone maintenance: a randomized controlled trial. Paper presented at the meeting of the Association for Behavior Analysis. Toronto; 2002.

188. Orsillo SM, Batten SV. Acceptance and commitment therapy in the treatment of posttraumatic stress disorder. Behav Modif 2005; 29(1):95–129.

189. Schelling G, Kilger E, Roozendaal B, et al. Stress doses of hydrocortisone, traumatic memories, and symptoms of posttraumatic stress disorder in patients after cardiac surgery: a randomized study. Biol Psychiatry 2004; 55(6):627–633.

190. Schelling G, Roozendaal B, De Quervain DJ. Can posttraumatic stress disorder be prevented with glucocorticoids? Ann NY Acad Sci 2004; 1032:158–166.

191. Schelling G, Briegel J, Roozendaal B, et al. The effect of stress doses of hydrocortisone during septic shock on posttraumatic stress disorder in survivors. Biol Psychiatry 2001; 50(12):978–985.

192. Prins A, Kimerling R, Cameron R, et al. PTSD Screen Paper Presentation at the 15th Annual International Society for Traumatic Stress Studies 1999, Miami, FL, 1999.

193. O'Reilly SM, Grubb N, O'Carroll RE. Long-term emotional consequences of in-hospital cardiac arrest and myocardial infarction. Br J Clin Psychol 2004; 43(Pt 1):83–95.

194. Momartin S, Silove D, Manicavasagar V, et al. Comorbidity of PTSD and depression: associations with trauma exposure, symptom severity and functional impairment in Bosnian refugees resettled in Australia. J Affect Disord 2004; 80(2–3): 231–238.

195. Momartin S, Silove D, Manicavasagar V, et al. Dimensions of trauma associated with posttraumatic stress disorder (PTSD) caseness, severity and functional impairment: a study of Bosnian refugees resettled in Australia. Soc Sci Med 2003; 57(5):775–781.

196. Cardozo BL, Bilukha OO, Crawford CA, et al. Mental health, social functioning, and disability in postwar Afghanistan. JAMA 2004; 29(5):575–584.

197. Gregurek R, Pavic L, Vuger-Kovacic H, et al. Increase of frequency of post-traumatic stress disorder in disabled war veterans during prolonged stay in a rehabilitation hospital. Croat Med J 2001; 42(2):161–164.

198. Oquendo M, Brent DA, Birmaher B, et al. Posttraumatic stress disorder comorbid with major depression: factors mediating the association with suicidal behavior. Am J Psychiatry 2005; 162(3):560–566.

199. Martz E. Do post-traumatic stress symptoms predict reactions of adaptation to disability after a sudden-onset spinal cord injury? Int J Rehabil Res 2004; 27(3):185–194.

200. Jaycox LH, Marshall GN, Schell T. Use of mental health services by men injured through community violence. Psychiatr Serv 2004; 55(4):415–420.

201. Kleinpell R, Silva N, Tully MJ, Hancock B. The use of a web-based education program to promote family member satisfaction with ICU care. Crit Care Med 2005; 33(12) suppl (261S).

202. Zatzick DF, Russo JE, Katon W. Somatic, posttraumatic stress, and depressive symptoms among injured patients treated in trauma surgery. Psychosomatics 2003; 44(6):479–484.

203. Andreski P, Chilcoat H, Breslau N. Post-traumatic stress disorder and somatization symptoms: a prospective study. Psychiatry Res 1998; 79(2):131–138.

204. Tagay S, Herpertz S, Langkafel M, et al. Trauma, post-traumatic stress disorder and somatization. Psychother Psychosom Med Psychol 2004; 54(5):198–205.

205. Boscarino JA. Posttraumatic stress disorder and physical illness: results from clinical and epidemiologic studies. Ann N Y Acad Sci 2004; 1032:141–153.

206. Schuder SE. stress-induced hypocortisolemia diagnosed as psychiatric disorders responsive to hydrocortisone replacement. Annals NY Acad Sci 2005; 1057:466–478.

207. Weis F, Kilger E, Roozendaal B, et al. Stress doses of hydrocortisone reduce chronic stress symptoms and improve health-related quality of life in high-risk patients after cardiac surgery: A randomized study. J Thorac Cardiovasc Surg 2006; 131(2):277–282.

208. Anisman H, Griffiths J, Matheson K, Ravindran AV, Merali Z. Posttraumatic stress symptoms and salivary cortisol levels. Am J Psychiatry 2001;158:1509–1511.

66

Rehabilitation for Trauma and Critical Care

J. C. Heygood

Division of Occupational Therapy, Department of Rehabilitation Services, UC San Diego Medical Center,
San Diego, California, U.S.A.

Kerrie Olexa

Division of Physical Therapy, Department of Rehabilitation Services, UC San Diego Medical Center,
San Diego, California, U.S.A.

INTRODUCTION

Patients who survive massive trauma and critical illness must not only overcome the initial injury but also the profound debilitation of many other organ systems during their recovery. For example, orthopedic spine injuries may cause paralysis (with its multiple ramifications); pulmonary contusions may lead to severe acute respiratory distress syndrome and prolonged ventilatory dependence; and hemorrhagic pancreatitis will often cause anemia, as well as metabolic and nutritional complications. Organ systems not directly injured by the trauma may also become impaired following critical illness. For example, renal failure may develop from radio-contrast dye, hypotension, aminoglycosides, or immunosuppressant therapy. ICU psychosis may result from sleep deprivation and drug withdrawal, or the administration of multiple psychoactive compounds. Even in excellent specialized trauma units, critically ill patients may develop derangements in the hematological, endocrine, metabolic, and immunological systems. Furthermore, all patients confined to bedrest for prolonged periods of time will suffer deconditioning of cardiovascular and musculoskeletal systems and become susceptible to decubitus ulcers, deep venous thrombosis (DVT), muscle weakness, and joint contractures. All of these systems must be rehabilitated for optimum outcomes to occur.

☛ **The overall goal of rehabilitation is to achieve maximum restoration of the patient's physical, psychological, social, vocational, recreational, and economic functions within the limits imposed by the trauma, critical illness, or any other pre-morbid deconditioning that may have occurred.** ☛ Successful rehabilitation requires a dedicated multidisciplinary team working together toward the above stated goal. This multidisciplinary team includes the physicians, nurses, physical therapists (PTs), occupational therapists (OTs), speech and language pathologists, respiratory therapists, social workers, psychiatrists, vocational counselors, and the patient and family.

This chapter focuses upon the key role played by PT and OT teams during rehabilitation from trauma and critical illness. The review begins by defining the scope of practice for both PTs and OTs. Next, the consequences of prolonged bedrest and deconditioning are discussed. The methodology utilized to complete a formal PT and OT needs assessment, as well as the criteria for monitoring and discharge planning are then discussed. Specific rehabilitation for various organ system injuries are also provided, as are important age-specific guidelines. The psychological hurdles that must be overcome for successful rehabilitation in the intensive care unit (ICU) are thoroughly presented, and factors affecting overall patient outcomes are summarized thereafter. Recently developed and emerging ideas for rehabilitation are presented in "Eye to the Future" section. The benefits of early rehabilitation following trauma and critical care are emphasized throughout this text.

PHYSICAL AND OCCUPATIONAL THERAPIES DEFINED
Physical Therapy

☛ **PT involves the identification, prevention, correction, and rehabilitation of acute or prolonged movement dysfunction of any etiology.** ☛ The musculoskeletal, neuromuscular, and cardiopulmonary systems are most often impacted by trauma and/or critical illness (1). PTs assess the physiological factors that may contribute to any movement dysfunction, as well as the previous and current levels of gross motor function. The involvement of the various impairments is considered, while formulating goals and treatment plans that are instituted by the primary PT and the PT assistant. Just as in other specialties, the realm of rehabilitation medicine is replete with specific jargon and a large list of commonly employed abbreviations (Table 1). The ultimate PT goal is to maximize patients' gross motor function and achieve independent functional mobility. As integral members of the ICU team, PTs provide input to the primary service and critical care physicians through direct communication, during rehabilitation rounds, and through documentation, thus ensuring maximum progress for the patient.

Initiation of the PT process in the ICU is analogous to "jump-starting a car's battery," in order to prepare the patient for more aggressive PT in the future. Patients who are unable to actively participate in PT cannot be treated as aggressively as interactive patients. However, treatment goals will be established to prevent the secondary complications of prolonged bedrest. After ensuring maximum range of motion (ROM), contracture prevention, and caregiver education, the PT's next goal is rehabilitation of the patient's gross motor skills. In the ICU setting, these skills relate to functional mobility, including rolling, moving to and from supine and sitting, and transfers from bed to chair and back. In many instances, the initiation of gait training coincides with recommendations for the use of support devices such as an ankle foot orthotic. Assistive devices may be issued for out of bed activities.

Table 1   Common Physical Therapy and Occupational Therapy Abbreviations

Abbreviation	Definition
Weight-bearing status:	
NWB	Non-weight bearing
TDWB	Touch-down weight bearing (<10%, unless otherwise stated)
PWB	Partial weight bearing (25 or 50%, unless otherwise stated)
WBAT	Weight bearing as tolerated
FWB	Full weight bearing
Adaptive equipment:	
w/c	Wheelchair
FWW	Front wheeled walker
PUW	Pick-up walker
PFW	Platform walker
HW	Hemi-walker
AC or CR	Axial crutches
QC	Quad cane
SPC	Single-point cane
BSC or 3:1	Bedside commode/"three-in-one" commode
Miscellaneous:	
A&Ox4	Alert and oriented to person, place, time, and situation
ADL	Activity of daily living
OOB	Out of bed
WFL	Within functional limits
HEP	Home exercise program
CI	Contraindicated

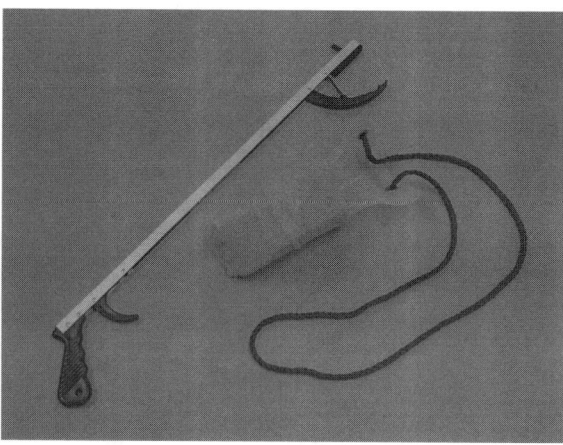

Figure 1   Reacher and sock aide: Both devices are commonly used by patients who are unable or instructed not to bend down during lower body dressing. The reacher can also be used to grab items that are low, high, or outside of the patient's base of support to prevent the need for reaching.

Occupational Therapy

☞ **OT primarily focuses upon improving patients' abilities to perform activities of daily living (ADLs) and functional mobility.** ☞ "Occupation" is defined as "specific 'chunks' of activity within the ongoing stream of human behavior, which are named in the lexicon of the culture (2)." In the context of a hospital, the patients' occupations are often limited to basic ADLs such as dressing, bathing, grooming, and self-feeding. Occupational therapists (OTs) use such occupations as therapeutic modalities to allow their patients to regain function, strength, and independence. Important functional mobility addressed by OTs in this setting include: transferring to and from a toilet, moving into and out of a bathtub or shower, as well as sitting and standing while performing ADLs. Other functional activities commonly addressed by OTs include: household management, driving safety, recreation, and work tasks, in addition to addressing various cognitive and psychosocial deficits. Adaptive equipment can be issued to expedite patients' progress toward regaining functional independence. Two commonly employed adaptive equipment devices (the reacher and the sock aide) assist patients with lower body dressing (Fig. 1). Because trauma and critical illness often lead to functional decline in numerous areas, OTs help foster maximal progress toward independence by employing these and other adaptive devices.

Patients in the ICU benefit from early OT intervention by promoting patient participation in ADLs, functional mobility, and cognitive or perceptual activities. OTs can help patients with tasks as simple as face washing or feeding, or with transferring to and from a bedside commode. These seemingly trivial activities provide major benefits to critically ill patients by helping them feel more independent. Additionally, the light exercise helps prevent further decline caused by inactivity. The OTs also address fine motor and eye-hand coordination, cognitive impairments, and visual/perceptual deficits, as they are all important components contributing to patients' functional decline. OT assistants also work closely with patients, expanding the range of patient care and providing key information in collaboration with the therapist for setting treatment priorities or revising goals.

Splinting is another important focus of OT. Splints maintain the body in a functional position and prevent the development of contractures. This is especially important for minimally-conscious or sedated patients who are immobile, as they present a higher risk for developing contractures and skin breakdown. Splints can be pre-fabricated or custom-made from thermoplastic or other materials. Splints are most commonly used to protect or support the hands, wrists, and ankles. However, splints can be fabricated for almost any joint, including the neck, knees, elbows, and shoulders. Note that there is some crossover between the interventions performed by OTs and PTs, however the final balance of roles and responsibilities is often institution-dependent.

CONSEQUENCES OF PROLONGED BED REST AND INACTIVITY

For over sixty years, research has shown that prolonged bedrest is detrimental to a satisfactory post-surgical recovery. Indeed, as early as 1944, a study published in the *Journal of the American Medical Association* stated that physicians should "always consider complete bedrest as a highly unphysiologic and definitely hazardous form of therapy, to be ordered only for specific indications and discontinued as early as possible (3)." The sooner bedrest is discontinued and rehabilitation ordered, the better the patient's prognosis unless the patient has an unstable spine or other injuries requiring temporary immobility.

Table 2 Preventative Measures to Combat Sequelae of Prolonged Bedrest

Organ system	Potential results of prolonged bedrest and inactivity	PT and OT preventative measures
Cognitive	Decreased cognitive function, confusion, hallucinations	Exercise, activity, daytime orientation
Psychiatric	Depression, anxiety, apathy, decreased pain tolerance	Exercise, activity, sitting, social interaction
Respiratory	Decreased oxygen saturation, pneumonia	Sitting, standing, activity, deep breathing
Cardiovascular	Increased heart rate, decreased aerobic capacity, orthostatic hypotension, DVT, PE	Exercise, AROM, standing, activity, compression devices
Muscular	Weakness, decreased muscle mass, muscle atrophy	AROM, exercise, stretching, activity
Skeletal	Decreased bone density, osteoporosis/osteopenia, fractures	Standing, exercise, weight-bearing, activity
Joints	Contractures, osteoarthritis	AROM, PROM, stretching, splinting
Skin	Pressure ulcers, tissue ischemia	Frequent turning, positioning, splinting

Abbreviations: PT, physical therapy; OT, occupational therapy; DVT, deep venous thrombosis; PE, pulmonary embolism; AROM, active range of motion; PROM, passive range of motion.

☞ **Patients relegated to extended bedrest suffer more secondary disabilities and require longer recovery periods than patients who are mobilized out of bed early.** ☞ Table 2 provides a summary of conditions resulting from prolonged bedrest and inactivity, along with preventive measures that can be employed by PT and OT. Common morbidities of chronic confinement to bed include musculoskeletal and cardiovascular deconditioning. Other common problems include contractures, decubitus ulcers, and DVTs. Accordingly, it is important to order rehabilitation for patients early in their hospital stay.

Musculoskeletal Weakness

The wasting and other ramifications of muscle disuse are dramatic and may be long lasting. Within just four hours of strict bedrest, muscles begin to atrophy, exhibiting decreased mass, cell diameter, and number of cell fibers (4). Several studies regarding the effects of bedrest have confirmed that decreased activity in the ICU negatively affects a patient's functional status. In fact, muscle strength declines 1% to 1.5% per day following strict bedrest, and up to 40% after only one week (5–9).

Antigravity muscles, involved in activities such as standing and ambulation, face the highest rate of atrophy for patients on bedrest and without appropriate rehabilitation, these muscles may never return to their original strength (4). Patients subjected to prolonged bedrest are also at increased risk for pathological musculoskeletal damage from falls, especially if standing or ambulating before muscles and bones have sufficiently recovered (4). Osteoporosis is also exacerbated with prolonged bedrest, due to a lack of weight-bearing exercise. This further subjects patients to an increased risk of fractures upon resuming activity (10). Finally, ICU patients may develop new onset neuromuscular disorders, secondary to their critical illness (11). These myopathies, neuropathies, and neuromuscular junction disorders further contribute to the general wasting that occurs with bedrest. These lesions are reviewed in depth in Volume 2, Chapter 6.

Cardiovascular Deconditioning

Cardiovascular deconditioning is another common accompaniment of prolonged inactivity, reflected by an increase in both the resting heart rate and the heart rate associated with activity. An increase of one half beat to several beats per minute at rest and more than 30–40 beats per minute

during activity can be expected after just a few weeks of inactivity (12,13). Although less dramatic than skeletal muscle atrophy, the cardiac muscle is also subject to atrophy from inactivity. Decreased ventilatory capacity as a result of bedrest and pulmonary pathology further impairs aerobic capacity (10).

However, it is the vascular and orthostatic control systems which are most affected by bedrest. Within only a few days of bedrest, the cardiovascular system adjusts to the decreased work required to pump blood throughout the body due to elimination of gravity's effects. Lying in a horizontal position allows the blood volume to diminish, and the vasculature and responsiveness to decrease. This tends to cause orthostatic hypotension when the patient eventually sits up or stands. Although this is reversed with activity over time, recovery often takes twice as long as it took to develop (14). Symptoms of hypotension are disconcerting and makes the debilitated patient feel lightheaded, and they naturally seek to return to a supine position, which will only lengthen the recovery process further. Encouraging patients to perform simple ADLs themselves can help begin to reverse the inevitable cardiovascular deconditioning and orthostatic hypotension which occur with prolonged critical illness.

Contractures and Pressure Ulcers

Prolonged bedrest is also a leading factor in the development of joint contractures and skin breakdown (especially in neurologically impaired patients). Contractures limit recovery and contribute to further morbidity. However, they can be prevented if aggressive ROM and splinting programs are initiated early (15). The most common sites for decubitus ulcers are the coccyx, greater trochanters, and heels (10).

Joints should be fully ranged at least twice a day to prevent contracture development. Active range of motion (AROM) is preferred, as this also serves to maintain strength and motor control; however, passive range of motion (PROM) is still effective for patients who are unable or for whom active movement is contraindicated (15). Passive stretching minimizes muscle atrophy and stimulates growth by stabilizing muscles in lengthened positions (16). As part of their treatment plans, PTs and OTs educate patients, nurses, families, and other caregivers about proper PROM and AROM techniques. When patients are taught to perform PROM by themselves, this is referred to as self ROM (SROM). After performing the ROM exercises, the therapist places the patient in an optimal static position to reinforce the positive aspects of treatment. For example, after cervical stretching of a patient with neck contractures, towel rolls are placed to maintain the neck in an optimal neutral alignment.

Ranging joints and extremities and frequently changing the patients' positioning play important roles in the prevention of decubitus ulcers by stimulating circulation (4). Frequent turning for bed-confined patients and those who are unable to move themselves helps minimize the constant pressure on bony prominences. At a minimum, patients should be turned from side to back to opposite side every two hours, using foam wedges and pillows to maintain appropriate positions; special mattresses are also beneficial for optimizing pressure-relief. Splinting also helps maintain a functional position and optimal tendon stretch, and also helps protect skin from breaking down.

Deep Venous Thrombosis and Pulmonary Embolism

Pulmonary embolism is a leading cause of death in trauma patients directly related to inactivity and consequent DVT formation (17). In fact, one study revealed that 13% of bedridden patients developed DVTs (18). For this reason, DVT prevention is critical, with a combined prophylactic approach of anticoagulation, lower extremity compression (through the use of support hose and/or sequential compression devices), and mobilization. Studies have shown that early ambulation for the majority of patients with DVTs is safe (19). Furthermore, ambulation also serves to reduce pain, swelling, and venous stasis associated with DVTs by increasing blood circulation, provided that patients are anticoagulated, and have compression bandages (20,21). Properly elevating a patient's heels—either on pillows or through the use of pressure-relieving orthotics—is another important maneuver, as it returns blood to the central circulation and may aid in decreasing DVTs. Encouraging mobility through early ambulation, therapeutic exercises, and out-of-bed activities help to prevent the development of DVTs by increasing circulation. Refer to Volume 2, Chapter 56 for additional discussions on the ramifications of DVT.

Other Complications

Development of aspiration pneumonia and urinary tract infections are additional complications that are commonly associated with complete bedrest in debilitated patients (3,10,22). Additionally, depression and other mood disorders may result from lengthy hospital stays. Learned helplessness is a common condition seen in long-term ICU patients, in which patients become accustomed to others doing even simple tasks for them, such as rolling, feeding, or hygiene (10). Another important complication is the development of an "ICU psychosis" which is characterized as decreased orientation and increased confusion, anxiety, and agitation. When severe, these patients may require antipsychotic medications. The elderly, those who have been sleep deprived, and those withdrawing from alcohol and other drugs are most frequently affected.

All of the above conditions can significantly lengthen a patient's stay in the hospital and prolong overall recovery. By eliminating or reducing the duration of bedrest, patients experience a more rapid recovery with fewer complications. Commencing rehabilitation services while in the ICU improves the outcome and better prepares patients for transferring to a general surgical floor and continuing therapy as they progress, thus resulting in shorter duration

of hospitalization. ☞ **Ordering PT and OT early in patients' hospitalization will likely decrease medical and functional complications because patients will be stronger, more active, and mentally more interactive, leading to better outcomes.** ☞

REHABILITATION NEEDS ASSESSMENT AND MONITORING
Initial Evaluation

Beginning with the initial evaluation, therapists review the patient's needs and rehabilitation expectations from a holistic perspective. The patient's current injuries and illnesses are assessed, noting neurological function, stability of the musculoskeletal system, and cognitive abilities. The patient's prior level of function (PLOF), including any previously needed supportive equipment (e.g., a walker or cane), is considered in order to set realistic goals. The patient's living situation is also evaluated to determine what assistance will be available after discharge and if caregiver or family training will be necessary.

Assessments are made for ROM, strength, sensation, endurance, tone, coordination, and pain. Balance is measured statically and dynamically for both sitting and standing. Mobility tasks are broken down into the basic elements of rolling, transitioning to and from supine, sitting, and standing, as well as transferring to a chair and toilet, gait, and wheelchair mobility. Patients also perform several ADLs, including grooming and hygiene tasks, upper and lower body dressing and bathing, toileting, and self-feeding. To assess cognition, therapists grade patients' orientation, safety and body awareness, judgment, and attention to detail. Refer to Tables 3–6 for examples of objective PT/OT assessment scales used at the UCSD Medical Center.

Once objective data are gathered, goals are set with patient and family input to establish treatment priorities. Appropriate treatment plans are then established to reach

Table 3   UCSD Grading Scale for Motor Strength

Numeric grade	Letter grade	Abilities of patient
5	N	Full available ROM against gravity and max resistance
4	G	Full ROM against gravity and mod resistance
3+	F+	Full ROM against gravity and min resistance
3	F	Full ROM against gravity; no added resistance
3−	F−	Greater than 50% ROM against gravity; no resistance
2+	P+	50% or less ROM against gravity; no resistance
2	P	Full ROM with gravity eliminated; no resistance
2−	P−	Only a portion of ROM; gravity eliminated
1	T	Contraction can be palpated; no observable movement
0	0	Contraction cannot be palpated; no observable movement

Abbreviations: N, normal; G, good; F, fair; P, poor; T, trace; ROM, range of motion; max, maximal; mod, moderate; min, minimal.

Table 4 UCSD Grading Scale for Sensation

Numeric grade	Definition	Abilities of patient
N	Normal	Able to correctly respond 100% of the time
I	Impaired	Able to correctly respond with inconsistency or incorrect responses
0	Absent	Unable to feel, respond, or patient appears to be guessing

Table 6 UCSD Grading Scale for Independence Levels

Grade	Assistance required
I	Independent
Mod I	Modified independent
S	Supervision
SBA	Stand-by assist
CGA	Contact-guard assist
Min A	Minimum assist (<25% needed)
Mod A	Moderate assist (25–50% needed)
Max A	Maximum assist (50–75% needed)
Dep	Dependent (needs >75% assist)

these goals. Goals and treatment plans are modified as needed throughout the treatment sessions. Patient and family education begins during the initial evaluation and continues throughout all treatment sessions. Common goals for patients in an ICU setting include: sitting at the edge of the bed unsupported for 15 minutes, transferring to a chair with moderate assistance and sitting up for two hours, performing grooming tasks independently while seated, and performing simple exercise programs with assistance of the nurse or family.

Treatment Frequency and Monitoring

Treatment frequency is determined primarily by the patient's need for and ability to participate in therapy. At UCSD, both PT and OT typically treat patients once a day, five days a week. Patients with neurological or orthopedic conditions often require more intensive rehabilitation, and

are therefore seen twice a day and/or on weekends. Patients who are unable to fully participate in daily rehab program, such as those who cannot follow commands or are on strict bedrest, may only be seen by a PT and/or OT professional two to three times a week. However, a plan of care for ROM and positioning is developed with nurses and family members so that these patients can receive daily therapy from the start. Before decreasing treatment frequencies for patients, therapists train family or staff until they can independently perform the exercise programs. Non-responsive patients who are unable to actively participate and need only occasional monitoring until becoming more alert and medically stable are typically followed once a week by PT and/or OT while ICU nurses continue established ROM and splinting programs to prevent secondary complications from developing. Table 7 lists the types of ROM programs.

During treatments, therapists and assistants monitor the patient's abilities and future rehab needs. Pain and vital signs are assessed before, during, and after treatments, with activities and exercise programs graded accordingly. When pain is a limiting factor for progressing in therapy, patients should be offered pre-therapy analgesia (in coordination with the medical staff). Whenever possible, treatments are spread throughout the day, such as having OT in the mornings to address self-care and PT in the afternoons for gait training. This allows patients to rest between treatment sessions so that they can benefit most from the therapy.

Therapists caring for ICU patients must possess an understanding of various monitors and lines. Frequently used monitors include pulse oximetry, arterial lines,

Table 5 UCSD Grading Scale for Balance

Grade	Static abilities of patient	Dynamic abilities of patient
G+	Takes max challenges, maintains through max excursions of active trunk motion	Maintains through max excursions of active trunk motion
G	Takes mod challenges in all directions	Maintains through mod excursions of active trunk motion (i.e., weight-shifting)
G−	Maintains position with min challenges	Maintains through min excursions of active trunk motion
F+	Maintains position without supervision or cuing	Maintains within base of support
F	Maintains without assistance but unable to take challenges; requires supervision or cuing	N/A—cannot move within base of support without losing balance
P+	Needs min assist to maintain	N/A
P	Needs mod assist to maintain	N/A
P−	Needs max assist to maintain	N/A
U	Needs total assist to maintain sitting without back support	N/A

Abbreviations: TG, good; F, fair; P, poor; U, unable; max, maximal; mod, moderate; min, minimal; N/A, not applicable.

Table 7 Range of Motion

Type	Definition	How produced
Passive range of motion (PROM)	When no voluntary movement by the muscle is involved	External force (i.e., mechanical device, third party, or one of patient's functioning body parts)
Active-assistive range of motion (AAROM)	When a primary contractile muscle uses an external force	Primary contractile muscle and external force
Active range of motion (AROM)	Active contraction of the muscle without an external force	Primary contractile muscle

electrocardiography, intracranial pressure (ICP) measurement devices, intravenous lines, catheters, drains, chest tubes, and naso-gastric or gastric feeding tubes. Caution must also be taken when a patient has a tracheostomy or is orally intubated and on a ventilator, especially during upper body activity. Care is exercised so that tubes and lines are not pulled during activity or by an agitated or confused patient. Information obtained from the monitors can be used to assess cardiopulmonary status and levels of pain, which is especially useful for the minimally-conscious patient who is unable to communicate. For example, an increase in heart rate, blood pressure, or ICP can indicate pain, fear, or anxiety. Similarly, a decrease in oxygen saturation can indicate excessive stress of the activity. Therapists use this information in the clinical decision-making process to determine when and how to progress the patient's plan of care.

Therapeutic Progression

Therapists try to create a "just right challenge" for their patients (23). Grading treatment activity throughout the session assures that the patients' abilities are challenged but not overly exceeded. This concept refers to balancing the challenge of the task with the person's ability to perform that task. Finding the "just right challenge" ensures that patients do not become either frustrated by failure or bored by not being challenged at all.

With practice, performing activities should become easier as patients' skills improve, allowing the tasks to become more demanding. For example, a common goal in the ICU is for patients to be able to transfer from supine to sitting with only supervision and without using the bed rails. With patients' first attempts at this task, therapists will allow them to pull on the bed rail for rolling to the side and for pushing up when coming to a sitting position. Once this is mastered, patients are encouraged not to use the rail. The ultimate goal is to increase patients' independence without relying on an assistive device, such as the bed rail. Requesting patients to sit up without using the rail during the initial treatment is often too challenging, causing great frustration, a high level of anxiety, and an increased fear of falling out of bed without the protection of the rail. The use of the rail allows patients to learn proper bed mobility techniques (e.g., log-rolling), while having more assistance and security. This is an example of how therapists use graded challenges and assistive devices in the therapeutic progression.

Rehabilitation and Discharge Planning

✐ **Discharge planning considerations are deliberated during the initial rehab evaluation, even for ICU patients. The more time the patient, family, and medical team have to prepare, the more successful the discharge plan.** ✐ Therapists help to determine whether a patient will likely be safe to return home after being discharged from the hospital. If not, the patient may require continued therapy at an acute rehabilitation facility, a skilled nursing facility, or may need placement at an assisted living or board and care facility. If the patient is being discharged home, therapists help to determine appropriate equipment needs (refer to Figs. 2 and 3 for examples of commonly-issued durable medical equipment). Table 8 lists common discharge destinations from the acute hospital and their rehabilitation criteria.

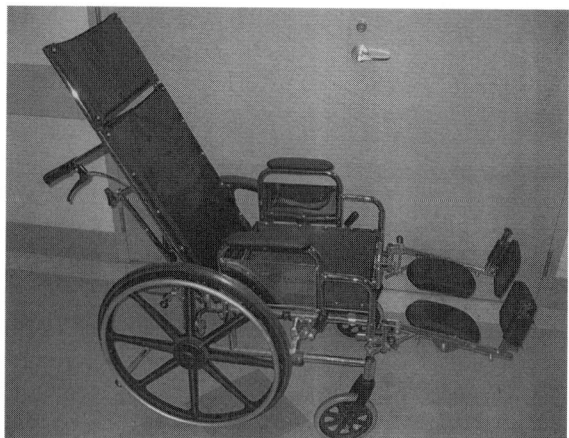

Figure 2 Reclining wheelchair.

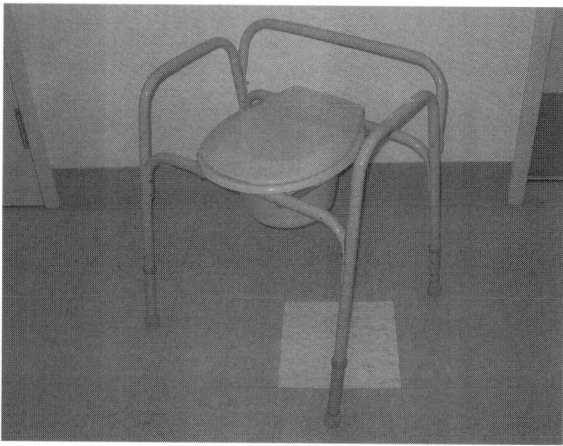

Figure 3 Bedside commode, also known as a 3:1 (three-in-one) commode—named for its multiple uses as a portable commode, raised toilet seat, and shower seat.

Table 8 Common Discharge Destinations and Rehabilitation Criteria

Destination	Rehabilitation criteria
Acute rehabilitation facility	Patient must be able to tolerate 3+ hours/day of aggressive therapies
Skilled nursing facility (SNF)	Therapy often averages 1–2 hours/day
Transitional care unit (TCU)	Intermediate level between acute rehab and SNF
Board and care or assisted living facilities	May or may not offer skilled PT/OT services
Home with home health PT/OT	Patient must be home-bound; therapies often 2–3 visits/week for short period
Home with outpatient PT/OT	Able to go into the community; therapy frequency and duration vary
Home with no needs	Patient is usually independent or at PLOF

Abbreviations: PT, physical therapy; OT, occupational therapy; PLOF, prior level of function.

INJURY-SPECIFIC REHABILITATION CONSIDERATIONS

Brain Injury

Once the brain-injured patient is medically stable and a physician's order is received, therapists perform their evaluations. The Glasgow Coma Scale is useful for assessing coma following head injuries. However, once patients are awake, a higher level of cognitive function needs to be determined. ☞ **The Rancho Los Amigos Cognitive Scale provides the most useful and reproducible categorization of cognitive and behavioral status for patients who are awake and interacting with their environment (24).** ☞ The Rancho Los Amigos Cognitive Scale (Table 9) is composed of 10 levels (24). Each level describes a patient's behavior as the patient progresses from a coma state through and beyond a confused state.

The initial goal of rehab following brain injury is the prevention of secondary complications of inactivity while the patient is recovering. As patients progress into less confused states, therapists provide a daily routine and structured environment while addressing the cognitive and behavioral dysfunctions as they relate to sensorimotor function. Treatments are influenced by cognitive and behavioral status and are focused on improving behavioral management, motor learning, motivation, attention, memory, and motor control.

Consistency in PT/OT training helps improve progress made in rehabilitation from cognitive and behavioral dysfunction. If possible, the same therapist should treat the patient throughout the hospitalization. Therapists must set limits and provide the patient with clear feedback, as well as redirect the patient's attention from sources of anxiety and frustration. Whenever appropriate, therapists include the patient's interests and/or hobbies in the treatment to promote self-motivation.

The quality of therapy sessions can be improved by reducing outside noise, clutter, light, and the number of persons in the room. At UCSD, a "quiet room" has been designated for patients with brain injuries to facilitate rehabilitation therapy. Soothing music can also quell agitation, and help to focus (the use of music for relaxation is discussed in more detail later in this chapter). Familiar objects and photographs of family members provide a sense of security and assist in facilitating earlier thoughts and memories and should be liberally used in the patient's room.

Conversely, sensory-deprived patients who are categorized with low response levels on the Rancho scale, often benefit from intensive stimulation. One way to facilitate this is by optimizing the patient's environment. For example, altering the position of the bed so activity and patient's interests (e.g., watching television and talking to family and medical staff) take place on the affected, injured, and/or hemiplegic side of the body. Encourage head turning and looking toward the affected side. By using this approach, the affected side is forced to react, thereby increasing sensory stimulation to that side.

Properly positioning patients in bed plays an important role in their functional outcome. In patients with hemiplegia, lying on the affected side may reduce spasticity by elongating the structures of that side, providing added sensory input, and increasing body awareness. ADL performance is also improved because the more skillful hand is free to move and perform activities, (e.g., adjusting the sheets for comfort). Figure 4 illustrates proper bed

Table 9 Rancho Los Amigos Levels of Cognitive Functioning

No.	Response level	Behavior	Dependency
I	None	Total absence of response to visual, auditory, tactile, or painful stimuli	Total dependence
II	Generalized	Response to repeated auditory or painful stimuli with associated physiological changes, gross body movement, or vocalization	Total dependence
III	Localized	Recognition of auditory or visual stimuli demonstrated by turning of the head or movement of the eyes; inconsistently responds to simple commands	Total dependence
IV	Confused/agitated	Alert, heightened state of activity; performance of motor activities without purpose; aggressive or exaggerated behavior; poor short-term memory	Maximal assistance
V	Confused, inappropriate, nonagitated	Lack of orientation to person, place, or time; ability to consistently respond to simple commands	Maximal assistance
VI	Confused, appropriate	Inconsistently oriented to person, time, or place; ability to attend to familiar task in non-distracting environment for 30 min with moderate redirection	Moderate assistance
VII	Automatic, appropriate	Consistently oriented to person, place; moderate assist to orientation to time; minimal supervision for new learning; unable to think about consequences of an action	Minimal assistance
VIII	Purposeful, appropriate	Consistently oriented to person, place, and time; independently attends to and completes familiar tasks for 1 hour in distracting environment; requires no assistance with newly-learned tasks; self-centered	Stand-by assistance
IX	Purposeful, appropriate	Use of memory devices to recall daily schedules; ability to think about consequences of decisions with assistance when requested	Stand-by assistance on request
X	Purposeful, appropriate	Ability to handle multiple tasks simultaneously in all environments and to recognize consequences of actions; social interaction behavior is consistently appropriate	Modified independence

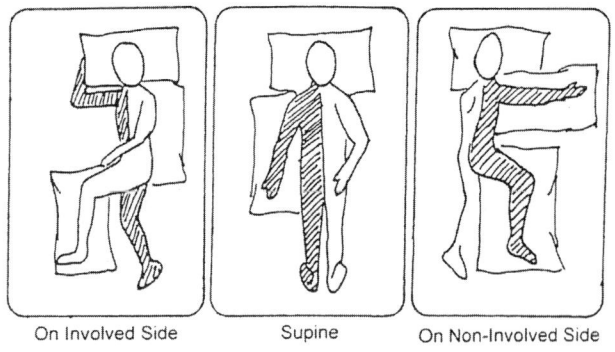

On Involved Side Supine On Non-Involved Side

Figure 4 Proper bed positioning for patients with hemiplegia. The right side is the hemiplagia-involved (*stippled*) side. *Source*: From the International Clinical Educators, Inc.

positioning for hemiplegic patients. The supine position should be avoided as much as possible because it enhances abnormal reflex activity due to tonic neck and labyrinthine reflexes (22).

Spinal Cord Injury
Assessment
🖝 Therapists should perform a standardized American Spinal Injury Association (ASIA) evaluation within the first 72 hours of admission following spinal cord injury (SCI). 🖝 The ASIA evaluation quantifies both sensory and motor abilities of the patient (Fig. 5) (25). Sensation is assessed through light touch and pin prick, and motor function is assessed through manual muscle testing. This standardized assessment is used to objectively determine the level of SCI. It also predicts the patient's functional expectations based on that particular level of injury. Refer to

Table 10 for a summary of UCSD's critical path for the treatment of patients with acute spinal cord injury (SCI).

Pre-stabilization Phase
Patients with an unstable spine who are awaiting surgical stabilization or receipt of an orthotic device are referred to as "pre-stabilization." An activity level of strict bedrest is appropriate during this phase. Treatment in the pre-stabilization phase involves patient and family education in the areas of therapeutic exercise, positioning, and splinting (if needed). One common spine stabilizing brace is the thoracic-lumbar-sacral orthotic (TLSO). The patient is taught AROM exercises and to be the "director" of his/her own care, informing family and staff when and how to perform PROM and positioning. At UCSD, patients are initially placed on a rotating bed, which provides positional changes mechanically while maintaining spinal alignment. Resting hand splints or hand rolls are issued as needed for patients with a high level of SCI. Short opponent splints may be used to facilitate grasp for patients with at least a fair-plus grade in the manual muscle testing in the wrist extensors. Ankle splints are issued to maintain ankle alignment as well as prevent pressure sores from developing at the heels.

Post-stabilization Phase
Once the spine is stable, the patient can begin functional mobility and self-care training. The activity level should be definitively declared by physician's orders as "spine cleared/OK for out of bed." The patient is often transferred from the rotating bed and issued a bed with a mattress with pressure-relief mechanisms. The initial functional mobility goals are rolling and tolerating an upright/vertical posture. Rolling improves bed mobility and prepares the patient for self-pressure relief and lower body dressing in bed. A gradual progression into the vertical position is

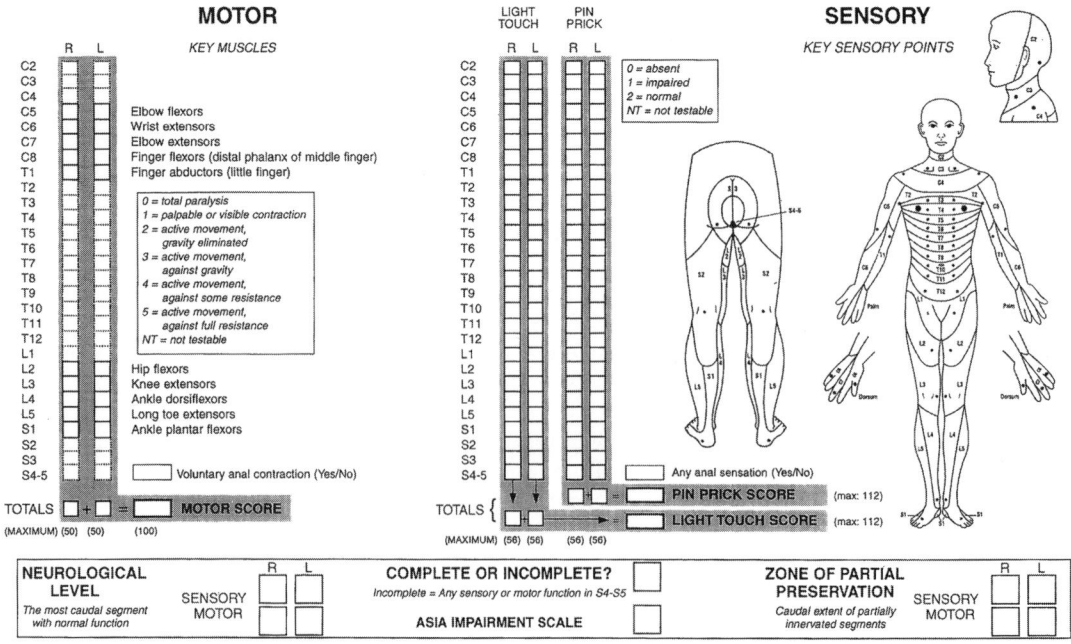

Figure 5 American Spinal Injury Association scale for assessing level of sensory and motor spinal cord injury.

Table 10 Critical Path for Rehabilitation Following Acute Spinal Cord Injury

Area	Pre-stabilization	Post-stabilization days 1–3	Post-stabilization days 4–7
Evaluation	Complete ASIA evaluation	Clarify orders and complete second ASIA evaluation	Reassess as needed
Equipment required	Foot-drop and wrist splints and communication devices as needed	Issue an abdominal binder and ace wraps for BLE; adapt call light as needed; cardiac chair and reclining wheelchair with removal armrests and elevating leg-rests	Continue with necessary equipment
Caregiver and patient education	Education in skin integrity/breakdown; rehab expectations; issue and educate on PROM booklet	Education on pressure relief techniques (1 min every hour or 30 sec every 30 min)	Continue as tolerated
Treatment	Initiate PROM	Initiate dependent transfers to cardiac and/or wheelchair; begin BUE and BLE exercises including ROM and hamstring stretches	For C1-C3 SCI levels, continue exercise program and initiate mouth/neck therapeutic exercise. For C4-T3 SCI levels, same as above and progress to mat activities For T4-L5 SCI levels, same as above and progress to ambulation

Abbreviations: ASIA, American Spinal Injury Association; BLE, bilateral lower extremities; PROM, passive range of motion; min, minutes; sec, seconds; BUE, bilateral upper extremities; ROM, range of motion; SCI, spinal cord injury.

most effective. This progression begins by just elevating the head of bed to 30 degrees, and then to 60 degrees. Once a patient can tolerate this position for approximately two hours, then the next step is sitting at the edge of bed followed by transferring into a reclining wheelchair.

When a patient begins the functional activity of sitting, lower extremity ace wraps and an abdominal binder are issued to the patient. Ace wraps are bandaged around the legs to increase venous return and decrease the possibility of postural hypotension. The abdominal binder improves the resting position of the diaphragm (making it more domed), thus increasing the excursion of the diaphragm during ventilation and increasing both vital capacity (VC) and maximum inspiratory force (MIF). The abdominal binder will typically increase these weaning parameters (VC and MIF) by 15% in patients with C5-6 SCI (26). The abdominal binder may also help maintain blood pressure in some patients. If a patient is having difficultly with this progression of upright/vertical sitting, the use of a tilt table is recommended (26).

Most patients with SCIs are discharged to acute rehabilitation facilities. There, they continue to receive intensive therapies to achieve their maximum functional outcome. Table 11 lists functional outcomes for spinal cord injuries that patients should achieve when medical issues are stable and they have received optimal rehab.

Mechanical Principles

In the SCI population, some joints require increased flexibility while others benefit from increased tightness. Within the shoulder joint, PT and OT aim to increase extension and external rotation to ease transfers and seated self-care activities. Full elbow extension and triceps strength are necessary in order to use the locking technique to achieve the goal of independent sitting. Intact wrist extensors and normal range is crucial for the locking technique and tenodesis. To promote tenodesis, the long finger flexors must be of mild to moderate tightness. Lumbar tightness is encouraged, as this helps with transfers, lower extremity dressing, and balance activities. The primary ROM goal for the hips is full extension for a greater and more normalized gait pattern. Hamstring flexibility to 110–120 degrees is recommended for long-sitting activities such as lower body dressing and floor transfers. Full dorsiflexion of the ankles

Table 11 Functional Outcomes for Spinal Cord Injuries

Level of SCI	Transfers	Activities of daily living	Wheelchair
C1-3	Dependent	Dependent	Electric with head controls
C4	Dependent	Limited independence using mobile arm supports and environ-mental control units	Electric with head or breathing controls
C5	Dependent	Independent with set-up	Electric with joystick
C6	Independent with slide board	Independent with universal cuff	Manual
C7-T3	Independent without slide board	Independent	Manual
T4-L5	Independent; may progress to ambulation with orthotics and/or assistive device	Independent	Manual

will allow for a normalized placement of patients' feet on footplates of the wheelchair.

Mechanical principles are used to increase functional mobility in the SCI patient. Agonist muscles are used to compensate for weakened deinverted muscles. For example, the tightness of the long finger flexors allows for tenodesis grasp. Momentum is the "throwing" of a particular body part to complete a functional activity when it cannot be completed by going against gravity to place it in a particular area (27). Unweighing is a mechanical principle by which a body part is used to advance another body part. For example, the patient bears weight on the right hip while the therapist unweighs the left hip in order to scoot in sitting. Head-hip relationship is implemented when the therapist repositions the hips by actively moving the head and shoulders in opposite directions; this eases dependent transfers of a patient into and out of a wheelchair (27,28). All of these learned techniques take time and dedicated training by the PT and OT.

Orthopedic Trauma

☞ **Although a period of immobilization via traction or casting is necessary for the recovery of certain injuries and surgical repairs, therapy should be initiated as soon as medically appropriate.** ☞ Early ranging will maximize joint ROM, ensure smooth tendon gliding, prevent or minimize adhesions from developing, provide sensory re-education and desensitization, and improve overall motor function. Exercises, with or without resistance, will strengthen both affected and unaffected muscles. Educating the patient, family, and staff in the proper techniques is critical for the success of home exercise programs, as they should be performed several times each day for an optimal outcome. To prevent secondary injuries from developing, therapy should be consulted to range and/or strengthen noninvolved joints while others are immobilized.

Edema management is important to a successful rehab program. The most effective method for preventing and/or minimizing edema is through extremity elevation. Positioning the arm or leg on pillows, wedges, or other elevation devices above the level of the heart while in bed not only helps with reducing or minimizing edema, but also provides support to minimize strain placed on the proximal joint. The use of a sling can help avoid keeping one's hand in a dependent position while out of bed; this can also increase the patient's comfort during ambulation. Patients are encouraged to perform frequent AROM, and this is taught early in most therapy programs and practiced several times a day to decrease edema. Other methods used for effective edema reduction include PROM, retrograde massage, and the use of compression devices.

Axial Spine Considerations

Within the trauma setting, many patients are diagnosed with axial spine injuries. Treatment for this population is similar to that of spinal cord-injured patients with respect to protecting the fracture site(s). Often, orthotic devices such as a TLSO are prescribed for stabilization. For these patients, an additional goal for donning and doffing the brace is created. Patients are educated about the necessary precautions to protect their spine, which may include but are not limited to avoidance of bending, lifting, or twisting. To maintain these spine precautions, an assistive device called a reacher may be needed for lower body dressing and for picking objects off the floor, as well as for reaching items overhead (Fig. 1). Patients are also taught to limit sitting to

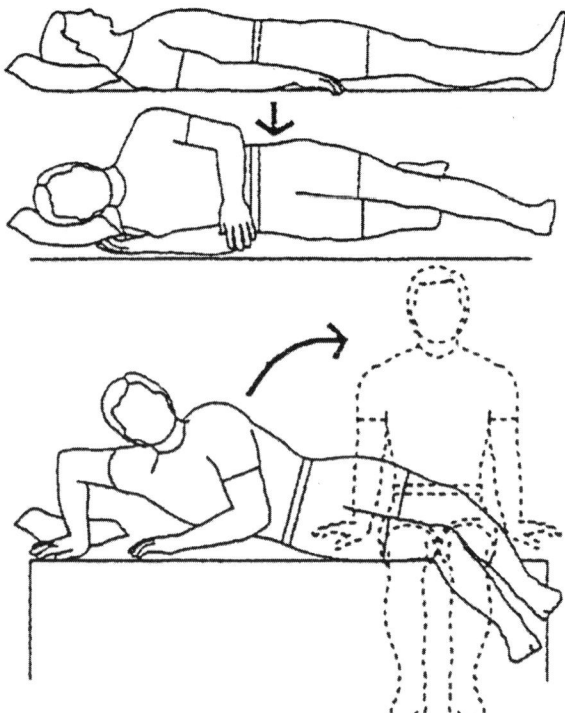

Figure 6 Log-rolling technique: this is often the most effective method for a patient to safely get into and out of bed in order to protect the spine and/or minimize abdominal pain or trauma. The patient will roll to his side and push himself up with his arms while lowering his legs simultaneously. This procedure is reversed for moving from sitting to supine.

15–30 minutes at a time (this may vary with different procedures or surgeons). Therapists also instruct the patient in specific techniques to protect the spine while getting into and out of bed, referred to as log-rolling. Refer to Figure 6 for an illustration and description of this technique.

Lower Extremity Considerations

Ambulation goals are initiated as soon as possible. Many studies have shown that early ambulation is critical to a good recovery. Conversely, prolonged bed rest is detrimental to recovery following hip fractures, particulary in the frail. A recent study of elderly patients following hip fracture demonstrated that early ambulation and progressive weight bearing after surgery was associated with less morbidity and improved ambulatory status (29). Another study suggested that twice-daily treatments during the first post-operative week following hip fractures increases the odds of regaining independent bed mobility and ambulation with a walker, as well as the likelihood of being discharged directly to home (30).

Weight-bearing status is an important consideration that varies depending upon the surgical procedure and type of injury. For example, nonweight-bearing is common for non-surgical calcaneal fractures, whereas weight bearing as tolerated is common for minor pelvic fractures. The use of assistive devices is necessary to maintain lower extremity weight-bearing restrictions during out of bed activity and ambulation. Refer to Figure 7 for examples of commonly used assistive devices for ambulation. The use

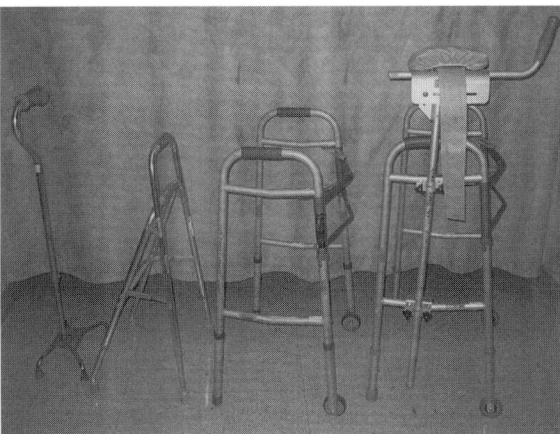

Figure 7 Example of various ambulation devices: left to right—quad cane, hemi-walker, front-wheeled walker, and front-wheeled walker with platform attachment.

of a platform walker for ambulation allows the patient to maintain weight-bearing precautions on the distal upper extremities.

Upper Extremity Considerations

Patients with upper extremity injuries will most likely need OT for proper ROM, strengthening, and positioning techniques, as well as fine-motor coordination and ADLs. Splinting is an effective method for providing proper hand position. Splints can be used to support joints, tissues, and bones as they heal or facilitate and maintain increased ROM. Collaboration between the OT and the surgeon is essential for the use of proper postoperative splints.

The most commonly issued splint for the ICU patient is the resting hand splint (Fig. 8). This splint allows for wrist extension and metacarpophalangeal (MP) joint flexion, thus placing ligaments and tendons in the wrist, hand, and fingers in maximal stretch and reducing the likelihood of contractures. Additionally, slight interphalangeal (IP) joint flexion of the fingers and carpometacarpal and

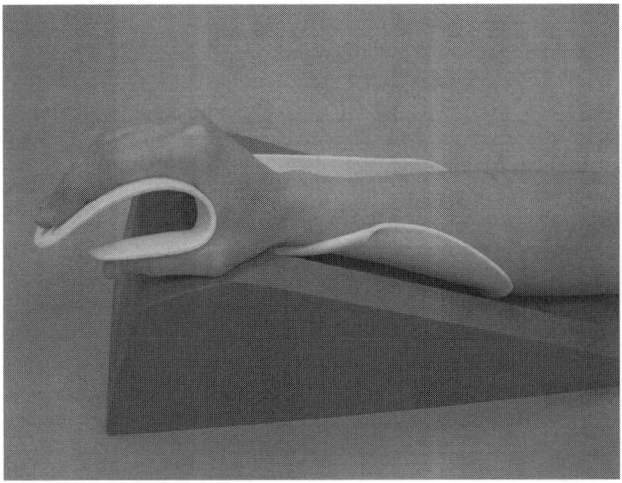

Figure 8 Resting hand splint. This device places the hand in the so-called "position of function" with the wrist in moderate extension, the metacarpophalyngeal (MP) joint in flexion, and the fingers in only mild flexion to maintain stretch on aggregate flexor and extensor tendons and limit contractures of prolonged disuse.

MP opposition of the thumb maintain the hand in the most functional position. Soft, off-the-shelf wrist cock-up splints are another frequently used option for providing wrist extension in patients who do not require finger or thumb support. This is a more economical approach and preferred by some patients because of their smaller size and padding for comfort. However, custom-made splints provide added support and comfort if properly fit. A large variety of splints are commercially available and even more splinting options are possible for the experienced splinter.

Once splints are issued, OTs then educate patients, staff, and families regarding correct protocols for donning and doffing the splints. Most often, splints are to be worn for two hours and removed for two hours throughout the daytime, and worn at night. Immobilization splints are usually worn at all times and removed only for hygiene and/or wound inspection, if cleared by the physician. Skin is inspected each time the splints are removed to assess for redness or pressure spots to ensure proper fit of the splint and to prevent skin breakdown. To combat stiffness, joints should be fully ranged upon splint removal when indicated.

Hand injuries are often associated with profound psychological effects on patients. Because most injuries to the hand are quite traumatic, patients can develop a post-traumatic stress disorder (PTSD) regarding the event that led to their injury (31). The hand is one of the most important body parts for performing daily activities and, therefore, the loss of hand function can significantly affect the patient's personal, professional, and social life. Therapists endeavor to reassure and educate patients and caregivers that these conditions can improve or be coped with when the therapy program is properly applied.

Amputations

☞ **Patients admitted for elective amputations should be introduced to therapy pre-operatively.** ☞ Table 12 shows a summary of the critical path for acute lower extremity amputations used at UCSD (because upper extremity amputations are more rarely performed, the focus of this section is on the lower extremity). During the pre-surgical phase, the PT prescribes an individualized exercise program in order to prepare the patient for the post-operative phase. The exercise program consists of strengthening both the upper and lower extremities, as well as continued functional mobility, which increases endurance and allows for bilateral lower extremity weight-bearing. These important considerations are not often practical or available for traumatic amputations.

Post-operatively, PT is resumed and OT is initiated to address ADL needs such as modified dressing techniques. Patient education and positioning of the residual limb is a key component in the postoperative PT program. Positioning assists in the prevention of joint contractures and the shortening of soft tissues. Prone lying is highly encouraged in order to prevent hip flexion contractures; however, special consideration should be taken with geriatric patients and patients with multiple injuries. A patient unable to lie prone should lie supine with his hip in extension against a supporting surface. In side–lying, the PTs can also perform stretches in order to increase hip extension. A pillow should not be placed under the knee for prolonged durations due to the increase in flexion moment, which leads to knee or hip flexion contractures. The patient who remains in a seated position, may use another supporting surface, such as a chair, to maintain knee extension. A patient seated with the knee flexed for a prolonged period of time may develop a

Table 12   Critical Path for Rehabilitation Following Acute Lower Extremity Amputation

Area	Day 1	Days 2–4	Days 4–6
Evaluation	Complete evaluation	Re-evaluate patient	Re-evaluate patient
Equipment needs	Establish need for assistive devices and adaptive equipment	Re-evaluate need for assistive devices and adaptive equipment	Re-evaluate need for assistive devices and adaptive equipment
Caregiver/patient education	Initiate home exercise program and family training	Continue with home exercise program and family training	Continue with home exercise program and family training
Treatment	Begin functional mobility and edge of bed self care skills training	Progress functional mobility and advance self care skills to sitting at sink	Progress functional mobility and advance self care skills to standing at sink

flexion contracture and increased edema in the residual limb due to its dependent position. These complications delay the patient's fitting for a prosthesis.

Skin care is another important factor in the education of the amputee, especially if the patient suffers from diminished lower extremity sensation. Proper hygiene should be exercised to prevent skin breakdown in the uninvolved leg. This involves daily foot inspections, thorough washing of the foot, and careful selection of footwear. The skin should be kept clean and dry at all times. It is imperative that the patient also conducts daily inspections of the residual limb with a mirror, looking for signs of infection or drainage at the incision site. Friction massage therapy should be utilized daily to mobilize adherent scar tissue and to desensitize to touch and pressure.

It is recommended that the amputee keep the residual limb elevated to prevent increased swelling. Patients not fitted with a rigid cast can also use an elastic wrap called a "stump shrinker" to reduce the size and control edema. It should be worn at all times, except when bathing. An alternative technique to reduce edema is to use an ace wrap, which can begin to shape and shrink the tissue and control swelling in order to prepare the residual limb for a prosthetic fitting. The residual limb should be re-wrapped every 3–4 hours, or more frequently if the wrap becomes loose. When wrapping, always use diagonal turns, providing greater distal than proximal pressure to facilitate fluid return back into the body circulation, and ensure there are no wrinkles or bulges, which can cause tissue ischemia (32).

The main goal of pre- and post-operative amputation therapy in an acute care setting is to allow the patient to be functionally independent prior to the possible use of a prosthetic device. It is recommended that patients attend a support group whenever possible to address the emotional impact associated with losing a limb. With proper psychological support and routine follow-up PT, a patient with an amputation can return to an active lifestyle with or without a prosthetic device.

Burns

More than 50,000 patients are admitted to burn units each year in the United States (33). Burn victims face a variety of complications related to their injury. These complications include, but are not limited to: decreased strength, ROM, endurance, mobility, and independence with ADLs.

The initial role of the therapists is to establish a functional baseline within the first 24–48 hours (or after resuscitation is finished) to compare with the patient's status as complications or limitations in the functional abilities arise. The initial evaluation and follow-up treatments

can be performed in coordination with the burn technicians during dressing changes to allow therapists to better observe the skin's mobility. Although the patient may be unresponsive, sedated, and/or on paralytics, therapy is vital to prevent complications of immobility. In this stage of rehab in the ICU, OTs fabricate splints for both upper and lower extremities to assist graft stabilization and/or wound closure, and to prevent contractures or damage to anatomical structures.

Also in this stage, therapists educate caregivers and the burn team members on proper positioning, splinting, ROM, and scar management to the involved and uninvolved joints (see Table 13 for rehabilitation guidelines following grafting). ☞ **The success of the burn patient's recovery relies greatly on their positioning in and out of bed. It is important to note that a position of comfort is, unfortunately, one that will facilitate contractures.**☜ For example, allowing a burn patient's extremities to remain flexed can lead to contractures of flexor tendons.

Edema control is another crucial focus of therapy for burn patients because edema directly affects function, especially for the hand. If edema persists, it may lead to such problems as adaptive shortening, adhesions, and eventually to a loss of function (34–36). Coban self-adhesive wrap is frequently used to control edema, as well as to conform and compress the scarring (37). The use of Coban does not impede grip strength, hand mobility, or the patient's ability to perform self-care tasks (38).

As the patient weans off paralytics and increased active participation in the exercise program is evident, therapists should reassess the treatment plan. They perform a functional mobility and ADL assessment, as well as reassess the previous splinting, scar management, and therapeutic exercise programs. Prior to beginning weight-bearing activities, such as tilt table and/or gait training, the lower extremities may be wrapped with circumferential graded passive supports such as ace wraps. The ace-wrapping supports the new grafts, promotes venous return, and assists in the reduction of pain. If the patient cannot tolerate the upright position required to begin gait training due to orthostatic hypotension or increased pain in the lower extremities, a tilt table treatment can assist in preparing the patient for walking.

Burn patients are at risk for hypertrophic scarring. This abnormal tissue produces excessive amounts of collagen, minimal elastin, and may form thick rope-like bands. The scars may contract over joints, greatly limiting ROM and functional use. Scar management is critical to minimize the effects of hypertrophic scars. Modalities may include aggressive stretching, splinting, Compression garments (e.g., Jobst® compression stockings and gloves). Close attention should be paid to scarred areas for up

Table 13 Critical Path for Rehabilitation Following Acute Burn Injury

Area	Admission	Pre-treatment	Post-treatment
Assessment	Complete a burn evaluation	Re-evaluate patient's progress and needs	Re-evaluate patient's progress and needs
Positioning and splinting	Issue splints and wearing schedule	Monitor effects of splints and make adjustments as needed	Monitor effects of splints and make adjustments as needed
ADLs	Determine deficits and establish treatment plan	Initiate activities designed to maximize self-care	Encourage active movement and ADLs with grafted extremity in accordance with post-op orders
Mobility	Determine ROM and mobility deficits; establish and implement treatment plan	Continue therapeutic exercise program and training for bed mobility, transfers, and gait	Advance treatment program to maximize mobility and ambulation in accordance with post-op orders
Strength	Instruct patient in exercise program	Monitor exercise program	Progress to independent exercise program
Scar management	Determine need for and initiate pressure management and proper skin care	Monitor changing needs for pressure management and instruct in proper skin care	Progress to independent pressure management and skin care

Abbreviations: ADLs, activities of daily living; ROM, range of motion.

to four years post-burn to minimize contractures and deformity. Surgical contracture release may be needed for more severe cases. Every patient who is hospitalized for the treatment of a burn should be referred for follow-up rehab upon discharge in order to achieve and maintain the ultimate goal of independence.

Transplants

Most patients who have received organ transplants are quite deconditioned before their transplants as a result of organ failure, and therefore have lengthy recoveries. Pre-transplant therapies should be ordered when patients are admitted to the hospital so that they may be as strong as possible before undergoing surgery and become introduced to the therapy process. After the transplant, therapists continue working with the patient to return to his/her PLOF.

Mobilizing transplant patients as early as possible is important for their overall recovery. Sternal precautions are followed for patients who have received heart and lung transplants, avoiding strenuous movements to stretch the chest wall before the sternum has healed. All transplant patients must avoid resistive exercises and heavy lifting for several weeks or months following surgery. Patients are taught log-rolling techniques for bed mobility to minimize abdominal strain or pain at the incision sites (refer back to Fig. 6). Abdominal binders are frequently used for additional support and comfort.

At UCSD, the standard discharge goal for patients following liver transplants is to be able to walk at least 50 feet, climb one flight of stairs, and perform simple ADLs with no more than minimal assistance (39). Following discharge, most patients go to an acute rehab facility if needed and then home with their families.

Minimally Conscious Patients
Range of Motion, Positioning, and Caregiver Training

For minimally-conscious patients, ROM should be performed to each joint at least twice a day to prevent the development of contractures. Most family members are eager to learn how they can help their loved one, and therapists can teach them appropriate ranging and positioning techniques. In the absence of family or visitors, nurses need to be more proactive with rehab. Family involvement in therapy sessions has many benefits. They feel they are contributing to the patient's well being (which they are). Moreover, knowledge of proper techniques may also prevent potential injury from accidentally moving a limb in a contraindicated method or an unnatural position. The importance of passive stretching at end range when the patient is at risk for or has a contracture is also stressed to family members who may otherwise not perform the stretches properly. Families and caregivers are also trained in safe transfer techniques (utilizing mechanical lifts if necessary) and proper body mechanics while ranging and transferring the patient.

OT Assessment for Splinting

Some patients may require splints if they are unable to move a limb. Often, a patient's hands are closed at rest, which may result in shortening of flexor tendons, thereby preventing full finger or wrist extension. OTs can issue splints to ensure proper positioning and prevent contractures. Ankle splints are also commonly needed to prevent or combat foot drop contractures. Patients on chronic bedrest commonly develop a shortening of the heel cords due to a lack of stretching through standing. This is further exacerbated by sheets and blankets pressing down on their toes causing further plantar flexion at the ankles. ✄ **Consulting OT for splinting will ensure that minimally-conscious patients are properly positioned and do not develop contractures.** ✄

AGE-SPECIFIC CONSIDERATIONS
Pediatric Patients

Pediatric patients are more likely to present with a higher anxiety level than adults, as they are too young to fully understand what is happening around them. The ICU is a scary place for most patients, and especially so for a child with multiple IVs, monitors, and many physicians, nurses, and other medical professionals entering the patient's room at all hours (Table 14).

Bringing in stuffed animals or other toys from home can provide a sense of familiarity and comfort. Working with and training parents and family members are critical for pediatric therapists. This helps the patient feel more

Table 14 Pediatric Considerations for Physical and Occupational Therapy

Age	Focus	Perceptions	Approaches	Possible adverse effects of hospitalization
Infants (newborn to 1 yr)	Bonding, trust formation, sensorimotor integration	Entire body feels and responds to pain, perceives world as uncaring if cries not attended, reacts with appetite and play	Consistent caregiver, eye-contact, smiles, maintain parent contact, stroking, holding, singing	Separation from parents may cause anxiety, inactivity may delay gross and fine motor skills
Toddlers (1–3 yrs)	Autonomy, gross and fine motor, exploration	Punishment, separation anxiety, regression with stress	Explain who you are and what you are doing, focus on what toddler can do to help, give choices when appropriate, establish routines	Increased dependence on parents, separation anxiety, delayed toilet-training, regressive behavior (may want a bottle)
Preschoolers (3–6 yrs)	Fantasy, motor skills, social skills, very independent	Punishment, fear of bodily harm or intrusive procedures	Same as toddler, use play as outlet for fear and anger, praise accomplishments	Parents become overprotective, regressive in behavior, lack of exposure to new experiences, bed wetting, eating and sleeping problems
School-age adolescents (6–13 yrs)	Separation from mother as individual, social/peer development,	Fear of mutilation, loss of control, or uncontrolled pain	Allow decisions when appropriate, explain what is affected, encourage peer support, offer coping methods and activities that promote mastery	Loss of body control
Adolescents (13–19 yrs)	Independence, role exploration, acquiring values	Views treatment as intimidation, loss of independence, body image is critical, idealistic	Give clear and detailed explanations, allow decisions, elicit input into treatment plans	Fears about ability to function in school, sense of isolation, fewer peer opportunities, resents loss of control

comfortable with the PT/OT process, partly because the therapy is provided by familiar individuals rather than by strangers. Finally, the developmental level of the child must also be considered when constructing treatment plans and goals.

Geriatric Patients

As with children, special considerations must be made when working with geriatric patients, especially in the ICU. Therapy treatments are often less aggressive than for younger, typically healthy patients, as they often have secondary diagnoses that must be accounted for during therapy (Table 15). Older patients have significantly more comorbidities than younger or middle-aged patients (Volume 1, Chapter 37). Incidence of comorbid diseases rises from 9% for patients under age 45 to 65% for patients over 75 years (40). The most common comorbidities include diabetes, coronary artery disease, cirrhosis, chronic renal failure, and chronic obstructive pulmonary disease (15). Therapists also consider the presence of dementia when working with older patients. Presence of comorbidities likely extends the length of stay in the ICU and the patient's overall hospitalization.

Geriatric patients rarely function at a fully independent level even prior to hospitalization. It would therefore not be appropriate for therapists to set goals of complete independence for these patients. Caregiver/family training is an important component of PT/OT treatment sessions, as they must show that they are able to care for the patient appropriately and safely at home.

PSYCHOLOGICAL REHABILITATION

☞ **The psychological component of rehabilitation is just as important as the physical component.** ☞ One must need a "drive" or motivation to recover to achieve and improve one's overall functional mobility and self-care. This is especially true for trauma patients because they need to overcome several psychological ramifications from being a victim of a traumatic event. A large number of trauma patients suffer from psychological problems that may have lead to the event. For example, alcohol abuse may contribute to the mechanism of injury such as a fall that causes a subdural hematoma, a motor vehicle accident that results in multiple orthopedic injuries, or chronic conditions such as liver disease, which may require a transplant.

Common psychological reactions of an ICU patient resulting from traumatic events and/or loss of functional independence include confusion, frustration, apathy, depression, worthlessness, denial, anger, and PTSD. Indeed, many hospitalized trauma survivors develop acute stress disorder or PTSD (refer to Volume 2, Chapter 65). In addition, over 30% of patients in the ICU suffer significant anxiety (41). These reactions must be taken into account when the PT and OT create individualized plans of care for the ICU patient.

OUTCOME PREDICTION

☞ **Continuity of care for rehabilitation begins in the ICU and is continued until after the patient is discharged.** ☞ The goal

Table 15 Adult Considerations for Physical and Occupational Therapy

Age	Cognitive changes	Approaches	Possible adverse effects of hospitalization
Young adults (19–45 yrs)	Mental abilities peak during twenties, reasoning, and information recall	Watch body language as a cue for feelings, allow for as much decision-making as possible, explore impact of hospitalization to work/job	Actual or perceived anticipation of harm, anxiety of the unknown, threats to physical self-image, change in role as a provider, loss of control
Middle adults (46–60 yrs)	Mood swings, decreased short-term memory and synthesis of new information	Allow choices and decision-making in plan-of-care, explore relationship of illness to body image, encourage as much self care as possible	Anxiety for an unidentified threat, threats to physical image and change in functional ability, fear of death, perception of aging, losing independence
Older adults (>60 yrs)	Decreased ability to respond to internal and external environment, decreased short-term memory	Teach stress reduction strategies, encourage social interactions	Aggressive or hostile behavior, withdrawal, non-compliance, apathy, dependency, shock, denial, information-seeking

of overall independence is not always met prior to discharge from the hospital, partly due to third-party payer restrictions. Patients often require continued rehabilitation after discharge to continue progressing toward independence (Table 8).

EYE TO THE FUTURE
Kinesio Taping

Kinesio Taping, developed by Dr Kenzo Kase, was first introduced to the United States in 1995 as a modality treatment for PT and OT. This treatment approach is based on providing a supportive exoskeleton during rehab while healing occurs and the muscles regain strength (42). The tape affects the skin, muscles, lymphatics, and joints (Fig. 9). In the skin, the tape relates sensory stimuli to mechanical receptors, decreases inflammation, and decreases pressure chemical receptors. The tape improves contraction of weak muscles and reduces muscle fatigue and over-contraction, in addition to relieving pain. In the lymphatic system, blood and lymphatic circulation improve. The tape promotes

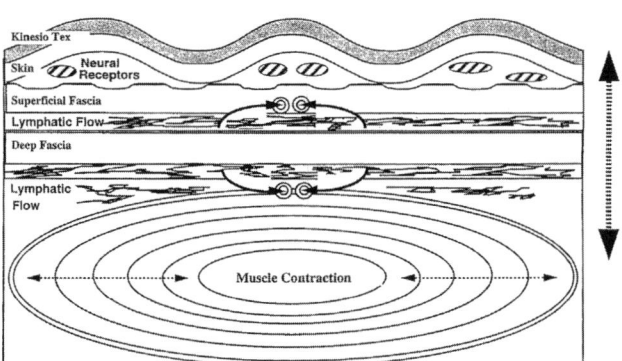

Figure 9 Kinesio taping graphical representation of blood, lymphatic, and interstitial fluid mobilization. Taped areas form convolutions, which intermittently increase, then decrease the space between skin and muscles, serving as a pump, which promotes the flow of lymphatic and interstitial tissue into capillaries, and back to the blood stream. *Source*: Adapted from Ref. 42.

lymphatic drainage from the extremity and reduces excess inflammatory chemical substances in the tissue. The tape is also believed to adjust joint misalignments caused by spasm/shortened muscle, thus improving AROM. Kinesio Taping is used in conjunction with therapeutic exercise programs and manual therapeutic techniques in order to assist the patient in achieving his/her goals to maximize functional independence with minimal pain.

Body Weight Support Treadmill Training

Body weight support treadmill training (BWSTT) is a treatment intervention used to assist patients in more quickly achieving ambulation goals. The BWSTT is composed of the following parts: harness, groin piece, overhead straps, unweighting scale, adjusting handes, and a height adjuster. The idea to use this intervention with diagnoses of stroke and SCI was first introduced by Finch et al. and Barbeau and Blunt (43,44). Researchers have found that the spinal locomotor pools are highly responsive to phasic segmental sensory inputs as well as demonstrated motor learning during step training (45).

In patients post-stroke, BWSTT is shown to be more effective than treadmill training without any weight support, and treadmill training is more effective than conventional over ground gait training (46,47). A three-month study demonstrated that the BWSTT group continued to have increased motor recovery and ambulation speeds than the non-BWSTT group (47). Step training with BWSTT is most effective when stroke patients ambulate at speeds close to normal over ground walking velocities (48). For example, a speed of 2.0 mph on the treadmill is more effective than training at speeds less than 2 mph (48). It also recommended 40% body weight support, as this was found to be the most effective amount of support (47). In studying EMG recordings of the paretic limbs of patients post-stroke, Hesse et al. found that they were more phasic and had more symmetrical patterns following BWSTT, than over ground training (49). In patients with incomplete SCI, Wernig et al. found that BWSTT was most effective in progressing patient's ambulation (50). Prior to this study, 38 of 44 patients used a wheel chair. After BWSTT, 38 patients were able to ambulate with either a cane or a walker (50). In patients with Parkinson's disease, BWSTT assists in the improvement of short step length (51). Further studies are required to determine the effectiveness of BWSTT for other neurological diagnoses.

Neuromuscular Electrical Stimulation

Neuromuscular electrical stimulation (NMES) is used as a therapeutic modality to increase muscle size and strength. This is especially useful during spinal cord injury rehabilitation, but it can also be used for post-surgical recovery (52,53). NMES can be utilized for maintaining and/or improving muscular contractions for patients restricted to bedrest (54). Other uses for NMES include maintenance or increase of ROM and substitution for various orthoses (52).

NMES uses pulses of current to activate the larger, fast-twitch muscle fibers, causing them to contract. These muscles can significantly atrophy during prolonged periods of immobilization or bedrest and are difficult to strengthen through exercise alone. Studies have shown that muscle atrophy can be prevented through the use of NMES (52). When nerves are impaired and active motion is limited, NMES can help to increase the movements. Some common indications for applying NMES are weakened wrist and finger extensors, in order to improve fine-motor coordination; and shoulder subluxation, to correct and maintain proper joint alignment (54,55). This modality is more commonly used in out-patient programs; however, it can also be a useful tool for therapists in the acute setting to address problems before they worsen or become chronic, thus complicating recovery.

Complementary and Alternative Therapies

Various complementary and alternative therapeutic techniques can be implemented to promote relaxation for hospitalized patients. This is especially important for patients in the ICU, because of the "white noise," and frequent sleep-disturbing intrusions that are more common in the ICU than on general medical floors. The use of multiple monitors, IV machines, and ventilators, coupled with less privacy and numerous professionals entering the room around the clock can heighten anxiety and diminish rest. Patients with acute neurological injuries are also easily over-stimulated and cope better when relaxation techniques are utilized.

One calming technique utilized at UCSD involves dedicating programming on television sets located in patients' rooms. Each television set has one station that plays relaxing music and displays calming scenery 24 hours a day. This allows patients, families, or staff to "drown out" noxious noises so the patient can relax, sleep, or otherwise focus on something other than pain and the hospital environment. Focusing on music has been shown to reduce the effects of unwanted stimuli while stimulating endorphins, which produce pleasurable feelings (56). This noninvasive intervention is an excellent adjunct to therapy treatments, especially while performing ROM.

Relaxed patients typically have reduced perceptions of pain, thus facilitating better stretching by reducing resistance to passive movements. Easily distracted patients can also focus better on cognitive activities and require fewer cues for redirection when listening to relaxing background music. Music can also be a useful relaxation and distraction tool to offset painful or stressful activities such as dressing changes or wound care as an alternative to increasing pharmacologic dosages for improved pain control (57). The Joint Commission on Accreditation of Health Care Organizations (JCAHO) has recommended that facilities implement non-pharmacological treatments such as music therapy to complement traditional methods of post-surgical pain control (58).

Animal-assisted therapy is another novel intervention known to help patients cope with painful and unpleasant conditions. Pet therapy involves visits from specially trained animals (typically dogs) that serve to improve patients' cooperation in cognitive or physical training. These animals also serve to combat the stresses and anxieties of hospitalization, improving patients' mood, and decreasing loneliness (59–61).

Pets can be used during PT and OT treatments to motivate patients to participate in therapeutic activities. For example, patients may be encouraged to sit up or use their injured arm to pet the animal. In addition to pet therapy visits, similar benefits can be gained from visitations by the patients' own pets (however, personal pets must be certified free of disease and vaccinated). At UCSD, volunteers take Polaroid photos of the pet therapy visits, providing mementoes of pleasurable events during their hospitalization. Pet visits can be permitted for ICU patients typically with a physicians' order, as long as they meet the medical criteria (not immuno-suppressed, allergic to animals, or have a communicable disease or unexplained fever). Having pets visiting the units can be a positive experience for patients, families, and staff members, which is important in such a highly stressful environment.

SUMMARY

Early rehabilitation is essential for optimal treatment of trauma and critical care patients. The sooner therapy is initiated, the less likely patients will decline in the ICU and will therefore have better outcomes. Important points to consider when ordering therapy include a clear summary of all injuries and medical conditions, and the expected goals of rehabilitation. Additionally, the orthopedic surgeons and/or neurosurgeons should clearly declare the stability of the spine, pelvis, and extremities to both the trauma team and the PT/OT consultant. A daily review of weight bearing restrictions and/or other precautions regarding physical movement of the spine or extremities is useful and should be reflected in the patient's activity orders.

Activity orders must further indicate whether patients are cleared for edge of bed, out of bed to chair, out of bed with assistance, or out of bed as tolerated. Out of bed orders should be written as soon as the patient is medically appropriate. Spine precautions must be cleared prior to therapy or out of bed orders to ensure that the patient is safe to participate in therapy programs. Orders for weight-bearing (for each involved extremity), type and wearing schedule for orthotic devices (e.g., if a specific back brace is required when out of bed), other specific precautions or contraindications (e.g., following anterior or posterior hip replacement surgeries), any ROM limitations, and any other critical information necessary for therapists to treat the patient appropriately and effectively must be included with the therapy orders. If in doubt, consult PT and/or OT for a patient evaluation.

An individualized plan of progressive exercise initiated as soon as possible in the recovery process is the best way to ensure the total recovery of the patient in the least amount of time and with fewest complications (4).

KEY POINTS

🖙 The overall goal of rehabilitation is to achieve maximum restoration of the patient's physical, psychological, social, vocational, recreational, and economic functions within the limits imposed by the trauma, critical illness, or any other pre-morbid deconditioning that may have occurred.

🖙 Physical therapy (PT) involves the identification, prevention, correction, and rehabilitation of acute or prolonged movement dysfunction of any etiology.

🖙 Occupational therapy (OT) primarily focuses upon improving patients' abilities to perform activities of daily living (ADLs) and functional mobility.

🖙 Patients relegated to extended bedrest suffer more secondary disabilities and require longer recovery periods than patients who are mobilized out of bed early.

🖙 Ordering PT and OT early in a patients' hospitalization will likely decrease medical and functional complications because patients will be stronger, more active, and mentally more interactive, leading to better outcomes.

🖙 Discharge planning considerations are deliberated during the initial rehab evaluation, even for ICU patients. The more time the patient, family, and medical team have to prepare, the more successful the discharge plan.

🖙 The Rancho Los Amigos Cognitive Scale provides the most useful and reproducible categorization of cognitive and behavioral status for patients who are awake and interacting with their environment (24).

🖙 Therapists should perform a standardized American Spinal Injury Association (ASIA) evaluation within the first 72 hours of admission following spinal cord injury (SCI).

🖙 Although a period of immobilization via traction or casting is necessary for the recovery of certain injuries and surgical repairs, therapy should be initiated as soon as medically appropriate.

🖙 Patients admitted for elective amputations should be introduced to therapy preoperatively.

🖙 The success of the burn patient's recovery relies greatly on their positioning in and out of bed. It is important to note that a position of comfort is, unfortunately, one that will facilitate contractures.

🖙 Consulting OT for splinting will ensure minimally-conscious patients are properly positioned and do not develop contractures.

🖙 The psychological component of rehabilitation is just as important as the physical component.

🖙 Continuity of care for rehabilitation begins in the ICU and is continued until after the patient is discharged.

REFERENCES

1. Black KS, Campbell MK. Physical therapy. In: Nickel VL, Botte MJ, eds. Orthopaedic Rehabilitation. 2nd ed. New York: Churchill Livingstone 1992:27–40.
2. Yerxa EJ, Clark F, Frank G, et al. An introduction to occupational science, a foundation for occupational therapy in the 21st century. Occupational Therapy in Health Care 1989; 6:1–17.
3. Dock W. The evil sequelae of complete bedrest. JAMA 1944; 125(16):1083–1085.
4. Kasper CE, Talbot LA, Gaines JM. Skeletal muscle damage and recovery. Am J Crit Care 2002;13(2):237–247.
5. Bloomfield SA. Changes in musculoskeletal structure and function with prolonged bedrest. Med Sci Sports Exerc 1997; 29(2):197–206.
6. Deitrick DE, Whedon GD, Shorr E. Effects of immobilization upon various metabolic and physiologic functions of normal men. Am J Med 1948; 4:1033–1038.
7. Fowles JR, Sale DG, MacDougal JD. Reduce strength after passive stretch of the human plantar flexors. J Appl Physiol 2000; 89(3):1179–1188.
8. Honkonen SE, Kannus P, Natri A, Latvala K, Jarvinen MJ. Isokinetic performance of the thigh muscles after tibial plateau fractures. Int Orthop 1997; 21(5):323–326.
9. Muller EA. Influence of training and of inactivity on muscle strength. Arch Phys Med Rehabil 1970; 51:449–462.
10. Mahoney JE. Immobility and falls. Acute Hospital Care 1998: 14(4)699–726.
11. Lorin S, Nierman DM. Critical illness neuromuscular abnormalities. Crit Care Clin 2002; 18:553–568.
12. Greenleaf JE. Energy and thermal regulation during bedrest and spaceflight. J Appl Physiol 1989; 67(2):507–516.
13. Saltin B, Blomqvist G, Mitchell JH, Johnson RL, Wildenthal K, Chapman CB. Response to exercise after bedrest and after training. Circulation 1968; 38(5):VII1–VII78.
14. Taylor HL, Henschel A, Brozek J, Keys A. Effects of bedrest on cardiovascular function and work performance. J Appl Physiol 1949;2:223–229.
15. Tisherman SA, Darby J, Peitzman AB. Intensive care unit: structure, role, and function in a trauma center and regional system. Surg Clin North Am 2000; 80(3):783–790.
16. Herbert RD, Balnave RJ. The effect of position of immobilization on resting length, resting stiffness, and weight of the soleus muscle of the rabbit. J Orthop Res 1993; 11(3): 358–366.
17. Hoyt DB, Hollingsworth-Fridlund P. Trauma surgery and trauma nursing. In: Nickel VL, Botte MJ, eds. Orthopaedic Rehabilitation. 2nd ed. New York: Churchill-Livingstone; 1992:95–103.
18. Kierkegaard A, Norgren L, Olsson, CG, et al. Incidence of deep vein thrombosis in bedridden non-surgical patients. Acta Med Scand 1987; 222:409–414.
19. Aldrich D, Hunt DP. When can the patient with deep venous thrombosis begin to ambulate? Phys Ther 2004; 84:268–273.
20. Partsch H. Therapy of deep vein thrombosis with low molecular weight heparin, leg compression and immediate ambulation. Vasa 2001; 30:195–204.
21. Partsch H, Blattler W. Compression and walking versus bedrest in the treatment of proximal deep venous thrombosis with low molecular weight heparin. J Vascular Surgery 2000; 32:861–869.
22. Davies PM. Steps to follow, a guide to the treatment of adult hemiplegia. Berlin: Springer, 1994.
23. Jacobs K, Jacobs J, eds. Quick reference dictionary for occupational therapy. Thorofare, New Jersey: Slack, 2001.
24. Hagen C. Rancho Los Amigos cognitive scale (1982). Hagen C. In: Herndon RM, (1997). Handbook of clinical neurologic scales. New York: Dernos Vermande. Pg.195:207–208. Revised scale 1997 by Hagen C.
25. American Spinal Injury Association/International Medical Society of Paraplegia: International standards for neurological and functional classification of spinal cord injury patients. Chicago: ASIA, 2000.
26. Luce JM. Spinal cord injury. In: Luce JM, and Pierson DJ, eds. Critical Care Medicine. Philadelphia: W.D. Saunders Co. 1988:438.
27. Yarkony GM, ed. Spinal cord injury: medical management and rehabilitation (Rehabilitation Institute of Chicago manual). Rockville, Maryland: Aspen Systems Corporation., 1994.
28. Somer MF. Spinal cord injury: functional rehabilitation. Norwalk, Connecticut: Appleton & Lange, 1992.
29. Koval KJ, Skovron ML, Aharanoff GB, et al. Ambulatory ability after hip fracture: a prospective study in geriatric patients. Clin Orthop 1995; 310:150–159.
30. Guccione AA, Fagerson TL, Anderson JJ. Regaining functional independence in the acute care setting following hip fracture Phys Ther 1996; 76(8):818–826.

31. Grunert BK, Devine CA. Psychologic effects of upper extremity disorders. In: Mackin EJ, Callahan AD, Skirven TM, Schneider LH, Osterman AL, eds. Rehabilitation of the Hand, and Upper Extremity. 5th ed. St. Louis: Mosby, 2002;1088–1096.

32. Karacoloff LA, Hammersley CS, Schneider FJ. Pre-prosthetic program in lower extremity amputation: a guide to functional outcomes in physical therapy management. Gaithersburg, MD: Aspen Publishers, 1992;11–23.

33. American College of Surgeons Committee on Trauma. Resources for the optimal care of the injured patient. American College of Surgeons Committee on Trauma, Chicago, 1998;55.

34. Howell JW. Management of the burned hand. In: Richard RL, Staley MJ, eds. Burn care and rehabilitation: principles and practice. Philadelphia: FA Davis, 1994;531–532.

35. Laseter G. Management of the stiff hand: a practical approach. Orthop Clin North Am 1983; 14:749–765.

36. Saunders S. Physical therapy management of hand fractures. Phys Ther 1989; 69:1065–1076.

37. Ward RS, Reddy R, Brockway C, Hayes-Lundy C, Mills P. Uses of coban self-adherent wrap in management of post-burn hand grafts: case reports. J Burn Care Rehabil 1994; 15:364–369.

38. Lowell M, Pirc P, Ward RS, et al. Effect of 3M Coban self-adherent wraps on edema and function of the burned hand: a case study. J Burn Care Rehabil 2003; 24(4):257–258.

39. University of California Regents. UCSD guide for post liver transplant care. San Diego: University of California, San Diego Medical Center. 2003.

40. Milzman DP, Boulanger BR, Rodriquez A, Soderstrom CA, Mitchell KA, Magnant CM. Pre-existing disease in trauma patients: a predictor of fate independent of age and ISS. J Trauma 1992; 32:236–243.

41. Jones C, Skirrow P, Griffiths RD, et al. Rehabilitation after critical illness: a randomized, controlled trial. Crit Care Med 2003; 31(10):2456–2461.

42. Kase K. Illustrated Kinesio Taping. Ken'i kai information. Albuquerque: New Mexico, 2000;6–11.

43. Barbeau H, Rossignol S. Recovery of locomotion after chronic spinalization in the adult cat. Brain Res 1987; 412:84–95.

44. Finch L, Barbeau H, Arsenault B. Influence of body weight support on normal human gait: development of gait retraining strategy. Phys Ther 1991; 71:842–855.

45. Edgerton VR, Roy RR, de Leon RD, Tillakaratne N, Hodgson JA. Does motor learning occur in the spinal cord? Neuroscientist 1997; 3:287–294.

46. Richards CL, Malouin F, Wood-Dauphinee S, Williams JI, Bouchard JP, Brunet D. Task-specific physical therapy for optimization of gait recovery in acute stroke patients. Arch Phys Med Rehabil 1993; 74:612–620.

47. Visintin M, Barbeau H, Korner-Bitensky N, Mayo NE. A new approach to retrain gait in stroke patients through body weight support and treadmill stimulation. Stroke 1998; 29:1122–1128.

48. Sullivan K, Knowlton B, Dobkin B. Step training with body weight support: effect of treadmill speed and practice paradigms on poststroke locomotor recovery. Arch Phys Med Rehabil 2002: 83:683–691.

49. Hesse S, et al. Treadmill walking with partial body weight support versus floor walking in hemiparetic subjects. Arch Phys Med Rehabil 1999; 80:421–427.

50. Wernig A, Nanassy A, et al. Laufband (treadmill) therapy in incomplete paraplegia and tetraplegia. J Neurotrauma 1999; 16(8):719–726.

51. Miyai I, Fujimoto Y, UedaY. Long-term effect of body weight-supported treadmill training in Parkinson's disease: a randomized controlled trial. Arch Phys Med Rehabil 2002; 83:1370–1373.

52. Baldi JC, Jackson RD, Moraille R, Mysiw WJ. Muscle atrophy is prevented in patients with acute spinal cord injury using functional electrical stimulation. Spinal Cord 1998; 36(7):463–9.

53. Hangartner TN, Rodgers MM, Glaser RM, Barre PS. Tibial bone density loss in spinal cord injured patients: effects of FES exercise. J Rehabil Res Dev 1994; 31(1):50–61.

54. Michlovitz SL. Ultrasound and selected physical agent modalities in upper extremity rehabilitation. In: Mackin, E.J., Callahan, A.D., Skirven, T.M., Schneider, L.H., Osterman, AL, eds. Rehabilitation of the hand and upper extremity. 5th ed. St. Louis: Mosby, 2002; 1745–1763.

55. Wang RY, Chan RC, Tsai MW. Functional electrical stimulation on chronic and acute hemiplegic shoulder subluxation. Am J Phys Med Rehabil 2000; 79(4):385–94.

56. Schiedermayer D. Music therapy for the relief of postoperative pain. In: The physician's guide to alternative medicine, Volume II. Atlanta: American Healthcare Consultants. 2000; 295–297.

57. Fratianne RB, Prensner JD, Huston MJ, Super DM, Yowler CJ, Standley JM. The effect of music-based imagery and musical alternate engagement on the burn debridement process. J Burn Care Rehabil 2001; 22(1):47–53.

58. Good M, Anderson GC, Stanton-Hicks M, Grass JA, Makii M. Relaxation and music reduce pain after gynecologic surgery. Pain Manag Nurs 2002; 3(2):61–70.

59. Cole K, Garlinski A. Animal assisted therapy in the intensive care unit? a staff nurse's dream comes true. Nurs Clin North Am 1995; 30(3):529.

60. Connor K and Miller J. Help from our animal friends. Nurs Manage 2000; 31:42–46.

61. Titler MG. Family visitation and partnership in the critical care unit. In: Chulay M, Molter N, eds. Protocols for practice: creating a healing environment. Aliso Viejo: Am. J. Crit. Care 1998; 1–46.

62. Lee R. Guided imagery of supportive therapy in cancer treatment. In: The Physician's Guide to Alternative Medicine, Volume II. Atlanta: American Healthcare Consultants. 2000; 261–264.

67

Ethical and Legal Issues in Trauma and Critical Care

John M. Luce

Department of Medicine and Anesthesia, UC San Francisco School of Medicine, San Francisco General Hospital,
San Francisco, California, U.S.A.

INTRODUCTION

Patients with trauma and critical illness present physicians and other health professionals with a host of ethical considerations. Ethical behavior is aspired to by the vast majority of physicians and health care workers around the world. Although there is broad agreement on fundamental principles, complex ethical dilemmas can arise in clinical practice that challenge even the most erudite and ethically sophisticated of clinicians.

The fields of ethics and law have occasionally been outpaced by the rapid technological changes in health care. Consequently, disagreement and uncertainty can occur when formulating clinical decisions, which uphold legal and ethical precepts. The situation is complicated further by the global mobility of patients and family members—some countries, the interpretation of ethical issues have been enshrined in local and national law. As might be expected, the legal interpretation of ethical issues tends to reflect the values of individuals and the society to whom these laws apply.

☞ **Important ethical issues in trauma and critical care include medical decision-making, informed consent, resuscitation, brain death, organ transplantation, the withholding and withdrawal of life support, and the allocation of medical resources.** ☞ These issues are addressed in this chapter after providing a background to the field of biomedical ethics. The relationships between ethical and legal considerations are discussed with specific reference to the American and British case law. In the "Eye to the Future" section, suggestions are provided regarding how this field may evolve in coming years.

BACKGROUND TO BIOMEDICAL ETHICS
Ethical Principles

Beauchamp and Childress (1) have described four ethical principles that govern the attitudes and behaviors of physicians and other health professionals. In addition to influencing professional standards, these four principles (based on Western philosophical thought) inform most health care law. The oldest ethical principle is *beneficence*: acting to benefit patients by sustaining life, treating illness, and relieving pain. A correlative principle is *nonmaleficence*: refraining from causing harm as per the dictum of *"primum non nocere"* (*"first, cause no harm"*). A third principle, which has increasingly gained importance in the United States and some other countries, is that of *autonomy*: respecting the patient's right to self-determination. A fourth ethical principle, enumerated by Beauchamp and Childress, is *distributive justice*: the fair, equitable, and appropriate allocation of medical services in society. Underlying these ethical principles are the covenantal virtues of *trust* (or fidelity), as articulated in the Hippocratic Oath (Fig. 1) (2), and *honesty*, the obligation to tell the truth (not explicitly referred to in the Hippocratic Oath). Patients have the right to expect that all physicians and health care workers will be honest and trustworthy at all times.

An additional ethical principle increasingly emphasized over the last decade is that of *confidentiality*: the respect of privileged patient information (this concept is explicitly mentioned in the in the Hippocratic oath). The four ethical principles of Beauchamp and those additional precepts addressed in the Hippocratic oath (trust and confidentiality) are summarized in Table 1.

The Fiduciary Relationship

The first three ethical principles outlined above also constitute the foundation of the fiduciary relationship through which physicians hold a special relationship of trust, confidence, and responsibility and, as such, are expected to serve the best interests of their patients. Such a relationship is expected by society, because patients are assumed to be vulnerable and medically naïve compared to physicians (and other health professionals) who possess superior medical knowledge. In keeping with the principles of beneficence and nonmaleficence, physicians and other knowledgeable health practitioners may feel compelled to decide what is best for their patients. The principle of autonomy, which respects the individual's right to self-determination, is viewed ethically and legally as having priority, even if the patient's choice is contrary to that of the practitioner (3).

☞ **In keeping with the principle of autonomy when capable of rational informed decision-making, patients should always be allowed to define their own interests.** ☞

Increased Legal Emphasis upon Confidentiality

Confidentiality in health care involves the respect of privileged patient information. Respect for confidentiality is firmly established in codes of ethics and in law. As an element of the principles of fidelity (promise keeping), confidentiality is an essential component of trust as part of the fiduciary relationship. The Hippocratic Oath explicitly demands that physicians respect their patient's confidences.

Confidentiality is linked with rights to privacy and is prescribed in law, including the 1996 Health Insurance Portability and Accountability Act (HIPAA), which was passed as Public Law 104–191 by the 104th congress. The HIPAA regulations call for series of privacy standards to be met in all patients, including trauma and critically ill (4).

I swear by Apollo the physician and by Asclepius and by health [the God Hygieia] and Panacea and by all the Gods as well as Goddesses, making them judges [witnesses], to bring the following oath and written covenant to fulfillment, in accordance with my power and my judgment:

To regard him who has taught me this techné [art and science] as equal to my parents, and to share, in partnership, my livelihood with him and to give him a share when he is in need of necessities, and to judge the offspring [coming] from him equal to [my] male siblings, and to teach them this techné, should they desire to learn [it], without fee and written covenant, and to give a share both of rules and of lectures, and of all the rest of learning, to my sons and to the [sons] of him who has taught me and to the pupils who have both made a written contract and sworn by a medical convention but by no other.

And I will use regimens for the benefit of the ill in accordance with my ability and my judgment, but from [what is] to their harm or injustice I will keep [them].

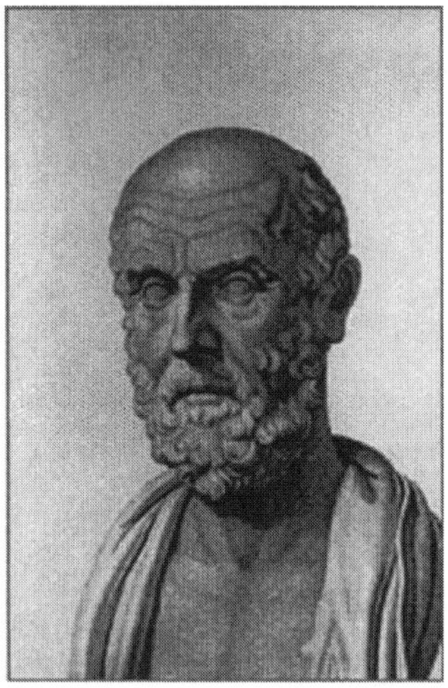

And I will not give a drug that is deadly to anyone if asked [for it], nor will I suggest the way to such a counsel. And likewise, I will not give a woman a destructive pessary. And in a pure and holy way I will guard my life and my techné. I will not cut, and certainly not those suffering from stone, but I will cede [this] to men [who are] practitioners of this activity.

Into as many houses as I may enter, I will go for the benefit for the ill, while being far from all voluntary and destructive injustice, especially from sexual acts both upon women's bodies and upon men's, both of the free and of the slaves. And about whatever I may see or hear in treatment, or even without treatment, in the life of human beings —things that should not ever be blurted outside — I will remain silent. Holding such things to be unutterable [sacred, not to be divulged]. If I render this oath fulfilled. And if I do not blur and confound it [making it to no effect] may it be [granted] to me to enjoy the benefits both of life and of techné, being held in good repute among all human beings for time eternal. If, however, I transgress and perjure myself, the opposite of these.

Figure 1 Classical version of Hippocratic Oath—as translated and relayed by Miles SH: The Hippocratic Oath and the Ethics of Medicine. Oxford University Press, 2004.

Special Circumstances of Trauma and Critical Illness

The fiduciary relationship is relatively easy to maintain when patients have minor or chronic illnesses and are seen in primary physicians' offices or in hospital rooms. Disagreements about what is best for patients can be discussed unhurriedly in such settings, and both parties have ample opportunity to engage in deliberate conversation regarding the plan of care and treatment goals. Such relationships are more difficult to establish in the emergency department (ED), the Trauma Resuscitation Suite (TRS), the operating room (OR), and the Surgical Intensive Care Unit (SICU). One reason that the fiduciary relationship may be compromised during critical illness is that primary physicians usually have to share responsibility for their patients with specialists or, in many cases, transfer it entirely. In this process, physicians who have no prior familiarity with the patients must develop new fiduciary relationships of their own.

At the same time, the ethical principles outlined earlier can be more complex and difficult to apply in the ED, the OR, or the SICU than in other settings. Beneficence and non-maleficence often collide when critical care technologies that support life also cause pain or loss of dignity. Autonomy is more difficult to preserve when patients are unresponsive, because their prior wishes are unknown and the pace of medical intervention is accelerated. Finally, the interests of patients and society may clash over issues such as the triage of multiple trauma victims and the continuation of life support in the face of a poor prognosis or limited space in the SICU.

MEDICAL DECISION MAKING
Competent Patients

In the United States and some other countries, most medical decisions are made jointly by patients and their physicians. Some patients may make unilateral decisions; others may prefer to let physicians decide for them in some, if not all circumstances. Nevertheless, most mentally competent

Table 1 Principles of Biomedical Ethics

Principle	Explanation
Honesty	Perhaps the paramount ethical principle. In past eras (of paternalism), honesty with patient regarding his or her condition may have been a secondary concern; whereas, beneficence and nonmaleficence were held as more important.
Beneficence	Acting to benefit patients and promote good"cure sometimes, relieve often, "comfort always."
Nonmaleficence	Avoiding injury or harm *primum non nocere* "first do no harm."
Autonomy	*Auto* = self, *nomy* = govern: Respecting a patients' right to self-determination.
Distributive justice	Allocating resources fairly, and allowing equal access to health care.
Confidentiality	Information gained as part of the doctor/patient relationship is privileged and not to be shared with a third party without the consent of the patient.

patients seek physicians' opinions, weigh the medical options available to them, and either accept or reject their physicians' recommendations.

The propriety of competent patients to make medical decisions is supported by the ethical principle of autonomy and by the legal rights of consent and refusal, which have been contained for centuries within British and American common law. In keeping with this legal tradition, court decisions, such as that in *Bartling v. Superior Court* (5) and *Bouvia v. Superior Court* (6) in California, have established that competent patients have the right to accept or refuse any and all medical treatments, including those that are potentially life saving. Similarly, in its *Cruzan* (7) decision, the U.S. Supreme Court confirmed that competent patients have such a right under the 14th Amendment to the Constitution.

Use of Surrogates for Incompetent Patients

Some previously competent patients remain so following trauma and/or throughout a critical illness and, therefore, can participate in medical decisions. However, many critically ill patients are decisionally incapacitated due to illness-related factors. When patients are incompetent to begin with, or are unable to communicate because they are comatose or sedated, their surrogates may become involved in the decision-making process. The proper role for the surrogates is to represent patients' interests and previously expressed wishes. Surrogates are less helpful when they represent their own interests or speak only from their own points of view. Failure of surrogates to fully comprehend the patient's clinical condition can also impair their ability to fully convey the patient's true beliefs about decision-making.

The legal authority to use surrogates in making medical decisions for incompetent patients was established in the United States with the case of *in re Quinlan* (8), in which the New Jersey Supreme Court allowed a parent to exercise the incompetent daughter's right of refusal through the mechanism of substituted judgment. The U.S. Supreme Court, in its *Cruzan* (7) decision, allowed the states to require "clear and convincing evidence" of patients'

wishes before allowing surrogates to refuse life-sustaining interventions for them. Nevertheless, the U.S. Supreme Court did not mandate that other states adopt this strict standard, and states other than New York (9) and Missouri (10) generally do not inhibit surrogates from exercising the rights of consent and refusal on behalf of the incompetent.

☞ **The most ideal surrogates are those who have been designated by patients before or during their critical illness to make medical decisions in the event of incapacity.** ☜ In California and many other states, such surrogates may be granted a durable power of attorney for health care (DPAHC) (11). Proxy directives of this sort are legally binding so long as patient's interests are being protected. Properly executed DPAHCs are more helpful than living wills and other instructional directives, most of which are either too broadly or too narrowly drawn (12).

Proxy and instructional directives are prepared for the most part by patients with chronic illness who anticipate further decomposition. Yet, only a minority (<20%) of such patients draw up directives despite passage of the Federal Patient Self-Determination Act of 1990, which requires that healthcare institutions inquire whether patients have advance directives, and help them to obtain such directives if they have not already done so (13). Living wills and DPAHCs are even more rarely thought of by healthy persons, even though they may become trauma victims. As a result, unofficially designated surrogates, usually spouses, parents, children, or siblings must make decisions for patients, usually in a shared decision-making model with physicians.

States vary in their processes and rules for medical surrogacy. In general, these variations fall into two categories: rules for determining the surrogate decision-makers and rules stipulating what surrogates can decide. Rules involving the first category are addressed by family consent laws. Thus, many states, including Illinois, Ohio, Virginia, and Washington, have enacted statutes that allow close family members to act on behalf of incompetent patients when the patients have not delegated this responsibility before losing competence. All of the statutes prescribe a hierarchy of family members and require agreement among members at the highest available class in the hierarchy (14). With respect to what surrogates are allowed to decide, differences also exist between various states.

In the *Wendland* case (15), the California Supreme Court unanimously decided to restrict sharply the authority of a patient's wife, who was also her husband's conservator, to limit life-sustaining interventions in the face of opposition from the patient's mother. In this case, the patient was conscious, and expected to survive for many years if the interventions were continued.

In contrast, Terri Schiavo was a woman who remained in a persistent vegetative state after suffering cardiac arrest. Mrs. Schiavo had been sustained by artificial hydration and nutrition through a feeding tube for 15 years. In the *Schiavo* case (16), the husband served as her surrogate and expressed her wishes that life-supporting therapy (in this case, food and water) be withheld, despite vehement disagreement from Terri's parents. The parents were waged in a legal battle to continue the tube feedings and obtained surrogacy rights for over a decade.

The Pinellas County Circuit Court initially ruled in favor of the husband citing a previous decision by the Florida Supreme Court in *Re: Guardianship of Estelle M. Browning* (17). Judge Greer and the Circuit Court held that Michael Schiavo (Terri's husband) was the proper surrogate, that prior to developing anoxic encephalopathy (and while mentally competent) Terri Schiavo had made credible and reliable statements regarding her wishes that she not be kept alive by tubes if she entered a chronic vegetative state. The court was also satisfied that Mrs. Schiavo was in such an irreversible and chronic vegetative state (18).

Subsequently, the case was appealed numerous times; eventually going to the Florida District Court, which also held in favor of the spouse's right to serve as the proper surrogate, conveying Terri Schiavo's wishes not to remain in a persistent vegetative state. This ruling was further upheld by the district court of appeals and ultimately the U.S. Supreme Court.

Unlike most incompetent patients for whom decisions must be made about life-sustaining interventions, in the *Wendland* case (15), the patient was conscious and was expected to survive for many years as long as the interventions were continued. If the *Wendland* ruling were extended to others like the *Schiavo* case, where the patient was in a chronic vegetative state, patients could be subjected to burdensome interventions that offer little clinical benefit, which they might not have ever wanted. In the *Schiavo* case (16), the court ruled differently and held that the husband was the proper surrogate to convey her wishes that she not remain in a persistent vegetative state.

In English law, the surrogate situation is different. No one may give consent on behalf of an incompetent adult. If the patient, when competent, made his wishes known and the circumstances are unchanged, those wishes must be respected. The only exception to this rule is when patients are detained under the Mental Health Act of 1983 (19). If the patient is incompetent and has not made his or her wishes known, it is generally accepted that life-saving treatment may be given if physicians and surrogates agree that such treatment is essential and in the patient's best interest. If there is time and the decision is difficult, guidance may be sought from the High Court. Examples of High Court involvement include separation of conjoined twins when one is almost certain to die and withdrawal of feeding for patients with severe brain damage.

When Surrogates Are Lacking

Legal guidelines are less clear for cases in which incompetent patients lack surrogates. Two states—Connecticut (20) and Hawaii (21)—allow physicians to make decisions for incompetent patients based on wishes expressed by the patients to the physicians when the patients were competent. However, no state explicitly authorizes unilateral decision-making by physicians based on any other standard, including the patients' best interests. As such, where patients have not stated otherwise, physicians can make decisions they consider in the patients' best interests under the principle of beneficence, especially when urgent decisions must be made.

An alternative approach is for physicians to ask the court to appoint conservators or other advocates to help preserve the autonomy of their patients. This approach is cumbersome and time-consuming, and conservators often rely upon the physicians to make medical decisions because the conservators are seldom experts in health care. In certain situations, and time permitting, this approach may be justified. Otherwise, rather than make unilateral decisions, physicians are best advised to review these decisions with their colleagues or consult with members of the institutional ethics committee. Such review is in keeping with good medical practice, even though it has no legal standing.

☞ **Physicians may make decisions they consider in a patient's best interests in an emergency, unless the patient has stipulated otherwise.** ☜

INFORMED CONSENT
Forms of Consent

The ethical principle of autonomy is contained in the concept of informed consent, which Beauchamp and Childress (1) define as "... an autonomous authorization by individuals of a medical intervention or of involvement in research." According to these authors, consent can only be informed if patients or their surrogates are competent insofar as they can understand what they are being asked to do. In addition, information that is material to them and their situations must be disclosed to them. They must also be able to deliberate about this information. Finally, they must be free of undue influence or coercion in giving consent. In health care decision-making, a fully informed, capable, and freely consenting patient (or surrogate) has the right to make an autonomous decision (Table 2). In certain situations, the state has the right to override the principle of autonomy as discussed later in this chapter.

Beauchamp and Childress (1) note that informed consent differs from other forms of consent, including implicit consent. Implicit consent exists when approval of one medical procedure is implicit in approval of another; for example, consent to anesthesia may be implicit in consent to surgery. Another form of consent is implied consent. Consent may be implied in emergency situations, wherein physicians feel obligated to provide medically necessary treatment when patients or surrogates have not expressed their wishes. The rationale for treatment in such situations is that patients or surrogates would consent if they could be informed and that harm would result if care were delayed (3).

The practice of trauma and critical care medicine frequently involves the institution of emergency life saving treatment, and physicians frequently use implied consent to justify invasive treatments, including immediate surgery. Although this may be appropriate in true emergencies, informed consent should be sought prior to procedures whenever possible, even if it requires an extensive family search or the appointment of a conservator or other advocate to protect patient interests. ☞ **If a true emergency exists, then consent may be considered to be implied.** ☜

Evolution in the Concepts and Standards of Informed Consent

The concept of informed consent is supported by the rights of consent and refusal that are inimical to British and

Table 2   Required Elements of Informed Consent

Requirement	Explanation and examples
Competence	Patients or surrogates can understand what is asked of them (legal status).
Full disclosure	Information that is material to patients and their situation is disclosed to them.
Specificity	Consent for each component of healthcare and each procedure (no blanket consent).
Freedom of coercion	Patients or surrogates are free of coercion. Patients or surrogates can deliberate.

American common law, as discussed earlier. Common and constitutional law also have held that physicians have a number of professional duties to patients, including the duty to do good (i.e., beneficence) and avoid harm (i.e., nonmaleficence). Failure to fulfill these duties is a tort, which may result in punishment under the criminal law or in an obligation to compensate patients monetarily under civil law (22).

Modern considerations for informed consent emanate from the ethical principle of autonomy. However, until the 20th century medical paternalism prevailed. Indeed, the concept of consent was not even mentioned in the first medical ethics code of the American Medical Association (AMA) in 1847 (Table 3). The ethical paradigms of consent evolved as society changed, but also changed in response to legal decisions.

The legal obligation of clinicians to obtain consent before treating patients was established by several landmark rulings in the United States in the early 20th century. In the first case, *Schloendorff v. Society of New York Hospitals* (23), which occurred in 1914, the Court of Appeal of New York determined that "Every being of adult years and sound mind has the right to determine what should be done with his own body; and a surgeon who performs an operation without his patient's consent commits an assault, for which he is liable in damages, except in cases of emergency when the patient is unconscious, and when it is necessary to operate before consent can be obtained."

Only assent (the agreement to proceed) was required for an operation at that time; no true consent was needed until the late 1950s. In 1957, the case of *Salgo v. Trustees of Leland Stanford Hospital* (24) involved a patient, Mr. Salgo, who underwent transabdominal aortography that resulted in paralysis, a known risk of the procedure of which he was not informed. Mr. Salgo contended that he would not have consented to the procedure had he known about the

risk. The judge ruled in favor of Mr. Salgo, and clarified difference between assent and consent (which is legally required), when he stated: "A physician violates his duty to his patient and subjects himself to liability if he withholds any facts which are necessary to form the basis of an intelligent consent by a patient to a proposed treatment."

The next step in the progression of consent rulings occurred in 1960 with the case of *Natanson v. Kline* (25), in which a patient, (Ms. Natanson) sustained radiation burns while undergoing radiation treatment for a tumor, a known complication for which she was not informed. This decision established the "Professional Practice Standard" later known as the "Reasonable Doctor Standard." The Judge asserted that disclosure to a patient should be to the extent "a reasonable practitioner would make under the same or similar circumstances."

The "reasonable doctor standard" prevailed until the case of *Canterbury v. Spence* (26) in 1972, which involved a patient (Mr. Canterbury) who sustained quadriplegia during a cervical laminectomy, a known but uncommon complication. In this case, Mr. Canterbury was not informed of the possibility of this complication because it was not customary local practice to do so. Mr. Canterbury sued, and the court agreed that the "reasonable doctor" threshold was too low. The Court held that disclosure to a patient should include all material that a "reasonable person" would consider important for decision making. So was born the "reasonable patient standard" which is used today.

In another case, *Cobbs v. Grant* (27), the Supreme Court of California clarified in 1972 that the battery theory of *Schloendorff* (23) "should be reserved for these circumstances where a doctor performs an operation to which the patient has not consented." Other actions may constitute negligence, especially if a patient is harmed and a physician did not uphold his/her duty, for example, if physicians applied an intervention that caused harm without "reasonable disclosure of the available choices with respect to the proposed

Table 3 Historical Standards and Landmark Legal Cases that Impacted or Altered the Ethical Paradigms Underpinning Informed Consent

Era	Prevailing ethical principles of era	Examples of societal focus or legal cases prompting ethical paradigm shift
Antiquity	Paternalism	"Conceal most things from the patient while you are attending to him ... revealing nothing of the patient's future or present condition," Hippocrates.
Late 19th century	Paternalism	"Consent" not even mentioned in first American medical ethics code, American Medical Association, 1847.
Early 20th century	Assent = consent	"Surgery without consent = assault" (23).
Mid 20th century	Autonomy but, only assent (agreement to have a procedure) was required.	Increased emphasis on civil and consumer rights in the United States and western countries led to increased emphasis on autonomy.
Mid 20th century	Full disclosure (not defined)	Must provide all facts required to form an intelligent decision (24).
Mid 20th century	Full disclosure (Reasonable Dr Std)	Disclosure should be to the same extent "a reasonable practitioner would make under the same or similar circumstances" (25).
Mid-late 20th century	Full disclosure (Reasonable Pt Std)	Disclosure should include all material a "reasonable person" would consider important (26).
Mid-late 20th century	Full disclosure (Reasonable Pt Std) Ruling clarified breech of duty.	Clarifies difference between battery (operation without consent) versus negligence (improper treatment) versus dereliction of duty (failure to provide indicated treatment or information) (27).
Late 20th century to current	Full disclosure (Clarifies fiduciary duty of M.D. during medical research)	Physician must disclose conflicts of interest that can affect patient care (31).

therapy and the dangers inherently and potentially involved in each."

With the continuing escalation in medical technology, physicians have the duty to be knowledgeable of the latest treatment options, and the most potentially beneficial treatments should be made known to the patient, even if the physician disclosing the information cannot personally provide them (due to training or resource availability).

Consent for Clinical Research

In recent years, the same legal principles and precedents that deal with informed consent for treatment have been applied to clinical research. Research conducted by institutions that receive federal funding is governed by the Code of Federal Regulations (CFR) for the protection of human subjects. According to the 1991 version of the CFR (28), "... no investigation may involve a human being as a subject in research unless the investigator has obtained the legally effective informed consent of the subject or the subject's legally authorized representative."

Most states have not clarified which surrogates are legally authorized to represent subjects in issues regarding research. However, the California Health and Safety Code recently was amended to allow agents pursuant to an advanced directive, conservators or guardians, and family members to provide consent for subjects who are incompetent and cannot consent for themselves. If a subject is in a non-ED environment, consent may be sought from available surrogate decision-makers in descending order of legal priority. In an ED environment, any available surrogate may give consent. In both environments, when two or more proxies are present and at least one disagrees with the participation of the subject in the medical experiment, surrogate consent is not valid (29).

Recognizing that surrogates are not always available, the 1991 CFR also permits that consent be waived if "(i) the research involves no more than minimum risk to the subjects, (ii) the waiver ... will not adversely affect the right and welfare of the subjects, (iii) the research could not practically be carried out without the waiver ..., and (iv) whenever appropriate, the subjects will be provided with additional pertinent information after participation." The definition of "minimum risk" here is that "... the probability and magnitude of harm or discomfort anticipated in the research are not greater in and of themselves ... than those encountered in daily life or during the performance of routine physical or psychological examinations or tests."

Although the 1991 CFR provides some latitude in enrolling incompetent subjects without available surrogates, its definition of minimal risk was interpreted by some to preclude investigations of emergency interventions such as cardiopulmonary resuscitation. This situation led trauma and critical care investigators to enroll patients under a "deferred consent mechanism" which the government declared inappropriate. They then argued that the minimal risk standard should be changed to allow incompetent patients access to potentially beneficial treatment in clinical trials.

In response to these arguments, the 1991 CFR was revised in 1996 to allow research to be conducted in emergency situations without patient or surrogate consent if the following provisions are met: (i) the human subjects are in a life-threatening situation, (ii) obtaining consent is not feasible, (iii) participation in the research holds the prospect of direct benefit to the subject, (iv) the clinical investigation could not practically be carried out without the waiver,

(v) the proposed investigation plan defines the length of the potential therapeutic window (during which the surrogate will be contacted for consent), (vi) the Institutional Review Board (IRB) has revised and approved informal consent procedures, and (vii) consultation (will occur) with representatives of the communities in which the clinical investigation will be conducted and from which the subjects will be drawn (30).

The 1996 CFR revisions were rapidly implemented by most IRBs. However, there has been variability on how the IRBs ensure that investigators consult "with representations of the communities in which the clinical investigations will be conducted and from which the subjects will be drawn ...." The 1996 CFR did broaden patient access to clinical research in areas restricted by the 1991 CFR to include trauma and cardiopulmonary arrest while also protecting patient autonomy.

Many critical care interventions have yet to be subjected to prospective randomized, controlled trials. This is partly due to the reluctance of physicians to participate in trials that involve current practices that they believe are beneficial. However, new and unproven treatments, such as the use of hypothermia for head injury, and the introduction of new drugs, such as activated Protein C, have and should continue to be subject to rigorous scientific testing before their generalized introduction. It may not be possible to reduce current costs without depriving some patients of beneficial treatment, but critical care physicians can fulfill their obligation to individual patients and society by only offering interventions that are of proven or likely benefit.

Another important ethical conflict that can arise during the consent of subjects for clinical studies is that of financial or intellectual rights conflict. For example, a physician scientist investigating the clinical efficacy of a device or drug that is produced by a company in which he or she holds stock, or receives research funds from, should be fully disclosed to the potential study subject (31). This information should also be disclosed on any publications that result from the research.

Patients with Unusual Beliefs: The Example of Jehovah's Witnesses

Physicians and other health professionals occasionally seek consent from patients whose personal beliefs appear unusual or unreasonable. Some of these patients clearly are incompetent to make medical decisions due to drug use, delirium, and chronic neurologic or psychiatric conditions such as schizophrenia. Other patients, however, are capable of making decision but refuse medical interventions because of beliefs to which adherence is not ipso facto a sign of incompetence. Among these patients are herbalists, advocates of faith healing, followers of homeopathy rather than allopathic medicine, Christian Scientists who prefer care from practitioners within their faith, and Jehovah's Witnesses who refuse blood and blood products. Because obtaining consent for transfusions is common during the management of trauma and critical illness, and because Jehovah's Witnesses are representative of patients with unusual beliefs, they will be discussed here.

In general, Jehovah's Witnesses believe that blood contains the essence of life and that the mingling of one's blood with that of another is prohibited by the Bible (32). Whereas the biblical passage on which this belief is based refers to the art of drinking blood, its interpretation by Jehovah's Witnesses precludes the receipt of whole blood, red blood cells, platelets, and plasma, though not necessarily of clotting factors or plasma proteins such as albumin. Jehovah's Witnesses also have accepted preblood loss hemodilution with a continuously flowing circuit, but not an extracorporeal circuit with a heart-lung or dialysis machine that may be "tainted" by blood from another. Their beliefs hold that exposure to another's blood risks eternal damnation and ostracism from one's family and other members of the faith, instead of eternal life after death and resurrection. As a result, saving the life of a Jehovah's Witness may condemn that person not only to a life not worth living but also salvation unrealized.

As an affirmation of their faith, Jehovah's Witnesses may be asked on an annual basis to sign a wallet-sized advance directive called a "blood card" to document their informed refusal of blood and blood products in emergency situations (33). When seen in an ED or in other areas of the hospital, they may be surrounded by family and other members of the faith who try to reinforce their resolve to forgo transfusions. Although such reinforcement may be effective, not all Jehovah's Witnesses ultimately refuse blood and blood products. A recent study (34) of 58 trauma victims who were Jehovah's Witnesses revealed that four patients were given blood and three were given autotransfusions that were potentially "tainted." Documented consent to receive blood was found in the charts of two of these patients. This situation and others has reinforced the need to question Jehovah's Witness patients individually (apart from family and friends) to ensure autonomous, uncoerced decision-making.

Court decisions such as that *in re Estate of Brooks* (35) have stated "... even though we may consider (an individual's) beliefs unwise, foolish, or ridiculous, in the absence of an overriding danger to society we may not permit interference therewith ... for the sole purpose of compelling (an individual) to accept medical treatment forbidden by (his or her) religious principles, and previously refused by (him or her) with full knowledge of the probable consequences." Such decisions and the ethical principles of autonomy they reflect mandate that Jehovah's Witnesses, who are competent and can articulate their wishes, may refuse blood and blood products in both emergency and elective circumstances.

The law is less clear regarding emergencies in which wishes cannot be articulated by patients, and the exhortations of family and members of the faith or a "blood card" must be relied on. Some physicians would prefer not to treat patients without a court order in such situations, even though a delay might mean death. Most would rely on legal precedents such as *in Re The Estate of Varrell Dorne* (36), in which the Pennsylvania Supreme Court said that "... when there is an emergency calling for an immediate decision, nothing less than a fully conscious contemporaneous decision by the patient will be sufficient to override evidence of medical necessity."

Neither in emergencies nor elective circumstances do Jehovah's Witnesses have an ethical or legal right to prohibit the administration of blood or blood products to their children if these treatments are needed to sustain life. This principle was established in the 1944 case of *Prince v. Commonwealth of Massachusetts* (37) which did not involve transfusions. The court held that "Patients may be free to be martyrs themselves. But it does not follow that they are free in identical circumstances to make martyrs of their children." In all cases since *Prince*, the courts have agreed that children should receive transfusions if they are medically indicated. Indeed, many physicians will give blood and blood products to the critically ill children of Jehovah's Witnesses before the court order is granted. According to Jonsen (38), the courts likely would judge in the same way if the life of a viable fetus were in question.

Above and beyond the ethical issues, management of Jehovah's Witnesses may not require transfusions at all. It is our duty as health-care providers to keep abreast of medical developments that allow us to treat Jehovah's Witnesses in a manner that not only saves life but also respects their religious beliefs. Experience with these patients, among others, has demonstrated that patients with trauma and other conditions may tolerate hemoglobin levels in the range of 5 gm/DL (39). Such tolerance may be enhanced by decreasing the patients' metabolic rate with hypothermia, sedatives, and neuromuscular blocking agents; and by increasing oxygen delivery to the tissues with volume expansion and by dissolving more oxygen in blood by providing a higher inspired oxygen fraction. Red blood cell production can be maximized in Jehovah's Witnesses and other patients with erythropoetin. Red blood cell loss may be minimized by discouraging unnecessary phlebotomies, using hemodilution and hypotensive anesthesia, administering DDAVP, and employing blood salvage devices in surgery. Finally, patients may benefit by the development of practical blood substitutes some day (40,41).

✍ **Consent is required from Jehovah's Witnesses for transfusion in elective situations but may not be needed in emergencies, unless the patients refuse this therapy.** ✍

RESUSCITATION
Evolution of Hospital Resuscitation Policies

Cardiopulmonary resuscitation (CPR) is a potentially lifesaving medical intervention. It must be applied rapidly to be effective, so physicians and other health professionals who perform CPR have little time to consider the consequences of their actions. In addition, patients who require CPR often have not thought out their preferences for or against their therapy. For these and other reasons, CPR was applied universally after its introduction in the 1960s. Subsequently most hospitals adopted policies that advocated CPR in all circumstances, and most practitioners felt obligated to administer CPR to everyone.

Eventually, however, physicians appreciated that not all patients, especially those with terminal illness, want to be resuscitated. Cardiopulmonary resuscitation also was shown to be ineffective in many critically ill inpatients (42). As a result, hospital CPR policies became discretionary rather than universal. Physicians today are advised to ensure the ethical principle of autonomy by obtaining informed consent from patients or surrogates regarding CPR. ✍ **In situations where patients (or surrogates acting on the patient's wishes) do not want CPR performed, valid Do Not Attempt Resuscitation (DNAR) orders should be written in the medical record.** ✍

Although obtaining consent is appropriate, it may be difficult to do after trauma and during critical illness. Some patients are hospitalized in these circumstances because they already have been resuscitated, with or without their permission, and their caregivers are hesitant not to use CPR again. Physicians also may be reluctant to raise the issue of resuscitation because of concern that patients might feel abandoned if the possibility of not being resuscitated is brought up. In fact, because they associate the ED, the OR, and the

SICU with maximum support, many physicians consider it illogical, if not unethical, to ever follow or write DNAR orders in these settings.

Do-Not-Attempt-Resuscitation Orders in the Emergency Department, the Operating Room, and the Surgical Intensive Care Unit

Despite these sentiments, and despite the fact that DNAR orders frequently are overruled in other areas of the hospital (43), they generally should be respected and may even be initiated in the ED, the OR, and the SICU. Regarding the first location, increasing numbers of patients in community facilities such as nursing homes now have DNAR orders, and emergency medical services in many states have developed policies enabling their personnel to accept DNAR orders for patients transported by ambulance (44). Most EDs have similar policies that limit resuscitation if patients or surrogates so request. At the same time, although the ED is not an ideal place to discuss DNAR orders with patients and families, DNAR orders are written in some EDs when the patient's condition warrants withholding of CPR to honor their wishes (45).

The OR is a difficult environment for implementation of DNAR orders, in part because of the intimate relationship between the practice of anesthesia and resuscitation itself. Because of this relationship, some (46) have argued that when a patient's DNAR order does not preclude surgery and there is a reasonable chance of achieving the patient's treatment objectives, a preexisting DNAR order should be suspended perioperatively. Others (47) have stated that the patient's right to refuse treatment outweighs physicians' concern about the possibility of perioperative mortality. Procedure-specific DNAR order forms that allow for surgery but not for prolonged intubation thereafter have been developed. These forms have facilitated the institution of certain beneficial procedures within limits they find acceptable. Such forms avoid an all-or-none approach and allow individualization of patients' values and goals (48).

Procedure-specific DNAR orders also are appropriate in the SICU, where they are used with increased frequency (49). Patients who require the SICU for monitoring or therapeutic purposes but are unlikely to benefit from CPR are potential candidates for such DNAR orders. An example here might be a person who needs intensive nursing care but who should not be resuscitated in the event of a cardiopulmonary arrest because they have an underlying irrecoverable malignancy. Another situation in which DNAR orders are called for in the SICU involves patients, including those with multiple organ system failure, in whom further care is considered non-beneficial. In such patients, DNAR orders frequently represent a philosophic turning point in attitude on the parts of physicians and families from restorative to palliative care (50). ☞ **Procedure-specific DNAR orders are useful in many hospital environments, including the ED, the OR, and the SICU.** ☞

Must Resuscitation Always Be Attempted?

Even if DNAR orders are appropriate in the ED, the OR, and the SICU, it is not clear whether or at what point patients and their surrogates should be offered CPR. Some physicians believe that CPR always should be offered and would do so at the earliest opportunity if the issue has not been raised outside the hospital. Others (51) have argued that CPR, like renal dialysis and other technologies, may be potentially more burdensome than beneficial and is not a

required option if a patient's condition becomes so grave that CPR would be futile. "Slow codes," during which physicians pretend to perform CPR but do not attempt aggressively to bring patients back to life have been pursued as a means of limiting resuscitation without actually obtaining DNAR orders (52). Most hospital policies do not allow this; rather, efforts must be made to identify the patient's wishes (or surrogate's decision) beforehand to avoid CPR in futile or unwanted circumstances.

Unilateral DNAR orders written by physicians represent another way of withholding treatment they consider futile in some circumstances. Although physicians are not obligated to provide treatment they believe to be futile, unilateral orders, in conflict with the patient's wishes (or those of the surrogate) violate the principle of autonomy. Physicians should transfer care of the patient to another doctor, rather than unilaterally make decisions in conflict with the patient or their surrogate. Actions may be called futile when they are incapable of achieving a desired goal.

If CPR cannot possibly restore life in a given patient, the procedure may be considered physiologically futile and may be foregone unilaterally by physicians (53). However, if CPR may succeed in restoring the patient's life but physicians consider the patient's life not worth living, the procedure itself is not physiologically futile and, therefore, should not be foregone without the patient's or surrogate's consent. The concept of futility invoked in the latter case is vague and value-ridden, and it fails to provide an ethically coherent rationale for limiting life-sustaining treatment (49). Like the "slow code" approach, DNAR orders written unilaterally by physicians violate the principle of autonomy. They also preclude important discussions between practitioners, patients, and surrogates, undermining the practice of informed consent that is essential to the fiduciary relationship.

WITHHOLDING AND WITHDRAWAL OF LIFE SUPPORT
History and Present Practice

The DNAR order is a specific example of withholding treatment. The withholding and withdrawal (WH/WD) of life support are processes by which various medical interventions either are not given to or are removed from patients with the expectation that they probably will die from their underlying disease, or from an acute intercurrent process, thus avoiding an anticipated slow, painful, and sometimes undignified death.

These processes were uncommon in American hospitals until approximately 20 years ago, largely because physicians and health-care institutions felt obligated to preserve life whenever possible, regardless of the human and economic costs. In recent years, however, this obligation has been challenged, just as hospital expenses have been scrutinized. Clinical research (54,55) has revealed that many patients do not survive critical illness or do so only after prolonged pain and suffering. Patients and providers alike have questioned the advisability of supporting life in all circumstances. Legal cases have promoted patient and surrogate autonomy in decision-making, and the advent of medical cost-consciousness has restrained the application of therapies that merely prolong death with little hope of long-term cure or recovery (56). As a result of these and other factors, physicians (especially intensivists), with the implicit or explicit support of the hospitals in which they practice, have become increasingly involved in managing death in the ICU (57).

The first major observational study (58) of how critically ill patients die was conducted in 1987–1988 in two medical-SICUs at hospital affiliated with the University of California, San Francisco. During this one-year period, 13% of the patients admitted to the ICUs died. Of the patients who died, 51% did so after a decision had been made to limit treatment, and DNAR orders were written for almost all of them. A study (59) performed five years later in the same two ICUs revealed that, of the 13% of patients who died over a one-year period, a decision was made to WH/WD of life support from 90%, compared with 51% in the first study. Again, DNAR orders were written for almost all of the patients.

Following these studies, a national survey (60) of end-of-life care was conducted in 131 ICUs from 110 institutions in 38 states. Of all the patients admitted to these ICUs over a six-month period, 9% died. Of the patients who died, only 20% did so despite full support including attempted CPR. On the other hand, 24% did so after receiving full support but not CPR; 14% had life support withheld; 36% had life support withdrawn; and 6% were declared brain-dead. Thus, of the patients who died in the ICU and were not brain-dead, 74% received less than full support. Their percentage probably would have been higher if the study included patients who died shortly after being transferred out of the ICU with no provision for readmission.

One striking finding of the national survey was the wide variation in end-of-life care practices: the range of proportions of death preceded by failed CPR was 4% to 79%; for DNAR status the range was 0% to 83%; and for WH/WD of life support the range was 0% to 67% and 0% to 79%, respectively. This considerable variation could not be explained by the types of ICUs, the kinds of hospitals, or their geographic regions. However, a pattern was observed in the two states with strict legal standards for care limitation by surrogates: ICUs in New York and Missouri had lower proportions of deaths preceded by withdrawal of support than did the mid-Atlantic and Midwest regions, in which these states are located.

Although the national survey did not demonstrate changes in ICU deaths over time, as the studies from the University of California, San Francisco did, it suggested that limits to life support have become so commonplace in the United States as to represent a de facto standard of end-of-life care for critically ill patients. Nevertheless, the extreme variation in the categories of ICU death underscores the absence of a true consensual approach to end-of-life care attitudes and practices. Hopefully, consensus can be reached by the development of guidelines on limiting treatment when appropriate. Such guidelines are contained within recent position papers by professional societies (61,62) which have emphasized the need for improving the quality of end-of-life care in the ICU (see Volume 2, Chapter 69).

⚔ **Most patients who die in ICUs in the United States do so during the WH/WD of life support.** ⚔

Justification of the Withholding and Withdrawal of Life Support and the Administration of Palliative Care

In the United States, the WH/WD of life support is legally justified by the theories of informed consent and refusal discussed earlier. To reiterate, a series of court cases, including *Bartling* (5) and *Bouvia* (6) in California, have established that competent patients may refuse life-sustaining treatment, a position upheld by the U.S. Supreme Court in *Cruzan* (10). The use of surrogates to exercise the right of refusal for incompetent patients was facilitated in New Jersey under *Quinlan* (8) and has been adopted by most state. Exceptions are Missouri and New York, which require clear and convincing evidence of patients' wishes before they become incompetent.

Although state courts generally have allowed surrogates to request that life-sustaining treatment be foregone on behalf of incompetent patients, the patients themselves usually have been severely compromised in that they are both critically and terminally ill. The recent case of *Wendland v. Wendland* (15) suggests that surrogates may not be allowed to forego treatment for patients who are less severely compromised. In this case, the California Supreme Court reasoned that a conservator could not discontinue tube feeding from a patient who, although unable to feed himself, control his bowels or bladder, or communicate consistently, nevertheless was conscious and able to follow commands. Furthermore, although the patient had expressed some sentiments before he became incapacitated that he would not want to be supported indefinitely, the court felt that those statements were not clear and convincing, and because the comments did not address his current condition they were not necessarily intended to direct his medical care.

The ruling in *Wendland* need suggest no more than that American courts are willing to apply a clear and convincing evidence standard in cases involving patients who are not terminally ill. Nevertheless, some physicians may fear that the same standard will be more broadly applied to critically ill patients and consider it legally prudent to continue life-sustaining interventions regardless of the patients' circumstances. Continuing interventions violates the fiduciary relationship, however, if the burdens imposed by these interventions outweigh their benefits (63). In this regard, *Wendland* is best interpreted as a reminder that, in considering WH/WD of life support, the courts are most interested in what patients or their surrogates desire.

Underscoring this idea is the fact that courts have almost uniformly ordered treatment when asked to resolve disputes between families who favor treatment and physicians who oppose it on the grounds of futility. Judges seem unwilling to cause the death of a patient, as was seen in the case of *Baby K* (64), where the court refused to approve an advance physician decision to withhold life support over an anencephalic child's mother's negation. However, judges and juries seem equally reluctant to punish physicians who act carefully and within professional standards in refusing to provide treatment that they consider inappropriate. In this regard, the only clear legal rule on medically futile treatment is the traditional malpractice test, which measures a physician's treatment decisions against the relevant standard of medical care and then requires that any substandard care causes the patient injury.

The issue of malpractice was raised in *Gilgunn v. Massachusetts General Hospital* (65), in which a Massachusetts jury imposed no liability on a hospital or the physicians who issued a DNAR order and removed the ventilator from a critically ill patient over the objections of her daughter. *Gilgunn* conforms to a trend in futility cases in which physicians are likely to get better results when they refuse to provide nonbeneficial treatment and then defend their actions in court as being consistent with professional standards rather than seeking advance permission from a court to withhold care.

Despite the outcome of *Gilgunn* and studies showing that physicians frequently limit treatment they consider futile, unilateral actions based on futility generally are undesirable. Such actions certainly may be ethical in that they are supported by the principles of beneficence and nonmaleficence. Nevertheless, autonomy remains the first ethical principle for removing life-sustaining treatment, even though most critically ill patients must exercise their autonomy through surrogates. Ethics here reflect law, because informed consent and refusal are the primary legal theories that underlie this practice. Unilateral action also can be risky: disagreements between families and physicians can increase the potential for lawsuits.

In addition to ruling on the issue of surrogate refusal in *Cruzan*, the U.S. Supreme Court recently provided guidelines for administering palliative care. This provision comes for the *Glucksberg* (66) and *Vacco* (67) cases, in which the Court drew distinctions between physician-assisted suicide and WH/WD of life support. In *Vacco*, the court wrote "Everyone, regardless of physical condition, is entitled, if competent, to refuse life-saving medical treatment; no one is permitted to assist a suicide." "When a patient refuses life-sustaining medical treatment, he dies from an underlying disease or pathology; but if a patient ingests lethal medication prescribed by a physician, he is killed by that medication."

Administering Sedatives and Analgesics for Palliative Care

Although the Supreme Court condemned the administration of sedatives and analgesic to achieve physicians-suicide in *Glucksberg* and *Vacco*, it sanctioned palliative care for critically ill patients, even to the point of terminal sedation, if informed consent is obtained and the care does not contradict the rule of double effect. This rule, which derives from medieval Catholic theology, distinguishes between intended and foreseen consequences. Under it, acts such as giving drugs that lead to morally good effects, such as the relief of pain, are permissible even if they produce morally bad effects, such as the hastening of death, provided that only the good effect is intended. The bad effect may also not be a means to the good effect, and the good effect must outweigh the bad one.

The rule of double effect is limited in that it comes from a single religious tradition. More important, the rule overlooks the complexity of human intention and does not recognize that the patient's consent to an action that causes death may be more important than a physician's intent (68). The complexity of human intent was demonstrated in a study by Wilson et al. (69) from the University of California, San Francisco in which some physicians ordered and nurses administered benzodiazepines and opioids primarily to prevent pain and dyspnea (but occasionally to also treat family members anxiety or even to hasten death) during the WH/WD of life support from SICU patients. A subsequent survey by Asch (70) revealed that 16% of a sample of critical care nurses felt they had engaged in assisted suicide or euthanasia when trying to relieve suffering, often without physicians' knowledge.

Just as some physicians and nurses have mixed motives in caring for dying patients, so do some family members want to ease pain and hasten death simultaneously when their loved ones are suffering. That such motivation is widespread presumably accounts for the fact that few

healthcare professionals who are suspected of participating in assisted suicide or euthanasia have been punished through the criminal justice system (71).

Although the Supreme Court found no constitutional right to physician-assisted suicide in *Glucksberg* and *Vacco*, it nevertheless allowed states to authorize this practice. Experience in the state of Oregon, which permits physicians to prescribe lethal doses of controlled substances to terminally ill patents, suggests that physician-assisted suicide is not widespread and this practice rarely occurs in SICUs. In Oregon, most patients who request prescriptions for potentially lethal medications do so, because of concern about loss of autonomy and not because of uncontrollable pain (72). ☞ **The WH/WD of life support and the provision of palliative care have both been sanctioned by the U.S. Supreme Court.** ☞

Satisfying Ethical and Legal Requirements

The foregoing of life-sustaining therapy is only legally justified if such therapy is unwanted by the patient or surrogate, or deemed futile by the treating physicians. Accordingly, therapy should only be withheld or withdrawn with the consent of patients or their surrogates. When futility is the reason for withholding or withdrawal of treatment, this should not occur without patients' or surrogates' knowledge, or over their objections. Indeed, even if they practice in hospitals that have developed futility policies, physicians should recognize that such policies serve primarily as vehicles for reinforcing joint decision-making between health professionals and patients and their surrogates, not as devices for enforcing decisions made by physicians unilaterally (73). Where surrogates are lacking, or patients cannot make decisions, physician practice should be guided by their best understanding of what the patients would have wanted, or in the absence of such understanding, on what they believe to be in the patient's best interest.

Because the goal of palliative care is to provide comfort, measures that do not relieve suffering but merely hasten death should be avoided. Although most patients die within 24 hours after life support is withheld or withdrawn, the dying process may last for several days. Whatever time is required for death to occur, the palliative measures undertaken and their tempo should be dictated by objective manifestations of patient distress whenever possible. For example, physicians should order sedatives and analgesics for patients who can benefit from these agents, and initial doses should be substantial (as many of these patients may be tolerant of these drugs). However, dosages should not so large as to suggest they are given primarily to cause death (when dose is reviewed in the context of the patient's history and current clinical condition). Instead, the drug dosages should be titrated upward or downward in response to physiological manifestations of pain and discomfort, such as grimacing or hypertension, and ideally according to written protocols (see Volume 2, Chapter 69).

☞ **Neuromuscular blocking (NMB) drugs that could prevent spontaneous breathing should never be administered during the withholding or withdrawal of ventilatory support.** ☞ Otherwise, the caring physician and nurses will not be able to ensure that the patient died peacefully with a minimum of pain or anxiety. In patients already receiving these agents, restoration of neuromuscular function should be documented in all situations prior to withdrawing mechanical ventilation. Some have advocated allowing NMB drugs during withdrawal of ventilatory support, claiming that waiting for the drugs to wear off would unduly burden the patient (74). However, examples of why this would be burdensome were not provided by authors, and most clinicians do not adhere to this practice. Increasingly, processed electroencephalograph monitoring devices such as bispectral index monitors are being employed to supplement clinical assessment for maximizing the likelihood that the patient does not suffer during the withdrawal of futile life support (75). Injections of potassium chloride have no place during the WH/WD of life support, because they do not contribute to patient comfort and suggest a primary intention of hastening death.

Because mechanical ventilation is one of the therapies most frequently withdrawn from patients, and because its withdrawal may cause discomfort, physicians should pay particular attention to how the ventilator is withdrawn. Some practitioners prefer rapid extubation, whereas others use "terminal weaning" in which supplemental oxygen and positive end expiratory pressure are discontinued before the ventilator is withdrawn, and the patient usually remains intubated throughout the procedure. Either approach is ethically or legally justified even if death is unintentionally hastened, provided that informed consent has been obtained, and the patient receives sedation and/or analgesia titrated to minimize suffering.

Finally, because intent can be conveyed in words as well as through actions, the goal of palliative care and the means of achieving that goal should be spelled out in the medical record. In their notes, physicians should document how decisions were made to forego life-sustaining treatment, how consent was obtained from the patient or surrogate, and how the process of achieving patient comfort was conducted. In their notes, nurses should describe what steps they took to achieve the goals of palliative care, including an indication for all sedatives and analgesics they have administered. The ethical and legal requirements for the withholding or withdrawal of therapy are summarized in Table 4.

🖝 **When life support is withheld or withdrawn, palliative care should be provided so that patient suffering is avoided and ethical and legal requirements are satisfied.** 🖝

BRAIN DEATH AND ORGAN TRANSPLANTATION
Definition of Death
Death once was defined as the cessation of cardiopulmonary functions, in keeping with the concept that life is made possible by the flow of vital fluids (also see Volume 2, Chapters 16 and 68). However, the advent of CPR and postresuscitation life support in survivors of "sudden death" rendered this traditional definition obsolete, and brought about the realization that the brain is the only organ whose function cannot be replaced by medical intervention. At the same time, the development of organ transplantation required that death be legally redefined, so that physicians who remove organs from patients whose cardiopulmonary function is being supported following irreversible brain damage are not accused of murder. Here again, as in other areas of critical care medicine, technological advances outpaced existing philosophical paradigms and prompted ethical and legal change (3).

At present, in the United States, death is defined as the total and irreversible loss either of cardiopulmonary function or the function of the entire brain and brain stem (76). Death by neurologic criteria, which also is known as brain death, must be distinguished from other conditions in which patients merely appear to be dead. These conditions include transient coma, in which cerebral hemispheric function may be lost only temporarily; the persistent vegetative state, in which cerebral hemispheric function is lost for at least a month but brainstem function remains intact; and the locked-in state, in which cerebral hemispheric function is preserved but patients cannot move (77). Other conditions such as the Guillain-Barre syndrome and encephalitis may also mimic brain death, but the loss of brain stem reflexes and the ability to breathe do not result from irreversible structural brain damage and are recoverable.

Determination of Whole Brain Death
The determination of death by whole-brain and brainstem criteria is thoroughly reviewed in Volume 2, Chapter 16. The following summary briefly highlights the key principles. The initial requirements for the determination of brain and brainstem death includes the demonstration of coma, which is characterized by lack of alertness and awareness and signifies the loss of cerebral hemispheric function; and the documentation of absent corneal, oculovestibular, oropharyngeal, and ventilatory reflexes, indicating loss of function of the brain stem (Table 5).

The patient must be in an unresponsive coma and apneic on a ventilator. A diagnosis compatible with irreversible structural brain damage leading specifically to death of the brain stem must have been made. All drugs that can cause reduced consciousness including alcohol, analgesics, and sedatives must have been excluded as a potential cause of coma. In addition, electrolyte abnormalities, metabolic derangements, and hypothermia must have been excluded as a cause of coma. Furthermore, drugs that compromise the ability to breathe such as muscle relaxants must have been reversed or allowed to wear off.

The final step in the determination of brain death frequently is apnea testing (fully described in Volume 2, Chapter 16). In brief, such testing involves giving intubated

Table 4 Satisfying Ethical and Legal Requirements During the Withholding and Withdrawal of Life Support

---

Withhold or withdraw life support only with the consent of patients or surrogates

Involve patients or surrogates in decisions regarding how life support is withheld or withdrawn

Administer sedatives and analgesics to relieve suffering, not to hasten death, in whatever dosages are necessary

Do not use neuromuscular blocking drugs when the ventilator is withdrawn

Do not give potassium chloride or other agents that do not contribute to patient comfort

Document decisions and actions in the medical record

Eliminate unnecessary treatments which increase suffering or burden

Table 5 Determination of Brain Death

Lack of potential reversible causes of coma, for example, hypothermia, drugs, metabolic derangements, etc.

Lack of alertness and awareness

Lack of corneal, oculovestibular, oropharyngeal, and ventilatory reflexes

Lack of ventilatory efforts during apnea testing

patients insuflated oxygen through the endotracheal tube and observing them for respiratory efforts while they are not mechanically ventilated and while allowing the arterial carbon dioxide tension to rise from a normal level to at least 60 mmHg. Brain death is confirmed if patients do not make ventilatory efforts during apnea testing.

If the patient's surrogates have been prepared for this confirmation, accept the fact that the patient is dead, and agree with discontinuation of support, mechanical ventilation need not be reinstated unless organ transplantation is planned. In this case, cardiopulmonary function will be maintained temporarily, prior to organ procurement. Although it is useful in certain circumstances, laboratory confirmation of brain death by cerebral blood flow studies in adults is not generally required (78).

Surrogate approval is not required before brain death is determined in either group because such determination is a medical issue. Nevertheless, approval should be sought before such determinations, because apnea testing is not riskfree and subsequent decision-making regarding organ procurement also should be known. Furthermore, although there are good reasons to honor patients' previously expressed desires to donate organs despite surrogates' wishes to the contrary, most physicians find it difficult to do so and guidelines from Regional Organ Procurement Agencies require surrogate consent.

Finally, it is important to note that brain death need not be determined before the withholding or withdrawal of life support, which represents the forgoing of unwanted treatment in living patients. Indeed, most patients from whom life support is withheld or withdrawn are not brain-dead.

Brain Stem Death: The British Alternative to Brain Death

Some countries accept the determination of irreversible loss of brain stem function only as an alternative cause of death rather than requiring death of the entire brain and brainstem. England is an example and has a strict Code of Practice that describes how and when the diagnosis can be made. The diagnosis is made in two stages by two senior doctors. First, the same set of preconditions must be met, as required in the United States. Brain death should not be declared in patients whose central nervous systems are depressed by hypothermia, metabolic abnormalities, or drugs. Only if these preconditions are fully met may the doctors proceed to the second stage and perform the tests. The tests are designed to demonstrate the absence of cranial nerve (II–X) reflexes bilaterally and to confirm apnea in the presence of a $PaCO_2$ of 60 mmHg (or an increase of 20 mmHg). If after meeting the preconditions and performing the tests, the diagnosis of brain stem death is made, the entire process is repeated. Although the second set of tests is required to confirm the diagnosis, legally death is deemed to have occurred at the time the first set of tests was completed.

The British Code of Practice is based on the belief that the brain stem is the part of the brain that is vital for integrated functioning. Not only is the brain stem essential for the transmission of afferent information and the responses to this information but also it contains nuclei that control cardiovascular, respiratory, and thermoregulatory functions.

Promoting Organ Transplantation

The major limitation to more widespread transplantation in most countries is physician reluctance to discuss this issue with the surrogates of patients such as trauma victims who, by virtue of their young age and lack of chronic disease, are ideal organ donors (see Volume 2, Chapter 16). Although this reluctance is understandable with families whose religious or cultural values prohibit organ donation (e.g., gypsies and some Asians) (see Volume 2, Chapter 68), many people are consoled by the knowledge that their loved ones are helping to keep others alive through the gift of their organs. With this in mind, many states have adopted legislation that requires discussion of transplantation with the surrogates of patients who are likely to be brain-dead. Physicians, who hold such discussions are not subject to legal liability in the United States (79).

ALLOCATING MEDICAL RESOURCES
Physicians as Patient Advocates

A historical view, which can be traced to Hippocrates, holds that physicians own a duty only to their patients (80). This concept of duty is supported by the ethical principles of beneficence, nonmaleficence, and autonomy. It also is reflected in the fiduciary relationship through which physicians are expected to maintain their patients' medical interests in trust. According to one author (81), "... physicians are required to do everything that they believe may benefit each patient without regard to costs or other social considerations. In caring for an individual patient, the doctor must act surely as that patient's advocate, against the apparent interests of society as a whole, if necessary."

A corollary to this concept of duty is the idea that physicians cannot be providers and rationers of healthcare service simultaneously. Although they may advise society about certain issues, including the allocation of scarce or costly medical resources, physicians must not bring such issues to the bedside. In one author's (81) words, "... it may be difficult for doctors to separate their roles as citizens and expert advisors from their role in the practice of medicine as unyielding advocates for the health needs of individual patients." When practicing medicine, doctors cannot serve two masters. It is to the advantage both of society and of the individuals it comprises that physicians retain their historic single-mindedness. However, physicians can and should help save money and resources by knowing the approximate costs of various therapies and diagnostic tests, and choosing the ones which are the most cost-effective.

The single master view of medicine has prevailed over time for several reasons. One is that the fiduciary relationship traditionally has allowed physicians' broad discretion in determining what their patients' interests are. At the same time, while operating under the principles of beneficence, nonmaleficence, and autonomy, physicians have encouraged patients to expect, if not demand, that everything possible be done on their behalf. Of course, under fee-for-service reimbursement, physicians have benefited financially from the tests they have ordered for patients and the procedures they have performed on them. As a result, physicians who have advocated for the health needs of individual patients have also acted, whether they know it or not, as advocates for themselves.

Another reason for the prevalence of the single master view of medicine is that it and the ethical principles supporting it have not conflicted until recently with the principle of distributive justice, under which medical resources are to be allocated fairly, according to need, and to patients most likely to benefit from them. Until the last half of the 20th century, physicians had relatively few diagnostic and thera-peutic services to offer patients, and hospitals were viewed primarily as places to die. However, healthcare has become more promising with new developments, such as trauma services, new operative techniques, and critical care facili-ties. It also has become more expensive and, arguably, less available to the uninsured.

That over 45 million Americans lack health insurance makes the single master view of medicine seem somewhat incomplete. Indeed, the principle of distributive justice demands that physicians not only serve individual patients but also strive to improve access for all. It also requires that the interests and needs of all patients be balanced. To meet this requirement, physicians cannot hoard critical care resources solely for their own patients. They also cannot waste resources that are of limited benefit or benefit only a few patients. The responsibility for conserving medical resources is shared both by ICU directors and by the physicians who care for patients in the ICU.

Rationing Resources and Managed Care

Ideally, the judicious allocation of critical care resources will prevent their rationing either at the bedside or as a result of social policies. The United States has no acknowledged policy on rationing medical services; instead, the govern-ment and private insurance companies simply refuse to pay for them. One current manifestation of this "policy" is managed care, which is widely identified as a tool for increasing corporate profits by denying medical services. Managed care organizations commonly pay physicians through capitation rather than fee-for-service, and they have induced them to do less for patients through the use of incentive plans that reward physicians for using fewer and less costly services. In the process, managed care has made patients suspicious of the physicians and the health-care institutions they once relied on (82).

Fortunately, the interference of managed care organiz-ations into the physician–patient relationship has lessened in recent years, largely in response to protests from both physicians and patients. Physicians also have learned how to act as fiduciaries under capitation, just as they have learned how to provide cost-conscious care without overt rationing. Whether such rationing ever becomes common-place remains to be determined. One reason it might become commonplace is the perception that healthcare costs can be reduced by limiting intensive care at the end of life.

Can Health Care Costs Be Reduced by Limiting Intensive Care at the End of Life?

Because the terminally ill are often hospitalized and may be candidates for intensive care and because the ICU is particu-larly resource-intensive, reducing the use of the ICU among such patients appears to present unique opportunities for cost reduction. The quality of these patients' end-of-life care also may be improved if those who would benefit more from palliation than from heroic restorative efforts were identified early, and the patients received this treat-ment in places other than the ICU.

The major reason that cost reduction might be possible in the ICU is that critical care is so expensive (see Volume 2, Chapter 68). Of the $989 billion spent on health care in the United States in 1995, hospitals costs were around $350 billion. Assuming that ICU costs were 20% of hospital costs, they amounted to $70 billion or 1% of the Gross

Domestic Product. The costs of ICU care are higher today not only because total hospital costs are higher but also because ICU costs represent a larger fraction of hospital costs, inasmuch as a greater percentage of hospitalized patients are cared for in the ICU (83).

In addition to its high cost, sufficient geographic variation exists in the use of intensive care to suggest that this treatment is overutilized in some institutions. On average, patients who die in the ICU are more expens-ive (unless they die quickly, e.g., head injury) than those who live, and sustaining their lives may not be cost-effec-tive. Furthermore, cost-reduction strategies are possible in the ICU. In support of this idea, investigators (84) retro-spectively identified ICU patients who either died during admission or within three months of discharge and were in the upper 25% of all critically ill patients in terms of resource use. Were such recipients of "poten-tially ineffective care" identified and their ICU stays restricted to five days, the investigators estimated, charges at the study hospital could have been decreased by $1.8 to $5 million a year.

Although limiting potentially ineffective care is appealing, shortening stays in the ICU may not reduce costs unless beds are taken out of circulation, personnel are relocated, and other fixed costs are decreased. Although patients who die in the ICU generally are more expensive than those who survive on an individual basis, the most expensive patients are those with indeterminate outcomes, who defy prognostication. The most cost-ineffective care actually is provided to a small number of patients; whereas the majority of patients benefit from ICU care. Furthermore, although the study of potentially ineffective care suggested that considerable savings could be realized if such patients were identified and their ICU stays reduced, a follow-up study (85) suggested that efforts to decrease access to the ICU might actually increase overall mortality. Finally, even if terminal care were provided in hospice rather than the ICU, the savings would be minimal over the patients' last year of life (86).

Clearly, ICU costs can be saved by not opening beds in the first place, as is the approach taken in countries with limited healthcare resources (87). Yet the price of such ration-ing would be to dash the expectations of patients and surro-gates and sacrifice lives that could be saved or at least prolonged through ICU admission. This idea of not provid-ing critical care services has proven to be politically unten-able in the United States, and has led to growing dissatisfaction in other countries (88).

In the final analysis, healthcare costs cannot be reduced appreciably by limiting intensive care at the end of life. That said, providing timely and intensive pal-liative care is desirable in its own right, independent of economic implications. In countries with adequate medical resources such as the United States, all critically ill patients should receive a trial of intensive care unless they or their surrogates specify otherwise, or if, in the absence of available information in the patients' wishes, such care can be deemed to not to be in their best inter-ests. When restorative efforts fail, they should give away to a palliative approach if patients or surrogates agree, not because the approach will save money, but because palliation will be of the greatest benefit to the patient in achieving the goal of a comfortable and dignified death, regardless of its impact on healthcare costs. ☞ **Improving care, rather than reducing costs, is the most appropriate reason to provide palliative treatment.** ☞

EYE TO THE FUTURE

The basic principles of biomedical ethics presumably will remain the same in the foreseeable future, but they will be increasingly adopted throughout the world in developing nations. For example, the principle of autonomy is becoming more and more accepted outside the United States and Canada. For example, in Western Europe, where physicians traditionally (paternalistically) made most decisions regarding the WH/WD of life support, patients and families increasingly are involved in decision-making (89). In other countries predominated by religious or tribal traditions, paternalism will likely persist in the near future.

The principle of distributive justice is receiving more attention in the United States and elsewhere, and it will receive even more as biomedical ethics continue to evolve. A growing burden of acute traumatic illnesses and of chronic conditions, such as obesity and diabetes, in developed countries, coupled with the advancing age of the populations of these nations, should increase the demand for medical services within them. At the same time, poor economic conditions should create difficulties in meeting the demand, especially as technological innovations occur. The problem of equitable distribution of limited resources is common in underdeveloped nations, where morbidity and mortality from infectious diseases and illness caused by poverty is all but overwhelming. Increasingly, distribution schemes—in a word, rationing—may need to be followed in more affluent countries if distributive justice is to be realized.

Clarification of patient outcomes and what constitutes futility are important considerations that impact ethical decision-making in the SICU (90). Increasing emphasis on outcomes research should continue to clarify disease processes that are treatable versus those that are irrecoverable (with current technology) for which further therapy is futile.

SUMMARY

Traumatized and critically ill patients present many ethical issues to physicians and other health professionals. These patients should be encouraged to define their own interests whenever possible. Unfortunately, many patients cannot make decisions about clinical care or research participation for themselves, so surrogates must do so for them. Patient autonomy is contained in the concept of informed consent, and may be considered to be implied for clinical purposes in situations where a true emergency exists. Consent cannot necessarily be considered to be implied in patients with known (but unusual) beliefs, such as Jehovah's Witnesses, unless the patients have clearly stipulated beforehand. Procedure-specific DNAR orders are useful in the ED, the OR, and the SICU. Brain death demonstrated by the absence of cerebral and brainstem function or, in some countries (i.e., U.K.), brain stem death, are vital diagnoses made in critical care areas because they (*i*) are essential to the concept of a dignified death and (*ii*) contribute to the salvage of life brought about by organ transplantation.

Most patients who die in ICUs do so during the WH/WD of life support. ✍ **The WH/WD of life support and the provision of palliative care have both been sanctioned by the U.S. Supreme Court.** ✍ While the administration of sedatives at the time of WH/WD of life support is ethically

quite different than prescribing lethal drugs for the sole goal of assisting suicide, a recent (Jan 17, 2006) six to three decision by the U.S. Supreme court to upheld the 1997 Oregon Death With Dignity Act has an effect on the former (91). The significance of this ruling in terms of the WH/WD of life support is (*i*) the courts affirmed the patients right to self determination, (*ii*) physicians are empowered to prescribe drugs at the end of life according to their judgment as regulated by states (rather than federal) oversight, and (*iii*) had the decision not been upheld, it would have likely had a chilling effect on the compassionate administration of sedatives and analgesics to dying patients during the WH/WD of therapy. In the words of Quill and Meier (92), who raised concerns if the Court ruled the other way: "physicians may become hesitant to prescribe the best available medications to manage the pain, agitation, and shortness of breath that sometimes accompany the end stages of illness. As a result, they may, in essence, abandon patients and their families in their moment of greatest need."

Life support should be WH/WD and palliative care should be provided at the request of patients or their responsible surrogates when treatment is physiologically futile. The ethical and legal requirements are summarized Table 4. Improving care, rather than reducing costs, is the most appropriate reason to provide palliative care.

KEY POINTS

- ✍ Important ethical issues in trauma and critical care include medical decision-making, informed consent, resuscitation, brain death, organ transplantation, the withholding and withdrawal of life support, and the allocation of medical resources.
- ✍ In keeping with the principle of autonomy when capable of rational informed decision-making patients should always be allowed to define their own interests.
- ✍ The most ideal surrogates are those who have been designated by patients before or during their critical illness to make medical decisions in the event of incapacity.
- ✍ Physicians may make decisions they consider in a patient's best interests in an emergency, unless the patient has stipulated otherwise.
- ✍ If a true emergency exists, then consent may be considered to be implied.
- ✍ Consent is required from Jehovah's Witnesses for transfusion in elective situations but may not be needed in emergencies, unless the patients refuse this therapy.
- ✍ In situations where patients (or surrogates acting on the patient's wishes) do not want CPR performed, valid Do Not Attempt Resuscitation (DNAR) orders should be written in the medical record.
- ✍ Procedure-specific DNAR orders are useful in many hospital environments, including the ED, the OR, and the SICU.
- ✍ Most patients who die in intensive care units in the United States do so during the WH/WD of life support.
- ✍ The WH/WD of life support and the provision of palliative care have both been sanctioned by the U.S. Supreme Court.
- ✍ Neuromuscular blocking (NMB) drugs that could prevent spontaneous breathing should never be administered during the withholding or withdrawal of ventilatory support.
- ✍ When life support is withheld or withdrawn, palliative care should be provided so that patient suffering is

avoided and ethical and legal requirements are satisfied.

☞ Improving care, rather than reducing costs, is the most appropriate reason to provide palliative treatment.

REFERENCES

1. Beauchamp TL, Childress JF. Principles of Biomedical Ethics. 4th ed. New York: Oxford University Press, 1994.
2. Miles SH. The Hippocratic Oath and the Ethics of Medicine. New York: Oxford University Press, 2004.
3. Luce JM. Ethical principles in critical care. JAMA 1990; 263:696–700.
4. PL 104-191, HR 3103.
5. Bartling v. Superior Court, 163 Cal. App. ed 190, 209 Cal. Rptr. 200 (1984).
6. Bouvia v. Superior Court, 179 Cal. App. 3d 1127, 225 Cal. Rptr. 297 (1986).
7. Cruzan v Director, Missouri Department of Health, 497DS 261 (1990).
8. In re Ouinlan, 755 A2A 647 (NJ), cert denied, 429 US 922 (1976).
9. In re: O'Connor, 72 N.Y. 2d 517, 531 N.E. 2d 607,534 N.Y.S. 2d 886 (1998).
10. Cruzan v. Harmon. 760 S.W. 2d 408 (Mo. 1988) (en banc).
11. Steinbrook R, Lo B. Decision making for incompetent patients by designated proxy. N Engl J Med 1984; 310:1598–1601.
12. Raffin TA. Value of the living will. Chest 1980; 90:444–446.
13. Greco PJ, Schulman KA, Lavisso-Mourey R, Hansen-Flaschen J. The Patient Self-Determination Act and the future of advance directives. Ann Intern Med 1991; 115:639–643.
14. Luce JM, Alpers A. End-of-life care: What do the American courts say. Crit Care Med 2001; 29:N40–N45.
15. Wendland v Wendland, 26 Cal. 4th 519, 28 P. 3d 151 (2001).
16. Quill TE. Terri Schiavo—A Tragedy Compounded. N Engl J Med 2005; 352:1630–1633.
17. In re: Guardianship of Estelle M. Browning v. Herbert, No. 74,174 (S. Ct. Fla., 1990).
18. In re: The Guardianship of Theresa Marie Schiavo, Incapacitated. In the Circuit Court for Pinellas County, Florida, Probate Division File No. 90-2908GD-003.
19. Mental Health Act of 1983—Available at the UK Department of Health Webpage: http://www.dh.gov.uk/ PublicationsAndStatistics/Legislation/ActsAnctBills/ActsAndBills/Article/fs/en? CONTENT_ID = 4002034&chk = lmZd%2Bu (accessed Mar 16, 2006).
20. Conn. Gen. Stat. Ann: 199–571.
21. Haw. Rev. Stat. 327D-21.
22. Faden RR, Beauchamp TL. A History and Theory of Informed Consent. New York: Oxford University Press, 1986.
23. Schloendorff v Society of New York Hospital, 211 NY 125, 105 NE 92, 1914.
24. Salgo v. Leland Stanford etc. Bd. Trustees (1957) 154 CA2d 560.
25. Natanson v. Kline, 350 P.2d 1093 (1960).
26. Canterbury v. Spence., 464 F.2d 772 (DC Cir. 1972).
27. Cobbs v Grant, 8 Cal 3d 229, 502 P. 2d1, 1972.
28. Title 45, U.S. Code of Federal Regulations (CFR), part 46. Protection of Human Subjects.45CFR46.116. Available at: http:// ohrp.usophs.dhs.gov/human subjects /guidance/45cfr46.htm
29. Luce JM. California's new law allowing surrogates consent for clinical research involving subjects with impaired decision-making capacity. Intens Care Med 2003; 29(6):1024–1025.
30. Moore v. The Regents of the University of California, 793 P.2d 479 (Cal 1990).
31. Moore v Regents of University of California, CA 1990.
32. Layon AJ, D'Amico R, Caton D, Mollet CJ. And the patient chose: medical ethics and the case of the Jehovah's Witness. Anesthesiology 1990; 73:1258–1262.
33. Muramoto O. Recent development in medical care of Jehovah's Witnesses. West J Med 1999; 170:297–301.
34. Victorino G, Wisner DH. Jehovah's Witnesses: unique problems in a unique trauma population. J Am Coll Surg 1997;184: 458–468.
35. In re Estate of Brooks, 32 Ill. 2d 361,372–373 (Ill. App. LT. 1ST District; 1965).
36. Re Estate of Darrell Dorne, 534 A. 2d 452 (Pa. 1987).
37. Prince v. Commonwealth of Massachusetts, 321 U.S. 158 (1944).
38. Jonsen AR. Blood transfusions and Jehovah's Witnesses. Crit Care Clin 1986; 2(1):91–100.
39. Viele MK, Weiskopf RB. What can we learn about the need for transfusion from patients who refuse blood? The experience with Jehovah's Witnesses. Transfusion 1994; 34(5):396–401.
40. Mann MC, Votto J, Kambe J, McNamee MJ. Management of the severely anemic patient who refuses transfusion: lessons learned during the care of a Jehovah's Witness. Ann Intern Med 1992; 117:1042–1048.
41. Akingbola OA, Custer JR, Bunchan TE, Sedman AB. Management of severe anemia without transfusion in a pediatric Jehovah's Witness patient. Crit Care Med 1994; 22(3):524–528.
42. Beddell SE, Delbanco TL, Cook EP, Epstein FH. Survival after cardiopulmonary arrest in the hospital. N Engl J Med 1983; 309:569–576.
43. Heffner SE, Barbieri C. Compliance with do-not-resuscitate orders for hospitalized patients transported to radiology departments. Ann Intern Med 1998; 124:801–805.
44. Sachs GA, Miles SH, Levin RA. Limiting resuscitation: emerging policy in the emergency medical system. Ann Intern Med 1991; 114:151–154.
45. Wrenn K, Brody SL. Do-not-resuscitate orders in the emergency department. Am J Med 1992; 92:129–133.
46. Cohen CB, Cohen PJ. Do not resuscitate orders in the operating room. N Engl J Med 1991; 325:1879–1882.
47. Walker RM. DNR in the OR: resuscitation as an operative risk. JAMA 1991; 261:2407–2412.
48. Truog RD, Waisel DB, Burns VP. DNR in the OR: a goal-directed approach. Anesthesiology 1999; 90:289–295.
49. Hayes RL, Zimmerrnan JE, Wagner DP, et al. Do-not-resuscitate orders in intensive care units: current practices and recent charges. JAMA 1993; 270:2213–2217.
50. Luce JM, Prendergast TJ. The changing nature of death in the ICU. In: Curtis RJ, Rubenfeld GD, eds. Managing Death in the Intensive Care Unit: the Transition from Cure to Comfort. New York: Oxford University Press, 2001.
51. Blackhall LJ. Must we always use CPR? N Engl J Med 1987; 317:1281–1285.
52. Gazelle G. The slow code-should anyone rush to its defense? N Engl J Med 1998; 338:467–469.
53. Waisel DB, Truog RD. The cardiopulmonary resuscitation—not indicated order: futility revisited. Ann Intern Med 1995; 122:304–308.
54. Rubenfeld GD, Crawford SW. Withdrawing life support from mechanically ventilated recipients of bone marrow transplants: a case for evidence-based guidelines. Ann Intern Med 1996; 125:625–633.
55. Wachter RM, Luce JM, Safrin S, Berrios DC, Charlebois E, Scitovsky AA. Cost and outcome of intensive care for patients with AIDS, *Pneumocystis carinii* pneumonia and severe respiratory failure. JAMA 1995; 273:230–235.
56. Cher DJ, Lenert LA. Method of Medicare reimbursement and the rate of potentially ineffective care of critically ill patients. JAMA 1997; 278:1001–1007.
57. Karlawish JHT, Hall JB. Managing death in the intensive care unit. Am J Respir Crit Care Med 1997; 155:1–2.
58. Smedira NG, Evans BH, Grais LS, et al. Withholding and withdrawal of life support from the critically ill. N Engl J Med 1990; 322:309–315.
59. Prendergast TJ, Luce JM. Increasing incidence of withholding and withdrawal of life support from the critically ill. Am J Respir Crit Care Med 1997; 155:15–20.
60. Prendergast TJ, Claessens MT, Luce JM. A national survey of end-of-life care for critically ill patients. Am J Respir Crit Care Med 1998; 158:1163–1167.
61. Faber-Langendoen K, Lanken PN, for the ACP-ASIM End-of-Life Care Consensus Panel. Dying patients in the intensive care unit: forgoing treatment, maintaining care. Ann Intern Med 2000; 133:886–893.

62. Truog RD, Cist AFM, Brackett SE, et al. Recommendations for end-of-life care in the intensive care unit: the ethics committee of the society of critical care medicine. Crit Care Med 2001; 29:2332–2348.

63. Lo B, Dornbrand L, Wolf LE, Graman M. The Wendland case-withdrawing life support from incompetent patients who are not critically ill. N Engl J Med 2002; 346:1489–1493.

64. In the Matter of Baby K, 16F, 3d 590 (4th in. 1994).

65. Gilgunn v Massachusetts General Hospital, Noi92-480 (Mass. Super. Ct Civ ction Suffolk So. April 22, 1995).

66. Washington v Glucksberg, 521 US 702 (1997).

67. Vacco v Quill, 521 US 793 (1997).

68. Quill TE, Dresser R, Brock RW. The rule of double effect—a critique of its role in end-of-life decision making. N Engl J Med 1997; 337:1768–1771.

69. Wilson WC, Smedira NG, Fink C, Luce JM. Ordering and administration of sedatives and analgesics during the withholding and withdrawal of life support from critically ill patients. JAMA 1992; 267:949–953.

70. Asch DA. The role of critical care nurses in euthanasia and assisted suicide. N Engl J Med 1996; 334:1374–1379.

71. Alpers A. Criminal act or palliative care? Prosecutions involving the care of the dying. J Law Med Ethics 1998; 26:308–331.

72. Sullivan AD, Hedberg K, Fleming DW. Physician-assisted suicide in Oregon—the second year. N Engl J Med 2000; 342:598–604.

73. Halevy A, Brody BA. A multi-institutional collaborative policy on medical futility. JAMA 1998; 276:571–574.

74. Truog RD, Bums JP, Mitchell C. Pharmacologic paralysis and withdrawal of mechanical ventilation at the end of life. N Engl J Med 2000; 342:508–511.

75. Barbato, M: Bispectral index monitoring in unconscious palliative care patients. J Palliat Care 2001; 17(2):102–108.

76. President's Commission for the Study of ethical problems in Medicine and Biomedical and Behavioral Research. Guidelines for the determination of death. JAMA 1981; 246:2184–2186.

77. The Multi-Society Task Force on PVS. Medical aspects of the persistent vegetative state. N Engl J Med 1994; 330:1491–1508, 1572–1579.

78. Kelly BJ, Luce JM. Neurologic criteria for death. In: Parillo JE, Bone RC, eds. Critical Care Medicine: Principles of Diagnosis and Management. St Louis: Mosby, 1995.

79. Caplan AL. Ethical and policy issues in the procurement of cadaver organs for transplantation. N Engl J Med 1984; 311:981–983.

80. Luce JM. The changing physician-patient relationship in critical care medicine under health care reform. Am J Respir Crit Care Med 1994; 150:266–270.

81. Levinsky NG. The doctor's master. N Engl J Med 1984; 311:1573–1575.

82. Luce JM. Making decisions about the forgoing of life-sustaining therapy. Am J Respir Crit Care Med 1997; 156:1715–1718.

83. Luce JM, Rubenfeld GD. Can health care costs be reduced by limiting intensive care at the end of life? Am J Respir Crit Care Med 2002; 165:750–754.

84. Esserman L, Belkova J, Lenert L. Potentially ineffective care: a new outcome to assess the limits of critical care. JAMA 1997; 274:1544–1551.

85. Cher DJ, Lenert A. Method of Medicare reimbursement and the rate of potentially ineffective care of critically ill patients. JAMA 1997; 278:1001–1007.

86. Emanuel ES. Cost savings at the end-of-life: what do the data show? JAMA 1996; 275:1907–1914.

87. Zimmerman JE, Knaus WA, Judson JA, et al. Patient selection for intensive care: a comparison of New Zealand and United States hospitals. Crit Care Med 1988; 16:318–326.

88. Donelan K, Blendon RJ, Schoen C, Davis K, Binns K. The cost of health system change: public discontent in five nations. Health Aff (Millwood) 1999; 18:206–216.

89. Pochard F, Azoulay E, Chevret S, et al. French intensivists do not apply American recommendations regarding decisions to forgo life-sustaining therapy. Crit Care Med 2001; 29(10):1887–1892.

90. Truog RD, Brett AS, Frade J. The problem with futility. N Engl J Med 1992; 326:1560–1564.

91. Annas GJ. Congress, controlled substances, and physician-assisted suicide—elephants in mouseholes. N Engl J Med 2006; 354(4):1079–1084.

92. Quill TE, Meier DE. The big chill—inserting the DEA into end-of-life care. N Engl J Med 2006; 354:1–3.

68

End of Life: Spiritual and Cultural Considerations

Anne J. Sutcliffe

Department of Anesthesia and Critical Care, Alexandra Hospital, Redditch, U.K.

William C. Wilson

Department of Anesthesiology and Critical Care, UC San Diego Medical Center, San Diego, California, U.S.A.

Catherine McCoy-Hill

School of Nursing, Azusa Pacific University, Azusa, California, U.S.A.

INTRODUCTION

Before mass emigration and global travel were the norm, it was common for members of the caring professions to share the same background and belief systems as their patients. Today, however, most countries contain populations from numerous ethnicities, cultures, and religions, with varying legal experiences and degrees of trust of the medical professions (Table 1).

Religious and cultural influences permeate all segments of society, including medical decision-making. Physicians, whether consciously or unconsciously, conform to values and behaviors reflecting family and society, as well as professional standards. Personal influences often affect one's interactions with patients and general approach to practice, yet these tendencies are not necessarily apparent to the practitioner.

Most clinicians are cognizant that patients possess their own belief systems; however, the need to respect these differences and incorporate them into patient decision-making still requires emphasis from time to time. Religious and cultural backgrounds tend to be the most significant influences underlying patient and family belief systems in terms of life, death, brain death, medical futility, organ donation, and trust in doctors. Accordingly, understanding these considerations can aid the traumatologist/intensivist in avoiding or rectifying ethical dilemmas due to these factors that complicate end of life decision-making and care.

This chapter addresses these considerations and provides cultural and religious guideposts for readers who may, or may not, be familiar with the general principles and ethical beliefs underlying most of the world's organized religions. In addition, other cultural influences that relate to specific geographic regions or are unique to certain ethnic groups are reviewed. ☞ **Medical goals in end of life care must be responsive to the needs and preferences of individuals within their sociocultural, religious, and family contexts.** ☜

FACTORS INFLUENCING END OF LIFE DECISION MAKING
Culture and Custom

Culture can be defined as the ideas, customs, and art of a society. The term is also used to describe a particular society at a particular point in time. Customs tend to be activities that are long established. Although cultures change over time, current thinking within a given culture is often influenced by customs established in an earlier era and passed down over generations. ☞ **Cultures tend to embrace specific beliefs, perceptions, and values. These cultural norms and values strongly influence how individuals and groups think about death, dying, and end of life issues.** ☜

Cultural development has historically been slow to evolve, and was deeply enmeshed in the context of community, family, and religious values. However, with the global society, cultural transformations occur far more quickly and are more readily influenced by changing societal, legal, and ethical norms. For example, in the Western world, medical behavior has been altered by pressure from patient advocates and bioethicists. These forces have altered Western culture from a custom of medical paternalism to an ethic of patient autonomy (the principle that underlies the ethical concepts of informed consent, and use of advanced directives). ☞ **The ethnicity, culture, and religion of patients and families strongly influence bioethical differences regarding end of life issues. Likewise, the ethical and legal climate within countries influences physician practices and medical decision-making surrounding end of life care.** ☜

Decision-making by individuals is not a feature of all cultures even in the Western world. For example, in Italy, paternalism is still an accepted method of practice in some provinces. Hispanic cultures also place important emphasis on patriarchal decision-making within the family. In some North American native populations such as the Inuit, Cree, Navajo, and Dene, decision-making is often situational, and always dependent on the values of the individual within the context of family and community (1).

In Eastern cultures, including members of the Hindu, Muslim, and Sikh religions, decision-making involves not only the individual but also the family. In Japan, the culture of medical paternalism existed until very recently and is only just beginning to change (2). Japanese attitudes regarding disclosure, decision-making roles, and end of life choices reflect a shifting emphasis toward autonomy, much as has occurred in the United States in recent generations.

Table 1 Factors Influencing Decision Making Related to
Death, Dying, End of Life Care, and Organ Donation

Factor	Description
Culture	Values, beliefs, ideas, customs, and art of a society
Religion	Worship or belief in a supernatural power(s) or divine transcendent being(s)
Law	Rules regulating members of a society or community typically within political borders of authority
Trust in the medical profession	Varies according to cultural and religious customs and among groups within society, depending on their personal or aggregate recent experience

Religion

Religion can be described as a specific part of culture and custom. Religion is the worship of or belief in a supernatural power or powers. "Life" after death is a key feature of most organized religions. This often involves beliefs about the soul or spirit of a person that survives even though the biological body has died. Interestingly, the soul/spirit is often thought to embody the individual's personality, intellect, will, and emotions, features that scientists attribute to the brain (see philosophical discussion in Volume 2, Chapter 16). Some theologians view spirituality as a global concept which encompasses the transcendent values that promote human fulfillment and connectedness with others as well as with a transcendent being or higher power.

The relationship between the soul and the body of the deceased varies across different religions and cultures (Table 2). For Christians, Jews, and Muslims, the soul is thought to leave the body to be reunited with their God in the afterlife. For Hindus, Sikhs, and Buddhists, the soul is

Table 2 Religious Views on Organ Donation

Religion	Donation allowed (yes/no)	Explanations and comments (regarding the official position of the religion)
AME Zion	Yes	Supported as an act of love and charity.
Amish	Yes	Supported when organs are likely to benefit recipient. Reluctant if outcome is questionable.
Assembly of God	Yes	No official position—decision up to the individual.
Baptist	Yes	Individual decision, but considered charitable.
Brethren	Yes	Considered a charitable act as long as donor death is not hastened, and tissue not from an unborn child.
Buddhist	Yes	Individual decision, but considered honorable.
Roman Catholic	Yes	Support and encourage donations as an act of charity.
Christian Church[a]	Yes	Support and encourage organ donation.
Church of Christ	Yes	No prohibitions—decision up to the individual.
Christian Science	Yes	No official position—decision up to the individual.
Episcopal	Yes	Supported and viewed as part of their ministry.
Greek Orthodox	Yes	Not opposed as long as organs used to better human life (i.e., for transplantation or research).
Gypsies	No	Not a formal religion, rather a grouping of ethnicities, with common folk beliefs against organ donation.
Hindu	Yes	No prohibitions—decision up to the individual.
IC Evangelical	Yes	No official position—decision up to the individual.
Islam	Yes	Most Islamic scholars believe transplantation is noble.
Jehovah's Witness	Yes	Individual decision—all blood must be removed from organs and tissues before transplantation.
Judaism	Yes	All four branches (orthodox, conservative, reform, and reconstructionist) support donation.
Lutheran	Yes	Support and encourage organ donation.
Mennonite	Yes	No official position—decision up to the individual.
Mormon	Yes	No opposition—decision up to the individual.
Pentecostal	Yes	No official position—decision up to the individual.
Presbyterian	Yes	Supports and encourages organ donation.
Shinto	No	Injuring a corpse is a serious crime in Shinto folk beliefs. Thus, families may be reluctant to donate.
Quakers	Yes	No official position—decision up to the individual.
Unitarian	Yes	Supported and viewed as an act of love.
United Church of Christ	Yes	Support and encourage organ donation.
United Methodist	Yes	Encourages members to become card carrying organ and tissue donors.

[a]Disciples of Christ.
Abbreviations: AME, African Methodist Episcopal; IC Evangelical, Independent Conservative Evangelical.
Source: From Refs. 2, 7–15, 19–24.

seen as reincarnated as a new life in another body. Gypsies believe that the spirit of the person remains on earth for a year after biological death, and requires its earthly body to wander freely. Many Japanese believe that the dead body must be in perfect condition or the soul will be unhappy in the next world. They also believe, as do others, that the dead person's spirit can communicate with the living and that the sadness of the dead person's soul can affect family members. ⚻ **Historically, members of those religions and cultures that believe that the body is needed even after death have been less likely to accept organ donation than those who believe the soul leaves the physical body following death and no longer needs it.** ⚻

Law

Laws are rules regulating what may or may not be done by members of a society or community. Usually, laws reflect the cultural and religious beliefs of the majority of individuals in the community to which they apply. As such, laws tend to change over time in line with changing societal beliefs and moral values. Consequently, a law that is right for one generation or century may not be right for the next. Similarly, various countries, or locales within countries, change their beliefs at differing paces, so laws that work well in a cosmopolitan European capital, may not function well in Saudi Arabia, or in a small village in the Amazon rain forest.

Trust in the Medical Profession

Trust implies confidence in the truthfulness, honesty, and reliability of a person. Specifically, the relationship between physicians and their patients is based on trust. The patient's trust in his or her doctor places an obligation on the physician to care for the patient based on the highest medical and ethical standards. ⚻ **Death is the final diagnosis. Patients, their relatives, and their religious and societal mentors honor doctors by trusting them to accurately declare when biological life has ended.** ⚻ Trust is expected as a moral imperative, despite the fact that physicians, scientists, clergy, and bioethicists continue to struggle with the precise definition of death in the context of medical advances (as discussed subsequently).

DIAGNOSIS OF DEATH

The diagnosis of biological death is made when clinical examination and appropriate tests have been performed

(see Volume 2, Chapter 16 for specific clinical determinants and confirmatory studies). These may include tests to identify irreversible cessation of heart beat, irreversible cessation of breathing, or irreversible cessation of brain (and/or brain stem) function. The tests are chosen to demonstrate that certain criteria have been fulfilled. It is argued, however, that criteria for death cannot be definitively determined until death is better defined, the definition which itself relies on resolving philosophical and biological concepts of death (3).

Concept of Human Death

Biologically, death marks the transition of the human body from the living to the nonliving state. An alternative concept of human death is loss of personhood. Inevitably, personhood means different things to different people, but usually loss of consciousness is a key element. Philosophers have stipulated that sentient death occurs when self-awareness is permanently lost, that social death occurs when a person has lost his or her role in society and lastly, sociological death where a person is cut off from his community (4). Examples include people exiled because they have betrayed their country, or people who are legally declared dead in the absence of a body because they have been missing for many years. ⚻ **Ultimately, medical goals in end of life care must be responsive to the needs and preferences of individuals within their sociocultural, religious, and family contexts.** ⚻

Definition of Death

Defining death is both complex and controversial. This is because a single definition cannot include all the concepts of death described earlier. From a religious or cultural perspective, the definition of death as the end of a particular biological life is acceptable but incomplete, because it ignores other important events that occur when a person dies (Table 3).

The nascent idea of brain death emerged as physicians and families grappled with the reality that medical technology had advanced beyond the philosophical constructs available. In particular, a definition of brain death was needed to account for the fact that brain necrosis could occur despite continued tissue perfusion, due to artificial support of heart and lungs. From a medical perspective, defining death of an individual as the biological event that marks the transition from being alive to being dead is hard to argue against, but is incomplete because it does not provide any actual criteria for being dead.

Table 3 Religious and Cultural Events After Biological Death

Event	Religion or culture	Comments
The soul is reunited with a deity	Christians, Jews, and Muslims	Body no longer relevant.
Soul is reincarnated in a new body	Hindus, Sikhs, and Buddhists	Body is no longer relevant. The soul lives on in numerous bodies until nirvana is achieved. Quality of the soul's next biological life is influenced by deeds in the previous life.
Soul exists on earth after biological death	Gypsies and Japanese	A whole body is needed if the soul is to wander freely and be happy.
Spirit exists on earth after biological death	Aboriginal groups	Spirit beings need a whole body. They often play a role in the decision-making of the living.
Immortality	Various	As illustrated by beliefs about the soul but also biological/conceptual for example, living on in our children.

Thus, some suggest that death be defined as "permanent cessation of the critical functions of the organism as whole" (3). In this definition, critical functions are divided into three groups. These groups are the vital functions of spontaneous breathing, autonomic cardiovascular control, and integrative functions such as neuroendocrine feedback loops and consciousness that allow the organism to respond to essential needs such as hydration and nutrition. Inevitably this definition, and others similar to it, facilitate acceptance of the brain death concept.

Criteria for Pronouncing a Patient Dead

When a definition of death is agreed upon, criteria can be listed to show that the definition has been fulfilled. In the medical context, criteria have been described for cardiorespiratory death, brain death, brain stem death, and neocortical death (5). ✝ **Currently, cardiorespiratory and brain death are diagnosed widely and brain (and brain stem) death are accepted in most modern societies.** ✝

In ancient times the criteria for death, such as lack of breathing associated with a cold body, were common to all cultures and religions. More recently, cessation of heartbeat has been an additional criterion. Acceptance of cardiac arrest as a new criterion was facilitated because irreversible cardiac and respiratory arrest are normally so closely linked that in both practical and philosophical terms, the moment of death is unchanged. Consequently, religious teaching and traditional beliefs remained valid, according to the accepted criteria.

Tests Confirming the Criteria for Death

In past times, it was relatively easy to sense breathing and skin temperature. Nevertheless, there is evidence that the ancient Greeks and Romans delayed burial for several days, perhaps because they needed to be certain that death had occurred. The advent of cardiac arrest as a criterion began the process whereby the recognition of death was removed from the population as a whole, and became the province of doctors and nurses. However, advances in resuscitation and the advent of the diagnosis of brain death have meant that physicians are now the only ones formally able to diagnose death. Furthermore, the brain dead person no longer "looks dead" according to traditional criteria. Consequently, although all religious and cultural groups still discuss the concept and definition of death, they rely on physicians—not only to decide what exams and tests are necessary to diagnose biological death, but also to perform those tests. It is freely acknowledged that events such as the soul leaving or entering a new relationship with the body is not amenable to naturalistic tests.

✝ **Tests currently used to establish that death has occurred do not pinpoint the actual moment of death. Only when irreversible cardiac or respiratory arrest is witnessed is the time of death known.** ✝ Even then, a period of delay can occur, allowing for resuscitation attempts before death is diagnosed formally. Current criteria and tests diagnose the state of being dead, not the moment of death. In critically ill and patients, death may proceed more as a process than an event (6). Death of the person often proceeds as a process is in accordance with current definitions, which describe the sequential loss of several vital organ systems.

In the United Kingdom death is defined as death of the brain stem (see Volume 2, Chapter 16). The U.S. definition is based on "whole brain" death. The diagnosis of brain death has clinical criteria (sufficient in the majority of cases) and confirmatory tests (occasionally required to expedite diagnoses), both of which are completely reviewed in Volume 2, Chapter 16. However, both the brain stem and the cortex undergo a dying process. After the function of certain critical cells is lost, breathing and cardiovascular control becomes erratic, brain stem reflexes are lost one by one, and, finally, control of body temperature is lost. The dying process is even more complex for the whole brain, as additional cells and pathways are involved.

Until scientists and doctors define more precisely which critical functions determine death, death will always be a process and not an event. This is one reason why it has been so difficult for religious leaders to incorporate concepts of brain death into their teachings. Perhaps more precision in the use of words is needed and acknowledgment that diagnosis in its current form specifies the condition of being dead, not the actual moment of death itself.

RELIGIOUS CONTROVERSIES
Written and Oral Tradition

Most religions rely on texts that record the thoughts of prophets who lived in an era when absence of breathing was the main criterion for death. ✝ **Modern medicine has developed to the point where it has become very difficult for religious leaders to interpret ancient religious texts in a manner meaningful to contemporary society.** ✝ A review of the extensive literature illustrates how difficult it is for religious groups to reach a consensus view on the definition of death, and explains why although most major religious groups support organ transplantation programs and tacitly accept the diagnosis of brain death there is still debate about the meaning and definition of death. Written texts provide a common basis for discussion but are open to a variety of interpretations. Furthermore, societal changes and attitudes toward death continue to evolve, along with changes in the practice of medicine.

Aboriginal tribes throughout the world rely on oral tradition. Oral history changes as it passes down the generations, and ethics are best understood as a process rather than correct interpretation or a unified code (1). Spirit Beings participate in decision-making. We can only speculate about whether this very different ethical approach makes the task of decision-making, in relation to brain death and organ donation, easier or more difficult. Given the intense and intricate discussions still ongoing in many religious and cultural groups, the following sections are an interim but honest attempt to summarize the issues they face. For a greater understanding of the ethical views held by the major organized religions, the reader is referred to a recent series on end of life issues for various religions published in Lancet (7–13).

Life as a Valuable Gift

✝ **Although all religions celebrate life, attitudes regarding both life and death and how it occurs vary.** ✝ Most religions teach that life is sacred and that killing is wrong. Most also believe that life is a gift which must be valued. Suicide and euthanasia are therefore, generally forbidden. Buddhist belief is complex. Experience is divided into five skandhas. In Buddhism, the teaching of nonself (anatman) asserts that in the five skandhas, no independent self or soul can be found. Thus, Buddhists are encouraged to be compassionate, to meet death mindfully, to look beyond their own needs, and to serve the needs of everyone in society. Thus, although a dignified death is an acceptable personal goal, suicide in the interests of others is not only accepted but also considered laudable, if the person's motives are pure and in accordance with Buddhist teaching (14). Judaism also forbids killing. Some Jewish leaders argue that accepting donated organs would make the recipient an accessory to murder of the donor. Others, however, teach that the organ would have been removed anyway, and so as long as there is more than one potential recipient, a Jew may accept an organ if it is offered (15). Most Jewish scholars now believe that organ donation is acceptable, providing the donation does not hasten the death of the donor, or in any other way cause pain or suffering. Other groups, such as the Jehovah's Witnesses (JWs), forbid the transfusion of blood products. They believe that death from profound anemia or lack of clotting factors is Jehovah's will. Clinicians from other cultural or religious traditions find this attitude hard to accept and some might interpret this particular religious teaching as tantamount to suicide (see Volume 2, Chapter 67 for ethical issues involved in the care of JW patients).

Within the medical community, there are those who believe that brain death is not death (16). Others argue that the diagnosis of brain death is a strategy that is used solely to facilitate transplantation programs (17). They suggest that the diagnosis should be abandoned, and those patients with devastating brain damage, or who are nearing death for other reasons, should be allowed to donate organs before they die from irreversible cardiorespiratory arrest. This is likely to be interpreted as killing or suicide by some religious groups and would be unacceptable to them.

Religion and Organ Donation

➤ **Almost all religious groups have leaders who encourage the altruistic donation of organs for the benefit of others and tacitly accept the diagnosis of brain death.** ➤ These recommendations have not been achieved easily. It is clear that within many religious groups, guidance has been provided in an inconsistent and piecemeal way. For example, Muslims follow the teachings of Islam but are divided into Shi'a and Sunni branches. Jurists from the Shi'a branch have ruled that organ donation by brain dead patients is acceptable, but their rulings were made at different times in Iran, Egypt, Saudi Arabia, Singapore, and the United Kingdom. The Sunni branch has made similar rulings but generally later than the Shi'a branch (18). For Hindus, conscious death at home is the ideal. An unknown Hindu author has written "under no circumstances should organs be removed for use by others" (19). In contrast, a leading Hindu neurosurgeon has advocated acceptance of brain death and organ donation (20). The Sikh religion teaches that a person's soul is their real essence, and encourages followers to serve god by helping others. Because the body is of minor importance compared to the soul, organ donation is encouraged (21). Senior Rabbis from the Jewish community disagree about the definition of death according to religious texts. There is debate about whether breathing alone or heartbeat and breathing must have stopped. Another requirement is that the person must be "comparable to a dead man who does not move his limbs." Spastic movement, which is not normal, is acceptable to some. Yet others argue that even if the limbs do not move, a beating heart's movements are not spastic and therefore death can only be declared when there is no rhythmic heart beat (15). Consequently, the majority of Rabbis support organ donation, though a few do not.

In all these religious groups, acceptance of brain death and organ donation appears to have been achieved more quickly in some countries than others. This suggests that cultural and religious factors have a significant influence. In Japan, for example, the diagnosis of brain death and organ donation are very recent developments. Cultural rather than religious beliefs seem to have been the major barrier to acceptance (2). In particular, medical paternalism has led to mistrust of doctors by patients.

IMPLICATIONS OF RELIGIOUS AND CULTURAL DIVERSITY

Bioethical attitudes are influenced by religion and culture. ➤ **Ethical behavior accepted as the norm in Western countries may not be appropriate for minority groups within in these countries or in Eastern countries where the majority religion and culture is fundamentally different.** ➤ References to attitudes among the Japanese and North American native populations have already been made and are good examples. Whatever their ethnic origin, most individuals conceptualize death in a complex manner that is both personal and within cultural and spiritual contexts. In addition to biological and religious concepts of death, other ill-defined concepts exist. An illustration is the fear of elderly Westerners that their body will not be found for several days after death that suggests that life in their abstract thought somehow extends beyond biological life (4). Another example is the pressures on Western women to bear children, which may be linked to the concept of "living on in our children." Although biological transfer of genes is real, whether this really represents continuation of our personhood in our dependants is debatable.

All cultures and religions have rules, customs, and beliefs that require individuals to lead a "good" life. Most also describe a "good" death and require that the dead and dying are treated with dignity and respect for their values and beliefs. ➤ **As medical practitioners, we can facilitate a "good" death by recognizing that our patients' beliefs may differ from our own, and by attempting to elucidate what patients (or their families) believe is right for them, without imposing our own ethical values.** ➤ Recent correspondence in the British Medical Journal serves as a timely reminder that even within the medical profession, the definition of a "good" death varies enormously (22). Discussions with families about death and organ donation should occur in the context of their beliefs rather than ours. ➤ **Many intensive care units have access to support from a variety of religious communities, as well as social and spiritual care services and ethics committees whose assistance can be extremely helpful in facilitating appropriate end of life discussions (see Volume 2, Chapter 69).** ➤

In regard to organ donation, all the major religions allow, and most support, organ donation after death (Table 2). Often, however, these teachings do not filter down to the church membership (18). Educational material provided by transplant organizations (which includes religion-based recommendations) needs to be specifically targeted to relevant groups to enhance understanding.

The media can also have a profound effect on societal attitudes. Some years ago in Britain, a sensational television program purporting to show patients living normal lives after brain stem death had been mistakenly diagnosed led to an almost total cessation of the U.K. kidney transplantation program. Although the claims were later retracted, the accompanying publicity was minimal and it took many months for public confidence to return. Conversely, publicity about individual children nearing death because a suitable donor cannot be found usually leads to a flood of offers of organs.

Varying interpretations of a "good" death have already been described. Many religions encourage believers to aspire to a dignified death and teach respect for the body after death. To most, a dignified death implies that futile medical intervention should not proceed for long periods, and that patients should not suffer, justifying the use of sedation and analgesia at the time of withholding or withdrawing of nonbeneficial medical therapy. Additionally, it is incumbent on the medical profession therefore to ensure that suffering is not prolonged and the diagnosis of death is made promptly.

Not all brain dead patients become organ donors. However, ventilation and other life support should be discontinued as soon as brain death is declared if the patient is not an organ donor. The exception to this rule occurs when a patient dies so quickly that family has not had the opportunity to pay last respects. In this setting, a modest prolongation of mechanical ventilation of the deceased is acceptable. When patients have irrecoverable injuries or medical conditions, but are not brain dead, critical care practitioners may withhold or withdraw treatment reflecting ethical principles of autonomy (patient, family, or surrogate), beneficence, and nonmaleficence, as well as legal directives. Because the decision to withhold or withdraw treatment is based on medical opinion, some families may not agree, may believe it is unacceptable, or may cling to the hope that the patient will recover. Discontinuing ventilation in the presence of brain death is different than withdrawing ventilation, because the decision to discontinue is based on a diagnosis made by applying strict criteria rather than on the physicians' opinion of futility. However, families may still challenge the diagnosis and request that the diagnosis be confirmed by an independent physician.

In the truly brain dead patient, the heart usually stops after a couple days. In some patients, however, the heartbeat may continue for more than a few days, albeit at a slow rate, as other organs begin to fail and die cell by cell. Doctors who practiced in the era when discontinuation of futile treatment was not ethically or legally acceptable still remember the smell of putrefaction that surrounded these patients (due to generalized tissue necrosis and liquefaction). Such deaths were neither dignified nor "good." If brain death is abandoned as a definition of death, it is probable that some patients will be denied a dignified death. Thus, it is imperative that the apparently incontrovertible link between the diagnosis of brain death and organ transplantation is severed. This suggestion has been made before (23) (see Volume 2, Chapter 16).

EYE TO THE FUTURE

Advances in trauma care have already reduced the pool of potential organ donors and have triggered the development of alternative donation techniques. There is increasing interest in obtaining organs for transplantation from living relatives or nonheart beating donors. As techniques develop, the need for brain dead donors may diminish. Gene therapy will revolutionize many aspects of treatment for an enormous variety of diseases. This too may reduce the need for organ donors. Gene therapy and cell transplants may also alter outcomes from brain injury and irreversible brain injury may eventually become reversible.

✋ As medicine advances, and more and more parts of the biological organism (including the brain) become treatable or replaceable, the need for a precise definition of biological death becomes increasingly important. ✋ Although this is the remit of scientists and doctors, we should learn the lessons of the past. The adoption of brain death as a medical diagnosis and its effects on cultural and religious communities serve as a good example. As we strive to define biological death more precisely, we must facilitate a concurrent dialogue with philosophers, theologians, and cultural leaders so that society as a whole participates in the debate. Although the diagnosis of biological death is a task allocated to physicians, we must recognize that the diagnosis has implications that extend far outside of our realm of expertise (24).

It is clear from the available literature that the knowledge and wisdom of numerous senior individuals throughout the world have contributed to the debate about brain death and organ donation. Consensus opinion has evolved within various groups, but international consensus has not yet been achieved. It is equally clear that within the medical profession, the procedures for diagnosing brain (and brainstem) death have been agreed by committee. A relatively limited number of individuals have contributed in the literature to the discussion about the definition of death. For such an important subject, perhaps we are right to rely on experts. However, physicians are called on to diagnose death, and for our patients, this is the final and most significant involvement we will ever have in their care. More individuals from diverse backgrounds will need to contribute to the debate to achieve a broader consensus on the biological definition of death.

SUMMARY

Culture creates unique patterns of beliefs and perceptions, and cultural norms and values profoundly influence how individuals and groups think about death, dying, and issues surrounding the end of life. Religious traditions, as well as one's individual spirituality, also significantly influence attitudes and beliefs about death and the existence of an afterlife. Furthermore, societal changes and attitudes toward death continue to evolve, along with changes in the practice of medicine.

These ideas are inextricably linked to the meaning of death and what defines a "good death." Although definitions vary among philosophers, theologians, and some clinicians, it is clear that a dignified death is a goal sought by all. Physicians, by virtue of their role, are entrusted to make what is a final diagnosis—the diagnosis of a patient's death, based on clinical and legal standards, in accordance with moral/ethical principles. ✋ Currently, cardiorespiratory and brain death are diagnosed widely, and brain (and brain stem) death are accepted in most modern societies. ✋ The diagnoses of brain- and brain-stem death are essential to the concept of a dignified death, and contribute to the salvage of life brought about by altruistic organ donation for the benefit of others in society.

As medical practitioners, the most important contribution we can make in facilitating a "good" death is by recognizing that the values and beliefs of our patients may differ from our own, and by attempting to elucidate what patients (or their families) believe is right for them, without imposing our own biases and belief systems. Ultimately, medical goals in end of life care must be responsive to the needs and preferences of individuals within their sociocultural, religious, and family contexts.

KEY POINTS

✍ Medical goals in end of life care must be responsive to the needs and preferences of individuals within their sociocultural, religious, and family contexts.

✍ Cultures tend to embrace specific beliefs, perceptions, and values. These cultural norms and values strongly influence how individuals and groups think about death, dying, and end of life issues.

✍ The ethnicity, culture, and religion of patients and families strongly influence bioethical differences regarding end of life issues. Likewise, the ethical and legal climate within countries influences physician practices and medical decision-making surrounding end of life care.

✍ Historically, members of those religions and cultures that believe that the body is needed even after death have been less likely to accept organ donation than those who believe the soul leaves the physical body following death and no longer needs it.

✍ Death is the final diagnosis. Patients, their relatives, and their religious and societal mentors honor doctors by trusting them to accurately declare when biological life has ended.

✍ Ultimately, medical goals in end of life care must be responsive to the needs and preferences of individuals within their sociocultural, religious, and family contexts.

✍ Currently, cardiorespiratory and brain death are diagnosed widely and brain (and brainstem) death are accepted in most modern societies.

✍ Tests currently used to establish that death has occurred, do not pinpoint the actual moment of death. Only when irreversible cardiac or respiratory arrest is witnessed is the time of death known.

✍ Modern medicine has developed to the point where it has become very difficult for religious leaders to interpret ancient religious texts in a manner meaningful to contemporary society.

✍ Although all religions celebrate life, attitudes regarding both life and death and how it occurs vary.

✍ Almost all religious groups have leaders who encourage the altruistic donation of organs for the benefit of others and tacitly accept the diagnosis of brain death.

✍ Ethical behavior accepted as the norm in Western countries may not be appropriate for minority groups within in these countries or in Eastern countries where the majority religion and culture is fundamentally different.

✍ As medical practitioners, we can facilitate a "good" death by recognizing that our patients' beliefs may differ from our own, and by attempting to elucidate what patients (or their families) believe is right for them, without imposing our own ethical values.

✍ Many ICUs have access to support from a variety of religious communities, as well as social and spiritual care services and ethics committees whose assistance

can be extremely helpful in facilitating appropriate end of life discussions (see Volume 2, Chapter 69).

✍ As medicine advances, and more and more parts of the biological organism (including the brain) become treatable or replaceable, the need for a precise definition of biological death becomes increasingly important.

REFERENCES

1. Ellerby JH, McKenzie J, McKay S, Gariepy GJ, Kaufert JM. Bioethics for clinicians. 18. Aboriginal Cultures. CMAJ 2000; 163:845–850.

2. Morioka M. Bioethics and Japanese culture. Eubious J Asian Int Bioethics 1995; 5:87–90.

3. Bernat JL. A defence of the whole-brain concept of death. Hastings Cent Rep 1998; 2:14–23.

4. Kalish RA. Life and death: dividing the invisible. Soc Sci Med 1968; 2:249–259.

5. Bernat JL. How much of the brain must die in brain death? J Clin Ethics 1992; 3:21–28.

6. Pallis C, Harley DH. ABC of brainstem death. 2nd ed. London: BMJ Publishing Group, 1996:55.

7. Firth S. End-of-life: A Hindu view. Lancet 2005; 366(9486): 682–686.

8. Sachedina A. End-of-life: the Islamic view. Lancet 2005; 366(9487):774–779.

9. Dorff E. End-of-life: Jewish perspectives. Lancet 2005; 366(9488):862–865.

10. Keown D. End of life: the Buddhist view. Lancet 2005; 366(9489):952–955.

11. Engelhardt TH Jr, Smith Iltis A. End-of-life: the traditional Christian view. Lancet 2005; 366(9490):1045–1049.

12. Markwell H. End-of-life: a Catholic view. Lancet 2005; 366(9491):1132–1135.

13. Baggini J, Pym M. End of life: the humanist view. Lancet 2005; 366(9492):1235–1237.

14. Hughes JJ, Keown D. Buddhism and medical ethics: a bibliographic introduction. J Buddhist Ethics 1995; 2-ISSN: 1076–9005.

15. Breitowitz YA. The brain death controversy in Jewish Law [accessed 6/30/2005]. Available from: http://www.usisrael.com/jsource/Judaism/braindead.html

16. Shewmon DA. Recovery from brain death: a neurologist's apologia. Linacre Quarterly 1997; 64:30–96.

17. Truog RD, Robinson WM. Role of brain death and the dead-donor rule in the ethics of organ transplantation. Crit Care Med 2003; 31:2391–2396.

18. Syed J. Islamic views on organ donation. J Transpl Coord 1998; 8:157–163.

19. Anon. The Hindu ideal of conscious death [accessed 14/10/2003]. Available from: http://www.globalideasbank.org/soonlat/SL-5.html

20. Ganapathy K. Death redefined. The Hindu, Sunday, November 12th, 2000 [accessed 6/30/2005]. Available from: http://www.hindu.com/2000/11/12/stories/13120461.htm

21. UK Transplant. Sikhism and organ donation [accessed 6/30/2005]. Available from: http://www.uktransplant.org.uk/ukt/how_to_become_a_donor/religious_perspectives/leaflets/sikhism_and_organ_donation.jsp

22. Multiple authors. Letters. Br Med J 2003; 327:1047–1048.

23. Hauerwas S. Religious concepts of brain death and associated problems. Ann NY Acad Sci 1978; 315:329–338.

24. Wijdicks EFM. Brain death worldwide: accepted fact but no global consensus in diagnostic criteria. Neurology 2002; 58:20–25.

69

Palliative Care During the Withholding or Withdrawal of Life Support

William C. Wilson
Department of Anesthesiology and Critical Care, UC San Diego Medical Center, San Diego, California, U.S.A.

Catherine McCoy-Hill
School of Nursing, Azusa Pacific University, Azusa, California, U.S.A.

Anne J. Sutcliffe
Department of Anesthesia and Critical Care, Alexandra Hospital, Redditch, U.K.

INTRODUCTION

The withholding (WH) and withdrawal (WD) of life support (LS) are processes by which various medical interventions either are not given to patients or are removed from them with the expectation that the patients will die from their underlying disease, or from an acute intercurrent process. Life-sustaining treatment includes, among other therapies, mechanical ventilation, vasoactive drugs, chemotherapy, antibiotics, renal dialysis, artificial nutrition, and hydration. ☞ **Consistent with the principle of autonomy, it is medically ethical to WH/WD-LS whenever it is unwanted, or no longer desired, by the patient or his/her surrogate.** ☞

The WH/WD-LS is also appropriate when further treatment is deemed futile (1). A therapy is defined as futile when it has no realistic chance of providing benefits that the patient has the capacity to appreciate. This definition encompasses treatment that merely preserves permanent unconsciousness, or cannot end permanent dependence on medical care only available in an intensive care unit (ICU) (2). It is important to recognize that treatments which are futile in terms of overall outcome can, and often do, produce measurable improvements in individual physiological parameters. The key aspect of these improvements is that when they are futile, their sole function is that of delaying the dying process. Futile treatments do not contribute to cure or palliation of the underlying disease processes.

The concept of futile treatment is not new (1,2). However, significant controversy surrounds this topic when one tries to quantify futility (3–7). One recent study retrospectively evaluated Acute Physiologic and Chronic Health Evaluation (APACHE) scores and found a good correlation with outcomes; however, no specific futility threshold was identified (8). ☞ **Recent thinking emphasizes the notion that futility occurs when the burden of treatment far exceeds any anticipated benefit to the patient.** ☞ The concept of futility is important when balancing the ethical principles of beneficence (the obligation of physicians and nurses to endeavor to benefit the patient) and nonmaleficence (the obligation of caregivers to "not cause harm"). Medical futility occurs when a medical treatment has an inordinately greater burden (harm) than good.

Palliative care has been defined by the World Health Organization (WHO) in 1990 as "the active total care of patients whose disease is not responsive to curative treatment" (9). In the critical care unit, the administration of sedatives and analgesics represent one of the pillars of palliative care, aimed at mitigating unnecessary pain and suffering. In addition, meticulously maintaining the patient's cleanliness and appearance, among other aspects of comfort care, are essential to respecting the patient. Providing this level of attention to the patient also fulfills the need of the family to see that their loved one is cared for at the highest level, even at the time of death. Palliative care is multidisciplinary and is provided from the moment WH/WD-LS has been decided until the end of life (EOL), and is also extended to families in bereavement.

The WH/WD-LS and the implementation of palliative care in critical care settings have evolved over the past several decades. When initial recommendations for discontinuing ventilator support were made in the early 1980s, the provision of sedatives, analgesics, and other elements of palliative care were variable and not well studied.

Currently, one in five Americans (>500,000 people) die in an ICU every year, and of this group the majority die following decisions to limit or forego life-sustaining therapy (10–12). Initiatives addressing palliative care in the critical care setting have expanded recently in the wake of numerous studies and several major consensus publications focused on efforts to improve EOL care in the ICU (12–16).

Although many ICU clinicians deal with EOL considerations in an optimal fashion, the landmark SUPPORT study, among others, demonstrated that many critically ill patients at the EOL receive care that is incongruent with their wishes, and that some still die suffering needlessly prolonged and painful deaths (17–19). To address these issues, the Society of Critical Care Medicine (SCCM), published "Recommendations for End-of Life Care in the Intensive Care Unit" in 2001. This report identified the humanistic competencies, technical knowledge, and clinical skills required to ensure patient comfort during the WH/WD-LS (15). Recently, the Robert Wood Johnson Foundation (RWJF) "ICU Peer Workgroup Promoting Excellence in End of Life Care Project" proposed a set of essential EOL care domains as a national agenda for practice, education, and research to improve care of patients dying in ICUs (Table 1) (16). Additional information can be found regarding the "Promoting Excellence"

Table 1 Quality Indicators for Palliative Care in the Intensive Care Unit

Quality indicator	Examples/comments
Patient and family centered decision-making	Decision-making should be in accordance with the patient's wishes.
	Surrogates must not interject their own philosophical beliefs, may need guidance in reaching decisions, and should not be made to feel responsible for the patient's death, if/when they decide to WH/WD-LS.
	It is appropriate for physicians to recommend WH/WD-LS when further treatment is considered futile.[a]
	Methods of WH/WD-LS vary according to patient's condition and family wishes, but usually involves removal of mechanical ventilation (i.e., terminal weaning vs. extubation).
	Physicians should address conflict issues early, directly, and compassionately.
Communication with patients, family, and multidisciplinary team members	Goals of care should be clear, and the WH/WD-LS plan coordinated with the multidisciplinary team.
	The medical record should explicitly document the rational and plan for WH/WD-LS.
	The family should be prepared for what to expect.
Continuity of care across clinicians and settings	Consider nontransfer status of patient to maintain continuity of care in ICU.
	Maintain plan of care with new clinicians if transfer required or requested by family.
	Request palliative care, ethics consultations, and support service referrals (e.g., social services, pastoral care) as indicated.
Symptom management during WH/WD-LS	Analgesia and sedation should be provided to maximize comfort, and avoid distress (e.g., pain, dyspnea, anxiety, agitation) during preparation for and during the process of WH/WD-LS.
	Opioids and benzodiazepenes (or propofol) provide analgesia and sedation.
	NMBAs should be strictly avoided in order best avoid masking patient discomfort.
	Clear guidelines must be stipulated for PRN indications and dosage titration of opioids and sedatives for nursing staff.
	Interventions that cause patient discomfort should be discontinued/avoided.
Emotional and practical support for families	Comfort care and patient dignity should be maintained during WH/WD-LS.
	Privacy and unrestricted family visitation are important aspects.
	Environmental stressors of ICU should be reduced: avoid unnecessary monitoring, alarms, and imposing equipment.
	Ensure practical support needs for the family are met.
	Meticulously attend to patient's physical comfort, hygiene, and appearance.
	Facilitate cultural and spiritual EOL rituals.
Institutional support systems	Consider use of standardized order sets for WH/WD-LS and "comfort care" orders.
	Develop ICU policies/protocols for WH/WD-LS and interdisciplinary accountability according to best practices.
	Establish mechanisms for ongoing support and education of novice and seasoned clinicians regarding palliative ICU care.

[a]Futility is defined within the chapter.
Abbreviations: EOL, end-of-life; ICU, intensive care unit; NMBAs, neuromuscular blockade agents; PRN, pro re nada as needed; WH/WD-LS, withholding or withdrawal of life support.
Source: From Ref. 16.

project at the following web address: www.promotingex-cellence.org.

This chapter reviews the legal and ethical justification for the provision of sedatives and analgesics during WH/WD-LS, as well as the indications and decision-making process. The techniques utilized are variable, and are ethically acceptable only if the primary goals of maximizing patient comfort, avoiding suffering, and promoting patient dignity and respect are observed. Some guidelines in this regard are offered. In addition, various techniques for optimizing the management of symptoms, as well as for promoting a caring environment are emphasized.

LEGAL AND ETHICAL JUSTIFICATION
Legal Principles of Informed Consent and Right to Refuse Medical Treatment
In health care decision-making, a fully informed, capable, and freely consenting adult has the legal right to decide whether to accept (consent to) or refuse any and all medical treatments, including those where death is a consequence. The legal and ethical justifications for the WH/WD-LS rest on the principles of informed consent and autonomy. In terms of consent to treatment, or the WH/WD-LS, patients must be fully informed of the expected benefits and burdens of treatment. Accordingly, when further provision of life-sustaining therapy is unlikely to benefit the patient, physicians are ethically required to inform the family or surrogate(s) of the patient's prognosis and initiate palliative care discussions (when appropriate). The legal foundations of informed consent are further discussed in Volume 2, Chapter 67.

Ethics
Autonomy (Right to Self-Determination)
The principle of autonomy from the Greek, *auto* = self and *nomy* = govern, respects the freedom and right of self-determination in decisions affecting the individual. Regard for autonomy honors the patient's right to choose to limit

or forgo life-sustaining therapy. The majority of patients dying in ICUs must exercise their autonomy through surrogate decision makers (20,21), since less than 5% have adequate decision-making capacity and an estimated 10%–15% (even less in trauma patients) have existing advanced directives (see Volume 2, Chapter 67)

In the Case of Futility: Balancing Beneficence with Nonmaleficence

✍ When futile conditions are recognized by the care team, physicians are obligated to convey this information to the family to ensure full disclosure of medical information, a necessary prerequisite to shared decision-making. ✍

When there is little hope of meaningful recovery the WH/WD-LS is consistent with the ethical principles of beneficence and nonmaleficence. The principle of beneficence requires physicians to "do good" and take actions that benefit or contribute to the welfare of the patient. The principle of nonmaleficence is based on the dictum *primum non-nocere* "above all do no harm." This principle obliges physicians to inform patients/families and act with diligence in avoiding therapy known to cause suffering or harm in cases where treatment has no realistic chance of providing benefit that the patient has the capacity to appreciate, that is, futile therapy. Under these circumstances, physicians should also suggest that the emphasis of treatment be shifted from an intent to cure to a focus of comfort.

Although no consensus has been achieved on the definition of what constitutes medical futility, futile conditions do occur regularly in critically ill-trauma and postsurgical patients, and most intensivists incorporate some form of this concept into their decision-making regarding the aggressiveness of therapy and during deliberations regarding the WH/WD-LS. Accurate prognostication of individual patient outcomes is both difficult and controversial, and the probability of survival is only one of several factors (i.e., clinical judgment and experience) used in determining the appropriateness of treatment (22–24).

Use of Sedatives and Analgesics: Ethical Principle of Double Effect

✍ The ethical principle of "double effect" when used to justify comfort care conveys that analgesics and sedatives can have the dual effect of relieving suffering as well as hastening death, and that the administration of these drugs is ethically appropriate if the primary goal is to provide symptom control (e.g., relief of pain and suffering), even if death, a secondary, unintended effect is hastened in the process (25–27). ✍ The fundamental difference between symptom management during the WH/WD-LS and euthanasia is based on what is intended (palliation) versus what is foreseen, but not the primary intent (death).

Ethical Equivalence of Withholding and Withdrawal

Distinctions between the WH and the WD of treatment have been made by some physicians who have felt justified in not initiating treatment, but not comfortable with the discontinuation of life-sustaining therapy. **✍ From an ethical perspective there is no difference between the WH and the WD of treatment that only prolongs life without a realistic chance of cure, and such distinctions are morally irrelevant. ✍** Accordingly, when treatment is not wanted by the patients (or surrogates), is contrary to the patient's

values, and/or is unwarranted due to medical futility, it is ethically and legally permissible to WH or WD treatment. The moral equivalence of WH and WD also permits the initiation of life saving interventions and time-limited trials of therapy, with subsequent discontinuation of treatment, if later determined to be futile.

✍ It is important to recognize that it is never an emergency to WH/WD-LS. ✍ Although discussions may be urgent and intense, particularly when families and/or the care team are in disagreement, it is nearly always best to continue supportive care until consensus can be reached. An additional reason to briefly continue supportive care arises when families are en route to the hospital from out of town and wish to be with the patient as he/she expires. In this instance, it is best to maintain life support for the patient until the family is present and prepared to discontinue LS.

SHARED DECISION MAKING BETWEEN PHYSICIANS AND SURROGATES

Most clinicians and family members advocate a shared decision-making model of mutual negotiation between the physician(s), patient, surrogates, and the medical team caring for the patient as the best approach for deciding when to limit or forgo life-sustaining therapy. When the patient's previous wishes are unknown, the goal is to act in accordance with the best-known evidence.

Family members acting as surrogates should not make decisions according to their own values, but rather acting as the patient's advocate, in accordance with the wishes of the patient they represent.

As families look to physicians for guidance, it is entirely appropriate to make recommendations to surrogates, and it should be considered a disservice to the patient and family not to do so. This advice is first focused on the best judgment in terms of likely outcomes with continued treatment in terms of meaningful recovery and final rehabilitation potential.

With regard to the order of events during the WH/WD-LS, limiting options to the most relevant approaches is most appropriate during initial discussions. Confusing families with a diffuse array of unguided options is often more likely to overwhelm them during the stressful deliberations. However, when families express preferences of how the WH/WD-LS should proceed, these wishes should be incorporated into the plan of care whenever possible.

In addition, it is critical for physicians to impart to family members that making the decision to WH/WD-LS when indicated is not analogous to active euthanasia or causing death, but rather that the decision allows the patient to die naturally without further prolonging unnecessary, and potentially painful, treatment through the institution or continuation of life support.

Finally, once the decision has been made to pursue palliative care goals, discussions regarding the WH/WD-LS should conclude with affirmation of the active interventions that will be provided to ensure the patient's comfort and meet the family's needs. Before leaving from these discussions, family members should be invited to ask any final questions and/or to make any other requests known.

Preparing Family and Loved Ones

The emotional burdens and uncertainty family members experience over decisions to withdraw life-sustaining treatment are well known. Research exploring the process has shown that as families come to terms with the patient's prognosis, consideration is given to what the patient would have wanted, and eventually hopes are redirected from cure to a comfortable and dignified death for their loved one. Family preparation needs to center on support and guidance, affirmation of the appropriateness of their decisions, and reassurance that the patient's suffering will be minimized (28–33).

☞ **Family members should not be left to feel alone with the burden or guilt that their decisions are responsible for ending a loved one's life. Clinicians can effectively guide families through the process of reorienting goals from therapeutic to comfort care through honest, timely, and compassionate communication (28).** ☞

To diffuse the burden of guilt, as much as possible, it is important for loved ones to feel that the patient is making the decision. Accordingly, it is important to emphasize that the WH/WD-LS never means the withdrawal of care. Assurance that quality care will continue to be provided, focusing on the patient's comfort and dignity is imperative. ☞ **Families also need to be assured that WH/WD-LS is legally permissible and ethically humane, and that the administration of sedatives and analgesics is not analogous to euthanasia.** ☞ When the decision-making process is handled sensitively by clinicians, the family is usually able to develop a sense of satisfaction from doing what they perceive as right and noble (e.g., carrying out the patient's wishes and limiting unnecessary suffering) (31,34–36).

Developing Consensus and Conflict Resolution

Emphasizing that it is the patient's preferences which are paramount is often helpful in gaining consensus from all those involved in decisions to forgo further treatment. This requires explicit discussion and effective communication, often over the course of several days. Multidisciplinary family conferences, led by the attending physician, are extremely valuable to consensual decision-making and the prevention of conflict between clinicians and surrogates. When the decision to pursue comfort care is made, a consensus regarding the plan for how life support will be withdrawn is essential.

When conflicts arise, specific issues of misunderstanding (e.g., values conflicts, inadequate knowledge) should be elicited and dealt with accordingly to reduce discordant expectations. Skillful negotiation resolves most conflicts including futility disputes. In situations where conflict with families is ongoing or anticipated, early ethics consultation is often helpful. When there is dissention within the family, which is often due to prior unresolved issues, emotional support from the social worker or spiritual care services, if appropriate, can be invaluable. When conflicts exist among interdisciplinary team members, it is important to clarify goals of care before the family becomes involved in the discussions so that efforts are coordinated, and family members are not burdened by divergent medical views. One member of the medical team should serve as the main spokesperson with the family; this is traditionally the attending physician or his/her designate, and should not be left to house staff or junior clinicians.

PROCESS OF WITHHOLDING OR WITHDRAWAL
Transition from Life-Sustaining Care to Comfort Care

Management goals in the transition from life-sustaining treatment to comfort care should focus on ensuring that the patient and family are prepared, patient suffering is avoided, and that death occurs in the best manner possible within the ICU, thus preserving the patient's dignity, respect, and comfort. As such, only interventions aimed at achieving the goals of comfort care should be pursued; all previous therapies or procedures that do not specifically contribute to the patient's comfort should be avoided or discontinued.

Documentation of DNaR and Withdrawal of Life Support Orders

Do not attempt resuscitation (DNaR) orders are one form of withholding life support intervention. Often in the critical care setting, the determination of DNaR precedes the decision to withdraw other life support measures (e.g., mechanical ventilation, vasopressors, etc.). As such, DNaR orders alone carry no implications regarding other EOL treatment plans, and therefore must be specified separately. DNaR order protocols require the stipulation of whether all resuscitative efforts are to be withheld, or attempted with limitations (e.g., medication or defibrillation only).

☞ **With the decision to WH/WD-LS, all orders should be rewritten to reflect that the intent of treatment has shifted to providing comfort care to the patient, without regard to physiologic stability.** ☞ Documentation should be explicit regarding the patient's condition, the agreed on goals of care, and the procedure for WH/WD-LS, including the plan for the assessment and management of symptoms. ICU nurses should be given latitude in pharmacologic dosing with clear guidelines for PRN indications and dosage adjustment (e.g., pain, dyspnea, anxiety, and agitation). Several authors have recommended the use of standardized order sets (37), though this practice is not currently in widespread use. If needed, palliative care or pain management consultation can be sought. This is done proactively in some institutions. Appropriate multidisciplinary consultation for support services for example, social work and pastoral care should also coincide with orders for WH/WD-LS.

Confirming Patient Preparation

☞ **Before any active WH/WD-LS, the patient needs to be started on sedatives and analgesics and made comfortable as assessed by the bedside nurse and/or attending physician.** ☞ If neuromuscular blockade agents (NMBAs) were used to this point, they must be stopped. Suggestions for sedatives and analgesics to achieve this goal are detailed subsequently.

Although the vast majority of patients have already lost consciousness, by the time WH/WD-LS is considered, any conscious patient should be prepared for what they will experience.

Ensuring Family Preparation

The patient's family and loved ones require particular preparation and ongoing support during the transition process. Anticipatory guidance in relation to the dying process, for example, how the patient will look, and in general terms, the patient's expected length of survival (though rarely predictable), can help prepare family members for what to expect. Specific needs and wishes regarding the moment of death should be clarified; though most family members wish to be present, this is neither universal nor always possible. Postponing withdrawal to await the arrival of geographically distant loved ones when requested is another important consideration since WH/WD-LS is never an emergency. Adherence to the planned time of WD is essential, as families should not be burdened with the emotional upheaval of waiting due to competing clinician time demands.

Cultural and religious traditions have a significant influence on the experience of death. ☞ **Traditional rituals or practices should be respected and allowed to occur whenever possible, as their observance in preparation for death is frequently a source of comfort for the patient/family.** ☞ Cultural and spiritual values and beliefs may differ markedly from those of clinicians, emphasizing the importance of elucidating patient/family goals and preferences before the process of WH/WD-LS (see Volume 2, Chapter 68).

Clinician presence and time spent with the family to learn about the patient as an individual is invaluable. ☞ **Encouraging reminiscence of positive life experiences and important relationships in the patient's life often helps to facilitate the family's grieving process at the EOL.** ☞

Before withdrawal of therapy it is also important to discuss with families what will happen after the patient's death. Consideration should be given to issues such as death notification procedures, autopsies, handling of the body, and resources for funeral arrangements.

Technical Details of Withdrawing Therapy

The withdrawal of life support is a clinical procedure and deserves the same level of physician preparation and involvement as any other medical intervention. Physicians need to decide which life support measures will be WH/WD, in what sequence, and by whom. This decision-making should be in accordance with family preference. However, since families are seldom experienced in this regard, clinicians should facilitate the process by supplying options that are most suitable to a peaceful death.

☞ **Discussions with families regarding the WH/WDLS should not be left to novice clinicians.** ☞ This is the time when experienced senior clinicians are required. However, most families are agreeable for novice clinicians to sit in on discussions for the purposes of training, especially if the novice is known to them or has already participated in the patient's care. ☞ **The family should be reassured that clinicians will remain available and that their loved one will be kept comfortable and free of pain, suffering, or any distress throughout the entire process.** ☞

Considerations for Therapy Withdrawal

When determining which therapies to withdraw, physicians should be guided by the goals of care, that is, mitigation of patient suffering and needs of the family, rather than a prescribed pattern. In general, once the decision to WH/WD-LS has been made, all focus should be on maintaining the patient's comfort. Owing to their lack of impact on the dying process, it generally is best to WH/WD all drugs and therapy except for the administration of sedatives and analgesics, unless other agents are needed for symptom palliation (e.g., antiemetics, seizure prophylaxis).

Occasionally, the family will ask that certain therapies, for example, enteral nutrition and hydration, continue to be administered, and that treatments be WH/WD in a stepwise fashion. When this approach is used, the ordering sequence should be prioritized such that any treatment that is

potentially uncomfortable be WH/WD first. The only therapy that should be considered for a staged WH/WD is ventilator support, because absence of nearly any other therapy is not associated with pain or discomfort (38). Indeed, the gradual WH/WD of other therapies risks exposure of the patient to additional suffering, and is not legally necessary or ethically appropriate. There is no ethical reason for gradual withdrawal, and a valid ethical case against gradual withdrawal can be made on the grounds that partial treatment strategies or stepwise withdrawal when death is inevitable may expose the patient to further suffering, and prolong the family's grief as well (38).

Abrupt Ventilator Withdrawal vs. Terminal Weaning

Several methods of withdrawal from mechanical ventilation can be used depending on the patient's clinical condition and physician experience. In terminal weaning, the endotracheal tube is left in place following stepwise reductions in ventilatory support, which can take place gradually or rapidly. In some cases, extubation follows the wean. Terminal extubation entails a rapid cessation of mechanical ventilation and artificial airway removal. Arguments in favor of extubation following rapid weaning focus on the removal of unnecessary equipment, maximization of comfort, and reducing the prolongation of dying as well as the family's anguish. Those who favor of terminal weaning reason that it minimizes dyspnea, and prevents airway obstruction (19,39). Limited data are available to justify one method over the other for any particular set of clinical circumstances. Accordingly, practice patterns vary widely in terms of approach at WH/WD-LS, with most studies demonstrating that terminal weaning is currently more common, although this is changing. However, terminal weaning lasting for many hours should be avoided as it only prolongs the dying process. Regardless of the method employed, patient comfort and support of the attendant family are the primary concerns. Dyspnea and anxiety should always be anticipated, and patients should be appropriately medicated with sedatives or analgesics before the initiation of WH/WD-LS (14,15,40).

Recommended Approaches

The optimal approach to WH/WDLS will vary between institutions, physicians, patients, and clinical circumstances. However, several key principles (Table 2) should be observed regardless of the specific details. These considerations have been articulated in other sections of this chapter. Above all else, providing a humane environment for the patient and family and ensuring that the patient is allowed to die with respect, dignity, and with the least discomfort possible represents the optimal approach.

The optimal approach also requires that the family is involved in the decision-making process to WH/WD-LS. Once the plan has been decided, it should be clearly articulated to the nursing staff, documented in the patient record, and corresponding orders should be written. Patients on NMBAs should have these discontinued, and those not receiving sedatives or analgesics should have these started, with orders to select and titrate dosing as required to prevent symptoms of dyspnea, pain, or anxiety.

The environment should be made conducive to the WH/WD-LS, with particular attention to comfort and esthetic elements. A private room, soft lighting, and reduced noise are often comforting, as are presence of photographs and other meaningful mementos of the patient's life.

Table 2   Key Considerations During the Withholding or Withdrawal of Life Support in the Intensive Care Unit

Key consideration	Examples/comments
Ensure family agreement and preparation	Ascertain consensus and acceptance of transition to palliative care goals. Explicitly address and attempt to resolve any conflicts before WH/WD-LS.
	Once the decision has been made to WH/WD-LS, family preparation centers on support and guidance during the process.
	Reassurance that the patient's comfort and dignity will be maintained is critical to the family's well-being.
	Specific needs and preferences regarding the time of death (e.g., wish to be present) should be elicited and accommodated whenever possible.
Document orders are written for WH/WD-LS	Distinguish DNaR orders from WH/WD-LS orders; DNaR orders alone carry no implications regarding other EOL treatment plans, and must be specified distinctly.
	Documentation should be explicit regarding the patient's condition, the agreed on goals of care, and the procedure for WH/WD-LS.
Confirm patient preparation (including adequate analgesia/sedation)	Initial IV bolus dosing and continuous IV infusion of analgesics and sedatives should be started before the active WH/WD-LS, and PRN bolusing to treat any symptoms of distress is optimal.
	Provision of adequate dosages of opioids and benzodiazepenes will provide effective analgesia and sedation in virtually all patients.
Physical care and comfort of the patient	Remove invasive lines and discontinue interventions that may cause discomfort to the patient.
	Disable audible monitors and alarms (except at central station).
	Disable pacemakers and automatic internal (or external) cardiac defibrillators.
	Allow family to participate in care of patient as desired; encourage physical touch/contact.
	Respond to family member's concerns regarding patient comfort as often they are able to accurately interpret patient behaviors indicative of distress.
Appropriate setting, quality, and continuity of care	Transfers out of the ICU should be the exception, rather than the norm; ICU care ensures lower nurse: patient ratios, close surveillance, and availability of multiple resources for aggressive symptom management.
	If transfer is required or requested, assure family members that continuity in the plan of care will be maintained. New clinicians should be introduced to the family, and transfer protocols clearly specified.
Privacy and environmental modifications	Ensure privacy of family for personal expressions of words, emotions and cultural/spiritual rituals.
	Modify environment to reduce noise, soften lighting, and make as comfortable as possible. Remove unnecessary machines/technology.
Multidisciplinary support	Maintain clinician access and close presence to inform and support family members during the dying process.
	Offer support services (pastoral care, ethics consultation, bereavement specialists) as appropriate.

Abbreviations: DNaR, do not attempt resuscitation; EOL, end-of-life; ICU, intensive care unit; IV, intravenous; PRN, pro re nata as needed; WH/WD-LS, withholding or withdrawal of life support.

For some patients and families, playing calming music can also help transform the environment and keep the emphasis on pleasant, loving memories. Visitation policies should be liberalized, allowing loved ones who wish to be present to remain with the patient during the WH/WD-LS.

☞ **Throughout the entire WH/WD-LS the patient should be as clean and meticulously cared for as possible.** ☞ This helps the family and loved ones remember the dying patient in a more positive way and to ensure that the patient's dignity at the time of WH/WD-LS. Moreover, this also communicates to the family that the medical and nursing staff care for, respect, and share their concerns for the patient.

Once all the arrangements previously described are complete, the patient should optimally have all tubes removed, except for the infusion line for sedatives or analgesics, and drainage tubes that may result in obstructive symptoms and pain without their presence. Alarms on all ventilator devices, infusion pumps, and monitors should be disabled. The monitor screen at the bedside should also be turned off, although an ECG or pulse oximetry signal transmitted to the central nursing station can give helpful

clues about the speed of the patient's decline. In addition, pacemakers and automatic internal cardiac defibrillators should be deactivated.

It is important for the bedside nurse to keep a watchful eye over the patient to check for signs of inadequate sedation and analgesia as well as monitoring for the cessation of ventilatory efforts, and cardiac function. The nurse's presence at the bedside during this time can be an invaluable source of information and emotional support for family and loved ones.

Last, the ventilation should be discontinued and, when sedation and analgesics are optimally titrated, the ETT should also be removed providing that removal is not expected to lead to stridor or immediate partial/complete airway obstruction. Often, careful positioning of the patient in the "recovery position" can reduce symptoms of airway obstruction. The benefit of removal of the ETT is that the patient will appear more natural and like themselves. In the case of patients with expected stridor or obstruction following extubation despite adequate positioning, the ETT should remain in place, with the patient removed from the ventilator circuit and placed on humidified room air.

SYMPTOM MANAGEMENT
Administration of Sedatives and Analgesics

There is no sound rationale for withholding analgesia or sedation when the goal is comfort and symptom relief. During the WH/WD-LS, conventional administration rules do not apply and optimal dosing is determined by the control of symptoms (e.g., pain, agitation, and dyspnea), without concern for cardiopulmonary side effects of the drugs, regardless of the dosage required. **When administered in adequate dosages, opioids and benzodiazepines (or propofol) provide adequate analgesia and sedation in virtually all patients during the WH/WD-LS.** Anticipatory dosing should also occur whenever the patient has any presumptive reason for distress. Medical orders should clearly specify the intended use for analgesia and sedation, guided by the principle of double effect.

Opioids provide the foundation of pharmacologic management during the WH/WD-LS by providing analgesia, some sedation, and blunting of respiratory and cough responses. In most cases morphine is the ideal opioid because it is easily titratable with rapid onset of action and few adverse effects; fentanyl and hydromorphone are equally effective. Fentanyl is less likely to cause histamine-related effects and is useful in patients allergic to morphine, although it produces less sedation. Meperidine should be avoided because its active metabolite normeperidine can theoretically produce seizures. Age, organ system function, and prior use of opioids (opioid naive vs. tolerant) also necessitate dose adjustment. Occasionally nonopioids are used adjuvantly to manage concomitant inflammatory or neuropathic pain.

Benzodiazepenes are indicated for sedation and anxiolysis, are synergistic with opioids, and have useful anterograde amnesic effects and anticonvulsant properties. Benzodiazepines are generally preferable to antipsychotics (e.g., haloperidol). However, propofol can be used as well. As with opioids, benzodiazepenes or propofol are optimally administered by continuous IV infusion with bolus dosing as needed for symptom control and drug level maintenance. Haloperidol is generally not required at this juncture in patient care.

Neuromuscular blockade agents should be avoided or discontinued before the WH/WD-LS as there is no therapeutic purpose for paralytic use during ventilator withdrawal. NMBAs mask assessment of patient distress, making it impossible to determine the efficacy of analgesics and sedatives in achieving comfort, and may cause suffering without adequate analgesia (12,14,15,38,41).

Physiologic assessment tools, sedation scales, and so on are useful (though not always reliable in unconscious patients) to quantify evaluation of pain or other distress (see Volume 2, Chapter 5). In addition, family members are often able to accurately interpret patient behaviors associated with pain or anxiety and should be encouraged to share opinions and concerns regarding symptom management with the nursing staff.

Nonpharmacologic Management of Pain and Suffering

Palliative care in the ICU involves more than analgesia and sedation. **Nonpharmacologic management of suffering involves discontinuation of "routine" interventions in the ICU that cause unnecessary discomfort to the patient.** Any treatment that is not essential to achieving comfort should be stopped; this includes blood draws, diagnostic exams, painful wound care, and repeated vital sign monitoring.

Aggressive pulmonary hygiene including endotracheal suctioning should be avoided unless it aids in comfort, although this is rare. In contrast, gentle suction of secretions from the mouth of a recently extubated patient can reduce the noise of breathing. Noisy breathing is distressing for families and loved ones who often refer to it as "the death rattle" which is historically associated with a prolonged and painful death.

Invasive lines, for example, Swan Ganz catheters, arterial lines, ICP monitoring devices, and so on, can be removed and monitor alarms disabled. Environmental stressors such as excessive noise, light, and activity should be minimized. Removal of restraints, equipment, and lowering of bedrails allows loved ones more intimate contact with the patient (12,15,35,41).

Even though family members may be fully cognizant of the withdrawal process, they are often reluctant to touch the patient. This is probably a consequence of their previous experience when active care was still in progress and they may have been fearful of dislodging vital monitoring devices or equipment. **During the WH/WD-LS process, family members should be explicitly informed that it is entirely permissible, and usually beneficial, to touch and hug the patient, if this is their wish.**

Physical Care and Comfort of the Patient

Attentiveness to the physical care of the patient is important from a patient comfort perspective, as well to assure family and loved ones that the patient is receiving excellent care from clinicians. Meticulous attention to the patient's physical comfort, hygiene, and appearance conveys caregiver respect and protects dignity. To meet both, patient and family needs, ICU staffing patterns should reflect requirements for higher, not lower, intensity and acuity in the nursing care needs of dying patients.

PROVIDING A CARING ENVIRONMENT
Appropriate Settings, Quality, and Continuity of Care

When death is imminent in critically ill-ventilator dependent patients, it is recommended that the patient remain in the ICU for comfort care; transfers should be the exception, rather than the norm. This ensures continuity of caregivers, higher nurse: patient ratios, and availability of multiple resources needed when aggressive symptom management or close surveillance is required (e.g., ventilator or vasopressor withdrawal). Efforts should be made to adapt the ICU environment to provide a comfortable, private, and less technology dominant setting.

If the family requests transfer, or when needs may be more effectively met in another setting, the patient can be transferred out of the ICU, especially if not ventilator dependent. When the patient is transferred to a new location, it is imperative that the transition to floor care (or although rare for critically ill patients, to a hospice environment), be as seamless as possible. In circumstances where a new set of clinicians must be involved, introductions should be made to family members, and transfer protocols should include a detailed report of the patient's status to ensure the plan of care will not be disrupted. The receiving clinicians must be made specifically aware of the rationale for WH/WD-LS as well as the agreed on plans for implementation so that continuity of care is maintained.

Ensuring Patient and Family Preferences for Privacy

Family members should be allowed to spend as much as they wish with the dying patient with unrestricted visiting hours. Although preferences for the level of involvement in care vary, family members can be allowed to participate in care at a level which they feel most comfortable. Private time spent together as a loved one is dying is, for many families, a time of reflection and reconciliation.

Providing Emotional and Physical Comfort to Family and Loved Ones

The support and presence of clinicians, especially the ICU nurse, is vital to the family's emotional well-being during this vulnerable time. Distress is reduced when the family is kept informed of the withdrawal process, and expressed concerns are assiduously addressed (28,42,43). Private space for families away from the general visitors waiting room to eat, rest, make phone calls, and so on, is important to provide respite and accommodate practical support needs (see Volume 2, Chapter 64).

Multidisciplinary Support

↗ The combined efforts of a multidisciplinary team including nurses, physicians, social workers, and spiritual care providers are essential to providing comprehensive palliative care in the SICU. ↗ No one discipline can address the multidimensional needs of patients and families, and each offers expertise in achieving the goals of care. Ideally, clinicians involved in the patient's care should be available at the time of death to support bereaved family and loved ones.

Emotional Support for the Clinical Staff

The death of any patient is often difficult for medical staff to reconcile, particularly if that patient has already been subject to intensive efforts directed at saving life. Other factors that tend to make it more difficult than usual for caregivers is when the dying patient is young, was talking or active for some portions of the critical care management, and when the patient has an unforeseen sudden catastrophic event, such as a massive pulmonary embolus.

Although one's professional responsibility is concerned primarily with the care of the patient and family, the emotional needs of colleagues, particularly those who are inexperienced, should also be considered. Senior clinicians should ensure that there is a mechanism for dealing with the impact of the death of a patient on those staff members who have been involved in the patient's care.

EYE TO THE FUTURE

Although WH/WD-LS is common practice for general intensive care patients, its application and benefits are less well studied in trauma populations (44). The unexpected, often tragic nature of life-threatening injury and the fact that trauma patients tend to be young and previously healthy complicate the traditional notions of palliative care and create enormous levels of stress and uncertainty in both family members and clinicians. Although increasing attention is being given to palliative care, current models do not always fit the clinical realities of a trauma/surgical ICU. At present there is a dearth of studies specifically addressing EOL issues in trauma populations, and hopefully more will come in the future.

Much remains to be learned regarding best methods of WH/WD-LS and optimizing comfort of the dying patient, as well as the most effective intervention strategies to support grief-stricken family members through the process of decision-making and the transition to EOL care following trauma. Because death is inevitable the culture of the trauma service necessitates an expansion of the mission and focus from one solely aimed at saving lives to one which also addresses the physical and emotional EOL issues for those patients who will not survive their injuries.

Palliative care must not be considered as a sequel to "failed" intensive care but rather an integrative component of caring for critically ill and injured patients (45). Further research is needed to explore trauma-specific intervention strategies regarding WH/WD-LS, and to identify the most effective quality measures for improving palliative care in trauma populations.

Although this is changing, trauma care providers have had little formal education in the principles and skills of palliative care. Numerous efforts are underway such as those by the SCCM, RWJF, and the AMA Education for Physicians on End-of-Life Care (EPEC) Project. California has led the way by enacting law AB487, which requires all MDs to take 12 hours of continuing medical education in pain management and palliative care by Dec 31, 2006.

Furthermore, in the clinical setting, experienced critical care practitioners have many opportunities which enable them to serve as role models and mentors to junior clinicians, in teaching and demonstrating the knowledge and skill sets required to provide excellent palliative care in the ICU.

SUMMARY

As most patients who die in an ICU do so following WH/WD-LS, compassionate clinical management of death is an important goal. As providers of EOL care, trauma surgeons and critical care clinicians must be knowledgeable and skilled in both the humanistic competencies of shared decision-making surrounding EOL issues and the technical competencies required to provide quality palliative care to patients and their families during this stressful time.

Legal and ethical justification for WH/WD-LS rests on the principles of informed consent and patient autonomy. In ICU patients, this right is most often exercised through surrogates (usually a family member or other loved one) acting on behalf of and in accordance with the patient's values and beliefs.

When medical futility is evident, it is incumbent on physicians to inform and advise surrogates of the limitations of medical treatment and technology. In preparing families for EOL decision-making, clinicians must recognize the emotional toll involved and be prepared to guide them through the difficult process, avoiding undue guilt or burden. A shared model of decision-making is the optimal approach.

When hope for recovery is ended, and the decision to WH/WD-LS has been made by families and the medical staff, the focus of patient care changes from curative interventions to comfort care, where the primary goal is the provision of nonpainful supportive measures and the elimination of needless suffering and distress. Adequate analgesia and sedation is achievable in virtually all patients during the WH/WD-LS, and based on the principle of double effect, no maximum dose of analgesics or sedatives exists when the intent is to relieve pain or suffering.

Families and loved ones of dying patients require the utmost support and compassionate care from clinicians. Care provided to the patient which emphasizes comfort, dignity, and respect is vital to achieving this end. Individual preferences and spiritual and cultural values and traditions should be honored. All families should also be offered supportive services from multidisciplinary experts in pastoral care, ethics, and social services during this vulnerable time, as well as being provided with information on referral sources for bereavement support (see Volume 2, Chapter 64).

KEY POINTS

- Consistent with the principle of autonomy, it is medically ethical to WH/WD-LS treatment whenever it is unwanted, or no longer desired by the patient or his/her surrogate.
- Recent thinking emphasizes the notion that futility occurs when the burden of treatment far exceeds any anticipated benefit to the patient.
- When futile conditions are recognized by the care team, physicians are obligated to convey this information to the family to ensure full disclosure of medical information, a necessary prerequisite to shared decision-making.
- The ethical principle of "double effect" when used to justify comfort care conveys that analgesics and sedatives can have the dual effect of relieving suffering as well as hastening death, and that the administration of these drugs is appropriate if the primary goal is to provide symptom control (e.g., relief of pain, and suffering), even if death is hastened in the process (25–27).
- From an ethical perspective there is no difference between the WH and the WD of treatment which only prolongs life without a realistic chance of cure, and such distinctions are morally irrelevant.
- It is important to recognize that it is never an emergency to WH/WD-LS.
- Family members should not be left to feel alone with the burden or guilt that their decisions are responsible for ending a loved one's life. Clinicians can effectively guide families through the process of reorienting goals from therapeutic to comfort care through honest, timely, and compassionate communication (28).
- Families also need to be assured that withdrawal is legally permissible and ethically humane, and that the administration of sedatives and analgesics is not analogous to euthanasia.
- With the decision to WH/WD-LS, all orders should be re-written to reflect that the intent of treatment has shifted to providing comfort care to the patient, without regard to physiologic stability.
- Before any active WH/WD-LS, the patient needs to be started on sedatives and analgesics and made comfortable as assessed by the bedside nurse and/or attending physician.
- Traditional rituals or practices should be respected and allowed whenever possible, as their observance is in preparation for death is frequently a source of comfort for the patient/family.
- Encouraging reminiscence of positive life experiences and important relationships in the patient's life often

helps to facilitate the family's grieving process at the EOL.
- Before withdrawal of therapy it is also important to discuss with families, what will happen after the patient's death.
- Discussions with families regarding the WH/WDLS should not be left to novice clinicians.
- The family should be reassured that clinicians will remain available and that their loved one will be kept comfortable and free of pain, suffering, or any distress throughout the entire process.
- Throughout the entire WH/WD-LS the patient should be as clean and meticulously cared for as possible.
- When administered in adequate dosages, opioids and benzodiazepines (or propofol) provide adequate analgesia and sedation in virtually all patients during the WH/WD-LS.
- Nonpharmacologic management of suffering involves discontinuation of "routine" interventions in the ICU that cause unnecessary discomfort to the patient.
- During the WH/WD-LS process, family members should be explicitly informed that it is entirely permissible, and usually beneficial, to touch and hug the patient, if this is their wish.
- The combined efforts of a multidisciplinary team including nurses, physicians, social workers, and spiritual care providers is essential in providing comprehensive palliative care in the SICU.

REFERENCES

1. Schneiderman LJ, Jecker NS, Jonsen AR. Medical futility: its meaning and ethical implications. Ann Intern Med 1990; 112:949–954.
2. Luce JM. Making decisions about the forgoing of life-sustaining therapy Am J Respir Crit Care Med 1997; 156(6):1715–1718.
3. Schneiderman LJ, Jecker NS, Jonsen AR. Medical futility: response to critiques. Ann Intern Med 1996; 125:669–674.
4. Schneiderman LJ, Jecker NS, Jonsen AR, et al. Abuse of futility. Arch Int Med 2001; 161(1):128–130.
5. McGee DC, Weinacker AB, Raffin TA. The patient's response to medical futility. Arch Intern Med 2000;160:1565–1566.
6. Curtis JR, Patrick DL, Caldwell ES, Collier AC. The attitudes of patients with advanced AIDS toward use of the medical futility rationale in decisions to forgo mechanical ventilation. Arch Intern Med 2000; 160:1597–1601.
7. Rubenfeld GD, Crawford SW. Withdrawing life support from mechanically ventilated recipients of bone marrow transplants: A case for evidence-based guidelines. Ann Intern Med 1996; 125:625–633.
8. Afessa B, Keegan MT, Mohammad Z, et al. Identifying potentially ineffective care in the sickest critically ill patients on the third ICU day. chest 2004; 126(6):1905–1909.
9. World Health Organization Definition of Palliative Care [accessed 5-17-06]. Available from the WHO website: http://www.who.int/cancer/palliative/definition/en/
10. Prendergast TJ, Luce JM. Increasing incidence of withholding and withdrawal of life support from the critically ill. Am J Respir Crit Care Med 1997; 155:15–20.
11. Angus DC, Barnato AE, Linde-Zwirble WT, et al. Use of intensive care at the end of life in the United States: An epidemiologic study. Crit Care Med 2004; 32:638–643.
12. Brody H, Campbell ML, Faber-Langendoen K, et al. Withdrawing intensive life-sustaining treatment: Recommendations for compassionate clinical management. NEJM 1997; 336(9):652–657.
13. Faber-Langendoen K, Lanken PN for the ACP-ASIM End-of-Life Care Consensus Panel. Dying patients in the intensive

care unit: Forgoing treatment, maintaining care. Ann Int Med 2000; 133:886–893.

14. Hawryluck LA, Harvey WRC, Lemieux-Charles L, et al. Consensus guidelines on the use of analgesia and sedation in dying ICU patients. BMC Ethics 2002; 3:3. Published online 2002 August 12. doi: 10.1186/1472-6939-3-3. Available from: http://www.bmccentral.com

15. Truog RD, Cist AFM, Brackett SE, et al. Recommendations for end of life care in the intensive care unit: The Ethics Committee of the Society of Critical Care Medicine. Crit Care Med 2001; 29:2332–2348.

16. Clarke EB, Curtis JR, Luce JM, et al. Quality indicators for end of life care in the intensive care unit. Crit Care Med 2003; 31(9):2252–2262.

17. The SUPPORT Principal Investigators. A controlled trial to improve care for seriously ill hospitalized patients. The Study to Understand Prognoses and Preferences for Outcomes and Risks of Treatments (SUPPORT). JAMA 1995; 274:1591–1598.

18. Levy MM. End of life care in the intensive care unit: Can we do better? Crit Care Med 2001; 29(2)(suppl):N56–N61.

19. Nelson JE, Danis M. End of life care in the intensive care unit: Where are we now? Crit Care Med 2001; 29(2)(suppl):N2–N9.

20. Thompson BT, Cox PN, Antonelli M, et al. Challenges in end of life in the ICU: Statement of the 5th International Consensus Conference in Critical Care: Brussels, Belgium, April 2003: executive summary. Crit Care Med 2004; 32:1781–1784.

21. Luce JM, Alpers A. Legal aspects of withholding and withdrawing life support from critically ill patients in the United States and providing palliative care to them. Am J Respir Crit Care Med 2000; 162(6):2029–2032.

22. American Medical Association Council on Ethical and Judicial Affairs. Medical futility in end of life care: Report of the Council on Ethical and Judicial Affairs. JAMA 1999; 281(10):937–941.

23. The Ethics Committee of the Society of Critical Care Medicine. Consensus statement of the Society of Critical Care Medicine's Ethics Committee regarding futile and other possibly inadvisable treatments. Crit Care Med 1997; 25(5):887–891.

24. Way J, Back AL, Curtis JR. Withdrawing life support and resolution of conflict with families. BMJ 2002; 325:1342–1355.

25. Hawryluck LA. Analgesia and sedation in the ICU: the ethics and law. Clin Pulm Med 2004; 11:237–241.

26. Wilson WC, Smedira NG, Fink C, et al. Ordering and administration of sedatives and analgesics during the withholding and withdrawal of life support from critically ill patients. JAMA 1992; 267(7):949–953.

27. Quill TE, Dresser R, Brock, DW. The rule of double effect: A critique of its role in end of life decision-making. NEJM 1997; 337:1768–1771.

28. McHale-Weigand DL. Withdrawal of life-sustaining therapy after sudden, unexpected life-threatening illness or injury:

Interactions between patient's families, healthcare providers, and the healthcare system. Am J Crit Care 2006; 15(2):178–187.

29. Cook D, Rocker G, Marshall J, et al. Levels of care in the intensive care unit: A research program. Am J Crit Care 2006; 15(3):269–278.

30. Kirchhoff KT, Walker L, Hutton A, et al. The vortex: Families experiences with death in the intensive care unit. Am J Crit Care 2002; 11:200–209.

31. Boyle DK, Miller PA, Forbes-Thompson SA. Communication and end of life in the intensive care unit: Patient, family, and clinician outcomes. Crit Care Nurs Quart 2005; 28(4):302–316.

32. Tilden VP, Tolle SW, Garland MJ, Nelson CA. Decisions about life-sustaining treatment. Arch Int Med 1995; 155:633–638.

33. Swigart V, Lidz C, Butterworth V, et al. Letting go: Family willingness to forgo life support. Heart Lung 1996; 25(6):483–494.

34. Danis M, Federman D, Fins JJ, et al. Incorporating palliative care into critical care education: Principles, challenges, and opportunities. Crit Care Med 1999; 27(9):2005–2013.

35. Prendergast TJ, Puntillo KA. Withdrawal of life support: Intensive caring at the end of life. JAMA 2002; 288(21):2732–2740.

36. Fins JJ, Solomon MZ. Communication in intensive care settings: The challenge of futility disputes. Crit Care Med 2001; 29(2)(suppl):N10–N16.

37. Treece PD, Engelberg RA, Crowley L, et al. Evaluation of a standardized order form for the withdrawal of life support in the intensive care unit. Crit Care Med 2004; 32(5):1141–1148.

38. Rubenfeld GD. Principles and practice of withdrawing life-sustaining treatments. Crit Care Clin 2004; 20:435–451.

39. Faber-Langendoen K, Lanken PN. Dying patients in the intensive care unit: Forgoing treatment, maintaining care. Ann Int Med 2000; 133(11):886–893.

40. Zawistowski CA, DeVita MA. A descriptive study of children dying in the pediatric intensive care unit after withdrawal of life-sustaining treatment. Ped Crit Care Med 2004; 5(3):216–223.

41. Curtis JR. Interventions to improve care during the withdrawal of like-sustaining treatments. J Pall Med 2005; 8(suppl 1):S116–S129.

42. Borneman T, Brown-Saltzman K. Meaning in illness. In: Ferrell B, Coyle N, eds. Textbook of Palliative Nursing. New York: Oxford University Press, 2001:382–394.

43. Pitorak EF. Care at the time of death: How nurses can make the last hours of life a richer, more comfortable experience. Am J Nurs 2003; 103:42–52.

44. Watch LS, Saxton-Daniels S, Schermer CR. Who has life-sustaining therapy withdrawn after injury? J Trauma 2005; 59(6):1320–1327.

45. Mosenthal AC, Murphy PA. Trauma care and palliative care: Time to integrate the two? J Am Coll Surg. 2003; 197(3): 509–516.

70

Critical Care Rounds, Notes, and Use of Consultants

José A. Acosta
Division of Trauma and Critical Care, Department of Surgery, Naval Medical Center San Diego,
San Diego, California, U.S.A.

William C. Wilson
Department of Anesthesiology and Critical Care, UC San Diego Medical Center, San Diego, California, U.S.A.

Raul Coimbra
Division of Trauma, Burns, and Critical Care, Department of Surgery, UC San Diego Medical Center,
San Diego, California, U.S.A.

INTRODUCTION

The training of medical students, interns, and residents in busy trauma and critical care services are generally focused on the basic science principles and clinical treatment guidelines required to manage severely injured patients. Often missing in the curriculum is expert guidance regarding the most efficient methods of data collection, patient presentation on rounds, and clear note writing. This chapter provides guidance in these areas, and also suggests techniques for obtaining appropriate assistance and input from consultant specialists.

PREROUNDING

Some of the most tedious and at times stressful portions of a young physician's life on a trauma and critical care service are spent chasing down information and evaluating patient conditions in preparation for the subsequent presentation of this data on attending rounds. Some of this stress is natural and unavoidable due to the numerous tasks that need to be accomplished during the typically short time window. However, the guidance summarized in this chapter provides some structure to these activities and, if followed, should help to facilitate the process. ☞ **In general, the resident should collect and organize the information in the same way that he/she plans to present the data on rounds.** ☞

Much of the information can be collected (and arranged) prior to the morning "preround scramble." For example, the night before, the resident can compile lists of information to be presented (listed subsequently) on a card or piece of paper, organized in the same order as it will be used for presentation in the morning. All the information that is known to have occurred since the last attending rounds and not expected to change can be included in these lists, leaving blank spots for the new data (which can be obtained in the morning).

Data that can often be chronicled in the evening prior to rounds include: (*i*) radiographic and other imaging results, including computed tomography (CT), magnetic resonance imaging (MRI), and ultrasound (U/S); (*ii*) laboratory studies ordered and completed that day, such as gram stain and culture data; (*iii*) progress made during spontaneous breathing trials of weaning patients, along with weaning parameters; (*iv*) tolerance of enteral nutrition, and so on. These precollected data points only need brief verification in the morning. Items that are expected to change and need to be evaluated in the morning include: (*i*) the physical examination, with particular focus on the neurological, and cardiopulmonary status; (*ii*) fluid balance; (*iii*) laboratory results from the morning blood draws; (*iv*) morning radiographs, and so on. Asking the bedside nurse about the important events that transpired through the evening and speaking directly to the various consulting teams will also help fill in the blanks.

☞ **New computerized patient information systems allow automatic incorporation of vital signs, laboratory, and even radiographic reports into templates that can be used for prerounding.** ☞ Often rounds can be expedited by printing these templates first thing in the morning, and transcribing (or appending) the precollected data from the prior day to the prerounding template. In order to make these written notes useful for rounds and subsequent note writing, they must be organized according to a logical scheme, generally in the same order as it will be used for the presentation itself.

PRESENTATION ON ROUNDS

Because of the limited time available for rounds, typically one and half hours to review up to 20 critically ill patients, no longer than five minutes should be routinely spent presenting the data and summarizing your assessment and plans for any one particular patient. Accomplishment of this goal requires that data be transmitted to the team in an accurate, timely, and concise yet comprehensive manner. This requires a high level of sophistication of the resident, as well as hard work. More extensive discussion on specific patients can occur at case conferences, during patient management tasks. On any given day expect that some percentage of patients will require more in-depth discussion, further evaluation, and management discussion time during attending rounds.

Table 1 Elements for Presentations in the SICU

Topic	Relevant data	Details required

Identification	Identify patient
	    Reason for admission
	    Days in the SICU
		Detailed

Past medical problems	Conditions medications	Detailed first day and then abbreviated

Specificity of presentation
    (trauma patient)
	Mechanism of injury
	Full admission trauma evaluation listing the GCS
	    and VS in TRS, as well as ABG, Hct
	Full list of imaging studies involving head, C-spine,
	    chest, abdomen, pelvis, and extremities
		Detailed first day—only refer to pertinent
		    studies as appropriate subsequently
		    (note this is the tertiary survey
		    of the trauma patient)

Specificity of presentation
    (other surgical Hx)
	Chief complaint
	History of present illness
	    Work up
		Detailed first day only abbreviated
		    subsequently

Past medical problems	Conditions Medications	Detailed first day and then abbreviated

Systematic review	Significant events since last rounds
	    System by system review to include physical exam
	        and relevant medications
		Detailed

Current medications
    and prophylaxis
	Discussion of medications not discussed in
	    systems review
	Discussion of need for deep venous thrombosis and
	    gastrointestinal bleeding
		Detailed

Assessment	Identification of problems	Detailed
Plans	Recommendations of management of problems	Detailed

Abbreviations: ABG, arterial blood gas; C-spine, cervical spine; GCS, Glasgow Coma Scale; Hct, hematocrit; SICU, surgical intensive care unit; TRS, trauma resuscitation suite; VS, vital signs.

Many different models are available for presentation of critically ill patients, which can vary in sequence but are similar in content (1,2). The six elements that should be present in surgical intensive care unit (SICU) patient presentation, corresponding with the six steps of the presentation, are summarized in Table 1.

Step 1—Identification of the Patient

All presentations in the SICU should begin with identification of the patient. The most up-to-date diagnoses and problems should be presented up front, just as if one is reading the headline of a newspaper. **☞ Identification of the patient should explain to all the team members exactly what is wrong with the patient (i.e., why the patient is here) and where the team is in the work up of, or therapy for, the patient's pathological conditions. ☞**

An example of a good identification (for a new trauma admission) is as follows: Mr. "X" is a 70-year-old man with steroid dependent chronic obstructive pulmonary disease (COPD) who was a restrained passenger in a motor vehicle collision yesterday. He is now postoperative day #1, status post exploratory laparotomy and splenectomy.

Step 2—History of Present Illness (Includes the Trauma Workup)

Following the identification for a new patient, a focused but complete history of present illness (HPI) is provided that includes only the pertinent data (positive and negative studies). In the case of a trauma patient, pertinent prehospital details as well as the radiographic and laboratory results of the primary (see Volume 1, Chapter 8) and secondary (see Volume 1, Chapter 14) surveys of the trauma evaluation are

presented on the first day. In addition, operative and nonoperative interventions are described and any pertinent changes in neurological or cardio-pulmonary stability that occurred during the procedures are noted; the operative estimated blood loss (EBL) and resuscitation fluids are also presented when significant.

Pertinent trauma evaluation data includes mental status in the trauma bay (head CT if altered), results of chest X-ray (CXR), pelvic, and cervical spine (C-spine) radiographs or CT results and the methods used to objectively evaluate the abdomen [focused abdominal sonography for trauma (FAST) versus CT versus diagnostic peritoneal lavage (DPL)] (Table 1). Trauma patients will require a detailed and accurate list of all injuries enumerated at this time. An abbreviated version is presented on subsequent days. This subsequent day list should be a short summary of all known injuries presented either with the most significant injuries first, or a listing of injuries in a head to toe fashion.

Step 3—Past Medical–Surgical History

Often large portions of data from the past Medical–Surgical history (PMHx) are missing in the obtunded trauma patient upon initial presentation. Young healthy patients usually have an insignificant PMHx and in this population the missing information is often of little consequence. However, with the increasing number of elderly patients presenting with trauma, the PMHx can be particularly pertinent. Accordingly, efforts should be made to call family or primary physicians to obtain such data in these individuals.

In one or two sentences, the presenter should list the known medical problems as well as prior surgeries, trauma, and often pre-existing conditions (e.g., missing kidney, prior stroke, etc.). An abbreviated version of this step (including a list of all significant ongoing medical or surgical problems) should be presented daily. This practice, in concert with listing all known injuries as mentioned in step 2, serves to remind members of the team of: (*i*) the original injuries or pathology; (*ii*) the current status of treatment; along with (*iii*) the possible confounding issues that help put the patient's response to therapy into proper context. Any new information obtained about the patients PMHx should also be presented at this time, and on subsequent days.

Step 4—Current Review of Systems

The next phase in the critical care presentation of trauma patients involves a stepwise update of the patient's current physiological status in terms of each major organ system. The presenter should provide a clear picture of the current condition, along with any important perturbations that have occurred since the last rounds. ☞ **The systematic review of the patient's various organ systems should proceed methodically, but with only the detail required to provide the listeners with a clear understanding of the patient's status.** ☞

The systems review is usually best accomplished using a format that covers each organ beginning with the most important, the brain (Table 2). The review then proceeds with the other systems: cardiovascular, pulmonary, and so on, providing a head to toe review.

Medications relevant to each organ system are typically listed during that portion of the presentation. For example, during the neurological presentation, sedative, analgesics, neuromuscular blockade, seizure prophylaxis, mannitol, and so on, are mentioned; during the cardiovascular report, inotropes, vasodilators, and pressors are discussed; during the hematological discussion anticoagulation drugs employed therapeutically [or for deep venous thrombosis (DVT) prophylaxis] are usually mentioned. Any new findings on the physical exam, as well as laboratory or imaging data, is also reported when the relevant organ system is discussed.

Table 2 Systems Review of Patients in the Surgical Intensive Care Unit

System	Physical examinations	Monitoring/lab values	Medications/therapy
Neurologic	GCS Ox3 Pupils RASS Motor and sensory CN I–XII	ICP measuring devices Pain and anxiety level	Analgesic Anxiolysis Paralytics Osmotic agents Antiseizure
Cardiovascular	Auscultation Murmurs Skin perfusion Pulse character	Mean arterial pressure ECG Pulmonary pressure monitoring Troponin	Pressors Inotropes Vasodilators
Pulmonary	Breath sounds Secretions Ventilatory pattern	Level of support (ventilation mask, FIO_2, V_T, PEEP) PIP, ABG results	
GI	Inspection (distension) Auscultation Palpation	Nasogastric tube output Bowel movements (constipation or diarrhea) Laboratory (amylase, lipase, LFT's, etc.)	Motility agent Nutrition (enteral or parenteral laxatives) Antidiarrheals
GU	Is & Os	Electrolytes to include BUN and creatinine	Diuretics IV fluilds
ID	T_{MAX} Line (peripheral and central)	WBC Culture results Sputum Lines Blood CSF Urine Wounds	Antibiotics GM + coverage GM − coverage Anerobe coverage Antifungal/antiviral Total days therapy
Hematology	Blood Hematomas Telangiectasias	Hematocrit Coagulation profile	Heparin, FFP SCDs
Endocrine	Goiter, etc.	Glucose, TFTs	Insulin, synthroid

Abbreviations: ABG, arterial blood gas; BUN, blood urea nitrogen; CN, cranial nerves; CSF, cerebral spinal fluid; ECG, electrocardiogram; FFP, fresh frozen plasma; FIO_2, forced inspiratory oxygen; GCS, Glasgow Coma Scale; GM−, gram-negative; GM+, gram-positive; GU, genitourinary; ICP, intracranial pressure; ID, infectious diseases; LFT, liver function tests; Is & Os, Inputs and Outputs; Ox3, oriented x person, place, time; PEEP, positive end expiratory pressure; PIP, peak inspiratory pressures; RASS, Richmond agitation sedation scale; SCDs, sequential compression devices; TFTs, thyroid function tests; T_{MAX}, maximum temperature; V_T, tidal volume; WBC, white blood cell count.

Neurological

In terms of neurological examination, the highest level of functioning is reported, along with any alteration or new deficits discovered since admission or the last rounds. Patients who are awake are described in terms of alertness and orientation. Those who are comatose are assigned a Glasgow Coma Score (GCS). Those with intracranial pressure (ICP) monitoring devices, and/or ventriculostomy outputs should have those values reported at this time, along with the cerebral perfusion pressure (CPP) when relevant. A pupillary exam is also reported along with the infusion doses of sedatives, analgesics, and neuromuscular blockade drugs (if used), as these will affect both the neurological exam and CPP indices.

Patients who are sedated but not comatose are reported in terms of their pain score and a sedation agitation score such as the Richmond Agitation Sedation Scale (RASS) further described in Volume 2, Chapter 5. Patients with subarachnoid hemorrhage may require nimodapine and triple H (hypervolumia, hemodilution, and hypertensive) therapy. Those patients receiving seizure prophylaxis medication should have dosing and blood levels reported, along with mention of any recognized seizure-like activity since admission, or the last rounds. Patients with spinal cord injury are described in terms of motor and sensory level per the American Spinal Injury Association (ASIA) guidelines (also see Volume 1, Chapters 16 and 26, and Volume 2, Chapter 13).

Cardiovascular

The presenter should declare the type of electrocardiogram rhythm (sinus or otherwise) manifested by the patient's heart. This along with the heart rate (HR) and blood pressure (BP) constitutes the minimal cardiovascular (C/V) data that must be presented for each patient. Those with peripheral vascular disease or limb injuries should have mention of the pulse presence and character, capillary refill, and color/warmth of the skin on the extremities. Patients who are hemodynamically unstable and/or with invasive monitoring of filling pressures and hemodynamics should have that data reported in a logical and coherent fashion.

In the case of invasive monitoring, it is often useful to report pressures in sequence from the right side to the left side of the heart, followed by the cardiac output ($\dot{Q}$) and derived variables [e.g., central venous pressure (CVP), pulmonary artery (PA) pressure, wedge, $\dot{Q}$, systemic vascular resistance (SVR), pulmonary vascular resistance (PVR), etc.]. The type and quantities of vasopressors and inotropes, should also be provided during the cardiovascular report so that the hemodynamic data can be interpreted within the proper context. Patients who have had U/S evaluations, troponin values, or other C/V data performed should have those results reported at this time. For patients who are hemodynamically stable and off inotropes, the preceding statement alone can in many times suffice, allowing the presenter to proceed to the next system which may be more relevant for that patient.

Pulmonary

If the patient is oxygenating and ventilating adequately on room air (RA), little more needs to be said, other than the RR and pulse oximetry saturation level on RA. Patients receiving mechanical ventilatory support but still oxygenating adequately should have a brief mention of the mode of ventilation, forced inspiratory oxygen (FIO_2), RR, tidal volume (V_T), level of positive end expiratory pressure (PEEP), as well as a report of the pH, PaO_2, and $PaCO_2$ achieved on those settings, for evaluation of the ventilation settings. Whenever patients are oxygenating and ventilating without significant support, (i.e., $PaO_2 > 60$ mmHg, on $FIO_2 < 40$ and PEEP ≤ 5) then progress in weaning status should be reported. Minimal data regarding suitability for weaning involves the RR/V_T achieved during any spontaneous breathing trials that were tolerated (Volume 2, Chapter 28).

In contrast, the patient with severe acute respiratory distress syndrome (ARDS) will require a detailed review of ventilatory settings beyond the FIO_2, RR, V_T, and PEEP, including peak inspiratory pressures (PIP), lung compliance, I:E ratio, $\dot{V}_E$, and so on. The associated arterial blood gas (ABG) is more carefully scrutinized in this condition, as is the CXR, and discussions of confounding oxygenation issues are appropriate at this time. Any relevant bronchoscopy, pulmonary secretion or chest tube data should also be offered at this time.

Gastrointestinal/Splanchnic

The gastrointestinal (GI) system is typically reviewed here (Table 2). Pertinent positives include tolerance of enteral nutrition and naso-gastric tube (NG) outputs (if NPO and/or receiving parenteral nutrition). Prealbumin values should be reported every couple days until in the normal range is achieved, then evaluated and reported weekly thereafter (also see Volume 2, Chapter 31). Other considerations regarding the patient's nutritional status can be mentioned as well [e.g., results of metabolic cart, respiratory quotient (RQ), etc.].

GI stress ulcer prophylaxis can be mentioned here or later (when institutional protocols are reviewed). Liver function tests—amylsase and lipase when pertinent—are mentioned in the GI presentation only when pertinent [e.g., following liver transplant (LFTs), pancreatitis (amylase)]. Patients with hepatic encephalopathy may have their dosing of lactulose and neomycin (or rifaxamine) mentioned in the neuro section, or here in the GI review. Plans for paracentesis are usually mentioned here or below with the fluid management presentation.

Genitourinary-Fluid Status, Electrolytes, Blood Urea Nitrogen/Cr

The fluid, electrolytes, and genito-urinary data is generally presented next. Most important of which includes the $24°$ inputs and outputs (Is and Os) from various sites, of which the amounts and type of fluids infused are important, and the outputs from urinary catheters, naso-gastric (N-G) or oro-gastric (O-G) tubes, chest tubes, and other drains as well as stool are all important.

The daily assessment of blood urea nitrogen (BUN), creatinine, electrolytes, and glucose are monitored closely in critically ill patients. Abnormalities should be reported and corrective measures suggested. Some individuals may prefer to discuss glucose levels and insulin administration later in the review of endocrine considerations. Patients with oliguria (see Volume 2, Chapter 40) may have fractional excretion of sodium (FeNa) reported, and dialytic therapies are mentioned at this juncture.

Infectious Disease

The infectious disease (ID) considerations are reviewed daily in all patients following trauma, surgery, or critical illness. The presenter should start by reporting the maximum temperature (T_{MAX}) and the white blood cell (WBC) count along with a differential (if known). This is followed by a report of gram stain and culture data from likely or known sources of infection including sputum, blood, invasive lines, and wounds. Urine is also reported and although commonly colonized, the urinary tract is an infrequent source of infection and fever in SICU patients, whereas the most common sources of infection in trauma and critical care followed by wound infections are lungs and invasive lines.

After presenting the culture data, the current antibiotics should be reported. A useful organization for presentation of antibiotics is to discuss them in terms of gram positive, gram negative, and anaerobic coverage. Patients receiving antifungal therapy will have this discussed after the bacterial considerations are dealt with. Rarely atypical organisms, viral, and/or parasite coverage is pertinent in trauma or postsurgical patients, but if so, these values are also mentioned. Each antibiotic being used should be reported in terms of the organism(s) it is covering and the number of days it has been used thus far, as well as the total number of days of therapy planned.

Hematological

The hematological data presentation begins with a report of the current hematocrit (Hct), platelet counts, and coagulation values—for example, protime (PT), partial thromboplastin time (PTT), and the international normalization ratio (INR). The number of transfusions of blood, platelets, fresh frozen plasma (FFP), or other components that were infused since the last rounds is also summarized. Any ongoing sources of blood loss is also mentioned (e.g., Jackson-Pratt drains, wound vac outputs, concerns about nonoperative spleen or liver injury, GI bleed, etc.). Because all trauma and critically ill patients are at risk for thromboembolic complications, the current method of DVT and/or pulmonary embolis (PE) prophylaxis is often mentioned here or later in a catch-all category.

Endocrinological

The need for insulin therapy should be addressed in patients with elevated serum glucose levels. Most SICUs are now following aggressive insulin infusion protocols with targeted glucose levels between 80 and 120 mg/dL (see Volume 2,

Chapter 60). A review of other pertinent endocrinological issues is also provided at this time, if not already mentioned. For example, patients with steroid requirements, thyroid, or other endocrine issues may have those discussed here.

The suggested data in Table 2 does not fully represent the minimal data on a simple patient, or the maximal data on a complicated patient, but rather the commonly evaluated parameters that must be known to the presenter on a daily basis. The amount of data that should be provided on rounds depends upon myriad pertinent factors for that patient. The residents will need to learn what is relevant, and the considerations will vary over time.

Step 5—Review of Missed Drug or Therapeutic Measures

A review of all medications and therapies not previously discussed should be quickly carried out next. Drug discussions should include the name of the medication, route of administration, dose, indication, and therapeutic endpoint. The participation of a pharmacist during this phase of the patient presentation can greatly enhance the management of SICU patients (3).

☞ **Most attending will take some time to review and ensure that various institution-specific protocols of care are being adhered to.** ☞ Others will prefer that each protocol based treatment is mentioned during the review of systems. In either case a discussion of DVT prophylaxis should determine whether or not it is indicated and possible therapies such as heparin, coumadin, sequential compression devices (SCDs), and inferior vena caval (IVC) filters.

In those patients receiving stress ulcer prophylaxis, the route of the medication and dose should be reviewed. All patients in the ICU should have the head of the bed elevated, unless clinically contraindicated, in an attempt to decrease aspiration pneumonia (4). A recently proposed mnemonic to cover these areas utilizes the acronym FAST HUGS (Feeding, Analgesia, Sedation, Thromboembolic prophylaxis, Head-of-bed elevation, stress Ulcer prevention, and Glucose control—Table 3) to review the commonly accepted beneficial therapies used in the SICU (Fig. 1) (4).

Other considerations such as extremity management of casts, traction, or fitting for orthotics or braces should be discussed. The results of occupational therapy, physical

Table 3 The Seven Components of the Fast Hug Approach

Component[a]	Consideration for SICU/trauma team
Feeding	Can the patient be fed orally? If not, begin enteral nutrition. If not tolerated or contraindicated, consider starting parenteral nutrition, and (unless contraindicated) trophic tube feeds.
Analgesia	All trauma and critically ill patients should receive adequate analgesia.
Sedation	Patients who require sedation should receive it, but excessive sedation should be avoided; "calm, comfortable, collaborative" is typically the best level.
Thromboembolic prevention	All should receive SCDs and LMWH unless unable (e.g., 4 extremity casts) or contraindicated (e.g., DVT), those at high risk contraindications should also receive LMWH. Those with contraindications and prolonged high risk should be considered for IVC filter placement.
Head of the bed elevated	Optimally, 30° to 45°, unless contraindications (e.g., threatened cerebral perfusion pressure) untreated spine injury.
Stress Ulcer prophylaxis	H₂RA, PPIs, gastric feedings, control of anxiety
Glucose control	Within limits defined in each ICU

[a]Other components to consider include surveillance for causes of fever, mechanical ventilation in patients with ARDS using lung protective strategies (V_T 6–7 cc/kg, PEEP as required to keep lungs open), review of decubitus ulcers, aggressive PT/OT, use of splints and orthotics in patients with chronic neurologic ailments to prevent tendon contractures. Daily spontaneous breathing trials for patients on mechanical ventilation, and so on.
Abbreviations: DVT, deep venous thrombosis; H₂RAs, histamine 2 receptor antagonists; ICU, intensive care unit; IVC, inferior vena cava; LMWH, low molecular weight heparins; PPIs, proton pump inhibitors; SCDs, sequential compression devices; SICU, surgical intensive care unit; V_T, tidal volume.
Source: Adapted from Ref. 4.

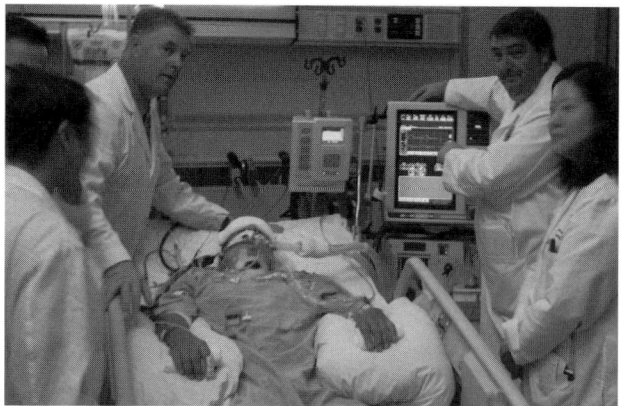

Figure 1 Attending rounds at UCSD Medical Center. Dr. W. C. Wilson (*top left*), and Dr. R. Coimbra (*top right*) demonstrate to residents and fellow that the Fast Hug concepts (Feeding, Analgesia, Sedation, Thromboembolic prophylaxis, Head-of-bed elevation, stress Ulcer prevention, and Glucose control), are being employed in a 38 year old male admitted to the intensive care unit three days prior following a traumatic brain injury, left pulmonary contusion, and splenectomy.

therapy, or the need to order these or other rehabilitation-related treatments or devices should be considered, along with plans for discharge and/or placement.

Step 6—Assessment and Plans

At this point, an overall assessment of the patient (brief sentence) followed by a summary of each significant problem suffered by the patient should be enumerated, and recommendations should be made to address each significant problem. This provides for an organized systems approach to the presentation, yet a problem-oriented assessment and management review at the end.

The critical care resident should also be aware of the assessment and plans being made by the other consulting services (e.g., neurosurgery plans to remove a ventriculostomy, renal wants to stop continuous veno-veno hemodialysis (CVVHD), critical trauma team wants to wean to a trach collar, ID wants different antibiotics, etc.). However, it is the presenting resident's assessment and plans that are most important to the critical care attending. When these are contrary to the assessment and plans of another team, particular energy must be put forth to diplomatically arrive at a cooperative management plan that addresses all

concerns. The final plans should be clear, and the rationale should be provided.

Finally, the presenter should note that very few patients will require long descriptions of data for each organ system. ☞ **The skillful presenter will separate the important/essential information from the mass of normal, or insignificant data generated daily.** ☞ Only the relevant information should be presented, and all of this should occur in less than five minutes, including the brief assessment and specific recommendations for each of the patient's active problems. The plans or recommendations for therapy are the most important aspect of the presentation and becomes easier if the preceding information is collected and presented in a logical and organized way. The time spent by the resident organizing and reprioritizing patient care issues as conditions change will improve presentation quality as well as patient care.

CRITICAL CARE NOTES

Notes are required for the documentation of events (for later review), and are also important for communication between teams. ☞ **If notes are too extensive they tend not to be read; if they are too short, they tend not to contain enough data to convince team members of the logic underlying the plans.** ☞ In the current era of computerized records, increasing amounts of redundant information is often included.

The authors believe that information which is already a part of the pertinent medical record (e.g., SICU flow charts of parameters) does not bear significant repetition. Rather, the notes should highlight pertinent positives, include all relevant data that would otherwise be missing from the automated record, and should also emphasize the assessment and plans for the patient. The notes should be placed in the record in a timely manner (immediately after important procedures, surgeries, or events), should always include the date, time, and signature, and also should be most clear as to both recommendations and rationale.

SICU notes should clearly identify the service and level of training (e.g., medical student, intern, resident, attending, etc.) of the individual writing the note, and include the following seven elements (as summarized in Table 4): (*i*) identification, (*ii*) title (e.g., Post op day #2, S/P exploratory laporatomy and spleenectomy), (*iii*) mention of significant events, (*iv*) systems approach patient status (abbreviated from the amount delivered on rounds). In hospitals where only one team is caring for critically ill patient, and there is no automated information in the chart, then all

Table 4 Critical Care Note Format

Element	Topic	Examples/comments
I	Identification	R-4 resident critical care note
II	Title	Post-op day #2 S/P exploratory laparotomy and splenectomy Post-op day #1 S/P take back for bleeding
III	Significant events	Patient has been hemodynamically unstable requiring large quantities of blood products due to mesenteric bleeding
IV	Systems review	Neuro, C/V, pulmonary, GI, GU, ID, heme, endo, extremity, and skin
V	Assessment	Initially unstable due to missed mesenteric bleeding vessel, now repaired and stable
VI	Plans	As appropriate for each system problem
VII	Documentation and authentication	Time, date, and signature

of the information provided in the above presentation sections will need to be included in the note. However, in situations where much data is automatically placed in the chart via computerized systems (including vital signs, trends, and laboratory information), this information should not be duplicated in the note. Instead, the usual SICU note should only chronicle the important data points along with the two following elements: (*v*) assessment; and (*vi*) plans. Finally, documentation with time, date, and authentication with signature are required components.

In some settings items 4, 5, and 6 may be coupled together for brevity and to minimize repetition of information already in the chart. Whenever significant events occur, the additional elaboration of items 4, 5, and 6 is required. Finally, all notes must be dated, timed, and signed by the author. The author should also provide a stamp or printing of their name and contact information (pager number), so that questions can subsequently be asked in case of confusion.

ASSISTANCE FROM CONSULTANTS

✍ **When consultants are needed to assist the critically ill patients with the care of trauma, a clear focused question should be asked of them.** ✍ Rather than asking for a blanket cardiology evaluation, ask the cardiology consult team the specific question you need assistance with. For example, the best method to convert the atrial fibrillation, or does this patient require U/S evaluation of pump function, and so on. Whenever possible, direct communication between the SICU team member and the consultant should be carried out. Optimally, the SICU team member will be present during the consultant's exam and chart review as well, to both provide and receive information. This person-to-person conversation will help prevent miscommunication and lead to better patient care. Whenever, the SICU team member cannot be at the bedside during the consultant's evaluation, a clear note should be left in the chart citing the key questions for which the consultant's help is requested.

CONFLICT RESOLUTION

Conflicts between the teams occur in all aspects of medicine from time to time. These disputes should not be played out in the medical chart or on teaching rounds, and especially not at the patient's bedside. When one team disagrees with another, a calm and civil discussion needs to occur regarding the interpretation of the patient status and goals of therapy envisioned by one team and compared to that of the other team. The critical care team is often charged with helping the other various consulting teams sort out their differences. In the case of the trauma patient, the trauma service will usually have the final say on the management of their patient, but they often need help from the others; thus, relations need to be unstrained and dialogue needs to be collegial and open.

OPEN VS. CLOSED INTENSIVE CARE UNITS

Recent studies have reviewed the advantages and disadvantages of closed versus open ICUs (5–7). In closed units patients are managed by the critical care team who serve as the patient's primary physicians. The data suggests that closed ICUs may improve patient outcome and decrease time spent on the ventilator. This type of approach is gaining popularity and tends to decrease the amount of consults obtained in the ICU. However, for trauma and the usual post surgical patient, important information and expertise belongs to the primary surgical team who admitted the patient. Hence, a comanagement model with the critical care team closely managing sedation, analgesia, fluids, acute hemodynamic, and ventilator considerations as well as other critical care-related support supervision such as enteral nutrition, and so on, is probably the best model. Thus open units will continue to be used in most trauma and SICUs in the near future.

EYE TO THE FUTURE

The challenges for physicians taking care of critically ill patients have become increasingly complex. The accumulation of large volumes of data from each patient can, from time to time, overwhelm the practitioner. As we continue to learn about the pathophysiology of critical illness, computerized filtering systems will likely be used to help filter out noise, target early treatment goals, and help minimize complications.

Handheld computer technology that allows real time updating is now widely used (8). These systems can be connected by wireless network to the SICU patient data systems and, if properly formatted, to portable digital assistants (PDAs), which can decrease the amount of prerounds time spent acquiring data, and with the proper software, can also help to organize it. This computer technology may be able to prompt the practitioner when an opportunity arises to follow best practices clinical guidelines and also decrease the time of order entry (9).

The use of picture archiving communication system (PACS) is now widely available and this has decreased the time needed to look for hardcopy films (10). The next step will be to have this information available in a handheld format, using high resolution data compression files.

Physician extenders such as nurse practitioners and physician assistants will play a greater role in the management of patients in the ICU (11). The health care providers will help bridge the gap left behind in academic medical centers with the 80 hour work week for residents. This contribution to patient care will likely provide improved continuity of care, better dissemination of information to family members, and improved compliance with best practice guidelines.

SUMMARY

The accurate distribution and presentation of information between the SICU team members is both an art and science. This is a skill that takes time to acquire. Although, the acceptable format can vary between attendings and institutions, the basic elements should remain. These include identification of the patient, a systematic review of the patient, assessment, and a plan for management.

Understanding the scientific foundations underlying the pathophysiology of various problems in trauma and critical care helps the presenter organize the data into a cogent format. Being cognizant of the needs to be complete while at the same time succinct helps motivate the presenter to carefully organize the contents. Presenting with a spirit of enthusiasm and sincere interest in the patient also helps other team members to focus and pay attention.

Consultants should be asked to participate in a patient's care when appropriate and to answer specific management questions. The daily note should avoid redundancy but provide enough information to serve as a guide to other consultants and team members as to the patient's condition and management strategy.

KEY POINTS

✍ In general, the resident should collect and organize the information in the same way that he/she plans to present the data on rounds.

✍ New computerized patient information systems allow automatic incorporation of vital signs, laboratory, and even radiographic reports into templates that can be used for prerounding.

✍ Identification of the patient should explain to all the team members exactly what is wrong with the patient (why the patient is here) and where the team is in the workup of, or therapy for, the patient's pathological conditions.

✍ The systematic review of the patient's various organ systems should proceed methodically, but with only the detail required to provide the listeners with a clear understanding of the patient's status.

✍ Most attending will take some time to review and ensure that various institution-specific protocols of care are being adhered to.

✍ The skillful presenter will separate the important/essential information from the mass of normal, or insignificant data generated daily.

✍ If notes are too extensive they tend not to be read; if they are too short, they tend not to contain enough data to convince team members of the logic underlying the plans.

✍ When consultants are needed to assist with the care of trauma and critically ill patients, a clear focused question should be asked of them.

REFERENCES

1. Dodek PM, Raboud J. Explicit approach to rounds in an ICU improves communication and satisfaction of providers. Intensive Care Med 2003; 29:1584–1588.
2. Elliot DL, Hickam DH. Attending rounds on in-patient units: differences between medical and non-medical services. Med Educ 1993; 27:503–508.
3. Leape LL, Cullen DJ, Clapp MD, et al. Pharmacist participation on physician rounds and adverse drug events in the intensive care unit. JAMA 1999; 282:267–270.
4. Vincent JL. Give your patient a fast hug (at least) once a day. Crit Care Med 2005; 33:1225–1229.
5. Ghorra S, Reinert SE, Cioffi W, et al. Analysis of the effect of conversion from open to closed surgical intensive care unit. Ann Surg 1999; 229:63–71.
6. Carson SS, Stocking C, Podsadecki T, et al. Effects of organizational change in the medical intensive care unit of a teaching hospital: a comparison of "open" and "closed" formats. JAMA 1996; 24:322–328.
7. Topeli A, Laghi F, Tobin MJ. Effect of closed unit policy and appointing an intensivist in a developing country. Crit Care Med 2005; 33:299–306.
8. Lapinsky SE, Wax R, Showalter R, et al. Prospective evaluation of an internet-linked handheld computer critical care knowledge access system. Crit Care 2004; 8:R414–R421.
9. Thompson W, Dodek PM, Norena M, Dodek J. Computerized physician order entry of diagnostic tests in an intensive care unit is associated with improved timeliness of service. Crit Care Med 2004; 32:1306–1309.
10. Watkins J, Weatherburn G, Bryan S. The impact of a picture archiving and communication system (PACS), upon an intensive care unit. Eur J Radiol 2000; 34:3–8.
11. Nishimura RA, Linderbaum JA, Naessens JM, et al. A nonresident cardiovascular inpatient service improves residents' experiences in an academic medical center: a new model to meet the challenges of the new millennium. Acad Med 2004; 79:426–431.

71

Economics of Trauma and Critical Care

Pedro Alejandro Mendez-Tellez and Todd Dorman

Departments of Anesthesiology, Adult Critical Care Medicine, and Surgery, School of Medicine,
Johns Hopkins University, Baltimore, Maryland, U.S.A.

INTRODUCTION

The United States operates a health care system that is unique among nations. It is the most expensive of systems, outstripping by over half the health care expenditures of any other country (1). U.S. Health care expenditures continue to rise. The growth in national health care spending is principally due to new technologies and medications, the aging of the population, and the increasing number of uninsured and under-insured. Globally, health care costs are also on the rise. However, most countries around the world are able to deliver health care to their citizens for a fraction of what is spent in the U.S. (2).

A large portion of U.S. health care funding pays for the care of critically ill and injured patients. ☞ **Even though intensive care unit (ICU) beds account for about 10% of all inpatient hospital beds, critical care expenditures account for 15–20% of inpatient costs (3), and near 1% of the gross domestic product (GDP).** ☞

Trauma care is also extremely resource-intensive. Severely injured patients consume one-third of all hospital days utilized for trauma care, almost 70% of all days in the ICU, and they account for 45% of the total charges generated (4).

Health care financing impacts the delivery of critical and trauma care. As critical and trauma care consume increasing portions of the national health care resources, factors that maximize health and societal benefits, such as resource allocation, economic impact, and costs, have become more relevant (5).

This chapter provides the reader with an overview of health care economics and the costs and funding of trauma and critical care. It also introduces some of the economic tools used for assessing the value of medical practices, including cost-effectiveness analyses.

HEALTH CARE ECONOMICS

☞ **The costs of health care in the U.S. have been rising sharply over the past four decades and currently consume approximately 15% of the GDP.** ☞ In 1960, the national health care bill totaled a mere $26.9 billion. Between 1966, (when the Medicare and Medicaid programs began), and 1993, health care expenditures increases averaged 11.7% annually, inflating the national health care bill to $895.1 billion by 1993. Over the period of 1993–1997, the rate of growth in health-care spending was unusually slow, averaging only five percent per annum as a result of low general and medical-specific inflation, the growth and impact of managed care, and the capacity of health care plans to negotiate "discounts" from provider systems (6). Despite the downward trend in the rate of growth of health care spending, U.S. health care costs surpassed $1 trillion by 1996. It is estimated that the costs of health care will double to an astronomical $2.2 trillion by 2008 (6,7).

The proportion of the GDP consumed by health care has been rising almost linearly since 1960, when the U.S. spent 5.1% of its GDP on health expenditures. By 1993, the percentage of the GDP spent had already exceeded 13% and by 2002, it was 14.9% (6). Projections indicate that the share of GDP spent on health care will rise to 16.2% by 2008 (7).

By comparison, in 1998, when the U.S. spent 14% of its GDP on health care, other industrialized countries such as Germany, France, the United Kingdom, Canada, and Japan spent a substantially less (i.e., 7–10%) of their GDP on health care (Fig. 1). In Taiwan, which has a national health-care system, individuals pay an average of $20.00 per month for full coverage (including maternity care, dental, vision, and all medical visits) (2). This is approximately 1/20 of the cost to U.S. individuals for the same coverage (2). The $400 to $500 per month that is paid by the average U.S. citizens for their health care insurances is "out-of-pocket," or, is paid by their employer. These huge healthcare expenditures paid by employers are the principle reason many U.S. jobs have moved overseas to countries like India, China, Russia, and Mexico (2).

Aging of the U.S. population, new technologies, a growing number of uninsured and "under-insured," and the expectation (and perception) by the U.S. citizens and foreign nationals living in the U.S. that they receive the highest level of health care constitute the most important demographic, cultural or psychological factors that are continually driving up costs.

Ageing is important because of the comorbid disease "burden," such that when these patients become ill, the severity of the illnesses increase, and resource consumption also increases (see Volume 1, Chapter 37). The introduction of new medical technologies (drugs, devices, procedures) always seem to come at a high price. Most experts attribute the continued rise in health care expenditures as a percent of GDP in the U.S. to the impact of technological changes. The uninsured and under-insured also contribute to rising health care costs because they seldom seek preventative care, and instead wait for interventions involving acute high resource-consuming care episodes (6).

☞ **For the past three decades, the U.S. government has attempted (ineffectively) to reduce the growth of**

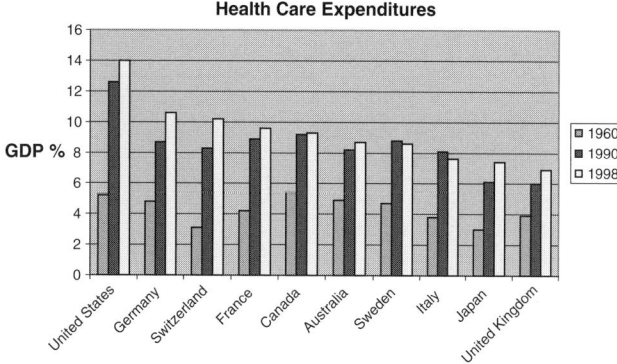

Figure 1   Health care expenditures. *Source*: From Ref. 51.

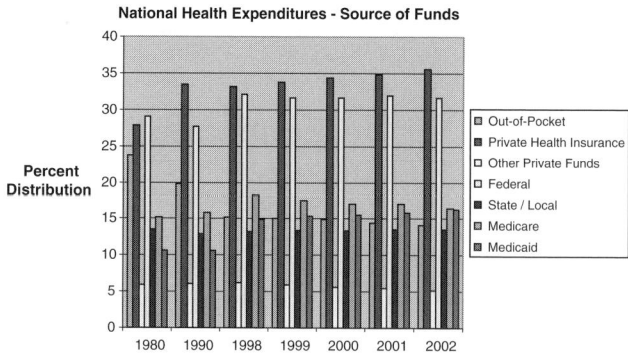

Figure 2   National health expenditures: *Source*: From Ref. 52.

health-care expenditures. ☞ The extraordinary increases in health care costs that financially threaten the purchasers of health care services (individuals and businesses) led in the mid 1980s to the implementation of several measures aimed at restraining the rising health costs such as price control and the prospective payment system.

Since these initial measures failed to control the rising costs of health care, the federal government then chose to control health expenditures with a number of mechanisms loosely referred as "managed care," including a wide-range of government subsidies and programmes made available to assist the development of these entities. Managed care organizations (MCOs) were originally successful in controling health care costs by reducing fees paid to providers, and by participating in the decision-making process of health care [i.e., denying services to enrollees that did not meet (arbitrary) benchmark criteria, and delaying services to those that did qualify, i.e., "queuing"]. More recently, premiums are increasing and MCOs no longer seem capable of controlling the rise in health care expenditures. This is partly due to the consumer revolt regarding denied and delayed services, as well as other factors such as realization of an increasing proportion of funds devoted to administrative overhead, salaries and bonuses paid to executives, and distribution of profits to publicly listed MCOs.

The Role of Government

Health care expenditure funding is not distributed evenly. The government finances the Medicare and Medicaid programmes as well as the Veteran's Administration Hospital system, the Department of Defense military care system, the Public Health Service, and the Indian Health Service (8). In 1997, public funding financed nearly 47% of the health care bill. Other funding sources include private health insurance and out-of-pocket consumers. In 1997, private health insurance and out-of-pocket consumers funded 32% and 17% of health care spending, respectively (9). Though the total funds spent have increased, these percentages have remained fairly stable over the last decade (Fig. 2).

Medicare

☞ **The Medicare program is by far the largest and most influential health insurance program.** ☞ The original congressional act provided health care insurance for the elderly who were eligible for social security. Before the establishment of Medicare, only about half of those who were 65 years of age or older had health insurance. By 1970, 97% of

older Americans were enrolled in the program. Today, the Medicare program covers nearly 40 million people, including persons over the age of 65 years, many disabled persons of all ages, and persons with chronic renal failure (CRF). Currently, Medicare insures one of every seven Americans. By 2030, the program is projected to cover 77 million people (i.e., more than one of every five Americans) and will consume 4.4% of the GDP (9,10).

Medicare consists of two related insurance programs. The Medicare Hospital Insurance Fund, also known as "Part A," covers inpatient services, skilled nursing care, and home health care, and is funded by compulsory federal payroll taxes on employers and employees. Payroll taxes raised $115 billion in 1997 (88% of the Trust Fund). Medicare "Part B," the Supplemental Medical Insurance Program, covers physician fees, outpatient hospital services (emergency room visits, and ambulatory surgery, as well as laboratory and other diagnostic tests) and durable medical equipment. Medicare pays 80% of the approved amount of "Part B" services in excess of an annual deductible. Medicare "Part B" is funded by general federal tax revenues that are appropriated by Congress, and by premiums paid by the beneficiary.

Since the late 1970s, slowing the growth of Medicare spending has been a sustained priority for legislators. In the 1980s, Medicare shifted from a cost-based system to one in which payments were predetermined (9). These and other cost-containment efforts slowed the growth rate of expenditures for some time, yet costs have continued to rise.

In another cost-containment effort, Medicare beneficiaries have been allowed to enroll in private health maintenance organizations (HMOs) and private fee-for-service plans (e.g. "Medicare Plus," or "Medi-Gap" Choice plans) instead of remaining exposed to traditional fee-for-service payments. In 1997, the program expanded the types of plans that could participate in Medicare and to further reform the payment system.

Medicare's benefit package has been termed "inadequate" because it leaves beneficiaries liable for nearly half the cost of their acute care and also grossly underpays doctors for their care. Beneficiaries have to rely on supplemental policies, because Medicare is an inefficient method of care delivery. Currently, over 85% of the beneficiaries have supplemental insurance. Medicaid, (possessed by 15% of Medicare beneficiaries) and employer-sponsored retirement benefits (used by one-third of beneficiaries) fill in part of the "gap" in coverage. Private supplemental plans (e.g. Medi-Gap), which serve about one-fourth of beneficiaries, are increasingly perceived as unaffordable for those with an average income (9).

When the Medicare program became operational in 1966, its primary orientation was the treatment of acute, episodic illness. Medicare maintained this orientation for 40 years despite the trend of people living longer with chronic diseases. The Medicare Prescription Drug Improvement and Modernization Act of 2003 took the first step at re-orienting Medicare toward the care of chronic conditions (11). It provides seniors, and those with disabilities a prescription drug benefit, but has also added costs to the program (11). The initial three diseases to be covered (beyond CRF) are diabetes (DM), chronic obstructive pulmonary disease (COPD), and congestive heart failure (CHF).

The modernization program will be implemented in two phases. Phase one utilizes a pilot study (certain states and regions were selected on December 8, 2004) that will be responsible for providing services to all Medicare beneficiaries who have DM, CHF, or COPD in those locales. Payments in Phase 1 are dependent on improvements in "quality of care," "satisfaction" of beneficiaries and providers, and a success in lowering costs. Phase 2 (scheduled to begin in 2007), is expected to expand nationally, if Phase 1 is successful (11).

Although the Medicare Modernization Act is the first step toward reform and the cost-effective treatment of beneficiaries with multiple chronic conditions, additional changes in financing will be required. In 2001, out-of-pocket spending by Medicare beneficiaries increased by an average of nearly $400 for each additional chronic condition (Fig. 3) (11). To cover these costs for the chronically ill, some have suggested restructuring the cost-sharing arrangements in fee-for-service Medicare by "shifting" costs to the less ill. Alternatively, lowering other fixed costs may be more palatable (and resource preserving), such as developing a national electronic medical record to the secure data repository that can be accessed when trauma patients or other emergency patients enter the hospital and are unable to provide their past medical history. These and other technology-driven strategies purported to be "cost-savers" constitute the only currently identified techniques that will both improve medical care and reduce costs in the near term.

Medicaid

Medicaid provides supplemental federal funding to states operating approved medical-assistance plans. Medicaid is a federal-state funded health insurance program for certain low income citizens, as well as other individuals in need. Unlike Medicare, eligibility for Medicaid is "means-tested"

(i.e., there are financial criteria for enrollment); like Medicare, however, ♂ **Medicaid is an individual legal entitlement. Medicaid is the single largest source of financial support for community health services to low income patients.** ♂ It coves over 45% of inpatients in public hospitals, and more than one-third of patients who obtain care at federally-funded community health centers.

There are two basic criteria for eligibility: financial need and a federally recognized eligibility category. Both criteria should be met for enrollment. Each state independently establishes eligibility criteria within those general federal guidelines; sets the type, amount, and duration of services; sets the rate of reimbursement; and administers its program. Medicaid policies of eligibility, services and payments are complex and vary considerably among states.

In 1998, obstructive pulmonary covered over 40 million people, one of every 10 people under the age of 65 years, including nearly 30 million pregnant women, parents under the age of 65 years, and children, as well as more than 11 million persons with disabilities and elderly persons who had low incomes or who were impoverished because of medical expenses.

By 2004, Medicaid was helping to finance long-term health care for more than 55 million low-income children and parents, people with severe disabilities, and elderly at an annual cost of $300 billion to the federal and state governments (12). The program now provides health coverage for one in four U.S. children, as well as coverage for illegal aliens. Although children and their parents account for the majority of enrollees, elderly and those with disabilities account for 70% of the expenditures (Fig. 4).

The program's impact on certain sectors of the health care system is enormous: in 1998, Medicaid paid the costs of one-third of all births in the United States, nearly half of all nursing home care, and health care for 25% of children under the age of five years. The Medicaid program actually pays for much of the care for elderly and disabled Medicare beneficiaries, who also qualify for Medicaid on the basis of poverty.

Federal financing of state Medicaid plans is open-ended. Each participating state is entitled to payments up to a federally-approved percentage of state expenditures, and there is no limit on total payments to any state.

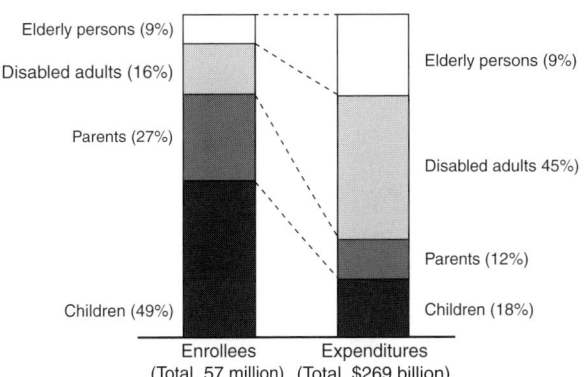

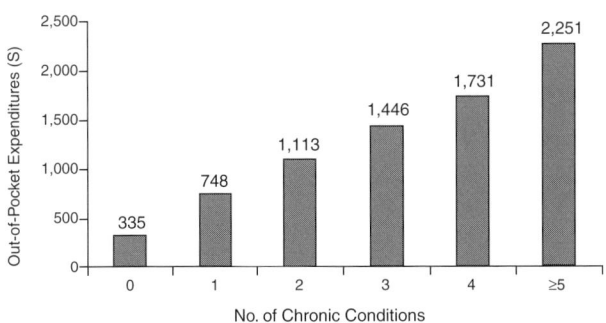

Figure 3 Annual out-of-pocket spending by Medicare Beneficiaries in 2001 according to number of chronic conditions. *Source*: From Ref. 53.

Figure 4 Medicaid enrollees and expenditures in 2004 according to enrollment group. The graph shows values estimated by the Kaiser Commission on Medicaid and the Uninsured on the basis of data from the Congressional Budget Office and the Centers for Medicare and Medicaid Services, 2005. Totals may not add to 100% because of rounding. *Source*: From Ref. 54.

Payments are calculated based on a federal formula linked to state revenue, and ranged from 50% to 80% of approved state medical expenditures. In 2000, Medicaid accounted for 50% of total state health care costs.

Between 2000 and 2005, individual states began to more aggressively restrain Medicaid spending by limiting prescription drug coverage, provider payments, and eligibility. Several states have restructured their programs. Utah created a new primary care benefit package that does not include hospital or specialty care. Tennessee and Missouri are contemplating plans that would drop 200,000 and 90,000 adults, respectively (12). Connecticut and Minnesota are petitioning the federal government for permission to extend the period of time that must elapse before Medicaid begins to cover nursing home fees. California, Georgia, Kentucky, and New Hampshire are all preparing to reduce spending on acute care by adding new premiums, raising cost-sharing premiums, and by limiting coverage for prescription drugs (12).

Centers for Medicare and Medicaid Services (CMS)

In 1965, the Social Security Act established both Medicare and Medicaid. Medicare was a responsibility of the Social Security Administration (SSA) while federal assistance to the State Medicaid Programs was administered by the Social and Rehabilitation Service (SRS). SSA and SRS were agencies in the Department of Health, Education, and Welfare (HEW). In 1977, the Health Care Financing Administration (HCFA) was created under HEW to effectively coordinate Medicare and Medicaid. In 1980, HEW was divided into the Department of Education and the Department of Health and Human Resources (HHS). In 2001, the Health Care Financing Administration (HCFA) became known as the CMS (10,13).

☞ **CMS was established as a federal agency that administers several programs including Medicare, Medicaid, State Children's Health Insurance Program (SCHIP), Clinical Laboratory Improvement Amendments of 1988 (CLIA) and Health Insurance Portability and Accountability Act of 1996 (HIPAA).** ☞ CMS oversees the reimbursement of health care providers and hospitals under Medicare and Medicaid, including promulgating the regulation for physician documentation, and charging submission and payment. Most insurers adopt CMS/HCFA's standards and regulations for physician reimbursement. A thorough knowledge of these standards and regulations is therefore mandatory for successfully billing (and receiving payments from) Medicare, as well as most other insurers (10).

Employer-Sponsored Health Insurance Plans

Collectively, private employers and employees are the most important purchasers of health care through the insurance premiums they pay together for coverage (1). The premiums that finance coverage are paid in "Part B" by the employee. Much of the private insurance bill (usually 80% or more), however, is paid for by employers through their employee benefits packages. Approximately 70% of the non-elderly U.S. population is covered by some form of private medical insurance.

As medical costs go up, health insurance costs also rise and businesses owners must either pass on higher premium and co-payment costs to their employees, raise their prices (potentially impairing their competitive position in the marketplace), or reduce their profit margin (unpopular with stockholders). Like the government, businesses can also negotiate lower prices with health care providers and/ or health insurance plans.

"Managed care" is a generic term that embraces a wide spectrum of health insurance systems that integrate the financing and delivering of health care. Managed care organizations contract with doctors and hospitals to provide comprehensive care to enrolled members for a fixed, prospectively set premium. These MCOs also shop their services to various employers. Employer-sponsored health insurance plans include traditional indemnity plans, health maintenance organizations (HMOs), preferred-provider organizations (PPOs), and point-of-service plans (14,15).

In the traditional indemnity plan, patients would choose their physicians from among all those in the community. After receiving treatment, a bill was then submitted to the insurer. Insurers would in turn pay "usual and customary" fees set by the local physicians in each community.

In the early 1980s, insurers were permitted to contract with selected providers. With this new option, insurers were able to exclude providers that did not accept their rules and fee schedules. Insurers began to build physician networks such as PPOs to care for their enrollees. As managed care and the demand for expanded services grew, insurers broadened the network of preferred providers to include some coverage from providers who were not part of the network, leading to the development of "point-of-service plans."

More recently, insurers have begun to offer "multi-tiered" plans which give patients three different options: full coverage in an HMO with a limited number of providers; access to a PPO, with slightly higher co-payments; and use of out-of-network providers, with the highest co-payments (i.e., traditional indemnity) (14).

The Uninsured and Underinsured

As previously discussed, the U.S. health care system is a mixed system of public and private insurance. Most working-age persons receive insurance through their employers. Medicare provides health care to all persons over 65 years of age as well as to persons with disabilities or end-stage renal disease, and Medicaid covers low-income individuals

Apart from those covered by private or public plans lays a substantial population without any health insurance (16). Data from the U.S. Census Bureau indicate that 45 million people had no health insurance of any kind during a typical month in 2003, representing 15.6% of the U.S. population (17). The great majority of uninsured individuals either work for small employers who do not offer health insurance benefits or, more commonly, cannot afford the premiums of the plan(s) that are offered (18). About 80% of the underinsured are either workers or live in families with workers. They typically have low-wage jobs or work in small businesses in which the employer does not offer health insurance, or, if it is offered, they decide not to purchase it (often due to high cost, and competing needs for their wages) (16).

Underinsurance has a significant impact on the "working poor" by presenting them with the burden of paying out a substantial proportion of their family's income for health insurance premiums and out-of-pocket medical costs (deductibles, co-payments, and uninsured care) (18). The underinsured are much more likely to delay or forgo needed treatment, have their conditions diagnosed at a later stage, and to be admitted to the hospital for avoidable conditions (16).

Some states have experimented with expanded coverage through their Medicaid programs to help the uninsured poor (such as the Oregon Medicaid program). For the foreseeable future, however, it does not appear that the federal government is inclined to comprehensively address this problem (18).

THE ECONOMICS OF CRITICAL CARE

Over the past four decades, intensive care medical advances have markedly improved our ability to treat the critically ill and the injured (18). During this time, the demand for ICU services has grown dramatically. However, the care of critically ill patients has consumed a disproportionately large fraction of the health care resources (7). Even though ICUs contain only 5–10% of total hospital beds, they account for 15–20% of total hospital costs, which in turn comprise about 38–40% of all U.S. health care expenditures (19). Thus, in the U.S., critical care costs alone comprise over one percent of the GDP.

The resources used to care for ICU patients includes the physical plant, equipment, supplies, professional staff, and all of its support services and personnel. Modern ICUs provide three major types of services: (*i*) active treatment, which includes life-supporting therapies or techniques; (*ii*) ICU monitoring and nursing and technological services that are observational rather than therapeutic; and (*iii*) standard floor care services that are not unique or limited to ICUs (20).

✐ **Critical care costs are mainly generated by human resources, expensive drugs, and newer technologies, all promising to prolong the lives of critically ill and severely injured patients.** ✐ The largest fraction of ICU costs goes to personnel-related expenditures. Human resources account for approximately 64% of total ICU cost per stay. The largest personnel component in terms of number and costs is critical care nursing. There is an enormous salary expenditure due to the high nurse:patient ratio. Nursing salary expenditures approximate 65% of the typical critical care human resource budget (8). Accordingly, efforts to control ICU costs necessitate consideration of organizational costs, supplies, and most importantly, staffing.

Technologies such as mechanical ventilation, hemodynamic monitoring and hemodialysis require costly equipment in conjunction with specialized personnel. Other technology-intensive "capital resources" include diagnostic imaging and laboratory testing equipment (3). Similarly, critically ill patients receive a wide variety of medications, and an ever-increasing number of particularly costly innovative treatments. Pharmaceuticals comprise some 7.4% of ICU budgets (8). Today, critical care is caught between an increasing demand for services and constrained global resources. Until recently, much of ICU care was excluded from economic scrutiny. Times are changing. There is a strong perception that ICU care can become a financial burden to the institution. ICU costs are high and the majority of such health care resources are consumed by a remarkably small segment of the population. Furthermore, the true impact and efficiency of the delivery of such services has yet to be defined. Lastly, ICU care is perceived as a way for "prolonging the inevitable" in many patients, and thus representing a "waste of resources" to some commentators (21).

Budgeting and Revenues for the ICU

Financial resources directed to the ICU are usually allocated through the hospital or organizational budgetary process. The ICU budget may be entirely related to known, estimated, or pre-negotiated input costs (human and capital resources), and the ICU may operate as a budget or cost center. In other words, the budgeted revenue is the estimated amount required to pay for the services the hospital wishes to deliver. In other circumstances, the ICU budget may be allocated as a profit center, in which all corresponding revenues and expenditures are accounted for and the ICU is expected to achieve a designated financial performance (8).

The "DRG System" attempts to predict resource consumption in a defined patient population, using variables such as diagnoses, operative procedures, complications, comorbidities, and discharge status (8). Reimbursement for a patient's hospital stay is fixed through diagnosis-related groups (DRGs). DRG weights (or relative values) do not directly include ICU utilization. One DRG using more ICU days than another is meant to be reflected in the relative values attributed to the entire stay; the ICU component is not separated out. However, substantial data support inequities in the DRG system for reimbursement of patient care in the ICU. For certain patient types (and corresponding DRGs), the ICU generates large losses, especially in elderly patients and those with prolonged ventilatory management (8).

Economic Analysis Models Used for Critical Care

Traditionally, decision-making in critical care has focused on "patient outcomes" (such as treatment effectiveness, morbidity, and mortality). Because of increasing pressure to reduce the growth of health care expenditures, considering only "patient outcomes" as a decision-making tool is no longer acceptable to health care financing entities. To achieve the most effective care, physicians must now regard outcomes not only from a clinical perspective, but also with integrated consideration of resource allocation, length of stay, patient satisfaction, and economic impact and costs, among other factors (5).

Delivering "cost-effective care" is becoming a qualifier to compete. As critical care consumes an increasing proportion of health care resources, economic analyses must be incorporated into clinical decision-making to help make resource allocation decisions (22,23). Physicians now need to become educated on how to accurately analyze these situations.

The purpose of economic analysis is to demonstrate a more beneficial use of critical care resources (22,23). Traditional cost analysis (i.e., comparing which option is cheaper) did not take patient outcomes into account. More recently, methodologies measuring both outcomes and costs have been developed. These methodologies attempt to measure and compare different interventions by counting and combining costs with real data from patient outcomes (5).

Four different types of economic evaluations are quoted: cost-effectiveness, cost-utility, cost-benefit, and cost minimization analyses. Even though these analyses all

Table 1 Comparison of Various Economic Evaluation Models

Economic analysis model	Numerator	Denominator (net benefits)	Example
Cost-effectiveness	Costs (dollars)	Specific measure of effectiveness (years of life saved)	Thrombolysis for acute myocardial infarction
Cost-utility	Costs (dollars)	A common utility metric (QALYs)	Prophylaxis against recurrence of PUD
Cost-benefit	Costs (dollars)	Costs (dollars)	Use of aminoglycoside dose-monitoring program for burn patients with gram-negative sepsis
Cost-minimization	Costs (dollars)	None	Antibiotic therapy for ICU patients with low risk of nosocomial pneumonia

Abbreviations: QALY, quality-adjusted life year; PUD, peptic ulcer disease; ICU, intensive care unit.

have costs in the numerator, the denominator is different (Table 1) (25).

Cost-Effectiveness Analysis

In general, cost-effectiveness is defined as cost divided by net benefits. The numerator (cost) is expressed in a reference currency (such as dollars), and the denominator (net benefits) is expressed as beneficial outcomes minus adverse outcomes. Although the primary goal of cost-effectiveness is to maximize benefits in relation to available resources, cost-effectiveness is also a reflection of health care quality (24).

Cost-effectiveness analysis (CEA) is the most common type of economic assessment, probably because the outcome data (effectiveness) in such analyses are relatively simple to calculate, and often comprise clinical measures of health that are routinely collected in clinical trials (e.g., percentage deduction in blood pressure, reduced incidence of hip fracture). To improve comparability between studies, generic measures of outcome are sometimes used, such as life-years saved or disability-days avoided (21).

CEA attempts to link the economic consumption and clinical utility in one "summary" measure. In CEA, the added costs and health outcomes of multiple interventions are used to calculate a cost-effectiveness ratio (9). Essentially, CEA estimates the incremental cost required to improve the clinical outcome by 1 unit. Lower ratios imply improved cost effectiveness, as fewer resources are expended to procure the desired level of benefit (21).

Cost-Utility Analysis

Cost-utility analysis (CUA) is identical to CEA, except that the outcomes are measures in terms of a single composite index that combines length of life with quality of life [quality-adjusted life-year (QALY)] and this measure is preference based (14). This is very useful, as many patients discharged from ICU may require extensive intervention and their quality of life may be very low (such as ongoing dialysis, home ventilation, or full nursing support in a specialist facility) (25).

Cost-Benefit Analysis

CEA and CUA aid in decision-making and are generally used to compare treatment alternatives (25). Cost-benefit analysis (CBA) has a broader scope than both CEA and CUA, and differs mainly in that its outcome measures are defined in monetary terms (14). There are two ways to assign economic values to health consequences. "Willingness-to-pay" (WTP) is the most popular way of expressing cost-benefit in a healthcare environment and can be inferred from decisions that people make about trade-offs between health and money. Alternatively, quantifying human capital attaches a value to health such as those people working in an economy versus those consuming health care resources through chronic disability.

The CBA determines the net social benefit of a program and then determines the overall costs of the program. The incremental effects of a program is calculated as the benefits minus the costs, with both expressed in monitary terms (5).

Cost-Minimization Analysis

If there are equivalent outcomes for two different interventions, costs are compared in cost-minimization analysis (CMA), a type of CEA. The fundamental assumption of CMA is that outcomes as measured by clinical benefit or use are equivalent (5). CMA looks only at resources used and assumes that the clinical benefit is self-evident (21).

As hospital budgets tighten, economic analyses will help hospitals and ICU managers maximize health benefits while minimizing waste for any given resource (21). Implementation of cost-effective strategies will ensure the best outcomes by providing evidence-based care and by reducing costs through controlling variability and implementing cost-effective interventions (5).

Cost-Containment in Critical Care

Critical care resources are finite, and therefore limited. A significant limiting factor in the availability of critical care services is related to their extraordinary costs. Much of the pressure for rationing is brought about because of the cost. Demonstration of effective containment of these costs would do much to allay the perceived needs for rationing of this form of care.

Cost containment can be defined as either (*i*) preventing further increases in cost, (*ii*) slowing the rate of rise, or (*iii*) actually decreasing the costs. Cost containment can be achieved by limiting the use of critical care, by improving the efficiency with which it is delivered (changes in process), or by limiting other inputs. Conceptually, there are four major ways to control medical spending: (*i*) control prices, (*ii*) control volume of care provided, (*iii*) control the total budget available to pay for care, and (*iv*) shift costs to another payer (18).

✐ **Two of the most important price control initiatives in medicine have been the Medicare Hospital Prospective Payment System and the Medicare Fee Schedule for**

physicians. ☞ In 1983, Medicare replaced its retrospective cost-based hospital reimbursement system with a prospective payment system noted above, the DRG system. The DRG system was designed to promote efficiency and cost-containment in hospital-based care. While it has helped to control Medicare costs, it has not reduced overall U.S. health care costs, possibly because of substantial cost-shifting by hospitals to the private insurance sector (18). Under DRGs, hospitals have been severely under-reimbursed for all types of patients requiring ICU care. Additionally, under DRGs, critically ill patients who are transported to tertiary care centers place the accepting institutions at financial risk because allotted reimbursements to the accepting institution are substantially below the costs that are generated (26).

Recognizing the importance that physicians play in health care expenditure (i.e., physicians have control over patient care–procedures, length of stay, hospital admission), a physician payment system based on the use of a "resource-based relative value scale" (RBRVS) was introduced in 1992. The Medicare Fee Schedule has three components: (*i*) a measure of the total work (incorporating both time and complexity) involved in each physician service, and standardized across all specialties, (*ii*) a practice expense to cover the cost of running an office, and (*iii*) an amount to cover malpractice insurance costs. The Medicare Fee Schedule classifies all physician services using the American Medical Association's Current Procedural Terminology (CPT) codes. Each CPT code has an associated "relative value units" (RVUs) weight. The RVU weights are multiplied by a national conversion factor to generate the actual physician fee associated with a particular service. Even though efforts at price controls seem attractive for effective cost-containment because they are less expensive, they generally do not achieve control of costs because of compensatory responses by providers (e.g., cost-shifting to other sectors) (18).

Volume controls include programs to limit utilization rates, for example, the widespread use of expensive technologies or extra hospital beds. Limits can be operationalized using either a regulatory approach [such as certificate of need (CON) programs] or a budgetary approach. Utilization review protocols attempt to discern which expensive care items, and how many days of ICU care are medically necessary (18).

☞ **Budgetary controls are simpler to employ than either price- or volume-control approaches.** ☞ In Canada, for example, hospitals have global annual budgets. How the money is spent is decided by each hospital. If the budget is exceeded, there are no guarantees that the shortfall will be covered (18); in many cases certain types of care are no longer delivered during the remainder of that fiscal period.

Finally, payers can control their costs by "cost-shifting" to other willing (or unwitting) payers. For example, as health insurance premiums rise, employers can choose to shift a greater proportion of these costs to employees. Hospitals and doctors who earn less money caring for Medicare patients can try to make up short falls in some instances by charging more to private insurance patients. Alternatively, insurance companies can choose to offer limited or no coverage for certain pharmaceuticals, shifting the full cost of expensive new medicines directly to patients (8).

THE ECONOMICS OF TRAUMA CARE

Trauma care is resource-intensive. The 2001 National Trauma Data Bank (NTDB) Report found that severely injured patients consumed one-third of all hospital days

utilized for trauma care. They also consumed almost 70% of all days in the ICU, and accounted for 45% of the total charges generated. Even patients with less severe injuries, (although requiring only 21% of all ICU days), utilized more than half of all hospital days, and accumulated charges almost equal to those of the more severely injured (4). Hospital charges varied widely from stab wounds not requiring ICU care (average per case $6373) to major burns requiring ICU care (average per case $49,600). The total estimate hospital charges for the entire group of trauma patients was more than $3 billion (4).

Trauma Systems

Trauma systems are designed to provide an organized and coordinated response to injury (22). Their goal is to deliver prompt, high-quality, and cost-effective care for seriously injured patients. Fully operational trauma systems ensure a continuum of care involving public access to the system, out-of-hospital emergency medical services, and timely triage and transport to definitive acute care and rehabilitation (27). When a trauma care system is established, severely injured patients in the region are triaged and transported to the regional trauma center, a designated hospital offering the expertise of trauma care professionals available 24 hr per day. Trauma centers require other support elements including emergency operative capabilities, intensive care, and rehabilitation (28,29).

In 1976 the American College of Surgeons Committee on Trauma (ACS/COT) published criteria for categorizing hospitals according to the resources required to provide various levels of trauma care. Yet, uniform implementation of regional trauma systems in the U.S. has been somewhat limited because of financial considerations. A 1987 report found that less than 25% of the U.S. geographical area was served by a trauma system (19). Those areas not served were primarily in the Midwest, the Rocky Mountain region, and other rural areas (29).

A 2002 national inventory of hospital trauma centers found that the number of trauma centers has more than doubled since 1991. In 2002, there were 1154 trauma centers in the U.S., including 190 level I centres and 263 level II centres (27). The number of level I and II centers per million population ranged from 0.19 to 7.8 by state, and all but one state (Arkansas) have at least one level I or II trauma center (27).

The number of states that formally designate or certify trauma centers has also increased. In 2002, a total of 35 states and the District of Columbia had developed formal designations or certified trauma centers. Fifteen states were yet to establish their own trauma systems (27,30). Poor access to trauma systems is particularly pronounced in the more rural areas of the country (27). Despite the growth in trauma systems there is still a wide disparity in trauma center distribution and variation in both the availability and configuration of trauma resources (27,30).

Financial considerations have factored in on the slow development of trauma systems in some (especially the geographically isolated) regions. Increasing numbers of uninsured, declining reimbursement for both physicians and hospitals, soaring malpractice premiums, and new limits on resident-physician hours have contributed to a tenuous environment for trauma centers (27).

Unlike other medical centers, trauma centers care for a disproportionately high number of patients unable to pay for their care. Young adults and the poor make up a high proportion of these critically ill, injured patients. These patients are less likely to have insurance coverage or be eligible for public assistance programs. Trauma centers care for the sickest and most expensive injured patients (28). However, said this, geographic location and demographics of the local trauma (i.e., MVC vs. "knife and gun" vs. "work-related" trauma) generally determines the profitability. In certain locations, trauma centers are the most profitable service within a given hospital system.

Regional variations in the implementation of trauma centers has also been due, in part, to the lack of strong evidence of trauma center effectiveness coupled with high costs associated with verification of trauma center capabilities. Hospitals have difficulty justifying the expense of maintaining trauma centers without strong evidence of their effectiveness. The National Study on the Costs and Outcomes of Trauma (NSCOT) was designed to address these limitations and determine differences in outcomes and costs associated with treatment at level I trauma centers and non-trauma center hospitals.

In their first report, MacKenzie et al. (50) examined the differences in mortality in 18 level I trauma centers and 51 non-trauma center hospitals located in 12 states. ☞ **The results of the NSCOT study showed that the overall risk of dying is significantly lower in trauma centers versus non-trauma centers and argues for continued efforts at regionalization.** ☞ The risk of dying within one year after injury was significantly lower in trauma centers (10.4%) versus non-trauma centers (13.8%) (relative risk = 0.75; 95% confidence interval: 0.60–0.95). The effects of trauma centers on mortality were seen primarily for patients with AIS scores of four or higher. The study has also highlighted the difficulty in improving mortality outcomes for elderly trauma patients. Trauma center effects were larger for younger patients, less than 55 compared to those 55 and older, although differences in relative risks by age were not statistically significant except for mortality at 365 days (50). An important limitation to the study was the smaller number of older patients with severe injuries.

Financing Trauma Care

"Regionalization" is the economic foundation for trauma systems. Regional trauma systems control the number of trauma centers serving a geographic area. Regionalization is intended to limit the duplication of services while achieving both high quality and cost-effective care; major savings can be achieved if the number of hospitals providing trauma care is limited and coordinated. Furthermore, the expertise of trauma care professionals is concentrated in fewer hospitals (28,29), resulting in optimization of facilities, practitioners, and patients.

Trauma care is also frequently financed by "non-traditional" funds. These funds include publicly sponsored programs for the elderly, disabled, and underprivileged, as well as an extensive array of health insurers and managed care plans, workers compensation programs, automobile insurance systems, additional taxes, and cost-shifting measures, such as public lotteries, tobacco, or motor vehicle registration surcharges.

Public funds secure full and unimpeded access for the uninsured. Some states support trauma care for all indigent patients with special funding, such as Medicaid payments. Other states and counties provide specific funding to trauma centers to offset the burden posed by uninsured, underinsured, or indigent patients (28).

An intervention aimed to support regional trauma systems is the functional monopoly of the market granted by state governments. Trauma systems with an optimum number of designated trauma centers and with enforced triage systems are examples of a publicly granted monopoly (28).

Motor vehicle accidents account for a large proportion of the trauma population. Auto insurance plays an important role in financing trauma care. Each year, U.S. automobile insurance pays approximately $14 billion for the care of trauma victims. The amount of these funds reaching trauma centers varies considerably depending on the given state's automobile insurance system. Furthermore, since auto insurance has defined coverage limits, a "first-come, first-paid" system develops whereby transport services and the transferring hospital will be paid before the trauma center and physicians caring for such patients (28). To some extent this is also a function of effectiveness and timeliness of the business unit responsible for submitting the bills for payment—whoever submits their changes first will be more likely to be paid.

The NTDB (31) published an updated analysis of 430,557 records from 130 trauma centres in the United States for the period of 1994–2001. Self-pay was the largest source of payment for hospital charges (20.81%), followed by Medicare (17.43%), commercial insurance (14.52%), managed care (13.34%), and Medicaid (10.81%). Automobile insurance was the source of payment for less than 5% of cases (Fig. 5) (31).

Cost-Containment and Managed Care

Cost-containment, through careful utilization monitoring and cost control, is an important goal for MCOs. Unlike other illnesses where the costs of health care fall within predictable limits, trauma has a wide spectrum of severity and associated costs. Trauma occurs suddenly and unpredictably, eliminating the planning review and approval process that are important components for cost containment (32).

☞ **An element of cost containment is lost when MCO patients are injured and transported to non-participating institutions (33).** ☞ Trauma victims meeting specific injury criteria are triaged to regional trauma centers directly from the scene or are transferred from local hospitals after stabilization. Managed care organizations have no power in determining the patient's destination, so treatment is often provided at out-of-network facilities. This out-of-network status for MCO injured patients enables trauma centers the possibility for extensive cost-shifting. Cost-shifting, or charging insured patients more for the uncompensated costs of treating uninsured and under-reimbursed patients, has become a fundamental trauma center financing mechanism (33,34). Trauma centers often increase charges to the out-of-network providers to push pricing and revenue well beyond the level required to meet costs. Cost shifting is particularly prevalent in regions where uncompensated care is high.

A measure to bring costs under better control is repatriation. Repatriation is the act of transferring an acute care patient from a non-participating institution to an institution with MCO contract to reduce the cost of out-of-system care (32). In most cases, the repatriation process results in transfer from a designated trauma center to a non-trauma center, potentially resulting in the delivery of substandard trauma care. The value of

Source of Payment for Hospital Charges

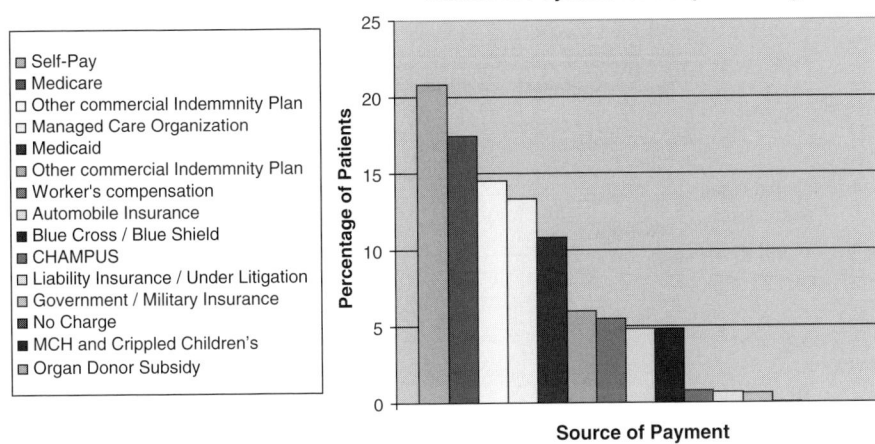

Figure 5   Source of payment for hospital charges. *Source*: From Ref. 55.

repatriation as a cost-effective measure has been questioned. Repatriation may actually increase costs, presumably because of unnecessary or repeated studies done by the receiving institution (32). Moreover, besides the possibility of delayed and/or substandard care, such practices place the medical professionals caring for these patients in an awkward position. This repatriation doctrine can also raise the specter of quasi-criminal activities by MCOs by unduly influencing emergency medical decisions, in effect "practicing medicine without a license."

A major concern for MCOs is that the costs for trauma care cannot be controlled and are often excessive. Specific concerns range from patients with minor injuries being transported by air, over-triaging, excessive utilization of ancillary tests and ICUs, and high costs for treating patients with minor injuries. MCO responses include payment denial and reduction in payment schedules, immediate or early repatriation, and initiatives to limit triage of patients into trauma systems (28,32).

Although regionalized trauma care systems have been shown to improve outcome, such systems have been developed at high expense. The financial burden imposed to trauma centers not only originates from uncompensated care. Causes of underfunding include (*i*) more self-pay patients compared with other hospitalized patients (possibly as an inter-relationship to "trauma prone" behavior of such individuals), (*ii*) a reduced bill-collection ratio for patients covered by Medicare and Medicaid, (*iii*) the inability to shift cost to other payers, and (*iv*) inappropriate assignment and poor definition of DRGs for Medicare prospective payment (35,36).

Costs and Cost-Effectiveness of Trauma Care

Trauma systems can reduce trauma deaths (37–41). Ten years following initial trauma system implementation, mortality due to traffic crashes began to decline; about 15 years following trauma system implementation, mortality was reduced by 8% (42). Similarly, preventable death rates declined significantly after implementation of a regional trauma system (37,43).

Although several studies have reported the costs of trauma (44–46), the cost-effectiveness of trauma systems has not been properly evaluated. In 1988, the costs for the care of 597 injured patients ranged from $5446 to $24,107

(44). Within each body region, both length of stay and hospital charges increased as a function of injury severity (44,47). The direct and indirect costs of trauma were estimated in $11 billion per year (45). Similarly, a study of 12 trauma centers and 43,219 patients in the state of New York, where trauma patients were categorized according to DRGs for comorbidities and complications, it was reported that the trauma cases cost 27.5 million dollars more than non-trauma patients in the same DRG designations (46). The implication is that the care of the injured is inherently more costly.

However, these studies did not provide any measurement of the "value of health" that resulted from the economic expenditures. None of these studies conformed to standard economic models for the evaluation of medical technologies (47). The use of quality-adjusted life years (QALYs) is now considered an integral component of all economic models of health care evaluation (47). Consequently, any economic evaluation of trauma care that does not incorporate an estimate of QALYs is less useful (47).

Séguin et al. (47) demonstrated the potential benefits of using both costs and QALYs in performing economic evaluations of trauma care. Cost-effectiveness was determined by estimating the incremental cost/QALY attributable to treatment at a trauma center. Their results suggested that tertiary trauma care is cost-effective and less costly than treatment programs for other diseases when the QALY gained is included in the evaluation.

☞ **Future economic evaluations of trauma care must include both measurement of costs as well as estimates of QALYs gained to truly determine whether trauma care is cost-effective.** ☞ Only by capturing the "health state achieved" through estimation of QALYs gained from a given health-care technology, can a meaningful denominator be derived for the economic cost of trauma care (the numerator) (47).

EYE TO THE FUTURE

Over the next decade, it is anticipated that the growth in health care spending will continue to increase. The government can not sustain these costs indefinitely. Indeed, between 1980 and 1998 national health expenditures in

National Health Expenditures 1980-2002

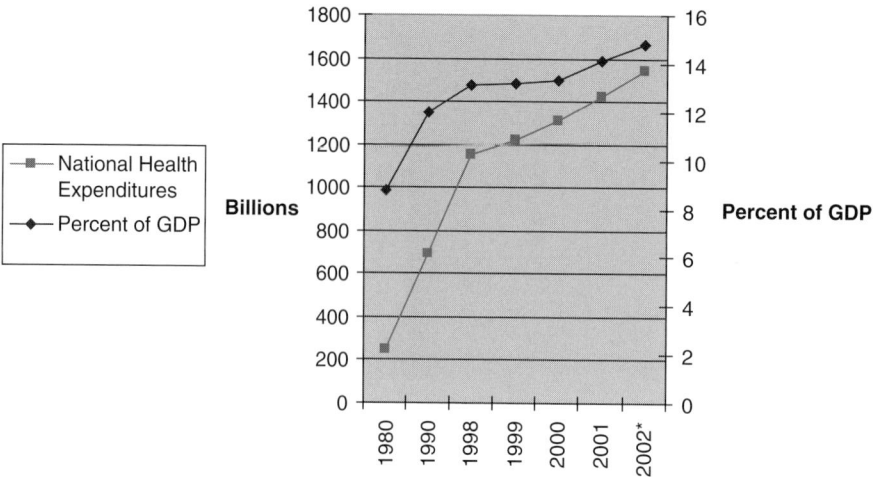

Figure 6   National Health Expenditures 1980–2002. *Abbreviation*: GDP, gross domestic product, the total value of final goods and services produced in the United States. *Source*: From Ref. 56.

the U.S. were skyrocketing both in terms of dollars spent and as a percentage of the GDP (Fig. 6). Since 1998, the expenditures have continued to increase, but at a less rapid rate. Immense pressures are now being exerted on all governmental agencies to limit these expenditures; similar forces are being felt by corporations, in the private sector, and by the consumers. Thus, there will be significant impetus placed upon providing care at lower costs.

Key developments in the health care sector that will likely affect the (rate of) growth in health spending include (*i*) the impact of managed care, (*ii*) the role of the private health insurance, (*iii*) the effect of a rising uninsured population, (*iv*) the impact of the Balanced Budget Act (BBA) of 1997 on Medicare and Medicaid spending, (*v*) the growth or contraction in real capita income, (*vi*) the economy-wide inflation, and (*vii*) demographics such as the aging and overall growth of the U.S. population (7).

Changes in the various health care financing systems must occur. A medical financing system that meets the basic needs of the entire U.S. population will require the efficient use of health care expenditures, while at the same time ameliorating medical care inflation and encouraging innovation, productive competition, and progress toward quality cost-effective health care (48). Neither the current market-driven system nor Medicare and Medicaid programs meet these requirements (48).

Cost-effective analyses will play an increasingly important role in the evaluation of medical care. A new cost-effective health care system is needed to balance quality, choice, and access to care. As with other health-care services, trauma and critical care will have to be measured by new standards of cost-effectiveness. Economic evaluations will be crucial when evaluating the efficacy of existing and future changes in trauma and critical care management, as well as to provide necessary information for policy decisions about ongoing resource allocation in these areas (47).

A specific focus on critical care medicine is crucial because of the disproportional spending in that arena (49). Similarly, mechanisms for accurate cost-allocation and cost-accounting will need to be implemented. These mechanisms will maximize health benefits and minimize waste for any

given resource. Finally, the health care industry will need to implement cost-effective strategies that ensure the best outcome by providing evidence-based care, while reducing costs and controlling variability (5).

SUMMARY

The health care system in the U.S. remains a "paradox of excess and deprivation." The U.S. spends more on medical services than any other nation in the world (24). A large percentage is spent on under-insured and uninsured patients, another large percentage is spent on research and development of new medical technologies.

Unlike other developed nations that rely on centralized planning for provision of health care, the U.S. depends on a mixed health care system of public and private insurance (26). Most working-age Americans effectively purchase health care through their employers (at group discount rates). Medicare provides health insurance to individuals over 65 years of age and to persons with disabilities or end-stage renal disease, whereas Medicaid covers low-income individuals (24). On the other hand, a growing number of individuals in the U.S. either lack health insurance or possess minimal, often standard, coverage. It has been broadly reported that over 40 million persons in the U.S. are uninsured or underinsured (24).

U.S. health care is being reshaped. Over the last decade, U.S. health care has undergone major changes in modes of delivery and payment (7). In the private sector, managed care has been somewhat successful in containing costs, at least in the short term. On the other hand, public health spending growth has exceeded private health spending growth by a substantial margin (7).

Health care spending will continue to impact the delivery of critical and trauma care. As critical and trauma care consume increasing portions of the national health-care expenditures, practitioners, patients, and families must consider not only outcomes but resource allocation, economic impact, and costs. Appropriate use of evidence-based care and economic analyses will provide high-quality care and will ensure the best outcomes by reducing costs and implementing cost-effective interventions (5).

Finally, little will likely change without an acceptance or realization by large segments of the U.S. population that certain patients (e.g. illegal aliens, the elderly, and the chronically ill) consume a grossly disproportionate share of the resources with respect to their contributions to the financing system.

KEY POINTS

✍ Even though ICU beds account for about 10% of all in-patient hospital beds, critical care expenditures account for 15 to 20% of inpatient costs (3), and near 1% of the GDP.

✍ The costs of health care in the US have been rising sharply over the past four decades and currently consume approximately 15% of the GDP.

✍ For the past three decades, the U.S. government has attempted (ineffectively) to reduce the growth of health-care expenditures.

✍ The Medicare program is by far the largest and most influential health insurance program.

✍ Medicaid is the single largest source of financial support for community health services to low income patients.

✍ CMS was established as a federal agency that administers several programs including: Medicare, Medicaid, State Children's Health Insurance Program (SCHIP), Clinical Laboratory Improvement Amendments of 1988 (CLIA) and Health Insurance Portability and Accountability Act of 1996 (HIPAA).

✍ Critical care costs are mainly generated by human resources, expensive drugs, and newer technologies, all promising to prolong the lives of critically ill and severely injured patients.

✍ Two of the most important price control initiatives in medicine have been the Medicare Hospital Prospective Payment System and the Medicare Fee Schedule for physicians.

✍ Budgetary controls are simpler to employ than either price- or volume-control approaches.

✍ The results of the NSCOT study showed that the overall risk of dying is significantly lower in trauma centers versus non-trauma centers and argues for continued efforts at regionalization.

✍ An element of cost containment is lost when MCO patients are injured and transported to non-participating institutions (33).

✍ Future economic evaluations of trauma care must include both measurement of costs as well as estimates of QALYs gained to truly determine whether trauma care is cost-effective.

REFERENCES

1. Iglehart JK. The American health care system. NEJM 1999; 340:70–76.
2. Editorial Commentary Business Factor. Org - December 13, 2004. Available at the Business Factor. Org website (Accessed Nov. 13, 2005 at http://www.businessfactor.org/001765.html).
3. Hassan E. Future advances in health care and their impact on intensive care unit services. New Horizons 1999; 7:173–175.
4. http://www.facs.org/ntdbreport2001/index.html.
5. Pines JM, Fager SS, Milzman DP. A review of costing methodologies in critical care studies. J Crit Care 2002; 17(3): 181–187.
6. Cowan C, Catlin A, Smith C, Sensenig A. National health expenditures 2002. Health care Financing Review 2004; 25(4):143–166.
7. Smith S, Heffler SK, Stephen C, Kent C, Freeland M, Seifert ML et al. National health projections through 2008. Health Care Financing Review 1999; 21(2):211–237.
8. Noseworthy TW, Phillip J. Economics of critical care. In: Hall JB, Schmidt GA, Wood L, eds. Prin Crit Care 1998:17–23.
9. Moon M. Medicare. New England J Med 2001; 344(12):928–931.
10. Center for medicare and medicaid services 2003. http://cms.hhs.gov/.
11. Anderson GF: Medicare and Chronic Conditions. New England J Med 2005; 353(3):305–309.
12. Rowland D: Medicaid - Implications for the Health Safety Net. New England J Med 2005; 353(14):1439–1441
13. HIPPA Insurance Reform. http://cms.hhs.gov/hippa/.
14. Dudley RA, Luft HS. Managed care in transition. New England J Med 2001; 344(14):1087–1092.
15. Rice T, De Lissovoy G, Gabel J, Ermann D, Abbruscato CR. The State of PPOs: Results from a National Survey. Vol. 2. Healtlh Aff 2003; 25–40.
16. Oberlander J. The US health care system: On a road to nowhere? CAMJ 2002; 2(167):163–168.
17. Thorpe KE. Election 2004: Protecting the uninsured. New England J Med 2004; 351(15):1479–1481.
18. Mark DB. Economics issues in clinical medicine. Harrison's Online 2001.
19. Gipe BT. Financing critical care medicine in 2010. New Horizons 1999; 7:184–197.
20. Zimmerman JE. Managing the internal evaluation process. In: Sibbald WJ, Massaro T, eds. The Business of critical care: A textbook for clinicians who manage special care units. Armonk, NY: Futura Publishing Company, 1996.
21. Oliver A, Healy A, Donaldson C. Choosing the method to match the perspective: economic assessment and its implications for health-services efficiency. Lancet 2002; 359:1771–1774.
22. Understanding costs and cost-effectiveness in critical care. Report from the second American Thoracic Society workshop on outcomes research. A J Respir Crit Care Med 2002; 165:540–550.
23. Pronovost P, Angus DC. Economics of end-of-life care in the intensive care unit. Crit Care Med 2001; 29:N46–N51.
24. Rhodes RS, Rice CL. Elements of cost-effective nonemergency surgical care. In: Wilmore DW, Cheug LY, Harken AH, Holcroft JW, Meakins JL, Soper NJ, eds. ACS Surgery: Principle and Practice. New York, NY: WebMD Corporation, 2002: 519–533.
25. Critical care medicine tutorials: The cost of critical care 2002. http://www.ccmtutorials.com/organization/index.htm.
26. Chalfin D, Fein A. Critical care medicine in managed competition and a managed care environment. New Horizons 1994; 2(3):275–282.
27. MacKenzie EJ, Hoyt D, Sacra JC, Jurkovich GJ, Carlini AR, Teitelbaum SD, Teter H. National inventory of hospital trauma centers. JAMA 2003;289:1515–1522.
28. Rosenbaum S. Medicaid. New England J Med 2002; 346(8): 635–640.
29. Bazzoli G. Factors that enhance continued trauma center participation in trauma systems. J Trauma 1996; 41:3.
30. Trunkey DD. Trauma centers and trauma systems. JAMA 2003; 289:1566–1567.
31. http://www.facs.org/dept/trauma/ntdbannualreport2002.pdf
32. Gabel J, Levitt L, Pickreign J, Whitmore H, Holve E, Hawkins S et al. Job-based health insurance in 2000: Premiums rise sharply while coverage grows. Health Affairs 2000; 19(5): 144–151.
33. Mackersie RC. Trauma and managed care. In: Current therapy of trauma. 4th edn. Donald D Trunkey, Frank R Lewis, eds. St. Louis, Mo; London: Mosby, 1999: 18–22.

34. Eastman AB, Bishop GS. The economics of trauma care. In: Current therapy of trauma. 4th edn. Donald D Trunkey, Frank R Lewis, eds. St. Louis, Mo; London: Mosby, 1999: 27–35.

35. Baker SP, Whitfield R, O'Neill B. Geographical variations in mortality from motor vehicles crashes. New England J Med 1987; 16(22):1384–1387.

36. Eastman AB. An analysis of the critical care problem of trauma center reimbursement. J Trauma 1991; 31:292–297.

37. Cales RH. Trauma mortality in Orange County: the effect of implementation of a regional trauma system. Ann Emerg Med 1984; 13:1–10.

38. Shackford SR, Mackersie RC, Hoyt DB, et al. Impact of a trauma system on outcome of severely injured patients. Arch Surg. 1987; 122:523–527.

39. Stewart TC, Lane PL, Stefanits T. An evaluation of outcomes before and after trauma center designation using Trauma and Injury Severity Score analysis. J Trauma 1995; 39:1036–1040.

40. Rutledge R, Fakhry SM, Meyer A, Sheldon GF, Baker C. A analysis of the association of trauma centers with per capita county trauma death rates. Ann Surg 1993; 218:512–524.

41. Mullins RJ, Mann NC, Hedges JR, Worrall W, Jurkovich GJ. Preferential benefit of implementation of a statewide trauma system in two adjacent states. J of Trauma 1998; 44:609–617.

42. Nathens AB, Jurovich GJ, Cummings P, Rivara FP, Maier RV. The effect of organized systems of trauma care on motor vehicle crash mortality. JAMA 2000; 283:1990–1994.

43. Shackford SR, Hollingsworth-Fridlund P, Cooper GF, et al. The effect of regionalization upon the quality of trauma care as assessed by concurrent audit before and after institution of a trauma system: a preliminary report. J Trauma 1986; 26:812–820.

44. MacKenzie EJ, Siegel SH, Shapiro S, et al. Functional recovery and medical costs of trauma: an analysis by type and severity of injury. J Trauma 1988; 28:281–295.

45. MacKenzie EJ, Morris JA, Smith GS, et al. Acute hospital costs of trauma in the United States: implications for regionalized systems of care. J Trauma 1990; 30:1096–1103.

46. Joy SA, Lichtig LK, Knauf RA, et al. Identification and categorization of and cost for care of trauma patients: a study of 12 trauma centers and 43,219 statewide patients. J Trauma 1994; 37:303–308.

47. Seguin J, Garber BG, Coyle D, Herbert PC. An economic evaluation of trauma care in a Canadian lead trauma hospital. J Trauma 1999; 47:S99–S103.

48. Austin GE, Burnett RD: An innovative proposal for the health care financing system of the United States. Pediatrics 2003; 111:1093–1097.

49. Chalfin DB, Cohen II, Lambrinos J: The economics and cost-effectiveness of critical care medicine. Intensive Care Med 1995; 21:952–961.

50. MacKenzie EJ, Rivara FP, Jurkovich GJ, et al. A national evaluation of the effect of trauma-center care on mortality. New England J Med 2006; 354:366–378.

51. Iglehart JK. Revisiting the Canadian health care system. NEJM 2000; 342:2007–2012.

52. http://www.cms.hhs.gov/statistics/nhe/projections-2002/default.asp

53. Medical Expenditure Panel Survey of 2001 Medical Expenditure Panel Survey. Rockville, MD: Agency for Healthcare Research and Quality, 2001.

54. Medical Expenditure Panel Survey of 2001 Medical Expenditure Panel Survey. Rockville, MD: Agency for Healthcare Research and Quality, 2001.

55. http://www.facs.org/dept/trauma/ntdbannualreport2002.pdf

56. http://www.cms.hhs.gov/statistics/nhe/projections-2002/default.asp

72

Remote Management of Trauma and Critical Care

José Manuel Rodríguez-Paz and Todd Dorman
Departments of Anesthesiology, Adult Critical Care Medicine, and Surgery,
School of Medicine, Johns Hopkins University, Baltimore, Maryland, U.S.A.

Joseph F. Rappold
Division of Trauma and Critical Care, Department of Surgery, Naval Medical Center San Diego, San Diego, California, U.S.A.

INTRODUCTION

In 1966, a report was published by the National Research Council, entitled "Accidental Death and Disability—The Neglected Disease of Modern Society" (1). This publication led to the passage of the 1966 Highway Safety Act, and subsequently to the establishment of the Emergency Medical Services (EMS) program by the Department of Transportation. In 1976, the American College of Surgeons (ACS) Committee on Trauma (COT) recommended guidelines for designing and implementing trauma centers be adopted (2). Since then, trauma centers have been established in numerous communities. A recent meta-analysis of level I trauma centers have shown a 15% improvement in patient outcomes since the implementation of these facilities (3). Numerous reasons are responsible for the improved outcomes, including the requirement to have an attending trauma surgeon present within 15 min of a seriously injured patient's arrival to the Emergency Department (ED) (4,5). Similarly, a high-intensity model of critical care staffed by intensivists has been shown to decrease morbidity and mortality, and length of stay in both in the SICU and in the hospital overall (6–10).

♂ **The regionalization of trauma care has improved overall outcome, but not solved the significant problem of providing high-level trauma and critical care services to remote locations, where organized trauma systems do not exist.** ♂ To further complicate the problem, an estimated third of the U.S. population reside in rural areas (11). This population shares more than 50% of the deaths from motor vehicle collisions (MVCs), and a rural trauma patient is twice as likely to die as an urban victim wounded by a similar mechanism of injury (12). Delays in therapy have been proven to worsen outcomes in trauma patients (especially in cases of injuries to the spinal cord, brain, and internal organs).

The flow of injured patients is of even greater complexity in military trauma. Currently, approximately 77% of all deaths occur on the battlefield before an injured soldier reaches a medical treatment facility (MTF), while only 23% who expire die of wounds after reaching a MTF (13). These data demonstrate improvements in management and coordination of patient care in the current conflicts compared to past wars. However, more needs to be done, and telemedicine can play an increasing role in the future.

Even modern, adequately staffed triage systems can be inadequate in disaster situations where patient numbers can overload existing resources. Current established level I trauma centers can have as many as half of their admissions resulting from transfers from other institutions (14). In the case of critical care, as many as 90% of adults in intensive care units (ICUs) do not have a high-intensity physician staffing model with trained intensivists (15,16), and this is more of a problem, but not exclusive, to smaller communities.

♂ **A potential solution to delivering trauma and critical care to remote locations and to address shortages of subspecialty-trained physicians is the use of telemedicine.** ♂ Telemedicine holds the significant advantage of resolving the issue of delivering care to these distant locations, while at the same time maintaining the current structure and organizations of advanced trauma centers and ICUs. Telemedicine brings expert physicians (whether trauma surgeon or intensivists) to the site of the emergency via advanced telecommunication systems and can allow them to evaluate patient data and direct care more effectively than would occur with nontrained personnel that might respond to the trauma scene. The goal of any trauma and intensive care delivery system is not only a reduction in mortality and morbidity associated with the injury or critical illness, but also to prevent further injuries due to treatment errors. The use of telemedicine can accomplish these goals by permitting better triage and prioritization of care, avoiding delay of care in those patients in remote areas that need it the most, and optimizing the available resources.

In 1997, the telemedicine report to the U.S. Congress established that "Telemedicine can mean access to health care where little had been available before. In emergency cases, this access can mean the difference between life and death. In particular, in those cases where fast medical response time and specialty care are needed, telemedicine availability can be critical" (17).

The topics that will be examined in this chapter include the historical uses of telemedicine through 2006, the definition and technical aspects of telemedicine, as well as the current applications of telemedicine in trauma and critical care, with particular attention focused on telemedicine considerations for remote and austere locations. Financial and legal issues have slowed the forward progress of telemedical advancements; accordingly, these considerations are also explored.

☞ **Military research has helped develop many aspects of telemedicine, and the direct applications to both military and civilian care are enormous.** ☞

This chapter discusses how advanced technology has been used in military planning and the execution of battle-field maneuvers. However, many currently available telemedical applications have yet to be fully deployed in trauma care in the combat zone, or at level II military treatment facilities (MTFs).

Historically, medical care improves after the initiation of each major military campaign, but further development tends to regress with contraction of responsibilities. Current U.S. and coalition military medical leaders are committed not only to revising this trend but also to expediting the application of currently available telemedicine technologies, increasing future development, and improving maintenance of institutional memory about the needs of the injured soldier during war. Indeed the application of telemedical technologies has improved significantly in both Afghanistan and Iraq over the last year. One of us (JRR) has been to Iraq twice in the last two years and witnessed significant improvements in the intelligent use of these technologies, as will be described herein.

HISTORY

Since 1920, when S.G. Brown was able to demonstrate the first "electrical stethoscope and telephone relay" in London at a distance of over 50 miles (17), numerous examples of telemedicine techniques have been employed. In 1950, the first application capable of transferring radiograms across standard telephone lines was created. In 1959 the University of Nebraska College of Medicine was able to use, for the first time, video communications for a telemedical consultation (18). During the 1960s an escalation of telemedicine techniques occurred. One such example includes a project carried out by NASA and Lockheed Corporation, called STARPAHC (Space Technology Applied to Rural Papago Advanced Heath Care), in which remote health care was provided to the Papago Indian reservation in Arizona by two Native American paramedics employing radiographic and electrocardiographic (ECG) peripherals transmitted via microwave system to a Public Health Service facility (19,20). This study was designated to pilot equipment planned for use to provide medical services to astronauts while on their missions. In 1968 medical data [such as ECGs, blood pressure (BP) readings, stethoscope sounds, and blood smear images] were transmitted between first-aid stations at Boston's Logan Airport and physicians at the Massachusetts General Hospital (MGH) (21).

In the late 1970s, Canada was already testing a satellite transmission system for telemedical use in remote provinces. At the same time, in the U.S., several states began establishing large statewide networks to connect large centers of knowledge with government and rural communities, thus creating an information highway that serves multiple purposes and includes large medical centers.

In the late 1980s the Picture Archival and Communication Systems (PACS), a system that could transmit radiographic images over telephone lines, became very popular among radiology departments. Also by then, the U.S. Navy was testing a system for the support of personnel onboard ships and at remote locations. However, PACS was first clinically available in the United States and United Kingdom in the early 1990s. It has taken until now for PACS technology to become widely available worldwide.

In 1982, Grundy et al. (22) reported a direct association between reduced mortality and a higher proportion of recommendations enacted by using a real-time, interactive video consultation between the University Hospital of Cleveland and the ICU at Forest City Hospital of Cleveland. Other examples of the use of telemedicine techniques for trauma care included the 1988 Spacebridge Project. Established by NASA, it provided real-time connectivity between physicians in the U.S. and Armenian surgeons after an earthquake that caused more than 150,000 casualties.

More recently, in 1998, a research project carried out by NASA and Yale University allowed monitoring the medical conditions and vital signs of climbers on Mount Everest using radio transmitters and audio and video data via a satellite link (23).

☞ **Computer-assisted surgical robotics is a technological area whose immense potential will likely facilitate telemedicine applications for trauma in the near future.** ☞ Computer-assisted surgical robotics began to be utilized clinically in 1999, the year the *da Vinci*® Surgical System (Intuitive Surgical, Inc., Sunnyvale, CA) was introduced. The original, prototype for the *da Vinci* System was developed in the late 1980s at a former Stanford Research Institute under contract to the U.S. Army. Today, Intuitive Surgical is the global leader in the rapidly emerging field of robotic-assisted minimally invasive surgery (MIS) (clinical applications are discussed further below). As of April 2006, nearly 300 *da Vinci* Systems have been installed in hospitals worldwide.

DEFINITIONS AND TECHNIQUES

The American Telemedicine Association defines telemedicine, telehealth or e-health as "the use of medical information exchanged from one site to another via electronic communication for health and education of the patient or health care provider and for the purpose of improving patient care." ☞ **Telemedicine connects two physically separated locations (which can be positioned anywhere on the globe), and facilitates the sharing of clinical information between health care providers (or between patient and provider) for the diagnosis and/or management of medical and surgical conditions.** ☞

There are two major categories of telemedicine interactions: Pre-recorded ("store-and-forward"), also known as *asynchronous* telemedicine, and "real time" or *synchronous* telemedicine. In the asynchronous mode, static images or audio-video clips can be sent either physically or via electronic means to a remote storage device. Once at the storage site (file cabinet, or on-line server with remote download capabilities), the information can be subsequently sent over numerous modes of delivery or stored for analysis when convenient. The second form of telemedicine data transfer involves "real-time" interactions, also known as interactive or *synchronous*. Both types are utilized, and will be discussed below.

☞ **Telemedicine can be used in a variety of situations from consultative care, triage, and direct patient care, to image transfer and continuing medical education.** ☞ The routine use of telemedicine techniques has been around for quite some time. The everyday use of phone communication and the use of facsimiles have been part of the routine way of communication between health providers for many years.

The high-speed development of personal computers and the increasing capabilities of mainframe supercomputers have fostered capabilities not previously available. The development of communication tools [e.g., e-mail, and internet protocols (IPs) that allow streaming voice and data] have permitted and improved the methodology for the transmission of both text and images in most medical environments (from small offices to state-of-the-art medical facilities). Also, real-time interactive, multipoint videoconferencing with application sharing has become commonplace and technically easier to use. Furthermore, the development of wireless technologies (from cellular phones to satellite-based technologies) have permitted the transmission of all this information from remote locations that would otherwise lack the standard hardwire technology that would allow routine communication.

TECHNICAL ASPECTS/PHYSICAL CHARACTERISTICS
Central Consultation Unit (Command Module)

The central consultation station can be physically located anywhere on the globe. It should be ergonomically arranged with a user-friendly interface, which should include video and voice communication, as well as text messaging capabilities. Computer-based patient data evaluation tools should also be employed (e.g., assisted diagnosis, linkage to databases, etc.). Generally this receiver station consists of a dedicated workstation which can be used by the medical expert to handle and record all the data, and should be able to transmit back all of the information needed. Security and confidentiality are also critical issues in the design of these units, which require encryption coding.

The specific computer-based elements needed for each telemedicine application varies, but when dealing with trauma or critically ill patients, the system requires capability to handle real-time, synchronous interactive videoconference. In contrast, routine care for less acute patient care situations may only need data sent to the clinician via a store-and-forward technology.

The software used in this workstation should be able to work in a stand-alone fashion, capture, display, and transmit data to multiple sites using asynchronous protocols (two-way communication in which a time delay between transmission and reception is allowed). These systems also need to support all required hardware devices and have a simple interface.

Ideally these software applications should be capable of real-time screening and interpretation of certain types of data that it handles. For example, ECG recordings or rhythm strips should yield an instantaneous diagnosis to both the remote site and at the command module. Discussion on management can then proceed while a simultaneous text message of ACLS® protocol recommendations are displayed on a running header display on the video monitor. In addition, the drug recommendations and the detection of any errors are important and necessary tools.

Another type of peripheral device that could be useful in this setting includes telemanipulators that enhance the ability of the physician to perform tissue manipulation on the patient (surgical procedures) from a distance, via

multisensory input that recreates remote tactile and visual environments. These devices are similar to some of the operating room robotic devices presently in use today (as will be discussed in greater detail below) (24).

Data Transmission Media

The main characteristic that defines the quantity of data that can be transmitted over a line or other medium is bandwidth. Bandwidth is defined as the information-carrying capacity of the information transport medium, and is normally expressed in bits per second (bps). The bandwidth requirements increases with the complexity of the task; a telephone/fax transmission takes only approximately 100 kbps or (0.1 Mb)/sec whereas virtual presence or telepresence (the highest end in telemedicine) takes 100,000 kbps or (100 Mb)/sec.

Two important basic concepts in telecommunications that limit bandwidth in various systems are that (*i*) the slowest part of the connection determines the real throughput rate, and (*ii*) once approximately 20% of the available bandwidth is consumed by usage, degradation in performance is observed. In addition, the link ideally should have a minimal delay factor or latency, which in some cases, such as satellite communications, could be as long as 1 to 2 seconds.

Transmission over conventional telephone lines and utilizing standard modems are the simplest way to send information. These systems are referred to as plain old telephone service (POTS). They provide data transmission at a maximum rate of 64 kbps. Although their major advantages include low cost, near ubiquitous availability, and high levels of international standardization, the major disadvantage is their low bandwidth. This becomes especially problematic when trying to transmit data-dense applications such as real-time data.

More modern telephone lines include digital networks and asymmetric digital submission lines. The digital networks include Integrated Services Digital Networks (ISDNs) which are protocols permitting the delivery of high bandwidth data to homes and offices by standardizing high-speed digital transmission, allowing integrated transmission of video, data, and voice. Normally it requires installation of special input and output devices. Digital subscriber lines (DSL) or T1 lines (24 channel, high-capacity circuit for data, voice, and video transmission) provide a rate of transmission of from 1.5 to 2.0 megabytes (Mb)/sec and offer some increase in bandwidth.

The highest end bandwidths occur through fiber optic networks (i.e., OC3 fiber optic cable connection, a 243-channel, high capacity circuit—up to 155 Mb/sec—for data, voice, and video transmission), and satellite [i.e., Low Earth Orbiting Satellites (LEOS), Advanced Communications Technology Satellite (ACTS)] that can deliver up to 1 billion bits/sec. The major disadvantage of these networks is their cost, limited range, and lack of international standardization. In addition, in the case of satellites, bandwidth may not always be immediately available. However, there is an increasing array of satellites in orbit, with increasing opportunities; these can be tracked by anyone with a computer by logging in to the NASA website (http://science.nasa.gov/temp/StationLoc.html).

A common solution to the use of large and expensive bandwidths is the compression of the data before transmission. Two basic algorithms are available: lossy and lossless (25). The difference between the two algorithms is based in whether or not data are lost during transmission. The higher the quality of data (i.e., lossless), the more expensive is the compression technology.

New compression technologies and greater bandwidth opportunities are being made available; projects like Internet Two and Next Generation Internet (NGI) may fill holes left by the current technology. The National Library of Medicine has ongoing research projects in the specific applications and uses of NGI in medical applications, including trauma. Another alternative is the asynchronous transfer modes (ATM), one the newest high-speed ways of telecommunication. Its advantage is that offers high-quality and low-decay conditions ideal for high-speed communications.

Remote Unit and Systems

The remote system consists principally of telemedicine peripheral devices. These devices are used to acquire patient data (e.g., vitals, image, video). They need to be portable, lightweight and easy to use with sufficient power autonomy. They also require a user-friendly interface. The system must allow bi-directional audio and visual communication (transmission of critical biosignals, images of the patient, and other vital data, including radiographs).

Typical examples of telemedicine peripherals are analog-based audio stethoscopes, digital BP meters, video otoscopes, etc. More advance technology includes devices like the FDA, approved remote "Life Support for Trauma and Transport®" (LSTAT®) (Fig. 1). This device is a self-contained stretcher platform designed for in the field stabilization and transport of severely injured patients. This LSTAT® incorporates a series of monitors which allows a remote team to follow respiratory and hemodynamic data, blood chemistry, mechanical ventilator settings, inhaled and exhaled O_2 and CO_2 values, infusion pumps for drugs and intravenous fluids, etc. The LSTAT® also incorporates an automated external defibrillator. The LSTAT® can be linked to a prepared medical facility while the patient is transported, allowing for both remote monitoring as well as remote manipulation of care (including all of the above mentioned support systems).

TRAUMA APPLICATIONS
Currently Employed Remote Trauma Applications

It is not unusual that most current emergency department Trauma Resuscitation Suites (TRSs) are connected via simple models of telemedicine with prehospital providers to assist in trauma care and to initiate triage long before the trauma or patient arrives to those facilities. Emergency telemedicine has been evolving during the past few years and has become a common interactive video application used in telemedicine.

In most rural or remote facilities teleradiology utilizing PACS technology is a common standard procedure. Also in this setting, teleconferencing both for consultation or education are common techniques used to take care of patients. For example, the St. Francis Hospital in Tulsa has, besides the teleradiology services, developed a system by which emergency medicine physicians are available for consultation with other practitioners located in small surrounding rural hospitals (26). This system has been shown to improve specific areas of patient care, especially the triage of critically ill patients, decreasing the transfer rate of patients who did not actually require a higher level of care

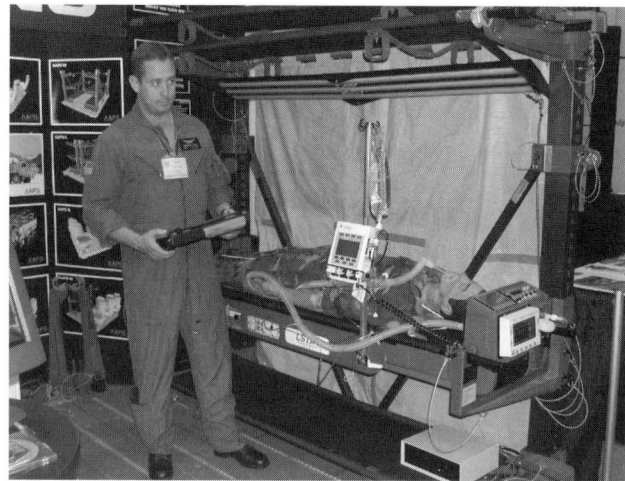

Figure 1   Life Support for Trauma and Transport (LSTAT®). The patented LSTAT system is an individualized, portable, networked ICU and surgical table in a patient-care platform. Integrated within the LSTAT system are a state-of-the-art defibrillator, ventilator, suction, three-channel fluid and drug infusion pump, point-of-care blood chemistry analyzer, and patient monitoring subsystems. The platform, which is only 5 inches thick, also incorporates on-board power and oxygen subsystems. The medical subsystems are further integrated into an on-board computer that captures, stores, and transmits continuous, real-time, multi-device, multi-parameter, time-synchronized patient data. Patient data is also available at bedside on a handheld secondary display (with optional wireless capability) and over numerous patient data information systems, including over the Internet through secure web sites that protect patient privacy. Information about the platform itself (battery status, oxygen supply, device health, etc.) is also available to a distant monitoring center. *Source*: Photo courtesy of Integrated Medical Systems, Inc., Signal Hill, California, U.S.A.

and thus resulting in better utilization of the available emergency services.

This sort of model has also been used in the United Kingdom (27,28) where Armstrong and colleagues have reported a successful initial experience with a system that linked the emergency department of a large tertiary care hospital with a small rural facility in Scotland, via a land integrated digital network and also a satellite link, to diagnose and manage mild to moderately injured patients. In another study, low cost ISDN videoconferencing units were successfully installed in England, in what is called minor injuries units (MIUs). In that study, the researchers found no difference in diagnosis or management in over 45 patients seen during a period of six months (mostly with fractures, soft-tissue injury, and suspected fractures), but there was a significant reduction in patients transferred to higher level of care centers (29).

A preliminary follow up study of this experience performed by Tachakra et al. (30) showed that it is clinically safe and effective. This successful system of telemedicine applied to minor injuries prompted the opening of over 20 MIUs around the U.K. There are several case reports of describing the successful diagnosis of patients with severe undetected injuries admitted to remote/rural facilities that were properly diagnosed by an experienced specialist via telemedicine (i.e., spinal cord compression) (31).

Multiple evaluations have been done to validate the different telemedicine technologies when used in a trauma setting. The great majority of these studies showed that clinical data in trauma patients can be successfully obtained by standard video and audio telemedicine technologies (32–35).

The current concept of advance trauma care is based on a team approach, and the role of the team leader (an ATLS® trained physician) is considered crucial for the success of this model. Several studies have investigated the effect of physically removing the team leader from the TRS and evaluated whether this role could be assumed by a remote ATLS® trained physician via telemedicine (36). In London a resuscitation room in a community hospital was linked via a teleconferencing system using three ISDN lines linking three cameras working at 384 kbps to a trauma center (36). Fifteen scenarios from the ATLS Course Manual were analyzed. The researchers found no statistical differences when they compared primary survey, resuscitation, and secondary survey performed via telemedicine or standard care. ✎ **The role of trauma leader can be safely provided by a traumatologist not physically present in TRS settings where the trauma training of the other team members is insufficient but telecommunication understanding is adequate (36).** ✎

Subsequently, the same group studied this model using real patients (37). In this study, two separate rooms were linked using a telemedicine videoconferencing system in a London ED. Two hundred patients with minor to moderate injuries admitted to the ED were evaluated by the remote attending physician. The study evaluated a series of physical parameters associated with the clinical exam and found that the quality of treatment offered compared well with face-to-face consultation. Similar results were found in a pilot study in Houston (Ben Taub General Hospital) where researchers found >90% accuracy between remote clinical data (using video technology) and that assessed via standard techniques in almost half of the ATLS® clinical variables evaluated; however, it was <70% accurate in another 15 variables in the assessment of acute trauma resuscitations (32). The ATLS® clinical variables included in this study were demographics, primary and secondary survey, initial and subsequent vital signs, physical exam (including advanced diagnostic tools like diagnostic peritoneal lavage), data (radiographs, MRI, CT, ECG), and diagnosis and disposition (32). Authors concluded that the remote supervision of trauma care by the trauma leader can provide accurate and safe evaluation and stabilization of injured patients.

Following these findings, the same team studied seventeen trauma victims who were randomly selected to have their assessment done via telemedicine (38), using a closed circuit analog television system linking several trauma rooms to a centralized trauma command center. The majority of victims had sustained blunt injuries (mostly MVCs). Immediately after arrival to the ED, an attending trauma surgeon located in the remote centralized trauma coordinator's office was called and was in direct communication with the third-year surgical resident via a wall-mounted video camera (which provided a full room view), microphone, and a hands-free telephone worn by the resident (via a dedicated telephone line).

The study evaluated 44 specific ATLS variables, with concurrent assessment by the attending surgeon as they occurred. Then, an independent party compared the assessment done remotely with that recorded in the clinical chart, and discrepancies were noted. All patients survived their injury and were subsequently discharge alive. On two occasions, two simultaneous resuscitations were performed. On average, the remote evaluations included 28 of the 44 variables. The variables that showed the highest degree of concordance were demographics (92%), primary survey (76%), initial vital signs (70%), and secondary physical exam and diagnosis (76%). Technical difficulties with the communication link happened in only one instance. This study confirms the feasibility of remote evaluation of trauma patients under controlled circumstances.

Another example of the use of telemedicine for real-time video consultation for remote trauma care was reported by Rogers et al. (39). They described the use of a videoconferencing system via a dedicated ISDN line that linked four community hospitals in rural Vermont and New York with trauma surgeons located at their homes. Over a period of eight months, 26 telemedicine consults were completed. In general, the patients included in the telemedicine project were more severely injured and had higher mortality than the general trauma population. The types of trauma in this study included MVCs (50%), followed by all-terrain vehicle (ATV) accidents and pedestrians struck by vehicles. In two cases, the telemedicine intervention was considered lifesaving. In approximately 50% of the patients the recommendation made by the trauma surgeon was to transfer the patient to the trauma center (secondary to the lack of neurosurgeon or orthopedic surgeon in the referring facility) and in another 25% of the cases the recommendation was to keep the patient in the referring facility. Other interventions included recommending placement of chest tube, CT scan, diagnostic peritoneal lavage (DPL), and transfusion.

Telemedicine has also been studied for the provision of emergency orthopedic care. In a study done over two years in North Dakota (40), orthopedic surgeons performed over ninety teleconsultations, mostly evaluation and treatment of fractures, swollen joints and infections. In this study, a level II trauma center was connected to three rural facilities staffed with primary care providers via a network with a two-way videoconferencing system and computer software that enabled the physicians located at both locations to send and receive graphics, slides, radiographs, patient information, and other data. The orthopedic teleconsultations were done by board-certified orthopedic surgeons and divided into emergent (23%), urgent (39%), and scheduled consults.

No adverse outcomes were detected and there were no major discrepancies in diagnosis between radiographs read during teleconsultation and after the fact. Of all the consults, 68% of the patients remained in the rural facility and one procedure was performed via teleconsultation (removal of a pin by the primary care physician). The orthopedic surgeons rated the technology utilized as satisfactory or excellent. In another study by the same group (41), a series of 100 patients were included in consecutive teleconsults between a Level II Trauma Center and three rural sites staffed by primary care providers via a video teleconferencing system and a T1 communications network. The majority of patients included in this study (60%) were considered urgent. Half of the consults were done with orthopedists but emergency medicine physicians and neurosurgeons were also consulted.

The most common reason for trauma teleconsults in this study was diagnosis and treatment of extremity and pelvic trauma. Radiological images were sent (via PACS) for interpretation and the hardcopies were reviewed *a posteriori* by a radiologist to confirm diagnosis. No significant discrepancies were found between the two modes of interpretation. Almost 70 patients in the study stayed in their local community for further care. Since these studies were published, the Dakota Telemedicine System (DTS) has extended specialty telecare to several rural hospitals, and performs on average 25 teleconsults every month (42).

A prospective controled trial completed in New Jersey by Brennan et al. (43) studied management at two EDs [one defined as low volume (rural), and the other as high volume (suburban)] where the physicians and nurses were trained in telemedicine techniques. Fifteen patient scenarios were studied in 104 patients, who were randomized to either a control group ("high-volume"—suburban on site physician) or an experimental group ("low-volume"—rural with remote physician access via telemedicine system).

The experimental group consisted of patients who had arrived to the "high-volume" ED. Once the patient was managed via telemedicine, he or she was re-evaluated by the "in-situ" physician. The outcomes measured included diagnosis, treatment and return visits, need for additional care, as well as patient, physician, and nurse satisfaction. Although a range of medical and trauma conditions were evaluated, the most common diagnosis seen was extremity injuries (62% of patients). None of the variables studied showed any significant difference between the control or experimental groups and the level of patient and physician's satisfaction was rated as very satisfying.

More recently, the Southern Arizona Teletrauma and Telepresence (SATT) Program was launched by the Section of Trauma and Critical Care at the University of Arizona Medical Center (UAMC), the only Level 1 Trauma Center in Southern Arizona (44). The SATT program was developed to assist trauma patients in rural communities. Using advances in technology, SATT provides a live consultation link including videoconferencing, telemetry, digital radiographs, and ultrasound (via PACS) between the trauma team at UAMC and rural emergency departments in the southern section of the state. The SAAT program has been found to save both lives and resources, and is being expanded (44).

Burn assessment is an area of trauma management where frequent discrepancies can contribute to both delayed appropriate transport to a burn center as well as overuse of air transport resources (45). The ability to evaluate burn patients by telemedicine has the potential to assist decisions regarding transfer, avoid errors in initial care, and reduce costs. Saffle et al. are currently developing and testing such a system (45).

Evolving Applications in Trauma Care

Another potential remote management application for trauma care involves expansion of the Telemedicine Emergency Neurosurgical Network (TENNS) project, which was created to facilitate decision-making by neurosurgeons before the patient was transported to tertiary facilities (46). The TENNS project could be expanded to facilitate the placement of burr holes in craniotomy patients whose outcomes would be improved by emergent decompression and stabilization prior to transfer to a level I facility. This system might save lives when transport times exceed some threshold time limit (e.g., 1–2 hours) as set by the supervising neurosurgical team.

A similar project that could have trauma applicability is the use of wireless technology in ambulances to see what impact telemedicine has on stroke mortality. The pilot project has been conducted with the intention of diminishing the time between onset of ischemic stroke and initiation of therapy. This project, funded by the National Library of Medicine and carried out by the University of Maryland Hospital and BDM Federal, Inc., enables video images, audio, vitals signs, and ECG rhythm to be transmitted from a moving ambulance through an off-the-shelf digital wireless telephone system using a commercial telephone service. The data is reviewed in real time by a tertiary care center (neurologists) via workstations. The intention of the research team is to conduct a pilot study to investigate whether early treatment via telemedicine significantly reduces morbidity and mortality of strokes. Results of this project are still pending.

The camera-phone has recently been studied as a tool for remote evaluation regarding the replantation potential of completely amputated fingers. The pilot study demonstrated that the camera-phone (Fig. 2) is both feasible and valuable for remote evaluation of replantation potential of completely amputated fingers and holds significant promise for future clinical application with the advent of further-evolving technology (47). The technology holds promise in avoiding both missed opportunities to replant digits, and unnecessary patient transfer by providing useful information.

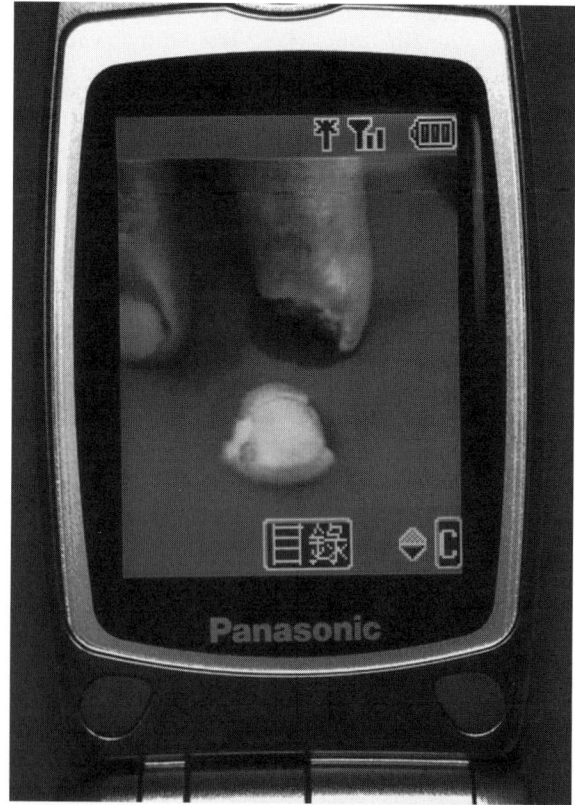

Figure 2 Camera phone image of severed fingertip. The camera-phone has been utilized as a tool for remote evaluation regarding injuries from remote locations. In this case, the replantation potential of amputated digits is evaluated. *Source*: From Hsieh C-H, Jeng S-F, Chen C-Y, et al.: Teleconsultation with Mobile Camera-Phone in Remote Evaluation of Replantation Potential. J Trauma 2005; 58(6):1208–1212.

Telepresence trauma surgery is the ultimate management modality tested to date in the field of telemedicine. Telepresence surgery has been used in the past and there are numerous instances (48–54) in which this technique has been successfully used since Dr. Mouret performed the first video-assisted laparoscopy in France in 1987, which has since revolutionized MIS.

☞ **The application of telepresence in trauma surgery has evolved to include use of the *Da Vinci*® computer-assisted robotics system.** ☞ This device utilizes a telemanipulator (Fig. 3A) permitting the remotely located trauma surgeon a stereoscopic (three dimensional) video display of the remote operative field (Fig. 3B) where the computer-assisted robotic device employs surgical instrumentation with far greater dexterity and degrees of freedom than standard MIS surgical techniques. The remote telemanipulator workstation site is typically linked to the robotic device by coaxial cable, though fiber optic cables or computer uplinks could also provide the needed bandwidth.

During initial experimentation using an early prototype of the *Da Vinci*® system, surgeons repaired vascular anastomoses and other procedures following multiple trauma in animals (55). Anesthetized swine were operated upon, and surgeons performed two-layer closure gastrotomies, cholecystectomies, and hemorrhage control from liver lacerations (55). Although the *Da Vinci*® system was used to perform all of these surgeries, it increased the time for completion of surgical maneuvers (like tying knots) and procedures by up to 3 times. This prototype

(A)

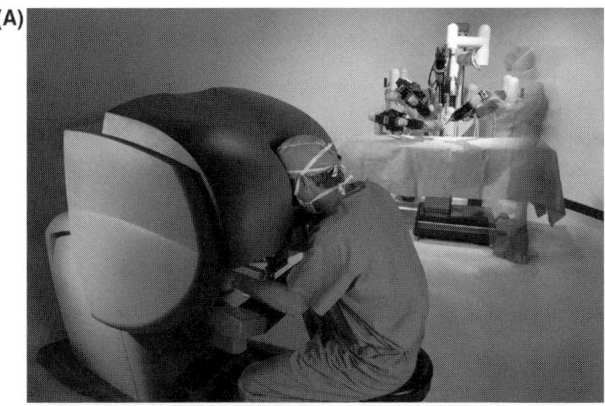

(B)

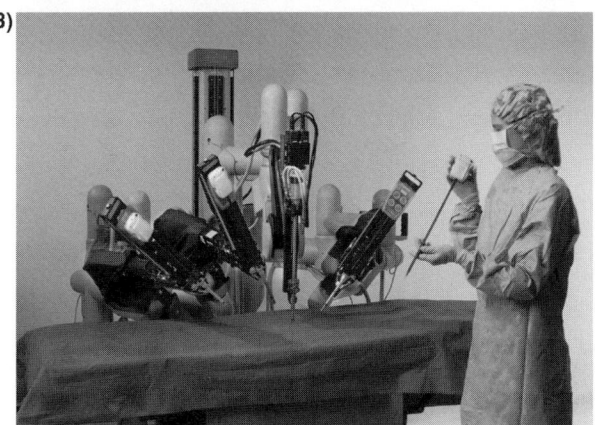

Figure 3 Da Vinci® surgical system. This device utilizes a telemanipulator workstation (**A**), and a remote computer assisted robotic device (**B**). *Source*: Photos courtesy of Intuitive Surgical, Inc., Sunnyvale, California, U.S.A.

demonstrated that robotic manipulations of surgical instruments could be precisely carried out, and that complete surgical procedures could be accomplished without complications. Several subsequent studies demonstrated that general surgical procedures can be performed successfully using telemanipulators (56–58).

More recently the Academic Robotics Group prospectively studied 211 robotically assisted operations in patients to assess the safety and utility of the FDA-approved *da Vinci*® robotic system (59). A variety of procedures were undertaken, including 69 antireflux operations, 36 cholecystectomies, and 26 Heller myotomies (59). Of direct interest to trauma surgery (although these were performed electively) included a variety of relevant procedures: 17 bowel resections, 15 donor nephrectomies, 14 left internal mammary artery mobilizations, seven splenectomies, six adrenalectomies, and three exploratory laparoscopies. There were eight (4%) technical complications, none of which caused harm to the patient, and only two of which required conversion to standard laparoscopy (none required open laparotomy). The robotic-assisted surgery was demonstrated to be safe and effective with expectation that the technology will rapidly expand into other realms (including urgent and remote assistance in surgery) (59).

The current version of the *da Vinci*® system allows seven degrees of freedom, and has improved stereoscopic (three dimension) visualization of the operative field. Although there is an initial steep learning curve (60,61), the development of the *da Vinci*® device, along with tools for laparoscopic splenectomy that isolate and seal the large blood vessels surrounding the spleen, have reduced intraoperative bleeding and minimized conversions to open splenectomy (62). Improvements in optics and instrumentation, as well as robotic technology, will further facilitate the acceptance of laparoscopic splenectomy (62) and increase the likelihood that these devices will someday be utilized in remote locations, and ultimately even in austere battlefield situations.

☞ **The theoretical goal of minimally invasive computer-assisted robotic techniques in trauma is that they will be applied in resuscitative (including damage-control) surgery as a potential method to stabilizing selected patients.** ☞ The drawback at the present time is that this technology is too slow for acute hemorrhage, and massive bleeding will likely eliminate visualization. In addition, the current technology requires high bandwidth in order to provide instantaneous throughput and to display real-time operative field visualizations. More safety and efficacy studies need to be conducted before these procedures can be initially used in trauma patients.

Telemedicine was recently utilized during the care of victims in the Indian Ocean Tsunami (Dec. 26, 2004), and was reported in a case involving a young tsunami victim who subsequently developed a brain abscess (63). A clinical-response team at the MGH was formed to work with Project HOPE (Health Opportunities for People Everywhere) volunteers along with the U.S. Navy Ship (U.S.N.S.) Mercy T-AH19 in Operation Unified Assistance, off the coast of Banda Aceh, Sumatra, Indonesia. The ability to transmit high-level digital images from the Navy ship to the conference of faculty in Boston, and for the clinicians in the Indian Ocean to engage in a real-time consultative conference with their Boston counterparts, helped make a diagnosis and formulate a plan of therapy (63).

Telemedicine can also be used for the follow-up of trauma patients. In a study done by Boulanger et al. in

Kentucky (64), 22 trauma patients (average ISS on admission of 18) were followed after discharge from a trauma center at a Teletrauma Clinic run by a registered nurse at a remote location via a T1 line and a videoconferencing system with multiple peripheral devices (cameras with macro lenses, electronic stethoscope, ENT scopes). Both surgeons and patients showed high degrees of satisfaction with this method of follow-up care, and there was a significant reduction of traveled miles by the patients for follow-up care.

CRITICAL CARE APPLICATIONS

As mentioned previously, the first example of telemedicine applied to critical care was published in Critical Care Medicine in 1982 (22). In that article, Dr. Grundy at Case Western Reserve University published an article reporting provision of daily consultations between university-based intensivists and a smaller inner city hospital without intensivists on staff via telemedicine. Rounds started at the nurse's station where the nurse reported directly to the intensivist. After reviewing each case, and if possible after interacting with the patient, recommendations were made. The outcomes measured were mortality and estimated patient disability at discharge. Considering the technology used in 1982, the results were quite good, with the system being functional 85% of the time. The system allowed the intensivist at Case Western to gather enough information to provide consultation, including physical findings (such as ventilatory chest patterns and mental status). In approximately 78% of the cases recommendations were made, although recommendations were carried out in only 30% of the cases. The investigators were able to demonstrate a correlation between increased survival rate and fewer disabilities in those cases in which the recommendations were carried out.

Data regarding telemedical applications in the ICU that are used continuously and interactively have recently entered the literature (65–68). Real-time bi-directional data and video conferencing using personal computers and a telephone access system allowed a group of University-affiliated intensivists, located at home, to monitor and manage from a distance a community-based teaching hospital 10-bed Surgical Intensive Care Unit. At the remote location, a roll-about videoconferencing unit was available and allowed the follow-up and management of patients by using video conferencing and computer-based data transmission. The study compared a 16-week period of study with seasonally matched adult patients from the previous year. The primary outcome measured was ICU and hospital mortality, and the secondary outcome was length of stay and costs. Every day an intensivist was responsible for the management of the ICU patients. Each day after reviewing all the data available, the intensivist formulated a plan and discussed this with the surgical team. Approximately every two hours after the initial assessment and plan, the intensivist reviewed all the available data for each patient and, if needed, changes were made by discussing the data with the available team. The study showed a statistically significant 68% reduction in APACHE III-adjusted ICU mortality and in-hospital mortality (34%), with a reduced number of ICU complications (44%) and a decreased length of stay in the ICU (30%) in the experimental group. Additionally, this study showed a 33% reduction in total ICU costs. The most likely cause of reduced mortality is attributed to the decreased number of adverse effects associated to medical errors.

One of the earliest efforts to apply the concepts of telemedicine to critically ill patients was developed by Breslow and Rosenfeld in 1998 with the founding of a venture-backed company, VISICU, Inc. (Baltimore, MD). A recent study from Sentara Health System in Virginia utilizing a telemedicine system provided by VISICU provides insight into the future of critical care (67). The study included more than 600 patients discharged from 16 ICU beds during a six-month period. These units included a general ICU (10 beds) and a vascular ICU (six beds), which were wired into a remote VISICU monitoring site (eICU). This system permitted the remote intensivist not only to detect deviations from normal or early pathology at the beginning of a disease process, but also to make interventions that otherwise would have to wait for the physical presence of a physician in the ICU (i.e., weaning mechanical ventilation during the night or making adjustment in medications).

The study compared patients discharged from the same units before the implementation of this new system to the cohort cared for with the new system. The study showed a 30% reduction in the mortality rate in the ICU, which represents approximately 60 lives saved per year or one person per week. The study also showed a 17% average reduction in length of stay for both the ICU and subsequent recovery on a regular floor. The added benefit of the system implemented is that, despite the initial expense, it produced an annualized net financial benefit of approximately three million U.S. dollars. These savings included an increased patient turnover rate (20%) secondary to the reduction of ICU days and increased number of patients admitted to the ICU.

In a more recent study by Breslow et al. a total of 2140 patients receiving eICU care for 19 hr/day were evaluated with similar positive results (69). The remote care program used intensivists and physician extenders to provide supplemental monitoring and management of ICU patients for 19 hr/day (noon to 7 am) from a centralized, off-site facility (eICU). ☞ **The addition of supplemental, telemedicine-based, remote intensivist programs has been associated with both improved clinical outcomes and hospital financial performance.** ☞ The magnitude of the improvements was similar to those reported in studies examining the impact of implementing on-site dedicated intensivist staffing models.

FINANCIAL AND LEGAL CONSIDERATIONS
Centers for Medicare and Medicaid Services (Previously HCFA) Requirements

As of 1999, the Health Care Financing Administration (HCFA and now CMS) started reimbursing physicians for telemedical care for Medicare patients, though the acceptable reimbursable conditions are restricted to only a few specific conditions. These include: that the patient must be located in a rural area, that the referring physician must be present, and that part of the reimbursement that the consultant physician receives needs to be remitted to the referring physician. The type of technology used is limited only to real-time interactions and excludes store-and-forward technology. However, effective as of October 2001, Medicare has expanded its coverage of telemedicine services to include broader geographical areas and physician services (70).

On the other hand, some health insurance providers have seen the benefits of the use of telemedicine and have started reimbursing for some telemedicine services, and in some states laws have been passed that require reimbursement of telemedicine services. ☞ **Effective as of October 2001, Medicare has expanded its coverage of telemedicine services to include broader geographical areas and physician services (70).** ☞

Medical Guidelines and Technical Standards

Guidelines help physicians by being tools that help in decision-making in improving patient's outcomes. The establishment of telemedicine guidelines has the additional benefit of being a framework that offers better quality and improves these systems during their early development (operational and technical guidelines), facilitates the establishment of clinical research, and reduces risk of litigation. At present, there are very few clinical telemedicine guidelines applicable to trauma care. These include limited guidelines for the handling of emergencies that the British Association for Accident and Emergency Medicine has established (71). These guidelines cover teleconsultation protocols, drugs use, radiographic evaluation, and management protocols, and applies to all minor injury units linked to their nearest Accident and Emergency facility.

Establishing technical standards has also become very important. The available standards for telemedicine techniques are based on the definition of the International Telecommunication Union (ITU) for videoconferencing, including the H.320 standard using ISDN and the more recent H.323 standard using IP networks (72). Another set of standards are included in the DICOM standard (Digital Imaging and Communications in Medicine) widely recognized for medical imaging communication (transmission of X-ray images and other medical image types). DICOM defines a standard network interface and data model allowing interoperability between equipment from different manufacturers. Interoperability using standards will facilitate telemedicine growth, whereas proprietary systems serve as short term solutions, but limit growth over the long term.

Legal Aspects

Most of the legal aspects of telemedicine include licensure of physicians, hospital credentialing, clinical privileges, patient confidentiality, and liability. This is not different when applied to trauma and intensive care.

Universal clinical privileges do not exist in the U.S. In some cases, some state licensure statutes have provisions that allow a licensed physician to request consult from an out-of-state physician. Unfortunately most licensure boards do not allow practicing out-of-state physicians to provide telemedicine services unless they hold a valid license for that state. Moreover, this is not a problem exclusive to physicians but also to nurses, physician assistants, and nurse practitioners. There have been several attempts to address this problem but they have been unsuccessful to date. ☞ **The Joint Commission on Accreditation of Hospitals (JCAHO) has recently dictated a requirement of credentialing in hospitals, which are establishing telemedicine care.** ☞ The physician that practices in that institution, via telemedicine or not, needs to go through the process of credentialing approved for the institution.

Patient confidentially must also be addressed and maintained. The regulation of transmission of information and establishing protocols that keep information safe and confidential, especially the information sent over e-mail and through internet access, is crucial to maintain the success of this technology.

Liability is also another issue that has affected the development of telemedicine technology in the areas of trauma and critical care. This is especially true in the area where more patient-physician interactions have been particularly significant, and for high risk conditions where prompt and accurate diagnoses are most critical. Interestingly, new technologies (e.g., real-time interactive videoconference) could conceivably decrease liability if full consensus is gathered from the group, even if it later turns out not be the best choice.

MILITARY CONSIDERATIONS
Initial Trauma Medevac and Resuscitation

The ongoing wars in both Afghanistan and Iraq have once again placed the U.S. military at the forefront of the telemedicine revolution. Ranging from the conveyance of patient information between far-forward positions and more sophisticated levels of medical care to the tactical decision making regarding site location for forward surgical teams, etc., the Department of Defense (DoD) has put into place a series of telemedicine systems.

☞ **Much more can and must be done to utilize current technological capabilities to improve medical communication between levels of care.** ☞ These capabilities can assist providers with both the transfer of information as well assisting those providers with the expertise of medical experts in the initial management of complex wartime casualties.

Currently the bulk of initial care provided to U.S. and Coalition forces is done at Level I and II Medical Treatment Facilities (MTFs) which are often located in very isolated and austere environments (see Volume 1, Chapter 5). Rapid telecommunication systems are in place that allow providers at these locations to request and obtain the assistance of more experienced and seasoned personnel for the initial triage and treatment of these casualties. This is mostly in the form of secure satellite communication systems, but can also include technology as simple as cellular phones (when discussed information is not necessarily privileged). Although the technology now exists, the use of video conferencing between the level II [Army Forward Surgical Team (FST) or Marine Forward Resuscitative Surgery System (FRSS)] MTFs, and the higher level III Combat Support Hospital (CSH) is not yet available in most austere environments. Accordingly providers in these locations have had to adapt and change as the battle space evolved.

Communications Between Levels of Care for Patient Transport

Logistics communications between MTFs at various levels of care is of the highest quality, thus casualty evacuation (casevac) and patient transport is highly coordinated. The reader can review current methodologies involving casevac to a FST or FRSS (level II MTF) or to a CSH (Level III MTF) and the use of U.S. Air Force Critical Care Air Transport Teams (CCATTs) in Volume 1, Chapter 7. However, transmission of patient management information from the initial level II field surgery facility to the next level of care, often a level IV facility, can still improve, though improvements have occurred during the campaigns in Iraq and Afghanistan.

As recently as one to two years ago, the mechanism for sending injured soldier medical information between the

FST or FRSS and higher levels of care was provided by writing brief descriptions of operative findings on transfer papers, and by writing directly on the patient's skin or bandages (as shown in Volume 1, Chapter 7). Although this practice is helpful, and continues, the development of the Combat Trauma Record (a simple two page document) has significantly improved the transfer of information. In addition, several new-technology-based techniques have been employed by industrious military physicians and core men to obtain and package digital information to be transported with the patient. For example, digital photos of wounds and operative findings, are now routinely placed on transportable digital media and transferred with the wounded soldier to the next level of care.

Because the digital media can become lost or destroyed during transport, an additional improvement in care would occur if the digital data were transmitted digitally in real time to high capacity servers for storage, along with real-time relay of information to the expected destination. Dedicating portions of the satellite bandwidth for real-time video and voice conferencing and transmission of radiographs via PACS, etc. is another important idea that could improve care.

As patients are subsequently moved through the evacuation chain, more sophisticated means of telemedicine are now being utilized. Weekly patient care conferences as well as weekly morbidity and mortality conferences are held via real-time video teleconferencing between Iraq, Germany, and military medical facilities within the continental United States. These real-time, interactive events have greatly enhanced patient care and facilitated feedback to providers in the field who in the past never had feedback on the patients they initially helped stabilize, treat, and operate upon.

As discussed above, these sophisticated telemedicine devices come at a price, and that is the bandwidth required to achieve them. This is of particular concern in the military as medical providers are often at odds with the war-fighters over access to limited bandwidth. With improved technology and communication systems there will hopefully come a time where both the medical community and the operational forces will have unlimited access to real-time bandwidth which will allow the simultaneous care of patients as well as the ability to execute the military campaign.

EYE TO THE FUTURE

The greatest technical problem inhibiting the growth of telemedicine today is the lack of cost-effective, dependable technology with enough bandwidth to transmit the amount of information needed for acute care in real-time. Wider availability of high-speed fiber optic lines and even satellite communications will facilitate not only the diffusion and use of existing technologies but the development and application of advanced technological telemedicine modalities, like the use of telepresence technology. The development of new networks systems like Second Generation Internet (SGI) may solve some of these problems. Current technologies such as global position satellites (GPS) can help locate EMS personnel and transport devices, facilitating more efficient deployment. The application of artificial intelligence to supplement technological advances will likely lead to the next breakthrough in medical applications (74).

Another area where advancement will occur is in the realm of distant anesthetic management of trauma and critically ill patients. Indeed a recent report from Virginia Commonwealth University (VCU) shared anesthetic management decision-making between the home institution and Ecuador (75). Airway management, dysrhythmias, and oxygen saturation-related decision-making was made from the distant location over a 64 kbps satellite linked data line.

Public and health care perception must also improve, especially for the application of remote care systems in emergency situations such as trauma and critical care. Additional studies are needed. These studies should include standard outcomes as well as patient, family, and provider satisfaction data.

Regulations will continue to limit advancement of this field. Federal and private reimbursement issues will need to be continually addressed. In order to promote that change in mentality, more research needs to be done to study the cost-effectiveness of the application of telemedicine techniques when compared to conventional trauma and critical care.

The gaps between bench discovery and bedside application must continue. Those who focus on implementing the enormous capabilities of digital technologies in the realm of trauma and critical care will close an important technology gap. It must be recognized that initial systems will require significant capital outlay, but will return a priceless dividend of lives and limbs saved.

SUMMARY

Optimal care to trauma and critically ill patients requires an organized approach with dedicated resources delivered by specialty-trained professionals. Telemedicine applications in trauma and critical care are being developed and studied. At present, limited research exists to support a wholesale adoption of this technology. Based on presently available data, telemedicine has incredible untapped potential for augmenting care in emergency circumstances, especially in the areas of trauma in critical care and in the follow-up of that care. Regionalization of care and application of these technologies is beginning to demonstrate significant advantages to remote locations and those that are otherwise understaffed with specialized health care providers. It is quite encouraging that the presently limited available data from application of these technologies into the ICU has been able to demonstrate improvement in the quality of care while reducing costs and resource utilization. These improvements have been realized despite the usual steep learning curve and, in many circumstances, limited resources.

Telemedicine has been used in many instances for education, image transfer, second opinions, consultative care, and direct acute care. In these domains there is growing evidence that these systems are effective at improving care to patients located in remote areas. Clearly, more work needs to be done to improve not only the technological aspects of telemedicine but also the human aspects of delivering this type of care, at the practitioner, organizational, and governmental levels.

Some have likened the use of outside physicians for night-time coverage (e.g., NightHawk radiological oversight) of patients as a form of outsourcing (73). Yet, in many cases the doctors serving in foreign countries are U.S. trained, or possess a similar level of certification. American radiology departments will likely rely in increasing numbers on NightHawk services from foreign countries, because as one hemisphere of the globe sleeps the other is awake; hence, a natural reciprocation of responsibilities avails itself. The next critical element in wider utilization of these services rests in the realm of certification and credentialing. Providing levels of training and oversight (quality control) are similar within institutions; distant radiologists or other physicians should be capable of providing the same level of care. A system of reciprocity is being developed to confirm that levels of expertise are at a high level for those making diagnosis from distant shores.

The establishment of accepted standards including medico-legal and regulatory issues need to be accomplished in order to have a working and efficient system. The future of these systems seems to grow in potential importance given the shortage of specialty-trained physicians like intensivists and the present trend for fewer surgical trainees to enter specialty training tracks. Given the lack of availability of specialty-trained physician groups in remote areas, health care decision makers should be strongly embracing telemedical approaches to better leverage care by such highly skilled and trained individuals.

KEY POINTS

✍ The regionalization of trauma care has improved overall outcome, but not solved the significant problem of providing high-level trauma and critical care services to remote locations where organized trauma systems do not exist.

✍ A potential solution to delivering trauma and critical care to remote locations and to address shortages of subspecialty-trained physicians is the use of telemedicine.

✍ Military research has helped develop many aspects of telemedicine, and the direct applications to both military and civilian care are enormous.

✍ Computer-assisted surgical robotics is a technological area whose immense potential will likely facilitate telemedicine applications for trauma in the near future.

✍ Telemedicine connects two physically separated locations (which can be positioned anywhere on the globe), and facilitates the sharing of clinical information between health care providers (or between patient and provider) for the diagnosis and or management of medical and surgical conditions.

✍ Telemedicine can be used in a variety of situations from consultative care, triage, and direct patient care, to image transfer and continuing medical education.

✍ The specific computer-based elements needed for each telemedicine application varies, but when dealing with trauma or critically ill patients, the system requires capability to handle real-time, synchronous interactive videoconference.

✍ The main characteristic that defines the quantity of data that can be transmitted over a line or other medium is bandwidth.

✍ The role of trauma leader can be safely provided by a traumatologist not physically present in the TRS in locations where the trauma training of individuals is insufficient, but telecommunication understanding is adequate (36).

✍ The application of telepresence in trauma surgery has evolved to include use of the *Da Vinci*® system computer-assisted robotics.

✍ The theoretical goal of minimally invasive computer-assisted robotic techniques in trauma is that they will be applied in resuscitative (including damage-control) surgery as a potential method to stabilizing selected patients.

✍ The addition of supplemental, telemedicine-based, remote intensivist programs has been associated with both improved clinical outcomes and hospital financial performance.

✍ Effective as of October 2001, Medicare has expanded its coverage of telemedicine services to include broader geographical areas and physician services (70).

✍ The Joint Commission on Accreditation of Hospitals (JCAHO) has recently dictated a requirement of credentialing in hospitals, which are establishing telemedicine care.

✍ Much more can and must be done to utilize current technological capabilities to improve medical communication between levels of care.

REFERENCES

1. National Research Council. Accidental death and disability: The neglected disease of modern society. Washington, D.C.: National Academy of Sciences, 1966.
2. Committee on Trauma, American College of Surgeons. Optimal hospital resources for care of the seriously injured. Bull Am College Surgeons 1976; 61(9):15–22.
3. Celso B, Tepas J, Langland-Orban B, et al. A systematic review and meta-analysis comparing outcome of severely injured patients treated in trauma centers following the establishment of trauma systems. J Trauma 2006; 60(2):371–378.
4. Rogers FB, Simons R, Hoyt DB, et al. In-house board-certified surgeons improve outcome for severely injured patients: a comparison of two university centers. Trauma 1993; 34(6):871–875.
5. Mullins RJ, Veum-Stone J, Hedges JR, et al. Influence of a state-wide trauma system on location of hospitalization and outcome of injured patients. Trauma 1996; 40:536–546.
6. Vincent JL. Need for intensivists in intensive-care units. Lancet 2000; 356:695–696.
7. Blunt MC, Burchett KR. Out-of-hours consultant cover and case-mix-adjusted mortality in intensive care. Lancet 2000; 2000(356):735–736.
8. Pronovost PJ, Jenckes MW, Dorman T, Garrett E, Breslow MJ, Rosenfeld BA, et al. Organizational characteristics of intensive care units related to outcomes of abdominal aortic surgery. JAMA 1999; 291:1310–1317.
9. Pronovost PJ, Waters J, Dorman T. Impact of critical care physician workforce for intensive care unit physician staffing. Curr Opin Crit Care 2001; 7(6):456–459.
10. Pronovost PJ, Angus DC, Dorman T, Robinson KA, Dremsizov TT, Young TL. Physician staffing patterns and clinical outcomes in critically ill patients: a systematic review. JAMA 2000; 288(17):2151–2162.
11. U.S. Congress Office of Technology Assessment. Rural Emergency Medical Services: Special Report. OTA-H-445. 1989.
12. Rogers FB, Shackford SR, Osler TM, Vane DW, Davis JH. Rural trauma: the challenge for the next decade. Trauma 1999; 47(4):802–821.
13. Holcomb JB, Stansbury LG, Champion HR, et al. Understanding combat casualty care statistics. J Trauma 2006; 60(2):397–401.
14. Ovadia P, Szewczyk D, Walker K, Abdullah F, Schmidt-Gillespie S, Rabinovici R. Admission patterns of an urban level I trauma center. Am J Med Qual 2000; 15:9–15.
15. Groeger JS, Strosberg MA, Halpern NA, et al. Descriptive analysis of critical care units in the United States. Crit Care Med 1992; 20:846–863.

16. Angus DC, Kelley MA, Schmitz RJ, et al. Current and projected workforce requirements for care of the critically ill and patients with pulmonary disease. JAMA 2000; 284:2762–2770.

17. Abbruscato CR. A brief history of the telestethoscope. Telemedicine 1997; 6(5):16.

18. Crump WJ, Pfeil T. A telemedicine primer: an introduction to the technology and an overview of the literature. Arch Family Med 1995; 4(9):796–803.

19. Allely EB. Synchronous and asynchronous telemedicine. J Med Syst 1995; 19:20.

20. Ausseresses AD. Telecommunications requirements for telemedicine. J Med Syst 1995; 19:143.

21. Goldberg MA. Teleradiology and telemedicine. Radiol Clin North Am 1996; 34(3):647–665.

22. Grundy BL, Jones PK, Lovitt A. Telemedicine in critical care: problems in design, implementation, and assessment. Crit Care Med 1982; 10:471–475.

23. Angood PB. Telemedicine, the Internet, and world wide web: overview, current status and relevance to surgeons. World J Surg 2001; 25:1449–1457.

24. Cleary K, Nguyen C. State of the art in surgical robotics: clinical applications and technology challenges. Computer Aided Surgeon 2001; 6(6):312–328.

25. Makris L, Kopsacheillis EV, Strintzis MG. Hippocrates: an integrated platform for telemedicine applications. Med Inform 1998; 23:265.

26. Swart D. The Saint Francis emergency room telemedicine system: marriage of technology and business models. Telemed Today 1997; 5:28–29.

27. Armstrong IJ, Haston WS. Medical decision support for remote general practitioner using telemedicine. J Telemed Telecare 1997; 1:27–34.

28. Tachakra S, Sivakumar A, Everand R, Mullett S, Freij R. Remote trauma management setting up a system. J Telemed Telecare 1996; 2:65–68.

29. Beach M, Goodall J, Miller P. Evaluating telemedicine for minor injuries units. J Telemed Telecare 2000; 6(1):90–92.

30. Tachakra S, Loane M, Uche CU. A follow-up study of remote trauma teleconsultations. J Telemed Telecare 2000; 6(330): 334.

31. Patterson VH, Craig JJ, Wootoon R. Effective diagnosis of spinal cord compression using telemedicine. Br J Neurosurg 2000; 14:552–554.

32. Aucar JA, Villavicencio RT, Wall MJ, Liscum KR, Granchi TS, Mattox KL. Evaluation of clinical data by remote observation in trauma. Proc AMIA Ann Fall Symp 1997; S68:408–412.

33. Aucar, et al. Evaluation of clinical data by remote observation in trauma. AMIA 1999; 25:617–623.

34. Brebner JA, Ruddick-Brakken H, et al. Evaluation of a pilot telemedicine network for accident and emergency work. J Telemed Telecare 2002; 8:5–6.

35. Xiao Y, MacKenzie C, Orasanu J, Spencer R, Rahman A, Gunawardane V. Information acquisition from audio-video-data sources: an experimental study on remote diagnosis. Telemedicine 1999; 2:139–155.

36. Tachakra S, Jaye P, Bak J, Hayes J, Sivakumar A. Supervising trauma life support by telemedicine. J Audiovisual Medica Medicine 2000; 6(S1):7–11.

37. Tachakra S, Lynch M, Stinson A, et al. A pilot study of the technical quality of telemedical consultations for remote trauma management. J Audiovisual Media Medicine 2001; 24:16–20.

38. Aucar JA, Eastlack R, Wall MJ, et al. Remote clinical assessment for acute trauma: an initial experience. Proc AMIA Symp 1998; 550:396–400.

39. Rogers FB, Ricci M, Caputo MSS, et al. The use of telemedicine for real-time video consultation between trauma center and community hospital in a rural setting improves early trauma care: preliminary results. Trauma 2001; 51:1037–1041.

40. Lambrecht CJ, Canham WD, Gattey PH, McKenzie GM. Telemedicine and orthopaedic care. Clin Orthopaedics Related Research 1998; 348:228–232.

41. Lambrecht CJ. Telemedicine in trauma care: description of 100 trauma teleconsults. Telemedicine 1997; 3:265–268.

42. Lambrecht CJ. Telemedicine in trauma care. Telemedicine Today 1998; 6(1):25.

43. Brennan JA, Kealy JA, Gerardi LH, Shih R, Allegra J, Sannipoli L, et al. Telemedicine in the emergency department: a randomized controlled trial. Telemedicine Today 1999; 5:18–22.

44. Latifi R, Peck K, Porter JM, et al. Telepresence and telemedicine in trauma and emergency care management. Stud Health Technol Inrom 2004; 104:193–199.

45. Saffle JR, Edelman L, Morris SE: Regional air transport of burn patients: a case for telemedicine? J Trauma 2004; 57(1): 57–64.

46. Kirkpatrick AW, Brenneman FD, McCallum A, et al. Prospective evaluation of the potential role of teleradiology in acute interhospital trauma referrals. Trauma 1999; 46:1017.

47. Hsieh C-H, Jeng S-F, Chen C-Y, et al. Teleconsultation with mobile camera-phone in remote evaluation of replantation potential. J Trauma 2005; 58(6):1208–1212.

48. Link RE, Schulam PG, Kavoussi LR. Remote monitoring and assistance during laparoscopy. Urol Clin North Am 2001; 28:177–178.

49. Cadeddu JA, Stoianovici D, Kavoussi LR. Robotic surgery in urology. Urol Clin North Am 1998; 25:75–85.

50. Rassweiler J, Binder J, Frede T. Robotic and telesurgery: will they change our future? Curr Opin Urol 2001; 11(3): 309–320.

51. Schlag PM, Moesta KT, Rakovsky S, Graschew G. Telemedicine: the new must for surgery. Arch Surg 1999; 134:1216–1221.

52. Cadiere GB, Himpens J, Vertruyen M, Favretti F. The world's first obesity surgery performed by a surgeon at a distance. Obes Surg 1999; 9:206–209.

53. Cubano M, Poulose BK, Talamini MA, et al. Long distance telementoring: a novel tool for laparoscopy aboard the USS Abraham Lincoln. Surg Endosc 1999; 13(7):673–678.

54. Endean ED, Mallon LI, Kwolek CJ, Schwartz TH. Telemedicine in vascular surgery: Does it work? Am Surg 2001; 67: 334–341.

55. Bowersox JC, Cordts PR, LaPorta AJ. Use of an intuitive telemanipulator system for remote trauma surgery: an experimental study. Am Coll Surg 1998; 186:615–621.

56. Bowersox JC, Shah A, Jensen J, Hill J, et al. Vascular applications of telepresence surgery: initial feasibility studies in swine. Vasc Surg 1996; 23:281–287.

57. Shennib H, Bastawisy A, McLoughlin J, Moll F. Robotic computer assisted telemanipulation enhances coronary artery bypass. Thorc Cardiovasc Surg 1999; 117:310–313.

58. Talamini MA, Campbell K, Stanfield C. Robotic gastrointestinal surgery: early experience and system description. Laparoendosc Adv Surg Tech A 2002; 12(4):225–223.

59. Talamini MA, Chapman S, Horgan S, Melvin WS. The Academic Robotics Group. A prospective analysis of 211 robotic-assisted surgical procedures. Surg Endosc 2003; 17(10):1521–1524.

60. Hernandez JD, Bann SD, Munz Y, et al. The learning curve of a simulated surgical task using the *Da Vinci* telemanipulator system. Br J Surg 2002; 89:17–18.

61. Hernandez JD, Bann SD, Munz Y, et al. Qualitative and quantitative analysis of the learning curve of a simulated surgical task on the *Da Vinci* system. Surg Endosc 2004; 18:372–378.

62. Bellows CF, Sweeney JF. Laparoscopic splenectomy: present status and future perspective. Expert Rev Med Dev 2006; 3(1): 95–104.

63. Kao AY, Munandar R, Ferrara SL, et al. Case 19-2005—A 17-year-old girl with respiratory distress and hemiparesis after surviving a tsunami. N Engl J Med 2005; 352:2628–2636.

64. Boulanger B, Kearney P, Ochoa J, et al. Telemedicine: a solution to the follow-up of rural trauma patients? J AM Coll Surg 2001; 192:447–452.

65. Dorman T. Remote access to critical care. Curr Opin Crit Care 2000; 6(4):304–307.

66. Rosenfeld BA, Dorman T, Breslow MJ, et al. Intensive care unit telemedicine: alternate paradigm for providing continuous intensivist care. Crit Care Med 2000; 28(12): 3925–3931.

67. Becker C. Remote Control. Specialists are running intensive-care units from remote sites via computers, and at least one health system with the eICU is reaping financial rewards—and saving lives. Mod Health 2002; 32(8):40–42.

68. Celi LA, Hassan E, Marquardt C, Breslow M, Rosenfeld B. The eICU: it's not just telemedicine. Crit Care Med 2001; 8:N183–N189.

69. Breslow MJ, Rosenfeld BA, Doerfler M, et al. Effect of a multiple-site intensive care unit telemedicine program on clinical and economic outcomes: an alternate paradigm for intensivist staffing. Crit Care Med 2004; 32:31–38.

70. http://cms.hhs.gov/state/telelist.asp

71. http://www.baem.org.uk/tele.htm

72. http://www.itu.int/itudoc/itu-t/rec/h/h320.html

73. Wachter RM: The "Dis-location" of U.S. Medicine—The implications of medical outsourcing. N Engl J Med 2006; 354:661–665.

74. Hanson WC, Marshall BE: Artificial intelligence applications in the intensive care unit. Crit Care Med 2001; 29(2):427–435.

75. Cone SW, Gehr L, Hummel R, et al. Case report of remote anesthetic monitoring using telemedicine. Anesth Analg 2004; 98:386–388.

73

Hyperbaric Oxygen Therapy in Trauma and Critical Care

Enrico M. Camporesi

Department of Anesthesiology and Critical Care, University of South Florida College of Medicine, Tampa, Florida, U.S.A.

Irving "Jake" Jacoby

Hyperbaric Medicine Center, Department of Emergency Medicine, UC San Diego Medical Center, San Diego, California, U.S.A.

INTRODUCTION

Hyperbaric oxygen (HBO$_2$) therapy is a growing specialty in medicine that overlaps many other specialties due to the ever-increasing understanding of the numerous physiologic effects of O$_2$ under pressure. The increasing elucidation of HBO$_2$ mechanisms of action has increased the therapeutic application of this treatment by specially trained physicians around the globe. This chapter provides an overview of HBO$_2$ therapy, including the basic science, physiology, and the clinical indications relevant to the fields of trauma and critical care.

Hyperbaric medicine is a relatively new field of medicine that has been recently reviewed from a historical perspective (1). However, a couple landmark developments deserve special note. Its beginnings were in non-scientifically-based air compression chambers, starting in the 17th century. Initial treatments for Caisson's Disease during the construction of underwater tunnels in New York City and in Europe were with compressed air. Several unusual large chambers were built in the early 20th century, including the 6-story high "Steel Ball Hospital," built by Cunningham in Cleveland (1,2). This edifice did not survive, however, due to lack of scientific grounding in indications and procedures at that time.

Modern HBO$_2$ therapy had its beginnings in 1955 with the work of Churchill–Davidson, who attempted to use HBO$_2$ to potentiate radiation therapy in cancer patients (3), and with Boerema, at the University of Amsterdam, who during that same year proposed using HBO$_2$ in cardiac surgery to prolong tolerance of circulatory arrest by patients (4). It was a logical step for Brummelkamp at the University of Amsterdam to consider the possibility of inhibiting anaerobic infections with O$_2$ under pressure, and the first published report of use of HBO$_2$ for gas gangrene was reported in 1961 (5). Treatment of carbon monoxide (CO) poisoning was also first reported in 1961 (6).

Since that time, hyperbaric medicine has developed into a full-fledged medical discipline, with specialty journals, fellowships, and board certification for physicians within the last decade. The Hyperbaric Therapy Committee of the Undersea and Hyperbaric Medical Society (UHMS) meets and reviews all submitted indications for HBO$_2$ therapy, and that list is updated approximately every three years (7). There are currently 13 UHMS-approved indications for HBO$_2$ therapy (Table 1).

GENERAL PRINCIPLES

☞ **HBO$_2$ therapy is defined as the therapeutic administration of O$_2$ at pressures greater than one atmosphere at sea level.** ☞ One atmosphere of pressure, expressed in millimeters of mercury (mmHg), corresponds to 760 mmHg, and in units of atm abs, "atmospheres absolute," units commonly used in HBO$_2$ therapy, is 1 atm abs. The concentration of O$_2$ in air is approximately 21%, therefore, the partial pressure of dry O$_2$ (PO$_2$) is 160 mmHg at 1 atm abs (0.21 × 760 mmHg = 160 mmHg). The remaining component (79% of air) is mainly Nitrogen (N$_2$) and other trace inert gases. Together, they exert a partial pressure of approximately 600 mmHg at 1 atm abs (0.79 × 760 mmHg = 600 mmHg). The partial pressure of water vapor (P$_{H_2O}$) in air is variable and depends on both temperature and humidity. At 37°C and 100% humidity, conditions commonly found in the lung, P$_{H_2O}$ is 47 mmHg. This value is unchanged at 2 and at 3 atm.

The PO$_2$ in dry air is increased to approximately 479 mmHg when the pressure is raised to 3 atm abs (3 × 760 mmHg × 0.21 = 479 mmHg). If the concentration of O$_2$ is then increased to 100%, PO$_2$ at 3 atm abs increases approximately to 2280 mmHg (3 × 760 mmHg × 1.00 = 2280 mmHg).

In the alveoli, carbon dioxide (CO$_2$) as well as H$_2$O vapor is added to inspired gases, reducing the initial partial pressure of any inspired gas to the alveolar level. The typical alveolar partial pressure of CO$_2$ (P$_{ACO_2}$) is 40 mmHg and is usually closely regulated by subjects and patients around this value, despite changing the ambient pressure. The alveolar P$_{H_2O}$, as mentioned above, is unchanged at 47 mmHg. By using the "alveolar gas equation" one can calculate approximate alveolar partial pressures of O$_2$ (P$_{AO_2}$), at various chamber pressures:

$$P_{AO_2} = (P_B - P_{H_2O}) \, FI_{O_2} - P_{ACO_2},$$

where P$_B$ = ambient pressure or chamber pressure, FI$_{O_2}$ = fractional concentration of inspired O$_2$ and the approximation is represented by the assumption that the respiratory quotient is equal to 1. P$_{AO_2}$ is usually 110 mmHg while breathing air at 1 atm abs [P$_{AO_2}$ = (760 − 47)0.21 − 40 = 110] and increases to 2193 mmHg while breathing 100% O$_2$ at 3 atm abs [P$_{AO_2}$ = (2280 − 47)1.00 − 40 = 2193].

While the P$_{AO_2}$ increases in proportion to the increase in ambient pressure, the arterial PO$_2$ (Pa$_{O_2}$) will vary according

Table 1   Undersea and Hyperbaric Medical Society Approved Indications for Hyperbaric Oxygen Therapy

Decompression sickness
Air or gas embolism
Carbon monoxide poisoning alone or complicated by cyanide
    poisoning
Clostridial myositis and myonecrosis (gas gangrene)
Crush injury, compartment syndrome and other acute traumatic
    ischemias
Enhancement of healing in selected problem wounds
Exceptional anemia
Intracranial abscess
Nonclostridial necrotizing soft tissue infections
Chronic refractory osteomyelitis
Delayed effects of radiation (soft tissue- and osteo-radionecrosis)
Threatened skin grafts and flaps
Thermal burns

Source: From Refs. 7 and 61.

Table 2   Approximate Values of Alveolar Oxygen Pressure, After Correction for Water Vapor Pressure and CO_2 Pressure, Assuming a Respiratory Quotient of 0.8

Environmental pressure (atm abs)	Alveolar PO_2 (mmHg) breathing air (21% O_2)	Alveolar PO_2 (mmHg) breathing 100% O_2
1	102	673
2	262	1433
3	422	2193

to the degree of pulmonary dysfunction present. The [a/A] O_2 ratio has been utilized and verified in healthy subjects and in patients with varying pulmonary problems as a predictor of arterial oxygenation at increased inspired oxygen concentrations up to 2.8 atm abs (8). When arterial O_2 tension (PaO_2) approaches 1200 mmHg, about 4% vol of O_2 are dissolved in plasma and can provide for the total metabolic requirements of the tissues. The oxygen dissolved in plasma diffuses first from the capillaries, and constitutes the majority of the (a–v) difference required by tissue consumption.

☞ **Treatment with HBO$_2$ is empirically limited to a maximum tolerated inspired PO$_2$ and the total time of exposure.** ☞ Normally 100% O_2 is administered at pressures no greater than 3 atm abs ($PO_2 = 2280$) and only for intervals no longer than 20–25 min. "Air breaks," intermittent periods of air breathing, of 5 to 10 min, are administered between intervals if therapy is required to exceed these times. Air breaks reduce periodically the inspired PO_2, thereby minimizing the acute onset of central nervous system O_2 toxicity and delaying the development of pulmonary O_2 toxicity. Some typical values commonly found in a hyperbaric environment are summarized in Table 2.

MULTIPLACE VS. MONOPLACE HYPERBARIC CHAMBERS

The traditional method of administering HBO$_2$ therapy is with a multiplace chamber that accommodates two or more individuals. Size may vary from small, often portable two-man chambers used for transporting patients in the field, to several feet in diameter, in which up to a dozen or more patients may be comfortably admitted, in addition to tenders, nurses, and physicians. This type of multiplace chamber is usually compressed with air, while the patient breathes oxygen either with a head tent, facemask, or through a tracheal tube. ☞ **Because of the immediate access to the patient by accompanying personnel, monitoring is commonly simplified with multiplace HBO$_2$ chambers.** ☞ Intravenous lines can be inserted at any time during treatment and airway control can be provided. Surgery has even been performed inside multiplace hyperbaric chambers. On the other hand, setting up and

maintaining these chambers is complex. They have a large space requirement for installation and are costly.

The other type of chamber is the monoplace. This type of chamber is large enough to accommodate only one patient. The chamber wall in several types is manufactured of clear plastic, facilitating close observation of the patient. The chamber is compressed with 100% O_2. The advantage of monoplace chambers is their relatively low cost and ease of installation. The chamber may be put into use by connecting the oxygen inlet to the hospital supply, with modification to accommodate large flow rates. Operation of the chamber is relatively simple. The disadvantage is the lower flexibility and the treatment pressure range, which most often cannot exceed 3 atm abs. Inside a monoplace chamber monitoring is more remote, and emergency care of the airway cannot be provided. ☞ **Development of a tension pneumothorax, although rare, could be fatal in a monoplace chamber because of the impossibility of inserting a chest tube prior to decompression.** ☞ Nevertheless, monoplace technology now permits intravenous fluid administration from the outside of the chamber, invasive intravascular monitoring, and mechanical ventilation. Most chambers are now equipped with a mask system (called BIBS or "built in breathing system") from which the patient may breath air and receive air breaks. Critically ill patients can routinely be treated in monoplace chambers if the experience of the personnel warrants it.

TRAUMA AND HBO$_2$

HBO$_2$ can be utilized in the treatment of several clinical situations associated with acute trauma. Therapy with HBO$_2$ is effective by elevating total pressure in body compartments in gas embolic disease and increasing oxygen tensions in blood and tissues. Of particular note is the possibility of pulmonary venous emboli that can occur following both penetrating and severe blunt thoracic trauma. The institution of HBO$_2$ therapy in this patient population is complicated due to the other common competing problems. However, in the case of severe pulmonary venous air entry and subsequent systemic arterial embolization to important structures (e.g., brain, heart, and other viscera), HBO$_2$ therapy can be life saving.

In addition, HBO$_2$ exposure has been associated with intense vasoconstriction, resulting in reduction or resolution of edema in compartment syndrome, while nutrient blood flow is preserved (7). Several post-traumatic infectious syndromes appear to benefit from HBO$_2$, as elevated O_2 tension is bactericidal toward a variety of micro-organisms (5).

AIR AND GAS EMBOLISM

Air or gas can gain entry into the intravascular spaces more often than is currently recognized. Embolism can occur as a complication during a medical diagnostic or therapeutic procedure (9) or during accidental rapid decompression (10). The latter has been traditionally associated with scuba divers, but it can also occur in aviators, typically pilots of high performance military aircraft (11). During scuba dives, and usually in an inexperienced diver, embolism can happen with a rapid ascent from a dive, while breathing compressed gas and while breath-holding during ascent.

Pulmonary barotrauma can then occur, forcing gas into pulmonary capillaries, producing an arterial gas embolus (AGE). An iatrogenic embolism can occur during almost any invasive medical procedure penetrating tissue and bone and can produce either an AGE and/or a venous gas embolus (VGE). Included in such procedures are head, neck, or thoracic surgery; cardiopulmonary bypass (12); penetrating chest injury; needle or catheter placement for monitoring (13), diagnostic (14–16), or therapeutic purposes (17–21); renal dialysis (22); obstetric or gynecologic manipulation (23); and urologic procedures (24). In recent years several reports of forced air embolism have been published following use of rapid infusers, and steps have been taken to better detect the potentially lethal air bubbles in an effort to decrease the embolic risk (25).

Venous gas embolism occurs when the partial pressure of the intravascular offending gas exceeds the ambient pressure. As little as $5\ cmH_2O$ pressure difference between the atmosphere and the intravascular space is enough to entrain large volumes of air (26). Many of these bubbles are clinically "silent" as they cause no symptoms to the patient. These are however detectable by Doppler ultrasound (27). The technology has been applied clinically to study decompression sickness and monitor cardiopulmonary bypass and intracranial surgery.

However, the ability of the pulmonary vasculature to eliminate venous air emboli is limited (28). Transpulmonary passage of venous air emboli seems to be related to air infusion rates; if they are kept below a threshold value, the lungs can clear gaseous emboli. It also appears that vascular pressures have an important role in the passage of gas emboli through the pulmonary circulation. An infusion rate of 0.30 ml/kg/min in dogs is a threshold above which the lung capillaries can no longer clear the air embolus to the alveoli (29).

Intravascular gas can produce injury by two mechanisms. Intravascular bubbles cause a mechanical obstruction to blood flow and induce intravascular thrombosis through platelet aggregation and activation of other hemostatic mechanisms, mainly fibrin deposition. Manifestations of gas emboli are varied and depend on their size and location, the volume of gas entrained, speed of the event, position of the patient, and whether the main location is intra-arterial or intra-venous. These undesirable occlusive processes inevitably result in organ or tissue ischemia (30). AGE commonly produce clinical symptoms in the cerebral and spinal cord circulations as well as in the coronary circulation. Usual CNS symptoms include sudden dizziness, nausea, sensory or motor deficits, visual disturbances, confusion, coma, and seizures. Cardiac symptoms include ischemic chest pain and electrocardiographic changes associated with ischemia. VGE may produce pulmonary symptoms such as chest pain, coughing, dyspnea, and hemodynamic instability, including hypotension, tachypnea, pulmonary edema, or cardiac arrest. Elevation of CPK enzyme levels is reportedly a very frequent accompaniment to air emboli (31).

Mortality and morbidity can be significant. The diagnosis of air or gas embolism may be difficult, unless air entry is actually witnessed, or gas is found on aspiration from a central line, or the bubbles are visualized via ultrasonic imaging. Rarely is the diagnosis made by auscultation alone through the classic "millwheel murmur." New Doppler and neuroimaging modalities, particularly magnetic resonance imaging (MRI), have greatly added to the diagnostic armamentarium; however, both have limitations. The Doppler devices can alert that air emboli are occurring, but in general are more qualitative than quantitative. In addition, these devices do not determine the precise target tissue, or the severity of ischemia affecting that tissue. ☞ **MRI is the most sensitive in detecting focal cerebral ischemia due to air embolism.** ☞ A study by Warren et al. has determined that MRI is more sensitive than computed tomography scanning in this situation (27).

HBO_2 therapy has the ability to increase both tissue perfusion and tissue O_2 tensions and is therefore the treatment of choice for air or gas embolism. Rapidly increasing the ambient pressure decreases bubble volume immediately via the reduction in actual bubble volume, improving blood flow to the affected area. Increasing pressure by only 760 mmHg or to 2 atm abs decreases bubble volume by 50%; increasing pressure to 3 atm abs decreases bubble volume to 33% of the original volume. As the patient is also ventilated with 100% O_2, the largest gradient is created for inert gases present in the bubble (N_2 if the embolus is air) to be reabsorbed. In cases involving emboli to the cerebral and spinal cord circulations, hyperoxic vasoconstriction may decrease edema and improve the survival of marginally viable or ischemic tissue. Various treatment protocols have been used. These include the use of O_2 at 2.8 atm abs or compressed air or Nitrox (50% O_2 and 50% N_2) at 6 atm abs utilizing U.S. Navy Table 6 or 6A, repeating the treatment until no further improvement can be demonstrated (32).

DECOMPRESSION SICKNESS

☞ **Decompression sickness (DCS), also known as caisson disease, or the bends, is the clinical syndrome occurring during decompression.** ☞ Bubbles of N_2 form intravascularly and in tissues. The details on formation and growth of these bubbles are still unknown. However, bubbles form when the speed of decompression exceeds the rate at which perfusion can carry the dissolved gas to the lungs for exchange. Bubbles may form in any part of the body, producing a variety of signs and symptoms. Table 3 identifies the "no decompression" time limits for divers breathing compressed air and provides a frame for decompression-free limits in human diving at sea level.

The clinical presentation of DCS can vary widely from patient to patient; therefore a high index of suspicion and a history of decompression are essential to making a diagnosis. Correct diagnosis is vital; without treatment, permanent

Table 3   No-Decompression Limits for
Sport Divers Breathing Compressed Air

Depth	No decompression limit
40 feet	200 min
50 feet	100 min
90 feet	30 min
100 feet	25 min
130 feet	10 min

neurological deficits can ensue in previously healthy patients. So-called Type I DCS or the "bends" occurs in over 90% of cases and includes joint pain and cutaneous rashes. Typically this syndrome is characterized by deep, dull pain occurring in any joint. Type II DCS occurs in over 25% of cases and is characterized by primarily CNS effects with a predominance of spinal cord involvement. Dizziness, nausea, behavioral changes, visual disturbances, seizures, and coma are common presentations. Motor and/or sensory deficits, paraplegia, bowel or bladder incontinence, and loss of sexual function usually indicate spinal cord involvement.

A more careful neurological exam and a more attentive physician can often elicit significant subtle symptoms early in the disease.

In approximately 22% of all the sport divers presenting with DCS, peripheral nervous system symptoms are present. These may include low back pain, paresthesias, weakness, or proprioceptive deficits. Rarely do labyrinthine effects such as nystagmus, vertigo, nausea, and vomiting occur. When they do, treatment should be initiated as soon as possible to prevent permanent damage. More serious cardiorespiratory symptoms, pulmonary edema, shock, and death depict a wide spectrum of problems (33).

Various factors predispose to decompression sickness. Included are: cramped position during or after decompression, a recent strain or sprain of a muscle or a joint, hard exercise during or after decompression, hyperthermia, postalcoholic state, age over 40, and hypercarbia. One study found that in 23 divers with serious decompression sickness the incidence of a patent foramen ovale was 40% as compared to 5% in 176 normal volunteers. It has been hypothesized that the presence of a patent foramen ovale allowed otherwise innocuous venous gas bubbles to enter the arterial circulation and produce symptoms (33).

☞ **The definitive treatment for DCS is recompression in a HBO$_2$ chamber, and is the standard of care for patients suffering from decompression sickness and arterial gas embolism.** ☞ Often there is a need to transport a patient a long distance to the nearest hyperbaric chamber. The ambient pressure during transport should be maintained as high as possible by utilizing pressurized or low-flying aircraft (best at less than 1000 feet). In the meantime 100% O$_2$ should be administered via a tight-fitting face mask or endotracheal tube to hasten the elimination of N$_2$. Fluid resuscitation with intravenous crystalloid or colloid solutions are used also to aid in the elimination of N$_2$ as well as to maintain tissue perfusion. Hypotonic fluids should be avoided in cases of pulmonary involvement because they will add to any pulmonary edema present.

Whenever cerebral or spinal cord edema is suspected, the use of steroids should be considered, even if it may take several hours to be effective. Though steroids have been shown in animal studies to increase the risk of oxygen toxicity this has not been proven to be clinically significant in human studies. Also, hyperglycemia has been shown to augment neurologic injury due to ischemia (34). Therefore, glucose-containing fluids should not be used for resuscitation.

The clinical severity of the illness, clinical response to treatment, and residual symptoms after HBO$_2$ treatments will dictate the choice of treatment tables and the number of such treatments required. U.S. Navy Table 6 is most often used to treat severe DCS symptoms (with compression to 2.8 atm abs), whereas, U.S. Navy Table 5 is utilized for less severe symptoms (32).

Multiple treatments may be given until there is no further clinical improvement. Best results occur when the patient is treated as soon as possible. This is especially true when treating labyrinthine DCS. However, even after a delay of several days, treatment can still be effective. Finally, treatments are continued until no further improvement is seen in the patient. Altitude DCS is similar to diving DCS in pathophysiology and clinical presentation. Return to sea level and oxygen breathing are usually sufficient to treat mild cases. Compression in a hyperbaric chamber may be required with more serious presentations. ☞ **HBO$_2$ treatment of decompression sickness and arterial gas embolism is very cost-effective in today's medical climate of cost control given the alternative of permanent spinal cord, brain or peripheral nerve damage, or death.** ☞

CARBON MONOXIDE TOXICITY

Toxicity due to CO occurs commonly during traumatic events when patients are exposed to fire, explosions, or the emission of gases from combustion engines. The presentation is often nonspecific, as a variety of symptoms can manifest. Exposure is most often accidental, occurring in the absence of other trauma, during cold weather. Sources of CO toxicity include motor vehicle exhaust, space-heaters, industrial furnaces, and house fires. Increasing recognition of CO poisoning is occurring following disasters, particularly in the recovery phase after floods (35,36) and hurricanes (37–39), generally due to powered pressure washers and generators used indoors or in proximity to open doors or windows.

Classic presentation includes headache, nausea, vomiting, hypotension, syncope, vasomotor collapse, behavioral abnormalities, seizures, and coma. In acute exposures carboxyhemoglobin (Hb-CO) levels of 10% to 20% are often asymptomatic, while levels of 50% to 60% are found frequently in comatose victims. In chronic exposure, as measured in hours, Hb-CO levels that are normally survivable can become lethal, and the initial values do not correlate well with clinical findings or outcome. This is because blood levels do not accurately reflect the amount of intracellularly bound CO. This was observed in a study by Norkool and Kirkpatric, who found, in patients admitted to care after a prolonged exposure, that the mean Hb-CO levels in those who survived (29.3%) did not differ significantly from those who died (30.8%) (40). Neuropsychiatric abnormalities are often present, but may be subtle and may require psychometric testing for detection (41). ☞ **In judging the severity of CO intoxication it is important to account for the duration of exposure, the activity of the victim during exposure, and the time from exposure to**

assessment. ☞ Recently it has been shown that intracellular binding of carbon monoxide to cytochrome oxidase in mitochondria may occur in vivo (42). This may contribute to tissue hypoxia by causing a persistent disruption of intracellular respiration.

Oxygen therapy either via hyperbaric or via face mask/endotracheal route is the therapy of choice in CO intoxication. It improves tissue oxygenation by decreasing the half-life of Hb-CO, by increasing the amount of oxygen physically dissolved in solution, and by hastening the liberation of CO from cytochromes. The half-life of Hb-CO is inversely related to the inspired oxygen partial pressure. Thus HBO_2 causes carboxyhemoglobin dissociation faster than normobaric oxygen (43). Prior to instituting HBO_2, patients should receive 100% O_2 via a tight-fitting face mask or an endotracheal tube. Transfer to a hyperbaric chamber should be accomplished as soon as possible. In patients with the history of exposure, with Hb-CO levels greater than 25%, therapy should be guided by the presence of neurologic symptoms, circulatory or respiratory collapse, and ischemic changes on the electrocardiogram. The recommended therapy is at 2.5 to 3.0 atm abs for up to 90 min. Treatment is guided by the severity of symptoms and response to therapy. Follow-up treatments may be administered 12 to 24 hrs later in those who presented with severe manifestations or in those with persistent symptoms. This treatment paradigm is supported by an excellent randomized clinical study (44).

The use of HBO_2 for CO intoxication during pregnancy has been described. Recent literature presented a case of maternal CO intoxication leading to signs of fetal distress, reviewed the pertinent literature, and concluded that short hyperoxic exposures during therapy can be well tolerated by the fetus in all stages of development. Therefore, HBO_2 may reduce the risk of death to the mother and deformity or death to the fetus. ☞ **HBO_2 therapy is not only safe to use during pregnancy but is very beneficial, when used for standard indications (45).** ☞

ACUTE INFECTIONS
Clostridial Myonecrosis

Clostridial myonecrosis, commonly known as gas gangrene, is a dramatic necrotizing infection characterized by rapidly spreading muscle necrosis (46). Diabetic or debilitated patients with traumatic, contaminated, or ischemic wounds are particularly at risk. Compound fractures and the presence of foreign bodies in the wound also increase risk. The most common organism implicated in causing clostridial myonecrosis is *Clostridium perfingens*. *Clostridium novii*, *C. septicum*, *C. histolyticum*, *C. fallax*, *C. sordellii*, and *C. bifermentans* have also been cultured from involved wounds. *C. perfingens* is an anaerobic, spore-forming, gram positive rod found abundantly in the soil and in the normal flora of the gastrointestinal tract. Despite being an anaerobic organism it can grow freely in O_2 tensions up to 30 mmHg (similar to body tissue oxygen tensions) and under certain conditions up to 70 mmHg. By providing an area of low O_2 tension, the clostridial spores can develop into a major infectious threat.

The pathophysiology of clostridial myonecrosis is related to the production of exotoxins of which 20 types have now been identified. Nine of these are seen in clinical clostridial myonecrosis and myositis (47). It also causes serious side effects via cytolysins and promotes direct vascular injury at the site of infection. Usually in the area immediately surrounding the infected wound the patient complains of extreme pain, and exaggerated swelling, brownish skin discoloration, gas production, and a brownish sweet-smelling drainage are present. Some systemic effects of alpha-toxin include septic shock, hemolysis-causing anemia, renal failure, disseminated intravascular coagulation, cardiotoxicity, and neurologic abnormalities. The clinical course is characterized by rapid deterioration if early treatment is not initiated.

The rationale for HBO_2 in this type of infection is based on the fact that anaerobic organisms lack antioxidant enzymes (superoxide-degrading enzyme, dismutase; and hydrogen peroxide-degrading enzyme, catalase). This enables oxygen to be lethal for anaerobic organisms (48). HBO_2 at 2 to 3 atm abs by increasing tissue oxygen tensions above 30 mmHg has been demonstrated to stop spore germination and to inhibit bacterial growth in a bacteriostatic fashion. In an inoculum of tissues from rats exposed to 3 atm abs for one and one-half hours it was found that the production of alpha-toxin could be inhibited but the toxin already produced was still stable in this environment (49). HBO_2 also induces hyperoxic-vasoconstriction that has also been demonstrated to decrease edema and improve perfusion to swollen ischemic tissue. HBO_2 is recommended as adjuvant therapy in addition to surgical debridement and broad spectrum antibiotics. Mortality rates with gas gangrene have ranged as high as 30% to 50% prior to the addition of HBO_2. However, since the addition of HBO_2, both mortality and morbidity have decreased significantly. In 1983 a study covering 20 years of experience found the overall mortality rate to be 20% (50). Mortality directly attributed to gas gangrene was reported to be 10.6%. Therapy with HBO_2 produced the best results when begun within 24 hrs of diagnosis. HBO_2 decreased the amputation rate when surgery was the primary therapy from 50% to 24% when used in addition to surgery. Similar findings have been supported in other studies.

Other Necrotizing Infections

Although clostridial myonecrosis is the most common and lethal of the necrotizing infections, other anaerobic and aerobic gas-forming organisms are capable of causing clinical syndromes similar to gas gangrene. Most often these infections occur in debilitated patients with either traumatic or surgical wounds. These conditions favor local tissue hypoxia and encourage bacterial growth. Prognosis with these infections is closely related to any coexisting disease present. Crepitant anaerobic cellulitis is a gas-producing infection involving the soft tissues without muscle involvement. This disease is neither a cellulitis produced by anaerobes nor a Clostridial toxin-induced disease. The onset of infection after a traumatic injury, usual to the lower extremities, is gradual. Systemic involvement is low. Mortality is lower than in other disease entities in this group at 10% to 15%. Bacteroides, Peptostreptococcus, Enterobacteriaceae, and Clostridium species are frequently isolated from the wounds. Progressive bacterial gangrene begins as an indurated site slowly progressing to painful ulcerating lesions involving the skin and subcutaneous tissues of the abdominal and thoracic walls. Usually it takes about two weeks to develop after a traumatic injury or surgery. Mortality ranges between 10% and 25%.

The synergistic action of anaerobic streptococci with *Staphylococcus aureus* or Enterobacteriaceae is the cause of this syndrome. Necrotizing fasciitis was first described by Meleny in 1924. It was called hemolytic Streptococcal gangrene. It is a common clinical entity involving deep infection of subcutaneous tissues (51). It has a high mortality, averaging 40%. Necrotizing fasciitis is characterized by extensive necrosis of the superficial and deep fascia, and in the pure form does not involve muscle. However, it is not uncommon to have spread to ischemic muscles (myonecrosis) in numerous clinical settings.

The necrotizing fasciitis infection spreads through tissue planes. The sine qua non of necrotizing fasciitis is the rapid spread of the disease along fascial planes with ensuing necrosis of the superficial skin above. Fournier's Gangrene is a necrotizing fasciitis involving the perineum or scrotal areas. Systemic toxicity is marked. Anaerobic organisms (Bacteroides, Peptostreptococcus, and Fusobacterium species) as well as aerobic organisms (*S. aureus*, *Streptococcus pyogenes*, and Enterobacteriaceae) have been isolated from these infections.

↗ **HBO$_2$ is recommended as adjuvant therapy following emergency surgical debridement and antibiotics for most necrotizing infections.** ↗ HBO$_2$ is effective because of the direct lethal effect of O$_2$ on anaerobic and microphilic aerobic organisms. Also, the neutrophil myeloperoxidase-hydrogen peroxide-halide system that is postulated to aid in bacterial cell wall destruction may be another important oxygen dependent system contributing to the success of HBO$_2$. Prophylactic antibiotics in addition to HBO$_2$ produced an additive effect in the reduction of infectious necrosis (52). The recommended therapy involves twice daily treatments at 2.0 to 2.5 atm abs for 90 to 120 min until the patient's condition stabilizes. After that, treatments can be reduced to once a day.

ACUTE ISCHEMIC PROCESSES

↗ **Acute ischemic processes that are amenable to HBO$_2$ include crush injury and compartment syndrome.** ↗ Crush injury is defined as a severe diffuse trauma involving two or more different tissues. Various degrees of tissue and microvascular damage occurs producing edema and swelling. The result is ischemia from poor perfusion to the involved area. Compartment syndrome occurs commonly in the anterior compartment of the leg and volar aspect of the forearm. Ischemia is produced by a similar mechanism in that edema and swelling, confined by fascia compartments leads to decreased perfusion. Vasodilation from local tissue hypoxia leads to further swelling and decreased perfusion.

Muscle necrosis can occur ultimately causing fibrous tissue deposition and contractures. HBO$_2$ promotes hyperoxic-vasoconstriction which reduces swelling and edema and improves local blood flow and oxygenation. It also increases tissue oxygen tensions and improves the survival of marginally viable tissue. At the time of surgical debridement, prior treatment with HBO$_2$ aids in the demarcation of nonviable tissue. Best results, again, are obtained when therapy is begun early. Twice daily treatments at 2.0 to 2.5 atm abs for 90 to 120 min are recommended for five to seven days with frequent examinations of the affected area.

MASSIVE BLOOD LOSS

Only when blood transfusion is unavailable (usually due to a major blood typing incompatibility) or has been refused (due

to religious reasons as with a Jehovah's Witness) should HBO$_2$ be use to treat exceptional anemia. The rationale for using HBO$_2$ is based on the fact that life can be supported solely by O$_2$ physically dissolved in plasma when 100% O$_2$ at 3 atm abs is administered. HBO$_2$ used in this rare circumstance can only sustain a patient temporarily until compatible blood is available or until there is sufficient time for erythropoiesis. A summary of several treatments spanning several years of practice has been published by Hart et al. (53).

THERMAL BURNS

↗ **HBO$_2$ therapy in the treatment of burns in the absence of CO intoxication is controversial.** ↗ The rationale is that burn wounds are often characterized by edema, increased vascular permeability, stasis of circulation, and intravascular coagulation. Thus tissue surrounding a burn is prone to hypoxia, infection, poor wound healing, and scar formation. HBO$_2$, by several mechanisms described above, can decrease tissue hypoxia surrounding a burn, correcting many of these shortcomings directly. HBO$_2$ therapy can maintain microvascular integrity, minimize edema and provide the vital oxygen needed for tissues to heal and become viable once again (54). HBO$_2$ therapy minimized white blood cell adherence to endothelial cell walls, preventing the cascade causing vascular damage (55). Thus HBO$_2$ has a beneficial effect on the microcirculation. Also, burns are often complicated by smoke inhalation, CO intoxication, and cyanide toxicity. These complications should be suspected in all unconscious patients rescued from fires.

EYE TO THE FUTURE

Many effects of HBO$_2$ therapy remain to be elucidated. As time goes on, it is expected that additional studies will clarify the effects of HBO$_2$ therapy for additional clinical situations.

In the field of diving medicine, newer areas of interest include exploration of whether the addition of adjunctive drugs might enhance the response of Type II decompression sickness to HBO$_2$. Drugs currently under investigation for this application include lidocaine and steroids (56,57).

The use of HBO$_2$ for chronic refractory osteomyelitis raises the question of whether there are other roles for HBO$_2$ in bone healing. Hyperbaric oxygen affects the activity levels of both osteoblasts and osteoclasts, and there might be a role for HBO$_2$ in accelerating bone healing, particularly for nonunions. One particular area that is intriguing is in the setting of open fractures of the tibia, which have a predilection for developing osteomyelitis. Could there be a role for HBO$_2$, for instance, in prophylaxis to prevent osteomyelitis and mal-union in the setting of trauma?

The addition of brain abscess as an approved indication in the last UHMS hyperbaric therapy committee report also suggests the issue of whether enough data can be acquired to demonstrate effectiveness in other infectious diseases, such as mucormycosis (58), actinomycosis, anaerobic liver abscesses, and other infections. Although several case reports of activity in some of these clinical scenarios exist, true randomized controlled studies to demonstrate effectiveness are still lacking, but are sorely needed. A case registry for cases of mucormycosis is currently attempting to track cases of mucormycosis for further outcome study. A recent evidence-based report on the benefits and risks of HBO$_2$ therapy for brain injury, cerebral palsy, and stroke has been issued (59), also demonstrating the need for further studies.

Although hyperbarics has a demonstrated beneficial effect on many nonhealing diabetic and other hypoxic wounds, current Medicare coverage limits reimbursement to Wagner 3 or greater wounds in diabetics, thus limiting the physician's ability to get appropriate treatment for their patients with recalcitrant wounds. Better, more definitive studies, especially cost-effectiveness studies, are still needed in this arena to justify appropriate medical treatment in this particular patient population. Progress is being made at the cellular level in understanding the mechanisms affecting white blood cell adhesion (60).

Hyperbaric medicine remains a fertile ground for augmenting medical care in many specialties, and opportunities for significant contributions in basic and clinical studies abound. Future demonstration of additional physiologic effects of clinical importance is likely.

SUMMARY

This chapter reviews basic physical and physiological principles of HBO$_2$ therapy. Specifically reviewed are traumatic syndromes that are amenable to therapy with HBO$_2$. Included are: bubble-mediated diseases (air and gas embolism, decompression syndrome), toxicosis (CO toxicity), acute infections (clostridial myonecrosis and other necrotizing infections), acute ischemic processes (crush injury, compartment syndrome), and syndromes requiring special considerations (exceptional blood loss, thermal burns). Basic physiological considerations and practical issues of clinical treatment in the hyperbaric environment are discussed.

KEY POINTS

- HBO$_2$ therapy is defined as the therapeutic administration of O$_2$ at pressures greater than atmospheric at sea level.
- Treatment with HBO$_2$ is empirically limited to a maximum tolerated inspired PO$_2$ and the total time of exposure.
- Because of the immediate access to the patient by accompanying personnel, monitoring is commonly simplified with multiplace HBO$_2$ chambers.
- Development of a tension pneumothorax, although rare, could be fatal in monoplace chamber because of the impossibility of inserting a chest tube prior to decompression.
- MRI is the most sensitive in detecting focal cerebral ischemia due to air embolism.
- Decompression sickness (DCS), also known as caisson disease, or the bends, is the clinical syndrome occurring during decompression.
- The definitive treatment for DCS is recompression in a hyperbaric chamber, and is the standard of care for patients suffering from decompression sickness and arterial gas embolism.
- HBO$_2$ treatment of decompression sickness and arterial gas embolism is very cost-effective in today's medical climate of cost control given the alternative of permanent spinal cord, brain or peripheral nerve damage, or death.
- In judging the severity of CO intoxication it is important to account for the duration of exposure, the activity of the victim during exposure, and the time from exposure to assessment.
- HBO$_2$ therapy is not only safe to use during pregnancy but is very beneficial, when used for standard indications (45).
- HBO$_2$ is recommended as adjuvant therapy following emergency surgical debridement and antibiotics for most necrotizing infections.
- Acute ischemic processes that are amenable to HBO$_2$ include crush injury and compartment syndrome.
- HBO$_2$ therapy in the treatment of burns in the absence of CO intoxication is controversial.

REFERENCES

1. Kindwall EP. A history of hyperbaric chambers. In: Kindwall EP, Whelan HT, eds. Hyperbaric Medicine Practice, 2nd Edition. Flagstaff, AZ: Best Publishing Co., 1999:1–21.
2. Haux GFK. History of Hyperbaric Chambers. Flagstaff, AZ: Best Publishing Co., 2000:38.
3. Churchill-Davidson I, Sanger C, Thomlinson RH. High-pressure oxygen and radiotherapy. Lancet 1955; 1:1091–1095.
4. Boerema I, Kroll NG, Meijne NG, et al. High atmospheric pressure as an aid to cardiac surgery. Arch Chir Neder 1956; 8:193–211.
5. Brummelkamp WH, Hogendijk J, Boerema I. Treatment of anaerobic infections (clostridial myositis) by drenching the tissues with oxygen under high atmospheric pressure. Surgery 1961; 49:299–302.
6. Smith G and Sharp GR. Treatment of coal gas poisoning with oxygen at 2 atmospheres pressure. Lancet 1962; 1:816–819.
7. Feldmeier JJ (ed). Hyperbaric Oxygen Therapy 2003: Indications and Results: The Hyperbaric Oxygen Therapy Committee Report. Kensington, MD: Undersea and Hyperbaric Medical Society, 2003:141.
8. Moon RE, Camporesi EM, Shelton DL. Prediction of Arterial PO$_2$ during hyperbaric treatment. 9th International Symposium on Underwater and Hyperbaric Physiology, Undersea and Hyperbaric Medical Society, Bethesda, MD, 1987:1127–1131.
9. Peirce EC. Cerebral gas embolism (arterial) with special reference to iatrogenic accidents. Hyperbaric Oxygen Rev 1980; 1(3):161–184.
10. Davis JC, Elliott DH. Treatment of decompression disorders. In: Bennett PB, Elliott DH (eds). The Physiology and Medicine of Diving. 3rd ed., London: Bailliere, Tindall, 1982:473–486.
11. Kumar K, Waligora JM, Calkins DS. Threshold altitude resulting in decompression sickness. Aviat Space Environ Med 1990; 61:685–689.
12. Stoney WS, Alford WC Jr, Burrus GR, Glassford DM Jr, Thomas CS Jr. Air embolism and other accidents using pump oxygenators. Ann Thorac Surg 1980; 29(4):336–340.
13. Vesely TM. Air embolism during insertion of central venous catheters. J Vasc Interventional Radiol 2001; 12:1291–1295.
14. Ashizawa K, Watanabe H, Morooka H, Hayashi K. Hyperbaric oxygen therapy for air embolism complicating CT-guided needle biopsy of the lung. AJR 2004; 182:1606–1607.
15. Emby DJ, Arnold BW, Zwiebel WJ. Percutaneous transthoracic needle biopsy complicated by air embolism. AJR 2003; 181:279–280.
16. Mokhlesi B, Ansaarie I, Bader M, Tareen M, Boatman J. Coronary artery air embolism complicating a CT-guided transthoracic needle biopsy of the lung. Chest 2002; 121:993–996.
17. Jones PM, Segal SH, Gelb AW. Venous Oxygen embolism produced by injection of hydrogen peroxide into an enterocutaneous fistula. Anesth Analg 2004; 99:1861–1863.

18. Haller G, Faltin-Traub E, Faltin D, Kern C. Oxygen embolism after hydrogen peroxide irrigation of a vulvar abscess. Br J Anaesth 2002; 88:597–599.

19. Balki M, Manninen, PH, McGuire GP, El-Beheiry H, Bernstein M. Venous air embolism during awake craniotomy in a supine patient: Aeroembolie veineuse pendant la craniotomie chez un patient en decubitus dorsal. Can J Anaesth 2003; 50: 835–883.

20. Faure EAM, Cook RI, Miles D. Air embolism during anesthesia for shoulder arthroscopy. Anesthesiology 1998; 89:805–806.

21. Moskop RJ Jr, Lubarsky DA. Carbon dioxide embolism during laparoscopic cholecystectomy. South Med J 1994; 87:414–415.

22. Baskin SE, Wozniak RF. Hyperbaric oxygenation in the treatment of hemodialysis-associated air embolism. NEJM 1975; 293:184–185.

23. Fong J, Gadalla F, Gimbel AA. Precordial Doppler diagnosis of haemodynamically compromising air embolism during caesarian section. Can J Anaesth 1990; 37:262–264.

24. Joliffe MP, Lyew MA, Berger IH, Grimaldi T. Venous air embolism during radical perineal prostatectomy. J Clin Anesth 1996; 8:659–661.

25. Avula RR, Kramer R, Smith CE. Air detection performance of the Level I H-1200 fluid and blood warmer. Anesth Analg 2005; 101:1413–1416.

26. Hallenbeck JM, Bove AA, Moquin RB, Elliott DH. Accelerated coagulation of whole blood and cell-free plasma by bubbling in vitro. Aerospace Med 1973; 44:712–714.

27. Warren LP, Djang WT, Moon RE, et al. Neuroimaging of scuba diving injuries to the CNS. AJNR 1988; 9:933–938.

28. Massey EW, Shelton DL, Moon RE, Camporesi EM. Hyperbaric treatment of iatrogenic air embolism. Abs. Undersea and Hyperbaric Medical Society Annual Scientific Meeting, 1989.

29. Lanier WL, Stangland KL, Scheithauer BW, Milde JH, Michenfelder JD. The effects of dextrose infusion and head position on neurologic outcomes after complete cerebral ischemia in primates: examination of a model. Anesthesiology 1987; 66:39–48.

30. Barak M, Katz Y. Microbubbles: pathophysiology and clinical implications. Chest 2005; 128:2918–2932.

31. Smith RM, Neuman TS. Elevation of serum creatine kinase in divers with arterial gas embolization. N Engl J Med 1994; 330:19–24.

32. U.S. Navy Diving Manual. Revision 5, Volume 5: Diving medicine and recompression chamber operations, Document SS521-AG-PRO-010, Naval Sea Systems Command, 15 August 2005. Available at: http://www.supsalv.org/00c3_publications.asp?destPage=00c3&pageId=3.9

33. Moon RE, Camporesi EM, Kisslo JA. Patent foramen ovale as a risk factor for decompression sickness in compressed air divers. Lancet 1989; I:513–514.

34. Drummond JC, Moore SS. The influence of dextrose administration on neurological outcome after temporary spinal cord ischemia in the rabbit. Anesthesiology 1989; 70:64–70.

35. Daley WR, Shireley L, Gilmore R. A flood-related outbreak of carbon monoxide poisoning—Grand Forks, North Dakota. J Emerg Med 2001; 21(3):249–253.

36. Jacoby I. Mitigating medical maladies in disasters. J Emerg Med 2001; 21(3):285–287.

37. CDC. Carbon monoxide poisoning from hurricane-associated use of portable generators—Florida 2004. Morbid Mortal Weekly Rep 2005; 54(28):697–700.

38. CDC. Carbon monoxide poisoning after Hurricane Katrina—Alabama, Louisiana and Mississippi, August–September 2005. Morbid Mortal Weekly Rep 2005; 54(39):996–998.

39. CDC. Carbon monoxide poisoinings after 2 major hurricanes—Alabama and Texas, August–October 2005. Morbid Mortal Weekly Rep 2006; 55(9):236–239.

40. Norkool DM, Kirkpatrick JN. Treatment of acute carbon monoxide poisoning with hyperbaric oxygen: A review of 115 cases. Ann Emerg Med 1985; 14:1168–1171.

41. Myers RAM, Bray P. Delayed treatment of serious decompression sickness. Annals Emerg Med 1985; 14(3):254–257.

42. Piantadosi CA. Carbon monoxide, oxygen transport, and oxygen metabolism. J Hyperbaric Med 1987; 2(1):27–44.

43. Pace N, Strajman F, Walker EL. Acceleration of carbon monoxide elimination in man by high pressure oxygen. Science 1950; 111:652–654.

44. Weaver LK, Hopkins RO, Chan KJ, Churchill S, Elliot CG, Clemmer TP, Orme JF Jr, Thomas FO, Morris AH. Hyperbaric oxygen for acute carbon monoxide poisoning. N Engl J Med 2002; 347(14):1057–1067.

45. Van Hoesen KB, Camporesi EM, Moon RE, Hage ML, Piantadosi CA. Should hyperbaric oxygen be used to treat the pregnant patient for acute carbon monoxide poisoning? A case report and literature review. JAMA 1989; 261(7):1039–1043.

46. Bakker DJ. Clostridial myonecrosis. In: Davis JC amd Hunt TK (eds) Problem Wounds, Elsevier, New York, 1988:153–172.

47. Demello FJ, Hashimoto T, Hitchcock CR, Haglin JJ. The effect of hyperbaric oxygen on the germination and toxin production of Clostridium perfringens spores. In: Wada J, Iwa T (eds) Proceedings of the Fourth International Congress on Hyperbaric Medicine, Williams & Wilkins, Baltimore, 1970:276–281.

48. McCord JM, Keele BB Jr, Fridovich I. An enzyme-based theory of obligate anaerobiosis: The physiologic function of superoxide dismutase. Proc Nat Acad Sci USA 1971; 68(5):1024–1027.

49. Van Unnik AJM. Inhibition of toxin production in Clostridium perfringens in vitro by hyperbaric oxygen. Antonie Van Leeuwenhoek 1965; 31:181–186.

50. Hart GB, Lamb RC, Strauss MB. Gas gangrene. J Trauma 1983; 23(11):991–1000.

51. Mader JT. Mixed anaerobic and aerobic soft tissue infections. In: Davis JC and Hunt TK (eds) Problem Wounds: The Role of Oxygen, Elsevier, New York, 1988:173–186.

52. Knighton DR, Halliday B, Hunt TK. Oxygen as an antibiotic: A comparison of the effects of inspired oxygen concentration and antibiotic administration on in vivo bacterial clearance. Arch Surg 1986; 121:191–195.

53. Hart GB, Lennon PA, Strauss MB. Hyperbaric oxygen in exceptional acute blood-loss anemia. J Hyperb Med 1987; 2(4):205–210.

54. Grossman AR, Hart GB, Yanda RL. Thermal burns. In: Davis JC, Hunt TK (eds) Hyperbaric Oxygen Therapy. Bethesda (MD), Undersea Medical Society, 1977:267–279.

55. Cianci P, Lueders H, Lee H, et al. Adjunctive hyperbaric oxygen reduces the need for surgery in 40–80% burns. J Hyperb Med 1988; 3(2):97–101.

56. Mitchell SJ. Lidocaine in the treatment of decompression illness: A review of the literature. Undersea Hyperbaric Med 2001; 28(3):165–174.

57. Cogar WB. Intravenous lidocaine as adjunctive therapy in the treatment of decompression illness. Ann Emerg Med 1997; 29(2):284–286.

58. Gonzalez CE, Rinaldi MG, Sugar AM. Zygomycosis. Infect Dis Clin No Am 2002; 16(4):895–914.

59. McDonagh M, Carson S, Ash J, et al. Hyperbaric Oxygen Therapy for Brain Injury, Cerebral Palsy, and Stroke. Evidence Report/Technology Assessment No. 85 (Prepared by the Oregon Health and Science University Evidence-based Practice Center under Contract No. 290-97-0018). AHRQ Publication No. 03-E050. Rockville, MD: Agency for Healthcare Research and Quality. September 2003. Available at http://www.ahrq.gov/clinic/epcsums/hypoxsum.htm, accessed 5–23–06.

60. Thom SR, Mendiguren I, Hardy K, et al. Inhibition of human neutrophil beta-2-integrin-dependent adherence by hyperbaric O_2. Am J Physiol 1997; 272:C770–C777.

61. http://www.uhms.org/indications/indications.htm

74

Severity of Illness Scoring for Trauma and Critical Care

Raul Coimbra and Tercio de Campos

Division of Trauma, Burns, and Critical Care, Department of Surgery, UC San Diego Medical Center, San Diego, California, U.S.A.

Catherine McCoy-Hill

School of Nursing, Azusa Pacific University, Azusa, California, U.S.A.

INTRODUCTION

The management of trauma and critical care consumes a significant portion of the healthcare budget and has become progressively more complex. Numerous conditions remain associated with high mortalities despite intensive resource allocation. Accordingly, traumatologists and intensivists are increasingly challenged to measure and improve outcomes. Governmental agencies, accrediting bodies, and third-party payers increasingly evaluate performance for quality outcomes as well as cost-effectiveness. Consumers seeking quality healthcare have greater access than before to hospital quality data and performance indicators (mortality rates, lengths of stay, complication rates, volumes etc.), which compare outcomes across institutions and providers. Accordingly, clinicians and researchers want to evaluate and improve the quality of care delivered and identify "best practices" in the treatment of their patients.

Two of the early pioneers of trauma and critical care scoring research, Champion (1) and Knaus (2), were instrumental in forming many of the initial ideas. These early investigators developed and tested scoring and mortality prediction models that have proven valid in outcomes studies and serve as the foundations for the tools that are used currently. Subsequent contributions to their creative visions have helped promote injury severity and critical illness scoring models into increasingly refined and accurate measurement devices.

This chapter begins by reviewing the purpose of scoring systems in terms of their utility in clinical decision-making, and for facilitating comparisons between various treatment units and institutions. Trauma scoring systems are only briefly surveyed, because the topic is extensively reviewed in Volume 1, Chapter 4, of this textbook along with trauma triage. Critical care scoring systems are presented in greater detail with an effort to illuminate the clinically relevant elements of the most commonly utilized scoring instruments.

Because multiple organ dysfunction (MOD) syndrome is responsible for a large fraction of the morbidity that occurs in critically ill patients and also represents the most common scenario for irrecoverable states (i.e., futile therapy) from which medical therapy is withheld or withdrawn, organ injury scoring is also reviewed.

A comparison between the various scoring systems is provided as a mechanism to further amplify their strengths and weaknesses. The Eye to the Future section provides some provocative ideas about the future of scoring systems and emphasizes the need for unification of these schemes; the first steps of which have been taken by the American College of Surgeons National Trauma Databank (NTDB) (3), the Society of Critical Care Medicine's "Project Impact" (4), and the Intensive Care Audit and Research Centre (INARC) in the United Kingdom (5).

PURPOSE AND UTILITY OF SCORING SYSTEMS

Prior to the implementation of critical illness scoring systems, it was difficult to determine if mortality outcome variance across surgical intensive care units (SICUs) and Trauma Units was related to treatment effects or a difference in the patient case mix. Mortality rate (MR) and length of stay (LOS) as single indices used to assess SICU performance offered only a rudimentary analysis for comparison and demonstrated the need for case-adjusted data for accurate quantitative risk assessment and outcome comparisons (6).

Trauma scoring systems were developed for both triage purposes and outcomes research (as fully described in Volume 1, Chapter 4), whereas, SICU scoring systems are designed to estimate the probability of in-hospital death of patients admitted to an SICU, based on severity-adjusted mortality measures.

☞ **All scoring systems represent quantitative classification schemes and most use multiple logistic regression methodology applied to prospectively collected data sets of demographic, physiological, and clinical variables.** ☞ From this, standard mortality ratios (SMRs) can be calculated by dividing the observed mortality rate by the mortality rate predicted using the specific patient-related variables. The SMR can be used as a risk-adjusted measure for probability estimates and for comparisons of SICU performance over time, as well as for cross-comparative analyses. These tools provide reasonably accurate prediction in acutely ill patients of the severity, prognosis, and expected course of disease, with mortality outcomes usually measured as death before discharge from hospital after intensive care (7,8).

Although their primary purpose is to predict mortality, scoring systems have been used on broader scales to research and analyze other outcomes (e.g., LOS, readmission rates etc.), address cost-benefit analyses, evaluate resource utilization, and improve care through comparative evaluation of treatment effectiveness and benchmarking for continuous quality improvement. Predictions of mortality or prolonged stay in the ICU are also of potential benefit for triage, resource allocation, and patient-family counseling as adjuncts (not substitutes) to clinical judgment. Severity scores are frequently used in research trials to stratify patients and establish group similarities (9).

⚲ **While scoring systems are useful for research and comparing SICU performance with respect to endpoints such as mortality and LOS, their usefulness is less clear in medical decision-making or prognostic estimations for individual patients.** ⚲ Controversy exists about the utility of mortality prediction models as decision support tools due to differences in the accuracy in probability estimates for group versus individual outcomes. Other limitations of models which may result in under- or overestimations of probability include: (*i*) degradation of reliability over time due to changes in population characteristics and/or advances in treatment, (*ii*) "goodness of fit" calibration and discrimination issues affecting internal and external validation, (*iii*) errors in data collection (manual or electronic) and/or misinterpretation of scoring rules (human factors), (*iv*) lag time issues, (*v*) statistical problems related to sample size, selection, weighting of variables and so on, and (*vi*) individual patient-related confounds (e.g., presence of outliers) (10,11).

Although mortality outcome predictions will never be entirely accurate, ICU scoring systems, as with trauma scoring systems, are nevertheless extremely useful tools to classify and quantify severity of illness and to predict outcomes for groups of patients. The use of common terminology (e.g., SMR) enables comparisons between patient groups, individual units, and among ICUs. Such outcome comparisons are essential to research and in the evaluation and improvement of ICU care and organization.

TRAUMA SCORING SYSTEMS

Numerous well-functioning trauma scoring systems and prediction models based on anatomical injury and physiological impairment (or combinations thereof) are in current use (1,12–17). These tools are useful for: (*i*) triage and prehospital treatment, (*ii*) injury severity description, (*iii*) assessment and documentation using common terminology, (*iv*) quality of care and patient outcome evaluation, (*v*) trauma system evaluation and comparison, (*vi*) trauma epidemiology, and (*vii*) trauma research and funding. The most commonly used trauma scoring tools are highlighted in this section.

Trauma Score and Revised Trauma Score (TS, RTS)

The coefficient values assigned reflect each parameter's ability to affect outcome, with the highest assigned weight given to the GCS, reflecting increased impact that head injuries have on outcome compared to the initial SBP or RR. The RTS values range from 0 to 7.8, with a higher value indicating increased probability of survival (P_s) (12).

The RTS is limited by exclusion of age and other comorbidities that affect outcome (13). The TS and the RTS are simple to use, accurate, and have been incorporated into the trauma score-injury severity score (TRISS) methodology (described in Volume 1, Chapter 4).

Organ Injury Scale

The Organ Injury Scale (OIS) was developed by the American Association for the Surgery of Trauma (AAST) in 1987 (14) as a tool to devise injury severity scores (ISSs) for individual organs using common nomenclature to describe injuries. The classification scheme provides detailed anatomic descriptions, scaled from one to six [one representing the least, and five the most severe that is salvageable; the value of six denotes the organ is nonsalvageable (in the case of a liver or cardiac trauma this also connotes lethality)] (14). Injuries may also be divided by mechanism (blunt versus penetrating) or by injury description (e.g., hematoma, laceration, and contusion), and grades are advanced for multiple injuries to the same organ.

The first OIS version covered liver, spleen, and kidney injuries. Since 1987, several revisions have occurred and other organs were added. There now exist OIS characterizations for lung, heart, chest wall, diaphragm, abdominal, vascular, ureter, bladder, and urethra, as well as the original three organs. These OIS schemes continue to be updated periodically. These scales are provided throughout this text in other chapters covering the affected organs. The OIS differs from the AIS, which is also anatomically based, but is designed to reflect the impact of a specific organ injury on patient outcome.

Abbreviated Injury Scale

The abbreviated injury scale (AIS) is an anatomically based global scoring system that classifies each injury in various body regions, using a six-point ordinal scale to rank injury severity (15). The AIS was initially developed in 1969 as a uniform tool to categorize and quantify blunt injuries sustained in motor vehicle collisions (MVCs) by a consortium of automobile insurance firms along with the American Medical Association (15). The AIS has since expanded considerably and is revised and updated every five to ten years.

The AIS is the most frequently modified and commonly used anatomical scoring system, and continuously expands to accommodate changing clinical demands. The AIS is a component of the ISS described subsequently. Limitations of AIS are mainly related to describing physiologically based injuries and in specifying wounds. It cannot accurately describe all fractures and locations (e.g., anterior, posterior, bilateral), contusions commonly seen together in the same region (e.g., rib fractures and pulmonary contusions), near drowning, hypo- and hyperthermia, or inhalation injuries. Despite their limitations, both the AIS and the OIS provide reasonably accurate rankings of injury severity in trauma patients.

Injury Severity Score

The Injury Severity Score (ISS) is an anatomical scoring system introduced by Baker et al. in 1974 (16). It was developed as an extension of AIS as an ordinal summary severity score for patients with multiple injuries. ⚲ **ISS correlates with hospital stay, morbidity, mortality, and other measures of trauma severity and is the most widely accepted severity of injury index in use today.** ⚲

Each injury is assigned an AIS code and classified in one of six body regions, as follows: (*i*) head/neck, (*ii*) face, (*iii*) thorax, (*iv*) abdomen, (*v*) extremities (including pelvis), and (*vi*) external (15). The highest scores from the three most severely injured regions are squared, and then added together to provide the ISS score (i.e., ISS = $a^2 + b^2 + c^2$) (16). Any injury assigned the AIS score six is automatically given the maximal ISS score of 75. ISS values range from zero (no injuries) to 75 (incompatible with life). An example ISS calculation and expected outcomes based upon the ISS encountered are provided in Volume 1, Chapter 4 (Tables 4–6).

Limitations of the ISS include its one-dimensional representation of wide varieties of injuries of the polytrauma patient. Equal (correctly evaluated) AIS scores in different body regions can give the identical ISS scores, but represent a wide range of injuries with vastly different outcomes. Furthermore, multiple injuries in the same body region are (by convention) not taken into consideration, as ISS uses only the highest, rather than the overall, score from the body region (18). Any error in AIS scoring decreases the subsequent ISS precision (19–21). Age and comorbidity are not taken into account, and severe neurological trauma is undervalued (22).

Despite these shortcomings, the ISS remains the most widely accepted severity of injury index for multiple trauma, and its value correlates with mortality. When the ISS ≤15 there is less than 10% risk of mortality; ISS = 17 is critical with values greater than 17 denoting severe injury; and mortality increases linearly with ISS >25 (Volume 1, Chapter 4). Although ISS has not incorporated multiple injuries in the same region, a modified version, the "new ISS" (NISS), statistically outperforms the ISS, is easier to use, and provides a more accurate prediction by calculating the three highest AIS scores regardless of body regions (17,23–25).

CRITICAL CARE SCORING SYSTEMS

The most commonly used mortality prediction models in critical care include the acute physiology and chronic health evaluation (APACHE) score, and the subsequent upgrades, APACHE II*, APACHE III, and APACHE IV. Other clinically useful scoring systems for critical care include the simplified acute physiology score (SAPS), SAPS II*, SAPS III, and the mortality probability model (MPM) and MPM II*. The most commonly used versions are signified by the affixed asterisk* (6,9).

The primary differences in scoring systems are based on the number and types of patient characteristics selected and the assignment of their relative weights as covariates, as well as the inclusion/exclusion criteria and timing of assessment. In general, these instruments use clinical and physiological data collected on the first day of ICU admission to predict mortality risk. ☞ **The APACHE II/III/IV, SAPS II/III, and MPM II are considered "third generation" scoring systems based on their use of multiple regression statistical techniques (7,8).** ☞

Acute Physiology and Chronic Health Evaluation

The first widely used severity of illness classification system for critical care was the APACHE score, published in 1981 by Knaus and colleagues at the George Washington University Medical Center (2). The APACHE score was developed based on the evaluation of 805 patient admissions in two

U.S. ICUs, taking into account three patient factors: disease, reserve, and severity, all of which were treatment independent. The original APACHE consisted of two parts: the acute physiology score (APS), which indicated the degree of physiologic derangement, and a chronic health evaluation (CHE), which was considered an indicator of physiologic reserve before the acute illness onset. Thirty-four physiological variables were selected (by expert panel) and assigned relative weights, using the worst value for each variable within the first 32 hours following ICU admission. The CHE component classified patients into four categories (A for excellent health, to D for severely failing health). Results from the initial study population and others demonstrated high correlations between APS scores and the probability of death; however, with the CHE, only class D was found to be an independent predictor of mortality. Despite its relatively good correlation with mortality, criticisms of the APACHE included the large number of variables (34) needed to calculate scores, making it difficult to use clinically, as well as the restrictive time frame of 32 hours allowed for data collection. Use of APACHE is no longer recommended because of its outdated database (26).

APACHE II was found to be easier to use than the original APACHE and soon became the most widely utilized and studied prediction tool worldwide. The current criticisms of APACHE II are: (*i*) its risk predictions are based on old data from 1979 to 1982, (*ii*) the system was not designed to predict outcome for individual patients and particular diseases, (*iii*) variations in timing of ICU admission (e.g., ED vs. floor transfer) cause errors in prediction, (*iv*) the included diagnostic categories do not accurately account for the diversity of conditions that lead to ICU admissions, and most importantly, (*v*) the predictive database includes relatively few surgical and trauma patients. Indeed there is widespread agreement that APACHE II underestimates mortality in surgical patients (27,28). APACHE II also lacks a component to assess accurately the full extent of acute trauma-related illness in formerly healthy individuals, as opposed to patients with more chronic conditions.

☞ **APACHE III is more predictive than APACHE II due to modifications (increased size and representativeness of the database, and expansion of diagnosis to include more complex injury characterizations).** ☞ APACHE III (Table 1) was released in 1991 to address many of the above detailed shortcomings of its predecessor. APACHE III has numerous additional advantages over APACHE II scoring as it controls for selection and lead-time bias (difference between hospital/ICU admit dates) through the inclusion of weights for ICU readmissions as well as patient location and LOS prior to ICU admission. In addition, APACHE III has a proprietary "clinical support package" which includes the ability to derive ICU core measure outcomes [e.g., deep venous thrombosis (DVT), ventilator associated pneumonia (VAP), and stress ulcer disease (SUD) prophylaxis], as well as software linkages to the Society of Critical Care Medicine's *Project Impact* (Cerner Corporation, Kansas City, MO) (4). With the release of the third version, Knaus and colleagues (developers of the various APACHE versions) recommended that APACHE II, with its outdated reference data (based on 1979–1982) be abandoned, and that APACHE III (based on 1988–1990 reference data) be utilized instead (29).

Major drawbacks to APACHE III relate to its complexity, user difficulty, and cost. APACHE III has not gained wide acceptance because it is less freely available (licensing fees)

Table 1   Acute Physiology and Chronic Health Evolution III Variables and Definitions

Acute physiology score (0–252 points)	Points
Mean blood pressure	0–23
Respiratory rate adjusted for mechanical ventilation	0–18
Temperatures	0–20
Pulse	0–17
Neurologic status	0–48
24-hrs urine output	0–15
Hematocrit	0–3
White blood cell count	0–19
Arterial pH adjusted for PCO_2	0–12
Arterial PO_2 or A-aDO_2 if ventilated	0–15
Serum sodium	0–4
Serum albumin	0–11
Serum glucose	0–9
Serum creatinine	0–10
Blood urea nitrogen	0–12
Serum bilirubin	0–16

Age, in years (0–24 points)	
≤44	0
45–59	5
60–64	11
65–69	13
70–74	16
75–84	17
≥85	24

Chronic health condition[a] *(0–23 points)*	
AIDS	23
Hepatic failure	16
Lymphoma	13
Metastatic cancer	11
Leukemia/multiple myeloma	10
Immunosuppression	10
Cirrhosis	4

[a]Excluded for elective surgery patients.
Source: From Ref. 29.

than APACHE II (in public domain). It has, therefore, been slow to receive validation studies (although this is beginning to change). Several large population studies have shown APACHE III to underestimate mortality (30). Like APACHE I & II, version III lacks specificity with trauma patients and has not been convincingly validated in trauma populations (31). Another problem with APACHE scoring is that 24-hour physiological data used to derive APACHE II and APACHE III scores can be treatment-dependent and therefore may reflect poor clinical management rather than sicker patients (32).

☞ **APACHE IV was released in 2005 using data from 116,209 admissions to 104 ICUs at 45 hospitals during 2002 and 2003.** ☞ While predictor variables are similar to APACHE III, new variables have been added including impact of sedation on the GCS, ventilator status, thrombolysis and so on. In addition, different statistical modeling techniques are used (33).

Simplified Acute Physiology Score

In 1984, another predictive scoring system was created in France, based on the evaluation of 679 consecutive patients

in eight French ICUs. Named the SAPS, it promoted a simplified version of APACHE taking into account 14 biologic and clinical variables (34).

SAPS II (Table 2) was updated in 1993 by Le Gall et al. based on a large European/North American multicenter study with a cohort of almost 13,000 patients from 137 hospitals (110 in Europe; 27 in N.A.). SAPS II includes 17 variables: 12 physiologic (weighted according to their degree of deviation from normal), as well as age, type of admission (medical and scheduled/unscheduled surgery), and three variables related to particular diseases (acquired immunodeficiency syndrome, metastatic cancer, and hematologic malignancy). SAPS II scores range from 0 to 163 points (up to 16 for physiology, up to 17 for age, and up to 30 for underlying diagnosis). As with APACHE II, summed scores are converted to probability scores using logistic regression to predict mortality. ☞ **SAPS II is the most widely used mortality prediction tool in European ICUs (35).** ☞

One major problem with this scoring system is that sedated patients do not have their GCS calculated. While many ventilated patients are sedated, the neurological evaluation is not considered for the calculations (36). SAPS II has also been shown to underestimate mortality in trauma patients (37). A recently published paper has described an expanded and updated version of SAPS II (with updated statistics and inclusion of more routine data variables), which has shown better calibration and discrimination in SMR calculations across populations (38).

The main advantage of the SAPS II score is the ease of data collection. Furthermore, this scoring system is calculated directly from the logistic regression equation without needing to add points or make other corrections (6). Overall SAPS II has shown reasonable accuracy in stratifying the risk of death in a wide range of disease states and clinical settings and is predictive in nontrauma surgical patients (39). In comparison studies with APACHE II, SAPS II showed good overall linear correlation on aggregate data; however, significant disparities exist with predicted mortalities on individual patients (40).

☞ **A latest version (SAPS III) has been recently released with 2002 data from 22,791 patients in 309 participating ICUs worldwide.** ☞ SAPS III conceptually dissociates evaluation of the individual patient from evaluation of the ICU. For individual patient assessment, the system separates the relative contributions of chronic health status or previous therapy, circumstances related to ICU admission, and degree of physiologic dysfunction. Equations are also customized to four areas of the world (North America, Europe, Australia, and South America) for regional and/or global reference comparisons. No comparison between SAPS III and other scores are available to date (41,42). As with the APACHE versions, trauma patients are generally under scored.

Mortality Prediction Model

The first model developed using multiple regression techniques was the Mortality Prediction Model (MPM), published in 1985 by Stanley Lemeshow, Professor of Biostatistics at the University of Massachusetts (Table 3) (43–45).

The MPM system, unlike the APACHE and the SAPS systems, was designed to measure mortality risk at later times after ICU admission (i.e., at 24, 48, and 72 hrs) (46). Major advantages of the MPM system are that multiple diagnoses can be included (rather than a single, most severe condition) and adjustments can be made in conditions

Table 2 Simplified Acute Physiology Score II Variables and Definitions

Variable	Definition	Points
Age	Age (in years) at last birthday	0–18
Heart rate	Use the worst value in 24 hrs, either low or high heart rate: if it varied from cardiac arrest (11 points) to extreme tachycardic (7 points), assign 11 points	0–11
Systolic blood pressure	Use the same method as for heart rate: e.g., if it varied from 60 mm Hg to 205 mm HG, assign 13 points	0–13
Body temperature	Use the highest temperature	0–3
PaO_2/FIO_2	If ventilated or continuous pulmonary artery pressure, use the lowest value of the ratio	0–11
Urinary output	If the patient is in the intensive care unit for <24 hrs, make the calculation for 24 hrs: e.g., 1 L in 8 hrs = 3 L in 24 hrs	0–11
Serum urea or serum urea nitrogen level	Use the highest value in mmol/L for serum urea and in mg/dL for serum urea nitrogen	0–10
WBC count	Use the worst (high to low) WBC count	0–3
Serum potassium level	Use the worst (high or low) value in mmol/L	0–3
Serum sodium level	Use the worst (high or low) value in mmol/L	0–5
Serum bicarbonate level	Use the lowest value in mEq/L	0–6
Bilirubin level	Use the highest value in μmol/L or mg/dL	0–9
Glasgow Coma Scale	If the patient is sedated, record the estimated Glasgow Coma Scale score before sedation	0–26
Type of admission	Unscheduled surgical[a], scheduled surgical[b], or medical[c]	8,0, or 6
AIDS	Yes, if HIV-positive with clinical complications such as *Pneumocytis carinii* pneumonia, Kaposi's sarcoma, lymphoma, tuberculosis, or *Toxoplasma* infection	17
Hematologic malignancy	Yes, if lymphoma, acute leukemia, or multiple myeloma	10
Metastatic cancer	Yes, if proven metastatic by surgery, CT, or any other method	9

[a]Patients added to operating room schedule within 24 hrs of the operation.
[b]Patients whose surgery was scheduled at least 24 hrs in advance.
[c]Patients having no surgery within 1 week of admission to intensive care unit.
Abbreviations: AIDS, acquired immunodeficiency syndrome; CT, computed tomography; FIO_2, fraction of inspired oxygen; HIV, human immunodeficiency virus; SAPS, simplified acute physiology score; WBC, white blood cells.
Source: From Ref. 35.

Table 3 Mortality Probability Models Variables and Definitions

MPM II Model at admission (MPM0)	MPM II Model at 24 (MPM24), 48 (MPM48), and 72 (MPM72) hrs
Age	Variables obtained at admission
Coma or deep stupor	Age
Heart rate	Cirrhosis
Systolic blood pressure	Intracranial mass effect
Chronic renal insufficiency	Metastatic neoplasm
Cirrhosis	Medical or unscheduled surgery admission
Metastatic neoplasm	Variables obtained in 24 hrs
Acute renal failure	Coma or deep stupor
Cardiac dysrhythmia	Creatinine > 2.0 mg/dL
Cerebrovascular incident	Confirmed infection
Gastrointestinal bleeding	Mechanical ventilation
Intracranial mass effect	PaO_2 < 60 mm Hg
Cardiopulmonary resuscitation	Prothrombin time >3 secs above standard
Mechanical ventilation	Urine output <150 mL in 8 hrs
Medical or unscheduled surgery admission	Vasoactive drugs >1 hrs intravenously

Source: From Ref. 44.

considered and in weightings which can be altered from admission to other time points, reflecting differing impacts on mortality. As a result of timing intervals, however, treatment-related factors can significantly influence mortality predictions.

Therapeutic Intervention Scoring System

The Therapeutic Intervention Scoring System (TISS) was developed in 1974 by Cullen et al. (47). It is based on the fact that therapeutic interventions are more common and extensive in patients with more advanced disease (48). TISS was developed to quantify severity of illness among intensive care patients based on the type and amount of treatment received. The underlying philosophy is that the sicker the patient, the greater the number and complexity of treatments. By quantifying this, a (rough) measure of illness severity can be obtained. Initially the system scored 76 therapeutic interventions. However, due to its complexity, the TISS-28 was proposed, reducing the variables from 76 to 28 (49). This score considers seven main parameters: basic activities, ventilatory (e.g., mechanical ventilation), cardiovascular (e.g., vasoactive drugs), renal (e.g., dialysis), neurologic (e.g., ICP monitoring), and metabolic support (e.g., parenteral nutrition), in addition to specific interventions, with each of the variables divided in subitems (Table 4). In a comparison between patients in a surgical ICU, the simplified version (TISS-28) was shown to be easier and more accurate than the TISS-76.

Table 4   Therapeutic Intervention Scoring System Variables and Definitions

	Points
Basic activities	
Standard monitoring. Hourly vital signs, regular registration and calculation of fluid balance	5
Laboratory, biochemical, and microbiological investigations	1
Single medication. Intravenously, intramuscularly, subcutaneously, and/or orally (e.g., gastric tube)	2
Multiple intervention medication. More than one drug, single shots, or continuously	3
Routine dressing changes. Care and prevention of decubitus and daily dressing change	1
Frequent dressing changes. Frequent dressing change (at least one time per each nursing shift) and/or extensive wound care	1
Care of drains. All (except gastric tube)	3
Ventilatory support	
Mechanical ventilation. Any form of mechanical ventilation/assisted ventilation with or without positive end-expiratory pressure, with or without muscle relaxants; spontaneous breathing with positive end-expiratory pressure	5
Supplement ventilatory support. Breathing spontaneously through endotracheal tube without positive end-expiratory pressure; supplementary oxygen by any method, except if mechanical ventilation parameters apply	2
Care of artificial airways. Endotracheal tube or tracheostomy	1
Treatment for improving lung function. Thorax physiotherapy, incentive spirometry, inhalation therapy, intratracheal suctioning	1
Cardiovascular support	
Single vasoactive medication. Any vasoactive drug	3
Multiple vasoactive medications. More than one vasoactive drug, disregard type and doses	4
Intravenous replacement of large fluid losses. Fluid administration $>3L/m^2/$day, disregard type of fluid administered	4
Peripheral arterial catheter	5
Left atrium monitoring. Pulmonary artery flotation catheter with or without cardiac output measurement	8
Central venous line	2
Cardiopulmonary resuscitation after arrest; in the past 24 hrs (single precordial percussion not included)	3
Renal support	
Hemofiltration techniques. Dialytic techniques	3
Quantitative urine output measurement (e.g., by urinary catheter à demeure)	2
Active diuresis (e.g., furosemide >0.5 mg/kg/day for overload	3
Neurologic support	
Measurement of intracranial pressure	4
Metabolic support	
Treatment of complicated metabolic acidosis/alkalosis	4
Intravenous hyperalimentation	3
Enteral feeding. Through gastric tube or other gastrointestinal route (e.g., jejunostomy)	2
Specific interventions	
Single specific interventions in the intensive care unit. Naso or orotracheal intubation, introduction of pacemaker, cardioversion, endoscopies, emergency surgery in the past 24 hrs, gastric lavage. Routine interventions without direct consequences to the clinical condition of the patient, such as radiographs, echography, electrocardiogram, dressings, or introduction of venous or arterial catheters, are not included	3
Multiple specific interventions in the intensive care unit. More than one, as described above	5
Specific interventions outside the intensive care unit. Surgery or diagnostic procedures	5

Source: From Ref. 49.

TISS scores, though not widely used to quantify severity of illness, have shown usefulness in identifying ICU acuity, staffing needs, and cost (50).

ORGAN DYSFUNCTION SCORING SYSTEMS

The idea of developing an organ-dysfunction score was first reported by Baue in 1975 (51). Most organ dysfunction scores include the evaluation of six organ systems: the central nervous, cardiovascular, respiratory, hepatic, renal, and hematological systems. ☞ **The advantage of organ dysfunction scores is that they allow the analysis of the function of** different and specific organs, making possible comparisons between patients with the same disease processes. ☞ In addition, these scores can be used to assess response to treatment and monitor recovery or deterioration of specific organs during the evolution of the patient's disease process in ICU, with data collected on admission and usually daily thereafter. The three most widely utilized organ injury scoring systems are reviewed subsequently.

Sequential Organ Failure Assessment (SOFA) Score

The sepsis-related organ failure assessment (SOFA) was developed by the European Society of Intensive Care Medicine in 1994 (52). It was renamed to Sequential Organ Failure

Table 5 Sepsis-Related Organs Variables and Definitions

	Score				
	0	1	2	3	4
Respiration PaO2/FiO2 (Torr)	>400	301–400	201–300	101–200 with respiratory support	≤100 with respiratory support
Coagulation Platelets (x10^3/mm^3)	>150	101–150	51–100	21–50	≤20
Liver Bilirubin (mg/dL)	<1.2	1.2–1.9	2.0–5.9	6.0–11.9	≥12.0
Cardiovascular Hypotension	No	MAP <70 mmHg	Dopamine≤5 or dobutamine (any dose)	Dopamine>5 and ≤ 15 or epi ≤ 0.1 or norepi ≤0.1	Dopamine >15 or epi >0.1 or norepi >0.1
Central nervous system Glasgow Coma Scale Score	15	13–14	10–12	6–9	3–5
Renal Creatinine (mg/dL) or urinary output	<1.2	1.2–1.9	2.0–3.4	3.5–4.9 or 200–500 mL/day	≥5.0 or <200 mL/day

Source: From Ref. 53.

Assessment (SOFA), which remains the current terminology (Table 5), after the verification that it could be also used for nonseptic patients. This scoring system includes six organ systems (central nervous, cardiovascular, pulmonary, hepatic, renal, and hematological system) and takes into account the worst values on each day using a scoring system that ranges from 0 (normal) to 4 (most abnormal). The aggregate score [total maximum SOFA score (TMS)] is calculated by summing the worst scores for each of the organ systems during the ICU stay. TMS scores can be used to quantify and evaluate the patient's organ dysfunction over time. Janssens et al. demonstrated that the SOFA score is a valid and reliable tool to access the severity of organ dysfunction not only in septic patients, but also in surgical, trauma, and medical cardiovascular patients (53).

SOFA is a simple and effective instrument for use in the evaluation of organ dysfunction/failure and the effects of cumulative insult by assessing degree of dysfunction already present on admission, as compared to maximum and delta SOFA scores. Serial assessment of organ dysfunction during the first few days of ICU admission may be a particularly good indicator of prognosis (54).

Multiple Organ Dysfunction (MOD) Score

The MOD score is another system based on organ dysfunction that was published in 1995 by Marshall and colleagues (Table 6) (55). This system evaluates the same six organ systems as the SOFA score. Raw values for each of the component variables are obtained daily. The range of the most representative values for each organ system is graded from 0 (normal function) to 4 (markedly deranged function) on a daily basis. Scores are calculated at the same point in time each day (first morning values) to avoid capturing momentary changes in physiologic variables. The overall score varies from 0 to 24 points and correlates well with ICU mortality. The major difference between the SOFA and MOD scores lies in the variables used to define cardiovascular dysfunction.

The MOD and SOFA scores have been used to assess and document specific organ function, taking into account

Table 6 Multiple Organ Dysfunction Variables and Definitions

	Score				
	0	1	2	3	4
Respiration PaO2/FiO2 (Torr)	>300	226–300	151–225	78–150	≤77
Coagulation Platelets (x10^3/mm^3)	>120	81–120	51–80	21–50	≤20
Liver Bilirubin (μmol/L)	≤20	21–60	61–120	121–240	>240
Cardiovascular (Pressure adjusted rate)	≤10	10.1–15.0	15.1–20.0	20.1–30.0	>30
Central nervous system Glasgow Coma Scale Score	15	13–14	10–12	7–9	3–6
Renal Creatinine (μmol/L)	≤100	101–200	201–350	351–500	>500

Source: From Ref. 55.

the time and course of a patient's condition during an entire ICU stay, and to correlate these to expected outcome. The SOFA score incorporates both physiologic measures and measures of therapeutic intervention (e.g., need for mechanical ventilation, inotropic or vasopressin support), whereas MOD scoring is independent of treatment. Most comparison studies have shown little practical difference between SOFA and MOD scores; however, in most studies the SOFA cardiovascular score has shown better performance.

Logistic Organ Dysfunction (LOD) Score

The Logistic Organ Dysfunction (LOD) scoring system was published in 1996 by LeGall and colleagues using methodology similar to that used with SAPS II. The LOD score takes into account both the relative severity among organ systems and the degree of severity within a system. The LOD is a global score that can be calculated to summarize the combined effect of dysfunction among several organs. Logistic regression techniques are used to determine severity levels and relative weights (according to prognostic significance) for the LOD score and its conversion to a probability of mortality (56).

INTENSIVE CARE UNIT SCORING SYSTEM COMPARISONS

✎ **Third generation ICU scoring systems (APACHE II/III, SAPS II, and MPM II use statistical modeling techniques to select and weigh variables and generate prognostic information.** ✎ APACHE and SAPS collect data within 24 hours of admission and, with MPM II, data is collected serially to 72 hours post admission. These tools are comparable and produce similar results with regard to discrimination (identifying survivors versus nonsurvivors). Wide variations exist, however, in calibration (difference between observed and predicted mortality).

Several large U.S. and European comparative studies with third generation models have shown that each of the models provide reasonable discrimination. Large discrepancies were found across the models evidenced by significant variations in SMR. Studies on sub-groups of patients confirm these findings. Though these models clearly show better performance than earlier generations, their discriminative accuracy (sensitivity/specificity) remains inconsistent across populations (31,57,58).

A study comparing APACHE II, MPM II, and SAPS II demonstrated that MPM II and APACHE II models presented very similar mean predicted mortality and were closer to the observed mortality than SAPS II (59). Another comparison of four scores: APACHE II, SAPS II, MPM0 and MPM24 in 969 patients showed that prediction of mortality was good in all four scoring systems, although it was better with APACHE II and MPM0. When divided into disease sub-groups, MPM0 and MPM24 overestimated mortality in the nonoperative trauma group, whereas SAPS II underestimated mortality in medical patients other than those admitted for cardiovascular, respiratory, and neurological problems (60).

Due to several scoring systems available, there is a need to evaluate these scores to determine which is more accurate to a specific ICU population. In the past 10 years, the APACHE II was the system most commonly used and evaluated (Fig. 1) (31).

In a comparison between five scores including APACHE II, APACHE III, a U.K. version of APACHE II, SAPS II, and MPM II at admission (MPM0) and at 24 hrs

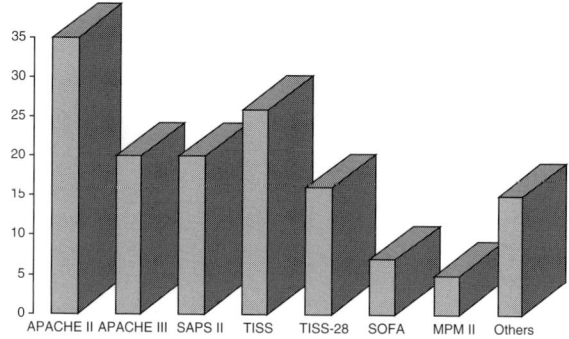

Figure 1 Severity of illness scoring systems: frequency of use and evaluation. *Abbreviations*: APACHE, acute physiology and chronic health evolution; MPM, multiple organ dysfunction; SAPS, simplified acute physiology score; SOFA, sepsis-related organs; TISS, therapeutic intervention system.

(MPM24), data on 10,393 patients in 22 ICUs in Scotland was analyzed (Table 7). It was concluded that SAPS II demonstrated the best overall performance, but APACHE II was the most appropriate model for comparisons of mortality rates between ICUs. APACHE III underestimated the mortality (Table 1) (31).

Each of the three organ scoring systems has generally been shown to have reasonable discrimination and calibration; in one study all three were also comparable to APACHE III in predicting mortality (61–63). However, in a recent large Canadian study by Zygun et al. comparing SOFA with MODS, it was found that neither discriminated or calibrated well with multisystem patients (12% were trauma patients), questioning the ability to use these scoring system predictively in patients with multisystem organ dysfunction at their current level of development (64). Differences between prognostic and organ dysfunction scores are summarized in Table 8 (61).

EYE TO THE FUTURE

Recent years have shown significant improvement in the sophistication, accuracy of illness, injury scoring tools, and mortality prediction models. However, given the rapid changes in the treatment of critically ill and injured patients, many challenges remain in the evaluation of outcomes aimed at improving the quality and consistency of ICU care. ✎ **Innovations in managing the magnitude of data necessary for predictive accuracy in risk adjustment (essential to the performance of prognostic models) will parallel a continually increasing ability to automatically capture and retrieve demographic and clinical data.** ✎ Statistical techniques utilizing "artificial intelligence" or neural networks are proceeding to the next level of development, whereby continuous updating of databases and "real time" recalibration of variables is possible. Multicenter linkages with updated national databases (e.g., NTDB, "Project Impact," and INARC) and global data collaboration efforts are one step in this direction whereby information from multiple institutions can be analyzed centrally and strengthened through data volumes and wider geographic inputs. Recently, newer disease-specific and customized mortality prediction models have been utilized which show better "goodness of fit" than generic models when applied to

Table 7   Hosmer-Lemeshow Goodness-of-Fit Statistics for All Models

	Predicted deciles of mortality (%)	Observed survivors	Expected survivors	Observed deaths	Expected deaths	GOF statistic and *df*
APACHE II	0 < 4	958	959.63	27	025.37	
	4 < 8	919	925.57	66	059.43	
	8 < 12	887	889.95	98	095.05	
	12 < 17	847	846.67	138	138.33	
	17 < 23	796	792.41	189	192.59	
	23 < 31	710	722.93	275	262.07	
	31 < 40	658	637.11	327	347.89	
	40 < 52	599	532.13	386	452.87	
	52 < 69	451	396.72	534	588.28	*df* = 8
	69 < 100	203	186.50	780	796.50	36.39[a]
APACHE III	0 < 2	1010	1023.32	23	009.68	
	2 < 3	986	1009.26	47	023.74	
	3 < 5	952	992.35	81	040.65	
	5 < 8	913	966.27	120	066.73	
	8 < 13	856	927.62	177	105.38	
	13 < 20	791	869.41	242	163.59	
	20 < 30	678	779.37	355	253.63	
	30 < 45	575	649.89	458	383.11	
	45 < 68	384	454.68	649	578.32	*df* = 8
	68 < 100	141	173.18	888	855.82	331.65[a]
UK APACHE II	0 < 8	952	933.29	33	51.71	
	8 < 13	938	875.75	47	109.25	
	13 < 18	880	829.17	105	155.83	
	18 < 24	839	777.24	146	207.76	
	24 < 31	813	714.64	172	270.36	
	31 < 39	720	645.39	265	339.61	
	39 < 48	670	565.16	315	419.84	
	48 < 59	574	466.89	411	518.11	
	59 < 73	424	343.37	561	641.63	*df* = 8
	73 < 100	218	163.55	765	819.45	307.51[a]
SAPS II	0 < 3	1011	1018.09	22	014.91	
	3 < 5	992	994.20	41	038.80	
	5 < 9	958	962.54	75	070.46	
	9 < 14	897	919.84	136	113.16	
	14 < 20	841	862.12	192	170.88	
	20 < 29	792	784.72	241	248.28	
	29 < 41	681	676.18	352	356.82	
	41 < 58	559	534.23	474	498.77	
	58 < 80	415	333.42	618	699.58	*df* = 8
	80 < 100	145	108.92	892	928.08	57.75[a]
MPM$_0$	0 < 3	991	1013.51	48	025.49	
	3 < 6	950	991.01	89	047.99	
	6 < 9	923	960.37	116	078.63	
	9 < 14	856	920.19	183	118.81	
	14 < 20	819	863.52	220	175.48	
	20 < 26	761	803.75	278	235.25	
	26 < 37	695	718.79	344	320.21	
	37 < 53	636	570.85	403	468.15	
	53 < 75	457	377.37	582	661.63	*df* = 8
	75 < 100	250	131.27	792	910.73	307.47[a]
MPM$_{24}$	0 < 4	715	714.19	19	019.81	
	4 < 7	675	694.97	59	039.03	
	7 < 11	662	670.26	72	063.74	
	11 < 16	590	636.51	144	097.49	
	16 < 22	568	596.65	166	137.35	
	22 < 30	500	545.46	234	188.54	
	30 < 40	495	479.72	239	254.28	
	40 < 53	397	395.13	337	338.87	
	53 < 71	310	278.27	424	455.73	*df* = 8
	71 < 100	179	119.80	558	617.20	101.87[a]

[a]$p < 0.001$.

Abbreviations: APACHE, acute physiology and chronic health evaluation; *df*, degrees of freedom; MPM, mortality probability model; SAPS, simplified acute physiology score.

Source: From Ref. 31.

Table 8 Differences Between Prognostic and Organ Dysfunction Scores

	Prognostic scales: severity of illness scores	Outcome measures: organ dysfunction scales
Uses	Prognostication; risk stratification	Outcome measurement; evaluation of clinical course over time
Timing of ascertainment	Early during ICU stay	Following resuscitation; at any time during
Selection of variables	Physiologic measures	Measures of physiology or therapeutic response stable, representative values
	Worst values	
	Selected to maximize	Selected to reflect clinical construct
	Predictive capability	
Calibration	Maximize prediction	Maximize description

Abbreviation: ICU, intensive care unit.
Source: From Ref. 6.

subgroups of ICU patients. This trend of adapting models to unique patient populations is likely to continue and improve their value as benchmarks. While specificity and qualification of variables improve accuracy, there remains a need for uniform and compatible reporting methods and languages for research, and broader comparison across ICUs. The expanded utilization of multiple models and combinations, as well as integration with other disease-specific classification measures and with ICD-10 codes, will enhance predictive capabilities and help to identify the most clinically relevant variables and endpoints.

Restricting parameters to measures of mortality and LOS do not, for trauma and ICU survivors, address many of the patient-centered outcomes of ICU performance such as quality of life and functional status following illness or injury. A greater focus on multidimensional outcomes is emerging, and the evaluation methodologies to assess these outcomes must be broad enough to capture these constructs without losing precision. In other words, our tools need continual refinement in order to capture the complex and meaningful variables associated with illness and injury and their consequences.

Lastly, comparative information about ICU and trauma outcomes is critical, but in and of itself insufficient, if not matched by methods to determine the structures and practice patterns that ultimately influence and contribute to improving the quality of patient care (65).

SUMMARY

Characterization of injury and illness severity are essential to the scientific study of trauma and critical care. A number of severity scoring systems and prediction models have been developed which are designed to quantify severity, prognosis, and course of disease. They also serve the purposes of assessing therapies, comparing quality outcomes, and of evaluating performance within and across centers and patient populations.

Accuracy of injury scoring tools reflects their ability to describe the patient's anatomic and physiologic injury. With the increasing sophistication of these measures they have assumed a major role in trauma practice and outcomes studies.

Critical care prognostic scoring systems are used to characterize ICU patient populations and predict (albeit imperfectly) mortality (9). Although increasingly sophisticated, prognostic models exhibit a level of

uncertainty, and an understanding of their limitations is essential for their appropriate selection and use in individual ICUs. ✍ **Clearly no single "gold standard" model exists which can be applied to all populations and types of ICUs.** ✍ Currently these systems should not be used to prognosticate individual patients or used solely in decisions regarding futility of care.

Scoring models for organ dysfunction such as the SOFA, MOD, and LOD systems are utilized to assess risk in patients with severe illnesses (e.g., sepsis and ARDS) and those with several impaired organ systems. Although methodological differences exist between the various organ dysfunction scales (Table 8), each of these has shown predictability within its realm of evaluation. In addition, these are easy to use, relying on objective and easily accessible clinical data to evaluate patient outcomes. Yet, none of these organ dysfunction scoring systems is specific for the trauma patient.

Other scores can be utilized to assess the severity of specific disease processes. Examples include the Hunt–Hess classification of subarachnoid hemorrhage, the GCS (also a component of other scores), the Murray lung injury severity score for ARDS, NYHA classification, and Child's classification of chronic liver disease (66). These scores have the advantage of focusing on a specific aspect of each disease, and can be used to supplement the overall severity score to evaluate that particular organ for a patient.

KEY POINTS

✍ All scoring systems represent quantitative classification schemes, most of which use multiple logistic regression methodology applied to prospectively collected data sets of demographic, physiological, and clinical variables.

✍ While scoring systems are useful for research and comparing SICU performance with respect to endpoints such as mortality and LOS, their usefulness is less clear in medical decision-making or prognostic estimations for individual patients.

✍ ISS correlates with hospital stay, morbidity, mortality, and other measures of trauma severity, and is the most widely accepted severity of injury index in use today.

✍ The APACHE II/III/IV, SAPS II/III, and MPM II are considered "third generation" scoring systems based on their use of multiple regression statistical techniques.

☞ APACHE III is more predictive than APACHE II due to modifications (increased size and representativeness of the database, and expansion of diagnoses to include more complex injury characterizations).

☞ APACHE IV was released in 2005 using data from 116,209 admissions to 104 ICUs at 45 hospitals during 2002–2003.

☞ SAPS II is the most widely used mortality prediction tool in European ICUs.

☞ A latest version (SAPS III) has been recently released with 2002 data from 22,791 patients in 309 participating ICUs worldwide.

☞ The advantage of organ dysfunction scores is that they allow the analysis of the function of different and specific organs, making possible comparisons between patients with the same disease processes.

☞ Third generation ICU scoring systems (APACHE II/III, SAPS II, and MPM II use statistical modeling techniques to select and weigh variables and generate prognostic information.

☞ Innovations in managing the magnitude of data necessary for predictive accuracy in risk adjustment (essential to the performance of prognostic models) will parallel a continually increasing ability to automatically capture and retrieve demographic and clinical data.

☞ Clearly no single "gold standard" model exists which can be applied to all populations and types of ICUs.

REFERENCES

1. Champion HR, et al. Assessment of injury severity: the triage index. Crit Care Med 1980; 8:201–208.
2. Knaus WA, Zimmerman JE, Wagner DP, et al. APACHE-acute physiology and chronic health evaluation: a physiologically based classification system. Crit Care Med 1981; 9(8):591–597.
3. National Trauma DataBank—2005 Report. From the American College of Surgeons Website (Accessed March 31, 2006, at http://www.facs.org/trauma/ntdb.html).
4. Project IMPACT, CCM. Website (Accessed March 31, 2006, at http://www.cerner.com/piccm/).
5. Intensive Care National Audit & Research Centre (ICNARC) Website (Accessed March 31, 2006, at http://www.icnarc.org/)
6. Herridge MS. Prognostication and intensive care unit outcome: the evolving role of scoring systems. Clin Chest Med 2003; 24(4):751–762.
7. Mourouga P, Goldfrad C, Rowan KM. Does it fit? Is it good? Assessment of scoring systems, Curr Opin Crit Care 2000; 176–180.
8. Glance LG, Osler TM, Dick A. Rating the quality of intensive care units: is it a function of the intensive care unit scoring system? Crit Care Med 2002; 30(9):1976–1982.
9. Mendez-Tellez PA, Dorman T. Predicting patient outcomes, futility, and resource utilization in the intensive care unit: The role of severity scoring systems and general outcome prediction models. Editorial. Mayo Clin Proc 2005; 80:161–163.
10. Young JD. Severity scoring systems and the prediction of outcome from intensive care. Curr Opin Anesth 2000; 13(2):203–207.
11. Randolph AG, Guyatt GH, Calvin J, et al. Understanding articles describing clinical prediction tools. Crit Care Med 1998; 26:1603–1612.
12. Champion HR, et al. A revision of the trauma score. J Trauma 1989; 29:623–629.
13. Demetriades D, Sava J, Alo K, et al. Old age as a criterion for trauma team activation. J Trauma® Injury, Infection, and Critical Care 2001; 51(4):754–756; discussion 756–757.
14. Moore EE, Shackford SR, Pachter HL, et al. Organ injury scaling: spleen, liver, and kidney. J Trauma 1989; 29(12):1664–1666.
15. Committee on Medical Aspects of Automotive Safety: Rating the severity of tissue damage. JAMA 1971; 215:277–280.
16. Baker SP, O'Neill B, Haddon W, Long WB. The injury severity score: a method for describing patients with multiple injuries and evaluating emergency care. J Trauma 1974; 14(3):187–196.
17. Frankema SPG, Steyerberg EW, Edwards MJR, van Vugt AB. Comparison of current injury scales for survival chance estimation: an evaluation comparing the predictive performance of the ISS, NISS, and AP Scores in a Dutch Local Trauma Registration. J Trauma 2005; 58(3):596–604.
18. Boyd C, Tolson MA, Copes WS. Evaluating trauma care: The TRISS method. J Trauma 1987; 27(4):370–378.
19. Morgan TO, Civil ID, Schwab CW. Injury severity scoring: influence of timing and nurse raters on accuracy. Heart Lung 1988; 17(3):256–261.
20. Zoltie N, de Dombal FT. The hit and miss of ISS and TRISS. Yorkshire Trauma Audit Group (BMJ) 1993; 9:307(6909): 906–909.
21. Osterwalder JJ, Riederer M. Quality assessment of multiple trauma management by ISS, TRISS or ASCOT? Schweiz Med Wochenschr 2000, 130(14):(Abstract).
22. Miltzman DP, Boulanger BR, Rodriguez A, et al. Pre-existing disease in trauma patients: a predictor of fate independent of age and injury severity score. J Trauma 1992; 32(2):236–43; discussion 243–244.
23. Brenneman FD, Boulanger BR, McLellan BA, Redelmeier DA. Measuring injury severity: time for a change? J Trauma 1998; 44(4):580–582.
24. Sacco WJ, MacKenzie EJ, Champion HR, et al. Comparison of alternative methods for assessing injury severity based on anatomic descriptors. J Trauma 1999; 47(3):441–446.
25. Osler T, Baker SP, Long W. A modification of the injury severity score that both improves accuracy and simplifies scoring. J Trauma 1997; 43(6):922–925; discussion 925–926.
26. Wong DT, Knaus WA. Predicting outcome in critical care: the current status of the APACHE prognostic scoring. Canadian J Anesth 1991; 38:374–383.
27. Knaus WA, Draper EA, Wagner DP, Zimmerman JE. APACHE II: a severity of disease classification system. Crit Care Med 1985; 13(10):818–829.
28. Civetta JM, Hudson-Civetta JA, Nelson LD. Evaluation of APACHE II for cost containment and quality assurance. Ann Surg 1990; 53:266–276.
29. Knaus WA, Wagner DP, Draper EA, et al. The APACHE III prognostic system. Risk prediction of hospital mortality for critically ill hospitalized adults. Chest 1991; 100(6):1619–1636.
30. Ho KM, Dobb GJ, Knuiman M, et al. A comparison of admission and worst 24-hr Acute Physiology and Chronic Health Evaluation II scores in predicting hospital mortality: a retrospective cohort study. Crit Care 2005; 10(1):R4.
31. Livingston BM, MacKirdy FN, Howie JC, et al. Assessment of the performance of five intensive care scoring models within a large Scottish database. Crit Care Med 2000; 28(6):1820–1827.
32. Ihnsook J, Myunghee K, Jungsoon K. Predictive accuracy of severity scoring system: a prospective cohort study using APACHE III in a Korean intensive care unit. Int J Nurs Stud 2003; 40(3):219–226.
33. Zimmerman JE, Kramer AA, McNair DS, et al. Acute Physiology and Chronic Health Evaluation (APACHE) IV: Hospital mortality assessment for today's critically ill patients. Crit Care Med 2006 Mar 14; Publish ahead of print [Epub ahead of print].
34. Le Gall JR, Loirat P, Alperovitch A, et al. A simplified acute physiology score for ICU patients. Crit Care Med 1984; 12(11):975–977.
35. Le Gall JR, Lemeshow S, Saulnier F. A new Simplified Acute Physiology Score (SAPS II) based on a European/North American multicenter study. JAMA 1993; 22–29; 270(24):2957–2963.
36. Fery-Lemonnier E, Landais P, et al. Evaluation of severity scoring systems in ICUs-translation, conversion and definition ambiguities as a source of inter-observer variability in Apache II, SAPS and OSF. Intensive Care Med 1995; 21(4):356–360.

37. Apolone G, Bertolini G, D'Amico R, et al. The performance of SAPS II in a cohort of patients admitted to 99 Italian ICUs: results from GiViTI. Gruppo Italiano per la Valutazione degli interventi in Terapia Intensiva. Intensive Care Med 1996; 22(12):1368–1378.

38. Le Gall JR, Neumann A, Hemery F, et al. Mortality prediction using SAPS II: An update for French intensive care units. Crit Care 2005; 9(6):R645–R652.

39. Vosylius S, Sipylaite J, Ivaskevicius J. Evaluation of intensive care unit performance in Lithuania using the SAPS II system. Eur J Anaesthesiol 2004; 21(8):619–624.

40. McNelis J, Marini C, Kalimi R, et al. A comparison of predictive outcomes of APACHE II and SAPS II in a surgical intensive care unit. Am J Med Qual 2001; 16(5):161–165.

41. Metnitz PG, Moreno RP, Almeida E, et al. SAPS 3 Investigators. SAPS 3—From evaluation of the patient to evaluation of the intensive care unit. Part 1: Objectives, methods and cohort description. Intensive Care Med 2005; 31(10):1336–1344.

42. Moreno RP, Metnitz PG, Almeida E, et al. SAPS 3 Investigators. SAPS 3—From evaluation of the patient to evaluation of the intensive care unit. Part 2: Development of a prognostic model for hospital mortality at ICU admission. Intensive Care Med 2005; 31(10):1345–1355.

43. Lemeshow S, Teres D, Pastides H, et al. A method for predicting survival and mortality of ICU patients using objectively derived weights. Crit Care Med 1985; 13(7):519–525.

44. Lemeshow S, Teres D, et al. Mortality Probability Models (MPM II) based on an international cohort of intensive care unit patients. JAMA 1993; 270(20):2478–2486.

45. Lemeshow S, Klar J, Teres D, et al. Mortality probability models for patients in the intensive care unit for 48 or 72 hr: a prospective, multicenter study. Crit Care Med 1994; 22(9):1351–1358.

46. Rue M, Artigas A, Alvarez M, et al. Performance of the Mortality Probability Models in assessing severity of illness during the first week in the intensive care unit. Crit Care Med 2000; 28(8):2819–2824.

47. Cullen DJ, Civetta JM, Briggs BA, Ferrara LC. Therapeutic intervention scoring system: a method for quantitative comparison of patient care. Crit Care Med 1974; 2(2):57–60.

48. Fortis A, Mathas C, Laskou M, et al. Therapeutic Intervention Scoring System-28 as a tool of post ICU outcome prognosis and prevention. Minerva Anaesthesiol 2004; 70(1–2):71–81.

49. Miranda DR, de Rijk A, Schaufeli W. Simplified Therapeutic Intervention Scoring System: the TISS-28 items-results from a multicenter study. Crit Care Med 1996; 24(1):64–73.

50. Lefering R, Zart M, Neugebauer EA. Retrospective evaluation of the simplified Therapeutic Intervention Scoring System (TISS-28) in a surgical intensive care unit. Intensive Care Med 2000; 26(12):1794–1802.

51. Baue AE. Multiple, progressive, or sequential systems failure. A syndrome of the 1970s. Arch Surg 1975; 110(7): 779–781.

52. Vincent JL, Moreno R, Takala J, et al. The SOFA (Sepsis-related Organ Failure Assessment) score to describe organ dysfunction/failure. On behalf of the Working Group on Sepsis-Related Problems of the European Society of Intensive Care Medicine. Intensive Care Med 1996; 22(7):707–710.

53. Janssens U, Graf C, Graf J, et al. Evaluation of the SOFA score: a single-center experience of a medical intensive care unit in 303 consecutive patients with predominantly cardiovascular disorders. Sequential Organ Failure Assessment. Inten Care Med 2000; 26(8):1037–1045.

54. Ferreira FL, Peres Bota D, Bross A, et al. Serial evaluation of the SOFA score to predict outcome in critically ill patients. JAMA 2001; 286:1754–1758.

55. Marshall JC, Cook DJ, Christou NV, et al. Multiple organ dysfunction score: a reliable descriptor of a complex clinical outcome. Crit Care Med 1995; 23(10):1638–1652.

56. Le Gall JR, Klar J, Lemeshow S, et al. The Logistic Organ Dysfunction. A new way to assess organ dysfunction in the intensive care unit. JAMA 1996; 276(10):802–810.

57. Moreno R, Morais P. Outcome prediction in intensive care: results of a prospective, multicentre, Portuguese study. Intensive Care Med 1997; 23(2):177–186.

58. Glance LG, Osler T, Shinozaki T. Intensive Care unit Prognostic scoring systems to predict death: a cost-effectiveness analysis. Crit Care Med 1998; 26(11): 1842–1849.

59. Patel PA, Grant BJ. Application of mortality prediction systems to individual intensive care units. Intensive Care Med 1999; 25(9):977–982.

60. Arabi Y, Haddad S, Goraj R, et al. Assessment of performance of four mortality prediction systems in a Saudi Arabian intensive care unit. Crit Care 2002; 6(2):166–174.

61. Marshall JC. Risk prediction and outcome description in critical surgical illness. In: Norton JA, Bollinger RR, eds. Surgery Basic Science and Clinical Evidence. New York: Springer-Verlag; 2001:306.

62. Pettila V, Pettila M, Sarna S, et al. Comparison of multiple organ dysfunction scores in the prediction of hospital mortality in the critically ill. Crit Care Med 2002; 30(8):1913–1914.

63. Timsit JF, Fosse JP, Troche G, et al. Calibration and discrimination by daily Logistic Organ Dysfunction scoring comparatively with daily Sequential Organ Failure assessment scoring for predicting hospital mortality in critically ill patients. Crit Care Med 2002; 30(9):2003–2013.

64. Zygun DA, Laupland KB, Fick GH, et al. Limited ability of SOFA and MOD scores to discriminate outcome: a prospective evaluation in 1,436 patients. Can J Anesth 2005; 52:302–308.

65. Rotondi AJ, Angus DC, Sirio CA. Assessing intensive care performance: A new conceptual framework. Curr Opin Crit Care 2000; 6:155–157.

66. Tsai MH, Chen YC, Ho YP, et al. Organ system failure scoring system can predict hospital mortality in critically ill cirrhotic patients. J Clin Gastroenterol 2003; 37(3):251–257.